NEONATOLOGY

GORDON B. AVERY, M.D., Ph.D.

Professor and Interim Chairman
Department of Pediatrics
George Washington University School of Medicine and Health Sciences
Chief of Medicine
Physician-in-Chief
Children's National Medical Center
Washington, District of Columbia

MARY ANN FLETCHER, M.D.

Associate Professor of Pediatrics and of Obstetrics and Gynecology
George Washington University School of Medicine and Health Sciences
Associate Director, Newborn Service
George Washington University Medical Center
Washington, District of Columbia

MHAIRI G. MACDONALD, M.B.Ch.B., F.R.C.P.(E), D.C.H.

Professor of Pediatrics
George Washington University School of Medicine and Health Sciences
Vice-Chairman, Department of Neonatology
Children's National Medical Center
George Washington University School of Medicine and Health Sciences
Director, Neonatal Intensive Care Unit
Children's National Medical Center
Washington, District of Columbia

with 104 contributors

NEONATOLOGY

Pathophysiology and Management of the Newborn

FOURTH EDITION

J. B. Lippincott Company, Philadelphia

Acquisitions Editor: Richard Winters
Sponsoring Editor: Kimberley Cox
Project Editor: Molly E. Dickmeyer
Indexer: Julia Figures
Design Coordinator: Kathy Kelley-Luedtke
Interior Designer: Maria Karkucinski
Cover Designer: Larry Pezzato
Production Manager: Caren Erlichman
Production Coordinator: Sharon McCarthy
Compositor: Bi-Comp, Incorporated
Printer/Binder: Walsworth Publishing Company

4th Edition

6 5 4 3 2 1

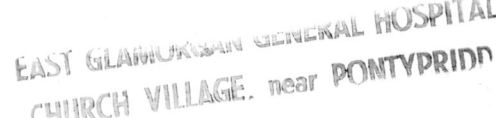

Library of Congress Cataloging-in-Publication Data
Neonatology : pathophysiology and management of the newborn / [edited by] Gordon B. Avery, Mary Ann Fletcher, Mhairi G. MacDonald ; with 104 contributors.—4th ed.
p. cm.
Includes bibliographical references and index.
ISBN 0-397-51101-9
1. Infants (Newborn)—Diseases. 2. Neonatology. I. Avery, Gordon B. II. Fletcher, Mary Ann. III. MacDonald, Mhairi G.
[DNLM: 1. Infant, Newborn, Diseases—physiopathology. 2. Infant, Newborn, Diseases—therapy. 3. Prenatal Diagnosis. WS 420 N441 1994]
RJ254.N46 1994
618.92'01—dc20
DNLM/DLC
for Library of Congress 92-48398
CIP

The authors and publisher have exerted every effort to ensure that drug selection and dosage set forth in this text are in accord with current recommendations and practice at the time of publication. However, in view of ongoing research, changes in government regulations, and the constant flow of information relating to drug therapy and drug reactions, the reader is urged to check the package insert for each drug for any change in indications and dosage and for added warnings and precautions. This is particularly important when the recommended agent is a new or infrequently employed drug.

CONTRIBUTORS

HOMAS E. ADRIAN, PH.D., M.R.C., Path.
rofessor of Physiology and Head
ivision of Physiology
reighton University School of Medicine
maha, Nebraska

. J. S. ANAND, M.B.B.S., D. Phil.
ssistant Professor of Anesthesia and Pediatrics
mory University School of Medicine
ttending Intestivist
ivision of Critical Care Medicine
epartment of Pediatrics
enrietta Egleston Hospital for Children
tlanta, Georgia

ATHRYN D. ANDERSON, M.D.
rofessor of Surgery
niversity of Southern California
urgeon-in-Chief
hildren's Hospital
os Angeles, California

OBERT J. ARCECI, M.D., Ph.D
ssistant Professor
ediatrics and Pediatric Hematology/Oncology
arvard Medical School
ana-Farber Cancer Institute
he Children's Hospital
oston, Massachusetts

OHN H. ARNOLD, M.D.
structor in Anaesthesia (Pediatrics)
arvard Medical School
ssistant in Anesthesia
ssociate Director, Multidisciplinary Intensive Care Unit
ssociate Medical Director, Respiratory Care Department
hildren's Hospital
oston, Massachusetts

ORDON B. AVERY, M.D., Ph.D.
rofessor and Interim Chairman
epartment of Pediatrics
eorge Washington University School of Medicine
d Health Sciences
hief of Medicine
hysician-in-Chief
hildren's National Medical Center
ashington, District of Columbia

DAVID A. BECKMAN, Ph.D.
Associate Professor of Pediatrics
Jefferson Medical College
Thomas Jefferson University
Philadelphia, Pennsylvania

EDWARD F. BELL, M.D.
Professor of Pediatrics
Director, Division of Neonatology
University of Iowa
Iowa City, Iowa

JOSEPH A. BELLANTI, M.D.
Professor of Pediatrics and Microbiology
Director, International Center for Interdisciplinary Studies of Immunology
Georgetown University Medical Center
Director, Division of Allergy, Immunology and Virology
Departments of Pediatrics and Laboratory Medicine
Georgetown University Hospital
Washington, District of Columbia

FORREST C. BENNETT, M.D.
Professor of Pediatrics
University of Washington School of Medicine
Director, High Risk Infant Follow-up Program
Child Development and Mental Retardation Center
Seattle, Washington

JUDY C. BERNBAUM, M.D.
Associate Professor of Pediatrics
The University of Pennsylvania School of Medicine
Director, Neonatal Follow Up Program
The Children's Hospital of Philadelphia
Philadelphia, Pennsylvania

VICTOR BLANCHETTE, M.D., M.R.C.P.(U.K.), F.R.C.P.(C)
Hematologist/Oncologist
The Hospital for Sick Children
Associate Professor
Department of Pediatrics
University of Toronto
Toronto, Ontario, Canada

CARL L. BOSE, M.D.
Associate Professor
Department of Pediatrics
University of North Carolina
School of Medicine
Neonatologist
North Carolina Children's Hospital
University of North Carolina Hospitals
Durham, North Carolina

MICHAEL BOYAJIAN, M.D.
Assistant Professor, Surgery and Pediatrics
George Washington University School of Medicine and Health Sciences
Chairman, Plastic and Reconstructive Surgery
Children's National Medical Center
Washington, District of Columbia

T. BERRY BRAZELTON, M.D.
Clinical Professor of Pediatrics Emeritus
Harvard Medical School
Founder and Chief, Child Development Unit
Children's Hospital
Boston, Massachusetts

ROBERT L. BRENT, M.D., Ph.D., D.Sc.(Hon)
Distinguished Professor
Louis and Bess Stein Professor of Pediatrics
Radiology and Anatomy
Jefferson Medical College
Chairman of Pediatrics
Thomas Jefferson University Hospital
Philadelphia, Pennsylvania
Chairman of Pediatrics
A.I. Dupont Institute
Wilmington, Delaware

LUC P. BRION, M.D.
Associate Professor of Pediatrics
Albert Einstein College of Medicine
Associate Director of Newborn Services
Bronx Municipal Hospital Center
Bronx, New York

RICHARD L. BUCCIARELLI, M.D.
Professor and Associate Chairman
Department of Pediatrics
Associate Executive Director
Institute for Child Health Policy
University of Florida
Gainesville, Florida

BARBARA K. BURTON, M.D.
Professor and Head
Division of Genetics and Metabolism
Department of Pediatrics
University of Illinois College of Medicine
Director, Center for Medical and Reproductive Genetics
Michael Reese Hospital and Medical Center
Chicago, Illinois

GEORGE CASSADY, M.D.
Clinical Professor
University of California San Francisco
San Francisco, California

DENNIS T. CROUSE, M.D., Ph.D.
Assistant Professor of Pediatrics
Division of Neonatology
University of Alabama at Birmingham
University Hospital
Birmingham, Alabama

JONATHAN M. DAVIS, M.D.
Associate Professor of Pediatrics
State University of New York at Stony Brook
School of Medicine
Director of Neonatology and Newborn Medicine
Director, Pulmonary Research Institute
Winthrop-University Hospital
Mineola, New York

JOHN DOYLE, M.D., F.R.C.P.(C)
Hematologist/Oncologist
The Hospital for Sick Children
Associate Professor
Department of Pediatrics
University of Toronto
Toronto, Ontario, Canada

ARIE DRUGAN, M.D.
Department of Obstetrics and Gynecology
Rambam Medical Center
Haifa, Israel

CHESTER M. EDELMANN, JR., M.D.
Professor of Pediatrics
Senior Associate Dean
Albert Einstein College of Medicine
Attending Pediatrician
The Jack D. Weiler Hospital of the Albert Einstein College of Medicine
Bronx Municipal Hospital Center
Bronx, New York

MAUREEN EDWARDS, M.D., M.P.H.
Associate Professor of Pediatrics and of Obstetrics and Gynecology
George Washington University School of Medicine and Health Sciences
Director of Newborn Service
George Washington University Medical Center
Washington, District of Columbia

MARTIN R. EICHELBERGER, M.D.
Professor of Surgery and Pediatrics
George Washington University School of Medicine and Health Sciences
Director, Emergency Trauma Services and Pediatric Surgeor
Children's National Medical Center
Washington, District of Columbia

GLORIA D. ENG, M.D.
Professor of Pediatrics and Medicine
George Washington University School of Medicine and Health Sciences
Senior Attending Staff
Department of Physical Medicine and Rehabilitation
Children's National Medical Center
Washington, District of Columbia

IARK I. EVANS, M.D.
rofessor and Vice-Chief of Obstetrics and Gynecology
rofessor of Molecular Biology, Genetics and Pathology
/ayne State University
irector, Division of Reproductive Genetics
irector, Center for Fetal Diagnosis and Therapy
utzel Hospital
etroit, Michigan

IURRAY FEINGOLD, M.D., Ph.D.(Hon)
rofessor of Pediatrics
oston University School of Medicine
hysician-in-Chief
ational Birth Defect Center
oston, Massachusetts

ICHAEL F. FLANAGAN, M.D.
ssistant Professor of Pediatrics
artmouth Medical School
ssistant in Pediatric Cardiology
artmouth-Hitchcock Medical Center
anover, New Hampshire

NNE B. FLETCHER, M.D.
rofessor of Pediatrics
eorge Washington University School of Medicine
and Health Sciences
hairman, Department of Neonatology
hildren's National Medical Center
eorge Washington University School of Medicine
and Health Sciences
ashington, District of Columbia

ARY ANN FLETCHER, M.D.
ssociate Professor of Pediatrics and of Obstetrics
and Gynecology
eorge Washington University School of Medicine
and Health Sciences
ssociate Director, Newborn Service
eorge Washington University Medical Center
ashington, District of Columbia

ISHARA J. FREIJ, M.D.
hief, Division of Infectious Diseases
epartment of Pediatrics
illiam Beaumont Hospital
oyal Oak, Michigan
inical Associate Professor of Pediatrics
ayne State University School of Medicine
etroit, Michigan

AVID S. FRIENDLY, M.D.
ofessor of Ophthalmology
eorge Washington University School of Medicine
and Health Sciences
hairman of Ophthalmology
hildren's National Medical Center
ashington, District of Columbia

ONALD C. FYLER, M.D.
ofessor of Pediatrics (Emeritus)
sociate Chief of Cardiology (Emeritus)
rvard Medical School
ston, Massachusetts

PENNY GLASS, Ph.D.
Associate Professor of Pediatrics
George Washington University School of Medicine
and Health Sciences
Director, Center for Child Development
Children's National Medical Center
Washington, District of Columbia

PAUL P. GRIFFIN, M.D.
Professor of Orthopedic Surgery
Medical University of South Carolina
Medical University Hospital
Charleston, South Carolina

PHILIP C. GUZZETTA, M.D.
Professor and Chairman
Division of Pediatric Surgery
University of Texas Southwestern Medical School
Chief, Division of Pediatric Surgery
Parkland Memorial Hospital
Chief of Surgical Service
Children's Medical Center of Dallas
Dallas, Texas

MORDECHAI HALLAK, M.D.
Assistant Professor
Department of Obstetrics and Gynecology
Wayne State University
School of Medicine
Hutzel Hospital
Detroit, Michigan

MICHAEL R. HARRISON, M.D.
Professor of Surgery and Pediatrics
Chief, Division of Pediatric Surgery
Director, Fetal Treatment Center
University of California San Francisco
School of Medicine
Chief, Division of Pediatric Surgery
University of California San Francisco Medical Center
San Francisco, California

EDMUND HEY, D.M., D. Phil.
Consultant Pediatrician
Princess Mary Maternity Hospital
Newcastle-upon-Tyne, England

ALAN HILL, M.D., Ph.D.
Professor and Head
Division of Neurology
University of British Columbia
Head, Division of Neurology
British Columbia's Children's Hospital
Vancouver, British Columbia, Canada

W. ALAN HODSON, M.M.Sc. M.D.
Professor of Pediatrics
University of Washington School of Medicine
Seattle, Washington

PROFESSOR DR. MED WOLFGANG HOLZGREVE
Geschaffsf. Oberarit und Leiterdes
Bereichs Ultrasora Lund Pranatale Medizin
Tentrum Fur Fraueheilkunde
West F. Wilhelms—Universitat Munster
Albert-Schweitzer
Germany

NELSON B. ISADA, M.D.
Assistant Professor
Department of Obstetrics and Gynecology
Divisions of Reproductive Genetics and Maternal-Fetal Medicine
Wayne State University
Hutzel Hospital
Detroit, Michigan

BEVERLY JOHNSON, B.S.N., M.A.
Coordinator
Perinatal Education Exchange Program
Children's National Medical Center
Washington, District of Columbia

LAUREN A. JOHNSON, M.D.
Instructor in Pediatrics
George Washington University School of Medicine and Health Sciences
Postdoctoral Fellow in Neonatal–Perinatal Medicine
Children's National Medical Center
George Washington University Hospital
Washington, District of Columbia

MARK P. JOHNSON, M.D.
Assistant Professor
Department of Obstetrics, Gynecology, Molecular Biology, Genetics, and Pathology
Wayne State University
Associate Director
Division of Reproductive Genetics
Hutzel Hospital
Detroit, Michigan

GEORGE W. KAPLAN, M.D., M.S.
Clinical Professor of Surgery and Pediatrics
University of California at San Diego
School of Medicine
Chief of Pediatric Urology at San Diego
Children's Hospital of San Diego
San Diego, California

JOAN McGREGOR KELLY, M.D.
Assistant Professor of Pediatrics
George Washington University School of Medicine and Health Sciences
Assistant Director of Pediatric Medical Education
Holy Cross Hospital of Silver Spring
Associate Physician, Department of General Pediatrics
Children's National Medical Center
Silver Spring, Maryland

ALLEN P. KILLAM, M.D.
Professor of Obstetrics and Gynecology
Associate Professor of Pediatrics
Duke University Medical Center
Durham, North Carolina

WINSTON W. K. KOO, M.B.B.S, F.R.A.C.P.
Associate Professor of Pediatrics, Obstetrics and Gynecology
The University of Tennessee Memphis
The Health Science Center
Staff Neonatologist
The Regional Medical Center at Memphis
Crump Women's Hospital
Perinatal Center
Memphis, Tennessee

SHARON KOVZELOVE, R.N.
Director, Critical Care Nursing
The Children's Hospital of Philadelphia
Philadelphia, Pennsylvania

DIANE BEHAN LOISEL, R.N.C., N.N.P.
Neonatal Nurse Practitioner
Children's National Medical Center
Washington, District of Columbia

JOSE L. LUCENA, M.D.
Fellow, Division of Neonatal-Perinatal Medicine
Wayne State University
School of Medicine
Children's Hospital of Michigan
Hutzel Hospital
Detroit, Michigan

MHAIRI G. MACDONALD, M.B.Ch.B., F.R.C.P.(E), D.C.H.
Professor of Pediatrics
George Washington University School of Medicine and Health Sciences
Vice-Chairman, Department of Neonatology
Children's National Medical Center/George Washington University School of Medicine and Health Sciences
Director, Neonatal Intensive Care Unit
Children's National Medical Center
Washington, District of Columbia

M. JEFFREY MAISELS, M.B., B.Ch.
Clinical Professor of Pediatrics
Wayne State University School of Medicine
University of Michigan Medical Center
Chairman, Department of Pediatrics
William Beaumont Hospital
Royal Oak, Michigan

FRANK A. MANNING, M.D., M.S.C.(OXON) F.R.C.S.
Professor and Chairman
Department of Obstetrics and Gynecology
University of Manitoba
Winnipeg, Manitoba, Canada

ANDREW M. MARGILETH, M.D.
Clinical Professor of Pediatrics
University of Virginia Medical Center
Charlottesville, Virginia
Associate Staff Physician
Mary Washington Hospital
Fredericksburg, Virginia

iEORGE H. MCCRACKEN, JR., M.D.
'rofessor of Pediatrics
he Sarah M and Charles E Sealy Chair in Pediatric Infectious Diseases
niversity of Texas Southwestern Medical Center at Dallas
ttending Physician
hildren's Medical Center
arkland Memorial Hospital
allas, Texas

'HOMAS H. MILHORAT, M.D.
'rofessor and Chairman
epartment of Neurosurgery
tate University of New York Health Science Center at Brooklyn
eurosurgeon-in-Chief
niversity Hospital
ings County Hospital and Long Island College Hospital
rooklyn, New York

OHN I. MILLER, M.D.
ssistant Professor, Department of Neurosurgery
UNY-Health Science Center at Brooklyn
irector, Division of Pediatric Neurosurgery
UNY-University Hospital of Brooklyn
ings County Hospital
rooklyn, New York

HOMAS MOSHANG, JR., M.D.
rofessor of Pediatrics
niversity of Pennsylvania School of Medicine
irector of Endocrinology/Diabetes Ambulatory Clinics
hildren's Hospital of Philadelphia
hiladelphia, Pennsylvania

OHN STEPHEN NAULTY, M.D.
linical Professor of Anesthesia and of Obstetrics
niversity of Pennsylvania
chool of Medicine
hairman, Department of Anesthesia
ennsylvania Hospital
hiladelphia, Pennsylvania

ICHOLAS NELSON, M.D.
rofessor of Pediatrics
ne Pennsylvania State University
ollege of Medicine
.S. Hershey Medical Center
ershey, Pennsylvania

URT D. NEWMAN, M.D.
ssociate Professor of Surgery and Pediatrics
eorge Washington University School of Medicine and Health Sciences
tending Surgeon
hildren's National Medical Center
ashington, District of Columbia

DWARD S. OGATA, M.D.
ofessor of Pediatrics and Obstetrics and Gynecology
aymond and Hazel Speck Berry Professor of Neonatology
ce Chair, Department of Pediatrics
orthwestern University Medical School
ead, Division of Neonatology
ildren's Memorial Hospital and Prentice Women's Hospital of Northwestern Memorial Hospital
icago, Illinois

WILLIAM OH, M.D.
Professor and Chairman
Department of Pediatrics
Brown University School of Medicine
Chief of Pediatrics
Rhode Island Hospital
Women and Infants Hospital
Providence, Rhode Island

ENRIQUE M. OSTREA, JR., M.D.
Professor of Pediatrics
Wayne State University
School of Medicine
Chief of Pediatrics
Hutzel Hospital
Detroit, Michigan

RODERIC H. PHIBBS, M.D.
Professor of Pediatrics
Associate Staff Member
Cardiovascular Research Institute
University of California San Francisco
San Francisco, California

GABRIELLA PRIDJIAN, M.D.
Assistant Professor of Obstetrics and Gynecology
Tulane University Medical School
New Orleans, Louisiana

PETER PRYDE, M.D.
Fellow
Department of Obstetrics and Gynecology
Division of Reproductive Genetics
Wayne State University School of Medicine
Hutzel Hospital
Detroit, Michigan

GLORIA S. PRYHUBER, M.D.
William Cooper Proctor Research Scholar
University of Cincinnati College of Medicine
Children's Hospital Medical Center
Cincinnati, Ohio

YUNG-HAO PUNG, M.D., M.P.H.
Assistant Professor of Pediatrics
Georgetown University School of Medicine
Attending Physician
Division of Allergy and Immunology
Department of Pediatrics
Georgetown University Medical Center
Washington, District of Columbia

MARY E. REVENIS, M.D.
Assistant Professor of Pediatrics
George Washington University School of Medicine and Health Sciences
Assistant Director of the Nursery
Attending Neonatologist
Children's National Medical Center
Washington, District of Columbia

WARD R. RICE, M.D., Ph.D.
Associate Professor of Pediatrics
University of Cincinnati College of Medicine
Children's Hospital Medical Center
Cincinnati, Ohio

WARREN N. ROSENFELD, M.D.
Professor of Pediatrics
SUNY at Stony Brook
Chairman, Department of Pediatrics
Winthrop-University Hospital
Mineola, New York

THOMAS M. ROUSE, M.D.
Department of Pediatric Surgery
Methodist Hospital of Indiana
Indianapolis, Indiana

LISA M. SATLIN, M.D.
Assistant Professor
Albert Einstein College of Medicine
New York, New York
Attending Physician
Weiler Hospital of the Albert Einstein College of Medicine
Bronx Municipal Hospital
Bronx, New York

JOHN W. SCANLON, M.D.
Professor of Pediatrics
Georgetown University School of Medicine
Director, Neonatology
Columbia Hospital for Women
Washington, District of Columbia

BARBARA SCHMIDT, M.D., M.Sc., F.R.C.P.(C)
Staff Neonatologist
Chedoke McMaster Hospital
Associate Professor
Department of Pediatrics
McMaster University
Hamilton, Ontario, Canada

JAY J. SCHNITZER, M.D., Ph.D.
Instructor in Surgery
Harvard Medical School
Assistant in Surgery
Massachusetts General Hospital
Boston, Massachusetts

JEFFERY E. SELL, M.D.
Director, Heart Transplant Program
Assistant Professor of Surgery and Pediatrics
George Washington University School of Medicine and Health Sciences
Attending Cardiovascular Surgeon
Children's National Medical Center
Washington, District of Columbia

JOHN L. SEVER, M.D., Ph.D.
Professor of Pediatrics, Obstetrics and Gynecology, Microbiology, and Immunology
George Washington University School of Medicine and Health Sciences
Infectious Diseases Department
Children's National Medical Center
Washington, District of Columbia

VIVIAN SHATZ, B.S.N., R.N.C.
Clinical Nurse Educator
George Washington University Hospital
Washington, District of Columbia

THOMAS H. SHEPARD, M.D.
Professor of Pediatrics
Adjunct Professor, Obstetrics, Gynecology, and Environmental Health
University of Washington
School of Medicine
Seattle, Washington

BILLIE LOU SHORT, M.D.
Professor of Pediatrics
George Washington University School of Medicine and Health Sciences
Director of ECMO Program
Children's National Medical Center
Washington, District of Columbia

MARIA ASUNCION SILVESTRE, M.D.
Senior Research Fellow
Division of Neonatal-Perinatal Medicine
Wayne State University
Attending Neonatologist
Children's Hospital of Michigan
Hutzel Hospital
Detroit, Michigan

PAUL S. THORNTON, M.B., B.Ch., M.R.C.P.I.
Instructor of Pediatrics
University of Pennsylvania School of Medicine
Endocrine Fellow
The Children's Hospital of Philadelphia
Philadelphia, Pennsylvania

SHARON M. TOMASKI, M.D.
Fellow
Department of Otolaryngology
Children's National Medical Center
Washington, District of Columbia

WILLIAM E. TRUOG, M.D.
Professor of Pediatrics
University of Washington
School of Medicine
Attending Neonatologist
University of Washington Medical Center
Children's Hospital Medical Center
Seattle, Washington

REGINALD C. TSANG, M.D.
Professor of Pediatrics, Obstetrics and Gynecology
University of Cincinnati Medical Center
Children's Hospital Medical Center
Executive Director, Perinatal Research Institute
Vice Chair, Academic Affairs and Research
Cincinnati, Ohio

JON A. VANDERHOOF, M.D.
Professor and Chairman
Department of Pediatrics
Creighton University
Director, Joint Section of Pediatric Gastroenterology and Nutrition
Creighton University/University of Nebraska Medical Center
Chief of Pediatrics
St. Joseph Hospital
Omaha, Nebraska

JOSEPH J. VOLPE, M.D.
Bronson Crothers Professor of Neurology
Harvard Medical School
Neurologist-in-Chief
Children's Hospital
Boston, Massachusetts

ROBERT M. WARD, M.D.
Associate Professor, Pediatrics
University of Utah School of Medicine
Medical Director
Newborn Critical Care Services
Primary Care Medical Center
Salt Lake City, Utah

BARBARA B. WARNER, M.D.
William Cooper Proctor Research Scholar
University of Cincinnati College of Medicine
Children's Hospital Medical Center
Cincinnati, Ohio

HOWARD J. WEINSTEIN, M.D.
Associate Professor of Pediatrics
Harvard Medical School
Director, Pediatric Bone Marrow Transplant Program
Children's Hospital and Dana-Farber Cancer Institute
Boston, Massachusetts

SUSAN E. WERT, Ph.D.
Research Associate, Department of Pediatrics
Division of Neonatology and Pulmonary Biology
University of Cincinnati College of Medicine
Research Scholar
Director, Morphology Core
Division of Pulmonary Biology
Children's Hospital Research Foundation
Cincinnati, Ohio

JEFFREY A. WHITSETT, M.D.
Professor of Pediatrics
University of Cincinnati College of Medicine
Director, Division of Pulmonary Biology
Children's Hospital Medical Center
Cincinnati, Ohio

JUDYTH BROWN WIGGINS, R.N., B.S.N., C.N.N.P.
Neonatal Nurse Practitioner
Children's National Medical Center
Washington, District of Columbia

TERENCE L. ZACH, M.D.
Assistant Professor of Pediatrics
Creighton University
Omaha, Nebraska

BARBARA J. ZELIGS
Research Associate
Department of Pediatrics
Georgetown University School of Medicine
Washington, District of Columbia

ALVIN ZIPURSKY, M.D., F.R.C.P.(C)
Hematologist/Oncologist
The Hospital for Sick Children
Professor
Department of Pediatrics
University of Toronto
Toronto, Ontario, Canada

PREFACE

As this textbook arrives at a fourth edition, the specialty of neonatology has moved through its infancy, childhood, and adolescence to a robust adulthood. Far and away the largest boarded subspecialty of pediatrics, neonatology still occupies about one sixth of the training time of pediatric residents. A similar prominence is found in the table of contents of research publications and among the platform presentations at national meetings. The six to eight billion dollars annually expended on neonatal intensive care in the United States represent an appreciable part of the total health budget.

At the same time, neonatology as a specialty has become somewhat disorganized and fragmented. Deregionalization has led to the establishment of Level II units in many community hospitals and a distinction between academic and community-practice neonatologists. Technology has been more highly dispersed. On the other hand, specialization to a remarable degree has taken root among neonatologists in academic centers. Once generalists who gave age-specialized intensive or comprehensive care to newborns, neonatologists, in their research and special competence roles, are now segregated into multiple sub-sub-specialties. At research meetings, gastrointestinal nutrition, cardiopulmonary conditions, growth and development, metabolism, genetic diseases, nephrology, hematology, and neurology each may have separate sections—all addressing the neonate.

The fourth edition of *Neonatology* attempts to address this current state of affairs. The book is still centered on the pathophysiology and management of the major disease processes affecting the neonate. "General Considerations," including the organization of perinatal care, moral and ethical issues, and specific aspects of the intensive care nursery environment, are addressed in an opening section. The crucial transitions of the newborn period are discussed in major sections entitled "The Fetal Patient" and "Transition and Stabilization." The special vulnerability of "The Low-Birth-Weight Infant" is acknowledged in a section comprised of chapters on the small-for-gestational-age infant, the premature infant, and the infant born of a multiple gestation. The largest section, entitled "The Newborn Infant," discusses disease entities, which are mostly classified along disciplinary or organ system lines. Final sections address "Pharmacology" and issues "Beyond the Nursery," such as discharge planning, care after discharge, and developmental outcome.

Two coeditors, Mhairi MacDonald, M.B.Ch.B., F.R.C.P.(E), D.C.H., and Mary Ann Fletcher, M.D., have joined me in bringing out this new edition, now with 61 chapters. Virtually all chapters have been extensively rewritten, and 10 entirely new chapters have been added. The changing perinatal health-care environment is addressed in new chapters on regionalization, resource issues, and transport. Developments in maternal–fetal medicine are described in chapters on fetomaternal interaction and pharmacology, fetal development, and multiple gestation. Important breakthroughs in neonatal pulmonology, such as surfactant therapy, are covered in new chapters on acute and chronic lung disease and on extracorporeal membrane oxygenation. The effects of treatment on the development of the vulnerable neonate are addressed in chapters on the neonatal intensive care environment and development of the sick neonate, anesthesia and pain control, and infants of drug-abusing mothers. Follow-up issues are discussed further in new chapters on discharge planning, care after discharge, and developmental outcome.

It is our hope that those who use this book will find that it brings together in one place the work of countless specialists whose collective efforts advance neonatology at such a breathless pace. No textbook is a substitute for journals and scientific meetings, where new ideas constantly emerge. But as a broad representation of the state of the art, a textbook provides a platform on which to stand while we struggle to find new concepts and better ways to care for newborn infants and their families.

Gordon B. Avery, M.D., Ph.D.

PREFACE TO THE FIRST EDITION

Neonatology means knowledge of the human newborn. The term was coined by Alexander Schaffer, whose book on the subject, *Diseases of the Newborn*, was first published in 1960. This book, together with Clement Smith's *Physiology of the Newborn Infant*, formed cornerstones of the developing field. In the past 15 years, neonatology has grown from the preoccupation of a handful of pioneers to a major subspecialty of pediatrics. Knowledge in this area has so expanded that it now seems important to collect this material into a multiauthor reference work.

Although the perinatal mortality rate has declined over the past 50 years, the best presently attainable survival rates have not been achieved throughout the world, and indeed the United States lags behind 15 other countries, despite its vast resources. New knowledge and improvement in the coordination of services for mother and child are needed to drive down perinatal mortality further. And finally, far greater emphasis must be placed on morbidity, so that surviving infants can lead full and productive lives. One hopes that in the future the yardstick of success will be the quality of life and not the mere fact of life itself.

In this past decade, neonatology, as a recognized subspecialty of pediatrics, has come into being around the intensive care–premature nursery. Needless to say, the problems of prematurity are far from solved. But neonatology is ripe for a broadening-out from its prematurity–hyaline membrane disease beginnings. The newborn is heir to so many problems and his physiology is so unique and rapidly changing that all conditions of the newborn should come within the concern of the new and expanding discipline of neonatology. It has long since become standard practice to admit to premature nurseries other high-risk infants such as those of diabetic or toxemic mothers. Here the criterion is the need for intensive care. However, the neonatologist's specialized knowledge should give him a significant role in the care of other infants in the first 2 to 3 months of life, whether or not they require intensive care, and whether or not they are readmitted for problems unrelated to prematurity and birth itself. Detailed knowledge of newborn physiology can assist in the management of congenital anomalies, surgical conditions of the neonate, failure to thrive, nutritional problems, genetic, neurologic, and biochemical diseases, and a host of conditions involving delayed maturation. Thus one can conceive of a subspecialty sharply limited in age to early infancy, but broad in its study of the interaction of normal physiology and disease processes.

Neonatology must also grow in its relationship to obstetrics and fetal biology. In the best centers, an active partnership has developed between obstetrics and pediatrics around the management of high-risk pregnancies and newborns. Sometimes training has been cooperative, but in only a few instances have basic scientists concerned with fetal biology been brought into this effort. Important beginnings have been made in studying the fetomaternal unit, such as the endocrine studies of Egon Diczfalusy, the cardiopulmonary studies of Geoffrey Dawes, and the immunologic studies of Arther Silverstein. But fundamental processes such as the controls of fetal growth and the onset of labor are not understood at this time. Centers or institutes bringing together workers of diverse points of view are needed to wrestle with the profound problems of fetal biology. At the clinical level, the interdependence of obstetrics and neonatology is obvious. As an ultimate development, these two specialities may one day be joined as a new entity, perinatology, at least at the level of training and certification. In the meantime, far greater mutual understanding and daily interaction are needed for the optimal care of mothers and their infants.

This book is organized around problems as they occur, as well as by organ systems. It hopes to achieve a balance between presentation of the basic science on which rational management must rest, and the advice concerning patient care which experts in each subarea are qualified to give. Individual chapter authors have approached their subjects in varying ways, and no attempt has been made to achieve a completely uniform format. In some instances, there is overlap of subject material, but the somewhat different viewpoints presented, and the desire to spare the reader hopscotching through the book after cross references, have persuaded me to leave small overlaps undisturbed.

It is appreciated that no volume such as this can have more than a finite useful lifetime. Yet while its currency lasts, I hope it will serve as a practical guide to therapy and an aid in the understanding of pathophysiology for those active in the care of newborns.

Gordon B. Avery, M.D., Ph.D.

CONTENTS

Part One: General Considerations

Part Two: The Fetal Patient

Part Three: Transition and Stabilization

Part Four: The Low-Birth-Weight Infant

Part Five: The Newborn Infant

Part Six: Pharmacology

Part Seven: Beyond the Nursery

Appendices

NEONATOLOGY

Part One

GENERAL CONSIDERATIONS

Neonatology: Pathophysiology and Management of the Newborn, Fourth Edition,
edited by Gordon B. Avery, Mary Ann Fletcher, and Mhairi G. MacDonald.
J.B. Lippincott Company, Philadelphia © 1994.

chapter 1

Neonatology: Perspective in the Mid-1990s

GORDON B. AVERY

ʀapid change has characterized neonatology since he name was coined in 1960 by Alexander Schaffer. ›tructurally, it can be compared with a tree (Fig. 1-1). ts "roots"—obstetrics, pediatrics, and physiology—›egan at the turn of the century. A sturdy "trunk" ıas developed in the intensive care nurseries (ICNs) ›cattered across the United States and around the vorld. The "branches" have spread so widely that it s difficult for a single person to be expert in all the ıreas of activity required for a tertiary neonatology ervice. Important interactions have gone beyond alied disciplines such as obstetrics, anesthesiology, ardiology, radiology, and surgery. Neonatologists oday struggle with hospital administrators, pediatric raining program directors, legislatures, Congress, he courts, the federal government, malpractice lawers, right-to-life groups, and ethicists in an effort to letermine their proper roles and limits. Caught in a ross fire between strenuous cost-containment meaures and regulations mandating the vigorous treatnent of all newborns regardless of prognosis, many ıeonatologists wonder when a stable situation will e reached. Yet stimulating growth has occurred—nainly since 1960.

HE ROOTS

)ne of the main roots from which neonatology grew vas supplied by obstetricians such as Pierre Budin nd Sir Dugald Baird, who were interested in the babies they delivered and not merely in the immediate welfare of the mother. It may be a serious oversimplification to imply that in former times, obstetricians were content if the baby was liveborn. Childbirth, however, was the cause of a significant number of maternal deaths and for many was a fearful experience. Premature infants were expected to die, as were most neonates with malformations. There was a feeling that natural selection should be allowed to discard the "runt of the litter," as suggested by the designation of prematures as "weaklings." It was Budin and his pupil Couney who pioneered incubator care of premature infants and thus helped change some of the early, pessimistic attitudes toward these babies.

Another significant root of neonatology can be found in the "quiet premature nursery," such as that run by Julius Hess and Evelyn Lundeen in Chicago in the early 1900s.[1] Only premature infants were admitted to these nurseries, and gentleness with minimal intervention was the policy. To prevent infection, staff wore gowns, caps, and masks and set up a scrub routine that excluded parents and minimized traffic in the area. Feedings of breast milk by eyedropper were delayed for up to 72 hours, and the infants were handled as little as possible. Yet the supportive conditions needed to allow the body to recover, as described by Florence Nightingale, were present: "warmth, rest, diet, quiet, sanitation, space, and others."[2] Perhaps some of the high-tech nurseries of today could benefit from an infusion of this superb nurturing orientation.

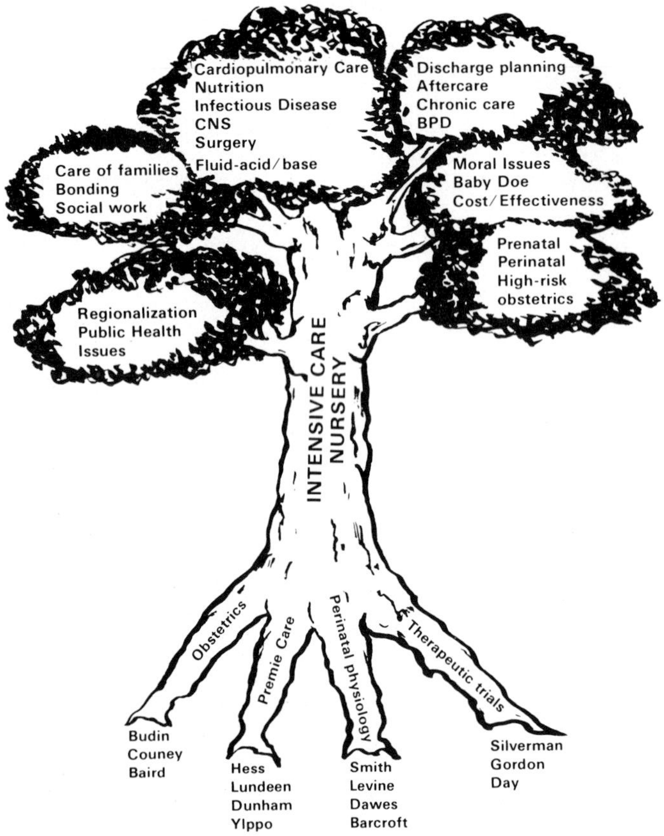

FIG. 1–1. The neonatal–perinatal tree shows the root, trunk, and branches of the specialty.

Physiology is a tap root of neonatology. Advances in neonatal care rest directly on descriptions of the changing body processes of the newborn infant. Men such as Barcroft and Dawes began delineation of fetal circulation and placental function. These studies in turn led to the establishment of the fetal lamb model, which subsequently was widely exploited. Neonatal metabolic, gastrointestinal, respiratory, and central nervous system functions were studied by Levine, Smith, Peiper, and others. The 1945 publication of the first edition of Clement Smith's textbook, *Physiology of the Newborn Infant*, was a signal event in our evolving ability to care for sick newborns in a rational manner.[3]

A final anchoring root of neonatology is the therapeutic trial. Innumerable traditional teachings about premature infants have eventually been proved false. Without scientific testing as a guide, neonatologists would constantly be off course. As it is, several dangerous misadventures have been averted by clinical trials. An example is prophylactic sulfonamide treatment of premature infants, which was found to cause increased kernicterus.[4] Silverman, Gordon, and Day were pioneers who insisted on rigor in such trials.

THE TRUNK

The ICN is the institution that forms the sturdy trunk of endeavors in neonatology. The ICN is a therapeutic environment, a collection of equipment, and a multidisciplinary team that is guided by dedicate leadership, by a group of specific protocols, and by body of relevant scientific knowledge. It is the ICN a an integrated organism, rather than any single pe son or collection of people, that takes care of the sic neonate—in a sense, this is holistic medicine turne inside out. The ICN has proved very effective in th care of desperately ill babies, but its rationale remain difficult to explain to hospital administrators, insu ance companies, and congressmen.

Over the years, there has been a steady increase i the intensity of illness observed in the ICN. With thi rise has come an increase in the number and variet of personnel and the amount of technically sophist cated equipment. In the 1950s, premature care was major concern. The principal interventions were re suscitation, thermoregulation, careful feeding, sim ple and exchange transfusion, and supportive care c respiratory distress. By the 1960s, electronic monitor came into use, and blood gases began to be mea sured. Feedings were aided by nasogastric tubes, an increased laboratory monitoring became possible Antibiotics became available for treatment of neonat sepsis.

By the 1970s, the use of umbilical catheters an arterial pressure transducers was routine, and resp rator therapy of hyaline membrane disease began t succeed. Nutritional support for sick infants wa aided by transpyloric feeding tubes and finally b complete intravenous alimentation. Microchemistr ests for most necessary parameters became widely vailable. Neonatal surgery was shown to be feasible or many congenital abnormalities, including serious ardiac defects. With the 1980s came the advent of omputed tomography and ultrasonography. Significant concern centered around ventricular hemorrhages and consequent post-hemorrhagic hydrocephlus in small premature infants. Transcutaneous lectrodes became available first for measurement of xygen and then for carbon dioxide. Pulse oximetry ncreasingly has been used for continuous physiogic monitoring. Nutritional and metabolic supports vere significantly refined. Surfactant replacement as reduced the severity of lung disease in premature nfants. Extracorporeal membrane oxygenation peritted the survival of some previously unsalvageable nfants. In the 1990s, magnetic resonance imaging improved visualization of lesions, and positron emision tomography and magnetic resonance spectrospy promise to reveal the physiology of the intact rain. As survival has become common for infants vho weigh as little as 600 g at birth, increased attenon has swung to assuring intact survival, and the 990s have been dubbed the decade of the brain.

HE BRANCHES

ERINATALOLOGY

body of specialized knowledge, a group of subspealized professionals, the advent of technically adanced equipment, and the formation of special care nits all contributed to the development of neonatogy. In obstetrics, these same elements came toether about 10 years later and resulted in the spealty of maternofetal medicine. Perinatologists eveloped high-risk prenatal clinics and special delivy facilities for unstable patients. A steadily growing ody of literature from animal and clinical investigaons allowed improved management of pregnancy mplications and monitoring of fetal status. Ultranography allowed the detection of fetal abnormalies and determination of fetal size, anatomy, activity, eathing, and response to stress. For the first time, others were given drugs designed to treat fetal contions, and intrauterine transfusions were performed in cases of threatened hydrops. Fetal surgery as yet to find its proper place, but prenatal shunts ave been inserted for hydrocephalus, obstructed inary tracts have been drained, and repair of diaragmatic hernia has been attempted.

In many major teaching hospitals, perinatal obstet: and neonatal services have joined forces to form rinatal centers. Often with codirectors from the o disciplines, these centers fostered cooperation in e best interests of the high-risk patient. Integrated anning and management in optimal cases consisted a high-risk prenatal clinic, timing and management labor and delivery, resuscitation, and intensive care in the nursery. Statistics on morbidity and mortality, reviewed in periodic joint conferences, permit constant refinement of policy and technique. These centers have been the locations of training programs in both perinatology and neonatology and the sources of important research. They have demonstrated the best survival rates for small prematures and other categories of infants at highest risk, and they provide the standard by which perinatal care is judged.

The natural alliance between perinatal obstetrics and neonatology is so great that some have suggested that it receive department status within the medical complex. In some ways, the perinatal center accomplishes this on an *ad hoc* basis. But perinatologists and neonatologists are parts of traditional departments of obstetrics and pediatrics, with surgical and medical orientations, respectively. Allocation of resources and ranking of faculty occur predominantly through the parent departments, where the priorities of the chairmen are paramount.

REGIONAL CONNECTIONS

The medical community found that to optimize function of the perinatal center, it was necessary to form complex relationships among hospitals and community resources (see Chap. 3). First neonatal and then maternal transport services were developed to move patients safely and efficiently to the center and back. Hot lines were established to provide consultation and bed allocation, which could be coordinated through a single phone number. Affiliations for continuing education were formed, and standard protocols for referral were worked out. In some instances, exchange of personnel and joint review of statistics helped cement the connection.

Government agencies extended a helping hand in this networking. Some state legislatures were convinced early of the public health advantage of regional systems. The government began to award grants to perinatal centers to underwrite some of the cost of outreach and system activities. Training and research grants from the federal government often were given to the same perinatal centers and served to buttress the resources of these centers. With passage of the National Health Planning and Resources Development Act (Public Law 93-641) in 1974, the federal government mandated regional planning of expensive resources in the interest of efficiency and economy. Designation of care levels I, II, and III was adopted, and publication of regional plans for perinatal care became widespread.

Unfortunately, during the 1980s, regionalization suffered striking reversals. The mandated state health planning mechanisms were emasculated. Hospitals became increasingly competitive and wished to offer full services to prepaid health plans. Large numbers of neonatologists moved into suburban hospitals and set up level II nurseries. The result was a decentralization of perinatal high-risk care, with loss of efficiency and economy of scale.

Finally, I wish to call attention to the involvement of neonatologists in a mixture of educational, administrative, and political activities that have been very taxing and time consuming. Although neonatology training has emphasized bedside care, a business school or public health degree would be directly useful to today's neonatologist. A thorough training in counseling, group dynamics, and law also would be invaluable.

ETHICS

During the newborn period, babies with congenital malformations, asphyxia, and extreme immaturity are seen. Modern powerful life-support systems provide the technology for relatively prolonged continuation of futile care. These circumstances have thrust neonatologists into the center of a national debate on medical ethics. In the midst of all this, neonatologists must keep their heads and care for babies and their families as best they can. Chapter 2 deals extensively with the moral issues raised by neonatal intensive care.

CARE OF THE FAMILY

In general, there has been striking improvement in care of the distressed families of critically ill newborn infants. Formerly excluded from the ICN because of fear of infection, parents are brought to the bedside and encouraged to touch their babies. Limited sibling visitation often is permitted. Nurses help parents get used to intrusive medical equipment and, as soon as possible, parents perform simple caretaking procedures with their child. Social workers, parent support groups, chaplains, and literature for parents have become increasingly available. Starting with the work of Klaus and Kennell, a growing body of publications has appeared that suggests that bonding of parents to the newborn infant is important to later functioning of the family unit. The change of the title of Klaus and Kennell's monograph from *Maternal–Infant Bonding* in 1976 to *Parent–Infant Bonding* in 1982 reflects recognition of the role of fathers in the parenting of neonates.[5,6]

HOME CARE

The aftercare of discharged high-risk newborns has become an increasingly important area of concern for neonatologists. Although many problems are quickly resolved and require only routine follow-up, a significant number of babies with chronic problems are taken home from the ICN. As a small premature infant approaches discharge, it becomes clear that parent instruction, sleep apnea testing, cardiopulmonary resuscitation training, concern with feeding and growth, schedules for testing sight, hearing, and speech, physical medicine, and developmental psy chology foreshadow a first year of life crowded with clinic visits and special needs. Infants with chroni lung disease not uncommonly go home on oxyge therapy, multiple medications, and special feedin regimens. During the first year or two of life, inter current infections may require several readmissions The best outcomes have been achieved with earl diagnosis of developmental difficulties and the mobi lization of community resources. All this necessitate input from a physician with appreciation of th stormy neonatal period and an understanding of th continuing problems of infants born prematurel with other perinatal insults. Often, a multidisciplin ary team at the tertiary center collaborates with th family's pediatrician to provide this special care. Al though oriented to neonatal intensive care, neonatc logists have begun to assume responsibility in thi aftercare.

THE INTENSIVE CARE NURSERY AS A SPACE STATION

The quiet, simple, gentle premature nursery of 5 years ago has been transformed into a bustling spac station. Suspended halfway up a tall building, to often it is drenched in bright light and alive wit activity throughout the night. The tiny baby in th incubator is dwarfed by a procedure light, a res pirator, a multichannel monitor, four intravenou pumps, and a transcutaneous oxygen module. Th baby's chest is covered with electrodes, and tube lead into and out of his or her body at several point Eight to twelve electrical cords, two oxygen lines, an a suction catheter attach to the bedside console. Me ications and flush solutions are drawn up in syringe close at hand. A resuscitation bag is at the head of th baby's bed in case he or she should stop breathin Alarms sound, knots of people move busily abou and large machines are pushed among the incuba tors. Ultrasonographic elements are touched to th infant's head, chest, and abdomen. Images flash on screen and are recorded on tape for later analysi House officers speak rapidly in an acronymic cod barely intelligible to residents who graduated 2 yea previously. Hess and Lundeen, coming some morn ing for a visit, might wonder if they had missed th address and arrived on the wrong planet!

At such a bedside, today's neonatologist must cop with a constantly enlarging body of new literature o cardiopulmonary physiology, nutritional and meta bolic support, new antibiotics and infectious diseas conditions, ventricular hemorrhage and asphyxi syndromes, and surgical, genetic, and cardiac prob lems. It is no longer possible for a physician to rea all the new publications, even when restricted to th area of neonatology. New therapeutic approach are proposed much faster than they can be teste in an orderly way; many such theories never will b tested.

IMPLICATIONS FOR THE FUTURE

The field of neonatology will never again return to the quiet premature nursery of Hess and Lundeen, but we must conserve some of the gentleness and nurturing qualities of that era.

Neonatology is now, and hereafter will be, a team activity. We must therefore care for our teams with skill and make them effective instruments.

The ICN is embedded in a community to which it must be related in an efficient and systematic way. We can ill afford to begrudge the time it takes to maintain regional systems.

The government is involved with neonatal intensive care more than with most other areas of medicine. Regional systems, Medicaid regulations, Baby Doe regulations, cost-containment measures, and maternal and child health programs all bring neonatologists in contact with government agencies. Neonatologists will need to become diligent and skillful advocates, negotiators, and lobbyists.

Within medical centers, relationships among the hospital, the medical school, and the neonatologists as a practice group are changing. A satisfactory support base must be developed for activities split among patient care, teaching, administration, research, and advocacy.

Some specialization within neonatology is inevitable. No one person can be at the forefront in all the branches of the field.

Neonatology training programs should include opportunities to gain knowledge and skill in the business aspects of nursery and practice management, in administrative and negotiating techniques, and in public health and regional planning.

Despite all this complexity, the final need is for calm and simplicity. Within health care systems, in the last analysis, we meet others one by one. Patient care can never be better than the quality of individual human encounters. Today, our ideal role model could still be Evelyn Lundeen putting tiny hats on premature infants to keep their heads warm.

REFERENCES

1. Hess JH, Lundeen EC. The premature infant: its medical and nursing care. Philadelphia: JB Lippincott, 1941.
2. Nightingale F. Notes on nursing: what it is and what it is not. (A facsimile of the first edition printed in London, 1859, with a foreword by Annie W. Goodrich.) Philadelphia: JB Lippincott, 1969.
3. Smith CA. The physiology of the newborn infant. Springfield, IL: Charles C Thomas, 1945.
4. Silverman WA, Anderson DH, Blanc WA, Crozier DN. A difference in mortality rate and incidence of kernicterus among premature infants allotted to two prophylactic antibiotic regimens. Pediatrics 1956;18:614.
5. Klaus MH, Kennell JH. Maternal–infant bonding. St Louis: CV Mosby, 1976.
6. Klaus MH, Kennell JH. Parent–infant bonding. St Louis: CV Mosby, 1982.

Neonatology: Pathophysiology and Management of the Newborn, Fourth Edition
edited by Gordon B. Avery, Mary Ann Fletcher, and Mhairi G. MacDonald
J.B. Lippincott Company, Philadelphia © 1994

chapter 2

The Morality of Drastic Intervention

GORDON B. AVERY

A decade after the Baby Doe regulations of 1983, we still have not decided as a society how to set limits on the use of drastic life support systems in the newborn. There are those who believe that anticipated quality of life cannot enter into care decisions in critically ill infants; that, short of cessation of the heartbeat, every possible therapy should be used. Some people deplore the suffering of marginally viable prematures, and consider the huge expenditure of resources for their care a violation of distributive justice. Often, the decision-making process among parents, medical teams, hospital ethics committees, and external review mechanisms such as the courts is tense. The final area of societal ambivalence is that there is an enormous bias to save life during the medical crisis in the nursery, yet there is paltry provision of aftercare and support for families with damaged and disabled children.

BABY DOE AND BEYOND

The federal government passed the Baby Doe regulations in 1983 in reaction to the decision to withhold lifesaving surgery for esophageal atresia in a child with Down syndrome.[1] The regulations were written with the assumption that physicians and even parents could not be trusted to give needed care, that withholding of indicated treatment was widespread, and that the Federal Government needed to protect the civil rights of handicapped newborns. These regulations presumed to draw their authority from Section 504 of the Rehabilitation Act of 1973, which is a law written to protect the civil rights of handicappe people. Pursuant to these regulations, signs in nu series invited anonymous tips to a central numbe resulting in numerous hasty and badly conducted ir vestigations with not a single instance of treatmen withholding found or corrected. The regulation were challenged in court and were ruled to have bee illegally promulgated.

Revised regulations and another index case—th of Baby Jane Doe—followed.[2] In this case, which ir volved a child with spina bifida, a lawyer who nev knew the child or family pursued them through th New York court system and finally to the Suprem Court while attempting to force surgery for the chil While the state proceeding was still in progress, th Department of Health and Human Services requeste access to Baby Jane Doe's medical records. The hosp tal refused to release the patient records, arguing th a cause of action did not exist and that the privacy patient records should govern. Without the family plaintiffs or access to the medical record, the Surgeo General was unable to make a judgment as whether there was a credible case. The courts in eac instance ruled that the medical record need not released without parental consent or prior eviden of abuse or neglect.

The federal child abuse laws were amended in 19 to deal with the potential withholding of indicate medical treatment.[3] The final wording of this amen ment was the result of delicate compromise involvi many participants, including a group of Senators, t American Academy of Pediatrics, and right-to-li groups. Withholding of indicated medical treatme as held to be a form of child abuse and was enforceble under this legislation. An area for judgment was arefully preserved, however. Medical treatment is ot mandated if it is not medically indicated, if it erely prolongs the act of dying, if it is futile, if it fails ameliorate all of the infant's life-threatening conditons, or if it is virtually futile and under the circumances inhumane. In the wake of this legislation, eonatologists and their medical teams, families, initutional ethics committees, and the community ave had to decide these issues. However, the reponsibility for making these decisions has returned rgely to the family and the medical team, backed up y hospital ethics committees, which have become creasingly common.

Brain death is fairly well accepted as grounds for rminating life-support in older patients. The criteria r brain death are harder to agree on in the newborn, owever, because of reported recoveries after relavely prolonged periods of unresponsiveness and at electroencephalograms. Further, the prognosis of evastatingly poor quality of life or persistent vegetave state often engenders the question of withdrawg support because these drastic measures are dged virtually futile and under the circumstances humane. The Catholic Church has taken the posion that care that is excessively burdensome need ot be given.[4]

In the case of the extremely premature infant, some eople feel that the lower limits of viability are delineed by the smallest recorded survivor (<400 g)[5]; hers would choose the size at which a significant oportion of survivors occurs (*i.e.*, 600–800 g). Most ates require the report of a live birth if the infant is yond a certain weight or gestation age, and some quire it if the slightest sign of life is detected (*e.g.*, a int heartbeat, a gasp). Yet, once the infant is delived, the area for choice among management alternaes remains great.

THICAL ISSUES

rmal ethical principles have gradually been applied the special circumstances of critically ill newborns. e first and generally preeminent principle is *indilual beneficence*, or in some cases its inverse, *nonmaicence*. This principle requires that medical decins be made so as to do good for and avoid doing rm to the patient. Where healing and recovery are ssible, this almost always means giving indicated atment. When recovery is uncertain or unlikely, en suffering is intense, and when quality of life in e best circumstances is anticipated to be barely ore than vegetative, the beneficence of prolonged d invasive life-support systems is debatable. eonatologists are as often criticized for failing to andon ill-advised drastic interventions as they are aised for occasional remarkable successes. Neonaogists should consider themselves in their primary role as servants, albeit technically sophisticated ones, of the babies and their families, rather than as professors, scientific innovators, medical team leaders, or keepers of outcome statistics.

A second ethical principle is justice, a sense of fairness to all. A particular concern is *distributive justice*. This principle requires that scarce resources be allocated for the maximum common good and not be overly consumed by a favored minority. A single infant may require a million dollars or more for an initial hospitalization, tie up a critical care bed for 6 months, and require burdensome and expensive aftercare indefinitely. The Office of Technology Assessment estimated that neonatal intensive care cost about $4 billion dollars nationally in 1986.[6] Health resources are not infinite, and we have begun to resort to *de facto* rationing in this country, mostly by insurance status and ability to pay. Some jurisdictions, however (*e.g.*, Oregon) have begun to withdraw public support for extremely expensive procedures that are deemed of marginal utility. In the next few years, federal and state regulations, curtailment of reimbursement by third-party payers, and economic stresses on medical institutions will bring the messy considerations of cost and resource use alongside the more humane consideration of individual beneficence. In considering distributive justice, however, the neonate has the potential of a whole lifetime and amazing powers of recovery, as compared with some instances of merely prolonging the dying of the elderly.

A third ethical principle is that of *individual autonomy*. According to this principle, an adult patient may decide against treatment, even when it is medically indicated and effective. Here the right of a person to make his or her own decisions is the primary consideration. But babies are unable to express autonomy, so an appropriate surrogate must exercise this option on their behalf. Who is the appropriate surrogate? The first answer is the parents, who are authorized by law to give consent for medical treatment, are presumed to have a close and loving relationship with the child, and are personally affected by the baby's outcome and therefore a closely interested party. In most instances, parents are given great leeway in deciding on medical treatment for their infants. But the judgment of parents is sometimes suspect. They may be unable to understand the medical complexities of the alternative choices. They may be too emotionally distressed to think rationally. They may be drugged, intoxicated, psychotic, or unavailable. Occasionally, their desire to avoid dealing with a handicapped child may lead to the request that indicated and effective therapy not be given.

In such instances, the medical team may be more directive but cannot actually go against a parent's request without a court order. Institutional Ethics Committees are designed to bring a broader and more dispassionate view to difficult situations in medical ethics. Health professionals who are not part of the responsible medical team, allied disciplines (*e.g.*, social workers, religious and community representatives, lawyers), and even parents who have experienced neonatal critical care in their own children, may bring a collective wisdom to these dilemmas. These committees normally are advisory rather than vested with direct, decision-making authority, but there is considerable moral weight in the group's recommendation. In some cases, experienced patient advocates are brought in to mediate between caregivers and parents on behalf of the infant. The courts may become arbiters where a standoff between parents and hospital staff cannot be resolved. Unfortunately, the judicial system is slow, conservative, and sometimes unrealistic and insensitive. As a final backstop against abuse, they are absolutely necessary, but as a front-line resource for making case-by-case medical care decisions, the courts are a clumsy and unresponsive mechanism.

CONSIDERATIONS IN THE DECISION-MAKING PROCESS

A decision of whether or not to withhold or withdraw life-sustaining therapy is an intensely human transaction. All the faculties—mind, emotions, experience, and personal values—come into play. The issues are so complex that detailed reference to policy and precedent cannot resolve most cases. Therefore, the integrity of the process is the single most crucial factor. No single set of rules prevails, but some of the considerations below have proved humane and beneficial in my institution.

The parents always must be involved. If a critical decision point is approaching, they should be given the background as the situation evolves so that they are not suddenly thrust into a crisis with decision-making responsibility and no preparation. The neonatologist should wait, listen carefully, and give the parents more than one opportunity to say what may be extraordinarily difficult to express in words. We should understand that they are ambivalent and may have strong feelings on both sides of the question. This passion and subjectivity has been used as an argument to take parents out of prime responsibility; however, deep caring also is a priceless gift that parents may bestow. Amita Sarin, the mother of a severely handicapped premature child, has spoken eloquently regarding the role of the parent in such situations:

> Indeed, it is up to the "emotionally involved" to say when it is enough. In fact, let society be grateful for the "emotional involvement" and the passion that cause parents to turn their lives inside out to care for severely ill or disabled children . . . I know what it is like to see something terrible happen to someone you love; what it is like to love someone to whom very few other people can relate . . . I have to provide a counterpoint to the medical, objective, legal, logical, tangible and scientific by continuing to espouse the intangible, instinctive, intuitional, emotional—b championing the subjective.[7]

The medical team must go through a thoughtf and sensitive process to be ready to participate i dialogue with the parents. Science should be used t go as far as current knowledge will permit in makir diagnoses and prognoses before dealing with th unknown. Appropriate consultation should be ob tained. As issues become increasingly ethical rath than scientific, views should be solicited from a those closely involved, whether junior or senior pra titioners and whether physician, nurse, or allie health professional. Consensus generation may re quire multiple discussions, but it is vital to mora and function in the intensive care nursery, where a tachment and stress in caregivers are real and ong ing. Individual nurses are very involved with the patients and often become proxy mothers whose pa ticipation and understanding is crucial.

Both uncertainty and authority must be handle with care. The extremes are to be avoided—dogm tism in the face of uncertainty, or spreading out confusing carpet of conflicting and unintegrated fac and alternatives. The authoritarian physician who an nounces decisions and is patronizing to the paren deserves the criticism he or she often receives toda however, the physician who leaves parents alone struggle with impossible choices and refuses to mak a recommendation and share the agony of terrib dilemmas and awful uncertainty also is cheating h or her patients. Parents can accept the failure of on plan and its replacement by another. They cann accept a situation in which the team has given u and there is no plan. Even the withdrawal of respir tor support is not the termination of care; it is th redirection of care toward new goals: minimizing th baby's pain and discomfort, affirming his or her di nity and worth, supporting the family, and settir the stage for eventual healing and recovery.

UNRESOLVED ISSUES

Society in the United States is rife with unresolv conflicts over critically ill newborns. We require i tensive care in all but the most extreme circu stances, yet we give scant support to families wi lifelong responsibility for severely damaged or hanc capped children. We spend billions on neonatal i tensive care, yet we fail to provide the prenatal ca and general support for childbearing women th substantially reduces prematurity and poor pre nancy outcomes elsewhere in the industrializ world. We celebrate the most expensive high-tec nology treatments, yet a substantial part of our pop lation is uninsured and unable to pay for even t most basic medical care. Some families have e hausted the lifetime maximum of insurance benef for their child and are subsequently bankrupt by co tinuing medical expenses. This burden falls most cr lly on middle-class families, because they are ineligi-le for many government programs and may lose neir savings, their possessions, and their other chil-ren's college support to medical bill collectors. Med-cal malpractice suits, court decisions, and public out-ry are crude, blunt instruments for setting these natters straight. Perhaps the ethical imperative is to ay, "With these resources, we must do better!"

EFERENCES

Nondiscrimination on the basis of handicap, interim final rule. Federal Register. March 7, 1983;48:9630.

2. U.S. Court of Appeals (2nd Cir 1984).
3. Child Abuse Prevention and Treatment Act and Child Abuse Prevention and Treatment and Adoption Reform Amendments, Amendment No. 3385. Congressional Record—Senate S8951–S8956, January 29, 1984. 45 C.F.R. Part 1340 (1990).
4. Pius XII. The prolongation of life. The Pope Speaks 1958;4:395.
5. Ginsberg HG, Goldsmith JP, Stedman CM. Survival of a 380-g infant. N Engl J Med 1990;322:1753.
6. U.S. Congress, Office of Technology Assessment. Neonatal intensive care for low birthweight infants: costs and effectiveness. Office of Technology Assessment, Washington, DC, December, 1987.
7. Sarin A. Championing the subjective: my role on the ethics forum. In: Ethicscope. Washington, DC: Office of Ethics, Children's National Medical Center, Spring, 1990.

Neonatology: Pathophysiology and Management of the Newborn, Fourth Editio
edited by Gordon B. Avery, Mary Ann Fletcher, and Mhairi G. MacDonal
J.B. Lippincott Company, Philadelphia © 199

chapter 3

Neonatology in the United States: Scope and Organization

RICHARD L. BUCCIARELLI

The footprint of neonatal and perinatal medicine has changed enormously since its recognition as a distinct subspecialty in 1975. The development of technologies as complex as extracorporeal membrane oxygenation and as simple as the administration of exogenous surfactant have resulted in the survival of many infants who would have succumbed to their illnesses a few years ago.

Unfortunately, these and other technologic advances of the 1980s have been countered by trends in American society that have diminished the impact of this progress. The United States lags further behind many less wealthy countries in measurements of perinatal outcome than it did 20 years ago. The record numbers of women and children living in poverty, the ever-growing financial and geographic barriers to the access to prenatal care, the inability to decrease the numbers of low-birth-weight (LBW) infants, the increased incidence of perinatally acquired immune deficiency syndrome and other sexually transmitted diseases, the crack cocaine epidemic, and the record numbers of children born to children stand in the way of achieving the goals of lowering infant mortality and preventing the morbidities associated with prematurity.

The United States' dismal performance compared with other nations is not because of an unwillingness to commit significant financial and human resources to perinatal care. In 1985, expenditures for obstetric and neonatal care exceeded $15 billion, and at current rates of medical inflation, that figure approached $2 billion by the end of 1992. In addition to these hug expenditures, the United States continues to inve vast amounts of capital in neonatal intensive car units (NICU) as almost every hospital in the natio joins the race to compete for a franchise to care fc infants with special care needs. Fellowship progran in neonatal and perinatal medicine continue to pro duce physicians with the expertise to care for th most complex patients and with the vision to develo new technologies for the future. Entire new profes sions, such as neonatal nurse practitioners (NNP and neonatal developmental interventionists, hav grown out of the increased neonatal manpow needs in acute and long-term care settings.

How can these levels of commitment to obstetr and neonatal care be reconciled with a LBW rate th exceeds that of Romania and Kuwait? With all these efforts, why does the United States have a infant mortality rate (IMR) greater than that of Sing pore and just less than that of Cuba?

The answers to these and similar questions appe to be in the realization that past efforts have conce trated on developing the world's most sophisticate high-tech neonatal care without investing equal tin and effort in attempting to understand the societ issues responsible for producing high-risk infant Our nation has developed a superb ability to care fo the individual high-risk infant after delivery but h failed to develop systems that integrate resources rovide efficient, cost-effective prenatal care that ould prevent significant human suffering and save ast economic resources.

In this chapter, the current size and scope of the ractice of neonatology in the United States is re- iewed, while the concentration is on how resources re used to deliver neonatal care.

IZE AND SCOPE OF NEONATOLOGY N THE UNITED STATES

EONATAL HOSPITAL CAPACITY

ecause there is no national data base defining or nventorying special care neonatal beds, the exact ca- acity for the provision of NICU services in the Jnited States is unknown. One of the largest avail- ble data sets on this topic was compiled by the American Hospital Association in 1989.[1] Hospitals vith established NICUs served as the basis for the nalysis. Services were classified as NICU or normal ursery. There was no attempt to subdivide NICU ervices into level II (*i.e.*, intermediate care) or level I (*i.e.*, intensive, critical care). Using these data and ata from a similar survey conducted in 1985, the National Perinatal Information Center (NPIC) calcu- ated regional hospital NICU capacity, occupancy ates, and trends (Fig. 3-1; Table 3-1).[1] Normal nur- ery services were excluded from analysis. In 1988, 03 (27%) of surveyed hospitals reported that they rovided NICU care, a 17.8% increase from 1985. hese 703 hospitals accounted for 11,020 NICU beds nd a total of more that 2.8 million inpatient days, vhich is an increase of 19.9% and 26.7% from 1985. his trend toward more hospitals offering NICU ser- ices is continuing, with 1990 estimates placing the number of NICUs in the nation at 792, an increase of 89 (13%) over 1988 levels.[3] Many of these units developed in the southern United States, where a large number of NICU beds already existed and where the occupancy rates were among the lowest.[1–3]

Because the need for beds is related to several factors, a more meaningful way to analyze bed capacity is to compare regional NICU bed rates, which normalize the number of NICU beds for the number of live births (*i.e.*, NICU bed rate = number of NICU beds/1000 live births) in that region. When regional NICU bed rates were calculated using 1988 data, two points became evident. First, there appeared to be a uniform NICU bed rate in all major geographic regions of the country. Second, the calculated average national NICU bed rate of 2.90 per 1000 live births and each of the regional NICU bed rates (range, 2.54–3.28) exceeded the NICU bed rate of 1.5 to 2.0 per 1000 live births projected by the Committee on Fetus and Newborn (COFN) of the American Academy of Pediatrics and others as necessary to meet the nation's NICU needs.[4–7] Regional NICU occupancy rates remained surprisingly low (U.S. mean, 71.26%; range, 61.8%–83.07%) despite an increase of 5.7% over 1985. Both of these facts suggest existing excess capacity within the neonatal health care delivery system.

This concept of excess bed capacity may seem surprising, because most regional level III centers, even in the southern United States, run average occupancy rates in excess of 95%, leading many to suggest and advocate even more capacity within the system. Several factors may explain these apparent discrepancies. First, available data suggest that most excess capacity appears to be in level II units that care for moderately ill neonates, but most level III units, which care for the most complex patients, remain at

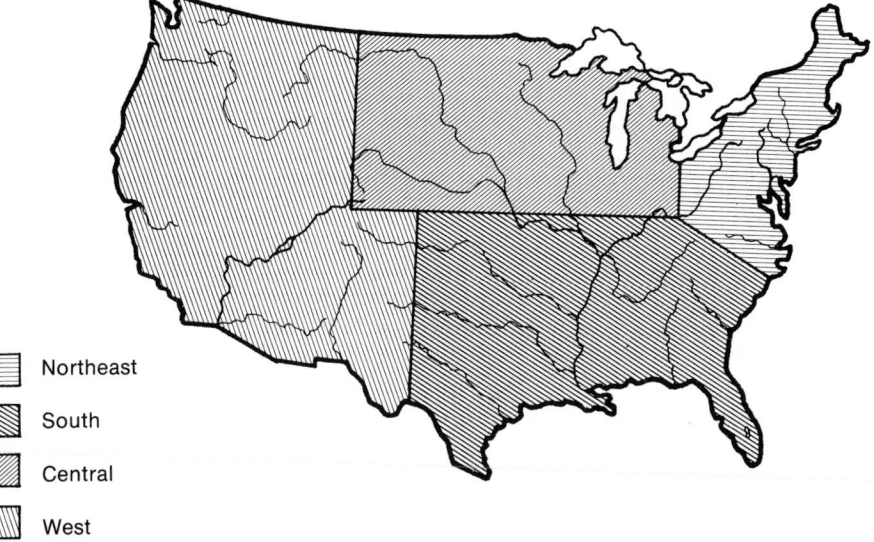

G. 3–1. Regional boundaries sed in analysis of changes in neo- atal intensive care unit services etween 1985 and 1988. (Adapted om National Perinatal Informa- on Center Newsletter. American ospital Association survey data pes, 1985–1988. 1990;Fall:1.)

TABLE 3–1
CHANGES IN NEONATAL INTENSIVE CARE SERVICES FROM 1985 TO 1988

Characteristic Analyzed	Year	Area Analyzed				
		Northeast	South	Central	West	Total United States
Hospitals reporting NICU beds	1985	110	205	151	131	597
	1988	123	261	158	161	703
	% change	11.8%	27.3%	4.6%	22.9%	17.8%
NICU beds	1985	1,842	2,971	2,578	1,801	9,192
	1988	2,051	3,871	2,894	2,204	11,020
	% change	11.3%	30.3%	12.3%	22.4%	19.9%
NICU bed rate*	1985	2.71	2.35	2.89	2.26	2.53
	1988	2.77	2.97	3.28	2.54	2.90
	% change	2.3%	26.4%	13.3%	12.2%	14.7%
NICU Inpatient days	1985	542,261	629,022	623,615	466,678	2,261,576
	1988	621,884	873,605	756,508	614,282	2,866,279
	% change	14.7%	38.9%	21.3%	31.6%	26.7%
NICU occupancy rates	1985	80.65%	58.0%	66.3%	70.99%	67.41%
	1988	83.07%	61.8%	71.6%	76.36%	71.26%
	% change	3.0%	6.6%	8.1%	7.6%	5.7%
Births	1985	680,420	1,262,765	891,345	796,431	3,630,961
	1988	740,465	1,302,047	883,146	868,711	3,794,369
	% change	8.8%	3.1%	0.9%	9.1%	4.5%

* NICU bed rate = number of NICU beds/1000 live births.
NICU, neonatal intensive care unit.
From American Hospital Association survey data tapes, 1985–1988. National Perinatal Information Center Newsletter 1990:1.

or near capacity. Second, although the total NICU bed rate appears to be equally distributed among large geographic sections of the country, regional variability in the availability of resources could result in some centers being used at or above capacity while others experience low occupancy rates.

Excess capacity within a geographic area is likely to have a negative impact on the delivery of neonatal health care in two ways. First, because neonatology is a capital-intensive service, excess capacity leads hospitals to become highly competitive for revenue positive patients. Patients are revenue positive because they are only moderately ill and are responsible for actual costs that are less than recoverable charges or are patients with significant third-party support. Most patients meeting one or both of these criteria are more often found in community level II units rather than in the urban level III units. Because the excess capacity appears to be in facilities designed to care for this type of patient, competition is keen and results in more pressure on urban level IIIs to care for smaller, more expensive patients who are often underfunded or unfunded. The combination of sicker patients requiring more expensive resources and the decreased ability to recover actual costs has placed many urban level III units in financial jeopardy.

Second, because the guidelines for the use of special care nurseries are vague and because many neonatologists extol the virtues of close observation (*e.g.*, infants of diabetic mothers without hypoglycemia, neonates with suspect sepsis, neonates with low initial Apgar scores), excess capacity creates a situation that drives hospital- and physician-induced demand for NICU services, which leads to greater use with little or no improvement in outcome, resulting in unnecessary cost escalations for the whole system.

In 1988, there was a 5.7% increase in the NICU occupancy rate despite a 19.9% increase in beds at a time when the LBW rate remained stable and there was only a modest increase of 4.5% in births.[8] The stable LBW rates suggest that many of the additional NICU admissions were of larger, term or near-term infants. Because there are no data to suggest that the intensity of care increased between 1985 and 1988, any increase in the length of stay during this time may be related to availability of resources rather than objective need. Both of these observations raise the possibility that excess capacity can become an engine driving resource consumption and cost without improving outcome.

NEONATAL MANPOWER: NEEDS AND ASSESSMENT

NEONATOLOGIST

In 1975, 355 physicians were certified by the American Board of Pediatrics' Sub-Board of Neonatal and Perinatal Medicine as the first neonatologists in the

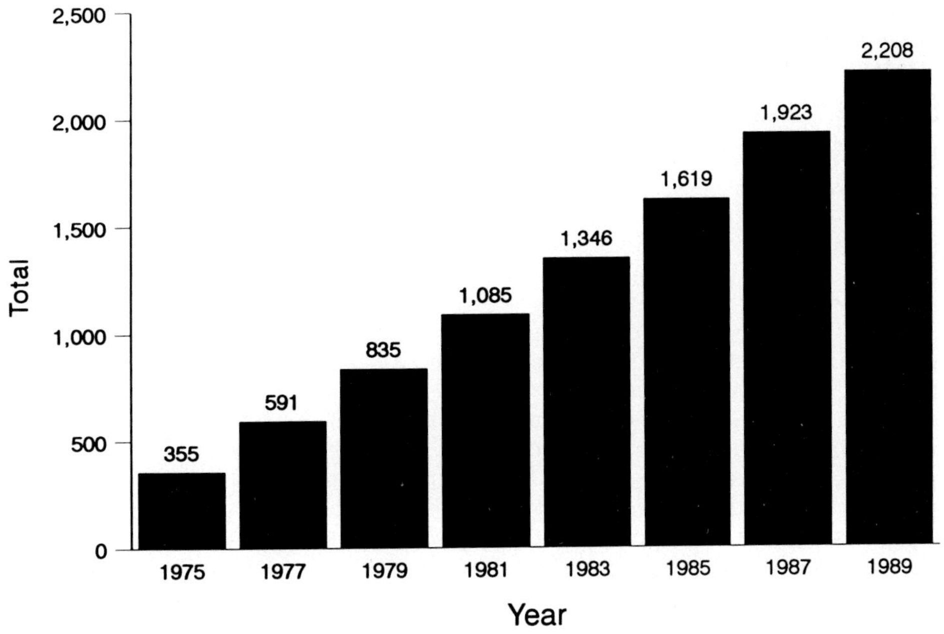

FIG. 3–2. Cumulative total of neonatologists who successfully completed certification by the American Board of Pediatrics Sub-board of Neonatal and Perinatal Medicine (Personal communication, October 1991).

United States. Since then, an average of 264 new neonatologists have been certified each time the certification examination has been given (Fig. 3-2). As of 1989, 2208 neonatologists were certified, and the attrition rate, once thought to be high, has been only 1% to 2% over a 5- to 10-year period.[3,9*] It is estimated that there are 1533 physicians actively engaged in the practice of neonatology as board-eligible physicians who have not successfully completed sub-board certification requirements or as pediatricians with special training in neonatology who concentrate their efforts on caring for neonates with special needs. The total number of physicians providing care to high-risk neonates is estimated to be 3764.[3] These data suggest that the physician manpower capacity for providing level II and level III NICU care has more than doubled since 1985.[10]

In 1982, the Residency Review Committee of the Accreditation Council for Graduate Medical Education of the American Medical Association (ACGME) began certifying fellowship training programs in neonatology. Certified programs require 3 years of training in an environment that fosters the development of clinical and research skills and exposes the neonatal fellow to other important aspects of neonatal care, including transport, long-term follow-up, and the organization of perinatal care.[11] Initially, 114 programs submitted applications for review. From this group, approximately 90 were approved, and there are currently 103 approved training programs in neonatal–perinatal medicine with an estimated 433 fellows in training.[3,11]

*Gagnan D, personal communication, November 1991.

The concerns about physician manpower devoted to neonatology, its distribution, and the effect on regionalization has been raised several times. In its 1985 statement on manpower, the COFN estimated that 1479 neonatologists were needed to provide special care services for a population of 3.8 million live births (*i.e.*, neonatologists/live births = 1/2569).[6] In 1983, Merenstein and Rhodes conducted an extensive national telephone survey of the numbers and distribution of practicing neonatologists and found the average ratio of neonatologists to live births in the United States was 1:2547, a figure close to the estimated needs.[7] Although the distribution of neonatologists varied greatly among regions (*i.e.*, from a high of 1:1860 in the Mid-Atlantic states of NY, NJ, and PA to a low of 1:3217 in the Mountain states of ID, WY, CO, NM, AR, UT, and NE), the actual infant mortality in each region was similar, suggesting that neonatal outcome may be the result of factors other than the availability of specialized neonatal care. These data combined with the increasing number of positions available for neonatologists led the COFN to conclude that "trends in the recruitment of neonatologists appeared to be based more on institutional entrepreneurial efforts than patient need, were not consistent with the concept of regionalization and would result in the fragmentation of perinatal care."[6,10]

The ratio of neonatologists to live births is 1:1596, implying, if there are no other significant changes in the neonatal patient population, that the supply of neonatologists was almost twice the capacity necessary to care for the needs of the 4.1 million live births in 1991. This excess in neonatal manpower, in combination with the excess in NICU capacity, magnifies the potential for competition and enhances the probability of the unnecessary use of resources.

PEDIATRICIANS

Providers other than neonatologists have emerged as important members of the neonatal care team. The role and supply of these specialists must be considered in any discussion of manpower in neonatology because they undoubtedly affect the projection of needs.

The ACGME requires a certified pediatric residency program to offer a minimum of 4 months and a maximum of 6 months of training in neonatal intensive care.[11] It appears that pediatricians should be well trained in the practice of neonatology, and data suggest that many would like to have the opportunity to practice those skills after completion of their training. This concept is supported by the original recommendations of the Committee on Perinatal Health, the American Academy of Pediatrics, the American College of Obstetricians and Gynecologists, and others.[5,12–15] Although the role and level of activity of pediatricians in the care of sick neonates varies from region to region, most agree that pediatricians should be considered a key resource in the delivery of normal newborn care and in level II units, providing stabilization and acute care to the newly born infant and participating in the long-term care and follow-up of NICU graduates. Involvement of the local pediatrician in the continuing care of convalescing infants reserves level III resources for more acutely ill patients and may be cost effective.[16]

The role of the pediatrician in NICU care and in the delivery room has been significantly restricted for many reasons, including medical liability and the need for maintaining special skills. Many programs are reassessing the time commitments to neonatal training as part of the general pediatric residency. Any reduction in time devoted to training in neonatal care will probably cause the pediatrician to feel less qualified to treat critically ill neonates and withdraw further from neonatology, resulting in more positions for neonatologists in community hospitals and more residents entering neonatal fellowship programs.

NEONATAL NURSE CLINICIANS AND NURSE PRACTITIONERS

Additional valuable members of the neonatal care team are the neonatal nurse clinician (NNC) and NNP. These extended care givers have proven to be of considerable benefit in providing acute and long-term neonatal care under the supervision of a neonatologist or, in some level II units, under the supervision of a pediatrician.[17] Nationwide, there are approximately 1612 licensed NNCs and NNPs.[3] These professionals have been effective in providing continuity of care to some of the more complex, chronically ill patients and their families. In many instances, their roles are evolving from the practice of acute-care inpatient neonatology into case management and long-term follow-up after discharge.

Because most NNCs and NNPs function as neonatologist extenders rather than as nurses, their impact on neonatal practice raises many questions.[18] However, they are well established as members of the neonatal care team and future reductions in the availability of residents in the NICU will make these professionals even more valuable to the level III centers. Their presence affects neonatal physician requirements, further adds to existing excess capacity, and should be considered as part of health care planning.

NEONATAL RESPIRATORY THERAPISTS

Special care nurseries depend on respiratory therapists for assistance with the ventilation and the respiratory support of its patients. These specialists have the responsibility for monitoring and maintaining ventilators and administering inhaled medications. In some units, they perform blood gas determinations. They are often valued members of the neonatal transport team, assisting in the stabilization and treatment of the critically ill neonate before and during transport.

NEONATAL INTENSIVE CARE UNIT NURSES

The duties of NICU nurses vary from unit to unit and region to region. Most units use their talents in roles considerably broader than that of nurses 20 years ago. In addition to traditional bedside nursing, the NICU nurse is responsible for continuous monitoring and assessment of the patient and has the responsibility to initiate resuscitative efforts in emergencies. The NICU nurse is the main communication link between the patient and parents and often a major source of strength and support. Like respiratory therapists, NICU nurses have proven their value as key members of neonatal transport teams. The development of regional level III centers could not have occurred without the development of neonatal transport teams and the unique contributions of NICU nurses.

NEONATAL SOCIAL WORKERS

The admission of any infant to the NICU produces anxiety and stress for the parents and family. Neonatal social workers provide the emotional support necessary to allow these families to survive the ups and downs of the NICU. Because many infants are transported great distances and families are separated during the hospitalization of the neonate, social workers provide the support needed to keep families together emotionally. More NICU social workers are becoming responsible for coordinating discharge planning, serving as case managers for the family after disharge, and providing assistance with the transition rom the hospital to the home.

IEONATAL DEVELOPMENTAL INTERVENTIONAL SPECIALISTS

Several studies indicate the benefit of developmental ntervention on the long-term outcome of NICU graduates.[19–21] The long-term developmental needs of the xtremely LBW infant often require a mixture of expertise in dealing with sensory and motor deficits. deally, these needs are supplied by persons trained n early childhood development with an understanding of occupational and physical therapy and expertise in teaching infants and children with hearing and isual impairment. Few formal training programs exist, and most receive on-the-job multidisciplinary raining as members of the neonatal developmental ollow-up team. In many cases, they can supply eeded developmental services previously unavailable and can serve as valuable case managers for infants with special needs and their families after discharge. Caution must be used so that they do not eplace the need for pediatric follow-up, further isolating the pediatrician from participating in the care f the NICU graduate and adding to the existing excess capacity in this field.

OTHER MEMBERS OF THE NEONATAL CARE TEAM

n addition to the direct members of the NICU team, nany other ancillary services are needed to care for ne high-risk infant in level II and level III care units. These services include the need for a broad spectrum f imaging services (*e.g.*, radiology, ultrasound, magnetic resonance imaging), microlaboratory techniques, nutritional consultation, and pharmacokinetic support. Ideally, each of these programs should nclude someone with special training or interest in ne needs of critically ill neonates. Level III NICU apabilities should have full pediatric subspecialty upport, including pediatric cardiology, surgery, and eurology and neurosurgery.[13]

The delivery of neonatal intensive care requires nore than just hospital beds and a neonatologist. It equires a complete team made up of many highly killed professionals dedicated to the care of the critically ill neonate and his or her family during the hospital stay and for years after discharge.

IGH-TECH NEONATAL CARE

CUTE CARE COSTS

Estimates suggest that the 1992 national expenditures or perinatal care will approach $24 billion. Most of hese resources are spent on acute high-tech care of he LBW infant, with average daily charges easily eaching $1200 to $1500 for hospital services and an additional $240 to $300 each day for physician services.[22]

Actual expenditures are hard to compute accurately because there is no national data base containing information on total public, private, hospital, and physician expenditures that allows these analyses. Most published data are limited to individual hospital, state, or regional experiences. In many instances, estimates of disease- and patient-specific expenditures are based on small sample sizes, resulting in wide variations within and between studies. Expenditure comparisons are further complicated by regional variations in costs, charges, and standards of care and differences in patient population demographics and intensity of illness. Most published data are from urban level III NICUs or state-funded perinatal programs, which include a high percentage of publicly funded patients. Because these patients often represent the highest perinatal risks, disease-specific expenditures may be skewed by over-representation of the most complex patients in the data base, resulting in higher cost estimates. Most data bases include little private-sector spending, resulting in incomplete information.

One of the largest, most complete perinatal fiscal data sets available in the United States is the State of Florida's Regional Perinatal Intensive Care Center (RPICC) data base. Established in 1974 and maintained by Florida's Department of Health and Rehabilitative Services, Children's Medical Services, this data set includes hospital and physician total expenditures associated with the provision of high-risk perinatal care in the state's ten RPICCs.[23] This system was designed as an on-line interactive system for data entry and retrieval of patient information, program management, and patient monitoring. It has been adapted to perform electronic billing for hospital and physician services based on the state's prospective payment model for hospital, obstetric, and neonatal services. This prospective payment program, implemented in July 1985, uses 15 obstetric care groups and 15 neonatal care groups (NCGs) as a basis for determining reimbursement for services rendered to the state's fiscal year 1990 (FY 1990) 5016 program Medicaid-sponsored patients (Fig. 3-3).[24–26]

All patients admitted to the state's ten RPICCs are entered into the data base. After assignment into one of the NCGs, approved reimbursement is calculated. The calculated approved reimbursement was the basis for hospital payment until 1988 and remains the basis for physician payment for services rendered on behalf of program patients. Reimbursement for services rendered on behalf of nonprogram patients is provided independently of this system. No aggregate data are available detailing total expenditures for nonprogram patients, but the use of state-approved reimbursement based on the NCG allows estimation of the impact of these patients on consumption of resources in providing neonatal care in the State of Florida. State-approved reimbursement data appear

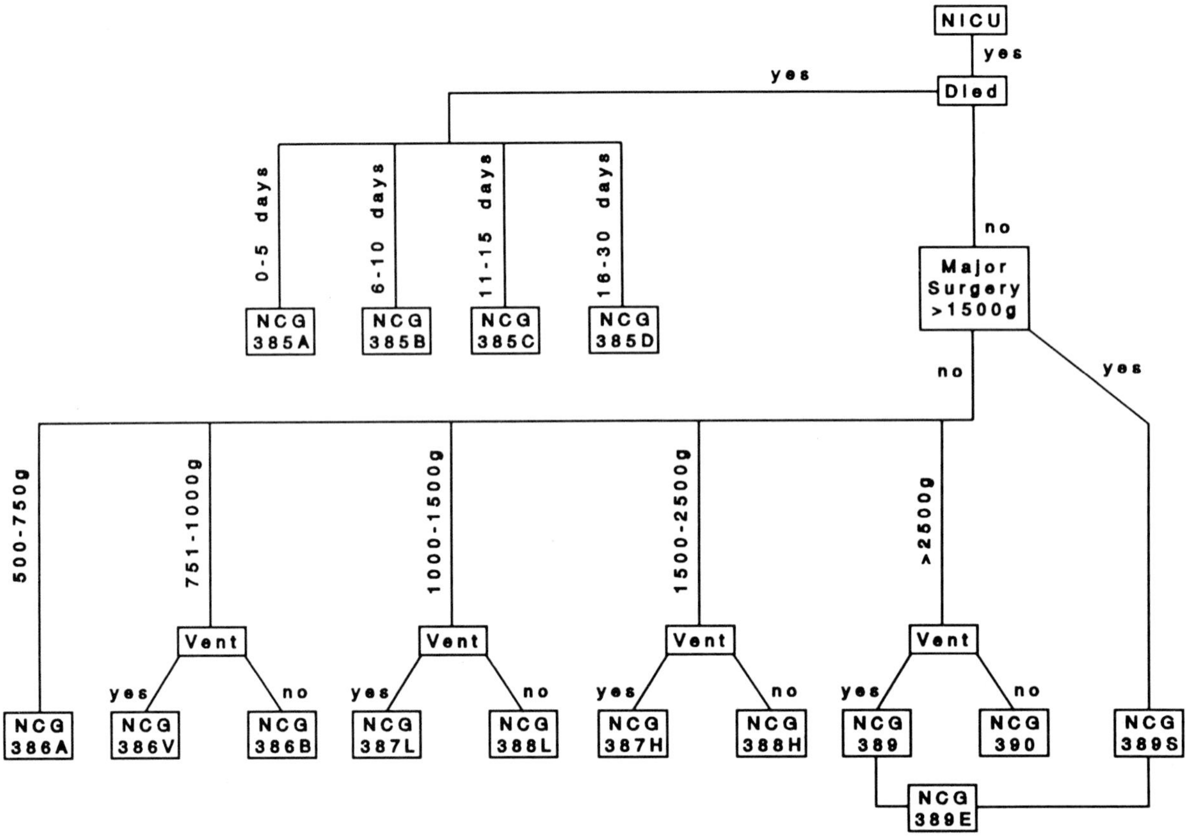

FIG. 3–3. Florida neonatal care groups (NCGs). Categories are based on federal diagnostic-related grips and subdivided into cells according to birth weight.

NCG 385:	Death (A, 0–5 days; B, 6–10 days; C, 11–15 days; D, 16–30 days)
NCG 387L:	1000- to 1500-g birth weight
NCG 387H:	1500- to 2500-g birth weight
NCG 386A:	500- to 750-g birth weight
NCG 386B:	751- to 1000-g birth weight
NCG 389:	>2500-g birth weight

Neonatal care groups serve as a basis for reimbursement for neonatal physicians only. Consultative subspecialty care is reimbursed independent of NCG. Neonatal care groups served as the basis for hospital reimbursement from 1987 to 1990. (E, ECMO; NICU, neonatal intensive care unit; S, surgery; V, ventilated; from State of Florida Department of Health and Rehabilitative Services. Children's Medical Services regional perinatal intensive care program (RPICC) handbook. Tallahassee: State of Floride Department of Health and Rehabilitation Services, 1991.)

to be reasonable proxies for true costs, because charges are influenced by hospital and physician pricing practices (*e.g.*, cost shifting due to uncompensated care, differences in accounting), but NCG-approved reimbursement is based on clinical condition and calculated against a state standard.

Review of published RPICC data indicates that the State of Florida–approved reimbursement for perinatal care totaled $59.1 million in FY 1986. Hospital reimbursement amounted to $32.9 million for neonatal intensive care and $9.4 million for obstetric services, and neonatal and obstetric physician reimbursement accounted for $12.4 million and $4.4 million, respectively (Table 3-2).[26,27] The average hospital RPICC-approved reimbursement was $10,95 per neonate and $2842 per woman, with an averag physician reimbursement of $4128 per neonate an $1000 per obstetric patient. The FY 1990 data indicat the level of approved reimbursement has increase 79% to $19,657 per neonate for hospital services an that neonatal physician-approved reimbursement de creased by 7%. Average hospital-approved reim bursement for obstetric care increased by 25% t $3542 for hospital services, and obstetric physicia approved reimbursement increased by 34%.

The highest levels of approved reimbursement i the NICU payment system are for the treatment c extremely low-birth-weight (ELBW) infants (<1000 g

TABLE 3–2
APPROVED REIMBURSEMENT BY NEONATAL CARE GROUPS FOR REGIONAL PERINATAL INTENSIVE CARE CENTER IN FLORIDA

Factors In Reimbursement	FY 1986	FY 1990	Percent Change
Number of Patients			
Neonatal component	3,000	5,016	67%
Obstetrical component	3,311	8,259	149%
Total	6,311	13,275	110%
RPICC Approved Reimbursement			
Neonatal component	$45,257,737	$117,885,460	160%
Obstetrical component	$13,808,705	$40,307,977	192%
Total	$59,066,442	$158,253,437	168%
RPICC Approved Reimbursement			
Hospital			
Neonatal component	$32,872,681	$98,601,231	200%
Obstetric component	$9,411,721	$29,257,364	211%
Physician			
Neonatal component	$12,385,056	$19,284,229	56%
Obstetrical component	$4,396,984	$11,110,613	153%
Average RPICC Approved Reimbursement per Patient			
Hospital			
Neonatal component	$10,957	$19,657	79%
Obstetric component	$2,842	$3,542	25%
Physician			
Neonatal component	$4,128	$3,844	7%*
Obstetric component	$1,000	$1,345	34%

* Decrease.
FY, fiscal year; RPICC, Regional Perinatal Intensive Care Center.
Data from State of Florida Department of Health and Rehabilitative Services. Children's Medical Services regional perinatal intensive care center program (RPICC) handbook. Tallahassee: State of Florida Department of Health and Rehabilitative Services, 1991.

having respiratory distress syndrome and requiring mechanical ventilation.[28] Average FY 1990 total entitlement for this group exceeded $89,700 per surviving infant, representing a 64% increase from the FY 1986 level of $54,670. Because the number of surviving ELBW infants increased from 232 in FY 1986 to 335 in FY 1990, total entitlement for this group increased from $12.7 million to $30.1 million, representing 28% of total FY 1986 entitlement and 25% of FY 1990 (Table 3-3). The disproportionate impact of this group of patients is appreciated in realizing that, although these infants are responsible for using just over 25%

TABLE 3–3
FLORIDA NEONATAL CARE GROUP ENTITLEMENT FOR REGIONAL PERINATAL INTENSIVE CARE OF SURVIVING EXTREMELY-LOW-BIRTH-WEIGHT INFANTS

Entitlement Factors	FY 1986	FY 1990	Percent Change
Number surviving	232	335	44%
Average entitlement for each surviving ELBW* infant	$54,670	$89,721	64%
Total entitlement for each surviving ELBW infant	$12,683,510	$30,056,401	137%
Total neonatal program entitlement	$45,257,737	$117,885,460	160%
Percent of total entitlement committed to surviving ELBW infants	28%	25%	3%†

* ELBW infants weigh 1000 g or less at birth.
† Decreased.
ELBW, extremely-low-birth-weight; FY, fiscal year.
Data from State of Florida Department of Health and Rehabilitative Services. Children's Medical Services regional perinatal intensive care center program (RPICC) handbook. Tallahassee: State of Florida Department of Health and Rehabilitative Services, 1991.

of total program resources, they make up less than 7% of the total NICU population served. These data are supported by similar relative expenditures and trends reported by other authors, although actual dollar amounts vary among studies.[28,29]

COSTS AFTER DISCHARGE

Because the ELBW infant is at high risk for long-term sequelae, the resources dedicated to providing acute care must be supplemented with the continued investment of resources for long-term follow-up. With the realization that long-term outcome of the ELBW infant is enhanced by developmental follow-up, including multidisciplinary intervention programs, postdischarge costs per NICU graduate are substantial. Shankaran and associates reported 1988 expenditures for NICU graduates with no disabilities to be in the range of $31.00 per month, predominantly for primary health care but also for limited occupational and physical therapy and neurologic and ophthalmologic follow-up. These expenditures increase to $86.50 per month for infants with mild developmental or physical residuals and to $108.90 per month for infants with severe disabilities receiving care in the home (Table 3-4).[30] In both cases, additional costs were related to the need for extensive occupational and physical therapy. The costs of neurologic follow-up were less but significantly greater for severely damaged infants than for normal infants. In this study, the cost of institutional care for an NICU graduate up to 3 years of age exceeded $1200 per month ($43,200/36 months).

As more and more ELBW infants survive, their impact on the educational system is becoming more significant. In an attempt to assess the long-term educational needs of these infants, Walker and associates estimated the 1982 costs of early intervention (*i.e.*, from 0–3 years of age) and transitional education (*i.e.*, from 3–5 years of age) for mild or moderately handicapped ELBW infants (*i.e.*, Bayley Development Quotient of 80–85 for mild and 65–80 for moderate) to be $13,800 per year for each survivor, with a 1982 total lifetime cost of $24,177 (Table 3-5). The educational costs of the severely handicapped exceed $22,000 per year and $192,000 at 1982 value of lifetime costs.[31]

COST-EFFECTIVENESS OF NEONATAL CARE

When long-term cost–benefit ratios were calculated in the 1970s and early 1980s, provision of neonatal care appeared extremely cost effective. This is still true, because good neonatal care decreases the incidence of significant morbidity in almost all weight groups. However, the increased number of surviving ELBW infants with their financial, social, and educational impacts have led several researchers to raise significant ethical and moral questions about future directions in therapy. Two studies designed to address the cost-benefit ratio of neonatal care showed significant savings for infants with birth weights greater than 1000 g. The treatment of neonates between 500 and 999 g showed a loss, questioning the economic value of treating this group of patients.[31,32]

Although the cost-benefit ratio for ELBW infant is questionable, ethical and moral decisions about the

TABLE 3–4
OUTPATIENT COSTS AFTER NEONATAL INTENSIVE CARE UNIT DISCHARGE

Cost Components	Group* A (n = 23)	B (n = 15)	C (n = 22)	F Value	Significant Comparisions
Total outpatient costs	31.2 (22.9)	86.5 (93.4)	108.9 (58.7)	9.8	A < B^b; A < C^c
Specialized services	10.7 (8.9)	9.1 (.57)	9.3 (6.3)	0.3	NS
Primary health care	0.7 (2.4)	14.1 (15.8)	18.9 (21.9)	8.2	A < B^a; A < C^c
Occupational or physical therapy	0.5 (1.4)	4.1 (9.1)	6.6 (8.7)	4.4	A < C^b
Neurology					
Ophthalmology	3.6 (7.4)	4.8 (5.7)	5.6 (1.7)	0.6	NS
Emergency room	1.1 (2.9)	0.8 (1.5)	1.7 (2.8)	0.5	NS

* Group A children had no developmental disabilities; group B children were mildly developmentally disabled; and group C children were moderately or severely developmentally disabled. Results are mean dollars per infant per month with standard deviations in parentheses. Analyses of variance by groups were done for outpatient costs. Significant comparisons: $^a p < 0.5$, $^b p < 0.01$, $^c p < 0.001$. Scheffe tests were performed on pairwise comparisons.

From Shankaran S, Cohen SN, Linver M, Zonia S. Medical care costs of high-risk infants after neonatal intensive care: a controlled study. Pediatrics 1988;81:372.

TABLE 3–5
LONG-TERM EDUCATIONAL NEEDS OF NEONATAL INTENSIVE CARE UNIT GRADUATES WEIGHING LESS THAN 1000 g AT BIRTH

	Moderately Handicapped		Severely Handicapped	
	Annual Costs/ Survivor	1982 Value	Annual Costs/ Survivor	1982 Value
Early intervention (0–3 y)	$1,800	$4,902	$1,800	$4,902
Transitional (3–5 y)	$12,000	$19,275		
Meeting Street School (3–21 y)			$12,000	$121,175
Group home residence (21 y to death)			$10,000	$66,193
1982 value of total lifetime costs		$24,177		$192,270

From Walker DB, Feldman A, Vohr BR, Oh W. Cost-benefit analysis of neonatal intensive care for infants weighing less than 1,000 grams at birth. Pediatrics 1984;74:20.

treatment of the extremely premature infant have not kept pace with technology. Our nation has only recently been willing to admit that even the richest country in the world cannot afford to buy all that science has to offer. Some states are beginning to respond to this reality and make prospective decisions based on economics and on ethical and social considerations.[32,33] Prioritizing therapies and rationing resources will be discussed more in years to come.

MISSED OPPORTUNITIES

One cannot consider the magnitude of these costs and the amount of human suffering involved in the delivery of a high-risk infant without wondering why America continues to expend enormous resources on postnatal care when one-half of the number of ELBW deliveries could be avoided with early prenatal care.[34] The benefit of $900 of prenatal care instead of $89,000 for each surviving LBW infant is obvious. In 1985, the Institute of Medicine reported that for every $1.00 spent on prenatal care, $3.00 were saved in the first year and $10.00 more saved over a lifetime.[35] In considering the long-term costs associated with the ELBW group of patients and the effects of medical inflation, the benefits of early prenatal care are staggering.

MAJOR PAYERS FOR NEONATAL CARE

There are four groups of major payers of neonatal care: private health insurance, public programs including Medicaid and other state and local programs, special perinatal demonstration projects both public and private, and uninsured, self-paying. None of the major payers completely cover the costs of high-risk obstetric and neonatal care, especially for the complicated ELBW infant. A significant portion of this uncompensated care is shifted to other payers in the form of increased charges. One study suggested that as much as 27% of total costs of NICU care in the State of Florida is shifted to paying patients who are responsible for generating 60% of total revenues while accounting for only 33% of costs.[36] As insurance premiums skyrocket (*i.e.*, 25%/year) and public funding for prenatal care becomes more limited, attempts to limit cost shifting will increase.

PRIVATE HEALTH INSURANCE

Although private health insurance is the financial foundation of the current health care system in the United States, coverage for pregnant women and their neonates is more limited than for any other segment of the population and is being continually eroded. Only 67% of civilian women of child-bearing age and only 61% of the 3.9 million infants under 1 year of age are insured privately.[37] These rates are well below the 85% to 87% coverage for the general population. More than one-half of women covered under group insurance policies received coverage as a dependent of their employed husband. This is of major concern because employer-based coverage of dependents has decreased by almost 20% during the last decade, leaving many working families totally uncovered for prenatal care and for all types of neonatal care, preventive and catastrophic.[38] Even among policies that include dependent coverage, few cover the prenatal and newborn costs related to the 500,000 annual deliveries of teenage pregnancies.[39] Neglecting this segment of the population produces significant financial barriers to care for these teens and increases the chance of high-risk delivery.

To counter escalating costs, most insurers introduced substantial cost-sharing requirements (*e.g.*, deductibles, co-payments), leaving even the insured family directly responsible for a significant portion of the costs of their infant's care. In the case of high-risk neonatal care, obligation for copayments can be financially devastating. For example, a 20% copayment responsibility on a combined hospital and physician bill for a LBW infant of $125,000 results in a family responsibility of $25,000, an amount that would be impossible for most families to pay.

In an attempt to counter the erosion of prenatal coverage, many states have passed mandates requiring obstetric and neonatal benefits for families and for teens living at home. Despite being cognizant of the long-term benefits of prenatal care, many insurance companies and employers see mandated coverage for dependents, particularly the high-risk neonate, as adding significantly to the cost of insurance, making it unaffordable to employers and middle-class Americans. Instead of recognizing the long-term benefits of access to prenatal care and the financial burden of neonatal intensive care, they are opting for short-term reductions in premiums by attempting to overturn these and other state mandates.[40] If these attempts are successful, coverage will be further eroded, increasing the number of uninsured and placing more financial pressure on other payers.

MEDICAID

The largest public program for the financing of prenatal and neonatal care is Medicaid. Authorized as Title XIX of the Social Security Act in 1965, Medicaid is a federal-state public partnership that finances care for 26 million low-income persons who are elderly, blind, disabled, or members of families with children.[41] During the past several years, the federal-state match has remained relatively constant, with federal funds accounting for an average of 56.9% of total FY 1989 program expenditures. The exact level of federal funding is determined from a formula reflecting the state's per capita income and varies between 50% and 80% of the state's total Medicaid expenditures.[42]

In 1989, 48% of the targeted population consisted of pregnant women and children; however, only 13% of the $89 billion in total program expenditures were directed toward them. In FY 1989, pregnant women and children received less than 5% of total federal spending, 20% of the amount spent on the population older than 65 years of age.[42] The more than 3.9 million children younger than 1 year of age did worse, receiving only 3.8% of all Medicaid spending for an average of $1697 per infant.[43] Approximately 15% of all Medicaid-sponsored deliveries require NICU care, a rate three times those with other sources of payment.[26]

With the exception of the matching requirements for federal funds and the required compliance with an increasing number of federal mandates, each state has the responsibility for developing and administering its own Medicaid program, including setting eligibility and coverage standards within broad federal guidelines. As a result, there is considerable variation among states in eligibility requirements, range of services offered, limitations on services, and reimbursement policies. Although an average 51% of the nation's poor receive Medicaid services, the portion of this population eligible for Medicaid varies by state from a low of 17% to a high of 83%. Specific data on women and infants are not available.[44]

Until recently, Medicaid's financial eligibility criteria were linked to eligibility for cash assistance programs, particularly Aid to Families with Dependent Children. Because eligibility criteria for these programs were set so low, most women and children living at or below the federal poverty level (FPL) did not qualify for coverage. Congress has been successful in breaking this link and extending Medicaid coverage to more women and children in need. All states are required to extend Medicaid benefits to pregnant women and children younger than 6 years of age with family incomes below 133% of the FPL and have the option of extending benefits to pregnant women and infants younger than 1 year of age with family incomes below 185% of FPL.

In 1986, Medicaid was the source of payment for 648,000 births, 17% of the nation's deliveries.[45–47] By 1990, as a result of program expansions and the worsening national economy, Medicaid was the source of payment for 25% to 30% of U.S. deliveries and the resultant neonates and still reached only one-half of those in need.[47,48] These expansions combined with increased spending on the disabled elderly have resulted in enormous growth of the Medicaid program (*i.e.*, from $23 billion in FY 1980 to $104 billion in FY 1992), resulting in added financial stress for states already hard hit by a sluggish economy.[47,48] In FY 1990–FY 1991, 40% of all of the State of Florida's new general revenue was required to cover federally mandated Medicaid expenditures.[49]

Because reporting systems for hospital and physician services vary greatly among states, it is not possible to assess what percentage of hospital and physician fees are paid by Medicaid. However, FY 1990 Medicaid reimbursement covered only 55% of the total obstetric and neonatal hospital and physician charges in the State of Florida, a state with one of the highest reimbursement rates. Because of these levels of reimbursement, Florida's public hospitals lost $16.5 million while providing neonatal intensive care in 1985.[36] This low level of reimbursement is one of the reasons why many hospitals and physicians refuse to care for Medicaid patients, producing significant barriers to the access to prenatal care and resulting in more high-risk deliveries.[50–53] Because most Medicaid-sponsored pregnant women and their infants are cared for in large urban hospitals or teaching centers, increased volume and intensity combined with low reimbursement is placing an increasingly disproportional load on these centers, threatening their very existence.

TITLE V MATERNAL AND CHILD HEALTH BLOCK GRANT PROGRAM

Located within the Health Resources and Services Administration (HRSA) of the Department of Health and Human Services (HHS), the Maternal and Child Health (MCH) Block Grant Program was authorized by Title V of the Social Security Act to provide grants to states for a variety of preventive and primary care services to women and children, including prenatal care, immunizations, and rehabilitative services for children with special needs.[41] Although FY 1991 funding for this program exceeded $550 million, it accounts for only 0.3% of the HHS budget.[48] Current funding levels are so low that less than one-half of eligible women are able to receive adequate prenatal care under the program. The MCH Block Grant Program has received little to no increase in funding and frequently had to be saved from the threat of significant budget cuts, situations well known to all major block grant programs.

COMMUNITY HEALTH CENTERS, MIGRANT HEALTH CENTERS, AND THE NATIONAL HEALTH SERVICE CORPS

As part of HRSA, $600 million for community health centers, migrant health centers, and programs of the National Health Service Corps are directed toward providing primary preventive care, including prenatal and well-child care for those served in urban community health centers and in rural areas of the United States.[48] Chronically underfunded, these programs have seen little increase in funding the last few years and have been targets for reductions or eliminations of programs.

SPECIAL DEMONSTRATION PROJECTS

Because the financial and personal consequences of LBW infants and the positive influence of early prenatal care are well known, many public (*e.g.*, state, county, and municipal governments) and private (*e.g.*, March of Dimes, Robert Wood Johnson, Pew Foundation) organizations have dedicated significant resources to study how to reach high-risk populations more effectively to reduce the high mortality and morbidity related to premature deliveries. Although most of these projects are small and contribute little to covering the total costs of perinatal care, many are highly successful and result in significant overall savings for individual patients. A major problem with these projects is that targeted patients are highly selected, making it difficult to apply program results to larger populations. Most programs are funded for a limited time, creating the problem of how to continue to provide services after funding has expired.

UNINSURED, SELF-PAYING PATIENTS

Most of the uninsured, self-paying patients cannot afford to pay for any type of medical care. They contribute little to the financing of perinatal care used by themselves and their families. This inability to pay results in such a potent barrier to access that one-third of all pregnant women in the United States receive inadequate neonatal care. Being uninsured is the greatest barrier to receiving prenatal care, and it results in the highest risk for delivering a LBW infant, approximately three times the rate for women with minimal prenatal care.[52] In 1989, an estimated 6 million women of childbearing age had no health insurance coverage, public or private, and an additional 5 million women had private, employer-based coverage without maternity benefits.[53] Coverage for maternity benefits appear to be even worse than these figures suggest, because it is estimated that as many as 20 million women have their insurance interrupted for at least 2 months over a 24-month period. Data indicate that 26% of women are uninsured when they conceive, and 15% are uninsured when they deliver, leaving an estimated 800,000 pregnant women with no maternity coverage and over 70,000 births without the benefit of any prenatal care.[43]

MAJOR MEASURES OF OUTCOME

INFANT MORTALITY RATE

The IMR is defined by the National Center for Health Statistics and by the World Health Organization as the number of deaths occurring within the first year of life per 1000 live births. Infant mortality can be further divided into neonatal mortality (*i.e.*, death before 29 days of age) and postneonatal mortality (*i.e.*, death between 29 days and 1 year of age). Neonatal mortality is generally the result of factors related to pregnancy and birth, and postneonatal mortality is generally the result of environmental factors (*e.g.*, trauma, infection, nutrition, sudden infant death syndrome).[54]

After more than a decade of significant progress, the improvement in the IMR in the United States slowed significantly during the 1980s, and there was no statistical difference in IMRs between 1987 and 1988, the last year for which final national statistics were available (Fig. 3-4). The 1988 U.S. IMR of 9.95 deaths per 1000 live births ranked ninteenth in the world, just behind Italy and just ahead of Israel (Table 3-6).[39] Provisional estimates for 1989 and 1990 indicate that the U.S. IMR has again begun to drop. If trends continue, the 1989 U.S. IMR should be 9.73 per 1000 live births. The anticipated 6.2% decline in infant mortality would be the largest proportional decline since 1977. Most of this decline was due to an 8% decrease in the neonatal component; the postnatal rate declined by only 4.3%. Any potential exuber-

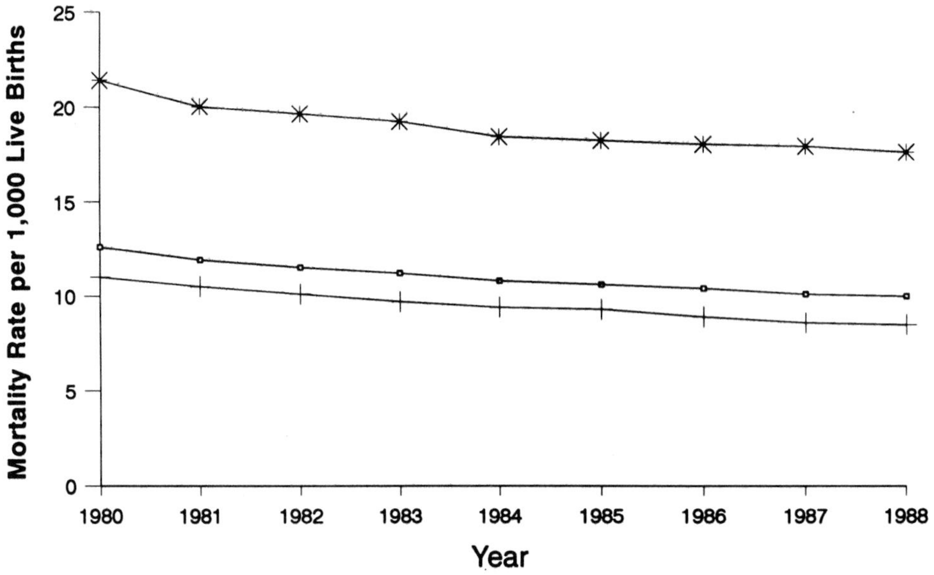

FIG. 3–4. Infant mortality rates in the United States from 1980 to 1988 by race. Infant mortality constitutes deaths that occur before 1 year of age (□, all races; *, African Americans; +, Caucasians; from Wegman M. Annual summary of vital statistics—1990. Pediatrics 1991;88:1081, and U.S. Department of Health and Human Services. Perinatal mortality, sect 3. Vital statistics of the United States—1988. vol. 2. pt A. Hyattsville, MD: U.S. Government Printing Office, 1991.)

ance over these facts should be tempered by the realization that Japan, with the world's best IMR of 5 per 1000 live births, ranked just behind the United States at number seven in the world in 1950.

The greatest improvements in the overall IMR between 1985 and 1988 occurred in Caucasian children, with a decrease of 8.6%, compared with that of 3% for African Americans. This discrepancy is even more obvious in the differences in IMRs in 1987 among races across the United States and in various cities (Table 3-7).[55] Overall, the IMR of African Americans and all minorities ranges between 1.5 and 2.0 times that of Caucasians. The best urban African-American and minority IMRs are still worse than the worst IMRs for urban Caucasians.

TABLE 3–6
INFANT MORTALITY RATES AND RANKINGS FOR 1988

Rank	Nation	Rate*
1	Japan	5
2	Finland	6
2	Sweden	6
4	Canada	7
7	Hong Kong	8
7	France	8
15	Singapore	9
15	United Kingdom	9
19	Italy	10
19	United States	10
23	Israel	11
24	Czechoslovakia	12

* Infant (<1 year of age) deaths per 1,000 live births
From Children's Defense Fund. S.O.S. America! A children's defense budget. Washington, DC: Children's Defense Fund, 1990:160.

NEONATAL MORTALITY RATE

Although IMR reflects the general health of a community, separate examination of early and late infant deaths can further pinpoint problems. The neonatal mortality rate (NMR) equals the number of deaths occurring at less than 29 days after birth per 1000 live births. These account for about 67% of all infant deaths. One-half of all neonatal deaths can be attributed to four leading causes:

1. LBW
2. Acute perinatal asphyxia
3. Congenital anomalies
4. Perinatal infections.[56]

Between 1985 and 1988, neonatal mortality declined more than five times as fast as postneonatal mortality. The 1989 and 1990 provisional rates of 6.2[illegible] deaths per 1000 live births and 5.74 deaths per 1000 live births are thought to be a reflection of the marked improvement in death related to perinatal conditions that declined by 8.5% in 1990 and an additional 6.37% in 1990. Included in this category are deaths related to respiratory distress of the newborn. Between 198[illegible] and 1990, deaths due to respiratory distress syndrome decreased by 33%, leading some to relate this improvement to the widespread availability of exogenous surfactant products. African American and minority NMRs parallel the IMR and are considerably higher than Caucasian NMRs, with a African American–Caucasian ratio for NMR greater than the IMR African American–Caucasian ratio of 2.13 compared with 2.07 (Fig. 3-5; Table 3-8).[54]

TABLE 3–7
KEY INFANT MORTALITY RATE INDICATORS FOR UNITED STATES CITIES, 1987

Indicator	Total	Large Cities	Medium Cities	Small Cities
Infant Mortality Rate (Infant Deaths/1000 Live Births)				
All races	10.1	13.2	11.6	12.8
Caucasians	8.6	9.6	9.7	10.3
African Americans	17.9	19.4	18.0	21.3
Non-Caucasians	15.4	16.9	16.1	20.9
Low Birth Weight (%)				
All races	6.9	9.2	8.5	7.5
Caucasians	5.7	6.3	6.4	6.0
African Americans	12.7	13.2	13.2	12.7
Non-Caucasians	13.3	12.1	11.8	11.3

Large cities, 500,000 or more population; medium cities, 250,000–499,999 population; small cities, 100,000–249,999 population.
From Children's Defense Fund. Maternal and child health in America. Special report three. Washington, DC: Children's Defense Fund, 1991:20.

PERINATAL MORTALITY RATE

The perinatal mortality rate (PMR) is defined by the National Center for Health Statistics as the number of late fetal deaths (*i.e.*, fetal deaths of 28 weeks or more of gestation) plus early neonatal deaths (*i.e.*, deaths of infants 0–6 days of age) per 1000 live births.[55] Because there is no uniform international definition of fetal deaths, international comparisons of PMR are difficult to interpret.

Most fetal deaths are a result of chronic asphyxia (60%–70%); congenital malformations (20%–25%); superimposed complications of pregnancy, such as placental abruption, Rh isoimmunization, diabetes mellitus, and intrauterine infection (5%–10%); and unexplained deaths (5%–10%).[57] Although the incidence of congenital malformations has remained relatively constant over the last few years, improvements in the management of pregnancy-related complications combined with improved early neonatal survival has resulted in a significant decrease in PMR to 9.7 deaths per 1000 live births for 1988.[55] Race variations in PMR are identical to those seen in IMR and NMR (Fig. 3-6).

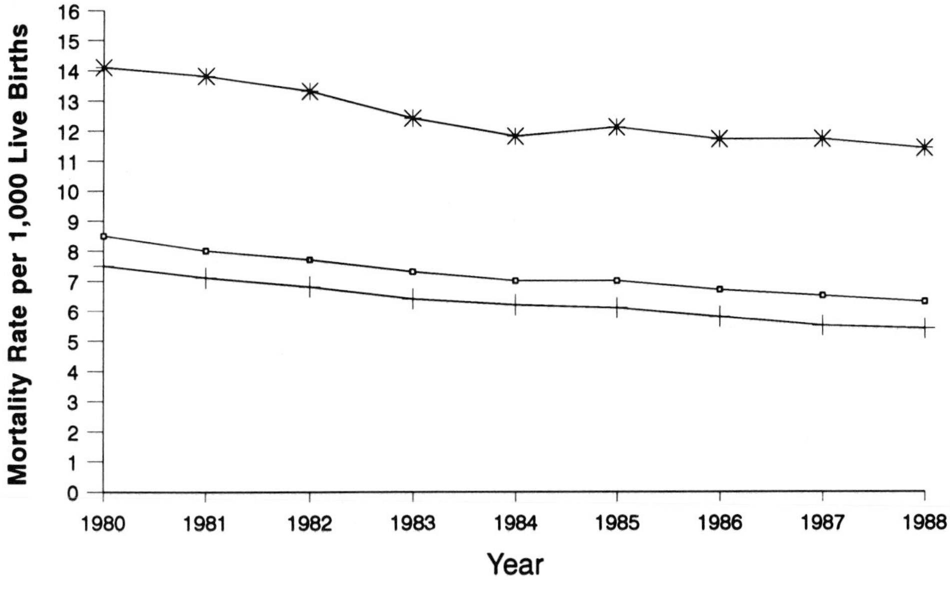

FIG. 3–5. Neonatal mortality rates in the United States from 1980 to 1988 by race. Neonatal mortality constitutes deaths that occur before 29 days of age. (□, all races; *, African Americans; +, Caucasians; from U.S. Department of Health and Human Services. Perinatal mortality, sect 3. Vital statistics of the United States—1988. vol. 2. pt. A. Hyattsville, MD: U.S. Government Printing Office, 1991.)

TABLE 3–8
INFANT MORTALITY RATES BY AGE AND RACE

Group Analyzed	1990*	1989*	1988	Percent Decline				
				1985	1980	1960	1940	1940–1988
Total†	908.0	973.3	995.3	10.6	12.6	26.0	47.0	78.8
Caucasians			851.1	9.3	11.0	22.9	43.2	80.3
African Americans			1762.0	18.2	21.4	44.3	72.9	75.8
African Americans–Caucasians ratio			2.07	2.0	1.9	1.9	1.7	
<29 days of age	574.7	625.0	631.5	7.0	8.5	18.7	28.8	78.1
Caucasians			536.6	6.1	7.5	17.2	27.2	80.3
African Americans			1145.1	12.1	14.1	27.8	39.9	71.3
African Americans–Caucasians ratio			2.13	2.0	1.9	1.6	1.5	
Postneonatal	333.3	348.3	363.7	3.7	4.1	7.3	18.3	80.1
Caucasians			314.5	3.2	3.5	5.7	16.0	80.3
African Americans			616.8	6.1	7.3	16.5	33.0	81.3
African Americans–Caucasians ratio			1.96	1.9	2.1	2.9	2.1	

* Provisional data, estimated from a 10% sample of deaths. Rates for 1990, 1989, and 1988 are per 100,000 live births; rates for 1940–1985 are per 1000 live births.
† Includes races other than Caucasian and African American.
Data from the National Center for Health Statistics.
From Wegman M. Annual summary of vital statistics—1990. Pediatrics 1991;88:1081.

MAJOR MORBIDITIES

LOW BIRTH WEIGHT

Low birth weight is responsible for 60% of the U.S. IMR and carries a 40-fold increased risk of death in the first month of life and a twofold to threefold increase in the chance of long-term disability. Considering these realities, the prevention of LBW has been one of the nation's top priorities in its effort to reduce infant mortality and morbidity. Despite this focus, no progress has been made in reducing the incidence of LBW over the last decade. The 1989 LBW rate of 7% is identical to that of 1979 and places us twenty-eighth among the world's countries. Spain's LBW rate of 1% is the world's best, and Japan, which leads the world in infant mortality, ranks fifth with a rate of 5% (Table 3-9).[39]

Like other measures of perinatal outcome, LBW rates are disproportionately higher in large cities and in the urban African-American population.[73] In 1987, cities with populations of 100,000 or more accounted for 33% of all LBW nationally, but they were respon-

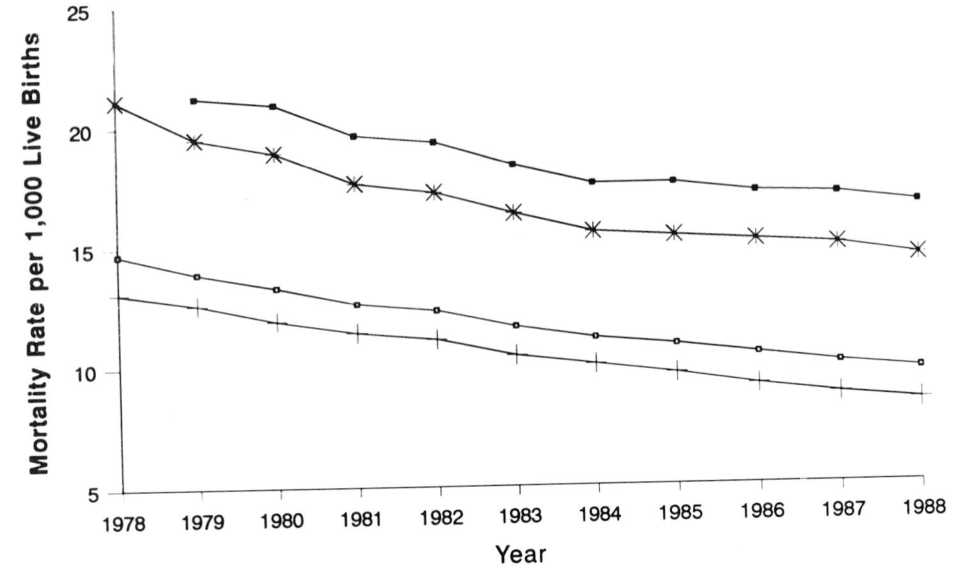

FIG. 3–6. Perinatal mortality in the United States from 1978 to 1988 by race. Perinatal mortality constitutes fetal death before 28 weeks of gestation plus infant deaths at 0 to 6 days of age. (□, all races; ■, African Americans; *, all other non-Caucasians; +, Caucasians; from U.S. Department of Health and Human Services. Perinatal mortality, sect 3. Vital statistics of the United States—1988. vol. 2. pt. A. Hyattsville, MD: U.S. Government Printing Office, 1991.

TABLE 3–9
LOW-BIRTH-WEIGHT RATE FOR 1982 THROUGH 1988 AND WORLD RANKINGS FOR SELECTED COUNTRIES

Rank	Nation	Percentage
1	Spain	1
2	Finland	4
2	Sweden	4
2	Ireland	4
6	Jordan	5
6	Japan	5
6	Egypt	5
6	Hong Kong	5
16	Hungary	6
16	Czechoslovakia	6
16	USSR	6
16	Oman	6
16	Canada	6
29	Italy	7
29	United Kingdom	7
29	United States	7
29	Yugoslavia	7
29	Chile	7
29	Kuwait	7

From Unicef and Children's Defense Fund. The state of America's children. Washington, DC: Children's Defense Fund, 1991:139.

sible for only 14.4% of all U.S. births. In the nation as a whole, African American infants born in urban areas are at least twice as likely as Caucasian infants to have LBWs (see Table 3-5).

The birth weight of U.S. infants is related to several important maternal demographic characteristics (Fig. 3-7). The lowest incidence of LBW is seen in married Caucasian women between 25 and 29 years of age, who completed at least 16 years of school and who received prenatal care starting in the first trimester. The highest risks occur in unmarried African American women who attended school for fewer than 12 years and received late or no prenatal care. Although maternal age was not a factor in LBW rates among African Americans, the LBW rate for Caucasians younger than 20 years of age was almost twice the rate for women 25 to 29 years of age.[56]

The benefit of early prenatal care is seen in both Caucasians and African Americans, with the incidence of LBW decreasing for each group when prenatal care is initiated in the first trimester, rather than late or not at all. Data from Western Europe, where early prenatal care is available and is used by most women, suggest that the United States LBW rate could be halved with a minimal investment in prenatal care.[32]

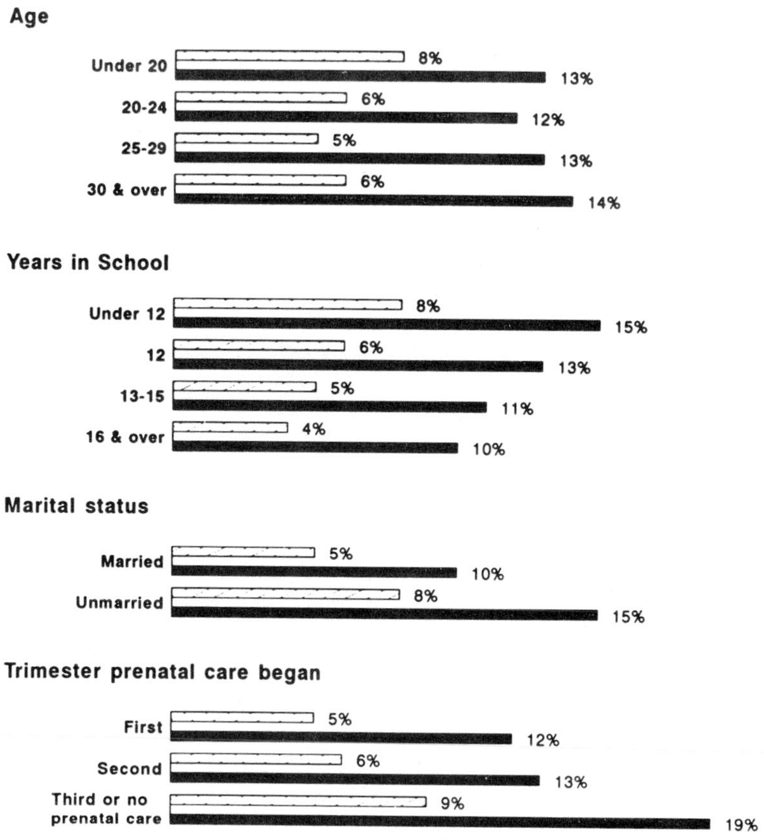

FIG. 3–7. Low-birth-weight rate by race for selected maternal characteristics in 1988. (□, Caucasians; ■, African Americans; from Robert Wood Foundation. Challenges in health care: perspective 1991. Princeton, NJ: RWJ Foundation, 1991:35.)

NEURODEVELOPMENTAL SEQUELAE

With survival rates approaching 95% for premature infants weighing between 1500 and 2500 g and 80% for those between 1000 and 1499 g, the incidence and magnitude of the neurodevelopmental sequelae related to the treatment of premature and critically ill neonates has become increasingly important. Although abnormalities vary with gestational age, population demographics, and length of follow-up, most sequelae are seen in the smallest infants, often those weighing less than 1500 g. Caution must be used in interpreting short-term NICU follow-up data, because minor neuromuscular abnormalities seen in the immediate neonatal period may not persist, and significant abnormalities in cognitive function may not be detectable until the infant is older and more sophisticated testing can be performed.

Grogaard and associates reported an 18% incidence of major handicaps in very-low-birth-weight infants (VLBW; infants <1500 g) at 18 months' follow-up.[58] Cerebral palsy was found in 7.6%, and 6.5% were mentally retarded with developmental quotients of less than 70. Severe retinopathy of prematurity existed in 5.5%, with neurosensory hearing loss occurring at a similar frequency of 5.4%. Further analysis of the data from two treatment periods (*i.e.*, 1976–1980 and 1981–1985) showed that the incidence of major handicaps were reduced to less than one-half: 12.1% of the infants treated during the later period, demonstrated major sequelae compared with 27.2% of those treated between 1976–1980. Similar improvements were seen in ELBW infants, with a 37.3% incidence of major sequelae between 1976 and 1980 decreasing to 15.9% between 1981 and 1985.

Although the absolute number of VLBW and ELBW infants with major sequelae have increased, proportionally more VLBW and ELBW infants are surviving intact. Teplin and associates found an 18% incidence of moderate or severe handicaps in infants weighing less that 1001 g at 6 years of follow-up, but 46% had no functional disability, and 36% had only mild residua.[59]

Certain sociodemographic variables (*e.g.*, race, family income, mother's marital status, age, educational level) have a significant effect on the mental development of NICU survivors. In a study of 6281 NICU graduates followed for as long as 48 to 60 months, Resnick and associates found that mental developmental performance decreased significantly between first testing at 12 months and second testing at 24 months. The greatest decrease was seen in non-Caucasian populations, and although Caucasian infants stabilized or improved between 24 and 48 to 60 months, non-Caucasians continued to decline four additional DQ points. Multivariant analysis showed these declines were more closely related to the maternal sociodemographic factors than to birth weight or NICU course.[60] This same group extended their analysis to 457 NICU graduates attending public school and found strong correlations among poverty, race and academic performance in school. The NICU medical course and treatment correlated with school performance only in those graduates with significant sensory (*e.g.*, blind, hearing impaired) or motor (*e.g.*, cerebral palsy) handicaps.[61]

EXPOSURE TO SUBSTANCE ABUSE

The use of alcohol and illicit drugs during pregnanc is increasing at an alarming rate. Few data are avail able concerning the use of alcohol during pregnancy but several researchers report perinatal cocaine expo sure rates between 0.4% and 27%, depending on th region of the country and population demograph ics.[62–67] Myriad neonatal complications have been re ported as a result of cocaine exposure, ranging fror none to antenatal cerebral infarction (Table 3-10). Th long-term neurodevelopmental effects of perinatal i licit drug exposure are just now being carefully stud ied.

In addition to these physical and social implication of perinatal cocaine abuse, the direct fiscal costs to th health care system are enormous. One report esti mated the short-term initial hospitalization costs c treating infants of cocaine-exposed pregnancies a $5110 per patient and a yearly cost of $1,057,921.0(more than twice the costs for control infants.[68]

REGIONALIZATION: A CONCEPT IN EVOLUTION

Regionalization of perinatal care has been lauded b many as the single most important factor influencin the birth-weight-specific neonatal mortality. Outline in 1977 by the Committee on Perinatal Health of th

TABLE 3–10
EFFECTS OF COCAINE ON THE NEONATE

Common Complications	Rare Problems
Intrauterine growth retardation	Antenatal cerebral infarction
Microcephaly	Birth defects secondary to vasoconstriction
Prematurity	Myocardial infarction, ischemic changes
Infections, especially STDs	Necrotizing enterocolitis
Neurobehavioral abnormalities	
Neurophysiologic abnormalities	
Poor feeding	
Small CNS bleeds	

CNS, central nervous system; STD, sexually transmitted di ease.

From Dixon SD, Bresnahan K, Zuckerman B. Cocaine babie meeting the challenge of management. Contemp Pedia 1990;June:70.

National Foundation of the March of Dimes in its landmark report, *Toward Improving the Outcome of Pregnancy: Recommendations for the Regional Development of Maternal and Perinatal Health Services*, this concept served as the guide for the development of perinatal services for the last two decades.[69] The Committee's concept of regionalization was based on the geographic concentration of neonatal intensive care services supported by cooperative arrangements among hospitals within a region to provide, as a network, the necessary levels of care defined in the document as level I, II, and III services.

Although quite intuitive and logical, this concept of cooperation is rather foreign to the American health care system, which is built on the philosophy of free market, free enterprise, and competition.[70] The level of planning and cooperation necessary to make regionalization work is often resisted by all levels of health care providers.

How did regionalization take hold? Many observers think that it came at the right time, when knowledge of high-risk mothers and neonates was rapidly advancing. It came when the transfer of technology was confined to larger urban teaching hospitals and academic centers. It came at a time when other hospital services were running at near capacity.

Under the plan, regions were not defined strictly by geography, but by tradition and the organizational skills of the early leaders in neonatology. This informal approach to the organization of perinatal care worked well as long as cooperation was seen as mutually beneficial to all involved. In the late 1970s and early 1980s, the health care environment began to change dramatically. In an extensive study of the evolution of the regionalization of perinatal care in the United States, the NPIC identified changes in the financing of health care as key to the initiation of changes in the regional network.[70] The fragile alliance built on cooperation was being replaced by a drive for competition.

Medicare's replacement of fee-for-service reimbursement with a prospective payment system caused hospital inpatient census to drop as adult care was shifted to the outpatient clinics and ambulatory surgical centers. Declining hospital margins with excess capacity in the form of empty beds began to drive competition. The diffusion of technology into the community in conjunction with increased numbers of available neonatologists made competition for neonatal patients a possibility. Managed care plans captured an increasing share of the traditional indemnity plan markets and required hospitals to be full-service providers, making competition a reality. Obstetric and newborn services, once seen as avoidable losses, became a requirement of participation.

In some parts of the country, other factors hastened the move to competition. The medical liability crisis of the 1980s and the huge legal awards for poor neonatal outcome, particularly in the southern United States, increased the desire to have a neonatologist present at almost every delivery. At the same time, the presence of a hospital-based neonatologist presented the opportunity and the necessity to expand neonatal services beyond the delivery room to cover costs of the neonatologist and to present appropriate challenges to him or her and the nursery staff. In other regions, the overcrowding of level III units and the need to back transport convalescing neonates provided additional opportunity for community hospitals to begin neonatal programs. The differences in the levels of care, as defined by the Committee and by the American Academy of Pediatrics, became blurred and merged.

Some say these changes have resulted in better obstetric and neonatal care available at less expensive community hospitals, reducing the need for transporting critically ill infants over long distances. High-quality care received locally is less stressful on the family, involves the pediatrician in follow-up, and preserves the regional center's resources for the sickest, most complex patients.

These could be positive changes if all hospitals and programs operated on a level playing field, but they do not. Most level II units are not able or willing to provide the same full service of neonatal care provided in regional centers. Even the moderately ill infant often requires multiple consultations from neurologists, pediatric cardiologists, and pediatric surgeons. In many cases, these support subspecialists are not available in level II units, leading to delays in diagnosis and therapy and the eventual transfer of the patient for further evaluation. Few level II units are willing to provide unrefundable services, such as social workers and parent support groups, or to develop the appropriate follow-up programs.

The erosion of regionalization threatens the financial stability of regional centers. Competition for funded patients intensifies the burden of caring for the poor, a burden already carried disproportionately by urban regional centers. Even if community level II units are willing to carry their share of unfunded patients, the association of poverty with prematurity results in a higher number of unfunded patients needing complex care available only at regional centers.[36,71] The need to cross-subsidize increasing amounts of uncompensated care makes urban regional centers uncompetitive in managed care markets, completing a scenario that places many urban level III centers in serious financial jeopardy.[72]

The evolution being experienced in the perinatal health care system of the United States is often referred to as deregionalization. This movement is characterized by less cooperation and more emphasis on competition. Viewed in this way, deregionalization is a step backward and if uncontrolled could have a significant negative impact on perinatal outcome.

The development of regional NICUs has been instrumental in decreasing weight-specific infant mortality. However, most agree that neonatal intensive care is much less cost effective than prevention in the form of teenage family planning, supplemental nutrition programs, and early prenatal care.[74,75] Local, state, and federal governments are more willing to pay for expensive acute intensive care than less expensive prenatal care. Even though the value of prenatal care is well known and espoused in many public forums, it is difficult to obtain and maintain funding for it. It seems that the public is more willing to invest in expensive acute care with its immediate gains rather than invest in the nation's future by supporting prenatal care. Contrast the difficulty in obtaining stable public subsidy for prenatal care with the newly born infant's immediate access to acute care almost without regard to gestational age, weight, or amount of resources consumed.[75] Health care professionals must join in the effort to provide a more universal, efficient, and cost-effective, and humane perinatal health care system.

REFERENCES

1. American Hospital Association. Survey of obstetric and newborn services—1989. Chicago: Hospital Data Center and the Section for Maternal and Child Health, 1990:1.
2. National Perinatal Information Center. American Hospital Association survey data tapes 1985–1988. National Perinatal Information Center Newsletter, 1990;Fall:1.
3. Ross Laboratories. Survey of Neonatal Intensive Care Centers. Columbus, OH: Ross Laboratories, 1990.
4. American Academy of Pediatrics' Committee on Fetus and Newborn and Section on Perinatal Pediatrics. Estimates of need and recommendations for personnel in neonatal pediatrics. Pediatrics 1980;65:850.
5. American Academy of Pediatrics' Committee on Fetus and Newborn. Level II units. Pediatrics 1980;65:810.
6. American Academy of Pediatrics' Committee on Fetus and Newborn. Manpower needs in neonatal pediatrics. Pediatrics 1985;76:132.
7. Jury AG, Gherman S. Total population estimate of newborn special-care bed needs. Pediatrics 1985;75:993.
8. Children's Defense Fund. The state of America's children. Washington, DC: Children's Defense Fund, 1991;139.
9. American Board of Pediatrics. Sub-board of neonatal and perinatal medicine report, 1990.
10. Merenstein GB, Rhodes PG, Little GA. Personnel in neonatal pediatrics: assessment of numbers and distribution. Pediatrics 1985;76:454.
11. Accreditation Council for Graduate Medical Education. 1991–92 directory of graduate medical education program. Chicago, IL: American Medical Association, 1991.
12. Merenstein GB. The pediatrician's role in the level II nursery. Pediatr Ann 1988;17:453.
13. Frigoletto FD, Little GA, eds. Guidelines for perinatal care. 3rd ed. Washington, DC: American Academy of Pediatrics and American College of Obstetrics and Gynecology, 1992.
14. Committee on Perinatal Health. Toward improving the outcome of pregnancy: recommendations for the regional development of maternal and perinatal service. White Plains, NY: The National Foundation—March of Dimes, 1976.
15. Avery GB. The pediatrician and neonatology today. Pediatr Ann 1988;17:7.
16. Bose CL, La Pine TR, Jung AL. Neonatal back-transport cost effectiveness. Med Care 1985;23:14.
17. Martin RG, Fenton LJ, Leonardson G, Reid TJ. Consistency o care in an intensive care nursery staffed by nurse clinicians Am J Dis Child 1985;139:169.
18. Cassidy G. Through the looking glass—or look before yo leap. Pediatrics 1982;70:1001.
19. Resnick MB, Eyler FD, Nelson RM, Eitzman DV, Bucciarel RL. Developmental intervention for low birth weight infants improved early developmental outcome. Pediatrics 1987;80:68
20. Leib SA, Benfield G, Guidubaldi J. Effects of early interventio and stimulation on the preterm infant. Pediatrics 1980;66:83.
21. Achenbach TM, Phares V, Howell CT, Rauh VA, Nurcombe B Seven-year outcome of the Vermont Intervention Program fo low-birth-weight infants. Child Dev 1990;61:1672.
22. Resnick MB, Eitzman D, Dickman H, Ariet M, Ausbon W Data base management system for Children's Medical Service Regional Perinatal Intensive Care Centers program. J Fla Me Assoc 1983;70:718.
23. Resnick MB, Ariet M, Carter RL, et al. Prospective pricin system by diagnosis-related groups: comparison of federal di agnosis-related groups with high-risk obstetric care groups Am J Obstet Gynecol 1987;156:567.
24. Resnick MB, Ariet M, Carter RL, et al. Prospective pricin system for tertiary neonatal intensive care. Pediatrics 198 78:820.
25. Resnick MB, Ariet M, Carter RL, et al. Prospective pricin model for neonatologists and obstetricians in tertiary care cen ters. Pediatrics 1988;82:442.
26. State of Florida Department of Health and Rehabilitative Ser vices. Children's Medical Services regional perinatal intensiv care center program (RPICC) handbook. Tallahassee: State o Florida Department of Health and Rehabilitative Services 1987.
27. State of Florida Department of Health and Rehabilitative Ser vices. Children's medical services regional perinatal intensiv care program (RPICC) handbook. Tallahassee: State of Florid Department of Health and Rehabilitative Services, 1991.
28. Walker DB, Vohr BR, Oh W. Economic analysis of regionalize neonatal care for very low-birth-weight infants in the state c Rhode Island. Pediatrics 1985;76:69.
29. Boyle MH, Torrance GW, Sinclair JC, Horwood SP. Economi evaluation of neonatal intensive care of very-low-birth-weigh infants. N Engl J Med 1983;308:1330.
30. Shankaran S, Cohen SN, Linver M, Zonia S. Medical care cos of high-risk infants after neonatal intensive care: a controlle study. Pediatrics 1988;81:372.
31. Walker DB, Feldman A, Vohr BR, Oh W. Cost-benefit analysi of neonatal intensive care for infants weighing less than 100 grams at birth. Pediatrics 1984;74:20.
32. United States Congress, Office of Technology Assessmen Neonatal intensive care for low birth weight infants: cost an effectiveness. Health technology case study 38. Washingtor DC: U.S. Printing Office, 1987.
33. Kitzhaber JA. The Oregon model. In: The Richard and Lind Rosenthal lectures. Improving access to affordable health car Washington, DC: Institute of Medicine, 1990;69.
34. Developmental Disabilities Planning Council State of Florid Florida's children, their future is in our hands: the report of th Task Force for Prevention of Developmental Handicaps. Tall hassee: The Florida Developmental Disabilities Plannin Council, 1991:11.
35. Committee to Study the Prevention of Low Birth Weight. Pr venting low birthweight. Washington, DC: National Academ Press, 1985.
36. Imershein AW, Turner C, Wells JG, Pearman A. Covering th

costs of care in neonatal intensive care units. Pediatrics 1992;89:56.
37. Foley JD, Employee Benefit Research Institute. Uninsured in the United States: the nonelderly population without health insurance—analysis of the March 1990 current population survey. Special Report SR-10. Washington, DC: Employee Benefit Research Institute, 1991.
38. American Academy of Pediatrics. Children first: a legislative proposal. Washington, DC: Department of Government Liaison, 1991.
39. Children's Defense Fund. S.O.S. America! A children's defense budget. Washington, DC: The Children's Defense Fund, 1990:160.
40. Gabel JR, Jensen GA. The price of state mandated benefits. Inquiry 1989;26:419.
41. Ford M. Medicaid: FY 1991 budget and child health initiatives. CRS issue brief. Washington, DC: Library of Congress, 1990.
42. Hewlett SA. When the bough breaks. New York: Basic Books, 1991:169–192.
43. American Academy of Pediatrics. Medicaid State Reports, FY 1989. Washington, DC: American Academy of Pediatrics Department of Research, 1991.
44. Tharpe KI, Siegal J, Dailey T. Including the poor: the fiscal impacts of Medicaid expansions. JAMA 1989;261:1003.
45. Howell EM, Ellwood MR. Medicaid and pregnancy: issues in expanding eligibility. Fam Plann Perspect 1991;23:123.
46. Kenney AM, Torres A, Ditts W, Macias J. Medicaid expenditures for maternity and newborn care in America. Fam Plann Perspect 1986;18:103.
47. Kent C, ed. Medicaid under the microscope. Medicine and health perspectives. Washington, DC: Faulkner and Gray, 1991.
48. Wiener JO, ed. Medicare and health perspectives. Bush budget: something new for '92. Washington, DC: Faulkner and Gray, 1991.
49. Clarke GJ. Overview of the Medicaid program: presentation to the State of Florida House Health Care Committee. Tallahassee: State of Florida Department of Health and Rehabilitative Services, 1991.
50. Rich S. More pediatricians spurn Medicaid cases. Washington Post 1991:6a.
51. Rich S. State Medicaid payments faulted as too low. Washington Post 1991:3a.
52. National Commission on Children. Beyond rhetoric: a new American agenda for children and families. Washington, DC: National Commission on Children, 1991:122.
53. Tuckson R. Testimony before the Committee on Labor and Human Resources, U.S. Senate, regarding the need for health care reform. Washington, DC: March of Dimes Birth Defects Foundation, June, 1991.
54. Wegman M. Annual summary of vital statistics—1990. Pediatrics 1991;88:1081.
55. United States Department of Health and Human Services. Perinatal mortality, sec 3. Vital statistics of the United States—1988, vol II, part A. Hyattsville, MD: U.S. Department of Health and Human Services, 1991.
56. The Robert Wood Foundation. Challenges in health care: perspective 1991. Princeton, NJ: RWJ Foundation, 1991.
57. Gabbe SG. Antepartum fetal evaluation. In: Gabbe SG, Niebyl JR, Simpson JL, eds. Obstetrics normal and problems pregnancies. New York: Churchill Livingston, 1986;271.
58. Grögaard JB, Lindstrom DP, Parker RA, Culley B, Stahlman MT. Increased survival rate in very low birth weight infants (1500 grams or less): no association with increased incidence of handicaps. J Pediatr 1990;117:139.
59. Teplin SW, Burchinal M, Johnson-Martin, N, Humphry RA, Kraybill EN. Neurodevelopmental, health, and growth status at age 6 years of children with birth weights less than 1001 grams. J Pediatr 1991;118:768.
60. Resnick MB, Stralka K, Carter RL, et al. Effects of birthweight and sociodemographic variables on mental development of neonatal intensive care unit survivors. Am J Obstet Gynecol 1990;162:374.
61. Resnick MB, Roth J, Ariet, M, et al. Educational outcome of neonatal intensive care graduates. Pediatrics 1992;89:373.
62. Chasnoff IJ, Burns WJ, Schnoll SH, Burns KA. Cocaine use in pregnancy. N Engl J Med 1985;313:666.
63. Chasnoff IJ. Drug use in women, establishing standard of care. Ann N Y Acad Sci 1989;562:208.
64. Frank DA, Zuckerman BS, Amaro H, et al. Cocaine use during pregnancy: prevalence and correlates. Pediatrics 1988;82:888.
65. Pietrantoni M, Knuppel RA. Alcohol use in pregnancy. In: Chasnoff IJ, ed. Clinical perinatology. Philadelphia: WB Saunders, 1991;93.
66. Dixon SD, Bresnahan K, Zuckerman B. Cocaine babies: meeting the challenge of management. Contemp Pediatr 1990; 7(6):70.
67. Chasnoff IJ, Bussey ME, Savich R, Stack CM. Clinical and laboratory observations. J Pediatr 1986;108:456.
68. Chiu TTW, Vaughn AJ, Carzoli RP. Hospital costs for cocaine-exposed infants. J Fla Med Assoc 1990;77:897.
69. Committee on Perinatal Health. Toward improving the outcome of pregnancy. White Plains: The National Foundation March of Dimes, 1977.
70. Gagnan DE. Regionalization: a movement in transition. Natl Perinat Assoc Bull 1988;2:4.
71. Handler A, Rosenberg D, Driscoll M, Cohen M, Swift E, Garcia P, Cohn J. Regional perinatal care in crisis: a case study of an urban public hospital. J Public Health Policy 1991;12:184.
72. Gagnan DE, Allison-Cook S, Schwartz RM. Perinatal care: the threat of re-regionalization. Pediatr Ann 1988;17:447.
73. Children's Defense Fund. Maternal and child health in America. Special report three. Washington, DC: Children's Defense Fund, 1991:20.
74. Stahlman MT. Improving health care provision to neonates in the United States. Am J Dis Child 1991;145:510.
75. Rosenblat RA. The perinatal paradox: doing more and accomplishing less. Health Aff 1989;8:159.

Neonatology: Pathophysiology and Management of the Newborn, Fourth Edition,
edited by Gordon B. Avery, Mary Ann Fletcher, and Mhairi G. MacDonald.
J.B. Lippincott Company, Philadelphia © 1994.

chapter 4

Perinatal Outreach Education

MHAIRI G. MACDONALD
BEVERLY JOHNSON

> We may, then, say that the product of the hospital in medical education, like the product in the number of cases treated, depends on whether or not the cases are well treated.[1]

It has been estimated that biomedical knowledge doubles every 8 to 10 years.[2] Unless the health practitioner keeps abreast of the rapidly advancing knowledge and can apply it to those areas in which he or she is specialized, his or her professional obligation to the patient is not met. The critical factor in providing perinatal care of high quality consists not of modern facilities or electronic equipment but of trained and experienced personnel who are able to provide the best professional techniques of obstetric and newborn care within a coordinated regional perinatal care system. Tertiary care centers in a regionalized perinatal system are expected to provide leadership in establishing and executing educational programs to maintain this high standard of care.[3,4]

THE TEAM CONCEPT

In no other area of medicine is the team concept of care more important than in perinatal medicine.[5] The first essential message of the perinatal outreach program is that modern perinatal care is so complex, and scientific advances in the field occur so rapidly, that optimal patient care requires a highly organized team approach. The educational program should benefit all members of the team, including physicians, nurses, social workers, respiratory therapists, laboratory technicians, x-ray technicians, nutritionists, patient transport personnel, and hospital administrators. The pool of available teachers for the program must represent expertise in all these areas; thus, key health care personnel and administrators at the tertiary center must be committed to the concept of outreach education.

The following basic educational needs should be met:

- updated science and techniques necessary to provide optimal patient care
- ability to screen for high-risk states
- knowledge of how to develop a patient health care plan
- definition of responsibility as a member of a health care team
- recognition of the role and ability of other team members
- ability to integrate the skills of other team members into care.

In a regionalized system, the perinatal care team at an individual hospital develops objectives and functional capabilities related to the level of perinatal care that the hospital is providing. Although it is likely that an individual team will be able to meet the needs of most of its patients, it can be anticipated that patients with problems that are not managed routinely will present for care. Health care teams at all levels of the perinatal care system must have four essential features:

1. The ability to perform necessary emergency care
2. Knowledge of the capabilities of perinatal health care teams at other centers
3. Free communication with these centers
4. Methods for interaction that benefit the patient.

In a coordinated delivery system, it should be possible for the referring and receiving teams to share the responsibility for the patient. Because each team becomes responsible not only to itself but to other institutions and teams within the region, the educational content of any training program should include the following:

- study and use of common terminology
- communication methods, including optimal documentation of patient care
- how to use consultants
- emergency care and stabilization
- transport of the high-risk perinatal patient
- how to maintain continuity of care
- methods of evaluating the quality of the patient care provided.

Outreach education is a two-way process. Tertiary center staff should recognize the strengths of the community hospital, particularly in the area of family-centered care. For reinforcement of the interinstitutional team concept, information is offered in a noncritical fashion, with an emphasis on information exchange among institutions. Specialized personnel at the tertiary center should be easily accessible for consultation at all times.

PROGRAM DEVELOPMENT

Ideally, planning, implementation, and evaluation of outreach education should be a cooperative effort involving representatives from local tertiary centers, community hospitals, and health agencies. The tertiary center functions as a role model insofar as assessment, communication, research, and education are concerned; however, staff at the tertiary center must be open to suggestions and criticism from the community.

ADMINISTRATIVE CONSIDERATIONS

Although the administrative structure of an individual program will vary somewhat according to the hospital area that is to be serviced, there are certain administrative considerations vital to the success of any program. The key management figure is the program coordinator. The coordinator is usually a nurse who has a friendly, open, and noncondescending attitude toward participants in the educational program. It is important that the coordinator has had recent and preferably ongoing hands-on experience in either high-risk obstetrics or neonatal intensive care. Understandably, there is likely to be considerable resistance to educational programs that are provided by personnel viewed as not having up-to-date patient care experience. In addition, the coordinator should have considerable organizational abilities and be very familiar with educational resources within the region to be served and the particular aspects of the educational process that are specifically related to adult peer education.

The job description for the coordinator includes the following:

Plan, implement, and evaluate educational programs for individual hospitals with the outreach team.
Act as the primary liaison with the transport team.
Participate in the teaching of educational programs.
Maintain contact with and serve as educational resource consultant to perinatal staff at the community hospital.
Provide ongoing feedback to the community hospitals about the program.
Revise program structure and content with program director or directors as needed, based on evaluation of need at individual hospitals.
Prepare an annual report for the program.
Collaborate in fund-raising activities.
Assist in the production of the newsletter.

It is desirable that the directorship of the program reflect both the obstetric and neonatal aspects of perinatal care. This can be achieved by codirectors who are subspecialized in these areas. Other personnel might include a clinical nurse educator, preferably with clinical expertise that complements that of the nurse coordinator.

GEOGRAPHIC, DEMOGRAPHIC, AND CULTURAL CONSIDERATIONS

It is important to be aware of some of the basic geographic parameters of the region to be served.[6] How many miles does it encompass? Is it urban or rural? In some parts of the country, climate may impede travel during parts of the year. Local demographic data also are vital. How many deliveries occur at each hospital? What is the number of high-risk births per year? How many mothers or infants are transported? What is the socioeconomic status of the patient population? Are there cultural factors (*e.g.*, large numbers of immigrants who receive little prenatal care) that affect perinatal mortality and morbidity statistics? What health care resources are available in the community? Is health care provided mainly by physicians in private practice, by resident physicians, by nurse midwives or practitioners? Are there affiliate relationships between institutions that may be used to enhance communication? How active are the maternal–child health departments of the city, county, or state? Are there active childbirth education groups or health care promotion groups? Are there people or groups resistant to regional education and organizational concepts? Do hospital administrators support outreach efforts?

EDUCATIONAL RESOURCES

Existing educational resources in the community should be identified, such as the physical facilities and educational aids that are available at the community hospitals. Resources and expertise should be shared. Staff from both the community hospitals and the tertiary center should be encouraged to donate their time to the pool of available teachers. In areas in which there are several tertiary centers, all efforts should be made to eliminate counterproductive interinstitutional competition. The benefits of this type of cooperation include improved regional communication, a significantly larger pool of teaching staff, and better use of all educational resources.

It should be recognized, however, that the quality of the educational programs and advice (*e.g.*, helping to develop patient management protocols) provided must be monitored by the director of the outreach education program. It is theoretically possible that an educational program, and thus the hospital supporting the program, might be held liable for the results of poor instruction.[7]

ASSESSMENT OF HEALTH EDUCATION NEEDS

Initial assessments of health education needs may take the form of site visits, which provide information on physical facilities, equipment, personnel, policies, and procedures.[6] Provision of opportunities for personal contact between tertiary center staff and community hospital personnel helps these people ascertain attitudes and feelings and identify facilities and needs. Although site visits may be expensive and time consuming, the opportunity to develop relationships may outweigh the costs.

Alternatively, needs may be assessed by questionnaire. This method costs less and reaches a greater number of people in a shorter time. Questionnaires, however, may be viewed as impersonal, may not be returned, and tend to reflect only the opinions of the people who complete them.

The transport team can provide a valuable resource for needs assessment.[8] During transportation activities, staff from the referring hospital interact directly with staff from the referral center. This provides an opportunity to develop the close relationships necessary for a successful outreach program, and permits direct observation of the resources and needs of the community hospital. Repeated visits to a referring institution allow the members of the transport team to identify educational needs clearly. Periodic retrospective review of transport logs also may aid in identifying the needs of individual hospitals. Perhaps most important, the interaction between the transport personnel and the community hospital staff, at the time of patient transport, offers a unique opportunity for direct educational exchange that cannot be duplicated in another setting.

A combination of assessment techniques may be the most effective method. In outreach education, as in any educational modality designed for adults, participation in the assessment process enhances the probability that education will produce a change in behavior.

EDUCATIONAL CONTENT AND FORMAT

To effect change, the educational program should increase knowledge, improve clinical proficiency, and influence attitudes. The program content should be tailored to the needs of the individual community hospital. It is essential, however, that planners balance interest with need. For example, although it is important for staff at community hospitals to be informed of the availability and the general concept of programs, such as extracorporeal membrane oxygenation and *in vitro* fertilization, it is not necessarily appropriate for the tertiary center to provide extensive in-depth education on these topics to every hospital. If individual hospitals are not fulfilling basic needs for patients in areas such as thermoregulation, resuscitation, and stabilization, outreach educators should address these needs as priorities. The frequency with which these core areas of the curriculum are repeated will depend primarily on the frequency with which personnel at a given institution are required to deal with a particular high-risk situation. As a rule, the less frequently a high-risk situation is encountered, the more frequently the pertinent educational program should be repeated. The outreach team also must provide more sophisticated programs for those hospitals whose staff members are better versed in basic knowledge.

Before the format for an educational presentation is chosen, some practical points should be considered.

The community hospital staff should have input into the topic and mode of presentation.[9]

The environment must be conducive to learning. The term "outreach," meaning that staff members from the tertiary center go out to the community hospital, takes into account the fact that people are more comfortable and more able to learn in familiar surroundings. The room used for teaching should be comfortable and accessible to staff on duty, and it should have adequate lighting, blackboards, and audiovisual equipment.

Timing is important. Time away from patient care must be considered and the duration of individual sessions limited as necessary. For staff who work in shifts, programs presented around shift changes may be more convenient and attractive. Programs designed primarily for physicians often are optimally scheduled to coincide with their regular staff meetings. Scheduling for the speakers should take into consideration any travel time involved.

Individual participants will not all have the same learning processes.

It has been observed that nurses listen differently or more effectively to another nurse than to a physician and that nurses do not participate actively in discussions when physicians attend the same conference. In addition, it has been observed that physicians are reluctant to receive education from nursing staff and to participate in educational programs that include nurses. This type of behavior is counterproductive to the team concept of perinatal care. However, although every effort should be made to avoid the separation of programs for nursing and support personnel from programs for physicians, it is realistic to expect that some of the educational material will have to be presented in a format tailored specifically to the needs of an individual professional group.

There are three major approaches to outreach education. The first has been described by Kattwinkle and colleagues.[10] This method depends on the education at the tertiary center of a key liaison person from each community hospital. This person also is taught how to supervise the use of workbooks and self-instructional materials by perinatal personnel at their own institution. The second method is based on the media library. The educational program is presented on tape and videocassettes that are purchased or rented by the participating hospitals.[11] The last method—and by far the most time-consuming—involves face-to-face contact between educators and personnel at the community hospitals.

A combination of all three methods is probably optimal. There is evidence that the behavior of health professionals cannot be altered without some face-to-face contact.[12–16] On-site educational efforts at community hospitals also help make tertiary center personnel more approachable to the community center staff and thus help develop a better communication system between hospitals. Tertiary center staff are able to collect direct information on activities and problems at a given institution, which can then be used for program modification.

The format selected for the presentation of educational material also may be tailored to the needs and desires of the participating hospitals. Choices include lectures, demonstrations, workshops, informal discussions, case presentations, and ward rounds (Tables 4-1 and 4-2).

The transport conference has proved very popular and effective (Table 4-3).[17] The key aspects of this type of program are travel of the center team to the community hospital, a discussion based on the maternal, fetal, and infant patient population referred during a recent time period, and encouragement of active participation by both center and community hospital personnel. Leadership comes from the center, but a local health professional is involved as a facilitator. The discussion centers on the management of specific cases and their outcome.

A program of nurse exchange between perinatal care centers and community hospitals allows direct observation of or participation in the care of patients.

TABLE 4–1
FORMATS FOR PERINATAL OUTREACH EDUCATION

Format	Description
Lecture	A planned didactic presentation of a specific subject by a knowledgeable professional; usually 45–50 min long, with 10–15 min for discussion
Conference	A formal interchange of views in a 1- to 2-d program devoted to specific aspects of perinatal care
Seminar	A short, 15- to 20-min lecture followed by an informal discussion of the topic by participants; optimal group size is 15–20
Workshop	A seminar emphasizing practical skills
Programmed instruction	A self-instruction program that provides immediate feedback
Independent learning modules	A self-instruction program involving audiovisuals and programmed instruction
Discussion groups	A group of people meet informally to discuss patient topics of mutual concern
Case presentations	A detailed presentation and discussion of specific cases (*e.g.*, patients transported to a referral center or patients of special clinical interest)
Traineeship or clerkship	A clinical program of any duration that provides for demonstration and return demonstration of patient care skills; usually combines clinical and theoretical components
Exchange program	A short-term clinical experience that allows staff from a community hospital to observe or participate in care of patients at a tertiary center and also provides an opportunity for tertiary-center staff to observe or provide care at a community hospital; participation in ward rounds contributes a didactic component

TABLE 4–2
HOW TO ORGANIZE A CONFERENCE

1. Start well ahead of the anticipated date—allow 4–6 mo for planning.
   a. Select topic.
   b. Determine format (*e.g.*, lecture, workshop, group discussion)
   c. Select date and place. Keep in mind conflicts with other programs, transportation, parking, and room allocation.
   d. Create list of speakers.
   e. Determine appropriate fees.
2. Contact speakers by phone and letter. Obtain confirmation. Send them a brief outline and objectives and obtain their curricula vitae.
3. Design brochure and contact printer. Allow 2 weeks for printing. Mail brochures 8–10 wk before conference to allow time for scheduling.
4. Plan and arrange for coffee breaks and lunches.
5. Apply for continuing medical and nursing education credits at least 60–90 d before program. Objectives, outlines, bibliography, evaluation, and curriculum vitae for speakers are needed to apply for educational credits. Contact local medical school and state nursing association for their requirements.
6. Make sure that audiovisual equipment is available and that speakers are familiar with it.
7. Delegate several people to register participants on the day of the conference. Explain to participants the evaluation forms, pre- and posttests, panel discussions or small group workshops, and how to find restrooms and telephones.
8. Designate a moderator to keep speakers within time limits.
9. Hold a postsession review with the planning committee to go over program evaluations and to elicit constructive suggestions for the next program.
10. Anticipate problems. Keep in mind "Murphy's Law"—if something can go wrong, it will!

Advice should be sought from hospital attorneys if hands-on care by participants is planned. The hospital may be held responsible for the patient care provided by the participants, under the ostensible agency theory.[18]

In laboratories, personnel can sharpen clinical skills in resuscitation, endotracheal intubation, monitoring, placement of intravenous lines, and other activities that require practice (Fig. 4-1; Table 4-4).

The consciousness-raising aspect of the evaluation component of the educational program also may be a valuable educational tool if the data generated are made available to the health professionals who are creating them.[14–16]

TABLE 4–3
BASIC ORGANIZATION OF A TRANSPORT CONFERENCE

Activity	Participants
Explain format	Director, outreach education program Nurse coordinator
Select patients for discussion 3–4 wk before conference	Nurse coordinator Physician from perinatal program Community hospital nurses and pediatricians
Present clinical history through time of transport to referral center	Community hospital physician or nurse
Present clinical history from transport to disposition from intensive care nursery	Member of the perinatal center staff
Discuss clinical details at community hospital and referral center, with information on findings at follow-up if available	Community hospital staff Perinatal center staff
Make a didactic presentation on a specific topic (optional)	Member of the outreach education teaching pool
Complete conference evaluation forms	Community hospital staff
Process continuing education certificates within 2–4 wk of conference	Nurse coordinator

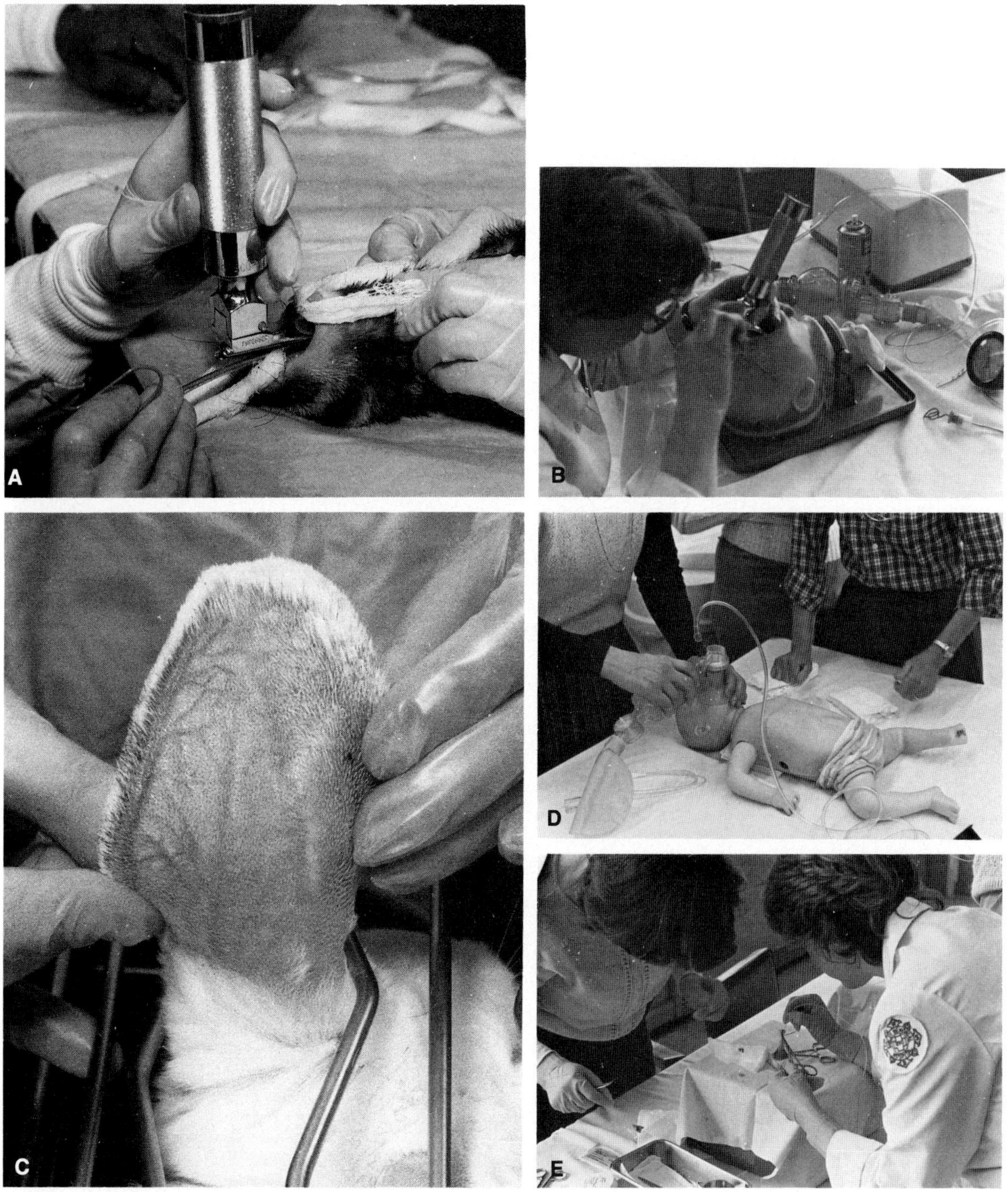

FIG. 4–1. Teaching models (**A**) A ferret is used to demonstrate endotracheal intubation. (**B**) An infant intubation model (Resusci Intubation Model, Laerdal Medical, Armonk, NY) is used to practice endotracheal intubation. A viewing port in the back of the head allows demonstration of anatomic relationships. (**C**) A rabbit's ear has been shaved to demonstrate vessels for intravenous placement. (**D**) A resuscitation model (Resusci Baby, Laerdal Medical) is used to practice bag and mask ventilation. (**E**) An umbilical cord is used to practice catheter insertion. The cord is placed in an infant feeding bottle, filled with normal saline, and supported inside a cardboard box. The end of the cord projects through a cut nipple.

TABLE 4–4
SOME TEACHING MODELS USED IN PERINATAL OUTREACH EDUCATION

Mannequins (Small Dolls With Soft Vinyl Skin)

To teach tracheotomy care:
- Create a hole in the doll's neck with a sharp instrument—a corkscrew works well.
- Insert a size 1 or size 0 tracheotomy tube.
- Tie the ties and use as a model to teach proper suctioning and skin care techniques.

To teach umbilical catheter management[19]:
- Puncture the doll's anterior abdomen using a 16-gauge medicut needle.
- Insert needle through the doll's front and back, then remove.
- Thread an umbilical catheter through from front to back.
- Insert blunt needles onto catheter at both ends. An IV bag containing water tinted with red food coloring can be attached to the posterior end of the catheter to simulate blood.

To teach technique for drawing samples for blood gases:
- Insert a three-way stopcock into the umbilical catheter anteriorly and attach IV bag and tubing.

This system also can be used to teach arterial and venous blood pressure monitoring by transducer.
- To simulate arterial pressure, wrap a blood pressure cuff around the partially filled IV bag and inflate to 60–70 torr.
- For a venous line, inflate to 5–10 torr.

Resusci Head*

The model head used for endotracheal intubation (see Fig. 4-1*B*) can be modified to teach orogastric and nasogastric feeding by attaching a reservoir to the esophageal opening.

Rabbits

To teach placement of chest tubes[20]:
- Anesthetize a rabbit weighing approximately 2.0 kg using xylazine, 8.8 mg/kg IM. Wait 10 min, then administer ketamine HCl, 50 mg/kg IM.
- Place the rabbit on its back and shave or clip the chest hair as closely as possible. Use a commercial depilatory to remove remaining hair.
- Restrain the rabbit's fore- and hindpaws securely.
- Surgically drape the rabbit.
- Place electrodes on the chest wall for attachment to a cardiorespiratory monitor. Changes in ECG tracing due to the pneumothorax can then be demonstrated.
- Insert chest tube.

To demonstrate placement of peripheral intravenous needles and cannulae, see Figure 4-1*C*.

Weanling Kittens

To teach endotracheal intubation[21,22]:
- Use kittens weighing 1–1.5 kg.
- Withhold food 8 h before intubation; however, allow water intake.
- Give ketamine HCl 20 mg/kg IM.
- Wait 10 min for full effect of ketamine HCl.

Examine larynx after every four or five attempts at intubation. If the laryngeal area is traumatized, allow 7–10 d for recovery.

Ferrets

To teach endotracheal intubation[23]:
- Withhold food 8 h before intubation; however, allow water intake.
- Give ketamine HCl, 5 mg/kg IM, and acepromazine maleate, 0.55 mg/kg IM, and allow to take effect.
- Maintain anesthesia with 40% of original dose IM as needed. If necessary, control sneezing with 0.5 mg/kg IM of diphenhydramine.
- Apply bland ophthalmic ointment to eyes to prevent dessication.

Examine larynx for signs of trauma, as for kittens, and allow recovery between training sessions. Evidence of trauma was noted in 100% of ferrets after ten intubations.[23]

Placenta and Cord

To teach insertion of intravenous infusion lines and umbilical vessel catheters[24,25]:†
- Preserve placenta and cord by freezing in *individual* containers.
- Allow 3–4 h for thawing before use.
- Use vessels on the fetal surface of the placenta to demonstrate insertion of peripheral intravenous needles and cannulae. Blood drawing also can be demonstrated.
- Cut a 15-cm length of cord to demonstrate the anatomy of the umbilical stump and the technique for arterial and venous catheterization. The cord may be placed in an infant's feeding bottle that contains saline. One end of the cord then protrudes through a suitably cut nipple and can be pulled out of the bottle for each attempt at the procedure.

* Laerdal Medical, Armonk, NY.

† Use of this model is not recommended unless human immunodeficiency virus and hepatitis B virus status of source is known.

IARKETING AND FINANCIAL RESOURCES

\ successful perinatal outreach education program narkets itself by its high standard of performance. uccess is facilitated by measures that reinforce pro-ram identity and cohesiveness, such as use of a logo nd publication of a regular newsletter.

Significant financial support, in addition to that de-ived from the tertiary center, often is required. This eed has been emphasized by the radical changes in he reimbursement system for hospitals and physi-ians that have occurred in the past decade in the Jnited States.[26,27] These changes are designed to con-ain immediate costs for acute care and do not give riority to preventive measures with a view to reduc-ng future costs; they have impeded, rather than en-anced the organization of facilities providing perina-al care into effective regional networks. In some reas of the United States, at least part of the financial upport for the local perinatal outreach education rogram has been supplied by the local state health epartment. Community hospitals can be asked to ontribute financial support once the program is ac-epted and established in the community.

ROGRAM EVALUATION

n 1973, Caplan stated that "we live in a 'Prove it!' ge."[28] Today, his comment is even more relevant. \n effective way to examine cost-effectiveness of erinatal education, so that adequate support for hese programs will continue to be a priority of the ertiary perinatal center, has yet to be defined. Unfor-unately, evaluation of the impact of perinatal out-each education in terms of increasing knowledge nd changing health care practices has proved ex-remely difficult.[9,10,29–31] Changes effected by continu-ng education on the behavior of health professionals are particularly hard to document. Measures of short-term changes in cognitive knowledge do not offer a true assessment of whether or not the participant will retain and use knowledge to modify patient care and improve patient outcome. Changes in the behavior of health care givers eventually should be reflected in changes in the local perinatal mortality rate; however, this rate is influenced by many other factors and changes slowly. The collection of as many as 7 to 10 years of postprogram mortality data may be neces-sary before any significant change can be detected. A decrease in perinatal morbidity is likely to be a more sensitive indicator of behavioral change on the part of health care providers, but is more difficult and expen-sive to measure. Changes in health care practice are reflected, however, in the frequency with which vital procedures are performed; changes in the number of appropriately indicated transfers to, and consulta-tions with, the tertiary perinatal center; and the con-dition of high-risk mothers and high-risk neonates on arrival at tertiary centers. Qualitative changes in the relationship between the referral and community hospital due to positive contacts between personnel are illustrated in Figure 4-2.

Although it seems reasonable to consider orga-nized, high-quality, ongoing postgraduate education desirable, particularly in a field that is advancing as quickly as perinatal medicine, financial support for health care programs will be increasingly determined by analysis of their cost-effectiveness. In addition, lack of meaningful program evaluation data will im-pede the search for, and implementation of more ef-fective methods. Problems with the utility and com-parability of data and the cost of the evaluation process for perinatal outreach education suggest that a nationally sponsored multiinstitutional evaluation may be indicated. This project would be intended to determine the most cost-effective method of provid-ing outreach education to hospital regions that are disparate both geographically and demographically.

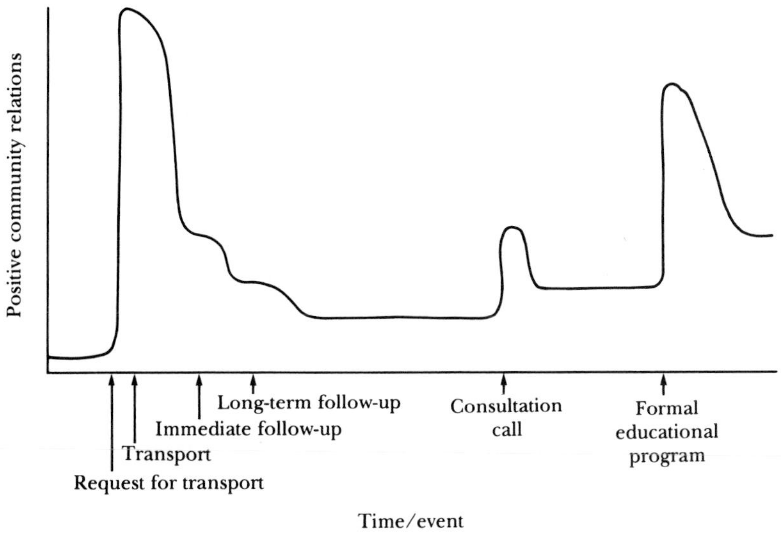

IG. 4–2. Many specific events may impact n the relations between the referral center nd referring hospitals. (From MacDonald IG, Miller MK, eds. Emergency transport f the perinatal patient. Boston: Little, rown & Co., 1989:58.)

REFERENCES

1. Codman EA. The product of a hospital. Surg Gynecol Obstet 1913;18:491.
2. Cooper JAD. Continuing education: what do we mean by it, and why is it important? J Med Educ 1974;49:617.
3. Ryan GM. Toward improving the outcome of pregnancy: recommendations for the regional development of perinatal health services. J Obstet Gynecol 1975;46:375.
4. Schneider JM. Attitudes and organization of the Medical Center. In: Duxbury M, Graven S, Redmann R, Sommers J, eds. Proceedings of the conference on outreach programs: their integral parts and processes. White Plains, New York: The National Foundation March of Dimes, 1978:7.
5. Pernoll ML. Perinatal educational demands. Clin Perinatol 1976;3:453.
6. Little GA. Establishing and maintaining relationships with community hospitals and health professionals. In: Duxbury M, Gnaven S, Redmann R, Sommers J, eds. Proceedings of the conference on outreach programs: their integral parts and processes. White Plains, New York: The National Foundation March of Dimes, 1978:16.
7. Air Shields, Inc. v Spears, 590 SW2d 574, 578 (Tex Civ App 1979).
8. Bose CL. An overview of the organization and administration of a perinatal transport service. In: MacDonald MG, Miller MK, eds. Emergency transport of the perinatal patient. Boston: Little, Brown & Co., 1989:34.
9. Sibley NC, Sackett DL, Neufeld V, et al. A randomized trial of continuing medical education. N Engl J Med 1982;306:511.
10. Kattwinkle J, Cook LJ, Nowcek GA, et al. Improved perinatal knowledge and care in the community hospital through a program of self-instruction. Pediatrics 1979;64:451.
11. Weinberg AD, McNamara DG, Christiansen CH, et al. Cardiopulmonary diseases in newborns: a study in continuing medical education. J Med Educ 1979;54:230.
12. Avorn J, Soumeri SB. Improving drug-therapy decisions through educational outreach. N Engl J Med 1983;308:1457.
13. Pinkerton RE, Tinanoff N, Willms JL, et al. Resident physician performance in a continuing education format. JAMA 1980; 244:2183.
14. Kessner DM. Diffusion of new medical information (editorial Am J Public Health 1981;71:367.
15. Stross JK, Harlan WR. The dissemination of new medical info mation. JAMA 1979;241:2622.
16. Innui TS, Yourtee EL, Williamson JW. Improved outcomes i hypertension after physician tutorials: a controlled trial. An Intern Med 1976;84:646.
17. Philip AGS, Little GA, Lucey JF. The transport conference as teaching strategy. Perinatology—Neonatology 1984;8:63.
18. Ginzburg HM. Legal Issues in medical transport. In: Ma Donald MG, Miller MK, eds. Emergency transport of the per natal patient. Boston: Little, Brown & Co., 1989:155.
19. Carey B, Larson B, Goold G. A neonatal teaching tool: workin with umbilical catheters. Matern Child Nurs J 1980;5:393.
20. Alden E, Jennings P, Hoffman J, Alden E. Tension pneum thorax: a teaching model. Pediatrics 1976;58:861.
21. Calderwood HW, Ravin MB. The cat as a teaching model f endotracheal intubation. Anesth Analg 1972;51:258.
22. Jennings PB, Alden ER, Brenz RW. A teaching model for ped atric intubation utilizing ketamine sedated kittens. Pediatri 1974;53:283.
23. Powell D, Gonzales C, Gunnels R. Use of the ferret as a mod for pediatric endotracheal intubation training. Lab Anim S 1991;41:86.
24. Clark TA, Levy L, Mannino F. Use of the placenta as a teachin model. Pediatrics 1978;62:234.
25. Clarke TA, Levy L, Mannino F. Teaching models in neonat logy. Perinatology—Neonatology 1980;4:51.
26. Gagnon DE. Perinatal systems: are they in jeopardy? Perinat Press 1983;7(9):131.
27. Imershein AW, Turner C, Wlls JG, et al. Covering the cost care in neonatal intensive care units. Pediatrics 1992;89:56.
28. Caplan RM. Measuring the effectiveness of continuing medic education. J Med Educ 1973;48:1150.
29. Kattwinkel J, Nowacek GA, Cook LJ, et al. Perinatal outreac education: a continuation strategy for a basic program. Am Perinatol 1984;1:335.
30. Harlan WR, Hess GE, Borer RC, et al. Impact of an educatio program on perinatal care practices. Pediatrics 1980;66:893.
31. Maisels MJ, Morrow D, Fernsler S, et al. Care of low-birt weight and sick newborn infants in community hospitals: e fect of an education program. Am J Perinatol 1984;1:247.

Neonatology: Pathophysiology and Management of the Newborn, Fourth Edition,
edited by Gordon B. Avery, Mary Ann Fletcher, and Mhairi G. MacDonald.
J.B. Lippincott Company, Philadelphia © 1994.

chapter 5

Neonatal Transport

CARL L. BOSE

n 1900, the development of the first mobile incubator or the care of "weakly and prematurely born infants" was described by Dr. Joseph DeLee, of the Chicago Lying-In Hospital.[1] This incubator was used o transport "these delicate infants from distant parts f the city and suburbs."[1] The development of this evice represented a recognition of the need to create controlled environment for the transport of infants hat simulated the inpatient environment. The first eport of an organized transport program in the nited States appeared in 1950.[2] This program was eveloped by the New York Department of Health in onjunction with area hospitals. This remarkable sysem, created long before the evolution of neonatal ntensive care, incorporated many of the features of odern neonatal transport programs. These included round-the-clock staffing by specially trained nurses, edicated vehicles, a clerk to receive referral calls, nd equipment developed specifically for neonatal ansport. During a 2-year period, this program transorted 1209 patients, of whom 194 weighed less than 000 g.[3]

Regionalization of perinatal care had two effects on ansport. First, the number of infants requiring ansport was minimized by shifting the hospital of irth to a center capable of delivering neonatal intenve care. Second, the responsibility for transporting nfants shifted to tertiary centers. For example, in 976 in North Carolina, fewer than 40% of very-lowirth-weight (VLBW) infants were delivered in level I hospitals; approximately 30% were delivered in vel I hospitals (Fig. 5-1). By 1982, after the evolution f an organized program of regionalized perinatal care, more than 70% of VLBW infants were delivered in level III hospitals. The remainder, however, continue to be delivered in community hospitals illequipped to manage high-risk infants. In the past 5 years, the percentage of VLBW infants delivered in level III centers has changed little.

The advantages of intrauterine transport of high-risk infants by transfer of the mother compared to neonatal transport after delivery have been documented.[4–6] Whether the continued delivery of VLBW infants in hospitals incapable of providing intensive care results from a conscious choice on the part of obstetric caretakers or is unavoidable and results from unpredictable, emergent events in the intrapartum period is unknown. It is clear, however, that even in regionalized perinatal programs in which prenatal risk assessment is routine, neonatal transport of some VLBW infants still will be necessary. Illness in the neonate may not be predictable based on prenatal risk factors or may result from a problem arising too late in the intrapartum period to effect transfer of the mother. For these reasons, it can be concluded that regionalized perinatal care does not eliminate the need for neonatal transport. Neonatal transport is a necessity and should be an integral part of all regionalized perinatal care programs.

Neonatal transport to a tertiary care center can be performed by either the community hospital referring the patient (one-way transport) or by the tertiary center receiving the patient (two-way transport). In most perinatal regions, two-way transport is preferable for economic and other reasons.[7] Two-way transport may also result in improved survival.[8,9] For these rea-

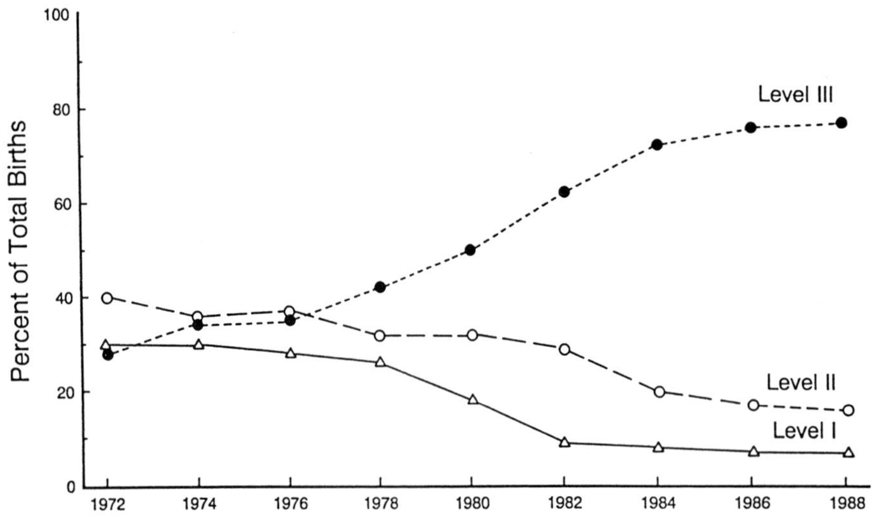

FIG. 5–1. Percentage of live birth of infants with birth weights les than 1500 g born in level I, II, and II hospitals in North Carolina fron 1972 to 1988. (Richard Nugent M.D., personal communication 1989.)

sons, the responsibility of tertiary centers to provide two-way neonatal transport has been generally accepted and is recommended by the American Academy of Pediatrics.[10]

ORGANIZATION AND ADMINISTRATION

ADMINISTRATIVE PERSONNEL

Transport programs have components that generally can be categorized into those related to medical care and those related to transportation, communications, and finances, the nonmedical components. The medical components of a transport program must fall under the direction of a physician who is credentialed to supervise the patients served by the program. Direction of the nonmedical components of the program often is the responsibility of a member of the hospital administration (Fig. 5-2). This division of responsibility may create problems when the interests of variou components compete; in practice, however, the divi sion is rarely this precise. Rather, a collaborative ef fort exists that takes advantage of the availability an expertise of professionals in all disciplines. A brie discussion of each of the potential contributors to th administration of a transport program follows.

HOSPITAL ADMINISTRATOR

A hospital administrator generally is responsible fo those aspects of the program that are not directl related to patient care. Many decisions on the opera tion of a program require an analysis of costs an benefits. Whereas medical personnel generally are re lied on to provide an estimate of benefit, the hospita administrator must assess financial impact. There fore, the hospital administrator should be prepared t receive advice from medical personnel and develo the nonmedical components of the program in con sideration of the financial resources of the institution

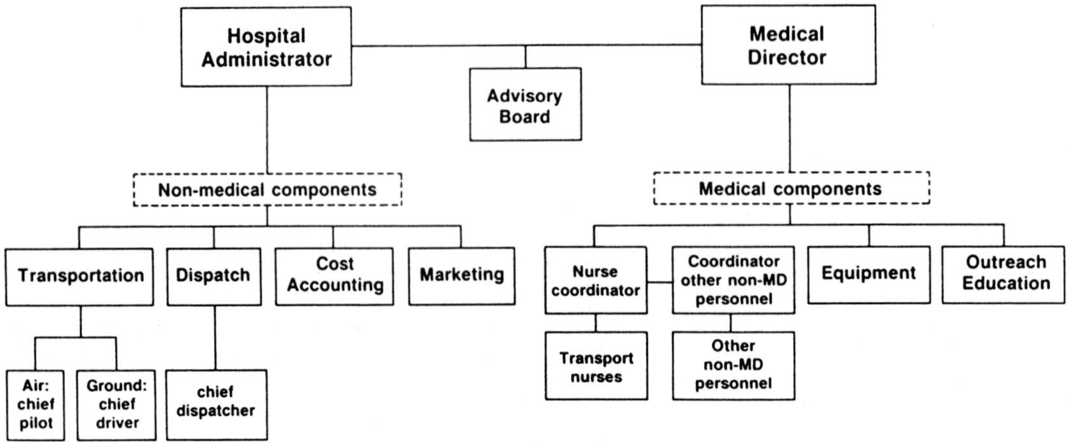

FIG. 5–2. The administrative structure of a typical neonatal transport program.

MEDICAL DIRECTOR

The medical director of a neonatal transport program usually is a neonatologist who has expertise or a special interest in transport. The medical director is ultimately responsible for the quality of care provided by the transport team; this is particularly true if physicians do not participate directly in transport. The medical director is responsible for developing training programs and treatment protocols. The medical director, in conjunction with the coordinator of nonphysician personnel, must ensure that all personnel have completed training requirements successfully and have satisfied the regulations of the agencies that govern the various professional groups. The director also must develop and maintain a system for reviewing the quality of care provided during transport.

COORDINATOR OF NONPHYSICIAN PERSONNEL

Each group of professionals (*e.g.*, nurses and respiratory therapists) on the transport team should have a person who is designated as the coordinator of that group. The coordinator should supervise the selection and training of personnel and develop a system of peer review. This person should be responsible for scheduling and identifying needs of team members. It also is advisable to designate a single person to coordinate team activities who will interface closely with the medical director. Most often, this person will be the nurse coordinator of the team.

CONSULTING NEONATALOGISTS AND OTHER SUBSPECIALISTS

During the transport of a patient, it is important, and often mandated by law, that a physician provide consultation to the transport team. The logical person to provide such consultation is the one who will receive the patient on return to the tertiary center. This person often already has discussed the patient's care with the referring physician and made suggestions about interim care. Given this broad consultative role to both the referring physician and to the transport team, the consultant should be a person with extensive training, at a level in excess of that available in the community hospital. For this reason, the consultant usually should be a neonatologist or comparably trained subspecialist, or a postdoctoral fellow. In addition, the consultant must be aware of the handicaps and hazards imposed by the transport environment and must be familiar with the operational aspects of the program.

THE ADVISORY BOARD

A transport program should be considered an extension of the inpatient unit to which it delivers patients. Therefore, the operation of the program should be reviewed periodically by representatives of all of the services that interface with the inpatient unit. These representatives might include the following:

- Medical Director of the Neonatal Intensive Care Unit (NICU)
- Director of the Neonatal Division
- Respiratory Therapy Administrator
- Nursing Administrator
- Outreach Education Coordinator
- Director of Public Relations
- representatives of other hospitals to which patients are transported.

Advice should be solicited from this group about all major changes in the program because of the impact these changes may have on their respective services.

THE TRANSPORT TEAM

A variety of personnel participate in the inpatient care of infants; all should be considered candidates for caretakers during neonatal transport. These personnel include the following:

- neonatologists
- neonatal fellows
- pediatric housestaff
- nurse practitioners
- transport nurses
- NICU staff nurses
- respiratory therapists.

The selection of the type of personnel used by each program usually is based on the unique aspects of that program; however, some general principles apply that determine the relative desirability of various professionals. As the number of transports increases, it becomes less practical to send physicians on transport. Neonatologists rarely have sufficient time to devote to frequent transports, and reimbursement usually is not adequate to support a neonatologist's professional effort. Although participation in transport can be very educational, in high-volume programs, time spent on transport by housestaff and fellows often competes with other aspects of training. In addition, the interest in participation and expertise may vary considerably among trainees. This is a particular problem when participation is mandated. For these reasons, most high-volume programs have chosen to use nonphysician personnel as attendants during transport.

The use of neonatal nurse practitioners offers an attractive alternative to physician attendance.[11] Nurse practitioners generally are highly skilled and provide a consistency of expertise not usually encountered in other professional groups. They are licensed in most states to perform all the diagnostic and therapeutic procedures required during transport. The greatest disadvantage to the use of neonatal nurse practitioners in some regions is their scarcity and their relatively high salaries. Also, they are rarely trained, or willing, to transport patients other than neonates.

As an alternative to nurse practitioners, many centers have chosen to train NICU staff nurses to participate in transport. This often is a very practical alternative because salaries of staff nurses are less than those of practitioners, and they generally are more available. In addition, in most states, they are permitted to perform invasive procedures as an extension of their inpatient nursing role under guidelines and protocols approved by the boards of nursing. Therefore, they can be trained to provide all the care required by a critically ill neonate during transport. This training often is extensive, however, because most staff nurses lack the cognitive knowledge necessary to diagnose problems, in addition to lacking experience in performing invasive procedures. This extensive training period must be considered when estimating the cost of using staff nurses compared to nurse practitioners. The requirement of training is particularly burdensome when the turnover rate of personnel is high.

Most patients transported to NICUs either have respiratory failure requiring mechanical ventilation or are receiving supplemental oxygen. For this reason, respiratory therapists should be considered when selecting transport personnel. Their expertise in the use and maintenance of respiratory care equipment is extremely valuable. Physicians and nurses rarely have acquired this expertise. The therapists' ability to adapt this equipment to the unique environment of transport can be lifesaving, particularly in circumstances when unexpected events occur. The only disadvantage of using therapists is the narrow focus of their usual training. They rarely are prepared to assist with aspects of care beyond respiratory therapies. This disadvantage can be minimized by cross-training them to perform tasks generally assigned to physicians and nurses.

Eliminating physicians from attendance during transport can create problems that must be anticipated. Advisory personnel at the tertiary center, particularly physicians, often are unwilling to endorse a patient care program that does not mandate initial evaluation by a physician. This resistance usually stems from a concern for the well-being of the patient, and can be overcome by the selection and training of competent nonphysician personnel. The support and endorsement of an involved medical director also may be critical. A similar attitude may prevail in community hospitals. Referring physicians may find it unacceptable to relinquish care of a critically ill patient to nonphysician personnel. In an environment in which tertiary centers compete for patients, this may be a motivation for maintaining physician attendance during transport. Most referring physicians, however, are concerned only about transferring their patients in a safe and timely fashion. Anecdotal experience[12] and one controlled study[13] suggest that properly selected and trained nurses provide a satisfactory level of care during transport. Once a nonphysician team demonstrates its competence and efficiency, the concerns of most referring physicians will vanish. Because the use of specially trained nonphysician personnel represents both a safe and economic alternative to physician participation in neonatal transport, most programs now rely on nonphysician personnel for patient care.

Transport personnel must be proficient in cognitive knowledge of neonatal diseases, principles of management of acute problems, and technical skills. The method and extent of training necessary to reach proficiency will depend on the type of personnel; however, the pattern of preparation will be similar for all professionals. Cognitive knowledge is best provided in didactic sessions in conjunction with self-study exercises. Management principles also may be taught in a didactic setting, but refinement of these skills usually requires repeated experiences in the inpatient setting. Laboratory simulation of technical skills, such as intubation, umbilical catheterization, and thoracostomy tube placement, provide a good introduction to these procedures. These skills can then be refined in the inpatient setting under supervision. Demonstration of proficiency in these areas should be ensured by examination or observation by a qualified supervisor. After this initial preparation, a period of training should be provided during which the trainee accompanies a more experienced team member on transport. Final certification of competence should be awarded by both the medical director and the coordinator for the trainee's professional group.

COMMUNICATION

The success or failure of many transport programs depends on the quality of the communication system that supports the program.[14] The communication system serves two basic functions: to provide a point of access for the physician referring a patient and to coordinate the activities of the transport team. A single call by the referring physician should provide access to all of the services of the tertiary center related to neonatal care. The use of a toll-free hot line often associated with a memorable acronym is favored by some centers.[15] An alternative is to request that referring physicians call the NICU directly. If consultation is requested, the referring physician should be connected in a timely fashion with a consultant of appropriate training. If transfer is requested and deemed appropriate, an available bed in the NICU of the tertiary center, or an alternate center if necessary, should be identified. Without further calls by the referring physician, the transport team should be dispatched.

In many parts of the country, locating an available and appropriate site of care is difficult because of a severe shortage of NICU beds or the lack of availability of subspecialty support in some centers. These regions often benefit from an organized system of identifying available resources. Several such programs exist, and are of two varieties. In some areas, sophisticated computerized communications networks linking neighboring centers have been developed.[16] An alternative is the use an operator-assisted central referral or bed locator system. These systems speed the referral of patients and relieve both referring physicians and the physician at the tertiary center of the burden of placing numerous calls to locate a bed.

Once a bed has been located and the decision has been made to transport the patient, the role of the communications system shifts to that of dispatching the team and disseminating information about the transport. In this role, the system is best served by a communication center that is staffed and equipped for emergency medical service functions. The referring hospital should be informed of the estimated time of arrival and of any necessary preparations for the arrival of the vehicle. The receiving unit should be notified and be provided with any information necessary for admission of the patient.

During the conduct of the transport, periodic communication between the dispatch center and the vehicle operator is advisable. In so doing, unexpected delays or mishaps are promptly identified and appropriate action taken. When the transport team does not include a physician, the team should have the capability of communicating directly with the consulting physician at all times. This level of communication is mandated by the nurse practice acts in some states. This is a trivial problem while the team is in the referring hospital, but it can present a challenge during transit. This problem usually can be solved by the acquisition of sophisticated, and expensive, telecommunications equipment. Unfortunately, this substantial investment is essential for the operation of a safe, efficient program.

Many communication centers are equipped with automated devices that record all communications. Although not essential, the recordings made by these devices may be valuable educational tools, and often are critical if a medicolegal question arises.

FINANCIAL CONSIDERATIONS

Subjecting a transport program to periodic cost–benefit analyses is a critical aspect of the program's operation. The following elements should be included in the cost of operation:

- Medical components
  - Nonphysician personnel salaries
  - Salary support of the medical director
  - Equipment and supplies
  - Medication
  - Expenses related to education of personnel
- Nonmedical components
  - Administrative overhead
  - Vehicle operation and maintenance
  - Communications
  - Educational and marketing material.

Identifying the costs associated with the program may be difficult if its operation is financially integrated into the operation of the NICU. For example, personnel costs often are difficult to quantify because, except in very high-volume programs, transport personnel usually contribute to inpatient services during transport duty time. Therefore, the cost assigned to the transport program should be discounted based on this contribution. The proportion of time devoted by the medical director is even more difficult to quantify, and often is ignored in the financial analysis. The cost of equipment is most easily separated from the cost of inpatient services because transport equipment rarely is used for purposes other than transport. Included in estimates of equipment costs should be allowances for depreciation and maintenance.

The nonmedical components of a program often are more costly than the medical components because of expenses related to transportation. This is particularly true when air transportation is used. The expense of transportation can be minimized by sharing resources with other hospitals or agencies. Ground ambulances may be shared with local emergency medical service agencies or be used for convalescent transport. Aircraft sometimes can be used by a consortium of hospitals. The major disadvantage of this approach is the possibility of a vehicle being unavailable at the time of a request for transport. The potential for this occasional conflict may be far outweighed by the cost reductions, however.

The net costs of a program are determined by subtracting costs from revenues, which come from three general sources: reimbursement, support from governmental agencies, and support from other extramural organizations.[17] In the past decade, support from government and charitable organizations has diminished. Hospitals are increasingly dependent on reimbursement to support transport programs. Unfortunately, the costs of a transport program nearly always exceed the revenues. Subsistence of the program therefore depends on subsidy by the sponsor hospital.

The decision to fund a transport program usually is based on a favorable cost–benefit analysis, and benefit is extremely difficult to define. Medical personnel typically define benefit in terms of medical outcomes, morbidity and mortality. Although there has been a number of studies that support the use of hospital-based transport programs for adult patients based on improved morbidity and mortality,[18,19] these studies are not necessarily applicable to neonates. In an attempt to quantify the benefits of a neonatal transport program, the most prudent approach may be to scrutinize carefully the type of patients being transported to ensure that they are likely to benefit from transport. The number of these patients, combined with other benefits to the institution, such as improved public relations and recruitment of patients, provides an estimate of the benefit to the sponsor institution.

This estimate must then be weighed against the net costs.

TECHNICAL ASPECTS

THE TRANSPORT ENVIRONMENT

The principles of care provided during transport are not different from the principles of inpatient care. Any differences in practices arise from the unique features of the transport environment.[20] The following features may distinguish the environment in transport vehicles from the inpatient environment:

- excessive noise
- vibration
- improper lighting
- variable ambient temperature and humidity
- changes in barometric pressure
- confined space
- limited support services.

A detailed discussion of the impact of each of these features is beyond the scope of this chapter. A brief discussion of the most important problems follows.

High sound levels are already inherent to the NICU; although dependent on the type of vehicle, levels recorded during transport are significantly higher (Fig. 5-3).[21,22] Brief exposure to these levels probably has little long-term effect on the caretakers; however, repeated exposure over time may result in hearing loss. High-frequency range hearing loss is a well-recognized occupational hazard of pilots. Personnel should protect themselves from exposure by using sound-attenuating devices. The effects of exposure to high sound levels on the neonate are not known. The possibility of physiologic changes, however, is suggested by studies of hospitalized infants.[23] Probably the most significant problem resulting from high sound levels is the inability to use auscultation to assess the patient. This handicap must be recognized before transport. Alternative methods for assessing heart rate and respiratory sufficiency must be available during transport.

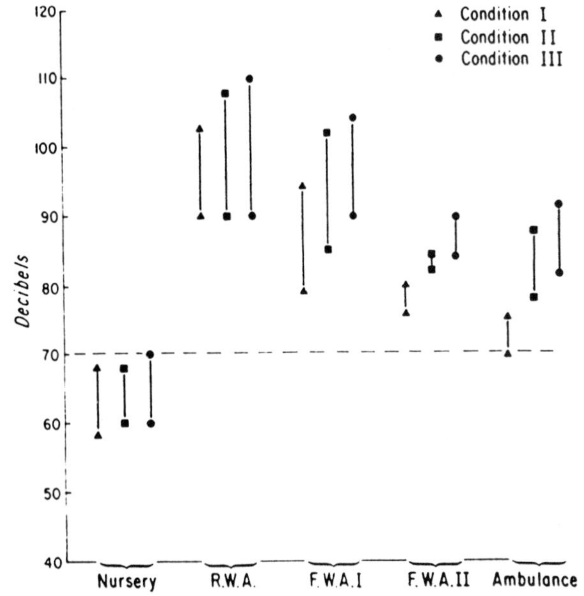

FIG. 5–3. Sound levels in various transport vehicles and in the neonatal intensive care unit. Measurements were made under three conditions: Condition I, inside the isolette with the portholes closed; condition II, inside the isolette with the portholes open; condition III, outside the isolette. (FWAI and FWAII, two types of fixed-winged aircraft; RWA, rotary-winged aircraft; from Shenai J. Sound levels for neonates in transit. J Pediatr 1977;90:812.)

Exposure to vibration is a problem unique to the transport environment.[24] The physiologic consequences of this exposure are not known. Animal studies[25,26] and investigation using healthy adults[26] suggest that effects on the autonomic and central nervous system may occur. Whether these effects are a hazard to a critically ill patient is unknown. The effects on personnel may be less profound but are potentially more important. For example, a typical helicopter transport results in vibration exposure associated with reduced efficiency.[27] The overt symptoms of motion sickness resulting from low-frequency vibration may be incapacitating. A more subtle manifestation of motion sickness, termed the sopite syndrome, may also affect personnel.[28] The symptoms associated with this syndrome include drowsiness, inability to concentrate, and disinclination to communicate with others.

The effect of vibration on equipment also constitutes a major problem. Monitor artifact is a common phenomenon. Personnel should be familiar with monitor artifact and with the use of alternative monitoring techniques. The selection of equipment should be made in consideration of resistance to the effects of vibration. Premature failure of equipment should be anticipated, and preventive maintenance should be on an accelerated schedule. The problem of early obsolescence should be anticipated when transport budgets are developed.

An appreciation of the problems created by the transport environment and plans to minimize these problems are essential for safe transport. Some general principles include the following:

Prepare the transport vehicle. The vehicle should be retrofitted to simulate the inpatient environment as much as is possible and practical. This generally requires that supplemental lighting, sound insulation, and a regulated heating–cooling system be added.

Assess and stabilize the patient extensively before transport. Most neonates have problems that can be managed adequately by the transport team. Rarely is there urgency in returning to the tertiary center. Therefore, time spent in the community hospital preparing the patient for transport is not time wasted. This stabilization will prepare the patient for the most risky period of transport, the time in transit between hospitals.

Monitor electronically all possible physiologic parameters. Because of the dynamic nature of the diseases in most transported patients and the inability to assess patients by physical examination, electronic monitoring is critical to the identification of significant changes in physiology.

Anticipate deterioration. All possible forms of deterioration should be anticipated before transport; strategies to support the patient in the event of deterioration should be planned. Application of this principle often results in the performance of procedures or therapies that may not be necessary in the inpatient setting. For example, intubation and ventilation may not be necessary for mild degrees of respiratory failure or apnea in the hospitalized patient but may be advisable before transport because of the difficulty of intubation during transport.

EQUIPMENT

Before the 1970s, transport equipment generally was fabricated from equipment acquired from the NICU. Although this equipment often was designed with great ingenuity, failures or inadequacies often occurred. In the past two decades, considerable effort has been devoted to the development of devices specifically for neonatal transport, resulting in greater safety.

The following is a list of the major pieces of equipment used during transport:

Essential equipment
- Portable isolette
- Mechanical ventilator

TABLE 5–1
NEONATAL NURSING PACK

Equipment	Amount	Equipment	Amount
Procedure tray, sterile	1	Buretrol	1
Omphalocele bag, sterile	1	Disposable transducer	1
Dextrostix bottle	2	Scissors	1
Sterile lancets	5	Hemostat	1
Blood culture bottle	1	Tape measure	1
Angiocaths		K-Y jelly	2
18 g	2	Disposable BP cuffs	
22 g	2	sizes 2, 3, 4, and 5	1 each
Intraosseous needles	2	Pacifier	1
Blood collection tubes	6	Bulb syringe	1
IV limb board	2	Sterile gauze	2
Rubber bands	6	Stopcocks	2
Safety pins	6	Extension tubing	1
Tape		Trocars	
Silk	1 roll	10 Fr	2
Dermaclear	1 roll	12 Fr	2
Stethoscope	1	Digital thermometer	1
IV fluids		Umbilical catheters	
$D_{10}W$	1 500 mL bag	3.5 Fr	2
D_5W	1 500 mL bag	5.0 Fr	2
NS	1 500 mL bag	Heimlich valves	2
Masks	2	Blood component filter set	2
Syringes		Alcohol and Betadine swabs	10 each
20 mL Luer Lok	2	IV extension T-connectors	2
60 mL Luer Lok	4	Butterfly needles	
Transilluminator	1	19 g	2
Gloves, sterile		23 g	2
size 6½	2 pairs	25 g	6
size 7½	2 pairs	Syringes	
Suction catheters, sterile		10 ml	4
size 6 Fr	2	3 ml	6
size 8 Fr	2	1 ml	9
Stockinette for caps	2	Needles, 19 g	10
Cotton balls	4	Angiocath, 24 g	9
Feeding tubes		Purple adapters, blunt needles	2
8 Fr	2	Replogle, 10 Fr	2
5 Fr	2		

- Cardiorespiratory monitor
- Blood pressure transducer
- Transcutaneous O_2 monitor or pulse oximeter
- Intravascular pumps
- Air–oxygen blender

Desirable equipment

- Body temperature monitor
- Transcutaneous CO_2 or end-tidal CO_2 monitor
- Noninvasive blood pressure monitor
- Suction apparatus
- Airway humidification system.

Although these devices can be purchased individually and either carried separately or attached to the isolette, it usually is advisable, and often more economic, to purchase a modular isolette that includes many of the devices listed above. Modular transport isolettes have been designed to minimize space and weight. They also use a common battery power supply for most devices. Several of these isolettes ar commercially available. The logical choice for eac program often depends on the size, weight, and heat ing capability of the unit.

Accessory equipment and supplies can be divide into respiratory care supplies and medical–nursin supplies. These supplies can be divided in this man ner and carried in packs or equipment bags (Tables 5 1 through 5-4). They should be organized in a recog nized and reproducible fashion. This technique wi aid in rapidly locating a needed item, and assist i restocking after use. It also is helpful to separate med ications into an accessory pack.

TRANSPORT VEHICLES

An essential component of neonatal transport i rapid, safe transportation. The types of vehicles i use include standard ambulances, specially prepare

TABLE 5–2
NEONATAL RESPIRATORY THERAPY PACK

Equipment	Amount	Equipment	Amount
Exterior Pockets		**Interior of Bag (*Continued*)**	
Oxygen tubing	3	Silicone adapter	2
Pediatric simple mask	1	O_2 flowmeter nipple	2
Infant nasal canula	1	One-way valve	1
Aerosol tubing	1	Gould transducer dome	1
Complete ventilator set-up with exhalation valve (plus one in isolette)	1	Set of EKG lead wires	2
		25 g ½-in butterfly	2
Spare Cavitron exhalation valve	1	Septisol	1 can
Isolette bag	1	Pressure manometer	1
Face bucket	1	Albuterol	1
Treatment setup	1	Tape measure	1
Space blanket	1	Infant MVB bag with O_2 tubing (plus one in isolette)	1
Head block	1		
Pulse oximeter sensors (N-25 and I-20)	2 each	Infant oral airway	2
		Small child oral airway	2
Interior of Bag		Suction catheters, 5 Fr, 6 Fr, and 8 Fr	1 each
Airway Supplies		C-size batteries for laryngoscope	2
Laerdal masks		Normal saline vials	4
#0	2	Silk tape	1 roll
#1	2	Dermaclear tape	1 roll
#2	1	Oxygen connectors	2
Infant McGill forceps	1	Hemostat	1
Laryngoscope handle with #0 and #1 Miller blades	1 each	Infant BP cuff (small, medium, and large)	1 each
		Oxygen analyzer membrane kit	2
Set of endotracheal tubes with stylets		Briggs T-adapters	2
Other Equipment		15-mm adapter	2
Benzoin applicators	6	Right-angle adapter	2
Alcohol preps	4	O_2 connectors (NCG, OES, P-B)	1 each
Adjustable wrench	1	Air connectors (NCG, P-B)	1 each
E-tank wrench	1	EKG lead pads	3
Cable ties	10	3-way stopcock	2
Scissors	1	E-Z Heat hot packs	4
9-volt battery	2	Stethoscope	1
Assorted laryngoscope bulbs	4	Alupent	1
Adjustable venturi	2	1-mL syringe	2

BP, blood pressure; EKG, electrocardiogram; MVB, manual ventilation bag.

ABLE 5–3
EONATAL MEDICINE PACK

Drug	Amount
Isotonic saline vials, 20 mL	4
Heparin	1
Sodium chloride (2%)	1
Dilantin	2
Narcan	2
Regitine	1
Epinephrine 1 : 1000, 1 mL	1
Epinephrine 1 : 1000, 30 mL	1
Ampicillin	
250 mg	1
500 mg	1
Gentamicin	1
Calcium gluconate	1
Dobutamine	1
Norcuron	1
$D_{50}W$	1
Calcium chloride Bristojet	1
Atropine Bristojet	1
Tubex	1
Exosurf	2
Sterile water vials, 20 mL	4
Heparin lock flush	2
KCl	1
Decadron	1
Lasix	1
Lacrilube	1
Lidocaine 1%	1
Digoxin	1
Clindamycin	1
Aminophylline	1
Dopamine	1
Pavulon	1
Epinephrine 1 : 1000 Bristojet	1
Sodium bicarbonate	1
Cardiac lidocaine Bristojet	1
Albumin 25%	2
Vitamin K	1
Neonatal Narcotic Pack	
Morphine	2
Chloral hydrate supp.	1
Versed	1
Phenobarbital	3
Valium	1
Fentanyl	1
For Personal Use	
Aspirin	12
Tylenol	12
Antivert	
12.5 mg	6
25 mg	6
Scopolamine discs	6

round ambulances, helicopters, and fixed-wing air-aft. The selection of one or more of these vehicles to ıpport a neonatal transport program usually is ased on resources, geography, and practical issues ıch as the use of the vehicle by other hospital-based ervices.

Ambulances are the least costly and most available; owever, they generally require modest retrofitting to make them acceptable for neonatal transport. Extensive retrofitting, including the addition of radiant heat and a blood gas analyzer, improves patient care capabilities but dramatically increases costs and decreases the vehicle's usefulness for other services. The major disadvantage of ground ambulance transport is the long travel time compared to air transport. This disadvantage can be prohibitive if frequent long transports are anticipated.

Helicopters minimize transit time, and for distances between hospitals of up to 150 miles, usually provide the fastest service. The major disadvantages of helicopter transportation are the constraints of the patient care environment (*e.g.*, limited space, high noise and vibration) and the high cost of operation. Although the impact of the former can be minimized, the cost of helicopter transportation usually cannot be justified unless the vehicle can be shared by other emergency medical services.

Fixed-wing aircraft are less costly, roomier, less noisy, and faster than helicopters. Because they must travel between airports, however, at least two additional transfers are required. These shuttles between the hospital and airport often are troublesome and may increase the likelihood of mishap. For these reasons, transportation by fixed-wing aircraft usually is advantageous only for distances between hospitals in excess of 150 miles.

RECORD KEEPING

Transport programs traditionally have developed record-keeping systems that are unique and distinct from the inpatient record. The accurate, thorough record of each transport is essential for several reasons. As a part of the medical record, it provides permanent documentation of the care rendered. As such, it should adhere to the standards of record keeping of the sponsor institution. The record also is a valuable tool for quality assurance and education. The critical components of a typical transport record include the following:

- consultation–referral form
- transport record
- parental consent form
- billing slip.

QUALITY ASSURANCE

Review of the performance of a transport program should be a continual process and involve two strategies. First, all activities of the program should be reviewed periodically to ensure that standard operating procedures are being observed. This involves the review of details including medical record keeping, communication protocols, vehicle operation safety, equipment maintenance, and adherence to medical care protocols. These reviews are best conducted by people directly related to each activity. Second, the

TABLE 5–4
BACK TRANSPORT PACK

Equipment or Drug	Amount
Equipment	
Dextrostix bottle	1
Lancets, sterile	5
Stethoscope	1
Syringes	
1 mL	3
3 mL	3
10 mL	3
20 mL	1
60 mL	1
Needles, 19 g	10
Nonsterile gloves	4 pairs
Bulb syringe	1
Feeding tubes	
5 Fr	1
8 Fr	1
Butterfly needles	
23 g	2
25 g	2
ET tubes, 2.5 through 5.0	2 of each
Stylettes	4
Laryngoscope and blades	1
Face masks, assorted sizes	3
Face tent	1
Manual ventilation bag	1
Nebulizer set-up	1
Venturi tubing	1
Oxygen tubing	2
Nasal canula	4
IV fluid, D_5W	1 100-mL bag
Alcohol and Betadine swabs	10 each
Thermometers	2
Suction catheters	
6 Fr	2
8 Fr	2
10 Fr	1
Yankauer	1
Equipment (*Continued*)	
Oximeter probes	1
Monitor electrodes	6
K-Y jelly	1
Hot packs	
Small	2
Large	1
Silver thermal hats	
Small	1
Large	1
IV tubing	1
IV arm board	1
Rubber bands	6
Intraosseous needle	1
BP cuffs of various sizes	1 each
Scissors	1
Hemostat	1
T connector	2
Angiocath, 24 g	4
Safety pins	6
Tape	2 rolls
Benzoin	1
Medications	
Isotonic saline	2
Heparin flush	2
Sodium bicarbonate	1
Epinephrine 1 : 10,000 Bristojet	
Atropine Bristojet	1
Sterile water	2
Dextrose 50%	1
Calcium gluconate	1

BP, blood pressure.

medical care provided by the team should be scrutinized to determine if quality care is being rendered. It is not adequate merely to demonstrate that medical care protocols are being properly executed. An equally important issue is whether the appropriate protocol was selected. For nonphysician teams, this level of review should be conducted by the medical director or a physician designate. All aspects of care, including data collection, formulation of problems, monitoring, performance of procedures, and patient outcome should be reviewed.

Quality assurance activities should be closely linked to education and research. Review of individual transport records can be an extremely valuable method of identifying transport personnel in need of further education and training. The compilation o reviews and the monitoring of patient outcomes pro vide an assessment of the efficacy of existing proto cols and procedures, and may identify a need to alte program activities. In addition, new therapies an equipment can be evaluated using existing qualit assurance techniques.

Although transport programs traditionally hav not been closely scrutinized by regulatory agencies as the number of programs increases and standard become better defined, review by these agencies i inevitable. Guidelines for developing quality assur ance programs, not specific to transport, have bee published.[29,30] A more helpful guide has been pro duced by the Association of Air Medical Services.[31]

PSYCHOSOCIAL CONSIDERATIONS

PSYCHOLOGICAL IMPACT ON THE FAMILY

There is virtually no way to eliminate the parental anxiety associated with neonatal transport; there are a few techniques, however, that may help families in coping with this anxiety. The transport team should provide the family with as much information as possible on the nature of their child's illness, the therapies and equipment that will be used, the NICU to which the infant will be transported, and the professionals who will provide care. A member of the referring hospital staff should be in attendance during this discussion to prepare them for dealing with questions that arise after the departure of the transport team. This information should be provided both verbally and in written form. Audiovisual aids also may assist in the dissemination of this information. The transport team of the University of North Carolina Hospitals distributes a videotape to community hospitals in their area, which is made available to families of transported infants. It describes and pictures the NICU, providing a more comprehensive view of the NICU milieu compared to the information provided at the time of transport. This technique is particularly effective with illiterate parents, or those with little understanding of the hospital environment.

It is almost always advisable to arrange contact between parents and infant before departure from the referring hospital. Visitation should be encouraged even during the transport of a critically ill infant or when parents are reluctant to view their child. A photograph of the infant should be left with the family. Immediately on arrival in the receiving hospital, the transport team should call the family to reassure them that their child has arrived safely. The transport team should alert the NICU staff to any unusual problems with the parents' preparedness to cope with their child's illness.

RELATIONSHIPS WITH REFERRING HOSPITAL PERSONNEL

Transporting a neonate from a community hospital to a tertiary center has the potential to improve dramatically the relationship between institutions or to cause irreparable damage to the relationship. Each transport represents an opportunity for success or failure. To ensure success, referring personnel must have easy access to the service. The team should respond in a reasonable period of time. Rapidity of response is often critical from a public relations standpoint, even when the infant's medical condition does not mandate speed. All reasonable efforts should be made to minimize the time between the request and arrival in the referring hospital.

Even the most responsive service will fail to satisfy personnel in the referring hospital if the team does not conduct itself appropriately. The team must understand the psychological milieu surrounding a transport. The event is often emotionally charged because of the acute nature of the infant's illness. Emotions may be fragile because of feelings of inadequacy on the part of referring hospital personnel. These feelings seem to arise even when excellent, comprehensive care is provided. Referring hospital personnel may be very sensitive to criticism; any critique of care, unless requested, should be deferred until a later time. The team should appreciate the contribution made by the referring staff. They should seek information about the history and condition of the infant before their arrival. They should ask for assistance when practical. The team should explain the need for performing all procedures. This is particularly important when referring personnel have made the decision not to perform a procedure because of their lack of understanding of the transport environment. Nonphysician teams must avoid conflicts with referring physicians over the need for therapies or procedures. Any disagreements should be resolved through discussion between the referring physician and the consultant in the tertiary center.

Communication should not end with the departure of the transport team from the referring hospital. It is incumbent on the tertiary center staff to provide comprehensive follow-up to the referring hospital caretakers. Failure to provide follow-up is one of the most common criticisms of tertiary centers. There are several critical points in time at which information should be provided. A call should be made by the receiving physician within 24 hours of the transport. Plans for further follow-up can be established at that time. Referring hospital personnel should be notified immediately on the death of a patient. Failure to fulfill this obligation may result in embarrassment and anger toward the tertiary center. It also is imperative that the referring physician be contacted in advance of discharge of the patient.

LEGAL CONSIDERATIONS

The medicolegal climate in which perinatal medicine is practiced has changed dramatically in the past several decades. Litigation of malpractice suits involving perinatal caretakers is common. Transport personnel, by contrast, usually have avoided legal entanglements. It is unlikely, however, that this trend will continue. Neonatal transport is more closely associated with inpatient intensive care and less likely to be considered an emergency service providing extraordinary care under adverse conditions. A standard of care is expected by other medical professionals; a good outcome usually is expected by families.

Although there are few regulations and almost no case law defining legal obligations of transport services, understanding the principles that are likely to govern legal decision making will help guide programs in establishing sound practices, those that are most likely to limit risk of litigation.[32] The principles of respondent superior define the hospital as the party responsible for governing the protocols and procedures followed by its personnel.[33] These principles, no doubt, apply to mobile services as well as inpatient care. Therefore, the hospital that sponsors a transport program is responsible for selecting and training the personnel, and defining their scope or practice. Logically, the medical director, as the medical professional delegated to ensure the quality of care, also is liable for the governance of the team. Team members assume personal liability only if they perform outside their enfranchised scope of practice.

The method used for selecting, training, and certifying personnel should be documented. Similarly, protocols and procedures should be recorded and approved by the medical director. Activities of nonphysician personnel that exceed their usual scope of practice in the inpatient setting should be approved by the respective governing bodies (*e.g.*, board of nursing). All documentation should be kept on permanent file.

During the conduct of a transport, the team should adhere to established protocols and procedures unless the patient's needs dictate an abridgement of usual standards. In this situation, advice from a consulting physician should be sought. Recommendations by this person should be recorded in the patient record.

Special problems arise during interstate transport when medical professionals are not licensed in the state of the referring or receiving hospital.[34] Although some neighboring states have established reciprocal relationships regarding licensure, this is not routine. Unfortunately, there is no simple solution to this problem.

NEONATAL BACK TRANSPORT

Overcrowding of level III centers is a major problem in many regions of the country. One strategy for managing this problem has been to transport convalescing infants to level I or level II hospitals before discharge home. This strategy often is referred to as back transport. The benefits of back transport include the following:

- reserves level III center resources for critically ill patients[35]
- improves use of level I and level II center resources and helps prepare their personnel for the care of acutely ill patients
- familiarizes primary care physicians with infants before discharge home
- improves relationships between level III and level I and II hospitals
- improves family visitation and promotes family–infant bonding[36]
- reduces the total cost of medical care.[37,38]

There also are potential disadvantages associated with back transport, including the following:

- parental anxiety and loss of continuity of care, caused by the change of caretakers[36]
- hazards and cost of transport
- lack of reimbursement by third-party payers for the transport[38]
- the occasional requirement for readmission to the level III center
- loss of the opportunity by level III personnel to participate in convalescent care.

Back transport should be considered an option for all infants who no longer require the unique resources of the level III center, and for whom the level III center is not the site of primary care.[39]

REFERENCES

1. Cone TE. History of the care and feeding of the premature infant. Boston: Little, Brown & Co, 1985:46.
2. Losty MA, Orlofsky I, Wallace H. A transport service for premature babies. Am J Nurs 1950;50:10.
3. Wallace HM, Losty MA, Baumgartner L. Report of two years experience in the transportation of premature infants in New York City. Pediatrics 1952;22:439.
4. Modanlou HD, Dorchester W, Freeman RK, et al. Perinatal transport to a regional perinatal center in a metropolitan area: maternal versus neonatal transport. Am J Obstet Gynecol 1980;138:1157.
5. Sachs BP, Marks JS, McCarthy BJ, et al. Neonatal transport in Georgia: implications for maternal transport in high-risk pregnancies. South Med J 1983;76:1397.
6. Merenstein GB, Pettett G, Woodall J, et al. An analysis of air transport results in the sick newborn: II. Antenatal and neonatal referrals. Am J Obstet Gynecol 1977;128:520.
7. Bose CL. Organization and administration of a perinatal transport service. In: MacDonald MG, Miller MK, eds. Emergency transport of the perinatal patient. Boston: Little, Brown & Co, 1989:43.
8. Hood JL, Cross A, Hulka B, et al. Effectiveness of the neonatal transport team. Crit Care Med 1983;11:419.
9. Chance GW, Matthew JD, Gash J, et al. Neonatal transport: a controlled study of skilled assistance. J Pediatr 1978;93:662.
10. American Academy of Pediatrics, Committee on Fetus and Newborn, and American College of Obstetricians and Gynecologists, Committee on Obstetrics. Maternal and fetal medicine: guidelines for perinatal care. Evanston, IL: American Academy of Pediatrics and American College of Obstetricians and Gynecologists, 1983:45.
11. Mitchell A, Watts J, Whyte R, et al. Evaluation of graduating neonatal nurse practitioners. Pediatrics 1991;88:789.
12. Pettett G, Merenstein GB, Battaglia FC, et al. An analysis of air transport results in the sick newborn infant: part I. The transport team. Pediatrics 1975;55:774.
13. Thompson TR. Neonatal transport nurses: an analysis of their role in the transport of newborn infants. Pediatrics 1980;65:887.
14. Conn AKT, Bowen CY. The communications network for perinatal transport. In: MacDonald MD, Miller MK, eds. Emergency transport of the perinatal patient. Boston: Little, Brown & Co, 1989:92.

15. Perlstein PH, Edwards NK, Sutherland JM. Neonatal hot line telephone network. Pediatrics 1979;64:419.
16. Bostick JS, Hsiao HS, Lawson EE. A minicomputer-based perinatal/neonatal telecommunication network. Pediatrics 1983; 71:272.
17. Risemberg HM. Financing a perinatal transport program in the United States. In: MacDonald MA, Miller MK, eds. Emergency transport in the perinatal patient. Boston: Little, Brown & Co, 1989:85.
18. Baxt WG, Moody P. The impact of rotorcraft aeromedicine emergency care service on transport mortality. JAMA 1983; 249:3047.
19. Elliot JP, O'Keeffe DF, Freeman RK. Helicopter transportation of patients with obstetric emergencies in an urban area. Am J Obstet Gynecol 1982;143:157.
20. Bose CL. The transport environment. In: MacDonald MG, Miller MK, eds. Emergency transport of the perinatal patient. Boston: Little, Brown & Co, 1989:194.
21. Shenai J. Sound levels for neonates in transit. J Pediatr 1977; 90:811.
22. Campbell AN, Lightstone AD, Smith JM, et al. Mechanical vibration and sound levels experienced in neonatal transport. Am J Dis Child 1984;138:967.
23. Gadeke R, Doring B, Keller R, et al. The noise level in a children's hospital and the wake-up threshold in infants. Acta Paediatr Scand 1969;58:164.
24. Shenai JP, Johnson GE, Varney RV. Mechanical vibration in neonatal transport. Pediatrics 1981;68:55.
25. Floyd WN, Broderson AB, Goodno JF. Effects of whole body vibration on peripheral nerve conduction time in the rhesus monkey. Aerospace Medicine 1973;44:281.
26. Clark JG, Williams JD, Hood WB, et al. Initial cardiovascular response to low frequency whole body vibration in humans and animals. Aerospace Medicine 1967;38:464.
27. Adey WR, Winters WD, Kado RT, et al. EEG in simulated stresses of space flight with special reference to problems of vibration. Electroencephalogr Clin Neurophysiol 1963;15: 305.
28. Graybiel A, Knepton J. Sopite syndrome: a sometimes sole manifestation of motion sickness. Aviat Space Environ Med 1976;47:873.
29. Council on Medical Services. Guide for quality assurance. JAMA 1988;259:2572.
30. Joint Commission on the Accreditation of Hospitals and Health Organizations. Examples of monitoring and evaluation in emergency services. Chicago: JCAHHO, 1988:13.
31. Eastes L, Jacobson J, eds. Quality assurance in air medical transport. Orem, UT: WordPerfect Publishers, 1990.
32. Ginzburg HM. Legal issues in medical transport. In: MacDonald MG, Miller MK, eds. Emergency transport of the perinatal patient. Boston: Little, Brown & Co, 1989:152.
33. Tonsic v Wagner, 458 Pa 246, 329 A2d 497 (1974).
34. Brimhall DC. The Hospital administrator's perspective. In: MacDonald MG, Miller MK, eds. Emergency transport of the perinatal patient. Boston: Little, Brown & Co, 1989:147.
35. Jung AL, Bose CL. Back transport of neonates: improved efficiency of tertiary nursery bed utilization. Pediatrics 1983; 71:918.
36. Meyer CL, Mahan CK, Schreiner RL. Retransfer of newborns to community hospitals: questionnaire survey of parents' feelings. Perinatology Neonatology 1982;6:75.
37. Bose CL, LaPine TR, Jung AL. Neonatal back transport: cost effectiveness. Med Care 1985;23:14.
38. Phibbs CS, Mortensen L. Back transporting infants from neonatal intensive care units to community hospitals for recovery care: effect on total hospital charges. Pediatrics 1992;90:22.
39. Lynch TM, Jung AL, Bose CL. Neonatal back transport: clinical outcome. Pediatrics 1988;82:845.

Neonatology: Pathophysiology and Management of the Newborn, Fourth Edition,
edited by Gordon B. Avery, Mary Ann Fletcher, and Mhairi G. MacDonald.
J.B. Lippincott Company, Philadelphia © 1994.

chapter 6

The Intensive Care Nursery

DIANE BEHAN LOISEL
SHARON KOVZELOVE
VIVIAN SHATZ

ORGANIZATION

The organization of today's neonatal intensive care unit (NICU) requires a complex array of interdependent multidisciplinary professionals. The effectiveness of any organization further demands that the professionals collaborate, communicate, and remain flexible to the ever-changing needs of the patients they serve. Providing the necessary leadership and direction for the successful management of both human and technological resources will be one of the many challenges that professionals engaged in neonatal intensive care will need to meet if they are to survive amidst increasing economic and societal pressures.

MEDICAL DIRECTOR

The medical director is responsible for the clinical, administrative, and educational aspects of the NICU. The role of the medical director involves the development and implementation of unit policy, education of the unit staff, and management of the quality assurance–improvement programs.[1] These activities must be coordinated with the nursing director or nursing manager as part of the strategic planning and daily management of the NICU. The medical director is vital to the successful implementation of change and in developing innovative patient care programs.[2]

NURSING DIRECTOR

The role of the nursing director or nurse manager is defined as the coordination and integration of human and material resources. The responsibilities include the evaluation of clinical practice in the NICU, the development of the professional nursing and ancillary staff, and management of the fiscal resources that promote efficient patient care outcomes in the critical care environment.[3,4]

One of the primary responsibilities of the nursing director is to establish the mechanism for decision making in the unit. Since the mid-1980s, there has been increasing emphasis on the shared governance approach for professional accountability in the health care environment.[5-7] Successful implementation of this form of decentralized decision making will require the nurse manager to be the catalyst for innovative change. Requisite leadership skills include the ability to adapt rapidly to change within the critical care setting and to cultivate this behavior among the professional staff. In addition to the governance structure, the nursing director must be involved in the development and implementation of the nursing care delivery model in the NICU. Standards of neonatal nursing practice must be firmly established to provide a consistent approach to care. Hospitals are redesigning their operations around consumer expectations and technology.[8]

As a result, the nursing director will be expected to develop a patient care model that promotes collaboraion and respect between departments, improves communication within the organization, increases he productivity of the staff, and involves staff at every step in the process.[9]

PERSONNEL

The duties and responsibilities of the personnel who provide care in the NICU are diverse and encompass clinical, educational, and managerial roles. The professional staff nurse in the NICU can be identified by a variety of titles (*e.g.*, primary nurse, patient care coordinator, charge nurse, case manager, clinical nurse). Clinical career ladders in many settings have evolved to encourage and promote advancement at he bedside.[10,11] In the NICU, the common thread for all nursing activity is the provision of care from admission through discharge with the goal of providing continuity for the patient and family. The neonatal clinical nurse specialist is designated to provide leadership and development for the staff around the advanced clinical aspects of care, consultation, collaboration with the medical staff involved in patient care, and leadership in the arena of clinical research. The neonatal clinical educator develops a comprehensive orientation program, and is responsible for ongoing staff development and inservice programs.

Neonatal nurse practitioners and transport nurses are responsible for total patient management under he supervision of the medical staff. These expanded oles have become critical to the effective functioning of a neonatal department. In the NICU, it is highly desirable to provide 24-hour coverage for each of hese roles. These nurses provide significant continuity of care for the infants and families while also serving as clinical experts for the nursing staff and junior medical staff.

Another nursing role that is essential in the NICU is that of the discharge planning coordinator. Every staff nurse is responsible for planning the discharge of the patient and family. The medical and financial complexity that is involved, however, requires that one primary person take the initiative to coordinate he multidisciplinary plan.

The respiratory therapist in the NICU is responsible for the overall management of ventilatory equipment and respiratory protocols in the unit. It is necessary to provide adequate coverage in the NICU on a full-time basis. Respiratory therapists contribute to he daily management of the infant and should be involved routinely in the development of unit policies hat affect their department. In addition, qualified aboratory technicians must be on duty 24 hours a day to provide rapid analysis of blood gases and other critical diagnostic studies.

Additional ancillary roles have become vital to the efficient functioning of the NICU. The nursing assistant or patient care assistant in the critical care unit has assumed even greater significance as the supply of registered nurses has been outdistanced by demand.[12] Although it is recognized that the specific job functions are task oriented and limited in scope, the nursing assistive personnel are able to run errands, manage the unit supplies, and assist with routine care needs. The role of the unit clerk cannot be underestimated in the fast-paced environment of the NICU unit. The management of all nonclinical aspects of care such as ordering supplies, maintenance of equipment, documentation of patient orders, and the coordination of all communication is the unit clerk's responsibility. These roles support the professional nurse in providing care and also provide an avenue for recruitment into the profession.[13]

The care of the parents and family during the hospitalization of a critically ill infant can become a difficult challenge to the entire staff. In addition to dealing with the medical needs of the infant, the NICU staff also must confront the social problems that exist in the community at large. The social worker is instrumental in providing the necessary interventions on behalf of both the staff and family.

COMMUNICATION

The nature of the work in a NICU places both the staff and the family in crisis situations on a daily basis. These daily stressors, coupled with the number of people who need to relate to one another while providing care, almost guarantee that communication will at best be a challenge and at worst become a process requiring conflict management. Open communication fosters cooperative problem solving, free flow of accurate information, and, ultimately, improved decision making at all levels within the organization.[14] To achieve these goals, trust must be established by the medical and nursing leaders. If the leaders promote an attitude of openness, honesty, and direct communication, the staff will then be able to model their own behavior accordingly and collaborate effectively in reaching consensus.

Communication takes place by a variety of mechanisms; both formal and informal means are used in the daily management of unit activity. In both cases, the attention given to the manner in which the message is delivered must be equal to that given to the message itself. The unit leaders need to develop effective communication skills and must be willing to try a variety of approaches.

PHYSICAL ENVIRONMENT: SPACE AND EQUIPMENT

Creating the optimal physical environment for the neonate and the staff is one of the most difficult challenges for hospital administrators, physicians, and nurse executives (see Chap. 8). A growing body of research, however, indicates that the developmental outcome for fragile preterm infants is potentially at risk if care is not taken to reduce or eliminate excessive noise and overstimulation in the NICU environment.[15]

The design of a NICU requires long-term commitment by both administration and staff. If done correctly, the product can be spectacular. The planning process is critical to the outcome; to reach the goal, everyone must participate at each phase along the way. There are excellent resources from the literature that specifically provide insight into critical care unit design.[16,17]

Maintaining the technology-dependent environment of the NICU within the economic climate of health care today poses a significant challenge to the entire health care team. Products and equipment are constantly changing to keep up with biomedical advances in the field. Decisions about the purchase of new equipment must be approached with nursing, biomedical, and medical input. Purchasing departments within the institution need to create systems for timely evaluation and introduction of new products.[18] A clear mechanism is needed at the unit level to coordinate the many requests from vendors as well as from staff for evaluation of new equipment. The nursing staff needs to be a part of the final decisions, through unit committees or through staff representation at the institutional level.[19,20]

POLICIES AND PROCEDURES

The nursing director is responsible for ensuring that appropriate policies and procedures are in place in the NICU so that high-quality patient care is delivered. The extent to which the policies are successfully implemented and supported rests largely with the nursing staff. It is therefore imperative that staff have the responsibility to develop protocols and contribute to their revision and implementation within the unit. Appropriate consultation with medical staff must be ensured by the nursing director, as well as communication with the other departments that come into contact with the NICU.

The policies should minimally cover admission to the unit, general safety practices, emergency protocols, visitation of parents and siblings, infection control, medication administration, and NICU routine care practices. In addition to these, specific clinical procedures and protocols should be in place to assist the staff in the delivery of patient care.[21,22]

INFECTION CONTROL

Infants in the NICU are at risk for the development of nosocomial infections. There are precautions and standards of practice aimed at the prevention and spread of neonatal nosocomial infections within the intensive care unit.[23] In addition, the 1988 *Guidelines for Perinatal Care* provides clear and specific direction for the basic management and practice of infection control.[23a]

The practice of good handwashing technique cannot be overemphasized to all personnel who com into the NICU. This is essential and needs to be moni tored regularly through the quality assurance mech anisms in the unit. It is helpful to place automati timers at the entry sinks of the unit so that the appro priate scrub can be maintained. Particular attentio must be paid to keeping the baby's immediate envi ronment as clean as possible. The isolette must b changed at least once per week. Soiled linen, equip ment, and supplies should be disposed of in a timel manner.

The effectiveness of cover gowns as a protectiv measure for controlling the spread of infection is nc confirmed; however, the traditional practice con tinues in most NICUs. It should be emphasized tha the personnel who come into direct contact with th infant should keep any clothing on the arms pushe above the elbow, remove all jewelry, and ensure tha hands, wrists and forearms have been washed wit an antimicrobial soap before and after each contac with an infant. While holding a baby outside of th isolette, a barrier (*e.g.*, cover gown, baby blanket chux) should be used to protect the clothes of th person holding the infant.[24]

Routine surveillance by the nurse epidemiologist i an essential element in monitoring nosocomial infec tions within the NICU. A clear procedure for trackin suspected or confirmed infections should be estab lished. In addition, all nursing and medical staff pre senting with symptoms of contagious illnesses (*e.g.* upper respiratory infections, diarrhea, sore throats must not handle infants. Communicable disease should be reported to the Epidemiology or Infectiou Disease Department in a prompt manner.

STAFFING

Traditionally, NICUs have had a staff composed en tirely of registered nurses. As health care costs esca late and reimbursement declines, staffing patterns ul timately will be forced to change. Creative strategie can be used to support the goal of quality patient car while at the same time providing structured opportu nities for students and ancillary staff to become a pa of the health care team.

In addition to coverage for direct patient care, th nurse manager often will need to consider the impac of special programs within the unit (*e.g.*, transpo staff, neonatal nurse practitioners, extracorpore membrane oxygenation specialists). All of thes groups must be integrated into the framework of th NICU environment and participate in management the unit as a singular staff.

Data collection is essential for the nurse manager t plan both day-to-day operations and long-term goals Methods to obtain average daily census, length c stay in the NICU by diagnostic grouping, annual ac missions, transports, and required hours of care ar needed. Patient classification systems are one way t identify patient acuity and nursing requirements.

The nurse manager must devise tracking systems, preferably computerized ones, that will assist in program planning. Success in managing this highly complex environment will depend on the ability to remain open to a variety of alternative patterns and to include the staff in the decision-making process at every level.

BASIC CARE OF THE SICK NEONATE

ADMISSION TO THE NURSERY

Resuscitation and stabilization generally begin in the delivery room. During admission to the nursery, the nurse obtains baseline data on the patient and further stabilizes the infant. The data obtained include vital signs, weight, laboratory values, physical assessment, and maternal and delivery history. The first few hours after admission are used by the nurse to meet immediate needs such as thermoregulation, monitoring glucose and fluid needs, and assessing respiratory requirements. The nurse implements the physician's orders and continues to assess the patient's response to these interventions.

Documentation of the admission process is different in each intensive care nursery (ICN), but all will include physical assessment, psychosocial history, delivery and transport history, and stabilization procedures. From this documentation a data base, nursing problem list, and nursing care plan are developed.

Admission to an ICN can be a very confusing period for the family of an ill neonate. The nursery environment is a high-tech area with unfamiliar equipment and busy personnel. Time must be taken to establish a relationship between the infant's team of physicians and nurses and the parents. The parents' initial perception may be colored by the high activity level and they often do not follow detailed explanations. The first family visits should focus on the child rather than the equipment and numbers on the monitors. The health care professional can assess the amount of information the family is ready to hear and understand, during each subsequent visit.

SETUP OF THE BEDSIDE ENVIRONMENT

The equipment necessary for an admission to the nursery can be set up before the admission, with beds of different levels of acuity prepared, based on the infant's needs. All bedsides should include the following equipment:

- radiant warmer or isolette, prewarmed with humidity, and K-pad (American Medical Systems, Indianapolis, IN) for infants weighing 1000 g or less
- oxygen source, resuscitation bag capable of providing 100% oxygen, and appropriate sized mask
- ventilator, laryngoscope, and endotracheal tubes of all sizes
- suction equipment with suction set at 80 to 100 cm H_2O, catheters of appropriate size, and sterile gloves
- monitoring equipment, including cardiorespiratory monitor with indwelling blood pressure monitoring ability, pulse oximeter, and stethoscope
- gastric tube
- blood glucose monitoring equipment
- intravenous (IV) equipment and solutions
- supplies for drawing lab studies (*e.g.*, syringes, tubes).

The equipment should be placed at the bedside to allow for easy retrieval during the admission and to allow visualization of the monitors and the patient. Overstocking the bed with equipment does not make the admission easier if it is hard to find the essential equipment among the clutter.

SAFETY AND MONITORING

Hospital personnel are responsible for ensuring a safe and therapeutic environment for the infant and family. Name cards must be on the beds to identify patients, and two identification bands should be worn by the infant. These should be documented as present every shift and checked before any procedure with the infant.

At the beginning of each shift, the nurse checks each of his or her patients' equipment and supplies to make certain they are properly functioning and that all alarms are set appropriately. All IV infusions are checked against the physician's orders and the site of the infusion is checked every hour by the nurse. The infusion chamber is filled with no more than 10 mL plus 3 hours' worth of fluids, to prevent fluid overload in the event of pump malfunction.

Any time the door of an isolette is opened the infant must be attended. A heat source with a measured safety distance from the patient is used. Eye shields are placed over the infant's eyes for protection from the light.

THERMOREGULATION

It is of primary importance for all neonates to be maintained within a neutral thermal environment (see Chap. 25). Charts demonstrating neutral thermal environment based on gestational age, weight, and days of life are available and can be placed in the nursery for quick reference.[26] An infant's axillary temperature should be maintained between 36.4°C and 37.2°C. If the temperature is above or below this range, the temperature should be monitored every 15 minutes until it returns to normal. Recording the isolette temperature and servo control set point, in addition to the patient's temperature, may help differentiate fever from equipment malfunction.

Hypothermia often can be a sign of sepsis in the infant and may be the only early warning sign. A hypothermic infant should be allowed to warm up gradually with the goal of increasing the infant's temperature 0.5°C each hour. Interventions to warm an infant include dressing the infant, warming the air around the isolette with a heat lamp, decreasing the amount of time the isolette doors are opened, postponing a procedure if the condition warrants, placing a K-pad or warming mattress under the infant, wrapping the isolette in tin foil, and increasing humidity. The consequences of hypothermia in the ill neonate can include apnea, bradycardia, hypoglycemia, poor perfusion, increased respiratory distress, acidosis, and, without intervention, death.

Many nursing interventions can aid in the prevention of hypothermia. Conductive heat loss can be decreased by warming surfaces the infant comes in contact with (*e.g.*, scales), covering radiograph plates with a sheet, and replacing wet linen immediately. Reduction in convective losses can be achieved by keeping the isolette door closed, using a heat lamp when the door is open, and keeping porthole sleeves in place. Bathing infants under 1000 g in the isolette, using bed scales, adding humidity to isolettes, and heating inspired oxygen will minimize evaporative heat loss. Radiant loss is decreased by keeping the isolette away from drafts, keeping infants in open cribs away from windows, using double-walled isolettes or plastic shields, and placing hats on the infants' heads. Using a K-pad under a sheet for infants under 1000 g can significantly decrease temperature fluctuations.

Hyperthermia is seen most often in neonates with sepsis or neurologic impairment. It also may occur as a side-effect of medication, from malfunctioning warmers, or extraneous heat sources (*e.g.*, heat lamps, phototherapy lights). To cool a hyperthermic infant, remove excess clothing, sponge with tepid water, and medicate per physician orders.

DAILY CARE

Daily care of the neonate focuses on caregiving activities but incorporates the needs of the patient and family for psychosocial support, information, and nurturing. The frequency with which vital signs are assessed is based on the acuity and need of the individual patient. An apical heart rate is taken, noting extra heart sounds. Upper and lower extremity pulses should be palpated and capillary filling time assessed. Respiratory rate can be visualized or auscultated. Breath sounds should be assessed for equality, rhythm, and the presence of abnormal breath sounds, such as rales and wheezes. The infant should be observed for signs of respiratory distress, such as nasal flaring, retractions, unequal chest expansion, and cyanosis. Blood pressure may be monitored continuously with an indwelling arterial catheter and transducer or intermittently with an extremity cuff. Cuff size, in relation to the size of the extremity, affects the blood pressure reading. The correct-sized cuff, covering no more than two-thirds of the upper arm or lower leg, should therefore be used.

Infants generally are bathed once a day, preferably at a time when the parents can interact with their infant. The infant should be bathed in a warm environment, free of drafts, with warm water and a mild soap. Sponge baths are given until the cord falls off. The cord and surrounding area should be examined carefully for redness, drainage, or foul odor; if present, these should be reported to the physician. The umbilical cord is cleaned with alcohol after the bath and with every diaper change. Care must be taken not to dislodge any indwelling umbilical lines.

The skin of a premature or ill neonate is very susceptible to injury and irritation from lead patches, skin probes, tape, and Betadine. The skin should be examined carefully every shift and any breakdown, rashes or reddened areas documented. Very-low-birth-weight (VLBW) infants can have semipermeable transparent dressings applied to chest, back, thighs and forearms to prevent skin breakdown. Lotions and powders are not used routinely in neonates unless a specific condition warrants. The perineal area should be cleaned with every diaper change and examined for rashes. Mouth care with sterile water should be given frequently to intubated infants and to those who are not receiving any nutrition orally. This is a task most parents will enjoy doing for their child.

The infant should be weighed daily at approximately the same time each day, with the same scale, and before feeding. It often is convenient to weigh at the same time the bath is given. Head circumference should be measured weekly and the results charted on a graph. Length is an important indicator of growth and also is obtained and charted weekly.

NUTRITIONAL SUPPORT

Most infants in the ICN receive several forms of nutritional support during their stay in the nursery. This support ranges from IV therapy through central lines to oral feedings of their mothers' breast milk. Each form of nutritional support has both risks and benefits that must be weighed to determine which type of caloric supplementation is best with the current status of the patient (see Chap. 24).

Before initiating a feeding, the nurse must assess the infant for signs and symptoms of distress or illness that may indicate an alternative method of nutritional support. The nurse also must assess readiness for oral feeding by gestational age, suck–swallow coordination, and amount of respiratory distress. Tachypnea, with a respiratory rate of over 60, may contraindicate nipple feeding due to the risk of aspiration. Infants with low body temperature may be less willing to bottle feed. During the feeding the nurse continues to assess the patient's stability and observes for signs of stress. He or she provides feedback to the physician and input into feeding plans.

BREAST MILK

Mothers who wish to breast-feed their infant often are unable to do so in the ICN due to the prematurity or illness of their infant. It is the responsibility of staff to find ways to encourage and support the mother who desires to breast-feed her child. Nurseries can make available a breast pump to allow mothers to collect and store their milk. Breast milk may be stored in a freezer at −18°C to −20°C for 3 to 6 months. After this, the milk's taste may change and the infant may not be willing to drink it.[27] Breast milk may be stored in the refrigerator at 4°C for 24 hours once it is thawed or pumped. At approximately 33 to 34 weeks of gestation the infant can begin going to the breast at least once a day. Providing privacy screens and dimming the lights offers the mother an atmosphere more conducive to breast-feeding and may help with her initial attempts.

GAVAGE AND TRANSPYLORIC FEEDING

When an infant is unable to nipple feed due to prematurity or illness, intermittent or continuous gavage or continuous transpyloric feedings are used. Gavage feedings also may be used to supplement oral feedings in the infant learning to nipple feed or who tires easily with feedings. The characteristics and volume of residuals should be examined and then they should be replaced: discarding residuals can cause electrolyte imbalance. Residuals greater than one-fourth of the total feeding should be reported and discussed with the physician. A gavage feeding is administered by gravity, over a time period equal to the amount of time an oral feeding would take. The infant should be held upright or positioned right side down during the feeding. Offering a pacifier during the gavage feeding for nonnutritive sucking has been shown to aid infants in preparation for bottle feeding.[28] Continuous gavage feeding is done with a pump to infuse the feeding slowly over a given time period. Residuals are checked every 3 to 4 hours and amounts up to 1 hour's worth of feeding are acceptable. This is the method of choice for very small infants and for infants who do not tolerate larger bolus volumes.

Duodenal or jejunal feedings may be administered when infants do not tolerate gastric feedings or when transpyloric feedings are preferred because of intubation or continuous positive airway pressure. After initial placement, the tube aspirates are checked for a *p*H of 7 and the tube position is confirmed radiographically. Transpyloric feedings are administered by continuous infusion pump. The transpyloric tube is not aspirated for residuals but gastric residuals are checked every 3 to 4 hours.

GASTROSTOMY

Gastrostomy tube feeding is most common among surgical patients or infants discharged home on tube feedings. Before feeding, the tube is aspirated or drained by gravity to detect any residuals. The feeding is given by gravity with the tube held approximately 10 cm above the patient. The time should approximate that of an oral feeding. The tube is externally vented after the feeding to allow for burps and to avoid regurgitation.

TOTAL PARENTERAL NUTRITION GIVEN THROUGH CENTRAL LINES

Total parenteral nutrition (TPN) supplies calories, proteins, essential fatty acids, vitamins, and minerals when enteral feedings are contraindicated or just being initiated (see Chap. 24). Total parenteral nutrition may be infused through peripheral IV lines or through central catheters. Central catheters are needed to infuse higher concentrations of dextrose. The central catheter may be surgically placed directly into a major vein or percutaneously inserted into a smaller vein and threaded centrally. Generally, only TPN is infused through a central line. Nursing responsibilities include sterile central line dressing changes, monitoring serum glucose, urine specific gravity, *p*H, and dipsticks, and observing for signs and symptoms of sepsis.

MONITORING FOR TOLERANCE

Any type of feeding regimen, whether enteral or parenteral, can lead to complications. The patient must be monitored continually for signs of intolerance. The nurse assesses intake and output, performs daily weights, and ensures the prescribed amount of fluid is administered. Daily and weekly laboratory studies are conducted to monitor nutritional status. Before each feeding, vital signs, abdominal girth, residuals, activity level, and stools are examined and recorded. Abnormal signs are reported. Increased abdominal girth may be an early sign of feeding intolerance, and the infant should be checked for tenderness, guarding, and blood in the stool. Residuals of formula left in the stomach from a previous feeding also may indicate intolerance of the feeding regimen. Change in activity level may indicate sepsis or feeding intolerance.

MEDICATIONS

In the newborn and young infant, the metabolism, excretion, distribution, and pharmacologic effects of medications are affected to a large degree by the amount of organ maturation. Organ immaturity puts the premature infant at high risk for accentuation of medication effects due to increased half-life of the drug in the body.[29] Many organ systems are affected by the medications administered in the nursery, of which there is a diverse array. Each nursery should have current guidelines for medication administration, encompassing routes of administration, compatibility, methods of dilutions, length of time for administration, dosage, and people responsible for giving medications. Before administering any drug, the nurse should be aware of the indication for its use and any possible drug interaction or potentiation with the current drug regimen. Oral medications may be given by mixing them with a small amount of formula and allowing the infant to nipple feed, by slowly injecting the medication into the cheek and allowing the child to swallow, or by injecting the medication directly into the stomach through the gastric tube. Some oral preparations are thick or unpleasant and the premature infant who is just beginning to nipple feed may have difficulty taking them by mouth. Some cause gastric irritation and place the infant at risk for feeding intolerance. These should not be given until the infant reaches full enteral intake.

Parenteral medications all have specific methods of dilution and length of time for administration. Some have special requirements for the vial or syringe in which they are mixed; some will bind to the plastic in syringes or IV tubing. Before and after administering IV medications, the line should be flushed with normal saline to determine patency and prevent mixing of incompatible solutions. Some drip medications may lose their potency after a period at room temperature. Be aware of these drugs and change the solutions as indicated by the pharmacy. Monitor the infant closely after administration of any medication for adverse effects.

NURSING RECORDS AND CHARTING

Nursing documentation of daily care is generally done on a flow record, with hourly documentation as well as shift assessments. Further documentation is recorded in progress notes. Some hospitals require progress notes with each shift for each patient, whereas others require notes to be written only if an assessment or problem cannot be documented on the flow record. Initial documentation by the nurse begins with the transport or resuscitation record. From this point on, the nurse records patient data on the flow record, writes an admission assessment, interviews the family, and formulates a problem list and a nursing care plan. The problem list and care plan should be discussed with the parents and agreed-on goals and plans formulated. Medications and treatments are charted on the flow record or separate medication administration sheets. Charting throughout the shift is more accurate than waiting until the end of the shift and trying to recall all that has transpired.

NURSING THE INFANT WITH SPECIAL PROBLEMS

THE TINY PREMATURE INFANT

The prognosis for infants with birth weights of 750 g or less and gestational ages of 26 weeks or younger is uncertain. Some centers report improved outcomes,[30] but substantial mortality and morbidity continues in others.[31] What is certain is that these extremely-low-birth-weight infants have very unique nursing care needs.

These infants are born with surfactant-deficient lungs, insufficient respiratory drive, underdeveloped respiratory muscles, and compliant chest walls. They also have a high incidence of patent ductus arteriosus. All this contributes to ventilator dependence. Surfactant replacement improves the biochemical deficiency but cannot speed the growth and development of supporting structures. Such immature lungs are at enormous risk for ventilator-induced tissue damage and subsequent bronchopulmonary dysplasia.

The skin of these tiny infants is translucent and lacks subcutaneous fat deposits. It is relatively incapable of holding in heat or water. To decrease heat and water losses, double-walled isolates or heat shields, Saran blankets (Dow Chemical, Indianapolis, IN), and head caps are imperative. These infants should not be nursed under radiant warmers, where further insensible losses would occur. Drugs and chemicals used for skin preparation can be easily absorbed and cause toxicity. If used, they must be removed thoroughly. Abrasions and tears in the skin develop easily. Removal of tape used to affix monitoring and lifesaving devices also can remove the epidermis. To minimize this occurrence, skin barriers (*e.g.*, Hollihesive, Hollister, Libertyville, IL) under the tape are recommended. Transcutaneous oxygen monitors, which can cause burns, are contraindicated.[32]

The skin of the premature infant is a poor barrier against infection. This, in addition to their extremely immature immune systems, makes these babies very vulnerable to infections. In particular, fungal sepsis occurs more frequently in premature infants than in full-term infants.

Hyperglycemia is common, even when the infant is on modest glucose infusions. Insulin drips may be required to improve glucose tolerance and enhance the administration of calories. They must be titrated very carefully and slowly to prevent rebounding.

Caring for these infants is a challenge. They may become apneic and bradycardic when their isolettes are approached. Their nervous systems cannot self-regulate to stimulation. Vital sign and color changes occur in response to the slightest amount of touch, noise, or light.[33,34] Repeated hypoxic events, precipitated by exposure to various stimuli, may adversely nfluence brain development. Nurses have an obliga- ion to protect these babies; this should include limit- ng negative environmental stressors, encouraging elf-regulating behaviors, and educating oneself to ecognize behavioral patterns and cues.[35] Structuring aregiving and the environment to each infant's indi- idual needs can assist immature neonates to main- ain state control, to self-regulate, and to have a righter developmental outcome.[36] Table 6-1 contains uggested admission orders for infants weighing less han 1000 g.

ESPIRATORY CARE

Vhen caring for an infant in respiratory distress, the urse must be knowledgeable about the newborn dis- ases that cause respiratory symptoms, and be famil- ar with the equipment used to treat these infants. He r she also must be skilled in physical assessment, ecognition of distress, and administration of respira- ory physical therapy.

HEST PHYSIOTHERAPY

hest physiotherapy (CPT) involves positioning, per- ussion, and vibration. It aids ventilation and perfu- ion, removal of infectious or aspirated debris, and ne prevention or treatment of atelectasis.

Postural changes facilitate the movement of secre- ons with the aid of gravity. This can be accom- lished by placing the infant prone with frequent po- ition changes, and by positioning to drain specific bes (Fig. 6-1). To be effective, the position should be eld for 5 to 10 minutes. It may only be feasible to rain one or two lobes per treatment. Note the eated lobes and the infant's tolerance to the proce- ure; if the baby is unstable, concentrate only on af- cted areas.[37]

Percussion transmits pressure through a column of r to loosen secretions in the larger airways. It is done with a cupped device (*e.g.*, cupped hand, commercially available percussor, neonatal face mask, or other padded apparatus). The specified area is tapped at a rate of three to four beats per second for 30 to 60 seconds.[37,38]

Vibration is done after, or in place of, percussion—some premature infants will not tolerate both. It thins mucus and mobilizes secretions in the smaller airways so they can be removed by coughing or suctioning. It can be performed using the fingertips, a mechanical vibrator, or padded electric toothbrush.[37] The vibrations are applied to the affected area during expiration, held during inspiration, for approximately 2 to 3 minutes.[38]

ABLE 6–1
UGGESTED ADMISSION ORDERS OR INFANTS WEIGHING LESS THAN 1000 g

Place in isolette
Use in-isolette scale when available
Weigh daily
Irradiate all blood products
Use protective isolation
Use Saran blanket (Dow Chemical, Indianapolis, IN)
Place hat on infant's head
Use light filter or glasses to protect eyes
Keep lights dimmed as much as possible
Protect eyes at all times from heat and treatment lights

Adapted from the neonatal intensive care unit admission or- ers, Children's National Medical Center, Washington, DC.

SUCTIONING

Suctioning removes the loosened secretions and maintains a patent airway. Suctioning through an endotracheal tube is a sterile procedure. Usually, normal saline, 0.25 to 0.5 mL, is instilled and the patient is mechanically or manually ventilated for a few breaths. A transcutaneous oxygen monitor or pulse oximeter should be used to evaluate the need for additional oxygen, and to prevent hyperoxygenation. The catheter is passed, without suction, to the end of the endotracheal tube (Fig. 6-2), suction is applied, and the catheter is removed with a twisting motion. Suction with the head positioned midline. The catheter should not pass the end of the tube onto the carina. Gently hyperinflate the lungs between passes and at the end of the procedure to restore the functional residual capacity and prevent atelectasis. To avoid hypoxia, atelectasis, and other complications (*e.g.*, tissue damage, changes in heart rate, alterations in cerebral blood flow), limit suction time to 5 to 10 seconds per pass. Chart the infant's tolerance to the procedure, and the color and consistency of the secretions. Routine CPT and suctioning should be avoided—need should be determined on an individual basis.[37,39]

NEURAL TUBE DEFECTS

A myelomeningocele or encephalocele results from failure of the neural tube to close. The infant with a neural tube defect usually presents with a visible sac along the spinal cord.

The primary nursing goal is to maintain the integrity of the sac. If the sac is leaking, prevention of infection is a priority. A warmed, sterile, normal saline-soaked dressing is applied to the defect and covered with clear plastic wrap to decrease evaporative fluid losses. Nursing the infant prone with a roll under the hips provides proper orthopaedic alignment of the lower extremities and protects the defect. Lumbosacral lesions are at risk for stool contamination but

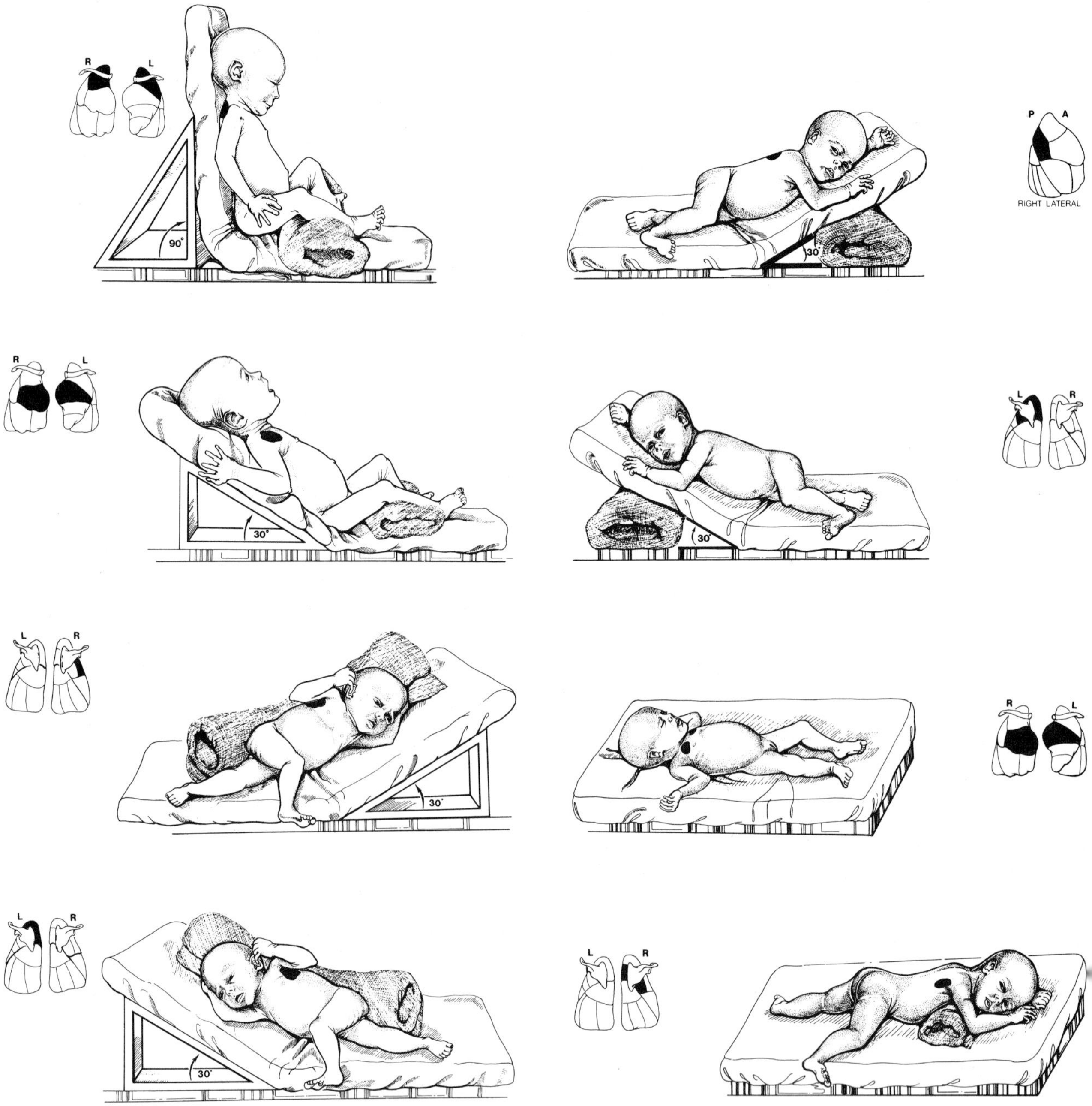

FIG. 6–1. Postural drainage positions. Insets indicate the segments drained while in each position. Shading on the infant indicates the area for chest percussion and vibration. (From Fletcher MA, MacDonald MG, Avery GB, eds. Atlas of procedures in neonatology. Philadelphia: JB Lippincott, 1983.)

placing a plastic flap (*e.g.*, Steri-Drape, 3M, St. Paul, MN) along the bottom of the dressing can avert this.[40]

Temperature regulation, fluid and antibiotic administration, and a baseline neurologic assessment are additional nursing responsibilities. The latter includes measuring the head circumference, fontanelle, and sutures; assessing the quality of the cry, suck, and grasp; and noting the position and movement of all extremities. The infant must be watched for signs of hydrocephalus. Bowel and bladder functio should be observed.[40]

Surgery usually is performed within 48 hours. A ter surgery, the infant is nursed prone with the hea of the bed elevated. This protects the surgical site an helps reduce intracranial pressure. Contamination (the surgical site by urine and stool must be min mized. Postvoid catheterizations may be ordered t measure residual urine caused by swelling in the in

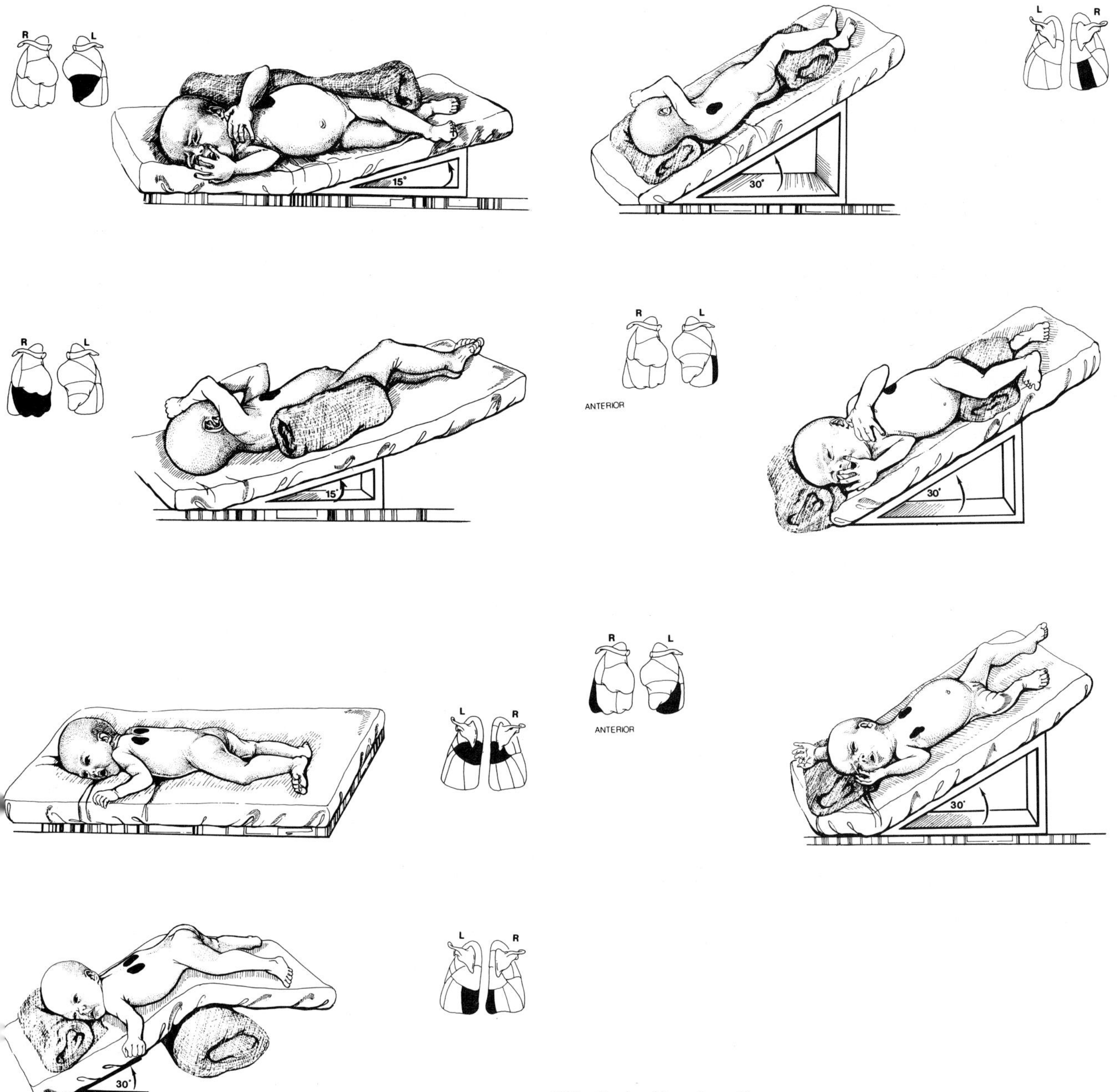

FIG. 6–1. *(Continued)*

mediate postoperative period. It is quite common for hese infants to have neurogenic bladder stasis, requiring routine catheterizations or urinary diversion. Monitoring continues for symptoms of sepsis and neningitis (*e.g.*, temperature instability, apnea, lethırgy). An associated Arnold–Chiari malformation nay present with airway or swallowing difficulties.[40] These patients require extensive follow-up by a multilisciplinary team.

ABDOMINAL WALL DEFECTS

The nursing care of an infant with an omphalocele is quite similar to the care required by an infant with gastroschisis. Infants with omphaloceles, however, may have heart disease or other associated defects. Those with gastroschisis often are premature.

The eviscerated organs or sac should be covered with warm, normal saline-soaked, sterile towels and

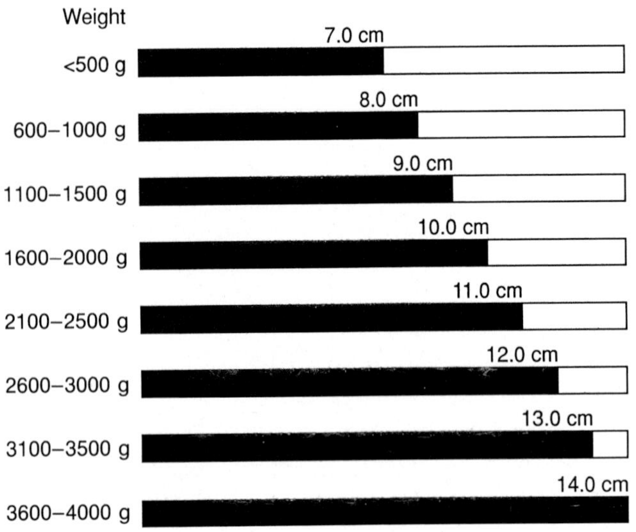

FIG. 6–2. Safe length at which a catheter can be inserted for endotracheal suctioning can be determined by the infant's weight. Measure catheter along the appropriate line for weight. Add the length of endotracheal tube that is sticking out of the mouth. This is the maximum safe distance for insertion of a suction catheter through an endotracheal tube. (From Anderson K, Chandra R. Pneumothorax secondary to perforation of sequential bronchi by suction catheters. J Pediatr Surg 1976;11:687.)

the baby's trunk covered with plastic wrap or placed inside a commercially available bowel bag. This decreases fluid and heat loss from the large surface area of exposed bowel. These babies need to be nursed in a side-lying position to prevent pressure on the organs. A double-lumen nasogastric tube with low, intermittent suction is necessary for gastrointestinal decompression. Antibiotics are given to prevent infection, and the defect is closed as soon as possible. If primary closure cannot be accomplished, the organs are placed inside a Silastic silo that is sutured to the skin. The surgeon reduces the silo daily until all the organs have been returned to the abdominal cavity. A second surgery is performed to close the skin.[41]

After surgery, the pressure of the organs on the inferior vena cava and fluid third spacing may impair venous return, causing poor perfusion and a metabolic acidosis. If venous return is impaired, IV fluids should not be administered in the lower extremities. The infant needs to be monitored closely for signs of hypovolemia (*e.g.*, intake and output, urine specific gravity, blood pressure). Gastric drainage should be replaced to prevent electrolyte imbalance. Respiratory distress frequently occurs due to the increased abdominal pressure and elevation of the diaphragm. Mechanical ventilation usually is required. Raising the head of the bed may provide some relief.[41]

When feedings are begun, observe for abdominal distention, gastric residuals, vomiting, and diarrhea. Recovery may be complicated by intermittent bowel obstruction, adhesions, ileus, or malabsorption problems.[41]

TRACHEOSTOMY

The nursing care of an infant with a tracheostomy is threefold. It involves maintaining a patient airway, preventing infection, and providing good peristomal skin care.

When the tracheostomy is performed, stay sutures are placed through the soft tissue in the neck and taped to the infant's chest. They are used to hold the stoma open, should the tracheostomy tube accidentally be dislodged. The tracheostomy tube is not changed for the first 7 days, while the tract is healing. The surgeon usually does the first tube change and removes the sutures. Subsequently, the tracheostomy tube is changed routinely once a week. A spare tracheostomy tube, the size of the existing tube, one a size smaller, an obturator, and a hemostat always should be at the bedside. If the tube becomes occluded with secretions or falls out, emergency replacement is necessary and lifesaving.

Secretions have to be kept loose and mobilized. This requires constant humidity, adequate hydration, CPT, and frequent suctioning. In small infants, too much humidity can cause overhydration, resulting in edema and rales. The nurse should observe the color and consistency of drainage. Any purulent secretions from the tracheostomy tube or around the stoma may indicate an infection. Peristomal care should be done routinely several times a day with half-strength hydrogen peroxide. Change moist or crusty ties to prevent skin irritation. Position the infant carefully, protecting the tracheostomy opening from occlusion.[42]

ENTEROSTOMY

Placing an ostomy appliance on an infant, especially a premature one, can be quite a challenge for the neonatal nurse. Proper application is essential, however, to prevent skin irritation, breakdown, and infection.

Fresh stomas are covered with Vaseline or Xeroform gauze (Baxter Healthcare, Deerfield, IL) to prevent irritation and sticking of dressings. The gauze is changed frequently so the color of the stomas and drainage can be assessed. The stomas should be pink. Blackened areas may indicate tissue ischemia or necrosis.

After 48 hours, a collection device can be applied. A correct fit will prevent spillage onto the skin. Ileostomy drainage is especially corrosive because of its enzymes. Before applying the appliance, wash the peristomal skin with warm water and pat dry. Do not apply ointment or cream; they will prevent the appliance from sticking properly. Place a skin shield such as Stomahesive (Bristol-Myers Squibb, Princeton, NJ) or Hollihesive securely around the base to protect the skin. Apply a clear pouch, allowing visualization of the drainage and stoma. One without a precut opening can best be cut to fit the individual stoma. Empty the contents frequently and rinse the pouch, as needed, with warm water. Leave the pouch in place unless it is leaking. Frequent changes add to skin irritation and breakdown. An enterostomal therapist, if available, can assist with specific techniques and individual patient problems.[43]

FEEDING PROBLEMS

It is difficult to administer adequate fluids and calories enterally to premature infants. Their small stomach capacity, incompetent esophageal cardiac sphincter, delayed gastric emptying, and poor gag reflex puts them at high risk for aspiration. They also have decreased absorption of some nutrients, necessitating small, dilute feedings.[44]

Premature infants are at quite a disadvantage when it comes to oral feedings. They usually have been given little opportunity for positive oral stimulation. They have poor suck–swallow reflexes and are unable to coordinate sucking, swallowing, and breathing. Their rooting reflex may be absent. Reduced buccal sucking pads and inability to cup their tongue makes compressing the nipple and directing the flow of milk difficult. They lack the physiologic flexion needed to support their tongue and jaw, and have weak perioral muscle tone, which limits sucking strength and endurance.[45,46]

Infants under 32 to 34 weeks of age should be gavage fed and offered a pacifier during the feeding. Sucking a pacifier has been found to help weight gain and the development of an effective suck.[47] When oral feedings are begun, hold the infant in a flexed posture with the head slightly forward. Nipple feed only when the baby is alert. Choose a nipple that fits the individual infant's sucking strength and ability to handle volume. Remain calm and relaxed, and resist the temptation to prod. Prodding does not allow the infant to learn to feed and increases the risk of aspiration. The nurse can assist by using his or her fingers to support the cheeks and the base of the tongue (*i.e.*, finger midway between the chin and the throat).[45] Stop the feeding if choking, gasping, cyanosis, apnea, bradycardia, or behavioral signs of stress occur. Observe for evidence of intolerance of the feedings (*i.e.*, reducing substances, blood, or both in the stools; abdominal distention; vomiting; diarrhea; gastric residuals).

Sick or recovering term infants also may have decreased strength and tone resulting in poor feeding behavior. They benefit from the same techniques and patience afforded a premature infant.

SKIN CARE

The transparent, gelatinous skin of the premature infant has a decreased capacity to perform critical functions such as temperature regulation, fat storage, water and electrolyte balance, and resistance to infection. It is susceptible to irritation, trauma, and infection.[32]

The bond between the dermis and epidermis is so weak that the epidermis is easily removed when adhesive tape, electrodes, and the like are lifted. Tape therefore should be kept to a minimum. If taping is necessary, Hollihesive can be used under it as a skin barrier. Transcutaneous PO_2 monitors should not be used on the VLBW infant. The electrodes can burn and tear the skin. Tape should be removed carefully with warm water and cotton balls. The increased permeability of premature infants' skin puts them at risk for toxicity from adhesive removers and alcohol.[32]

A bactericidal acid surface normally is present on an infant's skin. Bathing with alkaline soaps destroys this acid mantle. It may take more than an hour for the acid *p*H of the skin to return. It is important to avoid these soaps and to limit the frequency of bathing when possible.[32]

Frequent turning, water beds, and sheepskin can be used to minimize pressure sores. Egg crate pads should be used with caution, because a premature infant may not be able to clear his or her nose when lying prone. A semipermeable membrane (*e.g.*, Opsite, Smith & Nephew Medical, Lachine, Quebec, Canada; Tegaderm, 3M) is useful as a protective covering or second skin. It decreases irritation at pressure points (*e.g.*, knees, elbows), protects wounds from infection, facilitates wound healing, and significantly reduces transepidermal water loss. Humidifying the environment also will decrease insensible water loss and prevents the skin from drying, cracking, and peeling. The integrity of the skin usually improves by 2 weeks of age.[32]

Nurses must take an active role in protecting this vital organ. Preventing trauma, decreasing exposure to toxic substances, and maintaining the normal skin *p*H should be part of daily care.

DISCHARGE PLANNING

Discharge planning (see Chap. 59) begins during the parents' first visit to the baby's bedside. The initial planning may be very informal. By the questions the parents ask, the ICN staff begins to plan with them how and when their child will go home. Planning continues as the infant's condition stabilizes and the parents begin to feel more confident that their child will come home. As the infant's condition improves and the parents are able to participate in more caregiving activities, formal discharge teaching should begin. Each parent is ready at a different point and the nurse should decide with the parent when to begin discharge teaching. Knowing a projected discharge date is helpful. It is best if a specific nurse (*i.e.*, primary nurse/care manager) who will arrange and be responsible for discharge teaching is identified to the parents. Teaching should be individualized and allow each parent to learn in her or his own way. It should occur over a sufficient time period and allow time for the parents to demonstrate what they have learned. Information provided should be both verbal and visual, with written materials supplied as references for the parents.

A discharge teaching care plan should be available in the nursery. This can be reviewed with the parents, and specific areas of emphasis outlined. It should include the basics of newborn care: temperature taking, bathing, stooling and urination patterns, feeding, and dressing. Specific discharge teaching for the premature infant often will include medication administration, home monitoring and CPR, oxygen administration and treatments, and special feeding techniques and restrictions. Before the day of discharge, all appointments should be made and confirmed with the parents, equipment should be in the home, and teaching completed. Teaching new information on the day of discharge is rarely successful because the parents do not have time to incorporate the new information.

Parents with infants going home on monitors often benefit from spending a night rooming in with their child in the hospital. Giving parents time to practice and feel comfortable with their child, and the care they must give, leads to a more successful discharge.

REFERENCES

1. Society of Critical Care Medicine. Guidelines for categorization of services for the critically ill patient. Crit Care Med 1991; 19:279.
2. Turner SO. Dealing with medical staff: it's time to do it differently. Nursing Management 1990;21(12):52.
3. Ward CW, Cardin S. Selecting competent critical care nurse managers. In: Cardin S, Ward CW, eds. Personnel management in critical care. Baltimore: Williams & Wilkins, 1989:4.
4. Pilette PC, Kirby KK. Expectations and responsibilities of the nursing director role. Nursing Management 1991;22(3):77.
5. Porter-O'Grady T, Finnegan S. Shared governance for nursing: a creative approach to professional accountability. Rockville, MD: Aspen Systems, 1984:79.
6. Porter-O'Grady T. Creative nursing administration: participative management into the 21st century. Rockville, MD: Aspen Systems, 1986:83.
7. Wake MM. Nursing care delivery systems: status and vision. J Nurs Adm 1990;20(5):47.
8. Strasen L. Redesigning hospitals around patients and technology. Nursing Economics 1991;9:233.
9. Madden MJ, Lawrenz E. Work redesign. In: Mayer GG, Madden M, Lawrenz E, eds. Patient care delivery models. Rockville, MD: Aspen Systems, 1990:4.
10. Vanevenhoven RA, Stull MK, Pinkerton SE. The nursing shortage and staff nurse retention. In: Stull MK, Pinkerton SE, eds. Current strategies for nurse administrators. Rockville, MD: Aspen Systems, 1988:76.
11. Hesterly S, Sebilia AJ. Recognizing clinical excellence. J Nurs Adm 1986;16(12):34.
12. Secretary's Commission on Nursing. Final report. vol. 1. Rockville, MD: U.S. Department of Health and Human Services, 1988:5.
13. Hayne AN, Bailey ZW. Nursing administration of critical care. Rockville, MD: Aspen Systems, 1982.
14. Carr N. Trust relationships. In: Pinkerton SE, Schroeder P, eds. Commitment to excellence: developing a professional nursing staff. Rockville, MD: Aspen Systems, 1988:12.
15. Cole JG, Begish-Duddy A, Judas ML, et al. Changing the NICU environment: the Boston City Hospital model. Neonatal Network 1990;9(2):15.
16. Swain TJ, ed. Critical care unit design. Critical Care Nursing Quarterly 1991;14(1):1.
17. Thomas KA. Design issues in the NICU: thermal effects of windows. Neonatal Network 1990;9(4):23.
18. Myers S. Material management: nurses' involvement. Nursing Management 1990;21(8):30.
19. Stahler-Wilson JE, Worman FR. A product nurse specialist: the compleat clinical shopper. Nursing Management 1991; 22(11):36.
20. McConnell EA. Key issues in device use in nursing practice. Nursing Management 1991;22(11):32.
21. Hines C, Hansen A. CNMC neonatal intensive care unit. In Hines C, Hansen A, eds. PRN float nurse handbook. Washington, DC: 1992.
22. Kovzelove SM, Fletcher A. In: CNMC neonatal intensive care unit standard of care manual. Washington, DC: Children's National Medical Center, 1989.
23. Garner JS, Jarvis WR, Emori TG, et al. CDC definitions for nosocomial infections, 1988. Am J Infect Control 1988;16(3) 128.

23a. Frigoletto FD, Little GA, eds. Guidelines for perinatal care. Elk Grove, IL: American Academy of Pediatrics, 1988.

24. Thigpen JL. Responding to research: realistic use of scrub clothes and cover gowns. Neonatal Network 1991;9(5):41.
25. Jennings BW, Rea RE, Antopol BB, et al. Selecting, implementing, and evaluating patient classification systems: a measure of productivity. Nursing Administration Quarterly 1989;14(1):24
26. Slopes J, Ahmed I. Range of initial temperatures in sick and premature newborn babies. Arch Dis Child 1966;41:417.
27. Lawrence RA. Breastfeeding: a guide for the medical profession. St. Louis: CV Mosby, 1989.
28. Measel CP, Anderson GC. Non nutritive sucking during tube feeding: effect on clinical course in premature infants. J Obstet Gynecol Neonatal Nurs 1979;8:265.
29. Waechter EH, Phillips J, Haladay B. Nursing care of children 10th ed. Philadelphia: JB Lippincott, 1985.
30. Ferrara T, Hoekstra R, Graziano E, et al. Changing outcome of extremely premature infants (≤26 weeks' gestation and ≤750 gm): survival and follow-up at a tertiary center. Am J Obstet Gynecol 1989;161:1114.
31. Hack M, Fanaroff A. Outcomes of extremely-low-birth-weight infants between 1982 and 1988. N Engl J Med 1989;321:1642.
32. Kuller J, Tobin C. Skin care management of the low-birthweight infant. In: Gunderson L, Kenner C, eds. Care of the 24–25 week gestational age infant (small baby protocol). Petaluma, CA: Neonatal Network, 1990.
33. Southwell S. Respiratory management. In: Gunderson L, Kenner C, eds. Care of the 24–25 week gestational age infant (small baby protocol). Petaluma, CA: Neonatal Network, 1990.
34. Linton P. Behavioral development of the premature infant. Perinatology Neonatology 1986;10:27.
35. VandenBerg K. Behaviorally supportive care for the extremely premature infant. In: Gunderson L, Kenner C, eds. Care of the 24–25 week gestational age infant (small baby protocol). Petaluma, CA: Neonatal Network, 1990.
36. Als H. Individualized behavioral and environmental care for the VLBW preterm infant at high risk for bronchopulmonary dysplasia: NICU and developmental outcome. Pediatrics 1986 78:1123.

37. Merenstein G, Gardner S. Handbook of neonatal intensive care. St. Louis: CV Mosby, 1989:376.
38. Fletcher M. Respiratory physical therapy. In: Fletcher M, MacDonald M, Avery G, eds. Atlas of procedures in neonatology. Philadelphia: JB Lippincott, 1983:234.
39. Hodge D. Endotracheal suctioning and the infant: a nursing care protocol to decrease complications. Neonatal Network 1991;9:7.
40. Cotten J. A comprehensive nursing approach to the neonate with myelomeningocele. Neonatal Network 1984;2:7.
41. Frentner S. Abdominal wall defects: omphalocele and gastroschisis. Neonatal Network 1987;6:29.
42. Fuller R. Optimizing care for the infant with a tracheostomy. Neonatal Network 1986;5:55.
43. Lund C, Alterescu V. Skin care in the intensive care nursery: part III. Stoma care. Neonatal Network 1984;3:28.
44. Harper R, Yoon J. Handbook of neonatology. Chicago: Year Book, 1987:94.
45. Shaker C. Nipple feeding premature infants: a different perspective. Neonatal Network 1990;8:9.
46. VandenBerg K. Nippling management of the sick neonate in the NICU: the disorganized feeder. Neonatal Network 1990; 9:9.
47. Bernbaum J, Pereira G, Watkins J, et al. Nonnutritive sucking during gavage feeding enhances growth and maturation in premature infants. Pediatrics 1983;71:41.

Neonatology: Pathophysiology and Management of the Newborn, Fourth Edition,
edited by Gordon B. Avery, Mary Ann Fletcher, and Mhairi G. MacDonald.
J.B. Lippincott Company, Philadelphia © 1994.

chapter 7

Family-Centered Nursing Care in the Intensive Care Nursery

JUDYTH BROWN WIGGINS

Extensive study and observation during the last decades have provided a wealth of information about the effects of illness and separation not only on the infant, but also on his or her family. As early as 1907, in his book *The Nursling*, Pierre Budin, the father of neonatology, made the very cogent observation that ". . . a certain number of mothers abandon the babies whose needs they have not had to meet, and in whom they have lost all interest. The life of the little one has been saved, it is true, but at the cost of the mother."[1] Budin encouraged mothers to participate in care and to breast-feed their infants. Unfortunately, this aspect of infant care did not find its way into nurseries being established in the United States. With rare exceptions, most hospitals, concerned with preventing infection, excluded parents completely. This exclusion lasted well into the 1960s. By then it was becoming apparent that infants who had been separated from their parents for an extended period after birth were far more likely to return to the hospital later as ill-thriving or battered children.[2]

Fortunately, intensive care nurseries (ICNs) now encourage parents to visit with no concomitant increase in infection. But even with open visiting policies, the birth and hospitalization of a premature or otherwise ill newborn is emotionally stressful and disruptive of the natural course of events surrounding birth. Before this disruption can begin to be understood, some aspects of normal maternal–infant attachment must be considered.

MATERNAL–INFANT ATTACHMENT

Klaus and Kennell define attachment, bond or love as a "unique relationship between two people that is specific and endures through time."[3] They go on to describe a mother's attachment to her child as "perhaps the strongest bond in the human and the wellspring for all the infant's subsequent attachments. Throughout his lifetime, the strength and character of this attachment will influence the quality of all future bonds to other individuals."[3]

The foundations of this attachment are laid long before conception. Parents bring to a pregnancy the total of many years of accumulated experience that helps shape their perception of pregnancy, of parenting, and of their new infant. Multiple factors are at work, going back to the care each parent received from his or her own parents, the foundation for all subsequent nurturing experiences. Parental attitudes are further shaped by lifelong experiences of caring and by cultural and social values. Experiences with previous pregnancies and childbirth as well as events during the present pregnancy are significant.

Once pregnancy is confirmed, multiple factors in the mother's life and relationships influence her acceptance of the pregnancy and the fetus growing inside her. Quickening generally marks the beginning of a mother's perception of the fetus as a separate individual. Hopes and plans, fears and fantasies intermingle as pregnancy progresses. A picture of the ıoped-for, normal baby forms in the mother's mind s she prepares for labor and delivery. Most pregnant vomen, however, also have conscious or uncon-cious fears of producing a dead or deformed child. 'hese fears and the anxiety they provoke are normal nd may actually work to prepare the mother for the djustments and demands that lie before her.[4]

Ideally, labor and delivery proceed as parents and bstetrician had planned. Newton and Newton ound that mothers were most likely to be very leased with their infants at first sight if they were alm and relaxed during labor and had good rapport vith their attendants.[5] Much has been written about "sensitive period"[5a] in the mother in the hours im-ıediately after birth and its importance in the estab-shment of a bond from parent to infant.[5b,5c,5d] Stud-:s indicate that prolonged early contact of mother nd newborn has significant effects and benefits. ven with a normal birth, new parents face the task f resolving the discrepancy between features of the eal baby and the fantasized ideal. Time spent to-ether in the first hours and days of life allows this ısk to be accomplished. Any circumstance that dis-ıpts this period, such as premature birth, birth of an l or malformed infant, restrictive hospital practices, r even deep maternal anesthesia, will affect the onding process. But, as Klaus and Kennel wisely bserve,

> in spite of a lack of early contact experienced by parents in hospital births in the past 20–30 years, almost all these parents became bonded to their babies. The human being is highly adaptive, and there are many fail-safe routes to attachment. . . . If the health of the mother or infant makes this [early, prolonged contact] impossible, then discussion, support, and reassurance should help the parents appreciate that they can become as completely attached to their infants as if they had the usual bonding experience, although it may require more time.[6]

RANSFER

'hen an infant is born prematurely or with a prob-m, the nurse plays a vital role not only in the stabili-ıtion and possible transfer of the baby, but also in roviding the parents with baseline information out their newborn child. Through a comprehensive terview with the parents about the history of the regnancy, the astute nurse can start to gain a sense the parents' attitudes about the pregnancy itself ıd will be able to pass on information relevant to ırental adjustment to the health care team. Once ırents have been told that there is something wrong ith their infant, they will most likely be in a state of ıock and begin to experience anticipatory grief. The pected healthy, full-term infant has been replaced a small, sick infant. They may be hesitant to see eir infant, as a means of preparing themselves for e loss.

It is very important that the nurse ensure that the parents see and touch and, whenever possible, hold their infant. Taking the time to ask the parents if they have named their baby and thereafter referring to him or her by name help reinforce the identity of the infant. Encouraging parents to look at, touch, and hold the infant and stressing the baby rather than the equipment helps the parents deal with the infant in a more realistic way. He or she starts to become a real person rather than a fetus inside the mother's womb or a small, helpless thing attached to numerous wires and tubes. Taking several Polaroid pictures of the infant to leave with the parents is especially important if he or she is being transferred to another hospital. Pointing out the various physical characteristics of the baby that are similar to those of the parents, such as hair color or facial features, will help reinforce to his or her parents that he or she is uniquely theirs.

ADMISSION TO THE NEONATAL INTENSIVE CARE UNIT

INTRODUCTION TO THE UNIT

There is much anxiety surrounding the illness of a newborn and the separation it necessitates. Added to this shock is the adjustment to the complex and often frightening ICN. Obviously it is the staff's responsibility to reach out to these new parents with information and reassurance. Many nurseries accomplish this formally with an introductory letter or booklet designed to orient parents to this busy new place. This booklet may contain a statement of the staff's philosophy and concern. Other information includes maps of the physical layout of the hospital, with the locations of the ICN, chapel, and cafeteria. Also included are names and phone numbers of social workers and chaplains. Visiting policies are explained, and strict infection control measures are outlined. The roles of the physicians, nurse practitioners, and staff nurses are explained, and telephone contact is strongly encouraged. There also is a valuable section containing a description, with pictures, of the specialized equipment that will be used with many of the infants.

Equally important is the informal, personal orientation parents receive when they first visit. Parents always should be made to feel welcome. Who does the initial orientation often depends on when the parents appear and who is available to speak to them. Ideally, the parents can speak with their infant's primary physician and nurse and identify them as the best sources of ongoing, comprehensive information. Regardless of who speaks with the parents, it is essential that parents' reactions and concerns be recorded and communicated.

THE ROLE OF THE FATHER

If delivery has been at a perinatal center, the effects of maternal–infant separation obviously can be lessened.[7] In cases where the infant is transferred to another hospital, the father usually will be the first visitor. His normal daily pattern of activities will be severely disrupted; he typically will be visiting the baby, reporting the infant's condition back to his convalescing wife, and working an 8-hour day. He also may have concerns about the care of other children. Fathers frequently report frustrations with limited visiting and telephone policies at hospitals of birth. The father often shares his wife's dismay that she cannot visit her child with him.[8] During this time problems can arise with fathers trying to shield their wives from what may seem to be the too-harsh reality of their child's condition. Most nurseries make it clear from the outset that they withhold no information from either parent. Parents report over and over that knowing the facts, no matter how difficult, is better than not knowing what is really going on.

THE ROLE OF THE MOTHER

Meanwhile, the mother, in another part of the hospital, or in another hospital perhaps hundreds of miles away, has her own unique problems. Along with her husband, she is experiencing anticipatory grief, but if she cannot see and touch her child, her fears and fantasies only intensify her feelings. Many mothers wish to be moved from the postpartum unit to convalesce. Others prefer to stay, and postpartum nurses need to be sensitive to what a particular mother would rather do. But regardless of where she is, the mother needs frequent information about the baby. Ideally, she will feel comfortable calling several times a day, but if she does not call, the staff must be aware of this and call her. It must be determined why she has not called. Is she just afraid she will bother the staff, or is she overwhelmed and detaching herself from her infant? She may be compromised by other emotional or physical problems. Simple shyness can be overcome, but more serious problems will necessitate counseling with a social worker.

Ideally, most phone conversations will be with the same nurse who knows both the baby and the mother. But this one nurse cannot always be available. In a busy unit, especially if a nurse is speaking to a mother for the first time, there is a tendency to forge ahead with a barrage of facts and figures. Most telephone conversations will be more beneficial if the nurse starts out by asking what the parent understands about the baby or what the baby's condition was the last time the parent called. This encourages two-way conversation and helps bring misperceptions to light. It must be remembered that tone of voice is just as important as the facts communicated to the parents. Small gestures may mean a lot to the mother. The nurse should call the baby by name and stress his or her individuality and, along with the ventilator settings, mention his or her temper or dimples or silky hair. It is just as important to tell parents what is "right" about their baby as to tell them what is "wrong." The nurse also should ask how the parent is feeling, eating, and sleeping. The most important and often the most difficult thing to do when speaking with a parent is not to sound rushed.

THE MOTHER'S VISIT

Regardless of their obstetricians' recommendations, most mothers will visit their child immediately on discharge. Through telephone conversations, husband's reports, and pictures, a mother is somewhat prepared. Although many mothers are physically uncomfortable and emotionally overwrought during their first visit, most report that only after an introduction to the nursery and their baby can they begin to cope with the baby's illness.[9] The staff must think of the mother's physical well-being, because she is preoccupied with her infant. Provision of a wheelchair to get to the nursery and a comfortable seat at the bedside are helpful. Simple explanations of equipment will be needed initially, but the nurse should be sensitive to what is preoccupying the mother. She should be allowed silence to look, touch, and think. The simple question, "Well, what do you think of your daughter?" can yield much information. The nurse should promise to repeat information and reanswer questions as often as necessary, and, again, should stress the son or daughter, not the equipment or disease.

As parents continue to visit, they will benefit from the nurse's input on the special needs and limitations of their medically fragile infant. A healthy, full-term newborn infant orients to a high-pitched voice, sucks vigorously at the breast, attends with interest to a human face, molds to a caress and tightly grasps an adult's finger.[10] A high-risk infant, on the other hand, sleeps more,[11] is more difficult to arouse, and, once aroused, more difficult to soothe.[12] He or she is less apt to orient to a face or voice, and his or her grasping and sucking responses are weaker.[13] Thus, even with continuous access to the premature infant, it is more difficult for most mothers to establish a mutually rewarding flow of interactions. Parental interactions often will need to be structured early on so that negative consequences of behavior are not initiated (*e.g.*, apnea, bradycardia, desaturations). As time goes by and the infant is more available for interaction (*e.g.*, holding, feeding), the nurse can teach and encourage parents to increase their participation.[10]

CARE OF THE PARENTS OF THE CRITICALLY ILL CHILD

The birth of a premature or critically ill child immediately engulfs his or her parents in feelings of anxiety and guilt. The perfect, smiling baby they expected i not the baby they have. Their child is ill, needs intensive care, may be damaged, and may even die. Parents of a premature infant have difficulty accepting that their child actually has been born. The grieving process begins as shock and denial set in. Later, parents can recall little of what was told to them during the first hours and days after their child's birth. They do, however, remember the gentle, patient willingness of the staff to repeat information over and over to them.

The first step in acceptance of this unexpected stranger comes as parents see and touch their child. At this time, the mother in particular will begin to experience feelings of guilt and inadequacy, fearing something she did or did not do produced the prematurity or illness. If she cannot verbalize this fear, staff can help by asking her what she understands about why the child is premature or ill. Her answer can provide the opportunity to correct misconceptions and to reassure her.[9]

Anxiety is the obvious and intense emotion experienced by parents during this time. During the uncertain days when even survival is in question, parents will experience anticipatory grief. This is a reaction felt before the loss of a loved object. It is characterized by sadness, loss of appetite, inability to sleep, increased irritability, preoccupation with thinking about the baby, and feelings of guilt and anger. Episodes of crying, praying for the baby, depression, disbelief, thinking that the baby might die, and wanting to be left alone all are perfectly normal. Parents are enormously relieved when assured that all of these painful emotions are to be expected.[14] Staff must allow parents to cry and be angry at what has happened to them. The expression of their emotions may even mean angry criticism and distrust of the staff. Tolerance and understanding of this behavior are difficult but productive, and gratitude certainly will be expressed later.[14]

Although each infant's course and his parents' reactions to this course differ somewhat, all families are placed in a crisis situation when their newborn is critically ill. Caplan and colleagues define crisis as a time-limited period of disequilibrium or behavioral and subjective upset precipitated by an inescapable demand or burden to which the person is temporarily unable to respond adequately.[15] During this period of tension, the person grapples with the problem and develops novel resources by calling on internal reserves and making use of the help of others. These resources are then used to handle the precipitating factor, and the person once more achieves a steady state. Unlike developmental crises such as changing jobs or homes, the birth of a premature or ill child is an acute, unpredictable crisis that involves the pain and possible death of a loved one.[15]

Caplan and colleagues have identified three very useful categories of grappling behavior that parents will use as they struggle to achieve a steady state. After studying the responses and outcomes of 86 families to the births of premature, ill infants, they further divided these categories to identify behavior that portends a healthy or unhealthy outcome.[15]

1. Cognitive grasp of the crisis situation
   - Healthy outcome. Parents continually survey the situation and gather as much information as possible about the baby and the causes and manifestations of the prematurity or illness. Their perceptions of the child are based on reality and minimally distorted by irrational fantasies.
   - Unhealthy outcome. Parents do little active searching for evidence on which a current assessment of the situation and a judgment about outcome or plans for handling it can be made. They suppress thoughts about danger or burden. Outcome is considered in terms of a global belief: "All will be well," or "Luck will be bad." These beliefs depend more on inner fantasies than on appraisal of external realities.
2. Handling of feelings
   - Healthy outcome. Parents show continual awareness of negative feelings throughout the crisis, with free verbal and nonverbal expression of these feelings in interaction with others. Occasionally, at peak periods of stress, there will be temporary use of the defenses of denial, suppression, and avoidance, but anxiety, depression, and frustration soon give way to awareness, and a conscious attempt is made to master these feelings alone and with the help of others.
   - Unhealthy outcome. Parents make little or no verbal admission of negative feelings and pretend to be cheerful, denying discomfort. Often, the only negative feeling that is given open and continual expression is blaming others.
3. Obtaining help
   - Healthy outcome. Parents actively seek help within the family or community with tasks associated with care of their child. They also seek support and special attention to reassure, share anxieties, and relieve guilt.
   - Unhealthy outcome. Parents are reluctant or unable to seek or accept help. They do not help each other in any consistent way, and when they do it is maladaptive grappling (*i.e.*, urging denial, stimulating blaming oneself or others, bickering).

These grappling behaviors are used by parents as they move through what Caplan and associates call the four major psychologic tasks necessary to master this painful situation and provide a healthy parent–infant relationship in the future.[15]

1. Anticipatory grief involves withdrawing from the idea of the expected child. While parents hope for survival, they prepare emotionally for death. Emotions must be expressed, and attach-

ment to the real baby begun. This response occurs regardless of separation. While Klaus and Kennel suggest that early contact and frequent visits accelerate both parents' dissipation of grief and their acceptance of their small baby,[16] Taylor and Hall report that the grief response occurs even when mothers are delivered at a perinatal center and allowed unrestricted access to the ICN.[7]

2. The mother must face her feelings of failure. She will struggle with these feelings until the chances for survival seem secure.
3. Characteristically, there is a point at which the mother really begins to believe the baby will survive. This may be due to an increase in weight, a change in feeding, a change in activity or appearance, or a change in the nurse's behavior.
4. The final task is learning how to care for her particular infant with his or her unique needs and personality. This comes with time, supervised experience participating in care, and lots of encouragement. Discharge jitters can be minimized for parents and staff if assessment and teaching are started as soon as survival seems certain.

CARE OF THE PARENTS OF AN INFANT WITH A CONGENITAL DEFECT

Perhaps one of the most difficult tasks for medical personnel is helping parents of an infant with a congenital defect deal with the reality and accept their infant.

It generally is accepted that parents must be told there is something wrong with their child as soon as a reliable diagnosis is made. Parents can easily sense a problem through the attitude and actions of the staff; they will lose trust in the staff if they are ignored or told that nothing is wrong.

The task of telling parents about the baby with an anomaly is, by its nature, very difficult and unpleasant. D'Arcy interviewed a large group of mothers about how, when, and from whom they first learned of their children's defects and found the following to be true:

> . . . mothers attached great importance to the approach and general attitude of the medical and nursing staff who told them about their babies, particularly if they learned soon after the baby's birth. Very often [the mother] could not remember exactly what had been said, but she could always recall whether the informant had an understanding approach and seemed aware of her suffering. Mothers who were hurt by seeming lack of sympathy towards them tended to attribute the abruptness to lack of feeling of the informant rather than the likely cause—the difficulty of imparting such information. Most mothers were impressed by the kindness and sympathy extended to them by medical and nursing staff. Small acts of kindness were remembered years after the event.[17]

Peggy Muller Miezio, who is a nurse and the mother of a daughter born with spina bifida, points out the truth can be told gently and matter-of-factly, without use of the professional's own reactive adjectives. "I know this will be a shock to you, but your child has a condition called spina bifida. She has problems with nerve damage to the lower legs, bladder and bowel and she also has a build-up of fluid in her head called 'hydrocephalus.'" Miezio contrasts this with, "This child will always be a hopeless cripple; she will never walk or run or have bowel or bladder control, and she may be retarded as well." All aspects of the situation need to be explained in terms the parent can understand, but never with the underlying spoken or unspoken message that the child is worthless or hopeless. Miezio urges caregivers to remember that the whole truth must include not only the problems of the child but also what is positive about the situation. Assure the parents, for example, that their son has a strong cry or enjoys being held and cuddled. Other positive aspects of the situation include what treatments are possible for the child and what supports (*e.g.*, parent groups) are available for the parents. Parents also need to have a sense of what constructive action can be taken. This can be as simple and basic as "What this baby needs now is to be held and fed and loved," if no immediate surgical or medical treatments are needed. Last, the parents need and deserve the caregiver's expressions of compassion and recognition that this is indeed a severe blow.[18]

The medical staff must be aware of and sensitive to the multiple factors that make up the crisis of the birth of a child with a congenital defect. The emotional responses that parents exhibit may be prolonged. Shock and denial are followed by overwhelming grief, not unlike that expressed when a loved one dies. The anticipated perfect child is "dead." Anger also is present—anger directed toward self, family members, the medical and nursing staff, and God. Fear of the unknown, of complicated and extended health care, and of financial burden often compounds the anger. Parents experience a sense of guilt and personal responsibility at having produced a less-than-perfect child. They grieve because of the pain they foresee for the child. It is not uncommon for parents to experience depression characterized by a physical and emotional retreat and withdrawal. Patience, kindness, and understanding together constitute some of the best medicine the staff can offer.

While dealing with all these conflicts, the parents are confronted with the tasks of reorganization and attachment. If the attitude of the medical personnel has been reassuring and accepting, the parents will find it easier to believe in their self-worth and ability and the worth of their infant.

:ARE OF THE PARENTS)F A CHRONICALLY ILL CHILD

'arents of infants who are chronically ill may be the nost demanding and frustrating. Their infant usually ıas survived an acute crisis, and the parents have aced shock, denial, and anger and are trying to re- olve and reorganize their lives in relation to their hild. These parents are left in a kind of limbo, not :nowing for certain whether their child will improve ignificantly and be able to grow and develop, con- inue to maintain a state of chronic illness for an inde- erminate period of time, or die.

The parents may exhibit anger and hostility toward he staff as they see other infants admitted and dis- harged repeatedly while their child remains behind. 'eelings that the staff are not doing enough to help heir infant recover may be manifested by direct accu- ations of poor medical or nursing care or, con- 'ersely, by attempts to bribe staff members with raise or gifts in an effort to get what they believe will e better care.

Parents of a chronically ill child need consistent aretakers and communicators. They need calm, pa- ient, understanding personnel to listen quietly to heir fears and anxieties without responding person- lly to accusations. These parents need to be guided o evaluate their infant's progress over a span of time, erhaps weekly or longer rather than daily, to help elieve their feelings of frustration.

Parents may go through a period of time when they isit continually and then suddenly not visit at all for while. This seemingly erratic visiting pattern is typi- al of parents who are saturated and overwhelmed vith frustration and need a break to refresh and reor- anize themselves. The staff should be understand- ıg and supportive of the parents' behavior, and con- istent staff members such as the primary physician nd nurse should call the parents to touch base with hem and let them know of any changes.

When parents do visit, they need to be encouraged ɔ hold, cuddle, and provide tender loving care for heir infant. They should be allowed to diaper and ed their baby if possible and to participate in as ıuch care as they can. Reinforcing to parents their bility to love and care for their baby enables them to ain some sense of control and purpose during this ɔng ordeal.

)ISCHARGE TEACHING

'HE NURSE'S ROLE

:arly in the sick infant's course, it is not at all unusual ɔr a mother to experience puzzling feelings of resent- ıent and jealousy toward the nurses who care for er child. The nurses are doing what she expected to e doing—caring for her child—and for the time be- ıg they are doing a more competent job than she feels she can. Successful discharge teaching will facilitate the transition from these feelings of inadequacy and competition to feelings of self-assurance and attachment. Discharge is most satisfying and successful if done by one nurse who has come to know the infant and parents well over some time. A comfortable relationship must be established between mother and nurse to foster the learning experience. Written tools and instructions are useful only when accompanied by a personal relationship, enabling appreciation of the uniqueness of each mother and infant.[9]

READINESS TO LEARN

As described earlier, there is a definite progression in the nature and amount of physical contact a mother has with a newborn and the extent of the self-involvement she feels in his or her care. This progression is interrupted when the infant is premature or ill. By encouraging gradual participation in the baby's care as appropriate, the nurse helps reestablish this progression. Mothers have been known to call and interrupt their husbands at work to announce they have changed the diaper for the first time under their ventilator-bound son. It is essential that a mother understands that her presence and participation in care is very important to her ill infant's well-being. Furthermore, she needs to be assured that, with a little practice, she will get to know her baby better than anyone else and do the best job of all.

WHAT THE MOTHER NEEDS TO KNOW

All nursery nurses have known the frustration and confusion of discharging an infant they do not know well to a poorly prepared mother in a flurry of last-minute instructions. Early on in the hospitalization, once survival is certain, one nurse needs to assume responsibility for planning teaching. In my nursery, this is the primary nurse working with a unit-based discharge nurse and, if needed, the hospital's home care team. The primary nurse determines what this particular mother needs to know and do before she can successfully take her infant home. Every mother needs to learn how to feed, bathe, handle, and dress her child. There often are additional specific teaching needs (*e.g.*, use of an apnea monitor, gastrostomy care, administration of medications). Appropriate medical follow-up and, if needed, home nursing visits also must be arranged with the parents' input. It is useful for the nurse to begin explaining these tasks to the mother in simple terms long before discharge. The mother needs gentle reassurance that she will be comfortable with all tasks before discharge. Finally, the nurse should work out a timetable for learning with the mother. In this way, even the mother of a small, sick infant, weeks from discharge, can set goals for herself and begin to feel that her ordeal will have an end point.

Teaching will be most successful if two principles are remembered. First, a mother will learn best from one sympathetic, supportive nurse with whom she has a continuous relationship. Second, an anxious mother can misunderstand even the clearest and simplest instructions. She needs the opportunity to ask questions freely and digest material gradually over time.[9]

It is useful to have a written plan to document discharge teaching and to enable associate nurses to participate in teaching in an organized manner. This plan may be written in the patient's care plan, or a specific discharge tool may be used.[19]

Finally, many mothers benefit from a night of rooming in with their infant in a private hospital room before discharge. In my nursery, mothers are offered the opportunity of spending a night in the parent room. This affords mothers a time, usually about 12 hours, during which they can assume total care of their infants, with nursing assistance and supervision only if needed. Discharge jitters are inevitable no matter how prolonged and thorough the teaching. Only the experience of total responsibility for her infant's care will dissolve these jitters.

Most mothers report that they do not feel the baby is really theirs until they are home.[20]

CARE OF THE PARENTS OF A DYING INFANT

Despite growing medical knowledge and aggressive, sophisticated care, death comes to our nurseries. Engel states:

> Death is an intensely poignant event which touches the deepest sources of human anguish, one which each of us yearns to be spared. Yet, as doctors and nurses, it is our constant companion. How can we protect ourselves from such repeated, personal suffering? One way is to develop a shell, to insulate ourselves, to avoid engagement, to make out it does not occur or it is not our concern.[14]

Another more difficult way is to become engaged, empathizing and sticking with a family through the illness, death, and the aftermath. Only in this way can nurses bring tenderness and meaning to death amidst machines.

As has been stated, from the time the infant becomes ill, parents will experience anticipatory grief, with sadness, loss of appetite, inability to sleep, increasing irritability, and feelings of grief and anger. They are withdrawing from the expected child and getting to know the actual child while anticipating his or her death.

Death may come within hours of birth, after several long, nightmarish days, or after months of roller-coaster vigil. Each child, family, and story is different. Often, survival is uncertain and even the staff cannot predict whether or when an infant will die. The importance of staff support during this time of uncertainty has been discussed in previous sections.

AS DEATH APPROACHES

It is not often that staff and family recognize the inevitability of death at the same time. The staff has had the experience of previous deaths and can recognize the clinical changes that mean death is likely. Although parents may see the changes and hear the prognosis, real acceptance on their part can take a long time. It is difficult to find anything positive or reassuring to say to parents who are desperately grasping at straws, and staff may try to avoid anything but superficial conversation with them. Understandably, parents can perceive this change in the staff's attitude as rejection or abandonment. At this critical time, they need to feel the support of those they have come to identify as primary caregivers and emotional supports. Frequent communication of information, concern for parents' well-being, and gentle repetition of the medical situation must continue. Parents need to be allowed to hope and to ventilate feelings of anger, bewilderment, and sadness. Often they hesitate to share their feelings with busy staff. Understandably, they fear that showing anger could alienate staff and affect their infant's care. For these reasons and many others, a social worker needs to be involved in helping the parents of a critically ill or dying child.

Once staff believes an infant will die, it is only natural that they may find themselves giving less vigorous care or pulling away. Attempts to detach from the infant can be manifested by not wanting to care for the baby or needing a break. Staff also may be angry about the situation. Anger and guilt come as caregivers face their inability to cure. The staff needs opportunities to express these feelings; if left unrecognized, they can become burnt out. Caregivers must be especially mindful that these feelings can be misdirected toward the parents when they do not behave as the health care professional feels they should. Sometimes the caregiver feels angry if the parents do not call or visit as often as the caregiver thinks they should and fancies that he or she is more caring than the parents. Other times, the caregiver may criticize the parents' denial and blind hope when they will not listen to dismal predictions.

THE ACTUAL DEATH

Whenever possible, parents must be notified when death seems imminent. Some parents will very much want to be at their child's bedside. Although their grief is painful, being there is all they feel they can do. Sensitivity on the staff's part is essential in helping these parents relate to their infant at this time. Every effort should be made to facilitate parent caretaking activities, such as holding, diapering, or just stroking and talking, if parents desire. Obviously, no parent should be made to feel guilty if these activities are too difficult to face. Some parents' intense grief makes it impossible for them to even come to the hospital at the time of death.

In still other cases, mothers, particularly those with older infants, are placed in the difficult competitive position of giving up to nurses the caretaking they gave in the past. Engel stresses the need for staff to recognize and respect the mother's need to minister to her own child, yet be sensitive when she needs relief.[14] In these cases, mothers' attempts to cope will swing from tender bedside care to frantic, inappropriate bedside activity, from exaggerated praise and gratitude to doctors and nurses to harsh criticism and complaints, from tearful sentimentality to philosophic resignation. Both the mother who cannot bear to leave her child and the mother who cannot bear to enter her child's room are suffering and need opportunities to share feelings and thought.[14]

TAKING LEAVE

Near the time of the baby's death, and certainly afterward, parents need a private area to confer with staff, meet with other family members, or be alone. News of the death is best given in a private area where parents can behave naturally and, if possible, with other support people present. Numb shock may last minutes or hours before it gives way to tears and overwhelming sadness. Parents may not even remember what is said to them. Anyone who has sat with parents at this difficult time knows the gnawing feeling of not knowing what to say. Actually, once the simple facts have been gently given, it is best to allow the parents time to react and think. Silences that feel uncomfortable to the caregiver are not so to parents. Their minds and emotions are racing, and, if the caregiver sits quietly, time will bring questions and reactions from them that otherwise would not have been anticipated. Parents should be given the opportunity to take leave of their son or daughter as they wish. Often they will want to hold and be alone with their infant after death. They may ask for or should be offered the opportunity to take pictures. A lock of hair can be saved, footprints can be taken, and the hat or a blanket used for the baby can be given to the parents.

Various alternatives for burial arrangements need to be simply explained. At this time, permission for autopsy usually is requested. Printed material written especially for the parents, grandparents, friends, and siblings of infants who have died is available and can be given to parents to take home to read at a later time. Once these details have been dealt with, parents often are eager to leave. This is only the beginning of their grief and should never be the last contact with the hospital. Each nursery has different arrangements concerning who will stay in touch with parents. Someone should call them within several days to see how they are doing. Often, after the funeral is over and family and friends are gone, the parents' thoughts begin to clear. Questions can be answered and misconceptions clarified. Well-meaning relatives and friends often will try to erase the memory of the baby by dismantling the nursery, by not talking about the baby, or by reassuring the parents that they can always have another baby. Parents are invariably relieved to hear a nurse, as a professional and a friend, confirm their own feelings that although they may have other children, no one will ever take this child's place. Also, if their child has been hospitalized his or her entire life, other family members did not have the same opportunity to watch the parents interact with their child that the staff did. The caregiver is in a unique position to commend the parents on their obvious love for their child and their faithfulness in calling and visiting even when it was frightening and painful. Finally, we as health care professionals can reassure them that the somatic upheavals of sleeplessness, loss of appetite, crying, bizarre dreams, and so on, are entirely normal and will subside with time. Follow-up conferences need to be routinely scheduled to continue to help parents and detect any pathologic problems. Parents should always feel free to call nursery staff, if only just to talk about the baby with someone who knew him or her. Beware of arbitrarily assigning a specific period of time as a normal period of grieving. Mourning may last a year or more. For years to come, painful memories will return unexpectedly. The parents may go on to have other children, but no child will ever truly take the place of the child they lost.

REFERENCES

1. Budin P. The nursling. London: Caxton Publishing, 1907.
2. Klaus MH, Kennell JN. Parent–infant bonding. St. Louis: CV Mosby, 1982:35.
3. Klaus MH, Kennell JN. Parent–infant bonding. St. Louis: CV Mosby, 1982:3.
4. Brazelton TB. Effect of maternal expectations on early infant behavior. Early Child Development 1973;2:259.
5. Newton N, Newton M. Mothers' reactions to their newborn babies. JAMA 1962;181:206.

5a. Klaus MH, Kennell JH. Maternal-infant bonding. St. Louis: CV Mosby, 1976:50.

5b. Klaus MH, Jerauld R, Kreger NC, et al. Maternal attachment: importance of the first postpartum days. N Engl J Med 1972;286:400.

5c. Lozoff B, Brittenham GM, Trause MA, et al. The mother-newborn relationship. Limits of adaptability. J Pediatr 1977; 91:1.

5d. deChateau P. Effects of hospital practices on synchrony in the development of the infant-parent relationship. Semin Perinatol 1979;3:45.

6. Klaus MH, Kennell JN. Parent–infant bonding. St. Louis: CV Mosby, 1982:6.
7. Taylor PM, Paul BL. Parent–infant bonding: problems and opportunities in a perinatal center. Semin Perinatol 1979;3:1.
8. Benfield DG, Leib SA, Rector J. Grief response of parents fol-

lowing referral of the critically ill newborn. N Engl J Med 1976;294:975.

9. Prugh DG. Emotional problems of the premature infant's parents. Nurs Outlook 1953;1:461.
10. Ross GS. Parental responses to infants in intensive care: the separation issue reevaluated. Clin Perinatol 1980;7:47.
11. Saint-Ann Dargassies S. Neurological development in the full-term and premature neonate. New York: Excerpta Medica, 1974.
12. Howard J, Parmelee AH Jr, Kopp CB, et al. A neurological comparison of pre-term and full-term infants at term conceptional age. J Pediatr 1976;88:995.
13. Kurtzberg D, Vaughan HG Jr, Daum C, et al. Neurobehavioral performance of low birthweight infants at 40 weeks conceptional age: comparison with normal full-term infants. Dev Med Child Neurol 1979;21:590.
14. Engel G. Grief and grieving. Am J Nurs 1964;64:93.
15. Caplan G, Mason EA, Kaplan DW. Four studies of crisis in parents of prematures. Community Mental Health Journal 1965;1:149.
16. Klaus MH, Kennell JN. Parent–infant bonding. St. Louis: CV Mosby, 1982:287,160.
17. D'Arcy E. Congenital defects: mother's reactions to first information. Br Med J 1968;3:796.
18. Miezio PM. Parenting children with disabilities: a professional source for physicians and guide for parents. New York: Marcel Dekker, 1983.
19. Cagen J, Meier P. A discharge planning tool for use with families of high-risk infants. Journal of Obstetric and Gynecologic Nursing 1979;8:146.
20. Richards MPM. Possible effects of early separation on later development of children: a review. Clinics in Developmental Medicine 1978;68:12.

Neonatology: Pathophysiology and Management of the Newborn, Fourth Edition,
edited by Gordon B. Avery, Mary Ann Fletcher, and Mhairi G. MacDonald.
J.B. Lippincott Company, Philadelphia © 1994.

chapter 8

The Vulnerable Neonate and the Neonatal Intensive Care Environment

PENNY GLASS

Environmental factors in the neonatal intensive care unit (NICU) have major implications for the care of the sick newborn infant. Advances in medical technology during the last three decades are credited with dramatic reductions in mortality, with the point of 50% survival decreasing from birth weight of 1500 g in 1970 to less than 700 g in 1990. Morbidity among survivors, however, is a problem of increasing proportions. The rate of major morbidity has remained fairly stable, around 10%, and yet this focus on major morbidity has overlooked the much larger number of children born prematurely who have learning disabilities at school age. Broad evidence implicates the environment in the NICU as a factor in neonatal morbidity. Abnormal sensory input can be a source of potentially overwhelming stress and, at a sensitive period during development, can modify the developing brain. The NICU environment therefore assumes a crucial role in the care of the sick newborn infant.

Preterm birth is the most common single risk factor for developmental problems in childhood, and learning disability is the most pervasive developmental problem. This is a catch-all term, but includes children of low average or otherwise normal intelligence who have deficits in language, visual perception, or visuomotor integration, deficiencies in attention span, hyperactivity, or social immaturity. Such children require either special services to function in a regular classroom, or placement in a special class. Reports of school-age children who were of very low birth weight indicate that as many as one-half have learning disabilities.[1–8] Such deficits may originate from overt damage to the brain or from a more general disturbance in brain organization.

Throughout infancy, both behavioral and neurologic differences exist between full-term and preterm infants, even when matched for conceptional age. The latter often exhibit manifestations of altered brain organization, including disrupted sleep, difficult temperament, both hyperresponsivity and hyporesponsivity to sensory input, prolonged attention to redundant information, inattention to novel stimuli, and poor quality of motor function.[9–15] These precursors of learning problems in school are not fully explained by either the severity of illness among the preterm infants or by later conditions in the home environment.[10]

The sensory environment in the NICU is different in virtually every respect, both from the environment of a fetus *in utero* and from that of a full-term newborn at home. The NICU experience contains frequent aversive procedures, excess handling, disturbance of rest, noxious oral medications, noise, and bright light. These conditions are sources of stress and anomalous sensory stimulation, both of which may affect morbidity.

The immediate effects of stress are autonomic instability, apnea–bradycardia, vasoconstriction, and decreased gastric motility. Cortisol, adrenaline, and catecholamines are secreted during stress as part of an intricate hypothalamic–pituitary–adrenocortical system.[16,17] High levels of these hormones interfere with tissue healing. Even medical complications commonly associated with prematurity *per se*, such as bronchopulmonary dysplasia and necrotizing enterocolitis, may be in part stress-related diseases.[18]

Sensory input is essential during maturation. Most of the cortex is part of one of the sensory systems. Abnormal experience, both depriving and overstimulating, can modify the developing brain. The most vulnerable period occurs during rapid brain growth and neuronal differentiation.[19,20] The timing of these events for the human fetus corresponds to 28 to 40 weeks of gestation.[21] It is assumed that for the fetus the optimal sensory environment is within the womb.

The potential impact of the anomalous NICU environment on the vulnerable newborn infant has raised unabated concerns for over a decade.[22–28] A more optimal NICU environment might reduce iatrogenic morbidity and improve the outcome of sick neonates; however, the parameters are not yet well defined. This chapter summarizes the maturation of each sensory system during late fetal development, with particular reference to evidence for the prenatal onset of function; compares the intrauterine and NICU sensory experience; and critiques techniques of developmental intervention.

NEONATAL SENSORY SYSTEMS: DEVELOPMENT, DISORDERS, ENVIRONMENT, AND INTERVENTION

Maturation of all the sensory systems begins during the latter part of embryogenesis; however, the process is neither unitary nor fixed. Within each system some reciprocity between structure and function probably exists. To some extent, sensory input drives maturation.[29] In addition, the rate of maturation of each sensory system varies, with the onset of function generally in the following order: tactile, vestibular, gustatory–olfactory, auditory, and visual.[30] The senses also are interrelated—stimulation of more mature senses (*e.g.*, tactile, vestibular) influences development of later-maturing ones (*e.g.*, visual).[31] This hierarchical organization and integration of sensory function is widely recognized and lends two guiding principles for developmental intervention in the NICU: stimulation of the senses should begin with the most mature; and optimal stimulation for initial postnatal development resembles the sources naturally available to the fetus and infant—those that come from the mother. State organization will be described first, since it is a predominant neurophysiologic index of central nervous system (CNS) maturation and a marker of reactivity to environmental input.

STATE ORGANIZATION

State can be organized into five discrete stages of sleep or wake:

1. Quiet sleep
2. Active rapid-eye-movement (REM) sleep
3. Awake, inactive
4. Awake, active
5. Crying.

The infant's ability to maintain a given state as well as the smooth transition across different states reflects a level of brain maturation.

In the preterm, differentiation of sleep and wake periods are not readily apparent before 28 weeks of gestation, either behaviorally or by electroencephalographic (EEG) pattern. Subsequently, behavioral organization appears, followed by maturation of differentiated EEG patterns. The beginning of attention within periods of spontaneous awake activity is reported around 32 weeks of gestation.[32] Concordance of eye movement, EEG pattern, respiration, and behavioral parameters during sleep is evident by 36 weeks of gestation. Parallel fetal states also have been described.[33] More than 50% of sleep at this age is Active REM, diminishing with maturation. The amount of Quiet sleep increases with maturation.

Active REM sleep is accompanied by physiologic instability, including periodic respirations and associated fluctuations in oxygen saturation and blood pressure, as well as increases in cerebral blood flow and oxygen metabolism in the brain. This state decreases with maturation and with sedation. Even so, Active REM sleep may have an important beneficial affect on brain development through endogenous stimulation.[34]

Sleep–wake cycles occur approximately every 3 to 4 hours. During sleep, a Quiet–Active REM cycle occurs every 50 to 60 minutes in a newborn, compared to 90 minutes in an adult. These cycles represent only one of the endogenous rhythms that emerge in development.[35,36]

Responsivity of the infant is state dependent. When awake, body movement impedes the infant's ability to attend to visual or auditory input; thus, normal sensory responsivity is facilitated during awake, inactive periods. During sleep, reactivity to sound and touch is greater in Active REM than Quiet sleep.[37]

Disturbance in sleep can have biologic consequences for the neonate. Secretion of cortisol and adrenaline is inhibited during sleep. Growth hormone, which is released during Quiet sleep, increases protein synthesis and mobilization of free fatty acids for energy use.[38,39] Thus, sleep, particularly Quiet sleep, facilitates healing and can even be a response to stress. Neonates are noted to have a prolonged period of Quiet sleep after painful procedures.[16]

TACTILE SYSTEM

The cutaneous system includes sensation of pressure, pain, and temperature. Only pressure will be discussed here; pain is discussed in Chapter 58. Receptors in the skin respond to pressure, and then transmit impulses to the spinal cord through the dorsal root, ascending in the posterior tract and terminating in the gray matter of the cord. At this point, connecting fibers decussate and continue in the ventral spinothalamic tract to the medulla and the thalamus, terminating in the postcentral gyrus of the cortex. Representation here is somatotopic and contralateral to the stimulated side.

DEVELOPMENT

Like the vestibular system, the tactile sense develops early in fetal life and is thought to play a particularly pervasive role in the early development of the organism. Receptor cells are present in the perioral region in the fetus by the eighth week of gestation and spread to all skin and mucosal surfaces by the twentieth week. The cortical pathway is intact by 20 to 24 weeks of gestation, and some myelin is present at that time. Response to tactile stimulation has been observed by ultrasound as early as 8 weeks of conceptional age.[40,41] Response to stroking of the lip is first, followed by a response to stimulation of the palms. Most of the body is sensitive to touch by 15 weeks.[42]

Tactile threshold is very low in the preterm infant. It is more related to postconceptional age (PCA) than to natal age but increases by term. Infants younger than 30 weeks PCA respond by an unequivocal leg withdrawal to pressure of a 0.5 g von Frey hair applied to the plantar surface of the foot, compared to 1.7 g pressure by 38 weeks PCA.[43] A qualitative shift occurs around 32 weeks PCA. Infants under than 32 weeks PCA respond to repeated stimulation with sensitization and a diffuse behavioral response. In contrast, infants after this age show habituation to the same stimuli.

DISTURBANCES

Classic studies by Harlow and Harlow demonstrated the profound importance of contact comfort in development.[44] The tactile hypersensitivity or tactile defensive behavior contained in clinical reports of preterm infants and children may be a manifestation of overt brain damage or disordered sensory integration. It is seen in some infants who otherwise appear normal. Behaviorally, this appears as an infant's overreaction to touch, usually in specific areas of the body. Some infants are intolerant of food with texture. With oral hypersensitivity, the infant may gag or retch when touched even around the outside of the mouth. Infants also may be hypersensitive to touch on their extremities, with exaggerated hand and toe grasp or leg withdrawal. An extreme case was a 2-month-old (corrected age) infant who when supine arched his buttocks off the table surface in response to his legs being grasped. Later manifestations of tactile sensitivity may appear as an intolerance for handling play materials of certain textures. In one extreme example, a 1-year-old infant would gag when grasping dry macaroni. Some children are intolerant of normal clothing or do not like body contact. Such aversion affects parent–infant bonding. The link between early tactile disturbances and learning disabilities at school age is indicated by excessive attention to the feel of objects rather than to their functional attributes.

INTRAUTERINE EXPERIENCE

The fetus is housed in a thermoneutral, fluid-filled space that is a source of cutaneous input throughout the body surface. Fetal movement provides tactile self-stimulation. As term approaches and the intrauterine space becomes more constraining, the posture of flexion evokes body-on-body tactile feedback.

After a normal term birth, a ventral–ventral position is preferred by both mother and infant, with touch followed by slow stroking.[45] Traditionally, the infant is then swaddled and held.

TOUCH AND HANDLING IN THE NICU

After premature birth, tactile input is radically altered. The extrauterine fetus is typically nursed naked, with the exception of maybe a diaper and a hat. The surface of the mattress generally is unyielding. She or he is exposed to air currents, cold stress, tape, instruments, handling by caregivers, and painful stimuli. Pressure is not uniform.

The type and frequency of tactile stimulation imposed on a preterm newborn in the NICU would be overwhelming even for a healthy adult. Over a 2-week period, a sick neonate may be handled by more than ten different nurses, in addition to physicians, occupational or physical therapists, laboratory and x-ray technicians, and finally the parent.[46] Handling occurs more often among the sickest infants, is typically related to procedures, is generally disturbing, and often is painful. In spite of wide attention in the literature over the last decade to the consequences of excess handling in the NICU, the amount has not decreased from 1976 to 1990, even among the more severely ill infants.[46a] On the average, sick preterm newborns are handled more than 150 times a day, with less than 10 minutes of consecutive uninterrupted rest.[26] The biologic and immunologic consequences of disturbing sleep were described earlier.[35–39]

Excess handling has other significant physiologic consequences for the sick neonate. Blood pressure changes, alterations in cerebral blood flow, and decreased transcutaneous partial pressure of oxygen ($TcPO_2$) are associated with noxious procedures, handling, or crying.[47–51] Fluctuations in blood pressure may contribute to intracranial hemorrhage in the unstable preterm infant.[52] Importantly, when caretakers monitor the infant's level of oxygenation during procedures, the severity of hypoxemic episodes can be significantly reduced.[47] Thus, the amount and type of handling may have direct detrimental consequences for the vulnerable neonate.

In addition to the hemodynamic impact of obviously noxious procedures described earlier, more benign manipulations, such as those that occur during neurodevelopmental assessment, also may adversely affect the preterm infant.[25,51] Decreased plasma growth hormone has been reported after administration of the Brazelton neonatal assessment scale (NBAS) to preterm infants at 36 weeks PCA.[53] Even at the time of discharge, the evaluation was associated with elevated cortisol levels.[17,54] It is not clear whether these effects were from the neurodevelopmental assessment or from the stress associated with crying, which normally occurs during administration of the NBAS. Handling could be stressful even for stable preterm infants.

TACTILE INTERVENTION IN THE NICU

Intervention studies in the tactile modality encompass both the reduction of general handling and the provision of planned touch experiences. Touch may be pressure alone or may include stroking. The distinction is an important one. As part of an individualized approach to developmental care for acutely ill preterm infants, Als and her associates provided "minimal handling" and clustering of routine procedures, as well as positive tactile input and containment from bunting, rolls, positioning, and the like.[55] The immediate goal was to stabilize autonomic function, state, and motor organization in a hierarchical manner. Stimulation of interactive processes occurred last. Outcome was improved for her intervention group compared to a nonintervention group. Her technique has had a major impact on developmental intervention as a whole, although it is not possible to isolate which aspect of this multimodal approach was effective.

More specifically, Jay evaluated the effects of planned, gentle, tactile contact for 12-minute periods four times a day for preterm infants on mechanical ventilation.[56] This intervention, which consisted of hands-on contact but not stroking or manipulating, was associated with a lower fraction of inspired oxygen (FiO_2) after 5 days compared to a similar nonintervention group. Hands-on contact is most effective in responding individually to an infant but would be more appropriate if not temporally regimented.

In apparent contrast, Field and associates initiated a touch intervention that differed from that of Jay and Als in important respects: the infants were recruited when "stable and growing" rather than during an acute period; the treatment provided three 15-minute periods a day of massage (*i.e.*, stroking and passive limb movement) for a 10-day treatment period.[57,58] The massaged infants showed a greater weight gain, even though the groups did not differ in formula intake. These early effects on growth are thought to be mediated by induction of catecholamine release.[53] The massaged infants also spent more time awake, showed better performance on the Brazelton neonatal assessment, were discharged home 6 days sooner, and had better performance on developmental assessment at 8 months past term. In related research, the tactile intervention group performed better on later tests of auditory and visual function than preterm infants who did not receive the intervention.[13,59] Finally, preterm infants will seek and maintain greater contact if the tactile source contains rhythmic stimulation.[60] These findings provide strong support for intervention in the tactile modality.

Although overall effects of tactile intervention have been strong, the response of individual infants is variable and deserves attention. For example, an increase in periods of oxygen desaturation during parent touch, compared to baseline, has been reported.[61] A number of infants have responded with apnea and bradycardia to the type of intervention described by Field and colleagues.[57,58] This physiologic response may occur after the intervention. It is not clear whether the intervention itself was excessive or whether the abrupt shift after the cessation of tactile input leads to an unexpected physiologic response. Individual differences exist among caregivers that also affect the infants' response to the stimulation. Finally, the distinction between touch, stroking, and massage is probably important.

All of these issues advise against standardized protocols of stroking or massage for all preterm infants. When any form of tactile and kinesthetic intervention is applied, the caregiver should continue to monitor the infant's physiologic and behavioral responses before onset, during, and after the cessation of the intervention. Consistency of contact across caregivers would help.

Soft swaddling or clothing may provide tactile input in a more sustained fashion than periodic hands-on contact. Arguments that this obscures the view of the infant and interferes with temperature regulation by servocontrol simply argue against servocontrol rather than against covers. Clothing or swaddling could actually dampen the fluctuations in temperature that occur during incubator care and inhibit exaggerated movement or agitation, which in itself may be stabilizing. Creative swaddling with crisscrossed strips and Velcro could allow for more visualization of the infant.

Thus, the amount and type of stimulation are important and change with acuity, maturation, and the response by the infant. Parents need specific guidance and modeling from the beginning. The general order of tactile intervention might be: *if acutely ill*, minimal handling, containment (*e.g.*, swaddling rolls), gentle touch (*e.g.*, warm hand) without stroking; *when medically stable*, holding, rocking gently, and stroking. Minimal handling protocols have a definite place in the NICU but not as the end point. It also is important during the hospital stay to help the infant develop increased tolerance for social contact and gentle handling, especially as discharge approaches. Systematic desensitization may even be necessary.

Nonnutritive Sucking. Nonnutritive sucking (NNS) represents an early endogenous rhythm and a manifestation of sensorimotor integration.[62] It is reported in the fetus[63] and observed in the preterm newborn at least by 28 weeks of gestation. Increase in the number of sucks per burst occurs with maturation. Duration of the burst appears fairly stable across ages.

Nipples used for NNS abound, varying in size, configuration, consistency, and utility. A feeding nipple is not designed for NNS and is inappropriate. It readily collapses; the infant experiences little resistance to his or her suck and may loll the device. Gauze inserted in the nipple may absorb oral secretions and breed bacteria. In larger infants, the nipple is unsafe because of possible aspiration. A variety of commercially available pacifiers should be available in any NICU to suit the individual needs of each infant. Some neonates who are hypersensitive to touch in the perioral region often respond first to their hands swaddled near their face.

Nonnutritive sucking experience may facilitate important physiologic and behavioral mechanisms and even reduce cost of care. Infants provided with NNS during gavage feeding have shown significantly improved gastrointestinal transit time, greater suck pressure, more sucks per burst, and fewer sporadic sucks. They initiated bottle feeding earlier, showed better weight gain, and thereby shorter hospital stay.[64,65] Having a pacifier continuously available, however, may not be beneficial and may in fact encourage inappropriate sucking patterns, particularly in the chronically ill neonate.

Nonnutritive sucking can act as organizer or facilitator. It has been shown to decrease motor activity and increase quiet states in stable preterm infants.[66] It dampens an infant's behavioral response after a painful procedure such as circumcision or heelstick,[67,68] although it does not appear to dampen the cortisol response.[17] It is noteworthy that sucking on a pacifier before the onset of repeated painful procedures such as heelsticks may be inappropriate, because simple aversive conditioning to the pacifier could occur.

VESTIBULAR SYSTEM

The vestibular system responds to movement as well as directional changes in gravity and is situated in the nonauditory labyrinth of the inner ear. The three fluid-filled semicircular canals lie at right angles to each other, one for each major plane of the body. The ampulla, located at the end of each canal, contains hair fibers in a sac or cupula. Motion of the body or head causes pressure changes that move the cupula, which stimulates the hair cells and transmits an impulse along the vestibular portion of the VIIIth nerve to the vestibular nuclei of the medulla. The vestibular organs consist of the utricle and saccule, which respond to changes of head position involving linear motion. The macula, a thickening in the wall of the utricle and saccule, contains hair cells sensitive to position of the head. Impulses from the macula transmit along the vestibular nerve to the medulla and cerebellum. From there, information is transmitted to motor fibers going to the neck, eye, trunk, and limb muscles. There are no connections to the cortex.[69]

DEVELOPMENT

Initial vestibular development is concurrent with auditory development, emanating from the same otocyst early in gestation. The three semicircular canals begin to form before 8 weeks of gestation, reaching morphologic maturity by 14 weeks, and full size by week 20.[29] The vestibular sacs probably develop at the same time. Response to vestibular stimulation has been observed by 25 weeks of gestation.[42] The traditional vertex presentation of the fetus at term gestation is thought to occur from fetal activity in response to vestibular input.

DISTURBANCES

Considerable research with animals has demonstrated the importance of both tactile and vestibular input.[44,70] Lack of normal vestibular stimulation in the developing organism is thought to affect general neurobehavioral organization.[31] Children who were born preterm are reported to have deficits in balance at preschool age,[8] but this is not necessarily a vestibular problem.

INTRAUTERINE EXPERIENCE

The fetus experiences both contingent and noncontingent vestibular stimulation that varies during gestation. From the beginning of embryonic life, the fluid environment of the womb provides periodic oscillations and movements that emanate from normal movements of the mother as well as activity of the fetus itself. Reports by mothers of fetal movement occur around 16 weeks. After 28 weeks of gestation, there is a decrease in the relative amount of amniotic fluid, and thus the movement of the fetus becomes partially constrained by the more limited physical space. Vestibular experience is then less contingent on self-activation and more related to normal maternal activity and position change. In general, maternal activity level slows as parturition approaches.

After birth, the infant is held. Movement is slow from maternal breathing and shifting. Change of position is gradual. Vestibular stimulation affects state—moving to upright increases arousal; monotonous side-to-side rocking, walking, and parental pacing reduce the level of arousal.

EXPERIENCE IN THE NICU

Vestibular stimulation after preterm birth is limited to efficient manipulation or turning of the neonate by the caregiver. It certainly lacks any of the temporal qualities or contingencies that the maternal environment may have provided. Spontaneous limb movement generally is diffuse, often unrestricted, and typically disorganizing in its effect.

INTERVENTION IN THE NICU

Like the tactile sense, the early development of the vestibular system provides a theoretical basis for primary intervention with preterm neonates. In an early study, Neal demonstrated that daily rocking facilitated the development of preterm infants.[59] More recent attempts simulate the intrauterine environment and provide compensatory vestibular stimulation. An oscillating waterbed was devised, which moved with the rhythm of maternal respirations but with an amplitude less than 2.5 mm at the surface of the unoccupied waterbed. The safety of this paradigm as well as efficacy in reduction in apnea of prematurity has been well demonstrated.[71] Furthermore, the infants on waterbeds demonstrated more organized sleep state and motor behavior, decreased irritability, enhanced visual alertness, and improved somatic growth.[71–74]

Difficulty in nursing sick infants on an oscillating surface may have precluded more widespread adoption of the waterbed. An infant's own movement may induce more than optimal movement, as for example an infant with gastroesophageal reflux; however, some babies are still likely to benefit. At the least, it would seem prudent to provide a trial on a waterbed for a nonventilated infant with apnea of prematurity before introduction of pharmacologic intervention.

Other sources of vestibular stimulation, such as rocking chairs, swings, and hammocks have not been formally investigated. Rocking chairs probably belong in any nursery. Swings are questionable, given the excessive upright position of the baby and the standard rate of oscillation (*i.e.*, too fast). A crib has been devised that provides controlled motion similar to a woman walking; the motion may be individually controlled and faded.[75] It appears to be effective in modulating fussiness in full-term infants and is currently being tested with preterm infants.

Positioning. The physical position of an infant is part of the NICU tactile–vestibular experience. Nursing sick preterm infants has routinely been with the infant in supine, which may simplify management but may not be advantageous for the infant. For example, Yu and colleagues demonstrated that gastric emptying was facilitated in either prone or right lateral positions compared to supine or left lateral.[76] This was particularly significant for the sick preterm who already showed a delay in gastric emptying. Prone position, compared to supine, is associated with more Quiet sleep and less Active sleep or crying. Quiet sleep is in turn associated with improved lung volume, more stable respiration, less apnea, and improved PaO_2.[77,78] Finally, prone position compared to supine is associated with a higher PaO_2 among healthy preterm infants and, even more significantly, in those with respiratory distress syndrome.[78,79] The evidence would suggest that, when possible, the sick preterm infant should be nursed in a prone or in the right lateral position.

When preterm infants return for neurodevelopmental follow-up, parents often complain that their baby's feet turn out. In fact, the legs are more often externally rotated at the hip. Grenier has described hip deformities on roentgenograms for preterm infants after prolonged nursing in a frog-leg position.[80] Winging of the scapula also is frequent in the preterm infant.

Proper support of the trunk and limbs in prone or supine positions lessen this extreme rotation and may diminish orthopaedic or neuromuscular complications. In prone, placing the infant on a small folded strip could allow better adduction of the shoulders and hips. In side lying, it may be easier to position the infant in soft flexion. Gentle containment of the limbs usually can be managed with strips of soft cloth across the upper arm and thigh. Some movement should be allowed within a controlled range. If the supine position is unavoidable, then a posture of physiologic flexion also would be desirable, with particular attention to shoulders and hips. Maintenance of postures can be facilitated by nesting the infant in soft rolls. Some modification with each infant is necessary.

For older, more medically stable preterm infants, infant seats often are used as an alternative to continuous lying in bed. The infant should be swaddled and nested, the angle probably should be no more than 30°, and the length of time limited. Oxygen desaturation has been reported in stable preterm infants placed in car seats.

Kangaroo Care. Kangaroo care is a technique that evolved primarily in South America.[81] The infant is clad only in a diaper and placed under the mother's clothing between her breasts, remaining there according to the mother's comfort, and feeding on demand. The technique provides fairly sustained multimodal stimulation: tactile, vestibular, proprioceptive, olfactory, and auditory. It appears to be safe for larger preterm infants or those who are medically stable. Temperature regulation in the infant does not appear to be a problem, but needs to be carefully monitored on an individual basis. It seems to have the greatest benefit in terms of facilitating and maintaining lactation and enhancing maternal sense of competency for these infants. Fathers enjoy the experience as well. The studies, however, are of insufficient sample size to evaluate whether morbidity, such as intracranial hemorrhage, is increased. More data are needed among stable infants before kangaroo care should be attempted with very-low-birth-weight infants or those requiring mechanical ventilation.

CHEMICAL SENSES

The chemoreceptors include taste and olfaction. Taste receptors are in the taste buds, which are located primarily in the papillae of the tongue but also are found on the soft palate and epiglottis.[29,82] Taste stimuli (*i.e.*, sweet, sour, bitter, salt) transmit to the brain stem with a primary branch to the hypothalamus. Cortical regions are involved in learned taste preferences. The olfactory receptors are located in the lining of the olfactory epithelium in the posterior portion of the nasal passage. The afferent pathway has no cortical projection area, but is direct to the limbic system.

DEVELOPMENT OF TASTE

The chemoreceptors are well developed within the first trimester.[29,82] Taste buds appear around 8 to 9 weeks of gestation. The receptors are present at least by the sixteenth week of gestation, and increase by term to adult levels. During the second one-half of gestation, morphologic changes occur that continue after term. By term, taste is sufficiently sensitive to detect a 0.1 mol/L concentration of NaCl in water.[83] Postnatal development is associated with changes in taste preferences and sensitivity.

Taste discrimination has been measured by differential consumption, autonomic responses, and facial expressions. Full-term neonates as well as anencephalic infants demonstrate differential behavioral responses to sweet, bitter, sour, and salty.[84] In a behavior described as "savoring," normal newborns discriminate between different concentrations of sucrose and even among various sugars.[83] Taste discrimination has been demonstrated in the preterm infant, who will pucker with a sour taste.[84] Finally, taste receptors are functional before birth. It is well known that the human fetus swallows amniotic fluid. Injection of distinct tastes into the amniotic fluid of pregnant women between 34 and 39 weeks of gestation altered fetal swallowing behavior, which increased with the sweeter taste and decreased with bitter.[29]

DEVELOPMENT OF OLFACTION

The olfactory epithelium is evident around 5 weeks in the lining of the posterior nasal passage. Nerve fibers and cells form the olfactory nerve, which extends from the epithelium to the ventral wall of the forebrain. At that time, the olfactory bulb develops.[29] No information exists about the functional onset of human olfaction, but it is thought to be present prenatally, having been demonstrated in a rat model. Rat fetuses exposed to citral in the amniotic fluid will selectively attach postnatally to a nipple of the same scent.[85]

Prenatal olfactory function also is inferred from the sophistication present by term, including behavioral discrimination, preference, and conditioning to olfactory stimuli. For example, 1-week-old infants will reliably turn their head away from a noxious smell.[86] In response to a series of pleasant or aversive odors, infants less than 12 hours old will exhibit different facial expressions that are discriminable by adults.[84] Infants under 1 week of age reliably prefer the odor of their mother's breast pad to the breast pad of another mother.[87] Neonates who were given a period of familiarization to a novel odor subsequently demonstrated a preference for that odor, whereas infants exposed to it for the first time did not.[88] Finally, classical conditioning to a novel olfactory stimulus has been empirically demonstrated within the first 48 hours after term birth.[89] Given ten 30-second pairings of citrus odor with stroking, neonates the following day showed increased activity and head turning in the presence of the citrus but not to a novel odor.

DISORDERS

Feeding disorders are reported commonly among preterm infants, particularly those with chronic lung disease. The cause generally is attributed to frequent stressful procedures around the mouth as well as poor coordination of suck–swallow–breathing. No systematic research, however, has been done to address whether deficits in taste or smell are present. The injury could be either peripheral or central. Certainly in adults, loss of the sense of smell radically affects eating habits. Significantly, olfaction also is considered an important aspect of maternal–infant bonding and may even be mutual.[88]

INTRAUTERINE EXPERIENCE

The amniotic fluid is a complex solution of suspended particulate and dissolved odorants that changes in volume and chemical composition during the pregnancy.[29,90] The fluid is swallowed by the fetus, bathing taste and olfactory receptors. The fetus contributes to the chemical status through urination, oral mucosa, lung secretions, and the mother contributes to the chemical status through hormones. It is not known whether these chemical changes are sufficient to overcome adaptation effects in the receptor cells, although the normal episodic closing of the mouth would change the oral environment sufficiently to stimulate the cells.[29]

EXPERIENCE IN THE NICU

The environment in the NICU has not been described previously in terms of gustatory or olfactory content, but it clearly is not well adapted here. Stimulation of taste receptors in sick as well as extremely premature neonates is absent. Oral feeding is initiated as soon as the preterm infant has a reasonably coordinated suck–swallow reflex, often by 32 to 34 weeks of gestation. The chemical composition of the breast milk or formula is different from amniotic fluid or colostrum. The addition of oral medications, electrolyte supplements, as well as common changes in formula composition and concentration, introduce wide variability. Noxious-tasting medication repeatedly administered orally and temporally associated with feeding could lead to aversive conditioning. More research in this area would be clinically productive. Quite obviously, avoiding aversive experiences would likely benefit feeding behavior. Finally, in contrast to the healthy full-term neonate, preterm infants lack a stable olfactory source that would be provided by sustained body contact of a consistent caretaker.

INTERVENTION IN THE NICU

The chemoreceptors present a potential avenue for intervention that has not been explored. For example, the evidence with full-term infants described earlier would suggest a period of familiarization with the odor of breast milk or formula before introduction of oral feeding.[88] Familiarization with the odor of medications before ingestion may even help. Similarly, small tastes of formula before the introduction of the nipple may foster behavioral organization and facilitate the onset of feeding.[90] Finally, like breast milk from the source, the feeding should be at body temperature rather than the typical room temperature.

Positive stimulation of taste receptors may have applications beyond basic feeding. Recent studies in the fetal rat model demonstrated that intraoral infusion of milk stimulates the endogenous opioid systems and raises the threshold to noxious tactile stimuli, whereas intragastric infusions do not.[90] Furthermore, parallel research with human infants has suggested that sucrose on the tongue may modulate the response to pain through endogenous opioid release.[91] All these considerations suggest that gut priming probably should not bypass the mouth entirely; colostrum may have an unsuspected role in initiation of feeding; and surfactant replacement may have a broader role than pulmonary function alone.

AUDITORY SYSTEM

The auditory system is composed of both peripheral and central components.[92–94] Sound waves are conducted through the auditory canal and physically displace the tympanic membrane. Movement of the membrane is amplified by the ossicles in the middle ear and transmitted to the oval window. This action displaces fluid in the cochlea. A mechanical disturbance differentially displaces hair cells at a specific place on the basilar membrane of the cochlea, as a function of both frequency and intensity of the sound. These hair cells are the sensory receptor cells of the ear. The complex neural impulse thus generated proceeds to the auditory cortex via the cochlear nucleus, superior olivary nucleus, inferior colliculus, and medial geniculate body. The primary cortical reception area is the Herschl gyrus in the temporal region. Approximately 60% of the nerve fibers from each ear transmit to the contralateral hemisphere. The initial development of the central component of the auditory system is independent of peripheral maturation; however, once the auditory pathway is complete, the absence of auditory stimulation will cause cortical neuronal degeneration.[94]

DEVELOPMENT

The development of the auditory system begins around 3 to 6 weeks of gestation.[94,95] Although the adult dimensions of the external auditory canal, tympanic membrane, and middle ear cavity will not be attained until 1 year after birth, all the major structures of the ear are essentially in place by 25 weeks of gestation. The ossicles have evolved from a thickening of mesenchymal tissue and are of adult proportions, although residual mesenchyme may diminish auditory thresholds. The cochlear nucleus has reached adult proportions and differentiated sufficiently to be functional by this time, although microscopically the cochlea still is not mature even at term. The hair cells are fully present and in a process of differentiation. The frequency-specific place on the basilar membrane is shifting during this period of development.[94] The afferent pathway from the cochlea to the auditory cortex is complete, and even myelination of the auditory pathway is present.

With regard to function, both cortical auditory evoked responses (CAER) and brain stem auditory evoked responses (BAER) can be elicited by 25 to 28 weeks.[96,97] The morphology is different from the full-term infant's, and the latency is prolonged. A blink response to vibroacoustic stimulation has been obtained in human fetuses of 24 to 25 weeks of gestational age. A more complex behavioral response to sound occurs at least by 28 weeks, but readily fatigues. The maximum rate of electrophysiologic change occurs in the CAER and BAER between 28 and 34 weeks of gestation. Orienting behavior to soft sound can be elicited by this time.

Maturation of the fetal auditory system is marked by an increase in the spectral sensitivity, in both lower and higher frequencies, and a decrease in auditory threshold.[92–94] The range of auditory sensitivity initially is fairly restricted: from 500 to 1000 Hz in the third trimester, compared to around 500 to 4000 Hz at term, and an adult range of 30 to 20,000 Hz. Changes in auditory threshold are related to maturation of both peripheral and central components. Auditory thresholds in a preterm infant at 25 weeks of gestation have been obtained with a 65-dB stimulus, compared to 25 dB at term.

Evidence for a functional auditory system in the fetus is strong. Specific anatomic sites are present in the cortex that are responsible for processing complex sounds, such as language. A biologic predisposition to respond to the specific acoustic patterns of speech is present in neonates. For example, they have lower thresholds for sound within the most important range for speech perception (*i.e.*, 500–3000 Hz).[98] Within this frequency range, they respond differently to speech and nonspeech stimuli. There are even hemispheric differences in auditory evoked potentials that support this language sensitivity.[99] Finally, healthy full-term neonates demonstrate a preference for sound they were exposed to *in utero*. Research has shown that 2- to 4-day-old neonates prefer heartbeat sounds and placental sounds to noise; female to male voice; their mother's voice compared to another female voice; and a recording of a story read by their mother prenatally to a recording of a story read by their mother that was not read prenatally.[100–104]

DEFICITS

Preterm infants are at increased risk for sensorineural hearing loss as well as developmental language disorders. In a follow-up study of preterm infants, Schulte and colleagues reported sensorineural hearing loss in over 10%, compared to 0.5% reported among children in general.[20] Language disorders may be receptive or expressive problems. Auditory processing deficits include difficulty in discrimination of speech sounds, and disorders involving syntax, semantics, or auditory memory. These deficits are the result of direct damage to central structures as well as incidental to more general brain dysfunction. They occur in children with normal hearing thresholds and otherwise normal intelligence. They occur more commonly among children born preterm.[105]

INTRAUTERINE EXPERIENCE

Development of this sophisticated auditory system occurs within a uterine environment that contains rhythmic, structured, and patterned sound emanating predominantly from the mother. Internal sounds include maternal respirations, borborygmi, placental and heart rhythms, and the like. Maternal speech transmits both externally and internally. Prosody (*i.e.*, intonation, rhythm, stress) is probably the most salient aspect of speech available to the fetus. The intensity of internally recorded sound within the amniotic fluid is approximately 70 to 85 dB, with a predominance of low frequency (Fig. 8-1).[106] External sound also is transmitted to the fetus, but is attenuated by the time it reaches the intrauterine cavity, more so at higher frequencies (*i.e.*, 70 dB at 4000 Hz) than lower frequencies (*i.e.*, 20 dB at 50 Hz).[107] Given these considerations, the fetus probably is minimally exposed to frequencies above 1000 dB.[108] The available frequencies *in utero* also parallel cochlear development.[101]

The auditory environment in the womb likely provides the substrate for normal development of the sensory system, but defining the acoustic properties of the sound actually transmitted to the inner ear of the intrauterine fetus is problematic. The fluid-filled womb would alter the conductive property of the middle ear; data are unavailable. The best guess generally is that fetal hearing is limited to bone conduction. Hearing thresholds are elevated in the prematurely born infant, but no unequivocal data are available on the actual hearing thresholds of the fetus *in utero*.

After a normal full-term birth, the auditory environment is quiet by contrast. This may serve to increase the salience of the human voice. Early speech to the neonate is subdued.

NICU ENVIRONMENT

The acoustic environment in the NICU differs from the intrauterine environment in peak intensity, spectral characteristics, and pattern (see Fig. 8-1). Ambient noise is generated by motors, fans, ventilator equipment, personnel, telephones, alarms, hand-washing areas, trash lids, pagers, intercoms, and carts, to name a few. The intensity of background noise is around 50 to 60 dB and therefore not louder than *in utero*, although episodic bursts of higher intensity (*i.e.*, >100 dB) occur. It would appear (see Fig. 8-1) that speech input for the neonate is selectively masked by the NICU auditory environment.

The auditory environment is different for babies nursed in open beds or in incubators. To some degree, the incubator may partially attenuate high-frequency room noise (see Fig. 8-1), but produces its own background noise level for the baby within (*i.e.*, 50–70 dB). In addition, the infant in an incubator may be subjected to the closing of porthole doors, an object being placed on the top surface, or rapping on the incubator to stimulate an infant who is apneic or bradycardic, which may peak over 100 dB.[74]

EFFECT OF THE NICU ENVIRONMENT

Exposure to aberrant noise levels in the NICU may cause sensorineural damage, induce stress, and contribute to language or auditory processing disorders in the preterm neonate. Schulte and colleagues reported nearly 12% hearing loss in a follow-up of preterm infants.[20] Damage to the outer hair cells of the cochlea of neonatal guinea pigs has been reported after exposure to noise of similar intensities and frequencies found in the NICU.[109] These researchers

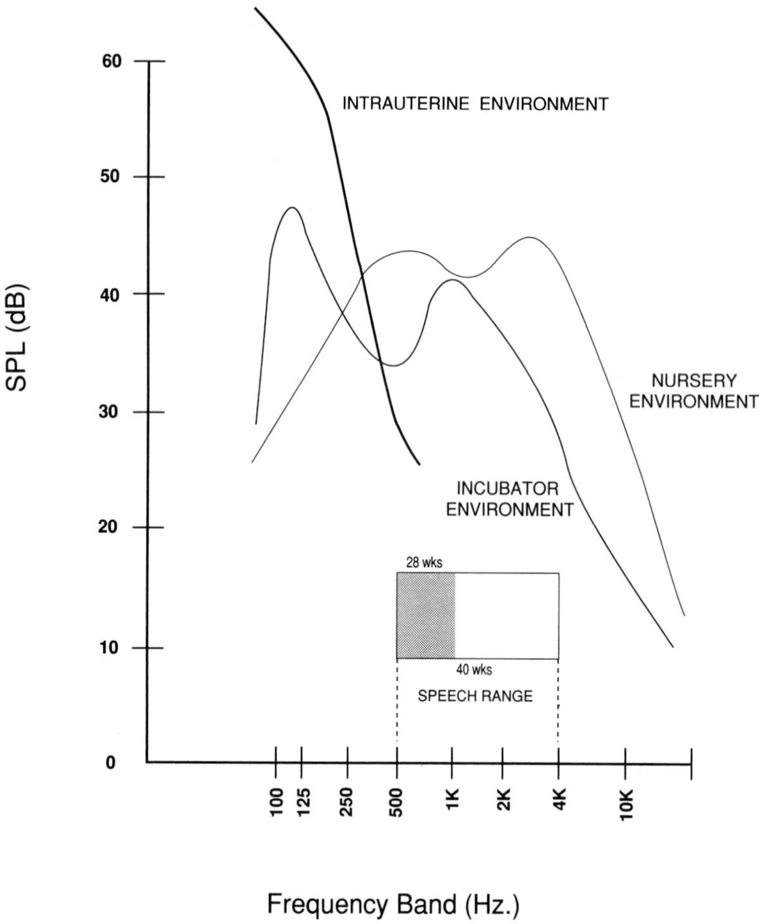

FIG. 8–1. Comparison of the frequency-specific auditory environment of the fetus *in utero* and the preterm infant in the neonatal intensive care unit. (Data from Walker D, Grimwade J, Wood C. Intrauterine noise: a component of the fetal environment. Am J Obstet Gynecol 1970;109:91, and Otho Boone, personal communication, December 1992.)

found no correlation between hearing loss and duration of exposure to incubator noise, but did report an association between hearing loss and a measure of severity of illness. Although not stated, more severely ill neonates may be exposed to increased NICU noise compared to healthy preterm infants. In other research, the combination of noise and ototoxic drugs commonly given to sick preterm infants (*e.g.*, aminoglycosides, diuretics) was found to have a potentiating effect on hearing loss.[110,111] The data further suggest that the immature cochlea may be more susceptible to damage than the mature one. Increased susceptibility is coincident with the final stages of anatomic development and differentiation of the cochlea.[112] Given these data, incubator manufacturers have lessened the noise level emitted by the incubator motor, but limits on the environmental source of noise in the NICU itself are few.

In addition to possible sensory nerve damage, loud noise could have physiologic consequences in the newborn preterm infant in the form of stress, with alterations in corticosteroid levels and autonomic changes. Decreases in oxygen tension recorded by transcutaneous monitors as well as increases in intracranial pressure and in peripheral vasoconstriction are reported in preterm infants after exposure to sudden noise.[113] Finally, sleep is disrupted by intermittent noise in the NICU.

The NICU auditory environment also could contribute to language problems in preterm children through direct damage to auditory structures by noise, neuronal loss, or disruption of sensory integration due to limited speech or patterned stimulation. Delayed CAER among healthy preterm infants have been reported, as well as deficits in brain stem response when linguistic stimuli were used.[105,114] The fetal as well as the preterm environment likely plays an important role in the normal development of the auditory system.

INTERVENTION IN THE NICU

Auditory intervention in the NICU includes efforts both to reduce ambient noise and to induce patterned auditory input. Personnel in the NICU generally have made focused efforts to lower the level of noise in the environment. Quiet times during each shift are prevailing and radios are less constant. Evidence would suggest caring for the smallest and sickest preterm infants inside an incubator, as a shield against environmental noise. The steady incubator noise may induce sleep in the preterm.[37] At some point, however, the continuous white noise in the incubator masks more socially relevant auditory stimuli and thus the incubator becomes a source of sensory deprivation. Prolonged housing in this environment would be inappropriate. Thus, weight and temperature cannot be the only criteria for weaning from the incubator. The precise timing is unknown; a gradual transition always would be appropriate.

There are no known studies that have measured the effect of decreasing the level of ambient noise reaching the infant by occluding the infant's ears, but caution here is warranted. Auditory input could be particularly critical for hearing-impaired infants. Preterm infants' auditory thresholds generally are not tested until near the time of discharge. Thus, if attenuation is practiced, the safer device would model that provided by the womb, where higher frequencies are selectively attenuated. Without this approach, speech sounds would also be dampened. The strategy is therefore potentially harmful. On the other hand, short-term occlusion might be appropriate during a brief, acute phase of illness. This should be studied empirically in a sufficient sample, with both short-term and long-term consequences carefully evaluated using speech stimuli in addition to hearing thresholds.

Auditory stimulation, as a single modality, has been studied in the preterm infant. Schmidt and associates reported that auditory stimulation in the form of a heartbeat lengthened the duration of the first Quiet sleep period; Quiet sleep is a more stabilized state that reflects CNS maturity.[37] In one of the earliest studies, Katz reported using auditory stimulation in the form of recorded maternal speech played to healthy preterm infants of 28–32 weeks of gestation until each reached 36 weeks PCA.[115] Compared to controls, the intervention group showed better neuromotor development and improved auditory and visual responses. This study highlights once more that the effects of an intervention may not be limited to the stimulated sense.

Some NICUs have urged using sound as a protective window for the infant—when music is played, the infant will not be disturbed. This approach responds to the potential for conditioning in the preterm infant. Soothing sound is soft, simple, repetitive, and harmonic, with a limited dynamic range. Nonetheless, speech and nonspeech stimuli differentially stimulate the cerebral hemispheres.[99] Availability of speech sounds may be particularly critical.

VISUAL SYSTEM

The visual system is the most extensively studied sensory system, and therefore the mechanisms are better understood. The eye is considered a window to the brain, as it contains two-thirds of the afferent nerve fibers in the CNS. Light energy is transmitted through the cornea, pupil, lens, and optic media to the retina. There it bypasses the retinal blood vessels, a layer of ganglion cells, and a layer of bipolar cells, before it finally reaches the outer segments of the photoreceptors (*i.e.*, rods and cones). Light is absorbed by the photoreceptors in a photochemical response that converts the radiant energy to an electrical impulse. The amount of light energy necessary to stimulate a single photoreceptor cell is extremely small—one quantum.[116] In the absence of a light stimulus, retinal firing still occurs in the form of a tonic discharge. Some processing occurs even at the level of the retina.[116] The impulse travels to the ganglion cells, the optic nerve, and through the lateral geniculate nucleus to the occipital cortex. Fibers from the medial portion of each retina decussate, whereas those from the lateral one-half do not. Thus, information from either the left or right visual field will fall on the contralateral portion of each retina and be transmitted to the same hemisphere of the brain. Representation in the cortex is topographic, but upside-down and reversed.

DEVELOPMENT

The eye is an outgrowth of the brain from the early embryonic stage. By 24 weeks of gestation, gross anatomic structures are in place and the visual pathway is complete. As shown in Table 8-1, the visual system is undergoing extensive maturation and differentiation between 24 and 40 weeks of gestation. Corresponding functional visual responses have been elicited in the preterm infant.[10,32,117–122]

Immature function is present by 24 to 28 weeks of gestation. A visual evoked response (VER) to bright light can be obtained, but it consists of a long-latency negative wave that readily fatigues. A behavioral response to bright light consists of lid tightening, but the response also fatigues quickly. The refractive error is about −5 diopters. Important functional changes occur between 30 to 34 weeks of gestation. The morphology of the VER is more complex with the addition of a positive wave, and the latency decreases. The pupillary reflex is more efficient. A bright light will cause immediate lid closure, and the response sustains. The eyes may open spontaneously, and the infant may even briefly fixate. This has been described as the beginning of "attention."[32] Attention as such may be best elicited with a large, high-contrast form held closer to the eyes than would be necessary at term, and under conditions of low illumination (*i.e.*, 5 foot-candles [ftc]). By 36 weeks, the VER resembles that of a full-term infant, but the latency is still longer for the preterm infant and remains so. Spontaneous eye opening has even been observed on fetal ultrasound. Although alertness still is less sustained than at term, the preterm infant now shows a spontaneous orientation toward a soft light and can track an object horizontally and vertically. Additionally, the infant prefers pattern to a nonpatterned surface, in a manner similar to a full-term infant. The refractive error is near zero.

TABLE 8–1
MATURATION OF THE FETAL EYE IN THE THIRD TRIMESTER

Fetal Eye Components	26–28 Weeks of Gestation	30–32 Weeks of Gestation	34–36 Weeks of Gestation
Eyelid	Fused early in development, now reopens	Less translucent	
Pupil	Tunica vasculosa lentis begins to atrophy	Fully atrophied by end of period	Few remanants
	No reflex present	Sluggish reflex	Complete reflex
Lens	Second of four-layer nucleus forming	Second complete, third begins	
Media	Cloudy	Clears	
	Hyaloid system begins to regress	Hyaloid almost disappeared	Some remanants may still be present
Retina	Rod differentiation begins	Complete except for fovea, cone differentiation begins	Cone number in fovea increases
	Vascularization just beginning	Nasal portion nearly complete	Temporal region nearly fully vascularized
Visual cortex	Rapid dendritic growth and differentiation	Marked development of dendritic spines and synapses	Morphologically now similar to full term

By term birth, the visual system still is immature relative to the other sensory systems, with considerable development still to occur over the next 6 months.[123] Full-term infants have a less dense optic media and macular pigmentation than adults. The newborn eye transmits more short-wavelength light than an adult by a factor of four.[83] Color vision probably is present. Newborns are photophobic, and thus visual attention is facilitated under low illumination (*i.e.*, approximately 5 ftc). Acuity estimates are in the range of 20/200 Snellen equivalents. The refractive error is slightly hyperopic (*i.e.*, +1 diopter).

The newborn can attend to form, object, and face. Specifically, he or she can fixate a high-contrast form (*i.e.*, 1/16-inch wide line at a distance of 1 foot) as well as show preference for patterns along dimensions of brightness and complexity. She or he will track a bright object horizontally across midline and somewhat vertically. Attention to the human face by a neonate can been explained as a predisposition to respond to contrast (*e.g.*, eyes, open mouth) or to edge (*e.g.*, hairline), to slow movement (*e.g.*, nodding), and to contingent stimulation (*e.g.*, adult captures the infant's gaze). In any event, this behavior is powerfully adaptive.

DEFICITS

It generally is agreed that the visual system of the preterm infant is particularly susceptible to insult. The most well known visual problem is retinopathy of prematurity (ROP), which is a proliferative vascular disease of multifactorial origin, most strongly associated with degree of immaturity of the retina.[124,125] Visual disorders other than ROP also commonly are associated with prematurity, including thicker lenses, poorer visual acuity, higher incidence of astigmatism, and high myopia, strabismus, and anisometropia.[126,127] For example, among a sample of 5-year-old low-birth-weight children, 35% lacked stereopsis and 25% had less than 20/20 corrected acuity in both eyes.[127] Among the very-low-birth-weight sample, over 60% had one or more visual defects. In addition to these visual problems, the preterm infant also has difficulty processing visual information at a more cognitive level. Measures of visual attention, pattern discrimination, visual recognition memory, and visuomotor integration repeatedly indicate particular vulnerability for the preterm infant on visually mediated tasks.[9,12,13,128,129]

INTRAUTERINE ENVIRONMENT

The womb generally is dark, but under certain conditions light can transmit to the fetus. A behavioral response by a fetus to light has been described.[130] Transmission through all the tissue is limited to small amounts of red, or long-wavelength, light. Probably only 2% of incident light reaches the uterus.* In later pregnancy, the head of the human fetus is in the vertex position, the neck is flexed, and the face posterior, thereby diminishing exposure. It is unlikely that light exposure is a necessary condition for the fetus, or that periodic exposure to low levels of long-wavelength light is harmful. Aspects of the light–dark cycle that reach the fetus probably are mediated more by maternal sources such as rest–activity cycles and hormones, than by light directly.

After birth, ambient light increases markedly, although typically the room is kept dim and cycled

*Sliney D, personal communication, June 1992.

with dark to some extent. In dim light, the newborn is more likely to open his or her eyes. A prolonged wake period linked to catecholamine release occurs during this transition to extrauterine life.

NICU ENVIRONMENT

Modern intensive care nurseries are brightly lit environments with ambient light in excess of standard office lighting for adults (Fig. 8-2). The general range reported has been 30 to 150 ftc, with peaks over 1500 ftc from sunlight.[131,132] The intensity of ambient illumination for any individual infant is determined by the location of the crib in a room, the number of overhead light units, the size, location, and compass direction of windows, the season of the year, and even the prevailing weather conditions (*i.e.*, sunny *versus* hazy). The duration of exposure generally is 24 hours a day over the length of hospital stay, which is a function of degree of immaturity and medical complications. Thus, light exposure is greater for those most vulnerable to visual problems.

In addition to ambient light, preterm infants are routinely exposed to supplementary sources, such as the bili-light, the heat lamp, and the indirect ophthalmoscope. The standard double-bank phototherapy unit produces 300 to 400 ftc of illumination. The Mini Bili-Lite has an intense beam, estimated at over 10,000 ftc. Infants' eyes are routinely patched under phototherapy; however, in some cases the eye pads are inadequate or may slip off. A commonly used heat lamp consists of one or two infrared bulbs that produce an intensity over 300 ftc at an infant's face. Exposure time varies but is typically longer for younger and sicker infants. The eyes of infants are not typically covered while under the heat lamp.

Finally, an indirect ophthalmoscope is used for the routine eye examinations to rule out ROP. Exposure for 2 minutes, which is the approximate time of retinal examination, at maximum power has been estimated as equivalent to exposure at 2000 ftc for 3 hours.[133] Extra precautions for protecting the infant's dilated eyes from ambient or supplementary sources of light before and after the eye examination are not routine. For the smallest infants, the addition of a heat lamp during the examination often is necessary to maintain the baby's temperature.

PHOTOTOXICITY IN ANIMALS

Animals exposed to similar levels of light have sustained damage to their photoreceptors, pigment epithelium, and choroid.[133,134] Phototoxicity is a consequence of a photochemical effect but may be exacerbated by heat. The effectiveness of light in producing retinal damage is proportional to its efficiency in bleaching rhodopsin. A level of 100 ftc bleaches rhodopsin to 80% in approximately 10 minutes. Continuous illumination is more potent than cyclic, but intermittent exposure may be cumulative.

Factors that enhance photochemical damage to the animal retina strikingly parallel the perinatal course of the preterm infant.[131] Retinal damage in animals is facilitated by maintenance of the animal in constant dark before light exposure; by an increase in body temperature; by conditions of hyperoxia, hypoxia, or ischemia; and by retinal disease. Finally, light and oxygen may have a synergistic effect on ROP.[135] In spite of all these considerations, safety standards have not yet been determined.

PHOTOBIOLOGIC EFFECTS OF LIGHT IN THE NICU

Mounting data indicate that light has potent biologic effects that are not routinely considered in standard NICU care. An association between light and ROP was first suggested by Terry in 1946.[136] Potential mechanisms to account for phototoxicity as one of the contributing factors in ROP have been proposed and

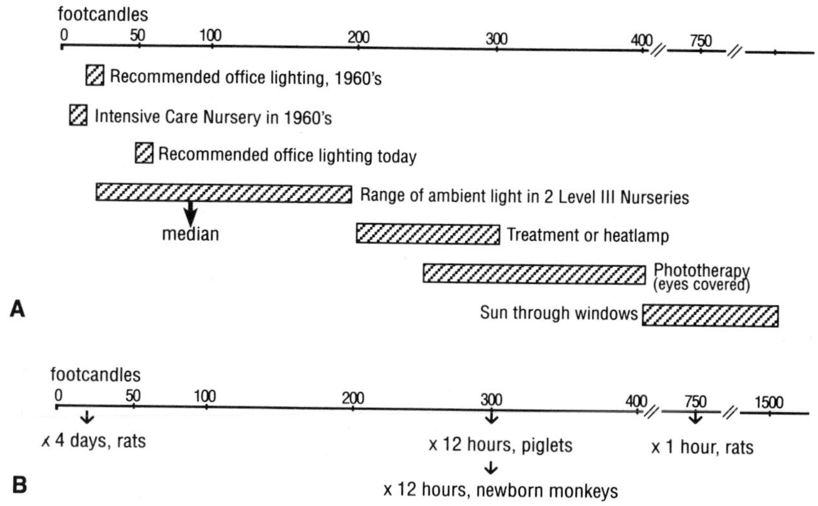

FIG. 8–2. (A) Levels of light exposure in the intensive care nursery. (B) Light exposure and retinal damage in animals. (From Glass P, Avery GB, Subramanian KL, et al. Effect of bright light in the hospital nursery on the incidence of retinopathy of prematurity. N Engl J Med 1985;313:401.)

are consistent with the oxygen toxicity hypotheses: damage to endothelial cells, alteration of normal retinal metabolism, disruption of the normal regenerative process of the retina, and the generation of free radicals.[131,135,137–140] Preliminary evidence with preterm infants supports an association between light and ROP. In a prospective but nonrandomized study, preterm infants for whom the light levels were reduced had a lower incidence of ROP compared to a similar group of preterm infants exposed to standard bright levels of nursery light.[141] The same effect was found in both nurseries studied. Similar findings were reported by Hommura and colleagues,[142] although not by Ackerman and associates,[143] who used historical controls. The light hypothesis is supported by converging evidence that showed increased ROP in the region of the retina more exposed to light—specifically, more in the regions around 3 o'clock and 9 o'clock compared to the superior and inferior regions.[144] There is no evidence that light is a necessary condition for ROP or that maintaining a preterm infant in the dark will completely prevent it.

Photobiologic effects are not limited to the retina. Elevated room light or phototherapy may cause degradation of riboflavin and vitamin A, common components of total parenteral nutrition.[145] Solutions containing these vitamins may be covered at the source, but tubing often is not shielded. Light in the visible spectrum penetrates the skin and may thereby alter more than the bilirubin concentration in the blood. Riboflavin levels were reduced *in vivo* among infants undergoing phototherapy.[146] Thrombocytopenia (*i.e.*, platelets $< 150{,}000/mm^3$) was more than tripled among preterm infants exposed to phototherapy light.[147] *In vitro* experiments demonstrated an inhibition in the normal constriction of immature lamb ductal rings exposed to ambient laboratory light.[148] Subsequently, Rosenfeld and associates found a significant reduction in the occurrence of patent ductus arteriosus among preterm infants whose chests were shielded from exposure to phototherapy light.[149]

LIGHT AND BEHAVIOR

Bright light in an infant's face is a source of stress that is easily demonstrated. Even routine ambient light level affects sleep and wake states in preterm infants. Lower ambient light is associated with significantly less Active REM sleep and significantly more Quiet sleep among preterm infants at 35 to 36 weeks of PCA.[150] Lower ambient light also is associated with increased eye opening and awake periods. Light level influences an infant's response to sound. Under bright light, an infant shows an aversive response to a tone, whereas under a dim light the same tone elicits an orienting response.[151] Dimming the light has a quieting effect on caregivers, who are apt to behave as though someone were sleeping.

INTERVENTION IN THE NICU

The optimal level of NICU lighting has not been determined; however, no study supports the safety of current light levels. It would therefore be prudent to limit ambient nursery light to necessary levels and shield the infant's eyes and chest from ambient as well as supplementary sources. Shading does not mean occluding. Evidence does not suggest that infants eyes should be patched beyond what is necessary for phototherapy. Prolonged patching may be detrimental, both in terms of stimulus deprivation and possible effects on corneal growth.

Opportunities for spontaneous eye opening under dim (*i.e.*, 5 ftc) or dark conditions ought to be provided. Visual attention is facilitated under these conditions. Animal studies would also suggest that dim–dark cycling may be beneficial for regeneration after retinal damage.

A day–night cycling regimen in the intermediate care nursery before hospital discharge affects behavior.[152] Infants in the cycled nursery showed improved sleep patterns both in the hospital and after discharge, spent less time feeding, and gained more weight; however, light, noise, and handling all were reduced at night in the experimental unit. That does not negate the effect, but the necessity of entrainment of preterm infants to light–dark cycles is not supported. Rest–activity cycles may be more potent. Biologic rhythms are much more complex.[35,36]

The question then becomes whether to provide patterned stimulation. An infant's ability to respond to a level of stimulation does not necessarily mean that he or she should be stimulated at that level. For example, infants are more likely to respond to a louder sound, yet psychologists do not recommend higher-intensity noise just because the baby hears it better. Likewise, babies attend more to high-contrast black-and-white stimuli than to pastels, but that does not necessarily mean that the baby should be stimulated with the stronger visual pattern either. Prolonged or obligatory visual attention is not a preferred behavior. Given that the visual system is the least mature, the most parsimonious approach would be to provide stimulation of the other senses first. Then the most appropriate visual stimulus to begin with is probably the human face, which bears no resemblance to strong black-and-white patterns.

GENERAL PRINCIPLES

A central issue in developmental intervention is whether to conceptualize the preterm infant as an extrauterine fetus and therefore attempt to reproduce the intrauterine environment, or whether by dint of being born, the system now requires other forms of stimulation to foster the unique development of the preterm infant. To some extent this is a nonissue:

abrupt change to extrauterine life in altricial species has most always been modulated by the mother. The aversive conditions found in the NICU would not be conducive for development for even the healthiest full-term infant. Further research is not necessary to determine whether excess handling, noise, and bright light ought to be reduced. The NICU environment is a potential source of stress and overt damage to the preterm brain. Research is needed to establish safety limits, rather than to study whether or not aversive conditions do harm.

Sensory deprivation also can affect development. Research still is necessary to determine the optimal type, timing, duration, and level of stimuli; however, basic guiding principles for developmental intervention do exist:

Preterm infants are not a homogeneous group. Thus, determining the appropriate level of stimulation is based on an understanding of developmental neurophysiology and evaluation of an individual infant's medical status, neurologic maturation, physiologic stability, and social and physical needs.

Sensory development is not a unitary process. The hierarchical organization and integration of function among the sensory systems provides the conceptual framework for developmental intervention. Thus, intervention should begin with the most mature system, should support the normal maturational process, and should not attempt to accelerate that process.

The model of optimal stimulation for early development lies in the sources naturally available to the fetus and infant (*i.e.*, the mother). The optimal NICU model would thus begin with the intrauterine conditions, then parallel and extend the transition period that occurs immediately after a normal term birth.

A general algorithm therefore seems possible:

For any infant, provide protective care, minimal handling, undisturbed rest, dim, and quiet. Provide for stabilization of autonomic, state, and motor processes through positioning and containment. Model supportive touch.

Consider the role of olfaction and taste.

If the infant is medically stable, introduce graded tactile–vestibular and auditory input before visual. Introduce stimulation at lower intensity first, and only if no major medical changes are occurring simultaneously.

Monitor and modify the program.

Decreasing aversive conditions such as bright light, noise, and handling in the NICU, as well as enhancing comfort through touch, holding, positioning, and containment, not only benefit the infant but communicate directly to parents.

ACKNOWLEDGMENTS

I thank Susan Lydick, M.A., for substantial contributions to this chapter by providing research, suggestions, and encouragement, and R. D. Walk, Ph.D., my mentor.

REFERENCES

1. Hack M, Breslau N, Weissman B, et al. Effect of very low birth weight and subnormal head size on cognitive abilities at school age. N Engl J Med 1991;325:231.
2. Hunt J, Cooper BA, Tooley WH. Very low birth weight infants at 8 and 11 years of age: role of neonatal illness and family status. Pediatrics 1988;82:596.
3. McCormick MC, Gortmaker SL, Sobol AM. Very low birth weight children: behavior problems and school difficulty in a national sample. J Pediatr 1990;117:687.
4. Klein N, Hack M, Gallaher J, et al. Preschool performance of children with normal intelligence who were very low birth weight infants. Pediatrics 1985;75:531.
5. Ross G, Lipper EG, Auld PAM. Educational status and school-related abilities of very low birth weight premature children. Pediatrics 1991;88:1125.
6. Vohr BR, Garcia Coll CT. Neurodevelopmental and school performance of very low birthweight infants: a seven-year longitudinal study. Pediatrics 1985;76:345.
7. Volpe JJ. Cognitive deficits in premature infants. N Engl J Med 1991;325:276.
8. Sostek AM. Prematurity as well as IVH influence development outcome at five years. In: Friedman S, Sigman M, eds. Preterm birth and psychological development. 2nd ed. New York: Academic Press, 1992.
9. Kopp C, Sigman M, Parmelee A, et al. Neurological organization and visual fixation in infants at 40 weeks conceptional age. Dev Psychobiol 1975;8:165.
10. Parmelee AH, Sigman M. Development of visual behavior and neurological organization in preterm and fullterm infants. In: Minnesota symposium on child psychology. vol. 10. Minnesota: University of Minnesota Press, 1976.
11. Sostek AM, Quinn PO, Davitt MX. Behavior, development and neurologic status of premature and full-term infants with varying medical complications. In: Field TM, Sostek A, Goldberg S, et al, eds. Infants born at risk. New York: Spectrum, 1979:281.
12. Caron A, Caron R. Processing of relational information as an index of infant risk. In Friedman S, Sigman M, eds. Preterm birth and psychological development. New York: Academic Press, 1981:219.
13. Rose SA. Enhancing visual recognition memory in preterm infants. Dev Psychol 1980;16:85.
14. Garcia-Coll C. Behavioral responsivity in preterm infants. Clin Perinatol 1990;17:113.
15. Sigman M. Early development of preterm and fullterm infants: exploratory behavior in eight-month olds. Child Dev 1976;47:606.
16. Gunnar M, Hertsgaard L, Larson M, et al. Cortisol and behavioral responses to repeated stressors in the human newborn. Dev Psychobiol 1991;24:487.
17. Gunnar MR. Reactivity of the hypothalmic-pituitary-adrenocortical system to stressors in normal infants and children. Pediatrics 1992;90:491.
18. Gorski PA. Developmental intervention during neonatal hospitalization. Pediatr Clin North Am 1991;38:1469.

19. Weisel TN, Hubel DH. Single cell response in striate cortex of kittens deprived of vision in one eye. J Neurophysiol 1963; 26:1003.
20. Schulte FJ, Stennert E, Wulbrand H, et al. The ontogeny of sensory perception in preterm infants. Eur J Pediatr 1977; 126:211.
21. Dobbing J. Later development of the brain and its vulnerability. In: Davis JA, Dobbing J, eds. Scientific foundations of paediatrics. London: Heinemann, 1974:565.
22. Field T. Supplemental stimulation of preterm infants. Early Hum Dev 1980;4:301.
23. Cornell EH, Gottfried AW. Intervention with premature human infants. Child Dev 1976;47:32.
24. Lawson KR, Daum C, Turkewitz G. Environmental characteristics of the neonatal intensive care unit. Child Dev 1977; 48:1633.
25. Gorski PA. Premature infant behavioral and physiological responses to caregiving interventions in the intensive care nursery. In: Call JD, Galenson E, Tyson RL, eds. Frontiers of infant psychiatry. New York: Basic Books, 1983:256.
26. Korones S. Iatrogenic problems in intensive care. In: Moore TD, ed. Report of the sixty-ninth Ross Conference on pediatric research. Columbus, OH: Ross Laboratories, 1976:94.
27. Korner AF. Preventive intervention with high-risk newborns: theoretical, conceptual, and methodological perspectives. In: Osofsky JD, ed. Handbook of infant development. 2nd ed. New York: John Wiley & Sons, 1987:1006.
28. Avery GB, Glass P. The gentle nursery: developmental intervention in the NICU. J Perinatol 1989;9:204.
29. Bradley RM, Mistretta CM. Fetal sensory receptors. Physiol Rev 1975;55:352.
30. Gottlieb G. The psychobiological approach to developmental issues. In: Mussen PH, ed. Handbook of child psychology. vol. II. 4th ed. Toronto: John Wiley & Sons, 1983:1.
31. Turkewitz G, Kenny PA. The Role of developmental limitations of sensory input on sensory/perceptual organization. J Dev Behav Pediatr 1985;6:302.
32. Hack M, Mostow A, Miranda S. Development of attention in preterm infants. Pediatrics 1976;58:669.
33. Nijhuis JG, Prechtl HFR, Martin CB, et al. Are there behavioural states in the human fetus? Early Hum Dev 1982;6:177.
34. Guilleminault C. Sleep and breathing. In Guilleminault C, ed. Sleeping and waking disorders: indications and techniques. Menlo Park, CA: Addision-Wesley, 1982:155.
35. Glotzbach SF, Rowlett EA, Edgar DM, et al. Light in the newborn nursery: chronobiologic issues. Sleep Res 1991;20:457.
36. Mirmiran M, Kok JH. Circadian rhythms in early human development. Early Hum Dev 1991;26:121.
37. Schmidt K, Rose SA, Bridger WH. Effect of heartbeat sound on the cardiac and behavioral responsiveness to tactual stimulation in sleeping preterm infants. Developmental Psychology 1980;16:175.
38. Adam K, Oswald I. Sleep helps healing. Br Med J 1984; 289:1400.
39. Sassin JF, Parker DC, Mace JW, et al. Human growth hormone release: relation to slow-wave sleep and sleep-waking cycles. Science 1969;165:513.
40. Humphrey T. Correlation between appearance of human fetal reflexes and development of the nervous system. Prog Brain Res 1964;4:93.
41. Birnholtz JC, Farrell EE. Ultrasound images of human fetal development. American Scientist 1984;72:608.
42. Hooker D. The prenatal origin of behavior. New York: Hafner, 1969.
43. Fitzgerald M, Shaw A, MacIntosh N. Postnatal development of the cutaneous flexor reflex: comparative study of preterm infants and newborn rat pups. Dev Med Child Neurol 1988;30:520.
44. Harlow H, Harlow M. The effects of rearing conditions on behavior. Bull Menninger Clin 1962;26:213.
45. Klaus MH, Kennell JH. Maternal–infant bonding. St. Louis: CV Mosby, 1976.
46. Tribotti SJ. Effects of gentle touch on the premature infant. In: Gunzenhauser N, ed. Advances in touch: new implications in human development. Skillman, NJ: Johnson & Johnson Consumer Products, 1990:80.
46a. Eyler FD, Woods NS, Behnke M, et al. Changes over a decade: adult-infant interaction in the NICU. Unpublished manuscript, 1992.
47. Long JG, Philip AGS, Lucey JF. Excessive handling as a cause of hypoxemia. Pediatrics 1980;65:203.
48. Murdoch DR, Darlow BA. Handling during neonatal intensive care. Arch Dis Child 1984;59:957.
49. Peabody JL, Lewis K. Consequences of newborn intensive care. In: Gottfried AW, Gaiter JL, eds. Infant stress under intensive care: environmental neonatology. Baltimore: University Park Press, 1985:201.
50. Perlman JM, Volpe JJ. Suctioning in the preterm infant: effects on cerebral blood flow velocity, intracranial pressure, and arterial blood pressure. Pediatrics 1983;72:329.
51. Speidel BD. Adverse effects of routine procedures on preterm infants. Lancet 1978;2:864.
52. Volpe JJ. Intraventricular hemorrhage and brain injury in the premature infant: diagnosis, prognosis, and prevention. Clin Perinatol 1989;16:387.
53. Schanberg S, Field T. Maternal deprivation and supplemental stimulation. In: Field T, McCabe P, Schneiderman N, eds. Stress and coping across development. Hillsdale, NJ: Erlbaum, 1988:3.
54. Kuhn CM, Schanberg SM, Field T, et al. Tactile-kinesthetic stimulation effects on sympathetic and adrenocortical function in preterm infants. J Pediatr 1991;119:434.
55. Als H, Lawhon G, Brown E, et al. Individualized behavioral and environmental care for the very low birth weight preterm infant at high risk for bronchopulmonary dysplasia: neonatal intensive care unit and developmental outcome. Pediatrics 1986;78:1123.
56. Jay S. The effects of gentle human touch on mechanically ventilated very short gestation infants. Doctoral dissertation, University of Pittsburgh, Pittsburgh, PA, 1982.
57. Field TM, Schanberg SM, Scafidi F, et al. Tactile/kinesthetic stimulation effects on preterm neonates. Pediatrics 1986;77: 654.
58. Scafidi FA, Field TM, Schanberg SM, et al. Massage stimulates growth in preterm infants: a replication. Infant Behavior and Development 1990;13:167.
59. Neal MV. Vestibular stimulation and developmental behavior of the small premature infant. Nursing Research Report 1968;3:1.
60. Thoman EB, Ingersoll EW, Acebo C. Premature infants seek rhythmic stimulation, and the experience facilitates neurobehavioral development. J Dev Behav Pediatr 1991: 12:11.
61. Harrison LL, Leeper JD, Yoon M. Effects of early parent touch on preterm infants' heart rates and arterial oxygen saturation levels. J Adv Nurs 1990;15:877.
62. Hack M, Estabecek M, Robertson S. Development of sucking rhythm in preterm infants. Early Hum Dev 1985;11:133.
63. Birnholz J, Stephens J, Faria M. Fetal movement patterns: a possible means of defining neurologic developmental milestones in utero. AJR 1978;130:537.
64. Bernbaum JC, Pereira GR, Watkins JB, et al. Nonnutritive

sucking during gavage feeding enhances growth and maturation in premature infants. Pediatrics 1983;71:41.

65. Field T, Ignatoff E, Stringer S, et al. Nonnutritive sucking during tube feedings: effects on preterm neonates in an intensive care unit. Pediatrics 1982;70:381.
66. Woodson R, Drinkwin J, Hamilton C. Effects of nonnutritive sucking on state and activity: term-preterm comparisons. Infant Behavior and Development 1985;8:435.
67. Dixon S, Syder J, Holve R, et al. Behavioral effects of circumcision with and without anesthesia. J Dev Behav Pediatr 1984; 5:246.
68. Field T, Goldson E. Pacifying effects of nonnutritive sucking on term and preterm neonates during heelstick procedures. Pediatrics 1984;74:1012.
69. Geldard FA. The human senses. New York: John Wiley & Sons, 1967.
70. Mason WA. Wanting and knowing: a biological perspective on maternal deprivation. In: Thoman EB, ed. Origins of infant's social response. Hillsdale, NJ: Erlbaum, 1979:225.
71. Korner AF. The use of waterbeds in the care of preterm infants. Journal of Perinatology 1986;6:142.
72. Cordero L, Clark DL, Schott L. Effects of vestibular stimulation on sleep states in premature infants. Am J Perinatol 1986;3:319.
73. Kramer LI, Pierpont ME. Rocking waterbeds and auditory stimuli to enhance growth of preterm infants. J Pediatr 1976;88:297.
74. Pelletier JM, Short MA, Nelson DL. Immediate effects of waterbed flotation on approach and avoidance behaviors of premature infants. In: Vestibular processing dysfunction in children. Haworth Press, 1985:81.
75. Gatts J, Winchester S, Fisle K. The safety of part intrauterine analog transition environment: a literature review and discussion. Neonatal Intensive Care 1992;5:51.
76. Yu VYH. Effect of body position on gastric emptying in the neonate. Arch Dis Child 1975;50:500.
77. Henderson-Smart DJ, Read DJ. Depression of intercostal and abdominal muscle activity and vulnerability to asphyxia during active sleep in the newborn. In: Guilleminault C, Dement W, eds. Sleep apnea syndromes. New York: Alan R Liss, 1978:93.
78. Martin RJ, Herrell N, Rubin D, et al. Effect of supine and prone positions on arterial oxygen tension in the preterm infant. Pediatrics 1979;63:528.
79. Wagaman MJ, Shutack JG, Moomijian AS, et al. The effects of different body positions on pulmonary function in neonates recovering from respiratory disease (abstract). Pediatr Res 1978;12:571.
80. Grenier A. Prévention des déformations précoches de hanche chez les nouveau-nés à cerveau lésé: maladie de Little sans ciseaux? Ann Pediatr (Paris) 1988;35:423.
81. Anderson GC. Current knowledge about skin–skin (kangaroo) care for preterm infants. Perinatol 1991;11:216.
82. Mistretta CM, Bradley RM. Development of the sense of taste. In: Blass EM, ed. Handbook of behavioral neurobiology. vol. 8: developmental psychobiology and developmental neurobiology. New York: Plenum Press, 1986:205.
83. Werner JS, Lipsitt LP. The infancy of human sensory systems. In: Gollin ES, ed. Developmental plasticity: behavioral and biological aspects of variations in development. New York: Academic Press, 1981:35.
84. Steiner JE. Human facial expressions in response to taste and smell stimulation. Adv Child Dev Behav 1979;13:257.
85. Pedersen PE, Greer CA, Shepherd GM. Early development of Olfactory function. In: Blass EM, ed. Handbook of behavioral neurobiology. vol. 8: developmental psychobiology and Developmental Neurobiology. New York: Plenum Press, 1986: 163.
86. Rieser J, Yonas A, Wikner K. Radial localization of odors by human newborns. Child Dev 1976;47:856.
87. Macfarlane JA. Olfaction in the development of social preferences in the human neonate. In: Parent–infant interaction: Ciba Foundation Symposium 33. Amsterdam: Elsevier, 1975: 103.
88. Porter RH, Balogh RD, Makin JW. Olfactory influences on mother–infant interaction. In: Rovee-Collier C, Lipsitt LP, eds. Advances in infancy research. Camden, NJ: LP Ablex Publication, 1988:39.
89. Sullivan RM, Taborsky-Barba S, Mendoza R, et al. Olfactory classical conditioning in neonates. Pediatrics 1991;87:511.
90. Smotherman WP, Robinson SR. Dimensions of fetal investigation. In: Smotherman WP, Robinson SR, eds. Behavior of the fetus. Caldwell, NJ: Telford, 1988:19.
91. Blass EM, Hoffmeyer LB. Sucrose as an analgesic for newborn infants. Pediatrics 1991;87:215.
92. Aslin RN, Pisoni DB, Jusczyk PW. Auditory development and speech perception in infancy. In: Mussen PH, ed. Handbook of child psychology. vol. 11. 2nd ed. New York: John Wiley & Sons, 1983:573.
93. Hecox K. Electrophysiological correlates of human auditory development. In: Cohen LB, Salapatek P, eds. Infant perception: from sensation to cognition. Perception of space, speech, and sound. vol. II. New York: Academic Press, 1975: 151.
94. Rubel EW. Auditory system development. In: Gottlieb G, Krasnegor N, eds. Measurement of audition and vision in the first year of postnatal life: a methodological overview. Camden, NJ: Ablex Publishing, 1985:53.
95. Parmelee HP, Sigman MD. Perinatal brain development and behavior. In: Mussen PH, ed. The handbook of child psychology. 2nd ed. vol. 2. New York: John Wiley & Sons, 1983:95.
96. Birnholz JC, Benacerraf BR. The development of human fetal hearing. Science 1983;222:516.
97. Querleu D, Renard X, Boutteville C, et al. Hearing by the human fetus? Semin Perinatol 1989;13:409.
98. Berg, KM, Smith M. Behavioral thresholds for tones during infancy. J Exp Child Psychol 1983;35:409.
99. Molfese D, Freeman R, Palermo D. Ontogeny of brain lateralization for speech and non-speech stimuli. Brain Lang 1975; 2:356.
100. Fifer W, Moon C. Psychobiology of newborn auditory preferences. Semin Perinatol 1989;13:430.
101. Fifer WP, Moon C. Auditory experience in the fetus. In: Smotherman WP, Robinson SR, eds. Behavior of the fetus. Caldwell, NJ: Telford Press, 1888:175.
102. DeCasper AJ, Fifer WP. Of human bonding: newborns prefer their mothers' voices. Science 1980;208:1174.
103. DeCasper AJ, Spence MJ. Prenatal maternal speech influences on newborn's perception of speech sounds. Infant Behavior and Development 1986;9:133.
104. Spence M, DeCasper A. Newborns prefer a familiar story over an unfamiliar one. Infant Behavior and Development 1987;10:133.
105. Kurtzberg D, Stapells DR, Wallace IF. Event-related potential assessment of auditory system integrity: implications for language development. In: Vietze PM, Vaughan HG, eds. Early identification of infants with developmental disabilities. Philadelphia: Grune & Stratton, 1988:160.
106. Gerherdt K. Characteristics of the fetal sheep sound environment. Semin Perinatol 1989;13:362.
107. Armitage SE, Baldwin BA, Vince MA. The fetal sound of sheep. Science 1980;208:1174.

108. Walker D, Grimwade J, Wood C. Intrauterine noise: a component of the fetal environment. Am J Obstet Gynecol 1970; 109:91.
109. Douek E, Dodson HC, Bannister LH, et al. Effects of incubator noise on the cochlea of the newborn. Lancet 1976;2:1110.
110. Falk SA. Combined effects of noise and ototoxic drug. Environ Health Perspect 1972;2:5.
111. Walton JP, Hendricks-Munoz K. Profile and stability of sensorineural hearing loss in persistent pulmonary hypertension of the newborn. J Speech Hear Res 1991;34:1362.
112. Carlier E, Pujol R. Supra-normal sensitivity to ototoxic antibiotic of the developing rat cochlea. Arch Otorhinolaryngol 1980;226:129.
113. Long JG, Lucey JF, Philip AGS. Noise and hypoxemia in the intensive care nursery. Pediatrics 1980;65:143.
114. Salamy A, Mendelson T, Tooley WH, et al. Differential development of brainstem potentials in healthy and high-risk infants. Science 1980;210:553.
115. Katz V. Auditory stimulation and developmental behavior of the premature infant. Nurs Res 1971;20:196.
116. Gregory RL. Eye and brain: the psychology of seeing. 4th ed. Princeton: Princeton University Press, 1990.
117. Dreyfus-Brisac C. Neurophysiological studies in human premature and fullterm newborns. Biol Psychiatry 1975;10: 485.
118. Mann I. Development of the human eye. New York: Grune & Stratton, 1964.
119. Purpura DP. Morphogenesis of visual cortex in the preterm infant. In: Brazier MAB, ed. Growth and development of the brain: nutritional, genetic, and environmental factors. International Brain Research Organization Monograph Series. New York: Raven Press, 1975:1.
120. Dubowitz LM, Dubowitz V, Morante A, et al. Visual function in the preterm and fullterm newborn infant. Dev Med Child Neurol 1980;22:465.
121. Miranda SB. Visual abilities and pattern preferences of premature infants and full-term neonates. J Exp Child Psychol 1970;10:189.
122. Senecal J, Defawe G, Roussey M, et al. Le comportement visuel du premature. Arch Fr Pediatr 1979;36:454.
123. Abramov I, Gordon J, Hendrickson A, et al. Light and the developing visual system. In: Marshall J, ed. Vision and visual dysfunction. Boca Raton, FL: CRC Press, 1991.
124. James L, Lanman J. History of oxygen therapy and retrolental fibroplasia. Pediatrics 1976;57:590.
125. Lucey J, Dangman B. A reexamination of the role of oxygen in retrolental fibroplasia. Pediatrics 1984;73:82.
126. Fledelius T. Prematurity and the eye. Acta Ophthalmol 1976; 128:3.
127. Hoyt C. Long-term visual effects of short-term binocular occlusion of at-risk neonates. Arch Ophthalmol 1980;98:1967.
128. Sigman M, Parmelee A. Visual preferences of four month old premature and fullterm infants. Child Dev 1974;45:959.
129. Siegel L. The prediction of possible learning disabilities in preterm and fullterm children. In: Field T, Sostek A, eds. Infants born at risk: physiological, perceptual, and cognitive processes. New York: Grune & Stratton, 1983:295.
130. Brazelton TB, Field TM. Introduction. In: Nigunzehauser, ed. Advances in touch: new implications in human development. Skillman, NJ: Johnson & Johnson Consumer Products, 1990.
131. Glass P. Light and the developing retina. Doc Ophthalmol 1990;74:195.
132. Landry RJ, Scheidt PC, Hammond RW. Ambient light and phototherapy conditions of eight neonatal care units: a summary report. Pediatrics 1985;75:434.
133. Lanum J. The damaging effects of light on the retina: empirical findings, theoretical and practical implications. Surv Ophthalmol 1978;22:221.
134. Williams TP, Baker BN, eds. The effects of constant light on visual processes. New York: Plenum Press, 1980.
135. Ham WT, Mueller HA, Ruffolo JJ. Mechanisms underlying the production of photochemical lesions in the mammalian retina. Curr Eye Res 1984;3:165.
136. Terry L. Retrolental fibroplasia. J Pediatr 1946;29:770.
137. Dorey CK, Delori FC, Akeo K. Growth of cultured RPE and endothelial cells is inhibited by blue light but not green or red light. Curr Eye Res 1990;9:549.
138. Riley PA, Slater TF. Pathogenesis of retrolental fibroplasia. Lancet 1969;2:265.
139. Stefansson E, Wolbarsht ML, Landers MB. In vivo O_2 consumption in rhesus monkeys in light and dark. Exp Eye Res 1983;37:251.
140. Zuckerman R, Weiter JJ. Oxygen transport in the bullfrog retina. Exp Eye Res 1980;30:117.
141. Glass P, Avery GB, Subramanian KN, et al. Effect of bright light in the hospital nursery on the incidence of retinopathy of prematurity. N Engl J Med 1985;313:401.
142. Hommura S, Usuki Y, Takei K, et al. Ophthalmic care of very low birthweight infants, report 4: clinical studies of the influence of light on the incidence of ROP. Nippon Ganka Gakkai Zasshi 1988;92:456.
143. Ackerman B, Sherwonit E, Williams J. Reduced incidental light exposure: effect on the development of retinopathy of prematurity in low birth weight infants. Pediatrics 1989; 83:958.
144. Fielder AR, Robinson J, Shaw DE, et al. Light and retinopathy of prematurity: does retinal location offer a clue? Pediatrics 1992;89:648.
145. Bhatia J, Mims L, Roesel R. The effect of phototherapy on amino acid solutions containing multivitamins. J Pediatr 1980; 96:284.
146. Sisson T. Advances in phototherapy of neonatal hyperbilirubinemia. In: Helene C, Charlier M, Montenay-Garestier T, et al, eds. Trends in photobiology. New York: Plenum Press, 1982:339.
147. Maurer H, Fratkin M, McWilliams N, et al. Effects of phototherapy on platelet counts in lowbirthweight infants and on platelet production and life span in rabbits. Pediatrics 1976; 57:506.
148. Clyman RI, Rudolph AM. Patent ductus arteriosus: a new light on an old problem. Pediatr Res 1978:12:92.
149. Rosenfeld W, Sadhev S, Brunot V, et al. Phototherapy effect on the incidence of patent ductus arteriosus in premature infants: prevention with chest shielding. Pediatrics 1986; 78:10.
150. Glass P, Sostek A. Sleep organization in preterm infants: the effect of nursery illumination. Presented at the International Conference of Infancy Studies, New York, New York, April 21, 1984 (poster session).
151. Haith MM. Rules that babies look by. Hillsdale, NJ: Erlbaum, 1980.
152. Mann NP, Haddow R, Stokes L, et al. Effect of night and day on preterm infants in a newborn nursery: randomised trial. Br Med J 1986;293:1265.

Part Two

THE FETAL PATIENT

Neonatology: Pathophysiology and Management of the Newborn, Fourth Edition,
edited by Gordon B. Avery, Mary Ann Fletcher, and Mhairi G. MacDonald.
J.B. Lippincott Company, Philadelphia © 1994.

chapter **9**

Prenatal Diagnosis in the Molecular Age

NELSON B. ISADA
MARK P. JOHNSON
PETER PRYDE
MARK I. EVANS

The modern era of molecular and biochemical genetics commenced with the observations of Sir Archibald Garrod at the turn of the twentieth century.[1] He proposed that four diseases, namely alkaptonuria, albinism, cystinuria, and pentosuria, resulted from inherited disorders of chemical metabolism, and further suggested that these disorders, which he called "inborn errors of metabolism," represented only a small fraction of every human's "chemical individuality" that had gone awry.[1]

Advances in biochemistry have confirmed Garrod's concepts by characterizing the structural protein abnormality or enzymatic defect of many disorders. Other advances in molecular genetics have allowed precise identification of the defect in the deoxyribonucleic acid (DNA) message, sometimes before the protein defect itself is known.[2] This knowledge has direct and immediate applications in the field of prenatal diagnosis.[3]

This chapter will discuss gene organization, mutations and polymorphism analysis, molecular diagnostic techniques, DNA cloning, an approach to disorders diagnosable by molecular genetics, biochemical disorders not amenable to DNA technology or better studied by protein chemistry techniques, and carrier screening.

GENE ORGANIZATION

The Watson–Crick double-helix model of DNA organization is well known.[4] DNA conveys information encoded by a series of four nucleotides: adenine (A), thymine (T), cytosine (C), and guanine (G), connected sequentially on two strands. The two strands are complementary to each other, with nucleotide base pairs (bp) being formed by hydrogen bonding between adenine–thymine and guanine–cytosine. Eukaryotic DNA is located in the nucleus and organized into structures called chromosomes. During interphase, chromosomes are not visible by light microscopy. They become visible only when the genetic content has doubled, and the chromosomes have condensed before mitosis. Chromosomal material is organized into euchromatin and heterochromatin. The former is vigorously transcribed into ribonucleic acid (RNA). Heterochromatin is relatively inactive. An example of heterochromatin is the inactivated X chromosome.

An unexpected discovery made in the 1970s was that some regions of the eukaryotic chromosome do not code for any known protein.[5] Specifically, these noncoding regions (*i.e.*, introns), were noted to be interspersed within coding regions (*i.e.*, exons; Fig.

9-1).[6,7] Exons carry information to direct the assembly of amino acids into a protein, whereas introns do not. Messenger RNA (mRNA) acts as an intermediate molecule to convey information encoded by the DNA by a process called translation. Posttranslational modification of mRNA takes place such that introns are removed. After further biochemical modifications, the mRNA passes out of the nucleus into the cytoplasm, where protein-synthesizing organelles are located.

About 60% of the human genome comprises regions of unique nucleotide sequences that presumably code for proteins.[8] It is estimated that there are 50,000 to 100,000 expressed genes and proteins active in humans; however, expressed genes make up less than 10% of total genomic DNA. A significant portion of the human genome, perhaps about 40%, contains repetitive DNA sequences.[9] Various terms are used for the different classes of repetitive DNA sequences found in humans. Highly repetitive sequences are found in the chromosome region adjacent to centromere. These are simple sequences repeated thousands of times, present in more than 10^4 copies and comprising about 20% of the genome. These repeating simple sequences have compositions unlike most of the organism's DNA, are several hundred bp long, and are easily separated by centrifuging slightly fragmented DNA through a cesium chloride density gradient. DNA separated by this process is called satellite DNA, because the centrifuged DNA forms a main band and several satellite bands above and below the main band. In humans, four satellite bands comprise about 6% of the total DNA, with each band representing tandem repeat sequences. Blocks of satellite DNA are readily localized to regions around the centromeres of metaphase chromosomes by *in situ* hybridization. Satellite DNA should not be confused with satellites, a cytogenetic term referring to the segment of an acrocentric chromosome distal to short arm, separated by a constriction. Other classes of repetitive DNA, which may overlap, are moderately repetitive DNA, which are gene-sized in length, repeated $\sim 10^1$ to $\sim 10^3$ times, and comprise about 20% of genome (*i.e.*, one-half of the ~40% that is repetitive DNA); a variable number of tandem repeat sequences, which are stretches of DNA in which a short nucleotide sequence is tandemly repeated 20 to 100 times, the exact number varying from person to person; alphoid DNA, which are chromosome-specific, repeated monomeric 170-bp units located in centromeric regions; and *Alu* sequences, which are highly repetitive sequences not clustered around centromeres, but instead more evenly distributed throughout the genome and interspersed within longer stretches of unique or moderately repetitive DNA. In humans, most such 300-bp sequences belong to a single group called the *Alu* family. Most contain a single cleavage site near the middle for the restriction enzyme *Alu* I, derived from the bacterium *Arthrobacter luteus* (see Restriction Fragment Length Polymorphism Analysis). Almost one million *Alu* sequences are present in the human genome, accounting for 3% to 6% of the total DNA. Each individual human has a unique amount of repetitive DNA. This genetic fingerprint has been used for paternity testing and forensic analysis.

A discovery involving repeat sequences has demonstrated an association between triplet repeat mutations and human disease. In this situation, a sequence of three repeated nucleotides has been found in normal people; when these sequences are found to be increased, there is an increased likelihood of clinical morbidity. This has been described in the fragile X syndrome, a common form of heritable male mental retardation, where a polymorphic sequence of -CGG- repeats on the X chromosome is increased from a mean of 29 repeats to over 200 repeats in affected males. The reasons for this association are not yet known. This triplet expansion also has been found in association with congenital myotonic dystrophy and spinal–bulbar muscular atrophy (*i.e.*, Kennedy disease), in which increases in -GCT- and -CAG- repeats, respectively, have been found.[10,11]

Regulation of gene expression occurs at many levels. Substrate concentrations have been shown both to enhance and repress specific enzymes, especially in bacteria. In eukaryotes and prokaryotes, a region separate from a given gene but still involved in regulation of expression is called a promoter, which binds RNA polymerase and initiates transcription (see Fig. 9-1).[6,7] Exons carry information to direct the assembly of amino acids into a protein, whereas introns do ryotes, such an area or box contains a common or consensus nucleotide sequence, CAAT, and is called a CAAT box. A conserved area associated with RNA polymerase positioning contains repeated sequences of the nucleotides thymine and adenine, and is called a TATA box.

Extranuclear DNA found in mitochondria (mtDNA) is inherited independently of nuclear DNA,

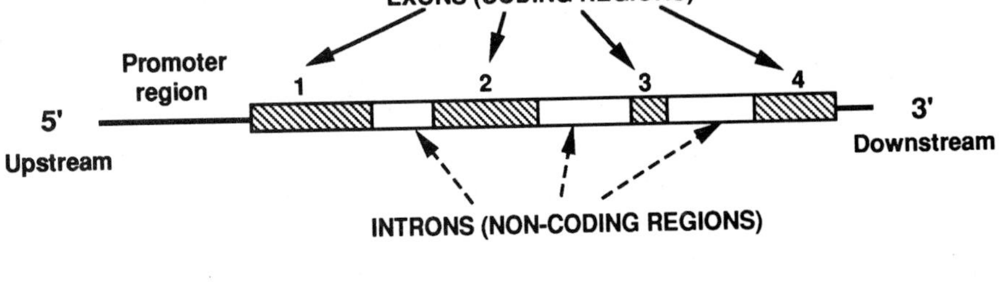

FIG. 9–1. An idealized representation of mammalian gene structure shows the promotor region, exons, and introns.

is 16.5 kb in length, contains no introns, and is organized as a double-stranded circle, a configuration similar to that in photosynthetic eubacteria, suggesting that mitochondria probably were acquired by endosymbiosis. Of further interest, mtDNA is subject to a relatively high rate of mutation compared to nuclear DNA and is inherited maternally, the paternal spermatic mitochondria being excluded from the oocyte at the time of fertilization. A variety of neonatal and pediatric disorders, predominantly neuromuscular, have been associated with mtDNA deletions and mutations.[12] mtDNA polymorphisms also have enhanced the studies of potential human origins and migration patterns.[13]

MUTATIONS AND POLYMORPHISMS

Many types of mutations can affect a gene. The DNA within a gene contains information for the final sequence of a protein and also signals for the correct expression and processing of mRNA. If the actual coding region is altered, then the resultant protein may be changed. These alterations can be in the form of deletions that may be many kilobases or as small as a single base, inversions or translocations that produce no net nucleotide changes, but potential or actual protein changes, or single-base changes. Even a change at the junction of a coding and noncoding region can result in abnormal mRNA formation. Defects in the promoter region may result in too little or too much expression of mRNA, which will be reflected in abnormal protein synthesis. A deletion of all or part of the gene will result almost always in the disruption of normal gene expression. One example of molecular pathology can be seen in Tay–Sachs disease in the Ashkenazi Jewish population.[14] In the severe infantile type, a mutation at an exon–intron splice site in the α-subunit has been identified (*i.e.*, G $\rightarrow$ C transversion); another mutation is a four-base insertion in exon 11 of the α-subunit causing a frameshift mutation and marked reduction in mRNA.[15,16] Another example is the identification of the mutation most commonly found in cystic fibrosis (CF) in people of northern European ancestry. There is a phenylalanine deletion in the CF transmembrane regulator (CFTR) protein at a critical adenosine triphosphate binding site, arising from a deletion of three amino acids, two of which code for phenylalanine. This is called the DF 508 mutation and accounts for approximately 70% of CF mutations in people of northern European ancestry, with the remaining 30% being a heterogeneous assortment of other mutations.[17–19]

Mutations are possible for practically all loci. Genes not found associated with mutations *in vivo* include those whose products are so vital that any change would probably result in lethality early in development (*i.e.*, housekeeping genes). Possible examples of this type include enzymes coded by nuclear or possibly mtDNA that catalyze critical steps in aerobic metabolism. Genes not associated with clinical mutation include those whose protein products are coded by repetitive DNA, whereby the remaining DNA can compensate. For example, ribosomal RNA (rRNA) genes are so abundant that the deletion that occurs when acrocentric chromosomes fuse, as in a Robertsonian translocation, has no phenotypic effect. Other mutations unassociated with clinical disease can occur in noncoding areas such as introns, or in other unexpressed areas of the genome such as pseudogenes, which are duplicated sequences similar to normally expressed genes, but contain no introns.

A variety of approaches have been used to detect mutations. Optimally, determination of DNA structure and sequence, followed by elucidation of gene structure and organization in the normal allele, are completed before beginning a search for specific defects. Only about 5% to 10% of clinically significant mutations, however, are due to gross alterations in gene structure detectable by Southern blot analysis of genomic DNA, leaving unknown the remaining 90%. The problem is compounded by normal variation in the nucleotide sequence (*i.e.*, polymorphisms). Thus, when variations from the normal sequence are found, additional analysis is required before these changes can be construed as being a disease-causing mutation.

LINKAGE ANALYSIS

Linkage analysis is a very powerful technique that can be used to follow genetic disorders throughout a family, and to localize specific genes by closer mapping of linked markers to a putative disease gene.[20] Linkage analysis can be used for genetic diagnosis when the precise nucleotide mutations are not known. As mentioned previously, there is a variety of genetic differences among individuals for a given trait, called polymorphisms, spread throughout the entire human genome. The functions of these polymorphisms are not always known. Many are associated with bacterial endonuclease cleavage sites, described later. Linkage analysis has proven and continues to be an extremely powerful tool in mapping the human genome.[21–25]

A standard principle of classic Mendelian inheritance states that inherited traits sort independently. This is not always the case, however; some traits or characteristics associate more frequently than can be accounted for by chance. With the discovery of chromosomes, the idea arose that multiple traits could be carried on one chromosome. This implied that the closer together two genetic traits were on a chromosome, the more likely they would be to segregate together during meiosis and the less likely crossing-over would occur between them. When genes are in such close proximity that crossing-over rarely occurs, such as for hemophilia A and color blindness, the two sites are said to be linked.[26] Any polymorphism that is found to be linked with the trait of interest is termed informative. Unfortunately, family studies are not always informative because molecular or clinical polymorphisms are not always present.

The degree of linkage can be described mathematically by a number called the logarithm of the ODds (LOD) score, developed in 1955 by Morton.[27] The LOD can be thought of as the likelihood that two given traits are linked. It can be derived from recombinations observed between clinical or biochemical traits from pedigree analysis, or from molecular polymorphisms.[28] The probability of recombination during meiosis between two loci is quantified by a term called the recombination fraction (*i.e.*, theta or q), the maximum being 0.5. The LOD score is derived from various values of q. Viewed simplistically, the higher the LOD score, the higher the likelihood of linkage. Because this number is used on a logarithmic scale, each integer increase reflects a tenfold increase in likelihood of linkage. A LOD score of 4 suggests that there is linkage between two polymorphisms, the odds of random association being 10,000 to 1. A LOD score of zero suggests no linkage, and that the two traits are on different chromosomes or are far apart on the same chromosome. Tight linkage indicates little or no recombination, and suggests an actual physical proximity of two polymorphisms, measured in physical map distances, with the common unit of genetic distance reported as centimorgans. Linkage disequilibrium describes closely linked genes that occur more frequently than would be expected from random distribution, suggesting nonrandom or nonequilibrium mating, or some survival advantage from natural selection. Examples of linkage disequilibrium include the carrier states for sickle-cell disease and thalassemia, where those affected have increased resistance to certain types of malarial infections.

RESTRICTION FRAGMENT LENGTH POLYMORPHISM ANALYSIS

Bacteria possess enzymes that recognize and cleave DNA at specific sites. Presumably, these enzymes evolved as a defense against hostile invading DNA, as might occur with bacteriophages. Because these cleavage sites are quite specific, that is, are restricted to specific palindromic sequences four to ten nucleotides in length, these enzymes are called restriction endonucleases. When these enzymes are added to eukaryotic DNA, the resultant mixture contains a variety of DNA fragments of different sizes, which can be separated by gel electrophoresis and transferred for analysis by Southern blotting. Each enzyme cuts an individual's DNA according to the positions of the cleavage sites, with every person having his or her own unique pattern of cleaved DNA fragments. Thus, people are polymorphic for the resulting lengths of DNA fragments, which vary between which of the different restrictor enzymes are used and the distribution of cleavage sites. Many of these recognition site polymorphisms are neutral and represent normal inherited variability. These characteristics have given rise to the term restriction fragment length polymorphisms (RFLPs), which refer to the polymorphic patterns observed in specific nucleotide sequences that are cleaved by bacterial restriction enzymes (Fig. 9-2). The resultant mixture of DNA fragments can be separated and further characterized by gel electrophoresis, Southern blotting, and oligonucleotide probes.[29]

DNA alterations that affect a RFLP site by either creating a new site for endonuclease cleavage or by eliminating a previously existing one can be detected on Southern blot as a result of changes in the size of the DNA fragment associated with this site.[30] If, by chance, either a mutation or normal sequence corresponds to an RFLP site, this situation can be exploited for allele identification using linkage analysis. An initial use of such mapping involved the Huntington disease locus, as yet undefined.[31] Another early application was for prenatal identification of the sickle-cell mutation in the β-chain of hemoglobin.[32–35] For example, the restriction enzyme *Dde* I, derived from the bacterium *Desulfovibrio desulfuricans*, recognizes the nucleotide sequence -CTNAG- (where N indicates that any nucleotide may occupy that position) that occurs within the hemoglobin A (-CTGAG-) and hemoglobin C (-CTAAG-) gene, but not within hemoglobin S (-CTGTG-). In hemoglobin S, the nucleotide thymine is substituted for adenine, which is not recognized and thus not cleaved by *Dde* I. This results in a much larger RFLP fragment that can be recognized on Southern blot. Initially, this technology used unamplified DNA and Southern blot transfer. Target gene sequences can now be preamplified a million-

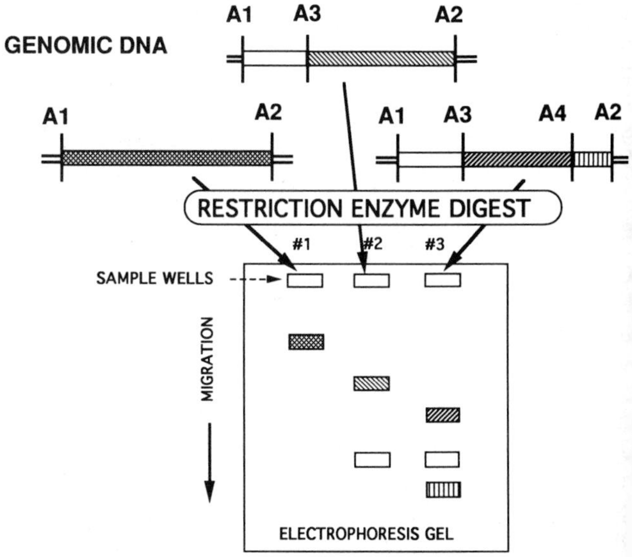

FIG. 9–2. Restriction fragment length polymorphisms. Lane 1, A1 and A2 present; lane 2, A1–A3 present; lane 3, A1–A4 present; A1–A5, hypothetical polymorphisms.

fold by polymerase chain reaction (PCR; see below) and cut by restriction endonucleases, which greatly facilitates target sequence recognition. This approach is potentially useful in prenatal diagnosis, particularly when the quantity of clinical material is limited.

MOLECULAR DIAGNOSTIC TECHNIQUES

Because DNA is present in each cell nucleus, any nucleated cell theoretically is suitable for DNA analysis regardless of whether the gene in question is being transcribed and expressed. Thus, leukocytes, amniocytes, and chorionic villi all are candidate cells for DNA analysis. Restriction fragment length polymorphisms analysis was described earlier. Several other methods also are used for DNA diagnosis (*i.e.*, Southern blot, oligonucleotide probe, PCR). Northern blotting is used for RNA analysis.

SOUTHERN BLOT

Southern blot is a standard method for DNA analysis in both the clinical and basic science settings. In the Southern blot technique, named after the investigator Edwin Southern, double-stranded DNA is digested by a restriction endonuclease (see below) chosen because of its ability to detect a DNA polymorphism that may or may not have any clinical significance.[36] After endonuclease digestion, the resulting DNA fragments are separated using gel electrophoresis. The DNA in the gel is then denatured to generate single-stranded DNA molecules. DNA fragments are then transferred from the gel to nylon filter paper (*i.e.*, blotting), and specific filter-bound DNA fragments can then be detected by hybridization. A radiolabeled DNA or RNA probe is used that has sequence homology to the DNA fragment of interest, usually 200 to 2000 bases long. Subsequent autoradiography produces a radiographic film with banding patterns that indicate the hybridization locations on the filter that reflect the fragment sizes of the DNA sequences homologous to that particular probe (Fig. 9-3).

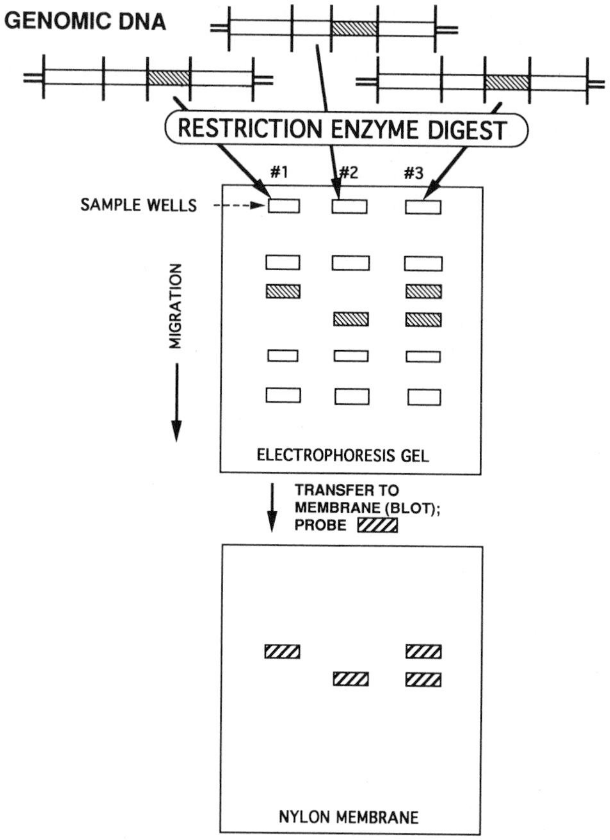

FIG. 9–3. Southern blot for a hypothetical autosomal recessive disorder. Lane 1, unaffected; lane 2, affected; lane 3, carrier.

OLIGONUCLEOTIDE PROBE ANALYSIS

Oligonucleotide probe analysis is similar to Southern blot analysis in that DNA is digested and electrophoresed in a gel. It differs in that a shorter probe, known as an oligonucleotide probe, is used for hybridization. Each oligonucleotide probe is biochemically synthesized and is about 20 bases in length. Because of their short length, they will not hybridize to genomic DNA sequences that differ by even a single nucleotide from the probe sequence. Thus, these probes are useful because they can detect very subtle variations in genomic sequences, but only if the specific nucleotide alterations in genomic DNA are known.

This approach for mutation detection involves direct DNA analysis using sequence-specific oligonucleotides. These specific oligonucleotides were first used for detection of the single-base mutations found in sickle-cell disease, the first "molecular disease" described.[37–39] For the purposes of routine mutation screening, this method is useful only if the gene for the disorder under consideration has been sequenced and involves a small number of mutant alleles. This is important because the oligonucleotides that are complementary and specific for the mutation in question must be synthesized before testing. These nucleotide sequences can be synthesized to recognize the normal gene sequence, or ones that have specific nucleotide changes. Therefore, if a normal oligonucleotide sequence fails to recognize and hybridize to the gene in question, then a change in its sequence must be present. In contrast, if the oligonucleotide probe is constructed to complement a specific mutation, then recognition and hybridization of this probe implies that the mutation is present in that gene. Some diseases that can be detected in this manner include sickle-cell disease, CF, β-thalassemias, Tay–Sachs disease, and Gaucher disease, where the nucleotide abnormalities for the more commonly occurring mutations are already known.

POLYMERASE CHAIN REACTION

The PCR has revolutionized the field of molecular genetics.[40–43] This procedure allows *in vitro* amplification of minute amounts of DNA to generate sufficient quantities of signal to make detection by more traditional methods possible. This procedure makes use of a relatively heat-stable bacterial enzyme, *Taq* I, derived from a thermoacidophilic bacterium, *Thermus aquaticus*. If the target nucleotide sequence is known, a specific set of oligonucleotides, called primers, can be synthesized to encompass the target sequence. The target DNA, oligonucleotide primers, *Taq* I polymerase, and free nucleotides are placed in solution. This reaction mixture is further heated to allow already denatured DNA to anneal with the oligonucleotides, between which the polymerase synthesizes complementary strands (Fig. 9-4). Repeated cycles of heating and cooling result in cyclic primer sequence synthesis, leading to annealing and amplification of the target sequence, since each set of DNA strands gives rise to two additional sets of sequence templates in each cycle of the reaction. This process can be automated to allow 20 to 30 cycles, which can produce more than a millionfold duplication of the target sequence within hours. Modifications of this process can be performed to allow the following:

- analysis of RNA
- analysis of multiple DNA areas (*i.e.*, multiplex PCR)
- selective amplification of one strand instead of both (*i.e.*, asymmetric PCR)
- simultaneous use of one primer set within another to increase specificity (*i.e.*, nested PCR)
- simultaneous use of two different primer sets, one of which selects for a normal sequence and the other for a mutant sequence (*i.e.*, competitive oligonucleotide priming)
- simultaneous use of a known amount of a second, easily identified target DNA to measure the amount of original DNA (*i.e.*, semiquantitative PCR).

Many technical difficulties must be addressed to eliminate both false-positive and false-negative results. Problems with reagent or reactant contamination can lead to false-positive results and require that appropriate control methods be performed simultaneously to verify positive PCR results. Other problems such as primer instead of target amplification and nonspecific amplification must be recognized and eliminated.

NORTHERN BLOT

Northern blotting is used for RNA analysis. The general principles of the technique are similar to those for Southern blotting. RNA analysis requires prompt specimen processing and committed laboratory reagents and instruments because of ubiquitous ribo-

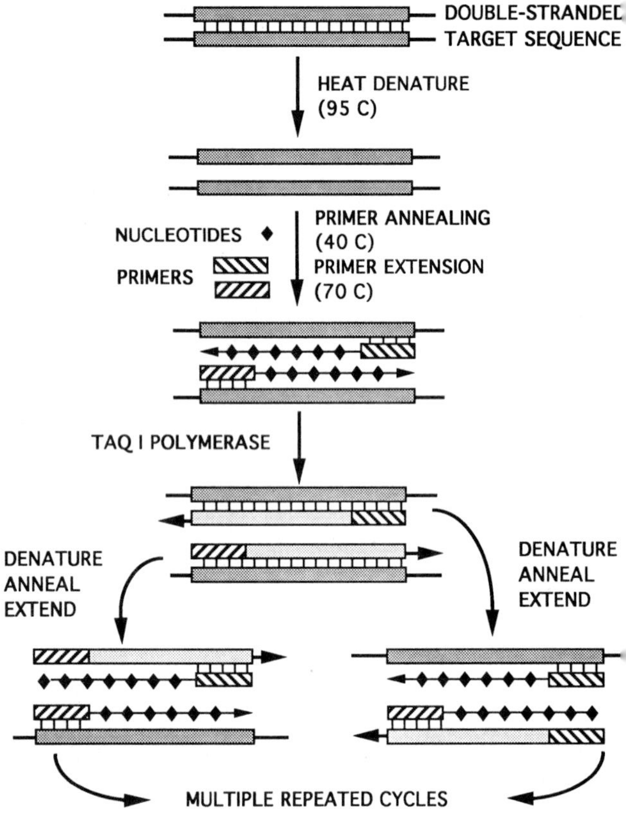

nucleases, present even on finger surfaces. Examination of the size and amount of a mRNA transcript is a useful initial step in evaluating mutations of genes that are expressed in cells or tissues, especially those that are expressed clinically. Fibroblasts and lymphocytes are good sources of mRNA. Hepatic or muscle tissue is useful if available. Placental tissue can be used if maternal cell contamination can be avoided. Of the cell's total RNA, only 1% to 2% is mRNA, which is highly unstable at room temperature because of tissue RNases. The remainder of the RNA is mainly rRNA and transfer RNA (tRNA). Once isolated, the mRNA is denatured, separated by agarose gel electrophoresis, transferred to a membrane filter, and analyzed by hybridization of a specific fluorescent or radiolabeled probe.

For most diseases studied at the molecular level, about 5% to 10% of patients have no detectable mRNA for the gene product in question; 10% to 20% have reduced but detectable amounts of normal mRNA; and about 5% have some alteration in mRNA size. The approximately 50% remaining have normal amounts of normal-sized mRNA. Given this information, it is possible to deduce the general type of mutation at the DNA level, such as large or total gene deletions, which are suggested by a total absence of mRNA; mutations in promoter regions, which are suggested by reduced amounts of normal mRNA, mutations at exon–intron junctions, which are suggested by changes in mRNA size; or point mutations, which are suggested by normal-sized mRNA but abnormally functioning proteins.

DEOXYRIBONUCLEIC ACID CLONING

The initial step in the study of a gene is now the isolation of a DNA molecule complementary to its mRNA, called cDNA. cDNA contains no intronic sequences. Using cDNA, many molecular investigations of the corresponding gene become possible. The first step in cDNA cloning is the isolation of mRNA from a particular cell or tissue that contains a significant amount of the desired mRNA. A retroviral enzyme, reverse transcriptase, is used to synthesize cDNA from the mRNA. Because the cell or tissue mRNA contains transcripts of many genes, the resultant pool of cDNAs will be heterogeneous and must be sorted out. The cDNAs are inserted into a vector to form what is called a cDNA library. A second type of chromosome library, called a genomic library, is composed of fragments of native genomic DNA and contains introns and other noncoding regions. Vectors include viruses that can replicate within bacteria, such as bacteriophage λ, or autonomous, self-replicating, circular DNA molecules found in bacteria called plasmids. Another vector that combines properties of plasmids and bacteriophage λ are called cosmids. Cosmids are plasmid vectors into which larger fragments of DNA can be cloned. The term cosmid is derived from the presence of internal cohesive end sites (cos) that have been inserted into a plasmid. Cos are nucleotide sequences from bacteriophage λ between which DNA sequences are normally expressed as capsule proteins. In cosmids, these sequences can be replaced with other nucleotide sequences, which can then be expressed and concentrated *in vitro*.

An alternative approach to cDNA cloning uses mRNA itself instead of cDNA. Using mRNA is advantageous because the mRNA pool, although heterogeneous, is not nearly so complex as a corresponding pool of genomic DNA fragments that contains a mixture of introns, nonexpressed genes, and DNA from noncoding regions. Methods of cDNA cloning to detect the presence of a specific cDNA segment include screening a cDNA library with synthetic oligonucleotide probes and screening a bacteriophage λ library with antibodies directed against the protein of interest. Using the first approach, a set of radiolabeled oligonucleotide probes is synthesized with sequences complementary to those predicted for the mRNA from the amino acid sequence found in the protein. These oligonucleotides are used to probe a DNA library that contains bacterial colonies infected with bacteriophage λ. With the second approach, antibodies against the protein of interest are used to detect a corresponding protein expressed by cDNAs inserted into bacteriophage λ.

cDNAs for many genes have been cloned using these approaches. Nucleotide sequencing is the first step in the analysis of a cDNA. With this information, the investigator can identify potential sites of restriction endonuclease cleavage, examine the deduced amino acid sequence to verify correspondence with the protein of interest, and identify regions of homology with other proteins, which can suggest evolutionary relationships and previously unrecognized functions. In addition to providing nucleotide and amino acid sequence information, these cDNAs can be used as hybridization probes to characterize and quantitate corresponding mRNA in cells and tissues from patients with a variety of diseases.

This process by which DNA analysis leads to an identifiable protein abnormality has been called "reverse genetics," or, more recently, "positional cloning."[44,45] Several hundred genes associated with human disease have been identified. In some, the protein defect has been identified, such as with CF, and the identification of the triple-nucleotide/single–amino-acid deletion in the CFTR protein. For some diseases, the gene and protein are better characterized, such as for neurofibromatosis type 1 (NF-1).[46] For most human diseases, however, the genes have yet to be cloned and protein defects defined, as with Huntington disease.

PRENATAL DIAGNOSIS

MOLECULAR BIOLOGY

Prenatal diagnosis has been successfully accomplished by analysis of fetal DNA extracted from a variety of samples.[47] In the initial cases, the fetus was at risk for having a hemoglobinopathy, such as sickle-cell anemia or thalassemia,[33,48–50] in which the specific protein, mRNA, and DNA defects were known. Since that time, the number of genetic disorders in which DNA technology can be applied for prenatal diagnosis continues to grow geometrically. In addition to the hemoglobinopathies, a partial list of other potentially prenatally diagnosable defects that can be evaluated by molecular genetic techniques include Duchenne muscular dystrophy (DMD),[51–54] CF, fragile X syndrome,[10,11] infantile myotonic dystrophy, hemophilias A and B,[55,56] congenital adrenal hyperplasia,[57] Tay–Sachs disease,[58] NF-1,[59,60] and ornithine transcarbamylase (OTC) deficiency.[61–64]

If the molecular abnormality of the abnormal gene is known, RFLP analysis or oligonucleotide probes can be used. Polymerase chain reaction also can be used to amplify known regions, and the resultant product analyzed by Southern blot. Polymerase chain reaction is especially useful when using milligram amounts of clinical material obtained at the time of chorionic villus sampling (CVS), amniocentesis tissue culture, or cordocentesis. If the exact gene abnormality and location is not known, linkage analysis with

RFLPs can be performed as an indirect method if family members are informative; this means that an affected family member must be available and willing to be tested. Occasionally, a patient may have a previously undescribed molecular pathologic condition, and the standard probes and markers are not helpful. This situation invariably lengthens the time to diagnosis. Other difficult situations arise when a disease appears in a family of a particular ethnic group where the molecular pathologic condition differs from that in other ethnic groups with a known molecular pathologic condition. An example of this situation is an African–American couple who have a child with CF, in whom studies for the DF 508 mutation, most commonly found in northern Europeans, are negative. Despite these problems, as more genes are cloned and more chromosomal markers identified, this approach to prenatal diagnosis will become more common. The further applications of invasive fetal diagnostic modalities are discussed in Chapter 12.

BIOCHEMISTRY

Biochemical assays remain an important aspect of prenatal diagnostic testing, even with the tremendous advances in molecular genetics. These assays include assessment of gene products such as enzymes, receptors, and transport proteins, and metabolites such as amino acids, organic acids, vitamins, and hormones. Prenatal diagnosis of biochemical defects may be made by assay of fetal tissue, fetal cells, or tissue culture supernatant if the particular product is produced solely or primarily by the gene in question, and the product already is known to be expressed in the fetal specimen to be analyzed. Enzyme assays can be performed using tissue, extracts from cultured fetal cells, or from live cells kept in tissue culture. Biochemical tests for the diagnosis of metabolic disorders consist of identification of abnormal metabolites or abnormal levels of metabolites that reflect a metabolic block. Ultimately, the goal is identification, quantitation, and characterization of the defective or deficient gene product that is responsible for the metabolic block. When the underlying biochemical defect is known and is expressed in accessible fetal tissue (*e.g.*, chorionic villi, fetal muscle, liver) or cells (*e.g.*, trophoblasts, amniocytes, fetal erythrocytes and leukocytes), prenatal diagnosis can be approached by analysis of the enzyme or other protein product that has been shown to be primarily involved.

Definitive biochemical diagnosis of an inherited metabolic disorder must be based on a clear-cut distinction between the values of affected and unaffected fetuses. In genetic disorders, there is potential for overlap between the normal and heterozygous ranges of enzyme activities. This arises mainly as a result of the wide variation found in the activity of almost any biologic enzyme in the normal population. Because variability due to different mutations and different genomic backgrounds exists among families, additional testing of leukocytes or cultured skin fibroblasts from presumably unaffected parents and siblings can provide valuable information. In addition to the benefit in interpretation of prenatal results, such studies may provide a reliable means for identification of other carriers among members of the extended family.

The fetus also can be assessed indirectly by determination of maternal serum enzyme activities during pregnancy. For example, the normal increase in serum hexosaminidase A seen in pregnancy appears to be of fetal origin.[65,66] Therefore, unchanged levels in pregnancies at risk for Tay–Sachs disease may indicate an affected fetus.

For many inherited metabolic disorders or inborn errors of metabolism, biochemical means of prenatal diagnosis are available or are theoretically possible. For an autosomal recessive disease, the assay used should discriminate among homozygous affected, heterozygous unaffected, and homozygous normal fetuses. Assays for detection of autosomal dominant diseases such as some of the porphyrias usually are capable of identifying affected homozygotes, but sometimes fail to differentiate conclusively affected heterozygotes from unaffected fetuses. X-linked disorders present unique difficulties in heterozygote detection, which arise because of random X inactivation. Depending on the ratio of an active mutant X to normal X in tissues involved in the pathogenesis of the disease, a female heterozygous for an X-linked disorder may be clinically normal, or may have mild or even severe disease manifestations. To complicate matters further, measured enzymatic activities also vary depending on the ratio of mutant to normal X chromosomes that are active in the analyzed specimen—chorionic villi, for example. Occasionally, the activity levels in chorionic villi may not correlate with clinical expression. Males, on the other hand, have only one X chromosome, and are either hemizygous affected with deficient enzyme activity or hemizygous normal with activity in the normal range. Thus, prenatal biochemical assessment of X-linked disorders is less complicated if the fetus is male.

FETAL SAMPLES AND TISSUE PROCESSING

The use of direct and cultured fetal specimens for prenatal evaluation of metabolic disorders ideally requires the availability of normal control preparations. This applies to readily obtainable specimens such as chorionic villus tissue, cultured trophoblasts, cultured amniotic fluid cells, and amniotic fluid supernatant, as well as to those obtained by more invasive procedures such as fetal blood sampling and fetal liver and muscle biopsies. Except for trophoblasts and amniotic fluid cells that can be maintained in culture, availability of fresh controls is often a problem, and in most instances long-term frozen controls with partial loss of activity must be used. There are other potential pitfalls that seem specific for each of these tissue, cell, and fluid types. All samples should be analyzed as soon as possible, except those requiring initial tissue culture. Chorionic villi, fetal tissue biopsies, cell pellets, amniotic fluid supernatant, and fetal serum or plasma that are not used for tissue culture can be kept frozen and shipped on dry ice. Cell cultures and tissue for cell culture, however, should be shipped at room temperature or wet ice, depending on the circumstances. Whenever possible, appropriate controls matched by gestational age should accompany the samples to be analyzed.

Extraction and analysis of labile enzymes is especially difficult because test results are very sensitive with respect to the duration of homogenization or sonication. Using fresh chorionic villi or amniocytes or freshly harvested trophoblasts helps preserve the activity of such labile enzymes.[67]

Elevated concentrations of amino acids and organic acids in amniotic fluid serve as preliminary indications for several inherited disorders such as amino and organic acidopathies and urea cycle defects. In most cases, however, final diagnosis is made by measuring the actual gene products responsible for the metabolic block. Identification and quantitation of amino acids and organic acids in physiologic fluids and in reaction mixtures are performed by an amino acid analyzer and gas chromatography, respectively. Quantities are determined by the ratio between the peak area found in the sample compared to known controls. Organic acids also must be extracted before their subsequent separation and quantitation by gas chromatography.

In the case of chorionic villus sampling, it is crucial to obtain samples that are of fetal origin only and in which maternal cells are either completely absent or extremely rare. The use of frozen controls may adversely affect the interpretation of results by causing false-negative diagnoses, especially when the enzyme in question is very labile, such as sialidase in sialidosis, or when the normal activity levels in chorionic villi are extremely low, as for α-iduronidase in mucopolysaccharidosis I. Specific problems also may be encountered because of different distribution of enzymes and isozymes.[68] The characteristic presence of high levels of arylsulfatase-C activity in chorionic villi hampers the differential detection of arylsulfatases-A in metachromatic leukodystrophy and -B in mucopolysaccharidosis VI when villi are used.

For most first-trimester prenatal tests, the recommended practice is to use fresh chorionic villi for preliminary evaluation followed by subsequent analysis of cultured trophoblasts for confirmation of the diagnosis. One exception is with nonketotic hyperglycinemia. Although the glycine–serine ratio in amniotic fluid is elevated in this disease, there is a significant overlap with normal values. The potential for prenatal diagnosis of this disorder would rely exclusively on the results obtained in fresh chorionic villi because the glycine cleavage system is not expressed in amniotic fluid cells or trophoblasts, but is detectable in fresh tissue.[69,70]

Amniotic fluid supernatants should be aliquoted into multiple vials to avoid the loss of activity that occurs with repeated freezing and thawing. Determinations of amniotic fluid concentrations of specific metabolites, as well as enzymes and other proteins, usually serve as supporting evidence in prenatal diagnoses. The final diagnosis should rely preferably on demonstration of the underlying biochemical defect in fetal cells or tissue. The variability in enzyme activities or in the levels of other proteins and metabolites frequently observed in cultured amniotic fluid cells and trophoblasts can be minimized by a careful choice of control cells.

Fetal blood sampling and fetal liver and muscle biopsy should be considered only in the absence of other alternatives because of the higher risk for pregnancy loss with these invasive procedures. Fetal blood sampling by cordocentesis has a wide variety of potential applications because both fetal cells and serum can be obtained. Fetal muscle biopsy has been used in rare cases of DMD, when molecular analysis of trophoblasts, amniocytes, or fetal leukocytes is nondiagnostic and family studies are uninformative. An *in utero* fetal muscle biopsy can be performed in the middle of the second trimester to assess dystrophin levels in myoblasts by *in situ* hybridization. Absence of dystrophin suggests an affected fetus. Fetal liver biopsy also can be performed for certain rare enzyme deficiencies. For example, in one type of glycogenosis, glucose-6-phosphatase is decreased; this enzyme is expressed only in fetal liver and kidney. In the absence of direct DNA techniques, the only option available for prenatal diagnosis is fetal liver biopsy in which glucose-6-phosphatase activity can be measured. Fetal liver biopsy also is applicable in rare cases of OTC deficiency where family studies are uninformative and known deletions cannot be detected.[61]

MOLECULAR AND BIOCHEMICAL TESTING FOR CARRIER SCREENING

Carrier screening usually is limited to populations or ethnic groups at increased risk for a diagnosable disease. The ultimate benefit of carrier detection programs is the identification of couples at risk before they have an affected child, empowering them with reproductive choices. For example, carrier detection for Tay–Sachs disease is offered routinely to all people of Ashkenazi Jewish descent, in whom the combined frequency for the two common mutations in the α-subunit gene of hexosaminidase is 1 in 31.[71] Hexosaminidase A levels can be assayed enzymatically in serum, plasma, or leukocytes, and compared to a constant value of thermostable hexosaminidase B. Pregnant women should have only the leukocyte assay performed, because of problems with false-negative or indeterminate results in serum or plasma.[65] Screening also is offered to people of French–Canadian background, in whom the clinical disease is similar and the carrier frequency high, but the mutation different (*i.e.*, 7.6-kb deletion in the α-subunit).

In people of African descent, sickle-cell screening is offered routinely. Sickle-cell screening usually is performed by a biochemical assay assessing hemoglobin solubility; positive results are followed up by electrophoresis to characterize the hemoglobin type. In unusual cases, the exact nucleotide defect can be characterized using techniques described earlier.

Biochemical screening programs for Tay–Sachs disease and sickle-cell disease, when coupled with appropriate counseling, generally are well received by patients. In contrast, the recent molecular and biochemical characterization of the molecular defect causing CF has not resulted in widespread implementation of screening programs, even though CF is a common genetic disease (1 in 2000–3000) with a relatively high heterozygote frequency in American Caucasians (1 in 25). The controversy surrounding widespread implementation of CF screening arises because of a variety of factors.[72,73] First, only about 70% of carriers are positive for the most common mutation (*i.e.*, ΔF 508). As a result, this requires screening for multiple mutations, which is performed with PCR and oligonucleotide probes specific for known CF mutations. Using probes for 12 mutations, about 85% of carriers can be identified. If screening were to be implemented, there is no consensus on who should be screened and when this screening should take place. Some options include testing the fetus at the time of genetic testing for other indications, testing the mother alone, or testing both parents. Another factor affecting implementation of screening programs is the clinical variability of the disorder. In contrast to the infantile form of Tay–Sachs disease, CF morbidity can range from debilitating pulmonary disease and death in childhood to minimal symptomatology and survival into adulthood, which correlates with the type and magnitude of the molecular defect.[17] Also to be considered is the increased clinical burden on existing genetics services for appropriate pretest and posttest counseling. A final objection is the potential counseling difficulty arising when the fetus is found to have only one positive allele for a known CF mutation, and linkage analysis cannot be applied because there is no index case. Although the likelihood of an affected fetus is low, the possibility cannot be entirely ruled out, and the parents are left with an ambiguous result.[74]

There are pilot studies examining different screening approaches and their resultant impacts on patient choices and their understanding of counseling and the implications of screening. Some centers already offer parental and fetal CF screening to all patients having genetic counseling and procedures for other indications. Despite the difficulties outlined above, it is our belief that maternal and possibly fetal antenatal screening for CF, using PCR and oligonucleotide probes to detect multiple mutations, will eventually become a routine practice because of heightened public awareness and continued improvements in molecular technology.

THE FUTURE OF MOLECULAR BIOLOGY

The knowledge explosion in molecular biology has revolutionized medical practice. Prenatal diagnosis has benefited enormously, because bench discoveries rapidly result in clinical applications. Development of PCR, increasingly sophisticated electrophoretic methods, positional cloning,[44] recognition of new genetic causes of human disease such as triplet repeats,[10,11] uniparental disomy,[75,76] genetic imprinting[77,78] and microsegmental aneusomy,[79] all have had direct and immediate impact on the practice of reproductive genetics. Advances in chromosome painting and *in situ* hybridization potentially allow cytogenetic diagnoses within 24 to 48 hours.[80] There is increased use of antenatal genetic screening as more disease-causing genes are cloned and sequenced, and their function characterized. Finally, the prospect of embryonic or fetal gene diagnosis and therapy, along with the *in utero* creation of a transgenic human may not be as far in the future as many believe or fear.[81,82] The medical community must address the applications of these technologies and the attendant myriad social, legal, and ethical issues.

REFERENCES

1. Garrod AE. The Croonian lectures. Lancet 1908;2:1.
2. Caskey CT. Disease diagnosis by recombinant DNA methods. Science 1987;236:1223.
3. King CR. Prenatal diagnosis of genetic disease with molecular genetic technology. Obstet Gynecol Surv 1988;43:493.
4. Watson JD, Crick FHC. Molecular structure of nucleic acids: a structure for deoxyribose nucleic acid. Nature 1953;171:737.
5. Berget SM, Moore C, Sharp PA. Spliced RNA segments at the 5′-terminus of late adenovirus 2 m RNA. Proc Natl Acad Sci USA 1977;74:3171.
6. Gilbert W. Why genes in pieces? Nature 1978;271:501.
7. Gilbert W. Genes-in-pieces revisited. Science 1985;228:823.
8. Cooper DN, Smith BA, Cooke HJ, et al. An estimate of unique DNA sequence heterozygosity in the human genome. Hum Genet 1985;69:201.
9. Miller DA, Choi YC, Miller OJ. Chromosome localization of highly repetitive human DNAs and amplified ribosomal DNA with restriction enzymes. Science 1983;219:395.
10. Caskey CT, Pizzuti A, Ying-Hui Fu, et al. Triplet repeat mutations in human disease. Science 1992;256:784.
11. Richards RI, Sutherland GR. Heritable unstable DNA sequences. Nature Genetics 1992;1:7.
12. Wallace DC. Mitochondrial DNA mutations and neuromuscular disease. Trends in Genetics 1989;5:9.
13. Cann RL, Stoneking M, Wilson AC. Mitochondrial DNA and human evolution. Nature 1987;325:31.
14. Petersen GM, Rotter JI, Cantor RM, et al. The Tay-Sachs dis-

ease gene in North American Jewish populations: geographic variation and origin. Am J Hum Genet 1983;35:1258.
15. Myerowitz R, Costigan C. The major defect in Ashkenazi Jews with Tay-Sachs disease is an insertion in the gene for the a-chain for β-hexosaminidase. J Biol Chem 1988;263:18587.
16. Ohno K, Suzuki K. A splicing defect due to an exon-intron junctional mutation results in abnormal β-hexosaminidase X-chain in RNAs in Ashkenazi Jewish patients with Tay-Sachs disease. Biochem Biophys Res Commun 1988;153:463.
17. Cutting GR, Kasch LM, Rosenstein BJ, et al. Two cystic fibrosis patients with mild pulmonary disease and nonsense mutations in each CFTR gene. N Engl J Med 1990;323:1685.
18. Cutting GR, Kasch LM, Rosenstein BJ, et al. A cluster of cystic fibrosis mutations in the first nucleotide-binding fold of the cystic fibrosis conductance regulator protein. Nature 1990; 346:366.
19. Kerem E, Corez M, Kerem BS, et al. The relationship between genotype and phenotype in cystic fibrosis: analysis of the most common mutation (ΔF508). N Engl J Med 1990;323:1517.
20. Smith CAB. The development of human linkage analysis. Ann Hum Genet 1986;50:293.
21. Botstein D. 1989 Allen Award address. Am J Hum Genet 1990; 47:887.
22. Botstein D, White RL, Skolnick M, et al. Construction of a genetic linkage map using restriction fragment length polymorphisms. Am J Hum Genet 1980;32:314.
23. Cavalli-Sforza LL, King MC. Detecting linkage for genetically heterogeneous diseases and detecting heterogeneity with linkage data. Am J Hum Genet 1986;38:599.
24. White R, Lalouel J-M. Sets of linked genetic markers for human chromosomes. Ann Rev Genet 1988;27:259.
25. White R. 1989 Allen Award address. Am J Hum Genet 1990; 47:892.
26. Haldane JBS, Smith CAB. A new estimate of the linkage between the genes for color-blindness and hemophilia in man. Annals of Genetics Eugenics 1947;14:10.
27. Morton NE. Sequential tests for the detection of linkage. Am J Hum Genet 1955;7:277.
28. Risch N. Genetic linkage: interpreting LOD scores. Science 1992;255:803.
29. Antonarakis SE, Phillips JA III, Kazazian HH Jr. Genetic diseases: diagnosis by restriction endonuclease analysis. J Pediatr 1982;100:845.
30. Gusella JF. DNA polymorphism and human disease. Ann Rev Biochem 1986;55:831.
31. Gusella JF, Wexler NS, Conneally PM, et al. A polymorphic DNA marker genetically linked to Huntington disease. Nature 1983;306:234.
32. Antonarakis SE, Kazazian HH Jr, Orkin SH. DNA polymorphism and molecular pathology of the human globin gene clusters. Hum Genet 1985;60:1.
33. Boehm CD, Antonarakis SE, Phillips JA, et al. Prenatal diagnosis using DNA polymorphisms: report on 95 pregnancies at risk for sickle-cell disease or beta thalassemia. N Engl J Med 1983;308:1054.
34. Embury SH, Scharf SJ, Saiki RK, et al. Rapid prenatal diagnosis of sickle cell anemia by a new method of DNA analysis. N Engl J Med 1987;316:656.
35. Weatherall DJ, Old JM, Thein SL. Prenatal diagnosis of the common haemoglobin disorders. J Med Genet 1985;22:422.
36. Southern EM. Detection of specific sequences among DNA fragments separated by electrophoresis. J Mol Biol 1975;98:503.
37. Pauling L, Itano HA, Singer SJ, et al. Sickle cell anemia, a molecular disease. Science 1949;110:543.
38. Rossiter BJF, Caskey CT. Molecular scanning methods of mutation detection. J Biol Chem 1990;265:12753.
39. Saiki RK, Chang CA, Levenson CH, et al. Diagnosis of sickle cell anemia and beta thalassemia with enzymatically amplified DNA and non-radioactive allele-specific oligonucleotide probes. N Engl J Med 1988;319:537.
40. Ehrlich HA, Gelfand D, Sninsky JJ. Recent advances in the polymerase chain reaction. Science 1991;252:1643.
41. Mullis KB, Falloona FA. Specific synthesis of DNA in vitro via a polymerase-catalyzed chain reaction. Methods Enzymol 1987;155:335.
42. Saiki RK, Gelfand DH, Stoffel S, et al. Primer-directed enzymatic amplification of DNA with a thermostable DNA polymerase. Science 1988;239:487.
43. Scharf SJ, Horn GT, Erlich HA. Direct cloning and sequence analysis of enzymatically amplified genomic sequences. Science 1986;233:1076.
44. Collins FS. Positional cloning: let's not call it reverse anymore. Nature Genetics 1992;1:3.
45. Ruddle FH. The William Allan Memorial Award address: reverse genetics and beyond. Am J Hum Genet 1984;36:944.
46. Xu G, O'Connell P, Viskochil D, et al. The neurofibromatosis type 1 gene encodes a protein related to GAP. Cell 1990;62:599.
47. Antonarakis SE. Diagnosis of genetic disorders at the DNA level. N Engl J Med 1989;320:153.
48. Kan YW. The William Allan Memorial Award address: thalassemia: molecular mechanism and detection. Am J Hum Genet 1986;38:4.
49. Kazazian HH Jr, Boehm CD. Molecular basis and prenatal diagnosis of beta-thalassemia. Blood 1988;72:1107.
50. Saiki RK, Scharf S, Faloona F, et al. Enzymatic amplification of β-globin genomic sequences and restriction site analysis for diagnosis of sickle cell anemia. Science 1985;230:1350.
51. Gillard EF, Chamberlain JS, Murphy EG, et al. Molecular and phenotypic analysis of patients with deletions within the deletion-rich region of the Duchenne muscular dystrophy (DMD) gene. Am J Hum Genet 1989;45:507.
52. Hoffman EP, Fischbeck KH, Brown RH, et al. Characterization of dystrophin in muscle-biopsy specimens from patients with Duchenne's or Becker's muscular dystrophy. N Engl J Med 1988;318:1363.
53. Kunkel LM. Analysis of deletions in DNA from patents with Becker and Duchenne muscular dystrophy. Nature 1986;322: 73.
54. Multicenter Study Group. Diagnosis of Duchenne and Becker muscular dystrophies by polymerase chain reaction: a multicenter study. JAMA 1992;267:2609.
55. Antonarakis SE. Molecular genetics of hemophilia A and B. Adv Hum Genet 1988;17:27.
56. Kogan SC, Doherty M, Gitschier J. An improved method for prenatal diagnosis of genetic diseases by analysis of amplified DNA sequences: application to hemophilia A. N Engl J Med 1987;317:985.
57. Pang S, Pollack MS, Marshall RN, et al. Prenatal treatment of congenital adrenal hyperplasia due to 21-hydroxylase deficiency. N Engl J Med 1990;322:111.
58. Grabowski GA, Kruse VR, Goldberg JE, et al. First-trimester prenatal diagnosis of Tay-Sachs disease. Am J Human Genet 1984;36:1369.
59. Cawthon RM, Weiss R, Yu G, et al. A major segment of the neurofibromatosis type 1 gene: a DNA sequence, genomic structure, and point mutations. Cell 1990;62:193.
60. Viskochil D, Buchberg AM, Yu G, et al. Deletions and a translocation interrupt a cloned gene at the neurofibromatosis type 1 locus. Cell 1990;62:187.
61. Holzgreve W, Golbus MS. Prenatal diagnosis of ornithine transcarbamylase deficiency utilizing fetal liver biopsy. Am J Hum Genet 1984;36:320.

62. Kwok SCM, Ledley FD, Dilella AG, et al. Nucleotide sequence of a full-length complementary DNA clone and amino acid sequence of human phenylalanine hydroxylase. Biochemistry 1985;24:556.
63. Nussbaum RL, Boggs BA, Beaudet AL, et al. New mutation and prenatal diagnosis in ornithine transcarbamylase deficiency. Am J Hum Genet 1986;38:149.
64. Woo SLC, Lidsky AS, Guttler F, et al. Cloned human phenylalanine hydroxylase gene allows prenatal diagnosis and carrier detection of classical phenylketonuria. Nature 1983;306:151.
65. Ben-Yoseph Y, Pack BA, Thomas PM, et al. Maternal serum hexosaminidase A in pregnancy: effects of gestational age and fetal genotype. Am J Med Genet 1988;29:891.
66. Navon R, Leibokowicz I, Adam A. Fetal hexosaminidase A in mother's serum: pitfalls in carrier detection and prospects for prenatal diagnosis of GM 2 gangliosidoses. Am J Hum Genet 1987;40:60.
67. Ben-Yoseph Y, Evans MI, Bottoms SF, et al. Lysosomal enzyme activities in fresh and frozen chorionic villi and in cultured trophoblasts. Clin Chim Acta 1986;161:307.
68. Giles L, Cooper A, Fowler B, et al. Aryl sulphatase isozymes of chorionic villi: implications for prenatal diagnosis. Prenat Diagn 1987;7:245.
69. Applegarth DA, Levy HL, Shih VE, et al. Prenatal diagnosis of nonketotic hyperglycinemia. Prenat Diagn 1986;6:257.
70. Hayasaka K, Tada K, Fueki N, et al. Feasibility of prenatal diagnosis of nonketotic hyperglyanemia: existence of the glycine cleavage system in placenta. J Pediatr 1987;110:124.
71. Triggs-Raine BL, Feigenbaum ASJ, Natowicz M, et al. Screening for carriers of Tay-Sachs diseases among Ashkenazi Jews. N Engl J Med 1990;323:6.
72. Caskey CT, Kaback MM, Beaudet AL. The American Society of Human Genetics statement on cystic fibrosis screening. Am J Hum Genet 1990;46:393.
73. Wilfond BS, Fost N. The cystic fibrosis gene: medical and social implications for heterozygote detection. JAMA 1990;263:2777.
74. Beaudet AL, Feldman GL, Fernback SD, et al. Linkage disequilibrium, cystic fibrosis, and genetic counseling. Am J Hum Genet 1989;44:319.
75. Knoll JH, Nichols RD, Magenis RE, et al. Angelman and Prader-Willi syndromes share a common chromosome 15 deletion but differ in parental origin of the deletion. Am J Med Genet 1989;32:285.
76. Spence JE, Perciaccante RG, Greig GM, et al. Uniparental disomy as a mechanism for human genetic disease. Am J Hum Genet 1988;42:217.
77. Nicholls RD, Knoll JH, Butle MG, et al. Genetic imprinting suggested by maternal heterodimory in nondeletion Prader-Willi syndrome. Nature 1989;342:281.
78. Reck W. Genomic imprinting and genetic disorders in man. Trends in Genetics 1989;5:331.
79. Schmickel RD. Contiguous gene syndromes: a component of recognizable syndromes. J Pediatr 1986;109:231.
80. Kuo WL, Tengin H, Seqranes R, et al. Detection of aneuploidy involving chromosomes 13, 18 or 21, by fluorescence in situ hybridization (FISH) to interphase and metaphase amniocytes. Am J Hum Genet 1991;49:112.
81. Gordon JW. Micromanipulation of embryos and germ cells: an approach to gene therapy? Am J Med Genet 1990;35:206.
82. Handyside AH, Kontogianni EH, Hardy K, et al. Pregnancies from biopsied human preimplantation embryos sexed by Y-specific DNA amplification. Nature 1990;344:768.

Neonatology: Pathophysiology and Management of the Newborn, Fourth Edition,
edited by Gordon B. Avery, Mary Ann Fletcher, and Mhairi G. MacDonald.
J.B. Lippincott Company, Philadelphia © 1994.

chapter **10**

Developmental Pathology of the Embryonic and Previable Fetal Periods

Thomas H. Shepard

Growth and pathologic changes during the embryonic and previable fetal period generally have been neglected by pathologists and other scientists, because the material is difficult either to obtain or to interpret after postmortem changes. Observations on early forms of congenital defects or on a number of syndromes uniquely found during this biologic continuum can lead to a better understanding of the cascade of events that precedes the final manifestations of the more common abnormalities. With the widespread use of prenatal ultrasound, there is need for prenatal standards with which to evaluate the fetus. Most of the normal and pathologic data given in this chapter were developed over 30 years by myself and my collaborators in the Central Laboratory for Human Embryology at the University of Washington. The standards given here for organ weights, placental weights, and crown–rump, foot, and umbilical cord lengths are very difficult or impossible to locate in existing texts on fetal pathology.[1–12] Similarly, accurate fetal standards improve the neonatologist's ability to determine pathologic events and causes of prenatal deaths. There are a number of new hypotheses presented in this chapter, with supporting information and attempted differentiation from generally accepted theories.

MEASUREMENTS AND AGES OF THE EMBRYO AND FETUS

EMBRYONIC PERIOD

This period spans 52 to 60 days from fertilization through completion of major organogenesis. By the end of the embryonic period, the embryo measures 27 to 32 mm in crown–rump length, most of the organs have their final shape and location, and bone formation has commenced. At the end of the embryonic period, it usually is possible to identify the species. Human embryonic development is divided into 23 well defined stages that often are referred to as Streeter horizons (Table 10-1). A scanning electron micrograph of the face of a human embryo at 42 days estimated age (*i.e.*, stage 18) is shown in Figure 10-1.

Considerable error and confusion arises over the age of embryos. Fertilization or ovulation age is about 14 days less than menstrual age, the age from onset of the last normal menstrual period. Many peer review articles fail to distinguish between the two ages. A further problem is introduced by the use of weeks rather than days because of the significant changes that can occur within a single week. During week 4 (*i.e.*, 21–28 days after fertilization), major changes oc-

TABLE 10–1
LANDMARKS OF HUMAN EMBRYONIC DEVELOPMENT

Age* (days)	Crown–Rump (mm)	Streeter Stage	Characteristic Features
0–1.5		1	One-celled egg
1.5–3.0		2	Segmenting egg, 2–16 cells
4–5		3	Free blastocyst
6.0		4	Implanting ovum
7–11		5	Ovum implanted but avillous
12–14		6	Primitive villi, distinct yolk sac, primitive streak
15–16		7	Branching villi, axis of germ disk defined
17–18		8	Hensen node, primitive groove
19–21		9	Neural folds, elongated notochord, somites appear
22–23(29)†		10	Early somites (*i.e.*, 4–12) present, neural folds begin fusion, S-shaped heart, two branchial bars, posterior neuropore closing
23–25(31)	1.5	11	Paired somites, formation and closure of anterior neuropore, perforation of oral membrane begins
25–27(31)	3–5	12	Paired somites, three branchial bars posterior neuropore closing
26–28(32)	4–6	13	Limb buds become conspicuous
28–30(34)	4–8	14	Indentation of the lens vesicle metanephros developing
30–32(36)	6–10	15	Closed lens vesicle, heart chambers emerging arm buds regionally subdivided
32–34(38)	7–12	16	Eye pigment, prominent olfactory pits, auricular hillocks
34–36(40)	10–14	17	Face appearing, cartilage in ribs, finger rays
36–38(42)	12–17	18	Gender difference in gonad develops, nipples appear, rudimentary ear, interventricular septum complete, müllerian ducts developing rapidly, toe rays
38–40(45)	16–21	19	Point system of Streeter, head straightens, cloaca divided
40–42(46)	19–23	20	Vascular plexus above ear, perforation of anal membrane
42–44(48)	20–25	21	Vascular plexus halfway to vertex, hands approach each other
44–46(52)	23–27	22	Vascular plexus three-fourths of the way to vertex, overlapping hands
46–48(55)	27–32	23	Scalp plexus close to vertex, end of embryonic period and horizons

* Streeter's ages (from ovulation) were obtained by comparison with timed monkey matings. Specimens were fixed in formalin. Data from Streeter GL. Developmental horizons in human embryos: age groups XI to XXIII. Washington, DC: Carnegie Institution of Washington, 1951.

† Fertilization ages in parentheses are calculated from menstrual histories of women undergoing therapeutic abortions. The specimens were fixed. Data from Iffy L, Shepard TH, Jakobovits A, et al. The rate of growth in young human embryos of Streeter's horizons XIII to XXIII. Acta Anat 1967;66:178, and Shiota K, Fischer B, Neubert D. Variability of development in the human embryo. In: Neubert D, Merker H-J, Hendrickx AG, eds. Nonhuman primates: developmental biology and toxicology. Wien, Berlin: Ueberreuter Wissenschaft, 1988.

cur in the embryo. For instance, all neurulation and doubling of length is accomplished; assigning an event to this week of time rather than day lacks precision. Two other problems with assignment of embryonic age usually are not fully recognized. First, many descriptions of human embryonic events use the timing given by Streeter and his associates even though the data are based on timed rhesus monkey embryos, which grow more rapidly than humans.[13,14] At the early limb bud stage, the human embryo is approximately 5 days older than the monkey, and by the end of the embryonic period, the difference is about 8 days.[15–17] A second problem is that the variability in age of an embryo belonging to a particular stage is greater than supposed, probably by as much as 10 days. This variability, although often observed, has been attributed to inaccuracy in dates of the last normal menstrual period. It is an interesting observation that if the dates reported are plotted against the day of the month, an inordinate number of them fall o the first or fifteenth of the month, probably due t rounding by the patient or questioner. Even in a care ful analysis of staged embryos with known, isolate copulation date, Shiota and colleagues found wid variation in age, with a standard deviation of 4 to days.[18] The reason for this wide variation could b differences in times of ovulation, fertilization, or in plantation, or possibly in the rate of growth. Sinc ovulation is fairly constant, and sperm may b present for immediate fertilization at the time of ovu lation, it might be suspected that the time of implar tation is the most variable biologic event. It is strang that a biologic event of this magnitude still shrouded in some mystery.

The period or window of vulnerability for terat genic activity of an agent is commonly assigned as time span of a number of days. At the end of this tim period, the morphogenetic event is completed an

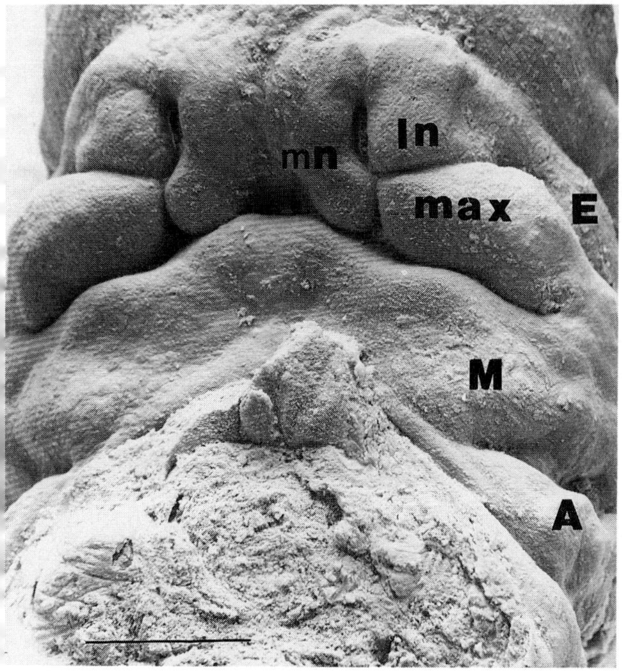

FIG. 10–1. Facial fusion in a stage-17 human embryo at 42 days from estimated fertilization. (A, auricular hillocks; E, eye; ln, lateral nasal process; M, mandible; max, maxillary process; MN, medial nasal process; bar = 250 μm; specimen H-10,804 courtesy of Central Laboratory for Human Embryology, University of Washington, Seattle, WA.)

any change is assumed to be due to disruption of the structures. In *in vitro* cultures of rat and mouse embryos, it is common in the same litter to find a difference in somite number of three to five. The response on exposure to an agent may be markedly dissimilar in two experimental groups of embryos that differ by only two to three somites or a few hours.[19,20] This difference helps explain how identical twins may vary strikingly in their response to a teratogenic exposure. This most exquisite timing obviously creates further problems for the clinical investigator studying the time effects of teratogens on humans.

FETAL PERIOD

The fetal period extends from the end of the embryonic period until birth. Several methods for fetal measurements can be used. The crown–rump length is a favorite measurement because it is simple, accurate, and reproducible. The crown–rump length *versus* age is shown in Figure 10-2. In early embryonic stages, until the embryo converts from dorsiflexion to ventroflexion at about day 25, crown–rump length is not helpful, but subsequently, it often is measured to within 0.1 mm. For older specimens, the measurement is made in the prone position. The data reported here are collected from fetal specimens before fixation because fixation slightly reduces the length and sometimes causes reduction by flexion. The crown–heel measurement, although useful after

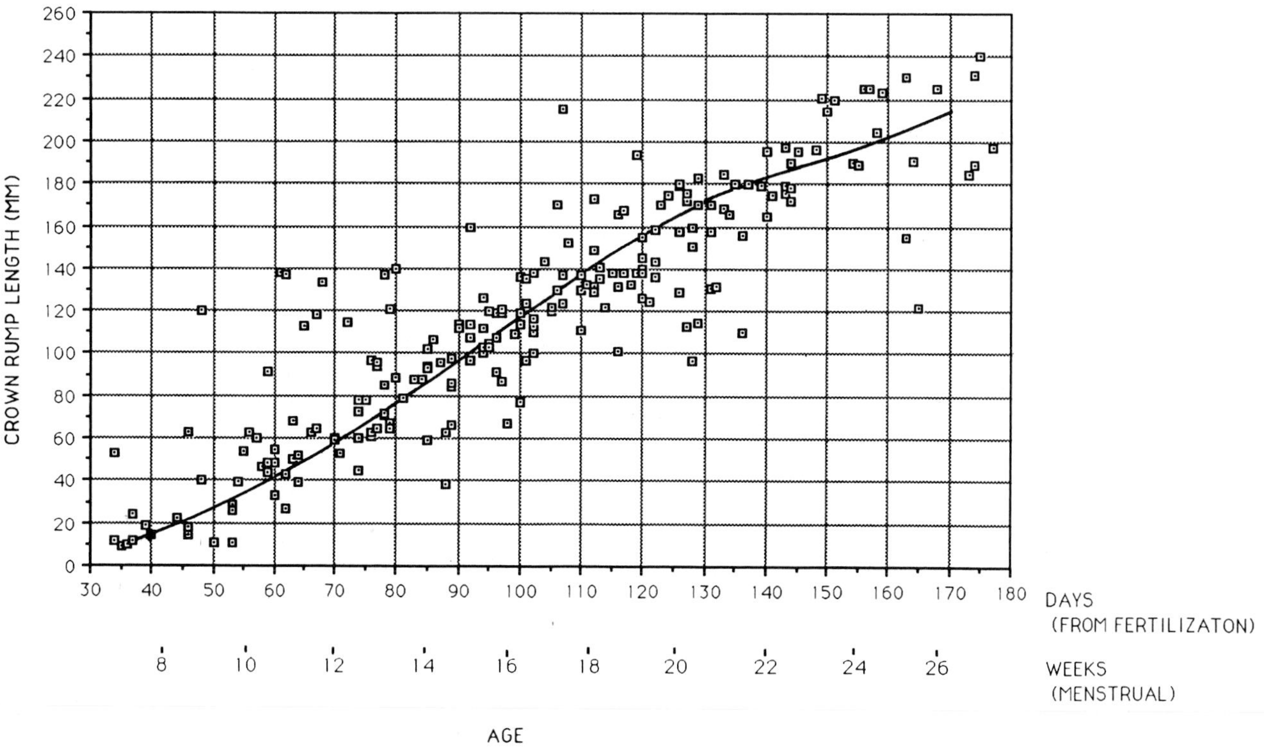

FIG. 10–2. Crown–rump length *versus* age. The tick marks for weeks indicate the last day of the week.

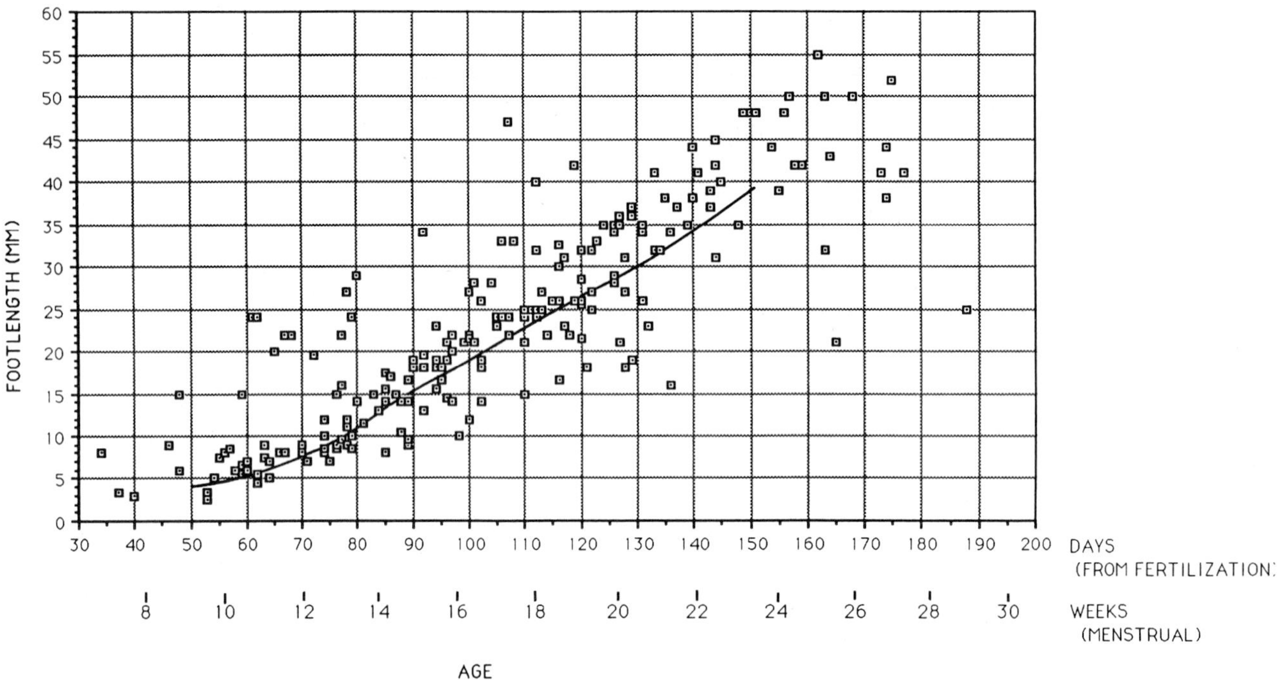

FIG. 10–3. Foot length *versus* age. The tick marks for weeks indicate the last day of the week.

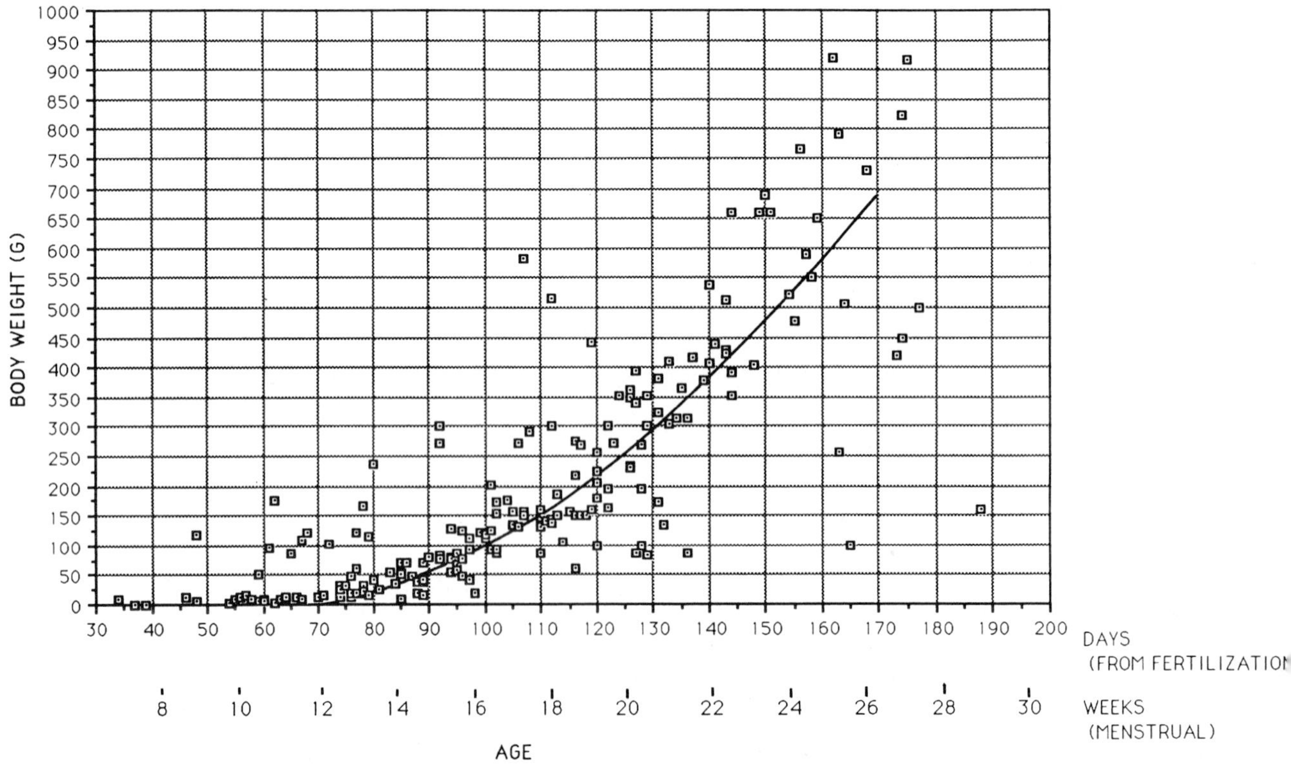

FIG. 10–4. Body weight *versus* age. The tick marks for weeks indicate the last day of the week.

midgestation, adds error by increasing the number of angles to be straightened (*i.e.*, hip, knee, and ankle). After fixation, crown–heel measurement is inaccurate, whereas crown–rump measurement is feasible. After the embryonic period, the greatest foot length is of particular help in estimating the crown–rump length and age of disrupted specimens (Fig. 10-3). Because the elements of foot length are mostly bony skeleton, the measurement changes little with fixation. Body weight is used for fetal measurements (Fig. 10-4). Because the water content of the younger embryo is 93% or more, exposure to air rapidly dehydrates and damages an embryo. Fixation in formalin increases the weight gradually by about 10%, so this increase returns the specimen toward its true embryonic weight after about 2 weeks.

LANDMARKS OF FETAL DEVELOPMENT

The normal herniation of the gastrointestinal tract is sometimes seen on ultrasound and may be confused with omphalocele. The retraction of the gut from the cord is complete by 64 days from fertilization, or the start of the eleventh menstrual week.[21] The final fusion of the posterior palate occurs between 60 and 65 days after fertilization, which is a few days after the eyelids have fused at about 60 days from fertilization. The average time for opening of the eyelid is stated to be the sixth month, but the precise week is variable. The testes become extraperitoneal during the seventh month.[22]

ORGAN AND PLACENTAL WEIGHTS

The means and 95th percentiles of various fetal organ weights are essential information for an approach to the study of fetal pathology. These data for organ weights of fetuses with normal autopsies, drawn from over 500 specimens with body weights between 25 and 1000 g,[23,24] are given in Table 10-2. These figures are similar to those reported in another, smaller study by Globus and associates.[25] In Figure 10-5, the percentages of organ weights to body weights are shown. The relative weight of the brain, liver, and heart remain constant, whereas a slight increase in kidney weight and a drop in lung and adrenal weight are evident. Thymus and spleen weights increase

Text continued on page 116

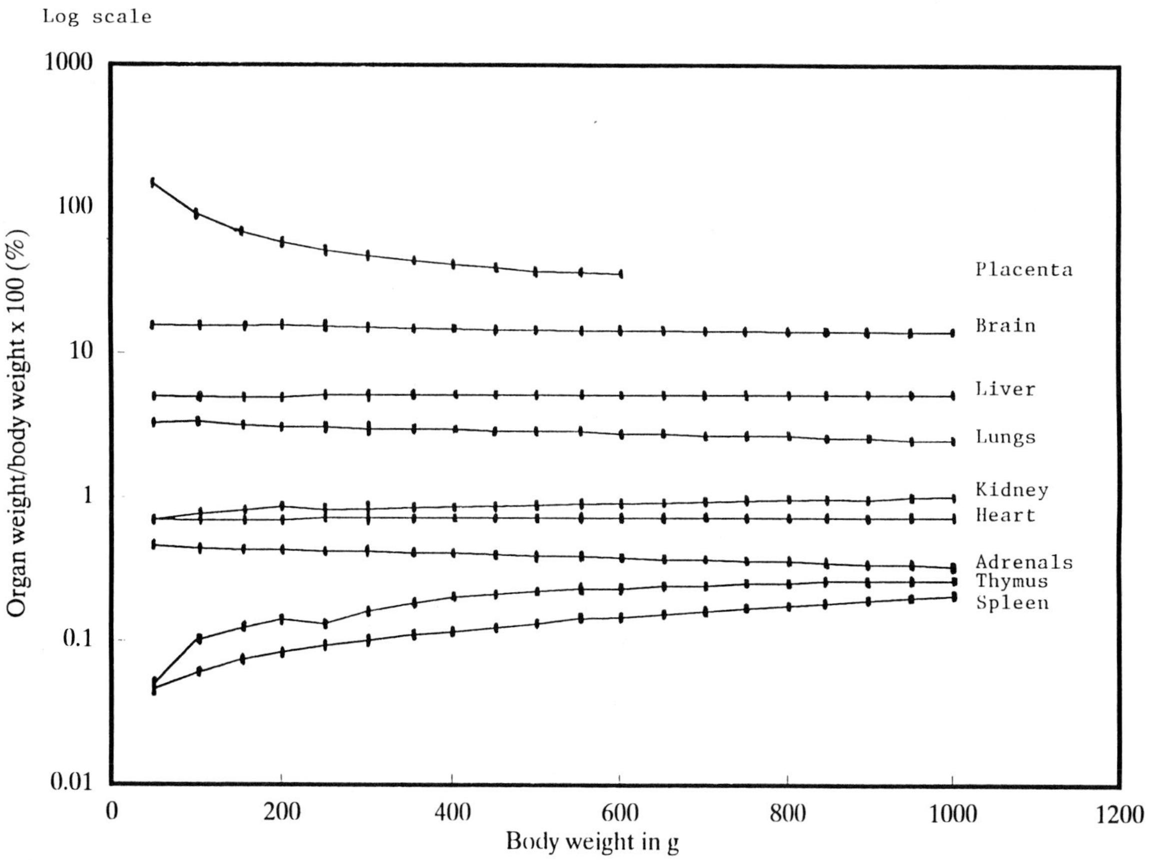

FIG. 10–5. Ratio of organ and placenta weights to body weight × 100 on log scale, *versus* body weight (see Table 10-2). (Data from Shepard TH, Barr M, Fellingham GW, et al. Organ weight standards for human fetuses. Pediatr Pathol 1988;4:513, and Shepard TH, FitzSimmons J, Fantel AG, et al. Placental weights of normal and aneuploid early human fetuses. Pediatr Pathol 1989;9:425.)

TABLE 10–2
FETAL ORGAN WEIGHTS AND RANGES BY BODY WEIGHT IN GRAMS

Body Weight	Placenta	Thymus	Spleen	Liver	Kidneys	Adrenals	Lungs	Heart	Brain
25	45.8 (18.8–72.8)	0.018 (0–0.038)	0.01 (0–0.02)	1.28 (0.76–1.81)	0.165 (0.075–0.255)	0.11 (0.05–0.17)	0.79 (0.39–1.19)	0.175 (0.085–0.27)	3.84 (2.6–5.0)
50	74.1 (28.6–132.6)	0.025 (0–0.077)	0.023 (0.003–0.04)	2.51 (0.76–1.81)	0.35 (0.19–0.52)	0.23 (0.11–0.35)	1.64 (0.87–2.42)	0.35 (0.18–0.52)	7.66 (6.3–9.1)
75	86.6 (34.6–138.6)	0.068 (0.01–0.127)	0.04 (0.009–0.07)	3.75 (2.25–5.25)	0.55 (0.3–0.8)	0.33 (0.14–0.52)	2.51 (1.21–3.84)	0.52 (0.27–0.78)	11.5 (8.7–14.3)
100	92.5 (40.5–144.5)	0.099 (0.018–0.136)	0.059 (0.017–0.1)	4.98 (2.98–6.98)	0.76 (0.42–1.1)	0.44 (0.19–0.69)	3.42 (1.62–5.22)	0.69 (0.35–1.03)	15.3 (11.5–19.1)
125	98.5 (46.5–150.5)	0.135 (0.04–0.23)	0.08 (0.03–0.13)	6.22 (3.7–8.75)	0.98 (0.55–1.4)	0.546 (0.24–0.86)	4.36 (2.1–6.6)	0.86 (4.4–1.29)	19.1 (14.7–23.5)
150	104.5 (52.5–156.5)	0.175 (0.06–0.29)	0.11 (0.04–0.17)	7.46 (4.5–10.5)	1.22 (0.71–1.7)	0.65 (0.28–1.03)	4.74 (2.69–6.8)	1.04 (0.53–1.55)	23 (17.2–28.8)
175	110.5 (56.5–161)	0.22 (0.08–0.36)	0.135 (0.06–0.21)	8.69 (5.2–12.2)	1.46 (0.86–2.1)	0.75 (0.31–1.19)	5.5 (2.9–8.1)	1.21 (0.61–1.81)	26.8 (20.3–33.3)
200	116.5 (64.5–168.5)	0.27 (0.11–0.43)	0.166 (0.08–0.25)	9.93 (5.5–14.3)	1.72 (1.15–2.3)	0.86 (0.36–1.36)	6.25 (3.3–9.2)	1.38 (0.81–1.96)	30.7 (25–36.3)
225	122.5 (70.5–174)	0.35 (0.1–0.6)	0.187 (0.097–0.28)	11.6 (6.6–16.6)	1.83 (1.8–2.58)	0.96 (0.4–1.5)	6.99 (3.8–10.2)	1.62 (0.97–2.27)	34.8 (28.8–40.7)
250	128.4 (76.4–180)	0.326 (0.1–0.68)	0.23 (0.13–0.32)	12.9 (7.64–18.1)	2.05 (1.23–2.87)	1.06 (0.43–1.68)	7.72 (5.5–15.5)	1.8 (1.06–2.54)	38.1 (31.1–45.6)
275	134.4 (82–186.4)	0.4 (0.1–0.79)	0.26 (0.15–0.49)	14.2 (8.45–20)	2.27 (1.33–3.2)	1.15 (0.47–1.84)	8.43 (4.4–12.4)	1.98 (1.2–2.76)	41.5 (33.0–50.0)
300	140.4 (88.4–192.4)	0.48 (0.1–0.89)	0.3 (0.17–0.55)	15.5 (9.2–21.7)	2.5 (1.5–3.5)	1.25 (0.5–2.0)	9.14 (4.8–13.5)	2.16 (1.26–3.06)	44.9 (36.0–53.0)
325	146.4 (94.4–198.4)	0.54 (0.1–0.99)	0.34 (0.06–0.62)	16.7 (9.74–23.7)	2.73 (1.6–3.8)	1.34 (.54–2.1)	9.97 (5.4–14.6)	2.34 (1.3–3.3)	48.2 (38.2–58.2)
350	152.4 (100.4–204)	0.63 (1.3–1.13)	0.38 (0.08–0.68)	18 (10.5–25.5)	2.96 (1.8–4.1)	1.43 (0.6–2.3)	10.5 (5.5–15.5)	2.52 (1.5–3.6)	51.6 (41.1–62.1)
375	158.3 (106–210)	0.71 (0.19–1.23)	0.42 (0.1–0.73)	19.3 (11.3–27.3)	3.2 (1.95–4.45)	1.53 (0.59–2.46)	11.2 (5.8–16.2)	2.7 (1.6–3.8)	55 (43.5–66.5)
400	164.3 (112–216)	0.79 (0.21–1.36)	0.46 (0.12–0.8)	20.6 (12.1–29.1)	3.44 (2.0–4.8)	1.62 (0.6–2.6)	11.9 (6.1–17.6)	2.87 (1.7–4.1)	58.3 (46.3–70.3)

425	170.3 (118–223)	0.87 (0.26–1.47)	0.5 (0.14–0.87)	21.9 (12.9–30.9)	3.68 (2.2–5.2)	1.7 (0.64–2.8)	12.5 (6.3–18.8)	3.06 (1.76–4.4)	61.7 (48.7–74.7)
450	176.3 (124–228)	0.94 (0.29–1.6)	0.55 (0.15–0.95)	23.2 (13.5–32.8)	3.92 (2.4–5.4)	1.79 (0.7–2.9)	13.2 (6.6–19.8)	3.24 (1.9–4.6)	65 (52.5–78.5)
475	182.3 (130–234)	1.02 (0.34–1.7)	0.6 (1.8–1)	24.5 (14.5–34.5)	4.17 (2.6–5.8)	1.88 (0.69–3.1)	13.8 (6.9–20.7)	3.42 (2.0–4.9)	68.4 (54.4–82.4)
500	188.3 (136–240)	1.1 (0.4–1.95)	0.65 (0.21–1.1)	25.7 (15–36.5)	4.42 (2.77–6.1)	1.96 (0.73–3.2)	14.5 (7.1–21.8)	3.6 (2.1–5.1)	71.8 (56.8–86.8)
525	194 (142–246)	1.17 (0.4–1.95)	0.7 (0.25–1.16)	27 (15.8–38.3)	4.67 (2.9–6.4)	2 (0.75–3.33)	15.1 (7.5–22.7)	3.78 (2.18–5.38)	75.2 (59.7–90.7)
550	200 (148–250)	1.25 (0.46–2)	0.78 (0.3–1.26)	28.3 (16.3–40.3)	4.93 (3.05–6.8)	2.12 (0.76–3.48)	15.7 (7.7–23.7)	3.96 (2.31–5.6)	78.5 (62–95)
575	206 (154–258)	1.33 (0.5–2.1)	0.81 (0.31–1.31)	29.6 (17–42.2)	5.2 (3.2–7.2)	2.2 (.81–3.6)	16.3 (8.1–24.6)	4.14 (2.4–5.9)	81.9 (64.9–98.9)
600	212 (160–264)	1.4 (0.56–2.25)	0.87 (0.35–1.39)	30.9 (18–43.8)	5.46 (3.45–7.47)	2.28 (0.78–3.78)	16.9 (8.2–25.5)	4.32 (2.53–6.11)	85.3 (67–103)
650		1.56 (0.64–2.5)	0.99 (0.44–1.55)	33.5 (19.7–47.2)	5.99 (3.79–8.19)	2.43 (0.81–4.05)	18 (8.6–27.5)	4.67 (2.72–6.62)	92 (73–111)
700		1.7 (0.72–2.7)	1.12 (0.505–1.73)	36 (21–51)	6.54 (4.14–8.94)	2.58 (0.83–4.3)	19.2 (9–29.3)	5.03 (2.93–7.13)	98.7 (77.7–119.7)
750		1.87 (0.84–2.9)	1.26 (0.61–1.19)	38.6 (23.1–54.1)	7.1 (4.57–9.63)	2.71 (0.85–4.57)	20.2 (9.3–31.2)	5.39 (3.13–7.64)	105.5 (83.5–127.5)
800		2.02 (0.88–3.16)	1.4 (0.7–2.1)	41.3 (25.3–59.3)	7.68 (5–10.4)	2.85 (0.85–4.85)	21.3 (9.8–32.8)	5.75 (3.4–8.1)	112 (88.7–135.7)
850		2.18 (0.97–3.4)	1.55 (0.81–2.29)	43.7 (25.3–62)	8.27 (5.4–11.2)	2.97 (0.86–5.1)	22.3 (9.9–34.7)	6.11 (3.56–8.67)	119 (94–144)
900		2.33 (1.03–3.6)	1.71 (0.91–2.51)	46.3 (27–65.6)	8.67 (5.6–11.7)	3.1 (0.84–5.34)	23.2 (10–36.7)	6.47 (3.77–9.2)	125.7 (99–152)
950		2.48 (1.13–3.83)	1.88 (1.04–2.72)	48.9 (28.6–69.2)	9.48 (6.3–12.7)	3.2 (0.83–5.6)	24 (10.3–38)	6.83 (4–9.7)	132.4 (105–160)
1000		2.64 (1.22–4.1)	2.05 (1.16–2.9)	51.5 (30.4–72.5)	10.1 (6.7–13.5)	3.32 (0.8–5.8)	25 (10.5–39.5)	7.2 (4.2–10.2)	139 (110–168)

Data are means of 95% confidence level.

Data from Shepard TH, Barr M, Fellingham, GW, et al. Organ weight standards for human fetuses. Pediatr Pathol 1988;4:513, and Shepard TH, FitzSimmons J, Fantel AG, et al. Placental weights of normal and aneuploid early human fetuses. Pediatr Pathol 1989;9:425.

during this period. Placental weights for fetuses up to 500 g body weight are shown in Figure 10-6.[26] These specimens were obtained from fetuses with normal autopsies and recorded in the fresh state after removal of maternal clots and the umbilical cord.

Cord lengths are shown in Figure 10-7.[27] Cord lengths from fetuses weighing up to 500 g fit into the lower levels of the cord lengths reported for older fetuses.[28] Umbilical length is believed to be increased by fetal movement and decreased by fetal inactivity.[1] Fujinaga and colleagues have questioned this association because some fetuses with oligohydramnios and presumed decreased activity have unusually long cords.[27] More information on movement by fetuses with oligohydramnios is needed. Fetuses with trisomy 18 and anencephaly tend to have short cords, as do fetuses with body wall fixation from amniotic bands.

Because the limit of extrauterine viability is considered by some to be when the fetus weighs about 500 g, some means of specific growth parameters at this stage are given. The 500-g fetus is approximately 158 days from conception, or about 21 menstrual weeks of age. The average crown–rump length is 203 mm, crown–heel length 295 mm, and foot length 42 mm. The head circumference is about 20 cm (Fig. 10-8). The external biparietal diameter is 5.5 cm.

Standards for bone length and measurement by ultrasound are available (see Chap. 13).[29,30] The length of the long bones in control and trisomy 21 fetuses has been reported by FitzSimmons and associates and Benacerraf and colleagues.[31,32] Some disproportionate reduction in femur and humerus length has been reported for trisomy 21, but the variation is not consistent enough to be of practical use in prenatal diagnosis. The classification and pathology of short-limbed dwarfism in the fetus has been reviewed by Yang,[33] and prenatal diagnosis by ultrasound examination is fully covered by Mahony.[30]

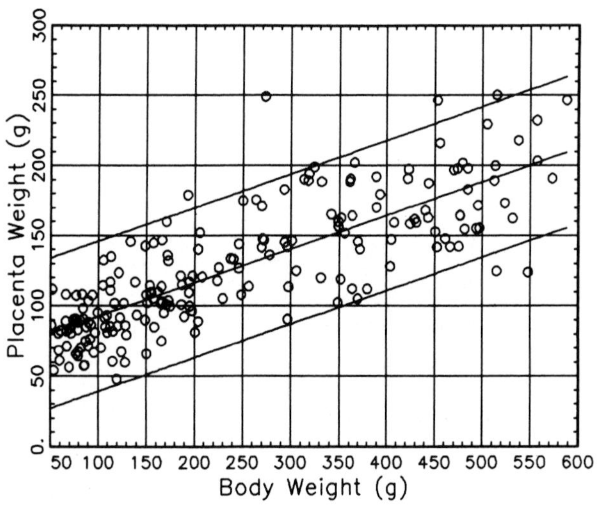

FIG. 10–6. Placenta weight *versus* body weight. (From Shepard TH, FitzSimmons J, Fantel AG, et al. Placental weights of normal and aneuploid early human fetuses. Pediatr Pathol 1989;9:425.)

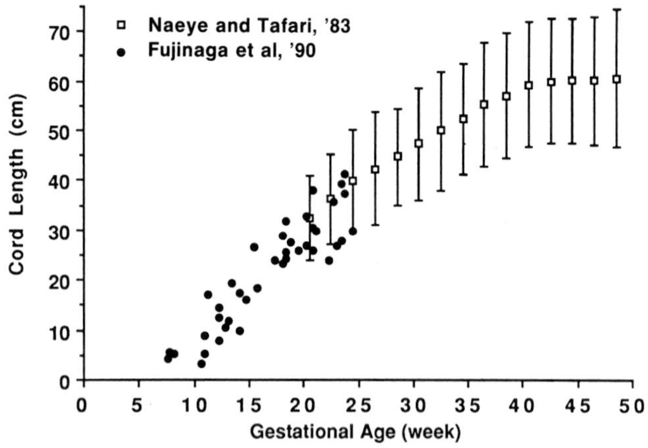

FIG. 10–7. Cord length *versus* menstrual age. (Data from Fujinaga M, Chinn A, Shepard TH. The umbilical cord length in human and rat fetuses: normal and pathologic condition. Teratology 1990;41:333, and Naeye RL, Tafari N. Noninfectious disorders of the placenta, fetal membranes and umbilical cord. In: Risk factors in pregnancy and disease of the fetus and newborn. Baltimore: Williams & Wilkins, 1983;145.)

PATHOLOGIC MECHANISMS IN THE EMBRYO AND FETUS

Cellular and humoral mechanisms for defense in the fetus have been described, but less so for the embryo, particularly in the primate. Data from experimental models in small rodents exposed to teratogens suggest that the embryonic defense mechanism is based strictly on local or cellular reaction rather than the systemic response of chemical attractants, vascular changes, and mobilization of an immune cellular system. Instead of the usual major response, the embryo relies on a very active, local phagocytosis. Almost every embryonic cell, including the neuroblast, has the ability to convert to a phagocytosing cell. This activity allows for the cleanup of dead cells and, to some extent, the phagocytosed material may allow the recipient cells to grow and multiply more rapidly. Although a hypothesis, there is good experimental evidence for this rapid, local cleanup by surviving cells. If the embryo survives this process, there is a deficit of cells that causes parts of the embryo to be incomplete or absent. Because there is no acute-phase injury response with leukocytes and then fibroblast repair, the embryo's only "scar" is represented by missing tissue.

A number of examples of this embryonic defense mechanism are available. Rat embryos exposed to riboflavin deficiency and deprivation of electron transport activity are characterized at birth by absent digits

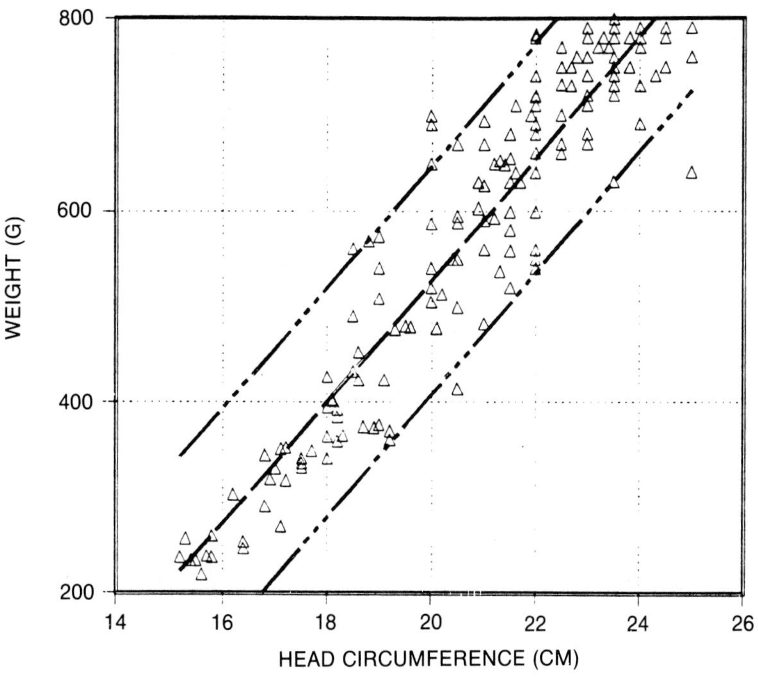

FIG. 10–8. Head circumference (cm) *versus* weight (g). Dashed lines enclose 95% confidence interval. (Data from Mark Elliot, M.D., unpublished medical school thesis, University of Washington, Seattle, WA, 1986.)

and short mandibles.[34,35] On embryonic days 12 and 13, major areas of the precursors of these two organs contain large areas of cell necrosis. With phagocytosis by day 15, the necrotic areas disappear; the resulting lack of cells produces reductions in the number of digital rays and the length of the mandible. A photomicrograph showing phagocytosis on day 14 is presented in Figure 10-9. Some of the remaining digital rays appear thicker than normal as a result of absence of interdigital mesenchyme and fusion of two rays. A similar cellular reaction (*i.e.*, oligosyndactylism) has been shown in a mutant mouse.[36] Extensive cell death has been found in the central nervous system in limbs of rat embryos exposed to another teratogen, hydroxyurea.[37] Cell death also is a prominent feature in embryos exposed to hyperthermia.[38] In these studies, there has been no evidence such as perivascular accumulation of phagocytes that would suggest the cells arrive through the vascular system. In addition, inflammatory cells are not present within the vascular system. Restorative and compensatory growth by damaged mammalian embryos has been reviewed by Snow,[39] but he seems not to have realized the importance of local phagocytosis. Programmed cell death (*i.e.*, apoptosis) is a normal mechanism of developmental sculpturing, difficult to differentiate at times from cell death due to toxic agents.

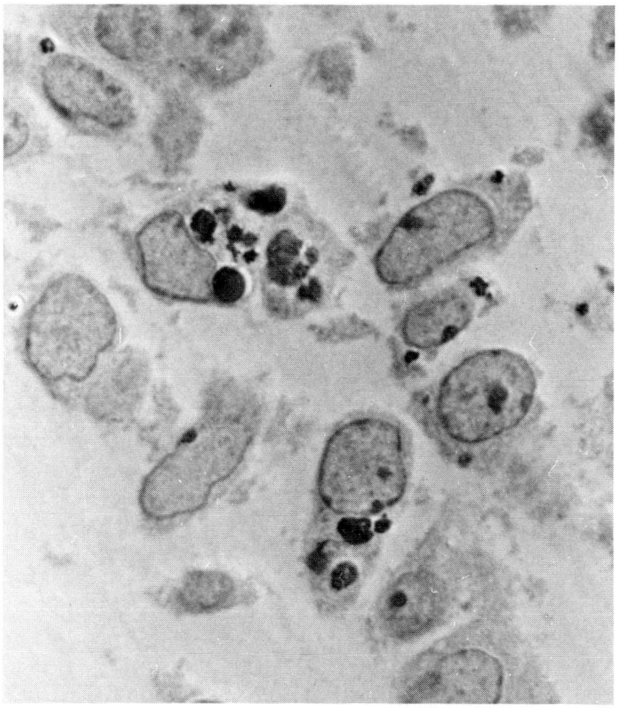

FIG. 10–9. Three cells contain numerous dark-staining ingested particles in mesenchyme of the upper extremity of a riboflavin-deficient embryo. (Plastic embedded, 1-μm thickness, toluidine blue stain, original magnification × 2450; from Shepard TH, Lemire RJ, Aksu O, et al. Studies of the development of congenital anomalies in embryos of riboflavin-deficient, galactoflavin-fed rats: I. Growth and embryonic pathology. Teratology 1968;1:75.)

Other cellular mechanisms such as delay in differentiation or decrease in mitotic rate can account for congenital defects of embryonic origin. One of the best-studied examples is facial clefting in the genetically susceptible, inbred mouse strain A/J. Detailed studies showed that the nasal and maxillary processes were smaller and more separated than in controls, and their increased distances prevented normal closure.[40] The role of glucocorticoids and epidermal growth factor as well as other growth factors has been under study. Evidence that retinoic acid causes palatal teratogenesis through embryonic growth factors has appeared.[41,42] The role of defective morphogenetic tissue interactions in the pathogenesis of malformations has been thoroughly reviewed by Saxen[43] and Bernfield.[44]

During the second one-half of pregnancy, inflammatory response matures gradually toward the limited reaction found in newborns. In fetal and neonatal rats, Dixon produced burns using an electrically heated needle.[45] On days 16.5 and 17.5 of 21-day gestations, mesenchymal reaction without blood vessel reaction occurred, whereas on day 18, vascular congestion and mononuclear infiltrates were found. On day 19, 2 days before birth, polymorphonuclear cells began to increase. In a study of guinea pig fetuses, histocytes were the reactive cells during the first one-half of gestation.[45] In a study of monkey fetuses receiving various subcutaneous injections, small mononuclear cells appeared after treatment with turpentine at 90 days.[47] At 150 days, the response was mostly mononuclear, with occasional polymorphonuclear cells present in addition to edema and fibrin. In human fetuses with congenital syphilis or toxoplasmosis, plasma cells and lymphocytes were found to be increased after week 24.[48] Plasma cells were not found in normal fetuses and an inflammatory response to syphilis was absent in fetuses of less than 5 months' gestation.

Studies of peripheral blood from human fetuses indicate very low leukocyte precursor counts ranging from 20 to 50 to 500 per mm^3 between the twelfth to sixteenth menstrual week and increasing to around 2000 to 5000 per mm^3 by the twentieth week.[49,50] Lymphocyte counts reach 2000 to 5000 and monocytes are from 100 to 2000 per mm^3 by the twentieth week.[49] The hemoglobin is 6 to 8 g/dL and the hematocrit between 20% to 30% at 10 weeks. Hemostasis in the early fetus is practically nonexistent.[51] In fetuses of a crown–rump length of 80 mm or less, whole blood clotting times are at infinity and no platelets are seen. Overall, these ontogenetic events reflect the phylogenetic pattern in which vessel contraction, platelet reactions, and fibrin formation are thought to have evolved successively. The fetal level for serum proteins is 3.60 $\pm$ 1.0 g/dL and the albumin is 1.90 $\pm$ 0.66 g/dL in fetuses with crown–rump lengths of 102 to 213 mm.[52] This borderline low level in normal fetuses may help explain the frequent appearance of edema in fetuses with a variety of disease states.

A rather convoluted set of classifications purporting or implying mechanisms has been developed for congenital defects.[53–55] A *deformation* is a physical change in form, shape, or position caused by mechanical forces secondary to restricted intrauterine motion (*e.g.*, clubfoot). Application of a countering force usually corrects the deformation. A *disruption* is a congenital defect resulting from an extrinsic breakdown in or interference with an originally normal developmental process; an amniotic band malformation, for example, would fit into this group. In most of these cases, the pathogenetic effect would be initiated after the window of vulnerability and cell death usually would be a feature. A final major classification is the *developmental field defect,* which implies a basic embryologic problem. Congenital defect syndromes could result from field defects either in contiguous (*i.e.*, monotopic) or distantly located (*i.e.*, polytopic) structures. The concept of field defects is interesting, but does not help much in the current understanding of developmental pathology. Without a real understanding of normal embryologic controls, it is difficult to postulate abnormal ones. These fields should be better defined by knowledge of specific cascades of known developmental genes, some of which may belong to the homeobox group. For example, the congenital Beckwith–Weidemann syndrome has been closely linked to paternal disomy on chromosome position 11p15.5, which is the domain of an important embryonic growth factor, insulinlike growth factor 2.[56–58] This example links embryonic growth factors to congenital defects and, in addition, to certain childhood neoplasms that have been shown to be linked with this biologic control mechanism.

POSTMORTEM ARTIFACTS

Postmortem artifacts represent one major reason for lack of interest in prenatal pathology of the abortus. Separating from true pathology the effects of autolysis resulting from long uterine retention has vexed many workers in this field. It is possible to calculate the gestational age of the conceptus from menstrual history and from the crown–rump or foot lengths of the embryo or fetus. The former presumably represents the period of time during which the embryo or fetus remained *in utero*, whereas the latter represents time of growth, assuming reasonably normal growth rates. The discrepancy between the two sets of ages gives a crude estimation of the period of time *in utero* after death.

When this estimation was done for 30 specimens in my collection, the average discrepancy was approximately 24 days—that is, 3 weeks intervened between the death of the conceptus and its expulsion. An extreme example was that of a woman who had rubella during early pregnancy. After 8 months of pregnancy, she miscarried a fetus measuring 140 mm in crown–rump length. This length corresponds to an estimated gestational age of approximately 112 days, giving a discrepancy of around 14 weeks between fetal demise and expulsion. Rubella virus was cultured from the placenta.

I have found it useful to categorize abortuses by

TABLE 10–3
CLASSIFICATION OF POSTMORTEM EFFECTS IN ABORTUSES

Grade I	Grade II	Grade III
Fresh: (0–12 h postmortem), glistening, hydrated	Grossly normal: (≥12 h postmortem), not grey or tan	Macerated: (≥ 2–3 days postmortem) gray or tan
Skin intact except for occasional neck tears	Some peeling of skin, slight posterior nuchal edema	Collapsed head and chest
Blood unclotted usually	Blood clotted	Old blood in tissues has greenish cast
Heart muscle irritable	No heart irritability	
Liver firm	Liver soft	Liver liquified
Subcutaneous hemorrhage of vertex indicates viability at time of passage	No subcutaneous hemorrhage if stillbirth	
Extremities firm and of normal configuration	Rigor of extremities	Soft, misshapen extremities
Mitotic figures in tissue: cortex of kidney and ependymal zone of nervous system	No mitotic figures	Many necrotic cells

their degree of postmortem change, using the scheme presented in Table 10-3. The three classes span the range from those with no postmortem change and numerous mitotic figures in tissues throughout the body, to severely macerated ones with collapsed head and chest and liquified liver. The collapsed head may even be mistaken for hydrocephalus in extreme cases. Postmortem changes are associated with increased friability of tissues and this may lead to tearing of the abdomen at the point of insertion of the umbilical cord. This tearing may be misdiagnosed as gastroschisis or omphalocele. Similar changes occur less frequently in the cervical area. The normally fused eyelids may open. The skin of the fingers may slough, mimicking syndactyly. Developmental inconsistencies may result. Most frequently, circular pigmentation of the iris is observed in an embryo when physiologic coloboma would still be expected. In these instances, I believe that certain developmental processes, once begun, will continue despite relative hypoxia or other necrotic changes of the conceptus.

DEFECT RATES

The congenital defect rates in spontaneous abortuses are approximately 20%, which is about ten times higher than in the newborn. Based on a 20-year study of 1124 spontaneously aborted specimens, 214 (19.0%) had either a localized defect or identifiable syndrome.[59] No trend or change over time was noted in the type of defect or the incidence. Compared to ten other studies, where the rate varied between 4.8% to 39.8%, the differences are explained mostly in methods of defining defects, the ages of the conceptuses, and in selection by the referral system.[58]

The type of congenital defect present is very different among spontaneous abortuses, therapeutic abortuses, and newborns. In Table 10-4, it can be seen that structural defects of the brain are about 44 per 1000 spontaneous abortuses, compared to 2 to 4 and 0.3 to 0.9 in the therapeutic and newborn groups, respectively. The spontaneous abortion group also contains a very high proportion of sirenomelia, heart

TABLE 10–4
DEFECT RATES PER 1000 CASES IN EACH GROUP: SPONTANEOUS ABORTUSES, VOLUNTARY TERMINATION ABORTUSES, AND NEWBORNS

Defect Type	Spontaneous Abortuses	Voluntary Termination Abortuses	Newborns
Brain structure	44	2–4	0.3–0.9
Cleft lip, cleft palate, or both	25.8	5.8	1.0–2.7
Heart defect	130		5
Cyclopia	5–18	2.1	0
Polydactyly	0.6–1.3	2.8	0.5–1.4
Sirenomelia	4.0		0
Chromosomal	500–600 (early) 200–300 (late)	28	6

Data from references 59 through 66.

defects, amniotic band syndrome, and cleft lip and palate (see Table 10-4). In contrast, the frequency of polydactyly does not differ significantly among the three groups.

The most notable difference is in the rate of chromosomal aneuploidy. Approximately 75% of structurally abnormal embryos and fetuses never reach the viable stage, and Warkany has suggested that more attention be paid to the natural screening process whereby these defective fetuses are lost.[67] Warkany coined a name for study of the process: "terathanasia."[67]

PATHOGENESIS OF SELECTED SYNDROMES

Direct examination of embryonic and fetal material from specimens that ultimately would have had various malformations is a valuable source for creating and testing hypotheses about pathogenesis. The following comments on a selected few syndromes are based on over 12,000 specimens selected during a 30-year period. Most of the material has been published, but the proposed mechanisms have not always been given prominence. Three books specializing in descriptions of spontaneous abortion material are available,[3,12,68] as well as other textbooks dealing with neonatal and fetal pathology.[3–13]

AMNIOTIC BAND DISRUPTION SYNDROMES

A spectrum of congenital amniotic band syndromes ranges from a single constriction of a digit to more severe distortions of the body wall, face, and brain. It usually is sporadic, with a rate of 1 to 3 per 10,000 newborns.[69,70] The bands are made up of amniotic cells with a fibrous core.[1] I agree with Jones and Gilbert–Barness and Opitz that the type of involvement relates to the period of development in which the insult occurs.[55,71] Figure 10-10 illustrates the various anatomic associations in this group. My collection of 42 cases contains an overabundance of the more se vere types due to a bias in referral. The involvemer of the skull occurred in 19 cases and was combine with facial disruption in 18. The facial features wer remarkably similar to one another, with a distortin band extending through the face deep into the nas pharynx. The premaxillary portion of the palate wa displaced rostrally, whereas the palatal shelves wer elevated and either touching or fused (Fig. 10-11 The brain lesion has been called pseudoanencephaly the band attachments appear in the area of the fore brain. During the midsomite stages (*i.e.*, stages 11 12), the two surfaces most likely to adhere to a ban are the cephalic edges of the closing neuropore an the breakdown areas of the oral plate. Filaments c tissue have been observed extending from the perfo rating oral plate and, in animal embryos, surface ruf fles have been described on the edges of the neura fold. The hypothesis is that strands in the amnioti fluid attach to these two areas and subsequently, b traction, deform the structures. In the four cases I'v seen that had head and face attachments, there wa involvement of the upper extremity only; this coul have been initiated at a later period when the arm had grown long enough to tangle in the bands fror the face and head. It is noteworthy that no combina tions of skull and extremity or face and extremit were found. This may support a separation in time c the two events. Ventral body wall defects are calle cyllosomus or pleurosomus, depending on whethe the abdominal or pleural cavity, respectively, is in volved. Only 4 of the 21 cases of ventral body wa defect were isolated.

One aspect of embryonic development that ma play an important role in this malformation sequenc has been mostly neglected. The space between th amnion and chorionic base (*i.e.*, exocoelom) is fille with a very sticky substance. The stickiness of thi jellylike material is illustrated in Figure 10-12. The ge liquifies after formalin fixation or simple overnigh storage in refrigeration, which may account for wh so little attention has been given it in the literature

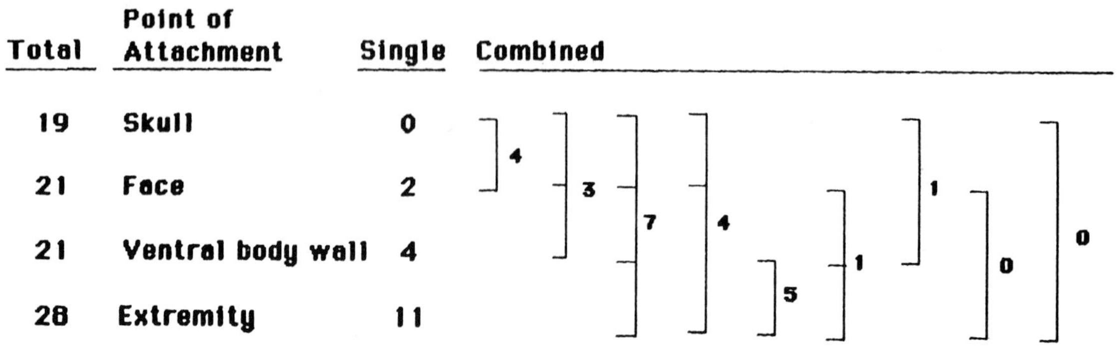

FIG. 10–10. Anatomic associations of 42 cases of amniotic band disruption were collected over 27 years in the Central Laboratory for Human Embryology (University of Washington, Seattle, WA.)

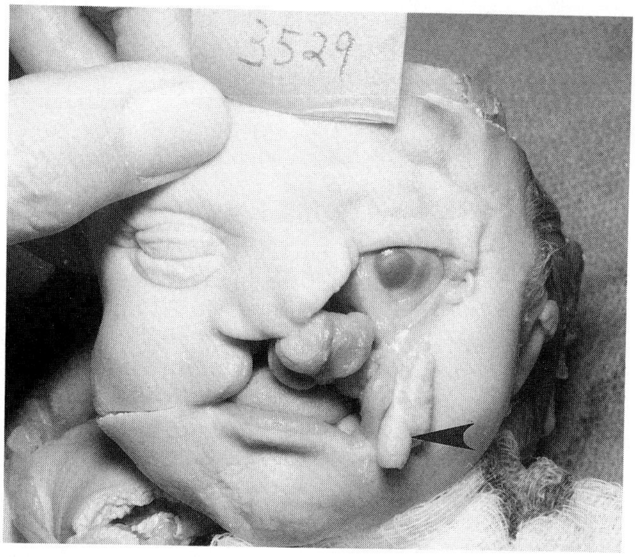

FIG. 10–11. Facial features of amniotic band disruption. The premaxilla is displaced rostrally, and a deep cleft exists between the lateral and medial nasal processes. A partial proboscis (*arrow*) is located on top of the maxillary region. The palatal shelves were touching posteriorly. (Specimen H-3529, courtesy of Central Laboratory for Human Embryology, University of Washington, Seattle, WA.)

This cavity becomes obliterated when the expanding amniotic cavity contacts the chorion toward the end of the embryonic period. The presence of such a sticky material separated from the embryo by only a single epithelial layer of the amnion makes it tempting to hypothesize that it may be important in pathogenic events that lead to amniotic band disruption.

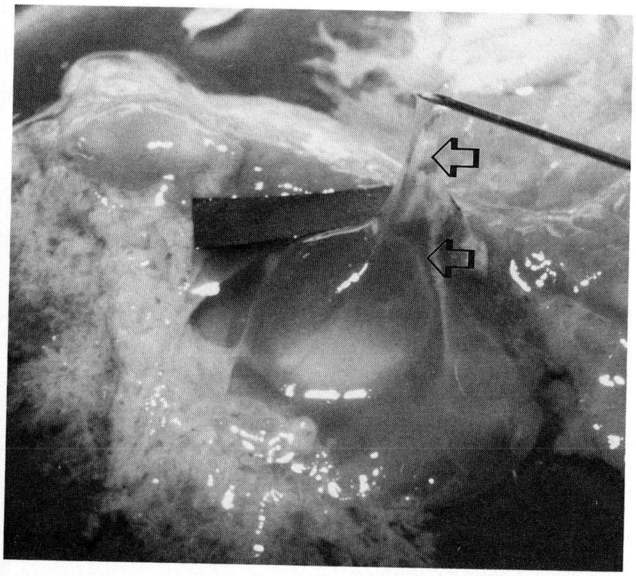

FIG. 10–12. Exocoelomic jelly (*arrows*) adheres tenaciously to a needle. Placental villi (*left*) can be seen, and the amniotic cavity is visible behind the jelly.

TRISOMY 21

The absence or subtlety of the gross findings at autopsy of fetuses with Down syndrome is disconcerting to the clinicians who diagnose and manage the cases. Simian creases and occasionally facial features may be present, but the middle fifth phalanx usually is triangular in outline, causing radial deviation (*i.e.*, clinodactyly). This shape difference is present even in the cartilaginous stage before ossification. In reported autopsies, 4 of 13 Down syndrome fetuses were found to have atrioventricularis communis.[72] Detailed studies of the histology of the brains from trisomy 21 fetuses have failed to identify any abnormalities.[73] These mild or absent abnormalities may indicate that the trisomy of chromosome 21 does not interfere with development until late fetal development or postnatal life. If true, the syndrome might be significantly ameliorated by any therapy that could

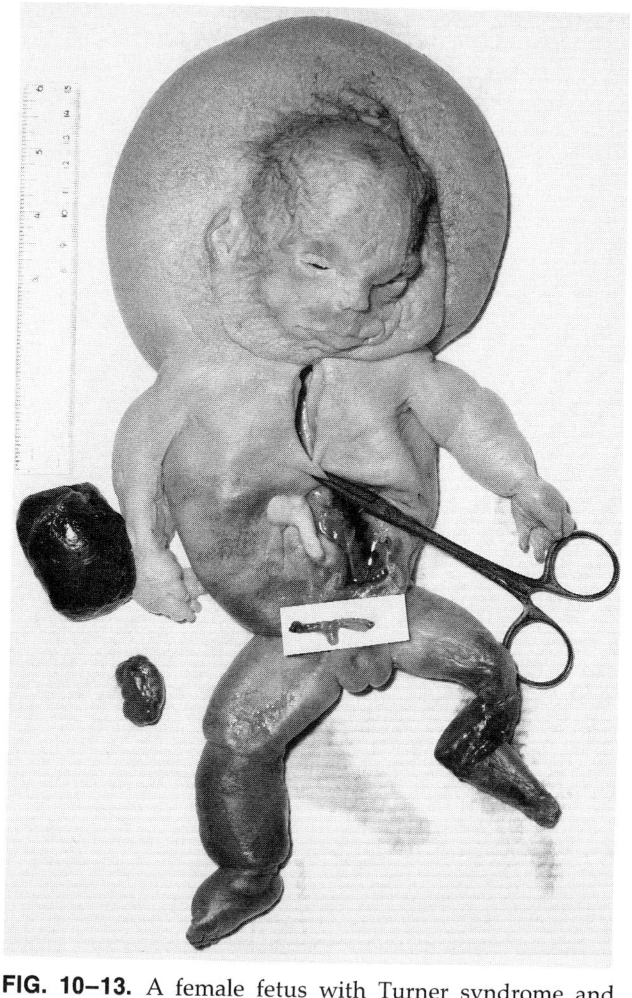

FIG. 10–13. A female fetus with Turner syndrome and monosomy X shows a large nuchal cystic hygroma and generalized edema. The ears are displaced on the hygroma. The ovaries were grossly normal. (Specimen H-588, courtesy of Central Laboratory for Human Embryology, University of Washington, Seattle, WA.)

prevent the later genetic expression of an extra chromosome 21.

TURNER SYNDROME WITH X MONOSOMY

The phenotype of cystic hygroma with generalized edema in a female fetus often is associated with X monosomy, but a number of other etiologies have been recognized (Fig. 10-13).[74] By calculating from life tables, it has been estimated that of all human fertilizations, about 3% may have X monosomy.[65] Because over 99% of these fail to reach term, it is not surprising that numerous examples are seen among aborted fetuses. Many are early, blighted embryos that do not have the Turner phenotype and are chromosomally identified.

The cause of the edema and cystic hygroma has been postulated to be a defect in the development of lymphatic drainage.[75,76] An alternative hypothesis supported by finding extremely low fetal serum albumin levels may be that the edema is secondary to low osmotic pressure in the vascular system, leading to dilation of the developing lymphatic system.[52] This hypothesis requires the assumption that the control of the osmotic pressure is different in the fetus because newborns and infants with Turner syndrome gradually clear their edema and do not have albumin-low serum. Most of the congenital defects in Turner syndrome can be explained by the effect of deformation from the edematous structures during either early or late fetal development. These are outlined in Figure 10-14, and discussed further by Shepard and Fantel.[77]

RENAL HYPERTROPHY IN THE FETUS

In fetuses with unilateral renal agenesis, kidney weight is significantly increased.[78] In addition, with oligohydramnios, renal weights may be significantly increased.[79] The fetus does not depend on renal excretion for clearing metabolic wastes, so this source seems an unlikely cause of hypertrophy. These findings lead to the question of whether there is a fetal control mechanism for increasing renal size and a humeral response from the amniotic cavity when oligohydramnios occurs.

URETHRAL VALVE AND PRUNE-BELLY SYNDROMES

This sequence of congenital defects has become better understood by the observation that the absence of abdominal musculature follows muscle cell necrosis caused by pressure from an enlarged bladder.[80,81] Ex-

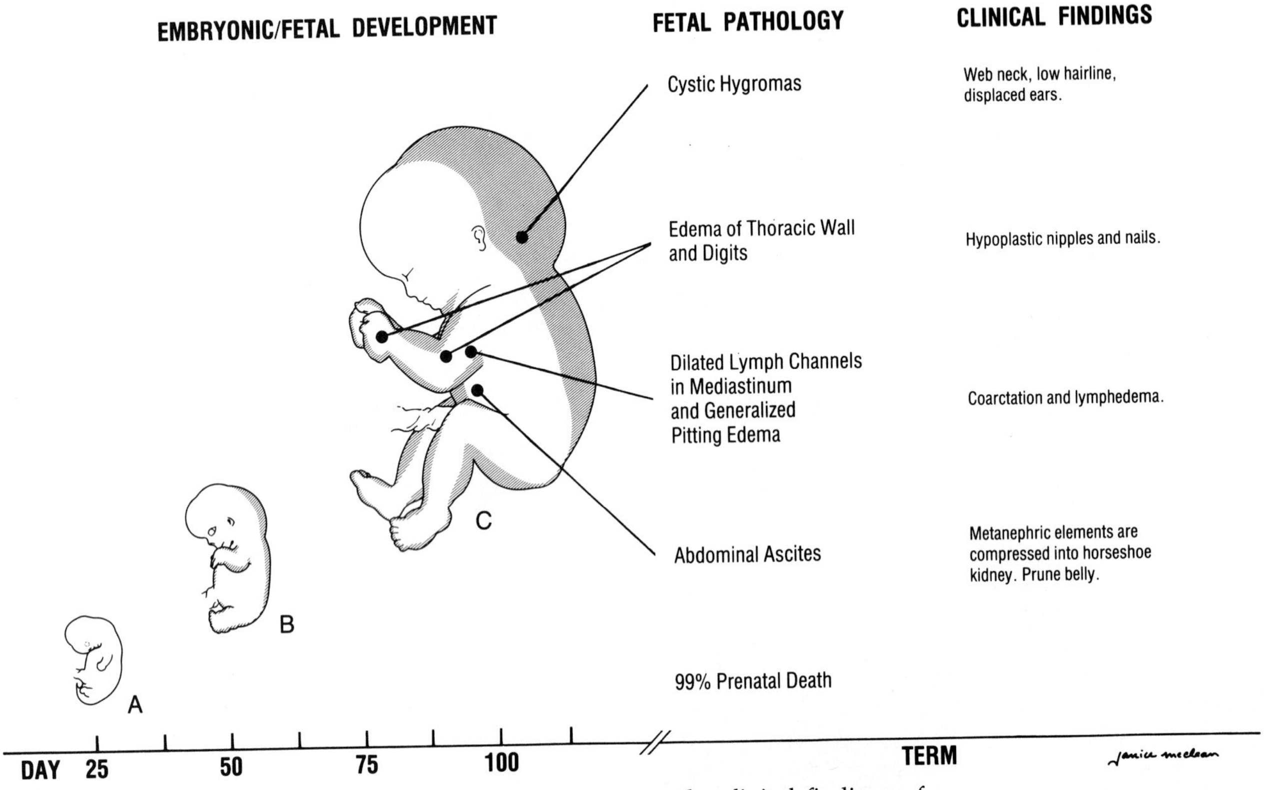

FIG. 10–14. The edema of a monosomy-X fetus can produce the clinical findings of Turner syndrome. (From Shepard TH, Fantel AG. Pathogenesis of congenital defects associated with Turner's syndrome: the role of hypoalbuminemia and edema. Acta Endocrinol 1986;112[Suppl279]:440.)

cept for occasional cases of cloacal dysgenesis, nearly all are male fetuses and the obstruction appears in the prostatic urethra close to the prostatic utricle (male uterus).[7] This is the area where the müllerian ducts fuse. If the fusion of the müllerian ducts were to be displaced ventrally on the cloaca, it is conceivable that valvelike folds might develop and obstruct the flow of urine. More detailed studies of young fetuses with this syndrome are indicated.

FETAL PATHOLOGY ASSOCIATED WITH COCAINE

Many publications have described dysfunction of the central nervous system in the newborn exposed to cocaine, but there are no neuropathologic studies.[82,83] In brain examinations of three human fetuses, Kapur and colleagues found hemorrhages that were localized mainly to the germinal matrix.[84] This type of lesion is similar to the pathologic condition that develops postnatally in very small premature infants with central nervous system complications. Webster and associates have described a similar finding in cocaine-exposed rat fetuses.[85] Accordingly, it might be expected that cocaine exposure could produce a wide spectrum of developmental defects, including spastic diplegia as seen in surviving premature infants. Because premature birth often occurs with cocaine exposure, it will be difficult to separate the effects of prematurity from drug effects.

Coronary occlusion in a fetus exposed to cocaine has been reported and there is evidence that the resulting infarct altered development, producing a three-chambered heart.[86] In retrospective series, congenital heart disease has been found to be increased,[88–91] but in a rigorous unpublished epidemiologic study, no increase in the rate of trilocular hearts was found over time in cocaine-exposed offspring in the Atlanta, Georgia area. Because cocaine seems to cause deficits in uterine and fetal blood supply and oxygen transport, this teratogen is one that has a window of vulnerability extending throughout the entire gestation.[91]

ACKNOWLEDGMENTS

I thank numerous fellows and associates for their contributions to the data and concepts contained in this chapter. The entire period of study was supported by the National Institutes of Health (grant HD 00836). John Rajan and Julie Pascoe-Mason ably helped with preparation of the manuscript and data.

REFERENCES

1. Benirschke K, Kaufmann P. The pathology of the human placenta. 2nd ed. New York: Springer-Verlag, 1990.
2. Gompel C, Silverberg S. Pathology in gynecology and obstetrics. 3rd ed. Philadelphia: JB Lippincott, 1985:3.
3. Kalousek DK, Fitch N, Paradice BA. Pathology of the human embryonic and previable fetus: an atlas. New York: Springer-Verlag, 1990.
4. Macgregor AR. Pathology of infancy and childhood. Edinburgh: E & S Livingston, 1960.
5. Morrison JE. Foetal and neonatal pathology. 2nd ed. London: Butterworths, 1963.
6. Polin RA, Fox WW. Fetal and neonatal physiology. Philadelphia: WB Saunders, 1991.
7. Potter EL, Craig JM. Pathology of the fetus and the infant. 3rd ed. Chicago: Year Book, 1975.
8. Reed GB, Claireaux AE, Bain AD. Disease of the fetus and newborn: pathology, radiology and genetics. St. Louis: CV Mosby, 1989.
9. Warkany J. Congenital malformations. Chicago: Year Book, 1971.
10. Wigglesworth JS, Singer DB. Textbook of fetal and perinatal pathology. Oxford: Blackwell Scientific Publications, 1991.
11. Willis RA. The borderline of embryology and pathology. 2nd ed. London: Butterworths, 1962.
12. Winter RM, Knowles SAS, Beiber FR, et al. The malformed fetus and stillbirth: a diagnostic approach. Chichester: John Wiley & Sons, 1988.
13. Streeter GL. Weight, sitting height, head size, foot length and menstrual age of the human embryo. Contributions to Embryology 1920;55(11):143.
14. Streeter GL. Developmental horizons in human embryos: age groups XI to XXIII. Washington, DC: Carnegie Institution of Washington, 1951.
15. Iffy L, Shepard TH, Jakobovits A, et al. The rate of growth in young human embryos of Streeter's horizons XIII to XXIII. Acta Anat 1967;66:178.
16. Nishimura H, Tanimura T, Semba R, et al. Normal development of early human embryos: observation of 90 specimens at Carnegie stages 7 to 13. Teratology 1974;10:1.
17. O'Rahilly R, Müller F. Developmental stages in human embryos. Washington, DC: Carnegie Institution of Washington, 1987.
18. Shiota K, Fischer B, Neubert D. Variability of development in the human embryo. In: Neubert D, Merker H-J, Hendrickx AG, eds. Non-human primates: developmental biology and toxicology. Wien, Berlin: Ueberreuter Wissenschaft, 1988.
19. Morris GM, New DAT. Effect of oxygen concentration on morphogenesis of cranial neural folds and neural crest in cultured rat embryos. Journal of Embryology and Experimental Morphology 1979;54:17.
20. Shum L, Saddler TW. Biochemical basis for D, L-beta-hydroxybutyrate induced teratogenesis. Teratology 1990;42:553.
21. Cry DR, Mack LA, Shoenecker SA, et al. Potential pitfalls in diagnosis of fetal abdominal wall abnormalities: sonographic detection of normal fetal bowel migration. Radiology 1986;161:119.
22. Kogan BA. Testicular descent. In: Polin RA, Fox WW, eds. Foetal and neonatal physiology. Philadelphia: WB Saunders, 1991:1871.
23. Tanimura T, Nelson T, Hollingsworth RR, et al. Weight standards for organs from early human fetuses. Anat Rec 1971; 171:227.
24. Shepard TH, Barr M, Fellingham GW, et al. Organ weight standards for human fetuses. Pediatr Pathol 1988;4:513.
25. Golbus MS, Berry LC Jr. Human fetal development between 90 and 170 days postmenses. Teratology 1977;15;103.
26. Shepard TH, FitzSimmons J, Fantel AG, et al. Placental

weights of normal and aneuploid early human fetuses. Pediatr Pathol 1989;9:425.
27. Fujinaga M, Chinn A, Shepard TH. The umbilical cord length in human and rat fetuses: normal and pathologic condition. Teratology 1990;41:333.
28. Naeye RL, Tafari N. Noninfectious disorders of the placenta, fetal membranes and umbilical cord. In: Risk factors in pregnancy and disease of the fetus and newborn. Baltimore: Williams & Wilkins, 1983;145.
29. Goldstein I, Reece A, Hobbins JC. Sonographic appearance of the fetal heel ossification centers and foot length provide independent markers for gestational age assessment. Am J Obstet Gynecol 1988;159:923.
30. Mahony BS. The extremities. In: Nyberg DA, Mahony BS, Pretorius DH, eds. Diagnostic ultrasound of fetal anomalies: text and atlas. Chicago: Year Book, 1990:492.
31. FitzSimmons J, Droste S, Shepard TH, et al. Long bone growth in fetuses with Down syndrome. Am J Obstet Gynecol 1989; 161:1174.
32. Benacerraf BR, Gelman R, Frigoletto FD. Sonographic identification of second trimester fetuses with Down's syndrome. N Engl J Med 1987;317:1371.
33. Yang SS. The skeletal system. In: Wigglesworth JS, Singer DB, eds. Textbook of fetal and perinatal pathology. Oxford: Blackwell Scientific Publications, 1991:1171.
34. Shepard TH, Lemire RJ, Aksu O, et al. Studies of the development of congenital anomalies in embryos of riboflavin-deficient, galactoflavin-fed rats: I. Growth and embryonic pathology. Teratology 1968;1:75.
35. Aksu O, Mackler B, Shepard TH, et al. Studies of mechanisms underlying the development of congenital anomalies in embryos of riboflavin deficient, galactoflavin-fed rats: II. Role of the terminal electron transport systems. Teratology 1968; 1:93.
36. Milaire J. Aspects of limb morphogenesis in mammals. In: DeHaan RL, Ursprung H, eds. Organogenesis. New York: Holt Rinehart and Winston, 1965:283.
37. Scott WJ, Ritter EJ, Wilson JB. DNA synthesis inhibition and cell death associated with hydroxyurea teratogenesis in rat embryos. Dev Biol 1971;26:306.
38. Mirkes PE. Effects of acute exposure to elevated temperatures on rat embryo growth and development in vitro. Teratology 1985;32:259.
39. Snow MHL. Restorative growth in mammalian embryos. In: Kalter H, ed. Issues and reviews in teratology. vol. 1. New York: Plenum Press, 1983:251.
40. Trasler DG. Pathogenesis of cleft lip and its relation to embryonic face shape in A/J and C57 BL mice. Teratology 1968;1:33.
41. Pratt RM, Chung SK, Grove RI. Role of glucocorticoids and epidermal growth factor in normal and abnormal palatal development. Curr Top Dev Biol 1984;19:81.
42. Abbott BD, Birnbaum LS. Retinoic acid-induced alterations in the expression of growth factors in embryonic mouse palatal shelves. Teratology 1990;42:597.
43. Saxen L. Abnormal cellular and tissue interactions In: Wilson JG, Fraser FC, eds. Handbook of teratology. vol. 2. New York: Plenum Press 1977;171.
44. Bernfield M. Developmental biology: preventive medicine for neonatology. Pediatr Res 1990;27(Suppl 6):21.
45. Dixon JB. Inflammation in the foetal and neonatal rat: local reaction to skin burns. J Pathol Bacteriol 1960;80:73.
46. Wohlwill F, Bock HE. Weitere Untersuchungen uber Entzundungen der Placenta and fetal Sepsis: Zuglerch ein Beitrag zur Kenntnis der fetalen Entenndurg. Beitr Pathol Anat 1930; 85:469.
47. Schwartz LW, Osburn BI. An ontogenic study of the acute inflammatory reaction in the fetal rhesus monkey. Lab Invest 1974;441.
48. Silverstein AM, Lukes RJ. Fetal response to antigenic stimulus: I. Plasmacellular and lymphoid reactions in the human fetus to intrauterine infection. Lab Invest 1962;11:918.
49. Playfair JHL, Wolfendale MR, Kay HEM. Leucocytes of peripheral blood in the human fetus. Br J Haematol 1963;9:336.
50. Thomas DB, Yoffey JM. Human foetal haemopoiesis: 1. cellular composition of foetal blood. Br J Haematol 1962;8:290.
51. Bleyer WA, Hakami N, Shepard TH. Development of hemostasis in the human fetus and newborn infant. J Pediatr 1971;79:838.
52. Shepard TH, Wener MH, Myhre SA, et al. Lowered plasma albumin in fetal Turner's syndrome: how does this relate to the edema. J Pediatr 1986;108:114.
53. Spranger JW, Benirschke K, Hall JG, et al. Errors in morphogenesis; concepts and terms: recommendations of an International Working Group. J Pediatr 1982;100:160.
54. Perrin E VDKB, Gilbert-Barness EF. Congenital anomalies and dysmorphology. In: Reed CB, Claireaux AE, Bain AD, eds. Disease of the fetus and newborn: pathology, radiology and genetics. St. Louis: CV Mosby, 1989:75.
55. Gilbert-Barness EF, Opitz JM. Congenital anomalies: malformation syndromes. In: Wigglesworth JE, Singer DB, eds. Textbook of fetal and perinatal pathology. vol. 1. Oxford: Blackwell Scientific Publications, 1991:381.
56. Ferguson-Smith AC, Cattanach BM, Barton SC, et al. Embryological and molecular investigations of parental imprinting on mouse chromosome 7. Nature 1991;351:667.
57. Little M, Van Heyningen V, Hastie N. Dads and disomy and disease. Nature 1991;351:609.
58. Henry I, Bonaiti-Pellie C, Chehensse V, et al. Uniparental paternal disomy in a genetic cancer predisposing syndrome. Nature 1991;351:665.
59. Shepard TH, Fantel AG, FitzSimmons J. Congenital defect rates among spontaneous abortuses: twenty years of monitoring. Teratology 1989;39:325.
60. Fantel AG, Shepard TH. Morphological analysis of spontaneous abortuses. In: Bennett MJ, Edmonds DK, eds. Spontaneous abortion. Oxford: Blackwell Scientific Publications, 1987:8.
61. Chinn A, FitzSimmons J, Shepard TH, et al. Congenital heart disease among spontaneous abortuses and stillborn fetuses: prevalence and associations. Teratology 1989;40:475.
62. Nishimura H, Yamamura H. Comparison between man and some other mammals of normal and abnormal developmental processes. In: Nishimura H, Muller R, eds. Methods for teratological studies in experimental animals and man. Tokyo: Igaku Shoin, 1969:223.
63. Neel JV. A study of major congenital defects in Japanese infants. Am J Hum Genet 1958;10:398.
64. McIntosh R, Merritt K, Richard MR, et al. The incidence of congenital malformations: a study of 5964 pregnancies. Pediatrics 1954;14:505.
65. Boué J, Boué M, Lazar P. Retrospective and prospective epidemiological studies of 1,500 karyotyped spontaneous human abortions. Teratology 1975;12:11.
66. Alberman ED, Creasy MR. Frequency of chromosomal abnormalities in miscarriages and perinatal deaths. J Med Genet 1970;14:313.
67. Warkany J. Terathanasia. Teratology 1978;17:187.
68. Bennett MJ, Edmonds DK. Spontaneous and recurrent abortion. Oxford: Blackwell Scientific Publications, 1987.
69. Torpin R. Fetal malformations caused by amnion rupture during gestation. Springfield, IL: Charles C. Thomas, 1968.

70. Garza A, Cordero JF, Mulinare J. Epidemiology of the early amnion rupture spectrum of defects. Am J Dis Child 1988; 142:541.
71. Jones KL. Smith's recognizeable patterns of human malformations. 4th ed. Philadelphia: WB Saunders, 1988.
72. Stephens TD, Shepard TH. The Down syndrome in the fetus. Teratology 1980;22:37.
73. Schmidt-Sidor B, Wisniewski KE, Shepard TH, et al. The brain growth in Down syndrome subjects: 15–22 weeks of gestational age and birth to 60 months. Clin Neuropathol 1990; 9(4):181.
74. Beiber FR, Petres RE, Beiber JM, et al. Prenatal detection of a familial nuchal bleb simulating encephalocele. Birth Defects 1979;15:51.
75. van der Putte SCJ. Lymphatic malformation in human fetuses. Virchows Arch [A] 1977;376:233.
76. Alvin A, Diehl J, Lindsten J, et al. Lymph vessel hypoplasia and chromosome aberrations in six patients with Turner's syndrome. Acta Derm Venereol (Stockh) 1967;47:25.
77. Shepard TH, Fantel AG. Pathogenesis of congenital defects associated with Turner's syndrome: the role of hypoalbuminemia and edema. Acta Endocrinol 1986;(Suppl)112:279:440.
78. Hartshorne N, Shepard TH, Barr M. Compensatory renal growth in human fetuses with unilateral renal agenesis. Teratology 1991;44:7.
79. Hickok DE, McLean J, Shepard TH, et al. Unexplained second trimester oligohydramnios: a clinical pathological study of a new syndrome. Am J Perinatol 1989;6:8.
80. Pagon RA, Smith DW, Shepard TH. Urethral obstruction malformation complex: a cause of abdominal muscle deficiency and the prune belly. J Pediatr 1979;94:900.
81. Monie IW, Monie BJ. Prune belly syndrome and fetal ascites. Teratology 1979;19:111.
82. Vandstra ES, Burkett G. Maternal-fetal and neonatal effects of in utero cocaine exposure. Semin Perinatol 1991;15:288.
83. Scanlon JW. The neuroteratology of cocaine: background, theory and clinical implications. Reproductive Toxicology 1991; 5:89.
84. Kapur RP, Shaw CM, Shepard TH. Brain hemorrhages in cocaine exposed fetuses. Teratology 1991;44:11.
85. Webster WS, Brown-Woodman DDC, Lipson AH, et al. Fetal brain damage in the rat following prenatal exposure to cocaine. Neurotoxicol Teratol 1991;13:621.
86. Shepard TH, Fantel AG, Kapur RP. Fetal coronary thrombosis as a cause of single ventricular heart. Teratology 1991;43:113.
87. Neerhof MG, MacGregor SN, Retsky SS, et al. Cocaine abuse during pregnancy: peripartum prevalence and perinatal outcome. Am J Obstet Gynecol 1989;161:633.
88. Little B, Snell LM, Klein VR, et al. Cocaine abuse during pregnancy: maternal and fetal implications. Obstet Gynecol 1989; 73:157.
89. Bingol N, Fuchs M, Diaz V, et al. Teratogenicity of cocaine in humans. J Pediatr 1987;110:93.
90. Lipshultz SE, Frassica JJ, Orav EJ. Cardiovascular abnormalities in infants prenatally exposed to cocaine. J Pediatr 1991; 118:44.
91. Woods JR, Plessinger MA. Effect of cocaine on uterine blood flow and fetal oxygenation. JAMA 1987;257:957.

Neonatology: Pathophysiology and Management of the Newborn, Fourth Edition,
edited by Gordon B. Avery, Mary Ann Fletcher, and Mhairi G. MacDonald.
J.B. Lippincott Company, Philadelphia © 1994.

chapter 11

Fetomaternal Interactions: Placental Physiology and Its Role as a Go-Between

Gabriella Pridjian

Far from the primitive exchange organ in lower animals, the human placenta has evolved into a highly sophisticated interface between mother and fetus. As the gatekeeper for maternofetal interactions, its functions are diverse and essential.

HUMAN PLACENTATION

Based on the modified classification of Grosser, which separates placentas by the numbers of layers interfacing the maternal and fetal circulations, the human placenta is hemomonochorial, with only the syncytiotrophoblast, fetal connective tissue, and fetal capillary endothelium forming the barrier between the two circulations (Fig. 11-1).[1] The human placenta, with this most intimate interface, is similar to that of the guinea pig and the monkey.

Placentation in other animals is different, and there is great variation in mammalian placentation. For example, the ovine placenta is epitheliochorial. The maternal blood in the sheep does not directly bathe the syncytiotrophoblast, but is delivered to that cell by maternal capillaries. Between maternal and fetal circulations is the maternal capillary endothelium, maternal connective tissue, syncytiotrophoblast, fetal connective tissue, and fetal capillary endothelium. Although the sheep is an excellent model to study certain aspects of maternofetal physiology, ovine placental transport data, especially of diffusional substances, is not applicable to the human. For example, the ovine placenta is almost impermeable to diffusional transfer of the ketone body β-hydroxybutyrate, but human placenta is permeable to this ketone body, which has been implicated with the fetal distress accompanying diabetic ketoacidosis.[2] Unless otherwise specified, the discussion that follows pertains to human placentation.

The human placenta is discoid and made up of 8 to 10 cotyledons. Fetal blood is supplied to the placenta by two umbilical arteries and drained by one umbilical vein. On the fetal surface of the placenta, the umbilical arteries, crossing over fetal veins, decrease in caliber and increase in divisions as they travel toward the placental edges and dive deeply into the placental disc to supply individual cotyledons. Within the substance of the placenta, the caliber of the arteries decreases until only fetal capillaries exist at the level of the terminal villi. The fetal capillaries are dilated, providing a broad surface area for maternofetal transfer. The maternal blood supply to the placenta originates from the uterine artery, which divides into spiral arteries and percolates through the intervillous space, bathing the terminal villi.

PLACENTAL TRANSFER

The fetus depends almost exclusively on the placenta for nutritional, respiratory, and excretory functions. The placenta, growing steadily as gestation progresses, parallels fetal growth. Studies of placental

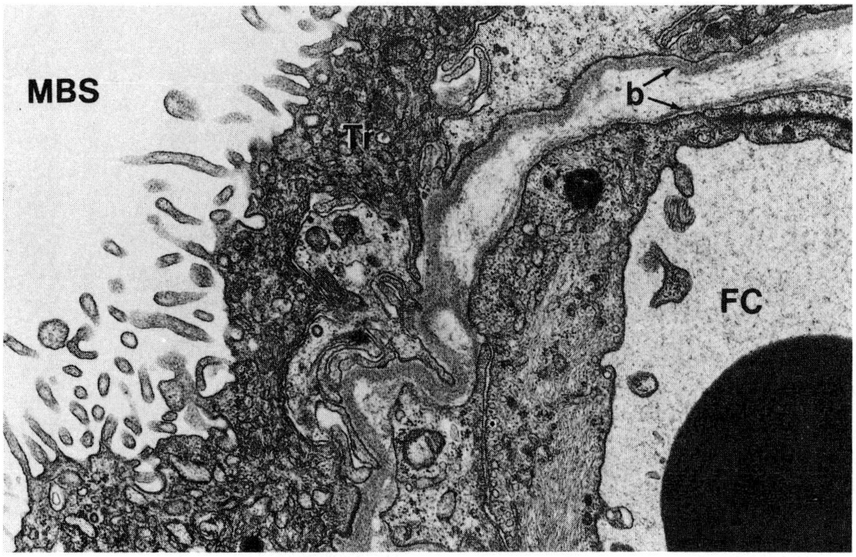

FIG. 11–1. Electron micrograph of the placental barrier of the human hemomonochorial full-term placenta. Notice the numerous endocytotic vesicles in various stages of formation located on the maternal-side brush border membrane of the syncytiotrophoblast. (MBS, maternal blood space or intervillous space; Tr, syncytiotrophoblast with microvillous brush border membrane; bar = 0.5 μm; from Thornberg KL, Faber JJ. Placental physiology. New York: Raven Press, 1983:19.)

growth and physiology in disease states suggest that placental growth and size are determined by the fetus and modulated by maternal factors. Normal placental-to-fetal weight ratios are approximately 1:6. As the placenta grows, villous processes increase in number as fetal vasculature expands, and by the third trimester, a large surface area is available to the maternal and fetal circulations.

Most placental transport is transcellular. Although the placenta is often thought of as a "separating membrane," it is actually a series of membranes. The most efficient areas for maternofetal exchange are the epithelial plates, which consist of thinly stretched, attenuated villous tissue separating maternal blood in the intervillous space from fetal blood in the fetal sinusoids. To cross epithelial plates from the maternal to the fetal side, a substance must traverse the brush border membrane of the syncytiotrophoblast, the cellular plasma of this cell, the basal membrane of the syncytiotrophoblast, the maternal side of the fetal capillary endothelial cell and the fetal side of the same endothelial cell. The microvillous brush border membrane of the syncytiotrophoblast appears to be the membrane most involved in regulation of transport, especially of active or carrier mediated transport. Although there is considerable knowledge of transport mechanisms at the microvillous brush border of the syncytiotrophoblast (*i.e.*, maternal side), less is known about transport through the basal membrane of that cell (*i.e.*, fetal side) or through the fetal capillary endothelial cell. Certain diffusible substances traverse the trophoblast and endothelial cell intact for release on the fetal side; some substances may be partially or completely metabolized by the placenta; and others may be involved in intricate transport systems (Fig. 11-2).

SIMPLE DIFFUSION

Many nutrients, metabolites, and excretory products cross the placenta by diffusion. Diffusion of substances in the placenta depends on multiple factors; these are summarized in Table 11-1.

The amount of a nutrient delivered to the placenta is directly proportional to its concentration in the maternal blood stream, which depends on nutritional intake and gastrointestinal absorption. Famine, maternal gastrointestinal diseases that interfere with absorption, or maternal pulmonary diseases that interfere with alveolar exchange may significantly affect blood concentrations and transfer and accrual of fetal fuels. A lack of fetal fuels produces fetal and placental growth restriction. Abnormalities in maternal homeostatic mechanisms may produce either an insufficiency or an abundance of nutrients. For example, in poorly controlled diabetes, maternal hyperglycemia, hyperaminoacidemia, and hypertriglyceridemia allow unrestrained nutrient delivery to the fetus with excessive growth of fetal organs, body fat, and the placenta.[3]

Delivery of a nutrient to the placenta is directly proportional to blood flow in the intervillous space. Maternal blood volume gradually increases to 30% to 40% above prepregnancy volume, with 40% directed to the uterus and placenta. Maternal cardiac disease with lower cardiac output may result in fetal and placental growth restriction. Even in healthy women, maternal position influences blood flow to the uterus. Normal pregnant women have an 18% lower cardiac output in the standing position compared with lying on their sides, perhaps explaining why women who stand at work throughout their pregnancy have newborns of lower birth weight.

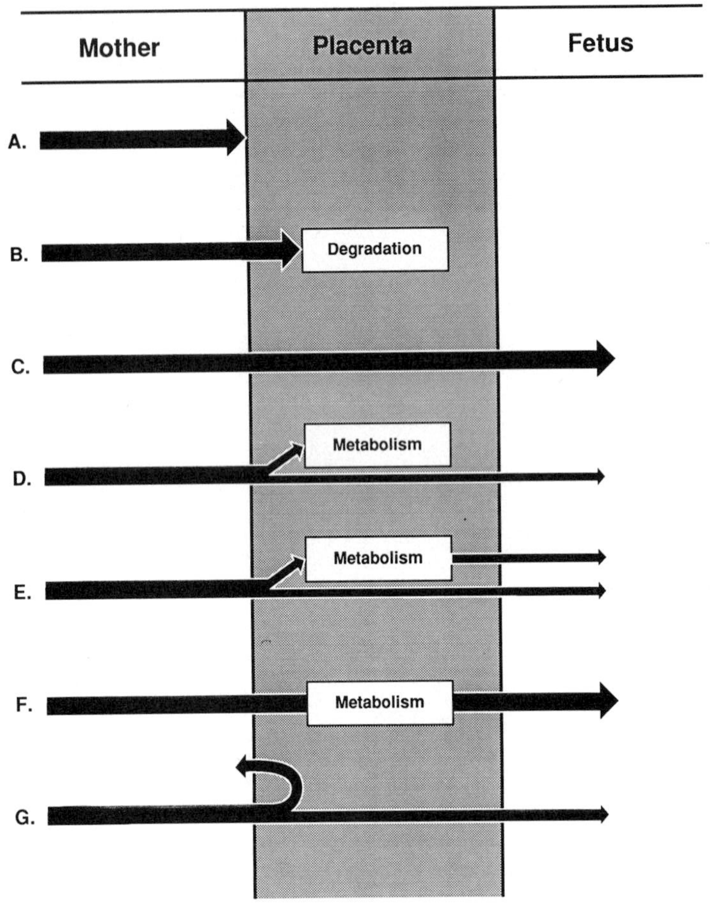

FIG. 11–2. Patterns of maternofetal transport. (**A**) Minimal or no placental uptake and no fetal transfer (*e.g.*, succinylcholine, highly charged quaternary ammonium compounds). (**B**) Placental uptake, degradation, and no fetal transfer (*e.g.*, insulin). (**C**) Placental uptake and transfer predominantly unmodified to the fetus (*e.g.*, betahydroxybutyrate, bilirubin). (**D**) Placental uptake, partial use, and transfer to the fetus (*e.g.*, oxygen, glucose, amino acids, free fatty acids). (**E**) Uptake, partial metabolism, and transfer to the fetus (*e.g.*, cyclosporine). (**F**) Uptake, modification, and transfer to the fetus (*e.g.*, 25-hydroxyvitamin D_3, of which most undergoes 1α-hydroxylation in the placenta to form 1,25-dihydroxyvitamin D_3). (**G**) Carrier-coupled uptake with release of the ligand to the fetal side and regeneration of the carrier on the maternal side (*e.g.*, transferrin–iron complex).

TABLE 11–1
FACTORS AFFECTING THE PLACENTAL TRANSFER OF A DIFFUSIBLE SUBSTANCE

Maternal Factors	Placental Factors	Fetal Factor
Amount Delivered to the Intervillous Space Blood concentration Exogenous and endogenous supplies Homeostatic mechanisms Arteriovenous mixing in the intervillous space Flow rate in intervillous space Hemodynamic factors in mother Local circulatory factors Shunting	**Transfer Physiology** Area of diffusing membrane(s) Diffusion resistance Characteristics of transferred material (size, charge, polarity, shape) Characteristics of membrane (physiochemical composition, fluidity) Diffusion pressure across each placental cell membrane Maternofetal concentration gradients Placental cellular production or use Maternofetal blood flow characteristics; intervillous flow	**Amount Delivered to the Fetal Capillaries** Blood concentration Fetal metabolic production or gastrointestinal absorption Prior placental transfer Flow rate in the fetal capillaries Hemodynamic factors in fetus Local circulatory factors Shunting

Fetal factors influencing diffusion are those that affect nutrient delivery to the fetal side of the placenta. The concentration of a substance in the umbilical artery depends on the amount of prior placental transfer, absorption from swallowed amniotic fluid, and fetal metabolism. Fetal blood flow to the uterus depends on fetal cardiac output and placental vascular tone. Normally, fetal vessels on the chorionic plate are maximally dilated, providing the least resistance to flow.

Numerous placental factors influence diffusion. The number of branching structures of the placental villus and amount of dilatation of the fetal capillaries regulate transfer surface area. Overall, transfer is governed by the quantity of epithelial plates, the specialized regions of enhanced diffusion where the interhemal barrier is less than a few microns. The geometric interrelation of the maternal and fetal placental blood circulations influences diffusion. The most efficient pattern of blood flow for exchange is countercurrent flow; the direction of flow in the maternal vessels is the reverse of that in the fetal vessels, as seen in the guinea pig placenta or human kidneys. A concurrent flow pattern is the least efficient for transfer. The human placenta has an intervillous pool flow system in which fetal capillaries in terminal villi are bathed in a maternal blood reservoir continuously filled by arteries and drained by veins (Fig. 11-3). Concurrent and countercurrent flows exist in areas of uneven distribution of flow (*i.e.*, shunting), where a portion of the villus is well supplied by maternal blood but poorly supplied by fetal blood; in other areas, the opposite occurs.

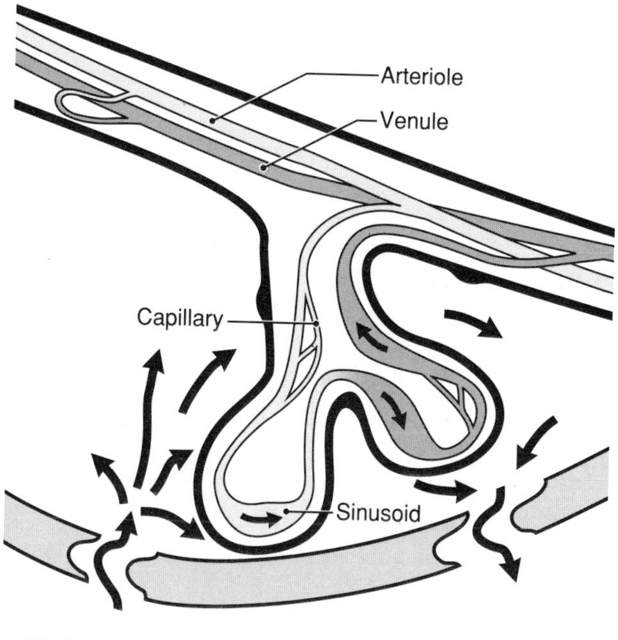

FIG. 11–3. Areas of concurrent and countercurrent flow exist in the intervillous pool flow system of the human placenta.

Stereochemical characteristics of a substance are major factors in transferability. Small, compact, nonpolar, lipophilic substances are most efficiently transferred. The placenta is relatively impermeable to large, polar molecules that do not have specific transport systems or carrier proteins or are able to take advantage of an analogous transport system to aid in their transfer. For example, because succinylcholine is a highly charged molecule, there is minimal placental uptake and transfer to the fetus. However, cyclosporine, a lipophilic drug, is readily taken up by the placenta, partially metabolized, and quickly transferred to the fetus, producing fetal cyclosporine levels of about 50% of maternal levels.[4] Bioactive cyclosporine metabolites in cord blood supersede maternal levels.

Alpha-fetoprotein (AFP), a 70-kd fetal protein, does not transfer to the maternal side in appreciable amounts despite large quantities in fetal blood. Maternal AFP is derived from transplacental transfer from fetal blood and transmembrane (*i.e.*, chorioamnion) transfer from amniotic fluid. The fetal blood AFP level at 17 weeks of gestation is approximately 3 mg/mL when the maternal blood level is about 0.1 μg/mL, resulting in a fetomaternal gradient of about 30,000 to 1. The low level of fetomaternal transplacental transfer allows detection of elevated maternal serum levels from transmembrane (*i.e.*, amniochorion) transfer of abnormally high amniotic fluid AFP, which provides the basis of maternal serum AFP screening for neural tube defects. False-positive elevations of maternal serum AFP (*i.e.*, high maternal serum value with a structurally normal fetus) suggest placental microabruptions or loss of integrity of the maternofetal barrier and forecast a higher rate of fetal morbidity.

Membrane characteristics regulate transport. The fluidity of the membrane, determined by the degree and character of membrane-incorporated phospholipids, influences transfer of certain substances. Diseases, such as diabetes, may influence membrane fluidity.[5]

The major driving force in favor of transfer by diffusion is the concentration gradient across the placenta; the resistance to diffusion is dictated by the nature of the molecule. The principles of diffusion of molecules that are generally applicable to biologic membranes hold true in the placenta, although specifics remain to be defined.

Availability of a substance for diffusional transfer across the placenta is not always related to blood levels of that substance, because many metabolites, nutrients, and drugs that are poorly water soluble are protein bound. Although proteins aid in delivery of these substances to the placenta, they may actually hinder transfer. It is the free, unbound, or soluble fraction of a substance that is available for transfer. Conversely, high-affinity carrier proteins on the receiving side of the placenta drive diffusional transfer to their side by decreasing a ligand's free fraction and increasing its maternofetal gradient.

Oxygen, for example, is 98% bound to hemoglobin. It is the transplacental difference in the partial pressure (PO_2) of dissolved oxygen that determines the diffusion pressure. The more oxygen-avid fetal hemoglobin counterbalances the resistance to transfer from the maternal circulation. The O_2 content (*i.e.*, dissolved and hemoglobin-bound O_2) of the blood on each side of the placental membrane is determined principally by different affinities of maternal and fetal hemoglobin for oxygen. In humans, the fetal oxyhemoglobin dissociation curve is displaced leftward of the maternal curve, facilitating a much greater uptake of oxygen by fetal blood at the placental capillary level than would be possible otherwise. At any given PO_2, a much higher O_2 content is achieved in fetal blood than in maternal blood. The O_2 content in the umbilical vein (14.5 mL/dL) is as high as that of the uterine artery (15.8 mL/dL) despite an umbilical venous PO_2 of only 27 torr (Table 11-2). Relatively high fetal blood O_2 content confers on the fetus the ability to deliver sufficient oxygen to peripheral tissue despite low PO_2. Low PO_2 may be essential to fetal physiologic adaptation to maintain high pulmonary vascular resistance and to keep the ductus arteriosus open.

The excretion of bilirubin provides an example of fetomaternal interaction using specific permeability properties of the placenta to accomplish a given objective.[6] Before birth, elimination of bilirubin from the fetus is by diffusional transfer through the placenta to the mother. The placenta is extremely permeable to unconjugated bilirubin but relatively impermeable to bilirubin–glucuronide (*i.e.*, conjugated bilirubin). In the fetus, because of minimal bilirubin glucuronyltransferase, hepatic conjugation of bilirubin is suppressed. Because fetal bilirubin is predominantly unconjugated and highly lipid soluble, it diffuses freely from the fetal to the maternal side. After transfer to the mother, it is efficiently conjugated and excreted (Fig 11-4).

In mothers with erythrocyte hemolysis and unconjugated hyperbilirubinemia, there may be elevated bilirubin in amniotic fluid due to diffusional transfer of maternal bilirubin to the fetal compartment. The falsely elevated amniotic fluid Δ-OD450 may incorrectly suggest fetal erythrocyte hemolysis.

FACILITATED DIFFUSION

Most substances cross the placenta by simple diffusion. Maternal glucose, the principal substrate for oxidative metabolism in the fetus, is a water-soluble, polar molecule that crosses the placenta by facilitated diffusion, which is a gradient-dependent, receptor-mediated, saturable process.

Transfer of glucose by facilitated diffusion is supported by guinea pig (*i.e.*, hemomonochorial) and human placental studies in which glucose transports more readily than other carbohydrates (*e.g.*, fructose), even though these carbohydrates' physiochemical properties predict equal transfer by simple diffusion. In the human placenta, preferential transfer of D-glucose (over L-glucose) exists. Transfer stereospecificity implies a carrier-mediated process that provides the fetus with the appropriate isomer for metabolism. The presence of glucose transporter genes in the placenta that code for glucose transporter proteins confirms indirect experimental evidence for the existence of a membrane-bound D-glucose carrier protein.[7] Under physiologic and pathologic human conditions, the carrier protein for glucose is not saturated, and the amount transferred to the fetus is directly related to the amount supplied to the placenta. Using vesicles made from the microvillous membrane of the human syncytiotrophoblast, Johnson and Smith showed maternofetal facilitated glucose transport with a K_m six times higher than the maternal blood glucose concentration.[8]

ACTIVE TRANSPORT

To provide appropriate fuels for fetal growth, specific energy-requiring transport mechanisms in the microvillous surface aid in transfer of substances that are not readily lipid soluble and are required in large amounts by the fetus.

Most amino acids cross the placenta by an active transport mechanism.[9–11] Active amino acid uptake

TABLE 11–2
NORMAL OXYGEN VALUES IN MATERNAL AND FETAL BLOOD

Oxygen Measurements	Uterine Artery	Uterine Vein	Umbilical Vein	Umbilical Artery
PO_2 (torr)	95	40	27	15
Hemoglobin O_2 saturation (%)	98	76	68	30
O_2 content (mL/dL)	15.8	12.2	14.5	6.4
Hemoglobin (g/dL)	12.0	12.0	16.0	16.0

Adapted from Longo L. Disorders of placental transfer. In: Assali NS, ed. Pathophysiology of gestation. New York: Academic, 1972;2:11.

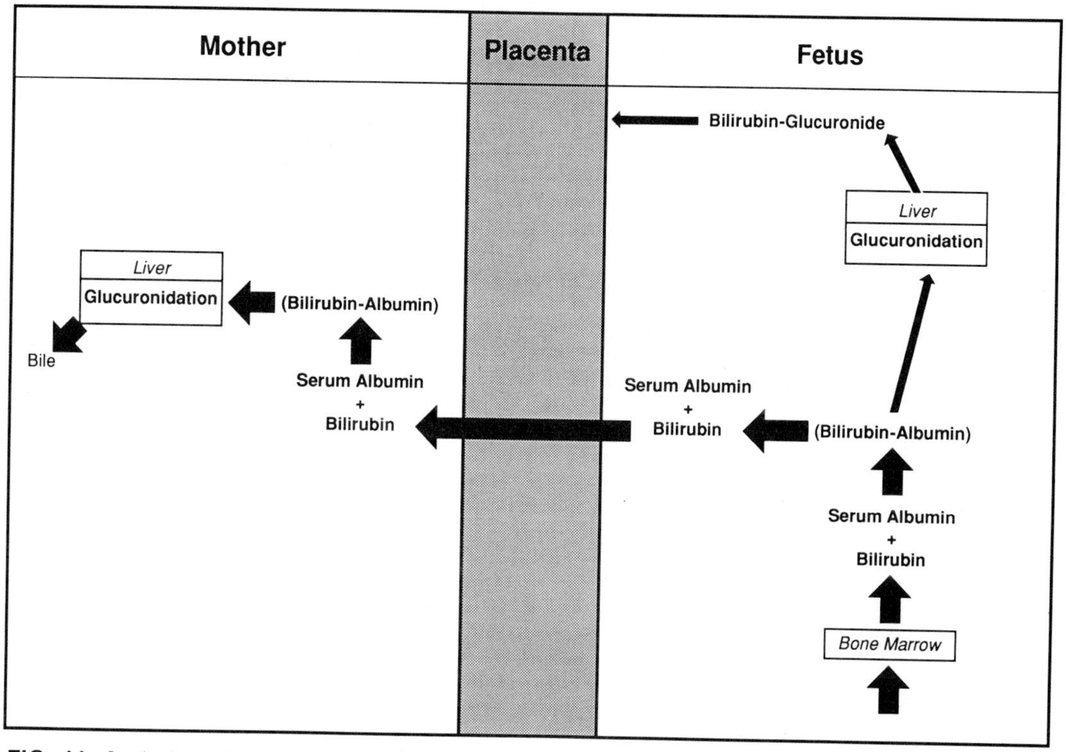

FIG. 11–4. Antepartum excretion of bilirubin. Fetal bilirubin is transferred from fetal serum albumin through the placenta to maternal serum. It is then conjugated with glucuronic acid by the maternal liver and excreted into the bile. Fetal glucuronidation is suppressed. The placenta is relatively impermeable to the glucuronide.

has two major purposes: placental production of peptide hormones and their transfer to the fetus. Transfer from maternal to fetal circulation is especially important for the essential amino acids required for fetal growth, including the adult essential amino acids histidine, isoleucine, leucine, lysine, methionine, phenylalanine, threonine, tryptophan, and valine; and the proposed fetal essential amino acids cysteine, tyrosine, histidine, and taurine. Early in development, before maturation of fetal metabolic systems, all amino acids are essential to the fetus. Fetal amino acid levels are 1.5- to 5-fold higher than maternal levels, confirming a transport process against a concentration gradient.

Placental transfer of amino acids is stereospecific, with the natural L form preferred. Transport of amino acids by animal cells is mediated by specific carrier systems that have overlapping substrate reactivities. In human villous tissue fragments, three carrier systems exist for neutral amino acids.[12] System A is sodium dependent, reversible at low *p*H, and most reactive with amino acids that have short, polar, or linear side chains (*e.g.*, alanine, glycine). System L is sodium independent and most reactive with large, apolar, branched-chain and aromatic amino acids (*e.g.*, leucine, isoleucine, tyrosine, tryptophan, valine, phenylalanine, methionine, glutamate). The ASC system is sodium dependent and is involved in transport of alanine and cysteine. Evidence suggests that a B system exists in placenta for taurine transport.[13] Taurine, although produced by the maternal liver from cysteine and methionine, is essential for fetal neurologic development but is not produced by the fetus.

Certain drugs cross the placenta by active transport. Zidovudine (formerly called azidothymidine [AZT]), which is used for treating human immunodeficiency virus (HIV), has been found in the perfused human placental model to cross from the maternal to the fetal side by energy-dependent transport.[14] Because zidovudine is a thymidine analog, it may take advantage of placental thymidine transport systems. Zidovudine levels are higher in cord blood than in maternal blood, suggesting transport against a concentration gradient and an active transport mechanism. This finding has several implications for the fetus. Maternal administration of zidovudine may become therapy for fetal HIV or prevention of vertical transmission to the fetus. Erythrocyte aplasia, a side-effect of zidovudine therapy, may develop in fetuses of mothers undergoing treatment, potentially leading to fetal hydrops due to severe fetal anemia. The effectiveness of zidovudine in treatment or prevention of HIV in the fetus has not been determined.

Iodide, calcium, and phosphorus are transported to the fetal side of the placenta by an energy-requiring process. Binding proteins within the trophoblast may be involved in calcium transport. Maternofetal transport of ascorbic acid is accomplished more efficiently than expected if by simple diffusion, and fetal levels are at least three times maternal levels, suggesting an active transport mechanism.

RECEPTOR-MEDIATED ENDOCYTOSIS

Although many large protein molecules cross the placenta by pinocytosis in extremely small quantities, specific receptor-mediated processes expedite transfer of certain larger substances that are required by the fetus. The receptor-rich microvillous brush border of the syncytiotrophoblast and the numerous coated micropinocytotic vesicles found just beneath it provide anatomic evidence for receptor-mediated endocytosis.[15] The receptors involved in this process, found on the surface of the syncytiotrophoblast, are thought to extend through the glycocalyx layer of the cell membrane and bind to the protein clathrin to form a membrane complex. After the ligands are bound to their receptors, aggregation and internalization occurs to form a cytoplasmic-coated vesicle (Fig. 11-5). Destiny of the contents of the vesicles depends on the ligand.

Maternal immunoglobulins are transferred to the fetus by receptor-mediated endocytosis. IgG subclass 1 and 3 and IgA are known to cross the placenta. Once internalized, the intact immunoglobulin molecules within the vesicles are delivered from the cytoplasm of syncytiotrophoblast through the capillary endothelial cell and into the fetal circulation.[16,17] Antenatal fetal transfer of maternal IgG antibodies may interfere with antibody-based diagnostic testing in the fetus, necessitating analysis of fetal-specific IgM antibody. Developmentally, the transfer of maternal IgG to the fetus is probably protective and beneficial, but this transfer backfires in some situations, such as immune fetal hydrops (*i.e.*, erythroblastosis fetalis) and alloimmune fetal thrombocytopenia. By receptor-mediated endocytosis, anti-D or another blood group antibody crosses the placenta to cause fetal hemolytic anemia, and anti-PLA1 crosses the placenta to cause fetal thrombocytopenia.

Transfer of transferrin–iron complex into the placental syncytiotrophoblast occurs through receptor-mediated endocytosis. Brush border membrane transferrin-specific receptors on the maternal side of the syncytiotrophoblast bind transferrin–iron complex, and aggregate and internalize it to form vesicles of transferrin–iron complexes. In the cytoplasm, the complexes dissociate to form apotransferrin and ferrous iron. Apotransferrin is recycled to the maternal circulation, and ferrous iron is transiently stored as ferritin and released to the fetal circulation to be made into a complex with fetal transferrin. No maternal transferrin or placental ferritin is transferred to the fetus.[18] Maternofetal iron transport is independent of maternal levels.

Uptake of low-density lipoprotein cholesterol (LDL) from maternal blood for progesterone synthesis by the placental trophoblast is accomplished through receptor-mediated endocytosis. Specific receptors that have a high affinity for LDL but not for high-density lipoprotein (HDL) are located on the microvillous brush border of the syncytiotrophoblast. Low-density lipoprotein binds to its receptor and is actively internalized. Within the cytoplasm, LDL vesicles fuse with lysosomes, where enzyme hydrolysis of cholesterol esters releases cholesterol for mitochondrial synthesis of progesterone.

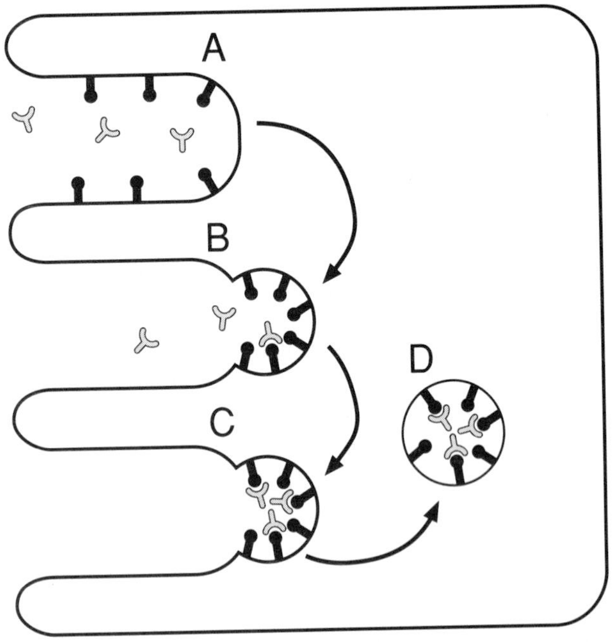

FIG. 11–5. Receptor-mediated endocytosis. The placental syncytiotrophoblast with the microvillous maternal border (see Figure 11–1) has (**A**) specific receptors, located in the microvillous projections (**B**) clustering in intervening pits on exposure to specific ligand in the maternal bloodstream. Endocytosis occurs. (**C**) The receptor–ligand complexes and associated cell wall invert to form (**D**) an endocytic vesicle that is internalized. The destiny of the vesicle depends on the ligand.

OTHER MECHANISMS OF TRANSFER

A variety of other mechanisms of transfer are probably functional in the human placenta. Large protein molecules may cross the placental membranes by a slow, non–receptor-mediated process of pinocytosis. Ions may cross placental membranes with the aid of ion pumps. Evidence suggests that small molecules and ions may cross through intercellular channels.

PLACENTAL METABOLISM

The placenta is a highly metabolic organ. Oxygen is consumed at a rate of 10 mL/minute/kg, representing the amount of maternal oxygen needed to supply the placenta and fetus for metabolic functions. Approximately 20% of placental oxygen uptake is used by the placenta; the remainder diffuses to the fetus. Glucose, the principle metabolic carbon source of the placenta, is converted to lactate or oxidized to CO_2. Placental tissue requires energy for maintenance of active transfer systems, hormone production, and substrate metabolism.

PLACENTA AS AN ENDOCRINE ORGAN

It is the placenta that maintains the maternal milieu most favorable for pregnancy by elaboration of large amounts of steroid and peptide hormones, which are required to maintain the fetoplacental unit. Generally, placentally produced steroid hormones, but not peptide hormones, cross to the fetal side.

HUMAN CHORIONIC GONADOTROPIN

Sensitive techniques demonstrate that the secretion of human chorionic gonadotropin (hCG) begins during implantation, when the cytotrophoblast differentiates into the syncytiotrophoblast. Although the messenger RNA for hCG can be found in the cytotrophoblast, this cell is thought not to be the origin of this peptide hormone, but only gains the ability to secrete hCG after it differentiates into a syncytiotrophoblast. The maternal plasma hCG level rises after implantation, peaks by 10 menstrual weeks of pregnancy, and declines to a nadir in the second trimester, after which levels remain low. (Fig. 11-6).

The only well-established role of hCG is continued stimulation of the ovarian corpus luteum to produce 17-hydroxyprogesterone for maintenance of the pregnancy. Although placental production of progesterone occurs early in gestation, the transition to placental autonomy from the ovary occurs between 10 and 12 menstrual weeks. Before this transition, loss of the corpus luteum results in loss of the pregnancy unless exogenous progesterone is administered. Primary control of trophoblastic hCG production has not been determined, but hormonal modulation is apparent.[19] There may be a role for hCG in the autocrine and paracrine control of production of other placental hormones. Proposed roles for hCG include the immunologic protection of the trophoblast and regulation of placental progesterone production. Falling levels of hCG before 10 menstrual weeks heralds pregnancy loss and is associated with miscarriage or ectopic gestation. Higher than normal hCG levels are seen with multiple gestations, hydatidiform mole, choriocarcinoma, and fetal triploidy when associated with molar changes of the placenta.

HUMAN PLACENTAL LACTOGEN

Human placental lactogen (hPL) is a single-chain polypeptide that has about 85% similarity to human growth hormone. The quantity of hPL synthesized by

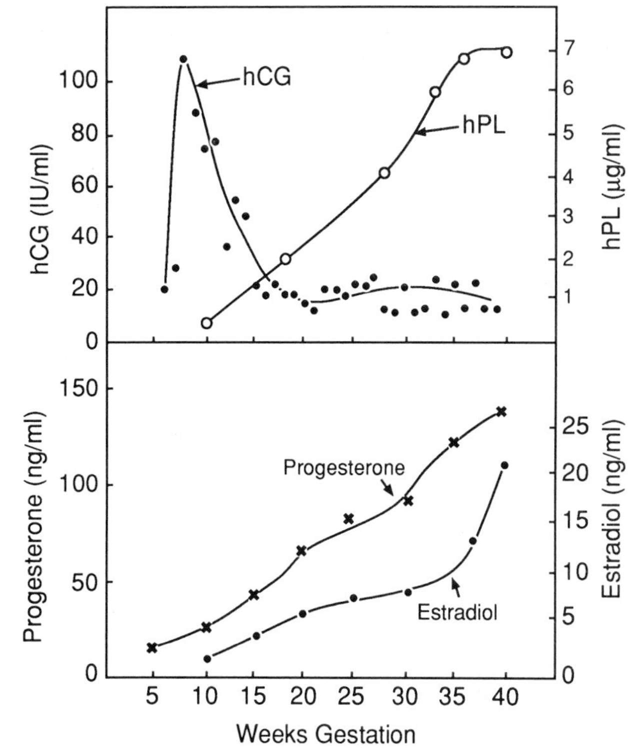

FIG. 11–6. Maternal blood levels of the major hormones produced by the placenta throughout pregnancy. (Data from Ashitaka Y, Nishimura R, Takemori M, Tojo S. Production and secretion of hCG and hCG subunits by trophoblastic tissue. In: Segal S, ed. Chorionic gonadotropins. New York: Plenum Press, 1980;151, Selenkow HA, Varma K, Younger D, White P, Emerson K Jr. Patterns of serum immunoreactive human placental lactogen and chorionic gonodotropin in diabetic pregnancy. Diabetes 1971;20:696, and Speroff L, Glass RH, Kase NG. Clinical gynecologic endocrinology and infertility. 4th ed. Baltimore: Williams & Wilkins, 1989.)

the placental syncytiotrophoblast parallels placental mass, reaching its peak at term and falling dramatically after delivery of the placenta.

Functionally, hPL can be considered a fetal growth hormone, because it maintains the maternal metabolic milieu optimal for delivery of nutrients to the fetus. Despite its name, hPL has not been demonstrated conclusively to exert a lactogenic effect in humans. The physiologic role of hPL appears to be in shifting the pattern of maternal energy metabolism during pregnancy from carbohydrate to one that depends on fat. The hormone promotes adipolysis and increases free fatty acid availability for maternal metabolism, saving glucose and amino acids for transfer to the fetus. Free fatty acids do not cross the placenta as readily as amino acids and glucose.

Human placental lactogen has antiinsulin effects thought to be mediated by the elevated free fatty acids, which promote peripheral tissue resistance to insulin. The subsequent increased pancreatic production of insulin leads to down regulation of peripheral insulin receptors.

Maternal blood levels of hPL correlate with placental function. It was once thought that low hPL levels could predict pregnancies with deteriorating placental function and those with fetal compromise.[20] Unfortunately, hPL levels are not as clinically useful as other methods. Similarly, elevated maternal hPL levels were thought predictive of gestational diabetes or outcome in preexisting diabetes, but large biologic variations in maternal levels preclude its use in prediction or diagnosis. There are no clinical applications for hPL levels at this time.

ESTROGEN

Estrogen production by the syncytiotrophoblast requires an elaborate concerted effort by the mother, fetus, and placenta (Fig. 11-7). Because there is no activity of 17-hydroxylase and 17,20-desmolase in the human placenta, estrogen precursors must be obtained from the fetal adrenal gland. The placenta produces three major estrogens—estradiol (E2), estriol (E3), and estrone—which are secreted predominantly into the maternal circulation. Maternal estrogen levels increase with gestational age.

Little is known about the specific functions of estrogen during pregnancy. Estrogens effect many general changes in the mother to prepare for and maintain pregnancy. The uterine myometrium responds exquisitely with increased protein synthesis and cellular hypertrophy. Estrogens cause vascular relaxation and increased blood flow to the uterus. Uterine contractility is increased by estrogens, supporting a role in the onset of parturition. Placental sulfatase deficiency, an X-linked fetal disorder, is associated with low estrogen levels. Except for dysfunctional labor, women with these fetuses have normal pregnancies. Fetuses with this disorder may develop ichthyosis later in life.

A specific role for estrogens in the fetus has not been determined. The fetal liver can metabolize E3 to estetrol (E4), which binds to fetal estrogen receptors but has no estrogenic activity, protecting fetal tissue from massive amounts of free estrogen.

PROGESTERONE

The placental syncytiotrophoblast produces progesterone from maternally derived LDL cholesterol (Fig. 11-8). Fetal contribution to progesterone synthesis is minimal. Maternal progesterone levels increase with gestational age. The major role of progesterone is to maintain the pregnancy. Early production of progesterone is by the ovarian corpus luteum. After a transition period of shared function between 6 and 12 weeks of gestation, the placenta becomes the dominant producer of progesterone, and the pregnancy continues even if the corpus luteum is removed. Low levels of progesterone may be associated with first-trimester pregnancy loss.

The most important role of progesterone may be that of principal substrate for fetal adrenal gland production of glucocorticoids and mineralocorticoids. Progesterone may have a role in parturition and in

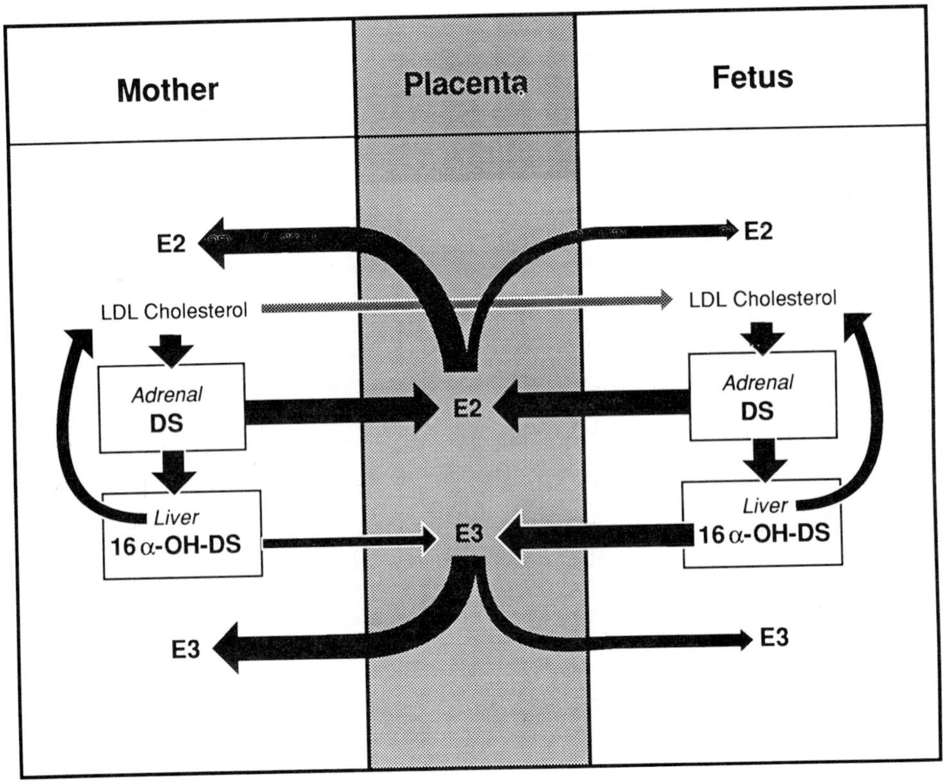

FIG. 11–7. Placental estrogen synthesis from fetal and maternal precursors. After 20 weeks of gestation, the fetal compartment supplies most steroid precursors for placental estrogen production. The fetal adrenal uses low-density lipoprotein cholesterol, produced by the fetal liver or transferred from the maternal compartment, to synthesize dehydroepiandrosterone sulfate (DS). Dehydroepiandrosterone sulfate is converted to 16 α-OH-DS in the fetal liver. Dehydroepiandrosterone sulfate and 16 α-OH-DS undergo placental metabolism to estradiol (E2) and estriol (E3), respectively, which are released predominantly on the maternal side.

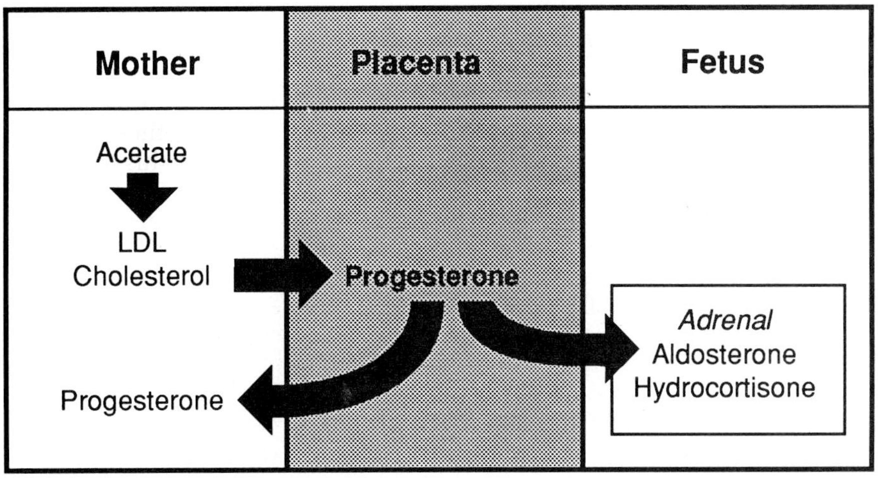

FIG. 11–8. Placental progesterone synthesis depends only on maternal precursors.

suppressing the maternal immunologic response to fetal antigens.

OTHER HORMONES

The placenta secretes a large number of proteins and peptide hormones into the maternal circulation, including human chorionic thyrotropin, chorionic adrenocorticotropic hormone, gonadotropin-releasing hormone, thyroid-releasing factor, corticotropin-releasing factor, and somatostatin. The exact functions of these hormones are unknown. Investigators have suggested that corticotropin-releasing factor may be involved in the onset of labor.[21]

AMNIOTIC FLUID

Formation and circulation of the amniotic fluid reflect intimate and dynamic maternal and fetal interactions. Amniotic fluid is ultimately derived from maternal water. Very early in pregnancy, amniotic fluid is cellular transudate with the same tonicity but lower protein content than maternal plasma. By at least 8 gestational weeks, when the maternal and fetal blood circulations are well established, most amniotic fluid water is thought to be derived from maternal plasma water by direct transfer from the maternal circulation to fetal capillaries in response to osmotic and hydrostatic forces. Once circulating in the fetus, water is filtered and excreted by the urinary system into the amniotic cavity. By 8 gestational weeks, the urethra is patent, and the fetal kidneys begin to form urine; by 10 to 11 weeks, a fetal bladder can be seen ultrasonographically. Concurrently, the fetus begins to swallow. Swallowed amniotic fluid is reabsorbed into the fetal circulation to be reexcreted by the kidneys, or transferred across the placenta to the mother. By the end of the first trimester, the amniotic fluid circulation has been established. Before fetal skin keratinization at 22 weeks, additional water transfer can occur directly through the highly permeable fetal skin.

Prolactin, produced by the decidualized endometrial cells, enters the amniotic cavity in large amounts by direct transport across the fetal membranes. Although undefined, amniotic fluid prolactin may have a role in regulating amniotic fluid volume.[22]

The content of amniotic fluid changes over gestation. The early electrolyte content is similar to that of extracellular fluid. As the kidneys become functional, fetal urine electrolytes and excretory products become major components. As gestation progresses, the fetal kidneys mature and are better able to retain electrolytes and produce more dilute urine. At 20 weeks, the sodium content of amniotic fluid is 136 mEq/L and the osmolality is 276 mOsm/L; at 40 weeks, the sodium content is 124 mEq/L and the osmolality is 258 mOsm/L.

Amniotic fluid contains excretory products of the fetus and maternal products that can diffuse directly across the fetal membranes from the maternal compartment. In addition to electrolytes and proteins, amniotic fluid contains carbohydrates, amino acids, urea, creatinine, lactate, pyruvate, lipids, enzymes, hormones, and various other metabolites reflective of the fetal milieu. Their presence and the presence of desquamated fetal cells allows diagnosis of many fetal abnormalities by biochemical and genetic analysis of amniotic fluid (see Chap. 12). Amniotic fluid also contains fetal pulmonary fluid. The usefulness of the lecithin–sphingomyelin ratio in predicting maturity of the fetal lungs has its basis in contributions from this fluid. In fetal sheep, there is constant outpouring of pulmonary fluid into the trachea.[23]

Although the range of normal amounts of amniotic fluid varies and depends on gestational age, abnormal volumes often herald fetal structural or growth abnormality. Maternal factors can affect amniotic fluid volume. Maternal plasma volume correlates with amniotic fluid volume. In hypovolemic mothers, expansion of plasma volume with albumin increases amniotic fluid volume.[24] Maternal use of diuretics may influence amniotic fluid volume indirectly by decreasing maternal intravascular volume and directly by increasing fetal micturition after transplacental passage.

FETAL MEMBRANES

The fetal amnion and chorion, although simple in anatomic design, are intricately involved in fetomaternal interactions. The thin, avascular layer of epithelial cells that makes up the amnion arises from fetal ectodermal cells, and the chorion, several layers thick, arises from extraembryonic somatic mesoderm and a trophoblast layer. The trophoblast layer in the area of the chorion that is destined to be the fetal surface of the term placenta undergoes rapid proliferation and branching into villi. By 8 menstrual weeks, the trophoblast layer of the remaining chorion becomes compressed, attenuated, and microscopic. These microscopic cells are intimately intermingled with the outermost maternal layer, the decidua or gestational endometrium, to allow paracrine interaction of these cells.

Paracrine interactions of the fetal chorionic cells with maternal decidual cells may be involved in the control of maternal production of prolactin and amniotic fluid volume regulation. In 1977, Riddick reported that decidua, an exclusively maternal cell line, synthesized and secreted a biologically active prolactin similar to pituitary prolactin.[25] These investigators were able to show that decidually produced prolactin crossed the amniochorion and entered the amniotic cavity intact. Prolactin receptors have been found in the chorion but not in amnion. Transport studies with tritiated water suggest that the net transport of water by the chorioamnion with adherent decidua is greatest in the fetomaternal direction, suggesting a net outflow of water from the amniotic fluid compartment to maternal circulation.[26] Lower osmolality in the amniotic fluid compartment favors movement of water from the amniotic cavity to the maternal compartment. Amniotic fluid prolactin decreases the permeability of the chorioamnion to water. Decidual prolactin production may be under amnion-derived prostaglandin control. Indomethacin was shown to inhibit decidual prolactin production.[27] Clinically, indomethacin has been associated with oligohydramnios and has been used to treat polyhydramnios.[28]

The cells of the amnion, rich in esterified arachidonic acid, are active in prostaglandin metabolism and are at least indirectly involved in cervical ripening and the onset or maintenance of labor. Initiation of human labor may involve autocrine and paracrine mechanisms within the fetal membranes and possibly maternal decidua, resulting in amnion cell production of prostaglandin E_2 (PGE_2), a potent cervical-ripening and uterotonic agent.[29] Although amnion cell production of PGE_2 has been associated with initiation and maintenance of labor, control of its production is less well understood.

The role of the amnion in the onset of preterm labor is of interest. In preterm labor associated with intraamniotic infection, significant amounts of interleukin-1 activity has been found in the amniotic fluid.[30,31] Interleukin-1, of monocyte–macrophage origin, functions as a mediator of fever and has a central role in the acute-phase response to infection and tissue injury. Interleukin-1 can stimulate PGE_2 biosynthesis by human amnion and may serve as the signal for initiation of labor in cases of intrauterine or systemic infection.[32] Investigators suggest that other cytokines play a role affecting the common pathway of amnion cell production of PGE_2 and subsequent labor.[33]

The chorioamnion produces a variety of other hormone products, including prorenin and renin, E2, progesterone, and hCG, although the rate of production of these hormones is less than that of their renal and placental counterparts. Neither the primary signals regulating secretion of these substances from the chorioamnion nor their specific targets have been elucidated.

UMBILICAL CORD

The umbilical cord contains one fetal artery and two fetal veins, which are supported and protected by Wharton jelly, a gel-like connective tissue composed of a ground substance of open-chain polysaccharides in a network of collagen and microfibrils.[34] Externally, the cord is covered by amnionic but no chorionic epithelium. The length of the umbilical cord ranges from 30 to 100 cm (mean, 55 cm) with reported extremes from 0 to 155 cm. Fetuses with no umbilical cords have a severe, fatal abdominal wall defect due to failure of formation of the body stalk. The association of short cords and low IQ raises the question of whether the length of the cord is determined by fetal movement mediated by antenatal neurologic function. Fetuses with long cords are more likely to have cord entanglement. Short cords are more likely to stretch and avulse during descent of the fetus, resulting in signs of fetal distress during expulsion or hemorrhage at birth.

The normal umbilical cord increases in circumference with gestation until term, when the average circumference is 3.8 cm.[35] Although excessive Wharton jelly (*i.e.*, thick cords) has not been associated with fetal abnormalities, lack of this connective tissue has. Thin cords are frequently seen with growth-retarded fetuses and may be associated with cord strictures, umbilical vessel rupture, or thrombi.[36] Thin cords are more likely to allow symptomatic external compression, stretch, or occlusion of umbilical vessels. Resolution of umbilical venous bleeding after percutaneous umbilical blood sampling is facilitated by Wharton jelly surrounding the vessel.

PLACENTAL PHYSIOLOGY IN DISEASE STATES

PREECLAMPSIA AND HYPERTENSIVE DISORDERS OF PREGNANCY

Preeclampsia, a hypertensive disease unique to pregnancy, has its genesis in the placenta. It is more common in women with multiple-gestation (*i.e.*, multiple placentas) and molar pregnancies (*i.e.*, excessive trophoblastic tissue), and it abates after delivery of the placenta. Altered placentation may be responsible for maternal vasospasm, the basic physiologic abnormality in preeclampsia. Vascular constriction in most maternal organs results in hypoperfusion of the uterus and placenta, making the fetus at risk for intrauterine growth restriction, placental abruption, and fetal death.

Placentas of preeclamptic women have a significantly lower total volume and volume of parenchymal and villous surface area than placentas of normal controls.[37] There is a greater proportion of centrally located, infarcted areas due to poor intervillous maternal circulation. Histologically, cellular degenerative changes are found.[38] An abundance of syncytial budding is common in histologic sections and teased preparations of villi. Budding, or knotting of the placental syncytiotrophoblasts, consists of bunching of the cytoplasm of these cells with aggregation of nuclei, a histologic finding suggestive of perfusional compromise.

The maternal vascular response to placentation is inadequate in women who develop preeclampsia.[39] Normally, with trophoblastic invasion, spiral arteries of the placental bed lose their muscular and elastic components, which are replaced by a fibrinoid layer of irregular thickness. The uteroplacental arteries become sinusoidally distended from their origin in the myometrium through the decidua into the intervillous space, allowing optimal blood flow for maternofetal exchange. In preeclamptic pregnancies, the myometrial segments and some of the decidual segment of spiral arteries show no evidence of trophoblast-induced physiologic distention. Some spiral arteries show absence of physiologic changes throughout the entire length, suggesting a complete lack of invasion by trophoblasts (Fig. 11-9). Invasive trophoblasts from preeclamptic placentas have disorganized expression of adhesion molecules.[40] In particular, preeclamptic trophoblasts lack normal expression of integrin, a surface molecule important in trophoblast adherence and invasion into the endometrium. Disorganized trophoblastic integrin formation may be responsible for the poor endometrial and myometrial invasion seen in preeclampsia.

Certain spiral arterioles at the implantation site undergo acute atherosis. Initially, fibrinoid degeneration and mural thrombosis of decidual vessels occurs. The vessel wall then becomes replaced by fibrin, and the intima is replaced by cholesterol-laden macrophages. Eventually, fibrinoid necrosis and total obstruction of the lumen leads to loss of maternal blood flow, which is possibly responsible for placental infarcts.[41]

There are no microscopic or macroscopic placental changes that are pathognomonic for preeclampsia. The pathologic changes in placentas of preeclamptic women that suggest the disease are indistinguishable from those of women with lupus anticoagulant syndrome, suggesting a shared physiology. In the lupus anticoagulant syndrome, autoimmune antiphospholipid antibodies, detectable in the maternal blood stream, are associated with maternal arterial and venous thrombosis, recurrent miscarriage, early-onset preeclampsia, placental and fetal growth restriction, and fetal death. Placentas from these women,

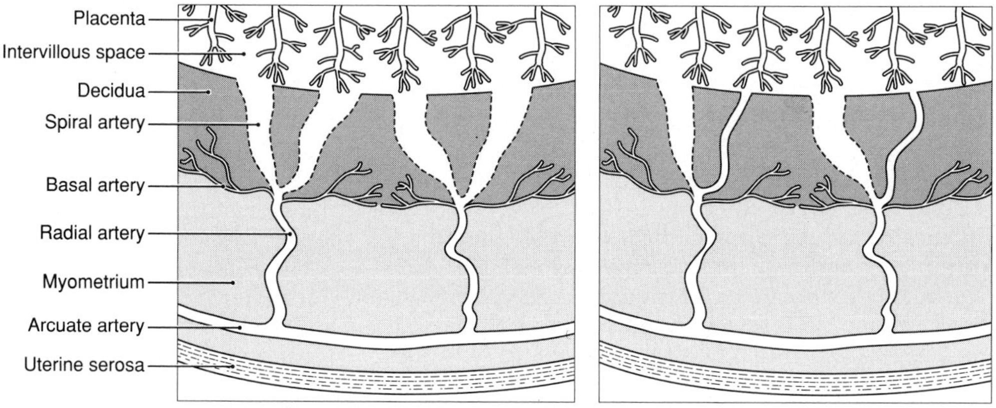

FIG. 11–9. Maternal blood supply to the placenta in normal pregnancy (*left*) and preeclampsia (*right*). Notice the lack of normal physiologic dilation of radial arteries and of some decidual segments of spiral arteries in preeclampsia. (Adapted from Khong TY, De Wolf F, Robertson WB, Brosens I. Inadequate maternal vascular response to placentation in pregnancies complicated by preeclampsia and by small-for-gestational age infants. Br J Obstet Gynaecol 1986;93:1049.)

whether or not they show signs of overt preeclampsia, have infarctions, fibrosis, a decrease in vasculosyncytial membranes, and an increase in syncytial knots.[42]

Preeclampsia is a disease resulting from abnormal maternoplacental interaction. The cause of preeclampsia is unknown. One of the most attractive pathogenetic mechanisms is that of an immune-mediated disease, supported by similarities with the lupus anticoagulant syndrome. However, in preeclampsia, neither the exact antigenic stimulus nor the antibody response has been defined, although the former is probably derived from trophoblasts.

Preeclampsia may be caused by placental production of a circulating humoral factor, perhaps immunologic, that affects prostaglandin homeostasis. Prostaglandins are involved in normal vasodilation of pregnancy. Prostacyclin (PGI_2), because of its potent effect in relaxing vascular smooth muscle and lowering systemic arterial pressure, is thought to be most involved. Prostacyclin is produced in vascular endothelial cells and is thought to exert its effect on vascular smooth muscle in a paracrine fashion. Prostacyclin is an inhibitor of platelet aggregation and an inhibitor of uterine contractility. The combined effects of this prostaglandin prevent maternal hypertension, prevent platelet aggregation, and promote uteroplacental blood flow. Thromboxane, produced predominantly by platelets, is a powerful vasoconstrictor, stimulator of platelet aggregation, and stimulator of uterine contractility, favoring maternal hypertension, decreased uteroplacental blood flow, and intrauterine growth restriction.

Abnormal prostaglandin homeostasis has been found in preeclampsia.[43] Excessive placental production of thromboxane and insufficient production of PGI_2 result in an abnormally high ratio of thromboxane to PGI_2. Prostacyclin production is decreased in umbilical arteries, placental veins, and uterine vessels. Thromboxane production is increased in placental tissue and in circulating platelets from preeclamptic women with infants who are small for gestational age.[44]

Higher thromboxane-to-PGI_2 ratios in the uterine vessels may be responsible for the abnormal maternal vascular response to placentation. Thromboxane in relative excess may decrease fetal blood flow to the placenta and cause shunting in the cotyledons; the umbilical arteries respond to these prostaglandins.[45] Antiprostaglandin therapy in the form of low-dose aspirin for prevention or treatment of preeclampsia is based on aspirin's selective inhibition of thromboxane production. Initial clinical trials using low-dose aspirin have been successful.[46]

Compared with normal placentas, placental findings in women with chronic or essential hypertension vary from lower total volume, lower parenchymal tissue, and infarcts to normal volumes and large, villous surface areas. Findings differ with various degrees of severity of disease and lack of differentiation between chronic hypertension and chronic hypertension with superimposed preeclampsia.

DIABETES

Just as the infant of a diabetic mother can be macrosomic, growth restricted, or normally grown, the diabetic placenta can have various findings. Some investigators have associated these findings with severity of maternal diabetes, especially the duration and complications of the disease, and others with degree of glycemic control.

Placentas of diabetic mothers without significant vascular disease (*i.e.*, White's class A–D) differ from normal by having more parenchymal and villous tissue, a higher cellular content, and a larger surface area of exchange between mother and fetus in terms of peripheral villous and capillary surface areas and intervillous space volume.[47–49] These larger placentas are able adequately to support growth of large fetuses. Placentas of diabetic mothers with appropriate-for-gestational-age newborns are morphologically closer to control, nondiabetic placentas. It is the placentas of macrosomic infants that are heavier, due predominantly to a significant accumulation of nonparenchymal and parenchymal tissue. These placentas have retarded maturation of surface areas of terminal villi. Grossly, they appear large, thick, and plethoric. Microscopically, focal immaturity (*i.e.*, dysmaturity) and villous edema are found.

The excessive growth and dysmaturity of these placentas suggest an accelerated growth process or a loss of the normal growth process that occurs in placentas of healthy women. Because the placenta is essentially a fetal organ different from other fetal organs only in that it is subject to more direct maternal modulation, it is not surprising that macrosomic fetuses have large placentas. The major mechanism for organ enlargement or macrosomia in the fetus of a diabetic mother involves anabolic metabolism of excess glucose and its deposition as glycogen and fat. The placenta of a macrosomic infant of a diabetic mother has neither excessive fat nor glycogen, suggesting a different mechanism by which the fetus (or mother) increases placental size and surface areas of terminal villi to maintain fetal nutrition, understanding that the size of the placenta and quality and topography of the transfer surface regulate nutrient availability to the fetus.

Placental cells respond to maternally or fetally produced hormones directly by alterations in growth and indirectly by elaboration of certain substances that control their own growth. Insulin and its associated family of growth-promoting peptide hormones, such as insulinlike growth factor I (IGF-I) and insulinlike growth factor II (IGF-II), have been implicated in affecting placental function in endocrine, autocrine, and paracrine fashion. These growth factors may be involved in excessive placental growth in the diabetic placenta.

Insulin receptors have been localized to the apical brush border of the syncytiotrophoblast (bathed in maternal blood).[50] Maternal insulin binds to these receptors, is internalized, and eventually degraded by this cell. Investigators using the *in vitro* perfused human placental cotyledon model have shown that placental facilitated uptake and metabolism of glucose does not appear to be regulated by insulin.[51] The lack of insulin regulation of glucose transport in the intact placenta correlates with glucose transporter genes in placenta, *GLUT1* and *GLUT3*, both thought to code for insulin-unresponsive glucose transporter proteins.[7] Why then is there active insulin uptake by the placental syncytiotrophoblast? Insulin, more likely fetal but possibly maternal, may have growth-promoting activity in the placenta and thereby effect placental size.

The placental trophoblast microvillous brush border membrane contains specific heterotetrameric IGF-I receptors that have been found in trophoblasts as early as 6 weeks of gestation.[52] This somatomedin has been measured in placental explant cultures and placental fibroblast culture fluid and is thought to be involved in control of placental growth.[53] Maternal serum IGF-I levels and the ratio of cord serum IGF-I to its binding protein correlate with birth weight.[54] Cord serum IGF-II levels are 50% higher in infants of diabetic than in those of nondiabetic mothers.

Because fetal macrosomia in diabetic pregnancies cannot always be prevented despite excellent maternal blood glucose control, attention has been turned to excessive placental transfer of fetal fuels other than glucose. Some investigators suggest a greater diffusional transfer of free fatty acids in diabetic pregnancies, probably related to greater maternal availability (*e.g.*, maternal hyperlipidemia in diabetic pregnancies) and greater placental transfer surface.[55] Excessive placental transfer of insulin-secretagogue amino acids (*e.g.*, arginine) may also be responsible for fetal hyperinsulinemia and macrosomia.

Placentas of diabetic women with vascular complications (*e.g.*, nephropathy, retinopathy, heart disease, White's class F, R, or H) frequently have infarcts and are associated with growth-retarded fetuses. The weights of the placentas of these diabetic women are lower than normal gestational age–matched placentas. There have been no specific placental findings to explain the higher stillborn rate in macrosomic fetuses of diabetic mothers.

ERYTHROBLASTOSIS

Erythroblastosis fetalis, or hemolytic disease of the newborn, is a condition in which specific IgG antibodies formed by the mother against erythrocyte antigens of the fetus cross the placenta by receptor-mediated endocytosis and coat fetal erythrocytes, causing their splenic sequestration, intravascular hemolysis, anemia, and unconjugated hyperbilirubinemia. Unconjugated bilirubin is easily transported to the maternal side, conjugated, and excreted by the mother. Anemia stimulates fetal hematopoiesis, especially in the liver and spleen, resulting in release of immature erythrocyte precursors into fetal blood. Severe fetal anemia causes fetal and placental hydrops, and often hypoproteinemia and thrombocytopenia. The placenta of newborns with erythroblastosis fetalis is pale and enlarged, displaying villous immaturity, edema, and an increase in Hofbauer cells (*i.e.*, macrophages). Erythrocyte precursors are found in the vascular spaces. The severity of placental changes parallels the severity of fetal disease. There is ultrasonographic evidence of reversal of placental thickening and edema as fetal hydrops improves with treatment.

Placental changes are secondary to the disease process and do not contribute to its formation. Hydropic placentas from fetuses with erythroblastosis fetalis are indistinguishable from those with other causes. In placentas of newborns with erythroblastosis fetalis, compensatory placental hematopoiesis, specifically in the villous stroma, is suggested because numerous erythrocyte precursors are found packed in fetal villous sinusoids mimicking *de novo* erythrocyte synthesis in the placenta. No specific erythrocyte synthesis occurs in the placenta.

Hydropic placentas produce elevated titers of hCG. Serum levels of this hormone are significantly above normal in women with hydropic fetuses and placentas.[56] It is unclear whether this is due to overproduction of the hormone or normal production by larger placental cell mass. Other placental hormones, including hPL, are found in elevated quantities in serum of women with hydropic placentas.

Preeclampsia occurs frequently in mothers with fetal and placental hydrops. Reversal of preeclamptic signs and symptoms has been observed after fetal and placental hydrops resolved spontaneously or was reversed by fetal transfusion.[57] Because hydropic placentas release greater amounts of placental hormones into the maternal circulation, this finding gives credence to a humoral placental product theory for the cause of preeclampsia.

TWIN-TO-TWIN TRANSFUSION SYNDROME

Abnormal placental physiology due to congenital placental vascular malformations in monozygotic twins is the basis of twin-to-twin transfusion syndrome.

Although dizygotic twinning always involves separate placentas and membranes (*i.e.*, diamnionic dichorionic), monozygotic twinning results in separation ranging from complete separation of the placentas and membranes (*i.e.*, diamnionic dichorionic) to shared placentas and chorion (*i.e.*, diamnionic monochorionic) to shared placentas, chorion, and amniotic cavity (*i.e.*, monoamnionic monochorionic) to shared fetal tissues (*i.e.*, monoamnionic conjoined).

Twin-to-twin transfusion syndrome is a disease of

monochorionic twins. Extraembryonic somatic mesoderm lining the extraembryonic cavity of the developing embryo gives rise to the chorion and to the mesenchymal core of the placental villus and associated fetal vessels. Monozygotic twins who share chorions (*i.e.*, monochorionic) also share fetal circulations by vascular connections. Fetal vascular anastomoses are almost never found on placentas of dichorionic twins, but they are usually found on those of monochorionic twins.[58]

In monochorionic twin placentas, the normal 1:1 ratio between the artery supplying and the vein draining a cotyledon is lost. Haphazard vascular patterns exist (Fig. 11-10). Certain cotyledons are supplied from a single or anastomotic artery from both twins and are drained by one or two veins. Others are supplied by an artery of one fetus and drained by a vein of the other. Drainage by the vein of the opposite fetus may not be obvious when capillaries join the venous system in a neighboring cotyledon before surfacing as a contralateral fetal vessel. An intertwin arteriovenous shunt should be suspected when an artery diving into a cotyledon is not accompanied by an adjacent emerging vein.

The most common fetal vascular anastomosis on the surface of the placenta is artery to artery, occurring in two-thirds of monochorionic placentas.[59] Vein-to-vein anastomoses are the least common, occurring in only 1 of 20 monochorionic placentas. Arteriovenous anastomosis, or arterial supply with contralateral fetal venous drainage of a cotyledon, which occurs in about two-thirds of monochorionic placentas, is thought to be the most common placental lesion leading to inequality of blood flow and twin transfusion syndrome. Placental injection studies using contrast have been performed to ascertain vascular anastomosis, but injection studies only demonstrate the presence of anastomosis and do not establish overall inequality of flow.

In twin-to-twin transfusion syndrome, blood from the donor twin flows to the recipient cotwin through intertwin placental vascular connections. Remaining anastomoses are insufficient to allow return of the lost blood volume, and an imbalance of blood flow exists. The donor twin becomes hypovolemic, anemic, malnourished, growth restricted, and responds with oliguria (*i.e.*, oligohydramnios) and, in severe cases, anuria (*i.e.*, ahydramnios). The recipient twin becomes hypervolemic and plethoric, develops cardiomegaly and polyuria (*i.e.*, polyhydramnios), and, if severe, develops cardiac failure and hydrops fetalis. Grossly, the placental portion of the donor twin is anemic, pale, and usually smaller than that of the cotwin. If hydrops has not yet occurred, the recipient twin's placental portion is red, thick, and congested. After hydrops ensues, the placenta becomes pale from villous edema. Microscopically, anemia and villous immaturity are found in the donor's placental portion and polycythemia and congestion in that of the recipient.

Despite the high frequency of cross-placental vascular anastomoses in monochorionic placentas, the incidence of clinically evident twin-to-twin transfusion syndrome is only 5% to 10%. In some twin pairs, intertwin vascular connections may produce a chronic twin transfusion syndrome in which the larger twin responds with cardiac hyperplasia and hypertrophy.[60] Cardiac hyperplasia may be compensatory, and certain sets of monochorionic twins may withstand the vascular inequalities throughout gestation (*i.e.*, subclinical twin-to-twin transfusion syndrome). In others, the pumping capabilities of the enlarged heart are exceeded, and cardiac failure occurs. It is tempting to speculate that as the heart enlarges and fails, delicate pressure-flow characteristics in the placental vasculature are disrupted, exacerbating shunting to the recipient twin.

Twin-to-twin transfusion syndrome is a condition

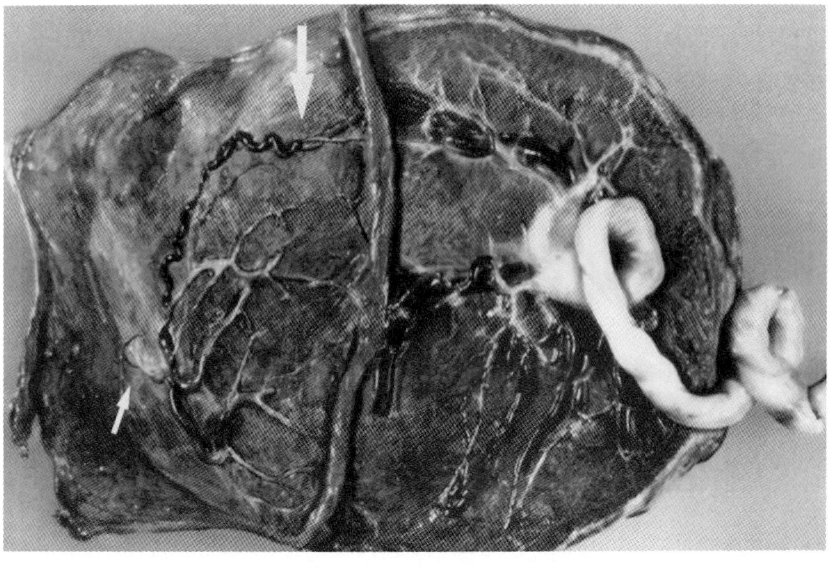

FIG. 11–10. Diamnionic, monochorionic twin placenta, with the intervening amnion rolled in the center. Notice the haphazard vascularization (*large arrow*). The velamentous cord insertion (*small arrow*) of the smaller twin of this discordant pair is not an unusual finding in monochorionic twins.

that begins early in embryonic vascular development. Benirschke described the youngest example, a pair of aborted twin embryos measuring 7 and 8 cm (10 weeks of gestation) in which the heart of the donor twin was one-half the size of that of the recipient.[61] Intertwin vascular distribution established early in the embryonic period may control intertwin placental mass distribution. Inequality in placental mass distribution may have an early, direct effect on fetal growth, causing significant growth restriction in one fetus.

Antenatal ultrasonographic evaluation of the number of layers in intervening membranes has allowed diagnosis of chorionicity with high sensitivity and positive predictive value.[62] The obstetrician can confirm chorionicity and assess placental vascular patterns immediately after delivery of the twin placenta and should impart this information to the pediatrician.

Some antenatal treatment approaches for twin transfusion syndrome attempt to reverse the abnormal placental physiology. Selective termination of one fetus, usually the donor, prevents further transfusion to the recipient. This treatment introduces risks to the living twin from passage of emboli from the dead twin through anastomotic channels (*i.e.*, twin embolization syndrome). Serial amniocentesis to decompress the polyhydramniotic sac of the recipient twin has reversed twin-to-twin transfusion syndrome in a few cases.[63] Loss of amniotic fluid pressure on a large placental vascular anastomosis allows changes in fetal blood flow. After amniotic fluid decompression of severe polyhydramnios, ultrasonographically observed placentas appear thickened and less stretched. Fetoscopic laser occlusion of placental vessels, reported by De Lia and associates, may prove to be the most logical therapy, because treatment is directed at the cause of the problem.[64] At the time of delivery, the placenta is two discs, separated by an area of infarcted cotyledons previously supplied by the coagulated vessels.

Acute transplacental fetus-to-fetus bleeding can occur in monochorionic twins and is distinct from twin transfusion syndrome. Acute fetus-to-fetus bleeding occurs in placentas with medium- or large-caliber vascular anastomosis when loss of established pressure-flow relations occurs. For example, the death of one twin of a monochorionic pair may allow large shifts of blood from the living twin to the deceased cotwin. Shifts may be sufficient to cause anemia and hydrops fetalis in the surviving twin. If the deceased cotwin was the growth-retarded donor of a twin-to-twin transfusion pair, paradoxical plethora of the donor twin may occur.

Acute transplacental fetal bleeding may occur at the time of labor. For example, during the uterine contractions, umbilical cord compression may occur to a sufficient degree that it diminishes umbilical venous return but not arterial perfusion. The resulting higher resistance in the placental venous system of the cord-compressed twin favors return of blood to the cotwin. Acute intraplacental fetal bleeding may occur after delivery of the first fetus. Loss of established placental pressure-flow relations after clamping of the umbilical cord favors intraplacental pooling of the second twin's blood through anastomoses resulting in hypovolemia. Acute transplacental fetal bleeding can create disparate newborn hematocrits that do not reflect hematocrit levels during fetal life.

REFERENCES

1. Ramsey EM. The placenta: human and animal. New York: Prager Publishers, 1982;49.
2. Pridjian G, Moawad AH, Whitington PF. Handling of beta-hydroxybutyrate in the human placenta. Abstract 268. In: Scientific program and abstracts. St Louis: Society for Gynecologic Investigation, 1990:230.
3. Lind T, Aspillaga M. Metabolic changes during normal and diabetic pregnancies. In: Reece EA, Coustan DR, eds. Diabetes mellitus in pregnancy: principles and practice. New York: Churchill Livingstone, 1988;75.
4. Venkataramanan R, Koneru B, Wang CCP, Burckart GJ, Caritis SN, Starzl TE. Cyclosporine and its metabolites in mother and baby. Transplantation 1988;46:468.
5. Neufeld ND, Corbo L. Increased fetal insulin receptors and changes in membrane fluidity and lipid composition. Am J Physiol 1982;243:E246.
6. Dancis J. Aspects of bilirubin metabolism before and after birth. Pediatrics 1959;24:980.
7. Kayano T, Fukumoto H, Eddy RL, et al. Evidence for a family of human glucose transporter-like proteins. J Biol Chem 1988; 263:15245.
8. Johnson LW, Smith CH. Monosaccharide transport across microvillous membrane of human placenta. Am J Physiol 1980; 238:C160.
9. Yudelivech DL, Sweiry JH. Transport of amino acids in the placenta. Biochem Biophys Acta 1985;822:169.
10. Miller RK, Berndt WO. Characterization of neutral amino acid accumulation by human term placental slices. Am J Physiol 1974;227:1236.
11. Schneider H, Mohlen KH, Dancis J. Transfer of amino acids across the in vitro perfused human placenta. Pediatr Res 1979;13:236.
12. Enders RH, Judd RM, Donohue TM, Smith C. Placental amino acid uptake. III. Transport systems for neutral amino acids. Am J Physiol 1976;230:706.
13. Hibbard JU, Pridjian G, Whitington PF, Moawad AH. Taurine transport in the in vitro perfused human placenta. Pediatr Res 1990;27:80.
14. Fortunato SJ, Bawdon RE, Swan KF, Sobhi S. Transfer of azidothymidine (AZT) across the in vitro perfused human placenta. Abstract 3. In: Scientific program and abstracts. San Diego: Society for Gynecologic Investigation, 1989:82.
15. Ockleford CD, Whyte A. Differentiated regions of human placental cell surface associated with the exchange of materials between maternal and fetal blood. The structure, distribution, ultrastructural cytochemistry and biochemical composition of coated vesicles. J Cell Sci 1977;25:293.
16. McNabb T, Koh TY, Dorrington KJ, Painter RH. Structure and function of immunoglobulin domains V. Binding of immunoglobulin G and fragments to placental membrane preparations. J Immunol 1976;117:182.
17. Niezgodka M, Mikulska J, Ugorski M, Boratynski J, Lisowski J.

Human placental membrane receptor for IgG-1. Studies on the properties and solubilization of the receptor. Mol Immunol 1981;18:163.
18. Okuyama T, Tawada MD, Furuya H, Villee CA. The role of transferrin and ferritin in the fetal-maternal-placental unit. Am J Obstet Gynecol 1985;152:344.
19. Ringler GE, Kallen CB, Strauss JF. Regulation of human trophoblast function by glucocorticoids: dexamethasone promotes increased secretion of chorionic gonadotropin. Endocrinology 1989;124:1625.
20. Cohen M, Haour F, Dumont M, Bertrand J. Prognostic value of human chorionic somatomammotropin plasma levels in diabetic patients. Am J Obstet Gynecol 1973;115:202.
21. Riley SC, Walton JC, Herlick JM, Challis JRG. The localization and distribution of corticotropin-releasing hormone in the human placenta and fetal membranes throughout gestation. J Clin Endocrinol Metab 1991;72:1001.
22. Ross MG, Ervin MG, Leake RD, Oakes G, Hobel C, Fisher DA. Bulk flow of amniotic fluid water in response to maternal osmotic challenge. Obstet Gynecol 1983;147:697.
23. Adams FH, Fujiwara T. Surfactant in fetal lab tracheal fluid. J Pediatr 1963;63:537.
24. Goodlin RC, Anderson JC, Gallagher TF. Relationship between amniotic fluid volume and maternal plasma volume expansion. Am J Obstet Gynecol 1983;146:505.
25. Riddick DH, Kusmik WF. Decidua: a possible source of amniotic fluid prolactin. Am J Obstet Gynecol 1977;127:187.
26. McCoshen JA. Associations between prolactin, prostaglandin E_2 and fetal membrane function in human gestation. In: Mitchell BF, ed. The physiology and biochemistry of human fetal membranes. Ithaca, NY: Perinatology Press, 1988;117.
27. Maslar I, Rosenberg S, Riddick D. Diminished prolactin production by human endometrium exposed to drugs which inhibit prostaglandin synthetase. Abstract 277. In: Scientific program and abstracts. Denver: Society for Gynecologic Investigation, 1980:277.
28. Mamopoulos M, Assimakopoulos E, Reece EA, Andreou A, Zheng XZ, Mantalenakis S. Maternal indomethacin therapy in the treatment of polyhydramnios. Am J Obstet Gynecol 1990; 162:1225.
29. Okazaki T, Casey ML, Okita JR, MacDonald PC, Johnston JM. Initiation of human parturition, XII Biosynthesis and metabolism of prostaglandins in human fetal membranes and uterine decidua. Am J Obstet Gynecol 1981;139:373.
30. Romero R, Mazor M. Infection and preterm labor. Clin Obstet Gynecol 1988;31:553.
31. Romero R, Brody DT, Oyarzun E, et al. Infection and labor III. Interleukin-1: a signal for the onset of parturition. Am J Obstet Gynecol 1989;160:1117.
32. Romero R, Duram S, Dinarello C, Oyarzun E, Hobbins JC, Mitchell MD. Interleukin-1 stimulates prostaglandin biosynthesis by human amnion. Prostaglandins 1989;37:13.
33. Romero R, Avila C. Santhanam U, Sehgal PB. Amniotic fluid interleukin 6 in preterm labor: association with infection. J Clin Invest 1990;85:1392.
34. Benirschke K, Kaufmann P. Pathology of the human placenta. 2nd ed. New York: Springer-Verlag, 1990;182.
35. Silver RK, Dooley SL, Tamura RK, Depp R. Umbilical cord size and amniotic fluid volume in prolonged pregnancy. Am J Obstet Gynecol 1987;157:716.
36. Robertson RD, Rubinstein LM, Wolfson WL, et al. Constriction of the umbilical cord as a cause of fetal demise following midtrimester amniocentesis. J Reprod Med 1981;26:325.
37. Boyd PA, Scott A. Quantitative structural studies on human placentas associated with preeclampsia, essential hypertension and intrauterine growth retardation. Br J Obstet Gynaecol 1985;92:714.
38. Cibils LA. The placenta and newborn infant in hypertensive conditions. Am J Obstet Gynecol 1974;118:256.
39. Khong TY, De Wolf F, Robertson WB, Brosens I. Inadequate maternal vascular response to placentation in pregnancies complicated by preeclampsia and by small for gestational age infants. Br J Obstet Gynaecol 1986;93:1049.
40. Zhou Y, Damsky CH, Chiu K, Roberts JM, Fisher SJ. Preeclampsia is associated with abnormal expression of adhesion molecules by invasive cytotrophoblasts. J Clin Invest 1993;91: 950.
41. Zeek PM, Assali NS. Vascular changes in the decidua associated with eclamptogenic toxemia of pregnancy. Am J Clin Pathol 1950;20:1099.
42. Out HJ, Kooijman CD, Bruinse HW, Derksen RH. Histopathological findings in placentae from patients with intrauterine fetal death and antiphospholipid antibodies. Eur J Obstet Gynecol Reprod Biol 1991;41:179.
43. Walsh SW. Preeclampsia: an imbalance in placental prostacyclin and thromboxane production. Am J Obstet Gynecol 1985;152:335.
44. Wallenburg HC, Rotmans N. Enhanced reactivity of the platelet thromboxane pathway in normotensive and hypertensive pregnancies with insufficient fetal growth. Am J Obstet Gynecol 1982;144:523.
45. Tuvemo T. Role of prostaglandins, prostacyclin, and thromboxanes in the control of the umbilical-placental circulation. Semin Perinatol 1980;4:91.
46. Schiff E, Peleg E, Goldenberg M, et al. The use of aspirin to prevent pregnancy-induced hypertension and lower the ratio of thromboxane A2 to prostacyclin in relatively high risk pregnancies. N Engl J Med 1989;321:351.
47. Teasdale F. Histomorphometry of the placenta of the diabetic woman. Class A diabetes mellitus. Placenta 1981;2:241.
48. Teasdale F. Histomorphometry of the human placenta in class B diabetes mellitus. Placenta 1983;4:1.
49. Teasdale F. Histomorphometry of the human placenta in class C diabetes mellitus. Placenta 1985;6:69.
50. Deal CL, Guyda HJ. Insulin receptors of human term placental cells and choriocarcinoma (JEG-3) cells: characteristics and regulation. Endocrinology 1983;112:1512.
51. Challier JC, Hauguel S, Desmaizieres V. Effect of insulin on glucose uptake and metabolism in the human placenta. J Clin Endocrinol Metab 1986;62:803.
52. Grizzard JD, D'Ercole AJ, Wilkins JR, Moats-Staats, Williams JR. Affinity-labeled somatomedin-C receptors and binding proteins from the human fetus. J Clin Endocrinol Metab 1984;58:535.
53. Fant M, Monro H, Moses AC. An autocrine/paracrine role for insulin-like growth factors in the regulation of human placental growth. J Clin Endocrinol Metab 1986;63:499.
54. Hall K, Hansson U, Lundin G, et al. Serum levels of somatomedins and somatomedin-binding protein in pregnant women with type I or gestational diabetes and their infants. J Clin Endocrinol Metab 1986;63:1300.
55. Thomas CR. Placental transfer of non-esterified fatty acids in normal and diabetic pregnancy. Biol Neonate 1987;51:94.
56. Hatjis CG. Nonimmunologic fetal hydrops associated with hperreactio luteinalis. Obstet Gynecol 1985;65(Suppl):11.
57. Pryde PG, Nugent CE, Pridjian G, Barr Jr M, Faix RG. Spontaneous resolution of nonimmune hydrops fetalis secondary to parvovirus B19 infection. Obstet Gynecol 1992;79:869.
58. Robertson EG, Neer KJ. Placental injection studies in twin gestation. Am J Obstet Gynecol 1983;147:170.

59. Benirschke K, Kaufmann P. Pathology of the human placenta. 2nd ed. New York: Springer-Verlag, 1990;658.
60. Pridjian G, Nugent CE, Barr M. Twin gestation: influence of placentation on fetal growth. Am J Obstet Gynecol 1991; 165:1394.
61. Benirschke K. Prenatal cardiovascular adaptation, comparative pathophysiology of circulatory disturbances. In: Bloor CM, ed. Advances in experimental medicine and biology. New York: Plenum Press, 1972;22:3.
62. D'Alton ME, Dudley DK. The ultrasonographic prediction of chorionicity in twin gestation. Am J Obstet Gynecol 1989; 160:557.
63. Elliott JP, Urig MA, Clewell WH. Aggressive therapeutic amniocentesis for treatment of twin-twin transfusion syndrome. Obstet Gynecol 1991;77:537.
64. De Lia JE, Cruikshank DP, Keye WR. Fetoscopic neodymium:YAG laser occlusion of placental vessels in severe twin-twin transfusion syndrome. Obstet Gynecol 75:1046.

Neonatology: Pathophysiology and Management of the Newborn, Fourth Edition,
edited by Gordon B. Avery, Mary Ann Fletcher, and Mhairi G. MacDonald.
J.B. Lippincott Company, Philadelphia © 1994.

chapter 12

Prenatal Diagnosis: Procedures and Trends

ARIE DRUGAN
NELSON B. ISADA
MARK P. JOHNSON
MORDECHAI HALLAK
MARK I. EVANS

The culturing and karyotyping of amniotic fluid fibroblasts became feasible in the mid-1960s, and initiated the era of prenatal diagnosis of fetal genetic disorders.[1] After the first diagnosis of a fetal chromosome anomaly by amniocentesis,[2] the diagnosis of an enzyme deficiency in amniotic fluid cells was reported by Nadler in 1968.[3] Thereafter, collaborative studies established the safety and accuracy of midtrimester amniocentesis,[4,5] so that this technique became a routine part of prenatal care in high-risk patients and the gold standard against which other procedures for prenatal diagnosis have been compared.

The results of amniocentesis generally were not available, however, until about 20 weeks of gestation. At this gestational age, the termination of a malformed, albeit otherwise wanted pregnancy, frequently is emotionally traumatic as well as more dangerous to the mother than a first-trimester pregnancy termination.

Improvement in ultrasound machinery and expertise allowed physicians to invade the intrauterine environment with earlier, more accurate, and safer guided procedures for diagnosis of fetal congenital anomalies. In the late 1980s, attempts to move prenatal diagnosis into the first trimester were made, introducing chorionic villus sampling (CVS) and early amniocentesis. Chorionic villus sampling usually is performed between 9 and 12 weeks of gestation so that results are available by the end of the first trimester. The accuracy and safety of CVS are very comparable to those of amniocentesis,[6,7] and the early results allow patients privacy in reproductive decisions and an earlier and safer termination of pregnancy if so opted. An alternative to CVS has been offered by early amniocentesis performed between 10 and 14 weeks of gestation.[8] A trend toward increasing preference on the part of patients for first-trimester prenatal diagnosis procedures has been observed.[9]

The need for rapid karyotyping may arise when fetal anomalies are observed on ultrasound in the second trimester, near the legal limit for termination of affected pregnancies. In those cases, the diagnostic options are late CVS,[10] or cordocentesis and karyotyping of fetal blood lymphocytes. Other tests that may be performed on blood obtained by cordocentesis include hematologic, acid–base balance, and immunologic status of the fetus.[11]

PRENATAL DIAGNOSIS IN THE FIRST TRIMESTER

CHORIONIC VILLUS SAMPLING

The first attempts at first-trimester prenatal diagnosis were made in the Soviet Union and China in the early 1970s, mainly for fetal gender determination.[12] It was not until 1983, however, that laboratory techniques to obtain karyotypes adequate for interpretation from chorionic villi were developed by Simoni and Brambati in Milan,[13] who also reported the first diagnosis of trisomy 21 by the direct method 5 hours after CVS was performed.[14] Over the years, the quality of chromosome preparation from CVS material has improved considerably, approaching the banding quality obtained from amniocytes or blood karyotypes.[15] The clinical procedure also has been refined, with the use of real-time ultrasound guidance and malleable catheters for villi aspiration. The use of variable approaches (*i.e.*, transcervical *versus* transabdominal) depending on placental location has improved the yield and safety of CVS.[16,17]

Chorionic villus sampling can be offered to almost every patient who needs prenatal diagnosis. The most common indication for CVS is advanced maternal age, which accounts for 70%–80% of cases.[9,16] Other indications for fetal karyotyping include a previous child with chromosome anomalies or a parent carrier of a balanced translocation or inversion. Normal ranges of lysosomal enzymes in fresh and cultured villi also have been established, allowing for the diagnosis of disorders such as Tay–Sachs or the mucopolysaccharidoses.[18] Chorionic villus sampling is particularly suitable for DNA molecular prenatal diagnosis of classic genetic disorders. The amount of DNA obtained from even a few villi is much larger than that contained in amniocytes from 40 mL of amniotic fluid. Molecular approaches are discussed in Chapter 9.

TECHNICAL ASPECTS

Chorionic villus sampling procedures, whether transcervical, transabdominal or transvaginal, are most commonly performed between 9 and 12 weeks of gestation (Fig. 12-1). After 13 weeks, the procedure usually is best done transabdominally.[19] Fetal viability and gestational age always must be confirmed before the procedure. The major determinant of approach is placental location. Fundal placentas are most commonly an indication for the transabdominal approach; however, other factors may dictate the preferable approach to CVS in specific cases. Thus, transcervical or transvaginal CVS should be avoided in patients with active vaginal or cervical infection (*e.g.*, herpes), whereas the transabdominal approach should be avoided in cases with interposed bowel or with marked uterine retroversion.[19] After CVS, fetal heart activity should be verified, and Rh immuno-prophylaxis should be administered to Rh-negative patients.

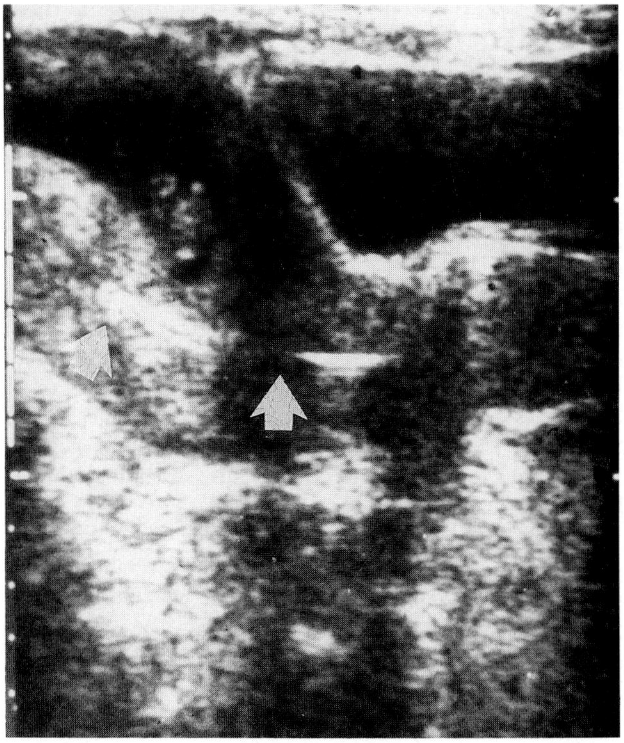

FIG. 12–1. In transcervical chorionic villus sampling (CVS), the CVS catheter (*arrows*) is guided through the cervical canal and into the placenta.

Despite the growing tendency of American and European centers to use the transabdominal approach for CVS,[20,21] in our experience, transabdominal sample size usually has been lower than that obtained transcervically.[22] Proficiency in both types of procedures is necessary, however. Transabdominal CVS is the procedure of choice for cases with anterior fundal placentas, whereas transcervical CVS should be performed when the placenta is posterior and low-lying. In general, tailoring the type of procedure to placental location is expected to reduce complication rates after CVS.[16,23]

Transvaginal transmural CVS should be reserved to a very limited number of cases in which the placenta is posterior, the uterus is retroverted and retroflexed, and the cervical canal points toward the mother's abdomen. In those cases, the procedure can be performed transvaginally with a needle guided by transabdominal or transvaginal ultrasound.[24,25]

SAFETY

The safety of CVS must be judged from the perspective of the natural pregnancy loss rate in the first trimester. Simpson calculated the likelihood of spontaneous abortion in women at 8 to 11 weeks of a viable gestation to be 3% to 5%, and increasing with maternal age.[26] Both the Canadian and the American collaborative studies documented an excess loss rate in the CVS group of 0.6% to 0.8%, which is not significantly different than the loss rate in the amniocentesis group.[6,7] Fundal placental location, three catheter insertions, and obtaining small amounts of villi have been significantly associated with pregnancy loss after CVS. These factors may reflect technical difficulty during the procedure.[19]

Concerns over the safety of CVS have been raised by Firth and Burton.[27,28] In two small series of procedures done by relatively inexperienced physicians, they claimed a 1% risk of limb reduction defects (LRDs) following CVS. In contrast, evaluation of over 125,000 cases from experienced centers worldwide reveals that the incidence of LRDs or any other defects is identical to that of the background population (Table 12-1). Furthermore, closer assessment of cases of LRDs has shown that several had unreported familial factors.[29] There may be a very slightly increased risk with CVS procedures done at 6 to 7 weeks of gestation as opposed to the usual time of 9 to 12 weeks of gestation or by inexperienced personnel, but the data suggest that CVS is otherwise safe and effective.

FETOMATERNAL TRANSFUSION

Another concern for CVS is the potential for fetomaternal transfusion. Transiently rising maternal serum α-fetoprotein (AFP) levels after CVS have been reported.[30] The increase is correlated to sample size, but not to CVS technique, whether transabdominal or transcervical.[31] The calculated mean volume of transfused fetal blood was 5.4 mL. Others have reported the volume of fetomaternal transfusion after CVS to reach 21% of fetoplacental blood volume.[32] Thus, Rh isoimmunization should be considered a relative contraindication to CVS.

CHROMOSOMAL ANALYSIS

Two types of cells are observed in chorionic villi. The outer layer consists of cytotrophoblasts, which divide spontaneously, and is used for direct evaluation of metaphases. The inner mesenchymal core is used to initiate long-term cultures and usually is more representative of fetal karyotype. Overall, cytogenetic results are obtained by either direct analysis, long-term culture, or both in 99.6% of cases in which villi are obtained.[15] Results of direct analysis are equivocal in 1% to 2% of cases, but questions raised usually are resolved by long-term CVS or amniotic cell cultures.[19] Most commonly, an abnormal direct result that proves to be normal on long-term culture will not be confirmed in karyotypes obtained from amniocytes or fetal lymphocytes. The more rare situation is a normal direct result followed by an abnormal result in long-term culture, with the abnormality being confirmed in fetal tissue in one-half of those cases.[15] Maternal cell contamination has been observed in 1.9% of long-term cultures, but did not contribute to diagnostic error in any case.[19]

Chromosomal mosaicism in CVS material affects about 1.2% to 2.5% of cases (average 1.3%), and is more common in direct preparations than in long-term culture.[32] Mosaicism was restricted to extraembryonic tissue in 70% to 80% of cases. Despite the fact that mosaicism was confined to the placenta, however, follow-up of these cases documented a significantly elevated fetal loss rate (16.7%), mostly in the second and third trimesters, suggesting that such placental mosaicism is not entirely benign.[33] Intrauterine growth retardation (IUGR) also appears to be more common in this situation.[34] Trisomy 3 mosaicism is one of the most common types observed in placental cells.[32]

The diagnosis of mosaicism in CVS presents difficulties in genetic counseling because it implies uncertainty with respect to fetal phenotype and genotype. The accuracy of diagnosis by CVS may be increased by using both direct preparation and long-term culture. When further evaluation is needed, level II ultrasonographic screening for anomalies and amniocentesis is adequate for follow-up. In our experience, however, the frequency of mosaicism in amniotic fluid cultures is not significantly different from that observed in CVS (0.35% *versus* 0.56%, respectively).[35] Cordocentesis may be used in such cases to verify mosaicism in fetal blood.[36] Even if fetal blood karyotype is normal, however, there still will remain a small chance that mosaicism is confined to specific fetal tissues, as observed in trisomy 20 mosaicism.

TABLE 12–1
INCIDENCE OF LIMB REDUCTION AFTER CHORIONIC VILLUS SAMPLING

Number of CVS cases	124,556
Number of limb reduction cases	74
Observed frequency	5.94/10,000
Expected frequency	5.97/10,000

* All fetuses were ≥6 weeks of gestational age.

Unpublished data through December 1992, courtesy of Ronald Wapner, M.D., Thomas Jefferson School of Medicine, Philadelphia, PA.

EARLY AMNIOCENTESIS

Early amniocentesis refers to aspiration of amniotic fluid for analysis before 15 weeks from the last menstrual period. Because many obstetricians are familiar with the technique of amniocentesis, it was assumed incorrectly that the early procedure would exhibit the same safety and accuracy as when performed in midtrimester.[32,37] With improved ultrasound technology and increasing experience with ultrasound-guided needle manipulations, earlier amniocentesis appeared to be an attractive alternative to CVS late in the first trimester. The procedure is relatively simple; using continuous ultrasound guidance and aseptic technique, a 22-gauge needle is inserted into a pocket of fluid, and about 1 mL of fluid per week of gestation is aspirated into a 20-mL syringe (Fig. 12-2). Tenting of membranes ahead of the needle is relatively common in early amniocentesis, because membranes are not yet adhering to the uterine wall. In our experience, aspiration of fluid is hampered by tenting of membranes in about 5% of early procedures, but the procedure still is successful.[9]

Complications of early amniocentesis include bleeding, uterine cramping, leakage of fluid, and infection, as observed sometimes after amniocentesis performed at later gestational ages. Rupture of membranes after early amniocentesis was observed in 2.5% of cases in Penso and Frigoletto's series.[37] The total unintentional loss rate after early amniocentesis is reported in the literature to be between 1.4% to 4.2% (Table 12-2); however, not all of these losses could be related causally to the early procedure.[37–42] There seems to be a trend in all series toward increased loss rates after amniocentesis performed at 11 or 12 weeks of gestation[37]; however, there are many caveats to be considered. A 14-week amniocentesis is not comparable to a 9-week CVS. It has become abundantly clear that the principal determinant of total fetal loss after any procedure is the gestational age. Our experience shows procedure-related losses of amniocentesis and CVS to be nearly identical.

In comparison with CVS, early amniocentesis has a lower rate of pseudomosaicism and maternal cell contamination. A concern has been raised, however, about culture failure after early amniocentesis. In our experience, culture failure rate is 1 in 700 after midtrimester amniocentesis, but about 1% after early procedures, and nearly 5% at under 12 weeks.[22,43] This rate is somewhat lower than the 1.6% rate of culture failure reported by Stripparo and colleagues,[39] but higher than 0.32% reported by Elejalde and associates.[43]

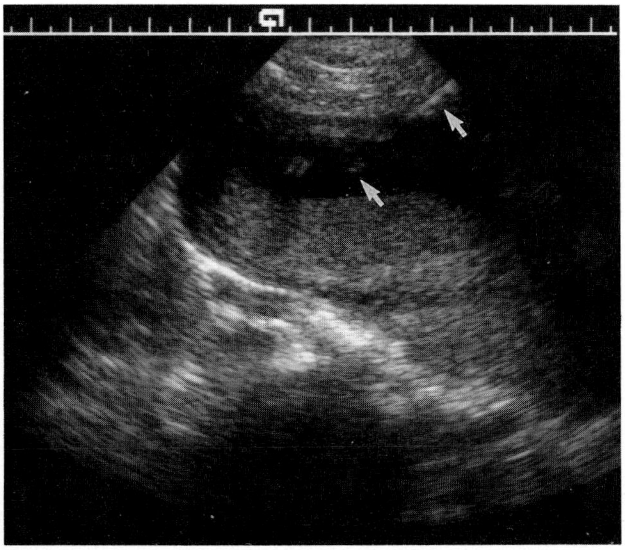

FIG. 12–2. In early amniocentesis, the needle (*arrows*) is inserted through the uterine wall and into the amniotic cavity.

TABLE 12–2
RATE OF PREGNANCY LOSS AFTER EARLY AMNIOCENTESIS

Author	Loss Rate*
Penso and Frigoletto[37]	3.8%
Hanson et al.[38]	2.3%
Stripparo et al.[39]	3.1%
Nevin et al.[40]	1.4%
Dunn and Godmilow[41]	4.2%
Elejalde et al.[42]	1.6%

* Mean 2.7% ± 1%.

Early amniocentesis also may permit the diagnosis of fetal structural anomalies through analysis of amniotic fluid AFP and acetylcholinesterase (AChE). Alpha-fetoprotein peaks in amniotic fluid at 12 to 13 weeks of gestation and then gradually declines, similar to fetal serum.[44,45] High amniotic fluid AFP levels have been observed with fetal neural tube defects (NTD) or omphalocele even in these early samples, and low amniotic fluid AFP values accompanied some conceptions diagnosed as aneuploid, as seen in samples of amniotic fluid obtained at midtrimester, but the data still are questionable as to accuracy. The interpretation of amniotic fluid AChE results is, however, more complex. Acetylcholinesterase usually is analyzed on gel electrophoresis as a bimodal result, either positive or negative. In early amniotic fluid samples, a faint, inconclusive band is frequently observed. This finding seems, however, to be associated with fetal anomalies only in a minority of cases, in contrast to the same AChE result in amniotic fluid samples from midtrimester.[46] Thus, it appears that in early amniotic fluid samples a negative AChE result may be reliable in the setting of elevated amniotic fluid AFP, but the interpretation of a positive AChE may necessitate quantitative evaluation of band density.[47]

CHORIONIC VILLUS SAMPLING *versus* EARLY AMNIOCENTESIS IN FIRST-TRIMESTER PRENATAL DIAGNOSIS

Most procedures for prenatal diagnosis are performed for relatively low-risk indications (*e.g.*, advanced maternal age, a previous child with chromosome anomalies, parental translocation or inversion). Prenatal diagnosis in the first trimester enables us to reassure most patients with normal results 6 to 9 weeks earlier than would be possible with midtrimester amniocentesis. Although still at risk for miscarriage, patients undergoing CVS for prenatal diagnosis show a sharp drop in anxiety levels immediately after receiving results, whereas patients undergoing amniocentesis remain anxious longer.[48] In the few unfortunate cases that are diagnosed as abnormal, the mother can have a less traumatic and less risky first, rather than second-trimester termination of pregnancy[49]; however, which of the two procedures available for prenatal diagnosis is preferable in the first trimester? The only prospective, randomized study that compares CVS and early amniocentesis in the first trimester is that by Byrne and associates, which suggests that the two techniques can be comparable in terms of accuracy and successful results.[50] Early amniocentesis is a viable alternative to CVS in the first trimester. The possibility of analyzing amniotic fluid AFP and AChE also is tempting, especially for patients at high risk for NTD per family history and for diabetics. It should be noted, however, that amniocentesis at 12 weeks or earlier is associated with significantly more culture failures and pregnancy loss than observed later in gestation. Moreover, concerns have been raised that removal of amniotic fluid so early in gestation may affect fetal lung development and function. Thus, our opinion is that CVS is the procedure of choice before 12 weeks of gestation, for karyotyping as well as for DNA molecular analysis. On the other hand, early amniocentesis may be preferable in certain biochemical disorders and in situations in which CVS may not truly represent fetal tissue. An example of the latter situation is a twin pregnancy with fused placenta—sampling the placenta in such a case will not discriminate one fetal karyotype from the other, but with early amniocentesis, the needle can be clearly identified in the separate sacs (Fig. 12-3).

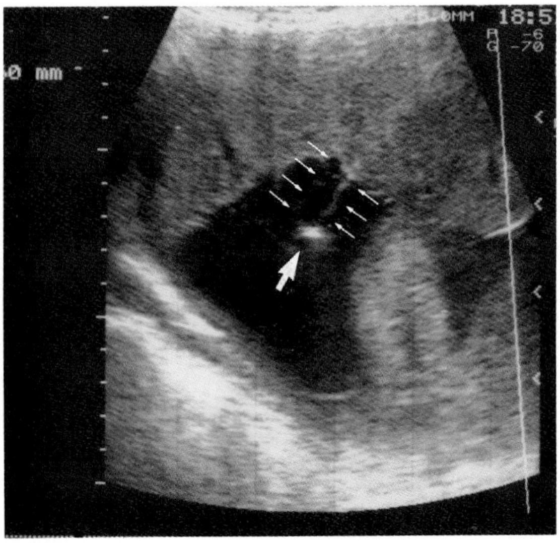

FIG. 12–3. In cordocentesis, the umbilical cord insertion in the placenta (*small arrows*) must be located. The needle tip (*bright spot*) is placed in the umbilical vein (*large arrow*).

PRENATAL DIAGNOSIS IN THE SECOND AND THIRD TRIMESTERS

MIDTRIMESTER AMNIOCENTESIS

Midtrimester amniocentesis is the oldest, most commonly performed procedure for prenatal diagnosis. It also is considered the gold standard to which other procedures for prenatal diagnosis are compared. Indications for genetic amniocentesis include increased risk for chromosome anomalies or for structural anomalies that may be associated with elevated AFP (Table 12-3). In addition, some metabolic genetic disorders may be diagnosed by measurement of precursor levels in cell-free fluid or by enzyme activity in cultured amniocytes.[51]

For cytogenetic studies, amniocytes are removed from amniotic fluid by centrifugation and cultured in flasks or on cover glasses to grow in monolayers. Dividing cells are arrested in metaphase, when chromosomes are maximally condensed, using agents such as colcimide that prevent spindle formation. The cells are then harvested, placed in hypotonic saline, which causes intracellular swelling and better spreading of the chromosomes during slide preparation, and, after fixation, the chromosomes are stained by Giemsa or quinacrine for microscopic analysis. The use of triple gas incubators, specific growth media (*e.g.*, Chang) that enhance cellular proliferation, and *in situ* culture on cover glass have shortened considerably the sampling–harvesting interval; in most laboratories, the results are available within 2 weeks. Additional improvement is obtained by computerized cytoanalyzers that expedite recognition of metaphase spreads and obviate the need for darkroom and photography.

TECHNICAL ASPECTS

Amniocentesis should be performed by an obstetrician trained and experienced in the procedure. Genetic counseling and a detailed ultrasound examina-

TABLE 12–3
INDICATIONS FOR GENETIC AMNIOCENTESIS

Increased risk of chromosome anomalies
Advanced maternal age
Previous offspring with chromosome anomalies
Parental balanced translocation or inversion
Ultrasound diagnosis of fetal anomalies
Abnormal maternal serum screening
Previous offspring with neural tube defect or ventral wall defect
Parents carriers of Mendelian disorders
Biochemical diagnosis:
Precursor levels in cell-free fluid (*e.g.*, 17-OH progesterone in congenital adrenal hyperplasia)
Enzymatic activity in amniocytes (*e.g.*, Tay–Sachs disease)
Molecular DNA diagnosis (*e.g.*, sickle-cell anemia)

tion to evaluate gestational age, placental location, and amount of amniotic fluid and to exclude fetal anomalies are prerequisites to amniocentesis. After sterile preparation of the skin, a draped sterile ultrasound transducer is used to locate a suitable pocket of fluid. Then, under continuous ultrasound guidance, a 20- to 22-gauge, 3.5-inch-long spinal needle is inserted in a single smooth motion into the pocket of fluid. When the needle, which is visualized on ultrasound as a bright spot, is placed satisfactorily into the pocket of amniotic fluid, the stylet is removed, and a 5-mL syringe is used to aspirate the first 2 to 3 mL of fluid, which is then discarded. This is done to minimize the risk of contamination from maternal cells collected in the path of the needle. Twenty to 30 mL of amniotic fluid is then gently aspirated, transferred into sterile tubes, and transported at room temperature to the laboratory for processing.[52,53]

In Rh-negative patients, the risk of Rh isoimmunization probably is increased by transplacental passage of the needle.[53] The risk of Rh isosensitization after amniocentesis in Rh-negative women with Rh-positive fetuses has been estimated to increase by 1% above the background risk of Rh isoimmunization during pregnancy for these patients.[54] Thus, the patient's blood type and antibody status should be known before amniocentesis, and unsensitized Rh-negative women should receive Rh immunoprophylaxis after the procedure.

SAFETY AND COMPLICATIONS

Amniocentesis is a relatively safe procedure when performed by trained personnel. The procedure-related pregnancy loss rate in experienced hands is 0.2% to 0.5% over and above the spontaneous loss rate at 16 weeks of gestation, which is estimated at 2% to 3%.[51] Pregnancy loss rates seem to be associated with the number of failed needle insertions at the same session and with vaginal bleeding after amniocentesis. Gestational age at the time of amniocentesis, volume of fluid removed, and repeat amniocentesis at a different session after a failed attempt do not seem to correlate with increased risk of pregnancy loss.[55] Leakage of amniotic fluid through the cervix is a relatively frequent complication affecting approximately 1% to 2% of patients after amniocentesis, but it usually is of minor long-term consequence. In most cases, it resolves with bed rest for 48 to 72 hours.[56] On the other hand, prolonged amniotic fluid leakage, although rare, may lead to severe oligohydramnios, which can result in fetal pressure deformities (*i.e.*, arthrogryposis) and to pulmonary hypoplasia.[57] Even patients with complete absence of fluid after amniocentesis, however, may reaccumulate amniotic fluid and go on to have normal outcomes.[58] Thus, as long as there is no evidence of infection, expectant management for at least several days seems prudent. The risk of severe amnionitis endangering maternal health appears to be very low, around 0.1%.[51] Likewise, fetal injury by the needle should be very rare with ultrasound-guided amniocentesis.

Cytogenetic analysis of amniotic fluid cells reflects fetal status accurately in over 99% of cases, but mosaicism sometimes may confuse the interpretation of results. In our experience, the frequency of results needing further investigation is similar in cultures from amniocentesis and from CVS.[35] Differentiation between cytogenetic abnormalities that truly reflect fetal chromosome aberrations from those that are the result of laboratory artifacts may be difficult. One or more hypermodal cells are identified in 2% to 3% of all amniocyte cultures and usually will be associated with a normal phenotype.[59] True fetal mosaicism should be considered when hypermodal cells are identified in different culture flasks or in separate colonies in the same culture flask. The frequency of hypermodal cells in one or more colonies from the same flask is 0.7%. Hypermodal cells with the same abnormality originating from multiple culture flasks are observed in 0.2% of amniotic cultures.[60,61] Even in the latter situation, however, the abnormality in culture may not represent true fetal mosaicism, as observed by Gosden and colleagues.[36] Fetal blood sampling for karyotype should help to avoid termination of pregnancy of some normal fetuses in these cases.

LATE CHORIONIC VILLUS SAMPLING

The techniques of transabdominal CVS to obtain fetal karyotype from analysis of chorionic villi in the first trimester also have been applied successfully in the second and third trimesters. Nicolaides and associates first reported six successful human placental biopsies at 14 to 37 weeks of gestation, and suggested that CVS should not be confined to the first trimester.[62] Chieri and Aldini performed transabdominal placental biopsy and amniocentesis in 220 patients at midtrimester; 210 of the procedures were indicated for advanced maternal age.[63] A villi sample adequate for analysis (>2 mg) was obtained in 90.9% of cases. The success rate was 94% with an anterior or fundal placenta, and 83.8% with a posterior placental location. In the latter situation, the approach to the placenta was transamniotic. Cytogenetic results were obtained in 95% of samples. No discrepancy could be found between cytogenetic results obtained in villi or in amniotic fluid, and when fetal anomalies were observed on CVS they were acted on without waiting for corroboration from the amniotic fluid culture.[63] It was apparent from that study that despite the decrease in mitotic index with placental aging, direct results could be obtained even with small amounts of placental tissue, as also observed by Saura and colleagues.[64] Moreover, the risk of maternal cell contamination in late CVS samples actually may be lower than that observed in the first trimester because of less direct contact between villi and decidua at later gestational age.[65] Thus, placental biopsies in the second and third trimesters are technically feasible procedures for prenatal diagnosis, with results apparently as accurate as those of amniocentesis. The major advantage of late CVS is the possibility of obtaining rapid results in situations where such information is needed for decisions about pregnancy termination or fetal therapy. Such situations would include the ultrasound diagnosis of fetal anomalies late in the second trimester, close to the legal limit in gestational age after which termination of pregnancy is no longer possible. In the third trimester, knowing the fetal karyotype in pregnancies complicated by severe IUGR or fetal anomalies on ultrasound may influence the mode of delivery; the management of intrapartum fetal distress, which is a common phenomenon in fetuses with chromosome anomalies; or the decision for surgical intervention within the first few hours after birth.

The collaborative results of 2058 late CVS procedures performed at 24 centers were reported by Holzgreve and colleagues.[10] A fetal karyotype was obtained in 96% of procedures. The frequency of abnormal chromosome results was 21% when fetal anomalies were observed on ultrasound, and 6.2% with normal ultrasound findings. The pregnancy loss rate, excluding terminations, was 10.3% in the group with abnormal ultrasound findings, and 2.3% in the normal ultrasound group. Holzgreve and associates further presented their own data on 301 CVS procedures in the second and third trimester, 225 (74.7%) of which were performed for abnormal ultrasound scans.[66] Karyotyping was successful in 99% of cases. The rate of chromosome anomalies was 20% in the group with abnormal ultrasound, and increased to 38% when the ultrasound findings included abnormalities of amniotic fluid volume. Thus, late CVS is apparently a safe and accurate procedure for rapid fetal karyotyping, and is especially suitable in situations in which oligohydramnios prevents an easy access to the cord for blood sampling.

CORDOCENTESIS

Freda and Adamson originally attempted to access the vascular system of the fetus for treatment of Rh isoimmunization by hysterotomy and fetal exposure.[67] This method soon was abandoned because of the unacceptably high risk for the mother and fetus. Subsequently, the development of fiberoptics allowed the introduction of fetoscopy to visualize and sample vessels on the chorionic plate or the umbilical cord.[68,69] Although the risk of maternal compromise with this method was relatively small, the high rate of pregnancy loss associated with fetoscopy (*i.e.*, up to 11.3%) was considered a major disadvantage.[70]

Introduced by Daffos and associates in 1983 for the diagnosis of fetal infections,[71] percutaneous ultrasound-guided umbilical blood sampling rapidly gained wide acceptance. In experienced hands, the risk of fetal loss is relatively small, about 1%.[72] Other complications, usually associated with excessive needle manipulations, include hematoma of the umbilical cord and placental abruption.[11] Maternal complications also are negligible, although one case of life-threatening amnionitis has been reported.[73] It appears that the risks are higher when the mother is obese, the placenta is posterior, and when the sampling is performed relatively early in gestation (*i.e.*, before 19 weeks).[72]

Parental counseling before cordocentesis should include the risk of that pregnancy being affected by the conditions considered and the yield of information of fetal blood sampling in such a situation. The risk and potential complications of the procedure itself also should be discussed. A detailed ultrasound examination should be performed before cordocentesis for evaluation of gestational age, placental location, and the diagnosis of fetal anomalies. Fetal blood can be obtained by puncture of the fetal heart, the intrahepatic part of the umbilical vein, or by puncture of an umbilical vessel close to its placental insertion, the latter being by far the most common site for cordocentesis. When the placenta is anterior or lateral, the needle is introduced transplacentally into the umbilical cord (see Fig. 12-3). In cases with a posterior placenta, the needle is introduced transamniotically and the cord is punctured close to its placental insertion. Different guidance techniques (*i.e.*, fixed needle guides *versus* freehand), needles of lengths varying from 8 to 15 cm and gauges varying from 20 to 27, and differing patient preparation protocols are used by various centers. Nicolaides and colleagues advocate an outpatient setting in the ultrasound department, without need for maternal fasting, sedation, tocolytics, antibiotics, or fetal paralysis for the procedure (Table 12-4).[74]

Molecular diagnoses now are available for many of the mutations resulting in thalassemia, sickle-cell disease, and hemophilia A and B, enabling diagnosis in the first trimester by CVS, with blood sampling performed only in noninformative cases or with ambiguous results. Cordocentesis is, however, necessary for the diagnosis and management of von Willebrand disease and of congenital alloimmune thrombocytopenia.[75] In alloimmune thrombocytopenia, cordocentesis allows the determination of fetal platelet phenotype and count. A low fetal platelet count in this situation can be treated by weekly infusion of platelets until delivery.[76,77]

In Rh isoimmunization, fetal blood sampling is performed for immediate confirmation of fetal antigenic status, obviating the need for further intervention in the Rh-negative fetus. If the fetus is Rh positive, cordocentesis enables a more accurate assessment of fetal anemia and an immediate rise in fetal erythrocyte count on correction by intravascular transfusion. From case-control studies, it appears that intravascular correction of fetal anemia is more efficient and less risky to the mother and fetus than the intraperitoneal approach at all gestational ages or levels of disease severity.[78,79] Moreover, in cases with cardiac decompensation in which the fetus may be compromised by

TABLE 12–4
INDICATIONS FOR CORDOCENTESIS

Prenatal diagnosis of inherited blood disorders
Hemoglobinopathies (*e.g.*, homozygous thalassemia, sickle-cell disease)
Coagulopathies (*e.g.*, hemophilia A and B, von Willebrand disease)
Prenatal diagnosis of metabolic disorders
Fetal infections
Toxoplasmosis—specific IgM or DNA hybridization
Rubella—specific IgM
Cytomegalovirus—specific IgM, blood cultures
Varicella zoster virus—specific IgM
Human parvovirus (B19)—viral DNA
Human immunodeficiency virus—specific IgM
Rapid fetal karyotyping
Late booking or failed amniocentesis
Suspected fetal mosaicism on amniocentesis
Abnormal maternal serum screening
Ultrasound diagnosis of fetal malformations
Evaluation of the small for gestational age fetus
Acid–base status
Oxygenation
Assessment and treatment of fetal anemia
Diagnosis and treatment of fetal thrombocytopenia

Adapted from Nicolaides KH, Sniders RJM. Cordocentesis. In: Evans MI, ed. Reproductive risks and prenatal diagnosis. Norwalk, CT: Appleton & Lange, 1992:201.

the volume overload needed to correct the severe anemia, better results were obtained by intravascular exchange transfusion.[80] It should be noted, however, that cordocentesis may enhance maternal sensitization more than does amniocentesis, especially if blood sampling is performed by a transplacental approach.[81] Rh immunoprophylaxis should be offered to all Rh-negative, nonsensitized patients with an Rh-positive fetus undergoing cordocentesis.

The diagnosis of fetal infection is based commonly on the demonstration of the agent-specific IgM in fetal blood, since the large molecule IgM does not cross the placenta. Fetal blood sampling should be scheduled to allow enough time from initial exposure for IgM to appear after immunocompetence develops in the fetus. For first-trimester exposures, the best time for cordocentesis is probably around 22 weeks gestation. In specific cases, *in utero* treatment also is available. Thus, after toxoplasmosis infection in the mother, and demonstration of IgM specific for toxoplasmosis in fetal blood, antibiotic treatment with spiramycin reduced significantly the risk of congenital toxoplasmosis as well as the risk of late sequelae.[82] Cordocentesis has been used for repeated blood transfusions *in utero* to hydropic fetuses with hemolytic anemia caused by parvovirus B19 infection.[83]

Cordocentesis also has been used for the evaluation of the small-for-dates fetus. Severe, early-onset, IUGR commonly is associated with fetal chromosome anomalies. Cordocentesis allows for rapid fetal karyotyping, which can be available within 48 to 72 hours. Other abnormalities observed in blood samples from IUGR fetuses with normal chromosomes include hypoxemia, hypercapnia, lactic acidemia, leukopenia, thrombocytopenia, and disturbed carbohydrate, lipid, and protein metabolism.[81] Several studies have compared the prediction of fetal acidosis by Doppler or biophysical profile with cord blood gases. Weiner demonstrated a statistically significant correlation between an increased umbilical systolic to diastolic ratio (>3.5) and fetal hypoxia and acidemia in cord blood.[84] This relationship was even more significant with absent or reversed diastolic flow. In another study, the biophysical profile significantly correlated with changes in cord *p*H, including, to some extent, the degree of fetal acidemia.[85] In the situation of severe IUGR with equivocal biophysical score and umbilical blood flow studies, however, the availability of fetal PO_2 and *p*H may provide additional and crucial information in the balance between the risk of premature delivery and the risk of leaving the fetus to grow in a hostile intrauterine environment.

REFERENCES

1. Steel MW, Breg WR. Chromosome analysis of human amniotic fluid cells. Lancet 1966;1:383.
2. Jacobson JB, Barter RH. Intrauterine diagnosis and management of genetic defects. Am J Obstet Gynecol 1967;99:795.
3. Nadler HL. Antenatal detection of hereditary disorders. Pediatrics 1968;42:912.
4. Medical Research Council. Diagnosis of genetic disease by amniocentesis during second trimester of pregnancy. Ottawa, Ontario: Medical Research Council, 1977.
5. National Institute of Child Health and Human Development Amniocentesis Registry, 1978. The safety and accuracy of midtrimester amniocentesis. DHEW Publication No. (NIH) 78–190. Washington, DC: United States Department of Health, Education and Welfare, 1978.
6. Canadian Collaborative CVS–Amniocentesis Clinical Trial Group. Multicenter randomized clinical trial of chorionic villus sampling and amniocentesis. Lancet 1989;1:1.
7. Rhoads GG, Jackson LG, Schlesselman SE, et al. The safety and efficacy of chorionic villus sampling for early prenatal diagnosis of cytogenetic abnormalities. N Engl J Med 1989; 320:609.
8. Hanson FW, Happ RL, Tennant FR, et al. Ultrasonography-guided early amniocentesis in singleton pregnancies. Am J Obstet Gynecol 1990;162:1376.
9. Evans MI, Drugan A, Koppitch FC, et al. Genetic diagnosis in the first trimester: the norm for the 90's. Am J Obstet Gynecol 1989;160:1332.
10. Holzgreve W, Miny P, Schloo R, et al. "Late CVS" international registry: compilation of data from 24 centers. Prenat Diagn 1990;10:159.
11. Hoskins IA. Cordocentesis in isoimmunization and fetal physiologic measurement, infection and karyotyping. Curr Opin Obstet Gynecol 1991;3:266.
12. Kazy Z, Rozovsky IS, Balchaten VA. Chorion biopsy in early pregnancy: a method of early prenatal diagnosis for inherited disorders. Prenat Diagn 1982;2:39.

13. Simoni G, Brambati B, Danesino C, et al. Efficient direct chromosome analyses and enzyme determinations from chorionic villi samples in the first trimester of pregnancy. Hum Genet 1983;63:349.
14. Brambati B, Simoni G. Letter to the editor. Lancet 1989;1:583.
15. Ledbetter DH, Martin AO, Verlinsky Y, et al. Cytogenetic results of chorionic villus sampling: high success rate and diagnostic accuracy in the United States Collaborative Study. Am J Obstet Gynecol 1990;162:495.
16. Copeland KL, Carpenter RJ, Penolio KR, et al. Integration of the transabdominal technique into an ongoing chorionic villus sampling program. Am J Obstet Gynecol 1989;161:1289.
17. Jahoda MGJ, Pijpers I, Reuss A, et al. Transabdominal villus sampling in early second trimester: a safe sampling method for women of advanced age. Prenat Diagn 1990;10:307.
18. Evans MI, Moore C, Kolodny F, et al. Lysosomal enzymes in chorionic villi, cultured amniocytes, and cultured skin fibroblasts. Clin Chim Acta 1986;157:109.
19. Simpson JL. Chorionic villus sampling. Semin Perinatol 1990; 14:446.
20. Brambati B, Oldrini A, Lanzani A. Transabdominal villus sampling: a free hand ultrasound guided technique. Am J Obstet Gynecol 1987;157:134.
21. Smidt-Jensen S, Hahnemann N. Transabdominal fine needle biopsy from chorionic villi in the first trimester. Prenat Diagn 1984;4:163.
22. Evans MI, Quigg MH, Koppitch FC, et al. First trimester prenatal diagnosis. In: Evans MI, Fletcher JC, Dixler AO, et al, eds. Fetal diagnosis and therapy: science, ethics and the law. Philadelphia: JB Lippincott, 1989:17.
23. Brambati B, Lanzani A, Tului L. Transabdominal and transcervical chorionic villus sampling: efficiency and risk evaluation of 2411 cases. Am J Med Genet 1990;35:160.
24. Ghirardini G, Popp WL, Camurri L, et al. Vaginosonographic guided chorionic villi needle biopsy. Eur J Obstet Gynecol Reprod Biol 1986;23:315.
25. Sidransky E, Black SH, Soenksen DM, et al. Transvaginal chorionic villus sampling. Prenat Diagn 1990;10:583.
26. Simpson JL. Incidence and timing of pregnancy losses: relevance to evaluating safety of early prenatal diagnosis. Am J Med Genet 1990;35:165.
27. Firth HV, Boyd PA, Chamberlain P, et al. Severe limb abnormalities after chorionic villus sampling at 56-66 days' gestation. Lancet 1991;337:762.
28. Burton BK, Schulz CJ, Burd LI. Limb anomalies associated with chorionic villus sampling. Obstet Gynecol 1992;79:726.
29. Schloo R, Miny P, Holzgreve W, Horst J, Lenz W. Distal limb deficiency following chorionic villus sampling? Am J Med Genet 1992;42:404.
30. Blakemore KJ, Baumgarten A, Schonfeld Dimaio M, et al. Rise in maternal serum alpha-fetoprotein concentration after chorionic villus sampling and the possibility of isoimmunization. Am J Obstet Gynecol 1986;155:986.
31. Shulman LP, Meyers CM, Simpson JL, et al. Fetomaternal transfusion depends on amount of chorionic villi aspirated but not on method of chorionic villus sampling. Am J Obstet Gynecol 1990;162:1185.
32. McGowan KD, Blackemore KJ. Amniocentesis and chorionic villus sampling. Curr Opin Obstet Gynecol 1991;3:221.
33. Johnson A, Wapner RJ, Davis GH, et al. Mosaicism in chorionic villus sampling: an association with poor perinatal outcome. Obstet Gynecol 1990;75:573.
34. Kalousek DK, Dill FJ. Chromosomal mosaicism confined to the placenta in human conceptions. Science 1983;221:665.
35. Wright DJ, Brindley BA, Koppitch FC, et al. Interpretation of chorionic villus sampling laboratory results is just as reliable as amniocentesis. Obstet Gynecol 1989;74:739.
36. Gosden C, Rodeck CH, Nicolaides KH. Fetal blood sampling in the investigation of chromosome mosaicism in amniotic fluid cell culture. Lancet 1988;1:613.
37. Penso CA, Frigoletto FD. Early amniocentesis. Semin Perinatol 1990;14:465.
38. Hanson FW, Zorn EM, Tennant FR, et al. Amniocentesis before 15 weeks gestation: outcome, risks and technical problems. Am J Obstet Gynecol 1987;156:1524.
39. Stripparo I, Buscaglia M, Longatii L, et al. Genetic amniocentesis: 505 cases performed before the sixteenth week of gestation. Prenat Diagn 1990;10:359.
40. Nevin J, Nevin NC, Dornan JC, et al. Early amniocentesis; experience of 222 consecutive patients from 1987–1988. Prenat Diagn 1990;10:79.
41. Dunn LK, Godmilow L. A comparison of loss rates for first trimester chorionic villus sampling, early amniocentesis and midtrimester amniocentesis in a population of women of advanced maternal age [abstract]. Am J Hum Genet 1990;47(Suppl):A273.
42. Elejalde BR, de Elejalde MM, Acuna JM, et al. Prospective study of amniocentesis performed between weeks 9 and 16 of gestation: its feasibility, risks, complications and use in early genetic amniocentesis. Am J Med Genet 1990;35:188.
43. Rooney DE, MacLachlan N, Smith J, et al. Early amniocentesis: a cytogenetic evaluation. Br Med J 1989;299:25.
44. Drugan A, Syner FN, Greb A, et al. Amniotic fluid alphafetoprotein and acetylcholinesterase in early genetic amniocentesis. Obstet Gynecol 1988;72:33.
45. Crandall BF, Hanson FW, Tennant F, et al. Alpha-fetoprotein levels in amniotic fluid between 11 and 15 weeks. Am J Obstet Gynecol 1989;160:1204.
46. Drugan A, Syner FN, Belsky RL, et al. Amniotic fluid acetylcholinesterase: implications of an inconclusive result. Am J Obstet Gynecol 1988;159:469.
47. Burton BK, Nelson LH, Pettenati MJ. False positive acetylcholinesterase with early amniocentesis. Obstet Gynecol 1989;74:607.
48. Robinson GE, Garner DM, Olmsted MP, et al. Anxiety reduction after chorionic villus sampling and genetic amniocentesis. Am J Obstet Gynecol 1988;159:953.
49. Gosden CM. First trimester fetal karyotyping: CVS or early amniocentesis (editorial)? Ultrasound in Obstetrics and Gynecology 1991;1:233.
50. Byrne D, Marks K, Azar G, et al. Randomized study of early amniocentesis versus chorionic villus sampling: a technical and cytogenetic comparison of 650 patients. Ultrasound in Obstetrics and Gynecology 1991;1:235–40.
51. Drugan A, Johnson MP, Evans MI. Amniocentesis. In: Evans MI, ed. Reproductive risks and prenatal diagnosis. Norwalk, CT: Appleton & Lange, 1992:191.
52. Hanson FW, Tennant FR, Zorn EM, et al. Analysis of 2136 genetic amniocenteses: experience of a single physician. Am J Obstet Gynecol 1985;152:435.
53. Golbus MS, Stephens JD, Cann HM, et al. Rh isoimmunization following genetic amniocentesis. Prenat Diagn 1982;2:149.
54. Murray JC, Karp LE, Williamson RA, et al. Rh isoimmunization as related to amniocentesis. Am J Hum Genet 1983;16:527.
55. NICHD National Registry for Amniocentesis Study Group. Midtrimester amniocentesis for prenatal diagnosis: safety and accuracy. JAMA 1976;236:1471.
56. Crane JP, Rohland BM. Clinical significance of amniotic fluid leakage after genetic amniocentesis. Prenat Diagn 1986;6:25.
57. Nimrod C, Varela-Gittings F, Machin G, et al. The effect of

very prolonged membrane rupture on fetal development. Am J Obstet Gynecol 1984;148:540.
58. Gold R, Goyert G, Schwartz DB, et al. Conservative management of midtrimester post amniocentesis fluid leakage. Obstet Gynecol 1989;74:745.
59. Simpson JL. Amniocentesis: what it can tell you and what it can't. Contemporary Obstetrics and Gynecology 1988;31:33.
60. Hsu LYF, Kaffe S, Perlis ET. Trisomy 20 mosaicism in prenatal diagnosis: a review and update. Prenat Diagn 1987;7:581.
61. Worton RG, Stern RA. A Canadian collaborative study on mosaicism in amniotic fluid cell cultures. Prenat Diagn 1984;4:131.
62. Nicolaides KH, Soothill PH, Rodeck CH, et al. Prenatal diagnosis: why confine chorionic villus (placental) biopsy to the first trimester? Lancet 1986;1:543.
63. Chieri PR, Aldini AJR. Feasibility of placental biopsy in the second trimester for fetal diagnosis. Am J Obstet Gynecol 1989;160:581.
64. Saura R, Longy M, Horowitz J, et al. Direct chromosome analysis in the second and third trimesters by placental biopsy in 30 pregnancies. Br J Obstet Gynecol 1989;96:1215.
65. Ganshirt-Ahlert D, Pohlschmidt M, Gal A, et al. Transabdominal placental biopsy in the second and third trimester of pregnancy: what is the risk of maternal contamination in DNA diagnosis? Obstet Gynecol 1990;75:320.
66. Holzgreve W, Miny P, Gerlach B, et al. Benefits of placental biopsies for rapid karyotyping in the second and third trimesters (late chorionic villus sampling) in high risk pregnancies. Am J Obstet Gynecol 1990;162:1188.
67. Freda VJ, Adamson KJ. Exchange transfusion in utero. Am J Obstet Gynecol 1964;89:817.
68. Hobbins JC, Mahoney MJ. In utero diagnosis of hemoglobinopathies: technique for obtaining fetal blood. N Engl J Med 1974;290:1065.
69. Rodeck CH, Cambell S. Umbilical cord insertion as source of pure fetal blood for prenatal diagnosis. Lancet 1979;1:1244.
70. Ward RHT, Modell B, Fairweather DVI. Obstetric outcome and problems of midtrimester fetal blood sampling for antenatal diagnosis. Br J Obstet Gynaecol 1981;88:1073.
71. Daffos F, Cappella-Pavlovsky M, Forestier F. Fetal blood sampling via the umbilical cord using a needle guided by ultrasound: report of 66 cases. Prenat Diagn 1983;3:271.
72. Nicolaides KH, Sniders RJM. Cordocentesis. In: Evans MI, ed. Reproductive risks and prenatal diagnosis. Norwalk, CT: Appleton & Lange, 1992:201.
73. Wilkins I, Mezrow G, Lynch L, et al. Amnionitis and life threatening respiratory distress after percutaneous umbilical blood sampling. Am J Obstet Gynecol 1989;160:427.
74. Nicolaides KH, Soothill PW, Rodeck CH, et al. Ultrasound guided sampling of umbilical cord and placental blood to access fetal well being. Lancet 1986;1:1065.
75. Bussel JB, Berkowitz RL, McFarland JG, et al. Antenatal treatment of neonatal thrombocytopenia. N Engl J Med 1988;319:1374.
76. Nicolini U, Rodeck CH, Kochenour NK, et al. In utero platelet transfusion for allo-immune thrombocytopenia. Lancet 1988;2:506.
77. Murphy MF, Pullon HWH, Metcalfe P, et al. Management of fetal allo-immune thrombocytopenia by weekly in utero platelet transfusions. Vox Sang 1990;58:45.
78. Keckstein G, Stoz F, Tschurtz S, et al. Intrauterine treatment of severe fetal erythroblastosis: intrauterine transfusion with ultrasonic guidance. J Perinat Med 1989;17:341.
79. Harman CR, Bowman JM, Manning FA, et al. Intrauterine transfusion: intraperitoneal versus intravascular approach: a case control comparison. Am J Obstet Gynecol 1990;162:1053.
80. Poissonier MH, Brossard Y, Demedeiros N, et al. Two hundred intrauterine exchange transfusions in severe blood incompatibilities. Am J Obstet Gynecol 1989;161:709.
81. Weiner CP, Grant S, Hudson J, et al. Effect of diagnostic and therapeutic cordocentesis on maternal serum alpha-fetoprotein concentration. Am J Obstet Gynecol 1989;161:706.
82. Daffos F, Forestier F, Capella-Pavlovsky M, et al. Prenatal management of 746 pregnancies at risk for congenital toxoplasmosis. N Engl J Med 1988;318:271.
83. Peters MT, Nicolaides KH. Cordocentesis for the diagnosis and treatment of human fetal parvovirus infection. Obstet Gynecol 1990;75:501.
84. Weiner CP. The relationship between the umbilical artery systolic/diastolic ratio and umbilical blood gas measurements in specimens obtained by cordocentesis. Am J Obstet Gynecol 1990;162:1198.
85. Ribbert LSM, Sniders RJM, Nicolaides KH, et al. Relationship of fetal biophysical profile and blood gas values at cordocentesis in severely growth retarded fetuses. Am J Obstet Gynecol 1990;163:569.

Neonatology: Pathophysiology and Management of the Newborn, Fourth Edition,
edited by Gordon B. Avery, Mary Ann Fletcher, and Mhairi G. MacDonald.
J.B. Lippincott Company, Philadelphia © 1994.

chapter 13

Ultrasonography

FRANK A. MANNING

High-resolution, dynamic ultrasonographic systems permit detailed examination of the fetus' structures, activities, and environment. Because it provides cross-sectional visualization of internal fetal anatomy, ultrasonography may, in some respects, provide more information on the fetus than can be gained by physical examination of the newborn. The data base from ultrasonography on normal and abnormal fetal characteristics is growing exponentially.

Because most of the improvement in perinatal survival is due to advances in neonatal care, the relative contribution of fetal deaths to overall perinatal mortality is increasing. From 80% to 90% of all fetal deaths occur among structurally normal fetuses. Approximately 75% of these deaths are due to fetal asphyxia of a subacute or chronic nature often associated with impaired growth, and the remaining 25% are due to either acute asphyxia or acquired fetal disease. When fetal assessment based on dynamic ultrasonography is used in large populations, congenital anomalies account for more than 60% of fetal deaths, compared with an expected rate of 10% to 15% in an untested population.[1] Detailed assessment by ultrasonography improves recognition of the fetus at risk for intrauterine compromise and can guide management such that the majority of these patients are delivered before an insult becomes lethal.

ASSESSMENT OF FETAL AGE, GROWTH, AND MATURITY

Virtually all perinatal management decisions hinge on an accurate assessment of fetal age. As neonatal survival statistics continue to improve at progressively earlier gestational ages and weights, the clinical significance of accurate gestational dating becomes even greater. The extremes of error in this age determination are a recognized cause of preventable perinatal mortality and morbidity. Overestimation of fetal age can result in iatrogenic prematurity, whereas underestimation of age, as with a growth-retarded fetus, can result in an otherwise preventable fetal death.

Determination of fetal age based on obstetric historical or clinical data can be accurate, but, in at least 40% of patients, the estimation of gestational age is difficult.[2] The introduction of ultrasound-derived fetal morphometric data to the gestational age equation can greatly enhance the accuracy of determination. The fetal morphometric variables used to assess age are selected primarily because of the ease and reproducibility of the unique and precise relationship with age. For example, fetal biparietal diameter (BPD) measurement is a common ultrasonographic marker of age because this measurement was one of the only fetal indices that could be measured with primitive ultrasonographic instruments (*e.g.*, A-scan).[3] A unique relationship between BPD and fetal age has not been established, however, and indeed the measure is not used postnatally to assess age. With more sophisticated ultrasonographic equipment, more fetal indices are included in age estimates (*e.g.*, fetal femur length, abdominal circumference). Because fetal growth involves all organ systems, it is likely that measurements of any given fetal variable will bear some relationship to gestational age. Major areas of active investigation are the selection of new indices of age and the study of the association among recognized variables for age determination. Neonatologists have known for some time that neonatal age is best determined by consideration of morphometric, functional, and behavioral characteristics (*i.e.*, Dubowitz score).[4] Functional studies of the fetus to determine gestational age (*e.g.*, fetal breathing patterns) are at the investigational stage, and fetal behavioral studies to determine gestational age are nonexistent. Estimation of age is improved with consideration of an array of fetal morphometric indices, particularly when these are determined serially over an expanded time scale.[5]

SPECIFIC METHODS OF DETERMINING FETAL AGE

TRANSVAGINAL SCANNING: AN ADJUNCT TO FIRST-TRIMESTER ASSESSMENT

In the first trimester, fetal imaging using a transabdominal approach often is difficult because the uterus and its contents are in the maternal pelvis and, as a result, the ultrasound image obtained is subject to shadowing produced by the bony pelvis and the maternal bowel. The development of transvaginal ultrasound transducers has greatly enhanced visualization of the fetus in the first trimester. This method is based on introduction of a modified probe into the maternal vagina in close proximity to the uterus and fetus. By this method it is possible to obtain high-quality fetal images permitting accurate fetal morphometric and morphologic assessment from as early as 6 weeks of gestation.

CROWN–RUMP MEASUREMENT

The relationship between crown–rump length and gestational age of fetuses aborted before 12 weeks of gestation is very precise.[6] Similar measurements may be obtained accurately *in utero* with conventional ultrasonographic instruments. Crown–rump length is the most accurate determinant of gestational age, yielding an average error of ± 3 days.[7] Crown–rump length can be converted to gestational age using standard nomogram tables or, in clinical practice, by adding 6.5 to the measured length and expressing the sum in weeks. This crown–rump length determination is difficult after 12 weeks of gestation, thus limiting its usefulness.

FETAL BIPARIETAL DIAMETER

The fetal BPD is a purely obstetric measurement referring to the transverse diameter of an oval plane that passes through the upper midbrain at the level of the thalamic nuclei and the septum cavum pellucidum. Within this oval plane are observed the lateral walls of the midportion of the lateral ventricles, the anterior and posterior continuation of the falx cerebri, and usually a portion of the middle cerebral artery within the cerebral cortex (Fig. 13-1). By convention, the diameter is measured from the external surface of the proximal parietal bone (near table) to the inner surface of the distal parietal bone (far table). It is critical to measure the bony confines of diameter and not the soft tissue, because the latter may vary with the extent of fetal scalp soft tissue and hair and with the type of ultrasonographic instrument used.

Fetal BPD bears a direct but less than precise relationship with age (Table 13-1). A fetal BPD can be measured from as early as 12 weeks of gestation. In general, the earlier the gestational age at which the measurement occurs, the greater the predictive accuracy of the measurement. Predictive error with the BPD generally derives from two sources. First, there may be inherent errors in the actual measurement because of improper selection of the measurement plane, which in turn is due either to angulation of the ultrasonic beam or to calibration errors within or between ultrasound instruments.[8] The second major source of predictive error is failure to consider normal distribution patterns within a population. Variations in BPD are normal phenomena and the limits of normal distribution increase with advancing gestational age. Thus, a single BPD measured before 16 weeks of

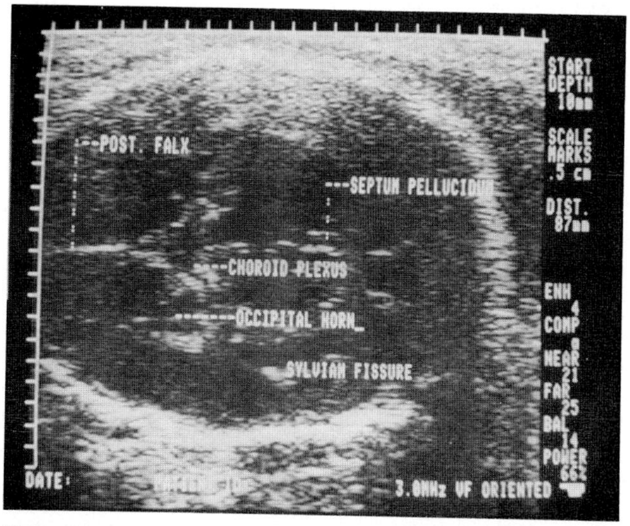

FIG. 13–1. Fetal biparietal diameter (BPD) can be determined with a linear array dynamic ultrasonic method (ADR Model 4000, ADR Ultrasound, Tempe, AZ). The BPD measurement of this fetus is 87 mm.

TABLE 13–1
RELATION BETWEEN SELECTED FETAL INDICES AS MEASURED BY ULTRASOUND AND GESTATIONAL AGE AS DETERMINED BY MENSTRUAL WEEKS

Menstrual Age (wk)	Biparietal Diameter (cm)	Head Circumference (cm)	Abdominal Circumference (cm)	Femur Length (cm)
12	2	7.1	5.6	0.8
13	2.3	8.4	6.9	1.1
14	2.7	9.8	8.1	1.5
15	3	11.1	9.3	1.8
16	3.3	12.4	10.5	2.1
17	3.7	13.7	11.7	2.4
18	4	15	12.9	2.7
19	4.3	16.3	14.1	3
20	4.6	17.5	15.2	3.3
21	5	18.7	16.4	3.6
22	5.3	19.9	17.5	3.9
23	5.6	21	18.6	4.2
24	5.8	22.1	19.7	4.4
25	6.1	23.2	20.8	4.7
26	6.4	24.2	21.9	4.9
27	6.7	25.2	22.9	5.2
28	7	26.2	24	5.4
29	7.2	27.1	25	5.6
30	7.5	28	26	5.8
31	7.7	28.9	27	6.1
32	7.9	29.7	28	6.3
33	8.2	30.4	29	6.5
34	8.4	31.2	30	6.6
35	8.6	31.8	30.9	6.8
36	8.8	32.5	31.8	7
37	9	33.1	32.7	7.2
38	9.1	33.6	33.6	7.3
39	9.3	34.1	34.5	7.5
40	9.5	34.5	35.4	7.6

From Hadlock FP, et al. Computer assisted analysis of fetal age using multiple fetal growth parameters. J Clin Ultrasound 1983;11:313.

gestation may carry a predictive accuracy of ± 7 days, whereas the same measurement done at 40 weeks of gestation has a predictive accuracy of ± 21 days.[9] Consideration of biologic variation in the relationship between BPD and gestational age cannot be overemphasized because it is possible to create iatrogenic fetal or neonatal morbidity when obstetric decisions are based on mean values rather than on the range of normal values.

Serial estimation of BPD improves the predictive accuracy of the technique.[10] Assignment of growth percentiles to BPD measurements (*i.e.*, the growth-adjusted sonographic age method) is an alternative means of improving the predictive accuracy of fetal age estimates by BPD.[11]

FEMUR LENGTH DETERMINATION

Femur length, as measured by ultrasonography, is an alternative means of pregnancy dating (see Table 13-1).[12] Femur length, defined as the greatest distance between the greater trochanter and the distal end of the femur, may be determined from as early as 12 to 14 weeks of gestation (Fig. 13-2). As with BPD measurement, gestational age prediction from femur length is subject to error arising from measurement difficulties and biologic variation. Often, it may be difficult to define the lower end of the femur, especially when calcification of a distal femoral epiphysis occurs (see Fig. 13-2). Unlike BPD, however, femur length nearly always can be measured. The predictive accuracy of femur length for gestational age ranges from an average of ± 1 week at 12 to 16 weeks of gestation to an error as great as ± 3 weeks at 36 weeks of gestation and beyond.[5] The relationship of femur length to crown–heel length of the fetus appears to be relatively precise, yielding in late gestation an average error of prediction of ± 1.5 cm.[13] This latter observation may become important in calculation of a fetal ponderal index.

FETAL WEIGHT ESTIMATES

An accurate and reproducible method of determining fetal weight would have major clinical advantages in assessment of fetal age, growth, and maturity and in

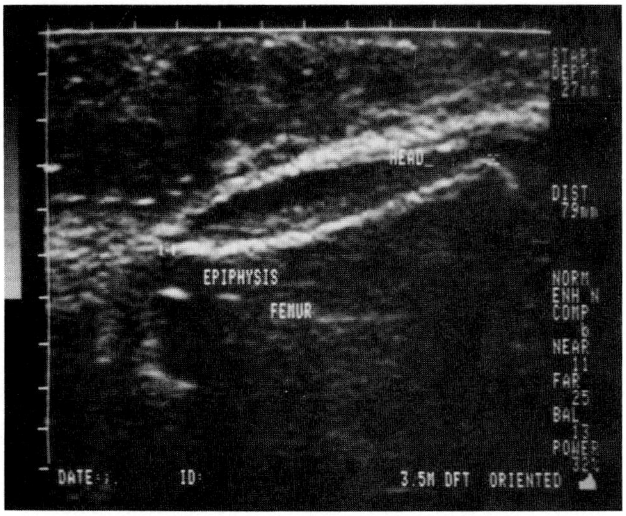

FIG. 13–2. A longitudinal scan of the fetal thigh demonstrates femur length of 79 mm, which is consistent with a gestational age of 32 weeks. Note the well-formed, calcified, proximal tibial epiphysis. Femur length is measured from the greater trochanter to the distal end of the developing femur.

determination of the risks of neonatal morbidity and mortality. Ultrasonographic estimates of fetal weight may be derived from a single measurement such as thoracic diameter, BPD, or abdominal circumference,[14,15] or by a combination of measurements such as abdominal circumference and BPD.[16]

The concept of estimation of fetal age based on a composite assessment of multiple fetal morphometric variables has become standard practice in modern perinatal medicine, and the reliance on a single variable to determine fetal age is no longer an accepted practice. Given the number of fetal morphometric variables that can be measured, there are many algorithms available. Most centers now rely on a combination of head size (*i.e.*, either BPD or head circumference), femur length, and abdominal circumference. This combination yields an estimate error (2 SD) that varies directly with true age and ranges from as little as ±1.46 weeks between 24 and 30 weeks of gestation to as great as 2.34 weeks at 36 weeks of gestation and beyond.[17]

All ultrasonographic methods for weight estimation assume a constant relationship between the variable measured and fetal volume over a wide age and weight range, and also assume fetal density constant and equal to that of water (*i.e.*, 1 g/mL). The validity of either assumption may be seriously challenged. Both of these basic assumptions have been examined using serial estimates of volume in living and dead perinates.[18] In a human neonate, the mean newborn density as measured by a water displacement method is 0.919 g/mL, but in my studies ranged from 0.833 g/mL to 1.1 g/mL.[18] Density varied within the neonate: 0.571 g/mL for the head and 1.118 g/mL for the remainder of the body.[18] Furthermore, on average, the mass of the head represented 19% of the total mass of the perinate, whereas the trunk and extremities accounted for 81% of neonatal mass. It follows that in fetuses with growth disorders such as macrosomia or intrauterine growth retardation (IUGR), in which the relationship of head mass to body mass is known to vary, significant inaccuracy in estimation of fetal volume and weight may be expected. Most reported methods of fetal weight estimation by ultrasonographic morphometry report average head estimates within a normal population and do not account for these density and volume considerations.

All ultrasonographic methods for fetal weight estimations contain inherent error. The most accurate but least practical method requires detailed fetal scanning for estimation of fetal volume; in a human neonate, with direct measurement, this method yields an error of ± 8.2% of actual body weight.[18] In general, less tedious methods yielding larger errors of estimation are used in clinical practice. Measurement of abdominal circumferences at a transverse plane passing through the midportion of the fetal liver (Fig. 13-3) yields an average error of weight estimate of 18.2% over a wide range of birth weights.[15] Alternatively, BPD and abdominal girth may be used in combination to estimate weight, yielding a similar error (20%).[19] The absolute estimated error decreases as birth weight decreases.

Because fetal weight estimates remain relatively imprecise, estimation of fetal age based on estimates of weight is not a useful clinical method. Determina-

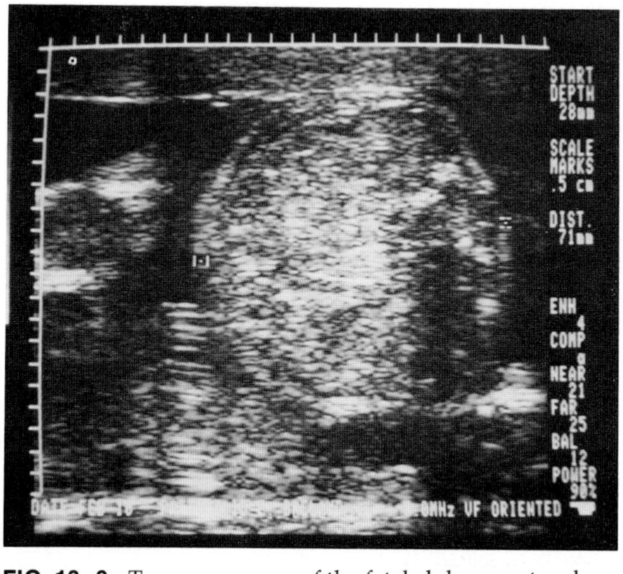

FIG. 13–3. Transverse scan of the fetal abdomen at a plane passing through the midportion of the fetal liver just above the insertion of the umbilical vein. Note the echodense fetal spine at approximately 1 o'clock and the heavy acoustic shadow. Fetal liver tissue demonstrates the characteristic granular echodense pattern, and a slight rim of normal peritoneal fluid is visible. Abdominal diameter in two perpendicular planes is 71 mm; abdominal circumference is 22.3 cm (πd). Estimated fetal weight is 1100 ± 165 g.

tion of incremental fetal weight change with serial ultrasonographic methods, however, is an effective tool in detecting abnormalities of fetal growth.[5] Within the accepted range of error of estimation, fetal weight determination also is useful in determining the probability of perinatal survival.

ASSESSMENT OF FETAL GROWTH

Abnormalities of fetal growth commonly are associated with increased risks of perinatal death or damage, with the risk being greatest at the extremes of the newborn weight distribution curve. Recognition of fetuses whose weight has exceeded the limits of normal distribution or in whom growth rates are such that the limits will be exceeded with time is a key preventive step in improving perinatal outcome. The rate of growth in the normal fetus is not constant, but varies with gestational age, being best described by an increasing exponential curve in the first trimester, a linear curve in the second and most of the third trimester, and a decreasing exponential curve after 36 weeks of gestation.[20] Studies suggest that fetal growth remains linear from 12 weeks until 42 weeks of gestation.[21] Serial ultrasonographic estimates of single or combined morphometric indices may be used to plot fetal growth. These measures include fetal BPD, femur length, and abdominal circumference and may include weight estimates derived from a combination of these variables.

ABNORMALITIES OF FETAL GROWTH

Intrauterine Growth Retardation. Intrauterine growth retardation, when used synonymously with small-for-gestational-age (SGA), is defined as a birth weight equal to or less than the 10th percentile for gestational age and gender. There is an important distinction between stricter definitions of IUGR and SGA—a fetus may have a relative degree of IUGR but still be above the 10th percentile for his gestational age, so not truly SGA. All birth weight distribution curves are derived from data in liveborn infants. Because stillbirths are not included in the calculation of these curves, birth weight percentile curves may not truly reflect fetal weight distribution curves. The population of SGA perinates whose weight at a given gestational age falls below the 10th percentile is heterogeneous, with normal small fetuses representing approximately 60% of the group, fetuses with associated congenital anomalies accounting for approximately 15% of the population, and fetuses with true growth impairment (*i.e.*, dysmaturity, IUGR) composing the remaining 25% of the population. Recognition of these subgroups of IUGR perinates is of critical clinical importance because perinatal management strategies vary radically. Thus, the normal small perinate is not at increased risk and therefore does not require intervention, whereas the perinate with true growth impairment may be at extreme risk and require urgent intervention. The problem is compounded when gestational age of the fetus is in doubt. Differentiation of these subgroups with ultrasonography remains imprecise and is an area of active investigation.

Several ultrasonographic methods for detecting the IUGR fetus have been described, but, for the most part, are useful only in detecting the more severe disease states. A slowing of the rate of head growth, as measured by BPD, may be inherent with severe IUGR,[22,23] as may slowing of femur growth.[24] Unfortunately, neither of these measurements is sensitive enough for detection of earlier disease. Growth-adjusted sonographic age determination based on either BPD or abdominal circumference has been proposed.[8,25] This method, based on serial ultrasonographic observations, assumes that fetal growth remains within a narrow percentile band and that deviation from this individual growth band may be an early sign of growth disorders.[26] Serial estimation of abdominal circumference or fetal weight or both is an alternative method for identifying IUGR. Unfortunately, in view of the inherent error with weight estimation and the normal distribution of data points within a given population, the method is useful only at the extreme deviation or only after frequent observations over a prolonged time (*i.e.*, several weeks). Comparison of morphometric variables for a given fetus to detect asymmetry of growth may be useful in establishing the diagnosis of severe dysmature IUGR. Altered head–abdomen ratios, resulting from loss of liver mass with normal or near-normal head growth is a frequent finding in severe IUGR, but again lacks the specificity needed to detect less severe disease states.[27,28] Consideration of fetal proportion—that is, total length as reflected by femur length, and total mass as reflected by head and abdominal circumferences—may prove valuable in the detection of IUGR. The concept of a fetal ponderal index requires extensive clinical testing.[29]

Detection of functional sequelae of dysmature IUGR represents an alternative and ancillary means of assessing the presence and severity of disease. Oligohydramnios is a clinical hallmark of prolonged or repetitive episodes of uteroplacental insufficiency and most likely results from diminished production of fetal urine and pulmonary fluid during episodes of fetal hypoxemia.[30] Amniotic fluid is recognized readily with ultrasonography, and total volume may be assessed subjectively or by the semiquantitative method of measuring the vertical diameter of the largest visible pocket of amniotic fluid (Fig. 13-4).[31] In fetuses assessed for suspected IUGR, the diagnosis may be confirmed in more than 96% of cases if the largest pocket of fluid measures 1 cm or less in the vertical axis.[31] Unfortunately, a lesser degree of disease may not be associated with oligohydramnios (Table 13-2).[32]

Finally, the evaluation of immediate fetal condition may be a useful adjunct in the diagnosis of IUGR. It

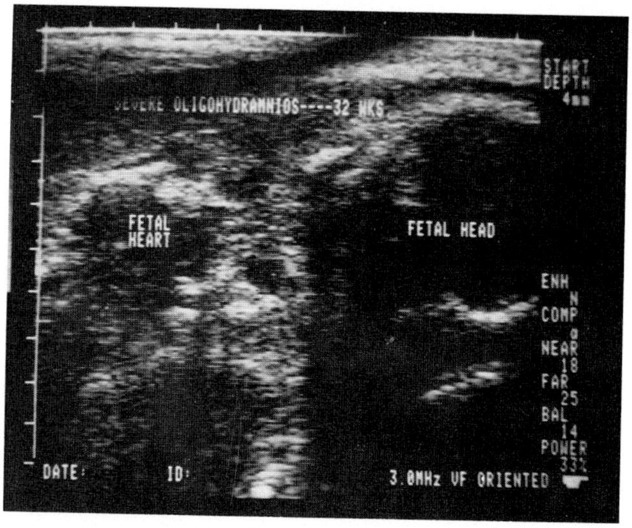

FIG. 13–4. Severe oligohydramnios at 32 weeks of gestation as determined with a linear array ultrasonic method. Note the loss of clear discrimination of fetal structures, a characteristic ultrasonic sign of diminished fluid. The fetal head is deeply flexed on the thorax. There are no pockets of fluid measuring more than 1 cm in the vertical axis. At delivery, the infant weighed 1070 g and exhibited the classic signs of dysmature intrauterine growth retardation.

may be argued that, provided the fetus on serial assessment exhibits no signs of asphyxial compromise, continued observation may be reasonable. Fetal biophysical profile scoring (BPS) appears to be a very reliable method of detecting fetal asphyxia.[1] Regardless of which method is used to detect IUGR, ongoing assessment of fetal well-being appears to be a critical aspect of continuing clinical management.

Macrosomia. Neonates whose birth weights exceed the 90th percentile for gestational age and gender are termed large-for-date, or macrosomic. Like fetuses with IUGR, this group of large infants is heterogeneous, being composed of normal large infants and infants with abnormally excessive growth. Most, but not all, of the infants in the latter group are associated with abnormalities in maternal glucose homeostasis. The perinatal complications common to macrosomic infants may be divided into two groups: intrapartum obstetric complications related purely to perinatal mass such as birth injury, and complications resulting from maternal diabetes, the most common of which is early neonatal hypoglycemia. Ultrasonographic methods for detection of macrosomia are similar to those described for identification of IUGR (*i.e.*, serial assessment of linear growth variables and the interrelationship of these variables within a given fetus). In addition, the evaluation of fat deposition may be a useful adjunct. Prominent malar fat pads (*i.e.*, the cherub sign) and folding of the posterior cervical skin (*i.e.*, the dragon sign) are common findings in a macrosomic infant (Fig. 13-5).

FETAL MATURITY

Ultrasonographic assessment of fetal maturity affects perinatal decision making in two general categories. The first is the determination of whether a fetus has reached an age and weight at which neonatal survival is possible. Such estimates are critical for fetuses at extreme risk in balancing the risk of fetal death against the risk of neonatal death. Fetal age and weight determinations, combined with frequent ultrasonographic assessment of immediate health (*i.e.*, fetal BPS), are used in making these difficult clinical decisions. Second, fetal maturity estimations are used to determine in more elective clinical circumstances that the risk of neonatal morbidity is minimal.

Fetal maturity estimates by ultrasonographic determination of morphometric indices of fetal age and weight and evaluation of placental architecture have been suggested as alternative methods for timing of

TABLE 13–2
RELATION BETWEEN QUALITATIVE AMNIOTIC FLUID VOLUME AND INTRAUTERINE GROWTH RETARDATION*

qAFV	Number of Live Births	Number IUGR	Percentage IUGR
Normal	7327	348	4.74†
Marginal	155	31	20†
Decreased	57	22	38.6†
Total	7539	401	5.32

* Live births only.
† $p < 0.001$ between normal qAFV and marginal qAFV and between normal qAFV and decreased qAFV groups only.
IUGR, intrauterine growth retardation; qAFV, qualitative amniotic fluid volume.
From Chamberlain PF, Manning FA, Morrison I, et al. Ultrasound evaluation of amniotic fluid volume: I. The significance of marginal and decreased amniotic fluid to perinatal outcome. Am J Obstet Gynecol 1984;150:245.

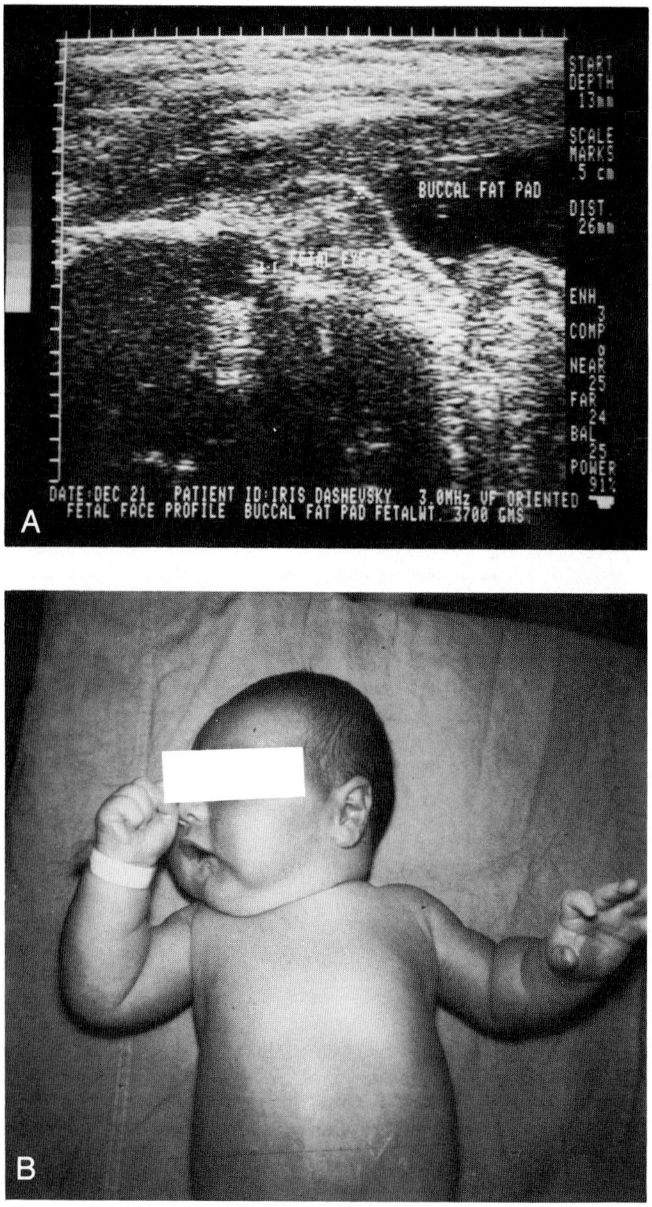

FIG. 13–5. (A) Facial profile of a macrosomic infant was obtained with a linear array ultrasonic method. Note the prominent malar fat pads known as the cherub sign. **(B)** A side view of the infant's face at delivery demonstrates the overt malar fat pads observed *in utero*. These findings are characteristic of the macrosomic infant.

TABLE 13–3
CORRELATION BETWEEN PLACENTAL GRADE AND LECITHIN–SPHINGOMYELIN RATIO IN 563 PATIENTS*

	Grade 0	Grade 1	Grade 2	Grade 3
L/S ratio ≥2	1	108	244	121
L/S ratio <2	5	50	25	9
Total	6	158	269	130
Proportion with L/S ratio ≥2	16.7%	68.4%	90.7%	93.1%

* The relationship between ultrasound grading of placental architecture and fetal pulmonary maturity as determined by amniotic fluid phospholipid determination.

L/S, lecithin–sphingomyelin ratio.

From Harman CR, Manning FA, Stearns E, et al. The correlation of ultrasonic placental grading and fetal pulmonic maturity in five hundred and sixty-three pregnancies. Am J Obstet Gynecol 1982;143:941.

TABLE 13–4
CORRELATION BETWEEN PLACENTAL GRADE AND PRESENCE OF PHOSPHATIDYL GLYCEROL*

	Grade 0	Grade 1	Grade 2	Grade 3
PG present	1	43	143	75
PG absent	5	63	39	25
Total	6	106	182	100
Proportion with PG-positive results	16.7%	40.6%	78.6%	75%

* The relationship between ultrasound grading of placental architecture and fetal pulmonary maturity as determined by amniotic fluid phospholipid determination.
PG, phosphatidyl glycerol.
From Harman CR, Manning FA, Stearns E, et al. The correlation of ultrasonic placental grading and fetal pulmonic maturity in five hundred and sixty-three pregnancies. Am J Obstet Gynecol 1982;143:941.

elective delivery. Such methods have the advantage of avoiding the recognized risks of amniocentesis, but, to be of practical value, these measures must have a predictive accuracy equal to or greater than that accepted for amniotic fluid analysis. Studies on elective deliveries based on age determination by BPD or weight estimates from BPD and abdominal circumference, in general indicate excellent results.[33–35] The inherent error of age estimates common to all methods necessitates caution, however. Grading of placental maturity based on ultrasonographic evaluation of placental architecture has been proposed as a useful measure of fetal maturity. In a retrospective analysis, Granum and Hobbins noted that in 23 fetuses with the most mature degree of placental maturation (*i.e.*, grade 3 placenta), all exhibited a mature lecithin–sphingomyelin (L/S) ratio.[36] In a prospective study, Harman and coworkers were unable to confirm the precise relationship, noticing that 7% of patients with a grade 3 placenta were identified with an immature L/S ratio (Tables 13-3 and 13-4).[37] In view of these latter findings, the value of ultrasonographic grading of placental maturity to determine fetal maturity may be seriously questioned.

IDENTIFICATION OF CONGENITAL ANOMALIES

The term "congenital anomaly" refers to a large spectrum of developmental defects ranging from inconsequential to major lethal disorders. In my study population in the province of Manitoba, congenital anomalies complicate from 1.5% to 1.8% of all pregnancies, and in 0.3% to 0.5% of pregnancies the anomaly may be major and potentially lethal. The advent of high-resolution dynamic ultrasonography has produced profound changes in recognition and management of fetal anomalies. In theory, all anomalies that exhibit macroscopic anatomic change in organ structure and most anomalies that are associated with functional change in major organ systems may now be recognized *in utero* with ultrasonography (Fig. 13-6). If the anomaly or its effects are visible to the naked eye, the potential exists for ultrasonographic diagnosis *in utero*. In excess of 90% of all major anomalies are recognized with a prospective ultrasonography screening program.[38] Because the manifestation of anomalies becomes more apparent with advancing gestational age, the diagnostic accuracy increases with gestational age.

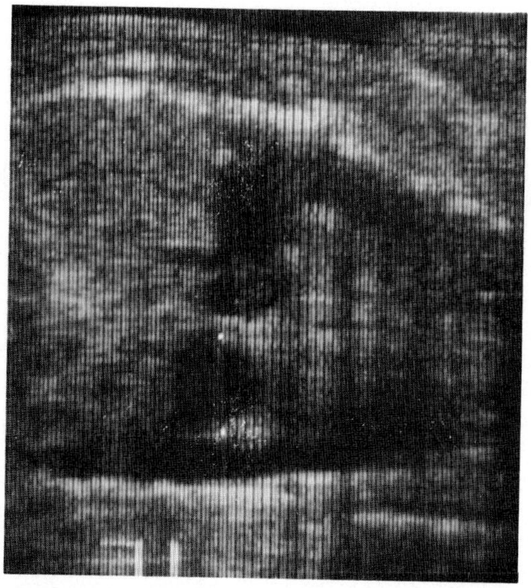

FIG. 13–6. A longitudinal scan of the fetal thorax and abdomen in the coronal plane obtained with a linear array ultrasonic method demonstrates bilateral fetal pleural effusion. Fetal lung tissue is highlighted because of the surrounding pleural fluid. Bilateral thoracentesis was performed immediately at delivery, and the infant survived. The diagnosis of chylothorax subsequently was confirmed.

The clinical impact of this ever-improving ability to recognize anomalies on the practice of perinatal medicine is enormous. Prenatal diagnosis now permits consideration of prognosis, disease progression, and therapeutic intervention. Because the presence of a fetal anomaly may influence both fetal and maternal risk of morbidity and mortality, it is necessary, in clinical terms, to move beyond the mere recognition of an anomaly to its classification to guide clinical management. Factors to be considered include gestational age, deleterious functional effect of the disorder, if any, and ultimate fetal and neonatal prognosis with or without therapy (see Chap. 14).

Several general principles need to be considered in using ultrasonographic technique to diagnose anomalies. A comprehensive and organized anatomic review is essential, followed by evaluation of amniotic fluid volume, cord position and structure, and placental position and structure. In addition to performing the anatomic screen, a functional review should be performed, noting movement characteristics, heart rate and rhythm, and so on. Second, because some anomalies may not become evident until later in gestation (*e.g.*, progressive hydrocephalus), follow-up evaluation of the fetus at risk is critical. Finally, in the event that a suspicion of anomaly is raised, a detailed and repeated evaluation certainly is required.

DETECTION OF FETAL ASPHYXIA

Fetal asphyxia, due to dysfunction of the fetoplacental unit, is a major cause of morbidity and mortality among perinates. Recognition of this complication is extremely important because expeditious delivery may result in intact survival. The characteristic biophysical responses of the fetus to an asphyxial insult appear to be similar to those observed in the newborn, being primarily a loss of activity and function due to central nervous system (CNS) depression and cardiovascular decompensation. Acute fetal asphyxia is relatively uncommon except in obstetric emergencies such as cord prolapse or major abruption of the placenta. Therefore, most asphyxiated fetuses exhibit both subacute and chronic signs of the disease process. In the human fetus suffering from uteroplacental insufficiency, it is likely that hypoxemic episodes are intermittent, being induced during periods of uterine contraction. In the intervening periods, the fetus is likely to be normoxic or exhibit a minor compensated hypoxemia. The signs associated with hypoxemia will therefore depend on the duration of the disease, its progression, and the frequency of contraction-induced hypoxemic episodes.

Cumulative chronic effects of intermittent hypoxemia on fetal condition may be recognized by ultrasonographic evaluation. These effects include impaired fetal growth (*i.e.*, dysmaturity, IUGR) and include the very important sign of oligohydramnios. The latter, readily recognized by ultrasonography, is most likely a result of hypoxia-induced reflex redistribution of cardiac output.[30] The finding of oligohydramnios always must be considered indicative of fetal asphyxia unless absent renal function (*e.g.*, renal agenesis) or rupture of membranes can be demonstrated (see Table 13-2).

Alterations of acute biophysical responses occur during episodes of fetal hypoxemia. Fetal breathing movements and gross body movements are profoundly reduced or disappear during hypoxemia in chronically instrumented fetal lambs.[39,40] Similarly, fetal muscle tone is reduced, and heart rate responses to movement (*i.e.*, accelerations) are lost during hypoxemia in the human.[41] Because spontaneous CNS rhythms or maternal depressant medication also may alter CNS state and therefore fetal biophysical activities, however, it is important that these causes be ruled out in the inactive fetus. Medication can be eliminated by reviewing maternal history and CNS rhythms by extending the observation period beyond the normal duration of fetal CNS states (*i.e.*, 20 to 40 minutes).

FETAL BIOPHYSICAL PROFILE

A combination of five ultrasound-monitored fetal biophysical variables—fetal breathing movements, gross body movements, tone, heart rate reactivity, and semiquantitative amniotic fluid volume determination—is used to assess fetal risk of asphyxia.[42] Each variable may be coded as normal or abnormal, according to fixed and tested criteria (Table 13-5), and then assigned an arbitrary score of 2 when normal and 0 when abnormal. Observation of each variable should be continued until normal criteria are met or until at least 30 minutes of continuous observation elapse. The composite score of these variables, termed a BPS, provides the most accurate guide for differentiation of the normal from the compromised fetus. In a preliminary blinded study of high-risk patients, the perinatal mortality ranged from 0 per 1000 when all variables were normal (BPS of 10) to as high as 600 per 1000 when all variables were abnormal (BPS of 0).[42] This method of fetal risk assessment has been used in a prospective clinical study of 12,620 referred high-risk patients at the Women's Hospital of Manitoba.[1] The total number of tests done on this population was 25,670 (mean, 2.1 tests per patient). In this prospective study, intervention was based on abnormal score results (BPS $\leq$ 4) or initiated when oligohydramnios was observed in suspected cases of intrauterine growth retardation or in postdates patients (Table 13-6). Perinatal mortality and morbidity in the study population was compared with that in an untested historical controlled population. The cumulative results of this study are encouraging. Gross perinatal mortality fell to 7.37 per 1000, representing a drop in excess of 68%, and corrected perinatal mortality fell to 3.53 per 1000, a reduction in excess of 68%

TABLE 13–5
BIOPHYSICAL PROFILE SCORING: TECHNIQUE AND INTERPRETATION

Biophysical Variable	Normal*	Abnormal†
FBMs	At least one episode of FBM of at least 30-sec duration in a 30-min observation period	Absent FBM or no episode of ≥30 sec in 30 min
Gross body movement	At least three discrete body or limb movements in 30 min: (episodes of active continuous movement are considered a single movement)	Two or fewer episodes of body or limb movements in 30 min
Fetal tone	At least one episode of active extension with return to flexion of fetal limb(s) or trunk; opening and closing of hand considered normal tone	Either slow extension with return to partial flexion or movement of limb in full extension or absent fetal movement
Reactive FHR	At least two episodes in 30 min of FHR acceleration of ≥15 bpm of at least 15-sec duration associated with fetal movement	Less than two episodes of acceleration of FHR or acceleration of <15 bpm in 30 min
Qualitative AFV	At least one pocket of AF that measures at least 2 cm in two perpendicular planes	Either no AF pockets or a pocket <2 cm in two perpendicular planes

* Score = 2.
† Score = 0.
AF, amniotic fluid; AFV, amniotic fluid volume; bpm, beats per minute; FBM, fetal breathing movement; FHR, fetal heart rate.
From Manning FA, Morrison I, Lange IR, et al. Fetal assessment based on fetal biophysical profile scoring: experience in 12,620 referred high risk pregnancies: I. Perinatal mortality by frequency and etiology. Am J Obstet Gynecol 1985;151:343.

compared with control. The stillbirth rate in the tested population fell to 1.9 per 1000, compared with a rate of 8.8 per 1000 in the control population. The false-negative test rate—that is, death of a structurally normal fetus within 1 week of a normal test result (BPS ≥ 8)—is recorded at 0.685 per 1000.[1] Clinical studies from other centers have reported similar results with this method.[43]

Accurate differentiation of the normal fetus from the compromised one has a profound affect on planning prenatal care and on the timing and indication for intervention. Assurances of continued fetal well-being for a finite period can prevent early intervention in high-risk cases and thereby reduce neonatal morbidity. In contrast, in the fetus exhibiting abnormal biophysical variables in whom the risk of still-

TABLE 13–6
BIOPHYSICAL PROFILE SCORING: MANAGEMENT PROTOCOL

Score	Interpretation	Management
10	Normal infant, low risk for chronic asphyxia	Repeat testing at weekly intervals; repeat twice weekly in diabetics and patient ≥42 weeks of gestation
8	Normal infant, low risk for chronic asphyxia	Repeat testing at weekly intervals; repeat testing twice weekly in diabetics and patients ≥42 weeks of gestation; oligohydramnios is an indication for delivery
6	Suspicion of chronic asphyxia	Repeat testing in 4–6 h; deliver if oligohydramnios present
4	Suspicion of chronic asphyxia	If ≥36 weeks of gestation and favorable, deliver; if <36 weeks of gestation and L/S <2, repeat test in 24 h; if repeat score ≤4, deliver
0–2	Strong suspicion of chronic asphyxia	Extend testing time to 120 min; if persistent score ≤4, deliver, regardless of gestational age

L/S, lecithin–sphingomyelin ratio.
From Manning FA, et al. Fetal assessment based on fetal biophysical profile scoring: experience in 12,620 referred high risk pregnancies: I. Perinatal mortality by frequency and etiology. Am J Obstet Gynecol 1985;151:343.

birth is greatly increased, early delivery and immediate neonatal care may be initiated. The degree to which fetal condition may be assessed by currently available ultrasonographic methods is primarily limited by the practical constraints of testing time. The variables used in formulating the fetal BPS were selected because of ease and rapidity of measurement; however, these five variables reflect only a portion of the dynamic biophysical data base that may be accumulated with dynamic ultrasonography. Variables such as CNS state change, rapid eye movement state, fine coordinated movement, peristalsis of fetal gut, fetal cardiac output and blood pressure, and umbilical vessel flow rates may add to the evaluation of immediate fetal condition.

The detection by ultrasonography of obstetric conditions predisposing the fetus to acute asphyxia is an area of active investigation. Cord prolapse, a clinical event often associated with disastrous perinatal consequences, may be one cause of acute fetal asphyxia whose risk may be identified before clinical occurrence (Fig. 13-7). Such recognition sets the stage for preventive management. Lange and coworkers reported accurate prenatal diagnosis of cord presentation, the precursor to cord prolapse, using ultrasonographic techniques in late pregnancy.[44] Similarly, abruptio placentae, a pathologic event that in full expression is a major cause of perinatal morbidity and mortality, may be recognized in earlier and less severe forms by ultrasonography (Fig. 13-8). Evidence is accumulating to indicate that abruption, rather than a catastrophic and sudden pathologic entity, may be a chronic, progressive disorder that is characterized by segmental placental structure and membrane disruption ultimately leading to full-fledged clinical abruption. Further work is needed to define the value of these observations in preventative clinical management.

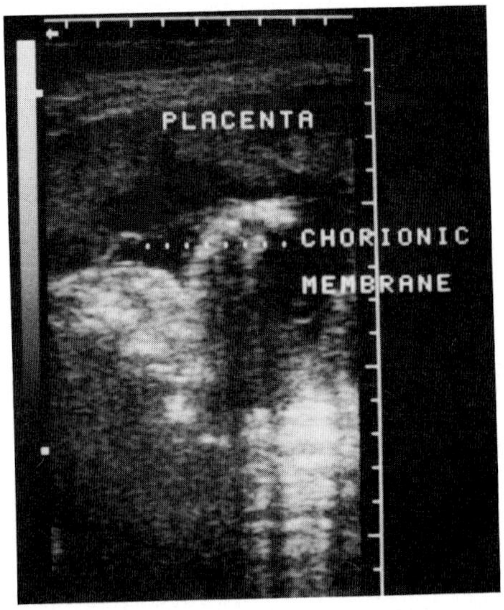

FIG. 13–8. A linear array ultrasonographic scan demonstrates a fresh intracotyledonary bleed. The developing hematoma appears echolucent and is confined to a discrete area within a single cotyledon. The fetal membranes are lifted off the placenta. Mild abruption was confirmed at delivery.

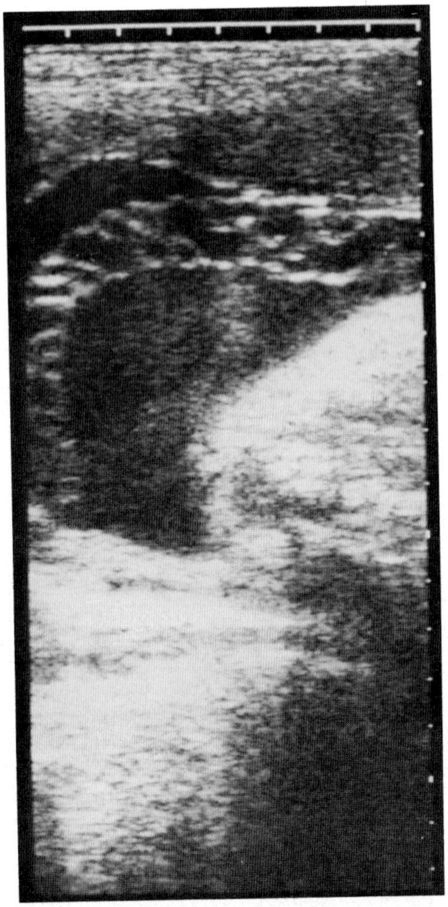

FIG. 13–7. Longitudinal scan of the lower uterine segment in the midline sagittal plane demonstrates cord presentation. Note that the umbilical cord extends below a fetal limb and across the entire inferior aspect of the lower uterine segment. Cord presentation was confirmed by vaginal examination and delivery was by cesarean section.

DOPPLER ASSESSMENT OF BLOOD VELOCITIES IN FETAL UMBILICAL VESSELS

Measurement of the spectrum of blood flow velocities in the umbilical artery and intrafetal vessels has gained popularity as a method for assessing fetal health. The method is based on directing a pulsed or continuous beam of high-frequency ultrasound (*i.e.*, 2.25–5.0 MHz) toward the fetal vessels and recording the frequency shift (*i.e.*, Doppler effect) in the returning echoes as a result of the flow in the target vessel. By this method, blood flow toward the transducer causes an increase in frequency of the returning echoes, whereas flow away from the transducer causes a relative decreasing echo frequency. The frequency spectrum of the echoes is displayed on the ultrasound screen. The method is not accurate for the measurement of absolute flow but does give an accurate reflection of the relative resistance to flow. The frequency spectrum obtained is analyzed by comparing the systolic to diastolic flow velocities and is expressed as either the ratio of the difference between peak systolic and diastolic flow velocity over the mean flow velocity (*i.e.*, the pulsatility index), the difference between peak systolic and diastolic flow over the peak systolic flow (*i.e.*, the Pourcelot index), or more simply as the ratio of the peak systolic to diastolic flow (*i.e.*, the S/D ratio); the latter method is the one most commonly used.

The major clinical application of this method of fetal assessment has been in the measurement of flow velocities in the umbilical artery. In a normal pregnancy, the placental resistance declines slowly with advancing gestational age, manifested in the umbilical artery by a decrease in the peak systolic flow velocity and an increase in diastolic flow velocities. Consequently, the umbilical artery S/D ratio declines, slowing with advancing gestational age.[45] In pregnancies complicated by the loss of the normal placental microvasculature (*e.g.*, preeclampsia, IUGR), there is an increase in placental vascular resistance that becomes manifest by an increase in the systolic flow velocities and a decrease in the diastolic component, resulting in an increase in the S/D ratio. With severe disease, there may be a complete absence of the diastolic component and the S/D ratio becomes infinite. When the placental resistance becomes massively increased, blood flow in the umbilical artery during diastole may reverse in direction in a rebound effect, giving rise to the ominous pattern of reversed diastolic flow velocities.

Initially, it was hoped that monitoring of the umbilical artery flow velocity waveforms would give an accurate estimate of fetal condition and might be used to time intervention for the compromised fetus. As clinical experience with the method has increased, it has become apparent that the relationship between placental resistance and fetal condition is subject to considerable variation. There is no direct correlation between these parameters of flow velocity and fetal blood gas status.[46] Accordingly, the use of this measure to detect fetal asphyxia is without clinical merit. In contrast, there is a clear association between changes in the umbilical artery velocity waveform and the risk of chronic fetal disease, an association that results from the relationship of increased placental resistance to both an increased risk of fetal disease and a change in the umbilical artery flow velocity waveforms.[47] As a result, the contemporary application of this measure is to aid in the identification of the fetus at increased risk and to guide the frequency and intensity of application of other more specific measures of fetal condition such as the fetal BPS or antepartum fetal heart rate testing. Intervention solely on the basis of an abnormal umbilical artery velocity waveform is not indicated. The interval between the appearance of the abnormality in the flow velocity and the development of abnormalities in the fetal condition, as reflected by the fetal BPS, can be as long as 3 weeks. In a study of 26 immature fetuses (*i.e.*, ≤28 weeks of gestation) with absent diastolic flow velocities in the umbilical artery, the interval between recognition of the abnormal flow velocity pattern and deterioration of the fetal BPS averaged 15 days.[48] The hope that alterations in the umbilical artery velocity waveform might be used to differentiate accurately the fetus with growth retardation secondary to placental disease from the fetus with growth retardation secondary to intrinsic fetal disease or anomaly has not been sustained. The incidence of anomaly among fetuses with absent diastolic flow velocity has been reported to be significantly increased, and is on average about 25%.[49]

DOPPLER ASSESSMENT OF BLOOD VELOCITIES IN OTHER VESSELS

Measurement of flow velocity waveforms in the uterine artery holds promise as a method for early recognition of the pregnancy at risk for preeclampsia and IUGR long before there are any clinical signs of the disease process.[50] If studies of the use of low-dose aspirin in pregnancy prove to be effective in preventing or ameliorating this common disease, the use of uterine flow velocity assessment may become an important part of early pregnancy assessment. It also is possible to measure flow velocities of intrafetal vessels, including the carotid, middle cerebral, and renal arteries.[51,52] Although experimental, these measures hold promise as means of assessing the distribution of fetal blood flow in health and disease and may ultimately prove useful in assessing the fetal cardiovascular adaptive responses to chronic hypoxemia. Color flow mapping of the Doppler flow velocity waveforms makes it possible to assess the intracardiac blood flow characteristics. Although an exciting technical advance, the practical application of color Doppler in modern perinatal medicine remains unproven.

ANTEPARTUM FETAL BLOOD SAMPLING

In 1983, Daffos and colleagues reported the use of an ultrasound-guided technique to obtain a pure fetal blood sample from the umbilical vein of an undelivered fetus.[53] The applications of this now common technique are broad indeed and range from rapid determination of the fetal karyotype, assessment of biochemical and endocrine status of the fetus at risk for various inherited metabolic disorders, determination of hemoglobin structure in fetuses at risk for inherited hemoglobinopathies, the determination of erythrocyte and platelet membrane antigen status in fetuses at risk for alloimmune disorders, and, in the affected fetus, the determination of the presence and severity of disease, and the determination of the blood gas, acid–base, and biochemical status in the fetus at risk for antepartum asphyxial disease. By this method it is possible prenatally to measure all the blood and plasma components that may be part of the assessment of a newborn. As a result of this advance, yet one more of the barriers that separate the practice of fetal and neonatal medicine has been withdrawn.

The technique is based on the use of high-resolution dynamic ultrasound to direct a needle through the tissues of the maternal abdomen and uterus to a relatively fixed portion of the umbilical vein, either where it enters the placenta (Fig. 13-9) or where it exits from the fetal abdomen. Confirmation of appropriate needle placement is obtained by observing the turbulence created by injection of a small bolus of normal saline into the vessel and by immediate analysis of a fetal blood sample (Fig. 13-10). In experienced hands, the method will yield a pure fetal venous or arterial blood sample in almost all cases and may be used from as early as 16 weeks of gestation. The procedure is invasive and not without fetal risk. Complications include fetal death, which occurs at a frequency of approximately 1 per 500 procedures, and fetal hemorrhage either into the amniotic fluid, the cord substance (*i.e.*, cord hematoma), or into the maternal circulation (*i.e.*, transplacental hemorrhage). Maternal risks with the procedure are exceedingly

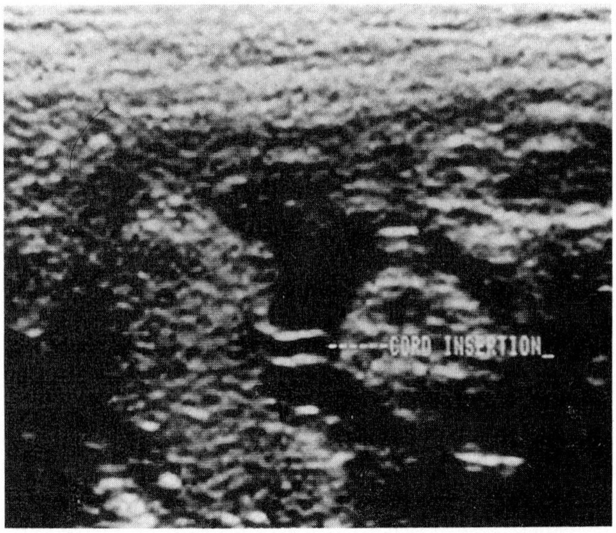

FIG. 13–9. A real-time ultrasound image shows the insertion of the fetal umbilical cord into the substance of the placenta. The cord in this position is relatively stable, and it usually is possible to place a needle in the umbilical vein with minimal difficulty.

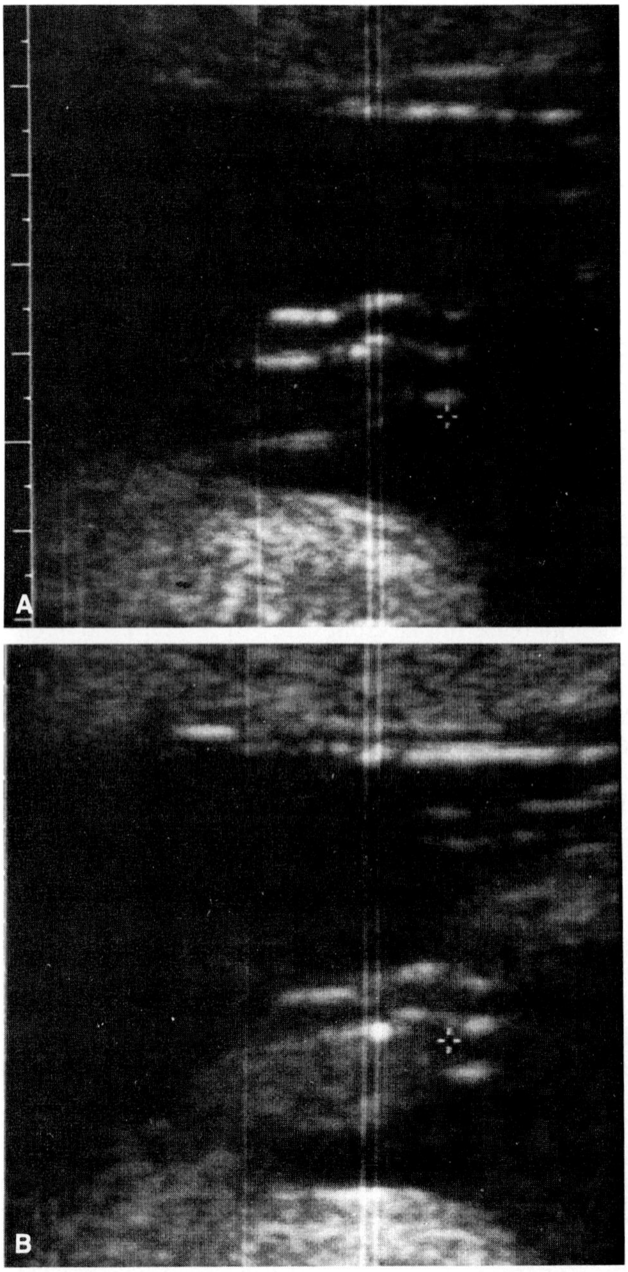

FIG. 13–10. **(A)** A section of umbilical cord downstream from the site where a needle (*) has been placed into the umbilical vein. The superior parallel lines are produced by the relatively echogenic umbilical artery walls. The inferior echolucent (*i.e.*, dark) portion is the umbilical vein. **(B)** The second image was taken just after injection of ~0.5 mL of normal saline into the umbilical vein. The brightness in the umbilical vein occurs because of turbulence created by the saline bolus. This simple test confirms immediately that the needle is in the umbilical vein.

rare but include the risk of infection, placental abruption, and hemorrhage. Accordingly, the use of this procedure should be reserved for those fetuses in whom the benefits exceed the procedural risk by a considerable margin and for whom there are no other reasonable means of obtaining the critical information.

It is possible to detect fetal hypoxemia by fetal blood sampling[54]; nomograms describing the normal values and changes with gestational age of the fetal PO_2, PCO_2, *p*H, lactate, and blood glucose have been published.[55,56] The application of blood gas determination by the invasive method of cordocentesis in the management of the high-risk fetus is uncertain. Undoubtedly, these results add to the understanding of the effects of hypoxemia and asphyxia on the fetus and aid in describing the range of human fetal adaptation to conditions of impaired oxygen delivery to tissues. There is no convincing evidence, however, that these direct measures are superior to the estimates of fetal condition and risk that may be obtained by measuring fetal biophysical variables using the noninvasive dynamic ultrasound methods. Accordingly, intervention on the basis of abnormal blood gas values in the presence of a normal antepartum fetal heart rate record or a normal fetal BPS is not recommended.

The advantages of the ability to gain access to the fetal circulation are not restricted to diagnosis alone but also include the prospect of replacement therapy in various fetal diseases. There is now overwhelming clinical evidence to suggest the treatment of the anemic fetus with alloimmune disease by direct intravascular transfusion is the method of choice. It is likely that in the future other fetal conditions may be treated by direct intravascular therapies (see Chap. 14).

ASSESSMENT OF ISOIMMUNIZATION SYNDROMES

The characteristic ultrasonographic features of the isoimmunized fetus include morphologic changes in the placenta and umbilical cord as well as alterations in amniotic fluid volume. With mild disease, the placenta becomes thickened, and its normal ultrasonographic architecture disappears; with more severe disease, cotyledon structure and chorionic plate are obliterated, and the placenta takes on a ground-glass appearance. The umbilical vein becomes progressively larger as disease advances. Fetal morphologic changes are specific and well recognized, including hepatosplenomegaly, increased abdominal circumference, and the appearance of peritoneal fluid (*i.e.*, ascites) and pleural fluid (Fig. 13-11). Scalp, abdominal wall, and limb edema are late signs indicating severe disease (*i.e.*, hydrops fetalis). Alterations in amniotic fluid volume are frequently seen, with hydramnios the most common finding. In my experience, oligohydramnios in the Rh-isoimmunized fetus is an ominous sign. Fetal biophysical variables such as gross body movement, tone, breathing movements, and heart rate reactivity, when coupled with qualitative determination of amniotic fluid volume, are very useful in evaluation of the immediate condition of the Rh-isoimmunized fetus. In a fetus with mild to moderate disease, BPS usually is normal, but in more advanced disease, an abnormal BPS is almost a constant finding. A persistently abnormal BPS (*i.e.*, ≤4) is associated with a very poor prognosis.[57]

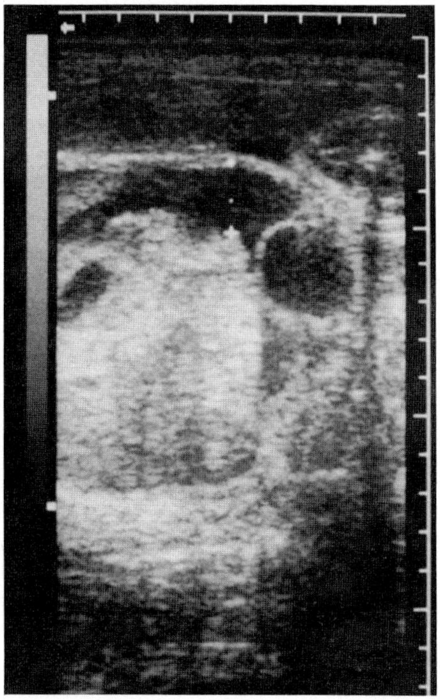

FIG. 13–11. A longitudinal scan of a fetus in the midline sagittal plane was obtained with a linear array ultrasonic method. Gross fetal ascites is evident, but abdominal wall edema and limb edema (*upper right*) are absent. Massive hepatomegaly filling most of the fetal abdomen is evident. The cystic lower abdominal structure is a normal fetal bladder as outlined by peritoneal (*i.e.*, ascitic) fluid.

Ultrasound is extremely useful in guiding therapy in the Rh-isoimmunized fetus. Fetal intrauterine transfusion is the therapy of choice in the immature fetus but may be associated with a traumatic death rate of up to 5%.[58] Ultrasonographic guidance and fetal localization at the time of fetal transfusion can reduce the probability of inadvertent fetal trauma and subsequent compromise.[57] Similarly, because peritoneal absorption of fetal erythrocytes may be monitored accurately with ultrasonography (Fig. 13-12), ultrasonographic assessment plays a critical role in the timing of subsequent transfusions. Before dynamic ultrasonographic assessment, timing of subsequent intraperitoneal transfusion in Rh-isoimmunized fetuses was empirical. The timing of repeat

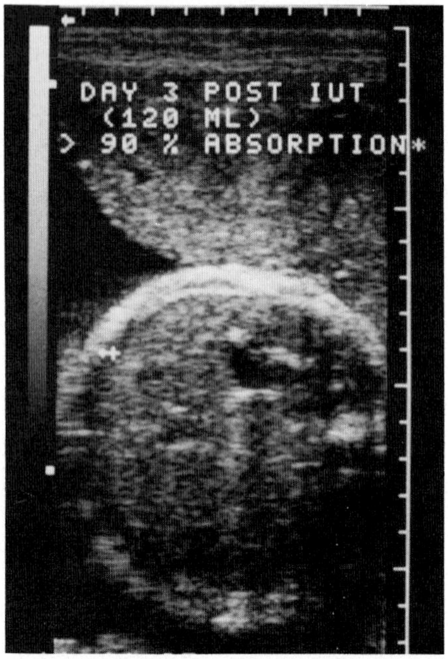

FIG. 13–12. A transverse scan of a fetal abdomen at the midhepatic portion was obtained with a linear array ultrasonic method. The fetal spine is located at approximately 3 o'clock. Note the small residual rim of intraperitoneal blood persistent at day 3 after intrauterine transfusion of 120 mL of tightly packed O-negative blood. Rapid absorption of transfused blood, as in this case, denotes an excellent prognosis, despite the residual placental edema.

transfusions now is based on the ultrasonographically determined rate of disappearance of transferred erythrocytes, the rate and extent of ascitic fluid accumulation, and the degree of placenta and scalp edema.

The treatment of the severely affected alloimmune fetus has been done through direct intravascular fetal transfusion via a needle placed under ultrasound guidance into the umbilical vein at or near its insertion into the placenta. There are obvious advantages to this technique—the needle used for direct intravascular transfusion is much smaller (*i.e.*, 22-gauge), and therefore the risk of trauma is less. The blood, given directly to the fetus, can be observed to reach the fetus, thereby eliminating the risks of failure to absorb the blood, with the fetus benefiting almost immediately from the therapy. Based on a comparative study, it is evident that the intravascular method of transfusion is far superior to the intraperitoneal method and should be the method of choice.[59] The intraperitoneal route is reserved for those patients in whom, for technical reasons, access to the umbilical vein is not possible. Perinatal survival is improved with the use of intravascular transfusion and overall survival exceeds 90%. The improvement in overall survival has been primarily the result of salvage of fetuses with severe disease. The survival rate of hydrops with aggressive intravascular transfusion can exceed 85%,[60] and this study included two grossly hydropic fetuses with an initial hematocrit of less than 3%.

SUMMARY

The relative explosion of information on fetal condition that may be garnered through dynamic ultrasonography has profoundly influenced the practice of perinatal medicine. It is becoming ever more possible to extend the principles of extrauterine neonatal examination to the fetus by use of this tool. Serious complications such as developmental anomalies, multiple pregnancy, intrauterine asphyxia, and growth abnormalities may now be recognized more frequently and more accurately than was possible in the past. Recognition of risk conditions such as abruption, cord prolapse, and some forms of anomaly is fostering the concept of preventive fetal care. Obstetric care always has been hampered by inability to examine the intrauterine patient. The ability to indirectly see the fetus and to examine its morphology, function, and environment is likely to be viewed in years to come as the quantum leap of perinatal medicine.

REFERENCES

1. Manning FA, Morrison I, Lange IR, et al. Fetal assessment based on fetal biophysical profile scoring: experience in 12,620 referred high risk pregnancies: I. Perinatal mortality by frequency and etiology. Am J Obstet Gynecol 1985;151:343.
2. Dewhurst CJ, Beasley JM, Campbell S. Assessment of fetal maturity and dysmaturity. Obstet Gynecol 1972;113:141.
3. Donald I. Ultrasound in obstetrics. Br Med Bull 1968;24:71.
4. Dubowitz LMS, Dubowitz V, Goldberg C. Clinical assessment of gestational age in the newborn infant. J Pediatr 1970;71:1.
5. Hadlock FP, Deter RL, Harrist RB. Computer assisted analysis of fetal age using multiple fetal growth parameters. J Clin Ultrasound 1983;11:313.
6. Hellman LM, Kobayashi M, Fillisti L, et al. Growth and development of the human fetus prior to the twentieth week of gestation. Am J Obstet Gynecol 1969;1034:789.
7. Robinson HP, Fleming JEE. A critical evaluation of sonar crown–rump length measurement. Br J Obstet Gynaecol 1975; 82:702.
8. Sabbagha RE, Hughey M. Standardization of sonar cephalometry and gestational age. Obstet Gynecol 1978;52:402.
9. Campbell S, Newman GB. Growth of the fetal biparietal diameter during normal pregnancy. Br J Obstet Gynaecol 1971;78: 513.
10. Sabbagha RE, Turner JH, Rockette H, et al. Sonar BPD and fetal age: definition of the relationship. Obstet Gynecol 1974; 43:7.
11. Sabbagha RE, Hughey M, Depp R. Growth adjusted sonographic age (GASA): a simplified method. Obstet Gynecol 1978;51:383.

12. Queenan JT, O'Brien GD, Campbell S. Ultrasound measurement of fetal limb bones. Am J Obstet Gynecol 1980;138:297.
13. Manning FA, Lange IR, Morrison I, et al. Calculation of fetal length in utero: an ultrasound method. Proc SOGC, Vancouver BC, June, 1983.
14. Iannirubertо A, Gibbons JM. Predicting fetal weight by ultrasonic B-scancephalometry: an improved technique with disappointing results. Obstet Gynecol 1971;37:689.
15. Campbell S, Wilkin D. Ultrasound measurement of fetal abdominal circumference in the estimation of fetal weight. Br J Obstet Gynaecol 1975;82:689.
16. Warsof SL, Gohari P, Berkowitz RL, et al. The estimation of fetal weight by computer assisted analysis. Am J Obstet Gynecol 1977;128:881.
17. Deter RL, Harrist RB, Birnholz JC, et al. Evaluation of fetal dating studies. In: Hedlock F, Deter RL, eds. Qualitative obstetrical ultrasonography. New York: John Wiley & Sons, 1986:33.
18. Thompson TR, Manning FA. Estimation of volume and weight of the perinate: relationship to morphometric measurement by ultrasonography. J Ultrasound Med 1983;2:113.
19. Shepard MJ, Richards VA, Berkowitz RL, et al. An evaluation of two equations for predicting fetal weight by ultrasound. Am J Obstet Gynecol 1982;142:47.
20. Lubchenco LO, Harsman C, Presser M, et al. Intrauterine growth as estimated from live born weight data at 24 to 42 weeks of gestation. Pediatrics 1963;32:793.
21. Deter RL, Harrist RB, Hadlock FP, et al. Longitudinal studies of fetal growth with the use of dynamic image ultrasonography. Am J Obstet Gynecol 1982;143:545.
22. Campbell S. Fetal growth. Clin Obstet Gynecol 1974;1:41.
23. Persson PH, Grennert L, Gennssar G, et al. Diagnosis of intrauterine growth retardation by serial ultrasonic cephalometry. Acta Obstet Gynecol Scand Suppl 1978;178:40.
24. O'Brien GD, Queenan JT. Ultrasound fetal femur length in relation to intrauterine growth retardation. Am J Obstet Gynecol 1982;144:33.
25. Tamura RK, Sabbagha RE. Percentile ranks of sonar fetal abdominal circumference measurements. Am J Obstet Gynecol 1980;138:475.
26. Sabbagha RE. Intrauterine growth retardation: antenatal diagnosis by ultrasound. Obstet Gynecol 1978;52:252.
27. Campbell S. Ultrasound measurement of the fetal head to abdomen circumference ratio in assessment of growth retardation. Br J Obstet Gynaecol 1977;84:165.
28. Wladimiroff JW, Bloemsma CA, Wallenburg HCS. Ultrasound assessment of fetal head and body sizes in relation to normal and retarded fetal growth. Am J Obstet Gynecol 1978;131:857.
29. Sabbagha RE. Intrauterine growth retardation: avenues of future research in diagnosis and management by ultrasound. Semin Perinatol 1984;8:31.
30. Cohn HE, Sacks EJ, Heyman MA, et al. Cardiovascular responses to hypoxemia and acidemia in fetal lambs. Am J Obstet Gynecol 1974;120:817.
31. Manning FA, Hill LM, Platt LD. Qualitative amniotic fluid volume determination by ultrasound: antepartum detection of intrauterine growth retardation. Am J Obstet Gynecol 1981;1139:254.
32. Chamberlain PF, Manning FA, Morrison I, et al. Ultrasound evaluation of amniotic fluid volume: I. The significance of marginal and decreased amniotic fluid volume to perinatal outcome. Am J Obstet Gynecol 1984;150:245.
33. Goldstein P, Gershenson D, Hobbins JC. Fetal biparietal diameter as a predictor of mature L/S ratio. Obstet Gynecol 1976;48:667.
34. Strassner HT, Plat LD, Whittle M, et al. Amniotic fluid phosphatidylglycerol and real-time ultrasonic cephalometry. Am J Obstet Gynecol 1979;135:804.
35. Golde SH, Platt LD. The use of ultrasound in the diagnosis of fetal lung maturity. Clin Obstet Gynecol 1984;27:391.
36. Grannum PAT, Hobbins JC. The ultrasound changes in the maturing placenta and their relationship to fetal pulmonic maturity. Am J Obstet Gynecol 1979;133:915.
37. Harman CR, Manning FA, Stearns E, et al. The correlation of ultrasonic placental grading and fetal pulmonic maturity in five hundred and sixty-three pregnancies. Am J Obstet Gynecol 1982;143:941.
38. Manning FA, Lange IR, Morrison I. Congenital anomalies and the role of ultrasound. In: Persaud TVN, ed. Advances in the study of birth defects. Vol 5. Genetic disorders, syndromology and prenatal diagnosis. Lancaster, England: MTP Press, 1981:175.
39. Boddy K, Dawes GS. Fetal breathing. Br Med Bull 1976;31:3.
40. Natale R, Clewlow F, Dawes GS. Measurement of fetal forelimb movements in the lamb in utero. Am J Obstet Gynecol 1981;140:545.
41. Brown R, Patrick J. The non-stress test: how long is enough. Am J Obstet Gynecol 1981;141:646.
42. Manning FA, Platt LD, Sipos L. Antepartum fetal evaluation: development of a fetal biophysical profile score. Am J Obstet Gynecol 1980;136:787.
43. Baskett TF, Gray JH, Prewett ST, et al. Antepartum fetal assessment using a fetal biophysical profile score. Am J Obstet Gynecol 1983;148:630.
44. Lange IR, Manning FA, Morrison I, et al. Cord prolapse: is antenatal diagnosis possible? Am J Obstet Gynecol 1985;151:1083.
45. Giles WB, Trudinger BJ, Cook CM. Umbilical artery velocity time waveforms in pregnancy. J Ultrasound Med 1982;1:9.
46. Morrow R, Richie K. Doppler ultrasound and fetal velocimetry and its role in obstetrics. Clin Perinatol 1989;16:771.
47. Trudinger BJ, Cook CM, Giles WB, et al. Fetal umbilical artery velocity waveforms and subsequent neonatal outcome. Br J Obstet Gynaecol 1991;98:378.
48. Tsang H, Manning F. Combined use of the fetal biophysical profile score and umbilical artery flow velocity waveform assessment in the management of the very premature growth retarded fetus. Am J Obstet Gynecol 1993 (in press).
49. Rochelson B, Schulman H, Farmakides G, et al. The significance of absent end diastolic velocity in umbilical artery velocity waveforms. Am J Obstet Gynecol 1987;156:1213.
50. Campbell S, Griffin DR, Pearce FMF. New Doppler ultrasound technique for assessing uteroplacental blood flow. Lancet 1983;1:675.
51. Wladimiroff JW, Wijingaard JAGW, Degani S. Cerebral and umbilical blood flow velocity waveforms in normal and growth retarded pregnancies. Obstet Gynecol 1987;69:705.
52. Veille JC, Kanaan C. Duplex Doppler ultrasonographic evaluation of the fetal lamb artery in normal and abnormal fetuses. Am J Obstet Gynecol 1989;161:1502.
53. Daffos F, Capella-Pavlovsky M, Forestier F. Fetal blood sampling via the umbilical vein using a needle guided by ultrasound: report of 66 cases. Prenat Diagn 1983;3:271.
54. Soothill PW. Cordocentesis: role in the assessment of fetal condition. Clin Perinatol 1989;16:755.
55. Soothill PW, Nicolaides KH, Rodeck CH, et al. The effect of gestational age on blood gas and acid base values in the human pregnancy. Fetal Therapy 1986;1:168.
56. Nicolaides, KH, Economides DL, Soothill PW. Perinatal asphyxia, hyperlacticacidemia, hypoglycemia and erythroblastosis in growth retarded fetuses. Br Med J 1987;1:1051.

57. Bowman JM, Manning FA. Intrauterine fetal transfusions: Winnipeg, 1982. Obstet Gynecol 1983;61:203.
58. Manning FA, Harman CR. Fetal transfusion in operative obstetrics. In: Iffy CD, Apuzzio JJ, Vintzileos AM, eds. New York: McGraw-Hill, 1992:80.
59. Harman CR, Bowman JM, Manning FA, et al. Intrauterine transfusion—intraperitoneal versus intravascular approach: a case-control study. Am J Obstet Gynecol 1990;162:1053.
60. Harman CR. Fetal monitoring in the alloimmunized pregnancy. Clin Perinatol 1989;16:691.

Neonatology: Pathophysiology and Management of the Newborn, Fourth Edition,
edited by Gordon B. Avery, Mary Ann Fletcher, and Mhairi G. MacDonald.
J.B. Lippincott Company, Philadelphia © 1994.

chapter 14

Fetal Therapy

MARK I. EVANS
MICHAEL R. HARRISON
MARK P. JOHNSON
WOLFGANG HOLZGREVE

The whole process of prenatal diagnosis is full of irony—not only from the perspective of the abortion debate, but also because of the inherent potential for conflict between mother and fetus. The development of interventive fetal therapies serves simultaneously to heighten and diminish the ethical arguments in abortion *versus* fetal rights debates. The development of fetal therapy closes the logical loop of diagnosis leading to treatment for fetuses with anomalies.

Several questions arise when a potentially correctable fetal anomaly is diagnosed[1]:

What is the natural outcome of this anomaly?
Will additional or irreversible damage be caused to the fetus if repair procedures are delayed until after birth?
Is it possible to correct the anomaly or its consequences *in utero*?
Will the procedure change the natural outcome?
What is the risk to the mother and the fetus?

Surgical intervention *in utero* should be considered only if:

The natural history of the anomaly frequently is associated with a severe neonatal handicap or early death.
There is evidence from animal models that the natural history of the anomaly can be significantly changed by the surgical procedure.
The risk to the mother is relatively small, as proven in a rigorous animal model (*e.g.*, the nonhuman primate).

As fetal therapy has developed, approaches have been compartmentalized either by fetal disease as such or by the specific modality of treatment. We have found the latter approach to be more useful, and divide interventive fetal therapies into percutaneous *in utero* surgical procedures, open fetal surgical procedures, and noninvasive medical therapies.

PERCUTANEOUS SURGERY

Fetal surgery is not new. The first attempts were transfusions for hemolytic anemias by Liley in the early 1960s.[2] With the increasing sophistication of ultrasound, the development of intravascular transfusions and prevention of Rh disease with RhoGam (Ortho Diagnostic Systems, Raritan, NJ), fetal death or severe complications from fetal anemia are much less common than a generation ago.[3] The role of fetal transfusion is discussed elsewhere in this volume (see Chap. 13).

VENTRICULOMEGALY

Much of the focus in the early 1980s of the potential for fetal therapy centered on obstructive ventriculomegaly (Fig. 14-1).[4] Interest in this disorder emerged from the relative ease in diagnosing such anomalies by ultrasound and the success rates of a simple shunting procedure performed in the neonate. The concept of interventive surgical therapy in the fetus, as developed in animal models, was that early shunting of ventriculomegaly *in utero* might prevent the irreversible damage caused by prolonged increased intracranial pressure.

In humans, however, the results achieved with ventriculoamniotic shunts seem at first glance to be very disappointing. As of March 1993, 45 cases of fetal ventriculomegaly treated *in utero* by chorionic ventriculoamniotic shunts have been reported to the International Fetal Registry.[5] In most instances, the shunting was performed on a fetus presumed to have ventriculomegaly–hydrocephalus secondary to aqueductal stenosis. The mean gestational age at diagnosis was 25 ± 2.73 weeks (range, 18–31 weeks), and the mean age at treatment was 27 ± 2.6 weeks (range, 23–33 weeks). The duration of effective therapy cannot be determined from registry data because objective means of assessment of shunt function are not available. Of 41 fetuses with hydrocephalus treated by ventriculoamniotic shunting, 34 have survived (83%). Of the seven deaths that occurred, four could be attributed directly to trauma at the time of placement of the shunt or to premature labor and delivery occurring within 48 hours of shunt placement. The crude mortality rate for the procedure thus is 9%. The 38 surviving infants have been followed on average for 12.2 ± 5.8 months (range, 6–36 months). Of the 34 surviving fetuses, 14 (33.5%), all with aqueductal stenosis, are reported as normal at follow-up evaluation. The remaining 24 survivors all have exhibited varying degrees of neurologic handicap; most of these children (18 of 34 survivors, 53%) are classified as having severe handicaps. These infants all exhibited gross delay in reaching developmental milestones, and the tested development quotient was always less than 60. Five of these infants have cortical blindness, three have seizure disorders, and two have spastic diplegia. Outcome among survivors was related principally to the primary etiology of obstructive hydrocephalus. Aqueductal stenosis of uncertain etiology was the most common etiologic factor for obstructive hydrocephalus (28 of 41 cases, 68%), and the only intact survivors were found in this group.

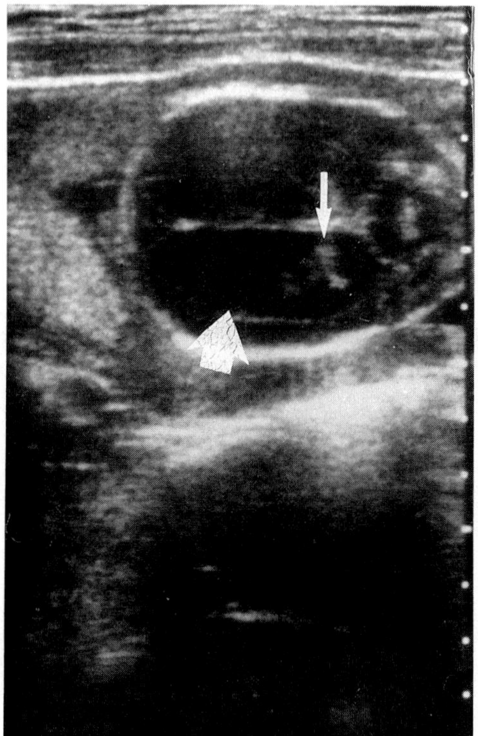

FIG. 14–1. Ultrasound reveals ventriculomegaly in an 18-week fetus. The lateral ventricles (*thick arrow*) and the choroid plexus (*thin arrow*) are visible.

The results of ventriculoamniotic shunting for fetal ventriculomegaly have been disappointing,[6] and consequently there has been a *de facto* moratorium in place since the early 1980s. The hope, which was to take fetuses who otherwise would be severely impaired by ventriculomegaly and circumvent irreversible damage by intrauterine surgical treatment, was substituted in a few instances with survival of severely affected infants who otherwise would have died.

Despite the poor outcomes in treated fetuses, abandonment of the concept of *in utero* shunting for ventriculomegaly must be reconsidered for several reasons.[7] Analysis of the reported cases in the registry of ventriculoamniotic shunt placement performed in the 1980s shows that selection criteria were not always used appropriately, and fetuses with ventriculomegaly associated with other severe anomalies (*i.e.*, holoprosencephaly or autosomal trisomies) also were given intrauterine treatment despite the fact that even with therapy the prognosis was extremely poor.

Current reports demonstrate that the natural history of fetal ventriculomegaly also is dismal (Table 14-1).[7] The major prognostic determinants are the association with other intracranial or extracranial malformations. Additional malformations are found in 70% to 85% of fetuses with ventriculomegaly, and all such cases suffer high perinatal mortality or severe morbidity. Even if a diligent search for additional malformations is performed by combining a detailed ultrasound study of the fetus with amniocentesis for karyotype and amniotic fluid α-fetoprotein and acetylcholinesterase, 20% to 40% of abnormalities would not be detected, even by experienced personnel.

The obvious candidates for *in utero* ventricular shunting are the fetuses with isolated progressive ventriculomegaly. These are limited in number by the

TABLE 14–1
VENTRICULOMEGALY: GROUPS AND OUTCOMES

CATEGORY	TREATMENT	OUTCOME
Ventriculomegaly with other anomalies	No	90%–100% Severe
Ventriculomegaly with other anomalies	Yes	70%–90% Moderate–severe
Isolated ventriculomegaly, nonprogressive	No	80% Normal
Isolated ventriculomegaly, progressive	Yes	50%–80% Moderate–severe

high rate of associated anomalies and by the relative failure to exclude additional malformations prenatally. The severity of ventriculomegaly, however, is not always predictive of outcome or even of the need for postnatal shunt, because ventriculomegaly may not be associated with elevated intracranial pressure.

Considering the uncertainty and difficulty of accurate prenatal diagnosis, intrauterine treatment of fetal ventriculomegaly remains a controversial and highly experimental procedure that is moribund because a *de facto* moratorium is in place. When the option in midtrimester is between termination of pregnancy or inactive observation of progressive dilatation of the ventricles, however, placement of a ventriculoamniotic shunt should present a third option in select isolated cases. Given the small number of good candidates and the need to develop a new shunt catheter (none is available), a future study should be performed in one of the select centers experienced in the technical aspects of ventriculoamniotic shunt placement that might resolve the questions of its efficacy and usefulness for the prevention of long-term sequelae in obstructive ventriculomegaly–hydrocephaly.

OBSTRUCTIVE UROPATHY

The widespread use of obstetric ultrasonography and the increase in resolution and technical expertise permit more frequent recognition of obstructive uropathies earlier in pregnancy (Fig. 14-2). The development of high-resolution ultrasound has allowed detection of numerous parenchymal and collecting system abnormalities of the fetal urogenital system.[8] Several reports have addressed the poor prognosis of fetuses with persistent urinary obstruction, particularly with oligohydramnios and resultant pulmonary hypoplasia.[9,10] Poor prognosis is associated with persistent obstruction that results in reflux of urine, which eventually can destroy the renal parenchyma and not allow pulmonary development because of severe oligohydramnios.[11,12] Retrograde pressure forms behind the obstruction and accelerated reflux causes increasing dilation of the urinary system with progressive hydronephrosis and compression of renal parenchyma.[9] As documented in animal studies, hydronephrosis predisposes to dysplastic degeneration within the renal parenchyma.[13,14] The severe oligohydramnios associated with bilateral urinary tract obstruction results in pressure deformities of the face and limbs, and pulmonary hypoplasia. Paradoxically, neonatal death is caused by respiratory insufficiency and not renal failure. The timing of onset and the degree of obstruction are crucial determinants in the development of irreversible renal and pulmonary damage, with onset before 22 weeks of gestation associated with poorer outcome if intervention is not attempted.[15–17]

PREDICTORS OF REVERSIBLE DISEASE

Prenatally, several parameters have been used in the evaluation of renal function in fetuses with obstructive uropathy, including amniotic fluid volume, ultrasound appearance of kidneys, and biochemical composition of fetal urine. It must be remembered that

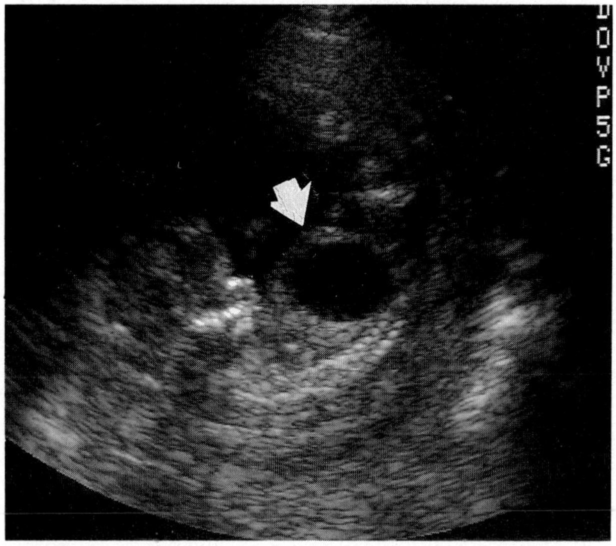

FIG. 14–2. Ultrasound reveals a distended bladder (*arrow*) in a fetus at week 13 of gestational age.

information about renal function derived from urinary metabolites remains controversial.

In a retrospective study of 40 fetuses with obstructive uropathy, Crombleholme and coworkers reported that urine sodium of less than 100 mmol/L was associated with good renal function.[18] Similarly, Grannum and colleagues measured urinary sodium in 12 fetuses with obstructive uropathy and demonstrated that the 4 fetuses with urine sodium under 100 mmol/L had either normal neonatal renal function or no evidence of renal dysplasia, whereas the 8 fetuses with urine sodium over 100 mmol/L had renal dysplastic changes.[19]

In contrast, Wilkins and colleagues and Elder and associates reported that fetal urine electrolytes in their studies were not accurate predictors of outcome.[20,21] Thus, in their combined series of 13 fetuses with obstructive uropathy, only four of the seven with urinary sodium over 100 mmol/L had poor outcome or histologic evidence of renal dysplasia, and only one of the six fetuses with urinary sodium under 100 mmol/L had good renal function after birth. One possible explanation for the apparent discrepancy in results is that in these studies no consideration was given to the gestational age at which the fetuses were sampled because another study has demonstrated that the composition of fetal urine changes with gestational age.[22]

In the antenatal evaluation of obstructive uropathy, the ultrasonographic finding of multicystic kidneys is associated with renal dysplasia; abnormal urinary biochemistries merely confirm the underlying poor renal function. In contrast, both the degree of pelvicalyceal dilation and amount of amniotic fluid volume present in hydronephrosis are poor predictors of outcome. In these cases, urodochocentesis or pyelocentesis with measurement of sodium, calcium, urea, and creatinine provide useful information for more accurate assessment of underlying renal function and subsequent counseling of the parents. Fetal urinary biochemistry provides a rational basis for selecting patients who may benefit from vesicoamniotic shunting or other intrauterine urinary diversion procedure and allows evaluation of the effectiveness of such therapeutic interventions. Poor renal function can be inferred reliably when high urinary sodium, calcium, and sodium–calcium levels, and low urea and creatinine are found in percutaneously aspirated fetal urine.

Urine Biochemistry. Mueller and Dumez have evaluated multiple urinary parameters and found sodium, β_2-microglobulin, NH_3, and creatinine to be good predictions of renal function and long-term outcome (Table 14-2).[14] Data from Detroit suggest that a single fetal urine test may be insufficient to declare irreversible damage.[17] After decompression, improvement in urine biochemistry or its failure to improve as shown in serial measurements may be more representative of ultimate outcome. Decompression by either percutaneous needle aspiration or *in utero* shunting is warranted in carefully selected cases and can save fetuses who would otherwise very likely be doomed. We believe that serial urine aspirations for biochemical profile are an essential part of the evaluation of obstructive uropathies. The initial urine obtained by percutaneous bladder aspiration represents urine that has been present in the bladder over a period of time.

Karyotyping. Intrauterine treatment should be reserved for cases with bilateral urinary tract obstruction, demonstrated reasonable renal function, decreased amniotic fluid volume, and no associated life-threatening anomalies.[17] Cytogenetic anomalies and congenital malformations of other systems are diagnosed in about 15% of cases of fetal obstructive uropathy. The evaluation should include fetal karyotype, echocardiography, and a detailed ultrasound examination to assess renal size and parenchymal thickness as well as to detect dysplastic changes, bladder filling, and additional malformations.[17] Different types of chromosomal abnormalities seem to relate to different patterns of renal defects. In mild

TABLE 14–2
FETAL URINE BIOCHEMISTRY

	Dead	Alive	Good Function	Poor Function
Na (mmol/L)	112	53	46	57
Ca (mg/dL)	1.99	0.93	0.67	1.27
PO_4 (mg/24 h)	1.40	0.28	0.08	0.51
GLU (mg/dL)	2.89	0.38	0.19	0.65
NH_3 (mg/L)	192	654	767	493
CR (mg/dL)	5.61	8.65	9.20	8.00
TP (mg/dL)	1.18	0.04	0.02	0.06
β_2-MICRO (mg/dL)	16.0	3.16	1.02	5.7

GLU, glucose; CR, creatinine; TP, total protein; β_2-MICRO, β_2-microglobulin.
From Mueller F, Dumez Y. Contribution of biochemistry to prenatal diagnosis of obstructive uropathies. Am J Human Genet 1991;49(4):175.

hydronephrosis, the most common chromosome abnormality is trisomy 21, whereas in moderate to severe hydronephrosis, multicystic kidneys, or renal agenesis, the most common abnormalities are trisomies 18 and 13. If fetal visualization is hampered by severe oligohydramnios, artificial installation of fluid by amnioinfusion will improve sonographic visibility and fetal assessment. The observation of fetal behavior (drinking, filling of the stomach and bladder) makes the study of fetal anatomy more accurate.

SHUNT PROCEDURES

Most placements of vesicoamniotic shunts have been performed percutaneously using ultrasonographic guidance.[17] A double-coiled nylon catheter has been used in most cases with good results. One-way valve catheters are not necessary because the pressure in the obstructed bladder usually exceeds that in the amniotic fluid and there is no apparent harm in amniotic fluid entering the fetal bladder (Figs. 14-3 and 14-4).

The function of these shunts, however, may be impaired by occlusion or displacement, necessitating close observation and replacement of a nonfunctioning shunt. When weeks to months of continuous drainage are required, some favor open surgical decompression by bladder marsupialization or bilateral ureterostomies; however, this would involve an increased risk to both mother and fetus.

OUTCOME

The fetal surgery registry coordinated by Dr. Frank Manning of the University of Manitoba lists 98 cases as of March 1992, treated by indwelling shunts. The longest follow-up is over 11 years and the overall survival has been 40.8%. Particularly at the beginning of the series, a number of patients were inappropriately chosen for surgery, which considerably lowers the survival statistics. For example, several fetuses were shunted before the elucidation of a chromosome abnormality. When appropriately stratified by etiology, survival reaches as much as 70% for a male fetus with a posterior urethral valve (Tables 14-3 through 14-5).

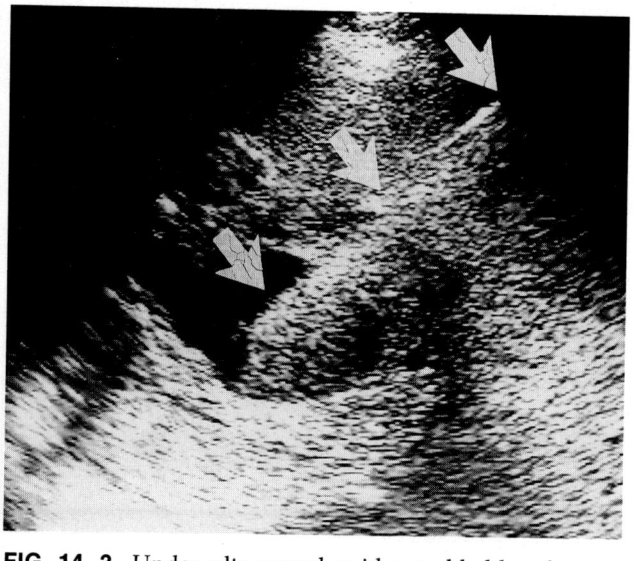

FIG. 14–3. Under ultrasound guidance, bladder shunt is introduced percutaneously (*arrows*) into the fetal bladder.

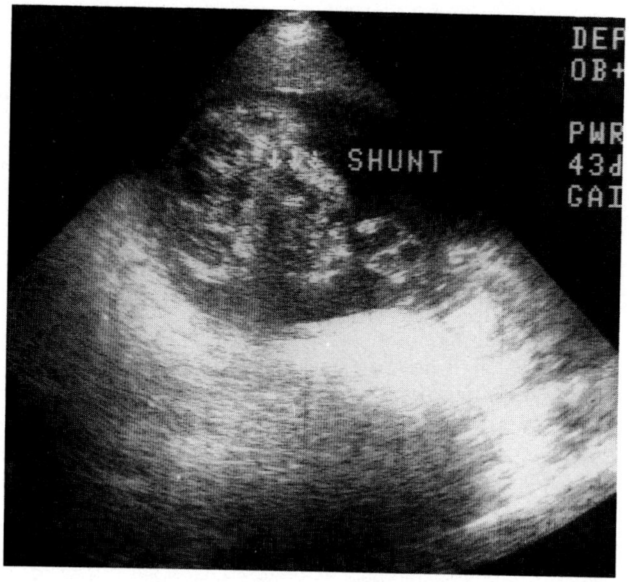

FIG. 14–4. Ultrasound shows the bladder shunt in place (*arrows*). The distal portion is within the bladder, and the proximal portion is free in the amniotic cavity, where it drains fetal urine.

Attempts to develop more accurate assessments of the degree and reversibility of renal compromise, specific etiologies, and likelihood for successful prenatal or postnatal treatment have been thwarted by a poor understanding of normal fetal urine biochemistry. Such confusion has been compounded further by conflicting inferences about the significance of different biochemical parameters in compromised situations. Originally, it was suggested that a urine sodium of greater than 100 mEq/L indicated irreversible renal damage. Mueller and Dumez have proposed that β_2-microglobulin might be a more sensitive indicator and have further demonstrated gestational age variations for several fetal urine parameters.[13,14] No parameter or combination, however, is believed to offer satisfactory evidence of long-term renal competence or compromise, and the search goes on to find more specific markers.[17]

The many patients who have undergone successful shunting procedures are a testimonial to the potential benefits of early, aggressive evaluation of fetal renal function and for fetal treatment in selected cases of obstructive uropathies (see Figs. 14-3 and 14-4). Our data also suggest that placement of a suprapubic fetal bladder shunt need not be considered the rule in pri-

TABLE 14–3
FETAL OBSTRUCTIVE UROPATHY: PRIMARY DIAGNOSIS* AND OUTCOME IN 98 CASES

Primary Diagnosis	Number of Cases	Percentage of Total	Number of Survivors	Percentage Survival by Diagnosis
Posterior urethral valve syndrome	31	31.6	22	70.96
Karyotype abnormality	7	7.14	0	0
Renal dysplasia by ultrasound	6	6.12	0	0
Urethral atresia	8	8.2	1	12.5
Prune-belly syndrome	5	5.10	4	80
Unknown	1	1.00	1	100
Cloacal anomalies	1	1.00	0	0
Ureteropelvic function obstruction	2	2.04	2	100
Unknown etiology	37	37.8	10	27
Total	98	100.0	40	40.8

* Total of 11 new cases: six cases of posterior urethral valve—five survived, one therapeutic abortion performed at 21 weeks for persistent oligohydramnios; two cases of urethral atresia (*i.e.*, neonatal death renal dysplasia and respiratory failure); one case of cloacal anomalies resulting in neonatal death; and two cases in which diagnoses were not available. One of the patients with urethral atresia had Down syndrome.

From the Fetal Surgery Registry, courtesy of Frank Manning, M.D., University of Manitoba, Canada. Data was gathered until March 1993.

TABLE 14–4
FETAL OBSTRUCTIVE UROPATHY: OUTCOME AS RELATED TO GESTATIONAL AGE AT DIAGNOSIS AND AT TREATMENT

	At Initial Diagnosis			At Treatment		
Gestational Age (wk)	Number of Patients	Number of Survivors	Percentage Surviving	Number of Patients	Number of Survivors	Percentage Surviving
<20	36	12	33.3	27	8	37.8
20–22	10	5	50.0	9	3	33.3
22–24	15	5	33.3	15	3	20.0
24–26	10	4	40.0	13	4	30.8
26–28	8	5	62.5	11	9	81.8
28–30	5	2	20.0	8	5	62.5
30–32	6	4	66.7	7	3	66.7
>32	8	3	37.5	8	5	62.5
Total	98	40	40.8	98	40	40.81

From the Fetal Surgery Registry, courtesy of Frank Manning, M.D., University of Manitoba, Canada. Data was gathered until March 1993.

TABLE 14–5
FETAL OBSTRUCTIVE UROPATHY: CLASSIFICATION OF 58 DEATHS BY PRIMARY ETIOLOGY

	Time of Death			
Etiology of Death	Stillbirth	Postnatal	**Total Number of Deaths**	**Percentage of All Deaths**
Elective termination	15	0	15	25.9
Associated anomalies	1	0	1	1.7
Procedure related	3	2	5	8.6
Pulmonary hypoplasia	0	34	34	58.6
Renal disease	0	3	3	5.2
Total	19	39	58	100.0

* From the Fetal Surgery Registry, courtesy of Frank Manning, M.D., University of Manitoba, Canada. Data was gathered until March 1993.

mary treatment of obstructive uropathies.[17] The clinician must consider alternatives, keeping in mind the long-term problems associated with an indwelling catheter (obstruction, displacement, anatomic damage, and iatrogenic ventral wall defects) before committing a fetus to such therapy.

Furthermore, not only does fetal renal function seem to improve after percutaneous fine needle bladder decompression, but in a number of cases the underlying etiology apparently resolved because megalocystis did not redevelop. This has led to our hypothesis that the release of the intravesicular pressure may allow the posterior urethral valves to fall open, or may relieve the pressures that led to a functional obstruction due to a secondary spasm of the bladder neck.

In those instances in which abnormal fetal urine biochemistry failed to improve despite decompression and the relief of obstruction, the prognosis was confirmed on follow-up as dismal and the outcome poor.

The exact benefits and risks of decompression are unclear. It is certain that correction of oligohydramnios is critical to pulmonary development. Without a reasonable amniotic fluid volume, pulmonary hypoplasia and no subsequent chance for survival can be expected.

Whether decompression prevents, reverses, or merely forestalls renal damage cannot yet be concluded. We believe that serial evaluation probably is better than a single measurement, particularly if values are abnormal. It seems reasonable that the relief of obstruction would allow a rapidly developing fetal organ either to regenerate or at least not suffer further damage.

With increasing ultrasound and biochemical sophistication, it is obvious that most of the initial early attempts at fetal urinary diversion were performed on poorly chosen patients. There is a need to start afresh in creating a data base to evaluate the natural history, pathophysiology, and possibilities for intervention.

Recently, Crombleholme and associates have analyzed the data from the San Francisco program.[18] They categorized patients on the basis of a normal karyotype, normal ultrasound, and urine biochemistry. They used a sodium under 100 mEq/L, an osmolality of no more than 210 mOsm/L, and a chloride of less than 90 mEq/L as indicators that the prospect for acceptable renal function was "good."[18] Survival was better with *in utero* intervention in both their good and poor groups (89% *vs.* 70%, and 30% *vs.* 0%, respectively), but no single factor was indicative of prognosis.[18]

No one center is likely to have enough cases to develop universal criteria, and therefore a flexible approach based on each center's experience will be required until there are more definitive data. Our data and others suggest an approach to the management of obstructive uropathy. Some points follow directly from the data but others are still speculative because all studies, including our own, are to some degree uncontrolled.[13–23]

The list below summarizes the shared conclusions and approaches of the major investigators in the field to the evaluation of fetuses with obstructive uropathies.[17]

Urinary tract decompression has a place in the management of isolated distal obstruction in fetuses who do not have underlying irreversible renal pathologic conditions.

Decompression with restoration of amniotic fluid volume should improve pulmonary status, but the reversibility of damaged renal parenchyma after decompression is unclear.

Early, aggressive identification of potential candidates for shunting is appropriate in obstructive uropathies. The mere drainage of urine may suffice to relieve a urethral obstruction and should be the first interventive therapy attempted.

Experience with very early gestational ages both for needle decompression and bladder shunting is encouraging and suggests that the earlier a pathologic condition can be reversed, the greater the potential for return to normality.

A single evaluation of fetal urine may not correctly reflect current or future renal function. Relief of obstruction may bring about improved parameters from which speculation about the resilience of fetal renal tissues can occur.

It is not yet possible to distinguish factors concerning the amelioration of lung pathologic conditions for those fetuses that show improved renal function and are therefore candidates for vesicoamniotic shunting. Improvement of amniotic fluid volume after decompression or shunting likely will prove to be an important element in fetal lung development and maturation.

Iatrogenic abdominal wall defects may be a complication of urinary shunts secondary to the active or passive fetal displacement of the indwelling catheters.

Fetuses with persistent megalocystis, but whose biochemical parameters after initial decompression improved on successive aspirations (sodium < 100, osmolality < 200), probably represent the group most likely to require and benefit from further invasive interventive fetal therapy.

CONDITIONS THAT CAUSE INTRATHORACIC OR MEDIASTINAL COMPRESSION

Intrauterine intrathoracic and mediastinal compression by conditions such as cystic adenomatoid malformation and pleural effusions can lead to the development of hydrops and polyhydramnios, which are associated with a high risk of premature delivery and intrauterine or neonatal death.

Isolated pleural and pericardial effusions or pulmonary cysts in the fetus may either resolve spontaneously or they can be effectively treated after birth. Nevertheless, in some cases where onset is early in gestation, or progression is rapid, severe and chronic compression of the fetal lungs can result in pulmonary hypoplasia and subsequent neonatal death. In others, mediastinal compression may lead to the development of hydrops and polyhydramnios, which, as mentioned, are associated with a high risk of premature delivery and perinatal death.

The data from fetuses with isolated idiopathic pleural or pericardial effusions suggest that certainly in some cases, short-term decompression by thoracocenteses or temporary drainage may disrupt the underlying pathologic condition. In most cases, however, the fluid reaccumulates within 24 hours, requiring repeated procedures that are likely to be more traumatic than thoracoamniotic shunting.

Thoracoamniotic shunting also is an effective and apparently safe method for chronic drainage of fetal pleural effusions or pulmonary cysts. It can reverse idiopathic nonimmune fetal hydrops, resolve polyhydramnios and thereby reduce the risk of preterm delivery, and may also prevent pulmonary hypoplasia. Nevertheless, in a high proportion of nonimmune hydropic fetuses (50% in our series), thoracoamniotic shunting did not prevent their ultimate death due to the underlying disease responsible for the hydrops.

OPEN SURGERY

Although the percutaneous approach under ultrasonographic guidance seems to be the preferred method for placing a shunt in a hollow enlarged viscus, the correction of more complex fetal anomalies requires more extensive and invasive surgery on both mother and fetus.[23] The feasibility of open fetal surgery was demonstrated anecdotally in the 1960s when an open technique was used for intrauterine exchange transfusions in erythroblastosis fetalis. Preterm labor and abortion, however, made this initial experience so discouraging that direct extrauterine exposure of the fetus was abandoned for over a decade.[23] In the late 1970s and early 1980s, interest in open fetal surgery was revived by two factors. Prenatal diagnoses of several simple, anatomic defects (*e.g.*, fatal pulmonary hypoplasia secondary to urinary tract obstruction or diaphragmatic hernia) were being made more easily and earlier. At the same time, neonatologists and pediatric surgeons were coming to grips with the futility of attempting to salvage these babies after birth. It became increasingly apparent that the only way to salvage fetuses with these lesions was by open extrauterine fetal surgery.

In the early 1980s, the fetal therapy group at the University of California, San Francisco, studied the

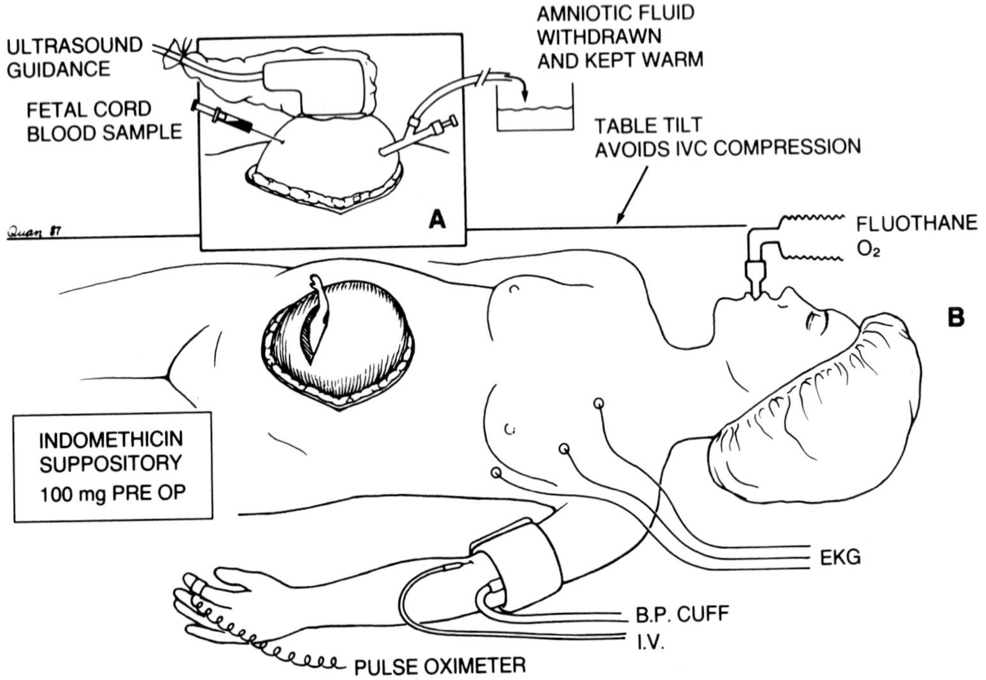

FIG. 14–5. Maternal positioning and monitoring during fetal surgery. **(A)** After laparotomy and uterine exposure, the placenta is localized by ultrasound, fetal blood is withdrawn, and amniotic fluid is preserved. **(B)** Maternal positioning includes tilting to avoid compression of the inferior vena cava by the gravid uterus. The hysterotomy is made away from the placenta, and only the fetal anatomy is exposed. Maternal monitoring consists of heart rate, electrocardiogram, blood pressure, and pulse oximetry. (From Longaker MT, Golbus MS, Filly RT, et al. Maternal outcome after open fetal surgery. A review of the first 17 human cases. JAMA 1991;265:739.)

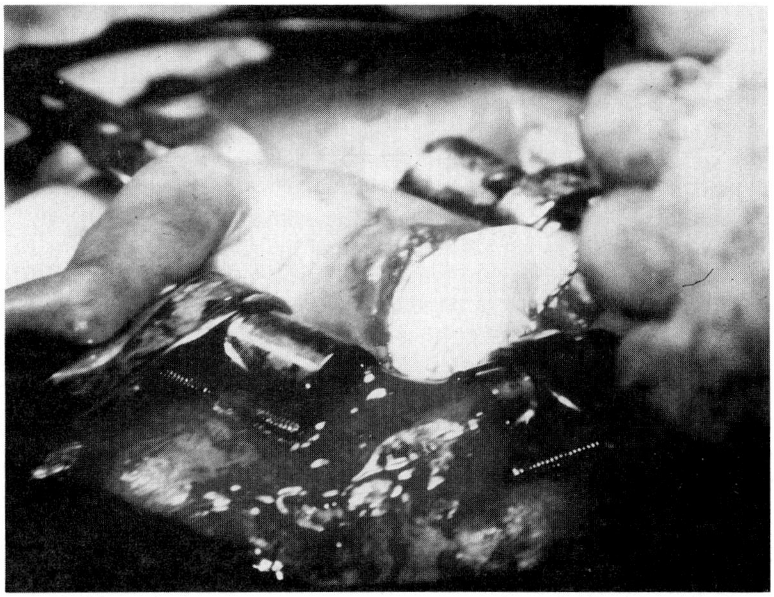

FIG. 14–6. The fetus is exteriorized from the uterus in open fetal surgery.

pathophysiology of diaphragmatic hernia and hydronephrosis in animal models, defined the natural history and outcome of diaphragmatic hernia and obstructive uropathy in human fetuses, and developed the anesthetic, pharmacologic, and surgical techniques in the nonhuman primate necessary to make open fetal surgery safe for both mother and fetus.[24]

Throughout the 1980s and early 1990s, the San Francisco group has performed over two dozen open fetal surgeries for obstructive uropathies, congenital diaphragmatic hernias, and congenital cystic adenomatoid malformations of the lung. Creating vesicostomies for obstructive uropathy and lobectomies for cystic adenomatoid malformations has been quite successful, with salvage of most of these severely affected fetuses. Repair of congenital diaphragmatic hernias (CDH), however, has proven deceptively difficult (Figs. 14-5 and 14-6). Despite extensive work in animal models, the first attempts failed due to unforeseen technical problems. The most difficult was the unexpected finding of significant amounts of liver as well as bowel in the chest cavity. The bowel could be reduced without difficulty; however, when attempts were made to reposition the liver back into its normal intraabdominal position, the umbilical vein would kink, leading to vascular collapse.[23] Eventually, the presence of a significant proportion of the liver in the chest became an exclusion criterion, and subsequently patient number 7 proved to be the first successful delivery of a viable infant after this revolutionary new surgery (see Figs. 14-5 and 14-6).[25] Since then, in patients who meet the new criteria, the survival rate has been about 50%.*

* Adzick NS, personal communication, June 1992.

There is considerable controversy as to the efficacy of open fetal surgery for CDH because survival rates by concurrent therapy (*i.e.*, postnatal extracorporeal membrane oxygenation) and surgery vary from 5% to 50%. It is clear that the only way to resolve the question of the role of prenatal surgery in CDH will be to perform randomized, controlled studies of fetal surgery *versus* postnatal treatment.

A major side benefit of the fetal surgery program has been the discovery that fetal wounds seem to heal without a scar. Extensive work now suggests that the mechanism by which the fetus heals is fundamentally different from adult healing in the organization of collagen deposition and the composition of the extracellular matrix, especially with regard to hyaluronic acid.

There are several potential uses for the knowledge gained from the study of fetal wound healing. Scarless healing would allow plastic surgeons to do less obtrusive reconstructive and plastic repairs. In the future, craniofacial malformations and some types of cleft lip and palate may be corrected early *in utero* to take advantage of rapid scar-free healing and the prevention of secondary disruption sequences in these disorders.

MEDICAL THERAPY

Although surgical experiments, particularly the first successes of open fetal surgery,[25] have gained more notoriety in the lay media, some of the most significant advances in fetal therapy have been pharmacologic. Medical fetal therapy has been effective in two main areas, the prevention of external genital masculinization in female fetuses affected with 21-hydroxylase deficiency (congenital adrenal hyperplasia,

[CAH]) and the correction of fetal cardiac arrhythmias than can lead to nonimmune fetal hydrops and fetal death. The pharmacology of the fetus can be altered in some other areas, although the usefulness of such alterations is less well established. The correction of fetal cardiac arrhythmias has been accomplished in hundreds of cases.

The spectrum of pharmacologic interventions includes attempts in which there have been documented reversals of pathophysiology, prevention of structural anomalies, and biochemical alterations of questionable clinical significance. With evolving sophistication of diagnostic techniques, there is an increasing confidence in the ability to transfer agents into the fetus. The debate now moves to when and who to treat, and the best way to treat the fetus (*i.e.*, either indirectly through the mother and placenta, or directly into the fetus by injection or through cordocentesis).

CONGENITAL ADRENAL HYPERPLASIA

The fetal adrenal gland can be suppressed pharmacologically by maternal replacement doses of dexamethasone.[26,27] In CAH caused by 21-hydroxylase deficiency, impaired metabolism in the pathway between cholesterol and cortisol creates excess 17-OH progesterone, which is shunted through other pathways into the production of androstenedione and androgens. Consequently, genetically normal females are exposed to excess androgens and can be masculinized. The subsequent abnormal differentiation can vary from clitoral hypertrophy to complete formation of a phallus and apparent scrotum.

In an attempt to prevent this birth defect, Evans and colleagues first administered dexamethasone, a fluorinated steroid, to an at-risk mother beginning on the tenth week of gestation. Maternal estriol and cortisol values indicated rapid and sustained fetal and maternal adrenal gland suppression. This fetus ultimately turned out to be a carrier for 21-hydroxylase deficiency.[26] After the initial observation of Evans and colleagues, Forrest and David used the same protocol of 0.25 mg of dexamethasone four times daily beginning at 9 weeks to treat several fetuses, and demonstrated that fetuses known to be clinically affected with CAH were spared external congenital masculinization.[27] To date, several infants with classic CAH, who clearly would have been masculinized, have been born with normal genitalia.[28,29] In a few cases, some masculinization still has been observed after this regimen beginning at 9 weeks. Current protocol, therefore, is to begin therapy at 7 weeks, although there have been too few cases to assess this modification.[28,29] These events represent the first prevention of a birth defect and may serve as a model for other attempts at pharmacologic fetal therapy. One interesting element to this first case was the fact that therapy had to begin long before a diagnosis was possible. With the autosomal recessive genetics of CAH, only one of eight pregnancies would be expected to benefit (females with CAH). With the availability of a molecular probe for the CAH gene,[30] a nearly definitive diagnosis may be possible by DNA analysis of chorionic villi in the first trimester, although, still, the diagnosis is possible only several weeks after the initiation of steroid therapy.

The fundamental principles addressed in such attempted prevention of masculinization are logically extended to other medical fetal therapies. The concepts of a thoroughly informed consent procedure, thorough documentation of progress, and high-risk obstetric management generally have been followed by subsequent investigators in this field.

CARDIAC THERAPY

The treatment of fetal cardiac anomalies is an extensive topic that ranges far beyond the space available here; however, just as cardioversion is performed neonatally with pharmacologic agents targeted to the specific arrhythmia, the same approach is applicable to the fetus. The major difference, of course, is the indirect route the drug must take to the fetus, first having to go through the mother, and thus being exposed to degradation by the maternal liver.

RHYTHM AND RATE

Early in gestation, the fetal heart rate averages 140 beats per minute (bpm) and as the fetus approaches 40 weeks gestation, the mean heart rate is more in the range of 120 bpm. Although early in gestation there is very little variability in heart rate, the fetus develops beat-to-beat variability as it matures concomitant with the development of parasympathetic innervation to the sinus node. Sinus arrhythmia may occur in the later stages of pregnancy. As a general rule, fetal tachycardia is defined as heart rates greater than 180 bpm, with bradycardia being less than 100 bpm.

Benign arrhythmias are common and do not require any intervention. Sinus bradycardia is the most common of these rhythms and occurs often early in pregnancy.[31] It also is noted frequently during abdominal ultrasonography because the umbilical cord may be compressed or placental blood flow compromised by the gravid uterus compressing the maternal vena cava and aorta when the mother is lying supine during examination. This type of intermittent sinus bradycardia is benign. It must be distinguished from apparent slow heart rate caused by blocked premature atrial contractions. A fetal echocardiogram is helpful in distinguishing the two. Sinus bradycardia that is not intermittent is unusual, but can be associated with severe fetal compromise and may represent a preterminal event. There is no treatment *per se* for persistent sinus bradycardia, although the mother and the fetus should be observed carefully for untoward events.

Atrial and ventricular ectopic beats generally are benign. Atrial ectopy is far more common than ventricular and is more likely to occur in the latter third of pregnancy. Ectopic beats are not uncommon during labor and generally are not associated with physiologic or anatomic abnormalities. As mentioned previously, this rhythm should be distinguished from sinus bradycardia. Although it has been reported that fetal atrial ectopy can lead to supraventricular tachycardia, this is not generally accepted.

More significant fetal arrhythmias may lead to hydrops fetalis.[32] Approximately 30% of nonimmune hydrops is related to a cardiac disorder, and one-half of these may be related to a fetal arrhythmia. It generally is thought that intermittent arrhythmias alone do not result in hydrops. Hydrops fetalis, however, is a true fetal emergency, and thus efforts to diagnose a particular arrhythmia and institute treatment are extremely important.

Specific arrhythmias appropriate for treatment include complete atrioventricular block and atrial and ventricular tachycardias. Agents for treatment have evolved over time, paralleling the development of cardiac agents in adults. A major debate exists as to whether newer, longer-acting drugs should be injected directly into the fetus or through cordocentesis, obviating the need for transplacental transfer in which incomplete passage is known to occur. Furthermore, direct injection would reduce the risk of maternal toxicity, which is a major factor to consider in *in utero* treatment. Also, as noted earlier, a significant percentage of maternally administered drug can be lost through the first and subsequent passages through the maternal liver.

NEURAL TUBE DEFECTS

There are historical data in humans suggesting increased neural tube defect (NTD) frequencies in subjects with poor dietary histories or with intestinal bypasses. Smithells and associates originally suggested that vitamin supplementation—and perhaps folate alone—could reduce the frequency of NTD recurrence in families with one or more prior affected children.[33] Pooled data from investigations in different centers using Smithell's mixture of vitamins and minerals showed that NTD recurrence in the offspring of women treated with vitamin supplements was about 0.7%, whereas recurrence in women who did not receive supplements was about 4.6%.[34–36] In 1991, the seemingly definitive study was published showing conclusively that there is a definite reduction in recurrence risks from the use of preconceptual and early gestation folic acid supplementation in patients with histories of offspring affected by NTD.[37]

GENE THERAPY

The drugs of fetal therapy of the late 1990s likely will be replacement genes. Gene introduction by infection with genes integrated into retroviral vectors could be applied at extremely early stages; there are at least two examples in animal models where such transfer of genes into the preimplantation embryo has resulted in correction of a genetic defect. One involved genetic correction of hypothalamic hypogonadism in mice using a cloned GnRH gene; in the other, normal, cloned mouse, normal β-globin genes were introduced into pronucleate eggs and the subsequent hematologic manifestations of murine thalassemia were reduced or eliminated in the resultant offspring. The frequency of success with these approaches is low, and in the thalassemia model, the hemoglobin regulation was not fully normalized. Using viral vector insertional conversion also carries the risk of insertional mutagenesis, in which a normal functioning gene is lost or its function altered because of the insertion of the vector DNA into the host genome within that gene. These studies only begin to show the possible potential of this powerful technology.

Advances in molecular genetics and recombinant DNA technology have been dramatic, and have led to the development of sensitive diagnostic techniques for a continuously increasing number of single-gene disorders.[38] Cutting DNA with restriction endonucleases and analysis of restriction fragment length polymorphisms (RFLP), sequence-specific DNA isolation techniques, and cloning of single-stranded DNA have allowed the formation of highly specific gene probes. These have increased not only the accuracy of diagnosis of abnormal conditions, but also the basic understanding of normal gene function and regulation, with specific emphasis on the understanding of the development of the mechanisms of cancer and its potential treatment. The next natural step in this evolving technology was the development of techniques to introduce purified or cloned gene sequences into cultured cells, and, eventually, living animals to correct single-gene defects. Once these techniques were established in animal systems, attention could then be directed to their application in the treatment and prevention of single-gene disorders in the human.

Gene therapy has attracted the attention of the medical community and the lay media. The possibility of treating severe disorders that are not amenable to any other mode of treatment is obviously appealing to the medical community, especially when children are affected. Public acceptance, however, is limited by valid concerns about ethical issues surrounding still undeveloped methods and endangered by pseudoscientific publications on the potential to change traits,[39] appearance, and behavior. As a result, controversy persists over the advantages and dangers of gene therapy. Gene therapy, however, is not one uniform issue, and different levels of gene therapy will have definite and different potential advantages and dangers.

Approaches to gene therapy can be divided initially into three concepts:

1. Modification of existing material
2. Removal of material
3. Addition of material.

Addition of material is the most promising approach for stable correction of defects. Anderson defines three potential levels of genetic engineering and therapy[40]:

1. *Somatic cell gene therapy*: a gene is inserted into the cells of an affected person to correct a genetic disorder in that person only.
2. *Germ line gene therapy*: insertion of a gene into the germ cells of an affected person to correct a disorder in the patient and his or her offspring.
3. *Enhancement genetic engineering*: insertion of a gene into a normal person, intended to enhance a desirable known characteristic.

A consensus among active workers in the field exists that human gene therapy will be feasible and should be applied to at least some serious genetic disorders.[40] It also generally is held that human gene therapy should not be applied at this time to germ cells, but only to somatic cells that cannot transmit the altered genetic material to subsequent generations.[40] The first target of human gene therapy would, therefore, be the somatic cell. Clinical studies of adults with terminal diseases are under way and there are proposals to begin treatment of children with life-threatening diseases such as adenosine deaminase deficiency. Because 90% of adult cells already are present at the time of birth, however, it seems to make much more sense to try to insert these cells *in utero*—as early as possible to increase the proportion of cells that can take up the material.

In addition, early progenitor cells such as stem cells would carry the advantage of reduced antigenicity and the ability to give rise to multiple differentiated cell lines that carry and express a normal gene product. Hematopoietic stem cells can be obtained from first-trimester fetal livers obtained at the time of elective pregnancy termination, homogenated and enriched for stem cell components, and used as donor material for potential fetal transplant. If obtained before 14 weeks of gestation, these stem cells carry no antigenic markers that would elicit an immunologic response and lead to graft rejection. Also, if transplanted to a recipient fetus before 14 weeks of gestation, persistent tolerance to these cells may be established in the recipient fetus, resulting in dramatically reduced risk of graft-*versus*-host disease and rejection.

Fetal-to-fetal hematopoietic stem cell transplantation research is under way and has primarily focused on hemoglobinopathies and severe immune deficiency disorders. Once established and the immunologic postulates proven valid, this approach may hold great promise in the potential treatment of inborn errors of metabolism due to single-gene enzymatic deficiencies. Such treatment would change the course of history in the treatment of genetic disorders and would dramatically change the clinical course for these otherwise severely afflicted people facing devastating medical diseases.

REFERENCES

1. Evans MI, Drugan A, Manning FA, et al. Fetal surgery in the 1990s. Am J Dis Child 1989;143:1431.
2. Liley AW. Intrauterine transfusion of foetus in haemolytic disease. Br Med J 1963;2:1107.
3. Berkowitz RL, Chitkara U, Goldberg JD, et al. Intrauterine transfusion in utero: the percutaneous approach. Am J Obstet Gynecol 1986;154:622.
4. Clewell WH, Johnson ML, Meier PR. A surgical approach to the treatment of hydrocephalus. N Engl J Med 1982;306:1320.
5. Manning FA, Harrison MR, Rodeck C, et al. Special report: catheter shunts for fetal hydronephrosis and hydrocephalus: report of the International Fetal Medicine and Surgery Society Registry. N Engl J Med 1986;315:336.
6. Berkowitz RL, Tertora M, Hobbins JC, et al. The management of fetal hydrocephalus. Am J Obstet Gynecol 1985;151:993.
7. Drugan A, Krause B, Canady A, et al. The natural history of prenatally diagnosed ventriculomegaly. JAMA 1989;261:1785.
8. Callan NA, Blakemore K, Park J, et al. Fetal genitourinary tract anomalies: evaluation, operative correction, and follow-up. Obstet Gynecol 1990;75:67.
9. Helin I, Persson PH. Prenatal diagnosis of urinary tract abnormalities by ultrasound. Pediatrics 1986;78:879.
10. Smith D, Egginton JA, Brookfield DSK. Detection of abnormality of fetal urinary tract as a predictor of renal tract disease. Br Med J 1987;294:27.
11. Wilson RD, Morrison MG, Wittmann BK, et al. Clinical follow-up of fetal urinary tract anomalies diagnosed prenatally by ultrasound. Fetal Therapy 1988;3:141.
12. Fremond B, Babut JM. Obstructive uropathies diagnosed in utero: the postnatal outcome—a study of 43 cases. Prog Pediatr Surg 1986;19:160.
13. Dumez Y, Revillon Y, Dommergues M, et al. Long-term predictive value of fetal renal function. Presented at the 5th Meeting of the International Fetal Medicine and Surgery Society, Bonn, Germany, June, 1988.
14. Mueller F, Dumez Y. Contribution of biochemistry to prenatal diagnosis of obstructive uropathies. Am J Human Genet 1991;49(4):175.
15. Adzick NS, Harrison MR, Glick PL, et al. Fetal urinary tract obstruction: experimental pathophysiology. Semin Perinatol 1985;9:79.
16. Weiner C, Williamson R, Monsib MS, et al. In utero bladder diversion problems with patients selection. Fetal Therapy 1986;1:196.
17. Evans MI, Sacks AJ, Johnson MP, et al. Sequential invasive assessment of fetal renal function and the intrauterine treatment of fetal obstructive uropathies. Obstet Gynecol 1991; 77:545.
18. Crombleholme TM, Harrison MR, Golbus MS, et al. Fetal intervention in obstructive uropathy: prognostic indicators and efficacy of intervention. Am J Obstet Gynecol 1990;162:1239.
19. Grannum PA, Ghidini A, Scioscia A, et al. Assessment of fetal renal reserve in low level obstructive uropathy. Lancet 1989;1:281.
20. Wilkins IA, Chitkara U, Lynch L, et al. The non-predictive value of fetal urinary electrolytes: preliminary report of outcomes and correlations with pathologic diagnosis. Am J Obstet Gynecol 1987;157:694.
21. Elder JS, O'Grady JP, Ashmead G, et al. Evaluation of fetal renal function: unreliability of fetal urinary electrolytes. J Urol 1990;144:574.
22. Nicolaides KH, Cheng HH, Snijders RS, et al. Fetal urine biochemistry in the assessment of obstructive uropathy. Am J Obstet Gynecol 1992;166:932.

23. Jennings RW, Adzick NS, Harrison MR. The fetus as a surgical patient. In: Evans MI, ed. Reproductive risks and prenatal diagnosis. Norwalk, CT: Appleton & Lange, 1992:311.
24. Harrison MR, Bressack MA, Chung AM, et al. Correction of congenital diaphragmatic hernia in utero: II. Simulated correction permits fetal lung growth with survival at birth. Surgery 1980;88:260.
25. Harrison MR, Adzick NS, Longaker MT, et al. Successful repair in utero of a fetal diaphragmatic hernia after removal of herniated viscera from the left thorax. N Engl J Med 1990; 322:1582.
26. Evans MI, Chrousos GP, Mann DL, et al. Pharmacologic suppression of the fetal adrenal gland: attempted prevention of 21-hydroxylase deficiency congenital adrenal hyperplasia in utero. JAMA 1985;253:1015.
27. Forrest M, David M. Prenatal treatment of congenital adrenal hyperplasia due to 21 hydroxylase deficiency. 7th International Congress of Endocrinology Abstract 911, Quebec, Canada, 1984.
28. Shulman DI, Mueller OT, Gallardo LA, et al. Treatment of congenital adrenal hyperplasia in utero. Pediatr Res 1989; 25(4):2.
29. Pang S, Pollack MS, Marshall RN, et al. Prenatal treatment of congenital adrenal hyperplasia due to 21-hydroxylase deficiency. N Engl J Med 1990;322:111.
30. Phillips JA III, Burr IM, Orlando P, et al. DNA analysis of human steroid 21-hydroxylase genes on congenital hyperplasia. Am J Hum Genet 1985;37:A171.
31. Allen LD. Fetal arrhythmias. In: Long WA, ed. Fetal and neonatal cardiology. Philadelphia: WB Saunders, 1990: 170.
32. Allen LD, Crawford DG, Sheridan R, et al. Aetiology of non-immune hydrops: the value of echocardiography. Br J Obstet Gynaecol 1986;93:223.
33. Smithells RW, Sheppard S, Schorah CJ, et al. Vitamin supplementation and neural tube defects. Lancet 1981;1:425.
34. Milunsky A, Jick H, Jick SS, et al. Multivitamin/folic acid supplementation in early pregnancy reduced the prevalence of neural tube defects. JAMA 1989;262:2847.
35. Mills JL, Rhoads GG, Simpson JL, et al. The absence of a relation between the periconceptional use of vitamins and neural tube defects. N Engl J Med 1989;321:430.
36. Mulinare J, Cordero JF, Erickson JD, et al. Periconceptional use of multivitamins and the occurrence of neural tube defects. JAMA 1988;260:3141.
37. MRC Vitamin Study Research Group. Prevention of neural tube defects: results of the Medical Research Council Vitamin Study. Lancet 1991;338:131.
38. Caskey CT, Rossiter BJF. Molecular methods of disease diagnosis. In: Evans MI, ed. Reproductive risks and prenatal diagnosis. Norwalk, CT: Appleton & Lange, 1992:265.
39. Anderson WF. Human gene therapy: scientific and ethical considerations. J Med Philos 1985;10:275.
40. Anderson WF. Gene therapy. In: Evans MI, Fletcher JC, Dixler AO, et al, eds. Fetal diagnosis and therapy: science, ethics, and the law. Philadelphia: JB Lippincott, 1989:421.

Neonatology: Pathophysiology and Management of the Newborn, Fourth Edition,
edited by Gordon B. Avery, Mary Ann Fletcher, and Mhairi G. MacDonald.
J.B. Lippincott Company, Philadelphia © 1994.

chapter 15

The Impact of Maternal Illness

ALLEN P. KILLAM

There has been a steady decrease in perinatal death rates over the past 25 years.[1] Although most of the improved perinatal survival resulted from improved survival of newborns in intensive care units, improved obstetric care and maternal health has lessened the impact of maternal illness on fetal health and neonatal outcome.[2–5] The impact of maternal illness on the fetus may be direct, as in altered growth rates or induction of anomalies, but the concern for maternal and fetal well-being that influences the timing and method of delivery may have greater consequences. For instance, fetal macrosomia in diabetic mothers may lead to cesarean delivery for cephalopelvic disproportion or Erb palsy from shoulder dystocia during a difficult vaginal delivery.[6,7] Severe preeclampsia may threaten the life of a mother seriously enough to force her to be delivered more than 10 weeks prematurely. Vaginal delivery of very-low-birth-weight babies may increase the risk of intraventricular hemorrhage, but cesarean delivery may increase the risk to a critically ill mother.[5] As the gestational age for neonatal viability decreases and perioperative maternal intensive care lessens the risks in cesarean delivery, the timing and method of delivery for pregnancies complicated by maternal disease shifts to increasing reliance on cesarean delivery of extremely premature babies, approaching the gestational age at which abortion is an option. Development of a health care system for pregnant women that is readily accessible, friendly, and includes effective screening for complications followed by appropriate referral for tertiary care, must be a high priority. This chapter discusses maternal illnesses that may affect the developing fetus and outlines strategies for lessening their impact on perinatal outcome.

PRENATAL RISK SCREENING

An increasing number of maternal and fetal conditions that adversely affect outcome may be detected with prenatal screening techniques, and the course of many of these conditions may be altered favorably by timely intervention.[8–10] The most frequent and important risk to the fetus is preterm birth. Techniques to identify the population at risk for preterm labor and rupture of the fetal membranes plus interventions to prevent them deserve the most attention, but drug abuse and perinatal infections are increasing as separate threats that require specific interventions. Universal screening for gestational diabetes and α-fetoprotein testing for neural tube defects and chromosomal abnormalities are widely practiced. Ultrasonic examinations for multiple gestations, fetal defects, altered fetal growth, and mistaken dates of conception frequently are offered. How to apportion available dollars and health care provider time is an important consideration, but frequently the success or failure of prenatal care depends on early access to care and patient compliance.

PRETERM LABOR SCREENING AND INTERVENTION

For obvious reasons, there has been considerable effort to determine the most effective combination of historical and physical factors that would identify the risk a pregnant patient has for preterm labor.[11,12] When applied to different obstetric populations, the best that screening programs can achieve is to identify a high-risk group comprising 10% to 15% of the total population, that will include one-half of the patients who ultimately would deliver prematurely.[13,14] By virtue of their past obstetric experience, multiparous patients can be screened more accurately than nulliparous women. Patients with multiple gestation or incompetent cervix are at obvious risk for prematurity and in indisputable need of special care. The population at high risk for prematurity on the basis of multiple social factors (*e.g.*, poverty, non-Caucasian race, teenage pregnancy, sexual promiscuity) are more difficult to separate into the groups who will deliver early and those who will not.[15–18] Furthermore, patients from publicly funded, urban high-risk clinics do not appear to benefit from special prematurity prevention clinics as much as those attending private obstetric clinics.[19]

Exactly which factors, when subjected to a multivariate analysis, have significant correlation with preterm delivery varies from study to study. Prognostic factors associated with preterm labor include the following:[19a]

- prior preterm delivery
- multiple gestation
- three or more first-trimester abortions
- previous second-trimester abortion
- cervical incompetence
- abdominal surgery during current pregnancy
- uterine or cervical anomalies (*e.g.*, DES exposure)
- placenta previa
- premature placental separation, spontaneous or drug induced (*e.g.*, cocaine use)
- fetal abnormality
- hydramnios
- serious maternal infection
- second-trimester bleeding
- cervical effacement or dilatation of more than 50% or 1 cm
- prepregnancy weight less than 45 kg (100 lbs)
- single parent
- no prenatal care.

This is similar to the list of 18 significant factors selected by Holbrook and associates from a total of 37 potentially significant factors.[13] Several factors included in the technical bulletin but not found to be significant by Holbrook and colleagues include placenta previa, single parent, and low prepregnancy weight. Neither included very low socioeconomic status or strenuous job activity. Smoking was not included in the technical bulletin, but was concluded to be a significant factor for risk screening for preterm labor by Holbrook and colleagues. It is obvious that an ideal list of factors for preterm labor screening that will suit all populations has not been devised and widely accepted.

Perhaps even more controversial is the efficacy of various interventions such as bed rest and tocolytic medications.[20–25] One hopeful development is the advent of home uterine monitoring.[26–34] In some high-risk populations such as prior preterm delivery, home monitoring appears to allow earlier and thus more successful intervention by identifying preterm labor earlier than does intensive education and self-reporting. The application of home uterine monitoring is steadily expanding as evidence of its efficacy mounts, but a national consensus on the proper use of the device is lacking.[26]

Much of the reason why tocolytic medication has not easily been proven to lower prematurity rates in spite of the widespread use in large populations has stemmed from either its use in patients not truly at risk for preterm delivery, or the fact that preterm labor has advanced too far before therapy is started. One general approach to increasing the accuracy of predicting those patients as high risk for preterm labor is to identify a biochemical marker for preterm labor, avoiding much of the subjective and inaccurate predictions of risk. Fetal fibronectin in vaginal and cervical secretions shows promise as an accurate predictor of preterm delivery and perinatal mortality.[35] Amniotic fluid interleukins also may prove to be accurate predictors of risk, in so far as they relate to the role of infection in the pathogenesis of preterm labor and delivery.[20] The presence of fetal breathing detected by ultrasound is unusual in a patient in true and progressing labor.[20] Amniotic fluid volume is a good predictor of the length of time after premature rupture of the fetal membranes until delivery occurs.

Failure to reaccumulate fluid generally indicates a shorter interval until spontaneous premature labor begins, whereas some reaccumulation suggests resealing and a longer interval.

The presence of either polyhydramnios or oligohydramnios before rupture suggests higher risk for preterm labor.[21]

SCREENING FOR PERINATAL INFECTIONS

It has been estimated that 25% of premature labor is caused by genital infections. The exact role of infection in causing preterm delivery is poorly understood. Although several organisms are clearly associated with preterm labor and preterm, premature rupture of the fetal membranes, no single organism or group of organisms has been proven to cause preterm labor consistently.[36–50] The types of infection associated with preterm labor also are common in patients who deliver at term. Organisms that cause neonatal sepsis are found regularly in the vagina of asymptomatic pregnant women; and the amniotic fluid of women not in preterm labor may contain the same variety of organisms present in amniotic fluid of women who are in preterm labor, making it impossible to predict which pregnancies will be affected. Organisms commonly present in infected amniotic fluid or in fetal membranes of women with intact membranes at the onset of preterm labor include the following:

Ureaplasma urealyticum
Mycoplasma hominis
Fusobacterium sp.
Bacteroides sp.
Capnocytophagia sp.
Clostridium sp.
Peptostreptococcus sp.
Escherichia coli.

Detection of many of these organisms requires special microbiology techniques not practical for screening.

One prevailing scenario for how bacterial infection causes preterm delivery starts with subclinical infection of fetal membranes, usually extending from the cervical canal. The ascending infection weakens the membranes, causing their preterm premature rupture, just as the infection may stimulate premature labor by causing the formation of prostaglandin through phospholipase A^2 or the formation of interleukins by inflammatory leukocytes.

Due to the polymicrobial nature of the infections involved in preterm labor, protocols for prophylactic, broad-spectrum antibiotic regimens have been tried for patients believed to be at high risk for preterm labor of infectious etiology. Treatment of apparently idiopathic preterm labor frequently includes antibiotic therapy in part to prevent neonatal sepsis caused by group B streptococci,[51] but also in part because antibiotics may be effective in delaying labor in patients with intact membranes who present in preterm labor.

Although screening for all the organisms associated with either preterm labor or rupture of fetal membranes may not help prevent preterm labor, screening for and treating bacterial vaginosis may be very worthwhile.[52–54] One-half of the patients with bacterial vaginosis are asymptomatic, whereas others complain of a foul discharge and discomfort. The diagnosis of bacterial vaginosis is established by a microscopic examination of the vaginal secretions, revealing both the presence of clue cells, which are epithelial cells with granular cytoplasm and a typical irregular rough border, plus a proliferation of small coccobacilli replacing the larger, normally predominant lactobacilli. The slide of vaginal secretions can be dried and stained for later evaluation or examined immediately as a wet prep. Additional evidence of bacterial vaginosis can be obtained by treating the vaginal secretions with 10% KOH, which releases a fishy odor (*i.e.*, the whiff test) or by finding a vaginal *p*H of over 4.5, but examination of the microscopic slide is sufficient to establish the diagnosis. Culturing the vaginal bacterial flora does not aid the diagnosis of bacterial vaginosis, because the diagnosis is established by these simple laboratory tests. A variety of organisms are involved in this condition, formerly called nonspecific vaginitis. *Bacteroides* sp. and other anaerobic organism such as *Peptococcus* and *Peptostreptococcus* sp. are believed to be the primary organisms involved. *Gardnerella vaginalis* may proliferate over a thousandfold to become the predominant organism. *Mobiluncus* and *Mycoplasma* spp. frequently are identified when a patient has bacterial vaginosis. The presence or absence of any one of these organisms does not alter the diagnosis or the prognosis for the patient.

The presence of bacterial vaginosis doubles the risk for premature delivery and treating the vaginosis appears to reduce this risk. Because it is not possible to identify which organism or organisms cause the membranes to rupture or labor to start prematurely, there is confusion as to which antibiotic is the best choice for therapy. In nonpregnant patients, metronidazole has been the treatment of choice. In pregnant patients, clindamycin per vagina, orally, or intravenously if the patient is hospitalized in preterm labor, has been used successfully. Ceftriaxone or another yet to be identified broad-spectrum antibiotic may prove to be more successful in preventing prenatal loss in patients with bacterial vaginosis or chronic inflammation of the fetal membranes and underlying maternal tissue in the upper cervix or uterine cavity.

Trichomonas vaginitis also is associated with a higher risk of preterm labor in the absence of additional vaginal infections, and for this reason it is logical to treat this condition when a pregnant woman complains of vaginitis with trichomonads visible in a wet mount of her vaginal secretions. Out of concern for possible teratogenesis from metronidazole use during the first trimester of pregnancy, many obstetricians are reluctant to use it until after the thirteenth week. There is no other therapy available for trichomonal vaginitis with the therapeutic efficacy of metronidazole. Urinary tract infections also should be screened for and treated aggressively because of their possible involvement in preterm labor.[55,56]

Screening for and treating all infections to lower the incidence of preterm labor may be controversial, but screening for several specific infections is an accepted obstetric practice because of the clear role these infections play in damaging the developing fetus or newborn. These screening tests include the immune status for rubella,[57] the presence of hepatitis B surface antigen,[58–60] antibodies against syphilis,[61] and, with consent, human immunodeficiency virus (HIV). In high-risk populations, skin tests for tuberculosis are recommended. After a maternal exposure to other specific infections known to affect the fetus seriously, serologic tests are need to determine the immune status of the mother or to document that a recent infection has occurred. Serious infections include parvovirus B19 (*i.e.*, fifth disease),[62–66] which causes fetal hydrops from aplastic anemia but only rarely causes fetal anomalies. The varicella-zoster virus may cause a severe, life-threatening illness in susceptible mothers, congenital anomalies in the fetus, and severe neonatal varicella if the baby is born 3 days before or 5 days after the rash develops in the mother.[67] Lyme disease may cause fetal death or congenital anomalies if the mother is actively infected with *Borellia*.[68–71] Routine screening for cytomegalovirus (CMV) and toxoplasmosis is not recommended because of the difficulties in interpreting any results.[72,73] Many clinics taking care of populations at high risk for sexually transmitted diseases such as unmarried teenagers also routinely test for gonorrhea and chlamydia.[74] Listeriosis may cause fetal death and serious maternal illness.[75,76]

The best way to screen for group B streptococcal colonization of the pregnant woman's vagina remains controversial. Once a positive vaginal culture for group B streptococcus has been obtained, there is general agreement to treat the mother with 2 g of ampicillin every 4 to 6 hours during labor.[77,78] Women with a previous baby affected with group B streptococcus and women with premature labor or premature rupture of the fetal membranes are routinely cultured for group B streptococcus and treated either until the culture is found to be negative or only after the culture is reported to be positive. Routine culturing of all low-risk pregnant patients has its proponents, but 20% of all pregnant patients will be positive. In low-risk populations, the attack rate is 1%. Treatment of vaginal carriers frequently fails and a significant number of women with negative cultures before 30 weeks of gestation will be positive for group B streptococcus at delivery.[79] Treating 20% of the obstetric population with antibiotics would be expensive and expose them to potentially serious side-effects. Some medical groups routinely screen pregnant patients for group B streptococcus, but only treat those with risk factors before labor. All women with positive cultures at any time during their pregnancy are treated during labor. Rapid screening tests for vaginal group B streptococcal colonization have lacked the sensitivity to gain wide acceptance.[80]

Women who have had a genital herpes simplex infection during the current pregnancy are no longer cultured for herpes weekly the last 6 weeks of gestation, because the result of the last weekly culture does not alter the odds that the culture at delivery will be positive (1.2% if negative *versus* 1.4% if positive).[81] It has been estimated that 15,000 otherwise unnecessary cesarean deliveries were done each year during the 1980s to salvage approximately 8 babies from death due to herpes septicemia. Women with recent primary herpes or evidence of active lesions are delivered by cesarean section. All women suspected of having had genital herpes at any time during the current pregnancy are cultured when admitted in labor. Prophylactic acyclovir for the mother or the newborn is controversial but appears to have few, if any, side-effects.[81]

PRENATAL SCREENING FOR DRUG ABUSE

Routine screening for drug abuse may help reduce the risk to the developing fetus and afford some protection to the child,[82] but the threat of detection and subsequent legal action has driven many pregnant women away from effective prenatal care. The drug-abusing community's perception of how helpful and confidential prenatal screening is should be a major consideration when deciding when to order a drug screen, how permission is obtained, who is told the results, and how the positive results are used.[83,84] There is little doubt that a drug screen should be ordered when there is a strong suspicion of drug use.[85] The patient should be informed the test is being done in a manner that is not punitive or condemning, but rather offered as an attempt to help lessen the effect of drug use on the fetus and the mother.[84] Regular prenatal care and enrollment in a drug rehabilitation program can serve as a sanctuary against punitive action as well as being medically useful.

Cocaine is the most commonly abused substance.[85] Estimates based on a combination of universal anonymous screening and self-reporting are in the neighborhood of 10%, but the incidence varies widely and other substances such as alcohol usually are taken in addition to cocaine. Cocaine abuse can easily escape detection if a woman has the financial resources to sustain her habit without engaging in illegal behaviors such as prostitution and drug trafficking. The effect of cocaine abuse on the fetus is determined by the pattern of abuse, any other drugs that are used in addition to cocaine, and the associated high-risk lifestyles that make the mother prone to multiple infections, trauma, neglect, and malnutrition. Cocaine alone can cause preterm labor, preterm premature rupture of the fetal membranes,[86–89] intrauterine growth retardation (IUGR), placental abruption, asphyxia, major congenital anomalies,[90–92] and neurobehavioral problems,[93–95] which may include sudden infant death syndrome as well as learning disabilities. Methamphetamine or "ice" mimics the effect of cocaine with a catecholamine rush, diminished perfusion of vital organs, and euphoria. Its duration of action is much longer than that of cocaine, making it preferable to some abusers.

Heroin, other narcotics, and barbiturates are more likely to cause obvious and longer-lasting changes in a woman's mental status and are more likely to cause clinically significant withdrawal syndromes in both the mother and her baby.[96] The fetal alcohol syndrome is a persistent problem and may complicate the effect of other drugs that are abused. Marijuana alone in moderate amounts may not have a major effect on fetal development, but its use frequently is associated with a pattern of other drug abuse.[97]

From 25% to 46% of pregnant women smoke tobacco, even though it is well advertised that smoking lowers birth weight and perinatal survival. The adverse effect of smoking is more pronounced in women over 35 years of age compared with women under 20 years of age. Chronic hypertension also intensifies the adverse effects of smoking, especially placental abruption and placenta previa. Tobacco smoking decreases placental perfusion and interferes with oxygen transport by hemoglobin. Babies are smaller, and placentas are larger. Prematurity is more frequent and more babies die when women smoke. The effect is dose dependent. All women should be strongly urged to stop smoking and avoid passive exposure while pregnant.[98,99]

HYPERTENSION

The effect of the different hypertensive disorders on the developing fetus varies with the type and severity of the disorder as well as the gestational age at which it becomes a problem.[99] Transient hypertension or mild preeclampsia developing late in the third trimester are unlikely to affect fetal outcome. Mild chronic hypertension slightly increases the risk of IUGR and placental abruption.[100] More severe degrees of chronic hypertension, especially if associated with superimposed preeclampsia in the second trimester, may have profound effects on the fetus, including fatal placental abruption and neonatal death after planned preterm delivery necessary to protect the mother's life.[101,102]

Coincidental chronic hypertension in pregnant women usually is essential in nature. Pheochromocytomas are rare (*i.e.*, 1 per 5000 pregnancies), and if undiagnosed they are very dangerous to both the mother and her fetus. Hypertension associated with renal and vascular diseases, or with advanced stages of diabetes, usually carries a poor fetal prognosis because of placental insufficiency, planned and unplanned preterm delivery, and frequent fetal death.

Preeclampsia–eclampsia and the less severe forms of pregnancy-induced hypertension not associated with proteinuria represent unique conditions to pregnancy that disappear when the pregnancy terminates. Preeclampsia, defined by the triad of hypertension, proteinuria, and edema beginning in the second one-half of pregnancy, may in fact be two separate conditions.[103,104] The classic preeclampsia occurs in primigravidas, usually is not manifest until after 34 weeks of gestation, and does not affect fetal growth or outcome until after hypertension has developed. Preeclampsia in previously normotensive primigravidas is unlikely to recur,[105,106] but it occurs in families in an inheritance pattern strongly suggesting a single-gene defect.[107–109] On the other hand, preeclampsia developing in second or later pregnancies is more likely to be associated with an underlying chronic vascular disease, to recur in subsequent pregnancies, and to affect fetal growth and well-being before there is a significant rise in blood pressure. Understanding of the etiology and pathogenesis of preeclampsia has expanded over the past decade. There are a number of characteristics of pregnancy-induced hypertension that set it apart from chronic hypertension in nonpregnant women:

- abnormal trophoblast invasion
- inadequate placental perfusion
- thromboxane excess
- platelet aggregation and coagulation abnormalities
- endothelial damage
- vascular hyperreactivity
- genetic predisposition
- immunologic phenomenon
- calcium intracellular excess and dietary deficiency.

In preeclamptic patients, the cytotrophoblasts from the anchoring villi fail to invade all of the spiral uterine arteries in the decidua basalis or to invade the walls of uterine arteries in the underlying myometrium, and therefore do not establish good perfusion, in contrast to what happens in patients not destined to become preeclamptic.[110–112] Later in pregnancy, the inadequately perfused placenta appears to set in motion a series of pathophysiologic conditions that lead to the clinical expression of the disease. As pregnancy progresses to its second one-half, placental perfusion is compromised further by aggregation of platelets, fibrin clots, vasospasm, and multiple placental infarcts.[113,114] Although patients destined to become hypertensive in the third trimester do not experience an increase in their blood pressure during the first two trimesters, they can be identified by an increased sensitivity to vasoconstrictors such as angiotensin II,[100,115] decreased calcium excretion in the urine,[116–118] and altered calcium flux in platelets by the beginning of the second trimester.[119]

Preeclamptic patients produce excessive thromboxane in relation to their prostacyclin production.[120,121] This imbalance leads to platelet aggregation, vasospasm, clot formation, and diminished placental perfusion. Knowledge of this unique characteristic of preeclampsia has led to the use of low-dose aspirin to delay or prevent the onset of the clinical manifestations of preeclampsia.[122] The ideal dose of aspirin is in the range of 60 to 80 mg daily. The standard adult analgesic dose, which is ten times greater, blocks both prostacyclin and thromboxane production, whereas the low dose of aspirin leaves prostacycline production mostly intact while blocking 80% of the thromboxane production, restoring the imbalance of preeclampsia to a more normal state. A metaanalysis of six early clinical trials indicates that prophylaxis with low-dose aspirin prevents 65% of clinical preeclampsia while causing no apparent harm to the mother or her fetus.[123] Particularly encouraging is the fact that low-dose aspirin appears to be most effective in preventing the more severe proteinuric forms of pregnancy-induced hypertension and in reducing the incidence and severity of IUGR. There also is mounting evidence that 1.5 to 2.0 g of supplemental calcium per day will reduce the incidence of preeclampsia, especially in patients who consume 600 mg or less calcium in their diet.[124] Calcium supplementation also may reduce the incidence of preterm labor in some high-risk populations.[125]

Low-dose aspirin therapy and calcium supplementation are expected to be effective only if begun during the second trimester, before the onset of clinical signs of preeclampsia. Bed rest is effective in reversing the hypertension of preeclampsia and may improve perinatal mortality by more than 20-fold compared to patients who fail to comply with bed rest supervised in a hospital setting.[126] When severe preeclampsia develops early in pregnancy, judicial use of antepartum testing for fetal well-being and maturity helps time the delivery to achieve the best fetal outcome without unduly risking the mother's health.

DIABETES

Before the availability of insulin it was unusual for women with diabetes to conceive and survive and even less likely for the fetus to survive. The effects of diabetes on the fetus are well known and include the following:

- fetal death
- fetal macrosomia and birth trauma
- cardiac, gastrointestinal, and skeletal congenital anomalies
- respiratory distress syndrome
- hypoglycemia
- hypocalcemia and decreased magnesium levels
- polycythemia and hyperbilirubinemia
- perinatal asphyxia
- IUGR.

The physiologic derangements in a pregnant diabetic that produce the problems enumerated above include hyperglycemia, vascular disease, and ketoacidosis. If a diabetic woman's blood sugars can be maintained at normal levels throughout her pregnancy, will this completely eliminate all of the risk to the fetus? Obviously, advanced renovascular disease, especially with superimposed preeclampsia, will place the fetus at high risk for poor placental perfusion, IUGR, and preterm delivery regardless of how well the maternal blood sugar is controlled. There is good evidence that maintaining a diabetic's blood sugar in the normal range from before conception through the first trimester reduces the incidence of congenital anomalies to levels similar to those in nondiabetics.[127–131] There may be a threshold level of blood glucose above which the fetus is at increasing risk for congenital anomalies.[130] Because of their excessive body fat contributing to greater anatomic diameters, macrosomic infants of diabetic mothers are at greater risk for birth trauma than babies weighing the same born to nondiabetic women. Good glycemic control in diabetic mothers reduces the incidence of fetal macrosomia and obesity.[132–134] The incidence of low blood sugar, calcium, and magnesium in the neonate is reduced by good control of maternal blood sugars in the later weeks of pregnancy, with the last 48 hours being the most critical.[135] High maternal blood glucose levels result in high fetal metabolic rates because the fetus is unable to regulate glucose transport across the placenta, even when the amount of glucose coming across the placenta far exceeds its metabolic needs. Fetal hyperglycemia results in lowered tissue oxygen levels from the excessive metabolic rate. Chronically low tissue oxygen levels increase erythropoietin production and erythrocyte mass, leading to polycythemia and hyperbilirubinemia in the newborn.[136] Good control of a diabetic mother's blood glucose virtually eliminates these complications. In labor, or during febrile illnesses and other crises, it is very important to keep a diabetic mother's blood glucose as near normal as possible to reduce fetal oxygen consumption when the margin of safety is particularly low.

Home blood glucose monitoring has allowed pregnant diabetics to maintain tight glucose control without risking serious hypoglycemia. Routine testing of all pregnant women with 1-hour blood glucose levels after ingesting 50 g of glucose at 26 weeks of gestation or earlier in high-risk patients permits detection and treatment of gestational diabetics with diet and, when needed, with insulin.[137] Frequent antepartum testing for fetal well-being and, when needed, testing for fetal lung maturity help determine the best time for delivery and may allow the mother to deliver after 38 weeks of gestation by the vaginal route.[138]

THYROID DISEASE

Thyroid disease is a relatively rare condition in pregnant patients in part because significant thyroid disease markedly reduces fertility.[139] Thyroid-stimulating hormone and the hormones that the thyroid gland produces do not cross the placenta in significant amounts. Thyroid-releasing hormone easily can cross the placenta intact and influence fetal thyroid function if the fetus has functioning pituitary and thyroid glands.[140,141] Iodine readily crosses the placenta, so sustained high levels of maternal intake may cause marked fetal goiter and hypothyroidism. Although iodine deficiency is extremely rare in the United States, in other areas of endemic goiter and maternal hypothyroidism from severe iodine deficiency, fetal loss can be as high as 30% from miscarriages and fetal deaths.[142,143] In addition, congenital anomalies, goiter, cretinism, prolonged jaundice, impaired brain function, and hypothyroidism occur in the offspring. Maternal hypothyroidism in the presence of adequate iodine in the diet can seriously affect fetal outcome, although pregnancy rarely occurs in significantly hypothyroid patients. Some mothers with hypothyroidism have been found to have immunoglobulins with thyroid growth-blocking effects that may suppress the fetal thyroid.[144,145]

Maternal hyperthyroidism, if accompanied by fever, tachycardia, agitation, tremor, or disorientation, may be a serious threat to the health of the mother and child. Hyperemesis may be brought on by hyperthyroidism and resist treatment until the thyroid disease is brought under control. The autoimmune thyroid-stimulating antibodies of Graves disease cross the placenta in sufficient quantities to produce fetal and neonatal hyperthyroidism.[144] If a mother with Graves disease has been previously treated with surgery, she may be euthyroid without taking any antithyroid drugs. She may have high levels of thyroid-stimulating immunoglobulins, however, which cross the placenta and cause fetal and neonatal problems unless the mother is treated with antithyroid drugs such as propylthiouracil to protect the baby.[146]

LUPUS AND OTHER AUTOIMMUNE DISEASES

Lupus erythematosus may become a serious maternal illness with severe renal, vascular, and cardiac impairment causing increased fetal loss and IUGR. Even in the absence of maternal signs or symptoms and often before an established diagnosis, the fetus may be seriously affected by maternal autoantibodies.[147–149] Classic examples of fetal impact are congenital heart block and the anticardiolipid or lupus anticoagulant syndrome.[150] After an adverse fetal outcome due to lupus, the offending autoantibody can be identified in the mother's serum. These autoantibodies may be present in women with clinical lupus as well as in apparently healthy women.[151]

Autoimmune and isoimmune thrombocytopenia may result in fetal intracranial hemorrhage. Benign thrombocytopenia of pregnancy in women with normal platelet counts before pregnancy is not associated with fetal complications, but if maternal platelet counts were depressed before pregnancy, fall below 100,000/mL, or if free antiplatelet antibody is present in maternal serum, vaginal delivery is considered unsafe unless a direct fetal platelet count is over 50,000. Pregnant women with other autoantibodies causing maternal hemolytic anemia, granulocytopenia, or myasthenia gravis may deliver a fetus with similar difficulties until the passively acquired autoantibodies gradually disappear over the next 6 months. Autoantibodies affecting the fetal thyroid have been discussed previously.

The treatment of the different autoimmune diseases varies with the type and severity of the illness. Adrenal corticosteroids have been the mainstay in the treatment of many of these conditions.[152] Large doses of intravenous γ-globulin have been used when life-threatening autoimmune diseases have not responded to more conventional therapy, sometimes resulting in direct fetal improvement. In the lupus anticoagulant syndrome, low-dose aspirin may improve fetal outcome, but treatment decisions in this condition are hampered by the lack of randomized, placebo-controlled studies as well as a lack of understanding of which antibodies are merely associated with the syndrome and not pathogenic and what substance is directly responsible for the condition.[153]

INFECTIOUS DISEASES

The role of infections in preterm labor and screening practices for infections that may affect the fetus have been discussed previously. An important infection affecting the long-term health of both mother and her fetus is HIV.[154] It is estimated that 1 to 8 of every 1000 pregnant women in the United States carry the virus that causes aquired immunodeficiency syndrome (AIDS) and will eventually die of the disease. Approximately 30% of them will transmit the virus to their fetus,[154] with the same fatal result.[155] In developed countries, women previously had been spared from the disease, but as heterosexual spread of the virus is becoming increasingly more common,[156–158] the prevalence is rapidly approaching the 1–1 gender ratio found in central Africa. Asymptomatic HIV infection does not appear to influence the course of a pregnancy, nor does pregnancy alter the course of the disease.[154] Clinical maternal AIDS infection exposes the fetus to a greater risk for a number of secondary infections such as hepatitis, CMV, toxoplasmosis, and tuberculosis.[159,160] Transmission of HIV to the fetus is probably more common in women with symptomatic AIDS.[154]

Hepatitis B is several times more prevalent than AIDS and is more likely to infect the fetus, especially if the mother is e-antigen–positive at birth. About 5% of fetuses will get hepatitis B from their mother during the first trimester, and as many as 90% will get it around the time of birth unless they are vaccinated within 12 hours. Vaccination with hepatitis B immune globulin and the antigen prevents approximately 90% of neonatal hepatitis B.[58]

Congenital syphilis has increased rapidly since the last part of the 1980s. Because of the high incidence of congenital syphilis in infants born to mothers who tested negative in the first one-half of pregnancy, many clinics are retesting obstetric patients in the third trimester. If a pregnant woman who is allergic to penicillin gets syphilis, she should be desensitized and given penicillin since the fetus cannot be treated adequately with erythromycin.[61]

Acute febrile illnesses from whatever cause can affect the fetus in several ways. The temperature elevation increases the metabolic rate of the fetus at a time when there may be diminished perfusion of the fetus and lowered oxygen saturation in the mother.[161,162] Pregnancy makes a woman more susceptible to adult respiratory distress syndrome with pyelonephritis and other infections.[161] Pregnancy also worsens the course of influenza, coccidiomycosis, mycoplasma, and tuberculosis, as well as other infections. In general, acute infections increase the risk of preterm labor, at least in part due to increased levels of prostaglandin production.[162] Peritonitis from a ruptured appendix or other causes almost always initiates labor within a day or two.[163]

CANCER

The only malignancies that are known to have metastasized to the fetus and persisted are malignant melanoma,[164] and members of the leukemia–lymphoma group.[165] A pregnant patient with cancer often is faced with difficult choices because of the threat to her life if she is not diagnosed and treated promptly with major surgery and chemotherapeutic drugs that carry considerable risk to the fetus.[166] There often is a reluctance on the part of the mother or her physicians to administer the usual therapeutic measures while she is still pregnant. Diagnostic radiographs do not have a significant adverse effect on the fetus. Therapeutic irradiation has been given to a pregnant patient's chest, head, or extremity without obvious fetal effect.[166,167] Major surgery outside of the mother's abdomen carries little risk to the fetus and agents used for regional and general anesthesia are unlikely to have a permanent effect on the fetus. Most chemotherapeutic agents can be given safely after the first trimester,[168] but folic acid antagonists should not be given early in pregnancy.[169,170] Preterm delivery as early as 32 to 34 weeks after giving betamethasone to help mature the fetal lungs may be a logical approach in some women with advanced malignancies.

ORGAN TRANSPLANTS

Obstetricians treating high-risk patients are seeing increasing numbers of pregnant women who have had organ transplants, including heart, lung, liver, pancreas, kidney, and various combinations of the above. There are over 2000 women who have delivered a baby after having a renal transplant.[171] Fetal outcome generally is very favorable if the kidney is functioning well 2 years after the transplant, and the patient's general health is good.[172–176] Successful pregnancy is possible after heart and multiple organ transplants, but there are too few to reach many conclusions except that the immunosuppressive drugs have not had significant adverse fetal effects.[177–179] A Pittsburgh group reported 20 pregnancies in 17 women with liver transplants. Two babies were liveborn and ten of the women were still living. Preeclampsia, anemia, and preterm delivery rates were high.

HEART DISEASE

With improving care, more women with congenital, and to a lesser degree, acquired heart disease are becoming pregnant.[180] With congenital heart disease, there is a risk for recurrence in the fetus as well as the hemodynamic consequences for the fetus.[181] In Marfan and some cases of Ehlers–Danlos syndromes, the risk of occurrence in fetus is 50%. If the mother has a cyanotic congenital heart defect, as many of 15% of her newborns may have a heart defect. Heart diseases with particularly poor fetal outcomes include cyanotic heart disease with high maternal hematocrits,[180] conditions with pulmonary hypertension,[182] cardiomyopathies, and arrhythmias with frequent episodes of symptomatic hypotension. In general, infants born to mothers with impaired cardiac function will be small for dates.[183]

There are case reports of successful heart surgery, sometimes with cardiopulmonary bypass during pregnancy, resulting in a viable, normal-appearing fetus.[180] A myocardial infarction during pregnancy carries a relatively poor prognosis for the mother, but the author has been associated with three successful pregnancies in patients who had prior coronary artery bypass surgery. Asymptomatic women whose last myocardial infarction was more than 2 years before their pregnancy have done well as a group.

MALNUTRITION

It is certain that chronic prolonged maternal starvation followed by poor nutrition in infancy adversely affects the growth and mental potential of a child. After the 1944 to 1945 period of severe malnutrition in The Netherlands, fetal size was reduced,[183] but mental performance at age 18 years was not altered.[184] In cases of acute malnutrition in previously well nourished mothers, resulting from hyperemesis gravidarum,[185] acute illnesses, surgery, bowel obstruction, and so forth, eventual fetal outcome usually is very favorable. Churchill reported that diabetic and nondiabetic pregnant patients who become ketonuric had babies with lower intelligence quotients compared to case controls who never had ketonuria.[186] Other studies have not confirmed this observation.

Folic acid supplementation may reduce the risk of recurrence of neural tube defects. Iron deficiency anemia in the mother may reduce the iron stores of her infant.[186] Calcium-deficient mothers may be at increased risk for preeclampsia and preterm births compared to controls who take 1.5 to 2.0 g/day of calcium supplement. Obligate vegetarians who do not eat eggs or milk products and do not supplement their diet with vitamin B_{12} have babies with reduced B_{12}

stores.[187] If they exclusively breast feed, their babies may have severe B_{12} deficiency syndromes, including coma.[187]

In general, food supplement programs in humans are hard to evaluate because of compliance problems and the length of gestation compared to animal models. Maternal weight gain of less than 4.9 kg (10 lbs) during pregnancy, especially in underweight women, is associated with smaller babies at birth.[188] Failure to gain weight or loss of weight in the third trimester is associated with adverse fetal outcome. When this occurs in women with no external limits to their caloric intake, such as famine, poverty, or medical illness, it is more likely that poor fetal growth and development causes the women to gain less weight, rather than poor caloric intake causing fetal growth retardation. The defective growth would more likely be caused by poor placental function if the newborn has no defect in its postnatal growth and development, as evidenced by the success of low-dose aspirin in increasing fetal growth when fetal growth retardation was detected at the beginning of the third trimester.

SUMMARY

Modern medicine, when applied appropriately, lowers the risk to the developing fetus. Although maternal health in general may be improving, women with major diseases are attempting pregnancies often at older ages than before. New threats such as HIV are appearing and there are resurging numbers of diseases that were uncommon in the past. Preterm delivery remains the greatest threat to fetal outcome. The neonatologist's understanding of the causes of preterm labor and their ability to predict and prevent premature births is evolving slowly. As treatment of prematurity becomes more successful, congenital anomalies and births before 26 weeks of gestation are accounting for an increasing percentage of perinatal morbidity and mortality, making these two groups the major challenges for the next decade.

REFERENCES

1. Editorial. Statistics from Division of Vital Statistics, National Center for Health Statistics, CDC: Infant mortality—United States, 1988. JAMA 1991;266:1912.
2. McCormick MC. The contribution of low birth weight to infant mortality and childhood mortality. N Engl J Med 1985; 312:82.
3. United States Department of Health and Human Services, National Institutes of Health. Final Mortality Statistics. Washington, DC: 1988.
4. Dolfus C, Patetta M, Siegel E, et al. Infant mortality: a practical approach to the analysis of the leading causes of death and risk factors. Pediatrics 1990;86:176.
5. Sachs BP, Ringer SA. Intrapartum and delivery room management of the very low birthweight infant. Clin Perinatol 1989;16:809.
6. Keller JD, Lopez-Zeno JA, Dooley SL, et al. Shoulder dystocia and birth trauma in gestational diabetes: a five-year experience. Am J Obstet Gynecol 1991;165:928.
7. Langer O, Berkus MD, Huff RW, et al. Shoulder dystocia: should the fetus weighing ≥ 4000 grams be delivered by cesarean section. Am J Obstet Gynecol 1991;165:831.
8. Hobel C, Youkeles L, Forsythe A. Prenatal and intrapartum high risk screening: II. Risk factor reassessed. Am J Obstet Gynecol 1979;135:1051.
9. Sokol RJ, Rosen MG, Stojkov J, et al. Clinical application of high risks covering on an obstetric service. Am J Obstet Gynecol 1977;128:652.
10. Herron MH, Katz M, Creasy RK. Evaluation of a preterm birth prevention program: preliminary report. Obstet Gynecol 1982;59:452.
11. Creasy RK, Merkatz IR. Prevention of preterm birth: clinical opinion. Obstet Gynecol 1990;76(Suppl 1):2.
12. Lumley J. Review article: the prevention of preterm birth: unresolved problems and work in progress. Aust Paediatr J 1988;24:101.
13. Holbrook RH, Laros RK Jr, Creasy RK. Evaluation of a risk-scoring system for prediction of preterm labor. Am J Perinatol 1989;6:62.
14. Creasy RK. Preventing preterm birth. N Engl J Med 1989; 325:727.
15. Main DM, Gabbe S, Richardson D, et al. Can preterm deliveries be prevented? Am J Obstet Gynecol 1985;151:892.
16. Morrison JC. Preterm birth: a puzzle worth solving. Obstet Gynecol 1990;76(Suppl 1):5.
17. Sinclair JC. Epidemiology of prematurity. International Journal of Technology Assessment in Health Care 1991;7(Suppl 1):2.
18. Savitz DA, Blackmore CA, Thorp JM. Epidemiologic characteristics of preterm delivery: etiologic heterogeneity. Am J Obstet Gynecol 1991;164:467.
19. Wilkins I, Creasy RK. Preterm labor. Clin Obstet Gynecol 1990;33:502.
19a. American College of Obstetrics and Gynecology. Preterm labor. ACOG technical bulletin. no. 133. Washington, DC: ACOG, 1989:1.
20. Turnbull AC. The early diagnosis of impending premature labour. Eur J Obstet Gynecol Reprod Biol 1989;33:11.
21. Veille JC. Management of preterm premature rupture of membranes. Clin Perinatol 1988;15:851.
22. Gilstrap LC, Brown CEL. Prevention and treatment of preterm labor in twins. Clin Perinatol 1988;15:71.
23. Besinger RE, Niebyl JR. The safety and efficacy of tocolytic agents for the treatment of preterm labor. Obstet Gynecol Surv 1990;45:415.
24. Graber EA. Dilemmas in the pharmacological management of preterm labor. Obstet Gynecol Surv 1989;44(7):512.
25. King JF, Grant A, Keirse MJNC, et al. Beta-mimetics in preterm labour: an overview of the randomized controlled trials. Br J Obstet Gynaecol 1988;95:211.
26. Meis PJ, Ernest JM, Moore ML, et al. Regional program for prevention of premature birth in northwestern North Carolina. Am J Obstet Gynecol 1987;157:550.
27. Katz M, Gill PJ, Newman RB. Detection of preterm labor by ambulatory monitoring of uterine activity: a preliminary report. Obstet Gynecol 1986;68:773.
28. Morrison JC, Martin JN, Martin TW, et al. Prevention of preterm birth by ambulatory assessment of uterine activity: a randomized study. Am J Obstet Gynecol 1987;156:536.

29. Iams JD, Johnson FF, O'Shaughnessy RW. A prospective random trial of home uterine activity monitoring in pregnancies at increased risk of preterm labor: part II. Am J Obstet Gynecol 1988;159:595.
30. Editorial. Sounding board: home monitoring of uterine activity: does it prevent prematurity? N Engl J Med 1991;325:1374.
31. Morrison JC, Martin JN Jr, Martin RW, et al. Cost effectiveness of ambulatory uterine activity monitoring. Int J Gynaecol Obstet 1989;28:127.
32. Morrison JC, Pittman KP, Martin RW, et al. Cost/health effectiveness of home uterine activity monitoring in a Medicaid population. Obstet Gynecol 1990;76(Suppl 1):76.
33. Mou SM, Sunderji SG, Gall S, et al. Multicenter randomized clinical trial of home uterine activity monitoring: for detection of preterm labor. Am J Obstet Gynecol 1991;165:858.
34. Kosasa TS, Abou-Sayf FK, Li-Ma G, et al. Evaluation of the cost-effectiveness of home monitoring of uterine contractions. Obstet Gynecol 1990;76(Suppl 1):71.
35. Lockwood CJ, Senyei AE, Dische MR, et al. Fetal fibronectin in cervical and vaginal secretions as a predictor of preterm labor. N Engl J Med 1991;325:669.
36. Romero R, Mazor M, Wu YK, et al. Infection in the pathogenesis of preterm labor. Semin Perinatol 1988;12:262.
37. Dodson MG, Fortunato SJ. Microorganisms and premature labor. J Reprod Med 1988;33(Suppl):87.
38. Gibbs RS. Subclinical infection as a cause of preterm delivery. Pediatr Infect Dis J 1990;9:777.
39. McGregor JA, French JI, Lawellin D, et al. Preterm birth and infection: pathogenic possibilities. Am J Reprod Immunol Microbiol 1988;16:123.
40. Witkin S, McGregor JA. Infection-induced activation of cell-mediated immunity: possible mechanism for preterm birth. Clin Obstet Gynecol 1991;34:112.
41. McGregor JA. Prevention of preterm birth: new initiatives based on microbial–host interactions. Obstet Gynecol Surv 1988;43:1.
42. Romero R, Mazor M. Infection and preterm labor. Clin Obstet Gynecol 1988;31:553.
43. Casey ML, Cox SM, Word RA, et al. Cytokines and infection-induced preterm labor. Reprod Fertil Dev 1990;2:499.
44. Ohlsson A, Wang E. An analysis of antenatal tests to detect infection in preterm premature rupture of the membranes. Am J Obstet Gynecol 1990;162:809.
45. Romero R, Sirtori M, Oyarzun E, et al. Infection and labor: V. Prevalence, microbiology and clinical significance of intraamniotic infection in women with preterm labor and intact membranes. Am J Obstet Gynecol 1989;161:817.
46. McGregor JA, French JI. *Chlamydia trachomatis* infection during pregnancy. Am J Obstet Gynecol 1991;164:1782.
47. Andriole VT, Patterson TF. Epidemiology, natural history and management of urinary tract infections in pregnancy. Med Clin North Am 1991;75:359.
48. Romero R, Mazor M, Oyarzun E, et al. Is genital colonization with *Mycoplasma hominis* or *Ureaplasma urealyticum* associated with prematurity/low birth weight. Obstet Gynecol 1989; 73:532.
49. Gibbs RS, Duff P. Progress in pathogenesis and management of clinical intraamniotic infection. Am J Obstet Gynecol 1991;164:1317.
50. Romero R, Mazor M, Wu YK, et al. Is there an association between colonization with group B streptococcus and prematurity? Semin Perinatol 1988;12(4):262.
51. Romero R, Mazor M, Oyarzun E, et al. Is there an association between colonization with group B streptococcus and prematurity. J Reprod Med 1989;34:797.
52. Swedberg JA. Bacterial vaginosis: etiology, association with preterm labor, diagnosis and management. Compr Ther 1989; 15:47.
53. Martius J, Eschemback DA. The role of bacterial vaginosis as a cause of amniotic fluid infection, chorioamnionitis and prematurity: a review. Arch Gynecol Obstet 1990;247:1.
54. Thomason JL, Gelbart SM, Scaglione NJ. Bacterial vaginosis: current review with indications for asymptomatic therapy. Am J Obstet Gynecol 1991;165:1210.
55. Patterson TF, Andriole VT. Bacteriuria in pregnancy. Infectious Disease Clinics of North America 1987;1:807.
56. Hooton TM. The epidemiology of urinary tract infection and the concept of significant bacteriuria. Infection 1990;28(Suppl 2):40.
57. Morgan-Capner P. Viral infection in pregnancy. Br J Hosp Med 1991;45:150.
58. Ramia S, Arif M. Perinatal transmission of hepatitis B virus infection: a recommended strategy for prevention and control: a review. Br J Obstet Gynaecol 1991;98:141.
59. Norkrans G. Epidemiology of hepatitis B virus (HBV) infections with particular regard to current routes of transmission and development of cirrhosis and malignancy. Scand J Infect Dis 1990;69:43.
60. Koretz RL. Universal prenatal hepatitis B testing: is it cost-effective? Obstet Gynecol 1989;74:808.
61. Zenker PN, Rolfs RT. Treatment of syphilis, 1989. Rev Infect Dis 1990;12(Suppl 6):590.
62. Levy M, Read SE. Erythema infectiosum and pregnancy-related complications. Can Med Assoc J 1990;143:849.
63. Torok TJ. Human parvovirus B19 infections in pregnancy. Pediatr Infect Dis J 1990;9:772.
64. Gurevich I. Fifth disease and other parvovirus B19 infections. Heart Lung 1991;20:342.
65. Frickhofen N, Young NS. Persistent parvovirus B19 infections in humans. Microbial Pathogenesis 1989;7:319.
66. Feder HM, Anderson I. Fifth disease: a brief review of infections in childhood, in adulthood, and in pregnancy. Arch Intern Med 1989;149:2176.
67. Prober CG, Gershon AA, Grose C, et al. Consensus: varicella-zoster infections in pregnancy and the perinatal period. Pediatr Infect Dis J 1990;9:865.
68. Edly SJ. Lyme disease during pregnancy. NJ Med 1990;87:557.
69. Smith LG, Pearlman M, Smith LG, et al. Lyme disease: a review with emphasis on the pregnant woman. Obstet Gynecol Surv 1991;46:125.
70. MacDonald AB. Gestational Lyme borreliosis: implications for the fetus. Rheum Dis Clin North Am 1989;15:657.
71. Duffy J. Lyme disease. Ann Allergy 1990;65(7):1.
72. Frenkel JK. Toxoplasmosis in human beings. J Am Vet Med Assoc 1990;196:240.
73. Jeannel D, Costagliola D, Niel G, et al. What is known about the prevention of congenital toxoplasmosis? Lancet 2 1990; 336:359.
74. United States Department of Health and Human Services. Sexually transmitted diseases: treatment guidelines. MMWR 1989;38:1.
75. MacGowan AP, Cartlidge PHT, MacLeod F, et al. Maternal listeriosis in pregnancy without fetal or neonatal infection. J Infect 1991;22:53.
76. Bergstron S. Genital infections and reproductive health: infertility and morbidity of mother and child in developing countries. Scand J Infect Dis Suppl 1990;69:99.
77. Gotoff SP, Boyer KM. Prevention of group B streptococcal early onset sepsis: 1989. Pediatr Infect Dis J 1989;8:268.
78. Boyer KM, Gotoff SP. Prevention of early onset group B streptococcal disease with selective intrapartum chemoprophylaxis. N Engl J Med 1986;314:1665.

79. Regan JA, Klebanoff MA, Nugent RP. The epidemiology of group B streptococcal colonization in pregnancy. Obstet Gynecol 1991;77:604,.
80. Isada MB, Grossman JH. Rapid screening test for the diagnosis of endocervical group B streptococci in pregnancy: microbiologic results and chemical outcome. Obstet Gynecol 1987;10:139,.
81. Brown ZA, Benedetti J, Ashley R, et al. Neonatal herpes simplex virus infection in relation to asymptomatic maternal infection at the time of labor. N Engl J Med 1991;324:1247.
82. Phibbs CS, Bateman DA, Schwartz RM. The neonatal costs of maternal cocaine use. JAMA 1991;266:1521.
83. Evans AT, Gillogley K. Drug use in pregnancy: obstetric perspectives. Clin Perinatol 1991;18:23.
84. Connolly WB Jr, Marshall AB. Drug addiction, pregnancy, and childbirth: legal issues for the medical and social services communities. Clin Perinatol 1991;18:147.
85. Chasoff IJ, Burns WJ, Schnoll SH, et al. Cocaine use in pregnancy. N Engl J Med 1985;313:666.
86. MacGregor SN, Keith LG, Bachicha JA, et al. Cocaine abuse during pregnancy: correlation between prenatal care and perinatal outcome. Obstet Gynecol 1989;74:882.
87. Petitti DB, Coleman C. Cocaine and the risk of low birth weight. Am J Public Health 1990;80:25.
88. Zuckerman B, Frank DA, Hingson R, et al. Effects of maternal marijuana and cocaine use on fetal growth. N Engl J Med 1989;320:762.
89. Acker D, Sachs DP, Tracey KJ, et al. Abruptio placentae associated with cocaine use. Am J Public Health 1990;80:25.
90. Bingol N, Fuchs M, Diaz V, et al. Teratogenicity of cocaine in humans. J Pediatr 1987;110:93.
91. Chavez GF, Mulinare J, Cordero JF. Maternal cocaine use during early pregnancy as a risk factor for congenital urogenital anomalies. JAMA 1989;262:795.
92. Jones KL. Developmental pathogenesis of defects associated with prenatal cocaine exposure: fetal vascular disruption. Clin Perinatol 1991;18:139.
93. Neuspiel DR, Hamel SC, Hochberg E, et al. Maternal cocaine use and infant behavior. Neurotoxicol Teratol 1991;13:229.
94. Hume RF, O'Donnell KJ, Stanger CL, et al. In utero cocaine exposure: observations of fetal behavioral state may predict neonatal outcome. Am J Obstet Gynecol 1989;161:685.
95. Neuspiel DR, Hamel SC. Cocaine and infant behavior. J Dev Behav Pediatr 1991;12:55.
96. Hoegerman G, Scholl S. Narcotic use in pregnancy. Clin Perinatol 1991;18:51.
97. Day NL, Richardson GA. Prenatal marijuana use: epidemiology, methodologic issues, and infant outcome. Clin Perinatol 1991;18:77.
98. Abel EL. Smoking during pregnancy: a review of effects on growth and development of offspring. Hum Biol 1980;52:593.
99. Killam AP. Tobacco smoking. In: Gleicher N, ed. Principles of medical therapy in pregnancy. New York: Plenum Press, 1984:114.
100. Wellen I. The infant mortality in specific hypertensive disease of pregnancy and in essential hypertension. Am J Obstet Gynecol 1953;66:36,.
101. Sibai BM, Mercer B, Sarinoglu G. Severe preeclampsia in the second trimester: recurrence risk and long-term prognosis. Am J Obstet Gynecol 1991;165:1408.
102. Sibai BM, Taslimi M, Abdella TN, et al. Maternal and perinatal outcome of conservative management of severe preeclampsia in midtrimester. Am J Obstet Gynecol 1985;152:32.
103. Odendaal HJ, Pattison RC, Dutoit R. Fetal and neonatal outcome in patients with severe preeclampsia before 34 weeks. S Afr Med J 1987;71:555.
104. Chesley L. Hypertensive disorders in pregnancy. In: Gleicher N, ed. Principles of medical therapy in pregnancy. New York: Plenum Press, 1985:751.
105. Davey DA, MacGillivray I. The classification and definition of the tensive disorders of pregnancy. Am J Obstet Gynecol 1988;148:892,.
106. Long PA, Abell DA, Beischer NA. Parity and preeclampsia. Aust NZ J Obstet Gynaecol 1979;19:203.
107. Campbell DM, MacGillivray I, Carr-Hill R. Preeclampsia in second pregnancy. Br J Obstet Gynaecol 1985;92:131.
108. Sutherland A, Cooper DW, Howie PW, et al. The incidence of severe preeclampsia among mothers and mother-in-law of preeclamptics and controls. Br J Obstet Gynaecol 1981;88:785.
109. Kilpatrick DC, Liston WA, Gibson F, et al. Association between susceptibility to preeclampsia within families and HLA DR4. Lancet 1989;2:1063,.
110. Sibai BMN, El-Nazer A, Gonzalez-Ruiz AR. Severe preeclampsia-eclampsia among mothers and mother-in-law of preeclamptics and controls. Br J Obstet Gynaecol 1981;88:785.
111. Brosens IA. Morphological changes in the uteroplacental bed in pregnancy hypertension. Clin Obstet Gynaecol 1977;4:583.
112. Kong TY, DeWolf F, Robertson WB, et al. Inadequate maternal vascular response to placentation in pregnancies complicated by preeclampsia and by small-for-gestational age infants. Br J Obstet Gynaecol 1986;93:1049.
113. Shanklin DR, Sibai BM. Ultrastructural aspects of preeclampsia: I. Placental bed and uterine boundary vessels. Am J Obstet Gynecol 1989;161:735.
114. Frusca T, Morassi L, Percorell S, et al. Histological features of uteroplacental vessels in normal and hypertensive patients in relation to birthweight. Br J Obstet Gynaecol 1989;96:835.
115. Sheppard BL, Bonnar J. An ultrastructural study of uteroplacental spiral arteries in hypertensive and normotensive pregnancy and fetal growth retardation. Br J Obstet Gynaecol 1981;88:695.
116. Gant NF, Daley GL, Chand S, et al. A study of angiotensin II response throughout primigravid pregnancy. J Clin Invest 1973;52:2682.
117. Taufield PA, Ales KL, Resnick LM, et al. Hypocalciuria in preeclampsia. N Engl J Med 1987;316:715.
118. Rodriguez MH, Masaki DI, Mestman J, et al. Calcium/creatinine ratio and microalbuminuria in the prediction of preeclampsia. Am J Obstet Gynecol 1988;159:1452.
119. Macintosh MC, Hutchesson AC, Duncan SL, et al. Hypocalciuria and hypertension in pregnancy: a prospective study. (Abstract) Br J Obstet Gynaecol 1989;96:1243.
120. Zemel MB, Zemel PC, Berry S, et al. Altered platelet calcium metabolism as an early predictor of increased peripheral vascular resistance and preeclampsia in urban black women. N Engl J Med 1990;323:434.
121. Goodman RP, Killam AP, Brash AR, et al. Comparison of production during normal pregnancy and pregnancy complicated by hypertension. Am J Obstet Gynecol 1982;142:817.
122. Walsh SW, Parisi VM. The role of arachidonic acid metabolites in preeclampsia. Semin Perinatol 1986;10:335.
123. Imperiale TF, Petrulis AS. A meta-analysis of low-dose aspirin for the prevention of pregnancy-induced hypertensive disease. JAMA 1991;266:260.
124. Belizan JM, Villar J, Gonzalez L, et al. Calcium supplementation to prevent hypertensive disorders of pregnancy. N Engl J Med 1991;325:1399.
125. Repke JT, Villar J. The role of dietary calcium in pregnancy-induced hypertension. Clin Nutr 1989;8:169.
126. Gilstrap LC, Cunningham FG, Whalley PF. Management of pregnancy-induced hypertension in the nulliparas patient remote from term. Semin Perinatol 1978;2:73.

127. Kitzmiller JL, Gavin LA, Gin GD, et al. Preconception care of diabetes: glycemic control prevents congenital anomalies. JAMA 1991;265:731.
128. Gabbe SG. Congenital anomalies among infants of diabetic mothers. Obstet Gynecol Surv 1977;32:125.
129. Cousins L. Congenital anomalies among infants of diabetic mothers: etiology, prevention, diagnosis. Am J Obstet Gynecol 1983;147:333.
130. Mills JL, Baker L, Goldman AS. Malformations in infants of diabetic mothers occur before the seventh gestational week: implications for treatment. Diabetes 1979;28:292.
131. Miller E, Hare JW, Cloherty JP, et al. Elevated maternal hemoglobin A_{1c} in early pregnancy and major congenital anomalies in infants of diabetic mothers. N Engl J Med 1981;304:1331.
132. Pedersen J. The pregnant diabetic and her newborn. 2nd ed. Baltimore: Williams & Wilkins. 1977.
133. Jovanovic-Peterson L, Peterson CM, Reed FG, et al. Maternal postprandial glucose levels and infant birth weight: the Diabetes in Early Pregnancy study. J Obstet Gynecol 1991; 164:103.
134. Sosenko JM, Kitzmiller JL, Fluckiger R, et al. Umbilical cord glycosylated hemoglobin in infants of diabetic mothers: relationships to neonatal hypoglycemic, macrosomia, and cord serum C-peptide. Diabetes Care 1982;5:566.
135. Karlsson K, Kjellmer I. The outcome of diabetic pregnancies in relation to the mother's blood sugar level. Am J Obstet Gynecol 1972;112:213.
136. Shannon K, Davis JC, Kitzmiller JL, et al. Erythropoiesis in infants of diabetic mothers. Pediatr Res 1986;30:161.
137. Gabbe SG, Mestman JH, Freeman RK, et al. Management and outcome of class A diabetes mellitus. Am J Obstet Gynecol 1977;127:465.
138. Cousins L. Pregnancy complications among diabetic women: review 1965–1985. Obstet Gynecol Surv 1987;42:140.
139. Becks GP, Burrow GN. Thyroid disease and pregnancy. Med Clin North Am 1991;75:121.
140. Morreale de Escobar G, Obregon MJ, Escobar de Rey F. Fetal and maternal thyroid hormones. Horm Res 1987;26:12.
141. Rodin A, Rodin AD. Thyroid disease in pregnancy. Br J Hosp Med 1989;41:234.
142. Balen AH, Kurtz AB. Successful outcome of pregnancy with severe hypothyroidism: case report and literature review. Br J Obstet Gynaecol 1990;97:536.
143. Hetzel BS, Mano MT. A review of experimental studies of iodine deficiency during fetal development. J Nutr 1989; 119:145.
144. Salvi M, How J. Pregnancy and autoimmune thyroid disease. Endocrinol Metab Clin North Am 1987;16:431.
145. Dussault JH, Rousseau F. Immunologically mediated hypothyroidism. Endocrinol Metab Clin North Am 1987;16:417.
146. Bruinse HW, Vermeulen-Meiners C, Wit JM. Fetal treatment for thyrotoxicosis in non-thyrotoxic pregnant women. Fetal Therapy 1988;3:152.
147. Siamoopoulos-Mavridou A, Manoussakis MN, Mavridia AK, et al. Outcome of pregnancy in patients with autoimmune rheumatic disease before the disease onset. Ann Rheum Dis 1988;47:982.
148. Feinstein DI. Lupus anticoagulant, thrombosis, and fetal loss. N Engl J Med 1985;313:1348.
149. Lockshin MD, Druzin ML, Goei S, et al. Antibody to cardiolipin as a predictor of fetal distress or death in pregnant patients with systemic lupus erythematosus. N Engl J Med 1985;313:152.
150. Nossent HC, Swaak TJ. Systemic lupus erythematosus: VI. Analysis of the interrelationship with pregnancy. J Rheumatol 1990;17:771.
151. Rote NS, Dostal-Johnson D, Branch DW. Antiphospholipid antibodies and recurrent pregnancy loss: correlation between the activated partial thromboplastin time and antibodies against phosphatidylserine and cardiolipin. Am J Obstet Gynecol 1990;163:575.
152. Lockshin MD, Druzin ML, Qamar T. Prednisone does not prevent recurrent fetal death in women with antiphospholipid antibody. Am J Obstet Gynecol 1989;160:439.
153. Petri M, Golbus M, Anderson R, et al. Antinuclear antibody, lupus anticoagulant, and anticardiolipin antibody in women with idiopathic habitual abortion: a controlled, prospective study of forty-four women. Arthritis Rheum 1987;30:601.
154. MacGregor SN. Human immunodeficiency virus infection in pregnancy. Clin Perinatol 1991;18:33.
155. Friedland IR, Snipelisky M. Vertically transmitted HIV-1 infection in children. S Afr Med J 1991;79:157.
156. Allen JR, Setlow VP. Heterosexual transmission of HIV: a view of the future. JAMA 1991;266:1695.
157. Allen S, Lindan C, Serufilira A, et al. Human immunodeficiency virus infection in urban Rwanda: demographic and behavioral correlates in a representative sample of childbearing women (editorial). JAMA 1991;266:1657.
158. Padian NS, Shiboski SC, Jewel NP. Female-to-male transmission of human immunodeficiency virus (editorial). JAMA 1991;266:1664.
159. Cotton P. Medicine's arsenal in battling "dominant dozen," other AIDS-associated opportunistic infections. JAMA 1991; 266:1476.
160. Working group on HIV testing of pregnant women and newborns. HIV infection, pregnant women, and newborns: a policy proposal for information and testing. JAMA 1990; 264:2416.
161. Pearlman M, Faro S. Obstetric septic shock: a pathophysiologic basis for management. Clin Obstet Gynecol 1990;33:482.
162. Clark SL. Shock in the pregnant patient. Semin Perinatol 1990;14:52.
163. McGee TM. Acute appendicitis in pregnancy. Aust NZ J Obstet Gynaecol 1989;29:378.
164. Ho VC, Sober AJ. Therapy for cutaneous melanoma: an update. J Am Acad Dermatol 1990;22:159.
165. Caligiuri MA, Mayer RJ. Pregnancy and leukemia. Semin Oncol 1989;16:388.
166. van der Vange N, van Dongen JA. Breast cancer and pregnancy. Eur J Surg Oncol 1991;17:1.
167. Barnavon Y, Wallack MK. Management of the pregnant patient with carcinoma of the breast. Gynecol Obstet 1990;171:347.
168. Turchi JJ, Villasis C. Anthracyclines in the treatment of malignancy in pregnancy. Cancer 1988;61:435.
169. Doll DC, Ringenberg S, Yarbro JW. Management of cancer during pregnancy. Arch Intern Med 1988;148:2058.
170. Williams SF, Birtan JD. Cancer and pregnancy. Clin Perinatol 1985;12:609.
171. Davison J, Lindheimer M. Pregnancy in women with renal allografts. Semin Nephrol 1984;4:240.
172. Penn I, Makowski E, Harris P. Parenthood following renal transplantation. Kidney Int 1980;18:221.
173. Davison J, Lind T, Uldall P. Planned pregnancy in a renal transplant recipient. Br J Obstet Gynaecol 1976;83:518.
174. Lewis G, Lamont C, Lee H, et al. Successful pregnancy in a renal transplant recipient taking cyclosporin A. Br Med J 1983;186:603.
175. Rudolph J, Shwihizir R, Barius S. Pregnancy in renal transplant patients: a review. Transplantation 1979;27:26.
176. Parsons V, Bewick M, Elias J, et al. Pregnancy following renal transplantation. J R Soc Med 1979;72:815.

177. Cote C, Meuwissen H, Pickering R. Effects on the neonate of prednisone and azathioprine administered to the mother during pregnancy. J Pediatr 1974;85:324.
178. Saarikoski S, Sappala M. Immunosuppression during pregnancy: transmission of azathioprine and its metabolites from mother to the fetus. Am J Obstet Gynecol 1973;115:1100.
179. Price H, Salaman J, Laurence K, et al. Immunosuppressive drugs and the fetus. Transplantation 1976;21:294.
180. McFaul PB, Dornan JC, Lamki H, et al. Pregnancy complicated by maternal heart disease: a review of 519 women. Br J Obstet Gynaecol 1988;95:861.
181. Commentary. The next lady has a heart defect. Br J Obstet Gynaecol 1987;94:97.
182. Gleicher N, Midwall J, Hochberger D, et al. Eisenmenger's syndrome and pregnancy. Obstet Gynecol Surv 1979;34:721.
183. Smith CA. Effects of maternal undernutrition upon the newborn infant in Holland (1944–1947). Am J Obstet Gynecol 1947;30:229.
184. Stein Z, Susser M, Saenger G, et al. Nutrition and mental performance. Science 1972;178:708.
185. Gross S, Librach C, Cecutti A. Maternal weight loss associated with hyperemesis gravidarum: a predictor of fetal outcome. Am J Obstet Gynecol 1989;160:906.
186. Churchill JA, Berendes HW, Nemore U. Neuropsychological deficits in children of diabetic mothers. Am J Obstet Gynecol 1977;165:257.
187. Rios E, Lipschitz DA, Cook JD, et al. Relationship of maternal and infant iron stores as assessed by determination of plasma ferritin. Pediatrics 1975;55:694.
188. Higginbottom MC, Sweetman L, Nyhan WL. A syndrome of methylmalonic aciduria, homocystinuria, megaloblastic anemia and neurologic abnormalities in a vitamin B_{12}-deficient breast-fed infant of a strict vegetarian. N Engl J Med 1978;299:317.
189. Eastman NJ, Jackson E. Weight relationships in pregnancy: I. The bearing of maternal weight gain and pre-pregnancy weight on birth weight in full term pregnancies. Obstet Gynecol Surv 1968;23:1003.

Neonatology: Pathophysiology and Management of the Newborn, Fourth Edition,
edited by Gordon B. Avery, Mary Ann Fletcher, and Mhairi G. MacDonald.
J.B. Lippincott Company, Philadelphia © 1994.

chapter 16

Effects of Prescribed and Self-Administered Drugs During the Second and Third Trimesters

DAVID A. BECKMAN
ROBERT L. BRENT

This chapter summarizes the known effects of some frequently used medications on the fetus. It is accepted that every drug administered or taken by a pregnant woman presents the mother with both risks and benefits. The controversies in this field primarily are related to the risks of these drugs.

Most human teratogens affect the embryo during a very narrow period of early embryonic development, as illustrated by the short period that the human embryo is susceptible to the limb reduction defects caused by thalidomide (Table 16-1). There are a few teratogens and many fetotoxic agents, however, that have deleterious effects during the second and even the third trimester.

Teratogenic agents that produce permanent cell deletion, vascular disruption, necrosis, specific tissue or organ pathology, physiologic decompensation, or severe growth retardation have the potential to cause deleterious effects throughout gestation. In addition, sensitivity of the fetus for induction of mental retardation and microcephaly is greatest at the end of the first and the beginning of the second trimester. Other permanent neurologic effects can be induced in the second and third trimesters. Known teratogens that affect the developing fetus beyond the period of organogenesis (*i.e.*, 18–40 days for major malformations, excluding genital malformations and cleft palate, which have longer periods of sensitivity) are listed in Table 16-2.

Drugs that are administered in the third trimester may not have teratogenic effects but may have the potential for fetopathic effects. The classic example of a drug that presents little risk to the developing embryo during organogenesis but can affect the near-term fetus if high doses are used is aspirin. It is possible that many antiinflammatory drugs present a similar risk.

Some drugs that are used commonly in the third trimester and their risks to the fetus and pregnant women are discussed in this chapter. Table 16-3 summarizes the acute effects on the fetus of drugs used during the second and third trimester and around the time of delivery.

ALCOHOL

Jones and colleagues described a fetal alcohol syndrome (FAS) in children with intrauterine growth retardation, microcephaly, mental retardation, maxillary hypoplasia, flat philtrum, thin upper lip, and reduction in the width of palpebral fissures as well as

TABLE 16–1
SENSITIVITY OF THE HUMAN TO LIMB REDUCTION DEFECTS CAUSED BY THALIDOMIDE BY DEVELOPMENTAL STAGE

Developmental Stage (Days Gestation)	Limb Reduction Defect
24–29	Amelia, upper limbs
21–26	Thumb aplasia
24–33	Phocomelia, upper limbs
23–34	Hip dislocation
27–31	Amelia, lower limb
25–31	Preaxial aplasia, upper limb
28–33	Preaxial aplasia, lower limb
28–33	Phocomelia, lower limb; femoral hypoplasia; girdle hypoplasia

Adapted from Brent RL, Holmes LB. Clinical and basic science lessons from the thalidomide tragedy: what have we learned about the causes of limb defects? Teratology 1988;38:241.

cardiac abnormalities.[1] Many of the children of alcoholic mothers had FAS and all of the affected children evidenced developmental delay.[2]

A period of greatest susceptibility and a dose–response relationship have not yet been established. Although we are reluctant to claim that malformations are due to single exposures to alcohol in the human, binge drinking early in pregnancy has been suggested to be associated with neural tube defects.[3] Actually, the neural tube defect, if real, is a minor risk when compared to the risk of decreased brain growth and differentiation that results from high levels of alcohol consumption during the second and third trimesters. Chronic consumption of 6 oz of alcohol per day constitutes a high risk, whereas FAS is not likely when the mother drinks fewer than two drinks equivalent to 2 oz of alcohol per day.[4] Reduction of alcohol consumption at any time in pregnancy reduces the severity of FAS but may not significantly reduce the risk of some degree of physical or behavioral impairment. The human syndrome is likely to involve the direct effects of alcohol and the indirect effects of genetic susceptibility and poor nutrition.

Sulik and Johnston have reported an animal model exhibiting craniofacial features in the mouse similar to those characteristic of FAS in humans.[5] Chernoff showed that the incidence of congenital defects and the maternal alcohol level were inversely related to the maternal alcohol dehydrogenase levels in three mouse strains.[6] It has been suggested that inhibition of cell growth is the primary effect of alcohol, resulting in developmental abnormalities.[7] Developmental delay in the central nervous system, especially in the midbrain, may cause abnormal patterns of innervation with resulting detrimental effects on learning and behavior. Acetaldehyde has been shown to be embryotoxic, but its role in producing teratogenesis is questionable.[8]

Although alcoholic mothers frequently smoke and consume other drugs, there is little doubt from the human and animal data that alcohol ingestion alone can have a disastrous effect on the developing embryo or fetus. As summarized by Schardein, the incidence of FAS in children born to alcoholic women is about 2.5%.[9] It has been estimated that up to 5% of congenital malformations may be due to prenatal alcohol exposure,[10] and that FAS appears to be the leading known cause of mental retardation. There are at least several hundred children born each year with full FAS and probably several thousand children born with fetal alcohol effects.[11]

TABLE 16–2
HUMAN TERATOGENS THAT CAN AFFECT THE FETUS IF EXPOSED AFTER THE FIRST TRIMESTER

Alcohol
Angiotensin-converting enzyme inhibitors
Androgens, high-dose
Anticonvulsants, chronic administration
Cocaine
Diethystilbestrol
Infectious diseases (*e.g.*, toxoplasmosis, syphilis, rubella, Venezuelan equine encephalitis, herpes simplex)
^{131}I, antithyroid drugs (*i.e.*, propylthiouracil)
Radiation, high-dose
Tetracycline
Warfarin

ANGIOTENSIN-CONVERTING ENZYME INHIBITORS

Angiotensin-converting enzyme (ACE) is a dipeptidyl-carboxypeptidase that catalyzes the conversion of the biologically inactive decapeptide angiotensin I to the active octapeptide angiotensin II. Angiotensin II is one of the most potent vasoconstrictors known. Captopril and enalapril, competitive inhibitors of ACE, are used to treat resistant hypertension.

Adverse effects on the fetus of a pregnant woman treated with captopril beginning at week 26 of gestation were first reported in 1981.[12] Oligohydramnios was detected 2 weeks later and a cesarean delivery was performed in week 29 due to fetal distress. The infant was anuric and hypotensive and died on the seventh postpartum day. The kidneys and bladder were normally developed but had hemorrhagic foci in the renal cortex and medulla. There have been several reviews and reports of oligohydramnios or neonatal anuria, pulmonary hypoplasia, mild to severe intrauterine growth retardation, persistent patent ductus arteriosis, renal tubular dysplasia, and fetal death associated with maternal therapy with ACE inhibitors.[13]

TABLE 16–3
DRUGS LIKELY TO BE USED NEAR DELIVERY AND THEIR ACUTE EFFECTS ON THE FETUS

Indication	Drug	Comments	Dose
Reduce respiratory distress in premature infant	Glucocorticoids Betamethasone	No adverse fetal effects reported	12 mg IM q 12 h × 2 doses
	Dexamethasone	No adverse fetal effects	5 mg IM q 12 h × 4 doses
	Hydrocortisone	No adverse fetal effects	500 mg IV q 12 h × 2 doses
	Methylprednisone	No adverse fetal effects	125 mg IM q 12 h × 2 doses
Prevention or reduction of intraventricular hemorrhage in premature infant	Phenobarbital	No adverse fetal effects	500–780 mg IV over 30 min
	Indomethacin	Increased risk of oligohydramnios, reduced fetal renal function, constriction of ductus arteriosus, fetal hydrops	Therapeutic dose is controversial but higher than the 25 mg q 6 h used for treatment of polyhydramnios
Polyhydramnios	Indomethacin	Risk for adverse fetal effects (oligohydramnios) not as great as with higher doses	25 mg q 6 h
Fetal dysrhythmia	Digoxin	No adverse fetal effects	0.25–0.75 mg q 8 h PO; If digoxin is ineffective, however, second-line drugs may be acceptable (*e.g.,* quinidine, procainamide, verpamil, and propranolol)
Prophylaxis against Rh immunization	Rh immunoglobulin	No adverse fetal effects	300 μg IM at 28 weeks of gestation
Sexually Transmitted Diseases			
Syphilis			
<1-y duration	Penicillin G benzathine	No adverse fetal effects	2.4 million U IM once
Undetermined duration	Pencillin G benzathine	No adverse fetal effects	2.4 million U IM weekly for 3 wk
Gonorrhea	Ceftriaxone and Doxycycline	No adverse fetal effects	100 mg q 12 h PO for 7 d
Chlamydia	Erythromycin base or stearate	Possible increased risk of cholestatic hepatitis	500 mg q 6 h PO for 7 d
Congenital adrenal hyperplasia	Dexamethasone	No adverse fetal effects	0.25 mg IM 1 6 h
Fetal thyrotoxicosis and hyperthyroidism	Propylthiouracil	Thioamides may cause fetal goiter but dose can be adjusted to minimize this effect	
Biotin-responsive multiple carboxylase deficiency	Biotin	No adverse fetal efects	10 mg/d PO
Vitamin B_{12}–responsive methylmalonic acidemia	Cyanocobalamin	No adverse fetal effects	5 mg/d IV
Prevention of neural tube defects	Folic acid	The efficacy of folic acid supplementation for reducing the risk of neural tube defect recurrence may be limited to a select portion of the population; there are no adverse fetal effects	1–5 mg/d PO
Preeclamspia, idiopathic placental insufficiency, some immunologic states, increased platelet aggregation	Aspirin	No increased risk for maternal or fetal bleeding	60–150 mg PO

Animal studies have shown that ACE inhibitors cross the placenta and affect the fetus but are not teratogenic during the period of early organogenesis.[13] There are five case reports, however, of skull bone (*i.e.*, calvarial) hypoplasia in the human fetus of mothers who had received ACE inhibitors.[13–15] Barr summarized the fetopathic properties of a very effective and otherwise safe group of antihypertensive agents.[15] He reported a patient exposed to an ACE inhibitor that was administered throughout pregnancy. Oligohydramnios was diagnosed at 20 weeks of gestation. Anuria, growth retardation, and calvarial hypoplasia were observed in the neonate. The infant died from oligohydramnios-associated pulmonary hypoplasia.

Animal studies and human case reports suggest that ACE inhibitors do not cause congenital malformations by interfering with organogenesis but nevertheless can deleteriously affect the developing mammalian fetus. Animal studies indicate that ACE inhibitors, although not teratogenic during the period of early organogenesis, can reduce uterine blood flow in the pregnant guinea pig and can inhibit fetal ACE activity.[16,17] Broughton Pipkin and associates observed a high rate of perinatal mortality in pregnant sheep and rabbits treated with captopril.[18] Evidence suggests that fetal and neonatal mortality, oligohydramnios, neonatal anuria, intrauterine growth retardation, renal tubular dysplasia, and calvarial hypoplasia are related to severe fetal hypotension during the second and third trimester. Although the fetopathic risk appears to be low, the effects are severe. It can be inferred that adverse fetal effects will be applicable to all ACE inhibitors that cross the placenta, because the fetal effects are plausibly explained by the direct therapeutic effectiveness of these drugs. Although there was some controversy in the early literature as to whether captopril and enalapril crossed the placenta in some species, data indicate that ACE activity was reduced in neonates treated with captopril and enalapril, thus indicating that both cross the human placenta.[19,20] Although there appears to be a consensus pertaining to the fact that the ACE inhibitors may present little or no reproductive risk during the first trimester, there is controversy regarding the magnitude of the risk during the later stages when the fetus is at risk.

The severe skull hypoplasia is a unique feature of this syndrome and may be explained readily by the combination of low fetal blood pressure, poor peripheral perfusion of the superficial tissues, and oligohydramnios. The special vulnerability of the skull may be due to the fact that the uterine musculature can exert pressure directly on the skull because of the oligohydramnios. Because the skull also is poorly perfused due to fetal hypotension, one can envision why the calvaria fail to ossify properly. There may be other explanations forthcoming to explain the calvarial hypoplasia. Infants who present in breech may be at even greater risk when also exposed to the ACE inhibitors because the skull will have a greater likelihood of direct contact with the uterus, and the brain is much more vulnerable to injury due to the marked reduction in the calvaria.

Angiotensin-converting enzyme inhibitors are effective and important therapeutic agents for the treatment of hypertension. There is no reason to change their use in women of reproductive age because the therapy can be changed during the first trimester if the woman becomes pregnant. A rational, deliberative plan to switch over to a secondary regimen should be undertaken shortly after pregnancy has been diagnosed. Certainly it would be medically inappropriate to suggest the interruption of a wanted pregnancy because of a presumed teratogenic risk due to exposure early in pregnancy, because these drugs do not appear to interfere with early organogenesis at therapeutic doses. Angiotensin-converting enzyme inhibitors are agents that interfere with normal fetal development, but whose major effects are due to chronic exposure during the fetal stages and not to exposures during early organogenesis.[13,14] Thus, the ACE inhibitors can be added to that category of teratogens, such as warfarin and radioactive iodine, that are relatively safe during early periods of gestation and present a greater risk after organogenesis.

COCAINE

The contribution of drug abuse to the incidence of congenital malformations is difficult to assess because street drugs are of variable potency and purity, abusers neglect health care and nutrition, the frequency of multiple drug abuse is high, and there is a high incidence of infections and venereal disease among drug abusers. There does not appear to be a significant increase in teratogenic risk associated with the abuse of narcotics, marijuana, benzodiazepines, barbiturates, amphetamines, or toluene. There is, however, increased fetal wastage, intrauterine growth retardation, and complications of pregnancy associated with abuse of these drugs. Cocaine is an important exception because, along with increased perinatal morbidity, the available evidence indicates that cocaine produces various types of vascular disruption and therefore has teratogenic potential.

Cocaine (benzoylmethylecgonine) is prepared from the leaves of the plants *Erythroxylon coca* and, to a lesser extent, *Truxillo coca*. Illicit cocaine in powder form is a water-soluble salt, cocaine hydrochloride, that may be adulterated by sugars, stimulants, or local anesthetics.[21] Cocaine has a half-life of about 40 to 60 minutes after intravenous or intranasal administration. Crack cocaine is the alkaloidal form that, when smoked, produces a rapid increase in blood concentration and half-life similar to those obtained with intravenous administration.[21,22] Since cocaine is lipid soluble, has a low molecular weight, and is a weak base, it is not surprising that it crosses the placenta by diffusion.[23] Cocaine is metabolized primarily by plasma and liver cholinesterase to water-soluble metabolites (*i.e.*, benzoylecgonine and ecgonine methyl ester) that are excreted in the urine. Fetuses and pregnant women have low plasma cholinesterase activity and therefore are likely to be more sensitive to the effects of cocaine than nonpregnant adults.[21] Cocaine abusers often abuse more than one substance, suffer from malnutrition, and neglect prenatal medical care. Cocaine use during pregnancy has been associated with preterm labor and delivery, fetal loss, and fetal abnormalities, including decreased birth weight, microcephaly, urinary tract malformations, and neurobehavioral abnormalities.[14,24]

The initial effects of cocaine include hypertension, tachycardia, mydriasis, and hyperpyrexia. Temperatures rise as high as 45°C during acute intoxication. These sympathomimetic effects of cocaine are mediated by the inhibition of presynaptic catecholamine reuptake. Placental vasoconstriction and increased uterine contractility have been reported in pregnant women using cocaine.[14] Cocaine has been shown to decrease uterine blood flow in animal studies,[25] and to produce congenital malformations after administration during midgestation in the rat.[26] A reduction in uterine blood flow due to the vasoconstrictive action of cocaine may cause hypoxia and infarction in the developing fetus.[27]

There is a substantial body of evidence indicating the vascular pathogenesis of major malformations that could be induced, not only during organogenesis, but also during later stages of development in experimental animals and in the human.[28–30] It is likely that the adverse fetal effects associated with maternal cocaine use are due to both the vasoconstriction of uterine blood vessels and to local vasoactive effects in the fetus.[24,25,27] Localized hemorrhagic and cavitary lesions as well as a generalized cerebral injury have been reported in fetuses of animals exposed to cocaine and in newborns of chronic cocaine abusers.[14]

Although vasoconstrictive action on uterine and fetal blood vessels could explain the observed malformations associated with exposure to cocaine, cocaine does not cause a morphologically specific syndrome analogous to FAS. Malformations with a vascular disruptive pathogenesis vary too widely between patients to constitute a syndrome. Nevertheless, all of the reported fetal effects associated with exposure to cocaine appear to be various types of vascular disruptive phenomena (*e.g.*, congenital limb amputations, cerebral infarctions, certain types of visceral and urinary tract malformations). Experimental animal studies and human epidemiology indicate that the risk of major malformations from cocaine is low but the malformations may be severe.

ANTIBIOTICS

The incidence of intraamniotic infection is about 1% of all pregnancies and 3% to 40% of women with ruptured membranes for 24 hours or more.[31] Intraamniotic infection is associated with increased morbidity in the newborn, including pneumonia and sepsis. There also is a significant increase in perinatal mortality associated with intraamniotic infection, although this is due in part to prematurity.

Increased neonatal mortality and morbidity, especially from group B streptococcal infection, can be largely prevented by intrapartum chemoprophylaxis. Intrapartum antibiotics for acute intraamniotic infection can effectively eliminate positive blood cultures for group B streptococci.[32] Neonatal sepsis also is significantly reduced if mothers receive antibiotics intrapartum rather than after cord clamping.[33]

CEFTRIAXONE PLUS DOXYCYCLINE

Untreated *Neisseria gonorrhoeae* infection can lead to serious consequences for the infected woman. Treatment with ceftriaxone (250 mg intramuscularly once) plus doxycycline (100 mg orally twice a day for 7 days) has no reported adverse effects on the fetus.

PENICILLIN

The incidence of infection with *Treponema pallidum* in pregnant women is increasing, accompanied by an increase in the occurrence of congenital syphilis. Penicillin G benzathine, 2.4 million units intramuscularly once, is an effective treatment for maternal infections of less than 1 year. For infections of longer or undetermined duration, or when associated with human immunodeficiency virus infection, penicillin G, 2.4 million units intramuscularly weekly for 3 weeks, is needed. There are no adverse fetal effects with either regimen; none have been reported for any penicillins.

TETRACYCLINES

Tetracyclines are known to cause discoloration of the deciduous teeth, but short-term exposure to the usual therapeutic doses near the time of delivery does not pose an increased risk to the fetus.

ERYTHROMYCIN

As is the case with other sexually transmitted diseases, chlamydial infection is on the increase. The infant most likely acquires chlamydial infection during parturition at an incidence of approximately 50%. Erythromycin, 500 mg four times daily for 7 days, is an effective prenatal treatment; however, there may be an increased risk of cholestatic hepatitis.

STREPTOMYCIN AND KANAMYCIN

The aminoglycosides streptomycin and kanamycin have been associated with ototoxicity.[34,35]

CEPHALOSPORINS

The cephalosporins containing N-methylthiotetrazole have been associated with testicular toxicity in experimental animals. More data are needed to determine whether this association indicates a potential fetal hazard in the human.

It appears that acute exposure to antibiotics in usual therapeutic doses poses little significant risk to the fetus, especially compared to the potentially devastating effects of neonatal sepsis.

ANTIHYPERTENSIVES

CLONIDINE

Clonidine exerts its hypotensive effect by a direct α-adrenergic agonist action in the central nervous system. It appears to be relatively safe during pregnancy, but there are few available data.[36]

HYDRALAZINE

Hydralazine is a vasodilator often used in combination with methyldopa for the treatment of preexisting hypertension in pregnancy, and is considered to be safe. Although there is one report of fetal thrombocytopenia,[37] over 120 normal pregnancies have been reported.[38]

METHYLDOPA

Methyldopa is the safest antihypertensive drug available for use during pregnancy.[39] Methyldopa is a centrally acting adrenergic antagonist with no reported adverse effects on the fetus or on mental and physical development.[36]

NIFEDIPINE

Nifedipine is a calcium channel blocker used for the treatment of preterm labor with no reported adverse effects.[40] The potential for adverse effects with its long-term use in the treatment of hypertension is unknown.

PROPRANOLOL

Propranolol is a β-blocker useful in treating preexisting hypertension during pregnancy. There is well founded concern, however, that prolonged use may cause major growth retardation.[41]

ASPIRIN

Aspirin acts principally by inhibiting prostaglandin synthesis by irreversibly acetylating and inactivating fatty acid cyclooxygenase. Low-dose aspirin (60–150 mg) is used clinically in the prevention or treatment of preeclampsia, intrauterine growth retardation, immunologic states associated with an increased risk of fetal loss, and maternal conditions resulting from increased platelet aggregation.

Preeclampsia is associated with vasospasm, increased platelet activation, coagulation, and pregnancy-induced hypertension. Although there is some evidence that aspirin may prevent or treat preeclampsia, the effective minimum dose is undetermined; the decreased incidences of preeclampsia, hypertension, and fetal death are not statistically significant in all reports.[42]

There is some evidence that aspirin combined with dipyridamile may prevent or ameliorate intrauterine growth retardation associated with idiopathic uteroplacental insufficiency.[43] Aspirin alone (150 mg/day) improved fetal growth in fetuses with high, but not extreme, umbilical artery systolic–diastolic ratio.[44] Third-trimester exposure to low daily doses of aspirin was not associated with adverse fetal outcome in these studies.[43,44]

High fetal losses are associated with lupus anticoagulant antibodies, anticardiolipin antibodies, and systemic lupus erythematosus. Surviving fetuses experience an increased incidence of growth retardation, fetal distress, and preterm delivery. Low-dose aspirin (60–80 mg/day) in combination with prednisone (20–80 mg/day) improve pregnancy outcome and greatly reduce thrombosis.[42]

Case reports suggest that 75 to 300 mg of aspirin per day in combination with dipyridamole might reduce the risk of late fetal loss in patients with arterial thromboembolism, thrombotic thrombocytopenia purpura, and idiopathic or essential thrombocythemia.[42]

Although doubts over the safety of aspirin during pregnancy have been expressed, aspirin use during the first trimester is not associated with an increased teratogenic risk.[45] Third-trimester exposure to 80 mg per day or less is not associated with an early constriction of the ductus arteriosus.[46] Much larger doses of aspirin during the third trimester have been associated with an increased length of gestation, duration of labor, frequency of postmaturity, and blood loss at delivery,[47] and justify careful fetal surveillance.

Another question is the potential for increased fetal and maternal bleeding associated with low-dose aspirin use near the time of delivery or higher doses used to treat preterm labor. Jankowski and associates reported a study involving 25 women threatened with premature delivery who were given 3.6 g of oral aspirin per day for 4 successive days within 10 days before delivery.[48] They and others found no adverse effect on maternal bleeding at delivery, fetal hemorrhage, or circulatory disorders.

DIGOXIN

Digoxin (0.25–0.75 mg orally every 8 hours) is the drug used most often to correct fetal tachyarrhythmias with no substantiated adverse fetal effects.[49] The possibility of any adverse side-effects, however, must be balanced with the fetal prognosis if the dysrhythmia persists or is likely to lead to fetal cardiac failure.

GLUCOCORTICOIDS

Glucocorticoids (*i.e.*, dexamethasone, betamethasone, hydrocortisone, methylprednisone) are effective in reducing the incidence of respiratory distress syndrome in premature newborns by inducing early lung maturation,[50] as first hypothesized by Liggins and Howie.[51] Endogenous glucocorticoids mediate normal pulmonary maturation. Exogenous glucocorticoids are used to stimulate the production of surfactant. The adverse fetal effects observed in experimental animals exposed to pharmacologic doses are not seen in humans at therapeutic levels.[50]

It has been reported that antenatal thyroid-releasing hormone combined with glucocorticoid therapy enhances the lung maturation achieved with glucocorticoids alone, but this effect must be confirmed.[52]

Dexamethasone is used to suppress the fetal adrenal gland in cases of congenital adrenal hyperplasia.[53] 21-Hydroxylase deficiency impairs the conversion of cholesterol to cortisol and results in excess 17-hydroxyprogesterone, which in turn results in excess levels of androgens. The masculinization of female fetuses with congenital adrenal hyperplasia varies from clitoral hypertrophy to formation of a phallus. Maternal replacement doses of dexamethasone, 0.25 mg 4 times a day beginning at 9 weeks of gestation, suppress both the maternal and fetal adrenal glands and prevent masculinization in most patients. The efficacy of the same regimen initiated at 7 weeks of gestation is being evaluated (see Chap. 14).[54]

INDOMETHACIN

Oral administration of the prostaglandin synthetase inhibitor, indomethacin (25 mg every 6 hours), is effective in the treatment of polyhydramnios that is either idiopathic or related to maternal diabetes mellitus. The reduction in renal prostaglandin levels achieved using indomethacin would reduce the inhibitory action of the E prostaglandins on the antidiuretic effect of arginine vasopressin and result in decreased urine production by the fetal kidneys. Oligohydramnios, constriction of the ductus arteriosus (prostaglandins are necessary to maintain the patency of the fetal ductus arteriosus), and fetal hydrops are potentially serious side-effects of indomethacin and warrant careful fetal surveillance.[55]

The efficacy of antepartum therapy with indomethacin to prevent intraventricular hemorrhage is controversial. The cord levels achieved after doses used to treat preterm labor (25 mg every 6 hours) are far below those that are likely to provide protection against intraventricular hemorrhage. Even these lower doses, however, are associated with a 10% incidence of impaired fetal renal function and oligohydramnios and a 50% incidence of ductus arteriosus constriction.[56]

PHENOBARBITAL

In two prospective studies of patients in high-risk groups for neonatal intraventricular hemorrhage, intravenous phenobarbital administered antenatally resulted in a significant reduction in the incidence of severe cases of intraventricular hemorrhage by increasing cerebral vascular resistance.[57] Phenobarbital reduces peak arterial blood pressure, thereby reducing the risk of intraventricular hemorrhage, one of the leading complications of the very-low-birth-weight preterm infant.[58] The early neonatal period probably is too late a time for the initiation of intravenous phenobarbital to derive the potential benefits of this therapy.

Although antenatal administration of vitamin K may not reduce the risk of intraventricular hemorrhage, vitamin K therapy combined with phenobarbital appears to improve the outcome compared to phenobarbital alone.[57]

RH IMMUNE GLOBULIN

After exposure to Rh(D)-positive erythrocytes, usually resulting from a fetal transplacental hemorrhage that occurs to some degree in 75% of pregnancies,[59] the Rh(D)-negative mother becomes Rh immunized. Rh immunization during a previous pregnancy results in brain damage of various degree or death in an Rh(D)-positive newborn in approximately 50% of cases.[59] Once maternal Rh immunization has developed, it cannot be treated effectively, but it can be prevented by antenatal prophylaxis with 300 μg of Rh immune globulin at 28 weeks of gestation.[59] No adverse fetal effects to immunoprophylaxis have been reported.

SMOKING AND NICOTINE

Approximately 30% of all women of childbearing age smoke, and about 25% of all women will continue smoking after they become pregnant.[60] Evidence in humans indicates that smoking affects the fetus directly in a dose-related manner, and that probably more than one component of smoke is involved.[61] Although smoking is associated with intrauterine growth retardation, a variety of maternal and placental complications, fetal death, and increased postnatal morbidity, there is no proven relationship between smoking and specific malformations or malformations in general. One study suggests that infants of women who smoked throughout pregnancy experience an increase in mortality that continues until at least 5 years of age.[62] Because of the large number of pregnant women who smoke and the documented effects of smoking on the fetus, it can be said that smoking presents a significant risk to the fetus for growth retardation and spontaneous abortion.

THIOAMIDES

Fetal thyrotoxicosis is induced by thyroid-stimulating immunoglobulins produced in euthyroid or hypothyroid women. The adverse fetal effects (*e.g.*, craniosynostosis, intellectual impairment, increased mortality) are caused by excess fetal thyroid hormone production.

Thioamides include all the antithyroid drugs used clinically. The thioamides block thyroid hormone synthesis by inhibiting the oxidation of iodide or iodotyrosyl. Unlike other thioamides, propylthiouracil also inhibits the peripheral deiodination of thyroxine to triiodothyronine. All thioamides are associated with a significant risk of fetal goiter and teratogenesis.[9] In the case of propylthiouracil, however, the fetal goiter can be reduced with intraamniotic injections of thyroxine,[63] which also prevents other abnormalities caused by inhibition of fetal thyroid function.

TOCOLYTICS

Fetal distress can result from uterine hypertonus, umbilical cord compression, premature rupture of the fetal membranes, oligohydramnios, placental abruption, and uteroplacental insufficiency. In some cases of severe fetal hypoxemia or acidosis, prompt delivery may be recommended. If immediate surgery is not feasible, however, tocolytics may help to reduce fetal distress until delivery is possible.

In cases of hypoxemia due to reduced blood flow to the fetus, inhibiting uterine activity should increase the delivery of oxygen to the fetus by increasing uterine and intervillous perfusion. In addition to inhibiting uterine activity, β-adrenergic agonists both increase maternal cardiac output and dilate uterine vessels, resulting in a further increase in placental perfusion.

Ritodrine, a β_2-adrenergic receptor agonist, may be administered as an intravenous bolus for acute fetal distress.[64] Ritodrine's mechanism of action leads to a reduction in the intracellular calcium available for smooth muscle contraction.

Terbutaline sulfate, a nonspecific β-adrenergic agonist, is associated with a higher incidence of cardiovascular side-effects than ritodrine with prolonged use.

When the use of β-adrenergic agonists is contraindicated in cases of intraamniotic infection, uncontrolled maternal thyroid disease, diabetes mellitus, and cardiovascular disease, magnesium sulfate may be used as a tocolytic agent. Although its mechanism of action is unknown, it results in an uncoupling of the actin–myosin interaction in smooth muscle.[65] An advantage of magnesium sulfate tocolysis is the absence of cardiovascular side-effects.

The data on the fetal effects of tocolytic agents are restricted to case reports, but there are no reports of adverse fetal outcome resulting from exposure to therapeutic doses of terbutaline,[66] ritodrine,[67] or magnesium sulfate.[68] Infants born immediately after use of magnesium sulfate for controlling some of the symptoms of preeclampsia may be vasodilated, sedated, and have reduced respiratory drive and decreased bowel motility. For this reason, tocolytic therapy with magnesium sulphate usually is stopped as long before delivery as possible to allow fetal placental clearance.

TRANQUILIZERS

The minor tranquilizers as a group are probably the most frequently prescribed therapeutic agents. Within this group, the propanediol carbonates and the benzodiazepines, the two most widely used classes,[9] have been associated with teratogenic effects. The strongest association has been between diazepam and cleft lip with or without cleft palate, but even this association is not likely to be causal.[69] Because these drugs are widely used, even a small increased risk would be expected to result in more reported adverse effects than has been the case. Continued surveillance is warranted because so many pregnancies are exposed to these drugs.

VITAMINS

BIOTIN

Biotin-responsive multiple carboxylase deficiency is an inborn error of metabolism in which there is a severe reduction in the activities of the mitochondrial biotin-dependent carboxylase enzymes. Affected people exhibit dermatitis, severe metabolic acidosis, and a characteristic pattern of organic acid excretion. Metabolism in these patients is restored to normal levels by biotin supplementation. Prenatal administration of 10 mg per day of oral biotin initiated during the third trimester prevented neonatal complications with no adverse fetal effects.[70]

FOLIC ACID

The relationship between folic acid supplementation and a reduction in the incidence of neural tube defects has not been settled. Smithells and colleagues suggested that folic acid supplementation can reduce the frequency of neural tube defect recurrence in families with prior affected children.[71] Studies have both supported[72] and not supported[73] the hypothesis. Problems in study design, recall error, and patient selection restrict comparisons among these studies.

If folic acid supplementation does in fact reduce the incidence of neural tube defects, the effective dose has not been established. Oral doses of 1 to 5 mg per day have had no adverse effect on the fetus.

VITAMIN B_{12}

Ampola and colleagues were the first to report prenatal treatment of a vitamin-responsive inborn error of metabolism.[74] Their report involved a fetus with a vitamin B_{12}-responsive variant of methylmalonic acidemia, a metabolic disease involving a functional deficiency in the coenzymatically active form of vitamin B_{12}. Oral cyanocobalamin (10 mg per day) initiated at 32 weeks of gestation, resulted in only a slight increase in maternal serum B_{12} level. Oral therapy was therefore stopped at 34 weeks of gestation, and 5 mg per day of intravenous cyanocobalamin was initiated. This regimen produced a progressive increase in maternal serum B_{12} and a decrease in urinary methylmalonic acid excretion. The infant had no acute neonatal complications after delivery at 41 weeks.

REFERENCES

1. Jones KL, Smith DW, Ulleland CN, et al. Pattern of malformation in offspring of chronic alcoholic mothers. Lancet 1973;1:1267.
2. Jones KL, Smith DW. The fetal alcohol syndrome. Teratology 1975;12:1.
3. Graham JM Jr. The effects of alcohol consumption during pregnancy. In: Marois M, ed. Prevention of physical and mental congenital defects. Part C: basic and medical science, education, and future strategies. New York: Alan R Liss, 1985:335.
4. Streissguth AP, Landesman-Dwyer C, Martin JC, et al. Teratogenic effects of alcohol in humans and laboratory animals. Science 1980;209:353.
5. Sulik KK, Johnston MC. Acute ethanol administration in an animal model results in craniofacial features characteristic of the fetal alcohol syndrome. Science 1982;214:936.
6. Chernoff GF. The fetal alcohol syndrome in mice: maternal variables. Teratology 1989;22:71.
7. Kennedy LA. The pathogenesis of brain abnormalities in the fetal alcohol syndrome: an integrating hypothesis. Teratology 1984;29:363.
8. Blakely PM. Experimental teratology of ethanol. In: Kalter H, ed. Issues and reviews in teratology. vol. 4. New York: Plenum Press, 1988:237.
9. Schardein JL. Chemically induced birth defects. New York: Marcel Dekker, 1985:879.
10. Hanson JW, Jones KL, Smith DW. Fetal alcohol syndrome. JAMA 1976;235:1458.
11. Brent RL. Editorial: teratologists, the fetal alcohol syndrome and alcohol addiction: are we doing enough? Teratology 1990;41:491.
12. Guignard JP, Burgener F, Calame A. Persistent anuria in neonate: a side effect of captopril. Int J Pediatr Nephrol 1981;2:133.
13. Brent RL, Beckman DA. Angiotensin-converting enzyme inhibitors, an embryopathic class of drugs with unique properties: information for clinical teratology counselors. Teratology 1991;43:543.
14. Beckman DA, Brent RL. Teratogenesis: alcohol, angiotensin converting enzyme inhibitors, and cocaine. Curr Opin Obstet Gynecol 1990;2:236.
15. Barr M. Fetal effects of angiotensin converting enzyme inhibitor. Teratology 1990;41:537A.
16. Davidson D, Stalcup SA, Mellins RB. Captopril administration to the pregnant guinea pig inhibits fetal angiotensin converting enzyme activity. Pediatr Res 1981;15:658.
17. Ferris TF, Weir EK. Effect of captopril on uterine blood flow and prostaglandin E synthesis in the pregnancy rabbit. J Clin Invest 1982;71:809.
18. Broughton Pipkin F, Symonds EM, Turner SR. The effect of captopril (SQ 14,225) upon mother and fetus in the chronically cannulated ewe and in the pregnancy rabbit. J Physiol 1982;323:415.
19. Guignard JP. Drugs and the neonatal kidney. Dev Pharmacol Ther 1982;4(Suppl 1):19.
20. Schubiger G, Flury G, Nussberger J. Enalapril for pregnancy-induced hypertension: acute renal failure in a neonate. Ann Intern Med 1988;108:215.
21. Johanson C-E, Fischman MW. The pharmacology of cocaine related to its abuse. Pharmacol Rev 1989;41:3.
22. Fischman MW. Behavioral pharmacology of cocaine. J Clin Psychiatry 1988;49(Suppl):7.
23. American Society for Pharmacology and Experimental Therapeutics and Committee on Problems of Drug Dependence. Scientific perspectives on cocaine abuse. Pharmacologist 1987; 29:20.
24. Chasnoff IJ, Lewis DE, Griffith DR, et al. Cocaine and pregnancy: clinical and toxicological implications for the neonate. Clin Chem 1989;35:1276.
25. Woods JR, Plessinger MA, Clark KE. Effect of cocaine on uterine blood flow and fetal oxygenation. JAMA 1987;257:957.
26. Webster WS, Brown-Woodman PDC, Lipson AH. Teratogenic properties of cocaine in rats. Teratology 1989;40:263.
27. Chavez GF, Mulinare J, Cordero JF. Maternal cocaine use during early pregnancy as a risk factor for congenital urogenital anomalies. JAMA 1989;262:795.
28. Franklin JB, Brent RL. The effect of uterine vascular clamping on the development of rat embryos three to fourteen days old. J Morphol 1965;115:273.
29. Webster WS, Lipson AH, Brown-Woodman PDC. Uterine trauma and limb defects. Teratology 1987;35:253.
30. Hoyme HE, Jones KL, Van Allen MI, et al. The vascular pathogenesis of transverse limb reduction defects. J Pediatr 1982; 101:839.
31. Cox SM, Williams ML, Leveno KJ. The natural history of preterm ruptured membranes: what to expect of expectant management. Obstet Gynecol 1988;71:558.
32. Gilstrap LC, Leveno KJ, Cox SM, et al. Intrapartum treatment of acute chorioamnionitis: impact on neonatal sepsis. Am J Obstet Gynecol 1988;159:579.
33. Sperling RS, Ramamurthy RS, Gibbs RS. A comparison of intrapartum versus immediate postpartum treatment of intra-amnionic infection. Obstet Gynecol 1987;70:861.

34. Donald PR, Sellars SL. Streptomycin ototoxicity in the unborn child. S Afr Med J 1981;60:316.
35. Good RG, Johnson GH. The placental transfer of kanamycin during late pregnancy. Obstet Gynecol 1971;38:60.
36. Redman CW. Treatment of hypertension in pregnancy. Kidney Int 1980;18:267.
37. Widerlov E, Karlman I, Storsater J. Hydralazine-induced neonatal thrombocytopenia. (Letter) N Engl J Med 1980;301:1235.
38. Bott-Kanner G, Schweitzer A, Reisner SH, et al. Propranolol and hydralazine in the management of essential hypertension in pregnancy. Br J Obstet Gynaecol 1980;87:110.
39. NHBPEP Working Group. NHBPEP Working Group report on high blood pressure in pregnancy. Public Health Service, National Institutes of Health Publication No. 91-2039. Bethesda, MD: National Institutes of Health, 1991.
40. Constantine G, Beevers DG, Reynolds AL, et al. Nifedipine as a second line antihypertensive drug in pregnancy. Br J Obstet Gynecol 1987;94:1136.
41. Witter FR, King TM, Blake DA. Adverse effects of cardiovascular drug therapy on the fetus and neonate. Obstet Gynecol 1981;58:100.
42. Barton, J.R, Sibai, B.M. Low-dose aspirin to improve perinatal outcome. Clin Obstet Gynecol 1991;34:251.
43. Wallenburg HCS, Rotmans N. Prevention of recurrent idiopathic fetal growth retardation by low-dose aspirin and dipyridamole. Am J Obstet Gynecol 1987;157:1230.
44. Trudinger BJ, Cook CM, Giles WB, et al. Low-dose aspirin in pregnancy. Lancet 1989;1:410.
45. Werler MM, Mitchell AA, Shapiro S. The relation of aspirin use during the first trimester of pregnancy to congenital cardiac defects. N Engl J Med 1989;321:1639.
46. McParland P, Pearce JM, Chamberlain GVP. Doppler ultrasound and aspirin in recognition and prevention of pregnancy-induced hypertension. Lancet 1990;335:1552.
47. Lewis RB, Schulman JD. Influence of acetylsalicylic acid, an inhibitor of prostaglandin synthesis, on the duration of human gestation and labour. Lancet 1973;2:1159.
48. Jankowski A, Skublicki S, Wichlinski LM, et al. Clinical-pharmacokinetic investigations of acetylsalicylic acid in cases of imminent premature delivery. Journal of Clinical and Hospital Pharmacy 1985;10:361.
49. Pinsky WW, Rayburn WF, Evans MI. Pharmacologic therapy for fetal arrhythmias. Clin Obstet Gynecol 1991;34:304.
50. Collaborative Group on Antenatal Steroid Therapy. Effect of antenatal dexamethasone administration in the prevention of respiratory distress syndrome. Am J Obstet Gynecol 1981; 141:276.
51. Liggins GC, Howie RN. A controlled trial of antepartum glucocorticoid treatment for prevention of the respiratory distress syndrome in premature infants. Pediatrics 1972;50:515.
52. Morales WJ, O'Brien WF, Angel JL, et al. Fetal lung maturation: the combined use of corticosteroids and thyrotropin-releasing hormone. Obstet Gynecol 1989;73:111.
53. Evans MI, Chrousos GP, Mann DW, et al. Pharmacologic suppression of the fetal adrenal gland in utero: attempted prevention of abnormal external genital masculinization in suspected congenital adrenal hyperplasia. JAMA 1985;253:1015.
54. Evans MI, Schulman JD. In utero treatment of fetal metabolic disorders. Clin Obstet Gynecol 1991;34:268.
55. Moise KJ. Indomethacin therapy in the treatment of symptomatic polyhydramnios. Clin Obstet Gynecol 1991;24:310.
56. Moise KJ, Huhta JC, Sharif DS, et al. Indomethacin in the treatment of premature labor: effects on the fetal ductus arteriosus. N Engl J Med 1988;319:327.
57. Morales WJ. Antenatal therapy to minimize neonatal intraventricular hemorrhage. Clin Obstet Gynecol 1991;34:328.
58. Morales WJ. Effect of intraventricular hemorrhage on the one-year mental and neurologic handicaps of the very low birth weight infant. Obstet Gynecol 1987;70:111.
59. Bowman JM. Antenatal suppression of Rh alloimmunization. Clin Obstet Gynecol 1991;34:296.
60. Prager K, Malin H, Speigler D, et al. Smoking and drinking behavior before and during pregnancy of married mothers of liveborn and stillborn infants. Public Health Rep 1984;99: 117.
61. Naeye RL. Effects of maternal cigarette smoking on the fetus and placenta. Br J Obstet Gynaecol 1978;85:732.
62. Rantakallio P. The effect of maternal smoking on birth weight and the subsequent health of the child. Early Hum Dev 1978;2:371.
63. Clewell WP. In utero treatment of thyrotoxicosis. In: Evans MI, Fletcher JC, Ditlen AO, et al, eds. Fetal diagnosis and therapy: science, ethics, and the law. Philadelphia: JB Lippincott, 1984;124.
64. Smith CV. Reversing acute intrapartum fetal distress using tocolytic drugs. Clin Obstet Gynecol 1991;34:353.
65. Caritis SN, Darby MJ, Chan L. Pharmacologic treatment of preterm labor. Clin Obstet Gynecol 1988;31:635.
66. Egarter CH, Husslein PW, Rayburn WF. Uterine hyperstimulation after low-dose prostaglandin E_2 therapy: tocolytic treatment in 181 cases. Am J Obstet Gynecol 1990;163:794.
67. Mendez-Bauer C, Shekarloo A, Cook V, et al. Treatment of acute intrapartum fetal distress by B_2-sympathomimetics. Am J Obstet Gynecol 1987;156:638.
68. Reece EA, Chervenak FA, Romero R, et al. Magnesium sulfate in the management of acute intrapartum fetal distress. Am J Obstet Gynecol 1984;148:104.
69. Safra MJ, Oakley GP. Valium: an oral cleft teratogen? Cleft Palate J 1976;13:198.
70. Roth KS, Yang W, Allan L, et al. Prenatal administration of biotin: biotin responsive multiple carboxylase deficiency. Pediatr Res 1982;16:126.
71. Smithells RW, Sheppard S, Schorah CJ, et al. Apparent prevention of neural tube defects by periconceptional vitamin supplementation. Arch Dis Child 1981;56:911.
72. MRC Vitamin Study Research Group. Prevention of neural tube defects: results of the Medical Research Council vitamin study. Lancet 1991;338:131.
73. Mills JL, Rhoads GG, Simpson JL, et al. The absence of a relation between the periconceptional use of vitamins and neural tube defects. N Engl J Med 1989;321:430.
74. Ampola MG, Mahoney MJ, Nakamura E, et al. Prenatal therapy of a patient with vitamin B responsive methylmalonic acidemia. N Engl J Med 1975;293:313.

Neonatology: Pathophysiology and Management of the Newborn, Fourth Edition, edited by Gordon B. Avery, Mary Ann Fletcher, and Mhairi G. MacDonald. J.B. Lippincott Company, Philadelphia © 1994.

chapter 17

Obstetric Anesthesia

JOHN STEPHEN NAULTY

Obstetric anesthesia has, since its inception in the nineteenth century, been a controversial practice. This controversy has arisen from the very nature of obstetric anesthesia, which is the administration of powerful and potentially dangerous drugs to the parturient. These interventions may be beneficial, as in cesarean section, and usually are benign, but occasionally they are deleterious to the fetus. Thus, when considering the administration of an anesthetic during the puerperium, the physician must assess the risk–benefit ratio for both mother and fetus. It is the goal of the practitioner of obstetric anesthesia to devise and use techniques that maximize the pleasurable aspects of parturition while minimizing the risks to both mother and fetus. This chapter introduces the neonatal practitioner to the scientific background and techniques of modern obstetric anesthesia and discusses the effects of these techniques on the fetus and neonate.

THE PAIN OF PARTURITION

NEUROTRANSMISSION

It appears that the sensation of pain arises from stimulation of various receptors in an area where trauma is produced. Each type of receptor gives rise to a characteristic pattern of impulses; this pattern is modulated by the nature and intensity of the initiating stimulus. Nervous impulses arising from these receptors travel as packets of neural firings, which are conducted on both small myelinated and unmyelinated nerves. These packets seem to have a range of frequency response and duration that is relatively specific for the type of pain experienced. The packets of neural firings are analogous to the digital "words" that form the basis for computer software.

The afferent nerve fibers carrying the encoded information from noxious stimuli are somatic and visceral sensory fibers. These fibers enter the spinal cord primarily through the dorsal roots that correspond to the embryonic dermatomes from which the involved tissues developed. The somatic and visceral afferent sensory fibers from the uterus and cervix travel with the sympathetic nervous supply to the uterus. These fibers pass through the paracervical tissue with the uterine artery and then through the inferior, middle, and superior hypogastric plexuses to the sympathetic chain. Nerve impulses from the uterus and cervix then enter the spinal cord through the tenth, eleventh, and twelfth thoracic nerves. Somatic impulses differ from visceral impulses in both the "word structure" and rapidity of conduction, and these different syntaxes and pathways produce two very different types of pain sensation. Somatic pain (*e.g.*, incisional pain, second-stage labor pain) is well localized, described as "sharp," is carried by rapidly conducting fibers, and is typically associated with high rates of firing of the conducting neurons. Visceral pain (*e.g.*, uterine contractions in the first stage of labor) is poorly localized, described as "dull and aching," is carried by slower-conducting fibers, and is associated with lower-frequency firing of both conducting and internuncial neurons. It appears that these two types of pain-information–bearing impulses also differ in their neuropharmacology, as will become evident when the roles of different analgesics in the control of these two types of pain are discussed.

On entering the central nervous system (CNS), the pain-information–bearing impulses undergo a complex modulatory process in the posterior horn of the spinal cord. Although this process is not completely understood, it is clear is that many neurotransmitters, notably enkephalins, endorphins, and polypeptides such as substance P, serotonin, γ-aminobutyric acid, dopamine, and epinephrine,[1] all participate in the processing of pain impulses by these interneurons, and play a role in whether a painful stimulus ultimately will produce the sensation of pain. If sufficient inhibitory modulation takes place, the sensation will be perceived as a sensory modality other than pain, that is pressure or pruritus. On the other hand, excitatory modulation produces disproportionate responses to otherwise ordinary stimuli, such as are found in causalgia and similar hyperesthetic syndromes.

It has become evident that applying either local anesthetics, inhibitory neurotransmitters, or analogues thereof (*e.g.*, notably opioids), or antagonists of excitatory neurotransmitters (*e.g.*, clonidine) to the spinal cord or elsewhere in the CNS can diminish the transmission of pain to consciousness. It is this realization that forms the physiologic and pharmacologic basis for the application of narcotics and other drugs to the CNS and, in particular, to the spinal cord through epidural injections to produce analgesia.

If this polysynaptic modulation in the dorsal horn permits upward transmission of impulses whose information content is "pain," then these impulses will exit from the dorsal horn and will travel rostrally, primarily through the neospinothalamic and paleospinothalamic tracts. These impulses can then stimulate the reticular formation and tegmental tract in the brain stem, where they will evoke the typical reflex responses to pain. These responses include tachycardia, hyperventilation, increased blood pressure, and release of catecholamines and hypothalamic hormones. The nervous impulses then continue upward to the ventral posterolateral nucleus of the thalamus. From there, fibers project to the sensory cortex for localization and discrimination of pain. It is important to note that nerve fibers also arise from the medulla, thalamus, and cortex and project to the dorsal horn of the spinal cord. There they participate in the release of the above-mentioned neurotransmitters and modulation of pain impulses entering the spinal cord, creating a feedback loop whereby pain may provide analgesia for itself. This feedback system seems to be particularly effective during pregnancy; pain thresholds are roughly two to three times higher for pregnant than for nonpregnant subjects. This decrease in pain threshold probably is due to elevations in the concentrations both of progesterone or its metabolites and of CSF and spinal cord inhibitory neurotransmitters such as endorphins and enkephalins. Progesterones have a generalized stabilizing effect on neural tissue.[2] Endorphins and enkephalins cause down-modulation of noxious impulses received in the dorsal horn.[3]

REFLEX EFFECTS

In addition to the subjective sensation of pain, nerve impulses of labor pain lead to stimulation of the autonomic nervous system and create reflex cardiovascular, respiratory, endocrine, and musculoskeletal effects.

CARDIOVASCULAR

Cardiovascular sympathetic nervous system stimulation may cause an increase in cardiac output by as much as 60% during labor.[4] Tachycardia, hypertension, and arrhythmias may develop. Uterine blood vessels have been shown to be particularly sensitive to sympathetic tone. Shnider and colleagues have demonstrated that experimentally produced pain can reduce uterine blood flow in pregnant ewes by release of endogenous catecholamines.[5] Fetuses of mothers who receive no analgesia have been found to have higher concentrations of lactate and lower *p*H in their blood at birth.[6]

RESPIRATORY

Hyperventilation is a common response to painful stimulation. Arterial carbon dioxide is severely reduced in some patients during labor. The resultant respiratory alkalosis may produce fetal hypoxia by shifting the maternal oxyhemoglobin dissociation curve to the left,[7] leading to decreased oxygen release at the placenta.[8]

ENDOCRINE

Catecholamines are released in large amounts during painful uterine contractions. Endogenous pain-controlling substances, such as endorphins and enkephalins, also are released from the placenta, fetus, and CNS during labor.[9]

MUSCULOSKELETAL

Maternal skeletal muscle expulsive efforts (*i.e.*, "bearing down") may become an uncontrollable urge as a result of labor pain. Obstetric anesthesia has been shown to control these reflexes and to decrease the metabolic acidosis that may result from excessive muscular efforts.[10]

ADMINISTRATION OF OBSTETRIC ANESTHESIA

BENEFITS

Properly performed obstetric analgesia not only reduces the psychological or subjective component of pain but also may prevent reflex effects that are particularly dangerous for some patients. For example, patients with severe mitral regurgitation may undergo cardiac decompensation and congestive heart failure as a result of sympathetic stimulation. Decreasing this stimulation with obstetric anesthesia may prevent these adverse effects.

METHODS

The impulses arising from labor pain may be blocked in many ways, so numerous methods of pain relief have been developed. Selection of any given technique depends on the stage of labor, maternal condition, fetal condition, and experience of the anesthesiologist and obstetric team. In the first stage of labor, paracervical, paravertebral, epidural, and spinal anesthetics may be used to prevent noxious impulses from either entering or ascending the spinal cord. The sensation of pain also may be blocked by systemic analgesia with narcotics or by inhalation analgesia. Finally, the motivational–affective component of pain may be blocked with psychological methods, hypnosis, or acupuncture. These techniques may be continued in the second stage of labor. In addition, the pudendal nerve may be blocked to relieve perineal pain.

CURRENT PRACTICE

Obstetric anesthesia traditionally has been a problem for many anesthesia departments. Because of unpredictable and widely fluctuating manpower requirements, many anesthesia departments cannot or will not provide 24-hour obstetric anesthesia coverage. The American Society of Anesthesiologists viewed this as an undesirable development and, in 1978, published a paper that stated that parturients were entitled to the same level of anesthetic care as elective surgical patients.[11] This care should include the availability of a full-time anesthesiologist with modern equipment for administering anesthetics and monitoring the parturient. In 1970, a survey by the American College of Obstetricians and Gynecologists revealed that in only 37% of hospitals were obstetric anesthetics administered by personnel who were specifically trained in anesthesia.[12] A similar study in 1980 showed slight progress, and in 1990, 67% of hospitals were providing adequate anesthetic coverage of the obstetric suite.[13] It is hoped that the rapidly expanding interest in regional anesthetic techniques, pain control, and perinatal medicine will produce continued improvement in this chronic staffing problem. In another survey, anesthesia was deemed directly responsible for 8% of 950 maternal deaths in the United States.[14] More than two-thirds of these deaths were judged to have been preventable. Similar results have been obtained in Great Britain,[15] with the most common causes of anesthetic mishap in the obstetric suite being unfamiliarity with the pathophysiology of obstetric disease and the use of unfamiliar techniques in the parturient. Obviously, the practitioner who wishes to provide adequate care for the parturient should have an easy familiarity with the techniques commonly used in obstetric anesthesia and should practice these techniques regularly. For example, if obstetric epidural anesthesia is administered infrequently, the technique will be considerably less familiar than in a busy obstetric service administering many thousands of such anesthetics each year. John Bonica stated, "In case there is a choice between poorly administered anesthesia and no anesthesia, the latter should be selected."[14] This is no less true today. Many of the techniques of obstetric anesthesia have applications in general operating rooms; these techniques should be practiced first in a general setting with a premedicated, cooperative patient before they are attempted on an obstetric patient, who frequently is uncooperative because of severe, acute pain.

ENDOGENOUS ANALGESIA

Several techniques have been developed to produce analgesia by using the body's own analgesic system. It appears that all these methods of analgesia rely on the enhancement of release of inhibitory neurotransmitters in the CNS that attenuate the response to noxious stimuli and produce analgesia. Some of these techniques produce an analgesia that is reversible with naloxone,[16] implicating release of endorphins as part of their mechanism of action. Such techniques include the various forms of psychoprophylaxis,[17] acupuncture,[18] transcutaneous nerve stimulation,[19] hypnosis, and accupressure. These techniques are quite effective in approximately 30% to 50% of pregnant women,[20] particularly for relatively low intensities of pain of short duration.[21] They cannot provide intense analgesia for longer periods of time but, if used in conjunction with other forms of pain therapy, their effectiveness appears to be enhanced. Psychoanalgesia, however, is not without risk. The breathing techniques of psychoanalgesia are designed to minimize hyperventilation, but some parturients do hyperventilate and lower their arterial carbon dioxide tensions to as low as 12 to 15 torr. Extremely low carbon dioxide tension displaces the maternal oxyhemoglobin dissociation curve to the left and interferes with placental oxygen exchange. Neonates of hyperventilating parturients are more acidotic than those born of a control group who do not hyperventilate.[22] These adverse effects can be prevented with adequate obstetric analgesia. For example, Zador and Nillson found that fetal acid–base balance during prolonged labor was better maintained in patients receiving epidural anesthesia than in patients receiving either no analgesia or small doses of systemic narcotic drugs.[23]

Psychoanalgesic techniques require a high level of personal concentration and are not entirely reliable. Some enthusiasts of psychoanalgesic techniques promote them as being applicable to all deliveries. Therefore, a woman who experiences severe pain during parturition and wishes further anesthesia may feel as if she has failed.[24] When interviewing her before initiating an analgesic technique, it is important to stress that not all patients find psychoanalgesia techniques adequate and that further anesthetic intervention is not uncommon. Appropriately applied drug therapy appears to be an increasingly popular and certainly the most effective means of providing analgesia.

OBSTETRIC ANALGESIA WITH DRUGS

Labor pain inadequately controlled with techniques of endogenous analgesia will require additional analgesic intervention. These techniques include intramuscular, intravenous (IV), and inhalation administration of sedative or analgesic drugs and perineural application of local anesthetics or narcotics.

INTRAVENOUS AND INTRAMUSCULAR MEDICATIONS

The systemic administration of sedatives, tranquilizers, and narcotics to the parturient is the most frequently used method of obstetric analgesia. In the past, large doses of these drugs were used to create the state of twilight sleep. Increasing realization of the adverse effects of excessive medication on both mother and fetus has led to a reduction in dosage of these drugs. In addition, better understanding of maternal uptake, distribution, and placental transfer has improved methods of administration and timing of these drugs in labor. Current practice uses small doses of minimally depressant drugs administered intravenously early in labor for the least placental transfer to produce a minimally depressed neonate. The major groups of drugs used today are sedative–tranquilizers, narcotic analgesics, and dissociative anesthetics.

SEDATIVE–TRANQUILIZERS

Sedatives and tranquilizers are administered to the parturient to diminish the adverse motivational–affective component of labor pain. Examples of such drugs are barbiturates, phenothiazines, and benzodiazepines.

Barbiturates. Secobarbital (Seconal) and pentobarbital (Nembutal) have been used in obstetrics. Owing to their prolonged effects, they are used today principally during the early latent phase of labor when delivery is not likely to occur before 12 to 24 hours. Barbiturates have been described as having an "antianalgesic effect,"[25] and may convert a minimally uncomfortable, controlled patient into a hyperventilating, confused, and unmanageable one. For this reason, they are used rarely today.

Phenothiazines. Promethazine (Phenergan) and propiomazine (Largon) are the drugs in this class commonly used in obstetrics. Hydroxyzine (Vistaril), although not a phenothiazine, has similar properties. These drugs are useful for relieving anxiety and thus modifying the response to painful stimulation. They are less likely than the barbiturates to cause antianalgesia, and they potentiate the actions of the narcotic analgesics. In addition, they are useful in controlling nausea and vomiting, which may be severe enough in some labors to produce maternal dehydration. In the recommended dosages (promethazine, 50 mg; propiomazine, 20 mg; hydroxyzine, 50–100 mg), these drugs appear to have minimal depressant effects on both mother and fetus.[26]

Benzodiazepines. Diazepam (Valium) and midazolam (Versed) are among the most widely prescribed drugs in the world, and it is not surprising that they have been used as anxiolytic agents in obstetrics. Their use is controversial, but they can reduce maternal anxiety, decrease narcotic dosage, and treat convulsions associated with local anesthetic toxicity or eclampsia. When used in small doses (2.5–10 mg IV diazepam; 0.25–1 mg midazolam), no significant adverse fetal or neonatal effects have been noted.[27]

NARCOTICS

Narcotics, one of the earliest groups of pain relievers used in obstetrics, are today still the most commonly used obstetric analgesics. Indeed, with some of the most recent developments in narcotic pharmacology, these drugs also are one of the most exciting subjects of obstetric analgesic research.

Basic Pharmacology. The narcotic analgesics act by stimulating opiate receptors that are found in many locations throughout the CNS. These drugs act by binding onto the receptor and altering its conformation.[28] More than one type of opiate receptor exists, each with particular drug affinities and responses.[29] Thus, to describe the pharmacology of a narcotic drug adequately, the type of opiate receptors it affects (*i.e.*, receptor specificity) and in what way it affects these receptors (*i.e.*, agonist–antagonist activity) must be described (Table 17-1).

TABLE 17–1
AGONIST–ANTAGONIST ACTIVITY, TYPE OF ANALGESIA PRODUCED, AND EFFECTS ON CO_2 RESPONSE

Receptor Type	Agonists	Antagonists	Analgesia	CO_2 Response
μ	Morphine Meperidine Fentanyl	Naloxone Naltrexone	Somatic = visceral depression Spinal cord = brain	 Linear dose response
κ	Nalbuphine Butorphanol	Naloxone (high doses)	Visceral > somatic Spinal cord > brain	Depression Nonlinear dose response
δ	Enkephalins	Nalmephene (high doses)	Somatic > visceral	No effect

Opiate Receptor Specificity. All the details of the nature and specificity of opiate receptors have not been elucidated. The preponderance of opiate receptors in the brain and spinal cord that produce analgesia are the μ-receptors.[30] These receptors also probably are responsible for narcotic respiratory depression, and may affect thermoregulation. Examples of μ-stimulating narcotic drugs are morphine, meperidine, sufentanil, and fentanyl.

Kappa- and δ-receptors are found predominantly in the spinal cord, and, when stimulated, seem to potentiate spinal analgesia.[31] They also seem to be responsible for the sedative and dysphoric reactions seen with narcotics that stimulate these receptors, such as pentazocine. Sigma opiate receptors are found primarily in smooth muscle, and are responsible for some significant side effects of opiates, such as nausea, vomiting, and urinary retention. The specificity of these opiate receptors is far from absolute, and their classification is based on relative binding of various drugs. Thus, a drug that is described as a μ-stimulating drug, such as morphine, merely binds most strongly to μ-receptors; it is perfectly capable of producing some effect at other receptor sites.

Agonist–Antagonist Activity. The alteration in conformation of an opiate receptor that is produced by the application of a narcotic drug is capable of changing neural transmission, probably at synaptic junctions. Drugs that bind to the receptor and cause this change in neural pain sensitivity (*i.e.*, analgesia) are called agonists. Examples of such drugs are morphine, alphaprodine, meperidine, and fentanyl. There is another class of narcotic drugs that binds to the receptor—in most cases very avidly—but does not seem to cause the conformational change in the receptor to produce analgesia. Because of their high affinity for the receptor, these drugs are capable of displacing the agonist drugs from the receptor and reversing their effects; therefore, they are known as narcotic antagonists (*e.g.*, naloxone, naltrexone). There is a third possible interaction with the receptor: agonist–antagonist. In this interaction, similar to that with antagonists, the drugs have a high affinity for the receptor and competitively displace the pure agonist drugs from the receptor. Unlike the pure antagonists, however, these drugs are capable of producing some analgesic effect themselves. Examples of the agonist–antagonist drugs are levallorphan, pentazocine, nalbuphine, and butorphanol. It is interesting that these drugs are typically κ-receptor agonists and μ-receptor antagonists; it is tempting to view this receptor specificity as the explanation for their peculiar actions.[32]

Peripartum Pharmacology. Narcotics used in obstetrics to relieve labor pain should not also produce adverse effects on either mother or baby. All narcotic drugs readily cross the placental barrier and can exert neonatal effects in normal doses. To achieve maternal analgesia without neonatal depression, it must be kept in mind that choices concerning the method of administration, appropriate drug, and the appropriate patient are important variables.

Method of Administration. Narcotics can be given intramuscularly, intravenously, or intrathecally. In choosing a method of administration, the well-being of both the mother and the baby must be considered.

Intramuscular. Intramuscular administration is technically easy but leads to uneven analgesia, late respiratory depression, and profound neonatal effects if not properly timed.[33] For these reasons, many centers have abandoned this method.

Intravenous. This method frequently is used to provide analgesia in labor. The effects of an IV injection of narcotic are more predictable, making timing of doses easier. Achievement of a steady blood level of narcotic sufficient to provide analgesia is difficult, however, with the parturient frequently suffering either underdosage or overdosage. Continuous IV infusion of short-acting narcotics (*e.g.*, alfentanil) or self-administration of IV narcotics may overcome this limitation[34,35] Patient-controlled analgesia (PCA) is becoming a very popular method of IV administration of these drugs, because the patient seems to be able to titrate her dose to the minimum required for analgesia with the lowest blood levels of narcotics, and hence considerably less placental transfer.[36]

Intrathecal. The epidural injection of opiates alone has proven to be of limited utility for the relief of labor pain. Intraspinal opiates first were demonstrated to be capable of producing profound analgesia in humans in 1979.[37] Shortly thereafter, several researchers attempted to apply this technique for the relief of labor pain. In one study, high doses of morphine (7.5 mg) provided satisfactory analgesia for 6 hours in only the first stage of labor,[38] whereas 2 to 5 mg produced satisfactory analgesia in fewer than one-half of the patients.[39] In fact, the results with even the higher doses of morphine did not differ significantly from those found using natural childbirth techniques.[20] Also, the long time of onset of 1 hour or more proved to be a significant problem. Subarachnoid (*i.e.*, spinal) injections of fentanyl, meperidine, and sufentanil through an indwelling spinal catheter have been more promising; however, these are experimental techniques that should not be applied indiscriminately to patients in labor.

Epidural morphine and fentanyl have been used to produce incomplete but adequate analgesia for labor in patients with conditions in which the use of local anesthetics was thought to be contraindicated (*e.g.*, Eisenmenger syndrome, cystic fibrosis, pulmonary hypertension).[40] Generally, however, even when rapidly acting, lipid-soluble drugs (*e.g.*, meperidine, fentanyl), have been used, epidural narcotics used as the sole analgesic drug have proven to be inferior to dilute concentrations of local anesthetics.[41] Adding epinephrine to the narcotic solution appears to increase the incidence of satisfactory analgesia, but not sufficiently to make this a reliable technique.[41] The chief limitation of these drugs seems to be that they can reduce visceral pain such as that occurring in the first stage of labor, but they are not as effective in the treatment of somatic pain such as that experienced in the second and third stages of labor. In contrast, local anesthetics produce better somatic than visceral analgesia.

Drug Selection. An ideal narcotic for perinatal use would provide the following:

- good analgesia
- no maternal respiratory depression
- no other maternal side effects (*e.g.*, nausea, pruritus, dysphoria)
- no short-term or long-term neonatal effects
- no adverse effects on mother–infant interactions.

No drug or technique provides all these ideal effects. The drugs that most closely approach this goal are the agonist–antagonist drugs, such as butorphanol and nalbuphine.[42]

Patient Selection. Narcotic drugs can provide analgesia only and cannot take the place of major regional anesthetic techniques when these are indicated. Narcotics should not be used when it is necessary to prevent deleterious effects arising from the reflex responses to labor pain, as in patients with severe cardiac disease. Narcotics are most useful in primiparae in early labor, as adjuncts to major regional anesthetics for uncontrollable patients, and in multiparae with relatively short, predictable labors with minimal pain. When administered intrathecally, they are useful primarily in the first stage of labor; they do not always provide adequate analgesia for operative obstetric procedures.[41] In summary, narcotic analgesics are a class of drugs that have had a major role in reducing the discomfort of labor and that may play an even larger role if improved methods of administration and more suitable drugs can be found. Their major role lies in their use as potentiators of local anesthetics for epidural analgesia, as will be discussed below.

GENERAL ANALGESIA AND ANESTHESIA

The extension of the concept of systemic medication for the relief of labor pain is general analgesia and anesthesia. General analgesia consists of administration of subanesthetic concentrations of inhalation agents (*e.g.*, nitrous oxide) that produce analgesia roughly equivalent to that provided by narcotic analgesics. The goal of general analgesia is that the patient remain awake and cooperative while maintaining protective laryngeal reflexes. General anesthesia broadens the scope of inhalation analgesia and provides profound analgesia, amnesia, hypnosis, and muscle relaxation. Various types of general anesthesia and analgesia are available through a wide variety of drugs. The techniques commonly applied to obstetrics include intermittent inhalation analgesia, dissociative general analgesia and general endotracheal anesthesia supplemented with neuromuscular blockers.

INTERMITTENT INHALATION ANALGESIA

This technique, first applied by Simpson in 1847, consists of the inhalation by the parturient of subanesthetic concentrations of anesthetic agents. This technique may have an advantage over the use of narcotics because of the rapid onset and reversibility of the analgesia produced. The technique is simple in concept—the parturient self-administers an anesthetic agent from an inhaler device during contractions. A major hazard of the technique is its apparent simplicity, because the understaffing of many obstetric units may lead to inadequate observation of the parturient. The hazard exists because the physiology of the pregnant state predisposes the patient to overdose with inhalation anesthesia.[43] In pregnancy, the functional residual capacity of the lungs is reduced, and alveolar ventilation is increased. When combined with the reduced anesthetic requirements noted in pregnancy,[44] this physiologic condition leads to a rapid induction of an unconscious, anesthetized state rather than the desired analgesic state. Thus, the major risk of inhalation analgesia is inadvertent overdosage with loss of consciousness and protective laryngeal reflexes. Maternal regurgitation, vomiting, and aspiration may then lead to airway obstruction, asphyxia, and aspiration pneumonitis. It is estimated that approximately 5% to 15% of maternal deaths in the United States are attributable to anesthesia, with one-half of these being the sequelae of aspiration. If the parturient is observed carefully, the risks of overdosage are minimized.

DISSOCIATIVE ANALGESIA

The intramuscular or IV administration of low-dose ketamine (Ketalar) produces a state known as dissociative analgesia. This state is characterized by an intense analgesia and amnesia, without loss of consciousness or protective airway reflexes.[45] This is accompanied by a dreaming phenomenon, which may be unpleasant. Used in doses less than 1 mg/kg, ketamine provides adequate analgesia for vaginal delivery and episiotomy repair. Airway protection cannot be guaranteed, however, so aspiration may occur. This technique is best reserved for situations in which more reliable and safer techniques are contraindicated.

GENERAL ENDOTRACHEAL ANESTHESIA

General anesthesia is used in obstetric practice for both vaginal delivery and cesarean section. It should be used with endotracheal intubation because of the risks of aspirating gastric contents. The technique consists of the administration of a combination of a muscle relaxant, a sedative–hypnotic drug, a narcotic or inhalation agent, and nitrous oxide. General anesthesia frequently is chosen for use in emergency obstetrics because of its rapid and predictable action. Properly used, general anesthesia is safe, with certain limitations that will be considered in the discussion of fetal effects of anesthesia.

MAJOR REGIONAL ANALGESIA AND ANESTHESIA

In many centers, regional analgesia and anesthesia for labor and delivery is the technique of choice. The parturient remains awake and cooperative, the risks of aspiration are minimized, and excellent, predictable analgesia can be provided. The commonly used methods of major regional anesthesia for parturition are subarachnoid (*i.e.*, spinal) block and peridural (*i.e.*, caudal or lumbar epidural) block.

Types

Subarachnoid Block (Spinal Anesthesia). Spinal anesthesia usually is administered immediately before delivery. A small dose of a local anesthetic (*e.g.*, tetracaine, 4 mg; lidocaine, 25–50 mg; bupivacaine, 3–5 mg) dissolved in a hypertonic dextrose solution is injected into the subarachnoid space with the patient in the sitting position. Injection produces immediate analgesia of the lumbosacral nerve roots and provides excellent anesthesia for episiotomy, forceps application, and delivery. Larger doses frequently are used to produce anesthesia for cesarean delivery (Table 17-2).

Peridural Block (Caudal, Epidural Anesthesia). Peridural block usually is performed early in labor, as soon as a satisfactory progress of labor is established (*i.e.*, usually 3 to 4 cm of cervical dilation in nulliparae, less in multiparae). A needle is placed by a variety of techniques in the potential space just outside the dura (*i.e.*, the peridural space). A plastic catheter is then introduced through the needle, the needle is removed, and local anesthetic solutions are injected through the catheter. Analgesia may be attained and continued throughout the active phase of labor and delivery.

The mechanism by which epidural injections of local anesthetic drugs produce analgesia is only poorly understood, but most authorities agree that their prime mechanism of action is to decrease both the number and frequency of afferent nerve firings in the vicinity of the spinal cord. Local anesthetics are most effective at reducing or eliminating somatic pain. An inevitable consequence of their action also is a decrease in efferent nerve activity, leading to motor

TABLE 17–2
COMMON DRUGS FOR OBSTETRIC SPINAL ANESTHESIA

Local Anesthetic	Concentration	Onset	Duration (min)
Lidocaine–glucose	5% Lidocaine, 7.5% glucose	Rapid	45–60
Bupivacaine–glucose	0.75% Bupivacaine, 8.25% glucose	Intermediate	60–90
Tetracaine–glucose	0.5% Tetracaine, 5% glucose	Slow	90–120
Tetracaine–procaine	0.5% Tetracaine, 10% procaine	Rapid	90–120

blockade. The ideal choice of a local anesthetic for labor would be one that provides safe, excellent analgesia and sensory blockade while preserving motor function. Bupivacaine and ropivacaine are the local anesthetics that provide maximum sensory block with minimum motor block. The drugs commonly used for labor and delivery are described in Table 17-3.

Maintenance

Local anesthetics usually were injected into the epidural space by intermittent bolus injections for labor analgesia; however, an increasing realization of the hazards of this method of administration, combined with the development of reliable and inexpensive infusion pumps, has produced a widespread interest in the use of truly continuous epidural infusion techniques for the relief of labor pain. Several investigators have demonstrated that the use of continuous infusions of local anesthetics produces more reliable pain relief with similar or lower blood levels of local anesthetics than intermittent boluses of these drugs.[46,47] Most important, the possibility of disastrous complications of total spinal anesthesia or massive intravascular injections with cardiovascular collapse secondary to large doses of local anesthetics is decreased. If an epidural catheter enters an epidural vein during continuous infusion, the analgesia merely ceases without producing neurologic or cardiovascular toxicity that dictates the mode of delivery.[48] If the catheter enters the subarachnoid space instead, then the level of sensory and motor blockade increases slowly without the sudden onset of complete subarachnoid blockade that may occur with bolus techniques.[49]

The choice of drug for continuous infusion remains controversial. Solutions of lidocaine, bupivacaine, and chloroprocaine all have been used successfully to produce labor analgesia.[50,51] In addition, considerable controversy exists over the concentration and volume required as a loading dose before inception of the continuous infusion. The common practice of initiating epidural local anesthetic blockade with a high concentration of local anesthetic (*e.g.*, 0.5% bupivacaine) may be no more effective than using a slightly larger volume of a lower concentration of local anesthetic (*e.g.*, 0.125% bupivacaine), except that the higher concentration will provide a slightly faster onset of analgesia in some cases.[52] Also, the volume of local anesthetic required for continuous infusion may be less than that currently recommended. In an interesting study, Gambling used a PCA pump and allowed the patient to determine her own optimal dosing schedule of small epidural boluses of local anesthetic.[53] There was a wide individual variation in dose requirements, but the mean dose of local anesthetic was significantly lower in the patients using PCA pumps. More investigation will be required before the optimal drug, dose, and method of infusion is established. A promising technique that is the use of extremely dilute concentrations of local anesthetics (*e.g.*, 0.03% bupivacaine) combined with a lipid-soluble opiate such as fentanyl or sufentanil. The analgesia produced by this combination of epidural local anesthetics and opiates can be profound. In general, patients who receive epidural injections of local anesthetics and narcotics report more rapid onset of analgesia, more profound analgesia, longer durations of analgesia, but less motor block than patients receiving either drug alone. Therefore, it is common to see patients who have received both local anesthetics and narcotics in labor, and their effects on the fetus must be discussed.

Complications

Hypotension. Hypotension secondary to sympathetic blockade is the most common complication of major regional block for parturition.[46] Prophylactic measures include adequate hydration, avoidance of the supine position, and displacement of the uterus off the abdominal great vessels. Hypotension is much less common when combinations of opiates and local anesthetics are used. Should hypotension occur, however, treatment includes further IV fluids, more uterine displacement, and vasopressor administration (*e.g.*, ephedrine, 10–20 mg). If treated promptly,

TABLE 17–3
COMMON DRUGS FOR OBSTETRIC EPIDURAL ANESTHESIA

Local Anesthetic	Concentration	Onset	Duration (min)	Toxic Plasma Concentration (μg/mL)	Indications	Contraindications
Mepivacaine	1.5%–2%	Intermediate	60–90	>5	Postpartum operations	Fetal toxicity
Lidocaine	1.5%–2%	Rapid	45–60	>5	Elective cesarian-section	Fetal distress
Ropivacaine	0.5%	Intermediate	90–120	>4		
Bupivacaine	0.5%	Slow	90–120	>1.5 (less in pregnancy)	Slow onset cesarian section	Rapid injection
Chloroprocaine (*i.e.*, ester)	2%–3%	Rapid	30–45	?	Emergency cesarian-section	Esterase deficiency

hypotension does not produce fetal depression or morbidity.

Convulsions. High blood levels of local anesthetics may produce excitation of the CNS, seizures, and cardiovascular depression. High levels may result from overdosage or inadvertent intravascular injections. If either occur, the mother should have an airway secured and be given oxygen and small doses of barbiturates or diazepam. The circulation must be maintained with cardiopulmonary resuscitation if required. Resuscitation and support of the mother will reestablish uterine blood flow and allow adequate fetal oxygenation and excretion of local anesthetic.[54] Unless the mother cannot be resuscitated, delivery of the fetus should be delayed because the neonate has an extremely limited ability to excrete local anesthetics and may have convulsions for many days.[55]

Hypoventilation. At any time during subarachnoid or peridural anesthesia, an excessive level of neural blockade may develop, leading to blockade of the motor nerves to the respiratory muscles. Treatment consists of endotracheal intubation and ventilation with oxygen. This complication must be anticipated at all times during major regional anesthesia because its onset may be insidious and go unnoticed until severe hypoxic damage occurs to both mother and fetus.

MINOR REGIONAL ANESTHESIA

Other regional anesthetic techniques have been used for parturition. These techniques, including paracervical and pudendal blocks and local perineal infiltration, are used commonly by obstetricians. Paracervical block is useful in the first stage of labor; pudendal block and local infiltration are useful for delivery. Analgesia is not as profound as during major regional block, but complications such as hypotension and hypoventilation are avoided. Convulsions, however, may occur as a result of these techniques with local anesthetics. In addition, paracervical block is associated with a high incidence of fetal bradycardia after the block. The etiology of this phenomenon is unclear but probably involves a combination of decreased uterine blood flow secondary to the vasoconstrictor properties of local anesthetics and high fetal levels of local anesthetic. Because the fetal bradycardia is associated with increased neonatal morbidity and mortality, this block is rarely performed and should be used only in low-risk pregnancies.[56]

FETAL AND NEONATAL EFFECTS OF OBSTETRIC ANESTHESIA

Maternal anesthetics may affect the fetus and neonate adversely by two mechanisms. First, drugs administered to the mother may diffuse from the maternal circulation to the fetal circulation, causing direct drug effects. These are drug-specific effects, predictable from the pharmacology of the anesthetic, with treatment dependent on the particular drug. Second, an anesthetic drug or technique may affect the fetus indirectly, producing the signs and symptoms of fetal distress and asphyxia; treatment is based on restoring placental exchange, perfusion, and gas exchange. These two types of adverse interactions may coexist in the same patient, exerting both effects in the neonate.

DIRECT EFFECTS

When a drug is present in sufficient concentration in the fetus, it will exert direct pharmacologic effects. Serial dilutions and protein–tissue binding protect the fetus from the effects of anesthetic drugs administered to the mother. If an excessive amount of any anesthetic drug is administered, or if with even a small amount some of the serial dilutions are bypassed by IV injection of local anesthetics or direct injection into the uterine artery or fetus in paracervical blocks, the drug may exert profound effects. The effects observed vary with the specific drug concerned.

SEDATIVE–TRANQUILIZERS

Barbiturates. These drugs are highly lipid-soluble drugs that rapidly cross the placenta and produce a dose-related global depression in the neonate. Their primary use occurs in low dosage for general anesthesia during cesarean section (*e.g.*, thiopental, 4 mg/kg). Maternal protein binding and maternofetal organ uptake usually prevent significant depression of the neonate. Neonatal depression is found with higher dosages of barbiturates (*e.g.*, thiopental, 8 mg/kg), however, which must be treated by cardiorespiratory supportive techniques until the neonate can excrete the drug. This process may take up to 2 days.[57]

Phenothiazines. These drugs rapidly cross the placenta and have been noted to cause a decrease in fetal beat-to-beat variability. When used in the recommended dosages, however, these drugs do not seem to cause neonatal depression, at least as measured by Apgar scores. An inadvertent overdosage of these medications should be treated similarly to barbiturate-induced depression.

Benzodiazepines. The most commonly used member of this drug group, diazepam (Valium) rapidly crosses the placenta, yielding approximately equal maternal and fetal blood levels within minutes of IV administration.[58] In addition, the neonate has a limited ability to excrete diazepam, so the drug and its active metabolite may persist in significant amounts in the neonate for a week.[59] The drug may produce hypotonia, lethargy, and hypothermia when used in large maternal doses (30 mg)[43]; however, when used in small doses (2.5–10 mg IV), minimal sedation and hypotonia have been observed. It would appear, then, that low-dose diazepam is a safe anxiolytic drug, but that particular attention must be paid to providing a warm environment for these infants for at least 36 hours after delivery.

Narcotics. After maternal administration, the lipid-soluble, poorly ionized narcotic analgesics rapidly enter the fetal circulation. Their chief fetal effect is a dose-related respiratory depression, as evidenced by a rightward shift in the carbon dioxide response curve. The degree of depression is a function of the amount of drug administered, the timing, and the route of administration. Intramuscular administration appears to be associated with a high incidence of neonatal depression 2 to 4 hours after injection, which is the usual time when delivery may be expected. In addition, some narcotics, most notably meperidine, have active metabolites that prolong their fetal effects far longer than the action of the parent drug. Therefore, intramuscular injection of meperidine largely has been replaced by IV injection, which produces peak neonatal depression at 30 to 60 minutes postinjection, a time when delivery is less likely. If a neonate is suspected of narcotic-related depression, the administration of naloxone (Narcan, 0.02 mg/kg IV) will produce a reversal of the drug depression within 1 to 2 minutes and will last 1 to 2 hours. The indiscriminate use of naloxone in the immediate neonatal period should be discouraged, however, because neonatal cyanosis or sudden death have been reported with the use of narcotic antagonists in addicted fetuses or in neonates who did not have narcotic-induced respiratory depression. When in doubt, bag and mask ventilation is probably a safer alternative than narcotic antagonists. If using naloxone, the anesthesiologist must be aware that narcotic-induced (*e.g.*, meperidine) respiratory depression has been reported to last up to 5 hours, so renarcotization may develop in the infant.

GENERAL ANESTHETICS

Inhalation Agents. Placental transfer of inhalation agents is rapid because these are nonionized, highly lipid-soluble substances of low molecular weight. The fetal concentrations of these agents depend directly on the concentration and duration of anesthetic in the mother. If excessive concentrations of anesthetic are given for inordinately long times, neonatal anesthesia, evidenced by flaccidity, cardiorespiratory depression, and decreased tone, may be anticipated.[60,61] It cannot be overemphasized that if the neonatal depression is due to transfer of anesthetic drugs, the infant is merely lightly anesthetized and should respond easily to simple treatment measures. Treatment should include effective cardiopulmonary resuscitation, which allows excretion of the inhalation anesthetic by the infant's lungs. Rapid improvement of the infant should be expected, and, if not forthcoming in 5 to 10 minutes, a search for other causes of depression should begin.

NEUROMUSCULAR BLOCKERS

Nondepolarizing Neuromuscular Blockers. Under normal circumstances, the poorly lipid soluble, highly ionized, nondepolarizing neuromuscular blockers (*e.g.*, D-tubocurarine, pancuronium, atracurium, vecuronium) do not cross the placenta in amounts significant enough to cause neonatal muscle weakness.[62] This placental impermeability is only relative, however, and when large doses are given over long periods of time, as in the treatment of maternal tetanus or status epilepticus, neonatal neuromuscular blockade can occur.[63]

Depolarizing Neuromuscular Blockers. Succinylcholine, normally hydrolyzed in maternal blood by the enzyme pseudocholinesterase, usually does not interfere with fetal neuromuscular activity. If the hydrolytic enzyme is present either in low concentrations,[64] or in a genetically determined atypical form,[65] prolonged maternal and neonatal respiratory depression secondary to muscular paralysis can occur.

Diagnosis and Treatment of Neonatal Neuromuscular Blockade. The diagnosis of neonatal depression secondary to neuromuscular blockade may be made on the basis of the maternal history (*e.g.*, prolonged administration of neuromuscular blockers, history of atypical pseudocholinesterase), the response of the mother to neuromuscular blocking drugs, and the physical examination of the newborn. The paralyzed neonate will have normal cardiovascular function and good color, but no spontaneous ventilatory movements, muscle flaccidity, and no reflex responses. The anesthesiologist can place a nerve stimulator on the neonate and demonstrate the classic signs of neuromuscular blockade.[66] Treatment consists of respiratory support until the drug is excreted by the neonate, taking up to 48 hours. Reversal of nondepolarizing relaxants with cholinesterase inhibitors may be attempted (*e.g.*, neostigmine, 0.06 mg/kg), but adequate respiratory support should be the mainstay of treatment.

LOCAL ANESTHETICS

The local anesthetic drugs in common use are divided into two groups: ester and amide. They differ in their mode of metabolism and in their fetal effects.

Esters. Esters are broken down in the maternal blood by pseudocholinesterase, the same enzyme responsible for the hydrolysis of succinylcholine. If normal levels of enzyme are present, the half-life of these drugs in the maternal serum is extremely short (*e.g.*, 21 seconds for 2-chloroprocaine), so the amount available for placental transfer is limited.[67] If the enzyme is deficient or atypical, more local anesthetic is available for diffusion across the placenta, and fetal seizures and cardiorespiratory depression can occur.

Amides. The primary metabolic pathway for the excretion of amide drugs is through the liver. This is a much slower process than the hydrolysis of esters, so significant maternal blood levels of these drugs may be produced during regional anesthesia. These drugs are arranged in Table 17-3 in the order of their placental permeability, with mepivacaine exhibiting the most placental transfer and bupivacaine and ropivacaine the least.[68] In addition, bupivacaine and etidocaine are highly protein-bound in maternal tissues and serum, decreasing placental transfer. Mild forms of local anesthetic overdose are exhibited by decreases in neonatal neuromuscular tone, similar to that seen with magnesium. If a direct intravascular or intrafetal injection of any of the local anesthetics occurs, significant depression can develop, exhibited by bradycardia, ventricular arrhythmias, and severe cardiac depression with acidosis.

Treatment of Toxicity. The most important principle to follow if large amounts of any local anesthetic reach the fetus during regional anesthesia is not to attempt to deliver the baby immediately. If maternal cardiorespiratory support is provided, these reactions will be brief and the local anesthetic that has reached the fetus will diffuse back to the mother, where the drugs can be redistributed, metabolized, and excreted by her. If immediate delivery is effected, this important route of excretion is lost. If maternal cardiorespiratory collapse occurs, however, then immediate delivery must be performed to ensure the survival of the neonate and facilitate maternal cardiopulmonary resuscitation. In this instance, because the neonate has an extremely limited ability to metabolize and excrete amide local anesthetics, prolonged seizures and cardiorespiratory depression can be expected.

INDIRECT EFFECTS

In addition to the specific effects of the drugs mentioned above, interference with normal placental gas exchange can occur with all obstetric anesthetic techniques, adversely affecting the fetus and neonate. There are several mechanisms by which this interference can occur.

DECREASED ARTERIAL OXYGEN CONTENT

Any technique that produces maternal hypoxia will decrease maternofetal oxygen exchange and produce fetal distress. Examples of this phenomenon include overdosage with narcotics or inhalation analgesia, total spinal anesthesia, or the maternal aspiration of vomitus.

DECREASED SYSTEMIC PERFUSION

Uteroplacental blood flow depends on an adequate maternal cardiac output and perfusion pressure. Anesthetic techniques that interfere with maternal cardiovascular integrity can produce fetal depression by several mechanisms:

- Decreased cardiac output secondary to decreased venous return, caused by vena cava compression by the gravid uterus (*i.e.*, supine hypotension syndrome), or from venodilation and bradycardia secondary to the sympathectomy accompanying spinal or peridural block
- Decreased cardiac output secondary to myocardial depression, usually produced by an overdose of potent inhalation anesthetic or local anesthetic drug
- Decreased systemic blood pressure caused by the sympathectomy of high-spinal or peridural anesthesia.

UTERINE ARTERIAL VASOCONSTRICTION

Some local anesthetic drugs, notably lidocaine and mepivacaine, can cause constriction of uterine artery segments.[69] This is thought to be at least part of the etiology of fetal bradycardia after paracervical block and IV injections of local anesthetics. The use of vasopressors to treat hypotension secondary to the sympathectomy of regional anesthesia also can cause uterine vasoconstriction. Drugs with primarily α-adrenergic activity should be avoided in treating hypotension because the uterine arterial vasoconstriction they provide worsens uterine blood flow. Drugs such as ephedrine and mephentermine will have primarily β-effects, restoring blood flow to normal values in this situation.

INCREASED UTERINE TONE

An increase in uterine muscular tone can decrease uteroplacental perfusion by impeding venous outflow from the intervillous space.[70] High levels of local anesthetics (*e.g.*, after intravascular injection) or of α-adrenergic vasopressors may produce increased myometrial tone and fetal distress, particularly when combined with oxytocin stimulation.

The most commonly observed effect of obstetric analgesia–anesthesia on the fetus is a transient decrease in fetal heart rate secondary to decreased uterine perfusion. This may occur in the absence of hypotension, and is thought to be secondary to a decrease in cardiac output secondary to decreased preload and contractility. It may be sufficient to produce transient fetal distress if placental perfusion is sufficiently impaired. The diminution in preload occurs as a response to the vasodilation brought about by sympathetic nervous blockade, but the decrease in myocardial contractility is more likely than not due to the effects of local anesthetics on the myocardium.

This effect is most pronounced with bupivacaine and less so with lidocaine and chloroprocaine.

DIAGNOSIS AND TREATMENT OF INDIRECT FETAL DEPRESSION

The decreases in uteroplacental perfusion caused by the above-mentioned mechanisms all lead to signs of fetal distress detectable by fetal monitoring. When any obstetric anesthetic technique is used, it is imperative that continuous fetal heart rate monitoring likewise be initiated. Detection of decreased beat-to-beat variability, late decelerations, or prolonged fetal bradycardia should prompt a search for the cause. Treatment should then be directed at correcting the cause, by increasing cardiac output or systemic blood pressure with appropriate vasopressors, changing maternal position, administering oxygen, and decreasing oxytocin infusions.

REFERENCES

1. Watkins DE. Multiple endogenous opiate and non-opiate analgesia systems: evidence of their existence and clinical implications. Ann NY Acad Sci 1986;467:273.
2. Flanagan HL, Datta S, Lambert DH, et al. Effect of pregnancy on bupivacaine induced conduction blockade in the isolated rabbit vagus nerve. Anesth Analg 1987;66:123.
3. Sander HW, Gintzler AR. Spinal cord mediation of the opioid analgesia of pregnancy. Brain Res 1987;408:389.
4. Ueland K, Hansen J. Maternal cardiovascular dynamics: II. Posture and uterine contractions. Am J Obstet Gynecol 1969; 103:1.
5. Shnider SM, Wright RG, Levinson G, et al. Uterine blood flow and plasma norepinephrine changes during maternal stress in the pregnant ewe. Anesthesiology 1979;50:524.
6. Myers RE. Maternal psychologic stress and fetal asphyxia: a study in the monkey. Am J Obstet Gynecol 1975;122:47.
7. Motoyama EK, Rivard G, Acheson F, et al. Adverse effect of maternal hyperventilation on the fetus. Am J Obstet Gynecol 1975;122:47.
8. Ralston DH, Shnider SM, De Lorimer AA. Uterine blood flow and fetal acid-base changes after bicarbonate administration in the pregnant ewe. Anesthesiology 1974;40:348.
9. Gintzler AR. Endorphin-mediated increases in pain threshold during pregnancy. Science 1980;210:193.
10. Pearson JF, Davies P. The effect of continuous epidural analgesia on maternal acid-base balance and arterial lactate concentration during the second stage of labour. J Obstet Gynecol Br Commonw 1973;80:225.
11. American Society of Anesthesiologists. Guidelines for anesthetic practice. Chicago: American Society of Anesthesiologists, 1979.
12. American College of Obstetricians and Gynecologists. National survey of maternal care. Chicago: The American Society of Obstetricians and Gynecologists, 1970.
13. American College of Obstetricians and Gynecologists. National survey of maternal care. Chicago: The American Society of Obstetricians and Gynecologists, 1990.
14. Taylor ES, ed. Beck's obstetrical practice and fetal medicine. 9th ed. Baltimore: Williams & Wilkins, 1971:607.
15. Ministry of Health. Report on confidential enquiries into maternal deaths in England and Wales 1985–1987. London: Her Majesty's Stationery Office, 1990.
16. Bragin RE. Opioid and catecholaminergic mechanisms of different types of analgesia. Ann NY Acad Sci 1986;467:331.
17. Lamaze F. Painless childbirth: psychoprophylactic method. London: Burke, 1958.
18. Abouleish E. Acupuncture in obstetrics. Anesth Analg 1975; 54:82.
19. Tyler E, Caldwell C, Ghia JN. Transcutaneous nerve stimulation: an alternative approach to the management of postoperative pain. Anesth Analg 1982;61:449.
20. Scott DB. Effect of psychoprophylaxis (Lamaze preparation) on labor and delivery in primiparas. N Engl J Med 1976;294:1205.
21. Doering SG, Entwisle DR. Preparation during pregnancy and ability to cope with labor and delivery. Am J Orthopsychiatry 1975;45:825.
22. Saling E, Ligidas P. The effect on the fetus of maternal hyperventilation during labour. J Obstet Gynaecol Br Commonw 1969;76:877.
23. Zador G, Nillson BA. Low dose intermittent epidural anesthesia with lidocaine for vaginal delivery. Acta Obstet Gynecol Scand Suppl 1974;34:17.
24. Wahl CW. Contraindications and limitations of hypnosis in obstetric analgesia. Am J Obstet Gynecol 1960;16:210.
25. Dundee JW. Alterations in response to somatic pain associated with anesthesia: II. The effect of thiopentone and pentobarbitone. Br J Anaesth 1960;32:407.
26. Powe CE, Kiem IM, Fromhagen C, et al. Propiomazine hydrochloride in obstetrical analgesia. JAMA 1962;181:290.
27. McAllister CB. Placental transfer and neonatal effects of diazepam when administered to women just before delivery. Br J Anaesth 1980;52:423.
28. Pert C, Synder S. Opiate receptor: its demonstration in nervous tissue. Science 1973;179:1011.
29. Yaksh AR. Opioid receptor systems and the endorphins: a review of their spinal organization. J Neurosurg 1987;67:157.
30. Yaksh TL. Spinal opiate analgesia: characteristics and principles of action. Pain 1981;11:293.
31. Schmauss C, Yaksh TL. In vivo studies on spinal opiate receptors mediating antinociception. J Pharmacol Exp Ther 1983; 228:1.
32. Bullingham RE, McQuay HJ, Moore RA. Clinical pharmacokinetics of narcotic agonist-antagonist drugs. Clin Pharmacokinet 1983;8:139.
33. Shnider SM, Moya F. Effects of meperidine on the newborn infant. Am J Obstet Gynecol 1960;89:1009.
34. Bower S, Hull C. Comparative pharmacokinetics of fentanyl and alfentanil. Br J Anaesth 1982;54:211.
35. Bennett RL, Batenhorst RL, Bivins BA, et al. Patient-controlled analgesia. Ann Surg 1982;195:700.
36. McIntosh DG, Rayburn WF. Patient-controlled analgesia in obstetrics and gynecology. Obstet Gynecol 1991;78:1129.
37. Wang JK, Nauss LE, Thomas JE. Pain relief by intrathecally applied morphine in man. Anesthesiology 1979;50:149.
38. Booker PD, Wilkes RG, Bryson THL, et al. Obstetric pain relief using epidural morphine. Anaesthesia 1980;35:377.
39. Husemeyer RP, O'Connor MC, Davenport HT, et al. Failure of epidural morphine to relieve pain in labor. Anaesthesia 1980; 35:161.
40. Robinson DE, Leicht CH. Epidural analgesia with low dose bupivacaine and fentanyl for labor and delivery in a parturient with severe pulmonary hypertension. Anesthesiology 1988; 68:285.
41. Skjolderbrand A, Garle M, Gustaffson LL, et al. Extradural pethidine with and without adrenaline during labor:wide variation in effect. Br J Anaesth 1982;54:415.

42. Hodgkinson R, Hoff RW, Husain FJ. Double blind comparison of maternal analgesics and neonatal behavior. J Int Med Res 1979;7:234.
43. Cohen S. Inhalation analgesia and anesthesia for vaginal delivery. In: Snider SM, Levinson G, eds. Anesthesia and obstetrics. 3rd ed. Baltimore: Williams & Wilkins, 1993:194.
44. Palahnuik RJ, Shnider SM, Eger II. Pregnancy decreases the requirement for inhaled anesthetic agents. Anesthesiology 1974;41:82.
45. Galloon S. Ketamine for obstetric delivery. Anesthesiology 1976;44:522.
46. Rosenblatt R, Wright R, Denson D, et al. Continuous epidural infusions for obstetric analgesia. Reg Anaesth 1983;8:10.
47. Hicks JA, Jenkins JG, Newton MC, et al. Continuous epidural infusion of 0.075% bupivacaine for pain relief in labour: a comparison with intermittent top-ups of 0.5% bupivacaine. Anaesthesia 1988;43:289.
48. Dathis F, Macheboeuf M, Thomas H, et al. Epidural analgesia with a bupivacaine-fentanyl mixture in obstetrics: comparison of repeated injections and continuous infusion. Can J Anaesth 1988;35:116.
49. Li DF, Rees GA, Rosen M. Continuous extradural infusion of 0.0625% or 0.125% bupivacaine for pain relief in primigravid labour. Br J Anaesth 1985;57:264.
50. Abboud TK, Afrasiabi A, Sarkis F, et al. Continuous infusion epidural analgesia in parturients receiving bupivacaine, chloroprocaine, or lidocaine: maternal, fetal, and neonatal effects. Anesth Analg 1984;63:421.
51. Chestnut DH, Bates JN, Choi WW. Continuous infusion epidural analgesia with lidocaine: efficacy and influence during the second stage of labor. Obstet Gynecol 1987;69:323.
52. MacLeod DM, Tey HK, Byers GF, et al. The loading dose for continuous infusion epidural analgesia: a technique to reduce the incidence of hypotension. Anaesthesia 1987;42:377.
53. Gambling DR, Yu P, Cole C, et al. A comparative study of patient controlled epidural analgesia (PCEA) and continuous infusion epidural analgesia (CIEA) during labour. Can J Anaesth 1988;35:249.
54. Morishima HO, Adamsons K. Placental clearance of mepivacaine following administration to the guinea pig fetus. Anesthesiology 1967;28:343.
55. Ralston DH, Shnider SM. The fetal and neonatal effects of regional anesthesia in obstetrics. Anesthesiology 1978;48:34.
56. Thiery M, Vroman S. Paracervical block analgesia during labour. Am J Obstet Gynecol 1972;113:988.
57. Fox FS, Smith JB, Namba Y, et al. Anesthesia for cesarean section. Am J Obstet Gynecol 1979;133.15.
58. Cree IE, Meyer J, Hailey DM. Diazepam in labour. Br Med J 1973;4:251.
59. Scher J, Hailey DM. The effects of diazepam on the fetus. J Obstet Gynaecol Br Commonw 1972;79:635.
60. Moya F. Volatile inhalation agents and muscle relaxants in obstetrics. Acta Anesthesiol Scand Suppl 1966;25:368.
61. Marx GF, Joshi CW, Orkin LR. Placental transmission of nitrous oxide. Anesthesiology 1970;32:429.
62. Kivalo I, Saaroski S. Placental transmission and foetal uptake of C-dimethyltubocurarine. Br J Anaesth 1972;44:557.
63. Older PO, Harris JM. Placental transfer of tubocurarine. Br J Anaesth 1968;40:459.
64. Shnider SM. Serum cholinesterase activity during pregnancy, labor and puerperium. Anesthesiology 1965;26:355.
65. Brada A, Haroun S, Bassili M, et al. Response of the newborn to succinylcholine injection in homozygotic atypical mothers. Anesthesiology 1975;43:115.
66. Ali HH, Savarese JJ. Monitoring of neuromuscular function. Anesthesiology 1976;45:216.
67. O'Brien JE, Abbey V, Hinsvark O, et al. Metabolism and measurement of 2-chloroprocaine, an ester-type local anesthetic. J Pharm Sci 1979;68:75.
68. Hyman MD, Shnider SM. Maternal and neonatal blood concentrations of bupivacaine associated with obstetrical conduction anesthesia. Anesthesiology 1971;34:81.
69. Greiss FC, Still JG, Anderson SG. Effects of local anesthetic agents on the uterus vasculature and myometrium. Am J Obstet Gynecol 1976;124:889.
70. Vasicka A, Kretchmer H. Effect of conduction and inhalation anesthesia on uterine contractions. Am J Obstet Gynecol 1961;82:600.

Part Three

TRANSITION AND STABILIZATION

Neonatology: Pathophysiology and Management of the Newborn, Fourth Edition,
edited by Gordon B. Avery, Mary Ann Fletcher, and Mhairi G. MacDonald.
J.B. Lippincott Company, Philadelphia © 1994.

chapter 18

Physiology of Transition

NICHOLAS NELSON

By the end of normal-term gestation, the fetus and its lungs are well prepared to assume responsibility for extrauterine gas exchange. The alveoli are developed by week 25 of gestation, and, by week 35, the type II great alveolar pneumocyte has begun to produce adequate quantities of the surface-active material on which alveolar stability will later depend, once air breathing commences. *In utero*, the alveoli are open and stable at nearly the normal neonatal lung volume because they are filled with a fetal lung liquid, probably produced by ultrafiltration of pulmonary capillary blood, as well as secretion by alveolar cells.[1]

The pulmonary and bronchial circulations are well developed and thoroughly admixed by multiple connections at the alveolar level. This combined circulation is characterized by high pressure and low flow, because of a high degree of both passive and active pulmonary vascular resistance. The passive resistance most likely relates to compression of pulmonary capillaries by the fetal lung liquid,[2] but there also is a high degree of active vasomotor tone resulting from the hypoxic level (*i.e.*, PO_2 of 25 torr) of the pulmonary venous stream.[3–6] This hypoxic increase in active pulmonary vasomotor tone is a dominant feature in the behavior of the pulmonary vasculature at all stages of development, but is more active in the fetus because of a relatively much larger vascular muscle mass than in the adult.[7,8] These features are responsible for the key characteristic of the fetal circulation—namely, that pulmonary vascular resistance greatly exceeds systemic resistance (Table 18-1), so that nearly 50% of the fetal cardiac output perfuses the placenta, whereas only 5% to 10% perfuses the lung (Tables 18-2 and 18-3). With the onset of inflation and ventilation of the lung at birth, these resistances will reverse, and it is the success of this reversal that principally determines the success of the cardiopulmonary adaptation to birth.

The neuromuscular controls of respiration also are laid down well before even premature birth. The fetus spends nearly 30% of its time engaged in a rapid, discoordinate form of panting—paradoxical motions of the chest and abdominal wall[9,10] associated with the rapid, irregular, and low-voltage electrocortical activity seen in active rapid eye movement (REM) sleep.[11,12] In the human fetus near term, as much as 600 mL of amniotic fluid per day is inhaled through such activity[13]; a lot of this volume is swallowed.[14] These breathing movements can even modulate blood flow through the fetal ductus arteriosus.[15] Thus, the "first breaths of life" is perhaps an inaccurate label, albeit a dramatic underscoring of the events that mark the perinatal shift from placental to pulmonary gas exchange and from liquid to gaseous ventilation.

THE FIRST BREATHS

The passive phase of these events during vaginal birth is shown in Figure 18-1, wherein the thoracic cage is compressed to pressures of 30 to 160 cm H_2O during passage through the birth canal, sometimes producing forcible ejection of as much as 30 mL of tracheal fluid through the airways.[16] The subsequent recoil of the chest wall after birth of the trunk may

TABLE 18–1
HEMODYNAMIC CHARACTERISTICS OF THE PERINATAL CIRCULATION

	Resistance (torr × L^{-1} × kg × min)			Conductance (mL × kg^{-1} × min × $torr^{-1}$)		
	Fetal Sheep	Neonatal Sheep	Neonatal Human	Fetal Sheep	Neonatal Sheep	Neonatal Human
Pulmonary	530	85	140	1.9	11.8	7.1
Ductus	30	810		33.3	1.2	
Systemic	170	220	300	5.9	4.5	3.3

Data from references 151 through 157.

produce a small passive inspiration of air, perhaps accompanied by active glossopharyngeal forcing of some air into at least the proximal airways and introduction of some blood into pulmonary capillaries (*i.e.*, "capillary erection").[17] Thus, an air–liquid interface is established within the larger airways of the lung, and with it are established the surface retractive forces that would tend to collapse the smaller airways and alveoli, were it not for the presence of surface-active material in the alveolar lining layer.

The functional life cycle of this surface-active material is shown in Figure 18-2.[18,19] The effective spreading and stabilization of the phospholipid monolayer, which is principally dipalmitoyl lecithin, is coming to be understood as the special purview of several lung-specific proteins. Of these surfactant proteins (Table 18-4), SP-A, SP-B, and SP-C are concerned especially with secretion and metamorphosis of the surface-active material from its intracellular storage sites (*i.e.*, the lamellar bodies) to the tubular myelin of the hypophase, en route to the phospholipid interface. At that interface, an interaction of charges among the basic arginine and lysine residues of SP-B apparently helps to resist surface tension by increasing the lateral stability of the phospholipid monolayer.[20] The critical concentration of surfactant in the lung liquid necessary to lower surface tension is about 3 mg/mL,[21] but much higher concentrations appear necessary for alveolar stability in the premature infant.[18] It appears that the respiratory distress syndrome may involve some sort of difficulty in the movement of phospholipid into tubular myelin, a process apparently facilitated by SP-A and SP-B.[22]

The first opening of the alveoli and lung will be made easier if some fetal lung liquid is retained in at least the smaller airways of the lung before the first active breaths are taken (Fig. 18-3).[23] The reason for this is that inflation of the lung by air from the totally

TABLE 18–2
DISTRIBUTION OF CARDIAC OUTPUT*

	Full-Term Fetal Lamb			Human	
	Resistance (torr/mL/kg/min)	Conductance (mL/kg/min/torr)	F_{CO}	Fetus F_{CO}	Adult F_{CO}
Vital Organs					
Brain	3.3	0.3	0.03	0.14	0.14
Heart	2.5	0.4	0.04	0.02	0.05
Lung	2	0.5	0.05	0.1	1
Placenta	0.25	4	0.4	0.33	0
Metabolic Organs					
Liver	0.56	1.8	0.18		
Gut	2	0.5	0.05	0.08	0.23
Spleen	5	0.2	0.02	0.02	
Kidney	5	0.2	0.02	0.05	0.22
Adrenal				0.04	
Carcass	0.27	3.7	0.37		
Bone					0.14
Muscle					0.18
Skin					0.04

* Values calculated from assumed mean blood pressure of 55 torr.
F_{CO}, fractional cardiac output.
Data from references 158 through 163.

TABLE 18–3
ORGAN BLOOD FLOW

Tissue	Fetal Sheep (mL/kg body weight/min)	Fetal Human (mL/kg body weight/min)	Fetal Sheep (mL/100 g tissue/min)	Fetal Human (mL/100 g tissue/min)	Adult Human (mL/100 g tissue/min)	
					Rest	Maximum
Vital Organs						
Brain	16.5	51	132	25	50	130
Heart	22	7.3	291	165	70	400
Lung	27.5	36.3	126			
Placenta	220	120	130	11		
Metabolic Organs						
Liver	99		20		50	250
Gut	27.5	29	69	101	40	200
Spleen	11	7.3	240			
Kidney	11	18.2	173	155	400	550
Adrenal		14.5		340		
Carcass	204		26		2.5	260
Bone					3	15
Muscle					3	60
Skin					10	150
Total cardiac output (both ventricles)	550	363				

Data from references 158 through 162 and 164.

collapsed and gas-free state (see Fig. 18-3, dashed line) requires the exertion of considerable distending pressure across the lung—10 cm H_2O pressure is shown here, but levels up to 80 cm H_2O are not uncommon for the first full expansion—so that the spontaneous occurrence of alveolar rupture in full-term infants with healthy lungs becomes understandable. Note that filling with liquid (see Fig. 18-3, solid line) requires rather less force than inflation with air because of the lack of an air–liquid interface. Note also that the deflation curve in air is not superimposable on its inflation curve (*i.e.*, hysteresis), because mobilization and orientation of alveolar surfactant molecules during deflation decrease alveolar surface tension as the alveolar surface contracts. Thus, the transpulmonary (*i.e.*, alveolus to intrapleural space) distending pressure required to maintain lung volume at 30 mL diminishes from 10 to nearly 0 cm H_2O.

STIMULI FOR BREATHING

The precise reason or reasons for the first extrauterine inspirations probably will remain somewhat obscure because the unfamiliar stimuli to which the newborn infant is suddenly subjected are multiple: cold, light, noise, gravity, and pain, all in addition to the hypercapnea, respiratory acidosis, and hypoxia, collec-

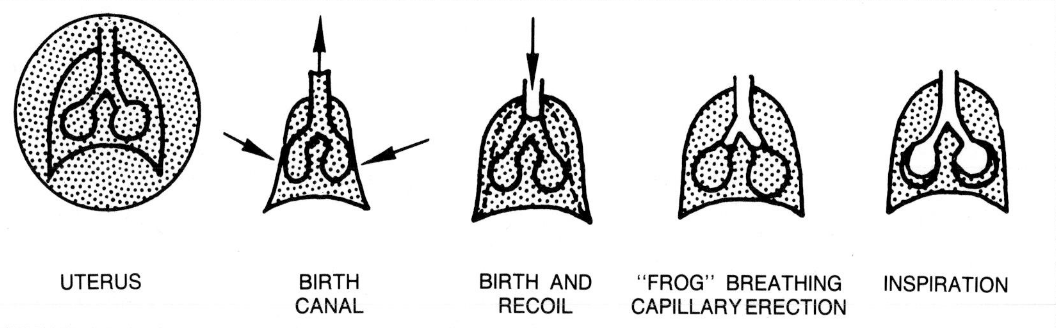

FIG. 18–1. Mechanical events of the first breaths. (From Smith CA, Nelson NM. Physiology of the newborn infant. 4th ed. Springfield, IL: Charles C. Thomas, 1976:123.)

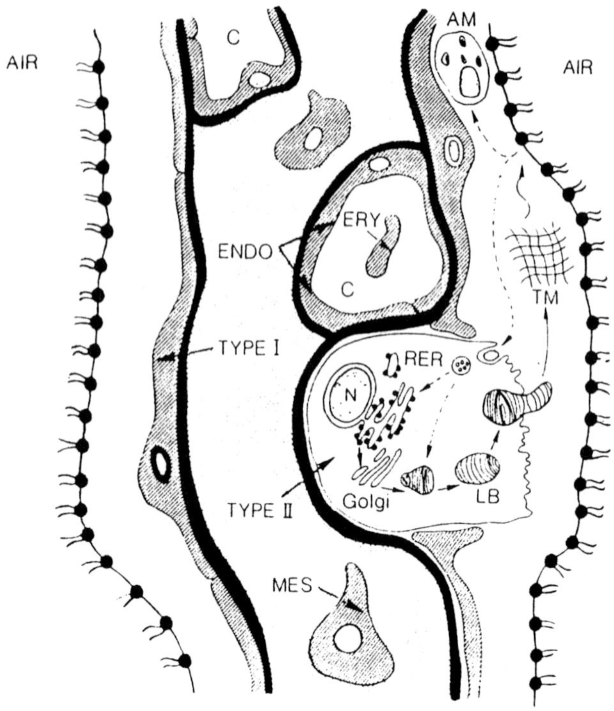

FIG. 18–2. Schematic cross section of an alveolar wall. Surface-active material is a translation product that moves from the rough endoplasmic reticulum (RER) to storage in the lamellar bodies (LB) before being excreted into the hypophase as tubular myelin (TM), a process requiring lung-specific surfactant proteins (*i.e.*, SP-A, SP-B, SP-C). The monolayer–air interface is indicated by the two-tailed hydrophobic ends of the phospholipid molecules, whose orientation is stabilized by SP-B. (AM, alveolar macrophage; C, capillary; ENDO, endothelial cell; ERY, erythrocyte; MES, mesenchymal cell; N, nucleus; TYPE I, type I pneumocyte; TYPE II, type II pneumocyte; from Haagsman HP, van Golde LMG. Synthesis and assembly of lung surfactant. Annu Rev Physiol 1991;53:441.)

tively called asphyxia, that result from normal labor and its accompanying intermittent restriction of maternal placental perfusion.

The possible interplay of these stimuli around the respiratory center is shown in Figure 18-4. The animal fetus at term has been demonstrated to be responsive to all these stimuli, although there are certain inconsistencies. Thus, the fetal carotid body (*i.e.*, the peripheral chemoreceptor) responds to hypoxia and to hypercapnia, particularly oscillatory hypercapnia; neuronal traffic from these influences regularly is recordable along the carotid sinus nerve.[24] Moreover, although the acidity of the fetal cerebrospinal fluid, like that of the adult, appears to be regulated at *p*H levels lower than those of blood, the fetal central chemoreceptor responds but poorly to the normal ventilatory drive of cerebrospinal fluid acidosis.[25] Throughout all these observations, the fact has been noted that the animal fetus will not breathe when warm and submerged, despite the presence of chemi-

TABLE 18–4
PULMONARY SURFACTANT PROTEINS

	SP-A	SP-B	SP-C	SP-D
Chromosome Number	10	2	8	
Gene				
Length (kilobases)	5	6	3	
Content (exons)	11	11		
Translation Product				
Weight (kilodaltons)	26	40	20	
Length (amino acids)	248	381	197	
Monomer				
Weight (kilodaltons)	28	9	4	43
Length (amino acids)		79	35	
Polarity	Hydrophilic	Hydrophobic	Hydrophobic	Hydrophilic
Function				
Feedback inhibition	+			
SAM ≥ monolayer	+	+		
Stabilize monolayer		+		

+, present; SAM, surface-active materials.
Data from Hawgood S, Shiffer K. Structures and properties of the surfactant-associated proteins. Annu Rev Physiol 1991;53:375, and Mendelson CR, Boggaram V. Hormonal control of the surfactant system in fetal lung. Annu Rev Physiol 1991;53:415.

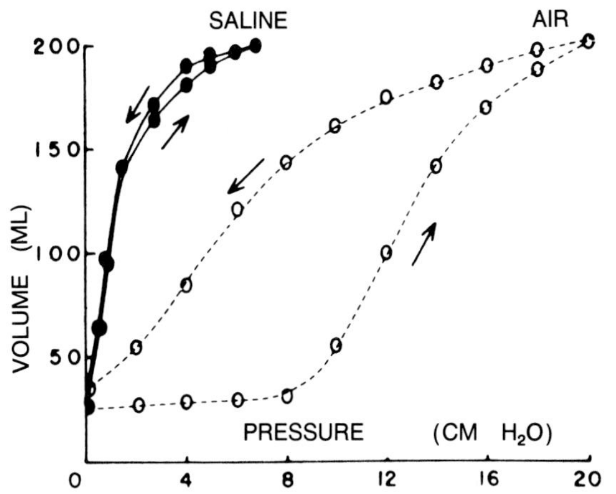

FIG. 18–3. Pressure–volume curves after air versus liquid expansion of the lung. (From Radford EP. In: Remington JW, ed. Tissue elasticity. Washington, DC: American Physiological Society, 1957.)

cal stimuli for respiration, whereas when chilled and exposed, the fetus will breathe, despite the lack of chemical stimuli for respiration. The possibility thus arises of a well tuned fetal respiratory center, quite responsive to the usual chemical stimuli, that is repressed *in utero* but derepressed by delivery.[26]

The unaroused or perhaps repressed fetus is apneic and appears to have his or her respiratory rhythm generator switched off in expiration—that is, the inspiratory neurones are inhibited, and the expiratory neurones are in tonic discharge.[27] In this state, the respiratory centers appear unresponsive to chemical or sensory stimuli. This refractory state can result from vagal (*i.e.*, pulmonary stretch afferents)[28] or superior laryngeal (*i.e.*, laryngeal taste afferents)[29,30] discharge in states of experimental manipulation, but in the normal fetus it may more likely represent a hypoxic repression of facilitation from suprapontine centers. In any case, states of fetal arousal (*e.g.*, REM sleep) appear to be linked, possibly through the reticular formation, to a rhythmic, alternating discharge of inspiratory and expiratory neurones. The accentuation of fetal hypoxia by disruption of placental gas exchange during normal birth produces a gasping respiratory effort with resultant improved cerebral oxygenation, accompanied by decreasing tonic discharge of expiratory neurones. These effects, coupled with the general sensory arousal of birth, evidently are sufficient to restore the inherent rhythmicity of discharge in the respiratory centers.[31]

Figure 18-4 represents imaginary cross connections that could explain these phenomena of possible interaction. This interactional concept portrays the inspiratory and expiratory centers as mutually inhibitory and, moreover, affected by neighboring neuronal traffic from both above and below. Thus, the general tone of the respiratory neurons may well be enhanced or facilitated by nonrespiratory environmental stimuli, such as heat or cold, pain, change in position or pressure, noise, and light.

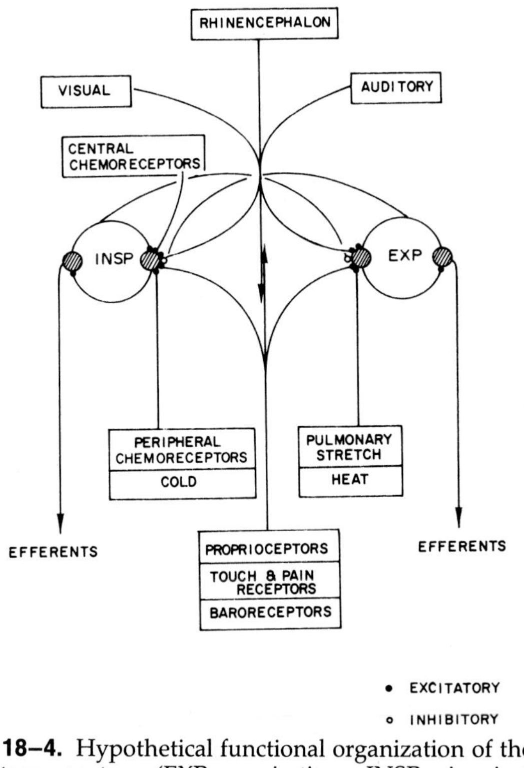

FIG. 18–4. Hypothetical functional organization of the respiratory center. (EXP, expiration; INSP, inspiration; adapted from Burns BD. The central control of respiratory movements. Br Med Bull 1963;19:7.)

PULMONARY ADAPTATION

In any case, the first active breaths of air, once taken and sustained, set in motion a nearly inexorable chain of events that:

1. Converts the fetal to the adult circulation
2. Empties the lung of liquid
3. Establishes the neonatal lung volume and the characteristics of pulmonary function in the newborn infant.

These events are outlined in Figure 18-5, and will be analyzed separately later in this chapter, although they occur concurrently. The upper left corner of Figure 18-5 is a reprise of the events diagrammed in Figure 18-1. Air entry into the respiratory system establishes the lung retractive forces of surface tension (see Fig. 18-3), with the consequent development of negative intrapleural and interstitial pressure, because the overlying chest wall resists collapse. These events, along with the increase in alveolar oxygen tension, are solidly established fact and are indicated as such by the solid boxes of Figure 18-5; less well established events are indicated by dashed boxes. The final and most dramatic events in the sequence are the great increases in blood and lymph flow through the lung that follow the onset of ventilation.

As lung liquid is ejected from the airways and alveoli, retractive forces become established, hydrostatic

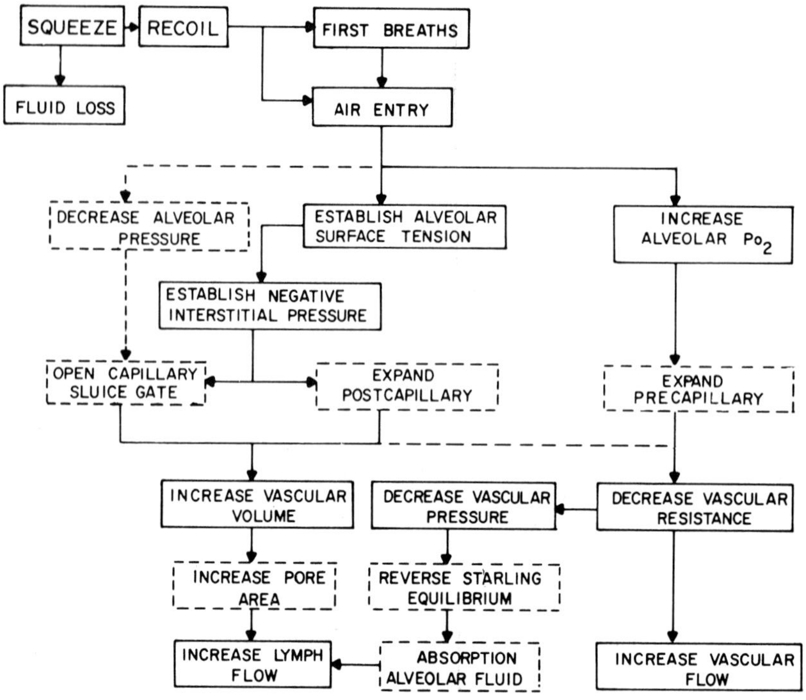

FIG. 18–5. The sequence of events following the onset of ventilation. (From Smith CA, Nelson NM. Physiology of the newborn infant. 4th ed. Springfield, IL: Charles C. Thomas, 1976:131.)

alveolar pressure on the pulmonary capillaries decreases, and these compressible vessels with tone open the "sluice gate" of the "alveolar waterfall" of blood flow through the lung.[32] Moreover, the increasing pulmonary venous oxygen tension of the air-breathing newborn serves to decrease active vasomotor tone in the precapillary pulmonary arterioles. Thus, for both reasons, intralumenal hydrostatic capillary pressure (Pc) rises as pericapillary interstitial alveolar pressure (Pif) decreases and Starling's equilibrium is perturbed, so that capillary fluid tends to transude into the interstitium,[33] and alveolar fluid also may well be directly absorbed into the interstitial spaces at the alveolar corners.[34] Starling's equilibrium can be expressed as the following equation:

$$\text{Fluid transfer} = k([Pc - \pi pl] - [Pif - \pi if]),$$

where k is the filtration constant relating to pore size, πpl is plasma osmotic pressure, and πif is interstitial osmotic pressure. Positive values for fluid transfer indicate transudation, and negative values indicate fluid absorption. These events are marked by a decrease in total plasma volume, which reaches its nadir at 2 to 8 hours after birth, and by a dramatic increase in lung lymph drainage, beginning promptly on ventilation and subsiding by about 6 hours of age.[35] During this early period after birth, lymphatic distention in the lung has been demonstrated both histologically and radiologically,[36,37] but the role of atrial natriuretic factor in these fluid movements is uncertain.[38] It is of obvious clinical interest that infant rabbits delivered by cesarean section and immature lamb fetuses are both slow to clear their lung liquid—the one, presumably, denied the thoracic squeeze of vaginal birth, and the other influenced by higher alveolar surface tensions because of lack of adequate alveolar surface-active material.[39]

Infants born by cesarean section, especially where not preceded by labor, are less asphyxiated and less energized by surges of cortisol and catechols than are their vaginally delivered cohorts[40–42]; their lungs are wetter as well,[43–46] although cesarean birth is not prerequisite to "transient tachypnea" of the newborn, which is clinically ascribed to slow clearance of fetal lung liquid.[47]

CIRCULATORY ADAPTATION

The magnitude of the passive and active increase in pulmonary blood flow after inflation and ventilation of the lung is shown in the experimental data of Figure 18-6. If the lung is inflated from the fetal state and ventilated with a gas mixture that does not change the fetal composition of the blood gases (*i.e.*, pH 7.35, PCO_2 45 torr, PO_2 25 torr), an increase in pulmonary vascular conductance (*i.e.*, decrease in resistance) can be achieved, as shown by the increasing flow–pressure slopes of the two curves on the right in Figure 18-6. This increase in conductance most likely is caused by the expansion of collapsible pulmonary capillaries, as well as those vessels that are anatomically tethered to the pulmonary parenchyma. Then, as the blood gas composition is changed by the increase in PO_2 and decrease in PCO_2 similar to ventilation with air, further increases in vascular conductance are achieved, as shown in the pair of curves on the left in Figure 18-6.

The decrease in pulmonary vascular resistance thus set in motion,[48] combined with the increase in periph-

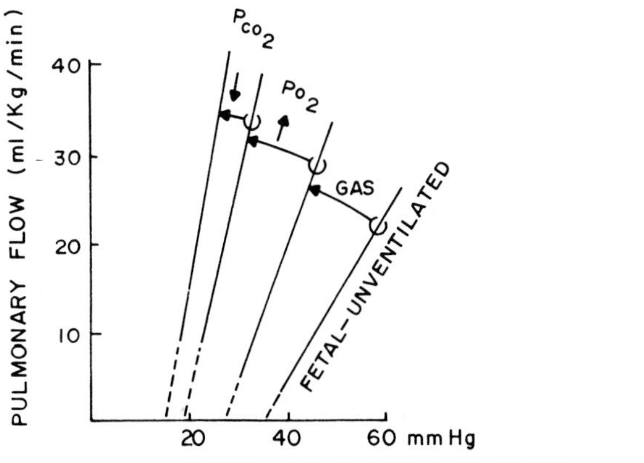

FIG. 18–6. Pulmonary vascular conductance increases with the onset of ventilation. Separate curves depict the contributions of gaseous inflation, increased PO_2 and decreased PCO_2. (Adapted from Strang LB. The lungs at birth. Arch Dis Child 1965;40:575.)

eral vascular resistance that follows increasing oxygenation, the loss of the umbilical circulation, and the cold shock of birth, leads to closure of the foramen ovale within minutes of birth (Fig. 18-7). The ductus arteriosus, however, remains open for some hours, and, because systemic resistance is now higher than pulmonary resistance—the reverse of the fetal circumstance—blood flow through the ductus also reverses, now passing left to right. This is the transitional phase of the perinatal circulation, during which there may be reversion to the fetal pattern at any time that pulmonary vascular resistance should again rise higher than peripheral vascular resistance.[49] During this phase, there also is a considerable increase in the volume load presented to the left ventricle, because of the vast increase in left ventricular input (*i.e.*, pulmonary venous return).[50] The ductus arteriosus constricts under the influence of prostaglandins interacting with rising oxygen tension in the blood coursing through it.[51,52] This normally begins at about 4 to 12 hours postnatally and is completed by around 24 hours of age.[53]

These events are diagrammed in Figure 18-8, along with blood flow data in mL/kg/minute taken from experiments in fetal sheep. In this diagram, parallel electrical generators have diodes to direct the flow of electrons, just as the ventricles have valves to direct the flow of blood. The electrical symbol for resistance indicates relative resistances in the pulmonary and systemic circuits. The large circle in the center of the pulmonary circuit represents the expanding and established alveolus. The diagrammatic sequence makes obvious the conversion of the central circulation from that of two ventricles connected in parallel circuits, where volume loads may be unequal, to connection in series where the right ventricular output must equal left ventricular input, and thus, output, except for some small amount of blood stored in the capacitance vessels (*i.e.*, capillaries and veins) of the pulmonary circulation.

Much of the increase in peripheral vascular resistance is a result of the cessation of the umbilical circulation. The umbilical arteries constrict vigorously un-

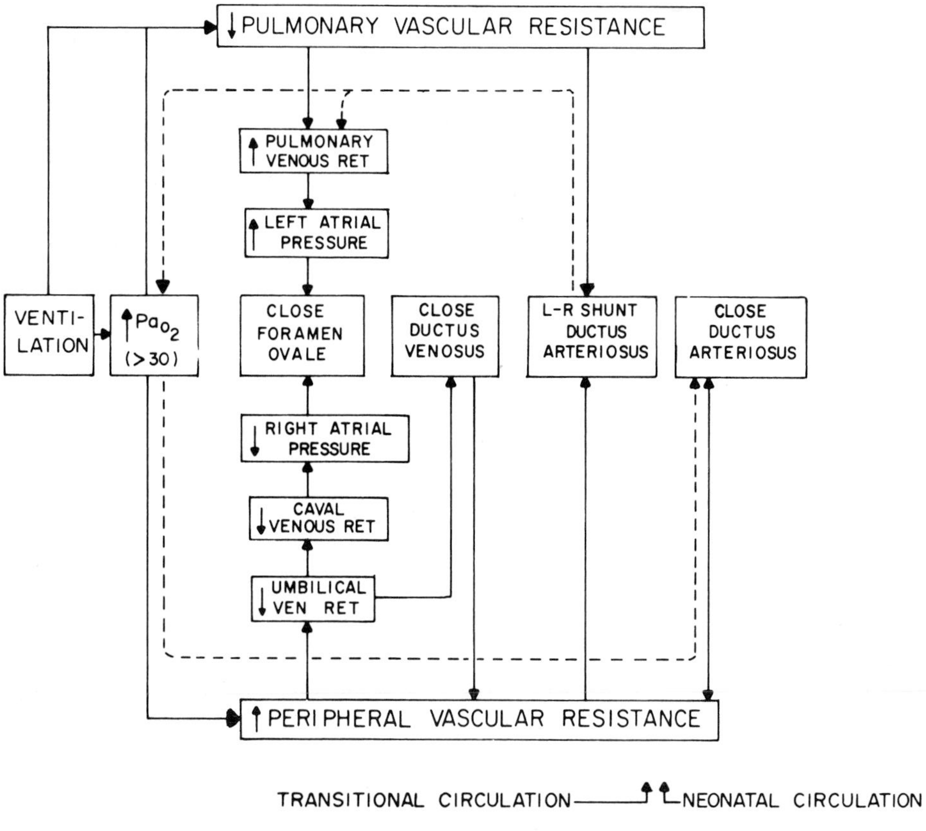

FIG. 18–7. The perinatal circulation converts with the onset of ventilation. (L–R, left-to-right; RET, return; VEN, venous; from Smith CA, Nelson NM. Physiology of the newborn infant. 4th ed. Springfield, IL: Charles C. Thomas, 1976:144.)

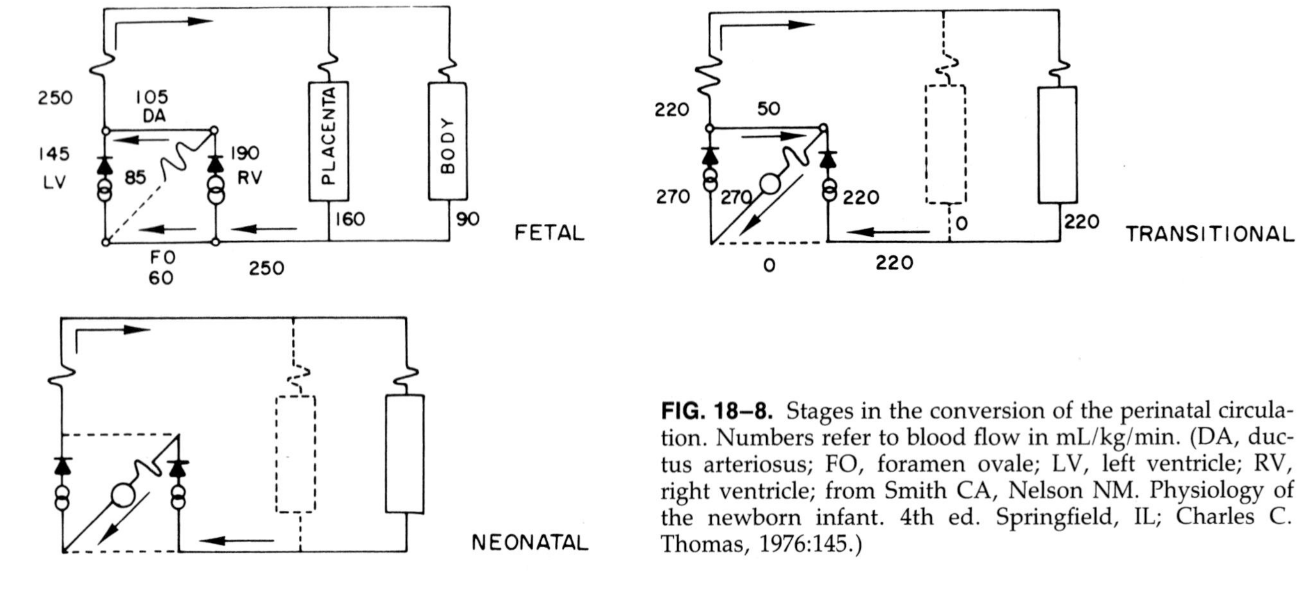

FIG. 18–8. Stages in the conversion of the perinatal circulation. Numbers refer to blood flow in mL/kg/min. (DA, ductus arteriosus; FO, foramen ovale; LV, left ventricle; RV, right ventricle; from Smith CA, Nelson NM. Physiology of the newborn infant. 4th ed. Springfield, IL; Charles C. Thomas, 1976:145.)

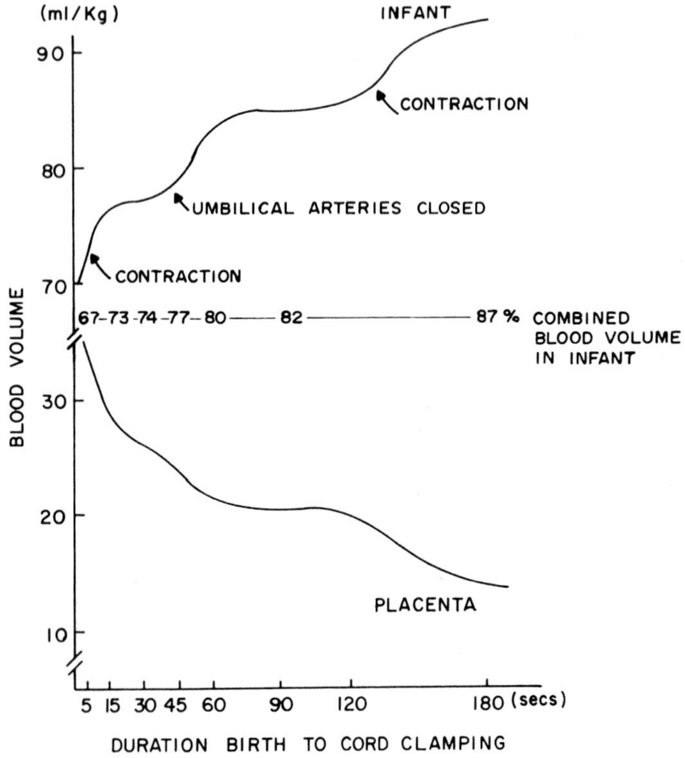

FIG. 18–9. The placental transfusion: sequence of events during the first 3 minutes of life. (From Smith CA, Nelson NM. Physiology of the newborn infant. 4th ed. Springfield, IL: Charles C. Thomas, 1976:139.)

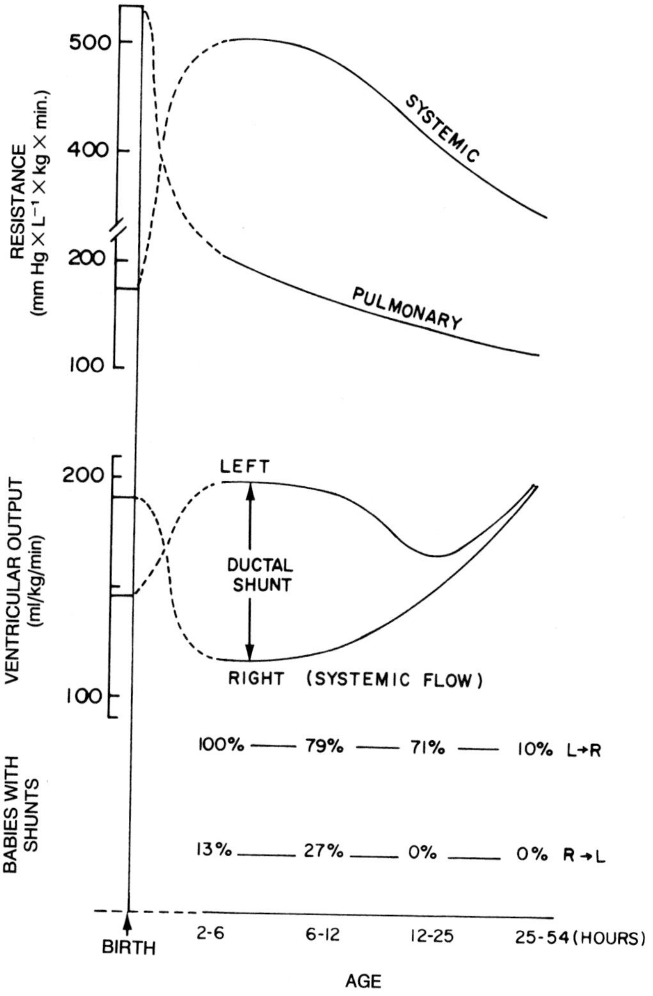

FIG. 18–10. Perinatal hemodynamics in the human show changes in vascular resistance, ventricular output, and shunting. (From Smith CA, Nelson NM. Physiology of the newborn infant. 4th ed. Springfield, IL: Charles C. Thomas, 1976:148, and data from references 188 and 189.)

der the influence of increased oxygenation and, particularly, in response to longitudinal stretch on the umbilical cord. The balance of umbilical arterial inflow to and umbilical venous outflow from the placenta, aided by the positive force of uterine contractions and the negative force of neonatal thoracic inspiration,[54–56] determines the course of the transfusion of blood from the placenta to the infant, as shown in Figure 18-9. The umbilical arteries close very rapidly, in advance of closure of the umbilical vein, resulting in an average net transfer of about 15 to 20 mL/kg of blood to the infant within 3 minutes, if he or she is held below the introitus with the cord untouched. If it is recalled that the primitive maternal posture for childbearing was kneeling rather than the lithotomy position of modern obstetrics, some insight can perhaps be gained into the nature and origin of this placental transfusion.

Apart from those shown in Figure 18-9, there are little human data to document these events, but those that are available are shown in Figures 18-10 and 18-11. Measurements of output from both ventricles, together with appropriate pressure data, permit calcu-

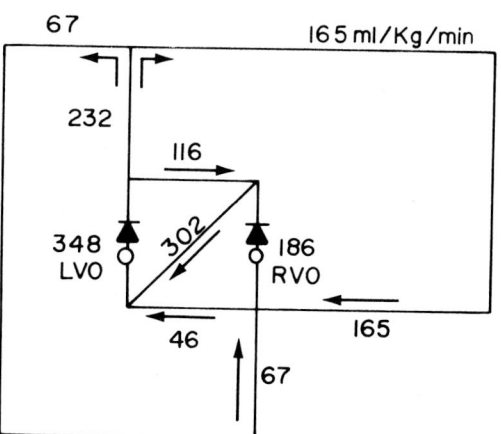

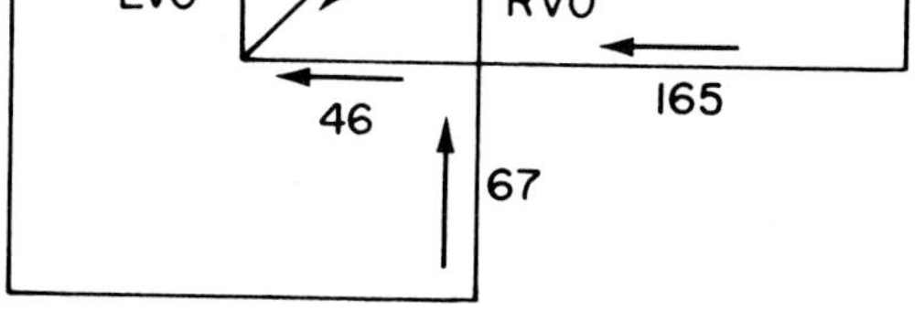

FIG. 18–11. The human perinatal transitional circulation is divided into cerebral blood flow (*left*) and carcass blood flow (*right*). Flow data are given in mL/kg/minute. (From Smith CA, Nelson NM. Physiology of the newborn infant. 4th ed. Springfield, IL: Charles C. Thomas, 1976:175, and data from references 188 and 189.)

lation of the resistances shown in Figure 18-10; the fetal data are taken from sheep. The dominant events depicted include the following:

- the rise and subsequent fall in systemic resistance
- the vast decrease in pulmonary resistance
- the large, albeit transient, increase in left ventricular volume and pressure work
- the decrease in right ventricular pressure work and transiently, volume work
- closure of the ductus arteriosus and equalization of ventricular volume work between 12 and 14 hours
- closure of the foramen ovale in the first minutes and hours after birth.

Human flow data during the transitional phase of the perinatal circulation are shown in Figure 18-11; they document that the left ventricle is pumping nearly two times the volume load of the right ventricle.[50,57,58]

It is pressure work, however, that chiefly determines the behavior of the electromotive forces of the beating heart—the QRS loop remains unchanged from its rightward-dominant vector orientation over the first days of life. This is a reflection of the dominance of right-over-left ventricular muscle mass, as a result of the chronic cor pulmonale of the fetal state, and will shift only slowly to the left-dominant picture of the adult over the first 3 to 6 months of life, as the ventricles become remodeled in response to decreasing right-ventricular pressure work and increasing left-ventricular pressure work. The only perinatal electrocardiographic indication of these shifting pressure–volume loads on the ventricles is the change in orientation of the T-vector: leftward inferior and anterior at birth; rightward inferior and anterior at transition (about 6 hours); leftward inferior and posterior at restitution (12 to 24 hours).

METABOLIC ADAPTATION

Many of the same stimuli that elicit the first breaths—the asphyxia of labor by diminution of placental perfusion, the cold shock of ejection from the womb, and the subsequent independent forage for fuel and oxygen mandated by separation from the placenta—all comprise the principal metabolic perturbations of birth: hypoxia, hypothermia, and hypoglycemia.[59,60] These combined assaults have been likened to ejection from a warm and friendly neighborhood pub into cold, midwinter streets—naked and without a free lunch. Each of these assaults separately can elicit a surge of catechols (*i.e.*, epinephrine, norepinephrine) from their stores in the adrenal and aortic paraganglia (*e.g.*, organ of Zuckerkandl) into the general circulation (Fig. 18-12), for distribution to the target tissues that will sustain the infant until his or her mother can reassume her responsibilities for warmth and nutrition. The immediate eightfold surge in thyroid-stimulating hormone seen in Figure 18-12 is principally the result of the cold shock of delivery, but also may be driven by the many ectopic (*i.e.*, nonhypothalamic) sources of thyroid-releasing hormone built up by the fetus.[61]

Three important enzymes are activated by this surge of catechols. First, hepatic phosphorylase becomes engaged in glycogenolysis, the average infant having sufficient glycogen stores to sustain blood glucose levels during the first 12 hours of postpartum

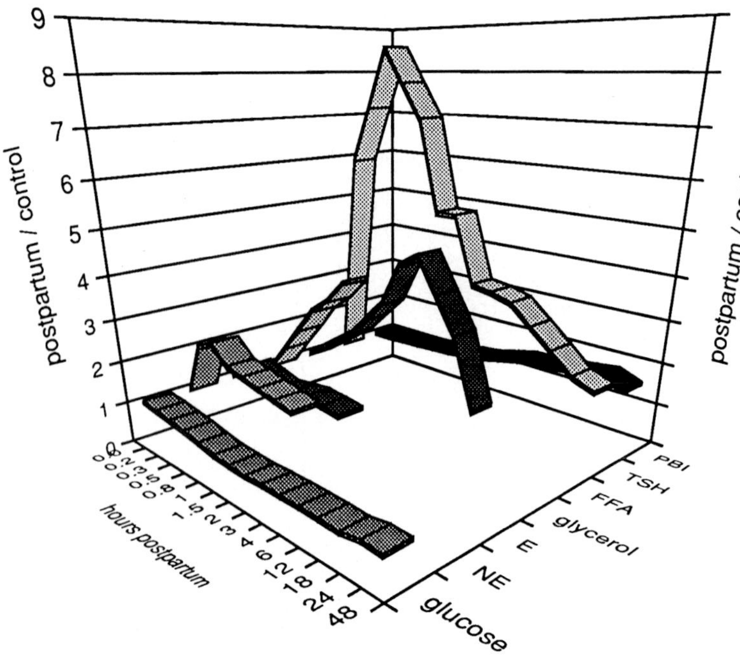

FIG. 18–12. Postnatal changes in metabolism. The value scale is the ratio of postpartum to prepartum (*i.e.*, fetal) levels of each of these moieties. (E, epinephrine; FFA, free fatty acids; NE, norepinephrine; PBI, protein-bound iodine, which is roughly equivalent to the sum of thyroxine and triiodothyronine; TSH, thyroid-stimulating hormone; data from references 40, 61 through 63, 82, and 192 through 198.)

fasting. Next, lipase in adipose tissue commences hydrolyzing stored fat into glycerol and free fatty acids, which thus are made available to gluconeogenesis as a fail-safe source of glucose. This rapid progression from carbohydrate to adipose energy sources, during a transient period of neonatal starvation, can be monitored by the respiratory quotient (*i.e.*, ratio of CO_2 production to O_2 consumption), which descends from 1.0 toward 0.7, until successful suckling completes the conversion from placental to peroral energy assimilation. Finally, deiodinase converts thyroxine to triiodothyronine with particular exuberance in brown adipose tissue. This specialized fat of the newborn serves as an "electric blanket" of nonshivering thermogenesis, because its triiodothyronine stimulates a protein, thermogenin, whose location and action are unique to brown fat; thermogenin diverts the energy of the protons within the mitochondrial respiratory chain to the production of heat, rather than its usual storage as adenosine triphosphate.[40,62,63] Thus does the stressed but sessile newborn bend the biology of fight-or-flight to his or her particular metabolic need.

PULMONARY MECHANICS

Figure 18-13 shows that the first breath (I) begins with no air volume and no transpulmonary pressure gradient. As the chest wall, including the diaphragm, expands, the transpulmonary distending pressure increases until it overcomes surface tension in the smaller airways and alveoli, usually at transpulmonary pressures lower than 25 cm H_2O (see Fig. 18-3).[64] At this point, actively inspired air begins to enter and does so with increasing ease as alveolar dimensions

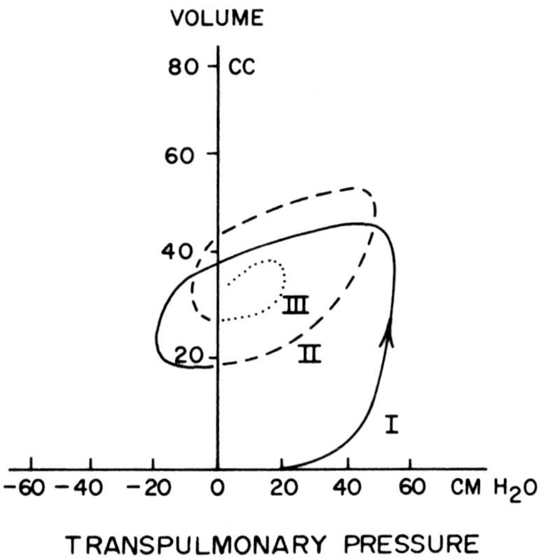

FIG. 18–13. Pressure–volume curves of the first three extrauterine breaths. (From Smith CA, Nelson NM. Physiology of the newborn infant. 4th ed. Springfield, IL: Charles C. Thomas, 1976:125.)

increase. The reason is contained in the Laplace relation:

$$P = 2T/R.$$

This equation states that if wall tension (T) of a spherical surface remains constant, the distending pressure (P) required to maintain equilibrium will decrease as the spherical radius (R) increases. An appropriate analogy is the increasing ease with which a child's balloon is inflated, once first expanded.

At the maximum inspiratory level, which is about 45 mL of air in this example, breath I is actively exhaled—note that transpulmonary pressure in Fig. 18-13 is negative—but not to 0 volume. Evidently with great rapidity the alveolar lining layer, containing surface-active material, is able to stabilize alveolar surfaces so that surface tension decreases as alveolar dimensions decrease. Thus, both T and R decrease together in the Laplace relation, so that the transpulmonary pressure required to maintain inflation is relatively stable and of small dimensions. These dimensions are indicated in Figure 18-14, which compares the pressure–volume characteristics of the infant lung, chest wall and diaphragm, and total respiratory systems to those of the adult. Notable is the fact that, whereas the relaxation pressure curves for the lung alone are remarkably similar across the age span, the infant's chest wall is almost infinitely distensible (*i.e.*, compliant).[65] This results in large part, of course, from the nonossification of the infant thorax—a matter of thoughtful convenience during the high extrinsic pressures of vaginal birth. Indeed, even the adults of diving species, also subjected to high extrinsic thoracic pressures, have chest walls as compliant as that of the newborn human. It is the opposition, however, of the retractive forces of the somewhat expanded lung against the expansive forces of the somewhat compressed chest wall that determines the rest (*i.e.*, end-expiratory) volume of the total respiratory system, and the higher the compliance (*i.e.*, nonstiffness) of the chest wall, the lower will be the rest volume. Note in Figure 18-14 that the infant's rest volume is a good deal closer to the residual or closing volume of the lung than is the case in the adult. Moreover, the transpulmonary pressure at rest also is lower in the infant. This tenuous situation is detailed further in Figure 18-15, wherein it is seen that some smaller airways of the infant actually can close within the range of the normal tidal volume and trap gas in the infant lung's periphery, so that it does not communicate with the trachea.[66] Through measurement of total thoracic gas volume, in comparison to functional residual capacity, as much as 6 mL/kg of lung volume may be measured as trapped in the first 2 weeks of life.[67]

The facts that such gas trapping is the more frequently observed in the first few postnatal days and that intrapleural negative pressure increases to adult levels by 16 days after birth suggest a developmental change in respiratory system equilibrium perhaps too

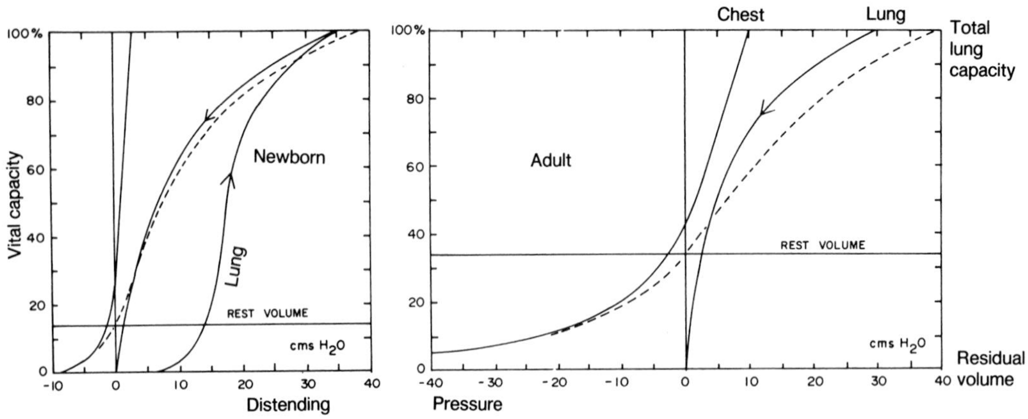

FIG. 18–14. Comparative mechanics of the infant and adult lung. (From Smith CA, Nelson NM. Physiology of the newborn infant. 4th ed. Springfield, IL: Charles C. Thomas, 1976:205.)

rapid to be accounted for by ossification of the thoracic cage.[68,69] It may be that this developmental change actually involves increasing tonus in the intercostal muscles (see below). This would serve to decrease the compliance of the chest wall such that the rest volume of the lung may increase to a level at which smaller airways no longer collapse during quiet breathing.

Moreover, in the first few hours and days of life, the resourceful infant keeps his or her functional residual capacity safely above the lung's rest volume by maintaining inspiratory muscle tone throughout a significant portion of passive expiration,[70–72] and by laryngeal adductive "braking" of the expiration through a series of passive "minigrunts."[73–77] Thus, the infant preserves the stability of his or her lung volume in a resistance–compliance (*i.e.*, larynx–lung and chest wall) circuit, just as the energy of the heart beat is stored in the elastic walls of the great vessels and then steadily discharged through the circulation, under control of the peripheral vascular resistance. The basic difference is that blood flow is direct current, whereas gas flow is alternating current.

The larynx and pharynx also must interlock the infant's epiglottis and palate to allow simultaneous nursing and breathing by providing an interruption of diaphragmatic action during a swallow.[78] These airway-protective mechanisms also can produce an early infantile form of breath-holding spells (*i.e.*, "squirming Valsalva") during motor activity[79]; they are chemoreflexive in nature, generally inhibit ventilation, and frequently are marked by bradycardia.[80,81]

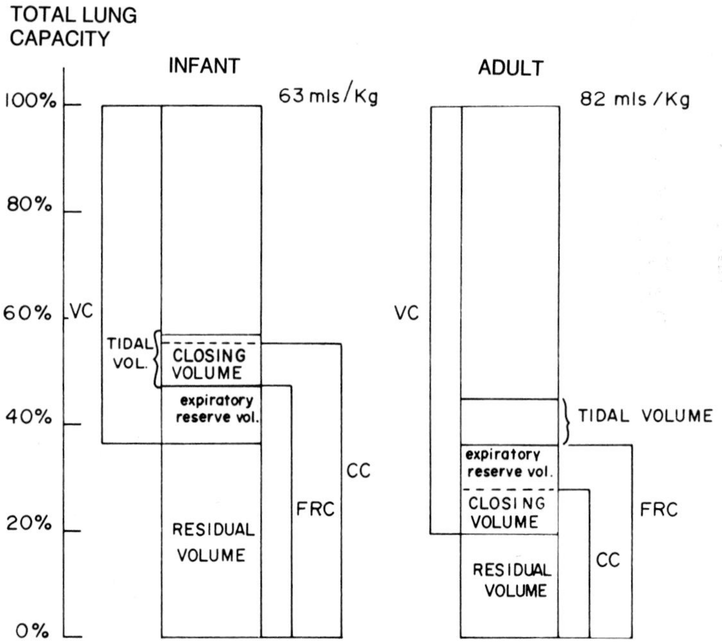

FIG. 18–15. Static lung volumes of the infant and adult. (CC, closing capacity; FRC, functional residual capacity; VC, vital capacity; from Smith CA, Nelson NM. Physiology of the newborn infant. 4th ed. Springfield, IL: Charles C. Thomas, 1976:207.)

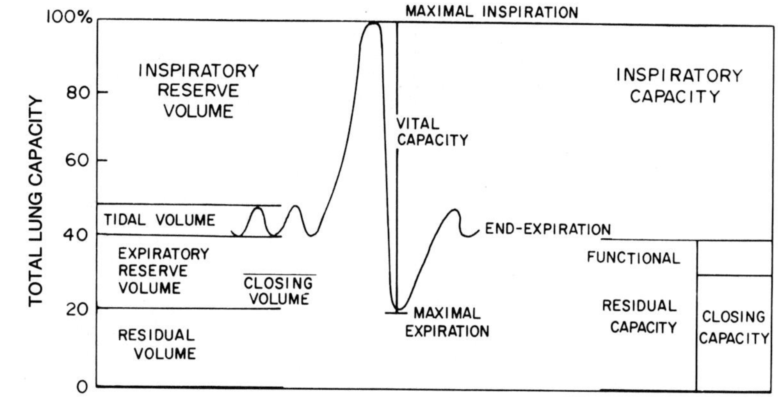

FIG. 18–16. Static lung volumes. A standard spirogram is shown for reference. (From Smith CA, Nelson NM. Physiology of the newborn infant. 4th ed. Springfield, IL: Charles C. Thomas, 1976:206.)

Despite these qualifications, the standard static lung volumes as defined by Figure 18-16 have been measured frequently and reproducibly by many investigators of the newborn, and are shown in Table 18-5. Infants delivered by elective cesarean section initially have a decreased lung gas volume, presumably because they have been denied the partial purging of fetal lung liquid provided by thoracic compression during passage through the birth canal.[44,82]

The decreased total, inspiratory, and vital lung capacities in the infant compared to the adult (see Table 18-5) may indicate an imperfect leverage exerted by a too-compliant chest wall on the underlying lung. The higher residual volume and lower expiratory reserve volume of the infant may be related to gas trapped behind smaller closed airways. In any event, the first few days of life, especially in the premature infant, are marked by disturbances in efficient gas exchange requiring simultaneous and nearly equal ventilation and perfusion. These disturbances can be ameliorated by stabilization of the chest wall.[83] Indeed, the prone position appears most conducive to efficient gas exchange—there is decreased resistance with increased compliance,[84] tidal volume,[85] and arterial oxygenation.[86] This apparently occurs because the prone position stabilizes the chest wall by coupling the rib cage to the abdomen so as to diminish the inefficient chest distortions of paradoxical respiration.[87]

TABLE 18–5
STATIC LUNG VOLUMES

	Infant (mL/kg)	Adult (mL/kg)
TLC	63	82
IC	33	52
TGV	30–36	30
FRC	30	30
VC	30–40	66
CC	35	23
VT	6	7
ERV	7	14
CV	12	7
RV	23	16
ERV/FRC	0.23	0.47
RV/TLC	0.37	0.20
FRC/TLC	0.48	0.37
VT/FRC	0.20	0.23

CC, closing capacity; CV, closing volume; ERV, expiratory reserve volume; FRC, functional residual capacity; IC, inspiratory capacity; RV, residual volume; TGV, thoracic gas volume; TLC, total lung capacity; VC, vital capacity; VT, tidal volume.
Data from references 148 and 166 through 173.

It has become apparent that the stability of the chest wall, as well as many other integrative functions involving the respiratory system, depends on the sleep state of the infant.[88–96] Active REM sleep is the dominant state in the newborn and is one of relative arousal, characterized by intense low-voltage and fast electrocortical and reticular activity. It is associated with sucking, swallowing, increased cerebral blood flow,[97] and esophageal peristalsis, as well as glottic closure.[98,99] Proprioceptive reflexes generally are depressed, with resultant loss of postural tone. The precise mode of this depression is incompletely understood, but appears, peripherally at least, to involve an inhibition of monosynaptic muscle spindle (*i.e.*, γ-loop) reflexes, which sense increased local muscular loads and, in response, increase α-motoneuron discharge.[88,89] Inhibition of the γ-loop reflex apparently results in loss of intercostal muscle tone during REM sleep, so that stiffness (*i.e.*, elastance) of the thoracic cage decreases and diaphragmatic contraction causes inward motion of the ribs during inspiration, producing paradoxical respiration (Fig. 18-17). This limits the effectiveness of the diaphragm as a generator of force.[100,101] Such deformation is capable of triggering the intercostal phrenic inhibitory reflex, resulting in the early termination of such an inspiration.[102–104] Thus, respiration in REM sleep is irregular and more rapid than in quiet sleep. Tidal volume is unchanged, but mean inspiratory air flow (*i.e.*, tidal volume divided by inspiratory duration) is increased, as is minute volume. This is, however, a fatiguing form of respiration,[105] the more so for the premature

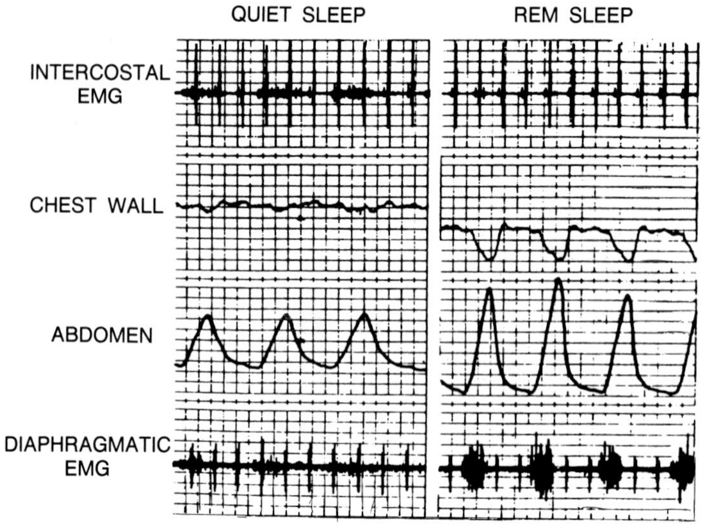

FIG. 18–17. Paradoxical respiration occurs in rapid-eye-movement (REM) sleep. As the abdomen expands (*i.e.*, upward deflection) and the diaphragm descends, the chest wall is drawn inward (*i.e.*, downward deflection). Large, brief electromyographic (EMG) spikes are an electrocardiographic artifact. Note the tonic discharge of the intercostal EMG throughout inspiration in quiet sleep, compared to brief, low-voltage, phasic intercostal EMG and intense phasic diaphragmatic EMG in REM sleep. (From Muller N, Gulston G, Cade D, et al. Diaphragmatic muscle fatigue in the newborn. J Appl Physiol, 1979;46:688.)

infant whose respiratory muscle fibers resist fatigue poorly.[106–108] He or she is especially ill-equipped, therefore, to compensate for extra respiratory loads during REM sleep.[109] The Hering–Breuer reflex, especially strong in the premature, fosters recruitment of intercostal neurones under respiratory loads, but this reflex is inhibited during REM sleep. The diminished lung volume and arterial oxygenation observed in REM sleep thus become more understandable.[110]

All these inefficiencies of chest wall performance render suspect the traditional assessment of pleural pressure by monitoring esophageal pressure, especially in the preterm infant.[111] Since nearly all the data in Table 18-6 were gained from studies of esophageal

TABLE 18–6
FORCES THAT OPPOSE BREATHING

	Infants		Adults	
Elastic Recoil (V_L/C_L)	1.5 cm H_2O		1.5 cm H_2O	
Volume (V_L)	0.1 L		2.1 L	
Compliance (C_L)—total	0.0026 L/cm H_2O	0.029 L/cm H_2O/L lung volume	0.100 L/cm H_2O	0.03 L/cm H_2O/L lung volume
Chest wall	0.0236 L/cm H_2O	0.262 L/cm H_2O/L lung volume	0.200 L/cm H_2O	0.06 L/cm H_2O/L lung volume
Lung tissue	0.0050 L/cm H_2O	0.055 L/cm H_2O/L lung volume	0.200 L/cm H_2O	0.06 L/cm H_2O/L lung volume
Flow Resistance (R × F)	0.4 mean/1.9 max cm H_2O		0.4 mean/1.9 max cm H_2O	
Mean (pulmonary) resistance	35 cm H_2O/L/sec			
Inspiratory (total) resistance	69 cm H_2O/L/sec	100% total resistance	5.5 cm H_2O/L/sec	100% total resistance
Chest wall		26% total resistance		16% total resistance
Pulmonary	25–50 cm H_2O/L/sec		4.5 cm H_2O/L/sec	
Nose	10 cm H_2O/L/sec	21% total resistance	2.8 cm H_2O/L/sec	54% total resistance
Mouth–airway	16 cm H_2O/L/sec	34% total resistance	1.6 cm H_2O/L/sec	29% total resistance
Lung tissue	9 cm H_2O/L/sec	19% total resistance	0.1 cm H_2O/L/sec	1% total resistance
Expiratory (*i.e.*, total) resistance	97 cm H_2O/L/sec			
Chest wall				
Pulmonary	35–70 cm H_2O/L/sec			
Gas Flow (Mean)	0.030–0.050 L/sec			
Inspiration	0.048 L/sec			
Expiration	0.037 L/sec			

Data from references 166, 168, 170, 172 and 174 through 177.

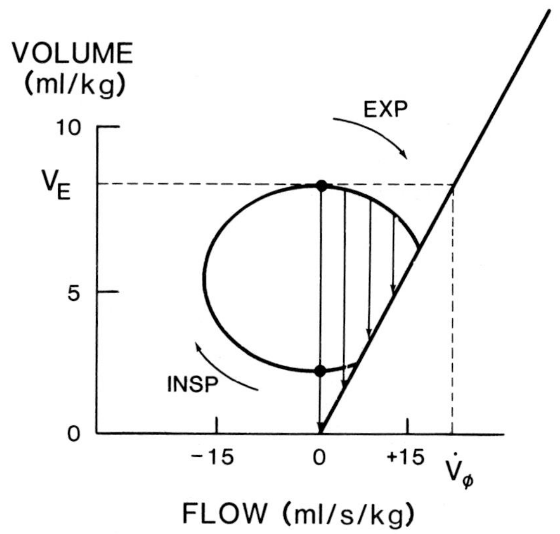

FIG. 18–18. In the flow–volume loop, the slope of the linear portion of passive expiration is the time constant (i.e., resistance × compliance) of the respiratory system. The vertical distance from any point on the loop to the linear passive phase represents inspiratory muscular activity. (VE, inspiratory volume; $\dot{V}_0$, peak expiratory flow.)

pressure, it is fortunate that an impeccable method (*i.e.*, passive expiratory flow–volume plot) is now available for remeasurement of passive respiratory mechanics (Fig. 18-18).[70,112,113]

During quiet breathing, the infant's ventilatory efforts are opposed by several forces: the resistance of the lung and chest wall to stretch (*i.e.*, elastic recoil), the resistance to movement (*i.e.*, flow resistance) of air and tissue, and the inertial resistance offered by air and tissue at rest to any large change in their state of motion. An equation of motion states the relations among these variables:

$$P = V/C + R \times F,$$

where P is the muscular force, measured as transpulmonary pressure, applied to the respiratory system; V is the volume of gas in the system; C is the distensibility or compliance of the system; V/C is the force of elastic recoil; R is the flow resistance; F is air flow; and R × F is the force required to overcome the resistance to flow. During quiet breathing the inertial resistance is negligible.

These forces are set out in Table 18-6, wherein it is apparent that the muscular force to be generated by both infant and adult in fact are quite comparable (*i.e.*, about 2 cm H_2O). Nonetheless, there are certain notable differences, including the lower proportional nasal resistance of the newborn. The much higher chest wall compliance of the newborn is, again, most striking.

The product of the total compliance and resistance of the system is its time constant: an expression of how rapidly the system, once perturbed by an active inspiration, will passively return to its rest position under the force of elastic recoil operating against flow resistance. This time constant is about 0.15 to 0.20 seconds in the infant and 0.55 seconds in the adult, so that the resting respiratory rate of the infant, which is 30 to 50 breaths per minute, is appropriately about twice that of the adult, which is 20 breaths per minute. Further, any entity that reduces the total compliance (*i.e.*, increases the stiffness) of the system (*e.g.*, fluid in the lung) must decrease the time constant and thus increase the resting respiratory rate.

PULMONARY VENTILATION

It is this higher ventilatory rate that is chiefly responsible for the higher minute ventilation, alveolar ventilation, wasted ventilation, and oxygen consumption (normalized for body weight) of the infant (Table 18-7). Yet, when compared on the basis of body surface area, which is generally held as a better basis for metabolic comparisons, the infant and adult are, again, strikingly similar.

TABLE 18–7
PULMONARY VENTILATION

	Infant	Adult	Units
Respiratory frequency (f)	34–35	13	bpm
Tidal volume (V_T)	6–8	7	mL/kg
Alveolar volume (V_A)	3.8–5.8	4.8	mL/kg
Dead space volume (V_D)	2.0–2.2	2.2	mL/kg
Minute ventilation ($\dot{V}_E$)	200–260	90	mL/kg/min
Alveolar ventilation ($\dot{V}_A$)	100–150	60	mL/kg/min
Wasted (*i.e.*, dead space) ventilation ($\dot{V}_D$)	77–99	30	mL/kg/min
Dead space/tidal volume (V_D/V_T)	0.27–0.37	0.3	
Oxygen consumption ($\dot{V}_{O_2}$)	6–8	3.2	mL/kg/min
Ventilation equivalent ($\dot{V}_A/\dot{V}_{O_2}$)	16–23	19–25	
Alveolar ventilation ($\dot{V}_A$)	2.3	2.4	$L/m^2/min$

bpm, breaths per minute.
Data from references 166, 168, 170, 176 and 178.

The chemical and neuronal drivers of neonatal respiration are becoming better defined, but a number of mysteries remain. It is now clear that the respiratory centers of the newborn respond normally to CO_2 and that their response becomes more powerful with increasing postconceptional age.[114,115] Conceivably, this increasing respiratory response may be, in the human, the result of a postnatal increase in excitatory respiratory neuronal synapses and consequent respiratory motor activity, as noted in other species.[116]

Responses to O_2 are more complex, probably because they involve suprapontine centers in the brain, as well as the peripheral chemoreceptors. Short-term (*i.e.*, less than 90 seconds) responses are like those in the adult, with hyperoxia producing immediate hypoventilation,[117,118] whereas hypoxia produces immediate hyperventilation,[119,120] thus demonstrating the presence of functional peripheral chemoreceptors.[121]

Prolonged (*i.e.*, 2 to 3 minutes) hypoxia or hyperoxia, however, soon leads to reversal of both these responses (Fig. 18-19). Postulated but unproved explanations for the biphasic hyperoxic response include cerebral vasospasm and CO_2 carriage impaired by O_2-saturated hemoglobin, leading to local accumulation of carbonic acid and consequent direct stimulation of the respiratory centers.[122] It also seems possible that the biphasic hypoxic response represents impaired facilitation by higher centers of possibly inadequate synaptic contacts among the respiratory motor neurons (see Fig. 18-4). It may even prove to be that such a hypoxic lack of neuronal facilitation of quantitatively marginal respiratory synapses is responsible for fetal respiratory quiescence apart from the fetal "respiration" seen to accompany the intense reticular activity of REM sleep. The interactional effects of CO_2 and O_2 breathing are, again, similar to the adult's (*i.e.*, hypoxic enhancement of CO_2 responses, presumably caused by peripheral chemoreceptor discharge), provided the experiments are short-term.[119]

It is the tidal volume that is unsustained during hypoxia,[123] despite the normal increase in brain blood flow also seen in adults,[124–126] possibly because of diaphragmatic fatigue. In any case, however denied the ability to maintain ventilation during hypoxia, the newborn acclimatizes by decreasing his or her oxygen consumption, just as do hibernating species and those at high altitudes.[127–129] If the hypoxia is chronic, the newborn acclimatizes by stimulated growth of the respiratory system.[130]

The association of chemical drives to ventilation,[131] and neuromuscular modulation of ventilation have come to be analyzed in the following equation[132]:

$$\dot{V}_E = V_T/T_I \times T_I/T_{TOT},$$

where $\dot{V}_E$ is total instantaneous ventilation and V_T is the tidal volume of each breath. T_I is the duration of a given inspiration, and T_{TOT} is the duration of the complete breath (*i.e.*, inspiration + expiration). V_T/T_I is the mean inspiratory gas flow per breath and a representative sum of chemical stimulation (*i.e.*, principally CO_2 and H^+) and neuronal modulation (*i.e.*, peripheral chemoreceptor signals, rapidly adapting vagal fiber signals from irritant receptors in the tracheobronchial epithelium, facilitative and inhibiting influences from suprapontine centers) of the inherent rhythmicity of respiratory neuronal discharge (see Fig. 18-4),[133] as well as its neuromuscular expression

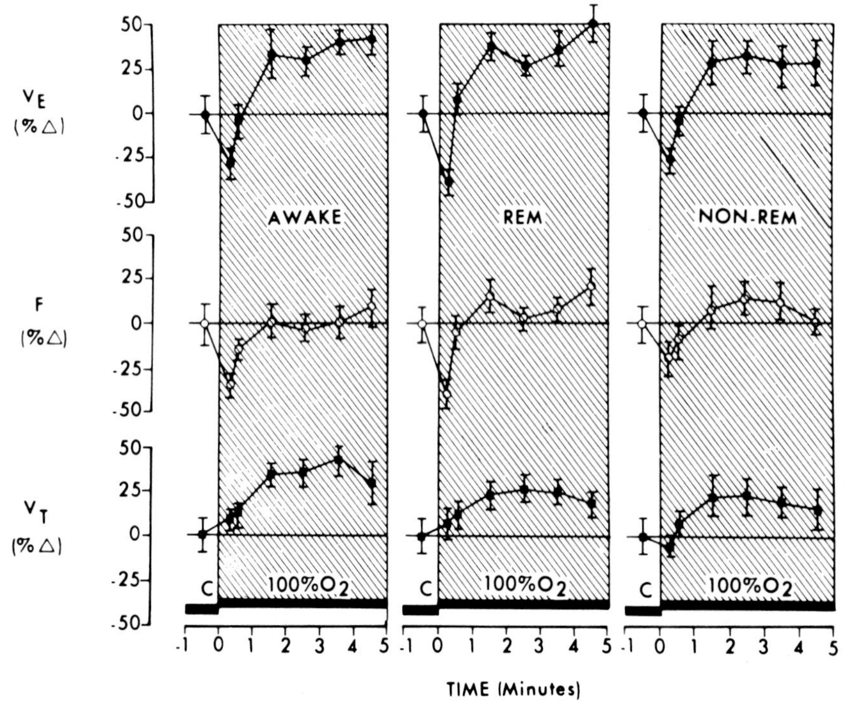

FIG. 18–19. Biphasic ventilatory responses to hyperoxia in the human newborn. The immediate ventilatory decrease in hyperoxic environments (*i.e.*, normal adult peripheral chemoreceptor response) is not sustained. (From Rigatto H, Kalapesi Z, Leahy FN, et al. Ventilatory response to 100% and 15% O_2 during wakefulness and sleep in preterm infants. Early Human Dev 1982; 7:1.)

in gas flow. The firing of these neurons requires a critical spatial and temporal summation of input impulses such that their resting potential may be raised above the firing threshold. T_I/T_{TOT} represents the duty cycle, which determines the duration of firing of inspiratory neurons (*i.e.*, T_I) or of expiratory neurons (*i.e.*, $T_E = T_{TOT} - T_I$). These controls of frequency largely rest in the pulmonary submucosal stretch receptors (*i.e.*, slow-adapting vagal fibers).[134]

All these relations have come under intense scrutiny in the newborn through detailed and critical analysis of the Hering–Breuer reflexes.[132,134–138] These are very well developed in the premature in quiet sleep and allow him or her to recruit intercostal neurons when presented with a respiratory load (*e.g.*, airway obstruction).[139] They are not, however, active during REM sleep. With maturation, the strengths of these reflexes clearly decrease.[135,137,138] It seems possible, therefore, that maturational increases in respiratory neuronal synapses (*i.e.*, dendritic arborization) may render the respiratory centers less susceptible to the influences of vagal stretch and irritant receptors. As higher volitional centers develop to modulate an increasingly robust group of respiratory neurons, it appears that more primeval modulation through the vagus becomes less necessary to maintain constancy of ventilation under varying respiratory loads (*e.g.*, speech, posture).

Although none of this increasing attention to the role of such factors as the central nervous system or sleep state has produced a definitive explanation of the periodic respiration and apnea characteristic of the immature infant, it may at least have increased the quality of the speculations. Although earlier studies were conducted without knowledge of sleep state, there is strong evidence that hypoxia inhibits respiration in the newborn infant and that hyperoxia decreases the frequency of periodic respiration in the premature infant, despite its other dangers.[140,141] In animals subjected to preterminal asphyxia, the evidence suggests that suprapontine centers become hypoxically depressed, allowing activity of the respiratory neurons to be unmodulated from above, and therefore responsive only to negative feedback from the peripheral chemoreceptors and vagal stretch receptors.[142,143] In such situations, any defect in the feedback loop can lead to oscillatory behavior.[133,144,145] In REM sleep, there are many such opportunities for disruption of feedback loops because of erratic respiratory timing. Premature infants, in addition, have in-phase oscillations of tidal volume and respiratory frequency during periodic breathing, suggesting an unstable total ventilation whereby CO_2 is either overblown or excessively retained.[144] Thus, the ancient observations that periodic respiration of the premature is relieved by O_2 breathing, which restores suprapontine facilitative neural influences, or CO_2 breathing, which increases pontine respiratory activity, become more understandable. Drugs such as caffeine and theophylline appear to facilitate respiration by increasing reticular activity, similar to that in REM sleep.

VENTILATION–PERFUSION IMBALANCE

Exchange of respiratory gases between the tissues and the environment is, of course, the basic purpose of respiration, both cellular and pulmonary. Thus, it is obvious that adequate pulmonary respiration will be to no avail if the intervening circulation cannot carry and release oxygen to the tissues. Just as this principle applies to adequate distribution of arterialized blood to tissues, so also must the distribution of venous blood flow be well matched to gaseous flow throughout the alveoli. Any inhomogeneity of the flow of gas and blood through the lungs must serve to reduce the efficiency of gas exchange. Such inhomogeneities are expressed most frequently as the ratio of ventilation to perfusion (V/Q) within given groups of alveoli. Whereas the overall V/Q of the normal lung is nearly 1, there is a vast range of possible ratios from 0, indicating a shunt, to infinity, indicating a dead space. Available estimates for V/Q ratios in the term newborn human at about 24 hours of age are shown in Table 18-8. It would appear from this that most ventilated areas are reasonably well perfused (*i.e.*, little dead space or wasted ventilation), whereas significant perfusion is directed to atelectatic alveoli or is totally shunted around the lung. Probably little of this shunt flow passes through the foramen ovale, and rather more passes right-to-left across the ductus arteriosus, even after reversal of dominant flow during the transitional phase of circulatory conversion. This occurs because of phasic pressure differences across the ductus during the cardiac cycle, with the mean pressures on the pulmonary and systemic sides being essentially balanced for the first several hours (see Fig. 18-10). An undocumentable amount of desaturated blood also may be shunted across the lung to the left atrium by way of bronchopulmonary anastomoses.

ALVEOLAR–ARTERIAL PRESSURE GRADIENTS

Such gas–blood flow variations essentially are responsible for the gas pressure differences established in the lung (Table 18-9), and the approximate relative contributions of the several components to the total alveolar–arterial oxygen differences ($AaDO_2$) can be estimated by measuring CO_2 and N_2 differences (Table 18-10). Thus, the portion of the $AaDO_2$ attributable to high V/Q areas (*i.e.*, dead space component) is reflected in the arterial–alveolar carbon dioxide difference ($aADCO_2$), whereas that which is attributable to low V/Q areas (*i.e.*, distribution component) is reflected in the arterial–alveolar nitrogen difference ($aADN_2$). The summed effects of direct venoarterial

Text continued on page 242

TABLE 18–8
DISTRIBUTION OF PULMONARY VENTILATION AND PERFUSION IN THE INFANT

Type of Alveolus	Percent Total Ventilation		Percent Total Perfusion		$V_A/\dot{Q}_C$
Anatomically shunted	20		10		0
Atelectatic, perfused	0		15		0
Trapped gas, perfused	0		10		0
Silent (*i.e,* atelectatic, nonperfused)	0		0		0
Low $V_A/\dot{Q}_C$ areas	2		5		0.4
Normal $V_A/\dot{Q}_C$ areas	68	75	58	65	1.2
High $V_A/\dot{Q}_C$ areas	5		2		2.5
Dead space (*i.e.,* ventilated, nonperfused)	5		0		∞
Diffusion block	<1		<1		

$\dot{Q}_C$, perfusion; V_A, pulmonary ventilation.
Data from references 168, 170, 179 through 181.

TABLE 18–9
RESPIRATORY GAS EXCHANGE AND PRESSURES OF ADULTS AND INFANTS

	Adult	Infant
Flows		
Alveolar ventilation (V_A)	60 mL/kg/min	120 mL/kg/min
Pulmonary capillary flow ($\dot{Q}_C$)	75 mL/kg/min	200 mL/kg/min
Ventilation/perfusion ratio ($V_A/\dot{Q}_C$)	0.8	0.6
Venous Admixture		
Low $V_A/\dot{Q}_C$ flow/total flow ($\dot{Q}_0/\dot{Q}_T$)	0.02	0.10–0.20
Shunt flow/total flow ($\dot{Q}_s/\dot{Q}_T$)	0.05	0.05–0.15
Alveolar Gases		
Oxygen (PAO_2)	105 torr	105 torr
Carbon dioxide ($PACO_2$)	40 torr	35 torr
Nitrogen (PAN_2)	568 torr	573 torr
Arterial Gases		
Oxygen (PaO_2)	95 torr	80 torr
Carbon dioxide ($PaCO_2$)	41 torr	36 torr
Nitrogen (PaN_2)	575 torr	583 torr
Gas Differences		
Oxygen ($AaDO_2$)	10 torr	24 torr
Carbon dioxide ($aADCO_2$)	1 torr	1 torr
Nitrogen ($aADN_2$)	7 torr	10 torr

Data from references 168, 170, 179, 180, and 182.

TABLE 18–10
RESPIRATORY GAS DIFFERENCES OF ADULTS AND INFANTS

	Total Difference ($AaDO_2$)	=	Diffusion Component ($AcDO_2$)	+	Dead Space Component ($aADCO_2$)	+	Distribution Component ($aADN_2$)	+	Shunt Component ($caDO_2$)
Adult	10 torr	=	<I	+	1	+	7	+	2
Infant	25 torr	=	<I	+	1	+	10	+	14

$aADN_2$, arterial–alveolar N_2 difference; $aADCO_2$, arterial–alveolar CO_2 difference; $AaDO_2$, alveolar–arterial O_2 difference; $AcDO_2$, alveolar–capillary O_2 difference; $caDO_2$, capillary–arterial O_2 difference.
Data from references 168, 179 through 181, and 183.

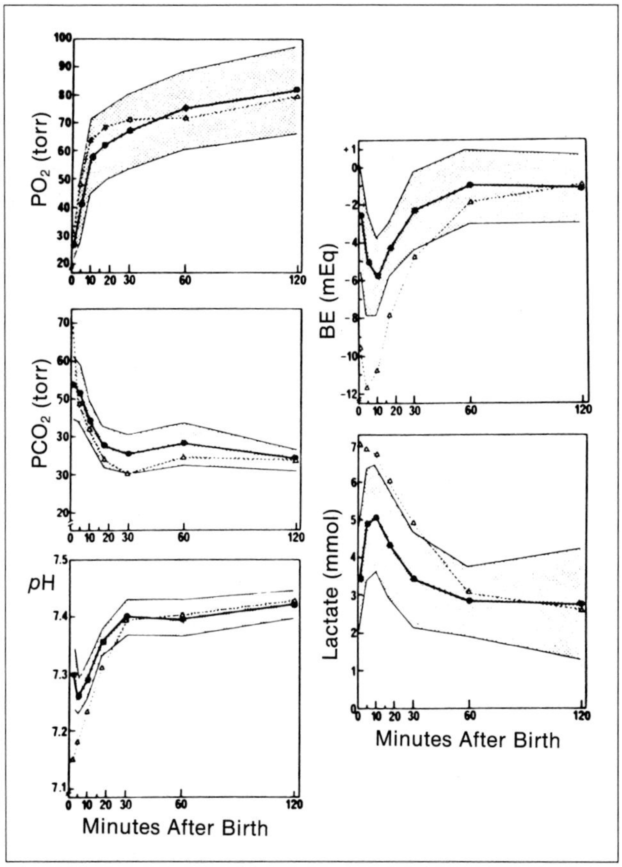

FIG. 18–20. Arterial blood gas changes in the first hours of life. (●, mean values for normal full-term infants; △, means for infants with fetal distress; *shaded zones*, ± 1 standard deviation; from Tunell R, Gopher D, Persson B, et al., The pulmonary gas exchange and blood gas changes in connection with birth. In: Stetson JB, Surger PR, eds. Neonatal intensive care. St Louis: Warren H. Green, 1976.)

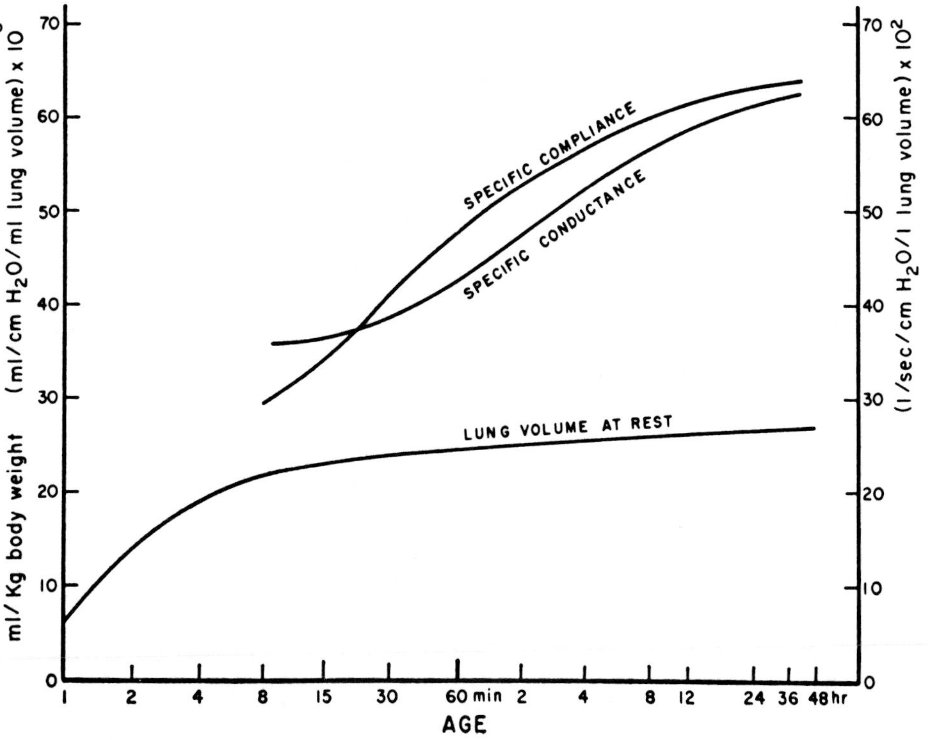

FIG. 18–21. Postnatal changes in pulmonary mechanics. (From Nelson NM. Neonatal pulmonary function. Pediatr Clin North Am 1966;13:769.)

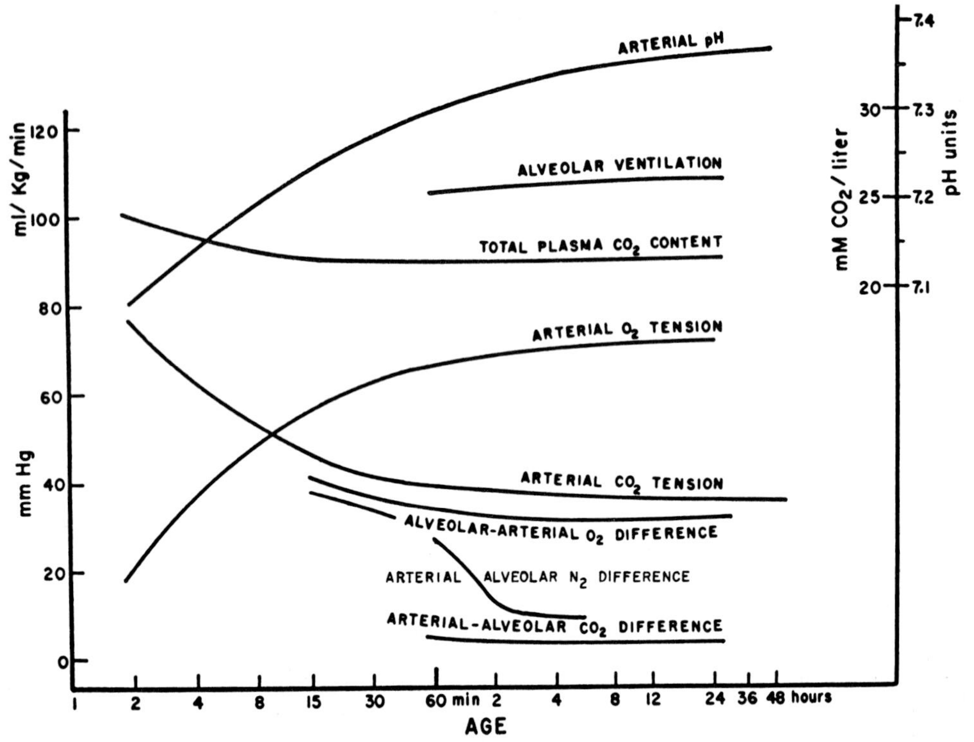

FIG. 18–22. Postnatal changes in blood gases. (From Nelson NM. Neonatal pulmonary function. Pediatr Clin North Am 1966;13:769.)

shunting and perfusion of atelectatic lung can be estimated separately in this manner. There are certain differences between the full-term and premature infant, with the premature tending to have a higher degree of venous admixture, owing to increases in both true anatomic shunts and virtual shunts (*i.e.*, low V/Q areas).[146–148] This possibly is related to alveolar instability, because the magnified blood gas differences of premature infants diminish if the chest is stabilized at higher lung volume,[83] and they also diminish during the first 2 weeks of life.

INTEGRATION AT BIRTH

Figure 18-20 allows an appreciation of just how rapidly the full-term newborn establishes respiration and recovers from the asphyxiating influence that is normal vaginal birth.

Finer indications of the components of this achievement are shown in Figure 18-21. The normal lung volume at rest (*i.e.*, functional residual capacity) essentially is established by 8 to 10 minutes, albeit some of the dependent airways may be in intermittent collapse, as previously seen. The specific compliance (*i.e.*, compliance normalized to lung volume) takes rather longer to achieve maximum. This most likely represents the rather slow clearance of fetal lung liquid from the parenchyma by way of the lymphatics. The airway conductance, which is the reciprocal of resistance, increases somewhat slowly, and may also represent the clearance of fluid and mucus from airways and alveoli. If so, it should be possible to document a decrease in specific compliance and conductance in those infants believed to have transient tachypnea of the newborn.[47]

Figure 18-22 traces the development of respiratory gas pressure differences at the onset of respiration and indicates that, even as early as at 60 minutes of age, there is insignificant wasted ventilation (*i.e.*, minimal $aADCO_2$). The large (*i.e.*, 35 torr) $AaDO_2$ in the first 2 hours, however, appears to be attributable mainly to perfusion of poorly ventilated areas of the lung (*i.e.*, higher $aADN_2$).[149] Subsequently, as lung volume becomes firmly established[150] and compliance improves as fluid clears around 2 to 4 hours of age, low V/Q areas evidently become better ventilated as the $aADN_2$ decreases. The high $AaDO_2$ remaining thus appears to be attributable exclusively to direct venoarterial shunting or to the perfusion of persistently atelectatic areas of the lung.

REFERENCES

1. Higuchi M, Murata Y, Miyake Y, et al. Effects of norepinephrine on lung fluid flow rate in the chronically catheterized fetal lamb. Am J Obstet Gynecol 1987;157:986.
2. Walker AM, Ritchie BC, Adamson TM, et al. Effect of changing lung liquid volume on the pulmonary circulation of fetal lambs. J Appl Physiol 1988;64:61.

3. Stenmark KR, James SL, Voelkel NF, et al. Leukotriene C4 and D4 in neonates with hypoxemia and pulmonary hypertension. N Engl J Med 1983;309:77.
4. Cassin S, Stenmark KR, Gause G, et al. Leukotrienes and prostaglandins in fetal lung liquid. J Appl Physiol 1990;68: 2214.
5. Pearce WJ, Longo LD. Developmental aspects of endothelial function. Semin Perinatol 1991;15:40.
6. Fineman JR, Soifer SJ, Heymann MA. The role of pulmonary vascular endothelium in perinatal pulmonary circulatory regulation. Semin Perinatol 1991;15:58.
7. Haworth SG, Hall SM, Chew M, et al. Thinning of fetal pulmonary arterial wall and postnatal remodelling: ultrastructural studies on the respiratory unit arteries of the pig. Virchows Arch [A] 1987;411:161.
8. Spitzer AR, Davis J, Clarke WT, et al. Pulmonary hypertension and persistent fetal circulation in the newborn. Clin Perinatol 1988;15:389.
9. Patrick J, Natale R, Richardson B. Patterns of human fetal breathing activity at 34 to 35 weeks' gestational age. Am J Obstet Gynecol 1978;132:507.
10. Boddy K, Mantell CD. Observations of fetal breathing movements transmitted through maternal abdominal wall. Lancet 1972;2:1219.
11. Merlet C, Hoerter J, Devilleneuve C, et al. Mise en evidence des mouvements respiratoires chez le foetus d'agneau in utero au cours du dernier mois de la gestation. C R Acad Sci [D] 1970;270:2462.
12. Dawes GS, Fox HE, Laduc BM, et al. Respiratory movements and rapid-eye-movement sleep in the foetal lamb. J Physiol 1972;220:119.
13. Duenhoelter JH, Pritchard JA. Fetal respiration: quantitative measurements of amniotic fluid inspired near term by human and rhesus fetuses. Am J Obstet Gynecol 1976;125:306.
14. Wolfson VP, Laitman JT. Ultrasound investigation of fetal human upper respiratory anatomy. Anat Rec 1990;227:363.
15. van Eyck J, van der Moooren K, Wladimiroff JW. Ductus arteriosus flow velocity modulation by fetal breathing movements as a measure of fetal lung development. Am J Obstet Gynecol 1990;163:558.
16. Saunders RA, Milner AD. Pulmonary pressure/volume relationships during the last phase of delivery and the first postnatal breaths in human subjects. J Pediatr 1978;93:667.
17. Mortola JP, Fisher JT, Smith JB, et al. Onset of respiration in infants delivered by cesarean section. J Appl Physiol 1982;52: 716.
18. Notter RH, Shapiro DL. Lung surfactants for replacement therapy: biochemical, biophysical, and clinical aspects. Clin Perinatol 1987;14:433.
19. Haagsman HP, van Golde LMG. Synthesis and assembly of lung surfactant. Annu Rev Physiol 1991;53:441.
20. Cochrane CG, Revak SD. Pulmonary surfactant protein B (SP-B): structure-function relationships. Science 1991;254: 566.
21. Kobayashi T, Shido A, Nitta K, et al. The critical concentration of surfactant in fetal lung liquid at birth. Respir Physiol 1990;80:181.
22. Hawgood S, Shiffer K. Structures and properties of the surfactant-associated proteins. Annu Rev Physiol 1991;53:375.
23. Faridy EE. Air opening pressure in fetal lungs. Respir Physiol 1987;68:293.
24. Purves MJ, Biscoe TJ. Development of chemoreceptor activity. Br Med Bull 1966;22:56.
25. Hodson WA, Fenner A, Brumley G, et al. Cerebrospinal fluid and blood acid-base relationships in fetal and neonatal lambs and pregnant ewes. Respir Physiol 1968;4:322.
26. Rigatto H. Control of ventilation in the newborn. Annu Rev Physiol 1984;46:661.
27. Bystrzycka E, Nail BS, Purves MJ. Central and peripheral neural respiratory activity in the mature sheep foetus and newborn lamb. Respir Physiol 1975;25:199.
28. Purves MJ. Onset of respiration at birth. Arch Dis Child 1974; 49:333.
29. Lee JC, Stoll BJ, Downing SE. Properties of the laryngeal chemoreflex in neonatal piglets. Am J Physiol 1977;233:R30.
30. Harned HS, Myracle J, Ferreiro J. Respiratory suppression and swallowing from introduction of fluids into the laryngeal region of the lamb. Pediatr Res 1978;12:1003.
31. Chernick V. Fetal breathing movements and the onset of breathing at birth. Clin Perinatol 1978;5:257.
32. Permutt S, Riley KL. Hemodynamics of collapsible vessels with tone: the vascular waterfall. J Appl Physiol 1963;18:924.
33. Raj JU, Hazinski TA, Bland RD. Effect of hypoxia on lung lymph flow in newborn lambs with left atrial hypertension. Am J Physiol 1988;254:H487.
34. Bland RD. Dynamics of pulmonary water before and after birth. Acta Paediatr Scand Suppl 1983;305:12.
35. Egan EA, Olver RE, Strang LB. Changes in non-electrolyte permeability of alveoli and the absorption of lung liquid at the start of breathing in the lamb. J Physiol 1975;244:161.
36. Aherne W, Dawkins MJR. The removal of fluid from the pulmonary airways after birth in the rabbit, and the effect on this of prematurity and prenatal hypoxia. Biol Neonate 1964;7: 214.
37. Fletcher BD, Sachs BE, Kotas RV. Radiologic demonstration of postnatal liquid in the lungs of newborn lambs. Pediatrics 1970;46:252.
38. Castro R, Ervin MG, Ross MG, et al. Ovine fetal lung fluid response to atrial natriuretic factor. Am J Obstet Gynecol 1989;161:1337.
39. Bland RD, Carlton DP, Scheerer RG, et al. Lung fluid balance in lambs before and after premature birth. J Clin Invest 1989;84:568.
40. Lagercrantz H, Marcus C. Sympathoadrenal mechanisms during development. In: Polin RA, Fox WW, eds. Fetal and neonatal physiology. Philadelphia: WB Saunders, 1992:160.
41. Kaneoka T, Ozono H, Goto U, et al. Plasma noradrenalin and adrenalin concentration in feto-maternal blood: their relation to feto-maternal endocrine levels, cardiotocographic and mechanoradiographic values, and umbilical arterial blood biochemical profiling. J Perinat Med 1979;7:302.
42. Grawjer LA, Sperling MA, Sack J, et al. Possible mechanisms and significance of the neonatal surge in glucagon secretion: studies in newborn lambs. Pediatr Res 1977;11:833.
43. Milner AD, Saunders RA, Hopkin IE. Effects of delivery by caesarean section on lung mechanics and lung volume in the human neonate. Arch Dis Child 1978;53:545.
44. Milner AD, Vyas H. Lung expansion at birth. J Pediatr 1982; 101:879.
45. Boon AW, Milner AD, Hopkin IE. Lung volumes and lung mechanics in babies born vaginally and by elective and emergency lower segmental cesarean section. J Pediatr 1981;98: 812.
46. Cassady G. Effect of cesarean section on neonatal body water spaces. N Engl J Med 1971;285:887.
47. Avery ME, Gatewood OB, Brumley G. Transient tachypnea of newborn. Am J Dis Child 1966;111:380.
48. Skinner JR, Boys RJ, Hunter S, et al. Non-invasive assessment of pulmonary arterial pressure in healthy neonates. Arch Dis Child 1991;66:386.
49. Musewe NN, Poppe D, Smallhorn JF, et al. Doppler echocardiographic measurement of pulmonary artery pressure from

ductal Doppler velocities in the newborn. J Am Coll Cardiol 1990;15:446.
50. Stopfkuchen H. Changes of the cardiovascular system during the perinatal period. Eur J Pediatr 1987;146:545.
51. Starling MD, Elliot RB. The effects of prostaglandins, prostaglandin inhibitors and oxygen on the closure of the ductus arteriosus, pulmonary arteries and umbilical vessels in vitro. Prostaglandins 1974;8:187.
52. Sharpe GI, Larsson KS. Studies on closure of the ductus arteriosus: X. In vitro effects of prostaglandins. Prostaglandins 1975;9:703.
53. Milne MJ, Sung RYT, Fok TF, et al. Doppler echocardiographic assessment of shunting via the ductus arteriosus in newborn infants. Am J Cardiol 1989;64:102.
54. Creasy RK, Drost M, Green MV, et al. Effect of ventilation on transfer of blood from placenta to neonate. Am J Physiol 1972;222:186.
55. Marquis L, Ackerman BD. Placental respiration in the immediate neonatal period. Am J Obstet Gynecol 1973;117:358.
56. Phillip AGS, Teng SS. Role of respiration in effecting placental transfusion at cesarean section. Biol Neonate 1977;31:219.
57. Rein AJJT, Sanders SP, Colan SD, et al. Left ventricular mechanics in the normal newborn. Circulation 1987;76:1029.
58. Baylen BG, Agata Y, Padbury JF, et al. Hemodynamic and neuroendocrine adaptations of the preterm lamb left ventricle to acutely increased afterload. Pediatr Res 1989;26:336.
59. Ogata ES. Carbohydrate metabolism in the fetus and neonate and altered neonatal glucoregulation. Pediatr Clin North Am 1986;33:25.
60. Lagercrantz H, Slotkin TA. The "stress" of being born. Sci Am 1986;254:100.
61. Fisher DA, Polk DH. Fetal and neonatal thyroid physiology. In: Polin RA, Fox WW, eds. Fetal and neonatal physiology. Philadelphia: WB Saunders, 1992:1842.
62. Nedergaard J, Cannon B. Brown adipose tissue: development and function. In: Polin RA, Fox WW, eds. Fetal and neonatal physiology. Philadelphia: WB Saunders, 1992:314.
63. Power GG. Fetal thermoregulation: animal and human. In: Polin RA, Fox WW, eds. Fetal and neonatal physiology. Philadelphia: WB Saunders, 1992:477.
64. Milner AD, Saunders RA. Pressure and volume changes during the first breath of human neonates. Arch Dis Child 1977;52:918.
65. Davis GM, Coates AL, Papageorgiou A, et al. Direct measurement of static chest wall compliance in animal and human neonates. J Appl Physiol 1988;65:1093.
66. Ratjen F, Zinman R, Stark AR, et al. Effect of changes in lung volume on respiratory system compliance in newborn infants. J Appl Physiol 1989;67:1192.
67. Geubelle F, Francotte M, Beyer M, et al. Functional residual capacity and thoracic gas volume in normoxic and hyperoxic newborn infants. Acta Paediatr Belg 1977;30:221.
68. Krauss AN, Auld PAM. Pulmonary gas trapping in premature infants. Pediatr Res 1971;5:10.
69. Agostoni E, Mead J. Statics of the respiratory system. In: Fenn WO, Rahn H, eds. Handbook of physiology. vol. 1. Washington, DC: American Physiological Society, 1964:387.
70. Mortola JP, Milic-Emili J, Noworaj A, et al. Muscle pressure and flow during expiration in infants. Am Rev Respir Dis 1984;129:49.
71. Stark AR, Cohlan BA, Waggener TB, et al. Regulation of end-expiratory lung volume during sleep in premature infants. J Appl Physiol 1987;62:1117.
72. Colin AA, Wohl MEB, Mead J, et al. Transition from dynamically maintained to relaxed end-expiratory volume in human infants. J Appl Physiol 1989;67:2107.
73. Kosch PC, Hutchison AA, Wozniak JA, et al. Posterior cricoarytenoid and diaphragm activities during tidal breathing in neonates. J Appl Physiol 1988;64:1968.
74. Harding R. Function of the larynx in the fetus or newborn. Ann Rev Physiol 1984;46:645.
75. Reed WR, Roberts JL, Thach BT. Factors influencing regional patency and configuration of the human infant upper airway. J Appl Physiol 1955;58:635.
76. Wise PH, Krauss AN, Waldman S, et al. Flow-volume loops in newborn infants. Crit Care Med 1980;8:61.
77. Kosch PC, Davenport PW, Wozniak JA, et al. Reflex control of expiratory duration in newborn infants. J Appl Physiol 1985;58:575.
78. Wilson SL, Thach BT, Brouillette RT, et al. Coordination of breathing and swallowing in human infants. J Appl Physiol 1981;50:851.
79. Abu-Osba YK, Brouillette RT, Wilson SL, et al. Breathing pattern and transcutaneous oxygen tension during motor activity in preterm infants. Am Rev Respir Dis 1982;125:382.
80. Wennergren G, Hertzberg T, Milerad J, et al. Hypoxia reinforces laryngeal reflex bradycardia in infants. Acta Paediatr Scand 1989;78:11.
81. Mortola JP, Rezzonico R. Ventilation in kittens with chronic section of the superior laryngeal nerves. Respir Physiol 1989;76:369.
82. Vyas H, Milner AD, Hopkin IE, et al. Role of labour in the establishment of functional residual capacity at birth. Arch Dis Child 1983;58:512.
83. Thibeault DW, Poblete E, Auld PAM. Alveolar-arterial O_2 and CO_2 differences and their relation to lung volume in the newborn. Pediatrics 1968;41:574.
84. Vanderghem A, Beardsmore C, Silverman M. Postural variations in pulmonary resistance, dynamic compliance, and esophageal pressure in neonates. Crit Care Med 1983;11:424.
85. Hutchinson AA, Ross KR, Russell G. The effect of posture on ventilation and lung mechanics in preterm and light-for-date infants. Pediatrics 1979;64:429.
86. Martin RJ, Herrell M, Rubin D, et al. Effect of supine and prone positions on arterial oxygen tension in the preterm infant. Pediatrics 1979;63:528.
87. Fleming PJ, Muller ML, Bryan MH, et al. The effects of abdominal loading on rib cage distortion in premature infants. Pediatrics 1979;64:425.
88. Bryan AC, Bryan MH. Control of respiration in the newborn. Clin Perinatol 1978;5:269.
89. Bryan MH, Knill RL, Bryan AC. Chest wall instability and its influence on respiration in the newborn infant. In: Stern L, Fries-Hansen B, Kildeberg P, eds. Intensive care in the newborn. New York: Masson, 1976.
90. Finer NN, Abroms IF, Taeusch HW. Ventilation and sleep states in newborn infants. J Pediatr 1976;89:100.
91. Harding R, Johnson P, McClelland ME, et al. Laryngeal function during breathing and swallowing in foetal and newborn lambs. J Physiol 1977;272:14PP.
92. Hathorn MKS. The rate and depth of breathing in new-born infants in different sleep states. J Physiol 1974;243:101.
93. Bolton DPG, Herman S. Ventilation and sleep state in the new-born. J Physiol 1974;240:67.
94. Frantz ID, Adler SM, Abroms IF, et al. Respiratory response to airway occlusion in infants: sleep state and maturation. J Appl Physiol 1976;41:634.
95. Haddad GG, Lai TL, Epstein MAF, et al. Breath-to-breath variations in rate and depth of ventilation in sleeping infants. Am J Physiol 1982;243:R164.
96. Knill R, Andrews W, Bryan AC, et al. Respiratory load compensation in infants. J Appl Physiol 1976;40:357.

97. van Eyck J, Wladimiroff JW, van den Wijngaard JAGW, et al. The blood flow velocity waveform in the fetal internal carotid and umbilical artery: its relation to fetal behavioural states in normal pregnancy at 37 weeks. Br J Obstet Gynaecol 1987;94: 736.
98. Durand M, Leahy FN, MacCallum M, et al. Effect of feeding on the chemical control of breathing in the newborn infant. Pediatr Res 1981;15:1509.
99. Read DJC, Henderson-Smart DJ. Regulation of breathing during different behavioral states. Annu Rev Physiol 1984;46:675.
100. Le Souef PN, Lopes JM, England SJ, et al. Effect of chest wall distortion on occlusion pressure and the preterm diaphragm. J Appl Physiol 1983;55:359.
101. Homma Y, Wilkes D, Bryan MH, et al. Rib cage and abdominal contributions to ventilatory response to CO_2 in infants. J Appl Physiol 1984;56:1211.
102. Knill R, Bryan AC. An intercostal-phrenic inhibitory reflex in human newborn infants. J Appl Physiol 1976;40:352.
103. Hagan R, Bryan AC, Bryan MH, et al. Neonatal chest wall afferents and regulation of respiration. J Appl Physiol 1977;42:362.
104. Tusiewicz K, Moldofsky H, Bryan AC, et al. Mechanics of the rib cage and diaphragm during sleep. J Appl Physiol 1977;43:600.
105. Lopes JM, Muller NL, Bryan MH, et al. Synergistic behavior of inspiratory muscles after diaphragmatic fatigue in the newborn. J Appl Physiol 1981;51:547.
106. Keens TG, Bryan AC, Levison H, et al. Developmental pattern of muscle fiber types in human ventilatory muscles. J Appl Physiol 1978;44:909.
107. Guslits BG, Gaston SE, Bryan MH, et al. Diaphragmatic work of breathing in premature human infants. J Appl Physiol 1987;62:1410.
108. Le Souef PN, England SJ, Stogryn HAF, et al. Comparison of diaphragmatic fatigue in newborn and older rabbits. J Appl Physiol 1988;65:1040.
109. Praud J, Egreteau L, Benlabed M, et al. Abdominal muscle activity during CO_2 rebreathing in sleeping neonates. J Appl Physiol 1991;70:1344.
110. Henderson-Smart DJ, Read DJC. Reduced lung volume during behavioral active sleep in the newborn. J Appl Physiol 1979;46:1081.
111. Le Souef PN, Lopes JM, England SJ, et al. Influence of chest wall distortion on esophageal pressure. J Appl Physiol 1983; 55:353.
112. Le Souef PN, England SJ, Bryan AC. Passive respiratory mechanics in newborn and children. Am Rev Respir Dis 1984; 129:552.
113. Gerhart T, Reifenberg L, Duara S, et al. Comparison of dynamic and static measurements of respiratory mechanics in infants. J Pediatr 1989;114:120.
114. Frantz ID, Adler SM, Thach BT, et al. Maturational effects on respiratory responses to carbon dioxide in premature infants. J Appl Physiol 1976;41:41.
115. Cosgrove JF, Neunburger N, Bryan MH, et al. A new method of evaluating the chemosensitivity of the respiratory center in children. Pediatrics 1975;56:972.
116. Suthers GK, Henderson-Smart DJ, Read DJC. Postnatal changes in the rate of high frequency bursts in inspiratory activity in cats and dogs. Brain Res 1977;132:537.
117. Reinstorff D, Fenner A. Ventilatory response to hyperoxia in premature and newborn infants during the first three days of life. Respir Physiol 1972;15:159.
118. Krauss AN, Tori CA, Brown J. Oxygen chemoreceptors in low birth weight infants. Pediatr Res 1973;7:569.
119. Albersheim S, Boychuk R, Seshia MMK. Effects of CO_2 on immediate ventilatory response to O_2 in preterm infants. J Appl Physiol 1976;41:609.
120. Rigatto H, Kalapesi Z, Leahy FN, et al. Ventilatory response to 100% and 15% O_2 during wakefulness and sleep in preterm infants. Early Hum Dev 1982;7:1.
121. Walker DW. Peripheral and central chemoreceptors in the fetus and newborn. Annu Rev Physiol 1984;46:687.
122. Haddad GG, Mellins RB. Hypoxia and respiratory control in early life. Annu Rev Physiol 1984;46:629.
123. Rigatto H, Wiebe C, Rigatto C, et al. Ventilatory response to hypoxia in unanesthetized newborn kittens. J Appl Physiol 1988;64:2544.
124. Longo LD, Pearce WJ. Fetal and newborn cerebral vascular responses and adaptations to hypoxia. Semin Perinatol 1991;15:49.
125. Darnall RA, Green G, Pinto L, et al. Effect of acute hypoxia on respiration and brain stem blood flow in the piglet. J Appl Physiol 1991;70:251.
126. Suguihara C, Bancalari E, Hehre D. Brain blood flow and ventilatory response to hypoxia in sedated newborn piglets. Pediatr Res 1990;27:327.
127. Duara S, Neto GS, Gerhardt T, et al. Metabolic and respiratory effects of flow-resistive loading in preterm infants. J Appl Physiol 1991;70:895.
128. Gleed RD, Mortola JP. Ventilation in newborn rats after gestation at simulated high altitude. J Appl Physiol 1991;70:1146.
129. Downing SE, Chen V. Myocardial hibernation in the ischemic neonatal heart. Circ Res 1990;66:763.
130. Okubo S, Mortola JP. Respiratory mechanics in adult rats hypoxic in the neonatal period. J Appl Physiol 1989;66:1772.
131. Moss IR, Inman JG. Neurochemicals and respiratory control during development. J Appl Physiol 1989;67:1.
132. Wyszogrodski I, Thach BT, Milic-Emili J. Maturation of respiratory control in unanesthetized newborn rabbits. J Appl Physiol 1978;44:304.
133. Haddad GG, Mellins RH. The role of airway receptors in the control of respiration in infants: a review. J Pediatr 1977;91: 281.
134. Olinsky A, Bryan MH, Bryan AC. Influence of lung inflation on respiratory control in neonates. J Appl Physiol 1974;36:426.
135. Olinsky A, Bryan MH, Bryan AC. Response of newborn infants to added respiratory loads. J Appl Physiol 1974;37:190.
136. Taeusch HW, Carson S, Frantz ID, et al. Respiratory regulation after elastic loading and CO_2 rebreathing in normal term infants. J Pediatr 1976;88:102.
137. Kirkpatrick SML, Olinsky A, Bryan MH, et al. Effect of premature delivery on the maturation of the Hering-Breuer inspiratory inhibitory reflex in human infants. J Pediatr 1976;88: 1010.
138. Adler SM, Thach ET, Frantz ID. Maturational changes of effective elastance in the first 10 days of life. J Appl Physiol 1976;40:539.
139. Moomjian AS, Schwartz JG, Wagaman MJ, et al. The effect of external expiratory resistance on lung volume and pulmonary function in the neonate. J Pediatr 1980;96:908.
140. Rigatto H, Brady JP. Periodic breathing and apnea in preterm infants: II. Hypoxia as a primary event. Pediatrics 1972;50:219.
141. Fenner A, Schalk U, Hoenicke H, et al. Periodic breathing in premature and neonatal babies: incidence, breathing pattern, respiratory gas tensions, response to changes in the composition of ambient air. Pediatr Res 1973;7:174.
142. Guntheroth WG, Kawabori I. Hypoxic apnea and gasping. J Clin Invest 1975;56:1371.
143. Lawson EE, Thach BT. Respiratory patterns during progressive asphyxia in newborn rabbits. J Appl Physiol 1977;43:468.
144. Waggener TB, Frantz ID, Stark AR, et al. Oscillatory breath-

ing patterns leading to apneic spells in infants. J Appl Physiol 1982;52:1288.
145. Fleming PJ, Goncalves AL, Levine MR, et al. The development of stability of respiration in human infants: changes in ventilatory responses to spontaneous sighs. J Physiol 1954; 347:1.
146. Parks CR, Woodrum DE, Alden ER, et al. Gas exchange in the immature lung: I. Anatomical shunt in the premature infant. J Appl Physiol 1974;36:103.
147. Koch G. Lung function and acid-base balance in the newborn infant. Acta Paediatr Scand Suppl 1968;181:5.
148. Dahms BB, Krauss AN, Auld PAM. Pulmonary function in dysmature infants. J Pediatr 1974;84:434.
149. Bolton DPG. Diffusional inhomogeneity: gas mixing efficiency in the newborn lung. J Physiol 1979;286:447.
150. Sandberg K, Sjoqvist BA, Hjalmarson O, et al. Analysis of alveolar ventilation in the newborn. Arch Dis Child 1984;59: 542.
151. Arcilla RA, Oh W, Wallgren G. Quantitative studies of the human neonatal circulation: II. Hemodynamic findings in early and late clamping of the umbilical cord. Acta Paediatr Scand 1967;179:25.
152. Assali NS. Some aspects of fetal life in utero and the changes at birth. Am J Obstet Gynecol 1967;97:324.
153. McMurphy DM, Heymann MA, Rudolph AM, et al. Developmental changes in constriction of the ductus arteriosus: responses to oxygen and vasoactive agents in the isolated ductus arteriosus of the fetal lamb. Pediatr Res 1972;6:231.
154. Wallgren G, Hanson JS, Lind J. Quantitative studies of the human neonatal circulation: III. Observations of the newborn infant's central circulatory responses to moderate hypovolemia. Acta Paediatr Scand Suppl 1967;179:45.
155. Wallgren G, Lind J. Quantitative studies of the human neonatal circulation: IV. Observations on the newborn infant's peripheral circulation and plasma expansion during moderate hypovolemia. Acta Paediatr Scand Suppl 1967;179:57.
156. Wallgren G, Hanson JS, Tabakin BS, et al. Quantitative studies of the human neonatal circulation: V. Hemodynamic findings in premature infants with and without respiratory distress. Acta Paediatr Scand Suppl 1967;179:71.
157. Drayton MR, Skidmore R. Ductus arteriosus blood flow during first 48 hours of life. Arch Dis Child 1987;62:1030.
158. Dawes GS. Fetal and neonatal physiology. Chicago: Year Book, 1968.
159. Folkow B, Neil E. Circulation. London: Oxford University Press, 1971.
160. Harned HS. Respiration and the respiratory system. In: Stave U, ed. Physiology of the perinatal period. New York: Appleton-Century-Crofts, 1970.
161. Rudolph AM, Heymann MA. The circulation of the fetus in utero: methods for studying distribution of blood flow, cardiac output and organ blood flow. Circ Res 1967;21:163.
162. Rudolph AM, Heymann MA. Circulatory changes during growth in the fetal lamb. Circ Res 1970;26:289.
163. Rudolph AM, Heymann MA, Teramo KAW, et al. Studies on the circulation of the previable human fetus. Pediatr Res 1971;5:452.
164. Reed KL, Anderson CF, Shenker L. Fetal pulmonary artery and aorta: two-dimensional Doppler echocardiography. Obstet Gynecol 1987;69:175.
165. Mendelson CR, Boggaram V. Hormonal control of the surfactant system in fetal lung. Annu Rev Physiol 1991;53:415.
166. Chu J, Clements JA, Cotton EK, et al. Neonatal pulmonary ischemia. Pediatrics 1967;40:709.
167. Mansell A, Bryan AC, Levison H. Airway closure in children. J Appl Physiol 1972;33:711.
168. Nelson NM. Neonatal pulmonary function. Pediatr Clin North Am 1966;13:769.
169. Phelan PD, Williams HE. Ventilatory studies in healthy infants. Pediatr Res 1969;3:425.
170. Polgar G, Promadhat V. Pulmonary function testing in children: techniques and standards. Philadelphia: WB Saunders, 1971.
171. Lacourt G, Polgar G. Development of pulmonary function in late gestation: the functional residual capacity of the lung in premature children. Acta Paediatr Scand 1974;63:81.
172. Milner AD, Saunders RA, Hopkin IE. Tidal pressure/volume and flow/volume respiratory loop patterns in human neonates. Clinical Science and Molecular Medicine 1978;54:257.
173. Tunell R, Gopher D, Persson B. The pulmonary gas exchange and blood gas changes in connection with birth. In: Stetson JB, Surger PR, eds. Neonatal intensive care. St. Louis: Warren H. Green, 1976:99.
174. Lacourt G, Polgar G. Interaction between nasal and pulmonary resistance in newborn infants. J Appl Physiol 1971;30: 870.
175. Sharp JT, Druz WS, Balagot RC, et al. Total respiratory compliance in infants and children. J Appl Physiol 1970;29:775.
176. Davis GM, Bureau MA. Pulmonary and chest wall mechanics in the control of respiration in the newborn. Clin Perinatol 1987;14:551.
177. Mortola JP. Dynamics of breathing in newborn mammals. Physiol Rev 1987;67:187.
178. Lees MH, Way RC, Ross BB. Ventilation and respiratory gas transfer of infants with increased pulmonary blood flow. Pediatrics 1967;40:259.
179. Corbet AJS, Ross JA, Beaudry PH, et al. Effect of positive-pressure breathing on $aADN_2$ in hyaline membrane disease. J Appl Physiol 1975;38:33.
180. Corbet AJS, Ross JA, Beaudry PH, et al. Assessment of ventilation-perfusion inequality by $aADN_2$ in newborn infants. Biol Neonate 1979;36:10.
181. Krauss AN, Klain DB, Auld PAM. Carbon monoxide diffusing capacity in newborn infants. Pediatr Res 1976;10:771.
182. Avery ME, Fletcher BD. The lung and its disorders in the newborn infant. 3rd ed. Philadelphia: WB Saunders, 1974.
183. Nourse CH, Nelson NM. Uniformity of ventilation in the newborn infant; direct assessment of the arterial-alveolar N_2 difference. Pediatrics 1969;43:226.
184. Smith CA, Nelson NM. Physiology of the newborn infant. 4th ed. Springfield, IL: Charles C. Thomas, 1976.
185. Radford EP. In: Remington JW, ed. Tissue elasticity. Washington, DC: American Physiological Society, 1957.
186. Burns BD. The central control of respiratory movements. Br Med Bull 1963;19:7.
187. Strang LB. The lungs at birth. Arch Dis Child 1965;40:575.
188. Rasmussen K. Quantitative blood flow in the fetal descending aorta and in the umbilical vein in normal pregnancies: longitudinal and cross-sectional studies. Scand J Clin Lab Invest 1987;47:319.
189. Mandelbaum VHA, Alverson DC, Kirchgessner A, et al. Postnatal changes in cardiac output and haemorrheology in normal neonates born at full term. Arch Dis Child 1991;66:391.
190. Winberg P, Jansson M, Marions I, et al. Left ventricular output during postnatal circulatory adaptation in healthy infants born at full term. Arch Dis Child 1989;64:1374.
191. Burnard ED, Granang A, Gray RE. Cardiac output in the newborn infant. Clin Sci 1966;31:121.
192. Padbury JF, Agata Y, Ludlow J, et al. Effect of fetal adrenalectomy on catecholamine release and physiologic adaptation at birth in sheep. J Clin Invest 1987;80:1096.
193. Padbury JF, Polk DH, Newnham JP, et al. Neonatal adapta-

tion: greater sympathoadrenal response in preterm than full-term fetal sheep at birth. Am J Physiol 1985;248:E443.
194. Broberger U, Hansson U, Lagercrantz H, et al. Sympatho-adrenal activity and metabolic adjustment during the first 12 hours after birth in infants of diabetic mothers. Acta Paediatr Scand 1984;73:620.
195. Faxelius G, Lagercrantz H, Yao A. Sympathoadrenal activity and peripheral blood flow after birth: comparison in infants delivered vaginally and by cesarean section. J Pediatr 1984; 105:144.
196. Hagnevik K, Faxelius G, Irestedt L, et al. Catecholamine surge and metabolic adaptation in the newborn after vaginal delivery and caesarean section. Acta Paediatr Scand 1984;73: 602.
197. Fisher DA, Klein AH. Thyroid development and disorders of the thyroid in the newborn. N Engl J Med 1981;304:702.
198. Cornblath M, Reisner SH. Blood glucose in the neonate and its clinical significance. N Engl J Med 1965;273:378.
199. Muller N, Gulston G, Cade D, et al. Diaphragmatic muscle fatigue in the newborn. J Appl Physiol 1979;46:688.

Neonatology: Pathophysiology and Management of the Newborn, Fourth Edition,
edited by Gordon B. Avery, Mary Ann Fletcher, and Mhairi G. MacDonald.
J.B. Lippincott Company, Philadelphia © 1994.

chapter 19

Delivery Room Management

RODERIC H. PHIBBS

Much of newborn intensive care is emergency medicine that requires rapid institution of appropriate diagnostic and therapeutic procedures. This is particularly true immediately after birth, when the newborn infant may have cardiac arrest and apnea. The procedures undertaken to restore life constitute resuscitation, from the Latin *resuscitate*, "to arouse again," and include those actions necessary to help an infant make the transition from dependent fetal life to independent neonatal life. Skillful resuscitation of the asphyxiated newborn infant can prevent brain damage and minimize subsequent neonatal disease. There is a high risk of asphyxia during labor, delivery, and the first minutes after birth. This is so because of the arrangement of the fetal circulatory pathways and because the newborn infant must successfully inflate his or her lungs and rearrange his or her circulation immediately after birth. Failure of either to occur leads to asphyxia. A rational approach to resuscitation must be based on the physiologic changes in the circulatory and respiratory systems that occur normally as the newborn infant adapts to extrauterine life. The physiology of transition, discussed in Chapter 18, should be understood before reading this chapter.

PATHOPHYSIOLOGY OF INTRAPARTUM ASPHYXIA AND RESUSCITATION

Asphyxia occurs when the organ of gas exchange fails. When this occurs, arterial carbon dioxide partial pressure ($PaCO_2$) rises; arterial oxygen partial pressure (PaO_2) and *p*H fall. Despite the low PaO_2, tissues continue to consume O_2. When the PaO_2 is very low, anaerobic metabolism occurs and large quantities of metabolic acids are produced. These are partly buffered by the bicarbonate in the blood.[1]

The human infant is particularly vulnerable to asphyxia in the perinatal period. During normal labor, transient hypoxemia occurs with uterine contractions, but the healthy fetus tolerates this well. There are five basic causes of asphyxia during labor and delivery:

1. Interruption of umbilical blood flow (*e.g.*, cord compression)
2. Failure of gas exchange across the placenta (*e.g.*, placental abruption)
3. Inadequate perfusion of the maternal side of the placenta (*e.g.*, severe maternal hypotension)
4. An otherwise compromised fetus who cannot further tolerate the transient, intermittent hypoxia of normal labor (*e.g.*, the anemic or growth-retarded fetus)
5. Failure to inflate the lungs and complete the change in ventilation and lung perfusion that must occur at birth.

The last cause may occur because of airway obstruction, excessive fluid in the lungs, or weak respiratory effort. Alternatively, it may occur as a result of fetal asphyxia from one of the first four causes, because fetal asphyxia often leads to an infant who is acidotic and apneic at birth.

The umbilical cord blood *p*H, partial pressure of oxygen (PO_2), partial pressure of carbon dioxide

(PCO_2), and the calculated base excess are standard measures of fetal asphyxia.[2,3] With fetal acidosis, the *p*H can vary over a wide range. Consequently, it is important to remember that *p*H is a logarithmic function of hydrogen ion concentration. A decrease of 0.3 *p*H units from 7.40 to 7.10 indicates only a 40 nmol/L increase in hydrogen ion (*i.e.*, from 40 to 80 nmol), whereas a 0.3 decrease from 7.10 to 6.80 indicates an increase of 80 nmol/L (*i.e.*, from 80 to 160 nmol). The gradient in blood gas tensions between umbilical artery and vein gives some indication of placental perfusion at the time of birth. The slower the flow of fetal blood through the placenta, the more complete the equilibration of gas tensions between fetal and maternal blood. For example, an arterial PO_2 of 25 torr with a venous PO_2 of 32 torr suggests good placental blood flow. An arterial PO_2 of 12 torr with a venous PO_2 of 45 torr suggests very slow flow. Metabolic acidosis suggests asphyxia, although some of the increased lactic acid in the blood may be due to reduced uptake of lactate by the asphyxiated liver rather than increased lactate production from anaerobic metabolism.[2,4] If asphyxia occurred just before birth, there may be lactic acid in the tissues that has not yet reached the central circulation. This will be detected only by blood gas measurements a few minutes after birth. If the fetus was asphyxiated an hour before delivery and recovered, that event will not be reflected in the umbilical cord blood gasses at birth. Other indicators of asphyxia include plasma hypoxanthine, which increases because of lack of aerobic metabolism, and plasma erythropoietin, which increases in response to fetal hypoxia.[5]

Asphyxia in the fetus or newborn infant is a progressive and reversible process. The speed and extent of progression are highly variable. Sudden, severe asphyxia can be lethal in less than 10 minutes. Mild asphyxia may progressively worsen over 30 minutes or more. Repeated episodes of brief, mild asphyxia may reverse spontaneously but produce a cumulative effect of progressive asphyxia. In the early stages, asphyxia usually reverses spontaneously if its cause is removed. Once asphyxia is severe, spontaneous reversal is unlikely because of the circulatory and neurologic changes that accompany it. Other sources provide a general review of these phenomena.[6]

Figure 19-1 schematically represents the sequence of pathophysiologic changes that accompany asphyxia. Although there are some quantitative differences between the changes that occur in the fetus and those in the newborn infant, the scheme generally applies to both. It is useful to consider the changes in both fetus and newborn infant together because many cases of neonatal asphyxia begin in the fetus and continue after birth. Cardiac output is maintained early in asphyxia, but its distribution changes radically. Selective regional vasoconstriction reduces blood flow to less vital organs and tissues such as gut, kidneys, muscle, and skin.[7] Blood flow to the brain and myocardium increases, thereby maintaining ade-

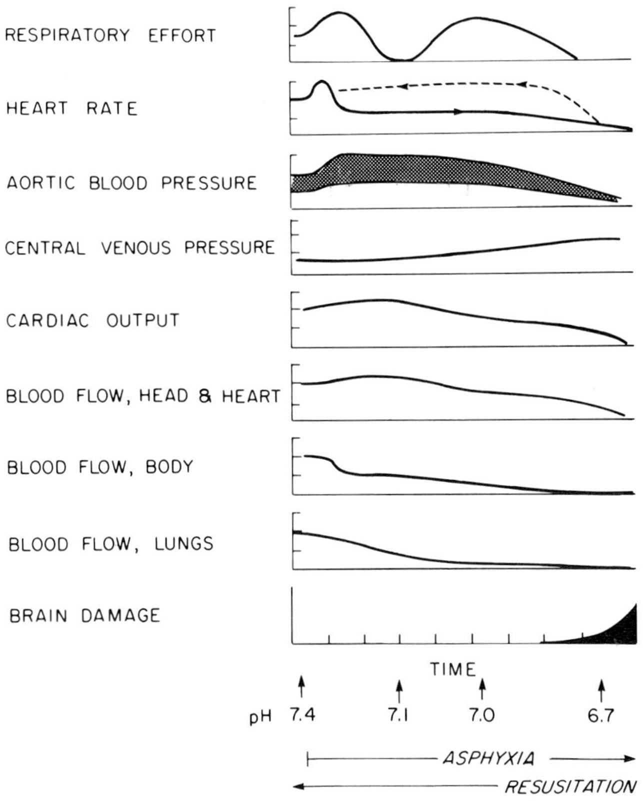

FIG. 19–1. The sequence of cardiopulmonary changes with asphyxia and resuscitation. If there is complete interruption of respiratory gas exchange, the entire process of asphyxia could occur in about 10 minutes. It could take much longer with an asphyxiating process that only partly interrupts gas exchange or one that does so completely but only for repeated brief periods. With resuscitation, the process reverses, beginning at the point to which the asphyxia has proceeded. (Adapted from Dawes G. Foetal and neonatal physiology. Chicago: Year Book, 1968:149.)

quate oxygen delivery despite reduced oxygen content of the arterial blood. Other organs and tissues must depend on increased oxygen extraction to maintain oxygen consumption.[8,9] Pulmonary blood flow is low in the fetus. It is decreased further by hypoxia and acidosis.[10] As a consequence of these adaptations, fetal oxygen consumption decreases.[11]

Early in asphyxia, newborns make vigorous attempts to inflate their lungs. If successful, the lungs become adequately ventilated and perfused, but the mere presence of gasping does not ensure that this will happen. As asphyxia becomes more severe, the respiratory center is depressed, and the chances of an infant's spontaneously establishing effective ventilation and pulmonary perfusion diminish.

If asphyxia progresses to the severe stage, oxygen delivery to the brain and heart decreases. The myocardium then uses its stored reserve of glycogen for energy. Eventually, the glycogen reserve is consumed and the myocardium is exposed simultaneously to progressively lower PO_2s and *p*Hs. The combined effects of hypoxia and acidosis lead to decreased myocardial function and decreased blood flow to the vital organs.[12,13] Brain injury begins late during this phase.[6]

This sequence of cardiovascular events is manifested by changes in heart rate and aortic and central venous pressures (see Fig. 19-1), all of which are measured easily in the newborn immediately after birth. The early bradycardia and hypertension are due to the reflexes that shunt blood away from nonvital organs. Early in asphyxia, central venous (*i.e.*, right atrial) pressure may rise slightly, owing to pulmonary hypertension and constriction of systemic capacitance vessels. When the myocardium finally fails, central venous pressure rises further, aortic pressure decreases, and heart rate is reduced further.

The initial adaptations of the systemic circulation to asphyxia are mediated by reflexes.[14] There also are major hormonal responses to asphyxia, including elevations in plasma corticotropin, glucocorticoids, catecholamines, arginine vasopressin, renin, and atrial natriuretic factor, and a decrease in insulin.[15,16] Some of these are important in maintaining the circulatory adaptations to asphyxia. Catecholamines, which come mainly from the adrenal medulla, maintain myocardial function in the presence of asphyxia, thereby increasing survival.[17,18] Arginine vasopressin helps maintain the hypertension, bradycardia, and redistribution of systemic flow.[19] Increased hepatic glycogenolysis helps maintain plasma glucose concentrations.[4]

The physiology of resuscitation is essentially a reversal of the pathophysiology of asphyxia. In Figure 19-1, which illustrates both processes, asphyxia proceeds from left to right, and resuscitation from right to left. It is crucial to determine where the infant is in this sequence of pathophysiologic events when resuscitation is started. If asphyxia has proceeded to myocardial failure, resuscitation must include restoration of cardiac output as well as establishment of effective ventilation and perfusion of the lungs. Generally, myocardial failure does not occur until both *p*H and PaO_2 are extremely low, approximately 6.9 and 20 torr, respectively. Cardiac output is reestablished through rapid correction of the severe hypoxia and acidosis. Until this is done, output must be maintained by cardiac massage. As soon as *p*H is raised to approximately 7.1 and PaO_2 to 50 torr, the myocardium responds rapidly, heart rate rises, aortic pressures rise, and pulse pressure widens, while central venous pressure falls. These changes indicate that cardiac massage can be stopped. At this point, the infant usually will be hypertensive because the vasoconstriction in nonvital organs still is present. This vasoconstriction is relieved only by continued adequate oxygenation and correction of acidosis. Pressures then will fall toward normal. The vasoconstriction also is manifested by intense pallor of the skin. As the vasoconstriction is relieved, the skin becomes pink and well perfused with rapid capillary refilling (*i.e.*, <2 seconds) when blanched by pressure. As peripheral flow improves, lactic acid sequestered in these tissues enters the central circulation and a large base deficit, which may have been corrected earlier, now reappears.

If asphyxia is only moderately severe, resuscitation begins in the middle of the sequence depicted in Figure 19-1. There is hypertension, indicating that the myocardium has not yet failed. Effective ventilation of the lungs with a high oxygen concentration may correct acidosis by lowering the $PaCO_2$, oxygenating the blood, and adequately dilating the pulmonary vascular bed. If significant acidosis persists after alleviation of the hypercarbia, however, alkali should be given to correct the metabolic component of the acidosis, relieve pulmonary vasoconstriction, and establish good pulmonary perfusion. Generally, raising *p*H to 7.25 is sufficient for this purpose, but there are some important exceptions discussed below in which a higher *p*H is needed to dilate the pulmonary vascular bed.

When the effects of asphyxia are alleviated, spontaneous respiratory efforts return. The duration between the onset of resuscitation and reappearance of spontaneous respiratory efforts is directly proportional to the amount of brain injury that has occurred.[6]

Onset of spontaneous respiratory efforts is not necessarily an indication to withdraw assisted ventilation. Often, there is residual atelectasis and the infant does not have strong, regular respiratory efforts. $PaCO_2$ may be normal and PaO_2 may rise to a high level with assisted ventilation. But when assisted ventilation is withdrawn, effective ventilation may decrease and the whole process of asphyxia reoccur. Such cases must be managed by gradual withdrawal of assisted ventilation and reduction of oxygen.

The blood volume of the asphyxiated infant may be abnormal. Intrapartum asphyxia alters the distribution of blood volume between infant and placenta at the time the cord is clamped. Asphyxia during labor usually shifts blood from the placenta to the fetus. There are certain situations, however, in which the infant's blood volume may be reduced. The most obvious of these is hemorrhage from the fetoplacental unit, which is manifested by vaginal bleeding. Three other conditions that shift blood volume from the fetus to the placenta are compression of the umbilical cord by the after-coming head in a breech delivery, in which umbilical venous flow is reduced selectively more than arterial flow; severe hypotension in the mother; and asphyxia occurring only at the end of labor.[20]

Initially, it may be difficult to determine whether or not blood volume is adequate in the asphyxiated newborn. There are two reasons for this. First, many of the circulatory responses to asphyxia are similar to those associated with loss of blood volume. Either asphyxia or hypovolemia may cause bradycardia, metabolic acidosis, poor peripheral perfusion indicated by pallor and slow capillary filling, and a large difference between core and skin temperature. A low aortic pressure could be due either to the end stage of asphyxia or to shock. Only changes in central venous pressure are in the opposite direction, and even here the coexistence of the two processes can have offsetting effects. Second, the circulatory changes during asphyxia and resuscitation may determine the adequacy or inadequacy of the circulating blood volume. If an infant is moderately asphyxiated, and has systemic and pulmonary vasoconstriction (see Fig. 19-1, center) and a small blood volume, aortic and central venous pressures will be nearly normal. Administration of a blood volume expander at this point would only overload the circulation. The effects of volume expansion would be even worse if the asphyxia were more severe and myocardial failure were present. Correction of asphyxia (see Fig. 19-1, left) relieves the vasoconstriction of resistance and capacitance vessels, and the small blood volume now becomes inadequate to support the circulation. Reperfusion of asphyxic and ischemic tissues also increases loss of intravascular water from these capillary beds, leading to edema and reduced plasma volume.[21]

During recovery from asphyxia, several metabolic abnormalities appear. There may be hypoglycemia due to depletion of carbohydrate reserves during the asphyxia. Hypoglycemia must be prevented because it can cause myocardial failure in a heart recently subjected to asphyxia.[22] Hyperglycemia due to excessive glucose administration similarly is dangerous during asphyxia because it worsens the acidosis by increasing lactic acid production.[23] Hypocalcemia also develops, possibly as a result of increased calcitonin release during asphyxia,[24] and can lead to myocardial failure.

Hyperkalemia occurs during asphyxia, when, in the process of buffering acidosis, H^+ enters the erythrocytes and K^+ is displaced from them. Although this increases plasma K^+ while the patient is asphyxiated, total body K^+ decreases as some of the K^+ is excreted by the kidney. On relief of asphyxia, the buffering processes are reversed and K^+ leaves the plasma and reenters the erythrocytes, leading to hypokalemia. An exception to this process is asphyxia that is so severe that it produces severe renal ischemia, anuria, and retention of potassium.

HIGH-RISK PREGNANCIES

Certain situations during pregnancy, labor, or delivery carry an increased risk of intrapartum asphyxia. If these high-risk deliveries are identified before birth, their progress during labor and delivery can be monitored and resuscitation can be initiated at birth. Tables 19-1 and 19-2 list some of the factors that alert the physician to a high-risk delivery. Optimal management of these cases requires good communication between obstetricians, anesthesiologists, and pediatricians. The physician responsible for care of newborn

TABLE 19–1
SOME FACTORS THAT PLACE THE NEWBORN INFANT AT HIGH RISK FOR ASPHYXIA

Maternal Conditions	Labor and Delivery Conditions	Fetal Conditions
Diabetes mellitus	Forceps delivery other than low-elective or vacuum-extraction delivery	Premature delivery Postmature delivery
Preeclampsia, hypertension, chronic renal disease	Breech or other abnormal presentation and delivery	Acidosis determined by fetal scalp capillary blood
Anemia (*i.e.*, hemoglobin <10 g/dL)	Cephalopelvic dysproportion: shoulder dystocia, prolonged second stage	Abnormal heart rate pattern or dysrhythmia
Blood type or group alloimmunization	Cesarean section	Meconium-stained amniotic fluid
Abruptio placentae, placenta previa, or other antepartum hemorrhage	Prolapsed umbilical cord	Oligohydramnios Polyhydramnios
Narcotic, barbiturate, tranquilizer, psychedelic drug use or alcohol intoxication	Cord compression (*e.g.*, nuchal cord, cord knot, compression by after-coming head in breech delivery)	Decreased rate of growth: uterine size or fetal size determined by ultrasonography
History of previous perinatal loss	Maternal hypotension or hemorrhage	Macrosomia
Prolonged rupture of membranes		
Lupus		Immaturity of pulmonary surfactant system
Maternal heart disease		Fetal malformations determined by sonography
Maternal fever or other evidence of amnionitis		Hydrops fetalis Low biophysical profile
Abnormal umbilical artery Doppler velocity		Multiple births; in particular, discordant, stuck, or monoamniotic

TABLE 19–2
FETAL HEART RATE PATTERNS ASSOCIATED WITH FETAL AND NEONATAL DISTRESS

Heart Rate Pattern	Fetal or Neonatal Problems
Severe (*i.e.*, <80 bpm), sustained bradycardia, with loss of variability	Fetal hemorrhage, fetal asphyxia
Sustained tachycardia, uncomplicated by other abnormal patterns	Infection, often with apnea
Late decelerations with loss of variability	Asphyxia
Severe, recurrent variable decelerations, with loss of variability	Asphyxia and possible hypovolemia
Sinusoidal	Severe anemia with asphyxia

bpm, beats per minute.

infants always should know of any patients with potential problems in the labor and delivery area.

RESUSCITATION OF THE ASPHYXIATED INFANT

If a severely asphyxiated infant is expected, a resuscitation team must be present at the birth. In almost all cases, good communication between obstetricians and pediatricians will provide timely notice of the impending delivery of an asphyxiated infant. The actual steps in the resuscitation fall into three major phases, and a typical division of duties among the team of skilled personnel is listed. One of these people should be experienced at tracheal intubation, ventilation of the lungs, and the general management of resuscitation, and one should be an experienced neonatal nurse. The extent of resuscitation needed can be determined only after the infant's condition is evaluated by someone with considerable clinical experience. The following list outlines the responsibilities of each member of the resuscitation team.

Member A:

1. Assess infant.
2. Manage airway and intubate the trachea if needed.
3. Provide manually assisted ventilation.
4. Secure endotracheal tube.

Member B:

1. Listen for heart rate, give cardiac massage if needed.
2. Auscultate chest to be sure endotracheal tube is in proper position and gas exchange is good.

(continued)

Member B:

3. Catheterize umbilical vessel or vessels and maintain patency of catheters.
4. Measure intravascular pressures, assess perfusion, sample blood for *p*H, PO_2, and PCO_2, and draw blood cultures.
5. Administer fluids and drugs.
6. Continue assessment of infant.

Member C:

1. Blot baby dry; apply electrocardiograph (ECG) monitor leads, radiant monitor servocontrol, and transcutaneous oxygen sensor.
2. Keep timed written record of resuscitation and vital signs and calls for Apgar scores at 1 and 5 minutes and every 5 minutes thereafter until the score is 7 or greater; time and record the rate and volume of infusions such as alkali and blood volume expanders.
3. Assist member A by providing endotracheal tube suction, adjusting the fraction of oxygen inspired (FiO_2), and helping to secure endotracheal tube.
4. Help member B by providing medications and blood volume expanders in sterile syringes; B is working in a sterile field early in resuscitation.
5. Monitor baby's temperature and capillary blood glucose.

Equipment and supplies for optimal resuscitation include the following:

- Resuscitation table with heat source to maintain normal body temperature
- Oxygen and air sources, oxygen–air blender, and infant ventilation systems; the standard infant anesthesia bag, with tailpiece and adjustable resistance and a Norman elbow, is the most versatile system for manual ventilation
- Airway suction system
- Infant face masks and endotracheal tubes from 2.5 to 4.0 mm internal diameter
- Laryngoscope with #1 Miller blade for full-term infants and a #0 blade for preterm infants; be sure the batteries and light bulb of the laryngoscope work
- Monitors
  - Heart rate by ECG
  - Transcutaneous oxygen saturation
  - Arterial and venous pressures with waveform displays; transducers can be connected to the catheters beforehand so that aortic pressure is displayed as soon as the umbilical artery catheter is inserted, and the venous waveform can be used to localize the catheter tip in the thoracic inferior vena cava[25]
  - Indirect blood pressure monitor
- Catheters and catheterization tray with instruments, sterile drapes, and sterile syringes for sampling blood and flushing the lines
- All emergency medicines and fluids

Tube thoracostomy tray with instruments and catheters from 10 to 14 Fr

Blood gas electrodes with a trained operator of the blood gas machines close enough to the resuscitation area so that results are available in under 5 minutes

In selected situations (see the following), it is useful to have present in the delivery room a unit of whole blood or packed erythrocytes that were cross-matched against the mother; this blood can be kept in a cold pack and returned to the blood bank if not used.

PHASE 1

CLINICAL ASSESSMENT OF SEVERITY OF ASPHYXIA

The Apgar score was the first attempt at a systematic assessment of birth asphyxia.[2,26] There is a loose correlation between low Apgar scores and umbilical cord blood gases. Some infants with severe acidosis, however, have normal Apgar scores and some with normal blood gases and *p*H have very low scores.[27,28] Maternal anesthetics, sedatives, maternal drugs, fetal sepsis, and central nervous system pathologic conditions can lower the Apgar score; extremely premature infants often have low scores without any other evidence of asphyxia.[29,30] Regardless of the cause, an Apgar score that remains low calls for action. The clinical significance of the Apgar score increases with time. Scoring should continue every 5 minutes until the score increases to 7 or above. The length of time it takes to reach a score of 7 is a rough indication of severity of asphyxia. Umbilical cord blood gases, discussed above, are useful measures of fetal asphyxia, but this information will not be available until a few minutes after birth, and resuscitation must be started before that. Thus, their main value is in guiding subsequent management of the infant.

It is essential to maintain body temperature. When the cord is clamped, blot the infant dry with a sterile towel to reduce evaporative heat loss and place him or her under a radiant heater on the resuscitation table.[31]

Next, clear the airway. Gently suction the oropharynx and nose. If the infant's respiration is vigorous, nothing more may be necessary. Attach ECG electrodes and pulse oximeter, and monitor the heart rate and oxygen saturations.

INITIATE VENTILATION

If the infant is apneic or the respiratory rate is slow and irregular, place a mask over the infant's face and ventilate with oxygen-enriched gas using intermittent positive pressure from the anesthesia bag while observing chest movements and the ventilation pressure on an aneroid manometer. Begin ventilation by slowly applying a pressure of 20 cm H_2O to the airway for term infants, and 30 cm H_2O to the airway for preterm infants. Maintain this inflating pressure for 1 to 2 seconds, then ventilate at a rate of 40 to 60 breaths per minute, using an inflation time of 0.25 to 0.5 seconds and just enough pressure to provide good expansion of the upper portion of the chest. Repeat the application of the initial inflating pressure pattern three to four times over the first 2 minutes. These prolonged breaths inflate regions of the lungs that were gasless and create the necessary functional residual capacity.[32] Figure 19-2 illustrates this process. If the stomach becomes inflated, pass an orogastric tube and apply suction.

In mildly asphyxiated infants, ventilation will produce a prompt increase in heart rate and the onset of regular, spontaneous respiration. If both do not occur, intubate the trachea and continue assisted ventilation. Tracheal intubation may induce severe bradycardia when the hypopharynx is stimulated, but heart rate should increase as soon as intubation is completed and assisted ventilation is begun. With severe asphyxia, the experienced resuscitator may prefer to intubate the trachea immediately. Ventilation through a properly positioned endotracheal tube is more effective than ventilation by mask and avoids distention of the stomach with gas. The less experienced physician who cannot intubate the trachea quickly, however, should use mask ventilation first, then intubate the trachea later if it still is necessary. Do not continue to attempt tracheal intubation for more than about 30 seconds. If unsuccessful in that time, ventilate the infant's lungs by mask for at least 1 minute before again attempting tracheal intubation. Intubate gently to avoid trauma to the hypopharynx and vocal cords. If a metal stylette is used to stiffen the tracheal tube during intubation, secure the stylette so the tip of the stylette is approximately 0.5 cm back from the tip of the tube. If the stylette extends beyond the tip of the endotracheal tube, it could traumatize the airway.

As a general guideline, use a 2.5-mm diameter endotracheal tube for babies weighing 1 kg or less, 3.0 mm for 1 to 1.5 kg, 3.5 mm for 1.5 to 2.5 kg, and 4.0 mm for larger babies (see Appendices F-3 and F-4). Some bigger babies need a tube one size smaller than that recommended for their weight. In general, gas should leak from the space between the endotracheal tube and the trachea when 15 to 30 cm of H_2O pressure is applied to the airway.

If the infant does not make strong respiratory efforts after initiating assisted ventilation, and the mother has received morphine or other narcotic within an hour before delivery, give naloxone hydrochloride, 0.1 mg/kg intravenously or intramuscularly.

BEGIN CARDIAC MASSAGE

If there is no electrical activity on the ECG, no audible heartbeat, or if the heart rate remains below 50 beats

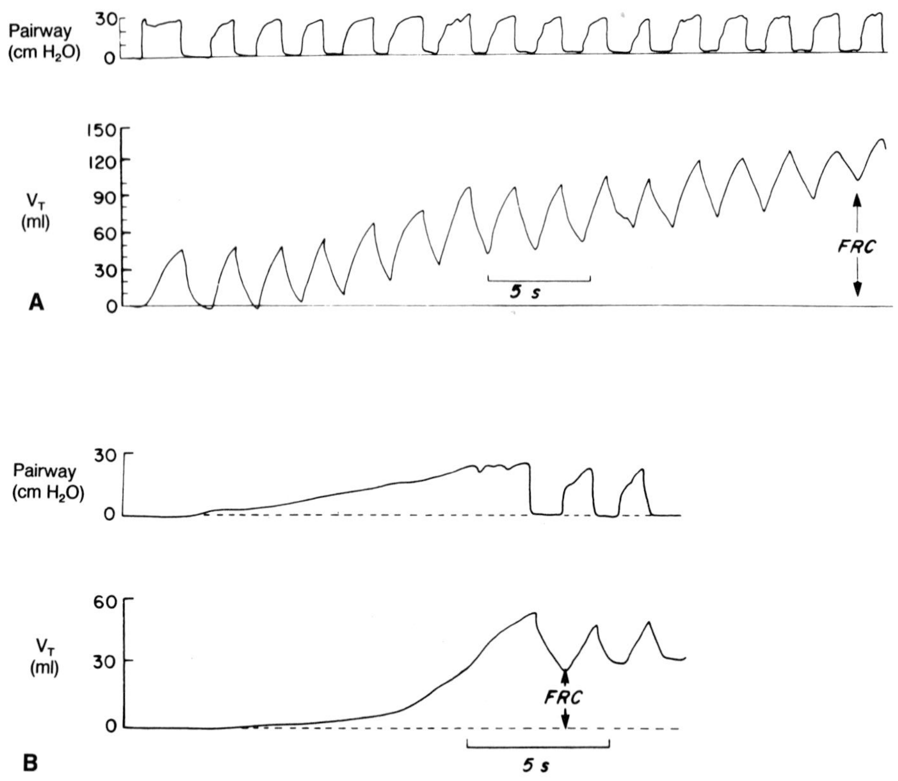

FIG. 19–2. Initial inflation of the lungs by assisted ventilation in two asphyxiated infants. **(A)** An inflation pressure of 30 cm H_2O is applied repeatedly for 1 to 2 seconds. For the first several breaths, the volume entering and leaving the lungs is the same. Then the volume out is slightly less than the volume in for several breaths, and this trapped gas begins to form the functional residual capacity (FRC). **(B)** The first inflation is with a pressure that is increased slowly up to 30 cm H_2O over 8 seconds and held at that pressure for 2 seconds. During exhalation, less gas leaves than what entered; therefore, some FRC has been generated with the first breath. (P_{air}, pressure applied to the airway; V_T, tidal volume; adapted from Boon AW, Milner AD, Hopkin IE. Lung expansion, tidal exchange, and formation of the functional residual capacity during resuscitation of asphyxiated neonates. J Pediatr 1979;95:1031, and Vyas H, Milner AD, Hopkin IE, et al. Physiologic responses to prolonged and slow-rise inflation in the resuscitation of the asphyxiated newborn infant. J Pediatr 1981;99:635.)

per minute after onset of assisted ventilation, begin cardiac massage. Give external cardiac massage by placing both hands around the infant's chest, with the fingertips over the back and the thumbs overlapping each other on the midsternum; then quickly press down firmly with both thumbs at a rate of 80 to 100 strokes per minute.[33] Increase the inspired oxygen to 100% and continue cardiac massage while proceeding with other resuscitative measures until the spontaneous heart rate rises above 100 and the arterial pressure is normal. If there is no spontaneous heart rate, give epinephrine (0.1 mL/kg of 1 : 10,000 solution) intravenously or through the endotracheal tube. It will be absorbed rapidly from the mucosa of the airway when given into the airway.[34] Most cases of presumed cardiac arrest actually are profound bradycardias that respond to effective ventilation alone or to ventilation and cardiac massage, or the latter plus epinephrine. The efficacy of massage and the return of adequate cardiac activity are best judged by monitoring aortic blood pressure. Massage can be discontinued for a few seconds to evaluate the spontaneous heart rate and blood pressure (Fig. 19-3). Infants who do not respond rapidly to these measures will require prompt correction of acidosis (see Correct Severe Metabolic Acidosis), atropine sulfate (0.01 mg/kg), and $CaCl_2$ (0.2 mL/kg of a 10% solution). Although epinephrine is recommended primarily to start the heart, it also is quite effective in correcting bradycardia. Rarely, persistent bradycardia requires treatment with isoproterenol, beginning with a dose of 0.1 μg/kg/minute.

CATHETERIZE AN UMBILICAL ARTERY AND DRAW A BLOOD SAMPLE

Measure *p*H, PaO_2, and $PaCO_2$ to evaluate the efficacy of ventilation. Depending on the values obtained, adjust ventilatory rate, pressure, and inspired oxygen accordingly. Measure hematocrit, connect the catheter to a precalibrated pressure transducer, and measure blood pressure. Alternatively, the catheter can be connected to the transducer ahead of time and the blood pressure displayed as soon as the catheter is passed into the aorta. This also reduces the risk of accidentally injecting air bubbles through the catheter into the infant's circulation while the catheter is being connected to the transducer.

It is important to obtain a measurement of *p*H and PCO_2 quickly. Although a venous blood gas analysis is not as representative as an arterial one, it will suffice as an initial measurement to detect severe acidosis and to determine whether or not PCO_2 is near the normal range. Venous PCO_2 is about 6 torr higher and *p*H about 0.06 units lower than in arterial blood.[25] If there will be a delay in placing an umbilical artery catheter, a line emergently placed in the lower portion of the umbilical vein will provide access until an arterial line is established.

CORRECT SEVERE METABOLIC ACIDOSIS

If the *p*H is less than 7.05 due to a mixed acidosis, or the base deficit is 15 mEq/L or more, correct the metabolic component of the acidosis with an infusion of either $NaHCO_3$ or tromethamine, depending on the $PaCO_2$. The immediate objectives are twofold: to reverse the myocardial failure and low cardiac output that occurs from acute metabolic, but not respiratory, acidosis[12,35,36]; and to relieve the intense pulmonary vasoconstriction that occurs with severe acidosis, particularly in full-term infants.[10,37,38] Metabolic acidosis causes greater pulmonary vasoconstriction than an equivalent degree of respiratory acidosis.[39]

Calculate the dose of buffer from the following formula:

$$\text{mmol buffer} = 0.3 \times \text{body weight (kg)} \times \text{base deficit (mEq/L)}.$$

Infuse at the rate of 1 mmol/L/kg/minute. $NaHCO_3$ comes as either a 1.0 or a 0.5 mol/L solution. Dilute

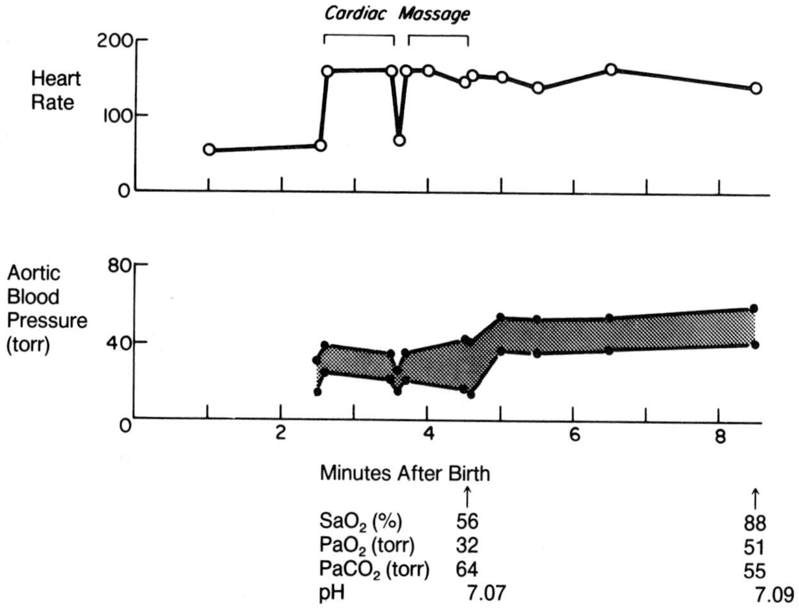

FIG. 19–3. Resuscitation and cardiac massage were performed on a 2.1-kg infant who was delivered by cesarean section due to signs of fetal asphyxia at week 34 of gestation. The infant was intubated and ventilated with 60% oxygen beginning 30 seconds after birth. An electrocardiogram was begun at 1 minute, and at 2.5 minutes an umbilical artery catheter connected to a pressure transducer and a recorder was passed into the descending aorta. Note persistent bradycardia despite assisted ventilation and low aortic pressure with narrow phasic pressure. Cardiac massage raised heart rate and pressure. When briefly discontinued after 1 minute, pressure and heart rate fell. After another minute of massage and assisted ventilation, good cardiac output had returned. This was manifested by a sustained higher heart rate and higher blood pressure with wider phasic pressure when massage was discontinued a second time at 5 minutes after birth. By 8.5 minutes, the infant was still acidotic, but there was adequate oxygenation and aortic pressure continued to rise. ($PaCO_2$, arterial carbon dioxide partial pressure; PaO_2, arterial oxygen partial pressure; SaO_2, saturation of arterial blood hemoglobin with oxygen.)

the former with sterile water, not a dextrose solution, to 0.5 or 0.3 mol/L. Tromethamine comes as a 0.3 mol/L solution that can be given without further dilution.

The ability of $NaHCO_3$ buffer to raise *p*H depends on the ability of the lungs to eliminate the CO_2 produced by the buffering process, as determined by the following equation:

$$H^+ + NaHCO_3 \rightleftarrows Na^+ + H_2CO_3 \rightleftarrows H_2O + CO_2.$$

Do not give $NaHCO_3$ unless ventilation is adequate and $PaCO_2$ low, normal, or declining toward normal. Continue ventilation during bicarbonate therapy to eliminate the excess CO_2 produced.

Some studies suggest that there is an association between rapid infusions of large volumes of concentrated sodium bicarbonate and intracranial hemorrhage in preterm infants. The hemorrhages might be caused by transient hypernatremia from too rapid an infusion, by an acute rise in $PaCO_2$ from inadequate ventilation during the $NaHCO_3$ infusion, or by the asphyxia for which the drug was given. Infusion of sodium bicarbonate into the inferior vena cava at the rate of 1 mEq/kg/minute, for a total dose of up to 5 mEq/kg, causes only a slight transient increase in arterial sodium concentration.

Tromethamine has the twofold advantage of reducing $PaCO_2$ and buffering metabolic acid. It is most useful for treating infants with severe mixed metabolic and respiratory acidosis and for situations of severe asphyxia with suspected extreme acidosis in which blood gas measurements are not available. Tromethamine may cause respiratory depression, so it should be used only in situations in which ventilation already is assisted. Tromethamine also may cause hypoglycemia. An earlier preparation of tromethamine was very hyperosmolar, highly alkalotic, and tended to sclerose vessels. These problems have been corrected in the 0.3 mol/L preparation, which is also adjusted to *p*H 8.6.[40] Figures 19-4 and 19-5 illustrate correction of acidosis in two very different situations.

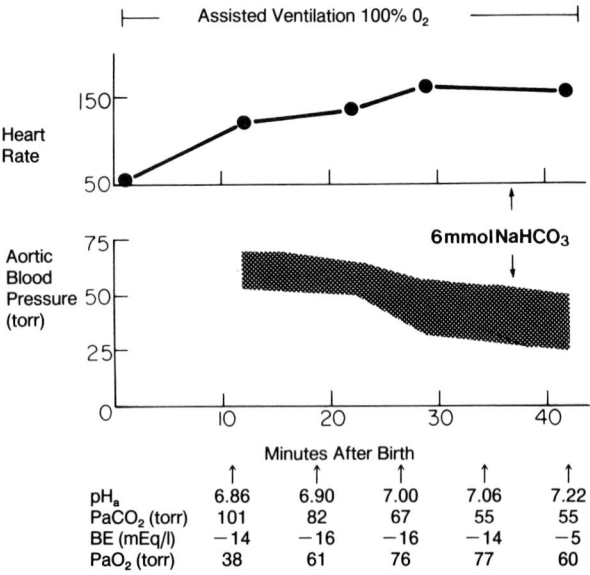

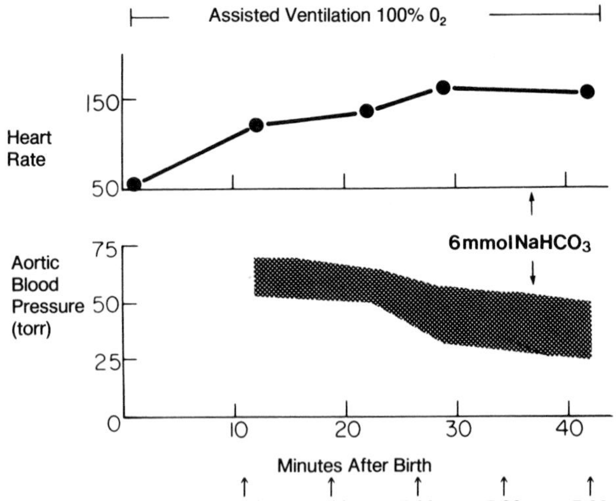

pH_a	6.86	6.90	7.00	7.06	7.22
$PaCO_2$ (torr)	101	82	67	55	55
BE (mEq/l)	−14	−16	−16	−14	−5
PaO_2 (torr)	38	61	76	77	60

FIG. 19–4. Changes occurred in heart rate, aortic blood pressure, and arterial blood gas tensions during the first 45 minutes after birth of a 1.2-kg premature infant with severe asphyxia complicated by bilateral pleural effusions. The child's trachea was intubated immediately after birth, and he was manually ventilated with 100% oxygen throughout this time. Note the severe mixed acidosis in the first blood gas measurement at 11 minutes after birth. Administration of $NaHCO_3$ at this point would have been inappropriate and ineffective because assisted ventilation had not yet achieved adequate elimination of CO_2. $NaHCO_3$ was given only after adequate CO_2 elimination was achieved. Note that there was no rise in the arterial carbon dioxide partial pressure ($PaCO_2$) after this, indicating that all the CO_2 produced during the buffering process was eliminated, and the only change was a reduction in base deficit from −14 to −5 mEq/L, which raised the *p*H from 7.06 to 7.22. Note the high initial aortic pressure, which was due to the vasoconstriction of asphyxia, indicating that myocardial failure had not yet developed. As asphyxia was relieved, aortic pressure fell to normal. (BE, base excess; PaO_2, arterial oxygen partial pressure.)

PHASE II

As soon as the infant's condition is stabilized, perform a thorough examination for major anomalies, dysmorphic features, abnormalities of intrauterine growth, and evidence of infection such as rashes and hepatosplenomegaly. It is easy to overlook a neural tube defect in a supine infant. A scaphoid abdomen and difficulty achieving adequate ventilation suggest a diaphragmatic hernia. If this is suspected and the lungs are being ventilated by a face mask, switch immediately to an endotracheal tube to prevent distention of the gastrointestinal tract, including the segment of bowel in the chest, and further restriction of ventilation. Insert an orogastric tube into the stomach and aspirate its contents. This reduces the risk of regurgitation and aspiration, which can happen despite the presence of an endotracheal tube. If the tube fails to enter the stomach, think of esophageal atresia and apply continuous suction to the tube. Suctioning of 20 mL or more fluid from the stomach suggests obstruction of the upper gastrointestinal tract. During resuscitation, an infant often will pass urine or meconium. Note and record this because the asphyxiated infant may not void or pass stool again for a day or longer.

REEVALUATE ASSISTED VENTILATION

Monitor for complications of assisted ventilation. The tube may be dislodged from the trachea and advance into the esophagus. Alternately, the tracheal tube may advance into the right main bronchial stem, leading to nonventilation of the entire left lung and the upper lobe of the right lung. This is the most

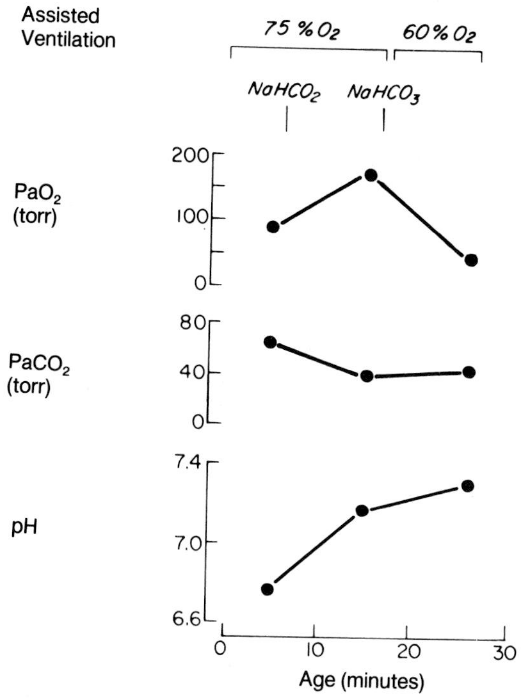

FIG. 19–5. Arterial blood gas tensions, *p*H, and therapy during the first 30 minutes after the birth of a 1.6-kg premature infant. There was severe mixed acidosis initially. The results in this case differ from those shown in Figure 19-4—assisted ventilation achieved effective CO_2 elimination early in this infant, and $NaHCO_3$ could be given earlier to begin correcting the metabolic component of the acidosis. The base excess on the first blood specimen was beyond the limits of calculation (more than −25 mEq/L). The first infusion of $NaHCO_3$ was given between 6 and 10 minutes. When the second sample was drawn at 15 minutes, the calculated base excess was −22 mEq/L. After the second infusion of $NaHCO_3$, the base excess was −6 mEq/L, and no more alkali was given. Note that arterial carbon dioxide partial pressure $PaCO_2$ fell between the first and second measurements when $NaHCO_3$ was given. (PaO_2, arterial oxygen partial pressure.)

common serious complication of tracheal intubation. Immediately after intubation, auscultate both sides of the chest to be sure the breath sounds are equal; reauscultate the chest every few minutes until the tube is removed or properly secured in position. The presence of reduced breath sounds in the left chest does not necessarily indicate partial ventilation of the left lung. In neonates, breath sounds can be transmitted from the opposite side of the chest and often can be heard over a lung that is completely collapsed. The breath sounds should be equal on both sides of the chest. If breath sounds are absent or diminished on the left side, slowly withdraw the endotracheal tube while continuing ventilation until breath sounds are equal. Some endotracheal tubes have centimeter marks on them to indicate the distance to the tracheal end of the tube. The tip of the tube generally will be in the midtrachea if the distance mark at the infant's lip is 7 cm in a 1-kg infant, 8 cm in a 2-kg infant, 9 cm in a 3-kg infant, and 10 cm in a 4-kg infant. In large preterm and full-term infants where a 3.0-mm or larger diameter endotracheal tube is appropriate (see Initiate Ventilation; see Appendices F-3 and F-4), right main bronchial stem intubation can be avoided by using a shouldered Cole endotracheal tube. When the proper-sized tube for the baby is used, the tube tip reaches the midtracheal region when the tube's shoulders abut the vocal cords. The shoulders prevent the tube from advancing into the bronchus. If the tube passes easily beyond the optimal distance (*i.e.*, it meets no resistance), one can be sure the tube is in the esophagus, not the trachea. Shouldered tubes do not work as well in smaller, preterm infants because the distal segment of the 2.5-mm diameter tube that is beyond the shoulders is long enough to reach the right main bronchial stem in the smallest infants. A shouldered tube cannot be used for long-term ventilation because it may traumatize the vocal cords, but it can be used safely for the first half-hour or hour of resuscitation. It then can be replaced with a straight tube when resuscitation is completed, should assisted ventilation still be required.

Aspirate the stomach during this phase of resuscitation. If a face mask was used for initial ventilation, the stomach will be distended with gas, which can restrict ventilation. On rare occasions, gastric distention caused by ventilation with a bag and mask may perforate the stomach. The resulting severe abdominal distention must be relieved to allow adequate ventilation.

During phase II, pulmonary function may change rapidly, leading to several complications. First, PaO_2 will rise and may reach dangerously high levels as ventilation and perfusion become better matched. Hyperoxia is managed better initially by reducing inspired oxygen concentration than by withdrawing ventilatory assistance. Second, improved ventilation may lead to acute hypocarbia, which will reduce cerebral and myocardial blood flow.[41–43] Correct hypocarbia by reducing the rate of assisted ventilation. Figure 19-6 illustrates these changes. Third, as lung compliance increases, the ventilatory pressure that was appropriate initially will become excessive. If the excess pressure is mild, the result will be hyperventilation and hypocarbia. If it is extreme, however, there will be tamponade of the pulmonary circulation and right-to-left shunting of blood at the atrial and ductal levels and low systemic blood flow. This phenomenon is manifested by a low aortic pressure, wide fluctuations in blood pressure in phase with the positive pressure ventilation, and arterial hypoxemia. This situation can be detected by briefly disconnecting the endotracheal tube from the ventilation system. Aortic pressure will rise within 2 to 3 seconds. If this occurs, restart ventilation using lower airway pressures. The hypoxia caused by the shunting of blood from right to left will improve quickly as the lungs are ventilated with lower pressures.

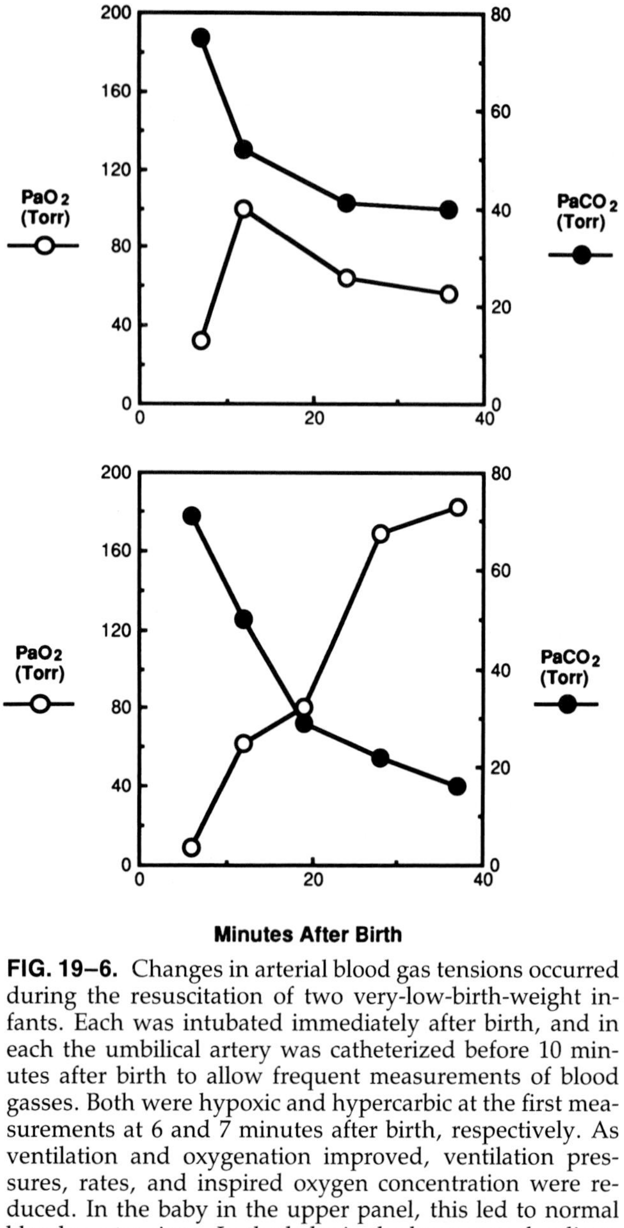

FIG. 19–6. Changes in arterial blood gas tensions occurred during the resuscitation of two very-low-birth-weight infants. Each was intubated immediately after birth, and in each the umbilical artery was catheterized before 10 minutes after birth to allow frequent measurements of blood gasses. Both were hypoxic and hypercarbic at the first measurements at 6 and 7 minutes after birth, respectively. As ventilation and oxygenation improved, ventilation pressures, rates, and inspired oxygen concentration were reduced. In the baby in the upper panel, this led to normal blood gas tensions. In the baby in the lower panel, adjustments were made too slowly, leading to hyperoxia and extreme hypocarbia. ($PaCO_2$, arterial carbon dioxide partial pressure; PaO_2, arterial oxygen partial pressure.)

Tension pneumothorax may occur during spontaneous or assisted ventilation of any infant. A tension pneumothorax of small or moderate size may interfere with ventilation and cause hypoxia and hypercarbia. Pneumothorax must be suspected whenever PaO_2 decreases despite a ventilation system that is functioning properly, a tracheal tube that is properly located in the trachea, and a properly functioning oxygen delivery system. Sometimes the diagnosis of pneumothorax is difficult to make by physical examination. Breath sounds may be unequal bilaterally, but often they are equal. The upper portion of the affected side of the chest tends to lag behind the unaffected side during inflation of the lungs. Transillumination with a cold fiberoptic light may cause the affected side to glow brightly; however, the absence of this sign does not rule out pneumothorax, particularly in the larger infant with a thicker chest wall. The diagnosis of pneumothorax can be made best by a chest radiograph, but this often is difficult to obtain quickly in the resuscitation area. The arterial and central venous pressures may not change with small pneumothoraces. If hypoxia and hypercarbia become severe, it may he necessary to perform a diagnostic thoracentesis with a small-gauge needle and syringe before there is time to obtain a radiograph.

The situation changes when a tension pneumothorax is large. Venous return to the heart and cardiac output may fall precipitously to extremely low levels. If blood pressure, PaO_2, and $PaCO_2$ are being measured, this critical situation will be diagnosed easily because the onset of hypoxia and hypercarbia will be accompanied by severe hypotension rather than the hypertension of asphyxia (see Fig. 19-1).[44] This situation requires as urgent treatment as cardiac arrest. One cannot wait for a confirmatory radiograph. Figure 19-7 illustrates the diagnosis and successful treatment of such a case. Satisfactory decompression of a tension pneumothorax usually requires insertion of a thoracostomy tube and continuous suction applied to the tube through an underwater suction system. Aspiration with a needle and syringe usually gives only very brief relief. While assembling equipment for decompression of the pneumothorax, however, insert a No.-22 gauge scalp infusion needle connected to a three-way stopcock and a 30-mL syringe. This is a convenient and relatively safe method for temporary decompression of the pneumothorax.

EVALUATE CIRCULATORY STATUS

The healthy newborn can compensate for loss of a large volume of blood. Asphyxia however, disrupts the newborn's ability to do so.[45] Most asphyxiated infants have a normal or greater than normal blood volume; only a few have a low blood volume.[20] Consequently, hypovolemic shock does not develop in most asphyxiated infants. Of the few infants in whom hypovolemic shock develops in the first hours after birth, however, almost all have had intrapartum asphyxia.[46] Blood volume expansion is essential for the infant who is in hypovolemic shock, but may be harmful for the asphyxiated infant who has a normal blood volume.

Because some circulatory changes due to asphyxia may either mimic or mask hypovolemic shock, it is impossible to identify those infants who need blood volume expansion until resuscitation has produced adequate oxygenation of arterial blood and a normal $PaCO_2$. Acute hypocarbia causes systemic hypotension,[47] and severe overventilation may reduce systemic blood flow (see Phase II). Neither of these states requires blood volume expansion.

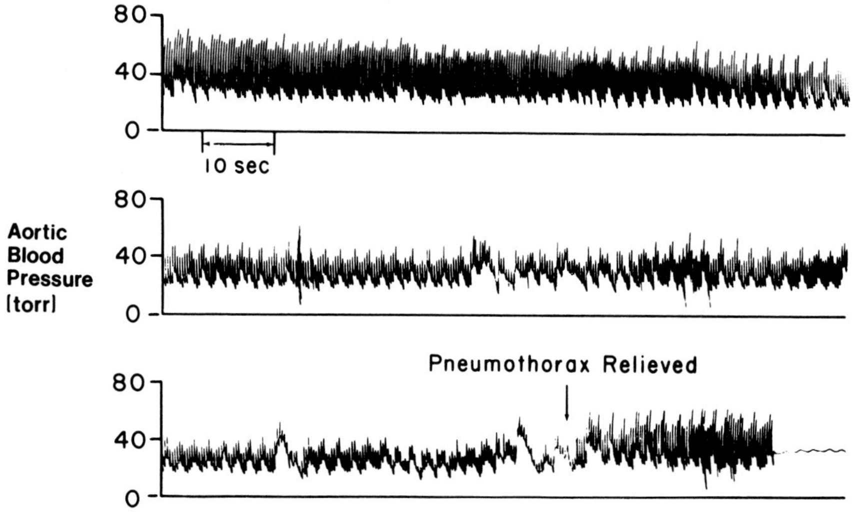

FIG. 19–7. Aortic blood pressure of a premature, 1.5-kg infant at 32 gestational weeks of age during development of a tension pneumothorax. This is a continuous tracing at 2 hours of age. Because the patient's condition was rapidly worsening, as shown by hypotension, a narrow pulse pressure, and rapidly increasing cyanosis despite assisted ventilation with 100% oxygen, thoracentesis of the right pleural cavity was done (*arrow*) before radiologic confirmation of the pneumothorax was obtained. About 50 ml of air escaped when the pleural cavity was opened. The patient's color improved, and blood pressure promptly returned to normal.

Signs that suggest an inadequate blood volume include the following: low aortic pressure and a narrow and abnormal aortic waveform (Figs. 19-8 and 19-9), falling hematocrit, persistent metabolic acidosis, low central venous PO_2 (*i.e.*, <30 torr) after correction of arterial hypoxia, cold extremities, and delayed (*i.e.*, ≥3 seconds) filling of capillaries in the skin after they have been blanched under pressure, provided that core temperature is normal. Tachycardia often is absent in the early stages of severe shock and may be present from too many other causes to be a useful sign.[48,49]

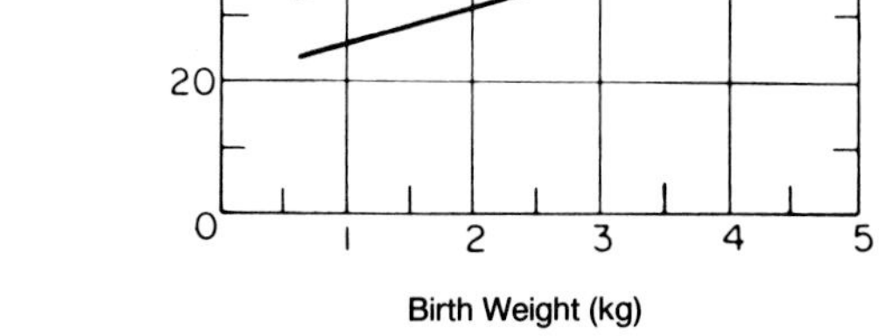

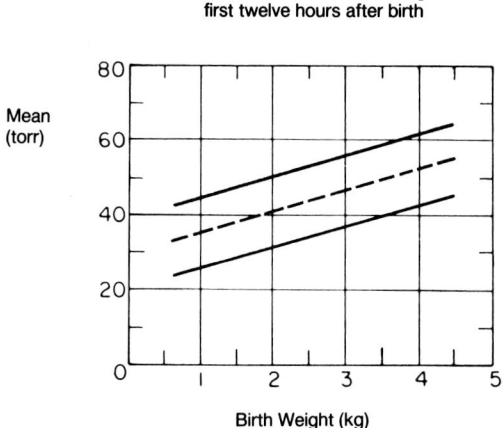

FIG. 19–8. Mean aortic blood pressure was obtained from an umbilical artery catheter. The dashed line is the average blood pressure at each birth weight, and the solid lines are the 95% confidence limits of this relationship. Blood pressure values below the lower confidence line are hypotensive. (From Versmold HT, Kitterman JA, Phibbs RH, et al. Aortic blood pressure during the first twelve hours of life in infants with birth weights 610–4220 grams. Pediatrics 1981;67:607.

If some findings suggest shock, but the diagnosis is uncertain, it is useful to connect a second catheter to a pressure transducer, insert the catheter into the umbilical vein, and use direct pressure monitoring to locate the position of the catheter tip in the inferior vena cava or right atrium.[25] Central venous pressure may be low or normal during hypovolemic shock, but it will be high with circulatory tamponade from excessive positive pressure ventilation, tension pneumothorax, or postasphyxial myocardiopathy. The findings of a low or normal central venous pressure in combination with signs of poor systemic perfusion support a trial of volume expansion. A low central venous oxygen content is a very sensitive, but nonspecific, indicator of increased oxygen extraction in the microcirculation in response to inadequate oxygen delivery from any cause. It is one of the earliest changes during hypovolemic shock.[50]

Hypovolemic shock is treated best with repeated small infusions of whole blood that has been cross matched against the mother before delivery and is available in the resuscitation area at birth.[51] Group O Rh-negative blood given to newborns without cross matching against the mother's serum occasionally has produced fatal transfusion reactions caused by incompatibility in minor blood groups, and should not be used. If only packed erythrocytes are available, give equal volumes of cells and a plasma substitute, such as 5% albumin or isotonic saline. If no erythrocytes are available, use a plasma substitute for initial resuscitation, then give packed cells as soon as they are available. This, however, is less effective than giving blood initially. The object of therapy is prompt restoration of adequate tissue perfusion. This must be done rapidly enough to avoid the cumulatively harmful effects of prolonged underperfusion of tissues. The latter can lead to the secondary effects of shock, including increased capillary permeability and pulmonary disease, which make therapy more difficult.

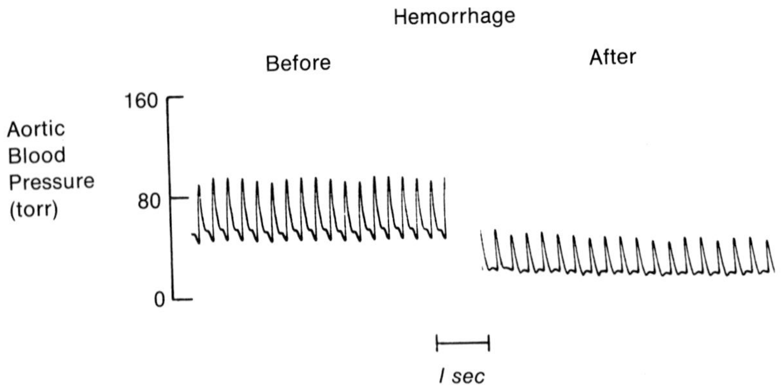

FIG. 19–9. Changes in aortic blood pressure during rapid hemorrhage in a newborn lamb. Blood pressure falls and pulse pressure (*i.e.*, systolic minus diastolic) narrows. Note the difference in waveform before and after hemorrhage. Before the hemorrhage, pressure continues to decrease after the dicrotic notch, indicating continued systemic flow during diastole. This disappears after hemorrhage, indicating little or no systemic flow during diastole. Heart rate has not yet increased but will do so later.

Excessive speed in volume replacement also is dangerous, however. Some vascular beds, such as that of the brain, vasodilate in response to systemic hypotension. If treatment produces an abrupt rise in systemic pressure, there is no time for this vasculature to partially constrict, and the higher pressure is transmitted to the capillaries, where it may cause capillary injury, edema, or hemorrhage. In most cases, shock can be treated with repeated infusions of 5 mL/kg blood given by a steady infusion over approximately 5 minutes. Observe the response to each infusion and stop therapy as soon as tissue perfusion is adequate. Usually, aortic pressure will rise after the first or first few infusions, but as these relieve systemic vasoconstriction, pressure falls again and further volume expansion may be required, provided other signs of poor perfusion persist. Occasionally, when there has been massive hemorrhage, volume may have to be replaced more rapidly. In such a case, monitor aortic pressure continuously to avoid abrupt rises in pressures. Figure 19-10 shows the course of successful treatment during the first hour of life in an infant who lost approximately 50% of his blood volume during delivery and also suffered asphyxia. Figure 19-11 shows the course in an infant in whom hypovolemia did not become evident until assisted ventilation relieved asphyxia and unmasked hypovolemia.

PHASE III

This is the time when infants with mild asphyxia will improve quickly, whereas those who were more severely asphyxiated may begin to manifest transient failure of various organ systems secondary to asphyxia. The clinical course of this organ failure is governed by the hierarchy for the preservation of organ blood flow during asphyxia. Thus, some evidence of renal injury may be seen after only moderate asphyxia. Myocardial failure will be seen only after more severe asphyxia, and hypoxic–ischemic encephalopathy usually will be seen only after the most severe asphyxia and in the presence of multiple organ system failure.[52]

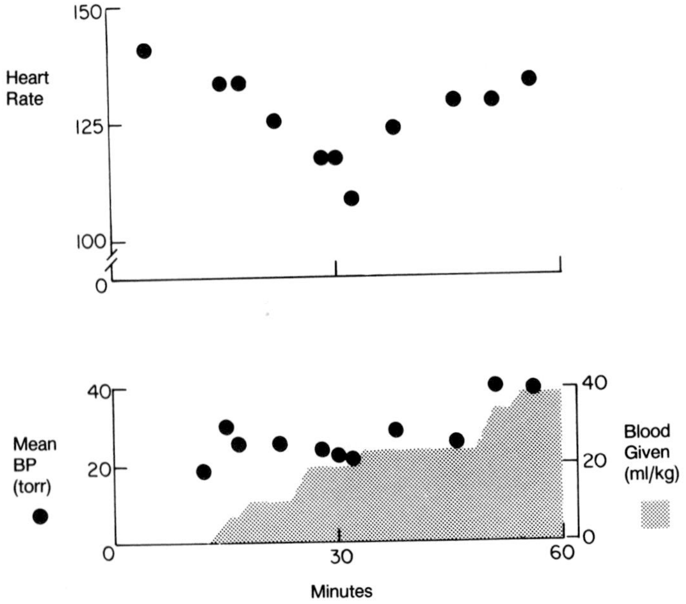

FIG. 19–10. Heart rate, aortic blood pressure, and blood volume replacement were monitored during the first hour after birth in a 2.8-kg infant who suffered massive blood loss when the anteriorly placed placenta was incised deeply at cesarean section delivery. The shaded area shows the cumulative volume of whole blood given expressed as mL/kg body weight. The final volume, which produced a normal aortic blood pressure and relieved signs of poor perfusion, was 40 mL/kg: approximately one-half the total blood volume for a normal newborn infant. The blood was given as a series of small transfusions guided by the changes in blood pressure. Note that the heart rate is not elevated at first, despite the extreme hypotension, and that subsequently heart rate does not consistently change in the opposite direction of blood pressure changes.

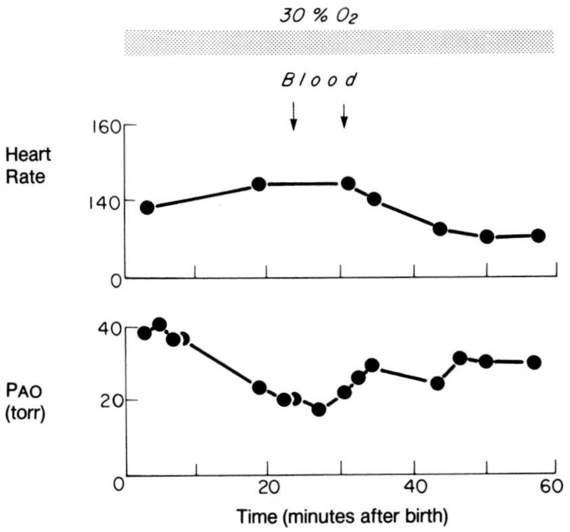

FIG. 19–11. Heart rate, aortic blood pressure (PAO), and therapy were monitored during the first hour after the birth of a 1.5-kg second twin delivered by cesarean section. There had been a large abruption of the placenta. Initially, the infant was hypoxic and acidotic, and aortic pressure was normal. As blood gas tensions normalized, aortic pressure fell and the infant continued to appear pale and poorly perfused. This probably is an example of the intense vasoconstriction of asphyxia keeping blood pressure at a normal level despite a subnormal blood volume. Relief of the asphyxia allowed sufficient vasodilation to unmask the hypovolemia.

ADJUST ASSISTED VENTILATION TO CHANGES IN PULMONARY FUNCTION

Pulmonary function will improve rapidly in many infants as compliance improves with absorption of lung water. Pulmonary perfusion will increase in response to a rising *p*H and PO_2. On the other hand, if ischemia has caused more severe asphyxia with lung injury, there may be continued respiratory distress that is indistinguishable from early hyaline membrane disease. This will require continued ventilatory assistance. Unlike hyaline membrane disease, however, this form of respiratory failure usually begins to improve within a few hours after birth,[53] whereas hyaline membrane disease due to immaturity of the surfactant system worsens over the first day after birth. When a fetus with immature lungs has suffered significant intrapartum asphyxia, the ensuing hyaline membrane disease generally will be more severe.[54] These divergent courses of respiratory distress are illustrated in Figure 19-12.

Infants with early-onset hyaline membrane disease should be given exogenous surfactant as soon as the condition is apparent and the endotracheal tube is in proper position with its tip above the carina. Early treatment with surfactant is more effective than treatment that has been delayed several hours. At this early stage in the infant's course, it often is impossible to distinguish between hyaline membrane disease, postasphyxial respiratory distress, and congenital pneumonia. This is not a reason to withhold surfactant treatment, because it has no adverse effect and may be of some benefit in some infants with other pulmonary disease.[55,56]

CARDIAC FUNCTION

Transient myocardial failure of 1 to 2 days of duration can occur after asphyxia.[22,57–59] The resulting circulatory failure is differentiated from that due to hypovolemic shock by an elevated central venous pressure. Postasphyxial myocardiopathy responds to a continuous infusion of dopamine with improved systemic perfusion and decreased central venous pressure. Start with a dose of 5 μg/kg/minute and increase the dose as needed to obtain adequate systemic perfusion pressures. If possible, correct hypoxia and acidosis to improve myocardial function before starting dopamine. If pulmonary vasoconstriction and hypertension coexist with systemic hypotension due to myocardial failure, venous-to-arterial shunting of blood through the foramen ovale and ductus arteriosus of-

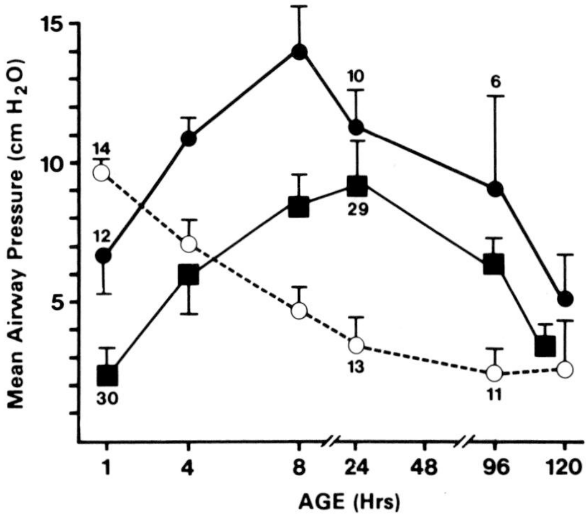

FIG. 19–12. The course of respiratory distress is characterized by changes in mean airway pressure in three groups of infants: those with severe perinatal asphyxia but no hyaline membrane disease, those with perinatal asphyxia plus hyaline membrane disease, and those with no perinatal asphyxia but hyaline membrane disease. In both groups with hyaline membrane disease, the disease worsens, as indicated by the increased mean airway pressure required over the first 24 hours. Those who also had asphyxia had more severe disease. Those with severe asphyxia but no hyaline membrane disease had a completely different course, with progressive improvement over the first 24 hours of life. (○, no respiratory distress syndrome—severe acidosis; ●, respiratory distress syndrome—severe acidosis; ■, respiratory distress syndrome—mild or no acidosis; from Thibeault DW, Hall FK, Sheehan MB, et al. Postasphyxial lung disease in newborn infants with severe perinatal acidosis. Am J Obstet Gynecol 1984;150:393.)

ten occurs. This leads to further systemic hypoxemia and worsening metabolic acidosis. When correcting acidosis in this situation, it is important to avoid hyperventilation, because hypocarbia constricts the coronary circulation and causes systemic hypotension[42,43,47] Some infants of poorly controlled diabetic mothers have a particularly severe form of myocardiopathy. The antecedents of this myocardiopathy are asphyxia plus hypoglycemia plus hypocalcemia, and all of these must be corrected to improve myocardial performance. See Chapter 35 for a discussion of the infant of a diabetic mother.

HEMATOLOGY

Consumption of coagulation factors may complicate severe asphyxia. This almost always is a transient process rather than continuing disseminated intravascular coagulation. Thrombocytopenia is the most consistent finding. In extreme cases, clinical bleeding occurs and requires replacement of platelets and plasma clotting factors. Other hematologic changes include a transient rise in the number of granulocytes, including immature forms, and in erythroid precursors in the peripheral blood. These can rise to very high concentrations and could be misleading when considering such diagnoses as infection and hemolytic anemia. If the changes are secondary to asphyxia, however, they will disappear in a few hours.

GLUCOSE

When hypoxia and acidosis have been relieved, begin a continuous infusion of 10% dextrose in water at 3 mL/kg/hour to maintain a normal concentration of blood glucose. This provides 5 mg glucose/kg/minute. Begin screening for hyperglycemia and hypoglycemia with repeated testing of capillary blood. Glucose infusions usually are not necessary until hypoxia is relieved. Hypoglycemia can be corrected by temporarily increasing the infusion rate of the 10% dextrose to 5 mL/kg/hour (8.4 mg/kg/minute), which is sufficient in all but the most extreme cases of asphyxia-induced hypoglycemia. Rapid infusions of more concentrated solutions of dextrose rarely are needed to correct hypoglycemia and can be dangerous because of their hyperosmolarity and their tendency to produce serious vascular injury. Care should be taken not to induce hyperglycemia during asphyxia, because this may worsen central nervous system damage.

FLUID AND ELECTROLYTES

Asphyxia causes renal ischemia.[60] Many asphyxiated infants are oliguric for the first day of life and have a rising serum creatinine. Very high serum creatinine concentrations in the first days of life, however, are not due to renal failure but to tissue necrosis after severe asphyxia. When urine output increases, there is transient hematuria and oliguria. With extreme asphyxia, corticomedullary hemorrhagic necrosis occurs and the renal failure is more severe. As renal function returns, sodium, potassium, and chloride can be added to parenteral fluids. As acidosis is corrected, extracellular potassium shifts back into cells and postasphyxial infants with good renal function may become hypokalemic. The usual maintenance amounts of electrolytes may be adequate to maintain serum electrolyte concentrations, but in many cases renal losses of electrolytes are very high during this diuresis, so it will be necessary to administer higher concentrations of electrolytes. When planning sodium requirements, take into account sodium given as $NaHCO_3$ during resuscitation and the NaCl in catheter-flush solutions. Infants who are asphyxiated often become hypocalcemic by the first day after birth. Serum ionized calcium should be measured and supplemental calcium given as needed.

GASTROINTESTINAL FUNCTION

During asphyxia, blood flow to the small and large bowels is reduced. Severe asphyxia may cause serious ischemic injury to these organs. Because of this, it may be advisable to delay enteral feedings for several days and continue intravenous fluids. Occasionally, acute necrotizing enterocolitis occurs when severely asphyxiated infants are fed in the first day or two after birth. This is particularly important in infants who also have suffered hypovolemic shock, since shock severely compromises intestinal blood flow.[61]

SPECIAL PROBLEMS

MECONIUM ASPIRATION

Meconium staining of amniotic fluid occurs in 10% to 15% of all deliveries.[62,63] Mature fetuses pass meconium in response to various stimuli, including asphyxia. Meconium staining diminishes with decreasing gestational age and is rare before 34 weeks of gestation, whereas it is quite common in postmature fetuses.[64] Infants can aspirate meconium into the airway by gasping, which may occur *in utero* in response to a variety of stimuli, including hypoxia, or by inhalation after delivery. Aspiration of meconium can cause pulmonary disease both by plugging of the airways and by producing a chemical pneumonitis. Clinical pulmonary disease is more likely if meconium staining occurs before the second stage of labor, if the meconium-stained fluid is thick with particulate matter, and if there is meconium below the vocal cords.[62,65] Many infants have meconium in the hypopharynx but none below the vocal cords, and disease is unlikely to develop in them. Some have no meconium in the hypopharynx but have meconium below the cords, and are at increased risk for pulmonary disease.

In some instances, asphyxia is present and requires resuscitation at birth; meconium aspiration syndrome follows immediately afterward. In other instances, infants are clinically well at birth and manifest symptoms of meconium aspiration syndrome during the first few hours after birth. Severe disease nonetheless can develop in infants with this more gradual onset of symptoms. Pulmonary air leaks are ten times as likely to develop in infants with meconium aspiration as in infants without meconium staining; the air leak often occurs during resuscitation. Pulmonary hypertension develops in some infants.[66]

Clearing thick meconium from the airway at birth reduces the risk and severity of disease. In vertex deliveries, suctioning the oropharynx after the head has been delivered, but before delivery of the shoulders, followed by prompt tracheal intubation and suctioning of the trachea once the baby is delivered, has reduced the incidence of clinical disease and reduced, but not eliminated, mortality from this disease.[62,63,67,68] These prophylactic procedures should be carried out in all cases of thick or particulate meconium. Some authors have questioned the need to intubate and suction meconium-stained infants who have Apgar scores of 9 and 10 at 1 minute and do not otherwise need resuscitation.[69] Severe and even fatal meconium aspiration syndrome, however, does develop in some of these babies who are not asphyxiated and are not intubated. Furthermore, intubation and suctioning carries very little risk when done properly.[66] The only reasonable exception to routine intubation and suctioning is the baby who struggles vigorously when laryngoscopy is attempted. An attempt to intubate such an infant is unlikely to be successful and may result in trauma to the upper airway or vomiting and aspiration of meconium-stained gastric contents.

Several measures should be taken to prepare for the delivery of a baby with meconium-stained amniotic fluid:

- Have a second person available to help with the suctioning.
- Have several endotracheal tubes available because the first tube used may become so obstructed with thick, tenacious meconium that it cannot be reused when necessary.
- Have oral suctioning ready on the resuscitation table.
- Have a manually operated meconium suction device that attaches to the endotracheal tube adapter and to a source of suction that will provide a negative pressure in the range of 80 to 120 torr.[70] This much pressure is needed to suck thick meconium through this system. The old practice of wearing a soft face mask and sucking on the endotracheal tube like a straw is unsafe and should not be used.

After delivery of the head, the obstetrician or a designated assistant should suction the oropharynx quickly while the chest is still compressed in the birth canal. Obviously, there will be cases in which this maneuver is not possible.

After the baby is delivered, do nothing that might stimulate him or her to cry or inhale. Intubate the trachea quickly. Ideally, this should be done without first suctioning the oropharynx, which often stimulates the infant to gasp. In some cases, however, large amounts of meconium in the oropharynx obstruct the view of the vocal cords so that intubation is impossible until the oropharynx is suctioned. If there is thick meconium staining but no meconium visible in the hypopharynx, it still is appropriate to intubate the trachea and suction because there may be significant amounts of meconium below the vocal cords. As soon as the endotracheal tube is inserted into the trachea, connect it to the suction apparatus, apply suction, and withdraw the tube while maintaining the suction. In many cases, meconium will not be drawn into the suction apparatus but a plug of meconium will be drawn into the tube, lodge there, and be seen only when the tube is removed. If more than a scant amount of meconium (*i.e.*, >½ mL) is obtained on the first suctioning, repeat the process until no more is seen. In some instances, there may be so much meconium in the airway that it still can be recovered after suctioning the trachea five or six times. During tracheal suctioning, a second person should monitor heart rate continuously. If significant sustained bradycardia develops, discontinue suctioning and give positive-pressure ventilation with oxygen.

After clearing the airway, proceed with resuscitation as with any other infant, paying particular attention to two problems. First, have a very high index of suspicion for a tension pneumothorax, which may occur early in the resuscitation. Second, be aware that intense pulmonary vasoconstriction is more likely to occur in these infants; when it occurs, it should be treated with more aggressive correction of metabolic acidosis than is necessary in other infants.

THE EXTREMELY-LOW-BIRTH-WEIGHT INFANT

Infants with birth weights less than 1250 g, and particularly those less than 1000 g, present a special set of problems. Hack and Fanaroff have pointed out the value of a well trained and experienced resuscitation team in the successful management of these infants.[71] One of the first problems to be faced with many of these infants is the issue of viability. This arises when the infant's birth weight and gestational age are in the range of 500 to 600 g and 23 to 24 weeks, respectively. There is understandable reluctance to subject an infant with no chance of long-term survival to hours and perhaps days of the discomfort of intensive care. It is even worse, however, initially to withhold resuscitation from an infant thought at first to be nonviable but then, because he or she continues to breathe and be vigorous, to resuscitate the infant, most likely after serious brain damage has occurred. In these borderline cases of uncertain viability, it is better to start with vigorous resuscitation. Yu and colleagues have pointed out that the infant's response to resuscitation is one of the determinants of viability.[72] This is illustrated in Figure 19-13. In such cases, it quickly will become evident that therapy is futile, so care can be withdrawn early.

The smaller the infant, the weaker the muscles of respiration and the less likely he or she will be able spontaneously to achieve adequate lung inflation and create an adequate functional residual capacity, even if the surfactant system has matured. Furthermore, lung inflation stimulates surfactant release from the type II alveolar cells.[73,74] This has led to the recommendation that all extremely-low-birth-weight infants should have their tracheas intubated at birth and have their lungs inflated. The findings of the only controlled trial of prophylactic intubation support this approach.[75] It may be that the same result can be achieved in very vigorous babies with the application of positive end-expiratory pressure.

Seriously consider prophylactic administration of surfactant to the extremely-low-birth-weight infant as soon as possible after birth unless there is evidence of a mature surfactant system.[76] Ventilation of a surfactant-deficient lung for as brief a period as 30 minutes produces the pathologic changes of hyaline membrane disease.[77] Surfactant administration is not a substitute for good resuscitation. A skillful, experienced resuscitation team often can give surfactant as a part of the initial resuscitation. If there is any question about the ability to do this, however, the initial phase of resuscitation should be completed first, then the surfactant given.

As pulmonary function improves and these smallest infants are weaned from assisted ventilation, it is important to remember that many of them cannot maintain an adequate functional residual capacity, even in the absence of lung disease, and progressive atelectasis gradually will develop unless end-expiratory distending pressure is applied to their lungs. Special attention also must be given to the inspired oxygen concentration as the infant's condition improves. The clinician's sense of time is distorted easily during a complex resuscitation and the ensuing period of recovery. What seems like minutes may be an hour or more, and failure to adjust inspired oxygen in a timely way may lead to prolonged hyperoxia.

The radiant heat required to maintain normal body temperature during resuscitation evaporates water from the infant's skin. This can produce very high insensible water losses from very premature infants. Once the endotracheal tube and catheter are in place and secured and other emergency procedures completed, cover the infant with a clear plastic wrap to reduce insensible water loss.

MULTIPLE BIRTHS

The five features of multiple births that complicate delivery room management are the following:

1. Increased incidence of preterm labor and delivery. This affects management only by increasing the number of personnel needed for resuscitation. The risk of intrapartum asphyxia is somewhat increased in the second-born of twins.
2. Increased incidence of congenital anomalies in monozygotic multiple births.

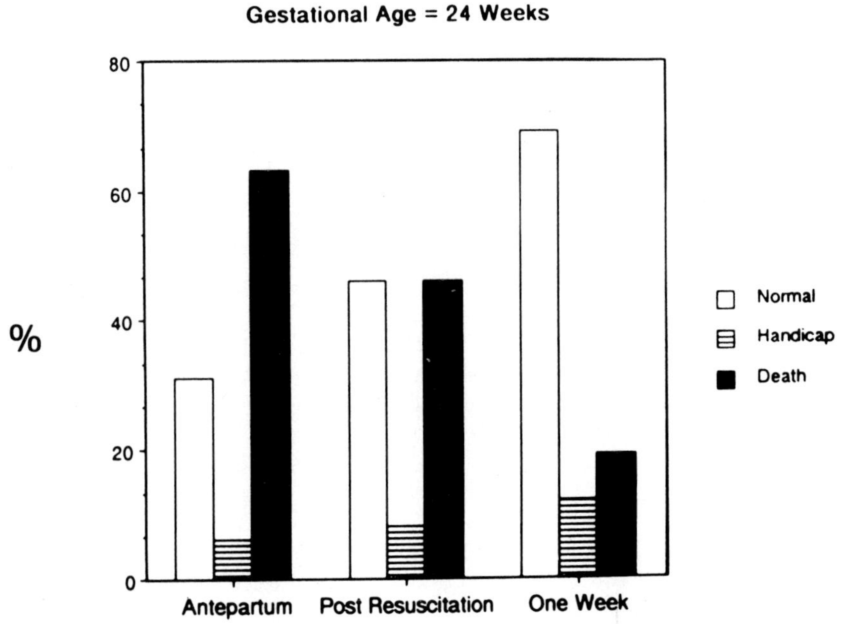

FIG. 19–13. Prognosis for infants born at an estimated 24 weeks of gestation. The prognosis is given three times: before birth, after resuscitation, and at 1 week after birth. The prognosis changes at the second and third points since it applies only to infants who survived to those points. (From Phibbs RH. Delivery room management of the extremely low birth weight infant. In: Cowett RM, Hay WW Jr, eds. The micropremie: the next frontier. Report of the 99th Ross Conference on Pediatric Research. Columbus, OH: Ross Laboratories, 1990.)

3. Increased risk of intrauterine growth retardation in one fetus in a multiple birth set because the placenta is unevenly shared. This results in the usual problems of small-for-gestational-age (SGA) infants, including intrapartum asphyxia, polycythemia, hypoglycemia, and pulmonary hemorrhage (see Chap. 26).
4. Twin-to-twin transfusion syndrome.
5. Stuck twin syndrome.

The twin-to-twin transfusion syndrome, which occurs in at least 5% of multiple pregnancies, results from vascular anastomosis between the circulations of monozygotic twins, primarily with monochorionic placentas. Both the degree of transfusion from one fetus to the other and the time course are quite variable, and determine the clinical problems at birth. Bleeding may have been relatively recent, or it may have begun in the second trimester and been longstanding at the time of birth. If the transfusion is primarily in one direction, the donor twin becomes anemic and the recipient twin polycythemic. With ongoing bleeding, the recipient grows normally while the donor becomes progressively smaller for gestational age. As the process becomes more severe, polyhydramnios develops in the recipient fetus and oligohydramnios in the donor. Ultimately, either twin may become hydropic, one from volume overload and the other from anemia. In severe cases, the donor twin may die and intravascular coagulation in the dead fetus can cause emboli that pass into the recipient's circulation. When embolization occurs, it commonly involves the brain, kidneys, and gastrointestinal tract of the recipient fetus. Recent embolization of the gastrointestinal tract may cause a bowel perforation, whereas early embolization causes an atretic area of the bowel.

When twins suffering from this syndrome are delivered, management during resuscitation may be extremely complicated. Fortunately, those responsible for the resuscitation of such babies usually are forewarned of the most severe cases. Findings in the mother should lead to close ultrasonic surveillance of the fetuses and prenatal recognition of the unidirectional twin-to-twin transfusion syndrome. The polycythemic baby needs to have his or her hematocrit reduced. Management of the anemic donor is less straightforward. Recent acute blood loss requires the same management as in any other hypovolemic baby. More often, the anemia has been prolonged and severe, so the donor's circulation may be compromised and may not tolerate blood volume expansion. In this case, the proper therapy is partial exchange transfusion with packed cells to raise the hematocrit to a normal level. Both arterial and central venous pressures should be monitored beginning immediately after birth (see Hydrops) to assess the circulatory status and make the correct adjustments in both hematocrit and intravascular volume. Have packed erythrocytes that are cross matched against the mother available in the resuscitation area. Rapidly measure hematocrit or hemoglobin in each twin and begin the appropriate therapy.

In monochorionic twins, the vascular anastomoses may be multidirectional so that the direction of flow is determined at least in part by the differences in circulatory resistance between the twins. Such twin-to-twin transfusions are not diagnosed so easily, nor are the hemoglobin measurements necessarily different at birth even when the blood volumes are.

The stuck twin syndrome is a poorly understood phenomenon thought to occur only in monochorionic twins. There is discordant growth with oligohydramnios in the SGA fetus and polyhydramnios in the appropriate-for-gestational-age fetus. The SGA fetus becomes compacted into a small volume within the uterus. Lung growth often is restricted, which leads to pulmonary hypoplasia that is lethal if severe. If mild, it requires positive-pressure ventilation at high pressures and rates. There usually are placental vascular anastomoses between the placentas, suggesting that this is a complication of the twin-to-twin transfusion syndrome. The hematocrits, however, often are nearly normal and similar in both twins. Preparations for delivery are the same as for the twin-to-twin transfusion syndrome.

BIRTH INJURY

Severe birth injury and intrapartum asphyxia often occur together. The main problem for delivery room management of these infants is significant hemorrhage from the traumatized tissues, which complicates the resuscitation (see Phase II). The blood loss almost always is internal, and therefore not immediately evident. Moderate blood loss can occur in fractured limbs or into the perineum in a difficult breech delivery. Sites for major blood loss include intracranial, mediastinal, and intraabdominal (*e.g.*, ruptured spleen, hepatic subcapsular hematoma). A subgaleal hematoma can produce a massive loss of blood volume because of the extremely large potential space. Any of these hematomas can contain several hundred milliliters of blood and are particularly dangerous because they can consume large quantities of coagulation factors and lead to generalized bleeding that perpetuates the hypovolemia. In severe cases, only early and extremely aggressive therapy can bring the situation under control. Treatment includes replacement of the lost blood volume and erythrocyte mass and, if there is depletion of clotting factors, very aggressive replacement of these factors with fresh frozen plasma, platelets and, on occasion, cryoprecipitate.

Early detection of internal hemorrhage from birth trauma is crucial. Abdominal distention and discoloration suggest intraabdominal bleeding, which easily is confirmed by aspiration of a small amount of blood from the peritoneal cavity. Control of intraabdominal bleeding may require surgery. Intracranial hemorrhage sufficient to cause hypovolemia usually is manifested by a bulging fontanelle and can be confirmed quickly by ultrasonography. Small intracranial hemorrhages also may cause circulatory instability through their effects on the autonomic nervous system. A mediastinal hematoma does not declare itself by any physical sign, but a chest radiograph often suggests its presence when the mediastinum is widened; if suspected, it can be diagnosed quickly by an ultrasound examination of the mediastinum. Early swelling of the back of the neck from a subgaleal hematoma may be hard to recognize, but an expanding subgaleal hemorrhage pushes the ears laterally and forward. This often is the earliest sign of this condition. Subgaleal hemorrhage, too, can be confirmed by ultrasound.

HYDROPS

Hydropic babies present a challenging set of problems for resuscitation. Usually, abnormal findings in the mother of a fetus with hydrops lead to an ultrasound diagnosis before delivery. Every effort should be made to establish the cause of the hydrops before delivery to help with preparations for managing the infant at birth. An ultrasound examination should be done or repeated just before delivery to assess the presence and size of pleural effusions. Assessment of fetal blood by percutaneous umbilical sampling is especially helpful for early management whenever feasible. Have whole blood or packed erythrocytes cross matched against the mother in the resuscitation area, even if the hydrops is not due to Rh disease or other alloimmune hemolysis, because many infants with nonimmune hydrops also are anemic at birth. More personnel are needed for management of these infants than for a routine resuscitation. One member of the resuscitation team should be prepared to perform paracentesis and thoracentesis as needed. The supplies needed for partial exchange transfusion and for paracentesis, plus specimen tubes for diagnostic studies, must be on hand. Two umbilical vessel catheters should be connected to pressure transducers and a recorder with one channel calibrated for arterial pressure and the other for venous pressure. There must be equipment for measuring hematocrit or hemoglobin near the resuscitation area, and someone should have the specific assignment of obtaining blood from the umbilical cord at birth and immediately making this measurement by 5 minutes after birth.

Lung inflation and ventilation often are difficult in hydropic infants because the lungs are compressed by the diaphragm, which is elevated by ascites and by large pleural effusions. There also is low compliance due to excessive lung water. Resuscitation usually requires tracheal intubation and ventilation with oxygen at high pressures. If the abdomen is distended with ascites, perform a paracentesis in the flank region to avoid puncturing a large liver or spleen. It is necessary to remove only enough fluid so that the abdomen is soft and the diaphragms move easily with inflation. If ventilation remains difficult and there are pleural effusions, these too should be reduced to allow ventilation. Even after fluid is removed from the abdomen and chest, many of these babies continue to require high pressures to provide adequate ventilation because of excess lung water, surfactant deficiency, and, in some cases of long-standing hydrops, pulmonary hypoplasia.[78]

While the baby is being ventilated and the effusions are being reduced, catheterize the umbilical artery and vein and measure blood gas tensions and *p*H and intravascular pressures to assess the state of the circulation. Anemia compromises tissue oxygenation and anemic hydropic infants usually do not respond well to resuscitative measures until their hematocrit is at least 30% to 35%.[79] Transfused blood is virtually 100% hemoglobin A, which transports oxygen much more efficiently after birth than hemoglobin F. How the anemia is corrected depends on the state of the circulation. Most infants with hydrops due to alloimmune disease have low or normal blood volumes.[80] The blood volumes of infants with nonimmune hydrops of various causes are unpredictable. If intravascular pressures indicate that blood volume is adequate, do a partial exchange transfusion and keep blood volume constant. If there is evidence of hypovolemia, infuse more blood than is withdrawn until intravascular pressures are normal. Alternately, infuse a bolus of packed erythrocytes, as is done for the treatment of hypovolemic shock. In most cases, evidence of hypovolemia does not appear until the asphyxia is relieved.[79] The most common sequence is a partial-exchange transfusion that keeps blood volume constant while raising hematocrit, and then repeated small infusions of packed erythrocytes and albumin or fresh frozen plasma to support the circulation. Do not give the plasma or albumin until the anemia is corrected. Fresh frozen plasma also partially corrects the hemostatic defects that often are present.[81] Most infants with alloimmune hydrops have very low concentrations of serum albumin and low plasma colloid osmotic pressures.[80,82] About one-half of those with nonimmune hydrops also are hypoalbuminemic. There has been concern that giving albumin and fresh frozen plasma to these infants during resuscitation would raise plasma colloid osmotic pressure enough to draw excessive volumes of fluid into the circulation and worsen pulmonary edema. In practice, however, this rarely occurs, and if it does, it can be managed by appropriate adjustments in assisted ventilation. Pulmonary vasoconstriction, which may occur in any asphyxiated infant, is particularly common in hydropic infants.[79,83] Therefore, if pulmonary perfusion has not improved after the initial steps in resuscitation, correct metabolic acidosis with alkali therapy. After resuscitation is complete, there usually is residual pulmonary disease that requires assisted ventilation. This may be transient respiratory distress, hyaline membrane disease, pulmonary hypoplasia, or some combination of these. Diuresis will improve lung function, and therapy with furosemide often is helpful.

REFERENCES

1. Torrance S, Wittnich C. The effect of varying arterial oxygen tension on neonatal acid-base balance. Pediatr Res 1992;31:112.
2. James LS, Weisbrot IM, Prince CE, et al. The acid-base status of human infants in relation to birth asphyxia and onset of respiration. J Pediatr 1958;52:379.
3. Yeomans ER, Hauth JC, Gilstrap LC, et al. Umbilical cord pH, PCO_2, and bicarbonate following uncomplicated term vaginal deliveries. Am J Obstet Gynecol 1985;151:798.
4. Rudolph CD, Roman C, Rudolph AM. Effect of acute umbilical cord compression on hepatic carbohydrate metabolism in the fetal lamb. Pediatr Res 1989;25:228.
5. Ruth V, Fyhrquist F, Clemons G, et al. Cord plasma vasopressin, erythropoietin and hypoxanthine as indices of asphyxia at birth. Pediatr Res 1988;24:490.
6. Dawes G. Fetal and neonatal physiology. Chicago: Year Book, 1968.
7. Cohn HE, Sacks FJ, Heymann MA, et al. Cardiovascular responses to hypokalemia and acidemia in fetal lambs. Am J Obstet Gynecol 1974;120:817.
8. Fisher DJ. Increased regional myocardial blood flows and oxygen deliveries during hypoxemia in lambs. Pediatr Res 1984; 18:602.
9. Boyle DW, Host K, Zerbe GO, et al. Fetal hind limb oxygen consumption and blood flow during acute graded hypoxia. Pediatr Res 1990;28:94.
10. Rudolph AM, Yuan S. Response of the pulmonary vasculature of hypoxia and H^+ ion concentration changes. J Clin Invest 1966;45:339.
11. Parer JT. The effect of acute maternal hypoxia on fetal oxygenation and the umbilical circulation in the sheep. Eur J Obstet Gynecol Reprod Biol 1980;10:125.
12. Fisher DJ. Acidemia reduces cardiac output and left ventricular contractility in conscious lambs. J Dev Physiol 1986;8:23.
13. Downing SE, Talner NS, Gardner TH. Influences of hypoxemia and acidemia on left ventricular function. Am J Physiol 1966;210:1327.
14. Itskovitz J, LaGamma EF, Bristow J, et al. Cardiovascular responses to hypoxemia in sinoaortic-denervated fetal sheep. Pediatr Res 1991;30:381.
15. Jones CT, Roebuck MM, Walker DW, et al. The role of the adrenal medulla and peripheral sympathetic nerves in the physiological responses of the fetal sheep to hypoxia. J Dev Physiol 1988;10:17.
16. Cheung CY, Brace RA. Fetal hypoxia elevates plasma atrial natriuretic factor concentration. Am J Obstet Gynecol 1988; 159:1263.
17. Fisher DJ. β-Adrenergic influence on increased myocardial oxygen consumption during hypoxemia in awake newborn lambs. Pediatr Res 1989;25:585.
18. Slotkin TA, Seidler FJ. Adrenomedullary catecholamine release in the fetus and newborn: secretory mechanisms and their role in stress and survival. J Dev Physiol 1988;10:1.
19. Perez R, Espinoza M, Riqueline R, et al. Arginine vasopressin mediates cardiovascular responses to hypoxia in fetal sheep. Am J Physiol 1989;256:R1011.
20. Linderkamp O, Versmold HT, Messow-Zahn K, et al. The effects of intrapartum and intrauterine asphyxia on placental transfusion in premature and full-term infants. Eur J Pediatr 1978;127:91.
21. Diana JN, Laughlin MH. Effect of ischemia on capillary pressure and equivalent pore radius in capillaries of the isolated dog hind limb. Circulation Res 1974;35:77.
22. Bucciarelli RL, Nelson RM, Egen EA, et al. Transient tricuspid insufficiency of the newborn: a form of myocardial dysfunction in stressed newborn. Pediatrics 1977;59:330.
23. Longstrath WJ Jr, Kwon JM, Zelenock GB, et al. Infusion of five percent dextrose increases mortality and morbidity following six minutes of cardiac arrest in resuscitated dogs. J Clin Care 1987;2:4.
24. Venkataraman PS, Tsang RC, Chen IW, et al. Pathogenesis of early neonatal hypocalcemia; studies of serum gastrin and plasma glucagon. J Pediatr 1987;110:599.
25. Kitterman JA, Phibbs RH, Tooley WH. Catheterization of umbilical vessels in newborn infants. Pediatr Clin North Am 1970;17:895.
26. Apgar V. A proposal for a new method of evaluation of the newborn infant. Anesth Analg 1953;32:260.
27. Sykes GS, Molloy PM, Johnson P, et al. Do Apgar scores indicate asphyxia? Lancet 1982;1:494.
28. Martin M, Paes BA. Birth asphyxia: does the Apgar score have diagnostic value. Obstet Gynecol 1989;72:120.
29. Meyer BA, Dickinson JE, Chambers C, et al. The effect of fetal sepsis on umbilical cord blood gases. Am J Obstet Gynecol 1992;166:2.
30. Catlin EA, Carpenter MW, Brann BS, et al. The Apgar score revisited: influence of gestational age. J Pediatr 1986;109:865.
31. Dahn LS, James LS. Newborn temperature and calculated heat loss in the delivery room. Pediatrics 1972;49:504.
32. Vyas H, Milner AD, Hopkin IE, et al. Physiologic responses to prolonged and slow-rise inflation in the resuscitation of the asphyxiated newborn infant. J Pediatr 1981;99:635.
33. Moya F, James L, Burnard L, et al. Cardiac massage in the newborn infant through the intact chest. Am J Obstet Gynecol 1962;84:798.
34. Lindemann R. Resuscitation of the newborn with endotracheal administration of epinephrine. Acta Paediatr Scand 1984; 73:210.
35. Downing ES, Campbell AGN, Racamora JM, et al. Influences of hypercapnia on cardiac function in the newborn lamb. Yale J Biol Med 1971;43:242.
36. Effron MB, Guarnieri T, Frederisken JW, et al. Effect of tris (hydroxymethyl) aminomethane on ischemic myocardium. Am J Physiol 1978;235:H167.
37. Chu J, Clements JA, Cotton E, et al. Pulmonary hypoperfusion syndrome. Pediatrics 1965;35:733.
38. Lewis AB, Heymann MA, Rudolph RA. Gestational changes in pulmonary vascular responses in fetal lambs in utero. Circ Res 1976;39:536.
39. Schreiber MD, Heymann MA, Soifer SJ. Increased arterial pH, not decreased $PaCO_2$, attenuates hypoxia-induced pulmonary vaso-constriction in newborn lambs. Pediatr Res 1986;20:113.
40. Wiklund L, Larsoquist, Skoog G, et al. Clinical buffering of metabolic acidosis: problems and a solution. Resuscitation 1985;279.
41. Wyatt JS, Edwards AD, Cape M, et al. Response of cerebral blood volume to changes in arterial carbon dioxide tension in preterm and term infants. Pediatrics 1991;29:553.
42. Kruyswijk H, Jansen BH, Muller EJ. Hyperventilation-induced coronary artery spasm. Am Heart J 1986;112:613.
43. Case RB, Felix A, Wachter M, et al. Relative effect of CO_2 on canine coronary vascular resistance. Circ Research 1978;42:410.
44. Ogata ES, Kitterman JA, Gregory GA, et al. Pneumothorax in idiopathic respiratory distress syndrome (IRDS): incidence and effect on vital signs, blood gases and pH. Pediatrics 1976; 58:177.

45. Morin F, Sola A, Brown C, et al. Hypoxia disrupts the newborn lamb's response to hemorrhage. Pediatr Res 1981;15:673.
46. Phibbs RH, Clements JA, Creasy RK, et al. Lung maturity, intrauterine growth, neonatal asphyxia and shock and the risk of hyaline membrane disease. Pediatr Res 1976;10:451.
47. Dale HH, Evans CL. Effects on the circulation of changes in carbon dioxide content of the blood. J Physiol 1922;56:125.
48. Sola A, Spitzer AR, Morin FC, et al. Effects of arterial carbon dioxide tension on the newborn lamb's cardiovascular responses to rapid hemorrhage. Pediatr Res 1983;17:70.
49. Meyers RL, Paulick RP, Rudolph CD, et al. Cardiovascular responses to acute, severe haemorrhage in fetal sheep. J Dev Physiol 1991;15:189.
50. Weil MH, Rackrow EC, Trevino R, et al. Difference in acid base state between venous and arterial blood during cardiopulmonary resuscitation. N Engl J Med 1986;315:153.
51. Paxton CL. Neonatal shock in the first postnatal day. Am J Dis Child 1978;132:509.
52. Perlman JM, Track ED. Renal injury in the asphyxiated newborn infant: relationship to neurologic outcome. J Pediatr 1988;113:875
53. Desmond MM, Kay JL, Megarity AL. The phases of transitional distress occurring in neonates in association with prolonged postnatal umbilical cord pulsations. J Pediatr 1959;55:131.
54. Thibeault DW, Hall TK, Sheehan MB, et al. Post-asphyxial lung disease in newborn infants with severe perinatal acidosis. Am J Obstet Gynecol 1984;150:393.
55. Segerer H, Stevens P, Schadow B, et al. Surfactant substitution in ventilated very low birthweight infants: factors related to response types. Pediatr Res 1991;30:6.
56. U.S. EXOSURF Pediatric Study Group. Effects of EXOSURF on infants with occult congenital pneumonia. Pediatr Res 1990;27:288A.
57. Burnard ED, James LS. Failure of the heart after undue asphyxia at birth. Pediatrics 1961;28:545.
58. Cabal LA, Devaskar U, Siassi B, et al. Cardiogenic shock associated with perinatal asphyxia in preterm infants. J Pediatr 1980;96:705.
59. Walther FJ, Siassi B, Ramadan NA, et al. Cardiac output in newborn infants with transient myocardial dysfunction. J Pediatr 1985;107:781.
60. Danial SS, Husain MK, Milliex J, et al. Renal response of fetal lamb to complete occlusion of umbilical cord. Am J Obstet Gynecol 1978;131:514.
61. Crissinger KD, Granger DN. Intestinal blood flow and oxygen consumption: responses to hemorrhage in the developing piglet. Pediatr Res 1989;2:102.
62. Gregory GA, Gooding C, Phibbs RH, et al. Meconium aspiration in infants: a prospective study. J Pediatr 1974;85:848.
63. Wiswell TE, Tuggle JM, Turner BS. Meconium aspiration syndrome: have we made a difference? Pediatrics 1990;85:5.
64. Matthews TG, Warshaw JB. Relevance of the gestational age distribution of meconium passage in utero. Pediatrics 1979;64:1.
65. Meis PJ, Hall M, Marshall JR, et al. Meconium passage: a new classification for risk assessment during labor. Am J Obstet Gynecol 1978;130:509.
66. Wiswell TE, Henley MA. Intratracheal suctioning, systemic infection, and the meconium aspiration syndrome. Pediatrics 1992;89:2.
67. Carson BS, Lasey BW, Bowes WA, et al. Combined obstetric and pediatric approach to prevent meconium aspiration syndrome. Am J Obstet Gynecol 1976;126:712.
68. Davis RO, Phillips JB, Harris BA, et al. Fatal meconium aspiration syndrome occurring despite airway management considered appropriate. Am J Obstet Gynecol 1985;151:731.
69. Linder N, Aranda JV, Tsur M, et al. Need for endotracheal intubation and suction in meconium stained neonates. J Pediatr 1988;112:613.
70. Kretlow RA. Handpowered apparatus for aspiration of meconium from the trachea. Pediatr 1987;70:642.
71. Hack M, Fanaroff AA. Changes in the delivery room care of the extremely small infant (less than 750 g): effects on morbidity and outcome. N Engl J Med 1986;314:660.
72. Yu VH, Lake HL, Bajuk B, et al. Prognosis for infants born at 23 to 28 weeks gestation. Br Med J 1986;293:1200.
73. Corbet A, Cregan J, Frink J. Distension-produced phospholipid secretion in postmortem in situ lungs of newborn rabbits. Am Rev Respir Dis 1983;128:695.
74. Massaro GD, Massaro D. Morphologic evidence that large inflations of the lung stimulate secretion of surfactant. Annual Review of Respiratory Disease [Am] 1983;127:235.
75. Drew JH. Immediate intubation at birth of the very low birth weight infant: effect on survival. Am J Dis Child 1982;136:207.
76. Kendig JW, Notter RH, Cox C, et al. A comparison of surfactant as immediate prophylaxis and as rescue therapy in newborns of less than 30 weeks gestation. N Engl J Med 1991;324:865.
77. Nilsson R, Grossman G, Robertson B. Lung surfactant and the pathogenesis of neonatal bronchiolar lesions induced by artificial ventilation. Pediatr Res 1978;12:249.
78. Chamberlain D, Hislop A, Hey E, et al. Pulmonary hypoplasia in babies with severe rhesus isoimmunization: a quantitative study. J Pathol 1977;122:43.
79. Phibbs RH, Johnson P, Kitterman JA, et al. Cardiorespiratory status of erythroblastotic newborn infants: III. Intravascular pressures during the first hours of life. Pediatrics 1976;58:484.
80. Phibbs RH, Johnson P, Tooley WH. Cardiorespiratory status of erythroblastotic newborn infants: II. Blood volume hematocrit and serum albumin concentrations in relation to hydrops fetalis. Pediatrics 1974;53:13.
81. Hey E, Jones P. Coagulation failure in babies with rhesus isoimmunization. Br J Haematol 1979;42:441.
82. Baum JD, Harris D. Colloid osmotic pressure in erythroblastosis fetalis. Br Med J 1972;1:601.
83. Phibbs RH, Johnson P, Kitterman JA, et al. Cardiorespiratory status of erythroblastotic infants: I. Relationship of gestational age, severity of hemolytic disease and birth asphyxia to idiopathic respiratory distress syndrome and survival. Pediatrics 1972;49:5.

Neonatology: Pathophysiology and Management of the Newborn, Fourth Edition,
edited by Gordon B. Avery, Mary Ann Fletcher, and Mhairi G. MacDonald.
J.B. Lippincott Company, Philadelphia © 1994.

chapter 20

Physical Assessment and Classification

MARY ANN FLETCHER

Physical assessment in neonates has two purposes. First, it is the unique process of determining anatomic normality for the first time in a new life. Second, it is the process of determining the state of health. Because many of the signs of normal transition mimic those of early disease, differentiating the markers of subtle illness from normal transitional variations is one of the more challenging aspects of neonatal physical diagnosis.

The first documentation of a neonatal examination occurs immediately after birth in the assigning of Apgar scores, which are actually encapsulated assessments of the cardiopulmonary and neurologic systems after inspection for color, heart rate, respiratory efforts, tone, and muscle activity. A cursory examination that includes designation of gender and inspection for major anomalies is an important part of all resuscitations. Any obvious abnormality merits more immediate evaluation, but the definitive examination in healthy infants should be completed after transition.

If an infant is discharged before resolution of jaundice or cardiovascular transition, reexamination during an early outpatient visit is indicated. During the first outpatient visit, the physician should fully reevaluate the infant, especially the systems not easily assessed during the first 2 days after birth.

NEWBORN HISTORY

It is tempting to start the physical examination of neonates before reviewing the histories and available laboratory information, especially if a parental historian is not at the bedside. A critical care situation may require the physician to initiate therapy and obtain a clinical response before completing the history and examination. Nonetheless, historic information is just as significant for neonates as it is for any other patient. Even if it is more practical to do the examination before the history, it is imperative to include all information in each newborn evaluation.

There are several elements of a newborn infant's history: maternal history, family history, the neonatal course, and placental examination.

Maternal history includes gravidity, parity, previous fetal losses; maternal illness before or during pregnancy; extent and location of prenatal care; labor and delivery history, including duration, assessments of fetal well-being, anesthesia, and route of delivery; drug, alcohol, and tobacco use; medication use; and vocation.

The family history includes current or significant medical illnesses in other family members, including siblings; physical traits or appearance, including birth weights of other siblings; consanguinity; social information, educational levels, vocations; and ethnic or racial background.

In determining the neonatal history, the examiner should document delivery room events; Apgar scores and resuscitation; and vital signs, feeding, and behavior since birth.

The placental examination, often more overlooked than history in evaluating neonates, provides crucial information about the gestation. Despite the fact that it may hold clues to diagnosis, the placental examination is too often an afterthought unless habit includes it as part of the available data for all deliveries. Several features of the placenta and cord should be assessed during gross examination at the time of delivery:

Placenta
- Size: ratio of fresh placental weight to infant weight is normally 1:6 in the last trimester; the placenta should have a uniform thickness throughout—depressions may be from abruption or infarction
- Color: pallor or plethora indicate fetal blood volume or hemoglobin status; staining by meconium or blood through the membranes or of the cord is of longer duration than if only superficial; cloudiness of fetal membranes; nodules on amnion indicate prolonged, extreme oligohydramnios and pulmonary hypoplasia; adherent clot suggests abruption
- Odor: essentially odorless except for slight odor of fresh blood; odor may indicate an infection
- Number of fetal membranes in multiple gestations

Cord
- Appearance: insertion site, intact, number of vessels, and pearly ivory color
- Length: normally 30 to 100 cm; shorter length suggests decreased fetal movement, often associated with failed or abnormal descent; a longer cord makes entanglement or prolapse more likely
- Diameter: at term, about 1.5 cm; relatively uniform throughout without strictures; firm Wharton jelly, with compression indicated by a thin cord.

GESTATIONAL AGE ASSESSMENT

For standard reporting of reproductive health statistics and as a prerequisite to determining normality, all infants should be classified by gestational age and birth weight.[1] Ultrasonography has improved accuracy of pregnancy dating, but discrepancies demand further evaluation. If there has been no prenatal care, physical assessment can help establish the gestational age.

There is recurring misuse of the terms preterm and post-term. A term infant is any infant whose birth occurs from the beginning of the first day of week 38 through the end of the last day of week 42 after the onset of the last menstrual period (*i.e.*, 260–294 days of gestation). A preterm infant is one born before 37 completed weeks (*i.e.*, before 260 days), and a post-term infant is one whose birth occurs from the beginning of the first day of week 43 (*i.e.*, after 294 days). Classifying infants born at term, preterm, or post-term helps to establish the level of risk for neonatal morbidity and long-term developmental problems.

ASSESSMENT TECHNIQUES

Estimation of gestational age by physical examination is possible because there is a predictable pattern of physical changes occurring throughout gestation. The most popular score for gestational age assessment was originally developed in part by Saint-Anne-Dargassies,[2] Amiel-Tison,[3] and Dubowitz;[4] it was then modified by Ballard.[5] Compared with reliable ultrasound dates, the earlier Ballard system tended to overestimate the age of premature infants and underestimate the age of post-term infants.[6] It was particularly inaccurate in very-low-birth-weight (VLBW) infants with a deviation of over 2 weeks.[7] Further modifications of the original scoring produced the New Ballard Score (NBS), which extended the range and accuracy of age assessment to within 1 week, decreasing many of the earlier problems (Fig. 20-1). Precision requires experience and consideration of the infant's history and condition in scoring. Examination as soon as possible after initial stabilization or by 12 hours increases the accuracy in gestations shorter than 38 weeks. The use of NBS is particularly attractive for neonates who are immature and instrumented, because it does not require lifting the infant. Although described separately from other components of the examination, the steps for assessing gestational age are done as part of the general physical examination and comprise a good portion of the neurologic evaluation.

NEUROMUSCULAR MATURITY

The resting posture, which is the posture assumed by an unrestrained, healthy infant, reflects a progressive increase in tone and flexion in a caudocephalad direction to a fully flexed pattern at term (see Fig. 20-1).

The square window is assessed by flexing the wrist and measuring the minimal angle between the palm and flexor surface of the forearm. The angle decreases with advancing gestational age. Conditions of marked intrauterine compression, such as severe oligohydramnios, increase wrist flexion. If an infant is born prematurely, he will not continue to develop as much wrist flexion after birth as he would had he stayed *in utero*.

The scarf sign, indicative of shoulder and superior axial tone, is assessed by pulling the hand across the chest to encircle the neck as a scarf and observing the position of the elbow in relation to the midline. There is decreased range and a higher score if there is marked obesity, chest wall edema, a fractured clavicle, an abnormally shortened humerus, or shoulder girdle hypertonicity. A brachial plexus injury produces a spuriously low score because of abnormally low muscle tone.

With the infant supine and head midline, arm recoil is assessed by first flexing the elbow and holding the arm against the forearm for 2 to 5 seconds. The elbow is then fully extended and released with observation of the time it takes for the infant to resume a

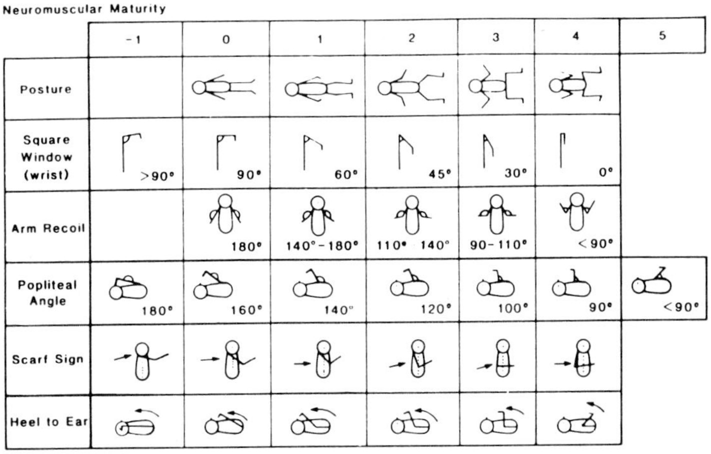

Physical Maturity

Skin	sticky friable transparent	gelatinous red, translucent	smooth pink, visible veins	superficial peeling &/or rash. few veins	cracking pale areas rare veins	parchment deep cracking no vessels	leathery cracked wrinkled
Lanugo	none	sparse	abundant	thinning	bald areas	mostly bald	
Plantar Surface	heel-toe 40-50 mm: -1 <40 mm: -2	>50mm no crease	faint red marks	anterior transverse crease only	creases ant. 2/3	creases over entire sole	
Breast	imperceptible	barely perceptible	flat areola no bud	stippled areola 1-2mm bud	raised areola 3-4mm bud	full areola 5-10mm bud	
Eye/Ear	lids fused loosely:-1 tightly:-2	lids open pinna flat stays folded	sl. curved pinna; soft; slow recoil	well-curved pinna; soft but ready recoil	formed & firm instant recoil	thick cartilage ear stiff	
Genitals male	scrotum flat, smooth	scrotum empty faint rugae	testes in upper canal rare rugae	testes descending few rugae	testes down good rugae	testes pendulous deep rugae	
Genitals female	clitoris prominent labia flat	prominent clitoris small labia minora	prominent clitoris enlarging minora	majora & minora equally prominent	majora large minora small	majora cover clitoris & minora	

Maturity Rating

score	weeks
-10	20
-5	22
0	24
5	26
10	28
15	30
20	32
25	34
30	36
35	38
40	40
45	42
50	44

FIG. 20–1. Assessment of maturity by the expanded Ballard Score. (From Ballard JL, Khoury JC, Wedig K, et al. New Ballard Score, expanded to include extremely premature infants. J Pediatr 1991; 119;418.)

flexed posture. Assessing recoil should not be done as part of testing traction or with a forceful extension as other responses may interfere with a normal reaction time. Any pathology affecting the motor strength of the arm will decrease this score as would a fetal position of fixed arm extension.

To determine the popliteal angle one should first flex the hips with the thighs along side the abdomen rather than against it. With the hips held in flexion, the knee is then extended as far as possible to estimate the popliteal angle. If an infant was a frank breech with legs extended, the popliteal angle will be greater than expected for age.

In the heel to ear maneuver, the legs are held together and pressed as far as possible toward the ears without lifting the pelvis from the table. The angle made by an arc from the back of the heel to the table decreases with maturity as long as the lower extremities were flexed in utero.

PHYSICAL MATURITY

As the skin develops, it gets progressively thicker, keratinized, and opaque so gestational age assessment depends on estimating how visible are the underlying vessels on the abdominal wall and how much cracking is present.

Lanugo, which is the fine hair evenly distributed over the body, first emerges at 19 to 20 weeks but for a few weeks is not readily apparent. Maximally apparent at 27 to 28 weeks, lanugo sheds first from the areas of greatest contact. Lanugo is distinct from the more pigmented body hair that may be quite prominent in infants of medium to dark complexion.

Assessment of the plantar surface includes measuring the foot as its length reliably corresponds to early gestational ages (see Chap. 10). With muscle activity and uterine compression, creases develop in the sole, progressing from the toes toward the heel. Inappropriate sole creasing is seen in infants with serious neuromotor deficit in the lower extremities (*e.g.*, decreased or deep vertical creasing) or with oligohydramnios (*e.g.*, increased creasing).

The breast develops with an increase in color and stippling of the areola and increase in the size of the breast tissue. Although the volume of the breast somewhat depends on nutrition and fat deposition, areolar development does not.

Ear cartilage becomes firmer with gestation if there is no continuous, extrinsic pressure and the auricular muscles have normal anatomy and activity. Unfusing of the eyelids can occur over several weeks, and a fused condition by itself is not a sign of extreme, nonviable immaturity. Opening starts by 22 weeks; complete unfusing is evident by 28 weeks.[5] The vessels in the anterior vascular capsule of the lens mature in a predictable enough pattern in the last trimester of gestation to augment assessment of gestational age between 27 and 34 weeks, but this method has a 2-week margin of error, 1 week greater than the NBS.[8]

Maturity of the external genitalia is one of the more reliable individual indicators of gestational age.[5] Due to timed descent in the third trimester, testicular progress through the canal into the scrotum is a gestational age marker. For the scrotum to develop fully into a pendulous, ruggated, term appearance, there has to have been testicular descension at some time, even if the sac is empty at the time of birth. The appearance of term female genitalia depends on fat deposition and is abnormally immature in a poorly nourished infant. Because the clitoris assumes its full size well before there is sufficient fat deposition to plump the surrounding structures, it often falsely appears hypertrophied in immature females.

INFLUENCES ON AGE ASSESSMENT RESULTS

If there is a discrepancy between expected and achieved scores, factors that influence the demonstrated findings should be sought before assigning gestational age. There is no significant difference among races in the dating scores other than what can be explained by individual variation.[9,10]

Resting posture reflects progressive flexion into the position assumed when a term fetus occupies virtually all available intrauterine space and is no longer in a freely floating state. To minimize the volume occupied, this flexion logically progresses in a caudal to cephalic sequence. Compression from oligohydramnios accelerates flexion; it gives an artificially advanced estimate of maturity. Conversely, poor fetal motor activity over a long period spuriously decreases estimated age. Fetuses with markedly decreased motor activity, poor swallowing, and polyhydramnios have decreased plantar and palmar horizontal creasing and inappropriately immature posturing. Any condition affecting the position or activity of the lower extremities, such as frank breech presentation with hyperextended knees or myelomeningocele with paresis, leads to an aberrantly lowered neuromotor score. Similarly, an infant who is hypotonic from illness or sedation has less flexion than normal for her true gestational age.

The uterine environment has less effect on the physical characteristics than on the neuromotor score.[9] Some physical maturity characteristics are affected by nutritional status (*e.g.*, amount of fat in breast tissue and in female genitalia). Ear recoil is decreased by compression.

GROWTH

MEASUREMENT TECHNIQUES

Infants weighing less than 2500 g are low birth weight regardless of gestational age. Very low birth weight refers to a weight less than 1500 g, and extremely low birth weight indicates an infant weighing less than 1000 g. Classification by these weight groups helps establish level of risk for neonatal and long-term morbidity and mortality.[11]

Of all measurements, crown–heel length is the most subject to variability, because it depends on achieving full extension of an infant who is more comfortable in flexion. The measurement is performed with the infant supine, the neck neutral, the leg fully extended, the ankle flexed. Deviation from an expected norm suggests remeasurement as a first step in evaluation.

If a crown–heel length falls below the percentiles for weight and head circumference, measuring the crown–rump length establishes leg and trunk proportionality, which may be abnormal in congenital dwarfisms. When anomalies of the lower extremities make crown–heel length implausible, the crown–rump measurement may be feasible. Crown–rump length is measured with the infant supine and the hips flexed 90°. Standards for separate lengths of upper and lower limbs are available.[12,13]

The head circumference is the largest dimension around the head obtained with a tape placed snugly above the ears; this is the occipital frontal circumference (OFC). Minor changes in head circumference occur over the first week after birth as scalp edema and molding resolve. If there is marked molding due to breech positions, the OFC may be as much as 2 cm higher than after molding resolves.

The OFC predictably falls on the same percentile curve as the length. If the OFC differs from length by more than one quartile, the cause should be sought, because head size in part reflects brain growth. The most frequent reason for a head percentile to exceed that of length is familial; the head circumference follows a persistently higher but consistent growth curve. In contrast, pathologic macrocephaly tends to cross to higher percentile curves as it progresses. A decreased rate of head growth, manifested by a flat curve or by dropping to a lower percentile, may indicate poor brain growth, atrophy, or premature cranial synostosis. The head circumference exceeds the abdominal circumference until 32 weeks. Between 32 and 36 weeks, the two circumferences are equivalent, and after 36 weeks, the abdominal circumference normally is greater.

INTERPRETATION OF GROWTH PARAMETERS

Interpretation of growth parameters requires plotting the measurements on percentile charts constructed from a similar race and environmental population. If birth weight falls between the 10th and 90th percentiles for a given gestational age, the infant is appropriate for gestational age; if less than the 10th percentile (>2 SD), the infant is small for gestational age (SGA); and if above the 90th percentile, the infant is large for gestational age (LGA). Some literature cites the 3rd and 95th percentiles (>3 SD) as outer limits, but for most clinical purposes, this broader range underselects for some at-risk infants. Accuracy in gestational age assessment is critical in determining if a weight is appropriate. Appropriate-for-gestational-age infants born at term are at lowest risk for problems associated with neonatal mortality and morbidity.[11]

If the three parameters of weight, length, and head circumference fall on the same curve, the infant is symmetric. He is asymmetric if the parameters are on different curves, usually with the weight lower. If an infant has either a slowing of intrauterine growth rate documented by serial fetal sonography or a presumed slowing by very low weight for length measurements, he or she is classified as having intrauterine growth retardation (IUGR). An infant can be IUGR without being SGA.

Infants who are SGA, IUGR, or LGA are at risk for perinatal and long-term problems. The problems encountered by SGA or IUGR infants are discussed in Chapter 26. The specific problems of infants of diabetic mothers are discussed in Chapter 35; however, several of the problems encountered by LGA infants include the following:

- Iatrogenic prematurity due to overestimation of gestational age by late size estimates
- Increased requirement for delivery by cesarean section
- Pulmonary hypertension
- Shoulder dystocia
- Birth injuries
    - Ecchymoses
    - Local fat necrosis associated with forceps applications
    - Cephalohematoma
    - Brachial plexus injuries
    - Paralysis of diaphragm
    - Fracture of clavicle or humerus
- Polycythemia
    - Jaundice
    - Hyperviscosity syndrome
    - Hypoglycemia
    - Seizures
    - Renal vein thrombosis
    - Increased total blood volume
- Poor feeding
- Hypoglycemia
    - Hyperinsulinemia
    - Polycythemia
    - Poor feeding.

EXAMINATION

EXAMINATION CONDITIONS

A routine neonatal examination, normally taking 5 to 10 minutes, should be in a quiet, warm environment. The room's light should be bright enough to detect skin markings and color but not so bright as to discourage open eyes. When an infant is ill, attention to optimizing his environment and recognizing the potential effect of the nursery surroundings on his state is fundamental.

Even healthy infants do not tolerate handling in extended examinations. The sicker or more immature they are, the less they tolerate manipulation. For all examinations, there must be the prevenient consideration that no harm should come by the process.

In routine care situations, having one or both parents present during an examination allows discussion about physical findings and offers the opportunity of pointing out behaviors that can help them better understand their infant. They can address directly any questions about history or therapy.

GENERAL ASSESSMENT

A neonatal physical examination includes the principles of inspection, palpation, percussion, and auscultation of each body system. Inspection plays the most important role and percussion the least. Unlike examinations of adults, there is less opportunity to progress through the systems in order and more need to proceed in whatever order is practical for the infant's state. For instance, it is important to observe the respiratory rate and pattern before touching the infant, and auscultating the heart precedes other handling if the infant is quiet. A systematic approach that includes all aspects while being efficient and nondisruptive is essential.

The specifics of neonatal examination are discussed in the following sections. Systems discussed in more detail in other chapters are given less emphasis in this chapter.

INSPECTION

Inspection begins before making any physical contact and from enough of a distance to encompass the infant as a whole. An immediate assessment of wellness comes from noting the state, color, respiratory effort, posture, and spontaneous activity.

STATE

Important indicators of infant well-being are the states or levels of arousal the infant achieves throughout the examination and throughout the day as described by the parent or nursing staff. These states were originally categorized by Prechtl and Beintema:[14]

- deep sleep
- light sleep
- awake, light peripheral movements
- awake, large movements, not crying
- awake, crying.

During examination, a healthy infant should demonstrate several levels of arousal. The most useful states for assessing an infant are those of light sleep and quiet awake, and irritating maneuvers are held until the conclusion of the assessment. What it takes to assist an infant in moving from one state to another or how well she does it without assistance is noteworthy. Because the deep sleep that follows a recent feeding may give an appearance of lethargy on arousal, knowing the feeding history and pattern is paramount to determining aptness of state.

Quieting an infant may require anything from stopping the handling to holding and talking to him. The amount of time spent in unstimulated crying is normally limited in the first 24 hours. Excessive crying, requiring more than routine consoling, particularly if there are no intervals of quiet alert states, indicates abnormal irritability.

COLOR

Color assessment includes judging perfusion and skin color for the presence of cyanosis, jaundice, pallor, plethora, or any unusual cast and evaluating the distribution and types of pigmentation.

RESPIRATORY EFFORT

The degree of respiratory effort is a primary indicator of how distressed or comfortable a newborn infant is, even if the cause of distress is not pulmonic. The physician can observe the respiratory rate, depth of excursions, use of accessory muscles with retractions or nasal flare, and any emitted sounds, such as grunting or whining. Understanding the infant's pattern of respiratory effort can suggest a specific illness and direct the examination. As the severity of a condition increases, these distinctions may be lost (Table 20-1).

TABLE 20–1
PATTERNS OF NEONATAL RESPIRATORY EFFORT*

Condition	Pattern Observed
Distal airway or lung parenchyma	Intercostal retractions, sternal retractions, flaring, tachypnea, grunt, increased work in breathing
Upper airway obstruction	Suprasternal retractions, subcostal retractions
Cardiac pattern	Tachypnea without effort, infant is quiet but not somnolent
Neurodepression	Poor effort compared with physiologic need, apnea
Metabolic or septic pattern	Tachypnea, apnea, lethargy, whining, minimal retractions

* Early in disease process, before patterns merge with multiple system involvement.

POSTURE

One of the more important clues to physical status is the resting posture assumed by an unrestrained infant. This posture reflects intrauterine positioning and general body tone, and it varies with gestational age (see Fig. 20-1). At term, the healthy infant lies with thighs partially abducted and the hips, knees, ankles, elbows, and shoulders comfortably flexed. While observing neck position, the examiner looks for symmetry between the sides and compares the upper and lower extremities. If there is lateral asymmetry and the head is turned to one side, there may be an asymmetric tonic neck reflex with the extremities on the mental side in extension and those on the occipital side in flexion. In that case, the head should be turned to the opposite side to verify that the asymmetry reverses.

If the fetal presentation is nonvertex or unknown or there is asymmetry or deformation, it is helpful to assist the infant in assuming a position reflecting his intrauterine attitude. The physician can fold the extremities into the fetal position by applying moderate pressure to a relaxed infant's feet while gently shaking his legs and by directing the arms toward the thorax through gentle pressure on the elbows.

SPONTANEOUS ACTIVITY

The examiner should observe what the infant does in light sleep and awake states. Does she stretch, move all extremities equally, open and close her hands, root and start sucking when something touches her face, and yawn with great facial expression, or does she lie quietly and move only in response to stimulation?

Premature infants spend more time sleeping but should have spontaneous activity and resting postures commensurate with their gestational age. Because they habituate and become disorganized and stressed quickly on handling, inspection before contact is important.

VITAL SIGNS

TEMPERATURE

It is unusual for neonates to develop fevers except in response to environmental temperature. If the infant's temperature remains elevated after the environment returns to normal, evaluation for infectious or neurologic causes is indicated. Infants often become hypothermic, usually in response to the environment, particularly if the infant remains quiet and does not cry vigorously.

Term infants sweat, albeit poorly, in response to thermal stress. Preterm infants develop a measurable response by 2 weeks of age.[15] Visible sweating at rest or on feeding in an afebrile infant is abnormal and may indicate distress, typically from cardiac disease.

RESPIRATORY RATE AND HEART RATE

Count the respiratory rate by looking at the upper abdomen for a full minute. As soon as an infant is touched, the respiratory rate and depth change. The normal respiratory rate is 30 to 60 inspirations per minute in a term infant, with lower rates occurring after cardiopulmonary transition. When awake, some normal infants breathe shallowly and rapidly but are able to slow sufficiently to feed well. Deep sleep is characterized by a more regular breathing pattern while the awake state has more bursts of rapid breathing.

The heart rate is 110 to 160 beats per minute in healthy term infants but may vary significantly during deep sleep or active awake states. Preterm infants have resting heart rates at the higher end of the normal range. Tachycardia, with a rate persistently greater than 160, may be a sign of many conditions, including central nervous system irritability, congestive heart failure, sepsis, anemia, fever, or hyperthyroidism.

BLOOD PRESSURE

The range of normal blood pressure in neonates depends on the method used for assessment and gestational age (see Appendix C-1). The values obtained by the blanching and flush methods are mean pressures and are lower than those registered by direct intravascular or Doppler monitoring. The flush method for obtaining mean pressure is easier in an active infant and requires only a sphygmomanometer. The Doppler methods, although providing diastolic and systolic pressures, require electronic equipment and a quieter patient. Two important elements for obtaining accurate blood pressures are a quiet infant and a properly sized cuff with a width 50% to 67% of the length of the arm.

For the flush method, the hand or foot is wrapped or squeezed firmly enough to blanch the skin.[16] The cuff is inflated, the wrapping removed, and the pressure slowly lowered until there is a flush of color, at which point the pressure is read.

FACIES

Assessment of facies includes looking for symmetry, size, shape, and the relations of all parts of the face and how the infant holds or uses them. An unusual appearance dictates analyzing the individual components of the facies to decide if the constellation represents malformation, deformation, a syndrome, or merely familial appearance.

HEAD AND NECK

Inspection of the head includes assessment of the shape and size relative to the rest of the body and face, distribution and character of the hair, and the underlying scalp.

Head circumference is discussed above. Even when the OFC is normal, it is important to notice if the size of the head seems appropriate to the size of the face.

The shape of the cranial vault reflects interaction of internal forces (*e.g.*, brain anatomy, volume, intracranial pressure) against external forces (*e.g.*, intrauterine and extrauterine molding, suture mobility). Normal intrauterine molding for a vertex presentation leads to a narrowed biparietal diameter and a maximal occipitomental dimension; after breech presentation, there may be marked accentuation of the occipitofrontal dimension with parietal flattening, an occipital shelf, and apparent frontal prominence. This normal breech shape requires differentiation from the abnormal occipital prominence found in posterior fossa masses (*e.g.*, Dandy–Walker malformation), frontal prominence due to increased cranial volume, or the boat-shaped scaphocephaly from synostosis of the sagittal suture. Normal molding resolves within a few weeks, but other aberrations progress. Pathologic conditions that prevented normal molding of the fetal head should be suspected in infants who failed to engage in vertex and descend in labor. These conditions are all unusual but important to detect as early as possible.

Isolated craniosynostosis occurs in 0.6 of 1000 live births with affected sutures found to be metopic in 50%, sagittal in 28%, coronal in 16.5%, and lambdoid in 5.5%.[17] Because plagiocephaly (*i.e.*, flattening) and torticollis often coexist, occipital flattening with contralateral frontal prominence dictates determining range of motion for the neck. The infant's head should turn as far as the shoulder in both directions—farther if it is premature. A unilateral epicanthal fold or asymmetry of the ears when viewed *en face* signals the need to view the head from the top and back to detect plagiocephaly.[18]

HAIR AND SCALP

The hair is inspected for color, texture, distribution, and directional patterns. Although hair color may change, there should be racial concordance. For example, reddish or blond hair in a dark-skinned infant may indicate albinism. Similarly, the hair color should be fairly uniform. Random patches of white hair are familial or sporadic and inconsequential, but white forelocks with other pigment defects and anomalies are associated with deafness and retardation.[19] The texture of hair at birth is relatively fine. Most of the conditions associated with abnormal textures or fragility appear some time later. With immaturity, the hair is even more fine and sparce.

The hair line may vary at the frontal margin, and normal but hirsute infants have hair well down the forehead but without synophrys (*i.e.*, grown-together eyebrows). The posterior hair line has a more consistent limitation, so that hair roots below the neck creases, particularly at the lateral margins, suggest syndromes associated with short or webbed necks.

Although neonatal hair initially appears quite disheveled, its growth direction normally is consistent. There is usually a single, parietal hair whorl, which is to the right of center. If there is more than one or if the whorl is frontal or central, there may be abnormal development of the underlying brain.[20] It is unusual for hair to be upswept at the neck or forehead except as an isolated cowlick. If there is extreme hair unruliness, particularly with unusual facies, microcephaly, or SGA, there may be poor brain growth of early fetal onset, which is typical of a number of genetic syndromes including Cornelia de Lange and Down syndromes.

Superficial ecchymoses and abrasions of the scalp are common after vaginal deliveries, especially after extraction by forceps or vacuum. Incision sites for fetal scalp electrodes or blood sampling should be small and inconsequential, although some require closure. A small defect of the scalp, *cutis aplasia,* that appears coincidentally at a potential monitoring spot may be confused with an electrode lesion, because it sometimes appears ecchymotic or blistered.

Many telangiectatic or staining lesions appear over the scalp, neck, and face, ranging from the superficial and transient flammeus nevus or stork bite to the more intense, permanent port wine stain. These and the common skin lesions are discussed in detail in Chapter 55. The light brown staining that develops after exposure to silver nitrate eye drops can be removed with alcohol; it disappears by 7 to 10 days.

Once an important part of the cranial examination, transillumination is now rarely used because only gross abnormalities are detectable and there are more precise diagnostic techniques. Transillumination remains an important adjunct to examining the chest, abdomen, and genitalia for fluid or air accumulations.

PALPATION OF THE HEAD

Palpation detects motility and firmness of adjacent bones, size of the sutures, and bony or dermal defects. Depending on the extent and direction of molding, there is variable overlap in the sagittal, coronal, or lambdoid sutures. With craniosynostosis, the fused sutures do not move freely when alternate sides are pressed. Any suture, particularly the metopic, may be normally wide in the absence of increased intracranial pressure; the exception is a wide lambdoid suture, which ordinarily indicates increased pressure. The sagittal and metopic sutures are normally wider in darker pigmented infants. Palpable tension in the anterior fontanelle is a late indicator of cranial hypertension. Palpation of the bones adjacent to the sagittal suture may reveal a give and return similar to that felt when pressing on an aluminum can. These softer areas, indicating craniotabes, occur most often in premature infants or in term gestations if the fetal head was compressed against the maternal bony pelvis for several weeks. Physiologic craniotabes resolve within a few weeks. Pathologic craniotabes occur in syphilis and rickets.

Measurement of the fontanelle is not helpful as part of a routine assessment, because the normal range in size varies widely and its reproducibility is poor. There is little clinical application for measurements in otherwise normal infants, because head growth can occur despite apparently closed fontanelles; the rate of closure is independent of other growth parameters and bone age.[21] Although aberrantly large fontanelles are seen in genetic syndromes and metabolic or endocrine diseases, they are not pathognomonic.

There are several other palpable findings on the head unique to the neonatal period. The most frequent, *caput succedaneum,* presents at birth and is initially most prominent over the presenting area. It represents edema of the scalp and, rarely, bleeding. The pitting edema can quickly shift to the dependent portion of the scalp.

Cephalohematoma is uncommon and rarely is present at birth. More typically, a cephalohematoma develops after delivery and expands during the first day as blood accumulates between the surface of a calvarial bone and its pericranial membrane.[22] The cephalohematoma is rounded and discrete, with boundaries limited by suture lines. Because of periosteal reflection at the margins, there is often a false sensation of bony depression. The blood contained in a cephalohematoma may take several weeks to resorb and prolongs neonatal jaundice. Unless there are neurologic indicators, radiographs to look for the occasional underlying skull fracture are not indicated.

The least frequent finding is a subgaleal hematoma, which may feel crepitant with less pitting than the edema of caput succedaneum. Because there is little anatomic restriction to subgaleal fluid accumulation, large volumes may redistribute and deplete total body volumes.

A thorough examination of the head includes auscultating for bruits over the temporal arteries and anterior fontanelle, particularly if there are conditions involving high-output cardiac failure or neuropathology.

The neck should be extended for maximal exposure to look for clefts or cysts. The isthmus of a normal thyroid is just palpable in the sternal notch on neck extension; rarely, midline enlargements represent a goiter. Other congenital neck masses include cystic hygroma, lymphangioma, and cervical teratoma.[23]

EYES

Examining the eyes of a neonate requires patience and a cooperative infant. Stimulating sucking may encourage spontaneous eye opening in dim light, but if the infant is crying inconsolably, delaying the examination is prudent. After ophthalmic prophylaxis, there may be enough edema of the lids to prevent opening without lid retractors. The neonatal eye examination is discussed in more detail in Chapter 53.

The emphasis of the neonatal eye examination is on the structure and appearance of the eye and its surroundings rather than assessment of visual acuity or extraocular muscle function. Observations include determining the relative size, shape, and position of the eye in its socket and demonstrating if the infant appears to have vision by reacting to light. Because measuring is reserved for eyes that appear abnormal, the examiner looks for symmetry and observes whether the eyes seem to fit their sockets. Both eyes should be the same size and sit neither too deeply nor too far forward. The size and shape of the socket needs to be related to the size and shape of the surrounding skull. Marked molding with depression of the forehead may make normal eyes appear to sit too far forward unless their position relative to the cheeks is considered. If the eyes are unequal, there should be a determination of which side is normal and whether one is too big or the other too small.

Chemical blepharoconjunctivitis, caused by silver nitrate, peaks on the second day of life with copious secretions and edema, but it is self-limited. Tearing or persistent eye crusting after the first 2 days requires evaluation for glaucoma, infection, corneal abrasion, mass lesions with obstruction of the nasolacrimal duct, or absence of the puncta. The signs of congenital glaucoma that may be noticed during the neonatal examination include photophobia, excessive tearing, cloudy cornea, or eyes that appear large.[24]

The pupil response to light requires a relatively dark room with only a moderately bright beam to avoid stimulating reflex eye closure. The pupil diameter decreases toward term as its response to light increases. Pupil reaction occurs consistently only after 32 weeks of gestation but may develop as early as 28 weeks of gestation. Pupils of term infants are anomalously dilated if their diameter is larger than 5.4 mm or anomalously constricted if smaller than 1.8 mm.[25]

Iris color is poorly defined at birth, but it should be circumferentially uniform. Because the corneas are cloudy in infants of less than 28 weeks of gestation, examination of the iris, pupils, and internal structures should be deferred until general cloudiness resolves.

A thorough fundoscopic examination with mydriasis is not routine, but there should be an attempt to detect cloudiness, masses, or large hemorrhages. The fundoscopic examination, using a small ophthalmoscopic beam, is best done while the infant sleeps, but the assessment of vision requires an alert, quiet infant.

The gemini red reflex (GRR) or choroidal light reflex is detected by examining both eyes simultaneously at a distance of 1 m. Because GRR requires the infant to fix both eyes on the light source and is best after mydriasis, it is difficult to accomplish in infants of only a few days of age; it is especially helpful after the first week in a term infant. From a wide beam on the ophthalmoscope, the circle of light covers much of the face. The focus is adjusted to give the brightest red glow. Asymmetry in the color, brightness, position, or presence of the glow is abnormal and warrants full ophthalmologic evaluation.[26]

EARS

The ear is examined for shape, size, position, the presence of a canal, and any extraneous tags or pits. The tympanic membranes are examined to evaluate sources of late neonatal infection. The shape of the external ear is determined in part by intrauterine forces and by the activity of extrinsic and intrinsic auricular muscles. Abnormal formation may be a sign of neuromuscular weakness or abnormalities in auricular muscles.[27] Position of the ears depends on how complete their cephalad migration and anterior rotation are and on how much molding or deformation there may be. The position at term should be similar on both sides with approximately one-third of the pinnae above a line extended from the medial canthus and base of the nose.

A behavioral reaction to a standardized sound excludes only gross bilateral deficits, but it should be elicited in all neonates. Assessment of hearing by evoked potential is specifically indicated in infants at risk for hearing deficits, particularly those with anomalies of the head and neck, a family history of childhood deafness, VLBW, severe asphyxia, fetal infection, meningitis, and after hyperventilation therapy and intracranial hemorrhage. Anomalies associated with hearing deficits include neural crest abnormalities, first or second branchial arch abnormalities, or syndromes known to be associated with hearing loss.

NOSE

The nose is assessed for shape, size, and patency and for the presence of swelling over the nasolacrimal duct, the size of the philtrum, and definition of the nasolabial folds. It should appear appropriately sized for the face when viewed laterally and *en face.*

Nasal deformation with asymmetry of the nares and apparent deviation occurs as part of facial compression and molding. The triangular cartilage may be dislocated during delivery, causing septal deviation, which requires surgical relocation during the first week. With depression of the tip of the nose, a dislocated septum appears more angled within the nares, but a normal septum merely compresses. After release, a dislocated septum does not return to normal.[28]

Nasal patency is assessed by free passage of a small catheter through both nares and into the stomach. Air flow is detected by holding a strand of thread in front of each nostril and observing fluttering with breathing.

Congenital obstruction of the nasolacrimal duct, usually symptomatic in the first days or weeks of life, presents with a large tear meniscus at the lower lid, tearing without stimulation, dried mucoid residue after a nap, or a discharge during waking. A distally obstructed nasolacrimal duct is diagnosed by pressing the finger over the lacrimal sac and sliding it along the course of the duct toward the eye to express material from the puncta. Dacryocystocele is a dilation of the lacrimal drainage system due to obstruction at its proximal and distal ends and filling of the enclosed space. Dacryocystoceles are observed at birth as tense, blue–gray cystic swellings about 1 cm in diameter, located just below the medial canthal tendon.[29]

MOUTH AND THROAT

The shape of the mouth is a marker of uterine position and neuromotor activity. For the mouth to develop properly, there must be muscle activity of the tongue against an intact hard palate. If not, the mandible recedes, and there is micrognathia; if the hard palate is intact but the tongue inactive, the hard palate may have a high arch or have prominent lateral palatine ridges.

Many common oral findings have counterparts in dermatology, and for the most part, they are benign (Table 20-2). The mouth should be observed with the infant at rest and crying. The shape and size of the mouth is best determined by looking at the mandible and how well it fits the maxilla. It should open at equal angles bilaterally. If the intrauterine position tilts the head laterally, there may be mandibular deviation so the jaw opens at an angle. Putting the infant in the fetal position may demonstrate an impression made by the shoulder under the temporomandibular angle. These deformations resolve spontaneously. Asymmetry on crying occurs with facial nerve pare-

TABLE 20–2
NEONATAL ORAL FINDINGS

Finding	Caucasians (%)	Non-Caucasians (%)	Comments
Palatal cysts (*e.g.*, Bohn nodules, Epstein pearls)	73–85	65–79	Yellow–white elevated cysts 1 mm in diameter; nests of epithelial cells in the midpalatal raphe at the fusion points of the soft and hard palates
Alveolar or gingival cysts	54	40	Appear similar to palatal cysts
Alveolar lymphangioma	0	4	Blue-domed, fluid-filled cysts in posterior portion quadrants; no more than 1 per quadrant; may cause discomfort during feeding if cysts are large
Alveolar eruption of cysts with or without teeth	<0.1	<0.1	Clear, fluid-filled cysts; mandibular central incisor; rates range from 1 : 2500 in Hong Kong to 1 : 3392 in Canada
Leukoedema	11	43	Filmy, white hue of mucosa, nonblanching of no significance compared with thrush
Median alveolar notch	16	26	Reduces when teeth erupt or persists as notch between central incisors
Ankyloglossia	~2	~2	Male–female ratio of 3 : 1; lingual frenum prevents protrusion of tongue, extends to papillated surface of tongue, or causes fissure in tip
Commissural lip pits	1	3	Blind-ended pits at corners of mouth; autosomally dominant; associated with preauricular pits; medial pits more syndromic
Thrush			Adherent white plaques on tongue and buccal and palatal surfaces; will scrape off; caused by *Candida* sp.
Bifid uvula	<1	<1	Associated with submucous cleft palate
Ranula	$\ll 1$	$\ll 1$	Cyst of sublingual salivary gland
Epulis	$\ll 1$	$\ll 1$	Large, pedunculated cyst of incisor region

Data from references 44 through 49.

sis, in which the nasolabial folds are asymmetric, or with absence of the depressor anguli oris muscle, in which the folds are symmetric. The muscle absence is palpable as a thinner lower lip.

The inside of the mouth should be assessed using a small tongue blade to visualize the tongue, buccal surface, palate, uvula, and back of the mouth; the gums and hard palate are best assessed with a gloved finger to feel for masses or submucous defects and to allow evaluation of sucking and of the gag reflex. If the tongue is too large, the mouth can not be closed completely in comparison to a protruding tongue associated with low tone and slack jaw or the darting tongue seen frequently in neonates with Down syndrome.

SKIN AND LYMPH NODES

The skin is assessed for general color, the presence of any extra markings or rashes, texture, turgor, edema or areas of induration, thickness of underlying fat, and maturity. Icterus progresses in a cephalocaudal pattern at a fairly predictable rate in the absence of phototherapy.[30] If any mark on the skin is considered to be a birth mark, there is rarely an infant born without several. In view of the many variations of normal and the important signs of other diseases or syndromes that are manifested on the skin, understanding the physical findings of the neonatal skin is fundamental. Details about dermal conditions are discussed in Chapter 55.

Lymph nodes are palpable in more than one-third of all neonates, most commonly in the inguinal region and independent of perinatal history. These nodes, from 3 to 12 mm in diameter, tend to persist.[31]

The most frequent, abnormal congenital lymphatic masses are cystic hygroma or cystic lymphangiomas, which are soft, compressible, and often poorly defined masses in almost any part of the body, but commonly occur in the head, neck, abdomen, and axilla. If markedly distended, they may transilluminate. Ultrasonography reveals their cystic anatomy. A discussion on the congenital abnormalities of the lymphatic system is available elsewhere.[32]

CHEST AND ABDOMEN

SIZE AND SYMMETRY

In term neonates, the chest circumference is 1 to 2 cm less than the head circumference; it is relatively smaller with lower gestational age. The thorax is normally symmetric and wider than its anteroposterior dimension. The ribs are compliant, and their shape is easily impacted by external and internal forces. Compression from the infant's own arm or a twin's body part may lead to marked asymmetry in thoracic shape and pattern on inspiration. By simulating the fetal position, the cause of deformation may become evident.

The abdomen is mildly protuberant compared with the chest. It should be softly rounded, with a diameter slightly greater above than below the umbilicus. The abdominothoracic relation is reversed in diaphragmatic defects, with herniation of abdominal contents into the thorax leaving a scaphoid abdomen. Supraumbilical fullness is increased in the presence of duodenal atresia with gastric distention or hepatomegaly, and infraumbilical fullness is increased with distention of the urinary bladder or in severe cases of IUGR with an abnormally small liver. Any significant abdominal visceral enlargement causes distention, as does forced depression of the diaphragm.

RETRACTIONS

Mild subcostal and intercostal retractions are common, even in healthy neonates because of their compliant chest walls. Suprasternal retractions, indicating proximal airway resistance, are normally less pronounced; supraclavicular retractions are never normal. In conditions notable for loss of lung volume and poor compliance, respiratory movements may become paradoxic (*i.e.*, seesaw), with a collapse of the chest wall on inspiration as the abdominal wall expands. With air trapping and increased thoracic volume, there is an increase in the anteroposterior dimension and abdominal distention if the diaphragm is depressed.

Because the diaphragm is the primary muscle of respiration with little contribution by accessory muscles, quiet respirations are abdominal with only mild subcostal retractions. The umbilical stump moves caudally in the midline with each contraction of the diaphragm. In the absence of abdominal abnormalities, any lateral deviation of the umbilicus with inspiration suggests a diaphragmatic paresis with the deviation toward the weak side. This sign is lost during mechanical ventilation. Albeit rare, neonatal diaphragmatic paresis occurs most often with brachial plexus injuries, and it should be sought if an arm is weak.

Neonatal lung sounds are relatively more tubular than vesicular because of better transmission of large airway sounds across a small chest. Changes in the pitch of the tubular sounds from one side to the other or between regions most likely represent main stem or conducting bronchial narrowing. The coarse crackle of distal airway opening is particularly common in neonates in whom there is a natural tendency in many conditions for microatelectasis. If heard at the end of inspiration, adventitial sounds represent more distal disease compared with those in beginning inspiration, which usually represent conducting airway secretions. A characteristic sound of crushing Styrofoam signals pulmonary interstitial emphysema.

Locating abnormal sounds requires listening over the extrathoracic airways, because these sounds may be transmitted well. If bowel sounds are heard, the examiner should differentiate direct transmission from herniated contents or referred abdominal sounds.

If there is stridor or wheezing, auscultation of the nose or throat may reveal a site of extrathoracic obstruction. Because there must be sufficient air flow to cause stridor or wheezing in the first place, stimulating the infant may accentuate an obstruction. If an endotracheal tube is in place and an air leak is present, a whistling sound corresponding to ventilator breaths may be evident in the periphery of the lung fields but is loudest over the upper trachea or outside the mouth.

CLAVICLES

The clavicles may be absent (*i.e.*, cleidocraniodysostosis) or fractured. If they are absent, the shoulders may be made almost to touch in the anterior midline. If carefully sought by radiographs or repeated examinations, fractures are found in at least 1.7% to 2.9% of term deliveries and more frequently on the right side.[33] They are usually silent until they develop a callus and mass over the fracture site at 2 to 3 weeks of age. If complete, the ends may be displaced and feel crepitant. An overlying hematoma may cause a visible fullness, there may be an associated brachial plexus injury or pseudoparesis, or the infant may not be willing to breast feed on one side because of discomfort with positioning. Standing at the foot of the infant, the physician feels each clavicle with the second and third fingers of the opposite hand and compares ease of outlining the borders, feeling for tenderness, swelling, and crepitation or eliciting pain with movement.

NIPPLES

The breasts of term male and female infants vary in diameter from 0.5 cm to several centimeters. Widely spaced nipples are features of a number of chromosomal abnormalities. The internipple distance varies with gestational age and body weight, but its relation to chest circumference is more constant. If the internipple distance in centimeters divided by the chest circumference in centimeters is greater than 0.28, the space is more than 2 standard deviations above the mean.[34] Larger breasts, influenced by maternal hormones, may secrete a thin, milky substance (*i.e.*, witches' milk) for a few days or weeks. Occasionally, a normal, transient bloody discharge may develop. Although the degree of enlargement may not be the same in both breasts, they should not be hot, red, or tender. Unless there are specific signs of inflammation, the breasts should be left alone.

Supernummary nipples occur in 1.2% to 1.6% of darkly pigmented infants; they are more unusual in lightly pigmented infants. These supernummary nipples, seen in the milk line below and medial to the true breast, are rudimentary, occasionally only distinguishable because of the presence of a small, pigmented mark or dimple. There is a suggested association of renal anomalies detectable on ultrasound or intravenous pyelography in Caucasian populations that is not confirmed in African-American population studies.[35,36]

UMBILICUS

The umbilicus is normally positioned approximately halfway between the xiphoid and the pubis. A caudally placed insertion occurs in conditions of caudal regression or underdeveloped lower body segment. The neonatal appearance of the umbilicus does not indicate what the adult appearance will be, because most are relatively protuberant with redundant skin. If the umbilical cord itself is broad or remains fluctuant after pulsations have stopped, there may be a herniation of abdominal contents into the cord.

PALPATION OF ABDOMEN

The infant tolerates palpation of the abdomen best when the organs are brought to the examining hand rather than the hand pushing into the abdomen and probing for the organs. Standing at the right side of the infant, with the left hand lifting the pelvis slightly off the mattress to relax the abdominal muscles, the examiner can keep the right hand flat and use the fingerpads rather than fingertips to palpate the abdominal organs. Palpation should start below the umbilicus and proceed upward. In some instances, it is helpful to palpate the abdomen with the infant in decubitus or prone positions, allowing the contents to fall toward the hand rather than being pushed away.[37] Palpation of the abdomen in ill neonates increases centrally measured blood pressure by as much as 25% above baseline.[38]

The liver is normally palpable 1 to 3.5 cm below the costal margin in the midclavicular line and across the midline as a left lobe that is distinguishable from the lobulated spleen that is felt more laterally. A left lobe larger than the right may reflect *situs inversus.* At term, the normal liver span, determined by percussing the upper and lower margins, is 5.9 ± 0.8 cm in the midclavicular line.[39] This varies by gestational age and weight. Estimation of hepatomegaly based on lower border estimation is inaccurate. A variation of percussion to outline the size of the liver or any solid mass is to scratch lightly across the skin surface while auscultating for changes in pitch with the diaphragm of the stethoscope held over the mass.

The normal edge of the liver is thin and soft, and the hepatic surface is smooth. A full or firm edge commonly represents a marked increase in total blood volume, increased extramedullary hematopoiesis, chronic infection, early cirrhosis, or an infiltrative process. Hepatomegaly is a late and inconstant finding in cardiac failure. Cardiac pulsations in the liver occur in right-sided obstructive cardiac lesions, but these hepatic pulsations should be differentiated from a normally transmitted cardiac impulse or respiratory excursions. In the first 24 to 48 hours after birth, the liver often decreases markedly in size, probably reflecting redistribution of circulating blood volume.

The kidneys are palpable if the abdomen is soft, and they are moderately firm and lobulated. An enlarged ureter simulates a filled large bowel, although it is less mobile.

An infant reveals tenderness by a grimace, cry, or drawing up of the legs. True guarding is unusual with poorly developed abdominal muscles. Rebound tenderness is difficult to detect, because infants are often too obtunded to show a reliable response in the presence of significant peritoneal disease. The presence of localized edema or discoloration of the abdominal wall is an important indicator of intraperitoneal disease. An unusual exception is ecchymosis caused by leaking of an umbilical vessel or urine edema from a patent urachus leaking into the subcutaneous space above the peritoneum. In either case, the dramatic findings are limited to the abdominal wall below the umbilicus.

A thin abdominal wall allows transillumination of fluid- or gas-filled masses to outline their position and size. Meconium-filled bowel loops do not transilluminate, but distended stomach, upper bowel loops, hydronephrotic kidneys or a distended bladder do. A transillumination pattern that shifts with patient rotation suggests free air.

Auscultation of the abdomen includes listening for pitch and activity of bowel sounds and for bruits. Bowel sounds tend to persist in neonates, even those with clinical ileus, and they reflect the degree of bowel motility; an absence of bowel sounds is always significant. Auscultation may reveal the presence of a bruit over the liver, indicating an arteriovenous fistula, or over the kidneys in the presence of renal artery stenosis.

CARDIOVASCULAR SYSTEM

The changes that occur in the cardiovascular system during the neonatal period complicate the cardiac examination until the pulmonic and systemic pressures have reversed their fetal associations, all communications have closed, and the left ventricle becomes predominant. Each aspect of examination from inspection through auscultation plays a role, but auscultating for murmurs is one of the least important aids in determining if a newborn infant has cardiac disease. The role for most clinicians in the newborn examination is not to determine precisely what the cardiac anatomy is but to rule out cardiac disease as part of a routine newborn examination and, in a symptomatic infant, to determine if the cause is cardiac. If so, the physician must determine the urgency of the condition by asking some basic questions. Is this a cardiac disease that could be fatal if not immediately treated (*e.g.*, ductal dependent lesions, cyanotic heart disease)? Is its presence aggravating or relieving other conditions (*e.g.*, patent ductus arteriosus in the presence of lung disease or pulmonary hypertension)? Is this something that requires following the patient and potential future intervention but is not emergent and should not interfere with newborn and parental adjustment?

Evaluation of the cardiovascular system begins in the delivery room with assessment of the Apgar scores and includes evaluation of heart rate, color, and respiratory effort. Frequently, a line of demarcation is observed, with the head, right arm, and right side of the chest pink and the rest of the infant pale or cyanotic before there has been functional closure of the ductus. With vigorous crying, its disappearance indicates an appropriate drop in pulmonary vascular resistance. Another reassuring milestone in cardiac transition often noticed at the first bath by nursing staff is a bright red flush over the entire body and extremities. This blush, reminiscent of cooked lobster, is distinguishable from the darker, ruddy, plethoric color of polycythemia, which is accentuated in the mucous membranes and less so on the palms and soles. The blush is not seen in infants with major cardiac disease. Specific points to be considered in the cardiac examination are outlined in Table 20-3.

GENITOURINARY SYSTEM

In the delivery room, one of the first documented observations of the neonate is assignment of gender. Genital abnormalities are relatively uncommon but cause significant parental stress. It is important to be able to distinguish the variations of normal that occur far more often than real pathologic malformations (see Chap. 43).

The male infant should be examined by stretching the penis for an expected penile length at term of at least 2.5 cm. The presence of chordae prevents complete stretching, but a twisted median raphe is of no significance. In obese infants, the shaft may be retracted and covered by suprapubic fat, appearing too small unless stretched. The meatal opening should be located, although completely retracting the foreskin is unnecessary.

The presence of both testes deep in the scrotal sac indicates term gestation. If a testis is not felt within the sac or canal, use a lubricated finger to sweep from the anterior iliac crest along the canal while palpating the scrotum. The volume of the testes should be estimated. Table 20-4 summarizes the normal values. If the scrotum or a testis is distended, transillumination may reveal a hydrocele. Discoloration suggests hematoma or torsion needing immediate surgical evaluation unless it represents only superficial ecchymosis after breech presentation. Hydrocele of the cord, a harbinger of inguinal hernia, is not likely to transilluminate but is easily felt.

Text continued on page 285

TABLE 20–3
NEONATAL CARDIAC EXAMINATION

Findings	Key Location	Points to Consider
Color	Over entire surface except presenting part; inside oral mucous membranes	Peripheral cyanosis may include area around mouth but not inside mucous membranes Prominent venous–capillary plexus around mouth and eyes simulates cyanosis Acrocyanosis of extremities reverses with warming Mild cyanosis may appear as pallor or mottling Infant with PDA runoff looks washed out, particularly in the feet.
Respiratory pattern	Lateral view of chest and abdomen Alae nasi	Most often have respiratory rate within normal range May be cyanotic but tachypneic without distress (*e.g.*, retractions, labored breathing) unless there is pulmonary edema or severe acidosis
Heart rate rhythm	PMI	Resting rate 120–130 (range, 100–150); higher second to the fourth weeks and in premature infants Most premature beats are transient and benign
Precordial bulge	Thorax compared side to side and to the abdomen	Thoracic asymmetry indicates bulge with AVM, tricuspid regurgitation (*i.e.*, Ebstein), tetralogy with absent PV, intrauterine arrhythmia, or myocardopathy Most commonly, asymmetry indicates pneumothorax, diaphragmatic hernia, atelectasis, or lobar emphysema
PMI	Left parasternal area	Visible until 4–6 hours of life during transition; beyond 12 hours, associated with volume overload lesions (*e.g.*, AP shunt, transposition) Normally more visible in premature infants but increases with PDA Abnormal to have PMI beyond 1–2 cm left of LSB at less than 1 week of age Right sided indicates dextrocardia *versus* shift due to intrathoracic pressures Absence of increased impulse with cyanosis indicates pulmonary atresia, tetralogy, tricuspid atresia Increase with cyanosis indicates transposition Thrill: gross insufficiency of atrioventricular valve, severe pulmonary stenosis, absent pulmonary valve
Blood pressure	Right arm and leg	Pressure in lower extremities is equal to or minimally higher than pressure in upper extremities in the first week Pressures are preserved by ductal flow in the presence of severe left sided obstructive disease Norms vary by age and method
Pulses	Right and left brachial and simultaneous femoral and right brachial	Look for equality of intensity and timing, synchronicity, slope of impulse curve, no delay in peak between preductal and postductal pulses Easily seen axillary pulses suggest runoff or wide pulse pressure

(*continued*)

AP, aortopulmonary; AV, atriventricular; AVM, arteriovenous malformation; BP, blood pressure; CHF, congestive heart failure; LSB, left sternal border; LA, left atrium; LV, left ventricle; MI, mitral insufficiency; PDA, patent ductus arteriosus; PMI, point of maximal impulse; PV, pulmonary valve; RA, right atrium; RV, right ventricle; S_1, first heart sound; S_2, second heart sound; S_3, third heart sound; S_4, fourth heart sound; TAPVR, total anomalous pulmonary venous return; VSD, ventricular septal defect.

From Johnson GL. Clinical examination. In: Long WA, ed. Fetal and neonatal cardiology. Philadelphia: WB Saunders, 1990:223, and Braudo M, Rowe RD. Auscultation of the heart—early neonatal period. Am J Dis Child 1961;101:575.

TABLE 20–3
NEONATAL CARDIAC EXAMINATION *(continued)*

Findings	Key Location	Points to Consider
Pulse pressure	Systolic minus diastolic BP	25–30 in term; 15–25 in preterm Narrow indicates myocardial failure, vasoconstriction, vascular collapse Widened indicates AV malformation, truncus arteriosus, AP window, PDA; may not be widened until pulmonary vascular resistance has dropped
S_1	Upper LSB	Usually single and relatively accentuated; audible split indicates Ebstein anomaly or slow heat rate; decreased with CHF, prolonged AV conduction
	Lower LSB	Increased accentuation with increased flow across AV valve indicates PDA, MI, VSD, TAPVR, AVM, tetralogy
S_2	Upper LSB	Two components should be heard by 6–12 hours of age Single sound indicates aortic atresia, pulmonary atresia, truncus arteriosus, transposition of great arteries Wide split indicates pulmonary stenosis, Ebstein anomaly, TAPVR, tetralogy, occasionally left-to-right atrial shunts Loud sounds indicate systemic or pulmonary hypertension
S_3 and S_4	Base or apex	S_3 indicates increased atrioventricular valve flow, PDA, CHF S_4 indicates severe myocardial disease with diminished LV compliance
Click	Lower LSB	Benign first several hours; abnormal after transition Dilation of great vessel indicates truncus arteriosus, tetralogy of Fallot, left- or right-sided ventricular outflow obstructions
Murmur	Precordium, back, under both axilla	Many serious cardiac malformations do not have their classical murmurs in early neonatal period but will have some combination of signs suggesting pathology; absence of murmur does not preclude presence of serious malformation (*e.g.,* transposition, TAPVR) At least 60% of infants have murmurs during the first 48 hours of life Quiet is necessary to auscultate murmurs; may need to disconnect the infant from the ventilator for a few beats Pathologic murmurs heard in the first hours of life indicate ventricular outflow obstruction
Venous pulse	Jugular vein, liver	Jugular a and v waves in sleeping infant In presence of cyanosis pulsating liver suggest RA or RV obstruction
Abdomen	Liver (left and right)	Span greater than 5.5 cm at term; late sign of congestive heart failure; presence of left-sided or central liver suggests likely cardiac anomaly
Edema	Presacrum, eyelids, legs and feet; Chest: hydrops	Causes are more often noncardiac except when associated with abnormalities of renal blood flow (*e.g.,* left-sided obstructions or severe hydrops associated with myocardiopathy such as severe anemia)

TABLE 20–4
NEWBORN GENITALIA

	Parameter	Normal Ranges	Abnormal Ranges
Penis	Length	3.5 cm	<2.5 cm
	Width	0.9–1.2 cm	
Testis	Volume	1–2 cm	
Anus			
Location, male	Anus to scrotum / Coccyx to scrotum	0.58 ± 0.06 cm	<0.46 cm
Location, female	Anus to fourchette / Coccyx to fourchette	0.44 ± 0.05 cm	<0.34 cm
Size	Diameter	7 mm + (1.3 × weight in kg)	
Masculinization (*i.e.*, labioscrotal fusion)	Anus to fourchette / Anus to clitoris	<0.5 cm	>0.5 cm

From Flatau E, Josefsberg Z, Resner SH, Bialik O, Laron Z. Penile size in the newborn infant. J Pediatr 1975;87:663, and Reisner SH, Sivan Y, Nitzan M, Merlob P. Determination of anterior displacement of the anus in newborn infants and children. Pediatrics 1984;73:216.

TABLE 20–5
NEONATAL NEUROLOGIC EVALUATION

Test	Technique	Normal for Term	Deviant for Term
Resting posture	Observe unswaddled infant without contact in quiet awake, quiet active, or light sleep states	Moderate flexion of four limbs, held off bed Equal side-to-side and upper-to-lower if head is in midline Extension of neck in face presentation or legs in breech presentation	Constant tight flexion Full extension, flaccid or forced Knees abducted to bed (*i.e.*, frog-leg) Elbows flexed with dorsum of hands on bed Tight, persistent fisting ATNR persistent ≥30 sec Strong lateral preference
State	Deep sleep Light sleep Awake, light peripheral movements Awake, large movements, not crying Awake, crying	Moves from one to the other with appropriate stimuli Self calms Modulated cry with expression	Is difficult to move from one to the other Stays too alert or cries without physical reason Does not come to fully awake state Weak or monotonous cry
Motor activity	Observe throughout physical examination	Appropriate for state of alertness Symmetric, fairly smooth Expressive face with yawn or cry	Bicycling, swatting without stimulus Asymmetric, weak Jittery while sucking Flat facial expression
Phasic (*i.e.*, passive) tone: resistance to movement	Measure resistance to extension (limb recoil) Scarf, heel to ear	Response appropriate for gestational age	Resists too much or too little Asymmetry
Tendon reflexes	Test patellar reflex with head midline	Patellar reflex only one reliably present at birth	Sustained clonus

(continued)

ATNR, asymmetric tonic neck reflex.

TABLE 20–5
NEONATAL NEUROLOGIC EVALUATION (*continued*)

Test	Technique	Normal for Term	Deviant for Term
Postural (*i.e.*, active) tone: resistance to gravity			
Traction response	Pull to sitting while grasping infant's hands	Infant pulls back with flexion at elbows, knees, and ankles Head comes with body with minimal lag and falls forward when sitting is obtained	Asymmetry in pulling back No resistance Full head lag Pull to stand instead Head does not fall forward as infant goes past upright
Vertical suspension	Suspend infant facing examiner with both hands in axillae	Infant supports himself then yields slowly Holds head erect, flexes hips, knees, ankles Eyes open	Infant falls through immediately Legs extend Eyes fail to open Infant fails to relax and fall through after 1 min
Horizontal suspension	Hold infant under chest and suspend in prone position Galant: stroke adjacent to spine Landau: stroke caudalcephalad along spine	Flexes arms, extends neck, holds back straight Curves toward side of stimulus Extends back, lifts head and pelvis, micturates	Hangs limply or excessively rigidly Asymmetric incurving Weak or absent response
Positive support	Hold infant to support trunk with feet touching firm, flat surface	Infant extends hips to bear his own weight and relaxes after 1 min	Infant fails to bear weight or extends too much or too long
Integrated reflexes			Unequal laterality
Moro reflex	Hold infant in supine position; support head and neck with hand; allow head to drop while still supporting it	Speading: arms abduct, extend; hands open Hugging: arms adduct and flex; hands close	Absence of spread Asymmetry Exaggeration with disorganization in state
Tonic neck reflex	Infant in supine, neutral position; turn head to one side; repeat opposite side	Mental extension, occipital flexion primarily of arms; does not remain in position for >30 seconds	Exaggerated response and stays in position >30 sec
Withdrawal reflex	Painful stimulus to one foot	Withdrawal of stimulated foot; variable extension of opposite leg	Absence of flexion in stimulated leg

ATNR, asymmetric tonic neck reflex.

The female genitalia should be inspected for size and location of the labia, clitoris, meatus, vaginal opening, and the relations of the posterior fourchette to the anus (see Table 20-4).

Virtually all female newborns have redundant hymenal tissue. Hymens tend be annular (80%) with a smooth or fimbriated edge and a central or ventrally displaced opening. Tags of tissue may extend from 1 to 15 mm beyond the rim of the hymen and occur in at least 13% of female neonates. These tags disappear within a few weeks. A complete review of the variations is available.[40]

Assessment for virilization in the female is difficult, because there are varying degrees of clitoral hypertrophy and labioscrotal fusion. With clitoral size fully developed by 27 weeks of gestation but with little deposition of fat in the labia, there is particular confusion about clitoral hypertrophy in premature infants. Masculinization causes posterior fusion of the labioscrotal folds independent of clitoral hypertrophy. The distance of the anus from the posterior fourchette varies by gestational age and body size, but its relation relative to other genital landmarks is more constant (see Table 20-4). Measurements are made with the hips flexed and the infant relaxed so the perineum does not bulge.

MUSCULOSKELETAL SYSTEM

Examination of the spine includes observation for abnormal curving and cutaneous manifestations of underlying deformities such as sacral agenesis or spina bifida. A pilonidal sinus is suspected if the bottom of a sacral pit is not visible or there is moisture in an otherwise dry area. Dark hair, overlying hemangioma, or pigmented nevus indicate a tethered cord. A palpable mass usually indicates a lipoma if it is covered with normal skin and moves with it. A sacrococcygeal teratoma tends to be just lateral to midline, and spinal dysraphism presents as a midline mass.

The physician assesses the extremities for symmetry, size and length, range of active and passive motion, and obvious deformity. The length of the upper extremities should allow the hands to reach to the upper thighs on extension. The muscles are not well defined but should not feel atrophic or fibrotic.

Hand examination consists of observing its activity and appearance, including the nails, the joints, and the palmar creases. The creases of the fifth digit should be parallel. If there is shortening of the midphalanx, the nonparallel creases mark a radial deviation, clinodactyly. Any curve less than 8° is normal. The hand maintains a constant enough proportion throughout life such that the distance from the tip of the index finger to the base of the thumb should be roughly one-half the distance of the index finger to carpal crease. If the thumb is proximally placed, the ratio will be greater than 0.58; if distal, it will be less than 0.43.[41] The thumb should reach just beyond the base of the index finger. See Figures 40-28 and 40-29 for total hand measurements.

The neonate's hips require reassessment with each visit because dislocations may not be detectable at each examination. If the femur freely dislocates, it may appear to jerk when the infant extends or flexes her hip. The legs should be symmetric in length on extension and with the knees flexed as the feet rest on the bed. If they are unequal, suggesting dislocation of the shorter leg (*i.e.*, Galeazzi sign), the next maneuver is to attempt reduction on the shorter side while stabilizing the pelvis (*i.e.*, Ortolani maneuver). With the hip and knee flexed, the thigh is grasped with the third finger over the greater trochanter and the thumb near the lesser trochanter. The other hand stabilizes the pelvis. As the thigh is abducted, pressure applied to the greater trochanter reduces the dislocated femoral head into the acetabulum with a clunking sensation. The commonly felt, benign clicks are distinct from the pathologic clunks, which often are seen as much as they are felt when the femoral head jerks. If the legs are of equal length, the first maneuver is to attempt to dislocate the head (*i.e.*, Barlow maneuver). With the hip and knee flexed, the thigh is grasped and adducted while applying downward pressure. If the hip dislocates, the Ortolani maneuver should reduce it. If the hip rides to the edge but not out of the acetabulum during the Barlow maneuver, it is subluxable. Even if dislocation is undetectable, there may be telescoping with free movement of the femur up and down, indicating some degree of instability.

NERVOUS SYSTEM

Neurologic evaluation begins with the initial observations made on approaching the infant and continues as the infant is positioned and stimulated for the remainder of the routine physical examination. Much can be learned about the neurologic state just by observing what the infant does on his own; little more is needed unless the observations indicate abnormality.

Jitteriness is a frequent finding in neonates that warrants special comment. It is characterized by rhythmic tremors of equal amplitude around a fixed

TABLE 20–6
ASSESSMENT OF CRANIAL NERVES

Cranial Nerve	Assessment	Pitfalls
I	Withdrawal or grimace to strong odor (*e.g.*, peppermint, oil of cloves)	Rarely tested clinically; rapid habituation
II	Behavioral response to light (*i.e.*, blink, fixing, following, turning to light source); searching nystagmus	Room too bright; infant too deeply asleep; overstimulation of other senses
III, IV, VI	Ocular movement, doll's eyes, oculovestibular response, pupil size, gemini red reflex	Should not force eyes to open; ocular alignment usually poor in neonates; light for pupil response causes eye closing
VII	Facial muscle tone at rest and during crying	Poor mouth opening due to absence of depressor anguli oris muscle
V, VII, XII	Sucking strength, rooting reflex	Gestational-age dependent; infant should be hungry
VIII auditory portion	Behavioral response to horn (*i.e.*, blink, widened eyes); quieting to voice	Room too loud; difficult to distinguish unilateral loss; rapid habituation
IX, X	Swallowing with normal gag	Irritated throat after suctioning
VII, IX	Facial expression to strong flavor	Rapid habituation
XII	Tongue fasciculation, thrust, ability to shape around nipple	Macroglossia

axis in an extremity or the jaw. It occurs more often if the infant is awake, after a startle, or after crying. Distinguishable from clonic–tonic seizure activity because it can be stopped by stimulating sucking, it is most often a physiologic activity. If it fails to cease during sucking, it may be a sign of hypoglycemia or hypocalcemia or of irritability associated with maternal drug abuse.[42,43]

The basics of the neonatal neurologic examination include assessment of state; spontaneous muscle activity for assessing amount, quality, and strength; passive and active muscle tone; and the functioning of the cranial nerves. The steps are described in Tables 20-5 and 20-6.

REFERENCES

1. American Academy of Pediatrics, Committee on Fetus and Newborn and American College of Obstetrics and Gynecology, Committee on Obstetrics. Maternal and fetal medicine. Guidelines for perinatal care. 3rd ed. Washington, DC: March of Dimes Birth Defects Foundation, 1992:254.
2. Saint-Anne-Dargassies S. La maturation neurologique des prématurés. Etudes Néonatales 1955;4:71.
3. Amiel-Tison C. Neurological evaluation of the maturity of newborn infants. Arch Dis Child 1968;43:89.
4. Dubowitz L, Dubowitz V, Goldberg C. Clinical assessment of gestational age in the newborn infant. J Pediatr 1970;77:1.
5. Ballard JL, Khoury JC, Wedig K, Wang L, Eilers-Walsman BL, Lipp R. New Ballard Score, expanded to include extremely premature infants. J Pediatr 1991;119:417.
6. Alexander GR, de Caunes F, Hulsey TC, Tompkins ME, Allen M. Validity of postnatal assessments of gestational age: a comparison of the method of Ballard et al and early ultrasonography. Am J Obstet Gynecol 1991;166:891.
7. Sanders M, Allen M, Alexander GR, et al. Gestational age assessment in preterm neonates weighing less than 1500 grams. Pediatrics 1991;88:542.
8. Hittner HM, Hirsch NJ, Rudolph AJ. Assessment of gestational age by examination of the anterior vascular capsule of the lens. 1977;91:455.
9. Constantine NA, Kraemer HC, Kendall-Tackett KA, Bennett FC, Tyson JE, Gross RT. Use of physical and neurologic observations in assessment of gestational age in low birth weight infants. J Pediatr 1987;110:921.
10. Stevens-Simon C, Cullinan J, Stinson S, McAnarney ER. Effects of race on the validity of clinical estimates of gestational age. J Pediatr 1989;115:1000.
11. Wilcox AJ, Russell IT. Birthweight and perinatal mortality: II. On weight-specific mortality. Int J Epidemiol 1983;12:319.
12. Sivan Y, Merlob P, Reisner SH. Upper limb standards in newborns. Am J Dis Child 1983;137:829.
13. Merlob P, Sivan Y, Reisner SH. Lower limb standards in newborns. Am J Dis Child 1984;138:140.
14. Prechtl H, Beintema D. The neurological examination of the full-term newborn infant. Clinics in developmental medicine no. 12. London: SIMP Heinemann, 1964.
15. Harpin VA, Rutter N. Sweating in preterm babies. J Pediatr 1982;100:614.
16. Goldring D, Wohltmann HJ. "Flush" method for blood pressure determinations in newborn infants. J Pediatr 1952;40:285.
17. Shuper A, Merlob P, Grunebaum M, Reisner SH. The incidence of isolated craniosynostosis in the newborn infant. Am J Dis Child 1985;139:85.
18. Jones MD. Unilateral epicanthal fold: diagnostic significance. J Pediatr 1986;108:702.
19. Waardenburg PJ. A new syndrome combining developmental anomalies of the eyelids, eyebrows and nose root with pigmentary defects of the iris and head hair and with congenital deafness. Am J Hum Genet 1951;3:195.
20. Smith DW, Gong BT. Scalp hair patterning as a clue to early fetal brain development. J Pediatr 1973;83:374.
21. Duc G, Largo RH. Anterior fontanel: size and closure in term and preterm infants. Pediatrics 1986;78:904.
22. Potter EL, Craig JM. Pathology of the fetus and the infant. 3rd ed. Chicago: Year Book, 1975:105.
23. Gundry SR, Wesley JR, Klein MD, Marr M, Coran AG. Cervical teratomas in the newborn. J Pediatr Surg 1983;18:382.
24. Crouch ER Jr. Pediatric vision screening: why? when? what? how? Contemp Pediatr 1991;Sept:9
25. Isenberg SJ. Clinical application of the pupil examination in neonates. J Pediatr 1991;118:650.
26. Adler R, Lappe M, Murphree AL. Pupil dilation at the first well baby examination for documenting choroidal light reflex. J Pediatr 1990;118:249.
27. Zerin M, Van Allen MI, Smith DW. Intrinsic auricular muscles and auricular form. Pediatrics 1982;69:91.
28. Silverman SH, Leibor SG. Dislocation of the triangular cartilage of the nasal septum. J Pediatr 1975;87:456.
29. Ogawa GSH, Gonnering RS. Congenital nasolacrimal duct obstruction. J Pediatr 1991;119:12.
30. Kramer LI. Advancement of dermal icterus in the jaundiced newborn. Am J Dis Child 1969;113:455.
31. Bamji M, Stone RK, Kaul A, Usmani G, Schacter FF, Wasserman E. Palpable lymph nodes in healthy newborn and infants. Pediatrics 1986;78:573.
32. Hilliard RI, McKendry JBJ, Phillips MJ. Congenital abnormalities of the lymphatic system: a new clinical classification. Pediatrics 1990;86:988.
33. Joseph PR, Rosenfeld W. Clavicular fractures in neonates. Am J Dis Child 1990;144:165.
34. Hassan A, Karna P, Dolanski EA. Intermamillary indices in premature infants. Am J Perinatol 1988;5:54.
35. Varsano IB, Lutfi J, Ben-Zion G, Mukamel MM, Grünebaum M. Urinary tract abnormalities in children with supernumerary nipples. Pediatrics 1984;73:103.
36. Robertson A, Sale P, Sathyanarayan. Lack of association of supernumerary nipples with renal anomalies in black infants. J Pediatr 1986;109:502.
37. Senquiz AL. Use of decubitus position for finding the "olive" of pyloric stenosis. Pediatrics 1991;87:266.
38. Sinkin RA, Phillips BL, Adelman RD. Elevation of systemic blood pressure in the neonate during abdominal examination. Pediatrics 1985;76:970.
39. Reiff MI, Osborn LM. Clinical estimation of liver size in newborn infants. Pediatrics 1983;71:46.
40. Berenson A, Heger A, Andrews S. Appearance of the hymen in newborns. Pediatrics 1991;87:458.
41. Merlob P, Mimouni F, Rose O, Reisner SH. Assessment of thumb placement. Pediatrics 1984;74:300.
42. Linder N, Moser AM, Asli I, Gale R, Livoff A, Tamir I. Suckling stimulation test for neonatal tremor. Arch Dis Child 1989;64:44.
43. Parker S, Zuckerman B, Bauchner H, Frank D, Vinci R, Cabral H. Jitteriness in full-term neonates: prevalence and correlates. Pediatrics 1990;85:17.
44. Jorgenson RJ, Shapiro SD, Salinas CF, Levin LS. Intraoral findings and anomalies in neonates. Pediatrics 1982;69:577.

45. Levin LS, Jorgenson RJ, Jarvey BA. Lymphangiomas of the alveolar ridges in neonates. Pediatrics 1976;58:881.
46. Monteleone L, McLellan MS. Epstein's pearls (Bohn's nodules) of the palate. J Oral Surg 1964;22:301.
47. King NM, Lee AM. Prematurely erupted teeth in newborn infants. J Pediatr 1989;114:807.
48. Leung AKC. Natal teeth. Am J Dis Child 1986;140:249.
49. Shprintzen RJ, Schwartz RH, Daniller A, Hoch L. Morphologic significance of bifid uvula. Pediatrics 1985;75:553.
50. Johnson GL. Clinical examination. In: Long WA, ed. Fetal and neonatal cardiology. Philadelphia: WB Saunders, 1990:223.
51. Braudo M, Rowe RD. Auscultation of the heart—early neonatal period. Am J Dis Child 1961;101:575.
52. Flatau E, Josefsberg Z, Resner SH, Bialik O, Laron Z. Penile size in the newborn infant. J Pediatr 1975;87:663.
53. Reisner SH, Sivan Y, Nitzan M, Merlob P. Determination of anterior displacement of the anus in newborn infants and children. Pediatrics 1984;73:216.

Neonatology: Pathophysiology and Management of the Newborn, Fourth Edition,
edited by Gordon B. Avery, Mary Ann Fletcher, and Mhairi G. MacDonald.
J.B. Lippincott Company, Philadelphia © 1994.

chapter 21

Behavioral Competence

T. BERRY BRAZELTON

It is important to assess the neonate's contribution to his or her new environment. The parents' inclination is to nurture newborns and to value their reactions to handling, voice, and vision; it is belittling to these reactions if physicians do not similarly value them. If we as physicians attend to them by changing neonatal nurseries and lying-in arrangements to value and capture the neonate's best periods of alert responsiveness, we place a stamp of approval on the parents' attention to their neonate and also on the newborn as an important, interactive person from the start. As physicians, we are providing new, confused parents with a way of communicating with their infants and showing them that the neonate can lead them when they are confused.

The demands of a complex, undirected society, coupled with the lack of support of new parents in our nuclear family system, leave most parents insecure and at the mercy of tremendous internal and external pressures. They have been told that their infant's outcome will be shaped by their parenting, but there are few stable cultural values on which they can rely for guidance in setting their course as new parents.

An infant is not as helpless as he or she appears to be. The infant comes well equipped to signal his or her needs and gratitude, can make choices about what to accept from his parents, and can shut out what isn't wanted in effective ways. The infant can be seen as a powerful force, stabilizing and influencing those around him or her.

Compared with newborns of other species, the human neonate is relatively helpless in motor capabilities and relatively precocious in sensory capabilities. This creates a motor dependence and a freedom for acquisition of the many patterns of sensory and affective information that are necessary for the child and adult human to master and survive in a complex world.

It is important to evaluate infants at risk as early as possible to permit the use of sophisticated preventive and therapeutic approaches when they can offer the most benefit. Premature and minimally brain-damaged infants seem to be less able to compensate in disorganized, depriving environments than well-equipped neonates, and the problems of the compromised infants with organization in development are compounded early.[1] If we are to improve the outcome for these children, assessment of the risk in early infancy should mobilize preventive efforts and programs for intervention.

We need more sophisticated methods of assessing neonates and of predicting their part in the possible failure of the environment–infant interaction. We need to be able to assess at-risk environments, because the scarcity of resources requires the selection of target populations for our efforts at early intervention. Minimally brain-damaged babies do make remarkable compensatory recoveries in a fostering environment.[2]

The behavioral responses of the neonate can be used to understand the organization of the central and autonomic nervous systems at birth. The individual differences in neonatal behaviors reflect the variations in genetic endowment and intrauterine influences. As the neonate responds to labor, delivery, and recovery in the new environment, we can begin to predict how new experiences and learning will affect him or her and how the infant will interact with the new environment.

NEONATAL BEHAVIORAL ASSESSMENT SCALE

To record and evaluate some of the integrative processes in neonatal behavior, my colleagues and I developed a behavioral evaluation scale that tests and documents the infant's changing state of consciousness and responses to various kinds of stimulation. The Neonatal Behavioral Assessment Scale (NBAS, Brazelton scale) was first published in 1973.[3] After modifications, the experiences of 10 years were summarized in a second edition in 1984.[4] Four centers and eight researchers contributed to the revised edition. The NBAS is in use in more than 600 locations. Training centers have been established in the United States, Europe, and Israel; and more than 248 published studies have appeared within the United States and in cross-cultural contexts.

CONCEPTUAL BASE

The original goal for the NBAS was to record the dimensions of state—autonomic, motor, sensory-receptive, and responsive—that were integrative and interactive with each other in the normal, healthy, full-term infant. The NBAS was seen not as a set of discrete stimulus–response presentations but was considered to be an interactive assessment in which the adult participant played a major role, facilitating the performance and organizational skills of the infant. We hoped to establish the infant's capacities for and limits in contributing to the caregiving environment. We expected to gain a deeper understanding of the meaning of infant behavior as it reflected the relative contribution of these developments. We conceived of a single assessment in the neonatal period as only one brief glimpse into the continuum of the infant's adjustment to labor, delivery, and the new environment. The test was expected to reflect the infant's inborn characteristics and the behavioral responses that had been shaped by the intrauterine environment. We hoped repeated examinations would demonstrate the infant's coping capacities and capacities for using his or her inner organization to experience, integrate, and profit developmentally from the environment's stimulation. We thought that serial examinations would reflect the interaction between the infant's inborn characteristics and the shaping of them in the first few weeks.

As we worked with the NBAS, several issues became clear. An assessment of the newborn presents an opportunity for looking forward into the baby's future and backward into the intrauterine experience. The intrauterine influences that shape newborn behavior are becoming more commonly recognized. The newborn's behavior at birth is phenotypic and genotypic, reflecting complex behaviors that are shaped by influences *in utero* that probably act in a synergistic fashion.

Any interpretation of reactions must be made with the understanding that the neonate's reactions to all stimuli depend on his or her ongoing state. The infant's use of state to maintain control of reactions to environmental and internal stimuli is an important mechanism and reflects his or her potential for organization. State no longer need be treated as an error variable; it instead sets a dynamic pattern to allow for the full behavioral repertoire of the infant. The NBAS tracks changes in state over the course of the examination and the lability and direction of these changes. The variability of state indicates the infant's capacities for self-organization; the child's ability to quiet himself and need for stimulation measure this adequacy.

The behavioral examination tests for neurologic adequacy with 20 reflex measures and for 28 behavioral responses to environmental stimuli, including the kind of interpersonal stimuli that mothers use in handling their infants. Best performance is accepted to overcome variability. In the examination, there is a graded series of procedures (*e.g.*, talking, hand on belly, restraint, holding, rocking) designed to soothe or alert the infant. His responsiveness to animate stimuli (*e.g.*, voice, face) and to inanimate stimuli (*e.g.*, rattle, bell, red ball, white light, temperature change) is assessed. Estimates of vigor and attentional excitement are measured, and an assessment is made of motor activity, tone, and autonomic responsiveness as the infant changes state. In addition, criteria to include three quantitative concepts have been added: cost to the neonate of the assessment, cost to the examiner of eliciting best performance, and quality of best performance.

With this examination, given on successive days, we have been able to outline the initial period of alertness immediately after delivery, the period of depression and disorganization that follows, and the curve of recovery to optimal function after several days. The period of depression and disorganization lasts 24 to 48 hours in infants with uncomplicated deliveries and no medication effects, but it persists for 3 to 4 days in infants compromised by medications given during the delivery. The curve of recovery may be the best single early predictor of individual potential function, and it seems to correlate well with the neonate's ability on retest at 30 days.[5]

CONTENT

The revised NBAS assesses the newborn's behavioral repertoire on 28 behavioral items, each scored on a nine-point scale. The NBAS measures the coping capacities and the adaptive strategies of the infant that emerge during recovery from the stresses of labor and delivery and adjustment to the demands of the extrauterine environment. This process of adaptation can be measured by studying patterns of change, called profile or recovery curves, over repeated Brazelton-type examinations.

The following items constitute the NBAS.[4] The numbers in parentheses refer to the optimal state for assessment, which are defined in the next section of this chapter.

- Response decrement to repeated visual stimuli, such as light (1,2,3)
- Response decrement to rattle (1,2,3)
- Response decrement to bell (1,2,3)
- Response decrement to tactile stimulation of the foot, such as a pinprick (1,2,3)
- Orienting response to inanimate visual stimuli (4,5)
- Orienting response to inanimate auditory stimuli (4,5)
- Orienting response to inanimate visual and auditory stimuli (4,5)
- Orienting response to animate visual stimuli, such as the examiner's face (4,5)
- Orienting response to animate auditory stimuli, such as the examiner's voice (4,5)
- Orienting response to animate visual and auditory stimuli (4,5)
- Quality and duration of alert periods (4,5)
- General muscle tone in resting and in response to being handled passively and actively (4,5)
- Motor maturity (4,5)
- Traction responses such as a pull-to-sit maneuver (4,5)
- Cuddliness—responses to being cuddled by examiner (4,5)
- Defensive movements—reactions to a cloth over the infant's face (3,4,5)
- Consolability with intervention of examiner (6 to 4,3,2)
- Peak of excitement and infant's capacity to control self (all states)
- Rapidity of buildup to crying state (all states)
- Irritability during the examination (all awake states)
- General assessment of kind and degree of activity (alert states)
- Tremulousness (all states)
- Amount of startle (3,4,5,6)
- Lability of skin color for measuring autonomic lability (from 1 to 6)
- Lability of states during entire examination (all states)
- Self-quieting activity—attempts to console self and control state (6 to 4,3,2,1)
- Hand-to-mouth facility (all states)
- Smiles (all states)

To be able to assess these patterns of change, at least two but preferably three or more examinations are needed for each infant. The first should be done on days 2 or 3, after the immediate stresses of labor and delivery have begun to wear off. The next examination is best performed at 7 to 14 days, and the third can be done at 1 month. Scores from the successive examinations establish a behavioral pattern of change over the first weeks of life. This pattern may be the most important measure for predicting later developmental outcome.

I believe that the behavioral items elicit important evidences of cortical control and responsiveness, even in the neonatal period. The neonate's capacity to manage and overcome the physiologic demands of this adjustment period to attend to, differentiate, and habituate to the complex stimuli of an examiner's maneuvers may be an important predictor of the baby's future central nervous system (CNS) organization. The curve of recovery of these responses during the first neonatal month is of more significance than the midbrain responses detectable in routine neurologic examinations.

Included in this examination are behavioral tests of important CNS mechanisms such as habituation or the neonate's capacity to shut out disturbing or overwhelming stimuli; choices in attention to various objects or human stimuli (*i.e.*, a neonate shows clear preferences for female rather than male voices and for human rather than nonhuman visual stimuli); and control of the neonate's state to attend to information from the environment (*e.g.*, effort to complete a hand-to-mouth cycle to attend to objects and people around him or her). All of these mechanisms are evidenced in the neonate, even in the premature infant, and are more predictive of CNS intactness than reflex responses.[6]

ASSESSMENT OF BEHAVIORAL STATES

There are predictable, directed responses from a neonate interacting socially with a nurturing adult or responding to an attractive auditory or visual stimulus. If positive rather than intrusive stimuli are used, the neonate has amazing capacities for alerting and attention and for suppressing interfering reflex responses to attend, and with predictable behaviors, the infant responds to and interacts with his or her environment from birth.[4] However, this predictability requires a knowledge of his ongoing state of consciousness.[7] State of consciousness, or the "state" of the infant, becomes a most important matrix for interpreting neonatal behavior. The infant's reactions to all stimuli, internal and external, depend on his ongoing state of consciousness. With state used as a matrix, behavioral responses become quite predictable.

State depends on physiologic variables, such as hunger, nutrition, degree of hydration, and the timing within the wake–sleep cycle of the infant. Our criteria for state throughout this chapter are based on the descriptions by Prechtl and Beintema.[7] If state is accounted for, most of the infant's reactions to negative and positive stimuli from internal and external sources are predictable. State becomes a matrix for understanding reactions. It qualifies stimulation as appropriate or inappropriate to the infant's organization. For almost any maturational level, the behavior produced by appropriate stimuli in appropriate states can demonstrate the complexity of an intact and adaptable CNS.

The matrix of state as a concept for organization in the neonate has become important since its use as a background for neurologic responses in Prechtl's assessment.[7] Within the context of the optimal state of alertness, Prechtl was able to demonstrate that the newborn could show better reflexive behavior and that the neurologic examination became a better predictive measure.[8]

If the sleeping or awake state of the baby is accounted for, an experienced examiner can make a fairly accurate prediction of how a baby will respond to any given stimulus. For example, within a deep sleep state, a baby responds slightly to a moderately loud, brief rattle; although breathing changes and blinking may occur, the child probably stirs very little. In lighter sleep, the infant may startle, may begin to rouse, and his or her face may become alert, with his or her respiratory patterns changing markedly. In a state between sleep and awake, the infant probably startles briefly, but the startle is followed by a slower movement of the arms and legs and a writhing of the trunk, and the child will open his or her eyes to look dully for the next stimulus. In a semi-alert state, the neonate becomes more alert, begins to move about, and may even search for the rattle, with respirations becoming slower and more regular. In a wide-awake state, a newborn infant often becomes quiet, looks surprised, but remains wide awake and alert; the child shifts his or her eyes and then head to turn toward the rattle as if searching for it. Unless it is a very loud or insistent rattle, he may not stop crying to respond to the sound when in a crying state. The state of arousal is a matrix for predictable responses and is the infant's way of defending himself from the world around him in the case of sleep states and of controlling arousal to attend to his environment in waking states. The parameters of state are relatively easy to determine by simple observation.[9] The categories of behavioral states are listed with their criteria for definition.

Quiet Sleep. The infant's eyes are firmly closed and still. There is little or no motor activity, with the exception of occasional startles or rhythmic mouthing. Respiration is abdominal and relatively slow (average, 36 breaths/minute), deep, and regular.

Active Sleep With Rapid Eye Movements. The infant's eyes are closed, and rapid eye movements (REMs) occur during a 10-second interval. Body activity can range from minor twitches to writhing and stretching. Respiration is irregular, costal, and generally faster than that seen in quiet sleep (average, 46 breaths/minute). Facial movements may include frowns, grimaces, smiles, twitches, mouth movements, and sucking, although face movements are not often seen in this category of active sleep.

Drowsy State. The infant's eyes may open and close or may be partially or fully open, but they are still and appear dazed. There may be some generalized motor activity, and respiration is fairly regular, but it is faster and more shallow than that observed in regular sleep.

Alert Inactivity. The infant's body and face are relatively quiet and inactive, and the eyes appear bright and shining.

Fussing. The characteristics of this state are the same as those for alert inactivity, but mild, agitated vocalizations are continuous, or one cry burst may occur.

Crying. The characteristics of this state are the same as those for alert inactivity, but generalized motor activity is more intense, and cry bursts are continuous.

SLEEP CYCLES

The length of sleep cycles (*i.e.*, active REM and quiet sleep) changes normally with maturation of the CNS. Term infants have regular cycles of 45 to 50 minutes, but immature babies have shorter, less-well-defined cycles. Newborn infants have as much active REM sleep in the first one-half of the deep period as in the second one-half. Initially brief sleep and wake patterns coalesce as the environment presses the neonate to develop diurnal patterns of daytime wakefulness and night sleep.[10] Appropriate feeding patterns, diet, absence of excessive parental anxiety, sufficient nurturing stimulation, and a fussing period before a long sleep have been implicated as reinforcing the CNS maturation necessary for the development of diurnal cycling of sleep and wakefulness.

Anders suggests that REM sleep is regulated by brain stem mechanisms that constitute an autoregulating and stimulating system of the CNS.[11] This state contributes to the growth and maintenance of neural tissue by cyclic excitatory activation of developing neuronal structures, which increases their differentiation. Without well-differentiated REM cycles, the neurophysiologic structures may be delayed in their development of differential responses. In immature organisms or neonates whose brain stems have been stressed by anoxia, maternal drugs, or other disorganizing factors, delays in differentiation of sleep states can be expected, and these infants may be at risk for prolonged CNS disorganization. Steinschneider suggested that this kind of sleep disorganization may be a predictor for the apneic attacks found in sudden infant death syndrome.[12]

CRYING

Crying serves many purposes in the neonate, not the least of which is to shut out painful or disturbing stimuli. Hunger and pain are responded to with crying, which brings the caretaker to the infant. There is a kind of fussy crying that occurs periodically throughout the day, usually in a cyclic fashion, that seems to act as a discharger of energy and an organizer of the states that ensue.[13] After a period of fussy crying, the neonate may be more alert, and she may sleep more deeply.

Crying seems to be an important behavior for organizing the day and for reducing disturbance within the CNS in the neonatal period. Most parents can differentiate cries of pain, hunger, and fussiness after 2 to 3 weeks and learn quickly to respond appropriately.[14] The cry is of ethologic significance for eliciting appropriate care for the infant.

Studies of the cry patterns of infants with various clinical syndromes or diseases suggest that there are cry features that differentiate damaged or sick infants from healthy controls.[15] The cry can be used to aid the differential diagnosis of certain diseases. Down syndrome is associated with a low-pitched, hoarse, guttural cry; a higher threshold for the production of the cry; and a longer latency from stimulation to cry onset. Infants with cri du chat syndrome and those with trisomy 13 have a fundamental frequency that is high-pitched, averaging 850 Hz, in contrast to the range of 400 to 600 Hz in healthy infants.

Lester found that malnourished infants had a longer cry duration, longer cry latency, higher fundamental frequency, lower amplitude of the fundamental frequency, and fewer harmonics than well-nourished infants.[16]

SENSORY CAPACITIES

VISUAL CAPACITY

The newborn is equipped at birth with the capacity for processing complex visual information and for demonstrating ocular movements to track an object in space. Even more important to her survival is the fact that she can defend herself from visual stimuli that may otherwise force her to make excessive demands on her immature physiologic system. When a bright light is flashed into a neonate's eyes, the pupils constrict, she blinks, her eyelids and whole face contract, and she withdraws her head by arching her whole body, often setting off a complete startle as she withdraws. Her heart rate and respirations increase, and there is an evoked response registered on her visual occipital electroencephalogram (EEG).

Repeated stimulation of this nature induces diminishing responses because of the infant's capacity to shut down responses. For example, in a series of 20 bright-light stimuli presented at 1-minute intervals, we found that the infant rapidly habituated and damped out the behavioral responses.[13] By the tenth stimulus, he had decreased not only his observable motor responses but also his cardiac and respiratory responses. The latency to evoked responses, as measured by EEG tracings, was increasing, and by the fifteenth stimulus, the EEG reflected the induction of a quiet, unresponsive behavioral state accompanied by trace alternans and spindles. The infant's capacity to shut out repetitious, disturbing visual stimuli protects him from having to respond to visual stimulation and frees his energy to meet physiologic demands.

This capacity of the neonate has been considered a kind of neurologic habituation and is present in neonates with intact CNSs.[17] The capacity to habituate to visual stimuli is decreased in immature infants.[18] It is affected by medication such as barbiturates given to mothers as premedication at the time of delivery. This led Brazier to postulate that the primary focus for this mechanism is in the reticular formation and midbrain.[19] The infant finally becomes deeply asleep with tightened, flexed extremities; has little movement except jerky startles; produces no eye blinks; has deep, regular respirations; and has a rapid, regular heart rate. This state of habituation seems to signal a defensive state against the assaults of the environment.

Any newborn baby in a bright, noisy nursery is likely to be in such a habituated state. She is unlikely to be responsive to loud noises or a flashlight if they are used as test stimuli, and testing her vision or hearing would require moving her to a darker, quieter room, where complex visual responses can be captured more easily and reliably. The only justification that I can find for those who claim that newborns cannot see or do not respond with real behavioral preference to various visual stimuli is that they have tested the infants in overlighted, inappropriate settings.

Just as he is equipped with the capacity to shut out certain stimuli, the newborn demonstrates the capacity to alert to, turn his eyes and head to follow, and fix on a stimulus that appeals to him. Fantz first pointed out neonatal preference for certain kinds of complex visual stimuli.[20] He found that sharply contrasting colors, larger squares, and medium-bright objects were appealing to the neonate and brought him to a prolonged, alert state of fixation. Fantz and others found that the neonate preferred an ovoid object and one in which there were eyes and a mouth. The kind of attention and the length of fixation were markedly reduced if mothers had been medicated before delivery.

Goren showed that, immediately after delivery, a human neonate would fix on a drawing that resembled a human face and follow it, with eyes and head turning for 180°.[21] A scrambled face did not demand the same kind of attention, nor did the infant completely follow the distorted face with her eyes and head; the head turned to follow only one-half of the arc. My colleagues and I found that the capacity of neonates to fix on and follow a red ball was a good predictive sign of neurologic integrity.[22] However, its absence is not a serious predictor, because it depends on whether the infant is in an alert state. Many conditions interfere with the neonate's capacity to come to an alert state: the CNS depression that follows delivery; hypoxia or any of the stresses of delivery; premedication given to the mother; transient effects of metabolic derangement or illness in the neonate; and normal conditions of hunger, fatigue, and an overly bright nursery. Newborns are capable of visual fixing and following during alert periods, and this may be a sensitive predictor of neurologic and visual integrity.[6]

Visual acuity of the newborn is still difficult to determine. Gorman and colleagues used the neonate's opticokinetic responses to a moving drum lined with stripes and found that 93 of 100 infants responded preferentially to stripes subtending a visual range of only 33.5 minutes of arc.[23] We found that premature infants were less reliable but could also fix on and follow the same lined drum.[22] Dayton and coworkers found at least 20/150 vision in newborns by this same technique.[24] Rather than being able to accommodate well, the infants have a fixed focal length of about 19 cm.[25] To capture visual interest, an examiner must present a bright object at this distance.

In one long-term study, Sigman and associates found that visual behavior may be one of the best predictors of an intact CNS in the neonate.[26] They found that summary scores on the neonate's neurologic examination were significantly related to the length of first fixation on a black-and-white checkerboard as a visual stimulus. This capacity to stare at a complex object was related to an alert state, and if infants could not be brought to such a state, the prediction was more ominous. The optimal response to visual stimulation in a neonate can be described as an initial alerting, attention that increases but that is followed by a gradual decrease in interest, and a final turning away from a monotonous presentation.

Several observers demonstrated that neonates prefer moving and somewhat complex visual patterns to stationary ones.[27] If the moving object can be moved slowly parallel to the natural, lateral movements of the eyes, it is more likely to capture the baby's interest. The duration and degree of his attention may be correlated with a middle range of complexity and the similarity of the target to the ovoid shape and the structures of the human face.

AUDITORY CAPACITY

The neonate's auditory responses are specific and well organized. Assessments are often not sensitive to the complexity of the newborn's behavior. For example, the loud clackers used on the Collaborative Project of the National Institute of Neurological Diseases and Blindness for early detection of CNS defects were ineffective in loud, noisy nurseries. A large percentage of the neonates tested in the first three days with this routine were unresponsive; they appeared to have shut out or habituated to the ambient auditory stimuli. Another approach under these conditions would have been to use a soft rattle in a quiet setting.

In response to an interesting auditory stimulus, such as a rattle, the infant moves from a sleeping state to an alert state. His breathing becomes irregular, his face brightens, and his eyes open, and when he is completely alert, his eyes and head turn toward the sound. In the case of a well-organized neonate, head turning is followed by a searching look on his face and scanning with his eyes to find a source for the auditory stimulus. To find out whether the neonate can respond this way, a full test of hearing should include several stimuli, animate and inanimate, with careful attention to the neonate's ongoing state of consciousness to ensure that the test breaks into his state.

Eisenberg determined the differential responses to different ranges of sound that are available to the infant.[28] In the range of human speech (*i.e.*, 500–900 Hz), the neonate inhibits motor behavior. She often demonstrates cardiac deceleration as evidence of attention and orients with head turning toward the source of sound. Outside this human range, there is a less complex behavioral response. The strikingly narrow range of stimuli for positive, attending responses can be demonstrated by linking devices for recording sucking to the auditory input.[29] Within this narrow human range, sucking ceases as an initial response to the stimulus and is followed by a burst–pause pattern of sucking, as if the infant is pausing to receive more of the interesting auditory input.

Various frequencies and intensities have different functional properties. High-frequency signals above 4000 Hz are more effective in producing a response, even in crying or sleep states, but they are likely to produce distress. Signals at lower intensities (*e.g.*, 35–40 dB) are effective inhibitors of distress, especially as continuous white noise.[30] White noise at these levels eventually induces a sleep state, even in a crying neonate. Kearsley demonstrated the importance of the rise time of the sound on the neonate's behavioral response.[31] Sounds with prolonged onset times and low frequencies produced eye opening and cardiac deceleration followed by an attentive look, and sounds with rapid onset and high frequency produced eye closing, cardiac acceleration, increased head movements, and aversion.

There is a series of regular steps in the neonate's behavioral response to an appropriate sound. As the sound is located, the cardiac rate increases and may be accompanied by a mild startle. If the auditory stimulus is attractive to the infant, his face brightens, his heart rate decelerates, his breathing slows, and he becomes alert and searches with his eyes until the source of the sound is localized to the *en face* midline of the baby. This behavior, which occurs as a response to an attractive auditory stimulus (*e.g.*, rattle, human voice), becomes a measure of the neonate's capacity to organize his central and autonomic nervous systems.

Habituation to repeated auditory stimuli becomes a further test of CNS function. If there is a damaged cortex, behavioral inhibition is not likely to occur. Bronstein and Petrova found that 2-hour-old to 8-day-old infants ceased sucking on a pacifier initially, but after repeated sounds of 60 to 70 dB, they resumed sucking.[32] Bridger found that the heart rate acceleration as an initial response to an auditory stimulus ceased after several trials, and the baby essentially habituated behaviorally and autonomically to this repetitive stimulus.[33] However, a change in frequency or a tonal change brought about an immediate increase in motor activity and a change in heart rate; this reaction represents dishabituation. Cardiac response can be used to study the infant's mental organization for repetitive, novel, and contingent responses.

Cairns and Butterfield documented the differences in the neonate's responses to human or nonhuman sounds by using a sucking paradigm to detect subtle information-processing differences (discussed in Sucking Capacity).[34] They believe that monitoring for a burst–pause pattern in sucking as one changes auditory stimuli can differentiate between CNS impairments of receptive processing from the kind of peripheral impairment that is found in nerve deafness of rubella, congenital malformations, hyperbilirubinemia, and other disorders.

OLFACTORY CAPACITY

Engen and associates demonstrated observable differentiated responses to odors in the neonate, concluding that the newborn is designed with a highly equipped sense of smell, ready to pick up the odors that help her adapt to her new world.[35] For example, she acts offended by acetic acid, asafetida, and alcohol in the neonatal period but is attracted to sweet odors of milk and sugary solutions. MacFarlane showed that 5-day-old neonates can reliably differentiate their own mothers' breast pads from those of other lactating mothers, although this power of discrimination was not present at 2 days of age.[36] They turn their heads toward their own mothers' breast pads with 80% reliability after controls for laterality are imposed. The neonate perceives the odor of her mother as a learned response by the fifth day.

TASTE CAPACITY

The newborn has fine differential responses to taste. Pratt and colleagues observed different sucking responses to sugar and decreased sucking to other tastes.[37] Johnson and Salisbury reported that a newborn's taste preferences are expressed in an even more complex fashion.[38] An infant is fed different fluids through a monitored nipple, and his sucking pattern is recorded. Saline causes such resistance that the baby is likely to aspirate. With a cow-milk formula, he will suck in a rather continuous fashion, pausing at irregular intervals. If breast milk then is fed to him by this same system, he will register his recognition of the change in taste after a short latency, and then suck in bursts with frequent pauses at regular intervals. The pauses seem to be directly related to the taste of breast milk, and his burst–pause pattern seems to indicate that he changes to a program for other stimuli (*e.g.*, social communication) to be added to the feeding situation during the pauses.

Procedures for recording various parameters of sucking behavior have documented the fine discriminations that infants make.[39] A suck apparatus connected to a polygraph has been used for recording the infant's sucking behavior under conditions in which the presentation of drops of fluid is contingent on that behavior. When sucking on a blank nipple, the infant sucks in short bursts separated by long pauses, and sucking within those bursts is quite rapid. When a sweet fluid (*e.g.*, 15% sucrose) is delivered contingent on sucking, the infant engages in more sucks per minute, invests more sucks per burst, takes shorter rest periods, and sucks more slowly within each sucking burst. Moreover, these parameters are affected by sweetness along a continuum from 0% through 15% sucrose and by the amount of fluid received per suck.[40] With increasing concentrations or increasing amounts of sucrose, infants tend to suck more slowly within bursts.

SENSITIVITY TO TACTILE STIMULI

The sensitivity of the infant to handling and to touch is apparent. A mother's first response to an upset baby is to contain him, to shut down his disturbing motor activity by touching or holding him. Fathers are more likely to tap in a playful, rhythmic fashion or to use tactile methods to excite the infant. Touch becomes a message system between the caregiver and the infant, for calming him and for exciting him to attend to cues. A patting motion of three times per second is soothing, but five to six times per second becomes an alerting stimulus.[41] As with auditory stimuli, the law of initial values seems to be important. When a baby is quiet, a rapid, intrusive tactile stimulus brings him up to an alert state. When he is upset, a slow, modulated tactile stimulus seems to reduce his activity.

Swaddling is used in many cultures to replace the important constraints offered first by the uterus and then by mothers and caretakers. As a restraining influence on the overreactions of hyperactive neonates, the supportive control that is offered by a steady hand on a baby's abdomen or by holding his arms so that he cannot startle reproduces the swaddling effects of holding or wrapping. This added control of disturbing motor responses allows the neonate to attend and interact with his environment.

If an infant cannot use soothing tactile stimuli to help him adapt his state behavior, the physician must consider a diagnosis of CNS irritability. A baby with CNS irritation from a bleed or from infection demonstrates constantly increasing irritability with stimuli, especially tactile. This response should signal the examiner to investigate the infant further for evidence of CNS difficulties.

SUCKING CAPACITY

An awake, hungry newborn exhibits active searching movements in response to tactile stimulation in the region around the mouth and even as far out on the face as the cheek and sides of the jaw and head. This is called the rooting reflex, and it is present in premature infants even before sucking itself is effective. Peiper described oral pads in the cheeks and mouth, which help maintain and establish negative pressure.[42] Sucking is facilitated by the thorax in inspiration and by fixing the jaw to maintain it between respirations.[42] A second mechanism, expressing, is made by the tongue as it moves up against the hard palate and from the front to the back of the mouth. Swallowing and respirations must be coordinated, and the depth and rate of respiration are handled differently in nutritive and nonnutritive sucking. Peiper argues for a hierarchic control of swallowing, sucking, and breathing, in which swallowing controls sucking and sucking controls breathing. The absence of coordination between these three systems in the neonate indicates discoordination within the CNS, which may occur in damaged or very immature infants.

Gryboski described a technique of monitoring three components of sucking with three transducers: a lapping mechanism at the front of the tongue, a milking action at the base of the tongue, and a suction component in the upper esophagus.[43] The timing of the three components becomes a measure of the maturity of the CNS of a premature infant. There is a latency before they become coordinated in an effective milking mechanism; the more prolonged the latency, the more immature is the baby. The examiner can feel these three components by placing a finger in the baby's mouth. A nurse who is familiar with premature infants can tell whether they are coordinated. If there is CNS irritation, the examiner can feel the disruption of the central processes that control these mechanisms by inserting a finger into the neonate's mouth, and when the infant is sucking, an examiner can determine for himself the presence and coordination of the three components. This is an easily available and valuable measure of the infant's stage of relative maturity and of his CNS coordination.

The infant sucks in a more or less regular pattern of bursts and pauses, with 5 to 24 sucks per burst.[44] The pause between bursts has been considered a rest and recovery period and a period during which cognitive information is being processed by the neonate. Kaye and Brazelton found that the pauses were important ethologically, because they are taken by mothers as signals to stimulate the infant to return to sucking.[45] Mothers tend to look down at, talk to, and stimulate a baby when he pauses in a sucking burst. The mother's jiggling actually prolongs the pause as the infant responds to the stimulating information given to him by his mother.

Sucking, because of the stability produced through central control early in gestation, is used by researchers to measure all sorts of behaviors in infants: sensory discrimination, conditioning, learning, orienting, and attention.[29,44,46] The importance of sucking as a way of self-regulation can be seen in a newborn as she begins to build from a quiet state to crying. Her attempts to achieve hand-to-mouth contact to keep her activity under control are fascinating. When she is finally able to insert a finger into her mouth, suck on it, and quiet herself, she seems rewarded. The sense of satisfaction and of gratification at having achieved this self-regulation are so striking that the watching adult can see that she has achieved a goal. Her face softens and alerts as she begins to concentrate on maintaining this kind of self-regulation. This is the most obvious evidence that the baby has goal-oriented behaviors that she can achieve for herself. A pacifier can achieve this same quieting in an upset baby, but a pacifier may not serve the self-regulating feedback system as richly as the baby's own maneuver.

Pairing sucking with other auditory, visual, or tactile modalities has been neglected in most neonatal nurseries. The variations and complexity of this system as it reflects CNS functions are well studied by psychologists and psychophysiologists.[47] For example, Cairns and Butterfield found that a neonate sucking on a nonnutritive pacifier presented a rich set of responses to human and nonhuman auditory signals.[34] After hearing a human voice, he would increase his sucking rate as a signal to bring it on again, and he could be conditioned in 20 minutes to suck harder or to pause to produce a second vocal signal. However, with white noise or pure-tone (*i.e.*, nonhuman) signals, he sucks less hard after the signal and learns to suck only to reduce the noise, not to repeat it or increase it.

If a human vocal sound was introduced to a neonate who was monitored by a nonnutritive pacifier, he began to produce a burst–pause pattern with prolonged pauses, as if he were waiting for the human signals to repeat themselves. Cairns and Butterfield suggest that pairing nonnutritive sucking with auditory stimulation can differentiate forms of CNS difficulty by the ability of the neonate to discriminate between paired signals that differ only in this way (*i.e.*, human *versus* nonhuman).[35] Cairn's group has been able to discriminate between the central and peripheral forms of impairment in auditory receptiveness that are the residua of rubella, hyperbilirubinemia, prematurity, and hypoxia.

Pairing two separate modalities of CNS function, such as sucking and sensory receptors, to test for fine discrimination tasks, for habituation and dishabituation to repetitive signals, and for conditioning and learning tasks suggests innovative methods for evaluating the neonate's CNS function.

ORGANIZATION OF MOTOR BEHAVIOR

One of the most neglected and illuminating sources of information about a neonate's status is gathered from simple observation of how he moves his extremities, what kind of movements he makes, and whether his movements are simple, random startles or purposeful. One of the most exciting behaviors that can be observed in the neonatal period is demonstrated by a well-organized newborn. As he begins to rouse from sleeping and when he begins to startle and become upset, he may attempt to bring his hand up to his mouth. In this effort, he may turn his head to one side, immediately controlling one side of his body by the central monitoring effects of the tonic neck reflex. The face and arm first extend and then slow down in extension. An observer can see the infant work to bring his hand up to his mouth. The infant's body begins to relax, his face softens, and he makes real efforts to insert his clenched fist. If these efforts are successful, he maintains a quiet state of semi-alertness, sucking loudly on the fist. Even if he cannot insert the hand or a finger, he remains in a rewarded peaceful state, ready to listen to a sound or look at a presenting stimulus. He has demonstrated to the observer that he can achieve a complex motor act by shutting out interfering reflex startles, completing a cycle of lateralizing his motor energy by bringing his hand up to his mouth, and using this activity to maintain a quiet and alert state, receptive to information from the environment. This complex behavior embedded in the goal-oriented achievement of wanting to listen or to look is powerful evidence in the neonate of optimal CNS organization.

When this behavioral organization is not observed in a particular interval, does it mean that the neonate cannot perform well? Not necessarily. Several conditions influence her performance:

- Ongoing state of arousal; if the child is too deeply asleep or too upset during an observation period, the likelihood of detecting organized behavior is reduced
- Environmental conditions (*e.g.*, too low or too high temperature, sound or light levels that reduce the child to a relative shutout state)
- Ongoing chemical or humoral imbalances (*e.g.*, mild dehydration, hypocalcemia, hypoglycemia), which render the child hypersensitive and jittery or too sleepy
- State of well-being (*i.e.*, illness, stress); relative motor disorganization may be a primary symptom of an impending illness
- Degree of recovery from the stresses of labor and delivery
- Perinatal stresses (*e.g.*, hypoxia, maternal medication).

Disorganization of motor activity may become an important symptom of stress in a neonate and should be assessed carefully. Repeated examinations as she recovers over the neonatal period are essential.

There are maneuvers that should be used for assessment of muscle tone and the balance of flexor and extensor muscles. The range that is possible for a given baby may be more important than any one sample of motor performance. The resting, spontaneous posture gives an idea of the preferred position. A normal full-term baby spontaneously prefers a position of flexion for both arms and legs. His extremities may extend from time to time, but he is usually found in flexed postures.

A baby who lies in full extension may be hypotonic. Hypertonicity is signaled by tightly flexed extremities with few spontaneous movements except brief, jerky startles. The examiner can determine in the first few minutes the most likely category to which the baby will be assigned. A few simple passive maneuvers of extending then flexing arms, legs, neck, and trunk confirm the degree of hypertonicity or hypotonicity. Hypertonicity is accompanied by jerky snapback of extremities or overshooting into tight flexion after the limbs are released. Hypotonicity is signaled by floppy, hyperextensive limbs, with little resistance or spontaneous movement after they are released. Organized reflex motor responses (*i.e.*, motor stepping, placing, and prone responses; crawling movements and attempts to lift the head; traction of his neck and shoulder; girdle musculature in a pull-to-sit maneuver) confirm and elaborate the infant's motor strength and the balance between flexor and extensor groups. Jerky, clonic movements and the snapback point to an imbalance of flexor and extensor muscle groups. Smooth movements of a neonate are an indicator of good balance between these groups and reveal a well-organized CNS.

Defensive reactions to a cloth over the face or to a painful stimulus to any part of the body elicit structured motor patterns, and the baby's effectiveness in approaching and removing an obtrusive stimulus becomes a way of testing intact motor pathways and their organization. For example, covering his face with a cloth elicits a series of motor maneuvers. He first roots, then twists his head from side to side, stretches his neck backward in active arching, and finally brings each arm up to swipe at the offending cloth. Many newborns effectively push the cloth off the face. These responses (*e.g.*, hand-to-mouth, defensive movements, other sequential motor acts) may be of equal value as elicited reflexes in assessing the upper extremities for neurologic adequacy.

LEARNING IN THE NEONATAL PERIOD

Because the neonate is equipped with remarkable capacities for responsiveness, we can improve assessments of CNS integrity at birth. Static neurologic assessments have not been particularly fruitful in predicting future function. Perhaps a model of assessment based on his capacity to use stimulation from the environment would offer us a better chance for predicting outcome.

CLASSIC CONDITIONING

One of the most obvious signs of newborn learning can be seen by use of classic conditioning techniques, in which the infant is presented with a neutral stimulus (*i.e.*, conditioning stimulus) in association with a stimulus effective in eliciting an observable response (*i.e.*, unconditioned stimulus). Over a series of presentations in which the stimuli are paired, the neutral stimulus comes to elicit the response under investigation and demonstrates the infant's capacity to retain these associations. Denisova and Figurin first demonstrated that newborns could be conditioned by being placed in the feeding position to which they had become accustomed.[48] After only a few days, they exhibited anticipatory sucking movements.

Lipsitt and Kaye used the presentation of a low-frequency, 93 dB tone in association with the insertion of a nipple in the mouths of infants 3 and 4 days of age.[49] To a control group, the tone and nipple were presented noncontiguously. On every fifth trial, the tone was presented alone as a test for conditioning, and after training was completed, all babies received a series of extinction trials with the test tone alone. Evidence was found for classic appetitive conditioning, although the effects of training did not manifest themselves until the extinction condition.

Papousek[50] and Siqueland and associates[51] studied the effect of contingent reinforcement of head turning to a touch at the side of the mouth. The stimulation produces the rooting reflex and head turning in 30% of preconditioning trials. After 5% dextrose solution was offered in response to successful head turning, the head turning was significantly increased by the reinforcement. Associating a tone with the positive condition enhanced head turning to a rate of 83%. If on alternate trials the head turns were not reinforced with dextrose solution, there was a gradual behavioral shift down to a rate of 30%. These studies demonstrated that reflexive behavior could be altered by contingent reinforcement.

EFFECTS OF STIMULATION ON RECOVERY

If these learning paradigms are capable of indicating sensory and neurologic integrity, perhaps a clinical test of the baby's future function could be based on a curve of behavioral improvement. Using the NBAS, we observed that there was a significant improvement over the first 10 days in major areas of behavior function in a low-risk group of babies.[52] The infants became more alert and capable of orienting to animate and inanimate stimuli. They turned significantly more to the voice and rattle and followed the human face and a red ball with significantly more head turning and alerting. Their motor maturity, muscle tone, and integrated motor performances also improved. On behavioral items reflecting their physiologic adjustments, such as startles and tremulousness, they improved significantly. This pattern of behavioral recovery based on the items of the NBAS can serve as an important system for evaluating CNS integrity and maturity.

There is increasing evidence that sensory input that is appropriate to the state of physiologic recovery of the neonate may further his weight gain, his sensory integrity, and his functional outcome. Unless we pay more attention to appropriate stimulation for the infant, we may be interfering with or retarding his optimal sensory development. Pettigrew found that for kittens specific visual input was necessary to develop the specificity of initially undifferentiated cells.[53] Blakemore and Cooper found that visual cortex neurons responded predominantly to stimuli that were equivalent to the environment in which the kittens were reared.[54] In both cases, these effects were found only after a given level of CNS maturity had been achieved. Before that time, exposure had no effect, because it did not appropriately fit the organism's level of development.

Most of the studies on early stimulation have not been individualized to the subjects. Evidence suggests that each premature or recovering neonate must be examined for the possibility of sensory overloading.[55] A premature infant responds to a soft rattle by turning his head away from the rattle and by other means of shutting it out, but a normal neonate turns toward the rattle and searches for the source of the sound.[55] The finely defined thresholds for appropriate sensory stimuli, as opposed to those that must be coped with or shut out, must be taken as seriously as whether or not we offer stimulation. In the recovery phase, a high-risk baby may be too easily overwhelmed, and routine stimulation may force him into an expensive coping model, but grading the stimuli to his particular sensory needs may further his recovery and his ultimate CNS outcome.

How can we tell when the infant is being overloaded? We can tell by watching his color changes, his kind of respirations, and his state of alertness and by looking for evidence of fatigue. Using Kearsley's ideas about the relative degree of attention to a stimulus as measured against physiologic demands, we have a clearly defined areas of "appropriate" and "inappropriate" properties of stimuli that can be applied to each neonate, permitting estimation of the amount and quality of stimulation that can be offered to every at-risk neonate without undue expense.[31]

The studies by Sander and associates show that the infant shapes his motility and his state behavior to the environment, particularly if it is sensitive to him and his needs.[56] Two models of regulation occurred with the neonates and caretakers they studied. The first consisted of basic regulation of endogenous biorhythmicity and was entrained by specific extrinsic cues in relation to the neonate's endogenous rhythm. Entrainment was most effective when the exogenous cue approximated the point in time at which a shift in the endogenous cycle was occurring. With the repeated establishment of contingent associations between state changes in the infant and specific configurations in caretaking events, entrainment was favored. The second model depended on the caretaker and infant achieving a regulatory balance based on mutual readiness of states, and with this, the stage was set to facilitate initial cognitive development. As the partners appreciated a mutual regulation of states of attention, they began to learn about and from each other, and a kind of reciprocity or affective interaction ensued.

These demonstrations of behavioral and sensory responsiveness can be used to assess the neonate and enable us to enhance the parent–infant interaction by sharing this assessment with the parent. The nonverbal communication between parent and infant in the initial stages of attachment is built on the infant's behavior. As pediatricians interested in enhancing the parent–infant bond, we would do well to observe, assess, and participate in the marvelous responsive capacities of the newborn infant.

REFERENCES

1. Greenberg NH. A comparison of infant-mother interactional behavior in infants with atypical behavior and normal infants. In: Hellmuth J, ed. Exceptional infant. vol 2. New York: Brunner Mazel, 1971:390.
2. Sigman M, Parmelee AH. Longitudinal evaluation of the preterm infant. In: Field TM, ed. Infants born at risk. New York: Spectrum, 1979.
3. Brazelton TB. Neonatal Behavioral Assessment Scale. Spastics international medical publications clinics in developmental medicine, monograph no. 50. Philadelphia: JB Lippincott, 1973.
4. Brazelton TB. Neonatal Behavioral Assessment Scale. 2nd ed. Spastics international medical publications clinics in developmental medicine, monograph no. 88. London: Blackwell Scientific Publications, 1984.
5. Brazelton TB, Nugent JK, Lester BM. Neonatal Behavioral Assessment Scale. In: Osofosky J, ed. The handbook of infant development. New York: Wiley & Sons, 1987.
6. Tronick E, Brazelton TB. Clinical uses of the Brazelton Neonatal Behavioral Assessment. In: Friedlander BZ, Sterritt GM, Kirk GE, eds. Exceptional infant. vol. 3. Assessment and intervention. New York: Brunner Mazel, 1975.
7. Prechtl H, Beintema O. The neurological examination of the full term newborn infant. London: William Heinemann, 1964.
8. Prechtl H, Dykstra J. Neurological diagnosis of cerebral injury in the newborn. In: Berge TS, ed. Proceedings of symposium on prenatal care. Groningen: Nordhoff, 1959.
9. Thoman EB. Early development of sleeping behavior in infants. In: Ellis NR, ed. Aberrant development in infancy. New York: John Wiley & Sons, 1975;123.
10. Michaelis R, Parmelee AH, Stern E, et al. Activity states in premature and term infants. Dev Psychobiol 1973;6:209.
11. Anders TF. Sleep and its disorders in infants and children: a review. Pediatrics 1972;50:312.
12. Steinschneider A. Nasopharyngitis and prolonged deep apnea. Pediatrics 1975;56:967.
13. Brazelton TB. Observations of the neonate. J Am Acad Child Psychiatry 1972;1:38.
14. Lester BM. The organization of crying in the neonate. Pediatr Psychol 1978;3:122.
15. Wasz-Hockert O, Lind J, Vuorenkoski V, et al. The infant cry. England: Lavenham, 1968.
16. Lester BM. Spectrum analysis of the cry sounds of well-nourished and malnourished infants. Child Dev 1976;47:237.
17. Ellingston RV. Cortical electrical responses to visual stimulation in the human infant. Electroencephalogr Clin Neurophysiol 1960;16:663.
18. Hrbek A, Mares P. Cortical evoked responses to visual stimulation in full term and premature infants. Electroencephalogr Clin Neurophysiol 1964;16:575.
19. Brazier MAB, ed. The central nervous system and behavior (translated). 2nd conf. New York: Josiah Macy Foundation, 1959.
20. Fantz RI. Visual perception from birth as shown by pattern selectivity. Ann N Y Acad Sci 1965;118:793.
21. Goren CC, Sarty, M, Wie PYK. Visual following and pattern discrimination by newborn infants. Pediatrics 1975;56:544.
22. Brazelton TB, Scholl MI, Robey JS. Visual responses in the newborn. Pediatrics 1966;37:284.
23. Gorman JJ, Cogan DG, Gellis SS. An apparatus for grading the visual acuity of infants on the basis of opticokinetic nystagmus. Pediatrics 1957;19:1088.
24. Dayton GO Jr, Jones MH, Aiu P, et al. Developmental study of coordinated eye movements in the human infant. Arch Ophthalmol 1964;71:856.
25. Haynes H, White BL, Held R. Visual accommodation in human infants. Science 1965;148:528.
26. Sigman M, Kopp CB, Parmelee AH, et al. Visual attention and neurological organization in neonates. Child Dev 1973;44:461.
27. Hershenson M. Visual discrimination in the human newborn. J Comp Physiol Psychol 1964;58:270.
28. Eisenberg RB. Auditory behavior in the human neonate: methodologic problems. J Aud Res 1965;5:159.
29. Lipsett EP. Learning in the human infant. In: Stevenson HW, Rheingold HL, Hess E, eds. Early behavior: comparative and behavioral approaches. New York: John Wiley & Sons, 1967:225.
30. Lipton EL, Steinschnieder A, Richmond J. Auditory sensitivity in the infant: effect of intensity on cardiac and motor responsivity. Child Dev 1966;37:233.
31. Kearsley RB. The newborn's response to auditory stimulation:

a demonstration of orienting and defensive behavior. Child Dev 1973;44:582.

32. Bronstein AI, Petrova EP. The auditory analyzer in young infants. In: Brackbill Y, Thompson GC, eds. Behavior in infancy and early childhood. New York: Free Press, 1967:163.
33. Bridger WH. Sensory habituation and discrimination in the human neonate. Am J Psychiatry 1961;117:991.
34. Cairns GF, Butterfield EC. Assessing infant's auditory functioning. In: Friedlander BZ, Sterritt GM, Kirk GE, eds. Exceptional infant. vol. 2. New York: Brunner Mazel, 1975:84.
35. Engen T, Lipsitt LP, Kaye H. Olfactory responses and adaptation in the human neonate. J Comp Physiol Psychol 1963; 56:73.
36. MacFarlane A. Parent-infant interaction. Oxford: Elsevier Press, 1975:103.
37. Pratt KC, Nelson AK, Sun KH. The behavior of the newborn infant. Ohio State University Student Contributions in Psychology. vol. 30. Ohio State University, 1930.
38. Johnson P, Salisbury DM. Parent-infant interaction. Oxford: Elsevier Press, 1975:119.
39. Lipsitt LP, Kaye H, Bosack TN. Enhancement of neonatal sucking through reinforcement. J Exp Child Psychol 1966;4:163.
40. Crook CK, Lipsitt LP. Neonatal nutritive sucking: effects of taste stimulation on sucking rhythm and heart rate. Child Dev 1976;47:518.
41. Brazelton TB, Tronick E, Adamson L, Als H, Wise S. Parent-infant interaction. Oxford: Elsevier Press, 1975:33.
42. Peiper A. Cerebral function in infancy and childhood. Nagler B, Nagler H, trans. New York: Consultant's Bureau, 1963.
43. Gryboski JD. The swallowing mechanism of the neonate: esophageal and gastric motility. Pediatrics 1965;35:445.
44. Kaye K. Infant sucking and its modification. In: Lipsitt LP, Spiker CC, eds. Advances in child development and behavior. vol. 3. New York: Academic Press, 1967.
45. Kaye K, Brazelton TB. The ethological significance of the burst-pause pattern in infant sucking. Presented at the Society for Research in Child Development, Minneapolis, April, 1971.
46. Haith MM, Kessen W, Collins D. Response of the human infant to level of complexity of intermittent visual movement. J Exp Child Psychol 1969;7:52.
47. Lipsitt LP. The study of sensory and learning processes of the newborn. Clin Perinatol 1977;4:163.
48. Denisova MP, Figurin NKL. Voprosu o pervykh sochetatelnykh pishchevykh refleksakh u grundykh detei. Vopr Genet Reflek Pedol 1929;1:81.
49. Lipsitt LP, Kaye H. Conditioned sucking in the human newborn. Psychosom Sci 1974;1:29.
50. Papousek H. Conditioned motor digestive reflexes in infants. II. A new experimental method for the investigation. Czekoslovakia Pediatrici 1960;15:981.
51. Siqueland ER, Lipsitt LP. Conditioned head turning in human newborns. J Exp Child Psychol 1966;3:356.
52. Tronick R, Wise S, Als H, et al. Regional obstetric anesthesia and newborn behavior: effect over the first 10 days of life. Pediatrics 1977;58:94.
53. Pettigrew JD. The effect of visual experience on the development of stimulus specificity by kitten cortical neurones. J Physiol 1974;237:49.
54. Blakemore C, Cooper GF. Development of the brain depends on the visual environment. Nature 1970;228:477.
55. Als H, Lester BM, Tronick E, Brazelton TB. Manual for the assessment of preterm infants' behavior (APIB). In: Fitzgerald HE, Lester BM, Yogman MW, eds. Theory and research in behavioral pediatrics. vol. 1. New York: Plenum Press, 1975.
56. Sander LW, Chappell PF, Gould SB, et al. An investigation of change in the infant-caretaker system over the first week of life. Presented at the Annual Meeting of the Society for Research in Child Development, Denver, 1975.

Neonatology: Pathophysiology and Management of the Newborn, Fourth Edition,
edited by Gordon B. Avery, Mary Ann Fletcher, and Mhairi G. MacDonald.
J.B. Lippincott Company, Philadelphia © 1994.

chapter 22

General Care

JOAN MCGREGOR KELLY

There are aspects of general care that apply to all newborns regardless of gestational age or medical condition. This chapter deals with the general care that newborns receive during the four phases of their hospitalization: delivery, transition, the hospital stay, and discharge. Infection control and general laboratory evaluation are also discussed.

DELIVERY ROOM CARE

RESUSCITATION

Neonatal resuscitation and the physiology of transition are discussed in Chapters 18 and 19. Practical recommendations regarding resuscitation in the delivery room can be found in the American Heart Association and American Academy of Pediatrics (AHA/AAP) Textbook of Neonatal Resuscitation.*

CORD CLAMPING AND CORD BLOOD COLLECTION

After delivery of the infant's head, the obstetrician must clear the infant's airway. During the 30 to 60 seconds of suctioning, usually before clamping the cord, the infant is held at the level of the introitus or abdomen to prevent a significant shift of his blood volume. Consequences of a significant shift toward the infant include polycythemia, circulatory volume overload, and hyperbilirubinemia, and these generally outweigh any potential advantage of augmenting the infant's iron reserve. Stripping the umbilical cord to enhance placental transfusion to the infant is reserved for infrequent instances of severe fetal hypovolemia. As soon as possible after suctioning, the cord is clamped and cut 4 to 5 cm from the infant's abdomen.[1] After the infant is dried and stabilized and if the umbilical base appears normal, an umbilical clamp is secured to the cord 1 to 2 cm distal to the abdominal wall, and any excess length is cut. If the base appears fuller than normal, suggesting an omphalocele, or if catheterization of umbilical vessels is likely, it is helpful to clamp the cord more distally. Notation should be made if fewer than three umbilical vessels exist.[2]

After delivery of the placenta, blood may be collected for laboratory tests by direct needle aspiration of the fetal vessels in the cord or on the fetal placental surface. Allowing placental blood to drip from the cord directly into laboratory tubes before placental delivery may contaminate the specimen if there is not a free flow. Fetal or placental blood should not clot for at least 15 minutes after cord clamping.

TEMPERATURE CONTROL

At delivery, the infant moves from a warm environment *in utero* into a much cooler delivery room. Although this immediate cold stress helps the infant initiate breathing, prolonged cold stress is dangerous.[3] Because the neonate is particularly vulnerable to hypothermia, she requires exquisite attention to her environmental support. She should be placed on

* P.O. Box 927, Elk Grove Village, IL 60009-0927.

a heated radiant warmer bed, dried with warm linens, and swaddled in clean ones, with a stockinet cap covering her head. If the parent holding the infant wishes to unwrap and inspect her, a radiant warmer should be placed over the parent and baby. Common potential sources of cold stress in the first few hours include cold oxygen used in resuscitation, unwarmed transport incubators, environmental drafts, and the initial weighing, bathing, and examination (see Chap. 25).

IDENTIFICATION AND SECURITY

Footprinting, palmprinting, or fingerprinting are the traditional methods of documenting a newborn's identity. Despite evidence that these methods are unreliable, local regulations may require them.[4] Before leaving the delivery room, each infant should be identified by wrist and ankle bands that indicate his mother's name and hospital identification number and the infant's hospital number and date of birth. The mother should wear a band with identical information; the father may do so as well. Any time an infant is released to a parent, the matching bands must be verified. Parents should verify the identity of anyone asking to take their infant from their room. Because of the variety of personnel and visitors in maternity, nursery, and postpartum areas, all hospitals should follow strict security precautions to ensure the safety of each newborn.

INFECTION CONTROL

Because bacterial and viral infections can be devastating to neonates, prevention and early detection are mainstays of general care. Meticulous attention to infection control is essential, because newborns are at risk for infections acquired from their mothers, their environment, and the personnel providing their care.

Careful hand washing is the mainstay of infection control. Before entering the nursery, personnel should scrub their hands and forearms to the elbows with a sponge and an antiseptic preparation such as iodophor, chlorhexidine, or hexachlorophene. Hands should be washed and dried before and after handling each baby and after touching any object likely to be contaminated.

If there is the potential for contact with blood or body fluids, personnel should protect themselves and other patients by following universal precautions. This means simply wearing gloves for diaper changes and phlebotomy. For more invasive procedures, gown, mask, goggles, and gloves are appropriate. Contaminated linens and clothing should be disposed of properly.

Cover gowns have traditionally been used in nursery and postpartum units, but gowning decreases neither bacterial colonization of the infant's nose or umbilicus nor the incidence of sepsis.[5] Gowns are valuable for protecting the caregiver's clothing and where universal precautions apply, but their routine use is unnecessary. The fact that ungowned visitors pose no greater risk to healthy newborns has also brought into question the traditional use of scrub attire in nurseries; it remains necessary for personnel who attend deliveries.

Providing each infant with his own clothing, diapers, and bulb syringe limits cross-contamination and essentially isolates each infant with his own equipment. It is common practice to wipe equipment such as stethoscopes with alcohol between uses on multiple infants. There is no convincing evidence that this decreases colonization or cross-contamination, but like gowning, if the practice reminds personnel to practice careful hand washing, it is valuable. Nursery linens and infant clothing may be routinely laundered; autoclaving is unnecessary.[6]

Separating infants into cohort groups by age, which allows complete cleaning of a nursery module as that cohort is discharged, is an effective means of preventing the spread of pathogens. Cohorting can be routine or instituted after an outbreak occurs.

ADMISSION PROCEDURES

After initial stabilization, bonding, and identification, the infant is transferred to an area where her adaptation to extrauterine life can be monitored while routine admission procedures are performed. This area may be in a specialized nursery, the routine care nursery, or the postpartum recovery room. Its staff should be attuned to the subtleties of newborn adaptation and familiar with aberrations of medical history, physical examination, or laboratory data that may necessitate immediate involvement of the infant's physician.

TRANSITION AND INITIAL PHYSICAL ASSESSMENT

The transition period classically refers to the first 6 to 12 hours of life, during which a healthy newborn goes through predictable patterns of alertness, vital sign changes, and gastrointestinal activity.[7] Sick, stressed, or premature infants do not follow the predictable patterns. Proper interpretation of the changing physical findings in the first few hours depends on familiarity with these normal patterns.

Increasingly, the term "transition" is used interchangeably with "adaptation." Physiologic adaptation to extrauterine life occurs over the first 24 hours and is considered complete when vital signs, feeding, and gastrointestinal and renal function are normal. Infants with delayed or prolonged transitions may have persistent tachypnea, delayed hunger and feeding, or difficulty maintaining their temperature. Differentiating an otherwise healthy infant with delayed transition from an ill infant with similar symptoms is sometimes difficult. Because time alone cures one and harms the other, it is crucial to make an accurate observation.

An initial assessment of the newborn includes measurement of vital signs (*e.g.*, heart rate, respiratory rate, temperature), body measurements (*e.g.*, weight, length, head circumference, sometimes chest and abdominal circumference), and a complete physical examination. Assessment of vital signs, behavior, and activity continues at least every half hour until remaining stable for 2 hours. Although the AAP suggests that the apparently normal infant should be examined by 12 to 18 hours of age by the responsible physician, many newborns are not seen by physicians until almost 24 hours of age.[8] There is much reliance on astute nurses whose experience and judgment are invaluable in the newborn's initial care.

VITAMIN K

Because of poor placental transport of vitamin K and an absence of intestinal flora to produce it, newborns have low levels of active vitamin K–dependent clotting factors. This insufficiency may present clinically as a spontaneous bleeding diathesis, notably as gastrointestinal, skin, or intracranial hemorrhage. Hemorrhagic disease of the newborn, a potentially lethal disorder, has an incidence of 0.25% to 1.7%; breast-fed infants and infants of mothers taking anticonvulsants are at highest risk.[9] Although effectively treated with vitamin K and blood products, the disease can be prevented by the administration of 0.5 to 1 mg of vitamin K, given intramuscularly within 1 hour of birth.[8] Oral vitamin K is effective, although there is no consensus on optimal dosage.[10] Careful documentation of vitamin K administration is important.

EYE PROPHYLAXIS

The prevention of neonatal gonococcal ophthalmia was the original impetus for newborn eye prophylaxis. *Chlamydia*, although causing a less serious ophthalmia, is the more prevalent ocular pathogen acquired by the newborn from the maternal genital tract. Penicillinase-producing gonococci (PPGC) are becoming prevalent. Acceptable agents for eye prophylaxis are 1% silver nitrate, 0.5% erythromycin, and 1% tetracycline.[11] Erythromycin and tetracycline have direct antibiotic effects; silver nitrate causes a chemical conjunctivitis, producing an inflammatory response with a secondary antibiotic effect. Each agent has limitations in its spectrum of activity. All are effective against sensitive gonococci; silver nitrate is the most effective against PPGC; no agent works particularly well against *Chlamydia*.[12]

All agents are instilled into the lower conjunctival sac, and the lids are massaged to distribute the medication. Excess medication can be wiped away, but the eyes should not be flushed. To allow for uninhibited mutual gazing and parent–infant bonding in the delivery room, eye prophylaxis may be delayed until admission to the nursery, where it can be carefully administered and documented. However, it should not be delayed longer than 1 hour.[11] Topical antimicrobial therapy is insufficient prophylaxis for infants of mothers with active gonococcal infections at delivery, and these infants must receive parenteral therapy as well.[11]

Although evidence suggests that ocular prophylaxis is not necessary for infants delivered by cesarean section after fewer than 3 hours of ruptured membranes, the AAP recommends prophylaxis for all infants, regardless of route of delivery.[13]

GENERAL LABORATORY EVALUATION

MATERNAL EVALUATION

Several screening blood tests are recommended for all pregnant women:[14]

- hemoglobin and hematocrit levels
- serologic test for syphilis (STS)
- blood group, Rh type, and indirect Coombs test
- rubella IgG
- hepatitis B surface antigen (HBsAg)
- α-fetoprotein.

In at-risk populations, screening for human immunodeficiency virus (HIV) and illicit drugs is routine, and STS in the third trimester and at delivery are recommended. The results of the tests should be available to the infant's caregivers as early diagnostic or therapeutic actions may be necessary. There should be a standard manner in which this information is transmitted to the infant's chart. Any other abnormalities or problems during the pregnancy should be also be noted on the chart.

NEONATAL EVALUATION

The value of routine laboratory evaluations on all patients admitted to hospitals is a subject of debate. Previous recommendations for newborns have included blood type and direct Coombs test, serologic test for syphilis, hemoglobin and hematocrit, glucose or rapid blood glucose screen, urinalysis, and the newborn metabolic screen. Of these, only the metabolic screen should be performed on every infant; other tests are necessary as indicated in the text that follows.

BLOOD TYPE AND COOMBS TEST

The infants at risk for hemolytic disease due to Rh type or major blood group incompatibility are Rh-positive infants of Rh-negative mothers and type A or B infants of type O mothers. The Rh status of any infant born to an Rh-negative mother should be determined to identify candidates for maternal immunoprophylaxis; even if an Rh-positive baby is unaffected by Rh disease, RhoGAM (*i.e.*, anti-Rh IgG) should be given to the mother postpartum to protect future Rh-positive fetuses. Blood typing all infants of type O mothers is more controversial. Infants with clinically significant hemolysis due to ABO incompatibility usually have only mild anemia; hyperbilirubinemia is the major problem. In the past, infants of type O mothers were observed for the development of jaundice; type and Coombs status were determined if jaundice occurred. Because of the current practice of discharging the mother and infant as early as 24 hours postpartum, further observation of the infant for jaundice is not feasible, and it is helpful to know the blood type of these infants before discharge. Direct Coombs-negative type A or B infants have hemoglobin values, reticulocyte counts, and bilirubin levels comparable to those of type O infants. Coombs-positive infants usually have lower hemoglobin values and higher reticulocyte counts and bilirubin levels, indicating more hemolysis.[15] Coombs testing should be done on the cord blood of all type A or B infants of type O mothers. Cord or serum bilirubin levels, hemoglobin and hematocrit testing, and reticulocyte counts are optional unless therapy for hyperbilirubinemia is likely or indicated.

GLUCOSE SCREENING

The incidence of hypoglycemia is decreasing as newborns are fed sooner after birth and as maternal diabetes is better controlled. Selected screening of infants who are at risk by virtue of history or size is appropriate.[16] Any infant with symptoms attributable to hypoglycemia should have a glucose test. Rapid glucose screening tests are technique dependent; those that use reagent strips demonstrating color change may be inaccurate at high hemoglobin and hematocrit levels. Abnormal results should be confirmed by standard whole blood glucose assays.

HEMOGLOBIN AND HEMATOCRIT DETERMINATIONS

There is little justification for routine hemoglobin and hematocrit determinations on a single infant with no evidence of anemia or polycythemia by history or physical examination.[17,18] Monochorionic twins, however, are at risk for twin-to-twin transfusion and its attendant complications; therefore same-gender twins should each have blood drawn for hemoglobin and hematocrit tests.[19]

NEWBORN SCREENING PROGRAMS

Programs are in place for neonatal screening for rare but potentially devastating disorders that are difficult to detect clinically, but for which there are dramatic benefits from early intervention. These disorders include phenylketonuria and congenital hypothyroidism. Most of the hospitals in the United States also screen for galactosemia, and some screen for other metabolic diseases and for hemoglobinopathies that are amenable to early preventive health measures.[20] The techniques and the timing for sampling vary; most programs require a sample shortly after birth and 2 weeks later. Because some assays measure metabolites of ingested substrates, it is advantageous to have feedings well established; blood is usually drawn on the morning of discharge. There should be a routine procedure in place for ensuring that each screen sample is drawn, with follow-up for abnormal results.

THE HOSPITAL STAY

The practice of an infant spending long periods of time in his mother's room (*i.e.*, rooming-in) has gained favor and forced reconsideration of practices based on fears of detriment to the infant not kept in a restricted nursery environment controlled for hygiene, attire, and visitors.[21] Rooming-in has become a necessity with the shortening of postpartum hospital stay, because new mothers staying in hospital only 24 to 36 hours simply cannot become comfortable with infant care if contact with their infants is limited.

Although relaxation of old restrictions allows infants to be outside the nursery, attention still must be given to providing a safe environment. Particular dangers are cold-induced stress, falls, and removal of the infant from the mother's care by unauthorized persons.

When the infant is with her mother, she should enjoy the same level of nursing care she would have within the nursery. This includes a general physical assessment and measurement of vital signs at least every 8 hours; recording of feeding volume, frequency, and behavior; recording of urine and stool output; cord and circumcision care; and any other procedures deemed necessary. The mother's assistance in all appropriate areas is desirable, because this helps ensure her competence in the care of her infant. The infant's bassinet should contain all clothing and equipment necessary for her care.

BATHING AND DRESSING

After achieving temperature stability, the infant with an apparently normal transition can be bathed. Although vernix has lubricating and antiinfectious properties that make its presence desirable, removing it for cosmetic purposes is routine. Bathing also removes gross maternal blood, minimizing exposure of the infant and his caregivers to blood-borne viruses such as hepatitis B virus (HBV), herpes simplex virus, and HIV. In infants whose maternal history is unclear or positive for one of these viruses, injections should be delayed until after the initial bath.

Warm water alone is sufficient for bathing most infants; a mild, nonmedicated soap or chlorhexidine gluconate may be used. Hexachlorophene, which can be absorbed through intact skin and cause neurotoxicity, is not recommended for routine bathing.[22] Care must be taken during bathing to minimize heat loss. After the bath, the infant is returned to the radiant warmer; when his temperature is stable, he is dressed in a diaper, shirt, and hat; wrapped in a double blanket; and transferred to an open bassinet. After 24 hours, most infants can maintain normal temperatures without a hat or second blanket.

Before discharge, the mother should understand how to bathe her baby safely. A mild soap and shampoo can be used sparingly.[23] Special baby soaps and lotions are expensive and unnecessary for infant skin care. Twice-weekly baths are usually sufficient. Overbathing dries and cracks skin; a mild hand lotion—not oil or ointment—can be applied if necessary.

Babies are often overdressed for their environments. The infant should be dressed in clothing that the parent would find comfortable, with one extra layer and a hat added in cool weather. Protection from direct and indirect sunlight is important, because infant skin burns easily.

Frequent diaper changing affords the best protection from diaper rash; creams, pastes, wipes, lotions, and powders are generally unnecessary. Warm water rinsing cleanses most soiled skin, with mild soap added as necessary. Diaper wipes are best reserved for times away from home when no sink is available. Air drying before rediapering helps keep the skin healthy. A product that adheres to the skin as a barrier to urine and stool should be applied to macerated skin; healthy skin needs nothing. Parents wishing to use powder should apply a nontalc, cornstarch type by hand; shaking the powder onto the baby may cause power-aspiration pneumonitis.[24] Neither cloth nor disposable diapers enjoy a clear advantage in maintaining infant skin health.

UMBILICAL CORD CARE

After the first bath, the umbilical cord and surrounding skin are treated topically to decrease invasive bacterial colonization. Acceptable agents include triple dye, alcohol, bacitracin, silver sulfadiazine, and povidone–iodine.[25,26] Thereafter, the cord remnant is left exposed outside the diaper to dry and mummify. The cord clamp can be safely removed after 24 hours.

Although it is unclear that any particular subsequent treatment shortens the time of cord attachment, it is common practice to wipe the cord at least daily, usually with alcohol.[26,27] The alcohol is applied underneath the dried cord to the still-moist areas. A mildly foul smell, slight oozing, a drop or two of blood, or a thin rim of erythema on the surrounding abdominal skin are normal.

FEEDING

Healthy infants tolerate feeding during transition; early feeding may prevent or minimize hypoglycemia. Vigorous infants without problems may nurse in the delivery room. Formula-fed infants are offered the first feeding after stabilization in the admission nursery. Because any newborn may have an uncoordinated suck and swallow reflex or an inapparent anomaly predisposing to aspiration, the formula-fed infant should take a few sips of sterile water before the formula. If aspirated, glucose water causes as severe a chemical pneumonitis as formula, and plain water is therefore recommended.[28] Subsequently, the infant can be fed room-temperature iron-fortified formula.[29] Breast-fed infants need not receive sterile water before the first nursing, because aspiration of colostrum is fairly benign.

Most mothers decide long before delivery whether they will breast or formula feed their infants.[30] Although breast milk is superior to formula, no mother should be subject to disapproval if she chooses to bottle feed. Because there remain many misunderstandings among first-time mothers about feeding, correcting misinformation is important.

On the first day of life, the breast-fed baby may latch onto the breast and nurse only briefly. Nursing becomes more vigorous in the second 24 hours, and by the third day, each session should last 10 to 15 minutes on each breast. Similarly, the formula-fed infant, who takes only 15 to 30 mL every 3 to 4 hours on day 1, increases to 75 to 90 mL by day 4 or 5.[31] Except when a more consistent glucose intake is required, babies should be fed on demand, when they are awake and hungry, rather than in accordance with a dictated schedule. There is no value in routinely supplementing the breast-fed infant with feedings of water, glucose water, or formula. In fact, this practice may discourage breast-feeding.[32]

Parents of bottle-fed infants should know how to prepare and store formula, know how to clean bottles and nipples, and understand the range of normal feeding volumes. Breast-feeding mothers need instruction about the mechanics of nursing, techniques for awakening and encouraging a sleepy baby, pumping and storing expressed milk, formula supplementation, and nutrition during lactation. Much of this instruction should occur prenatally, when the mother is interested and energetic. It should be supplemented in the hospital by nurses, physicians, or lactation specialists who can reinforce previous learning and ensure that the mother and her infant are doing well at discharge. Videotapes can supplement reading material. Mothers should know whom to contact and when to call if breast-feeding is not going well at home. Many pediatricians schedule office visits for breast-fed babies within a few days of discharge; by this time, mother's milk supply should be adequate to stop postnatal weight loss.

VOIDING AND STOOLING

Ninety-one percent of normal newborns void in the first 16 hours of life. Failure to do so by 24 hours should evoke concern but not panic.[33] An apparently well infant is unlikely to have serious disease and can be managed expectantly.[34] Similarly, 99% of term newborns pass a stool in the first 24 hours; 76% of premature infants do so, with 99% passing a stool by 48 hours.[33] As feeding is established, meconium stools give way to frothy, lighter transitional stools and then to a typical, seedy, yellow–green stool. Infants may produce stool in small quantities at each feeding because of the gastrocolic reflex; less frequent stools should be more voluminous. In the breast-fed infant, scanty, infrequent stools indicate poor caloric intake.[35]

BEHAVIOR

Sleeping, in approximately 4-hour cycles, occupies 20 to 22 hours of a typical newborn's day; the remainder is spent feeding and in the quiet alert state.[36] Crying is minimal. Parents may be concerned that their baby is inactive, particularly in the first 2 days. Despite extended sleeping, the newborn has a sophisticated array of behavioral responses to various stimuli, and certain aspects of later behavior patterns or personalities can be predicted by responses evoked on early examinations.[37] The knowledgeable caregiver can help strengthen the parent–infant bond by guiding the parents in choosing appropriate responses to their infant's behavioral cues (see Chap. 21).

JAUNDICE

Two-thirds of all babies appear jaundiced during their hospital stays.[38] Although the causes of jaundice are myriad and the pathophysiology complex, most jaundiced infants are normal, and their jaundice abates without ill effects.[39] Excess bilirubin resulting from hemolytic disease appears to be the only common cause of jaundice that should raise concern. The screening recommendations for Rh and ABO disease were discussed earlier. After hemolysis is excluded as a cause of moderate jaundice (bilirubin < 25 mg/dL) in a healthy, term infant younger than 1 week of age, further diagnostic and therapeutic procedures are unnecessary if there is follow-up to determine a return to normal.[40]

Jaundiced, breast-fed newborns have higher bilirubin levels than formula-fed infants.[41] This difference disappears if infants are nursed every 2 to 3 hours, rather than every 3 to 4 hours.[42] Frequent nursing has the added benefit of increasing the mother's milk supply and avoiding the problems caused by supplementation.[32,42]

RISKS OF PERINATALLY ACQUIRED INFECTION

SEPSIS

Neonatal sepsis is a relatively rare but potentially lethal disease. Conditions that place an infant at increased risk for sepsis include the following; many of these risk factors are additive:[43]

- prolonged rupture of the fetal membranes
- maternal chorioamnionitis, usually involving maternal fever, leukocytosis, uterine tenderness or irritability, purulent cervical discharge or foul-smelling amniotic fluid, or fetal tachycardia
- maternal colonization with group B streptococci
- prematurity
- maternal urinary tract infection
- perinatal asphyxia, unless clearly associated with a noninfectious cause, such as abruption
- male gender.

Infants who manifest even subtle clinical signs of sepsis deserve full evaluation and antibiotic therapy. Otherwise healthy infants with risk factors for sepsis pose a dilemma. Most of these clinically well infants are not infected, but because neonatal sepsis can be rapidly lethal, it must be promptly treated.

The laboratory evaluation of the possibly septic infant is complicated by several unique problems: low sensitivity of blood cultures; lack of cerebrospinal fluid pleocytosis in proven meningitis; variability of leukocyte counts; and the use of intrapartum antibiotics. There are several approaches to the evaluation and treatment of at-risk, asymptomatic neonates.[43,44] Although there is little agreement on the validity of specific approaches, especially when confounded by maternal antibiotics, an approach weighing risk factors and laboratory results is reasonable (Fig. 22-1).

POSITIVE MATERNAL SEROLOGIC TEST FOR SYPHILIS

As the prevalence of syphilis in the general population rises, so does the incidence of congenital syphilis. Recommendations for selected screening of pregnant women or infants at risk have failed to detect all infected infants. All mother–infant pairs should be screened. Because the STS (*i.e.*, Venereal Disease Research Laboratory [VDRL] test, rapid plasma reagin test) lacks specificity when performed on cord blood, this method of screening newborns is not recommended.[45] The Centers for Disease Control (CDC) recommends vigilance regarding the mother's STS:

> Pregnant women should be screened early in pregnancy. . . . In areas of high syphilis prevalence, or in patients at high risk, screening should be repeated in the third trimester and again at delivery. . . . An infant should not be released from the hospital until the serologic status of its mother is known.[46]

The CDC's recommendations for infant evaluation depend on the pediatrician's knowledge of the

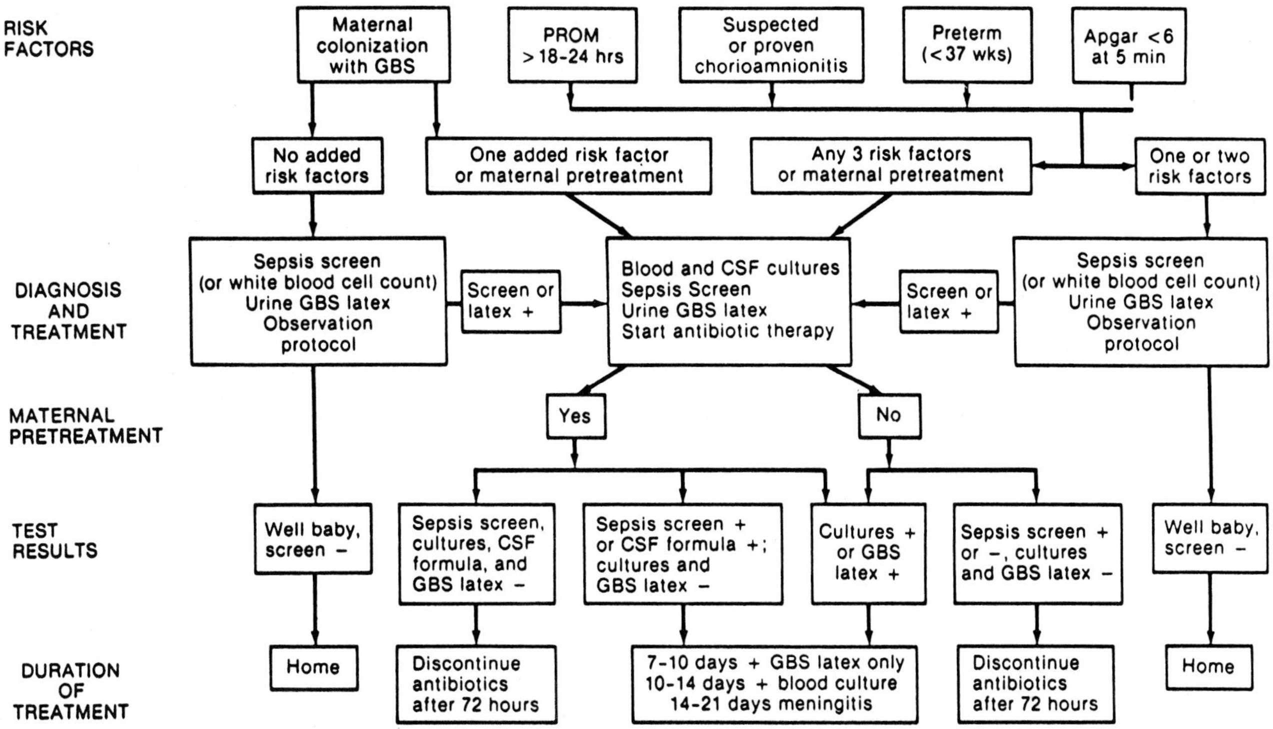

FIG. 22–1. Management of asymptomatic neonates at risk for sepsis. (+, positive; −, negative; CSF, cerebrospinal fluid; PROM, prolonged rupture of membranes; from Gerdes JS. Clinicopathologic approach to the diagnosis of neonatal sepsis. Clin Perinatol 1991;18:361)

mother's serologies and treatment throughout pregnancy. The physician should evaluate the infant if the mother has a positive STS confirmed by a treponemal test (*e.g.*, the fluorescent treponemal antibody absorption test) and was untreated, had poorly documented treatment, was treated with a drug other than penicillin, was treated within 1 month of delivery, or was treated adequately but did not demonstrate at least a fourfold fall in STS titer afterward, whether due to insufficient follow-up or treatment failure.[46]

Evaluation of the infant includes several measures:[46]

- complete physical examination
- STS (the same test performed on the mother so that titers can be compared)
- lumbar puncture for analysis of cells, protein, and VDRL
- long-bone radiographs
- any other test clinically indicated.

Differentiating between early infection and passive transfer of maternal antibody is problematic in the infant with an otherwise negative workup, because there is no reliable assay for IgM antitreponemal antibodies. The recommendations for treatment and follow-up are necessarily conservative. Moreover, excluding the diagnosis of neurosyphilis can be so difficult that therapy must be sufficient to treat it (see Chap. 48).

POSITIVE MATERNAL TEST FOR HEPATITIS B SURFACE ANTIGEN

The HBsAg-positive mother can transmit HBV perinatally to her newborn. The spectrum of disease manifestations in the infant range from asymptomatic seroconversion to fulminant, fatal hepatitis. Perinatally infected infants are at particular risk of becoming chronic carriers, and even if free of chronic hepatitis, they are at increased risk of developing later cirrhosis or hepatocellular carcinoma. Because immunoprophylaxis against HBV initiated at birth is 98% to 99% effective in preventing virus acquisition by the infant, identification of HBsAg-positive pregnant women is essential.[47] Confining testing to high-risk women (*e.g.*, Asian or African race, intravenous drug abuse, multiple sexual partners) misses 50% of those who are HBsAg-positive, and therefore, "routine screening is recommended for all women."[47]

Treatment of the infant whose mother is HBsAg-positive consists of immediate, thorough bathing; administration of 0.5 mL of hepatitis B immune globulin (HBIG) intramuscularly within 12 hours of birth; and the first dose of hepatitis B vaccine (0.5 mL, regardless of the product used) intramuscularly, concurrently with HBIG but at a different site. Subsequent doses of vaccine are given at 1 and 6 months of age.[47] No special isolation is necessary. Although HBV is found in breast milk, breast-fed infants, even if not receiving immunoprophylaxis, are not at increased risk of acquiring HBV infection, and breast-feeding is therefore allowed.[47]

A hepatitis B immunization series is recommended for all infants, including those of HBsAg-negative mothers. The first dose may be administered at birth, although alternate schedules are acceptable.[48] If the maternal HBsAg status is unknown at delivery, the infant should receive 0.5 mL of hepatitis B vaccine within 12 hours of birth. If the mother is subsequently found to be HBsAg-positive, HBIG should be given as soon as possible and no later than 7 days of age, and the vaccine series continued. If the mother is found to be HBsAg-negative, HBIG is unnecessary, and completion of the immunization series should follow recommended schedules and dosing.[48]

POSITIVE MATERNAL TEST FOR HUMAN IMMUNODEFICIENCY VIRUS

Vertical transmission of HIV from mother to infant occurs transplacentally and intrapartum, with an attack rate estimated at 30% to 35%, but perhaps as high as 50%, particularly with previous delivery of an infected infant.[49] Maternal antibodies are passively transferred to the infant and are detectable for 15 to 18 months. Diagnosis of HIV infection rests on sequential antibody testing of the infant to detect a rising titer. Amplification of HIV proviral DNA by means of the polymerase chain reaction may allow for diagnosis of infected infants shortly after birth. All exposed infants need comprehensive follow-up.

There are documented cases of infants acquiring HIV infection through breast-feeding. Though the AAP recognizes that the "additional risk, if any, of transmission of the virus to an infant through breast-feeding appears to be small," it recommends, "where alternative effective sources of feeding are available, an HIV-infected woman should be counseled not to breast feed."[49] No special isolation for mother or infant is necessary as long as universal precautions are followed.

MATERNAL DRUG USE

Maternal use of cocaine should be suspected if newborn infants have congenital anomalies, particularly those that can be explained by vascular disruption; irritability, abnormal behavior, seizures, or cerebral infarction; in all cases of placental abruption; and in cases of premature labor, unless otherwise explained.[50–52] Cocaine metabolites can be detected in neonatal urine after they have been cleared from maternal urine; a positive infant screen identifies drug use even if the maternal screen is negative. Cocaine-exposed infants do not go through a predictable pattern of drug withdrawal seen with opiate use. They are at risk for apnea, but there is no consensus regarding monitoring of these babies after discharge.[53]

The use of other illicit drugs and of alcohol abounds, with changes to new drugs occurring as interest and availability fluctuate. Suspicious maternal or infant behavior should prompt investigation of drug use. Social services support should be available for the drug-using mother and her infant. Chapter 57 provides a general discussion of drug withdrawal syndromes in the newborn, as do other sources.[54]

Mothers who use drugs are at increased risk for all sexually transmitted diseases.

THE POSTDATE INFANT

As the end of gestation approaches, the ability of the uteroplacental unit to nourish the fetus may deteriorate. The fetus may stop growing or lose weight. The fetus may respond to excessive hypoxia *in utero* by brisk hematopoiesis or may tolerate labor and delivery poorly, requiring nonroutine obstetric intervention or neonatal resuscitation. Postnatal sequelae can include polycythemia, hypoglycemia, meconium aspiration syndrome, and the various consequences of asphyxia, including persistent pulmonary hypertension.

MULTIPLE GESTATIONS

"We are faced with the undeniable fact that the human species is not designed to carry more than a single fetus *in utero* with any degree of biologic grace."[55] Twins have a mortality rate four times that of singletons, and that risk increases with increasing number of fetuses.[56] Most twin pairs are somewhat growth retarded; approximately one-half are also premature. Congenital anomalies may be more common in monozygotic twins than in singletons; these twins are also at risk for twin-to-twin transfusion and its consequences.[19] Parents of twins need special support; referring them to literature and support groups prenatally may help them recognize and cope better with the stresses of having two infants. Special help with breast-feeding may be necessary.[57] Caregivers must remember to assess and treat twins as individuals and should encourage the family to do so as well. Parents of a sick or dying twin grieve as deeply as do parents of singletons; that the other twin is alive and well does not diminish their grief and worry.[58]

CYANOTIC SPELL

Although the true incidence of the cyanotic or dusky spell in apparently well infants is unknown, personnel who work in well-baby nurseries see these episodes regularly. The otherwise healthy-appearing infant can have a problem as simple as spitting-up or one as potentially devastating as apnea, sepsis, or intracranial hemorrhage. Sorting through the various diagnostic possibilities demands an accurate description of the event, the activities immediately before and after it, and any intervention performed. Particular attention should be paid to the cardiac, respiratory, and neurologic examination of the infant. Continuous cardiopulmonary monitoring and pulse oximetry may be necessary to help define the problem and guide the workup.

CIRCUMCISION

Removal of the foreskin was almost routine in this country before the 1970s. In 1975, the AAP, although recognizing the sociocultural, cosmetic, and religious reasons for circumcision, found the evidence for its postulated medical benefits (*e.g.*, prevention of phimosis, balanitis, sexually transmitted diseases, and penile, prostatic, and cervical cancers) mostly unconvincing.

> A program of education leading to continuing good personal hygiene would offer all the advantages of routine circumcision without the attendant surgical risk.[59]

However, there is mounting evidence that uncircumcised males are at more risk for urinary tract infections and that lack of circumcision may enhance transmission of HIV. In 1989, the AAP relaxed its stance.

> Newborn circumcision has potential medical benefits and advantages as well as disadvantages and risks. When circumcision is being considered, the benefits and risks should be explained to the parents and informed consent obtained.[60]

The pendulum may swing back toward a policy of routine neonatal circumcision, but there is no consensus on this issue.[61]

Effective pain relief for circumcision can be provided by a dorsal penile nerve block, although this has potential risks.[62,63] The simple act of sucking on a pacifier, especially if sucrose flavored, appears to lessen the infant's pain during circumcision.[64]

The glans of the recently circumcised penis should be dabbed with petroleum jelly at each diaper change to prevent the friable mucosa from adhering to the diaper. A stuck glans can be atraumatically freed from the diaper by the application of warm water. The granulating tissue of the normal healing circumcision may be mistaken for pus. A swollen, oozing glans or an impaired urinary stream should prompt consultation with the physician.

An uncircumcised penis requires no special care. As the foreskin loses its adhesions to the glans, it can be retracted gently for cleansing. An excellent instructional pamphlet on care of the uncircumcised penis is offered to parents by the AAP.†

† P.O. Box 927, Elk Grove Village, IL 60009-0927.

DISCHARGE

CAR AND HOME SAFETY

Car safety should start before birth with parental acquisition of an approved child safety seat. Because these seats are often used improperly, hospital personnel should know the principles of their use and ensure that the babies discharged from their care are properly protected. Every hospital should have resources on site or readily available in the community for families without safety seats so that they may obtain them before discharge.

Literature or videotaped material regarding home safety for infants should be available to parents. Topics addressed should include burns, falls, aspiration and strangulation, bottle propping, and control of siblings and pets.

HOME ROUTINES AND VISITORS

Newborns do not have routines, which, combined with the recovering mother's fatigue, makes the first few weeks at home exhausting. Moreover, newborns are particularly susceptible to infection. For these reasons, parents should be discouraged from having a houseful of visitors or taking trips out of the home that could expose the infant to the general public. All energies should be directed at new baby care and feeding until the postpartum recovery is complete and a reasonably predictable feeding schedule established.

DISCHARGE TIME AND FOLLOW-UP

Discharge from the hospital should be dictated by the well-being of the mother and her infant, rather than by any other considerations. Both mother and infant should be sufficiently recovered from delivery so that continuous observation is no longer necessary; the mother should understand her postpartum care and be healthy enough to undertake it; and the parents should understand the care of their infant and how to obtain help if necessary. For the multiparous, vaginally delivered woman with a healthy, term infant and help at home, this length of time may be less than 24 hours. Obstetric, neonatal, and social considerations may preclude a rapid discharge.[65]

All infants should have follow-up arrangements documented before discharge. Those who are discharged within 24 hours of delivery should be examined within 2 to 3 days; others should be seen no later than 2 weeks of age. As with time of discharge, time for follow-up should be individualized, with consideration given for type of feeding, infant birth weight, maternal and infant blood types, parental experience, and the hospital duration and course.

REFERENCES

1. Cunningham FG, MacDonald PC, Gant NF. Williams obstetrics. 18th ed. Norwalk, CT: Appleton & Lange, 1989:307.
2. Froehlich LA, Fujikura T. Follow-up of infants with single umbilical artery. Pediatrics 1973;52:6.
3. Oliver TK Jr. Temperature regulation and heat production in the newborn. Pediatr Clin North Am 1965;12:765.
4. Thompson JE, Clark DA, Salisbury B, Cahill J. Footprinting the newborn infant: not cost effective. J Pediatr 1981;99:797.
5. Birenbaum HJ, Glorioso L, Rosenberger C, Arshad C, Edwards K. Gowning on a postpartum ward fails to decrease colonization in the newborn infant. Am J Dis Child 1990;144:1031.
6. Donowitz LG. Nosocomial infections in neonatal intensive care units. Am J Infect Control 1989;17:250.
7. Desmond MM, Franklin RR, Vallbona C, et al. The clinical behavior of the newly born. I: the term baby. J Pediatr 1963; 62:307.
8. AAP Committee on Fetus and Newborn and ACOG Committee on Obstetrics: Maternal and Fetal Medicine. Postpartum and follow-up care. In: Freeman RK, Poland RL, eds. Guidelines for perinatal care. 3rd ed. Elk Grove Village, IL: American Academy of Pediatrics and American College of Obstetricians and Gynecologists, 1992:91.
9. Lane PA, Hathaway WE. Vitamin K in infancy. J Pediatr 1985; 106:351.
10. Hathaway WE, Isarangkura PB, Mahasandana C, et al. Comparison of oral and parenteral vitamin K prophylaxis for prevention of late hemorrhagic disease of the newborn. J Pediatr 1991;119:461.
11. Committee on Infectious Diseases, American Academy of Pediatrics. Prevention of neonatal ophthalmia. In: Peter G, Lepow ML, McCracken GH Jr, Phillips CF, eds. Report of the committee on infectious diseases. 22nd ed. Elk Grove Village, IL: American Academy of Pediatrics, 1991:546.
12. Hammerschlag MR, Cummings C, Roblin PM, Williams TH, Delke I. Efficacy of neonatal ocular prophylaxis for the prevention of chlamydial and gonococcal conjunctivitis. N Engl J Med 1989;320:769.
13. Isenberg SJ, Apt L, Yoshimori R, McCarty JW, Alvarez SR. Source of the conjunctival bacterial flora at birth and implications for ophthalmia neonatorum prophylaxis. Am J Ophthalmol 1988;106:458.
14. AAP Committee on Fetus and Newborn and ACOG Committee on Obstetrics: Maternal and Fetal Medicine. Antepartum and intrapartum care. In: Freeman RK, Poland RL, eds. Guidelines for perinatal care. 3rd ed. Elk Grove Village, IL: American Academy of Pediatrics and American College of Obstetricians and Gynecologists, 1992:49.
15. Alter AA, Feldman F, Twersky J, et al. Direct antiglobulin test in ABO hemolytic disease of the newborn. Obstet Gynecol 1969;33:846.
16. Pagliaria AS, Karl IE, Haymond M, Kipnis DM. Hypoglycemia in infancy and childhood, part I. J Pediatr 1973;82:365.
17. Oski FA. The erythrocyte and its disorders. In: Nathan DG, Oski FA, eds. Hematology of infancy and childhood. 3rd ed. Philadelphia: WB Saunders Company, 1987:16.
18. Oh W. Neonatal polycythemia and hyperviscosity. Pediatr Clin North Am 1986;33:523.
19. McCulloch K. Neonatal problems in twins. Clin Perinatol 1988; 15:141.
20. Coen RW, Koeffler H. Primary care of the newborn. Boston: Little, Brown, 1987:167.
21. Committee on Fetus and Newborn, American Academy of Pediatrics. Postpartum (neonatal) sibling visitation. Pediatrics 1985;76:650.
22. AAP Committee on Fetus and Newborn and ACOG Committee on Obstetrics: Maternal and Fetal Medicine. Infection control. In: Freeman RK, Poland RL, eds. Guidelines for perinatal care. 3rd ed. Elk Grove Village, IL: American Academy of Pediatrics and American College of Obstetricians and Gynecologists, 1992:141.
23. Morelli JG, Weston WL. Soaps and shampoos in pediatric practice. Pediatrics 1987;80:634.
24. Mofenson HC, Greensher J, DiTomasso A, Okun S. Baby powder—a hazard! Pediatrics 1981;68:265.
25. Committee on Fetus and Newborn, American Academy of Pediatrics. Skin care of newborns. Pediatrics 1974;54:682.
26. Gladstone IM, Clapper L, Thorp JW, Wright DI. Randomized study of six umbilical cord care regimens. Clin Pediatr 1988;27:127.
27. Arad I, Eyal F, Fainmesser P. Umbilical care and cord separation. Arch Dis Child 1981;56:887.
28. Olson M. The benign effects on rabbits' lungs of the aspiration of water compared with 5% glucose or milk. Pediatrics 1970; 46:538.
29. Committee on Nutrition, American Academy of Pediatrics. Iron-fortified infant formulas. Pediatrics 1989;84:1114.
30. Sarett HP, Bain KR, O'Leary JC. Decisions on breast-feeding or formula feeding and trends in infant-feeding practices. Am J Dis Child 1983;137:719.
31. Driscoll JM Jr. Routine and special care. In: Fanaroff AA, Martin RJ, eds. Neonatal-perinatal medicine. 4th ed. St. Louis: CV Mosby, 1987:441.
32. Lawrence RA. Breast-feeding. Pediatr Rev 1989;11:163.
33. Clark DA. Times of first void and first stool in 500 newborns. Pediatrics 1977;60:457.
34. Moore ES, Galvez MB. Delayed micturition in the newborn period. J Pediatr 1972;80:867.
35. Lawrence RA. Infant nutrition. Pediatr Rev 1983;5:133.
36. Hack M. The sensorimotor development of the preterm infant. In: Fanaroff AA, Martin RJ, eds. Neonatal-perinatal medicine. 4th ed. St. Louis: CV Mosby, 1987:473.
37. Brazleton TB, Parker WB, Zuckerman B. Importance of behavioral assessment of the neonate. Curr Probl Pediatr 1976;7:1.
38. Maisels MJ, Newman TB. Jaundice in the healthy full-term infant: time for reevaluation. In: Klaus MH, Fanaroff AA, eds. 1990 Year book of neonatal and perinatal medicine. St. Louis: Mosby Year Book, 1990:iv.
39. Newman TB, Maisels MJ. Does hyperbilirubinemia damage the brain of healthy full-term infants? Clin Perinatol 1990; 17:331.
40. Oski FA. Hyperbilirubinemia in the term infant: an unjaundiced approach. Contemp Pediatr 1992;9:148.
41. Schneider AP II. Breast milk jaundice in the newborn. JAMA 1986;255:3270.
42. Yamauchi Y, Yamanouchi I. Breast-feeding frequency during the first 24 hours after birth in full-term neonates. Pediatrics 1990;86:171.
43. Gerdes JS. Clinicopathologic approach to the diagnosis of neonatal sepsis. Clin Perinatol 1991;18:361.
44. St. Geme JW Jr, Murray DL, Carter J, et al. Perinatal infection after prolonged rupture of membranes: an analysis of risk and management. J Pediatr 1984;104:608.
45. Committee on Infectious Diseases, American Academy of Pediatrics. Syphilis. In: Peter G, Lepow ML, McCracken GH Jr, Phillips CF, eds. Report of the committee on infectious diseases. 22nd ed. Elk Grove Village, IL: American Academy of Pediatrics, 1991:453.

46. Centers for Disease Control. 1989 sexually transmitted diseases treatment guidelines. MMWR 1989;38:9.
47. Committee on Infectious Diseases, American Academy of Pediatrics. Hepatitis B. In: Peter G, Lepow ML, McCracken GH Jr, Phillips CF, eds. Report of the committee on infectious diseases. 22nd ed. Elk Grove Village, IL: American Academy of Pediatrics, 1991:238.
48. Centers for Disease Control. Hepatitis B virus: a comprehensive strategy for eliminating transmission in the United States through universal childhood vaccination. MMWR 1991;40.
49. Committee on Infectious Diseases, American Academy of Pediatrics. AIDS and HIV infections. In: Peter G, Lepow ML, McCracken GH Jr, Phillips CF, eds. Report of the committee on infectious diseases. 22nd ed. Elk Grove Village, IL: American Academy of Pediatrics, 1991:115.
50. Hoyme HE, Jones KL, Dixon SD, et al. Prenatal cocaine exposure and fetal vascular disruption. Pediatrics 1990;85:743.
51. Chasnoff IJ, Griffith DR, MacGregor S, Dirkes K, Burns K. Temporal patterns of cocaine use in pregnancy. JAMA 1989;261:1741.
52. Chasnoff IJ, Bussey ME, Savich R, Stack CM. Perinatal cerebral infarction and maternal cocaine use. J Pediatr 1986;108:456.
53. Bauchner H, Zuckerman B. Cocaine, sudden infant death syndrome, and home monitoring. J Pediatr 1990;117:904.
54. Committee on Drugs, American Academy of Pediatrics. Neonatal drug withdrawal. Pediatrics 1983;72:895.
55. Hendricks CH. Twinning in relation to birth weight, mortality, and congenital anomalies. Obstet Gynecol 1966;27:47.
56. Ghai V, Vidyasagar D. Morbidity and mortality factors in twins. Clin Perinatol 1988;15:123.
57. Becker PG. Counseling families with twins: birth to 3 years of age. Pediatr Rev 1986;8:81.
58. Wilson AL, Fenton LJ, Stevens DC, Soule DJ. The death of a newborn twin: an analysis of parental bereavement. Pediatrics 1982;70:587.
59. Committee on Fetus and Newborn, American Academy of Pediatrics. Report of the ad hoc task force on circumcision. Pediatrics 1975;56:610.
60. Task Force on Circumcision, American Academy of Pediatrics. Report of the task force on circumcision. Pediatrics 1989;84:388.
61. Wiswell TE [letter], Schoen EJ [reply]. Circumcision. Pediatrics 1990;85:888.
62. Stang HJ, Gunnar MR, Snellman L, Condon LM, Kestenbaum R. Local anesthesia for neonatal circumcision: effects on distress and cortisol response. JAMA 1988;259:1507.
63. Schoen EJ [letter], Stang H, Snellman L [reply]. Dorsal penile nerve block for circumcision. JAMA 1989;261:701.
64. Blass EM, Hoffmeyer LB. Sucrose as an analgesic for newborn infants. Pediatrics 1991;87:215.
65. AAP Committee on Fetus and Newborn and ACOG Committee on Obstetrics: Maternal and Fetal Medicine. Postpartum and follow-up care. In: Freeman RK, Poland RL, eds. Guidelines for perinatal care. 3rd ed. Elk Grove Village, IL: American Academy of Pediatrics and American College of Obstetricians and Gynecologists, 1992:91.

Neonatology: Pathophysiology and Management of the Newborn, Fourth Edition,
edited by Gordon B. Avery, Mary Ann Fletcher, and Mhairi G. MacDonald.
J.B. Lippincott Company, Philadelphia © 1994.

chapter 23

Fluid and Electrolyte Management

EDWARD F. BELL
WILLIAM OH

Disorders of fluid and electrolyte balance are among the most commonly encountered problems in the care of newborn infants. Careful management of fluid and electrolyte intake can enhance the outcome of most critically ill or premature infants.

The goal of fluid and electrolyte management is to replace losses of water and electrolytes to maintain normal balance of these essential substances during growth and recovery from disease. A subsidiary aim in the first days of life is to allow successful transition from the aquatic environment of the fetus to the arid extrauterine milieu. The principles of fluid and electrolyte management in the neonatal period are similar to those established for older children, except for some variations and specific features of body composition, insensible water loss, renal function, and the neuroendocrine control of fluid and electrolyte balance.

To manage fluid therapy of newborns appropriately, the clinician should understand the normal physiologic mechanisms that govern water and electrolyte balance and the variations in these mechanisms that can occur in sick or premature infants. He or she should develop a systematic approach to the estimation of fluid and electrolyte requirements for correction of deficits and replacement of ongoing normal and abnormal losses. The results of fluid and electrolyte management must be carefully monitored so that the intakes of water and electrolytes can be adjusted as needed.

BODY COMPOSITION OF THE FETUS AND NEWBORN INFANT

CHANGES IN BODY WATER DURING GROWTH

The total body water (TBW) is divided into two major compartments, intracellular water (ICW) and extracellular water (ECW). The ECW is further divided into the interstitial water and the plasma volume, which is the intravascular component of the ECW. Figure 23-1 shows the approximate distribution of body water among these compartments in an infant at term.

In the early stages of fetal development, a large part of the body consists of water.[1] Total body water is estimated to be 94% of the body weight during the third month of fetal life. As gestation progresses, the TBW per kilogram of body weight declines. By 24 weeks, the TBW is approximately 86%, and by term, it is about 78% of body weight (Fig. 23-2). There are characteristic changes in the partition of body water between ECW and ICW during development. Extracellular water decreases from 59% of body weight at 24 weeks of gestation to about 44% at term, and ICW increases from 27% to 34% of body weight during the same period (Table 23-1).

After birth, TBW per kilogram of body weight continues to fall, primarily because of contraction of the ECW.[2,7–10] This mobilization of extracellular fluid is thought to be related to the concurrent improvement

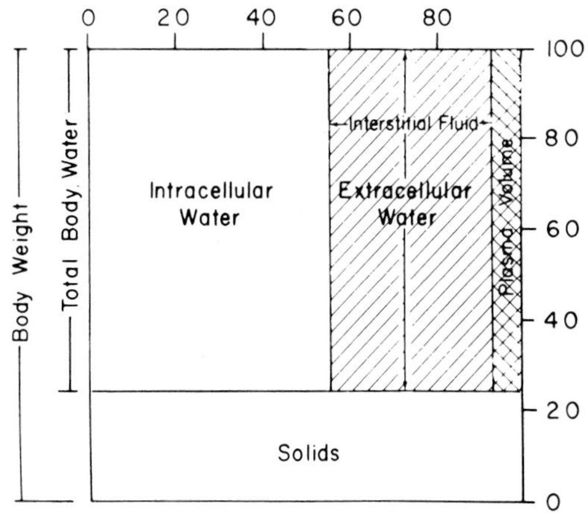

FIG. 23–1. Distribution of body water in a term newborn infant.

in renal function that occurs after birth.[11–13] Various studies have shown an increase, decrease, or no change in the ICW after birth. Intracellular water probably increases roughly in proportion to body weight in the first weeks of postnatal life.[2,9,10,14] Thereafter, ICW increases faster than body weight, and by 3 months, it exceeds ECW (see Fig. 23-2).[1,2] These postnatal changes in body water and its partition between ECW and ICW are influenced by the intake of water and electrolytes.[8,15] Failure to allow the normal postnatal contraction of ECW in premature infants may increase the risk of significant patent ductus arteriosus (PDA).[16]

SOLUTE DISTRIBUTION IN BODY FLUIDS

The major cation in the blood plasma is sodium (Fig. 23-3). Potassium, calcium, and magnesium constitute the balance of the cation fraction. The primary anion

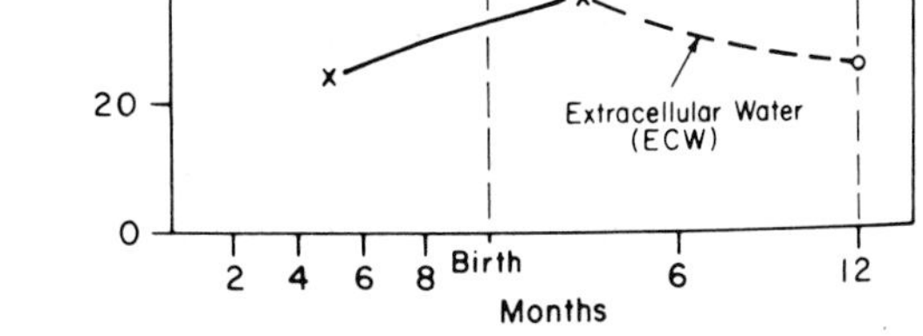

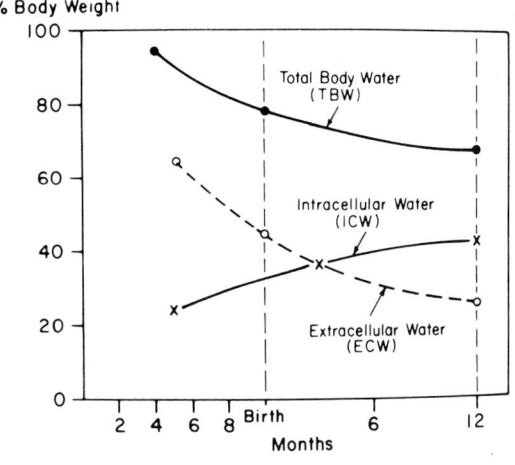

FIG. 23–2. Changes in body water during gestation and infancy. (Adapted from Friis-Hansen B. Changes in body water compartments during growth. Acta Paediatr Suppl 1957;110:1.)

is chloride, with protein, bicarbonate, and some undetermined anions constituting the balance of the anions. The interstitial fluid (*i.e.*, nonplasma ECW) has a solute composition that is similar to plasma, except that its protein content is lower. The ICW contains potassium and magnesium as its primary cations, and phosphate, both organic and inorganic, is the major anion, with bicarbonate contributing a smaller fraction.

The electrolyte composition of the body fluids of the newborn infant is largely determined by gestational age. Premature infants contain more sodium and chloride per kilogram of body weight than term infants because of their larger ECW (see Table 23-1).[3–5] Total body potassium content largely reflects ICW and is similar or slightly lower per kilogram of body weight in premature infants than at term.[3,6] These concepts are important for estimating electrolyte requirements during parenteral fluid therapy. Fetal fluid and electrolyte balance depends on maternal homeostasis and placental exchange; therefore, fluid and electrolyte status at birth is influenced by the maternal fluid and electrolyte management in labor.[17,18]

INSENSIBLE WATER LOSS

The loss of water by evaporation from the skin and respiratory tract is known as insensible water loss (IWL). About 30% of IWL normally occurs through the respiratory tract as moisture in expired gas, with the remaining 70% lost through the skin. Insensible water loss can be expressed in terms of body surface area (m^2) or weight (kg).[19–21] Insensible water loss depends more on surface area than weight, but it is commonly expressed per kilogram because weight is more easily determined than area.

Several factors influence IWL in a predictable manner (Table 23-2).[22–42] When expressed per kilogram of body weight, IWL is inversely proportional to birth weight and gestational age (Figs. 23-4 and 23-5).[22,25] Smaller, more immature infants have larger IWL per kilogram of body weight (Table 23-3). The same is true if IWL is expressed per square meter of body surface.[26] Therefore, although the greater IWL of smaller premature infants is partly due to the increased ratio of surface area of the skin and respiratory tract to body weight, it is also thought to be related to their thinner skin, greater skin blood flow, larger body water per kilogram of body weight, and higher respiratory rate.

FACTORS THAT INCREASE INSENSIBLE WATER LOSS

Any increase in ventilation volume per minute increases the respiratory IWL, as long as the water vapor pressure, or density, is less in the inspired gas than in the expired gas. This situation may occur in

TABLE 23–1
CHANGES IN BODY WATER AND ELECTROLYTE COMPOSITION DURING INTRAUTERINE AND EARLY POSTNATAL LIFE

Components	Gestational Age (wk) 24	28	32	36	40	1 to 4 Weeks After Full-Term Birth
Total body water (%)	86	84	82	80	78	74
Extracellular water (%)	59	56	52	48	44	41
Intracellular water (%)	27	28	30	32	34	33
Sodium (mEq/kg)	99	91	85	80	77	73
Potassium (mEq/kg)	40	41	40	41	41	42
Chloride (mEq/kg)	70	67	62	56	51	48

Data from references 1 through 6.

infants with cardiac disease, pulmonary dysfunction, or metabolic acidosis.

Environmental temperature above the neutral thermal zone increases IWL in proportion to the increment in temperature.[19,27,28] This effect can occur even without a rise in body temperature. A subneutral environmental temperature is not associated with reduced IWL, although metabolic heat production is increased.[28] Increased body temperature, whether caused by fever or environmental overheating, elevates IWL.[19,27]

Skin breakdown or injury disrupts the barrier against cutaneous evaporation and raises IWL. Skin trauma from thermal, chemical, or mechanical injury is common among critically ill, small, premature infants. Such injury may result from removal of tape or adherent monitoring devices or from prolonged skin exposure to disinfectant solutions. Insensible water loss is increased in conjunction with the skin manifestations of essential fatty acid deficiency,[43] a potential problem in infants receiving fat-free parenteral nutrition. Congenital skin defects, such as those seen in gastroschisis, omphalocele, and neural tube defects, are associated with increased IWL until surgically corrected.

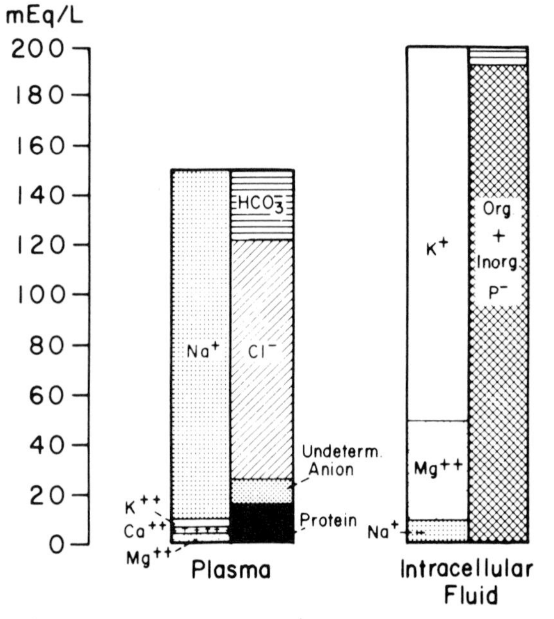

FIG. 23–3. Ion distribution in the blood plasma, which represents extracellular fluid, and in the intracellular fluid compartment.

Use of nonionizing radiant energy, in the form of either a radiant warmer or phototherapy, increases IWL by about 50%.[22,29–33] The mechanism of this increase in IWL with radiant energy is not well understood, but it may be related, at least in part, to increased skin blood flow.[44,45] The impact on IWL of phototherapy delivered by fiberoptic blankets or pads is not known, but it is probably less than with conventional fluorescent phototherapy lamps. In the case of radiant warmers, it is possible that IWL is higher, because absolute humidity (*i.e.*, water vapor pressure) is lower under radiant warmers than in incubators.[32] This may be true even though relative humidity is higher under radiant warmers, because the lower air temperature with radiant warmers means that the saturation pressure of water vapor is considerably lower with radiant warmers than in incubators (Table 23-4).[31,32] The effects on IWL of radiant warmers and phototherapy appear to be additive. The IWL with the combination is twice as large as in an incubator without phototherapy.[31]

Increased motor activity and crying raise IWL by as much as 70%.[19,34,35] This effect may be partly due to elevated minute ventilation.

FACTORS THAT REDUCE INSENSIBLE WATER LOSS

Increasing the humidity or water vapor pressure of inspired gas reduces respiratory IWL. The inspired humidity is raised by humidifying the air–oxygen mixture delivered to a head hood or directly to the infant's upper airway (*e.g.*, nasal cannula, face mask, endotracheal tube) if respiratory support is required. Increasing ambient humidity, as in an incubator, reduces total IWL by about 30%, but respiratory IWL is decreased more than cutaneous IWL.[19]

Plexiglas heat shields are effective in reducing the

TABLE 23–2
FACTORS AFFECTING INSENSIBLE WATER LOSS IN NEWBORN INFANTS

Factor	Effect on Insensible Water Loss
Level of maturity[22,24–26]	Inversely proportional to birth weight and gestational age (see Fig. 23-4)
Respiratory distress (*i.e.*, hyperpnea)	Respiratory insensible water loss increases with rising minute ventilation if dry air is being breathed
Environmental temperature above neutral thermal zone[19,27,28]	Increased in proportion to increment in temperature
Elevated body temperature[19,27]	Increased by as much as 300%
Skin breakdown or injury	Increased by uncertain magnitude
Congenital skin defects (*e.g.*, gastroschisis, omphalocele, neural tube defects)	Increased by uncertain magnitude until surgically corrected
Radiant warmer[22,29–32]	Increased by about 50%
Phototherapy[22,31,33]	Increased by about 50%
Motor activity and crying[19,34,35]	Increased by up to 70%
High ambient or inspired humidity[19,21]	Reduced by 30% when ambient vapor pressure is increased by 200%
Plastic heat shield[32,36,37]	Reduced by 10%–30%
Plastic blanket[38,39]	Reduced by 30%–70%
Semipermeable membrane[40,41]	Reduced by 50%
Topical agents[42]	Reduced by 50%

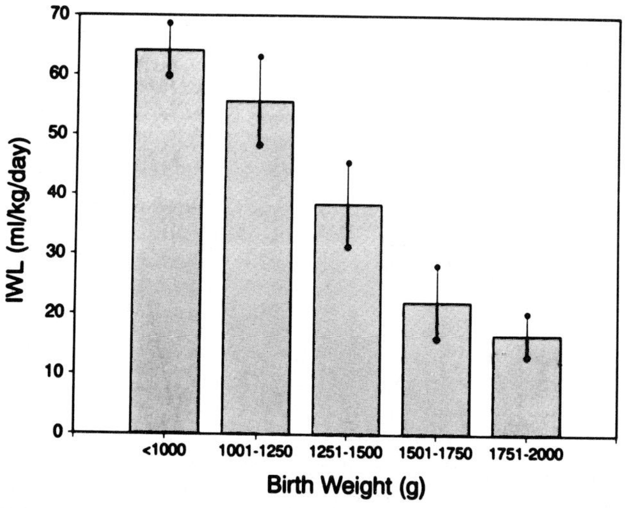

FIG. 23–4. Relation between insensible water loss (IWL) and birth weight of 5-day-old (mean) infants in incubators. (Data from Wu PYK, Hodgman JE. Insensible water loss in preterm infants: changes with postnatal development and non-ionizing radiant energy. Pediatrics 1974;54:704. From Shaffer SG, Weismann DN. Fluid requirements in the preterm infant. Clin Perinatol 1992;19:233.)

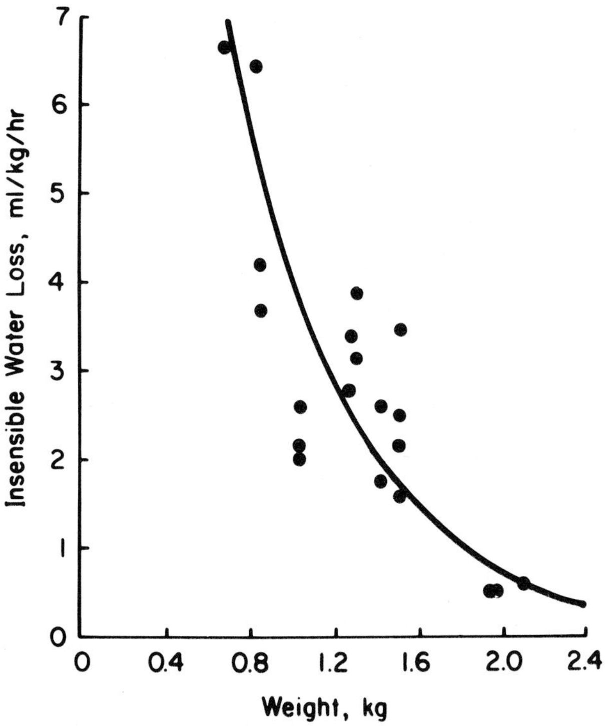

FIG. 23–5. Insensible water loss as a function of birth weight in premature infants nursed under radiant warmers. (Adapted from Costarino AT, Baumgart S. Controversies in fluid and electrolyte therapy for the premature infant. Clin Perinatol 1988;15:863.)

TABLE 23–3
AVERAGE INSENSIBLE WATER LOSS* OF PREMATURE INFANTS IN INCUBATORS

	Birth Weight Range (kg)					
Age (d)	0.50–0.75	0.75–1.00	1.00–1.25	1.25–1.50	1.50–1.75	1.75–2.00
0–7	100	65	55	40	20	15
7–14	80	60	50	40	30	20

* Insensible water loss is given in units of mL/kg/d.
Data from refeences 22, 24, 25.

IWL of small premature infants in incubators,[32,36] especially if the ends are at least partially closed to decrease air movement near the skin. Plexiglas heat shields are not effective for infants under radiant warmers,[32,37] because Plexiglas is opaque to the infrared energy produced by the radiant heaters. Thin barriers of saran wrap and other materials reduce IWL of infants under radiant warmers while allowing the infrared heat to reach the skin.[37] These heat shields presumably reduce IWL by limiting air movement and raising water vapor pressure near the infant's body surface.

Thin plastic blankets have reduced IWL by 30% to 70% for infants under radiant warmers and in incubators.[38,39] Semipermeable membranes and topical agents reduce IWL from the covered areas by an average of 50%.[40–42]

Knowledge of the factors that influence IWL is essential in estimating the water intake required by newborn infants. The IWL of premature and critically ill infants is especially susceptible to influence by these variables. These are the infants for whom precise maintenance of fluid and electrolyte balance is most important.

NEUROENDOCRINE CONTROL OF FLUID AND ELECTROLYTE BALANCE

The pituitary gland, the adrenal cortex, the parathyroid glands, and the heart are the major organs producing hormones involved in the regulation of water and electrolyte balance in the body. The basic mechanisms by which the antidiuretic hormone, arginine vasopressin (AVP), is produced and secreted by the posterior pituitary gland appear to be intact in newborn infants, even in those who are born prematurely.[46–48] It is not clear at what age precise quantitative hypothalamic control of AVP production is established.

Aldosterone is the most potent mineralocorticoid produced and secreted by the adrenal cortex. Its synthesis is regulated by the renin–angiotensin system, ACTH, and the plasma concentrations of sodium and potassium. These mechanisms appear to be intact in newborn infants, even those born prematurely.[49–53] However, increased sodium loss in the urine of premature infants who have high plasma concentrations of aldosterone and elevated urinary aldosterone excretion suggests that the renal tubule is less responsive in premature than in term infants.[51,52] Data suggest that the high plasma aldosterone concentrations enhance sodium reabsorption in the distal nephron under conditions of low sodium intake.[53]

Calcium concentration in the blood of newborn infants is regulated by the balance between parathyroid hormone (PTH), which is produced by the parathyroid glands, and calcitonin, which is produced in the thyroid. Serum PTH concentration is low at birth and rises slowly during the first few days in both full-term and premature infants.[54–56] The same pattern has been observed with serum calcitonin concentrations.[55,56] Tsang and colleagues found a gestational age-dependent rise in serum PTH during exchange transfusion with citrated blood in infants older than than 2 days of age.[57] However, Wieland and associates found serum PTH to fall during exchange transfusion due to removal of active PTH.[58] Intravenous calcium infusion to large premature and term infants caused elevation of serum calcitonin and a corresponding fall in serum PTH.[59] These data indicate that the hormonal regulation of calcium metabolism is basically intact in newborn infants, even those born prematurely.[54–59] Calcium metabolism is discussed further in the Chapter 36.

Atrial natriuretic factor (ANF) is present in the fetal heart early during development.[60] In the human fetus, cardiac atrial levels of ANF increase during gestation and, by the beginning of the third trimester, exceed adult human levels; during the same period,

TABLE 23–4
RELATIVE AND ABSOLUTE HUMIDITY RELATED TO INSENSIBLE WATER LOSS IN INCUBATORS AND UNDER RADIANT WARMERS

Factors Affecting Water Loss	Incubator	Radiant Warmer
Air temperature (°C)	35.0	27.6
Saturation pressure (torr)	42.1	27.7
Relative humidity (%)	31.4	39.0
Absolute humidity (torr)	13.2	10.8
Insensible water loss (mL/kg/h)	2.37	3.40

Data from Bell EF, Weinstein MR, Oh W. Heat balance in premature infants: comparative effects of convectively heated incubator and radiant warmer, with and without plastic heat shield. J Pediatr 1980;96:460.

fetal ventricular ANF levels decrease.[61] Fetal plasma ANF levels rise after birth, peaking at the time of maximal postnatal diuresis, usually 48 to 72 hours, and then returning to levels below those at birth.[63,64] Atrial natriuretic factor secretion is stimulated by volume loading,[65] and ANF levels correlate with atrial size.[66] Atrial natriuretic factor stimulates diuresis and natriuresis and seems to play an important role in the regulation of extracellular fluid volume in newborn infants.[66–68] However, studies of the effects of sodium supplementation on ANF levels and sodium excretion indicate that premature infants are less responsive to ANF than adults.[67]

RENAL FUNCTION IN RELATION TO FLUID AND ELECTROLYTE THERAPY

Most aspects of renal function are incompletely developed at birth, especially in premature infants.[12,69–73] Both glomerular and tubular functions increase with gestational age at birth and with postnatal age.[12,69–73] This development seems to depend most directly on postmenstrual age (*i.e.*, gestational age + postnatal age) and occurs at approximately the same rate, regardless of whether the infant has been born or is *in utero*.[70,71]

Despite the immaturity of some aspects of renal tubular function at birth, the tubules seem to respond to antidiuretic hormone from the first day of life, even in small premature infants.[47] However, the maximal urine concentration of premature infants, typically 600 mOsm/L, is less than that of term newborns (800 mOsm/L) or adults (1200 mOsm/L).[74,75] Both full-term and premature infants can excrete urine with osmolarity as low as 50 mOsm/L when challenged with an acute water load.[75–78] Although they can produce dilute urine, newborn infants cannot excrete a water load as rapidly as adults can.[76]

The limitations in renal function of premature infants contribute to the problems of fluid and electrolyte regulation in various disease states. The glomerular and tubular functions of premature infants allow them to handle some physiologic variations in water and electrolyte load, but imbalance readily occurs when errors are made in estimations of water and electrolyte needs, particularly those of very-low-birth-weight infants.

PRINCIPLES OF FLUID AND ELECTROLYTE THERAPY

As in older children, three steps should be followed in the management of infants with fluid and electrolyte disorders:

1. Estimate the deficits of fluid and electrolytes.
2. Calculate the amounts of fluid and electrolytes required for replacement of deficits, maintenance, and replacement of ongoing abnormal losses.
3. Monitor the adequacy of therapy.

ESTIMATION OF FLUID AND ELECTROLYTE DEFICITS

FLUID DEFICIT

A body water deficit can be estimated on the basis of the degree of dehydration. If serial body weight measurements are available, the acute weight loss is considered to represent the water deficit. During the first week of life, however, weight loss of as much as 15% occurs normally as a result of loss of ECW and tissue catabolism. Smaller infants lose a larger fraction of their weight, presumably because of their relatively larger ECW fraction and more negative protein and energy balance. Even small premature infants who can be enterally fed lose an average of 10% of their body weight during the first 5 days of life.[79] In infants weighing less than 1 kg who must be nourished intravenously, it is not uncommon to observe weight loss of 15% or even 20% without other evidence of significant dehydration. The precise amount of weight loss desired during the first week of life has not been established because of a lack of reliable physiologic data. In general, smaller infants are expected to lose larger fractions of their weight after birth. Term infants may lose a total of 5% to 10% of their birth weight, but premature infants may lose 10% to 20% without adverse consequences. For small premature infants, a weight loss of 2% to 3% per day is a reasonable target in the first week of life. Efforts to prevent any postnatal weight loss risk overhydration and problems with symptomatic PDA.[16] Beyond the first week of life, acute weight loss is considered an indication of nonphysiologic dehydration, and the calculated deficit of water should be replaced.

If an infant presents as an outpatient with dehydration, serial body weight data may not be available. In such cases, urine volume and concentration and physical signs can be used to estimate the degree of dehydration. Infants with 5% isotonic (*i.e.*, serum sodium concentration of 130–150 mEq/L) dehydration have dry mucous membranes, subnormal tear production with crying, flat or slightly sunken anterior fontanel when quiet and in the upright position, and oliguria. Infants with 10% isotonic dehydration have dry mucous membranes, a lack of tears, sunken eyes and fontanel, cool extremities, poor skin turgor, and oliguria. Infants with 15% isotonic dehydration have the aforementioned signs as well as signs of shock, such as hypotension, tachycardia, weak pulses, mottled skin, and altered sensorium. Infants with hypertonic dehydration (*i.e.*, serum sodium concentration > 150 mEq/L) have less severe symptoms than infants with isotonic dehydration who have lost the same fraction of body water; the intravascular volume is preserved better with hypernatremia than with isotonic dehydration. However, infants with hypotonic dehydration (*i.e.*, serum sodium < 130 mEq/L) may have more severe symptoms with the same degree of dehydration.

The usual clinical signs of dehydration are more difficult to evaluate in small premature infants. Their skin and mucous membranes may appear dry because of thermal or mechanical injury, particularly if the infants have been kept under radiant warmers. Skin turgor is harder to judge because of the lack of subcutaneous fat.

ELECTROLYTE DEFICITS

The nature and extent of electrolyte disturbances can often be determined by history and physical examination and by measurement of electrolyte concentrations in serum. Based on serum sodium concentration, electrolyte disturbances are divided into isotonic, hypotonic, and hypertonic abnormalities. The type of electrolyte disorder seen in a clinical situation depends on the cause of fluid and electrolyte abnormality. For example, severe acute diarrhea usually leads to isotonic dehydration. High IWL, occuring in small premature infants under radiant warmers, may result in hypernatremic dehydration. Inadequate replacement of salt losses from diarrhea may produce hypotonic dehydration.

Although it may be possible to anticipate the type of electrolyte disorder accompanying dehydration in some situations, confirmation must be made by measurement of serum electrolyte concentrations.

CALCULATION OF FLUID AND ELECTROLYTE REQUIREMENTS

After replacement of fluid and electrolyte deficits, the requirements of newborn infants for water and electrolytes are determined by the rates of loss of these substances from the body by various routes and by the net amounts retained by body tissues during changes in body weight and composition. Knowledge of the usual rates of loss and of expected changes in body weight and composition in the first postnatal days and during subsequent growth helps to estimate the water and electrolyte requirements of newborn infants. These estimates guide the management of fluid and electrolyte therapy.

REPLACEMENT OF FLUID AND ELECTROLYTE DEFICITS

The water deficit is calculated from the estimated degree of dehydration determined from measured body weight loss or determined by clinical examination. The rate and composition of initial fluid replacement depend on the severity of dehydration. As a rule, dehydration of acute onset and short duration requires more rapid correction. An exception to this rule is the case of hypertonic dehydration, in which rapid expansion of body water may cause brain swelling and convulsions. The deficit of electrolytes is calculated on the basis of the difference between total body solute expected before dehydration and that observed in the dehydrated state. Examples of such calculations in isotonic, hypotonic, and hypertonic dehydration are given in Table 23-5.

It is common to replace one-half of the water deficit over the first 8 hours and the other one-half over the next 16 hours. The sodium deficit is replaced over 24 hours. If the potassium deficit is large, it should be replaced over a longer period (*i.e.*, 48–72 hours) to be certain that the kidneys are functioning well and to avoid the possible cardiac effects associated with rapid potassium infusion. Initiation of potassium replacement is best deferred until urine flow is established.

TABLE 23–5
CALCULATION OF SODIUM DEFICIT

Type of Dehydration	Serum Sodium Concentration (mEq/L)	Calculation of Total Solute Deficit (mOsm/kg)*	Solute Deficit (mOsm/kg)	Sodium Deficit (mEq/kg)†
Isotonic (10%)	140	$(0.7 \times 280) - (0.6 \times 280)$	28	14
Hypotonic (10%)	127	$(0.7 \times 280) - (0.6 \times 254)$	44	22
Hypertonic (10%)	153	$(0.7 \times 280) - (0.6 \times 306)$	12	6

* Total solute deficit = $(TBW_e \times solute_e) - (TBW_o \times solute_o)$, where subscripts e and o indicate expected and observed, respectively. $TBW_e = 0.7$ L/kg; $TBW_o = 0.7 - 0.1 = 0.6$ L/kg; $solute_e = 140 \times 2 = 280$ mOsm/L, assuming total solute concentration in body water is twice the sodium concentration in serum; $solute_o$ = observed serum sodium × 2.

† Total solute deficit is assumed to be one-half sodium. Although the serum and extracellular water have lost this amount of sodium, only one-half of this amount has been lost to the environment; the other one-half has been exchanged for potassium in the cells. The potassium, in turn, has been lost from the body. Therefore, in practice only one-half the amount listed as a sodium deficit should be replaced with sodium; the other one-half should be given as potassium.

MAINTENANCE FLUID AND ELECTROLYTES

Insensible water loss, urine, fecal water, and water retained in new tissues during growth are the four components that must be considered in estimating the daily maintenance water requirement. Fecal water loss is approximately 5 to 10 mL/kg/day.[80] The water retained for growth is about 10 mL/kg/day, assuming a weight gain of 10 to 20 g/kg/day; 60% to 70% of which is water.[3] In the first week of life, fecal water loss is small, and no water is deposited in new tissues because growth has not yet begun. In fact, water is lost from body tissues during the period of physiologic extracellular dehydration. After growth begins, loss of fecal and growth water may require up to 20 g/kg/day of replaced fluid, but this amount is small compared with the IWL and urine water loss, the two major routes of water loss that must be considered in estimating the water intake required to maintain the desired water balance.

A small portion of the water required to replace these normal losses is derived from the oxidation of metabolic fuels (*i.e.*, carbohydrate, protein, fat). This water of oxidation consists of about 0.60 mL/g of carbohydrate oxidized, 0.43 mL/g protein, and 1.07 mL/g fat.[81] A newborn infant usually produces 5 to 10 mL/kg/day as water of oxidation. This amount is small enough to be neglected in most calculations but can be considered to offset the normal fecal water loss of 5 to 10 mL/kg/day.

For a term infant under basal conditions, IWL is approximately 20 mL/kg/day.[19] Urine volume depends on the excess of water intake over losses by other routes (*e.g.*, IWL, feces, growth), and urine concentration is determined by the urine volume and renal solute load. The range of urinary water loss within which the infant's immature kidneys can safely excrete the total renal solute load is determined by the limits of urine concentration (*i.e.*, volume = solute load/urine concentration).[82] A renal solute load of 15 to 30 mOsm/kg/day would require urine volume of 50 to 100 mL/kg/day to maintain an average urine concentration of 300 mOsm/L. This urine concentration is near the middle of the range of urine osmolarity that can be produced by the neonatal kidneys and allows a margin of safety for overestimation or underestimation of other water requirements.

In the first days of life, a term infant receiving intravenous fluid and electrolytes must excrete about 15 mOsm/kg/day, assuming that endogenous solute production and tissue deposition of solute are negligible. The urine volume of 50 mL/kg/day plus the IWL of 20 mL/kg/day yield a total maintenance water requirement of 70 mL/kg/day; this assumes growth and fecal water to be small enough to be negated by the water of oxidation. Allowing for a negative water balance of 10 mL/kg/day, the true water requirement at birth is about 60 mL/kg/day. With increasing postnatal age and enteral feedings, the renal solute load and fecal water loss increase, and water is deposited in new tissues as growth begins. By the second week of life, a growing term infant needs 120 to 150 mL/kg/day.

In premature infants, the maintenance water requirement is larger because of higher IWL.[22,24] The IWL component of maintenance water should be increased with decreasing birth weight or gestation.[83] During the first days of life, the renal solute load is less because little exogenous solute is provided. If 2 mEq of NaCl/kg/day (4 mOsm/kg/day) is administered and 8 mOsm/kg/day resulting from tissue catabolism is assumed to be excreted,[84] a urine volume of only 40 mL/kg/day is required to excrete this solute with a urine concentration of 300 mOsm/L. A small premature infant requires about 80 mL of water/kg/day on day 1 (*i.e.*, 60 IWL + 40 urine − 20 for negative balance). The water requirement for this same infant would be about 150 mL/kg/day in the second or third week (*i.e.*, 55 IWL + 85 urine + 10 feces + 10 growth − 10 oxidation). Very small (*i.e.*, < 1 kg), young infants may have considerably higher IWL, raising the total water requirement to 200 or 300 mL/kg/day or even higher. The minimal water intake of premature infants is higher than that of term infants because of the slightly lower urinary concentrating capacity.[74,75] However, the urine volumes (*i.e.*, 40–100 mL/kg/day) were selected to avoid taxing this limit of concentration and are not influenced by the effect of immaturity.

The allowance for IWL should be increased by about 50% for infants under radiant warmers or those receiving fluorescent phototherapy.[22,29–33] If both are used, the allowance for IWL should be increased by approximately 100%.[31] The effect of fiberoptic phototherapy blankets or pads on IWL is probably less than that of fluorescent phototherapy. The IWL of infants in incubators is increased if body or environmental temperatures are too high.[19,27,28] The IWL can be reduced by increasing the ambient or inspired humidity or by using certain types of heat shields, plastic blankets, semipermeable membranes, or topical agents such as paraffin (see Table 23-3).[19,21,32,36–42] The infant's maintenance requirements of sodium, potassium, and chloride can be estimated by adding the dermal, urinary, and fecal losses to the amounts retained in the body tissues during growth. The estimated requirements for sodium, potassium, and chloride are each between 2 and 3 mEq/kg/day.[85] Small premature infants may require additional sodium because of increased urinary excretion, especially during the second and third weeks of life.[73,86–89] The magnitude of urinary sodium excretion is inversely proportional to gestational age (Fig. 23-6).[69]

ONGOING ABNORMAL LOSSES OF FLUID AND ELECTROLYTES

Ongoing abnormal losses must be replaced concurrently with correction of established deficits and provision of maintenance fluid and electrolytes. Abnor-

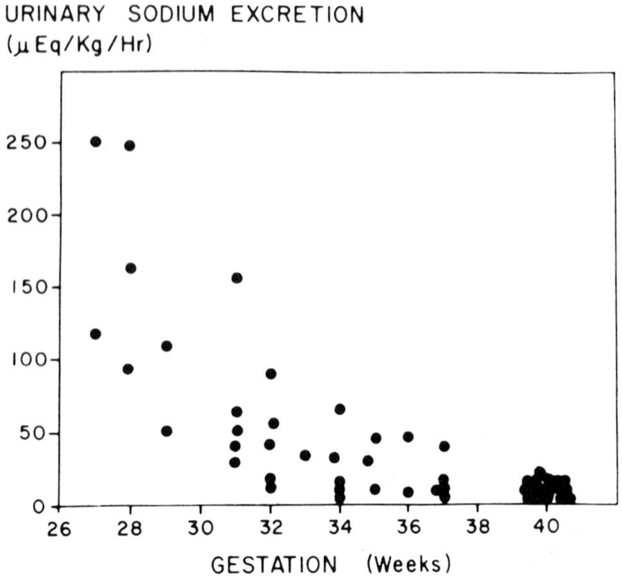

FIG. 23–6. Urinary sodium excretion in infants from 27 to 40 weeks of gestation. (Adapted from Siegal SR, Oh W. Renal function as a marker of human fetal maturation. Acta Paediatr Scand 1976;65:481.)

mal losses may occur with vomiting or diarrhea, ileostomy drainage, or removal by aspiration of gastrointestinal, pleural, peritoneal, or cerebrospinal fluid. The amount of extra water required can be estimated by carefully measuring the volume of the losses. The additional amounts of electrolytes required can be estimated by measuring their concentrations in an aliquot of fluid. The approximate electrolyte contents of several types of body fluid are shown in Table 23-6.

EXAMPLE FLUID AND ELECTROLYTE CALCULATION

Consider a 3-kg infant with 10% isotonic dehydration (*i.e.*, serum Na = 140 mEq/L). The calculations of fluid and electrolyte management for the first 24 hours are illustrated in Table 23-7. The infant should be given 27 mEq of sodium chloride in 600 mL of water containing 5% glucose over 24 hours. If the potassium deficit is to be corrected over 72 hours, 13 mEq of potassium chloride (21/3 + 6) should be given during the first 24 hours. This fluid can then be ordered as 5% dextrose with 45 mEq NaCl/L and 20 mEq KCl/L to be infused at 25 mL/hour. If the infant had significant metabolic acidosis as well, some or all of the sodium could be given as sodium bicarbonate or sodium acetate.

The initial glucose concentration of the infusate is determined by the estimated water requirement and the desired glucose intake, which is usually 5 to 8 mg/kg/minute. Smaller, more premature infants, because they require more water and may tolerate less glucose, are usually begun on fluids containing lower concentrations of glucose (*e.g.*, 5 g/dL); larger term or near-term infants require higher glucose concentrations (*e.g.*, 10 g/dL).

The fluid and electrolyte requirements of very small premature infants vary widely and are difficult to predict. Therefore, close monitoring of the fluid and electrolyte balance of these infants is especially important to detect any imbalance as soon as possible.

TABLE 23–6
ELECTROLYTE CONTENT OF BODY FLUIDS

Fluid Source	Sodium (mEq/L)	Potassium (mEq/L)	Chloride (mEq/L)
Stomach	20–80	5–20	100–150
Small intestine	100–140	5–15	90–120
Bile	120–140	5–15	90–120
Ileostomy	45–135	3–15	20–120
Diarrheal stool	10–90	10–80	10–110
Cerebrospinal fluid	130–150	2–5	110–130

TABLE 23–7
CALCULATION OF FLUID AND ELECTROLYTE INTAKE FOR A 3-KG INFANT WITH 10% ISOTONIC DEHYDRATION

	Water (mL)	Sodium (mEq)	Potassium (mEq)
Deficit	300*	21†	21†‡
Maintenance	300§	6	6
Ongoing losses	0	0	0
Total	600	27	27‡
Total/kg	200	9	9‡

* Water deficit of 0.10 × 3 kg.
† Electrolyte deficits are calculated as in Table 23-4 (*i.e.*, 14 mEq/kg × 3 kg divided between sodium and potassium).
‡ Potassium deficit should be replaced slowly, over 48 to 72 hours.
§ Maintenance water requirement is assumed to be 100 mL/kg/d.

MONITORING THE EFFECTIVENESS OF FLUID AND ELECTROLYTE THERAPY

During the course of parenteral fluid therapy, detailed and organized data collection is necessary for monitoring the adequacy of fluid and electrolyte intake. Data that should be collected and recorded regularly at designated intervals include water and electrolyte intake by all routes, measurable output of water and electrolytes, body weight changes, urine specific gravity or osmolarity, serum electrolyte and creatinine concentrations, and blood urea nitrogen (BUN). Clinical assessment should be made for the presence of dehydration, edema, or acute water overload. The associations among these data are shown in Figure 23-7. A calibrated infusion pump should be used to ensure reasonably accurate administration of prescribed parenteral fluids. Accurate measurement of urine volume is difficult in small infants. It is possible to collect urine from male infants by placing the penis into a test tube that is taped to the abdomen. Urine is then aspirated from the test tube with a catheter and syringe. Urine volume can be estimated by comparing the weights of dry and wet diapers, if the wet diaper is weighed soon enough to avoid evaporation.

Inadequate fluid may be administered if the fluid maintenance requirement is underestimated or if a preexisting deficit or ongoing loss is neglected or underestimated. Insufficient water intake reduces urine volume and increases urine concentration, and if these compensatory measures are inadequate, water is mobilized from body stores to provide for obligatory IWL and to allow solute excretion. This results in weight loss, clinical signs of dehydration, metabolic acidosis, and hemoconcentration. As serum osmolarity rises, neurologic sequelae of hypertonicity may occur. In severe cases, untreated dehydration may lead to decreased circulating blood volume, acute renal failure, and finally to death from cardiovascular collapse.

Excessive water intake leads to increased excretion of dilute urine. If these compensatory mechanisms are overtaxed, water is retained in the body, resulting in edema and weight gain. Rapid overhydration may produce congestive heart failure and pulmonary edema, particularly in ill infants with cardiopulmonary disorders. Even gradual daily administration of excess water (*i.e.*, in excess of that which is required or can be readily eliminated by the kidneys) may increase the risk of heart failure from PDA in premature infants.[16]

Urine specific gravity is a convenient and accurate guide to estimation of urinary solute excretion, because specific gravity generally correlates well with osmolarity.[90] Specific gravity is used routinely to monitor urine concentration, because it can be measured quickly at the bedside with a portable refractometer. Specific gravity should be recorded at least every 8 hours for infants who require parenteral fluid therapy.

If appropriate fluid therapy is being provided, body weight should be stable or slowly increasing after the first week of life. Urine specific gravity should be between 1.005 and 1.015, and there should be no evidence of fluid overload or dehydration. During the first week of life, loss of as much as 15% of body weight (1% to 3% per day) is considered normal if urine output is adequate and there is no acidosis or evidence of dehydration. This physiologic weight loss is at least partly the result of a postnatal fall in the ECW volume. Efforts to prevent this weight loss are ill advised and may produce fluid overload, edema, and hemodynamically significant PDA.

Routine measurement of serum electrolyte concentrations is the best way to monitor the body's electrolyte status and the adequacy or excess of electrolyte intake. It is not necessary to add sodium to the parenterally administered fluid during the first 24 hours of life, especially if it is anticipated that bicarbonate may be needed for the treatment of metabolic acidosis. It is advisable to determine the serum electrolyte concentrations soon after birth in infants who require parenteral fluids; if the mother received sodium-free fluid during labor, the infant may be hyponatremic[17,18] and require immediate addition of sodium to the prescribed fluid. If not required earlier, sodium in the form of sodium chloride, sodium acetate, or sodium bicarbonate should be administered at a dose of 2 to 3 mEq/kg/day, beginning with the second day of life. The acetate and bicarbonate salts are useful in infants with metabolic acidosis from renal immaturity or other causes.

During the first week of life, infants are in negative sodium balance because sodium is mobilized with

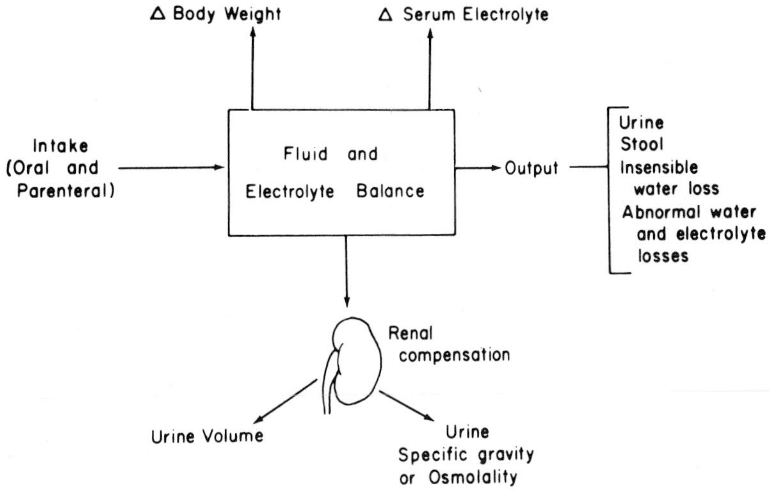

FIG. 23–7. A system of monitoring fluid and electrolyte therapy.

water from the extracellular compartment. This negative balance should be allowed as long as the serum sodium concentration remains normal. In the second and third weeks of life, small premature infants may require more sodium to replace the large amounts that are lost in the urine.[73,86–89]

Potassium supplementation (2 mEq/kg/day) may be started after the infant urinates unless the serum potassium concentration is elevated. In most infants, potassium should be added to the infused fluids by the second day. For very small, critically ill, premature infants, it is often wise to wait until the serum potassium falls below 4 mEq/L before administering potassium; these infants are at increased risk from hyperkalemia due to catabolism and release of potassium from cells as well as decreased renal potassium excretion.

Hyperkalemia is the most common life-threatening electrolyte disturbance in newborn infants. If an elevated serum potassium level is reported by the laboratory, it should not be attributed to *in vitro* hemolysis without verification of the result with another blood sample obtained with good technique to minimize hemolysis. If the serum potassium concentration is higher than 6 mEq/L, only potassium-free fluids should be administered. If the serum potassium concentration is higher than 7 mEq/L, rectal administration of a potassium-binding resin (*e.g.*, Kayexalate) should be considered. If a cardiac arrhythmia occurs in the presence of hyperkalemia, calcium, bicarbonate, and insulin with glucose should be given to protect the myocardium and to force potassium into body cells. In small premature infants, hyperkalemic arrhythmias include sinus bradycardia—especially if it occurs without hypoxia—and ventricular tachycardia.

Blood urea nitrogen and serum or plasma creatinine levels are useful for assessing renal function, although BUN may be elevated with dehydration. Normal plasma creatinine levels for premature infants have been established and are shown in Figure 23-8.[91]

ACID–BASE BALANCE

The physiologic buffer system, which is primarily bicarbonate and its weak acid counterpart carbonic acid, and the renal and respiratory compensatory systems are the major mechanisms responsible for the maintenance of normal acid–base equilibrium in the body fluids. Changes in the hydrogen ion concentration in body fluids follow the Henderson–Hasselbach equation:

$$pH = 6.1 + \log([HCO_3^-]/[H_2CO_3]),$$

in which 6.1 is the *p*K or dissociation constant for carbonic acid and H_2CO_3 is the concentration of carbonic acid.[92] It can be seen from this equation that any increase or decrease in the bicarbonate (HCO_3^-) concentration results in metabolic alkalosis or metabolic acidosis, respectively. Because H_2CO_3 is interchangeably linked to PCO_2 under the influence of carbonic anhydrase, any alteration in PCO_2 in body fluid alters *p*H. Hyperventilation, by reducing PCO_2, produces respiratory alkalosis, and hypoventilation with hypercarbia causes respiratory acidosis.

Metabolic alkalosis occurs with pyloric stenosis, because persistent vomiting results in the loss of hydrochloric acid and produces a relative excess of bicarbonate. Metabolic acidosis is most commonly seen as a consequence of lactic acid accumulation from anaerobic metabolism in hypoxic infants. Respiratory alkalosis may occur in an infant who is hyperventilated by a mechanical ventilator. Respiratory acidosis occurs as a result of hypercarbia in infants with respiratory distress syndrome (RDS) or other pulmonary disease.

In all types of acid–base disturbance, compensation by the lungs or kidneys occurs to restore the *p*H toward 7.4. Metabolic acid–base disorders are corrected by changes in ventilation, and respiratory disorders are compensated for by changes in renal bicarbonate excretion. If the compensation is adequate to correct the *p*H to normal, the acid–base disturbance is said to be compensated. For example, if an infant

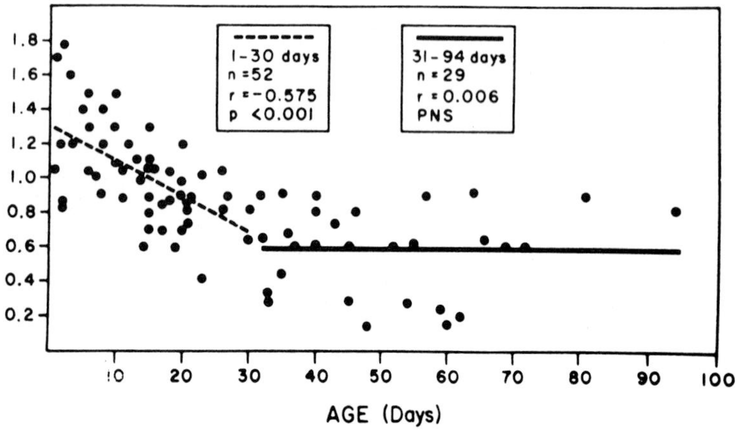

FIG. 23–8. Plasma creatinine levels of premature infants during the first 3 months of life. (From Stonestreet BS, Oh W. Plasma creatinine levels in low-birth-weight infants during the first three months of life. Pediatrics 1978;61:788.)

with RDS had a *p*H of 7.38, PCO_2 of 32 torr, bicarbonate concentration 18 mEq/L, and base excess of −5 mEq/L, the acid–base status would be called compensated metabolic acidosis. If the same infant had a *p*H 7.38, PCO_2 of 50 torr, bicarbonate concentration of 29 mEq/L, and base excess of +3 mEq/L, the acid–base status would be compensated respiratory acidosis.

FLUID AND ELECTROLYTE PROBLEMS ASSOCIATED WITH SPECIFIC CLINICAL CONDITIONS

EXTREME PREMATURITY

Infants born at gestational ages younger than 26 weeks present special problems in fluid and electrolyte management. These infants have large IWLs,[25,26] possibly more than 200 mL/kg/day if the infant is nursed under a radiant warmer and treated with phototherapy. The large IWL of extremely premature infants results from their meager skin barrier to evaporation and their larger ratio of surface area to body weight. The average water requirement for an infant with a birth weight between 500 and 750 g in the first week of life is estimated to be about 170 mL/kg/day if the infant is in an incubator with low ambient humidity and not treated with phototherapy; 210 to 220 mL/kg/day if a radiant warmer or fluorescent phototherapy is used; and 250 to 270 mL/kg/day if both a radiant warmer and phototherapy are used.[93]

Extremely premature infants, unless hyponatremic from maternal hypotonicity, should initially be started on electrolyte-free solutions of glucose (5 g/dL) in water. Sodium should be avoided because of the risk of hypernatremia from large IWL with inadequate free water replacement.[94] Sodium (2–3 mEq/kg/day) may be added on the second or third day if the serum sodium concentration is below 140 mEq/L. Extremely premature infants often have metabolic acidosis because of renal immaturity and transient renal tubular acidosis. Their maintenance sodium may be given as sodium bicarbonate or sodium acetate.

Hyperkalemia is a common problem in extremely premature infants during the first week of life. This dangerous condition results from potassium release from catabolized cells in the presence of immature distal renal tubular function.[95] Hyperkalemia is exacerbated if dehydration and oliguria occur as a result of inadequate water intake. No potassium should be given to extremely premature infants until the serum potassium concentration falls below 4 mEq/L. If the serum potassium concentration exceeds 7 mEq/L, rectal administration of a potassium-binding resin should be considered.

RESPIRATORY DISTRESS SYNDROME

The renal function of infants with RDS is similar to that of infants of the same gestational age without respiratory distress, if their cardiorespiratory status is not compromised.[96–98] If infants with RDS become hypoxic and acidotic, they may have decreased glomerular filtration (*e.g.*, inulin and creatinine clearance), renal blood flow (*e.g.*, *p*-aminohippuric acid clearance), and renal bicarbonate threshold.[97–100] It has been observed that clinical improvement in infants with RDS is accompanied by an increase in urine volume that occurs on the second and third days of life.[101] It is not clear whether this diuresis causes or is caused by the improving pulmonary function. It may be causally unrelated, because this is the time when all infants, especially premature infants, are in negative water balance[102] and undergo a contraction of the ECW.

In addition to the changes in renal function that may occur with pulmonary dysfunction resulting from severe RDS, positive-pressure ventilation may cause water retention through effects on renal function. Continuous positive airway pressure can decrease glomerular filtration rate, sodium excretion, and free water clearance without altering renal perfusion pressure.[103,104] Intermittent positive-pressure ventilation impairs water and sodium excretion by mechanisms that probably include increased aldosterone secretion and increased production of antidiuretic hormone.[105–107] It is possible for impaired filtration and solute excretion to result from decreased aortic pressure and renal perfusion if excessive mean airway pressures are used during ventilatory support.[108,109]

Infants with RDS and other pulmonary disorders may have increased secretion of antidiuretic hormone, especially if they develop pneumothorax.[48,110,111]

Patent ductus arteriosus is a problem that affects premature infants; those with RDS are more likely to develop cardiorespiratory signs related to PDA than those without RDS. In a randomized clinical trial, Bell and colleagues compared the effects of liberal and restricted water intake on the development of significant PDA in premature infants.[16] Infants with birth weights from 0.75 to 2.0 kg were randomly assigned to "high-volume" or "low-volume" water intake beginning on the third day of life and continuing until 30 days of age, until full enteral feedings were achieved or until congestive heart failure or dehydration occurred. The low-volume group received only enough water to meet average estimated requirements for urinary solute excretion, fecal loss, IWL, and growth; the high-volume group received an excess of at least 20 mL/kg/day. The mean water intake for the 85 infants in the low-volume group was 122 mL/kg/day (standard deviation, 14); for the 85 high-volume infants, it was 169 mL/kg/day (standard deviation, 20). The number with a typical PDA murmur (9 *versus* 35) and the number with congestive heart failure due to PDA (2 *versus* 11) were significantly lower in the low-volume group. Eleven of the 13 infants with hemodynamically significant PDA also had RDS, which was identified before enrollment in the study on day 3. There were more infants with dehydration in the low-volume group and more with necrotizing enterocolitis (NEC) in the high-volume group. Excessive water intake during the first few weeks of life was associated with a higher risk of morbidity from PDA in premature infants, especially those with RDS.

In a similar study by Lorenz and associates, premature infants were randomly assigned to one of two levels of water intake designed to produce different degrees of body weight loss during the first 5 days of life.[112] The group with lower water intake lost an average of 13% over 5 days, and the group with higher water intake lost 9%. There were no differences in clinical outcome, including the incidence of PDA. This result confirms that body weight loss of 10% to 15% during the first week of life is well tolerated, but it does not contradict the potentially detrimental effects of excessive water intake over a longer period.[16] The water intake of both groups in the study by Lorenz were considerably less than the high-volume intake associated with increased risk of PDA in the study by Bell and associates.[16,112]

Respiratory distress syndrome is commonly associated with a combined respiratory and metabolic acidosis resulting from hypercarbia and lactic acidemia. In severe RDS, in which the acidosis is primarily respiratory, assisted ventilation should be instituted. If the acidosis is primarily metabolic, the underlying cause should be identified and corrected; if this cannot be done, sodium bicarbonate may be given to correct the acidosis. There is little evidence to support the routine use of bicarbonate in infants with RDS.[113–116] Therefore, the current approach is to treat only significant metabolic acidosis, usually if the *p*H is below 7.25.

The dose of bicarbonate should be calculated from this equation:

$$NaHCO_3 \text{ dose} = \text{base deficit} \times \text{body weight} \times 0.5 \text{ L/kg}.$$

The 0.5 value in the equation is the volume of distribution (*i.e.*, bicarbonate space), which is confined mostly to the extracellular fluid compartment (see Fig. 23-3). There is some disagreement on the true bicarbonate space; the reported values range from 0.3 to 0.6 L/kg. The 0.5 value in the preceding equation applies to term infants; 0.6 L/kg should probably be used for premature infants because of their larger volume of ECW.[1]

The calculated bicarbonate dose should be diluted to a concentration of 0.5 mEq/mL and given intravenously at a rate no faster than 1 mEq/minute/kg of body weight. A slow infusion over 30 to 60 minutes is preferable, especially for premature infants, because it may reduce the risk of rapid osmolar changes in the intravascular and interstitial fluid compartments, which have been associated with intracranial hemorrhage in infants receiving bicarbonate.[117,118]

Tris[hydroxymethyl]aminomethane (THAM) has been used as a buffer in cases of severe metabolic acidosis with concurrent respiratory acidosis because it does not raise PCO_2 as bicarbonate does in infants with respiratory failure. It has been used in infants with metabolic acidosis and hypernatremia to avoid the additional sodium given with bicarbonate. However, the effect of THAM on *p*H is usually transient and requires large continuous doses that exceed its therapeutic safety. In addition, the osmotic effects of THAM are greater than the effects of sodium bicarbonate in doses that provide equivalent rises in blood *p*H and bicarbonate concentration.[119] If bicarbonate is used, the serum osmolarity can be indirectly estimated from serum sodium concentration, but with THAM, osmolarity must be measured directly. For these reasons, bicarbonate is preferred to THAM for treating acidosis in infants with RDS.

PERINATAL ASPHYXIA

Infants with hypoxia or ischemia of the brain and kidneys during the perinatal period may suffer brain or kidney injury. Increased secretion of AVP often accompanies hypoxic encephalopathy.[48,120,121] Moreover, acute renal failure may result from renal ischemia in these infants.[122,123] Both conditions cause oliguria and decrease the need for exogenous water. After birth asphyxia, it is advisable to restrict water intake in anticipation of possible increased AVP (*i.e.*, inappropriate antidiuretic hormone) secretion or acute renal failure. During the first 24 hours of life, the water intake for asphyxiated infants should be limited to IWL plus urine output minus about 20 mL/kg/day to allow some physiologic contraction of the ECW volume. If urine production is normal by the third postnatal day, water intake can be restored to a normal level.

During the oliguric phase of acute renal failure, potassium should not be administered unless the serum potassium concentration is less than 3.5 mEq/L. With acute renal failure due to hypoxia or ischemia, the initial period of oliguria may be followed by a diuretic phase with polyuria. If urine output increases and body weight falls below the expected level (*i.e.*, weight before fluid retention began), the intake of water must be increased to prevent dehydration. This diuretic phase may be accompanied by large losses of sodium and other electrolytes, which must be replaced.

CENTRAL NERVOUS SYSTEM INJURY

Infants with brain injury from other causes, such as intracranial hemorrhage or central nervous system infection, may also have oliguria and water retention because of inappropriate antidiuretic hormone secretion.[48,120]

SEPSIS AND NECROTIZING ENTEROCOLITIS

One study implicated overhydration as a factor in the pathogenesis of NEC, but this has not been confirmed.[16] Infants with septicemia who have meningitis may develop inappropriate antidiuretic hormone secretion, reducing their water requirements. Infants with septicemia or NEC may develop shock from endotoxin production or from hypovolemia due to loss of intravascular water and protein to the peritoneal and interstitial spaces or due to gastrointestinal bleeding. In infants with shock, it is essential to replace lost water and solutes in the form of blood products or other solute-containing fluids. Even if properly treated, septic shock may cause renal injury, which influences fluid management as discussed earlier.

PYLORIC STENOSIS

With pyloric stenosis, water, electrolytes, and hydrogen ions are lost from the stomach as a result of repeated vomiting. Infants with severe vomiting caused by pyloric stenosis have increased intracellular sodium and decreased potassium.[124] Infants with pyloric stenosis are likely to be dehydrated and have hypochloremic metabolic alkalosis and hypokalemia. The alkalosis may cause lethargy, hypoventilation, and, in severe cases, tetany.

Parenteral fluid therapy consists of replacing the deficits of water, potassium, and chloride. The chloride should initially be given as sodium chloride. Potassium chloride should be added after adequate urination has been established. Specific treatment of the metabolic alkalosis with acidic agents is usually unnecessary. In most cases, cessation of vomiting from withholding of oral intake, correction of dehydration, and replacement of chloride and potassium deficits restore the blood acid–base status to normal.

DIARRHEA

The principles of parenteral fluid therapy of diarrheal dehydration in the newborn infant are similar to those applied to older infants and children. Because of their limited renal concentrating ability, newborn infants are quicker to develop severe dehydration with hypovolemia and cardiovascular collapse. Rapid establishment of intravenous access for vascular expansion is of the utmost importance in newborn infants with moderate or severe dehydration from diarrhea. After stabilization, fluid and electrolyte deficits should be estimated as described earlier in this chapter. Water and electrolytes are given to correct established deficits, meet maintenance requirements, and counteract ongoing losses.

Metabolic acidosis is a frequent finding in diarrheal dehydration. During initial volume reexpansion, preexisting acidosis may worsen as the body bicarbonate is further diluted with bicarbonate-free replacement fluids. Prerenal azotemia is common with diarrheal dehydration. It is usually corrected spontaneously within several days as the infant is rehydrated.

Oral fluids and feeding should be withheld during recovery from diarrheal dehydration. Oral rehydration has been used successfully in older children with diarrhea, but there has been less experience with this technique in newborn infants.[125] Oral rehydration is not recommended for newborn infants in areas where adequate personnel and supplies are available to maintain parenteral infusions. The appropriate period of fasting depends on the severity and duration of the diarrheal episode. As a rule, a more severe, protracted bout requires a longer period of fasting. The number of diarrheal stools after the onset of fasting helps one determine the duration of fasting. Reintroduction of oral fluids should be carried out with extreme care. Aggressive refeeding may precipitate a recurrence of diarrhea or even protracted chronic diarrhea and malabsorption with consequent growth failure.

FLUID AND ELECTROLYTE MANAGEMENT OF NEONATAL SURGICAL PATIENTS

If a condition that requires surgery (*e.g.*, pyloric stenosis) results in dehydration and electrolyte or acid–base disturbance, the infant should be restored as nearly as possible to normal fluid, electrolyte, and acid–base status before surgery. Otherwise, the risks of anesthesia and surgery can be increased by dehydration, acidosis, alkalosis, or abnormal serum potassium concentration.

During surgery, the calculated fluid and electrolyte therapy should be continued with the same fluid composition and rate of infusion unless additional intraoperative losses require replacement. The anesthesiologist and surgeons should be apprised of the plan for parenteral fluid therapy to avoid errors resulting from lack of communication. The operative losses of fluid and blood should be recorded and replaced during surgery or immediately thereafter. During the initial postoperative period, some infants have reduced urine output as a result of fluid loss from the vascular compartment or increased secretion of antidiuretic hormone. The IWL may be reduced in the postoperative newborn infant; the reason for this is unknown.[126] The fluid provided for maintenance should be reduced during the immediate postoperative period. However, this reduction may be countered by the extra fluid required to replace abnormal operative and postoperative losses. A system of careful monitoring of fluid and electrolyte balance is essential in the surgical patient, as in other ill newborn infants.

TECHNICAL ASPECTS OF PARENTERAL FLUID THERAPY

BLOOD SAMPLING

Sampling of capillary blood by heel puncture is a safe and commonly used technique in newborn infants. Capillary blood is adequate for determination of serum electrolyte and BUN concentrations because most of these values agree closely with venous samples. Serum potassium concentration is slightly higher if obtained by heel puncture, but the difference is minimized if the blood flows freely from the puncture wound so that little squeezing is required. Blood flow can be enhanced by prior warming of the foot. Because the amount of blood obtained by heel puncture is limited, the neonatal service should be supported by a laboratory capable of performing the required analysis on blood samples of small volume.

Blood samples for blood gas and acid–base determination can be obtained by heel puncture. Their reliability is enhanced by warming the skin to 44°C, which reduces the arterial–capillary differences in blood gases and *p*H; however, PO_2 measurements on samples obtained by heel puncture tend to underestimate true arterial PO_2, especially in the hyperoxic range. It is usually possible to combine capillary acid–base and PCO_2 values with pulse oximetry or transcutaneous oxygen monitoring, avoiding the need for indwelling arterial catheters. However, indwelling umbilical or radial artery catheters are often used in infants who are extremely ill and require continuous blood pressure monitoring or high levels of oxygen and ventilatory support. Because indwelling arterial catheters are associated with serious thromboembolic complications, they should be removed as soon as possible. For occasional sampling of arterial blood, direct puncture and aspiration from a radial or temporal artery can be used. This procedure is fairly safe in skilled hands but can cause serious complications, such as arterial obstruction or nerve injury.

INTRAVENOUS FLUID INFUSION

With practice and skill, a small-gauge catheter or butterfly needle can be inserted into a peripheral vein in an extremity or the scalp. Shaving scalp hair to expose veins is distressing to many parents; the scalp should be used only if extremity sites have been exhausted and only after the procedure has been discussed with the parents. Plastic catheters offer the advantage of longevity, but they must be carefully inspected daily for evidence of infection at the insertion site. The site must be conscientiously monitored for evidence of extravasation that could injure subcutaneous tissues.

Techniques have been developed for percutaneous insertion of silicone elastomer (*i.e.*, Silastic) catheters into central veins of newborn infants.[127,128] These catheters can be used for long-term parenteral nutrition without the high risks of infection and thrombosis associated with surgically inserted central vein catheters.

Venous cutdown is seldom necessary if skilled personnel are available to insert and maintain standard intravenous needles. Cutdowns risk local infection or septicemia and permanent venous obstruction. Moreover, catheters inserted by cutdown usually do not last as long in newborn infants as they do in older children and adults. For these reasons, venous cutdown should be avoided in newborns whenever possible.

The umbilical vein is not suitable as a site for routine infusion of fluid, electrolytes, and nutrients because of the risks of infection, portal phlebitis, and liver damage. Its use should be reserved for central venous pressure monitoring and exchange transfusions. A possible exception is the use of umbilical vein catheters for fluid administration and blood sampling in extremely small premature infants in the first week of life. In such cases, a catheter with its tip in the inferior vena cava can be used for blood sampling, minimizing the need for peripheral venous or capillary blood sampling, which can be traumatic to the infant's tender skin and subcutaneous tissues. If an umbilical vein catheter is used in this way, it should be removed by the end of the first week of life, when the risks of infection and thrombosis probably surpass the advantages of continued catheter use.

The tibial bone marrow is a possible site for the emergency infusion of fluids and drugs.[129] This should be attempted only in a life-threatening situation where other routes of infusion are not possible.

With any route of parenteral fluid administration, a constant infusion pump and a volumetric chamber or syringe should be used to ensure a constant, precise rate of infusion. A fluctuating infusion rate may cause erratic blood glucose levels and overhydration or underhydration.

REFERENCES

1. Friis-Hansen B. Changes in body water compartments during growth. Acta Paediatr Suppl 1957;110:1.
2. Friis-Hansen B. Body water compartments in children: changes during growth and related changes in body composition. Pediatrics 1961;28:169.
3. Ziegler EE, O'Donnell AM, Nelson SE, Fomon SJ. Body composition of the reference fetus. Growth 1976;40:329.
4. Forbes GB, Perley A. Estimation of total body sodium by isotopic dilution. II. Studies on infants and children: an example of a constant differential growth ratio. J Clin Invest 1951; 30:566.
5. Cheek DB. Observations on total body chloride in children. Pediatrics 1954;14:5.
6. Romahn A, Burmeister W. Die Körperzusammensetzung während der ersten zwei Lebensjahre: Bestimmungen mit der Kalium-40-Methode. Klin Pädiatr 1977;189:321.
7. Cheek DB, Maddison TG, Malinek M, Coldbeck JH. Further observations on the corrected bromide space of the neonate

and investigation of water and electrolyte status in infants born of diabetic mothers. Pediatrics 1961;28:861.
8. Kagan BM, Stanincova V, Felix NS, Hodgman J, Kalman D. Body composition of premature infants: relation to nutrition. Am J Clin Nutr 1972;25:1153.
9. Shaffer SG, Bradt SK, Hall RT. Postnatal changes in total body water and extracellular volume in the preterm infant with respiratory distress syndrome. J Pediatr 1986;109:509.
10. Bauer K, Bovermann G, Roithmaier A, Götz M, Pröiss A, Versmold HT. Body composition, nutrition, and fluid balance during the first two weeks of life in preterm neonates weighing less than 1500 grams. J Pediatr 1991;118:615.
11. Oh W, Oh MA, Lind J. Renal function and blood volume in newborn infant related to placental transfusion. Acta Paediatr Scand 1966;55:197.
12. Aperia A, Broberger O, Elinder G, Herin P, Zetterström R. Postnatal development of renal function in pre-term and full-term infants. Acta Paediatr Scand 1981;70:183.
13. Guignard JP. Renal function in the newborn infant. Pediatr Clin North Am 1982;29:777.
14. Cassady G, Milstead RR. Antipyrine space studies and cell water estimates in infants of low birth weight. Pediatr Res 1971;5:673.
15. Stonestreet BS, Bell EF, Warburton D, Oh W. Renal response in low-birth-weight neonates. Results of prolonged intake of two different amounts of fluid and sodium. Am J Dis Child 1983;137:215.
16. Bell EF, Warburton D, Stonestreet BS, Oh W. Effect of fluid administration on the development of symptomatic patent ductus arteriosus and congestive heart failure in premature infants. N Engl J Med 1980;302:598.
17. Battaglia F, Prystowsky H, Smisson C, Hellegers A, Bruns P. Fetal blood studies. XIII. The effect of the administration of fluids intravenously to mothers upon the concentrations of water and electrolytes in plasma of human fetuses. Pediatrics 1960;25:2.
18. Tarnow-Mordi WO, Shaw JCL, Liu D, Gardner DA, Flynn FV. Iatrogenic hyponatraemia of the newborn due to maternal fluid overload: a prospective study. Br Med J 1981;283:639.
19. Hey EN, Katz G. Evaporative water loss in the new-born baby. J Physiol (Lond) 1969;200:605.
20. Sulyok E, Jéquier E, Prod'hom LS. Respiratory contribution to the thermal balance of the newborn infant under various ambient conditions. Pediatrics 1973;51:641.
21. Sosulski R, Polin RA, Baumgart S. Respiratory water loss and heat balance in intubated infants receiving humidified air. J Pediatr 1983;103:307.
22. Wu PYK, Hodgman JE. Insensible water loss in preterm infants: changes with postnatal development and non-ionizing radiant energy. Pediatrics 1974;54:704.
23. Shaffer SG, Weismann DN. Fluid requirements in the preterm infant. Clin Perinatol 1992;19:233.
24. Okken A, Jonxis JHP, Rispens P, Zijlstra WG. Insensible water loss and metabolic rate in low birthweight newborn infants. Pediatr Res 1979;13:1072.
25. Costarino AT, Baumgart S. Controversies in fluid and electrolyte therapy for the premature infant. Clin Perinatol 1988; 15:863.
26. Hammarlund K, Sedin G. Transepidermal water loss in newborn infants. III. Relation to gestational age. Acta Paediatr Scand 1979;68:795.
27. Rutter N, Hull D. Response of term babies to a warm environment. Arch Dis Child 1979;54:178.
28. Bell EF, Gray JC, Weinstein MR, Oh W. The effects of thermal environment on heat balance and insensible water loss in low-birth-weight infants. J Pediatr 1980;96:452.
29. Williams PR, Oh W. Effects of radiant warmer on insensible water loss in newborn infants. Am J Dis Child 1974;128:511.
30. Jones RWA, Rochefort MJ, Baum JD. Increased insensible water loss in newborn infants nursed under radiant heaters. Br Med J 1976;2:1347.
31. Bell EF, Neidich GA, Cashore WJ, Oh W. Combined effect of radiant warmer and phototherapy on insensible water loss in low-birth-weight infants. J Pediatr 1979;94:810.
32. Bell EF, Weinstein MR, Oh W. Heat balance in premature infants: comparative effects of convectively heated incubator and radiant warmer, with and without plastic heat shield. J Pediatr 1980;96:460.
33. Oh W, Karecki H. Phototherapy and insensible water loss in the newborn infant. Am J Dis Child 1972;124:230.
34. Day R. Respiratory metabolism in infancy and in childhood. XXVII. Regulation of body temperature of premature infants. Am J Dis Child 1943;65:376.
35. Zweymüller E, Preining O. The insensible water loss of the newborn infant. Acta Paediatr Scand Suppl 1970;205:1.
36. Fanaroff AA, Wald M, Gruber HS, Klaus MH. Insensible water loss in low birth weight infants. Pediatrics 1972;50:236.
37. Baumgart S, Fox WW, Polin RA. Physiologic implications of two different heat shields for infants under radiant warmers. J Pediatr 1982;100:787.
38. Marks KH, Friedman Z, Maisels MJ. A simple device for reducing insensible water loss in low-birth-weight infants. Pediatrics 1977;60:223.
39. Baumgart S. Reduction of oxygen consumption, insensible water loss, and radiant heat demand with use of a plastic blanket for low-birth-weight infants under radiant warmers. Pediatrics 1984;74:1022.
40. Knauth A, Gordin M, McNelis W, Baumgart S. Semipermeable polyurethane membrane as an artificial skin for the premature neonate. Pediatrics 1989;83:945.
41. Vernon HJ, Lane AT, Wischerath LJ, Davis JM, Menegus MA. Semipermeable dressing and transepidermal water loss in premature infants. Pediatrics 1990;86:357.
42. Rutter N, Hull D. Reduction of skin water loss in the newborn. I. Effect of applying topical agents. Arch Dis Child 1981;56:669.
43. Hartop PJ, Prottey C. Changes in transepidermal water loss and the composition of epidermal lecithin after applications of pure fatty acid triglycerides to the skin of essential fatty acid-deficient rats. Br J Dermatol 1976;95:255.
44. Oh W, Yao AC, Hanson JS, Lind J. Peripheral circulatory response to phototherapy in newborn infants. Acta Paediatr Scand 1973;62:49.
45. Wu PYK, Wong WH, Hodgman JE, Levan NE. Changes in blood flow in the skin and muscle with phototherapy. Pediatr Res 1974;8:257.
46. Leung AKC, McArthur RG, McMillan DD, Ko D, Deacon JSR, Parboosingh JT, Lederis KP. Circulating antidiuretic hormone during labour and in the newborn. Acta Paediatr Scand 1980;69:505.
47. Rees L, Brook CGD, Shaw JCL, Forsling ML. Hyponatraemia in the first week of life in preterm infants. Part I. Arginine vasopressin secretion. Arch Dis Child 1984;59:414.
48. Wiriyathian S, Rosenfeld CR, Arant BS Jr, Porter JC, Faucher DJ, Engle WD. Urinary arginine vasopressin: pattern of excretion in the neonatal period. Pediatr Res 1986;20:103.
49. Siegel SR, Fisher DA, Oh W. Serum aldosterone concentrations related to sodium balance in the newborn infant. Pediatrics 1974;53:410.
50. Dillon MJ, Rajani KB, Shah V, Ryness JM, Milner RDG. Renin and aldosterone response in human newborns to acute change in blood volume. Arch Dis Child 1978;53:461.

51. Aperia A, Broberger O, Herin P, Zetterström R. Sodium excretion in relation to sodium intake and aldosterone excretion in newborn pre-term and full-term infants. Acta Paediatr Scand 1979;68:813.
52. Sulyok E, Németh M, Tényi I, Csaba I, Györy E, Ertl T, Varga F. Postnatal development of renin-angiotensin-aldosterone system, RAAS, in relation to electrolyte balance in premature infants. Pediatr Res 1979;13:817.
53. Kojima T, Fukuda Y, Hirata Y, Matsuzaki S, Kobayashi Y. Effects of aldosterone and atrial natriuretic peptide on water and electrolyte homeostasis of sick neonates. Pediatr Res 1989;25:591.
54. David L, Anast CS. Calcium metabolism in newborn infants. The interrelationship of parathyroid function and calcium, magnesium, and phosphorus metabolism in normal, "sick," and hypocalcemic infants. J Clin Invest 1974;54:287.
55. David L, Salle B, Chopard P, Grafmeyer D. Studies on circulating immunoreactive calcitonin in low birth weight infants during the first 48 hours of life. Helv Paediatr Acta 1977;32:39.
56. Hillman LS, Rojanasathit S, Slatopolsky E, Haddad JG. Serial measurements of serum calcium, magnesium, parathyroid hormone, calcitonin, and 25-hydroxy-vitamin D in premature and term infants during the first week of life. Pediatr Res 1977;11:739.
57. Tsang RC, Chen IW, Friedman MA, Chen I. Neonatal parathyroid function: role of gestational age and postnatal age. J Pediatr 1973;83:728.
58. Wieland P, Duc G, Binswanger U, Fischer JA. Parathyroid hormone response in newborn infants during exchange transfusion with blood supplemented with citrate and phosphate: effect of iv calcium. Pediatr Res 1979;13:963.
59. David L, Salle BL, Putet G, Grafmeyer DC. Serum immunoreactive calcitonin in low birth weight infants. Description of early changes; effect of intravenous calcium infusion; relationships with early changes in serum calcium, phosphorus, magnesium, parathyroid hormone, and gastrin levels. Pediatr Res 1981;15:803.
60. Smith FG, Sata T, Varille VA, Robillard JE. Atrial natriuretic factor during fetal and postnatal life: a review. J Dev Physiol 1989;12:55.
61. Mercadier JJ, Zongazo MA, Wisnewsky C, et al. Atrial natriuretic factor messenger ribonucleic acid and peptide in the human heart during ontogenic development. Biochem Biophys Res Commun 1989;159:777.
62. Yamaji T, Hirai N, Ishibashi M, Takaku F, Yanaihara T, Nakayama T. Atrial natriuretic peptide in umbilical cord blood: evidence for a circulating hormone in human fetus. J Clin Endocrinol Metab 1986;63:1414.
63. Shaffer SG, Geer PG, Goetz KL. Elevated atrial natriuretic factor in neonates with respiratory distress syndrome. J Pediatr 1986;109:1028.
64. Liechty EA, Johnson MD, Myerberg DZ, Mullett MD. Daily sequential changes in plasma atrial natriuretic factor concentrations in mechanically ventilated low-birth-weight infants. Biol Neonate 1989;55:244.
65. Robillard JE, Weiner C. Atrial natriuretic factor in the human fetus: effect of volume expansion. J Pediatr 1988;113:552.
66. Bierd TM, Kattwinkel J, Chevalier RL, et al. Interrelationship of atrial natriuretic peptide, atrial volume, and renal function in premature infants. J Pediatr 1990;116:753.
67. Tulassay T, Rascher W, Seyberth HW, Lang RE, Tóth M, Sulyok E. Role of atrial natriuretic peptide in sodium homeostasis in premature infants. J Pediatr 1986;109:1023.
68. Kojima T, Hirata Y, Fukuda Y, Iwase S, Kobayashi Y. Plasma atrial natriuretic peptide and spontaneous diuresis in sick neonates. Arch Dis Child 1987;62:667.
69. Siegel SR, Oh W. Renal function as a marker of human fetal maturation. Acta Paediatr Scand 1976;65:481.
70. Leake RD, Trygstad CW, Oh W. Inulin clearance in the newborn infant: relationship to gestational and postnatal age. Pediatr Res 1976;10:759.
71. Arant BS Jr. Developmental patterns of renal functional maturation compared in the human neonate. J Pediatr 1978;92:705.
72. Ross B, Cowett RM, Oh W. Renal functions of low birth weight infants during the first two months of life. Pediatr Res 1977;11:1162.
73. Sulyok E, Varga F, Györy E, Jobst K, Csaba IF. Postnatal development of renal sodium handling in premature infants. J Pediatr 1979;95:787.
74. Hansen JDL, Smith CA. Effects of withholding fluid in the immediate postnatal period. Pediatrics 1953;12:99.
75. Calcagno PL, Rubin MI, Weintraub DH. Studies on the renal concentrating and diluting mechanisms in the premature infant. J Clin Invest 1954;33:91.
76. McCance RA, Naylor NJB, Widdowson EM. The response of infants to a large dose of water. Arch Dis Child 1954;29:104.
77. Leake RD, Zakauddin S, Trygstad CW, Fu P, Oh W. The effects of large volume intravenous fluid infusion on neonatal renal function. J Pediatr 1976;89:968.
78. Aperia A, Herin P, Lundin S, Melin P, Zetterström R. Regulation of renal water excretion in newborn full-term infants. Acta Paediatr Scand 1984;73:717.
79. Brosius KK, Ritter DA, Kenny JD. Postnatal growth curve of the infant with extremely low birth weight who was fed enterally. Pediatrics 1984;74:778.
80. Lemoh JN, Brooke OG. Frequency and weight of normal stools in infancy. Arch Dis Child 1979;54:719.
81. Williams GS, Klenk EL, Winters RW. Acute renal failure in pediatrics. In: Winters RW, ed. The body fluids in pediatrics. Medical, surgical, and neonatal disorders of acid-base status, hydration, and oxygenation. Boston: Little, Brown, 1973:523.
82. Gamble JL, Butler AM. Measurement of the renal water requirement. Trans Assoc Am Physicians 1944;58:157.
83. Bell EF, Oh W. Fluid and electrolyte balance in very low birth weight infants. Clin Perinatol 1979;6:139.
84. Sinclair JC, Driscoll JM Jr, Heird WC, Winters RW. Supportive management of the sick neonate. Parenteral calories, water, and electrolytes. Pediatr Clin North Am 1970;17:863.
85. Ziegler EE, Biga RL, Fomon SJ. Nutritional requirements of the premature infant. In: Suskind RM, ed. Textbook of pediatric nutrition. New York: Raven Press, 1981:29.
86. Roy RN, Chance GW, Radde IC, Hill DE, Willis DM, Sheepers J. Late hyponatremia in very low birthweight infants (< 1.3 kilograms). Pediatr Res 1976;10:526.
87. Engelke SC, Shah BL, Vasan U, Raye JR. Sodium balance in very low-birth-weight infants. J Pediatr 1978;93:837.
88. Rodriguez-Soriano J, Vallo A, Oliveros R, Castillo G. Renal handling of sodium in premature and full-term neonates: a study using clearance methods during water diuresis. Pediatr Res 1983;17:1013.
89. Al-Dahhan J, Haycock GB, Chantler C, Stimmler L. Sodium homeostasis in term and preterm neonates. I. Renal aspects. Arch Dis Child 1983;58:335.
90. Jones MD Jr, Gresham EL, Battaglia FC. Urinary flow rates and urea excretion rates in newborn infants. Biol Neonate 1972;21:321.
91. Stonestreet BS, Oh W. Plasma creatinine levels in low-birth-weight infants during the first three months of life. Pediatrics 1978;61:788.
92. Karlowicz MG, Simmons MA, Brusilow SW, Jones MD Jr. Carbonic acid dissociation constant in critically ill newborns. Pediatr Res 1984;18:1287.

93. Bell EF, Oh W. Nutritional support. In: Goldsmith JP, Karotkin EH, eds. Assisted ventilation of the neonate. 2nd ed. Philadelphia: WB Saunders, 1988:307.
94. Costarino AT Jr, Gruskay JA, Corcoran L, Polin RA, Baumgart S. Sodium restriction versus daily maintenance replacement in very low birthweight premature neonates: a randomized, blind therapeutic trial. J Pediatr 1992;120:99.
95. Gruskay J, Costarino AT, Polin RA, Baumgart S. Nonoliguric hyperkalemia in the premature infant weighing less than 1000 grams. J Pediatr 1988;113:381.
96. Siegel SR, Fisher DA, Oh W. Renal function and serum aldosterone levels in infants with respiratory distress syndrome. J Pediatr 1973;83:854.
97. Broberger U, Aperia A. Renal function in idiopathic respiratory distress syndrome. Acta Pediatr Scand 1978;67:313.
98. Tulassay T, Ritvay J, Bors Z, Büky B. Alterations in creatinine clearance during respiratory distress syndrome. Biol Neonate 1979;35:258.
99. Torrado A, Guignard JP, Prod'hom LS, Gautier E. Hypoxaemia and renal function in newborns with respiratory distress syndrome (RDS). Helv Paediatr Acta 1974;29:399.
100. Guignard JP, Torrado A, Mazouni SM, Gautier E. Renal function in respiratory distress syndrome. J Pediatr 1976; 88:845.
101. Langman CB, Engle WD, Baumgart S, Fox WW, Polin RA. The diuretic phase of respiratory distress syndrome and its relationship to oxygenation. J Pediatr 1981;98:462.
102. Bidiwala KS, Lorenz JM, Kleinman LI. Renal function correlates of postnatal diuresis in preterm infants. Pediatrics 1988;82:50.
103. Fewell JE, Norton JB Jr. Continuous positive airway pressure impairs renal function in newborn goats. Pediatr Res 1980; 14:1132.
104. Tulassay T, Machay T, Kiszel J, Varga J. Effects of continuous positive airway pressure on renal function in prematures. Biol Neonate 1983;43:152.
105. Cox JR, Davies-Jones GAB, Leonard PJ, Singer B. The effect of positive pressure respiration on urinary aldosterone excretion. Clin Sci 1963;24:1.
106. Bark H, LeRoith D, Nyska M, Glick SM. Elevations in plasma ADH levels during PEEP ventilation in the dog: mechanisms involved. Am J Physiol 1980;239:E474.
107. Hemmer M, Viquerat CE, Suter PM, Vallotton MB. Urinary antidiuretic hormone excretion during mechanical ventilation and weaning in man. Anesthesiology 1980;52:395.
108. Svenningsen NW, Andreasson B, Lindroth M. Diuresis and urine concentration during CPAP in newborn infants. Acta Paediatr Scand 1984;73:727.
109. Mullins RJ, Dawe EJ, Lucas CE, Ledgerwood AM, Banks SM. Mechanisms of impaired renal function with PEEP. J Surg Res 1984;37:189.
110. Paxson CL Jr, Stoerner JW, Denson SE, Adcock EW III, Morriss FH Jr. Syndrome of inappropriate antidiuretic hormone secretion in neonates with pneumothorax or atelectasis. J Pediatr 1977;91:459.
111. Stern P, LaRochelle FT Jr, Little GA. Vasopressin and pneumothorax in the neonate. Pediatrics 1981;68:499.
112. Lorenz JM, Kleinman LI, Kotagal UR, Reller MD. Water balance in very low-birth-weight infants: relationship to water and sodium intake and effect on outcome. J Pediatr 1982; 101:423.
113. Sinclair JC, Engel K, Silverman WA. Early correction of hypoxemia and acidemia in infants of low birth weight: a controlled trial of oxygen breathing, rapid alkali and assisted ventilation. Pediatrics 1968;42:565.
114. Hobel CJ, Oh W, Hyvarinen MA, Emmanouilides GC, Erenberg A. Early versus late treatment of neonatal acidosis in low-birth-weight infants: relation to respiratory distress syndrome. J Pediatr 1972;81:1178.
115. Corbet AJ, Adams JM, Kenny JD, Kennedy J, Rudolph AJ. Controlled trial of bicarbonate therapy in high-risk premature newborn infants. J Pediatr 1977;91:771.
116. Bell EF. Fluid therapy. In: Sinclair JC, Bracken MB, eds. Effective care of the newborn infant. New York: Oxford University Press, 1992:59.
117. Siegel SR, Phelps DL, Leake RD, Oh W. The effects of rapid infusion of hypertonic sodium bicarbonate in infants with respiratory distress. Pediatrics 1973;51:651.
118. Simmons MA, Adcock EW III, Bard H, Battaglia FC. Hypernatremia and intracranial hemorrhage in neonates. N Engl J Med 1974;291:6.
119. Heird WC, Dell RB, Price T, Winters RW. Osmotic effects of infusion of THAM. Pediatr Res 1972;6:495.
120. Moylan FMB, Herrin JT, Krishnamoorthy K, Todres ID, Shannon DC. Inappropriate antidiuretic hormone secretion in premature infants with cerebral injury. Am J Dis Child 1978; 132:399.
121. Speer ME, Gorman WA, Kaplan SL, Rudolph AJ. Elevation of plasma concentrations of arginine vasopressin following perinatal asphyxia. Acta Paediatr Scand 1984;73:610.
122. Dauber IM, Krauss AN, Symchych PS, Auld PAM. Renal failure following perinatal anoxia. J Pediatr 1976;88:851.
123. Anand SK, Northway JD, Crussi FG. Acute renal failure in newborn infants. J Pediatr 1978;92:985.
124. Benson CD, Lloyd JR. Infantile pyloric stenosis. Am J Surg 1964;107:429.
125. Pizarro D, Posada G, Mata L, Nalin D, Mohs E. Oral rehydration of neonates with dehydrating diarrheas. Lancet 1979; 2:1209.
126. Lister J. Insensible water loss in infants. J Pediatr Surg 1967; 2:483.
127. Dolcourt JL, Bose CL. Percutaneous insertion of silastic central venous catheters in newborn infants. Pediatrics 1982;70:484.
128. Sherman MP, Vitale DE, McLaughlin GW, Goetzman BW. Percutaneous and surgical placement of fine silicone elastomer central catheters in high-risk newborns. J Parenteral Enteral Nutr 1983;7:75.
129. Berg RA. Emergency infusion of catecholamines into bone marrow. Am J Dis Child 1984;138:810.

Neonatology: Pathophysiology and Management of the Newborn, Fourth Edition,
edited by Gordon B. Avery, Mary Ann Fletcher, and Mhairi G. MacDonald.
J.B. Lippincott Company, Philadelphia © 1994.

chapter 24

Nutrition

ANNE B. FLETCHER

FEEDING THE FULL-TERM INFANT

The science of feeding is not very old, and even today, much of what is practiced is based on what seems to work or not work. As Dr. Frank Oski pointed out, infant feeding practices are the longest, uncontrolled experiment lacking informed consent in the history of medicine.[1] Despite these reservations, it is likely that there are several correct ways to feed full-term and preterm infants.

SCHEDULING OF FEEDINGS

Because approximately 2000 feedings occur in the first year of life, it is best that they bring enjoyment to both mother and infant. In the first few days of life, full-term healthy infants feed at more frequent intervals until the sucking and swallowing mechanism is well developed and there is milk let-down. Thereafter, they usually settle into a schedule of every 3 to 4 hours, with sleep occurring about 60% of the time. Trying to wake an infant for feeding to create a better schedule will probably result in only small amounts of milk taken and tension in the caregivers. Infants needing a more controlled schedule are those with a poor suck and swallow reflex, chronic lung disease, or gastrostomies, for which careful calculations of intake are necessary to ensure growth. Breast-fed infants feed more frequently, often every 2 to 3 hours. Their intake is unknown but should be calculated by careful weighing before and after feedings only if the infant does not thrive. Feedings more frequent than every 2 hours should be discouraged.

For an obese infant, after the newborn period, the diet should be calculated and restricted in caloric intake. Low-caloric-density foods can be substituted (*e.g.*, vegetables substituted for fruits, dinners in place of pure meats), but skim milk should not be used in the first year of life. Even obese infants should receive at least 85 kcal/kg with a proper nutrient intake. As the infant gets older, the number of feedings decrease, and by 6 months, the number of meals should approach three to four daily.

BREAST *VERSUS* BOTTLE FEEDING

All healthy women should be helpfully encouraged to breast-feed their full-term infants. For various reasons, a woman may not want to do so; she should not be made to feel guilty. Breast-feeding declined through the late 1980s.[2] The largest decline was seen in young, unmarried, African-American women of lower income, although the decline was not limited to this group.

Despite the advent of modified cow-milk formula, no artificial formula has been found to equal breast milk. Since large numbers of women in industrial nations now breast feed, it appears that their infants have a lower incidence than formula-fed infants of gastrointestinal and nongastrointestinal diseases, including otitis media, bacteremia, pneumonia, meningitis, and urinary tract infection.[3,4] Infants in nonindustrial nations must still be breast-fed for survival.

The advantages of breast-feeding are many. Human milk is always at the correct temperature and requires no sterilization; the protein content is lower than in formula but of high quality, gives a small curd, and is easily digestible; the fats are well absorbed; the carbohydrate is relatively high in lactose but causes few problems; breast milk imparts a gram-positive intestinal flora rather than gram-negative; antibodies passed by way of the milk to the infant help prevent infection; the potential psychologic benefit to mother and child is obvious.

There are few instances in which breast-feeding should not be encouraged. Even temporary disorders, such as engorgement or mastitis, may be improved by continuing feeding. Breast-feeding is recommended for the first year of life, adding beikost (*i.e.*, solids) during the second 6 months. Certain diseases (*e.g.*, galactosemia, alactasia) call for formula substitutes containing no lactose. There are drugs taken by the mother that are contraindicated during breast-feeding (*e.g.*, amethopterin, bromocriptine, cimetidine, clemastine, cyclophosphamide, ergotamine, gold salts, methimazole, phenidione, thiouracil), and some agents merely require temporary cessation. For a complete listing, see the second edition of *Drugs in Pregnancy and Lactation.*[5]

Although mothers who are positive for hepatitis B antigen and those with cytomegalovirus infection may be at risk for transmission of these organisms through their breast milk, the risk does not seem to outweigh the benefits. The exact infectivity of seropositive mothers for human immunodeficiency virus-1 (HIV-1) is unknown. There is evidence that transmission is possible. IgG and IgA antibodies to HIV-1 are found in milk from seropositive women, indicating the virus can elicit a local immune response.[6] Whether the antibodies have any protective effect is unknown. In some instances, mothers are too sick to breast-feed; in others, drug intake (*e.g.*, cocaine, heroin, phencyclidine) may preclude breast-feeding. Although no definite recommendations can be made for an HIV-positive mother, caution should be taken.

Investigators from Finland have found slower gains in lengths in full-term infants exclusively breast-fed through the first year of life.[7] In the United States, limiting intake to breast milk without adding solids in the first year would be unusual and offers no advantages.

GUIDELINES FOR FORMULA SELECTION

A few basic guidelines should be considered in choosing the appropriate feeding for an infant. The diet should have the following characteristics:

- contain sufficient calories and essential nutrients
- be digestible
- contain a reasonable distribution of calories
- avoid potential problems suspected from a family history.

CALORIES AND ESSENTIAL NUTRIENTS

Underprovision of calories causes tissue breakdown, diverting other food substances into energy production. However, the traditionally taught caloric requirement of 120 kcal/kg/day may be an overestimation for some full-term infants. Adequate weight gains of as much as 30 g/day have been observed with as low as 90 kcal/kg/day, particularly in infants with decreased activity. Fluid volumes carrying these calories average 150 mL/kg, but the full-term infant fed *ad libitum* may exceed this. Both fluid and calories need to be calculated only for the newborn with poor or excessive weight gain if there is consideration of adjusting caloric concentration. Protein requirements for the normal full-term infant are probably overestimated at 2.2 g/kg/day. Essential nutrients for weight gain are contained in human milk and most commercially prepared infant formulas, with the occasional exception of some vitamins.

DIGESTIBILITY

A digestible diet should contain protein, carbohydrates, and fat in forms that have superior nutritive value and allow minimal fecal losses. Human milk still appears to be the best overall. Although its protein content is low (1.1%), the excellent lactalbumin–casein ratio (4:1) makes for small curds and easy digestibility. The variety of nucleotides may enhance the immune system, gut growth, and lipid metabolism.[8–11] Only Wyeth has added nucleotides to their infant formula. The modified cow milk in most routinely used infant formulas is an adequate source of nutrients. Some formulas have protein resembling that of breast milk (*e.g.*, 60% whey and 40% casein).

Although use of soy protein formulas produces adequate growth of full-term infants, these formulas contain only one-third of their available nitrogen as essential or semiessential amino acids.[12] For optimal growth, infants need approximately 10% more calories if they take soy formulas rather than human milk or bovine protein formulas. With soy formulas, because of binding with phytase, fat losses are increased in the stool, as are the losses of various minerals, vitamins, and trace elements. The predominant use of a soy formula has been in infants with presumed cow-milk allergy and in those who require a supplement to breast-feeding. Evidence suggests that serum IgG antibodies to soy proteins are formed as quickly or even more quickly than antibodies to cow-milk protein.[13] It is likely that IgE antibodies are more important in giving allergic manfestations. Soy formula should not be used without specific indications.

Casein hydrolysate formulas are satisfactory sources of nitrogen. Their osmolarity is low because glucose polymers have been substituted for sucrose, making them well tolerated. Their main use should be reserved for cow-milk or soy allergy. They are not needed for refeeding an infant after gastroenteritis, bowel surgery, or necrotizing enterocolitis. Anaphylaxis in response to hydrolysates has been reported.[14,15]

The most commonly used infant formulas contain lactose, glucose polymers, or a combination as their major carbohydrates. They are generally well tolerated. Infants fed human milk or formulas with added vegetable oils (*e.g.*, corn, coconut, soy, oleo), normally excrete less than 1 g fat/kg/day. Infants fed whole cow milk in many instances excrete fat in excess of 2 g/kg/day, and those fed evaporated milk without additional carbohydrates lose between 1 and 2 g/kg/day.[16] Fat absorption is least satisfactory in the first 10 days of life and then increases rapidly. Medium-chain triglyceride (MCT) oil has excellent absorption very early in life, although it may slow gastric emptying time. For the content of formulas, see Appendix E-4.

DISTRIBUTION OF CALORIES

An appropriate distribution of calories for good infant nutrition is 7% to 16% protein, 35% to 55% fat, and 35% to 65% carbohydrate. Most available infant formulas provide this distribution even if combined with various strained foods that are very low in fats. Only commercially prepared cow milk in regular or lowered fat concentrations, evaporated milk, and certain formulas designed for older infants (*e.g.*, Similac Advance, Gerber's Good Nature) have distributions of calories outside the optimal ranges, with a decrease in fat or carbohydrate and an increase in protein. In the late 1970s, Fomon and others reported that cow milk could be used without problems after the first 6 months of life as part of a mixed diet.[17] It was later shown that blood loss was still apparent through the gastrointestinal tract for infants on cow milk after 6 months of age.[18] Cow milk should be avoided as routine diet for infants younger than 1 year of age. The formulas for older infants and cow milk are also hazardous if abnormal losses are encountered (*e.g.*, diarrhea, vomiting, excessive temperature) because of their high solute load. The use of standard infant formula through the first year of life that is supplemented after 4 to 6 months with infant foods has been adequate, and there seems to be little use for formulas designed for the older infant.[19]

IRON FORTIFICATION

Iron deficiency has remained one of the most common causes of anemia in infancy and childhood despite widespread availability of iron-fortified formulas, supplements, and cereals. Although a full-term infant is born with adequate iron reserves, these stores begin to deplete at about 4 months of age, and deficiency appears between 6 and 9 months, particularly in lower socioeconomic groups. Without iron supplementation, there must be a large intake of commercial dried cereals, which are not well absorbed (see Appendix E-5).[20] The American Academy of Pediatrics (AAP) suggests 1 mg/kg/day for the full-term infant by 4 months of age and 2 mg/kg/day for preterm infants no later than 2 months of age.[21] Differing opinions exist about iron supplementation in the breast-feeding infant. By 6 months of age, breast-fed infants have decreased iron stores, and by 9 months, some become deficient.[22] In light of increasing reports of the effect of iron therapy on improvement of behavioral performance in nonanemic but iron-deficient infants and lowered mental and motor functioning in a 5-year follow-up of children who had hemoglobin levels less than or equal to 10.0 g/dL during infancy, it appears prudent to supplement breast-fed infants.[23,24]

Hesitation to give iron supplements or iron-fortified formulas has been based on poorly documented reports of gastrointestinal symptoms and low incidences of anemia in middle-class patients. However, controlled studies suggest no differences in symptoms between infants fed formulas with iron and those given formulas without iron.[25,26] Controversy also exists about whether administration of iron increases the risk of infection in the neonate, because iron saturates the binding sites of lactoferrin and interferes with its bacteriostatic function. It appears that the infection risk is more related to other factors, such as malnutrition and organisms to which an infant is exposed, than to iron, and I concur with the AAP recommendation for supplementation.

FLUORIDE SUPPLEMENTATION

Fluoride acts to strengthen dental enamel and is incorporated in the mineralization stage and through direct surface contact after eruption. Fluoride is well absorbed from foods, but best from sodium fluoride supplements.[27] Formula made with water fluoridated to levels of 3 ppm or higher provides the AAP recommendation of 0.3 to 0.7 mg/L/day. If the water contains less, 0.25 mg/day should be started in the first 2 weeks of life.[28] There is no indication that the preterm infant needs are any different. Any infant exclusively on human milk, ready-to-feed formula, or formula made with bottled water should receive fluoride supplementation.

MINOR PROBLEMS AND DIETARY MANIPULATION

The pediatrician frequently encounters spitting-up and changes in stool pattern in a bottle-fed infant. If there is sufficient growth, these problems do not merit formula changes. The physician can treat mild constipation by adding light or dark Karo syrup to the formula or prune juice or solid foods to the diet. Severe constipation requiring the constant use of suppositories should be investigated. Loose stools may be helped by elimination of some carbohydrate from the diet or by changing the carbohydrate source.

Many infants spit up small amounts of formula.

This can result from overfeeding, determined by a careful dietary history. The exact incidence of gastroesophageal reflux in infancy is unknown, but it is estimated to be very high. Medical treatment that includes prone positioning at a 30° angle, thickening of feedings, and perhaps the use of bethanechol or metoclopramide usually helps in all but the most severe cases. Projectile, bile-stained, or persistent vomiting with poor weight gain requires immediate investigation.

FEEDING THE PREMATURE INFANT

Although advances in management of premature infants have resulted in a lower mortality rate, feeding the premature infant still is a precise nursing and nutritional art because of the special liabilities of the infant. The aim of feeding should be to approximate intrauterine growth and mineral storage, a goal that is frequently impossible. The ideal growth rate remains unknown in the preterm extrauterine environment.

The premature infant faces several nutritional problems:

- poor suck and swallowing coordination until at least 34 weeks of gestation
- a relatively high caloric requirement with initially small gastric capacity
- poor gag reflexes, leading to aspiration
- immature and often incompetent esophagogastric sphincter, leading to reflux
- decreased intestinal enzyme secretion, which may affect nutrient absorption
- decreased secretion, absorption, and bile-acid pools
- decreased bowel motility, particularly if not fed enterally
- blunted gastrointestinal hormonal responses if given parenteral nutrition.

EARLY LOW-VOLUME FEEDING

The optimal time for initiating enteral feeding in the preterm infant is unknown. Larger, healthy infants weighing more than 1500 g can usually be fed within hours of birth after stabilization. The critical problem is when to feed a very-low-birth-weight (VLBW) infant weighing less than 1500 g and the micropremie weighing less than 1000 g. Caloric intake can easily be given early by means of parenteral nutrition, although gut villous involution can occur within 3 days in neonatal animals receiving intravenous calories.[29] There is no conclusive evidence that feeding should be delayed in viable premature infants. All unstable infants, whatever their size, should not be enterally fed until stable. After stabilization, minimal or low-volume feeds should be considered as soon as possible. Table 24-1 lists the evidence for early feeding. In several studies, infants fed earlier tended toward decreases in days to discharge, days on parenteral nutrition, and days to regain birth weight, and they showed no significant increase in necrotizing enterocolitis.[30–34]

SCHEDULING FEEDINGS

There is no evidence to suggest that the first few feedings of any infant must be sterile water or 5% dextrose, because it is aspirated gastric contents with acid that is harmful. Upper intestinal obstruction in the full-term infant is usually detected before the first feed. If not, a mature, normal infant is generally capable of protecting his airways should he experience emesis. Preterm infants older than 34 weeks of gestation are similar to full-term infants; those more immature have usually had radiographs that included the abdomen to rule out obstruction. Breast milk or the formula of choice may be given full strength for the full-term infant and generally one-quarter to one-half strength for the preterm infant at the first feed. Table 24-2 shows suggested intervals, amounts, and times to full feeds.

TABLE 24–1
EFFECT OF EARLY MINIMAL FEEDINGS IN PREMATURE INFANTS

Amount Fed	Demonstrated Effect*	Reference
Cumulative feeding, day 6 (well infant, 703 ± 33 mL; RDS infant, 400 ± 116 mL)	Increased plasma concentration of enteroglucagon, gastrin, GIP, motilin, neurotensin	30
12 mL/kg/d beginning day 8	Improved feeding tolerance, decreased gastric residuals, fewer days that feedings were discontinued, full feeds reached earlier	31
15–20 mL/kg/d beginning at 48 h	Full feeds reached earlier, fewer days under phototherapy, bilirubin lower at 2 wk, lower serum alkaline phosphatases	32
18 kcal/kg/d beginning at day 2	Improved weight gain, decreased gastric residuals, days feedings withheld	33, 34

* These effects are significant when compared with nonfed infants.
GIP, gastrointestinal peptide; RDS, respiratory distress syndrome.

TABLE 24–2
ORAL FEEDING SCHEDULE FOR THE LOW-BIRTH-WEIGHT INFANT

		≤ 1000 g		1001–1500 g		1501–2000 g		> 2000 g	
Time	**Substance***	Amount	Frequency	Amount	Frequency	Amount	Frequency	Amount	Frequency
First feeding	½-strength human milk or ¼-strength formula	1–2 mL/kg	1–2 h	2–3 mL/kg	2 h	3–4 mL/kg	2–3 h	10 mL/kg (full strength)	3 h
Subsequent feedings, 12–72 h	Formula or ½- to full-strength human milk	Increase 1 mL† every other feeding to maximum of 5 mL	2 h	Increase 1 mL† every other feeding to maximum of 10 mL	2 h	Increase 2 mL every other feeding to maximum of 15 mL	2–3 h	Increase 5 mL every other feeding to maximum of 20 mL	3 h
Final feeding schedule, 150 mL/kg	Full-strength formula or human milk	10–15 mL	2 h	20–28 mL	2–3 h	28–37 mL	3 h	37–50 mL, then *ad libitum*	3–4 h
Total time to full feeds			10–14 d or more for infants <750 g		7–10 d		5–7 d		3–5 d

* Supplemental IV fluids should be given to fulfill requirements of 140–160 mL/kg (urine specific gravities 1.008–1.010) and caloric requirements of 90–130 cal/kg.
† Strength should alternately be increased with volume.

Gastric capacities differ, but residuals should be measured before each feeding only in small preterm infants. If the amount retained in the stomach equals the anticipated feeding, nothing should be given. If there is less on isolated measurements, an additional increment to equal the desired total may be given with the refed residual aspirate. Because increasing residuals, with or without distention, may be an early indication of partial obstruction, ileus, or necrotizing enterocolitis, further feedings should be given only with caution.

SPECIAL REQUIREMENTS

A premature infant has a number of special requirements that differ from those of a full-term infant because the latter can usually be fed *ad libitum* with breast milk or formula with little need for special calculations.

ENTERAL ENERGY AND PROTEIN INTAKE

It has been difficult to settle on the ideal energy and protein allowances for preterm infants because of the many variables involved, including temperature stresses, activity, degree of illness, infection, malnutrition, and needs for catch-up growth. Data on adults suggest that nitrogen is used better in the presence of extra energy.[35] Studies in the 1960s and 1970s reported the most rapid weight gain of LBW infants with protein intakes between 3 and 5 g/kg/day.[36,37] Goldman and colleagues suggested that excess protein might be injurious to the developing nervous system.[38] Unfortunately, virtually all these studies contained a mixture of true preterm and small-for-gestational-age infants, whose requirements differ. Kashyap and associates studied three groups of true premature infants with various protein and energy intakes (Table 24-3).[39] The rates of weight gain and nitrogen retention in the high-protein groups were greater. In the group with the highest intake (3.9 g/kg/day) the excess gain was mainly fat. These data suggest an intake of at least 3 g/100 kcal/day (3.6 g/kg) or roughly 30 kcal/g of protein taken enterally is sufficient.

Schultze and colleagues showed similar results with excess energy contributing mainly to fat deposition and suggested that approximately 115 kcal/kg/day with protein intakes of 3.5 to 3.6 g/kg/day was adequate for the preterm.[40] Heird and colleagues published the following conclusions:[41]

> The LBW infant who can take feeds soon after birth requires a protein intake of at least 2.8 g/kg/day.
> LBW infants who do not receive protein in the first few days lose at least 1% of their endogenous protein stores daily. If protein intake is delayed, it must be increased to account for early losses.
> It appears that maintenance energy in LBW infants is 50 to 60 kcal/kg/day, and allowances for stress, loss through stool, and growth would require an additional 50 to 60 kcal/kg/day.[41] Barring any excess needs because of chronic disease or malabsorption, more than 120 kcal/kg/day is probably unnecessary.

There has been increasing interest in the use of preterm breast milk in neonatal intensive care units. Räihä and colleagues showed that the quality of protein (*i.e.*, whey *versus* casein) made a difference in serum amino acid levels, ammonia levels, urea nitrogen, and the incidence of acidosis.[42–45] Although these studies were of considerable importance, there was little focus on mineral status, lowered serum proteins in infants fed pooled breast milk, and less weight gain. Others have found that preterm infants fed pooled or preterm breast milk without fortification grew less well.[46–49]

Additional investigations focused on the increased protein content of preterm milk compared with full-term human milk (Table 24-4).[50–52] Only one study found no real increase when controlling for 24-hour volume.[53] Because of differences existing in collection of milk, foremilk and hindmilk, ongoing changes of the milk during subsequent weeks, and daily varia-

TABLE 24–3
PROTEIN AND ENERGY INTAKES IN LOW-BIRTH-WEIGHT INFANTS

Energy Intake Factors	Group 1 (n = 14)	Group 2 (n = 15)	Group 3 (n = 15)
Birth weight, median (g)	1390	1500	1460
Gestational age, median (wk)	32	32	32
Protein intake (g/kg/d)	2.8 ± 0.04	3.8 ± 0.04	3.9 ± 0.04
Energy (kcal/kg/d)	118 ± 1.7	119 ± 2.2	142 ± 2.4
Change in weight (g/kg/d)	16 ± 1.8	19.1 ± 3.2	21.5 ± 2.2
Head circumference at 2200 g (cm)	33 ± 0.79	32.7 ± 0.79	32.5 ± 0.53
Energy stored (kcal/kg/d)	50 ± 3.5	49 ± 5.7	69.8 ± 4.5

From Kashyap S, Schulze KF, Forsyth MS, et al. Growth, nutrient retention, and metabolic response in low birth weight infants fed varying intakes of protein and energy. J Pediatr 1988;113:713.

TABLE 24–4
NUTRIENT AND MINERAL CONTENT OF PRETERM MILK

Element*	Days 3–7	Day 21	Days 29–42	Days 57–98
Protein (g/dL)	3.24 ± 0.31	1.83 ± 0.14	1.31–1.81± 0.12	1.8 ± 0.07
Lactose (g/dL)	5.96 ± 0.2	6.49 ± 0.21		
Fat (g/dL)	1.63 ± 0.23	3.68 ± 0.4		
Energy (kcal/dL)	51.4 ± 2.4	65.6 ± 4.3		
Sodium (mEq/dL)	2.66 ± 0.3	1.3 ± 0.18	0.76 ± 0.09	0.55 ± 0.05
Chloride (mEq/dL)	3.16 ± 0.3	1.7 ± 0.17		
Potassium (mEq/dL)	1.74 ± 0.07	1.63 ± 0.09	1.1 ± 0.1	1.1 ± 0.1
Calcium (mg/dL)	20.3–26.3 ± 1.7	20.4 ± 1.5	24.6–26.2 ± 2.2	31.5 ± 1.3
Phosphorous (mg/dL)	9.5–14.6 ± 0.7	14.9 ± 1.3	13.3 ± 0.3	
Magnesium (mg/dL)	2.8 ± .1	2.4 ± 0.1	4.9 ± 0.1	

* Data from references 50, 51, and 52.

tion in nutrients, the content of preterm milk should never be taken for granted. Preterm infants receiving human milk, particularly, should be monitored for nutritional status.

CARBOHYDRATES

Carbohydrates, particularly glucose, is one of the body's main energy nutrients and is essential to the brain for normal metabolism. There is a need for glucose or galactose as lactose at all times, and yet there are no specific requirements. Carbohydrate intravenously promotes efficient nitrogen retention; the same could be expected of enteral intake.[54] Galactose is needed for glycogen storage and for provision of glucose during the fasting state. The preterm infant is much more likely to become hypoglycemic, so keeping within the suggested energy guidelines seems appropriate.

LIPIDS

Lipids, like carbohydrates, are a major source for growth, metabolism, and muscle activity. In 1929, the first fatty acid deficiency was described in rats on a fat-free diet. When given fat, symptoms of skin rash and growth delay disappeared.[55] It was not until the advent of fat-free parenteral nutrition that typical symptoms in neonates were seen. It now appears that two long-chain unsaturated fatty acids, linoleic acid (ω6 18:2) and α-linolenic acid (ω3 18:3), are essential for the preterm infant and that deficiency of the latter is subtle. Linoleic acid elongates and saturates to become the precursor of arachidonic acid; linolenic acid is metabolized to eicosapentaenoic acid (EPA) and docosahexaenoic acid (DHA) by the same mechanism. Eicosapentaenoic and DHA may provide structure to the phospholipid layer, influencing important membrane functions.[56] Docosahexaenoic acid and EPA is present in breast milk; formula-fed infants have levels that decrease slowly with time.[57] Uauy and colleagues studied 83 preterm infants weighing between 1000 and 1500 g who were given breast milk, preterm formula with only linoleic acid, preterm formula containing linoleic and linolenic acids, or an experimental preterm formula containing fish oil that supplemented EPA and DHA similar to quantities found in human milk.[58] After discharge, the infants received 5 months of full-term formulas with corresponding fatty acid intake. The infants fed formula with fish oil showed DHA levels similar to infants fed breast milk, and those fed the formula with linoleic and linolenic acids had lower levels, suggesting that they were not able to metabolize sufficient DHA. In addition, their retinal function was not as good as the other group.

The AAP suggests that 3% of energy intake should be linoleic acid.[59] The European Society for Pediatric Gastroenterology and Nutrition proposed that essential fatty acids (*i.e.*, both EFAs) be added to preterm infant formulas.[60] Uauy found that fish oil seems to be well tolerated by preterm infants. He makes the following recommendations for intake:

Total EFA content should be set at 4% to 5% of energy intake but may go as high as 12% safely with linoleic acid at 0.5 to 0.7g/kg/day and α-linolenic acid at 70 to 150 mg/kg/day.

Because enzymes to convert α-linolenic acid to DHA may be suboptimal, DHA at doses of 35 to 75 mg/kg/day should be given.

Linoleic acid intake should not exceed 12% of total energy, because an excess may inhibit the formation of linolenic acid. The ratio of ω6 to ω3 fatty acids should be in the range of 5:1 to 15:1.[56] It appears that formula manufacturers are considering this suggestion.

Carnitine synthesis may be limited in the preterm infant. It facilitates the transport of long-chain fatty acids across the inner mitochondrial membrane. Fortunately, breast milk has high levels of carnitine, and most formulas have been supplemented, and it is only an issue if infants receive carnitine-deficient total parenteral nutrition (TPN) solutions.

VITAMINS AND IRON

Although most formulas contain vitamins and are adequate for the full-term infant, preterm infants may require additional supplements. Table 24-5 shows the suggested intakes. Intramuscular vitamin K (0.5 to 1 mg) should be given to all infants at birth.

Vitamin E deficiency was first described in 1967 by Oski, who found preterm infants with an anemia unresponsive to iron, high reticulocyte counts, increased hydrogen peroxide hemolysis, and puffy feet.[61] Until 1985, it was generally accepted that 25 IU of vitamin E and 2 mg/kg/day of iron could be given simultaneously to the preterm infant. However, Gross and Gabriel showed that vitamin E levels were inadequate in preterm infants at 6 weeks of age if iron-fortified formulas were given but not if the infants were receiving preterm or mature human milk with iron.[62] Vitamin E levels should be followed weekly to biweekly and supplements given as needed. Up to 75 IU/day have been needed by some infants to maintain normal levels. Iron is started at 36 to 40 weeks except in the smallest infants (<1000 g) in whom iron and ferritin levels are checked before starting iron at approximately 40 weeks of corrected age. If iron and ferritin levels are sufficient, supplementation may be delayed if needed.

The relation of vitamin E to retinopathy of prematurity (ROP) in preterm infants weighing less than 1500 g has been an ongoing investigation for the past 20 years. Several studies showed a decrease in incidence and severity of ROP if large amounts of vitamin E were supplemented.[63–65] Subsequently, a large, controlled study showed no significant change in the incidence of ROP with prophylactic vitamin E but did show an increased incidence of necrotizing enterocolitis and retinal hemorrhages.[66] Another showed a decreased overall incidence of ROP but an increase in necrotizing enterocolitis and sepsis. Two studies have suggested that because regression of ROP is so common, prophylaxis is not reasonable.[66,67] Johnson and colleagues have suggested that treatment of ROP with vitamin E may be helpful and deserves further study.[68] After the intravenous E-Ferol (polysorbate 80) disaster, I cannot recommend maintaining high levels of vitamin E but do suggest keeping serum α-tocopherol levels between 1 and 2 mg/dL (10–20 μg/mL).[69–71]

Premature infants, particularly those who are critically ill, have low vitamin A levels. This is a result of their missing the last trimester of placental transfer compounded by the fact that vitamin A added to parenteral nutrition adheres to plastic tubing.[72,73] Vitamin A deficiency is characterized by reduced wound healing, increased squamous metaplasia in lung tissue, increased incidence of infection, night blindness, and xerophthalmia. In 1985, Shenai showed that infants with bronchopulmonary dysplasia (BPD) had lower plasma vitamin A levels than those with no lung disease.[74] A controlled study was subsequently performed in which infants with an estimated 90% risk of developing BPD were given 2000 IU of vitamin A intramuscularly on day 1 and then every other day for 14 doses. All infants received routine vitamin A with their parenteral or enteral nutrition. The control infants had an 85% incidence of BPD, and the treated infants had a 45% incidence. The need for ventilation on day 28 was decreased from 55% in the controls to 21% in the treated group; ROP decreased from 60% to 26%.[75] My colleagues and I found a decreased incidence of BPD at 36 weeks corrected age, but our study was performed with a less homogeneous population. Our infants received the same dosage as the prior study, but supplementation, given by injection or enterically, was continued until the infants had normal vitamin A levels or were discharged.[76] For the small preterm infant (<1250 g), I suggest starting early supplementation of vitamin A with close monitoring of serum levels to determine dosage.

TABLE 24–5
PRETERM VITAMIN SUPPLEMENTATION FOR HUMAN MILK AND FORMULAS

Source of Nourishment	Daily Supplement*
Enfamil Premature Formula† (Mead Johnson)	
Special care formula† (Ross Laboratories)	0.5 mL Poly-vi-sol
Human milk	1 mL Poly-vi-sol
Pregestimil, Nutramigen, Portagen	1 mL Poly-vi-sol

* At Children's National Medical Center, it has been found that very immature infants often need extra supplementation of vitamins A and E.
† Manufacturer states that no supplementation is needed.

SELECTION OF FEEDS FOR THE PREMATURE INFANT

Many formulas have been used at one time or another to feed the preterm infant. Some formulas are still used because they seem to work rather than because they have been examined carefully with regard to nutrient content and growth of the infant. There is no ideal formula, probably because there is disagreement over what the ideal is. In the United States, three manufacturers produce specially designed preterm formulas. These and other commonly used formulas are listed in Appendix E-4. All of them provide an acceptable distribution of calories and are tailored to the concentrating abilities of preterm kidneys. They have been modified in carbohydrate content to give lower osmolalities and in fat content to give better absorption. Premie SMA differs considerably in calcium and phosphorus content with levels lower than Enfamil Premature or Similac Special Care.

Preterm human milk with or without the use of

breast-milk modifiers deserves special comment. As can be seen in Table 24-4, preterm breast milk, compared with full-term breast milk, seems to be higher in protein during the first month; higher in sodium and chloride, which decrease during the first month; slightly lower in energy because of lower levels of lactose and fat, which rise during the same period; and stable in magnesium content. However, preterm, human milk remains low in calcium and phosphorus, and the supply of these minerals is inadequate, particularly for the infant weighing less than 1500 g. The immunologic elements are also altered in preterm milk but appear more than adequate to help protect the infant.[77]

The use of breast milk modifiers, particularly for recovering ill infants and infants weighing less than 1250 g, helps increase essential nutrient content while maintaining the distinct advantages of breast milk. Table 24-6 shows the two available modifiers. Enfamil Human Milk Modifier is a cow-milk whey protein and caseinate powder without fat that can be mixed 1 packet with 25 mL of human milk. Similac Natural Care is a liquid made from nonfat cow-milk protein with soy and coconut oils, which can be mixed in dilutions of 1:1, 1:2, or 1:3 with breast milk, depending on the ultimately desired concentration of nutrients, particularly protein, calcium, and phosphorus. In 1981, Reichman and colleagues showed that preterm infants fed a formula similar to human milk in amounts to maintain expected intrauterine weight gain had excess fat accretion.[78] Two years later, the same group showed normal nutrient accretion in infants fed their own mother's milk.[79] The earlier group of infants were given an average of 140 kcal/kg/day beginning at week 2, and the latter group received only 111 kcal/kg/day. This may have contributed to the excess fat accretion. It is appealing to use a modifier that does not contain extra vegetable oils because it may be better for the infant. For this reason, I use the powdered modifier, which also maintains the appearance of breast milk.

Fresh human milk is best for feeding the premature infant. However, fresh breast milk may be refrigerated only for as long as 24 hours before it is frozen. At −80°F, it can safely be stored for at least 3 months with maintenance of many of the growth factors, enzymes, IgA, and macromolecules. Live cells are destroyed.[80] Freezing at higher temperatures allows the lipases to begin digesting the fat. When prepared for a feeding, human milk should never be warmed in a microwave oven because uneven heating may cause severe burns.[81] It is better to defrost an 8-hour supply in the refrigerator and take each feeding out 1 hour before it is used. The milk may be further warmed in a tepid bath if necessary.

Better fat digestion and absorption have been seen

TABLE 24–6
HUMAN MILK FORTIFIERS

	Enfamil Human Milk Modifier*		
Contents	Without Human Milk	With Human Milk‡	**Similac Natural Care†**
Energy (kcal)	14	85.3	81
Protein (g)	0.7	2.53	2.2
Whey : casein	60 : 40	60 : 40	60 : 40
Fat (g)	<0.1	3.68	4.4 (soy, coconut oils)
CHO (g)	2.7	9.3	8.6
Vitamin A (IU)	780	970	75
Vitamin D (IU)	210	212	60
Vitamin E (IU)	3.4	3.66	1.58
Ca (mg)	90	108.4	171
P (mg)	45	59.9	85
Zn (mg)	0.71	0.85	1.2
Mn (μg)	9	0.14	10
Cu (μg)	80	108	203
Na (mg)	7	27	35
K (mg)	15.6	74.6	105
Cl (mg)	17.7	64.7	66
Osmolarity	120	265	300

* Mead Johnson Laboratories; per 4 packets of whey protein and sodium caseinate.
† Ross Laboratories; values per 1 dL undiluted nonfat cow milk protein; can be mixed 1 : 1, 1 : 2, or 1 : 3 with human milk.
‡ Based on analysis of human milk at 21 days after delivery; values per 1 dL; data from Atkinson SA, Bryan MH, Anderson GH. Human milk feeding in premature infants: protein, fat and carbohydrate balances in the first two weeks of life. J Pediatr 1981;99:617.

in LBW infants fed a mixture of fresh human milk and formula.[82] It is presumed that lingual and breast-milk lipases aid in the digestion of the fat in the formula. If formula supplementation rather than milk modifier is desired or necessary, combining human milk and formula appears preferable to giving them alternately. Because breast milk seems to stimulate or exaggerate the immune response of the infant intestine, it is important to determine if there is any history of milk allergy. This is also true for modifiers and cow-milk formula.

It is important to remember that if preterm human milk is given, the exact content of each feeding is unknown. Unless all hospital laboratories become equipped to analyze milk, monitoring of the infant's growth and nutritional status is imperative. If using a premature formula, the manufacturers suggest starting at one-quarter strength, and one-half strength is appropriate when starting human milk. Volumes and concentrations should be increased slowly and not simultaneously. For approximate feeding schedules, see Table 24-2.

Soy formulas are not recommended for use in premature infants without specific indications and then not for long durations.[83] Shenai[84] reported lower phosphorus levels in preterm infants fed soy formula, and Hillman[85] found osteopenia, hypocalcemia, and lower vitamin D levels.

There are only a few other formulas that are occasionally used in preterm infants; these include Portagen in infants with cholestasis because of its MCT content and Nutramigen or Pregestimil in infants with cow-milk intolerance or as a powder supplement to human milk–fed infants. There do not appear to be good reasons to use the latter formulas routinely for refeeding infants who have had abdominal surgery or are recovering from necrotizing enterocolitis.

The use of pooled breast milk for preterm infants is not recommended because the pool usually comes from full-term mothers; it is lower in protein and must be pasteurized at 62.5°C for 30 minutes. This results in a milk that is not nutritionally complete for the premature infant and has substantially fewer growth factors, enzymes, and immunologic elements.[80] Balance studies have shown that protein retention and fat absorption are much decreased with the use of pooled milk.[86] The results of infants fed banked breast milk have been inferior in terms of weight, length, head circumference, and length of hospitalization.[48,87] This may be because the infants fed the banked milk ingested fewer calories or because of changes in the milk due to processing. Lucas and colleagues found that when infants were assigned to receive preterm formula or banked breast milk as supplements to human milk feedings, those fed banked milk for more than 50% of their intake had a 5.3-point decrement in their IQs at 9 months of age. The difference is statistically, but arguably not clinically, significant.[88]

Dietary supplements are useful for specific conditions, but because they are not complete diets, care should be taken to provide all nutrients required for growth (Table 24-7). Medium-chain triglyceride oil and corn syrup solids (*i.e.*, glucose polymers) have frequently been used to supplement the diet of premature infants. Medium-chain triglyceride oil should be mixed thoroughly with the formula, because it has been reported to cause lipoid aspiration pneumonia if given alone and to adhere to feeding tubes.[89,90] Microlipid is an emulsion and mixes better with formulas.

Preterm infants, particularly those with BPD, often suffer nutritionally from the consequences of intensive care, and they may have larger energy needs while requiring fluid restriction. Supplements should be added one at a time as the infant is observed for intolerance. Basic protein, mineral, and vitamin requirements should be met before and after caloric supplements are added. It is usually advisable not to increase the energy content of a formula to more than 30 kcal/30 mL because of excess osmolar content.

SPECIAL FEEDING TECHNIQUES

GAVAGE FEEDINGS

Intermittent feedings by means of nasogastric or orogastric tubes are used in infants who cannot take oral feedings for limited periods of time but whose gastrointestinal tract is intact. Included in this group are infants with poor suck and swallow mechanisms who

TABLE 24–7
DIETARY SUPPLEMENTS

Substance	Contents	Uses
Casec powder	Casein hydrolysate: 88 g protein/100 g powder	Dietary supplement for protein
MCT oil	Medium chain triglyceride: 1 g = 8.3 kcal	Caloric supplement, malabsorption
Corn syrup solids	100% glucose polymers	Carbohydrate supplement: liquid (2 kcal/mL), powder (4 kcal/g)
Microlipid (emulsion)	4.5 kcal/mL 73.8 PUFA, linoleic acid 73.7%, linolenic acid 1.0%	Caloric supplement

have central nervous system depression or are younger than 32 weeks of gestation.

A 5-F (1.65-mm) or 8-F (2.6-mm) nasogastric tube is inserted through the nose or mouth into the stomach before feeding to avoid aspiration. Proper placement of tubing should be checked by aspiration of gastric contents. The formula should be run in by gravity, and the length of time for feeding should be equal to that allotted to oral feedings of a similar amount. I do not recommend feeding injected by syringe. Special tubes (*e.g.*, Argyle Indwell, Sherwood Medical, St. Louis, MO) may be kept in place for 30 days, and they eliminate repeated insertions and risks of vagal stimulation and bradycardia. Feeds are given every 2 to 4 hours, depending on the size of the infant and type of formula used (*e.g.*, if giving fresh breast milk, small frequent feedings are used). Hazards of this technique include partial airway obstruction, increased airway resistance, incompetence of the esophagocardiac sphincter when the tube is in place, excessive nasal secretions, and rarely, colonization with indwelling tubes, ulceration or perforation of the nasal septum, malplacement into the trachea, and perforation of the esophagus. Nasogastric tubes are more stable in position, but orogastric tubes cause less airway obstruction.

The beginning volume of constant drip feedings is about twice the amount calculated for starting bolus feeding. The amount is divided into an hourly rate. Constant feeds usually are not given at less than 0.5 mL/hour, and 1 mL/hour is preferable so that a feeding rather than an intravenous pump may be used.

CONTINUOUS ENTERAL GASTRIC OR TRANSPYLORIC FEEDINGS

Continuous enteral feedings by pump have increased in popularity over the years. Initially used in infants with tetanus, this form of feeding has become most useful in several categories of infants:

- VLBW infants who do not tolerate handling
- infants who have had necrotizing enterocolitis with or without short guts
- infants who are intolerant to bolus feeds
- infants who are chronically ventilator-dependent when continuous feedings may decrease oxygen consumption and increase absorption
- infants with severe apnea and bradycardia.

Toce demonstrated increased weight gain in infants weighing 1000 to 1249 g who were given continuous nasogastric feeds.[91] Grant found energy expenditure and oxygen consumption decreased.[92] Differences in hormonal secretion are also reported but do not seem to make a difference in weight gain.[93]

For transpyloric placement, the infant is positioned on his right side or prone. The tube is passed through the nostril into the stomach, allowing sufficient tube length. Small amounts of air are injected into the stomach while the infant sucks on a pacifier. The tube should move through the pylorus within the first one-half hour and give a return of bile-stained material. If there is no passage after several attempts, a dose of metachlopromide may be given one-half hour before placement, or the tube may be guided by fluoroscopy, with its concurrent radiation risks. The *p*H is tested at frequent intervals, and after a *p*H of 5 to 7 is attained, a flat plate of the abdomen is taken to determine placement. Location of the tip may be in the duodenum or jejunum. Transpyloric feeding has been my preference for feeding intubated infants to decrease the risk of aspiration.

After there is correct positioning, feedings may be started with quarter-strength formula or half-strength human milk. Feeding volumes are started at 1 to 2 mL/kg/hour. Feedings are increased in concentration and volume, as previously discussed, but remain continuous. Commonly used formulas may be used for these types of feeds, but hypertonic feedings should not be given. Constant drip of human milk poses a number of problems. It can be hung for only 4 hours at room temperature before bacterial counts begin to rise rapidly; therefore, milk may be lost in the tubing from the frequent and costly tubing changes. Because fat rises rapidly to the surface of the liquid, the infant may receive an unpredictable or insufficient quantity of fat unless the suspension is shaken fequently.[94] For these reasons, my colleagues and I may choose bolus feeds with human milk for ventilated infants. Gastric residuals should be checked with a nasogastric tube. I allow residuals equivalent to 1 to 2 hours of feedings if there are no other symptoms (*e.g.*, gastric distention, vomiting).

Transpyloric tubes have had their ups and downs in frequency of use, complications, and efficacy. Although better growth in premature infants has been reported, impaired assimilation of fat and potassium and increased bacterial contamination of the jejunum have been documented.[95–97] A few cases of duodenal and jejunal perforations, midgut volvulus, and necrotizing enterocolitis have occurred.

After using any tube feedings, oral feedings by nipple or breast-feeding should be instituted as soon as possible. Full-term infants who never suckle feedings during their first 2 months or preterm infants after 3 to 5 months may fail to learn to suck, become difficult feeders, and later fail to thrive. This is particularly true if there are other chronic problems. Tube-fed infants should be held and cuddled if their conditions permit. Non-nutritive sucking during tube feedings should be encouraged, because it accelerates maturation of the sucking reflex, decreases intestinal transit time, and causes a more rapid weight gain with decreased hospital stay.[98,99] Widström and colleagues reported better bowel motility, lower somatostatin levels, and increased gastric secretion. Stimulation of gastric function and facilitation of digestion may explain faster weight gain.[100]

GASTROSTOMY FEEDINGS

The use of a gastrostomy, first suggested in 1837, was successful in 1876. Enthusiasm for this technique has waxed and waned in the last 100 years, although it is the accepted mode of therapy for surgical patients for decompression, drainage, and feeding. Gastrostomy feedings are dripped in slowly by gravity over 30 minutes, and the tubing is left open and elevated above the abdominal wall as a pop-off valve. Residuals are checked before the next feeding. Elevate the reservoir no more than 10 to 12 cm above the stomach.

A number of small, uncontrolled studies suggested use of gastrostomies in small premature infants and claimed no major complications or increased mortality.[101,102] Vengusamy and colleagues reported a controlled study of premature infants weighing 750 to 1250 g.[103] Survival was significantly higher in the control group, and infection was more frequent in the gastrostomy group at autopsy. This high incidence of infection has not been confirmed in other series. Gastrostomy has proved useful for feeding infants with chronic lung disease with severe gastroesophageal reflux. A Nissen or Thal (*i.e.*, partial wrap) procedure is usually performed at the same time.

The rate of major complications of gastrostomy in surgical and nonsurgical infants is between 2.5% and 5.8%. Complications include intraabdominal leaks with peritonitis, leaks around the tube requiring surgical closure, and bleeding. Minor complications occur at a rate of 4.3% to 10.8% and include leaks not requiring surgery, delayed closure, and displacement of tube. The mortality rates directly attributed to gastrostomy reported in old studies were between 0.4% and 4.7%.[104,105] The current incidence is probably lower.

NUTRITIONAL MONITORING

Feeding a premature infant by any method is not without hazard. After the feedings begin, it is important to watch for milk tolerance, to see that there is continued growth, to monitor nutritional status, and to prevent complications. In a small, retrospective study in my institution, my colleagues and I found that infants who had systematic, nutritional monitoring were discharged 1 week earlier at the same weight with a greater length and higher albumin (Alb) levels than those who were not monitored.[106] Every infant is monitored with nutritional charts, and suggestions from the dietitians are at the bedside. The nutrition charts are part of the infant's permanent record. Table 24-8 shows what is considered to be adequate monitoring. Growth is assessed by the usual methods of weight, length, and head circumference and by comparing the rates to norms expected for gestational age. Although normal values for skin-fold thickness and mean arm circumference are available in growing premature infants, this monitoring is not routine.

Although zinc deficiency had been found in preterm infants after a 6 to 8 weeks of TPN and oral feeding, zinc levels are no longer routinely monitored because of higher levels now provided by both methods.[107] It is appropriate to measure zinc levels in infants with poor growth or extra losses through an ileostomy.

It is not unusual for an infant weighing less than 1500 g to have elevated alkaline phosphatase and lowered phosphorus levels. Hypomineralization of bones has been shown in LBW infants fed unfortified breast milk and continues to 25 weeks of age.[108] Fortification of formulas with extra calcium and phosphorus and of breast milk with fortifiers improves ossification and mineral retention.[109–111] However,

TABLE 24–8
NUTRITIONAL MONITORING IN PREMATURE INFANTS ON ENTERAL FEEDS

Tolerance		Status	
Parameter	Interval Measured	Parameter	Interval Measured
Stools		Anthropometric	
Reducing substances	Each stool	Weight	Daily
Hematest	Each stool	Height	Weekly
Consistency	Each stool	Head circumference	Weekly
Abdominal girth	Daily or as needed	Protein, calorie intake	Daily
Gastric residuals	Each feeding	Laboratory	
Vomiting	Each feeding	Prealbumin	Weekly (>1000 g)
		Albumin	Monthly
		Calcium, phosphorus	Weekly
		Alkaline phosphatase	Weekly
		Vitamins E, A	Weekly if abnormal, then biweekly

the amounts of calcium and phosphorus used in various studies and other confounding variables known to alter absorption and use have made it difficult to know exactly how much to add. Giles and colleagues showed that calcium best approached intrauterine accretion rates at an intake of 124.5 mg/dL/day. Phosphorus was absorbed well, regardless of calcium intake, although retention improved with increased calcium intakes.[112] Addition of calcium alone leads to hypercalciuria and excess fat excretion, and supplementation of phosphorus alone corrects hypophosphatemia but does not produce normal bone growth.[113] The physician must be aware of imposing excessive intake and its subsequent risks without adequate monitoring. Awareness of intake includes the effects of drug usage such as furosemide in infants with BPD, who show moderate hypercalciuria.[114] Gross has shown that normal, healthy preterm infants weighing less than 1600 g may not need any calcium or phosphorus supplementation.[115] In sick infants and those on soy formulas, the physician must still guard against rickets resulting from inadequate intake of phosphorus, vitamin D, and calcium.[116–119] Breast-fed infants of vegetarian mothers who have a high soy intake may also be vitamin D deficient.

By following serum prealbumin and Alb, the physician can monitor visceral protein status. Occasionally, in infants weighing less than 1000 g in the second week of life, serum Alb may fall low enough to cause edema followed by ascites, generalized anasarca, and renal failure. In these severe cases, I recommend infusing salt-poor 5% Alb (1 g/kg over 24 hours) until the Alb level is slightly greater than 2 g/dL. Infusion above this level is probably not helpful.

QUALITY OF GROWTH

Ideal standards of growth for premature infants are still controversial. Should one attempt to duplicate intrauterine growth? Is catch-up growth desirable? Is bigger better? Only in the past 10 to 12 years have there been attempts to examine nutrient accretion or quality of growth with different types of feedings. Reichman and others showed that formula-fed infants were able to gain weight at a rate comparable to that demonstrated by fetuses, retained protein appropriately, but accumulated fat at about three times the normal rate.[78] With mother's milk, accretion rates of fat and protein and growth rates were similar to those demonstrated by fetuses.[79] Logic dictates that it is better not to be small for gestational age by the time the infant reaches 40 weeks of gestation.

TOTAL PARENTERAL NUTRITION

The concept of TPN in infants is relatively new, although the giving of wines and oils by vein dates back to the mid-1660s.[120] The first serious attempts to give nutrition by vein, but without positive nitrogen balance, were undertaken by the Japanese in the 1920s with emulsified oils. In 1944, the first intravenous feeding of a complete diet in a 5-month-old patient with Hirschsprung disease was reported, with maintenance of the infant's weight.[121] The science of giving total calories and all essential nutrients by vein is at the point where sustained weight gain is possible for long periods.

TECHNIQUE

In 1968, Wilmore and Dudrick first described an aseptic technique for insertion of a Silastic catheter into the external or internal jugular vein.[122] Since that time, several different catheters and sites have been described. Perhaps the most commonly used catheters for central parenteral nutrition are the single-lumen Silastic Broviac or Hickman catheters. They have four features that enhance their usefulness:

1. The portion of the catheter extending from the patient and the Luer adapter piece have an outer coat of Silastic that decreases kinking.
2. The adapter piece of the catheter has a Luer lock connector that enables snug insertion of the intravenous tubing.
3. A Dacron sheath attached to the midpoint of the catheter that is placed subcutaneously stimulates fibrous adhesions that anchor the catheter securely.
4. The catheter is constructed so that it can be repaired easily.

These features lessen the incidence of catheter-related infection and dislodgement.[123] Double- and triple-lumen catheters allow administration of medications and parenteral nutrition through the same line but are not widely used in infants. Their size makes use in the very small premature infant questionable, and an increased incidence of infections has been reported. Percutaneously placed central catheters permit a central line without surgery; their complication rates appear to be no different from surgically placed lines.

Through a centrally placed catheter, hypertonic solutions may be slowly infused by pump. They are rapidly diluted, preventing sclerosis of veins and marked changes in blood sugar and serum osmolarity. To maintain its integrity, it is advisable not to use a single-lumen catheter to draw blood or to administer blood or medications; if it is necessary, use only with strict aseptic technique. External tubing should be changed daily. With good technique, a surgically placed catheter can remain in place for months.

Several studies looked at the use of the umbilical artery catheter (UAC) for infusion of parenteral nutrition and compared this with enteral feeds or tunneled jugular catheters.[124–127] All researchers found no difference in short-term comparisons between the two methods, except for Yu and colleagues,[125] who found fewer cases of necrotizing enterocolitis and better weight gain in the TPN group, and Hall and Rhodes,[126] who may have had more mortality in their arterial catheter group. Although Merritt and others caution against the use of UACs, I have used them on a short-term basis while blood gases are needed for management of respiratory distress and have had no major problems.[128–131] Better methods of TPN delivery need to be found.

INDICATIONS

Total parenteral nutrition is only indicated in infants whose bowel cannot be used by means of nasogastric or nasojejunal feeds for specific lengths of time or to augment insufficient enteric feeds. It is not indicated in the infant who is dying. Besides the specific indications listed here, I have felt it important to begin TPN if the infant will be receiving nothing orally for at least 2 to 3 days. This may result occasionally in a short, perhaps unnecessary, course.

There are definite indications for parenteral nutrition in infants:

- Surgical lesions
  - Omphalocele
  - Gastroschisis
  - Intestinal atresia with or without complicated anastomoses
  - Diaphragmatic hernias
  - Short bowel syndrome
  - Other abnormalities, including volvulus and Hirschsprung disease
  - Necrotizing enterocolitis
- Intractable, nonspecific diarrhea
- Infants on extracorporeal membrane oxygenation
- Premature infants in whom feedings not tolerated or in conjunction with increasing oral calories
- Chronically ill infants in whom feedings are not tolerated.

Total parenteral nutrition has reversed the high mortality rate from omphalocele, gastroschisis, and other severe surgical problems, for which oral feedings previously were delayed for as long as 4 to 5 weeks. Intensive care of premature infants has permitted survival of shocky, moribund babies, but among this group, an increased incidence of necrotizing enterocolitis has been observed. Oral feedings are not tolerated for 1 to 3 weeks, and TPN has often made the difference between life and death while the bowel heals.

Parenteral nutrition and prolonged catheterization have their complications, and the technique should be used only if ultimate survival of the child is expected and malnutrition would jeopardize recovery. Peripheral intravenous techniques alleviate some of the difficulties of central venous catheters, but they may also limit caloric intake because less concentrated solutions are tolerated and intravenous lines are more difficult to maintain.

INGREDIENTS AND REQUIREMENTS

Solutions for TPN may be tailored for each infant's specific requirements, or stock solutions can be used; both are successful. My colleagues and I prefer tailored preparations and think that their metabolic complications are fewer. No matter how they are made, laminar flow hoods should be used in their preparation, because these solutions readily support the growth of bacteria and fungi. Approximate total daily requirements are listed in Table 24-9.

PROTEIN

Protein deficiency in humans is known to produce poor growth, delayed wound healing, and generalized weakness. Exact intravenous requirements of amino acids are unknown. Kashyap found that infants weighing less than 1000 g lost more than 1% of endogenous protein on a daily basis if only glucose at 30 kcal/kg/day was given, a finding that provides impetus for giving early protein and calories.[132] When infants were given as little as 60 kcal/kg/day, but including 2.5 g/kg/day of amino acids, a positive nitrogen balance was achieved.[133] Zlotkin found that when energy intakes of greater than 70 kcal/kg/day were given to preterm infants, the major determinant of nitrogen retention was nitrogen intake. Protein intakes of 2.7 to 3.5 g/kg/day simulated fetal nitrogen accretion rates.[134] In full-term infants undergoing surgery, protein intakes of 2.3 to 2.7 g/kg/day with sufficient energy duplicated weight gain, and nitrogen retention observed in healthy infants fed human milk.[135] I have observed a marked decrease in serum Alb and prealbumins after surgery in full-term and preterm infants. The requirements may be higher, particularly in preterm infants. Daily parenteral in-

TABLE 24–9
DAILY REQUIREMENTS OF TOTAL PARENTERAL NUTRITION

Nutrient	Requirement
Protein	2.5–3.5 g/kg
Fat emulsion	2–4 g/kg (max 3 g/kg in infants < 2.5 kg)
Calories	90–110 kcal/kg
H_2O	125–150 mL/kg or as needed
Na	3–4 mEq/kg
K	2–3 mEq/kg
Ca	50–100 mg/kg, depending on size of infant
P	1–1.5 mM/kg
Mg	0.5–1 mEq/kg
Multivitamins (*e.g.*, MVI Pediatric)	10 mL (40%/kg/day)

takes of protein in amounts of 2.5 to 3.5 g/kg/day seem to prevent complications of protein overload and allow adequate growth if combined with sufficient energy.

The commercial parenteral amino acid solutions are not really ideal for the full-term or preterm newborn. The pediatric solutions introduced in the mid-1980s have improved choices with the addition of the semiessential amino acids taurine, water-soluble tyrosine, and L-cysteine available as an additive, along with the lowering of methionine, glycine, and phenylalanine. Wu showed that the use of Trophamine normalized blood amino acid levels to equal those of healthy full-term infants 2 hours after breast-feeding.[136] Helms and colleagues compared Trophamine with an adult solution in preterm infants requiring surgery and found significantly greater weight gain and nitrogen retention in the Trophamine group.[137] Helms also compared Trophamine with Aminosyn PF, another pediatric formulation, and found Trophamine to be superior in nitrogen balance.[138] However, a larger, multicentered trial comparing the two solutions showed similar nitrogen retention and weight gain.[139]

All pediatric protein solutions are not identical. Trophamine is higher in essential amino acids and in the proportion of branched-chain amino acids. When the nutrition group at Children's National Medical Center changed from Aminosyn to Trophamine in 1984, we compared total and direct bilirubin levels at 1 and 2 months of TPN in infants who had not been fed. Fifteen of 19 infants on Aminosyn had elevated direct bilirubin levels, but only 2 of 15 infants on Trophamine had elevated levels. The mean total–direct ratio of bilirubin at 2 months in the Aminosyn group was 7.8:3.6 mg/dL in 16 of the 17 patients still receiving nothing orally; in 7 of these infants in the Trophamine group it was 2.0:0.82 mg/dL, except for 2 infants with fungal sepsis and transiently elevated direct bilirubin levels. Mauer reviewed the charts of 100 patients on TPN with Trophamine for longer than 14 days and found no infants with elevated direct bilirubin.[140] Heird and associates studied 40 infants and children on Trophamine TPN for 5 to 21 days and found that, in contrast to the expected incidence of cholestasis of 30% to 50%, that mean after-study bilirubin levels were no different from those before the study. They thought that normalizing plasma amino acids or providing taurine may decrease the incidence of cholestasis.[141] Institutions should continue to study and monitor their infants for the solution that may be best for them. Table 24-10 compares some commonly used adult and pediatric solutions. For information regarding specialized solutions such as HepatAmine, BranchAmine, NephrAmine, and others, refer to the *American Hospital Formulary Service*.[141a] There is no convincing evidence that any of these formulas is preferable to more commonly used solutions in the neonate.

As with oral feedings, at least 25 nonprotein calories are needed for each gram of protein added to the solution. Complications of acidosis, azotemia, and hyperammonemia have markedly decreased with the pediatric solutions compared with the previously used adult amino acid solutions and protein hydrolysates.

A few amino acids merit special comment, particularly in regard to the extra requirements of stressed preterm infants. They are considered semiessential or necessary in greater quantity.

Cysteine was thought to be an essential amino acid for premature infants but was not available until the past few years because of its instability in parenteral nutrition fluids.[142] Although cysteine does not appear to affect growth or nitrogen balance, a more stable form now may be used in TPN solutions to improve the solubility of more calcium and phosphorus necessary for VLBW infants by increasing the acidity of the solution.[143]

Glutamine is a prevalent, free amino acid in plasma and intracellular pools. It is synthesized from glutamate and ammonia by glutamine synthetase with contribution from alanine pools. Glutamine is not in TPN amino acid solutions, because it previously had been classified as nutritionally nonessential. It has now been shown, principally in animal studies, that glutamine may have great importance for maintenance and growth of the intestinal villous surface with prevention of atrophy and may also improve intestinal immune function. L-Glutamine given to healthy adults orally and parenterally increases blood levels. It has been well tolerated and seems to have no toxic effect.[144] An excellent review of glutamine was provided in the proceedings of an International Glutamine Symposium.[145]

Taurine is a β-amino-sulfonic acid synthesized from cysteine that is abundantly available in its free form; it is not incorporated into proteins. Taurine is present in good quantities in human milk and has now been added to most formulas and pediatric amino acid solutions. Although it has been shown that severe retinal changes and blindness occur in cats fed a taurine-deficient diet, no real deficits have been shown in infants despite the fact they have low taurine levels.[146] Guertin and colleagues reported that guinea pigs given TPN without taurine had less bile flow and increased 7-ketolithocholate bile acid production, which can be toxic to the liver. Adding taurine reversed the process with an increase of taurine-conjugated bile acids.[147] The addition of taurine to TPN may be what has decreased cholestasis clinically. Tyson showed that orally supplemented preterm infants had higher taurine levels and more mature auditory evoked responses at 37 weeks of corrected age.[148]

CARBOHYDRATE

Glucose is the source of carbohydrate most commonly used in parenteral solutions. Although there are no stated requirements, small premature infants have relatively large needs because of their high

TABLE 24–10
COMPARISON OF COMMONLY USED AMINO ACID 10% SOLUTIONS

Solution Characteristics*	Aminosyn 11	Freamine 111	Travasol	Aminosyn PF	Trophamine†
Manufacturer	Abbot	McGraw	Clintec	Abbott	McGraw
Available solutions (%)	7, 8.5, 10	3, 6.9, 8.5, 10	5.5, 8.5, 10	7, 10	6, 10
Nitrogen (g/100 mL)	1.53	1.53	1.65	1.52	1.55
Total essential amino acids (mg/100 mL)	4580	4910	4530	4921	5740
Total nonessential amino acids (mg/100 mL)	5471	4770	5470	5008	4236
Total essential–total amino acid ratio (%)	45.6	50.7	45.3	49.6	52.3
Branched chain–total essential amino acid ratio (%)	47.2	46	42.2	36.6	57.5
Other components	No cysteine‡	Cysteine‡ < 20 mg/100 mL; no tyrosine, glutamic acid, or aspartic acid	No cysteine‡ glutamic acid, or aspartic acid	No cysteine‡ low tyrosine; contains taurine 70 mg/100 mL	Cysteine‡ < 16 mg/100 mL; contains taurine 250 mg/100 mL
*p*H	5–6.5	6.5	6	5.4	5.5
mOsm/L	873	950	1000	829	875

* Data partially taken from the American Hospital Formulary Service and published by authority of the Board of Directors of the American Society of Hospital Pharmacists; most solutions have some electrolyte supplementation.
† Pediatric formulations.
‡ Cysteine may be added to all preparations.

brain–liver weight ratios, but only limited quantities are tolerated.[149] Full-term newborn and older infants handle up to 14 mg/kg/minute without significant glucosuria, but all premature infants develop hyperglycemia and glucosuria with this same amount.[150] Amino acids given with glucose seem to decrease hyperglycemia, perhaps by increasing insulin secretion.

Other sources of carbohydrate include fructose, which is infrequently used but does not require or stimulate insulin secretion. It is relatively expensive and not as readily available. Galactose in conjunction with glucose has been used in small numbers of hyperglycemic LBW infants with subsequent normoglycemia, without signs of toxicity.[151] However, no attempt was made in the studies to achieve sustained growth with glucose–galactose mixtures.

Ethyl alcohol, 3 to 5 g/kg/day, has been used as a supplementary caloric source because it provides 7 kcal/g when metabolized. At this intake, liver functions have remained essentially normal in full-term infants, although elevated alcohol levels have been found in premature infants, even with low intake. Alcohol and amino acids are not sufficient for maintenance of positive nitrogen balance unless some other carbohydrate source is provided.

In my experience, virtually all infants weighing less than 800 g become hyperglycemic as full calories are approached between days 5 and 7, as do 40% of infants weighing between 800 and 1000 g. This happens despite the fact that glucose intake is carefully calculated and slowly increased. If glucose intake is decreased enough to reverse hyperglycemia, there is inadequate caloric intake. Hyperglycemia has been attributed to many factors, including decreased insulin production, peripheral insulin resistance, endogenous glucose production, immature hepatic enzymes, decreased or abnormal numbers of insulin receptor sites, and stress. During the late 1970s and mid-1980s, the few investigators who used exogenous insulin met with varying success.[152–154] Insulin recently has been used in premature infants with good outcomes and has allowed more energy intake.[155–157] Some clinicians question its use, and practice varies throughout the United States.[158]

My practice is to start glucose infusion at 6.5 mg/kg/minute and to increase by 2 mg/kg/day to lessen the incidence of hyperglycemia. If there is hyperglycemia, I use Humulin according to a sliding scale (Table 24-11). The first solution is used initially as the infant becomes hyperglycemic, and the second is used to facilitate weaning as hyperglycemia abates. Insulin is not used in infants with sepsis or shock. Some infants are more responsive to insulin than others, but few have had wide swings in their blood glucose levels. With this regimen, I have been able to give 85 to 90 kcal/kg/day by day 7 to 8 of feeding to these small, unstable infants.

FAT EMULSIONS AND ESSENTIAL FATTY ACIDS

Indications

Many oils have been employed to provide calories with various rates of success. The first attempt with some success in the United States was by L. Emmett Holt and associates in 1935. In the mid-1950s, Upjohn introduced Lipomul, the first commercially prepared fat emulsion. This preparation produced many problems, including a high percentage of febrile reactions and the overload syndrome, and it was removed from the market. In 1960, the Swedish soybean oil–egg emulsion called Intralipid was introduced and has been used widely and with great success in Europe, Canada, and the United States.

The syndrome of EFA deficiency includes decreased growth, scaly dermatitis, and various anatomic, degenerative, and pathophysiologic changes in many organs. The full syndrome is rare in infants on fat-free TPN, because it takes at least 6 weeks to develop, but infants develop plasma lipid changes of EFA deficiency within 1 week.[159,160]

Fat emulsions have added greatly to the efficiency of intravenous nutrition, and the advantages include the ability to give large amounts of energy in a small, isotonic volume; to give EFA; and to give less hypertonic solutions by a peripheral route, prolonging the viability of peripheral venous access.[161] There are several 10% and 20% fat emulsions on the market, of which Intralipid and the multiple Liposyn preparations are probably most widely used. Their contents and others are shown in Table 24-12. Although long-term studies in animals have not shown profound differences in tolerance of the various emulsions, the substances are somewhat different. For instance, if the physician believes that the ratio of linoleic acid to linolenic acid should ideally be 5:1, but no more than 15:1, Liposyn without linolenic acid may have too much linoleic acid in it. Liposyn II and III contain linolenic acid and are thought to be more comparable to Intralipid, as are other products. Because I have only used Intralipid, most of this discussion concerns the use of this product.

Term infants usually tolerate up to 4 g/kg/day of lipid emulsion. Infants younger than 32 weeks of gestation usually require lower intakes to avoid hyperlipemia. There are two conflicting studies that examined the effects of giving lipid to the LBW infant in the first 5 to 8 days. Hammerman compared two groups of infants weighing less than 1750 g (average weight, 1126 g). Group I was begun on TPN plus lipids as Vamin on day 3 of life. The fat emulsion was increased to 2.5 g/kg/day by day 5. Group II received TPN without Vamin for the first 5 days. Group I required ventilatory support for a mean of 37 days, and group II needed only 21 days. Supplemental oxygen was needed for 51 days and 28 in the two groups, respectively. There was a significant difference in the number of infants who received lipids who had stage III BPD and the need for going home in oxygen.[162] Gilbertson and associates studied two groups of infants weighing less than 1500 g. Intralipid was started at 1 g/kg/day on day 1 and increased to 3 g/kg/day by day 4 in the first group, but the second group did not receive Intralipid until after 8 days of age. There were no differences in the occurrence of adverse clinical events such as BPD, although time on ventilation and in oxygen were not reported. The patients who did not receive Intralipid for the first 8 days lost more weight.[163] More data are needed to determine when to start lipids in the VLBW infant. With proper monitoring, giving some lipid early seems reasonable.

TABLE 24–11
SLIDING SCALE FOR INSULIN ADMINISTRATION

Factors Affecting Dose	Solution 1 Initiating Dose (25 U in 50 mL)	Solution 2 Weaning Dose (12.5 U in 50 mL)
Insulin Concentration		
U/mL	0.5	0.25
U/0.1 mL	0.05	0.025
Blood Sugar		
< 150 mg/dL	0	0
150–200 mg/dL	0.1 mL/h	0.2 mL/h
200–250 mg/dL*	0.2 mL/h	0.4 mL/h

* If blood sugar is >250 mg/dL, give more insulin or decrease the glucose concentration.

TABLE 24–12
AVAILABLE FAT EMULSIONS

Preparation Characteristics	Intralipid	Liposyn II	Liposyn III	Nutrilipid
Manufacturer	Clintec	Abbott	Abbott	McGraw
Solutions available (%)	10, 20	10, 20	10, 20	10, 20
Fat source	Soybean	Safflower	Soybean	Soybean
Fatty acids				
Linoleic (%)	50	65.8	54.5	49–60
Linoleic–linolenic ratio	5.5	15.6	6.6	8.2–6.7
Linolenic (%)	9	4.2	8.3	6–9
Oleic (%)	26	17.7	22.4	21–26
Palmitic (%)	10	8.8	10.5	9–13
Stearic (%)	3.5	3.4	4.2	3–5
Egg phosphatides (g/100 mL)	1.2	1.2	1.2	1.2
Glycerol (g/100 mL)	2.25	2.5	2.5	2.21
*p*H	6–8.9	6–9	6–9	6–7.9
Calories (10–20%)/mL	1.1–2	1.1–2	1.1–2	1.1–2
mOsm/L	260	276	292	280–315

Intercurrent illness such as sepsis may cause hypertriglyceridemia in any infant who has previously tolerated fat. Elevated triglycerides have occurred with the use of steroids and aminophylline in chronically ill infants and in infants on long-term TPN, perhaps due to lack of carnitine.[164] Dahlström and others, although finding low blood and plasma carnitine levels in children receiving long-term TPN, found no increase in triglyceride levels.[165] Enhanced lipid use was observed in infants receiving L-carnitine during long-term parenteral nutrition, as evidenced by increased ketogenesis; there were no differences in triglyceride levels.[166] Carnitine-supplemented fat emulsion increased net retention of carnitine, suggesting its essential nature.[167] However, enhanced growth has not been shown by adding L-carnitine, and it is not commonly used.

Fat emulsions may be added to the nutritional support after significant early hyperbilirubinemia has resolved and if it is apparent that enteral nutrition will be delayed. Initial test doses are unnecessary. Infusion may be started at 0.5 g/kg/day and increased on successive days as clearance allows to 3 to 4 g/kg/day. At no time should more than 60% of calories be given as fat. If only EFA are needed, 0.5 to 1 g/kg/day (2%–4% of total calories) should be given.

Fat emulsions should be infused over 16 to 24 hours to allow metabolic clearing and should be run separately from any other intravenous solution so that the stability of the emulsion is not disturbed. It may be run through the same line near the infusion site by means of a Y-connector, but it should never be filtered. It appears that the mixing of emulsions and the amino acid plus glucose solution is safe, but the combination makes precipitates and other particles difficult to see.

In the last few years, mixtures of MCT and long-chain triglycerides have been tried in neonates. One study showed higher cholesterol levels with pure long-chain triglycerides emulsions.[168] Another showed higher triglyceride and fatty acid levels.[169] Additional studies are needed before these products are available.

Complications

Hyperlipidemia. Elevation of triglycerides and free fatty acids (FFAs) occurs if an infant's ability to metabolize fat is exceeded. This may be due to developmental insufficiency of lipoprotein lipase or its activator. Monitoring of triglyceride levels is important; measurement of FFAs also is possible but takes longer. Serum cholesterol rises because of infusion and because of endogenous production. It should be monitored periodically.

Displacement of Albumin-Bound Bilirubin by Free Fatty Acids. Intralipid itself has little negative effect on bilirubin binding to Alb. It is the FFAs, generated during hydrolysis of triglycerides, that compete for Alb. *In vivo* and *in vitro* studies indicate no negative effect on binding if the molar ratio of FFA to Alb is less than 6.[170] A study of infants weighing between 670 and 3630 g and given a fat emulsion in increasing amounts showed that the FFA–Alb ratios were usually less than 1, but always less than 3. The mean bilirubin levels were 5.8 mg/dL. The researchers stress that monitoring is essential because triglyceride levels are quite variable.[171] Even though FFA–Alb ratios are difficult to measure, the data suggest that what is generally given is in the safe range. There are also no reports indicating a higher incidence of kernicterus in infants given fat emulsions. In practice, the need to give nutritional support predominates unless bilirubin is near an exchange level and provided triglyceride levels are low.

Effects on Pulmonary Function. Arterial PO_2 values have been shown to decrease minimally during the first week of life when 1 g/kg of Intralipid was infused over 4 to 6 hours. This dose compares to 4 to 6 g/kg/day of Intralipid, which is higher than that usually given to premature infants. This drop in PO_2 may be due to changes in erythrocyte membrane structure or coating of the erythrocytes with lipid. Pulmonary blood flow can be reduced, possibly related to deposition of lipid in arterioles and capillaries or to release of prostaglandins. Fat embolism has occurred if rates of infusion were too high. The magnitude of the pulmonary problem is unknown, and unless further evidence becomes available, it can be stated that Intralipid probably enhances the survival of infants through better growth.

Decreased Reticuloendothelial Function. Chylomicrons are taken up by the reticuloendothelial system of the liver, lung, and other organs and, in theory, can interfere with fighting infection, particularly in an immunocompromised infant. Fat emulsions are good media for the growth of organisms, particularly fungi. However, their use is better than the alternatives of glucose overload or malnutrition.

Other Effects and Complications. Hepatic dysfunction, although observed with Intralipid, was seen in parenteral nutrition before its use. Thrombocytopenia has disappeared after fat administration; the significance of occasional eosinophilia is unknown.

Rarely, an infant may not tolerate intravenous fats, in which case, cutaneous application of sunflower seed oil may correct EFA deficiency.[172] Because this procedure is not uniformly effective, absorption must be documented by measurements of EFAs.[173] In certain infants, small amounts of oils sufficient to provide EFAs may be tolerated orally and absorbed even when other nutrients are not and must be given parenterally.

ELECTROLYTES, MINERALS, AND VITAMINS

Table 24-9 lists approximate estimates of electrolytes that are needed by premature infants, provided that there are no excessive losses for other reasons. Monitoring serum electrolytes helps prevent serious deficiencies.

Macrominerals. In managing TPN, the addition of calcium and phosphorus are the most difficult, mainly because of the high daily requirements, particularly in the VLBW infant. Calcium and phosphorus solubility is based on acidity of the solution, the percent protein solution, the ambient temperature, length of storage, and the order of calcium and phosphorus addition.[174] A ratio of these elements at 1.7:1 appears to give the best retention of both.[175] Acidity can be affected by the type of amino acid solution. Fortunately, Trophamine, although not quite as acidic as Aminosyn, has a low *p*H.[176] It can be further acidified by adding L-cysteine. L-Cysteine is usually added at a rate of 40 mg/g of protein; its use has resulted in cost containment by preventing precipitation.[177] The addition of phosphorus before calcium allows more of both to be added.[178,179] Calcium is often begun in TPN before the addition of phosphorus, and it can cause phosphaturia followed by hypercalcemia.[180] Although small amounts of calcium may be necessary in early TPN, serum phosphorus levels should be monitored and phosphorus added as soon as possible. To give larger quantities of calcium and phosphorus to premature infants, alternate infusion of each element has been tried. One study showed loss of the infused mineral and poor retention of both.[181] Another showed hypercalcemia after calcium was given and hyperphosphatemia after phosphorus was infused.[182] Giving both together is best for bone mineralization and can be accomplished with current solutions unless fluids or protein are restricted for some reason. The use of different calcium or phosphorus or monobasic phosphorus salts for increased solubility may allow more intake.[183–185] In piglets, calcium glycerophosphate was shown to give better retention than if usual salts were used.[186]

Overt rickets, once seen with some frequency, is now rarely observed, although osteopenia is still relatively common with a mild or moderate elevation of alkaline phosphatase. This is particularly true after prolonged TPN.

Knowledge of trace essential elements is increasing, and deficiencies of zinc, copper, and selenium have been described.[106,187–189] Potential deficiencies of chromium, manganese, and iodine are less well defined. Trace elements are now routinely added to TPN solutions. The report of the Subcommittee on Pediatric Parenteral Nutrient Requirements from the Committee on Clinical Practice Issues of The American Society for Clinical Nutrition has set guidelines for requirements for six trace elements (Table 24-13).[190] Selenium is generally added after 2 weeks of TPN, and iodine is added after 6 weeks. Thyroid studies should be performed before addition of iodine.

Vitamins. Vitamins play an extremely important role in bone metabolism, development of the eye, maintenance of erythrocytes, blood coagulation, and fat, carbohydrate, and protein metabolism. In 1981, a reasonably good pediatric vitamin preparation (*i.e.*, MVI Pediatric) was approved for use in infants and children younger than 11 years of age. This formulation was the result of the Nutrition Advisory Group of the Department of Food and Nutrition of the American Medical Association (AMA), which published their guidelines in 1975. In 1986, a subcommittee from the American Society for Clinical Nutrition

TABLE 24–13
SUGGESTED DAILY INTRAVENOUS INTAKE OF ESSENTIAL TRACE ELEMENTS

Element	Daily Intake
Zinc	
Premature	400 μg/kg
Full-term, <3 mo	250 μg/kg
Full-term, >3 mo	100 μg/kg
Copper*	20 μg/kg
Chromium†	0.20 μg/kg
Manganese*	1 μg/kg
Selenium†	2 μg/kg after 2 wk of parenteral nutrition
Iodine	1 μg/kg after 6 wk of parenteral nutrition; check thyroid function
Molybdenum†	0.25 μg/kg

* If evidence of liver damage appears, delete copper and manganese from total parenteral nutrition.
† Omit in patients with renal dysfunction.
Adapted from Greene HL, Hambidge KM, Schanler R, Tsang RC. Guidelines for the use of vitamins, trace elements, calcium, magnesium, and phosphorus in infants and children receiving total parenteral nutrition: report of the Subcommittee on Pediatric Parenteral Nutrient Requirements from the Committee on Clinical Practice Issues of the American Society for Clinical Nutrition. Am J Clin Nutr 1988;48:1324.

reviewed available data on the preparation to see if new guidelines should be given.[190] They made the following recommendations.

Guidelines set by the AMA 1975 report were adequate for short-term and long-term TPN, although the pediatric preparation had only been tested in medically stable infants and children.

Current data in preterm infants indicate that all vitamin levels are not maintained in an acceptable range. There is a need for a preterm supplementation.

Manufacturers are encouraged to develop a new formulation that separates water- and fat-soluble vitamins, and the latter should be available without the addition of emulsifiers, such as polysorbate.

Water- and fat-soluble vitamins should be tested in an intensive care setting to determine the most appropriate way of giving them, their bioavailability, and their possible photodegradation.[190]

Current recommendations are to give 40%/kg/day of the 10-mL vial of MVI Pediatric. The maximal dose is 1 vial.

Giving MVI Pediatric in the lipid emulsion has been tried with the hope of increasing delivery of vitamin A in particular. Plasma levels of vitamins A and D increased slightly over time, but unfortunately riboflavin levels increased 20 to 100 times the initial value. There were, however, no signs of toxicity.[191] Whether the emulsion protected against photodegradation is unknown. Because of fixed formulation, decreasing riboflavin would decrease the intake of the fat-soluble vitamins.

MANAGEMENT OF THE PATIENT

Fluids are initiated with intravenous glucose and small amounts of calcium. By day 2 or 3, glucose intake is at least at 6.5 mg/kg/minute in preterm infants and between 8 and 10 mg/kg/minute in full-term infants. In small infants, the aim has been to achieve a caloric intake of 55 to 60 kcal/kg/day by day 3, 70 to 75 kcal/kg/day by day 5, and 85 to 90 kcal/kg/day by day 7. Larger infants may tolerate a more rapid increase. After enough nonprotein calories (25–30 cal/g of protein) are being given, 0.5 to 1 g/kg of protein is started and increased gradually to full requirements. Protein should be started as early as possible. Intralipid is usually begun between 4 and 5 days. If hyperbilirubinemia persists, 0.5 g/kg of fat can be given for EFAs, and triglycerides should be monitored carefully. If triglycerides remain low (<50 mg/dL), fat may be increased slowly despite hyperbilirubinemia.

Monitoring for efficacy and potential toxicity is mandatory while administering TPN. The schedule presented in Table 24-14 is thought to be adequate and has been suggested with consideration of blood sampling in small infants. Increased surveillance of these parameters is indicated if abnormalities or symptoms are apparent. After the infant's TPN has been stabilized, an increase in serum glucose or triglycerides suggests that infection may be present. A central catheter need not be removed as soon as sepsis is suspected because there usually is time for evaluation of catheter sepsis during treatment. Paired quantitative Broviac and peripheral blood cultures may help delineate the problem.[192,193] Studies of children and infants have shown that sepsis may be treated with the catheter left in place.[194–196] Nahata and others found that catheter sepsis could be managed with appropriate antibiotics and suggested a trial should be given before removal.[196] Aschner and colleagues reported 64% colonization with *Malassezia furfur* in their hospitalized infants. These infants were usually older and of lower gestational age.[197] When *M. furfur* is cultured, fat emulsions should be stopped, and the catheter should be removed; if there are no symptoms, the infant may not require further treatment.

Most centers use heparin in TPN solutions in the concentration of 1 U/mL to keep central lines patent and reduce the formation of a fibrin sheath around the catheter. In 1986, it was reported that infants receiving heparin at 1 u/mL had a fourfold increase in the risk of germinal matrix intraventricular hemorrhage. A biased population of infants could not be ruled out, and a controlled clinical trial was suggested.[198] At that time, the heparin in TPN was decreased to 0.5 u/mL but the catheter occlusions increased. No controlled trial has been performed.

TABLE 24–14
SUGGESTED MONITORING FOR TOTAL PARENTERAL NUTRITION

Variable	First Week	Later
Growth		
Weight	Daily	Daily
Length and head circumference	Weekly	Weekly
Chemistry		
Na, K, Cl, CO_2	Daily until stable	Twice weekly
Glucose (Chemistrip bG)	Daily	Daily
Triglycerides	With each increase in IL	Twice weekly when stable
Ca (ionized Ca is most accurate)	Daily till stable	Weekly
P	Initially	Twice weekly for first week, then weekly
Albumin	Initially	Monthly
Prealbumin	Initially	Weekly (biweekly) in infants <1000 g
Alkaline phosphatase	Initially	Weekly
Bilirubin	Initially	Every 4 wk or PRN
Mg	Initially	Weekly
Ammonia	As needed	As needed
Gamma GT	Initially	Weekly
Alanine aminotransferase	As needed	Monthly
Amino acids	As needed	As needed
Zinc		Monthly
Serum osmolarity	Initially	Weekly
Vitamin A (if infant is <1300 g)	Weekly	Weekly while supplemented
Hematology		
Complete blood count	Initially	At least weekly
Type and screen	Initially	
Urinalysis		
Sugar	Each void	Each shift
Protein	Each void	Each shift
Specific gravity	Each void	Each shift

The use of heparin has possible benefits. One study of heparin use in adults showed a reduction of catheter-associated sepsis with low-dose heparin.[199] It is unknown whether the same effect occurs in infants. Heparin can lower triglyceride levels in preterm neonates but may only increase lipolysis, perhaps exceeding the capacity of the preterm to dispose of FFAs.[200,201]

Infants placed on TPN usually require it totally or partially for at least 2 to 3 weeks. Surgical infants with gastroschisis or omphalocele may require even longer periods of TPN. Even in very small infants, as long as the bowel is intact, minimal feeds should still be considered. Bowel function can be judged by the presence of bowel sounds, absence of distention, absence of bile stained residuals, and stooling. Usually passage of stools continues despite taking nothing orally because of normal intestinal secretions and sloughing of cells.

REFEEDING INFANTS

Refeeding an infant must progress with caution and depends on the initial reason for stopping feedings. Most infants can be started on half-strength, low-concentration regular formula or half-strength breast milk. Concentration and volume are increased slowly but not simultaneously. An infant with short gut or an ileostomy has particular difficulty in tolerating the last 25% of intake rather than the earliest feedings. It is important to continue intravenous calories until about 90% of caloric intake is enteric and the infant is gaining weight before removing central nutrition lines.

Occasionally, infants develop transient diarrhea during refeeding advances. Reducing concentration, decreasing volume, or interrupting feeding for a short period usually suffices. Monitoring for tolerance of formula should be performed as previously discussed.

COMPLICATIONS

Complication rates attributed to TPN in the early years were reported to be as high as 68.5%, with a mortality rate of 8.4%.[202] The success of TPN depends in part on skill and experience, and it should probably be used only in centers that have requisite support. With a multidisciplinary approach, including physicians, nutritionists, nurses, and pharmacists, the morbidity rate has dropped to less than 10%, and mortality is only rarely due to TPN itself. The following lists the complications of parenteral nutrition according to origin and in decreasing order of frequency:

Catheter-Related Complications

- Central
  - Sepsis
    - Bacterial
    - Fungal
  - Local skin infections
  - Hemorrhage
  - Improper placement
  - Dislodgement, occlusion
  - Superior vena cava syndrome
  - Extravasation of fluid
  - Pleural effusion
  - Pericardial effusion
  - Chylous effusion
  - Pneumothorax
  - Intracardiac thrombi, aseptic or septic
  - Cardiac endothelial damage and perforation
  - Fat embolism
  - Air embolism
  - Nerve injury
    - Brachial plexus
    - Phrenic nerve
- Peripheral
  - Slough
  - Local infection
  - Inadequate nutrition
  - Thrombophlebitis
  - Sepsis

Metabolic Complications

- Hyperglycemia
- Glucosuria
- Hypophosphatemia
- Elevated aluminum levels
- Elevated alkaline phosphatase
- Cholestasis
- Hyperlipidemia
- Hypocalcemia
- Acidosis
- Hypokalemia
- Radiographic bone changes
  - Osteopenia
  - Rickets
- Postinfusion hypoglycemia
- Gallstones or sludge
- Trace element deficiency
- Hepatic damage
  - Cirrhosis
  - Hepatoblastoma
- Abnormal aminograms

If placement is done with good technique and location of the tip is correct, catheter-related complications can be minimized. Sepsis is a major problem, particularly in infants weighing less than 1000 g who remain in neonatal intensive care units for prolonged periods. Metabolic complications are reduced by monitoring, but some may have long-term residua. Catheter occlusions occur despite good care. They have been attributed to blood clots, calcium and phosphorus precipitates, or infusion of drugs without proper clearing of the line. In my institution, if no precipitate is seen, urokinase (5000 u/mL) is used to dissolve blood or fibrin clots. Urokinase (0.2–0.5 mL) is instilled into the catheter for 30 minutes and then aspirated and flushed. If patency is not reestablished or if a precipitate is seen, 0.1 N HCl (0.2–0.5 mL) is instilled for 20 minutes. If patency is not reestablished after two attempts, the catheter is removed.[203] Patients have tolerated this well, and more than one-half of the catheters can be cleared.

The aluminum content of TPN solutions cannot be controlled. Aluminum is the third most abundant mineral on the face of the earth and contaminates much of what humans eat and drink. It was first associated with disease in the 1970s, when a syndrome of osteomalacia, encephalopathy, and hemolytic anemia was described in dialyzed patients.[204] Aluminum accumulates in the bones of preterm infants, and their blood levels are higher on TPN than controls.[205,206] Calcium and phosphorus salts and certain Alb solutions appear to be the biggest contaminants.[207] Aluminum damage has been hard to prove because the osteopenia seen in premature infants on TPN is probably due to inadequate intakes of calcium and phosphorus. There is pressure to ensure that manufacturers use appropriate control procedures and employ a standard unit of aluminum measurement.[208] Despite the lifesaving effect of TPN for many infants and the fact that there have been many improvements in the safety and efficacy of current solutions, essential nutritional elements may still be missing and problems remain.

Cholestasis, which used to affect 30% to 50% of infants on TPN for longer than 3 to 4 weeks, has been markedly reduced with pediatric amino acid solutions. Although an exact cause is unknown, limited oral intake with decreased bile flow, amino acid toxicity, immaturity of bile salt secretion, and sepsis have been implicated. The most common cause now appears to be sepsis. In some infants with continuing high direct bilirubin, liver biopsies show mild changes of cholestasis with hepatocellular injury compatible with the use of TPN. In other infants, paucity of the bile ducts and Alagille syndrome have been diagnosed. Although a few patients die after long-term TPN with cirrhosis, the incidence has markedly decreased, and it is rarely seen in neonatal intensive care units.

Hyperglycemia, glucosuria, hypophosphatemia, hyperlipidemia, hypocalcemia, acidosis, hypokalemia, and bone changes can be avoided with careful monitoring.

REFERENCES

1. Barness LA. Brief history of infant nutrition and view to the future. Pediatrics 1991;88:1054.
2. Ryan AS, Rush D, Krieger FW, Lewandowski GE. Recent declines in breast-feeding in the United States, 1984 through 1989. Pediatrics 1991;88:719.
3. Cunningham AS, Jelliffe DB, Jelliffe EFP. Breast-feeding and health in the 1980's: a global epidemiologic review. J Pediatr 1991;118:659.
4. Pisacane A, Graziano L, Mazzarella G, et al. Breast-feeding and urinary tract infection. J Pediatr 1992;120:87.
5. Briggs GG, Freeman RK, Yaffe SJ. Drugs in pregnancy and lactation. Baltimore: Williams & Wilkins, 1990.
6. Belec L, Bouquety JC, Georges AJ, et al. Antibodies to human immunodeficiency virus in the breast milk of healthy, seropositive women. Pediatrics 1990;85:1022.
7. Salmenpera L, Perheentupa J, Siimes MA. Exclusively breastfed healthy infants grow slower than reference infants. Pediatr Res 1985;19:307.
8. Carver JD, Pimentel B, Cox WI, Barness LA. Dietary nucleotide effects upon immune function in infants. Pediatrics 1991;88:359.
9. Quan R, Barness LA, Uauy R. Do infants need nucleotide supplemented formula for optimal nutrition? J Pediatr Gastroenterol Nutr 1990;11:429.
10. Uauy R, Stringel G, Thomas R, Quan R. Effect of dietary nucleosides on growth and maturation of the developing gut in the rat. J Pediatr Gastroenterol Nutr 1990;10:497.
11. Quan R, Uauy R. Nucleotides and gastrointestinal development. Semin Pediatr Gastroenterol Nutr 1991;2:3.
12. Graham GG, Placko RP, Morales E, et al. Dietary protein quality in infants and children. Am J Dis Child 1970;120:419.
13. Eastham EJ, Lichauco T, Grady MI, Walker, WA. Antigenicity of infant formulas: role of immature intestine on protein permeability. J Pediatr 1978;93:561.
14. Saylor JD, Bahna SL. Anaphylaxis to casein hydrolysate formula. J Pediatr 1991;118:71.
15. Ellis MH, Short JA, Heiner DC. Anaphylaxis after ingestion of a recently introduced hydrolyzed whey protein formula. J Pediatr 1991;118:71.
16. Fomon SJ, Ziegler EE, Thomas LN, et al. Excretion of fat by normal full-term infants fed various milks and formulas. Am J Clin Nutr 1970;23:1299.
17. Fomon SJ, Filer LJ, Anderson TA, Ziegler EE. Recommendations for feeding normal infants. Pediatrics 1979;63:52.
18. Ziegler EE, Fomon SJ, Nelson SE, et al. Cow milk feeding in infancy: further observations on blood loss from the gastrointestinal tract. J Pediatr 1990;116:11.
19. Fomon SJ, Sanders KD, Ziegler EE. Formulas for older infants. J Pediatr 1990;116:690.
20. Fomon SJ. Infant nutrition. 2nd ed. Philadelphia: WB Saunders, 1974.
21. American Academy of Pediatrics, Committee on Nutrition. Iron supplementation. Pediatrics 1976;58:765.
22. Pizarro F, Yip R, Dallman PR, et al. Iron status with different infant feeding regimens: relevance to screening and prevention of iron deficiency. J Pediatr 1991;118:687.
23. Oski FA, Honig AS, Helu B, Howanitz P. Effects of iron therapy on behavior performance in non-anemic iron deficient infants. Pediatrics 1983;71:877.
24. Lozoff B, Jimenez E, Wolf AW. Long-term developmental outcome of infants with iron deficiency. N Engl J Med 1991; 325:687.
25. Oski FA. Iron-fortified formulas and gastrointestinal symptoms in infants: a controlled study. Pediatrics 1980;66:168.
26. Nelson SE, Ziegler EE, Copeland AM, et al. Lack of adverse reactions to iron-fortified formula. Pediatrics 1988;81:360.
27. Casey CE, Walravens PA. Trace elements. In: Tsang R, Nichols B, eds. Nutrition during infancy St. Louis: CV Mosby, 1988:204.
28. American Academy of Pediatrics, Committee on Nutrition. Fluoride supplementation. Pediatrics 1986;77:78.
29. Hughes CA, Dowling RH. Speed of onset of adaptive mucosal hypoplasia and hypofunction in the intestine of parenterally fed rats. Clin Sci 1980;59:317.
30. Lucas A, Bloom SR, Aynsley-Green A. Gut hormones and "minimal enteral feeding." Acta Paediatr Scand 1986;75:719.
31. Slagle TA, Gross SJ. Effect of early low-volume enteral substrate on subsequent feeding tolerance in the very low birth weight infants. J Pediatr 1988;113:526.
32. Dunn L, Hulman S, Weiner J, Kliegman R. Beneficial effects of early hypocaloric enteral feeding on neonatal gastrointestinal function: preliminary report of a randomized trial. J Pediatr 1988;112:622.
33. Meetze W, Valentine C, Sacks J, et al. Effects of gastrointestinal (GI) priming prior to full enteral nutrition in very low birth weight (VLBW) infants. [Abstract] Pediatr Res 1990;27:287A.
34. Neu J, Valentine C, Mietze W. Scientifically-based strategies for nutrition of the high-risk low birth weight infant. Eur J Pediatr 1990;150:2.
35. Calloway DH, Spector H. Nitrogen balance as related to caloric and protein intake in active young men. Am J Clin Nutr 1954;2:405.
36. Davidson M, Levine SZ, Bauer CH, Dann M. Feeding studies in low-birth-weight infants. I. Relationships of dietary protein, fat, and electrolytes to rates of weight gain, clinical courses, and serum chemical concentrations. J Pediatr 1967; 70:695.
37. Kagan BM, Stanincova V, Felix NS, et al. Body composition of premature infants: relation to nutrition. Am J Clin Nutr 1972;25:1153.
38. Goldman HI, Liebman OB, Freudenthal R, Reuben R. Effects of early dietary protein intake on low-birth-weight infants: evaluation at 3 years of age. J Pediatr 1971;78:126.
39. Kashyap S, Schulze KF, Forsyth MS, et al. Growth, nutrient retention, and metabolic response in low birth weight infants fed varying intakes of protein and energy. J Pediatr 1988; 113:713.
40. Schulze KF, Stefanski M, Masterson J, et al. Energy expenditure, energy balance and composition of weight gain in low birth weight infants fed diets of different protein and energy content. J Pediatr 1987;110:753.
41. Heird WC, Kashyap S, Gomez MR. Protein intake and Energy Requirements of the Infant. Semin Perinatol 1991;15:438.
42. Räiha NCR, Heinonen K, Rassin DK, Gaull GE. Milk protein quantity and quality in low-birth-weight infants: I. Metabolic responses and effects on growth. Pediatrics 1976;57:659.
43. Rassin DK, Gaull GE, Heinonen K, Räiha NCR. Milk protein quantity and quality in low-birth-weight infants: II. Effects on selected aliphatic amino acids in plasma and urine. Pediatrics 1977;59:407.
44. Gaull GE, Rassin DK, Räiha NCR, Heinonen K. Milk protein quantity and quality in low birthweight infants: III. Effects on sulfur amino acids in plasma and urine. J Pediatr 1977;90:348.
45. Rassin DK, Gaull GE, Räiha NCR, Heinonen K. Milk protein quantity and quality in low birthweight infants: IV. Effects on tyrosine and phenylalanine in plasma and urine. J Pediatr 1977;90:356.
46. Davies DP. Adequacy of expressed breast milk for early growth of preterm infants. Arch Dis Child 1977;52:296.
47. Atkinson SA, Bryan MH, Anderson GH. Human milk feeding

in premature infants: protein, fat and carbohydrate balances in the first two weeks of life. J Pediatr 1981;99:617.
48. Tyson JE, Lasky RE, Mize CE, et al. Growth, metabolic response, and development in very-low-birth weight infants fed banked human milk or enriched formula. I. Neonatal findings. J Pediatr 1983;103:95.
49. Schanler RJ, Oh W. Nitrogen and mineral balance in preterm infants fed human milks or formula. J Pediatr Gastroenterol Nutr 1985;4:214.
50. Gross SJ, David RJ, Bauman L, Tomarelli RM. Nutritional composition of milk produced by mothers delivering preterm. J Pediatr 1980;96:641.
51. Schanler RJ, Oh W. Composition of breast milk obtained from mothers of premature infants as compared with breast milk obtained from donors. J Pediatr 1980;96:679.
52. Feeley RM, Eitenmiller RR, Jones JB, Barnhart H. Calcium, phosphorus and magnesium contents of human milk during early lactation. J Pediatr Gastroenterol Nutr 1983;2:262.
53. Anderson DM, Williams FH, Merkatz RB, et al. Length of gestation and nutritional composition of human milk. Am J Clin Nutr 1983;37:810.
54. Long JM, Wilmore DW, Mason AD, et al. Effect of carbohydrate and fat intake on nitrogen excretion during total intravenous feeding. Ann Surg 1977;185:417.
55. Burr GO, Burr MM. A new deficiency disease produced by rigid exclusion of fat from the diet. J Biol Chem 1929;82:345.
56. Uauy R, Treen M, Hoffman DR. Essential fatty acid metabolism and requirements during development. Semin Perinatol 1989;13:118.
57. Carlson SE, Rhodes PG, Ferguson MG. Docosahexaenoic acid status of preterm infants at birth and following feeding with human milk or formula. Am J Clin Nutr 1986;44:798.
58. Uauy R, Hoffman DR. Essential fatty acid requirements for normal eye and brain development. Semin Perinatol 1991; 15:449.
59. American Academy of Pediatrics, Committee on Nutrition. Nutritional needs of low birth weight infants. Pediatrics 1985;75:976.
60. European Society of Paediatric Gastroenterology and Nutrition (ESPGAN). Nutrition and feedings of preterm infants. Acta Paediatr Scand 1987;336(Suppl):3.
61. Oski FA, Barnes LA. Vitamin E deficiency: a previously unrecognized cause of hemolytic anemia in the premature. J Pediatr 1967;70:211.
62. Gross SJ, Gabriel E. Vitamin E status in preterm infants fed human milk or infant formula. J Pediatr 1985;106:635.
63. Johnson L, Schaffer D, Boggs TR. The premature infant, vitamin E deficiency and retrolental fibroplasia. Am J Clin Nutr 1974;27:1158.
64. Hittner HM, Godio LB, Rudolph AJ, et al. Retrolental fibroplasia: efficacy of vitamin E in a double-blind clinical study of preterm infants. N Engl J Med 1981;305:1365.
65. Hittner HM, Godio LB, Speer ME, et al. Retrolental fibroplasia: further clinical evidence and ultrastructural support for efficacy of vitamin E in the preterm infant. Pediatrics 1983; 71:423.
66. Phelps DL, Rosenbaum AL, Isenberg SJ, et al. Tocopherol efficacy and safety for preventing retinopathy of prematurity: a randomized, controlled, double-masked trial. Pediatrics 1987;79:489.
67. Johnson L, Bowen FW, Abbasi S, et al. Relationship of prolonged pharmacologic serum levels of vitamin E to incidence of sepsis and necrotizing enterocolitis in infants with birth weights of 1500 grams or less. Pediatrics 1985;75:619.
68. Johnson L, Quinn GE, Abbasi S, et al. Effect of sustained pharmacologic vitamin E levels in incidence and severity of retinopathy of prematurity: a controlled clinical trial. J Pediatr 1989;114:827.
69. Lorch V, Murphy D, Hoersten LR, et al. Unusual syndrome among premature infants: association with a new intravenous vitamin E product. Pediatrics 1985;75:598.
70. Martone WJ, Williams WW, Mortensen ML, et al. Illness with fatalities in premature infants: association with an intravenous vitamin E preparation, E-Ferol. Pediatrics 1986;78:591.
71. Balistreri WR, Farrell MK, Bove KE. Lessons from the E-Ferol tragedy. Pediatrics 1986;78:503.
72. Shenai JP, Stahlman MT, Chytil, F. Vitamin A delivery from parenteral alimentation solutions. J Pediatr 1981;99:661.
73. Riggle MA, Brandt RB. Decrease of available vitamin A in parenteral nutrition solutions. J Parenter Enteral Nutr 1986; 10:388.
74. Shenai JP, Chytil F, Stahlman MT. Vitamin A status of neonates with bronchopulmonary dysplasia. Pediatr Res 1985; 19:185.
75. Shenai JP, Kennedy KA, Chytil F, Stahlman MT. Clinical trial of vitamin A supplementation in infants susceptible to bronchopulmonary dysplasia. J Pediatr 1987;111:269.
76. Robbins ST, Fletcher AB. Vitamin A supplementation in very low birthweight infants. J Parenter Enteral Nutr (in press).
77. Goldman AS, Garza C, Nichols B, et al. Effects of prematurity on the immunologic system in human milk. J Pediatr 1982;101:901.
78. Reichman B, Chessex P, Putet G, et al. Diet, fat accretion and growth in premature infants. N Engl J Med 1981;305:1495.
79. Chessex P, Reichman B, Verellen G, et al. Quality of growth in premature infants fed their own mothers milk. J Pediatr 1983;102:107.
80. Bromberger P. Premature infants' nutritional needs. Part 2. Breast milk banking. Perinatol Neonatol 1982;10:35.
81. Pujczynski M, Rademaker D, Gatson RL. Burn injury related to improper use of microwave ovens. Pediatrics 1983;72:714.
82. Alemi B, Hamosh M, Scanlon JW, et al. Fat digestion in very low-birth-weight infants: effect of addition of human milk to low-birth-weight formula. Pediatrics 1981;68:484.
83. Committee on Nutrition. Soy protein formulas: recommendations for use in infant feeding. Pediatrics 1983;172:359.
84. Shenai JP, Jhaveri BM, Reynolds JW, et al. Nutritional balance studies in very low-birth-weight infants: role of soy formula. Pediatrics 1981;67:631.
85. Hillman LS, Hoff N, Martin LA, Haddad JG. Osteopenia, hypocalcemia, and low 25-hydroxyvitamin D (25-CHD) serum concentration with use of soy formula. [Abstract] Pediatr Res 1979;13:A448.
86. Atkinson SA, Bryan MH, Anderson GH. Human milk feeding in premature infants: protein, fat and carbohydrate balances in the first two weeks of life. J Pediatr 1981;99:617.
87. Cooper PA, Rothberg AD, Pettifor JM, et al. Growth and biochemical response of premature infants fed pooled preterm milk or special formula. J Pediatr Gastroenterol Nutr 1984;3:749.
88. Lucas A, Morley R, Cole TJ, et al. Early diet in preterm babies and development status in infancy. Arch Dis Child 1989; 64:1570.
89. Smith RM, Brumley GW, Stannard MW. Neonatal pneumonia associated with medium-chain triglyceride feeding supplement. J Pediatr 1978;92:801.
90. Mehta NR, Hamosh M, Bitman, J, Wood DL. Adherence of medium chain fatty acids to feeding tubes of premature infants fed formula fortified with medium-chain triglycerides. J Pediatr Gastroenterol Nutr 1991;13:267.
91. Toce SS, Keenan WJ. Enteral feeding in very-low-birth-weight infants. Am J Dis Child 1987;141:436.

92. Grant J, Denne SC. Effect of intermittent versus continuous enteral feeding on energy expenditure in premature infants. J Pediatr 1991;118:928.
93. Aynsley-Green A. Metabolic and endocrine interrelations in the human fetus and neonate. Am J Clin Nutr 1985;41:399.
94. Greer FR, McCormick A, Loker J. Changes in fat concentration of human milk delivery by intermittent bolus and continuous mechanical pump infusion. J Pediatr 1984;105:745.
95. Wells DH, Zachman RD. Nasojejunal feeds in low-birth-weight infants. J Pediatr 1975;87:276.
96. Roy RN, Pillnitz RP, Hamilton JR, Chance GW. Impaired assimilation of nasojejunal feeds in healthy low-birth-weight newborn infants. J Pediatr 1877;90:431.
97. Challacombe D. Bacterial microflora in infants receiving nasojejunal tube feeding. J Pediatr 1974;85:113.
98. Bernbaum JC, Pereira GR, Watkins JB, Peckham GJ. Nonnutritive sucking during gavage feeding enhances growth and maturation in premature infants. Pediatrics 1983;71:41.
99. Field T, Ignatoff E, Stringer S, et al. Nonnutritive sucking during tube feedings: effects on preterm neonates in an intensive care unit. Pediatrics 1982;70:381.
100. Widström AM, Marchini G, Matthieson AS, et al. Nonnutritive sucking in tube-fed preterm infants: effects on gastric motility and gastric contents of Somatostatin. J Pediatr Gastroenterol Nutr 1988;7:517.
101. Berg RB, Schuster SR, Colodny AH. The use of gastrostomy in feeding premature infants. Pediatrics 1964;33:287.
102. Tomsovic EJ, Barringer ML, Gay JH, et al. Feeding gastrostomy in small premature infants. Am J Dis Child 1966;112:56.
103. Vengusamy S, Pildes RS, Raffensperger J, et al. A controlled study of feeding gastrostomy in low birth weight infants. Pediatrics 1969;43:815.
104. Haws EB, Sieber WK, Kiesewetter WB. Complications of tube gastrostomy in infants and children. Ann Surg 1966;164:284.
105. Holder TM. Gastrostomy: its uses and dangers in pediatric patients. N Engl J Med 1972;286:1345.
106. Stave VS, Robbins S, Fletcher AB. A comparison of growth rates of premature infants prior to and after close nutritional monitoring. Clinical Proceedings of the Children's Hospital National Medical Center 1979;35:171.
107. Thorp JW, Boeckx RL, Robbins S, et al. A prospective study of infant zinc nutrition during intensive care. Am J Clin Nutr 1981;34:1056.
108. Abrams SA, Schanler RJ, Garza C. Bone mineralization in former very low birth weight infants fed either human milk or commercial formula. J Pediatr 1988;112:956.
109. Pettifor JM, Rajah R, Venter A, et al. Bone mineralization and mineral homeostasis in very low-birth-weight infants fed either human milk or fortified human milk. J Pediatr Gastroenterol Nutr 1989;8:217.
110. Greer FR, McCormick A. Improved bone mineralization and growth in premature infants fed fortified own mother's milk. J Pediatr 1988;112:961.
111. Rowe JC, Goetz CA, Carey DE, Horak E. Achievement of in utero retention of calcium and phosphorus accompanied by high calcium excretion in very low birth weight infants fed a fortified formula. J Pediatr 1987;110:581.
112. Giles MM, Fenton MH, Shaw B, et al. Sequential calcium and phosphorus balance studies in preterm infants. J Pediatr 1987;110:591.
113. Senterre J. Calcium and phosphorus balance in preterm infants fed human milk supplemented with vitamin D and minerals. In: Goldman AS, Atkinson SA, Hanson LA, eds. Human lactation 3: the effects of human milk on the recipient infant. New York: Plenum Press, 1987:71.
114. Rowe JC, Carey DE, Goetz CA, et al. Effect of high calcium and phosphorus intake on mineral retention in very low birth weight infants chronically treated with furosemide. J Pediatr Gastroenterol Nutr 1989;9:206.
115. Gross SJ. Bone mineralization in preterm infants fed human milk with and without mineral supplementation. J Pediatr 1987;111:450.
116. Rowe JC, Wood DH, Rowe DW, Raisz IG. Nutritional hypophosphatemic rickets in a premature infant fed breast milk. N Engl J Med 1979;300:293.
117. Lewin PK, Reid M, Reilly BJ, et al. Iatrogenic rickets in low birth weight infants. J Pediatr 1971;78:207.
118. Kooh SW, Fraser D, Reilly BJ, et al. Rickets due to calcium deficiency. N Engl J Med 1977;297:1264.
119. Kulkarni PB, Hall RT, Rhodes PG, et al. Rickets in very low birth weight infants. J Pediatr 1980;96:249.
120. Geyer RP. Parenteral nutrition. Physiol Rev 1960;40:150.
121. Helfrick FW, Abelson NM. Intravenous feeding of a complete diet in a child. J Pediatr 1944;25:400.
122. Wilmore DW, Dudrick SJ. Growth and development of an infant receiving all nutrients exclusively by vein. JAMA 1968;203:860.
123. Maksimak M, Ament ME, Fonkalsrud EW. Comparison of the pediatric Broviac Silastic catheter with a standard no. 3 French Silastic catheter for central venous alimentation. J Pediatr Gastroenterol Nutr 1982;1:227.
124. Higgs SC, Malan AF, Heese H DeV, et al. A comparison of oral feedings and total parenteral nutrition in infants of very low birthweight. S Afr Med J 1974;48:2169.
125. Yu VYH, James B, Hendry P, et al. Total parenteral nutrition in very low birth weight infants: a controlled trial. Arch Dis Child 1979;54:653.
126. Hall RT, Rhodes PG. Total parenteral alimentation via indwelling umbilical catheters in the newborn period. Arch Dis Child 1976;51:929.
127. Kanarek KS, Kuznick MB, Blair RC. Infusion of total parenteral nutrition via the umbilical artery. J Parenter Enteral Nutr 1991;15:71.
128. Merritt RJ. Neonatal nutritional support. Clin Consul Nutr Support 1981;1:10.
129. Kashyap S, Heird WC. Parenteral Nutrition. In: Nelson NM, ed. Current therapy in neonatal-perinatal medicine. St. Louis: CV Mosby, 1985:354.
130. Caeton JA, Goetzman BW. Risky business: umbilical arterial catheterization. Am J Dis Child 1985;139:120.
131. Cochran WD, Davis HT, Smith CA. Advantages and complications of umbilical artery catheterizations in the newborn. Pediatrics 1968;42:769.
132. Kashyap S. Nutritional management of the extremely-low-birth-weight infant. In: Cowett RM, Hay W, eds. The micropremie: the next frontier. Report of the 99th Ross Conference on Pediatric Research, 1990:115.
133. Anderson TL, Muttart ER, Bieber MA, et al. A controlled trial of glucose vs. glucose and amino acids in premature infants. J Pediatr 1979;94:947.
134. Zlotkin SH, Bryan MH, Anderson GH. Intravenous nitrogen and energy intakes required to duplicate in utero nitrogen accretion in prematurely born human infants. J Pediatr 1981;99:115.
135. Zlotkin SH. Intravenous nitrogen intake requirement in full-term newborns undergoing surgery. Pediatrics 1984;73:493.
136. Wu PYK, Edwards NB, Storm MC. Characteristics of the plasma amino acid pattern of normal term breast-fed infants. J Pediatr 1986;109:347.
137. Helms RA, Christensen ML, Mauer EC, et al. Comparison of a pediatric versus standard amino acid formulation in preterm

neonates requiring parenteral nutrition. J Pediatr 1987;110:466.

138. Helms, RA, Johnson MR, Christenson ML, et al. Evaluation of two pediatric amino acid formulations [abstract]. J Parenter Enteral Nutr 1988;12:4.

139. Adamkin DH, McClead R, Marchildon, M, et al. Multicenter comparative evaluation of Aminosyn PF (A) and Trophamine (T) in preterm infants [abstract]. J Parenter Enteral Nutr 1989;13:18.

140. Mauer EC, Penn D. Incidence of cholestasis in low birth weight (LBW) neonates on Trophamine [abstract]. J Parenter Enteral Nutr 1991;15:25S.

141. Heird WC, Dell RB, Helms RA, et al. Amino acid mixture designed to maintain normal plasma amino acid patterns in infants and children requiring parenteral nutrition. Pediatrics 1987;80:401.

141a. McEroy GK, Pharm D. American hospital formulary service. Bethesda, MD: The American Society of Hospital Pharmacists, 1993.

142. Pettei M, Abildskov K, Heird WC. Instability of cysteine HCl in total parenteral nutrition infusates. J Am Coll Nutr 1987;6:83.

143. Zlotkin SH, Anderson GH, Bryan MH. Cysteine supplementation to cysteine-free intravenous feeding regimens in newborn infants. Am J Clin Nutr 1981;34:914.

144. Ziegler TR, Benfell K, Smith RJ, et al. Safety and metabolic effects of L-glutamine administration on humans. J Parenter Enteral Nutr 1990;14:1375S.

145. Souba WW. Introduction. Proceedings of an International Glutamine Symposium. J Parenter Enteral Nutr 1990;14:39S.

146. Hayes KC, Carey RE, Schmidt SY. Retinal degeneration associated with taurine deficiency in the cat. Science 1975;188:950.

147. Guertin F, Roy CC, Lepage G, et al. Effect of taurine on parenteral nutrition-associated cholestasis. J Parenter Enteral Nutr 1991;15:247.

148. Tyson JE, Lasky R, Flood D, et al. Randomized trial of taurine supplementation for infants <1,300 gram birth weight: effect on auditory brainstem-evoked responses. Pediatrics 1989;83:406.

149. Hay WW. Fetal and neonatal glucose homeostasis and their relation to the small for gestational age infant. Semin Perinatol 1984;8:101.

150. Cowett RM, Oh W, Pollak A, et al. Glucose disposal of low birth weight infants: steady state hypoglycemia produced by constant intravenous glucose infusion. Pediatrics 1979;63:389.

151. Sparks JW, Avery BG, Fletcher AB, et al. Parenteral galactose therapy in the glucose intolerant premature infant. J Pediatr 1982;100:255.

152. Pollak A, Cowett RM, Schwartz R, Oh W. Glucose disposal in low-birth-weight infants during steady state hyperglycemia: effects of exogenous insulin administration. Pediatrics 1978;61:546.

153. Goldman SL, Hirata T. Attenuated response to insulin in very low birth weight infants. Pediatr Res 1980;14:50.

154. Vaucher YE, Walson PD, Morrow G. Continuous insulin infusion in hyperglycemic, very low birth weight infants. J Pediatr Gastroenterol Nutr 1982;1:287.

155. Binder ND, Raschko PK, Benda GI, Reynolds JW. Insulin infusion with parenteral nutrition in extremely low birth weight infants with hyperglycemia. J Pediatr 1989;114:273.

156. Collins JW, Hoppe M, Brown K, et al. A controlled trial of insulin infusion and parenteral nutrition in extremely low birth weight infants with glucose intolerance. J Pediatr 1991;118:921.

157. Kanarek KS, Santeiro ML, Malone JI. Continuous infusion of insulin in hyperglycemic low-birth-weight infants receiving parenteral nutrition with and without lipid emulsion. J Parenter Enteral Nutr 1991;15:417.

158. Schwartz R. Should exogenous insulin be given to very-low-birth-weight infants? [Editorial] J Pediatr Gastroenterol Nutr 1982;1:287.

159. White HB, Turner AC, Miller RC. Blood lipid alterations in infants receiving intravenous fat-free alimentation. J Pediatr 1973;83:305.

160. Friedman Z, Danon A, Stahlman MT, et al. Rapid onset of essential fatty acid deficiency in the newborn. Pediatrics 1976;58:640.

161. Phelps SJ, Cochran EC, Kamper CA. Peripheral venous line infiltration in infants receiving 10% dextrose, 10% dextrose/amino acids, 10% dextrose/amino acids/fat emulsion. [Abstract] Pediatr Res 1987;21:67A.

162. Hammerman C, Aramburo MJ. Decreased lipid intake reduces morbidity in sick premature neonates. J Pediatr 1988;113:1083.

163. Gilbertson N, Kovar IZ, Cox, DJ, et al. Introduction of intravenous lipid administration on the first day of life in the very low birth weight neonate. J Pediatr 1991;119:615.

164. Schmidt-Sommerfeld E, Penn D, Wolff H. Carnitine deficiency in premature infants receiving total parenteral nutrition: effect of L-carnitine supplementation. J Pediatr 1983;102:931.

165. Dahlström KA, Ament ME, Moukarzel A, et al. Low blood and plasma carnitine levels in children receiving long-term parenteral nutrition. J Pediatr Gastroenterol Nutr 1990;11:375.

166. Helms RA, Whitington PF, Mauer EC, et al. Enhanced lipid utilization in infants receiving oral L-carnitine during long-term parenteral nutrition. J Pediatr 1986;109:984.

167. Brasseur D, Johansson A, Goyens PL, et al. Carnitine (C) balance in the parenterally fed premature neonate receiving a new C-containing fat emulsion [abstract]. J Parenteral Enteral Nutr 1991;15:255.

168. Lima LAM, Murphy JF, Stansbie D, et al. Neonatal parenteral nutrition with a fat emulsion containing medium chain triglycerides. Acta Paediatr Scand 1988;77:332.

169. Bientz J, Frey A, Schirardin H, Bach AC. Medium chain triglycerides in parenteral nutrition in the newborn: a short term clinical trial. Infusionstherapie 1988;15:96.

170. Andrew G, Chan G, Schiff D. Lipid metabolism in the neonate. II. The effect of intralipid on bilirubin binding in vitro and in vivo. J Pediatr 1976;88:279.

171. Adamkin DH, Radmacher PG, Klingbeil RL. Use of intravenous lipid and hyperbilirubinemia in the first week. J Pediatr Gastroenterol Nutr 1992;14:135.

172. Friedman Z, Shochet SJ, Maisels MJ, et al. Correction of essential fatty acid deficiency in newborn infants by cutaneous application of sunflower-seed oil. Pediatrics 1976;58:650.

173. Hunt CE, Engel RR, Modler S, et al. Essential fatty acid deficiency in neonates: inability to reverse deficiency in topical applications of EFA-rich oil. J Pediatr 1978;92:603.

174. Dunham B, Marcuard S, Khazanie PG, et al. The solubility of calcium and phosphorus in neonatal parenteral nutrition solutions. J Parenter Enteral Nutr 1991;15:608.

175. Pelegano JF, Rowe JC, Carey DE, et al. Effect of calcium/phosphorus ratio in mineral retention in parenterally fed premature infants. J Pediatr Gastroenterol Nutr 1991;12:351.

176. Fitzgerald KA, MacKay MW. Calcium and phosphate solubility in neonatal parenteral nutrient solutions containing Trophamine. Am J Hosp Pharm 1986;43:88.

177. Schmidt GL, Baumgartner TG, Fischlschweiger W, et al. Cost containment using cysteine HCl acidification to increase calcium/phosphate solubility in hyperalimentation solutions. J Parenter Enteral Nutr 1986;10:203.

178. Venkataraman PS, Brissie EO, Tsang RC. Stability of calcium and phosphorus in neonatal parenteral nutrition solutions. J Pediatr Gastroenterol Nutr 1983;2:640.
179. Eggert LD, Rusho WJ, MacKay MW, et al. Calcium and phosphorus compatibility in parenteral nutrition solutions for neonates. Am J Hosp Pharm 1982;39:49.
180. Al-Jurf AS, Chapmann-Furr F. Phosphate balance and distribution during total parenteral nutrition: effect of calcium and phosphorus additives. J Parenter Enteral Nutr 1986;10:508.
181. Hoehn GJ, Carey DE, Raye JR, et al. Alternate-day infusion of calcium and phosphate in very low birth weight infants: wasting of the infused mineral. J Pediatr Gastroenterol Nutr 1987;6:752.
182. Kimura S, Nose O, Seino Y, et al. Effects of alternate and simultaneous administration of calcium and phosphorus on calcium metabolism in children receiving total parenteral nutrition. J Parenter Enteral Nutr 1986;10:513.
183. Henry RS, Jurgens KW, Sturgeon RJ, et al. Compatibility of calcium chloride and calcium gluconate with sodium phosphate in a mixed TPN solution. Am J Hosp Pharm 1980;37:673.
184. Hanning RM, Mitchell MK, Atkinson SA. In vitro solubility of calcium glycerophosphate versus conventional mineral salts in pediatric parenteral nutrition solutions. J Pediatr Gastroenterol Nutr 1989;9:67.
185. Chessex P, Pineault M, Brisson G, et al. Role of the source of phosphate salt in improving the mineral balance of parenterally fed low birth weight infants. J Pediatr 1990;116:765.
186. Draper HH, Yuen DE, Whyte RK. Calcium glycerophosphate as a source of calcium and phosphorus in total parenteral nutrition solutions. J Parenter Enteral Nutr 1991;15:176.
187. Sivasubramanian KN, Henkin RI. Behavioral and dermatologic changes and low serum zinc and copper concentrations in two premature infants after parenteral nutrition. J Pediatr 1978;93:847.
188. Heller RM, Kirchner SG, O'Neill JA, et al. Skeletal changes of copper deficiency in infants receiving prolonged total parenteral nutrition. J Pediatr 1978;92:947.
189. Lane HW, Barroso AO, Englert D, et al. Selenium status of seven chronic intravenous hyperalimentation patients. J Parenter Enteral Nutr 1982;6:426.
190. Greene HL, Hambidge KM, Schanler R, Tsang RC. Guidelines for the use of vitamins, trace elements, calcium, magnesium, and phosphorus in infants and children receiving total parenteral nutrition: report of the Subcommittee on Pediatric Parenteral Nutrient Requirements from the Committee on Clinical Practice Issues of the American Society for Clinical Nutrition. Am J Clin Nutr 1988;48:1324.
191. Boeckert PA, Greene HL, Fritz I, et al. Vitamin concentrations in very low birth weight infants given vitamins intravenously in a lipid emulsion: measurement of vitamins A, D, and E and riboflavin. J Pediatr 1988;113:1057.
192. Raucher HS, Hyatt AC, Barzilai A, et al. Quantitative blood cultures in the evaluation of sepsis in children with Broviac catheters. J Pediatr 1984;104:29.
193. Ruderman JW, Morgan MA, Klein AH. Quantitative blood cultures in the diagnosis of sepsis in infants with umbilical and Broviac catheters. J Pediatr 1988;112:748.
194. Prince A, Heller B, Levy J, et al. Management of fever in patients with central vein catheters. Pediatr Infect Dis 1986;5:20.
195. Hiemenz J, Skelton J, Pizzo P. Perspective on the management of catheter related infections in cancer patients. Pediatr Infect Dis 1986;5:6.
196. Nahata MC, King DR, Powell, DA, et al. Management of catheter-related infections in pediatric patients. J Parenter Enteral Nutr 1988;12:58.
197. Aschner JL, Punsalang A, Maniscalco WM, Menegus MA. Percutaneous central venous catheter colonization with *Malassezia furfur*: incidence and clinical significance. Pediatrics 1987;80:535.
198. Lesko SM, Mitchell AA, Epstein MF, et al. Heparin use as a risk factor for intraventricular hemorrhages in low-birth-weight infants. N Engl J Med 1986;314:1156.
199. Bailey MJ. Reduction of catheter-associated sepsis in parenteral nutrition using low-dose intravenous heparin. Br Med J 1979;1:1671.
200. Zarden H, Dhanireddy R, Hamosh M, et al. Effect of continuous heparin administration of Intralipid clearing in very-low-birth-weight infants. J Pediatr 1982;101:599.
201. Berkow SE, Spear ML, Stahl GE, et al. Total parenteral nutrition with intralipid in premature infants receiving TPN with heparin: effect on plasma lipolytic enzymes, lipids, and glucose. J Pediatr Gastroenterol Nutr 1987;6:581.
202. Heird WC, Driscoll JM, Schullinger JN, et al. Intravenous alimentation in pediatric patients. J Pediatr 1972;80:351.
203. Duffy LF, Kerzner B, Gebus V, Dice J. Treatment of central venous catheter occlusions with hydrochloric acid. J Pediatr 1989;114:1002.
204. Alfrey AC. Aluminum. Adv Clin Chem 1983;23:69.
205. Sedman AB, Klein GL, Merritt RJ, et al. Evidence of aluminum loading in infants receiving intravenous therapy. N Engl J Med 1985;312:1337.
206. Koo WWK, Kaplan LA, Bendon R, et al. Response to aluminum in parenteral nutrition during infancy. J Pediatr 1986;109:883.
207. Koo WWK, Kaplan LA, Horn J, et al. Aluminum in parenteral solutions—sources and possible alternatives. J Parenter Enteral Nutr 1986;10:591.
208. ASCN/A.S.P.E.N. Working Group on Standards for Aluminum Content of Parenteral Nutrition Solutions. Parenteral drug products containing aluminium as an ingredient or a contaminant: response to food and drug administration notice of intent and request for information. J Parenter Enteral Nutr 1991;15:194.

Neonatology: Pathophysiology and Management of the Newborn, Fourth Edition,
edited by Gordon B. Avery, Mary Ann Fletcher, and Mhairi G. MacDonald.
J.B. Lippincott Company, Philadelphia © 1994.

chapter 25

Thermoregulation

EDMUND HEY

Although it has always been considered a good thing to keep babies warm, a reasonable understanding of the physiology of temperature regulation in the newborn baby has only been achieved in the last 30 years. With this new knowledge, it is now possible to answer the question, "How warm is warm?" with much greater precision.

PHYSIOLOGY OF TEMPERATURE CONTROL

Adult mammals, including humans, have the attributes of homeotherms. Over a fairly wide range of environmental temperature, they maintain a remarkably constant deep body temperature, a vitally important aspect of sustaining a constant *milieu interieur.* Nonetheless, this homeothermy may be overwhelmed in extremes of cold or heat. Only since the early 1960s has it been demonstrated that the newborn baby has all the capabilities of a mature homeotherm, although the range of environmental temperature over which an infant can operate successfully is severely restricted. The newborn has several disadvantages in temperature regulation, including a relatively large surface area, poor thermal insulation, and small mass to act as a heat sink. The infant has little ability to conserve heat by changing posture and no ability to adjust his or her own clothing in response to thermal stress. Like the responses of the adult, those of a neonate may be jeopardized by illness and by adverse conditions such as hypoxia and drug intoxication. These responses and the factors limiting them make up the physiology of thermoregulation in the newborn.

As recently as 1957, there was little hard evidence that a baby in the first hours after birth was anything other than a temporary poikilotherm, although 15 years earlier, Day had shown that the thriving baby between 1 and 2 weeks of age had all the responses of a homeotherm.[1] In 1957 and 1958, Silverman and coworkers[2,3] deduced from their clinical trials that the newborn baby also had these responses, and in 1961, Brück[4] produced unequivocal physiologic evidence that these responses applied during the first hours after birth, even in prematurely born infants.

The baby produces heat as a result of metabolic activity (*i.e.,* basal metabolic rate). To maintain a constant body temperature, the neonate must dissipate this heat to the environment at a mean rate equal to that of his or her heat production. In cool conditions, the child must conserve heat; however, if, with maximal conservation, more heat is lost than produced, the infant must increase heat production (*i.e.,* display a metabolic response to cold). In a very warm environment, the infant must dissipate more heat by vasodilation and sweating. To achieve all this, the child must have a sensory system to appreciate temperature (*i.e.,* an affector arc), a central control system, and the means of adjusting heat production and dissipation (*i.e.,* an effector arc).

AFFECTOR ARC

As in the adult, cooling the skin produces a prompt and reproducible metabolic response in the baby, demonstrating the presence of skin receptors.[4] The trigeminal area of the face shows a marked sensitivity to heat and cold.[5] The existence of central (*i.e.,* thalamic) cold receptors is difficult to demonstrate with precision in the human baby, although they can be inferred from the modification of response at different deep body temperatures.

CENTRAL REGULATING MECHANISM

In adult and newborn animals, there is evidence of a complex central regulating mechanism in the area of the hypothalamus. In the human infant, the area can be inferred and confirmed by "experiments of nature," such as the studies of Cross and coworkers on an anencephalic infant.[6] The central thermostat is not, however, set at a fixed temperature; it undergoes cyclic changes, falls about 0.5°C with the onset of sleep, and is affected by pyrogens, drugs, and intrahypothalamic hormones such as noradrenaline.[7] Although set-point deviation can be considered a form of cold adaptation, there is no evidence to suggest that the set point of a newborn baby, around whom temperature is regulated, is normally different from that seen in later life.[8] This control center can be rendered partially or totally ineffective by various drugs and by disorders such as intracranial hemorrhage, gross cerebral malformation, trauma, and severe birth asphyxia.

EFFECTOR ARC

VASOMOTOR CONTROL

From birth, there is a well-developed ability to control skin blood flow, even in very small infants.[4,9] Despite this ability, a baby's total thermal insulation is poor compared with that of the adult.[10]

INCREASED HEAT PRODUCTION

The ability to increase heat production (*i.e.*, achieve a metabolic response to cold) is a consistent phenomenon in all healthy babies.[11,12] The heat may be produced by shivering and other muscular activity or by nonshivering thermogenesis. Large increases in heat production occur in babies in the absence of detectable shivering, although shivering may be observed at very low environmental temperatures (15°C). Brown fat is an important site of heat production in many newborn mammals.[13] Catecholamine-mediated nonshivering thermogenesis in brown fat represents a physiologic effector organ quantitatively important to cold-adapted animals, to hibernating animals, and to human newborns.[14]

The dependence of the newborn on brown fat nonshivering thermogenesis has important practical consequences, because this effector mechanism may be rendered useless by hypoxia, blockade by certain drugs, and nutritional depletion. Nonshivering thermogenesis in animals is reduced with increasing age, although it can be preserved by exposure to cold with *ad libitum* feeding, such as is used in producing a cold-adapted animal. In fasted newborn rabbits, brown fat deposits are maintained until death if the rabbits are kept warm (35°C), but they are depleted by the second day if the young rabbits are kept in a cool environment (30°C–25°C). When the metabolic response fails, brown fat and white fat are virtually depleted of lipid.[15]

No evidence is available to assess how long the response to cold stress lasts in the human baby or to what extent the human infant depends on nonshivering thermogenesis. Calculations based on estimates of the amount of brown fat in the human infant at birth suggest that restlessness and increased muscular activity may be at least as important as increased heat production within strategically situated deposits of brown fat in maintaining deep body temperature in cold surroundings.

SWEATING

Newborn term infants have six times as many functional sweat glands per unit area as adults, but the peak response of each gland is only about one-third that of an adult gland.[16] Although the baby's response to warm stress may be expected to exceed that of an adult, the full-term infant increases his or her insensible water loss only about fourfold, even when a warm environment has increased rectal temperature to 38°C.[17] This represents the dissipation of the infant's basal metabolic rate, and in a heat-gaining environment, the risks of hyperthermia are great. Babies born more than 8 weeks before term have virtually no ability to sweat, and even in a baby born only 3 weeks early, sweating is severely limited and largely confined to the head and face.[18] Sweat production matures relatively rapidly in the preterm baby after delivery. A 4-week-old baby born at 30 weeks of gestation can withstand heat stress better than a 2-day-old baby of 34 weeks of gestation.[19]

PHYSICS OF HEAT EXCHANGE

The baby, like any physical object, exchanges heat by conduction, convection, evaporation, and radiation. Table 25-1 shows the way heat loss is partitioned among these channels in the conditions that apply in a clinical warm-air incubator.[20] Because conduction depends on the thermal conductivity of the substance in contact with the body and because babies are usually laid on a mattress of low conductivity, thermal exchange through this channel is usually small. Convective exchange depends on air speed and air temperature, and the air conditions with radiation represent a major channel of heat loss, varying inversely with environmental air temperature. Evaporative loss depends on air speed and on the absolute humidity of the air.[21–23] This represents only a small fraction of all heat loss in a clothed baby or in a baby nursed in a regular warm-air incubator of moderate humidity. However, if an immature baby with a thin skin is nursed under a radiant overhead heater in an envi-

TABLE 25–1
EQUILIBRIUM VALUES FOR HEAT LOSS IN A 1-WEEK-OLD 2-KG BABY LYING NAKED ON A FOAM MATTRESS IN DRAFT-FREE SURROUNDINGS OF UNIFORM TEMPERATURE AND MODERATE HUMIDITY

	Environmental Temperature†		
Heat Loss*	30°C	33°C	36°C
Radiation	19 (43%)	12 (40%)	7 (24%)
Convection	15 (37%)	9 (33%)	5 (19%)
Evaporation	7 (16%)	7 (24%)	17 (56%)
Conduction	2 (4%)	1 (3%)	0 (1%)
Total	43	29	29

* Values for heat loss are given in units of kcal/m²·hour.
† Values in parentheses show the percent of total heat loss at that environmental temperature.
From Hey E. The care of babies in incubators. In: Hull D, Gairdner D, eds. Recent advances in paediatrics. London: Churchill, 1971.

ronment of low relative humidity, evaporation governs a major fraction of all heat loss. Because the latent heat of evaporation of water is large (*i.e.*, 540 cal/mL), a dry environment encouraging evaporation is cool, and a saturated environment preventing evaporation is warm. In environments warmer than the body, evaporation represents the only way in which heat can be dissipated. Drafts materially increase convective and evaporative losses.[22]

Radiant heat loss depends on the presenting surface area and geometry and on the surface temperature of the body compared with the temperature of the receiving surface. Table 25-1 shows how radiation accounts for a major proportion of all heat loss in a naked baby in an incubator.[24,25] The radiant receiving surface is the inside surface of the Perspex canopy of the incubator, which is opaque to the thermal radiation of the baby's skin at a wavelength of 9000 to 10000 nm. The temperature of the canopy is so affected by incubator air temperature and room temperature that the inside canopy temperature may be very different from the temperature set by the incubator thermostat (Fig. 25-1). Radiant exchange is profoundly affected by room temperature unless a second layer of Perspex is interposed between the baby and the canopy. This second layer is warmed by the incubator air, which is subject to the incubator's thermostat control.[26] The effect is shown in Figure 25-2. Heat can also be captured in incubators from radiant sources (*e.g.*, sunlight) that pass through the Perspex, creating a greenhouse effect.[25] Radiant sources can be used to heat a baby to counteract his or her heat dissipation.

In strictly scientific terms, no single temperature is a full statement of the thermal environment of the baby. However, in draft-free surroundings of moderate relative humidity, in which the temperature of the air, the conductive surfaces, and the radiant receiving surfaces are within a few degrees of each other, a single temperature, such as air temperature, is a reasonable reflection of the overall mean or operative environmental temperature.[20]

OPTIMAL THERMAL ENVIRONMENT

There are clinical consequences of environments that are too hot or too cold. In temperate zones, the more common failing in the past was to provide too little warmth. How warm is warm? With a better understanding of the physiology of the newborn, it is possible to answer this question more scientifically than in the past.

The neutral thermal environment is that range of thermal environment in which a baby with a normal body temperature has a minimal metabolic rate and

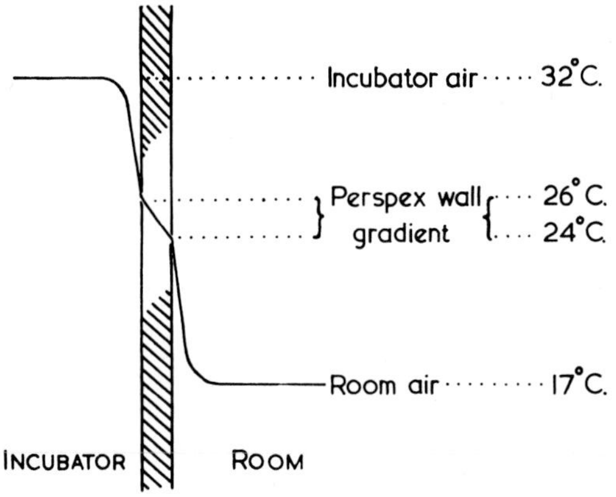

FIG. 25–1. The temperature gradient across the 9-mm Perspex wall of a typical incubator. (From Hey EN, Mount L. Temperature control in incubators. Lancet 1960;2;202.)

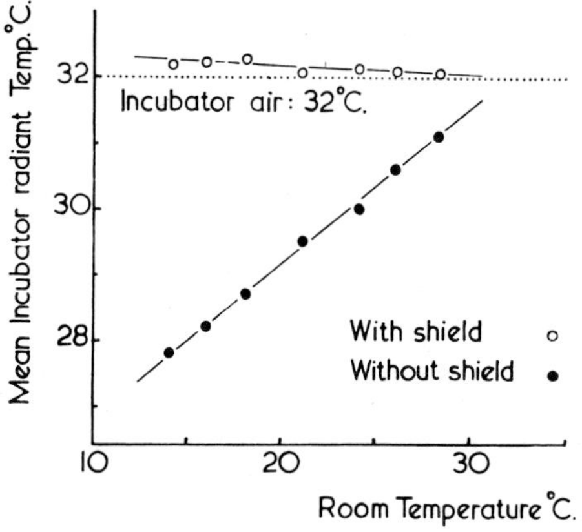

FIG. 25–2. The influence of room temperature on the mean temperature of the inner incubator wall to which a baby radiates heat. The incubator temperature was kept constant at 32°C. (From Hey EN, Mount L. Temperature control in incubators. Lancet 1966;2:202.)

can maintain a constant body temperature by vasomotor control and by posture.[27] Below this range, the lower end of which is called the critical temperature, a metabolic response to cold is necessary to replace lost heat. Above this range, skin water loss rises due to sweating, but the body temperature also soon rises, causing a further increase in basal metabolic rate. The neutral range represents the thermal range of minimal stress, and it is narrow for a naked baby. Nevertheless, estimates of the most likely temperature to provide neutral conditions for babies of differing weights and ages derived in the early 1970s (Fig. 25-3) seem to have withstood the test of time. The initial studies were conducted in a metabolic chamber, but similar results have been obtained from measurements made in commercial incubators under normal ward conditions.[10,28,29]

There are some important caveats for using the information summarized in Figure 25-3. The temperatures are appropriate only if the physical conditions defined in the legend apply. If relative humidity is high (*e.g.*, 75%), the temperature predicted should be decreased by 0.5°C for naked babies and 1°C for clothed babies. In a dry, nonhumidified incubator, the air temperature should be increased, especially if the baby has immature semipermeable skin.[19,23] If a single-wall incubator is used, an allowance of 1°C should be made for every 7°C by which room temperature is below the incubator air temperature.[24] These data are derived from healthy babies; if a low metabolic rate is expected in a baby (*e.g.*, very ill babies, infants with cyanotic heart disease), temperatures should be slightly higher. Conversely, in restless babies, babies with frequent seizures, and babies with large left-to-right shunts, slightly lower temperatures are appropriate.

Figure 25-3 emphasizes a number of important points. The neutral range is narrow for naked babies and falls only slightly with advancing age. All the temperatures are very warm by adult standards. There is no single environmental temperature that is appropriate for all sizes and conditions of babies. That which is appropriate for a lusty term infant is too cold for a tiny preterm infant, and that which is appropriate for the latter is too hot for the term infant. When a baby is clothed and in a crib, all avenues of heat dissipation are partially occluded; the temperatures required are lower, and the consequences of misjudgment are less.[30]

Figure 25-3 represents a scientifically based guess at an appropriate temperature for an untested baby. Because of the aforementioned caveats, it is necessary to monitor each baby's temperature.[31] This is a form of servocontrol, because the adult responsible adjusts the environmental temperature in response to a baby's temperature.

METHODS OF ACHIEVING THERMONEUTRALITY

SERVOCONTROL

Because of the narrowness of the optimal temperature range, many hospitals use servocontrolled heaters to regulate incubator air temperature with a

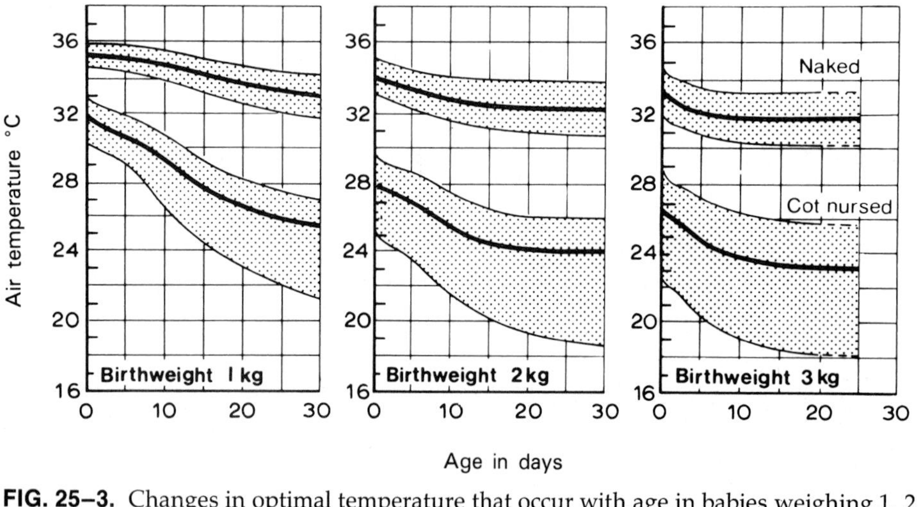

FIG. 25–3. Changes in optimal temperature that occur with age in babies weighing 1, 2, or 3 kg at birth. The dark line indicates the optimum, and the shaded area shows the range within which a baby can be expected to maintain a normal body temperature without increasing heat production or evaporative water loss by more than 25%. The upper range is for naked babies, and the lower is for cot-nursed babies. The operative temperature in these cases can be considered the same as air temperature in draft-free surroundings of approximately 50% humidity if the radiant receiving surfaces are the same temperature as the air (*i.e.*, with a second layer of Perspex interposed between the baby and the main incubator wall). (Adapted from Hey EN. The care of babies in incubators. In: Gairdner D, Hull D, eds. Recent advances in paediatrics. London: Churchill-Livingstone, 1971:171.)

sensing thermistor taped to the child's abdomen. However, when the effectiveness of servocontrol finally was studied some 20 years after the technique was first introduced, it was found to increase the instability of the environmental temperature.[32] Servocontrol devices can cause overheating if the skin sensor comes loose, obscure the signs of early septicemia, and possibly subject an infected infant with a raised thermoregulatory set point to marked cold stress.

For many years, it was conventional to maintain the abdominal skin at 36°C, and this is probably the ideal temperature for most babies older than a few weeks of age. In small babies, a temperature of 36.5°C is more frequently chosen. In very small babies with a high evaporative heat loss, abdominal skin temperature may appear to exceed rectal temperature when environmental humidity is low, partly because taping the thermistor to the skin locally reduces evaporative loss and produces a falsely high indication of true skin temperature.[33] A temperature of 36.8°C may be appropriate for these babies in the first few days of life.

SKIN WATER LOSS

Environmental humidity has only a modest effect on thermal balance in babies with a reasonably well-keratinized skin. The increase in evaporative heat loss that occurs after relative humidity falls 50% in a subthermoneutral environment can be counterbalanced by increasing the operative environmental temperature by something over 0.5°C. In warmer surroundings, spontaneous changes in skin blood flow and increased sweating maintain thermal equilibrium without any net change in heat balance.

Much more consideration must be given to evaporative water loss from the skin in babies of less than 31 weeks of gestation, especially in the first week of life, when water loss is often the single most important channel of obligatory heat loss from the skin.[18] Special nomograms have been produced for predicting the temperature most likely to offer thermal neutrality in such babies.[29] Halving this loss by increasing ambient humidity by 50% may have as potent an effect as increasing environmental temperature by almost 1.5°C, as Silverman showed in the first of his classic clinical trials of incubator management.[34,35] Placing a clear plastic drape or a Perspex radiant heat shield with closed ends over the baby works in much the same way by decreasing air movement and increasing the humidity of the microenvironment around the baby.[36]

Research has clarified many of the factors influencing skin water loss in the very premature baby. Inadequate keratinization leads to a high insensible water loss at birth in babies of less than 31 weeks of gestation, but permeability drops rapidly in the first 7 to 10 days after birth unless the skin becomes traumatized or secondarily infected. A 2-week-old baby born at 26 weeks of gestation loses much less water through the skin than a baby of 30 weeks of gestation in the first week of life (Fig. 25-4).[19]

Total insensible water loss increases as air speed increases and as the baby becomes active, partially because of increased respiratory loss. Skin water loss rises if abrasions traumatize the skin. Significant heat loss occurs if water or urine evaporate from the skin. Phototherapy causes an increase in skin blood flow and is thought to cause an increase in water loss from the skin, even if steps are taken to compensate for the change in the radiant environment, which is only partly due to increased fluid loss in the stool.[37–39] Overhead radiant heaters appear to have a similar effect, although much of the reported difference is due to differences in air speed and absolute humidity of the two environments, and the combination of phototherapy and direct radiant heat may be additive.[40,41] The reason for this reported increase is not known. Focal radiant heat may cause local sweating over the trunk, even in surroundings that left most of the body cool.

Important as it is to allow for evaporative heat loss when trying to optimize the thermal environment, it may be even more important to control fluid balance accurately in these babies. There is evidence that differences of as little as 2 mL/kg/hour in net fluid intake can significantly increase the risks of congestive failure due to patent ductus arteriosus and of necrotizing enterocolitis in babies weighing less than 1.5 kg with respiratory distress.[42,43] It may be hazardous to increase daily fluid intake more than 80 mL/kg above insensible water loss until respiratory problems have settled, particularly if there is reason to believe that the ductus arteriosus remains patent. Duct patency cannot be determined merely by listening.

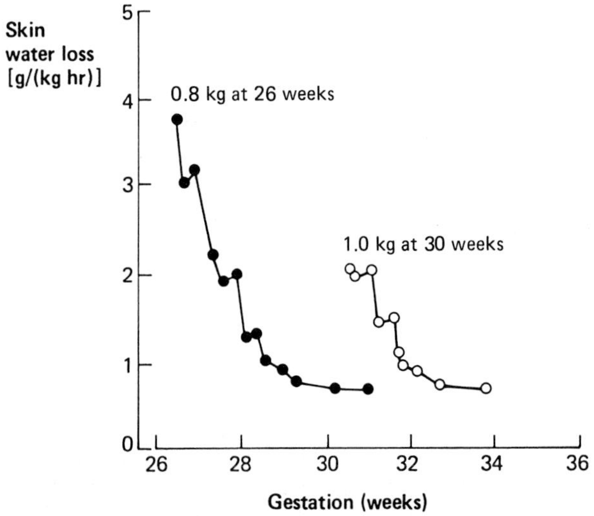

FIG. 25–4. Skin water loss falls rapidly in the first 2 weeks after birth as the skin becomes better keratinized. Enhanced skin maturation in response to premature delivery results in a 1-month-old baby born at 26 weeks of gestation having much more waterproof skin and sweat glands that are more functionally mature than a 1-week-old baby born at 30 weeks of gestation.

OVERHEAD RADIANT CRADLES

Overhead radiant heaters that put heat back into a baby while he or she is losing it by other means are important in intensive care situations in which free access to airways and umbilical vessels is essential. In these situations, ordinary monitoring of heat loss and heat gain is impossible, and monitoring the baby's temperature with a thermistor and a servocontrolled proportional heat control unit is the only practical way of ensuring heat balance. Such units have many advantages, but they make it difficult to predict or control evaporative heat loss in the smallest babies during the first few critical days of life. Servocontrolled radiant heat can compensate for the variation in evaporation and convective heat loss produced by stray drafts when a small baby is nursed in an open radiant cradle, but it cannot compensate for the variation in water loss, and this can be critical, as previously discussed. Perspex heat shields have been used to control these variable losses, but a transparent tented plastic drape appears more satisfactory because the direct transfer of radiant heat is largely blocked by Perspex.[44]

Ten years after radiant cradles were in widespread use, a metaanalysis of the available studies showed that the units provide a reasonably neutral environment, but there are no studies comparing the morbidity and mortality when such units are used in preference to closed incubators.[45] Although babies often have relatively cold extremities and may have a relatively high peripheral skin blood flow when nursed under a radiant cradle, there is little difference among the three basic ways of achieving thermoneutrality in a very immature baby immediately after birth (Fig. 25-5).[46] A radiant cradle may be the most convenient, but a well-humidified incubator may provide a more constant and predictable environment. Double glazing merely removes the need to increase incubator air temperature to compensate for the relatively high radiant loss of single-walled incubators.

IS A NEUTRAL TEMPERATURE OPTIMAL?

There are clinical consequences of allowing a baby to become too hot. Serious overheating can quickly cause heatstroke and death, and lesser degrees of stress can cause cerebral damage due to hypernatremic dehydration. Cold stress is more subtle in its consequences, unless it is severe enough to cause neonatal cold injury, but the need to increase heat production causes an increase in the baby's calorie requirements and in the need for oxygen, threatening the child's life if there is respiratory difficulty.[47]

In the 1950s, when hypothermia for organ surgery was in vogue, Silverman and associates[48] and Jolly and coworkers[49] conducted controlled trials on the effects of warmth, demonstrating a decrease in mortality with extra warmth. In Silverman's studies, survival rates in incubators maintained at 31.7°C were 93% for babies weighing more than 1500 g, 86% for babies between 1000 and 1500 g, and 50% for babies less than 1000 g; survival rates in cooler incubators (28.9°C) were 79% for babies more than 1500 g, 77% for babies between 1000 and 1500 g, and 14% for babies less than 1000 g. Warmth alone tripled the chances of survival of the very small babies. Other researchers showed the favorable effect of using the higher incubator temperature (31.5°C) plus supplementary radiant heat to maintain abdominal skin temperature at 36°C.[50,51]

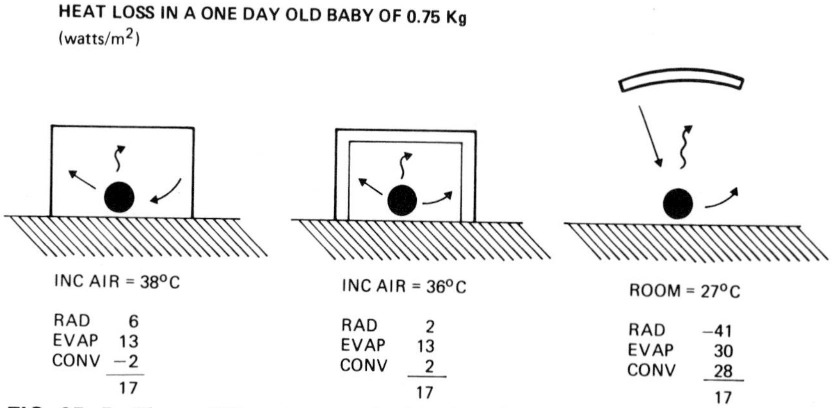

FIG. 25–5. Three different ways of achieving thermoneutrality can be used for a 1-day-old baby weighing 0.75 kg born at 28 weeks of gestation. Evaporative heat loss (EVAP) is high, even when the baby is nursed in a fully humidified incubator (75% relative humidity). This evaporative heat loss doubles when the baby is exposed under a radiant cradle in an unhumidified room (25% relative humidity) at 27°C. Uniform surroundings at 36°C provide thermoneutral conditions if the walls are the same temperature as the air in the incubator. Air temperature should exceed the baby's own deep-body temperature in a single-walled incubator (room temperature, 24°C [75°F]) to compensate for the continued radiant (RAD) and evaporative heat loss. (CONV, convection.)

Fluctuations in environmental temperature can precipitate apnea and affect overall mortality, and even routine nursing procedures cause marked temperature instability.[52,53] Nurses are rediscovering the advantages of cot nursing and finding that the temperature instability caused by nursing care is less in a lightly clothed cot nursed baby than it is in an unclothed baby in an incubator.[30,54] It is possible to care for most babies weighing 1.3 kg or more in a cot after the first 10 days if a heated mattress is used to provide supplementary warmth.[55]

It should not be assumed that because marked cold stress is hazardous to the ill, recently delivered, preterm baby, strict thermoneutrality necessarily provides optimal conditions for the small healthy preterm baby older than a few days of age.[27] Adults often are comfortable in an environment slightly cooler than the neutral range, and young animals often display a similar preference.[56] Nurses left to use their own judgment in selecting incubator temperature tend to make a similar choice, and apneic attacks appear to be less frequent when babies are nursed at the lower end of the thermoneutral range.[31,57] School children even think better in classrooms kept slightly below the thermal comfort zone![58]

Possible advantages of minimal cold stress to healthy thriving babies have been investigated by Glass, Silverman, and Sinclair.[59,60] In a controlled comparison of a group of babies servocontrolled at 35°C (as measured on abdominal skin) and another group servocontrolled at 36°C, there was minor growth retardation in the cool group that could be offset by increasing the feeds.[59] After 2 weeks, the babies in the cool group were better able to withstand minor cold stress—something they would have been intermittently subjected to if they had been nursed fully clothed in a cot rather than cared for naked in an incubator.[60]

RISK SITUATIONS

Immediately after birth, when a baby arrives naked, wet, and partially asphyxiated, there is a period in which body temperature falls abruptly unless very special precautions are taken. If the delivery room temperature is about 25°C, even a lusty baby producing a maximal metabolic response to cold cannot match the rate of heat loss (*i.e.*, 200 kcal/kg/minute). If the baby is small, ill, and asphyxiated, the rate of fall of body temperature is dramatic. Dabbing the infant dry to prevent evaporative loss and using a radiant heater to put some heat back into the child helps to decrease heat loss.[61] The period of time during which the baby is exposed to temperatures appropriate for adults must be minimized. Serious asphyxia may affect the baby's homeothermy for many hours after birth.[62,63] A good source of warmth not often used in sophisticated society is the baby's mother—a thermostatically controlled and affectionate heat sink.[64]

Other risk situations occur during major and minor surgery (*e.g.*, exchange transfusion), clinical examination, bathing, x-ray procedures, and transport. The risk of cooling associated with transporting a baby from one hospital to another is more obvious than the risk associated with transporting a baby down a hospital corridor or elevator. There is no panacea applicable to all situations, and control of only a single temperature in the environment is inadequate.

MONITORING BODY TEMPERATURE

Rectal measurement probably provides the best guide to core temperature; esophageal and tympanic membrane measurements are impractical except in a research setting. The deeper a rectal probe is inserted—up to a depth of 10 cm—the higher the temperature recorded; however, most of the change occurs in the first 4 cm. Axillary measurement can safely be used to rule out hypothermia if a low-reading thermometer is used. Axillary temperature is a close approximation to rectal temperature in most newborn babies, but it is easy to fail to recognize fever if the temperature is only measured in the axilla.[65,66] Although only two of the cases of traumatic rectal perforation in the world literature occurred in preterm babies, there is an understandable reluctance to take rectal temperature repeatedly. Skin thermistors make it possible to monitor the abdomen-to-foot skin temperature gradient continuously. They also make it possible to identify the environmental fluctuations caused by nursing care.

TRENDS IN THERMOREGULATION

The demonstration that adequate warmth can cut mortality in small babies by 25% is a powerful inducement to define what is meant by adequate warmth.[45] There have been several important advances in this area of thermoregulation since the early 1960s, and there is more to be learned—for example, about the boundary layer of air at the skin, its thermal consequences, and its aerodynamics. Some fascinating work is already in progress. The advantages of crib nursing are being rediscovered, and a move away from incubators can be expected.[55] The importance of environmental humidity in controlling water balance and in limiting evaporative heat loss has assumed a new meaning in the very preterm baby.[23,34] This consideration has sharpened the continuing debate between those who prefer to nurse ill babies within a conventional hot-air forced-convection incubator and those who prefer the freedom and accessibility offered by an open radiant cradle. Sophisticated studies and techniques of warming have identified the advantages of traditional methods such as swaddling and crib nursing, as advocated in this old quatrain:

Thou, Nurse, in swaddling Bands the Babe enfold,
And carefully defend its Limbs from Cold,
If Winter, by the chimney place thy Chair,
If Summer, then admit the cooling Air.

Moses was swaddled and placed in a basket on the Nile. The swaddling and the basket are again an acceptable modern practice; the advantages of the Nile as an enormous heat sink will no doubt be identified soon. I assume, however, that pediatric nurses can be relied on to remain in closer personal contact with the baby than Moses' mother and sister are said to have done.

REFERENCES

1. Day RL. Respiratory metabolism in infancy and in childhood. Regulation of body temperature of premature infants. Am J Dis Child 1943;65:376.
2. Silverman WA, Blanc WA. The effects of humidity on survival of newly born premature infants. Pediatrics 1957;20:477.
3. Silverman WA, Fertig JW, Berger AP. The influence of the thermal environment upon the survival of newly born premature infants. Pediatrics 1958;22:876.
4. Brück K. Temperature regulation in the newborn infant. Biol Neonate 1961;3:65.
5. Mestyan J, Jarai GB, Fekete M. The significance of facial skin temperature in the chemical heat regulation of premature infants. Biol Neonate 1964;7:243.
6. Cross KW, Gustavson J, Hill JR, Robinson DC. Thermoregulation in an anencephalic infant as inferred from its metabolic rate under hypothermic and normal conditions. Clin Sci Mol Med 1966;31:449.
7. Day RL. Regulation of body temperature during sleep. Am J Dis Child 1941;61:734.
8. Brück K. Which environmental temperature does the premature infant prefer? Pediatrics 1968;41:1027.
9. Hey EN, Katz G. The range of thermal insulation in the tissues of the newborn baby. J Physiol 1970;207:667.
10. Hey EN, Katz G, O'Connell B. The total thermal insulation of the newborn baby. J Physiol 1970;207:683.
11. Adamsons K, Gandy GM, James LS. The influence of thermal factors upon oxygen consumption of the newborn human infant. J Pediatr 1965;66:495.
12. Scopes JW. Metabolic rate and temperature control in the human baby. Br Med Bull 1966;22:88.
13. Hull D. Brown adipose tissue. Br Med Bull 1966;22:92.
14. Karlberg P, Moore RE, Oliver TK. The thermogenic response of the newborn infant to noradrenaline. Acta Paediatr Scand 1962;51:284.
15. Hardman MJ, Hey EN, Hull D. The effect of prolonged cold exposure on heat production in newborn rabbits. J Physiol 1969;205:39.
16. Foster KG, Hey EN, Katz G. The response of the sweat glands of the newborn baby to thermal stimuli and to intradermal acetylcholine. J Physiol 1969;203:13.
17. Hey EN, Katz G. Evaporative water loss in the newborn baby. J Physiol 1968;200:605.
18. Hammarlund K, Sedin G. Transepidermal water loss in newborn infants. III. Relation to gestational age. Acta Paediatr Scand 1979;68:795.
19. Rutter N, Hull D. Water loss from the skin of term and preterm babies. Arch Dis Child 1979;54:858.
20. Hey E. The care of babies in incubators. In Hull D, Gairdner D, eds. Recent advances in paediatrics. London: Churchill-Livingston, 1971:171.
21. Okken A, Blihjan C, Franz W, Bohn E. Effects of forced convection of heated air on insensible water loss and heat loss in preterm babies in incubators. J Pediatr 1982;101:108.
22. Thompson MH, Stothers JK, McLellan NJ. Weight and water loss in the neonate in natural and forced convection. Arch Dis Child 1984;59:951.
23. Saner PJJ, Dane HJ, Visser HK. Influence of variations in the ambient humidity on insensible water loss and thermoneutral environment of low birth weight babies. Acta Paediatr Scand 1984;73:615.
24. Hey EN, Mount LE. Heat losses from babies in incubators. Arch Dis Child 1967;42:75.
25. Wheldon AC, Rutter N. The heat balance of small babies nursed in incubators and under radiant warmers. Early Hum Dev 1982;6:131.
26. Hey EN, Mount LE. Temperature control in incubators. Lancet 1966;2:202.
27. Hey EN. Thermal neutrality. Br Med Bull 1975;31:69.
28. Bell FE, Weinstein MR, Oh W. Heat balance in premature infants: comparative effect of convectively heated incubator and radiant warmer, with and without plastic heat shield. J Pediatr 1980;96:460.
29. Sauer PJJ, Dane HJ, Visser HKA. New standards for neutral thermal environment of healthy very low birthweight infants in week one of life. Arch Dis Child 1984;59:18.
30. Hey EN, O'Connell B. Oxygen consumption and heat balance in the cot-nursed baby. Arch Dis Child 1970;45:241.
31. Rutter N, Brown SM, Hull D. Variation in the resting oxygen consumption of small babies. Arch Dis Child 1978;51:34.
32. Ducker DA, Lyon AJ, Ross Russell R, Bass CA, McInvosh N. Incubator temperature control: effect on the very low birthweight infant. Arch Dis Child 1985;60:902.
33. Belgaunkar TK, Scott KE. Effects of low humidity on small premature infants in servo-controlled incubators. I. Decrease in rectal temperature. Biol Neonate 1975;26:337.
34. Harpin VA, Rutter N. Humidification of incubators. Arch Dis Child 1985;60:219.
35. Silverman WA, Fertig JW, Berger AP. The influence of the thermal trial of non-thermal effect of atmospheric humidity on survival of infants of low birth weight. Pediatrics 1963;31:719.
36. Fanaroff AA, Wald M, Gruber HS, Klaus MH. Insensible water loss in low birth weight infants. Pediatrics 1972;50:236.
37. Oh W, Yao AC, Hansen JS, Lind J. Peripheral circulatory response to phototherapy in newborn infants. Acta Paediatr Scand 1973;62:49.
38. Oh W, Karecki H. Phototherapy and insensible water loss in the newborn infant. Am J Dis Child 1972;124:230.
39. Wu PYK, Moosa A. Effect of phototherapy on nitrogen and electrolyte levels and water balance in jaundiced preterm infants. Pediatrics 1978;61:193.
40. Wu PYK, Hodgman JE. Insensible water loss in preterm infants: changes with postnatal development and non-ionizing radiant energy. Pediatrics 1974;54:504.
41. Bell EF, Neidich GA, Cashore WJ, Oh W. Combined effect of radiant warmer and phototherapy on insensible water loss in low birth weight infants. J Pediatr 1979;94:810.
42. Bell EF, Warburton D, Stonestreet BS, Oh W. Effect of fluid administration on the development of symptomatic patent ductus arteriosus and congestive heart failure in premature infants. N Engl J Med 1980;302:598.
43. Bell EF, Warburn, D, Stonestreet BS, Oh W. High-volume fluid intake predisposes premature infants to necrotizing enterocolitis. Lancet 1979;2:90.
44. Baumgart S, Fox WW, Polin RA. Physiologic implications of

two different heat shields for infants under radiant warmers. J Pediatr 1982;100:787.
45. Sinclair JC. Management of the thermal environment. In Sinclair JC, Bracker MB, eds. Effective care of the newborn infant. Oxford: Oxford University Press, 1992.
46. Levison H, Linsao L, Swyer PR. A comparison of infra-red and convective heating for newborn infants. Lancet 1966;2:1346.
47. Mann TP. Hypothermia in the newborn. In Simpson K, ed. Modern trends in forensic medicine. London: Butterworths, 1966.
48. Silverman WA, Fertig JW, Berger AP. The influence of the thermal environment upon the survival of newly born premature infants. Pediatrics 1958;22:876.
49. Jolly H, Molyneaux P, Newell DJ. A controlled study of the effect of temperature on premature babies. J Pediatr 1962; 60:889.
50. Day RL, Caliguiri L, Kamenski C, Ehrlich F. Body temperature and survival of premature infants. Pediatrics 1964;34:171.
51. Buetow KC, Klein SW. Effects of maintenance of "normal" skin temperature of survival of infants of low birth weight. Pediatrics 1964;34:163.
52. Perlsven PH, Edwards NK, Alberto HD, Sutherland JM. Computer-assisted newborn inensive care. Pediatrics 1976; 57:494.
53. Mok Q, Bass CA, Ducker DA, McIntosh N. Temperature instability during nursing procedures in preterm infants. Arch Dis Child 1991;66:783.
54. Sarman I. Thermal responses and heat rates of low-birthweight premature babies during daily care on a heated water-filled mattress. Acta Paediatr 1992;81:15.
55. Sarman I, Tunell R. Providing warmth for preterm babies by a heated, water-filled mattress. Arch Dis Child 1989;64:29.
56. Hull J, Hull D. Behavioral thermoregulation in newborn rabbits. J Comp Physiol Psychol 1982;96:143.
57. Daily WJR, Klaus M, Meyer HBP. Apnea in premature infants: monitoring, incidence, heat rate changes and an effect of environmental temperature. Pediatrics 1969;43:510.
58. Auliciems A. Classroom performance as a function of thermal comfort. Int J Biometeorol 1972;16:233.
59. Glass L, Silverman WA, Sinclair JC. Relationship of thermal environment and calories intake to growth and resting metabolism in the late neonatal period. Biol Neonate 1969;14:324.
60. Glass L, Silverman WA, Sinclair JC. Effect of the thermal environment on cold resistance and growth of small infants after the first week of life. Pediatrics 1968;41:1033.
61. Dahm LS, James LS. Newborn temperature and calculated heat losses in the delivery room. Pediatrics 1972;49:504.
62. Stephenson JM, Du JN, Oliver TK. The effect of cooling on blood gas tension in newborn infants. J Pediatr 1970;76:848.
63. Gandy GM, Adamsons K, Cunningham N, et al. Thermal environment and acid-base homeostasis in human infants during the first few hours of life. J Clin Invest 1974;43:751.
64. Fardig JA. A comparison of skin-to-skin contact and radiant heaters in promoting neonatal thermoregulation. J Nurse Midwifery 1980;25:19.
65. Mayfield SR, Bhatia J, Nakamura KT, et al. Temperature measurement in term and preterm neonates. J Pediatr 1984; 104:271.
66. Keeley D. Taking infant's temperatures: forget the axilla—the rectum is better. Br Med J 1992;931:304.

Part Four

THE LOW-BIRTH-WEIGHT INFANT

Neonatology: Pathophysiology and Management of the Newborn, Fourth Edition,
edited by Gordon B. Avery, Mary Ann Fletcher, and Mhairi G. MacDonald.
J.B. Lippincott Company, Philadelphia © 1994.

chapter 26

The Small-for-Gestational-Age Infant

DENNIS T. CROUSE
GEORGE CASSADY

Nature is but a name for an effect.[1]

References to undergrown babies have appeared in the literature since the 1940s.[2] Söderling warned that maturity may not be judged properly by birth weight and observed that some low-birth-weight (LBW) infants were more advanced in motor ability, reflexes, alertness, and appetite than other infants of similar birth weight.[3] He suggested the need for different neonatal management for these "pseudopremature" infants.[3] In the 1960s, Gruenwald called attention to this common neonatal problem.[4–9] Reports that followed have employed a bewildering variety of terms to designate the fetus whose growth is impaired; these include pseudopremature, small-for-dates, dysmature, fetal-malnourished, chronic fetal distress, intrauterine growth-retarded (IUGR), hypotrophic, and small-for-gestational-age (SGA). The latter term is employed in this chapter.

CLASSIFICATION

A uniform definition of SGA has not emerged despite countless reports on this topic. The ideal definition would identify infants who are truly growth retarded and at risk for increased morbidity and mortality and exclude infants who have reached their genetic growth potential and are not at increased risk. The definition should contain three major components. First, the population studied should be defined in terms of race, gender, altitude, and genetic growth potential, among other demographic variables. Second, the growth variable measured should be clearly defined and reproducible (*i.e.*, birth weight, length, ponderal index [PI], head circumference [HC], length/HC). Third, the limits of normality in the population for the variable studied should be described in detail. Abnormal growth would be defined as that which is below these limits.

Historically, studies use arbitrary statistical limits based on population means (*e.g.*, <10th percentile, <3rd percentile, >2 SD below the mean) to define abnormal growth. However, 7% of the infants defined as abnormal by a 10% weight cutoff would be defined as normal by using less than 2 SD as the cutoff (*i.e.*, 2 SD below the mean corresponds to approximately 2.5%). This definition should be proven in a prospective trial to identify infants who are growth retarded and at risk. Most studies on this topic suffer from one or more major flaws in these requirements. For example, Lubchenco and colleagues define any infant whose birth weight is at the 10th percentile or less for his or her gestational age as SGA.[10] These Denver intrauterine growth curves were constructed with data from only Caucasian infants born at high altitude; use of the curves seldom takes into account the gender of the infant. Gruenwald, however, defines as SGA any infant whose birth weight is more than 2 SD below the mean for any given week of gestation, corresponding approximately to the third percentile on the intrauterine growth curves.[4–6] Although the data of Freeman and associates allow definition of such factors as race and gender, problems of population selection limit clinical use of these data.[11] These are only three examples from many studies that affect the correlation of birth weight with duration of gestation.

The minimal and maximal values for the 10th percentile of various studies that describe normal birth weight curves are presented in Figure 26-1.[12–24] Tenth percentile weights for Caucasian males from the Freeman data are presented for comparison.[11] Goldenberg and colleagues reviewed the literature and reported not only the difference in the birth weight values for the 10th percentile, but that the difference varied by gender.[25] This diversity underscores the uncertainty of the basic premise on which much of the presumed knowledge of the SGA infant is based.

Excluded from most studies are infants who have not reached their genetic growth potential but who are above these arbitrary statistical limits. For example, infants who have the potential to be large may manifest fetal wasting because of intrauterine events, but their weights may fall within the limits of normal. This group of infants would not be noticed as abnormal by the usual criteria. Some investigators have tried to make a distinction between the subset of infants who are SGA and the larger group of infants who have not reached their genetic growth potential. The latter infants are described as having IUGR; this group includes infants who are SGA and infants whose growth parameters are within the normal range but who have not reached their growth potential. The number of infants described as growth retarded would greatly increase if IUGR was used as the definition.

Premature infants present a perplexing problem in classification—they are not normal by virtue of their premature birth. Current data suggest that these infants are more likely to be undergrown than their unborn peers. As many as one-third may be SGA.[26,27] Normal intrauterine growth curves constructed with data from these infants may not be normal at all.

Birth weight below the 10th percentile is the usual criterion for defining SGA. This definition includes infants whose birth weight is below the 10th percentile due to fetal malnutrition or other intrauterine events, but it also includes infants who have reached their genetic growth potential, are normal, and happen to be lighter than 90% of the population. Ponderal index (PI = birth weight × 100/length^3) is another parameter that has been proposed to describe abnormal growth. The advantage of the PI is that race, gender, and gestational age do not affect the ratio for full-term infants. Use of the PI and birth weight define two populations: those who show growth impairment of both length and weight (*i.e.*, symmetric SGA), and those who show sparing of length and head growth with decreased weight (*i.e.*, asymmetric SGA). Timing of the insult is inherent in these descriptive terms, because symmetric growth retardation suggests an insult early in gestation, when cell division is predominate. The opposite is true for asymmetric growth retardation. Although the PI defines both symmetric and asymmetric growth retarded infants, sound pathophysiologic evidence is lacking to explain this finding.[28,29] We previously proposed that this might be an oversimplification of fetal growth and that more data were needed before this concept could be embraced. Data from Kramer and colleagues show that our skepticism was warranted; they studied 8719 neonates and found that a bimodal distribution of birth weight in growth-retarded infants was not present and that growth retardation was a continuum.[30] These researchers cautioned that their data applied to developed countries and that additional data are needed for developing

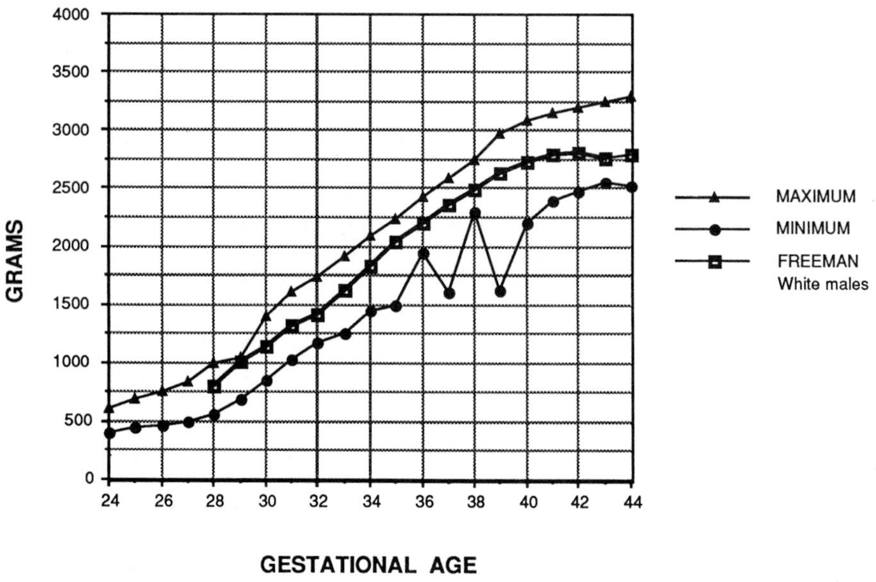

FIG. 26–1. Maximal and minimal values for the 10th percentile from pooled data describing normal birth weight curves. The 10th percentile from the Freeman birth weight curves is presented for comparison.

countries. Although these general views are eloquently expressed, currently popular, and logical on the surface, they still await scientific proof.[28,31,32]

The current definition of SGA is imprecise, and much work is needed if the complex issues that surround abnormal intrauterine growth are to be understood. Future studies cannot continue to perpetuate the design flaws of past work. A better definition of abnormal growth is needed if knowledge on which to base future therapies is to be abstracted from afflicted infants. Unfortunately, this becomes a circular argument; a better definition of abnormal fetal growth is needed to gain more knowledge about pathophysiology and morbidity, but a better understanding of the abnormal growth process is needed to construct a more specific definition.

INCIDENCE AND SIGNIFICANCE

Reports from developed Western nations indicate that about one-third of all infants with birth weights of less than 2500 g (*i.e.*, LBW) are not truly premature but are instead SGA. Evidence from developing countries suggests that a much higher proportion of their LBW babies may be SGA and that much of the variance in LBW rates may be due to population differences in the incidence of impaired fetal growth.[33] Evidence from developing countries over time also demonstrates that the incidence of SGA decreases as a country becomes more developed.[34] Caution must be used in interpretation of these reports because techniques for determining gestational age and fetal growth have changed over the same interval.

Smallness-for-gestational-age is second only to prematurity as a cause of perinatal death. Among preterm infants, the neonatal mortality is higher, but among SGA babies, there is a vastly increased fetal death rate. Risk of neonatal death is less for an SGA baby than for an appropriate-for-gestational-age (AGA) baby of similar weight but is greater than that for the normally grown baby of comparable gestational age. The major cause of death identified in most studies is asphyxia.[35] If the SGA baby lives, the quality of life may be compromised. The extrauterine growth rate may be slower, and catch-up growth may never occur.[36] Congenital anomalies occur more commonly, and suboptimal neurodevelopmental and physical growth has been found.

DIAGNOSIS

FETAL DIAGNOSIS

Multiple methods have been proposed in the search for early and precise diagnosis of impaired fetal growth. Retrospective methods or prospective studies with historic controls predominate but prospective trials are becoming more common in evaluating diagnostic methods for SGA. Diagnostic methods that have been described as useful range from maternal historic or clinical factors, through indicators of fetal well being, to ultrasound examination of fetal size and uteroplacental, or fetal blood flow. It is not surprising that the usefulness of these methods is uncertain and varies widely from one report to another.

Clinical assessment of risk factors in the maternal or pregnancy history may be useful in as few as one-third or as many as two-thirds of these cases.[37,38] History of maternal renovascular disease, multiple pregnancy, or previous SGA births accounts for most of these successful predictions. Such simple clinical methods as manual estimation of fetal weight, maternal assessment of fetal activity, and serial measurement of fundal height are lauded by some but condemned by others.[39–48] Physical examination of fundal height, the simplest of these screens, has a range of sensitivity of 56% in low-risk populations to 76% in high-risk populations.

Fetal heart rate monitoring is an example of clinical methodology that requires more expertise than the previously described tests. Late decelerations, absent short-term variability or intermittent variable decelerations that overshoot, decreased amplitude and frequency of accelerations or decelerations, nonstress Cardiff scoring more than 4, and decreased duration of accelerations and long-term variability in response to acoustic stimulation have been associated with growth retardation.[49–53]

The multiple biochemical indices and biophysical tests of fetoplacental function that have been proposed are summarized in Table 26-1, accompanied by calculated sensitivities and specificities.[54–78] Of particular interest are changes in amniotic fluid composition that may predict SGA. Presence of phosphatidylglycerol or a mature foam-stability test, despite a small fetus by ultrasonographic measurement, has been 80% to 100% diagnostic of SGA in several studies.[79–82] Amniotic fluid catecholamines are altered with SGA.[83] Low levels of C-peptide are associated with impaired fetal growth.[84] Measurement of amniotic fluid hydroxyproline as an index of fetal collagen turnover and growth activity makes physiologic sense, but it remains to be clinically proved.[85–87]

Studies of maternal blood and urine are easy and present a small risk to the mother and infant. Maternal serum α-fetoprotein is probably the most studied. Although many studies associate elevated serum levels of α-fetoprotein with growth retardation, few studies give information about the predictive value of this test.[78–90] Salafia and colleagues associated elevated maternal serum α-fetoprotein levels with growth retardation only when placental findings of chronic villitis or vascular changes were present.[91] Significantly lower serum cortisol levels are found in mothers who subsequently delivered SGA infants.[92] Unfortunately, the predictive value cannot be adequately ascertained because of multiple sampling on

TABLE 26–1
ESTIMATES OF DIAGNOSTIC UTILITY FOR SELECTED TESTS TO PREDICT SMALL-FOR-GESTATIONAL-AGE INFANTS BEFORE BIRTH

Reference	Measurement	Sensitivity (%)	Specificity (%)	Positive Predictive Values (%)	Negative Predictive Values (%)	Number of Patients	Number of SGA Patients (%)
43	Fundal height	56	85	21	96	753	7
44	Fundal height	73	79	60	88	138	30
45	Fundal height	36–76	60–94	20–41	60–94	381	12
46	Examination and history	50				226	100
47	Physical score	100	96	34	100	611	2
59	Nonstress test	52		50	81	102	26
57	Human placental lactogen	33				46	20
59	Human placental lactogen	55–70		45–50	85–86	102	26
60	Human placental lactogen	29–50	77–91	19–27	92–93	527	10
59	Serum estriol	70–75		29–38	79–86	102	26
59	Human placental lactogen and estriol	84		44	93	102	26
61	Glucose tolerance test	14–56	89	14–45	89–92	122	18
62	Glucose tolerance test	100	71	30	100	55	11
53	Glycoproteins	67	87	50	93	91	16
57	Glycoproteins	22				46	20
56	Cystyl aminopeptidase	82	71	72	81	186	48
57	Placental proteins	67				46	20
63	α-Fetoprotein	100		27		137	27
76	Dehydroepiandrosterone sulfate	95	93	76	99	102	20
77	Factor VIII	67	92	86	79	21	43
77	Amniotic fluid phosphatidylglycerol	77–93	28–52	49–55	75–84	99	43
81	Amniotic fluid phosphatidylglycerol	64	71	60	74	82	40
82	Amniotic fluid 3-methyl histidine	87	85	76	92	42	36
78	α-Fetoprotein	11	99	23	98	7049	12

SGA, small-for-gestational-age.

the same patients. Decreased amounts of urinary epidermal growth factor (EGF) has been identified in women who deliver SGA babies.[93] Although EGF is a mitogen for tissues of ectodermal and mesodermal origin, it is still speculative to equate decreased urinary amounts with fetal growth retardation.

Maternal hematologic abnormalities are found in women who deliver SGA infants. Decreased RNA polymerase content, impaired activation of fructose-1,6-phosphate, low levels of ATP, diminished levels of pyruvic and adenylic kinase, altered pyruvic kinase kinetics, and increased protein–DNA ratio are seen in leukocytes.[94–99] Many of these findings are present in fetal leukocytes and suggest diminished energy capacity.[94,95] Maternal monocytic changes also occur.[100] Plasminogen activator inhibitor type 2 is significantly decreased in normotensive and hypertensive women with growth-retarded infants.[101] Decreased levels of complement in maternal sera have been associated with placental lesions and SGA infants.[102] This evidence suggests that derangements of the maternal immune system may play a role in some cases of growth retardation presumably by adversely affecting the placenta.

Fetal blood has become more easily accessible with the advent of high-quality ultrasonography.[103] Some investigators advocate fetal blood sampling to measure *p*H, oxygen saturation, and lactate levels to detect fetal distress in infants with growth retardation, but others refute the utility of this effort.[104–106] Elevated lactate levels are found in maternal and umbilical arterial and venous blood samples at delivery from pregnancies that result in SGA infants.[107] The fetomaternal ratio and fetal plasma concentration of essential amino acids are decreased in growth-retarded infants, and this decrease is directly correlated with the degree of fetal hypoxemia.[108] The fetomaternal glucose ratio is increased.[109] Infusion of glucose into the umbilical vein of normally grown fetuses stimulates release of fetal insulin and a quick return of the fetal blood glucose to normal, but insulin is not released and the glucose remains elevated for a longer period of time in SGA infants.[110]

The most significant changes in the diagnosis of

growth retardation have come in the field of ultrasonography. The single most significant factor is the accuracy with which gestational age can be determined. Second-trimester ultrasonography is more reliable than neonatal dating by Dubowitz or Ballard scoring, and the results approximate gestational age determinations by reliable last menstrual date.[111] Fetal body growth parameters have been studied including biparietal diameter (BPD), HC and head area, abdominal circumference (AC) and area, trunk circumference and area, crown–rump lengths, femur length, and PI, as have fetal organ development (*e.g.*, liver, adrenal, cerebellum, kidney, distal femoral epiphyseal ossification center) and other physiologic parameters (*e.g.*, fetal blood flow, pulsatility of various fetal or umbilical vessels, cardiac output, fetal breathing movements). Changes in these parameters have been claimed to be useful in detection of impaired fetal growth.[112–145] Placental grading and amniotic fluid volume have been shown to have predictive value.[146,147] A combination of these measurements (*i.e.*, fetal growth profiles or fetal biometry) provides additional clues to body proportions and asymmetry of growth.[148,149] Most positive predictive values (PPV) for single determinants range from 17% for placenta grade to approximately 50% for BPD.[59,121,150] The PPV increases slightly when multiple determinants are used. The HC–AC ratio has a PPV greater than 50%.[151] Bergsjø and colleagues found that AC is strongly correlated to birth weight, but that a model that uses multiple parameters is a better predictor of SGA.[152] Benson and associates reported a combination of clinical and ultrasound data with a PPV of 82%.[153] Data from studies that used multiple physical measurements to determine fetal growth are listed in Table 26-2.[154–159]

Doppler studies of fetal or umbilical vessels are reported to be more predictive of growth retardation than physical growth parameters.[160,161] Increased systolic–diastolic ratios, absence of diastolic notch, and decreased or absent blood velocity are characteristics of flow that are associated with SGA infants.[160–167] Vessels studied include the fetal umbilical artery and vein, thoracic and abdominal aorta, pulmonary artery, cerebral arteries, internal carotid arteries, renal arteries, femoral and external iliac arteries, and maternal uterine arteries.[160–175] Predictive values of selected Doppler studies are presented in Table 26-3. An additional advantage of these methods is that the well-being of the fetus can be assessed and emergent interventions can be executed if the fetus is in extreme distress.[187,188]

Prenatal fetal ultrasound scans do have significant technologic problems. Fetal measurements may be altered if the fetus is compressed due to prolonged ruptured fetal membranes and oligohydramnios.[189] The tendency to embrace new technology should be avoided in the absence of definitive evidence of their superiority to standard methods.[190] For example, Cnattingius and colleagues demonstrated that the clinical utility of symphysial–fundal height measurements were better than the newer ultrasound BPD measurements.[191]

Several questions remain unanswered. At what gestational age should an ultrasound be performed? Should multiple exams be done? Warsof and associates suggest that 34 weeks, ±1 week, is the optimal time for routine screening.[192] Other investigators decree that earlier ultrasound examinations should be the rule.[193] What should gestational dating depend on, because gestational age dating becomes more inaccurate in the third trimester? Who should be screened? One-third of SGA infants are born to mothers with no identifiable risk factors. At what price—in dollars, facilities, and maternal inconvenience—is routine screening feasible? It is customary to screen private-paying patients for gestational age dating and for fetal gender determination, although these patients are not usually in the high-risk group.[194] Ringa and colleagues reviewed the literature and eloquently showed that most studies do not address whether ultrasound use affects fetal or maternal health.[195] Prospective, blinded, randomized studies are sorely needed.

NEONATAL DIAGNOSIS

Reduced birth weight for gestational age (*i.e.*, light-for-dates infants) is the simplest and oldest method of diagnosis; wasted or disproportionate growth, even if birth weight is within the range of normal, may be an important clue to disturbed fetal growth. Soft tissue wasting, diminished skin-fold thickness, decreased breast tissue, and reduced thigh circumference suggest recent wasting and are useful measurements for neonatal diagnosis.[196–201] Widened skull sutures with large fontanelles; shortened foot, femoral, and crown–heel length; and delayed development of epiphyses suggest longer-term failures in bone growth.[202–204] Head circumference may be reduced in some infants.[205]

Combinations of measurements, such as weight and HC, crown–heel length and HC, birth weight and crown–heel length, midarm circumference and HC, and midarm circumference and occipitofrontal circumference are being used more frequently to assess disproportionate patterns of fetal growth.[206–208] The height–weight ratio (*i.e.*, PI) is particularly popular. In full-term infants 48.5 or more cm in length, this ratio is not affected by race, gender, or gestational age. In preterm infants, it is affected by gestational age because of variations in soft tissue mass, especially fat. The term baby normally has a PI greater than 2.32.[209] Careful attention to these physical measures of the quality of fetal growth seems certain to expand knowledge of this condition.

Care must be exercised if Dubowitz or Ballard gestational screening is used. These screens consistently overestimate the gestational age in preterm infants by as much as 2 to 3 weeks.[111] Small errors in gestational

TABLE 26–2
ESTIMATES OF DIAGNOSTIC UTILITY OF ULTRASONOGRAPHY TO PREDICT SMALL-FOR-GESTATIONAL-AGE INFANTS BEFORE BIRTH

Reference	Measurement	Sensitivity (%)	Specificity (%)	Positive Predictive Values (%)	Negative Predictive Values (%)	Number of Patients	Number of SGA Patients (%)
114	CRL × TA	94	88			474	8
	HA–TA	44	91				
115	CRL × TA	100	78	71	100	21	71
113	BPD + AC	97				260	100
59	BPD + HPL	85		43	92	102	26
	BPD + estriol	85		37	90		
	BPD + estriol + HPL	95		40	96		
	BPD + estriol + HPL	50		93	86		
	BPD + NST	75		100	98		
79	BPD + PG	80	80	49	94	249	20
80	BPD + foam stability	100	86	84	100	38	42
		75	40	25	86	19	21
		80	40	42	79	57	35
118	BPD + AC	77	78	16	98	505	5
		83	78	17	99	441	5
		88	47	25	95	103	17
		82	66	33	95		
		82	84	50	96		
112	FL–AC	61				361	
138	FL–AC	70	64	18	95	322	10
		56	74	19	94		
141	FL–AC	47		23	89	204	15
	EFW	77		61	96		
142	DFEOC	97	83	71	99	226	8
143	FL–AC	30	91	14	96	1502	5
146	Com Bio	86	89	75	93	200	11
154	Fetal PI	77	82	36	96	113	12
155	FL–AC	27	66	60		101	66
	HC–AC	53	77	24			
	Chervenak score > 3	50	80	83			
	Antenatal IUGR score	66	49	49			
156	Bio + M-hyperox	56	94	83	80	52	35
157	FL–AC	53	73	22	92	121	12
	HC–AC	17	92	11	95		
	EFW	53	85	38	92		
158	IUGR score	75	98	86	97	356	11
159	Clinical score + BPD + TAD	61	98	62	98	1122	6

AC, abdominal circumference; Bio + M-Hyperox, biophysical profile with maternal hyperoxia; BPD, biparietal diameter; Com bio, computerized biophysical profile; CRL, crown–rump length; DFEOC, distal femoral extremity ossification center; EFW, estimated fetal length; FL, femur length; HA, head area; HPL, human placental lactogen; IUGR, intrauterine growth retarded; NST, nonstress test; PI, ponderal index; PG, phosphatidylglycerol; TA, trunk area; TAD, transverse abdominal diameter.

age determinations can have significant effects on SGA identification. Growth indices that are independent of gestational age are of particular interest for the diagnosis of growth retardation in preterm babies. Yogman and associates described the use of different reference standards (*i.e.*, gestational age relative to birth length, length for birth weight, and weight for HC) to diagnose alterations of growth in preterm infants.[210] Use of these indices reduced the variance between individual growth parameters and the differences seen with race.

Other neonatal or placental abnormalities may be identified that help in the diagnosis of growth retardation. Increased cardiothoracic ratio on a chest radiograph is associated with delayed growth in preterm infants.[211] Increased nucleated erythrocyte counts and ratios of elevated nucleated erythrocyte counts per 100 leukocytes are found in very-low-birth-weight infants who are SGA.[212] Placental pathologic analysis is helpful in determining the cause of growth retardation, especially in normotensive mothers.[213]

TABLE 26–3
ESTIMATES OF DIAGNOSTIC UTILITY OF DOPPLER TO PREDICT SMALL-FOR-GESTATIONAL-AGE INFANTS BEFORE BIRTH

Reference	Measurement	Sensitivity (%)	Specificity (%)	Positive Predictive Values (%)	Negative Predictive Values (%)	Number of Patients	Number of SGA Patients (%)
160	UA S–D	83	87	74	92	350	39
		79	93	83	91		
161	UA PI	76	100	100	55	53	79
	IC PI	79	91	97	56		
	UA/IC PI	84	91	97	63		
163	UA S–D	90	100	100	92	22	41
164	UTA S–D	81	90	86	86	71	20
	UTA notch	87	95	93	91		
169	Fetal aorta PI	50	97	93	69	159	47
176	UA PI	58	84	79	65	139	20
	UA BFC	89	58	35	96		
	Fetal aorta PI	40	87	76	57		
	Fetal aorta BFC	87	61	46	93		
177	Fetal aorta AEDF	73		85		608	
178	UTA S–D	66	64	45	81	68	31
	UA S–D	71	93	83	90		
	UTA + UA S–D	75	100	100	86		
179	Uteroplacental art RI	27	88	22	94	129	3
		18	90	19	90	157	1
180	UA S–D	55	90	77	77	48	38
	UA S–D + AC	44	90	73	73		
181	Uterplacental art RI	71		33		93	18
		56		29		43	21
182	UA S–D	29	74	11	91	518	10
		11	96	17	93	268	7
		19	96	30	92	470	9
		17	95	23	93	445	8
	Uteroplacental art	6	95	13	90	501	10
		6	92	5	93	254	7
		7	96	15	12	459	10
		9	96	16	92	432	8
183	UA S–D	50	87	38	92	146	47
184	UA S–D	45	89	58		168	25
	UA S–D + EFW	86	77	56			
185	UA S–D	49	94	81	77	127	35
	UA S–D + (AFV or FL–AC)	64	85	75	81		
186	UA S–D + NST	24	100	100	83	1000	25
	UA S–D + AFV	31	100	100	80		

AC, abdominal circumference; ADEF, absent end-diastolic flow; AFV, amniotic fluid volume; artery, art; BFC, blood flow class, EFW, estimated fetal length; FL, femur length; IC, internal carotid; NST, nonstress test; RI, resistive index; S–D, systolic–diastolic ratio; PI, pulsatility index; UA, umbilical artery; UTA, uterine artery.

CAUSES

Growth in the intrauterine environment can be divided into two time periods. The first one-half of gestation is characterized by cell proliferation and differentiation of a single cell to an intact fetus with complete organ systems. The second one-half of gestation is characterized by growth and the acquisition of body fat stores. Normal intrauterine growth for body weight, length, and specific organ weights progresses in an exponential fashion until about 34 weeks of gestation.[214] Thereafter, fetal growth and placental growth depart from this pattern.[215] During the first one-half of gestation, if there is a surfeit of nutrients from the placenta, fetal growth is limited in most instances by the inherent growth potential of the fetus. In the latter one-half of gestation, fetal growth is more influenced by limitations in nutrient support the fetus receives through the placenta. Two major factors influence fetal growth: the growth potential of the fetus and the nutrient support it receives from the mother.[216] Selected factors suggested to cause or accompany impaired fetal growth are shown in Figure 26-2.

ALTERED GROWTH POTENTIAL

Current writing continues to ignore the extraordinary variations in birth weight observed between populations. The classic study by Meredith reviews these data in detail and brings to attention the fact that mean birth weights may vary from 2400 g in New Guinea to 3800 g in the West Indies.[217] Even within the United States, the incidence of infants who are SGA varies greatly.[218] Of particular interest are data that demonstrate striking ethnic differences in birth weight, regardless of socioeconomic status or geographic location.[217–221] Whether these variations are the consequence of genetic factors or the mothers' own previous intrauterine experiences is unclear.[222,223] However, racial, ethnic, and population differences in expected birth weights at a given gestational age are considerable.

Retardation of growth *in utero* may be caused by factors inherent in the fetus itself. Subnormal embryonic growth may then be viewed as a form of maldevelopment. Examples include several genetically determined dwarfs, many chromosomal syndromes, certain sets of congenital anomalies and dysmorphic syndromes, some inborn errors of metabolism, and most fetal infections.[224–232] Susceptibility to the devastating effects of congenital infections and other teratogens is at its peak during the first 20 weeks of gestation because of the rapid cell proliferation and differentiation.[214] In some of these forms of SGA, reduced cell number has been demonstrated. These cruel experiments of nature provide us with several clues about fetal growth processes. For example, retarded fetal growth in the infant with intestinal or central nervous system anomalies—both of which preclude normal fetal swallowing—suggests that amniotic fluid is a very important source of nutrients.[215,233] The interrelations between impaired and abnormal fetal growth are complex, and differentiating between the two becomes more difficult as more is learned.[234]

Some fetuses may be destined to be small because of genetically determined maternal factors. For example, mothers who were SGA at birth are at a higher risk of delivering infants who are SGA.[235] Mothers who have delivered a previous SGA infant are at a higher risk of delivering a second growth-retarded infant.[236] These infants are at a significantly lower risk of sequelae than SGA infants born to mothers who delivered infants who were AGA.[236] These data suggest that some infants have a predetermined slower rate of growth and are otherwise normal, rather than having an abnormal growth rate due to maldevelopment, infections, or teratogens. More data are needed before conclusions can be made about these infants who may have constitutional growth impairment.

Thyroid hormone, pituitary growth hormone, adrenal hormones, and prolactin play important roles in postnatal growth, but they appear to have little consequence in terms of fetal growth.[237] A provocative report by Sato and colleagues described two infants

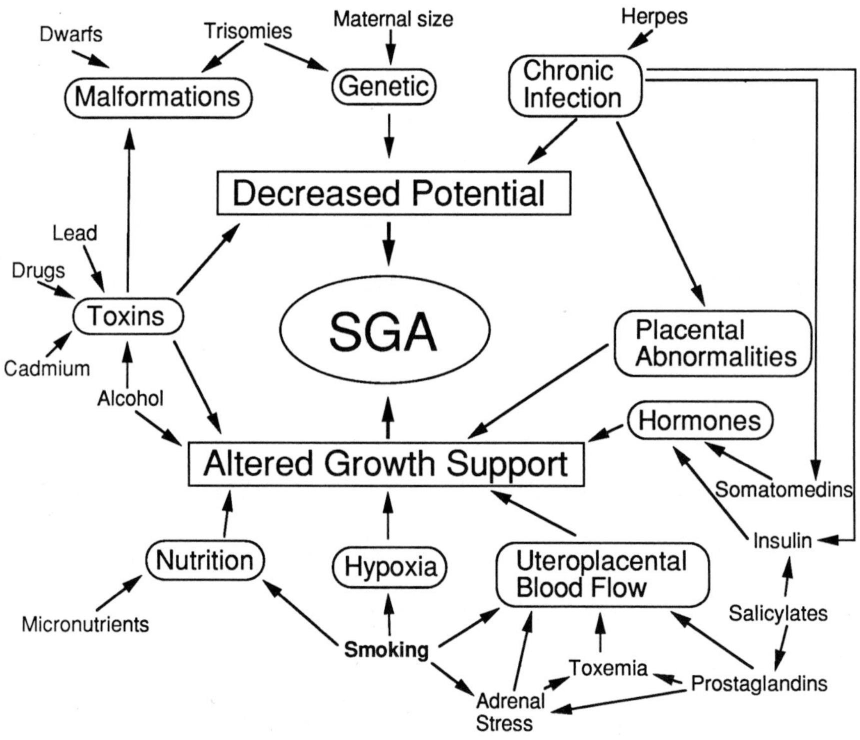

FIG. 26–2. Selected risk factors associated with impaired growth. (SGA, small for gestational age.)

who had growth retardation with subsequent short stature and hypothyrotropinemia with normal thyroid hormone levels.[238] These data suggest that thyroid-stimulating hormones may play a role in some instances of growth retardation. Elevated cortisol and 11-OH corticosteroids found at birth in SGA infants are probably related to prior fetal asphyxia.[239,240] The presence of profoundly impaired growth in infants with pancreatic agenesis provides a tantalizing glimpse of the importance of insulin in the growth process.[241] Some infants with insulin resistance caused by abnormalities in the quantity of insulin receptors have IUGR.[242] Although insulin affects fetal growth by an increase in glucose uptake and use and by an increase in fat synthesis and deposition, precise sequences for these events are poorly understood.

There is considerable evidence that insulin and insulinlike polypeptide hormones (*i.e.*, somatomedins) play a vital role in fetal growth.[241–250] The demonstration of somatomedins in placental tissue and cord blood provides even more convincing evidence of their involvement in fetal growth processes.[247–249] Moreover, reports of a significant relation between fetal levels of these substances and birth weight have led to speculation that disturbances in these substances, in their binding sites, or in their metabolism may be of considerable importance in the development of SGA infants.[248,250] Two somatomedins that have been associated with fetal growth are insulinlike growth factors-1 and -2 (IGF-1, IGF-2).[251,252] Fetal serum levels of IGF-1, but not IGF-2, are associated directly with fetal size.[253] Poor postnatal growth is associated with decreased levels of IGF-1.[254] The IGF-binding proteins have been found in placental tissue, suggesting a role for IGF in placental growth.[255] Human placental lactogen, which is diminished in some cases of growth retardation, stimulates the release of IGF-1 and IGF-2.[256,257] This area of study is likely to provide important clues about the regulation of fetal growth.

IMPAIRED SUPPORT FOR GROWTH

Adequacy of the nutrient supply line becomes the limiting factor during the third trimester. Multiple pregnancy is an example of a situation in which the fetus may have a normal growth potential but placental function becomes inadequate to meet the demands. Unrestricted growth of twins occurs until a cumulative weight of about 3000 g, and growth retardation begins at about 1500 g for each twin. The development of chronic fetal distress, with its attendant growth retardation, ultimately depends on the duration of intrauterine life beyond the capacity of the placenta to nurture. Placental insufficiency is recognized most often in post-term gestations, but it may occur at any time during gestation.

Maternal factors associated with subnormal birth weight include short stature, lower socioeconomic status, extremes of youth or age, primiparity or grandmultiparity, and low prepregnancy weight.[194] A metaanalysis of the literature between 1970 and 1984 demonstrates a host of factors that have a direct effect on fetal growth.[258] Although these factors, along with race, are usually accepted as interrelated in their affects on birth weight, Miller and associates provided convincing evidence that these variables alone do not produce an SGA infant.[259] There must be associated maternal behavioral problems, such as smoking, drug or alcohol abuse, or failure to seek available medical care. That these same factors may influence infant care after birth is suggested by evidence of "poor mothering" and other improper behavioral characteristics in some women who deliver SGA infants.[209,259] These observations suggest that growth impairment of the fetus in these circumstances may well be vulnerable to concerted maternal and medical interventions. The concept that maternal behavior during pregnancy may be a major factor in impaired fetal growth reshapes the view of the mother; rather than a passive conduit through which the ravages of disease and a hostile environment affect the fetus, she may be the cause of compromised fetal growth by her inappropriate actions or inactions.

The most commonly recognized associations with SGA are those that affect the fetus by way of the mother. Evidence that maternal actions can alter fetal growth is illustrated by the effects of maternal smoking. Maternal smoking profoundly hampers fetal growth, weight, length, and HC.[260–264] Deficient supply of nutrients or micronutrients has been proposed as causal, and caloric supplements have been suggested as useful.[265–267] Most information suggests little or no benefit from such therapy; in fact, there is recent convincing evidence for increased rather than decreased total caloric intake in smokers.[268–270] These observations suggest that complex factors of digestion, metabolism, or micronutrient and trace metal metabolism may be involved. Fetal hypoxia, carbon monoxide poisoning of hemoglobin, and vascular effects of nicotine have been proposed as causal factors in this association between maternal smoking and SGA fetuses.[271] The effects of smoking increase with age, because women older than 35 years of age who smoke have a significantly higher risk of having a growth-retarded or preterm infant compared with mothers who smoke and are 25 years of age or younger.[272] Although the exact sequence of events awaits precise definition, it is now certain that smoking is an important cause of impaired fetal growth. Equally important are observations that this cause is treatable; birth weights of babies born to smokers who abstained for the last one-half of pregnancy are essentially the same as those of babies whose mothers are nonsmokers.[273]

Impaired fetal growth has been linked to maternal therapeutic and recreational drug intake. Fetal growth retardation, microcephaly, intellectual deficiency, and altered facial features have been reported in as many as 1 of 10 infants exposed to hydantoin *in utero*.[274,275] Antimetabolites and alkylating agents may reduce birth weight.[276] The effects of narcotics are unfortunately common drug-related causes of SGA infants.[277–279] Current data suggest that 10% or more of women regularly abuse drugs during their pregnancy.[280] Cocaine is the most widely reported drug to have significant effects on fetal growth.[281–284] Some reports suggest that intrauterine cocaine exposure may be responsible for fetal anomalies by effecting fetal vascular disruption, but acceptance of this association awaits prospective data.[285–287] Maternal marijuana use is associated with SGA infants, possibly by causing fetal hypoxia.[284,288,289]

Alcohol is often abused but is more socially acceptable than narcotics.[290] In the United States, approximately 65% of fetuses are exposed to alcohol during gestation.[291] Although the harmful range remains uncertain, maternal alcohol intake during pregnancy has resulted in a consistent cluster of aberrations associated with markedly poor fetal growth, a condition called fetal alcohol syndrome.[290,292,293]

The effect of maternal nutrition during human pregnancy on birth weight of the fetus remains uncertain and highly controversial, despite a continual flow of published information on this topic. The emotional fervor with which this topic is discussed is puzzling, particularly in view of the serious flaws of experimental design that plague most available data on this subject.[263,294] War-related famines clearly affect birth weight.[295–298] During such calamities, however, poor nutrition is but one of many hurtful events; infertility and increased spontaneous abortions are the most common events. Birth weight is reduced only if starvation occurs during the last trimester of pregnancy. Infants born to mothers with anorexia nervosa show diminished weight gain during the third trimester, with catch-up growth occurring after birth.[299] Observations made during these studies confirm the concept of the fetus as a true parasite who lives well off maternal nutrient stores, despite serious decrements of maternal intake.

Controlled trials of nutritional supplementation during pregnancy have been reported.[300–302] In no study was clinically meaningful improvement in fetal weight found to follow maternal dietary intervention. Increase in fetal weights was modest but statistically significant in the studies from impoverished third-world countries; however, weights were unaltered and harmful effects possibly were observed in studies from the United States. The practical clinical value of even the higher weights is unclear, because the differences amount at most to a few ounces. In 1975, Sinclair and Saigal observed that "it is a central problem of perinatal medicine to know the relative contributions of heredity and environment to the variance in fetal growth rate, and among the environmental factors, to know the effect of maternal undernutrition."[303] The problem of clearly defining the weighted roles of nature and nurture in the SGA infant will remain unsolved until nonbiased studies of maternal nutrition and supplementation are performed.

An example of a well-meant social program that provides supplemental food to impoverished families to improve neonatal outcome is the Supplemental Feeding Program for Women, Infants, and Children (WIC) program in the United States. Graham stated in a review of this program, in regard to SGA infants, that "a significant role for undernutrition has never been established."[304] This program costs more than $3 billion each year without evidence of benefit. Programs such as this should not be instituted without hard evidence that they can be beneficial.

Disturbances in cation or trace metal metabolism have been found to accompany impaired fetal growth. Zinc depletion of maternal tissues, as assessed by leukocyte Zn levels, is related to poor fetal growth.[305,306] Certain data link zinc metabolism to fetal and neonatal growth, but whether this is a cause or effect is unclear.[307–310] Plasma copper levels have been found to be lower in SGA infants, perhaps because of diminished hepatic synthesis of ceruloplasmin. This suggests that hypocupremia is a consequence rather than a cause of SGA infants, as does the absence of the usual erythrocyte changes that accompany copper deficiency. In support of this skepticism is the observation that tissue copper content, which is independent of blood ceruloplasmin levels, is normal in SGA babies.[311] Increased maternal cadmium levels have been associated with impaired fetal growth in animals; levels are high in pregnant women who smoke, who give birth more commonly to SGA babies.[312,313] Hypocalcemia is common in SGA babies, probably as a secondary consequence of fetal asphyxia, and is probably of little clinical significance.[314,315] Magnesium deficiency often accompanies SGA; it has been shown to cause umbilical arterial spasm, suggesting the possibility of a causal association with SGA.[316]

A wide variety of anatomic abnormalities have been described in the SGA placenta.[317] It is probable that many of these (*e.g.*, gross or microscopic infarction, hemangiomas, aberrant cord insertion, single umbilical artery, umbilical vascular thrombosis) may directly impair fetal growth. Premature placental separation (*i.e.*, occult abruption), avascular terminal villi, and diffuse fibrinosis are factors that can reduce placental surface area for exchange and may cause SGA.[318] Interpretation of these findings is difficult. Placental tissue, as examined and analyzed at birth, is fetal tissue. As such, it shares the same reduced potentials for growth demonstrated by fetal tissue. An unpleasant intrauterine environment is likely to affect placental and fetal development. It is therefore not surprising that SGA babies have small placentas; in most instances, however, the fetal–placental weight ratio remains normal.

Maternal conditions that reduce uteroplacental blood flow (*e.g.*, pregnancy-induced hypertension or toxemia, chronic hypertensive vascular disease, primary cardiac or renovascular disorders) are consistently associated with SGA infants. Distal dilatation of the spiral arteries in the myometrium and decidua and the appearance of multinucleated cells and decreased musculoelastic tissue in their walls are normal events as gestation progresses. These changes are absent in two subpopulations of women: those with pregnancy-induced hypertension (*i.e.*, toxemia) and some of those who are normotensive but deliver SGA babies.[319] Intimal proliferation, fibrinoid degeneration of the media, and atherosclerosis in these vessels are associated and impaired fetal growth.[320–322] Another association between vascular compromise and birth of an SGA infant may be found in the provocative case report by Theobald, who described fetal death of an SGA baby in a mother with iliac artery hypoplasia and hypertension.[323] After denervation of the iliac vessels in this woman, subsequent pregnancies were accompanied by normal fetal growth and outcome. Diabetes mellitus may be accompanied by impaired fetal growth.[234,324] Past evidence of diminished clearance of radioactive sodium and confirming data from ^{131}I studies, especially coupled with the histopathologic vascular alterations in conditions associated with impaired fetal growth, provide impressive support for a causal role of impaired or improperly regulated uteroplacental blood flow in many instances of SGA.[325]

High altitude reduces birth weight.[326,327] Although some investigators believe that this effect is preventable and predictable, no one denies that women at high altitudes tend to bear smaller babies.[328,329] The assumption that diminished oxygen transport to the fetus is related to growth retardation may be correct. Mothers with hemoglobinopathies (*e.g.*, sickle-cell disease) commonly have SGA babies; whether mothers with nutritional or other forms of anemia do is unclear.[330–333] The maternal 2,3-diphosphoglycerate–hemoglobin ratio, an index of oxygen affinity, is correlated to fetal weight.[334] Infants born to asthmatic mothers are prone to growth retardation and may benefit from aggressive pulmonary care during gestation.[335,336]

Increased platelet activation and thromboxane A_2 production in normotensive and hypertensive pregnancies are linked to impaired fetal growth.[337,338] These and related findings point toward a defect in prostaglandin metabolism as causal for some SGA infants.[339–345] Work in this field deserves continued close attention.

COMPOSITIONAL CHANGES

ANIMAL STUDIES

Many of the clinical and pathophysiologic views of fetal growth have their origin in animal studies.[346–413] It is essential to understand the variations and limitations of the methods employed, the often distinctive and different developmental sequences in the models used, and the unique and sometimes alien composition of the animals compared.[414–416] Details from selected examples are summarized in Table 26-4. Some of these findings in animal models are similar to those observed in human SGA infants, but for most of the animal data, there are no matching observations in humans because the work has not yet been done.

Animal studies have used hamsters, rabbits, sheep, guinea pigs, mice, pigs, dogs, and monkeys, but the rat has been studied most frequently. Methods used to hamper fetal growth have included maternal administration of narcotics, bestatin that inhibits placental aminopeptidase, and immunosuppressants, such as alloxan, or narcotics; dietary restrictions from the time of conception through late pregnancy; administration of glucose epimers; fetal pancreatic and partial intestinal ablation; placental embolization with microspheres; partial surgical ablation of the placenta; ligation of placental vessels lead-

TABLE 26–4
ANIMALS STUDIED AND METHODS USED TO IMPAIR FETAL GROWTH

Animal	Procedure	References
Hamster	Maternal narcotics	346
Rabbit	Maternal or fetal narcotics; fetal alloxan	347–348
Sheep	Umbilical artery ligation; placental emboli with microspheres; alcohol; diet restriction; fetal pancreatic and partial intestinal ablation; partial placental ablation	349–360
Guinea pig	Diet restriction; placental emboli with microspheres	361–363
Pig	Natural runts	364–366
Monkey	Fetal streptozotocin; ligation of placental vessels	367–371
Mouse	Hyperbaric oxygen; superovulation; diet restriction	372–374
Rat	Immunosuppressants; posterm birth; unilateral renal artery constriction and contralateral nephrectomy; unilateral nephrectomy and contralateral heminephrectomy; narcotics; aspiration of fetal brain; decapitation; diet restriction; uterine vascular ligation (many variations); hyperbaric oxygen; fetal insulin infusion; ovariectomy	375–413

ing to the secondary placental disc; unilateral or bilateral uterine vascular clamping or ligation; unilateral maternal nephrectomy with contralateral renal artery constriction or contralateral nephrectomy; administration of low-dose x-rays; induction of post-term delivery; fetal administration of streptozotocin; and even decapitation or removal of fetal brain by aspiration. Natural runts have been studied. Timing of these insults has varied, and relation of this timing to specific developmental and growth sequences in animals and humans is often unclear.[414]

INFANT STUDIES

Comparison of an SGA infant to a preterm peer reveals a brain and heart that are large in proportion to the reduced body weight, but the liver, spleen, adrenals, placenta, and thymus are smaller.[224] The variety of compositional differences reported are summarized in Table 26-5.

The placenta has been well studied.[96,317–427] Enhanced protein synthesis, aromatizing capacity, and glycogen use have been found, and diminished oxygen consumption has been reported. Increased RNA polymerase activity and reduced RNA content have been found. Decreased DNA and nitrogen content are compatible with a reduced cell number in the organ. These placental findings are absent in some SGA babies, especially those with multiple malformations, reflecting the heterogeneity of causes and the pathophysiologic sequences leading to SGA infants.

Muscle composition has been studied.[428–435] Because of variations in patient selection and methods of analysis, widely discrepant results are available. It remains uncertain under which circumstances reduced cell size or number or both occur in muscles of human SGA infants. Visceral organs have received little attention, and results are scant.[431,433,436–438]

The brain has diminished cerebroside sulfatide content and galactolipid sulfotransferase enzyme activity, materials required for myelin formation. Because most myelin is formed after birth in humans, it is possible that these deficits may be reversible. Phospholipids and gangliosides, and neuronal tissue lipids are unaltered, but mucopolysaccharides are reduced.[439,440]

Body water content, distribution, and metabolism are altered. Water per kilogram is increased because of expanded extracellular and intracellular water, especially in the SGA infants with the most severe degrees of growth retardation and in those studied soon after birth.[441–448] Increased water turnover rates lead to prompt, downward adjustments toward normal within 4 to 6 hours of birth. These conclusions are primarily based on cross-sectional rather than serial studies. Sequential studies, accompanied by concurrent estimates of acid–base balance and other factors that affect cell water content, are required to validate and explain these observations.

TABLE 26–5
COMPOSITIONAL CHANGES IN SMALL-FOR-GESTATIONAL-AGE INFANTS

Organ	Finding
Placenta	Decreased or no change in weight
	Decreased or no change in DNA
	Decreased, increased, or no change in RNA; increased in RNA polymerase
	Increased or no change in RNA/DNA; no change in protein/DNA
	Increased or no change in N or protein
	Decreased glycogen; decreased glucose; increased glycogen use
	Decreased oxygen use
	Increased aromatization
	Increased protein synthesis from proline and leucine
	Decreased heat-stable alkaline phosphatase
	Decreased fibrinolysis (urokinase path)
Liver	Decreased weight
	No change in DNA
	No change in protein/DNA
	Decreased glycogen
Muscle	Decreased protein; decreased fat
	Decreased, increased, or no change in total water; increased ICW; increased or decreased ECW
	Increased, decreased, or no change in DNA; decreased RNA; decreased RNA/DNA; decreased protein/DNA
	Decreased Zn, K, Mg; increased Na
Brain	Decreased weight, especially cerebellar
	Decreased DNA in the cerebellum
	Decreased myelin lipids
	Decreased galactolipid sulfotransferase
	Decreased glucosaminoglycans
Water	Increased TBW; increased ECW; increased ICW; increased plasma volume
Heart	No change in DNA
	No change in protein/DNA
	Decreased sarcoplasm
	Decreased glycogen
Adrenal	Decreased fetal zone

ECW, extracellular water; ICW, intracellular water; TBW, total body water.

FUNCTIONAL CHANGES

Biochemical and metabolic consequences of impaired fetal growth have been studied extensively. Changes have been observed by several investigators, but the precise pathophysiologic sequences involved and the practical implications to the clinician are often unclear. Selected observations are summarized in Table 26-6.

Elevated blood levels of nitrogen products (*e.g.*, ammonia, urea, uric acid) may reflect diminished caloric reserves and a protein catabolic state.[449–451] Low

TABLE 26–6
BIOCHEMICAL AND METABOLIC CHANGES IN SMALL-FOR-GESTATIONAL-AGE INFANTS

Proteins and Collagen
Increased ammonia
Increased urea; increased uric acid
Decreased OH-proline turnover early; increased later
Increased uronic acid turnover
Decreased or no change in total protein
Decreased or no change in prealbumin
Decreased IgG
Increased IgM in some
Immunocompetence
Decreased humoral or cellular bactericidal capacity
Decreased phagocytic index
Decreased lysozyme
Decreased humoral and cellular immunocompetence
Hematology
Increased Hematocrit; increased RBC volume; increased fetal hemoglobin; increased erythropoietin
Increased viscosity
Decreased platelets
Increased PT, PTT
No change in retic count (% or absolute), but increased reticulocyte index
Carbohydrate and Fat Metabolism
Fetal or neonatal hypoglycemia
No change or increased glucose K_t
Decreased, increased, or no change in insulin
Low urinary adrenalin after hypoglycemia
Decreased or no change in β-hydroxybutyrate
No change or increased ketone bodies
Decreased, increased, or no change in FFA and glycerol
Decreased hepatic gluconeogenesis
Increased lactate and pyruvate
Increased alanine
Increased glucagon
Other
Decreased serum Ca^{2+}
Decreased, increased, or no change in amniotic fluid L–S ratio
Transient diabetes
Increased cortisol or 11-OH corticosteroids
No change or increased HGH
Decreased, increased, or no change in O_2 consumption

FFA, free fatty acids; K_t, rate constant for glucose metabolism; L–S, lecithin-to-sphingomyelin ratio; PT, prothrombin time; PTT, partial thromboplastin time; RBC, erythrocyte.

urine hydroxyproline–creatinine ratios at birth and a rapid rise in this ratio and in glycosaminoglycan excretion during the week after birth suggest that poor fetal growth has been replaced by rapid postnatal growth in SGA babies.[452–455] Although observations of reduced amniotic fluid hydroxyproline confirm these observations, there are some discrepancies.[85–87] Altered serum protein, prealbumin, and immunoglobulins are said to be low by most but not all investigators.[456–461] Investigators have found reduced humoral and cellular immunocompetence, but normal lymphocytic response to mitogens has been reported.[462–470] Whether these protein changes are caused by impaired placental transport or reflect impaired fetal production is unclear. Elevated IgM levels related to prior fetal infection are found in some SGA infants.[471]

Hematologic changes include an increased erythrocyte volume, which may be consequent to placental–fetal transfusion during episodes of fetal hypoxia or elevated erythropoietin levels after chronic hypoxia.[442–476] Increased viscosity is an expected and observed consequence of this polycythemia, and there is evidence for a relation between high hematocrits and coagulopathy in SGA babies.[477–480] Reticulocyte counts are unexpectedly normal, but the reticulocyte index, which corrects for the hematocrit, is elevated.[481]

Carbohydrate metabolism is seriously disturbed.[482–505] Although the rare SGA baby has a transient form of diabetes, the most common disturbance is hypoglycemia. The frequent occurrence of hypoglycemia before birth is often overlooked. Rapid disappearance rates for glucose are reported with normal insulinlike activity, but some researchers have found elevated insulin levels in selected babies. Failure of urine catecholamines to increase after hypoglycemia suggests a flawed adrenal medulla in some infants, but diminished insulin response to a glucose load points toward a defect in peripheral glucose use or a reduced insulin sensitivity in others. An unexpected absence of any relation between glucose and free fatty acid levels and observations of normal or reduced levels of β-hydroxybutyrate suggest defective lipolysis. However, elevated ketone and free fatty acid levels indicate appropriate use of alternative substrate lipids in response to hypoglycemia. The capacity for hepatic ketone synthesis is not fully developed at birth, and SGA babies may differ little from their normally grown peers in this regard. Observations that 3 to 4 g of glucose given to the mother in the hour before delivery prevents neonatal hypoglycemia and reduces the umbilical arteriovenous free fatty acid ratio suggest that incidental perinatal treatment rather than impaired fat use may explain some of these discrepancies. Reduced prostacyclin (PGI_2) production has been found, leading to the speculation that PGI_2 levels may serve as markers for essential fatty acid deficiencies.

A significant compromise in hepatic gluconeogenesis and glycogenolysis exists in many SGA infants.[500–505] An inverse relation of alanine to glucose levels in these babies, elevated concentrations of alanine and of all potential gluconeogenic amino acids entering the metabolic sequence at the level of pyruvate, and failure of alanine administration to provoke an appropriate increase in hepatic glucose output can be explained on the basis of a functional delay in development of a rate-limiting gluconeogenic enzyme in the liver.[500,502,503] The fact that oral fructose fails while galactose succeeds in raising glucose levels in SGA babies suggests that the flaw in gluconeogenesis may be at the level of hexose-1, 6-diphosphate.[504] Phosphoenolpyruvate carboxykinase has been suggested as the rate-limiting enzyme involved.[505]

Organ maturation in the SGA baby is usually equal to that of its AGA gestational peer. Exceptions include findings of diminished cardiac and hepatic glycogen, reduced myocardial fiber width, and a small fetal zone in the adrenal.[438] Pulmonary maturation may be enhanced or reduced.[506–510] Amniotic fluid lecithin–sphingomyelin ratios are lower before birth in some babies.[506,507] Although amniotic fluid lecithin is increased with acute pregnancy-induced hypertension, lower levels are found in chronic hypertensive states.[508,510]

Several investigators have found altered oxygen consumption.[511–517] An increased metabolic rate in these infants may be a consequence of imbalances between organs with a high oxygen use (*e.g.*, brain, the growth of which is least restricted in the SGA baby) and other organs with a lower consumption (*e.g.*, thymus, spleen, liver, in which weights are most reduced). Proper interpretation of these studies requires close attention to the relations among feeding, growth, and metabolic rate.[493] The oxygen dissociation curve is not shifted to the right so much in the SGA fetus as in the normally grown baby, perhaps because of an increased proportion of adult-type hemoglobin in these infants.[518] The clinical meaning of this observation is uncertain.

MANAGEMENT

The key to proper management is early diagnosis and meticulous fetal care. Unfortunately, the lock of ignorance has proved rusty, and this key often fails to fit the individual clinical situation. Nevertheless, proper attention to risk factors, careful clinical and chemical evaluation, and use of newer ultrasonographic techniques should enable detection of most SGA babies before birth. Although it is still unclear exactly what to do after the SGA baby is discovered, attention to correctable causes of impaired fetal growth should be the first order of business. Failing respiratory function of the placenta leading to asphyxial compromise or fetal death is characteristic; more than one-third of positive oxytocin challenge tests in one series were followed by the birth of an SGA infant.[519] Liberal and routine use of clinical tests of placental gas exchange (*e.g.*, stress and nonstress testing) may determine the degree of fetal compromise.[520] Fetal blood sampling may provide a direct way to detect and quantify fetal distress in infants who are SGA.[521] This insight provides the clinician a powerful tool to ensure that correct timing and planned preparation for delivery are accomplished.

The birth process represents an asphyxial stress to the normal fetus. The high frequency of intrapartum death, low Apgar scores, and meconium staining and aspiration syndrome vividly attest to the increased risks of labor for the SGA baby. Continuous electronic fetal monitoring by personnel who are able to interpret tracings properly and to intervene promptly in response to dangerous changes should be the rule and not the exception if impaired fetal growth is suspected. Chronic maternal oxygen administration, when severe IUGR is suspected, increases the mean blood velocity in the fetal aorta toward normal and results in a neonate with reduced complications at birth.[522] No randomized studies have been done. Transamniotic fetal feeding (TAFF) was proposed as a method to increase fetal nutrition by the provision of nutrients into the amniotic fluid that the fetus then swallowed.[523,524] Although initial reports looked promising, a randomized study in rabbits showed that TAFF did not result in appreciable weight gain, and adverse events were detected in some rabbits.[525]

Skilled resuscitation is essential for many of these babies; all necessary personnel and equipment must be available before delivery. The presence at each delivery of at least one person trained in the Neonatal Resuscitation Program is the goal of the American Academy of Pediatrics and American Heart Association. Achievement of this goal would ensure trained personnel at the delivery of growth-retarded babies. The critical importance of prompt clearing of meconium from the upper airways must be understood, and the skills required to intervene should be practiced and proved by those responsible at the birth of an SGA infant.[526–528]

Prevention of heat loss is important, because thermoregulation is compromised in these babies. Prompt and complete drying of the infant after birth is crucial. Radiant and convective heat losses may be reduced by the ability to reduce body surface area by a flexion posture of the extremities; in this way, the SGA infant has a thermal advantage over a preterm baby of comparable size. However, heat loss is increased compared with that observed in gestational peers because of diminished subcutaneous fat insulation, which allows increased heat exchange along the skin–air gradient. Meager fat stores deplete brown fat and prevent neonatal heat production if cold stress is prolonged.

The commonness of hypoglycemia demands meticulous and patterned monitoring of blood glucose in SGA babies. Low blood sugar may exist in the fetus or in the infant at birth, and providing glucose before delivery may prevent this problem. Failing this, serial sampling is required for prompt detection and intervention. Proof of the clinical utility of early enteral feeding in stabilizing blood glucose levels or the ability of hydrocortisone to correct the defective gluconeogenesis in these babies awaits prospective clinical trials.[529] Also ambiguous are the clinical implications of animal data showing reduced cerebrospinal fluid glucose despite elevated plasma pressors and catecholamines, vasopressin and endorphins, triglycerides, or the utility of plasma and urine xanthines in defining the severity of asphyxia in these infants.[530–537]

Before the infant's discharge from the nursery, a thorough search for anomalies should be made. This should include appropriate screening for intrauterine infections, most of which are clinically silent.

OUTCOME

An SGA infant who lives is said to be at increased risk for long-term neurologic and behavioral handicaps. Most of these infants, however, have no major handicaps. The striking heterogeneity of the SGA population has thwarted most attempts to relate the severity of the growth impairment to subsequent physical and intellectual growth.

The ultimate developmental prognosis basically depends on the cause for impaired fetal growth. Allen's excellent review summarizes the current knowledge in this field.[538] The SGA baby who is light and short has often suffered genetic, infectious, or other teratogenic insults in early fetal life. However, the SGA infant who is underweight but of normal length often represents a fetus with normal growth potential whose growth is impaired by an insult of limited severity and duration. The latter infant may have a happier outcome than the former, whose compromise may predate conception or may have begun in early fetal life.

A variety of acute perinatal events may affect outcome as well. Small-for-gestational-age infants are more vulnerable than most to perinatal complications, which have harmful influences on subsequent growth and development. Among these are perinatal asphyxia, meconium aspiration syndrome, hypothermia, polycythemia, and hypoglycemia. Asphyxia at birth may alone account for much of the handicap seen in some of these infants.[539–541]

Follow-up studies require meticulous design for results to be more than anecdotal.[542] There must be controls, matched at least for gender, gestational age, birth rank, socioeconomic status, and perinatal morbidity. The cause and degree of growth retardation must be accurately defined. Adequate numbers are required to provide sufficient predictive power. Factors of selection, details of perinatal care received, illnesses suffered, and treatments provided all must be precisely and completely described. Ideally, methods should be reproducible, employing hard data concerning motor and neurologic development, auditory and visual capabilities, electroencephalographic changes, and growth measurements, rather than using impressionistic soft data such as IQ or DQ tests, personality or behavioral deviations, speech development, and perceptual or reading disorders. The studies should be prospective; attrition rate should be so low that it cannot possibly affect the results; methods used should be standard, proven, and reproducible; and the examiners must be blind to whether the baby is a SGA infant or a control subject. Because there are no follow-up studies of SGA infants that meet even these minimal requirements, any views on outcome for these infants must be considered tentative and preliminary.

Morbidity and mortality are increased in SGA infants, especially in some subgroups.[543] Necrotizing enterocolitis is increased in SGA infants whose fetal aortic diastolic flow was absent.[544] Conversely, SGA infants whose diastolic flow was normal have very little risk of morbid events.[545] Small-for-gestational-age infants are more likely to require readmission to the hospital within 2 years of birth.[546] Death is more common among growth-retarded infants than their AGA peers, even if preterm birth is considered.[547] Death is increased for infants who are not identified before birth.[548] Sudden infant death may be more common in growth-retarded infants.[549,550]

There appears to be general agreement that many SGA babies will ultimately be slimmer and shorter than their gestational or weight peers.[17,62,539,551–561] However, not all investigators agree on this point.[562–566] The potential for catch-up growth may be influenced by the cause of retardation and by the neonatal events, especially nutrition, experienced by the baby.[567] Small-for-gestational-age infants with low PI appear capable of achieving normal weight and PI within 6 to 12 months of birth.[568–570] Small-for-gestational-age infants born with normal PIs often remain shorter and lighter with smaller HCs.[569,570] That such observations do not represent any universal truth is shown by studies in which SGA infants with low PIs, who may be expected to have the best potential for catch-up, are persistently shorter and lighter and have smaller HCs at 3 years and at 7 years after birth.[568,571] Twins whose weight was discordant by more than 20% were shown to achieve the same length and HC as their heavier sibs within 1 year but remained lighter.[572] Head circumference may grow in parallel with or faster than weight or height.[573–575] Acceleration of head growth may be more prominent in male SGA infants.[575] These studies show that the degree or nature of fetal growth impairment does not consistently predict postnatal growth achievements and that velocity of growth in the early months after birth may be an imprecise indicator of ultimate size.[31,551,553,555]

Delayed eruption of teeth and enamel hypoplasia have been found in SGA infants and appear related to impaired fetal skeletal growth.[558] Delayed humoral immunity and cellular immunity have occurred in some severely growth-retarded infants, and the increased incidence of postnatal infections in these infants has been thought to be responsible for subsequent growth problems.[576]

The role of preexisting or persistent hormonal defects in the postnatal growth processes of these infants is unclear. Insulin plays a critical role in fetal growth, and its role in catch-up growth appears to be equally important. A significant, positive correlation between linear growth velocity and insulin release after glucose load and the impact of insulin on growth patterns in transient neonatal diabetes suggest an important role for this hormone in the postnatal growth of SGA babies.[244,565,577] Evidence suggests an important role for somatomedins in fetal growth, and selected SGA infants have grown faster after growth hormone therapy.[247–580] Caution should be exercised, because final height may not differ with growth hormone therapy.[581]

Most studies demonstrate normal IQ and DQ results if infants with overt anomalies and clinically detectable congenital infections are excluded.[538–587] Major neurologic problems are infrequent in SGA infants, and data are conflicting about whether significant defects are present in the preterm, undergrown baby.[538–593] Decreased motor behavior, diminished Moro and grip release, delayed visually directed prehension, and abnormal visual and auditory brain stem evoked potentials have been observed, but what these findings mean for long-term outcome is uncertain.[594–599] Delayed language development was found at 3 years in full-term SGA infants.[600]

Several studies have shown the powerful influence of socioeconomic class on development of the SGA infant. Male offspring tend to have lower IQ scores and more behavior problems, but this is not always so.[474] The mother's education is the only factor that is significantly associated with preterm SGA infant's academic abilities.[601] Improper mothering behavior is common after the birth of an SGA infant, although these data are refuted by some.[602,603]

Behavioral changes are difficult to interpret.[554,604,605] Some researchers point to minor motor dysfunctions, subtle neurodevelopmental deficits, speech and language problems, attention deficits, hyperactivity, school failures despite normal intelligence, and increased fears, but others have found no real differences in motor or cognitive function, no developmental delays, and no language impairments.[40,538,587,606]

As more data become available, a widely variable but generally good outcome for SGA babies becomes more evident. This is due in part to improved maternal and neonatal care.[607,608] In addition to the normal infants who are included in the diagnosis because they are genetically small, a certain proportion of SGA infants have more of a constitutional growth delay and ultimately are normal. These infants are not doomed to damage by virtue of their poor fetal growth alone. Sensitive, meticulous fetal and neonatal management methods may reduce or prevent impairment in these infants.

REFERENCES

1. Cowper W. The Task. Book IV, The Winter Walk at Noon, line 223. New York: Clarke, Austin, 1850.
2. McBurney RD. The undernourished full-term infant: a case report. West J Surg 1947;55:363.
3. Söderling B. Pseudoprematurity. Acta Paediatr 1953;42:520.
4. Gruenwald P. Chronic fetal distress and placental insufficiency. Biol Neonate 1963;5:215.
5. Gruenwald P. Infants of low birth weight among 5,000 deliveries. Pediatrics 1964;34:157.
6. Gruenwald P. Growth of the human fetus: I. Normal growth and its variation. Am J Obstet Gynecol 1966;94:1112.
7. Gruenwald P. Growth of the human fetus: II. Abnormal growth in twins and infants of mother with diabetes hypertension, or isoimmunization. Am J Obstet Gynecol 1966; 94:1120.
8. Gruenwald P. The fetus in prolonged pregnancy. Am J Obstet Gynecol 1964;89:503.
9. Gruenwald P, Funakawa H, Mitani S, et al. Influence of environmental factors on foetal growth in man. Lancet 1967;1:1026.
10. Lubchenco LO, Hansman C, Dressler M, Boyd E. Intrauterine growth as estimated from liveborn birth-weight data at 24 to 42 weeks gestation. Pediatrics 1963;32:793.
11. Freeman MG, Graves WL, Thompson RI. Indigent negro and caucasian birth-weight, gestational age tables. Pediatrics 1970;46:9.
12. Parmelee AH, Stern E, Chervin G, Minkowski A. Gestational age and the size of premature infants. Biol Neonat 1964;6:309.
13. Thomson AM, Billewicz WZ, Hytten FE. The assessment of fetal growth. J Obstet Gynaecol Br Commonw 1968;75:903.
14. Pusey VA, Haworth JC. The relation between birth weight and gestational age for a Winnipeg hospital population. Can Med Assoc J 1969;100:842.
15. Rantakallio P. Groups at risk in low birth weight infants and perinatal mortality. Acta Paediatr Scand Suppl 1969;193:1.
16. Babson SG, Behrman RE, Lessel R. Fetal growth: liveborn birth weights for gestational age of white middle class infants. Pediatrics 1970;45:937.
17. Kloosterman GJ. On intrauterine growth: the significance of prenatal care. Int J Gynaecol Obstet 1970;8:895.
18. Penchaszadeh VB, Hardy JB, Mellits ED, et al. Growth and development in an "inner city" population: an assessment of possible biological and environmental influences. I. Intrauterine growth. Johns Hopkins Med J 1972;130:384.
19. Cheng MCE, Chew PCT, Ratnam SS. Birthweight distribution of Singapore Chinese, Malay and Indian infants from 34 weeks to 42 weeks gestation. J Obstet Gynaecol Br Commonw 1972;79:149.
20. Bjerkedal T, Bakketeig L, Lehmann EH. Percentiles of birth weights of single, live births at different gestation periods: based on 125,485 births in Norway, 1967 and 1968. Acta Paediatr Scand 1973;62:449.
21. Milner RDG, Richards B. An analysis of birth weight by gestational age of infants born in England and Wales, 1967. J Obstet Gynaecol Br Commonw 1974;81:956.
22. Brenner WE, Edelman DA, Hendricks CH. A standard of fetal growth for the United States of America. J Obstet Gynecol 1976;126:555.
23. Williams RL, Creasy RK, Cunningham GC, et al. Fetal growth and perinatal viability in California. Obstet Gynecol 1982;59:624.
24. Blidner IN, McClemont S, Anderson GD, Sinclair JC. Size-at-birth standards for an urban Canadian population. Can Med Assoc J 1984;130:133.

25. Goldenberg RL, Cutter GR, Hoffman HJ, et al. Intrauterine growth retardation: standards for diagnosis. Am J Obstet Gynecol 1989;161:271.
26. Tamura RK, Sabbagha RE, Depp R, et al. Diminished growth in fetuses born preterm after spontaneous labor or rupture of membranes. Am J Obstet Gynecol 1984;148:1105.
27. Secher NJ, Hansen PK, Thomsen BL, Keiding N. Growth retardation in preterm infants. Br J Obstet Gynaecol 1987; 94:115.
28. Villar J, Belizan JM. The timing factor in the pathophysiology of the intrauterine growth retardation syndrome. Obstet Gynecol Surv 1982;37:499.
29. Brans YW, Cassady G. Intrauterine growth and maturation in relation to fetal deprivation. In: Gruenwald P, ed. The placenta. Lancaster: Medical & Technical Publishing, 1975:307.
30. Kramer MS, McLean FH, Oliver M, et al. Body proportionality and head and length "sparing" in growth-retarded neonates: a critical reappraisal. Pediatrics 1989;84:717.
31. Parkinson CE, Wallis S, Harvey D. School achievement and behavior of children who were small-for-dates at birth. Dev Med Child Neurol 1981;23:41.
32. Kramer MS, Oliver M, McLean FH, et al. Impact of intrauterine growth retardation and body proportionality on fetal and neonatal outcome. Pediatrics 1990;86:707.
33. Villar J, Belizan JM. The relative contribution of prematurity and fetal growth retardation to low birth weight in developing and developed societies. Am J Obstet Gynecol 1982; 143:793.
34. Woo JSK, Li DFH, Ma HK. Intrauterine growth standards for Hong Kong Chinese. Aust N Z J Obstet Gynaecol 1986;26:54.
35. Lugo G, Cassady G. Intrauterine growth retardation: clinicopathologic findings in 233 consecutive infants. Am J Obstet Gynecol 1971;109:615.
36. Walther FJ. Growth and development of term disproportionate small-for-gestational age infants at the age of 7 years. Early Hum Dev 1988;18:1.
37. Tejani N, Mann LI, Weiss RR. Antenatal diagnosis and management of the small-for-gestational-age fetus. Obstet Gynecol 1976;47:31.
38. Galbraith RS, Karchmar EJ, Piercy WN, Low JA. The clinical prediction of intrauterine growth retardation. Am J Obstet Gynecol 1979;133:281.
39. Mathews DD. Maternal assessment of fetal activity in small-for-dates infants. Obstet Gynecol 1975;45:488.
40. Belizan JM, Villar J, Nardin JC, et al. Diagnosis of intrauterine growth retardation by simple clinical method: measurement of uterine height. Am J Obstet Gynecol 1978;131:643.
41. Beazley JM, Underhill RA. Fallacy of the fundal height. Br Med J 1970;4:404.
42. Ong HC, Sen DK. Clinical estimation of fetal weight. Am J Obstet Gynecol 1972;112:877.
43. Rosenberg K, Grant J, Tweedie I, et al. Measurement of fundal height as a screening test for fetal growth retardation. Br J Obstet Gynaecol 1982;89:447.
44. Quaranta P, Currell R, Redman CWG, Robinson JS. Prediction of small-for-dates infants by measurement of symphysial-fundal height. Br J Obstet Gynaecol 1981;88:115.
45. Calvert JP, Crean EE, Newcombe RG, Pearson JF. Antenatal screening by measurement of symphysis-fundus height. Br Med J 1982;2:846.
46. Rosenberg K, Grant JM, Hepburn M. Antenatal detection of growth retardation: actual practice in a large maternity hospital. Br J Obstet Gynaecol 1982;89:12.
47. Wennergren M, Karlsson K. A scoring system for antenatal identification of fetal growth retardation. Br J Obstet Gynaecol 1982;89:520.
48. Indira R, Oumachigui A, Narayan KA, et al. Symphysis-fundal height measurement—a reliable parameter for assessment of fetal growth. Int J Gynecol Obstet 1990;33:1.
49. Bekedam DJ, Visser HA, Mulder EJH, et al. Heart rate variation and movement incidence in growth-retarded fetuses: the significance of antenatal late heart rate decelerations. Am J Obstet Gynecol 1987;157:126.
50. Shields JR, Schifrin BS. Perinatal antecedents of cerebral palsy. Obstet Gynecol 1988;71:899.
51. Odendaal HJ, Kotz TJVW. Poor prognostic value of the basal fetal heart rate as observed during antenatal monitoring. Int J Gynaecol Obstet 1986;24:347.
52. Kidd LC, Patel NB, Smith R. Non-stress antenatal cardiotocography—a prospective blind study. Br J Obstet Gynaecol 1985;92:1152.
53. Gagnon R, Hunse C, Carmichael L, et al. Vibratory acoustic stimulation in 26- to 32-week small-for-gestational-age fetus. Am J Obstet Gynecol 1989;160:160.
54. Aickin DR, Duff GB, Evans JJ, Legge W. Antenatal biochemical screening to predict low birthweight infants. Br J Obstet Gynaecol 1983;90:129.
55. Tamsen L, Johansson SGO, Axelsson O. Pregnancy-specific B_1-glycoprotein (SP1) in serum from women with pregnancies complicated by intrauterine growth retardation. J Perinat Med 1983;11:19.
56. Gopalaswamy G, Balasubramaniam N, Kanagasabathy AS. Cystyl aminopeptidase in maternal serum for the antenatal recognition of fetal growth retardation. Aust N Z J Obstet Gynaecol 1983;23:79.
57. Wurz H, Luben G, Bohn H, et al. Concentration of placental protein 10 (PP10) in maternal serum and amniotic fluid throughout normal gestation and in pregnancy complicated by fetal growth retardation. Arch Gynecol 1983;233:165.
58. Simmonds RJ, Harkness RA, Coade SB. Increases in methylated nucleosides during human pregnancy. Adv Exp Med Biol 1984;165A:291.
59. Pavelka R, Schmid R, Reinold E. Evaluation of various monitoring techniques in late pregnancy to detect poor intrauterine fetal growth. Gynecol Obstet Invest 1982;13:65.
60. Lilford RJ, Obiekwe BC, Chard T. Maternal blood levels of human placental lactogen in the prediction of fetal growth retardation: choosing a cut-off point between normal and abnormal. Br J Obstet Gynaecol 1983;90:511.
61. Khouzami VA, Ginsburg DS, Daikoku NH, Johnson JWC. The glucose tolerance test as a means of identifying intrauterine growth retardation. Am J Obstet Gynecol 1981;139: 423.
62. Sokol RJ, Kazzi GM, Kalhan SC, Pillay SK. Identifying the pregnancy at risk for intrauterine growth retardation: possible usefulness of the intravenous glucose tolerance test. Am J Obstet Gynecol 1982;143:220.
63. Purdie DW, Young JL, Guthrie KA, Picton CE. Fetal growth achievement and elevated maternal serum alpha-fetoprotein. Br J Obstet Gynaecol 1983;90:433.
64. Chapman L, Burrows-Peakin R, Rege VP, Silk E. Serum cystine aminopeptidase and the small-for-dates baby in hypertensive pregnancy. Br J Obstet Gynaecol 1976;83:238.
65. Pathak S, Himaya A, Mosher R. The small-for-dates syndrome: some biochemical considerations in prenatal diagnosis. Am J Obstet Gynecol 1974;120:32.
66. Hensleigh PA, Cheatum SG, Spellacy WN. Oxytocinase and human placental lactogen for prediction of intrauterine growth retardation. Am J Obstet Gynecol 1977;129:675.
67. Spellacy WN. Human placental lactogen and intrauterine growth retardation. Obstet Gynecol 1976;47:446.
68. Daikoku NH, Tyson JE, Graf G, et al. The relative significance

of human placental lactogen in the diagnosis of retarded fetal growth. Am J Obstet Gynecol 1979;135:516.
69. Arias F. The diagnosis and management of intrauterine growth retardation. Obstet Gynecol 1977;49:293.
70. Burnard WP, Logan RW. The value of urinary oestriol estimation in predicting dysmaturity. J Obstet Gynaecol Br Commonw 1972;79:1091.
71. Campbell S, Kurjak A. Comparison between urinary oestrogen assay and serial ultrasonic cephalometry in assessment of fetal growth retardation. Br Med J 1972;4:336.
72. Petrucco DM, Cellier K, Fishtall A. Diagnosis of intrauterine fetal growth retardation by serial serum oxytocinase, urinary oestrogen, and serum heat stable alkaline phosphatase (HASP) estimations in uncomplicated and hypertensive pregnancies. J Obstet Gynaecol Br Commonw 1973;80:499.
73. Clemetson CAB, Churchman J. The placental transfer of amino-acids in normal and toxaemic pregnancy. J Obstet Gynaecol Br Commonw 1954;61:364.
74. Gordon YB, Grudzinskas JG, Jeffery D, et al. Concentration of pregnancy-specific β_1-glycoprotein in maternal blood in normal pregnancy and in intrauterine growth retardation. Lancet 1977;1:331.
75. Brock DHJ, Barron L, Jelen P, et al. Maternal serum-alphafetoprotein measurements as an early indicator of low birthweight. Lancet 1977;2:267.
76. Tanguy G, Zorn JR, Sureau C, Cedard L. Exogenous DHA-S half-life: a good index of intrauterine growth retardation. Gynecol Obstet Invest 1980;11:170.
77. Whigham KAE, Howie PW, Shah MM, Prentice CRM. Factor VIII related antigen/coagulant activity ratio as a predictor of fetal growth retardation: a comparison with hormone and uric acid measurements. Br J Obstet Gynaecol 1980;87:797.
78. Doran TA, Valentine GH, Wong PY, et al. Maternal serum alpha-fetoprotein screening: report of a Canadian pilot project. Can Med Assoc J 1987;137:285.
79. Gross TL, Sokol RJ, Wilson MV, Zador IE. Using ultrasound and amniotic fluid determinations to diagnose intrauterine growth retardation before birth: a clinical model. Am J Obstet Gynecol 1982;143:265.
80. Sher G, Statland BE, Knutzen VK. Identifying the small-for-gestational-age fetus on the basis of enhanced surfactant production. Obstet Gynecol 1983;61:13.
81. Gross TL, Sokol RJ, Wilson MV, et al. Amniotic fluid phosphatidylglycerol: a potentially useful predictor of intrauterine growth retardation. Am J Obstet Gynecol 1981;140:277.
82. Miodovnik M, Lavin JP, Gimmon Z, et al. The use of amniotic fluid 3-methyl histidine to creatinine molar ratio for the diagnosis of intrauterine growth retardation. Obstet Gynecol 1982;60:288.
83. Divers WA, Wilkes MM, Babaknia A, et al. Amniotic fluid catecholamines and metabolites in intrauterine growth retardation. Am J Obstet Gynecol 1981;141:608.
84. Lin CC, Moawad AH, River P, et al. Amniotic fluid C-peptide as an index for intrauterine fetal growth. Am J Obstet Gynecol 1981;139:390.
85. Wharton BA, Foulds JW, Fraser ID, Pennock CA. Amniotic fluid total hydroxyproline and intrauterine growth. J Obstet Gynaecol Br Commonw 1971;78:791.
86. Shah SI, Alderman M, Queenan JT, et al. Nondialyzable peptide-bound hydroxyproline in human amniotic fluid: an indicator of fetal growth. Am J Obstet Gynecol 1972;114:250.
87. Brans Y, Bailey P, Blake M, Cassady G. Urinary hydroxyproline/creatinine ratio and perinatal growth (abstract). Pediatr Res 1975;9:275.
88. Burton BK, Dillard RG. Outcome in infants born to mothers with unexplained elevations of maternal serum alpha-fetoprotein. Pediatrics 1986;77:582.
89. Killam WP, Miller RC, Seeds JW. Extremely high maternal serum alpha-fetoprotein levels at second-trimester screening. Obstet Gynecol 1991;78:257.
90. Katz VL, Chescheir NC, Céfalo RC. Unexplained elevations of maternal serum alpha-fetoprotein. Obstet Synecol Surv 1990;45:719.
91. Salafia CM, Silberman L, Herrera NE, Mahoney MJ. Placental pathology at term associated with elevated midtrimester maternal serum alpha-fetoprotein concentration. Am J Obstet Gynecol 1988;158:1064.
92. Phocas I, Sarandakou A, Rizos D. Maternal serum total cortisol levels in normal and pathologic pregnancies. Int J Gynaecol Obstet 1990;31:3.
93. Hofman GE, Rao CV, Brown MJ, et al. Epidermal growth factor in urine of nonpregnant women and pregnant women throughout pregnancy and at delivery. J Clin Endocrinol Metab 1988;66:119.
94. Metcoff J, Yoshida T, Morales M, et al. Biomolecular studies of fetal malnutrition in maternal leukocytes. Pediatrics 1971; 47:180.
95. Yoshida T, Metcoff J, Morales M, et al. Human fetal growth retardation: II. Energy metabolism in leukocytes. Pediatrics 1972;50:559.
96. Metcoff J, Wikman-Coffelt J, Yoshida T, et al. Energy metabolism and protein synthesis in human leukocytes during pregnancy and in placenta related to fetal growth. Pediatrics 1973;51:866.
97. Metcoff J. Maternal leukocyte metabolism in fetal malnutrition. Adv Exp Med Biol 1974;49:73.
98. Mameesh MS, Metcoff J, Costiloe P, Crosby W. Kinetic properties of pyruvate kinase in human maternal leukocytes in fetal malnutrition. Pediatr Res 1976;10:561.
99. Crosby WM, Metcoff J, Costiloe JP, et al. Fetal malnutrition: an appraisal of correlated factors. Am J Obstet Gynecol 1977;128:22.
100. Selvaggi L, Lucivero G, Iannone A, et al. Analysis of mononuclear cell subsets in pregnancies with intrauterine growth retardation: evidence of chronic B-lymphocyte activation. J Perinat Med 1983;11:213.
101. Estellés A, Gilabert J, España, et al. Fibrinolytic parameters in normotensive pregnancy with intrauterine fetal growth retardation and in severe preeclampsia. Am J Obstet Gynecol 1991;165:138.
102. Labarrere CA, Althabe OH. Intrauterine growth retardation of unknown etiology: II. Serum complement and circulating immune complexes in maternal sera and their relationship with parity and chronic villitis. Am J Reprod Immunol Microbiol 1986;12:4.
103. Sacher RA, Falchuk SC. Percutaneous umbilical blood sampling. Crit Rev Clin Lab Sci 1990;28:19.
104. Campbell S, Soothill PW. Role of fetal blood gas analysis in intrauterine growth retardation. Lancet 1990;336:1316.
105. Pardi G, Buscaglia M, Ferrazzi E, et al. Cord sampling for the evaluation of oxygenation and acid-base balance in growth-retarded human fetuses. Am J Obstet Gynecol 1987;157:1221.
106. Nicolini U, Nicolaidis P, Fisk NM, et al. Limited role of fetal blood sampling in prediction of outcome in intrauterine growth retardation. Lancet 1990;336:768.
107. Marconi AM, Cetin I, Ferrazzi E, et al. Lactate metabolism in normal and growth-retarded human fetuses. Pediatr Res 1990;28:652.
108. Economides DL, Nicolaides KH, Gahl WA, et al. Plasma amino acids in appropriate- and small-for-gestational-age fetuses. Am J Obstet Gynecol 1989;161:1219.

109. Nicolini U, Hubinont C, Santolaya J, et al. Maternal-fetal glucose gradient in normal pregnancies and in pregnancies complicated by alloimmunization and fetal growth retardation. Am J Obstet Gynecol 1989;161:924.
110. Nicolini U, Hubinont C, Santolaya J, et al. Effects of fetal intravenous glucose challange in normal and growth retarded fetuses. Horm Metab Res 1990;22:426.
111. Sanders M, Allen M, Alexander GR, et al. Gestational age assessment in preterm neonates weighing less than 1500 grams. Pediatrics 1991;88:542.
112. Hadlock FP, Deter RL, Harrist RB. Sonographic detection of abnormal fetal growth patterns. Clin Obstet Gynecol 1984; 27:342.
113. Kurjak A, Kirkinen P, Latin V. Biometric and dynamic ultrasound assessment of small-for-dates infants: report 260 cases. Obstet Gynecol 1980;56:281.
114. Neilson JP, Whitfield CR, Aitchison TC. Screening for the small-for-dates fetus: a two-stage ultrasonic examination schedule. Br Med J 1980;1:1203.
115. Neilson JP. Detection of the small-for-dates twin fetus by ultrasound. Br J Obstet Gynaecol 1981;88:27.
116. Sholl JS, Woo D, Rubin JM, et al. Intrauterine growth retardation risk detection for fetuses of unknown gestational age. Am J Obstet Gynecol 1982;144:709.
117. Lee JN, Chard T. Determination of biparietal diameter in the second trimester as a predictor of intrauterine growth retardation. Int J Gynaecol Obstet 1983;21:213.
118. Eik-Nes SH, Persson PH, Grottum P, Marsal, K. Prediction of fetal growth deviation by ultrasonic biometry. Acta Obstet Gynecol Scand 1983;62:117.
119. Kazzi GM, Gross TL, Sokol RJ, Kazzi NJ. Detection of intrauterine growth retardation: a new use for sonographic placental grading. Am J Obstet Gynecol 1983;145:733.
120. Kazzi GM, Gross TL, Sokol RJ. Fetal biparietal diameter and placental grade: predictors of intrauterine growth retardation. Obstet Gynecol 1983;62:755.
121. Patterson RM, Hayashi RH, Cavazos D. Ultrasonographically observed early placental maturation and perinatal outcome. Am J Obstet Gynecol 1983;147:773.
122. Hoddick WK, Callen PW, Filly RA, Creasy RK. Ultrasonographic determination of qualitative amniotic fluid volume in intrauterine growth retardation: reassessment of the 1 cm rule. Am J Obstet Gynecol 1984;149:758.
123. Manning FA, Hill LM, Platt LD. Qualitative amniotic fluid volume determined by ultrasound: antepartum detection of intrauterine growth retardation. Am J Obstet Gynecol 1981; 139:254.
124. Philipson EH, Sokol RJ, Williams T. Oligohydramnios: clinical associations and predictive value for intrauterine growth retardation. Am J Obstet Gynecol 1983;146:271.
125. Hill LM, Breckle R, Wolfgram KR, O'Brien PC. Oligohydramnios: ultrasonically detected incidence and subsequent fetal outcome. Am J Obstet Gynecol 1983;147:407.
126. Campbell S, Thomas A. Ultrasound measurement of the fetal head-to-abdomen circumference ratio in the assessment of growth retardation. Br J Obstet Gynaecol 1977;84:165.
127. Wittmann BK, Robinson HP, Aitchison T, Fleming JEE. The value of diagnostic ultrasound as a screening test for intrauterine growth retardation: comparison of nine parameters. Am J Obstet Gynecol 1979;134:30.
128. Sabbagha RE. Intrauterine growth retardation: antenatal diagnosis by ultrasound. Obstet Gynecol 1978;52:252.
129. Campbell S, Wilkin D. Ultrasonic measurement of fetal abdomen circumference in the estimation of fetal weight. Br J Obstet Gynaecol 1975;82:689.
130. Gohari P, Berkowitz RL, Hobbins JC. Prediction of intrauterine growth retardation by determination of total intrauterine volume. Am J Obstet Gynecol 1977;127:255.
131. Waldimiroff JW, Campbell S. Fetal urine production rates in normal and complicated pregnancy. Lancet 1974;1:151.
132. Campbell S, Dewhurst CJ. Diagnosis of the small-for-dates fetus by serial ultrasonic cephalometry. Lancet 1971;2:1002.
133. Murao F, Takamiya O, Yamamoto K, Iwanari O. Detection of intrauterine growth retardation based on measurements of size of the liver. Gynecol Obstet Invest 1990;29:26.
134. Chellani HK, Mahajan J, Batra A, et al. Fetal ponderal index in predicting growth retardation. Indian J Med Res 1990; 92:163.
135. Sato A, Yamaguchi Y, Liou SM, et al. Growth of the fetal kidney assessed by real-time ultrasound. Gynecol Obstet Invest 1985;20:1.
136. Reese EA, Goldstein I, Pilu G, Hobbins JC. Fetal cerebellar growth unaffected by intrauterine growth retardation: a new parameter of prenatal diagnosis. Am J Obstet Gynecol 1987;157:632.
137. Abramowicz JS, Jaffe R, Warsof SL. Ultrasonographic measurement of fetal femur length in growth disturbances. Am J Obstet Gynecol 1989;161:1137.
138. Hill LM, Guzick D, Thomas ML, et al. Thigh circumference in the detection of intrauterine growth retardation. Am J Perinatol 1989;6:349.
139. Devoe LD, Ruedrich DA, Searle NS. Value of observation of fetal breathing activity in antenatal assessment of high-risk pregnancy. Am J Obstet Gynecol 1989;160:166.
140. Benson CB, Doubilet PM, Saltzman DH, Jones TB. FL/AC ratio: poor predictor of intrauterine growth retardation. Invest Radiol 1985;20:727.
141. Geirsson RT, Patel NB, Christie AD. Efficacy of intrauterine volume, fetal abnominal area and biparietal diameter measurements with ultrasound in screening for small-for-dates babies. Br J Obstet Gynaecol 1985;92:929.
142. Giersson RT, Patel NB, Christie AD. Intrauterine volume, fetal abdominal area and biparietal diameter measurements with ultrasound in the prediction of small-for-dates babies in a high-risk obstetric population. Br J Obstet Gynaecol 1985; 92:936.
143. Batra A, Chellani HK, Mahajan J, et al. Ultrasonic variables in the diagnosis of intrauterine growth retardation. Indian J Med Res 1990;92:399.
144. Zilianti M, Fernandez S, Azuaga A, et al. Ultrasound evaluation of the distal femoral epiphyseal ossification center as a screening test for intrauterine growth retardation. Obstet Gynecol 1987;70:361.
145. Shalev E, Romano S, Weiner E, Ben-Ami M. Predictive value of the femur length to abdominal circumference ratio in the diagnosis of intrauterine growth retardation. Isr J Med Sci 1991;27:131.
146. Monaghan J, O'Herlihy C, Boylan P. Ultrasound placental grading and amniotic fluid quantitation in prolonged pregnancy. Obstet Gynecol 1987;70:349.
147. Varma TR, Bateman S, Patel RH, et al. Ultrasound evaluation of amniotic fluid: outcome of pregnancies with severe oligohydramnios. Int J Gynecol Obstet 1988;27:185.
148. Devoe LD, Castillo RA, Searle N, Searle JS. Prognostic components of computerized fetal biophysical testing. Am J Obstet Gynecol 1988;158:1144.
149. Manning FA, Harman CR, Morrison I, et al. Fetal assessment based on fetal biophysical profile scoring. Am J Obstet Gynecol 1990;162:703.
150. Chitlange SM, Hazari KT, Joshi JV, et al. Ultrasonographically observed preterm grade III placenta and perinatal outcome. Int J Gynecol Obstet 1990;31:325.

151. Benson CB, Doubilet PM, Saltzman DH. Intrauterine growth retardation: predictive value of US criteria for antenatal diagnosis. Radiology 1986;160:415.
152. Bergsjø P, Hoffman HJ, Davis RO. Preliminary results from the collaborative Alabama and Scandanavian study of successive small-for-gestational age births. Acta Obstet Gynecol Scand 1989;68:19.
153. Benson CB, Boswell SB, Brown DL, et al. Improved prediction of intrauterine growth retardation with use of multiple parameters. Radiology 1988;168:7.
154. Vintzileos AM, Lodeiro JG, Feinstein SJ, et al. Value of fetal ponderal index in predicting growth retardation. Obstet Gynecol 1986;67:584.
155. Hill LM, Guzick D, Belfar HL, et al. A combined historic and sonographic score for the detection of intrauterine growth retardation. Obstet Gynecol 1989;73:291.
156. Ruedrich DA, Devoe LD, Searle N. Effects of maternal hyperoxia on the biophysical assessment of fetuses with suspected intrauterine growth retardation. Am J Obstet Gynecol 1989;161:188.
157. Weiner CP, Robinson D. Sonographic diagnosis of intrauterine growth retardation using the postnatal ponderal index and the crown-heel length as standards of diagnosis. Am J Perinatol 1989;6:380.
158. Benson CB, Belville JS, Lentini JF, et al. Intrauterine growth retardation: diagnosis based on multiple parameters—a prospective study. Radiology 1990;177:499.
159. Rosendahl H, Kivinen S. Detection of small for gestational age fetuses by the combination of clinical risk factors and ultrasonography. Eur J Obstet Gynecol 1991;39:7.
160. Maulik D, Yarlagadda P, Youngblood JP, Ciston P. The diagnostic efficacy of the umbilical arterial systolic/diastolic ratio as a screening tool: a prospective blinded study. Am J Obstet Gynecol 1990;162:1518.
161. Degani S, Paltiely Y, Lewinsky R, et al. Fetal blood flow velocity waveforms in pregnancies complicated by intrauterine growth retardation. Isr J Med Sci 1990;26:250.
162. Schulman H, Ducey J, Farmakides G, et al. Uterine artery doppler velocimetry: the significance of divergent systolic/diastolic ratios. Am J Obstet Gynecol 1987;157:1539.
163. Lombardi SJ, Rosemond R, Ball R, et al. Umbilical artery velocimetry as a predictor of adverse outcome in pregnancies complicated by oligohydramnios. Obstet Gynecol 1989; 74:338.
164. Fleischer A, Schulman H, Farmakides G, et al. Uterine artery doppler velocimetry in pregnant women with hypertension. Am J Obstet Gynecol 1986;154:806.
165. Rochelson B, Schulman H, Farmakides G, et al. The significance of absent end-diastolic velocity in umbilical artery velocity waveforms. Am J Obstet Gynecol 1987;156:1213.
166. Cruz AC, Frentzen BH, Gomez KJ, et al. Continuous-wave doppler ultrasound and decreased amniotic fluid volume in pregnant women with intact or ruptured membranes. Am J Obstet Gynecol 1988;159:708.
167. van Vugt JMG, Ruissen KJ, Schouten HJA, et al. Umbilical artery blood velocimetry: a prospective longitudinal study in search of the intrauterine growth-retarded fetus. Early Hum Dev 1988;18:59.
168. Tonge HM, Wladimiroff JW, Noordam MJ, Van Kooten C. Blood flow velocity waveforms in the descending fetal aorta: comparison between normal and growth-retarded pregnancies. Obstet Gynecol 1986;67:851.
169. Laurin J, Marsál K, Persson PH, Lingman G. Ultrasound measurement of fetal blood flow in pedicting fetal outcome. Br J Obstet Gynaecol 1987;94:940.
170. Stewart PA, Wladimiroff JW, Stijnen T. Blood flow velocity waveforms from the fetal external iliac artery as a measure of lower extremity vascular resistance. Br J Obstet Gynaecol 1990;97:425.
171. Hecher K, Spernol R, Szalay S. Doppler blood flow velocity waveforms in the fetal renal artery. Arch Gynecol Obstet 1989;246:133.
172. Cartier MS, Doubilet PM. Fetal aortic and pulmonary artery diameters: sonographic measurements in growth-retarded fetuses. Am J Roentgenol 1988;151:991.
173. Satoh S, Koyanagi T, Fukuhara M, et al. Changes in vascular resistance in the umbilical and middle cerebral arteries in the human intrauterine growth-retarded fetus, measured with pulsed doppler ultrasound. Early Hum Dev 1989;20:213.
174. Arbeille P, Roncin A, Berson M, et al. Exploration of the fetal cerebral blood flow by duplex doppler—linear array system in normal and pathological pregnancies. Ultrasound Med Biol 1987;13:329.
175. Groenenberg IAL, Stijnen T, Wladimiroff JW. Blood flow velocity waveforms in the fetal cardiac outflow tract as a measure of fetal well-being in intrauterine growth retardation. Pediatr Res 1990;27:379.
176. Gudmundsson S, Marsál K. Blood velocity waveforms in the fetal aorta and umbilical artery as predictors of fetal outcome: a comparison. Am J Perinatol 1991;8:1.
177. Kirkinen P, Jouppila P, Huch R, Huch A. Blood flow velocity waveforms at late pregnancy and during labor. Arch Gynecol Obstet 1988;244:S19.
178. Kofinas AD, Penry M, Nelson LH, et al. Uterine and umbilical artery flow velocity waveform analysis in pregnancies complicated by chronic hypertension or preeclampsia. South Med J 1990;83:150.
179. Kurmanavichius J, Baumann H, Huch R, Huch A. Uteroplacental blood flow velocity waveforms as a predictor of adverse fetal outcome and pregnancy-induced hypertension. J Perinat Med 1990;18:255.
180. Kay HH, Carroll BB, Dahmus M, Killam AP. Sonographic measurements with umbilical and uterine artery doppler analysis in suspected intrauterine growth retardation. J Reprod Med 1991;36:65.
181. Jacobson S-L, Imhof R, Manning N, et al. The value of doppler assessment of the uteroplacental circulation in predicting preeclampsia or intrauterine growth retardation. Am J Obstet Gynecol 1990;162:110.
182. Newnham JP, Patterson LL, James IR, et al. An evaluation of the efficacy of doppler flow velocity waveform analysis as a screening test in pregnancy. Am J Obstet Gynecol 1990; 162:403.
183. Lowrey CL, Hensen BV, Wan J, Brumfield CG. A comparison between umbilical artery velocimetry and standard antepartum surveillance in hospitalized high-risk patients. Am J Obstet Gynecol 1990;162:710.
184. Berkowitz GS, Chitkara U, Rosenberg J, et al. Sonographic estimation of fetal weight and doppler analysis of umbilical artery velocimetry in the prediction of intrauterine growth retardation: a prospective study. Am J Obstet Gynecol 1988; 158:1149.
185. Divon MY, Guidetti DA, Braverman JJ, et al. Intrauterine growth retardation: a prospective study of the diagnostic value of real-time sonography combined with umbilical artery flow velocimetry. Obstet Gynecol 1988;72:611.
186. Devoe LD, Gardner P, Dear C, Castillo RA. The diagnostic values of concurrent nonstress testing, amniotic fluid measurement, and doppler velocimetry in screening a general high-risk population. Am J Obstet Gynecol 1990;163:1040.
187. van Vugt JMG, Ruissen CJ, Hoogland HJ, de Haan J. The blood flow velocity waveform index in the fetal thoracic aorta

and its ability to detect fetal compromise in the small for gestational age fetus. Eur J Obstet Gynecol 1988;27:105.
188. Trudinger BJ, Cook CM, Jones L. A comparison of fetal heart rate monitoring and umbilical artery waveform in the recognition of fetal compromise. Br J Obstet Gynaecol 1986;93:171.
189. Bottoms SF, Welch RA, Zador IE, Sokol RJ. Clinical interpretation of ultrasound measurements in preterm pregnancies with premature rupture of the membranes. Obstet Gynecol 1987;69:358.
190. Villar J, Belizan J. The evaluation of the methods used in the diagnosis of intrauterine growth retardation. Obstet Gynecol 1986;41:187.
191. Cnattingius S, Axelsson O, Lindmark G. The clinical value of measurements of the symphysis-fundus distance and ultrasonic measurements of the biparietal diameter in the diagnosis of intrauterine growth retardation. J Perinat Med 1985; 13:227.
192. Warsof SI, Cooper DJ, Little D, Campbell S. Routine ultrasound screening for antenatal detection of intrauterine growth retardation. Obstet Gynecol 1986;67:33.
193. Devore GR, Platt LD. Diagnosis of intrauterine growth retardation: the use of sequential measurements of fetal growth parameters. Clin Obstet Gynecol 1987;30:968.
194. Wen SW, Goldenberg RL, Cutter GR, et al. Intrauterine growth retardation and preterm delivery: prenatal risk factors in an indigent population. Am J Obstet Gynecol 1990;162:213.
195. Ringa V, Blondel B, Breart G. Ultrasound in obstetrics: so the published evaluative studies justify its routine use? Int J Epidemiol 1989;18:489.
196. Brans YW, Sumners JE, Dweck HS, Cassady, G. A non-invasive approach to body composition in the neonate: dynamic skinfold measurements. Pediatr Res 1974;8:215.
197. Roord JJ, Ramaekers LHJ. Quantifications of intrauterine malnutrition. Biol Neonate 1978;33:273.
198. Gampel B. The relation of skinfold thickness in the neonate to sex, length of gestation, size at birth, and maternal skinfold. Hum Biol 1965;37:29.
199. Oakley JR, Parsons RJ, Whitelaw AGL. Standards for skinfold thickness in British newborn infants. Arch Dis Child 1977; 52:287.
200. McGowan A, Jordan M, MacGregor J. Skinfold thickness in neonates. Biol Neonate 1975;25:66.
201. Petersen S, Gotfredsen A, Knudsen FU. Lean body mass in small for gestational age and appropriate for gestational age infants. J Pediatr 1988;113:886.
202. Philip AGS. Fetal growth retardation: femurs, fontanelles, and follow-up. Pediatrics 1978;62:446.
203. Woods DL, Malan AF, de V.Heese H. Patterns of retarded fetal growth. Early Hum Dev 1979;3:257.
204. de la Fuente AA, Dornseiffen G, van Noort G, Laurini RN. Routine perinatal postmortem radiography in a peripheral pathology laboratory. Virchows Arch [A] 1988;413:513.
205. Crane JP, Kopta MM. Comparative newborn anthropometric data in symmetric versus asymmetric intrauterine growth retardation. Am J Obstet Gynecol 1980;138:518.
206. Good F, Scott A, Ounsted M. A comparison of ratio and regression methods for assessing the proportionality of newborn babies. Early Human Dev 1980;4:347.
207. Georgieff MK, Sasanow SR, Chockalingham UM, Pereira GR. A comparison of the mid-arm circumference/head circumference ratio and ponderal index for the evaluation of newborn infants after abnormal intrauterine growth. Acta Paediatr Scand 1988;77:214.
208. Meadows NJ, Till J, Leaf A, et al. Screening for intrauterine growth retardation using ratio of mid-arm circumference to occipitofrontal circumference. Br Med J 1986;292:1039.
209. Miller HC, Merritt TA. Fetal growth in humans. Chicago: Year Book, 1979.
210. Vogman MW, Kraemer HC, Kindlon D, et al. Identification of intrauterine growth retardation among low birth weight preterm infants. J Pediatr 1989;115:799.
211. Bozynski MEA, Hanafy FH, Hernandez RJ. Association of increased cardiothoracic ratio and intrauterine growth retardation. Am J Perinatol 1991;8:28.
212. Philip AGS, Tito AM. Increased nucleated red blood cell counts in small for gestational age infants with very low birth weight. Am J Dis Child 1989;143:164.
213. Rayburn W, Sander C, Compton A. Histologic examination of the placenta in the growth-retarded fetus. Am J Perinatol 1989;6:58.
214. Vorherr H. Factors influencing fetal growth. Am J Obstet Gynecol 1982;142:577.
215. Brans YW, Cassady G. Fetal nutrition and body composition. In: Ghadimi H, ed. Total parenteral alimentation: premises and promises. Philadelphia: John Wiley & Sons, 1974.
216. Ounsted M, Ounsted C. On fetal growth rate: its variations and their consequences. Clinics in developmental medicine #46. Philadelphia: JB Lippincott, 1973.
217. Meredith HV. Body weight at birth of viable human infants: a worldwide comparative treatise. Hum Biol 1970;42:217.
218. Jason CJ, Samuhel ME, Glick BJ, Welsh AK. Geographic distribution of unexplained low birth weight. J Occup Med 1986;28:728.
219. Naylor AF, Myrianthopoulos NC. The relation of ethnic and selected socio-economic factors to human birth-weight. Ann Hum Genet 1967;31:71.
220. Handlesman Y, Davies AM. Birth weight in Israel, 1968–1970: II. The effect of paternal origin. J Biosoc Sci 1975;7:153.
221. Barron SL, Vessey MP. Birthweights of infants born to immigrant women. Br J Prev Soc Med 1966;20:127.
222. Johnstone F, Inglis L. Familial trends in low birth weight. Br Med J 1974;3:659.
223. Klebanoff MA, Graubard BI, Kessel SS, Berendes HW. Low birth weight across generations. JAMA 1984;252:2423.
224. Elliott K, Knight J, eds. Size at birth. Ciba Foundation symposium #27. Amsterdam: Elsevier, 1974.
225. Ounstead C. Effect of Y chromosome on fetal growth rate. Lancet 1970;2:857.
226. Cassady G. Anencephaly: a six year study of 367 cases. Am J Obstet Gynecol 1969;103:1154.
227. Cozzi F, Wilkinson AW. Intrauterine growth rate in relation to anorectal and oesophageal anomalies. Arch Dis Child 1969; 44:59.
228. Levy RJ, Rosenthal A, Fyler D, Nadas AS. Birth weight of infants with congenital heart disease. Am J Dis Child 1978; 132:249.
229. Donohue WL, Uchida I. Leprechaunism—a euphemism for a rare familial disorder. J Pediatr 1954;45:505.
230. Young DG, Wilkinson AW. Mortality in neonatal duodenal obstruction. Lancet 1966;2:18.
231. Rawls WE, Melnick JL. Rubella virus carrier cultures derived from congenitally infected infants. J Exp Med 1966;123: 795.
232. Siegal M, Fuerst HT. Low birthweight and maternal virus diseases. JAMA 1966;197:680.
233. Charlton V. Fetal nutritional supplementation. Semin Perinatol 1984;8:25.
234. Pedersen JF, Molsted-Pedersen L. Early growth delay predisposes the fetus in diabetic pregnancy to congenital malformation. Lancet 1982;1:737.
235. Klebanoff, MA, Meirik O, Berendes HW. Second-generation consequences of small-for-dates births. Pediatrics 1989;84:343.

236. Khoury MJ, Berg CJ, Calle EE. The ponderal index in term newborn siblings. Am J Epidemiol 1990;132:576.
237. Fisher DA. Intrauterine growth retardation: endocrine and receptor aspects. Perinat Clin 1984;8:37.
238. Sato T, Hashimoto H, Miyagawa K, Sonoda T. Euthyroid hypothryotropinemia in children of short stature. Endocrinol Jpn 1989;36:909.
239. Pichler E. 11-Hydroxycorticosteroids in maternal umbilical cord and neonatal plasma. Proceedings of the Second European Congress Perinatal Medicine, London, 1970. Basel: Karger, 1971:252.
240. Stern L, Sourkes TL, Raiha N. The role of the adrenal medulla in the hypoglycemia of foetal malnutrition. Biol Neonate 1967;11:129.
241. Hill DE. Effect of insulin on fetal growth. Semin Perinatol 1978;2:319.
242. Kadowaki T, Kadowaki H, Taylor SI. A nonsense mutation causing decreased levels of insulin receptor mRNA. Detection by a simplified technique for direct sequencing of genomic DNA amplified by the polymerase chain reaction. Proc Natl Acad Sci USA 1990;87:658.
243. Hill DJ, Milner RDG. Somatomedins and fetal growth. In: Elliott K, Whelan J, eds. The fetus and independent life. Ciba Foundation symposium #86. London: Pitman, 1981:124.
244. D'Ercole AJ, Underwood LE. Growth factors in fetal growth and development. In: Novy MJ, Resko JA, eds. Fetal endocrinology. New York: Academic Press, 1981:155.
245. D'Ercole AJ, Underwood LE, Groelke J, Plet A. Fetal growth retardation (FGR) and hyperinsulinism: evidence for an aberrant intracellular response to insulin (abstract). Pediatr Res 1977;11:513.
246. Schiff D, Colle E, Stern L. Metabolic and growth patterns in transient neonatal diabetes. N Engl J Med 1972;287:119.
247. Marshall RN, Underwood LE, Voina SJ, et al. Characterization of the insulin and somatomedin-C receptors in human placental cell membranes. J Clin Endocrinol Metab 1974; 39:283.
248. Svan H, Hall K, Ritzen M, et al. Somatomedin A and B in serum from neonates, their mothers and cord blood. Acta Endocrinol 1977;85:636.
249. Gsopodarowicz D. The role of growth factors in organ growth and differentiation. In: Jones CT, ed. Biochemical development of the fetus and neonate. Amsterdam: Elsevier Biomedical Press, 1982.
250. Foley TP, DePhilip R, Pericelli A, Miller A. Low somatomedin activity in cord serum from infants with intrauterine growth retardation. J Pediatr 1980;96:605.
251. Rechler MM, Yang YWH, Brown Al, et al. Insulin-like growth factors in fetal growth. In: Bercu BB, ed. Basic and clinical aspects of growth hormone. New York: Plenum Press, 1988: 233.
252. Gluckman PD, Brinsmead MW. Somatomedin in cord blood: relationship to gestational age and birth size. J Clin Endocrinol Metab 1976;43:1378.
253. Lassarre C, Hardouin S, Daffos F, et al. Serum insulin-like growth factors and insulin-like growth factor binding proteins in the human fetus. Relationships with growth in normal subjects and in subjects with intrauterine growth retardation. Pediatr Res 1991;29:219.
254. Thieriot-Prevost G, Boccara JF, Francoual C, et al. Serum insulin-like growth factor 1 and serum growth-promoting activity during the first postnatal year in infants with intrauterine growth retardation. Perdiatr Res 1988;24:380.
255. Fant M, Munro H, Moses AC. Production of insulin-like growth factor binding protein(s) (IGF-BPs) by human placenta: variation with gestational age. Placenta 1988;9:397.
256. Gluckman PD, Johnson-Barret JJ, Butler JH, et al. Studies of insulin-like growth factor I and II by specific radioligand assays in umbilical cord blood. Clin Endocrinol 1983;19:404.
257. Bagga R, Vasishta K, Majumdar S, Garg SK. Correlation between human placental lactogen levels and glucose metabolism in pregnant women with intrauterine growth retardation. Aust N Z J Obstet Gynaecol 1990;30:310.
258. Kramer MS. Intrauterine growth and gestational duration determinants. Pediatrics 1987;80:502.
259. Miller HC, Hassanein K, Hensleigh P. Effects of behavioral and medical variables on fetal growth retardation. Am J Obstet Gynecol 1977;127:643.
260. Stein ZA, Susser M. Intrauterine growth retardation: epidemiological features and public health significance. Semin Perinatol 1984;8:5.
261. Abel EL. Smoking during pregnancy: a review of effects on growth and development of offspring. Hum Biol 1980;52:593.
262. Murphy JF, Drumm JE, Mulcahy R, Daly L. The effect of maternal cigarette smoking on fetal birth weight and on growth of the fetal biparietal diameter. Br J Obstet Gynaecol 1980;87:462.
263. Picone TA, Allen LH, Schramm MM, Olsen PN. Pregnancy outcome in North American women: I. Effects of diet, cigarette smoking and psychological stress on maternal weight gain. Am J Clin Nutr 1982;36:1205.
264. Picone TA, Allen LH, Olsen PN, Ferris ME. Pregnancy outcome in North American women: II. Effects of diet, cigarette smoking, stress, and weight gain on placentas, and on neonatal physical and behavioral characteristics. Am J Clin Nutr 1982;36:1214.
265. Susser M. Prenatal nutrition, birthweight, and psychological development: an overview of experiments, quasi-experiments and natural experiments in the past decade. Am J Clin Nutr 1981;34:784.
266. Nilsen ST, Sagen N, Kim HC, Bergsjo P. Smoking, hemoglobin levels, and birth weights in normal pregnancies. Am J Obstet Gynecol 1984;148:752.
267. Papoz L, Eschwege E, Pequignot G, et al. Maternal smoking and birth weight in relation to dietary habits. Am J Obstet Gynecol 1982;142:870.
268. Haworth JC, Ellestad-Sayed JJ, King J, Dilling LA. Fetal growth retardation in cigarette-smoking mothers is not due to decreased maternal food intake. Am J Obstet Gynecol 1980;137:719.
269. D'Souza SW, Black P, Richards B. Smoking in pregnancy: associations with skinfold thickness maternal weight gain, and fetal size at birth. Br Med J 1981;282:1661.
270. Jacobs DR, Gottenborg S. Smoking and weight: the Minnesota Lipid Research Clinic. Am J Public Health 1981;71:391.
271. Mochizuki M, Maruo T, Masuko K, Ohtsu T. Effects of smoking on fetoplacental-maternal system during pregnancy. Am J Obstet Gynecol 1984;149:413.
272. Wen SW, Goldenberg RL, Cutter GR, et al. Smoking, maternal age, fetal growth, and gestational age at delivery. Am J Obstet Gynecol 1990;162:53.
273. Sexton M, Hebel JR. A clinical trial of change in maternal smoking and its effect on birth weight. JAMA 1984;251:911.
274. Hanson JW, Smith DW. The fetal hydantoin syndrome. J Pediatr 1975;87:285.
275. Gaily E, Granström M-L, Hiilesmaa V, Bardy A. Minor anomalies in offspring of epileptic mothers. J Pediatr 1988;112:520.
276. Warkany J, Monroe BB, Sutherland BS. Intrauterine growth retardation. Am J Dis Child 1961;102:249.
277. Wilson GS, Desmond MM, Verniaud WM. Early development of infants of heroin-addicted mothers. Am J Dis Child 1973;126:457.

278. Naeye RL, Blanc W, Leblanc W, Khatamee MA. Fetal complications of maternal heroin addiction: abnormal growth, infections and episodes of stress. J Pediatr 1973;83:1055.
279. Doberczak TM, Thornton JC, Bernstein J, Kandall SR. Impact of maternal drug dependency on birth weight and head circumference of offspring. Am J Dis Child 1987;141:1163.
280. Giacoia GP. Cocaine in the cradle: a hidden epidemic. South Med J 1990;83:947.
281. Hadeed AJ, Siegel SR. Maternal cocaine use during pregnancy: effect on the newborn infant. Pediatrics 1989;84:205.
282. Oro AS, Dixon SD. Perinatal cocaine and methamphetamine exposure: maternal and neonatal correlates. J Pediatr 1987; 111:571.
283. Little BB, Snell LM. Brain growth among fetuses exposed to cocaine *in utero*: asymmetrical growth retardation. Obstet Gynecol 1991;77:361.
284. Frank DA, Bauchner H, Parker S, et al. Neonatal body proportionality and body composition after *in utero* exposure to cocaine and marijuana. J Pediatr 1990;117:622.
285. Hoyme HE, Jones KL, Dixon SD, et al. Prenatal cocaine exposure and fetal vascular disruption. Pediatrics 1990;85:743.
286. Dixon SD, Bejar R. Brain lesions in cocaine and methamphetamine exposed neonates. Pediatr Res 1988;23:405A.
287. Chasnoff IJ, Chisum GM, Kaplan WE. Maternal cocaine use and genitourinary tract malformations. Teratology 1988; 37:201.
288. Day NL, Richardson GA. Perinatal marijuana use: epidemiology, methodologic issues, and infant outcome. Clin Perinatol 1991;18:77.
289. Fisher SE, Atkinson M, Chang B. Effect of Δ-9-tetrahydrocannabinol on the *in vitro* uptake of alpha-amino isobutyric acid by term human placental slices. Pediatr Res 1987;21:104.
290. Hanson JW, Jones KL, Smith DW. Fetal alcohol syndrome: experience with 41 patients. JAMA 1976;235:1458.
291. Sokol RJ, Bottoms SF. Practical screening for risk-drinking during pregnancy: diagnosis of alcohol abuse. Bocca Raton, FL: CRC Press, 1989:251.
292. Rosett HL, Weiner L, Lee A, et al. Patterns of alcohol consumption and fetal development. Obstet Gynecol 1983; 61:539.
293. Pietrantoni M, Knuppel RA. Alcohol use in pregnancy. Clin Perinatol 1991;18:93.
294. McDonald EC, Pollitt E, Mueller W, et al. The bacon chow study: maternal nutritional supplementation and birth weight of the offspring. Am J Clin Nutr 1981;34:2133.
295. Smith CA. Effects of maternal malnutrition on fetal development. Am J Dis Child 1947;73:243.
296. Smith CA. The effect of maternal undernutrition upon the newborn infant in Holland (1944–45). J Pediatr 1947;30:229.
297. Antonov AN. Children born during the siege of Leningrad in 1942. J Pediatr 1947;30:250.
298. Stein Z, Susser M. The Dutch famine, 1944–1945, and the reproductive process: I. Effects on six indices at birth. Pediatr Res 1975;9:70.
299. Treasure JL, Russell GFM. Intrauterine growth and neonatal weight gain in babies of women with anorexia nervosa. Br Med J 1988;296;1038.
300. Lechtig A, Habicht J-P, Delgado H, et al. Effect of food supplementation during pregnancy on birth weight. Pediatrics 1975;56:508.
301. Mora JO, deParedes B, Wagner M, et al. Nutritional supplementation and the outcome of pregnancy: I. Birth weight. Am J Clin Nutr 1979;32:455.
302. Rush D, Stein Z, Susser M. A randomized, controlled trial of prenatal nutritional supplementation in New York City. Pediatrics 1980;65:683.
303. Sinclair JC, Saigal S. Nutritional influences in industrial societies. Am J Dis Child 1975;129:54.
304. Graham GG. WIC—a fable for our time. Calif Pediatrician 1991;Fall:11.
305. Meadows NJ, Ruse W, Smith MF, et al. Zinc and small babies. Lancet 1981;2:1135.
306. Simmer K, Thompson PH. Zinc in the fetus and newborn. Acta Paediatr Scand 1985;319:158.
307. Jameson S. Effects of zinc deficiency in human reproduction. Linkoping University: Medical Dissertation no. 37, 1976.
308. Morriss FH, Caprioli RM. Techniques and investigation of trace element metabolism in the mother and fetus. In: Nathaniels PW, ed. Animal models in fetal medicine. Amsterdam: Elsevier Biomedical Press, 1982.
309. McMichael AJ, Dreosti IE, Gibson GT, et al. A prospective study of serial maternal serum zinc levels and pregnancy outcome. Early Hum Dev 1982;7:59.
310. Kynast G, Saling E. The relevance of zinc in pregnancy. J Perinat Med 1980;8:171.
311. Goel R, Misra PK. Plasma copper in fetal malnutrition. Acta Paediatr Scand 1982;71:421.
312. Kuhnert PM, Kuhnert BR, Bottoms SF, Erhard P. Cadmium levels in maternal blood, fetal cord blood, and placental tissues of pregnant women who smoke. Am J Obstet Gynecol 1982;142:1021.
313. Ahokas RA, Dilts PV, LaHaye EB. Cadmium-induced fetal growth retardation: protective effect of excess dietary zinc. Am J Obstet Gynecol 1980;136:216.
314. Tsang RC, Gigger M, Oh W, Brown DR. Studies in calcium metabolism in infants with intrauterine growth retardation. J Pediatr 1975;86:936.
315. Myers GJ, Cassady G. Neonatal seizures. Pediatr Rev 1983; 5:68.
316. Altura BM, Altura BT, Carella A. Magnesium deficiency-induced spasms of umbilical vessels: relation to pre-eclampsia, hypertension, growth retardation. Science 1983;221:376.
317. Altshuler G, Russell P, Ermocilla R. The placental pathology of small-for-gestational age infants. Am J Obstet Gynecol 1975;121:351.
318. Cefalo RC, Simkovich JW, Abel F, et al. Effect of potential placental surface area reduction on fetal growth. Am J Obstet Gynecol 1977;129:434.
319. Gerretsen G, Huisies HJ, Elema JD. Morphological changes of the spiral arteries in the placental bed in relation to pre-eclampsia and fetal growth retardation. Br J Obstet Gynaecol 1981;88:876.
320. Dixon HG, Browne JCM, Davey DA. Choriodecidual and myometrial blood-flow. Lancet 1963;2:369.
321. Sheppard BL, Bonnar J. An ultrastructural study of uteroplacental spiral arteries in hypertensive and normotensive pregnancy and fetal growth retardation. Br J Obstet Gynaecol 1981;88:695.
322. Nylund L, Lunell NO, Lewander R, Sarby B. Uteroplacental blood flow index in intrauterine growth retardation of fetal and maternal origin. Br J Obstet Gynaecol 1983;90:16.
323. Theobald GW. Sympathetic nerves and eclampsia. Br Med J 1953;1:422.
324. Naeye RL. Infants of diabetic mothers: a qualitative, morphologic study. Pediatric 1965;35:980.
325. Rosenfeld CR. Consideration of the utero-placental circulation in intrauterine growth. Semin Perinatol 1984;8:42.
326. Lichty JA, Ting RY, Bruns PD, Dyar E. Studies of babies born at high altitude: I. Relation to birth weight. Am J Dis Child 1957;93:666.
327. Yip R. Altitude and birth weight. J Pediatr 1987;111:869.
328. Cotton EK, Hiestand M, Philbin GE, Simmons M. Re-evalua-

tion of birth weights at high altitude: study of babies born to mothers living at an altitude of 3,100 meters. Am J Obstet Gynecol 1980;138:220.
329. Moore LG, Rounds SS, Jahnigen D, et al. Infant birth weight is related to maternal arterial oxygenation at high altitude. J Appl Physiol 1982;52:695.
330. Anderson M, Went LN, Maclver JE, Dixon HG. Sickle-cell disease in pregnancy. Lancet 1960;2:516.
331. Harrison KA, Ibeziako PA. Maternal anemia and fetal birthweight. J Obstet Gynaecol Br Commonw 1973;80:798.
332. Koller O, Sagen N, Ulstein M, Vaula D. Fetal growth retardation associated with inadequate haemodilution in otherwise uncomplicated pregnancy. Acta Obstet Gynecol Scand 1979; 58:9.
333. Fleming AF. Tropical obstetrics and gynaecology. 1. Anaemia in pregnancy in tropical Africa. Trans R Soc Trop Med Hyg 1989;83:441.
334. Brown EG, Memdoza GJB, Chervenak FA, et al. The relationship of maternal erythrocyte oxygen transport parameters to intrauterine growth retardation. Am J Obstet Gynecol 1990; 162:223.
335. Schatz M, Zeiger RS, Hoffman CP. Intrauterine growth is related to gestational pulmonary function in pregnant asthmatic women. Chest 1990;98:389.
336. Apter AJ, Greenberger PA, Patterson R. Outcomes of pregnancy in adolescents with severe asthma. Arch Intern Med 1989;149:2571.
337. Wallenburg HCS, Rotmans N. Enhanced reactivity of the platelet thromboxane pathway in normotensive and hypertensive pregnancies with insufficient fetal growth. Am J Obstet Gynecol 1982;144:523.
338. Wallenburg HCS, VanKessel PH. Platelet life span in pregnancies resulting in small-for-gestational age infants. Am J Obstet Gynecol 1979;134:739.
339. Demers LM, Gabbe SG. Placental prostaglandin levels in preeclampsia. Am J Obstet Gynecol 1976;126:137.
340. Pujkanen MD, Pitkanen Y, Ojala A, Hannelin H. Decrease of uteroplacental blood flow during prostaglandin F_2-alpha induced abortion. Prostaglandins 1975;9:61.
341. Terragno NA, Terragno A. Prostaglandin metabolism in the fetal and maternal vasculature. Fed Proc 1979;38:75.
342. Lewis PJ, Boylan P, Friedman LA, et al. Prostacyclin in pregnancy. Br Med J 1980;1:1581.
343. Zamorano B, Terragno A, McGiff JC, Terragno NA. A prostaglandin mechanism may contribute to the regulation of blood pressure in spontaneously hypertensive rats during pregnancy. Adv Prostaglandin Thromboxane Leukot Res 1980;7:807.
344. Goodman RP, Killam AP, Brash AR, Branch RA. Prostacyclin production during normal pregnancy and pregnancy complicated by hypertension. Am J Obstet Gynecol 1982;142:817.
345. Lewis PJ, Moncada S, O'Grady J, eds. Prostacyclin in pregnancy. New York: Raven Press, 1983.
346. Geber WF, Schramm LC. Postpartum weight alteration in hamster offspring from females injected during pregnancy with either heroin, methadone, a composite drug mixture or mescaline. Am J Obstet Gynecol 1974;120:1105.
347. Taeusch HW, Carson SH, Wang NS, Avery ME. Heroin induction of lung maturation and growth retardation in fetal rabbits. J Pediatr 1973;82:869.
348. Harding PGR, Young A, Possmayer F. The effect of hypoinsulinemia on the fetus (abstract). Clin Res 1975;23:611A.
349. Emmanouilides GC, Townsend DE, Bauer RA. Effects of single umbilical artery ligation in the lamb fetus. Pediatrics 1968;42:919.
350. Hobel CJ, Emmanouilides GC, Townsend DE, Yoshiro K. Ligation of one umbilical artery in the fetal lamb. Obstet Gynecol 1970;36:582.
351. Creasy RK, Barrett CT, de Swiet M, et al. Experimental intrauterine growth retardation in the sheep. Am J Obstet Gynecol 1972;112:566.
352. Creasy RK, deSwiet M, Kahanpää KV, et al. Pathophysiological changes in the fetal lamb with growth retardation. In: Foetal and neonatal physiology: proceedings of the Sir Joseph Barcroft Centenary Symposium. Cambridge: Cambridge University Press, 1973.
353. Pickart LR, Creasy RK, Thaler MM. Hyperfibrinogenemia and polycythemia with intrauterine growth retardation in fetal lambs. Am J Obstet Gynecol 1976;124:268.
354. Clapp JF, Szeto HH, Larrow R, et al. Fetal metabolic response to experimental placental vascular damage. Am J Obstet Gynecol 1981;140:446.
355. Block BSB, Llanos AJ, Creasy RK. Responses of the growth-retarded fetus to acute hypoxemia. Am J Obstet Gynecol 1984;148:878.
356. Potter BJ, Belling GB, Mano MT, Hetzel BS. Experimental production of growth retardation in the sheep fetus after exposure to alcohol. Med J Aust 1980;2:191.
357. Wallace LR. Effect of diet on fetal development (abstract). Proceedings of the Physiological Society 1945–1946;104:34P.
358. Wigglesworth JS. Foetal growth retardation. Br Med Bull 1966;22:13.
359. Liggins GC, quoted in Hill DE. Effect of insulin on fetal growth. Semin Perinatol 1978;2:319.
360. Alexander G. Studies on the placenta of the sheep (*Ovis aries* L.): effect of surgical reduction in the number of caruncles. J Reprod Fertil 1964;7:307.
361. Chase HP, Dabiere CS, Welch NN, O'Brien D. Intrauterine undernutrition and brain development. Pediatrics 1971; 47:491.
362. Widdowson EM. Harmony of growth. Lancet 1970;1:901.
363. Myers SA, Sparks JW, Makowski EL, et al. Relationship between placental blood flow and placental and fetal size in guinea pig. Am J Physiol 1982;243:12-H404.
364. Widdowson EM. Intrauterine growth retardation in the pig: I. Organ growth and cellular development at birth and after growth to maturity. Biol Neonate 1971;19:329.
365. Adams PH. Intrauterine growth retardation in the pig: II. The development of the skeleton. Biol Neonate 1971;19:341.
366. Dickerson JWT, Merat A, Widdowson EM. Intrauterine growth retardation in the pig: III. The chemical structure of the brain. Biol Neonate 1971;19:354.
367. Cheek DB, Hill DE. Changes in somatic growth after ablation of maternal or fetal pancreatic beta cells. In: Cheek DB, ed. Fetal and postnatal cellular growth. New York: John Wiley & Sons, 1975.
368. Myers RE, Hill DE, Holt AB, et al. Fetal growth retardation produced by experimental placental insufficiency in the rhesus monkey, I. Body weight, organ size. Biol Neonate 1971; 18:379.
370. Hill DE, Myers RE, Holt AB, et al. Fetal growth retardation produced by experimental placental insufficiency in the rhesus monkey, II. Chemical composition of the brain, liver, muscle and carcass. Biol Neonate 1971;19:68.
371. Hill DE. Experimental growth retardation in rhesus monkeys. In: Size at birth. Ciba Foundation symposium #27. Amsterdam: Excerpta Medica, 1974.
372. Meberg A. Transitory thrombocytopenia in newborn mice after intrauterine hypoxia. Pediatr Res 1980;14:1971.
373. Evans MI, Schulman JD, Golden L, Mukherjee AB. Superovulation-induced intrauterine growth retardation in mice. Am J Obstet Gynecol 1981;141:433.

374. Meberg A. Somatic growth and brain development: effects of intrauterine malnutrition and hypoxia in mice. Biol Neonate 1981;39:272.
375. Kwong MS, Moore TC, Lemmi CAE, et al. Histidine decarboxylase activity in fetal intrauterine growth-retarded rats. Pediatr Res 1976;10:737.
376. Scott JR. Fetal growth retardation associated with maternal administration of immunosuppressive drugs. Am J Obstet Gynecol 1977;128:668.
377. Bührdel P, Willgerodt H, Keller E, Theile H. The postnatal development of rats after preterm and post-term birth: I. Body weight. Biol Neonate 1978;33:184.
378. Bührdel P, Keller E, Willgerodt H, Theile H. The postnatal development of rats born preterm and post term: II. Liver, brain, heart and kidneys. Biol Neonate 1978;33:240.
379. Sybulski S, Toth A, Maughan GB. The influence of experimental renal hypertension on pregnancy in the rat. Am J Obstet Gynecol 1971;110:314.
380. Nitzan M, Ofloff S, Chrzanowska BL, Schulman JD. Intrauterine growth retardation in renal insufficiency: an experimental model in the rat. Am J Obstet Gynecol 1979; 133:40.
381. Zagon IS, McLaughlin PJ. Effect of chronic maternal methadone exposure on perinatal development. Biol Neonate 1977; 31:271.
382. Swaab DF, Honnebier WJ. The influence of removal of the fetal rat brain upon intrauterine growth of the fetus and the placenta and on gestation length. J Obstet Gynaecol Br Commonw 1973;80:589.
383. Wells LJ. Progress of studies designed to determine whether the fetal hypophysis produces hormones that influence development. Anat Rec 1947;97:409.
384. Chow BF, Lee CJ. Effect of dietary restriction of pregnant rats on body weight gain of the offspring. J Nutr 1964;82:10.
385. Adlard BPF, Dobbing J, Smart JL. An alternative animal model for the full-term small-for-dates human baby. Biol Neonate 1973;23:95.
386. Zamenhoff S, van Marthens E, Margolis FL. DNA (cell number) and protein in neonatal brain: alteration by maternal dietary protein restriction. Science 1968;160:322.
387. Venkatachalam PS, Ramanathan KS. Severe protein deficiency during gestation in rats on birth weight and growth of offspring. Indian J Med Res 1966;54:402.
388. Lee CJ, Chow BF. Protein metabolism in the offspring of underfed mother rats. J Nutr 1971;87:439.
389. Winick M. Cellular growth of the placenta as an indicator of abnormal fetal growth. In: Adamsons K, ed. Diagnosis and treatment of fetal disorders. New York: Springer-Verlag, 1968:83.
390. Winick M. Cellular changes during placental and fetal growth. Am J Obstet Gynecol 1971;109:166.
391. Brasel JA, Winick M. Maternal nutrition and prenatal growth. Experimental studies of effects of maternal undernutrition on fetal and placental growth. Arch Dis Child 1972;47:479.
392. Levitsky LL, Speck SM, Shulman R. Metabolic response to fasting in experimental intrauterine growth retardation: a comparison of two models. Biol Neonate 1976;30:11.
393. Franklin JB, Brent RL. The effect of uterine vascular clamping on the development of rat embryos three to fourteen days old. J Morphol 1964;115:273.
394. Brent RL, Franklin JB. Uterine vascular clamping: new procedure for the study of congenital malformations. Science 1960; 132:89.
395. Wigglesworth JS. Experimental growth retardation in the foetal rat. J Pathol Bacteriol 1964;88:1.
396. Dahlquist G, Persson B. Effect of intrauterine growth retardation on the postnatal development of D-β-hydroxybutyrate dehydrogenase activity in rat brain. Biol Neonate 1976;28:353.
397. Bernal A, Morales M, Feria-Velasco A, et al. Effect of intrauterine growth retardation on the biochemical maturation of brain synaptosomes in the rat. J Nutr 1974;104:1157.
398. Lugo G, O'Neil L, Cassady G. Carcass water, fat and chloride in the fetal growth retarded rat. Am J Obstet Gynecol 1971;110:358.
399. Hohenauer L, Oh W. Body composition in experimental intrauterine growth retardation in the rat. J Nutr 1969;99:23.
400. Brans YW, Ortega P. Water content and distribution in intrauterine growth-retarded newborn rats. Biol Neonate 1977; 31:166.
401. Nitzan M, Groffman H. Hepatic gluconeogenesis and lipogenesis in experimental intrauterine growth retardation in the rat. Am J Obstet Gynecol 1971;109:623.
402. Nitzan M, Groffman H. Metabolic changes in experimental intrauterine growth retardation in rats: blood glucose and liver glycogen in dysmature and premature newborn rats. Isr J Med Sci 1970;6:697.
403. Oh WH, D'Amodio MD, Yap LL, Hohenhauer L. Carbohydrate metabolism in experimental intrauterine growth retardation in rats. Am J Obstet Gynecol 1970;108:415.
404. Oh W, Guy JA. Cellular growth in experimental intrauterine growth retardation in rats. J Nutr 1971;101:1631.
405. Chanez C, Tordet-Caridroit C, Roux JM. Studies on experimental hypotrophy in the rat. II. Development of some liver enzymes of gluconeogenesis. Biol Neonate 1971;18:58.
406. Nitzan M, Groffman H. Glucose metabolism in experimental intrauterine growth retardation. *In vitro* studies with liver and brain slices. Biol Neonate 1971;17:420.
407. Roux JM, Jahchan T, Fulchignoni MC. Desoxyribonucleic acid and pyrimidine synthesis in the rat during intrauterine growth retardation: responsiveness of several organs. Biol Neonate 1975;27:129.
408. Roux JM, Tordet-Caridroit C, Chanez C. Studies on experimental hypotrophy in the rat. I. Chemical composition of the total body and some organs in the rat foetus. Biol Neonate 1970;15:342.
409. Friedler G, Cochin J. Growth retardation in offspring of female rats treated with morphine prior to conception. Science 1972;175:654.
410. Vileisis RA, Fain J, Oh W. Fatty acid synthesis in rat fetuses with intrauterine growth retardation. Metabol 1982;31:217.
411. Van Geijn HP, Kaylor WM, Nicola KR, Zuspan FP. Induction of severe intrauterine growth retardation in the Sprague-Dawley rat. Am J Obstet Gynecol 1980;137:43.
412. Gruppuso PA, Migliori R, Susa JB, Schwartz R. Chronic maternal hyperinsulinemia and hypoglycemia: a model for experimental intrauterine growth retardation. Biol Neonate 1981;40:113.
413. Croskerry PG, Smart JL, Charnock P. Unilateral ovariectomy during pregnancy in well-nourished and undernourished rats: effects on placenta and fetal body and brain growth. Biol Neonate 1981;40:46.
414. Dobbing J. The developing brain: a plea for more critical interspecies extrapolation. Nutr Rep Int 1973;7:401.
415. Dobbing J. The later growth of the brain and its vulnerability. Pediatrics 1974;53:2.
416. Evans MI, Mukherjee AB, Schulman JD. Animal models of intrauterine growth retardation. Obstet Gynecol Survey 1983; 38:183.
417. Rosado A, Bernal A, Sosa A, et al. Human fetal growth retardation. III. Protein, DNA, RNA, adenine nucleotides, and activities of the enzymes pyruvic and adenylate kinase in placenta. Pediatrics 1972;50:568.

418. Shanklin DR. The influence of placental lesions on the newborn infant. Pediatr Clin North Am 1970;17:25.
419. Gruenwald P. Fetal deprivation and placental pathology: concepts and relationships. In: Rosenberg HS, Bolande RP, eds. Perspectives in pediatric pathology, vol 2. Chicago: Year Book, 1975:101.
420. Tremblay PC, Sybulski S, Maughan GB. Role of the placenta in fetal malnutrition. Am J Obstet Gynecol 1965;91:597.
421. Sybulski S, Tremblay PC. Placental glycogen content and utilization *in vitro* in intrauterine fetal malnutrition. Am J Obstet Gynecol 1969;103:257.
422. Sybulski S. *In vitro* estrogen biosynthesis from testosterone by homogenates of placentas from normal pregnancies and pregnancies complicated by intrauterine fetal malnutrition and diabetes. Am J Obstet Gynecol 1969;105:1055.
423. Iyengar L. Chemical composition of placenta in pregnancies with small-for-date infants. Am J Obstet Gynecol 1973;116:66.
424. Winick M, Noble A. Cellular growth in human placenta. I. Normal placental growth. Pediatrics 1967;39:248.
425. Winick M. Cellular growth of human placenta. III. Intrauterine growth failure. J Pediatr 1967;71:390.
426. Dayton DH, Filer LJ, Canosa C. Cellular changes in the placentas of undernourished mothers in Guatemala. Fed Proc 1969;28:488.
427. Winick M. Cellular growth in intrauterine malnutrition. Pediatr Clin North Am 1970;17:69.
428. Naeye RL, Blanc WA. Pathogenesis of congenital rubella. JAMA 1965;194:1277.
429. Naeye RL. Unsuspected organ abnormalities associated with congenital heart disease. Am J Pathol 1965;47:905.
430. Cheek DB. Muscle cell growth in abnormal children. In: Cheek DB, ed. Human growth: body composition, cell growth, energy and intelligence. Philadelphia: Lea & Febiger, 1968:352.
431. Hill DE, Arellano C, Izukawa T, et al. Studies in infants and children with congenital rubella: oxygen consumption, body water, cell mass, muscle and adipose tissue composition. Johns Hopkins Med J 1970;127:309.
432. Brans Y, Ortega P, Bailey P. Water contents of human muscles in relation to fetal growth (abstract). Clin Res 1976; 24:72A.
433. Widdowson EM, Crabb DE, Milner RDG. Cellular development of some human organs before birth. Arch Dis Child 1972;47:652.
434. Cheek DBR, Graystone J, Mehrizi A. The importance of muscle cell number in children with congenital heart disease. Johns Hopkins Med J 1966;118:140.
435. Cheek DB, Brasel JA, Elliott D, Scott R. Muscle cell size and number in normal children and in dwarfs (pituitary, cretins, and primordial) before and after treatment (preliminary observations). Johns Hopkins Med J 1966;119:46.
436. Shelley HJ, Neligan GA. Neonatal hypoglycaemia. Br Med Bull 1966;22:34.
437. Naeye RL. Cardiovascular abnormalities in infants malnourished before birth. Biol Neonate 1965;8:104.
438. Naeye RL, Kelly JA. Judgement of fetal age: III. The pathologist's evaluation. Pediatr Clin North Am 1966;13:849.
439. Chase HP, Welch NN, Dabiere CS, et al. Alterations in human brain biochemistry following intrauterine growth retardation. Pediatrics 1972;50:403.
440. Vasan NS, Chase HP. Brain glycosaminoglycans (mucopolysaccharides) following intrauterine growth retardation. Biol Neonate 1976;28:196.
441. Cassady G. Body composition in intrauterine growth retardation. Pediatr Clin North Am 1970;17:79.
442. Cassady G. Plasma volume studies in low birth weight infants. Pediatrics 1966;38:1020.
443. Cassady G. Bromide space studies in infants of low birth weight. Pediatr Res 1970;4:414.
444. Cassady G, Milstead RR. Antipyrine space studies and cell water estimates in infants of low birth weight. Pediatr Res 1971;5:673.
445. Friis-Hansen B. Care and hazards of the small-for-dates infant. Proceedings of the Second European Congress of Perinatal Medicine, London, 1970. Basel: Karger, 1971:223.
446. Bhakoo ON, Scopes JW. Weight minus extracellular fluid as metabolic reference standard in newborn baby. Arch Dis Child 1971;46:483.
447. MacLennan AH, Millington G, Grieve A, et al. Neonatal body water turnover: a putative index of perinatal morbidity. Am J Obstet Gynecol 1981;139:948.
448. MacLennan AH, Hocking A, Seamark RF, et al. Neonatal water metabolism: an objective postnatal index of intrauterine fetal growth. Early Hum Dev 1983;8:21.
449. Marks JF, Kay J, Baum J, Curry L. Uric acid levels in full-term and low-birth-weight infants. J Pediatr 1968;73:609.
450. Rubaltelli FF, Formentin PA, Tato L. Ammonia nitrogen, urea and uric acid blood levels in normal and hypodystrophic newborns. Biol Neonate 1970;15:129.
451. Rubaltelli FF, Peratoner L. Ammonia nitrogen in "small-for-dates" newborn babies. Lancet 1969;1:208.
452. Younoszai MK, Kacic A, Dilling L, Haworth JC. Urinary hydroxyproline/creatinine ratio in normal term, pre-term and growth-retarded infants. Arch Dis Child 1969;44:517.
453. Younoszai MK, Haworth JC. Excretion of hydroxyproline in urine by premature and normal full-term infants and those with intrauterine growth retardation during the first three days of life. Pediatr Res 1968;2:17.
454. Klujber L, Maetyan G, Sulyok E, Soltesz G. Urinary hydroxyproline excretion in normally grown and growth retarded newborn infants. Biol Neonate 1972;20:196.
455. Klujber L, Sulyok E. Urinary glycosaminoglycan excretion in normally grown and growth retarded neonates. I. Total glycosaminoglycan excretion. Acta Paediatr Acad Sci Hung 1972;13:81.
456. Bazso M, Asztalos M, Kassai L. Serum proteins in foetal growth retardation. In: Horsky J, Stembra ZK, eds. Intrauterine dangers to the fetus. Amsterdam: Excerpta Medica Foundation, 1967:585.
457. Jacobsen BB, Peitersen B, Andersen HJ, Hummer L. Serum concentrations of thyroxine-binding globulin, prealbumin and albumin in healthy full-term, small-for-gestational age and preterm newborn infants. Acta Paediatr Scand 1979; 68:49.
458. Eggermont E, Socha J, Bhavani S, Carchon H. Plasma prealbumin in the newborn (letter). Acta Paediatr Scand 1979; 68:613.
459. Yeung CY, Hobbs JR. Serum gG-globulin levels in normal, premature, post-mature and "small-for-dates" newborn babies. Lancet 1968;1:1167.
460. Papadatos C, Papaevangelou G, Alexion D, Mendris J. Immunoglobulin levels and gestational age. Biol Neonate 1969; 14:365.
461. Papadatos C, Papaevangelou G, Alexion D, Mendris J. Serum immunoglobulin G levels in small-for-date newborn babies. Arch Dis Child 1970;45:570.
462. Yang SL, Lin CC, River P, Moawad AH. Immunoglobulin concentrations in newborn infants associated with intrauterine growth retardation. Obstet Gynecol 1983;62:561.
463. Catty D, Seger R, Drew R, et al. IgG-subclass concentrations

in cord sera from premature, full-term and small-for-dates babies. Eur J Pediatr 1977;125:89.
464. Hyvarinen M, Zeltzer P, Oh W, Stiehm ER. Influence of gestational age on serum levels of alpha-1-fetoprotein, IgG globulin, and albumin in newborn infants. J Pediatr 1973;82:43.
465. Prokopowicz J, Ziobro J, Iwaszko-Krawczuk W. Bactericidal capacity of plasma and granulocytes in small-for-dates newborns. Acta Paediatr Acad Sci Hung 1975;16:267.
466. Iwaszko-Krawczuk W, Propkopowicz J. Phagocytosis in small-for-dates newborns. Acta Paediatr Acad Sci Hung 1973;14:47.
467. Iwaszko-Krawczuk W. Serum lysozyme activity in small-for-dates newborn. Acta Paediatr Acad Sci Hung 1973;14:135.
468. Chandra RK. Immunocompetence in low-birth-weight infants after intrauterine malnutrition. Lancet 1974;2:1393.
469. Chandra RK. Fetal malnutrition and postnatal immunocompetence. Am J Dis Child 1975;129:450.
470. Pittard WB, Miller K, Sorensen RU. Normal lymphocyte responses to mitogen in term and premature neonates following normal and abnormal intrauterine growth. Clin Immunol Immunopathol 1984;30:178.
471. Alford CA, Schaefer J, Blankenship WJ, et al. A correlative immunologic, microbiologic and clinical approach to the diagnosis of acute and chronic infections in newborn infants. N Engl J Med 1967;277:437.
472. Haworth JC, Dilling L, Younoszai MK. Relation of blood-glucose to hematocrit, birth weight and other body measurements in normal and growth-retarded newborn infants. Lancet 1967;2:901.
473. Humbert JR, Abelson H, Hathaway WE, Battaglia FC. Polycythemia in small for gestational age infants. J Pediatr 1969; 75:812.
474. Oh W, Omori K, Emmanouilides GC, Phelps DL. Placenta to lamb fetus transfusion *in utero* during acute hypoxia. Am J Obstet Gynecol 1975;122:316.
475. Yao AC, Lind J. Blood volume in the asphyxiated term neonate. Biol Neonate 1972;21:199.
476. Finne PH. Erythropoietin levels in cord blood as an indicator of intrauterine hypoxia. Acta Paediatr Scand 1966;55:475.
477. Bergquist G. Viscosity of the blood in the newborn infant. Acta Paediatr Scand 1974;63:858.
478. Hakanson DO, Oh W. Hyperviscosity in the small-for-gestational age infant. Biol Neonate 1980;37:109.
479. Rivers RPA. Coagulation changes associated with a high haematocrit in the newborn infant. Acta Pediatr Scand 1975; 64:449.
480. Perlman M, Dvilansky A. Blood coagulation status of small-for-dates and postmature infants. Arch Dis Child 1975;50:424.
481. Lochridge S, Pass R, Cassady G. Reticulocyte counts in intrauterine growth retardation. Pediatrics 1971;47:919.
482. Chance GW, Bower BD. Hypoglycaemia and temporary hyperglycaemia in infants of low birth weight for maturity. Arch Dis Child 1966;41:279.
483. Gentz JCH, Cornblath M. Transient diabetes of the newborn. Adv Pediatr 1969;16:345.
484. Ongari MA, Ritter JM, Orchard MA, et al. Correlation of prostacyclin synthesis by human umbilical artery with status of essential fatty acid. Am J Obstet Gynecol 1984;149:455.
485. Phillips L, Lumley J, Paterson P, Wood C. Fetal hypoglycemia. Am J Obstet Gynecol 1968;102:371.
486. Melichar V, Novak M, Zoula J, et al. Energy sources in the newborn. Biol Neonate 1965;9:298.
487. De Leeuw R, de Vries IJ. Hypoglycemia in small-for-dates newborn infants. Pediatrics 1976;58:18.
488. Salle B, Ruitton-Uglienco A. Glucose disappearance rate, insulin response and growth hormone response in the small for gestational age and premature infant of very low birth weight. Biol Neonate 1976;29:1.
489. Horvath I, Toth P, Mehes K. The predictive value of glucose utilization rate in neonatal hypoglycaemia of small-for-gestational-age infants. Acta Paediatr Acad Sci Hung 1975;16:143.
490. Gentz JCH, Warrner R, Persson, BEH, Cornblath M. Intravenous glucose tolerance, plasma insulin, free fatty acids and β-hydroxybutyrate in underweight newborn infants. Acta Paediatr 1969;58:481.
491. Pildes RS, Patel DA, Nitzan M. Glucose disappearance rate in symptomatic neonatal hypoglycemia. Pediatrics 1973;52:75.
492. Madsen A. Spontaneous hypoglycaemia with convulsions and deficient adrenalin reaction. A case occurring in one of uniovular twins. Acta Paediatr Scand 1965;54:483.
493. Gentz J, Kellum M, Persson B. The effect of feeding on oxygen consumption, RQ and plasma levels of glucose, FFA, and D-β-hydroxybutyrate in newborn infants of diabetic mothers and small for gestational age infants. Acta Paediatr Scand 1976;65:445.
494. Melichar V, Novak M, Hahn P, Koldovsky O. Free fatty acid and glucose in the blood of various groups of newborns. Preliminary report. Acta Paediatr 1964;53:343.
495. Robertson AF, Sprecher HW, Wilcox JP. Total lipid fatty acid patterns of umbilical cord blood in intrauterine growth failure. Biol Neonate 1969;14:28.
496. Stanley CA, Anday EK, Baker L, Delivoria-Papadopolous M. Metabolic fuel and hormone responses to fasting in newborn infants. Pediatrics 1979;64:613.
497. Schiff D, Lowy C. Carbohydrate metabolism in the newborn. Lancet 1968;1:475.
498. Melichar V, Drahota Z, Hahn P. Ketone bodies in the blood of full term newborns, premature and dysmature infants and infants of diabetic mothers. Biol Neonate 1967;11:23.
499. Sabata V, Znamenacek K, Pribylova H, Melichar V. The effect of glucose in the prenatal treatment of small-for-dates fetuses. Biol Neonate 1973;22:78.
500. Pagliara AS, Karl IE, Haymond M, Kipnis DM. Hypoglycemia in infancy and childhood, part I. J Pediatr 1973;82:365.
501. Hay WW. Fetal and neonatal glucose homeostasis and their relation to the small-for-gestational-age infant. Semin Perinatol 1984;8:101.
502. Haymond MW, Karl IE, Pagliara AS. Increased gluconeogenic substrates in the small-for-gestational-age infant. N Engl J Med 1974;291:322.
503. Williams PR, Fiser RH, Sperling MA, Oh W. Effects of oral alanine feeding on blood glucose, plasma glucagon and insulin concentrations in small-for-gestational-age infants. N Engl J Med 1975;292:612.
504. Rautenbach M, Beyreiss K. Absorption rates of fructose and influence of fructose on the glucose blood level in preterm and term newborns appropriate for gestational age as compared to preterm and term newborns small for gestational age. Biol Neonate 1976;30:123.
505. Haymond M, Karl I, Pagliara A. Defective gluconeogenesis (GNG) in small-for-gestational-age infants (SGAI) (abstract). J Pediatr 1973;83:153.
506. Dewhurst CJ, Dunham AM, Harvey DR, Parkinson CE. Prediction of respiratory-distress syndrome by estimation of surfactant in the amniotic fluid. Lancet 1973;1:1475.
507. Dyson D, Blake M, Cassady G. Amniotic fluid lecithin/sphingomyelin ratio in complicated pregnancies. Am J Obstet Gynecol 1975;122:772.
508. Lindback T. Amniotic fluid lecithin concentrations in pregnancies complicated by hypertensive disorders and intrauter-

ine growth retardation. Acta Obstet Gynecol Scand 1976; 55:355.
509. Dahms BB, Krauss AN, Auld PAM. Pulmonary function in dysmature infants. J Pediatr 1974;84:434.
510. Gluck L, Kulovich MV. Lecithin/sphingomyelin ratios in amniotic fluid in normal and abnormal pregnancy. Am J Obstet Gynecol 1973;115:539.
511. Sinclair JC, Silverman WA. Intrauterine growth in active tissue mass of the human fetus, with particular reference to the undergrown baby. Pediatrics 1966;38:48.
512. Sinclair JC, Scopes JW, Silverman WA. Metabolic reference standards for the neonate. Pediatrics 1967;39:724.
513. Sinclair JC. Heat production and thermo-regulation in the small-for-dates infant. Pediatr Clin North Am 1970;17:147.
514. Scopes JW, Ahmed I. Minimal rates of oxygen consumption in sick and premature newborn infants. Arch Dis Child 1966; 41:407.
515. Bhakoo ON, Scopes JW. Minimal rates of oxygen consumption in small-for-dates babies during the first week of life. Arch Dis Child 1974;49:583.
516. Lees MH, Younger EW, Babson SG. Thermal requirements of undergrown human neonates. Biol Neonate 1966;10:288.
517. Rubecz I, Mestyan J. The partition of maintenance energy expenditure and the pattern of substrate utilization in intrauterine malnourished newborn infants before and during recovery. Acta Paediatr Acad Sci Hung 1975;16:335.
518. Ortner A, Zech H, Humpler E, Mairbaeurl H. May high oxygen affinity of maternal hemoglobin cause fetal growth retardation? Arch Gynecol 1983;234:79.
519. Freeman RK, Goebelsman U, Nochimson D, Cetrulo C. An evaluation of the significance of a positive oxytocin challenge test. Obstet Gynecol 1976;47:8.
520. Huddleston JF, Sutliff G, Carney FE Jr, Flowers CE. Oxytocin challenge test for antepartum fetal assessment: report of a clinical experience. Am J Obstet Gynecol 1979;135:609.
521. Cox WL, Daffos F, Forestier F, et al. Physiology and management of intrauterine growth retardation: a biologic approach with fetal blood sampling. Am J Obstet Gynecol 1988;159:36.
522. Nicolaides KH, Campbell S, Bradley RJ, et al. Maternal oxygen therapy for intrauterine growth retardation. Lancet 1987; 1:942.
523. Phillips JD, Diamond JM, Fonkalsrud EW. Fetal rabbit intestinal absorption: implications for transamniotic fetal feeding. J Pediatr Surg 1990;25:909.
524. Flake AW, Villa RL, Adzick S, Harrison MR. Transamniotic fetal feeding. II. A model of intrauterine growth retardation using the relationship of "natural runting" to uterine position. J Pediatr Surg 1987;22:816.
525. Flake AW, Villa-Troyer RL, Adzick NS, Harrison MR. Transamniotic fetal feeding. III. The effect of nutrient infusion on fetal growth retardation. J Pediatr Surg 1986;21:481.
526. Gregory GA, Gooding CA, Phibbs R, Tooley WH. Meconium aspiration in infants—a prospective study. J Pediatr 1974; 85:848.
527. Ting P, Brady JP. Tracheal suction in meconium aspiration. Am J Obstet Gynecol 1975;122:767.
528. Carson BS, Losey RW, Bowes WA, Simmons MA. Combined obstetric and pediatric approach to prevent meconium aspiration syndrome. Am J Obstet Gynecol 1976;126:712.
529. Sann L, Ruitton A, Mathieu M, Lasne Y. Effect of intravenous hydrocortisone administration of glucose homeostasis in small-for-gestational-age infants. Acta Paediatr Scand 1979; 68:113.
530. Holowach-Thurston J, Hauhart RE, Jones EM, et al. Decrease in brain glucose in anoxia in spite of elevated plasma glucose levels. Pediatr Res 1973;7:691.
531. Tsang R, Glueck CJ, Evans G, Steiner PM. Cord blood hypertriglyceridemia. Am J Dis Child 1974;127:78.
532. Anderson GE, Friis-Hansen B. Neonatal hypertriglyceridemia: a new index of antepartum-intrapartum fetal stress. Acta Paediatr Scand 1976;65:369.
533. Saugstad OD, Gluck L. Plasma hypoxanthine levels in newborn infants: a specific indicator of hypoxia. J Perinat Med 1982;10:266.
534. O'Conner MC, Harkness RA, Simmonds RJ, Hytten FE. The measurement of hypoxanthine, inosine and uridine in umbilical cord blood and fetal scalp blood samples as a measure of fetal hypoxia. Br J Obstet Gynaecol 1981;88:381.
535. Bistoletti P, Nylund L, Lagercrantz H, et al. Fetal scalp catecholamines during labor. Am J Obstet Gynecol 1983;147:785.
536. Stark RI, Wardlaw SL, Daniel SS, et al. Vasopressin secretion induced by hypoxia in sheep: developmental changes and relationship to beta-endorphin release. Am J Obstet Gynecol 1982;143:204.
537. Parboosingh J, Lederis K, Singh N. Vasopressin concentration in cord blood: correlation with method of delivery and cord *p*H. Obstet Gynecol 1982;60:179.
538. Allen MC. Developmental outcome and follow-up of the small-for-gestational-age infant. Semin Perinatol 1984;8:123.
539. Commey JOO, Fitzhardinge PM. Handicap in the preterm small-for-gestational-age infant. J Pediatr 1979;94:779.
540. Dweck HS, Huggins W, Dorman LP, et al. Developmental sequelae in infants having suffered severe perinatal asphyxia. Am J Obstet Gynecol 1974;119:811.
541. Babson SG, Henderson NB. Fetal undergrowth: relation of head growth to later intellectual performance. Pediatrics 1974;53:890.
542. Cassady G. Small premature intensive care: long-term results. J Perinat Med 1982;10:54.
543. Villar J, do Onis M, Kestler E, et al. The differential neonatal morbidity of the intrauterine growth retardation syndrome. Am J Obstet Gynecol 1990;163:151.
544. Hackett GA, Campbell S, Gamsu H, et al. Doppler studies in the growth retarded fetus and prediction of neonatal necrotizing enterocolitis, haemorrhage, and neonatal morbidity. Br Med J 1987;294:13.
545. Burke G, Stuart B, Crowley P, et al. Is intrauterine growth retardation with normal umbilical artery blood flow a benign condition? Br Med J 1990;300:1044.
546. Hakulinen A, Heinonen K, Jokela V, Launiala K. Prematurity-associated morbidity during the first two years of life. Acta Paediatr Scand 1988;77:340.
547. Van Heel IR-D, de Leeuw R. Clinical outcome of small for gestational age preterm infants. J Perinat Med 1989;17:77.
548. Wennergren M, Wennergren G, Vilbergsson G. Obstetric characteristics and neonatal performance in a four-year small-for-gestational-age population. Obstet Gynecol 1988;72:615.
549. Kraus J, Greenland S, Bulterys M. Risk factors for sudden infant death syndrome in the US collaborative perinatal project. Int J Epidemiol 1989;18:113.
550. Buck GM, Cookfair DL, Michalek AM, et al. Intrauterine growth retardation and risk of sudden infant death syndrome (SIDS). Am J Epidemiol 1989;129:874.
551. Fitzhardinge PM, Steven EM. The small-for-dates infant. I. Later growth patterns. Pediatrics 1972;49:671.
552. Beck GJ, VandenBerg BJ. The relationship of the rate of intrauterine growth of low-birth-weight infants to later growth. J Pediatr 1975;86:504.
553. Cruise MO. A longitudinal study of the growth of the low-birth-weight infants. I. Velocity and distance growth, birth to 3 years. Pediatrics 1973;51:620.
554. Low JA, Galbraith RS, Muir D, et al. Intrauterine growth

retardation: a preliminary report of long term morbidity. Am J Obstet Gynecol 1978;130:534.
555. Martell M, Falkner F, Bertolini LB, et al. Early postnatal growth evaluation in full-term, preterm and small-for-date infants. Early Hum Dev 1978;1:313.
556. Beargie RA, James VL, Greene JW. Growth and development of small-for-date newborns. Pediatr Clin North Am 1970; 17:159.
557. Fancourt R, Campbell S, Harvey D, Norman AP. Follow-up study of small-for-date babies. Br Med J 1976;1:1421.
558. Wedgwood M, Holt KS. A longitudinal study of the dental and physical development of 2–3-year-old children who were underweight at birth. Biol Neonate 1968;12:214.
559. Ounstead M. Post-natal growth of children who were S.F.D. and L.F.D. Dev Med Child Neurol 1971;13:121.
560. Piekkala P, Kero P, Sillanpää M, Erkkola R. The somatic growth of a regional birth cohort of 351 preterm infants during the first two years of life. J Perinat Med 1989;17:41.
561. Tenovuo A, Kero P, Piekkala P, et al. Growth of 519 small for gestational age infants during the first two years of life. Acta Paediatr Scand 1987;76:636.
562. Davies DP, Beverley D. Changes in body proportions over the first year of life: comparisons between "light-for-dates" and "appropriate-for-dates" term infants. Early Hum Dev 1979; 3:263.
563. Vohr BR, Oh W, Rosenfield AG, et al. The preterm small-for-gestational-age infant: a two-year follow-up study. Am J Obstet Gynecol 1979;133:425.
564. Chamberlain R, Davey A. Physical growth in twins, postmature and small-for-dates children. Arch Dis Child 1975;50: 437.
565. Colle E, Schiff D, Andrew G, et al. Insulin responses during catch-up growth of infants who were small for gestational age. Pediatrics 1976;57:363.
566. Drew JH, Bayly J, Beischer NA. Prospective follow-up of growth retarded infants and of those from pregnancies complicated by low oestriol excretion—7 years. Aust N Z J Obstet Gynaecol 1983;23:150.
567. Stanley OH, Speidel BD. "Catch-up" following severe intrauterine retardation of head growth. J Perinat Med 1985; 13:253.
568. Walther FJ, Ramaekers LHJ. Growth in early childhood of newborns affected by disproportionate intrauterine growth retardation. Acta Paediatr Scand 1982;71:651.
569. Villar J, Belizan JM, Klein RE. Heterogenous postnatal growth patterns of intrauterine growth retarded infants (IUGR). Am J Clin Nutr 1982;35:860.
570. Villar J, Belizan JM, Spalding J, Klein RE. Postnatal growth of intrauterine growth retarded infants. Early Hum Dev 1982;6:265.
571. Ounsted MK, Moar VA, Scott A. Children of deviant birthweight at the age of seven years: health, handicap, size and developmental status. Early Hum Dev 1984;9:323.
572. Philip AGS. Term twins with discordant birth weights: observations at birth and one year. Acta Genet Med Gemellol 1981;30:203.
573. Davies P, Davis J. Very low birth weight and subsequent head growth. Lancet 1970;2:1216.
574. Babson SG, Kangas J. Preschool intelligence of undersized term infants. Am J Dis Child 1969;117:553.
575. Ounsted M, Moar V, Scott A. Growth in the first year of life: effects of sex and weight for gestational age at birth. Dev Med Child Neurol 1982;24:356.
576. Saha K, Kaur P, Srivastava G, Chaudhury DS. A six-months' follow-up study of growth, morbidity and functional immunity in low birth weight neonates with special reference to intrauterine growth retardation in small-for-date infant. J Trop Pediatr 1983;29:278.
577. Schiff D, Colle E, Stern L. Metabolic and growth patterns in transient neonatal diabetes. N Engl J Med 1972;287:119.
578. Foley TP Jr, Thompson RG, Shaw M, et al. Growth responses to human growth hormone in patients with intrauterine growth retardation. J Pediatr 1974;84:635.
579. Lanes R, Plotnick LP, Lee PA. Sustained effect of human growth hormone therapy on children with intrauterine growth retardation. Pediatrics 1979;63:731.
580. Albertsson-Wikland K, in collaboration with the Swedish Pediatric Study Group for growth hormone treatment. Growth hormone secretion and growth hormone treatment in children with intrauterine growth retardation. Acta Paediatr Scand 1989;349:35.
581. Stanhope R, Ackland F, Hamill, et al. Physiological growth hormone secretion and response to growth hormone treatment in children with short stature and intrauterine growth retardation. Acta Paediatr Scand 1889;349:47.
582. Fitzhardinge PM, Steven EM. The small-for-dates infant. II. Neurological and intellectual sequelae. Pediatrics 1972;50:50.
583. Parmelee AH, Schulte FJ. Development testing of pre-term and small-for-date infants. Pediatrics 1970;45:21.
584. Vohr BR, Hack M. Developmental follow-up of low birth weight infants. Pediatr Clin North Am 1982;29:1441.
585. Westwood M, Kramer MS, Munz D, et al. Growth and development of full-term nonasphyxiated small-for-gestational-age newborns: follow-up through adolescence. Pediatrics 1983; 71:376.
586. Winer EK, Tejani NA, Atluru VL, et al. Four- to seven-year evaluation in two groups of small-for-gestational-age infants. Am J Obstet Gynecol 1982;143:425.
587. Low JA, Galbraith RS, Muir D, et al. Intrauterine growth retardation: a study of long-term morbidity. Am J Obstet Gynecol 1982;142:670.
588. Ellenberg JH, Nelson KB. Birth weight and gestational age in children with cerebral palsy seizure disorders. Am J Dis Child 1979;133:1044.
589. Nelson KB, Broman SH. Perinatal risk factors in children with serious motor and mental handicaps. Ann Neurol 1977;2:371.
590. Hagberg B. Epidemiological and preventive aspects of cerebral palsy and severe mental retardation in Sweden. Eur J Pediatr 1979;130:71.
591. Berg AT. Childhood neurological morbidity and its association with gestational age, intrauterine growth retardation and perinatal stress. Paediatr Perinat Epidemiol 1988;2:229.
592. Martikainen A. Growth and development at the age of 1.5 years in children with maternal hypertension. J Perinat Med 1989;17:259.
593. Kyllerman M. Dyskinetic cerebral palsy. II. Pathogenetic risk factors and intrauterine growth. Acta Paediatr Scand 1982; 71:551.
594. Schulte FJ, Schrempf G, Hinze G. Maternal toxemia, fetal malnutrition and motor behavior of the newborn. Pediatrics 1971;48:871.
595. Fredrickson WT, Brown JV. Gripping and Moro responses: differences between small-for-gestational-age and normal weight term newborns. Early Hum Dev 1980;4:69.
596. Paine PA, Pasquali L, Spegiorin C. Appearance of visually directed prehensive related to gestational age and intrauterine growth. J Genet Psychol 1983;142:53.
597. Stanley OH, Fleming PJ, Morgan MH. Abnormal development of visual function following intrauterine growth retardation. Early Hum Dev 1989;19:87.
598. Todorovich RD, Crowell DH, Kapuniai LE. Auditory responsivity and intrauterine growth retardation in small for

gestational age human newborns. Electroencephalogr Clin Neurophysiol 1987;67:204.
599. Rutstein RP, Wesson MD, Gotlieb S, Biasini FJ. Clinical comparison of the visual parameters in infants with intrauterine growth retardation vs. infants with normal birth weight. American Journal of Optometry and Physical Optics 1986;63:697.
600. Walther FJ, Ramaekers LHJ. Language development at the age of 3 years of infants malnourished *in utero*. Neuropediatrics 1982;13:77.
601. Roberston CMT, Etches PC, Kyle JM. Eight-year school performance and growth of preterm, small for gestational age infants: a comparative study with subjects matched for birth weight or for gestational age. J Pediatr 1990;116:19.
602. Leventhal JM, Berg A, Egerter SA. Is intrauterine growth retardation a risk factor for child abuse? Pediatrics 1987;79:515.
603. Miller HC, Hassanein K. Fetal malnutrition in white newborn infants: maternal factors. Pediatrics 1973;52:504.
604. Als H, Tronick E, Adamson L, Brazelton TB. The behavior of the full-term but underweight newborn infant. Dev Med Child Neurol 1976;18:590.
605. Michaelis R, Schulte FJ, Nolte R. Motor behavior of small-for-gestational-age newborn infants. J Pediatr 1970;76:208.
606. Walther FJ, Ramaekers LHJ. Developmental aspects of subacute fetal distress: behavior problems and neurological dysfunction. Early Hum Dev 1982;6:1.
607. Hogan G, Boylan P. The diagnosis of intrauterine growth retardation and its influence on perinatal outcome. Isr Med J 1987;80:63.
608. Unger C, Weiser JK, McCullough RE, et al. Altitude, low birth weight, and infant mortality in Colorado. JAMA 1988;259:3427.

Neonatology: Pathophysiology and Management of the Newborn, Fourth Edition,
edited by Gordon B. Avery, Mary Ann Fletcher, and Mhairi G. MacDonald.
J.B. Lippincott Company, Philadelphia © 1994.

chapter 27

The Very-Low-Birth-Weight Infant

JOHN W. SCANLON

To neonatologists with more than 20 years of experience, it is almost wondrous to discuss routine care for babies who weigh less than 1.5 kg at birth. The very-low-birth-weight (VLBW) baby (*i.e.*, <1.5 kg), the limit for intact survival 15 years ago, has been replaced by the extremely-low-birth-weight (ELBW) infant (*i.e.*, <1 kg) and the micropremie (*i.e.*, <800 g) as the neonatal intensive care unit (NICU) responds to these challenges. Perhaps no other area of medicine has undergone such a dramatic improvement in mortality and morbidity as newborn care has during the past 30 years. Table 27-1 provides an overview of the many vulnerabilities intrinsic to the very immaturely born.

EPIDEMIOLOGY

The hospital of birth has considerable impact on VLBW infant mortality. The level of available perinatal and neonatal hospital care directly influences survival.[1] The optimal circumstance for a threatened extremely immature delivery is for intrapartum management to occur in a hospital that can start aggressive, high-level neonatal care from the moment of birth.

Table 27-2 shows birth weight–specific mortality and morbidity by 250-g increments for ELBW and VLBW neonates from the Columbia Hospital for Women, a facility exclusively for women and infants. Table 27-3 describes the causes of death. There is an increase of almost 1 month in the mean estimated gestational age between the two middle 250-g categories. This documents the persistent lack of correlation between gestational age and birth weight for these categories. This phenomenon has a significant influence on obstetric decisions based on potential nonviability.

Although the national low-birth-weight (LBW) mortality rate is falling, the incidence of VLBW and ELBW births is not.[2] What has declined during the past 10 years is mortality for these LBW categories, producing a dramatic increase in survivors whose birth weights were between 500 and 1500 g.

Poverty influences VLBW epidemiology. Economic, educational, social, and environmental impoverishment have been repeatedly correlated with reproductive casualties involving immature births. Care must be exercised in interpreting statistics using weight criteria alone, because small-for-gestational-age (SGA) babies are frequently confounded with truly immature births. This can confuse the interpretation of factors that may be directly related to prematurity and thwarts attempts at prevention. Assessing the impact of smoking, teenage pregnancy, maternal nutrition, and prenatal care has been handicapped by confounding premature and undergrown groups.

Parents of an impending very immature birth often ask what the chances of living are. The query directly involves weight-specific survival statistics. Until 1991, most published studies reported small groups of infants or data collected over so many years that NICU care would have significantly changed. This problem was remedied by Phelps and her colleagues, who provided prospectively collected baseline demographic data from more than 6600 inborn neonates

TABLE 27–1
CONDITIONS THAT MAKE A VERY-LOW-BIRTH-WEIGHT INFANT MORE VULNERABLE THAN A FULL-TERM INFANT

Cardiovascular Immaturity	Vulnerable to ischemic injury because of NEC, periventricular leukomalacia, IVH; impaired response to critical postnatal adjustments to asphyxial, thermal, and environmental events
Reduced Metabolic Stores	Limited response to cold, infection, asphyxia; less stored lipid, metabolic fuel reserve, and insulation
Dermal Immaturity	Environmental substances and drugs pass into skin easily; water and heat exit
Pulmonary Immaturity	Anatomically and biochemically vulnerable to acute and chronic disorders of ventilation and oxygenation
Gastrointestinal Immaturity	Vascular and immunologic problems because of NEC, nosocomial gastrointestinal infections; enzymatic deficiency causes difficulty in acquiring nutrients; slow transit time, distention frequent
Hepatic Immaturity	More and higher jaundice; contributes to nutritional problem; retards drug metabolism
Immunologic Immaturity	Increased infection; graft *versus* host disease
Renal Immaturity	Handles transitional fluid and electrolyte fluxes less well; vulnerable to electrolyte imbalances and acid–base disturbances
Central Nervous System	PVH, IVH; functionally poor coordinated adaptation; limited behavioral repertoire with which to fine tune physiologic homeostasis to cold, light, and sound challenges
Endocrine System	Decreased adrenocortical and thyroid responses to illness, growth, and development

IVH, intraventricular hemorrhage; NEC, necrotizing enterocolitis; PVH, periventricular hemorrhage.

who weighed less than 1251 g at birth.[3] The babies in her study were born at 77 hospitals associated with 23 participating perinatal centers. Gestational age was assigned by treating neonatologists, using the best estimate from obstetric data and physical assessment of the baby. Ultrasound information was used if available. Infants with incomplete data or gestational age of less than 25 weeks were excluded. The average birth weight was about 900 g and gestational age of about 27.5 weeks. Approximately 20% were SGA infants. African-American women had ELBW deliveries more often than other groups. Forty percent of SGA infants were African American, although only 16% of all deliveries were to African-American mothers.[3]

The investigators determined the differential impact of gestational age and birth weight on survival. This was important because of confounding effects from gender, intrauterine nutrition, and race. When survival was considered by birth weight, female infants fared better than male infants in almost all 100-g incremental weight categories. After survival was analyzed by gestational age, gender differences diminished, but female infants still did better. African-American neonates had slightly improved survival rates. This beneficial effect also diminished after race-specific outcome was examined by gestational age.

Significant survival predictors were older gestational age, heavier birth weight, female gender, African-American race, singleton birth, and the absence of fetal malnutrition. Female neonates increased the odds of survival by 55%, and the survival rate of African-American neonates was increased by 28%. At term, Caucasian infants have lower mortality rates. Singletons had a 32% survival advantage over multiple births. SGA neonates had lower survival rates than AGA babies within each gestational age range. Any effects of the stress of fetal growth retardation did not improve the outcome for VLBW infants.

There was considerable variation in survival among perinatal centers. Even when improved outcome was thought to be explained by variances in hospital population, substantial differences still existed. The investigators suggested that various care practices were important, including applied research protocols, surfactant introduction, and improved maternal or prenatal health care.

Because gestational age is still the most important predictor of survival, improving the accuracy of its measurement during prenatal assessment assumes major importance. Adjusting for race, gender, and fetal nutrition also help to answer the critical obstetric question of whether the fetus can survive if born immediately.

PERINATAL RISKS

Many things place a woman at jeopardy for premature delivery. Socioeconomic impoverishment, inadequate housing, and poor personal and environmental hygiene increase fetal hazards. Nutritional inadequacies and diminished health care access are additional risks. To this list must now be added maternal cocaine abuse; the drugs stimulates uterine muscles and is associated with sudden placental abruption, vaginal bleeding, early delivery, and fetal demise.[4] Cocaine use is often associated with poverty, other drugs of abuse, and sexually transmitted diseases. America is witnessing a resurgence in congenital syphilis. The rates of sexually transmitted neonatal gonococcal disease, hepatitis, herpes simplex, human immunovirus, and group B β-hemolytic streptococci have risen. All occur with increased frequency in VLBW infants. The clinician must be aware of these threats when evaluating an extremely immature new-

TABLE 27–2
VERY-LOW-BIRTH-WEIGHT INFANT MORTALITY AT COLUMBIA HOSPITAL FOR WOMEN, 1988–1991

Birth Weight (g)	Total Births	Deaths (%)*	Average Gestational Age (wk)†
501–750	107	63 (59)	24.3
751–1000	88	12 (13)	25.17
1001–1250	76	6 (8)	29.1
1251–1500	105	2 (2)	30.9

* Deaths include all deaths before discharge and deaths after transfer for surgery.
† Gestational age was determined by best obstetric or clinical criteria.

born, because even careful history taking may not uncover these problems. Specific blood or urine tests may be necessary.

Intrapartum management impacts outcome. The obstetrician has to deal with potentially inaccurate fetal gestational age assessment in making management decisions. Presentation and mode of delivery may affect outcome. Cesarean section may be the optimal delivery mode for breech presentation during premature labor, but data do not indicate that operative delivery is the mode of choice for all premature infants.[5]

One complex, poorly illuminated issue is the interaction between infection and outcome after very immature birth. Neonatal sepsis is a risk to survival and intact outcome at all gestational ages. However, at any gestational age, there appears to be a positive correlation between outcome and maternal chorioamnionitis.[6] Accelerated pulmonary maturity, fetal hormonal response to stress, or other undocumented benefits have suggested that inflammatory changes in the chorioamnion or placenta may spare the resulting offspring. Studies about this topic are plagued with methodologic inconsistencies and confounding variables. Definitive data are not available.

The basic obstetric principle of minimizing perinatal asphyxia applies in managing preterm labor. For example, if there is profound maternal hypertensive

TABLE 27–3
CAUSES OF DEATH BY BIRTH WEIGHT AT COLUMBIA HOSPITAL FOR WOMEN, 1988–1991

Birth Weight (g)	Cause (Number of Patients)	Average Age (Range) in Days
<500	Extreme prematurity (34)*	<1 (<1–1)
	Congenital Infection (1)	<1
500–999	Extreme prematurity (20)*	<1 (<1–1)
	IRDS (19)	1.3 (<1–4)
	NEC (2)	48.6 (0.5–154)
	CNS (5)	
	BPD (5)	42 (14.5–150)
	Renal failure (2)	
	Congenital infection (2)	
1000–1499	IRDS (3)	4.7 (2–8)
	Pulmonary hypoplasia (2)	<1 (<1)
	CNS (1)	16 (4–28)
	Lethal malformation (1)	†
1500–1999	Lethal malformation (3)	†
	CNS (1)	
	NEC (1)	

* The diagnosis of extreme prematurity was given to infants thought too underdeveloped to treat (usually $\leq$ 23 weeks of gestation). Only 6 of 54 infants were supported by mechanical ventilation at any time.
† Age at death for some with malformations is unknown.
BPD, bronchopulmonary dysplasia or its complications; IRDS, idiopathic respiratory distress syndrome; CNS, lethal central nervous system injury; NEC, necrotizing enterocolitis.

disease complicated by renal, hepatic, or cardiac decompensation, skillful medical management and experienced judgment becomes mandatory for optimal fetal outcome. There are few data that address the topic of optimal obstetric anesthesia and maternal pain relief for extremely premature labor and delivery (see Chap. 17).[7] Characteristics of the specific labor and delivery, which consider individual risk factors and the urgency for fetal removal, must be weighed carefully. One cardinal rule is to minimize asphyxia; maintaining maternal and placental cardiovascular perfusion is another. Cord prolapse, an urgent, catastrophic event, dictates rapid delivery, most often operatively and usually under general anesthesia, regardless of gestational age. The use of ultrashort-acting narcotics and sedatives, the availability of pharmacologic reversal, and techniques for monitoring maternal hemodynamics are important considerations in delivering a very immature newborn.

DELIVERY ROOM RESUSCITATION AND STABILIZATION

Any baby born before 34 weeks of gestation requires a physician who has skill, experience, and specific training in comprehensive neonatal cardiorespiratory management. There should also be an experienced nurse or respiratory therapist present. Technical skills, including intubating a tiny larynx, catheterizing miniature umbilical vessels, experience with subdecimal drug dose calculations, and knowledge about critical care needs of very immature infants are the purview of neonatologists and the NICU staff. Gathering and recording pertinent perinatal and intrapartum history are routine tasks for the neonatal–perinatal specialist. Concerns about viability and ethical issues surrounding very premature birth are familiar to the NICU team.[8] This experience, coupled with emotional sensitivity, may be needed in the delivery room when a very premature delivery is at hand.

One exception to having a neonatologist present at every delivery of a very premature infant is when the obstetrician and parents have decided that the fetus is too immature to be deemed a viable newborn. This circumstance is confusing and problematic.[9,10] Antenatal gestational age prediction is often inaccurate, and nonviability is a murky term. Physicians, nurses, or parents may harbor distorted, unrealistic views about survival or neurologic outcome after premature birth.[11,12]

Reluctance to resuscitate the extremely immature neonate increases with exposure to the NICU during the 3 years of pediatric residency.[13] Attitudes, personal biases, and past experiences also influence treatment decisions. Parents' wishes, after consultation with the obstetrician and neonatologist, should dictate whether or not to initiate aggressive delivery room care if there is a presumption of nonviability. Current practice is to resuscitate most extreme premature infants in the delivery room, and then make decisions about further care based on continuously collected clinical information and detailed physician–parent discussions (see Chap. 2).

Any discussion about resuscitation and early treatment implicitly demands accurate, timely information sharing among obstetric and neonatology physicians and nursing personnel. The quality and quantity of this communication directly affects care. The presence and severity of fetal distress, intrauterine infection, therapeutic and illicit maternal drug exposure, and the mother's medical history and medical status are important facts for resuscitators and subsequent caretakers.

If possible, the extremely premature infant should be delivered in a facility that has an NICU staffed according to American Academy of Pediatrics (AAP) and American College of Obstetrics and Gynecology guidelines.[14] This implies trained, experienced physicians, nurses, and respiratory therapists available 24 hours daily and promptly available microsample laboratory and radiology services. These special needs are amply documented by the consistently better survival, at all birth weights, among inborn premature infants compared with those born elsewhere and transported after birth.

The Apgar score remains a useful, familiar set of vital signs on which to determine the severity of postnatal compromise or the response to resuscitation. However, the often hypotonic, vasoconstricted, poorly responsive VLBW neonate with respiratory distress uniformly has a low score if held to the same criteria as term infants. This fact diminishes the specificity of the Apgar score to define subtle physiologic disruptions. Heart rate, vascular perfusion (*i.e.*, capillary filling time), respiratory rate and effort, and a rough estimation of gestational age helps to guide resuscitation.

Various clinical assessments of gestational age based on physical and neurologic findings are available. The delivery room resuscitator, however, needs only a general sense of maturity during acute delivery room situations:

- 34 to 37 weeks of gestation—slightly preterm
- 30 to 34 weeks of gestation—preterm
- 26 to 30 weeks of gestation—very immature
- fewer than 26 weeks of gestation—possibly nonviable.

Few published physical or neurologic scores included sufficient babies weighing less than 1000 g or younger than 28 weeks of gestation to be reliable for determining extreme immaturity. Fused eyelids and gelatinous skin imply seriously threatened viability but are not consistent indicators. Ballard suggested that a foot length less than 50 mm differentiates extreme immaturity, with possible nonviability, from more mature ELBW infants.[15]

The basic principles of neonatal resuscitation appropriate for term infants apply to preterm infants with particular attention to supporting cardiac, pulmonary and thermoregulatory systems. It is important to perform serial measurements of blood pressure, continuous transcutaneous oxygen saturation, and body temperature during resuscitation and stabilization. Tables 27-4 and 27-5 describe normal blood pressure values.[16,17]

Delivery room resuscitation of the very premature newborn is a team event that requires preparation, anticipation, special skills, knowledge, and accurate communication. The following steps should be taken:

If the baby appears to be younger than 30 weeks of gestation or weighs less than 1 kg, intubate him or her promptly with a 2.5-F (0.8-mm) endotracheal tube to a depth of no more than 7 cm.

Ventilate the infant at approximately 60 breaths per minute using peak and end pressures of 20 and 5 cm H_2O, respectively, and 100% oxygen. Watch for adequate chest rise.

Intubate and ventilate the infant if his or her heart rate is less than 100 beats per minute for longer than 1 minute, regardless of gestational age.

Administer oxygen until complete assessment of cardiorespiratory status confirms normality.

Take axillary temperature every 3 to 5 minutes as a guide for supplemental warming.

After the infant is ready for transport to the NICU, parents should be informed, succinctly and humanely, about the care rendered and their baby's status. The location of the NICU and names of responsible physicians should be provided.

Potential complications, risks, or outcomes should be discussed later.

TABLE 27–4
MEAN BLOOD PRESSURE BY BIRTH WEIGHT AND POSTNATAL AGE

	Mean Blood Pressure (torr)*	
Birth Weight (g)	Postnatal Age 3 h	Postnatal Age 12 h
500	23 (35)	24 (36)
600	24 (35)	25 (36)
700	24 (36)	25 (37)
800	25 (36)	26 (37)
900	25 (37)	26 (38)
1000	26 (38)	27 (39)
1100	27 (38)	27 (39)
1200	27 (39)	28 (40)
1300	28 (39)	29 (40)
1400	28 (40)	29 (41)
1500	29 (40)	30 (42)

* Results in torr given as lower and upper 10th percentile.
From Weidling AM. Blood pressure monitoring in the newborn. Arch Dis Child 1989;64:444.

TABLE 27–5
BLOOD PRESSURE RANGES DURING THE FIRST 12 HOURS OF LIFE

Birth Weight of Infant	Blood Pressure (torr) Systolic	Diastolic	Mean
>1000 g	36–58	17–38	24–45
600–1000 g	35–55	14–35	10–28

From Versmold Am, Kitterman JA, Phibb RH, et al. Aortic blood pressure during the first 12 hours of life in infants with birthweight 610 to 4220 grams. Pediatrics 1981;67:607.

PULMONARY RESUSCITATION

Most babies born before 28 weeks of gestation and many delivered between 28 and 32 weeks need prompt tracheal intubation for intermittent positive-pressure ventilation (IPPV). Drew and colleagues showed that babies smaller than 1000 g at birth did better if their tracheas were intubated and IPPV commenced shortly after birth.[18] For most premature infants, an unshouldered 2.5-F (0.8-mm) endotracheal tube is easiest to insert and allows sufficient air leak to avoid overdistention of the lungs. If necessary, a larger tube can be inserted later.

The average lip–carina distance is about 6.5 cm for infants with birth weights less than 1000 g, 7.0 cm for those between 1000 and 1500 g, and 7.5 cm for those weighing more than 1.5 kg.[19] These lengths provide a rough estimate of the maximal insertion depth. However, the infant's clinical condition, response to mechanical ventilation, and adequacy of breath sounds are the most important criteria for determining when intubation is correct. For the ELBW baby, rapid establishment of an intrathoracic gas volume sufficient to achieve efficient ventilation, optimize compliance, and maintain appropriate pulmonary pressure–volume associations is critical.

Hoskyns and associates studied initial ventilatory response in infants of 25 to 36 weeks of gestational age who were intubated for resuscitation at birth.[20] Mean delivered inflation pressure was 30 cm H_2O at a rate of 30 breaths per minute. Inspiratory times were about 1 second. One-fourth of premature infants established an adequate tidal volume on their first breath. This proportion increased to one-third by the third breath. The best predictor for attaining adequate lung volume was the occurrence of gasping as inspiratory pressure was applied (*i.e.*, Head paradoxic reflex). This reflex was independent of inflation pressure or duration and occurred significantly less frequently among more premature infants. Asphyxia probably dampens this response.[21] A significant number of ELBW infants require ventilation for apnea rather than lung disease.

After several initial inflating breaths to establish adequate lung volumes, further mechanical ventilation is usually at peak pressures between 20 and 25 cm H_2O, a positive end-expiratory pressure of 5 cm H_2O, and respiratory rates up to 50 or 60 breaths per minute. Efficacy of ventilation is assessed by repeated physical examination (*e.g.*, chest rise, cyanosis abatement, adequate breath sounds) and by subsequent blood gas analysis in the NICU.

Hoskyns and colleagues, in evaluating bag and mask systems for term neonatal resuscitation, found a rigid bag preferable and decried the small bag size in popular use.[22] They recommended at least a 500-mL or 1-L bag as necessary to maintain proper end-expiratory pressure and a consistent tidal volume. Similar studies have not been carried out in immature newborns who may need even higher initial inflation pressures to overcome surfactant deficiency and to establish effective functional residual capacity.[23]

Premature infants chill more quickly than term infants. Special efforts are needed to prevent hypothermia during resuscitation. The optimal range for the VLBW infant's body temperature at birth is narrow, 36.5°C to 37°C (97.7°F–98.6°F). Premature infants whose body temperatures fall below 35.6°C (96°F) in the delivery room have a 55% mortality rate despite aggressive, expert care.[24] Assiduous drying, prewarming the crib mattress, using a mattress warming pad, an overhead radiant warmer, placing hot-water bottles, reducing air drafts, and careful attention to the transport incubator's heat loss are all important. Because overhead heaters may be blocked by resuscitators during acute care, special heating pads or water pillows, warmed before delivery, can be placed under the infant. Extra heat lamps may be necessary. Raising the ambient temperature in the delivery suite may be effective if there is an anticipated VLBW delivery. Warmed, humidified oxygen during mechanical ventilation is another aid to maintaining adequate neonatal care temperature in the delivery room, but most heating devices used in the delivery room neither heat nor warm delivered gases effectively.

One major advance in VLBW infant care has been the use of pulmonary surfactant for respiratory distress syndrome (RDS; see Chap. 29). Both synthetic and natural surfactants improve oxygenation, ventilatory requirements, and survival if given during diagnosed RDS.[25,26] Less clear is the role of surfactant in preventing RDS, because most published surfactant trials deal with rescue therapy for already established disease. There is some enthusiasm for prophylactically administering surfactant to ELBW infants in the delivery room to improve short term outcome and perhaps survival.[27] Extensive data supporting prophylactic efficacy are lacking and overtreating newborns who will never develop RDS could be frequent.

There are significant practical constraints to giving surfactant in the delivery room, including space and equipment. Following recommended dosing schedules requires weighing the infant. A scale in the delivery room, warmed and precisely balanced, is useful. Because dosing ranges are still being developed, estimating body weight is probably sufficient for the first dose if RDS risk is high. Merritt and associates suggest that surfactant should be reserved for rescue in established disease for babies older than 30 weeks of gestation.[28] They recommend prophylaxis for low-gestational-age newborns only if evidence of surfactant deficiency exists, such as no phosphatidyl glycerol in the amniotic fluid or respiratory distress starting from birth. Merritt cogently argues that proper antenatal care, selective maternal corticosteroid administration, and aggressive tocolysis may further reduce the need for surfactant. It appears that early surfactant treatment of RDS in the NICU is preferable to routine delivery room administration. Elective intubation in the delivery room solely to administer surfactant is not justified. Immediate intubation of ELBW infants to improve thoracic gas exchange may reduce the need for later surfactant rescue or provide a route for administration if a drug is needed. These issues are nicely summarized by Avery and Merritt.[29]

CARDIOVASCULAR RESUSCITATION

Very immature infants are often born with cardiovascular compromise due to acute placental dysfunction (*e.g.*, abruption, previa), perinatal asphyxia, infection, or other causes etiologically related to preterm delivery.

If cardiac activity is not evident by 10 minutes of age, despite external cardiac massage and drug resuscitation, the predicted outcome for the VLBW infant is bleak.[32] When a sustained heart rate is present but no spontaneous motor activity or respiratory efforts are apparent by 30 minutes, the likelihood of a normal outcome is minimal, regardless of gestational age.[33]

Obtaining an umbilical cord blood sample for sodium, potassium, chloride, blood urea nitrogen (BUN), and glucose concentrations is useful. Fluid and electrolyte disturbances are common among premature infants, particularly if the mother has received parenteral fluids and electrolytes, or has been given oxytocin, which has intrinsic antidiuretic hormone activity.[34] Additionally, if maternal glucose administration is too rapid, neonatal hypoglycemia may develop once the umbilical cord is severed.[35]

NUTRITIONAL AND METABOLIC SUPPORT

FLUIDS AND ELECTROLYTES

The initial fluid and electrolyte management of a VLBW infant is crucial and controversial. The incidence of certain morbid processes, particularly patency of the ductus arteriosus, renal failure, any pulmonary edema component of RDS, and chronic pulmonary disease, has each been linked to early fluid management problems. Hypernatremia, or at least a serum sodium level of more than 150 μmol/L, during the first 3 days of life has been associated with increased incidence and severity of intracranial hemorrhage.[36] Most recommended protocols for fluid management of VLBW infants employ data abstracted from full-term or more mature premature infants or from chronologically older infants. Early fluid and electrolyte administration for VLBW infants should strive to maintain electrolyte concentrations within physiologic limits and to ensure at least minimal urine output (0.5–1 mL/kg/hour). It should also provide adequate calories to maintain minimal cellular metabolism (approximately 40 kcal/kg).

To achieve these goals, accurate and precise serial measurements of body weight, serum electrolyte and glucose concentrations, arterial *p*H, urine output and occasionally urine electrolytes, and BUN are necessary. It is useful to estimate water insensibly lost to the environment. Open cribs, radiant warmers, auxiliary heating apparatus, and respiratory support equipment can influence insensible losses. The more immature the infant, the greater are its transdermal losses because of increased dermal permeability to water and the increased ratio of body surface area to mass. An important adjunct to initial fluid therapy is to minimize insensible water loss.

My colleagues and I suggest starting at 90 to 100 mL/kg/24 hours using an electrolyte-free solution of 5% glucose in water. This should avoid the twin pitfalls of dehydration and anuria. Adjust infusion rates and the infusate glucose concentration so that a minimum of 5 mg/kg/minute of glucose is provided. The maximal glucose infusion rate is below 8 mg/kg/minute. Measure capillary glucose frequently to maintain normoglycemia. An accurate in-bed scale is essential for frequent weighings with minimal disturbance to the VLBW infant.

It is my practice to measure serum glucose, sodium, potassium, chloride, and BUN as soon as possible after birth. Values change quickly after birth in VLBW infants, and maternal serum electrolyte concentrations are seldom available. Obtaining baseline measurements for VLBW infants within the first hour of life is prudent.

Water crosses the placenta more rapidly than sodium. Placental sodium permeability increases with gestational age. Rapid intravenous infusion of sodium-poor fluids to the mother during parturition may result in a net gain of free water to the fetus. This transplacental directional flux increases total fetal body water and may result in hyponatremia.

Early in the VLBW infant's course, hyponatremia is usually the result of superfluous water administration documented by body weight remaining the same or increasing. If fluid restriction does not correct hyponatremia, or if serial urine measurements show evidence of sodium wasting, sodium must be added to the intravenous solution.

Hypernatremia is most often caused by insufficient fluid provided to match insensible water loss. However, sodium infused in flush solutions, administered as bicarbonate buffer, or given as sodium salts in medications must be included in sodium intake calculations. Hypernatremia can be iatrogenic. Measurement of urine specific gravity has been a traditional NICU routine, but data suggest limited utility and accuracy for this value.[37] Determining serum and urine osmolarities can define the appropriateness of antidiuretic hormone secretion and whether hypernatremia is dehydrational or due to salt overload.

Potassium excretion is lower in preterm than in term infants. It is rarely necessary to supplement potassium during the first 48 hours of life in VLBW infants. Occasionally, maternal diuretic therapy, neonatal respiratory alkalosis due to forced mechanical hyperventilation, or neonatal diuretic administration may necessitate adding 1 to 3 mEq/kg/day.

Hyperkalemia is a serious problem in very immature infants, even if there has been no exogenous potassium administered. If severe hyperkalemia develops, measure the potassium concentration of all infusates, particularly blood used for exchange transfusion, to determine potassium load or excess intravenous potassium.[38] Renal function should also be assessed using BUN, creatinine, and creatinine clearance. The management of hyperkalemia in VLBW infants, including the use of $NaHCO_3$, insulin and glucose, or ion-exchange resins, is the same as in more mature newborns, but such practice is largely unsubstantiated by published data.

ACID–BASE BALANCE

The physiologic *p*H range in the VLBW infant's arterial blood is wider than at term because the bicarbonate threshold of the immature kidney may be as low as 14.5 μmol/L. This range narrows within the first month of life. The more immature the baby, the more likely is a lower average *p*H, but, very premature infants have been shown to lower their urine *p*H when plasma bicarbonate decreases.[39] Monitoring urine *p*H helps differentiate an inappropriate renal response to systemic acidosis.

Metabolic acidosis should always be evaluated. Possibilities include thermal stress, renal dysfunction, infection, and recent transfusion because the citrate buffer in transfused bank blood gives an initial acid load. As citrate is hepatically converted to bicarbonate, alkalosis occurs. Blood gases obtained during or in the immediate post-transfusion period reflect this. Nitrogen intake, particularly if excessive, also increases the tendency for metabolic acidosis. The late metabolic acidosis of prematurity has been related to nitrogen load or amino acid intake.

Various drugs, particularly diuretics and xanthines, may distort body fluid cation and anion concentrations. When these drugs are used during serum carbon dioxide elevation caused by hypoventilation, blood gas results are a confusing combination of metabolic alkalosis and respiratory acidosis. This is an important consideration in interpreting blood gas values in VLBW infants with chronic pulmonary disease.

CALCIUM AND PHOSPHOROUS HOMEOSTASIS

Nowhere is the murky distinction between normal as a statistical concept and normal as a biologic state more apparent than in considering calcium and phosphorous physiology in the very immature newborn. Almost two-thirds of premature neonates not given supplemental calcium have serum calcium levels below 7 mg/dL during their first 48 hours of life. This suggests that such a lower normal limit may be too high for this group of newborns. Early hypocalcemia is probably a manifestation of lost placental calcium transfer or insufficient fetal or neonatal tissue calcium mobilization.

Calcium supplementation for VLBW infants during their early course must be an exercise in clinical judgment. Even without bioelectric evidence of disturbed calcium-mediated cell membrane electrical activity, many clinicians routinely infuse calcium to babies whose serum calcium falls below 7 or 7.5 mg/dL. Intravenous calcium has significant risks, including serious cardiac dysrhythmias and tissue necrosis when extravasated. Although perhaps idiosyncratic and conservative, it is my practice not to supplement calcium unless the serum level falls below 6 mg/dL or there is electrocardiographic evidence of hypocalcemia. There are undoubtedly other valid approaches (see Chap. 36).

GLUCOSE

The normal biologic range of serum glucose values is lower in preterm than in term newborns.[40] Acutely, hepatic glucose clearance determines the blood sugar concentration. Hyperglycemia implies failure to regulate glucose production and increased serum osmolarity. The latter may disrupt fluid and electrolyte balance. A standard NICU practice is to measure capillary glucose values frequently with chemstrips and then validate low or high levels using laboratory testing. Many clinicians also order random blood glucose determinations. Such information allows manipulation of the glucose concentration of infused fluids to maintain euglycemia (40–120 mg/dL). In general, approximately 6 to 8 mg of glucose/kg/minute is appropriate. Calculations must include all glucose sources, including intravenous or arterial flushes, medication diluents, blood products, and pressor fluids (see Chap. 35).

NUTRITIONAL GOALS

Nutritional goals during the first 2 days of a VLBW infant's life include maintaining serum glucose in the normal range, keeping urine output between 1 and 3 mL/kg/hour, avoiding azotemia, and supplying sufficient calories (approximately 40 kcal/kg) to reduce or stop protein catabolism. Provision of lipid for cellular membrane maintenance and repair may also be attempted.

After vital signs, temperature, and respiratory and cardiovascular functions have stabilized, even if acute illness is ongoing, caloric increases for repair and recovery are the next step. Amino acid introduction, increasing lipid infusion, and pushing serum glucose limits can be attempted. Achieving these goals implies that nutrition is exclusively parenteral during stabilization and acute illness. As acute processes subside, the next goal is to introduce and increase oral alimentation as dependence on intravascular nutrition is reduced.

After resolution of acute neonatal illness, particularly respiratory, the major clinical emphasis shifts to providing adequate nutrition for growth and the development of internal organs, particularly the central nervous system. Somatic growth is typically measured by daily weight plus weekly length and head circumference values. Functional organ system maturity is somewhat more difficult to determine. Data suggest that 3 postnatal weeks is about the age when dermal maturity is achieved (*i.e.*, the epidermis cornifies).[41] Insensible water loss plus the inward transdermal movement of various drugs, dramatically declines at this time. The major nutritional limiting factor is the necessary administered volume to dilute nutrients.

Plotting the VLBW infant's ponderal data on standardized grids that display growth trajectories is important. Normative charts whose data were gathered at high altitude show considerably different curves for the three growth measures than do norms derived at sea level. Ethnic, racial, and gender differences are evident in growth patterns. A preterm infant's growth may reflect stalls or accelerations without apparent clinical consequence. Acute or daily swings in weight are almost always due to fluid balance variances.

If intravenous supplementation includes amino acids, lipids, multivitamins, electrolytes and minerals, the sobriquet total parenteral nutrition (TPN) is often applied. Using daily laboratory results, body weight, and intake and output data, additives can be tailored to meet specific needs. Total parenteral nutrition is an extension of earlier intravenous fluid prescriptions and follows the same principles.

In very small, sick babies, it is sometimes necessary to insert an indwelling venous line surgically to provide adequate nutrition. Surgically implanted catheters (*i.e.*, Hickman or Broviac) require the availability of a pediatric surgeon for placement, and they have significant infection rates. Percutaneous central venous lines have a rate of infections that is less than 2%.[42] Long-term placement of both types of catheters has been associated with colonization by coagulase-negative staphylococci, especially *S. epidermidis*.

The use of insulin to increase cellular glucose availability has been recommended (see Chap. 24). Personal experience is that risks from insulin overdosage outweigh its potential for enhanced calories. Similarly, the hemorrhagic risk of heparin, used to increase lipoprotein lipase activity, exceeds this drug's limited documented benefits to improve nutrition in most VLBW infants.

The early infusion of small amounts of intravenous lipids may provide essential fatty acids during acute illness and may even offer protection against oxidative injury.[43] Theoretically, fatty acids can displace bilirubin from albumin and potentially increase the risk of bilirubin toxicity. This has not been confirmed in humans. Early parenteral lipid may enhance caloric use and glucose homeostasis. I recommend starting lipids as early as the second day of life using a continuous 24-hour infusion of 0.5 g/kg/day. This can be slowly increased to 3 g/kg/day. Hourly rates below 0.12 g/kg/hour do not produce hyperlipidemia in VLBW infants.[44]

It is my recommendation that the gastrointestinal tract can and should be used as soon as the umbilical arterial catheter has been removed for 24 hours. This provides a richer, more specific source of nutritional materials for the VLBW infant than TPN alone and conditions the gut for oral alimentation.

To initiate oral feedings, start with sterile water followed by half-strength (0.33 cal/mL) premature formula or half-strength breast milk every 3 hours. I prefer to use intermittent nasogastric feedings (*i.e.*, gavage feeding). Except if there is reflux, regurgitation, or apnea associated with tube placement, intermittently placing a gavage tube seems preferable to an indwelling nasogastric or duodenal tube. A duodenal tube bypasses the stomach, where considerable lipid digestion occurs, and this route does not avoid esophageal reflux and regurgitation.

Increase the feeding volume until approximately one-half the total fluid intake is provided enterically. After the VLBW infant tolerates 0.33-cal/mL feedings for 48 hours and one-half the total fluid intake is oral, switch to 0.66-cal/mL special premature formula. Increase enteric volumes slowly (1–2 mL/feed) as parenteral fluids are decreased. Reducing the intravenous rate 1 mL/hour for every 3 mL increase in oral feeds maintains constant daily total fluids.

TEMPERATURE CONTROL

The very immature neonate is particularly vulnerable to high and low thermal challenges because of diminished subcutaneous fat, large surface to mass area, underdeveloped intrinsic central and peripheral temperature control mechanisms, and intercurrent illnesses. Providing an appropriate thermal environment is second in management importance only to maintaining respiratory sufficiency.

Until stabilized, most very premature infants should be managed on radiant warming tables to permit rapid caretaker access. Some babies, particularly micropremies weighing less than 800 g, may not be adequately warmed or maintained on these without additional heat sources. Creative techniques, including hot-water bottles and supplemental overhead warming lamps, may be necessary for their survival. My practice is to care for them on a warming table with an under-baby, servocontrolled, low-heat pad plus a clear plastic blanket or shield. Glad Wrap is pure polyethylene and offers no barrier to the passage of infrared radiation. Saran, Gold Seal, and some other clear plastics are made from complicated plastic polymers that may decrease transferred radiation by 50%. This probably holds only theoretic concern because of the massive radiant heat output from commercially available overhead warmers. Clear plastic wrap reduces convective and evaporative losses by minimizing air flow over the VLBW infant's skin surface. Warming infused fluids and blood and covering the baby's head and feet further reduce heat loss. Dermally applied clear surgical dressings decrease water and evaporative heat loss in ELBW infants and helps prevent skin breakdown.[45]

Premies cared for under radiant warmers have higher metabolic rates than incubator-managed infants because of the greater energy they expend in thermogenesis. This must be taken into account in determining caloric needs. Evaporative water losses diminish after the VLBW infant is moved from warmer to incubator, and fluid intake should be decreased accordingly.

Hyperthermia, like hypothermia, can be dangerous, even fatal. The VLBW infant poorly handles the accompanying heightened metabolic rate, metabolic acidosis, increased oxygen consumption, and loss of transdermal water. This may produce fatal multiple organ failure. Accurate, frequent body temperature measurements are essential to the care of VLBW infants.

For more than a century, the incubator has been an icon of intensive neonatal care for premature infants. Changes in design from convective to radiant heat sources, computerized servocontrols, lower air flow systems, convective warming, and double or heated wall incubators have improved but not changed the essential principles of a warm, safe house with good visibility from without. Plexiglass transmits visible light but blocks radiant heat. This barrier reduces radiant losses from the infant, but it renders extensive supplemental outside heating devices ineffective. Clear plastic wrap, caps and booties, extra blankets, frequent diaper changes to avoid wet skin, and proper humidification inside the incubator further decrease thermal losses.

During recovery, infants are frequently allowed out of incubators to be held and fed by caretakers and parents. This is a laudable practice as long as the infant maintains its body temperature. The optimal duration of outside contact and the need for supplemental warming can be determined by taking the baby's temperature before removal from and after return to the incubator.

JAUNDICE

An elevated serum bilirubin is almost universal in extremely premature newborns. Their hepatic capacity to take up, glucuronidate, and release conjugated bilirubin into the biliary ducts is underdeveloped. There also may be increased bilirubin load from bleeding in the skin, gastrointestinal tract, or brain. Enterohepatic recirculation of bilirubin may be increased by lack of bowel motility or ubiquitous antibiotic usage. Because of the notoriously increased neurologic morbidity among NICU graduates and autopsy evidence of kernicterus in very immature infants, there has been a remarkable lowering of criteria for initiating phototherapy and performing exchange transfusions for VLBW infants. There are few data to guide the clinician in this regard. An elevated bilirubin in a premature infant deserves the same evaluation recommended for a term infant.

Jaundice in the premature infant, by itself, may not be the significant morbid factor previously believed. Recent observations from the National Institutes of Health Collaborative Phototherapy Project[46] and from the Netherlands[47] support this bias. I do not routinely use phototherapy, even for the smallest premature infant, unless the total bilirubin is higher than 12 mg/dL. If serum bilirubin increases by more than 0.5 mg/dL/hour or if there is sufficient reason to anticipate a higher peak, such as bruising, infection, or hemolytic disease, phototherapy may be initiated at a lower level.

When phototherapy is used, particularly during the first week of life, the inherently elevated insensible water loss must be balanced by an increased fluid intake of approximately 20%. Safe eye patches are required for babies undergoing phototherapy.

PAIN CONTROL

Noxious sensations, including pain, arise in the skin and travel a highly interconnected path to their ultimate spinal and nervous system destinations. Newborns have the same or more pain endings per square millimeter of skin as adults do, and pain endings are ubiquitously present in fetal mucous membranes and integument midway through the second trimester.[48] Synapses between sensory neurons and spinal interconnections start to develop by the end of the first 3 months of intrauterine existence. These are complete by the start of the last trimester. At best, mature peripheral pain fibers are thinly myelinated. Most are unmyelinated. The lack of myelination is not a valid argument against neonatal pain appreciation. Central nervous system tracks that subserve pain pathways are completely myelinated by 30 weeks of intrauterine life. Corticothalamic interconnections, critical for higher central pain perception, are completed before 24 weeks of gestation. Descending inhibitory pain controllers are poorly developed in term neonates and even more so in those prematurely born.[49]

This leads to the intriguing and unsettling possibility that premature infants may be even more sensitive to pain than older children or adults. The issue of when in gestation a fetus develops the ability to centrally process afferent signals has been addressed by Tawia.[50] Based on a critical review of the fetal behavioral literature, 25 weeks seemed the earliest time that such sentience could occur anatomically. Thirty weeks seemed an even more reasonable postconceptional age for this functional capacity to be achieved.

Response to pain has subjective and objective (*i.e.*, physiologic) components. Although more easily measured, physiologic responses are nonspecific. They are, however, basic to an organism's survival. The landmark work by Anand and colleagues documented cardiovascular and metabolic disturbances due to inadequate neonatal pain relief during and after major surgery.[51] They demonstrated significant metabolic consequences from unanesthetized surgery and increased mortality. There is a hypermetabolic state during which cellular nutritional needs are not met by available caloric intake if pain relief is not provided. Many of their subjects were premature infants undergoing ductal ligation.

The fact that newborns, even very premature ones, have the ability to recognize painful tissue-damaging insults and respond to them should no longer be controversial. Such responses may be physiologically deleterious, produce complications, and impede recovery. They should be treated appropriately.

BEHAVIOR

Very-low-birth-weight infants have a unique generalized behavioral response during the first month of life that seems to conserve energy and protect them from the vicissitudes of excessive environmental stimuli. This has been called "protective apathy" by Tronick and colleagues, who evaluated infants weighing less than 1500 g at birth using a modified form of the Brazelton Neonatal Behavioral Assessment Scale.[55] During the first week of life, they found that infants were mainly in sleep states with no crying, few state changes, and blunted responsiveness. At 3 weeks, infants began to demonstrate wider state ranges, more excursions to alert states, and longer durations of wakefulness.

Compared with full-term infants, premature babies appear apathetic. They demonstrate less range in their states, appear stressed when alert, and require continuous manipulation to achieve an alert state. Premies exhaust after brief caretaker interaction and seem behaviorally disorganized. Unlike term infants, they are unable to use external stimulation to improve neurobehavioral organization. Perhaps by remaining inactive, generally unresponsive, and mostly asleep, premature infants conserve energy and maintain physiologic homeostasis. This apathetic behavior may be a protective mechanism that aids physical recovery, growth, and development.

MECHANICAL VENTILATION AND ITS COMPLICATIONS

An important concept underlying initial ventilator settings is to achieve chest rise and adequate gas exchange at lowest peak inspiratory and mean airway pressures. Ventilator adjustments based on invasive and noninvasive blood gas and *p*H values plus measurements of delivered volumes can be made as indicated. Oxygen saturation (SaO_2), transcutaneous partial pressures of oxygen (PO_2) and carbon dioxide (PCO_2), and invasive arterial blood gas monitoring provide information necessary to guide acid–base and respiratory management.

I prefer orotracheal to nasotracheal intubation for mechanical ventilation. An unshouldered 2.5-mm-diameter Portex tube is recommended for all VLBW and ELBW infants. Complications include repeated extubation events, anatomic pressure on the upper airway, and introduced infection. The former is statistically most common. There are various methods described for endotracheal tube fixation. I prefer a Logan Bow (Storz, St. Louis, MO) attached to the bony part of the infant's cheek using individually shaped moleskin.

It is not uncommon for the small premature baby's endotracheal tube to slide intermittently above and below its vocal cords. Under such circumstances, the baby may present with abdominal distention because some delivered breaths are aborted by the closed vocal cords. Ventilated gas then passes into the esophagus and stomach. Remember this possibility when evaluating a ventilated premature infant who has increased abdominal girth. Properly fixing the endotracheal tube to minimize motion cures this problem and prevents an inappropriate search for gastrointestinal disease.

In my experience, air leak syndromes occur in about 5% of mechanically ventilated VLBW infants. Some degree of pulmonary interstitial emphysema occurs in more. A delicate balance must be struck between maintaining acceptable blood gases and minimizing barotrauma. Volume overload, not excessive pressure, is what fractures lungs. Complications of mechanical ventilation and their relative occurrence in VLBW infants in my experience are listed in Table 27-6.

Weak respiratory muscles, a soft and compliant thorax, and blunted central respiratory drive are peculiar features of the ELBW infant. Even in the absence of severe lung disease, mechanical ventilation is frequently required to offset hypoventilation or apnea. The combined effects of inefficient respiratory apparatus, diminished energy reserves, the debilitating effects of other disease processes, and the physiologic cost of sustained ventilation conspire against the tiny premature. His resting lung volume is close to or overlaps his lung closing volume because of increased elastic recoil and diminished chest wall stability. Although continuous positive airway pressure (CPAP) restores a more physiologic lung volume, it confers additional respiratory load and resistance. The nasal prongs often used for CPAP are harder to maintain and confer increased airway resistance in the smallest neonates. All these considerations make ventilation of the ELBW infant an exacting process requiring the best of the neonatologist's science and art.

TABLE 27–6
COMPLICATIONS OF MECHANICAL VENTILATION OF VERY-LOW-BIRTH-WEIGHT INFANTS

Complication	Frequency
Acute	
Endotracheal tube misplacement	Common
Pulmonary interstitial air	Common
Pneumothorax	Infrequent
Pulmonary hemorrhage	Infrequent
Pneumonia	Infrequent
Pneumomediastinum	Rare
Pneumopericardium	Very rare
Chronic	
Bronchopulmonary dysplasia	Common
Nasopalatal abnormalities	Common
Pneumonia	Infrequent
Vocal cord abnormalities	Infrequent
Dental abnormalities	Infrequent, possibly underreported

NEONATAL DISORDERS

BRONCHOPULMONARY DYSPLASIA

Bronchopulmonary dysplasia (BPD) is a major cause of late mortality among VLBW and ELBW infants. Chapter 30 discusses this topic in more detail. It is sometimes surprising to witness a VLBW with BPD who is receiving diuretics and sodium supplementation at the same time. If diuretics work, this suggests that the mechanism is partly independent from an effect on fluid and electrolyte balance.

PATENT DUCTUS ARTERIOSUS

Anatomic and functional patency of the several fetal cardiovascular shunts, most notably the ductus arteriosus, is a particular problem for premature infants during the first week of life. Immaturity of the ductal closure mechanism, persistence of elevated pulmonary vascular resistance, and intercurrent illness and its management are held responsible for the patent ductus arteriosus (PDA). Depending on size and direction of blood flow, a PDA may seriously compromise the VLBW infant.

It is axiomatic that the clinician should minimize hypoxemic events and avoid fluid overload. Despite optimal care, early physical findings of PDA, such as hyperactive precordium, increased systolic and diastolic pressure differences, unexplained CO_2 retention, ventilator weaning reversal, or a murmur, should trigger investigation. Functional closure with indomethacin occurs in 60% to 80%, and there is an approximately 33% recurrence rate. The side-effects of indomethacin include reduced urine output and renal failure. Platelet dysfunction and a possibly increased infection rate have been reported. The usual dosage is 0.2 mg/kg every 12 hours for three doses. This has been modified to a lower dose spread over a longer period. For example, 0.1 mg/kg daily for 6 days has been proposed.[59] The incidence of renal, platelet, and infectious morbidities was reduced at lower, longer doses. Recurrence was also diminished if doses were given over 1 week.[60] There seem to be better closure rates and fewer complications if the drug is given over a longer time, but these studies involved relatively small subject numbers and unexplained population differences. Opinion is divided about the optimal gestational and postnatal ages for indomethacin administration. One study showed that indomethacin decreases cerebral blood flow, and another found that the drug reduced severe intraventricular hemorrhage (IVH).[61,62]

Definitive treatment of functionally significant PDA is surgical ligation. Morbidity from the operation and anesthesia should be considered. It may take considerable time for the overloaded pulmonary vasculature to return to normal after surgery. Patent ductus arteriosus closure does not cure underlying chronic lung disease.

APNEA AND BRADYCARDIA

Another problem for the VLBW infant is the occurrence of apnea and bradycardia. Among VLBW infants, there is a virtually 100% incidence of apnea (*i.e.*, >15 seconds of respiratory pause) starting from birth.[63] All VLBW infants have periodic breathing. If apnea is associated with hypoxemia or bradycardia, which implies myocardial hypoxia, it becomes necessary to evaluate and manage this problem. The premature infant responds to many illnesses with apnea. These include infections, seizures, hypoglycemia, hypocalcemia, hyponatremia, serious IVH, and anemia. Among mechanically ventilated babies, such response may manifest by requiring an increased ventilator rate or forced inspiratory oxygen. Specific therapy includes xanthines such as aminophylline or caffeine as first-line drugs. Therapeutic trough levels of aminophylline are 6 to 12 mg/dL. Because approximately 30% of VLBW infants methylate aminophylline into caffeine, therapeutic blood levels of aminophylline do not rule out toxic side-effects, but measuring serum caffeine or total xanthines can.

There is little agreement about the optimal hemoglobin level at which to maintain a premature infant. A cogent argument can be made that having adequate, even extra, erythrocyte oxygen carrying capacity may blunt the impact of hypoxemia on tissue hypoxia. Severity and frequency of significant apneic spells has been diminished by repeated booster transfusions in VLBW infants.[64]

Because most VLBW infants have periodic breathing and apneic spells from birth, unless history or laboratory tests suggest otherwise, an extensive search for other mechanisms is futile if nothing suggests associated disease.

Although most apnea of prematurity resolves between 34 and 36 postconceptual weeks, prolonged xanthine therapy is sometimes necessary. Occasionally, home monitoring for acute cardiorespiratory deceleration plus the use of drugs post discharge may be required. Recording the events associated with apnea and bradycardia at the cribside, studying airway gas flow during respiratory excursions, and looking for gastroesophageal reflux may add to the management of tiny babies with significant apnea and bradycardia. The obstructive component of apnea is probably related to central events that inappropriately close off the airway during inspiration. Controversy surrounds the role of gastroesophageal reflux in producing apnea.

It is my practice to care for all VLBW infants with apnea and bradycardia in the head-up position during the hour after feeding. Upper airway dysfunction during feeding may be one mechanism for feeding-associated apnea.[65] Because the frequency of apnea increases in non-REM sleep and most premature infants go into this state for 20 to 30 minutes after feeding, maintaining a head-up position has some salience for preventing reflux associated apnea.[66]

Aminophylline, which can only be used intravenously, or its oral analog theophylline, may be interchanged with caffeine. Caffeine has perhaps better gastrointestinal tolerance. Xanthines act centrally to increase medullary respiratory center and brain stem nuclei output. This increases minute ventilation. Xanthines may also reduce diaphragmatic muscle fatigue and stabilize upper airway muscles through a central response to hypercapnia. All xanthines increase the metabolic rate and potentially impair nutrition and decrease weight gain.

The infant's progress can be followed using time-trended heart rate and SaO_2 monitoring. Therapeutic failure or refractoriness is defined as apnea or bradycardia requiring aggressive resuscitation or that interferes with feeding, nutrition, or growth. Infants who do not respond or become refractory to xanthines can almost always be managed with doxapram (1–1.5 mg/kg/hour by continuous intravenous drip). This drug is thought to increase afferent input from carotid receptors.[67] Hypertension is an unwanted side-effect, and the drug can only be administered intravenously. Serious side-effects such as jitteriness, seizures and glucose intolerance occur, but less often.

By raising the low SaO_2 limit on the transcutaneous monitor, it is sometimes possible to reduce the number of apneic spells, even if increased supplemental oxygen becomes necessary. This may be explained by the paradoxic response of the immature infant's central nervous system to arterial hypoxemia. A premature infant may inhibit inspiration if its arterial PO_2 (PaO_2) drops.[67]

RETINOPATHY OF PREMATURITY

The incidence of retinopathy of prematurity (ROP) increases inversely with gestational age at birth. It is rarely detectable before 7 weeks of postnatal age. Some ROP seems unavoidable in the extremely premature infant.

Discussion about its pathophysiology and epidemiology occur elsewhere (see Chap. 53). Despite assiduous attention in the VLBW infant to optimizing oxygenation and the clinical testing of many antioxidants (*e.g.*, vitamin E, superoxide dismutase, selenium), the disease continues to occur. Widespread deployment of pulse oximetry, transcutaneous PO_2 and PCO_2 measurements, and repeated microsampling of arterial blood gases has not eliminated this problem.

Ophthalmologic examination around day 49 of life is important for all infants weighing less than 1500 g and for those who have received oxygen more than a few hours. Repeated ophthalmoscopic examinations continue until the retinal vasculature becomes mature. Follow-up depends on these findings.

NECROTIZING ENTEROCOLITIS

Necrotizing enterocolitis (NEC), a serious, sometimes fatal bowel disease, probably has many causes. It is associated with extreme immaturity, mesenteric vascular ischemia, feeding initiation, and the type of resident bacterial gut flora.

Necrotizing enterocolitis is a syndrome afflicting VLBW infants and particularly occurs around the start of enteral feedings. Although not a contagious process, there is probably an infectious component. Systemic bacterial and viral infections may start with gastrointestinal symptoms identical to the early findings of NEC.

The incidence of diagnosed NEC during the past 5 years at the Columbia Hospital for Women is shown in Table 27-7. Necrotizing enterocolitis–like entero-

TABLE 27–7
INCIDENCE OF NECROTIZING ENTEROCOLITIS BY BIRTH WEIGHT AND GESTATIONAL AGE AT COLUMBIA HOSPITAL FOR WOMEN, 1988–1992

	Total Number of Live Births			
Year	Birth Weight 0.5–1.5 kg	Gestational Age 31 wk	Number of Infants with NEC*	Incidence Per 1000 Very-Low-Birth-Weight Infants
1988	66	92	2	12
1989	93	118	0	0
1990	107	72	0	0
1991	74	59	1	7.5
1992	89	50	1	7
Total	429	391	4	4.8

* There was no NEC in infants who weighed between 1.501 and 2.500 kg or for those of gestational ages between 30 and 36 weeks.
NEC, necrotizing enterocolitis.

pathy is equally infrequent. I believe that several factors unique to managing VLBW and ELBW infants are responsible. Columbia Hospital does not accept neonatal transports. This limits the introduction of bacterial pathogens from other hospitals. Because the NICU bacteriologic experience is carefully reviewed, a minimal number of antibiotics are used, reducing the emergence of resistant bowel pathogens such as *Klebsiella* and *Pseudomonas* species. Babies with umbilical artery or venous catheters are not fed. Infusion through these vascular routes are limited to isotonic solutions. Prophylactic oral gentamicin has been my long-standing practice.

Regurgitation or vomiting, abdominal distention, diminished bowel sounds, apparent abdominal tenderness, grossly or occultly bloody stools, changing leukocyte counts, declining platelet count, or other evidence of bowel dysfunction herald the development of NEC. Each of these findings is nonspecific and may indicate several other processes. For example, rotavirus is a nonbacterial pathogen that can mimic NEC and produce classic symptoms. The traditional guaiac positive stool has been overrated as a predictor for NEC, as has the presence of reducing substances in the stool.

Feeding practices intended to reduce NEC risk vary among neonatologists. Some initiate feedings with 0.33-cal/mL feeds, and others use full-strength (*i.e.*, 0.66 cal/mL) formula. Because osmolar load in the gut may contribute to the development of NEC, diluting enteral medications, nutritional supplements, and feeds offers theoretic advantage.[68]

The utility of prophylactic oral gentamicin has been demonstrated in a random, controlled trial.[69] Subsequent investigators have confirmed and extended these findings. One major concern has been the emergence of antibiotic resistant gram-negative organisms. This has not occurred in my experience despite careful and repeated searches for such organisms. Parenteral gentamicin remains my first choice for suspected systemic gram-negative infections despite continued use of oral gentamicin to prevent NEC. The oral dose is 5 mg/kg/day, in two divided doses, continued for 21 days. There is little systemic absorption.[70] Most observed instances of NEC-like enteropathy occurred after oral gentamicin was discontinued or after inadvertent omission of the drug in otherwise eligible patients.

Another antiinfectious approach has been reported using the oral administration of immunoglobulin.[71] Six hundred milligrams of IgA–IgG was given for 28 days. There were no placebo controls. There was no NEC among immunoglobulin-treated babies, but NEC occurred in 7% of controls.

INFECTION AND ITS MANAGEMENT

The VLBW or ELBW neonate is spectacularly vulnerable to bacterial and viral infections before, during, and after birth. Perinatologists theorize that some premature births are caused by infection. Screening for congenital and intrapartum infections should be included in the initial evaluation of VLBW and ELBW infants.

Regular surveillance of NICU culture results can determine which perinatally acquired bacteria are most common in each institution and to what drugs these organisms are sensitive. Using such a system at Columbia Hospital, penicillin and gentamicin are administered for suspected intrauterine sepsis. A regimen of vancomycin plus gentamicin is used for nosocomial infection after considering prior NICU history and previous culture results.

Because many VLBW and ELBW infants remain in the NICU for long periods, some require basic immunization. The AAP's guidelines should be followed.[72] DPT and *Haemophilus* b conjugate vaccines should be given at the recommended chronologic age of 2 months and at a full dose of 0.5 mL intramuscularly. Babies with IVH who are neurologically stable should receive pertussis vaccine. Oral live polio vaccine should be given immediately before discharge to avoid viral shedding in the NICU.

PERIVENTRICULAR AND INTRAVENTRICULAR HEMORRHAGE

Bleeding into the germinal matrix formation, ventricles, or substance of the cerebral cortex occurs with unpredictable and considerable frequency in VLBW and ELBW neonates. Widespread availability of cribside ultrasonography has greatly facilitated diagnosis, staging, and follow-up.

From a clinical perspective, the smaller, sicker, premature infant, particularly if there is an abrupt downturn in vital signs or blood gases, should be suspected of having suffered intracranial hemorrhage. These babies should have cranial ultrasound scans at the time of these adverse events to use as a baseline; these scans should be performed again in 3 to 7 days. For less ill LBW infants, an ultrasound scan at 7 days should be routine. Depending on the presence and severity of hemorrhage, follow-up ultrasound scans may be performed.

Prevention or amelioration of brain damage is a goal in caring for an infant with intracranial hemorrhage. A host of agents, all with supporting rationales, have been tried, including the following:

- phenobarbital to decrease neural metabolism during periventricular and intraventricular hemorrhage (PIVH) genesis[73]
- vitamin E to retard cellular oxidant insults from injury-generated peroxides[74]
- indomethacin to diminish potentially damaging vascular effects from prostaglandins[75]
- tranexamic acid to reduce bleeding[76]
- ethamsylate to reduce 6-keto-PGF_1, a major prostanoid vasodilator[77]
- vitamin K to improve prothrombin times and reduce extension of bleeding[78]

- pancuronium to immobilize the infant and reduce sharp vacillations in blood pressure.[79]

All newborns should receive vitamin K. Very-low-birth-weight infants on TPN or antibiotics should receive additional doses. Vitamin E is commonly used in the NICU, and both vitamins have good safety records and supporting clinical data.[79,80] They are probably given to most VLBW infants. Ethamsylate, although highly regarded in Europe, has not found routine use in this country.[81] No large-scale, well-controlled trial about PIVH prevention has been published to inform clinicians about the safety or efficacy of PIVH preventive drugs.

As highly specialized, technologically complex care for VLBW infants has advanced, outcome observations have grown more and more sophisticated. Central nervous system imaging studies are available from birth to determine the impact and severity of PIVH.

Data about the school-age performance of former very immature babies are accumulating. Low and Papile looked at 6-year follow-up data.[82] They differentiated those with no PIVH from VLBW infants with mild forms of hemorrhage, such as minimal ventricular hemorrhage, with or without dilation and without periventricular leukomalacia. These babies were compared with a matched, longitudinally followed group of healthy, term infants. All were screened for PIVH between 5 and 10 days of age. All birth weights were less than 1.5 kg. Between 1 and 2 years of age, each VLBW infant was developmentally normal on routine neurologic and behavioral testing. Between 5 and 6 years of age, the children were assessed for cognitive performance, reading ability and skills, visual and motor integration, and several measures of motor and perceptual capability. There were significantly lowered scores among VLBW infants compared with term children. Children with mild forms of hemorrhage were significantly outperformed by their no-PIVH premature peers. Overall, VLBW infants scored significantly lower than normal on most individual neurobehavioral measurements and on combined test results. Children who had mild hemorrhages scored even lower.

These findings argue that, as a group, extremely immature babies function less well at visual, motor, and perceptual activities. Some have significant learning difficulties compared with full-term children after school age is reached. Even very mild forms of intracranial hemorrhage amplify these deficits when combined scores are analyzed (see Chap. 61).

COST OF CARE

It is very expensive to care for extremely immature humans. The costs for some surviving VLBW infants can bankrupt an average family. In 1985, surviving 1-kg babies averaged \$150,000 ± \$10,000 in hospital costs.[83] The post hospital bill during the first year of life averaged \$10,000 ± \$13,000. These are direct costs. Indirect expenses, including special child care, transportation to multiple diagnostic and therapy specialists, and missed working days, adds even more cost. Such expenditures are almost never reimbursable.

Tertiary NICU charges have been analyzed:[84]

- nursing, 40%
- room cost, 20%
- laboratory, 15%
- respiratory therapy, 15%
- supplies, 6%
- miscellaneous, 4%.

Physician fees were not included. These are regionally variable and may increase total expenses by 20% to 30%. Managed health care plan charges in the level III nursery were almost 2.5 times greater than those in the level II setting.

There are other nonfiscal costs for immature births. Family dissolution by divorce, suicide, and substance abuse (*e.g.*, alcohol, cocaine, heroin) frequently follow extremely immature births. Family disruption is enhanced by the vulnerability of many families to the same factors involved with socioeconomic impoverishment that were ongoing before the VLBW birth. The added stress of multiple medical problems, a potentially handicapped child, restricted social contacts, and hospital readmissions add to the burdens these parents bear.

In the Canadian system, where care is completely government funded, parents whose previous VLBW infants became handicapped said they still were glad their child had been saved and that they would make the same decision again.[85] They desired more input into decisions but would not request termination of life support. They wished to deal only with physicians and not with other caretakers during this process.

OUTCOME

A major issue is not whether very immature newborns can be saved, but whether or not they should be saved. The lower weight limit of human survival may not yet have been reached. The question remains: what happens to the survivors?

Escobar and colleagues performed a metanalysis of VLBW outcome studies published in English between 1960 and 1988 because of an apparent lack of consistent findings about this subject.[88] From more than 1100 literature references, 111 were found that met stringent criteria for adequacy. Studies that did not provide new data; were limited to only technical, ethical, economic or legal aspects; used pooled data; or did not provide subject numbers or reasons for exclusion were omitted. Of 1100 published reports, fewer than 10% were sufficiently robust to withstand met-analysis.

Some general conclusions were reached. The median incidence of cerebral palsy for all cohorts of LBW infants was approximately 7.7%. This rate showed little variation over time. The incidence of overall disability in VLBW survivors was estimated at approximately 25%. Because of the increased occurrence of disability in those studies that followed infants over longer periods, and because some neurologic or cognitive disabilities may not manifest until later in childhood, the average length of published follow-up (*i.e.*, about 3 years) may be too short to detect the most significant long-term impacts from VLBW. The ability to assess outcome for surviving LBW or VLBW infants has lagged behind the ability to resuscitate them.

What does all this mean? First, neonatologists are fooling themselves in attempting to predict final neurodevelopmental competence using current early developmental testing, although such assessments may be useful to sort infants into early intervention programs. Because early prognosis is generally inaccurate, it is not possible to predict which aspects of care might have been breached to produce an adverse outcome. This has great medical and legal salience. It is past time to conduct serious, multicenter, large population, carefully controlled studies to determine what does and does not make a difference in long-term outcome.

ACKNOWLEDGMENTS

I gratefully acknowledge the contributions of Kenneth L. Harkavy, M.D. and Kathleen B. Scanlon, M.S.N.

REFERENCES

1. Keirse MJNC. Preterm delivery. In: Chalmers J, Enkin M, Keirse MJNC, eds. Effective care in pregnancy and childbirth. Oxford: Oxford University Press, 1991:1277.
2. Raju TNK. An epidemiologic study of very low and very, very low birthweight infants. Clin Perinatol 1991;13:233.
3. Phelps DL, Brown DR, Tung B, et al. 28-Day survival rates of 6676 neonates with birthweights of 1250 grams or less. Pediatrics 1991;87:7.
4. Scanlon JW. The neuroteratology of cocaine: background, theory and clinical implications. Reprod Toxicol 1991;5:89.
5. Vasa R, Vidyasagas D, Winegar A, et al. Perinatal factors influencing the outcome of 501–1000 gram newborns. Clin Perinatol 1986;13:267.
6. Sweet RL. Perinatal infections: bacteriology, diagnosis, and management. In: Iffy L, Kaminetsky HS, eds. Principles and practices of obstetrics and gynecology. New York: John Wiley & Sons, 1981:1038.
7. Kierse MJNC. Preterm delivery. In: Chalmers J, Enkin M, Keirse MJNC, eds. Effective care in pregnancy and childbirth. Oxford: Oxford University Press, 1991:1282.
8. Scanlon JW. Should neonatologists do all newborn resuscitations? In: Van Zundert A, Ostheimer GW, eds. Pain relief and anesthesia in obstetrics. London: Churchill-Livingston, 1994.
9. Silverman WA. Setting a limit in the treatment of neonates: all or none? In: Duc G, Huch A, Huch R, eds. The very low birthweight infant. New York: Georg Thieme Verlag, 1990.
10. Milligan JE, Shennan AT, Hoskins EM. Perinatal intensive care: where and how to draw the line. Am J Obstet Gynecol 1984;148:499.
11. Lee SK, Penner PL, Cox M. Impact of very low birthweight infants on the family and its relation to parental attitudes. Pediatrics 1991;88:105.
12. Lee SK, Penner PL, Cox M. Comparison of the attitudes and health care professionals and parents toward active treatment of very low birthweight Infants. Pediatrics 1991;88:110.
13. Berseth CL, Kenny JD, Durand R. Longitudinal development in pediatric residents of attitudes toward neonatal resuscitation. Am J Dis Child 1986;140:766.
14. American Academy of Pediatrics/American College of Obstetrics and Gynecology. Guidelines for perinatal care. 2nd ed. Elk Grove Village, IL: American Academy of Pediatrics, 1988.
15. Ballard JL, Khoury JC, Wiedig K, et al. New Ballard score, expanded to include extremely premature infants. J Pediatr 1991;119:417.
16. Weidling AM. Blood pressure monitoring in the newborn. Arch Dis Child 1989;64:444.
17. Versmold AM, Kitterman JA, Phibb RH, et al. Aortic blood pressure during the first 12 hours of life in infants with birthweight 610 to 4220 grams. Pediatrics 1981;67:607.
18. Drew JH. Immediate intubation at birth of the very low birthweight infant. Am J Dis Child 1982;136:207.
19. Tochen ML. Orotracheal intubation in the newborn infant: a method for determining depth of tube insertion. J Pediatr 1979;95:1050.
20. Hoskyns EW, Milner AD, Boon AW, et al. Endotracheal resuscitation of preterm infants at birth. Arch Dis Child 1987;62:663.
21. Godfrey S. Respiratory and cardiovascular changes during asphyxia and resuscitation in fetal and newborn rabbits. Q J Exp Physiol 1968;53:97.
22. Hoskyns EW, Milner AD, Hopkins JE. A simple method of face mask resuscitation at birth. Arch Dis Child 1987;62:376.
23. Milner AD. Resuscitation of the newborn. Arch Dis Child 1991;66:66.
24. Bhat R, Zikos-Labropoulou E. Resuscitation and respiratory management of infants weighing less than 1000 grams. Clin Perinatol 1986;13:285.
25. Committee on Fetus and Newborn, American Academy of Pediatrics. Surfactant replacement therapy for respiratory distress syndrome. Pediatrics 1991;87:946.
26. Morley CJ. Surfactant treatment for premature babies: a review of clinical trials. Arch Dis Child 1991;66:445.
27. Enhorning G. Surfactant can be supplemented before the neonate needs it. J Perinat Med 1987;15:479.
28. Merritt TA, Hallman M, Vaucher Y, McFeeley E, Tubman TRJ. Impact of surfactant treatment in cost of neonatal intensive care. J Perinatol 1990;10:416.
29. Avery ME, Merritt TA. Surfactant replacement therapy. N Engl J Med 1991;324:910.
30. Greenberg MJ, Roberts JR, Baskin SI. Use of endotracheally administered epinephrine on a pediatric patient. Am J Dis Child 1981;135:767.
31. David R. Closed chest cardiac massage in the newborn infant. Pediatrics 1988;81:552.
32. Jaim L, Fene C, Vidyajagan D, et al. Cardiopulmonary resuscitation of apparently stillborn infants. J Pediatr 1991;118:778.
33. Levine MJ, Sands C, Gindulis H, et al. Comparison of two

methods of predicting outcome in perinatal asphyxia. Lancet 1986;1:67.
34. Grylack LJ, Chu SS, Scanlon JW. Use of intravenous fluids prior to cesarian section: effects on perinatal glucose, insulin and sodium homeostasis. Obstet Gynecol 1984;63:654.
35. Mendiola J, Grylack LJ, Scanlon JW. The effects of intrapartum maternal glucose infusion. Anesth Analg 1982;61:32.
36. Harkavy KL, Scanlon JW. Hypernatremia in the very low birthweight infant. Int J Pediatr Nephrol 1983;4:75.
37. Benitez OA, Benitez M, Stignen T, et al. Inaccuracy in neonatal measurement of urine concentration with a refractometer. J Pediatr 1986;108:613.
38. Scanlon JW, Krakaur RB. Hyperkalemia following exchange transfusion. J Pediatr 1980;96:108.
39. Sulyok E. The relationship between electrolyte and acid base balance in the premature infant during early postnatal life. Biol Neonate 1971;17:277.
40. Padbury JF, Ogata ES. Glucose metabolism during the transition to postnatal life. In: Polin RA, Fox WW, eds. Fetal and neonatal physiology. Philadelphia: WB Saunders, 1990:404.
41. Harpin VA, Rutter N. Barrier properties of the newborn infants' skin. J Pediatr 1983;102:419.
42. Chathas MK, Paton JB, Fisher DE, et al. Percutaneous central venous catheterization. Am J Dis Child 1990;144:1246.
43. Gilbertson N, Kovar JE, Cox DJ. Introduction of intravenous lipids on the first day of life in the very low birthweight neonate. J Pediatr 1991;119:615.
44. Brans Y. Tolerance of fat emulsions in very low birth weight neonates. Am J Dis Child 1988;142:145.
45. Krauth A, Gordin M, McNelis W, et al. Semipermeable polyurethane membrane as an artificial skin for the premature neonate. Pediatrics 1989;93:945.
46. Scheidt PC, Graubard BJ, Nelson KB, et al. Intelligence at six years in relations to neonatal bilirubin level. Pediatrics 1991;87:797.
47. Van de Bor M, Veen S, Ens-Pokkum , et al. Hyperbilirubinemia in preterm infants and neurodevelopmental outcome at 5 years of age. Pediatr Res 1990;27:259A.
48. Schuster A, Lenard HG. Pain in newborn and prematures: current practice and knowledge. Brain Dev 1990;12:459.
49. Fitzgerald M, Shaw A, MacIntosh N. The postnatal development of the cutaneous flexor reflex: a comparative study in premature infants. Dev Med Child Neurol 1988;30:520.
50. Tawia S. When is the capacity for sentience acquired during human fetal development. J Maternal Fetal Med 1992;1:153.
51. Anand KJS, Sippell WG, Aynsley-Green A. Randomization trial of fentanyl anesthesia in preterm babies undergoing surgery. Lancet 1987;1:423.
52. Purcell-Jones G, Dorman F, Sumner E. Paediatric anesthetist perception of neonatal and infant pain. Pain 1988;33:181.
53. Jacinto JS, Mondanlou HD, Crede M, et al. Renal calcification incidence in very low birthweight infants. Pediatrics 1988; 81:31.
54. Koo WKW, Sherman R, Succop P, et al. Fractures and rickets in very low birthweight infants. J Pediatr Orthop 1989;9:326.
55. Tronick EZ, Scanlon KB, Scanlon JW. Protective apathy: a hypothesis about the behavioral organization and its relation to clinical and physiological status of the preterm infant. Clin Perinatol 1990;17:125.
56. HIFI Study Group. High frequency oscillatory ventilation compared with conventional mechanical ventilation in the treatment of respiratory failure in preterm infants. N Engl J Med 1989;320:88.
57. Carlo WA, Siner B, Chatburn RL, et al. Early randomization intervention with high frequency jet ventilation in respiratory distress syndrome. J Pediatr 1990;117:765.
58. Kezler M, Donn SM, Bucciarelli RL, et al. Multicenter controlled trial comparing jet ventilation and conventional mechanical ventilation in newborn infants with pulmonary interstitial emphysema. J Pediatr 1991;119:85.
59. Rennie JM, Cook RWI. Prolonged low dose indomethacin for persistent ductus arteriosus of prematurity. Arch Dis Child 1991;66:55.
60. Hememan SC, Embruro JP. Prolonged indomethacin therapy for the prevention of recurrence of patent ductus arteriosus. J Pediatr 1990;117:771.
61. Mardoum R, Bejar R, Merritt TA, et al. Controlled study of the effects on indomethacin on cerebral blood flow velocities in newborn infants. J Pediatr 1991;118:112.
62. Badas HS, Green RS, Pourcyrous M, et. al. Indomethacin reduces the risk of severe intraventricular hemorrhage. J Pediatr 1989;115:631.
63. Barrington KJ, Finer NM. Periodic breathing and apnea in preterm infants. Pediatr Res 1990;27:118.
64. Joshi A, Gerhardt T, Shandloff P, et al. Blood transfusion effect on the respiratory patterns of preterm infants. Pediatrics 1987;80:79.
65. Duara S. Structure and function of the upper airway in neonates. In: Polin RA, Fox WW, eds. Fetal and neonatal physiology. Philadelphia: WB Saunders, 1990:827.
66. Altschuler SM. Pathophysiology of gastroesophageal reflux. In: Polin RA, Fox WW, eds. Fetal and neonatal physiology. Philadelphia: WB Saunders, 1990:1037.
67. Miller MJ, Martin RJ. Pathophysiology of apnea of prematurity. In: Polin RA, Fox WW, eds. Fetal and neonatal physiology. Philadelphia: WB Saunders, 1990:880.
68. White K, Harkavy KL. Hypertonic formula resulting from added oral medication. Am J Dis Child 1982;136:931.
69. Grylack LJ, Scanlon JW. A prospective controlled study of oral gentamicin in the prevention of necrotizing enterocolitis. Am J Dis Child 1978;132:1192.
70. Grylack LJ, Boehnert J, Scanlon JW. Serum concentration of gentamicin following oral administration in preterm newborn. Dev Pharm Therap 1982;5:47.
71. Eibl MM, Wolf HM, Fürnkranz H, et al. Prevention of necrotizing enterocolitis in low birthweight infants by IgA-IgG feeding. N Engl J Med 1988;319:1.
72. American Academy of Pediatrics. Report of the Committee on Infectious Diseases. 22nd ed. Elk Grove Village, IL: American Academy of Pediatrics, 1991:46.
73. Kuban KCK, Leviton A, Krishnamoorthy KS, et al. Neonatal intracranial hemorrhage and phenobarbital. Pediatrics 1986; 77:443.
74. Fish WH, Cohen M, Franzek D, et al. Effect of intramuscular vit E on mortality and intracranial hemorrhage in neonates of 1,000 grams or less. Pediatrics 1990;85:578.
75. Ment LH, Duncan CC, Ehrenkranz RA, et al. Randomized indomethacin trial for prevention of intraventricular hemorrhage in very low birthweight infants. J Pediatr 1985;107: 937.
76. Hensey OJ, Morgan MEI, Cooke RWI. Tranexamic acid in the prevention of periventricular hemorrhage. Arch Dis Child 1984;59:719.
77. Benson JWT, Drayton MR, Hayward C, et al. Multicenter trial of ethamsylate for prevention of periventricular hemorrhage in very low birthweight infants. Lancet 1986;2:1297.
78. Pomerance JJ, Teal JG, Gogolak JF, et al. Maternally administered antenatal vitamin K_1: effect on neonatal prothrombin activity, partial thromboplastin time, and intraventricular hemorrhage. Obstet Gynecol 1987;70:235.
79. Perlman JM, Goodman S, Kreusser KL, Volpe JJ. Reduction in intraventricular hemorrhage by elimination of fluctuating cere-

bral blood flow velocity in preterm infants with respiratory distress syndrome. N Engl J Med 1985;312:1353.
80. Fish WH, Cohen M, Franzek D. Effects of Intramuscular vitamin E on mortality and intracranial hemorrhage in neonates of 1,000 grams or less. Pediatrics 1990;85:578.
81. Benson JWT, Drayton MR, Hayward C, Murphy JF, et al. Multicenter trial of ethamsylate for prevention of periventricular haemorrhage in very low birthweight infants. Lancet 1986;2:1297.
82. Low J, Papile LA. Neurodevelopmental performance of very low birth weight infants with mild periventricular, intraventricular hemorrhage. Am J Dis Child 1990;144:1242.
83. Hernandez JA, Offult J, Butterfield LJ. The cost of care of the less than 1,000 gram infant. Clin Perinatol 1986;13:461.
84. Imershein AW, Turner C, Wells JG, et al. Costs of care in neonatal intensive care units. Pediatrics 1992;89:56.
85. Lee KS, Penner PL, Cox M. Impact of very low birthweight infants on the family and its relationship to parental attitudes. Pediatrics 1991;88:105.
86. Greenspan JS, Wolfson MR, Rubenstein SD, et al. Liquid ventilation of human preterm neonates. J Pediatr 1990;117:106.
87. Hoffman EL, Bennett FC. Birthweight less than 80 gram: changing outcomes and influences of gender and gestation number. Pediatics 1990;86:27.
88. Escobar GJ, Littenberg B, Petitti DB. Outcome among surviving very low birthweight infants: a meta-analysis. Arch Dis Child 1991;66:204.

Neonatology: Pathophysiology and Management of the Newborn, Fourth Edition,
edited by Gordon B. Avery, Mary Ann Fletcher, and Mhairi G. MacDonald.
J.B. Lippincott Company, Philadelphia © 1994.

chapter 28

Multiple Gestations

MARY E. REVENIS
LAUREN A. JOHNSON

The products of multiple gestations comprise a disproportionate number of admissions to neonatal intensive care units and suffer greater morbidity than do singletons, but there is relatively little space devoted to their problems in most textbooks of neonatology. A review of the major problems can help the clinician to anticipate the medical needs and to prepare the parents for what lies ahead. Although some of the problems occurring in higher multiples of gestation are unique or intensified as the numbers increase, most of the issues about twins discussed in this chapter apply to all multiple gestations.

EPIDEMIOLOGY

Twin deliveries represent approximately 1 of 100 live births in the United States. The actual rate of twin conceptions is much higher, because early fetal loss with a vanishing twin is far more common than clinically recognized.[1] In 1000 pregnancies studied early with ultrasonography, Landy found a twin conception rate of 3.29%, with subsequent reduction to a single fetus in 21.2% of those pregnancies.[1]

The incidence of higher multiple births is mathematically described by the Hellin–Zeleny law, which states that if twins occur at a frequency of 1/N, triplets occur at a frequency of $(1/N)^2$, quadruplets at $(1/N)^3$, and so on. Because most epidemiologic studies exclude data on twins with no live-born member, they grossly underestimate the incidence of multiple gestations.

Monozygotic twinning occurs at a fairly constant rate of 3.5 per 1000 live births, with limited variation among populations. The occurrence of monozygosity is not affected by environment, race, physical characteristics, or fertility. In contrast, rates for dizygotic twins vary greatly among populations, from 4 to 50 times per 1000 live births. In Scotland, the overall incidence of twins is 12.4 per 1000 live births; in Nigeria, it is 57.2 per 1000.[2] Japan has the lowest total rate of twins, with only 4.3 per 1000, most of which are monozygotic. Other factors that influence the incidence of dizygotic twinning include a maternally transmitted familial tendency, race, nutrition, parity, advanced maternal age, coital frequency, and seasonality. Twins are found most often in black populations and least often in Asians. Taller, heavier women bear twins at a rate 25% to 30% higher than short, undernourished women.[2] Parity is an independent risk factor, with multiparous women having a greater likelihood for multiple gestations.[3] Advanced maternal age predisposes to dizygotic twinning, with peak incidence at 37 years of age.[3] Coital frequency has a positive affect, with a high rate of twin conceptions within the first 3 months of marriage.[4] Another factor is the effect of the climatic seasons. In the Northern hemisphere, most dizygotic births are autumnal, reflecting more multiple ovulations during the winter and spring months. The seasonality of multiple births does not coincide with the peak months of singleton births.[5]

High circulating levels of follicle stimulating hormone (FSH) and luteinizing hormone (LH) lead to the release of more than one ovum per menstrual cycle, making multizygotic conceptions more likely. Conception stimulants such as clomiphene citrate (Clomid, Serophene), which act by stimulating endogenous secretion of gonadotropins, raise the incidence of multiple gestations by 6.8% to 17%; exogenous gonadotropins such as Pergonal (FSH and LH) or human chorionic gonadotropins (A.P.L., Follutein, Pregnyl, Profasi HP) may increase the incidence as much as 18% to 53.5%.[6] The women of the Nigerian Yoruba tribe, who have naturally elevated levels of FSH and LH, have a remarkably high rate of spontaneous, dizygotic twinning (*i.e.*, 1 in 20).[7] Martin examined another population and found that women with dizygotic twins have higher levels of FSH and estradiol than women bearing singletons.[8] A phenomenon likely due to increased pituitary gonadotropin release is the twofold higher incidence of twin conceptions in the 2 months after the cessation of oral contraceptives.[9] High FSH and LH levels probably account for the seasonal variation in twinning observed in many countries.[10,11]

ZYGOSITY

Zygosity is determined by the number of ova fertilized. Higher-order pregnancies may be monozygotic, dizygotic, or multizygotic. In 1955, Corner postulated that monozygotic twins develop by splitting of the conceptus at any time from day 2 after conception through days 15 to 17.[12] The timing of division determines whether monozygotic twins are dichorionic, monochorionic, or conjoined. Dizygotic or multizygotic gestations result if more than one ovum has undergone fertilization at the same coitus or even at different times or with different mates.

At birth, zygosity can be determined by gender differences or by direct placental examination. Other techniques have included blood typing, dermatoglyphics, and chromosome banding.[13,14] The most precise technique is DNA-variant restriction fragment length polymorphisms.[15] Because monozygotic twins carry significantly higher risks of morbidity and mortality prenatally and postnatally, establishing the zygosity of all multiple gestations is clinically important. More effort is going into determining zygosity prenatally using ultrasonography or genetic identification techniques.

PLACENTATION

The placenta from a twin gestation can be monochorionic or dichorionic, and if dichorionic, it can be fused or separated, making four types of placentation possible:

1. Diamnionic, dichorionic separate
2. Diamnionic, dichorionic fused
3. Diamnionic, monochorionic
4. Monoamnionic, monochorionic.

All dizygotic twins have a diamnionic, dichorionic placenta; all monochorionic twins are monozygotic. Zygosity should be determined the case of twins of the same gender if the placenta is not monochorionic, because these siblings may be monozygotic or dizygotic. Fusion of the placenta does not differentiate zygosity. Table 28-1 describes zygosity determination based on placental examination.

Benirschke described how to determine chorionicity of a fused placenta based on examination of the dividing membranes.[16] The amnion contains no blood vessels and is more transparent than the chorion, which contains fetal vessels and remnants of villous tissue. A monochorionic placenta is one in which the septum is composed of a thin, translucent amnion that can be easily separated and lifted from the chorionic plate. In a dichorionic placenta, the septum is thicker and more opaque. It does not separate as easily from the chorionic plate. Ultrasonography of the dividing membranes early in gestation is useful in some cases to determine the chorionicity, but it is not always technically feasible.[17,18]

A monochorionic, monoamnionic placenta is formed by division of the embryonal disc at 7 to 13 days, which is after differentiation of the amnion. Only 1% to 2% of monozygotic twins are monoamnionic; the fetal mortality rate is as high as 50%, primarily due to twisting, knotting, or entanglement of the umbilical cords.[19] Conjoined twins with their necessarily monoamniotic placenta result from the latest

TABLE 28–1
ZYGOSITY DETERMINATION

Clinical Finding	Percentage of Total Deliveries	Zygosity
Different genders	35	Dizygotic
Monochorionic placenta	20	Monozygotic
Same gender and dichorionic placenta	45	8% of monozygotic and 37% of dizygotic infants*

* Further differentiation can be obtained by genotyping.
From Cameron AH. The Birmingham twin survey. Proc R Soc Med 1968;61:229.

and incomplete splitting of the embryonic disc at days 13 to 15 of gestation. The monochorionic, diamnionic placenta with a dividing membrane consisting of two layers of amnion without an intervening chorion is formed at approximately 5 days of gestation. Dichorionic, diamnionic placentas are formed the earliest, within the first 3 days after conception.

ANTEPARTUM COMPLICATIONS

There are many complications of pregnancy that occur more frequently in multiple gestations. Preterm labor is the most frequent complication, occurring in 20% to 50% of multiple gestations, most likely due to uterine overdistention. Pregnancy-induced hypertension, antenatal and intrapartum hemorrhage, hyperemesis gravidarum, and premature rupture of membranes all occur at a higher rate.[20,21] Polyhydramnios, an almost expected complication of multiple gestations, is transient in pregnancies in which there are no other complications. If persistent, the polyhydramnios suggests abnormal fetal conditions, such as twin-to-twin transfusion syndrome (TTTS) or congenital anomalies.[22]

ANTENATAL MANAGEMENT

Recommendations for managing multiple gestations are controversial. The only unquestioned aspect of management is the benefit of early diagnosis, facilitating referral to an appropriate facility for high-risk infants. Antenatal management includes the following components:

- early diagnosis
- nutritional intervention
- cervical cerclage
- prophylactic tocolysis
- steroid stimulation of fetal lung maturity
- therapeutic amniocentesis
- multifetal reduction
- bed rest.

Bed rest beginning before 28 weeks is commonly advised to decrease perinatal mortality.[23] Betamethasone administration from 28 to 32 weeks of gestation is recommended by some practitioners to induce fetal lung maturity, even though the National Institutes of Health Collaborative Study showed no significant effect in twins. It is important to note that a relatively small number of twins were enrolled in that study.[24,25]

With the increased use of conception stimulants has come an increased number of gestations with multiple fetuses. The increased morbidity and mortality associated with these higher multiple gestations has led to the use of multifetal reduction as a means of improving pregnancy outcome. Reduction, most often to twins, is usually performed at 9 to 12 weeks of gestation.[26] Reduction of quadruplets to twins improves overall outcome, but reduction of triplets to twins does not markedly change outcome compared with nonreduced triplets.[27] Selective termination is employed during the second trimester in pregnancies in which one twin is discordant for a major genetic disease.[27,28]

LABOR AND DELIVERY

The total duration of labor in a twin gestation is similar to a singleton gestation, with some differences in the lengths of each stage. Friedman observed a shorter latent phase during twin labor but a longer active phase and second stage, probably due to dysfunctional labor in an overdistended uterus.[29]

There are many potential complications associated with delivery of multiple gestations, including malpresentation, cord prolapse, cord entanglement, vasa previa, locked twins, and fetal distress. Locked twins occur most often if the chins interlock to prevent expulsion or extraction of the first twin. Locking occurs at a rate of 1 per 817 twin gestations, and uterine hypertonicity, monoamnionic twinning, fetal demise, and decreased amniotic fluid are all contributing factors.[30]

The best method of delivery depends on the number of fetuses, the presentation of the first fetus, and the gestational age. Table 28-2 details the frequencies of each variation of presentation. If both twins are vertex, there is no evidence that cesarean section improves outcome.[31] In vertex–nonvertex twin gestations longer than 32 weeks, vaginal delivery is recommended.[32] Delivery of the nonvertex second twin can be by total breech extraction or external cephalic version under ultrasound guidance and epidural anesthesia.[33] If the first twin is nonvertex, delivery usually is by cesarean section.

Mode of delivery of the preterm multiple gestation depends on many factors, only one of which is the fetal presentation. If premature twins present in a vertex–vertex pattern without other complications, vaginal delivery results in an outcome similar to cesarean section.[34] Cesarean section is recommended for all other combinations of presentation if the gestational age is less than 34 weeks.[34] When these recom-

TABLE 28–2
TWIN PRESENTATION

Delivery (A–B)	Percentage of Total Deliveries
Vertex–vertex	42.5
Vertex–nonvertex	38.4
Nonvertex	19.1

From Chervenak FA. The controversy of mode of delivery in twins: the intrapartum management of twin gestation (part II). Semin Perinatol 1986;10:44.

mendations are followed, there is no effect of mode of delivery or birth order on the incidence of intracranial hemorrhage in very-low-birth-weight (VLBW) twins.[35,36]

MORTALITY

Multiple gestations account for 10% to 12% of perinatal deaths.[37] Mortality in twins is four times higher than for singletons, with perinatal mortality rates of 15% to 31%.[38,39] The increased frequencies of prematurity, preeclampsia, hydramnios, placenta previa, abruptio placentae, and cord prolapse contribute to the increased mortality. Of all intrauterine deaths in twins, 73.3% are associated with monochorionic placentation.[40–42]

The frequency of single fetal demise in multiple gestation is reported as 0.5% to 6.8%, although early ultrasonography suggests a much higher rate of early loss.[1,40–42] The causes of antepartum death include cord accidents, vascular anastomoses with overwhelming blood volume shifts, and velamentous insertion of the umbilical cord. Velamentous insertion, which makes the cord more vulnerable to trauma from twisting and compression, is 6 to 9 times more common with twin gestation and increases the risks for fetal distress and for vasa previa with fetal hemorrhage.[43]

After the demise of a fetal twin, the surviving fetus is at increased risk for distress, abnormal presentation, or dystocia with the mother at risk for toxemia or disseminated intravascular coagulation (DIC). In dichorionic twins, if the cause of death is intrinsic only to that fetus, complications to the surviving cotwin are rare except from spontaneous premature labor.[42] When one twin dies after at least 15 weeks of gestation in diamnionic pregnancies, a fetus papyraceous develops. The fetus loses all water content, becomes compressed, and because of oligohydramnios, may be mistakenly identified on sonography as a stuck twin. A retained twin may be large enough to hinder labor mechanically, necessitating cesarean section.[44] Before 15 weeks, the fetus is resorbed; this is called the vanishing twin phenomenon.

For most monochorionic twins, the death of one twin has little adverse effect on the surviving fetus.[45] However, if vascular connections are present, the surviving twin is at risk for complications related to interfetal blood exchange, including DIC from the release of thromboplastin by the dead twin. After the death of one twin, partial abruptio placenta, which separates further during labor, may cause asphyxia or demise of the other twin.[41] Fetal transfusion syndrome may be related to many of the antepartum deaths complicating twin pregnancy.[40–42,46]

The mortality of multiple gestations higher than two is greater than for twins because of smaller fetal size and placental or cord compromise from competition for space.[47] The perinatal mortality rate for triplet pregnancies is reported as 7% to 23%, and it is strongly related to gestational age at delivery.[48]

TWIN-TO-TWIN TRANSFUSION SYNDROME

Interfetal blood exchange occurs almost exclusively in monochorionic twins with circulations shared through vascular anastomoses that are present in most monochorionic placentas. Only 5% to 18% of these communications are sufficiently imbalanced to produce TTTS, but the actual rate would be higher if all cases of early fetal death of one twin were identified.[40,49,50] Vascular anastomoses and TTTS are rare in fused dichorionic placentas of dizygotic or monozygotic twins.[40,43,45,50]

Acute and chronic forms of TTTS have been described.[51,52] The onset of symptoms depends on what type of vessels are in communication, with an unbalanced, arteriovenous anastomosis and unidirectional shunt leading to the earliest and most profound symptoms. If anastomoses are balanced (*i.e.*, artery to artery, vein to vein), the onset and severity of symptoms depends on changes in perfusion pressures that may be temporary and vary throughout gestation or become problematic only after delivery or demise of one twin.

Chronic, unidirectional TTTS manifests at any time after 16 weeks and can occur when an arteriovenous anastomosis joins a high-pressure system with a low-pressure system. The donor twin becomes progressively anemic, hypovolemic, and growth retarded with oligohydramnios and is at risk for tissue hypoxia and acidosis from reduced perfusion.[46,53] The recipient twin becomes polycythemic and hypervolemic, with polyhydramnios developing from increased urine production to relieve the circulatory volume overload. Disparities in the weight of the heart and other viscera and in the size of glomeruli and of pulmonary and systemic arterioles have been reported.[46] Both twins are at risk for ischemia, thromboembolism, DIC, and death. In the donor twin, there is hypotension and poor tissue perfusion; in the recipient, there is also poor tissue perfusion from hyperviscosity and polycythemia. Although the net transfusion is in the direction of the recipient, thrombi can freely exchange in either direction through vascular anastomoses, resulting in infarcts or the death of either twin.

Manifestations of TTTS range in severity from mild differences in blood hematocrit to the extremes of anemia and polycythemia affecting the pair.[54,55] In the most severe cases, the growth-retarded donor twin may die of chronic hypoxia; the recipient develops congestive heart failure and hydrops and may die. Premature rupture of membranes, preterm labor, and delivery of compromised, premature infants are the usual sequelae. The perinatal mortality is 70% or more.[56,57] Prognosis is better if symptoms, diagnosis, and delivery occur at a later gestational age or if hydrops does not develop.

In rare cases, after death of one twin with TTTS, the polyhydramnios resolves, and a healthy survivor is born at a later time. However, compromising volumes of blood may be lost from the survivor into the dead twin. Other morbidity results from the release of thrombogenic material from degenerating fetal tissues, resulting in DIC, multiple infarcts, and tissue necrosis in the live twin.[40] Possibly relating to thromboembolic arterial occlusion, severe defects, such as porencephaly, multicystic encephalomalacia, renal cortical necrosis, infarcts of the spleen, cutis aplasia, small bowel atresia, colonic and appendiceal atresia with horseshoe kidney, hemifacial microsomia, and necrotic limb, have been observed in the survivor of monochorionic twins after one fetal demise.[40,42,57–60] An increased incidence of these defects is not reported in dichorionic twin survivors after the death of a co-twin.

One suggested criterion for diagnosing chronic TTTS is a hemoglobin difference between twins of 5 g/dL or more. In itself, this is not sufficient to establish TTTS, because large differences in hemoglobin concentration can also occur in separate, dichorionic placentas.[61] Tan diagnosed TTTS if a birth-weight difference of 20% and a hemoglobin difference of 5 g/dL or more was found.[51] However, a birth-weight difference of more than 20% occurs with similar frequency in monochorionic and dichorionic pregnancies; the smaller twin may have polycythemia, secondary to intrauterine growth retardation.[61] Fetal transfusion studies using adult cells as markers indicate significant interfetal blood exchange sufficient to cause discordant growth and amniotic fluid volumes occur far more often than differences in hemoglobin concentrations suggest.[62] Because TTTS in all degrees is limited to monochorionic placentations, differentiating the type of placenta and detecting vascular anastomoses is important.

Acardiac twinning (*i.e.*, reversed arterial perfusion syndrome) is a rare but interesting variation of TTTS, occurring in 1% of monozygotic twins.[63] The nonviable acardiac twin's survival depends on the existence of artery–artery and vein–vein anastomoses to the other twin.[64] The structurally normal, pump twin provides the circulation for itself and for its abnormal, acardiac twin, permitting slow growth of the abnormal twin. The reversed direction of flow in the umbilical arteries of the acardiac twin, demonstrable by ultrasonography, may be responsible for preventing normal anatomic differentiation.[65] Often assuming an amorphous shape, the cephalic pole is most severely affected, because it is the region most distal to the retrograde perfusion. The closer and better perfused lower part of the body is relatively spared.[64] The diagnosis of acardiac twinning can be suspected prenatally by absence or marked undergrowth of the heart, head, and trunk and by increased body soft tissue.[65] The acardiac twin is smaller than the pump twin, but the fetal skull and long bones may continue to grow slowly.[66] Frequent complications include congestive heart failure of the pump twin developing between 22 and 30 weeks of gestation with cardiomegaly, hepatomegaly, intrauterine growth failure, maternal hydramnios, preterm delivery, malpresentation, and fetal distress.[64,67] The mortality rate of the pump twin is 50% to 55%, primarily due to prematurity.[64,67]

An acute form of TTTS occurs with rapid transfer of blood through large superficial artery–artery or vein–vein anastomoses during labor and delivery, resulting in a hypovolemic donor and a hypervolemic recipient with similar birth weights.[51,52] The transfusion is from the first to the second twin during the delivery of the first twin. However, if the first cord clamping is delayed, blood from the undelivered twin can be transfused into the first infant. The potential for acute volume changes during labor and delivery of monochorionic twins contributes to their vulnerability, need for resuscitation, and volume management.

Antenatal management of the TTTS was previously limited to close observation and bed rest. Acute polyhydramnios, which often complicates TTTS, is managed with serial amniocenteses of enough amniotic fluid to lessen fetal symptoms.[68] In some instances, decreasing the polyhydramnios seems to stop or ameliorate the interfetal transfusion dramatically. Digoxin has been used successfully to treat cardiac failure in a recipient twin.[69] In severe TTTS, in which the death of both twins is anticipated, selective feticide has been used on the donor twin with survival of the recipient twin.[70]

STUCK TWIN

The stuck twin phenomenon occurs in a diamniotic pregnancy if there is a relatively acute onset of severe disparity in amniotic volumes, with one growth-retarded twin in an oligohydramniotic sac compressed against the uterine wall. If the oligohydramnios is severe enough, this twin may suffer all the complications of prolonged compression, including pulmonary hypoplasia, abnormal facies, and orthopaedic deformation. The other twin is in a distended, polyhydramniotic sac, adding to compression of the smaller twin.[71]

The stuck twin phenomenon occurs to some degree in as many as 35% of monochorionic diamnionic twin pregnancies, and it can develop in dichorionic pregnancies.[72] In monochorionic twins, the phenomenon may be related to TTTS. Other causes, regardless of placentation, include uteroplacental dysfunction, congenital infection, discordant aneuploidy, and structural malformations. Both twins are structurally normal in 95% of cases. Disparity in volumes of amniotic fluid can occur if one twin has structural anoma-

TABLE 28–3
BIRTH STATISTICS FOR MULTIPLE GESTATIONS

Number of Infants	Gestational Age (average in wk)	Birth Weight (average in g)	Reference
Twins	37.1	2390	110
Triplets	33.0	1720	111
Quadruplets	31.4	1482	112

lies that lead to polyhydramnios (*e.g.*, neural tube defect, upper gastrointestinal obstruction, congenital heart disease) or oligohydramnios (*e.g.*, ruptured amnion, urinary tract anomalies, growth retardation).[73] The onset is usually between 18 and 30 weeks of gestation.[72] Premature labor, possibly related to uterine distention from polyhydramnios and to preterm rupture of membranes, develops in most cases. Without intervention to reverse the fetal compression and uterine overdistention, the chance of survival of both twins is less than 20%.[74]

ASPHYXIA

Despite the clinical impression that the first-born twin (twin A) does better than the second-born twin (twin B), there is no demonstrable increase in neonatal death in the second-born twin.[31,39] Breech presentation is more frequent and large placental abruptions are more common in second twins.[39] Differences in the 1-minute Apgar score, umbilical venous *p*H, PO_2, and PCO_2 favor twin A, regardless of route of delivery, placentation, interval between twins, or presentation.[75] The second-born twin has potentially greater risk for hypoxia and trauma, regardless of the route of delivery, suggesting physiologic changes after the birth of the first twin. Findings in the venous blood gases suggest compromised intervillous placental blood flow after delivery of the first twin as a major factor.

In triplet pregnancies, although preterm labor is the most frequent complication and the most important factor in perinatal morbidity and mortality, the mode of delivery is also important. If delivery is by cesarean section, triplet C has a higher 5-minute Apgar score, and triplets B and C have increased survival compared with triplets of vaginal delivery.[76] If triplets are delivered by cesarean section, the three triplets have a similar acid–base status despite the finding of lower 1-minute Apgar scores for triplet C.[77] The influence of birth order on acid–base status becomes significant during vaginal births if there is a longer time *in utero* after delivery of triplet A. Triplets of more than 34 weeks of gestation and with birth weights above 2000 g for each fetus tolerate vaginal delivery more successfully than smaller triplets.[76]

GROWTH

Examination of fetuses between 8 and 21 weeks of gestation show similar weight–length ratios for singleton and twin fetuses.[78] Birth weights of live-born twins up to 30 weeks of gestation are slightly smaller but similar to singletons of the same gestational age, indicating that the growth rate is similar in twins and singletons until 30 weeks of gestation (Table 28-3).[79–81] After 30 weeks, the singleton fetus has accelerated, exponential growth, and twins fetuses have a more linear rate of growth.[82] Triplet growth was previously reported to decline progressively after 27 weeks of gestation.[47] Later studies indicate that growth of individual triplets and triplet sets remains linear throughout the third trimester.[83]

Better growth in the third trimester for multiple gestations reflects the positive impact of more aggressive maternal nutritional and obstetric care management. In a prospective study of nutritional intervention, the incidence of preterm delivery, low birth weight (LBW), and VLBW was lowered by 30%, 25%, and 50%, respectively, compared with twin pregnancies without nutritional intervention, but the rates of intrauterine growth retardation were not affected.[84]

Multiple gestations account for 17% of intrauterine growth retardation, with higher mortality rates for affected infants, particularly for the growth-retarded twin if only one is affected.[37,79,85] Monochorionic twins show greater degrees of intrapair variation in birth weight than dichorionic twins, and true intrauterine growth retardation occurs more often in monochorionic twins. The individual members of twin pairs are frequently discordant for the rate of growth due to TTTS, placental insufficiency, intrauterine crowding, or an unequal impact of maternal complications that impair growth, such as preeclampsia. Ultimately, the underlying factor in most instances is a limitation of intrauterine nutrition, which may be unequally shared by the fetuses.

The incidence of discordant fetal growth as measured by biparietal diameter increases significantly as gestation advances. It is important to differentiate discordant growth due to TTTS, in which both twins are at increased risk for morbidity and mortality often before the last trimester, from a twin gestation in which one fetus shows growth retardation, which usually becomes evident during the last trimester, and the other develops normally. With discordant growth not due to TTTS, the prognosis for the growth-retarded fetus depends on the severity of the growth failure and its cause, and the prognosis for the normally grown fetus may not be compromised. During the postnatal period, the smaller of discordant twins has an increased incidence of hypoglycemia and is more likely to have retarded growth and development during childhood.[86,87]

CONGENITAL ANOMALIES

Monozygotic twins have an increased frequency of congenital anomalies compared with dizygotic twins or singletons.[60] Monozygotic twins are frequently discordant for malformations or for the severity of a given malformation. Some structural defects are related to the monozygotic twinning process, such as conjoined twins or some amorphous twins. Early embryonic malformations and malformation complexes such as sirenomelia, holoprosencephaly, and anencephaly are increased in monozygotic twins, suggesting a common cause for monozygotic twinning and early malformation complexes. Structural defects that result from the disruption of previously normal tissues are associated with the exchange of circulation in monochorionic twins with vascular connections. Those defects in which a vascular disruptive cause has been suggested include central nervous system defects (*e.g.*, microcephaly, porencephalic cysts, hydranencephaly), gastrointestinal defects (*e.g.*, intestinal atresia), renal cortical necrosis, hemifacial microsomia, aplasia cutis congenital, and terminal limb defects.[58] Deformations due to crowding and constraint molding of the normal fetus *in utero* during late gestation are similar in type and frequency in dizygotic and monozygotic twins and include foot-positioning deformations.

Conjoined twins represent a unique structural defect of monozygotic monoamnionic twins. The nonseparated parts of the otherwise normal twins remain fused throughout the remaining period of development.[88] The incidence of conjoined twins is between 1 in 80,000 to 1 in 25,000 births, and 70% to 80% of these cases are female twins.[89] Approximately 40% are joined at the chest (*i.e.*, thoracopagus), 34% at the anterior abdominal wall (*i.e.*, xiphopagus or omphalopagus), 18% at the buttocks (*i.e.*, pygopagus), 6% at the ischium (*i.e.*, ischiopagus), and 2% at the head (*i.e.*, craniopagus). With ultrasonography, the diagnosis of conjoined twins can be established as early as week 12 of gestation.[90] Forty percent of conjoined twins are stillborn, and an additional 35% survive only 1 day.[91] Long-term survival with or without surgical separation depends on the anatomic site of attachment and the extent of shared organs.[92]

NEONATAL DISORDERS

HYALINE MEMBRANE DISEASE

Twins are at increased risk of developing hyaline membrane disease (HMD) due to the increase in preterm delivery.[38] Both twins are usually affected by HMD. However, if only one twin is affected, it is usually twin B, who had a lower Apgar score at 1 minute and a higher birth weight than twin A.[93] The greater risk to twin B is probably related to birth asphyxia.[93] Monozygotic twins are more often born prematurely and at an earlier gestational age than dizygotic twins, and they are more prone to develop HMD.

NECROTIZING ENTEROCOLITIS

Unique risk factors for the development of necrotizing enterocolitis (NEC) have not been identified for twins or higher multiple gestations, but as a group, they are at an increased risk due to the greater likelihood of prematurity and LBW. Comparisons of twins showed that the most significant factor in predicting the occurrence of NEC and the need for surgical intervention was a lower 1-minute Apgar score for the affected twins, predominantly twin B, compared with unaffected co-twins.[94] Samm found that, in all his case pairs, it was twin A who had developed NEC; in no case did only twin B have NEC.[95] In that study, the first-born infants were more stable, were fed sooner, and had feedings advanced more rapidly than the second-born twins, implicating feeding practices in the higher incidence of NEC for twin A.

GROUP B STREPTOCOCCAL INFECTION

The rate of early-onset group B streptococcal (GBS) disease in twin infants weighing less than 2.5 kg is five times higher than the rate in LBW singletons.[96] If just one of a pair of twins is infected or colonized with GBS *in utero*, it is most likely the twin positioned adjacent to the cervix, with the exposure due to ascending spread of GBS through the membranes. Spread of infection through the vascular connections between monochorionic twins has not been documented, although it is theoretically possible. However, spread of GBS from the amniotic fluid of an exposed twin to a co-twin may occur through intact dividing membranes.[97]

SUDDEN INFANT DEATH SYNDROME

Monozygotic and dizygotic twins are at some increased risk of sudden infant death syndrome (SIDS) compared with singletons, and this being especially true for LBW pairs.[98] If the birth weights of the twins differs significantly, it is usually the smaller twin who dies of SIDS.[98] For twins discordant for size, the risk of SIDS for the smaller of twins is greater than for LBW and premature singletons or other groups of infants at high risk for SIDS.[98] It is unusual for the surviving co-twin also to die of SIDS.

POSTNEONATAL CARE AND FOLLOW-UP

In addition to the long-term impact of some of the perinatal conditions previously mentioned, twins and higher multiples continue to be at risk for medical, developmental, and social problems beyond that experienced by singletons born at similar gestational ages. A brief list of factors that should be considered in following these patients is included to assist the clinician in anticipating the problems, many of which can be lessened by preventive measures, such as the following:

- parental stress of child-rearing[99,100]
- child abuse and neglect[100,101]
- intratwin favoritism[102]
- developmental delay (*e.g.*, performance below chronologic age, especially in language and speech)[103]
- mental retardation[104,105]
- cerebral palsy[104,106]
- growth delay.[107,108]

REFERENCES

1. Landy HJ, Weiner S, Corson SL, Batzer FR, Bolognese RJ. The "vanishing twin": ultrasonographic assessment of fetal disappearance in the first trimester. Am J Obstet Gynecol 1986; 155:14.
2. Nylander PPS. Biosocial aspects of multiple births. J Biosoc Sci Suppl 1971;3:29.
3. Bulmver MG. The effect of parental age, parity and duration of marriage on the twinning rate. Ann Hum Genet 1959; 23:454.
4. James WH. Dizygotic twinning, marital stage and status, and coital rates. Ann Hum Biol 1981;8:371.
5. Picard R, Fraser D, Hagay ZJ, Leiberman JR. Twinning in southern Israel. Seasonal variation and effects of ethnicity, maternal age and parity. J Reprod Med 1990;35:163.
6. Schenker JG, Yarkoni S, Granat M. Multiple pregnancies following induction of ovulation. Fertil Steril 1981;35:105.
7. Nylander PPS. Serum levels of gonadotrophins in relation to multiple pregnancy in Nigeria. J Obstet Gynaecol Br Commonw 1973;80:651.
8. Martin NG, Olsen ME, Theile H, et al. Pituitary-ovarian function in mothers who have had two sets of dizygotic twins. Fertil Steril 1984;41:878.
9. Bracken MB. Oral contraception and twinning: an epidemiologic study. Am J Obstet Gynecol 1979;133:432.
10. Timonen S, Carpen E. Multiple pregnancies and photoperiodicity. Ann Chir Gynaecol Fenn 1968;57:135.
11. Elwood JM. Maternal and environmental factors affecting twin births in Canadian cities. Br J Obstet Gynaecol 1978; 85:351.
12. Corner GW. The observed embryology of human single ovum twins and other multiple births. Am J Obstet Gynecol 1955;70:933.
13. Robertson JG. Blood grouping in twin pregnancy. J Obstet Gynaecol 1969;76:154.
14. McCracken AA, Daly PA, Zolnick MR, Clark AM. Twins and Q-banded chromosome polymorphisms. Hum Genet 1978; 45:253.
15. Hill AV, Jefreys AJ. Use of minisatellite DNA probes for determination of twin zygosity at birth. Lancet 1985;2:1394.
16. Benirschke K. Multiple pregnancy. In: Fox W, Polin R, eds. Fetal and neonatal physiology. Philadelphia: WB Saunders, 1991:97.
17. Barss VA, Benacerraf BR, Frigoletto FD. Ultrasonographic determination of chorion type in twin gestation. Obstet Gynecol 1985;66:779.
18. Winn HN, Gabrielli S, Reece EA, et al. Ultrasonographic criteria for the prenatal diagnosis of placental chorionicity in twin gestations. Am J Obstet Gynecol 1989;161:1540.
19. Timmons JD, De Alvarez RR. Monoamniotic twin pregnancy. Am J Obstet Gynecol 1963;86:875.
20. Newton ER. Antepartum care in multiple gestation. Seminars in Perinatology 1986;10:19.
21. Polin JI, Frangipane WL. Current concepts in management of obstetrics problems for pediatricians: II. Modern concepts in the management of multiple gestation. Pediatr Clin North Am 1986;33:649.
22. Hashimoto B, Callen PW, Filly RA, Laros RK. Ultrasound evaluation of polyhydramnios and twin pregnancy. Am J Obstet Gynecol 1986;154:1069.
23. Gilstrap LC, Hauth JC, Hankins GDV, Beck A. Twins prophylactic hospitalization and ward rest at an early gestational age. Obstet Gynecol 1987;69:578.
24. Loucopoulos A, Jewelewicz R. Management of multifetal pregnancies: sixteen years' experience at the Sloane Hospital for Women. Am J Obstet Gynecol 1982;143:902.
25. Collaborative Group on Antenatal Steroid Therapy. Effect of antenatal dexamethasone administration on the prevention of respiratory distress syndrome. Am J Obstet Gynecol 1981; 141:276.
26. Evans MI, Littmann L, King M, Fletcher JC. Multiple gestation: the role of multifetal pregnancy reduction and selective termination. Clin Perinatol 1992;19:345.
27. Melgar CA, Rosenfeld DL, Rawlinson K, Greenberg M. Perinatal outcome after multifetal reduction to twins compared with nonreduced multiple gestations. Obstet Gynecol 1991; 78:763.
28. Redwine FO, Hays PM. Selective birth. Semin Perinatol 1986; 10:73.
29. Friedman EA, Sachtelben MR. The effect of uterine overdistention on labor I. Multiple pregnancy. Obstet Gynecol 1964; 23:164.
30. Cohen M, Kome SG, Rosenthal AH. Fetal interlocking complicating twin gestation. Am J Obstet Gynecol 1965;91:407.
31. McCarthy BJ, Sachs BP, Layde PM, et al. The epidemiology of neonatal death in twins. Am J Obstet Gynecol 1981;141:252.
32. Adam C, Allen AC, Baskett TF. Twin delivery: influence of presentation and method of delivery on the second twin. Am J Obstet Gynecol 1991;165:23.
33. Chervenak FA. The controversy of mode of delivery in twins: the intrapartum management of twin gestation (part II). Semin Perinatol 1986;10:44.
34. Cetrulo CL. The controversy of mode of delivery in twins: the intrapartum management of twin gestation (part I). Semin Perinatol 1986;10:39.
35. Morales WJ, O'Brien WF, Knuppel RA, et al. The effect of mode of delivery on the risk of intraventricular hemorrhage in

nondiscordant twin gestations under 1500 g. Obstet Gynecol 1989;73:107.
36. Pearlman SA, Batton DG. Effect of birth order on intraventricular hemorrhage in very low birth weight twins. Obstet Gynecol 1988;71:358.
37. Manlan G, Scott KE. Contribution of twin pregnancy to perinatal mortality and fetal growth retardation: reversal growth retardation after birth. Can Med Assoc J 1978;118:365.
38. Ho SK, Wu PYK. Perinatal factors and neonatal morbidity in twin pregnancy. Am J Obstet Gynecol 1975;122:979.
39. Naeye RL, Tafari N, Judge D, Marboe CC. Twins: causes of perinatal death in 12 United States cities and one African city. Am J Obstet Gynecol 1978;131:267.
40. Benirschke K. Twin placenta in perinatal mortality. N Y State J Med 1961;61:1499.
41. Litschgi M, Stucki D. Course of twin pregnancies after fetal death in utero. Geburtschilfe Perinatol 1980;184:227.
42. D'Alton ME, Newton ER, Cetrulo CI. Intrauterine fetal demise in multiple gestation. Acta Genet Med Gemellol 1984; 34:43.
43. Benirschke K. Multiple gestation: incidence, etiology and inheritance. In: Creasy RK, Resnik R, eds. Maternal-fetal medicine. Philadelphia: WB Saunders, 1984:511.
44. Leppert PC, Wartel L, Lowman R. Fetus papyraceus causing dystocia: inability to detect blighted twin antenatally. Obstet Gynecol 1979;54:381.
45. Johnson SF, Driscoll SG. Twin placentation and its complications. Semin Perinatol 1986;10:9.
46. Naeye R. Human intrauterine parabiotic syndrome and its complications. N Engl J Med 1963;268:804.
47. McKeown T, Record RG. Observations on fetal growth in multiple pregnancy. Observations on fetal growth in multiple pregnancy in man. J Endocrinol 1952;8:386.
48. Egwuata VE. Triplet pregnancy: a review of 27 cases. Int J Gynaecol Obstet 1980;18:460.
49. Newton ER. Antepartum care in multiple gestation. Semin Perinatol 1986;10:19.
50. Robertson EG, Neer KJ. Placental injection studies in twin gestation. Am J Obstet Gynecol 1983;147:170.
51. Tan KL, Tan R, Tan SH, Tan AM. The twin transfusion syndrome. Clin Pediatr 1979;18:111.
52. Klebe JG, Ingomar CJ. The fetoplacental circulation during parturition illustrated by the interfetal transfusion syndrome. Pediatrics 1972;39:453.
53. Dudley DKL, D'Alton ME. Single fetal death in twin gestation. Semin Perinatol 1986;10:65.
54. Benirschke K, Driscoll SG. The pathology of the human placenta. New York: Springer-Verlag, 1967:87.
55. Fox H. Pathology of the placenta. Philadelphia: WB Saunders 1978:81.
56. Brennan JN, Diwan RV, Mortimer GR, Bellon EM. Fetofetal transfusion syndrome: prenatal ultrasonographic diagnosis. Radiology 1982;43:535.
57. Galea P, Scott JM, Goel KM. Feto-fetal transfusion syndrome. Arch Dis Child 1982;57:781.
58. Hoyme HE, Higginbottom MC, Jones KL. Vascular etiology of disruptive structural defects in monozygotic twins. Pediatrics 1981;67:288.
59. Mannino FL, Jones KL, Benirschke D. Congenital skin defects and fetus papyraceus. J Pediatr 1977;91:559.
60. Schinzel AAGL, Smith DW, Miller JR. Monozygotic twinning and structural defects. J Pediatr 1979;95:921.
61. Danskin FH, Neilson JP. Twin-to-twin transfusion syndrome: what are appropriate diagnostic criteria? Am J Obstet Gynecol 1989;161:365.
62. Fisk NM, Borrell A, Hubinont C, Tannirandorn Y, Nicolini U, Rodeck CH. Fetofetal transfusion syndrome: do the neonatal criteria apply *in utero*? Arch Dis Child 1990;65(Suppl 7):657.
63. Napolitani FE, Schreiber I. The acardiac monster. A review of the world literature and presentation of 2 cases. Am J Obstet Gynecol 1960;80:582.
64. Van Allen MI, Smith DW, Shepard TH. Twin reversed arterial perfusion (TRAP) sequence: a study of 14 twin pregnancies with acardius. Semin Perinatol 1983;7:285.
65. Billah KL, Shah D, Odwin C. Ultrasonic diagnosis and management of acardius acephalus twin pregnancy. Med Ultrasound 1984;8:108.
66. Stiller RJ, Romero R, Pace S, Hobbins JC. Prenatal identification of twin reversed arterial perfusion syndrome in the first trimester. Am J Obstet Gynecol 1989;160:1194.
67. Moore TR, Gale S, Benirschke K. Perinatal outcome of forty-nine pregnancies complicated by acardiac twinning. Am J Obstet Gynecol 1990;163:907.
68. Radestad A, Thomasses PA. Acute polyhydramnios in twin pregnancy: a retrospective study with special reference to therapeutic amniocentesis. Acta Obstet Gynecol Scand 1990; 69:297.
69. De Lia JE, Emery MG, Sheafor SA, and Hennison TA. Twin transfusion syndrome: successful *in utero* treatment with digoxin. Int J Gynaecol Obstet 1985;23:197.
70. Wittman BK, Farquaharson DG, Thomas WD, et al. The role of feticide in the management of severe twin transfusion syndrome. Am J Obstet Gynecol 1986;155:1023.
71. Urig MA, Clewell WH, Elliott JP. Twin-twin transfusion syndrome. Am J Obstet Gynecol 1990;163:1522.
72. Chescheir NC, Seeds JW. Polyhydramnios and oligohydramnios in twin gestations. Obstet Gynecol 1988;71:882.
73. Pretorius DH, Mahony BS. Twin gestations. In: Nyberg DA, Mahony BS, Pretorius DH, eds. Diagnostic ultrasound of fetal anomalies. Chicago: Year Book, 1990:592.
74. Mahony BS, Petty CN, Nyberg DA, et al. The "stuck twin" phenomenon: ultrasonographic findings, pregnancy outcome, and management with serial amniocenteses. Am J Obstet Gynecol 1990;163:1513.
75. Young BK, Suidan J, Antoine C, et al. Differences in twins: the importance of birth order. Am J Obstet Gynecol 1985; 151:915.
76. Deale CJC, Cronje HS. A review of 367 triplet pregnancies. S Afr Med J 1984;66:92.
77. Creinin M, MacGregor S, Socol M, et al. The Northwestern University triplet study. IV. Biochemical parameters. Am J Obstet Gynecol 1988;159:1140.
78. Iffy L, Lavenhar MA, Jakobovits A, Kaminetzky HA. The rate of early intrauterine growth in twin gestation. Am J Obstet Gynecol 1983;146:970.
79. Hendricks CH. Twinning in relation to birth weight, mortality, and congenital anomalies. Obstet Gynecol 1966;27:47.
80. Naeye RL, Benirschke K, Hagstrom JWC, Marcus CC. Intrauterine growth of twins as estimated from live born birthweight data. Pediatrics 1966;37:409.
81. Wilson RS. Twins: measures of birth size at different gestational ages. Ann Hum Biol 1974;1:57.
82. Arbuckle TE, Sherman GJ. An analysis of birth weight by gestational age in Canada. Can Med Assoc J 1989;140:157.
83. Jones JS, Newman RB, Miller MC. Cross-sectional analysis of triplet birth weight. Am J Obstet Gynecol 1991;164:135.
84. Dubois S, Dougherty C, Duquette MP, Hanley JA, Moutquin JM. Twin pregnancy: the impact of the Higgins Nutrition Intervention Program on maternal and neonatal outcomes. Am J Clin Nutr 1991;53:1397.
85. Powers WF. Twin pregnancy. Complications and treatment. Obstet Gynecol 1973;42:795.

86. Reisner SH, Forbes AE, Cornblath M. The smaller of twins and hypoglycemia. Lancet 1965;1:524.
87. Babson SG, Phillips DS. Growth and development of twins dissimilar in size at birth. N Engl J Med 1973;289:937.
88. Benirschke K, Temple WW, Bloor C. Conjoined twins: nosology and congenital malformations. Birth Defects 1978;16:179.
89. Rudolph AJ, Michaels JP, Nichols BL. Obstetric management of conjoined twins. Birth Defects 1967;3:28.
90. Schmidt W, Heberling D, Kubli F. Antepartum ultrasonographic diagnosis of conjoined twins in early pregnancy. Am J Obstet Gynecol 1981;139:961.
91. Edmonds LD, Layde PM. Conjoined twins in the United States, 1970–1977. Teratology 1985;25:301.
92. Filler RM. Conjoined twins and their separation. Semin Perinatol 1986;10:32.
93. De La Torre Verduzco R, Rosario R, Rigatto H. Hyaline membrane disease in twins. Am J Obstet Gynecol 1976;125:668.
94. Powell RW, Dyess DL, Luterman A, et al. Necrotizing enterocolitis in multiple-birth infants. J Pediatr Surg 1990;25:319.
95. Samm M, Curtis-Cohen M, Keller M, Harbhajan C. Necrotizing enterocolitis in infants of multiple gestation. Am J Dis Child 1986;140:937.
96. Pass MA, Khare S, Dillon HC. Twin pregnancies: incidence of group B streptococcal colonization and disease. J Pediatr 1980;97:635.
97. Benirschke K. Routes and types of infection in the fetus and the newborn. Am J Dis Child 1960;99:714.
98. Beal S. Sudden infant death syndrome in twins. Pediatrics 1989;84:1038.
99. Goshen-Gottstein ER. The mothering of twins, triplets and quadruplets. Psychiatry 1980;43:189.
100. Tanimura M, Matsui I, Kobayashi N. Child abuse of one of a pair of twins in Japan. Lancet 1990;336:1298.
101. Grouthuis JR, Altemeier WA, Rubarge JP, et al. Increased child abuse in families with twins. Pediatrics 1982;70:769.
102. Minde K, Corter C, Goldberg S, Jeffers D. Maternal preference between premature twins up to age four. J Am Acad Child Adolesc Psychiatry 1990;29:367.
103. Record RG, McKeown T, Edwards JH. An investigation of the differences in measured intelligence between twins and single births. Ann Hum Genet 1970;34:11.
104. Durkin MV, Kaveggia EG, Pendelton E, et al. Analysis of etiologic factors in cerebral palsy with severe mental retardation. Eur J Pediatr 1976;123:67.
105. Kragt H, Huisjes HJ, Touwen BCL. Neurobiological morbidity in newborn twins. Eur J Obstet Gynecol Reprod Biol 1985;19:75.
106. Petterson B, Stanley F, Henderson D. Cerebral palsy in multiple births in Western Australia: genetic aspects. Am J Med Genet 1990;37:346.
107. Silva PA. The growth and development of twins compared to singletons at ages 9 and 11. Aust Paediatr J 1985;21:265.
108. Morley R, Cole, TJ, Powell R, Lucas A. Growth and development in premature twins. Arch Dis Child 1989;64:1042.
109. Cameron AH. The Birmingham twin survey. Proc R Soc Med 1968;61:229.
110. Newton W, Keith L, Keith D. The Northwestern University multihospital twin study: IV. Duration of gestation according to fetal sex. Am J Obstet Gynecol 1984;149:655.
111. Sassoon DA, Castro LC, Davis JL, Hobel CJ. Perinatal outcome in triplet versus twin gestations. Obstet Gynecol 1990;75:817.
112. Collins SM, Bleyl BA. Seventy-one quadruplet pregnancies: management and outcome. Am J Obstet Gynecol 1990; 162:1384.

Part Five

THE NEWBORN INFANT

Neonatology: Pathophysiology and Management of the Newborn, Fourth Edition,
edited by Gordon B. Avery, Mary Ann Fletcher, and Mhairi G. MacDonald.
J.B. Lippincott Company, Philadelphia © 1994.

chapter 29

Acute Respiratory Disorders

JEFFREY A. WHITSETT
GLORIA S. PRYHUBER
WARD R. RICE
BARBARA B. WARNER
SUSAN E. WERT

Successful adaptation to air breathing at the time of birth is the culmination of an orderly process of growth and differentiation of pulmonary cells, leading to alveolar and capillary surfaces capable of providing oxygen and eliminating carbon dioxide. Failure to achieve adequate gas exchange at birth represents a major cause of perinatal morbidity and mortality. This chapter reviews the common disorders of neonatal respiratory adaptation, including respiratory distress syndrome (RDS), pulmonary meconium aspiration syndrome (MAS), pulmonary hypertension, pneumonia, air leak, pulmonary hemorrhage, and other causes of acute respiratory dysfunction in the perinatal period. The clinical manifestations and therapy of these disorders are discussed in the context of the morphologic, biochemical, and physiologic factors critical to normal pulmonary growth, maturation, and function in the newborn.

HUMAN LUNG DEVELOPMENT

Human lung development can be divided into five distinct stages of organogenesis.[1,2] The first is an early embryonic period (3–7 weeks of gestation), during which lung development is initiated and major airways are formed. The second is a pseudoglandular period (5–17 weeks of gestation), during which the bronchial tree and acinar tubules develop. The third is a canalicular period (16–26 weeks of gestation), during which vascularization of the surrounding mesenchyme with formation of the air–blood barrier occurs, and cytodifferentiation of bronchiolar and alveolar epithelial cells is initiated. The fourth is a saccular period (24–38 weeks of gestation), during which enlargement of the peripheral air spaces with development of primitive saclike alveoli and thick interalveolar septa occurs. The fifth is an alveolar period (36 weeks of gestation to 3 years of age), during which formation of thin secondary alveolar septa and remodeling of the capillary bed is initiated, giving rise to the mature alveolar organization of the adult lung (Fig. 29-1).

The human lung is a derivative of the primitive foregut and appears by 3 weeks (*i.e.*, 22 days) of gestation as an enlargement of the caudal end of the laryngotracheal sulcus located in the median pharyngeal groove, which is an outgrowth of the ventral wall of the primitive esophagus. During the fourth week (*i.e.*, 26–28 days) of gestation, the respiratory primordium enlarges and subdivides into the left and right main stem bronchi (see Fig. 29-1*A,B*). As the primitive lung continues to grow caudally, it expands

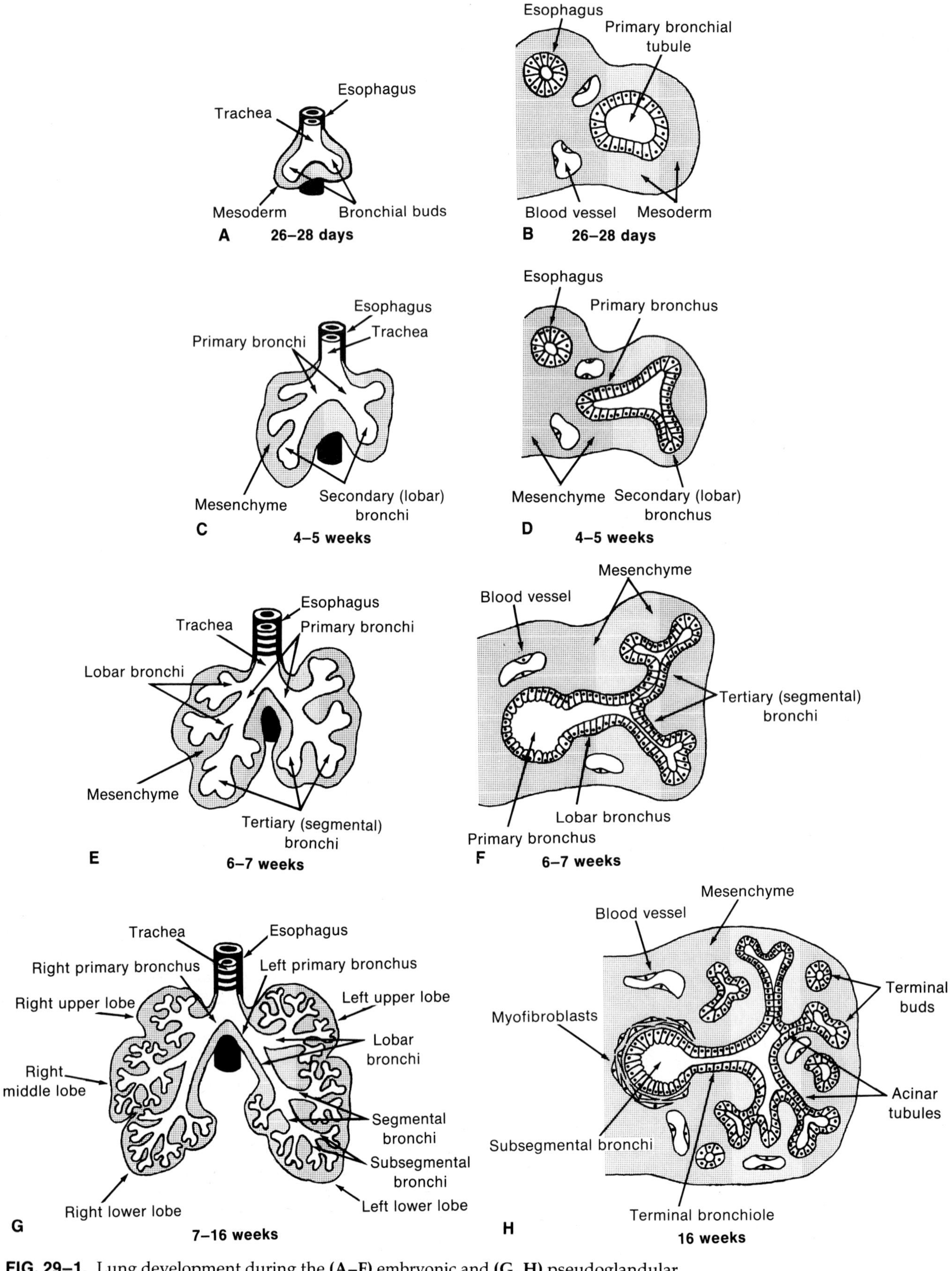

FIG. 29–1. Lung development during the **(A–F)** embryonic and **(G, H)** pseudoglandular stages of organogenesis. The overall branching pattern of the primitive lung (*left panels*) results in the development of the bronchial tree. The histological organization of the fetal lung becomes more complex as branching morphogenesis progresses through these stages (*right panels*).

into the mesenchyme surrounding the primitive foregut and becomes separated from the esophagus by a band of mesenchymal tissue called the tracheoesophageal septum. Between 4 and 5 weeks of gestation, the lobar buds arise as the left and right primary bronchi subdivide to produce the secondary, or lobar, bronchi (see Fig. 29-1*C,D*). Further subdivision of lobar bronchi into tertiary or segmental bronchi occurs during the sixth week of gestation, with the lung taking on a lobulated appearance as the segmental buds are formed (see Fig. 29-1*E,F*). The developing respiratory tract is lined by endodermally derived epithelium that forms conducting airways and alveoli. Surrounding mesoderm is composed of mesenchymal cells that differentiate into connective tissue components, such as blood vessels, fibroblasts, smooth muscle cells, and cartilage.

Preacinar blood vessels first appear at the end of week 4. Pulmonary arteries arise from the sixth pair of aortic arches and grow into the mesenchyme, where they accompany developing airways, segmenting with each bronchial subdivision. Pulmonary veins develop as outgrowths of the atrial portion of the heart and are enveloped by mesenchyme. Intraacinar arteries and veins develop later, in parallel with alveolar formation.

The pseudoglandular stage of fetal lung development extends from about 7 to 16 weeks of gestation and is marked by the formation of the bronchial portion of the lung. This occurs through a process known as branching morphogenesis, during which the segmental tubules of the developing lung undergo repetitive lateral and terminal dichotomous branching to form the primitive bronchial tree (see Fig. 29-1*G,H*). By week 16 of gestation, the segmental bronchi have subdivided to produce 16 to 25 generations of bronchial tubules ending in the terminal bronchioles. These bronchial tubules are lined initially by a pseudostratified columnar epithelium containing large pools of glycogen. A prominent basement membrane underlies the epithelium, and mesenchymal cells adjacent to these tubules differentiate into fibroblasts and become organized, aligning themselves in a circumferential orientation perpendicular to the long axis of the bronchial tubules. As branching progresses, pseudostratified columnar epithelium is reduced to a tall columnar epithelium, especially in distal regions of the bronchial tree. During this period, cytodifferentiation of the airway epithelium occurs in a centrifugal direction with ciliated, nonciliated, goblet, and basal cells appearing first in the more proximal airways. Cartilage, smooth muscle cells, and mucous glands are also found in the trachea during the pseudoglandular stage of development and extend as far as the segmental bronchi.

The canalicular stage of lung development extends from week 16 to 24 of gestation. By the end of week 16, the terminal bronchioles have divided into two or more respiratory bronchioles that have subdivided into small clusters of short acinar tubules and buds lined by cuboidal epithelium. These structures undergo further differentiation to become the adult respiratory unit, or pulmonary acinus, consisting of the alveolated respiratory bronchiole, alveolar ducts, and alveoli. Clusters of acinar tubules and buds grow further by lengthening, subdividing, and widening at the expense of the surrounding mesenchyme (Fig. 29-2*A*). This peripheral growth is accompanied by intraacinar capillaries, which align themselves around the air spaces, establishing contact with the overlying cuboidal epithelium. During this period, type II epithelial cell differentiation occurs in acinar tubules with formation of intracellular multivesicular bodies and, later, multilamellar bodies, the storage form of pulmonary surfactant phospholipids. Type I epithelial cell differentiation occurs in conjunction with the establishment of the air–blood barrier wherever endothelial cells of the developing capillary system come into contact with the overlying acinar epithelial cells.

During the saccular stage, which extends from week 24 to 38 of gestation, the terminal clusters of acinar tubules and buds begin to dilate and expand into thin, smooth-walled, transitory saccules and ducts that later become the true alveolar ducts and alveoli of the adult (Fig. 29-2*B*). During this period, there is a marked reduction in the amount of interstitial tissue. Intersaccular and interductal septa develop that contain a delicate network of collagen fibers and the intraacinar capillary bed. Near the end of this period, elastin is deposited in areas where future interalveolar septa will form. Increasing amounts of tubular myelin, the secretory form of pulmonary surfactant, are seen in the air spaces.

The alveolar period, which extends from 36 weeks of gestation to between 2 to 8 years of age, is the last stage of lung development and is marked by the formation of secondary alveolar septa partitioning the transitory ducts and saccules into true alveolar ducts and alveoli (Fig. 29-2*C,D*). This process of alveolarization greatly increases the surface area of the lung available for gas exchange. Between 20 to 70 million alveoli are formed before birth, and the postnatal formation of additional alveoli increases their number to between 300 to 400 million by 2 to 8 years of age. At the beginning of this period, the secondary interalveolar septa consist of short buds or projections of connective tissue that contain a double capillary network and interstitial cells that are actively synthesizing collagen and elastic fibers. By 5 months of age, these secondary interalveolar septa have lengthened and thinned and contain only a single capillary network. This suggests that alveolar formation occurs rapidly after birth and may be complete within the first 12 to 24 months of life. Further growth of the lung occurs by expansion and further subdivision of the alveolar spaces by tertiary interalveolar septa. From birth to adulthood, the conducting airways increase in length and diameter, while airspace and capillary volume increase coordinately at the expense of interstitial volume.

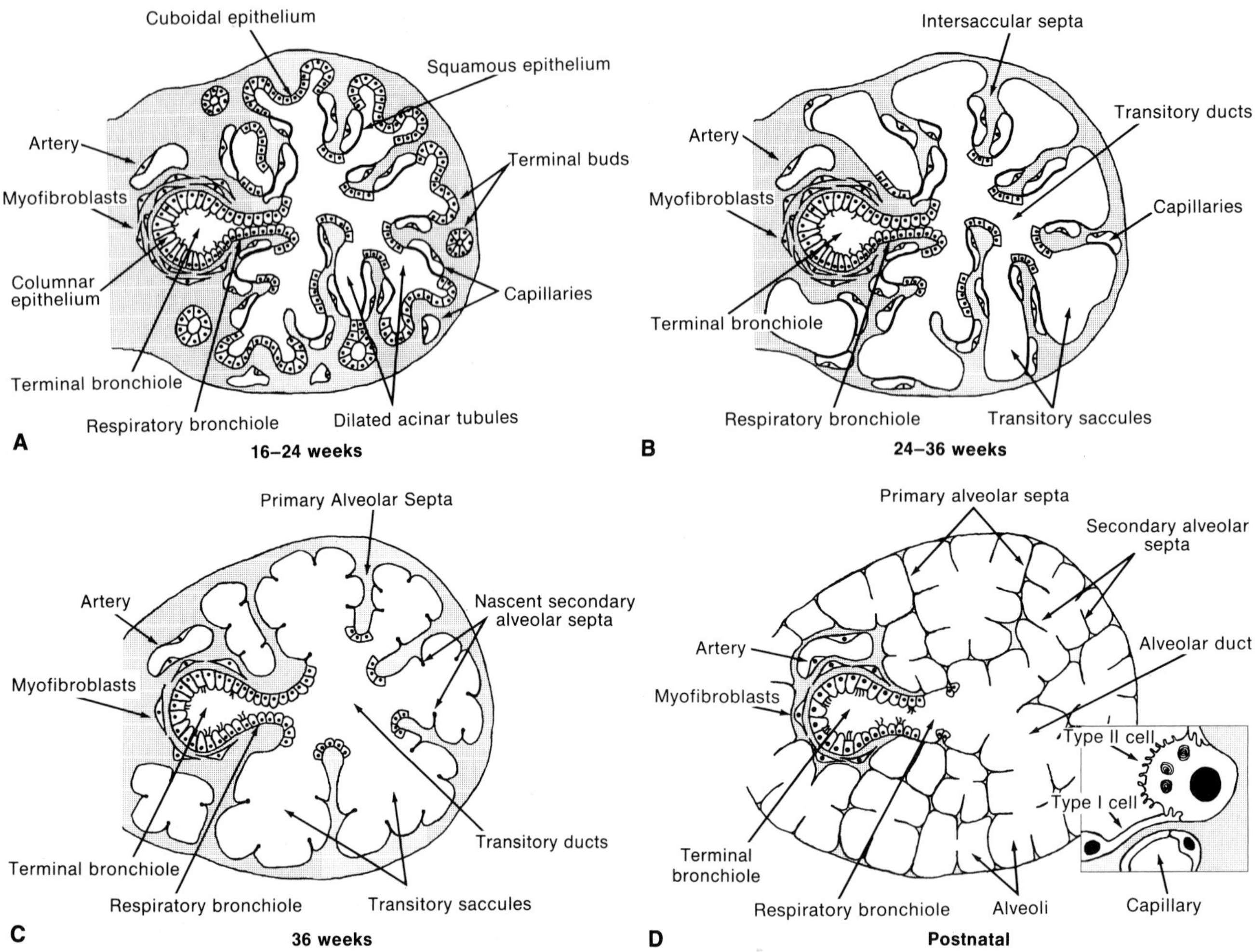

FIG. 29–2. Lung development during the **(A)** canalicular, **(B)** saccular, and **(C, D)** alveolar stages of organogenesis. Dramatic histological changes in tissue organization occur during these periods. The adult alveolar epithelium is composed of squamous type I cells and cuboidal type II cells (*inset*).

DEVELOPMENTAL ANOMALIES

Each of these stages of lung development comprises distinct changes in tissue organization and differentiation that are important for subsequent growth and maturation of the lung. Structural and functional defects in lung development at birth can often be traced to arrested or aberrant development during one of these periods of organogenesis. Developmental anomalies of the lung occur through defective division and differentiation of the lung bud or of the left or right bronchial bud. Pulmonary agenesis, bronchial malformations, tracheoesophageal fistulas, tracheomalacia, bronchomalacia, ectopic lobes, and congenital pulmonary cysts arise during the embryonic and pseudoglandular stages of lung development. Clinical disorders related to pulmonary hypoplasia and respiratory insufficiency are associated with later periods of development. Pulmonary hypoplasia can be caused by a reduction of space within the pleural cavity, usually as a consequence of another primary developmental defect, such as congenital diaphragmatic hernia, or by a reduction in the amount of amniotic fluid due to prolonged rupture of membranes or in association with renal dysgenesis (*i.e.*, Potter syndrome). Respiratory distress syndrome and bronchopulmonary dysplasia are associated with premature birth at a time when biochemical functions (*e.g.*, surfactant production) and structural functions (*e.g.*, elasticity) of the lung are still underdeveloped.

THE SURFACTANT SYSTEM

The unique physical–chemical boundary between the alveolar gases and the highly solvated molecules at the apical surface of the respiratory epithelium generates a region of high surface tension produced by the unequal distribution of molecular forces among water molecules at an air–liquid interface. Surface-active material at this interface in the alveoli provides surface tension, lowering activity that contributes to the remarkable pressure–volume associations characteristic of the lung. This surface-active material, called surfactant, has been subject to intense study in recent decades.[3-5]

Deficiency or dysfunction of pulmonary surfactant plays a critical role in the pathogenesis of respiratory diseases in the newborn period. Pulmonary surfactant exists in a variety of physical forms when isolated from the alveolar wash of the lung. These physical forms include lamellated and vesicular forms and highly organized tubular myelin. Tubular myelin is highly surface active and, although composed predominately of phospholipids, its unique structure depends on Ca^{2+} and lung surfactant proteins A (SP-A) and B (SP-B). Tubular myelin represents the major extracellular pool of surfactant from which a lipid monolayer is generated to produce an interface between the hydrated cellular surfaces and alveolar gas (Fig. 29-3). Lamellated and vesicular forms of surfactant represent nascent or catabolic forms of surfactant material; the latter is taken up by type II epithelial cells and recycled. SP-A, SP-B, and surfactant protein C (SP-C) play important roles in the organization and function of the surfactant complex regulating surfac-

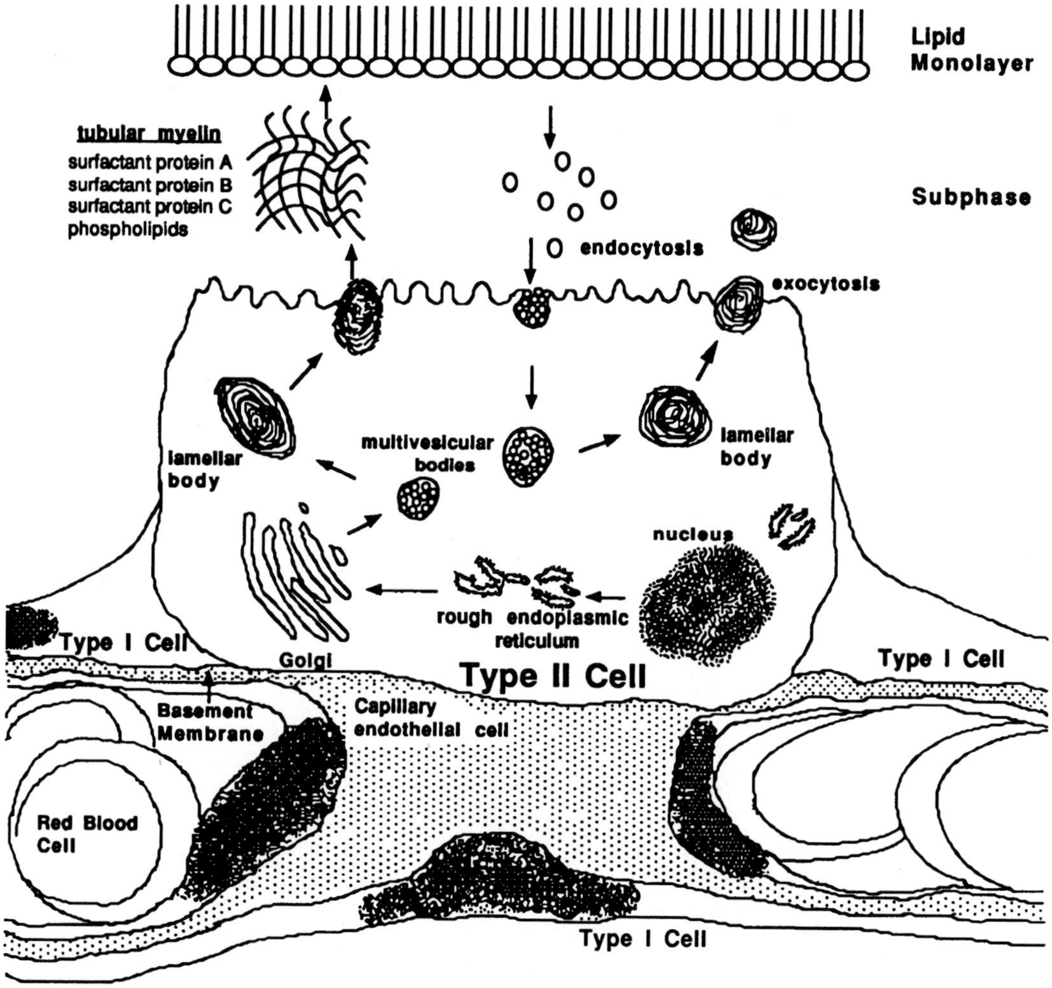

FIG. 29–3. Surfactant phospholipids are synthesized in the endoplasmic reticulum, transported through the Golgi apparatus to multivesicular bodies, and ultimately packaged in lamellar bodies before secretion. After exocytosis of the lamellar bodies, surfactant phospholipids are organized into a complex lattice called tubular myelin phospholipid that provides material for a monolayer at the air–fluid interface in the alveolus. Surfactant phospholipids and proteins are taken up by type II cells, probably transported by endosomal multivesicular bodies, and then catabolized or transported to lamellar bodies for recycling. Surfactant proteins are synthesized in polyribosomes and extensively modified in the endoplasmic reticulum, Golgi apparatus, and multivesicular bodies. Surfactant proteins are detected within lamellar bodies or in secretory vesicles closely associated with lamellar bodies before secretion into the alveolus.

tant recycling and secretion. Alveolar surfactant concentrations are tightly controlled by a variety of mechanisms that modulate lipid and protein synthesis, storage, secretion, and recycling.

COMPOSITION OF SURFACTANT

Pulmonary surfactant is composed primarily of the phospholipids phosphatidylcholine and phosphatidylglycerol (Fig. 29-4). These lipid molecules are enriched in dipalmitoyl acyl groups attached to a glycerol backbone that pack tightly and generate low surface pressures (Fig. 29-5). Rapid spreading and stability of pulmonary surfactant is achieved by the interactions of surfactant proteins and phospholipids. Surfactant is synthesized and secreted by type II epithelial cells in the alveolus. Synthesis of phosphatidylcholine, surfactant proteins, and lamellar bodies, an intracellular storage form of pulmonary surfactant, increases with advancing gestation. Lamellar bodies are secreted into the lung liquid that contributes to the amniotic fluid. The measurement of amniotic fluid phosphatidylcholine, disaturated phosphatidylcholine, posphatidylglycerol, or the surfactant proteins has provided useful biochemical markers that predict lung maturation and the adequacy of lung function at birth (*e.g.*, lecithin–sphingomyelin [L–S] ratio and phosphatidylglycerol values). Surfactant function can be assessed by a variety of physical and physiologic tests that generally measure its ability to reduce surface tension at an air–liquid interface and to spread rapidly during dynamic compression and expansion. The Wilhelmy balance, Langmuir trough, pulsating bubbleometer, and a variety of animal models have been used to assess the efficacy of surfactant and surfactant replacements.

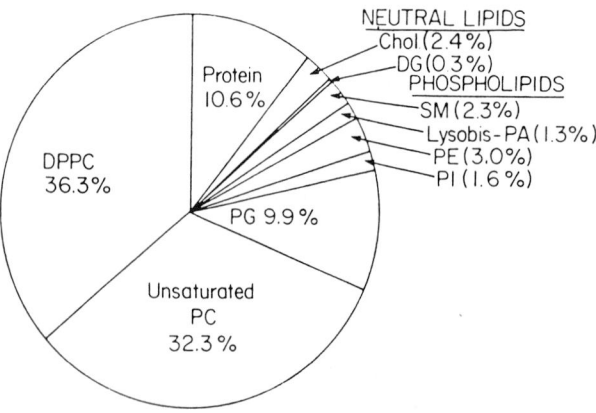

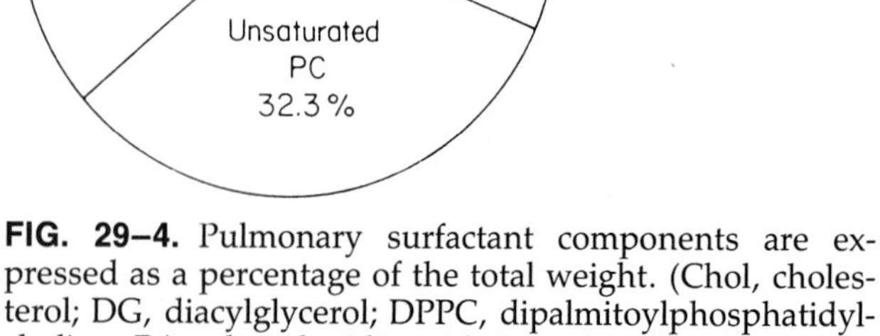

FIG. 29–4. Pulmonary surfactant components are expressed as a percentage of the total weight. (Chol, cholesterol; DG, diacylglycerol; DPPC, dipalmitoylphosphatidylcholine; PA, phosphatidic acid; PC, phosphatidylcholine; PE, phosphatidylethanolamine; PG, phosphatidylglycerol; PI, phosphatidylinositol; SM, sphingomyelin; adapted from Possmayer F. Pulmonary surfactant. Can J Biochem Cell Biol 1984;62:1121.)

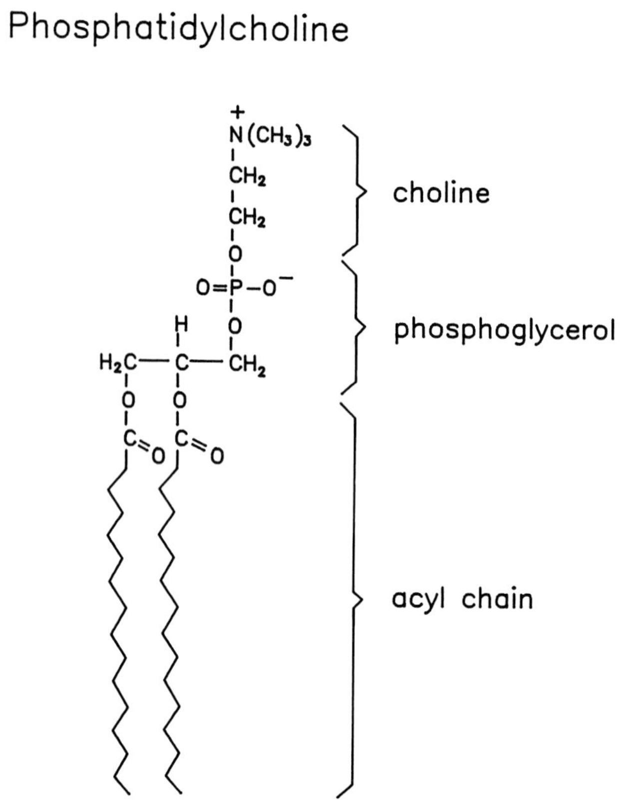

FIG. 29–5. Dipalmitoylphosphatidylcholine (DPPC) is the most abundant phospholipid in pulmonary surfactant. The acyl chains of DPPC pack tightly to form the surfactant monolayer, reducing surface tension in the alveolus.

CONTROL OF SURFACTANT SYNTHESIS AND SECRETION

Synthesis of pulmonary surfactant is closely linked to the morphologic and biochemical differentiation of alveolar type II cells in the peripheral respiratory epithelium. Interactions between mesenchymal and epithelial cells, mediated by direct cell–cell contact or by paracrine factors, contribute to the differentiation process. Endocrine factors also modulate the differentiation of type II epithelial cells and the synthesis of surfactant components. *In vivo* and *in vitro* evidence supports the role of glucocorticoids in the modulation of morphologic differentiation and production of phospholipids and surfactant proteins by the lung.

PHOSPHOLIPID SYNTHESIS

Phosphatidylcholine is produced by type II epithelial cells using extracellular substrate and the glycogen stores that accumulate in the pre–type II cells of the fetal lung. Metabolic pathways producing phosphatidylcholine depend on the production of phosphatidic acid and a glycerophosphate backbone (see Fig. 29-5); the latter is produced as an intermediate of the glycolytic pathway.[6] The synthesis of phosphatidylcholine involves the deacylation of phosphatidic acid and its reaction with cytidine diphosphocholine (CDP-choline).

Disaturated forms of phosphatidylcholine may be formed *de novo,* using disaturated acyl precursors or by remodeling (*i.e.,* salvage pathway) of phospholipids by deacylation and reacylation reactions. Production of CDP-choline is critical to phosphatidylcholine synthesis and is achieved by phosphorylation of choline and transfer to cytidine triphosphate in a reaction dependent on choline kinase and choline phosphate cytidylyltransferase. The activities of many of the enzymes in the synthetic pathway for phosphatidylcholine increase with advancing gestation in the lung, generally increasing in the last third of gestation.[6,7]

GLUCOCORTICOID ENHANCEMENT

A variety of hormonal factors influence the rate of production of the enzymes controlling phosphatidylcholine synthesis in the developing lung.[6,7] Glucocorticoids are the most clinically relevant and useful of these agents. Studies in fetal lambs and humans demonstrated that administration of glucocorticoid to the dam or mother resulted in precocious respiratory function in prematurely born offspring. The initial clinical studies of Liggins and Howie demonstrated that maternal administration of glucocorticoid decreased the incidence of respiratory distress in premature infants.[8] Although the precise mechanisms by which glucocorticoids induce pulmonary maturation and lung function in premature infants have not been discerned, increased phosphatidylcholine synthesis and morphologic remodeling of the alveolar architecture, including the thinning of interstitial components of the fetal lung, are observed after glucocorticoid treatment. Glucocorticoids regulate several genes that are associated with the differentiation of the fetal lung, including the genes encoding enzymes involved in the synthesis of phosphatidylcholine and the surfactant proteins. The effects of glucocorticoid on lung cell differentiation are mediated in part by glucocorticoid receptors, which when occupied by hormones, influence gene transcription and mRNA stability, altering the abundance of the proteins synthesized by pulmonary cells.

OTHER HORMONAL INFLUENCES

Thyroid hormones (*i.e.,* T_3, T_4), thyrotropin-releasing hormone (TRH), estrogens, prolactin, epidermal growth factor, β-adrenergic agents, and other agents that enhance cellular cAMP levels influence pulmonary maturation or biochemical indices of pulmonary maturation. T_3 and T_4 increase the synthesis of phospholipids in mammalian lung but do not readily cross the placenta. Recent studies of TRH support its role for prevention of chronic lung disease in premature infants. The mechanisms of action of TRH have not been clarified, but its action does not appear directly related to stimulation of surfactant synthesis.

SURFACTANT SECRETION

Surfactant is stored within type II cells in large lipid-rich organelles called lamellar bodies. Secretion of lamellar bodies occurs by a process of exocytosis that is regulated by a number of physical and hormonal factors. Stretch, the mode of ventilation, and the labor process enhance surfactant secretion and extracellular surfactant pool sizes at birth. Catecholamines, purinoceptor agonists (*e.g.,* adenosine triphosphate) that activate protein kinases, and Ca^{2+} ionophores enhance phospholipid secretion by type II cells *in vitro.*[6] SP-A, hyperglycemia and hyperinsulinemia inhibit surfactant phospholipid secretion. Newly secreted surfactant enters the extracellular space and undergoes dramatic structural reorganization to form tubular myelin, a process dependent on SP-A, Ca^{2+}, phospholipids, and SP-B. Phospholipids must move from tubular myelin to form a monolayer at the air liquid interface.

SURFACTANT RECYCLING

The process of inflation and deflation produces spent forms of surfactant phospholipids that are taken up by type II cells and reused. SP-A, SP-B, and SP-C enhance the reuptake of phospholipids *in vitro.* Surfactant phospholipid is reused at fast rates. In the adult rabbit lung, the half-life of surfactant phospholipids is approximately 8 hours, and in newborn animals, the half-life is 3.5 days. The intracellular and extracellular pools of surfactant are generally larger in the newborn animal than in adults. A relatively small fraction of the alveolar surfactant pool is cleared by catabolism and alveolar macrophages, with most of the surfactant phospholipid recycled by type II cells. Exogenously administered surfactant is reused efficiently by adult and newborn lungs.[9] The effects of surfactant replacement therapy are therefore related to the direct surface-tension–lowering properties of surfactant introduced into the airway and to the recycling of exogenous phospholipids by type II cells.

THE ROLE OF SURFACTANT IN LUNG DISEASE

Quantitative and qualitative abnormalities of pulmonary surfactant contribute to the pathogenesis of lung disease in the newborn infant. In premature infants, deficiency in surfactant production and secretion decrease intracellular and extracellular pools of surfactant, leading to alveolar surfactant insufficiency and atelectasis. Qualitative abnormalities of surfactant are also associated with many types of lung injury. Alveolar–capillary leak, hemorrhage, pulmonary edema, and alveolar cell injury fill the alveolus with proteinaceous material that inactivates surfactant. Serum and nonserum proteins, including albumin, fibrinogen, hemoglobin, and meconium, are potent inactivators of pulmonary surfactant *in vivo* and *in vitro*. SP-A, SP-B, and SP-C act synergistically to stabilize the surface properties of phospholipids in the presence of these inactivating proteins. Inhibitory factors associated with surfactant dysfunction in acute lung injury can be overcome by the administration of exogenous surfactants that contain the surfactant proteins.

SURFACTANT REPLACEMENT

The first successful surfactant replacement therapy in humans was reported by Fujiwara and colleagues in 1980.[10] Natural synthetic and semisynthetic surfactants have been successfully administered into the lungs of premature infants for treatment of RDS and are being tested for therapy of other lung diseases. Surfactant replacement has become standard for prevention and treatment of RDS. Animal surfactant preparations containing phospholipids, SP-B, and SP-C (*e.g.*, Survanta, Curosurf, Infrasurf) and synthetic preparations composed primarily of phospholipids mixed with spreading agents (*e.g.*, Exosurf) are in clinical use.[4,5] The surfactant preparations containing surfactant proteins provide highly surface active material to the alveolus. Surfactant replacement also contributes to the pool size of surfactant phospholipids, providing substrate for surfactant synthesis by means of the recycling pathways.

RESPIRATORY DISTRESS SYNDROME

Respiratory distress syndrome, previously called hyaline membrane disease, is a common cause of morbidity and mortality associated with premature delivery. Respiratory distress syndrome is a developmental disorder rather than a disease process *per se*, and it is usually associated with premature birth. The incidence and severity of RDS generally increases with decreasing gestational age at birth and is usually worse in male infants. Infants of diabetic mothers with poor metabolic control and infants born after fetal asphyxia, maternofetal hemorrhage, or in pregnancies complicated by multiple births are at higher risk for RDS. Respiratory distress syndrome affects approximately 20,000 to 30,000 infants each year in the United States and complicates approximately 1% of pregnancies. Approximately 50% of the infants born between 26 and 28 weeks of gestation develop RDS, and fewer than 20% to 30% of premature infants at 30 to 31 weeks have the disorder.

CLINICAL PRESENTATION

Infants with RDS present at birth or within several hours after birth with clinical signs of respiratory distress that include tachypnea, grunting, retractions, and cyanosis accompanied by increasing oxygen requirements. Physical findings include rales, poor air exchange, use of accessory muscles of breathing, nasal flaring, and abnormal patterns of respiration that may be complicated by apnea. Chest radiographs are characterized by atelectasis, air bronchograms, and diffuse reticular–granular infiltrates, often progressing to severe bilateral opacity characterized by the term "white-out" (Fig. 29-6). Radiographic patterns in RDS are variable and may not reflect the degree of respiratory compromise.

The infant attempts to maintain alveolar volume by prolonging and increasing expiratory pressures by breathing against a partially closed glottis, causing the grunting noise characteristic of RDS but often seen in other respiratory disorders. Increasing oxygen requirements and the need for ventilatory support often occur rapidly in the first 24 hours of life and continue for several days thereafter. The clinical course depends on the severity of RDS and the size and maturity of the infant at birth. In uncomplicated RDS, typically seen in more mature infants, recovery is rapid and infants generally no longer require oxygen or ventilatory support after the first week of life. The most premature infants are at greatest risk for severe RDS and frequently develop complications, including central nervous system (CNS) hemorrhage, patent ductus arteriosus (PDA), air leak, and infection, which contribute to prolonged requirements for oxygen and ventilatory support.

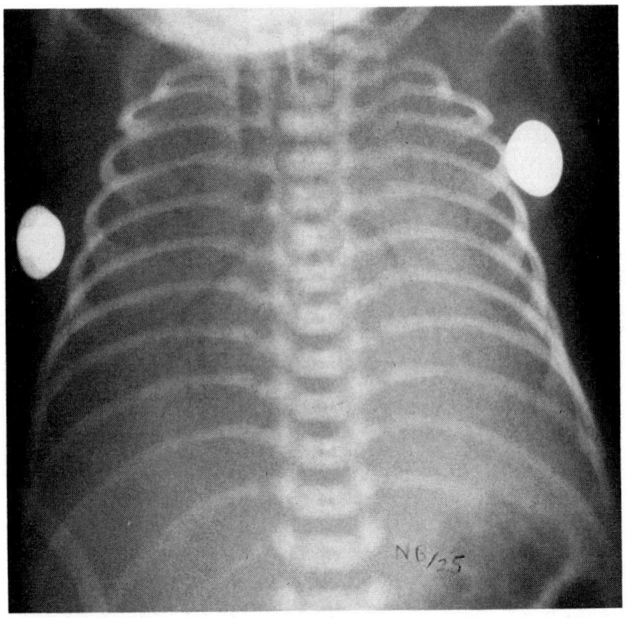

FIG. 29–6. This premature infant presented with grunting, retractions, and cyanosis after delivery. The diffuse reticular–granular opacification, air bronchograms, and decreased lung volumes in the chest x-ray film indicate respiratory distress syndrome.

PATHOLOGY

Pathologic findings early in the course of RDS include atelectasis, pulmonary edema, pulmonary vascular congestion, pulmonary hemorrhage, and evidence of direct injury to the respiratory epithelium (Fig. 29-7). Epithelial cell injury is especially evident in the bronchiolar region of the lung. Histologic findings include the presence of hyaline membranes, the characteristic eosinophilic material derived from bronchial and bronchiolar injury to epithelial cells. Alveolar spaces are generally not inflated, and at autopsy, the lungs of infants with RDS are often airless on passive deflation. Leukocytic infiltration is not observed early in the course of RDS unless complicated by infection. Pulmonary edema, hemorrhage, and hemorrhagic edema are common pathologic features in RDS, especially if the clinical course is further complicated by PDA and congestive heart failure.

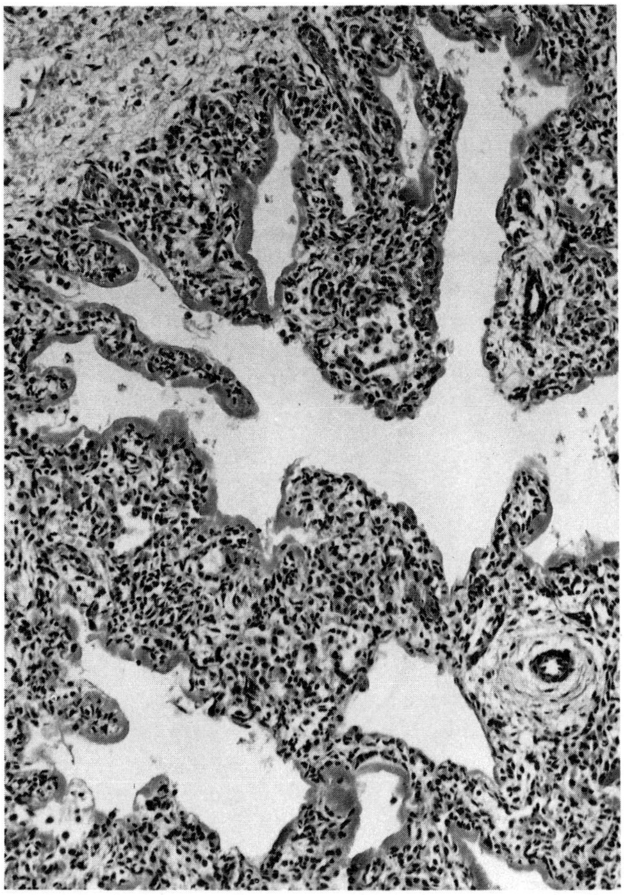

FIG. 29–7. Dilated air spaces, hyaline membranes, and extensive atelectasis are seen throughout the lung of an infant born at 28 weeks of gestation with severe respiratory distress syndrome. (Hematoxylin and eosin stain; original magnification × 250; courtesy of Edgar Ballard, Children's Hospital, Cincinnati, OH.)

PATHOPHYSIOLOGY

Avery and Mead first demonstrated the paucity of alveolar surfactant in the lungs of infants dying of RDS.[11] Quantitative and qualitative abnormalities of the pulmonary surfactant system are critical to the pathogenesis of RDS in premature infants. Lack of pulmonary surfactant leads to progressive atelectasis, loss of functional residual capacity, alterations in ventilation–perfusion ratio, and uneven distribution of ventilation. RDS is further complicated by the relatively weak respiratory muscles and the compliant chest wall of the premature infant that impair alveolar ventilation. Diminished oxygenation, cyanosis, and respiratory and metabolic acidosis contribute to increased pulmonary vascular resistance (PVR). Right-to-left shunting through the ductus arteriosus, foramen ovale, and intrapulmonary ventilation–perfusion mismatch further exacerbate hypoxemia.

PREVENTION

Although the incidence of premature birth in the United States (*i.e.*, approximately 7%) has not changed significantly in recent decades, the incidence of severe RDS has decreased at each gestational age as advances in maternal care and strict attention to avoidance of asphyxia and infection at birth have become standard treatment. Careful fetal monitoring, treatment of underlying maternal disorders, use of amniotic fluid L–S or other biochemical indicators of fetal lung maturity, and administration of tocolytics and maternal glucocorticoids have decreased the incidence of RDS. Surfactant replacement further decreases the incidence and severity of RDS. Rapid restoration of blood volume after hemorrhage and correction and avoidance of anemia, acidosis, and hypothermia improve the clinical outcomes in RDS. Positive-pressure ventilation and continuous positive airway pressure (CPAP) improve the course of severe RDS but do not prevent the disease itself.

TREATMENT

Postnatal therapy of RDS begins with careful assessment and resuscitation. Adequate ventilation, oxygenation, circulation, and temperature must be assured before transfer of the infant from the delivery room to the appropriate site of care. Surfactant replacement therapy may be initiated at birth in infants at risk for RDS or thereafter, as symptoms of RDS are established and the diagnosis of RDS is confirmed. Ventilatory management of neonatal respiratory disorders has been reviewed.[12]

Adequacy of ventilation and oxygenation must be established as soon as possible to avoid pulmonary vasoconstriction, further ventilation–perfusion abnormalities, and atelectasis. Positive-pressure ventilation, CPAP, and oxygen therapy may be required at any time during the course of RDS and must be readily available to the infant. Close monitoring of *p*H, oxygen saturation, PCO_2, and PO_2 by transcutaneous monitors and by arterial catheterization or sampling of arterialized capillary blood is critical in guiding mechanical ventilation and ambient oxygen requirements. Surfactant replacement therapy is provided through the endotracheal tube and is often used several times during the early course of RDS to maintain pulmonary function. Exogenous surfactants are given by intratracheal instillation of doses of approximately 100 mg of phospholipid per 1 kg of body weight.

Mild or moderate RDS can be managed by CPAP applied by mask, nasal cannula, nasal prongs, or endotracheal or nasopharyngeal tubes. In general, 3 to 6 cm of H_2O pressure is applied to the infant's airway. Oxygenation and effort of breathing are usually rapidly improved by CPAP. Rapid fluctuations in blood gases may occur, requiring careful monitoring of PCO_2 and PO_2. As forced inspiratory oxygen requirements decrease during recovery, airway pressure is decreased, and the infant is weaned to head hood or nasal cannula oxygen. Apnea, inadequacy of ventilation, atelectasis, mucous plugging, hyperaeration, or air leak may complicate the care of infants with RDS.

Careful attention to the mechanical details of the application of CPAP or mechanical respirators is required. Mandatory ventilation should be instituted well in advance of respiratory failure and severe respiratory acidosis to avoid severe hypoxemia and atelectasis. Ventilation is maintained through an endotracheal tube, which can be placed nasally or orally, for delivery of oxygen and positive pressure. Pressure-cycled ventilators are most frequently used in the NICU and are controlled by setting positive inspiratory pressure, rate, inspiratory–expiratory times, and positive end-expiratory pressures (PEEP). Volume-cycled ventilators, in which fixed volumes are delivered to define the respiratory cycle, are used less frequently in the newborn. As in all respiratory therapy, critical attention to adequacy of ventilation, as assessed by PO_2, PCO_2, *p*H, and transcutaneous oxygen saturation, is required on an almost continual basis to adjust to the rapid changes in respiratory status occurring in these critically ill infants. Barotrauma and oxygen toxicity to the lung represent significant pulmonary complications in the therapy of RDS. Excesses in ventilation, peak or mean airway pressure, and oxygen therapy should be avoided. Because hyperoxia is associated with retrolental fibroplasia, a major cause of blindness in premature infants, arterial PO_2 must be carefully monitored, generally maintaining PO_2 between 50 to 80 torr. Although other forms of ventilation such as high-frequency or jet ventilators have been used successfully for the treatment of RDS, these therapies should be considered experimental except for severely affected infants whose ventilation has not been supported by conventional mandatory ventilation and surfactant therapy.

COMPLICATIONS

Central nervous system hemorrhage, intraventricular hemorrhage (IVH), and PDA represent significant clinical problems affecting the care of infants with RDS. Patent ductus arteriosus and subsequent congestive heart failure and pulmonary edema further compromise respiratory function, decreasing pulmonary compliance and perhaps inactivating pulmonary surfactant. Prompt diagnosis and medical or surgical treatment of PDA is indicated during the treatment of RDS. Acute CNS hemorrhage is often associated with shock, pulmonary compromise, and pulmonary hemorrhage. Fluctuations in respiratory status may contribute to IVH and can be minimized by careful attention to respiratory care and by judicious use of sedation. Intravenous fluids and administration of oral feedings must be adjusted carefully during acute and convalescent care of infants with RDS. Excessive fluid administration impairs pulmonary function and increases the risk of PDA.

MECONIUM ASPIRATION SYNDROME

Meconium-stained amniotic fluid (MSAF) occurs in approximately 12% of live births. The cause, pathophysiology, and treatment of MSAF and MAS have been reviewed.[13–15]

Meconium first appears in the fetal ileum between 10 and 16 weeks of gestation as a viscous, green liquid composed of gastrointestinal secretions, cellular debris, bile and pancreatic juice, mucus, blood, lanugo, and vernix. Meconium is approximately 72% to 80% water. The dry weight composition consists primarily of mucopolysaccharides, with less protein and lipid. Although intestinal meconium appears very early in gestation, MSAF rarely occurs at less than 38 weeks of gestation. Incidence of MSAF increases thereafter, and approximately 30% of newborns have MSAF after 42 weeks of gestation. The increased incidence of MSAF with advancing gestational age probably reflects the maturation of peristalsis in the fetal intestine. Motilin, an intestinal peptide that stimulates contraction of the intestinal muscle, is in lower concentrations in the intestine of premature versus post-term infants. Umbilical cord motilin concentration is higher in infants who have passed meconium compared with infants with clear amniotic fluid. Intestinal parasympathetic innervation and myelination also increase throughout gestation and may play a role in the amplified passage of meconium in late gestation.

Passage of meconium may be a normal physiologic event, but it is associated with fetal asphyxia and decreased umbilical venous blood PO_2 (Fig. 29-8). The gasping respiratory efforts accompanying fetal asphyxia are thought to contribute to the entry of meconium into the respiratory tract, causing MAS. Experimentally, intestinal ischemia produces a tran-

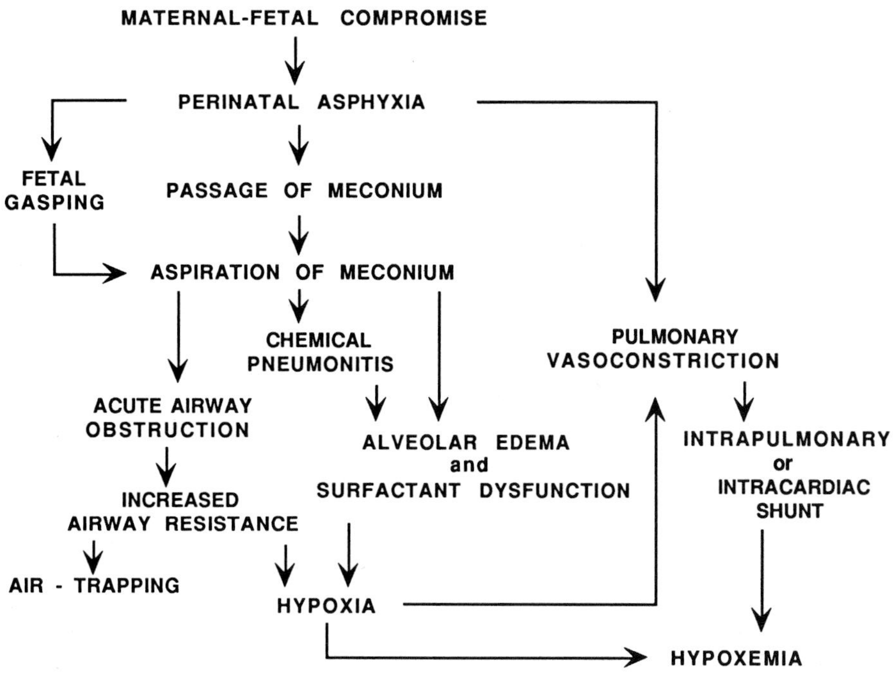

FIG. 29–8. Pathogenesis of meconium aspiration syndrome.

sient period of hyperperistalsis and relaxation of anal sphincter tone, leading to the passage of meconium. Intestinal ischemia is augmented in the fetus by the diving reflex that shunts blood preferentially to the brain and heart and away from the visceral organs during hypoxia.

An association between MSAF, fetal compromise, and perinatal morbidity has been clearly demonstrated. However, most infants with MSAF do not have lower Apgar scores, more acidosis, or clinical illness than infants born with clear amniotic fluid. When normal fetal heart rate patterns are observed in cases of MSAF, the neonatal outcome is generally comparable to deliveries with clear amniotic fluid. Neonatal outcomes of deliveries complicated by MSAF associated with fetal tachycardia and decreased fetal heart rate variability are similar to those of non–meconium-stained infants with similar abnormalities of fetal heart rate. Meconium staining may indicate fetal compromise and demands critical evaluation of fetal well-being. However, in infants with a normal fetal heart rate pattern, MSAF generally carries a low risk for perinatal morbidity.

CLINICAL PRESENTATION

Meconium found below the vocal cords defines MAS, which occurs in approximately 35% of live births with MSAF or in approximately 4% of all live births. Meconium aspiration syndrome describes a wide spectrum of respiratory disease, ranging from mild respiratory distress to severe disease and death despite mechanical ventilation. Meconium aspiration syndrome usually presents as respiratory distress and hypoxemia soon after birth. Pulmonary hypertension is frequently observed in infants with severe MAS.

The chest radiographs of infants with MAS demonstrate coarse infiltrates, widespread consolidation, or areas of hyperaeration (Fig. 29-9). Pleural effusions are detected in approximately 30% of infants with

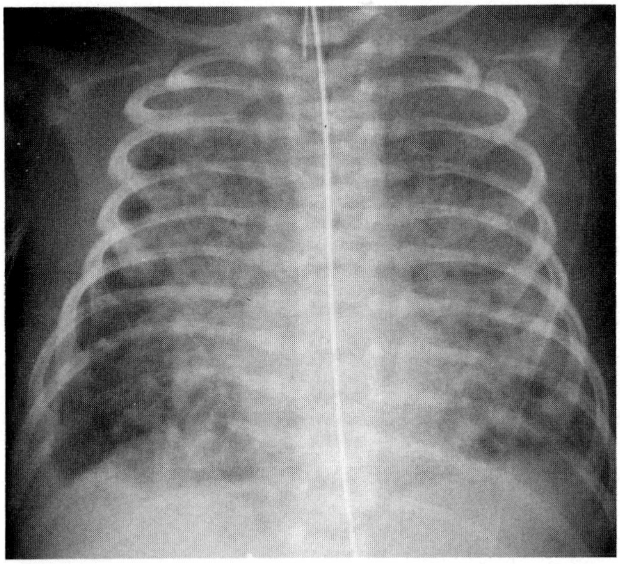

FIG. 29–9. This full-term infant was born with fetal bradycardia and thick meconium in the amniotic fluid. Cyanosis and respiratory distress were evident within minutes of delivery. The chest x-ray film demonstrates course, irregular infiltrates, hyperinflation (left and right diaphragms at ribs 10–11), and right pleural effusion indicative of meconium aspiration syndrome. Endotracheal and nasogastic tubes are in position.

MAS. Pneumothorax or pneumomediastinum occur in approximately 25% of severely affected infants. Chest radiographs are abnormal in more than one-half of infants with meconium detected below the vocal cords, but fewer than 50% of the infants with abnormal radiographs have significant respiratory distress. The severity of chest radiographic abnormalities may not correlate with the severity of clinical disease.

PATHOLOGY

Postmortem examination of lungs from infants with severe MAS reveals meconium, vernix, fetal squamous cells and cellular debris in the air spaces from the airways to the alveoli. An inflammatory response with polymorphonuclear leukocytes, macrophages, and alveolar edema may be observed, but large quantities of meconium may be present without histologic signs of inflammation. Hyaline membrane formation, pulmonary hemorrhage, and necrosis of pulmonary microvasculature and parenchyma can occur. Platelet-rich microthrombi in small arterioles and increased muscularization of distal arterioles have been described in some infants dying of MAS.

PATHOPHYSIOLOGY

The pulmonary abnormalities in MAS are related primarily to acute airway obstruction, decreased lung tissue compliance, and parenchymal lung damage (see Fig. 29-8). Instillation of meconium into adult rabbit and newborn dog tracheas causes acute mechanical obstruction of proximal and distal airways.[16] A ball-valve mechanism producing partial airway obstruction contributes to air trapping, which results in increased anteroposterior chest diameter, increased expiratory lung resistance, and increased functional residual capacity. Complete obstruction of small airways may result in regional atelectasis and ventilation–perfusion inequalities. Disruption of surfactant function by serum and nonserum proteins and fatty acids contributes to atelectasis, decreased compliance, and resulting hypoxia. In more than one-half of the infants with severe MAS, pulmonary hypertension with right-to-left shunting contributes to the characteristically severe hypoxemia. Perinatal asphyxia is a critical underlying factor in the pathogenesis of MAS, increasing the risks for pulmonary hypertension and meconium aspiration.

PREVENTION

Before the late 1970s, it was thought that aspiration of amniotic fluid and meconium occurred during the first few breaths after delivery. Therapy was aimed at preventing MAS at the time of delivery by DeLee suctioning of the nasopharynx before delivery of the shoulders and before the first breath. The trachea was immediately intubated and suctioned to limit aspiration of meconium from the oropharynx and trachea, a procedure that remains standard in most institutions. Mortality from MAS was decreased when the trachea was suctioned immediately after birth.[17] DeLee suctioning of the nasopharynx while the infant was at the perineum also decreased morbidity and mortality due to MAS.

Meconium aspiration syndrome continued to occur in infants who are adequately suctioned in the delivery room. Aspiration of meconium or amniotic fluid *in utero* probably occurred in some infants with MAS, particularly in those with perinatal asphyxia. Generally, fetal lung fluid flows outwardly from the lungs into the amniotic sac. However, studies with radiopaque contrast and ^{51}Cr-labeled erythrocytes injected into the amniotic sac demonstrated that some amniotic fluid enters the fetal lung in the nonasphyxiated human fetus. Fetal gasping may be a critical factor in entry of meconium into the lung before birth. Gasping associated with inhalation of amniotic fluid or meconium occurs in fetal lambs, rhesus monkeys, and humans in response to fetal asphyxia after compression of the umbilical cord or maternal aorta. Antenatal diagnosis and treatment of fetal asphyxia is therefore critical for prevention of MAS. Amnioinfusion, particularly in cases of oligohydramnios, may decrease morbidity related to MAS by decreasing cord compression and diluting the meconium, potentially minimizing its toxicity after aspiration.

Concerns about infection risks to delivery room staff and mechanical injury to the infant related to aggressive suctioning and intubation have been raised. The use of direct tracheal suctioning for all meconium-stained infants is undergoing reevaluation.[14,18] Meanwhile, clearing the airway and establishing respiration and oxygenation remain basic to the resuscitation of all infants.

TREATMENT

Postnatal therapy for MAS begins with continuous observation and monitoring of infants at risk. Pulmonary vasoconstriction is associated with MAS, and rapid correction of hypoxemia and acidosis is critical. Chest physiotherapy and suctioning may be useful if there is airway obstruction and the infant maintains adequate oxygenation during such therapy. Continuous monitoring of oxygenation by transcutaneous oxygen monitoring or pulse oximetry and assessment of PO_2, PCO_2, and *p*H by arterial catheterization should be used to guide the use of oxygen therapy and mechanical ventilation. The presence and severity of pulmonary hypertension should be evaluated. Mechanical ventilation to achieve respiratory alkalosis and infusion of sodium bicarbonate to produce a metabolic alkalosis may improve oxygenation.

VENTILATORY SUPPORT

Although improvement in oxygenation was observed in patients with MAS treated with 4 to 7 cm H_2O PEEP, further studies to confirm the safety and efficacy of positive end-expiratory pressure in MAS are needed. Mechanical ventilation is often required in severe MAS and must be managed carefully. Continuous positive airway pressure or PEEP may aggravate hyperinflation associated with MAS and should be used with caution. Pneumothorax or pneumomediastinum occur frequently during the course of MAS and may occur before the application of positive-pressure ventilation. Lengthening the expiratory time of the ventilatory cycle may minimize hyperinflation. Oscillation and high-frequency jet ventilation have been used in the treatment of MAS, but reports of their safety and efficacy in MAS are conflicting.

OTHER THERAPEUTIC CONSIDERATIONS

Therapy of the infant with MAS includes careful observation and vigorous treatment of other sequelae of neonatal asphyxia, including temperature instability, hypoglycemia, hypocalcemia, hypotension, and decreased cardiac function. Specific therapy directed to the sequelae from multiorgan hypoxemia and ischemia, including reduced renal function, reduced liver production of clotting factors, hypoalbuminemia, cerebral edema, and seizures, may be required.

Extracorporeal membrane oxygenation (ECMO) has been used successfully in treatment of severe MAS refractory to ventilatory therapy. Broad-spectrum antibiotics are routinely used in the therapy of MAS in infants with abnormal radiographic findings and respiratory distress. Treatment of acute MAS with glucocorticoids has not been beneficial. The use of exogenous surfactant for therapy of MAS is under active investigation.

PERSISTENT PULMONARY HYPERTENSION OF THE NEWBORN

Gersony and colleagues described hypoxemia in two infants with "persistent physiologic characteristics of the fetal circulation (PFC) in the absence of recognizable cardiac, pulmonary, hematologic, or central nervous system disease."[19] Because the placenta is no longer present and the ductus arteriosus may or may not be patent, the term persistent pulmonary hypertension of the newborn (PPHN) is now used to describe this disorder. The pathophysiology of PPHN is related to a failure to make the transition from high PVR and low pulmonary blood flow characteristic of the fetus to the relatively low PVR and high pulmonary blood flow of the postnatal infant. The clinical syndrome of PPHN has been reviewed.[20–22]

PATHOPHYSIOLOGY

The pathophysiology of PPHN can best be understood within the framework of the current knowledge of the transitional circulation. Normal transition occurs in four phases: the *in utero* phase, the immediate phase occurring in the first minutes after birth, the fast phase developing in the first 12 to 24 hours, and the final phase, which requires days or months to complete.

IN UTERO CIRCULATION

The *in utero* phase (*i.e.*, phase 1) is characterized by PVR that exceeds systemic vascular resistance, resulting in right atrial and ventricular pressures exceeding left atrial and ventricular pressures. As a result of this pressure differential, more than one-third of the oxygenated blood returning from the placenta through the inferior vena cava streams across the patent foramen ovale, is ejected from the left ventricle, and perfuses the head and neck vessels and the lower body. Venous blood returning through the superior vena cava preferentially flows into the right ventricle and main pulmonary artery. A small amount of this deoxygenated blood, comprising approximately 8% of the cardiac output with a PO_2 less than 20 torr, does perfuse the lungs, but because of elevated PVR, most is shunted across the PDA to mix with the blood returning in the inferior vena cava. The lower body is perfused with relatively less well oxygenated blood than the head and neck. Because of the large right-to-left shunt, blood bypasses the lungs *in utero*. Persistence of the elevated PVR after birth without the benefit of placental oxygenation results in the profound hypoxemia characteristic of PPHN. The mechanisms that maintain the fetal state of high PVR are under study. Pulmonary vasoconstriction induced by hypoxia, alterations in nitric oxide and arachidonic acid metabolism, and systemic acidosis probably contribute to physiologic abnormalities in PPHN.

IMMEDIATE PHASE

The second stage of normal transition, the immediate phase, is accomplished in the first minute after birth when the fluid-filled fetal lungs are distended with air during the first breath. A rapid decrease in PVR occurs with the mechanical distention of the pulmonary vascular bed, allowing more oxygenated blood to perfuse the lungs. The entry of air into the alveoli improves the oxygenation of the pulmonary vascular bed, further decreasing PVR.

FAST PHASE

The fast phase of the transitional circulation occurs for 12 to 24 hours after birth and accounts for the greatest reduction in PVR. The drop in PVR has been associated with the production of vasodilators, such as prostacyclin and endothelial-derived relaxing factor (*i.e.*, nitric oxide). Prostacyclin is produced in the neonatal lung in response to the initiation of ventilation. Pretreatment of the fetal lamb with cyclooxygenase inhibitor decreased prostacyclin production and prevented the late fall in PVR. The role of cyclooxygenase and prostacyclin in the transitional circulation may have clinical implications. Persistent pulmonary hypertension of the newborn has been observed in infants of mothers receiving aspirin or nonsteroidal antiinflammatory agents that inhibit cyclooxygenase activity. Pulmonary production of potent vasodilatory leukotrienes also occurs during the initiation of ventilation.

FINAL PHASE

The final phase of the neonatal pulmonary vascular transition involves remodeling of the pulmonary vascular musculature.[23] In the normal fetal and term lung, fully muscularized, thick-walled preacinar arteries extend to the level of the terminal bronchioles. Intraacinar and alveolar wall arteries are not muscularized. Within days after delivery, medial wall thickness of preacinar vessels smaller than 250 μm in diameter decreases, and within months, medial wall thickness of vessels larger than 250 and smaller than 500 μm also decreases. Hypoxia at birth prevents the remodeling of the smooth muscle of the preacinar bronchiolar arteries. High flow states and *in utero* hypoxia stimulate cells of the intraacinar and alveolar arteries to differentiate into smooth muscle and connective tissue, resulting in abnormally thickened and reactive arteriolar musculature. Increased muscularization of the pulmonary arteries has been described in infants dying of severe MAS with PPHN.

ETIOLOGY

Persistent pulmonary hypertension of the newborn has a variety of causes that can be classified by the predominant abnormality involved (Table 29-1). The clinician needs to recognize the subclasses of PPHN. Because of the availability of ECMO therapy, assessment of the clinical severity of PPHN helps determine the need for referral to tertiary care nurseries with ECMO capability.

CLINICAL PRESENTATION

Clinically, PPHN presents as labile hypoxemia that is disproportionate to the extent of pulmonary parenchymal disease. Infants with PPHN are commonly appropriate for gestational age and near term. The perinatal history frequently includes factors associated with perinatal asphyxia. Clinical symptoms include tachypnea, respiratory distress, and often rapidly progressive cyanosis, particularly in response to stimulation of the infant. The cardiovascular examination may be normal or may reveal a right ventricular heave, closely split or single loud S_2, and tricuspid regurgitation suggesting that pulmonary arterial pressure is equal to or greater than systemic arterial pressure. Differential diagnosis of PPHN includes severe pulmonary parenchymal disease, such as severe MAS, RDS, pneumonia, or hemorrhage, and congenital heart disease, such as transposition of the great arteries. Critical pulmonic stenosis, hypoplastic left ventricle, or severe coarctation should be considered in the differential diagnosis. Methods used to differentiate PPHN from pulmonary parenchymal disease or cardiac disease are outlined in Table 29-2.

The oxygenation of infants with severe pulmonary parenchymal disease generally improves after treatment with oxygen or mechanical ventilation. Infants with PPHN often have little or no parenchymal lung disease. They are easily ventilated but remain hypoxic despite high ambient forced inspiratory oxygen. Cyanotic congenital heart disease (CCHD) is usually associated with fixed, structural mixing of venous and arterial blood. In infants with CCHD, hypoxemia is generally unresponsive to increased exogenous oxygen or mechanical ventilation. Diagnosis of PPHN can be complicated by the coexistence of pulmonary hypertension, parenchymal lung disease, or CCHD. Echocardiography is useful in the diagnosis of structural heart disease in this clinical setting.

THERAPY

Supportive medical management includes correction of underlying abnormalities that may include polycythemia, hypoglycemia, hypothermia, diaphragmatic hernia, or CCHD. Metabolic acidosis and hypotension should be corrected by adequate replacement of intravascular volume and administration of sodium bicarbonate or pressors.

Specific therapy for PPHN is aimed at increasing pulmonary blood flow and decreasing right-to-left shunting. High ambient oxygen and mechanical ventilation are the pulmonary therapeutic interventions for treatment of PPHN. Ligation is not useful for treating PDA, and it may be detrimental. Cardiac failure may occur after PDA ligation as the right ventricle fails in the face of high afterload without the safety valve of the patent ductus. Because shunting between the pulmonary and systemic circulations depends on the relative pressures of each system, optimal therapy should decrease pulmonary artery pressure while increasing or not changing systemic arterial pressure and cardiac output.

Infants with severe PPHN are often sensitive to activity and agitation. Transcutaneous and intravascular monitoring equipment should be used and stimulation minimized during the care of these infants. Muscle relaxants (*e.g.*, pancuronium) and sedatives are frequently beneficial but should be used with caution because paralysis may further compromise ventilation and may mask clinical signs of respiratory insufficiency. Sedatives should be chosen to minimize cardiovascular side-effects. Infants with PPHN, especially if asphyxiated or septic, frequently develop systemic hypotension and signs of cardiac failure. Elevated right heart pressure due to increased PVR, poor venous return secondary to high intrathoracic pressures during mechanical ventilation, and previous asphyxia may contribute to myocardial dysfunction. The hematocrit should be maintained at or

TABLE 29–1
CLASSIFICATION SYSTEM FOR PERSISTENT PULMONARY HYPERTENSION OF THE NEWBORN

Pathology	Associated Diseases	Proposed Mechanisms	Prognosis
Functional vasoconstriction; normal pulmonary vascular development	Acute perinatal hypoxia Acute meconium aspiration Sepsis or pneumonia (especially group B streptococci) Respiratory distress syndrome Hypoventilation CNS depression Hypothermia Hypoglycemia	Response to acute hypoxia, particularly in the presence of acidemia	Good; reversible
Fixed decreased diameter; abnormal extension and hypertrophy of distal pulmonary vascular smooth muscle	Placental insufficiency Prolonged gestation *In utero* closure of ductus arteriosus Aspirin Nonsteroidal antiinflammatory agents Single ventricle without pulmonic stenosis Chronic pulmonary venous hypertension TAPVR Obstructive left-sided heart lesions Idiopathic diseases	Response to chronic hypoxia Excessive pulmonary blood flow *in utero* Elevated pulmonary venous pressure	Poor; fixed structural lesion
Decreased cross-sectional area of the pulmonary vascular bed	Space occupying lesions Diaphragmatic hernia Lung dysgenesis Pleural effusions Congenital lung hypoplasia Potter syndrome Thoracic dystrophies	Hypoplasia of alveoli and associated vessels	Poor; fixed structural lesion
Functional obstruction to pulmonary blood flow	Polycythemia Hyperfibrinogenemia	Increased blood viscosity	Good, unless chronic

CNS, central nervous system; TAPVR, total anomalous pulmonary venous return.

above 45%, and volume expanders, such as salt-poor albumin, Plasmanate, or normal saline, may be used to support the circulation. Dopamine and other pressors are commonly used for refractory hypotension.

RESPIRATORY AND METABOLIC ALKALOSIS

The often dramatic response of infants with PPHN to respiratory or metabolic alkalosis supports their use in the care of infants with severe PPHN. The degree of pulmonary parenchymal disease and risk of barotrauma may affect the clinical choice of inducing respiratory or metabolic alkalosis. It may be necessary to lower PCO_2 and raise the *p*H to 7.55 or above with hyperventilation and sodium bicarbonate to treat severe pulmonary vasoconstriction. Sustaining PCO_2 at less than 20 torr is not advocated. Excessive mechanical ventilation with over distention of the lung may increase right-to-left shunting. Pulmonary barotrauma associated with aggressive ventilation should not be underestimated. Hypocarbic alkalosis, by shifting the hemoglobin–oxygen dissociation curve, may also compromise the release of oxygen at the tissue level. Hyperoxia and hypocarbia may adversely affect cerebral blood flow. Weaning from ventilation and alkalinization must proceed with caution, because dramatic lability of PO_2 is often observed in infants with PPHN.

TABLE 29–2
DIAGNOSTIC EVALUATION OF SEVERE NEONATAL HYPOXEMIA

Test	Method	Result	Suggested Diagnosis
Hyperoxia	Expose to 100% FiO_2 for 5–10 min	PaO_2 increases to >100 torr	Pulmonary parenchymal disease
		PaO_2 increases to <20 torr	Persistent pulmonary hypertension or cyanotic congenital heart disease
Hyperventilation–hyperoxia	Mechanical ventilation with 100% FiO_2 and respiratory rate 100–150 bpm	PaO_2 increases to >100 torr without hyperventilation	Pulmonary parenchymal disease
		PaO_2 increases at a critical PCO_2, often to <25 torr	Persistent pulmonary hypertension
		No increase in PaO_2 despite hyperventilation	Cyanotic congenital heart disease or severe, fixed pulmonary hypertension
Simultaneous preductal–postductal PO_2	Compare PO_2 of right arm or shoulder to that of lower abdomen or extremities	Preductal $PO_2 \geq 15$ + postductal PO_2	Patent ductus arteriosus with right-to-left shunt
Echocardiography	M-mode	Increased RVPEP and RVET	Right ventricular systolic time interval ratio (RVSTI = RVPEP/RVET > 0.5) predicts PPHN
	Venous contrast injection	Simultaneously appears in PA and LA	Patent foramen ovale
	Two-dimensional echocardiography	Deviation of intraatrial septum to left; rule out congenital heart defect	Increased pulmonary arterial pressure
	Doppler	Failure of acceleration of systolic blood flow between large main pulmonary artery and small peripheral pulmonary artery	Suggests right-to-left PDA or intracardiac shunt

LA, left atrium; PA, pulmonary artery; PDA, patent ductus arteriosus; PPHN, persistent pulmonary hypertension of the newborn; RVET, right ventricular ejection time; RVPEP, right ventricular ejection period.

EXTRACORPOREAL MEMBRANE OXYGENATION

Extracorporeal membrane oxygenation has been useful for the treatment of severe PPHN refractory to medical management. The first newborn survivor of ECMO therapy was reported by Bartlett and colleagues in 1975.[24] In 1992, the National Registry of Neonatal ECMO reported an 87% survival rate for the 739 infants with the primary diagnosis of PPHN who were treated with ECMO.[25] Most of these infants met criteria for greater than 80% risk of mortality with conventional medical management. However, criteria used to determine risk of mortality vary from institution to institution and frequently are based on retrospective chart reviews, reflecting older methods of medical management. It is impossible to determine how these infants would have done with modern conventional therapy.

PULMONARY VASODILATOR THERAPY

Pharmacologic agents such as tolazoline and nitroprusside have been used for pulmonary vasodilation. Tolazoline has been used most commonly, but its vasodilatory effects are unpredictable, and systemic vasodilation is frequently observed. Inhalation of nitric oxide is undergoing clinical evaluation for the treatment of PPHN. Volume infusion and vasopressors should be readily available, if not used prophylactically, to treat systemic hypotension. Tolazoline has not been shown to influence survival of infants with PPHN.

LONG-TERM OUTCOME

Most infants treated for PPHN have few residual respiratory symptoms or neurologic or developmental sequelae by 1 year of age.[22,26] Infants with more severe parenchymal disease may have persistent or chronic tachypnea and bronchospasm. Infants with severe MAS and PPHN have an increased risk for chronic pulmonary sequelae. Continued oxygen therapy, bronchodilators, diuretics, and enhanced nutrition may be necessary to treat residual disease and establish adequate growth. Hearing, vision, and neurologic development should be followed closely in infants treated for PPHN, especially if severely asphyxiated.

PNEUMONIA

Pneumonia remains a significant cause of morbidity and mortality for preterm and term infants. The incidence of pneumonia in NICU patients exceeds 10%, and mortality of perinatally acquired pneumonia remains approximately 20%.[27] Pneumonia may be acquired transplacentally, during the birth process, or postnatally, and it is caused by a variety of pathogens, including viruses, bacteria, and fungi (Table 29-3). Unique environmental and host factors predispose the neonate to pulmonary infections. The increased susceptibility of neonates for pneumonia may be related to immaturity of mucociliary clearance, small size of the conducting airways, and lowered host defenses. Invasive procedures, such as tracheal intubation, barotrauma, and hyperoxic damage to the respiratory tract, may further impair resistance to pneumonia. The nosocomial flora of the hospital nursery, whether derived from nursery equipment or the unwashed hands of caregivers, are important vectors of pathogenic organisms.

TRANSPLACENTAL VIRAL PNEUMONIAS

Pneumonia acquired through the transplacental route is most commonly of viral origin. Rubella, varicella-zoster, cytomegalovirus (CMV), herpes simplex virus (HSV), and human immunodeficiency virus (HIV) are acquired by this route. Transplacentally acquired pneumonitis is also associated with adenoviral, enteroviral and influenza viral infections. Viral pneumonia is usually part of a systemic illness, reflecting hematogenous spread from the mother. Severity and onset of respiratory symptoms varies from respiratory failure at delivery to chronic pneumonia evolving months after birth.

Fetal infection may result from a primary maternal infection acquired during pregnancy or from reactivation of a latent infection. *In utero* transmission of rubella occurs as a result of primary infection acquired during pregnancy. Transmission of varicella-zoster, HSV, and CMV occurs as a result of primary or recurrent maternal infection. The timing of maternal infection in relation to birth is often a critical factor in outcome. Congenital varicella typically develops when primary maternal chickenpox occurs within the 21 days preceding parturition. If maternal varicella occurs less than 5 days before birth, antepartum transfer of maternal antibody to the fetus is minimal, increasing the risk of systemic varicella infection in the neonate. Varicella pneumonia usually presents 2 to 4 days after the onset of the exanthem. Although varicella pneumonia is often self-limited, it can cause significant mortality and morbidity. Treatment with

TABLE 29–3
PRIMARY PATHOGENS OF NEONATAL PNEUMONIA

Vector	Viruses	Bacteria	Other Agents
Transplacental	Rubella Varicella-zoster HIV CMV HSV	*L. monocytogenes* *M. tuberculosis* *T. pallidium*	
Perinatal	HSV CMV	Group B streptococci Gram-negative enteric (*i.e.*, *E. coli*, *Klebsiella*)	*C. trachomatis* *U. urealyticum*
Postnatal	CMV HSV Community based (*i.e.*, RSV, influenza, parainfluenza)	*S. aureus* *P. aeruginosa* *Flavobacterium* *S. marcescens*	*C. albicans*

HIV, human immunodeficiency virus; CMV, cytomegalovirus; HSV, herpes simplex virus; RSV, respiratory syncytial virus.

varicella-zoster immune globulin within 72 hours of birth improves clinical outcome in neonates exposed to varicella. Pneumonitis is not a common presentation in congenital CMV or herpes, but it is more common in perinatally acquired CMV and HSV. Pulmonary disease caused by transplacental transfer of the HIV virus generally presents after the neonatal period.

TRANSPLACENTAL BACTERIAL PNEUMONIAS

Transplacental bacterial infections are less common causes of pneumonia. *Listeria monocytogenes*, *Mycobacterium tuberculosis*, and *Treponema pallidum* are the most common organisms. Maternal listeriosis classically presents with a flulike syndrome, with fever and chills occurring up to 2 weeks before delivery. Preterm labor and meconium staining of amniotic fluid, even in preterm infants, are common. Early-onset listeriosis generally presents soon after birth with respiratory distress and pneumonia. Radiographic findings are nonspecific, consisting of peribronchial or widespread infiltrates. Congenital tuberculosis occurs most commonly in infants born to women with primary infections. Respiratory symptoms in neonatal tuberculosis typically present at 2 to 4 weeks of age. Transplacental transfer of *T. palladium* occurs most commonly during primary or secondary maternal infection, usually after 20 weeks of gestation. Pneumonia alba refers to the pale, firm, and enlarged lungs seen at autopsy in congenital syphilis. Although pulmonary involvement is uncommon, the recent increase in the incidence of primary and secondary syphilis should heighten physician awareness of all manifestations of congenital syphilis.

PNEUMONIA ACQUIRED IN THE PERINATAL PERIOD

Neonatal pneumonia is most commonly acquired during the process of labor and delivery. Infection occurs from organisms ascending from the genital tract after rupture of fetal membranes or acquired during passage of the infant through the birth canal. Respiratory symptoms are often present at delivery or have their onset in the first few days of life. Despite the abundance and heterogeneity of organisms in the genital tract, only a few commonly cause pneumonia.

In U.S. nurseries, group B streptococcus (GBS) is the most frequently identified organism causing neonatal pneumonia. The second largest group of organisms to produce early-onset sepsis or pneumonia are the gram-negative enteric bacilli: *Escherichia coli*, *Klebsiella*, *Enterobacter*, and *Proteus* species. Herpes simplex and CNV are the most common viral agents causing early-onset pneumonia. Pneumonia caused by *Chlamydia trachomatis*, usually begins at 2 to 8 weeks of age with upper respiratory tract symptoms, a staccato cough, and apnea. Antecedent conjunctival infection is common but not always observed. Interstitial pneumonitis and hyperinflation are associated with chlamydial pneumonia. *U. urealyticum* is a common inhabitant of the lower genital tract of women and is frequently associated with histologic evidence of chorioamnionitis. *U. urealyticum* is a cause of acute congenital pneumonia and has also been associated with chronic lung disease in infants.

PNEUMONIA ACQUIRED IN THE POSTNATAL PERIOD

Newborns exposed to respiratory equipment or humidified incubators are at risk for respiratory infection by *Pseudomonas* species, *Flavobacterium*, *Klebsiella*, or *Serratia marcescens*. Direct contamination by the hands of caretakers due to inadequate hand washing is associated with outbreaks of *Staphylococcus aureus* and gram-negative enteric organisms. Cytomegalovirus that is acquired postnatally through blood products or breast milk commonly presents as a pneumonitis. Onset of CMV disease is usually 4 to 12 weeks after exposure, presenting with tachypnea, cough, and upper respiratory symptoms.

Neonatal HSV infection is most often associated with HSV type II. However, data from the National Institute of Allergy and Infectious Disease indicate that 30% of symptomatic neonatal HSV infections were caused by HSV type I.[33] Postnatal infection from HSV generally occurs from orolabial, oropharyngeal or breast lesions. Community based respiratory pathogens, including respiratory syncyticial virus, influenza, parainfluenza, and enteroviruses, occur in the nursery. Pneumonia resulting from epidemic outbreaks of various enteroviral agents, including echovirus 22 and coxsackievirus type B, is often associated with other clinical manifestation of enteroviral disease. Risk factors for nosocomial fungal infections include very low birth weight, prolonged antibiotic therapy, intubation, central line catheter placement, intravenous alimentation, and corticosteroids. Pneumonia caused by *Candida albicans* usually presents in the context of disseminated disease.

PATHOLOGIC FINDINGS

Three common histopathologic patterns have been associated with neonatal pneumonia: hyaline membrane formation, suppurative inflammation, and interstitial pneumonitis. Hyaline membrane formation is a nonspecific response seen in lung injury associated with surfactant deficiency, pneumonia, and oxygen therapy. Damage to the alveolar epithelium results in cell necrosis and leakage of cell and serum proteins into the alveolar space. Hyaline membranes in neonatal pneumonia are often observed after GBS infection, but they are also associated with fatal pneumonia caused by *H. influenzae*, gram-negative enteric organisms, and viral agents. Bacteria are commonly seen within the hyaline membranes (Fig. 29-10). Dis-

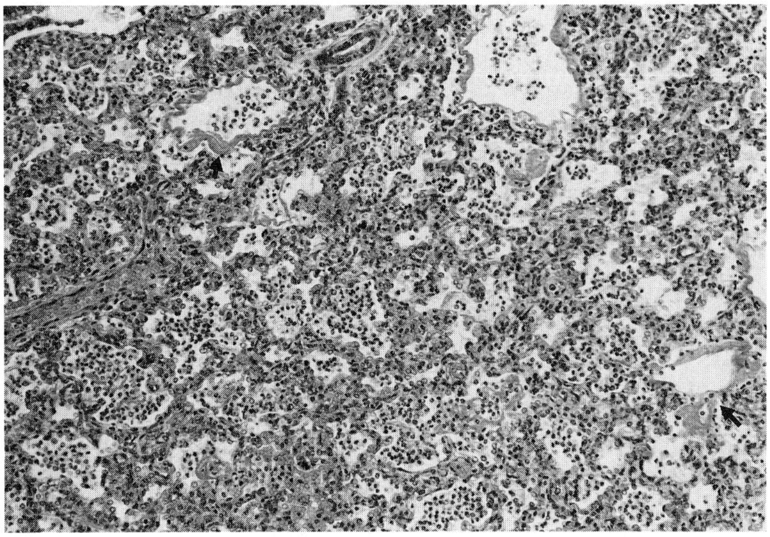

FIG. 29–10. Acute neutrophilic response with atelectasis and hyaline membranes (*arrows*) are seen in lung tissue from a full-term infant who died at 2 days of age of group B streptococcal pneumonia. (Hematoxylin & eosin stain; original magnification × 200; courtesy of Edgar Ballard, Children's Hospital, Cincinnati, OH.)

ruption of alveolar capillary permeability and cell injury results in leakage of proteins into the alveolus that further inactivate pulmonary surfactant, leading to atelectasis. The decreased compliance, atelectasis, and hypoxemia seen in pneumonia are often indistinguishable from findings in surfactant-deficient lungs in premature infants. The chest radiographic findings in RDS and neonatal pneumonia may be identical, although bronchopneumonia and pleural effusions are more common in GBS and other bacterial causes of neonatal pneumonia than in RDS.

SUPPURATIVE PNEUMONIA

Staphylococcus aureus, enteric bacilli, such as *Klebsiella pneumoniae*, *E. coli*, and *Pseudomonas* species, and fungi can cause suppurative pneumonia. An intense inflammatory response often occurs in the lungs during these bacterial infections. Necrosis of lung parenchyma, microabscess formation, and partial obstruction of terminal bronchioles results in thin-walled, air-filled pneumatoceles. Spontaneous rupture of these structures can produce pneumothorax. Microabcesses may consolidate into larger cavities or rupture to the pleural space causing empyema. Pneumonia may be focal or may consolidate to produce large confluent abscesses. Perfusion of consolidated lung tissue causes venous admixture and hypoxemia.

INTERSTITIAL PNEUMONITIS

Interstitial pneumonitis is typically caused by a virus and characterized by interstitial inflammation, edema, mononuclear infiltration, and septal hyperplasia. Alveolar spaces may remain uninvolved, but in severe cases, a serous exudate containing desquamated pneumocytes and macrophages may be associated with hyaline membrane formation. Septal wall necrosis may occur, adding a component of hemorrhage to the inflammatory exudate. Alveolar capillary block associated with the inflammation may impair respiratory function. Cytomegalovirus, HSV, varicella-zoster, rubella, HIV, enteroviruses, and the community-based pathogens, such as respiratory syncytial, influenza, and parainfluenza viruses, are commonly associated with interstitial pneumonitis.

GROUP B STREPTOCOCCAL PNEUMONIA

During the 1970s, GBS pneumonia emerged as the predominant pathogen causing neonatal sepsis and pneumonia. The incidence of GBS infection in the first week of life varies from 1.3 to 3 per 1000 live births. Despite increased awareness of the disease, GBS infection continues to be associated with mortality rates of 10% to 30%.[28]

Group B streptococci are commonly found in genital and intestinal flora of 10% to 20% of pregnant women. For women with positive GBS cultures at delivery, the infant colonization rate is approximately 50%. Of colonized infants, only 0.5% to 2% develop invasive disease. Risk of infection is inversely related to birth weight. Maternal factors increasing the risk of infection include the concentration of genital GBS and the level of maternal, type-specific GBS antibodies. Prolonged rupture of membranes (*i.e.*, >24 hours), chorioamnionitis, and use of fetal monitoring devices increase the risk of GBS disease.[28]

Intrapartum chemoprophylaxis may prevent early onset neonatal GBS disease. Efficacy of intrapartum treatment was demonstrated in high-risk pregnancies with documented prenatal GBS colonization and premature labor, rupture of membranes for more than 12 hours, or intrapartum fever. Boyer and colleagues demonstrated that intrapartum intravenous ampicillin followed by treatment of the infants with intramuscular ampicillin significantly reduced early-onset GBS disease.[29]

Early-onset GBS disease usually presents within the first week of life. Septicemia (30%–40%), meningitis (30%), and pneumonia (30%–40%) are the most common presentations. Regardless of the primary site of involvement, 90% of affected infants present with respiratory distress. Radiographic features of GBS infection may be indistinguishable from RDS, although pleural effusions may help differentiate GBS from RDS (Fig. 29-11). In two-thirds of affected infants, increased vascular markings or patchy infiltrates are observed on the initial chest radiographs. Respiratory distress in the absence of radiographic abnormalities may be associated with pulmonary vascular hypertension and hypoxemia. Late-onset GBS usually presents from 1 to 6 weeks after birth and is commonly associated with meningitis.

Respiratory failure in GBS pneumonia results from hyaline membrane formation, atelectasis, and pulmonary hypertension. Pulmonary hypertension is proposed to be mediated by high-molecular-weight polysaccharide exotoxin. In animals, infusion of GBS exotoxin results in an initial increase in pulmonary vascular pressures and fever, followed by a second phase characterized by granulocytopenia, granulocyte trapping in the lung, and increased pulmonary vascular permeability.[30]

Isolation of GBS from cultures of blood, cerebrospinal fluid, or suppurative foci (*i.e.*, pleural fluid) is diagnostic of GBS infection. Surface cultures of skin or mucous membranes may not be of clinical significance. Latex particle agglutination is a rapid diagnostic test that provides presumptive diagnosis of GBS disease pending the outcome of bacterial cultures. Antimicrobial therapy is usually instituted before an organism is identified and consists of a penicillin and an aminoglycoside. After the organism is identified and meningitis is excluded, therapy can continue with penicillin alone at 200,000 U/kg/day, usually for 10 to 14 days. Extensive supportive care, including oxygen, mechanical ventilation, and cardiovascular support, may also be required in treating an overwhelming infection.

HERPES SIMPLEX PNEUMONIA

The incidence of neonatal HSV is increasing in the United States, affecting 1500 to 2200 infants per year. Classification of HSV infection is based on the site and extent of involvement; HSV may be classified as a cutaneous infection; as encephalitic, with or without cutaneous infection; and as a disseminated infection. Mortality is highest among infants with disseminated disease. The mortality rate of infants with HSV pneumonitis is approximately 79%.[31] Transmission of HSV infection to the neonate is most frequently related to direct contact with virus at delivery. Most women delivering infants with symptomatic HSV disease shed virus asymptomatically at delivery, and fewer than 20% of these women reported a history of previous infection.[32] Whether the maternal infection is primary or recurrent is important in the pathogenesis of neonatal HSV infection. Infants of women with serologic evidence of a recent primary infection are more likely to develop disease than infants of women with recurrent herpes. Primary infections are associated with higher titers of viral shedding and with low levels of protective antibodies, placing the neonate at higher risk. Rupture of the amniotic sac for longer than 6 hours is associated with increased risk of neonatal HSV infection, although infection after cesarean section with intact membranes has also been reported.

Herpes simplex virus pneumonitis usually presents as part of a disseminated HSV infection. Many severely involved infants have no skin lesions. Infants

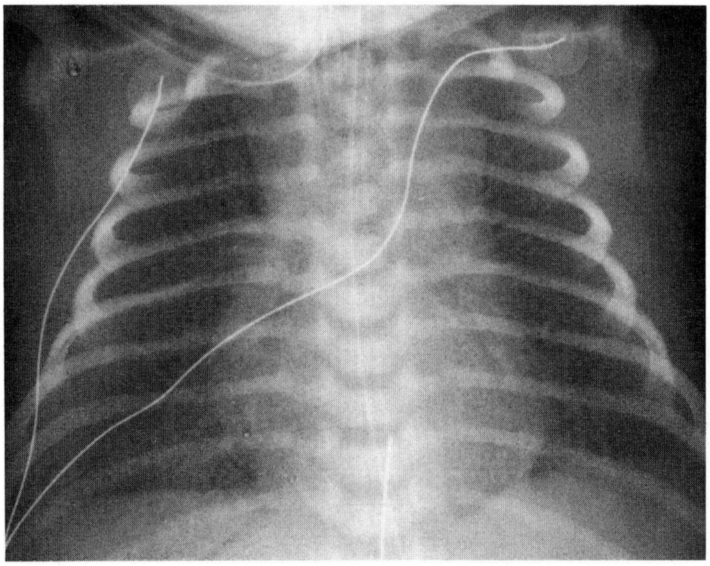

FIG. 29–11. A full-term infant of an uncomplicated pregnancy developed respiratory distress, cyanosis, and periods of apnea within 6 hours of life. The blood culture and urine latex particle agglutination assay were positive for group B streptococci. Diffuse reticulogranular pattern, air bronchograms, and right pleural effusion without significant volume loss are consistent with common radiologic features of group B streptococcal pneumonia.

typically develop signs of infection at 4 to 5 days of life. Fever, tachypnea, jaundice, and irritability, progressing to respiratory failure, shock, and disseminated intravascular coagulation are commonly seen. Diffuse interstitial pneumonitis and hemorrhagic pneumonitis are characteristic of HSV infection of the lung.

Isolation of HSV remains the definitive diagnostic method. Viral cultures should be obtained from skin lesions, cerebrospinal fluid, stool, urine, throat, nasopharynx, and conjunctiva. Hepatic dysfunction, neutropenia, bleeding diathesis, and interstitial pneumonitis are commonly associated with HSV but are not diagnostic. Serologic assays are not of clinical value, because they do not differentiate between antibodies to HSV types 1 and 2 or between maternal IgG and endogenously produced antibodies. Intranuclear inclusions and multinucleated giant cells observed in scrapings from cutaneous lesions are supportive but not diagnostic of HSV infection.

Early antiviral therapy decreases the progression from localized, cutaneous HSV infection to disseminated disease, and decreases the mortality from HSV infection. Vidarabine and acyclovir are now widely used in treatment of HSV infection in the neonate. Because of ease of administration, acyclovir is considered the treatment of choice.[33]

TRANSIENT TACHYPNEA OF THE NEWBORN

Transient tachypnea of the newborn (TTN) was first described in 1966 by Avery and colleagues in a group of 8 patients, 7 of whom were delivered vaginally at term.[34] All of the infants presented at or shortly after birth with grunting, retractions, and an increased respiratory rate. Respiratory rates of the original infants ranged from 80 to 140 breaths per minute, and the symptoms persisted for 2 to 5 days. These infants could be differentiated from infants with other acute lung diseases by their clinical course and radiographic findings. Although the precise cause of TTN remains unknown, it was originally postulated that infants with TTN had reduced lung compliance because of delayed resorption of lung fluid at the time of birth. Many clinicians support the original proposal of Avery and colleagues that TTN results from distention of interstitial spaces by fluid, leading to alveolar air trapping and decreased lung compliance. Since the original description, others have postulated that TTN may result from mild immaturity of the surfactant system. Lack of phosphatidylglycerol in amniotic fluid samples obtained from infants with TTN supports the latter concept.

The incidence of TTN is approximately 11 per 1000 live births. The risk factors for TTN include prematurity, maternal sedation, maternal fluid administration, maternal asthma, exposure to β-mimetic agents, and fetal asphyxia. Whether delivery by cesarean section predisposes the term infant for TTN is still debated.

Infants with TTN initially present with grunting, retractions, and increased respiratory rate. The symptoms of tachypnea may persist for several days, and most infants require less than 40% oxygen to maintain adequate systemic oxygenation. The radiographic findings in this disorder are ill defined but include increased central vascular markings, hyperaeration, evidence of interstitial and pleural fluid, prominent interlobar fissures, and cardiomegaly (Fig. 29-12). Because TTN is self-limited, no specific therapy is indicated, although adequate ventilation and oxygenation must be maintained. Because the symptoms of TTN are nonspecific and consistent with neonatal sepsis or pneumonia, most infants with TTN are evaluated for infection and are treated with broad-spectrum antibiotics pending a definitive diagnosis.

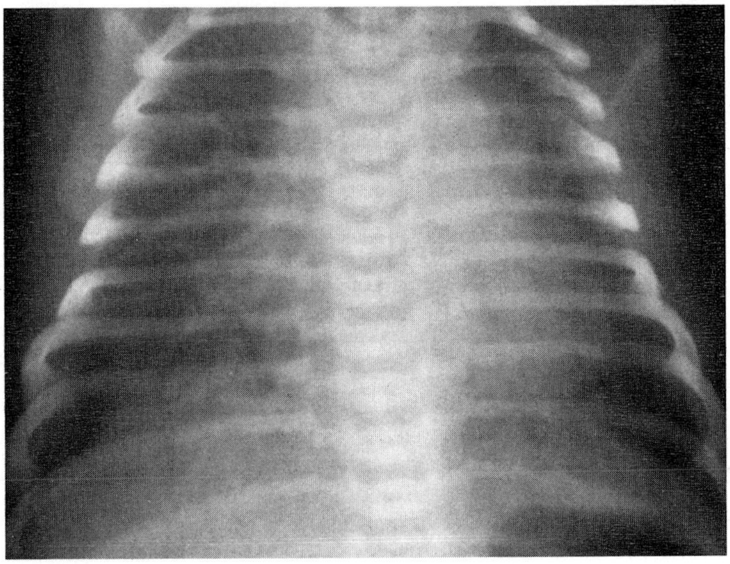

FIG. 29–12. This full-term infant was born by cesarean section and developed tachypnea and grunting that resolved 48 hours after birth. Perihilar vascular densities, streaky opacities of interstitial edema, fluid in the interlobar fissures, small pleural effusions, and cardiomegaly are observed on the radiograph. These features are indicative of transient tachypnea of the newborn.

PULMONARY HEMORRHAGE

Pulmonary hemorrhage in the newborn may vary from a focal, self-limited disorder to massive, lethal hemorrhage. The incidence of pulmonary hemorrhage in the neonatal period ranges from 0.8 to 1.2 per 1000 live births. Asphyxia, prematurity, intrauterine growth retardation, infection, hypothermia, oxygen therapy, severe Rh hemolytic disease, and coagulopathy are associated risk factors. In some studies, surfactant therapy has been associated with an increased incidence of pulmonary hemorrhage, although this remains controversial. Although disseminated intravascular coagulation may precede pulmonary hemorrhage, most infants with pulmonary hemorrhage do not have a coagulopathy. Pulmonary hemorrhage generally presents within the first week of life, and the mortality rate after pulmonary hemorrhage is estimated to be 75% to 90%. Although most infants who develop pulmonary hemorrhage have the predisposing factors of extreme prematurity and underlying asphyxia and stress, there are a few case reports describing previously healthy, term infants with pulmonary hemorrhage associated with an inborn error of the urea cycle and elevated blood ammonia.

CLINICAL FINDINGS

The observation that the hematocrit of lung effluent in pulmonary hemorrhage is lower than the hematocrit of blood supports the concept that most of these infants have hemorrhagic pulmonary edema. Neonatal pulmonary hemorrhage is therefore thought to result from shock, hypoxia, and acidosis, which lead to left ventricular failure and increased pulmonary capillary pressure with subsequent hemorrhagic pulmonary edema. Chest radiographic findings in pulmonary hemorrhage depend on whether the hemorrhage is focal or massive. Because blood or hemorrhagic edema fluid has tissue density, hemorrhagic tissue appears opacified. It is often difficult to differentiate focal hemorrhage from atelectasis or pneumonia by chest radiographs. In the case of massive pulmonary hemorrhage, the lungs can be atelectatic and opacified (*i.e.*, whited-out). The clinical course of massive pulmonary hemorrhage usually involves rapid deterioration of ventilatory function. Affected infants develop progressive hypoxia and hypercarbia with resultant respiratory acidosis and may rapidly succumb to this disorder.

TREATMENT

Early detection and aggressive intervention improves the outcome of massive pulmonary hemorrhage, an otherwise lethal syndrome. Positive-pressure ventilation and oxygen are critical components of therapy. Blood volume and hematocrit should be vigorously restored and maintained with erythrocyte transfusions. Careful correction of hypotension, hypoxemia, and acidosis is also indicated. Coagulation abnormalities should be assessed and may be corrected with fresh-frozen plasma or appropriate clotting factors. Pressors and diuretics are indicated if congestive heart failure develops.

AIR LEAKS

Air leaks include pneumothorax, pneumomediastinum, pneumopericardium, and pulmonary interstitial emphysema (PIE).

PATHOPHYSIOLOGY

Pulmonary interstitial emphysema, pneumomediastinum, pneumothorax, and pneumopericardium are closely related clinical entities. Air leak begins with formation of PIE in which alveoli rupture into the perivascular and peribronchial spaces. Air may be trapped in the interstitium of the lung, leading to PIE, but it may also dissect into the mediastinum along the perivascular and peribronchial spaces, producing pneumomediastinum. Mediastinal air ruptures into the pleural space, producing pneumothorax, or into the pericardial space, producing pneumopericardium. In some instances, air can form blebs on the surface of the lung that rupture to produce pneumothorax. Rupture of the lung directly into the pleural space is thought to occur rarely.

RISK FACTORS

Air leaks occur in 1% to 2% of all newborn infants, but they are thought to cause symptoms in only 0.05% to 0.07%. Mechanical ventilation and CPAP are important risk factors contributing to air leak in infants with lung disease. Summarizing data from 11 studies, Madansky found that air leak occurred in 12% of infants with RDS who were not on assisted ventilation, 11% of infants on CPAP, and 26% of infants on mechanical ventilation.[35] The incidence of air leak in infants admitted to the NICU is approximately 2% to 8%, but it is higher if only low-birth-weight infants are considered. As of 1986, of infants weighing 500 to 999 g at birth who developed air leak, 35% had PIE, 20% had pneumothorax, 3% had pneumomediastinum, and 2% had pneumopericardium.[36] Aspiration syndromes, including MAS, are frequently complicated by air leak.

RADIOGRAPHIC EVALUATION

The chest radiographs of infants with PIE have been described as demonstrating a salt-and-pepper pattern in which the radiolucent interstitial air is juxtaposed to lung parenchyma (Fig. 29-13). Radiolucent air is present in the pleural space in a pneumothorax. Because chest radiographs of neonates are usually per-

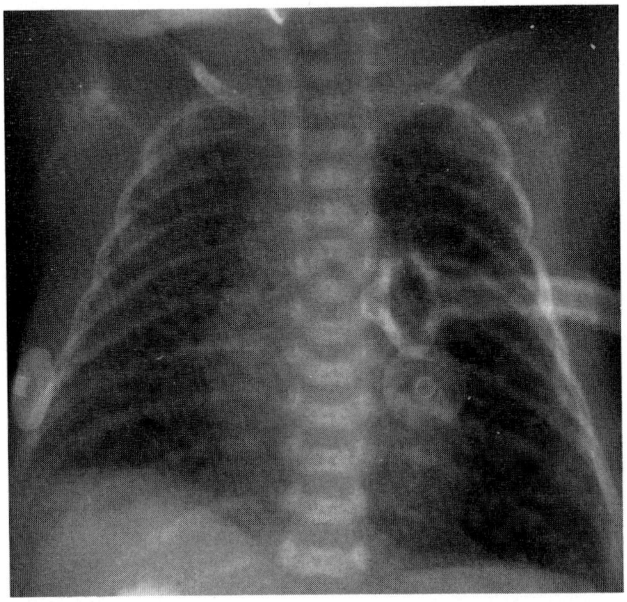

FIG. 29–13. Chest x-ray film of pulmonary interstitial emphysema (PIE). A premature infant with severe respiratory distress syndrome requiring mechanical ventilation developed worsening respiratory acidosis and hypoxia refractory to increased ventilatory support. An anteroposterior chest x-ray film demonstrates a salt-and-pepper pattern resulting from radiolucent interstitial air surrounding compressed lung tissue. A left chest tube was placed to treat pneumothorax, a common complication of pulmonary interstitial emphysema.

PNEUMOTHORAX, PNEUMOMEDIASTINUM, AND PNEUMOPERICARDIUM

Infants with pneumothorax often present with grunting, tachypnea, cyanosis, and retractions. Accumulated air may collapse the lung or shift the mediastinum to the side opposite the air leak. A shift of the trachea or point of maximal impulse and decreased breath sounds on the affected side may be found on clinical examination. Pneumothoraces fall into two major groups: spontaneous pneumothorax in otherwise healthy, full-term infants, which most often occurs within minutes of birth, and pneumothorax in infants with significant pulmonary disease, which frequently occurs several days after birth, during therapy for pulmonary disease.

Prompt recognition of air leak is essential for effective therapy. Unexpected changes in ventilatory requirements or status and abrupt fall in blood pressure, heart rate, respiratory rate, and PO_2 may indicate an air leak. Transillumination of the thorax can be useful in the diagnosis of pneumothorax and its response to therapy. Treatment of tension pneumothorax requires immediate surgical drainage and placement of a chest tube. For treatment of pneumothorax that does not involve tension or cardiovascular compromise, inhalation of 100% oxygen, usually for 6 to 12 hours, can be used in term infants as a nitrogen wash-out method. Premature infants formed in the supine position, pleural air of a pneumothorax may accumulate in the anterior chest and may be visible only on a cross-table lateral or decubitus radiograph. In a tension pneumothorax, the lung and mediastinal organs may be displaced away from the side of the pneumothorax (Fig. 29-14). The thymus may be outlined in pneumomediastinum, resulting in the pathognomonic sail sign seen on radiographs. Pneumopericardium results in a characteristic outline of the heart by radiolucent air.

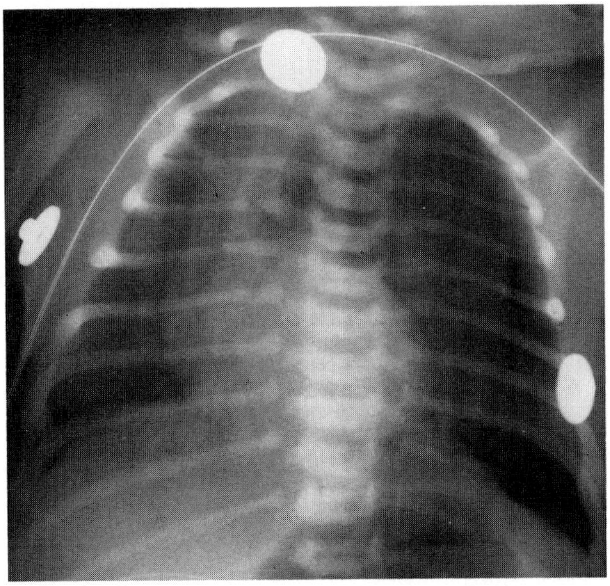

FIG. 29–14. A full-term infant born by a difficult breech delivery presented shortly after birth with crepitus in the neck area, tachypnea, grunting, and retractions. An anteroposterior chest x-ray film demonstrates bilateral pneumothorax under tension on the left. The heart and mediastinum are compressed and shifted to the right. The left pleural air herniates across the midline. The left diaphragm is depressed and inverted. Subcutaneous emphysema is seen in the soft tissues of the neck.

PULMONARY INTERSTITIAL EMPHYSEMA

Pulmonary interstitial emphysema occurs most frequently in smaller infants being treated by mechanical ventilation for primary lung disease. In this clinical setting, PIE is associated with a mortality rate of more than 50%. Unilateral PIE can be managed by placing the infant with the affected side down for 24 to 48 hours. Selective bronchial intubation and high-frequency or jet ventilation have been used to treat unilateral PIE. Careful attention to peak and mean inspiratory pressures may be beneficial in preventing and treating PIE. High-frequency ventilation may be helpful. Bronchopulmonary dysplasia is a frequent sequela in infants surviving PIE.

should not be treated with hyperoxia, because they are at risk for retrolental fibroplasia. Noncompromising pneumomediastinum and pneumopericardium can also be managed with 100% oxygen therapy. Tension pneumopericardium is life threatening, must be drained surgically, and is associated with a high incidence of morbidity and mortality.

REFERENCES

1. Burri PH. Postnatal development and growth. In: Crystal RG, West JB, Barnes PJ, Cherniack NS, Weibel ER, eds. The lung: scientific foundations. New York: Raven Press, 1991:677.
2. Randell SH, Young SL. Structure of alveolar epithelial cells and the surface layer during development. In: Polin RA, Fox WW, eds. Fetal and neonatal physiology. Philadelphia: WB Saunders, 1992:962.
3. Van Golde LMG, Batenburg JJ, Robertson B. The pulmonary surfactant system: biochemical aspects and functional significance. Physiol Rev 1988;68:374.
4. Whitsett JA. RDS in the premature infant. In: Crystal RG, West JB, Barnes PJ, Cherniack NS, Weibel ER, eds. The lung: scientific foundations. New York: Raven Press, 1991:1723.
5. Shapiro DL, Notter RH. Surfactant replacement therapy. New York: Alan Liss, 1989.
6. Rooney S. Regulation of surfactant associated phospholipid synthesis and secretion. In: Polin RA, Fox WW, eds. Fetal and neonatal physiology. Philadelphia: WB Saunders, 1992:986.
7. Ballard PL. Hormonal regulation of pulmonary surfactant. Endocr Rev 1989;10:165.
8. Liggins GC, Howie RN. A controlled trial of antepartum glucocorticoid treatment for prevention of the respiratory distress syndrome in premature infants. Pediatrics 1972;50:515.
9. Jobe A. Phospholipid metabolism and turnover. In: Polin RA, Fox WW, eds. Fetal and neonatal physiology. Philadelphia: WB Saunders, 1992:986.
10. Fujiwara T, Maeta H, Chida S, Morita T, Watabe Y, Abe T. Artificial surfactant therapy in hyaline membrane disease. Lancet 1980:55.
11. Avery ME, Mead J. Surface properties in relation to atelectasis and hyaline membrane disease. Am J Dis Child 1959;97:517.
12. Spitzer AR, Shaffer TH, Fox WW. Assisted ventilation: physiologic implications and application. In: RA Polin, WW Fox, eds. Fetal and neonatal physiology. Philadelphia: WB Saunders, 1991:894.
13. Bacsik RD. Meconium aspiration syndrome. Pediatr Clin North Am 1977;24:463.
14. Katz VL, Barnes WA. Meconium aspiration syndrome: reflections on a murky subject. Am J Obstet Gynecol 1992;166:171.
15. Holtzman RB, Banzhaf WC, Silver RK, Hageman JR. Perinatal management of meconium staining of the amniotic fluid. Clin Perinatol 1989;16:825.
16. Tran N, Lowe C, Swieni EM, Shaffer TH. Sequential effects of acute meconium obstruction on pulmonary function. Pediatr Res 1980;14:34.
17. Ting P, Brady JP. Tracheal suction in meconium aspiration. Am J Obstet Gynecol 1975;122:767.
18. Wiswell TE, Henley MA. Intratracheal suctioning, systemic infection and the meconium aspiration syndrome. Pediatrics 1992;89:203.
19. Gersony W, Duc G, Sinclair J. "PFC" syndrome. Circulation 1969;40(Suppl 111):87.
20. Clarke WR. The transitional circulation: physiology and anesthetic implications. J Clin Anesth 1990;2:192.
21. Hammerman C, Yousefzadeh D, Choi JH, Bui KC. Persistent pulmonary hypertension of the newborn. Managing the unmanageable? Clin Perinatol 1989;16:137.
22. Spitzer AR, Davis J, Clarke WT, Bernbaum J, Fox WF. Pulmonary hypertension and persistent fetal circulation in the newborn. Clin Perinatol 1988;15:389.
23. Rabinowitz M. Structure and function of the pulmonary vascular bed: an update. Cardiol Clin 1989;7:227.
24. Bartlett RH, Gazzanigo AB, Huxtable RF, Schippers HC, O'Connor MJ, Jeffries MR. Extracorporeal circulation (ECMO) in neonatal respiratory failure. J Thorac Cardiovasc Surg 1977;74:826.
25. ECMO Life Support Organization. ECMO registry. Ann Arbor, MI, 1992.
26. Ballard RA, Leonard CH. Developmental follow-up of infants with persistent pulmonary hypertension of the Newborn. Clin Perinatol 1984;11:737.
27. Dennehy PH. Respiratory infections in the newborn. Clin Perinatol 1987;14:667.
28. Baker JC, Edwards MS. Group B streptococcal infections. In: Remington JS, Klein JO, eds. Infectious diseases of the fetus and newborn infant. Philadelphia: WB Saunders, 1990.
29. Boyer KM, Gotoff SP. Prevention of early onset neonatal group B streptococcal disease with selective intrapartum chemoprophylaxis. N Engl J Med 1986;314:1165.
30. Rojas J, Stahlman M. The effect of group B streptococcus and other organisms on the pulmonary vasculature. Clin Perinatol 1984;11:591.
31. Whitley R, Arvin A, Prober C, et al. Predictors of morbidity and mortality among infants with herpes simplex virus infection. N Engl J Med 1991;324:453.
32. Whitley JR, Corey L, Arvin A, et al. Changing presentation of herpes simplex virus infection in neonates. J Infect Dis 1988;158:109.
33. Whitley R, Arvin A, Prober C, et al. A controlled trial comparing vidarabine with acyclovir in neonatal herpes simplex virus infection. N Engl J Med 1991;324:444.
34. Avery ME, Gatewood OB, Brumley G. Transient tachypnea of the newborn. Am J Dis Child 1966;111:380.
35. Madansky DL, Lawson EE, Chernick V, Taisusch HW. Pneumothorax and other forms of pulmonary air leak in newborns. Am Rev Respir Dis 1979;120:729.
36. Yu VYH, Wong PY, Bajuk B, Szymonowicz W. Pulmonary air leak in extremely low birthweight infants. Arch Dis Child 1986;61:239.

Neonatology: Pathophysiology and Management of the Newborn, Fourth Edition,
edited by Gordon B. Avery, Mary Ann Fletcher, and Mhairi G. MacDonald.
J.B. Lippincott Company, Philadelphia © 1994.

chapter 30

Chronic Lung Disease

JONATHAN M. DAVIS
WARREN N. ROSENFELD

Bronchopulmonary dysplasia (BPD) is a chronic lung disease that develops in newborn infants treated with oxygen and positive-pressure mechanical ventilation for a primary lung disorder. The introduction of new treatment modalities (*e.g.*, surfactant replacement therapy, high-frequency ventilation, extracorporeal membrane oxygenation), have significantly improved the outcome for many critically ill premature and term infants. As a result, more infants are surviving the newborn period and developing BPD. Approximately 7000 new cases of BPD occur each year, and approximately 10% to 15% of these infants die in the first year of life. Bronchopulmonary dysplasia has become an extremely important complication of neonatal intensive care and the most common form of chronic lung disease in infants.

The modern history of BPD began with Northway's observations in 1967.[1] This study documented the clinical course, radiographic findings, and histopathologic lung changes in a group of infants who had received oxygen and ventilatory support for treatment of respiratory distress syndrome (RDS) and established the term bronchopulmonary dysplasia. Although Northway originally postulated that oxygen toxicity caused BPD, the exact mechanisms causing the lung injury are complex and not completely understood.

Treatment with positive-pressure ventilation has been implicated in BPD, and factors such as oxygen toxicity, prematurity, genetic predisposition, inflammation, and excessive fluid administration may play important roles. Therapies for infants with BPD are directed toward improving the pathophysiologic abnormalities after they occur with oxygen and mechanical ventilation, fluid restriction, diuretics, bronchodilators, or steroids. Many different therapies can be used in these infants, often concurrently. The optimal treatment and prevention strategies have not been established.

There has been significant debate about the exact definition of BPD, further complicated because the nature of BPD has changed with the widespread use of surfactant and other therapeutic interventions. The current form of BPD appears to be much less severe than in the past. There has been a significant decrease in the number of infants with BPD who require tracheostomy and 6 months or longer of mechanical ventilation at home or in a chronic care facility.

This chapter reviews the definition and incidence of BPD, its pathogenesis, pathophysiologic changes, treatment strategies, and long-term outcome. Newly developed approaches for the prevention of BPD in high-risk infants are presented.

DEFINITION AND INCIDENCE

In the original description of BPD, Northway defined chronic lung changes in a group of premature neonates who survived artificial ventilation for treatment of RDS.[1] Northway reported 13 survivors of 32 neonates who had received mechanical ventilation.

These infants had an average gestational age of 34 weeks and birth weight of 2.2 kg, distinctly different from most patients who now develop BPD.

Northway's definition of BPD included radiologic, pathologic, and clinical criteria. Bronchopulmonary dysplasia was divided into four developmental stages. The acute stages (*i.e.*, I and II) were indistinguishable from RDS and were seen in the first 10 days of life. Stages III and IV marked the transition to the chronic stages of this disease; changes found in stage IV form the basis for the definition of BPD. This stage described abnormalities that persisted beyond 1 month of age (*i.e.*, 28 days) in patients who continued to require respiratory support (*i.e.*, ventilation or oxygen supplementation). Chest radiographs demonstrated cyst formation and hyperexpansion alternating with areas of atelectasis.

As the care of neonates has become more sophisticated and smaller, sicker infants have survived, the clinical and radiographic findings that define BPD have changed. With the introduction of surfactant replacement therapy, further changes in the definition of BPD will be necessary. Northway's original criteria depended heavily on a progression of radiographic changes, and clinical criteria were considered secondary. Further refinement was offered by Bancalari, whose criteria included ventilation for at least the first 3 days of life and respiratory symptoms (*e.g.*, tachypnea, auscultatory rales, retractions) at 28 days of life.[2] A need for supplemental oxygen to maintain a partial pressure (PO_2) greater than 50 torr and an abnormal chest radiograph at 28 days of life was also necessary. Tooley required that infants with BPD be older than 30 days of age and have radiographic abnormalities plus any one of the following: PO_2 less than 60 torr in room air, PCO_2 greater than 45 torr, or need for supplemental oxygen.[3]

Many infants who eventually develop chronic lung disease do not require prolonged mechanical ventilation, nor do they have radiographs consistent with those described by Northway, Bancalari, and Tooley. In contrast to the definitions that eliminated many infants who went on to develop chronic lung disease, several studies have used less stringent criteria. A study of techniques that may have influenced the development of BPD in eight neonatal centers defined BPD as the requirement for oxygen supplementation at 28 days of life.[4] A similar definition that excluded radiographic and clinical criteria was employed by Sinkin in his development of a predictive scoring system for BPD.[5] Shennan questioned the large number of normal neonates who would be included by this criterion and suggested that the need for additional oxygen at 36 weeks postconceptual gestational age may be a more accurate predictor of ultimate pulmonary outcome.[6]

The definition of BPD may need to be more flexible and not restricted to a single point in time to properly define the patients who develop long-term pulmonary sequelae. This may require inclusion of patients with abnormal radiographs who require oxygen therapy for respiratory support at 28 days and those who continue to require supplemental oxygen at 36 weeks postconceptual age.

The incidence of BPD depends on the definition used and the patient population studied. Several surfactant replacement trials have reported significantly improved survival for 750-g to 1500-g infants with RDS after surfactant replacement therapy.[7–15] This is true regardless of the type of the surfactant used (*e.g.*, human, synthetic, surfactant-TA). The incidence of BPD, defined as oxygen dependency at 28 days with appropriate radiographic findings, is in the range of 19% to 63% for the control groups in these studies. The surfactant treatment groups had a similar incidence of BPD, in the range of 11% to 57%. When the total number of patients in all these studies are combined, 402 (40%) of 1015 infants in the control groups and 396 (35%) of 1121 infants in the surfactant-treated groups survive with a diagnosis of BPD. A Chi-square analysis of these infants shows a significant reduction ($p < 0.05$) in the incidence of BPD when exogenous surfactant was used. It appears from these studies that the incidence of BPD will decrease after surfactant therapy; however, the prevalence, or total number of infants with BPD, will increase because of improved survival. Bronchopulmonary dysplasia will continue to be an important problem for the neonatologist and pediatric pulmonologist in the future. Further study of the mechanisms involved in the lung injury process and the development of possible prevention strategies are needed.

PATHOGENESIS

No single factor has been identified as the cause of BPD. Its origin is multifactorial and may depend on the nature of the injury, mechanisms of response, or the infant's inability to respond appropriately to the injury process.

Northway attributed the occurrence of BPD to prolonged hyperoxia in infants with RDS.[1] Since this original hypothesis, numerous causes have been proposed. Although some may have been previously implicated in the pathogenesis of BPD, the importance of others has been lessened with new developments in the treatment of premature neonates. For example, barotrauma from positive-pressure ventilation had been postulated to be a major factor in the pathogenesis of chronic lung disease, but new ventilatory techniques and the use of surfactant replacement therapy have markedly diminished the pressures needed to adequately ventilate neonates. Patent ductus arteriosus has been implicated, but current technology, which more rapidly detects and treats this problem, has decreased its relative role in BPD. These two factors were the focus of numerous intervention studies to decrease the incidence of BPD. Despite limiting their roles in this disorder, the prevalence of BPD is increasing, confirming the complexity of the disease process.

BAROTRAUMA

With the introduction of positive-pressure ventilation for the treatment of RDS, ventilatory pressures capable of causing pathologic changes were transmitted to the lung. Although the initial phases of lung injury in BPD are the result of the primary disease process (*e.g.*, RDS), superimposed positive-pressure mechanical ventilation appears to add to the lung injury and provoke a complex inflammatory cascade that ultimately leads to chronic lung disease.

The role of barotrauma in BPD depends on several factors, including the structure of the tracheobronchial tree and the physiologic effects of surfactant deficiency. With surfactant deficiency, surface tension forces are elevated, aeration is unequal, and most terminal alveoli are largely collapsed. The pressure needed to distend these poorly compliant saccules is high and transmitted to the terminal bronchioles and alveolar ducts. In the premature neonate, these airways are highly compliant and subject to rupture, as demonstrated by Ackerman.[16] Gas then dissects into the interstitium, where it is trapped, resulting in the development of pulmonary interstitial emphysema (PIE). The occurrence of PIE increases the relative risk of developing BPD sixfold. In contrast to the preterm infant, barotrauma in the term neonate may lead to direct rupture of the alveoli. The result is usually a pneumothorax, pneumomediastinum, or subpleural bleb caused by dissection of air into the perivascular sheath and then to the hilum.

Whether the acute injury that leads to the development of BPD is caused by direct barotrauma from prolonged ventilation or the toxic effects of oxygen supplementation is difficult to differentiate. Nilsson and colleagues showed that even brief periods of positive-pressure ventilation can cause bronchiolar epithelial damage in the lung.[17] The severity of the injury appears to correlate well with the amount of peak pressure used. Davis and associates demonstrated that short periods of positive-pressure ventilation with relatively low inspiratory pressure were associated with compromised cell integrity in the lung, resulting in increased permeability to albumin and other proteins.[18] Few other studies have been able to separate the relative contribution of barotrauma from oxygen toxicity. Davis and colleagues demonstrated that the physiologic, biochemical, cellular, and histologic changes of acute lung injury that precede the development of BPD were minimal in neonatal piglets subjected to positive-pressure ventilation with room air, but they were much more significant if 100% oxygen was used.[19] This suggests that the damaging effects of oxygen and mechanical ventilation are additive and possibly synergistic.

Strategies to prevent barotrauma and PIE have resulted in frequent and continuous changes in methods of ventilation. Early attempts at negative-pressure ventilation successfully minimized barotrauma, but this form of ventilation was impractical, difficult to control, and associated with other unique complications. Other ventilators, including high-frequency ventilators that employ rates from 120 to 1200 cycles/minute, have been developed. A major indication for their use is the prevention or treatment of pulmonary barotrauma. Results of a nationwide study failed to demonstrate that one particular high-frequency oscillator provided any advantage over conventional ventilation in the initial treatment of RDS.[20] Oscillators traditionally operate at higher mean airway pressures, which result in improved alveolar recruitment and oxygenation, but they may be associated with more barotrauma (*e.g.*, air leak, increased capillary permeability).[21] In contrast, high-frequency jet ventilation (HFJV) allows adequate gas exchange at lower peak inspiratory pressures.[22] A randomized, controlled trial demonstrated that complications of pulmonary barotrauma (*e.g.*, PIE, pneumothorax) resolved more rapidly in infants treated with HFJV than those treated with conventional ventilation.[23] However, animal studies examining the effects of HFJV on the lung have shown that neonatal piglets treated with 4 hours of HFJV had more significant inflammatory changes observed compared with those treated with conventional ventilation.[18] Further study is needed to define the effects of this type of ventilation on the lung and how it influences the development of acute and chronic lung injury.

The major advance in the prevention of pulmonary barotrauma has been the introduction of surfactant replacement therapy. Surfactant permits more equal distribution of pressures and ventilation to all saccules, prevents overdistention of air spaces and bronchioles, and stabilizes airways. A major benefit of surfactant therapy has been the reduction of ventilator pressures and pulmonary air leak.[7–15] However, BPD continues to be a serious problem, suggesting that barotrauma is only one of many factors involved in the pathogenesis of BPD.

OXYGEN AND ANTIOXIDANTS

Under normal conditions, a delicate balance exists between the production of free radicals and the antioxidant defenses that protect cells *in vivo*. Free radicals are molecules with extra electrons in their outer ring, and they are toxic to living tissues (Table 30-1). Oxygen has a unique molecular structure and is abundant within cells. It readily accepts free electrons generated by oxidative metabolism within the cell, producing free radicals. The balance may be disturbed by increased free-radical production under conditions of hyperoxia, reperfusion, or inflammation. Alternatively, free radicals can increase if an inability to quench production because of inadequate antioxidant defenses occurs. Damage caused by oxy-

TABLE 30–1
FREE RADICALS

Radical	Symbol	Antioxidant
Superoxide anion	O_2^-	Superoxide dismutase, uric acid, vitamin E
Singlet oxygen	$^1O_2$	β-carotene, uric acid, vitamin E
Hydrogen peroxide	H_2O_2	Catalase, glutathione peroxidase, glutathione
Hydroxyl radical	$OH^\cdot$	Vitamins C and E
Peroxide radical	$LOO^\cdot$	Vitamins C and E
Hydroperoxyl radical	LOOH	Glutathione transferase, glutathione peroxidase

L, lipid.

gen free radicals ranges from cell membrane destruction to the unraveling of nucleic acids.

The role of oxygen free radicals in lung injury has been demonstrated in numerous animal models. Increased oxidative stress results in injury unless the lung is able to compensate by proportionately increasing antioxidant defenses. At term, some species of neonatal animals can better tolerate a hyperoxic challenge than adults because of the ability to synthesize antioxidant enzymes. However, the premature neonate may be more susceptible to free-radical damage because adequate concentrations of these enzymes may be absent at birth. Frank and associates documented the development of the antioxidant enzymes superoxide dismutase (SOD), catalase, and glutathione peroxidase in the lungs of rabbits during late gestation (Fig. 30-1).[24] The 150% increase in these enzymes during the last 15% of gestation parallels the maturation pattern of pulmonary surfactant. These developmental changes in the fetal lung allow proper ventilation by reducing surface tension and provide for the transition from the relative hypoxia of intrauterine development to the oxygen-rich extrauterine environment. This increase in lung antioxidants has been documented in several other species.[25] Premature birth before the development of sufficient antioxidant enzymes may expose the neonate to supraphysiologic concentrations of oxygen and increase the risk for the development of BPD.

Further evidence for the role of free oxygen radicals in lung injury involves the ability to increase survival and prevent lung damage from prolonged hyperoxia by increasing the concentration of lung antioxidants. Rats exposed to sublethal concentrations of oxygen (85%) for 5 to 7 days were able to withstand exposure to normally lethal oxygen concentrations (>95%) later.[26] This protection was associated with increases in endogenous lung SOD, catalase, and glutathione peroxidase concentrations. Other animal studies have successfully prevented lung injury with antioxidant supplementation with SOD and catalase or by blocking the inflammatory response to free radicals.[27–29] These findings confirm the role of free oxygen radicals in the development of BPD.

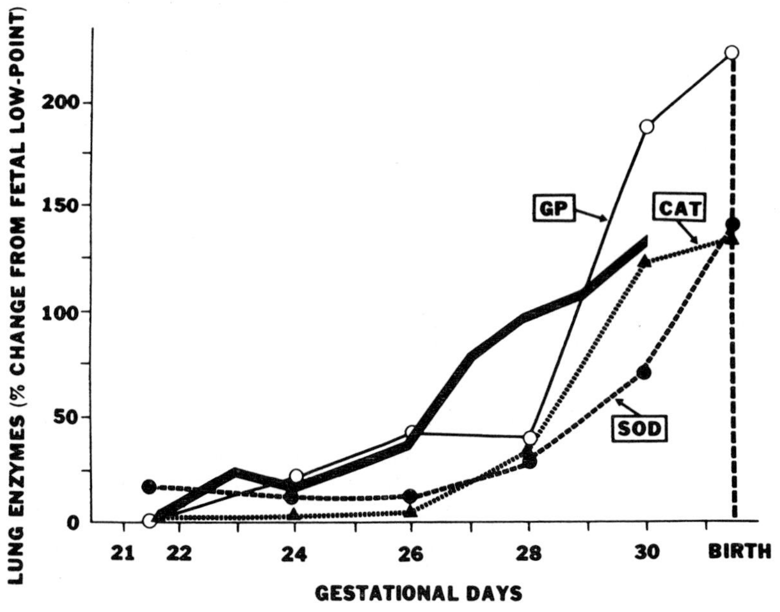

FIG. 30–1. Developmental changes in antioxidant levels and activity during gestation. The increases in superoxide dismutase (SOD), catalase (CAT), and glutathione peroxidase (GP) late in gestation are similar to those seen for pulmonary surfactant (*dark, thick line*). (From Frank L, Groseclose EE. Preparation for birth into an O_2 rich environment: the antioxidant enzymes in the developing rabbit lung. Pediatr Res 1984;18:240.)

To better understand the role of oxidant injury, it is important to understand the inflammatory response that it initiates. Oxygen radicals may first stimulate the inflammatory process. After the process is underway, more radicals can be generated by several reactions within the inflammatory cascade, thereby accelerating the damage by providing another source of these potentially dangerous molecules.

INFLAMMATION

Inflammation appears to play an important role in the pathogenesis of BPD and allows many factors to be unified into a single cause of this disease. Inflammatory mediators and cellular responses are outlined in Figure 30-2, and they have been found to be prominent in animal models of lung injury and in infants who develop BPD.

Bronchopulmonary dysplasia appears to begin as a cascade of destruction and abnormal repair that results in acute lung injury, which is followed by the development of chronic lung disease. The initial stimulus activating the inflammatory process in the lung may be free radicals secondary to oxygen therapy, pulmonary barotrauma, infectious agents, or other stimuli that result in the attraction and activation of leukocytes. This leukocyte infiltration appears to occur before the development of significant pathophysiologic abnormalities and has been demonstrated by tagging leukocytes with indium-111 and by inspection of tracheobronchial effluent and bronchoalveolar lavage.[30–32] Activated leukocytes are predominantly neutrophils and macrophages, both of which have the potential for further release of a variety of inflammatory mediators.[32–34]

Among the toxic products released are the lipid products from plasma membranes that are metabolized predominantly to arachidonic acid and lysoplatelet activating factor (see Fig. 30-2). Arachidonic acid may be catalyzed by lipoxygenase, giving rise to the eicosanoids (*i.e.*, cytokines) and leukotrienes. Alternatively, it may be altered by cyclooxygenase to produce thromboxane, prostaglandin, or prostacyclin. These products have potent vasoactive and inflammatory properties that have been seen in BPD. Stenmark and others have documented the presence of leukotriene B_4, platelet activating factor, thromboxane, and prostacyclin in tracheal aspirates of patients with BPD.[34,35] These agents and the activated leukocytes that accompany them cause significant pulmonary damage, including breakdown of capillary endothelial integrity and leakage of larger molecules (*e.g.*, albumin) into alveolar spaces. Albumin leakage and associated pulmonary edema have been postulated to be major factors in the development of BPD.[36] It appears that pulmonary edema may occur secondary to the inflammatory process rather than acting as a primary cause of BPD, as was originally suggested.

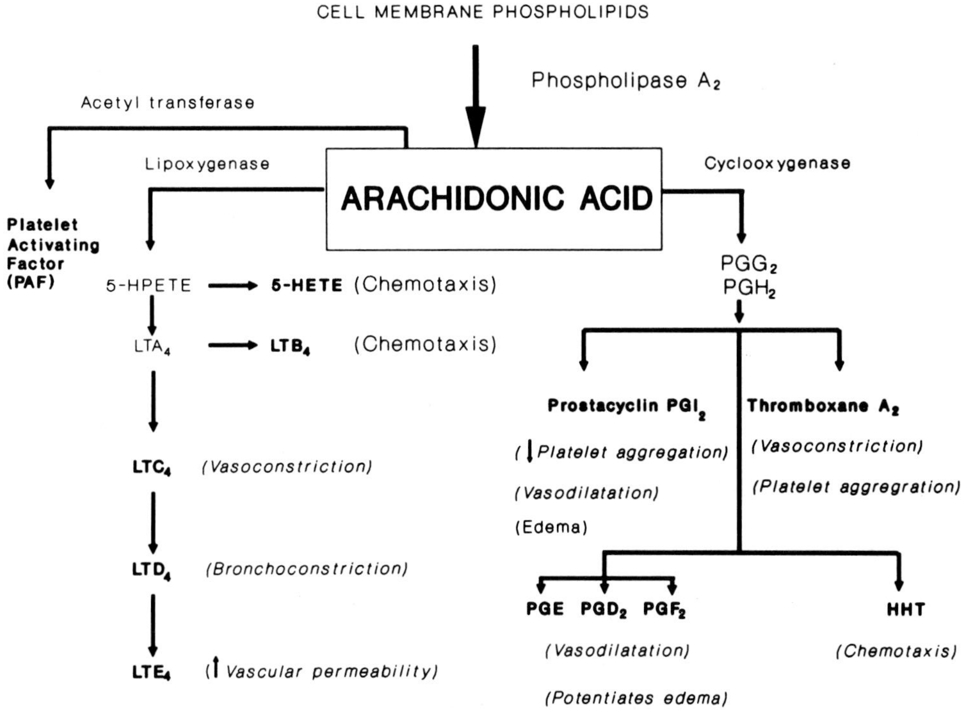

FIG. 30–2. Schematic representation of the metabolism of cell membrane lipids to arachidonic acid, which initiates the inflammatory cascade. The various metabolic pathways are shown with the agents that are produced and their function in the inflammatory process. (HETE, hydroxyeicosatetraenoic acid; HHT, heptadacatrienoic acid; HPETE, hydroxyperoxyeicosatraenoic acid; LT, leukotriene; PG, prostaglandin.)

The release of elastase and collagenase from activated neutrophils directly destroys the elastin and collagen framework of the lung. The breakdown products of collagen (*i.e.*, hydroxyproline) and elastin (*i.e.*, desmosine) have been recovered in the urine of infants who develop BPD.[37] The major defense against the action of elastase activity is α_1-proteinase inhibitor, which may be inactivated by oxygen radicals.[38] Increased elastase activity accompanied by compromised antiproteinase function may result in an imbalance of elastase and antiproteinase and enhance lung injury.[39] This imbalance has been demonstrated in tracheal aspirates and serum of neonates who develop BPD.[32,40,41]

As the acute cycle of injury continues with further production and accumulation of inflammatory mediators, significant injury to the lung can occur during a particularly critical period of rapid growth (*i.e.*, the six divisions from 24 to 40 weeks of gestation). It appears likely that this abnormal inflammatory process is primarily responsible for the acute and the chronic changes that occur in the lungs of infants with BPD. Additional evidence implicating the inflammatory process in BPD involves therapeutic interventions with antiinflammatory agents such as dexamethasone. Dexamethasone treatment interferes with the inflammatory process and is associated with significant improvements in clinical status and pulmonary mechanics.[42,43]

INFECTION

Ureaplasma urealyticum has been recovered from 44% of cervical cultures of pregnant women and implicated as a possible cause of chorioamnionitis, prematurity, and BPD.[44,45] Several studies have suggested a possible association between colonization with *Ureaplasma* and the development of BPD. Cassell and colleagues cultured tracheal aspirates and blood and found that BPD developed in 82% of infants (<1000 g) colonized with *Ureaplasma*, compared with 41% of those with negative cultures.[45] In animal studies, they were able to produce pneumonia in mice inoculated with *Ureaplasma*.[45] They postulated that chronic low-grade infection may result in the continued need for oxygen and ventilatory support. Others have suggested that infection acts as a stimulus for the inflammatory response, with recruitment of leukocytes and activation of the arachidonic cascade, ultimately leading to BPD.[46] Normal defense mechanisms against infection can be compromised in the lungs of chronically ventilated, premature infants. This makes them more susceptible to colonization and subsequent infection with a variety of infectious agents (*e.g.*, virus, bacteria, fungi) that may affect the severity of BPD.

NUTRITION

The nutritional status of the sick premature infant may play several roles in the development of BPD. Adequate calories and essential nutrients for growth may be lacking during a period of stress and growth; vital components for immunologic and antioxidant defenses may be inadequate; and the nutritional supplements provided may actually contribute to ongoing damage.

Premature infants have increased nutritional requirements because of increased metabolic needs and rapid growth requirements. Superimposed acute and chronic lung disease may further increase energy expenditures by 25% (*i.e.*, increased work of breathing) in infants with limited nutritional reserves.[47] If these increased energy needs are not met by exogenous sources, the infant will develop a catabolic state, which is probably a major contributing factor in the pathogenesis of BPD.[48] Inadequate nutrition, which could interfere with normal growth and maturation of the lung, may potentiate the deleterious effects of oxygen and barotrauma. Newborn rats with inadequate caloric intake have decreased lung weights, protein levels, and DNA content.[48] These abnormalities were even greater in pups who were nutritionally deprived at birth and exposed to hyperoxia.

Antioxidant enzymes may play a vital role in the protection of the lung and the prevention of BPD. Many of these enzymes have trace elements (*e.g.*, copper, zinc, selenium) that are an integral part of their structure. Deficiencies in these elements may compromise the premature infant's defenses and predispose the lung to further injury. Supplementation with these elements may provide protection to the lung and prevent hyperoxic lung injury.[49] The repair of elastin and collagen is limited in animals who are undernourished, and copper and zinc may be necessary for this repair.[50]

Vitamin deficiency has been postulated to be important in the development of BPD. Increasing serum levels of vitamin E, a natural antioxidant that prevents peroxidation of lipid membranes, was initially thought to prevent BPD.[51] However, data supporting this hypothesis came from a study in which infants were fed with vitamin E-deficient formulas. A second study in which control formulas contained minimal levels of vitamin E was unable to demonstrate any beneficial effects from additional vitamin E supplementation.[52] Some studies have demonstrated that vitamin E-deficient animals were more susceptible to lung damage and were protected by supplemental vitamin E administration.[53,54] Subsequent clinical trials have been unable to demonstrate any positive effect of supraphysiologic concentrations of vitamin E in the prevention of chronic lung disease.[55–57] Current nursery feeding and hyperalimentation regimens appear to provide adequate amounts of vitamin E for preterm and term infants.

Many vitamin E studies have measured polyunsaturated fatty acid (PUFA) concentrations in formula feedings. Infants fed formulas low in vitamin E, high in PUFA, or with a low vitamin E-to-PUFA ratio were more susceptible to developing BPD.[57] These researchers postulated that PUFAs were highly susceptible to lipid peroxidation by free radicals and might be a potential source of toxic products from oxidation. An opposing theory was proposed by Sosenko, who postulated that PUFAs may provide a sink for free radicals that could prevent injury in the lung.[58] Newborn rats fed diets high in PUFA (*e.g.*, safflower) and exposed to prolonged hyperoxia had a 60% higher survival rate at 7 days of age than the untreated animals. The role of these fatty acids in protecting the lung from hyperoxic lung injury and preventing BPD require further investigation.

Concentrations of vitamin A (*i.e.*, retinol) may be deficient in premature neonates younger than 36 weeks of gestation.[59–61] This vitamin appears to be important in maintaining cell integrity and in tissue repair. Its deficiency has been associated with changes in the ciliated epithelium of the tracheobronchial tree.[62] Hustead and associates demonstrated lower serum retinol levels in cord blood and at day 21 of life in infants who developed BPD.[61] Shenai and colleagues demonstrated lower plasma retinol concentrations in the first month of life in infants who subsequently developed BPD.[63] Despite adequate supplementation, some infants remain vitamin A deficient, presumably from increased absorption of parenteral vitamin A into the tubing of the intravenous administration set or due to higher nutritional requirements.[64]

Large volumes of intravenous fluids are often administered to premature infants to provide adequate fluid requirements (due to increased insensible water losses) and sufficient calories. An increased incidence of patent ductus arteriosus and BPD has been associated with excessive fluid administration.[65] Early closure of the ductus, using indomethacin or surgical ligation, has been associated with improvements in pulmonary function, but these approaches have not affected the incidence of chronic lung disease.[66] Van Marter reported that BPD was more likely to occur if neonates had received greater fluid volumes in the first days of life.[67] Excessive fluid may cause edema in an injured lung and increase oxygen and ventilator requirements and the subsequent risk of BPD.

GENETICS

Numerous investigators have observed that neonates were more likely to develop BPD if there was a strong family history of atopy and asthma. Nickerson and Taussig found a positive family history of asthma in 77% of infants with RDS who subsequently developed BPD, compared with only 33% who did not.[68] Bertrand evaluated the relation between prematurity, RDS, and need for mechanical ventilation to a family history of airway hyperactivity.[69] The severity of lung disease was directly related to the degree of prematurity and the duration of oxygen exposure. However, siblings and mothers of infants with the most significant lung disease had evidence of airway reactivity, suggesting that all three factors are involved in determining long-term outcome. When histocompatibility loci (HLA) were examined, Clark and associates found that only infants with HLA-A2 developed BPD, again suggesting that other underlying factors that are poorly understood may be important in the pathogenesis of BPD.[70]

PATHOPHYSIOLOGIC CHANGES

Infants with BPD demonstrate abnormal findings on clinical examination, chest radiograph, pulmonary function testing, echocardiogram, and morphologic examination of the lung. The severity of BPD is directly proportional to the degree of the pathophysiologic insult and can be assessed through all of these techniques. Determining the severity of BPD is complex and has been the subject of several workshops sponsored by the National Institutes of Health and many publications. Several scoring systems have been developed to address this important issue.

CLINICAL ASSESSMENT

A clinical scoring system to help evaluate the severity of BPD was developed by Toce and colleagues (Table 30-2).[71] Infants with BPD are tachypneic and may have intercostal and subcostal retractions. Accessory muscles may be used to assist with respiration. Infants can be hypoxic and hypercarbic and may grow poorly despite adequate caloric intake. The Toce system attempts to standardize clinical assessment, and a severity score can be assigned to each infant at 28 days of postnatal age and at 36 weeks of postconceptual age. The clinical assessment should be adjusted if infants are receiving multiple medications for their BPD (*e.g.*, diuretics, methylxanthines, and steroids), nasal continuous positive airway pressure, or positive-pressure mechanical ventilation.

RADIOGRAPHIC ABNORMALITIES

Radiographic abnormalities characteristic of BPD were first described by Northway and associates in 1967.[1] A staging system was employed that documented the progression of the disease process through four distinct stages. The first stage is similar to uncomplicated RDS and occurs in the first few days of life. The second stage is seen in the second week of life and involves pulmonary parenchymal opacity. Disease in this stage commonly appears as a diffuse, whited-out area associated with decreased lung volumes. It may be indistinguishable from diffuse pulmonary edema, congestive heart failure, patent ductus arteriosus, or fluid overload. During the third week of life, the diffuse haziness clears and is replaced by a bubbly appearance, as the infant enters stage III. Stage IV occurs after 1 month of life and is characterized by an inhomogeneous appearance associated with marked hyperinflation, bleb formation, irregular fibrous streaks, and cardiomegaly.

The radiographic progression of BPD is now seldom categorized by these four stages (Fig. 30-3). The

TABLE 30–2
BRONCHOPULMONARY DYSPLASIA CLINICAL SCORING SYSTEM

	Score*			
Variable	0 (Normal)	1 (Mild)	2 (Moderate)	3 (Severe)
Respiratory rate (average number/min)	<40	40–60	61–80	>80
Dyspnea (retractions)	0	Mild	Moderate	Severe
FiO_2 (PaO_2 50–70 torr)	0.21	0.22–0.30	0.31–0.50	>0.50
$PaCO_2$ (torr)	<45	46–55	56–70	>70
Growth rate (g/d)	>25	15–24	5–14	<5

* Score at 28 days of age or at 36 weeks postconceptual age. Score is a mean of four measures for respiratory rate, dyspnea, and FiO_2 obtained at 6-hour intervals. Growth rate represents average daily weight gain over a 7-day period before the assignment of the score. Highest score is 15. A score of 15 is assigned if the patient is receiving mechanical ventilation.

From Toce SS, Farrell PM, Leavitt LA, Samuels DP, Edwards DK. Clinical and radiographic scoring systems for assessing bronchopulmonary dysplasia. Am J Dis Child 1984;138:581.

radiographic classification of BPD was refined by Edwards and colleagues and then by Toce and associates to reflect the severity of the disease process (Table 30-3).[71,72] The system is based on the four most prominent radiographic findings in BPD, including lung expansion, emphysema (including bleb formation), interstitial densities, and cardiovascular abnormalities. The more severe the changes, the higher is the score, with a maximum possible score of 10. The occurrence of hyperinflation or interstitial abnormalities on chest radiograph appears to correlate well with the development of airway obstruction later in life.[73]

Computed tomography and magnetic resonance imaging may provide more detail of the pathologic process occurring in the lung. Computed tomography can reveal significant abnormalities that are not readily apparent on chest radiographs and can be important in determining ultimate pulmonary morbidity (Fig. 30-4).[74]

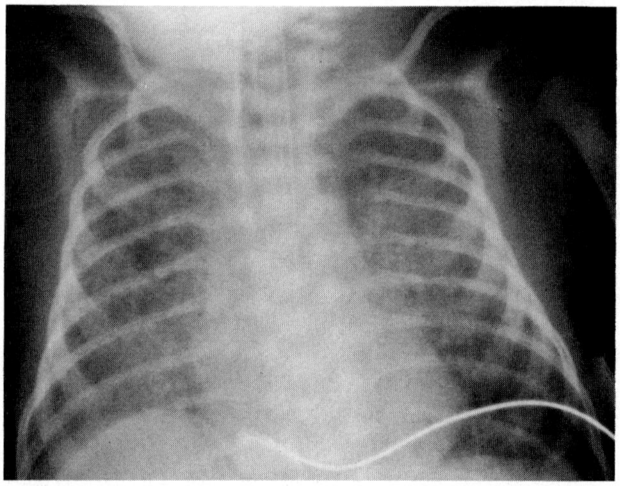

FIG. 30–3. Typical chest radiograph of a 1-month-old infant with bronchopulmonary dysplasia. The bilateral hazy appearance represents inflammatory exudate, edema, and atelectasis.

CARDIOVASCULAR CHANGES

The pulmonary circulation in infants with BPD can be abnormal, with endothelial cell degeneration and proliferation, medial muscle hypertrophy, peripheral extension of smooth muscle, and vascular obliteration.[75] These lesions are more significant in older infants dying of severe BPD. The vascular alterations lead to increased pulmonary vascular pressures and pulmonary vascular resistance with the development of cor pulmonale. Serial electrocardiograms may reveal evidence of right ventricular hypertrophy (*i.e.*, indirect evidence of pulmonary hypertension).[76] Echocardiograms may show elevated right ventricular systolic time intervals (RSTI) or, in more severe cases, left ventricular and septal wall thickening consistent with concentric left ventricular hypertrophy.[77] Cardiac catheterization may reveal elevated pulmonary vascular resistance and pulmonary vascular pressures.[78] Persistent right ventricular hypertrophy, elevated RSTI, or fixed pulmonary hypertension unresponsive to O_2 supplementation on cardiac catheterization have been associated with a poor prognosis.[78]

CHANGES IN PULMONARY MECHANICS

The development of computerized pulmonary function systems has enabled more accurate measurements of pulmonary mechanics in newborn infants with BPD. In the early stages of BPD, an increase in pulmonary resistance and airway reactivity can be demonstrated.[79] As the disease progresses in severity, airway obstruction can become more significant, with expiratory flow limitation seen on flow–volume

TABLE 30–3
ROENTGENOGRAPHIC SCORING SYSTEM FOR SEVERITY OF BRONCHOPULMONARY DYSPLASIA

	Score*		
Variable	0	1	2
Cardiovascular abnormalities	None	Cardiomegaly	Gross cardiomegaly or RVH or enlarged MPA
Hyperexpansion (anterior plus posterior rib count)	≤14	14.5–16	≤16.5, or flattened hemidiaphragms
Emphysema	No focal areas	Scattered, small, abnormal lucencies	≥1 Large bleds or bullae
Fibrosis or interstitial abnormalities	None	Interstitial prominence; few abnormal, streaky densities	Dense fibrotic bands, many abnormal strands
Subjective	Mild	Moderate	Severe

* Rib counts intersecting level of the dome of the right hemidiaphragm.
MPA, main pulmonary artery; RVH, right ventricular hypertrophy.
From Toce SS, Farrell PM, Leavitt LA, Samuels DP, Edwards DK. Clinical and radiographic scoring systems for assessing bronchopulmonary dysplasia. Am J Dis Child 1984;138:581.

curves (Fig. 30-5).[80] Airway constriction can occur secondary to hypoxia and can be demonstrated with cold air provocation testing.[81] The increased resistance may cause increased work of breathing and marked abnormalities in ventilation–perfusion matching. Functional residual capacity can be reduced initially because of atelectasis, but it can be elevated in later stages of BPD because of excessive air trapping and hyperinflation.

Two methods used to measure lung compliance include dynamic measurement and passive expiratory techniques after airway occlusion.[82] Both methods show a reduction of lung compliance in infants with BPD. The decrease in lung compliance appears to correlate well with morphologic changes in the lung (*e.g.*, atelectasis, edema, fibrosis). Compliance can be reduced because of increased resistance, with frequency dependence of compliance when infants are breathing rapidly.[83]

The use of pulmonary function testing to follow the progression of BPD and the response of the lung to various therapeutic interventions has become widespread, but care must be used in the interpretation of results because of inherent variability in the measurement and possible error from excessive chest wall distortion.[84–86]

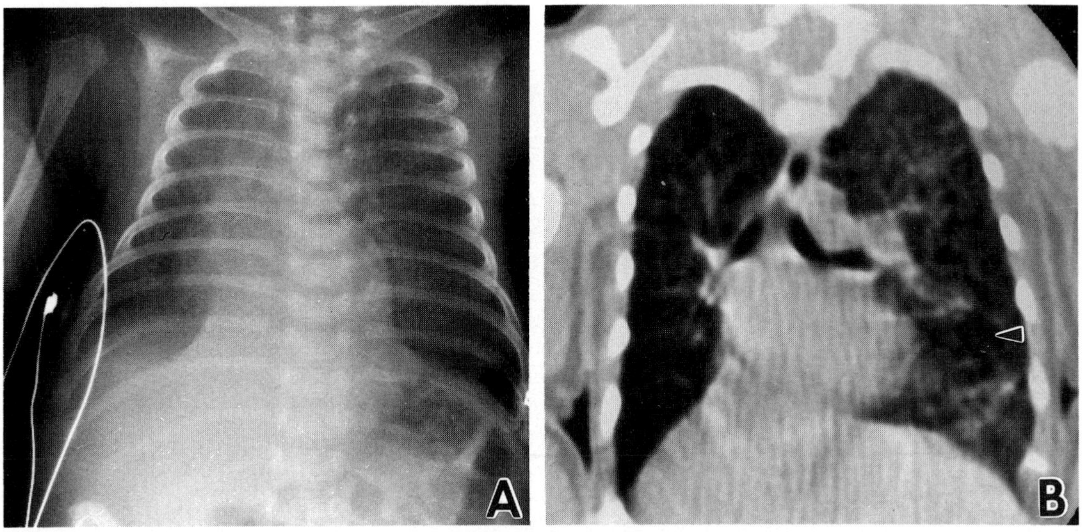

FIG. 30–4. **(A)** Chest radiograph of a 2-month-old infant with bronchopulmonary dysplasia, shows right- sided atelectasis and a shift of the mediastinum. The lung fields have a hazy appearance. **(B)** Computed tomography scan on the same infant. The major bronchi and areas of atelectasis are apparent. Fibrotic changes and a bleb are seen on the left (*arrow*).

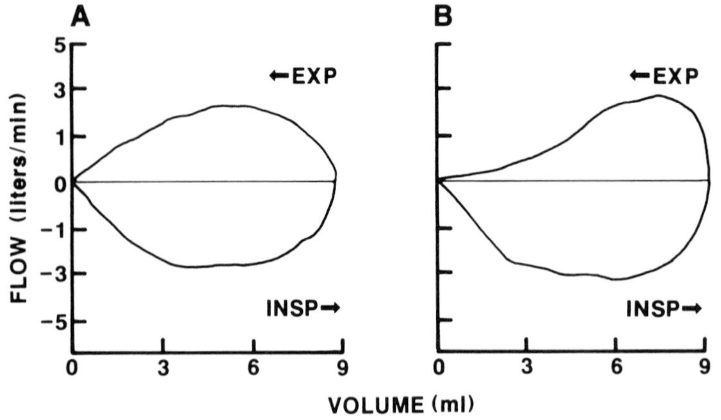

FIG. 30–5. **(A)** Normal flow–volume loop. **(B)** Expiratory flow limitation due to dynamic collapse of small airways during expiration. (INSP, inspiration; EXP, expiration.)

PATHOLOGIC CHANGES

AIRWAYS

The large upper airways (*i.e.*, trachea, main bronchi) of infants with BPD may reveal significant abnormalities, depending on the duration of intubation and positive-pressure ventilation. Grossly, mucosal edema or necrosis can be seen and may be focal or more diffuse.[87] Necrotic areas may break down into frank ulcerations. Many of these changes are similar to those seen in necrotizing tracheobronchitis. The earliest histologic changes include patchy loss of cilia from columnar epithelial cells. These cells may become dysplastic or necrotic, resulting in breakdown of the epithelial lining. Necrotic areas may involve the mucosa alone or extend into the submucosa. Infiltration of inflammatory cells such as neutrophils and lymphocytes into these areas may be prominent. Goblet cells may become hyperplastic, resulting in increased mucous production, which becomes mixed with dense cellular debris. Granulation tissue may develop in areas that have been damaged by the presence of the endotracheal tube or from repeated suctioning procedures. Mucosal cells may regenerate or ultimately be replaced by stratified squamous epithelium or metaplastic epithelium if the injury process continues (Fig. 30-6).

The most significant pathologic changes occurring in infants with BPD are seen in the terminal bronchioles and alveolar ducts. Hyaline membranes that appear during the acute phase of RDS become covered with a thin, dysplastic epithelial lining made up primarily of type II pneumocytes. These membranes may then become incorporated into the underlying airway. Edema, inflammation, exudate, and necrosis of epithelial cells can occur as the process continues. Necrotizing bronchiolitis may occur if the damage is

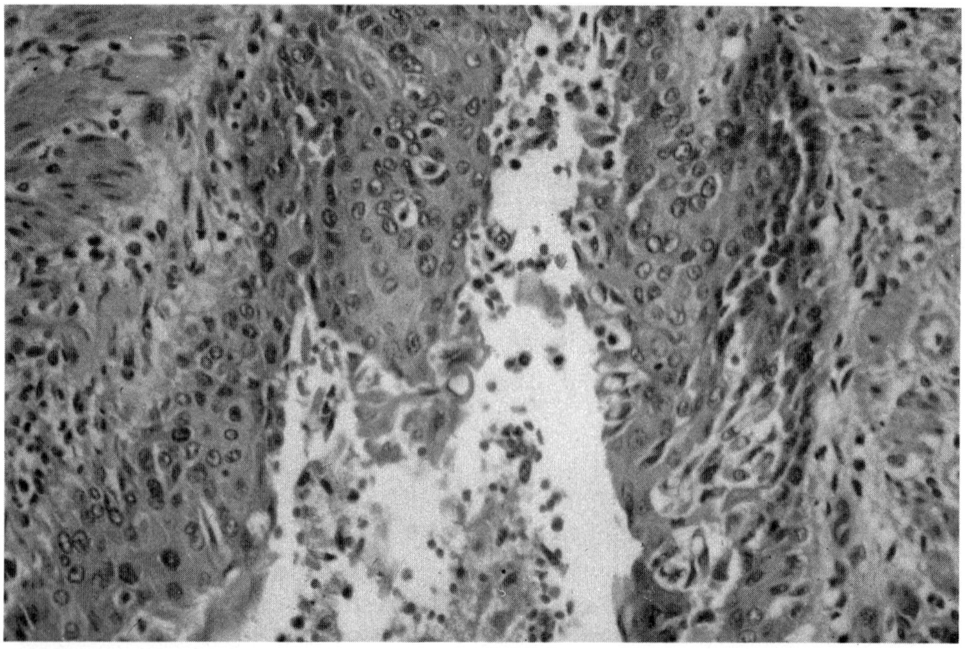

FIG. 30–6. Light micrograph from a 3-month-old infant with bronchopulmonary dysplasia shows squamous metaplasia and smooth muscle hypertrophy of a small airway. (Original magnification × 20.)

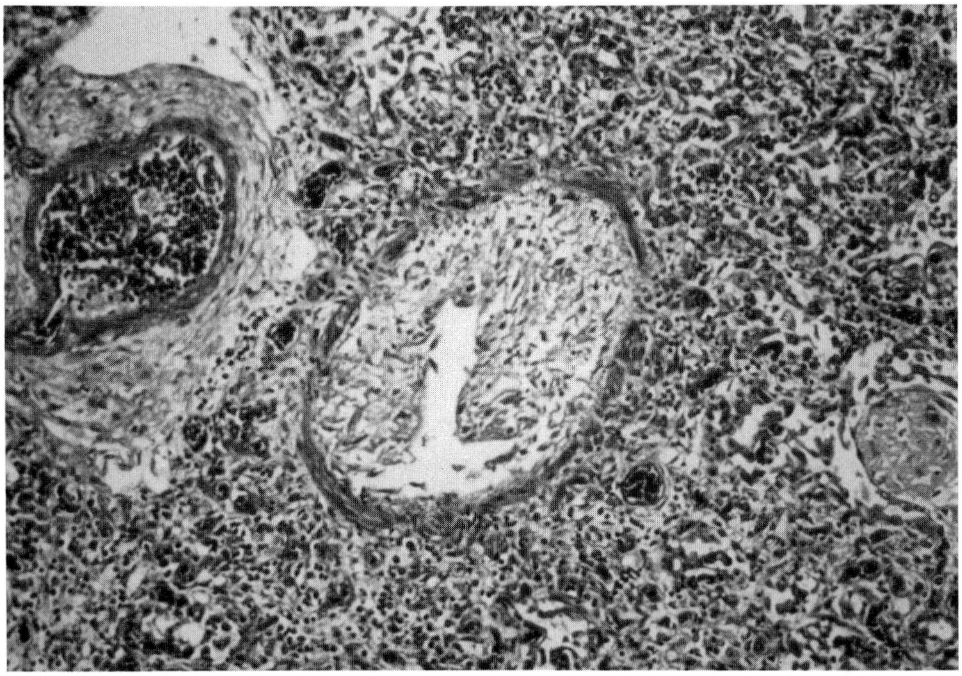

FIG. 30–7. Light micrograph from a 1-month-old infant with bronchopulmonary dysplasia, shows fibrosis of a small airway. (Connective tissue stain; original magnification × 10.)

particularly severe. Cellular debris, inflammatory cells, and proteinaceous exudate accumulate and obstruct many of the terminal airways; this process may actually be beneficial because it protects the distal alveoli from further damage from oxygen and mechanical ventilation. Fibroblast proliferation and activation in response to this insult may lead to peribronchial fibrosis and obliterative fibroproliferative bronchiolitis (Fig. 30-7). This causes narrowing of some small airways and further obstruction in others.

ALVEOLI

The earliest findings seen in the alveoli involve interstitial or alveolar edema. Focal areas of atelectasis, inflammation, exudate, and fibroblast proliferation develop later. As the disease progresses and becomes more severe, areas of atelectasis become more widespread and alternate with areas of marked hyperinflation (Fig. 30-8). These hyperinflated areas can become emphysematous blebs. Interstitial and alveolar fibrosis can become more widespread. Capillary beds can be severely damaged and, with medial muscle hypertrophy of pulmonary arterioles, these changes lead to marked pulmonary hypertension.

MANAGEMENT

The current approach to infants with BPD is multidisciplinary and directed toward improving the complex pathophysiologic abnormalities that have been previously described. The major treatment approaches are described in the following sections.

MECHANICAL VENTILATION

Positive-pressure mechanical ventilation has been implicated in the pathogenesis of BPD, but the benefits from continued ventilation outweigh the risks of continued progression of chronic lung damage. Arterial blood gases should be optimally maintained with a *p*H of 7.25 to 7.40, PCO_2 of 45 to 60 torr, and PO_2 of 55 to 70 torr.[88] The best method of assessing adequate oxygenation and ventilation is an arterial blood gas obtained from an indwelling arterial catheter when the infant is quiet. Intermittent arterial puncture may be accurate if obtained quickly or if local anesthesia is used, but it may not be representative if the infant is awake and agitated. Capillary blood gases should not be used to make significant therapeutic decisions because of wide variability and poor correlation with arterial blood gases.[89] However, if obtained properly (*i.e.*, after adequate warming and without squeezing the heel or finger), the *p*H and PCO_2 may correlate with arterial values. The use of pulse oximetry and transcutaneous CO_2 measurements can assist in ventilatory management and may reflect arterial values. End-tidal CO_2 measurements may not correlate well with arterial values in infants with significant ventilation–perfusion mismatch and chronic lung disease.

Because oxygen appears to cause more significant lung damage than mechanical ventilation in animals, sufficient mean airway pressure should be used to avoid atelectasis and if possible, maintain the fraction of inspired oxygen (FiO_2) at less than 0.5.[19] An inspiratory time of 0.5 to 0.6 seconds optimizes ventilation and improves pulmonary function.[90] Inspired gas

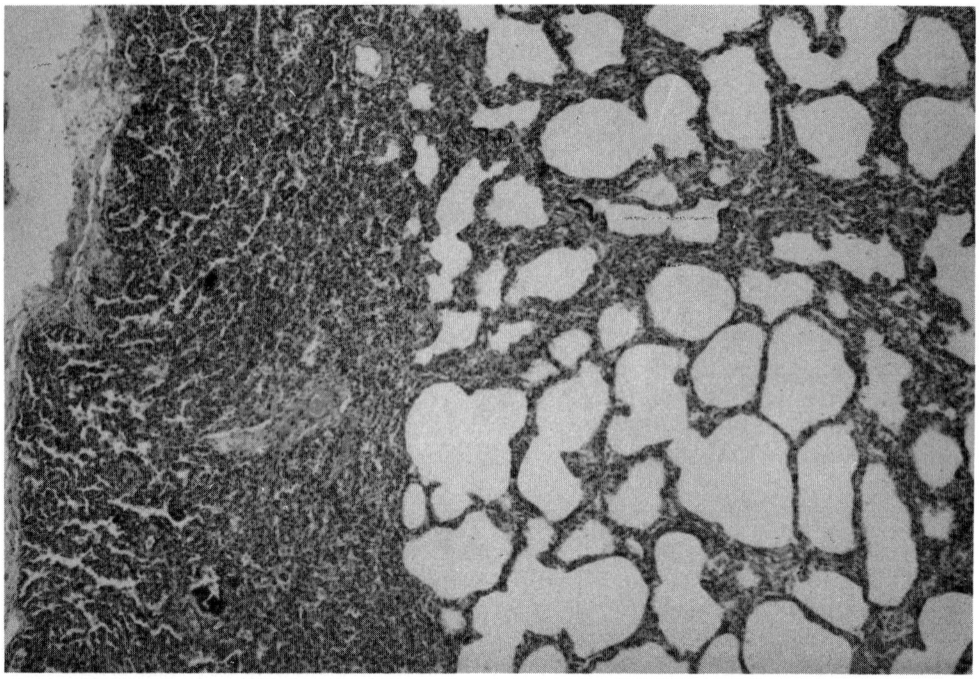

FIG. 30–8. Light micrograph from a 1-year-old infant with bronchopulmonary dysplasia, shows areas of atelectasis alternating with areas of hyperinflation. (Original magnification × 4.)

temperature should be maintained from 36.5°C to 37.5°C to ensure adequate humidity and minimize core temperature fluctuations and the progression of chronic lung disease.[91]

Weaning infants with BPD from mechanical ventilation is often difficult and should be done slowly. When peak inspiratory pressures have been reduced to approximately 20 cm H_2O and FiO_2 to less than 0.5 with acceptable blood gases, the ventilator rate should be reduced slowly to allow the infant to gradually breathe more independently. This is essential, because prolonged ventilation may be associated with atrophy of the muscle fibers of the diaphragm and increased diaphragmatic fatigue.[92] When infants have been weaned to a ventilator rate of 5 to 15 breaths per minute, infants should be extubated. The use of synchronized mechanical ventilation may reduce the work of breathing and facilitate weaning from mechanical ventilation. Analysis of pulmonary mechanics before extubation does not appear to be useful in determining optimal time of extubation because multiple factors (*e.g.*, central inspiratory drive, diaphragmatic endurance, chest wall stability) may be important.[93] Infants should not be weaned to continuous endotracheal tube positive airway pressure (CPAP), because increased airway resistance and work of breathing can cause fatigue, apnea, and CO_2 retention.[94] The use of methylxanthines before extubation or nasal CPAP just after extubation may facilitate successful extubation.[95,96] Higgins and colleagues demonstrated that infants weighing less than 1000 g were almost four times as likely to be successfully extubated on the first attempt when nasal CPAP was used compared with an oxyhood (76% *versus* 21%).[96] Chest physiotherapy and suctioning should be performed frequently to maintain a patent airway and prevent atelectasis.

Prolonged intubation and ventilation may be associated with the development of airway abnormalities (*e.g.*, subglottic stenosis, tracheomalacia).[97] These should be considered in infants who rapidly and repeatedly fail attempts at extubation. A bronchoscopic evaluation should be performed in these infants or in any infant intubated for more than 2 to 3 months who continues to require prolonged ventilation. Surgical intervention (*e.g.*, cricoid split, tracheostomy) should be performed as needed.

OXYGEN

In infants with BPD, chronic hypoxia results in pulmonary vasoconstriction, pulmonary hypertension, and the development of cor pulmonale. This contributes significantly to the morbidity and mortality of BPD. Elevated pulmonary artery pressures and pulmonary vascular resistance have been described in infants with BPD undergoing cardiac catheterization.[78,88,98] A significant reduction in pulmonary pressures were found when oxygen was administered, suggesting that oxygen acts as a pulmonary vasodilator. Ideally, PO_2 should be maintained between 55 to 70 torr and oxygen saturation (SO_2), as determined by pulse oximetry, between 90% and 95% in infants with BPD.

Pulse oximetry has become increasingly popular as a noninvasive method of neonatal oxygen monitoring. Pulse oximeters are most accurate when operating along the steep portion of the oxygen–hemoglobin dissociation curve and may be more reliable than PO_2.[99] Keeping the SO_2 between 90% to 95% should exclude values of PO_2 that are less than 45 torr and greater than 100 torr. Careful monitoring of oxygen status is essential, because hypoxia can cause pulmonary hypertension, increased airway constriction, and growth failure. Hyperoxia may worsen BPD or increase the risk of retinopathy of prematurity.[100] Oxygen can be administered through an endotracheal tube, hood, tent, or nasal cannula. Increased FiO_2 may be needed during periods of increased stress (*e.g.*, during feedings). Oxygen should be withdrawn gradually and may be required for months or years. Many infants are discharged from the neonatal intensive care unit and receive oxygen at home.

The use of booster transfusions to increase oxygen-carrying capacity in infants with BPD is controversial. Traditionally, hemoglobin is maintained from 12 to 15 mg/dL in oxygen-dependent infants with BPD. Alverson and associates demonstrated significant increases in oxygen content and systemic oxygen transport and decreases in oxygen consumption and oxygen use in infants with BPD after booster blood transfusion.[101] However, hemoglobin levels did not appear to correlate well with systemic oxygen transport and did not predict which infants would benefit physiologically from transfusion. Stefano and colleagues demonstrated a significant deterioration in pulmonary mechanics after booster transfusion in infants with BPD that was moderated by the use of furosemide.[102] The need for booster transfusion may be eliminated in the future if the development of human recombinant erythropoietin therapy is successful.[103]

NUTRITION

Because infants with BPD have increased metabolic demands, calories must be maximized to support tissue repair and growth. Enteral feedings with fortified breast milk or with premature formulas provide the best source of calories. Feedings should be given by intermittent or continuous gavage until the infant can be fed orally. Feedings can be concentrated to increase caloric density or glucose polymers (*i.e.*, polycose) and medium-chain triglycerides can be added to provide optimal calories while minimizing fluid intake. Infants may require 120 to 140 calories per 1 kg of body weight each day to gain weight (10–30 g/day). If fluid restriction interferes with the administration of adequate calories, a diuretic can be used to prevent fluid overload.

Intravenous nutrition should be started early to provide adequate sources of protein, fat, and carbohydrates. This may affect the ultimate outcome and severity of BPD, especially in the very-low-birth-weight infants. The early use of percutaneous Silastic central catheters has greatly enhanced the ability to provide more optimal calories to low-birth-weight infants.[104] Progressive increases in intravenous protein (*i.e.*, amino acid) concentrations should optimally provide 2.0 to 3.0 g of protein per 1 kg each day. The acid–base status of the infant should be monitored, because acid loads may not be well tolerated. Intravenous lipids (20% suspension) should be administered as a continuous infusion over 20 to 24 hours. Up to 3 g of lipids per 1 kg each day can be safely infused if serum triglyceride levels are closely followed. However, early administration of lipids may be associated with pulmonary vascular lipid deposition, hypoxia, and more severe BPD.[105] Intravenous glucose is a good source of calories, but excessive loads (>4 mg/kg/minute) may result in increased oxygen consumption, CO_2 production, and resting energy expenditures in infants with BPD.[106]

Adequate calcium and phosphorus intake is necessary, especially in infants receiving furosemide, to promote bone mineralization and prevent secondary hyperparathyroidism and rickets. Vitamins and trace metals should also be supplemented. Many premature infants are deficient in vitamin A, and adequate supplementation may promote tissue regeneration and growth in the lung and decrease the incidence and severity of BPD.[73] Physiologic or supraphysiologic doses of vitamin E do not appear to influence the course of BPD. Other investigators have not been able to demonstrate any beneficial effects of a combination of supplemental vitamins A and E for the prevention or treatment of infants with BPD.[107] Trace metals such as copper, zinc, and selenium are essential for the structure and function of antioxidant enzymes and should be provided.

MEDICATIONS

Many different types of drug therapies are used, often concurrently, to improve the clinical status of infants with BPD. The exact dosages, efficacy, mechanisms of action, pharmacokinetics, and side-effects have not been well established. The following sections update and summarize a previously published extensive review.[108]

DIURETICS

Furosemide (Lasix) is the treatment of choice for fluid overload in infants with BPD. It acts on the ascending loop of Henle and blocks chloride transport. Furosemide increases plasma oncotic pressure and lymphatic flow and decreases interstitial edema and pulmonary vascular resistance.[108,109] Several studies demonstrated that daily or alternate-day furosemide improves clinical respiratory status and pulmonary mechanics and facilitates weaning from mechanical ventilation in infants with BPD.[110–112] Side-effects include volume depletion, contraction alkalosis, hyponatremia, hypokalemia, chloride depletion, renal calculi secondary to hypercalcuria, cholelithiasis, osteopenia, and ototoxicity.[108] Supplemental potassium chloride is usually needed to prevent electrolyte depletion, but sodium chloride supplements should be avoided if possible. Long-term efficacy has not been determined.

The thiazides affect renal tubular excretion of electrolytes, but they are less potent than furosemide.[113] Potassium and bicarbonate (but not calcium) excretion accompany the sodium and chloride excretion produced by the thiazides. For this reason, the thiazides are usually given in conjunction with spironolactone (Aldactone), which is a competitive inhibitor of aldosterone. Spironolactone is a relatively weak diuretic that causes increased sodium, chloride, and water excretion, while potassium is spared. In several randomized, controlled trials, the combination of a thiazide diuretic and spironolactone resulted in increased urine output and improvements in pulmonary mechanics in infants with moderate BPD.[114,115] In contrast, Engelhardt and associates found that this combination of agents increased urine output in a manner similar to that seen with furosemide but had no effect on gas exchange or pulmonary mechanics in a similar population of infants with BPD.[116] Side-effects of the combination of a thiazide with spironolactone include azotemia, hyperuricemia, hyponatremia, hyperkalemia or hypokalemia, hyperglycemia, and hypomagnesemia.[108] Long-term studies comparing furosemide with thiazide–spironolactone therapy in BPD need to be performed. Diuretic dosing is shown in Table 30-4.

INHALED AGENTS

Isoproterenol is the most potent of the sympathomimetic amines that act exclusively on β-receptors. The β_1-effects target the heart and are chronotropic and inotropic. The β_2-effects cause relaxation of smooth muscle in airways, presumably through mechanisms that increase cyclic AMP. Isoproterenol aerosolization has been shown to cause short-term improvements in airway resistance, but not in lung compliance, in infants with BPD.[117] The duration of action is short (*i.e.*, 1 hour) because of rapid metabolism by the liver catechol-O-methyl transferase system (COMT). Because isoproterenol is not a selective β_2-agonist, side-effects such as tachycardia, hypertension, and hyperglycemia are frequent. A specific β_2-agonist is preferable in the treatment of infants with BPD.

Albuterol is a specific β_2-agonist that has become increasingly popular in the treatment of infants with

TABLE 30–4
COMMONLY USED MEDICATIONS FOR BRONCHOPULMONARY DYSPLASIA

Medication	Dosage
Diuretics	
Furosemide	0.5–2.0 mg/kg/dose IV or PO bid (qd in infants <31 wk postconceptual age)
Chlorthiazide	5–20 mg/kg/dose IV or PO bid
Hydrochlorthiazide	1–2 mg/kg/dose PO bid
Spironolactone	1.5 mg/kg/dose PO bid
Inhaled Agents	
Albuterol	0.02–0.04 mL/kg/dose of a 0.5% solution diluted to 1–2 mL with half-normal or normal saline q 4–6 h
Metaproterenol	0.1–0.25 mL (5–12.5 mg) of a 5% solution diluted to 1–2 mL with half-normal or normal saline q 6 h
Isoetharine	0.1–0.25 mL (1–2.5 mg) of a 1% solution diluted to 1–2 mL with half-normal or normal saline q 4–6 h
Isoproterenol	0.1–0.25 mL (0.5–1.25 mg) of a 0.05% solution diluted to 1–2 mL with half-normal saline q 3–4 h
Atropine, ipratropium bromide	0.025–0.08 mg/kg diluted to 1.5–2.5 mL in half-normal or normal saline q 6 h; doses of ipratropium up to 0.176 mg may be used
Cromylyn sodium	20 mg by inhalation q 6–8 h
Systemic Agents	
Aminophylline (IV), theophylline (PO)	LD 5 mg/kg; MD 2 mg/kg/dose q 8–12 h; serum levels of 5–15 mg/L
Caffeine citrate	LD 20 mg/kg; MD 5 mg/kg IV or PO q 24 h
Terbutaline	SC 5 μg/kg q 4–6 h
Dexamethasone	0.5 mg/kg/day IV or PO q 12 h for 3 days, decrease to 0.3 mg/kg/day for 3 days, then taper 10%–20% every 3 days
Albuterol	0.15 mg/kg/dose PO q 8 h

LD, loading dose; MD, maintenance dose; SC, subcutaneous.

BPD. Albuterol aerosolization has been associated with acute improvements in pulmonary resistance and lung compliance secondary to bronchial smooth muscle relaxation.[18] These changes in pulmonary mechanics returned to baseline by 4 hours after administration. The use of albuterol in conjunction with a muscarinic antagonist (*e.g.*, ipratropium bromide) may be more effective than either agent alone.[119] Albuterol is longer acting because it is resistant to metabolism by the COMT system. Side-effects are infrequent, but they can be similar to those seen with isoproterenol use. Tolerance may develop with prolonged usage, and long-term efficacy remains to be established. Albuterol appears to be the inhaled agent of choice in the treatment of reversible bronchospasm in infants with BPD. Metaproterenol (Alupent) and isoetharine (Bronkosol) are two other aerosolized selective β_2-agonists used in the treatment of BPD. Studies using both agents have shown short-term improvements in gas exchange and pulmonary mechanics in infants with BPD.[120,121] These two agents appear to be less β_2-specific than albuterol and may cause more cardiovascular side-effects.

Atropine is a competitive inhibitor of acetylcholine. In the lung, atropine decreases mucous secretion and transport in large airways and causes significant bronchial smooth muscle relaxation.[119] Two studies demonstrated significant improvements in pulmonary mechanics with atropine in infants with moderate BPD.[122,123] Side-effects are frequent and include tachycardia, decreased intestinal motility, tremors, and excessive dryness of respiratory secretions. Ipratropium bromide is a related muscarinic antagonist that is a much more potent bronchodilator than atropine. In infants with BPD, ipratropium causes a significant improvement in pulmonary mechanics that is similar to that seen after treatment with albuterol.[118] The combination of ipratropium and a β-agonist such as albuterol may be more effective than either agent alone.[119,124] Because aerosolized ipratropium is so poorly absorbed, it has significantly fewer side-effects than atropine. Long-term efficacy needs to be established. A selective β_2-agent should initially be used in infants with BPD; ipratropium can be added if clinical improvement is not seen. Ipratropium can be used alone if significant side-effects from β-agents occur.

Cromolyn has no direct bronchodilating effect but can be used to prevent bronchospasm in infants with BPD. Cromolyn inhibits the release of inflammatory mediators from mast cells.[125] Limited studies have shown a reduction in inflammatory mediators from tracheobronchial aspirates of chronically ventilated infants with BPD who were treated with cromolyn.[126] After nebulization, 8% to 10% of the total cromolyn dose is absorbed from the lungs. The dosage may need to be adjusted in infants with significant hepatic or renal dysfunction. An inhaled β-agonist can be given in conjunction with cromolyn with no apparent increase in toxicity. Side-effects are infrequent and include congestion, joint swelling, and rash.[108] Further short- and long-term safety and efficacy studies need to be performed before routine use of cromolyn can be recommended. Inhaled bronchodilator dosing is shown in Table 30-4.

SYSTEMIC BRONCHODILATORS

The methylxanthines (*e.g.*, caffeine, theophylline) are routinely used to increase respiratory drive and reduce the frequency of apnea in infants with apnea of prematurity.[92] They are also used in the treatment of infants with BPD. Measurements of pulmonary mechanics in infants with BPD have shown that caffeine and theophylline can reduce pulmonary resistance and increase lung compliance, presumably through a direct bronchodilator action.[127,128] These agents act as mild diuretics and improve skeletal muscle and diaphragmatic contractility. This is particularly important in chronically ventilated infants who may develop diaphragmatic atrophy and fatigue. Improved skeletal muscle contractility may stabilize the chest wall and improve functional residual capacity.[129] These actions may facilitate successful weaning from mechanical ventilation. There may be a synergistic effect if theophylline and a diuretic are used concurrently.[115]

The half-life of theophylline is 30 to 40 hours in newborns, and theophylline is metabolized primarily to caffeine in the liver and excreted in the urine. Adverse reactions include gastrointestinal (*e.g.*, gastroesophageal reflux, diarrhea), central nervous system (*e.g.*, agitation, seizures), cardiovascular (*e.g.*, tachycardia, hypertension), and endocrine (*e.g.*, hyperglycemia) disturbances.[108] The half-life of caffeine may be as long as 100 hours. It is excreted unchanged in the urine. Side-effects of caffeine are similar to theophylline but are rarely encountered. Caffeine is a safer drug with a wider therapeutic index and fewer side-effects than theophylline and may be a more appropriate adjunct in the treatment of apnea and BPD in preterm infants. Long-term comparative studies are needed.

Two other systemic β_2-agonists that act as bronchodilators include terbutaline and albuterol. Sosulski and colleagues demonstrated that subcutaneous terbutaline was associated with significant short-term improvement in clinical status and pulmonary mechanics in ventilator-dependent infants with BPD.[130] Stefano and associates demonstrated a 15% reduction in pulmonary resistance in infants with BPD with the use of oral albuterol.[131] Subcutaneous terbutaline and oral albuterol appear to offer no significant advantage to caffeine or theophylline as a primary therapy, but they may be beneficial as an adjunct to the methylxanthines in infants with BPD. Further long-term comparative studies are needed.

CORTICOSTEROIDS

Corticosteroids are synthesized by the adrenal cortex and are composed of mineralocorticoids that affect fluid and electrolyte balance and glucocorticoids that affect the metabolism of many tissues and possess potent antiinflammatory properties.[132] Dexamethasone is a synthetic corticosteroid that has been used in the prevention and treatment of BPD. Dexamethasone is thought to be effective in BPD because of its multiple pharmacologic effects, which include the following:

- stabilization of cell and lysosomal membranes
- increase in serum vitamin A concentration and surfactant synthesis
- stimulation of antioxidant enzyme activity
- inhibition of leukotriene and prostaglandin synthesis
- decrease in polymorphonuclear leukocyte recruitment to the lung
- breakdown of granulocyte aggregates with improvements in pulmonary microcirculation
- reduction in pulmonary edema
- enhancement of β-adrenergic activity.[133–140]

In infants with RDS who are at high risk for developing BPD, early dexamethasone treatment improves pulmonary mechanics, promotes more rapid weaning from oxygen and mechanical ventilation, minimizes lung injury, and improves neurodevelopmental outcome.[141] In infants with documented BPD, dexamethasone treatment acutely reduces inflammatory markers in the tracheobronchial aspirates, improves pulmonary mechanics and clinical pulmonary status, and facilitates weaning from mechanical ventilation.[42,43,142,143] Dexamethasone administration did not significantly improve survival, duration of oxygen treatment, or total length of hospital stay in any of the studies of infants with BPD.

Dexamethasone has a relatively long half-life (*i.e.*, 36–72 hours) and concurrent phenobarbital or phenytoin treatment may affect drug metabolism. If the drug is not effective after 4 to 5 days, it should be discontinued. The drug should be tapered slowly (*i.e.*, suppression of hypothalamic–pituitary–adrenal axis function), and if clinical deterioration occurs during the tapering process, a return to slightly higher doses may be effective with a subsequently slower tapering process. Some studies have not noted significant side-effects associated with dexamethasone use, but others have described poor weight gain, hyperglycemia, hypertension, osteoporosis, gastric ulcers, and an increased risk of sepsis.[108] Systemic steroids should be reserved for ventilator-dependent infants with moderate-to-severe BPD who are resistant to more conventional treatments. The use of inhaled, nonabsorbable steroids such as beclomethasone may be more effective and have fewer side-effects when used in the prevention and treatment of BPD.

PULMONARY VASODILATORS

Nifedipine is a calcium channel blocker that reduces pulmonary vascular pressures in some infants with BPD. A single oral dose of 0.5 mg/kg reduces pulmonary vascular resistance and improves cardiac output in older infants with severe pulmonary artery hypertension associated with BPD.[144] The effects of nifedipine appear to be greater than those observed after administration of 95% oxygen. The magnitude of the hemodynamic response appears to correlate well with plasma concentrations.[145] Pharmacokinetic studies suggest that a dose of 0.5 mg/kg every 6 hours provides optimal reduction in pulmonary pressures while avoiding side-effects such as systemic hypotension and decreased cardiac contractility. Nifedipine should be used cautiously, because verapamil, which is a closely related agent, has caused cardiac decompensation when used in infants with supraventricular tachycardia.[146] Long-term studies need to evaluate the safety and efficacy of nifedipine in infants with BPD and pulmonary hypertension.

ANTIBIOTICS

Increasing evidence suggests that infection with *Ureaplasma urealyticum* may be important in the pathogenesis and progression of BPD.[44,147,148] Clinical trials are underway to evaluate early treatment with erythromycin as a means of reducing the incidence and severity of BPD. Cultures of tracheal secretions should be performed intermittently to determine the types of colonizing organisms in chronically ventilated infants. If infants develop respiratory decompensation due to possible infection (*i.e.*, abnormal chest radiographs and complete blood count, positive Gram stain or cultures), appropriate broad-spectrum antibiotics should be used initially, with more specific antibiotic coverage determined after the organisms are isolated. Exposure of these infants to multiple courses of broad-spectrum antibiotics may place them at higher risk for the development of invasive fungal infections.

PHYSICAL THERAPY

Physical therapy may help overcome various types of motor deficits.[149] Infants with RDS and BPD are at increased risk for subsequent gross motor, fine motor, or cognitive developmental delays. To optimize ventilation, these infants use neck extension and accessory muscles. This produces abnormal posture of the neck, scapula, shoulder, and trunk. Efforts to reduce this abnormal posture and normalize tone should be provided in conjunction with a physical therapist. Infants are first positioned in a more neutral alignment. This is followed by strengthening of neck and trunk muscles, and independent movements and exploration of the environment through infant stimulation techniques are performed. A pacifier is used to facilitate and strengthen the suck reflex, especially when the infant is able to tolerate gavage feedings. When infants are orally fed, coordination of breathing, sucking, and swallowing may be difficult. Positioning the infants in natural flexion and using mandibular compression and cheek and upper palate stimulation may be helpful. Nasal oxygen is often necessary to assist the infant in feeding without tiring.

At the time of discharge, a comprehensive home therapy program is implemented. Nursing needs, home physical, and occupational or speech therapy are ordered as necessary. Reevaluation at appropriate intervals is scheduled in a neonatal high-risk follow-up program, with emphasis on the possible need for a future early-intervention program. These treatment programs emphasize teaching parents specific handling, positioning, and stimulation techniques. Normalizing muscle tone and posture and stimulating desired patterns of movements are the goals of these therapies.

OUTCOME

Most neonates who develop BPD ultimately achieve normal lung function and thrive. However, this group of neonates is at higher risk of dying in the first year of life or developing significant long-term complications. During infancy, continued normal lung growth should result in slow improvement of pulmonary function and weaning from mechanical ventilation or oxygen therapy. Later in childhood, other respiratory problems (*e.g.*, reactive airway disease) and abnormal neurologic development are additional complications that may occur and require careful follow-up.

MORTALITY

In Northway's original group of 32 patients, only 13 survived the first month of life.[1] Nine (69%) of these survivors developed BPD, and 5 died within the first year of life. The remaining 4 infants with BPD had persistent respiratory abnormalities that resolved slowly over time. Infants with BPD in this series died primarily of pulmonary hypertension and cor pulmonale. In contrast to this 66% mortality rate, other studies have shown a marked increase in the number of infants surviving with BPD, with mortality rates dropping to 30% to 40%.[150,151] Davidson followed a group of infants weighing less than 2500 g who were treated from 1983 to 1985 and found a mortality rate of 39% for infants with BPD in the first month of life.[152] Infants with BPD who survived to 1 month of age had a significantly higher (30%) chance of dying in the first year of life than infants surviving without BPD. Causes of death included ventilatory failure (5 patients), apnea (3 patients), and sepsis (1 patient). Abman studied a group of 64 patients who required mechanical ventilation for more than 30 days and found that 11 infants (17%) died, 7 of whom had sudden and unexpected deaths in the hospital with no apparent cause.[153] This description of sudden death occurring in hospitalized patients was similar to other reports of an increased incidence of sudden infant death syndrome in infants with BPD.[154] Gibson reported that 7 (47%) of 15 patients in their study who required more than 6 months of ventilation died at a mean age of 11.5 months.[155] This suggested that infants chronically ventilated for treatment of moderate or severe BPD have a higher risk of dying in the first year of life. Several surfactant replacement studies have demonstrated significantly improved survival, even of infants who develop BPD. Phibbs found a 32% incidence of BPD in his surfactant treatment and control groups.[156] There were no deaths from BPD in the surfactant-treated group, but 3 infants (25%) died in the control group. Merritt found similar rates of moderate or severe BPD in placebo and surfactant groups (9%).[8] Surfactant replacement therapy was able to significantly reduce mortality, especially from pulmonary complications. This confirms the observation that BPD is generally less severe than seen in the presurfactant era and is associated with a better outcome if it does develop.

PULMONARY FUNCTION

Although pulmonary function in most survivors with BPD improves over time with continued lung growth and permits normal activity, abnormalities detected by pulmonary function testing may remain. Follow-up studies of children with BPD have shown increased airway resistance and reactivity, decreased lung compliance, ventilation–perfusion mismatch, and blood gas abnormalities (*e.g.*, increased PCO_2) that may continue into later years.[157,158] Blayney investigated patients with BPD at 7 and 10 years of age and found that, although lung growth had occurred normally, residual volumes were increased, and forced expiratory volumes and flow rates were reduced.[159] Fifty percent of these children had a history of wheezing, suggesting airway hyperactivity. Significant improvement in pulmonary function occurred from years 7 through 10, indicating that pulmonary abnormalities from BPD persist well into childhood and continue to improve slowly over time. Hakulinen found lower airway conductance and increased residual volumes in children who had BPD.[160] The most significant abnormalities were found in children who had clinical respiratory symptoms, especially early in their childhood (≤2 years of age).

The longest follow-up of patients was reported by Northway, who studied patients until they were 25 years of age.[161] Although appearing clinically well, patients with BPD had continued evidence of pulmonary dysfunction, including airway obstruction and hyperactivity detected on pulmonary function testing and hyperinflation seen on chest radiographs.

The frequency of respiratory symptoms is increased in long-term survivors with BPD. Twenty-three percent of Northway's young adults with a history of BPD had chronic respiratory symptoms.[161] None of the infants with BPD reported by Bader required hospitalization after their second birthdays, but 80% still had frequent wheezing or pneumonias at 10 years of age.[157] Hakulinen found an increased need for hospitalization due to pulmonary problems for the first 2 years of life for his BPD survivors, but at 6 to 9 years of age, none had evidence of wheezing or distress.[160] It appears that abnormal pulmonary function and distress are greatest in the first 2 years of life, and survival beyond that age, although associated with persistent abnormalities on pulmonary function testing, permits children to function at normal capacity.

CARDIAC FUNCTION

Cardiac failure was found by Northway to be a major cause of morbidity and mortality in infants in his original study.[1] Cor pulmonale was found in 56% of his survivors, resulting in death in each case. The findings of abnormal muscularization of small pulmonary arteries (from chronic hypoxia) has been consistently identified in infants with severe BPD and may contribute to pulmonary hypertension.[75] Supplementation with oxygen to alleviate pulmonary hypertension has become a mainstay of therapy, and failure to respond is a poor prognostic sign.[88,98] In Northway's long-term follow-up of 26 patients with BPD, only 1 had evidence of right ventricular hypertrophy, suggesting that long-term survival is much improved if cor pulmonale can be prevented in infancy.[161]

INFECTION

Increased susceptibility to infection has been found in infants with BPD. Respiratory syncytial virus (RSV) is a major pathogen that causes illness and the need for rehospitalization and mechanical ventilation in children with BPD. Infants are more susceptible to RSV infection due to impaired lung defenses secondary to damaged lung tissue.[162,163] The prophylactic use of ribavirin at home is being studied as a way of preventing respiratory failure due to RSV infection in infants with BPD. Respiratory syncytial virus infection and its treatment may contribute to long-term pulmonary function abnormalities in infants with BPD.[164]

GROWTH AND NEUROLOGIC DEVELOPMENT

It is not surprising that the most critically ill and premature infants who develop BPD have an increased risk for growth failure and abnormal neurodevelopmental outcome. Infants with BPD have increased metabolic demands and caloric requirements and may grow poorly during infancy and childhood.[165–168] Markestad observed that children with improving respiratory function exhibited faster catch-up growth, and those with continued respiratory problems failed to do so.[169] Other studies have shown that a significant proportion of infants with BPD are consistently in the lower percentiles for height, weight, and head circumference.[170] This is frequently found during the first 2 years of life, when respiratory symptoms and illness may be prominent.[160]

Markestad and Fitzhardinge studied neurodevelopmental outcome and reported Bayley scores in 20 children with BPD at 2 years of age.[169] Twenty-five percent had major developmental delays, but they concluded that this poor outcome was related to perinatal events other than BPD. Similar conclusions were drawn by Luchi, who demonstrated that, although BPD may be associated with significant central nervous system dysfunction, common intracranial complications (*e.g.*, intracranial hemorrhage, periventricular leukomalacia) were stronger determinants of poor outcome.[171] It is not surprising that the smallest and sickest infants who develop significant BPD have a higher incidence of these neurologic complications.

Other studies have found that the severity of BPD is a major predictor of neurologic outcome. Meisels compared infants with BPD to those without significant lung disease and found that the development of BPD was associated with a significantly worse outcome.[172,173] Bozynski found that clinical pulmonary status and the need for chronic mechanical ventilation was consistently associated with a poorer neurodevelopmental outcome.[174] Vohr followed infants prospectively for as long as 24 months and found that only 24% of infants with BPD were neurologically normal with a mean mental developmental index of 65 ± 16.[175] In contrast, 86% of control infants had achieved normal developmental milestones and outcome. In a study of infants weighing less than 1500 g who had no major handicaps at 1 year of age, Williamson, using revised Gesell Development Schedules, found that disturbances in fine motor performance correlated with several perinatal factors, including BPD, intracranial hemorrhage, and total number of days hospitalized.[176] Vaucher compared outcome in surfactant-treated and control infants and found that, regardless of treatment group, treated infants who developed BPD were more likely to have neurodevelopmental abnormalities at 12 and 24 months of age.[177] Although the relative contribution of BPD to poor outcome remains undefined, it is associated with the sickest patients in the neonatal intensive care unit and consequently with a significant risk of poor neurodevelopmental outcome.

The introduction of surfactant replacement therapy has resulted in significantly improved survival and the development of less severe BPD. Follow-up studies suggest that the number of significant neurodevelopmental handicaps has not increased despite the survival of smaller, sicker infants and more BPD.

PREVENTION

A multidisciplinary approach to the prevention of BPD in infants is needed. The use of prenatal steroids in mothers at high risk of delivering a significantly premature infant appears to reduce the severity and incidence of BPD.[178] The early use of nasal CPAP in infants with respiratory distress may eliminate the need for mechanical ventilation in some infants and facilitate successful extubation in other low-birth-weight infants.[96] The use of exogenous surfactant replacement therapy in premature infants with significant RDS can reduce mortality and the severity and incidence of BPD, although the total number of survivors with BPD will increase. Exogenous surfactant may prevent acute and chronic lung damage in full-term infants with pneumonia or meconium aspiration syndrome.[179] Aggressive treatment of symptomatic patent ductus arteriosus may reduce the severity of BPD and should include fluid restriction, diuretics, indomethacin, or surgical closure. Prophylactic therapy directed at preventing the contribution of the ductus to BPD does not appear to be necessary.[66,180,181] Ventilator pressures and inspired oxygen concentrations should be reduced as low and as soon as possible to reduce barotrauma, air leak, and oxygen toxicity.

Aggressive nutritional support, initially with intravenous supplementation followed by enteral feeds when tolerated, is critical.[182] Adequate nutrition helps promote normal lung growth, maturation, and repair. It also protects the lung from the damaging effects of infection, hyperoxia, and barotrauma. Supplementation with vitamin A in sufficient quantities to establish normal serum retinol concentrations may reduce the incidence and severity of BPD.[183]

High-frequency ventilation provides adequate gas exchange at lower inspiratory pressures than conventional ventilation. The early use of high-frequency oscillatory ventilation in premature baboons reduced the incidence of RDS and decreased the severity of acute and chronic lung damage.[184] The collaborative high-frequency ventilation trial was unable to demonstrate a difference in the incidence of BPD in either treatment group.[20] There was no difference in pulmonary function studies between the two ventilation groups at the time of hospital discharge.[185] However, long-term studies of some of these infants revealed improved mechanics in infants who had received high-frequency ventilation, suggesting less lung damage occurred.[186] The early use of HFJV in newborn infants with significant RDS may reduce the severity or incidence of BPD. The combined use of HFJV and surfactant replacement may prevent significant lung damage in premature and term infants with significant lung disease unresponsive to surfactant replacement and conventional mechanical ventilation.[187] Two multicenter controlled trials are being performed to determine if surfactant therapy is more efficacious in preventing BPD when administered to preterm and term infants receiving high-frequency ventilation.

Extracorporeal membrane oxygenation is another technique that has gained widespread use in the treatment of infants older than 36 weeks of gestation with severe lung disease that is unresponsive to conventional forms of therapy.[188,189] This technique allows the lung to rest and repair itself while gas exchange is accomplished with the use of an external membrane oxygenator. The early use of ECMO before significant lung damage occurs may reduce BPD in some treated infants. Its use has been limited to term and near-term infants because of the necessity of anticoagulating treated infants. Future research that eliminates the need for anticoagulation and ligation of the carotid artery or jugular vein may allow ECMO to be used earlier, more safely, and in smaller infants.

In newborn piglets, prophylactic dexamethasone treatment appears to be effective in preventing acute lung injury caused by hyperoxia and mechanical ventilation, primarily by reducing the production of mediators chemotactic for neutrophils in the lung.[190] In infants, earlier use of dexamethasone has resulted in a lower incidence and severity of BPD without many associated side-effects.[141,191] Further prophylactic dexamethasone administration studies need to be performed to determine the optimal dose, timing, and duration of treatment to prevent BPD.

The most promising method for preventing the development of BPD appears to be prophylactic supplementation of human recombinant antioxidant enzymes. This seems to be a logical strategy in preventing BPD, because oxygen radicals appear to play a major role in the pathogenesis of lung injury and premature infants are known to be relatively deficient in these enzymes at birth. Several animal studies have shown that prolonged exposure to high-oxygen concentrations can cause severe lung damage and death, and systemic administration of antioxidants can prevent many of these complications.[192–196] In a pilot study using humans, Rosenfeld and colleagues showed that subcutaneous administration of bovine SOD decreased the severity of BPD in treated infants, although total duration of respiratory support was the same for the treated and control groups.[197] The development of human recombinant SOD and the ability to effectively deliver this enzyme directly to the lung may ultimately be effective in the prevention of BPD. The prophylactic use of a single intratracheal dose of human recombinant SOD appears to prevent significant lung injury from oxygen and mechanical ventilation in newborn piglets with no apparent associated toxicity.[29]

The exogenous SOD appears to localize in small, distal airways after administration, and significant quantities persist 48 hours after the dose is given (Fig. 30-9).[29] This is important because most of the initial histologic damage in BPD is seen in the terminal airways. Interest in exogenous SOD has increased because significant SOD activity has been demonstrated in natural lung surfactant (7 U/μmole phospholipid) and is absent in exogenous surfactant preparations.[198] Newer aerosolization techniques may lower effective doses and improve distribution of SOD.[199] National collaborative trials using prophylactic SOD in premature infants at high-risk for developing BPD may ulti-

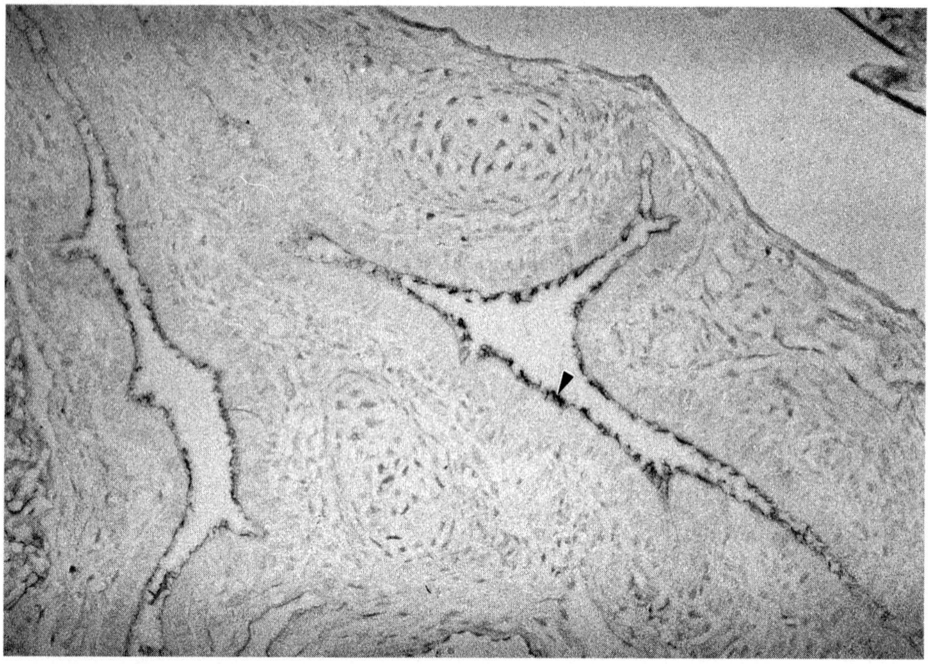

FIG. 30–9. Light micrograph from a neonatal piglet treated with intratracheal superoxide dismutase (SOD) followed by 48 hours of hyperoxia and hyperventilation. Immunocytochemistry was performed, staining human SOD black. Human SOD lines small airways (*arrow*) 48 hours after administration. (Original magnification × 20; from Davis JM, Rosenfeld WN, Sanders RJ, Gonenne A. The prophylactic effects of human recombinant speroxide dismutase in neonatal lung injury. J Appl Physiol 1993;74:2234.)

mately produce a therapy that can prevent or significantly ameliorate this important chronic lung disease.

REFERENCES

1. Northway WH Jr, Rosan C, Porter DY. Pulmonary disease following respirator therapy of hyaline-membrane disease. N Engl J Med 1967;76:357.
2. Bancalari E, Abdenour GE, Feller R, et al. Bronchopulmonary dysplasia: clinical presentation. J Pediatr 1979;95:819.
3. Tooley WH. Epidemiology of bronchopulmonary dysplasia. Pediatr 1979;95:851.
4. Avery ME, Tooley WH, Keller JG, et al. Is chronic lung disease in low birth weight infants preventable? A survey of eight centers. Pediatrics 1987;79:26.
5. Sinkin RA, Cox C, Phelps DL. Predicting risk for bronchopulmonary dysplasia: selection criteria for clinical trials. Pediatrics 1990;86:728.
6. Shennan AT, Dunn MS, Ohlsson A, Lennox K, Hoskins EM. Abnormal pulmonary outcomes in premature infants: prediction from oxygen requirement in the neonatal period. Pediatrics 1988;82:527.
7. Hoekstra RE, Jackson JC, Myers TF, et al. Improved neonatal survival following multiple doses of bovine surfactant in very premature neonates at risk for respiratory distress syndrome. Pediatrics 1991;88:10.
8. Merritt TA, Hallman M, Berry C, et al. Randomized, placebo-controlled trial of human surfactant given at birth versus rescue administration in very low birth weight infants with lung immaturity. J Pediatr 1991;118:581.
9. Soll RF, Hoekstra RE, Fangman JJ, et al. Multicenter trial of single-dose modified bovine surfactant extract (Survanta) for prevention of respiratory distress syndrome. Pediatrics 1990;85:1092.
10. Bose C, Corbet A, Bose G, et al. Improved outcome at 28 days of age for very low birth weight infants treated with a single dose of a synthetic surfactant. J Pediatr 1990;117:947.
11. Lang MJ, Hall RT, Reddy NS, et al. A controlled trial of human surfactant replacement therapy for severe respiratory distress syndrome in very low birth weight infants. J Pediatr 1990;116:296.
12. Liechty EA, Donovan E, Purohit D. Reduction of neonatal mortality after multiple doses of bovine surfactant in low birth weight neonates with respiratory distress syndrome. Pediatrics 1991;88:19.
13. Horbar JD, Soll RD, Schachinger H, et al. A European multicenter randomized controlled trial of single dose surfactant therapy for idiopathic respiratory distress syndrome. Eur J Pediatr 1990;149:416.
14. Fujiwara T, Konishi M, Chida S. Surfactant replacement therapy with a single postventilatory dose of a reconstituted bovine surfactant in preterm neonates with respiratory distress syndrome. Pediatrics 1990;86:753.
15. Long W, Thompson T, Sundell H, Schumacher R, Volberg F, Guthrie R. Effects of two rescue doses of a synthetic surfactant on mortality rate and survival without bronchopulmonary dysplasia in 700 to 1350 gram infants with respiratory distress syndrome. The American Exosurf Neonatal Study Group I. J Pediatr 1991;118:595.
16. Ackerman NB Jr, Carlson JJ, Keichl TJ, et al. Pulmonary interstitial emphysema in the premature baboon with hyaline membrane disease. Crit Care Med 1984;12:512.

17. Nilsson R, Grossman G, Robertson B. Lung surfactant and the pathogenesis of neonatal bronchiolar lesions induced by artificial ventilation. Pediatr Res 1978;12:249.
18. Davis JM, Metlay L, Dickerson B, Penney DY, Notter RH. Early pulmonary changes associated with high-frequency jet ventilation in newborn piglets. Pediatr Res 1990;27:460.
19. Davis JM, Dickerson B, Metlay L, Penney DP. Differential effects of oxygen and barotrauma on lung injury in the neonatal piglet. Pediatr Pulmonol 1991;10:157.
20. HiFi Study Group. High-frequency oscillatory ventilation compared with conventional ventilation in the treatment of respiratory failure in preterm infants. N Engl J Med 1989; 320:88.
21. Man GC, Ahmed IH, Logus JW, Man SFP. High-frequency oscillatory ventilation increases canine pulmonary epithelial permeability. J Appl Physiol 1987;63:1871.
22. Carlo WA, Chatburn RL, Martin RJ. Randomized trial of high-frequency jet ventilation versus conventional ventilation in respiratory distress syndrome. J Pediatr 1987;110:275.
23. Keszler M, Donn SM, Bucciarelli RL, et al. Multicenter controlled trial comparing high-frequency jet ventilation and mechanical ventilation in newborn infants with pulmonary emphysema. J Pediatr 1991;119:85.
24. Frank L, Groseclose EE. Preparation for birth into an O_2 rich environment: the antioxidant enzymes in the developing rabbit lung. Pediatr Res 1984;18:240.
25. Frank L. Developmental aspects of experimental pulmonary oxygen toxicity. Free Radic Biol Med 1991;11:463.
26. Crapo J, Barry B, Foscue H, Shelburne J. Structural and biochemical changes in rat lungs occurring during exposure to lethal and adaptive doses of oxygen. Am Rev Respir Dis 1980;122:123.
27. Turrens JF, Crapo JD, Freeman BA. Protection against oxygen toxicity by intravenous injection of liposome-entrapped catalase and superoxide dismutase. J Clin Invest 1984;73:87.
28. Padmanabhan RV, Gudapaty R, Liener JE, Schwartz BA, Hoidal JR. Protection against pulmonary oxygen toxicity in rats by the intratracheal administration of liposome-encapsulated superoxide dismutase or catalase. Am Rev Respir Dis 1985;132:164.
29. Davis JM, Rosenfeld WN, Sanders RJ, Gonenne A. The prophylactic effects of human recombinant superoxide dismutase in neonatal lung injury. Pediatr Res 1993;74:2234.
30. Rinaldo JE, English D, Levine J, Stiller R, Henson J. Increased retention of radiolabeled neutrophils in early oxygen toxicity. Am Rev Respir Dis 1988;137:345.
31. Merritt TA, Stuard IK, Puccia J, et al. Newborn tracheal aspirate cytology: classification during respiratory distress syndrome and bronchopulmonary dysplasia. J Pediatr 1981; 98:949.
32. Merritt TA, Cochrane CG, Holcomb K, et al. Elastase and α_1-proteinase inhibitor activity in tracheal aspirates during respiratory distress syndrome. Role of inflammation in the pathogenesis of bronchopulmonary dysplasia. J Clin Invest 1983;72:656.
33. Fantore JC, Feltner DE, Brieland DVM, Ward PA. Phagocytic cell-derived inflammatory mediators and lung disease. Chest 1987;91:428.
34. Stenmark KR, Eyzaguirre M, Westcott JY, Henson PM, Murphy RC. Potential role of eicosanoids and PAF in the pathophysiology of bronchopulmonary dysplasia. Am Rev Respir Dis 1987;136:770.
35. Holtzman, MJ. Arachidonic acid metabolism. Implications of biological chemistry for lung function and disease. Am Rev Respir Dis 1991;143:188.
36. O'Brodovich HM, Mellins RB. Bronchopulmonary dysplasia: unresolved neonatal acute lung injury. Am Rev Respir Dis 1985;132:694.
37. Bruce MC, Wedig KE, Jentoft N, et al. Altered excretion of elastin cross-links in premature infants who develop bronchopulmonary dysplasia. Am Rev Respir Dis 1985;131:568.
38. Ossanna PJ, Test ST, Matheson NR, Regiani S, Weiss SJ. Oxidative regulation of neutrophil elastase-alpha-1-proteinase inhibitor interactions. J Clin Invest 1986;77:1939.
39. Walti H, Tordet C, Gerbaut L, Saugier P, Moriette G, Relier JP. Persistent elastase/proteinase inhibitor imbalance during prolonged ventilation of infants with bronchopulmonary dysplasia: evidence for the role of nosocomial infections. Pediatr Res 1989;26:351.
40. Bruce M, Boat T, Martin CJ, et al. Protein inhibitors and inhibitor inactivation in neonatal airway secretions. Chest 1982; 81(Suppl):44.
41. Rosenfeld W, Concepcion L, Evans E, Jhaveri R, Sahdev S, Zabaleta I. Serial trypsin inhibitory capacity and ceruloplasmin levels in prematures at risk for bronchopulmonary dysplasia. Am Rev Respir Dis 1986;134:1229.
42. Yoder MC Jr, Chua R, Tepper R. Effect of dexamathasone on pulmonary inflammation and pulmonary function of ventilator-dependent infants with bronchopulmonary dysplasia. Am Rev Respir Dis 1991;143:1044.
43. Gerdes JS, Harris MC, Polin RA. Effects of dexamethasone and indomethacin on elastase, alpha-1-proteinase inhibitor, and fibronectin in bronchoalveolar lavage fluid from neonates. J Pediatr 1988;113:727.
44. Cassell GH, Waites KB, Crouse DT, et al. Association of Ureaplasma urealyticum infection of the lower respiratory tract with chronic lung disease and death in very-low-birth-weight infants. Lancet 1988;2:240.
45. Cassell GH, Waites KG, Crouse DT, et al. Association of ureaplasma urealyticum infection of the lower respiratory tract with chronic lung disease and death in very low birth weight infants. Lancet 1988;2:240.
46. Desilva NS, Quinn PA. Phospholipase A and C activity in ureaplasma urealyticum. J Clin Microbiol 1986;23:354.
47. Weinstein MR, Oh W. Oxygen consumption in infants with bronchopulmonary dysplasia. J Pediatr 1981;99:958.
48. Frank L, Groseclose EE. Oxygen toxicity in newborn rats: the adverse effects of undernutrition. J Appl Physiol 1982; 53:1248.
49. Forman HJ, Rotman EI, Fisher AB. Roles of selenium and sulfur-containing amino acids in protection against oxygen toxicity. Lab Invest 1983;49:148.
50. O'Dell BL, Kilburn KH, McKenzie WN, Thurston RJ. The lung of the copper deficient rat: a model for developmental pulmonary emphysema. Am J Pathol 1978;91:413.
51. Ehrenkranz RA, Bonta BW, Ablow RC, Warshaw JB. Amelioration of bronchopulmonary dysplasia after vitamin E administration: a preliminary report. N Engl J Med 1978;299: 564.
52. Ehrenkranz RA, Ablow RC, Warshaw JB. Effect of vitamin E on the development of oxygen-induced lung injury in neonates. Ann N Y Acad Sci 1982;393:452.
53. Ward JA, Roberts RJ. Vitamin E inhibition of the effects of hyperoxia on the pulmonary surfactant system of the newborn rabbit. Pediatr Res 1984;18:329.
54. Wender DF, Thulin GE, Smith GJW, Warshaw JB. Vitamin E affects lung biochemical and morphologic response to hyperoxia in the newborn rabbit. Pediatr Res 1981;15:262.
55. Hittner HM, Godio LB, Rudolph AJ, et al. Retrolental fibroplasia: efficacy of vitamin E in a double-blind clinical study of preterm infants. N Engl J Med 1981;305:1365.
56. Finer NN, Schindler RF, Grant G, et al. Effect of intramuscu-

lar vitamin E on frequency and severity of retrolental fibroplasia: a controlled trial. Lancet 1982;1:1087.
57. Saldanha RL, Cepeda EE, Poland RL. The effect of vitamin E prophylaxis on the incidence and severity of bronchopulmonary dysplasia. J Pediatr 1982;101:89.
58. Sosenko IR, Innis SM, Frank L. Intralipid increases lung polyunsaturated fatty acids and protects newborn rats from oxygen toxicity. Pediatr Res 1991;30:413.
59. Brandt RB, Mueller DG, Schroder JR. Serum vitamin A in premature and term neonates. J Pediatr 1978;92:101.
60. Shenai JP, Rush MG, Stahlman MT, Chytil F. Plasma retinol-binding protein response to vitamin A administration in infants susceptible to bronchopulmonary dysplasia. J Pediatr 1990;116:607.
61. Hustead VA, Gutcher GR, Anderson SA, Zachman RD. Relationship of vitamin A (retinol) status to lung disease in the preterm infants. J Pediatr 1984;105:610.
62. Anzano MA, Olson JA, Lamb AJ. Morphologic alterations in the trachea and the salivary gland following the induction of rapid synchronous vitamin A deficiency in rats. Am J Pathol 1980;98:7171.
63. Shenai JP, Chytil F, Stahlman MT. Vitamin A status of neonates with chronic lung disease. Pediatr Res 1985;19:185.
64. Hartline JL, Zachman RD. Vitamin A delivery in total parenteral nutrition solution. Pediatrics 1976;58:448.
65. Cotton RB. Contribution of the patent ductus arteriosus to lung injury. In: Merrritt TA, Northway WH, Boynton BR, eds. Bronchopulmonary dysplasia. Boston: Blackwell Scientific Publications, 1988;235.
66. Bancalari E, Sosenko I. Pathogenesis and prevention of neonatal chronic lung disease: recent developments. Pediatr Pulmonol 1990;8:109.
67. Van Marter LJ, Leviton A, Allred EN, Pagano M, Kuban KC. Hydration during the first days of life and the risk of bronchopulmonary dysplasia in low birth weight infants. J Pediatr 1990;116:942.
68. Nickerson BG, Taussig LM. Family history of asthma in infants with bronchopulmonary dysplasia. Pediatrics 1980;65:1140.
69. Bertrand JM, Riley P, Popkin J, Coates AL. The long-term pulmonary sequelae of prematurity: the role of familial airway hyperreactivity and the respiratory distress syndrome. N Engl J Med 1985;312:742.
70. Clark DA, Pincus LG, Oliphant M, Hubbell C, Oates RP, Davey FR. HLA-A2 and chronic lung disease in neonates. JAMA 1982;248:1868.
71. Toce SS, Farrell PM, Leavitt, LA, Samuels DP, Edwards DK. Clinical and radiographic scoring systems for assessing bronchopulmonary dysplasia. Am J Dis Child 1984;138:581.
72. Edwards DK. Radiographic aspects of bronchopulmonary dysplasia. J Pediatr 1979;95:823.
73. Mortensson W, Andreasson B, Lindroth M, Svenningsen N, Jonson B. Potentially of early chest roentgen examination in ventilator treated newborn infants to predict future lung function and disease. Pediatr Radiol 1989;20:41.
74. Lee H, Price A, Rosenfeld W. Increased detection of pathologic lung changes in infants with bronchopulmonary dysplasia using chest computerized tomography (abstract). Pediatr Res 1992;31:360A.
75. Abman SH. Pulmonary hypertension in infants with bronchopulmonary dysplasia: clinical aspects. In: Bancalari E, Stocker JT, eds. Bronchopulmonary dysplasia. Washington, DC: Hemisphere Publishing, 1988:221.
76. Harrod JR, L'Heureux P, Wagenstein OD, Hunt CE. Long-term follow-up of severe respiratory distress syndrome treated with IPPB. J Pediatr 1974;84:277.
77. Melnick G, Pickoff AS, Ferrer PL, et al. Normal pulmonary vascular resistance and left ventricle hypertrophy in young infants with bronchopulmonary dysplasia: an echocardiographic and pathologic study. Pediatrics 1980;66:589.
78. Berman W Jr, Yabek SM, Dillon T, Burnstein R, Corlew S. Evaluation of infants with bronchopulmonary dysplasia using cardiac catherization. Pediatrics 1982;70:708.
79. Goldman SL, Gerhardt T, Sonni R, et al. Early prediction of chronic lung disease by pulmonary function testing. J Pediatr 1983;102:613.
80. Tepper RS, Morgan WJ, Cota K, Taussig LM. Expiratory flow limitation in infants with bronchopulmonary dysplasia. J Pediatr 1986;109:1040.
81. Greenspan JS, De Giulio PA, Bhutani VK. Airway reactivity as determined by a cold air challenge in infants with bronchopulmonary dysplasia. J Pediatr 1989;114:452.
82. McCann EM, Goldman SL, Brody JP. Pulmonary function testing in the sick newborn infant. Pediatr Res 1987;21:313.
83. Gerhardt T, Bancalari E. Lung function in bronchopulmonary dysplasia. In: Bancalari E, Stocker JT, eds. Bronchopulmonary dysplasia. Washington, DC: Hemisphere Publishing, 1988:182.
84. Nickerson BG, Durano DJ, Kao LC. Short-term variability of pulmonary function tests in infants with bronchopulmonary dysplasia. Pediatr Pulmonol 1989;6:36.
85. LeSouef PN, Lopes JM, England SJ, Bryan MH, Bryan AC. Influence of chest wall distortion on esophageal pressure. J Appl Physiol 1983;55:353.
86. Hanrahan JP, Tager IB, Castile RG, Segal MR, Weiss WST, Speizer FE. Pulmonary function measures in healthy infants. Am Rev Respir Dis 1990;141:1127.
87. Stocker JT. Pathology of acute bronchopulmonary dysplasia. In: Bancalari E, Stocker JT, eds. Bronchopulmonary dysplasia. Washington, DC: Hemisphere Publishing, 1988:237.
88. Abman SH, Wolfe RR, Accurso FJ, Koops BL, Bowman M, Wiggins JW Jr. Pulmonary vascular response to oxygen in infants with bronchopulmonary dysplasia. Pediatrics 1985;75:80.
89. Courtney SE, Weber KR, Breakiel A, et al. Capillary blood gases in the neonate. Am J Dis Child 1990;144:168.
90. Goldman SL, McCann EM, Lloyd BW, Yup G. Inspiratory time and pulmonary function in mechanically ventilated babies with chronic lung disease. Pediatr Pulmonol 1991;11:198.
91. Tarnow-Mordi WO, Reid E, Griffiths P, Wilkinson AR. Low inspired gas temperature and respiratory complications in very low birth weight infants. J Pediatr 1989;114:438.
92. Aranda JV, Turmen T. Methylxanthines in apnea of prematurity. Clin Perinatol 1979;6:87.
93. Veness-Meehan K, Richter S, Davis JM. Pulmonary function testing before extubation in infants with respiratory distress syndrome. Pediatr Pulmonol 1990;9:2.
94. Kim EH. Successful extubation of newborn infants without pre-extubation trial of continuous positive airway pressure. J Perinatol 1989;9:72.
95. Viscardi RM, Raix RG, Nicks JJ, Grasela TH. Efficacy of theophylline for prevention of post-extubation respiratory failure in very low birth weight infants. J Pediatr 1985;107:469.
96. Higgins RD, Richter SE, Davis JM. Nasal continuous positive airway pressure facilitates extubation of very low birth weight neonates. Pediatrics 1991;88:999.
97. Miller RW, Woo T, Kelman RK, Slagle TS. Tracheobronchial abnormalities in infants with bronchopulmonary dysplasia. J Pediatr 1987;111:779.
98. Goodman G, Perkin RM, Anas NG, et al. Pulmonary hypertension in infants with bronchopulmonary dysplasia. J Pediatr 1988;112:67.

99. Ramanathan R, Durand M, Larrazabol C. Pulse oximetry in very low birth weight infants with acute and chronic lung disease. Pediatrics 1987;79:612.
100. Higgins RD, Phelps DL. Oxygen-induced retinopathy: lack of adverse heparin effect. Pediatr Res 1990;27:580.
101. Alverson DC, Isken VH, Cohen RS. Effect of booster transfusion on oxygen use in infants with bronchopulmonary dysplasia. J Pediatr 1988;113:772.
102. Stefano JL, Bhutani VK. Role of furosemide therapy after booster packed erythrocyte transfusion in infants with bronchopulmonary dysplasia. J Pediatr 1990;117:965.
103. Halperin DS, Wacker P, Lacourt G, et al. Effects of recombinant human erythropoietin in infants with anemia of prematurity: a pilot study. J Pediatr 1990;116:779.
104. Gilhooly J, Lindenberg J, Reynolds JW. Central venous silicone elastomer catheter placement by basilic vein cutdown in neonates. Pediatrics 1986;78:636.
105. Pereira GR, Fox WW, Stanley CA, et al. Decreased oxygenation and hyperlipemia during intravenous fat infusions in premature infants. Pediatrics 1980;66:26.
106. Yunis KA, Oh W. Effects of intravenous glucose loading on oxygen consumption, carbon dioxide production, and resting energy expenditure in infants with bronchopulmonary dysplasia. J Pediatr 1989;115:127.
107. Akramoff LA, Beharry K, Ling E, Papageorgiou A, Aranda JV. Combined vitamin A and E supplemental therapy for bronchopulmonary dysplasia (abstract). Pediatr Res 1992;31: 298A.
108. Davis JM, Sinkin RA, Aranda JV. Drug therapy for bronchopulmonary dysplasia. Pediatr Pulmonol 1990;8:117.
109. Bland RD, McMillan DD, Bressack MA. Decreased pulmonary transvascular fluid filtration in awake newborn lambs after intravenous furosemide. J Clin Invest 1978;62:601.
110. Engelhardt B, Elliott S, Hazinski TA. Short-and long-term effects of furosemide on lung function in infants with bronchopulmonary dysplasia. J Pediatr 1986;109:1034.
111. Kao LC, Warburton DW, Sargent CW, Platzker ACG, Keens TG. Furosemide acutely decreases airways resistance in chronic bronchopulmonary dysplasia. J Pediatr 1983;103:624.
112. McCann EM, Lewis K, Deming DD, Donovan MJ, Brady JP. Controlled trial of furosemide therapy in infants with chronic lung disease. J Pediatr 1985;106:957.
113. Weiner IM, Mudge GH. Diuretics and other agents employed in the mobilization of edema fluid. In: Gilman AG, Goodman LS, Rall TW, Murad F, eds. The pharmacological basis of therapeutics. New York: Macmillan, 1985:887.
114. Kao LC, Warburton DW, Cheng MH, Cedeno C, Platzker ACG, Keens TG. Effect of oral diuretics on pulmonary mechanics in infants with chronic bronchopulmonary dysplasia: results of a double blind crossover sequential trial. Pediatrics 1984;74:37.
115. Kao LC, Durand DJ, Phillips BL, Nickerson BG. Oral theophylline and diuretics improve pulmonary mechanics in infants with bronchopulmonary dysplasia. J Pediatr 1987; 111:439.
116. Engelhardt B, Blalock WA, DonLevy A, Rush M, Hazinski TA. Effect of spironolactone-hydrochlothiazide on lung function in infants with chronic bronchopulmonary dysplasia. J Pediatr 1989;114:619.
117. Kao LC, Warburton D, Platzker ACG, Keens TG. Effect of isoproterenol inhalation on airway resistance in chronic bronchopulmonary dysplasia. Pediatrics 1984;73:509.
118. Wilkie RA, Bryan MH. Effect of bronchodilators on airway resistance in ventilator-dependent neonates with chronic lung disease. J Pediatr 1987;111:278.
119. Weiner N. Atropine, scopolamine, and related antimuscarinic drugs. In: Gilman AG, Goodman LS, Rall TW, Murad F, eds. The Pharmacologic basis of therapeutics. New York: Macmillan, 1985:130.
120. Cabal LA, Larrazabal C, Ramanathan R, Durand M, Lewis D, Siassi B, Hodgman J. Effects of metaproterenol on pulmonary mechanics, oxygenation, and ventilation in infants with chronic lung disease. J Pediatr 1987;110:116.
121. Gomez-Del Rio M, Gerhardt T, Hehre D, Feller R, Bancalari E. Effect of a beta-agonist nebulization on lung function in neonates with increased pulmonary resistance. Pediatr Pulmonol 1986;2:287.
122. Logvinoff MM, Lemen RJ, Taussig LM, Lamont BA. Bronchodilators and diuretics in children with bronchopulmonary dysplasia. Pediatr Pulmonol 1985;1:198.
123. Kao LC, Durand DJ, Nickerson BG. Effects of inhaled metaproterenol and atropine on the pulmonary mechanics of infants with bronchopulmonary dysplasia. Pediatr Pulmonol 1989;6:74.
124. Brundage KL, Mohsini KG, Froese AB, Fisher JT. Bronchodilator response to ipratropium bromide in infants with bronchopulmonary dysplasia. Am Rev Respir Dis 1990;142:1137.
125. Douglas WW. Histamine and 5-hydroxytryptamine and their antagonists. In: Gilman AG, Goodman LS, Rall TW, Murad F, eds. The pharmacologic basis of therapeutics. New York: Macmillan, 1985;605.
126. Stenmark KR, Eyzaguirre M, Remigio L, Henson PM. Recovery of platelet activiating factor and leukotrienes from infants with severe bronchopulmonary dysplasia: clinical improvement with cromolyn treatment (abstract). Am Rev Respir Dis 1985;131:236.
127. Davis JM, Bhutani VK, Stefano JL, Fox WW, Spitzer AR. Changes in pulmonary mechanics after caffeine administration in infants with bronchopulmonary dysplasia. Pediatr Pulmonol 1989;6:49.
128. Rooklin AR, Moomjian AS, Shutack JG, Schwartz JG, Fox WW. Theophylline therapy in bronchopulmonary dysplasia. J Pediatr 1979;95:882.
129. Polgar G. Mechanical properties of the lung and chest wall. In: Thibeault DW, Gregory GA, eds. Neonatal pulmonary care. Norwalk: Apple-Crofts, 1986:49.
130. Sosulski R, Abbasi S, Bhutani VK, Fox WW. Physiologic effects of terbutaline on pulmonary function of infants with bronchopulmonary dysplasia. Pediatr Pulmonol 1986;2:269.
131. Stefano JL, Bhutani VK, Fox WW. A randomized placebo-controlled study to evaluate the effects of oral albuterol on pulmonary mechanics in ventilator-dependent infants at risk of developing BPD. Pediatr Pulmonol 1991;10:183.
132. Haynes RC, Murad F. Adrenocorticotropic hormone; adrenocortical steroids and their synthetic analogs: inhibitors of adrenocortical steroid biosynthesis. In: Gilman AG, Goodman LS, Rall TW, Murad F, eds. The pharmacologic basis of therapeutics. New York: Macmillan, 1985:1459.
133. Wilson JW. Treatment and prevention of pulmonary cellular damage with pharmacologic doses of corticosteroid. Surg Gynecol Obstet 1972;134:678.
134. Georgieff MK, Nammel MC, Mills MM, Gunter EW, Johnson DE, Thompson TR. Effect of post-natal steroid administration on serum vitamin A concentrations in newborn infants with respiratory compromise. J Pediatr 1989;114:301.
135. de Lemos RA, Shermeta DW, Knelson JH, Kotas R, Avery ME. Acceleration of appearance of pulmonary surfactant in the fetal lamb by administration of corticosteroids. Am Rev Respir Dis 1970;102:459.
136. Frank L, Lewis PL, Sosenko IRS. Dexamethasone stimulation of rat lung antioxidant enzyme activity in parallel with surfactant stimulation. Pediatrics 1985;75:569.

137. Hang SL, Levine L. Inhibition of arachadonic acid release from cells as the biochemical action of anti-inflammatory corticosteroid. Proc Natl Acad Sci USA 1976;73:1730.
138. Skubitz KM, Craddock PR, Hammerschmidt DE, Augusts JT. Corticortercoids block binding of chemotactic peptic to its receptor on granulocytes and cause disaggregation of granulocyte aggregates in vitro. J Clin Invest 1981;68:13.
139. Kusajima K, Wax SD, Webb WR. Effects of methylprednisolone on pulmonary microcirculation. Surg Gynecol Obstet 1974;139:1.
140. Townley RG, Reeb R, Fitzgibbons T, Adolphson RL. The effect of corticosteroid on the beta-adrenergic receptors in bronchial smooth muscle. J Allergy 1970;45:118.
141. Cummings JJ, D'Eugenio DB, Gross SJ. A controlled trial of dexamethasone in preterm infants at high risk for bronchopulmonary dysplasia. N Engl J Med 1989;320:1505.
142. Avery GB, Fletcher AB, Kaplan M, Brudno DS. Controlled trial of dexamethasone in respirator dependent infants with bronchopulmonary dysplasia. Pediatrics 1985;75:106.
143. Harkavy KG, Scanlon JW, Chowdhry PK, Grylack LJ. Dexamethasone therapy for chronic lung disease in ventilator and oxygen dependent infants: a controlled trial. J Pediatr 1989;115:979.
144. Brownlee JR, Beekman RH, Rosenthal A. Acute hemodynamic effects of nifedipine in infants with bronchopulmonary dysplasia and pulmonary hypertension. Pediatr Res 1988; 24:186.
145. Johnson CE, Beekman RH, Kostyshak DA, Nguyen T, Oh DM, Amidon GL. Pharmacokinetics and pharmacodynamics of nifedidine in children with bronchopulmonary dysplasia and pulmonary hypertension. Pediatr Res 1991;29:500.
146. Epstein ML, Kiel EA, Victorica BE. Cardiac decompensation following verapamil therapy in infants with supraventricular tachycardia. Pediatrics 1985;75:737.
147. Holtzman RB, Hageman JR, Yogev R. Role of Ureaplasma urealyticum in bronchopulmonary dysplasia. J Pediatr 1989; 114:1061.
148. Wang EE, Frayha H, Watts J, Hammerbert O, Chernesky MA, Mahony JB, Cassell GH. Role of Ureaplasma urealyticum and other pathogens in the development of chronic lung disease of prematurity. Pediatr Infect Dis J 1988;7:547.
149. Parker A. Expert handling. Nurs Times 1990;86:35.
150. Northway WH. Observations on bronchopulmonary dysplasia. J Pediatr 1979;95:815.
151. Myers MG, McGuinness GA, Lachenbruch PA, Koontz FP, Hollingshead R, Olson DB. Respiratory illness in survivors of respiratory distress syndrome. Am Rev Respir Dis 1986; 133:1011.
152. Davidson S, Schrayer A, Wielunsky E, Krikler R, Lilos P, Reisner SH. Energy intake, growth and development in ventilated very-low-birth-weight infants with and without bronchopulmonary dysplasia. Am J Dis Child 1990;144:553.
153. Abman SH, Burchell MF, Schaffer MS, Rosenberg AA. Late sudden unexpected deaths in hospitalized infants with bronchopulmonary dysplasia. Am J Dis Child 1989;143:815.
154. Werthammer J, Brown ER, Neff RH, et al. Sudden infant death syndrome in infants with BPD. Pediatrics 1982;69:301.
155. Gibson RL, Jackson JC, Twiggs GA, et al. Bronchopulmonary dysplasia: survival after prolonged mechanical ventilation. Am J Dis Child 1988;142:721.
156. Phibbs RH, Ballard RA, Clements JA. Initial clinical trial of Exosurf, a protein-free synthetic surfactant, for the prophylaxis and early treatment of hyaline membrane disease. Pediatrics 1991;88:1.
157. Bader D, Ramos AD, Lew CD, et al. Childhood sequelae of infant lung disease: exercise and pulmonary function abnormalities after bronchopulmonary dysplasia. J Pediatr 1987; 110:693.
158. Andreasson B, Lindroth M, Mortensson W, et al. Lung function eight years after neonatal ventilation. Arch Dis Child 1989;64:108.
159. Blayney M, Kerem E, Whyte H, O'Brodovich H. Bronchopulmonary dysplasia: improvement in lung function between 7 and 10 years of age. J Pediatr 1991;118:201.
160. Hakulinen AL, Heinonen K, Lansimies E, Kiekara O. Pulmonary function and respiratory morbidity in school-age children born prematurely and ventilated for neonatal respiratory insufficiency. Pediatr Pulmonol 1990;8:226.
161. Northway WH Jr, Moss RB, Carlisle KG, et al. Late pulmonary sequelae of bronchopulmonary dysplasia. N Engl J Med 1990;323:1793.
162. Groothuis JR, Gutierrez KM, Lauer BA. Respiratory syncytial virus infection in children with bronchopulmonary dysplasia. Pediatrics 1988;82:199.
163. Meert K, Heidemann S, Lieh-Lai M, Sarnaik AP. Clinical characteristics of respiratory syncytial virus infections in healthy versus previously compromised host. Pediatr Pulmonol 1989;7:167.
164. Gold DR, Tager IB, Weiss ST, et al. Acute lower respiratory illness in childhood as a predictor of lung function and chronic respiratory symptoms. Am Rev Respir Dis 1989; 140:877.
165. Kalhan SC, Denne SC. Energy consumption in infants with bronchopulmonary dysplasia. J Pediatr 1990;116:662.
166. Kao LC, Durand DJ, Nickerson BG. Improving pulmonary function does not decrease oxygen consumption in infants with bronchopulmonary dysplasia. J Pediatr 1988;112:616.
167. Kurzner SI, Garg M, Bautista DB, et al. Growth failure in infants with bronchopulmonary dysplasia: nutrition and elevated resting metabolic expenditure. Pediatrics 1988;81: 379.
168. Kurzner SI, Garg M, Bautista DB, Sargent C, Bowman CM, Keens TG. Growth failure in bronchopulmonary dysplasia: elevated metabolic rates and pulmonary mechanics. J Pediatr 1988;112:73.
169. Markestad T, Fitzhardinge PM. Growth and development in children recovering from bronchopulmonary dysplasia. J Pediatr 1981;98:597.
170. Yu VYH, Orgill AA, Lim SB, et al. Growth and development of very low birth weight infants recovering from bronchopulmonary dysplasia. Arch Dis Child 1983;58:791.
171. Luchi JM, Bennet FC, Jackson JC. Predictors of neurodevelopmental outcome following bronchopulmonary dysplasia. Am J Dis Child 1991;145:813.
172. Meisels SJ, Plunkett JW, Pasick PL, Stiefel G, Roloff DW. Effects of severity and chronicity of respiratory illness on the cognitive development of preterm infants. J Pediatr Psychol 1987;12:117.
173. Meisels SJ, Plunkett JW, Roloff DW, Pasick PL, Stiefel G. Growth and development of preterm infants with respiratory distress syndrome and bronchopulmonary dysplasia. Pediatrics 1986;77:345.
174. Bozynshi ME, Nelson MN, Genaze D, et al. Cranial ultrasonography in the prediction of cerebral palsy in infants weighing less than or equal to 1200 grams at birth. Dev Med Child Neuro 1988;30:342.
175. Vohr BR, Bell EF, Oh W. Infants with bronchopulmonary dysplasia. Am J Dis Child 1982;136:443.
176. Williamson WD, Wilson GS, Lifschitz MH, Thurber SA. Nonhandicapped very-low-birth-weight infants at one year of age: developmental profile. Pediatrics 1990;85:405.
177. Vaucher YE, Merritt TA, Hallman M, Jarvenpaa HL. Neuro-

developmental and respiratory outcome in early childhood after human surfactant treatment. Am J Dis Child 1988;142:92.
178. Van Marten LJ, Levitan A, Kuban KC, Pagano M, Allred EN. Maternal glucocorticoid therapy and reduced risk of bronchopulmonary dysplasia. Pediatrics 1990;86:331.
179. Auten RL, Notter RH, Kendig JW, Davis JM, Shapiro DL. Surfactant treatment of full-term newborns with respiratory failure. Pediatrics 1991;87:101.
180. Cassady G, Crouse DT, Kirklin JW, et al. A randomized, controlled trial of very early prophylactic ligation of the ductus arteriosus in babies who weighed 1000 g or less at birth. N Engl J Med 1989;320:1511.
181. Krueger E, Mellander M, Bratton D, Cotton R. Prevention of symptomatic patent ductus arteriosus with a single dose of indomethacin. J Pediatr 1987;111:749.
182. Frank L, Sosenko IR. Undernutrition as a major contributing factor in the pathogenesis of bronchopulmonary dysplasia. Am Rev Respir Dis 1988;138:725.
183. Shenai JP, Kennedy KA, Chytil F, Stahlman MT. Clinical trial of vitamin A supplementation in infants susceptible to bronchopulmonary dysplasia. J Pediatr 1987;111:269.
184. Gerstmann DR, deLemos RA, Coalson JJ, et al. Influence of ventilatory technique on pulmonary baroinjury in baboons with hyaline membrane disease. Pediatr Pulmonol 1988; 5:82.
185. Gerhardt T, Reifenberg L, Goldbert RN, Bancaleri E. Pulmonary function in preterm infants whose lungs were ventilated with high frequency oscillation. J Pediatr 1989;115:121.
186. Abbasi S, Bhutani VK, Spitzer AR, Fox WW. Pulmonary mechanics in preterm neonates with respiratory failure treated with high-frequency oscillatory ventilation compared with conventional mechanical ventilation. Pediatrics 1991;87:487.
187. Davis JM, Richter SE, Kendig JW, Notter RH. High frequency jet ventilation and surfactant treatment of newborns in severe respiratory failure. Pediatr Pulmonol 1992;13:108
188. O'Rourke PP, Crone RK, Vacanti JP, et al. Extracorporeal membrane oxygenation and conventional medical therapy in neonates with persistent pulmonary hypertension of the newborn: a prospective randomized study. Pediatrics 1989; 84:957.
189. Bartlett RH, Roloff DW, Cornell RG, Andrews AF, Dillon PW, Zwischenberger JB. Extracorporeal circulation in neonatal respiratory failure; a prospective randomzied study. Pediatrics 1985;76:479.
190. Davis JM, Whitin J. The prophylactic effects of dexamethasone in lung injury caused by hyperoxia and hyperventilation. J Appl Physiol 1992;72:1320.
191. Collaborative dexamethasone trial group. Dexamethasone therapy in neonatal chronic lung disease: an international placebo-controlled trial. Pediatrics 1991;88:421.
192. De Los Santos R, Seidenfeld JJ, Anzueto JF, Collins JF, Coalson JJ, Johanson WG, Peters JI. One hundred percent oxygen lung injury in adult baboons. Am Rev Respir Dis 1987;136:657.
193. Heffner JE, Repine JE. Pulmonary strategies of antioxidant defense. Am Rev Respir Dis 1989;140:531.
194. Jacobson JM, Michael JR, Jafri MH, Gurtner GH. Antioixdants and antioxidant enzymes protect against pulmonary oxygen toxicity in the rabbit. J Appl Physiol 1990;68:1252.
195. Tanswell AK, Freeman BA. Liposome-entrapped antioxidant enzymes prevent lethal O_2 toxicity in the newborn rat. J Appl Physiol 1987;63:347.
196. Walther PJ, Gidding CEM, Kuipers IM, et al. Prevention of oxygen toxicity with superoxide dismutase and catalase in premature lambs. Free Radic Biol Med 1986;2:289.
197. Rosenfeld W, Evans H, Concepcion L, Jhaveri R, Schaeffer H, Friedman A. Prevention of bronchopulmonary dysplasia by administration of bovine superoxide dismutase in preterm infants with respiratory distress syndrome. J Pediatr 1984; 105:781.
198. Matalon S, Holm BA, Baker RR, Whitefield MK, Freeman BA. Characterizations of antioxidant activities of pulmonary surfactant mixtures. Biochim Biophys Acta 1990;1035:111.
199. Lewis J, Ikegami M, Higuchi R, Jobe A, Absolom D. Nebulized vs. instilled exogenous surfactant in an adult lung injury model. J Appl Physiol 1991;71:1270.

Neonatology: Pathophysiology and Management of the Newborn, Fourth Edition,
edited by Gordon B. Avery, Mary Ann Fletcher, and Mhairi G. MacDonald.
J.B. Lippincott Company, Philadelphia © 1994.

chapter 31

Principles of Management of Respiratory Problems

W. ALAN HODSON
WILLIAM E. TRUOG

Respiratory diseases in the newborn have unique physiologic, anatomic, and clinical characteristics necessitating special techniques for management. Intensive respiratory care requires a highly skilled team of physicians, nurses, respiratory therapists and other support personnel, unique facilities, equipment, and a rapidly responding laboratory service. Diagnosis of the specific disorder can be made in most cases from clinical and radiographic information alone. Other laboratory aids, particularly blood gas tension and *p*H determinations, serve to assess the severity and in some cases pathophysiology of the disease. Knowledge of pathophysiology of pulmonary diseases and their differential impact on lungs of differing states of maturity is essential to the safe and efficacious application of special techniques of treatment.

There are standard principles of respiratory management:

- Establish airway.
- Ensure oxygenation.
- Assist ventilation.
- Assess adequacy of ventilation.
- Correct metabolic abnormalities.
- Alleviate the cause of distress.

Safe and effective assistance to oxygen delivery and carbon dioxide removal from the tissues is the goal of management. Inspired oxygen is administered in a carefully controlled fashion to provide adequate but not excessive blood oxygen tension levels. Mechanical assistance to ventilation may be required to treat hypoxemia, hypercarbia, or apnea. Hypotension, hypovolemia, hypothermia, metabolic acidosis, and anemia may accompany or exacerbate respiratory failure; correction of these abnormalities is vital to management. The patient's condition is evaluated continually, using clinical and laboratory data and electronic monitoring of vital signs. Management is altered promptly in accordance with the assessment, and the specific cause of the respiratory failure is determined and treated. This chapter focuses on techniques for rapid and accurate assessment of the adequacy of supplemental oxygen therapy and techniques used for respiratory assistance in the neonate (Table 31-1).

OXYGEN THERAPY

PHYSIOLOGIC CONSIDERATIONS

The goal of oxygen therapy is to provide adequate tissue oxygenation without undue risk of oxygen toxicity. An arterial partial pressure of oxygen (PaO_2) of 45 torr results in a saturation of fetal hemoglobin (HbF) of approximately 90%, and maintaining the PaO_2 above 50 torr should be sufficient for tissue oxygen needs. Mitochondrial PO_2 is about 2 torr. An ar-

TABLE 31–1
AVAILABLE FORMS OF RESPIRATORY ASSISTANCE

Spontaneously Breathing Infants
Supplemental oxygen
CPAP
Spontaneously but Ineffectively Breathing Infants
Low-rate IMV
Infant-triggered ventilation
Apneic Infants
Pressure control ventilation
Low-rate IMV
CPAP
Infants With Severe Hypoxemia and Hypercarbia
High-rate IMV
HFV
SIMV
ECMO
Experimental Forms of Sustaining Gas Exchange
Liquid ventilation
PAGE

CPAP, continuous positive airway pressure; ECMO, extracorporeal memrane oxygenation; HFV, high-frequency ventilation; IMV, intermittent mandatory ventilation; PAGE, perfluorocarbon-associated gas exchange; SIMV, synchronous intermittent mandatory ventilation.

bitrary ceiling of 80 torr is set to minimize the risk of retinopathy of prematurity (ROP) in infants weighing less than 1500 g at birth, although ROP may be unavoidable in certain extremely-low-birth-weight infants.[1-3] The rationale for maintaining the PaO_2 below 100 torr in larger infants is based on minimizing pulmonary oxygen toxicity. When administering oxygen, it is always useful to translate the percent of inspired oxygen to the corresponding partial pressure (PiO_2, $PiCO_2$). The gap between the alveolar partial pressure of oxygen (PAO_2) and the PaO_2 indicates the magnitude of the arterial O_2 gradient across the lungs and provides an indication of the magnitude of right-to-left shunting of blood. A simplification of the alveolar air equation provides an estimate of PAO_2 (*i.e.*, $PAO_2 = PiO_2 - PACO_2$).

Because the barometric pressure, minus water vapor pressure, is approximately 700 torr, the percent of inspired oxygen multiplied by 7 equals PiO_2 in torr (*e.g.*, 21% ≈ 147 torr, 50% ≈ 350 torr). Because $PACO_2$ $PaCO_2$ due to a usually insignificant arterial–alveolar CO_2 gradient ($aADCO_2$), $PaCO_2$ can be substituted for $PACO_2$, and PAO_2 can be derived. For example, if an infant is breathing 60% O_2, the measured PaO_2 is 70 torr and the $PaCO_2$ is 40 torr, the $PAO_2 = 420 - 40 = 380$ torr, and the alveolar–arterial gradient for O_2 ($AaDO_2$) is 310 torr. In an infant without lung disease or a significant right-to-left cardiac shunt, the $AaDO_2$ should not exceed 25 torr while breathing ambient air. Infants with severe hyaline membrane disease may have an $AaDO_2$ in excess of 500 torr while breathing 100% oxygen.[4]

OXYGEN DELIVERY

Each gram of HbF binds 1.37 dL of oxygen. The full-term newborn with a hemoglobin (Hb) of 17 g/dL binds and transports 23 dL of oxygen per 100 dL of blood. Less than 2% of transported O_2 is carried as oxygen dissolved in plasma. Normal tissue consumption extracts approximately 4 volumes percent (4 mL/100 mL) if oxygen consumption and cardiac output are normal. An anemic infant with a hematocrit of 21% (Hb = 7 g/dL) and 98% oxygen saturation (SaO_2) is able to transport 9.6 dL of oxygen per 100 dL of blood, which should be sufficient to meet the body tissue's oxygen needs. Several factors can adversely affect oxygen delivery, including decreased cardiac output, maldistribution of cardiac output, arterial vasoconstriction and shifts in the O_2 dissociation curve. Oxygen unloading in the tissues is increased with a shift to the right of the O_2 dissociation curve (*i.e.*, decreased O_2 affinity) facilitated by a local decrease in *p*H, increase in $PaCO_2$, and increase in temperature. Oxygen uptake depends on adequate alveolar ventilation ($\dot{V}_A$), an appropriate ventilation–perfusion match in the lungs, and absence of right-to-left shunting. Oxygen uptake or increased O_2 affinity of Hb (*i.e.*, shift of curve to left) is enhanced with alkalosis, decreased temperature, decreased 2,3-diphosphoglycerate, and HbF. The HbF as a proportion of total Hb decreases after birth, as HbA gradually increases.

ADMINISTRATION

The concentration, humidity, and temperature of inspired oxygen should be precisely controlled. Diluting or mixing chambers can deliver only an approximate O_2 concentration, and it is necessary to have a precise analysis of the O_2 concentration being delivered to the infant's airway. An incubator is ineffective in maintaining O_2 concentrations above 30%, because opening of the portholes causes considerable dilution. An oxygen hood or tent should be placed over the infant's head. Gas flow through the hood should be at least 2 L/minute to prevent CO_2 accumulation. Nasal prongs are the preferable route of humidified oxygen administration if there is need for chronic administration. The concentration and the rate of flow are varied, and the precise amount of oxygen delivered to the lungs by nasal prongs is difficult to determine. The concentration to be delivered should be determined by monitoring of peripheral SaO_2 and PaO_2. The O_2–air mixture should be warmed to the same temperature as the incubator air, which should be in the range of thermal neutrality (see Chap. 25).

A simple, effective method for heating and humidification is to bubble the gas mixture through water containing a heating device. The apparatus and water are replaced every 48 hours to prevent colonization with hydrophilic bacteria. This device should be equipped with a warning system to prevent overheating of the inspired air–oxygen mixture, which could lead to hyperthermia of the infant.

ASSESSMENT

Technologic advances in the assessment of tissue oxygenation have contributed to the management of respiratory failure. Pulse oximetry, in particular, has enabled on-line and noninvasive assessment of oxygenation, facilitating adjustments in respirator settings and inspired oxygen concentrations. The measurement of PaO_2 remains a necessary part of evaluating therapy to verify the values obtained by pulse oximetry or transcutaneous electrodes. Periodic evaluation of $PaCO_2$ is necessary, because it is the only true measure of the effectiveness of $\dot{V}_A$.

BLOOD SAMPLING

Capillary blood can be arterialized by warming a heal and the droplets collected rapidly to minimize exposure to room air. This sample provides useful information about *p*H and PCO_2; however, it is inadequate for PaO_2 assessment. Arterial blood must, therefore, be obtained by catheterization or direct puncture of a vessel. Sampling from the radial or posterior tibial arteries is preferred over the brachial and femoral arteries. The brachial artery is deeper and less well fixed than the radial artery. Risks of joint infection or of an occlusive hematoma make femoral artery puncture the least desirable. A 23- or 25-gauge scalp-vein needle is suitable for arterial puncture. The radial artery is identified by its location just lateral to the flexor carpi radialis tendon on the palmar surface of the wrist. It is sometimes useful to pinpoint its location by transillumination with a high-intensity lamp.[5] The skin is prepared with an antiseptic solution, and the artery is entered against the direction of flow at a 20° to 30° angle with the bevel of the needle facing upward. Blood should flow spontaneously or with gentle aspiration into the plastic tubing. After withdrawal of the needle, the site should be compressed for several minutes to prevent the formation of a hematoma. Repeated punctures can be made at the same site.

PERIPHERAL ARTERIAL CANNULATION

The choice of peripheral artery or umbilical artery catheterization is usually determined by the size of the infant, the anticipated duration of the cannulation, and the need for infusions of medications and parenteral nutrition including concentrated dextrose solutions. The infusions should not be given through a radial arterial cannula.

Percutaneous radial or posterior tibial artery cannulation often provides arterial access for several days. A 22-gauge cannula is passed through the artery after puncturing the skin with a 20-gauge needle. The stylet is removed and the cannula slowly withdrawn until the pulsatile flow of blood is observed. If the stylet has a lumen, the cannula is slowly advanced until blood emerges from the needle. The stylet needle is withdrawn and the catheter advanced into the artery approximately 1 cm. A continuous flush system must be attached to prevent clotting. Fixation of the catheter is sometimes difficult in small infants, requiring wedges, an arm board, and gentle taping. Attachment to a pressure transducer permits continuous monitoring of arterial blood pressure.

The major advantage of a peripheral arterial catheter is the avoidance of an umbilical artery cannulation and its high risk of thrombosis. There is an extremely low rate of complications with the use of peripheral cannulae. A right radial arterial catheter has the unique advantage of measuring preductal PaO_2, more accurately reflecting retinal PaO_2. The major disadvantage of small vessel cannulation is that hypertonic solutions may not be infused and dislodgement or thrombus formation usually limits its use to 2 or 3 days.

UMBILICAL ARTERIAL CANNULATION

The need to insert a cannula into the umbilical artery should be based on the infant's maturation, postnatal age, and the type, severity, and duration of the illness. Seriously ill infants weighing less than 1000 g at birth usually qualify. The high incidence of thrombus formation on the catheter tip, with its attendant risk of aortic obstruction and embolization to downstream tissues, must be weighed against the potential benefits to the infant. If only occasional samples are needed, arterial puncture is preferred. The catheter should be nonthrombogenic, transparent, radiopaque, and marked at 5-cm intervals. It should be nonkinking and have sufficient stiffness to permit easy insertion. Several types of catheters are commercially available including Silastic, polyvinylchloride, and silicone coated, although no obvious advantage in reducing thrombogenicity appears to exist.[6] Double-lumen catheters have the theoretic advantage of permitting uninterrupted infusion through one port and sampling blood from the other. Available umbilical catheters with a PO_2 electrode in the tip for continuous PaO_2 assessment may be useful in specific circumstances. However, their placement does not warrant removal of a functioning umbilical catheter for replacement with one with an indwelling PO_2 electrode.

Technique. The catheter is placed under aseptic technique, while the restrained infant is positioned on an open, radiantly heated table. Appropriate oxygen should be administered and the infant's condition closely monitored throughout the procedure, with constant evaluation of heart rate, respiration, and SaO_2 by pulse oximetry. Before antiseptic preparation of the umbilical area, the shoulder–umbilicus distance should be measured to determine the depth of catheter insertion. The distance to various levels within the aorta is estimated from data obtained and graphed by Dunn (Fig. 31-1).[7] A snug tie of umbilical tape is placed around the base of the cord to be tightened in the event of bleeding. The cord is then cut within 0.5 cm of the skin. The two arteries appear as small, whitish, thick-walled structures that are constricted, unlike the single vein.

The arterial lumen is gently dilated with iris forceps, first with one blade and then with both. Releasing tension on the inserted forceps produces gentle dilatation of the vessel; dilation should be maintained

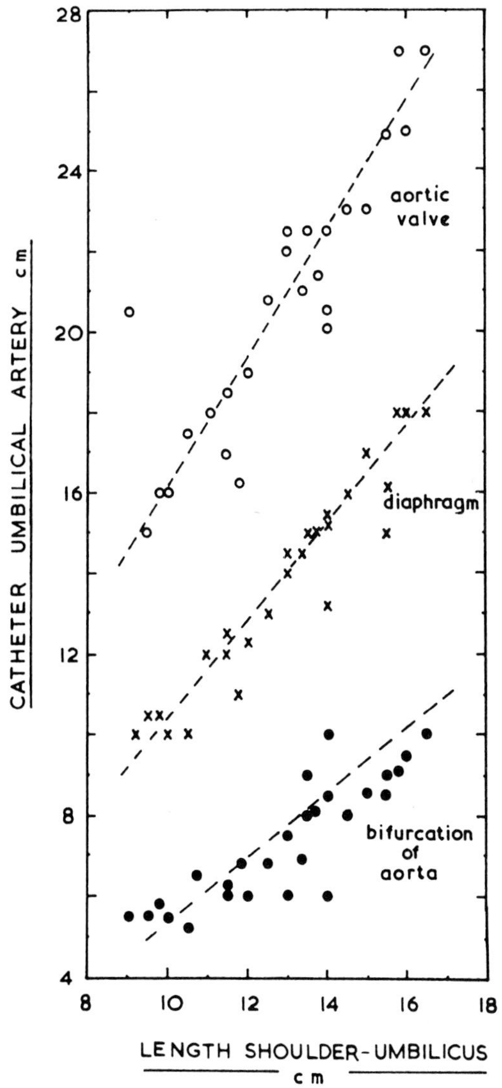

FIG. 31–1. Relation between the shoulder-to-umbilicus measurement and the length of umbilical artery catheter needed to reach the aortic bifurcation, diaphragm, and aortic valve. (From Dunn PM. Localization of the umbilical catheter by post-mortem measurement. Arch Dis Child 1966;41:69.)

for longer than 30 seconds. Probing too deeply with a sharp instrument may tear the arterial wall and allow the catheter to false track in the subintimal layer, as does inordinate manual pressure on the catheter after insertion has started. The saline-filled catheter is inserted in the lumen immediately on withdrawal of the iris forceps. It is advanced gently with a twisting motion using thumb and forefinger or the iris forceps. Slight traction on the cord may be necessary and resistance is often met at 1 to 2 cm. After overcoming this resistance, the catheter is advanced in a caudal direction, and further resistance may be encountered at the junction of the hypogastric artery at 5 to 6 cm. If the cannulation is not successful within a few minutes of the initial catheter tip insertion, cannulation of the second artery should be attempted. If cannulation is unsuccessful and a peripheral arterial cannulation is not feasible, a subumbilical cutdown may be indicated.[8] This procedure carries the risk of hemorrhage and accidental entry into the peritoneal cavity.

After the catheter is in the desired position, it is sutured in place. A purse-string suture through Wharton jelly can prevent bleeding from the other two vessels. The same suture or a second one should be passed through the skin margin to provide a secure anchor for the catheter. The suture is then wrapped around the catheter in two places: at the entrance into the vessel and 2 to 3 cm from the cord. A tape bridge incorporating the suture helps to prevent the catheter from moving in or out.

Location of the Catheter Tip. Two locations permit the catheter tip to reside at some distance from the orifice of a major branching artery, minimizing the risk of occlusion and thrombosis and permitting direct infusions of hypertonic solutions. These sites are the lower thoracic aorta between the ductus arteriosus (T4) and celiac artery (T11–T12), ideally resting between T7 and T10, and the lower abdominal aorta between the inferior mesenteric artery (L4) and the aortic bifurcation (Fig. 31-2). Three studies have compared the incidence of complications of "high" and "low" catheter placement.[9–11] Although there is no difference between groups and the rate of complications requiring catheter removal, there was a higher overall complication rate from the low-position catheters because of more episodes of blanching and cyanosis of the extremities. Thoracic placement allows greater leeway for catheter motion, but it carries the risk of embolization of clots from the catheter tip or surface into major down stream arteries. Because the estimate of catheter position is only approximate, it is necessary to confirm position by a thoracoabdominal radiograph soon after placement and before medications are infused. The vertebral landmarks and usual level of arterial branches are depicted in Figure 31-2. The catheter tip may enter and cross the ductus arteriosus if it is advanced above the level of T4. A frontal film is usually sufficient if care is taken to position the

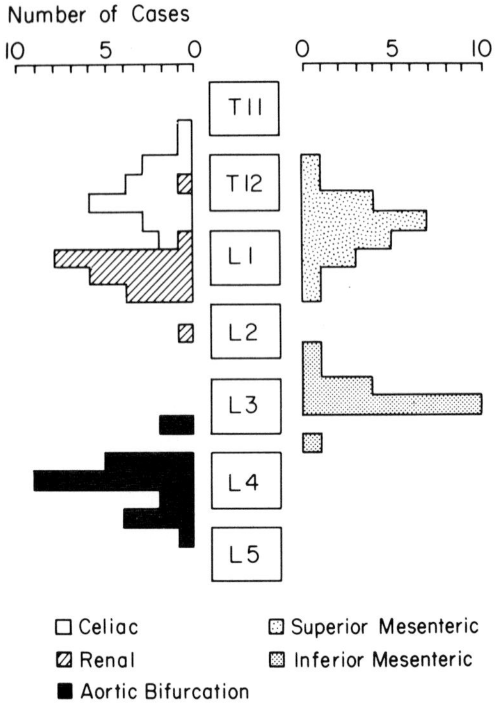

FIG. 31–2. Origins of the major arteries in relation to the vertebral bodies were determined by postmortem angiography on 27 full-term and premature infants. (Data courtesy of CB Graham, M.D., University of Washington, Seattle, WA.)

exterior portion of the catheter directly laterally in order to facilitate radiographic interpretation.

Management of Indwelling Catheters. Umbilical artery catheters should be flushed free of blood after each sampling. A continuous fluid infusion is the most satisfactory method for keeping the lumen clear. This is best accomplished with an infusion pump, because it is necessary to maintain an infusion pressure greater than aortic pressure. All or part of the infant's fluid requirements can be administered through the catheter, although the administration of medications and blood products may increase the risk of complications and shorten the life of the catheter. Heparin has been advocated as an additive to the fluid infusion or for periodic flushing of the catheter. However, this may induce inadvertent systemic heparinization and increase the infant's risk of severe hemorrhage. Keeping the catheter free of blood by flushing with any fluid should prevent clotting within the catheter lumen.

Evidence for clot formation within the catheter (*e.g.*, difficulty withdrawing blood, dampened blood pressure tracing) is an indication for its removal and possible replacement. A new catheter may be substituted. Under aseptic technique, the nonfunctional catheter is removed and the replacement catheter immediately inserted into the lumen before its closure. If the infant is older than 24 hours of age, successful cannulation of the second artery is improbable. A catheter may remain functional for 1 to 2 weeks and occasionally longer. It should be removed after the infant has demonstrated improvement, the frequency of blood gas measurements has decreased substantially, and systemic arterial pressure monitoring is no longer essential.

The cannula occasionally serves as the only route for parenteral nutrition or other infusions, and it may remain in place longer. Controversy exists about the risks of necrotizing enterocolitis if enteral feedings are instituted while the catheter is in place, but the evidence for causality is poor, and it is therefore appropriate to initiate feedings before catheter removal.

Catheter Removal. Withdrawal of the catheter over 5 to 10 minutes usually allows the artery to constrict and prevents significant bleeding. It is advisable to have a small artery forceps immediately available in the event of brisk bleeding. A purse-string suture or umbilical tape should be placed around the cord and immediately tightened after the catheter has been removed.

Complications. The complications of umbilical vessel catheterization are listed in Table 31-2. The most frequent problem is peripheral vasospasm asso-

TABLE 31–2
COMPLICATIONS OF UMBILICAL CATHETERIZATION

Complication	Incidence	Comment
Limb ischemia	<20%	Assess Doppler arterial and venous flow from femoral region to dorsalis pedis; if reflex and unilateral, apply warmth to contralateral extremity; if persistent (>15 min), remove catheter
Thrombosis	<90%	Assess by ultrasonographic study of aorta
Infection	Colonization: 57% Sepsis: 5%	Remove in presence of gram-positive blood culture if catheter was inserted more than 24 h previously; no relation to duration of catheter
Blood Loss	Rare	Connection to blood pressure transducer with alarm should prevent significant loss
Vascular perforation	Extremely rare	On removal, clamp for 5–10 min

ciated with blanching or patchy cyanosis of the distal leg, foot, or toes. If this does not improve with reflex vasodilation by warming of the contralateral leg or worsens over the next 15 to 20 minutes, the catheter should be removed. Assessment of peripheral arterial flow by Doppler stethoscope is often helpful in deciding about catheter removal. Some thrombosis at the catheter tip is inevitable. Fortunately, the rate of complications from thrombus formation is exceedingly low.

TRANSCUTANEOUS PO_2

Transcutaneous PO_2 should be used in conjunction with pulse oximetry. Most devices contain O_2 and CO_2 electrodes. Noninvasive PO_2 measurements continue to be helpful in certain situations, particularly if transcutaneous PCO_2 is also obtained. Calibration before use and correlation with an arterial sample is necessary, but the need for subsequent blood samples should be reduced.

The PaO_2 and transcutaneous PO_2 are not identical. Differences can be due to local O_2 consumption by the skin or by the electrode itself, heating of the skin, O_2 diffusion time, and response time of the electrode.[12] These differences, by acting in opposite directions, tend to cancel each other and fortuitously provide an accurate reflection of PaO_2.[13,14] Skin blood flow may be affected by vasopressor medications, hypotension, and shock.[15] Use of transcutaneous PO_2 can reduce the number of blood sampling procedures, particularly during a period when rapid changes in O_2 administration or mechanical ventilatory settings are taking place. Continuous monitoring for several hours also allows assessment of changes due to position, handling, suctioning, and feeding and for comparison with SaO_2 monitoring. Second-degree burns (*i.e.*, blistering) preclude its use for longer than 5 hours at a single site on the body. If longer use is required, the electrode site should be shifted every 3 to 4 hours and requires additional correlation with PaO_2. The short application time has made transcutaneous PO_2 monitoring less useful than oximetry for continuous assessment of oxygen over a period of many hours.

PULSE OXIMETRY

The introduction of pulse oximetry to the intensive care nursery has provided a safe, accurate, and noninvasive adjunct to the assessment of tissue oxygenation.[16] Although monitoring of SaO_2 by infrared devices has been available for longer than 20 years, it has not been sufficiently reliable for use in neonates until the development of the pulse oximeter, within the last 10 years. This device uses two electrodes and a small cuff that can be placed around a hand, foot, or toe without requiring heating or calibration. It has an extremely rapid response time. One electrode contains two diodes that emit light at two wavelengths: red at 660 nm and infrared at 940 nm. The other electrode senses the light from both of these diodes that has not been absorbed by blood or tissue. The relative concentration of HbO_2 and deoxyhemoglobin determines the amount of transmitted light, because different forms of Hb have markedly different absorption characteristics. The ratio of the amount of light absorbed at each wavelength is used to calculate an SaO_2 value. The pulsed element of the apparatus allows the instrument to differentiate added arterial blood oxygenation and absorption from tissue, and it subtracts the amount contributed by a constant venous and arterial blood flow. The instrumentation is sufficiently sensitive to detect less than 1% of the light transmitted. This discrete pulse signal undergoes large electronic amplification and is displayed as percent saturation. The displayed value usually represents an average of 5 to 7 seconds of sampling. The two electrodes must be placed on opposite sides of an arterial vessel and be protected from strong environmental light sources, such as radiant heaters, phototherapy lamps, and the sun.

The pulse rate must be accurate. Inaccuracies can result from movement artifact, particularly in very small infants. The accuracy of the pulse oximeter has been assessed in a variety of infants by comparing arterial and transcutaneous PO_2 measurements.[16] With PO_2 values greater than 40 torr, the saturation accurately reflects measurements of PO_2 obtained by catheter sample or by transcutaneous PO_2.[17]

A PaO_2 of 60 to 90 torr results in a saturation value of 94% to 98%, and changes of 1% to 2% usually reflect a PaO_2 change of 6 to 12 torr.[16] The point of inflection at which the hemoglobin–oxygen (HbO_2) dissociation curve steepens has considerable variability and depends on proportions of HbA, HbF, PCO_2, *p*H, and temperature. Generally, these variables are not so critical to the interpretation of the percent SaO_2 in arterial blood as they are to PaO_2. Below 40 torr, the SaO_2 falls below 90%. An alarm limit is usually set at 89%, although this lower limit may need adjustment. For example, if an infant has pulmonary hypertension, a PaO_2 below 50 torr may increase pulmonary vascular resistance, and the saturation may best be maintained above 94%. If the infant is acutely ill and unstable, a correlation with PaO_2, preferably obtained by a catheter blood sample, is indicated. Poor correlation with PaO_2 exists when the SaO_2 is above 98%, in which case the PaO_2 may be well above 100 torr. The data of Hay and colleagues suggest an appropriate goal is to maintain the saturation between 92% and 98% unless a specific clinical situation indicates otherwise.[16] Inaccuracies may reflect improper placement, movement, or peripheral ischemia.

NEAR-INFRARED SPECTROSCOPY

Application of some of the same principles of the unique light-absorbing properties of Hb and HbO_2 used in pulsed oximetry has led to a more sophisticated method of appraising tissue oxygenation by means of near-infrared spectroscopy. Near-infrared light penetrates the skin, bone, and various tissues and can be detected by electrodes placed on opposite sides of an infant's skull. This permits assessment of cerebral tissue O_2 use and alterations in cerebral blood volume. The increased wavelength of near-infrared light (*i.e.*, 700–1000 nm) results in less scattering and better transmission than visible light (*i.e.*, 400–700 nm). Hemoglobin, HbO_2, and cytochrome a, a_3 (cyt a, a_3) are the only substances that absorb near-infrared light. Cytochrome a, a_3 is at the terminal position of the respiratory chain. It exists as a complex, which is sometimes called cytochrome oxidase, and the complex is involved with more than 90% of cellular oxygen use. Hemoglobin and cyt a, a_3 change their absorption characteristics according to the degree of oxygenation. The wavelength at which maximal absorption occurs is different for HbO_2, deoxygenated Hb, total Hb, and reduced and oxygenated cyt a, a_3.[18] Using photomultiplication and algorithms, the degree of oxygenation can be determined. The total Hb (*i.e.*, Hb + HbO_2) is an indirect measure of blood volume. Reduced cyt a, a_3 mirrors changes in phosphocreatine as absorption changes at a slightly higher O_2 level than phosphocreatine and before there is a decrease in the amount of ATP. Quantification of reduced cyt a, a_3 should provide an early indication of insufficient mitochondrial oxygen.[19]

The small cranial size of the infant weighing less than 1500 g makes cross-temple spectroscopy feasible. Preliminary studies using experimental equipment are encouraging.[20,21] The light source at one temple is a fiberoptic bundle consisting of four laser diodes with different wavelengths. A second fiberoptic bundle on the opposite temple detects transmitted light of various wavelengths.[20,22] The amplified signals indicate the relative amounts of HbO_2 and cyt a, a_3, providing a continuous assessment of the trends in cerebral oxygenation and blood volume.[20–23] This important new mechanism of assessing brain oxygenation has the potential to provide new information on changes in cerebral blood flow and oxygenation resulting from infusions of drugs (*e.g.*, vasopressors, indomethacin), changes in position, nursing procedures, paralysis, apnea and bradycardia, shock, decreased blood pressure, patent ductus arteriosus, and intrathoracic pressure variations secondary to mechanical ventilation. Further refinement of equipment and verification of its accuracy in reflecting changes in cerebral blood flow and cerebral oxygenation are needed. This method of oxygen assessment has immense potential for use in the neonatal intensive care unit.

CONTINUOUS POSITIVE AIRWAY PRESSURE

Continuous positive airway pressure (CPAP) is a mode of respiratory assistance for spontaneously breathing infants (Table 31-3). Positive airway pressure may be administered through an endotracheal tube, a nasopharyngeal tube inserted into the posterior pharynx, or a short (0.3–0.5 cm) set of nasal prongs inserted to create a snug fit in the nares. In each case, the spontaneously breathing infant is exposed through CPAP circuitry to a constant stream of blended, warm, humidified O_2 and room air flowing through the device. Airway pressure is maintained in the range of 4 to 12 cm H_2O. Continuous positive airway pressure delivery systems include both nasal prongs, a means of stabilizing this device on the infant's head and a means of generating the positive pressure, usually by use of a retardation valve on the expiratory limb of the breathing circuit.

TABLE 31–3
CONTINUOUS POSITIVE AIRWAY PRESSURE

Indications
Spontaneously breathing infant with mild or moderate diffuse hyaline membrane disease
Very-low-birth-weight infant with apnea
Complications
Increased work of breathing, hypercarbic apnea
Air leak, especially pneumothorax
Nasal trauma

Although first introduced in 1971 and the subject of clinical trials thereafter, the technique was not unequivocally established to reduce mortality in babies with hyaline membrane disease.[24–26] The original rationale for CPAP was to attempt to overcome presumed diffuse atelectasis in the gas exchanging areas in the lungs of infants with hyaline membrane disease by preventing alveolar collapse in surfactant-deficient lungs. If this occurs, proportionate increases in end-expiratory lung volume and arterial oxygen levels could be expected. However, change in lung volume measured as functional residual capacity (FRC), change in level of distending pressure, and change in blood gas tensions bear inconsistent associations with each other.[27,28] More recent speculation regarding the mechanism of action of CPAP in hyaline membrane disease suggests that, rather than overcoming atelectasis, CPAP may be associated with improved gas flow to already ventilated areas of the lung, providing an explanation for the commonly found improvement in PaO_2. Indications and possible complications of CPAP are presented in Table 31-3.

In 1987, the role of nasal-prong CPAP as an alternative to endotracheal intubation and mechanical-assisted ventilation was suggested in a report by Avery and associates.[29] In this retrospective review of the outcome of infants weighing less than 1500 g at birth, one of the eight surveyed centers reported an equal mortality and substantially lower incidence of bronchopulmonary dysplasia, as assessed by supplemental oxygen or assisted ventilation needs at 1 month of age, compared with the other seven centers (Fig. 31-

3). The one distinguishing feature of neonatal respiratory treatment at this center (*i.e.*, Columbia University) compared with the others surveyed was extensive reliance on CPAP. This finding is compatible with the theory that cyclic positive-pressure ventilation is a major contributing factor to pulmonary injury in very-low-birth-weight infants. No prospective study of CPAP during the current era of widespread use of exogenous surfactant has been performed to confirm or refute this hypothesis.

Nasal-prong CPAP has been advocated in the treatment of idiopathic apnea of prematurity. The mechanism of action is not clear, and its use during this situation must be associated with extremely close monitoring because of the propensity of the technique to increase work of breathing and, under some circumstances, to elevate $PaCO_2$. Although application of CPAP by nasal prongs is a less invasive and a possibly less hazardous way of providing ventilatory assistance than intratracheal intubation and mechanical ventilation, its use is associated with complications (see Table 31-3). A particular risk is development of pneumothorax, perhaps due to localized overdistention of the lungs. Nonetheless, some larger premature infants with hyaline membrane disease may avoid intubation and assisted ventilation by application of CPAP. The use of CPAP in smaller infants is problematic because of the availability of an alternative therapy: delivery of exogenous surfactant through an intratracheal tube directly to the infant's lungs. Some infants may benefit from a course of brief intubation for delivery of exogenous surfactant, followed by application of CPAP delivered by endotracheal tube or by nasal prongs. The course would avoid the additional hazard of prolonged positive-pressure ventilation. Because of technical considerations (*e.g.*, small size of the nasal prongs), greater difficulty in providing a stabilization of the CPAP circuitry, and the more immature physiologic condition of the infant, extremely-low-birth-weight infants (<1000 g) have proven difficult to treat with CPAP alone.

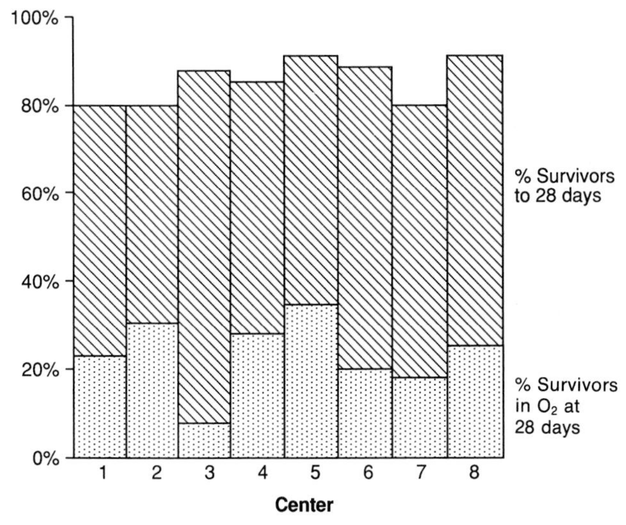

FIG. 31–3. Dotted areas indicate percentages of infants in oxygen at 28 days of age; cross-hatched areas indicate survivors without added oxygen at 28 days. Center 3 has the lowest percentage of infants who depended on oxygen and among the highest percentage of survivors. (Adapted Avery ME, Tooley WH, Keller JB, et al. Is chronic lung disease in low birth weight infants preventable? A survey of eight centers. Pediatrics 1987;79:26.)

ASSISTED MECHANICAL VENTILATION

INDICATIONS AND LIMITATIONS

The immature lung presents a special hazard in the application of assisted ventilation. Attempts to overcome respiratory failure by increasing $\dot{V}_A$ and optimizing ventilation–perfusion ($\dot{V}_A/\dot{Q}$) matching may injure epithelial and endothelial tissues. Most alveolization occurs postnatally, and the developing structures are less elastic and more vulnerable to barotrauma. Injury to the mesenchymal and epithelial tissues giving rise to alveolar septation may be irreversible. Studies in adult animals have demonstrated that otherwise healthy lungs can suffer injury, reflected by increased airway fluid and deterioration of gas exchange, if sufficient distending lung pressures are applied.[30] The particular problems of providing assisted ventilation are illustrated in Figure 31-4. Relative immaturity of distal bronchioles and respiratory ducts, coupled with fluid-filled and collapsed alveoli, create a set of conditions leading to overdistention of some areas with resultant ineffective gas exchange.

Great strides have been made in understanding how the immature lung differs from a mature lung in phospholipid and surfactant-associated protein biosynthesis. There are other factors unique to the immature lung that render it susceptible to injury, including incomplete development of the supportive net of collagen and elastin, incomplete development of the capillary bed in the gas exchange areas, relative instability of the chest wall and its inability to maintain expiratory lung volume at an adequate FRC, and immaturity of the neural control producing sustained spontaneous respiratory effort. The metabolic function of the pulmonary endothelium is not well studied in the immature infant, but it is probably deficient in metabolizing bioactive amines and peptides, especially given the limited pulmonary blood flow. Although detailed discussion of these areas is beyond the scope of this chapter, the clinician must have some understanding of these factors to understand the limitations and failures of assisted ventilation.

Assisted ventilation is used in neonates as immature as 24 to 25 weeks of gestation. Younger than this gestational age, the lung as an organ of gas exchange fails because of the profoundly immature state of the gas exchange surface area. If a consensus develops to

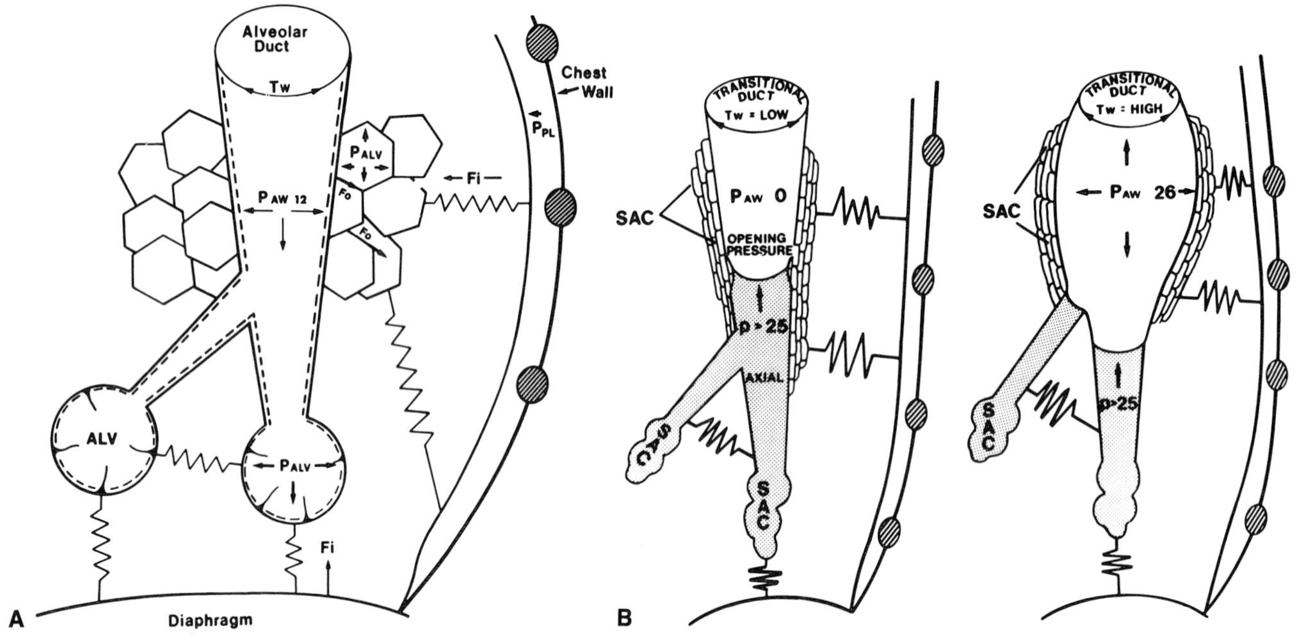

FIG. 31–4. **(A)** A mature alveolar duct and alveoli. (*Dotted line,* surfactant; P_{ALV}, alveolar pressure; P_{AW}, airway pressure; P_{PL}, pleural pressure; Fi, tissue force (stretched springs) acting inward; Fo, tissue force directed outward; Tw, wall tension or recoil pressure.) **(B)** The end-expiratory airway pressure (Paw) equals zero in an immature distal airway (*left*). The saccules (SAC) and airways contain fluid (*shaded area*). The axial airway is concave at the air–liquid interface due to the surface tension forces. The peripherol SAC are collapsed or fluid filled. The lax tissues are represented by relaxed springs. The inspiratory airway pressure (P_{Aw}) is equal to 26 cm H_2O (*right*). The distended distal airway has a high wall tension (Tw). The liquid front has been pushed peripherally, but the SAC are still not inflated. (From Thibeault DW. Mechanisms and pathobiologic effects of barotrauma. In: Merit TA, Northway WH Jr, Boynton BR, eds. Bronchopulmonary dysplasia. Contemporary issues in fetal neonatal medicine. Boston: Blackwell Scientific Publishers, 1988.)

attempt to sustain *ex utero* survival of fetuses of currently nonviable gestational age (*e.g.*, 20–22 weeks), alternative methods of gas exchange that do not rely on the lung must be devised.

ESTABLISHMENT OF AN ARTIFICIAL AIRWAY

PHYSIOLOGIC AND ANATOMIC AIRWAY PECULIARITIES

The newborn infant has distinct anatomic and physiologic characteristics of the airways and a strong preference for nasal breathing for the first few months of life.[31] Nasal or nasopharyngeal obstruction due to secretions, mucosal injury, or congenital abnormalities may produce respiratory distress. Approximately one-half of the infant's airway resistance occurs in the nose, although the narrowness of the lower respiratory tract results in a total airway resistance approximately 15 times greater than that of an adult.[32] Edema and inflammation can produce extremely high resistance to airflow in these narrow airways. During expiration, the airways become narrower, and resistance increases.

ENDOTRACHEAL INTUBATION

Route. Orotracheal and nasotracheal intubation may be used for prolonged mechanical ventilation of term and premature infants. The principal advantage of the nasal route is the stabilization of the tube afforded by the close fit within the naris, but the nasal passages may limit the size of tube that can be used. Necrosis of the nasal septum or the alae nasi can occur if circulation is impaired because the tube is too large. Orotracheal intubation is more easily and quickly accomplished and is indicated for delivery room and emergency situations. It is the preferred route for prolonged mechanical ventilation.

The endotracheal tube should allow a small air leak between the tube and the glottis. A tube that fits too snugly within the trachea is likely to cause pressure necrosis of the mucosa. If too large a leak is allowed, it may be difficult to achieve sufficient pressure for ventilation of noncompliant lungs. A tube with a 2.5-mm inner diameter usually fits infants weighing less than 1000 g; a 3-mm tube fits those from 1000 to 1500 g; a 3.5-mm tube fits those from 1500 to 2500 g; and a 4.0-mm tube fits larger infants.

Technique. Orotracheal intubation is a simple procedure that can be accomplished atraumatically within a few seconds. The necessary equipment consists of a straight-bladed laryngoscope, a suction catheter connected to a suction apparatus, an endotracheal tube of the appropriate size with an adapter for the bag or respirator, and an optical flexible Teflon introducer, bent to prevent its tip from protruding beyond the end of the endotracheal tube. The infant is ventilated with 100% oxygen by mask for a few breaths. A catheter to deliver oxygen can be taped to the laryngoscope blade to enhance oxygen delivery during intubation.[33] The physician straightens the infant's neck without hyperextension by placing a small towel under the shoulders, and the head is steadied by an assistant. The laryngoscope is held in the left hand between the thumb and first two fingers. The heel of the hand is placed against the infant's left cheek to provide stability. The blade is introduced into the right side of the mouth, and the tongue is deflected to the left as the blade is advanced into the vallecula, anterior to the epiglottis. The laryngoscope is lifted rather than rotated so that the larynx is elevated and the glottis is brought into view (Fig. 31-5). The pharynx is suctioned if necessary. The endotracheal tube is introduced into the mouth to the right of the laryngoscope and gently guided into the glottis under direct vision.

Placement of the nasotracheal tube is technically more difficult and often more time consuming than orotracheal intubation. It is best, particularly in a severely compromised infant, to have an orotracheal tube in place so that the infant can be ventilated while the nasotracheal tube is being positioned. The nasotracheal tube is inserted without an introducer through the naris and gently guided along the floor of the nose. The laryngoscope is placed in the mouth to the right of the orotracheal tube, and the tip of the nasotracheal tube is seen in the posterior pharynx. A Magill forceps is held in the right hand and introduced to the right of the laryngoscope. The nasotracheal tube is grasped a few millimeters back from its tip with the forceps, and the tip of the tube is elevated until it is almost at the glottis. It is helpful to have an assistant grasp the exterior end of the nasotracheal tube to assist in advancing it. The orotracheal tube is left in place until just before insertion of the nasotracheal tube in the glottis.

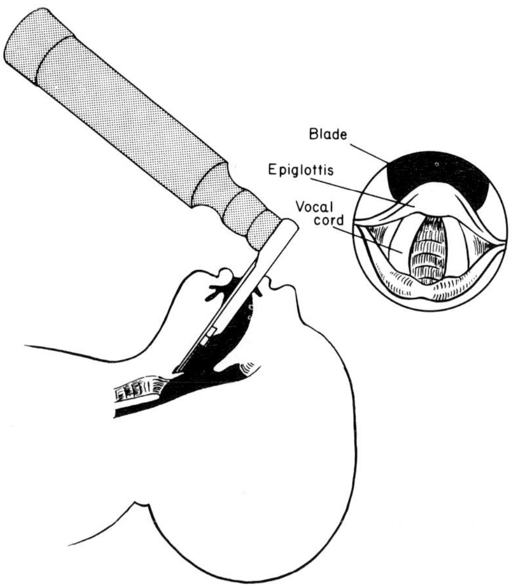

FIG. 31–5. Laryngoscopy for endotracheal intubation.

TABLE 31–4
DEPTH OF INSERTION OF AN OROTRACHEAL TUBE FROM THE LIPS OF A PREMATURE INFANT

Infant Weight (kg)	Depth of Insertion (cm)
1.0	7
2.0	8
3.0	9
4.0	10

Heart rate and, if possible, arterial SaO_2 should be monitored continuously during endotracheal intubation. If the heart rate falls, intubation should be deferred while the infant is ventilated with a resuscitation bag and face mask. Pretreatment with pancuronium bromide and atropine may minimize heart rate and intracranial pressure changes associated with endotracheal intubation, but further studies are needed to determine if minimizing these changes is useful clinically.[34,35]

Positioning. The length of the trachea from the vocal cords to the carina varies from about 3.6 cm in the smallest premature infants to 6 cm in large, term infants. Optimal positioning for the tip of an endotracheal tube is in the middle of the trachea, where it is least subject to dislodgement into the pharynx or displacement into a bronchus. The proper depth of insertion of an endotracheal tube, as determined by postmortem and radiographic measurements, is related to body weight.[36] Suggested depths of insertion for either orotracheal or nasotracheal intubation are given in Table 31-4.[36,37]

Immediately after intubation, the position of the tube should be confirmed by inspection and auscultation. Two common errors of tube placement are intubation of the esophagus and intubation of the right main-stem bronchus. The former should be suspected if insufflation through the tube produces abdominal distention with little chest expansion and if air movement is heard better over the stomach than over the chest. Breath sounds that are louder over the right chest than the left suggest that the tube is in the right main-stem bronchus. Auscultation, though helpful, is not reliable because breath sounds are well transmitted in a small chest. Frontal and lateral chest radiographs should be obtained immediately after intubation to confirm tube placement. The lateral view can differentiate between the trachea and the esophagus, and the frontal view shows the position of the tube in relation to the carina.

Care of Endotracheal Tubes. A tube in the trachea interferes with the physiologic mechanisms for clearance of respiratory secretions and may itself stimulate secretions. Meticulous care is needed to prevent accumulation and inspissation of secretions, which can obstruct the tube. Routine changing of the tube is unnecessary and subjects the infant to the repeated risk of trauma to the larynx and interruption of ventilation. The volume and quality of secretions vary with the type of pulmonary disease and with the individual patient. Suction frequency may vary from once each hour to fewer than 2 or 3 times per day. The tube need not be changed as long as it remains patent. However, the use of high-frequency jet ventilation necessitates changing the endotracheal tube to a special triple-lumen tube.

Another important aspect of the care of artificial airways is the provision of adequate humidification. The endotracheal tube bypasses the nasal and pharyngeal mucosa, which normally warms and humidifies inspired gases. If heat and humidity are not provided from an external source, drying of the lower airway mucosa, thickened secretions, and hypothermia may result. Inspired gases should be passed through a heated nebulizer so that they are delivered to the airway already warmed to a range of 32°C to 34°C and saturated with water vapor. A temperature probe with an audio alarm to detect overheating should be positioned in the inspiratory tubing near the infant. There is evidence that inadequate humidification contributes to the pathogenesis of acute and chronic pulmonary injury.[38]

MEANS OF PROVIDING VENTILATORY ASSISTANCE

Ventilators may be controlled by a preset volume, pressure, or time. Most commercially available neonatal ventilators operate by time cycling, with constant flow as the generated force. Volume-cycled respirators deliver the same volume with each breath regardless of the pulmonary resistance or compliance. The disadvantage of this type of ventilator is the risk of overdistending areas of the lung that are most compliant or delivering a high pressure to the lungs if compliance suddenly decreases. An unknown volume may be lost around the endotracheal tube. Pressure-cycled respirators regulate the volume of inspired gas delivered by setting a limit on the peak inspiratory pressure (PIP).

Time-cycled ventilators permit the limitation of peak pressure by a pop-off valve while delivering a constant flow. The flow rate, inspiratory time (T_I), and the inspiratory–expiratory (I–E) ratio can be adjusted. All types of respirators permit mixing of oxygen and air, temperature and humidity control, and limit alarms for all parameters. The ventilators should permit several types of respiratory patterns and ideally display PIP, mean airway pressure (P_{AW}), positive end-expiratory pressure (PEEP), I–E ratio, frequency, and T_I, because each variable may be important (Fig. 31-6).

The complex interplay of variables in those devices is not fully understood, and the optimal application of assisted ventilation at a specific point in the natural history of a specific disease is still a blend of experience, science, and art (Fig. 31-7).

INDICATIONS

The decision for initiation of assisted ventilation should be tailored for each baby with respect to underlying disease, birth weight, gestational age, postnatal age, chest radiograph, progression of clinical signs, serial arterial blood gas tension, and *p*H measurements. The criteria indicating a need for mechanical ventilation are difficult to define, and there is lack of unanimity about a particular threshold for PaO_2, $PaCO_2$, or fraction of inspired oxygen (FiO_2). In general, the PaO_2 should be maintained at or above 50 torr because of reasonable oxyhemoglobin saturation at this level, but the maximal level of inspired O_2 dictating intubation remains controversial. No rigid ceiling for $PaCO_2$ can be supported by morbidity or mortality data. A trend of rising $PaCO_2$ with concomitant decrease in *p*H and onset of apnea indicates a need for mechanical assistance.

After assisted ventilation is initiated, the generally accepted goals are to maintain the PaO_2 between 50

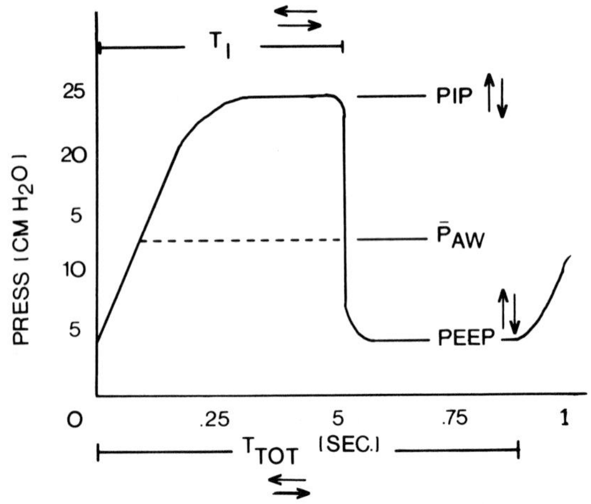

FIG. 31–6. Profile of a pressure waveform during mechanical ventilation. Bidirectional areas indicate some of the variables that can be altered to raise or lower main airway pressure. (PEEP, positive end-expiratory pressure; PIP, peak inspiratory pressure; T_I, inspiratory time; T_{TOT} duration of inspiration plus expiration.)

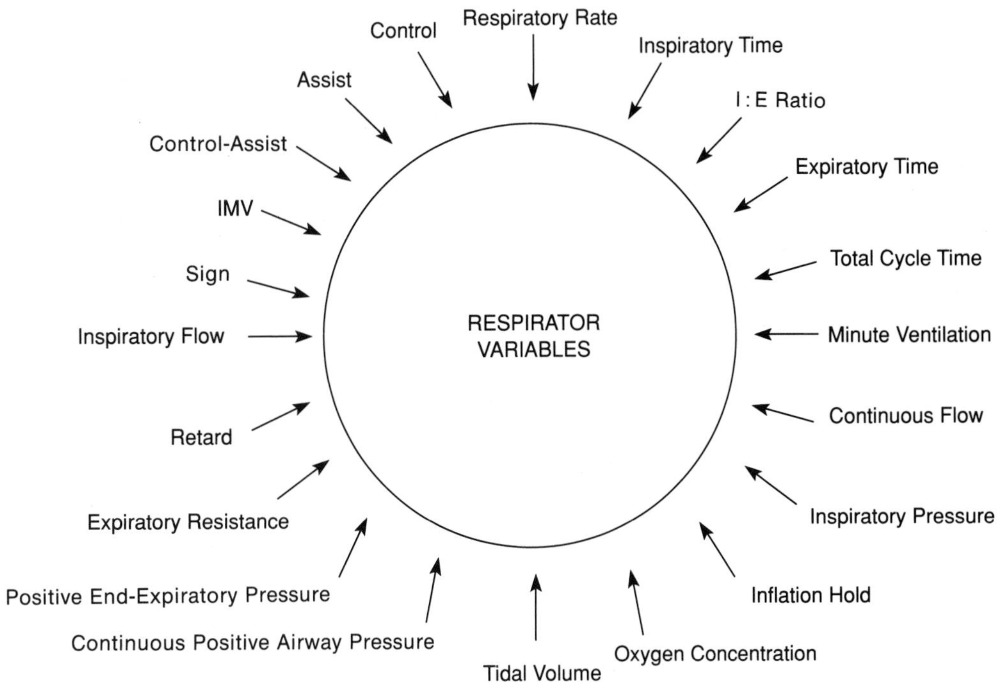

FIG. 31–7. Several respirator variables affect the efficiency of mechanical ventilation.

and 70 torr, $PaCO_2$ at 50 torr or less, and *p*H at 7.3 or more while minimizing PIP, $P_{AW[gas]}$, PEEP, and FiO_2. Because acute lung disease is usually more severe and protracted in the more immature infant, criteria for intervention for infants weighing less than 1000 g are stricter than those for larger infants. For example, a 750-g infant with hyaline membrane disease has a high probability of developing apnea, fatigue, or both, and most of these infants require assisted ventilation even if the FiO_2 is approximately 40%. A 2000-g infant with hyaline membrane disease has greater muscular and caloric reserve and is able to sustain rapid ventilatory rates and higher respiratory work for several days without assistance. With a normal $PaCO_2$, inspired O_2 may be increased to between 80% and 90% before intubation in some infants. The role of CPAP in the latter situation remains controversial, although it continues to be advocated in many centers.

PHYSIOLOGIC CONSIDERATIONS

A thorough understanding of the effects of mechanical ventilation on the lungs requires knowledge of respiratory mechanics, including pulmonary compliance and airway resistance, respiratory control mechanisms, and alveolar gas exchange in the infant.

Lung compliance (*i.e.*, change in lung volume per unit pressure change, in units of mL/cm H_2O) depends on the elastic properties of the tissue, which are influenced by the lung volume and abnormalities such as tissue inflammation and edema. Compliance is low if there is alveolar collapse or overdistention. Expansion from alveolar collapse requires inflation pressures of 12 to 20 cm H_2O. The lungs of infants with hyaline membrane disease have areas of collapse and overexpansion, and there is nonuniformity of compliance. Other conditions, such as pneumothorax, lobar atelectasis, consolidation, and pulmonary edema, decrease compliance. The degree of chest wall compliance is usually high and does not present a problem to mechanical ventilation.

Because the airway resistance (cm H_2O/L/second) is inversely related to the fourth power of the radius during laminar air flow, it is high in the infant, increasing with low lung volumes and with obstruction of the airway. High rates of air flow increase resistance by producing turbulence in the airways.

The rate at which lung areas inflate and deflate is determined by resistance and compliance. An increase in airway resistance increases the time required for air to reach the alveoli; a decrease in compliance results in less time required to reach equilibrium. The product of resistance and compliance is known as the pulmonary time constant. Changes in resistance or compliance can alter the pattern or distribution of ventilation, and recognition of the variations in the time constant (*e.g.*, short with poor compliance, prolonged with increased airway resistance) helps determine respirator settings.

Because hyaline membrane disease and its associated atelectasis should result in a fast time constant, rapid inspiratory and expiratory respirator times are permissible, and mean airway pressure should be increased to improve oxygenation. With meconium aspiration or airway edema, the time constant is slower, and sufficient time for expiration is important to avoid gas trapping, overdistention of the lungs, and possible air leak. If the expiratory time (T_E) is shorter than the time constant of the lung for expiration, overdistention results. If the time constants for the lung are longer than the imposed ventilator T_I, inadequate ventilation could result. Unequal time constants coexisting in different parts of the lung are most likely to occur if pulmonary abnormalities are unevenly distributed, as in pneumonia, meconium aspiration, pulmonary interstitial emphysema, pneumothorax, or bronchopulmonary dysplasia, in which case the optimal T_I or T_E becomes more difficult to determine and estimated adjustments may be necessary.

It is helpful to have an understanding of lung volumes when ventilating an infant. The tidal volume is approximately 8 mL/kg, with one-third consisting of dead space. Mechanical ventilators should permit a tidal volume in the range of 5 to 60 mL, depending on the size of the infant, with minimal apparatus dead space.

The circulatory effects of mechanically applied pressure to the alveoli are important but often overlooked. Normal breathing results in negative intrapleural pressures that enhance venous return and cardiac output, and positive-pressure breathing or negative pressure around the body impedes venous return and may diminish cardiac output unless the negative pressure is applied around the chest alone. Negative pressure does not impede venous return from the head. The duration of inspiration (*i.e.*, I–E ratio) influences the pulmonary capillary circulation and can effect pulmonary blood flow and gas exchange.

MANAGEMENT

The appropriate ventilator settings should allow the most effective gas exchange with the least risk of lung injury. Excess applied airway pressure or inspired oxygen concentration should be avoided. Less certain are the safe or tolerable limits of airway pressure, including the duration of its application during a respiratory cycle. The use of a prolonged T_I, a reversed I–E time ratio, or an inspiratory plateau may improve oxygenation, but at a cost of local overdistention and distal airway or alveolar lining injury. There are no carefully controlled clinical studies that substantiate that reversed I–E ratios ($T_I > T_E$), limitation of PIP, or any particular pattern of ventilation can reduce the incidence of bronchopulmonary dysplasia. Retrospective analysis associating high airway pressure with pathologic changes in the airways at postmortem examination does not differentiate cause and effect. Abnormal airways may have caused the use of high peak airway pressures for satisfactory gas exchange. It would seem wise to avoid the use of high airway pressures (>30 cm H_2O) unless manipulation of other variables, such as changes in PEEP, I–E ratio, and FiO_2, fails to improve gas exchange (see Fig. 31-6).

The most common need in hyaline membrane disease is for an increase in PaO_2; adjustments to correct an abnormal PCO_2 are often of secondary importance. The physician decides whether to increase FiO_2 or $P_{AW[gas]}$ by considering the prior settings and balancing the possible harmful effects of increasing $P_{AW[gas]}$ against those of increasing FiO_2, recognizing that threshold limits are arbitrary. If the FiO_2 is approaching 1.0, there is no choice but to increase $P_{AW[gas]}$. If PEEP is already 6 to 8 cm H_2O, the PIP or the T_I is increased. The use of PEEP helps to maintain patent small airways and prevent collapse to airlessness of those alveoli already open. Inspiratory pressures of greater than 15 cm H_2O are usually required to open collapsed or fluid-filled acinar areas. A combination of an increase in the I–E ratio with 6 cm H_2O PEEP may be optimal during the initial phase of assisted ventilation for hyaline membrane disease. With subsequent opening of air spaces, the optimal I–E ratio may need to be decreased. The use of an end-inspiratory pause or plateau should improve the distribution of inspired gas if there are regional differences in airway resistance (see Fig. 31-6). However, if the alveolar pressure exceeds capillary pressure, there will be tamponading of the pulmonary circulation and some wasting of ventilation to areas with little or no blood flow. Various effective approaches to assisted ventilation have been learned on larger babies with hyaline membrane disease; application of these lessons to the profoundly immature infant, now treated with surfactant, should be done with extreme caution.

Blood gas tensions should be measured 10 to 15 minutes after ventilatory settings are changed. If the PO_2 is below 50 torr or the PCO_2 is above 60 torr, adjustments may be made. However, it is recommended that the caregiver adjust only one variable at a time and reassess the resultant change in PO_2 and PCO_2. A marked increase in respiratory rate could have adverse effects on the PCO_2 by increasing dead-space ventilation. A moderate degree of hypercapnia (*e.g.*, 50–55 torr) should be well tolerated by the infant and should be accepted if modest changes in the respirator settings are unsuccessful.

Hypoxemia may persist during all combinations of respiratory settings in some conditions (*e.g.*, persistent pulmonary hypertension, persistent fetal circulation; Table 31-5). The physician should always consider the degree of air leak around the endotracheal tube when adjusting pressure and flow rates. Reevaluation of the infant for coexisting pulmonary vascular hypertension or structural or functional heart disease is then indicated. Attempts at relieving pulmonary vasoconstriction with induced alkalosis or agents such as tolazoline or the vasodilator prostaglandin E_1 are indicated.

If there is airway obstruction, as may occur with bronchopulmonary dysplasia or meconium aspira-

TABLE 31–5
MANAGEMENT CONSIDERATIONS

Accept suboptimal blood gas tensions and *p*H
Raise the hematocrit with packed erythrocyte transfusions
Reposition baby into prone position if supine or into left or right lateral positions
Consider use of paralysis or sedation; if infant is paralyzed, discontinue its use
Change to a larger size endotracheal tube to diminish air leak
Consider repeated doses of exogenous surfactant beyond 24 h of age
Change mode of ventilation to infant-triggered, high-frequency, or mandatory volume delivery system
Administer diuretic therapy to change pulmonary fluid concentration
Increase cardiac output by administration of vasopressor or positive ionotropic agents
Reevaluate cardiac hemodynamics and degree of pulmonary hypertension with initial or repeat echocardiography

tion, optimal ventilator settings may differ from those used for hyaline membrane disease. Because there is a relatively long time constant, the gas flow rate should not be too rapid, and there should be adequate time for expiration, which may need to be 2 to 3 seconds. The required PIP may be below 25 cm H_2O. The use of synchronous intermittent mandatory ventilation (IMV) or assisted control may be helpful in these circumstances.

ADJUNCTIVE MONITORS OF CONVENTIONAL VENTILATION

TIDAL VOLUME MONITOR

Application of hot wire anemometry or pneumotachography to neonatal ventilation systems allows measurement of inspiratory and expiratory tidal volumes, minute ventilation ($\dot{V}_E$), and air leak (*i.e.*, the difference between tidal volumes measured during inspiration and expiration) at any combination of ventilator settings. These measurements overcome a previous limitation found in time-cycled neonatal ventilators and allow a more rational selection of ventilatory settings, supplementing visual and auscultatory evidence of inadequate or excessive chest wall motion for assessing delivered tidal volume. It is possible to correlate the individual variable of tidal volume with the independently adjusted PIP, inspiratory gas flow rate, T_I, and PEEP. Knowledge of tidal volume from bedside measurements allows clinicians to determine the optimal PIP to achieve optimal tidal volume. This knowledge enables minimizing PIP, which otherwise may induce or exacerbate the small airway injury of bronchopulmonary dysplasia. However, knowledge of tidal volume and $\dot{V}_E$ does not provide knowledge of distribution of inspired ventilation and of $\dot{V}_A/\dot{Q}$ matching. Distribution of tidal volume may vary with the associated PIP; low PIP can result in tidal volume distribution only to already overinflated lung regions, resulting in worsened $\dot{V}_A/\dot{Q}$ matching, development or exacerbation of high $\dot{V}_A/\dot{Q}$ areas and worsening of arterial CO_2 retention, despite normal or elevated $\dot{V}_E$. Despite this limitation, use of tidal volume monitoring may permit ventilation at lower PIP, possibly reducing the incidence of pneumothorax or interstitial emphysema, complications which may increase the risk of bronchopulmonary dysplasia.[39]

MEASUREMENT OF LUNG RESISTANCE AND COMPLIANCE

Computerized analysis of bedside on-line measurements of compliance and resistance, using an esophageal catheter to estimate pleural and transpulmonary pressure, allows serial assessment of pulmonary mechanics. There is considerable intrapatient and interpatient variability in these measurements, rendering problematic their application to day-to-day management of the neonate.[40] The need to normalize resistance and compliance measurements by FRC and not by body weight, especially to compare results obtained at different times in the same patient, is critical for meaningful interpretation. This fact has been recognized by manufacturers, who have incorporated techniques for assessment of FRC into the bedside measurement of compliance and resistance. Techniques for measuring FRC use helium rebreathing or nitrogen wash-out. The lack of correlation between change in compliance and change in measurements of gas exchange efficiency in bronchopulmonary dysplasia and between change in compliance and change in FRC during hyaline membrane disease suggests that the usefulness of measurements of pulmonary mechanics in minute-to-minute management of assisted ventilation may be limited.[27,41] However, by correlating radiographic appearance, change in FRC, and change in specific compliance or resistance measurements, physicians should be able to individualize treatment better than with the use of currently available adjunctive therapies, which include inhaled or systemic bronchodilators of various classes and corticosteroids. Widespread use of lung volume-normalized pulmonary mechanics may yet produce improved long-term pulmonary outcome.

CO_2 MONITORING

Two relatively noninvasive techniques are available for monitoring PCO_2. End-tidal CO_2 monitoring allows a noninvasive estimate of breath-to-breath $PaCO_2$, because under many circumstances, end-tidal CO_2 is approximately equivalent to $PACO_2$ and $PaCO_2$. Changes in end-tidal CO_2 may provide a sensitive indication of underlying pathologic changes occurring in the infant's lung. The measuring device within the monitor is an infrared sensor. Now that the problems of additional dead space and the need for excessive amounts of continuous flow of expired gas through the device have been largely eliminated, the principal technical problem remaining with this device is its frequent occlusion with mucus and condensation within it. These limitations have so far precluded its widespread use in the smallest infants.[42,43]

Transcutaneous CO_2 monitoring, usually performed with a combined transcutaneous PO_2 skin electrode, is useful for acute management. This device measures CO_2 tensions at the surface of the epidermis, not the $PaCO_2$. Long-term use for weaning older infants from assisted ventilation has not proven useful because of decreased accuracy of the correlation.[44]

INTERACTIVE COMPUTER-ASSISTED MANAGEMENT

Carlo and associates developed a complex flow chart for automated management of changes in the ventilator.[45,46] The changes are based on common assumptions about current and safe means of increasing PaO_2 (*i.e.*, increasing FiO_2 and mean airway pressure) and decreasing $PaCO_2$ (*i.e.*, increasing $\dot{V}_E$ by increasing tidal volume or rate). In ventilator-treated infants suffering from hyaline membrane disease, the computer-assisted management succeeded more frequently than retrospective or prospective control groups in making a change in ventilator variables that restored acceptable blood gas tension measurements.[45] With the data obtained from continuous monitoring of end-tidal CO_2 and of SaO_2 coupled to currently available microprocessors, a new ventilator control system could maintain more precise control of FiO_2, PIP, and mean airway pressures. By so doing, use of such a device could limit the amount of time during which a baby receives excessive pressure support or inspired oxygen concentration.

PATIENT-INITIATED MECHANICAL VENTILATION

Patient-initiated ventilator-assisted tidal breathing is designed to improve interaction and reduce antagonism between spontaneously generated and mechanically generated breaths, as may occur with IMV, in which the baby's breaths are irrelevant to the evenly spaced and sized machine-generated breaths. Several assisted breathing techniques are available because of modifications of several neonatal ventilators. Pressure support ventilation allows a spontaneously breathing infant to trigger a flow of gas from the ventilator by initiating an inspiratory effort. Rapidly responding flow detectors in the airway sense the initiation of respiratory effort and initiate machine-generated inspiratory gas flow. This flow increases and maintains airway pressure at a preset level throughout inspiration. With another technique called synchronous intermittent mandatory ventilation (SIMV), spontaneous initiation of inspiration initiates the breath that would have been delivered by the ventilator using preset PIP, PEEP, and T_I.

Several infant ventilator systems have been adapted to provide some form of SIMV, and mechanical means have been developed of detecting onset of inspiration and conveying this signal to the ventilator. The Star-Synch Patient Triggered Ventilator (Infrasonics, San Diego, CA) incorporates a balloon-type sensor placed near the diaphragm on the anterior abdomen or on the flank. This sensor detects expansion of the abdominal wall at the onset of diaphragmatic contraction with initiation of spontaneous inspiratory effort. With a response time of 50 to 55 msec, the transducer signals the ventilator to initiate a synchronized breath. The infant can breathe at any frequency, but the predetermined numbers of machine-generated breaths are delivered only with the patient-generated signal. If hypoventilation or apnea occur, the machine reverts to the IMV mode. Malpositioning or dislodgement of the sensor results in nonsynchrony and decreased $\dot{V}_E$ if the IMV rate is set very low.

The Neonatal Ventilation Monitor (Bear Medical Systems, Riverside, CA) employs a hot wire anemometer in the breathing circuit on the inspiratory or expiratory circuit to detect changes in flow or pressure to measure tidal volume and to detect changes in air flow with initiation of patient-generated inspiration. This signal can be integrated through additional equipment to initiate a synchronized ventilator breath with a response time of 50 to 60 msec. In addition to SIMV, this system incorporates an assist–control mode, in which every patient breath can be assisted, and in the event of a period of apnea, the control or IMV part of this mode is available to continue to provide assisted ventilation. There is a minimal 250-msec exhalation time in the assist-control mode; no machine-assisted breath will be delivered if a patient inspiratory effort is sensed during this 250-msec window. Similar circuitry exists in the complex Servo 900C ventilator (Siemens Elma AB, Solna, Sweden), which is capable of operating in eight different gas delivery modes, and the newer Model 300 ventilators, both of which can be used with neonates with bronchopulmonary dysplasia. The advantages and disadvantages for neonates of each system are still being defined from bedside usage.

The particular appeal of SIMV and other assisted modes is their potential for limitation of lung overdistention and for prevention of ineffective or occluded breaths. These benefits accrue in assisted ventilation of term or older preterm infants, who have a more mature respiratory drive and tolerate IMV poorly. Interactive ventilator–patient modes may reduce problems of agitation, increased work of breathing, and need for sedation. By so doing, their use may contribute to reduced time of partial or complete dependency on ventilatory assistance. Only a few published reports are available for review, and they describe only small numbers of neonates treated with patient-triggered ventilation.[47,48] The sparse data available suggest inconsistent benefits. A comparison of gas exchange during total patient-initiated ventilation and during IMV in premature infants found modest improvement limited to infants older than 28 weeks of gestation who required initially only low ventilator rates.[49]

HIGH-FREQUENCY VENTILATION

PRINCIPLES OF USE

A clinical definition of a high-frequency ventilator includes the following features: machine-delivered breaths at least twice that of the most rapid, spontaneously generated breathing rate in an infant and a delivered tidal volume approximately equal to or less than the spontaneously generated or conventionally delivered tidal volume. In some cases, V_T is less than the dead space. A limited definition of high-frequency ventilation was adopted by the Food and Drug Administration several years ago when conventional mechanical ventilation for neonates was limited to a rate no greater than 150 breaths per minute. The neonatal high-frequency ventilator constituted machine-generated rates higher than 150 breaths per minute. Various types of high-frequency ventilation are illustrated (Fig. 31-8).

Attempts have been made to differentiate high-frequency ventilators based on several ventilator-specific factors.[50] Those factors are listed in Table 31-6. The distinction among the types of high-frequency ventilators may be relevant to the appropriate matching of any one type of high-frequency ventilator to a particular part of the natural history of a neonatal

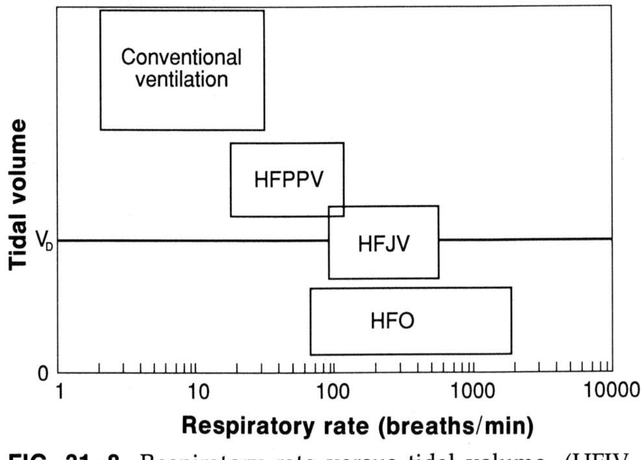

FIG. 31–8. Respiratory rate versus tidal volume. (HFJV, high-frequency jet ventilation; HFO, high-frequency oscillation; HFPPV, high-frequency positive-pressure ventilation; adapted from Slutsky AS. Non-conventional methods of ventilation. Am Rev Respir Dis 1988;138:176.)

TABLE 31–6
MEANS OF GAS EXCHANGE DURING HIGH-FREQUENCY VENTILATION

Facilitated or enhanced diffusion because of increased turbulence
Convective dispersion due to asymmetric velocity profiles
Direct alveolar ventilation
Axial distribution of transit times

pulmonary disorder. There is some agreement that certain forms of high-frequency ventilators are useful in treating certain neonatal air leak syndromes more rapidly and efficaciously than conventional mechanical ventilation. Beyond this principle, there is considerably less agreement about efficacy.

VENTILATION DEVICES AND THEIR INDICATIONS

Table 31-7 lists the three types of high-frequency ventilators that are available for clinical use in the United States. Other devices employing one of these patterns of high-frequency ventilation are available and in use in other nations.

High-frequency jet ventilation uses a high pressure gas source to generate a brief inspiratory flow of gas delivered near the end of a specifically designed endotracheal tube. Jet ventilators operate at 4 to 10 Hz. Clinical studies have demonstrated successful short-term treatment of hyaline membrane disease with high-frequency jet ventilation, but long-term outcome was the same as with conventional ventilation.[51] High-frequency jet ventilation has treated neonatal air leak syndromes more rapidly than the alternative of continuing conventional mechanical ventilation.[52] A hybrid device combining elements of jet and flow interruption to generate high-frequency ventilation, coupled with low-rate conventional ventilation, is available (Infrasonics, San Diego, CA). This device is operated at 10 to 15 Hz with pauses in the high-frequency ventilator operation during the conventional breath inspiratory phase of ventilation. When operated in its mixed conventional and high-frequency mode, this device generates high-pressure, short, and nonvariable inspiratory flow with a variable shut-off phase, allowing passive lung deflation. One attractive feature is the minimal patient disturbance involved in changing from high-frequency to conventional forms of ventilation. No published study has demonstrated that this device offers any significant advantage as primary or rescue therapy.

High-frequency oscillatory ventilation appears to be different from the other two types in that it delivers smaller tidal volumes at somewhat higher rates (see Table 31-7; see Fig. 31-8) and has an active expiratory phase. The Sensormedics high-frequency ventilator (Sensormedics, Anaheim, CA) has an additional

TABLE 31–7
HIGH-FREQUENCY VENTILATORS

	Flow Interruptor	Jet Ventilator	Oscillatory Ventilator
Commercially available device	Infant Star (Infrasonics, San Diego, CA)	Bunnell Life Pulse (Bunnell, Salt Lake City, UT)	Sensormedics (Sensormedics, San Antonio, TX)
Indications	Failure of conventional ventilation in VLBW infants, PIE	PIE, intractable air lead, failure of conventional ventilation	Primary or rescue treatment of respiratory failure; prevention of ECMO
Variables	Rate of conventional breaths, frequency of high-frequency	Inspiratory "on-time" rate temporarily 240–600 bpm.	Rate, mean airway pressure, I–E ratio
Expiratory phase	Passive (?)	Passive	Active
Special precautions	Not effective for infants >2 kg; no published trials	Needs special triple-lumen ETT with distal port for jet delivery	Rigid breathing circuit makes accidental dislodgment of ETT easy to occur

ECMO, extracorporeal membrane oxygenation; ETT, endotracheal tube; PIE, pulmonary interstitial emphysema; VLBW, very low birth weight.

feature of operating with varying T_I. This device has been licensed for use for primary initial treatment of assisted ventilation and for alternative therapy in intractable respiratory functions unresponsive to conventional mechanical ventilation in neonates.

EFFICACY

Development of high-frequency ventilation was spurred by the common development of bronchopulmonary dysplasia in low-birth-weight infants. The frequency of this complication is roughly inversely related to birth weight (Fig. 31-9). The alternative forms of high-frequency ventilation were tested to determine if they could reduce the incidence or severity of bronchopulmonary dysplasia, especially in low-birth-weight infants.

Two prospective, randomized, controlled studies were conducted using two different types of high-frequency oscillatory ventilation.[53,54] The rationale for these studies was that diminished cyclic distending pressures (*i.e.*, available with high-frequency oscillatory ventilation), compared with what is available using conventional mechanical ventilation, would be associated with fewer airway and cellular dysplastic changes of the lung and less frequent or severe bron-

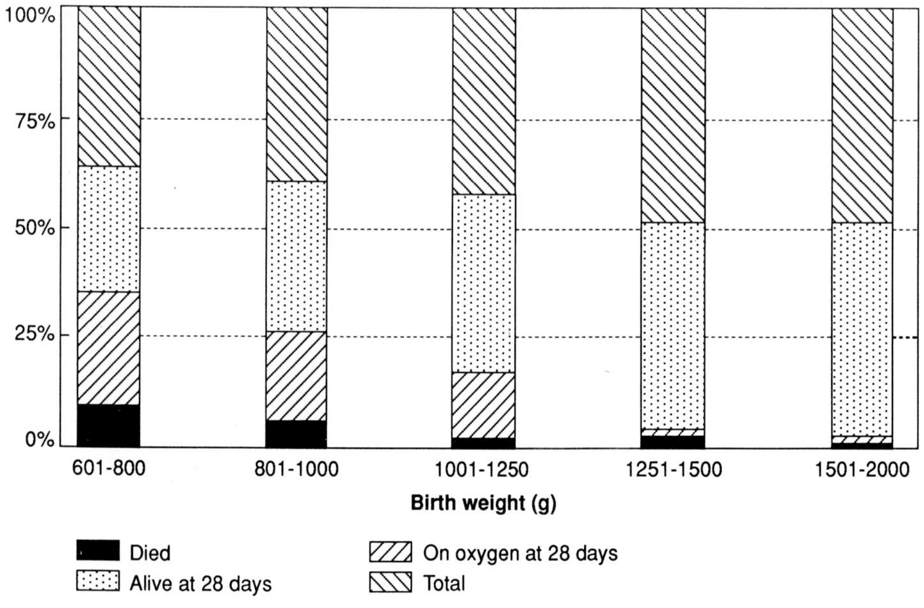

FIG. 31–9. The incidence of chronic lung disease by birth weight.

chopulmonary dysplasia. The conflicting conclusions of the two studies are shown in Table 31-8. The multicenter study demonstrated no change in incidence of bronchopulmonary dysplasia (*i.e.*, 40% of infants enrolled on each arm of the treatment group at 28 days).[53] The single-center San Antonio study demonstrated a significant decreased incidence (*i.e.*, from 65% to 30%) of bronchopulmonary dysplasia at 28 days. A number of significant differences limit comparing the two studies. For example, the HIFI study enrolled no babies with birth weights less than 750 g, and the San Antonio study enrolled babies with birth weights as low as 500 g. However, the mean birth weight of the enrolled patients in both arms of both studies was the same. The details of oscillatory ventilation are different between the studies. The HIFI study used a set frequency of 15 Hz and no single, tightly constrained pattern of suctioning nor any attempt to maintain elevated mean airway pressure. The San Antonio study used a frequency of 10 Hz, a shortened T_I, and an attempt early in the course of the disease to maintain elevated mean airway pressure. However, mean airway pressures in the two groups were similar when measured at 72 hours (*i.e.*, 8.9 cm H_2O in the HIFI and approximately 9.0 cm H_2O in the San Antonio study). Both studies were conducted without the use of exogenous surfactant in enrolled patients, a factor that limits the interpretation of these studies, because current practice typically includes early use of exogenous surfactant in many of the babies eligible for the two trials. In the evaluation of babies failing their ventilator of original assignment and crossing over in the HIFI study, approximately 50% in each group responded favorably to the change without regard to which device was used first.[53] These results suggest that high-frequency oscillatory ventilation can play a role in neonatal intensive care units, but the exact subset of infants who would maximally benefit from its use is still being defined.

One question raised, but not answered, by clinical studies of high-frequency oscillatory ventilation is the potential benefit gained by its application at birth. Although no studies have reported use of high-frequency oscillatory ventilation in this situation, two studies using premature primate models of hyaline membrane disease demonstrated improved gas exchange if high-frequency oscillatory ventilation was used without any prior conventional mechanical ventilation.[55,56] Jackson and colleagues found decreased proteinaceous alveolar edema and improved gas exchange after 6 hours of high-frequency oscillatory ventilation applied from the first breath (Fig. 31-10).[56] However, all animals in both treatment groups had evidence of pulmonary cellular injury. The finding of short-term benefit with concomitant cellular damage implies that high-frequency oscillatory ventilation used from birth could still be associated with signifi-

TABLE 31–8
USE OF HIGH-FREQUENCY OSCILLATORY VENTILATION TO PREVENT BRONCHOPULMONARY DYSPLASIA

	HIFI Study[53]	San Antonio Study[54]
Entry Criteria		
Weight range	750–2000 g	500–1750 g
Number enrolled	327 HFOV, 346 CMV	30 HFOV, 30 CMV
Mean birth weight	1.08 g	1.08 g
Postnatal age at entry	6 h	8 h
FiO_2	0.67 HFOV; 0.70 CMV	0.51 HFOV; 0.55 CMV
Death Before Discharge		
HFOV	19%	23%
CMV	19%	19%
BPD, Any Degree, at 28 Days		
HFOV	41%	30%*
CMV	40%	65%
Pneumothorax		
HFOV	26%	40%
CMV	24%	27%
Grade 3 or 4 IVH		
HFOV	26%*	20%
CMV	18%	23%

* $p < 0.05$ within the study.

BPD, bronchopulmonary dysplasia; CMV, conventional mechanical ventilation; HFOV, high-frequency oscillatory ventilation; IVH, intraventricular hemorrhage.

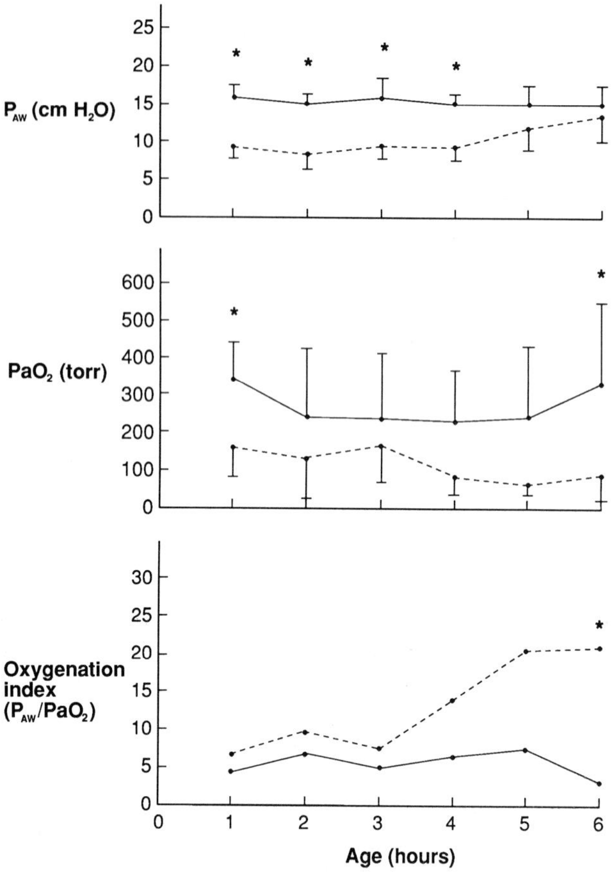

FIG. 31–10. Sequential measurements of mean airway pressure (P_{AW}) and arterial oxygen tension in 100% O_2 (mean ± SD). P_{AW} was initially higher in the high-frequency oscillatory-ventilated animals (*solid curve*), and PaO_2 was greater at the beginning and end of the study than in the conventionally mechanically ventilated (CMV) group (*broken curve*). Calculated oxygenation index was worse in the CMV group at the end of the experiment as a result of low oxygen tension despite high P_{AW}. Asterisks indicate statistical significance, $p < 0.05$. (Adapted from Jackson JC, Truog WE, Standaert TA, et al. Effect of high-frequency ventilation on the development of alveolar edema in premature monkeys at risk for hyaline membrane disease. Am Rev Respir Dis 1991;143:865.)

cant lung injury. These findings are consistent with the findings of Solimano and associates, who showed that fluid and protein leaks in preterm lambs still occurred although high-frequency oscillatory ventilation was applied from the first breath after delivery.[57]

A possible second indication for high-frequency ventilation is to preclude more invasive pulmonary support with extracorporeal membrane oxygenation (ECMO) to maintain gas exchange. A single study involving patients eligible for ECMO demonstrated that approximately one-half responded favorably to high-frequency oscillatory ventilation and did not need ECMO.[58] Most babies responding to high-frequency ventilation were larger infants suffering from severe hyaline membrane disease. Other acute pulmonary disorders, such as meconium aspiration pneumonia with severe airway obstructive changes as shown by chest radiography, may not respond as well to oscillatory ventilation.

COMPLICATIONS OF ASSISTED VENTILATION

AIRWAY-ASSOCIATED PROBLEMS

Acute and chronic complications of mechanical ventilation may develop in neonates (Table 31-9). All patients with tracheal intubation demonstrate some degree of mucosal injury, usually squamous metaplasia or mucosal necrosis.[59,60] In most infants, there seems to be spontaneous healing without significant sequelae. Hoarseness and stridor often occur after prolonged intubation but usually resolve in a few days. Persistent lesions may develop in some patients.[61] These complications include laryngomalacia and subglottic stenosis, occasionally requiring tracheostomy. Duration of intubation, pressure from oversized tubes, inadequate humidification, and airway pressure produced by the ventilator contribute to the development of laryngotracheal lesions.

The duration of intubation is dictated by the need for continued ventilatory support. In some infants requiring assisted ventilation longer than 3 to 6 months, tracheostomy tube placement may facilitate development of normal feeding patterns and social interaction and bypass already traumatized areas of the upper airway. However, infant tracheostomy is itself associated with a significant morbidity and mortality.[62] Complications can include fatal loss of airway after accidental extrusion of the tube, paratracheal soft tissue infection, severe paratracheal air leak resulting in inadequate generation of PIP, and tracheal cartilage softening, making decannulation difficult.

PULMONARY AIR LEAK COMPLICATIONS

Pulmonary air leak may occur as a complication of any of the life-threatening disorders of the newborn or as a result of their treatment. The air leak may consist of pulmonary interstitial emphysema, pneumomediastinum, pneumoperitoneum, pneumopericardium, or pneumothorax; pneumopericardium and pneumothorax usually require immediate treatment by evacuation of the free air.

Pneumothorax must be considered if there is abrupt worsening of the respiratory or circulatory status of an infant at risk. Unilateral hyperresonance, decreased breath sounds, a shift of the apical cardiac impulse, and skin mottling are useful clinical clues. High-intensity illumination may demonstrate the presence of a pneumothorax if the room can be adequately darkened.[63] A definite diagnosis often can be made only by radiographic examination. The volume

TABLE 31–9
COMPLICATIONS OF MECHANICAL VENTILATION

Acute Complications
Equipment failure
Failure of pressure in gas supply lines
Alarm failure, with failure of staff to realize ventilation is disconnected
Expiratory port occlusion producing inadvertent overdistention of lungs
Endotracheal tube connection failure
Dislodgement upward in pharynx
Occlusion of tip of endotracheal tube
Placement of tube tip beyond carina, providing only unilateral ventilation
Trauma to upper airway, including tracheal perforation
Equipment misuse
Hypoxemia or hyperoxemia from inappropriate use of oxygen
Arterial hypocarbia or hypercarbia from overventilation or underventilation
Overdistention with excessive ventilatory pressure; lung rupture
Other
Airway blockage by excessive secretions inadequately removed by suctioning
Trauma to airways by overvigorous suctioning
Pneumonia, produced by careless handling of equipment
Chronic Complications
Increased risk of chronic lung disease
Tracheal or subglottic stenosis
Nasal deformities with nasotracheal tube
Palatal deformities with endotracheal tube
Upper airway infections (*e.g.*, otitis media)
Excessive prolonged dependence on mechanical ventilation (*e.g.*, respiratory muscle impairment)

of the extrapulmonary air collection is not always a valid indication of tension. Interstitial emphysema, often a precursor of pneumothorax, causes the lung to remain partly expanded, even when intrapleural pressure is high.[64] Bilateral pneumothorax may lead rapidly to death and must always be considered in cases of severe deterioration.

Pneumothorax in otherwise asymptomatic infants often resolves without therapy. However, marked mediastinal shift, coexisting pulmonary disease, or use of mechanical ventilation indicate a need for evacuation of the air. Aspiration with a syringe and needle may be done as an emergency procedure but is rarely adequate by itself and should be followed with tube thoracostomy.

Thoracostomy tubes should be sterile and made of nonreactive rubber or plastic. The wall thickness should be sufficient to prevent kinking, and the lumen should be large enough to prevent occlusion by exudate. The presence of at least two holes in the tube reduces the likelihood of occlusion by tissue. Polyvinylchloride feeding tubes or 8-F (2.6-mm) to 10-F (3.3-mm) trocar catheters are suitable for thoracostomy use. The tube is inserted by grasping the tip with a clamp and pressing through a previously made incision through the pleura. Trocar catheters can be inserted after a skin incision has been made and can be Z-tracked over a rib for a better seal. However, the Z-tracked trocar catheters often require considerable force to insert, and lung puncture has been reported with their use. A novel approach to the placement of a catheter to minimize lung injury has been reported.[65] A pig-tailed catheter is inserted over the area of suspected air leak, and the tube is inserted and rotated to form a loop within the intrapleural space.

It is not usually practical to connect a suction apparatus to the tube before it has been secured, but the pneumothorax should be aspirated with a syringe and the tube occluded with a clamp or stopcock. A single suture is placed in the skin beside the tube; this suture can be used to tie the tube securely in place. The tube may become dislodged if care is not taken at this step. Taping alone is inadequate. Purse-string sutures tend to produce larger scars without providing much additional security against tube dislodgment.

The tube is connected to continuous suction at a negative pressure of 10 to 15 cm/H_2O with an underwater seal. A chest radiograph should be obtained soon after thoracostomy. If the pneumothorax has not been evacuated, the infant should be repositioned and the tube stripped, or if necessary, a second tube should be inserted.

A thoracostomy tube is left in place until air ceases to bubble from the tube and until the risk of recurrent pneumothorax is reduced (*i.e.*, until respiratory distress has subsided or mechanical ventilation is no longer required). The tube is then clamped. If there is neither clinical nor radiographic evidence of recurrent pneumothorax, the tube is removed and the skin incision promptly closed. Antibiotics are not used routinely, because the thoracostomy is performed under aseptic conditions.

Another form of leak, pneumopericardium, characteristically presents with sudden and profound hypotension, distant heart sounds, and rapid death. Emergency treatment consists of removing the air by insertion of a long catheter into the pericardial sac with a subxyphoid approach and constant application of gentle negative pressure on the plunger of the syringe. The tip of the catheter needle should be aimed toward the left midclavicular region, and the catheter tip should travel in a superficial plane toward the pericardial sac after penetrating the skin. An 18- or 20-gauge angiocath can be used for this purpose. There is a gush of air as the pericardial sac is entered and prompt relief of the hypotension. The catheter should be sutured into place and connected to underwater drainage because the pneumopericardium may recur. If it does, consideration should be given to replacement or repositioning of the tube under direct surgical observation. Despite these efforts, risk of mortality from pneumopericardium complicating respiratory distress remains very high.

MANAGEMENT OF SPECIFIC RESPIRATORY PROBLEMS

BRONCHOPULMONARY DYSPLASIA

Among the most frustrating problems in pediatric medicine is the treatment of premature infants who develop severe chronic lung disease, usually after severe hyaline membrane disease. Chronic lung disease, or bronchopulmonary dysplasia, is characterized by diffuse scarring in the lungs and produces, at its worst, areas of bullous emphysema interspersed with areas of pulmonary fibrosis. The incidence of bronchopulmonary dysplasia by birth weight at 28 days of postnatal life is shown in Figure 31-9. After bronchopulmonary dysplasia is fully developed, weaning from the ventilator can be difficult. Oximetry, occasional arterial blood gas or capillary blood gas tension assessments, and measurements of serum levels of bicarbonate as a rough indication of the degree of compensation for respiratory acidosis are helpful in guiding the weaning process.

Although mechanical features of the lung change with body and lung growth, these changes are of little practical concern in devising attempts to wean from the ventilator. Slow decreases in mandatory ventilatory rate are the most successful approach to weaning as persistence of abnormal lung mechanics necessitates high PIP to deliver an effective tidal volume. The infant's intermittent struggling against the ventilator is a common occurrence, especially if there is a tendency for bronchoconstriction and decreased ventilation—a factor that may relate to prognosis.[66] Sedating the infant during periods of extreme agitation helps to reduce the struggle against the ventilator and decreases oxygen consumption.

IDIOPATHIC APNEA

Recurrent apnea occurs in most very-low-birth-weight infants; its severity is usually in inverse proportion to gestational age, although there is considerable variability in incidence and severity. A single episode of severe apnea should be differentiated from recurrent apnea. A specific cause, such as hypocalcemia, seizures, central nervous central nervous system hemorrhage, and sepsis, should be determined and appropriately treated for solitary instances of apnea.

Determination of which infants with recurrent apnea require treatment with other than tactile stimulation depends on experienced nursing and medical staff and their clinical assessment of vital signs, including heart rate and color changes, and the degree of change in vital signs that occurs with apneic episodes assessed by cardiac, respiratory, and transcutaneous oxygen monitoring.

Most monitors depend on changes in thoracic impedance and can be set to alarm with limits set by duration of respiratory pause or a decrease in heart rate. Obstructive episodes of apnea are not necessarily detected; newer devices measuring end-tidal PCO_2 may prove to be more reliable. Detection of apnea by pressure-sensitive devices in an air- or water-filled mattress has not proved dependable. Observation of duration of episodes of apnea and heart rate changes can determine the most appropriate alarm settings for individual infants. Periodic dips in the heart rate to 80 beats/minute or less in healthy newborn infants is consistent with sinus bradycardia. Some infants need intervention after 10 to 15 seconds of apnea, and others tolerate longer pauses.

Most apneic episodes (*i.e.*, approximately 60% of cases) can be managed by tactile stimulation of the infant's extremities or stroking of the back, chest, and chin with the infant in a sitting position. If cyanosis occurs or bradycardia persists over the next 30 to 60 seconds, free-flow oxygen followed by bag and mask ventilation is indicated. Pulse-oximetry monitoring of SaO_2 is often helpful in these infants. Care should be taken not to increase the oxygen concentration above that already required by the infant.

If the frequency of apneic episodes increases to several per hour or if cyanosis develops, treatment with a methylxanthine drug (*e.g.*, theophylline, aminophylline, caffeine) is indicated. If severe apneic episodes persist, intubation and mechanical ventilation are necessary. Ventilator settings can be minimal; inspiratory pressure of 12 to 18 cm H_2O at a rate of 5 to 12 breaths/minute and physiologic levels of PEEP at 2 to 3 cm H_2O are usually sufficient. A physiologic level of 2 to 3 cm H_2O of CPAP has been advocated for the treatment of apnea.

MECONIUM ASPIRATION

Aspiration of meconium-contaminated fluid at or before birth may result in airway obstruction and pneumonitis with sufficiently severe hypoxemia or hypercarbia to require mechanical ventilation. This disorder may occur despite appropriate suctioning of the oropharynx of the infant as the head is delivered and suctioning the trachea of meconium while performing direct laryngoscopy.[67] The physician in the delivery room must balance the time involved in laryngoscopy and suctioning and its concomitant poor ventilation with the need to begin effective resuscitative efforts in an infant who is likely to be severely asphyxiated.

Ventilatory care is supportive during the fully developed syndrome. Because of the high resistance, it may be helpful to increase T_I above that used for treatment of hyaline membrane disease. However, T_E must be sufficiently long to avoid air trapping. Corticosteroids have no effect on the acute course or outcome of the disease.[68] Because meconium aspiration syndrome often occurs in full-term and post-term infants, the effectiveness of mechanical ventilation may be compromised by the infant's struggling and attempting to breathe against the ventilator. Sedation with or without respiratory paralysis (*e.g.*, pancuronium bromide, 0.05 to 0.1 mg/kg/dose) may be a useful adjunct for acute care. The risk of air leak is high in cases of meconium aspiration syndrome that require assisted ventilation. Prompt correction of air leak may help prevent intractable hypoxemia.

PERSISTENT PULMONARY HYPERTENSION

Persistent pulmonary hypertension may occur with little or no parenchymal lung disease or may occur secondary to severe parenchymal disease of any cause. Persistence or recurrence of right-to-left shunting through the ductus arteriosus, foramen ovale, or both occurs because of increases in the ratio of pulmonary to systemic vascular resistance. Hypoxemia results from the combination of these extrapulmonary and intrapulmonary shunts. This disorder usually occurs in full-term infants, sometimes after prenatal or intrapartum stress and sometimes associated with meconium aspiration. Treatment is directed at correcting hypoxemia by reducing the pulmonary hypertension and the right-to-left shunts.

It is a common practice in many nurseries to institute mechanical ventilation if the PaO_2 falls below 50 torr. Alkalinization through hyperventilation ($PCO_2 = 25 \pm 5$ torr) has been advocated, as has intravascular infusion of $NaHCO_3$ to raise *p*H to between 7.45 and 7.55 to reduce pulmonary vasoconstriction, although others report success treating the disorder without alkalosis.[69,70] No prospective study has defined the optimal approach. Alkalosis causes a left-shifted HbO_2 dissociation curve, increasing saturation with no change in concurrently measured PaO_2. Paralysis with pancuronium bromide and analgesia with intravenous morphine (0.1 mg/kg) may help. Positive end-expiratory pressure levels should probably remain below 5 cm H_2O in the absence of parenchymal lung disease to avoid further compromise to intraparenchymal blood flow. Peak inspiratory pressure and rate should be adjusted by frequent assessment of PCO_2. Continuous measurement of transcutaneous PCO_2 is useful in monitoring hyperventilation. Pulmonary vasodilators such as intravenous tolazoline (1–2 mg/kg over 10 minutes followed by 1–2 mg/kg/hour) have been used with variable success if the PaO_2 remains below 50 torr, indicative of persistent shunt.[71,72] Because systemic vasodilation may occur with tolazoline, the simultaneous administration of a systemic vasoconstricting agent (*e.g.*, dopamine) is usually required. It is reasonable to begin with 2 to 5 μg/kg/minute of dopamine and titrate with blood pressure to a maximum of less than 20 μg/kg/minute.

Other pulmonary vasodilating agents that may prove more specific and effective include nifedipine, a calcium channel blocker; prostaglandin I_2 (prostacyclin); prostaglandin E_1; and inhaled nitric oxide. None of these agents has undergone rigorous clinical testing in the treatment of persistent pulmonary hypertension in newborns.

The magnitude of the right-to-left ductal shunt and treatment efficacy can be assessed by the differential PaO_2 when sampled simultaneously in the right radial artery and the descending aorta or its distribution. The placement of two transcutaneous O_2 electrodes or saturation monitors in areas supplied by preductal and postductal blood flow is sometimes useful. The $PaCO_2$ is useful for adjusting PIP and frequency of the ventilator to assess the degree of hyperventilation. Echocardiography is essential for initial diagnosis to eliminate structural heart disease and for management of this syndrome by assessing myocardial contractility. Assessment of acute changes in pulmonary, ductal, and foramen ovale blood flow by Doppler echocardiography may help to evaluate treatment techniques.

PULMONARY HYPOPLASIA

The diagnosis of pulmonary hypoplasia is extremely difficult to make unless there is associated renal agenesis (*i.e.*, Potter syndrome). Chronic oligohydramnios resulting from prolonged rupture of the membranes has been associated with pulmonary hypoplasia due to intrauterine constraint and extrathoracic pressure or secondary to altered fetal lung liquid dynamics. There is no specific treatment other than that directed at respiratory failure, including supplemental oxygen and mechanical ventilation. Early occurrence of pneumothorax and intractable hypercarbia are early signs of pulmonary hypoplasia. High peak or mean pulmonary pressures are often necessary. Other associated congenital malformations should be considered, such as renal dysgenesis, phrenic nerve absence, diaphragmatic hernia, and vertebral and chromosomal anomalies.

PULMONARY EDEMA

The general edema of hydrops from isoimmune and nonimmune causes is recognized with increasing frequency because of the widespread use of fetal ultrasonography. Planned delivery can be scheduled to avert fetal demise. Pleural effusions often occur in a fetus with generalized edema, and these infants tend to be critically ill from the moment of birth. Treatment of hydropic infants manifesting respiratory distress should begin in the delivery room with immediate endotracheal intubation and, after stabilization of the airway, removal of the pleural fluid to permit lung expansion. This procedure is technically difficult if there is marked edema of the chest wall. A 22-gauge, short, beveled needle attached to a three-way stopcock and 50-mL syringe should be inserted at a 30° angle into the pleura just above the sixth or seventh rib in the midaxillary line. After satisfactory gas exchange occurs and the infant is stabilized, unilateral or bilateral thoracostomy tubes may be needed. Abdominal paracentesis may be necessary if diaphragmatic excursion appears to be impeded. Mechanical ventilation and other respiratory and metabolic support may be required for several days if pleural fluid continues to accumulate. Intravascular volume may shift rapidly, and hypervolemia, hypovolemia, hypoproteinemia, and electrolyte imbalance are common complications.

CONGENITAL DIAPHRAGMATIC HERNIA

Congenital diaphragmatic hernia occurs in about 1 of 2000 live births, and approximately one-half of these infants are diagnosed prenatally by ultrasound. This disorder produces immediate respiratory insufficiency in most infants. There is considerable controversy about the timing of surgery, application of ECMO, and definition of irreversible lung parenchymal or vascular hypoplasia.

Immediate management of the distressed infant includes intubation, placement of a gastric tube with suction, paralysis sedation, use of FiO_2 equal to 1.0, and attempts to maintain low mean and peak inspired pressures. A short T_I ($\leq$0.3 second) should be adequate to allow satisfactory gas exchange. Avoidance of intestinal distention with air and avoidance of parenchymal air leaks are the cornerstones of immediate management. Management thereafter should be coordinated by the primary care neonatologist and a pediatric surgeon well versed in neonatal pulmonary pathophysiology (see Chap. 44).

AREAS OF RESEARCH IN ASSISTED VENTILATION

One experimental approach to reducing the lung injury associated with gas ventilation is liquid ventilation. Lung injury may be the result of abnormal inflation patterns produced because of elevated alveolar surface tension. Liquid inflation of the lungs with saline eliminates the alveolar gas–lung liquid interface with its tendency to induce collapse and perhaps injury. However, saline is a poor carrier of oxygen. Liquid perfluorocarbon solutions are able to dissolve large volumes of oxygen and carbon dioxide at 1 atm. Perfluorocarbon solutions have been used as carriers for O_2 and CO_2 in moribund human infants and have been the subject of extensive experimental work in premature and full-term animals, including primates and lambs.[73,74]

Two methods of liquid ventilation are being tested. The first is total liquid ventilation, which employs a completely perfluorocarbon-filled ventilator circuit, and a membrane oxygenator to prime the inspired liquid flow. The second is perfluorocarbon-assisted gas exchange, in which a portion of the lung volume (*i.e.*, FRC) is filled with perfluorocarbon and the lungs are ventilated with conventional infant mechanical ventilators.[75] Liquid ventilation is an attractive form of pulmonary rescue because the perfluorocarbons used seem to be nontoxic and the technique, although experimental, is less invasive than ECMO. As with all forms of transpulmonary ventilation, the application of perfluorocarbon ventilation is limited by underlying anatomic conditions of immaturity in the fetal lung. The technique is not viewed as a means to extend downward the minimal gestational age at which a fetus can be delivered and maintain extrauterine survival.

MANAGEMENT IN THE INTENSIVE CARE SETTING

Management of respiratory problems requires specialized personnel and equipment. A physician skilled in neonatal intensive care techniques should be available within the unit at all times, and other specialists should be immediately accessible for consultation.

Nurses must be carefully trained in the techniques for the intensive care of infants. Necessary skills include application of ventilatory support equipment, recognition of equipment malfunction, airway management, assessment of ventilation, and use of monitoring equipment. Nurse–patient ratios vary from 1:1 to 1:3, depending on the severity of the illness. Infants who are receiving assisted ventilation usually require a nursing ratio of 1:1.

Respiratory therapists are critical to the effective use of respiratory equipment. Maintenance and calibration of all oxygen administration and oxygen-measuring devices require the presence of a respiratory therapist within the hospital at all times.

Equipment needs for neonatal intensive care include wall sources of compressed air and oxygen, oxygen dilutors, heating and humidification devices, and oxygen-monitoring systems with alarms. Critically ill infants need continuous monitoring of temperature, respiratory rate, and heart rate by electrical devices with alarm systems. In the acute phase of illness or if an umbilical or peripheral arterial catheter is in use, continuous blood pressure monitoring and oscilloscopic electrocardiographic display are available for all electrical equipment.

The parents of severely ill infants need understanding and support. They experience feelings of anxiety, fear, guilt, and hostility. Most families are ill equipped for the unexpected emotional and financial burden imposed by the child's hospitalization. A social worker should be available exclusively to the neonatal intensive care unit to provide assistance to parents by delineating parental concerns and helping coordinate communication with the medical and nursing staff and other hospital personnel.

The physical design of the intensive care unit must facilitate the management of acute respiratory problems. Each patient area should be large enough to accommodate the necessary personnel and the enormous amount of equipment without generating intolerable crowding. A small number of patients in each room facilitates parental visits and alleviates the overall level of stress. There is appropriate and growing concern that the proliferation of monitors and alarms is resulting in "monitor fatigue," with the risk that monitors become ignored.[76] Although neonatology is often thought of as an acute care specialty, it is more accurately categorized as a chronic care specialty, because of the many days and weeks of specialized care that small, sick infants require. Unfortunately, the physical design of most intensive care units has not caught up to that new reality, to the detriment of patients, family, and the staff.

Only after adequate attention is paid to these ancillary features of intensive respiratory care of the newborn can the optimal outcome expected for premature infants in this era be approached.

REFERENCES

1. Flynn JT, Bancalari E, Snyder ES, et al. A cohort study of transcutaneous oxygen tension and the incidence and severity of retinopathy of prematurity. N Engl J Med 1992;326:1050.
2. Lucey JF, Dangman B. A reexamination of the role of oxygen in retrolental fibroplasia. J Pediatr 1984;73:82.
3. American Academy of Pediatrics. Guidelines for perinatal care. 3rd ed. Elk Grove, IL: American Academy of Pediatrics, 1992: 201.
4. Thibeault DW, Hobel CJ, Kwong MS. Perinatal factors influencing the arterial oxygen tension in preterm infants with RDS while breathing 100% oxygen. J Pediatr 1974;84:898.
5. Wall PM, Kuhn LT. Percutaneous arterial sampling using transillumination. Pediatrics 1977;59:1032.
6. Jackson JC, Truog WE, Watchko JF, Mack LA, Cyr DR, van Belle G. Efficacy of thromboresistant umbilical artery catheters in reducing aortic thrombosis and other complications. J Pediatr 1987;110:102.
7. Dunn PM. Localization of the umbilical catheter by post-mortem measurement. Arch Dis Child 1966;41:69.
8. Clark JM, Jung AL. Umbilical artery catheterization by a cutdown procedure. Pediatrics 1977;59:1036.
9. Mokrobisky ST, Levine RL, Blumhagen JD, et al. Low positioning of umbilical artery catheters increases associated complications in newborn infants. N Engl J Med 1978;299:561.
10. Harris MS, Little GA. Umbilical artery catheters: high, low or no. J Perinat Med 1978;6:15.
11. Wesstrom G, Finnstrom O, Stenport G. Umbilical artery catheterization in newborns. 1. Thrombosis in relation to catheter tip and position. Acta Pediatr Scand 1979;68:575.
12. Cassady G. Transcutaneous monitoring in the newborn infant. J Pediatr 1983;103:837.
13. Graham G, Kenny MA. Assessment of transcutaneous oxygen measurements in a neonatal intensive care unit. Clin Chem 1980;26:629.
14. The Task Force on Transcutaneous Oxygen Monitors. American Academy of Pediatrics: report of consensus meeting, December 5–6, 1986. Pediatrics 1989;83:122.
15. Peabody JL, Gregory GA, Willis MM. Transcutaneous oxygen tension in sick infants. Am Rev Respir Dis 1978;118:83.
16. Hay WW, Thilo E, Curlander JB. Pulse oximetry in neonatal medicine. Clinics in Perinatology 1991;18:441.
17. Hay WW, Brockway J, Eyzaquirre M. Neonatal pulse oximetry: accuracy and reliability. Pediatrics 1989;83:717.
18. Chance B. Spectrophotometry of intracellular respiratory pigments. Science 1954;20:272.
19. Jöbsis FF. Noninvasive, infrared monitoring of cerebral and myocardial oxygen sufficiency and circulatory parameters. Science 1977;198:1264.
20. Brazy JE. Near-infrared spectroscopy. Clin Perinatol 1991; 18:519.
21. Wyatt JS, Cope M, Delpy DT, et al. Qualification of cerebral oxygenation and haemodynamics in sick newborn infants by near infrared spectrophotometry. Lancet 1986;2:1063.
22. Hampson NB, Camporesi EM, Stolp BW, et al. Cerebral oxygen availability by NIR spectroscopy during transient hypoxia in humans. J Appl Physiol 1990;69:907.
23. Wyatt JS, Cope M, Delpy DT, et al. Quantification of cerebral blood volume in human infants by near-infrared spectroscopy. J Appl Physiol 1990;68:1086.
24. Gregory GA, Kitterman JA, Phibbs RG, Tooley WH, Hamilton WK. Treatment of the idiopathic respiratory distress syndrome with continuous positive airway pressure. N Engl J Med 1971; 284:1333.
25. Rhodes PG, Hall RT. Continuous positive airway pressure delivered by face mask in infants with the idiopathic respiratory distress syndrome: a controlled study. Pediatrics 1973;52:1.
26. Belenky DA, Orr RJ, Woodrum DE, Hodson WA. Is continuous transpulmonary pressure better than conventional respiratory management of hyaline membrane disease? A controlled study. Pediatrics 1976;58:800.
27. Edberg KE, Sandberg K, Silberberg A, et al. Lung volume, gas mixing, and mechanics of breathing in mechanically ventilated very low birth weight infants with idiopathic respiratory distress syndrome. Pediatr Res 1991;30:496.

28. Richardson CP, Jung AL. Effects of continuous positive airway pressure on pulmonary function and blood gases of infants with respiratory distress syndrome. Pediatr Res 1978;12:771.
29. Avery ME, Tooley WH, Keller JB, et al. Is chronic lung disease in low birth weight infants preventable? A survey of eight centers. Pediatrics 1987;79:26.
30. Tsuno K, Prato P, Kolobow T. Acute lung injury from mechanical ventilation at moderately high airway pressures. J Appl Physiol 1990;69:956.
31. Rodenstein DO, Perlmutter N, Stanescu DC. Infants are not obligatory nasal breathers. Am Rev Respir Dis 1985;131:343.
32. Polgar G, Kong GP. The nasal resistance of newborn infants. J Pediatr 1965;67:557
33. Weng JT, Stark FI, Indyk L, et al. Oxygen supplementation during endotracheal intubation of the infant. Pediatrics 1977; 59:1042.
34. Fanconi S, Duc G. Intratracheal suctioning in sick preterm infants: prevention of intracranial hypertension and cerebral hypoperfusion by muscle paralysis. Pediatrics 1987;79:538.
35. Kelly MA, Finer NN. Nasotracheal intubation in the neonate: physiologic responses and effects of atropine and pancuronium. J Pediatr 1984;105:303.
36. Tochen ML. Orotracheal intubation in the newborn infant: a method for determining depth of tube insertion. J Pediatr 1979;95:1050.
37. Kohelet D, Goldberg A, Goldberg M. Depth of endotracheal tube placement in neonates. J Pediatr 1982;101:157.
38. Tarnow-Mordi WO, Reid E, Griffiths P, Wilkinson AR. Low inspired gas temperature and respiratory complications in very low birth weight infants. J Pediatr 1989;114:438.
39. Hodson WA, Truog WE, Mayock DE, et al. Bronchopulmonary dysplasia: the need for epidemiologic studies. J Pediatr 1979; 95:848.
40. Gerhardt TO, Bancalari E. Measurements and monitoring of pulmonary function. Clin Perinatol 1991;18:581.
41. Englehardt B, Elliot S, Hazinski TA. Short and long-term effects of furosemide on lung function in infants with bronchopulmonary dysplasia. J Pediatr 1986;109:1034.
42. Clark JS, Votteri B, Ariagno RL, et al. Non-invasive assessment of blood gases. Am Rev Respir Dis 1992;145:220.
43. Epstein MF, Cohen AR, Feldman HA, Raemer DB. Estimation of $PaCO_2$ by two non-invasive methods in critically ill newborn infants. J Pediatr 1985;106:282.
44. Rome ES, Stork EK, Carlo WA, Martin RJ. Limitations of transcutaneous PO_2 and PCO_2 monitoring in infants with bronchopulmonary dysplasia. Pediatrics 1984;74:217.
45. Carlo WA, Pacific L, Chatburn RL, et al. Efficiency of computer-assisted management of respiratory failure in neonates. Pediatrics 1986;78:139.
46. Carlo WA, Chatburn RL. Assisted ventilation of the newborn. In: Carlo WA, Chatburn RL, eds. Neonatal respiratory care. 2nd ed. Chicago: Year Book, 1988:320.
47. Greenough A, Greenall F. Patient triggered ventilation in premature neonates. Arch Dis Child 1988;63:777.
48. Greenough A, Pool J. Neonatal patient triggered ventilation. Arch Dis Child 1988;63:394.
49. Hird MF, Greenough A. Patient triggered ventilation using a flow triggered system. Arch Dis Child 1991;66:1140.
50. Slutsky AS. Nonconventional methods of ventilation. Am Rev Respir Dis 1988;138:175.
51. Carlo W, Chatburn R, Martin R, et al. Decrease in airway pressure during high frequency jet ventilation in infants with respiratory distress syndrome. J Pediatr 1984;104:101.
52. Keszler M, Donn SM, Bucciarelli RL, et al. Multi-center controlled trial comparing high frequency jet ventilation and conventional mechanical ventilation in newborn infants with pulmonary interstitial emphysema. J Pediatr 1991;119:85.
53. The HIFI Study Group. High-frequency oscillatory ventilation compared with conventional mechanical ventilation in the treatment of respiratory failure in preterm infants. N Engl J Med 1989;320:88.
54. Clark RH, Gerstmann DR, Null DM Jr, et al. Prospective randomized comparison of high-frequency oscillatory and conventional ventilation in respiratory distress syndrome. Pediatrics 1992;89:5.
55. Meredith KS, de Lemos RA, Coalson JJ, et al. Role of lung injury in the pathogenesis of hyaline membrane disease in premature baboons. J Appl Physiol 1989;66:2150.
56. Jackson JC, Truog WE, Standaert TA, et al. Effect of high-frequency ventilation on the development of alveolar edema in premature monkeys at risk for hyaline membrane disease. Am Rev Respir Dis 1991;143:865.
57. Solimano A, Bryan C, Jobe A, et al. Effects of high-frequency and conventional ventilation on the premature lamb lung. J Appl Physiol 1985;59:1571.
58. Carter MJM, Gerstmann DR, Clark MRH, et al. High-frequency oscillatory ventilation and extracorporeal membrane oxygenation for the treatment of acute neonatal respiratory failure. Pediatrics 1990;85:159.
59. Rasche RFH, Kuhns LR. Histopathologic changes in airway mucosa of infants after endotracheal intubation. Pediatrics 1972;50:632.
60. Klainer AS, Turndorf H, Wu WH. Surface alterations to endotracheal intubation. Am J Med 1975;58:679.
61. Porkin JL, Stevens MH, Jung AL. Acquired and congenital subglottic stenosis in the infant. Ann Otolaryngol 1976;85: 573.
62. Filston HC, Johnson DG, Crumrire RS. Infant tracheostomy. Am J Dis Child 1978;132:1172.
63. Kuhns LR, Bednorck FJ, Wyman ML. Diagnosis of pneumothorax or pneumomediastinum in the neonate by transillumination. Pediatrics 1975;56:355.
64. Ogata ES, Gregory GA, Kitterman JA, et al. Pneumothorax in the respiratory distress syndrome: incidence and effect on vital signs, blood gas and *p*H. Pediatrics 1976;58:177.
65. Jung AL, Nelson J, Jenkins MB, Hodson WA. Clinical evaluation of a new chest tube used in neonates. Clinical Pediatrics 1991;2:85.
66. Gibson RL, Jackson JC, Twiggs GA, et al. Bronchopulmonary dysplasia: survival after prolonged mechanical ventilation. Am J Dis Child 1988;142:721.
67. Wiswell TE, Henley MA. Intratracheal suctioning, systemic infection, and the meconium aspiration syndrome. Pediatrics 1992;89:203.
68. Yeh TF, Srinivasan G, Harris V, et al. Hydrocortisone therapy in meconium aspiration syndrome: a controlled study. J Pediatr 1977;90:140.
69. Ferrara B, Johnson DE, Chang PN, et al. Efficacy and neurologic outcome of profound hypocapneic alkalosis for the treatment of persistent pulmonary hypertension in infancy. J Pediatr 1984;105:457.
70. Drummond WH, Gregory GA, Heymann MA, et al. The independent effects of hyperventilation, tolazoline and dopamine on infants with persistent pulmonary hypertension. J Pediatr 1981;98:603.
71. Stevenson DK, Kosting DS, Dornall RA, et al. Refractory hypoxemia associated with neonatal pulmonary disease: the use and limitations of tolazoline. J Pediatr 1979;95:595.

72. Goetzman BW, Sunshine P, Johnson JD, et al. Neonatal hypoxia and pulmonary vasospasm: response to tolazoline. J Pediatr 1976;89:617.
73. Greenspan JS, Wolfson MR, Rubenstein SD, Shaffer TH. Liquid ventilation of human preterm neonates. J Pediatr 1990; 117:106.
74. Truog WE, Jackson JC. Alternative modes of ventilation in the prevention and treatment of bronchopulmonary dysplasia. In: Holtzman RB, Frank L, eds. Clinics in perinatology. Philadelphia: WB Saunders, 1992.
75. Fuhrman BP, Paczan RR, Francisis M. Perfluorocarbon associated gas exchange. Crit Care Med 1991;19:712.
76. Brams YW. Biomedical technology—to use or not to use. Clin Perinatol 1991;18:389.

Neonatology: Pathophysiology and Management of the Newborn, Fourth Edition,
edited by Gordon B. Avery, Mary Ann Fletcher, and Mhairi G. MacDonald.
J.B. Lippincott Company, Philadelphia © 1994.

chapter 32

Extracorporeal Membrane Oxygenation

BILLIE LOU SHORT

In 1944, Kolff and Berk observed that blood became oxygenated as it passed through cellophane chambers of their artificial kidney membrane.[1] This historic observation led to the recognition, by those involved in the fast-developing field of cardiopulmonary bypass, that blood could be oxygenated through a semipermeable membrane lung. In the bubble and disk oxygenators used during the early 1950s for open heart surgery, oxygen and blood were mixed directly. This mixing resulted in considerable damage to blood products and the potential for producing lethal fibrin emboli, making these systems unsuitable for prolonged clinical use.[2] For this reason, and in light of Kolff and Berk's findings, attention was directed to the development of semipermeable membrane oxygenators that separate blood and oxygen, decreasing or eliminating the risks of the earlier oxygenators.

The first membrane lung, using an ethylcellulose membrane, was described by Clowes in 1956 and was used successfully in open heart surgery 1 year later.[3] With this report began the study of prolonged cardiopulmonary bypass and the potential application of extracorporeal membrane oxygenation (ECMO) as an artificial lung.

The 1960s witnessed intensive research on materials and techniques.[2] Silicone polymers, available in thin sheets that enhanced gas transfer through membranes, began to be characterized and developed. The development of the Kolobow silicone membrane lung made the field of ECMO possible, and clinical trials, using prolonged bypass or ECMO as an artificial lung, began in the late 1960s.[2,4–6]

The concept of an artificial placenta, a device capable of continuing *ex utero* the gas-exchange functions of the placenta, developed in parallel with that of an artificial lung. In 1961, Callaghan and colleagues began using animal models of respiratory distress syndrome of the newborn to test the efficacy of an extracorporeal oxygenation circuit as an artificial placenta.[7] During the early 1960s, investigators, including Rashkind, White, Dorson, and Avery, used ECMO as an artificial placenta for premature infants.[8–10] Although the infants died, this was an extremely important period for the development and refinement of the mechanical and surgical techniques that lay the foundation for the subsequent success of ECMO.

It was not until ECMO therapy was applied to the term infant through the pioneering work of Dr. Robert Bartlett and colleagues that its full potential as a powerful therapy for infants in severe respiratory failure was recognized. In 1976, Bartlett and his associates reported the first neonatal ECMO survivor, a term infant with severe meconium aspiration syndrome (MAS).[11] During the next 10 years, neonatal ECMO was used to treat 99 term infants with respiratory failure in three centers in the United States, with an overall survival rate of 65%. Since then, ECMO therapy has developed explosively, and more than 7000 infants have been treated in more than 90 ECMO programs, with an overall survival rate of 82%.

Although ECMO has become accepted as an effective therapy and is being offered to an increasing number of infants, it remains in its infancy, with further development and potential applications yet to be

TABLE 32–1
RESULTS OF EXTRACORPOREAL OXYGENATION

Diagnosis	Survival After Therapy (%)
Meconium aspiration syndrome	93
Persistent pulmonary hypertension	87
Sepsis and pneumonia	77
Congenital diaphragmatic hernia	61
Respiratory distress syndrome	85
Total	82

Data from the Extracorporeal Life Support Neonatal Registry, 1992, for 5863 patients.

determined. The current status of ECMO resembles that of ventilator therapy for newborn infants 25 years ago.[12] Clinical applications, treatment strategies, and equipment are continually updated, and the procedure requires highly specialized personnel in constant attendance.

The most common use for ECMO is in the term or near-term infant with failure to oxygenate due to MAS, idiopathic persistent pulmonary hypertension (PPHN), congenital diaphragmatic hernia (CDH), sepsis and pneumonia, or hyaline membrane disease. Although overall survival is 82% nationally, the best results are for the MAS (93%) and PPHN (86%) groups (Table 32-1). The survival rate for the CDH population on ECMO has not increased over time and remains at 61% nationally, perhaps because of the heterogeneity of this group of infants, who have various degrees of pulmonary hypoplasia and pulmonary hypertension. Only 30% to 40% of the CDH population requires ECMO therapy, and survival in the group not requiring ECMO is close to 100%.[13] Therefore, with ECMO therapy, the overall survival rate has increased to over 70%. Use of ECMO before surgical repair of the diaphragmatic defect may help to further increase survival in the ECMO CDH population.[14,15]

INDICATIONS

One of the most controversial aspects of ECMO therapy has been the clinical criteria used to determine its use.[16–24] Because of the invasive nature of ECMO therapy and the potential risks associated with this therapy, the criteria are designed to select a population of infants who have an 80% or greater mortality risk with conventional therapy. Assumptions about the ability of ECMO to increase survival can only be true if the criteria are specific for this high-risk population. The ultimate test for the efficacy of ECMO and the predictability of ECMO criteria is a prospective, randomized trial. Although two randomized trials have been completed, most centers have used historic controls to develop their criteria.[16,17,20–22] In the prospective, randomized trial reported by O'Rourke and colleagues, a cross-over design was used which may have skewed the predictability of their criteria. However, the criteria used in O'Rourke's study, which were thought to predict an 80% mortality based on retrospective data, only predicted a 40% mortality when used prospectively.[22] It is imperative that all centers continually evaluate their criteria, especially as less-invasive therapies become available.

The potential risks associated with ECMO therapy include those associated with ligation of the carotid artery and jugular vein, prolonged exposure to systemic heparinization, alterations in pulsatile blood flow patterns, exposure to potential toxins such as aluminum and phthalate esters (*i.e.*, plasticizer) from the circuit, and others yet to be determined.[25,26] With its long-term outcome still unknown, use of ECMO should be limited to the term or near-term infant who has a 20% or less chance of survival with conventional therapy. Although criteria developed at other centers are available, these are based on the clinical management and patient populations in those centers and may not be valid when applied to patients in other institutions.[18,19,23] What is considered maximal conventional therapy (*e.g.*, hyperventilation) in one institution may not be used in others. Differences in patient populations, such as the percentage of patients who are inborn or outborn, may significantly alter applicability of criteria from one center to another. All ECMO centers should attempt to develop criteria based on their own management techniques and patient population.

Several important inclusion criteria for ECMO are based on known complications of the procedure. These are listed in Table 32-2.

AGE AND WEIGHT LIMITATIONS

The requirement for systemic heparinization of the ECMO patient places significant limitations on the population that can be treated. Use of ECMO in the late 1960s and early 1970s in premature infants weighing less than 2000 g or younger than 34 weeks of gestation resulted in a significant mortality rate because of intracranial hemorrhage (ICH).[13,27–29] This increased risk may be a result of the combination of systemic heparinization with a more direct effect of

TABLE 32–2
INCLUSION CRITERIA FOR EXTRACORPOREAL MEMBRANE OXYGENATION

Gestational age ≥34 wk or birth weight ≥2000 g
No significant coagulopathy or bleeding complications
No major intracranial hemorrhage
Mechanical ventilation provided for ≤10–14 d
Reversible lung disease
No major cardiac lesion

ECMO on the brain.[27,30] Concerns about an increased rate of ICH in the premature infant were corroborated by findings for infants weighing less than 2500 g at birth who received ECMO at Children's National Medical Center in Washington, D.C. This group had a 50% incidence of ICH, representing more than 50% of the major ICHs seen in the total patient population at the center.[28] My colleagues and I recommended that only infants weighing more than 2000 g at birth or older than 33 weeks of of gestational age be considered candidates for ECMO. New advances, such as heparin-bonded circuits and a better understanding of the effects of ECMO on the brain, may allow us to lower the gestational age cutoff in the future.[30,31]

HEMATOLOGIC LIMITATIONS

The requirement for systemic heparinization places the infant with a significant coagulopathy or with bleeding complications such as pulmonary hemorrhage at extreme risk. All attempts should be made to correct any coagulopathy before instituting ECMO. If the coagulopathy is severe and cannot be corrected with appropriate blood product replacement, the infant should not be considered for ECMO.

The septic infant is of particular concern because of the commonly associated coagulopathy. Although these infants are at an increased risk for bleeding complications on ECMO, correction of their coagulopathy and meticulous heparin management have resulted in successful treatment.[32]

The necessity for heparinization during ECMO precludes the treatment of any infant with a major ICH. Infants with grade I intraventricular hemorrhages or small parenchymal hemorrhages can be treated, if heparin management is monitored closely and activated clotting times (ACTs) are kept low (*e.g.*, 180–190 seconds).

PRIOR MECHANICAL VENTILATION

The limit of 10 to 14 days of assisted ventilation before ECMO therapy is imposed because of the probable development of chronic lung disease after aggressive assisted ventilation of this duration. Extracorporeal membrane oxygenation is unable to reverse this disease process within a safe period. After 14 days, the risk for complications related to the ECMO procedure itself, such as clot formation, nosocomial infections (*e.g.*, neck wound infections), and mechanical failures (*e.g.*, tubing ruptures) begin to increase. The maximal time that a patient can be kept on the ECMO circuit is unknown, but in view of the increasing risk of complications, most centers limit time on the circuit to less than 20 days. Infants with diseases, such as chronic lung disease, that do not improve in a short period should not be considered for ECMO unless there is a life-threatening underlying disease state, such as acute pulmonary hypertension, which can be rapidly reversed by ECMO.

CARDIOPULMONARY DISEASE

Candidates for ECMO must have reversible lung disease. Because of the cardiopulmonary support provided by this therapy, ECMO has allowed many infants thought to have irreversible lung disease to live. The diagnosis of irreversible lung disease has become progressively more difficult to make.[14,33,34]

Significant cardiac disease must be ruled out before ECMO, but infants with severe reversible lung disease superimposed on congenital heart disease may be candidates for ECMO support before cardiac surgery.

RISK ASSESSMENT AND MORTALITY CRITERIA

If the infant is failing maximal conventional therapy, ECMO should be considered. The next task is to predict which infants have an 80% mortality risk without ECMO.

Commonly used criteria (Table 32-3) are the alveolar–arterial oxygen gradient ($AaDO_2$), the oxygen index (OI), and arterial partial pressure of oxygen (PaO_2) levels less than 50 torr during a specific period.[16,17,20,21,35] The $AaDO_2$ can be calculated as follows:

$$AaDO_2 = P_B - 47 - PaCO_2 - PaO_2, \text{ when } FiO_2 = 1.00,$$

in which P_B is the barometric pressure and 47 is the water vapor pressure. The OI can be calculated with the following equation:

$$OI = \frac{MAP \times FiO_2 \times 100}{PaO_2},$$

in which MAP is the mean airway pressure.

Deciding when to transfer an infant to an ECMO center is a difficult task. Most infants with disorders treated by ECMO improve without ECMO. The referring physician must attempt to determine which infants are at high risk for failing maximal conventional therapy and do this before the infant becomes too moribund for transport. This is an enormous responsibility, which can be eased by early consultation with ECMO center personnel. Kanto and associates found

TABLE 32–3
NEONATAL EXTRACORPOREAL MEMBRANE OXYGENATION CRITERIA*

$AaDO_2$ 605–620 torr for 4–12 h
Oxygen index 35–60 for 0.5–6 h
PaO_2 35–50 torr for 2–12 h
*p*H <7.25 for 2 h with hypotension
Acute deterioration PaO_2 30–40 torr

* Criteria used only after maximal therapy instituted; 50% of centers use more than one criterion.

$AaDO_2$, alveolar–arterial oxygen gradient; PaO_2, arterial partial pressure of oxygen.

TABLE 32–4
AVERAGE VENTILATOR SETTINGS AND BLOOD GAS VALUES BEFORE EXTRACORPOREAL MEMBRANE OXYGENATION FOR SURVIVORS AND NONSURVIVORS

Ventilator and Blood Gas Parameters	Values for All Patients*	Values for Survivors	Values for Nonsurvivors
Rate (bpm)	97 ± 74	96 ± 74	99 ± 75
FiO_2	1.00	1.00	1.00
PIP (cm H_2O)	46 ± 11	46 ± 10	45 ± 12
PEEP (cm H_2O)	4 ± 3	4 ± 3	6 ± 3
MAP (cm H_2O)	19 ± 5	19 ± 5	19 ± 5
*p*H	7.39 ± .2	7.41 ± .2	7.29 ± .2†
PCO_2 (torr)	42 ± 24	39 ± 21	52 ± 32†
PO_2 (torr)	41 ± 32	41 ± 31	38 ± 32†

* Data from the Extracorporeal Life Support Neonatal Registry, July 1990. Data displayed as mean ± SD.
† $p < 0.05$, survivors *versus* nonsurvivors.
bpm, breaths per minute; FiO_2, forced inspiratory oxygen; MAP, mean airway pressure; PEEP, peak end-expiratory pressure; PIP, peak inspiratory pressure.

that 12% of their ECMO referrals died before arrival of the transport team or during interhospital transport.[36] Of these deaths, 32% occurred in infants with CDH, indicating that early referral of these patients is warranted. Data from the Children's National Medical Center show that approximately 20 infants per year (16% of ECMO referrals) died before or during transport. For the infants who died, the average peak inspiratory pressure (PIP) at the time of the referral call was 50 cm H_2O, with a PaO_2 of 28 torr, compared with 45 cm H_2O and 40 torr in ECMO survivors. Earlier transfer might have increased the likelihood of survival in these infants.

The typical ventilator settings and blood gas values before ECMO therapy are shown in Table 32-4. If possible, consultation for transfer should occur before reaching these ventilator settings and before the infant's PaO_2 falls below 40 torr. The presence of a respiratory acidosis, as shown in Table 32-4, is associated with a significant increase in mortality and is an indication for possible early transfer.

The infant with CDH is the most difficult to manage before ECMO and should be considered for early transfer to an ECMO center. Some centers exclude infants with CDH who have not had some period with a PaO_2 more than 100 torr, and other centers exclude CDH patients as candidates for ECMO because they do not have an arterial partial pressure of carbon dioxide ($PaCO_2$) less than 45 torr after maximal ventilation.[37–40] Most ECMO centers accept all comers, because survivors have been reported from both of the described exclusionary categories.[14,15,33,34]

The studies that are performed before transfer of a patient to an ECMO center include an echocardiogram to rule out heart disease; a cranial ultrasound scan to rule out significant ICH; coagulation studies, including a partial thromboplastin time, prothrombin time, fibrinogen level, fibrin degradation products, and platelet count; calcium and electrolyte levels; leukocyte count with a differential analysis; and hemoglobin and hematocrit levels. These studies help the team at the ECMO center determine whether the patient should be considered for ECMO and, if so, assist them in anticipating difficulties.

On admission to the ECMO center, it must be determined whether the patient is an appropriate ECMO candidate. The ultrasound examination of the central nervous system (CNS) is repeated to ensure that an ICH did not occur during transport. The cardiac evaluation is repeated if there is any residual question about the possibility of cardiac disease. Doppler flow techniques are used to document the severity of pulmonary hypertension. This information can be used later if the infant does not wean from ECMO appropriately. Serum electrolyte and calcium levels, hemoglobin and hematocrit, clotting studies including fibrinogen level, fibrin degradation products, partial thromboplastin and prothrombin times, platelet count, and a baseline ACT should be obtained on admission to detect abnormalities which require correction before ECMO.

Most ECMO candidates have received muscle relaxants before admission, making the neurologic status difficult to evaluate. It is imperative to obtain a complete perinatal history, including Apgar scores, history of resuscitation and seizure activity, and a description of the neurologic status of the infant before paralysis. Infants who have sustained severe neurologic damage should not be considered for ECMO.

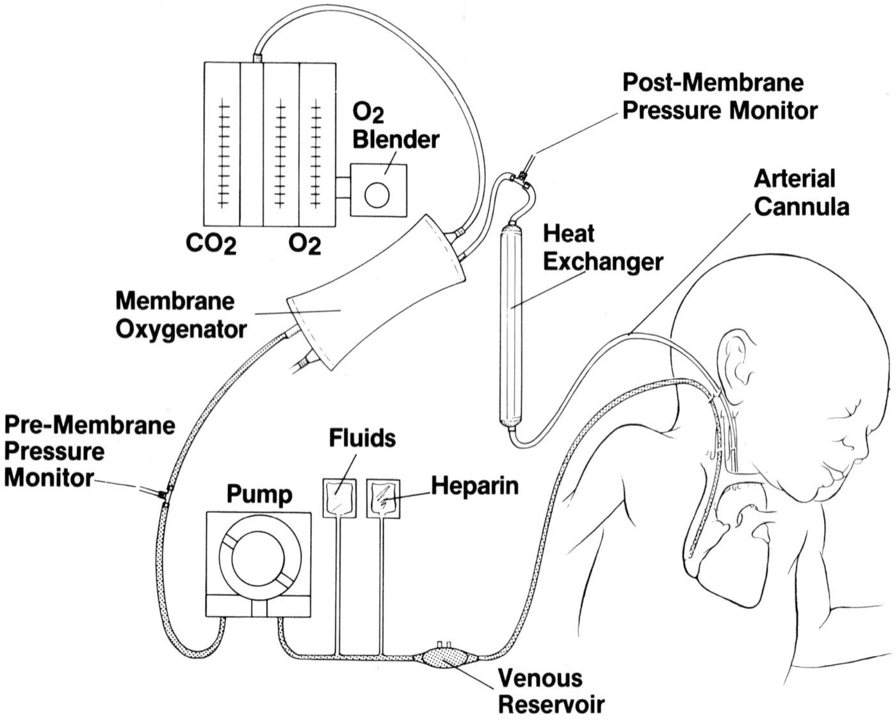

FIG. 32–1. Components of the venoarterial extracorporeal membrane oxygenation circuit. (From Short BL. Physiology of extracorporeal membrane oxygenation (ECMO). In: Polin RA, Fox WW, eds. Fetal and neonatal physiology. Philadelphia: WB Saunders, 1992:932.)

PROCEDURE

VENOARTERIAL METHOD

Venoarterial (VA) ECMO involves the use of two catheters: the venous outflow catheter in the right internal jugular vein with the tip in the right atrium and the arterial return catheter in the right carotid artery with the tip at the junction with the aortic arch. Blood is removed through the jugular catheter by means of gravity drainage into a venous reservoir (Fig. 32-1). Blood is pulled out of the reservoir by a roller occlusion pump and pushed through the membrane lung, where gas exchange occurs. Gas transfers across the silicone membrane lung into the blood because of pressure gradients, increasing the oxygen level and removing carbon dioxide (Fig. 32-2). Blood then enters the heat exchanger, where it is warmed to body temperature and returned to the infant through the arterial catheter.

This form of bypass provides support for the lungs and cardiac support. Although most infants requiring ECMO have only a pulmonary disorder, some have cardiac dysfunction secondary to severe hypoxia and require the cardiac support that VA ECMO provides. Oxygenation is achieved by allowing the pump to support as much of the cardiac output as is needed to oxygenate the infant, usually 120 to 150 mL/kg/minute in the first few days.

It is easy to support and oxygenate with VA ECMO, and it remains the gold standard for ECMO therapy. However, ligation of the carotid artery, al-

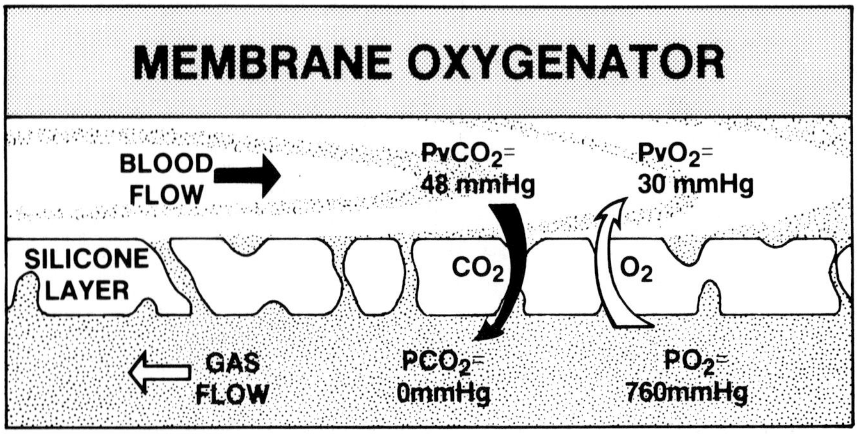

FIG. 32–2. The silicone membrane lung promotes gas transfer across a gradient for oxygen and carbon dioxide. The pore size does not allow blood products to cross. (From Short BL. In: Polin RA, Fox WW, eds. Fetal and neonatal physiology. Philadelphia: WB Saunders, 1992:932.)

teration of pulsatile arterial blood flow patterns, and the possibility that particles or air in the circuit may enter the cerebral or coronary circulations remain concerns.

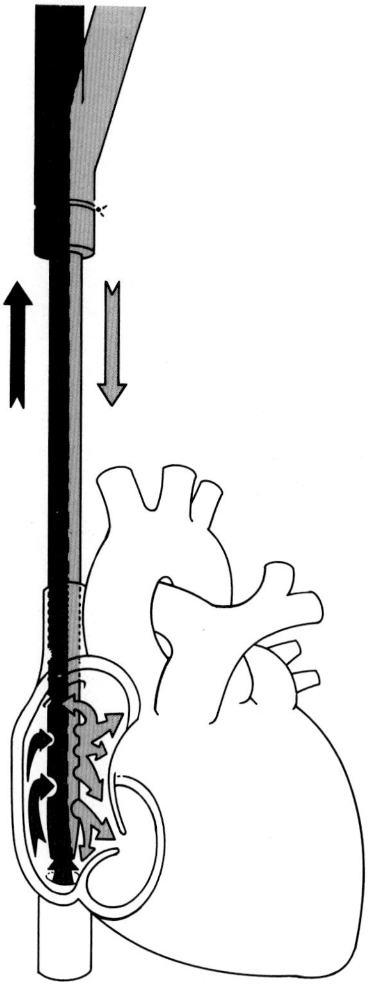

FIG. 32–3. The inflow and outflow characteristics of the venovenous catheter in the right atrium. (From Short BL, O'Brien A, Poindexter C, eds. CNMC ECMO training manual. 1993.)

VENOVENOUS METHOD

Venovenous (VV) techniques for ECMO have been developed because of the concerns about carotid ligation. Venovenous ECMO is currently achieved using a single double-lumen catheter placed through the internal jugular vein into the right atrium (Fig. 32-3).[41] This catheter has inflow and outflow ports that attach into the circuit. Because blood return and outflow occur in the right atrium, significant recirculation can occur, resulting in limited oxygenation with this technique (Fig. 32-4). Because the heart is the pump for VV ECMO, the use of this catheter depends on intact cardiac function. The advantages of this technique are the lack of necessity for ligation of the carotid artery, maintenance of normal pulsatile blood flow, and the theoretic advantage that particles entering the circuit enter the lungs, rather than the cerebral or coronary circulation. Disadvantages are the lack of cardiac support and limited oxygenation.

EQUIPMENT AND SYSTEMS

Most equipment currently used for ECMO therapy is modified cardiopulmonary bypass equipment designed for short-term use. To ensure safe and effective use of the ECMO equipment, the limitations of each piece of equipment must be understood and considered before its use for long-term bypass.

There is no single ECMO machine. Each ECMO center must design an ECMO system by using equipment evaluated and designed to meet space and other specific requirements of their center. Bioengi-

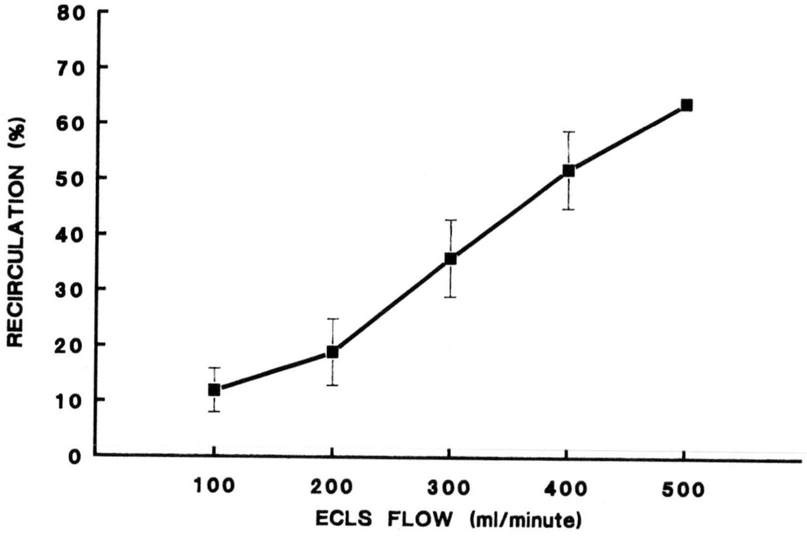

FIG. 32–4. Recirculation occurs with the use of the venovenous extracorporeal membrane oxygenation catheter. Flows greater than 400 mL/minute result in greater than 50% recirculation and decrease oxygenation at this point. (Data from Anderson HL, Otsu T, Chapman RA, Bartlett RH. Venovenous extracorporeal life support in neonates using a double lumen catheter. Trans Am Soc Artif Intern Organs 1989;35:650.)

neering experts and cardiopulmonary perfusionists should be consulted in the design and evaluation of the ECMO system. The basic equipment needed for a complete system is listed in Table 32-5.

Space requirements and the possible need to transport the patient on ECMO should be taken into consideration in the design of an ECMO system (Fig. 32-5; see Fig. 32-1). The system should be on a cart or other movable base. The nondisposable equipment required includes a roller occlusion pump, a water bath to maintain normothermic bypass temperatures, a venous return monitor (VRM), gas flow meters for CO_2 and O_2 delivery into the membrane lung, an in-line venous saturation monitor, and membrane pressure monitors. Necessary disposable equipment includes the ECMO catheters (*i.e.*, venous and arterial for VA ECMO; double-lumen venous for VV ECMO), tubing packs designed for the system, a venous reservoir, a heat exchanger, and a membrane lung.

Those involved in providing ECMO therapy must know the potential complications related to each piece of equipment, especially the thrombogenic characteristics and flow dynamics. Several of these concepts are discussed in this chapter; however, additional information can be found elsewhere.[42]

In VA ECMO, the venous catheter is the oxygenation catheter, because the rate of blood flow through this catheter determines the percentage of the cardiac output that is supported by the ECMO pump. Oxygenation is determined by the percentage of cardiac output passing through the ECMO membrane (*i.e.*, artificial lung) and bypassing the patient's lungs. If a small-gauge venous catheter is placed, minimal flow through the ECMO circuit occurs, and oxygenation may be compromised. Blood flow rates (Q) are directly proportional to the fourth power of the radius (r) of the tubing and inversely proportional to the length (L) of the tubing:

$$Q \propto r^4$$
$$Q \propto 1/L.$$

To maximize flow into the circuit, a relatively short venous catheter with as large a lumen as possible is used.

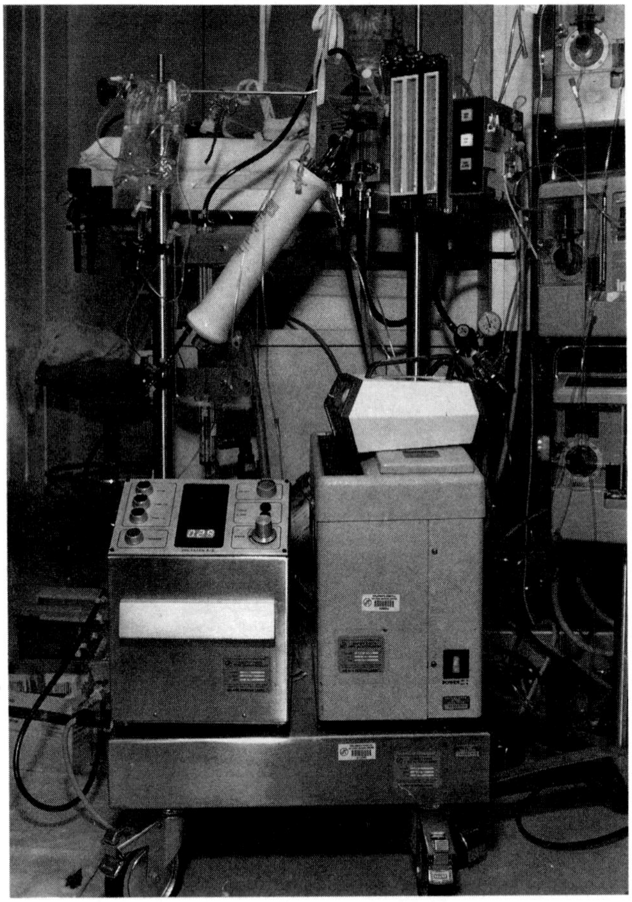

FIG. 32–5. The extracorporeal membrane oxygenation system used at the Children's National Medical Center has a modular design.

TABLE 32–5
EQUIPMENT FOR NEONATAL EXTRACORPOREAL MEMBRANE OXYGENATION

Roller occlusion pump
Pump base
Venous return monitor
Heating unit
Coagulation timer
Membrane mounting board
Oxygen blender
Carbon dioxide or carbogen tank
O_2 and CO_2 flowmeters
In-line temperature probes
In-line oxygen saturation monitor

The arterial catheter, which supplies return of flow from the circuit into the arch of the aorta, is the smallest-diameter component in the circuit and acts as the major resistance component in the circuit. A small arterial catheter may cause significant back pressure, resulting in restricted blood flow, hemolysis, or eventual rupture of the circuit. Resistance to flow depends on the dimensions and geometry of the tubing and the characteristics of the fluid used. Poiseuille's Law defines this concept by the following equation:

$$R = \frac{8\eta L}{\pi r^4},$$

in which $8/\pi$ is the constant of proportionality, L (cm) is the length of the tubing, η (*i.e.*, Poise = dyne − second/cm^2) is the coefficient of viscosity, and r (cm) is the radius of the tubing. The longer the tubing and the smaller the radius, the greater is the resistance. An 8-F (2.6-mm) catheter has much greater resistance than a 10-F (3.3-mm) catheter. A short, large-lumen catheter is ideal, but the size of catheter placed is limited by the diameter of the patient's carotid artery.[43]

The double-lumen catheter used in VV ECMO has a small lumen for blood return, which produces a relatively high back pressure in the circuit. Kinking of this catheter significantly increases circuit pressures and must be diligently avoided.

The VRM is an electronic device that monitors the blood flow from the patient into the ECMO circuit (see Fig. 32-1). The VRM functions as a servoregulator for the ECMO system and is designed to alarm and stop the pump if venous flow from the patient slows, ensuring that aortic blood input equals venous output. If a VRM system is not in place and venous return decreases without servoregulation, the roller pump continues to pump and causes the tubing to collapse, creating a negative pressure that pulls gas out of solution in the blood and air into the circuit at the connection points. The most common causes of loss of venous return are malplacement of the venous catheter (usually in the inferior vena cava), pneumothorax or pneumopericardium, unrecognized bleeding (*e.g.*, ICH, hemothorax), kinking of the venous catheter, or placing an anchoring suture too tightly around the catheter during cannulation.

The only membrane lung approved for long-term ECMO use is the silicone membrane lung made by Avecor (Minneapolis, MN). The 0.8-m^2 membrane is most commonly used for neonates, and can support oxygenation up to a Q of 1 L/minute. Carbon dioxide transfer is so efficient with this membrane that CO_2 must be added to the gases flowing into the membrane.

PATIENT MANAGEMENT

A team approach to the management of the ECMO patient is critical. Duties of the bedside nurse, respiratory therapist, and ECMO specialist should be clearly delineated to ensure efficient and effective care.[44]

DAILY MEDICAL MANAGEMENT

Most neonatal patients, with the exception of those with CDH, require ECMO support for 5 days. During this period, the patient who was in respiratory failure and dying before ECMO shows evidence of reversal of disease, can be slowly weaned off ECMO to minimal ventilator settings, and can usually be extubated within 24 to 48 hours after coming off the ECMO circuit. The rapidity of recovery is remarkable, given the severity of the illness suffered by these infants before ECMO. For this level of recovery to occur in such a short time, many physiologic changes must take place rapidly, making daily care of the infant a fine art. Routine care must incorporate the fact that these infants are systemically heparinized, and tasks such as suctioning of the airway should be done with caution.

As the lungs improve, less blood flow is required to pass through the artificial lung, and the ECMO blood flow can be reduced. In the first few days, a Q of 120 to 150 mL/kg/minute is required to oxygenate the infant.[45] With improvement of the infant's lungs, arterial blood gases improve, and the ECMO blood flow can be decreased by 10 to 20 mL/minute. The venous saturation of blood in the ECMO circuit can be monitored continuously, providing a representation of a mixed venous saturation level. However, this saturation is measured in blood from the right atrium, and right atrial blood saturation does not represent true mixed venous saturation if there are intracardiac shunts. Because most infants on ECMO develop left-to-right shunts, often occurring at the level of the foramen ovale, venous saturations must be interpreted in terms of other clinical signs. The following concepts must be understood:

$$C_VO_2 = CaO_2 - VO_2/\text{flow},$$
$$\text{Oxygen content} = \text{Hb} \times \%\ \text{saturation} \times 1.36 + 0.0031 \times PO_2,$$

in which C_VO_2 is venous oxygen content, CaO_2 is arterial oxygen content, VO_2 is oxygen consumption, and flow is cardiac output.

For venous oxygen saturation to represent a true indication of arterial oxygen content, several assumptions must be made: that the cardiac output remains stable, that hemoglobin concentrations remain stable, and that the metabolic rate of the patient does not change. Any one of these factors can cause a change in the venous saturation. Therefore, the patient should be carefully evaluated before using this parameter alone to wean the ECMO flows. Arterial blood gases are needed to determine the *p*H and $PaCO_2$ status of the patient and the membrane lung. If the arterial $PaCO_2$ of the membrane decreases below 35 torr during VA ECMO, a decrease in respiratory rate may result, because the brain detects the blood gas levels in blood from the membrane lung during VA ECMO. If the patient's respiratory rate falls and he or she is on low bypass, the result is a deterioration in blood gas status. The problem is corrected by increasing the CO_2 coming from the membrane to stimulate the infant to breath. A high membrane PCO_2 may indicate membrane failure and is an emergency, and a normal membrane PCO_2 with an abnormal patient PCO_2 indicates a change in the patient's clinical condition, such as development of pneumothorax or secondary pneumonia.

After being stabilized on ECMO, the infant is placed on lung-rest settings on the ventilator (*i.e.*, fraction of inspired oxygen [FiO_2] = 0.21, PIP = 15–18 cm H_2O; peak end-expiratory pressures [PEEP] = 5–6 cm H_2O; rate = 10–15 breaths per minute [bpm]). It is typical for the lungs to appear opaque on chest radiographs during the first 1 to 3 days of ECMO.[46–48] This is probably caused by the acute decrease in ventilatory settings, capillary leak, activation of complement as a result of interaction of blood products with the artificial surfaces in the circuit, and surfactant deficiency secondary to lung injury.[46,49,50] Lotze and associates showed that surfactant replacement therapy in infants on ECMO can decrease time on ECMO for all infants except those with CDH.[51] Lung compliance studies can help in predicting successful decannulation, especially in the infant who is borderline and when a decision is being made about removing an infant from ECMO because of complications.[47] A typical lung compliance curve is shown in Figure 32-6. An old-fashioned but effective technique for assessing pulmonary improvement is to hand-ventilate the infant daily. When the chest moves easily with a peak pressure of 20 cm H_2O or less, the infant can successfully come off ECMO.

Heparin is administered continuously into the ECMO circuit to prevent clotting.[44] Heparin management will vary, depending on events before and during ECMO. Optimal heparin management can achieve the level of heparinization needed to decrease the risk for fibrin and clot formation in the circuit while minimizing the risk for bleeding complications in the patient. Because heparinization must be evaluated rapidly and at the bedside, most centers use the ACT.[52] The ACT is determined in a system that uses activators, such as glass beads, to initiate the clotting cascade. The specimen is warmed to accelerate the clotting process. This test gives values of 80 to 120 seconds in a nonheparinized infant, compared with standard nonactivated bleeding time values of longer than 5 minutes.[53]

The primary cause of death in the ECMO population is ICH.[13,54] The risk factors associated with the development of an ICH include significant hypoxic or ischemic cerebral insult before ECMO, sepsis with coagulopathy, or gestational age less than 37 weeks. Initial heparin management is based on pretreatment risk factors. If there is a high risk for ICH before ECMO, the ACT is maintained between 180 and 200 seconds for at least the first 24 to 48 hours. Most intracranial bleeds occur during this period. If the infant is not at risk for ICH the ACTs are maintained between 200 and 240 seconds. The range can be narrowed, depending on the number of risk factors the infant has. The platelet count is maintained above 60,000/mm^3 in the noncomplicated case and between 100,000 and 150,000/mm^3 in a case complicated by bleeding.[42]

Fibrin formation is related to flow rate; if there are low Qs in the circuit, the heparin dose is increased to decrease the risk for clot formation. At the beginning of an ECMO run, blood flows are high and the ACTs can be maintained in a lower range. At the end of a run, the ACTs are increased, especially when the idling phase (*i.e.*, 60–80 mL/minute) is reached. When Q in the circuit is below 150 mL/minute, ACTs are increased to 220–240 seconds. Clinical factors that affect the ACT values are renal function (*i.e.*, heparin excretion is directly proportional to urine output), transfusion of unheparinized blood products or platelets, and a significant patent ductus arteriosus with a left-to-right shunt that may decrease renal blood flow.

Fluid requirements while on ECMO range from 80 to 120 mL/kg/day. Electrolyte requirements are significantly different from those before starting ECMO. Most infants require little sodium, usually 1 to 2 mEq/kg/day, and a large amount of potassium, usually 4 to 5 mEq/kg/day. The rationale for these requirements is unknown. Although renin levels increase on bypass, aldosterone levels decrease, and atrionaturetic peptide levels do not change.[55,56] Calcium requirements range from 20 to 40 mg of elemental calcium/kg/day.

Systemic hypertension is a common medical complication of ECMO. Hypertension (*i.e.*, mean blood pressure $>$ 65 torr for $>$ 3 hours) can affect as many as 70% of these patients. Hypertension usually develops shortly after cannulation and is transient, but 1% to 5% of infants require long-term antihypertensive therapy. The risk of ICH is increased by hypertension.[56] Although a subject of controversy, the

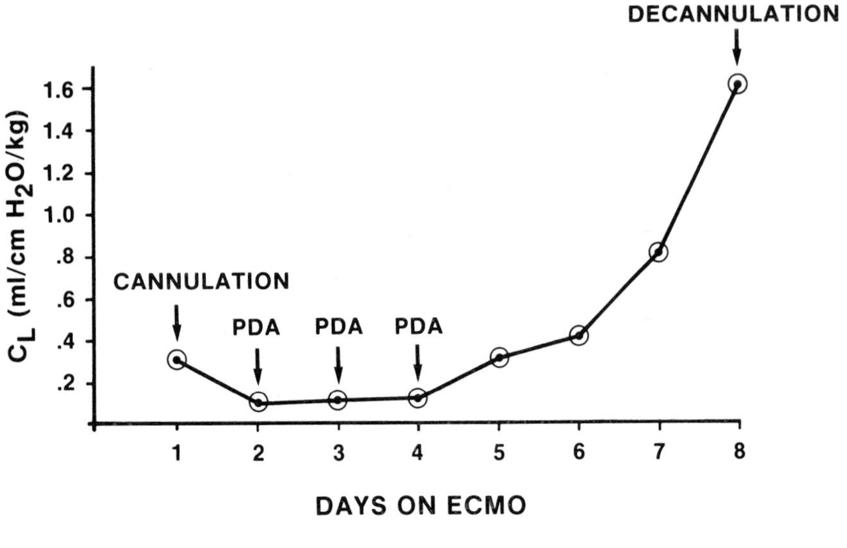

FIG. 32–6. The typical lung compliance curve for an infant with meconium aspiration syndrome on extracorporeal membrane oxygenation (ECMO). Infants in this study were successfully taken off ECMO if a lung compliance (C_L) of 0.8 mL/cm H_2O/kg was attained. (From Lotze A, Short BL, Taylor GA. Lung compliance as a measure of lung function in newborns with respiratory failure requiring extracorporeal membrane oxygenation. Crit Care Med 1987; 15(3):226.)

cause may be related to an increase in serum renin levels.[55–57] Fluid restriction and diuretic therapy may decrease the risk for prolonged hypertension.

Infants on ECMO commonly develop a left-to-right shunt across the patent ductus arteriosus, resulting in oxygenation difficulty.[45] Most of these shunts close with fluid restriction and diuretic therapy. Few patients require surgical intervention. Indomethacin should not be used in this population, because it decreases platelet aggregation. After the shunt closes, an immediate increase in the patient's PaO_2 is observed.

Cardiac stun is an interesting complication of ECMO therapy that also occurs in patients on cardiopulmonary bypass. Cardiac stun occurs in infants with severe hypoxia or in infants in whom the tip of the arterial catheter is placed too close to the coronary arteries.[57] This syndrome is characterized by a pulse pressure of 10 torr or less on ECMO, with the patient's PaO_2 equal to or within 50 to 100 torr of the pump PO_2 (*e.g.*, a pump PO_2 of 400 torr while on an FiO_2 of 1.00, with a patient PaO_2 between 300 and 350 torr). The electrocardiographic pattern is normal, indicating that electrical conduction is normal, but cardiac output is markedly reduced. The pathophysiology is not understood.[58,59] When data on infants with cardiac stun while on ECMO at the Children's National Medical Center were evaluated, there was a significant difference in pre-ECMO blood gases compared with infants who did not develop cardiac stun. Infants in stun were sicker before ECMO and had a higher incidence of death due to ICH, indicating the marked hypoxic–ischemic insult suffered by these patients before ECMO. Treatment of cardiac stun consists of maintaining ECMO Q high enough to supply appropriate cardiac output. Afterload reduction does not improve cardiac function in this population.[60] As stun resolves, the pulse pressure returns to normal, and the patient's PaO_2 no longer mirrors the pump PO_2.

Weaning from ECMO occurs slowly as the arterial blood gases and venous saturations improve. Idling flows (*i.e.*, 60–80 mL/minute) are continued for 6 to 8 hours and, if blood gases are normal during this period, most infants can be successfully taken off ECMO. A lung compliance measurement of at least 0.8 mL/cm H_2O/kg indicates that the infant can successfully come off ECMO (see Fig. 32-6).[47] Typical ventilator settings for infants after completing an ECMO course are FiO_2 of 0.30 to 0.40; rate of 30 to 40 bpm; PIP of 18 to 20 cm H_2O; and PEEP of 5 to 6 cm H_2O.

PATIENT CARE AFTER EXTRACORPOREAL MEMBRANE OXYGENATION

A neuromuscular blocking agent with an intermediate half-life is used at decannulation to help the patient breathe spontaneously as soon as possible after coming off ECMO. By the end of the ECMO run, it is common for the ECMO patient to require high $PaCO_2$ levels (*i.e.*, 45–55 torr) to stimulate respiratory drive. These levels of $PaCO_2$ should be continued after ECMO for the first 24 to 48 hours to continue to stimulate respiratory drive. Many of these infants have been receiving narcotics such as fentanyl and may need to be weaned slowly from this therapy to avoid withdrawal. PaO_2 levels of 60 to 70 torr are accepted, and every effort is made to wean the patient from the ventilator. The CDH patient is an exception; these patients require slower weaning to ensure that pulmonary hypertension does not reoccur.

Hemoglobin, hematocrit, calcium, and electrolyte measurements should be obtained 6 to 8 hours after ECMO. These can then be monitored every 24 hours or as clinically indicated. The platelet count should be followed closely (*i.e.*, values every 8 hours for 24 hours), because rebound thrombocytopenia may occur. Intravenous sodium is increased to 2 to 3 mEq/kg/day, and potassium supplementation is decreased to 1 to 2 mEq/kg/day.

After extubation, the infant usually requires oxygen therapy for another 5 to 7 days. Most ECMO infants feed poorly and may require feeding by tube for a few days. The cause of this problem is uncertain, but it is usually transient and does not indicate long-term developmental problems.

Because not all intracranial abnormalities are detected by ultrasound, a computed tomography or magnetic resonance scan is recommended before discharge.[54] A baseline hearing screen and a neurologic assessment are also recommended before discharge. All infants should be followed in a neonatal high-risk follow-up program.

Developmental outcome is encouraging, with most centers reporting that 60% to 70% of ECMO survivors are normal at 1 to 2 years of age.[61–63] Risk factors associated with poor outcome include finding a severe neuroimaging abnormality, chronic lung disease, prematurity, and β-streptococcal sepsis. The 10% to 15% of the ECMO-treated population who are considered suspect for abnormalities at 1 to 2 years of age require close follow-up, because a large percentage of these infants develop learning disabilities by 5 years of age.[64]

The need for carotid artery ligation for VA ECMO has caused concern that right-sided CNS lesions may result. Schumacher and colleagues reported right-sided CNS lesions in their ECMO population, but similar findings have not been reported by others.[54,65] Analysis of the first 360 patients treated at Children's National Medical Center did not reveal lateralizing hemorrhagic or nonhemorrhagic abnormalities, but there was a high incidence of posterior fossa hemorrhage, raising the concern that jugular venous ligation might increase venous back pressure and the risk of hemorrhage.[54,66] Data published by Taylor and Walker showed that decreased sagittal sinus blood flow velocity is associated with ICH (70%) in the ECMO population.[67] Whether this is cause or effect has yet to be determined. Many ECMO teams are now placing jugular bulb catheters in the right internal jugular vein to drain the venous outflow from the brain into the venous side of the circuit.

The infant with CDH may have unique long-term problems, including significant gastroesophageal reflux and chronic lung disease.[68] These infants require close follow-up in a multidisciplinary clinic to prevent problems such as failure to thrive and respiratory compromise.

SUMMARY

Care of the ECMO patient requires highly trained nurses, respiratory therapists, perfusionists, and physicians. The team must continually evaluate the treatment modalities and use the information to improve techniques and to define the indications for ECMO therapy. It has been estimated that only 1000 to 2500 term infants require ECMO each year in the United States.[69] The availability of ECMO therapy must be tailored to regional needs in an effort to maintain cost control and quality of care. Considering the developmental status of ECMO and with possible new and less invasive therapies, such as nitric oxide, appearing on the horizon, it is clear that not every neonatal intensive care unit should develop an ECMO program.[70]

REFERENCES

1. Kolff WJ, Berk HT. Artificial kidney: a dialyzer with a great area. Acta Med Scand 1944;17:121.
2. Kenedi RM, Courtey JM, Gaylor JDS, Gilchrsit T. Artificial organs. Baltimore: University Park Press, 1976:11.
3. Clowes GHA Jr, Hopkins AL, Neville WE. An artificial lung dependent upon diffusion of oxygen and carbon dioxide through plastic membranes. J Thorac Surg 1956;32:630.
4. Kolobow T, Stool EW, Sacko KL, Vurek GG. Acute respiratory failure, survival following ten days' support with a membrane lung. J Thorac Cardiovasc Surg 1975;69:947.
5. Zapol WM, Snider MT, Hil DJ, et al. Extracorporeal membrane oxygenation in severe acute respiratory failure: a randomized prospective study. JAMA 1979;242:2193.
6. Gille JP, Bagniewski AM. Ten years of use of extracorporeal membrane oxygenation (ECMO) in the treatment of acute respiratory insufficiency (ARI). Trans Am Soc Artif Intern Organs 1976;22:102.
7. Callaghan JC, delos Angeles J. Long-term extracorporeal circulation in the development of an artificial placenta for respiratory distress syndrome of the newborn. Surg Forum 1961; 12:215.
8. Rashkind WJ, Freeman A, Klein D, Toft RW. Evolution of a disposable plastic low volume, pumpless oxygenator as a lung substitute. J Pediatr 1965;66:94.
9. White JJ, Andrews HG, Risemberg H, et al. Prolonged respiratory support in newborn infants with a membrane oxygenator. Surgery 1971;70:288.
10. Dorson WJ, Baker E, Cohen ML, et al. A perfusion system for infants. Trans Am Soc Artif Intern Organs 1969;15:155.
11. Bartlett RH, Gazzaniga AB, Jefferies MR, et al. Extracorporeal membrane oxygenation (ECMO) cardiopulmonary support in infancy. Trans Am Soc Artif Intern Organs 1976;22:80.
12. Stahlman MT. Assisted ventilation in newborn infants. In: Smith GF, Vidyasagar D, eds. Historical review and recent advances in neonatal and perinatal medicine, vol II. Evansville, IN: Mead Johnson Nutritional Division, 21.
13. Stolar CJH, Snedecor SM, Bartlett RH. Extracorporeal membrane oxygenation and neonatal respiratory failure: experience from the extracorporeal life support organization. J Pediatr Surg 1991;26:563.
14. Breaux CW, Rouse TM, Cain WS, Georgeson KE. Improvement in survival of patients with congenital diaphragmatic hernia utilizing a strategy of delayed repair after medical and/or extracorporeal membrane oxygenation stabilization. J Pediatr Surg 1991;26:333.
15. Sanchez LS, O'Brien A, Anderson KD, et al. Best postductal PO_2 and PCO_2 do not predict outcome of CDH infants in extremis, stabilized with ECMO prior to surgical repair. Pediatr Res 1992;31:221A.
16. Bartlett RH, Roloff DW, Cornell RG, et al. Extracorporeal circulation in neonatal respiratory failure: a prospective randomized trial. Pediatrics 1985;76:479.
17. Beck R, Anderson KD, Pearson GD, et al. Criteria for extracorporeal membrane oxygenation in a population of infants with persistent pulmonary hypertension of the newborn. J Pediatr Surg 1986;21:297.
18. Cole CH, Jillson E, Kessler D. ECMO. Regional evaluation of need and applicability of selection criteria. Am J Dis Child 1988;142:1320.
19. Dworetz AR, Moya FR, Sabo B, et al. Survival of infants with persistent pulmonary hypertension without extracorporeal membrane oxygenation. Pediatrics 1989;84:1.
20. Krummel TM, Greenfield LJ, Kirkpatrick BV, et al. Alveolar-arterial oxygen gradients versus the neonatal pulmonary insufficiency index for prediction of mortality in ECMO candidates. J Pediatr Surg 1984;19:380.
21. Marsh TD, Wilkerson SA, Cook LN. Extracorporeal membrane oxygenation selection criteria: partial pressure of arterial oxygen versus alveolar-arterial oxygen gradient. Pediatrics 1988; 82:162.
22. O'Rourke PP, Crone RK, Vacanti JP, et al. Extracorporeal membrane oxygenation and conventional medical therapy in neonates with persistent pulmonary hypertension of the newborn: a prospective randomized study. Pediatrics 1989;84:957.
23. Wung JT, James LS, Kilchevsky E, James E. Management of infants with severe respiratory failure and persistence of the fetal circulation without hyperventilation. Pediatrics 1985;76: 488.
24. Hollenberg NK, Dzau VJ, Williams GH. Are uncontrolled clinical studies ever justified? N Engl J Med 1980;303:1059.
25. Kelly AT, Short BL, Rains TC, et al. Aluminum toxicity and albumin. Trans Am Soc Artif Intern Organs 1989;35:674.
26. Schneider B, Schena J, Troug R, et al. Exposure to di(2-ethylhexyl)phthalate in infants receiving extracorporeal membrane oxygenation. N Engl J Med 1989;320:1563.
27. Cilley RE, Zwischenferger JB, Andrews AF, et al. Intracranial hemorrhage during extracorporeal membrane oxygenation in neonates. Pediatrics 1986;78:699.
28. Revenis ME, Glass P, Short B. Mortality and morbidity among lower birth weight (2–2.5 kg) infants treated with extracorporeal membrane oxygenation (ECMO). J Pediatr 1992;121:452.
29. Toomasian JM, Snedecor SM, Cornell RG, et al. National experience with extracorporeal membrane oxygenation for newborn respiratory failure. Trans Am Soc Artif Intern Organs 1988;34:140.

30. Short BL, Walker LK, Bendu KS, Traystman RJ. Impairment of cerebral autoregulation during extracorporeal membrane oxygenation. Pediatr Res 1993;33:289.
31. Short BL, Walker LK, Gleason CA, et al. Effects of extracorporeal membrane oxygenation on cerebral blood flow and cerebral oxygen metabolism in newborn sheep. Pediatr Res 1990;28:50.
32. McCune S, Short BL, Miller MK, et al. Extracorporeal membrane oxygenation therapy in neonates with septic shock. J Pediatr Surg 1990;25:479.
33. Newman KD, Van Meurs KP, Short BL, Anderson KD. Extracorporeal membrane oxygenation and congenital diaphragmatic hernia—should any infant be excluded? J Pediatr Surg 1990;25:1048.
34. Van Meurs KP, Newman KD, Anderson KD, Short BL. Effect of extracorporeal membrane oxygenation on survival of infants with congenital diaphragmatic hernia. J Pediatr 1990;117:954.
35. Ortiz RM, Cilley RE, Bartlett RH. Extracorporeal membrane oxygenation in pediatric respiratory failure. Pediatr Clin North Am 1987;34:39.
36. Boedy RF, Howell CG, Kanto WP. Hidden mortality of ECMO. J Pediatr 1990;117:462.
37. Langham MR, Krummel TM, Bartlett RH, et al. Mortality with extracorporeal membrane oxygenation following repair of congenital diaphragmatic hernia in 93 infants. J Pediatr Surg 1987;22:1150.
38. Stolar C, Dillon P, Reyes C. Selective use of extracorporeal membrane oxygenation in the management of congenital diaphragmatic hernia. J Pediatr Surg 1988;23:207.
39. Howell CG, Hatley RM, Boedy FR, et al. Recent experience with diaphragmatic hernia and ECMO. Ann Surg 1990;211:793.
40. O'Rourke PP, Lillehei CW, Crone RK, Vacanti JP. The effect of extracorporeal membrane oxygenation on the survival of neonates with high-risk congenital diaphragmatic hernia: 45 cases from a single institution. J Pediatr Surg 1991;26:147.
41. Anderson HL, Otsu T, Chapman RA, Bartlett RH. Venovenous extracorporeal life support in neonates using a double lumen catheter. Trans Am Soc Artif Intern Organs 1989;35:650.
42. Short BL. Pre-ECMO considerations for neonatal patients. In: Arensman RM, Cornish D, eds. Extracorporeal life support. Cambridge MA: Blackwell Scientific, 1993.
43. Van Meurs KP, Mikesell GT, Seale SR, et al. Maximum blood flow rates for arterial cannulae used in neonatal ECMO. Trans Trans Am Soc Artif Intern Organs 1990;36:M679.
44. Short BL. Clinical management of the neonatal ECMO patient. In: Arensman RM, Cornish D, eds. Extracorporeal life support. Cambridge MA: Blackwell Scientific, 1993.
45. Martin GR, Short BL. Doppler echocardiographic evaluation of cardiac performance in infants on prolonged extracorporeal membrane oxygenation. Am J Cardiol 1988;62:929.
46. Taylor GA, Short BL, Kreismer P. Extracorporeal membrane oxygenation: radiographic appearance of the neonatal chest. Am J Radiol 1986;146:1257.
47. Lotze A, Short BL, Taylor GA. The use of lung compliance as a parameter for improvement in lung function in newborns with respiratory failure requiring extracorporeal membrane oxygenation. Crit Care Med 1987;15:226.
48. Keszler M, Subramanian KN, Smith YA, et al. Pulmonary management during extracorporeal membrane oxygenation. Crit Care Med 1989;17:495.
49. Lotze A, Whitsett JA, Kammerman L, et al. Surfactant protein A concentrations in tracheal aspirate fluid from infants requiring extracorporeal membrane oxygenation. J Pediatr 1990;116:435.
50. Anderson JM, Kottke-Marchant K. Platelet interactions with biomaterials and artificial devices. In: Williams DF, ed. Blood compatibility volume I. Boca Raton: CRC Press, 1987:127.
51. Lotze A, Knight GR, Martin GM, et al. Improved pulmonary outcome after exogenous surfactant therapy for respiratory failure in term infants requiring extracorporeal membrane oxygenation. J Pediatr 1993;122(2):261.
52. Hattersley P. Activated coagulation time of whole blood. JAMA 1966;196:436.
53. Kay LA, ed. Essentials of hemostasis and thrombosis. 2nd ed. New York: Churchill-Livingstone, 1988.
54. Taylor GA, Short BL, Fitz CR. Imaging of cerebrovascular injury in infants treated with extracorporeal membrane oxygenation. J Pediatr 1989;114:635.
55. Marinelli KA, Short BL, Martin GR, Goldstein D. Extracorporeal membrane oxygenation: its effect on renin, aldosterone and natriuretic peptide. Pediatr Res 1989;25:241A.
56. Sell LL, Cullen ML, Lerner GR, et al. Hypertension during extracorporeal membrane oxygenation: cause, effect and management. Surgery 1987;102:724.
57. Martin GR, Short BL, Abbott C, O'Brien AM. Cardiac stun in infants undergoing extracorporeal membrane oxygenation. J Thorac Cardiovasc Surg 1991;101:607.
58. Boedy RF, Goldberg AK, Howell CG, et al. Incidence of hypertension in infants on extracorporeal membrane oxygenation. J Pediatr Surg 1990;25:258.
59. Marban E. Myocardial stunning and hibernation. The physiology behind the colloquialisms. Circulation 1991;83:681.
60. Martin GR, Chauvin L, Short BL. Effects of hydralazine on cardiac performance in infants receiving extracorporeal membrane oxygenation. J Pediatr 1991;118:944.
61. Glass P, Miller M, Short B. Morbidity for survivors of extracorporeal membrane oxygenation: neurodevelopmental outcome at 1 year of age. Pediatrics 1989;83:72.
62. Schumacher RE, Palmer TW, Roloff DW, et al. Follow-up of infants treated with extracorporeal membrane oxygenation for newborn respiratory failure. Pediatrics 1991;87:451.
63. Towne BH, Lott IT, Hicks DA, Healey T. Long-term follow-up of infants and children treated with extracorporeal membrane oxygenation (ECMO): a preliminary report. J Pediatr Surg 1985;20:410.
64. Wagner A, Glass P, Papero P, Short B. Neurobehavioral status at age 5 of 42 ECMO-treated neonates. Pediatr Res 1992;31:262A.
65. Schumacher RE, Barks JDE, Johnston MV, et al. Right-sided brain lesions in infants following extracorporeal membrane oxygenation. Pediatrics 1988;82:155.
66. Bulas DI, Taylor GA, Fitz CR, et al. Posterior fossa intracranial hemorrhage in infants treated with extracorporeal membrane oxygenation: sonographic findings. Am J Roentgenol 1991;156:571.
67. Taylor GA, Walker LK. Doppler US evaluation of the intracranial venous system following ligation of the right jugular vein in infants treated with extracorporeal membrane oxygenation. Radiology 1992;183:453.
68. Van Meurs KP, Robbins ST, Karr SS, et al. Congenital diaphragmatic hernia: long-term outcome of ECMO-treated survivors. Pediatr Res 1991;29:A269.
69. Southgate WM, Howell CG, Kanto WP. Need for and impact on neonatal mortality of extracorporeal membrane oxygenation in infants of greater than 2500-gram birth weight. Pediatr 1990;86:71.
70. Frostell C, Fratacci MD, Wain JC, et al. Inhaled nitric oxide. A selective pulmonary vasodilator reversing hypoxic pulmonary vasoconstriction. Circulation 1991;83:2038.

Neonatology: Pathophysiology and Management of the Newborn, Fourth Edition,
edited by Gordon B. Avery, Mary Ann Fletcher, and Mhairi G. MacDonald.
J.B. Lippincott Company, Philadelphia © 1994.

chapter 33

Cardiac Disease

MICHAEL F. FLANAGAN
DONALD C. FYLER

During the past 10 years, the practice of neonatal cardiology has been revolutionized by advances made in diagnostic echocardiography. An infant suspected of having heart disease undergoes an echocardiographic examination, and based on the resulting anatomic diagnosis, a treatment program is devised that may include observation, use of pharmacologic agents, and surgical or catheter interventions. Because of greater diagnostic precision and improvements in surgical and catheterization treatments, overall mortality rates for managing neonates with cardiac disease have improved.

Discussion in this chapter is limited to the neonatal period; for further details about the cardiac problems of survivors, standard texts of pediatric cardiology should be consulted.[1–6] The patient experience presented in this chapter is derived from the Dartmouth-Hitchcock Medical Center and the Boston Children's Hospital. These two hospitals have diverse experience in this area; one is based on patients referred from its surrounding rural communities and the other is based on patients referred from other centers in a large metropolitan area.

INCIDENCE

The incidence of congenital heart disease has been most reliably estimated to be 7.5 per 1000 live births.[7] However, the statistic of most interest in planning services for babies with heart disease is the number who are ill enough to require some medical action. Considering only those sick enough to require cardiac catheterization or cardiac surgery or to have died with heart disease, there are approximately 2.7 sick cardiac infants per 1000 births.[8] Almost one-half of these infants are first seen before the second week of life. The prevalence of congenital heart disease as discovered by echocardiography in two institutions is shown in Table 33-1.

MORTALITY

Before the philosophy of aggressive intervention, Mitchell found that 2.3 of 1000 live births died with cardiac problems in infancy.[7] After a philosophy of aggressive palliation was adopted, the infant cardiac fatality rate fell to 0.8 of 1000 births.[8] Since then, the mortalities in neonates with specific cardiac lesions are improved, but the data required to calculate mortality per 1000 live births are not available for recent years. We think that survival figures are the best they ever have been, even though neonatal death from congenital heart disease accounts for most neonatal deaths in hospitals such as the Children's Hospital in Boston.

The importance of prematurity and of associated noncardiac anomalies in neonatal cardiac deaths has been emphasized and influences the potential for sal-

TABLE 33–1
ECHOCARDIOGRAPHIC DIAGNOSES IN THE FIRST MONTH OF LIFE

Diagnosis	Children's Hospital n = 1627 (%)	Dartmouth–Hitchcock n = 207 (%)
Ventricular septal defect	15	33
Valvar pulmonary stenosis	5	13
Atrial septal defect 2 secundum	5	10
Coarctation of the aorta	7	7
Cardiomyopathy	4	6
Tetralogy of Fallot	7	5
Transposition of the great arteries	17	4
Endocardial cushion defects	4	3
Hypoplastic left heart syndrome	7	2
Tricuspid atresia	2	2
Aortic stenosis	3	2
Malpositions	5	1
Total anomalous pulmonary veins	1	1
Truncus arteriosis	2	1
L-transposition of the great arteries	1	1
Tricuspid valve diseases	5	1
Pulmonary atresia and intact interventricular septum	2	
Single ventricle	1	
Other	7	8

Patients seen between 1986 and 1991. There were many infants with patent ductus arteriosus. These are not included because most were associated with respiratory distress syndrome. There were few with a diagnosis of normal heart, persistent fetal circulation, and rhythm problems. The marked difference between the two hospitals reflects the nature of their practices. The Children's Hospital in Boston has a large referral practice; and the Dartmouth–Hitchcock group has a community-based practice.

vaging infants with cardiac disease (Table 33-2).[8] In some situations, the mortality attributable to these problems is considerable.

SURVIVAL

With few exceptions, there is a cardiac operation or catheter intervention that can improve the quality of life or lengthen the life of a child with heart disease. Eighty-five percent of neonates survive 1 year (see Table 33-2), most can expect to survive into their teens or twenties, and many survive for several decades. For many years, it has been a matter of conviction among cardiologists that any improvement in survival was worth the effort, emotional drain, and cost, particularly because later progress in the field often allowed unexpected secondary interventions which provided even longer survival. The palliative shunt operations of 20 years ago unexpectedly produced candidates for later Fontan procedures. The central principle continues to be where there is life, there is hope.

An infant with an uncorrectable cardiac problem may survive because of a palliative operation but have no expectation of reaching adulthood. Similarly, the cardiac problem may be totally corrected, but in the process, the baby may suffer central nervous system damage. Correction of a cardiac defect in a child with crippling noncardiac anomalies can scarcely be categorized as salvaging the baby. However, with heroic treatment, a child may survive severe myocardial disease and be completely normal, and a cardiac operation can often cure the patient.

The pros and cons of treating a child who has crippling extracardiac defects must be discussed with the parents in understandable language. The long-range future of patients undergoing cardiac transplantation, Fontan operations, shunting operations, Senning operations, or intracardiac repair requires detailed discussion. These procedures have late complications. The possibility that brain injury or other injury may be acquired in the process of treatment should be understood. The expected physical capabilities of the patient after treatment should be delineated. After the physician is confident that the parents thoroughly understand the known facts, he or she is free to express an opinion about what may be best for the child. Almost invariably, the family, trusting their doctor, follows the advice.

The many surgical procedures and modifications of procedures, their early and late complications, and the management of those complications are beyond the scope of this book. Virtually all procedures have some late problems, often delayed until adulthood.

Confusing this situation is the inherent tendency of

TABLE 33–2
RANK ORDER OF CARDIAC DIAGNOSES AND FIRST-YEAR MORTALITY BY BIRTH WEIGHT

Birth Weight > 2.5 kg (n = 1552)			Birth Weight < 2.5 kg (n = 230)		
Frequency (%)	Diagnosis	Mortality (%)	Frequency (%)	Diagnosis	Mortality (%)
17	D-TGA	9	16	VSD	5
14	VSD	2	14	PDA	9
8	PDA	8	7	MYO	6
7	HLV	50	7	COARC	38
7	TF	16	6	TF	28
6	COARC	18	6	MAL	31
5	ASD2	1	6	TRI	8
5	PS	1	5	D-TGA	17
4	MAL	28	5	ASD2	0
4	TRI	1	4	PS	0/9
4	ECD	17	3	HLV	3/8
3	MYO	6	3	ECD	2/7
2	AS	26	2	TA	2/5
2	TA	19	2	TAPVR	2/5
2	TRUNC	24	2	AS	0/5
1	PA+IVS	14	2	TRUNC	2/5
1	TAPVR	11	1	SV	1/2
1	SV	31	1	PA+IVS	1/2
1	L-TGA	0/6	1	L-TGA	0/1
6	Other	16	8	Other	28
100	Total	13	100	Total	18

Data was based on 1843 infants younger than 1 month old who were examined by echocardiography between January 1986 and January 1991. Fifty-five of those with birth weights more than 2.5 kg and 6 of those with birth weights less than 2.5 kg had no heart disease. There were more babies with myocardial disease and ductus arteriosus and the first-year mortality was consistently higher in the low-birth-weight group.

AS, aortic stenosis; ASD2, atrial septal defect; COARC, coarctation of the aorta; D-TGA, D-transposition of the great arteries; ECD, endocardial cushion defects; HLV, hypoplastic left heart syndrome; L-TGA, L-transposition of the great arteries; MAL, malpositions; MYO, cardiomyopathy; PDA, patent ductus arteriosus; PA + IVS, pulmonary atresia and intact interventricular septum; PS, valvar pulmonary stenosis; SV, single ventricle; TA, tricuspid atresia; TAPVR, total anomalous pulmonary veins; TF, tetralogy of Fallot; TGA, transposition of the great arteries; TRI, tricuspid valve diseases; TRUNC, truncus arteriosus; VSD, ventricular septal defect.

pediatricians to consider the struggle to be won if the child can be coaxed to adulthood. The goal is to provide for a satisfying life for many years after childhood. Many children with cardiac disease survive to 20 years of age only to succumb in the next decade.

ETIOLOGY

Parents ask why their baby was born with a cardiac abnormality and whether it is likely to recur with a subsequent pregnancy. In most cases, the specific cause of the cardiac anomaly is unknown. Evidence suggests that extrinsic perturbations, genetic predisposition, and chance play roles.[5,9–12] Diagnostic frequency year by year, state by state, and hospital by hospital has been relatively constant, and any etiologic theory must account for this phenomenon.

Fetal exposure to specific environmental, pharmacologic, biochemical, and infectious factors may increase the risk for developing a cardiac abnormality (Table 33-3).[5,9,11–16] However, in individual cases, it is usually difficult or impossible to identify specific extrinsic factors.

Epidemiologic findings suggest that genetic factors play a role in isolated congenital malformations, but alone, they are not sufficient to explain causation in most cases. Rarely, all affected children in a family have the same cardiac defect. Few congenital cardiac diseases have clear mendelian inheritance, but hypertrophic cardiomyopathy is an exception. Approximately one-third of patients with congenital heart disease have a positive family history of congenital cardiac abnormalities. It is rare for both fraternal twins to have heart disease, but as many as 25% of identical twins both have cardiac abnormalities. The risk in siblings may be higher with some lesions, particularly left heart obstructive lesions, such as coarcta-

TABLE 33–3
POSSIBLE TERATOGENS FOR CONGENITAL HEART DISEASE

Environmental agents: high altitude,* trichloroethylene, irradiation
Drugs: ethanol*, hydantoin,* valproic acid,* trimethadione,* primidone,* carbamazepine,* lithium,* thalidomide,* retinoic acid,* antineoplastic agents (?), amphetamine, cocaine
Metabolic factors: maternal diabetes,* maternal phenylketonuria*
Immune factors: maternal autoimmune disease, including lupus erthematosus*
Infectious agents: rubella,* mumps (?), cytomegalovirus (?)

* It is generally accepted that these prenatal factors increase the risk for congenital heart disease.
Data from references 5, 9, and 11 through 16.

tion and hypoplastic left heart syndrome. If one parent has congenital heart disease, the risk to the offspring may be higher if the mother is the one affected.[2,11]

Some lesions are predominantly associated with the sex of the infant. Boys more commonly have coarctation of the aorta, aortic stenosis, and transposition of the great arteries, and girls are prone to have atrial septal defect and patent ductus arteriosus.

Approximately 8% to 13% of children with cardiac anomalies have inheritable syndromes with associated cardiovascular abnormalities (*e.g.*, Marfan syndrome), and 13% have chromosomal syndromes associated with cardiovascular malformation (Table 33-4).[5,9,11,15] The association of Down syndrome and heart anomalies, especially endocardial cushion defect, is common (Table 33-5). Clinical identification of a syndrome associated with congenital heart disease or vice versa should prompt an investigation for possible associated defects.

The tendency for various cardiac anomalies to occur together suggests common embryogenesis. For example, infundibular pulmonary stenosis is associated with ventricular septal defect, but valvar pulmonary stenosis is not. Similarly, the association of noncardiac anomalies and specific forms of heart disease (*e.g.*, asplenia, polysplenia) can be recognized. A single event may result in characteristic complex cardiac malformation by altering or killing embryonic primordial cells, such as in the neural crest or endocardial cushion, before formation of cardiac structures in the conotruncus or atrioventricular valves. Malformation of a specific structure may alter blood flow patterns and vascular growth downstream.[5,10–12,16] Certain cardiac lesions are associated with prematurity or low birth weight (see Table 33-2). Because closure of the ventricular septum may be delayed until the first months of life, it is not surprising that there is a somewhat greater incidence of ventricular septal defect among premature infants. The increased incidence of patent ductus arteriosus in prematurely born infants can be viewed as the result of birth long before the programmed time for closure of the ductus. Hypoxemia of pulmonary origin also promotes ductal patency.

TABLE 33–4
INCIDENCE OF SEVERE ASSOCIATED NONCARDIAC ANOMALIES AMONG 2220 INFANTS WITH HEART DISEASE

Diagnosis	Incidence (%)
Endocardial cushion defect	43
Patent ductus arteriosus	31
Ventricular septal defect	24
Malpositions	13
Tetralogy of Fallot	10
Coarctation of aorta	9
Pulmonary atresia with intact septum	1
D-Transposition of the great arteries	1

PHYSIOLOGY

Extensive information about the circulatory physiology of the fetus and newborn has accumulated. The works of Barcroft,[17] Dawes,[18] Lind,[19] and Rudolph[20] should be consulted for details, but the central features are discussed here.

FETAL CIRCULATION

The circulation before birth consists of parallel circuits (Fig. 33-1). Blood in the aorta may follow several routes to a capillary bed in the fetus or the placenta, back to the heart, passing through either ventricle, and out again to the aorta. The stream of newly oxygenated blood from the placenta passes through the umbilical vein, the ductus venosus, the inferior vena cava, and the right atrium. Unlike the circulation after birth, the streams of oxygenated and unoxygenated blood are not separated, although the more oxygenated blood from the inferior vena cava tends to be diverted through the foramen ovale into the left atrium. Blood from the left ventricle entering the ascending aorta and coronary and carotid circulations is somewhat higher in oxygen than that entering the descending aorta from the right ventricle by way of the ductus arteriosus.

Because of the parallel arrangement of the ventricles, the potential of each ventricle for pumping different amounts of blood exists. Normally, the volume pumped by the right ventricle is thought to be about 62% of the combined output of both ventricles. Because both ventricles pump against the systemic re-

TABLE 33–5
CONGENITAL DISORDERS ASSOCIATED WITH CARDIAC DISEASE

Disorder	Percent of Patients With Cardiac Disease	Types of Cardiac Abnormalities
Primary Isolated Cardiac Disorders		
Hypertrophic cardiomyopathy	100	Hypertrophic cardiomyopathy
Romano–Ward Syndrome	100	Prolonged QT interval, VT, sudden death
Autosomal Dominant Syndromes		
de Lange	30	VSD, ASD, PDA, AS, EFE
Holt–Oram cardiac–limb syndrome	100	ASD
Marfan syndrome	67–100	Aortic aneurysm, AR, MR, TR, prolapse, dysrhythmias
Noonan syndrome	67	PS, ASD, hypertrophic cardiomyopathy, VSD, PDA, LAD
Osler–Weber–Rendu hemorrhagic telangiectasia	15–25	Pulmonary and systemic arteriovenous malformations
Shprintzen velocardiofacial syndrome	80	VSD, TF, right aortic arch, aberrant left subclavian artery
Treacher Collins mandibulofacial dysostosis	Uncommon	ASD, VSD, PDA
Tuberous sclerosis	30	Cardiac rhabdomyomas
Autosomal Recessive Syndromes		
Carpenter syndrome	33	PDA, PS, VSD, TF, TGA
Ellis–van Creveld chondroectodermal dysplasia	50–60	Single atrium, primum ASD, COARC, small LV, CHF
Mucopolysaccharidosis	>50	Myocardial hypertrophy, coronary disease, AR, MR, TR, CHF
Pompe glycogenolysis type II	100	Myocardial hypertrophy, EFE, short PR, CHF
Smith–Lemli–Opitz syndrome, types I and II	20/100	VSD, PDA, ASD, TF
Thrombocytopenia with absent radii	33	ASD, TF
X-Linked Syndromes		
Duchenne muscular dystrophy	Common	Cardiomyopathy
Chromosomal Disorders		
Trisomy 21 (Down syndrome)	40–50	AV canal, VSD, PDA, ASD primum, TF
Trisomy 18 (Edward syndrome)	90–100	VSD, polyvalvular disease, ASD, PDA
Trisomy 13 (Patau syndrome)	80	PDA, VSD, ASD, detrocardia, COARC, AS, PS
XO (Turner syndrome)	45	COARC, bicuspid aortic valve, aortic aneurysm
Syndromes With Unknown Etiology		
Beckwith–Wiedemann syndrome	16–92	Cardiomegaly, ASD, VSD, PDA, TF
Cardiofacial (asymmetric crying facies) syndrome	5–10	VSD
CHARGE association	65–75	TF, DORV, ASD, VSD, PDA, COARC, AV canal
DiGeorge syndrome	50+	Interruped aortic arch, truncus arteriosus, TF
Goldenhar facioauriculovertebral spectrum	5–80	VSD, PDA, TF, CAORC
Rubinstein–Taybi syndrome	35	VSD, PDA, ASD, COARC, PS
VACTERL association	10	VSD, ASD, TF
Williams syndrome	50–80	Supravalvar AS, branch PS, VSD, hypoplastic aorta

AR, aortic valve regurgitation; AS, aortic stenosis; ASD, atrial septal defect; AV, atrioventricular; CHF, congestive heart failure; COARC, coarctation of the aorta; DORV, double-outlet right ventricle; EFE, endocardial fibroelastosis; LAD, left axis deviation; LV, left ventricle; MR, mitral valve regurgitation; PDA, patent ductus arteriosus; PS, pulmonary stenosis; TF, tetralogy of Fallot; TGA, transposition of the great arteries; TR, tricuspid valve regurgitation; VSD, ventricular septal defect; VT, ventricular tachycardia.

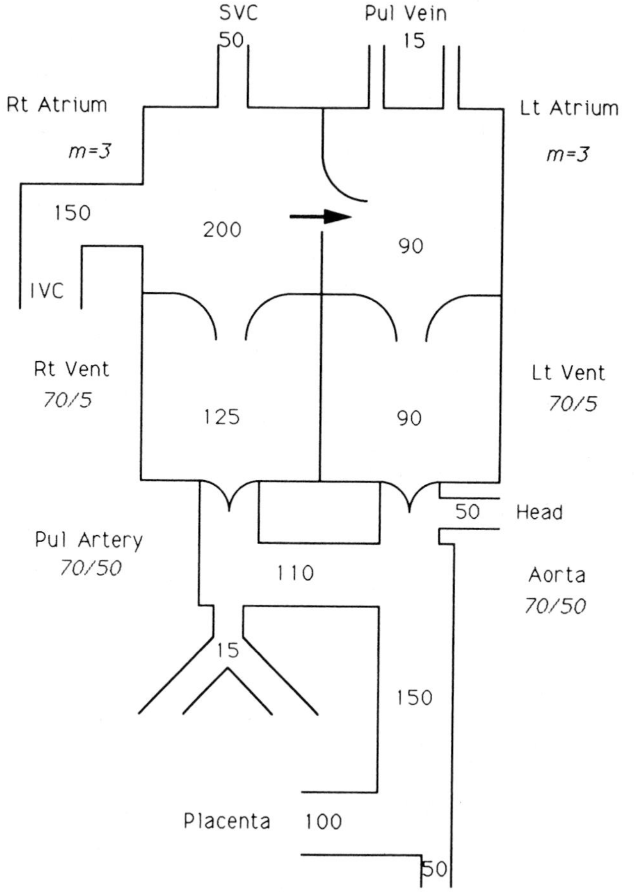

FIG. 33–1. Fetal circulation is in parallel, and the amount of blood handled by the left and right ventricles is 125 and 90 mL, respectively. Only 40 mL passes through the aortic arch to the descending aorta, and only a small fraction passes through the lungs. The numbers inside the diagram represent relative blood flow in mL; the numbers in italics are pressure measurements. (Modified from Rudolph AM. Congenital diseases of the heart. Chicago: Year Book, 1974.)

sistance, the level of pressure in the two ventricles is comparable. The resistance to blood flow through the lungs is relatively great; only minimal flow through the lungs occurs *in utero* and almost all of the right ventricular output into the pulmonary artery passes through the ductus arteriosus to the descending aorta.

The parallel arrangement of the ventricles allows fetal survival despite a wide variety of cardiac lesions. With total obstruction of either ventricle, the other ventricle assumes the entire cardiac output with surprising success. Reversal of the pulmonary arterial and aortic streams of blood, as occurs in transposition of the great arteries, produces no deleterious effect on the fetus. The birth weights of these babies are rarely less than average and often greater. Even lesions that cause increased fetal cardiac work, such as central nervous system arteriovenous fistulae, are tolerated well. The ability to withstand gross intrauterine circulatory abnormality is partially a result of simultaneous development of the anomaly and adaptation to it. Despite the remarkable ability to adapt, grow, and survive, the fetus is affected by limitations in myocardial contractility in direct proportion to their severity.

Because of the virtual exclusion of the lungs from the circulation, fetal congestive heart failure manifests as generalized edema. A fetus with myocardial dysfunction of any cause may be born with anasarca. The interplay between the metabolic effects of congestion in the fetus and the possible compensatory role of the placenta is not understood. Because lesions that may be expected to cause gross intrauterine difficulty are tolerated surprisingly well, the postulate that the placenta helps compensate for the metabolic abnormalities resulting from congestive heart failure is tenable.

CIRCULATORY ADJUSTMENTS AT BIRTH

With the first breath, the resistance to pulmonary blood flow drops sharply. The oxygen content of the left heart and systemic circulation rapidly reaches levels well above that of the fetal circulation. The oxygen saturation in the ascending fetal aorta is about 65%; immediately after birth, it rises to about 93%. The ductus venosus functionally closes, establishing the portal circulation as an independent loop between two capillary beds. With removal of the low resistance placenta, systemic resistance stabilizes at a higher level. The relative fall in the pulmonary resistance and rise in the systemic resistance results in a transitory left-to-right shunt through the ductus arteriosus.

The ductus becomes functionally closed toward the end of the first day of life, becoming anatomically obliterated at about 10 days of age. Even among cyanotic newborns who are duct dependent, the ductus may inexorably close, often severing the infant's only source of pulmonary blood flow (*e.g.*, pulmonary atresia). The mechanisms causing closure of the ductus arteriosus are not completely understood but involve decreased prostaglandins and increased blood oxygen. Prostaglandin levels in the blood decrease at birth due to removal of the placental source of production from the circulation and increase in perfusion of the lungs, where prostaglandins are metabolized. Persistent patency of the ductus arteriosus in the neonate with duct-dependent cardiovascular lesions can be achieved by infusion of prostaglandin E, and pharmacologic closure of the histologically normal duct in the preterm infant can be hastened by inhibition of prostaglandin synthesis with indomethacin.

At birth, the left ventricle abruptly becomes the sole supplier of systemic blood flow, and the volume that it pumps is fractionally increased. The left-to-right shunt through the ductus arteriosus adds further volume work, and the elevated systemic resistance must be overcome. Although this is a stressful time for the left ventricle, the magnitude of these suddenly acquired burdens is not so great that detectable left ventricular difficulties are seen normally, but any impairment of myocardial function may be magnified as a consequence. Myocardial disease as a cause of symptoms is more common in the first days of life than at any other time during infancy; 25% of infants with myocardial disease presented in the first week of life.[8] Hypoxic–ischemic myocardial dysfunction after delivery can be recognized by means of echocardiography. Recovery from severe left ventricular failure in the neonatal period is often surprisingly good.

At birth, the volume of blood to be pumped by the right ventricle decreases to the level of the systemic blood flow; right ventricular pressure falls as a result of the decrease in pulmonary resistance and closure of the ductus arteriosus. Although left ventricular work increases, right ventricular work decreases.

Before birth, the two ventricles share in supplying systemic blood flow and placental flow, and after birth, the two ventricles sequentially and independently handle the entire cardiac output. Effectively, each ventricle pumps blood in amounts comparable to those that it pumped *in utero,* despite a reduction by 50% in the amount of blood pumped through the aorta after removal of the placenta (Fig. 33-2). Although this arrangement results in each ventricle pumping comparable amounts of blood before and after birth, a central nervous system arteriovenous fistula, because of the shift from parallel to serial ventricular pumping, causes an acute increase in the volume of work for each ventricle, despite a constant flow through the fistula. These babies often die immediately after birth, despite normal growth *in utero.*

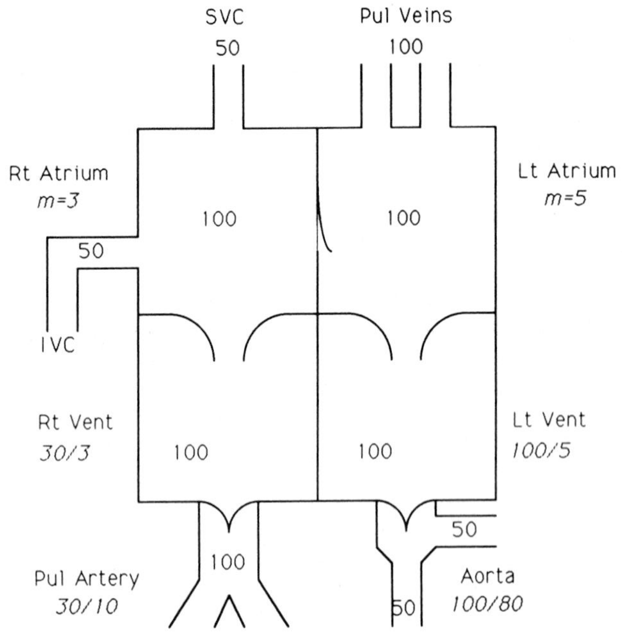

FIG. 33–2. Mature circulation is in series, and the amount of blood carried by the two ventricles is approximately the same as before birth. The lungs carry an amount equivalent to the cardiac output, as does the ascending aorta. The numbers inside the diagram represent relative blood flow in mL; the numbers in italics are pressure measurements.

Functional closure of the foramen ovale occurs soon after birth, largely as a result of increased left atrial volume and pressure secondary to the increased pulmonary venous return, to the ductal left-to-right shunt, and the developing differences in diastolic pressure of the two ventricles. Anatomic closure normally is delayed for months or years. Among infants with cardiac defects, lesions with increased right atrial pressure favor indefinite patency of the foramen ovale (*e.g.,* pulmonary stenosis), but abnormally increased left atrial pressure promotes early anatomic closure (*e.g.,* ventricular septal defect).

Before birth, the pulmonary arterioles are relatively muscular and constricted. With the first breath, total pulmonary resistance falls rapidly because of the unkinking of the vessels with expansion of the lungs and because of the vasodilatory effect of inspired oxygen. The muscular constriction relaxes, and gradually during the subsequent days and weeks, the muscular wall of the pulmonary arterioles thins. During the first weeks of life, the muscular arterioles retain a significant capacity for constriction. Pulmonary alveolar hypoxia normally produces an increase in pulmonary artery pressure at all ages, but in the young infant, the response is more profound and occurs more rapidly. The discovery of pulmonary hypertension equal to or greater than systemic pressure is a familiar observation in a sick baby.

PREMATURITY

The events at birth and in the neonatal period are modified in direct relation to the degree of prematurity. The muscular coat of the pulmonary arterioles develops late in gestation; the more premature the infant, the less muscular are the pulmonary arterioles at birth. The most notable consequence of this is that the difference between systemic and pulmonary resistance after birth is greater among premature than among normal infants. Shunting through a ductus arteriosus is often audible. The hypoxia so common among premature infants may be one of the factors that delays closure of the ductus, and as a result, ductal murmurs are more common. The propensity of the ductus to close at around 41 weeks after conception is clinically recognized. Among older infants with persistently patent ductus, the incidence of prematurity is greater than expected.

The prolonged ductal shunting in the premature infant would probably be of no consequence except that ductal shunting is often associated with respiratory distress. The ductal shunt causes increased pulmonary blood volume in an infant already severely ill with respiratory distress and sometimes causes left ventricular failure. Medical or surgical interruption of the ductus may have an appreciable effect on morbidity and mortality. However, it is our view that the ductus is rarely the sole problem in symptomatic neonates; it is instead an additional problem in an already serious situation. Patent ductus is found equally among premature male and female infants and is considered to be persistent patency of the normal ductus. Patent ductus unassociated with prematurity is an anomaly and is predominantly encountered in female infants (2:1).

RECOGNITION OF CLINICAL FEATURES

Only a few infants are born in hospitals equipped for all eventualities. To allow time for transfer to a specially equipped and staffed cardiac center, recognition that the baby has heart disease must be early enough to allow time for transportation, diagnostic workup, and treatment, including cardiac catheterization and surgery. The infrequent use of echocardiography to recognize heart disease in infants in remote areas has often been unsatisfactory. Cases of delayed transfer of babies because of erroneous diagnoses of inoperable congenital heart disease and erroneous reassurance that there is no significant lesion have been encountered. With limited experience in the diagnosis of congenital heart disease in neonates, it may be best to transport the infant to the nearest center for echocardiographic examination or to forward a tape of the examination for a second opinion if the echocardiographer is primarily experienced in examining adults.

AGE AT DISCOVERY

In New England in the 1970s, 35% of all infants who were suspected of having critical cardiac disease in the first year of life were admitted to a treatment center within the first week of life.[8] There is no comparable data for a recent period, but we suspect that there has been little change in the numbers since the advent of echocardiography. Because of the dramatic changes during the transition from fetal to extrauterine circulation in the first weeks of life, the danger of sudden deterioration requires that a confident diagnosis be established as early as is practicable.

MURMURS

Hearing a murmur is the most common means of recognizing infant heart disease. Evaluation includes assessment of the infant's well-being, respiratory work, precordial activity, perfusion, pulses and blood pressure in the extremities, splitting of the second heart sound, and murmur intensity, quality, and pitch. A chest radiograph and electrocardiogram (ECG) should be obtained. The murmurs of valvar regurgitation and stenosis are audible immediately after birth, and the murmurs of septal defects are usually delayed days, for as long as several months in the case of atrial septal defects. A two-dimensional echocardiogram is obtained if cardiac disease is suspected. This technique demonstrates the anatomic basis for the murmur, occasionally uncovering a potentially lethal lesion in advance of symptoms.

CYANOSIS

Much more threatening than a murmur is the presence of cyanosis. Cyanosis without pulmonary disease is almost invariably the result of a serious cardiac abnormality. Cyanosis may result from poor mixing of parallel circulation because of transposition of the great arteries; right-to-left shunting because of pulmonary outflow obstruction (*e.g.*, tetralogy of Fallot, critical pulmonary stenosis, tricuspid atresia); or intracardiac mixing (*e.g.*, total anomalous pulmonary venous connection, truncus arteriosus, single ventricle, hypoplastic left heart syndrome). Especially in the first week of life, cyanosis may be the sole evidence of an important cardiac lesion. One-third of infants with potentially lethal congenital heart disease have cyanosis as their major symptom; another one-third have cyanosis associated with respiratory symptoms.

Prompt cardiac evaluation of all cyanotic babies is mandatory, because most of these lesions are amenable to surgery. The clinical recognition of cyanosis is influenced by the baby's hemoglobin. An anemic infant may have severe arterial oxygen unsaturation without obvious cyanosis, and infants with polycythemia may appear cyanotic with normal arterial oxygen levels. Hypothermic infants may seem blue; babies viewed in fluorescent lighting may appear blue; and blue surroundings may make the estimation of cyanosis more difficult. Persistent cyanosis due to hypoglycemia or methemoglobinemia is rare.

RESPIRATORY SYMPTOMS

Cardiac disability may result in pulmonary vascular engorgement, pulmonary venous hypertension, and pulmonary edema. Grandmothers and multiparas often observe that the baby had always breathed too fast. There is no doubt that persistent respiratory rates of 60 per minute or greater, often with persistently increased depth of respirations, commonly precede hearing a murmur and may presage deterioration to gross dyspnea and congestive heart failure. Persistent tachypnea may be the first clue to heart disease or lung disease; a chest radiograph may provide the answer.

DIAGNOSTIC FEATURES

The number of cardiac lesions that cause serious disability among newborns is great (see Table 33-2); more than 100 physiologic entities are seen. Ventricular septal defects are the most common, but the largest category requiring hospitalization in the first 2 weeks of life is D-transposition of the great arteries. Among the lesions causing symptoms in this age group are coarctation of the aorta and the hypoplastic left heart syndrome.

AGE OF PRESENTATION

It is clinically useful to keep in mind the usual time of presentation of infants with various cardiac anomalies (Table 33-6). Although ventricular septal defect is by far the commonest congenital heart lesion discovered in neonates, transposition of the great arteries, coarctation of the aorta, and the hypoplastic left heart syndrome are the most common life-threatening anomalies presenting in the first week of life (see Table 33-2). Among those whose problem is cyanosis, transposition of the great arteries is the leading cause for admission through the third week of life; after that time, tetralogy of Fallot becomes the dominant cause of cyanosis for the rest of childhood. Among neonatal cardiac patients admitted because of respiratory symptoms, the hypoplastic left heart syndrome is the leading cause in the first week, complex coarctations lead in the second week, and thereafter, ventricular septal defect becomes the main cause for symptomatic admission (see Table 33-6).

TABLE 33-6
TOP FIVE DIAGNOSES PRESENTING AT DIFFERENT AGES

Diagnosis	Percent of Patients
Age on Admission: 0–6 Days (n = 537)	
D-Transposition of great arteries	19
Hypoplastic left ventricle	14
Tetralogy of Fallot	8
Coarctation of aorta	7
Ventricular septal defect	3
Others	49
Age on Admission: 7–13 Days (n = 195)	
Coarctation of aorta	16
Ventricular septal defect	14
Hypoplastic left ventricle	8
D-Transposition of great arteries	7
Tetralogy of Fallot	7
Others	48
Age on Admission: 14–28 Days (n = 177)	
Ventricular septal defect	16
Tetralogy of Fallot	7
Coarctation of aorta	12
D-Transposition of great arteries	7
Patent ductus arteriosus	5
Others	53

NONCARDIAC ANOMALIES AND LOW BIRTH WEIGHT

It is useful to know the relative frequency of the cardiac diagnostic possibilities among low birth weight babies (see Table 33-2) and among those who have other anomalies (see Tables 33-4 and 33-5). Among premature infants, patent ductus arteriosus, coarctation of the aorta, and ventricular septal defect are more commonly encountered. Chromosomal abnormalities and congenital syndromes may also be associated with cardiac malformations (*e.g.*, Down syndrome).

ACUTE LUNG DISEASE AND CARDIAC DISEASE

The differential diagnosis between primary lung disease and heart disease causing pulmonary edema is difficult. A chest radiograph may suggest lung disease, particularly if the findings are asymmetric, but in the presence of diffuse symmetrical changes possibly compatible with pulmonary edema, caution is necessary. Treatment for a pulmonary problem, with initial limited improvement in oxygenation, may confuse the picture. The correct diagnosis is delayed until the persistent poor response to oxygen and positive-pressure ventilation alerts the physician to the possibility that heart disease is the problem. Diagnoses such as transient tachypnea of the newborn or hyaline membrane disease in the full-term baby are particularly suspect.

The issue is most pressing when the infant is dyspneic and cyanotic. Although carbon dioxide retention is usually prominent among babies with primary lung disease, some severely cyanotic infants with pulmonary parenchymal disease have normal PCO_2 values. A time-honored test has been the response of the cyanosis to administration of 100% oxygen; cyanosis from cardiac causes is not significantly changed, but cyanosis with a pulmonary basis may disappear. Refinements of this test, through measurement of umbilical artery oxygen measurements while breathing 100% oxygen or room air, are useful. Difficulties arise when pulmonary and cardiac pathology coexists. For example, in the baby with both lung and heart disease or persistent pulmonary hypertension (PPHN) (see Chaps. 29 and 31) or the baby with heart disease causing pulmonary venous hypertension and pulmonary edema, results may be confusing. Arterial PO_2 measured from an umbilical artery catheter positioned in the descending aorta may detect right-to-left shunting through a ductus arteriosus caused by lung disease. Administration of oxygen may decrease pulmonary resistance and increase pulmonary flow, providing higher oxygen levels in a cyanotic child with a large pulmonary flow and congestive heart failure. Arterial PO_2 typically does not improve significantly in response to 100% oxygen in infants with PPHN. Comparison of the PO_2 measured in blood from the right radial artery or temporal artery with the PO_2 measured in blood from the umbilical arterial catheter may help to clarify the diagnosis in these conditions.

With the above exceptions, the infant who responds to breathing pure oxygen with a marked rise in arterial PO_2 to 250 torr or more has lung disease, and the infant who does not raise his preductal arterial PO_2 above 100 torr has heart disease. If doubt persists, the physician can make the diagnosis with two-dimensional echocardiography by establishing that the cardiac anatomy is normal or sufficiently abnormal to account for a critically ill baby.

Apparent diffuse pulmonary disease in a full-term baby, particularly if the chest radiograph is conceivably compatible with pulmonary edema, should be viewed with caution. Two-dimensional echocardiography usually solves the dilemma. Anomalous pulmonary venous drainage below the diaphragm (see Total Anomalous Pulmonary Veins) may be missed on electrocardiography.

CHRONIC PULMONARY HYPERTENSION AND COR PULMONALE

In the past, the term cor pulmonale was used to describe the circulatory physiology resulting from chronic lung disease, and pediatric cardiologists are using this terminology less often than previously. Cor pulmonale is the association of right ventricular hypertrophy with pulmonary hypertension secondary to ventilatory or pulmonary disease. It frequently presents as symptoms of congestive heart failure with pulmonary disease. Patients with cor pulmonale have a structurally normal heart and must be differentiated from those with pulmonary hypertension as a consequence of intracardiac shunts or pulmonary venous obstruction (*e.g.*, mitral stenosis, cor triatriatum). The most frequent cause in infants has been bronchopulmonary dysplasia, although a large number of other causes, including airway obstruction, central hypoventilation, pulmonary hypoplasia, and diaphragmatic abnormalities, also occur.

Pathophysiology. The pulmonary artery pressure is controlled by vascular resistance that is a function of the average luminal size and number of small pulmonary arteries. The number of vessels may be congenitally diminished by pulmonary hypoplasia or by acquired pulmonary parenchymal damage. The amount of small pulmonary artery musculature and the distance that it extends along the vessel determines the extent to which constriction may cause obstruction. The required muscle to prevent more than minimal pulmonary flow before birth is still present, although relaxed, after birth and can profoundly reconstrict with elevation of pulmonary resistance and pulmonary hypertension under the appropriate circumstances. The pulmonary vascular resistance is often labile with the potential for development of pulmonary hypertension above the level of normal systemic pressure for that patient.

The circumstances that may stimulate constriction include alveolar hypoxia (*e.g.*, perinatal asphyxia, pulmonary parenchymal disease, airway obstruction, high altitude), acidemia, increased pulmonary venous pressure (*e.g.*, left ventricular diastolic dysfunction), and bacteremia (*e.g.*, streptococcal infection). Polycythemia may also increase resistance. Increases in cardiac output with exertion, fever, or anemia can elevate pulmonary artery pressure beyond that caused by fixed resistance. For further discussion of acute PPHN, see Chapters 29 and 31.

Chronic pulmonary hypertension results in right ventricular hypertrophy and, if severe, right ventricular diastolic dysfunction and dilation. In addition to pulmonary hypertension, bronchopulmonary dysplasia also is frequently associated with systemic hypertension (see Chap. 30). The cause of the systemic hypertension is complex and may involve exposure to aortic catheters, reflex responses to pulmonary arterial hypertension, and altered pulmonary metabolism of vasoactive substances. Systemic hypertension causes left ventricular hypertrophy. Shifting of the interventricular septal position, caused by elevated intraventricular pressure and biventricular hypertrophy, may impair the diastolic compliance of both ventricles and lead to increased sensitivity to intravascular volume in the systemic and pulmonary circulations. Acute exacerbations of pulmonary hypertension may further increase the right ventricular diastolic pressure and shift the intraventricular septum leftward, leading to additional biatrial hypertension and edema.

The pulmonary hypertension and cardiac sequelae seen with bronchopulmonary dysplasia generally appear to resolve when the pulmonary parenchymal disease resolves. In contrast, permanent pulmonary vascular change (*i.e.*, Eisenmenger syndrome) occurs in patients with congenital heart disease after 1 or more years of exposure to a large left-to-right shunt with pulmonary artery hypertension.

Clinical Findings. Variable hepatomegaly and systemic venous congestion secondary to right atrial hypertension are predominant findings. Elevated left atrial pressure, especially in the presence of pulmonary parenchymal disease, may predispose to pulmonary symptoms and rales. The right ventricular impulse may be increased and the second heart sound loud and appear single. There may be a relatively soft murmur from tricuspid regurgitation, but a prominent murmur is not common and suggests possible congenital heart disease instead.

Two mechanisms produce cyanosis in patients with pulmonary hypertension with normally arranged cardiac structures. In the usual case of a patent foramen ovale (PFO), elevation of the pressure in the right atrium may allow right-to-left shunting and cyanosis. At first, this is likely to be transitory because right atrial pressure also depends on the level of exertion. Persistent cyanosis at rest, although not necessarily dangerous in itself, may suggest serious pulmonary hypertension if there is shunting right-to-left across the foramen ovale. Alternatively, cyanosis may be the result of alveolar dysfunction or intrapulmonary shunting with less than normal oxygen saturation in the pulmonary veins. In this case, cyanosis is a direct function of the extent of parenchymal involvement.

The degree of pulmonary artery hypertension and cardiac symptoms may vary with labile ventilatory or pulmonary conditions. The diagnosis of cor pulmonale may be justified with moderate elevation of pulmonary artery pressure because there may be the potential for symptomatic marked pulmonary hypertension on other occasions.

Infants with bronchopulmonary dysplasia appear to be at increased risk for sudden death. Multiple factors may contribute, including pulmonary hypertension.[5] Death from pulmonary hypertension is perhaps best documented in older patients with primary pulmonary hypertension. Some of these patients suddenly die, having been relatively well, often after episodes of fainting. The pulmonary hypertension can be acutely aggravated if there is alveolar hypoxia from mucus plugs, bronchospasm, upper airway obstruction, or intercurrent infection. Cardiac output is sharply limited by acutely elevated afterload; the patient collapses, and may develop fatal dysrhythmia. Babies with bronchopulmonary dysplasia are at risk for such problems. Patients who can develop a right-to-left shunt have a blow-off–valve effect that limits the height of the pulmonary pressure, providing some cardiac output while producing cyanosis.

Diagnostic Assessment. Noninvasive measurement of pulmonary artery pressure has been used as a method to follow the course of pulmonary parenchymal disease with pulmonary hypertension. The ECG signs of right ventricular hypertrophy have been useful in some patients, but in others, the electrical conductance anteriorly is altered by lung disease. A variety of echocardiographic methods, some remarkably precise, some not so accurate, and most applicable to particular circumstances, are discussed later in this chapter (see Echocardiography). No one technique in use is generally accepted and applicable in every patient. Sedation, often necessary for technically acceptable studies in older, active babies, may depress ventilation and should be used with caution. Externally measured pulmonary artery pressures are not precise, but they provide an estimation of the truth and should be used as such as a guide to therapy.

Treatment. The treatment of pulmonary hypertension secondary to pulmonary or ventilatory disease is directed primarily at the underlying disorder. Although oxygen in high amounts may be toxic, its judicious chronic use as a potent pulmonary vasodilator may be useful. Bronchodilators and diuretics may be helpful for treating pulmonary parenchymal disease. Digitalis has not been found to be beneficial in most infants with congestive symptoms. Nifedipine is useful in some older children with primary pulmonary hypertension, but its routine use in infants with bronchopulmonary dysplasia has not been established. With resolution of the underlying ventilatory disease, the pulmonary hypertension also resolves.

Differential Diagnosis. In patients with pulmonary hypertension, even those with lung disease, the presence of congenital heart disease should be sought. The absence of a loud murmur does not exclude a septal defect or patent ductus arteriosus in the presence of elevated pulmonary vascular resistance. Because many of the symptoms of cor pulmonale overlap those of congenital heart disease, echocardiography has been useful for excluding occult cardiovascular lesions that could lead to irreversible Eisenmenger syndrome. However, echocardiography used in cases of lung disease frequently faces the problem of poor ultrasound windows. These limitations should be realized, and the results correlated with other findings.

DIAGNOSTIC TOOLS

The clinical diagnosis of congenital heart disease frequently requires the use of ECG and chest radiographs. The transcutaneous measurement of partial pressure of oxygen or oxygen saturation is useful, particularly after the umbilical artery is no longer a source of arterial blood. A variety of instruments useful in measuring blood pressure are available.

ECHOCARDIOGRAPHY

Two-dimensional echocardiography with color Doppler ultrasound allows excellent analysis of the intracardiac anatomy in small infants.[21] Neonates are particularly good candidates for echocardiographic imaging because they are less active and have excellent echocardiographic imaging windows. Contrast echocardiography with injection of agitated saline or albumin into intravenous or umbilical artery catheters can serve as a useful adjunct to color Doppler to visualize the presence and direction of blood flow in patent ductus arteriosus, septal defects, systemic venous anomalies, and arteriovenous malformation. Pulsed and continuous wave Doppler techniques enable estimation of some physiologic parameters such as the pressure gradient across stenotic valves, septal defects, and patent ductus arteriosus. In the common case of tricuspid regurgitation, right ventricular peak systolic pressure may be estimated by Doppler measurement of the magnitude of the pressure gradient between the right ventricle and right atrium and the addition of right atrial V-wave pressure, whether assumed or directly measured through an umbilical vein catheter (usually 3–10 torr). Right ventricular systolic pressure relative to left ventricular pressure can also be qualitatively assessed by the curvature of the interventricular septum.

The shortening fraction of the left ventricular internal short axis dimension is used to assess left ventricular systolic function. The shortening fraction measures left ventricular performance, which is a function of contractility, afterload, preload, and heart rate. The relative end systolic wall stress velocity of fiber shortening is an index of contractility that can be measured using directed M-mode echocardiography, indirect central pulse tracing, and phonocardiography that in the physiologic range appears to be independent of preload and takes afterload and heart rate into account. Both techniques are impaired when right ventricular hypertension results in flattening of the interventricular septal curvature in systole.

CARDIAC CATHETERIZATION AND ANGIOGRAPHY

The miniaturization of standard catheterization and angiographic techniques for the study of infants was accomplished in the early 1970s. Infant cardiac catheterization has become a technical art demanding specific training and experience. The neonate undergoing study is ill, often critically ill, and may have a widely fluctuating physiologic state. The combinations of lesions encountered in this age group are large, and the natural mortality rate is high. To perform a therapeutic procedure or to extract the vital diagnostic information with the least danger to the patient requires vigilance against a multitude of treacherous pitfalls and a finely honed sense of the cost and benefit of each maneuver contemplated.

Catheterization is rarely used to learn the basic anatomy of the heart. It is used to perform specific therapeutic interventions or provide specific data unavailable through echocardiography that are useful in planning surgery. What is the pulmonary artery anatomy and pressure? What is the anatomy of systemic-to-pulmonary collaterals. Is catheter closure of the collaterals possible? What is the coronary anatomy? Is there a pressure gradient?

Catheterization for an acyanotic infant in congestive heart failure is better delayed until the pulmonary vascular resistance has decreased and the full effect of the medications has been appreciated. Duct-dependent infants with a closing ductus arteriosus are best managed with an infusion of prostaglandin E_1, begun before and continued throughout the catheterization.[22,23]

Death within 48 hours of cardiac catheterization is rare (0.1%) among children after the first months of life. Earlier in infancy, the risk is difficult to estimate because of the high natural mortality rates associated with the lesions encountered and the association of cardiac catheterization with cardiac surgery. In the first week of life, death within 48 hours of catheterization is 15 times greater than in the fourth week of life. The conclusion that this mortality parallels the natural mortality of the lesions is inescapable. Although this provides a universal excuse for a lamentable outcome, the potential for procedural error is undeniably greater in the sick newborn.[24]

If only unequivocally demonstrable damage to the infant is counted, the risk is quite small. We estimate the mortality rate directly attributable to cardiac catheterization to be 1% to 2% in the neonatal period. Morbidity, such as blood loss, electrolyte imbalance, angiographic myocardial stains, hypothermia, and acidosis, occurs during these studies and influences the outcome of subsequent cardiac surgery.

MAGNETIC RESONANCE IMAGING

Magnetic resonance imaging can detect intrathoracic structures, such as peripheral pulmonary arteries, systemic-to-pulmonary collateral vessels, and the postoperative aortic arch, that often are not adequately imaged by echocardiography. Use of the available diagnostic tools in conjunction with the history and physical examination enables precise diagnosis without resorting to diagnostic cardiac catheterization in most neonates.

MANAGEMENT PROCEDURES FOR SEVERE CARDIAC DISEASE

An infant in difficulty because of heart disease in the first days of life has the potential for rapid deterioration. Too often, the baby looks as though he will survive but is near death hours later. The earlier symptoms appear, the faster deterioration can take place. By the time the infant has reached 1 or 2 months of age, concern about sudden shifts in status is less warranted. The earlier an infant develops symptoms, the more rapidly the physician must respond.

Infants who present with severe cyanosis in the first days to 2 weeks of life may do so because right ventricular outflow is critically obstructed and pulmonary blood flow depends on a closing ductus arteriosus, or because the great arteries are transposed and require a ductus arteriosus for adequate mixing of the pulmonary and systemic circulations. Babies with congestive heart failure in the first week of life often have obstructed left ventricular or aortic outflow, with descending aortic flow supplied by a closing ductus arteriosus. In these babies, survival may depend on persistent patency of the ductus arteriosus; dependency should be suspected and prostaglandin E_1 therapy considered. If possible, echocardiography should be used to confirm a specific anatomic diagnosis, but this may not be available in many primary care facilities, and the infant's condition may prohibit transport to a facility where echocardiography is available. Duct dependency (*e.g.*, pulmonary atresia, hypoplastic left heart syndrome) or a lesion that is significantly worsening because of ductal closure (*e.g.*, D-transposition of the great arteries, critical pulmonary stenosis with $PO_2 < 25$, critical aortic stenosis, coarctation with congestive heart failure) can be suspected from a physical examination, ECG, and chest radiograph, and prostaglandin E_1 therapy can be initiated even if echocardiography is not available. The usual starting dose of 0.1 μg/kg/minute can frequently be reduced to 0.05 to 0.02 μg/kg/minute after stabilization. The occurrence of relatively common side-effects, particularly apnea, vasodilation with hypotension, and fever should be anticipated. Intubation of infants receiving prostaglandins before transport anticipates the risk of apnea.

Despite prostaglandin therapy, these critically ill infants may have low cardiac output that may respond to the correction of common metabolic perturbations including hypothermia, intravascular hypovolemia, hypocalcemia, and hypoglycemia, but frequently, inotropic support is needed (Tables 33-7 and 33-8). Placement of an umbilical venous catheter may allow measurement of central venous pressure to guide fluid therapy and permit administration of concentrated infusions of dextrose, calcium, and vasoactive amines. Hyperventilation should be avoided in babies with certain lesions in which the pulmonary and systemic circulations are in parallel, such as hypoplastic left heart syndrome. Hyperventilation and oxygen administration in these babies can drop pulmonary vascular resistance to low levels, resulting in runoff into the pulmonary vasculature, systemic hypotension, and low output. After appropriate steps to correct contributing metabolic abnormalities, fluid can be given in 5- to 10-mL/kg doses until adequate response is achieved or circulatory congestion occurs. Infusion of dopamine or dobutamine (5–20 μg/kg/minute) should be added to support pump function as needed. Higher doses or continuous infusion of epinephrine, amrinone, or isoproterenol can be considered to support refractory neonates until surgical palliation can be achieved. Digitalis preparations are much less desirable for acute inotropic support of crit-

TABLE 33–7
COMMON ORAL DRUGS FOR THE TREATMENT OF CONGESTIVE HEART FAILURE

Generic Drug	Proprietary Name	Form	Dose	Action	Toxicity
Digoxin	Lanoxin	Elixir: 50 μg = 0.05 mg/mL	Digitalizing dose: Premature, 20 μg/kg; Term, 30 μg/kg; Initial dose, ½; In 6 h, ¼; In 12 h, ¼; Maintenance dose: Premature, 3–4 μg/kg/12 h; Term, 4–5 μg/kg/12 h	Na–K ATPase inhibitor, increases contractility	Atrioventricular block (monitor ECG during loading), tachydysrhythmias, vomiting; use with caution in renal failure and myocarditis; decrease dose by one-half if used with quinidine
Furosemide	Lasix	Suspension: 10 mg/mL	1 mg/kg/12 h, PRN to 2.0 mg/kg/8 h	Loop of Henle Cl-pump inhibition, diuretic	Hyponatremia, hypokalemia, hypochloremic alkalosis, nephrocalcinosis
Chlorothiazide	Diuril	Suspension: 10 mg/mL	10–15 mg/kg/12 h	Blocks distal tubular Na reabsorption, diuretic	Hyponatremia, hypokalemia, hypochloremic alkalosis, hyperbilirubinemia, hyperuricemia, hyperglycemia
Spironolactone	Aldactone	Suspension: 5 mg/mL; Tablet: 25 mg	1–3 mg/kg/d, ¼ tab–½ tab, crushed, qod–qd	Blocks tubular aldosterone receptor, diuretic	Hyperkalemia
Captopril	Capoten	Tablet: 12.5 mg, 25 mg	0.2–1.0 mg/kg/8 h	Angiotensin-converting enzyme inhibition, decreases afterload	Hypotension, proteinuria, may cause hyperkalemia when given with spironolactone or potassium

ECG, electrocardiograph.

TABLE 33–8
INTRAVENOUS VASOACTIVE DRUGS

Drug	Dose (μg/kg/min)	Action	Preload	Systemic Resistance	Pulmonary Resistance	Contractility	Heart Rate	Use	Toxicity
Dopamine	2–5 5–20	D, β_1 D, β, α	+/− ↓ ↓	+/− ↓ ↓, ↑ ↑	0 ↑	↑ ↑ ↑	+/− ↑ ↑ ↑	↑ CO, ↑ BP	Tachycardia, dysrythmias, necrosis with extravasation, ↓ renal blood flow at higher doses
Dobutamine	2–20	β_1, mild B_2, α	+/− ↓	↓	↓	↑ ↑	↑	↑ CO	Tachycardia, dysrhythmias, necrosis with extravasation
Epinephrine	0.05–1.0	α, β_1, β_2	↓, ↑	↓, ↑ ↑	↓, ↑	↑ ↑ ↑	↑ ↑ ↑	↑ CO, ↑ BP, ↑ HR	Tachycardia, dysrhythmias, necrosis with extravasation, ↓ renal blood flow
Isoproteronol	0.05–2.0	β_1, β_2	↓	↓ ↓	↓	↑ ↑ ↑	↑ ↑ ↑	↑ CO, ↑ HR	Marked tachycardia, dysrhythmias, hypotension when volume depleted
Amrinone	5–10 (load: 1.0 mg/kg)	Phosphodiesterase inhibition	↓	↓ ↓	↓, ↑ ↑	↑	0	↑ CO	Thrombocytopenia, dysrhythmias
Nitroprusside	0.5–5	EDRF-like action	↓ ↓	↓ ↓ ↓	↓	0	↑	↑ CO, ↓ BP	Hypotension, V/Q mismatch, thiocyanate toxicity
Nitroglycerin	1–5	EDRF-like action	↓ ↓ ↓	↓ ↓	↓	0	↑	↑ CO, ↓ preload	Hypotension, V/Q mismatch, methemoglobinemia
Phenylephrine	0.5–4.0	α	↑	↑ ↑ ↑	↑	+/− ↑	+/− ↓	TF, cyanotic spells	Cardiac output, ↓ renal blood flow

+/−, may or may not; ↓, decrease; ↑, increase; α, alpha-adrenergic; β, adrenergic; BP, blood pressure; CO, cardiac output; D, dopaminergic; EDRF, endothelial-derived relaxing factor; HR, heart rate, TF, tetralogy of Fallot; V/Q, pulmonary ventilation–perfusion ratio.

ically ill infants who have variable renal and hepatic functions and electrolyte status. The acyanotic cardiac infant who develops symptoms of increased respiratory work and poor feeding after 2 to 4 weeks of life often has congestive heart failure due to decreasing pulmonary vascular resistance and increasing left-to-right shunt. Rarely, these infants have left-sided obstructive lesions or myocardial disease (*e.g.*, anomalous left coronary artery). In infants with isolated left-to-right shunts, a vigorous trial of diuretics, digoxin, and caloric supplementation may be rewarding. Afterload reduction may be beneficial in some infants (see Tables 33-7 and 33-8). Generally, the younger the baby, the more difficult it is to achieve persistent improvement.

THERAPEUTIC CATHETERIZATION

The creation of atrial septal defects, dilation of obstructed valves or vessels, occlusion of undesirable vessels, and myocardial biopsies are commonly performed in older children.[25,26] It is not unreasonable to assume that conditions such as pulmonary stenosis, coarctation of the aorta, aortic stenosis, and patent ductus arteriosus will soon be amenable to comparable treatment in the newborn period.

SURGERY

Heart disease in neonates is often life threatening and requires surgery. Early recognition, safe transport to a cardiac center, accurate diagnosis, and an experienced surgical team are needed for success. Anesthesiologists familiar with the problems of neonatal cardiac patients and a well-equipped intensive care unit with trained personnel contribute to successful management of these babies. The postoperative care requires fine adjustment of blood volume, body temperature, fluid, electrolyte balance, blood *p*H, PO_2, and PCO_2. Close cooperation between the cardiologists, intensivists, and surgeons responsible for the care of these infants is mandatory.

The timing of surgical intervention depends on the anatomic diagnosis and the likelihood of success. Only neonates who are in danger of death are candidates for immediate cardiac surgery.

In the past, there were two schools of thought concerning surgical management of infants critically ill with heart disease. The older view was that a life-saving, palliative operation should be done in infancy, followed months or years later with a reparative operation. This concept is being challenged by the conviction that single-stage repair should be used if possible. The justification for this view is the demonstrably acceptable mortality, avoidance of the double jeopardy of two cardiac operations, and the increasing evidence that early repair results in improved cardiac status and neurologic function.[27,28] Recent mortality data continue to support single-stage repair.

ACYANOTIC LESIONS

Lesions associated with normal pulmonary flow include coarctation of the aorta, aortic stenosis, myocardial disease, and tricuspid valve disease. Acyanotic lesions usually associated with increased pulmonary blood flow include ventricular septal defect, patent ductus arteriosus, atrial septal defect, endocardial cushion defects, L-transposition of the great arteries, and arteriovenous malformations.

COARCTATION OF THE AORTA

For clinical, prognostic, and probably etiologic reasons, coarctation of the aorta is best considered in two separate categories: simple and complex. Simple coarctation is usually a discrete constriction of the aortic isthmic area, occasionally associated with a patent ductus arteriosus inserting just at or below it. The complex malformation involves tubular hypoplasia of the aortic arch with or without discrete aortic narrowing, a patent ductus arteriosus, and one or more of the following lesions: ventricular septal defect, endocardial cushion defect, aortic stenosis, subaortic stenosis, mitral stenosis or regurgitation, hypoplasia of the left ventricle and ascending aorta, and endocardial fibroelastosis. This amalgam of left-sided involvement may be secondary to intrauterine low flow through the left heart, with consequent underdevelopment and hypoplasia extending from the left atrium to the aortic isthmus. The aortic arch may be atretic and completely interrupted as in DiGeorge syndrome. In simple and complex coarctations, there are great variations possible in the extent and location of the coarctation.

Coarctation occurs in 6% of newborns with heart disease (see Table 33-2). It is one of the common causes of congestive failure in the neonate (Tables 33-9 and 33-10). It is more common in male and premature infants. Girls sometimes have Turner syndrome. Among symptomatic infants, 82% have complex coarctation, and 18% have simple coarctation. Severe extracardiac anomalies, usually renal or gastrointestinal, occur in 6% of these patients.

PATHOPHYSIOLOGY

Simple Coarctation. The isthmus is normally smaller than the ascending or descending aorta in newborn infants with simple coarctation because only 25% of the combined ventricular output during fetal life passes through the isthmus into the descending aorta, whereas approximately 60% passes through the ductus arteriosus to the descending aorta. After birth, the isthmus gradually grows, but in simple coarctation, a curtainlike constricting band develops at the point of connection to the ductus arteriosus. The coarctation may become more severe in the neonatal period, as constriction of the adjacent ductal tissue occurs. During childhood, there may be

TABLE 33–9
FINDINGS IN ACYANOTIC 0- TO 2-WEEK-OLD NEONATES WITH CONGESTIVE HEART FAILURE*

Diagnosis	Physical Examination	Radiographic Findings	Electrocardiographic Findings
Coarctation	↓ Leg pulses and leg BP, soft SEM in back, +/− SRM, +/− click, S_3, +/− differential cyanosis, shocklike sepsis picture	↑ Heart size, pulmonary edema	+/− RVH, develops LVH, BVH
Critical aortic stenosis	Shock, ↓ pulses and perfusion, SEM, click, S_3, single S_2	↑ Heart size, pulmonary edema	LVH, T-wave abnormalities
Patent ductus arteriosus in premature infant	Heave, ↑ pulses, ↑ pulse pressure, continuous or SRM	↑ Heart size (LV, LA), ↑ pulmonary arterial markings	Develops RVH, LVH, BVH
Cardiomyopathy	↓ Pulses, ↓ perfusion, ↓ pulse pressure, ↑ HR, SRM	Large globular heart, pulmonary edema	↓ or ↑ voltage, T-wave changes, Q waves in ALCA
Critical pulmonary stenosis	SEM, click, single S_2, most have cyanosis	Normal or ↓ pulmonary arterial markings, RAE	QRS axis 0°–90°, +/− LVH, develops RVH
Systemic arteriovenous fistula	Heave, ↑ pulses, wide pulse pressure, soft SEM or SRM, bruit, shock, +/− cyanosis	↑ Heart size, ↑ pulmonary arterial markings	Develops RVH, LVH, BVH

* Congestive heart failure with cyanosis may be due to hypoplastic left heart syndrome, transposition of the great arteries, truncus arteriosus, total anomalous pulmonary venous connection, pulmonary atresia with tetralogy, tricuspid atresia, Ebstein malformation, or persistent pulmonary hypertension.

+/−, may or may not be present; ↓, decreased; ↑, increased; ALCA, anamolous left coronary artery; BVH, biventricular hypertrophy; HR, heart rate; LA, left atrium; LV, left ventricle; LVH, left ventricular hypertrophy; RAE, right atrial enlargement; RVH, right ventricular hypertrophy; S_2, second heart sound; S_3, third heart sound; SEM, systolic ejection murmur; SRM, systolic regurgitant murmur.

TABLE 33–10
FINDINGS IN ACYANOTIC 2- TO 8-WEEK-OLD NEONATES WITH CONGESTIVE HEART FAILURE*

Diagnosis	Physical Examination	Radiographic Findings	Electrocardiographic Findings
Ventricular septal defect*	Heave, harsh SRM, +/− S_3, +/− diastolic rumble, normal pulses	↑ Heart size (RV, LV, LA), ↑ pulmonary arterial markings	Develops RAE, RVH, LVH, BVH
Endocardial cushion defect	Same as ventricular septal defect, fixed split S_2	Same as ventricular septal defect	Left axis deviation, develops RAE, RVH, LVH, BVH
Atrial septal defect	Hyperdynamic precordium, soft SEM, fixed split S_2, +/− diastolic rumble	↑ Heart size (RV, normal LA and LV), ↑ pulmonary arterial markings	Develops RAD, RVH
Patent ductus arteriosus in full-term infants	Same as presentation at 0–2 weeks of age		
Cardiomyopathy	Same as presentation at 0–2 weeks of age		

* Murmur may be present earlier than 2 weeks of age, and congestive heart failure may occur earlier in premature infants.

+/−, may or may not be present; ↓, decreased; ↑, increased; BVH, biventricular hypertrophy; LA, left atrium; LV, left ventricle; LVH, left ventricular hypertrophy; RAD, right axis deviation; RAE, right atrial enlargement; RV, right ventricle; RVH, right ventricular hypertrophy; S_2, second heart sound; S_3, third heart sound; SRM, systolic regurgitant murmur.

progressive hypertrophy and endothelial thickening at the coarctation site, possibly engendered by high flow velocity at the narrowed point. Collateral circulation may be present at birth. In simple coarctation, the increased resistance to flow results in a pressure overload on the left ventricle to which a volume load may be added if there is a patent ductus arteriosus. With a gradual fall in pulmonary vascular resistance after birth, there is a reversal of flow through the ductus arteriosus from the aorta to the pulmonary artery, and a considerable left-to-right shunt may exist. If the increased pressure and volume load exceeds the ability of the heart to compensate by hypertrophy or dilation, congestive failure with diminution of systemic output ensues. Left ventricular end-diastolic pressure is elevated with consequent increase in left atrial filling pressure, increased pulmonary venous pressure, and development of pulmonary edema. The increased pulmonary venous pressure also produces pulmonary artery hypertension and right heart failure.

Complex Coarctation. Complex coarctation is characterized by pulmonary artery hypertension with a ductus arteriosus supplying the descending aorta, usually a large intracardiac left-to-right shunt, and increased pulmonary flow. The right-sided structures are dilated and hypertrophied. There is a pressure and volume overload on both ventricles and congestive heart failure. In cases of a large ventricular septal defect and patent ductus arteriosus, the systolic pressures in the pulmonary artery, descending aorta, ascending aorta, and right ventricle are identical. Peripheral pulse pressure is normal, and the pulses are equal throughout. With ductal closure or constriction, the femoral pulsations diminish. If the coarctation is severe, perfusion to the lower one-half of the body, previously supplied by the open ductus, is reduced, and manifestations of shock, renal and mesenteric hypoperfusion, and metabolic acidosis develop.

CLINICAL FINDINGS

Infants with isolated discrete coarctation may be asymptomatic, although some develop congestive heart failure, usually after the age of 1 month. The femoral pulses are absent or diminished and significantly delayed compared with brachial pulses. Left brachial pulses may be decreased if the left subclavian arises at or below the coarctation. Systolic blood pressure in the upper extremities is higher than in the lower extremities, but marked hypertension is uncommon. Pulse pressure in the lower extremities is narrow, often 10 to 15 torr. An ultrasonic flow probe or external blood pressure monitor may be helpful. S_3 is often prominent, and there may be an apical systolic ejection click. A systolic ejection murmur is usually heard best at the left interscapular area over the back, but it may be audible at the left upper sternal border. A continuous murmur suggests a left-to-right shunt across the ductus arteriosus. Manifestations of congestive heart failure are those of combined left and right heart failure. The chest radiograph shows cardiac enlargement and pulmonary venous congestion. The ECG usually reveals right ventricular hypertrophy in the early months and left ventricular hypertrophy later. Echocardiographic visualization of the aortic arch usually shows the site, length, and severity of coarctation and the aortic arch branching pattern. There is characteristically a constriction from the outer posterior curvature of the aortic wall, and an anterior periductal shelf may be identified. An instantaneous systolic gradient may be derived from the velocities across the coarctation but may underestimate the severity of the lesion if cardiac output is depressed. The descending aortic flow has a characteristically diminished systolic upstroke velocity and prolonged antegrade flow.

Infants with severe isolated and complex coarctation usually present with congestive heart failure in the early neonatal period. Generally, the younger the infant, the more severe and complex are the combined malformations. In addition to the findings described for simple coarctation, there is evidence of a large left-to-right shunt and pulmonary artery hypertension. Femoral pulsations may wax and wane, depending on ductal patency. This in itself is a useful diagnostic sign. A pansystolic murmur of a septal defect or mitral regurgitation may be found. Ductal closure may result in a critically ill baby with poor perfusion, metabolic acidosis, and possibly disseminated intravascular coagulation, necrotizing enterocolitis, and renal and hepatic dysfunction. The chest radiographs show considerable cardiac enlargement, pulmonary plethora, and edema (Fig. 33-3). The ECG shows right axis deviation, right atrial hypertrophy, right ventricular hypertrophy, and often diminished left ventricular forces. In addition to the aortic arch anatomy, echocardiography often reveals associated lesions, including mitral and aortic stenosis, ventricular septal defect, subaortic obstruction, and conotruncal abnormalities.

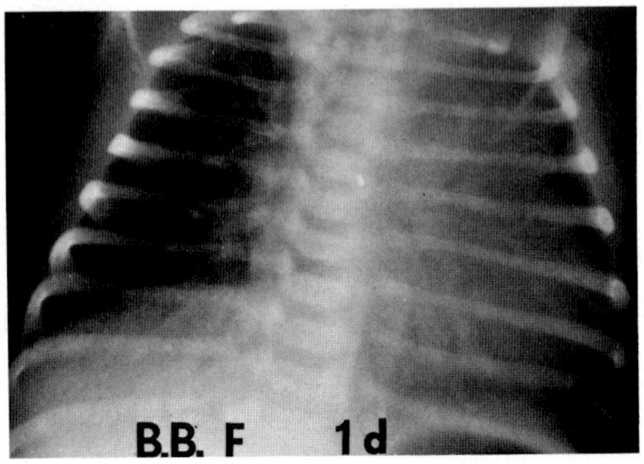

FIG. 33–3. A chest radiograph of a 1-day-old infant with complex coarctation of the aorta shows marked cardiac enlargement and pulmonary vascular engorgement.

TREATMENT

All neonates with congestive heart failure thought to have coarctation of the aorta should be promptly hospitalized, treated, and examined by echocardiography. Many infants with complex coarctation become symptomatic because of constriction of the ductus arteriosus. Prostaglandin E_1 infusion can dilate the ductus, restore systemic perfusion, improve metabolic abnormalities, and provide time to study the anatomy and arrange for surgery. Inotropic support with intravenous dopamine or adrenergic agents is often needed. In critically ill babies, there may be adverse ischemic consequences for the gastrointestinal, renal, hepatic, and coagulation systems. Echocardiography usually provides the anatomic detail needed for surgery. Cardiac catheterization, digital subtraction angiography, or magnetic resonance imaging (MRI) may be useful for additional delineation of the aortic arch and intracardiac anatomy.

After an initial period of clinical improvement, rapid deterioration may occur, and surgery should not be unduly delayed. The surgical procedures employed depend on the severity of the lesion and include resection of the coarctation with primary anastomosis, subclavian or prosthetic patch aortoplasty, or construction of a conduit from the ascending to descending aorta; division of the patent ductus arteriosus; and intracardiac repair or banding of the pulmonary artery if there is a large ventricular septal defect. In some older infants with simple coarctation who respond well to medical therapy, surgery may be delayed. The mortality rate for infants with complicated coarctation is 85% without surgery. Surgery increases the survival rate to 85%. Regardless of the type of coarctation, the mortality is related to age of presentation and is higher for those with duct-dependent descending aortic flow. The survivors need close medical supervision throughout childhood and may require other operations for various associated abnormalities at a later time. Those who undergo surgical coarctation repair early in infancy may develop restenosis later, which may require reoperation or catheter balloon dilation. The role of catheter balloon dilation of unoperated primary discrete coarctation is being investigated. It can offer palliation in the complex critically ill infant.

DIFFERENTIAL DIAGNOSIS

Aortic arch obstruction should be suspected in any critically ill term baby with a septiclike shock. A thorough examination, including careful palpation of all peripheral pulses and blood pressure measurement, should lead to the correct diagnosis. Infants presenting before 1 month of age usually have severe or complex coarctation. Complete interruption of the aortic arch is usually associated with a ventricular septal defect and a systemic patent ductus arteriosus and is clinically indistinguishable from complicated coarctation. It is frequently seen as part of DiGeorge syndrome, which may have additional manifestations of hypocalcemia, absent thymic shadow on the initial chest radiograph, and possible impaired immune response to transfused viable nonirradiated leukocytes. The presence of a ductus arteriosus supplying the descending aorta may be demonstrated by the finding of a lower arterial PO_2 in the legs than in the arms. The hypoplastic left heart syndrome produces a similar shocklike picture or congestive failure in the first week as the ductus arteriosus closes. In these patients, there is cyanosis, the peripheral pulses are diminished throughout, and the ECG shows marked diminution in left ventricular forces.

AORTIC STENOSIS

Symptomatic isolated aortic stenosis in infancy is rare and almost invariably valvar rather than supravalvar or subvalvar. Only the most severe aortic valve obstruction produces symptoms in early infancy. The symptoms are those of congestive heart failure, pulmonary edema, and sometimes peripheral vascular collapse. The baby may appear ashen and cyanotic if the pulmonary edema is severe. The cardinal features are tachypnea, a blowing stenotic murmur at the upper right or middle left sternal border, an apical early systolic click resembling a split S_1, cardiac enlargement and pulmonary venous congestion on chest radiographs, biventricular hypertrophy with T-wave changes on the ECG, and a deformed immobile aortic valve with commissural fusion on the echocardiogram. In severe aortic obstruction, transvalvar flow is diminished, and the systolic murmur and the Doppler-derived pressure gradient are of low amplitude and do not reflect the severity of the lesion. On the echocardiogram, the left ventricle appears hypertrophied and may have small or dilated internal dimensions and poor or hyperdynamic systolic function. Some patients may have coarctation and mitral valve abnormalities.

Initial treatment of critical stenosis consists of administration of inotropic support, oxygen, and frequently prostaglandin E_1, followed as soon as feasible by cardiac catheterization (Fig. 33-4) and balloon valvuloplasty or surgical valvotomy. Although most infants with critical aortic stenosis survive valvuloplasty or valvotomy, some have associated endocardial fibroelastosis or very small left ventricles that limit their survival. The asymptomatic infant with auscultatory findings of aortic stenosis and those after valvuloplasty require continued follow-up, because valvar aortic stenosis frequently recurs.

MYOCARDIAL DISEASE

Several diseases with different causes but with common clinical manifestations and pathophysiology affect the myocardium of the neonate (Table 33-11). These may be functionally grouped as dilated, hyper-

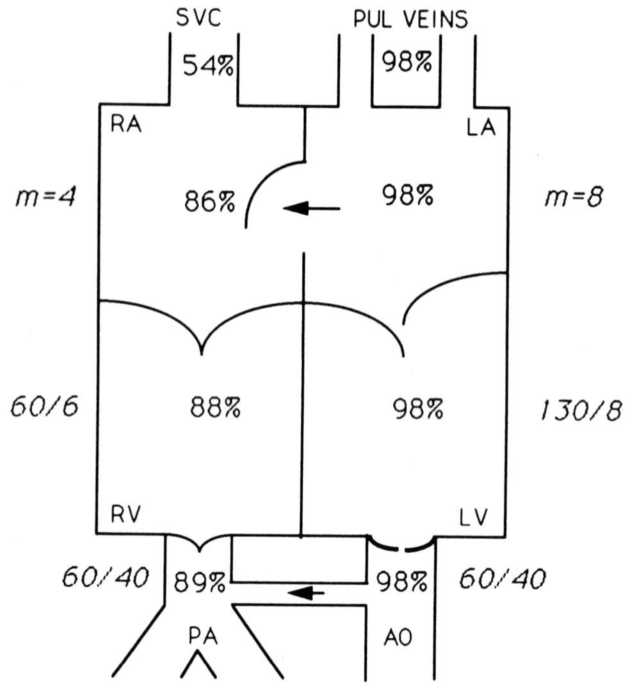

FIG. 33–4. This 1-month-old infant with valvar aortic stenosis had a systolic pressure gradient of 70 torr across the aortic valve. The blood passing from left to right through the ductus must return again through the aortic valve, with the excess flow compounding the obstruction. The large atrial shunt, whether a true anomaly or a sprung foramen ovale, elevated left atrial pressure. The percentages indicate oxygen saturation; the numbers in italics are pressure measurements.

trophic, and restrictive cardiomyopathy. The relatively rare primary myocardial disorders include viral myocarditis, neuromuscular diseases, nonobstructive and obstructive hypertrophic cardiomyopathies, and glycogen storage disease (*i.e.*, Pompe disease).

Dilated cardiomyopathies are characterized by cardiac dilation, diminished contractility, and congestive heart failure. There is frequently some insult to the myocardium that results in myocardial dysfunction, stunning, or necrosis, often with interstitial fibrosis leading to impaired systolic contractility and diastolic compliance. Ventricular dilation, as a result of the Frank-Starling phenomenon, and tachycardia occur in the attempt to maintain cardiac output despite diminished systolic shortening fraction. Pulmonary edema may develop, and cardiac output is often diminished. Unlike older children, neonates with dilated cardiomyopathy frequently have an identifiable cause.

A condition commonly encountered with neonatal cardiomyopathy is severe birth asphyxia. Hypoxemia and ischemia, often with pulmonary hypertension, lactic acidemia, hypercarbia, hypothermia, hypocalcemia, anemia, or polycythemia, may contribute to the myocardial dysfunction. Treatment consists of correction of coexistent metabolic abnormalities, supporting the myocardium with intravenous inotropic agents (*e.g.*, dopamine, dobutamine, epinephrine, amrinone), using antidysrhythmics as needed, and judiciously providing fluids to maintain cardiac output while minimizing edema. Other neonatal disorders associated with significant myocardial dysfunction are sepsis (*e.g.*, endotoxemia, exotoxemia) and persistence of fetal pulmonary hypertension. In addition to supportive measures, antibiotics, hyperventilation, paralysis, sedation, and vasodilators may be employed. In cases with severe but presumably self-limited cardiopulmonary failure refractory to conventional therapy, venoarterial extracorporeal membrane oxygenation (ECMO; see Chap. 32) has been used with success. Although serious complications continue to exist, ECMO has become a standard treatment for critically ill neonates with self-limited cardiopulmonary failure.

Neonatal viral myocarditis is an often fulminant disease frequently associated with hepatitis and encephalitis. The most commonly identified causes are rubella virus, echovirus, and Coxsackie virus, particularly type B. In individual cases, the cause is frequently not determined despite culturing of nasopharyngeal, tracheal, and stool swabs and serologic tests. The infection may be acquired perinatally or postnatally. Treatments including steroids, γ-globulin, in-

TABLE 33–11
NEONATAL CARDIOMYOPATHIES

Dilated Cardiomyopathies
Asphyxia-induced
Sepsis (*e.g.*, endotoxemia, exotoxemia)
Persistent pulmonary hypertension
Hypoglycemia
Hypocalcemia
Hypothermia
Polycythemia
Hypophosphatemia
Chloramphenicol
Adriamycin
Carnitine deficiency
Myocarditis (*e.g.*, coxsackie B, echo, rubella, and human immunodeficiency viruses)
Anomalous origin of left coronary artery
Tachycardia-induced
Arrhythmogenic right ventricular dysplasia
Maternal connective tissue disease (*e.g.*, systemic lupus erythematosus
Hypertrophic Cardiomyopathies
Maternal diabetes mellitus
Hypertrophic cardiomyopathy (*i.e.*, idiopathic)
Pheochromocytoma
Infiltrative Cardiomyopathies
Pompe glycogen storage disease
Mucopolysaccharidoses

terferon, and ribavirin have been under investigation in biopsy-proven myocarditides, but supportive measures are the mainstay of treatment. Several other viruses, bacteria, mycoplasma, rickettsiae, spirochetes, and fungi rarely cause myocarditis. Myocarditis because of an autoimmune reaction may occur with maternal lupus erythematosus. Maternal IgG Ro antibodies cross the placenta, bind to the fetal myocardium, and may block conduction or cause cardiomyopathy. Steroids may be beneficial in this disease.

The diagnosis of anomalous origin of the left coronary artery from the pulmonary artery should be considered in all children with dilated cardiomyopathy, particularly if there is an ECG pattern of anterolateral myocardial infarction. The anomalous origin of the left coronary artery can usually be seen on echocardiography, although angiography may be needed in some cases. Treatment is surgical and is usually successful.

Chronic supraventricular and ventricular tachycardia can lead to persistent myocardial dysfunction with the picture of cardiomyopathy.

Chronic therapy is supportive and aimed at control of the congestive heart failure and arrhythmias. Digitalization should be carried out with caution and orally if possible in infants with myocarditis, because they may be unduly susceptible to drug-induced dysrhythmias. Therapy should be maintained until cardiac enlargement subsides. Afterload reduction with angiotensin-converting enzyme (ACE) inhibitors can produce significant benefit. Cardiac transplantation may be considered if the course is fulminant.

Although sometimes a severe disorder in infants, the hypertrophic cardiomyopathy of infants of diabetic mothers is generally self-limited. Hypertrophic cardiomyopathy in infants of diabetic mothers is thought to be a result of a myocardial trophic response to fetal hyperinsulinemia provoked by transplacental passage of high maternal glucose loads. Clinical findings include a systolic ejection murmur and, rarely, evidence of congestive heart failure. There is an increased risk of structural heart disease (see Table 33-3). Echocardiography reveals left ventricular hypertrophy that is sometimes severe, usually with involvement of the septum, and occasionally with outflow obstruction (Fig. 33-5). Treatment is supportive. Digoxin may worsen outflow obstruction and is contraindicated if the obstruction is severe.

Idiopathic hypertrophic cardiomyopathy is a multigene disorder inherited as an autosomal condition with variable penetrance. This disorder is characterized by marked left ventricular hypertrophy associated with myocyte hypertrophy and disarray. There is a propensity for development of left ventricular outflow or intracavitary systolic gradients, symptoms of congestive heart failure due to poor diastolic chamber compliance, ventricular dysrhythmias, and sudden death. There can be significant progression with time, and a normal echocardiogram at birth may not exclude the possibility for phenotypic expression later in life. Those presenting at birth appear to have the poorest prognosis. Inotropic agents and diuretics are potentially harmful and generally not used. Calcium channel blockers decrease the systolic pressure gradient, improve diastolic compliance, and may improve survival in adults. Because of hazards associated with calcium channel blockers in infants, their use in infants less than 1 year of age remains investigational. Propranolol improves symptoms but has no effect on the progression of hypertrophy or survival. Ventricular septal myotomy or myomectomy may improve symptoms in those refractory to medical treatment. Holter monitoring for ventricular dysrhythmias should be routinely performed and amiodarone considered in those with ventricular tachycardia or syncope. Cardiac transplantation may be considered in severely affected refractory patients.

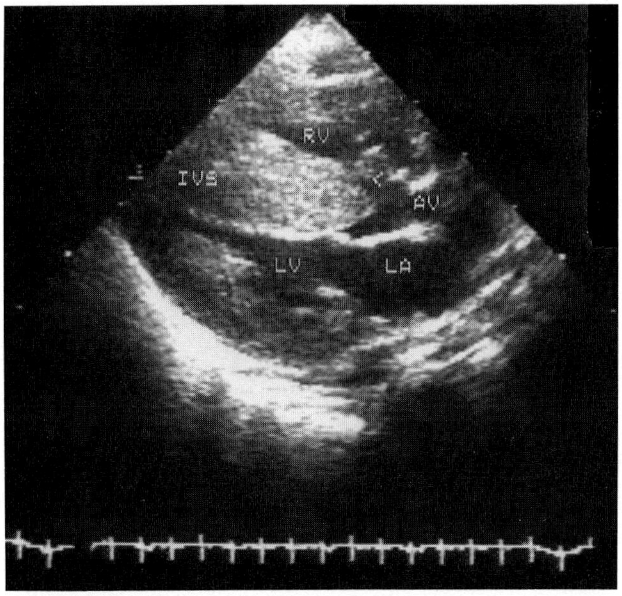

FIG. 33–5. Echocardiographic parasternal long axis view of a diabetic mother's infant with severe hypertrophic cardiomyopathy and subaortic ventricular septal defect. <, ventricular septal defect; AV, aortic valve, IVS, interventricular septum; LA, left atrium; LV, left ventricle; RV, right ventricle.)

Infiltrative disorders of the myocardium such as Pompe glycogen storage disease can present with clinical, ECG, and echocardiographic features resembling in many ways hypertrophic cardiomyopathy. Distinguishing features sometimes include skeletal muscular hypotonia, protruding tongue, short PR interval, left ventricular hypertrophy, and normal or diminished systolic function. Pompe disease is uniformly fatal.

TRICUSPID VALVE DISEASE

An abnormally functioning but anatomically normal tricuspid valve is a common finding in the newborn period. There may be right ventricular myocardial disease; perhaps asphyxial cardiomyopathy, which causes tricuspid regurgitation; or PPHN or pulmonary hypertension resulting from pulmonary parenchymal disease. Whether there is primary myocardial dysfunction or pulmonary hypertension and secondary right ventricular dysfunction, there is secondary tricuspid regurgitation of a normal tricuspid valve. If there is right ventricular diastolic dysfunction, there may be right-to-left shunting through a PFO. The explanation for a lower sternal murmur is documented by echocardiography and managed with observation, because tricuspid regurgitation of this type tends to regress as the underlying problem resolves.

VENTRICULAR SEPTAL DEFECT

Interventricular septal defects may be small or large, single or multiple, and isolated or associated with other cardiovascular malformations. They are an integral part of complex congenital heart disease lesions, such as tetralogy of Fallot, truncus arteriosus, double-outlet right ventricle, and atrioventricular canal, and they have been associated with virtually every other known congenital cardiac malformation. The defect occurs most commonly in the membranous septum, less often in the low portion of the muscular septum, rarely beneath the pulmonary valve, and rarely posteriorly adjacent to the tricuspid valve. Ventricular septal defects are the most common of the congenital cardiac lesions, and even though only 10% of ventricular septal defects cause symptoms, they remain the most common cause of congestive heart failure after the second week of life (see Tables 33-6 and 33-10). Extracardiac malformations occur in 24% of the patients.

PATHOPHYSIOLOGY

The common small ventricular septal defect does not produce symptoms, but a moderate or large defect in a neonate may cause significant hemodynamic alterations. If the defect is large, there is equilibration of right and left ventricular pressures and pulmonary hypertension. (Fig. 33-6) The decreasing pulmonary resistance after birth allows an increasing left-to-right shunt through the defect. The normal regression of pulmonary resistance in the first week of life is usually delayed in these babies. Nonetheless, sufficient reduction in pulmonary resistance occurs by the second week of life to cause symptoms in many patients. Others, presumably with smaller defects or further delay in the reduction of pulmonary vascular resistance, develop symptoms as late as 3 to 4 months of age.

Symptoms are the result of congestive heart failure or superimposed pulmonary problems such as pneumonia or atelectasis. Congestive heart failure is caused by the recirculation of large amounts of blood through the heart and lungs while simultaneously attempting to meet the demand for systemic flow.

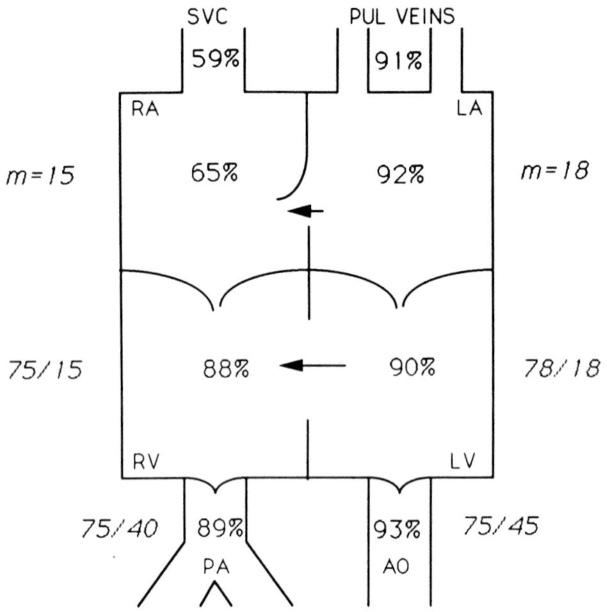

FIG. 33–6. A large ventricular septal defect in a 1-month-old baby allows equilibration of pressure between the two ventricles. With pulmonary resistance much less than systemic resistance, there is a very large left-to-right shunt that caused congestive heart failure, as evidenced by the elevated atrial pressures and the reduced pulmonary venous oxygen saturation because of pulmonary edema. The percentages indicate oxygen saturation; the numbers in italics are pressure measurements.

Mechanical pressure by enlarged structures, particularly the left pulmonary artery and atrium, may result in bronchial obstruction and pulmonary atelectasis. The added effect of pulmonary congestion, which produces decreased lung compliance, makes the infants with a large left-to-right shunt susceptible to recurrent respiratory airway obstruction and infections. Because pulmonary vascular resistance is lower in premature infants at birth, the development of symptoms from a ventricular septal defect occurs earlier.

Gradual improvement and diminution in pulmonary blood flow in an infant with a moderate or large ventricular defect may occur if there is an anatomic decrease in the size of the defect. Many defects spontaneously close and most—particularly muscular and membranous defects—become smaller with time. During childhood, but rarely in infancy, there may be progressive and irreversible development of anatomic obstructive changes in the pulmonary arterioles.

CLINICAL FINDINGS

A small ventricular septal defect is characterized by a readily audible harsh systolic murmur, which is loudest at the lower left sternal border. Infants with large septal defects develop congestive failure in the first few months of life with symptoms of tachypnea (*i.e.*, rate consistently ≥60), fatigue with feeding, decreased oral intake, excessive diaphoresis, and recurrent respiratory infections. Gross dyspnea is a late manifestation. Weight gain lags considerably behind height maturation. The infant often presents with a respiratory infection that may precipitate or mask underlying congestive failure. On examination, the infant is scrawny and tachypneic. The peripheral pulses are rapid and may be slightly bounding. The cardiac impulse is hyperdynamic. If pulmonary artery hypertension exists, the second heart sound may be single with an accentuated pulmonary closure. A gallop sound may be heard and is often associated with a mid-diastolic rumble. The systolic murmur is heard best at the lower left sternal border but is usually transmitted well to the entire precordium. There is hepatomegaly and frequently pulmonary wheezing and rales. Peripheral edema is rare.

A chest radiograph shows considerable cardiac enlargement, increased pulmonary blood flow, and sometimes pulmonary edema. The main pulmonary artery segment and left atrium are often enlarged. Atelectasis and parenchymal infiltrates are common. The ECG usually reveals left ventricular hypertrophy, and if the lesion is associated with pulmonary artery hypertension, right ventricular hypertrophy is detected. The echocardiogram can demonstrate the size, location, and number of ventricular septal defects. Associated lesions not appreciated on physical examination, including atrial septal defect, patent ductus arteriosus, coarctation of the aorta, and left and right ventricular outflow obstructions, are revealed by echocardiography. Right ventricular and pulmonary hypertension can be assessed from the curvature of the interventricular septum and by Doppler measurement of the instantaneous systolic pressure gradient across the defect. Some degree of tricuspid regurgitation often allows estimation of the right ventricular pressure from the pressure gradient between the right ventricle and right atrium. Large defects show evidence of left ventricular volume overload with large left atrial and left ventricular dimensions and hyperdynamic left ventricular function.

TREATMENT

An infant with a small ventricular septal defect requires no specific treatment but should be followed. Some infants with large defects have or develop progressive pulmonary stenosis that prohibits left-to-right shunting, cardiomegaly, and congestive heart failure. These babies may develop the features of the tetralogy of Fallot. Any evidence of increasing right ventricular hypertrophy on the ECG suggests the development of pulmonary stenosis or increasing pulmonary vascular resistance and the need for careful reevaluation. In infants with congestive heart failure, intensive medical therapy with the administration of digitalis and diuretics may produce considerable improvement. Systemic afterload reduction with ACE inhibitors (*e.g.*, captopril) may be beneficial in some refractory patients (see Table 33-7). If there are any pulmonary complications, antibiotics, bronchodilators, and pulmonary physiotherapy should be employed as appropriate. The use of high-caloric formulas may be helpful. The total *ad libitum* oral intake should not be restricted, because growth failure and small size are a common issue in these infants.

The infant who develops congestive failure or who has evidence of pulmonary artery hypertension may require cardiac catheterization to confirm the hemodynamics and determine the possible coexistence of other cardiac lesions. Palliative or corrective surgery is indicated if the infant does not grow despite intensive medical therapy after a reasonable period of observation, requires repeated hospitalizations for respiratory infections, or has persistent significant pulmonary artery hypertension after 6 months of age. Primary repair in infants entails cardiopulmonary bypass, possible deep hypothermic circulatory arrest, and in most patients, closure through the tricuspid valve. Some patients require right or left ventriculotomy. Of infants born with isolated, large defects requiring closure in the first year of life, 10% die, usually as a consequence of associated severe extracardiac congenital anomalies, pulmonary complications, or prematurity. The long-term prognosis after transatrial surgical closure of isolated ventricular septal defects in the first year of life is excellent, with essentially normal hemodynamics and a small risk for symptomatic dysrhythmias for most patients.

DIFFERENTIAL DIAGNOSIS

In the neonate, the murmur of a small ventricular septal defect may be difficult to differentiate from that caused by an obstructive lesion or atrioventricular valve regurgitation (*i.e.*, mitral or tricuspid regurgitation). Other malformations resulting in a large left-to-right shunt and congestive failure are often difficult to differentiate clinically and should be excluded by echocardiography (see Tables 33-9 and 33-10).

PATENT DUCTUS ARTERIOSUS

The ductus arteriosus, arising from the distal dorsal sixth aortic arch, is well developed by the sixth week of gestation and forms a bridge between the pulmonary artery and the dorsal aorta, inserting at the aortic isthmus. At term, it is a muscular contractile structure. In the full-term infant, functional closure occurs during the first day of life. Persistence of patency of the ductus arteriosus alone or in association with other cardiovascular lesions may produce no symptoms or severe hemodynamic changes, depending on its size.

Isolated patent ductus arteriosus, without hyaline membrane disease, is common, accounting for 3.9%

of all newborns symptomatic with heart disease.[8] It is more prevalent in female than male infants. Patent ductus arteriosus is a frequent complication of hyaline membrane disease in the premature infant, in surviving premature infants, and in infants born at high altitudes; in these patients, there is no sex difference. It is common in combination with other congenital heart lesions (*e.g.*, coarctation of the aorta, ventricular septal defect, vascular ring). It occurs in 60 to 70% of infants born with congenital rubella.

PATHOPHYSIOLOGY

At birth, ductal constriction is caused by multiple factors, the most important of which appears to be increased oxygen tension, the levels of circulating prostaglandins, and available ductus muscle mass. Prostaglandin E_1 is used to dilate a closing ductus in several forms of congenital heart disease in which patency of the ductus arteriosus is necessary to support pulmonary or systemic blood flow.[22,23] Delayed closure frequently occurs in premature infants with respiratory distress syndrome. Indomethacin, an inhibitor of prostaglandin synthesis, is used to promote closure of the ductus in this situation.[29,30] The ductus arteriosus that remains patent in the term infant is abnormal and not susceptible to pharmacologic closure.

Within the first hours after birth, with a fall in pulmonary vascular resistance and a rise in systemic resistance, a left-to-right shunt may develop through the ductus arteriosus. A small right-to-left or bidirectional shunt may occur. If spontaneous closure does not occur and the ductus is small, the left-to-right shunt remains small. However, a moderate-sized patent ductus arteriosus is usually associated with a significant left-to-right shunt, left ventricular volume overload, increased left ventricular end-diastolic volume and pressure, elevation of left atrial pressure, and the development of congestive heart failure. Increased pulmonary blood flow elevates the left ventricular stroke volume, increases systolic pressure, produces wide pulse pressure, and generates bounding peripheral pulsations.

The premature infant may fail earlier because of incomplete development of the medial musculature in the small pulmonary arterioles. The contractile function of the heart, required to handle the increased volume load, may be incompletely developed. Among those with respiratory distress syndrome, there may be an initial period of improvement as the pulmonary status improves, followed by clinical deterioration as left-to-right shunting through the ductus arteriosus increases.

A large patent ductus arteriosus produces pulmonary artery hypertension because the pressure is transmitted directly from the aorta to the pulmonary artery through the large defect. Those with moderate and large ducts are prone to the development of pulmonary vascular obstructive disease at a later age.

CLINICAL FINDINGS

In the neonate with a patent ductus arteriosus, as in all left-to-right shunts, the elevated but decreasing pulmonary vascular resistance determines the clinical manifestations. The classic continuous (*i.e.*, Gibson) murmur is heard infrequently, except in some small premature infants. There is usually a crescendo systolic murmur, often with clicks, sometimes detectably spilling into diastole. Often, S_2 is not clearly audible. The infant with a large patent ductus arteriosus has bounding peripheral pulses, wide pulse pressure, and hyperactive cardiac impulse at the apex. There may be an apical diastolic rumble. The child may have symptoms and signs of congestive heart failure, poor weight gain, and recurrent pulmonary infections. In a full-term infant with a large patent ductus arteriosus, overt failure usually does not develop until 3 to 6 weeks of age, but in premature infants, it may occur earlier.

The chest radiograph shows cardiac enlargement, pulmonary plethora, a prominent main pulmonary artery, and left atrial enlargement. The ECG reveals left ventricular hypertrophy, occasionally left atrial hypertrophy, and in severe failure, ST-T wave changes. Echocardiography demonstrates the ductus arteriosus, its size, and the direction of the flow across the defect. Disturbed flow in the pulmonary artery, seen best with color Doppler techniques, is particularly helpful in identifying a patent ductus arteriosus. Continuous-wave Doppler allows measurement of the pressure gradient across the defect and thereby, estimation of pulmonary pressure. Large defects show evidence of left heart volume overload and a large left atrium and left ventricle, and right ventricular hypertension with flattening of the interventricular septum curvature.

If there is associated pulmonary disease, the pulmonary resistance may be high, allowing only right-to-left shunting, which does not produce a murmur. Right-to-left ductal shunting also occurs with left heart obstructive lesions and coarctation of the aorta. If suspected, echocardiography should be used to exclude these lesions before treatment.

TREATMENT

The full-term and premature infant with a persistent patent ductus arteriosus and no evidence of cardiovascular embarrassment should be followed and catheter closure or surgical division of the ductus performed between 6 months and 1 year of age. Term infants with congestive heart failure should be digitalized, and if necessary, diuretics should be added. In the sick neonate, clinical differentiation from other lesions is often possible using echocardiography. Careful transfusion of packed erythrocytes in the anemic premature diminishes the left ventricular volume overload and may hasten ductal closure by increasing the arterial oxygen content.

Among preterm infants with significant patent ductus arteriosus, indomethacin treatment produces closure in approximately 85% of patients. Indomethacin can cause deterioration of renal and platelet function and should be avoided if there is significant renal dysfunction, thrombocytopenia, or bleeding. The ductus arteriosus occasionally reopens after initially successful indomethacin treatment and may respond to a second course of treatment. Failure of indomethacin does not adversely affect subsequent surgery.[31,32] Surgical interruption of the ductus arteriosus is indicated, regardless of age or weight in any infant with a persistent hemodynamically significant left-to-right shunt, particularly if there is pulmonary artery hypertension. Surgical mortality is low, and dramatic improvement often occurs. The procedure is performed using a left thoracotomy in the intensive care nursery or the operating room under intravenous or inhalation general anesthesia. Catheter closure is not yet technically achievable in neonates and preterm small infants.

DIFFERENTIAL DIAGNOSIS

The infant with congestive failure and a large left-to-right shunt caused by a ventricular septal defect may be clinically indistinguishable from the one with a large patent ductus arteriosus. Other lesions that may result in a large aortic runoff and mimic a patent ductus arteriosus include truncus arteriosus, hemitruncus (*i.e.*, right pulmonary artery from the ascending aorta), aortopulmonary window, aneurysm of the sinus of Valsalva, and a large systemic arteriovenous fistula, usually intracranial or hepatic (see Tables 33-9 and 33-10).

ATRIAL SEPTAL DEFECT SECUNDUM

Virtually all babies have a PFO at birth. Many PFOs become functionally closed within hours of birth, but most allow the passage of a catheter at least for the first months of life and sometimes for the rest of the person's life. This is important to the neonatologist, because umbilical vein catheters tend to follow the course of the circulation for the preceding 9 months and may pass through the foramen ovale into the left heart, providing erroneous measures of oxygen levels and allowing passage of undiluted intravenously injected materials straight to the brain, occasionally with disastrous results.

An opening in the atrial septum is a relatively common anomaly, but rarely causes symptoms or a murmur loud enough to attract attention in infants. Some of these defects are discovered because of concern initiated by extracardiac anomalies, and an echocardiogram is ordered. Others are discovered during workup for failure to thrive, but most are found because a murmur of pulmonary stenosis is heard. This murmur is thought to be produced by the excess flow across the pulmonary valve caused by the left-to-right shunt resulting from an atrial septal defect. Because there is rarely congestive heart failure, treatment consists of observation until the child is older, when if the defect persists, it may be closed by surgical or catheter techniques. Surprising numbers of these defects spontaneously close in the first years of life, raising the question about whether some were patent foramina ovale misinterpreted at echocardiography.

Rarely, a large atrial septal defect is associated with an early decrease in the pulmonary resistance and a large left-to-right shunt in the first months of life. Growth failure and congestive heart failure may raise the question of early cardiac surgery. This is a treacherous situation because any left-sided heart disease (*e.g.*, myocardial disease) may have upset the balance of bilateral atrial outflow resistance, causing the left-to-right shunt. Surgical closure of the defect may uncover the additional problem of myocardial failure, with a disastrous outcome. The simple rule of thumb is to undertake surgery for isolated atrial septal in early infancy with great caution.

ENDOCARDIAL CUSHION DEFECTS

Defects of endocardial cushion development may be partial, resulting in an ostium primum atrial defect, or complete, resulting in additional deficiency of the interventricular septum and a common atrioventricular valve (*i.e.*, complete atrioventricular canal). The atrioventricular valves, particularly the anterior mitral valve leaflet, are usually malformed, deficient, or abnormally attached to the ventricular septum. With ostium primum defect, there is usually a cleft in the mitral valve and frequently mitral regurgitation. In complete atrioventricular canal, the primitive atrioventricular valve floats like a sail over both ventricles. This malformation results in a large communication between the right and left atria and the right and left ventricles. Significant mitral incompetence or tricuspid incompetence is less common than in those with only an ostium primum defect. Occasionally, but more often in those without trisomy 21, the mitral valve has abnormal chordal attachments and is stenotic. The large atrioventricular valve is rarely primarily centered over one ventricle, and the contralateral ventricle is much smaller than normal. Endocardial cushion defects as primary lesions account for 4% of all newborns with serious heart disease (see Tables 33-1 and 33-2).

Forty percent of infants with Down syndrome have congenital heart disease, predominantly complete atrioventricular canals. Because babies who have Down syndrome have a tendency to underventilate, causing pulmonary venous oxygen unsaturation, they may have pulmonary hypertension that, associated with a common atrioventricular canal, may limit left-to-right shunting to amounts that do not produce a murmur (Fig. 33-7). All infants with Down syndrome should be examined for congenital heart disease. An ECG to show the leftward superior axis of

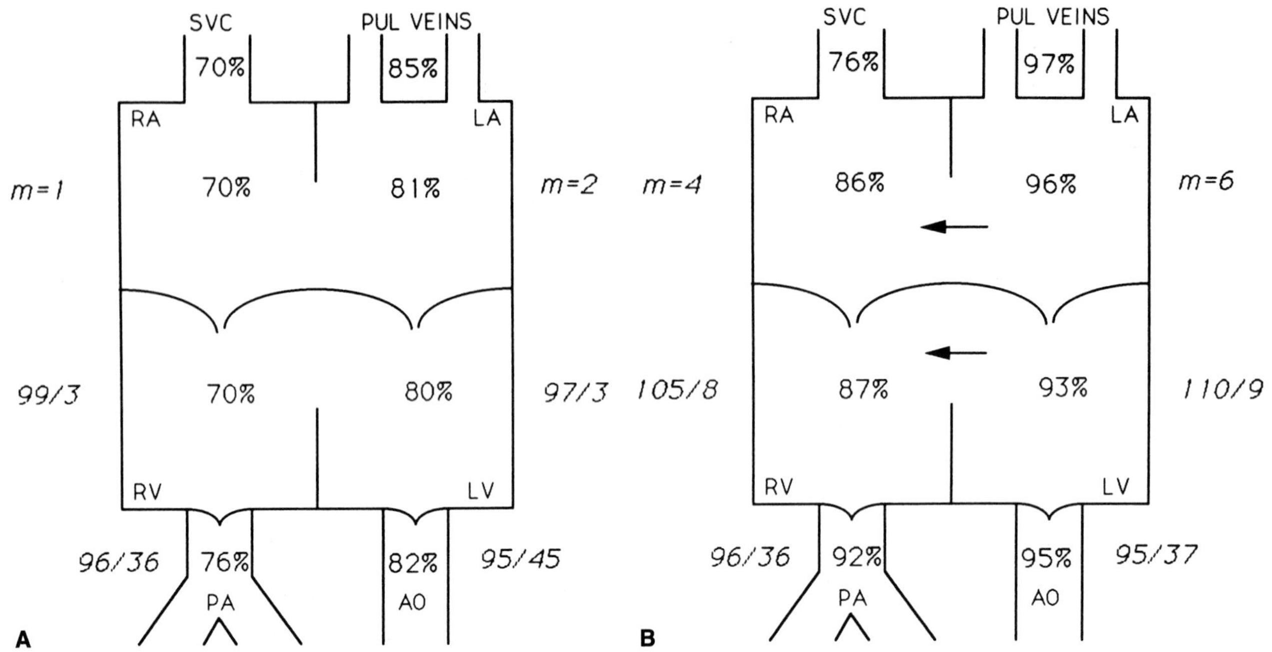

FIG. 33–7. **(A)** Atrioventricular canal in an asymptomatic girl with Down syndrome. There was no murmur. At catheterization of the girl at 6 months of age while breathing room air, the pulmonary resistance was high; there was no left-to-right shunt, and she had arterial oxygen unsaturation. **(B)** When breathing oxygen, a large left-to-right shunt developed and the estimated pulmonary resistance fell sharply. The percentages indicate oxygen saturation; the numbers in italics are pressure measurements.

the atrioventricular canal or an echocardiogram to show the anatomy is routinely required in the workup of these babies.

PATHOPHYSIOLOGY

The hemodynamic consequence of an ostium primum atrial septal defect is volume overload, which is caused by a left–to–right shunt across the atrial septal defect or regurgitation from the left ventricle to the right atrium through the cleft mitral valve. The large volume load, particularly if aggravated by an additional overload caused by mitral regurgitation, results in congestive heart failure, which is often severe. Streaming of inferior vena cava blood across the large, low-lying defect and cleft common valve leads to mild systemic arterial oxygen unsaturation. In complete atrioventricular canal, there is an additional left-to-right shunt through a ventricular septal defect and right ventricular and pulmonary artery hypertension at a systemic level. Infants with pulmonary artery hypertension are particularly susceptible to the development of pulmonary vascular obstructive disease and its complications in later childhood.

CLINICAL FINDINGS

Infants with ostium primum atrial septal defects who are symptomatic in the neonatal period usually have severe mitral regurgitation. Growth retardation may be marked, and weight lags considerably behind height maturation. Recurrent pulmonary infections are common. With atrioventricular canal, there is frequently mild cyanosis. Cardiac impulse is hyperdynamic, and S_1 is obscured by a loud pansystolic murmur audible at the apex or left sternal border. There is usually pulmonary hypertension, and the S_2 is accentuated. A loud S_3 and an apical middiastolic rumble are often heard. Occasionally, particularly among neonates with Down syndrome, there may be no perceptible auscultatory abnormality. The chest radiograph shows cardiac enlargement, sometimes out of proportion to the increased pulmonary vasculature, attributable to the large atria. The main pulmonary artery segment is prominent, and there is pulmonary vascular engorgement. The ECG characteristically shows a left superior QRS axis in the frontal plane, commonly 0° to −60° in primum defects and −60° to −100° in complete canal with a small Q wave in lead aVL. Significant right ventricular hypertrophy usually indicates right ventricular hypertension (Fig. 33-8). Echocardiography demonstrates the anatomic features relevant to surgical repair, including the anatomy of the atrioventricular valve with its chordal attachments, papillary muscles, ventricular relationships, and possible regurgitation or stenosis of the atrioventricular valves (Fig. 33-9). Patients with complete atrioventricular canals may require cardiac catheterization to determine the pulmonary vascular resistance and the presence of associated lesions. Se-

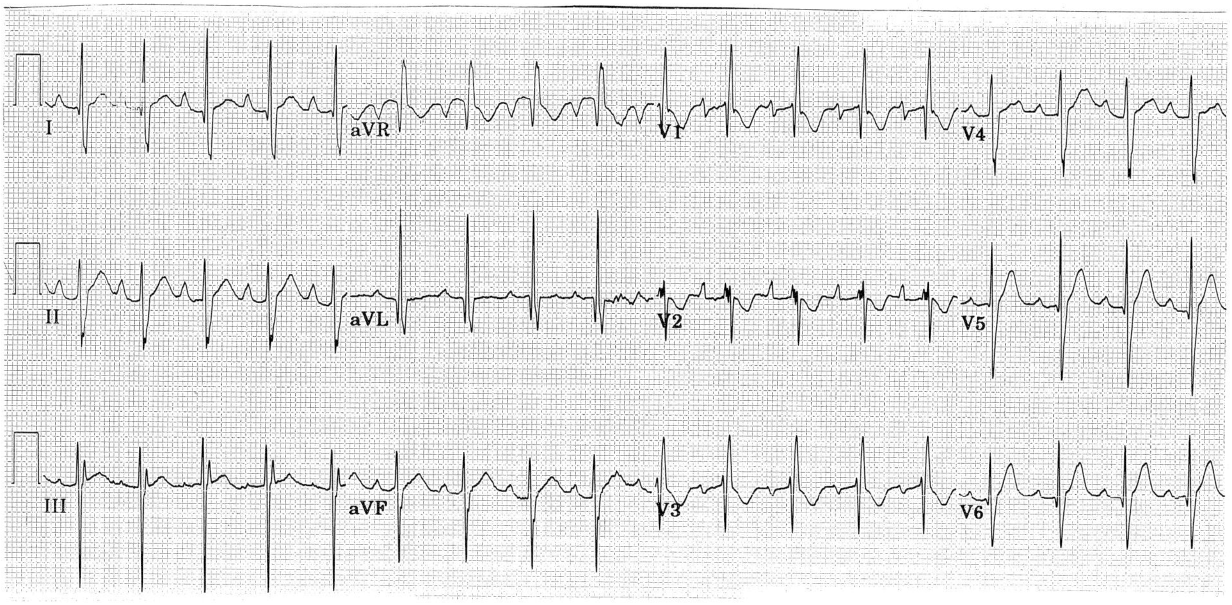

FIG. 33–8. Electrocardiogram of infant with endocardial cushion defect shows the characteristic left axis deviation.

lective left ventriculography in the case of complete atrioventricular canal shows a posterior inlet ventricular septal defect straddled by a common atrioventricular valve and a goose-neck sign in the left ventricular outflow. The latter results from diastolic anterior movement of the superior segment of the anterior mitral valve leaflet, producing an elongated and horizontal left ventricular outflow tract.

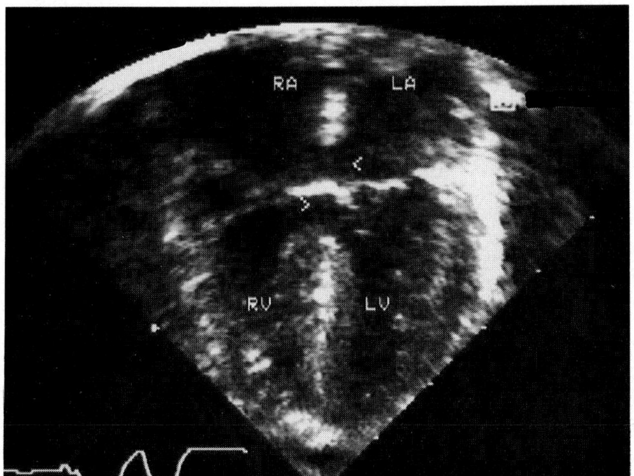

FIG. 33–9. Echocardiographic apical four-chamber view of an infant with trisomy 21 and complete atrioventricular canal defect. <, primum atrial septal defect; >, posterior inlet ventricular septal defect; LA, left atrium; LV, left ventricle; RA, right atrium; RV, right ventricle.

TREATMENT

In many patients, palliative or corrective surgery has to be performed in infancy because of refractory congestive heart failure or pulmonary hypertension. Treatment with digitalis and diuretics may result in sufficient improvement in growth and respiratory work to delay operative repair for several months. In some with refractory symptoms of congestive heart failure, afterload reduction may help. In infants with complete atrioventricular canals, there is pulmonary artery hypertension, and surgery is mandatory within the first year to prevent irreversible pulmonary vascular changes.

Primary complete repair is the preferred treatment. This entails cardiopulmonary bypass, atriotomy, patch closure of the atrial and ventricular septal defects, and attachment of the common valve leaflet to the patch or patches. In infants with refractory congestive heart failure weighing less than 2.5 to 3 kg or those with serious confounding noncardiac illness (*e.g.*, duodenal atresia), pulmonary artery banding may be helpful, with complete repair accomplished later. Children with isolated uncomplicated ostium primum atrial septal defects and few symptoms can undergo complete repair without cardiac catheterization at several years of age. The long-term prognosis after surgery is excellent. There is often some postoperative regurgitation of the atrioventricular valve, but in most infants, this is not a significant problem. Systemic vasodilators can reduce the volume of regurgitation and may help preserve ventricular function in patients with significant postoperative mitral regurgitation. Late dysrhythmias occasionally occur. When there is severe mitral regurgitation, closure of the septal defect with valvuloplasty may result in clinical improvement, but residual mitral regurgitation may later require valve replacement. Without surgery, the prognosis is poor. Only 50% of patients with endocardial cushion defects who become symptomatic in the first month of life survive beyond 1 year of age without surgical treatment, and many of these have considerable delays in growth.

L-TRANSPOSITION OF THE GREAT ARTERIES

In L-transposition of the great arteries with situs solitus, also called corrected transposition, the circulation is physiologically corrected. The systemic venous blood enters the right atrium and flows into a right-sided, morphologically left, ventricle and out to the pulmonary artery. Pulmonary venous blood returns to the left atrium and by way of the tricuspid valve into the left-sided, morphologically right, ventricle to the aorta. The aorta is abnormally positioned, anterior and usually to the left of the pulmonary artery. The hemodynamic changes in patients with L-transposition of the great arteries are caused by the commonly associated cardiac abnormalities that include ventricular septal defect (50%), single ventricle (42%), pulmonary stenosis or atresia (45%), and left atrioventricular valve regurgitation (23%). Conduction disturbances and arrhythmias, particularly complete heart block, are common, and this diagnosis should always be considered for a newborn with complete heart block. Medical management and surgery are directed toward correction or palliation of the associated cardiovascular malformations, such as closure of the ventricular septal defect, pulmonary valvotomy, and a cardiac pacemaker if needed.

ARTERIOVENOUS MALFORMATIONS

Malformation of the developing peripheral vascular system can result in abnormal connections of arteries, arterioles, and capillaries to the venous system (*i.e.*, arteriovenous fistulae) that create a large shunt. These fistulae can involve vessels of any size and location. Capillary hemangiomas involve ongoing abnormal neovascularization. Although most infants with arteriovenous malformations have no other cardiovascular anomaly, abnormal congenital systemic-to-pulmonary vascular corrections can occur with tetralogy of Fallot with pulmonary atresia, partial anomalous pulmonary venous connection (*i.e.*, scimitar syndrome), and bronchopulmonary sequestration. Some infants with prolonged respiratory disease complicated by pneumothorax requiring multiple chest tubes may develop collateral vessels from systemic arteries in the chest wall to the pulmonary arteries, resulting in a left-to-right shunt physiologically mimicking a patent ductus arteriosus but usually heard in a different location.

PATHOPHYSIOLOGY

Although most infants do not develop cardiovascular symptoms, a large systemic arteriovenous malformation can result in significant left-to-right shunt and congestive heart failure. Symptomatic babies usually have connections of relatively large arteries and veins in the cerebral or hepatic vasculature. Pulmonary arteriovenous malformations result in an intrapulmonary right-to-left shunt and cyanosis, but they do not produce congestive heart failure.

CLINICAL FINDINGS

Arteriovenous fistula is one of the few cardiovascular defects that may produce severe congestive heart failure in the first day of life. Cardiovascular shock may be the predominant clinical picture. There may be a hyperdynamic precordium and pulses, flow murmur, severe congestive heart failure, and cyanosis. Bruits over the fontanelle, posterior neck, or abdomen may be audible, and there may be an enlarged head or liver. Echocardiography can demonstrate biventricular dilation and sometimes an enlarged cava with increased flow. Arterial contrast injection demonstrates systemic arteriovenous fistulae. Systemic venous or pulmonary artery injection of contrast demonstrates pulmonary arteriovenous malformations. Ultrasonography, computed tomography, MRI, and angiography may be useful in finding and delineating the lesion.

TREATMENT

Malformations causing congestive heart failure usually do not spontaneously improve, except for capillary malformations that may respond to steroid or antiangiogenic drugs such as interferon. Large vessel malformations require mechanical occlusion. Surgery carries a considerable risk, and transcatheter occlusion with a variety of devices, including coils and detachable balloons, has been successful in many, usually older patients.

CYANOTIC LESIONS

The differential diagnosis of cyanotic heart disease includes many disorders (Table 33-12). Lesions usually associated with normal or decreased pulmonary flow include the tetralogy of Fallot, pulmonary stenosis, tricuspid atresia, pulmonary atresia with intact ventricular septum, and Ebstein disease. Cyanotic lesions usually associated with increased pulmonary vascular markings include D-transposition of the great arteries, hypoplastic left heart syndrome, total anomalous pulmonary veins, truncus arteriosus, single ventricle, and malpositions.

TABLE 33–12
DIFFERENTIAL DIAGNOSIS OF CYANOTIC HEART DISEASE

Diagnosis	Physical Examination	Radiographic Findings	Electrocardiographic Findings
Hypoplastic left heart syndrome	Single S_2, ↑ respiratory work, ↓ pulse amplitude, ↓ perfusion, +/− SRM	↑ Pulmonary arterial markings, cardiomegaly	↓ LV force usually, develops RAE, RAD, RVH
Transposition of great arteries (IVS, VSD)*	Split S_2, +/− murmur, +/− ↑ respiratory work (*i.e.*, peaceful cyanosis)	↑ Pulmonary arterial markings, +/− cardiomegaly with narrow mediastinum (*i.e.*, "egg on a string")	Develops RAE, RAD, RVH
Truncus arteriosus	Split S_2, multiple clicks, soft to loud SEM, +/− DRM, ↑ respiratory work	↑ Pulmonary arterial markings, cardiomegaly	Develops RAE, RAD, BVH
Total anomalous pulmonary venous connection	Narrow S_2 split, +/− murmur, ↑ respiratory work	↑ Pulmonary venous markings, ↑ diffuse interstitial markings	Develops RAE, RAD, RVH
Tricuspid atresia			
Without PS	Split S_2, heave, SRM	↑ Pulmonary arterial markings, cardiomegaly	Left axis deviation
With PS	Single S_2, SEM	↓ Pulmonary arterial markings, +/− cardiomegaly	
Tetralogy of Fallot			
With PS	Single S_2, SEM	+/− ↓ Pulmonary arterial markings, +/− boot-shaped heart	Develops RAE, RAD, RVH
With PA	Single S_2, continuous murmur, LSB back, axillae	↑, ↓ Pulmonary arterial markings and heart size	
Pulmonary stenosis (IVS or SV)	Single S_2, click, SEM	↓ Pulmonary arterial markings	In IVS QRS axis 0°–100°, develops RAE, RAD, RVH
Pulmonary atresia (IVS or SV)	Single S_2, soft SRM	↓ Pulmonary arterial markings	In IVS QRS axis 0–80°, ↓ RV forces, +/− develops Q waves
Persistent pulmonary hypertension	Narrow split or single S_2, ↑ S_2 loudness, +/− SRM	↓ Pulmonary arterial markings, +/− parenchymal infiltrates, +/− cardiomegaly	Develops RAE, RAD, RVH

* Single ventricle is usually associated with transposition of the great arteries, and in the absence of PS or PA, it presents similar to transposition with ventricular septal defects.

+/−, may or may not be present; ↓, decreased; ↑, increased; BVH, biventricular hypertrophy; DRM, diastolic regurgitant murmur; IVS, intact ventricular septum; LSB, left sternal border; LV, left ventricle; PA, pulmonary atresia; PS, pulmonary stenosis; RAD, right axis deviation; RAE, right atrial enlargement; RV, right ventricle; RVH, right ventricular hypertrophy; SEM, systolic ejection murmur; SRM, systolic regurgitant murmur; SV, single ventricle; VSD, ventricular septal defect.

TETRALOGY OF FALLOT

The tetralogy of Fallot is characterized by a large ventricular septal defect and infundibular pulmonary stenosis or pulmonary atresia. The right ventricular infundibulum is hypoplastic and narrow, and right ventricular hypertrophy is evident. There is often considerable valvar pulmonary stenosis, hypoplasia of the pulmonary arteries, a relatively large ascending aorta, and a right aortic arch (25%). In infants with pulmonary atresia, pulmonary perfusion occurs by way of a patent ductus arteriosus or by systemic to pulmonary arterial collateral vessels. Five percent of patients have abnormal coronary distribution that may influence later surgical correction. Tetralogy is one of the most common cyanotic congenital heart lesions presenting in the newborn period (see Tables 33-1 and 33-2) and is occasionally (10%) associated with severe extracardiac malformations.

PATHOPHYSIOLOGY

Depending on the severity of right ventricular outflow obstruction, there may be intracardiac left-to-right or right-to-left shunt and hypoxemia. Pressures equalize between the ventricles through the large septal defect. The amount of pulmonary blood flow depends on the severity of right ventricular outflow obstruction, the systemic vascular resistance, existence of a ductus arteriosus, and the possible presence of systemic to pulmonary arterial collateral supply to the lung. The extent of systemic venous admixture (*i.e.*, right-to-left shunt by way of the septal defect) is directly related to the severity of the pulmonary stenosis and inversely related to the systemic vascular resistance. The peripheral arterial oxygen saturation depends on the amount of venous admixture and the absolute pulmonary flow (Fig. 33-10). For example, in pulmonary atresia with a ventricular septal defect, the entire right heart output passes right to left through the ventricular defect, and pulmonary flow is supplied by a ductus arteriosus or collateral vessels and is usually less than normal. Cyanosis is the result. If the newborn has large aortopulmonary collateral vessels perfusing the lung, pulmonary blood flow may be large, and the infant may be barely cyanotic and rarely may have congestive heart failure.

Tetralogy of Fallot is a progressive lesion. Twenty-five percent of patients are clinically cyanotic at birth, 75% are affected by 1 year, and by 20 years of age, almost all have become cyanotic. Infundibular hypoplasia and stenosis is progressive, and with time, complete atresia can occur. A patent ductus arteriosus usually closes within the first week of life, resulting in severe and often sudden hypoxemia or cyanotic spells.

Hypoxemia, particularly of rapid onset such as during a hyperpneic spell secondary to a temper tantrum with infundibular spasm, to systemic vasodilation after meal or bath, or to constriction of a ductus arteriosus, may initiate a fall in systemic vascular resistance, metabolic acidosis, and further hypoxemia and hyperpnea. Hyperventilatory compensation for the metabolic acidosis may be ineffective because of inadequate pulmonary blood flow. The self-aggravating cycle of increasing hypoxemia and metabolic acidosis can produce coma and convulsions.

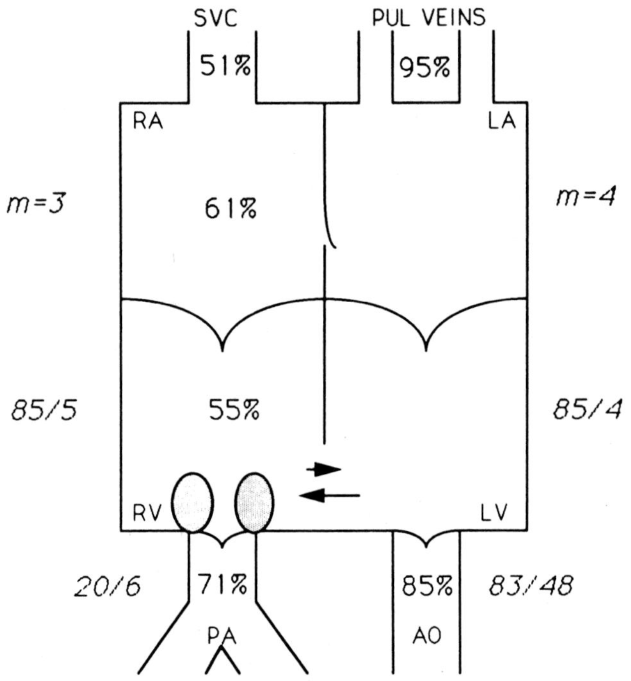

FIG. 33–10. This 4-year-old girl had mild cyanosis and a loud murmur audible at birth. She was found to have tetralogy of Fallot and was followed without medication. After recording the data above, she underwent successful repair. The percentages indicate oxygen saturation; the numbers in italics are pressure measurements.

CLINICAL FINDINGS

Various degrees of cyanosis and mild tachypnea are often observed soon after delivery. If hypoxemia is severe, the infant may be hypotonic and hypotensive with a slow heart rate. Hyperpneic spells characterized by a sudden onset of irritability, hyperpnea, and increasing cyanosis may develop. Spells may end in a loss of consciousness, seizures, cerebral injury, hemiparesis, or death. The disappearance of a previously heard right ventricular outflow systolic murmur with increased cyanosis suggests a spell and constitutes an indication for immediate therapy.

There is a systolic murmur at the left sternal border, and the second heart sound is single. In a newborn with pulmonary atresia, the systolic murmur is absent; there may be a constant apical systolic ejection click and prominent continuous murmurs of a patent ductus arteriosus or aortopulmonary collaterals, audible at the base, in the axillae, or over the back. A patent ductus arteriosus usually does not cause continuous murmur in the first months of life; therefore, the presence of murmurs with cyanosis and a single S_2 in a neonate strongly suggests tetralogy of Fallot with pulmonary atresia. Delay in height, weight, and skeletal maturation is common, but some infants flourish despite severe hypoxemia. Some young infants with the anatomic but acyanotic tetralogy of Fallot experience congestive heart failure, later recovering from congestion and becoming cyanotic. Rarely, congestive heart failure is seen in an infant with pulmonary atresia and very large aortopulmonary collaterals. Although subacute bacterial endocarditis and brain abscess are common in older children with tetralogy of Fallot, these complications are extremely rare in infancy. However, spontaneous cerebrovascular accidents are common, particularly in infants with severe hypoxemia and relative anemia (<6–8 g/dL of oxyhemoglobin).

The chest radiograph shows a normal-sized heart, sometimes with right ventricular enlargement resulting in an upturned apex and an absent or diminished main pulmonary artery segment (*i.e.*, boot-shaped heart), diminution of the pulmonary vasculature, and in 25%, the aorta arching to the right. The ECG demonstrates right axis deviation, right atrial hypertrophy, and right ventricular hypertrophy, but at birth, it may be difficult to differentiate from normally prominent right ventricular forces. The echocardiogram shows anterior, leftward deviation of the infundibular septum, creating subpulmonary stenosis and a malalignment ventricular septal defect with a large overriding aortic root (Fig. 33-11). Additional ventricular or atrial septal defects, central pulmonary artery hypoplasia, and coronary artery anatomy can often be assessed by echocardiography but may require cardiac catheterization. Determining the possible presence of distal pulmonary artery stenosis and the anatomy of systemic arterial to pulmonary arterial collaterals requires angiography.

TREATMENT

Treatment depends on the severity of the lesion. The newborn with tetralogy of Fallot and little or mild cyanosis should be carefully observed and repeated transcutaneous measurements of systemic oxygen saturation made until a stable level is apparent. Hyperpneic spells should be treated with oxygen, intramuscular or subcutaneous morphine sulfate (0.1 mg/kg), intravenous administration of saline boluses and sodium bicarbonate (approximately 1 mmol/kg), and if needed, phenylephrine (0.1 mg/kg subcutaneously; 5–20 μg/kg by intravenous bolus; 0.1–0.5 μg/kg/minute by intravenous infusion) titrated to elevate systemic vascular resistance and pressure. Prostaglandin E_1 may open a ductus arteriosus in the cyanotic newborn infant and improve pulmonary perfusion. Propranolol may be of some value in treating the infant with a reactive infundibulum. The hemoglobin concentration should be maintained high enough to permit adequate oxygen transport. The occurrence of a single hyperpneic spell is an indication for surgery, possibly as an emergency procedure.

In the past, critically ill infants who required surgery underwent palliative procedures, usually a shunt between the subclavian artery and branch pulmonary artery (*i.e.*, Blalock–Taussig). The shunt was ligated during a reparative operation when the child was older. Infants with uncomplicated tetralogy of Fallot requiring surgery now undergo one-stage reparative procedures with excellent results. The right ventricular outflow tract is enlarged with a pericardial patch, and the ventricular septal defect is closed with a Dacron patch. There are several potential sequelae, including late dysrhythmias, but most patients with uncomplicated tetralogy of Fallot have an asymptomatic long-term course. Those with anomalous origin of the left anterior descending coronary from the right coronary artery and those with pulmonary atresia and hypoplastic distorted pulmonary arteries may

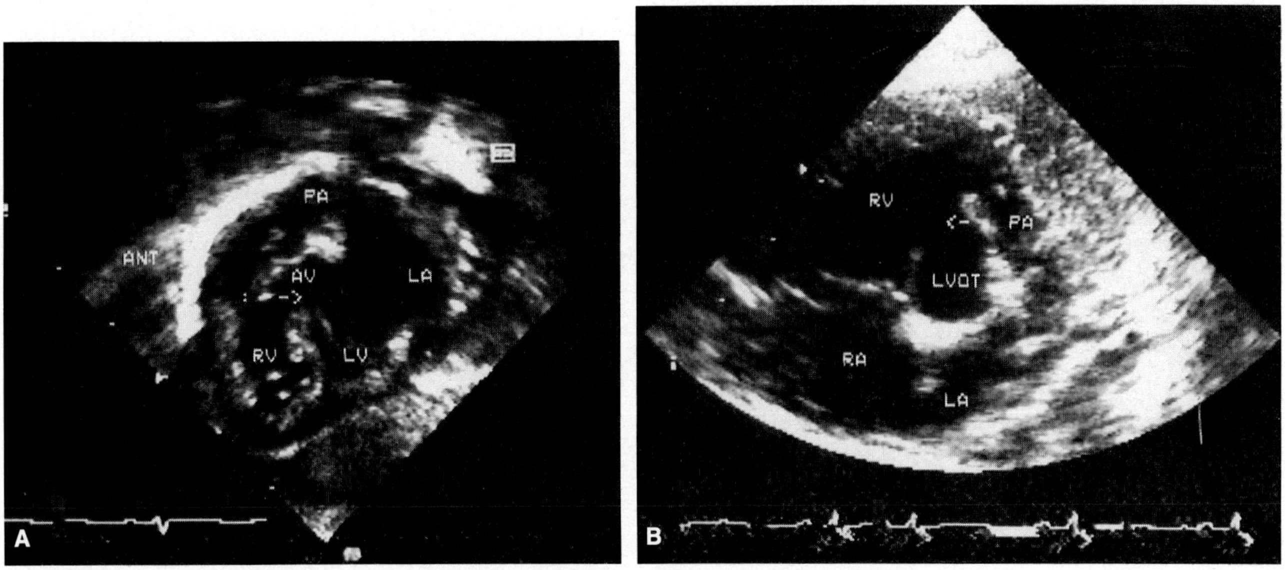

FIG. 33–11. Echocardiographic **(A)** subxiphoid and **(B)** parasternal short axis views of an infant with tetralogy of Fallot. Anterior deviation of the conal septum (*above the arrow*) is associated with malalignment ventricular septal defect and obstruction of the right ventricular outflow. (→, ventricular septal defect; :, narrowed right ventricular outflow; ANT, anterior; AV, aortic valve; LA, left atrium; LV, left ventricle; LVOT, left ventricular outflow tract; PA, pulmonary artery; RA, right atrium; RV, right venticle.)

require a palliative shunt with a more definitive repair, entailing a conduit from the right ventricle to the pulmonary artery when the child is older.

In general, the earlier severe hypoxemia develops, the more severe is the tetralogy of Fallot and the poorer the prognosis without surgery. The overall mortality rate without surgery is approximately 35% by 1 year of age.

DIFFERENTIAL DIAGNOSIS

The features of cyanosis, a harsh systolic ejection murmur, chest radiographic findings of diminished pulmonary vasculature with a normal-sized heart, and ECG evidence of right ventricular hypertrophy are characteristic of tetralogy of Fallot (see Table 33-12). The same findings with a continuous murmur suggest tetralogy of Fallot with pulmonary atresia. A few infants with tetralogy of Fallot and an underdeveloped pulmonary valve present with a characteristic to-and-fro murmur (*i.e.*, steam engine sound) and severe respiratory distress caused by bronchial or tracheal compression by aneurysmally dilated pulmonary arteries.

PULMONARY STENOSIS

Pulmonary stenosis is probably the most common form of congenital heart disease discovered by hearing a murmur. The abnormality is often a narrowing of the proximal pulmonary artery branches though minor obstructions at the pulmonary valve are equally common. Even minimal obstruction (<10 torr across the obstruction) produces a readily audible murmur, frequently resulting in a request for an echocardiogram. Rarely, valvar obstruction is severe enough to require intervention. Symptomatic peripheral pulmonary stenosis is rare and is usually associated with other problems, such as tetralogy of Fallot, Williams syndrome, and infants born of mothers with rubella.

The common valvar and proximal peripheral pulmonary artery obstructions are usually mild and can be located by echocardiography. Infundibular (*i.e.*, subvalvar) obstruction as an isolated lesion is rare; its presence usually indicates an associated ventricular defect. Severe valvar obstruction may occur with cyanosis (Fig. 33-12) because of right-to-left shunting through a foramen ovale or may present with the findings of right-sided congestive heart failure. If the obstruction is severe, the valve is immobile, and there is dilation and hypertrophy of the right ventricle; the velocity measured across the pulmonary valve by Doppler technique indicates a high pressure gradient.

Only reassurance and observation are required for the mild stenoses because progressive obstruction is rare. Moderate obstructions in early infancy become progressively worse with growth, and the patients should be periodically examined with this in mind.

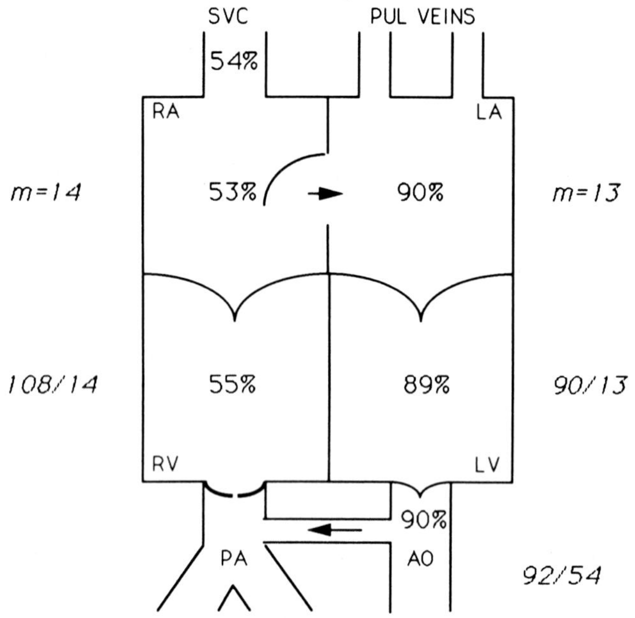

FIG. 33–12. This 3-day-old baby had cyanosis from birth. There was no murmur. At cardiac catheterization, the pulmonary valve was atretic. At surgery, a tiny orifice was found, and a valvotomy was done. The cyanosis resolved in 3 weeks, and at 5 years of age, balloon valvoplasty reduced the remaining pulmonary valve gradient to normal. The percentages indicate oxygen saturation; the numbers in italics are pressure measurements.

The severe obstructions are relieved by catheter balloon dilation or surgery. Bacterial endocarditis is rare, but the administration of antibiotics for prophylaxis prior to the procedure is recommended.

TRICUSPID ATRESIA

Tricuspid atresia is a relatively uncommon disease that is characterized by absence of the tricuspid valve. Except in rare cases, no valve exists, and tricuspid agenesis is therefore a more precise description of this anomaly.

PATHOPHYSIOLOGY

The entire systemic venous return (*i.e.*, cardiac output) enters the right atrium and exits through the foramen ovale to the left heart. The systemic and pulmonary venous streams are mixed in the left atrium. After passage to the left ventricle, the cardiac output passes to the aorta, and an amount equal to the pulmonary flow gains access to the pulmonary artery through a ventricular septal defect, a diminutive right ventricle, and various degrees of pulmonary stenosis. Flow to the pulmonary artery is limited by the size of the ventricular defect or the amount of pulmonary stenosis. Occasionally, the great vessels are transposed, with the aorta arising from the right ventricle, and the systemic output may be limited by the size of the ventricular defect. The level of cyanosis is determined by the amount of pulmonary blood flow. In early infancy, the pulmonary blood flow can be increased by a patent ductus arteriosus and subsequent Blalock–Taussig shunt. The ultimate goal is to provide the connections for Fontan physiology. Several methods of connecting the systemic venous return directly to the pulmonary arteries are used. In effect, the pulmonary circulation is supplied by passive flow, bypassing the heart. The normal postnatal elevation in pulmonary vascular resistance prevents this from being successful in young infants. In older children, these operations are surprisingly successful and last many years, although just how long remains to be determined.

CLINICAL FINDINGS

The babies are discovered to have cyanosis during the first months of life. Some have a systolic murmur; diastolic murmurs are rare. On chest radiographs, the heart is usually of normal size or minimally enlarged, and the pulmonary vasculature is diminished. Unlike most other cyanotic lesions, the ECG shows a leftward superior axis similar to endocardial cushion defects (see Fig. 33-10) but usually with diminished right precordial forces. The diagnosis is readily confirmed by echocardiographic identification of a diminutive right ventricle, an absent tricuspid valve, and right-to-left flow through the foramen ovale.

TREATMENT

Infants with severe obstruction of blood flow through the ventricular septal defect and right ventricle may require infusion of prostaglandin E_1 prior to palliative surgery. A shunt from an aortic branch to pulmonary artery allows an excessively cyanotic infant to grow. Sometime after the age of 1 to 3 years, variations on the Fontan operation are possible. About 75% of infants with tricuspid atresia survive with Fontan physiology.

Rarely, in an infant with a large ventricular defect and no pulmonary stenosis, the pulmonary blood flow may be excessive enough to cause congestive heart failure. Anticongestive medications are usually sufficient to allow growth, although a pulmonary artery banding procedure may be necessary to diminish pulmonary vascular pressure and resistance.

PULMONARY ATRESIA WITH INTACT VENTRICULAR SEPTUM

When the pulmonary valve is atretic and there is no ventricular septal defect, blood cannot pass through the right ventricle in the fetus, and the right ventricle cavity is frequently coarsely trabeculated and the size of a prune pit. There is membranous pulmonary valvar atresia and, in approximately one-third of the cases, associated infundibular stenosis, hypoplasia or atresia. The tricuspid valve annulus is small and may be stenotic or incompetent. There are often fistulous tracts connecting the right ventricular sinus to the distal coronary arteries, commonly with proximal coronary artery stenosis and myocardial fibrosis. The pulmonary arteries are of adequate size and are perfused through a patent ductus arteriosus or rarely through aortopulmonary collaterals. An interatrial communication is essential to survival. Pulmonary atresia with an intact ventricular septum is rarely associated with other cardiovascular or somatic malformations.

PATHOPHYSIOLOGY

The major hemodynamic consequences of pulmonary atresia with intact septum is the obligatory right-to-left passage of the total systemic venous return through the foramen ovale to the left atrium. A patent ductus arteriosus provides the only entrance to the pulmonary circulation. As it closes, pulmonary perfusion is greatly reduced and results in severe hypoxemia, metabolic acidosis, and death. The right ventricle, despite its severe hypoplasia and poor compliance, usually generates suprasystemic pressures. This is probably true *in utero* as well, and explains the frequent tricuspid incompetence with right atrial enlargement and the development of fistulae that drain blood from the right ventricle into the coronary artery.

Surgical establishment of continuity between the right ventricle and the pulmonary artery may result in sufficient decompression of the right ventricle to cause hypoperfusion of coronary beds supplied by fistulae from the right ventricle to coronary artery. There is often proximal coronary artery obstruction, in which case right ventricular decompression may reduce coronary blood flow enough to produce myocardial infarction. The size of the infarct and its impact directly correlate with the area of distribution of the coronary vessel involved.

CLINICAL FINDINGS

Most infants with pulmonary atresia are critically ill within the first week of life because of severe hypoxemia. With postnatal ductal constriction, severe cyanosis, hypotension, bradycardia, hypotonia, and marked acidosis occur. Signs of right-sided failure may develop but are usually absent. The precordium is quiet, and there is no thrill. S_2 is single, and there is often a pansystolic murmur of tricuspid incompetence. On the chest radiograph, the heart may appear mildly enlarged, the lung fields are ischemic, and the aortic arch is on the left (Fig. 33-13). The ECG usually reveals a QRS axis in the frontal plane between 0° and 80°, absent or diminished right ventricular forces, and a pattern of left ventricular hypertrophy.

An echocardiogram shows normal or somewhat enlarged left-sided structures, a small tricuspid valve

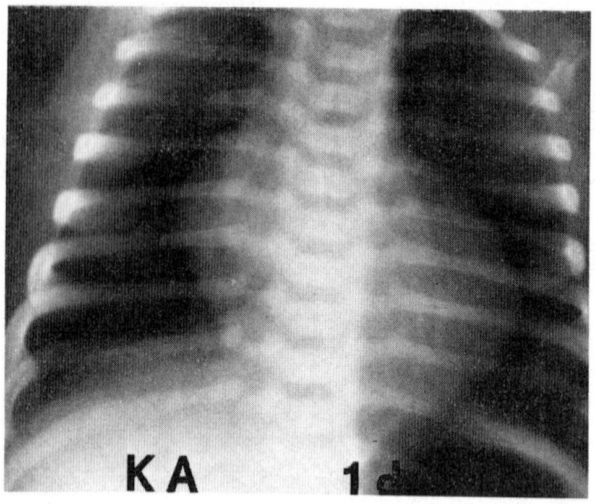

FIG. 33–13. A chest radiograph shows decreased pulmonary vascularity and mild cardiomegaly in a 1-day-old infant with pulmonary atresia and an intact ventricular septum.

and right ventricle, and atresia of the pulmonary valve. If there is membranous atresia of the pulmonary valve, the membrane moves like a true valve, and the diagnosis cannot be made with certainty without a Doppler flow examination. Color Doppler can help to delineate fistulas between the right ventricle and the coronary arteries. After the presumptive diagnosis is made, prostaglandins can be given to dilate the ductus arteriosus and increase pulmonary blood flow. There should be rapid improvement in oxygenation and relief of acidosis. Cardiac catheterization is indicated as soon as the diagnosis is made. Selective ventriculography and ascending aortography to delineate the coronary arteries are essential for planning surgery.

TREATMENT

After stabilization with prostaglandins, the treatment of choice is surgery, which is indicated as soon as feasible after the anatomy is established by catheterization. For infants with an adequately sized right ventricle, pulmonary valvotomy or valvectomy is performed. Some infants may require placement of a patch across the right ventricular outflow tract and valve annulus for adequate relief of obstruction. In infants with severe right ventricular hypoplasia and a noncompliant right ventricle, a systemic-to-pulmonary shunt also may be necessary for relief of hypoxemia. After a period during which the right ventricular capacity and compliance improves and the pulmonary vascular resistance decreases, these infants may no longer require shunts for maintenance of adequate pulmonary blood flow. Even infants with initially diminutive right ventricular chambers usually demonstrate some growth of the chamber if flow through the ventricle is provided by establishing continuity between the right ventricle and pulmonary artery. The right ventricle cannot be decompressed in infants who have fistulas between the right ventricle and coronary arteries and stenoses involving at least two separate proximal coronary vessels, without risk of fatal infarction. These infants may require a staged approach with an initial neonatal shunt and a later Fontan-type cavopulmonary anastomosis or transplantation. Without therapy, the malformation is usually fatal, and with surgical treatment, about 75% of these newborns survive to 1 year of age.

DIFFERENTIAL DIAGNOSIS

Pulmonary atresia with an intact septum should be differentiated from others causing severe cyanosis in the first week of life (see Table 33-12). Tetralogy of Fallot or pulmonary atresia with a ventricular septal defect and transposition of the great arteries with an intact ventricular septum are associated with ECG evidence of right ventricular hypertrophy. Infants with tricuspid atresia or endocardial cushion defect and pulmonary stenosis have a superior frontal plane axis on the ECG. Critical valvar pulmonary stenosis is accompanied by a systolic ejection murmur, congestive heart failure, moderate or marked cardiac enlargement, and right ventricular hypertrophy. Critical pulmonary stenosis with a diminutive right ventricle can be delineated by echocardiography. In Ebstein anomaly of the tricuspid valve, the precordium is quiet, and cardiac enlargement is severe (Fig. 33-14).

EBSTEIN DISEASE

Examples of Ebstein disease are encountered rarely in the newborn period. The septal leaflet of the tricuspid valve is displaced downward and adheres to the ventricular septum to various degrees. The result is a spectrum of dysfunctioning tricuspid valves that are regurgitant and sometimes stenotic. The dysfunction is compounded by the fact that the right atrium and right ventricle contract at different times, and there is an area of atrialized ventricle or ventricularized atrium, depending on the point of view. This discordant pumping of parts of each chamber contributes to the dysfunction. Those with severe prenatal tricuspid regurgitation often have massive cardiomegaly and may have pulmonary hypoplasia. The effective right ventricular volume is reduced, and there is limited passage of blood through the right ventricle. Some blood escapes through the PFO, causing cyanosis. The severity of the defect can be described by the degree of cyanosis that, in the newborn period, can be severe because of the concomitant unresolved elevation of the pulmonary vascular resistance left over from fetal life. As the newborn's pulmonary vascular resistance regresses, the cyanosis often improves, sometimes markedly, although babies with severe regurgitation and pulmonary hypoplasia have a high mortality rate. After surviving the newborn period, the course is determined by the degree of abnormality; some patients survive into late adulthood without important limitation, but others remain cyanotic and prone to arrhythmias.

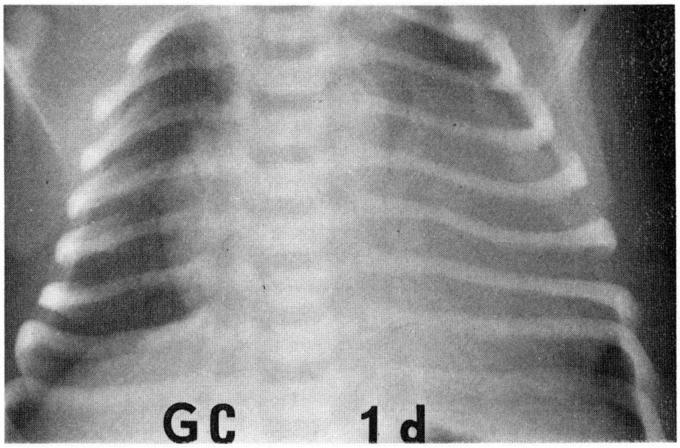

FIG. 33–14. A chest radiograph of a 1-day-old cyanotic infant with Ebstein anomaly of the tricuspid valve shows marked cardiomegaly.

Ebstein disease is recognized because of minimal systolic or diastolic murmurs, extra heart sounds, absent to severe cyanosis, and cardiomegaly that may vary from minimal to some of the largest hearts encountered in the newborn period (see Fig. 33-14). The diagnosis is established by echocardiography. Treatment is usually supportive. The pediatrician can recognize that the degree of displacement of the tricuspid valve may be so slight that the diagnosis becomes a matter of definition, which is not firmly established for this rare disease. The diagnosis of mild Ebstein disease may be erroneous and is of no known importance.

D-TRANSPOSITION OF THE GREAT ARTERIES

With transposition of the great arteries, the aorta arises from and above the right ventricle and the pulmonary artery from the left ventricle. In the commonest form, D-transposition, the aorta is anterior to and to the right of the pulmonary artery, rather than in its normal rightward and posterior position.

Transposition of the great arteries is one of the commonest congenital heart lesions presenting in the newborn period (see Tables 33-1 and 33-2) and is a frequent cause of death among unoperated neonates with congenital heart disease. The male–female ratio is 1.8:1, and the average birth weight is greater than that for other patients with congenital heart disease, although not for the general population. Transposition is frequently associated with other cardiac abnormalities, including ventricular septal defect, patent ductus arteriosus, hypoplastic right ventricle, and coarctation.

PATHOPHYSIOLOGY

The systemic and pulmonary circulations are normally in series with each other, but in complete transposition, the circulations are in parallel. Systemic venous blood returns to the right atrium, enters the right ventricle, and exits through the aorta. Pulmonary venous blood, coming from the lung, enters the left atrium and the left ventricle, and then returns to the pulmonary arteries and the lungs. Without some communication between the pulmonary and systemic circulations, survival is impossible; oxygenated blood cannot be delivered to the systemic circulation, nor can systemic venous blood pick up oxygen in the lung. An atrial communication, ventricular defect, or patent ductus arteriosus, singly or in combination, may provide for mixing between the circulations (Fig. 33-15). The foramen ovale and ductus arteriosus,

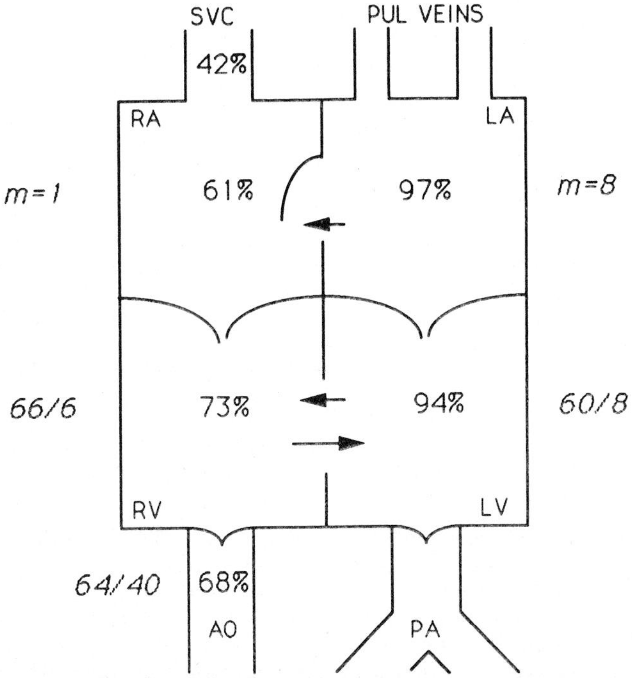

FIG. 33–15. Transposition of the great arteries with a single membranous ventricular septal defect in a 1-month-old baby who had mild cyanosis and controlled congestive heart failure. There is equilibration of pressure between the ventricles and elevation of left-sided diastolic pressures. After balloon septostomy, the arterial saturation rose to 75%. The percentages indicate oxygen saturation; the numbers in italics are pressure measurements.

both normally patent in the fetus, usually close soon after birth. Infants with transposition and intact ventricular septum become extremely cyanotic within the first few hours or days after delivery, as closure of the foramen ovale and ductus arteriosus occurs and mixing between the circulations diminishes (Fig. 33-16). The severe hypoxemia may lead to metabolic acidosis. Survival depends on prompt supportive medical care and reestablishment of patency of the ductus arteriosus and interatrial communication to improve mixing and oxygenation.

Infants born with transposition and a large ventricular septal defect are less cyanotic because the ventricular defect allows mixing. These babies may not be recognized in the newborn period but appear in subsequent months with congestive failure. The combination of a large pulmonary flow, pulmonary hypertension, and elevation of left atrial pressure leads to the development of congestive heart failure (see Fig. 33-15) and later pulmonary vascular obstructive disease. Anatomic changes during the first few months of life may result in important hemodynamic changes. A large ventricular septal defect may spontaneously diminish in size or close, reducing mixing and increasing hypoxemia. Increasing pulmonary stenosis may decrease pulmonary flow, and thereby improve congestive heart failure. Atrial septal defects created by balloon septostomy and those made by surgical septectomy may spontaneously diminish in size or close.

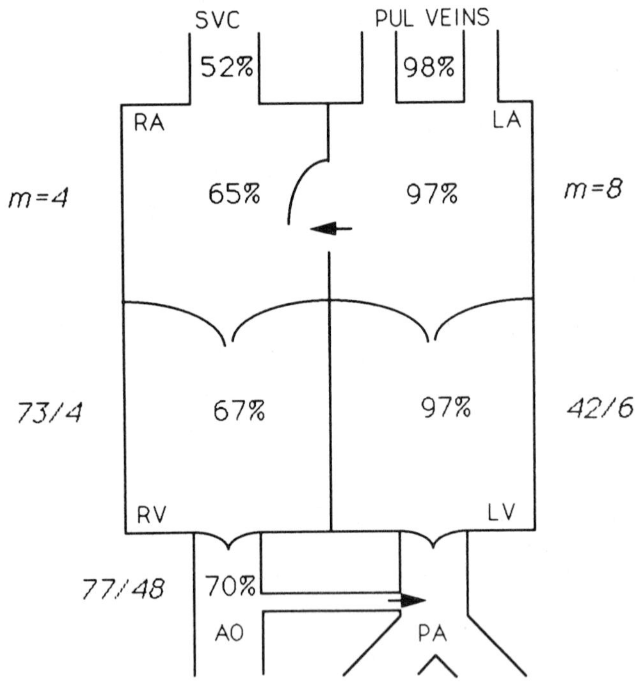

FIG. 33–16. Transposition with intact ventricular septum in a 1-day-old girl who was cyanotic at birth. At catheterization, she had less than systemic pressure in the left (*i.e.*, pulmonary) ventricle. The patent ductus arteriosus shunts blood into the pulmonary circuit, and the foramen ovale shunts an equal amount out of the pulmonary circuit. If this were not the case, blood would pile up on one side of the circulation in a matter of minutes. If the ductus spontaneously closed, the infant's condition would become precarious. If the ductus were dilated with prostaglandins, the infant would become pinker but might experience respiratory difficulty because of excess pulmonary flow. The percentages indicate oxygen saturation; the numbers in italics are pressure measurements.

CLINICAL FINDINGS

In infants with an intact ventricular septum, cyanosis accompanied by mild tachypnea develops soon after birth. Often the infants, though tachypneic, do not seem distressed (*i.e.*, peaceful cyanosis). The cardiac examination, chest radiograph, and ECG may be normal. The heart sounds are normal, and there may be no significant murmur. The ECG may show some excessive right ventricular forces.

On a plain chest radiograph, the heart and pulmonary vascularity may be initially normal, although at a few weeks of age, cardiac enlargement, a narrow mediastinum, and pulmonary plethora are detected. One of the most important diagnostic tests is the determination of arterial partial pressure of oxygen (PaO_2) in room air and after the inhalation of 100% oxygen for a 10-minute period. Failure of the PaO_2 (often <30 torr) to rise significantly is strong presumptive evidence for complete transposition. Failure to raise systemic arterial O_2 tension significantly is due to inadequate mixing between the pulmonary and systemic circulations. Subcostal echocardiography reveals that the great artery arising from the left ventricle has an abnormal superior course and then bifurcates into the right and left pulmonary artery. The right ventricle gives rise to a great artery that passes relatively straight superiorly to the posterior arching aorta (Fig. 33-17). The patency of the foramen ovale and ductus arteriosus and the coronary anatomy can be assessed.

An infant with transposition and a large ventricular septal defect usually presents with congestive failure and mild cyanosis between 3 to 6 weeks of age. Poor weight gain, tachypnea, and excessive diaphoresis are evident, and wheezing is common. A loud S_3 may produce a gallop rhythm, and there is a loud systolic murmur at the lower left sternal border, often associated with a mid-diastolic flow rumble. Rales may be audible in the lungs. The ECG reveals right axis deviation and right atrial and right ventricular hypertrophy. Infrequently, if the right ventricle is hypoplastic, right ventricular forces may be absent or reduced, and left ventricular hypertrophy is observed. The chest radiograph characteristically shows considerable cardiomegaly and pulmonary plethora. Echocardiography should identify the location of the ventricular septal defect and its relation to the great arteries and the atrioventricular valves and complex associated problems, including straddling or abnormal tri-

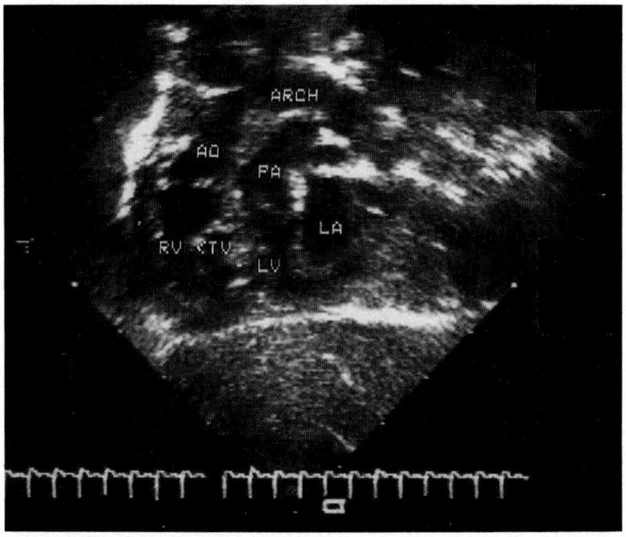

FIG. 33–17. Echocardiographic subxiphoid view of a neonate with transposition of the great arteries. (AO aorta; ARCH, aortic arch; LA, left atrium; LV, left ventricle; PA, pulmonary artery; RV, right ventricle; < TV, tricuspid valve.)

cuspid valve, hypoplastic right ventricle, valvar or subvalvar pulmonary stenosis, coarctation of the aorta, juxtaposition of the atrial appendages, and anomalous systemic or pulmonary venous drainage.

TREATMENT

After the diagnosis of transposition and intact ventricular septum is established by echocardiography, cardiac catheterization is scheduled. Infusion of prostaglandin E_1 to open and maintain patency of the ductus arteriosus may improve mixing and systemic oxygenation. Because prostaglandin E_1 may cause apnea and vasodilation, support with mechanical ventilation, volume infusion, and sometimes inotropic agents may be required. Some babies require, and most do better with, a widely open atrial defect. Balloon atrial septostomy usually results in considerable clinical improvement. The anatomy of the coronary arteries and associated lesions may also be established by catheterization. Echocardiography is also used and advocated by many. The type of surgical procedure employed depends on the associated cardiac defects. In recent years, there has been renewed interest in "anatomic repair" or arterial switch operations in neonates with uncomplicated transposition.[33,34] The aorta and pulmonary arteries are transected and the distal vessels rejoined to provide normal physiologic connections. A button of proximal aortic tissue surrounding each coronary artery origin is cut, and both coronaries with the surrounding aortic button are attached to the neoaorta. Although short-term results are similar to the Senning or Mustard atrial switch operations, midterm results suggest that it is superior to the atrial baffle procedures that have long-term difficulties with tricuspid valve and right ventricular function and dysrhythmias. Atrial baffle procedures are still used if there is difficult intracardiac or coronary anatomy.

Without therapy, 95% of infants born with transpositions die within 1 year. With aggressive medical and surgical treatment, mortality has been reduced to less than 10%.

DIFFERENTIAL DIAGNOSIS

Most infants with transposition and intact ventricular septum are readily recognized as cyanotic infants without significant murmurs and little respiratory distress. The diagnosis of transposition of the great arteries is rarely difficult and is confused only if other abnormalities, such as straddling tricuspid valve, hypoplastic right ventricle, coarctation of the aorta, or pulmonary stenosis, exist (see Table 33-12). Depending on the type and severity of the associated cardiac malformations, the clinical symptoms and findings in infants with complicated transposition of the great arteries may closely resemble those of almost any other cyanotic heart lesion.

The clinical picture in infants with transposition of the great arteries, ventricular septal defect, and pulmonary stenosis or atresia is virtually indistinguishable from that of tetralogy of Fallot or pulmonary atresia with a ventricular septal defect. If D-transposition of the great arteries is associated with a large ventricular septal defect and limited cyanosis, it is sometimes mistaken for other lesions with a large left-to-right shunt, such as a ventricular septal defect with normal aortic root or total anomalous pulmonary venous return without obstruction. The absence of cyanosis identifies the former, and echocardiography can differentiate all of these anomalies.

HYPOPLASTIC LEFT HEART SYNDROME

The hypoplastic left heart syndrome encompasses a variety of specific cardiovascular malformations producing similar hemodynamic and clinical manifestations, including aortic atresia, mitral atresia, premature closure of the foramen ovale, hypoplastic left ventricle with critical mitral stenosis, and aortic stenosis. Some cases of severe complex coarctation are also included in this category. The left heart chamber is usually very small, and endocardial fibroelastosis is common. Hypoplastic left heart syndrome occurs in 10.2% of infants with serious heart disease and is one of the most common lesions presenting in the first week of life (see Tables 33-2 and 33-6). It is less common in very premature infants (<1.85 kg). It is usually an isolated lesion, although it has been described in association with autosomal trisomy syndromes and in infants of diabetic mothers. Familial cases occur.

PATHOPHYSIOLOGY

Obstruction or atresia of the mitral or aortic valves limits or prevents flow through the left heart. The systemic venous return enters the right heart and is ejected into the pulmonary artery. The systemic circulation is largely or totally supplied by right-to-left flow through the ductus arteriosus. Blood traversing the lung enters the left atrium, flows through an interatrial defect or dilated PFO, and returns to the right atrium to join the incoming systemic venous return. Complete mixing takes place in the right atrium, with similar oxygen saturation measured in the right ventricle, pulmonary artery, and aorta. With little or no egress through the left heart, pulmonary flow must pass left-to-right through an interatrial communication. Any limitation of flow through the atrial septum produces pulmonary venous hypertension.

The maintenance of adequate systemic circulation requires patency of the ductus arteriosus. In aortic atresia, the ascending aorta, brachiocephalic vessels, and coronary arteries are perfused in a retrograde fashion with blood originating from the patent ductus arteriosus. Spontaneous constriction of the ductus results in low systemic blood flow, poor coronary perfusion, congestive failure, and shock with simultaneous flooding of the pulmonary circulation. Closure of the ductus leads to immediate death because of poor perfusion, metabolic acidosis, electrolyte imbalance, and coagulation abnormalities.

CLINICAL FINDINGS

These infants become symptomatic within the first week of life. Congestive failure and a shocklike picture may develop precipitously. The baby becomes ashen gray with poor peripheral perfusion, and all pulses are weak. Ductal constriction may be intermittent, with femoral pulses intermittently palpable. Symptoms and signs of congestive failure are associated with hypotension and, terminally, with bradycardia. S_2 is usually single, and a gallop is heard. The chest radiograph shows cardiac enlargement and pulmonary plethora, and the ECG usually demonstrates right axis deviation, right atrial hypertrophy, right ventricular hypertrophy, and markedly diminished or absent left ventricular forces. The diagnosis can be made with echocardiography by demonstrating a very small or unrecognizable left ventricle. The ascending aorta is small with retrograde flow in cases of aortic atresia, and there is frequently a discrete juxtaductal coarctation.

TREATMENT

Without surgery, the mortality rate is 98% by 1 year of age. There are a few survivors with mitral atresia or hypoplasia of the left ventricle with severe aortic or mitral stenosis. Advances in cardiac surgery have encouraged several approaches to infants with this condition. Palliative surgery can be performed in the newborn period after stabilization with prostaglandin E_1, inotropic agents, volume infusion, and bicarbonate. Hyperventilation (*i.e.*, arterial partial pressure of carbon dioxide [$PaCO_2$] < 40 torr) and unnecessary supplemental oxygen administration should be avoided, because these measures may lead to a decrease in pulmonary vascular resistance and preferential flow of the right ventricular output into the pulmonary vascular bed instead of across the ductus to the systemic vasculature, worsening the shock.

Surgical therapy consists of an attempt to convert the circulation to Fontan-type physiology or to transplant a new heart. A first-stage procedure anastomoses the transected main pulmonary artery to the aortic arch, ligates the ductus arteriosus, supplies perfusion to the distal oversewn pulmonary artery by creation of a modified Blalock–Taussig or direct central systemic to pulmonary artery shunt, and leaves an atrial septectomy to allow unimpeded pulmonary venous return to the right atrium. The long-term outlook depends on the ability of the right ventricle to support the systemic circulation while the pulmonary circulation is supplied relatively directly with systemic venous return through a cavopulmonary anastomosis at a second-stage Fontan-type procedure.[35] The perinatal and first-stage surgical mortality rate is between 25% and 40%, and overall during the first 5 years, it is as high as 50% to 75%. Long-range survival is undetermined.

Cardiac transplantation has been used as an alternative approach with good survival, but there is limited timely availability of neonatal donors and limited documentation of long-range survival.[36]

Neither reconstructive surgery leading to a Fontan procedure or cardiac transplantation can be viewed as curative. Both methods of treatment have high fiscal and emotional costs (see Chap. 34).

DIFFERENTIAL DIAGNOSIS

The clinical picture of the hypoplastic left heart syndrome may be simulated by respiratory distress syndrome, interrupted aortic arch, severe complex coarctation, early neonatal myocarditis, isolated critical valvar aortic stenosis, sepsis or some inherited metabolic disorders (see Table 33-12).

TOTAL ANOMALOUS PULMONARY VEINS

In the event of failure to connect the common pulmonary vein to the left atrium in the embryo, communications are established with available systemic venous channels that then drain the pulmonary veins. Anatomically abnormal drainage may be supracardiac (*i.e.*, into the right or left superior vena cava), intracardiac (*i.e.*, into the coronary sinus, right atrium), or subdiaphragmatic (*i.e.*, through the inferior vena cava or porta hepatis). Mixed sites of drainage occur in approximately 10% of these patients. A PFO or atrial septal defect is invariably present. Anomalous pulmonary venous return is often associated with heterotaxy.

Although total anomalous venous return accounts for only 2% of newborns with serious cardiac disease (see Table 33-2), it is an important lesion because it is potentially curable and often misdiagnosed as pulmonary disease.

PATHOPHYSIOLOGY

Infants with anomalous pulmonary venous drainage can be divided into two major categories on the basis of the hemodynamic changes produced: those with nonobstructed veins and those with obstructed veins. Nonobstructed pulmonary veins entering the systemic venous circulation or directly into the right heart result in a large left-to-right shunt, congestive heart failure, and pulmonary artery hypertension. Systemic output is maintained through an interatrial communication. Despite the obligatory right-to-left shunt through the atrium, the large pulmonary blood flow mixing with the systemic venous return at the right atrium allows a reasonable peripheral oxygen tension and produces only mild cyanosis.

If pulmonary venous return is obstructed, the circulatory effects are different. The obstruction may take the form of increased resistance to flow produced by a long, common, pulmonary venous channel or localized intrinsic or extrinsic obstruction. Subdiaphragmatic anomalous pulmonary venous return is usually obstructed by constriction of the ductus venosus, obstructing flow into the inferior vena cava (Fig. 33-18). Obstruction to supracardiac pulmonary venous return may occur because of compression of the common pulmonary venous channel between the left primary bronchus and left pulmonary artery or because of narrowing at the entry of the common pulmonary vein into the right superior vena cava. Obstruction at the foramen ovale is uncommon. After birth, significant resistance to flow through the pulmonary veins becomes evident, causing pulmonary venous hypertension, pulmonary edema, marked pulmonary artery hypertension, and severe cyanosis. The arterial oxygen tension is low because the contribution of fully oxygenated blood to the right atrial mixing is less than in the unobstructed form of this disorder.

CLINICAL FINDINGS

Infants with total anomalous pulmonary venous return without significant obstruction usually become symptomatic after the neonatal period, when the pulmonary vascular resistance decreases and a large left-to-right shunt and congestive heart failure develop. They are mildly cyanotic, often have congestive heart failure, and have a large heart revealed on chest radiographs.

Infants with obstructed pulmonary venous return are usually critically ill, cyanotic, and tachypneic within the first week of life. There is congestive heart failure and poor peripheral perfusion. Heart size, as seen on the chest radiograph, is often normal, and there is evidence of pulmonary edema. The clinical and the radiographic pictures may resemble hyaline membrane disease or diffuse pneumonia complicated by PPHN. The ECG shows right axis deviation, right atrial hypertrophy, and right ventricular hypertrophy. The findings on two-dimensional and color Doppler echocardiography include absence of pulmonary venous connections to the left atrium, right-to-left bulging of the interatrial septum, right-to-left interatrial shunt, and pulmonary venous confluence posterior to the left atrium connecting to a systemic venous channel. The diagnosis, especially if there is partial anomalous venous drainage below the diaphragm, may be missed altogether using echocardiography; however, this error is becoming less common with recent advances in instrumentation. The triad of severe cyanosis and a roentgenographic picture of a normal heart size associated with pulmonary edema is characteristic (see Fig. 33-18*A*). Surgical success is related to the anatomy (*e.g.*, results are poorest in the mixed variety) and to the age of onset of symp-

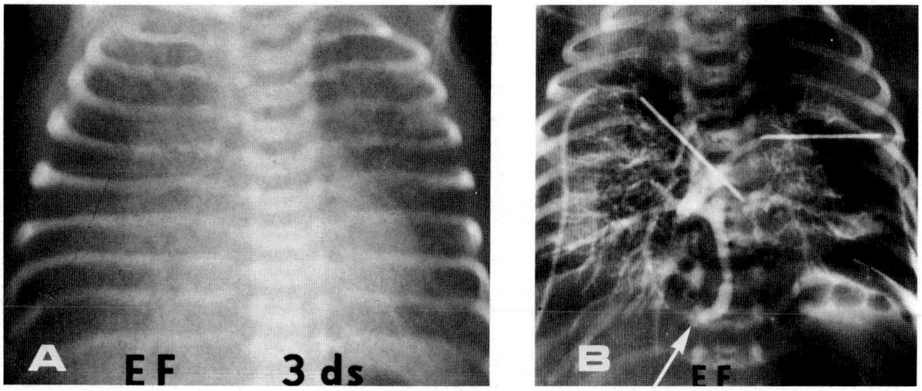

FIG. 33–18. (A) A chest radiograph of a 3-day-old infant with obstructed total anomalous pulmonary venous drainage shows a ground-glass appearance of the lungs and normal heart size. A similar clinical picture may be seen in respiratory distress syndrome. **(B)** Postmortem angiography shows obstruction of the common pulmonary venous channel below the diaphragm (*arrow*).

toms, as in patients with the infradiaphragmatic type. The success rate is better for infants with intracardiac drainage.

TREATMENT

The treatment of total anomalous pulmonary veins is surgical. Under deep hypothermic circulatory arrest, continuity or redirection of the pulmonary venous drainage into the left atrium is established. Although inotropic agents, diuretics, and supportive medical treatment are used, infants with severely obstructed anomalous venous return require immediate surgical intervention. Prostaglandin E_1 therapy is not beneficial and can lead to dramatic worsening of the pulmonary edema. In most patients, surgery can be done on the basis of information from echocardiography without the delays and risks involved with cardiac catheterization. If there are associated complex congenital anomalies (*e.g.*, heterotaxy syndrome) or intrinsic pulmonary vein stenosis is suspected, preoperative catheterization is needed. Those with unobstructed pulmonary veins and congestive heart failure with relatively normal pulmonary artery pressure may improve considerably on medical treatment, and corrective surgery may be delayed for a few weeks. Among those without additional lesions, the postoperative survivors have an excellent prognosis for a relatively normal life. A few infants develop pulmonary vein stenosis and dysrhythmias postoperatively, and close follow-up is mandatory for several years.

DIFFERENTIAL DIAGNOSIS

Respiratory distress syndrome and interstitial pneumonia were clinically indistinguishable from obstructed total anomalous pulmonary venous return until the advent of echocardiography. Any suggestion of an atypical course mandates echocardiography, particularly if there is equally diffuse involvement of both lungs and any suggestion of a murmur. Two-dimensional echocardiography shows the anomalous common venous connections and obstructions and other cardiac lesions are excluded.

TRUNCUS ARTERIOSUS

Failure of the truncus arteriosus to divide into the aorta and main pulmonary artery results in the clinical problem described as truncus arteriosus. The only arterial vessel arising from the heart is the truncus. There is one semilunar valve that may have extra valve leaflets and is often incompetent and rarely stenotic. The pulmonary arteries are supplied from the truncus by abnormal connections arising along the trunk. Classifications in vogue are based on the level at which the pulmonary vessels take off, but they are not especially pertinent to the physiology and the clinical picture. Almost universally, there is a ventricular septal defect, usually in the subaortic septum, similar to that seen in tetralogy of Fallot. There is a high incidence of associated extracardiac congenital anomalies (*e.g.*, DiGeorge syndrome).

PATHOPHYSIOLOGY

Because of the large ventricular defect and the common arterial trunk, the systemic and pulmonary venous returns are mixed, and the patient is cyanotic. The degree of cyanosis is determined by the pulmonary flow, which is a function of obstruction in the proximal pulmonary arteries. These obstructions are common, rarely severe, and located at the junction of the pulmonary artery and the trunk. If there is no obstruction, which is likely, there is excessive pulmonary flow, development of congestive heart failure, and poor survival without surgery. Without surgery, irreversible pulmonary vascular disease is likely to develop as early as the patient's first birthday. Congestive heart failure is less of a problem if there is branch pulmonary artery stenosis, although the degree of cyanosis is greater. The branch obstruction may cause problems after surgery.

CLINICAL FINDINGS

Infants with truncus arteriosus resemble those with ventricular defect more than the other cyanotic defects. Except cyanosis, which may be mild, development of symptoms is delayed until the pulmonary vascular resistance has resolved enough to allow a large pulmonary flow and the features of a left-to-right shunt. Tachypnea and the other signs of congestion predominate, although cyanosis may be recognized and documented in the first days of life. There is usually a murmur that sounds like a ventricular defect, the peripheral pulses are bounding, and other signs of an aortic runoff may be elicited. The S_2 is loud and single, and systolic clicks may be heard. On chest radiographs, the heart is enlarged, and the pulmonary vasculature is engorged. The EKG inexplicably varies, showing right, left, or combined ventricular hypertrophy.

TREATMENT

Anticongestive measures to control congestion and promote growth are rarely successful. Surgical correction is usually undertaken within the first 2 to 6 weeks of life. Although banding of the pulmonary arteries on both sides is possible and is sometimes the only choice, it is easy to understand the difficulty of applying bands on each side equally. For this reason and because of empirically poor results, most centers perform one-stage repair in infancy. This surgery consists of separating the pulmonary arteries from the trunk, establishing a conduit from the right ventricle to the pulmonary arteries, and closing the ventricular defect. It is too early to know the long-range outcome of this type of repair. The semilunar valve of the trunk is a known factor and may rarely be sufficiently incompetent to influence the outcome. Iatrogenic or natural branch pulmonary artery stenosis may be an important determinant of outcome.

SINGLE VENTRICLE

There are few patients who have only one ventricle. Most patients characterized as having a single ventricle have one dominant ventricle and a second diminutive structure that is often characterized as an outflow chamber. Because of the similarity to tricuspid atresia, some physicians have preferred the term univentricular heart to describe all patients with a functionally single ventricle, whether they have two atrioventricular valves, tricuspid atresia, or mitral atresia.

Seventy percent of these patients have a single left ventricle with a rudimentary right ventricular outflow chamber in the L-transposed position. The right ventricular outflow chamber leads to an anterior and leftward aorta, similar to that seen in corrected transposition. Pulmonary stenosis coexists in 50% of these patients. Almost any other cardiac anomaly may be associated with single ventricle.

PATHOPHYSIOLOGY

Depending on the presence of pulmonary stenosis, the clinical picture may be dominated by cyanosis or congestive heart failure, or the patient may be mildly cyanotic and otherwise asymptomatic. The problems peculiar to corrected transposition, such as the tendency to develop complete heart block or develop an incompetent atrioventricular valve (usually the left), are risks. The connection between the single ventricle and the outflow chamber (*i.e.*, ventricular defect) tends to get smaller with time in approximately 50% of patients. This has the physiologic effect of subaortic stenosis and must be considered in any management program.

CLINICAL FINDINGS

The patient usually is visibly cyanotic during the neonatal period. Sometimes those with excessive pulmonary blood flow, minimal cyanosis, and congestive heart failure present later because of growth failure or tachypnea. Most have systolic murmurs from pulmonary stenosis, atrioventricular valve regurgitation, or from other associated defects. The diagnosis is made by echocardiography. Cardiac catheterization is used preoperatively to confirm details that may influence surgical success.

TREATMENT

The ultimate goal of management is to provide a cavopulmonary or atriopulmonary anastomosis (*e.g.*, Fontan procedure). Rare patients who have perfectly balanced pulmonary and systemic circulations and are only mildly cyanotic and virtually asymptomatic fare well with no surgery for years. Most require a pulmonary artery band to limit pulmonary flow or a shunt procedure to increase pulmonary flow and arterial oxygenation until a Fontan procedure (*i.e.*, direct connection of systemic venous return to the pulmonary arteries) can be performed.

MALPOSITIONS

The term malposition is used to describe misplacement of the heart (*e.g.*, ectopia cordis), but it usually indicates concomitant heterotaxy (*i.e.*, discordant sidedness) and is used to describe patients with dextrocardia with situs solitus of the abdominal organs and levocardia with abdominal situs inversus (*i.e.*, isolated levocardia). Ambiguous location of the abdominal contents, as seen in the asplenia and polysplenia syndromes, is also described as malpositioning (Fig. 33-19). If the heart is displaced into the right chest because of pulmonary disease or diaphragmatic hernia or if there is total situs inversus (*i.e.*, situs inversus universalis), there is no heterotaxy. Because this form of dextrocardia is rare and it is not always immediately possible to be confident that all organs are inverse, dextrocardia with abdominal situs inversus is usually discussed with the malpositions. The discussion is brief, because situs inversus universalis is rare and the heart may be anatomically normal, unlike the more common forms of malposition.

For practical purposes, evidence of abnormal sidedness is primarily of consequence to the neonatologist and the pediatrician as a way to discover patients who have particularly difficult combinations of con-

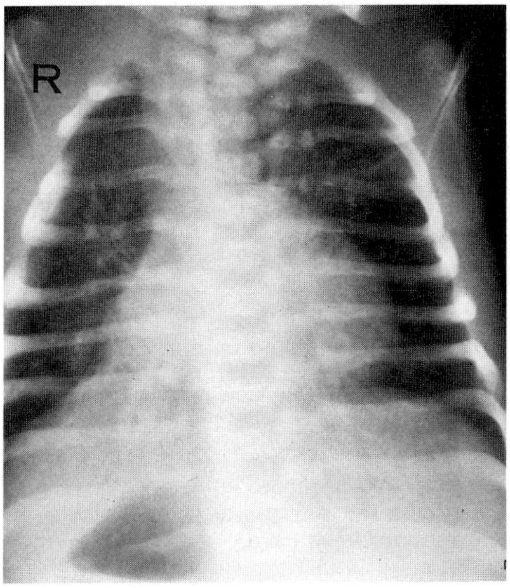

FIG. 33–19. A chest radiograph of a neonate with asplenia syndrome, tricuspid atresia, transposition of the great arteries, and a right aortic arch. The liver and stomach are on the right side.

genital heart lesions. Whether heterotaxy is discovered by physical examination because of abnormal sidedness of the abdominal contents or because the heart is located in the right chest on physical examination or chest radiographs, the result is the same. After the question has been raised and regardless of the clinical appearance of the baby, it is safest to proceed with a detailed workup. There is no consistent pattern of congenital cardiac defects associated with the different varieties of malposition that allows the physician to propose specific cardiac abnormalities based on the finding of dextrocardia or isolated levocardia. About all that can be confidently stated is that there is a high probability that life-threatening abnormalities exist and that the patient should be promptly turned over to a cardiac team that has the facilities and experience to handle the problem.

The cardiologists must sort out the combination of great vein, cardiac chamber, and great artery anomalies on a segment-to-segment basis, delineating the connections of the various segments of the heart. The cardiologist derives little diagnostic value from the nature of the malposition, other than to recognize that there is no practical alternative to painstaking and detailed evaluation of the cardiac anatomy and physiology using all the tools available. The combined information from echocardiography and cardiac catheterization is usually sufficient to propose a plan of surgical palliation, sometimes delaying full understanding of the anatomy until a later date.

Table 33-13 shows the anatomic abnormalities encountered in asplenic and polysplenic patients. Some combinations of defects encountered in these patients allow no potential for palliation or cure, but most can be palliated. The overall mortality rate tends to be high (see Table 33-2). Those with asplenia should receive lifetime prophylactic antibiotics because of their propensity for sepsis.

RHYTHM DISTURBANCES

Although any rhythm disturbance may occur *in utero* or in early infancy, those most commonly encountered include sinus tachycardia and bradycardia, premature atrial contractions, paroxysmal atrial tachycardia, and less commonly, atrial flutter and complete heart block. Atrial dysrhythmias are common, but those of ventricular origin are rare. In infants, wide-complex tachycardia is considered to be ventricular tachycardia, and digoxin is contraindicated. Acute life-threatening rhythm disturbances, such as ventricular fibrillation, ventricular tachycardia, sinus arrest, and extreme bradycardia, usually occur as a terminal event in a systemic illness or in association with severe hypoxemia, acidosis, electrolyte disturbance, or drug toxicity (*e.g.*, digitalis). Isolated ectopic atrial beats, atrial bigeminy, and nodal escape beats are only rarely associated with tachycardia and usually are of no serious consequence.

Tachydysrhythmias must be differentiated from sinus tachycardia, which can occur with serious illness, fever, anemia, or pain at rates up to 230 beats per minute (bpm). Faster rates and those with wide complex or an abrupt onset and termination are tachydysrhythmias. Sustained bradycardia at less than 70 bpm in neonates is abnormal. Noncardiac causes such as gastroesophageal reflux leading to vagal stimulation are common. Cardiac causes, including nonconducted atrial premature beats and second- or third-degree atrioventricular block, should be sought.

SUPRAVENTRICULAR TACHYCARDIA

Supraventricular tachycardia is a common rhythm disturbance in early infancy. It is frequently associated with an accessory atrioventricular bypass tract that is concealed during sinus rhythm because all conduction is passing through the normal pathway or

TABLE 33–13
COMMON ABNORMALITIES IN ASPLENIA AND POLYSPLENIA SYNDROMES

Asplenia	Polysplenia
Isolated levocardia or dextrocardia	Dextrocardia or levocardia
Visceral isomerism (midline liver and stomach)	Absent inferior vena cava (renal to hepatic segment)
Transposition of the great arteries	Endocardial cushion defect
Double-outlet right ventricle	Total anomalous pulmonary venous return
Total anomalous pulmonary venous return	Coronary sinus rhythm
Endocardial cushion defect	Bilateral hyparterial bronchi
Pulmonary atresia or pulmonary stenosis	
Single ventricle	
Bilateral superior vena cava	
Absent coronary sinus	
Ipsilateral inferior vena cava and abdominal aorta	
P-wave axis of atrial inversion	
Bilateral eparterial bronchi	
Bilateral trilobed lung	

manifested (*i.e.*, Wolff–Parkinson–White syndrome) because antegrade conduction in sinus rhythm passes to the ventricle through the bypass tract and the atrioventricular node. Other causes include reentry within dual atrioventricular nodal pathways, ectopic atrial foci and atrial flutter. Cardiac malformation (*e.g.*, Ebstein disease, corrected transposition of the great arteries), tumors, and myocarditis are predisposing factors in a few patients. Onset of the tachycardia at less than 4 months of age carries a better prognosis, and recurrence is unlikely after 1 year of age.

Electrocardiographically, the arrhythmia is characterized by a rate of over 230 bpm, abnormal or unidentifiable P waves that may be superimposed on the T waves, and normal QRS morphology with constant RR interval. The arrhythmia usually starts and ceases abruptly. The infant may be asymptomatic initially, but then he or she becomes irritable and fussy and refuses feeding. Congestive heart failure develops in approximately 20% after 36 hours and in 50% after 48 hours. Rapid bolus of intravenous adenosine (0.075 mg/kg, increased to 0.15 mg/kg if needed) is the treatment of choice for most infants. Adenosine rapidly and briefly blocks atrioventricular nodal conduction, interrupting atrioventricular bypass and atrioventricular node reentry tachycardias, and it effects brief, dramatic drops in heart rate and pressure with conversion. Side-effects appear to be rare.

Esophageal overdrive atrial pacing is also highly successful and offers the opportunity to obtain diagnostic atrial ECGs of the tachycardia and sinus rhythm. Intravenous verapamil should be avoided in infants younger than 1 year of age because of reports of cardiovascular collapse and profound bradycardia. Digoxin, preferably by the parenteral route if the infant is acutely ill, usually abolishes the arrhythmia within 6 to 12 hours. It has the advantage of improving myocardial contractility (Table 33-14). Vagal stimulation maneuvers (*e.g.*, ice to face, gagging) can be attempted while medications are being drawn up, but these are less often successful in neonates than older children. Synchronized direct current (DC) cardioversion with a DC defibrillator starting with 0.5–1.0 W-seconds/kg of body weight may be necessary for some infants refractory to adenosine if overdrive pacing is not readily available and prompt conversion is needed.

Because recurrence within 3 months is common, chronic preventative treatment is recommended. The recommended medications used in chronic management schemes differ among institutions. Without manifest Wolff–Parkinson–White syndrome, most physicians treat with digoxin, and if breakthrough occurs, they add or switch to propranolol followed by switching to oral verapamil, type IA agents (*e.g.*, quinidine, procainamide, disopyramide) or type IC agents (*e.g.*, flecainide) in various orders (see Table 33-14). The recommended schemes will change as more data about existing medications and new medications become available. If there is Wolff–Parkinson–White syndrome, most physicians will not use digoxin without electrophysiologic testing, because it may quicken antegrade conduction across the bypass tract in some patients. The administration of chronic suppressive medications such as propranolol or digitalis should be continued for approximately 6 months to 1 year after the last episode of arrhythmia. Esophageal electrophysiology studies with programmed atrial stimuli can be used to determine probability of recurrence on medications or after medications have been discontinued for those with reentry supraventricular tachycardia.

Infants with supraventricular tachycardia may be recognized *in utero* by a rapid fetal heart rate. If the arrhythmia has been present for some time, these infants may develop hydrops. *In utero*, the administration of digoxin, flecainide, or quinidine to the mother or procainamide or amiodarone directly into the umbilical vein may be effective.

ATRIAL FLUTTER

Atrial flutter is less common than other types of paroxysmal supraventricular tachycardia and may be idiopathic or associated with the same congenital heart lesions as those producing paroxysmal supraventricular tachycardia. Congestive heart failure is rare because some degree of atrioventricular block is present. The atrial rate may be 200 to 380 bpm. With a 2:1 block, the ventricular rate at the highest atrial rate would be 190 bpm, a rate insufficient to produce congestive failure in infancy. The rare infant without a block may have a rapid rate and shock. The ECG tracing reveals flutter waves, often seen best in leads II or V_1. The RR interval is constant unless the atrioventricular block changes. If the diagnosis is not certain from surface ECG, transesophageal atrial ECG can demonstrate the P waves, and intravenous adenosine may be used to alter transiently the atrioventricular block. The treatments of choice are overdrive atrial pacing from the esophagus or digoxin and, if necessary, cardioversion by DC countershock (initial dose = 5–10 W-seconds). Adenosine, although diagnostically helpful, does not convert atrial flutter. Maintenance therapy with digoxin should probably be continued for 6 months to 1 year. The addition of quinidine or propranolol may be necessary (see Table 33-14).

COMPLETE ATRIOVENTRICULAR BLOCK

In complete heart block, the ventricular rate is slower than and independent of the atrial rate. The arrhythmia is not infrequently recognized *in utero*. In approximately 50% of infants with congenital heart block, there is an associated cardiovascular malformation (*e.g.*, corrected transposition of the great arteries, ventricular septal defect, atrial septal defect). Myocarditis and fibrosis of the atrioventricular node or His

TABLE 33–14 NEONATAL ANTIDYSRHYTHMIC AGENTS

Drug	Currently Commonly Used	Group; Action	Oral Dose	Intravenous Dose	Theraputic Level	Indications	Contraindications	Toxicity
Adenosine	Yes	Purine, ↑ K conductance, transient AV node conduction block		0.075 mg/kg rapid IV push q 1 min PRN; ↑ to 0.15–0.25 mg/kg PRN		Rx-Rentry SVT, Dx Atrial flutter		Transient AV block, ↓ HR, ↓ BP, and flushing
Digoxin	Yes	Glycoside, "the leaf", Na-K ATPase inhibition, vagotonic	Load: 20–30 μg/kg divided in 3 doses Maintenance: 3–5 μg/kg/12 h; ↓ with renal–hepatic dysfunction	80% of oral dose	0.8–2.2 mg/ml	SVT, atrial flutter	AV Block, VT, many WPW	AV block, ↓ HR, tachydysrhythmias, vomiting, use with caution with renal failure, toxicity with hypocalcemia
Quinidine	Yes	IA; Na channel inhibition, ↓ conduction, slow repolarization	4–15 mg/kg/6 h; ↓ with renal–hepatic dysfunction		2–5 μg/ml	SVT, WPW with propranolol, PVC, VT	Long QT, known sensitivity, IV use, conduction block, myasthenia gravis	↓ Contractility, ↑ QT, VT, conduction block, vomiting, diarrhea, rash, blood dyscrasias, ↑ HR with atrial flutter without digoxin, ↑ digoxin level ↓ digoxin dose by one-half
Procainamide	Yes	IA	2.5–8 mg/kg/4 h	7 mg/kg over 1 h Infusion: 20–60 μg/kg/min	Procainamide* 4–10 μg/ml	SVT, WPW, PVC, VT	Conduction block, myasthenia gravis	Similar to quinidine, ↓ BP, lupuslike reaction, no effect on digoxin level
Disopyramide	No	IA	3.5–7.5 mg/kg/6 h		2–5 μg/ml	SVT, WPW, PVC, VT	Conduction block, myasthenia gravis	Similar to quinidine, ↓ contractility, anticholinergic, hypoglycemia, no effect on digoxin level
Lidocaine	Yes	IB; Na channel inhibition, ↓ refractoriness, ↓ APD		Bolus: 1 mg/kg/ 5–10 min Infusion: 20–50 μg/kg/min; ↓ with cyanosis, hepatic dysfunction	2–5 μg/ml	PVC, VT	Conduction block, ↓ junctional and ventricular escape rate	CNS reactions, seizure, ↓ BP, ↓ respiratory drive
Phenytoin	No	IB	2–3 mg/kg/12 h; ↓ with hepatic dysfunction	Load: 10 mg/kg Maintenance: same as oral	10–20 μg/ml	PVC, VT, digitalis intoxication	Not FDA approved for VT	CNS reactions, ↓ BP, blood dyscrasias, hepatic dysfunction, hypertrichosis, gingival hyperplasia, coarse facies, rash
Flecainide	No	IC; Na channel inhibition, ↓ conduction, ↓ automaticity	1–2.5 mg/kg/8 h; ↓ with renal, hepatic dysfunction		0.2–1.0 μg/ml	Refractory life-threatening SVT, PJRT, PVC, VT	Conduction block, hepatic dysfunction, myocardial dysfunction; not FDA approved for children, SVT	Occasional ↑ SVT frequency with WPW, ↑ pacing threshold and conduction block, VT, nausea, ↓ contractility
Propranolol	Yes	II: β-adrenergic receptor blockade, ↓ conduction ↑ refractoriness, ↓ automaticity	0.3–1.0 mg/kg/6 h; ↓ with chronic cyanosis, renal, hepatic dysfunction	0.02–0.10 mg/kg over 20 min		SVT, WPW, PVC, VT, hypertrophic cardiomyopathy, prolonged QT	Use with verapamil, bronchospasm, conduction block, CHF	↓ HR, conduction block, bronchospasm, ↓ BP, hypoglycemia, depression, ↓ cardiac reflexes with anesthesia
Amiodarone	No	III; prolong APD, ↓ conduction, ↓ automaticity	5 mg/kg/12 h for 1 wk, then 5 mg/kg/d; ↓ with hepatic dysfunction	Investigational	1–2 μg/ml	Refractory life-threatening SVT, VT, recurrent VF	Conduction block; not FDA approved for children	Extremely long half-life, corneal deposits, thyroid and hepatic dysfunction, pulmonary fibrosis, may ↑ conduction block and digoxin and quinidine levels, ↓ digoxin by one-half
Bretylium	No	III; inhibits norepinephrine release		Load: 5 mg/kg over 15 min Infusion: 20–50 μg/kg/min		Refractory VT, VF	Not FDA approved for children	Transient ↑ BP, dysrhythmia, then ↓ BP
Verapamil	No	IV; Ca channel blockade, ↓ conduction, ↑ refractoriness, ↓ automaticity	2–4 mg/kg/8 h; ↓ with hepatic or renal dysfunction, neuromuscular disease			Refractory SVT, hypertrophic cardiomyopathy, some PVC, VT	IV use, conduction dysfunction, CHF, many WPW, propranolol, muscular dystrophy, use with quinidine	↓ BP, ↓ HR, conduction block, myocardial depression, constipation, may ↑ digoxin level, ↓ digoxin dose one-third to one-half
Direct current cardioversion	Yes	Treatment of SVT Treatment of VT	0.5–1.0 W-sec/kg 1.0–2.0 W-sec/kg					

Continuous ECG monitoring should be done during initiation of antidysrhythmic therapy and with IV administration because of potential prodysrhythmia and conduction block.

* To differentiate from metabolite measured by some laboratories.

APD, action potential duration; AV, arteriovenous; BP, blood pressure; CHF, congestive heart failure; CNS, central nervous system; DX, diagnosis; FDA, Federal Drug Administration; HR, heart rate; PJRT, permanent junctional reciprocating tachycardia; PVC, premature ventricular contractions; Rx, treatment; SVT, supraventricular tachycardia; VF, ventricular fibrillation; VT, ventricular tachycardia; WPW, Wolff–Parkinson–White syndrome.

bundle are etiologic factors. There is an association between maternal connective tissue disorders, particularly systemic lupus erythematosus, and congenital complete heart block. Testing of the mother for antinuclear antibodies may be indicated. Complete heart block may occur as a complication of cardiac surgery, particularly in the correction of endocardial cushion defects, tetralogy of Fallot, and ventricular septal defects.

Most infants with congenital heart block and no other cardiac problems are asymptomatic and require no immediate therapy. Symptoms are usually related to the severity of the associated cardiovascular malformation and the degree of bradycardia. Infants without hemodynamically significant cardiac malformation tolerate bradycardia well, grow, and develop normally. Examination usually reveals cardiac enlargement due to an increased left ventricular end-diastolic volume. A systolic ejection murmur and apical mid-diastolic rumble are common. The ECG is usually characterized by normal atrial rate and P-wave configuration, independent ventricular rate with long but equal RR intervals, and abnormal or wide QRS complex. Syncopal (*i.e.*, Stokes–Adams) episodes may occur, but the initial episode is rarely fatal. The ventricular rate tends to decrease with increasing age. Patients with syncope or near syncope, congestive heart failure, or postsurgical block should be electrically paced with epicardial wires. Medical therapy with isoproterenol (Isuprel) or atropine or with a transcutaneous or transvenous pacemaker is helpful in the acute situation or in preparation for surgery.

REFERENCES

1. Keith JD, Rowe RD, Vlad P. Heart disease in infancy and childhood. 4th ed. New York: Macmillan, 1978.
2. Moss AJ, Adams FH, Emmanouilides GC, Riemenschneider TA. Heart disease in infants, children and adolescents. 4th ed. Baltimore: Williams & Wilkins, 1989.
3. Moller JH, Neal WA. Fetal, neonatal, and infant cardiac disease. Norwalk, CT: Appleton & Lange, 1989.
4. Garson A, Bricker JT, McNamara DG. The science and practice of pediatric cardiology. Philadelphia: Lea & Febiger, 1990.
5. Long WA. Fetal and neonatal cardiology. Philadelphia: WB Saunders, 1990.
6. Fyler DC. Nadas' pediatric cardiology. Philadelphia: Hanley & Belfus, 1992.
7. Mitchell SC, Korones SB, Berendes HW. Congenital heart disease in 56,109 births. Circulation 1971;43:323.
8. Fyler DC. Report of the New England Regional Infant Cardiac Program Pediatrics 1980;65(Suppl):375.
9. Ferencz C, Villasenor . Epidemiology of cardiovascular malformations: the state of the art. Cardiol Young 1991;1:264.
10. Kurnit DM, Layton WM, Matthysse S. Genetics, chance and morphogenesis. Am J Human Genet 1987;41:979.
11. Lacro RV. Dysmorphology. Nadas' pediatric cardiology. Philadelphia: Hanley & Belfus, 1992:37.
12. Pierpont MEM, Moller JH. The genetics of cardiovascular disease. Boston: Martinus Nijhoff, 1987.
13. Dawson BV, Johnson PD, Goldberg SJ, Ulreich JB. Cardiac teratogenesis of trichloroethylene and dichloroethylene in a mammalian model. J Am Coll Cardiol 1990;16:1304.
14. Goldberg SJ, Lebwitz MD, Graver EJ, Hicks S. An association of human congenital cardiac malformations and drinking water contaminants. J Am Coll Cardiol 1990;16:155.
15. Gorlin RJ, Cohen MM, Levin LS. Syndromes of the head and neck. 3rd ed. Oxford: Oxford University Press, 1990.
16. Smith DW, Jones KL. Recognizable patterns of human malformation: genetic, embryologic and clinical aspects. 3rd ed. Philadelphia: WB Saunders, 1982.
17. Barcroft J. Researchers of pre-natal Life. Oxford: Blackwell & Mott, 1944.
18. Dawes GS. Foetal and neonatal physiology: a comparative study of the changes at birth. Chicago: Year Book, 1969.
19. Lind J, Stern L, Wegelius C. Human and foetal neonatal circulation. Springfield, IL: Charles C Thomas, 1964.
20. Rudolph AM. Congenital diseases of the heart. Chicago: Year Book, 1974.
21. Sanders SS. Echocardiography. Nadas' pediatric cardiology. Philadelphia: Hanley & Belfus, 1992:159.
22. Olley PM, Coceani F, Bodach E. E-type prostaglandins: a new emergency therapy for certain cyanotic congenital heart malformations. Circulation 1976;53:728.
23. Lang P, Freed MD, Rosenthal A, et al. The use of prostaglandin E_1 in an infant with interruption of the aortic arch. J Pediatr 1977;91:805.
24. Braunwald E, Swan HJC. Cooperative study on cardiac catheterization. American Heart Association monograph no. 20. Circulation 1968;37(Suppl III):1.
25. Kan JS, White RI Jr, Mitchell SE, Gardner TG. Percutaneous balloon valvuloplasty: a new method for treating congenital pulmonary valve stenosis. N Engl J Med 1982;307:540.
26. Lock JE, Bass JL, Amplatrz K, et al. Balloon dilatation angioplasty or aortic coarctation in infants and children. Circulation 1983;68:109.
27. Borow K, Green LH, Castaneda AR, et al. Left ventricular function after repair of tetralogy of Fallot and its relationship to age at repair. Circulation 1980;61:1150.
28. Newburger JW, Silbert AR, Buckley LP, Fyler DC. Cognitive function and age at repair of transposition of the great arteries in children. N Engl J Med 1984;310:1495.
29. Friedman WF, Hirschklau MJ, Previtz MP, et al. Pharmacologic closure of patent ductus arteriosus in the premature infant. N Engl J Med 1976;295:526.
30. Heymann MA, Rudolph AM, Silverman NH. Closure of the ductus arteriosus in premature infants by inhibition of prostaglandin synthesis. N Engl J Med 1976;295:530.
31. Wagner HR, Ellison RC, Zierler S, et al. Surgical closure of patent ductus ateriosus in 268 preterm infants. J Thorac Cardiovasc Surg 1984;87:870.
32. Gersony WM, Peckham GJ, Ellison RC, et al. Effects of indomethacin in preterm infants with patent ductus arteriosus. Results of a national collaborative study. J Pediatr 1983;102: 895.
33. Jatene AD, Fontes VF, Paulista PP, et al. Anatomic correction of transposition of the great vessels. J Thorac Cardiovasc Surg 1976;72:364.
34. Castaneda AR, Norwood WI, Jonas RA, et al. Transposition of the great arteries and intact ventricular septum: anatomical repair in the neonate. Ann Thorac Surg 1984;38:438.
35. Norwood WI, Lang P, Hansen DD. Physiologic repair of aortic atresia—hypoplastic left heart syndrome. N Engl J Med 1984; 308:23.
36. Bailey LL. Role of cardiac transplantation in the neonate. J Heart Transplant 1985;4:506.

Neonatology: Pathophysiology and Management of the Newborn, Fourth Edition,
edited by Gordon B. Avery, Mary Ann Fletcher, and Mhairi G. MacDonald.
J.B. Lippincott Company, Philadelphia © 1994.

chapter 34

Cardiac Surgery

JEFFREY E. SELL

In the past 20 years, there has been considerable improvement in the techniques and technology of cardiac surgery. This has allowed increasing latitude in the approach to the treatment of the neonate with congenital heart disease. Many lesions that were in the past handled with an initial palliative procedure during the neonatal period are now completely reparable in infancy as a result of the safe application of cardiopulmonary bypass and deep hypothermic arrest.

The indications for surgical intervention in the first month of life are obstructed outflow from the heart, inadequate oxygenation, or congestive heart failure due to excessive pulmonary blood flow. The challenge of heart surgery for congenital defects is to assess the complex interplay of the anatomy and physiology, select the appropriate intervention and correct timing, and perform the procedure well.

PREOPERATIVE PREPARATION

A regionalized approach to perinatal medical care, with organized transport systems and outreach education programs, has optimized the resuscitation of newborns with critical congenital heart deformities and expedited the transfer of these infants to critical care nurseries. The most significant advancement in salvaging these extremely ill neonates was the introduction of prostaglandin E_1(PGE_1) therapy in the late 1970s.[1] Prostaglandin E_1 therapy allows the ductus arteriosus to be opened or kept open. In the case of obstruction of pulmonary blood flow resulting in cyanosis, the ductus can maintain pulmonary blood flow until the obstruction can be relieved or an appropriate shunt can be inserted. When systemic blood flow is obstructed, PGE_1 allows the support of the systemic circulation *via* the ductus arteriosus, and may relieve the obstruction temporarily, as in the case of coarctation. Thus, prostaglandin E_1 therapy allows perfusion of the critical organs and permits surgery to be delayed until organ function improves.

After the child's circulation is supported, acidosis must be corrected and cardiac output improved. This may require intubation, the administration of bicarbonate, and the addition of inotropic agents.

Most lesions requiring surgical intervention in the neonatal period can be adequately assessed with echocardiography. The anatomy of the lesion guides the appropriate preoperative course. In the case of transposition, it may be necessary to perform a balloon atrial septostomy to provide adequate mixing of oxygenated and deoxygenated blood. In many situations (*e.g.*, atrial and ventricular septal defects), no early surgical intervention is required. With proper stabilization and PGE_1 therapy if necessary, only the child with obstructed total anomalous pulmonary venous return must be rushed to the operating room. Optimal preoperative resuscitation leads to improved surgical outcome in most cases.

In no cardiac condition is preoperative preparation more important than it is for children with single ventricles. These so called "complete mixers" have a delicate balance of systemic and pulmonary blood flow.

Unlike the normal arrangement of in-series pulmonary and systemic circulation, these children have parallel circulation. As a result, the flow to various organ systems depends on the total cardiac output and the relative pulmonary and systemic resistances. The key to resuscitation of these neonates is to limit the pulmonary blood flow by various techniques, including intubation, hypoventilation, low fraction of inspired oxygen (FiO_2), and in some cases, positive end-expiratory pressure. Cardiac output can be increased with inotropic agents, and acidosis can be corrected. The renal and hepatic failure, which may result from closure of the ductus arteriosus, can usually be reversed with proper resuscitation. Surgery is performed when the child is in optimal condition.

Some children have uncorrectable lesions or lesions with relatively poor prognoses. In these situations, ethical considerations should guide discussion with the parents regarding the option of discontinuing support. This has been of particular concern for children with hypoplastic left heart syndrome. With continued improvements in the outcome of palliative approaches and of neonatal transplantation, the decision whether or not to intervene becomes more difficult. Socioeconomic considerations may become a significant issue in the United States as resources become limited.

After the child has been appropriately resuscitated, required surgery should be performed at the first available opportunity. In the case of neonates who will undergo heart transplantation, it is necessary to maintain vigilant support, because children on PGE_1 therapy are at significant risk for necrotizing enterocolitis, apnea, and infections. As many as 25% of neonates who are candidates for heart transplant die waiting for an organ to become available.

SURGICAL PRINCIPLES

The surgical procedures involved in congenital heart surgery are categorized in several ways. Open procedures employ the heart–lung machine. Closed procedures are those in which the child is not placed on bypass. Coarctation repair, ligation of patent ductus, and modified Blalock–Taussig shunts are examples of closed procedures.

Procedures that result in incomplete repair of a lesion (*i.e.*, operations that do not result in two in-series circulations with a ventricle in each circulation) are referred to as palliative. Children with palliative corrections have much more complicated postoperative courses and significantly higher mortality rates than patients with complete repairs.

The technology of cardiopulmonary bypass and myocardial preservation used in open procedures has undergone significant improvement. Current techniques use membrane oxygenators with low priming volumes. Cooling is an integral part of organ protection in all open heart procedures. In some complex congenital lesions, it is impossible to maintain flow from the oxygenator while the complicated repair is performed. In these cases, profound hypothermia is used to protect the child during a period of circulatory arrest. This procedure usually consists of cooling the child undergoing bypass to 18°C over a period of 20 minutes. At this temperature, complete circulatory arrest is usually well tolerated for as long as 60 minutes.

In the operating room, catheters can be placed in the right or left atrium or pulmonary artery for postoperative monitoring and blood drawing. Temporary wires may be placed on the atrium and ventricle for postoperative pacing or diagnostic purposes.

Cardiopulmonary bypass and hypothermia are not without risks. Bleeding is a significant concern in small circulations diluted by the pump prime. In many centers, fresh whole blood is thought to be the optimal blood product for expansion and reconstitution of intravascular volume and the clotting factors lost or impaired during bypass. Improved techniques of perfusion minimize the incidence of renal failure. Opening the circulatory system to air and artificial perfusion introduces a risk of neurologic sequelae. The incidence of significant symptomatic neurologic injury is less than 0.1% in most series. Because the infant is an adaptable patient and may functionally compensate for significant neurologic deficits, extensive randomized, controlled investigation is underway to determine more exactly the neurologic sequelae of open heart surgery. In deep hypothermic cases, there is a 10% incidence of postoperative seizures. These are not known to have any long-term impact, and they are usually treated for 3 to 6 months with phenobarbital without recurrence.

LESIONS WITH EXCESSIVE PULMONARY BLOOD FLOW

PATENT DUCTUS ARTERIOSUS

One of the earliest congenital lesions to be successfully repaired was the patent ductus arteriosus. With the development of catheter techniques for closure of a smaller ductus in older patients, most surgical cases are premature infants who have failed multiple courses of indomethacin therapy or in whom it is contraindicated. A ductal ligation is a closed procedure done from the left chest. The duct is ligated without division. Transient recurrent nerve paresis occurs in approximately 5% of cases; mortality approaches zero. Death is usually from respiratory causes related to excessive prematurity.

AORTOPULMONARY WINDOW

Aortopulmonary window consists of a communication between the aortic and pulmonary trunks beyond the level of the valve. There are two distinct semilunar valves, which distinguishes this lesion from truncus arteriosus, and ventricular septal defects are uncommon. This lesion often masquerades as a ductus arteriosus; it is important to differentiate the two. Repair of an aortopulmonary window requires cardiopulmonary bypass and is performed through a median sternotomy.

ATRIAL SEPTAL DEFECTS, VENTRICULAR SEPTAL DEFECTS, AND DEFECTS OF THE ATRIOVENTRICULAR SEPTUM

Septal defects as isolated lesions rarely require therapy in the first few weeks of life. Atrial septal defects of the secundum type or the sinus venosus type may rarely cause failure to thrive in the first year of life. If no other cause for failure to thrive can be found, these lesions should be surgically closed. Closure usually is performed before beginning school, at about 4 years of age. If the septal lesions are associated with left-sided obstructive lesions, such as coarctation, the risks associated with surgery are increased.

Ventricular septal defects are the most common lesions diagnosed between the ages of 7 days and 1 month of life. They are usually responsive to medical therapy, but if they are quite large, they may cause failure to thrive, increased pulmonary vascular resistance, and increased incidence of upper respiratory infections. The elevation in pulmonary vascular resistance is almost always reversible in the absence of trisomy 21, if repair is performed before 1 year of age. Some defects (*e.g.*, subpulmonary or supracristal defects) may deform the aortic cusps and result in aortic regurgitation. When this is detected by echocardiography, prompt surgical repair should be planned.

Repair of membranous and most muscular ventricular septal defects is performed though the right atrium. Occasionally, a transventricular approach is required. Subpulmonary ventricular septal defects are usually approached *via* the pulmonary artery. Patch closure is usually the procedure of choice. Pulmonary artery banding has been reserved for rare cases of multiple ventricular septal defects and cases of single ventricle. The mortality rate is less than 5% for complete repair in infancy, and the significant incidence of pulmonary artery distortion by pulmonary artery bands has greatly limited the use of the palliative banding approach.

Endocardial cushion defects or defects of the atrioventricular septum are more complicated due to the involvement of the atrioventricular valves. A primum atrial septal defect and cleft mitral valve is usually referred to as an incomplete or partial atrioventricular canal. Repair consists of closing the atrioventricular defect, always with a patch, usually of pericardium, and repairing the mitral valve. The latter is important if mitral regurgitation is found, because the mitral valve incompetence worsens with time, with the valve potentially becoming damaged beyond the point of repair. In the case of complete atrioventricular canal, there are atrial and ventricular components to the septal defect, and the common atrioventricular valve is quite abnormal. Repair of this lesion is undertaken in any symptomatic child on maximal medical support, usually before 6 months of age. There is no significant decrease in surgical mortality beyond 3 months of age, and in the case of trisomy 21, pulmonary hypertension may become irreversible by as early as 6 months of age. Repair consists of single- or double-patch closure of the septal defects, with reconstruction of the atrioventricular valve to form mitral and tricuspid components. Operative survival in most series is approximately 87%, and the most significant long-term concern is the mitral valve, which requires replacement in about 5% of patients.[2]

LESIONS WITH OBSTRUCTION TO PULMONARY BLOOD FLOW OR INADEQUATE OXYGENATION

CRITICAL PULMONARY STENOSIS AND PULMONARY ATRESIA WITH INTACT VENTRICULAR SEPTUM

Critical pulmonary stenosis and pulmonary atresia with intact ventricular septum (PA/IVS) comprise a spectrum of lesions involving probable late disruption of cardiac development. Their prognosis and surgical approach is mainly dictated by the effect of the obstruction on the development of the right ventricle.[3] In some cases, the right ventricle is well developed, with an inflow, a body, and an outflow portion. In PA/IVS, the right ventricle may be quite small or deformed, as in cases of pulmonary atresia with Ebstein anomaly. Children with critical pulmonary stenosis and a good right ventricle can be maintained on PGE_1 therapy and undergo balloon valvuloplasty. In cases such as dysplastic pulmonary valve, surgical valvectomy may be necessary. Severe subvalvar obstruction may require muscle resection or patching of the outflow tract.

For a child with PA/IVS, a transannular patch must be placed to provide outflow to the right ventricle. If the ventricle is quite small, a modified Blalock–Taussig shunt may be placed to ensure adequate saturation. This consists of a polytetrafluroethylene tube graft, 4 to 6 mm in diameter, from the subclavian artery to a branch pulmonary artery (Table 34-1). There is always an atrial septal defect with PA/IVS, and this is left as a "pop off" for the thick right ventricle. Sinusoids from a hypertensive right ventricle to the coronary circulation can occur in PA/IVS. If there is significant dependence of the coronary circulation on right ventricular sinusoids, transplantation should be considered.

TETRALOGY OF FALLOT WITH AND WITHOUT PULMONARY ATRESIA

Errors in infundibular septation with impingement on the right ventricular outflow constitute the spectrum of tetralogy of Fallot (TOF). The ventricular sep-

TABLE 34–1
COMMON SHUNTS USED TO TREAT CONGENITAL HEART DISEASE

Shunt	Blood Source	Conduit	Anastamotic Site
Modified Blalock–Taussig	Subclavian artery	PTFE	Branch pulmonary artery
Modified Waterston	Ascending aorta	PTFE	Branch pulmonary artery
Modified central	Ascending aorta	PTFE	Main pulmonary artery
Glenn	Superior vena cava	None	Branch pulmonary artery*
Bidirectional cavopulmonary	Superior vena cava	None	Branch pulmonary artery

* In the Glenn shunt procedure, the pulmonary artery is divided.
PTFE, polytetrafluroethylene.

tal defect is referred to as anterior malalignment, and the pulmonary arteries range from essentially normal in size to absent in the extreme cases of TOF with pulmonary atresia.

Tetralogy of Fallot with adequate-sized pulmonary arteries is usually repaired as a single-stage procedure in infancy, as soon as symptoms appear.[4] The procedure closes the ventricular septal defect and relieves the right ventricular outflow tract obstruction by dividing or resecting obstructing muscle bundles, with or without infundibular patching. Neonates seem to have the highest incidence of annular stenosis at the valve level, and they frequently require transannular patching.[5] The long-term effects of chronic pulmonary insufficiency seem to be minimal. Rarely is placement of a valved conduit necessary. The surgeon must relieve the obstruction sufficiently to decrease the right ventricular systolic pressure to less than 60% of systemic systolic pressure. If the right ventricle pressure is less than 40% of systemic pressure within 24 hours of the operation or the right ventricle outflow tract gradient on pullback is less than 40 torr, the risk of recurrent right ventricle outflow tract obstruction is low.[6]

The most important problem in TOF with pulmonary atresia is the pulmonary circulation. The central pulmonary artery may be absent, and the lung may be segmentally supplied by systemic collaterals, ductlike collaterals, and bronchial arteries. The goal of surgical therapy is twofold. The first goal is to achieve unifocalization—the centralization of as many pulmonary artery segments as possible into a common pulmonary source. Second, access to this common pulmonary source should be supplied to allow dilation of the branch pulmonary artery stenoses commonly seen with this disease. This is usually accomplished by a homograft conduit from the right ventricle. Closure of the associated ventricular septal defect can only be undertaken when net shunting of blood across the defect is from left to right, because suprasystemic pulmonary artery pressures may result. The early results of this multistaged approach are encouraging compared with the dismal results of the past.[7] These children require the most labor-intensive long-term therapies available for the treatment of congenital heart disease.

TRUNCUS ARTERIOSUS

Many authorities consider truncus arteriosus an extreme form of TOF. Therapy is dictated by the degree of failure and the semilunar valve or truncal valve function. Repair is usually undertaken before 3 months of age, but it is preferable to wait until the child is beyond the first month of life if symptoms allow. Complete repair consists of closure of the ventricular septal defect through the right ventricle, detachment of the pulmonary circulation from the trunk, and a conduit from the right ventricle to the pulmonary artery. Human homograft is the conduit of choice. The risks of this procedure depend on truncal valve function and the reactivity of the pulmonary vasculature. Complete sedation and paralysis is required in the early postoperative period to allow the pulmonary vasculature to relax and the reactivity to improve. The survival rate is between 80% and 90%, depending on many variables.

TRANSPOSITION OF THE GREAT ARTERIES

The most common congenital heart problem addressed in the first month of life, transposition of the great arteries, has undergone a significant change in surgical approach during the last decade. In this malformation, the aorta originates from the anterior right ventricle, and the pulmonary artery arises from the posterior left ventricle. Survival depends on communication between the two circulations at the atrial, ventricular, or ductal level. Approximately one-third of these children have ventricular septal defects. Infants can be supported with PGE_1 therapy, but early balloon atrial septostomy should be the rule. The coronary anatomy may be delimited at the time of catheterization, if necessary, but the coronaries often can be well defined by echocardiography.

The timing and selection of the operation are critical. Immediately after birth, the left ventricle is capable of producing systemic pressures. As the pulmonary resistance drops and the ductus closes, in the absence of an unrestrictive ventricular septal defect, the left ventricle loses its ability to function systemically by 2 weeks of age. The favored repair consists of switching the great arteries to their intended ventricles. This includes moving the coronaries from the sinuses of the anterior great vessel to the posterior great vessel. This operation results in better than 90% survival if done before the left-sided muscle mass decreases.[8]

The arterial switch operation has become the procedure of choice due to the long-term rhythm and venous obstruction problems encountered with the atrial switch operations (*i.e.*, Senning or Mustard procedures). The atrial operations are reserved for situations in which the coronary artery anatomy is unfavorable for arterial switch, usually intramural or single coronaries or the complicated cases in which the left-sided function is unfavorable for systemic use. Repair of a ventricular septal defect interferes with tricuspid valve function and makes this a particularly undesirable systemic atrioventricular valve. Arterial switch is therefore much more desirable in the case of transposition of the great arteries with ventricular septal defect. The survival rate in these cases is better than 95% in some series.

Late coronary artery loss has been seen in the arterial switch population, but the incidence is low, and ventricular function is not adversely affected in many cases. Supravalvar pulmonary stenosis seems to be a decreasing problem as the technical aspects of the operation improve.

TOTAL ANOMALOUS PULMONARY VENOUS CONNECTION

The failure of the pulmonary venous return to connect to the left atrium results in immediate cyanosis of the infant. The alternate routes of return to the heart and their approximate frequencies are supracardiac (40)%, infracardiac (25%), cardiac (25%), or mixed (10%). Therapy consists of reattaching the venous connections, usually a common focal pulmonary vein, to the left atrium. If the anomalous connection is unobstructed, the physiology is essentially one of common mixing, and repair may be undertaken electively after the fall of pulmonary vascular resistance. If the veins are obstructed, as is frequently the case for the infracardiac type, emergency repair is dictated. Severe pulmonary edema, which is the rule with obstructed veins, may be slow to clear postoperatively, and anastomotic problems should always be considered if lung field clearing does not occur. Branch pulmonary venous stenosis, unrelated to the surgical repair, occasionally complicates the postoperative course of these patients.

LESIONS WITH LEFT-SIDED OBSTRUCTION

CRITICAL AORTIC STENOSIS

The outcome of critical aortic stenosis, a relatively rare lesion, depends on left ventricular function and size and the anatomy of the valve. With a good left ventricle and a reasonable valve, balloon dilation is usually effective.[9] Rarely, these valves must be approached surgically for an open commissurotomy. The mortality of this lesion is significant. Maintenance on PGE_1 therapy may decrease the risk of catheter intervention. Children with small left ventricles fall into the category of hypoplastic left heart in terms of therapeutic consideration.

COARCTATION OF THE AORTA

Children with coarctation of the aorta, a relatively common anomaly, may present with a great range of problems, from late hypertension to early severe cardiac decompensation with low output. In the neonatal period, therapy consists of resuscitation with PGE_1 therapy. This can provide distal perfusion by means of the pulmonary artery and possibly open the area of the coarctation if significant ductal tissue is involved. Therapy is a matter of controversy. The subclavian flap angioplasty described by Waldhausen is effective in the neonatal period, with a reintervention rate of about 10% during the first 5 years of life.[10] Resection and end-to-end repair is used in many institutions. The initial reports showed reintervention rates as high as 25%, but the rate seems to be decreasing with increasing experience.[11] Patch angioplasty has been reserved for a few select cases with severe transverse arch problems because of the reports of late aneurysms. Primary catheter dilation of the neonatal coarctation is undergoing critical evaluation. Initial series showed a relatively high incidence of aneurysm, but more recent results look promising.

Coarctation is frequently associated with a ventricular septal defect. Most institutions have adopted the policy of approaching the coarctation first. If, after repair of the coarctation, the child fails to wean from mechanical ventilation or has other cardiac symptoms, catheterization is performed, and surgical repair of the ventricular septal defect is undertaken if appropriate.

HYPOPLASTIC LEFT HEART SYNDROME

This defect is the most commonly fatal cyanotic heart lesion in infancy. The lesion consists of a small, fibrotic left ventricle due to mitral or aortic atresia or stenosis. The lesion is a complete-mixing single-ventricle type and requires early resuscitation with PGE_1 therapy and control of pulmonary blood flow. Initial palliation has involved a procedure developed by Norwood, which consists of using the pulmonary artery for systemic outflow, augmenting the aortic arch, detaching the pulmonary circulation and supplying it by a shunt, and atrial septectomy.[12] This allows discontinuation of PGE_1 therapy and provides controlled pulmonary blood flow. The eventual goal is a modified Fontan-type repair with a single ventricle providing support to an in-series–type circulation.

Survival after the Norwood procedure has varied

widely among institutions, with many series reporting no long-term survivors.[13] Some series achieve a survival rate as high as 70% for first-stage survival.[14] The dismal results at many institutions led to the exploration of transplantation as a therapy for hypoplastic left heart syndrome. Volume loading a right ventricle, recurrent arch obstruction, pulmonary artery distortion, and pulmonary venous problems have plagued the short-term course of patients who are waiting for Fontan repair after the Norwood procedure, and a sizable number eventually fall outside the range of appropriate candidates for modified Fontan reconstruction.

Because of the lack of long-term success, many institutions have offered no therapy for hypoplastic left heart syndrome, and many fetuses diagnosed *in utero* with this lesion are aborted. More experience with transplantation and improved results with Norwood and modified Fontan procedures will help to clarify the selection of therapy for this lesion.[13]

INTERRUPTION OF THE AORTIC ARCH

Interrupted aortic arch is a ductal-dependent lesion that is almost always associated with a ventricular communication, usually of the posterior malalignment type. The type-B interruption, between the left carotid and left subclavian, is frequently associated with thymic aplasia and DiGeorge syndrome. Initial PGE_1 therapy and resuscitation is similar to management of hypoplastic left heart syndrome, but these children are usually quite amenable to a two-ventricle complete repair. Surgery is undertaken as soon as the child is favorably stabilized, and it consists of closing the ventricular septal defect and primarily reconstructing the aorta. The long-term survival rate is better than 80% for children without other deformities. Subaortic stenosis occasionally occurs within the first 3 years of life and is usually amenable to surgical repair. Arch stenosis has been successfully treated by balloon dilation in most cases.

LESIONS WITH SINGLE-VENTRICLE PHYSIOLOGY OR COMPLEX CONNECTIONS

Many children are born with lesions resulting in one usable ventricle. Tricuspid atresia, double-inlet left ventricle, and PA/IVS may all have essentially single left ventricle anatomy. Children with unbalanced atrioventricular canals and extreme errors in ventricular septation may have two ventricles, but lack the possibility of a two-ventricle repair. Initial care is the same as for all patients with parallel circulation: PGE_1 therapy until evaluation is complete, echocardiography, and control of systemic and pulmonary blood flow. Most of these cases can be categorized as unprotected pulmonary circulation, obstructed pulmonary outflow, or obstructed systemic outflow.

SINGLE VENTRICLE WITH OBSTRUCTED SYSTEMIC OUTFLOW

Patients may have an obstruction at the level of the subaortic region or at the level of primitive ventricular communication (*i.e.*, bulboventricular foramen). Coarctation is frequently associated with a single ventricle with obstructed systemic outflow. Therapy consists of augmenting the systemic outflow with the proximal pulmonary outflow as described by Stansel[15] and shunting the pulmonary circulation. Long-term therapy consists of a Fontan-type venous pulmonary direct connection.[16]

SINGLE VENTRICLE WITH OBSTRUCTED PULMONARY OUTFLOW

The therapy for patients with a single ventricle with obstructed pulmonary outflow depends on the degree of obstruction. In cases of complete ductal dependence, such as tricuspid atresia with pulmonary atresia, a neonatal modified Blalock–Taussig shunt is necessary. If there is mild or moderate pulmonary stenosis, it may be possible to follow the child closely without surgical intervention until cyanosis becomes a problem. In children younger than 6 months of age, a modified Blalock–Taussig-type shunt may be necessary. For those older than 6 months of age, a direct connection of the superior vena cava to the pulmonary artery may be performed (see Table 34-1). This bidirectional cavopulmonary shunt offers the advantages of sending unoxygenated blood to the lungs and decreasing the volume load on the single ventricle. In children who avoid intervention in the first year of life, it may be possible to proceed directly to a modification of the Fontan procedure, creating an in-series–type circulation.

SINGLE VENTRICLE WITH UNPROTECTED PULMONARY CIRCULATION

If there is unobstructed blood flow to both great arteries, it is necessary to protect the pulmonary circulation from the effects of high-pressure and high-flow circulation. The usual approach is pulmonary artery banding, although there are some advocates of pulmonary artery detachment and shunting. There is some concern that subaortic obstruction may be worsened by pulmonary artery banding, and this is a significant concern for patients with evidence of distal low flow, such as coarctation. Pulmonary artery bands may distort the pulmonary arteries, rendering them undesirable for Fontan-type repair.

COMPLEX HETEROTAXY

Lesions of the complex heterotaxy group consist of an array of cardiac lesions, usually grouped into the asplenia or polysplenia types. They are malformations related to errors in developmental left–right differentiation. The associated cardiac lesions are managed surgically as dictated by the anatomy. The splenic function must be assessed in all cases of heterotaxy, because poor splenic function, or splenic absence necessitates the institution of long-term antibiotic coverage, usually with amoxicillin. The presence of multiple small spleens does not guarantee adequate splenic function and may constitute functional asplenia.

POLYSPLENIA

Polysplenia is sometimes referred to as left atrial isomerism, and it is the more common form of heterotaxy. The most commonly reported cardiovascular abnormality in this group is azygous extension with interruption of the inferior vena cava. Common atrium and canal-type atrial defects are common in this group. Double-outlet right ventricle is a frequent finding. Univentricular connections are uncommon. Pulmonary stenosis or atresia is a commonly associated abnormality.

ASPLENIA

Asplenia is sometimes referred to as right atrial isomerism, and it constitutes about one-third of the cases of heterotaxy. Extracardiac anomalies of pulmonary venous connection are associated with this form of heterotaxy. Common atrium and atrioventricular canal-type defects occur in more than 90% of the patients. Approximately one-half of the patients have essentially a single-ventricle variant. Because of the greater complexity of these anomalies, more of these patients require surgery, and there is a higher overall mortality rate compared with patients with polysplenia.

CARDIAC TRANSPLANTATION IN THE NEONATE

During the last 10 years, increasing numbers of children are undergoing cardiac transplantation.[17] Ten years ago, cardiomyopathy was the single greatest indication for transplantation in children, but congenital cardiac lesion has replaced it as the most common indication. Most heart transplants are performed in the first months of life for children with congenital defects that are lethal or are associated with a very poor prognosis. The most frequent congenital lesions treated primarily with transplantation are hypoplastic left heart syndrome, imbalanced atrioventricular canal with dysfunctional atrioventricular valve, and PA/IVS with right ventricular-dependent coronary circulation. Secondary transplantation has been used to treat congenital lesions when surgical patients develop ventricular dysfunction or if other problems preclude further procedures (*e.g.*, a modified Fontan procedure). Many techniques have been developed to deal with the complex issues of situs and abnormalities of venous return, but the constant anatomic relationship of the aorta leaving the pericardium anterior to the pulmonary artery and the posterior positioning of the pulmonary veins make systemic venous connections the only severe challenge.

Results are varied, but they have shown improvement. Early results of neonatal cardiac transplantation reported a 60% 1-year survival rate.[18] This has improved to about 90% with increasing experience and improved technique.[19] Most institutions attempt to maintain growing infants on a nonsteroid regimen of immunosuppression. The introduction of FK506, which is in experimental stages, may significantly improve the pediatric results of this procedure.

The long-term outlook for the pediatric transplant patient is unclear. These children must go through the period of childhood illnesses with a suppressed immune system. Growth concerns continue to be important. The effect of long-term immunosuppression on the incidence of malignancy should be further delineated. Chronic rejection and the incidence of graft coronary artery problems (*e.g.*, graft atherosclerosis) may produce a sizable population requiring retransplantation.

POSTOPERATIVE CARE

With increasing complexity of operations at earlier ages, the intensity and importance of postoperative care cannot be underestimated. Most children require extensive monitoring, and the interplay of cardiac and respiratory care can make the critical difference in survival of an extremely sick neonate. A multidisciplinary team approach to the care of these infants, involving the surgeons, cardiologists, critical care physicians, and other subspecialty support, is vital. The most common cause of a poor postoperative course is problems with the operative repair. Echocardiographic evaluation and cardiac catheterization should always be considered early for neonates who do not make the expected postoperative progress. Any anatomic problems, whether relating to the repair or otherwise, should be addressed promptly with operative intervention if necessary.

Extracorporeal membrane oxygenation has been used for postoperative support of dysfunctional myocardium and occasionally as a bridge to transplant.[20,21] This continues to be a high-risk endeavor, and until its role in the treatment of postoperative cardiac patients is better delineated, it remains a modality limited to the tertiary care centers.

REFERENCES

1. Heymann MA. Pharmacologic use of prostaglandin E_1 in infants with congenital heart disease. Am Heart J 1981;101:837.
2. Pozzi M, Remig J, Fimmers R, Urban AE. Atrioventricular septal defects. J Thorac Cardiovasc Surg 1991;101:138.

3. Coles JG, Freedon RM, Lightfoot NE, et al. Long-term results in neonates with pulmonary atresia and intact ventricular septum. Ann Thorac Surg 1989;47:213.
4. Touati GD, Vouhe PR, Amodeo A, et al. Primary repair of tetralogy of Fallot in infancy. J Thorac Cardiovasc Surg 1990;99:396.
5. Di Donato RM, Jonas RA, Lang P, et al. Neonatal repair of tetralogy of Fallot with and without pulmonary atresia. J Thorac Cardiovasc Surg 1991;101:126.
6. Lang PE, Chipman CW, Siden H, et al. Early assessment of hemodynamic status after repair of tetralogy of Fallot: a comparison of 24 hour (intensive care unit) and 1 year postoperative data in 98 patients. Am J Cardiol 1982;50:795.
7. Millikan JS, Puga FJ, Danielson GK, et al. Staged surgical repair of pulmonary atresia, ventricular septal defect, and hypoplastic confluent pulmonary arteries. J Thorac Cardiovasc Surg 1986;91:818.
8. Norwood WI, Dobell AR, Freed MD, et al. Intermediate results of the arterial switch repair. J Thorac Cardiovasc Surg 1988;96:854.
9. Zeevi B, Keane JF, Castaneda AR, et al. Neonatal critical valvar aortic stenosis: a comparison of surgical and balloon dilation therapy. Circulation 1989;80:831.
10. Waldhausen JA, Nahrwold DL. Repair of warctation of the aorta with a subclavian flap. J Thorac Cardiovasc Surg 1966;51:532.
11. Sciolary C, Copeland J, Cork R, et al. Long-term follow-up comparing subclavian flap angioplasty to resection with modified oblique end-to-end anastomosis. J Thorac Cardiovasc Surg 1991;101:1.
12. Piggott JD, Murphy JD, Barber G, Norwood WI. Palliative reconstructive surgery for hypoplastic left heart syndrome. Ann Thorac Surg 1988;45:122.
13. Riemenschneider TA. Management of the hypoplastic left heart syndrome: a challenge to those who care for children with heart diseases. Am Heart J 1986;112:864.
14. Gustafson RA, Murray GF, Warden HG, et al. Stage I palliation of hypoplastic left heart syndrome: the importanceof neoaorta construction. Ann Thor Surg 1989;48:43.
15. Stansel HC Jr. A new operation for d-loop transposition of the great vessels. Ann Thorac Surg 1975;19:565.
16. Stein DG, Laks H, Drinkwater DC, et al. Results of total cavopulmonary connection in the treatment of patients with a functional single ventricle. J Thorac Cardiovasc Surg 1991;102:280.
17. Bailey LL, Assaad AN, Trimm RF, et al. Orthotopic transplantation during early infancy as therapy for incurable congenital heart disease. Ann Surg 1988;208:279.
18. Backer CL, Zales VR, Harrison HL, et al. Intermediate term results of infant orthotopic cardiac transplantation from two centers. J Thorac Cardiovasc Surg 1991;101:826.
19. Bailey L, Gundry S, Razzark A, Wang N. Pediatric heart transplantation: issues relating to outcome and results. J Heart Lung Transplant 1991; 11(Suppl):267.
20. Klein MD, Shaheen KW, Whittlesey GC, et al. Extracorporeal membrane oxygenation for the circulatory support of children after repair of congenital heart disease. J Thorac Cardiovasc Surg 1990;100:498.
21. Kanter KR, Pennington DG, Weber TR, et al. Extracorporeal membrane oxygenation for postoperative cardiac support in children. J Thorac Cardiovasc Surg 1987;93:27.

Neonatology: Pathophysiology and Management of the Newborn, Fourth Edition,
edited by Gordon B. Avery, Mary Ann Fletcher, and Mhairi G. MacDonald.
J.B. Lippincott Company, Philadelphia © 1994.

chapter 35

Carbohydrate Homeostasis

EDWARD S. OGATA

Glucose homeostasis results from the net balance between systemic organ requirements and the production and regulation of glucose. The neonate's ability to maintain glucose homeostasis is less than optimal because it is in a metabolic transition period. It has abruptly switched from intrauterine life, in which glucose and metabolic fuels are provided in a well regulated manner, to a situation where it is an intermittent meal eater. This necessitates regulation of exogenous glucose and production of endogenous glucose. As the capability to perform these functions continues to develop in the neonate, clinical disorders that can afflict the neonate may perturb this balance, resulting in hypoglycemia or hyperglycemia. In addition, antecedent intrauterine events can alter the development of glucoregulatory capabilities in the fetus, resulting in altered neonatal glucose homeostasis. Diabetes in pregnancy is the *sine qua non* of changes in maternal metabolism that affect fetal development and alter neonatal glucoregulation.

To understand the processes responsible for glucose homeostasis in the normal neonate, an understanding of the development of glucoregulatory capabilities in the fetus is necessary. This chapter reviews this information and its relation to the clinical disorders associated with altered neonatal glucose homeostasis. Information on the perinatal aspects of diabetes in pregnancy also is presented.

MATERNAL METABOLISM DURING PREGNANCY

Although the metabolic alterations that develop in the pregnant woman throughout gestation favor the growth and development of the fetus, the first half of gestation also is a critical period for maternal anabolism. The increased calories ingested by the woman during early gestation not only sustain fetal growth but facilitate maternal fat deposition. This is important preparation for the second half of gestation, a period of exponential fetal growth during which these maternal stores are mobilized to meet fetal needs. The storage of maternal energy stores is facilitated by the increased secretion of insulin that occurs in women with normal carbohydrate metabolism.[1–5]

From roughly midgestation onward, a number of anti-insulin factors develop in the mother to cause pregnancy to become a diabetogenic–like state. Human placental lactogen, progesterone, and estrogen, which directly antagonize maternal insulin, become increasingly available. In addition, insulin-degrading enzyme systems develop in the placenta that further deplete maternal insulin. These alterations guarantee metabolic fuel availability to the fetus during the postprandial state; the delay in clearance of glucose and other metabolic fuels from the maternal circulation due to blunting of insulin's effect allow a longer period for uptake by the uteroplacental circulation.[6–8] Preexisting maternal diabetes potentiates the effects of the antiinsulin factors, causing an excessive provision of glucose and other metabolic fuels to the fetus. This is the basic perturbation responsible for the problems of the infant of the diabetic mother (Fig. 35-1).[1,9]

Metabolic fuel availability is guaranteed to the fetus even during brief maternal fasting. After an overnight fast, pregnant women have significantly lower plasma glucose concentrations compared to fasted nongravid women[10,11]; however, glucose production in the mother is significantly increased.[12,13] This increased production ensures the provision of glucose to the fetus.

Prolonged maternal fasting does alter fuel provision to the fetus. As the fast progresses, maternal ketogenesis progressively increases.[11,14] The human fetal brain at early gestation can use ketones (Fig. 35-2).[15] This capability to use an alternative fuel may be harmful rather than beneficial to the fetus. Offspring of mothers who were ketotic during pregnancy appear to have an increased incidence of cognitive and psychomotor delay at 3 and 5 years of age.[16] Whether ketone use by the fetal brain was responsible for this is unknown. Equally unclear is the duration and degree of ketone exposure necessary to cause damage. Because of this uncertainty, maternal fasting, even forgoing breakfast, should be avoided during pregnancy.

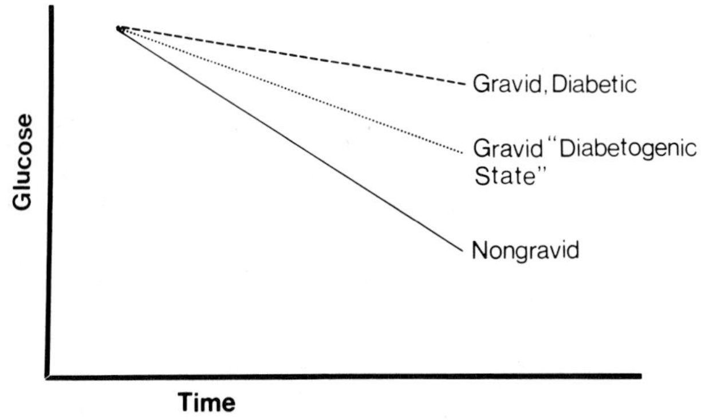

FIG. 35–1. Plasma glucose changes after glucose challenge in nongravid, gravid, and gravid diabetic women. Compared to the nongravid woman, the pregnant woman with normal carbohydrate metabolism demonstrates delayed glucose clearance from midgestation onward as a result of antiinsulin factors that develop during pregnancy. The delay in glucose clearance from the maternal circulation assures glucose provision to the fetus, particularly during the postprandial period. The blunting of maternal glucose clearance is exaggerated by the counterinsulin factors in the woman with diabetes mellitus. The decreased clearance of glucose and other metabolic fuels stimulates fetal insulin production and is responsible for many of the problems of the infant of the diabetic mother.

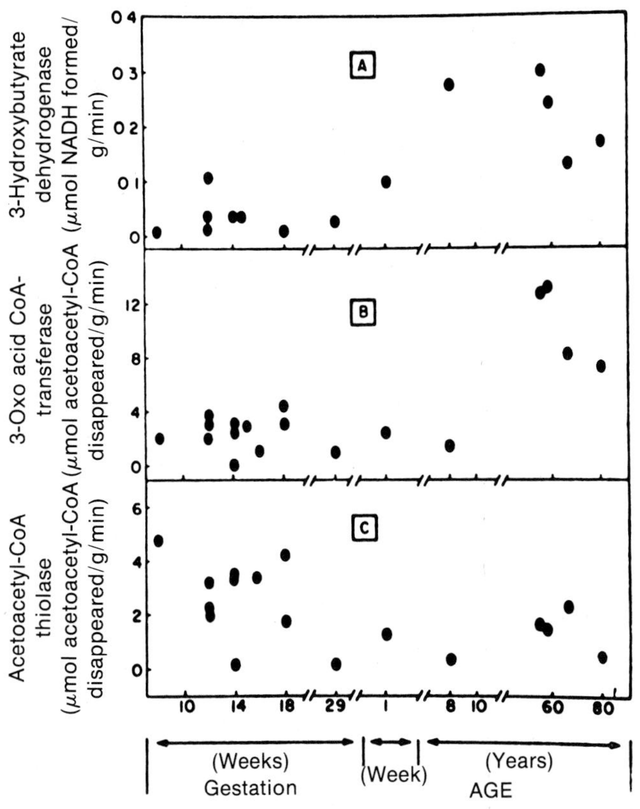

FIG. 35–2. Enzymatic activity of the three key enzymes necessary for the oxidation of ketones (*i.e.*, β-hydroxybutyrate and acetoacetate). The activities of these enzymes are present in substantial quantities in the human fetal brain during early gestation. (From Patel MS, Johnson CA, Rajan R, Owen OE. The metabolism of ketone bodies in developing human brain: development of ketone-body-utilizing enzymes and ketone bodies as precursors for lipid synthesis. J Neurochem 1975;25:905.)

DEVELOPMENT OF GLUCOSE-PRODUCING AND GLUCOREGULATORY CAPABILITIES IN THE FETUS

To understand the problems of neonatal glucose homeostasis, the development of glucose production and regulatory capabilities in the fetus must be understood.

GLYCOGEN

The third trimester of the human pregnancy is the first period in gestation during which some of the energy and substrate available to the fetus can be channelled from meeting needs for ongoing growth and development to energy storage. As the third trimester progresses, fat deposition and hepatic glycogen storage increase.[17] The human fetus can synthesize and mobilize glycogen and respond to the signals that regulate these processes as early as the ninth week of gestation.[18] Minute quantities of hepatic gly-

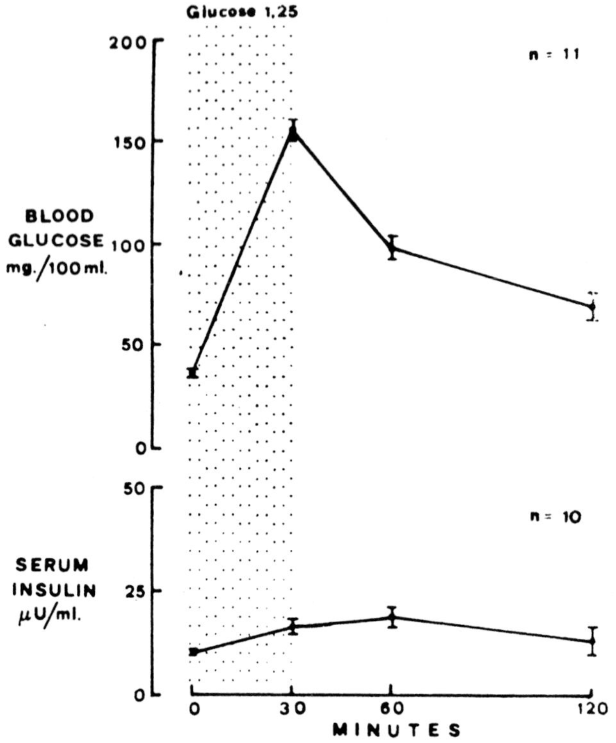

FIG. 35–3. Insulin secretion after glucose challenge in premature infants. Whereas normal adults secrete insulin briskly in response to glucagon, premature infants in the neonatal period secrete insulin only sluggishly. (From Grasso S, Messina A, Distefano G, et al. Insulin secretion in the premature infant: response to glucose and amino acids. Diabetes 1973;22:349.)

cogen are detectable in early gestation; however, the great bulk of hepatic glycogen accumulates during the third trimester.[18,19]

Several types of infants are at risk for neonatal hypoglycemia as a result of limited hepatic glycogen stores. Infants delivered prematurely have an abbreviated or no third trimester and thus have limited glycogen stores. Fetuses who are growth-retarded (*i.e.*, small for gestational age [SGA]) on the basis of limited metabolic fuel availability and diminished gaseous exchange (*i.e.*, uteroplacental insufficiency) will use these fuels for growth and not have glucose remaining for glycogen synthesis. Perinatal stress causes neonatal hypoglycemia in part because of catecholamine-stimulated mobilization of hepatic glycogen stores. This can occur at birth or during the antepartum period. In the latter situation, fetuses might recover from stress and be delivered without difficulty. As newborns, such infants have depleted glycogen stores and are at risk for hypoglycemia.

GLUCONEOGENESIS

For many years, it was believed that maternally derived glucose was the sole metabolic fuel for the fetus and that the fetus could not produce glucose. As indicated, the fetus can use other fuels such as the ketones and can under special circumstances mobilize hepatic glycogen. The fetus also can carry out gluconeogenesis to a limited degree, although it is likely that under normal circumstances it does not need to call on this function. Data from human abortus material have demonstrated that the four key gluconeogenic enzymes are demonstrable in fetal liver by 2 to 3 months of gestation.[20,21] The activities of these enzymes are believed to increase throughout gestation and the neonatal period. Thus, all newborns including the very premature probably have some degree of gluconeogenic capability.

ENDOCRINE REGULATION

Insulin and glucagon, important hormones for regulating glucose, can be measured in fetal plasma as early as 12 weeks of gestation.[22] Although plasma concentrations of these hormones are low, the relative content of these hormones in the fetal pancreas is quite high.[23,24] These high concentrations may result

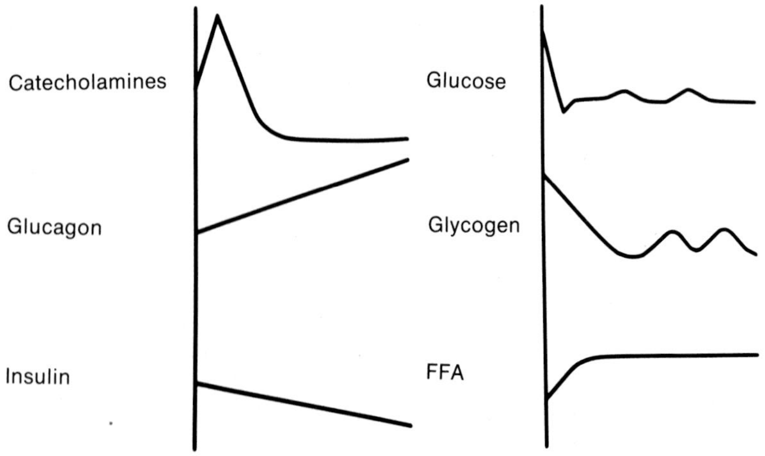

FIG. 35–4. Levels of hormone and metabolic fuels change after birth. At birth, the counterregulatory hormones (*i.e.*, catecholamines and glucagon) increase greatly, whereas insulin secretion decreases. Neonatal plasma glucose concentrations plummet as a result of cord clamping. The changes in counterregulatory hormones and insulin favor mobilization of glucose and fat and stimulate gluconeogenesis. These changes assure adequate neonatal glucose production. (FA, free fatty acids; from Ogata ES. Carbohydrate metabolism in the fetus and neonate and altered neonatal glucoregulation. Pediatr Clin North Am 1986;33:25.)

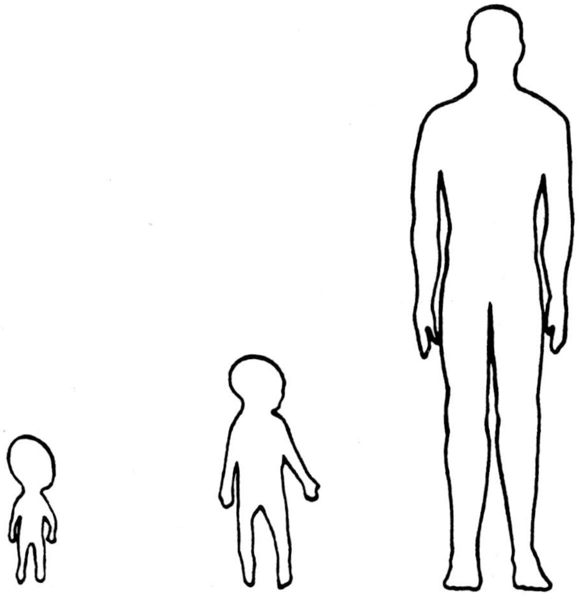

FIG. 35–5. Glucose turnover in premature and term neonates and the adult. When related to body weight, glucose turnover is greatest in the premature infant and least in the adult. The increased turnover in neonates is due in part to their relatively increased brain-to-body mass. (From Ogata ES. Carbohydrate metabolism in the fetus and neonate and altered neonatal glucoregulation. Pediatr Clin North Am 1986;33:25.)

from the limited ability of the fetal islets to secrete these hormones. Studies in premature and term infants in the newborn period indicate that their capacity to secrete these hormones in response to a glucose challenge is limited; this suggests that the fetus also has limited secretory capability (Fig. 35-3).[24–26] Of note, amino acids have a greater effect than glucose in stimulating insulin and limiting glucagon secretion.[27,28]

Insulin may be more important for enhancing growth than regulating metabolic fuels during fetal life. Insulin stimulates the growth of specific tissues (*e.g.*, adipose, hepatic, connective, skeletal, cardiac muscle).[29,30] Excessive insulin secretion during fetal life resulting from such conditions as maternal diabetes causes the disproportionate growth of insulin-sensitive tissues, resulting in macrosomia.[1,9,31,32] A lack of insulin, as in infants with transient neonatal diabetes mellitus, always is accompanied by fetal growth retardation.

Glucagon or a critical glucagon–insulin relation is important for inducing gluconeogenic enzymes. Glucagon stimulates the induction of gluconeogenic enzymes *in vitro* and *in vivo*.[33,34] Fetal plasma glucagon concentrations increase progressively during fetal life, and this is associated with a concomitant increase in gluconeogenic enzyme activity. At birth, plasma glucagon concentrations surge, coinciding with the rapid postnatal increase in gluconeogenic activity.[35] Insulin may modulate glucagon's effect because it can inhibit gluconeogenic enzyme induction.[34] Thus, a balance between these two hormones controls gluconeogenic enzyme induction during perinatal life.

Adrenergic mechanisms can stimulate hepatic glycogenolysis during fetal life, much as in the adult. As labor progresses, fetal sympathoadrenal activity increases, resulting in a considerable increase in circulating catecholamine levels.[36,37] Cord clamping triggers an increase in glucagon secretion.[38] As plasma glucose concentrations plummet with cord clamping,

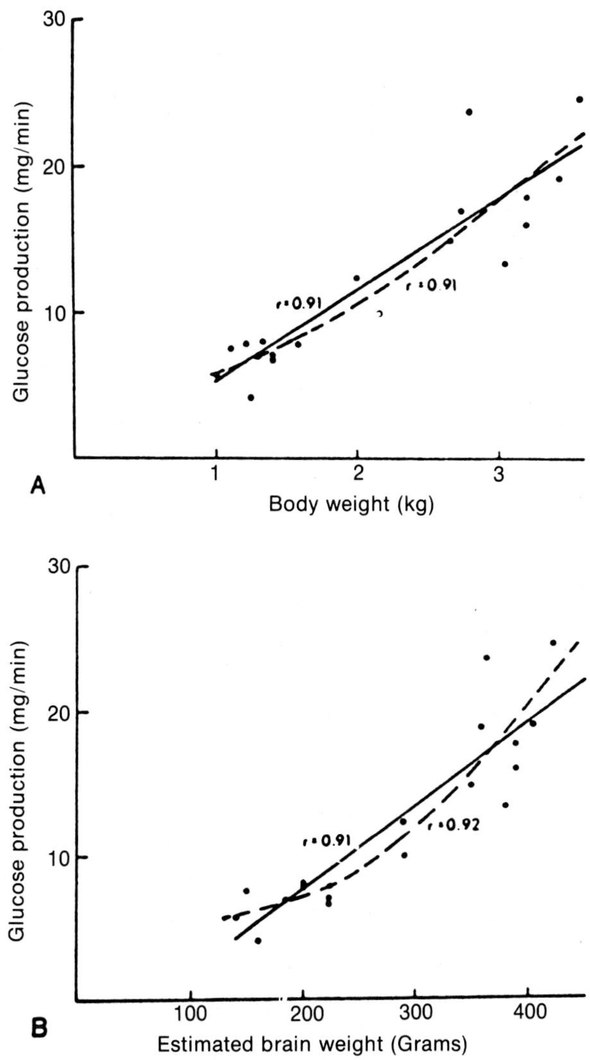

FIG. 35–6. Linear and curvilinear regression analyses indicate strong relations between glucose turnover and body mass, and glucose turnover and brain mass in newborn human infants. (From Bier DM, Leake RD, Haymond MW, et al. Measurement of "true" glucose production rates in infancy and childhood with 6,6 dideuteroglucose. Diabetes 1977;26:1016.)

insulin secretion slowly decreases. These adjustments, particularly the remarkable increase in catecholamine secretion, stimulate glycogenolysis and gluconeogenesis in the neonate (Fig. 35-4).

Islet cell function remains unresponsive for several weeks of neonatal life in term infants. Newborn infants increase insulin and limit glucagon secretion sluggishly in response to glucose challenge. Limited data indicate that these responses become adultlike between 1 to 2 weeks of life.[39] This adaptation is critically important because the neonate, unlike the fetus, must regulate glucose production and storage through feeding and fasting cycles. Little is known about the premature infant's ability to regulate glucose in the neonatal period. The ability to modulate insulin and glucagon secretion probably develops as the neonatal period progresses.

NEONATAL GLUCOSE REQUIREMENTS

The clinician makes a leap of faith in using the chemical or paper strip determination of plasma or blood glucose concentration to judge the adequacy of tissue glucose provision in the neonate. A normal plasma concentration is interpreted to mean that glucose supply to the brain and other organs is adequate for ongoing metabolic needs. To appreciate glucose requirements, glucose kinetics must be understood.

Glucose turnover represents the rate of production of glucose by the liver and other organs and the simultaneous use or uptake of glucose by the brain and other organs. Turnover is usually expressed as milligrams of glucose per kilograms of body weight per minute. Although stable isotope technology has allowed quantification of glucose turnover in neonates, this methodology cannot be directly applied for clinical purposes. Thus, the clinician must rely on the measurements of glucose concentrations, which are static, as representative of the dynamic rate of glucose production and use in a neonate. In general, plasma glucose concentrations roughly correlate with glucose turnover. Diminished plasma glucose concentrations suggest that glucose production is limited or that glucose use is increased (*i.e.,* need is outstripping production). Elevated plasma glucose concentrations suggest that either production is excessive or, more likely, that organ uptake and use are diminished. These are the dynamic physiologic conditions that define hypoglycemia and hyperglycemia.

In the neonate, glucose production correlates directly with brain and body mass, confirming the critical role of glucose as a metabolic fuel.[40–43] Glucose turnover for newborn infants when related to body mass significantly exceeds that of adults (Fig. 35-5). Premature infants have even greater turnover values than term neonates. This is due in part to the ratio of brain to body mass, which is greatest in premature infants and least in adults. These relations emphasize the importance of glucose as the primary fuel for the brain (Fig. 35-6).

NEONATAL HYPOGLYCEMIA

A variety of blood and plasma glucose concentration values based on screening of neonates or clinical experience have been recommended as values defining hypoglycemia.[44] All of these are somewhat arbitrary because they cannot be correlated directly with glucose use rate or severity of symptoms. Because plasma or blood glucose concentrations only roughly reflect glucose turnover, a plasma glucose concentration of less than 40 mg/dL should be used to define hypoglycemia. When glucose turnover is sufficient to meet the needs of the organism, concentrations usually exceed this value. It also is important to note that values somewhat less than 40 mg/dL still can be associated with adequate glucose provision.

The chemical definition of hypoglycemia must take into account the methodology of glucose determinations. Glucose concentration in whole blood is approximately 10% to 15% lower than in plasma. Delay in determination after blood sampling may result in glucose oxidation by erythrocytes, causing falsely low values. Although the use of paper strip methods to estimate glucose concentrations quickly is acceptable, their results should be corroborated by true chemical determinations.

The clinical manifestations of inadequate glucose provision to the neonatal brain range from no symptoms to lethargy or mild tremors to frank convulsions (Table 35-1). The degree of glucose limitation necessary to cause brain damage is unknown. The lack of clearly defined data on this problem and the prevailing opinion concerning the potentially damaging effects of hypoglycemia mandate that infants at risk be monitored and that asymptomatic and symptomatic infants be appropriately treated.

All conditions associated with the development of hypoglycemia in the neonate result from one or a combination of two basic mechanisms: inadequate production or excessive tissue use. Inadequate glucose production results from a lack of glycogen stores, an inability to synthesize glucose, or both (Fig. 35-7). Excessive tissue use results from increased insulin secretion. Table 35-2 categorizes infants at risk for hypoglycemia in relation to these basic mechanisms.

TABLE 35–1
SYMPTOMS OF HYPOGLYCEMIA

Jitteriness
Tremors
Apnea
Cyanosis
Limpness/lethargy

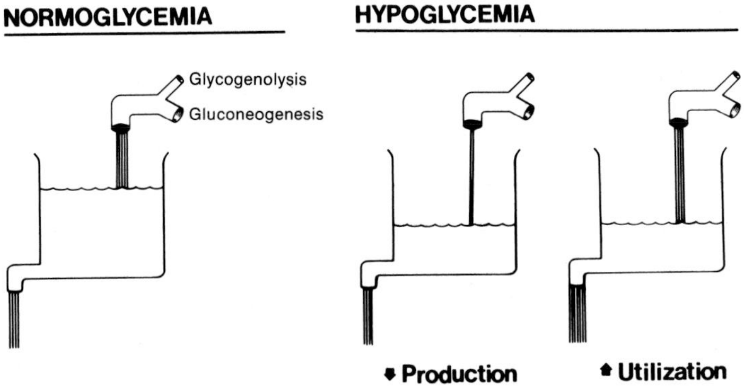

FIG. 35–7. The rates of glucose production and utilization are represented by the faucet and drain of the sink. The level in the sink is equivalent to plasma or blood glucose concentrations. If production from glycogenolysis and gluconeogenesis is adequate and use is not excessive, normoglycemia exists, and the plasma or blood glucose concentration (*i.e.*, the level in the sink) is normal. Hypoglycemia develops if production is inadequate to meet body needs or if use outstrips production. This results in decreased glucose concentrations (*i.e.*, diminished level in sink). (From Ogata ES. Carbohydrate metabolism in the fetus and neonate and altered glucoregulation. Pediatr Clin North Am 1986;33:25.)

INADEQUATE GLUCOSE PRODUCTION AS A RESULT OF LIMITED GLYCOGEN STORES

PREMATURE INFANTS

As indicated, the third trimester of pregnancy is an important period for hepatic glycogen deposition. An infant delivered prematurely without having had the benefit of part of or the entire third trimester will have limited hepatic glycogen stores. The greater the degree of prematurity, the less glycogen will be present. Small-for-gestational-age premature infants are at extremely high risk for development of hypoglycemia because available nutrients during intrauterine life are channeled toward growth, with little set aside for glycogen storage. For this reason, SGA premature infants have extremely limited glycogen stores.[45–47]

TABLE 35–2
INFANTS AT RISK FOR HYPOGLYCEMIA

Diminished Production
Limited glycogen
SGA
Prematurity
Birth stress
Glycogen storage disorders
Limited gluconeogenesis
SGA
Inborn errors
Increased Utilization
Hyperinsulinism
IDM
Beckwith–Wiedemann Syndrome
Nesidioblastosis or pancreatic adenoma
Erythroblastosis fetalis
Exchange transfusion, chlorpropamide, benzothiazides, β-sympathomimetics, malpositioned UA catheter
Unknown
LGA infants who are not IDM
Sepsis
Polycythemia or hyperviscosity syndrome
Congenital hypopituitarism

IDM, infant of diabetic mother; LGA, large for gestational age; SGA, small for gestational age; UA, umbilical artery.

INFANTS WHO HAVE SUFFERED PERINATAL STRESS

Infants who are stressed *in utero* are at increased risk for development of hypoglycemia as neonates. Hypoxia, acidosis, and alterations in fetal blood pressure and flow can stimulate catecholamine secretion *in utero*, which in turn will mobilize hepatic glycogen stores. In addition, hypoxia increases the rate of anaerobic glycolysis, thereby accelerating glucose use. These events deplete fetal glycogen stores and place the infant at risk for hypoglycemia after delivery.

GLYCOGEN STORAGE DISEASE

Intrinsic defects in glycogen synthesis, storage, or breakdown result in complex metabolic problems (see Chap. 39). Several types of glycogen storage disease (*i.e.*, Ia, I, VI, 0) have hypoglycemia as one of many associated complications.[44,48]

INADEQUATE PRODUCTION AS A RESULT OF LIMITED GLUCONEOGENESIS

SMALL-FOR-GESTATIONAL-AGE INFANTS

Full-term and premature SGA neonates are at great risk for development of hypoglycemia as a result of inadequate hepatic glycogen stores. With treatment, this usually is short-lived. Approximately 1% of SGA infants in whom hypoglycemia develops have a prolonged course requiring intravenous therapy for days. A delay in the induction of gluconeogenic capability probably is responsible for this prolonged hypoglycemia. These SGA neonates have elevated plasma concentrations of gluconeogenic precursors, suggesting an inability to convert exogenous gluconeogenic precursors such as alanine to glucose.[49,50]

In animal models of intrauterine growth retardation, the induction of one gluconeogenic enzyme, phosphoenolpyruvate carboxykinase, is delayed.[51,52] This occurs despite appropriate increases in glucagon and decreases in insulin; these relations should favor enzyme induction. Why some SGA infants fail to induce gluconeogenic capability is unclear. Corticosteroid therapy often was used in the past to treat prolonged hypoglycemia. The success of this practice probably was due in part to the ability of corticosteroids to induce hepatic gluconeogenic enzymes.

Many SGA infants have heightened metabolic requirements during the neonatal period. The mechanisms for this are not understood but may represent an attempt to compensate for the preceding intrauterine deprivation.[53] This may explain the increased glucose requirements demonstrated by some hypoglycemic SGA infants.

CONGENITAL ABSENCE OF GLUCONEOGENIC CAPABILITY

Unlike SGA infants in whom gluconeogenic capability eventually develops, a few infants have been reported who have permanent congenital lack of gluconeogenic enzymes.[54] A single infant who was unable to secrete glucagon also has been reported.[55]

EXCESSIVE TISSUE USE OR HYPERINSULINISM

A variety of disorders are associated with fetal and neonatal hyperinsulinism. In some disorders, the mechanisms for heightened β-cell function are well understood, whereas in others, the pathogenesis is unclear. In the former category are infants of diabetic mothers (IDM) and infants with altered pancreatic islets caused by conditions such as nesidioblastosis and pancreatic adenoma. Those for whom an etiology is not clear include infants with erythroblastosis and Beckwith–Wiedemann syndrome. The finding of a hypoglycemic infant who is macrosomic and requires high rates of glucose infusion (10–20 mg/kg body weight/minute) suggests a hyperinsulinemic state.

INFANTS OF DIABETIC MOTHERS

Infants of diabetic mothers are at great risk for development of hypoglycemia as a result of the carryover of the fetal hyperinsulinemic state into neonatal life. They have elevated plasma insulin concentrations and release insulin briskly in response to glucose challenge. The problems of the IDM are presented in the following sections.

NESIDIOBLASTOSIS AND ISLET CELL ADENOMA

These two accidents of development cause sustained hyperinsulinism and hypoglycemia during the newborn period. With nesidioblastosis, pancreatic ductular endocrine cells proliferate uncontrollably. These replace normal islet cells and also infiltrate acinar tissue. Islet cell adenomas occur less frequently than nesidioblastosis.[56–58] These disorders, however, cannot be clinically distinguished from one another because exuberant insulin secretion begins *in utero* and remains sustained throughout the neonatal period.

The diagnosis of either nesidioblastosis or islet cell adenoma should be considered whenever a macrosomic infant has hypoglycemia prolonged over several days, with elevated plasma insulin concentrations. Rebound hypoglycemia in response to excessive glucose administration is another characteristic. Increased insulin–glucose ratios and glucose requirements exceeding 10 mg/kg/minute suggest the possibility of either nesidioblastosis or islet cell adenoma. Both somatostatin and diazoxide have been used successfully to limit insulin secretion in patients with these conditions. Surgical excision offers definitive diagnosis and therapy.

UNEXPLAINED NEONATAL HYPERINSULINEMIA AND HYPOGLYCEMIA

Infants with Beckwith–Wiedemann syndrome, erythroblastosis fetalis, and those whose mothers have taken chlorpropamide or benzothiazides are at risk for development of hypoglycemia as a result of hyperinsulinism. In 1964, Beckwith and colleagues and Wiedemann independently reported the exophthalmos–macroglossia–gigantum syndrome. Such infants frequently have omphalocele, muscular macroglossia, macrosomia, and, neonatal hypoglycemia. The hypoglycemia and macrosomia are due to hyperinsulinism resulting from β-cell hypertrophy.[59–60] Some of the morbidity and mortality originally associated with this syndrome was due to unrecognized hypoglycemia. Thus, early recognition and prevention of hypoglycemia is mandatory.

Infants with erythroblastosis fetalis due to Rh incompatibility were reported in the past to be at risk for hypoglycemia due to hyperinsulinism from B-cell hyperplasia.[61] The mechanisms responsible for islet cell hyperplasia are unknown, although it was proposed that elevated plasma glutathione concentrations might stimulate the fetal β cell to increase insulin secretion.[62] The advent of direct intravascular transfusion of Rh-affected fetuses may reduce the risk of hypoglycemia. Severely affected Rh fetuses who receive serial intravascular transfusions by the percutaneous umbilical technique are normoinsulinemic despite originally having elevated glutathione concentrations. Hypoglycemia does not develop in them as neonates.[63]

It is important to note that infants undergoing exchange transfusion are at risk for development of hypoglycemia due to stimulation of insulin secretion by glucose in stored erythrocytes.[64] Checking for hypoglycemia during and after an exchange transfusion is therefore important.

Maternal use of chlorpropamide and benzothiazide can directly increase insulin secretion in the neonate.[65,66] Beta-sympathomimetic agents used to stop premature labor have been reported to cause neonatal hypoglycemia.[67] These drugs stimulate glycogen breakdown and gluconeogenesis in the mother and fetus.[68] Both the increased availability of maternal glucose and the β-sympathomimetic agent that crosses the placenta stimulate fetal insulin secretion, resulting in neonatal hyperinsulinism and hypoglycemia. For these reasons, infants whose mothers received tocolytic therapy shortly before delivery should be monitored for hypoglycemia.

Some debate exists as to whether glucose administered to the mother during labor and delivery stimulates fetal β-cell secretion and causes neonatal hyperinsulinism and hypoglycemia. Acute maternal glucose loading may stimulate fetal insulin secretion and increase the risk of neonatal hypoglycemia.[69] If glucose infusion is well controlled, the likelihood of this is minimized. Control of maternal glucose administration is particularly important in situations where the fetus is suspected of having heightened B-cell sensitivity (*e.g.*, maternal diabetes, Rh incompatibility), because under these circumstances even moderate excursions of glucose may stimulate fetal insulin secretion.

Malposition of the tip of an umbilical artery catheter at a level between the tenth thoracic and the second lumbar vertebrae may result in glucose-stimulated hyperinsulinism. Several infants have been reported in whom hypoglycemia was relieved only when the tip of umbilical artery catheter was repositioned. It has been proposed that glucose from the malpositioned catheter flows into the celiac axis, thereby stimulating insulin secretion.[70] Animal studies have confirmed this possibility,[71] which should be considered in unexplained cases of hypoglycemia.

Large-for-gestational-age (LGA) infants whose mothers do not have diabetes mellitus are at risk for transient hypoglycemia. This is particularly true of LGA infants of obese women.[72] The mechanisms responsible for hypoglycemia are unknown, although limited data suggest that hyperinsulinism is not a major factor.

Sepsis in a neonate often is heralded by hypoglycemia or hyperglycemia. The mechanisms for this are not understood. Several studies have indicated rapid glucose disposal rates after intravenous challenge in septic term neonates. Although this suggests a hyperinsulinemic state, insulin secretion in these neonates was normal.[73,74] The hyperglycemia and hypoglycemia that often precede the other signs of sepsis in premature infants may be catecholamine mediated.

Hypoglycemia is a well acknowledged complication of the neonatal polycythemia–hyperviscosity syndrome.[75] Although polycythemia is more likely to occur in SGA and LGA infants who are at risk for hypoglycemia for other reasons, hypoglycemia occurs at an increased rate in polycythemic appropriately grown infants. Animal studies have documented diminished cerebral glucose uptake with polycythemia; however, the mechanisms responsible for decreasing glucose provision are unknown.[76] The increased erythrocyte mass is not sufficient to reduce glucose availability. The diminished plasma volume resulting from polycythemia may limit glucose provision. These possibilities remain to be confirmed.

Congenital hypopituitarism is a rare disorder in the neonate resulting from a spectrum of developmental accidents.[77,78] Congenital absence of the anterior pituitary is the common cause of this disorder, although holoprosencephaly and optic disc dysplasia also have been associated. Affected males have microphallus, whereas females have normal external genitalia.[79] Neonatal hypoglycemia often develops and can be severe. The endocrine alterations resulting from congenital hypopituitarism are complex, and the mechanisms by which they cause hypoglycemia are not understood. Growth hormone is important in this regard because it can reverse hypoglycemia. As hypoglycemia can develop later in the postnatal period, infants should have growth hormone therapy initiated for the long term.

Infants who have suffered hypothermia (*i.e.*, environmental temperature below 90°F) are at increased risk for development of hypoglycemia.[80] This may result from increased availability of catecholamines,[81] which would deplete glycogen reserves. Tissue use of glucose also might be increased under these conditions.

Other unusual clinical conditions reported associated with hypoglycemia include salicylate administration,[82] congenital adrenal hyperplasia,[83] and trisomy 13 mosaicism.[84] The mechanisms for these phenomena are not known.

NEONATAL HYPERGLYCEMIA

Hyperglycemia occurs primarily in three major groups of infants: those who are very premature, those who have neonatal diabetes mellitus, and those who are septic. Altered glucoregulation due to sepsis was discussed in the preceding section (see Unexplained Neonatal Hyperinsulinemia and Hypoglycemia).

THE VERY PREMATURE INFANT

Advances in perinatal care have improved the survival rate of the very premature infant. With this, the problem of glucose intolerance has greatly increased because the risk of hyperglycemia is at least 18 times greater in infants weighing under 1000 g than in those weighing over 2000 g. Depending on the definition, age at screening, and type of intravenous solution administered, the incidence of hyperglycemia in very premature infants has been reported to range from 20% to 86%.[85,86] In general, the smaller and more premature an infant, the greater the likelihood that he or she will not tolerate exogenous glucose at maintenance rates (4–6 mg/kg/minute). It is not uncommon to administer glucose at 1 to 2 mg/kg/minute or less and still observe plasma glucose concentrations exceeding 200 mg/dL.

Several basic mechanisms probably are responsible for glucose intolerance in very premature infants. Many probably do not secrete glucoregulatory hormones appropriately. In addition, end organ response to these hormones may be blunted. Thus, endogenous glucose production may continue while tissue glucose uptake is limited despite intravenous glucose therapy. Limited data indicate that the premature infant will only slowly increase insulin secretion in response to glucose challenge.[87–90] The amount secreted may not be sufficient to regulate glucose. Such infants may[89] or may not[91] decrease glucagon in response to glucose. In addition, very premature infants can be resistant to insulin.[92] This resistance is accentuated by catecholamines, which often are quite elevated. These factors contribute to the limited ability of the premature infant to reduce glucose production in the same manner as the adult, when exogenous glucose is provided (Fig. 35-8).

NEONATAL DIABETES MELLITUS

This is a rare disorder characterized by hypoinsulinism, progressive wasting, polyuria, and glycosuria during the neonatal period. Such infants usually are not ketotic. Of note, they are always SGA.[93,94] The intrauterine growth retardation results from limited

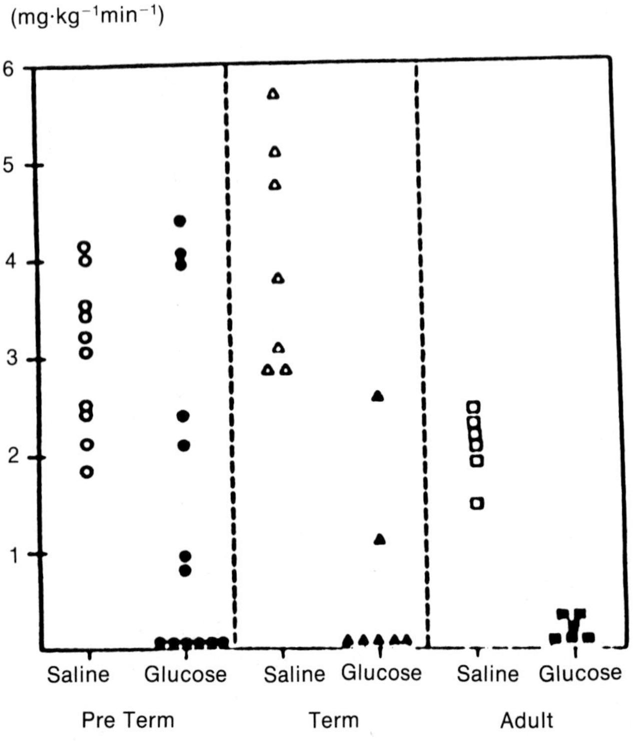

FIG. 35–8. Hepatic glucose production rates (GPR) in human premature neonates, full-term neonates, and adults during either saline (*open symbols*) or glucose (*closed symbols*) infusion. With glucose infusion, adults and full-term infants but not preterm infants reduce endogenous glucose production. Many preterm infants are apparently unable to regulate glucose production; this contributes to the development of hyperglycemia in these infants. (From Cowett RM, Oh W, Schwartz R. Persistent glucose production during glucose infusion in the neonate. J Clin Invest 1983; 71:467.)

fetal insulin secretion and exemplifies the importance of insulin as a fetal growth-stimulating hormone. This disorder may be heterogenous with respect to etiology. Synthesis of an abnormal poorly functioning insulin molecule or receptor deficiencies are other possible causes. Neonatal diabetes mellitus usually is transient; the early acute period calls for standard diabetic therapy (*i.e.*, monitoring caloric intake and administering exogenous insulin).

DIAGNOSIS AND TREATMENT

HYPOGLYCEMIA

All infants at risk for development of hypoglycemia should undergo frequent plasma glucose determinations. The commercially available paper strip indicators are widely used. Because their accuracy is fair, it is desirable to confirm values close to hypoglycemia or hyperglycemia with laboratory chemical determinations. Infants at risk for hypoglycemia should be checked at hourly intervals during the first 4 hours of life and then at 4-hour intervals until the risk period has passed. If an infant is feeding, blood sampling should be obtained before feeding. For IDMs and SGA infants, the screening should continue for at least 24 hours.

Infants who have borderline asymptomatic hypoglycemia, who do not have respiratory distress syndrome (RDS) or other serious disorders, and who are capable of enteral feedings may receive either 5% dextrose solution or formula as their initial treatment. In general, this approach can be used for infants at term who are LGA or SGA. However, because this mode of therapy is not always successful, plasma or blood glucose concentrations must be checked shortly after feeding.

Intravenous administration of glucose in a quantity sufficient to meet tissue requirements is the treatment of choice for hypoglycemia. The administration of 10% or 15% dextrose solution at 5 to 10 mL/kg body weight, followed by a continuous infusion at 5 to 6 mg/kg body weight/minute of glucose, will increase plasma glucose concentrations to 40 mg/dL or greater and acutely meet tissue requirements. The maintenance rates may require adjustment depending on the etiology of hypoglycemia.

Glucagon and epinephrine increase glucose production. Because both mobilize hepatic glycogen stores, their efficacy in treating hypoglycemia is variable, particularly in infants with limited hepatic stores. The numerous cardiovascular effects of epinephrine also limit its usefulness in infants.

Infants who are hypoglycemic for prolonged periods as a result of an inability to produce glucose can be treated with corticosteroids (hydrocortisone 5 mg/kg/day every 12 hours; prednisone 2 mg/kg/day orally). Steroids exert some of their effects by inducing gluconeogenic enzyme activity.

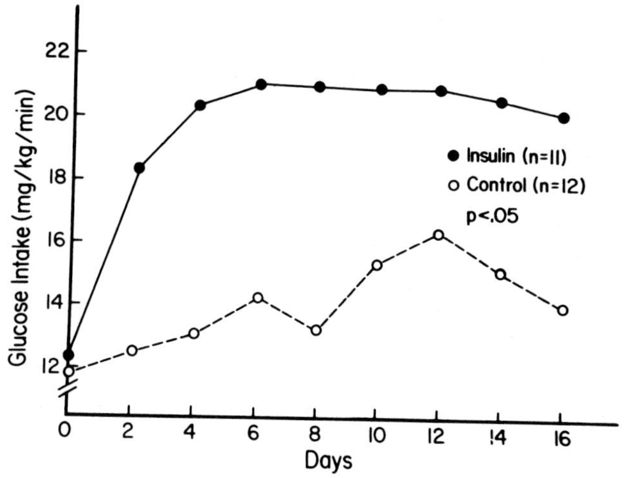

FIG. 35–9. Mean glucose infusion rates per day in insulin-treated (*solid line*) and control (*dashed line*) very-low-birth-weight infants. The controlled administration of insulin significantly increased glucose infusion from day 2 to 16.

HYPERGLYCEMIA

Hyperglycemia in low-birth-weight infants traditionally has been treated by reducing the rate of administration of exogenous glucose. This is something of a clinical paradox because such a reduction can theoretically limit glucose availability to the brain. Attempts in the past to provide exogenous insulin as a means to regulate glucose met with variable success, primarily because of technical difficulties in providing insulin.[92,95,96] New insulin delivery systems designed for children and adults provide the means to deliver minute amounts of insulin under controlled conditions. These systems have finely tuned programmable pumps and tubing that does not bind insulin.[97] Application of this technology has met with preliminary success.[98] Individualized continuous insulin infusion to infants at 26 weeks of gestation weighing 700 to 800 g enhanced glucose infusion and parenteral energy intake. Weight gain was significantly greater over 7 to 21 days, compared with infants managed conventionally (Fig. 35-9). If further studies confirm these observations and clarify the potential metabolic consequences of this therapy, this method may prove beneficial in treating hyperglycemia in low-birth-weight infants.

CONSEQUENCES

HYPOGLYCEMIA

The clinical manifestations of inadequate glucose provision to the brain range from no symptoms to mild tremors to seizures. The issue of potential long-term sequelae of hypoglycemia remains unclear. This issue is complicated by the fact that hypoglycemia often occurs in infants who have coexisting conditions that also can cause brain damage. The observations suggesting that asymptomatic hypoglycemia poses less of a risk compared to symptomatic hypoglycemia are limited, as are the observations that associate prolonged hypoglycemia with a greater risk of brain damage than brief hypoglycemia. Limited data suggest that seizures associated with hypoglycemia worsen prognosis.[99–108] Because of the uncertainty in this area, all hypoglycemic infants, symptomatic or not, should be appropriately treated.

HYPERGLYCEMIA

Hyperglycemia has been associated with an increased incidence of mortality, intracranial hemorrhage, and developmental delay in very premature infants. Whether hyperglycemia causes these problems or is merely associated with their development is unclear. Increased serum osmolarity resulting from hyperglycemia might disrupt cell–serum balance and cause cell injury.[85] In addition, hyperglycemia can alter cell glucose transport, which may perturb cell metabolic functions.

INFANTS OF DIABETIC MOTHERS

Table 35-3 lists the frequently occurring problems of the IDM categorized according to proposed mechanisms. The fetal and neonatal hyperinsulinism central to many of these problems results from exaggerated provision of maternal metabolic fuels to the fetus, resulting in pancreatic B-cell hypertrophy, hyperplasia, and hyperfunction.[1,9] The alterations in maternal metabolism resulting from diabetes mellitus that are responsible for these and other effects on the fetus have been reviewed.

ALTERED FETAL GROWTH

Macrosomia, a clinical term suggesting excessive weight for gestational age, is a well known characteristic of IDM (Fig. 35-10). Macrosomia in the IDM

TABLE 35–3
PROBLEMS OF THE INFANT OF A DIABETIC MOTHER

Macrosomia or birth stress
Hypoglycemia
Respiratory distress syndrome
Intrauterine growth retardation
Hypocalcemia
Hyperbilirubinemia
Polycythemia or hyperviscosity
Cardiomyopathy
Congenital anomalies
Hyperinsulinism
Altered metabolic fuels, uteroplacental insufficiency
Decreased parathormone
Increased erythrocyte destruction, bruising

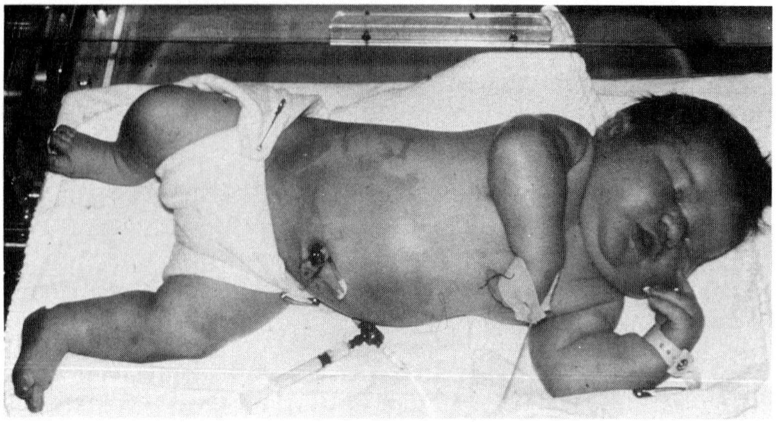

FIG. 35–10. A macrosomic infant of a diabetic mother (IDM) has head circumference and length that are at the 90th percentile; the IDM's body weight greatly exceeds the 90th percentile. The IDM has considerable fat deposition in the shoulder and intrascapular area.

results primarily from increased adiposity because IDMs have both adipocyte hyperplasia and hypertrophy.[109] Infants of diabetic mothers also have excess nonfatty tissue. The liver and heart often are enlarged and skeletal muscle increased. Much of this excess tissue is located in the shoulders and intrascapular area. As IDMs have normal brain growth, this results in a disproportionality between head and shoulder size and greatly increases the risk of shoulder dystocia (Fig. 35-11). This birth complication occurs far more frequently in macrosomic IDMs than in large infants of mothers who do not have diabetes. Macrosomia is responsible for the great risk of birth trauma, meconium aspiration syndrome, persistent pulmonary hypertension, and the high incidence of cesarean section delivery in IDMs.

As insulin has both mitogenic and anabolic effects in the fetus, the fetal hyperinsulinemic state is central to the development of macrosomia. The augmented production of insulin by the fetus stimulates the growth of insulin-sensitive tissues (*e.g.*, adipose, muscle, connective) to cause macrosomia. Hepatic glycogen storage is exaggerated. The effect of insulin probably is mediated to some extent through stimulation of insulinlike growth factors.[110] It is not surprising that head growth is normal in IDMs during intrauterine life because insulin does not stimulate brain growth to any great extent.

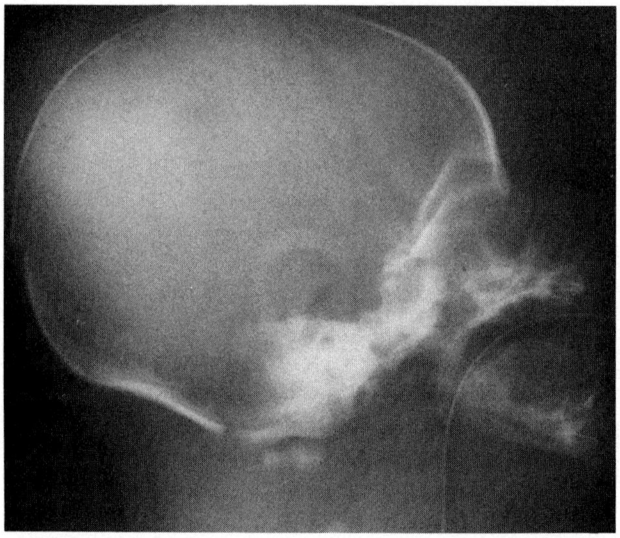

FIG. 35–11. Lateral skull and neck radiograph of an infant of a diabetic mother after a difficult vaginal delivery. Infants of diabetic mothers are at extreme risk for shoulder dystocia, which can result in severe complications, such as separation of the C1–C2 cervical spine.

The excess fat in IDMs develops during the third trimester; IDMs delivered before 30 weeks of gestation rarely are LGA. Serial fetal ultrasound measurements confirm that the fetal IDM does not exceed normal growth limits until 28 to 30 weeks of gestation.[31] Despite improved maternal therapy, 20% to 30% of insulin-dependent diabetic women continue to bear macrosomic infants.[111] Women with gestational diabetes, the mildest form of carbohydrate intolerance, have as great an incidence of macrosomia as women with preexisting diabetes.

Intrauterine growth retardation is another well known complication of diabetes in pregnancy. The development of growth retardation has been attributed to maternal vascular disease, causing uteroplacental insufficiency. More recent data suggest that growth retardation may result from alterations in maternal metabolic fuel availability during early gestation.

HYPOGLYCEMIA

Approximately 25% to 50% of all IDMs who manifest hypoglycemia will do so within the first 24 hours of life. Hypoglycemia is particularly likely to occur in macrosomic IDMs because hyperinsulinism is responsible for both fetal overgrowth and hypoglycemia (Fig. 35-12).[112] Several studies also suggest that these IDMs may fail to release glucagon or catecholamines in response to hypoglycemia.[113] These hormonal alterations result in both increased glucose clearance and diminished glucose production.

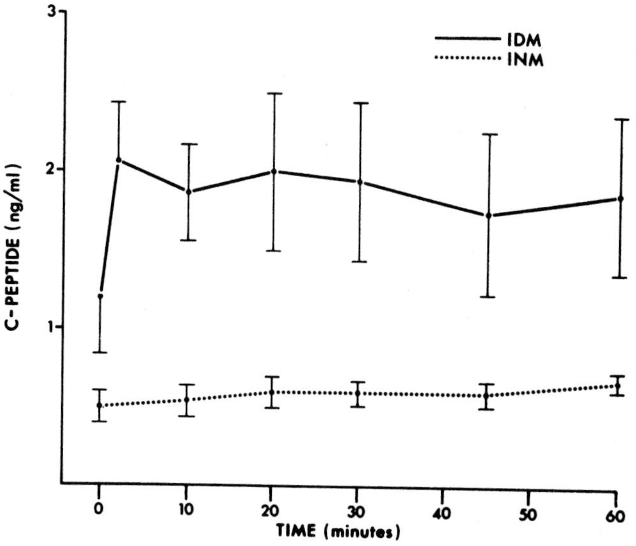

FIG. 35–12. Beta-cell response to intravenous glucose challenge in infants of diabetic mothers (IDMs) and infants of mothers with normal carbohydrate metabolism (INM). C-peptide is cleared from the proinsulin molecule when the β cell is stimulated to secrete insulin. The measurement of C-peptide represents insulin on an equimolar basis and is a more accurate measure of β-cell secretion than insulin in IDMs. Infants of diabetic mothers exuberantly secrete insulin in response to glucose challenge. This adultlike response differs greatly from the normally expected sluggish insulin response of the INM. The significantly increased insulin concentration in IDMs before glucose challenge (*i.e.*, 0 minutes) indicates that basal insulin secretion also is elevated. The increased β-cell function in IDMs is responsible for their high incidence of hypoglycemia.

HYPOCALCEMIA AND HYPOMAGNESEMIA

Hypocalcemia develops in 10% to 20% of IDMs during the neonatal period. This usually occurs in association with hyperphosphatemia and occasionally with hypomagnesemia. Parathormone concentrations are significantly lower in IDMs than in infants of normal mothers during the first 4 days of life (Fig. 35-13). This may be due to hypomagnesemia, which limits parathormone secretion even in the presence of hypocalcemia. Maternal hypomagnesemia, which may occur from increased renal loss due to diabetes, is believed responsible for fetal and neonatal hypomagnesemia.[114,115] Birth asphyxia, which frequently occurs in IDMs, also causes hypocalcemia.

HYPERBILIRUBINEMIA

Indirect hyperbilirubinemia develops in 20% to 25% of IDMs. Their carbon monoxide production is increased as a result of increased hemoglobin breakdown and bilirubin production.[116] The increased rate of erythrocyte breakdown in IDMs is probably due to altered erythrocyte membrane composition resulting from changes in maternal fuel availability. Polycythemia frequently occurs in IDMs, and the normal breakdown of this increased erythrocyte mass also causes hyperbilirubinemia. Macrosomic IDMs often are bruised at birth; the resultant resorption of blood also contributes to hyperbilirubinemia.

HYPERVISCOSITY

Infants of diabetic mothers have a 10% to 20% risk of being polycythemic and developing the neonatal hyperviscosity syndrome. Several factors are responsible for this. The hematocrit of umbilical cord blood at birth tends to be elevated, probably due to increased erythropoiesis.[117]

The increased incidence of renal vein thrombosis reported in IDMs probably is related to hyperviscosity, although this disorder does occur in IDMs with normal hematocrits.

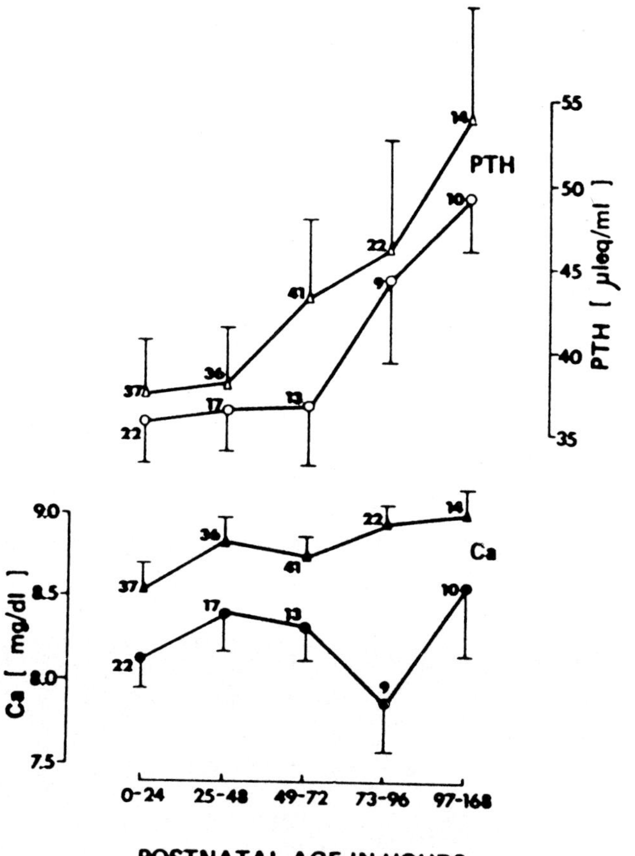

FIG. 35–13. Parathormone (PTH) and calcium concentration in infants of diabetic mothers (*circles*) and full-term control (*triangles*) infants. Infants of diabetic mothers have lower plasma calcium and PTH concentrations during the first 6 days of life. (From Schedewie HK, Odell WD, Fisher DA, et al. Parathormone and perinatal calcium homeostasis. Pediatr Res 1979;13:1.)

UNEXPECTED FETAL DEATH

In the past, a high incidence of unexpected fetal death occurred in late gestation. Improvement in metabolic control of maternal diabetes throughout pregnancy and new methods to assess fetal status have decreased the incidence of this tragic complication. The mechanisms of unexpected fetal death are not completely understood. In the fetal sheep, sustained hyperglycemia is associated with increased insulin secretion, elevated fetal oxygen consumption, acidosis, and death.[118] This could explain the association between poor maternal metabolic control and the increased risk of fetal death.

RESPIRATORY DISTRESS SYNDROME

Infants of diabetic mothers are at increased risk of developing RDS. In the past, IDMs have been at a fourfold to sixfold greater risk for RDS than infants of normal mothers.[119] This incidence has been reduced substantially by the recent emphasis on tight control of maternal metabolism. The increased risk of RDS in poorly regulated diabetic women is due in great part to fetal hyperinsulinism. Insulin adversely affects fetal lung maturation by inhibiting the development of enzymes necessary for the synthesis of the phospholipid components of surfactant.[120] Standard methods to assess fetal lung maturity antenatally may not be applicable to diabetic pregnancy. The measurement of phosphotidylglycerol has greatly improved this capability.

CARDIOMYOPATHY

Infants of diabetic mothers are at increased risk for various cardiomyopathies.[121] Many have thickening of the interventricular septum and the left or right ventricular wall. The increased cardiac muscle mass results from the fetal hyperinsulinemic state. Most of these infants are asymptomatic, and the thickening is detected by electrocardiogram or echocardiogram. In a small fraction of infants, outflow obstruction severe enough to cause left ventricular failure may occur. These abnormalities generally regress over 3 to 6 months, and the condition appears to have no permanent effect on the myocardium. Those infants with congestive heart failure who survive the initial period with medical management also improve spontaneously.

Occasionally, IDMs have severe congestive heart failure at birth. Frequently, these infants have suffered intrapartum asphyxia and are hypoglycemic and hypocalcemic. Such infants generally respond to assisted ventilation and correction of their metabolic abnormalities, and usually recover completely. It is unclear whether heart failure results from the combined effects of hypoglycemia, hypocalcemia, and asphyxia on an inherently normal myocardium, or whether the myocardium is abnormal and therefore more susceptible to failure.

CONGENITAL ABNORMALITIES

Major congenital malformations occur two to four times more frequently in IDMs than in infants born to nondiabetic women. Although many abnormalities occur in IDMs, ventricular septal defects, transposition of the great arteries, and the spinal agenesis–caudal regression syndrome occur with particular frequency (Fig. 35-14). Neural tube defects, gastrointestinal atresia, and urinary tract malformations also are relatively common. A transient anomaly unique to the IDM is known as the neonatal small left colon, microcolon, or lazy colon syndrome. This condition presents as gastrointestinal obstruction, and barium contrast studies suggest congenital aganglionic megacolon. Unlike infants with Hirschsprung disease, these infants have normal innervation of the bowel and ultimately have normal bowel function.

Poor control of maternal diabetes during the first trimester, a critical period of organogenesis, has been proposed as the mechanism for the increased incidence of malformations.[122,123] Infants of diabetic mothers with abnormalities have normal karyotypes.[124] *In vitro* studies using embryos of laboratory

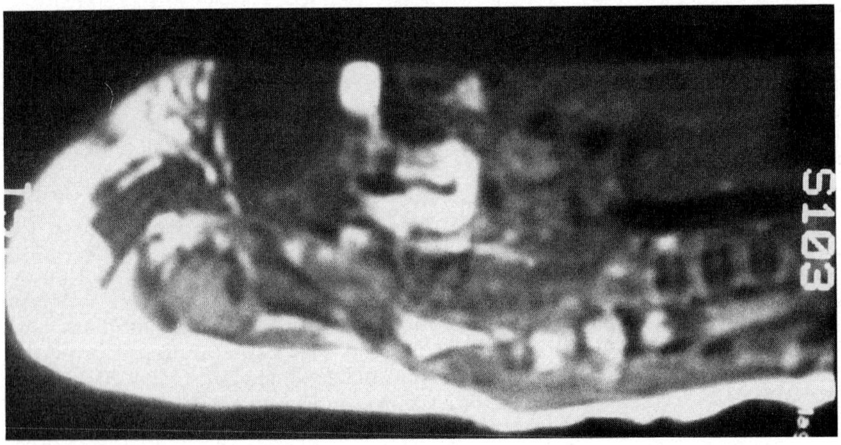

FIG. 35–14. Magnetic resonance image of an infant of a diabetic mother. The infant has spinal agenesis–caudal regression syndrome. The spinal cord is interrupted, and hip–femur relationships are malformed.

animals have demonstrated that altering metabolic fuels can produce profound malformations.[125] Clinical studies, however, have not confirmed a relation between birth defects and alterations in maternal metabolic variables.[126]

POSTNATAL PROBLEMS

Infants of diabetic mothers are at increased risk for development of obesity in later life, compared to infants of mothers with normal carbohydrate metabolism.[127] Studies suggest that *in utero* hyperinsulinism may be responsible for this postnatal phenomenon. Infants of diabetic mothers who become obese during childhood have the severest hyperinsulinism *in utero*.[128]

Whether maternal diabetes adversely affects the long-term cognitive development of the offspring remains unanswered. In the past, the increased incidence of birth trauma and neonatal disorders probably contributed to an increased risk of poor outcome. Studies suggest that altered maternal metabolic fuel availability also may have an effect. An inverse correlation has been reported between childhood IQ and degree of abnormality of second- and third-trimester maternal lipid metabolism.[129] This is consistent with the potential detrimental effect of ketones on fetal brain development.

A yet unanswered question is whether IDMs develop diabetes mellitus during postnatal life. Children and adults who were IDMs have an increased incidence of diabetes mellitus. Limited data suggest that offspring of fathers with insulin-dependent diabetes have a fivefold greater risk for development of diabetes mellitus than offspring of insulin-dependent diabetic mothers.[130] Although diabetes is in part a genetic disorder, it has not been possible to delineate precisely the mode of inheritance in IDMs. It is possible that the altered metabolic state of the diabetic pregnancy may modulate this genetic predisposition. Non–insulin-dependent diabetes mellitus occurs by age 20 years in 45.5% of IDMs of insulin-dependent diabetic mothers, but in only 8.6% and 1.4% of prediabetic and nondiabetic mothers, respectively.[131] The mechanisms by which alterations in maternal glucose and other metabolic fuels alter fetal B-cell function are unknown.

REFERENCES

1. Freinkel N. Banting lecture 1980: of pregnancy and progeny. Diabetes 1980;29:1023.
2. Hytten ET, Leitch I. The physiology of human pregnancy. 2nd ed. Oxford: Blackwell Scientific Publications, 1971.
3. Kalkhoff R, Schalch DS, Walker JG, et al. Diabetogenic factors associated with pregnancy. Trans Assoc Am Physicians 1974; 77:270.
4. Lind T, Billewicz WZ, Brown G. A serial study of changes occurring in the oral glucose tolerance test during pregnancy. Journal of Obstetrics and Gynaecology of the British Commonwealth 1973;80:1033.
5. Spellacy WN, Goetz FC. Plasma insulin in normal late pregnancy. N Engl J Med 1963;268:988.
6. Grumbach MM, Kaplan SL, Sciarra JJ, et al. Chorionic growth hormone prolactin (CGP) secretion, disposition, biologic activity in man, and postulated function as the "growth hormone" of the second half of pregnancy. Ann NY Acad Sci 1968;148:501.
7. Johansson EDB. Plasma levels of progesterone in pregnancy measured by a rapid competitive binding technique. Acta Endocrinol 1969;61:607.
8. Kalkhoff RJ, Kissebah AH, Kim HJ. Carbohydrate and lipid metabolism during normal pregnancy: relationship to gestational hormone action. Semin Perinatol 1978;2:291.
9. Pedersen J. The pregnant diabetic and her newborn. 2nd ed. Baltimore: Williams & Wilkins, 1977.
10. Bleicher SJ, O'Sullivan JB, Freinkel N. Carbohydrate metabolism in pregnancy: V. The interrelations of glucose, insulin and free fatty acids in late pregnancy and post partum. N Engl J Med 1964;271:866.
11. Felig P, Lynch V. Starvation in human pregnancy: hypoglycemia, hypoinsulinemia, and hyperketonemia. Science 1970; 170:990.
12. Kalhan SC, D'Angelo LJ, Savin SM, et al. Glucose production in pregnant women at term gestation: sources of glucose for human fetus. J Clin Invest 1979;63:388.
13. Ogata ES, Metzger BE, Freinkel N. Carbohydrate metabolism in pregnancy: XVI. Longitudinal estimates of the effects of pregnancy on D-(6^3H) glucose and D-(6-^{14}C) glucose turnovers during fasting in the rat. Metabolism 1981;30:487.
14. Scow RO, Chernick SS, Brinley MS. Hyperlipemia and ketosis in the pregnant rat. Am J Physiol 1964;206:796.
15. Patel MS, Johnson CA, Rajan R, et al. The metabolism of ketone bodies in developing human brain: development of ketone-body-utilizing enzymes and ketone bodies as precursors for lipid synthesis. J Neurochem 1975;25:905.
16. Churchill JA, Berendes HW, Nemore J. Neuropsychological deficits in children of diabetic mothers. Am J Obstet Gynecol 1969;105:257.
17. Shelley HJ. Glycogen reserves and their changes at birth and in anoxia. Br Med Bull 1961;17:137.
18. Schwartz AL, Rall TW. Hormonal regulation of incorporation of alanine-U-^{14}C into glucose in human fetal liver explants: effect of dibutyryl cyclic AMP, glucagon, insulin, and triamcinolone. Diabetes 1975;24:650.
19. Schwartz AL, Rall TW. Hormonal regulation of glycogen metabolism in human fetal liver. Diabetes 1975;24:1113.
20. Greengard O. Enzymatic differentiation of human liver: comparison with the rat model. Pediatr Res 1977;11:669.
21. Raiha HN, Lindros KO. Development of some enzymes involved in gluconeogenesis in human liver. Annales Medicinae Experimentalis et Biologiae Fenniae (Helsinki) 1964; 47:146.
22. Kaplan SL, Grumbach MM, Shepard TH. The ontogenesis of human fetal hormones: I. Growth hormone and insulin. J Clin Invest 1972;51:3080.
23. Assan R, Buillet J. Pancreatic glucagon and glucagon-like material in tissues and plasma from human fetuses 6 to 26 weeks old. In: Jonxis JH, ed. Metabolic processes in the fetus and newborn infant. Baltimore: Williams & Wilkins, 1971: 210.
24. Schaeffer LD, Wilder ML, Williams RH. Secretion and content of insulin and glucagon in human fetal pancreas slices in vitro. Proc Soc Exp Biol Med 1973;143:314.
25. Grasso S, Distefano G, Messina A, et al. Effect of glucose

priming on insulin response in the premature infant. Diabetes 1975;24:291.

26. Milner RDG. The development of insulin secretion in man. In: Jonxis JH, ed. Metabolic processes in the fetus and newborn infant, nutrition symposium. Baltimore: Williams & Wilkins, 1971:310.
27. Grasso S, Messina A, Distefano G, et al. Insulin secretion in the premature infant: response to glucose and amino acids. Diabetes 1973;22:349.
28. Wise JK, Lyall SS, Hendler R, et al. Evidence of stimulation of glucagon secretion by alanine in the human fetus at term. J Clin Endocrinol Metab 1973;37:345.
29. Hill DE. Effect of insulin on fetal growth. Semin Perinatol 1978;2:319.
30. Susa JB, McCormick KL, Widness JA, et al. Chronic hyperinsulinemia in the fetal rhesus monkey: effects on fetal growth and composition. Diabetes 1979;28:1058.
31. Ogata ES, Sabbagha R, Metzger BE, et al. Serial ultrasonography to assess evolving fetal macrosomia. JAMA 1980;243: 2405.
32. Pedersen J. Weight and length at birth of infants of diabetic mothers. Acta Endocrinol 1954;16:330.
33. Girard JF, Caquet D, Bal D. Control of rat liver phosphorylase and phosphoenolpyruvate carboxykinase activities by insulin and glucagon during the perinatal period. Enzyme 1973; 15:272.
34. Girard JR, Ferre A, Kervran A, et al. Role of the insulin/glucagon ratio in the changes of hepatic metabolism during development of the rat. In: Foa PP, Bajaj JS, Foa NL, eds. Glucagon: its role in physiology and clinical medicine. New York: Springer-Verlag, 1977:563.
35. Sperling MA, DeLamater PV, Phelps D, et al. Spontaneous and amino acid stimulated glucagon secretion in the immediate postnatal period: relation to glucose and insulin. J Clin Invest 1974;53:1159.
36. Padbury J, Agata Y, Ludlow J, et al. Effect of fetal adrenalectomy on catecholamine release and physiologic adaptation at birth in sheep. J Clin Invest 1987;80:1096.
37. Agata Y, Padbury JF, Ludlow JK, et al. The effect of chemical sympathectomy on catecholamine release at birth. Pediatr Res 1986;20:1338.
38. Grajwer LA, Sperling MA, Sack J, et al. Possible mechanisms and significance of the neonatal surge in glucagon secretion: studies in newborn lambs. Pediatr Res 1977;11:833.
39. Molsted-Pedersen L. Aspects of carbohydrate metabolism in newborn infants of diabetic mothers: II. Neonatal changes in K values. Acta Endocrinol 1972;69:189.
40. Bier DM, Arnold KJ, Sherman WR, et al. In vivo measurement of glucose and alanine metabolism with stable isotopic tracers. Diabetes 1977;26:1005.
41. Bier DM, Leake RD, Haymond MW, et al. Measurement of "true" glucose production rates in infancy and childhood with 6,6 dideuteroglucose. Diabetes 1977;26:1016.
42. Kalhan SC, Bier DM, Savin SM, et al. Estimation of glucose turnover and ^{13}C recycling in the human newborn by simultaneous [1-^{13}C] glucose and [6,6$^{2}H_2$] glucose tracers. J Clin Endocrinol Metab 1980;50:456.
43. Kalhan SC, Savin SM, Adam PAJ. Measurement of glucose turnover in the human newborn with glucose-1-^{13}C. J Clin Endocrinol Metab 1976;43:704.
44. Cornblath M, Schwartz R. Disorders of carbohydrate metabolism in infancy. 3rd ed. Boston: Blackwell Scientific Publications, 1991.
45. Pagliara AS, Karl IE, Haymond M, et al. Hypoglycemia in infancy and childhood: parts I and II. J Pediatr 1973;82:365, 558.
46. Ogata ES. Carbohydrate metabolism in the fetus and neonate and altered neonatal glucoregulation. Pediatr Clin North Am 1986;33:25.
47. Lubchenco LO, Bard H. Incidence of hypoglycemia in newborn infants classified by birth weight and gestational age. Pediatrics 1971;47:831.
48. Greene HL. Glycogen storage disease. Semin Liver Dis 1982; 8:291.
49. Haymond MW, Karl IE, Pagliara AS. Increased gluconeogenic substrates in the small-for-gestational-age infant. N Engl J Med 1974;291:322.
50. Mestyan J, Soltesz G, Schultz K, Horvath M. Hyperaminoacidemia due to the accumulation of gluconeogenic amino acid precursors in hypoglycemic small-for-gestational age infants. J Pediatr 1975;87:409.
51. Bussey ME, Finley S, LaBarbera A, et al. Hypoglycemia in the newborn growth-retarded rat: delayed phosphoenolpyruvate carboxykinase induction despite increased glucagon availability. Pediatr Res 1985;19:363.
52. Pollak A, Susa JB, Stonestreet BS, et al. Phosphoenolpyruvate carboxykinase in experimental intrauterine growth retardation in rats. Pediatr Res 1979;13:175.
53. Sinclair JC, Silverman WA. Intrauterine growth in active tissue mass of the human fetus, with particular reference to the undergrown baby. Pediatrics 1966;38:48.
54. Vidnes J, Sovik O. Gluconeogenesis in infancy and childhood: II. Studies on the glucose production from alanine in three cases of persistent neonatal hypoglycaemia. Acta Paediatr Scand 1976;65:297.
55. Vidnes J, Oyasaetor S. Glucagon deficiency causing severe neonatal hypoglycemia in a patient with normal insulin secretion. Pediatr Res 1977;11:943.
56. Garces LY, Drash A, Kenny FM. Islet cell tumor in the neonate. Pediatrics 1968;41:789.
57. Heitz PU, Kloppel G, Hacki WH, et al. Nesidioblastosis: the pathologic basis of persistent hyperinsulinemic hypoglycemia in infants. Diabetes 1977;26:632.
58. Salinas ED, Mangurten HH, Roberts SS, et al. Functioning islet cell adenoma in the newborn. Pediatrics 1968;41:646.
59. Beckwith JB. Macroglossia, omphalocele, adrenal cytomegaly, gigantism, and hyperplastic visceromegaly. Birth Defects 1967;5:188.
60. Wiedemann HR. E.M.G. syndrome and carbohydrate metabolism. Lancet 1968;2:104.
61. Barrett CT, Oliver TK. Hypoglycemia and hyperinsulinism in infants with erythroblastosis fetalis. N Engl J Med 1968; 278:1260.
62. Steinke J, Gries FA, Driscoll SG. In vitro studies of insulin inactivation with reference to erythroblastosis fetalis. Blood 1967;30:359.
63. Socol ML, Dooley SL, Ney JA, et al. Absence of hyperinsulinemia in isoimmunized fetuses treated with intravascular transfusion. Am J Obstet Gynecol 1991;165:1737.
64. Milner RDG, Chouksey SK, Assan R. Metabolic and hormonal effects of glucagon infusion in erythroblastotic infants. Arch Dis Child 1973;48:885.
65. Senior B, Slone D, Shapiro S, et al. Benzothiadiazides and neonatal hypoglycaemia. Lancet 1976;2:377.
66. Zucker P, Simon G. Prolonged symptomatic neonatal hypoglycemia associated with maternal chlorpropamide therapy. Pediatrics 1968;42:824.
67. Brazy JE, Pupkin MJ. Effects of maternal isoxsuprine administration on preterm infants. J Pediatr 1979;94:444.
68. Ogata ES. Isoxsuprine infusion in the rat: alterations in maternal, fetal and neonatal glucose homeostasis. J Perinat Med 1981;9:293.

69. Kenepp NB, Shelley WC, Gabbe SG, et al. Fetal and neonatal hazards of maternal hydration with 5% dextrose before caesarean section. Lancet 1982;1:1150.
70. Nagel JW, Sims S, Aplin CE, et al. Refractory hypoglycemia associated with a malpositioned umbilical artery catheter. Pediatrics 1979;64:315.
71. Cowett RM, Tenenbaum DG, Fatoba O, et al. The effects of arterial glucose infusion above the celiac axis in the neonatal lamb. Biol Neonate 1985;47:179.
72. Kliegman R, Gross T, Morton S, et al. Intrauterine growth and postnatal fasting metabolism in infants of obese mothers. J Pediatr 1984;104:601.
73. Leake RD, Fiser RH, Oh W. Rapid glucose disappearance in infants with infection. Clin Pediatr 1981;20:397.
74. Yeung CY, Lee VWY, Yeung CM. Glucose disappearance rate in neonatal infection. J Pediatr 1973;82:486.
75. Wiswell TE, Cornish JD, Northam RS. Neonatal polycythemia: frequency of clinical manifestations and other associated findings. Pediatrics 1986;78:26.
76. Rosenkrantz TS, Philipps AF, Skrzypczak PS, et al. Cerebral metabolism in the newborn lamb with polycythemia. Pediatr Res 1988;23:329.
77. Lovinger RD, Kaplan SL, Grumbach MM. Congenital hypopituitarism associated with neonatal hypoglycemia and microphallus: four cases secondary to hypothalamic hormone deficiencies. J Pediatr 1975;87:1171.
78. Johnson JD, Hansen RC, Albritton WL, et al. Hypoplasia of the anterior pituitary and neonatal hypoglycemia. J Pediatr 1973;82:634.
79. Kauschansky A, Genel M, Walker Smith GJ. Congenital hypopituitarism in female infants. Am J Dis Child 1979;133:165.
80. Bower BD, Jones LF, Weeks MM. Cold injury in the newborn. Br Med J 1972;1:303.
81. Schiff D, Stern L, Leduc J. Chemical thermogenesis in newborn infants: catecholamine excretion and the plasma nonesterified fatty acid response to cold exposure. Pediatrics 1966;37:577.
82. Pickering D. Neonatal hypoglycemia due to salicylate poisoning. Proc R Soc Med 1968;61:1256.
83. Gemelli M, De Luca F, Barberio G. Hypoglycaemia and congenital adrenal hyperplasia. Acta Paediatr Scand 1979;68:285.
84. Smith VS, Giacoia GP. Hyperinsulinaemic hypoglycaemia in an infant with mosaic trisomy 13. J Med Genet 1985;22:228.
85. Pildes RS. Neonatal hyperglycemia. J Pediatr 1986;109:905.
86. Dweck HS, Cassady G. Glucose intolerance in infants of very low birth weight: I. Incidence of hyperglycemia in infants of birth weights 1,100 grams or less. Pediatrics 1974;53:189.
87. Cowett RM, Oh W, Schwartz R. Persistent glucose production during glucose infusion in the neonate. J Clin Invest 1983;71:467.
88. Lilien LD, Rosenfield RL, Baccaro MM, et al. Hyperglycemia in stressed small premature infants. J Pediatr 1979;94:454.
89. Massi-Benedetti F, Falorni A, Luyckx A, et al. Inhibition of glucagon secretion in the human newborn by simultaneous administration of glucose and insulin. Horm Metab Res 1974;6:392.
90. Zarif M, Pildes RS, Vidyasagar D. Insulin and growth-hormone responses in neonatal hyperglycemia. Diabetes 1976;25:428.
91. Grasso S, Fallucca F, Mazzone D, et al. Inhibition of glucagon secretion in the human newborn by glucose infusion. Diabetes 1983;32:489.
92. Goldman SL, Hirata T. Attenuated response to insulin in very low birthweight infants. Pediatr Res 1980;14:50.
93. Gentz JCH, Cornblath M. Transient diabetes of the newborn. Adv Pediatr 1969;16:345.
94. Hutchinson JH, Keay AJ, Kerr MM. Congenital temporary diabetes mellitus. Br Med J 1962;2:436.
95. Vaucher YE, Walson PD, Morrow G. Continuous insulin infusion in hyperglycemic, very low birth weight infants. J Pediatr Gastroenterol Nutr 1982;1:211.
96. Binder ND, Raschko PK, Benda GI, et al. Insulin infusion with parenteral nutrition in extremely low birth weight infants with hyperglycemia. J Pediatr 1989;114:273.
97. Ostertag SG, Jovanovic L, Lewis B, et al. Insulin pump therapy in the very low birth weight infant. Pediatrics 1986;78:625.
98. Collins JW, Hoppe M, Brown K, et al. A controlled trial of insulin infusion and parenteral nutrition in extremely low birth weight infants with glucose intolerance. J Pediatr 1991;118:921.
99. Creery RDG. Hypoglycaemia in the newborn: diagnosis, treatment, and prognosis. Dev Med Child Neurol 1966;8:746.
100. Haworth JC. Neonatal hypoglycemia: how much does it damage the brain? Pediatrics 1974;54:3.
101. Haworth JC, McRae KN. Neonatal hypoglycemia: a six-year experience. Lancet 1967;87(2):41.
102. Haworth JC, Vidyasagar D. Hypoglycemia in the newborn. Clin Obstet Gynecol 1971;14:821.
103. Koivisto M, Blanco-Sequeiros M, Krause U. Neonatal symptomatic and asymptomatic hypoglycaemia: a follow-up study of 151 children. Dev Med Child Neurol 1972;14:603.
104. Pildes RS, Cornblath M, Warren I, et al. A prospective controlled study of neonatal hypoglycemia. Pediatrics 1974;54:5.
105. Pildes R, Forbes AE, O'Connor SM, et al. The incidence of neonatal hypoglycemia: a completed survey. J Pediatr 1967;70:76.
106. Raivio KO. Neonatal hypoglycemia: II. A clinical study of 44 idiopathic cases with special reference to corticosteroid treatment. Acta Paediatr Scand 1968;57:540.
107. Griffiths AD, Bryant GM. Assessment of effects of neonatal hypoglycaemia. Arch Dis Child 1971;46:819.
108. Lucas A, Morley R, Cole TJ. Adverse neurodevelopmental outcome of moderate neonatal hypoglycaemia. Br Med J 1988;297:1304.
109. Fee BA, Weil WB. Body composition of infants of diabetic mothers by direct analysis. Ann NY Acad Sci 1963;110:869.
110. D'Ercole AJ, Bose CL, Underwood LE, et al. Serum somatomedin-C concentrations in a rabbit model of diabetic pregnancy. Diabetes 1984;33:590.
111. Ogata ES, Freinkel N, Metzger BE, et al. Perinatal islet function in gestational diabetes: assessment by cord plasma C-peptide and amniotic fluid insulin. Diabetes Care 1980;3:425.
112. Sosenko IR, Kitzmiller JL, Loo SW, et al. The infant of the diabetic mother: correlation of increased cord C-peptide levels with macrosomia and hypoglycemia. N Engl J Med 1979;301:859.
113. Stern L, Ramos A, Leduc J. Urinary catecholamine excretion in infants of diabetic mothers. Pediatrics 1968;42:598.
114. Schedewie HK, Odell WD, Fisher DA, et al. Parathormone and perinatal calcium homeostasis. Pediatr Res 1979;13:1.
115. Noguchi A, Eren M, Tsang RC. Parathyroid hormone in hypocalcemic and normocalcemic infants of diabetic mothers. J Pediatr 1980;97:112.
116. Stevenson DK, Bartoletti AL, Ostrander CR, et al. Pulmonary excretion of carbon monoxide in the human infant as an index of bilirubin production: II. Infants of diabetic mothers. J Pediatr 1979;94:956.
117. Widness JA, Susa JB, Garcia JF, et al. Increased erythropoiesis and elevated erythropoietin in infants born to diabetic mothers and in hyperinsulinemic rhesus fetuses. J Clin Invest 1981;67:637.

118. Philipps AF, Dubin JW, Matty PJ, et al. Arterial hypoxemia and hyperinsulinemia in the chronically hyperglycemic fetal lamb. Pediatr Res 1982;16:653.
119. Robert MF, Neff RK, Hubbell JP, et al. Association between maternal diabetes and the respiratory distress syndrome in the newborn. N Engl J Med 1976;294:357.
120. Bourbon JR, Farrell PM. Fetal lung development in the diabetic pregnancy. Pediatr Res 1985;19:253.
121. Gutgesell HP, Speer ME, Rosenberg HS. Characterization of the cardiomyopathy in infants of diabetic mothers. Circulation 1980;61:441.
122. Miller E, Hare JW, Cloherty JP, et al. Elevated maternal hemoglobin A_{1C} in early pregnancy and major congenital anomalies in infants of diabetic mothers. N Engl J Med 1981;304:1331.
123. Fuhrmann K, Reiher H, Semmler K, et al. Prevention of congenital malformations in infants of insulin-dependent diabetic mothers. Diabetes Care 1983;6:219.
124. Simpson JL, Elias S, Martin AO, et al. Diabetes in pregnancy, Northwestern University Series (1977–1981): I. Prospective study of anomalies in offspring of mothers with diabetes mellitus. Am J Obstet Gynecol 1983;146:263.
125. Freinkel N, Lewis NJ, Akazawa S, et al. The honeybee syndrome: implications of the teratogenicity of mannose in rat embryo culture. N Engl J Med 1984;310:223.
126. Mills JL, Knopp RH, Simpson JL, et al. Lack of relation of increased malformation rates in infants of diabetic mothers to glycemic control during organogenesis. N Engl J Med 1988;318:671.
127. Vohr BR, Lipsitt LP, Oh W. Somatic growth of children of diabetic mothers with reference to birth size. J Pediatr 1980;97:196.
128. Metzger BE, Silverman BL, Freinkel N, et al. Amniotic fluid insulin concentration as a predictor of obesity. Arch Dis Child 1990;65:1050.
129. Rizzo T, Metzger BE, Burns WJ, et al. Correlations between antepartum maternal metabolism and child intelligence. N Engl J Med 1991;325:911.
130. Warram JH, Krolewski AS, Gottlieb MS, et al. Differences in risk of insulin-dependent diabetes in offspring of diabetic mothers and diabetic fathers. N Engl J Med 1984;311:149.
131. Pettitt DJ, Aleck KA, Baird R, et al. Congenital susceptibility to NIDDM: role of intrauterine environment. Diabetes 1988;37:622.

Neonatology: Pathophysiology and Management of the Newborn, Fourth Edition,
edited by Gordon B. Avery, Mary Ann Fletcher, and Mhairi G. MacDonald.
J.B. Lippincott Company, Philadelphia © 1994.

chapter 36

Calcium and Magnesium Homeostasis

WINSTON W. K. KOO
REGINALD C. TSANG

Calcium is the most abundant mineral in the body and, together with phosphorus, forms the major inorganic constituent of bone. Magnesium is the fourth most abundant mineral and is the second most common intracellular electrolyte in the body. After birth, 99% of total body Ca is in bones. The tissue distribution of Mg varies, according to the extent of bone mineralization and the rate of soft tissue growth. Near the end of the third trimester, however, about 60% of the body's Mg is in bone, 20% is in muscle, and most of the remainder is found in the intracellular space of other tissues. Although the major portions of Ca and Mg are found in the skeleton, both are essential to the function of soft tissues. It generally is agreed that about 80% of Ca and Mg accrue in the fetus between 25 weeks of gestation and term. During this period, the estimated daily accretion per kilogram fetal body weight is 2.3 to 2.98 mmol (92–119 mg) Ca and 0.1 to 0.14 mmol (2.51–3.44 mg) Mg. The peak accretion rates occur at 36 to 38 weeks of gestation. In newborn term infants, the total body Ca and Mg contents average approximately 28 g and 0.7 g, respectively.[1–5]

Serum or plasma is readily available for measurement of Ca and Mg, but the fraction of Ca and Mg in the circulation is less than 1% of their respective total body content. Disturbances in serum concentrations of Ca and Mg may be associated with disturbances of physiologic function. Chronic and severely lowered serum concentrations of these minerals also may reflect the presence of a deficiency state.

Serum Ca occurs in three forms: approximately 40% is bound predominantly to albumin; approximately 10% is chelated and complexed to small molecules such as bicarbonate, phosphate, or citrate; and approximately 50% is ionized. Complexed and ionized Ca are ultrafilterable.

Total Ca concentrations (tCa) in cord sera increase with increasing gestational age. Serum tCa may be as high as 3 mmol/L (1 mmol/L = 4 mg/dL) in cord blood of infants born at term, and they are significantly higher than paired maternal values at delivery. Serum tCa reach a nadir during the first 2 days after birth; thereafter, concentrations increase and stabilize to a level generally above 2 mmol/L. In infants exclusively fed human milk, the mean serum tCa increases from 2.3 to 2.7 mmol/L over the first 6 months postnatally. Serum tCa concentrations in infants and children generally remain slightly higher than adult values. Normally, serum tCa in children and adults remain stable, with a diurnal range of less than 0.13 mmol/L.[6–8]

Serum ionized calcium concentration (Ca^{2+}) is the best indicator of physiologic blood Ca activity. Measurement of serum Ca^{2+} is firmly established in clinical medicine, and the availability of highly reliable Ca^{2+} analyzers allows simple, rapid, and direct determination of Ca^{2+} in whole blood, plasma, and serum by ion-selective electrodes. Some differences exist in the reported values for circulating Ca^{2+} due to differences in the design of the reference electrode, formulation of calibrating solutions, and the lack of a reference system for Ca^{2+}.[9,10] Cord sera Ca^{2+} increases with increasing gestational age and is higher than values in paired maternal sera. With the use of newer ion-selective electrodes, serum Ca^{2+} averages 1.25 mmol/L with a 95% confidence limit of 1.1 to 1.4 mmol/L (4.5–5.6 mg/dL).[11] Serum Ca^{2+} concentrations in infants and children generally remain slightly higher than in adults. Clinical situations may affect the measured Ca^{2+} concentration. For example, the use of heparin may decrease Ca^{2+}, and the infant's blood *p*H is inversely related to Ca^{2+}. The effect of the latter may be minimized by the immediate analysis of the serum samples for Ca^{2+}. Freezing serum samples in 5% CO_2-containing tubes may minimize the impact of *p*H variations when storage exceeds 1 week.

The concentration of Ca^{2+} is critical to many important biologic functions, and there is a finely tuned regulation of extracellular Ca^{2+} concentration and maintenance of an extremely large Ca concentration gradient across the cellular plasma membrane. The Ca messenger system is a nearly universal means by which extracellular messengers regulate cell function. Many cellular enzyme cascades are activated by a transient increase in intracellular Ca^{2+} concentrations. In the cell, distribution of Ca is not uniform. The cytosolic compartment contains 50 to 150 nmol of Ca per liter of water; a larger intramitochondrial Ca pool contains 500 to 10,000 nmol of Ca per liter cell water. In contrast, the concentration of Ca^{2+} in extracellular fluid is 1 million nmol/L (1 mmol/L). There are at least two adenosine triphosphate–dependent mechanisms involved in the maintenance of the Ca concentration gradient across the plasma membrane. The measurement of intracellular Ca can be affected by some *in vitro* conditions,[12] and is not freely available.

Approximately 30% of serum Mg is in the protein-bound form, with the remainder in the ultrafiltrable portion. Seventy to 80% of ultrafiltrable Mg is in ionic form, the remainder being complexed to anions, particularly phosphate, citrate, and oxalate. Cord sera total Mg is higher than paired maternal values and remains slightly higher in infants and young children compared to adults, being 0.92 ± 0.13 mmol/L (2.2 ± 0.3 mg/dL, mean ± 2 SD) in children compared to approximately 0.88 ± 0.13 mmol/L (2.1 ± 0.3 mg/dL) in adults.[13]

The cellular Mg content of most tissues is 6 to 9 mmol/kg wet weight, and most of this Mg is localized in membrane structures (*e.g.*, microsomes, mitochondria, plasma membranes). The much smaller pool of free Mg in the cell is maintained at about 1 mmol/L and is in an exchanging equilibrium with the membrane-bound Mg. This unbound intracellular Mg has a critical role in cellular physiology and catalyzes enzymatic processes concerned with the transfer, storage, and use of energy.[14] Intracellular Mg usually remains stable despite wide fluctuations in serum Mg. In Mg-deficient states, however, the intracellular content of Mg can be low despite normal serum concentrations.[15,16]

Ion-selective electrodes are being used in the measurement of ionized Mg, and there are a number of methods available to determine the intracellular Mg concentrations.[17–19] The clinical value and application of ionized and intracellular Mg concentrations, however, have yet to be defined.

PHYSIOLOGIC CONTROL OF CALCIUM AND MAGNESIUM HOMEOSTASIS

Calcium continuously enters the extracellular fluid from gut and bone, but Ca concentration in the extracellular fluid is maintained relatively constant by the effects of interdependent hormonal mechanisms that regulate the influx and efflux of Ca between extracellular fluid, kidney, gut, and bone. Parathyroid hormone (PTH) and 1,25-dihydroxyvitamin D [$1,25(OH)_2D$] are the classic hormones that primarily regulate the extracellular fluid Ca concentration through their effects on kidney, gut, and bone (see Hormonal Control).[20,21] Other peptides, such as transforming growth factor-α, lymphotoxin, tumor necrosis factor, and interleukin-1α, may act in a paracrine (*i.e.*, cell-to-cell) or autocrine (*i.e.*, cell-to-own cell) fashion and may be important in influencing Ca flux under pathologic conditions such as humoral hypercalcemia of malignancy (HHM). Their role in Ca homeostasis under physiologic conditions is not known, however.

The kidney is a major regulator of extracellular fluid Ca concentration, primarily by modulation of Ca excretion (see Chap. 42). Altered renal regulation of Ca excretion is primarily responsible for the development of some hypercalcemic states, including familial, benign hypocalciuric hypercalcemia, or during chronic thiazide diuretic therapy. Its capacity in the acute regulation of extracellular fluid Ca concentration, however, may be overwhelmed when net Ca input into the extracellular fluid from the gut or bone exceeds the kidney's capacity for Ca excretion. The latter situation is exemplified best by hypercalcemia of malignancy. Conversely, in hypocalcemic states, the kidney cannot reduce Ca excretion sufficiently to prevent the occurrence of hypocalcemia.

The gut is important in chronic control of extracellular fluid Ca, primarily through dietary Ca load and the presence of hormonal stimulatory factors, including $1,25(OH)_2D$.[22] Gut hyperabsorption of Ca may be associated with hypercalciuria and nephrocalcinosis, but there is no major effect on the development of hypercalcemia.

There is exchange of Ca between the bone fluid and extracellular fluid across the bone lining cells, but in growing infants there is a net influx of extracellular fluid Ca to the bone for mineralization and skeletal growth.

Extracellular fluid Mg is primarily controlled by the kidney and gastrointestinal tract and appears closely linked to Ca, potassium, and sodium metabolism.[16,23,24] The production and secretion of the calciotropic hormones, PTH, and $1,25(OH)_2D$ may be affected (see Hormonal Control) by altered serum Mg concentrations, but the control of Mg homeostasis by calciotropic hormones under physiologic conditions appears to be limited.

The kidney is the main regulator of serum concentrations and total body content of Mg. Renal excretion of Mg normally increases in proportion to the load presented to the kidney. Renal Mg excretory capacity can be overwhelmed, however, especially in developmentally less mature kidneys as in the human infant and in the presence of a relatively high Mg load such as occurs in those receiving parenteral nutrition therapy.[25–27] Similarly, there is efficient renal Mg conservation, but it is insufficient to prevent hypomagnesemia in the presence of very low intake or excessive losses (*e.g.*, from the gastrointestinal tract).[25,28] Other factors, including sodium and Ca loading and loop diuretics, also increase Mg loss in the urine.[23,29,30]

Gastrointestinal absorption of Mg occurs in the small intestine, predominantly in the jejunum and ileum. Magnesium absorption occurs primarily by intercellular diffusion and solvent drag mechanisms, but decreased fractional absorption with larger intakes also is consistent with a facilitated diffusion or saturable component.[31] There is very little endogenous secretion of Mg, but gastrointestinal secretions contain large amounts of Mg, and increased secretory losses from gastrointestinal fistulas frequently result in Mg deficiency and hypomagnesemia.[28,32]

There is limited information on the exchange of Mg between bone and extracellular fluid, but with altered Mg status, particularly in hypomagnesemic patients, there is decreased Mg–Ca exchange at the bone surface and decreased release of bone Ca,[33,34] probably independent of decreased serum PTH concentrations.

HORMONAL CONTROL

Recent advances have better defined the available knowledge, particularly at the molecular level, of the classic hormones PTH, calcitonin (CT), and $1,25(OH)_2D$, which are important to mineral homeostasis. Newly discovered hormones, such as PTH-related protein, play a major role in tumor-associated hypercalcemic states and may further knowledge of mineral homeostasis under physiologic circumstances.

Parathyroid hormone is synthesized in the parathyroid gland. It is an 84-amino-acid polypeptide with a relative molecular mass (Mr) of 9500. In humans, the PTH gene, along with the genes for insulin, β-globulin, and CT, is located on the short arm of chromosome 11, and restriction site polymorphisms near the PTH gene have been detected.[35,36] The initial translational product of the mRNA is a 115-amino-acid prepro-PTH. Prepro-PTH then undergoes proteolytic cleavage to remove the amino-terminal signal sequence, on translocation across the membrane of the endoplasmic reticulum, to form pro-PTH. The prohormone-specific region is cleaved further during subsequent intracellular processing to generate the 84-amino-acid–secreted form of the intact hormone. The intact PTH molecule has a serum half-life of 5 to 8 minutes, undergoing a series of cleavages by hepatic Kupffer cells that results in the accumulation of biologically inert midregion and carboxyl-terminal fragments. The 1–34 fragment (*i.e.*, Mr 3500–4000) from the amino terminal of PTH appears to be the potent fraction for bioactivity. The inactive fragments are cleared from the blood virtually exclusively by glomerular filtration.

Current radioimmunoassay techniques for the measurement of PTH are directed at a specific sequence of the PTH molecule, hence the terms amino-terminal, midregion, and carboxyl-terminal assays. Normally, there are greater amounts of middle and carboxyl fragments than the intact hormone in the circulation, because of metabolic breakdown of the short-lived, intact hormone, coupled with glandular secretion of inactive fragments. Intact PTH and amino-terminal fragments constitute about 10% of PTH immunoreactivity in the peripheral circulation. Intact PTH, as measured by immunoradiometric assay (IRMA), offers the promise of being the most sensitive index of parathyroid gland secretory function.[37–39] Thus, consistency in the PTH assay methodology and serial measurements are critical to the interpretation of PTH measurements.

Parathyroid hormone concentrations in cord blood frequently are low and do not correlate with PTH concentrations in maternal sera,[7,8] although cytochemical assay suggests that bioactive PTH may be present at a higher level than immunoactive PTH in cord sera.[8,40] Serum PTH concentrations increase postnatally coincident with the fall in serum Ca in both term and preterm infants.[7,8,41] Serum PTH concentrations are similar for children and adults but increase in the elderly.[42–44] Serum concentrations of intact PTH as measured by IRMA showed no change during normal pregnancy.[7,45] In adults, serum intact PTH is present in picomolar concentrations. It has a significant circadian periodicity,[46–48] spontaneous episodic pulsatility with distinct peak properties,[47] and a significant temporal coupling with serum Ca^{2+} and phosphorus concentrations[47,48] and prolactin secretion.[46]

In physiologic terms, PTH is the most important regulator of extracellular Ca concentration, primarily through its effect on classic PTH target tissues, bone and kidney. It increases serum Ca concentration through mobilization of Ca from bone, probably synergistically with $1,25(OH)_2D$; increases renal distal tubular reabsorption of Ca but decreases proximal tubular reabsorption of sodium, Ca, phosphate, and bicarbonate; increases intestinal Ca absorption secondary to stimulating 1,25$(OH)_2$D production and probably also has a direct effect on intestinal Ca absorption.[6,20,49] Parathyroid hormone effects on end organ systems appear to be mediated through its binding to specific receptors,[50] signal transduction mediated by G proteins,[51,52] including both stimulatory and inhibitory responses, and functional response through activation of secondary messengers such as cyclic adenosine monophosphate (cAMP), inositol phosphate, and cytosolic Ca. Magnesium is required for PTH stimulation of adenylate cyclase. Other tissues such as skin fibroblasts, cardiac cells, and vascular smooth muscle are demonstrated to have PTH-sensitive adenylate cyclase, but the physiologic importance of PTH in these nonclassic target tissues is unknown.[53]

Extracellular Ca, in turn, is the most potent regulator of PTH secretion.[54,55] A decrease in serum Mg concentration also can stimulate PTH secretion,[56] although chronic hypomagnesemia inhibits secretion of PTH,[57] and possibly increases target tissue resistance to PTH.[33,57] The latter may be related to inactivity of adenylate cyclase, a Mg-requiring enzyme. Both hypercalcemia and hypermagnesemia are able to block PTH release.[58,59] Vitamin D metabolites, in particular 1,25$(OH)_2$D, can regulate PTH gene transcription and suppress PTH production.[60,61] Hyperphosphatemia stimulates PTH secretion, probably by lowering the serum Ca concentration.

Other systemic factors (*e.g.*, catecholamine, prostaglandins, growth hormone, CT, estrogen, progesterone, cortisol, and somatostatin) and local factors (*e.g.*, interleukin-1) modulate PTH secretion and function; However, their role in the regulation of Ca metabolism under physiologic conditions is not clear.[6,20]

Parathyroid hormone–related protein (PTHrP), also known as PTH-like peptide, PTH-like protein, and human humoral hypercalcemic factor, is thought to be the humoral mediator that is secreted by tumors in the syndrome of HHM. Parathyroid hormone–related protein has been purified and its amino acid sequence determined. Parathyroid hormone and PTHrP genes appear to be members of the same gene family. Parathyroid hormone–related protein cDNA encodes a 177-amino-acid protein consisting of a 36-amino-acid precursor segment and a 141-amino-acid mature peptide. The mature PTHrP contains several structural or functional domains. The 1–13 region of PTHrP is 70% homologous with the corresponding region of PTH. Both PTH and PTHrP appear to bind to the same G-protein–linked receptor. Synthetic and recombinant PTHrPs can mimic the effects of PTH on the classic PTH target organs, involving activation of adenylate cyclase and other second messenger systems.[50,62]

Parathyroid hormone–related protein gene expression is found in an extensive variety of normal endocrine and nonendocrine tissues. PTHrP biologic activity and immunoreactivity have been found in many tissues, including the human fetus by as early as 7 weeks of gestation, placenta, lactating breasts, and mammalian milk.[63–65] The exact physiologic role of PTHrP remains to be defined, although there is increasing evidence that its effects are predominantly local.[62,65]

Circulating immunoreactive PTHrP concentrations are low or undetectable in normal subjects. The 1–74 amino-terminal fragment of PTHrP appears to be specific for HHM, whereas the 109–138 carboxy-terminal fragment of PTHrP is elevated in the serum of patients with HHM or renal failure. The levels of PTHrP in these patients are similar to the concentration of PTH (*i.e.*, 10^{-12}–10^{-11} mol/L). The concentration of PTHrP in milk is an additional 100-fold higher.[64–66]

Calcitonin monomer is a 32-amino-acid peptide with a Mr of 3400. Its precursors are prepro-CT and pro-CT. The larger prohormones include peptides linked to the amino and carboxy terminals of the CT sequence (*i.e.*, flanking peptides). Calcitonin and equimolar amounts of non–CT-secretory peptides, corresponding to these flanking peptides, are generated during precursor processing. In addition, alternate processing of the initial gene transcript results in the production of another distinct RNA encoding precursor of CT gene–related peptide (CGRP). The latter is a 37-amino-acid peptide sequence (Mr 4000). Seventy-five amino-terminal residues of each preprohormone for CT and CGRP are predicted to be identical. Pro-CT is a 116-amino-acid peptide, whereas the pro-CGRP is a 103-amino-acid peptide. Bioactivity of human calcitonin (hCT) is present in the full 32-amino-acid structure or its smaller fragments, such as hCT 8–32 and hCT 9–32; the ring structure of CT enhances, but is not essential for, hormone action.[6,20,67,68]

The CT gene contains six exons and five introns with exon 4 coding for CT in the thyroid C cell and exon 5 coding for the CGRP in the central nervous system. Calcitonin gene transcription is positively regulated by cAMP, phorbol esters, and glucocorticoid hormones, and negatively regulated by 1,25$(OH)_2$D.[68–72] Secretion of CT is stimulated by an increase in serum Ca and Mg concentrations and by gastrin, glucagon, and cholecystokinin, along with several other structural analogues of these hormones (*e.g.*, pentagastrin, prostaglandin-E_2). Propranolol and adrenergic antagonists and somatostatin may inhibit the secretion of CT.[6,20,73] Calcitonin may activate the 1-hydroxylase system, which is independent of PTH, and increase 1,25$(OH)_2$D production,[74] whereas 1,25$(OH)_2$D affects CT gene expression in adult rats but is ineffective in 13-day-old suckling rats.[71] The latter observation may be related to fewer 1,25$(OH)_2$D receptors in C cells of immature rats.

Developmentally, CT-containing cells and parathyroid gland cells are thought to derive from the same tissue source as the neural crest. Calcitonin is secreted primarily from the thyroid C cells and also from many extrathyroidal tissues, including tissues with embryonic neural crest origin. Calcitonin gene–related peptide is found predominantly in nerve fibers in the central and peripheral nervous system, blood vessels, thyroid and parathyroid glands, liver, spleen, heart, lung, and possibly bone marrow. Both CT and CGRP are present in the fetus.

Circulating immunoreactive CT and CGRP are a heterogeneous mixture of different molecular forms and are recognized as long as the antigenic epitopes recognized by the antiserum are expressed. Sample preparation with initial extraction, gel chromatography, and high-pressure liquid chromatography separation can improve the sensitivity and specificity of the radioimmunoassays. Two-site immunometric assays may allow further refinement in sensitivity and specificity in the measurement of these hormones.[6,20,75,76]

In human adults, serum CT and CGRP concentrations are found in the picomolar range. Diurnal variability has been reported for serum CGRP but not for serum CT.[77–79] Serum CT concentrations are high at birth compared to paired maternal CT concentrations. Serum CT concentrations further increase during the first few days after birth and may reach levels fivefold to tenfold higher than adult CT concentrations. Serum CT concentrations decrease progressively during infancy; however, in preterm infants, the mean serum CT concentrations may remain twice the adult value up to several months postnatally. There is a small peak in serum CT concentration during late childhood.[6,20,43]

Calcitonin is a potent inhibitor of bone resorption and increases renal Ca excretion. There are distinct but overlapping effects of CT and CGRP. For example, CT has a potent hypocalcemic effect and inhibits bone resorption. Calcitonin decreases renal tubular reabsorption of Ca, Mg, phosphorus, and sodium and increases free water clearance in humans. In physiologic concentration, CT probably does not influence intestinal absorption of Ca and phosphorus. The net effect of CT is a lowering of serum Ca and phosphorus concentrations.[6,73] Thus, the bioactivity of CT frequently is opposite that of PTH; CT probably modulates the effect of PTH on organs. Calcitonin gene–related peptide primarily affects catecholamine release, vascular tone and blood pressure, and cardiac contractility, and the influence of CGRP on Ca and phosphorus homeostasis is minor compared to that of CT. However, amylin, a pancreatic islet–derived or synthetic 37-amino-acid peptide, is a member of the CGRP family with a potent hypocalcemic effect despite sharing only 15% of its amino acid sequence with human CT. The hypocalcemic effect of amylin is thought to be mediated by the CT receptors on osteoclasts and is 100-fold more potent than CGRP.[80] Both CT and CGRP inhibit gastric acid secretion and food intake. Calcitonin and amylin are used in the therapeutic management of hypercalcemia and pathologic states with increased bone resorption. Calcitonin also is useful as a tumor marker in the management of medullary carcinoma of the thyroid; however, the exact physiologic roles of CT, amylin, and CGRP remain to be defined.

Calcitonin function is mediated by binding to receptors linked to G protein and activation of adenylate cyclase and protein kinase.[69,81,82] The CT receptor shows sequence homology to the PTH/PTHrP receptor, indicating that the receptors for these hormones that regulate Ca homeostasis are part of a family of G-protein–coupled receptors.

The kidney appears to be the dominant organ in the metabolism of human CT. A small percentage of the metabolic clearance rate of CT in humans may be accounted for by enzymatic degradation in blood. Depending on the animal species, other sites such as liver, intestine, and bone may be involved in the metabolism of CT.

VITAMIN D

Dietary vitamin D (1 μg = 40 IU) is derived from plants as ergosterol (*i.e.*, vitamin D_2) and from animals as cholecalciferol (*i.e.*, vitamin D_3). In animals, vitamin D_3 can be synthesized endogenously in the skin after exposure to the ultraviolet B spectrum (*i.e.*, 280–300 nm) of sunlight.

In mammals, vitamins D_2 and D_3 appear to metabolize along the same pathway, and there is little functional difference between these metabolites. Vitamin D (Mr 384) undergoes several major metabolic conversion steps and under *in vivo* conditions produces at least 30 vitamin D metabolites, with and without putative functions. In the liver, vitamin D is 25 hydroxylated to 25-hydroxyvitamin D (25 OHD). Quantitatively, 25 OHD (1 nmol/L = 0.4 ng/mL) is the most abundant vitamin D metabolite in the circulation and is a useful index of vitamin D reserve. In the kidney, 25 OHD is hydroxylated further to $1,25(OH)_2D$, predominantly in the mitochondria of proximal tubules. $1,25(OH)_2D$ is the most active vitamin D metabolite and is critical to the maintenance of mineral homeostasis, in particular the prevention of hypocalcemia, rickets, and osteomalacia.[83,84]

Regulation of vitamin D 25 hydroxylase activity is limited. At high concentrations of vitamin D, the mitochondrial enzyme will form significant quantities of 25 OHD. The *in vivo* administration of $1,25(OH)_2D$ appears to decrease plasma concentration of 25 OHD.[85] Calcium deficiency appears to increase the metabolic clearance of 25 OHD.[86]

In contrast, the production of $1,25(OH)_2D$ is tightly regulated. Parathyroid hormone and deficiencies in Ca and phosphorus increase, whereas Ca, phosphorus, and 1,25$(OH)_2$D decrease the activity of the 25 OHD 1α hydroxylase enzyme and circulating 1,25$(OH)_2$D concentrations. Other factors, such as gender, pregnancy, steroids, prolactin, growth hormone, CT, and possibly thyroid hormone, also may increase circulating 1,25$(OH)_2$D. Magnesium is a cofactor of the 1α hydroxylase enzyme. Magnesium deficiency and hypomagnesemia in humans are associated with low serum 1,25$(OH)_2$D concentrations[57,87] and lower serum 1,25$(OH)_2$D response to low-Ca diet,[88] but do not appear to limit 1,25$(OH)_2$D production in animals.[89] In contrast to the rapid increase in PTH secretion and serum PTH concentrations, measurable alteration in serum 1,25$(OH)_2$D concentrations usually occurs hours after exposure to an appropriate stimulus.

Like other steroid hormones, 1,25$(OH)_2$D exerts its action through modulation of the cellular genome by binding to specific nuclear receptors present in numerous cell types. Through this mechanism, 1,25$(OH)_2$D may affect cell growth and differentiation and immune and endocrine function. Calcium homeostasis and bone mineralization are maintained by 1,25$(OH)_2$D through its effect on a number of target tissues, primarily by increasing vitamin D–dependent Ca absorption through the gut. The latter occurs as a result of increased transcription of mRNA for intestinal Ca-binding protein and other products. Additionally, 1,25$(OH)_2$D promotes bone resorption activities and releases bone Ca, thereby further increasing circulating Ca concentrations and acting on receptors of osteoblasts and osteocytes to promote bone remodeling.[83,84,90–92]

A rapid-onset (*i.e.*, within minutes after exposure to 1,25$[OH]_2$D), non–genomic-mediated action of 1,25$(OH)_2$D on intestinal Ca transport also has been demonstrated. The physiologic role of this nongenomic action and the genomic actions other than maintenance of Ca homeostasis and bone mineralization remain to be determined.[93]

Vitamin D receptors are up-regulated by 1,25 $(OH)_2$D at both the mRNA and protein levels. They also are increased during growth, gestation, and lactation, but show an age-dependent decrease in mature animals and humans[94]; presumably, this implies that vitamin D receptors may be up- or down-regulated, depending on Ca needs.

Quantitation of vitamin D and its metabolites has been achieved by several different methods. The more routine approaches include high-performance liquid chromatography with detection by ultraviolet absorbance or binding assays. Immunoassays based on antibodies raised to vitamin D metabolite conjugates also are available. Values from different laboratories cannot be compared without making direct comparison of their assay procedures. Interlaboratory coefficients of variation for the measurement of 25 OHD, 24,25$(OH)_2$D, and 1,25$(OH)_2$D may range between 35% and 52%.[95] Furthermore, differences between vitamins D_2 and D_3 in their affinity to the vitamin D binding protein and receptors and different chromatographic behavior on various preparative chromatographic systems demand that great care be taken with assay techniques when dealing with patients who have significant vitamin D_2 intake. To ensure reliable results, appropriate vitamin D standards must be used for standard curve generation when performing competitive protein binding assays of these compounds.

Maternofetal transfer of vitamin D and its metabolites varies, depending on the species. In humans, the cord serum vitamin D concentration is very low and may be undetectable, probably due to poor maternofetal crossover; the 25 OHD concentration is directly correlated with, but is lower than, maternal values, consistent with placental crossover of this metabolite; 1,25$(OH)_2$D concentrations also are lower than maternal values, but there is no agreement on the maternofetal relationship of this and other dihydroxylated vitamin D metabolites. *In vivo*, some placental crossover may occur after maternal exposure to pharmacologic doses of vitamin D or 1,25$(OH)_2$D. Seasonal and racial variations in what is presumably endogenously produced serum 25 OHD_3 concentrations, which are lower in winter and in African Americans, and 1,25$(OH)_2$D concentrations, which are higher in African Americans, in the mother may be reflected in cord serum values. It appears, therefore, that the human fetus receives the bulk of its vitamin D already metabolized to 25 OHD.[6,96]

Neonates, even the very-low-birth-weight infant, appear to have adequate capacity to absorb and metabolize vitamin D. In infants receiving standard supplementary vitamin D intake, circulating 25 OHD and 1,25$(OH)_2$D concentrations may be increased to levels comparable to, and sometimes exceeding, adult values. Circulating 25 OHD and 1,25$(OH)_2$D concentrations in infants also appear to be dependent on Ca and phosphorus intake.[6,25,26,96]

Parathyroid hormone and 1,25$(OH)_2$D, and possibly CT, appear to function closely to maintain a stable serum Ca concentration by intermodulation of their physiologic effects of each other. Parathyroid hormone serves as a component of rapid response to hypocalcemia, whereas 1,25$(OH)_2$D, with its major effect on elevating intestinal absorption of Ca, is responsible for a slower but more sustained contribution to the maintenance of normocalcemia. Calcitonin, on the other hand, appears to function in the opposite role to PTH but with the capacity to stimulate the production of 1,25$(OH)_2$D, and in theory may serve an additional regulatory role in the maintenance of Ca homeostasis. Magnesium functions primarily as a cofactor in the production of these hormones under normal circumstances, but, with the exception of Mg–PTH interaction, the interaction between Mg and these hormones during pathologic circumstances remains ill defined.

DISTURBANCES IN SERUM CALCIUM AND MAGNESIUM CONCENTRATIONS

HYPOCALCEMIA

Neonatal hypocalcemia may be defined as a serum total Ca concentration below 2 mmol/L (1 mmol/L = 4 mg/dL) in term infants and 1.75 mmol/L in preterm infants with Ca^{2+} below 0.75 to 1.1 mmol/L (3.0–4.4 mg/dL), depending on the particular ion-selective electrode used. These definitions are made from a clinical viewpoint, since serum Ca concentrations are maintained within narrow ranges under normal circumstances and the potential risk for disturbances of physiologic function increases as the serum Ca concentration further decreases. Physiologic dysfunction (*e.g.*, changes in cardiac contractility, blood pressure, and heart rate) may or may not be demonstrated in infants who have hypocalcemia or are undergoing Ca therapy.[97–99] Children with ionized hypocalcemia, however, are reported to have a higher mortality rate in a pediatric intensive care setting.[100]

Clinically, there are two peaks in the occurrence of neonatal hypocalcemia (Table 36-1). An early form typically occurs during the first few days of life, with the lowest concentrations of serum Ca being reached at 24 to 48 hours of age; late neonatal hypocalcemia occurs toward the end of the first week of life and generally presents as neonatal tetany. In some infants, however, the nadir of the serum Ca concentration may occur at less than 12 hours or not until some weeks after birth.

TABLE 36–1
CLINICAL CAUSES OF NEONATAL HYPOCALCEMIA

Early Occurrence
Prematurity
Birth asphyxia
Maternal insulin-dependent diabetes
Maternal hyperparathyroidism
Hypoparathyroidism* (sporadic or familial, gene mutation, autosomal dominant or sex-linked inheritance, DiGeorge syndrome)
In utero exposure to anticonvulsants (?)
Phototherapy (?)
Late Occurrence
Intake of high-phosphate milks or cereals
Phosphate enema
Intestinal calcium malabsorption
Hypoparathyroidism*
Hypomagnesemia
Decreased Ionized Calcium
Exchange transfusions with citrated blood
Intravenous lipid infusion (*i.e.*, increased free fatty acid)
Alkalosis
In utero exposure to narcotics (?)

* Hypocalcemia may be severe and prolonged, and present in later life.

Early neonatal hypocalcemia occurs primarily in preterm infants. The frequency of hypocalcemia varies inversely with birth weight and gestational age.[6,20,101] Over 50% of preterm very-low-birth-weight neonates may have hypocalcemia. Hypocalcemia also occurs in infants who have suffered birth asphyxia[102,103] and in infants of mothers with insulin-dependent diabetes.[104] Neonatal hypocalcemia usually is more severe and prolonged when associated with maternal hyperparathyroidism, fetal parathyroid hypoplasia or agenesis, or isolated hypoparathyroidism. The latter may be a part of the DiGeorge syndrome, which is characterized by the partial or complete absence of derivatives of the third and fourth pharyngeal pouches, and possibly the fifth pouch, and is often associated with defective development of the third, fourth, and sixth aortic arches (see Chap. 46). Clinical expression includes some combination of congenital heart disease, primarily involving the aortic arch, hypoparathyroidism, decreased T-cell number or function, and possibly thyroid C-cell deficiency.[105,106] Isolated hypoparathyroidism may be transient or permanent. Hypoparathyroidism may be present in a heterogenous group of disorders,[6,20,107,108] with differing Mendelian modes of inheritance, including autosomal dominant and X-linked; a familial point mutation in the signal peptide–encoding region of the prepro-PTH gene has been reported.[109] The use of phototherapy and maternal anticonvulsants is reported to be associated with neonatal hypocalcemia.[6,20]

Late neonatal hypocalcemia usually occurs toward the end of the first week of life and is less frequent than early neonatal hypocalcemia. Apart from phosphate imbalance from cow-milk–derived formulas or from early neonatal introduction of cereals, other clinical circumstances potentially associated with hypocalcemia may include intestinal malabsorption, hypomagnesemia, and hypoparathyroidism. In theory, the risk of neonatal hypocalcemia may be greater if there is preexisting maternal vitamin D deficiency.

The physiologic basis for the development of hypocalcemia is discussed earlier. The mechanisms of hypocalcemia are varied (Table 36-2), and each clinical condition may be associated with several factors that may contribute to hypocalcemia: for example, limited milk and Ca intake, in addition to transient limited increase in the serum PTH concentration, elevated serum CT concentration, and possibly end organ resistance to $1,25(OH)_2D$. These factors contribute to the development of hypocalcemia in the preterm infant. Alternately, a common basis may exist for the development of hypocalcemia in a number of clinical situations. For example, a predisposing factor to early neonatal hypocalcemia can be inadequate Ca intake when the placental supply of Ca to the neonate is abruptly discontinued at delivery. Postnatally, even if there is maximum intestinal absorption, Ca retention with milk feeding probably is only 15 mg/kg body

TABLE 36–2
MECHANISMS FOR THE DEVELOPMENT OF NEONATAL HYPOCALCEMIA

Agent	Problem	Clinical Association
Ca	Decreased intake or absorption	Prematurity; malabsorption syndrome
Ca^{2+}	Increased Ca complex	Chelating agent (*e.g.*, citrated blood for exchange transfusion, long-chain free fatty acid)
Mg	Decreased tissue store or absorption	Maternal hypomagnesemia; specific Mg malabsorption (rare)
P	Increased	Endogenous and exogenous (*e.g.*, dietary, enema) phosphate loading
*p*H	Increased	Respiratory or metabolic alkalosis (*i.e.*, shifts Ca from ionized to protein-bound fraction)
PTH	Decreased production	Maternal hyperparathyroidism; hypoparathyroidism; DiGeorge syndrome; hypomagnesemia
	Decreased parathyroid gland responsiveness	Hypomagnesemia
CT	Increased	IDM, birth asphyxia, prematurity
$1,25(OH)_2D$	Decreased end-organ responsiveness	Prematurity

CT, calcitonin; IDM, infant of an insulin-dependent diabetic mother; $1,25(OH)_2D$, 1,25-dihydroxyvitamin D; PTH, parathyroid hormone.

weight on the first day of life, rising to 45 mg/kg on the third day of life; these amounts are significantly lower than *in utero* Ca accretion rates.

Decreases in serum Ca^{2+} can occur without decreases in serum tCa. Agents that complex Ca in the blood would be expected to decrease ionized Ca. Such agents include citrate, which is used as an anticoagulant for blood storage. During exchange blood transfusion, Ca^{2+} can be decreased to 0.5 mmol/L, in spite of administration of conventional amounts of Ca (*i.e.*, 0.5–1 mL of 10% Ca gluconate for each 100 mL of blood exchanged) during the transfusion. Increased levels of long-chain free fatty acids also can complex Ca *in vitro* and lower ionized Ca. Alkalosis can result in shifts of Ca from the ionized state to the protein-bound fraction. Because alkalosis *per se* increases neuromuscular hyperirritability, the combination of decreased serum Ca^{2+} and alkalosis may precipitate clinical tetany in an infant with borderline serum Ca status. For reasons that are unclear, infants born to narcotic-using mothers have been reported to have a lower serum Ca^{2+} if they manifest withdrawal symptoms.[110]

DIAGNOSIS

The clinical manifestation of neonatal hypocalcemia in infants may be confused easily with other neonatal disorders (*e.g.*, hypoglycemia, sepsis, meningitis, anoxia, intracranial bleeding, narcotic withdrawal). The neonate with hypocalcemia also may be asymptomatic; the less mature the infant, the more subtle and varied are the clinical manifestations. Significant clinical signs are tremulousness, apnea, cyanosis, and seizures; infants also may be lethargic, feed poorly, vomit, and have abdominal distention. Frank convulsions are seen more commonly with late neonatal hypocalcemia. The degree of irritability of the infants does not appear to correlate with serum Ca values. The classic signs of peripheral hyperexcitability of motor nerves—carpopedal spasm (*i.e.*, spasm of the wrists and ankles) and laryngospasm (*i.e.*, spasm of the vocal cord)—are uncommon in newborn infants. Therefore, suspicion of hypocalcemia should be confirmed with the measurement of serum tCa and ionized Ca.

Diagnostic workup for hypocalcemia includes a history, physical examination, and relevant investigations (Table 36-3). At physiologic concentrations of hydrogen and potassium ion, tetany may develop in older infants at a Ca^{2+} of less than 0.8 mmol/L (3.2 mg/dL) and will almost always be manifested, with the possible exception of preterm infants, at a Ca^{2+} of less than 0.6 mmol/L (2.4 mg/dL). If serum albumin concentrations are normal, the corresponding serum tCa concentrations usually are less than 1.8 mmol/L (7.2 mg/dL). In the preterm infant, serum Ca^{2+} may not decrease to the same extent as total Ca, presumably related in part to the lower serum albumin concentrations or acidosis, which are found frequently in these infants. The standard nomogram relating serum tCa and total protein to ionized Ca has not been predictive of neonatal serum Ca^{2+}. The measurement of electrocardiographic QT intervals, corrected for heart rate, also is of little value for prediction of neonatal hypocalcemia.

Assays of calciotropic hormones and 25 OHD may be useful in the diagnosis of uncommon causes of neonatal hypocalcemia, such as primary hypoparathyroidism, malabsorption, and disorders of vitamin D metabolism. Other investigations listed in the tables may be important in the differential diagnosis and understanding of the mechanisms for hypocalcemia.

Confirmation of hypocalcemia as the cause of clinical symptomatology is the reversibility of clinical signs when serum tCa or ionized Ca has been increased to the normal range.

THERAPY

Any neonate with seizures should have blood drawn for diagnostic tests before therapy. Intravenous administration of Ca salts is the most effective and most rapid means of elevating serum Ca concentrations. Seizures suspected to be caused by hypocalcemia should be treated with intravenous 10% Ca gluconate (1 mL/kg) administered over 10 minutes with constant monitoring of the heart rate. Gradual or abrupt decrease in heart rate during the infusion is an indication to slow or stop the infusion. Intravenous Ca therapy may be complicated by acute hypercalcemia; extravasation of Ca solution leads to skin sloughs, tissue necrosis, and calcification. If umbilical venous catheters are used, the tips should not be intracardiac because of possible accidental administration of Ca directly into the heart. Direct admixture with bicarbonate or phosphate solution will result in precipitation.

There is little information on comparative efficacy of Ca preparations in the treatment of neonatal hypocalcemia. In neonates, 10% Ca gluconate (0.45 mmol [18 mg] elemental Ca/kg) can effectively increase serum Ca^{2+}, heart rate, and blood pressure.[97,98] In children, small equimolar doses (0.07 mmol [2.8 mg] elemental Ca/kg), 10% Ca chloride may result in higher mean arterial blood pressure with a slightly greater mean increase (0.06 mmol/L) in the measured serum Ca^{2+} compared to 10% Ca gluconate.[111] Thus, 10% Ca chloride (0.1–0.3 mL/kg) also may be used with the same precautions as above. Prolonged use of Ca chloride in high doses may be associated with acidosis and probably should be avoided. Subsequent Ca therapy will depend on symptomatic response to initial dose and repeated measurement of serum total concentration and Ca^{2+}.

After the resolution of the seizures, intravenous Ca solution may be continued at a dose of 1.87 mmol (75 mg) elemental Ca/kg/day until the serum Ca concentrations have remained consistently in the normal range. Thereafter, the intravenous Ca solution can be reduced in stepwise fashion (*i.e.*, 50% for 24 hours, 25% for another 24 hours, discontinuation). With intravenous therapy, bolus infusion may be associated with a transient slight decrease in blood *p*H and serum phosphorus.[112] Continuous infusion probably is more efficacious than intermittent therapy, since renal loss of Ca may be greater with the latter method.[113] Arterial infusion of Ca in high concentrations potentially is fraught with many dangers and should be avoided if possible. Anecdotal cases of massive sloughing of soft tissue in the area perfused by the peripheral artery receiving the infusion have been reported, and inadvertent administration into a mesenteric artery theoretically can lead to necrosis of intestinal tissues.

Oral Ca therapy in the same dosage (1.87 mmol [75 mg] elemental Ca/kg/day in four to six divided doses)

TABLE 36–3
DIAGNOSTIC WORKUP FOR HYPOCALCEMIA

History
Familial
Pregnancy (*i.e.*, maternal illness such as diabetes mellitus and hyperparathyroidism; intrapartum events; infant's gestational age)
Dietary intake of infant
Physical Examination
Jitteriness, apnea, cyanosis
Seizures
Associated features (*e.g.*, infant of a diabetic mother, prematurity, birth asphyxia, congenital heart defect)
Investigations
Serum Ca, Mg, P, Ca^{2+}, glucose
Vitamin D metabolites
Parathyroid hormone
Calcitonin
Acid–base balance
ECG (Q-Tc > 0.4 sec or Q-oTc > 0.2 sec)
Chest x-ray (*e.g.*, thymic shadow, aortic arch position)
Urine drug screen
Others (*e.g.*, malabsorption workup, lymphocyte count, T-cell numbers and function, maternal and family screening)

ECG, electrocardiogram
Adapted from Koo WWK, Tsang RC. Neonatal calcium and phosphorus disorders. In: Lifshitz F, ed. Pediatric endocrinology: a clinical guide. 2nd ed. New York: Marcel Dekker, 1990:569.

may be used for maintenance therapy. All Ca preparations are hypertonic, and there is a theoretic potential for precipitating necrotizing enterocolitis in infants at risk for this condition. Oral Ca preparations with a syrup base containing a high sucrose content may constitute a significant carbohydrate and osmolar load for very small infants and may be associated with an increase in frequency of bowel movements. Calcium syrup is concentrated; for example, Ca glubionate and Ca gluceptate have 2.88 and 2.25 mmol (115 and 90 mg) elemental Ca per 5 mL, respectively, if the infant is under fluid restriction.

The duration of supplemental Ca therapy varies with the course of hypocalcemia. Commonly, as little as 2 to 3 days of therapy is required, as illustrated by the treatment of early neonatal hypocalcemia. The requirement for Ca therapy may be prolonged, however, as in the case of hypocalcemia caused by malabsorption or hypoparathyroidism. The serum Ca concentrations should be measured twice daily during the first few days of treatment and for a day after discontinuation to detect any rebound phenomenon. A poor response to Ca therapy may be due to concurrent Mg deficiency (see Hypomagnesemia).

Vitamin D metabolites and exogenous PTH have been used in the treatment of neonatal hypocalcemia.[6,20] They offer no practical advantage in the treatment of acute hypocalcemia, however, and their use should be considered experimental. The vitamin D metabolite $1,25(OH)_2D$ is used commonly in the maintenance therapy for chronic conditions that cause hypocalcemia (*e.g.*, hypoparathyroidism).

The successful management of neonatal hypocalcemia also depends on the resolution, if possible, of the primary cause of hypocalcemia. For example, in phosphate-induced hypocalcemia, high-phosphate formulas and solids should be discontinued, and human milk or a low-phosphate formula should be substituted. Use of aluminum hydroxide gel to bind intestinal phosphate should be avoided because of potential risk for aluminum toxicity.

Neonatal hypocalcemia may resolve spontaneously. Thus, it is possible that asymptomatic neonatal hypocalcemia may not require treatment. Because of the major physiologic importance of Ca in all cellular systems, however, especially its role as a second messenger for the initiation of the intracellular enzymatic cascade, hypocalcemia potentially can alter important cellular functions and probably should be corrected. Treatment of asymptomatic hypocalcemia can be instituted with oral or intravenous Ca salts, using the regimen described earlier.

Pharmacologic prevention of neonatal hypocalcemia has focused primarily on the prophylactic use of Ca salts or the vitamin D metabolites. In newborn infants, Ca supplementation results in sustained lowering of serum intact PTH concentrations compared to unsupplemented controls.[41] This would suggest that Ca supplementation may decrease the metabolic stress from hypocalcemia and minimize the potential for depletion of tissue Ca stores. In low-birth-weight infants, continuous infusion of 0.025 to 0.038 mmol (1.0–1.5 mg) elemental Ca/kg/hour sustains low normal serum Ca concentrations; doses approximating the oral dose (1.8–2.0 mmol/kg/day [72–80 mg/kg/day]) may be needed in some infants and appear to be well tolerated in clinical practice. Vitamin D metabolites have been used in attempts to prevent neonatal hypocalcemia with variable degrees of success. In small preterm infants, serum Ca was normalized only at pharmacologic doses of $1,25(OH)_2D$. Early feeding and provision of Ca to the gut may be important in enhancing the ability of vitamin D metabolites to prevent neonatal hypocalcemia.

Thus, the most effective prevention of neonatal hypocalcemia includes prevention of prematurity and birth asphyxia, judicious use of bicarbonate therapy, and minimizing the occurrence of respiratory alkalosis from excessive mechanical ventilation. The practice of early feeding and, if necessary, oral or parenteral supplement of Ca salts also are useful measures. Maintenance of normal maternal vitamin D status with exogenous vitamin D supplement, if needed, may in theory be helpful in maintaining normal fetal vitamin D status and may secondarily prevent late hypocalcemia in some neonates.[6,20] Regular follow-up monitoring of serum Ca concentration and appropriate monitoring of underlying disease (*e.g.*, PTH concentrations) are necessary, since there are no definitive measures to determine whether an infant has a "transient" hypoparathyroidism that may last for several years,[107] or is at risk for "recurrence" of hypoparathyroidism and hypocalcemia, which has been reported to recur as late as adolescence.[108]

HYPERCALCEMIA

Hypercalcemia is present when serum tCa is more than 2.75 mmol/L (11 mg/dL) or when Ca^{2+} is more than 1.4 mmol/L (5.6 mg/dL). In pathologic hypercalcemia, elevation of serum Ca^{2+} usually occurs simultaneously with elevation of tCa; however, elevated tCa may occur without elevation of Ca^{2+}. Elevation of protein available to bind Ca (*e.g.*, prolonged application of tourniquet before venipuncture, transudation of plasma water into tissues, in adult patients with multiple myeloma, possibly in adrenal insufficiency) may result in elevation of serum tCa. A change in serum albumin of 1 g/dL generally results in a parallel change in tCa of about 0.2 mmol/L. Conversely, reduced albumin binding of Ca may result in normal serum tCa in the presence of elevated ionized Ca.

Hypercalcemia in infants is rare. It frequently is iatrogenic and may be discovered serendipitously on a routine panel of chemistry tests. Its onset may be at birth or delayed for weeks or months. The most common clinical cause of hypercalcemia in infants (Table 36-4) is a relative deficiency in the phosphate supply and hypophosphatemia, during inappropriate parenteral nutrition, or enteral human milk feeding in

TABLE 36–4
CLINICAL CAUSES OF NEONATAL HYPERCALCEMIA

Phosphate Deficiency
Parenteral nutrition
Very-low-birth-weight infants fed human milk or, less commonly, standard formula
Hypervitaminosis D
Excessive maternal vitamin D intake
Hyperparathyroidism
Congenital parathyroid hyperplasia
Maternal hypoparathyroidism
Uncertain Pathophysiologic Mechanism
Idiopathic infantile hypercalcemia
Severe infantile hypophosphatasia
Subcutaneous fat necrosis
Familial hypocalciuric hypercalcemia
Blue diaper syndrome
Congenital hypothyroidism
Congenital mesoblastic nephroma
Bartter syndrome variant
Other Causes of Chronic Maternal Hypercalcemia
Thyrotoxicosis
Chronic thiazide diuretic
Chronic lithium therapy
Vitamin A intoxication

preterm infants. Hypophosphatemia can result in elevated circulating 1,25$(OH)_2$D with attendant increased intestinal absorption of Ca. Phosphate deficiency results in increased bone resorption and decreased bone formation; Ca cannot be deposited in bone in the absence of phosphate and contributes to hypercalcemia. A number of other pathologic conditions associated with PTH or vitamin D may increase bone turnover, intestinal Ca absorption, and renal Ca absorption, and may result in hypercalcemia. Chronic excessive exposure to vitamin D or its metabolites secondary to the treatment of maternal hypocalcemic disorders or by self-medication may result in hypercalcemia of the mother and the neonate. Neonatal hyperparathyroidism may be congenital and inherited as an autosomal-dominant or autosomal-recessive trait or may be secondary to maternal hypoparathyroidism.[6,20]

Other causes of neonatal hypercalcemia in which no specific defect of vitamin D or PTH physiology has been demonstrated are listed in Table 36-4, such as idiopathic infantile hypercalcemia, often considered part of Williams syndrome. The major manifestations of the syndrome occur in varying combinations and include hypercalcemia, mental retardation, elfin facies, and supravalvular aortic stenosis. There also may be prenatal and postnatal growth failure. The presence of hypercalcemia in infants with Williams syndrome is variable and serum Ca may be normal, but the presence of nephrocalcinosis and soft tissue calcifications in some of these infants suggests that hypercalcemia may have occurred previously. An exaggerated response to pharmacologic doses of vitamin D_2 and a blunted CT response to Ca loading may contribute to the pathogenesis of hypercalcemia of idiopathic infantile hypercalcemia. No mutation of the CT/CGRP gene has been detected, however.[6,20,114,115]

Severe infantile hypophosphatasia is associated with hypercalcemia. It is a rare autosomal recessive disorder associated with severe bone demineralization, low serum alkaline phosphatase, and elevated urinary phosphoethanolamine. The condition may be lethal *in utero* or shortly after birth because of inadequate bony support of the thorax and skull.[116]

Neonates with extensive subcutaneous fat necrosis may develop hypercalcemia, usually occurring after a period of low or normal serum Ca concentrations. Increased prostaglandin-E activity, increased release of Ca from fat and tissues, and unregulated production of 1,25$(OH)_2$D from macrophages infiltrating fat necrotic lesions have been postulated to be responsible for the hypercalcemia in these conditions.[6,20,117]

Familial hypocalciuric hypercalcemia (FHH) has been reported in patients from 2 hours to 82 years of age. It usually is diagnosed in infants as part of a screening procedure after diagnosis of a family member with hypercalcemia or familial multiple endocrine neoplasia. Familial hypocalciuric hypercalcemia is inherited as an autosomal dominant trait with a high degree of penetrance. There usually is significant hypophosphatemia and a modest increase in serum Mg concentration. The pathophysiology of FHH is unknown, although functional parathyroid glands are needed for full expression, and the inheritance of FHH may be linked with specific HLA haplotype. There probably is no consistently increased tissue sensitivity to PTH.[118–121]

Blue diaper syndrome is a rare familial disorder, with malabsorption of tryptophan. The blue discoloration of the urine is due to the hydrolysis and oxidation of urinary indican, an end product of intestinal degradation of unabsorbed tryptophan and hepatic metabolism of its intermediate metabolites. Hypercalcemia and nephrocalcinosis usually do not manifest until some months after birth.[122]

Hypercalcemia may develop before and during thyroxine therapy of infants with congenital agoitrous hypothyroidism.[123] In theory, the deficient CT response to Ca loading or an increased degradation of CT from thyroxine therapy may be responsible for the hypercalcemia.[75,123] Congenital mesoblastic nephroma[124–126] and Bartter syndrome variant, which are associated with polyhydramnios, prematurity, nephrocalcinosis, and increased prostaglandin-E_2 excretion),[127,128] may be associated with hypercalcemia in infants. It is thought that causes of chronic maternal hypercalcemia, including maternal thyrotoxicosis, chronic thiazide diuretic, lithium therapy, and vitamin A intoxication, also may affect the newborn infants.[6,20,129]

DIAGNOSIS

Neonates with hypercalcemia may be asymptomatic and the diagnosis made on routine screening because of known predisposing factors, or the infants may have serious symptomatology requiring urgent treatment. Symptoms and signs frequently are nonspecific and include lethargy, irritability, polyuria, vomiting, constipation, dehydration, and failure to thrive. Hypertension, nephrocalcinosis, and band keratopathy of the limbus of the eye may be present in severely affected infants. Anatomic anomalies (*e.g.*, elfin facies, evidence of congenital heart disease) may be present on physical examination. A maternal dietary and drug history or history of polyhydramnios during pregnancy should be obtained, as should a family history for evidence of disturbed Ca metabolism (Table 36-5). Laboratory investigations are listed in Table 36-5.

THERAPY

Therapy of neonatal hypercalcemia includes management of specific underlying causes (*e.g.*, excessive vitamin D intake). Often, nonspecific therapy is the mainstay of therapy. Treatment for chronic conditions includes restriction of dietary intake of vitamin D and Ca and minimizing exposure to sunlight to lower endogenous vitamin D production. A low-Ca–low-vitamin D_3–low-iron infant formula is available for the management of hypercalcemia in infants (Calcilo XD, Ross Laboratories, Columbus, OH). This formula contains only trace amounts of Ca (<10 mg/100 kcal) and no vitamin D.

For short-term treatment of acute hypercalcemic episodes, expansion of the extracellular fluid compartment with 10 to 20 mL of 0.9% sodium chloride per kg intravenously, followed by an intravenous injection of a potent loop diuretic such as 2 mg of furosemide per kg, may be effective. Care should be taken to avoid fluid and electrolyte imbalance with careful monitoring of fluid balance and serum Ca, Mg, sodium, potassium, and osmolality at 6- to 8-hour intervals. Furosemide therapy may be repeated at 4- to 6-hour intervals. Prolonged diuresis also requires replacement of Mg losses. In patients with low serum phosphorus concentrations, phosphate supplements of 0.5 to 1.0 mmol of elemental phosphorus per kg per day in divided doses may normalize the serum phosphorus concentration and lower serum Ca concentrations; excessive amounts of phosphate may result in diarrhea and hypocalcemia and a theoretic possibility of metastatic calcification.

Minimal information is available on the use of hormonal and other drug therapy for neonatal hypercalcemia. Short-term treatment with salmon CT (4–8 IU/kg every 12 hours, subcutaneously or intramuscularly), prednisone (1–2 mg/kg/day), or a combination may be useful. Recombinant hCT, biphosphonates, and amylin may be useful.[80,130] Onset of action of these therapies is slow, and the hypocalcemic effect of CT may not occur. Rarely, parathyroidectomy may be necessary, although it is not always effective.[131] Indomethacin, a prostaglandin synthetase inhibitor, appears to be the specific agent of choice for Bartter syndrome variant. In some instances, neonatal hypercalcemia may resolve spontaneously. The need for treatment should be reassessed at regular intervals.

TABLE 36–5
DIAGNOSTIC WORKUP FOR HYPERCALCEMIA

History
Familial or maternal Ca or P disease
Difficult labor
Chronic excessive maternal or neonatal intake of vitamins D or A
Chronic maternal medications (*e.g.*, thiazide, lithium)
Physical Examination
Poor growth parameters
Lethargy, dehydration
Seizures, hypertension, band keratopathy (rare)
Associated features (*e.g.*, elfin facies, congenital heart disease, mental retardation, subcutaneous fat necrosis)
Investigation
Serum total Ca, Ca^{2+}, Mg, P, alkaline phosphatase, total protein, PTH, 25-OHD
Urine Ca, P, cAMP
Chest x-ray
X-ray hands
Renal function, abdominal ultrasound, ophthalmologic evaluation, ECG (*i.e.*, shortened QT interval)—to determine effect of hypercalcemia
Maternal Ca and P and other tests, as appropriate
Family screening depends on primary diagnosis

cAMP, cyclic adenosine monophosphate; ECG, electrocardiogram; 25-OHD, 25 hydroxyvitamin D; PTH, parathyroid hormone.

TABLE 36–6
CLINICAL CAUSES OF NEONATAL HYPOMAGNESEMIA

Decreased Magnesium Intake
Maternal magnesium deficiency
Small-for-gestational-age infants
Maternal insulin-dependent diabetes
Specific intestinal magnesium malabsorption (isolated, familial)
Extensive small intestine resection
Magnesium Loss
Exchange transfusion with citrated blood
Intestinal fistula or diarrhea
Hepatobiliary disorders
Decreased renal tubular reabsorption
Primary: hypokalemic alkalosis, hypomagnesemia with hypercalciuria or hypocalciuria
Secondary: extracellular fluid compartment expansion, osmotic diuresis
Drugs (*e.g.*, loop diuretic, aminoglycoside)
Other Causes
Increased phosphate intake
Maternal hyperparathyroidism

HYPOMAGNESEMIA

Hypomagnesemia is present when serum Mg is less than 0.06 mmol/L (1.5 mg/dL). Tissue Mg deficiency, however, may be present despite normal serum Mg concentrations (Table 36-6).[15,16]

Magnesium depletion in pregnant rats results in fetal mortality, malformations, hypomagnesemia, decreased skeletal Mg content, hemolytic anemia, and hypoproteinemia and edema.[132,133] Prolonged dietary Mg deprivation in human adults leads to personality change, tremor, muscle fasciculations, spontaneous carpopedal spasm and generalized spasticity, and hypomagnesemia, hypocalcemia, and hypokalemia.[32] Clinical manifestations in human congenital hypomagnesia (*i.e.*, fetal Mg depletion)[134] and neonatal hypomagnesemia are less well described.

Postnatally, hypomagnesemia occurs more frequently in infants with intrauterine growth retardation (IUGR) than in appropriate-for-gestational-age infants. Hypomagnesemia in IUGR occurs particularly in young, primiparous mothers, especially those who have toxemia of pregnancy.[135,136] The severity and prevalence of hypomagnesemia in infants of insulin-dependent diabetic mothers are directly related to the severity of maternal diabetes, which is thought to reflect the severity of maternal Mg deficiency. Hypomagnesemia in infants of diabetic mothers is associated with neonatal hypocalcemia and decreased parathyroid function.[104,136] Magnesium infusion in infants results in greater increases in serum Ca and PTH in those with initially low serum Mg concentrations,[137] and, in children with insulin-dependent diabetes, results in greater serum Ca and PTH responses than occur in normal control subjects.[88]

Specific intestinal malabsorption apparently predominates in males,[135,138,139] and hypocalcemia has occurred in all reported instances.

Intestinal resection, particularly of the jejunum and ileum, the major sites of Mg absorption, increases intestinal loss through ileostomy or fecal fistulas, and rapid intestinal transit time may lead to Mg deficiency.[28,135,140]

In the newborn period, exchange blood transfusions using citrate as anticoagulant result in complexing of citrate with Mg, which leads to hypomagnesemia, especially after multiple exchanges.[141]

Magnesium content in bile, gastric fluid, and pancreatic secretion varies from 0.2 to 5.0 mmol/L (0.5–12 mg/dL). Diarrheal Mg content may be as high as 7.1 mmol/L (17 mg/dL). Because the typical deficit required to produce symptomatic hypomagnesemia is approximately 0.5 to 1.0 mmol (12–24 mg) per kg of body weight, fluid losses from diarrhea or a chronic intestinal fistula may be associated with significant Mg loss.[28]

Infants with congenital biliary atresia and neonatal hepatitis may have low serum Mg concentrations.[142] This is thought to be due partly to increased aldosterone-related renal Mg losses.

Congenital primary defects in renal tubular reabsorption of Mg may occur,[143] and usually are associated with hypokalemic alkalosis with and without hypocalcemia. It may be classified further into hypercalciuric group consistent with the classic Bartter syndrome, which usually presents in infancy with failure to thrive and episodes of dehydration. A variant syndrome with hypocalciuria is thought to present later with short stature, substantially lower serum Mg, and more episodes of tetany.[144,145] Secondary defects in renal tubular reabsorption of Mg may result from extracellular fluid expansion due to excessive glucose, sodium, or fluid intake, or from osmotic diuresis. Loop diuretics such as furosemide and high doses of aminoglycosides such as gentamicin may cause magnesiuria.[146]

Increased phosphate intake may lead to decreased Mg absorption, and infants on high-phosphate milk preparations have lowered serum Mg concentrations. Further elevation of serum phosphate concentrations decreases serum Mg, possibly through the transfer of Mg from extracellular to intracellular sites. In infants with uremia, serum Mg concentrations may be decreased, possibly related to higher dietary phosphate.[147] Patients with renal failure, however, become hypermagnesemic at a Mg load that does not affect people with normal renal function.[148]

Negative Mg balance may occur with hyperparathyroidism.[149] Maternal hyperparathyroidism has been associated with neonatal hypomagnesemia.[150] In theory, negative maternal Mg balance in this situation may account for neonatal hypomagnesemia. Alternatively, neonatal hypoparathyroidism in this situation may lead to hypomagnesemia, since PTH has presumptive action on mobilization of bone Mg.

Symptoms and signs of hypomagnesemia, which often coexist with hypocalcemia, may be indistinguishable.[16,151] Serum Mg concentrations should be measured in infants at risk for hypomagnesemia and in any infant with hypocalcemia who is resistant to the usual therapy. When hypomagnesemia coexists with hypocalcemia, a trial infusion of 6 mg elemental Mg/kg over 1 hour with pre-Mg– and post-Mg–infusion measurement of total and ionized Ca and of PTH may be helpful in the diagnosis of the primary defect. An increase in serum PTH after Mg infusion is indicative of hypoparathyroidism secondary to Mg deficiency, whereas no change or a decrease in serum PTH supports the diagnosis of hypocalcemia unrelated to Mg deficiency.

Critical assessment of Mg deficiency is difficult, because more than 99% of total body Mg is found in intracellular fluids or is complexed in the skeleton. It has been proposed that high Mg retention after a Mg load may reflect Mg deficiency.[152] Infants generally retain large amounts of infused Mg, however, and there are large variations in response; the clinical utility of this test thus appears limited in infancy.

The treatment of choice for acute hypomagnesemic seizures is 50% Mg sulfate ($MgSO_4\,7\,H_2O$), 0.05 to 0.1 mL (0.1–0.2 mmol [2.5–5.0 mg] elemental Mg) per kg given intramuscularly or by slow intravenous infusion over 15 to 20 minutes. Repeat doses may be required every 8 to 12 hours. Possible complications of intravenous infusion include systemic hypotension and prolongation or even blockade of sinoauricular or atrioventricular conduction.

Concomitantly, oral Mg supplements can be started, if oral fluids are tolerated. Fifty percent Mg sulfate can be given at a dose of 0.2 mL/kg/day. In specific Mg malabsorption, daily oral doses of 1 mL/kg/day may be required. Daily serum Mg concentrations should be measured until values are stable, to evaluate efficacy and safety.[20,135] Oral Mg salts are not well absorbed, and large doses may cause diarrhea. The maintenance Mg supplement should be diluted fivefold to sixfold to allow for more frequent administration, maximizing gut absorption, and minimizing side-effects. Newer oral preparations of Mg (*e.g.*, Mg L-lactate dihydrate), especially those in a sustained-release form, may have greater bioavailability compared to other sources of Mg (*e.g.*, Mg oxide, hydroxide, citrate). Practical experience with the use of Mg salts other than Mg sulfate in infancy is extremely limited, however.

Potassium and zinc deficiency frequently occur in Mg-deficient states, especially when there are abnormal gastrointestinal losses or malabsorption. Appropriate replacement therapy is needed. Treatment of underlying disorders (*e.g.*, closure of gastrointestinal fistula) should be pursued actively.

HYPERMAGNESEMIA

Hypermagnesemia is present when serum Mg is more than 1.04 mmol/L (>2.5 mg/dL). It may result from a combination of excessive Mg load and a relatively low capacity for renal excretion of Mg. Neonatal hypermagnesemia most commonly occurs after maternal Mg sulfate administration for preeclampsia. In mothers given Mg sulfate, serum Mg concentrations have been reported from 1.1 to 5.8 mmol/L (2.6–14.0 mg/dL), with umbilical cord serum Mg concentrations from 0.83 to 4.8 mmol/L (2.0–11.5 mg/dL),[153,154] and concomitant maternal hypocalcemia also may occur secondary to decreased serum PTH concentrations.[59] Variations in parenteral Mg intake resulting from alteration in Mg content or the rate of infusion of parenteral nutrition fluids may result in hypermagnesemia, particularly in critically ill neonates.[25–27] The use of Mg-containing antacids or enemas can cause hypermagnesemia.[135,155,156] Prematurity and perinatal asphyxia may aggravate hypermagnesemia, presumably because of decreased renal Mg excretion (Table 36-7).[157]

In adults with hypermagnesemia, hypotension and urinary retention occur at serum Mg concentrations of 1.67 to 2.5 mmol/L (4.0–6.0 mg/dL), central nervous system depression, hyporeflexia, and electrocardiographic abnormalities (*i.e.*, increased atrioventricular and ventricular conduction time) at 2.5 to 5.0 mmol/L (6.0–12.0 mg/dL), and respiratory depression, coma, and cardiac arrest above 5.0 mmol/L (12.0 mg/dL).[148,155] In newborn infants, a delay in passage of meconium (*i.e.*, meconium plug syndrome) has been thought to be related to neonatal hypermagnesemia.[158] In pregnant and newborn rats and dogs, however, hypermagnesemia does not have an effect on intestinal motility or the consistency of meconium.[159] Most neonates with hypermagnesemia, particularly preterm infants, are asymptomatic, even at serum Mg concentrations of more than 1.25 mmol/L (3 mg/dL).[25–27,156] Clinical signs of neuromuscular depression with floppiness and lethargy may be the most frequent manifestation of neonatal hypermagnesemia. Clinical signs may not correlate with serum Mg concentrations, although there does appear to be a correlation with the duration of maternal Mg sulfate therapy,[154] possibly representing tissue Mg content. With judicious use of Mg sulfate in the mother, however, signs of Mg intoxication should be rare in the infant.[153]

Serum Ca concentrations may be normal, decreased, or increased in hypermagnesemic neonates.[157] Hypermagnesemia may suppress PTH and

TABLE 36–7
CLINICAL CAUSES OF NEONATAL HYPERMAGNESEMIA

Prematurity
Asphyxia
Maternal $MgSO_4$ administration
Neonatal Mg therapy
Parenteral nutrition
Antacid
Enema

$1,25(OH)_2D$ production and may result in lower serum Ca concentrations[59,157] and even rickets when maternal Mg therapy is prolonged (*e.g.*, tocolysis).[160] Hypermagnesemia, however, might in theory displace bound Ca and lead to elevation of serum Ca concentration.[161]

Calcium is a direct antagonist of Mg, and intravenous Ca given in the same dosage as for treatment of hypocalcemia may be useful for acute therapy. Loop diuretics (*e.g.*, furosemide) with adequate fluid intake may hasten Mg excretion.[16,23,146,151,155] Exchange blood transfusion with citrated blood is an effective treatment for severely depressed hypermagnesemic infants. Citrated donor blood is particularly useful because the complexing action of citrate will expedite removal of Mg from the infant. Peritoneal dialysis and hemodialysis may be considered in refractory patients. Supportive measures such as cardiorespiratory assistance and adequate hydration are needed.

SKELETAL MANIFESTATIONS OF DISTURBED MINERAL HOMEOSTASIS

The most frequent cause of skeletal abnormalities in infancy is nutritional deficiency (Table 36-8). True fetal or congenital rickets is rare. It may result from severe maternal nutritional osteomalacia associated with Ca and vitamin D deficiency,[162,163] maternal hypoparathyroidism[164] or hyperparathyroidism,[165] or prolonged maternal treatment with Mg sulfate[160] or phosphate-containing enemas.[166]

In the western world, rickets and osteopenia presenting during infancy occur most frequently in small preterm infants and may occur in more than 30% of extremely-low-birth-weight (<1 kg) infants.[3,167] The rate of occurrence depends on the nutrient intake and is associated most frequently with prolonged intake of soy formula, human milk, and low-Ca– and low-phosphorus–containing parenteral nutrition. In infants born at term, prolonged exclusive human milk feeding with limited exposure to sunshine, macrobiotic diet, and prolonged total parenteral nutrition are factors that contribute to the development of osteopenia and rickets.[163,168,169] The common underlying causes in preterm infants appear to be mineral deficiency, particularly Ca and phosphorus, whereas in term infants there is a relative lack of Ca intake in addition to vitamin D deficiency. Isolated nutritional deficiency of copper and ascorbic acid has been reported in preterm infants with clinical and radiographic manifestations similar to rickets.[3] Chronic diuretic therapy, commonly used in infants with bronchopulmonary dysplasia, and contamination of nutrients with toxins such as aluminum are added risk factors.[3,169] The extent, however, to which specific risk factors are responsible for the development of osteopenia and rickets is difficult to define in individual critically ill infants receiving multiple therapies and suboptimal nutritional support.

TABLE 36–8
RISK FACTORS FOR THE DEVELOPMENT OF OSTEOPENIA AND RICKETS IN INFANTS

In Utero
Severe maternal nutritional osteomalacia (*i.e.*, Ca and vitamin D deficiency)
Maternal hypoparathyroidism and hyperparathyroidism
Prolonged maternal Mg or phosphate treatment
Postnatal
Nutritional
Prolonged exclusive human milk feeding
Macrobiotic diet
Soy formula given to preterm infants
Prolonged total parenteral nutrition with low Ca and low P
Chronic loop diuretic therapy given to preterm infants
Aluminum contamination (?)
Inherited defects
Renal tubular disorder
Vitamin D or PTH metabolism disorder

PTH, parathyroid hormone.

Acquired and heritable forms of rickets that develop despite adequate availability of vitamin D usually are associated with renal tubular disorders and metabolic defects in vitamin D and PTH metabolism. These causes of rickets are rare, and their skeletal manifestations usually do not present before late infancy.[165,170–172]

Most cases of rickets and osteopenia are diagnosed incidentally during the investigation of complications such as fractures or conditions unrelated to the skeleton. The presence of osteopenia and rickets is confirmed by classic radiographic features such as generalized bone demineralization and widening, cupping, and fraying of the distal metaphyses. Classic features of rickets such as severe skeletal deformities, including kyphoscoliosis and bowing of the legs, may not be present if the diagnosis is made early in infancy before significant growth and weight-bearing have occurred. This is particularly true for the preterm infant whose skeletal problem typically is diagnosed between 2 and 6 months postnatally. Serial biochemical changes, including persistently low serum inorganic phosphate and serum alkaline phosphatase activity more than 5 times the normal adult range, may be helpful in the diagnosis. Measurement of serum 25 OHD as an indicator of vitamin D status also may be helpful. The use of photon absorptiometry allows a more accurate quantitation of the degree of bone mineralization, and serial measurements of bone mineral content may be useful to monitor the progress of bone mineralization during long-term follow-up.[3,169,173]

Osteopenia, rickets, and fractures in preterm infants appear to have become less frequent since the widespread use of high-Ca and high-phosphorus formulas designed specifically for preterm infants. The ingestion of the recommended daily amount of Ca and phosphorus should be adequate for otherwise healthy term infants.[174] A total daily intake of 400 IU vitamin D appears adequate to maintain normal vitamin D status in both preterm and term infants.[175–177] Preterm infants receiving mother's milk require supplementation with commercially available powder or liquid fortifier or liquid Ca and phosphorus preparation.[173]

The infant's mineral intake is monitored by maintaining a normal serum Ca, phosphorus, and alkaline phosphatase, while avoiding hypercalciuria (>0.15 mmol [6 mg] Ca/kg/day). Measurement of vitamin D metabolites such as 25 OHD and 1,25$(OH)_2$D and measurement of bone mineralization with standard skeletal radiographs or photon absorptiometry are needed if pathologic bone mineralization is suspected.

Rickets and fractures from nutritional deficiencies respond well to adequate nutrient intake. Short-term follow-up of these infants shows no major residual physical deformity. Skeletal maturation as assessed by ossification centers of the wrists for preterm infants is similar to term infants at 1 year of age.[167] There is a lack of information, however, on the long-term follow-up of these infants with regard to long-term bone mineralization and linear growth. Specific therapies are required for inherited renal tubular disorders and for disorders of vitamin D and PTH metabolism.

REFERENCES

1. Widdowson EM, McCance RA. The metabolism of calcium, phosphorus, magnesium and strontium. Pediatr Clin North Am 1965;12:595.
2. Ziegler EE, O'Donnell AM, Nelson SE, et al. Body composition of the reference fetus. Growth 1976;40:320.
3. Koo WWK, Tsang R. Bone mineralization in infants. Prog Food Nutr Sci 1984;8:229.
4. Greer FR, Tsang RC. Calcium, phosphorus, magnesium, and vitamin D requirements for the preterm infant. In: Tsang RC, ed. Vitamin and mineral requirements in preterm infants. New York: Marcel Dekker, 1985:99.
5. Ellis KJ, Shypailo RJ, Schanler RJ. Body elemental composition of the neonate: comparison with the reference fetus. FASEB J 1992;6:A1667.
6. Koo WWK, Tsang RC. Neonatal calcium and phosphorus disorders. In: Lifshitz F, ed. Pediatric endocrinology: a clinical guide. 2nd ed. New York: Marcel Dekker, 1990:569.
7. Saggese G, Baroncelli GI, Bertelloni S, et al. Intact parathyroid hormone levels during pregnancy, in healthy term neonates and in hypocalcemic preterm infants. Acta Paediatr Scand 1991;80:36.
8. Rubin LP, Posillico JT, Anast CS, et al. Circulating levels of biologically active and immunoreactive intact parathyroid hormone in human newborns. Pediatr Res 1991;29:201.
9. Bowers GN, Brassard C, Sena SF. Measurement of ionized calcium in serum with ion-selective electrodes: a mature technology that can meet the daily service needs. Clin Chem 1986;32:1437.
10. D'Orazio P, Bowers GN Jr. Design and preliminary performance characteristics of a newly proposed reference cell for ionized calcium in serum. Clin Chem 1992;38:1332.
11. Loughead JL, Mimouni F, Tsang RC. Serum ionized calcium concentrations in normal neonates. Am J Dis Child 1988;142: 516.
12. Ganz MB, Rasmussen J, Bollag WB, et al. Effect of buffer systems and pH_i on the measurement of $[Ca^{2+}]_i$ with fura 2. FASEB J 1990;4:1638.
13. Lowenstein FW, Stanton MF. Serum magnesium levels by age, sex and two racial groups in the United States, First National Health and Nutrition Examination Survey (NHANES I), 1971–1974. J Am Coll Nutr 1986;5:399.
14. Gunther T. Biochemistry and pathobiochemistry of magnesium. Artery 1981;9:167.
15. Elin RJ. Assessment of magnesium status. Clin Chem 1987;33: 1965.
16. Reinhart RA. Magnesium metabolism: a review with special reference to the relationship between intracellular content and serum levels. Arch Intern Med 1988;148:2415.
17. Handwerker SM, Altura BT, Royo B, et al. Ionized magnesium and calcium levels in human umbilical cord serum. FASEB J 1992;6:A1789.
18. Ryzen E, Servis KL, DeRusso P, et al. Determination of intracellular free magnesium by nuclear magnetic resonance in human magnesium deficiency. J Am Coll Nutr 1989;8: 580.
19. Elin RJ, Hosseini JM, Banks SM, et al. Precision of cellular magnesium assays. Clin Chem 1990;36:821.
20. Koo WWK, Tsang RC. Calcium and magnesium metabolism. In: Werner M, ed. CRC handbook of clinical chemistry. vol. 4. Orlando, FL: CRC Press, 1989:51.
21. Mundy GR. Calcium homeostasis: hypercalcemia and hypocalcemia. 2nd ed. Cory, NC: Martin Dunitz, 1990:17.
22. Bronner F. Current concepts of calcium absorption: an overview. J Nutr 1992;122:641.
23. Dirks JH. The kidney and magnesium regulation. Kidney Int 1983;23:771.
24. Whang R, Whang DD. Update: mechanisms by which magnesium modulates intracellular potassium. J Am Coll Nutr 1990;9:84.
25. Koo WWK, Fong T, Gupta JM. Parenteral nutrition in infants. Aust Paediatr J 1980;16:169.
26. Koo WWK, Tsang RC, Steichen JJ, et al. Parenteral nutrition for infants: effect of high versus low calcium and phosphorus content. J Pediatr Gastroenterol Nutr 1987;6:96.
27. Koo WWK, Tsang RC, Succop P, et al. Mineral vitamin D and high calcium and phosphorus needs of preterm infants receiving parenteral nutrition. J Pediatr Gastroenterol Nutr 1989;8:225.
28. Thoren L. Magnesium deficiency in gastrointestinal fluid loss. Acta Chir Scand 1963;306(Suppl):1.
29. Koo WWK, Tsang RC. Calcium, magnesium and phosphorus. In: Tsang RC, Nichols BL, eds. Nutrition in infancy. Philadelphia: Hanley & Belfus, 1988:175.
30. Senterre J, Salle B. Renal aspects of calcium and phosphorus metabolism in preterm infants. Biol Neonate 1988;53:220.
31. Hardwick LL, Jones MR, Brautbar, et al. Magnesium absorption: mechanisms and the influence of vitamin D, calcium, and phosphate. J Nutr 1991;121:13.
32. Shils ME. Experimental human magnesium depletion. Medicine 1969;48:61.
33. MacManus J, Heaton FW, Lucus PW. A decreased response to parathyroid hormone in magnesium deficiency. J Endocrinol 1971;49:253.
34. Graber ML, Schulman G. Hypomagnesemic hypocalcemia in-

dependent of parathyroid hormone. Ann Intern Med 1986; 104:804.
35. Kronenberg HM, Igarashi T, Freeman MW, et al. Structure and expression of the human parathyroid hormone gene. Recent Prog Horm Res 1986;42:641.
36. Meyers DA, Beaty TH, Maestri NE, et al. Multipoint mapping studies of six loci on chromosome 11. Hum Hered 1987;37:94.
37. Solal M-EC, Sebert J-L, Boudailliez B, et al. Comparison of intact, midregion, and carboxy terminal assays of parathyroid hormone for the diagnosis of bone disease in hemodialyzed patients. J Clin Endocrinol Metab 1991;73:516.
38. Cosman F, Shen V, Herrington B, et al. Response of the parathyroid gland to infusion of human parathyroid hormone-(1–34) [PTH-(1–34)]: demonstration of suppression of endogenous secretion using immunoradiometric intact PTH-(1–84) assay. J Clin Endocrinol Metab 1991;73:1345.
39. Nussbaum SR, Potts JT Jr. Immunoassays for parathyroid hormone 1–84 in the diagnosis of hyperparathyroidism. J Bone Miner Res 1991;6:S43.
40. Allgrove J, Adami S, Maning RM, et al. Cytochemical bioassay of parathyroid hormone in maternal and cord blood. Arch Dis Child 1985;60:110.
41. Dilena BA, White GH. The responses of plasma ionised calcium and intact parathyrin to calcium supplementation in preterm infants. Acta Paediatr Scand 1991;80:1098.
42. Specker BL, Lichtenstein P, Mimouni F, et al. Calcium-regulating hormones and minerals from birth to 18 months of age: a cross-sectional study: II. Effects of sex, race, age, season, and diet on serum minerals, parathyroid hormone, and calcitonin. Pediatrics 1986;77:891.
43. Fujisawa Y, Kida K, Matsudea H. Role of change in vitamin D metabolism with age in calcium and phosphorus metabolism in normal human subjects. J Clin Endocrinol Metab 1984;59: 719.
44. Insogna KL, Lewis AM, Lipinski BA, et al. Effect of age on serum immunoreactive parathyroid hormone and its biological effects. J Clin Endocrinol Metab 1984;53:1072.
45. Davis OK, Hawkins DS, Rubin LP, et al. Serum parathyroid hormone (PTH) in pregnant women determined by an immunoradiometric assay for intact PTH. J Clin Endocrinol Metab 1988;67:850.
46. Logue FC, Fraser WD, O'Reilly DSTJ, et al. The circadian rhythm of intact parathyroid hormone-(1-84): temporal correlation with prolactin secretion in normal men. J Clin Endocrinol Metab 1990;71:1556.
47. Kitamura N, Shigeno C, Shiomi K, et al. Episodic fluctuation in serum intact parathyroid hormone concentration in men. J Clin Endocrinol Metab 1990;70:252.
48. Calvo MS, Eastell R, Offord KP, et al. Circadian variation in ionized calcium and intact parathyroid hormone: evidence of sex differences in calcium homeostasis. J Clin Endocrinol Metab 1991;72:69.
49. Nemere I, Norman AW. Parathyroid hormone stimulates calcium transport in perfused duodena of normal chicks: comparison with the rapid effect of 1,25-dihydroxyvitamin D_3. Endocrinology 1986;199:1406.
50. Juppner H, Abou-Samra A-B, Freeman M, et al. A G protein-linked receptor for parathyroid hormone and parathyroid hormone-related peptide. Science 1991;254:1024.
51. Birnbaumer L. Transduction of receptor signal into modulation of effector activity by G proteins: the first 20 years or so. FASEB J 1990;4:3068.
52. Brown AM. A cellular logic for G protein-coupled ion channel pathways. FASEB J 1991;5:2175.
53. Gupta A, Martin KJ, Miyauchi A, et al. Regulation of cytosolic calcium by parathyroid hormone and oscillations of cytosolic calcium in fibroblasts from normal and pseudohypoparathyroid patients. Endocrinology 1991;128:2825.
54. Naveh-Many T, Silver J. Regulation of parathyroid hormone gene expression by hypocalcemia, hypercalcemia, and vitamin D in the rat. J Clin Invest 1990;86:1313.
55. Toffaletti J, Cooper DL, Lobaugh B. The response of parathyroid hormone to specific changes in either ionized calcium, ionized magnesium, or protein-bound calcium in humans. Metabolism 1991;40:814.
56. Rude RK, Oldham SB, Sharp CF Jr, et al. Parathyroid hormone secretion in magnesium deficiency. J Clin Endocrinol Metab 1978;47:800.
57. Fatemi S, Ryzen E, Flores J, et al. Effect of experimental human magnesium depletion on parathyroid hormone secretion and 1,25-dihydroxyvitamin D metabolism. J Clin Endocrinol Metab 1991;73:1067.
58. Brown EM, Chen CJ. Calcium, magnesium and the control of PTH secretion. J Bone Miner Res 1989;5:249.
59. Cholst IN, Steinberg SF, Tropper PJ, et al. The influence of hypermagnesemia on serum calcium and parathyroid hormone levels in human subjects. N Engl J Med 1984;310:1221.
60. Cantley LK, Russell JB, Lettieri DS, et al. Effects of vitamin D_3 25-hydroxyvitamin D_3 and 24,25-dihydroxyvitamin D_3 on parathyroid hormone secretion. Calcif Tissue Int 1987;41:48.
61. Russell J, Lettieri D, Adler J, et al. 1,25-dihydroxyvitamin D_3 has opposite effects on the expression of parathyroid secretory protein and parathyroid hormone genes. Mol Endocrinol 1990;4:505.
62. Stewart AF, Broadus AE. Clinical review 16: parathyroid hormone-related proteins: coming of age in the 1990s. J Clin Endocrinol Metab 1990;71:1410.
63. Moseley JM, Hayman JA, Danks JA, et al. Immunohistochemical detection of parathyroid hormone-related protein in human fetal epithelia. J Clin Endocrinol Metab 1991;73:478.
64. Law F, Moate PJ, Leaver DD, et al. Parathyroid hormone-related protein in milk and its correlation with bovine milk calcium. J Endocrinol 1991;128:21.
65. Anonymous. PTHrP: endocrine and autocrine regulator of calcium. Lancet 1991;337:146.
66. Bilezikian J. Parathyroid hormone-related peptide in sickness and in health. N Engl J Med 1990;322:1151.
67. Birnbaum RS, Mahoney W, Roos BA. Purification and amino acid sequence of a non-calcitonin secretory peptide derived from preprocalcitonin. J Biol Chem 1983;258:5463.
68. Fischer JA, Born W. Novel peptides from the calcitonin gene: expression, receptors and biological function. Peptides 1985;6 (Suppl 3):265.
69. Wallach S, Carstens JB Jr, Avioli LV. Calcitonin, osteoclasts, and bone turnover. Calcif Tissue Int 1990;47:388.
70. MacIntyre I. The calcitonin peptide family: relationship and mode of action. J Bone Miner Res 1992;16:160.
71. Besnard P, el M'Selmi A, Jousset U, et al. Effects of 1,25-dihydroxycholecalciferol and calcium on calcitonin mRNA levels in suckling rats. Mol Cell Endocrinol 1991;79:45.
72. Naveh-Many T, Raue F, Grauer A, et al. Regulation of calcitonin gene expression by hypocalcemia, hypercalcemia, and vitamin D in the rat. J Bone Miner Res 1992;7:1233.
73. Austin LA, Heath H III. Calcitonin, physiology and pathophysiology. N Engl J Med 1981;304:269.
74. Wongsurawat N, Armbrecht HJ. Calcitonin stimulates 1,25-dihydroxyvitamin D production in diabetic rat kidney. Metabolism 1991;40:22.
75. Zamboni G, Avanzini S, Giavarina D, et al. Monomeric calcitonin secretion in infants with congenital hypothyroidism. Acta Paediatr Scand 1989;78:885.
76. Zaidi M, Seth R, Girgis SI, et al. Development and perfor-

mance of a highly sensitive and specific two-site immunometric assay of calcitonin gene-related peptide. Clin Chem 1990; 36:1288.
77. Trasforini G, Margutti A, Portaluppi F, et al. Circadian profile of plasma calcitonin gene-related peptide in healthy man. J Clin Endocrinol Metab 1991;73:945.
78. De Los Santos ET, Mazzaferri EL. Calcitonin gene-related peptide: 24-hour profile and responses to volume contraction and expansion in normal men. J Clin Endocrinol Metab 1991; 72:1031.
79. Robinson MF, Body JJ, Offord KP, et al. Variation of plasma immunoreactive parathyroid hormone and calcitonin in normal and hyperparathyroid man during daylight hours. J Clin Endocrinol Metab 1982;55:538.
80. Wimalawansa SJ, Gunasekera RD, Datta HK. Hypocalcemic actions of amylin amide in humans. J Bone Miner Res 1992;7: 1113.
81. Lin HY, Harris TL, Flannery MS, et al. Expression cloning of an adenylate cyclase-coupled calcitonin receptor. Science 1991;254:1022.
82. Mbalaviele G, Jullienne A, de Vernejoul MC. Human umbilical cord blood monocytes express calcitonin receptors in culture in the presence of 1,25 dihydroxyvitamin D. J Clin Endocrinol Metab 1991;72:356.
83. Reichel H, Koeffler HP, Norman AW. The role of the vitamin D endocrine system in health and disease. N Engl J Med 1989; 320:980.
84. DeLuca HF, Krisinger J, Darwish H. The vitamin D system: 1990. Kidney Int 1990;38(Suppl 29):S2.
85. Bell NH, Shaw S, Turner RT. Evidence that 1,25-dihydroxyvitamin D_3 inhibits the hepatic production of 25-hydroxyvitamin D in man. J Clin Invest 1984;74:1540.
86. Clements MR, Johnson L, Fraser DR. A new mechanism for induced vitamin D deficiency in calcium deprivation. Nature 1987;325:62.
87. Rude RK, Adams JS, Ryzen E, et al. Low serum concentrations of 1,25-dihydroxyvitamin D in human magnesium deficiency. J Clin Endocrinol Metab 1985;61:933.
88. Saggese G, Federico G, Bertelloni S, et al. Hypomagnesemia and the parathyroid hormone–vitamin D endocrine system in children with insulin-dependent diabetes mellitus: effects of magnesium administration. J Pediatr 1991;118:220.
89. Weaver VM, Welsh J. 1,25 dihydroxycholecalciferol and the genesis of hypocalcaemia in magnesium-deficient chicks. Magnesium Research 1990;3:171.
90. Suda T, Shinki T, Takahashi N. The role of vitamin D in bone and intestinal cell differentiation. Annu Rev Nutr 1990;10: 195.
91. Dabek J. An emerging view of vitamin D. Scand J Clin Lab Invest 1990;50(Suppl 201):127.
92. Ozono K, Sone T, Pike JW. The genomic mechanism of action of 1,25-dihydroxyvitamin D_3. J Bone Miner Res 1991;6:1021.
93. Anonymous. Review: nongenomic effects of vitamin D. Nutr Rev 1991;49:306.
94. Ebeling PR, Sandgren ME, DiMagno EP, et al. Evidence of an age-related decrease in intestinal responsiveness to vitamin D: relationship between serum 1,25-dihydroxyvitamin D_3 and intestinal vitamin D receptor concentrations in normal women. J Clin Endocrinol Metab 1992;75:176.
95. Jongen MJM, Van Ginkel FC, van der Vijgh WJF, et al. An international comparison of vitamin D metabolite measurements. Clin Chem 1984;30:399.
96. Specker BL, Greer F, Tsang RC. Vitamin D. In: Tsang RC, Nichols BL, eds. Nutrition during infancy. Philadelphia: Hanley & Belfus, 1988:264.
97. Salsburey DJ, Brown DR. Effect of parenteral calcium treatment on blood pressure and heart rate in neonatal hypocalcemia. Pediatrics 1982;69:605.
98. Mirro R, Brown DR. Parenteral calcium treatment shortens the left ventricular systolic time intervals of hypocalcemic neonates. Pediatr Res 1984;18:71.
99. Venkataraman PS, Wilson DA, Sheldon RE, et al. Effect of hypocalcemia on cardiac function in very-low-birth-weight preterm neonates: studies of blood ionized calcium, echocardiography and cardiac effect of intravenous calcium therapy. Pediatrics 1985;76:543.
100. Broner CW, Stidham GL, Westenkirchner DF, et al. Hypermagnesemia and hypocalcemia as predictors of high mortality in critically ill pediatric patients. Crit Care Med 1990;18:921.
101. Nelson NA, Finnstrom O, Larsson L. Plasma ionized calcium, phosphate and magnesium in preterm and small for gestational age infants. Acta Paediatr Scand 1989;78:351.
102. Tsang RC, Chen I, Hayes W, et al. Neonatal hypocalcemia in infants with birth asphyxia. J Pediatr 1974;84:428.
103. Tsang RC, Steichen JJ, Chan GM. Neonatal hypocalcemia. Mechanism of occurrence and management. Crit Care Med 1977;5:56.
104. Mimouni F, Tsang RC, Hertzberg VS, et al. Polycythemia, hypomagnesemia and hypocalcemia in infants of diabetic mothers. Am J Dis Child 1986;140:798.
105. Burke BA, Johnson D, Gilbert EF, et al. Thyrocalcitonin-containing cells in the DiGeorge anomaly. Hum Pathol 1987;18: 355.
106. Keppen LD, Fasules JW, Burks AW, et al. Confirmation of autosomal dominant transmission of the DiGeorge malformation complex. J Pediatr 1988;113:506.
107. Bainbridge R, Mughal Z, Mimouni F, et al Transient congenital hypoparathyroidism: how transient is it? J Pediatr 1988; 111:866.
108. Kooh SW, Binet A. Partial hypoparathyroidism: a variant of transient congenital hypoparathyroidism. Am J Dis Child 1991;145:877.
109. Arnold A, Horst SA, Gardella TJ, et al. Mutation of the signal peptide-encoding region of the preproparathyroid hormone gene in familial isolated hypoparathyroidism. J Clin Invest 1990;86:1084.
110. Oleske JM. Experience with 118 infants born to narcotic-using mothers: does a lower serum ionized calcium level contribute to the symptoms of withdrawal? Clin Pediatr 1977;16:418.
111. Broner CW, Stidham GL, Westenkirchner DF, et al. A prospective, randomized, double-blind comparison of calcium chloride and calcium gluconate therapies for hypocalcemia in critically ill children. J Pediatr 1990;117:986.
112. Venkataraman PS, Sanchez GJ, Parker MK, et al. Effect of intravenous calcium infusions on serum chemistries in neonates. J Pediatr Gastroenterol Nutr 1991;13:134.
113. Brown DR, Salsburey DJ. Shortterm biochemical effects of parenteral calcium treatment of early onset neonatal hypocalcemia. J Pediatr 1982;100:777.
114. Russo AF, Chamany K, Klemish SW, et al. Characterization of the calcitonin/CGRP gene in Williams syndrome. Am J Med Genet 1991;39:28.
115. Pastores GM, Michels VV, Schaid DJ, et al. Exclusion of calcitonin/x-CGRP gene defect in a family with autosomal dominant supravalvular aortic stenosis. J Med Genet 1992;29:56.
116. Fraser D. Hypophosphatasia. Am J Med 1957;22:730.
117. Finne PH, Sanderud J, Asksnes L, et al. Hypercalcemia with increased and unregulated 1,25-dihydroxyvitamin D production in a neonate with subcutaneous fat necrosis. J Pediatr 1988;112:792.
118. Firek AF, Kao PC, Heath H III. Plasma intact parathyroid hormone (PTH) and PTH-related peptide in familial benign

hypercalcemia: greater responsiveness to endogenous PTH than in primary hyperparathyroidism. J Clin Endocrinol Metab 1991;72:541.

119. Firek AF, Carter WB, Heath H III. Cyclic adenosine 3′,5′-monophosphate responses to parathyroid hormone, prostaglandin E_2, and isoproterenol in dermal fibroblasts from patients with familial benign hypercalcemia. J Clin Endocrinol Metab 1991;73:203.
120. Auwerx J, Brunzell J, Bouillon R, et al. Familial hypocalciuric hypercalcaemia-familial benign hypercalcaemia: a review. Postgrad Med J 1987;63:835.
121. Sopwith AM, Burns C, Grant DB, et al. Familial hypocalciuric hypercalcemia: association with neonatal primary hyperparathyroidism and possible linkage with HLA haplotype. Clin Endocrinol 1984;21:57.
122. Drummond KN, Michael AF, Ulstrom RA, et al. The blue diaper syndrome: familial hypercalcemia with nephrocalcinosis and indicanuria. Am J Med 1964;37:928.
123. Tau C, Garabedian M, Farriaux JP, et al. Hypercalcemia in infants with congenital hypothyroidism and its relation to vitamin D and thyroid hormones. J Pediatr 1986;109:808.
124. Rousseau-Merck MF, Nogues C, Roth A, et al. Hypercalcemic infantile renal tumors: morphological, clinical, and biological heterogeneity. Pediatr Pathol 1985;3:155.
125. Ferraro EM, Klein SA, Fakhry J, et al. Hypercalcemia in association with mesoblastic nephroma: report of a case and review of the literature. Pediatr Radiol 1986;16:516.
126. Woolfield NF, Abbott GD, McRae CU. A mesoblastic nephroma with hypercalcaemia. Aust Paediatr J 1988;24:309.
127. Seyberth HW, Rascher W, Schweer H, et al. Congenital hypokalemia with hypercalciuria in preterm infants: a hyperprostaglandinuric tubular syndrome different from Bartter syndrome. J Pediatr 1985;107:694.
128. de Rovetto CR, Welch TR, Hug G, et al. Hypercalciuria with Bartter syndrome: evidence for an abnormality of vitamin D metabolism. J Pediatr 1989;115:397.
129. Larkins RG. Lithium and hypercalcemia. Aust NZ J Med 1991; 21:675.
130. Wisneski LA. Salmon calcitonin in the acute management of hypercalcemia. Calcif Tissue Int 1990;(Suppl)46:26.
131. Ross AJ, Cooper A, Attie MF, et al. Primary hyperparathyroidism in infancy. J Pediatr Surg 1986;21:493.
132. Dancis J, Springer D, Cohlan SQ. Fetal homeostasis in maternal malnutrition: II. Magnesium deprivation. Pediatr Res 1971;5:131.
133. Cosens G, Diamond I, Theriault LL, et al. Magnesium deficiency anemia in the rat fetus. Pediatr Res 1977;11:758.
134. Davis JA, Harvey DR, Yu JS. Neonatal fits associated with hypomagnesemia. Arch Dis Child 1965;40:286.
135. Tsang RC. Neonatal magnesium disturbances: a review. Am J Dis Child 1972;124:282.
136. Mimouni F, Tsang RC. Perinatal magnesium metabolism: personal data and challenges for the 1990s. Magnesium Research 1991;4:109.
137. Shaul PW, Mimouni F, Tsang RC, et al. The role of magnesium in neonatal calcium homeostasis: effects of magnesium infusion on calciotropic hormones and calcium. Pediatr Res 1987;22:319.
138. Paunier L, Radde IC, Kooh SW, et al. Primary hypomagnesemia with secondary hypocalcemia in an infant. Pediatrics 1968;41:385.
139. Stromme JH, Nesbakken R, Normann T, et al. Familial hypomagnesemia. Acta Paediatr Scand 1969;58:433.
140. Opie LH, Hunt BG, Finley JM. Massive small bowel section with malabsorption and negative magnesium balance. Gastroenterology 1964;47:415.
141. Bajpai PC, Sugden D, Stern L, et al. Serum ionic magnesium in exchange transfusion. J Pediatr 1967;70:193.
142. Kobayashi A, Shiraki K. Serum magnesium level in infants and children with hepatic diseases. Arch Dis Child 1967;42: 615.
143. Evans RA, Carter JN, George CRP, et al. The congenital "magnesium-losing kidney." Q J Med 1981;50:39.
144. Gitelman HJ. Hypokalemia, hypomagnesemia, and alkalosis: a rose is a rose—or is it? J Pediatr 1992;120:79.
145. Bettinelli A, Bianchetti MG, Girardin E, et al. Use of calcium excretion values to distinguish two forms of primary renal tubular hypokalemic alkalosis: Bartter and Gitelman syndromes. J Pediatr 1992;120:38.
146. Agus ZS, Wasserstein A, Goldfarb S. Disorders of calcium and magnesium homeostasis. Am J Med 1982;72:473.
147. Ghazali S, Hallett RJ, Barratt TM. Hypomagnesemia in uremic infants. J Pediatr 1972;81:747.
148. Randall RE, Cohen MD, Spray CC, et al. Hypermagnesemia in renal failure: etiology and toxic manifestations. Ann Intern Med 1964;61:73.
149. Hulter HN, Peterson JC. Renal and systemic magnesium metabolism during chronic continuous PTH infusion in normal subjects. Metabolism 1984;33:662.
150. Monteleone JA, Lee JB, Tashjian AH, et al. Transient neonatal hypocalcemia, hypomagnesemia and high serum parathyroid hormone with maternal hyperparathyroidism. Ann Intern Med 1975;82:670.
151. Levine BS, Coburn JW. Magnesium, the mimic/antagonist of calcium. N Engl J Med 1984;310:1253.
152. Byrne PA, Caddell JL. The magnesium load test: II. Correlation of clinical and laboratory data in neonates. Clin Pediatr 1975;14:460.
153. Stone SR, Pritchard JA. Effect of maternally administered magnesium sulfate on the neonate. Obstet Gynecol 1970;35: 574.
154. Lipsitz PJ. The clinical and biochemical effects of excess magnesium in the newborn. Pediatrics 1971;47:501.
155. Mordes JP, Wacker WEC. Excess magnesium. Pharmacol Rev 1978;29:273.
156. Brand JM. Hypermagnesemia and intestinal perforation following antacid administration in a premature infant. Pediatrics 1990;85:121.
157. Donovan EF, Tsang RC, Steichen JJ, et al. Neonatal hypermagnesemia: effect on parathyroid hormone and calcium homeostasis. J Pediatr 1980;96:305.
158. Sokal MM, Koenigsberger MR, Rose JS, et al. Neonatal hypermagnesemia and the meconium plug syndrome. N Engl J Med 1972;286:823.
159. Cooney DR, Rosevear W, Grosfeld JL. Maternal and postnatal hypermagnesemia and the meconium plug syndrome. J Pediatr Surg 1976;11:167.
160. Lamm CI, Norton KI, Murphy RJC, et al. Congenital rickets associated with magnesium sulfate infusion for tocolysis. J Pediatr 1988;113:1078.
161. Liu C-L, Mimouni F, Ho M, et al. In vitro effects of magnesium on ionized calcium concentration in serum. Am J Dis Child 1988;142:837.
162. Russell JGB, Hill LF. True fetal rickets. Br J Radiol 1974;47:732.
163. Zhou H. Rickets in China. In: Glorieux FH, ed. Rickets. New York: Raven Press, 1991:253.
164. Gradus D, Le Roith D, Karplus M, et al. Congenital hyperparathyroidism and rickets: secondary to maternal hypoparathyroidism and vitamin D deficiency. Isr J Med Sci 1981;17:705.
165. Hanukoglu A, Chalen S, Kowardski AA. Late onset hypocalcemia, rickets and hypoparathyroidism in an infant of a mother with hyperparathyroidism. J Pediatr 1988;112:751.

166. Rimensberger P, Schubiger G, Willi U. Congenital rickets following repeated administration of phosphate enemas in pregnancy: a case report. Eur J Pediatr 1992;151:54.
167. Koo WWK, Sherman R, Succop P, et al. Fractures and rickets in very low birth weight infants: conservative management and outcome. J Pediatr Orthop 1989;9:326.
168. Dagnelie PC, Vergote F, van Staveren WA, et al. High prevalence of rickets in infants on macrobiotic diets. Am J Clin Nutr 1990;51:202.
169. Koo WWK. Parenteral nutrition-related bone disease. JPEN J Parenter Enteral Nutr 1992;16:386.
170. Schutt-Aine JC, Young MA, Pescovitz OH, et al. Hypoparathyroidism: a possible cause of rickets. J Pediatr 1985;106:255.
171. Glorieux FH. Rickets, the continuing challenge. N Engl J Med 1991;325:1875.
172. Econs MJ, Drezner MK. Bone disease resulting from inherited disorders of renal tubule transport and vitamin D metabolism. In: Coe FL, Favus MJ, eds. Bone and mineral metabolism. New York: Raven Press, 1992:935.
173. Koo WWK, Tsang RC. Calcium, magnesium, phosphorus, and vitamin D. In: Tsang RC, Lucas A, Uauy R, et al, eds. Nutritional needs of the preterm infant: scientific practice and practical guidelines. Baltimore: Williams & Wilkins (in press).
174. National Research Council. Recommended dietary allowances. 10th ed. Washington, DC: National Academy Press, 1989:174.
175. Koo WWK, Sherman R, Succop P, et al. Sequential serum vitamin D metabolites in very low birth weight infants with and without fractures and rickets. J Pediatr 1989;114:1017.
176. Greer FR, Marshall S. Bone mineral content, serum vitamin D metabolite concentrations, and ultraviolet B light exposure in infants fed human milk with and without vitamin D_2 supplements. J Pediatr 1989;114:204.
177. Specker BL, Ho ML, Oestreich A, et al. Prospective study of vitamin D supplementation and rickets in China. J Pediatr 1992;120:733.

Neonatology: Pathophysiology and Management of the Newborn, Fourth Edition,
edited by Gordon B. Avery, Mary Ann Fletcher, and Mhairi G. MacDonald.
J.B. Lippincott Company, Philadelphia © 1994.

chapter 37

Gastrointestinal Disease

JON A. VANDERHOOF
TERENCE L. ZACH
THOMAS E. ADRIAN

Although most pediatric gastroenterologists are uncomfortable with primary care of the sick premature infant, they often are valuable consultants to the neonatologist. In evaluating a complex gastrointestinal or hepatobiliary problem, a gastroenterologist often uses an organ system-specific developmental pathophysiologic approach. In looking at a problem from a somewhat different perspective than the neonatologist, the opinion of the consultant may augment the analysis of the primary physician. It remains the responsibility of the neonatologist to put the consultant's view into perspective as it relates to the other complex problems of the sick infant.

The gastroenterologist also may offer his or her skills in invasive procedures to aid in the diagnosis of gastrointestinal and liver disease. Upper and lower gastrointestinal endoscopy, liver biopsy, rectal suction biopsy, and esophageal, antroduodenal, and anorectal motility studies, and even endoscopic retrograde cholangiopancreatography can be performed in term infants and, depending on the skill and training of the gastroenterologist, in premature infants as well.

Finally, in some institutions, gastroenterologists with special expertise in nutrition provide assistance in nutritional support of parenteral nutrition-dependent or malnourished infants. Their role becomes especially important in infants with gastrointestinal or liver disease who may require long-term follow-up, such as the infant with progressive liver disease, or home parenteral nutrition, such as the infant with short bowel syndrome.

DEVELOPMENT OF THE GASTROINTESTINAL TRACT

Subsequent to the development of the individual organs of the gastrointestinal tract, specialized features of the system begin to become apparent, mostly in the second and third trimester.[1] At approximately 14 weeks of gestation, differentiation of the pancreatic endocrine and exocrine tissues begins, and crypts and villi begin to form in the small intestine. A few weeks later, the colon, initially populated with villi similar to those in the small intestine, begins to develop its more characteristic surface with gradual loss of villi. As these morphologic changes occur, numerous functional processes begin, some of which mature early *in utero*, some only at birth, and some during the first year of life.

CARBOHYDRATE ABSORPTION

The functional maturation of the digestive process is complex.[2] There are marked differences in maturation of the digestive and absorptive processes of different nutrients (Table 37-1). In the neonate, most dietary carbohydrate is presented in the form of lactose, the predominant carbohydrate in virtually all

TABLE 37–1
DIGESTIVE AND ABSORPTIVE FUNCTION IN INFANTS RELATIVE TO ADULTS

Process	Premature Infant	Full-Term Infant	Adult
Salivary enzymes	Normal	Normal	Normal
Gastric acid production	↓	↓ To normal	Normal
Bile acid secretion	↓ ↓	↓	↓
Pancreatic enzyme production	↓ ↓	↓	Normal
Lactase production	↓	Normal	Normal
Sucrase and isomaltase production	Normal	Normal	Normal

↓, decreased.

mammalian milk. Lactose and other disaccharides are digested by enzymes located on the brush border membrane in mature enterocytes; those enterocytes located on the midportions and distal portions of the small intestinal villi. Component monosaccharides are released after hydrolysis by disaccharidases. Lactase hydrolyzes lactose to glucose and galactose, and both subsequently are transported by active carrier-mediated transport. Other disaccharidases include maltase, which hydrolyzes maltose to two glucose units, glucoamylase, which hydrolyzes glucose oligosaccharides to glucose monomers, and sucrase, which hydrolyzes sucrose to fructose and glucose. Sucrase is actually a double enzyme, the other part of the molecule being isomaltase, which hydrolyzes α-1–6 bonds of α-limit dextrins. Disaccharidase activities are highest in the proximal and midjejunum and decrease distally.

Lactase activity develops later in gestation than the other disaccharidases. Lactase activity is low until the final weeks of gestation. Although other disaccharidase levels can be detected somewhat earlier in gestation, and reach nearly adult levels between 26 and 34 weeks of gestational age, lactase levels are only 30% of full-term levels by that point in gestation. Because of the delayed maturation of lactase, specialized infant formulas for preterm infants have been designed with a significant percentage of carbohydrate presented as sucrose or glucose polymers rather than lactose. The predominant enzyme for digestion of starches and glucose polymers is pancreatic amylase, which is nearly absent during the first 4 to 6 months of life and gradually matures during the latter one-half of the first year. An alternative pathway must therefore exist for the digestion of these glucose polymers.[3,4]

Salivary glands produce an amylase that may be important in the digestion of complex carbohydrates in the newborn. This enzyme is detectable at 20 weeks of gestation and is present in significant quantities in premature infants. As with pancreatic amylase, however, the ability of the newborn to secrete salivary amylase is substantially reduced and matures throughout the first year of life. Salivary amylase is inactivated by gastric acid, but probably retains some activity in the stomach of premature infants. Glucoamylase is a brush border enzyme capable of digesting glucose units from the nonreducing ends of starch and dextrin. Glucoamylase is present in neonates and infants at 50% to 100% of adult levels.

Finally, it is probable that some malabsorbed carbohydrate is digested in the colon through the colon salvage pathway. Colonic anaerobic bacteria are capable of metabolizing carbohydrates to produce short-chain fatty acids that are then absorbed through the colonic mucosa. Considering the relative pancreatic insufficiency and lactase deficiency in the newborn infant, the colon salvage pathway may be an important mechanism by which infants absorb carbohydrates.

FAT ABSORPTION

Fat absorption is a complex process, primarily because fat is insoluble in the aqueous environment of the small intestinal lumen.[5] Solubilization, therefore, is an important part of the fat assimilation process.

The first phase of fat absorption is that of enzymatic digestion or lipolysis. Because most dietary fat is present in the form of triglycerides, otherwise known as triasylglycerols, these must first be hydrolyzed by pancreatic lipase. Phospholipids are hydrolyzed concurrently by pancreatic phospholipase. Colipase, a cofactor secreted by the pancreas, also is required, facilitating the action of lipase by binding to bile salt–lipid surfaces and improving the interaction of lipase with triglyceride. The efficiency of this process is augmented by the release of cholecystokinin (CCK) from the duodenal epithelium, which occurs in response to the presence of lipid and protein in the duodenum. Cholecystokinin stimulates pancreatic secretion, gallbladder contraction, and simultaneous relaxation of the sphincter of Oddi, to mix large quantities of bile acids and digestive juices with lipids. Pancreatic lipase levels are reduced in preterm infants and intrauterine growth-retarded infants, significantly impairing lipolysis.[6] Lingual lipase, secreted from the salivary glands, may facilitate lipolysis in the premature infant and partially compensate for the infant's relative pancreatic insufficiency.[7] Nonetheless, fat absorption is significantly impaired in newborn infants and, to a greater extent, in premature infants, due at least in part to pancreatic insufficiency.

Closely linked with the process of enzymatic digestion of fats is micellar solubilization by bile acids.[8] Bile acid molecules are complex structures with both hydrophobic and hydrophilic ends. Bile acids interface with lipids to render them water soluble by positioning the hydrophobic portion in close proximity to the lipid globules while allowing the hydrophilic portion to remain free to interact with the aqueous environment. Lipids then become enclosed in disc-shaped water-soluble micelles that contain fatty acids, monoglycerides, phospholipids, cholesterol, and fat-soluble vitamins.

Solubilization is particularly important because of the presence of the intestine's unstirred water layer. This stagnant layer of water overlies the microvillus membrane of the intestinal epithelial cells and is the primary barrier to lipid transport. The actual thickness of the unstirred water layer is complex and difficult to measure, but the layer is significantly reduced by the constant agitation of the fluid in the gastrointestinal tract due to gut motility and villus contraction. Because of the convolutions in the small intestine caused by the presence of villi and microvilli, the total surface area available to interface between the intestinal surface and the unstirred layer is much greater than the interface between the unstirred water layer and the aqueous intraluminal environment. Penetration through the unstirred layer by the disc-shaped micelles is the rate-limiting step for lipid absorption. Disease processes that increase the unstirred layer thickness will markedly inhibit fat absorption in much the same manner as disease states that render the supply of bile acids inadequate for micellar solubilization. Bile acids commonly are deficient in cholestatic liver diseases such as neonatal hepatitis or biliary atresia and in rare cases of congenital bile acid deficiency. Bile acids are deconjugated rapidly and reabsorbed in the presence of small intestinal bacterial overgrowth. Bile acid deficiency may therefore occur in patients with disorders that cause intestinal stasis and bacterial overgrowth such as short bowel syndrome. In disorders of mucosal injury, the unstirred layer thickness may be increased, making penetration of the fat-containing micelles difficult and further exacerbating fat malabsorption.

Bile acids are extremely important in the fat absorption process. In the absence of bile acids, only about one third of dietary triglycerides, a very small percentage of fatty acids, and virtually no cholesterol or fat-soluble vitamins are absorbed. Medium-chain triglycerides may be better absorbed because of their enhanced water solubility, which allows penetration of the unstirred water layer without micellar solubilization. In both preterm and term infants, bile acid synthesis is limited and the bile salt pool size is low.[9] Moreover, preterm infants may have an ineffective bile salt transport process in the distal ileum, resulting in impaired enterohepatic circulation of bile salts.[10] Consequently, the bile acid concentration may be less than adequate for the formation of micelles and solubilization of fat. Thus, penetration of the unstirred layer is less efficient in the term infant and further impaired in the preterm infant compared to adults.

After lipids are enclosed in the bile acid micelle and reach the lipid bilayer membrane of the small intestinal mucosal cell, absorption into the cell occurs by passive diffusion. Because of the convolutions of the gastrointestinal tract, a large surface area exists for lipid assimilation. In the absence of disease, this process progresses in the term and preterm infant relatively uninhibited. In disorders in which the absorptive surface area is reduced or damaged, however, such as short bowel syndrome or any form of diffuse enterocolitis, fat, carbohydrate, and, to a limited degree, protein are malabsorbed.

Within the enterocyte, monoglycerides and esterified fatty acids are immediately resynthesized to triglycerides. These triglycerides, along with apoproteins, phospholipids, free cholesterol, some diglycerides, and esterified cholesterol are stabilized within chylomicrons. The outer structure of the chylomicron then fuses with the basolateral membrane and is extruded into the lamina propria, where it is carried by the lacteals and lymphatic channels and deposited into the bloodstream.

PROTEIN ABSORPTION

The assimilation of protein begins in the stomach through the action of hydrochloric acid and pepsin. The maturational aspects of this process have been the subject of substantial study and some controversy. Conflicting data exist as to the status of acid secretion in the newborn infant. Newborn infants appear to be capable of secreting acid, although the process is somewhat immature.[11] In premature infants, it is probable that the process is impaired to a greater extent.[12] Pepsinogen, the proenzyme for pepsin, which facilitates protein digestion in the stomach, is secreted in preterm infants, but in much lower concentrations than in term infants.[13]

The gastric aspects of protein digestion are relatively inconsequential, compared to the much more complete process in the small intestine. Enterokinase, produced in the duodenal mucosa, activates the pancreatic proteolytic enzyme trypsinogen, converting it to trypsin, which then activates essentially all of the other enzymes involved in protein digestion. Enterokinase levels have been demonstrated in human fetuses as early as 21 weeks of gestation.[14] Enterokinase secretion is diminished during fetal development, however, and is only 10% of adult levels in the term newborn. In addition, pancreatic and duodenal proteolytic enzymes are present in preterm and term infants in lower concentrations than in older children and in adults. These enzymes initiate hydrolysis of proteins, and the hydrolysis process is completed by brush border and cytosolic peptidases. Protein is absorbed in the form of amino acids and dipeptides through active transport processes that appear to be well developed by 28 weeks of gestational age. Despite the relative immaturity of multiple phases of the protein assimilation process, both preterm and term infants are quite capable of absorbing adequate quantities of dietary protein. In small infants, the protein malabsorption resulting from mucosal injury is probably far less consequential than the malabsorption of the other major macronutrients.

MICRONUTRIENT ABSORPTION

Absorption of micronutrients matures at varying rates in infancy. Water is absorbed passively in response to sodium and other electrolytes, as it is in older children and adults.[15] Experimental evidence suggests that the intestinal epithelium may be more secretory during early infancy, and the increased susceptibility of infants to diarrheal disorders probably is at least partially related to this process.

Mineral absorption depends on the form in which the mineral is presented to the infant. Iron, for example, is absorbed extremely well from breast milk. Even the preterm infant is capable of absorbing nearly 50% of the iron in breast milk, whereas only a small percentage of iron is absorbed from cow-milk formulas, necessitating iron supplementation. Calcium and phosphorous also are well absorbed from breast milk.[16,17] Magnesium, copper, and, to a lesser extent, zinc are well absorbed by both term and preterm infants.[18] In general, minerals are absorbed somewhat better from breast milk than from cow milk. Most vitamins appear to be absorbed adequately in both term and preterm infants, although fat-soluble vitamin deficiency is common in disorders affecting fat absorption, especially disorders causing bile acid deficiency.

GUT MOTILITY

Although nutrient assimilation is heavily dependent on the development of digestive and absorptive function, actual feeding depends greatly on the maturation of gut motility.[19–21] Neuroblasts migrate in a cranial-to-caudal direction between weeks 5 and 12 of gestation. There is gradual maturation of gut motility throughout the fetal period and the first several years of postnatal life. In the fetus, normal propulsive motility in the gut probably does not appear until approximately 30 weeks of age. Interdigestive phenomena, known as migrating motor complexes, can be demonstrated by approximately 33 weeks of gestation. Motor activity in the neonatal gut differs significantly from that in adults, in that the propagation rate of the migrating motor complex is substantially slower in neonates, and the complex is not abolished by feeding as in older children.

Sucking and swallowing reflexes begin early during fetal development, but the maturation of the process is not completed until after birth. The fetus is able to swallow amniotic fluid as early as 11 to 12 weeks of gestation. Actual sucking probably does not occur until approximately 18 to 24 weeks. This type of sucking is termed nonnutritive sucking, differentiating it from the more effective nutritive sucking mechanism that develops by 34 to 35 weeks of gestation. The onset of nutritive sucking closely parallels a rapid increase in growth of the fetal stomach,[22] and the acquisition of mature patterns of gastric antral and small intestinal motility.

By the time a term infant is born, sucking movements are followed in an orderly progression by swallowing, esophageal peristalsis, relaxation of the lower esophageal sphincter, and relaxation of the gastric fundus. The first stage of swallowing is an involuntary reflex in both the term and preterm infant.

Some data suggest that nonnutritive sucking may play an important role in weight gain in preterm infants. The mechanism of this effect may be related to maturational changes in the infant gastrointestinal tract, and sucking may facilitate gastric emptying and other gastrointestinal functions, primarily through stimulation of secretion of gastrointestinal regulatory peptides.

Maturation of gastrointestinal motility may have important implications for a number of conditions. Gastroesophageal reflux is common in both term and preterm infants, and probably relates to diminished lower esophageal sphincter function or inappropriate relaxation of the lower esophageal sphincter, often in association with delayed gastric emptying. The maturation of both lower esophageal sphincter function and gastric emptying has been studied extensively, with somewhat equivocal results. Depending on the technique used to measure sphincter function, the lower esophageal sphincter tone has been shown to be either low or normal in both preterm and term infants.[23] Hypertonic carbohydrate solutions appear to delay gastric emptying in infants, much as they do in adults.

GASTROINTESTINAL HORMONES AND ENTERIC NEUROPEPTIDES

Gastrointestinal peptide hormones appear to play an important role in the structural and functional development of the gut, as well as in the control of alimentary functions. The function of a vast endocrine system is integrated with that of the enteric nervous system, which itself uses other regulatory peptides as local messengers.

Endocrine cells producing gastrin, somatostatin, motilin, and glucose-dependent insulinotrophic peptide (GIP) are detectable in the fetus at 8 weeks of gestation, with gastrin- and somatostatin-producing cells being most numerous.[24] By 14 weeks, all of the endocrine cell types are present in the intestinal mucosa, although the anatomic distribution is more widespread than that seen in the adult.[24] By the end of the second trimester, the distribution of gut endocrine cells resembles that of the adult.[24] Peptidergic nerves are first demonstrable in the myenteric plexus at about 12 weeks of gestation, correlating with the known developmental pattern of enteric nerve plexuses.[24] These enteric nerves then migrate through to the submucous plexus. By the third trimester, all of the regulatory peptide systems are well developed.[25] At birth, the molecular forms of the gastrointestinal regulatory peptides and their distribution in the gut are similar to those of the adult.[25]

Surges of gut hormones appear to be responsible for the marked growth and functional change that occur in the alimentary tract in early neonatal life. Substantial changes in gastrointestinal hormone secretion are seen during this period, triggered by the switch from intravenous to enteral feeding.[26]

Gastrin is an important regulator of gastric secretion and also is trophic to the gastric mucosa. At birth, cord blood levels of gastrin are already four or five times higher than those in the adult, and prefeed basal levels remain elevated for several weeks.[27,28] Furthermore, gastrin levels increase in response to the first milk feed.[29] After 3 or 4 weeks of life, basal gastrin levels decline, a change accompanied by development of marked feeding responses.[27,30] Gastric acid is detectable in the stomach at birth and reaches a peak in the first day or two of life.[28,31] Thereafter, acid output decreases for a period of about a month in spite of the hypergastrinemia and rapid growth of the stomach. It has been suggested that the lack of responsiveness to gastrin could be due to a lack of receptors in the oxyntic gland mucosa. Perhaps a more likely explanation, however, is that secretion is suppressed by an inhibitor, such as peptide YY (PYY) or neurotensin, thus enabling gastrin to stimulate growth of the gastric mucosa without hyperstimulation of acid secretion.[32,33]

Basal levels of the duodenal hormone, secretin, are higher at birth than in adults, and during the first 3 weeks of life a more marked postprandial response develops than is seen in the adult.[34] Because secretin is considered to be a major factor in triggering the neutralization of acid chyme entering the duodenum, the increase in circulating secretin levels may be of considerable importance in mucosal protection during this period. It is notable that the postnatal surge of secretin, unlike that of the other alimentary hormones, occurs even in the absence of feeding, indicating the importance of this mucosal cytoprotective function.[30]

Cholecystokinin, released from the upper small intestine, stimulates pancreatic enzyme secretion and contracts the gallbladder. In addition, CCK has marked trophic effects on the pancreas and appears to be responsible for regeneration after resection or acute pancreatitis.[35] The observed postnatal surge of plasma CCK concentrations may therefore be of importance in stimulating growth of this organ.[36]

Also released from the small intestine, motilin is a hormonal peptide with powerful motor functions. These motor functions include acceleration of gastric emptying and stimulation of the interdigestive myoelectric complexes during the interprandial period. Motilin concentrations are low in cord blood, but preprandial basal concentrations show a massive postnatal surge that peaks at around 2 weeks of postnatal life.[30] This peak is enhanced, but delayed, in preterm neonates. It is likely that this increase in circulating motilin concentrations is responsible for the known increase in motor activity of the gut that occurs during the neonatal period. Interdigestive motor complexes appear normal at birth in the term infant, but interdigestive cycles are incomplete in preterm neonates.[37] Premature babies exhibit abnormal motor activity, with periods of motor quiescence and nonpropagating contractions. Thus, motor activity is more immature in preterm infants than in term infants.[37] The relationship between maturation of the migrating motor complexes and the late postnatal surge of motilin in preterm neonates is not clear.

The jejunal hormone, GIP, is thought to be largely responsible for the postprandial increase in circulating insulin levels.[38] Basal GIP concentrations are low at birth and increase gradually throughout the first month of life, together with the development of a marked postfeeding GIP response similar to that seen in the adult after ingestion of a mixed meal.[30,39] The development of the GIP response to feeding in neonates is mirrored by the postprandial insulin response, which increases through the first month of life to maintain glucose homeostasis.[39]

Neurotensin is an ileal peptide that has inhibitory effects on gastric secretion and motility. Plasma neurotensin concentrations are higher in the neonate than in the adult, and an enhanced postprandial response develops in the first month of life.[40] Both reduction of gastric secretion and slowing of the rate of gastric emptying will decrease the rate at which acid chyme enters the duodenum and, therefore, will result in a more steady absorption of nutrients from the gut. Thus, neurotensin may be important in the adaptation of the neonate to enteral nutrition.

Peptide YY is an important hormone from the distal intestine that inhibits gastric emptying and slows small bowel transit.[41] Peptide YY also inhibits gastric and small bowel secretion, leading to an increase in net absorption.[32] Concentrations of PYY are elevated in cord blood and rise postnatally to a peak within the first 2 weeks postpartum.[33] At their peak, plasma PYY concentrations are about 50 times higher than fasting levels in normal adults.[33] There is evidence to suggest that gastric emptying and intestinal transit are rapid during the first week of life, both in term and preterm infants. The triggering mechanism for the changes that then take place is unknown, but it is likely that factors such as PYY play a role.[41] In addition, the very potent inhibitory effect of PYY on gastric secretion may account for the prevention of hypersecretion of acid during the early neonatal period, in spite of the marked hypergastrinemia.[32]

Plasma enteroglucagon concentrations show a very marked postnatal surge, which peaks within the first week and is associated with the development of a marked postprandial response.[27,30] As an increased rate of small intestinal mucosal growth is known to occur during this period, it can be speculated that the increase of this trophic hormone is important in neonatal alimentary maturation. The resulting mucosal growth increases the absorptive area for the uptake of nutrients from the gut lumen.

Temporally, the postnatal surges of gut hormones parallel the changes in gastrointestinal function that accompany the introduction of enteral feeding in the infant. It is therefore of considerable interest that these surges are not seen in infants who have never received enteral feeding.[30,42] Concentrations of all gut hormones, with the exception of secretin, remain low in infants receiving only parenteral nutrition.[30,42]

Precise mechanisms control the secretion of each gut hormone, and the amount of a particular peptide liberated by a meal is adequate to stimulate the appropriate digestive response.[43] For example, a meal rich in long-chain triglycerides will evoke a large CCK response, not seen with medium-chain fats.[44] The high circulating levels of CCK in turn stimulate the pancreatic enzyme secretion and, by gallbladder contraction, release the bile salts necessary for digestion of the long-chain fat. Medium-chain triglycerides, on the other hand, are rapidly hydrolyzed by lingual and gastric lipases; they are water soluble, do not require micelle formation, and are rapidly absorbed. Thus, bile salts and pancreatic enzymes are not required for digestion of medium-chain triglycerides, and a large CCK response is not seen when they are ingested.[44] The gut endocrine system, with its sparse distribution of overlapping cell types, is designed to produce an integrated digestive response to the discontinuous stimulation of ingested food.[43] Because the type of food presented can influence the integrated hormonal response, it is apparent that differences in nutrition in early neonatal life may result in changes in the growth and functional development of the neonatal alimentary tract.

Although the fetus makes little demand on its gastrointestinal tract, the situation changes dramatically at birth, when demand for nutrients necessitates the rapid maturation of the alimentary tract. This development of the gastrointestinal tract is characterized by the integrated maturation of its many functions. The observation, however, that premature infants make a satisfactory transition from intravenous nutrition through the placenta to extrauterine enteral feeding suggests that external influences can exert a substantial influence. The massive postnatal surges in circulating levels of hormones, which have trophic as well as secretory and motor functions, is compelling circumstantial evidence of a profound gut endocrine influence on alimentary development.[30] This is supported further by the observation that these hormonal surges are not seen in sick infants who are on parenteral nutrition and have not been fed orally.[42] It is likely that failure of secretion of trophic gut hormones is responsible for the hypoplastic gut and pancreas that accompany parenteral nutrition. Appropriate enteral stimuli or hormone replacement eventually may alleviate this problem.

ABNORMALITIES OF THE GASTROINTESTINAL TRACT

To avoid repetition, an attempt has been made to confine the abnormalities described in this section to those that might require consultation by a pediatric gastroenterologist. Some overlap with general surgery has been allowed, however, to avoid extensive cross-referencing (see Chap. 44).

ABDOMINAL WALL DEFECTS

Major defects of the abdominal wall, omphalocele and gastroschisis, are relatively uncommon malformations occurring in approximately 1 of 6000 live births.[45–47] In either case, a portion of the infant's gastrointestinal tract remains outside the abdominal cavity at birth. Omphalocele is a failure of the extraembryonic intestine to reenter the abdominal cavity through the umbilicus, a developmental anomaly that occurs between weeks 10 and 12 of gestational age. The defect therefore includes the umbilicus, and the viscera typically are covered with a peritoneal sac. Occasionally, the sac may rupture, making the disorder difficult to distinguish clinically from gastroschisis. Gastroschisis is an actual defect in the abdominal wall that occurs lateral to the umbilicus. The infant with gastroschisis has a normal umbilical cord not involved in the defect. Both defects may occur in the presence of other intestinal anomalies. Malrotation is present in association with omphalocele. Although intestinal atresias are more commonly found in gastroschisis, atresias may be associated with either anomaly. Abdominal wall defects frequently are diagnosed prenatally by fetal ultrasound. The preferred route of delivery remains controversial and may depend on the size of the defect.[48] Vaginal delivery may be acceptable for small defects, and cesarean section may be preferred in cases with large defects.[49]

Gastroschisis or omphalocele requires immediate pediatric surgical consultation. Fluid losses and hypothermia are of primary immediate concern, especially in the case of gastroschisis, since no membrane covers the bowel. Large fluid and heat losses are common and intravenous fluid replacement should be initiated immediately. The defect should be wrapped, using warm, sterile, moist saline gauze, with care taken to prevent twisting and infarction of the bowel.

Postoperative management includes sedation and mechanical ventilation for at least 48 to 72 hours because of increased intraabdominal pressure. During the postoperative period, gut motility is slow to return, especially in the case of gastroschisis. Patients with gastroschisis may demonstrate sluggish motility for up to 8 months, and a protracted course of parenteral nutrition commonly is required. Delayed onset of necrotizing enterocolitis (NEC) is not uncommon, and should be suspected if bloody stools are observed.

DISORDERS OF THE ESOPHAGUS

GASTROESOPHAGEAL REFLUX

Gastroesophageal reflux is the most common esophageal disorder in the neonatal period.[50] Gastric contents normally are retained within the stomach through the action of the lower esophageal sphincter, a zone of high pressure in the distal esophagus that remains tonically contracted except during deglutition.[51] The anatomy of the stomach and esophagus, and their relationship to the diaphragm and related structures, may play a secondary role in retaining gastric contents within the stomach. Although considerable controversy exists, there is evidence to suggest that the lower esophageal sphincter may be fully functional in the normal full-term infant. Some evidence suggests that sphincter pressure may be decreased, either continuously or intermittently, in infants with gastroesophageal reflux, facilitating reflux of gastric contents into the esophagus. There is considerable controversy over the incidence of reflux in the premature infant. Reflux appears relatively more common, but some data suggest that the lower esophageal sphincter may be competent. Delayed gastric emptying and other motility problems also may play a role in reflux in premature infants.

In adults and older children, chronic esophagitis due to reflux of acid into the distal esophagus is the major concern with gastroesophageal reflux. During the neonatal period, however, esophagitis rarely occurs. Reflux typically presents with continual regurgitation and spitting up or vomiting of small quantities of formula after eating, but also may present with apnea and bradycardia. Recurrent aspiration during reflux episodes may result in pneumonitis or exacerbation of preexisting neonatal pulmonary disease. If enough formula is regurgitated, the infant may fail to thrive. In neonates, reflux also may be associated with delayed gastric emptying. As in older children, reflux is encountered more frequently in infants with neurologic abnormalities.

Gastroesophageal reflux may exist as a primary disorder due to lower esophageal sphincter incompetence or intermittent relaxation, or may be a manifestation of another disorder. First of all, it must be realized that gastroesophageal reflux may occur physiologically in all infants, although not with the frequency and severity of pathologic reflux. Any disorder that limits gastric emptying or causes a partial proximal small intestinal obstruction, such as annular pancreas or pyloric stenosis, will result in some gastroesophageal reflux. Small bowel disorders, including milk protein enterocolitis or infectious enteritis, will cause vomiting and regurgitation—in essence, gastroesophageal reflux. Finally, a variety of systemic disorders, including certain inborn errors of metabolism, chronic infection, chronic renal disease, and increased intracranial pressure all may result in chronic emesis similar to gastroesophageal reflux. Drugs, such as xanthines, which may be given because of apnea or lung disease, decrease lower esophageal sphincter pressure and may exacerbate or even cause reflux.

Several diagnostic studies are available to diagnose gastroesophageal reflux in infants; however, these studies as a rule do not separate primary from secondary causes. For example, an infant with milk protein enterocolitis or pyloric stenosis will test positively for gastroesophageal reflux by any of the available studies. The most widely available test for reflux is an upper gastrointestinal series. An upper gastrointestinal series is preferable to a barium swallow, since the latter only examines esophageal motility. The stomach must be filled with barium to assess the patient accurately for reflux. Unfortunately, assessing a child for gastroesophageal reflux radiographically lacks sensitivity because of the short time interval during which the child is observed, and lacks specificity because of the likelihood of physiologic reflux occurring during performance of an upper gastrointestinal series. Therefore, the primary role of an upper gastrointestinal series is to exclude gastric outlet lesions such as pyloric stenosis or proximal small bowel partial obstructions such as duodenal webs or annular pancreas.

Twenty-four–hour *p*H monitoring is the most widely accepted means of assessing gastroesophageal reflux.[52] The *p*H probe is placed approximately 2 cm proximal to the lower esophageal sphincter, and distal esophageal *p*H is recorded over a 24-hour period. The infant must be bolus-fed during the study, to ensure adequate gastric distention to simulate the physiologic state. Considerable controversy exists over appropriate feeding for children during 24-hour *p*H monitoring. The inconsistency of acid secretion in small infants makes the procedure much less reliable during the neonatal period, and, consequently, simultaneous measurement of intragastric *p*H often is helpful in determining the validity of the study.

A ^{99}Tc scintiscan may be used to screen for gastroesophageal reflux, although this technique is not considered as reliable as 24-hour *p*H monitoring. The technique is useful, however, for measuring gastric emptying delay, which may coexist with gastroesophageal reflux in a number of infants. Endoscopy with biopsy is a useful technique for detecting reflux in older infants; however, endoscopic biopsies are less useful during the neonatal period because pathologic reflux has not had sufficient time to cause esophageal mucosal injury. In older children, the presence of intraepithelial eosinophils suggests reflux, but this sign cannot be relied on in neonates, and biopsy specimens frequently are normal.

Treatment of gastroesophageal reflux is based on the severity of symptoms. If the child is thriving well, and the major complaint is frequent regurgitation and spitting, the infant may be placed prone on an incline at approximately 30° with the head higher than the feet. It has been demonstrated that children positioned in this manner will reflux less frequently. Although it may take several weeks for symptoms to resolve, the risk of esophagitis is lessened and reflux tends to resolve more quickly. If the volume of reflux is severe and the infant is chronically irritable, has evidence of esophagitis, or is failing to thrive, then inhibition of gastric acid secretion with agents such as antacids or H_2 receptor antagonists may be necessary. Both cimetidine and ranitidine are available in liquid preparations, and work well. Data suggest that aluminum antacids may elevate serum aluminum levels in small infants.[53] Bethanechol, a parasympathomimetic agent, has been demonstrated to increase lower esophageal sphincter resting tone and improve weight gain in infants with failure to thrive secondary to gastroesophageal reflux.[54] Unfortunately, bethanechol may have associated central nervous system side-effects such as irritability and sleeplessness. Metoclopramide also has been used to treat gastroesophageal reflux in infants. The effectiveness of metoclopramide is controversial, and it probably is most helpful when delayed gastric emptying coexists with reflux. Some clinicians thicken infants' formula with cereal. Although this may reduce spitting, it usually does not reduce reflux or its complications and results in nutrient imbalance in the infant's carefully formulated diet.

Gastroesophageal reflux may be treated successfully with surgical fundoplication in approximately 95% of cases. The most common surgical procedures include the Nissen fundoplication, in which the stomach is wrapped and sutured 360° around the distal esophagus, and the Thal fundoplication, which consists of a 270° wrap. Complications, including gaseous distention of the stomach and dumping syndrome, may be less common with the Thal procedure. Indications for an operation for gastroesophageal reflux include recurrent aspiration pneumonia, failure to thrive secondary to severe vomiting unresponsive to in-hospital medical management, or apparent life-threatening apnea events associated with gastroesophageal reflux.[55]

Differential diagnosis of the typical neonate with chronic recurrent vomiting includes, in addition to gastroesophageal reflux, two major categories of disease. The first is upper gastrointestinal anomalies, including pyloric stenosis. Virtually all of these can be eliminated by upper gastrointestinal contrast studies; pyloric stenosis can be excluded adequately by ultrasonography in the hands of an experienced pediatric ultrasonographer. The second major diagnostic category is formula protein intolerance. Infants with formula protein intolerance commonly vomit, especially those with significant small bowel mucosal disease. Such infants often are irritable and usually have loose, Hematest-positive (Ames, Elkhart, IN) stools. Proctoscopic examinations of the rectum usually demonstrate colitis. This disorder is discussed in detail later in this chapter.

ESOPHAGEAL ANOMALIES

The other major category of esophageal disease that presents in the neonatal period is tracheoesophageal fistula or esophageal atresia.[56] These anomalies occur in approximately 1 in 4000 live births. In addition to a prenatal history of polyhydramnios, increased salivation with coughing, choking, and cyanosis shortly after birth should raise the suspicion of tracheoesophageal fistula–esophageal atresia. The most common variety is that of atresia with the distal esophageal pouch connected to the trachea through a fistula. Such infants frequently have a stomach distended with air, and respiratory symptoms due to tracheal aspiration of refluxed gastric acid. Immediate pediatric surgical consultation is required (see Chap. 44).

After surgery, gastroesophageal reflux is a virtual certainty. Patients with tracheoesophageal fistula or esophageal atresia have incompetent lower esophageal sphincter function as well as aperistaltic contractions in the midesophagus. Although swallowing usually proceeds without much difficulty, gastroesophageal reflux with chronic esophagitis and occasionally stricture formation are frequent long-term complications. Subsequent esophageal dilatations and fundoplication may be necessary.

DISORDERS OF THE STOMACH AND DUODENUM

CONGENITAL ANOMALIES

Congenital anomalies of the upper gastrointestinal tract frequently present with vomiting. The most common is pyloric stenosis, which occurs in approximately 1 in every 500 live births.[57,58] The disease is most common in Caucasian males. A positive family history often is present. Pyloric stenosis usually presents with nonbilious projectile vomiting during the third to fourth week of life. The disorder often is insidious in onset. After emesis, infants are hungry and will attempt to eat to compensate for malnutrition. Eventually, nutrition deteriorates and infants become dehydrated and alkalotic secondary to chronic vomiting of the acidic gastric contents. Unconjugated hyperbilirubinemia is present in a small percentage. Patients with pyloric stenosis have normal or firm stools, in contrast to infants with formula protein intolerance, who usually have loose stools with evidence of malabsorption, inflammation, or both. Serum electrolytes reveal potassium and chloride deficiency and metabolic alkalosis. Physical examination demonstrates visible peristalsis in the epigastric region. Careful palpation of the abdomen while feeding may reveal a pyloric olive. The olive can be felt best when the stomach is empty, particularly just after vomiting. Diagnosis usually is confirmed by an upper gastrointestinal series or ultrasonography, or in the case of ambiguity, both, before proceeding with surgical intervention.

Before operative correction of the pyloric stenosis, infants should be rehydrated intravenously and the electrolyte imbalance and alkalosis corrected. Surgical correction consists of longitudinal incision of the hypertrophied muscle (*i.e.*, pyloromyotomy). After the operation is completed, the patient usually can be fed within 6 to 12 hours. Pyloric stenosis has been noted to recur in rare cases. Nonoperative medical management of pyloric stenosis, consisting of anticholinergic drugs and small frequent feedings, occasionally may be helpful. This therapy, sometimes used in Europe, is rarely used in North America because of the excellent results of surgical intervention.

Other rare gastric anomalies also may present in the neonatal period. Various forms of gastric atresia or hypoplasia have been described, most of which present with vomiting at or shortly after birth. Congenital microgastria may occur in association with a variety of other anomalies, including limb abnormalities, asplenia, megaesophagus, situs inversus, midgut malrotation, and cardiac anomalies. After major reconstructive surgery of the stomach, prognosis may be quite good.

ACID PEPTIC DISEASE

Acid peptic disease may be seen in newborn infants.[59–61] Ulcers in children occur most commonly in the neonatal period or during the second decade of life. In newborn infants, ulcers, whether gastric or duodenal, usually present with hematemesis. Occasionally, blood loss may be substantial, manifested by symptoms of hypovolemia and shock. Differential diagnosis of hematemesis in the newborn includes swallowed maternal blood, or blood ingested from a cracked nipple through breast-feeding. In an otherwise stable infant, this differentiation can be made by assaying for fetal hemoglobin in the vomited gastric contents.

Diagnosis of peptic ulcer disease in the neonate requires endoscopy. Radiographic studies rarely are useful because the lesions are quite superficial and difficult to image radiographically. Endoscopy can be performed easily in a newborn infant by a skilled pediatric endoscopist using appropriate equipment. The smallest pediatric upper gastrointestinal endoscopes can be used safely in term infants, with little sedation and without general anesthesia. The minimum size of the infant that can be safely endoscoped varies with the skill of the endoscopist, but endoscopy often also can be performed safely in larger premature babies. A bronchoscope can be used in smaller infants, although the examination usually is unsatisfactory. Although ulcerations may be identified anywhere in the stomach and the duodenum, multiple superficial gastric lesions are most common in newborn infants. Ulcers may be primary, or secondary as in the case of drugs known to irritate the upper gastrointestinal tract, such as steroids or theophylline. Treatment with antacids, or preferably H_2 receptor antagonists such as cimetidine or ranitidine, for a period of 2 to 6 weeks results in complete healing of the lesion. Secondary ulcers may be treated in a similar fashion. In this instance, continuation of the offending agent requires careful assessment of the risk–benefit ratio, because lesions will heal more rapidly if the agents are discontinued.

Spontaneous gastric perforation is a rare occurrence in the newborn. It occurs most commonly during the first 5 days of life, especially in infants subjected to severe stress or hypoxia.[62] The constellation of symptoms typically includes a sudden deterioration in clinical status between the second and fifth day of life, characterized by refusal to eat, vomiting, abdominal distention, and respiratory distress. Free intraperitoneal air and fluid are demonstrable on plain radiographs of the abdomen. Immediate surgical consultation should be sought.

DISORDERS OF THE SMALL INTESTINE

CONGENITAL ANOMALIES

Of the various small intestinal disorders that present in the neonatal period, congenital anomalies that produce obstruction are likely to present earliest. Patients present with bilious vomiting, abdominal distention, and occasionally obstipation. Bilious vomiting associated with the passage of blood through the rectum suggests vascular compromise of the small intestine, necessitating immediate surgical intervention.

Malrotation or nonrotation of the gut is an anatomic defect produced by incomplete rotation and fixation of the embryonic intestine after return from its extraabdominal location at about week 10 of gestation.[63] During development, the intestine rotates 270° around the axis of the superior mesenteric artery to place the cecum in the right lower quadrant. When the cecum fails to rotate completely, the mesenteric attachment of the small intestine is limited to that supporting the superior mesenteric artery and vein. This permits the bowel to twist on itself and produces a midgut volvulus. In the malrotated colon, adhesive bands, otherwise known as Ladd bands, stretch anteriorly from the right peritoneal gutter over the duodenum, where they can produce obstruction. Rotational anomalies may be associated with other intestinal anomalies, usually duodenal stenosis or atresia or other small intestinal atresias. Cardiac, esophageal, urinary, and anal anomalies also may be present. Rotational abnormalities should be considered in the differential diagnosis of a high intestinal obstruction identified radiographically. Unfortunately, the diagnosis often is missed by plain abdominal radiographs because air may be present in several loops of bowel distal to the obstruction. Rotational abnormalities are identified more easily with an upper gastrointestinal series, or barium enema. The radiographic hallmark of malrotation is the identification of the cecum in the upper abdomen or to the left of the midline. Symptomatic rotational abnormalities require urgent surgical exploration, since a volvulus may result in loss of the entire midgut within hours of presentation due to vascular occlusion.

Jejunal or ileal atresias range from membranous obstructions to complete atresia. Atresias can be single or multiple.[64,65] An apple peel or Christmas tree deformity of the superior mesenteric artery results in an extensive jejunal atresia followed by multiple ileal atresias that are vascularly supplied by a branch of the ileocolic artery. Unlike duodenal atresia, relatively few anomalies are associated with ileal atresia. Cystic fibrosis, however, is present in approximately 20% of infants with jejunoileal atresia.

Small intestinal atresias in the neonatal period present with bilious vomiting. The degree of abdominal distention varies with the site of the atresia. If the atresia is distal, vomiting may be delayed for up to 24 hours after birth. Depending on the location of the atresia, varying numbers of dilated loops of bowel with air fluid levels may be present on abdominal radiographs. Because it is difficult to differentiate small intestine from colon on plain abdominal radiographs in newborns, a contrast enema should be performed to exclude colonic lesions and obstructions. Contrast enemas also are helpful in excluding disorders such as meconium plug syndrome or associated rotational abnormalities.

MECONIUM ILEUS

Meconium ileus occurs almost exclusively in patients with cystic fibrosis. It is caused by abnormally viscid mucus glycoprotein in meconium.[66] Approximately 10% to 20% of patients with cystic fibrosis have meconium ileus as the first sign of their disease. Pathologically, the lumen of the distal small intestine is obstructed by an accumulation of abnormal meconium. Infants present with bilious vomiting and abdominal distention during the first 2 days of life. A palpable sausagelike mass may be present, and rectal examination may identify hard, dry, gray-tan meconium. Abdominal radiographs demonstrate some evidence of complete obstruction, but the radiologic hallmark is the soap-bubble appearance of trapped air within the tenacious meconium in the distal small bowel. A water-soluble contrast enema occasionally is therapeutic in disrupting the meconium obstruction. Care should be taken to avoid dehydration, since contrast substances are hypertonic and can result in massive pooling of fluid within the bowel lumen. Surgical intervention is required if the contrast enema is unsuccessful.

Other disorders related to meconium may be seen in the neonatal period. Meconium peritonitis may occur when intrauterine bowel perforation, secondary to obstruction, has resulted in leakage of sterile meconium into the peritoneal cavity. Common causes include atresia, volvulus, stenosis, cystic fibrosis, meconium ileus, and Hirschsprung disease. Small flecks of intraabdominal calcification may be identified radiographically. Ascites occasionally occurs, but may resolve spontaneously unless secondary infection develops. In severe cases, meconium peritonitis can result in adhesions that require surgical intervention.

NECROTIZING ENTEROCOLITIS

Probably the most serious gastrointestinal disorder occurring in neonates is NEC.[67,68] Because NEC appears predominantly in sick, low-birth-weight infants, the incidence has increased in recent years as the mortality rate for the very-low-birth-weight infant has decreased. It has been estimated that 90% of cases occur in premature infants and that NEC may develop in 1% to 10% of infants hospitalized in neonatal intensive care units.[69] Significant intercenter differences in the prevalence of NEC have been reported.[70] The mortality rates vary from 10% to 50%. The age of onset of NEC is related to birth weight and gestational age. Smaller, more immature infants (<26 weeks of gestation) tend to have NEC at an older age than larger, more mature (>31 weeks of age) infants.[70] Thus, the more premature the infant, the longer the duration of risk.

The etiology of NEC is not fully known.[71] Multiple factors appear to be involved, including hypoxia, acidosis, and hypotension, which may lead to ischemic damage of the mucosal barrier of the small intestine.[72] Secondary bacterial invasion of the mucosa may be involved in the pathogenesis of pneumatosis intestinalis. Moreover, NEC has been observed to occur in epidemics in neonatal intensive care units, further supporting the role of microbial agents in pathogenesis. A number of conditions may predispose the larger infant to development of NEC, including cyanotic congenital heart disease, obstructive lesions of the systemic cardiac outflow (*e.g.*, hypoplastic left heart, coarctation of the aorta), polycythemia, umbilical catheters, exchange transfusions, perinatal asphyxia, maternal preeclampsia, and maternal use of cocaine. Infants with patent ductus arteriosus also seem to be at greater risk. In this case, oxygenated blood is shunted from the intestine. All of these factors suggest that mucosal injury and ischemia are important in the development of NEC. The role of inflammatory mediators, such as tumor necrosis factor-α and platelet-activating factor, and oxygen free radicals also have received attention.[73,74]

Rapid onset of enteral feeding may be a risk factor for NEC, because of changes in enteric blood flow and oxygen requirements during feeding.[75,76] Necrotizing enterocolitis is occasionally, but rarely, reported in infants who have never been enterally fed. Several factors related to enteral feeding have been studied and a number of theories have been proposed on how enteral feedings might precipitate NEC. Hyperosmolar formulas have been implicated in the production of NEC, but these formulas differed from standard formulas in other ways as well. In addition, most hyperosmolar formulas have been reformulated to minimize this risk. Formula feedings seem to predispose to NEC more than breast-feeding, suggesting that breast milk factors, including growth factors, antibodies, and cellular immune factors, might be protective. It also is likely that formula within the gastrointestinal tract may provide a substrate for bacterial proliferation. The role of bacterial invasion in this disease has been well recognized, but is likely to be a secondary event after compromise of the intestinal mucosal barrier.

The shunting of blood away from the intestine in a fashion similar to the diving reflex in aquatic mammals has been postulated as a potential mechanism for producing the initial gut ischemia. This reflex might occur in response to a hypoxic episode, and has been studied extensively in animal models.

The association of NEC with prematurity implicates immaturity of the intestinal mucosal barrier. A number of factors that affect the mucosal barrier are immature in premature infants, including acid output, intestinal motility, and enzyme production. Immaturity of the microvillus membrane itself, as well as differences in the mucus secreted by the small intestine, may play a significant role. The mucosal immune system is immature, and less secretory IgA is produced. Recent interest has arisen in the possible role of oral immunoglobulin administration for prophylaxis against NEC.[77]

The reported gastrointestinal hormone abnormalities in NEC patients are difficult to interpret because of the spectrum of ages at which the disease develops, the randomness of blood sample timing, and the variation in quantity of enteral feedings.[80] Concentrations of GIP, neurotensin, and enteroglucagon in infants with NEC are lower than those of fed normal infants of comparable age, but gastrin, motilin, and pancreatic polypeptide (PP) levels appear to be normal.[78]

Clinical presentations vary widely. Abdominal distention usually is one of the earliest and most consistent clinical signs. Other symptoms include bloody stools, apnea, bradycardia, lethargy, shock, and retention of gastric contents due to poor gastric emptying. Thrombocytopenia, neutropenia, and metabolic acidosis may develop during bowel ischemia. Not every patient has every sign, however, and clinical presentation may vary markedly. Diagnosis is confirmed by radiographic demonstration of pneumatosis intestinalis or portal hepatic venous air. Nonspecific radiographic findings include thickening of the bowel wall, dilated loops of bowel, and ascites. The presence of reducing substances in the stool, due to carbohydrate malabsorption, may be an early finding in NEC, as may increased α_1-antitrypsin levels, which indicate protein-losing enteropathy.

Suspicion of NEC dictates that all enteral feedings should be discontinued. An orogastric tube is placed routinely to relieve distention of the alimentary tract. Intravenous access must be secured to provide fluid and electrolytes and nutrition, since the patient will not be fed enterally for an extended period of time. Intravenous antibiotics are administered to provide coverage for enteric organisms. Inclusion of specific antianaerobic agents does not appear to be helpful.[79] The duration of oral intake restriction depends on the clinical status. Patients who merely have poor feeding with increased residuals, and the presence of minimal radiographic findings, may be fed within 48 to 72 hours. In the presence of pneumatosis intestinalis and marked abdominal distention, 2 weeks of parenteral nutrition may be required before judicious gradual reintroduction of enteral feedings is considered.

Throughout the course of the disease, frequent radiographic evaluation of the abdomen for evidence of intestinal perforation is required. Apnea, bradycardia, abdominal wall discoloration or edema, or a sudden increase in intraabdominal girth should give rise to the suspicion of bowel perforation. In the presence of perforation, surgical intervention should occur immediately.[80] Frequent laboratory evaluations include a complete blood count and platelet count to look for thrombocytopenia and neutropenia, both of which suggest deterioration. In infants with severe inflammation of the small intestine, large volumes of fluid and electrolytes or blood products may be required to maintain perfusion and blood pressure. This is especially true in infants in whom severe metabolic acidosis develops secondary to poor perfusion. Ventilatory support may be necessary.

Infants who require surgical intervention are at risk for short bowel syndrome and a variety of complications associated with total parenteral nutrition (TPN). In a number of infants, the mucosal inflammatory process may progress to transmural necrosis that may, if it does not lead to perforation, result in fibroblast proliferation, granulation tissue, and stricture formation. Stricture formation in the distal small intestine and colon is a relatively common complication following NEC. Some clinicians routinely study the gastrointestinal tract radiographically after NEC has been treated medically. It is not uncommon to find asymptomatic ileal stenosis or colonic stenosis in such patients. If symptoms of partial obstruction, such as abdominal distention, failure to thrive, or poor feeding develop in infants who have recovered from a bout of NEC, contrast studies are indicated.

SHORT BOWEL SYNDROME

Short bowel syndrome is defined as a malabsorptive state that occurs after bowel resection. Infants with short bowel syndrome fall into two categories: those with congenital anomalies (*e.g.*, gastroschisis, apple peel anomaly of the superior mesenteric artery, intestinal atresia) and anatomically normal patients who undergo bowel resection for NEC. The latter group tend to have fewer complications and a better prognosis, when equal lengths of residual small intestine remain.

After massive resection of the small intestine, the remaining small bowel undergoes an adaptation process characterized by epithelial hyperplasia.[81] Within 1 to 2 days after resection, enterocytes begin replicating in the crypts. Gradual morphologic changes occur in the small intestine, including a marked lengthening of villi that results in increased mucosal surface area. This is followed by an increase in absorptive capacity that eventually enables many to survive without parenteral nutrition. The adaptation process is gradual, however, and may require weeks to years.

The major gut hormone changes seen after ileal resection are marked increases in plasma levels of PYY, enteroglucagon, and motilin.[82,83] Increases of the putative trophic hormone, enteroglucagon, and of PYY, which inhibits gastric and small intestinal secretion and delays intestinal transit, are appropriate responses in this condition. Preservation, or even enhancement of the PYY response would be valuable in diminishing the rapid transit and diarrhea associated with this condition. Studies in experimental animals have revealed that improvements in transit and fluid absorption are temporally related to the increase in PYY response that occurs after bowel resection.[84]

Mucosal hyperplasia does not occur in the absence of enteral nutrition. In fact, mucosal atrophy may result if the patient is nourished only parenterally.[85] Enteral nutrition stimulates intestinal adaptation by several mechanisms.[86] Highly unsaturated long-chain fats stimulate intestinal adaptation to a greater extent than protein or carbohydrate; the mechanism by which this occurs is poorly understood. Nonetheless, careful attention to the provision of adequate enteral nutrition is important.

Management of the short bowel syndrome is a multistage process.[87] During the early postoperative period, use of parenteral nutrition and careful attention to fluid and electrolyte abnormalities are essential. High-volume ostomy losses must be replaced with a solution of comparable electrolyte content to obviate the need for frequent changes in electrolyte concentration in parenteral nutrition solutions.

The presence of an ostomy may create additional problems. These vary somewhat, depending on whether the ostomy is in the ileum, in which the volume output is likely to be much greater, or in the colon, in which stool consistency may vary markedly based on whether the ostomy was placed proximally or distally. If available, the services of an enterostomal therapist, with special training in rehabilitation of infants and children with ostomies, will assist the parents in understanding the implications of the ostomy. The ostomy should be placed away from sites such as the iliac crest, costal margin, or umbilicus so that ostomy appliances will fit easily.

Most ostomy devices consist of an adhesive, nonallergenic wafer device with a flange that allows the transparent drainage pouch to be secured to it over the stoma. The pouch is easily removed for draining by snapping it off the wafer, or it can be emptied through a drainage port at the bottom of the bag. When leakage occurs beneath the wafer, the device should be removed, and careful skin care around the ostomy is necessary. The skin should be washed gently with a soft cloth, moistened with mild soap and tepid water. The skin should then be dried thoroughly after cleansing. Many protective ointments and powders are available to apply around the stoma area to prevent skin breakdown. If skin irritation is present, tincture of benzoin or steroid preparations available in spray form may be used. The pouches often are reusable, and may be washed with mild soap and water and soaked in a deodorant solution to control odor problems. Appropriate teaching will prevent many of the other problems encountered by ostomy patients such as skin excoriation, minor stoma bleeding, stoma prolapse, and odor. Additional ostomy problems include prolapse and stenosis. The latter should be suspected in the presence of abdominal distention and vomiting. In either situation, the surgeon should be notified.

When enteral feeds are started, a slow continuous infusion of a dilute elemental formula generally works best. Formulations such as Alimentum (Ross Laboratories, Columbus, OH) or Pregestimil (Mead Johnson Laboratories, Evansville, IN), which contain significant quantities of long-chain fats, are ideal. These lactose-free preparations with hydrolyzed protein are rapidly absorbed, yet provide adequate stimulation of intestinal adaptation. Stool losses must be monitored carefully. A marked increase in fluid losses or significant evidence of carbohydrate malabsorption manifested by a low stool *p*H or positive stool-reducing substances are contraindications for further increasing the enteral infusion. Enteral infusions are increased as tolerated, and parenteral nutrition is decreased in a gradual isocaloric fashion. Patients can then be weaned to intermittent parenteral nutrition and prepared for home parenteral nutrition therapy.[88] Intermittent parenteral nutrition allows provision of parenteral nutrients at night, primarily for the convenience of caregivers. Parenteral nutrition initially is discontinued only for short periods of time, usually 4 to 6 hours, each day. In small infants, this usually is delayed until the patient can tolerate approximately 20% of calorie intake enterally to avoid hypoglycemia when he or she is not receiving parenteral nutrition. The duration of parenteral nutrition can be decreased gradually until all parenteral nutrition infuses over 10 to 12 hours at night. It is wise to taper the parenteral nutrition rates up and down when placing a patient on or off of parenteral nutrition, to prevent fluctuation in serum glucose levels.

Home parenteral nutrition has markedly reduced the cost of long-term management of short bowel syndrome patients and also has decreased family stresses and nosocomial infections.[89] It has become a standard therapy in patients with short bowel syndrome, and prolonged hospitalizations rarely are necessary. To minimize complications, careful training of home nursing personnel is essential and coordination of activity between physician and nursing staff must be tightly controlled.

Continuous enteral infusions are used in patients in short bowel syndrome for several reasons. The percentage of calories absorbed from the continuous infusion is greater than that possible with bolus feedings, because transport carrier proteins are continually saturated. Continuous infusion provides constant stimulation of mucosal adaptation and reduces the need for parenteral calories, decreasing the risk of parenteral nutrition liver disease. Children should be fed small quantities of formula orally, so as to learn to suck and swallow. Eventually, solids can be fed around the nasogastric tube. These manipulations often will speed the transition from continuous enteral to oral feeding later in the course of therapy.

Numerous chronic complications arise in the treatment of short bowel syndrome, including bacterial overgrowth, nutritional deficiency states, watery diarrhea, parenteral nutrition liver disease, and catheter-related problems. Bacterial overgrowth is defined as increased bacterial content in the small intestine.[90] Complications from bacterial overgrowth include increased malabsorption, D-lactic acidosis and colitislike or ileitislike syndrome. Normal small bowel bacterial counts vary from 10^3/mL proximally to much greater numbers in the ileum. Normal antegrade peristalsis and gastric and mucosal immune factors prevent excess bacterial proliferation. In short bowel syndrome, because of disruption of normal anatomy and motility, overgrowth is likely and bacterial counts usually exceed 10^5/mL. Bacterial overgrowth should be suspected whenever motility is slowed, bowel is dilated, or the ileocecal valve is absent. Organisms typically include facultative bacteria and anaerobes. Bacteria deconjugate bile salts, causing them to be reabsorbed, depleting the bile salt pool, impairing micelle solubilization, and resulting in steatorrhea and malabsorption of fat-soluble vitamins. More important, bacterial overgrowth causes mucosal inflammation, exacerbating malabsorption of all nutrients. Protein-losing enteropathy and loss of immunoglobulins may occur. Bacteria may compete with the host for nutrients, such as vitamin B_{12}.

Screening for bacterial overgrowth can be done with a fasting breath hydrogen or glucose breath hydrogen test, or by detecting the presence of indican in the urine. Measurement of breath hydrogen is a simple test in infants and children, although collection of samples in the neonate requires special care. A fasting breath hydrogen level greater than 42 ppm is seen only in small bowel bacterial overgrowth.[91] A breath hydrogen level greater than 20 ppm after the administration of 2 g/kg of oral glucose, with measurement at 15-minute intervals after ingestion, suggests bacterial overgrowth. Measurement of indican in the urine is a simple screening test for bacterial overgrowth, because bacteria convert dietary tryptophan to indican. Unfortunately, indicanuria may occur in other conditions, and the technique lacks sensitivity.[92] Bacterial overgrowth can be definitively diagnosed by culture of aspirates from the small intestine. Small intestinal biopsies demonstrating inflammatory changes suggest bacterial overgrowth.

Accumulation of D-lactate in the bloodstream results in neurologic symptoms varying from frank disorientation to coma.[93] Bacterial overgrowth may cause colitislike or ileitislike syndrome with large ulcerations characteristic of Crohn disease, but without granulomas.[94] Broad-spectrum oral antibiotics (*e.g.*, metronidazole, TMP-SMZ, gentamicin) and antiinflammatory agents often are beneficial. Broad-spectrum antimicrobial coverage should be directed at the organisms present, usually anaerobes. Antimotility agents may improve nutrient contact with the mucosa by lengthening transit time, but tend to exacerbate bacterial overgrowth and should be used with caution.

Secretory diarrhea may be a problem in some children with short bowel syndrome. This may be related to hypergastrinemia, which often occurs after resection. Because the tight junctions in the ileum are less permeable than the jejunum, the ileum plays a major role in fluid and electrolyte conservation, and ileal resections are more likely to result in major fluid and electrolyte losses than jejunal resections. Because most infants with NEC have ileal disease, this is a major problem in neonates after bowel resection. Ileal resection also results in malabsorption of bile acids, because the ileum is the primary site for bile acid reabsorption. Malabsorption of bile acids into the colon may cause fluid secretion and watery diarrhea, which may respond to a bile-acid–binding resin such as cholestyramine. Unfortunately, cholestyramine may further deplete the bile acid pool, exacerbating steatorrhea.

Nutritional deficiency states may occur after parenteral nutrition is discontinued, including deficiencies of fat-soluble vitamins A, D, and E, and the minerals iron, zinc, calcium, and magnesium.

Parenteral nutrition hepatobiliary tract disease is the major complication that may result in death in infants with short bowel syndrome.[89] The mechanism by which the liver injury occurs is unknown. In most instances, enteral administration of a significant percentage of calories, usually between 20% and 30% of total requirements, reduces the risk of parenteral nutrition liver disease.

Cholelithiasis develops in approximately 20% of infants receiving parenteral nutrition for short bowel syndrome because of malabsorption of bile acids, altered bilirubin metabolism, and gallbladder stasis. Cholangitis may occur in the presence of partial obstruction. Early cholecystectomy should be considered if patients are symptomatic with elevated direct bilirubin and liver enzymes.

Catheter-related infections and thrombosis are common in infants requiring long-term parenteral nutrition.[95] In our experience, catheter-related infections rarely are due to intestinal bacterial overgrowth and most commonly are related to catheter care technique. Diligent parental instruction in catheter care and in the signs and symptoms of sepsis is extremely important.

During later stages of therapy, additional surgery may be indicated.[96] One of the first questions usually concerns whether to close a stoma that was formed at the time of initial surgery. If the colon remains, and especially if ileum exists as well, reconnecting an ostomy may substantially conserve fluid and electrolytes, but also may result in perianal disease. In infants with dilated segments of proximal bowel, resecting a tight anastomosis or tapering the bowel to improve flow of luminal contents often reduces bacterial overgrowth. A number of procedures have been designed to slow transit time, including reverse segments of bowel, one-way valves, or colon interposition, but none is considered reliably effective, and all may increase bacterial overgrowth.

A procedure to increase the length of the bowel has been devised that involves transecting the bowel longitudinally, preserving the blood supply to both sides of the bowel, and creating a segment about twice the length and one-half of the diameter. This allows reducing the diameter of the bowel without any loss of mucosal surface area. Because it does not actually increase the mucosal surface area, it is indicated primarily to reduce bacterial overgrowth without losing absorptive surface in infants with dilated bowel. Our experience has been quite rewarding with this procedure, with 12 of 14 recent patients demonstrating significant improvement and several becoming independent of parenteral nutrition after surgery.[97] It should not, however, be performed in neonates, because it is successful only after significant bowel dilation has occurred.

Intestinal transplantation has become available, but remains experimental. Rejection and sepsis have been the major obstacles to success. Combined liver–bowel transplants in children with irreversible, severe TPN-associated liver disease and short bowel syndrome have achieved some success. Further experience with intestinal transplantation must be gained before its role in the treatment of short bowel syndrome can be determined.

It is possible for infants to survive without transplantation or permanent parenteral nutrition with surprisingly short segments of bowel.[98,99] As a general rule, patients with greater than 25 cm of bowel at the time of neonatal resection who have an ileocecal valve, or with greater than 40 cm of bowel at the time of neonatal resection who have no ileocecal valve, have a reasonable chance of eventually becoming independent of parenteral nutrition. The ileocecal valve appears to play a major role in determining the long-term prognosis, primarily because of its ability to exclude colonic bacteria from entering the small bowel and perhaps its ability to delay transit through the small intestine.

MUCOSAL INJURY DISORDERS

Because of the limited small intestinal reserve in small infants, small intestinal disease is perhaps most catastrophic in infancy. In small intestinal injury, all nutrients are malabsorbed. Most symptoms, however, are related to carbohydrate malabsorption because of the osmotic diarrhea produced when these malabsorbed molecules are broken down further by intestinal bacteria into smaller and smaller osmotically active particles. The osmotic gradient overrides the ability of the ileum and colon to reabsorb fluid effectively, and watery diarrhea ensues.

Measurement of stool *p*H and reducing substances is an ideal means to screen for small bowel mucosal disease in infancy. When carbohydrates are malabsorbed and broken down into organic acids by colonic bacteria, the stool *p*H drops below 5.5. Stool *p*H can be measured easily with litmus paper, simply by inserting the paper into the stool. Measurement of reducing substances in stool can be done by placing five drops of stool and ten drops of water into a test tube and dropping in a Clinitest (Ames, Elkhart, IN) tablet. Positive reducing substances in stool confirms the presence of carbohydrate malabsorption. Patients receiving formulas that are predominantly sucrose are less likely to demonstrate positive reducing substances in their stools because sucrose is a nonreducing carbohydrate.

INFECTIOUS DIARRHEA

During the neonatal period, infectious diseases of the small intestine are relatively uncommon. A number of viruses may cause diarrhea in small infants, including rotavirus, enteric adenoviruses, and enteroviruses. Viral gastroenteritis usually presents with watery stools with evidence of carbohydrate malabsorption. The predominant mucosal injury in viral gastroenteritis is in the proximal jejunum, where carbohydrates are absorbed. In contrast, bacterial pathogens generally produce more distal injury that involves the colon and results in Hematest-positive stools that contain leukocytes (Table 37-2). Bacterial causes of diarrhea include *Salmonella* sp, *Shigella* sp, invasive *Escherichia coli*, and *Campylobacter jejuni*. *Clostridium difficile* infection predominantly involves the large intestine, and in severe cases, produces pseudomembranous colitis. Infection with *C. difficile* usually follows a course of broad-spectrum antibiotics. Severe watery or bloody diarrhea and colonic perforation may occur. Diagnosis is difficult in neonates because a very high percentage of small infants carry *C. difficile* without evidence of disease.

HUMAN IMMUNODEFICIENCY VIRUS–ASSOCIATED DISEASE

Human immunodeficiency virus (HIV) in infants results in a variety of gastrointestinal problems. Failure to thrive is not uncommon. Chronic diarrhea and generalized lymphadenopathy often are present. Other common presentations include asymptomatic hepatosplenomegaly, which may occur in conjunction with severe interstitial pneumonia and hypergammaglobulinemia.

Chronic diarrhea in infants with acquired immunodeficiency syndrome (AIDS) presents a very difficult management problem. Diarrhea may result from opportunistic infections, tumors, including Kaposi sarcoma and lymphoma, and direct HIV infection of the gut. Opportunistic organisms include viral agents (*e.g.*, cytomegalovirus, rotavirus, herpes simplex, coxsackievirus, adenovirus), bacterial pathogens (*e.g.*, *Salmonella* sp, *Campylobacter*-like organisms, *Listeria* sp, *Mycobacterium avium-intracellulare*, *Plesiomonas shigelloides*), fungal pathogens (*e.g.*, *Candida* sp, *Aspergillus* sp), and parasitic pathogens (*e.g.*, cryptosporidium, *Strongyloides* sp, *Giardia* sp, amoebas, *Isospora belli*). A broad spectrum of endoscopic and histologic findings is possible because of the diverse nature of the disease. Extensive viral and bacterial cultures and examinations for ova and parasites are warranted in infants and children with AIDS.

Treatment consists of therapy directed at any specific infectious pathogen identified, coupled with use of parenteral and enteral nutrition. As in almost all chronic enteropathies, primary attention should be given to continuous enteral infusion with an elemental diet or protein hydrolysate formula. If malabsorption develops in the patient, as indicated by stools testing positive for reducing substances or manifesting a *p*H below 5.5, supplemental parenteral nutrition is needed to provide the remainder of caloric and other nutritional needs. The presence of a significant secretory component of the diarrhea may make treatment difficult, may complicate the use of continuous enteral infusion, and may require careful attention to intake and output of fluid and electrolytes to maintain biochemical homeostasis.

TABLE 37–2
SCREENING STOOL STUDIES IN INFECTIOUS DIARRHEA

	Bacterial	Viral
Clinitest	–	±
*p*H	≥5.5	≤5.5
Hematest	+++	–
Leukocytes	+++	–

–, negative; ±, negative or positive; +++, strongly positive.

HORMONAL CHANGES IN DIARRHEA

Infective diarrhea in infants is associated with a massive increase in circulating concentrations of motilin, enteroglucagon, and PYY.[100,101] These abnormalities resolve once the patients are better. The gut endocrine system in infants, however, responds in a manner different from that of adults. In infants with diarrhea, plasma motilin concentrations exceed those that are known to accelerate gastric emptying and increase small bowel motility.[101] Motilin is therefore likely to be involved in the motor abnormalities associated with this condition. A hormonally triggered increase in transit rate may constitute a defense mechanisms to rid the bowel of pathogens and secreted toxins. The extremely high enteroglucagon levels in neonatal infective diarrhea appear to be related to the extent of mucosal injury and its repair.[102] Measurement of selected gut hormones may give information on the extent of mucosal damage, or the presence of ongoing pathologic change.

FORMULA PROTEIN INTOLERANCE

One of the most common causes of chronic diarrhea in small infants is formula protein-induced enterocolitis.[103,104] Small bowel involvement (*i.e.*, enteritis), colon involvement (*i.e.*, colitis), or concomitant small bowel and colon involvement are possible with this disorder. Protein-induced mucosal injury has been reported with cow-milk protein, soy protein, breast milk, and even beef protein. We have observed infants who have manifested intolerance to protein hydrolysate formulas, and responded therapeutically to amino acid formulations such as Tolerex or Vivonex.

Infants typically present before 3 months of age with bright red blood in the stool, which may be normal or loose in consistency depending on the extent of inflammation. Sigmoidoscopic examination may reveal gross friability or may appear normal until the mucosa is wiped with a cotton swab, at which time the mucosa readily bleeds. Rectal biopsy confirms inflammation, with the combination of polymorphonuclear leukocytes and eosinophils in the lamina propria. Stools may test positive for occult blood and may contain leukocytes. If the inflammation extends into the small intestine, carbohydrate malabsorption may occur, infants will have watery diarrhea, and stools will be acidic (*p*H < 5.5) and test positive for reducing substances. Small intestinal biopsy will demonstrate varying degrees of mucosal injury, with shortening and blunting of the villi, inflammatory infiltrates, and an increase in mitotic activity in the crypts. Disaccharidase levels in the mucosal biopsies often are reduced.

Other symptoms that may occur as a result of formula protein-induced enterocolitis are vomiting and irritability. Infants with formula protein intolerance commonly vomit, especially those with small intestinal disease. It often is difficult to differentiate this disorder from gastroesophageal reflux, because both groups may present with irritability; however, babies with formula protein sensitivity commonly have loose stools and abnormal sigmoidoscopic examinations. This is an important distinction because the treatment is vastly different. Irritability, not dissimilar from infantile colic, may occur in infants with formula protein intolerance. In infantile colic, the irritability classically occurs at a specific time of the day and responds symptomatically to repetitive stimuli. Infants with irritability secondary to formula protein intolerance usually are inconsolably irritable, often feed poorly, have loose stools, spit up, and have abnormal sigmoidoscopic examinations or other evidence of small intestinal or colonic inflammation. A careful history and physical examination and appropriate laboratory studies can be quite specific in differentiating the two disorders.

Infants who manifest signs and symptoms of formula protein intolerance should be placed on a protein hydrolysate formula such as Nutramigen, Pregestimil, or Alimentum because a high percentage also will be intolerant of soy formula. A small percentage of infants who do not respond to these formulas may improve on an amino acid formulation such as Tolerex or Vivonex. These formulas are constituted for adults, and may not be appropriate for use in small infants. The addition of extra vitamins, minerals, and essential fatty acids should be considered if the formulas are to be used long-term. We frequently administer Tolerex diluted from normal adult strength (1 cal/mL) to 0.67 cal/mL and place the children on supplemental infant vitamins plus 5 to 10 mL of bolus safflower oil daily to prevent essential fatty acid deficiency.

Most infants with formula protein intolerance will outgrow their sensitivity by 1 year of age. Powell has described a specific challenge procedure to confirm the diagnosis of cow-milk protein intolerance.[105] Patients should not have received the suspected antigen for at least 2 weeks before testing and should be asymptomatic. A standard dose (100 mL of cow milk or soy formula) is administered and the child is monitored carefully for reaction. Stool specimens are analyzed for occult blood, leukocytes, and reducing sugars, and a leukocyte count is obtained 6 to 8 hours later. The test is considered positive if diarrhea develops within 24 hours, leukocytes or blood appear in stools, or the leukocyte count rises by over 4000 cells/mL over baseline. Approximately 20% of the infants have a delayed reaction. If the child originally had evidence of severe milk protein sensitivity, it is wise to hospitalize the infant, start with small volumes (5–10 mL) of formula, and gradually to increase the volume to avoid severe mucosal injury, anaphylaxis, and shock.

INTRACTABLE DIARRHEA OF INFANCY

A state of persistent diarrhea and malabsorption despite the institution of a protein hydrolysate formula and in the absence of infectious pathogens is referred to as intractable or protracted diarrhea of infancy.[106] These patients demonstrate a variety of histologic abnormalities on small intestinal biopsy, including blunting or flattening of the villi, increased mononuclear cells with occasional polymorphonuclear infiltrates, cuboidalization of the surface epithelium, and a mild to moderate increase in mitotic activity in the crypts. Histologic lesions vary substantially, however, and correlate poorly with ultimate prognosis.[107] Such infants have chronic weight loss and progressive malnutrition unless appropriate therapy is instituted. Initial therapy involves slow institution of a continuous enteral infusion of a diluted elemental formula such as Pregestimil or Alimentum.[108] The rate is rapidly advanced to approximately 150 mL/kg/day or more, provided the child is not on supplemental parenteral nutrition. The concentration of the formula is then sequentially advanced over 3 to 4 days, until the patient is tolerating full caloric requirements and gaining weight. During this time, stool *p*H and reducing substances are monitored and evidence of carbohydrate malabsorption suggests failure of enteral feedings. If this occurs, a period of parenteral nutrition is indicated, usually through a central venous catheter, with gradual reintroduction of enteral feedings by continuous infusion. In treating such infants, it is important to avoid using formulas that contain intact milk or soy protein, because the likelihood of protein sensitivity in such infants is high and further mucosal injury may result. Lengthy periods of parenteral or continuous enteral infusion may be necessary, but the ultimate prognosis is good.

In addition to intractable (*i.e.*, protracted) diarrhea associated with formula protein intolerance, other rare syndromes have been reported to result in mucosal injury and chronic diarrhea. One is congenital microvillus atrophy or microvillus inclusion disease, a disorder with hypoplastic atrophy of the villi and shortening or depletion of microvilli.[109] This disorder requires electron microscopic diagnosis and has a very poor prognosis. Severe protracted diarrhea also may be associated with autoimmune enteropathy; however, this disorder usually presents outside the immediate neonatal period.[110] Mucosal lesions are severe and the prognosis also is poor. Infants with this disorder often have multiorgan autoantibodies, including gut epithelium, and frequently have pancreatic involvement with hyperglycemia or hypoglycemia.

DISORDERS OF THE COLON

CONGENITAL ANOMALIES

There is substantial overlap in small bowel and colonic disease in neonates. Many of the congenital anomalies involve both the small and large intestine, and certain mucosal injury disorders, including formula protein enterocolitis and NEC, can involve both the small intestine and colon. There are some disorders that affect the colon primarily, however. Most are congenital and involve anatomic obstructions, such as atresias, or dysmotility, such as Hirschsprung disease.

ANATOMIC LESIONS

Colonic stenosis or atresia is a rare event, often associated with other skeletal anomalies. Colonic duplication also is a rare entity, which may present with delayed symptoms of obstruction. Duplications usually are cystic, gradually enlarging masses, located posterior to the rectum, which may be confused with tumors.[111]

MOTILITY DISORDERS

More frequent are the disorders that present with delayed passage of meconium secondary to dysmotility. Meconium plug syndrome is one such entity, in which inspissated meconium in the distal colon results in obstruction and dilatation proximally. Delayed passage of meconium is the presenting symptom, and barium enema examination reveals a large plug of meconium that often is evacuated after the barium enema. Normal feeding and stooling usually follows removal of the obstruction, but 20% to 30% of patients with meconium plug syndrome have Hirschsprung disease. If symptoms recur after removal of the meconium plug, rectal suction biopsy is indicated.

Delayed passage of meconium also may occur with the neonatal small left colon syndrome. Radiographic examination of these infants demonstrates normal to dilated proximal colon with constricted or smaller distal colon, with the constricted area usually beginning around the splenic flexure. The line of demarcation is much more abrupt than is seen in neonatal Hirschsprung disease. The disorder is more common in infants of diabetic mothers, as well as infants of mothers with hyperthyroidism. It usually resolves spontaneously, although placement of a colostomy may be necessary until normal motility returns. Colonic motility will eventually return, usually within 2 to 12 weeks, and the colostomy may be closed at that time.

Hirschsprung disease, or congenital aganglionic megacolon, occurs in approximately 1 in 5000 live births, more commonly in males than in females.[112] The risk of recurrence in families is reported to be as high as 10%, higher in infants with total aganglionosis. The frequency is ten times higher in infants with trisomy 21. The disease is caused by a congenital absence of the ganglion cells in both the submucous and myenteric plexuses. Ganglion cells regulate normal colonic peristaltic activity. The absence of ganglion cells results in an inability of the bowel to undergo coordinated relaxation. Impaired migration of neural crest cells into the distal colon is thought to be the mechanism through which Hirschsprung disease develops, although there is some controversy about this. The disorder almost always involves the distal rectum, but the extent varies substantially. There also is controversy as to whether or not skip areas can occur. A few such cases have been reported, but they appear to be extremely rare. In most instances, involvement does not extend proximal to the sigmoid colon. In very rare instances, the involvement may extend beyond the colon into the small intestine. The further the lesion extends, the more difficult the medical management becomes.

Most cases of Hirschsprung disease are not diagnosed in the neonatal period. When they are, the most common clinical presentation is delayed passage of meconium, with passage of the first stool beyond 24 hours of age. This presentation probably is common but often overlooked. Infants also may appear irritable, with poor feeding and failure to thrive—unfortunately, the typical presentation of a wide variety of small bowel and colonic disorders.

Some infants with Hirschsprung disease may present with a life-threatening complication—acute enterocolitis.[113] Toxic megacolon is common. Although enterocolitis may occur in the newborn period, it more commonly presents at 2 to 3 months of age. Mortality remains around 50%. The disorder presents with sudden or gradual onset of diarrhea, followed by bloody stools and eventually the clinical appearance of neonatal sepsis. The clinical overlap between infectious enterocolitis or formula protein-induced enterocolitis is such that Hirschsprung enterocolitis also must be considered in the differential diagnosis of these more common entities. Patients who present with bloody diarrhea in the neonatal period and have negative stool cultures, and who do not respond quickly to protein hydrolysate formula, need to have a rectal biopsy performed. If Hirschsprung disease is suspected, surgical consultation should be obtained immediately, and attempts should be made to decompress the colon with a rectal tube or rectal irrigation. A decompressing colostomy should be placed as soon as feasible.

Diagnosis of Hirschsprung disease usually rests with rectal suction biopsy. A small biopsy tube is inserted into the rectum and a small piece of tissue is removed from a point 2 cm proximal to the mucocutaneous junction. If the biopsy is obtained higher, patients with low-segment Hirschsprung disease may be missed, and if the biopsy is taken more distally it will be obtained in the hypoganglionic zone, an area in which ganglion cells are normally sparse, resulting in a false-positive biopsy for Hirschsprung disease. The biopsy must be deep enough to contain sufficient submucosa to identify ganglion cells. Superficial biopsies are inadequate to diagnose Hirschsprung disease. Because ganglion cells are sparse, the biopsy must be serially sectioned and 60 to 80 sections of tissue examined. Ganglion cells in newborns are somewhat immature and difficult to identify. Thus, a rectal suction biopsy is a reliable diagnostic tool, provided the biopsy is obtained from an appropriate location and depth and an experienced gastroenterologist or pathologist interprets the biopsy. If results are equivocal, a full-thickness biopsy may be performed to establish the diagnosis.

Diagnosis also can be made by inflating a balloon in the distal rectum and measuring relaxation of the internal anal sphincter, a process impaired in Hirschsprung disease. Although this technique is less commonly performed, those who are skillful in its use believe it is as reliable as rectal biopsy. In contrast, barium enema examination in the newborn is highly unreliable in the diagnosis of Hirschsprung disease because the transition zone has yet to develop. Therefore, proximal colonic dilation usually is not apparent in the neonate, and the clinician must look for irregular contractions in the rectosigmoid as the primary hallmark of Hirschsprung disease.

Treatment begins with placement of a decompressing colostomy proximal to the transition zone between ganglionic and aganglionic bowel. Definitive surgery usually is done at 8 to 12 months of age. A number of different operations have been devised in which the aganglionic bowel is removed and the ganglionic bowel attached into the distal rectum. Surgical treatment generally is successful in restoring long-term fecal continence.

Patients with total colonic Hirschsprung disease present major difficulties in postoperative fluid and electrolyte balance. Infants frequently require prolonged courses of parenteral nutrition. Parents should be warned about the protracted nature of the disease, and infants should be observed closely for fluid, electrolyte, and nutritional problems.

Several rare intestinal motility disorders present in the neonatal period. Transient hypomotility occurs in some premature infants, and is characterized by markedly delayed gastric emptying and absent or diminished small bowel motility. In most instances, these abnormalities gradually resolve with time; support with parenteral nutrition coupled with intermittent attempts at feeding is all that is indicated. Alterations in calcium and magnesium metabolism such as parathyroid dysfunction, or hypothyroidism can cause diminished motility, and these disorders should be excluded in infants with apparent motility disorders. Occasionally, infants with chronic idiopathic intestinal pseudoobstruction syndrome can present during infancy. This term applies to a number of neuropathic and myopathic disorders that result in chronic progressive gastrointestinal hypomotility. A variety of histologic lesions have been described, and the prognosis for improvement is poor. Occasionally, the disorder also may involve the urinary tract, with associated megalocystis and megaureter.

PANCREATIC DISORDERS

CYSTIC FIBROSIS

Disorders of the pancreas uncommonly present during the neonatal period. The most common is cystic fibrosis, which occurs in approximately 1 in 1600 Caucasian live births.[114] This autosomal recessive disorder usually presents later in childhood with failure to thrive or chronic pulmonary disease, but may present with meconium ileus in the neonatal period. After the obstruction has been relieved, therapy consists of compensating for the pancreatic insufficiency through use of elemental formulas such as Pregestimil or Alimentum that contain hydrolyzed protein as their protein source and medium-chain triglycerides as part of their lipid component. Medium-chain triglycerides do not require digestion by pancreatic enzymes for absorption and, consequently, may facilitate nutrient assimilation in infants with pancreatic insufficiency. Despite the use of elemental formulas, replacement pancreatic enzyme therapy from birth is necessary to aid the digestion of endogenously secreted proteins.

In children with pancreatic insufficiency due to cystic fibrosis the release of the pancreatic hormone PP is almost totally abolished.[115] Fasting PP levels are low and the normal response to milk feeding is absent.[115] Plasma insulin and GIP responses are significantly reduced in cystic fibrosis patients, compared to control subjects, even though the early glucose rise is greater in the former group.[115] Reduced GIP secretion in response to feeding may exacerbate the glucose intolerance that accompanies pancreatic destruction. Although plasma enteroglucagon concentrations are elevated in cystic fibrosis, levels of other hormones such as gastrin, secretin, motilin, and glucagon are quite normal.[115]

The second most common cause of pancreatic insufficiency in infancy is Shwachman syndrome, a disorder characterized by pancreatic insufficiency and bone marrow dysfunction with cyclic neutropenia.[116] This rare disorder should be considered in infants with steatorrhea and neutropenia. Extremely rare isolated defects in pancreatic enzyme secretion, including trypsinogen and lipase, also have been reported.

DISORDERS OF THE LIVER

The liver is a complex organ serving multiple metabolic functions. From a digestive standpoint, its primary function is that of an exocrine organ producing bile for the emulsification of fats. Postnatally, the liver receives its blood from two separate sources, approximately 25% from the hepatic artery, and 75% from the portal vein. The portal vein drains the splanchnic bed and allows the liver the opportunity to regulate and metabolize substances absorbed by the intestine and hormones produced in the gastrointestinal tract.

Bile is composed primarily of water. The concentration of solids in the bile are increased threefold by the gallbladder. The fetal liver is capable of synthesizing bile acids from cholesterol slowly, and the rate of synthesis increases progressively throughout gestation. The major bile salt in newborns is taurocholate. Conjugation of bile salts with glycine in preference to taurine gradually increases, and by adulthood, most bile salts are conjugated with glycine. The bile acid pool is very small in the preterm infant, but gradually increases in the newborn and matures throughout infancy. This relatively small bile acid pool results in reduced bile salt secretion and, in addition to the relative pancreatic insufficiency, plays a role in the less efficient absorption of fat in the newborn infant. Bile acids are reabsorbed in the ileum through an active transport mechanism. There is some passive transport of bile acids in the jejunum and colon as well. In the fetus, taurocholate is absorbed passively and active ileal transport appears after birth.

CHOLESTATIC LIVER DISEASE

Most liver diseases in the neonatal period present with cholestasis, or conjugated hyperbilirubinemia.[117,118] Although in older children and adults, elevation of the amino transferase (*i.e.*, transaminase) enzymes is considered the hallmark of hepatocellular injury, neonates may have significant hepatocellular injury even in the presence of normal amino transferase levels. There are many causes of prolonged conjugated hyperbilirubinemia in the neonatal period. These can be subdivided into general categories, including infectious disorders; toxic insults such as parenteral nutrition and sepsis; metabolic disorders; anatomic disorders, including congenital hepatic fibrosis and choledochal cyst; and idiopathic infantile cholangiopathies, including primarily biliary atresia and neonatal hepatitis.[119]

Neonatal Hepatitis and Biliary Atresia. After extensive evaluation of the infant with cholestasis, a diagnosis of either extrahepatic biliary atresia or idiopathic neonatal hepatitis is made in 70% to 80% of cases.[120,121] Current thinking suggests that neonatal hepatitis and biliary atresia form a continuum of a pathophysiologic process directed at various levels of the hepatobiliary tract. Inflammation in the bile duct epithelium may result in sclerosis and obliteration of the bile ducts and manifest itself as extrahepatic biliary atresia. Primary hepatocellular inflammation is more likely to result in neonatal hepatitis. Reovirus type III has been found in a number of infants with both idiopathic neonatal hepatitis and biliary atresia. This virus has been implicated as a causative agent in both disorders, although there is evidence that raises questions about this hypothesis.[122,123]

Idiopathic neonatal hepatitis is slightly more common than biliary atresia. Both sporadic and familial varieties exist. Neonatal hepatitis, unlike biliary atresia, is more common in low-birth-weight infants. Jaundice develops during the first week of life in most cases. A wide variety of clinical presentations may occur, from severe failure to thrive or fulminant hepatic failure to asymptomatic jaundice. Acholic stools are uncommon, but may occur if cholestasis is severe. Physical examination reveals a firm, enlarged liver and occasionally splenomegaly. The presence of other signs of congenital infection may point toward a more specific diagnosis. Liver biopsy may be helpful in making the diagnosis, but the histologic findings are relatively nonspecific. In most cases, neonatal hepatitis can be differentiated successfully from biliary atresia by percutaneous liver biopsy. Clinical management is directed toward nutritional support and medical management of clinical complications such as ascites or pruritus. The prognosis is variable, with one-half of the cases resolving with little or no sequelae. Life-threatening chronic liver disease may necessitate liver transplantation.

Extrahepatic biliary atresia accounts for about one third of cases of neonatal cholestasis. Familial cases are uncommon, as are cases in premature infants. Patients typically present with jaundice during the first or second week of life. Acholic stools are more common than in neonatal hepatitis. The liver is firm and enlarged, and splenomegaly may be present, as in neonatal hepatitis. Infants often appear clinically well, although progressive liver injury results in nutritional deficiencies, failure to thrive, and ascites.

Differentiation between neonatal hepatitis and biliary atresia has been the subject of controversy over the years. Serum amino transferase (*i.e.*, transaminase) levels are notoriously unreliable indicators of neonatal liver disease and may be normal even in some patients with neonatal hepatitis. Extremely elevated γ-glutamyl transferase levels are suggestive of the marked bile ductular proliferation found in biliary atresia.[124] Liver biopsy demonstrates inflammatory obliteration of the extrahepatic biliary tree, with bile stasis and bile ductular proliferation in the liver. Histologic features may overlap with neonatal hepatitis, particularly early in the course of the disease making it difficult to differentiate. Histologic transition from neonatal hepatitis to biliary atresia has been reported, and may be a relatively common phenomenon. The duodenal intubation and aspiration test is a simple, rapid, inexpensive method to check for patency of the extrahepatic biliary tree. Collection of 12 2-hour aliquots of duodenal drainage from a feeding tube placed in the duodenum over a 24-hour period suggests biliary atresia if no yellow fluid is present. Aspiration of bile-stained fluid from the duodenum suggests patency of the extrahepatic biliary tract. This test is sensitive and specific for the evaluation of infantile cholestasis.[125] The test has reliability comparable to or better than radionuclide imaging with scans, which may give abnormal results in neonatal hepatitis during periods of severe cholestasis. Reliability of the radionuclide studies may be improved by measurement of duodenal fluid counts collected by a simple string test.[126] The combination of liver biopsy and imaging study or duodenal drainage usually is used to determine whether the patient is more likely to have biliary atresia or neonatal hepatitis. If bile drainage cannot be confirmed or the typical histologic picture of neonatal hepatitis is not apparent on liver biopsy, then surgical exploration and intraoperative cholangiography usually is performed to establish a final diagnosis.

If the patient has biliary atresia, a hepatoportoenterostomy with Roux-en-Y enteroanastamosis (*i.e.*, Kasai procedure) is performed to attempt bile drainage. The Kasai procedure rarely alters the long-term outcome of biliary atresia,[127] but may delay the necessity of liver transplantation. For this reason, some advocate not performing a Kasai procedure. Most, however, believe that performing the procedure does not worsen the prognosis at transplant and may allow the child to live longer so that a more suitable liver donor may be located before transplantation. For those infants with progressive liver disease after the Kasai procedure, every attempt must be made to optimize their condition before transplantation. Deficiencies of the fat-soluble vitamins (*i.e.*, A, D, E, K) require supplementation. Nutritional deficiencies are treated by using formulas containing medium-chain triglycerides. Salt and protein restriction may become necessary, as liver failure progresses.

Hepatic transplantation is the definitive treatment for biliary atresia and results in long-term survival in 70% to 85% of infants.

Other Causes of Cholestasis. Rare causes of cholestasis must be excluded before confirming the diagnosis of neonatal hepatitis or biliary atresia (Table 37-3).[119] Infectious diseases such as cytomegalovirus, hepatitis B, HIV, rubella, herpes, toxoplasmosis, and syphilis should be excluded by standard serologic or culture techniques. Metabolic disorders to be considered include tyrosinemia, galactosemia, and hereditary fructose intolerance. Obtaining urine for reducing substances to exclude galactosemia and hereditary fructose intolerance, and succinyl acetone to exclude tyrosinemia should be done immediately. Anatomic disorders such as choledochal cysts can be diagnosed by ultrasonography. Other causes such as TPN cholestasis or sepsis should be considered, based on the clinical presentation.

TABLE 37–3
STEPS IN EVALUATING NEONATAL CHOLESTASIS

1. Determine that hyperbilirubinemia is predominantly direct
2. Exclude metabolic and infectious causes of cholestasis
3. Perform ultrasound to exclude anatomic lesions
4. Obtain percutaneous liver biopsy and hepatobiliary scan or duodenal drainage study
5. Explore whether studies suggest biliary atresia, and perform Kasai procedure if indicated

Occasionally, liver biopsy will demonstrate a marked reduction in the number of intrahepatic bile ducts, revealing a disorder known as paucity of the intrahepatic bile ducts or intrahepatic biliary hypoplasia. Some of these patients fall into the category of Alagille syndrome, also known as syndromatic paucity or arteriohepatic dysplasia.[128] These patients exhibit unusual facial characteristics, ocular abnormalities including posterior embryotoxon (*i.e.*, prominent Schwalbe line), pulmonic stenosis, and vertebral arch defects, including anterior vertebral arch fusion with butterfly vertebrae. Careful cardiac examination, examination of the eyes by an ophthalmologist, and radiographic examination of the lumbosacral spine should be obtained in patients with suspected Alagille syndrome who have a paucity of intralobular bile ducts. Prognosis for long-term survival in syndromatic patients is relatively good.

There are patients with nonsyndromatic paucity who have liver biopsy findings similar to those with Alagille syndrome. In general, these patients have a much poorer prognosis than those with syndromatic paucity. Life-threatening cirrhosis develops in many, and these patients may require hepatic transplantation. As in biliary atresia, liver transplantation has markedly changed the prognosis for these patients.

A number of infectious disorders, both viral and bacterial, may present during the neonatal period, and a specific diagnosis should be sought in such instances. Hepatitis B typically is found in infants whose mothers were infected during the third trimester. As many as 60% to 90% of infants born to hepatitis B surface antigen–positive mothers may be infected. Transmission from mother to infant most commonly occurs at the time of delivery. Mothers who are hepatitis B antigen–positive are at extremely high risk to transmit hepatitis B virus to their infants. In addition, mothers who are chronic carriers of hepatitis B surface antigen also may infect their infants. Most hepatitis B in infancy is asymptomatic. Abnormal liver tests develop at approximately 6 to 8 weeks of age, and may persist for up to a year. Nearly 50% of these children remain hepatitis B surface antigen–positive, and are at risk for developing hepatocellular carcinoma. Such children should be screened annually with α-fetoprotein levels for evidence of liver cancer, unless their hepatitis B surface antigen determinations revert to negative. Maternal screening for hepatitis B surface antigen is essential to prevent perinatal transmission of hepatitis B. Neonates born to mothers who are hepatitis B antigen–positive should receive hepatitis B hyperimmune globulin, 0.5 mL intramuscularly at the time of birth, and hepatitis B vaccine within 12 hours of birth. Booster immunizations with hepatitis B vaccine are recommended at 1 and 6 months of age.[129]

Several other viruses may produce hepatitis during the neonatal period. Hepatitis A may develop in infants of mothers with active icteric hepatitis A at the time of delivery. Hepatitis C, formerly known as parenterally transmitted non-A, non-B hepatitis, commonly is transmitted through blood contact and produces a clinical spectrum similar to hepatitis B. Serologic tests are available to detect hepatitis C, and its relationship to neonatal liver disease probably will be known in the near future. Other viruses, such as Epstein–Barr virus, cytomegalovirus, HIV, rubella, herpes simplex, coxsackievirus, and adenoviruses may cause a wide spectrum of neonatal liver disease.[130] In most instances, infection with these viruses results in spontaneous resolution without chronic injury.

Bacteria also may produce neonatal liver injury, because invasion of the liver may occur. Specific hepatic infection may result from certain bacterial diseases such as syphilis and listeriosis, as well as the parasitic disorder toxoplasmosis.

A number of metabolic diseases may present with neonatal cholestasis. The most common is α_1-antitrypsin deficiency. Alpha $_1$-antitrypsin is the major protease inhibitor in the hepatocyte. Deficiency of α_1-antitrypsin occurs in a number of inheritable phenotypes. These Pi or protease inhibitor phenotypes can be determined. Type ZZ produces the most complete deficiency state and most cases of liver disease. It is estimated that 10% to 20% of type ZZ patients develop liver disease.[131] Isolated cases of type MZ and MS also have been reported with liver injury.[132] The ZZ phenotype is inherited through an autosomal recessive mechanism and occurs in 1 in 2000 live births. Patients can be identified by the measurement of a very low α_1-antitrypsin level in the blood. Diagnosis is confirmed by the determination of the ZZ phenotype, plus the classic histologic findings of periodic acid-Schiff–positive, diastase-resistant granules on liver biopsy.

Liver disease may develop in patients with cystic fibrosis, although very few of these present during the neonatal period. Measurement of sweat chloride to exclude cystic fibrosis, however, should be part of the evaluation of neonatal liver disease.

Three metabolic diseases present with rather fulminant neonatal liver disease. These include galactosemia, hereditary fructose intolerance, and tyrosinemia. These disorders should be expected when coagulation abnormalities appear inappropriately severe relative to the apparent degree of liver disease. Patients with galactosemia have positive urinary reducing substances if they are being fed lactose at the time of screening. Patients with hereditary fructose intolerance also may test positive. Patients with tyrosinemia can be screened by measuring succinyl acetone content in the urine. Plasma and urine amino acids will demonstrate marked elevations of tyrosine, although this may be a nonspecific finding in any infant with neonatal liver disease. Patients with galactosemia respond to a galactose-free diet, and liver injury usually resolves spontaneously. Neonatal sepsis is a frequent occurrence in these infants and precautions should be taken. Patients with tyrosinemia commonly undergo progressive liver and renal dysfunction and are candidates for emergent liver transplantation once the diagnosis is made.

Several lipid storage diseases produce neonatal liver disease. Niemann–Pick disease, Wolman disease, cholesterol-ester storage disease, and Gaucher disease are included in this group. Most present with an insidious onset later in life.

A number of disorders exist in which peroxisomal dysfunction occurs. The most common is Zellweger syndrome, the cerebrohepatorenal syndrome. These patients present with cholestasis, hepatomegaly, hypotonia, and dysmorphic features, and may be diagnosed by demonstration of very-long-chain fatty acids in the serum.

Defects in the urea cycle may present with hyperammonemia during the first 2 days of life. A sepsislike picture with vomiting, lethargy, seizures, and coma suggests this diagnosis. The most common form is ornithine transcarbamylase deficiency. Serum ammonia levels are very high, provided the infant is being fed protein. Diagnosis depends on plasma and urinary amino acid levels, and liver biopsy must be assayed for specific enzymes (see Chap. 39). Protein intake should be restricted and liver transplantation should be considered. Transient hyperammonemia of the newborn also has been reported with spontaneous resolution and no long-term neurologic sequelae. Permanent resolution of the hyperammonemia usually occurs by 2 weeks of age.

Cholestasis may occur in any patient on chronic parenteral nutrition, but it is far more common in sick premature infants who receive parenteral nutrition for long periods of time.[133,134] The mechanism by which the liver injury occurs is unknown and perhaps multifactorial.[135] Several risk factors have been identified, however, including recurrent infections, prematurity, and lack of enteral feeding. Certain components of parenteral solutions have been implicated in causing liver injury. Excessive caloric administration may play a role. Certain amino acids may be more hepatotoxic, although many of these data are derived from animal studies. Higher doses of protein may result in a more rapid rise in bilirubin, but does not appear to alter ultimate risk of development of liver disease. Available intravenous lipid preparations do not appear to cause cholestasis, and may in fact be beneficial in this regard.

The reason premature infants are more susceptible to liver disease while on parenteral nutrition probably is related to developmental immaturity of several hepatobiliary processes. These infants have reduced and altered bile acid synthesis, decreased bile acid pool size, and therefore decreased intraluminal bile acids. Gallbladder function also is impaired. Bile acid reabsorption from the small bowel is underdeveloped. The premature liver also is less capable of detoxifying potentially toxic secondary bile acids.

Lack of enteral feeding definitely predisposes to parenteral nutrition cholestasis. Gastrointestinal hormones that stimulate bile flow depend on enteral feeding for their release. Reduced gut motility in the unused bowel may contribute to bacterial proliferation and the resultant production of toxic secondary bile acids. Infection, especially gastrointestinal, and gastrointestinal surgery may potentiate the liver injury through related mechanisms. Limited amounts of enteral feeding, as tolerated, may be very beneficial in preventing liver injury in the parenteral nutrition-dependent infant.

Diagnosis of parenteral nutrition liver disease depends on exclusion of other causes of cholestasis in the parenteral nutrition-dependent patient. Separation of this disorder from other causes of cholestasis is difficult using standard laboratory tests. Histologic study is nonspecific, but may be helpful in making the diagnosis.[136] The disease often is reversible once parenteral nutrition is discontinued. It occasionally may progress to cirrhosis, and hepatocellular carcinoma has been reported.

Treatment is best accomplished by discontinuing parenteral nutrition. If this cannot be accomplished, the following steps should be taken:

1. Reevaluate solutions to ensure they are appropriately formulated and balanced.
2. Use low-dose enteral feedings as tolerated to stimulate bile flow and gut motility.
3. Cycle the parenteral nutrition so that it is given over only part of the day.
4. Use amino acid solutions specially formulated for infants.

Other potential therapies, yet unproven, include choleretics such as phenobarbital or ursodeoxycholic acid, hormone stimulation of bile flow, and bowel prokinetic agents. Success with combined intestinal–liver transplants suggests that this procedure may play an important role in infants with end-stage parenteral nutrition liver disease.[137]

REFERENCES

1. Lebenthal E, Keung YK. Alternative pathways of digestion and absorption in the newborn. In: Lebenthal E, ed. Textbook of gastroenterology and nutrition in infancy. 2nd ed. New York: Raven Press, 1989:3.
2. Lebenthal E, Tucker N. Carbohydrate digestion: development in early infancy. Clin Perinatol 1986;13:37.
3. Cicco R, Holzman I, Brown D, et al. Glucose polymer intolerance in premature infants. Pediatrics 1981;67:498.
4. Lebenthal E, Lee PC. Alternate pathways of digestion and absorption in early infancy. J Pediatr Gastroenterol Nutr 1984;3:1.
5. Watkins JB. Lipid digestion and absorption. Pediatrics 1985; 75(Suppl):151.
6. Boehm G, Bierbach U, Seuger H, et al. Activities of lipase and trypsin in duodenal juice of infants small for gestational age. J Pediatr Gastroenterol Nutr 1991;12:324.
7. Jensen RG, Clark RM, de Jong FA, et al. The lipolytic triad: human lingual, breast milk and pancreatic lipases: physiological implications of their characteristics in digestion of dietary fats. J Pediatr Gastroenterol Nutr 1982;1:243.
8. Watkins JB, Ingall D, Szczepanik P, et al. Bile salt metabolism in the newborn. N Engl J Med 1973;288:431.
9. Balistreri WF, Heubi JE, Suchy FJ. Immaturity of the enterohepatic circulation in early life: factors predisposing to "physiologic" malabsorption and cholestasis. J Pediatr Gastroenterol Nutr 1983;2:346.
10. Acra SA, Ghishan FK. Active bile salt transport in the ileum: characteristics and ontogeny. J Pediatr Gastroenterol Nutr 1990;10:421.
11. Euler AR, Byrne WJ, Meis PJ, et al. Basal and pentagastrin stimulated acid secretion in human newborn infants. Pediatr Res 1979;13:36.
12. Hyman PE, Clarke DD, Everett SL, et al. Gastric acid secretory function in preterm infants. J Pediatr 1985;106:467.
13. Agunod M, Yamaguchi N, Lopez R, et al. Correlative study of hydrochloric acid, pepsin and intrinsic factor secretion in newborns and infants. Am J Digest Dis 1969;14:400.
14. Antonowicz I, Lebenthal E. Developmental pattern of small intestinal enterokinase and disaccharidase activities in the human fetus. Gastroenterology 1977;723:1299.
15. Younoszai MK, Sapario RS, Laughlin M, et al. Maturation of jejunum and ileum in rats: water and electrolyte transport during in vivo perfusion of hypertonic solutions. J Clin Invest 1978;62:271.
16. Southgate DAT, Widdowson EM, Smits BJ, et al. Absorption and excretion of calcium and fat by young infants. Lancet 1969;1:487.
17. Senterre J, Putet G, Salle B, et al. Effects of vitamin D and phosphorus supplementation on calcium retention in preterm infants fed banked human milk. J Pediatr 1983;103:305.
18. Voyer M, Davakis M, Antener I, et al. Zinc balances in preterm infants. Biol Neonate 1982;42:87.
19. Tomomasa R, Hyman PE, Itoh K, et al. Gastroduodenal motility in neonates: response to human milk compared with cow's milk formula. Pediatrics 1987;80:434.
20. Berseth CL. Gestational evolution of small intestine motility in preterm infants. J Pediatr 1989;115:646.
21. Worniak ER, Fenton TR, Milla PJ. The development of fasting small intestine motility in human neonates. In: Roman C, ed. Gastrointestinal motility. London: Lancaster Press, 1983: 265.
22. Nagata S, Koyanagi T, Horimoto N, et al. Chronological development of the fetal stomach assessed using real-time ultrasound. Early Hum Dev 1990;22:15.

23. Vanderhoof JA, Rappoport PJ, Paxson CL Jr. Manometric diagnosis of lower esophageal sphincter incompetence in infants: use of a small, single-lumen perfused catheter. Pediatrics 1978;62:805.
24. Buchan AMJ, Bryant MG, Polak JM, et al. Development of regulatory peptides in the human fetal intestine. In: Bloom SR, Polak JM, eds. Gut hormones. New York: Churchill-Livingston, 1981:119.
25. Bryant MG, Buchan AMJ, Gregor M, et al. Development of intestinal regulatory peptides in the human fetus. Gastroenterology 1982;83:47.
26. Lucas A, Bloom SR, Aynsley-Green A. Development of gut hormone responses to feeding in neonates. Arch Dis Child 1980;55:678.
27. Lucas A, Adrian TE, Christofides ND, et al. Plasma motilin, gastrin and enteroglucagon and feeding in the human newborn. Arch Dis Child 1980;55:673.
28. Euler AP, Byrne WJ, Cousins LM, et al. Increased serum gastrin concentrations and gastric hyposecretion in the immediate newborn period. Gastroenterology 1977;72:1271.
29. Aynsley-Green A, Lucas A, Bloom SR. The effects of feeds of differing composition on entero-insular hormone secretion in the first hours of life in human neonates. Acta Paediatr Scand 1979;68:265.
30. Lucas A, Bloom SR, Aynsley-Green A. Postnatal surges in plasma gut hormones in term and preterm infants. Biol Neonate 1982;41:63.
31. Miller BA. Observations on the gastric acidity during the first month of life. Arch Dis Child 1941;16:22.
32. Adrian TE, Savage AJ, Sagor GR, et al. Effect of peptide YY on gastric, pancreatic and biliary function in humans. Gastroenterology 1985;89:494.
33. Adrian TE, Smith HA, Calvert SA, et al. Elevated plasma peptide YY in human neonates and infants. Pediatr Res 1986;20:1225.
34. Lucas A, Adrian TE, Bloom SR, et al. Plasma secretin in neonates. Acta Paediatr Scand 1980;69:205.
35. Johnson LR. Regulation of gastrointestinal growth. In: Johnson LR, ed. Physiology of the gastrointestinal tract. 2nd ed. New York: Raven Press, 1987:301.
36. Calvert SA, Soltesz G, Jenkins PA, et al. Feeding premature infants with human milk or preterm milk formula: effects on postnatal growth, intermediary metabolism and regulatory peptides. Biol Neonate 1985;47:189.
37. Berseth CL. Gestational evolution of small intestine motility in preterm and term infants. J Pediatr 1989;115:646.
38. Sarson DL, Wood SM, Holder D, et al. The effect of glucose-dependent insulinotropic polypeptide infused at physiological concentrations on the release of insulin in man. Diabetologia 1982;22:33.
39. Lucas A, Sarson DL, Bloom SR, et al. Developmental aspects of gastric inhibitory polypeptide (GIP) and its possible role in the enteroinsular axis in neonates. Acta Paediatr Scand 1980;69:321.
40. Lucas A, Aynsley-Green A, Blackburn AN, et al. Plasma neurotensin in term and preterm neonates. Acta Paediatr Scand 1981;17:201.
41. Savage AP, Adrian TE, Carolan G, et al. Effects of peptide YY (PYY) on mouth to cecum transit time and on the rate of gastric emptying in healthy volunteers. Gut 1987;70:166.
42. Lucas A, Bloom SR, Aynsley-Green A. Metabolic and endocrine consequences of depriving preterm infants of enteral nutrition. Acta Paediatr Scand 1983;72:245.
43. Adrian TE, Bloom SR. Effect of food on the hormones of the gastrointestinal tract. In: Hunter JO, Jones V, eds. Food and the gut. Philadelphia: Baillière Tindall, 1985:13.
44. Isaacs PET, Ladas S, Forgacs IC, et al. A comparison of the effects of ingested medium- and long-chain triglyceride on gallbladder volume and the release of cholecystokinin and other gut peptides. Dig Dis Sci 1987;32:481.
45. Martin LW, Torres AM. Omphalocele and gastroschisis. Surg Clin North Am 1985;65:1235.
46. Meller JL, Reyes HM, Loeff DS. Gastroschisis and omphalocele. Clin Perinatol 1989;16:113.
47. Yazbeck S, Ndoye M, Khan AH. Omphalocele: a 25 year experience. J Pediatr Surg 1986;21:761.
48. Lewis DF, Towers DV, Garite TJ, et al. Fetal gastroschisis and omphalocele: is cesarean section the best mode of delivery. Am J Obstet Gynecol 1990;163:773.
49. Lenke RR, Hatch EI Jr. Fetal gastroschisis: a preliminary report advocating the use of cesarean section. Obstet Gynecol 1986;67:395.
50. Herbst JJ. Gastroesophageal reflux in infants. J Pediatr Gastroenterol Nutr 1985;4:163.
51. Werlin SL, Dodds WJ, Hogan WJ, et al. Mechanisms of gastroesophageal reflux in children. J Pediatr 1980;97:244.
52. Sondheimer JM. Continuous monitoring of distal esophageal pH: a diagnostic test for gastroesophageal reflux in infants. J Pediatr 1980;93:804.
53. Tsou VM, Young RM, Hart MH, et al. Elevated plasma aluminum levels in normal infants using antacids containing aluminum. Pediatrics 1991;87:148.
54. Strickland AD, Chang JHT. Results of treatment of gastroesophageal reflux with bethanechol. J Pediatr 1983;103:311.
55. Jolley SG, Halpern LM, Tunell WP, et al. The risk of sudden infant death from gastroesophageal reflux. J Pediatr Surg 1991;26:691.
56. Raffensperger JG. Esophageal atresia and tracheoesophageal stenosis. In: Raffensperger JG, ed. Swenson's pediatric surgery. 5th ed. Norwalk, CT: Appleton and Lange, 1990:697.
57. Benson CD, Lloyd JR. Infantile pyloric stenosis: a review of 1120 cases. Am J Surg 1964;107:429.
58. Dodge JA. Genetics of hypertrophic pyloric stenosis. Clin Gastroenterol 1973;2:523.
59. Nord KS. Peptic ulcer disease in the pediatric population. Pediatr Clin North Am 1988;35:117.
60. Drumm B, Rhoads JM, Stringer DA, et al. Peptic ulcer disease in children: clinical findings, and clinical course. Pediatrics 1988;82:410.
61. Murphy MS, Eastham EJ. Peptic ulcer disease in childhood: long-term prognosis. J Pediatr Gastroenterol Nutr 1987;6:721.
62. Bell JJ. Perforation of the gastrointestinal tract and peritonitis in the neonate. Surg Gynecol Obstet 1985;160:20.
63. Smith EI. Malrotation of the intestine. In: Welch KJ, Randolph JG, Ravitch MM, et al, eds. Pediatric surgery. 4th ed. Chicago: Year Book, 1986:89:882.
64. Grosfeld JL. Jejunoileal atresia and stenosis. In: Welch KJ, Randolph JG, Ravitch MM, et al, eds. Pediatric surgery. 4th ed. Chicago: Year Book, 1986:85:838.
65. Martin LW, Zerella JT. Jejunoileal atresia: a proposed classification. J Pediatr Surg 1967;11:399.
66. Holgersen LO, Stanly-Brown EG. Idiopathic post-operative intussusception in infants and childhood. Am Surg 1978; 44:305.
67. Brown EG, Sweet AY. Neonatal necrotizing enterocolitis. Pediatr Clin North Am 1982;29:1149.
68. Kliegman RM, Fanaroff AA. Necrotizing enterocolitis. N Engl J Med 1984;310:1093.
69. Hack M, Horbar JK, Malloy MH, et al. Very low birth weight outcomes of the National Institute of Child Health and Human Development Neonatal Network. Pediatrics 1991;87:587.
70. Uauy RD, Fanaroff AA, Korones SB, et al. Necrotizing entero-

colitis in very low birth weight infants: biodemographic and clinical correlates. J Pediatr 1991;119:630.
71. Kliegman RM, Walsh M. Neonatal necrotizing enterocolitis: pathogenesis, classification and spectrum of illness. Curr Probl Pediatr 1987;17:213.
72. Ballance WA, Dahms BB, Shenker N, et al. Pathology of neonatal necrotizing enterocolitis: a ten-year experience. J Pediatr 1990;117(Suppl 1, Pt 2):S6.
73. Kliegman RM. Neonatal necrotizing enterocolitis: bridging the basic science with clinical disease. J Pediatr 1990;117:833.
74. Caplan MS, Sun X-M, Hsueh W, et al. Role of platelet activating factor and tumor necrosis factor-alpha in neonatal necrotizing enterocolitis. J Pediatr 1990;116:960.
75. Anderson DM, Kliegman RM. The relationship of neonatal alimentation practices to the occurrence of endemic necrotizing enterocolitis. Am J Perinatol 1991;8:62.
76. Covert RF, Neu J, Elliott MJ, et al. Factors associated with age of onset of necrotizing enterocolitis. Am J Perinatol 1989; 6:455.
77. Eibl MM, Wolf HM, Furnkranz H, et al. Prophylaxis of necrotizing enterocolitis by oral IgA-IgG: review of a clinical study in low birth weight infants and discussion of the pathogenic role of infection. J Clin Immunol 1990;10(Suppl 6):72S.
78. Aynsley-Green A, Lucas A, Lawson GR, et al. Gut hormones and regulatory peptides in relation to enteral feeding, gastroenteritis, and necrotizing enterocolitis in infancy. Arch Dis Child 1990;(Suppl)117:24.
79. Faix RG, Polley TZ, Grasela TH. A randomized controlled trial of parenteral clindamycin in neonatal necrotizing enterocolitis. Pediatrics 1988;112:271.
80. Ross MN, Wayne ER, Janik JS, et al. A standard of comparison for acute surgical necrotizing enterocolitis. J Pediatr Surg 1989;24:998.
81. Dowling RH, Booth CC. Structural and functional changes following small intestinal resection in the rat. Clin Sci 1967; 32:139.
82. Adrian TE, Savage AP, Fuessl HS, et al. Release of peptide YY (PYY) after resection of small bowel, colon or pancreas in man. Surgery 1987;101:715.
83. Besterman HS, Adrian TE, Mallinson CN, et al. Gut hormone release after intestinal resection. Gut 1982;23:854.
84. Armstrong DN, Ballantyne GH, Adrian TE, et al. Adaptive increase in peptide YY and enteroglucagon after proctocolectomy and pelvic ileal reservoir reconstruction. Dis Colon Rectum 1991;34:119.
85. Wilmore DW, Dudrick SJ, Daly JM, et al. The role of nutrition in the adaptation of the small intestine after massive resection. Surg Gynecol Obstet 1971;132:673.
86. Vanderhoof JA. Short bowel syndrome. In: Lebenthal EB, ed. Gastroenterology and nutrition in early infancy. 2nd ed. New York: Raven Press, 1990:793.
87. Vanderhoof JA. Short bowel syndrome. In: Kassirer JP, ed. Current therapy in internal medicine. 3rd ed. Philadelphia: BC Decker, 1991:550.
88. Vanderhoof JA. Clinical management of the short bowel syndrome. In: Balistreri WF, Vanderhoof JA, eds. Pediatric gastroenterology and nutrition. London: Chapman and Hall, 1990:24.
89. Goulet OJ, Revillon Y, Jan D, et al. Neonatal short bowel syndrome. J Pediatr 1991;119(Suppl 1, Pt 1):18.
90. Gracey M. The contaminated small bowel syndrome: pathogenesis, diagnosis and treatment. Am J Clin Nutr 1979;32:234.
91. Perman JA, Modler S, Barr RG, et al. Fasting breath hydrogen concentration: normal values and clinical adaptation. Gastroenterology 1984;87:1358.
92. Aarbakke J, Schjonsby H. Value of urinary simple phenol and indican determinations of the stagnant loop syndrome. Scand J Gastroenterol 1976;2:409.
93. Hudson M, Packnee R, Mowat NA. D-lactic acidosis in short bowel syndrome: an examination of possible mechanisms. Q J Med 1990;74:157.
94. Taylor SF, Sondheimer JM, Sokol RJ, et al. Noninfectious colitis associated with short gut syndrome in infants. J Pediatr 1991;119:24.
95. Caniano DA, Starr J, Ginn-Pease ME. Extensive short-bowel syndrome in neonates: outcome in the 1980s. Surgery 1989; 105:119.
96. Thompson JS. Recent advances in the surgical treatment of the short-bowel syndrome. Surg Annu 1990;22:107.
97. Thompson J, Pinch L, Murray N, et al. Experience with intestinal lengthening procedures. J Pediatr Surg 1991;26:721.
98. Cooper A, Floyd TS, Ross AJ, et al. Morbidity and mortality of short bowel syndrome acquired in infancy: an update. J Pediatr Surg 1984;19:711.
99. Dorney SFA, Ament ME, Berquist WE, et al. Improved survival in very short small bowel of infancy with use of long-term parenteral nutrition. J Pediatr 1985;106:521.
100. Adrian TE, Savage AP, Bacarese-Hamilton AJ, et al. Peptide YY abnormalities in gastrointestinal disease. Gastroenterology 1986;90:379.
101. Besterman HS, Christofides ND, Welsby PD, et al. Gut hormones in acute diarrhea. Gut 1983;24:665.
102. Lawson GR, Nelson R, Domin J, et al. Gut regulatory peptides in acute infantile gastroenteritis. Arch Dis Child (in press).
103. Walker-Smith J, Harrison M, Kilby A, et al. Cow's milk-sensitive enteropathy. Arch Dis Child 1978;53:375.
104. Walker-Smith J. Cow's milk protein intolerance: transient food intolerance of infancy. Arch Dis Child 1975;50:347.
105. Powell GK. Milk- and soy-induced enterocolitis of infancy. J Pediatr 1978;93:553.
106. Avery GB, Villavicencio O, Lilly JR, et al. Intractable diarrhea in early infancy. Pediatrics 1968;41:712.
107. Goldgar CM, Vanderhoof JA. Lack of correlation of small bowel biopsy and clinical course of patients with intractable diarrhea of infancy. Gastroenterology 1986;90:527.
108. Orenstein SR. Enteral versus parenteral therapy for intractable diarrhea of infancy: a prospective, randomized trial. J Pediatr 1986;109:277.
109. Schmitz J, Ginies JL, Arnaud-Battandier F, et al. Congenital microvillous atrophy, a rare cause of neonatal intractable diarrhoea. Pediatr Res 1982;16:1014.
110. Unsworth J, Hutchins P, Mitchell J, et al. Flat small intestinal mucosa and autoantibodies against the gut epithelium. J Pediatr Gastroenterol Nutr 1982;1:503.
111. Holcomb GW III, Gheissari A, O'Neill JA Jr, et al. Surgical management of alimentary tract duplications. Ann Surg 1989;209:167.
112. Martin LW, Torres Am. Hirschsprung's disease. Surg Clin North Am 1985;65:1171.
113. Bill AJ, Chapman ND. The enterocolitis of Hirschsprung's disease: its natural history and treatment. Am J Surg 1962; 103:70.
114. Durie PR, Forstner GG. Pathophysiology of the exocrine pancreas in cystic fibrosis. J R Soc Med 1989;18(Suppl 16):2.
115. Adrian TE, McKiernan J, Johnstone DI, et al. Hormonal abnormalities of the pancreas and gut in cystic fibrosis. Gastroenterology 1980;79:460.
116. Aggett PJ, Cavanagh NPC, Matthew DJ, et al. Schwachman's syndrome. Arch Dis Child 1980;55:331.
117. Alagille D. Management of chronic cholestasis in childhood. Semin Liver Dis 1985;5:254.

118. Balistreri WF. Neonatal cholestasis. In: Lebenthal E, ed. Textbook of gastroenterology and nutrition in infancy. New York: Raven Press, 1981:1081.
119. Sokol RJ. Medical management of neonatal cholestasis. In: Balistreri WF, Stocker JT, eds. Pediatric hepatology. New York: Hemisphere Publishing, 1990:41.
120. Balistreri WF. Neonatal cholestasis: medical progress. J Pediatr 1985;106:171.
121. Balistreri WF. Neonatal cholestasis: lessons from the past, issues for the future. Semin Liver Dis 1987;7:61.
122. Morecki R, Glaser JH, Cho S, et al. Biliary atresia and reovirus type 3 infection. N Engl J Med 1982;307:481.
123. Morecki R, Glaser J. Reovirus 3 and neonatal biliary disease: discussion of divergent results. Hepatology 1989;10:515.
124. Maggiore G, Bernard O, Hadchouel M, et al. Diagnostic value of serum gamma-glutamyl transpeptidase activity in liver diseases in children. J Pediatr Gastroenterol Nutr 1991;12:21.
125. Faweya AG, Akinyinka OO, Sodeinde O. Duodenal intubation and aspiration test: utility in the differential diagnosis of infantile cholestasis. J Pediatr Gastroenterol Nutr 1991;13:290.
126. Rosenthal P, Miller JH, Sinatra FR. Hepatobiliary scintigraphy and the string test in the evaluation of neonatal cholestasis. J Pediatr Gastroenterol Nutr 1989;8:296.
127. Raffensperger JG. A long-term follow-up of three patients with biliary atresia. J Pediatr Surg 1991;26:176.
128. Alagille D, Odievre M, Gautier M, et al. Syndromic paucity of interlobular bile ducts (Alagille syndrome or arteriohepatic dysplasia): review of 80 cases. J Pediatr 1987;110:195.
129. Tajiri H, Nose O, Shimizu K, et al. Prevention of neonatal HBV infection with the combination of HBIG and HBV vaccine and its long-term efficacy in infants born to HBeAg positive HBV carrier mothers. Acta Paediatr Jpn (Tokyo) 1989; 31:663.
130. Hart MH, Kaufman SS, Vanderhoof JA, et al. Neonatal hepatitis and extrahepatic biliary atresia associated with cytomegalovirus infection in twins. Am J Dis Child 1991;145: 302.
131. Povey S. Genetics of alpha-1-antitrypsin deficiency in relation to neonatal liver disease. Mol Biol Med 1990;7:161.
132. Pittschieler K. Liver disease and heterozygous alpha-1-antitrypsin deficiency. Acta Paediatr Scand 1991;80:323.
133. Bell RL, Ferry GD, Smith EO, et al. Total parenteral nutrition-related cholestasis in infants. J Parenter Enteral Nutr 1986;10:356.
134. Merritt RJ. Cholestasis associated with total parenteral nutrition. J Pediatr Gastroenterol Nutr 1986;5:9.
135. Balistreri WF, Novak DA, Farrell MK. Bile acid metabolism, total parenteral nutrition, and cholestasis. In: Lebenthal E, ed. Total parenteral nutrition: indications, utilization, complications and pathophysiological considerations. New York: Raven Press, 1986:319.
136. Cohen C, Olsen MM. Pediatric total parenteral nutrition, liver histopathology. Arch Pathol Lab Med 1981;105:152.
137. Vanderhoof JA, Langnas AN, Pinch LW, et al. Short bowel syndrome: a review. J Pediatr Gastroenterol Nutr 1992;14: 359.

Neonatology: Pathophysiology and Management of the Newborn, Fourth Edition,
edited by Gordon B. Avery, Mary Ann Fletcher, and Mhairi G. MacDonald.
J.B. Lippincott Company, Philadelphia © 1994.

chapter 38

Jaundice

M. JEFFREY MAISELS

Jaundice is the most common and one of the most vexing problems that can occur in the newborn. Although most jaundiced infants are otherwise perfectly healthy, they make neonatologists anxious because bilirubin is potentially toxic to the central nervous system.

Jaundice occurs when the liver cannot clear sufficient bilirubin from the plasma. When the problem is excessive bilirubin formation or limited uptake and conjugation, unconjugated (*i.e.*, indirect-reacting) bilirubin appears in the blood. When bilirubin glucuronide excretion is impaired (*i.e.*, cholestasis), conjugated monoglucuronide and diglucuronide (*i.e.*, direct-reacting) bilirubin accumulate in plasma and, because of their solubility, also appear in the urine. Reverse-phase high-performance liquid chromatography permits the identification of an additional form of direct-reacting bilirubin, which appears to be formed nonenzymatically from conjugated bilirubin and is irreversibly bound to albumin (Fig. 38-1).[1,2] This fourth fraction—unconjugated, monoglucuronide, and diglucuronide being the first three—δ-bilirubin, reacts directly with the diazo reagent and is covalently bound to albumin to form a biliprotein.[3] Covalent bonds exist between atom pairs that can complete their electronic shells by sharing electrons. Covalent binding to albumin prevents filtration by the glomerulus; thus, δ-bilirubin does not appear in the urine but tends to form an increasing percentage of the total bilirubin during recovery from cholestatic jaundice.[2] The presence of this fraction explains the previously puzzling observation that, in some cases, during recovery from cholestatic jaundice, bilirubin disappears from the urine while the plasma remains icteric. In neonates with indirect hyperbilirubinemia, δ-bilirubin normally represents 5% or less of total bilirubin,[4,5] but in neonates with direct hyperbilirubinemia, 10% to 73% of total bilirubin may be present as δ-bilirubin.[4,5] The concentration of δ-bilirubin in the newborn appears to be related to the duration rather than the cause of the jaundice.[5] The fetus can also produce δ-bilirubin, which was found to represent 13% of total bilirubin at age 6 hours in an infant with neonatal giant-cell hepatitis.[5] Because of its tight binding to albumin, δ-bilirubin might prevent the binding of unconjugated bilirubin to albumin and potentially contribute to bilirubin toxicity.[5]

Other bile pigment species are also found in the blood of patients with cholestatic liver disease. Bilirubin glucuronides are prone to internal rearrangement (*i.e.*, acyl migration). In this reaction, the bilirubin moves rapidly back and forth from one OH group of the glucuronic acid to an adjacent group. Each glucuronide of bilirubin can therefore "spawn a whole family of new compounds that still contain the same proportions of bilirubin and sugar as the parent, but which are not, strictly speaking, glucuronides."[3] The blood from patients with cholestatic jaundice may therefore contain "bilirubin, bilirubin glucuronides, rearranged glucuronides, and biliproteins—not simply a trio, or quartet, but a whole orchestra of bilirubin derivatives in which the glucuronides are not necessarily predominant."[3] With the exception of bilirubin itself, all these substances react directly with the diazo reagent.

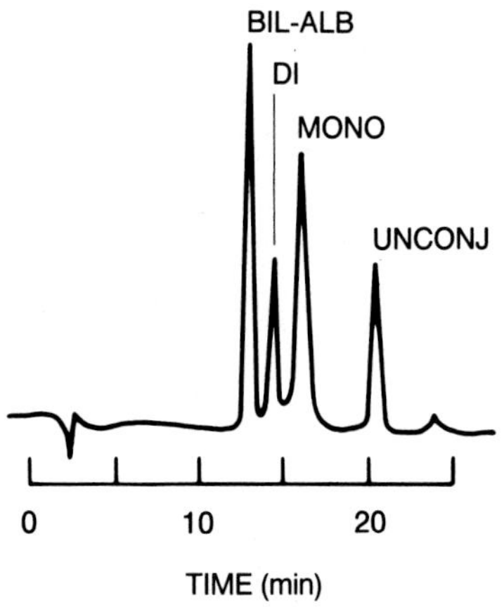

FIG. 38–1. A chromatogram of serum from an adult patient with cholestatic jaundice. (BIL-ALB, albumin-bound δ-bilirubin; DI, diconjugated bilirubin; MONO, monoconjugated bilirubin; UNCONJ, unconjugated bilirubin; from Weiss JS, Gautam A, Lauff JJ, et al. The clinical importance of protein-bound fraction of serum bilirubin in patients with hyperbilirubinemia. N Engl J Med 1983;309:147.)

In most jaundiced neonates, only unconjugated bilirubin is found in the blood, and the accumulated bilirubin is distributed by the circulation throughout the body and produces clinical jaundice. It is generally assumed that to cross intact cell membrane barriers, the bilirubin must be free, or dissociated, from its albumin binding. Unconjugated bilirubin also binds to certain membrane and cell phospholipids.[6]

In severe jaundice, crystals or precipitates of bilirubin may form,[7,8] which might contribute to the toxicity of the pigment. The total bilirubin space has not been measured in a newborn, but studies in normal adults suggest that it is at least twice the plasma volume.[9] In severe, prolonged jaundice, vast quantities of bilirubin are sequestered in the extravascular tissues—far more than can be accommodated in the plasma—and this is not reflected by the serum bilirubin concentration.[10,11]

FORMATION, STRUCTURE, AND PROPERTIES OF BILIRUBIN

Bilirubin is the end product of the catabolism of iron protoporphyrin or heme, of which the major source is circulating hemoglobin. The formation of bilirubin from hemoglobin involves removal of the iron and protein moieties followed by an oxidative process catalyzed by the enzyme microsomal heme oxygenase in which the α-methene bridge of the heme porphyrin ring is opened and carbon monoxide and biliverdin are formed (Fig. 38-2). The iron is salvaged and carbon monoxide excreted by the lungs, leaving the blue–green pigment biliverdin IXα. Biliverdin can be readily excreted in bile, but in mammals it is reduced to bilirubin by NADPH-dependent biliverdin reductase. Because it is derived from cleavage at the α position of the heme ring of ferroprotoporphyrin IX, the product thus formed is known as bilirubin IXα (see Fig. 38-2).

Why a readily excreted, nontoxic molecule (*i.e.*, biliverdin) is converted into a poorly excreted toxic molecule (*i.e.*, bilirubin) is not clear but might be explained by the fact that biliverdin is poorly transported by the placenta.[12] If biliverdin were the end product of heme catabolism, it would be trapped on the fetal side of the placenta, yielding fluorescent blue–green infants.[13] In addition, bilirubin appears to

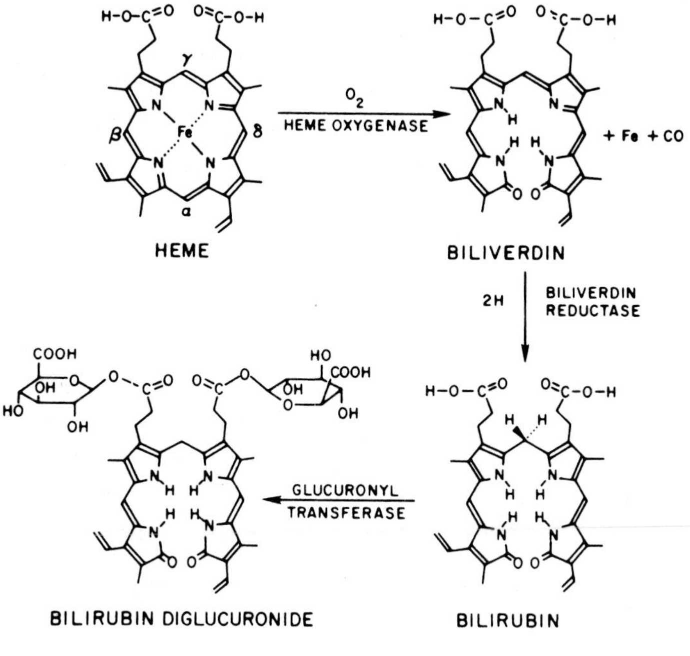

FIG. 38–2. Biosynthesis of bilirubin. (From Lightner DA, McDonagh AF. Molecular mechanisms of phototherapy of neonatal jaundice. Accounts of Chemical Research 1984;17:417.)

have an important role as an antioxidant, which may be beneficial to the newborn.[14]

A linear representation of bilirubin is shown in Figure 38-3. Trace amounts of other bilirubin isomers, including bilirubin IXβ, IXγ, IXδ, are found in human bile,[15] and bilirubin exists in the plasma in a variety of forms that determine its biologic properties. The ionic species of bilirubin are shown in Figure 38-4. Although these structures are conventionally illustrated in Figures 38-2 and 38-3, McDonagh points out that they "no more represent the shape of bilirubin than a snapshot of a baby represents its shape or weight. In fact, bilirubin, like a healthy, kicking infant, has no fixed shape. It is a flexible molecule that can assume a large number of shapes of different stability."[3]

X-ray diffraction studies[16] and nuclear magnetic resonance spectroscopy show one stable (*i.e.*, ridge-tile) conformation of bilirubin (Fig. 38-5). It is likely that this is the prevalent structure in plasma because it is consistent with the biologic properties of bilirubin. In this conformation, the bilirubin molecule is stabilized by the presence of intramolecular hydrogen bonds, and the hydrophilic polar COOH and NH groups are not available for the attachment of water. The hydrophobic hydrocarbon groups are on the perimeter, rendering the molecule insoluble in water but soluble in nonpolar solvents, such as chloroform.[3] Under these circumstances, bilirubin behaves like other lipophilic substances (*e.g.*, dioxin, polychlorinated biphenyls)—it is difficult to excrete but crosses biologic membranes, such as the placenta, blood–brain barrier, and hepatocyte plasma membrane, easily.[3] Brodersen questioned the long-held belief that bilirubin is lipophilic, although he found that bilirubin forms a complex with phosphatidylcholine (*i.e.*, lecithin), a major component of cell membranes.[17] McDonagh argues that the biologic properties are entirely consistent with those of a lipophil,[3,18] and this has been confirmed by recent studies.[19]

In an alkaline medium, after the structure is opened and the hydrogen-bonding groups are exposed (see Fig. 38-4), the molecule can form a soluble sodium or potassium salt. The addition of methanol or ethanol interferes with the hydrogen bonding and results in an immediate diazo reaction—the basis for the measurement of indirect bilirubin by the Van den Bergh reaction.

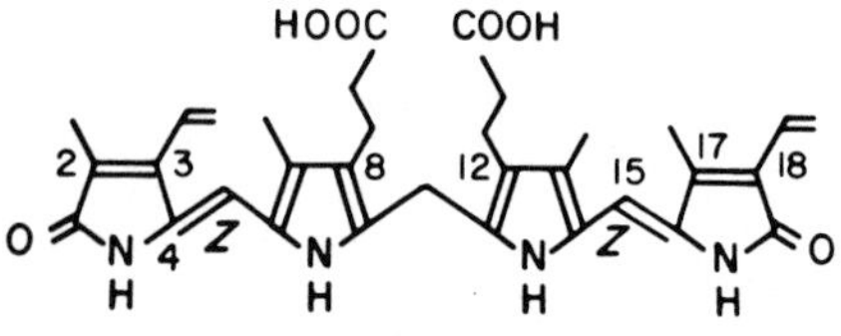

FIG. 38–3. The chemical structure of bilirubin. (From McDonagh AF, Lightner DA. "Like a shrivelled blood orange": bilirubin, jaundice and phototherapy. Pediatrics 1985;75:443.)

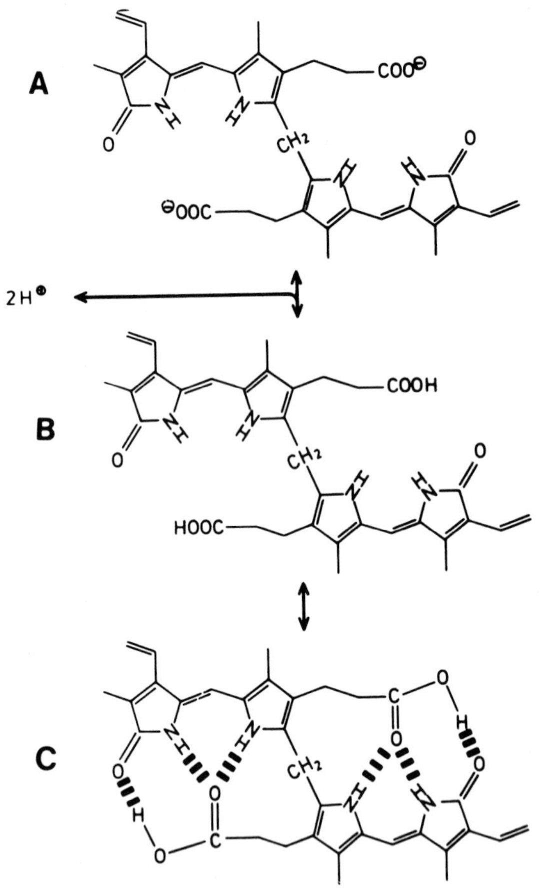

FIG. 38–4. Ionic species of bilirubin. **(A)** The dianion combines with two protons and forms **(B)** bilirubin acid, which is then stabilized internally by **(C)** the formation of intramolecular hydrogen bonds. (From Brodersen R. Binding of bilirubin to albumin. CRC Crit Rev Clin Lab Sci 1980;11:305.)

FETAL BILIRUBIN METABOLISM

BILIRUBIN IN AMNIOTIC FLUID

Bilirubin can be detected in normal amniotic fluid after about 12 weeks of gestation, but it disappears by 36 to 37 weeks. Increased levels of bilirubin in the amniotic fluid are observed in the presence of fetal unconjugated hyperbilirubinemia and can be used to predict the severity of Rh hemolytic disease (see Hemolytic Disease). Increased amniotic fluid bilirubin levels and bile acid concentrations are found in the presence of fetal intestinal obstruction if the obstruction occurs distal to the ampulla of Vater, but not in the presence of esophageal or pyloric atresia.[20–22]

It is not known precisely how bilirubin gets into the amniotic fluid. Suggested routes include tracheobronchial secretions; excretion by way of the mucosa of the upper gastrointestinal tract or the fetal urine and meconium; diffusion across the umbilical cord and fetal skin; and transfer from the maternal circulation. The most likely of these mechanisms appears to

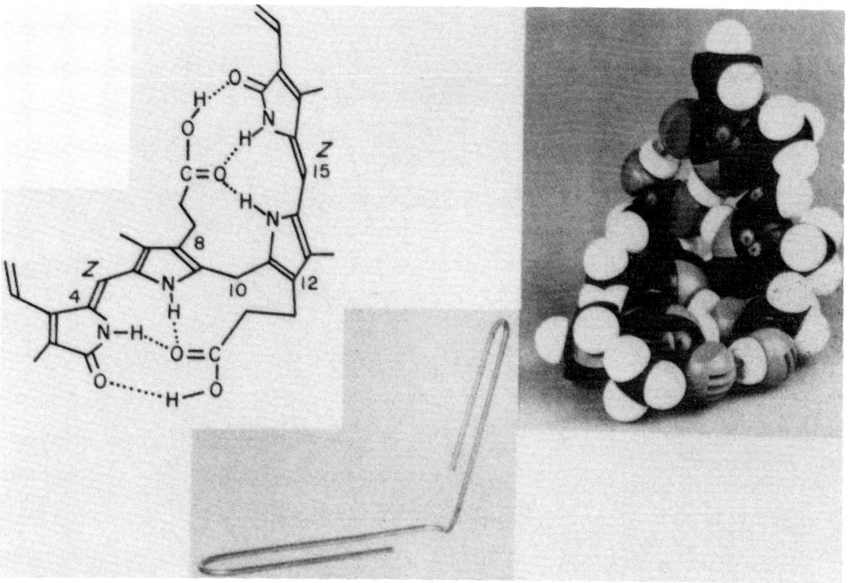

FIG. 38–5. Preferred conformation of bilirubin. Chemical structure (*left*). Bent paper clip analogy (*middle*). Space-filling molecular model (*right*). Each representation is asymmetric and has a nonsuperimposable mirror image, like a D- or L-amino acid. Only one of the two possible mirror-image forms is shown in each representation. (From McDonagh AF, Lightner DA. "Like a shrivelled blood orange": bilirubin, jaundice and phototherapy. Pediatrics 1985;75:443.)

be the first. Studies in rabbits demonstrate a correlation between increased serum unconjugated bilirubin concentrations and increased tracheal fluid bilirubin concentrations.[23]

BILIRUBIN PRODUCTION, HEPATIC FUNCTION, AND PLACENTAL TRANSFER

The rate of bilirubin production in the fetus has not been determined, but it is reasonable to assume that it is at least as great as that in the newborn (see Neonatal Bilirubin Metabolism).

In early fetal life, plasma albumin concentrations are low, but bilirubin binds to α-fetoprotein.[24] The ability of human fetal liver to remove bilirubin from the circulation and to conjugate bilirubin is severely limited, although some uridine diphosphoglucuronosyl transferase (UDPGT) activity can be detected by 16 weeks of gestation.[25,26] Until recently, a detailed analysis of the development of human hepatic UDPGT had not been performed because, before the introduction of high-pressure liquid chromatography, it was not possible to measure very low concentrations of bilirubin glucuronide. Onishi and colleagues studied the prenatal and postnatal development of UDPGT activity in the livers of fetuses after elective abortions, in preterm and full-term infants at autopsy, and in laparotomy samples obtained from infants and adults (Figs. 38-6 through 38-8).[26,27] Between 17 and 30 weeks of gestation, although UDPGT activity was only 0.1% of adult values, bilirubin glucuronide was detected, indicating that the UDPGT is active *in vivo.* Between 30 and 40 weeks of gestation, UDPGT activity in fetuses and in preterm and full-term newborns surviving less than 7 days increased tenfold to 1% of adult values (see Fig. 38-6). After birth, however, activity increased exponentially, reaching adult levels by 6 to 14 weeks (see Fig. 38-6). Marked postnatal development of UDPGT activity occurs in infants who survive more than 8 days and is independent of gestation (see Figs. 38-7 and 38-8).

Bilirubin pigment in fetal bile also has been studied in detail.[28] Until 14 weeks of gestation, no bile pigments are detectable. Between 14 and 15 weeks of gestation, bilirubin IXβ is the only bile pigment detected, and it is the predominant bilirubin up to 20 weeks of gestation; although between 16 and 17 weeks of gestation, some unconjugated bilirubin IXα is present. Between 20 and 30 weeks of gestation, bilirubin IXα glucuronide appears, and at 30 weeks of gestation, monoconjugates of bilirubin IXα are the predominant types of bilirubin present. In the full-term fetus, bilirubin IXα monoglucuronide is the major bilirubin derivative.

The major route of fetal bilirubin excretion is across the placenta. Because virtually all the fetal plasma bilirubin is unconjugated, it is readily transferred across the placenta to the maternal circulation, where it is excreted by the maternal liver.[29–32] Using high-performance liquid chromatography, Rosenthal measured serum bilirubin concentrations in umbilical arterial and venous blood in full-term infants at birth. In all samples, bilirubin consisted entirely of unconjugated pigment. The mean serum bilirubin level in umbilical arterial blood was 5.1 ± 1.8 mg/dL (86.6 ± 31.2 μmol/L), and it was 2.7 ± 0.7 mg/dL (45.6 ± 12.6 μmol/L) in umbilical venous blood. The bilirubin concentration in blood flowing from the fetus to the placenta was nearly twice that of blood returning from the placenta to the fetus, indicating that the placenta clears bilirubin efficiently from the fetal circulation. Mean maternal serum bilirubin concentrations were 0.5 ± .16 mg/dL (7.7 ± 2.8 μmol/L), confirming the

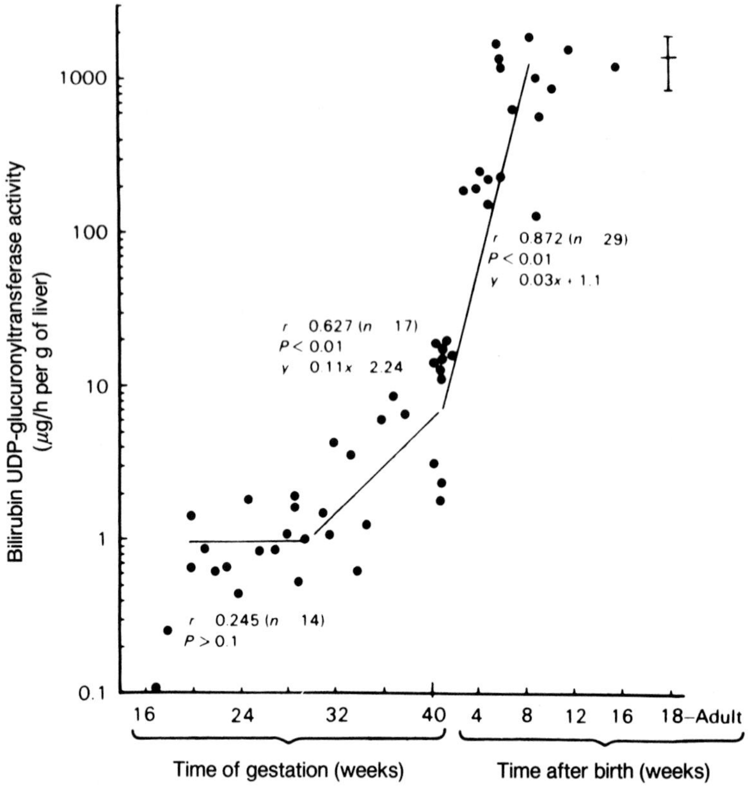

FIG. 38–6. Developmental pattern of human hepatic UDPGT activity. Samples were obtained from the livers of fetuses after elective abortions, at autopsy from premature and full-term newborns who survived less than 7 days, and from liver biopsies of infants, children, and adults undergoing laparotomy. Each point represents the activity of the liver homogenate of a single patient, but results for patients older than 18 weeks of age are shown as a mean ± SD. (From Kawade N, Onishi S. The prenatal and postnatal development of UDP-glucuronyl transferase activity toward bilirubin and the effect of premature birth on this activity in the human liver. Biochem J 1981;196:257.)

gradient of bilirubin flow from the fetus to the mother.[31] Thus, the newborn is rarely born jaundiced, except in the presence of severe hemolytic disease, when there may be an accumulation of unconjugated bilirubin in the fetus. Conjugated bilirubin is not transferred across the placenta, and it may also accumulate in the fetal plasma and other tissues.

MATERNAL HYPERBILIRUBINEMIA AND ITS EFFECT ON THE FETUS

Obstetricians and pediatricians occasionally are confronted with a pregnant mother who has hyperbilirubinemia as a result of hemolytic anemia or liver disease. Reported cases in the literature provide evidence for transfer of unconjugated bilirubin from the mother to her fetus. In four cases,[33–36] mothers developed cholestatic jaundice with elevations of both direct and indirect serum bilirubin concentrations. In all four, the indirect bilirubin levels in the umbilical cord blood were similar to the maternal serum level, with a difference of 1 to 3.8 mg/dL (17–65 μmol/L); large differences of 9.3 to 20.2 mg/dL (159–345 μmol/L) were found in the direct bilirubin levels. These data are consistent with the transfer of unconjugated but not conjugated bilirubin from mother to fetus. They do not, however, rule out the possibility that the elevation in maternal bilirubin concentration prevented the normal transfer of fetal unconjugated bilirubin across the placenta. In two pregnant mothers with homozygous sickle-cell anemia, the development of a crisis led to an acute elevation of indirect bilirubin to levels of 13 and 15 mg/dL (222 and 257 μmol/L), respectively, at the time of delivery.[37] Cord blood concentrations in these infants, however, were only 1.9 and 1.6 mg/dL (32 and 27 μmol/L), respectively. This suggests that transfer of bilirubin between the maternal and fetal circulations may be relatively slow. Of the cases described, two infants died. In one, the autopsy findings revealed no evidence of kernicterus.[35] The other infant expired on the first day, and clinical signs of kernicterus were said to have developed. No further clinical details were provided, however, nor was there any autopsy information.[34] The other infants survived. One was reported to be normal at 14 months of age,[36] and the other was followed only to age 3 months.[33] In the two infants whose mothers had only indirect hyperbilirubinemia, no follow-up data were provided. Thus, no conclusions can be reached regarding the possible effect of maternal hyperbilirubinemia on the developmental outcome of the offspring.

Maternal hyperbilirubinemia may have other adverse effects on reproduction. Of 28 pregnancies in women with Dubin–Johnson syndrome, only 9 resulted in normal deliveries and normal infants.[38] Whether this represents a causative association is speculative. The jaundiced female Gunn rat is frequently infertile, and plasma bilirubin levels are lower in those rats that do conceive.[39] Davis and colleagues fed activated charcoal to jaundiced Gunn rats and found that this was effective in reducing the

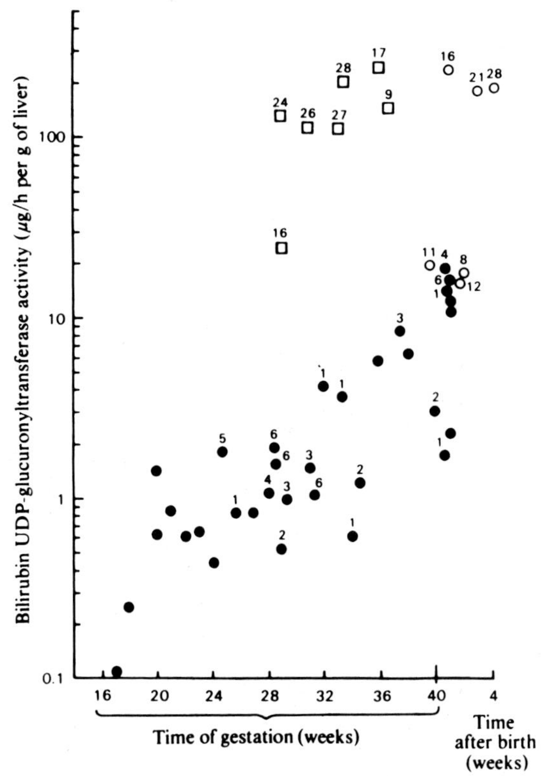

FIG. 38–7. Effect of premature birth on the development of UDPGT activity. Numbers beside symbols represent age in days at which death occurred. Note that after birth there is a rapid increase in UDPGT activity irrespective of gestational age. (●, fetuses and preterm and full-term infants who died within 7 days of birth; □, preterm infants who survived longer than 8 days; ○, full-term infants who survived longer than 8 days; from Kawade N, Onishi S. The prenatal and postnatal development of UDP-glucuronyl transferase activity toward bilirubin and the effect of premature birth on this activity in the human liver. Biochem J 1981;196:257.)

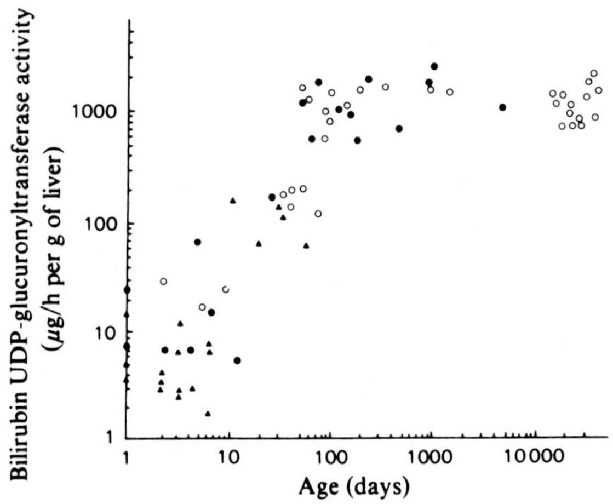

FIG. 38–8. Postnatal development of human hepatic UDPGT activity. (●, samples obtained at autopsy; ○, samples obtained after laparotomy; ▲, samples obtained from preterm infants; from Onishi S, Kawade N, Itoh S, et al. Postnatal development of uridine diphosphate glucuronyl transferase activity towards bilirubin and O-aminophenol in human liver. Biochem J 1979;194;705.)

plasma bilirubin levels by as much as 40%.[40] Forty-eight percent of charcoal-fed, *versus* 7% of control female rats, that were continuously mated produced a live litter. These findings support the possibility of an adverse effect of bilirubin on reproduction in the female Gunn rat.

NEONATAL BILIRUBIN METABOLISM

BILIRUBIN PRODUCTION

The normal destruction of circulating erythrocytes accounts for about 75% of the daily bilirubin production in the newborn. Senescent erythrocytes are removed and destroyed in the reticuloendothelial system, where the hemoglobin is catabolized and converted to bilirubin. One g of hemoglobin yields 35 mg of bilirubin.

A significant contribution (25% or more) to the daily production of bilirubin in the neonate comes from sources other than effete erythrocytes (Fig. 38-9). These sources are collectively known as the early-

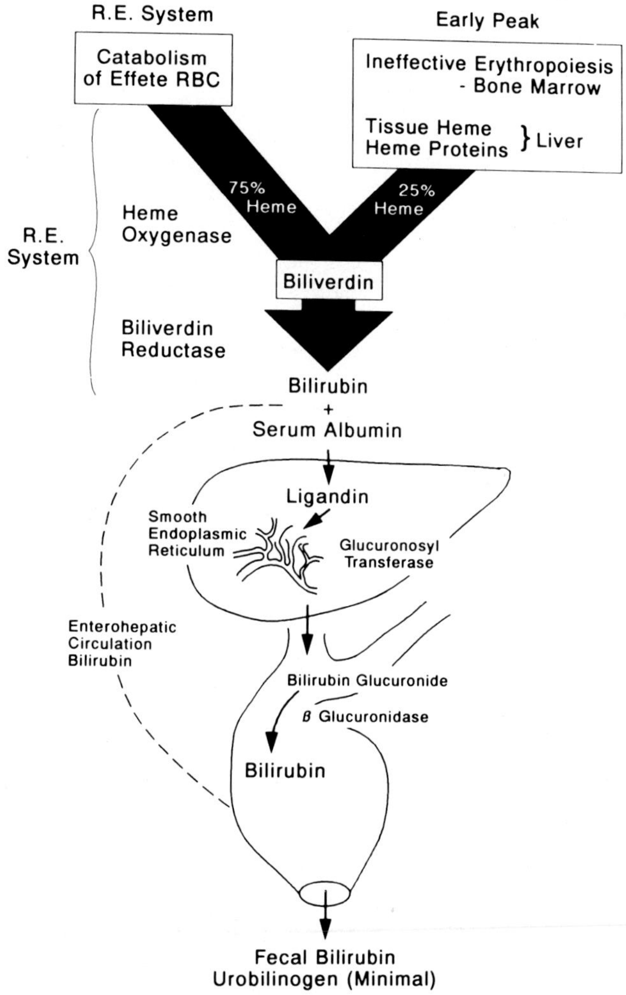

FIG. 38–9. Neonatal bile pigment metabolism. (R.E., reticuloendothelial; RBC, erythrocyte.)

labeled peak of bile pigment, a description based on the observation of an early peak of radioactivity that appears as labeled stercobilin in the stool within minutes to days after the administration of labeled glycine or δ-aminolevulinic acid.[41] This early bilirubin consists of two major components:

1. A nonerythropoietic component resulting from the turnover of nonhemoglobin heme protein and free heme, primarily in the liver
2. An erythropoietic component arising primarily from ineffective erythropoiesis and the destruction of immature erythrocyte precursors, either in the bone marrow or soon after release into the circulation.

TRANSPORT AND HEPATIC UPTAKE OF BILIRUBIN

Once bilirubin leaves the reticuloendothelial system, it is transported in the plasma and bound reversibly to albumin at a high-affinity primary binding site with a binding constant of 6.8×10^7 mol^{-1}.[42] At *p*H 7.4, the solubility of bilirubin is low—about 4 nm/L (0.24 mg/dL)—and at the bilirubin levels normally found in infants and adults, bilirubin must be bound to its carrier, albumin, so that the concentration of unbound (*i.e.*, free) bilirubin remains low.

The parenchymal cells of the liver have a selective and highly efficient capacity for removing unconjugated bilirubin from the plasma, but exactly how this is achieved remains controversial.[43] When the bilirubin–albumin complex reaches the plasma membrane of the hepatocyte, a proportion of the bilirubin, but not the albumin, is transferred across the cell membrane into the hepatocyte, where it is bound to soluble proteins (Fig. 38-10). The transfer of bilirubin from plasma to the liver cell is carrier-mediated.[43] Intracellularly, bilirubin binds, in part, to ligandin (*i.e.*, Y protein, glutathione S-transferase B) and possibly other cytosolic-binding proteins.[44]

Bilirubin flux across the hepatocyte membrane is bidirectional; in normal adults, about 40% of the bilirubin taken up by the hepatocytes in a single pass through the liver refluxes, unchanged, back into plasma.[44] Although ligandin does not appear to participate directly in the hepatic uptake of bilirubin, it probably decreases the efflux of bilirubin back into the plasma, thus increasing net hepatic uptake.[44] The administration of phenobarbital increases the concentration of ligandin and provides more intracellular

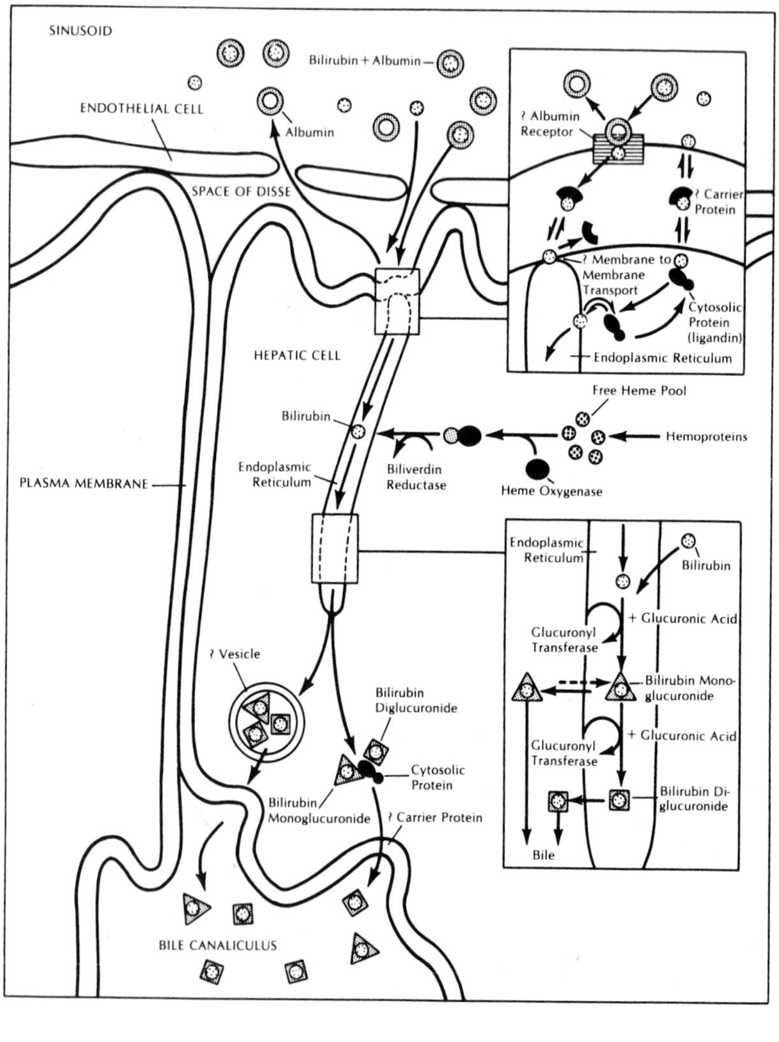

FIG. 38–10. Bilirubin transport and conjugation in the hepatocyte. Two mechanisms have been proposed for uptake of bilirubin from the extracellular environment: by means of an albumin receptor or directly. In either case, carrier protein may be involved in transmembrane passage (*upper box*). Transport into the endoplasmic reticulum is facilitated by complexing to ligandin, but direct membrane-to-membrane transfer also may occur. Cytosolic bilirubin is in equilibrium with endoplasmic reticulum bilirubin. The hypothesis of conjugation of insoluble bilirubin to polar glucuronides (*lower box*). Conjugated bilirubin may enter the bile canaliculi either by vesicular transport or by carrier-mediated transport. (From Gollan JL, Knapp AB. Bilirubin metabolism and congenital jaundice. Hosp Pract 1985;February:87.)

binding sites for bilirubin.[45] Bilirubin might also be transported intracellularly by direct membrane-to-membrane transfer (see Fig. 38-10).[44]

CONJUGATION AND EXCRETION OF BILIRUBIN

Because of its hydrogen-bonded conformation (see Formation, Structure, and Properties of Bilirubin), unconjugated (*i.e.*, indirect-reacting) bilirubin is nonpolar and insoluble in aqueous solutions at *p*H 7.4 and must be converted to its water-soluble conjugate (*i.e.*, direct-reacting bilirubin) before it can be excreted (see Fig. 38-10). This is achieved when bilirubin is combined enzymatically with a sugar, glucuronic acid, producing a new pigment that is more water-soluble and sufficiently polar to be excreted into the bile or filtered through the kidney. Esterification with glucuronic acid leads to the formation of one of the two isomers of bilirubin monoglucuronide (*i.e.*, C8 or C12) or diglucuronide, if esterification occurs in both the C8 and C12 positions of the carboxyl groups of the propionic acid side chains.[44]

Formation of the monoglucuronide is catalyzed by the enzyme hepatic urdine diphosphoglucuronosyl transferase (UDPGT), primarily located in the rough and smooth endoplasmic reticulum. The nomenclature for the bilirubin-conjugating enzyme has changed from uridine diphosphoglucuronyl transferase to UDPGT.[46] Bilirubin UDPGT belongs to a family of UDPGT isoenzymes that metabolize endogenous compounds and various food chemicals in most tissues.[47] This nomenclature is preferred because the enzyme that glucuronodates bilirubin catalyzes the transfer of a glucuronosyl group.

Conversion of both monoglucuronide isomers (*i.e.*, C8 and C12) to diglucuronide also is mediated by UDPGT, although the capacity of the enzyme system for *in vitro* diglucuronide formation appears to be much lower than that for monoglucuronide synthesis.[44] This may explain why patients with Gilbert syndrome or Crigler–Najjar type II disease have more monoglucuronide than diglucuronide present in their bile. Nevertheless, bilirubin diglucuronide is the major pigment found in normal human and rat bile. The reason for this is not clear, and the precise mechanism for the *in vivo* formation of bilirubin diglucuronide remains uncertain.

Rosenthal and colleagues used high performance liquid chromatography to measure serum bilirubin conjugates. In healthy adults, pregnant women at term, and in cord bloods from uncomplicated deliveries, total bilirubin concentrations did not exceed 2 mg/dL, and the bilirubin was entirely unconjugated.[48] In contrast, serum bilirubin concentrations in cord blood samples from infants with blood-group incompatibility and intrauterine hypoxia exceeded 2 mg/dL and contained conjugated bilirubin. These data confirm that in the presence of elevated bilirubin concentrations *in utero,* bilirubin UDPGT activity can be induced prematurely. In both premature and full-term infants, measurable amounts of esterified bilirubin appeared within 24 to 48 hours after birth. A distinct sequence of conjugating activity appears to occur, with monoconjugated bilirubin appearing in the serum during the first 24 to 48 hours followed by the diconjugated esters, which represent 21% of the total esters by the third day. The predominant bilirubin conjugate fraction observed is the C8 monoester. These conjugates are detectable once the total serum bilirubin level exceeds 2 mg/dL. Bilirubin esters were also detected in serum samples of a premature infant of only 25 weeks of gestation, and conjugated bilirubin levels were higher in the serum of full-term infants than premature infants.[48] The entire conjugated fraction, however, normally accounts for only 2% to 5% of the total bilirubin.

The fact that conjugates do not appear until the total serum bilirubin level increases suggests that bilirubin plays an important role in the initiation of its own conjugation after birth. The ratio of conjugated to total bilirubin remains constant during the period of physiologic jaundice. If cholestasis were present, the conjugated bilirubin fraction would be expected to increase progressively, but accumulation of conjugated bilirubin does not contribute significantly to physiologic jaundice. This differs from observations of bile acid transport in human newborns. Newborns have elevated serum bile acid concentrations, impaired bile acid uptake, and impaired transport and excretion of organic anions.[49]

TRANSFER OF BILIRUBIN INTO BILE AND INTESTINAL TRANSPORT

After conjugation, bilirubin is excreted rapidly into the bile canaliculi by the liver cell, a process that requires metabolic work for the active transport of bilirubin across a large concentration gradient (see Fig. 38-10). Canalicular excretion, like bilirubin uptake, appears to be a carrier-mediated process that is saturable and is rate-limiting in the overall transport of bilirubin from blood to bile.[44] Interference with this process is probably responsible for the hyperbilirubinemia associated with hepatocellular disorders such as hepatitis.

Once in the small intestine, conjugated bilirubin is not reabsorbed. In the healthy adult, it is largely reduced by the action of colonic bacteria to a series of colorless tetrapyrroles, collectively known as urobilinogen. The term stercobilinogen, synonymous with urobilinogen, is no longer used. An insignificant amount is hydrolyzed to unconjugated bilirubin and reabsorbed by way of the enterohepatic circulation. In the newborn, however, this enterohepatic circulation of bilirubin may be significant (see Physiologic Jaundice). In conditions involving high plasma bilirubin levels and poor hepatic excretion, there is a gradient for unconjugated bilirubin from the plasma to the intestinal lumen, and significant amounts of unconjugated bilirubin may be cleared by diffusion across the intestinal wall. Figure 38-9 summarizes bile pigment metabolism in the newborn.

Recent reviews of the chemistry and metabolism of bilirubin can be found elsewhere.[43,44,50,51]

PHYSIOLOGIC MECHANISMS OF NEONATAL JAUNDICE

INCREASED BILIRUBIN LOAD ON THE LIVER CELL

BILIRUBIN PRODUCTION

Measurements of carbon monoxide, which is produced in equimolar quantities with bilirubin, show that the normal newborn produces an average of 8 to 10 mg/kg (137–171 μmol/L) of bilirubin per day.[52,53] Similar rates of bilirubin production have been found in low-birth-weight infants.[52] This is more than twice the rate of normal daily bilirubin production in the adult and is explained by the fact that the neonate has a higher circulating erythrocyte volume, a shorter mean erythrocyte life span, and a larger early-labeled bilirubin peak. Bilirubin production decreases with increasing postnatal age but is still about twice the adult rate by age 2 weeks.[52]

ENTEROHEPATIC CIRCULATION

The newborn probably reabsorbs much larger quantities of unconjugated bilirubin, by way of the enterohepatic circulation, than does the adult. Infants have fewer bacteria in the small and large bowel and greater activity of the deconjugating enzyme, β-glucuronidase.[54,55] As a result, conjugated bilirubin, which is not reabsorbed, is not converted to urobilinogen but is hydrolyzed to unconjugated bilirubin, which is then reabsorbed, thus increasing the bilirubin load on an already stressed liver. Studies in newborn humans and monkeys suggest that the enterohepatic circulation of bilirubin is a significant contributor to physiologic jaundice.[56,57]

DECREASED CLEARANCE OF BILIRUBIN FROM THE PLASMA

UPTAKE

Ligandin, the predominant bilirubin-binding protein in the human liver cell, is deficient in the liver of newborn monkeys. It reaches adult levels by 5 days of age, coinciding with a fall in bilirubin levels and a normal hepatic uptake of sulfobromophthalein.[58] The administration of phenobarbital enhances hepatic uptake of sulfobromophthalein and simultaneously increases the concentration of ligandin.[59] Although this suggests that impaired uptake may contribute to the pathogenesis of physiologic jaundice, uptake does not appear to be rate-limiting during phase I (see Physiologic Jaundice)[56]; however, it may be important during phase II, the low-grade but more persistent stage of physiologic jaundice.

CONJUGATION

Deficient glucuronosyl transferase activity, with resultant impairment of bilirubin conjugation, has long been considered a major cause of physiologic jaundice. Studies in full-term newborn rhesus monkeys revealed virtually no hepatic glucuronosyl transferase activity in the first 24 hours.[56] Activity increased over the next 48 hours, coincident with a decline in serum bilirubin levels (*i.e.*, descending curve of phase I). By 48 hours, activity levels were close to those of the adult, but enzyme maturation in two premature infants was markedly delayed. In a single postmature monkey, activity at 4 hours of age was 10 times greater than that of full-term animals of comparable age. In human infants, the early postnatal increase in serum bilirubin appears to play an important role in the initiation of bilirubin conjugation.[48]

The administration of phenobarbital (5 mg/kg/day for 6 weeks) to pregnant monkeys and in similar dosage to their infants increased hepatic glucuronosyl transferase activity by almost threefold—sufficient to abolish completely phase I physiologic jaundice. Using high-pressure liquid chromatography, Onishi and colleagues studied the activity of UDPGT toward bilirubin in human subjects.[26,27] Liver samples were obtained from patients who underwent laparotomy or from autopsies of infants. In the first 10 days of life, UDPGT activity in full-term and premature neonates was usually less than 0.1% of adult values, although some infants showed activity between 0.1% and 1% (see Figs. 38-6 through 38-8). Thereafter, UDPGT activity increased at an exponential rate, reaching adult values by 6 to 14 weeks of age, after which it remained constant.[26] The postnatal increase in UDPGT activity was independent of the infants' gestation (see Fig. 38-7). These observations are consistent with the pivotal role of deficient glucuronosyl transferase activity and bilirubin conjugation in the first phase of neonatal jaundice.

EXCRETION

The absence of an elevated serum level of conjugated bilirubin in physiologic jaundice suggests that, under normal circumstances, the neonatal liver cell is capable of excreting the bilirubin that it has just conjugated. Nevertheless, the ability of the newborn liver to excrete conjugated bilirubin and other anions (*e.g.*, drugs, hormones) is more limited than that of the older child or adult and may become rate-limiting when the bilirubin load is significantly increased. Thus, when intrauterine hyperbilirubinemia occurs, usually as a result of isoimmunization, it is not uncommon to find an elevated serum level of conjugated bilirubin.[48]

EPIDEMIOLOGY OF NEONATAL JAUNDICE

Various factors in the epidemiology of neonatal jaundice are described in Table 38-1.

TABLE 38–1
EPIDEMIOLOGY OF NEONATAL JAUNDICE

	Effect on Neonatal Serum Bilirubin Levels		
Associated Factors	Increase	Decrease	No Effect
Race	East Asian Native American Greek	African American	
Genetic or familial	Previous sibling with jaundice		
Maternal	Primipara (?) Older mothers Diabetes Hypertension Oral contraceptive use at time of conception First-trimester bleeding Decreased plasma zinc level	Smoking	
Drugs administered to mother	Oxytocin Diazepam Epidural anesthesia Promethazine	Phenobarbital Meperidine Reserpine Aspirin Chloral hydrate Heroin Phenytoin Antipyrine Alcohol	Beta-adrenergic agents
Labor and delivery	Premature rupture of membranes Forceps delivery Vacuum extraction Breech delivery		Fetal distress Low Apgar scores
Infant	Low birth weight Prematurity Male gender Delayed cord clamping Elevated cord blood bilirubin level Delayed meconium passage Breast-feeding Caloric deprivation Larger weight loss after birth Low serum zinc and magnesium		
Drugs administered to infant	Choral hydrate		
Other	Altitude		

GENETIC, ETHNIC, AND FAMILIAL INFLUENCES

East Asian[60–65] and Native American[66–68] infants have mean maximal serum bilirubin concentrations that are significantly higher than those of Caucasian populations. Measurements of carbon monoxide production and blood carboxyhemoglobin levels suggest that increased bilirubin production is an important factor contributing to hyperbilirubinemia in these infants.[66,69,70]

In certain areas of Greece, there is a remarkably high incidence of idiopathic hyperbilirubinemia and an increased incidence of kernicterus.[71] Although glucose-6-phosphate dehydrogenase (G6PD) deficiency is more common in East Asian and Greek infants, it does not account for these startling differences in the incidence and severity of hyperbilirubinemia.[72] Japanese infants living in the United States have a much higher incidence of hyperbilirubinemia and higher mean bilirubin levels than do their American counterparts,[63,70] but infants born in Australia of parents who have emigrated from Greece do not have higher bilirubin levels than Australian infants.[73] Environmental rather than genetic factors appear to be important in this population. Black infants in the United States and in Great Britain have lower bilirubin levels than Caucasian infants (Table 38-2).[62,64,74,75]

Neonatal jaundice runs in families, which suggests that, to some extent, the risk of jaundice is genetically determined.[76–78] Khoury and colleagues studied 3301 infants and found that if previous siblings had a serum bilirubin level higher than 12 mg/dL (205 μmol/L) or higher than 15 mg/dL (257 μmol/L), the risk of similar bilirubin levels in subsequent siblings was 3.1 and 12.5 times greater, respectively, than in siblings of infants who did not have that degree of jaundice.[77] Nielsen and colleagues also found a highly significant

TABLE 38–2
EFFECT OF RACE ON THE INCIDENCE OF HYPERBILIRUBINEMIA

Peak Bilirubin Concentration (mg/dL)	Percentage East Asian	Caucasian	African American	References
≥10	49	20	12	Lin et al. 1985[64]*
≥12		13	7	Friedman et al. 1978[62]†
≥13	23	10	4	Newman 1990[75]‡
		6	4	Hardy 1979[74]
≥15	19	7	2	Lin et al. 1985[64]*

* About 7% of infants in this study were born at <37 weeks of gestation or weighed <2500 g.
† Includes preterm and low-birth-weight infants from total population of 12,461 (percentage unknown).
‡ All infants weighed ≥2500 g.

correlation between the peak bilirubin levels of siblings.[78]

MATERNAL FACTORS

SMOKING

Most studies suggest that infants of mothers who smoke during pregnancy have lower serum bilirubin levels than infants of nonsmokers,[64,79–83] but others have not found this.[76,84] Women who smoked at least one pack of cigarettes per day had a lower risk of having a child with hyperbilirubinemia than those who smoked less.[64] The data are confounded by the finding that women who smoke are much less likely to breast-feed[81] and that the incidence of breast-feeding is inversely related to the number of cigarettes smoked per day.[85] Breast-fed infants have higher serum bilirubin levels than bottle-fed infants (see Breast-Feeding and Jaundice).

DIABETES

As a group, infants of insulin-dependent diabetic mothers are more likely to become jaundiced than control infants,[81,86,87] but closer scrutiny suggests that hyperbilirubinemia in infants born to insulin-dependent diabetic mothers occurs mainly in those that are large for their gestational age[88,89] or have an increased birth weight–length ratio.[86] A direct relation has been found between the amount of carbon monoxide excreted—an index of bilirubin production—and the degree of macrosomia in these infants[90,91]; those who are large for their gestational age, but not those appropriate for their gestational age, have significantly higher bilirubin and carboxyhemoglobin levels than control infants.[89] These studies suggest that increased bilirubin production contributes to the hyperbilirubinemia of macrosomic infants of insulin-dependent diabetic mothers.

Ineffective erythropoiesis and polycythemia are probably responsible for the increased bilirubin production found in these infants. Infants of diabetic mothers have high erythropoietin levels and evidence of increased erythropoiesis[92]; as many as 24% of macrosomic infants of insulin-dependent diabetic mothers are polycythemic.[88] In addition, diabetic mothers have a threefold greater concentration of β-glucuronidase in their breast milk than nondiabetic mothers.[88] This enzyme enhances the enterohepatic circulation of bilirubin and could be an additional contributor to hyperbilirubinemia in breast-fed infants of insulin-dependent diabetic mothers.

OTHER FACTORS

Hyperbilirubinemia has been associated with primiparous mothers in some studies,[76,83] but not in others.[64,93] Gale and colleagues found a significant association between neonatal jaundice and increasing maternal age; teenage mothers had the lowest risk for hyperbilirubinemia.[76]

EFFECT OF EVENTS DURING LABOR AND DELIVERY

INDUCTION OF LABOR BY OXYTOCIN

The potential association between hyperbilirubinemia and the use of oxytocin to induce or augment labor has interested a surprising number of investigators, and several authors have reported an increased incidence of neonatal hyperbilirubinemia after induction of labor with oxytocin.[62,94–102] Caution must be exercised in interpreting positive results because of the possibility that the oxytocin-induced groups in these studies contained a greater number of less mature infants. Using linear logistic regression analysis in a prospective study of 739 infants, Lange and colleagues found a marginal effect of oxytocic agents but a highly significant influence of gestational age on the risk of jaundice.[103] Three controlled trials compared the incidence of hyperbilirubinemia in full-term infants after induction of labor with prostaglandin E_2 or oxytocin. There was a 30% increase in the incidence of jaundice, with bilirubin levels higher than 10 mg/dL (171–205 μmol/L) in infants of mothers who received oxytocin.[95,103–105]

The mechanism for the putative increase in serum bilirubin in association with oxytocin administration is unknown. It is possible that, in many cases, infants delivered after oxytocin induction are less mature than those delivered spontaneously. Others have suggested that hyperbilirubinemia is the result of hemolysis following erythrocyte swelling and loss of deformability.[94,106] Oxytocin is known to exert an antidiuretic effect, and it is commonly administered with relatively large quantities of electrolyte-free dextrose solutions. The infants born to these mothers show significant hyponatremia, hypoosmolality, and enhanced osmotic fragility of erythrocytes.[106] These infants also have lower hematocrits, decreased plasma haptoglobin, and increased plasma lactate dehydrogenase activity compared with those born after spontaneous labor.[94] With this hemolytic mechanism in mind, Johnson and colleagues administered minimal amounts of free water to mothers receiving oxytocin. They observed no hyperbilirubinemia in the infants.[107] The use of estradiol for cervical ripening has produced conflicting effects on serum bilirubin levels.[108,109]

ANESTHESIA AND ANALGESIA

Epidural anesthesia, specifically, bupivacaine, has been associated with neonatal jaundice in most studies[62,76,102,110] but not in others.[111] Anesthetic agents readily cross the placenta and produce measurable blood levels in the newborn.[112] Bupivacaine, but not lidocaine or mepivacaine, significantly reduced erythrocyte filterability *in vitro* and erythrocyte survival in the rat.[113] In a controlled trial, bupivacaine and lidocaine epidural anesthetics were compared; there was no difference in neonatal bilirubin levels.[114]

Johnson and colleagues[115] found a significant association between the maternal use of promethazine hydrochloride and the risk of neonatal jaundice. In other studies, maternal administration of promethazine, propiomazine, methotrimeprazine, meperidine, and chlorpromazine had no effect on neonatal bilirubin levels.[116–120]

OTHER DRUGS

Drew and Kitchen investigated the effect of the administration of various pharmacologic agents to the mothers of 1107 infants.[121] Administration of narcotic agents, barbiturates, aspirin, chloral hydrate, reserpine, and phenytoin–sodium was associated with lower serum bilirubin concentrations; the use of diazepam, which raised mean bilirubin levels by <1 mg/dL, and oxytocin led to higher bilirubin levels. Note that the finding of a lower bilirubin concentration in association with the administration of a drug could imply an adverse effect of the drug on bilirubin–albumin binding, with potentially deleterious results.[122–125] Antipyrine administered to mothers before delivery decreases neonatal bilirubin levels,[126] and infants of heroin-addicted mothers have lower bilirubin levels.[127] Phenobarbital, if given in a sufficient dose to the mother, lowers serum bilirubin levels significantly in the first week of life (see Pharmacologic Treatment).[71,128–131]

Singhi and colleagues randomly assigned mothers in labor to receive no fluids or intravenous dextrose water.[106] Serum bilirubin levels were significantly higher in the intravenous dextrose water group, and 60% of the jaundiced neonates in that group were considered to have frank hyponatremia. The mechanism here may be similar to that suggested for the use of fluids with oxytocin.

Controlled trials of the use of cimetidine[132] and intrapartum administration of vitamin K[133] to the mother have found no effect on neonatal jaundice.

The use of antenatal betamethasone to accelerate lung maturation did not increase neonatal serum bilirubin levels,[134] but antenatal dexamethasone was associated with an increase in the incidence of bilirubin levels higher than 15 mg/dL (257 μmol/L) in a group of premature infants.[135]

TOCOLYSIS

Beta-adrenergic agents used for tocolysis in labor are not associated with higher bilirubin levels[136] or an increase in bilirubin production.[137]

Because an increase in bilirubin production was observed in rats given nicardipine, women in preterm labor were randomly assigned to receive nifedipine or ritodrine[138] or ritodrine and terbutaline.[139] Carboxyhemoglobin levels in these infants[138] and the need for phototherapy[139] were similar.

DELIVERY MODE

Full-term Japanese infants delivered vaginally had significantly higher serum bilirubin levels throughout the first week of life than those delivered by cesarean section.[140] In a controlled trial, however, the incidence of hyperbilirubinemia was similar in low-birth-weight infants delivered vaginally or by cesarean section.[141] In the study by Yamauchi and Yamanouchi, infants born by cesarean section had significantly lower hematocrits than those born vaginally—probably due to the fact that placental transfusion is essentially absent in infants born by cesarean section.[140] When compared with forceps delivery, the use of vacuum extraction does not appear to increase the risk of jaundice,[142,143] although epidemiologic studies have found an association between vacuum extraction and hyperbilirubinemia.[76]

PLACENTAL TRANSFUSION AND HYPERVISCOSITY

The catabolism of 1 g of hemoglobin produces 35 mg (60 μmol) of bilirubin, so that it is reasonable to assume that a high hematocrit is a risk factor for neonatal jaundice. In controlled trials of the effect of exchange transfusion on hyperviscosity, infants with polycythemia and hyperviscosity were randomly assigned to receive either partial exchange transfusions or symptomatic treatment. The authors state that the mean bilirubin levels and the incidence of hyperbilirubinemia were similar in the treated and control infants, although serum bilirubin levels were not provided.[144–146]

The volume of placental transfusion is determined by the time of cord clamping as well as the distance that the infant is held below the introitus before the cord is clamped.[147] Controlled trials, in which full-term newborns were randomly assigned to have their cords clamped immediately or 5 minutes after delivery, showed mixed results.[148–150] In two studies,[148,149] infants were held 15 cm below the introitus before clamping. Neither study demonstrated any effect. In the study by Saigal and colleagues,[150] infants were held 30 cm below the introitus in the delayed group; this study showed the most significant effects in both full-term and preterm infants. Mean bilirubin levels at age 72 hours were 7.7 mg/dL (132 μmol/L) in the delayed-clamping group, compared with 3.2 mg/dL (55 μmol/L) in the early-clamping group. In preterm infants, 38% of infants in the delayed-clamping group had serum bilirubin levels that exceeded 15 mg/dL (257 μmol/L), compared with 6% in the early-clamping group.

CORD BLOOD BILIRUBIN LEVELS

The association between the level of bilirubin in the cord blood and the risk of hyperbilirubinemia in infants with Rh erythroblastosis is well known. In newborns with ABO incompatibility, a cord bilirubin level higher than 4 mg/dL (68 μmol/L) was highly predictive of a subsequent serum bilirubin level higher than 16 mg/dL (274 μmol/L).[151] Cord blood bilirubin levels are also related to subsequent bilirubin levels in infants without hemolysis.[115,152–155] Knudsen found that 36% of infants who required phototherapy had a cord blood bilirubin level higher than 2.3 mg/dL (14 μmol/L), compared with 4.1% of jaundiced infants who did not require phototherapy.[152] Knudsen and Lebech measured bilirubin concentrations in the mother and in the infant's umbilical cord blood at the time of delivery.[153] Compared with nonjaundiced infants, infants who subsequently became jaundiced had significantly higher transplacental bilirubin gradients and cord blood bilirubin levels, and the serum bilirubin levels in their mothers were also significantly greater. Measurements of serum albumin concentrations and reserve albumin concentration, which is a measurement of bilirubin-binding capacity, were similar in jaundiced and nonjaundiced infants, suggesting that the increased cord bilirubin in the infants who later became jaundiced was the result of either increased fetal bilirubin production or decreased removal of bilirubin from the maternal circulation, and not a difference in albumin binding.[152] Combining maternal and cord bilirubin levels at delivery provided a better prediction of neonatal jaundice than the cord bilirubin levels alone.[153]

NEONATAL FACTORS

BIRTH WEIGHT AND GESTATION

Low-birth-weight and decreasing gestational age are highly correlated with an increased risk for hyperbilirubinemia,[62,64,74,76,81,110] and infants who are only slightly premature are at significantly greater risk for hyperbilirubinemia than full-term infants. At 37 weeks of gestation, newborns were four times more likely to have a serum bilirubin level of 13 mg/dL (222 μmol/L) or higher than were those at 40 weeks of gestation.[76]

GENDER

As a group, male infants consistently have higher bilirubin levels than females.[62,64,76,81,156]

FEEDING, WEIGHT LOSS, AND CALORIC INTAKE

Caloric intake is known to affect bilirubin metabolism; decreased caloric intake is associated with increased serum bilirubin levels.[157,158] Early feeding might also decrease intestinal transit time and decrease the enterohepatic circulation of bilirubin. Low-birth-weight infants fed in the first few hours after birth have significantly lower serum bilirubin levels than those fed at 12 to 48 hours,[159–162] and an intake of 120 cal/kg/day for the first 5 days produces lower serum bilirubin levels than 60 cal/kg/day.[163] On the other hand, early intravenous feeding has little effect when compared with early or late oral feeding.[159,164,165] In the National Institute of Child Health and Human Development (NICHHD) phototherapy study, infants who received 90 or fewer cal/kg/day had significantly higher bilirubin concentrations than those fed more than 90 cal/kg/day, and phototherapy was less effective when calorie and fluid intakes were low.[166]

Consistent with the caloric effect on neonatal jaundice, a significant association has been found between hyperbilirubinemia and weight loss in the first few days after birth.[76,81,83,93,110,115,156,167]

Several mechanisms might explain the inverse association between caloric intake and serum bilirubin levels. In adults with a low-calorie intake, the predominant mechanism appears to be a decrease in hepatic clearance of bilirubin from the plasma.[168] Fasting- or insulin-induced hypoglycemia increases the activity of heme oxygenase and, possibly, bilirubin production, in rats,[169] but caloric deprivation in animals,[168] human adults,[170] and newborns[171] is not accompanied by an increase in carbon monoxide production. During fasting, nonesterified fatty acid (NEFA) levels increase and may impede hepatic clearance of bilirubin. Nonesterified fatty acids may affect bilirubin uptake by interfering with the receptors on the hepatic cell membrane.[172] Nonesterified fatty acids also compete with unconjugated bilirubin binding by ligandin[173] and may decrease bilirubin clearance by inhibiting glucuronosyl transferase activity.[174]

The effects of parenteral nutrition and protein intake on the development of cholestatic jaundice are well known. Compared with infants fed human milk or formula, those receiving intravenous glucose and amino acid solutions are more likely to develop conjugated hyperbilirubinemia.[175–177] A high-protein intake (3.6 g/kg/day *versus* 2.3 g/kg/day) is associated with higher peak direct serum bilirubin levels and earlier onset of cholestatic jaundice.[178]

TYPE OF DIET

When the diet of Gunn rats was changed from the standard laboratory diet to one composed predominantly of carbohydrate or protein, the plasma bilirubin concentration doubled over a period of 3 days. Rats fed a soybean oil lipid emulsion (*i.e.*, intralipid) showed a slight decrease in plasma bilirubin levels.[179]

Gourley and colleagues evaluated the effect of diet on fecal output and neonatal jaundice in infants fed human milk or infant formulas.[180] Infants who consumed a casein–hydrolysate formula had significantly lower bilirubin levels from days 10 through 18 than those fed standard casein or whey-predominant formulas. The cumulative stool output of the infants fed the casein–hydrolysate was lower than that of the infants fed the other formulas, suggesting that factors other than stool output and its effect on the enterohepatic circulation must explain these observations. The authors state that they have preliminary findings to indicate that casein–hydrolysate formula inhibits β-glucuronidase and may thus decrease the amount of bilirubin absorbed by the enterohepatic circulation.[180]

BREAST-FEEDING AND JAUNDICE

A strong association has been found between breast-feeding and an increased incidence of neonatal hyperbilirubinemia. In 1963, Newman and Gross,[181] and in 1964, Arias and colleagues,[182] described a syndrome of hyperbilirubinemia associated with breast-feeding. These infants, all full-term and healthy, had jaundice in the first week of life that did not resolve but persisted into the second and third week, achieving a maximal level of 10 to 30 mg/dL (171–513 μmol/L) by 10 to 15 days after birth. If breast-feeding continued, elevated levels persisted for 4 to 10 days, then declined slowly, reaching normal values by 3 to 12 weeks of age. If breast-feeding was interrupted, serum bilirubin levels fell within 48 hours. This condition became known as the breast-milk jaundice syndrome.

In addition to this syndrome, there is convincing epidemiologic evidence that serum bilirubin levels during the first 3 to 5 days after birth are significantly higher in breast-fed than in formula-fed infants. In a pooled analysis of 12 studies comparing bilirubin levels in over 8000 newborns, serum bilirubin levels of 12 mg/dL (205 μmol/L) or higher occurred in 12.9% of breast-fed infants and 4% of formula-fed infants ($p <$ 0.000001), and levels 15 mg/dL (257 μmol/L) or higher occurred in 2% of the breast-fed infants and in 0.3% of the formula-fed infants ($p <$ 0.000001).[183] Thus, breast-fed infants are about three times more likely to develop moderate jaundice and six times more likely to develop severe jaundice than formula-fed newborns. In a study of 2416 consecutive infants in a well-baby nursery, serum bilirubin levels of 13 mg/dL (222 μmol/L) or higher occurred in 9% of breast-fed and 2.2% of formula-fed infants. The corresponding percentages for bilirubin levels of 12 mg/dL (205 μmol/L) or higher were 3.6% for bottle-fed *versus* 12.1% for breast-fed infants ($p <$ 0.00001).[184] Table 38-3 and Figure 38-11 show the distribution of maximal serum bilirubin levels in a population of well, Caucasian newborns with birth weights greater than 2500 g. In these infants, the 95th percentile for maximal serum bilirubin before hospital discharge in the breast-fed group was 14.5 mg/dL (248 μmol/L), compared with 11.4 mg/dL (195 μmol/L) in the bottle-fed group. Eighty percent of the infants whose serum bilirubin concentrations were 13 mg/dL (222 μmol/L) or higher were breast-fed, compared with 47% of those whose maximal bilirubin level was lower than 13 mg/dL ($p <$ 0.00001).[184] Of the infants in whom no apparent cause for hyperbilirubinemia was found, 83% were breast-fed.

In a more recent study, 306 infants admitted to a pediatric ward within 21 days of birth with severe indirect hyperbilirubinemia were identified; the mean serum bilirubin level was 18.5 mg/dL (316 μmol/L).[185] Seventy-seven percent of these infants were fully breast-fed and 14% partially breast-fed. Average age at the time of readmission to hospital was 5 days; 91.5% were admitted in the first week, 8% between 8 and 14 days, and 0.5% after 14 days.[185]

The jaundice associated with breast-feeding may appear early (2–4 days of age) or later (4–7 days of age). The early-onset jaundice has been called breast-feeding jaundice syndrome, and the late-onset form has been called breast-milk jaundice syndrome.[186,187] So much overlap exists between these two entities, however, that the distinction between early- and late-onset breast-milk jaundice may be more artificial than real, although some feel that the two conditions can be distinguished by their pathophysiology.[186]

Evidence against two distinct syndromes comes from studies of the natural history of jaundice in the breast-fed infant. In addition to having higher bilirubin levels in the first 3 to 5 days, as a group, breast-fed infants have serum bilirubin levels that are higher than formula-fed infants for at least 3 to 6 weeks.[180,188–190] These infants are the same infants who have high bilirubin levels in the first week of life, so it is hard to believe that those still jaundiced at 2 to 3 weeks of age represent a distinct group, particularly since prolonged jaundice is common in the normal

TABLE 38–3
PERCENTILE RANKS FOR NEWBORN CAUCASIAN INFANTS WHO WEIGH MORE THAN 2500 g

	Maximal Serum Bilirubin					
	Breast-Fed Infants (n = 1260)		Bottle-Fed Infants (n = 1026)		Total Population* (n = 2297)	
Percentile	μmol/L	mg/dL	μmol/L	mg/dL	μmol/L	mg/dL
3	19	1.1	19	1.1	19	1.1
5	24	1.4	21	1.2	22	1.3
10	36	2.1	27	1.6	31	1.8
15	48	2.8	34	2	41	2.4
25	74	4.3	53	3.1	62	3.6
50	125	7.3	96	5.6	111	6.5
75	168	9.8	135	7.9	154	9
90	214	12.5	171	10	197	11.5
95	248	14.5	195	11.4	231	13.5
97	269	15.7	212	12.4	253	14.8
99	291	17	267	15.6	286	16.7

* Includes 11 infants who were both breast- and bottle-fed.
From Maisels MJ, Gifford KL, Antle CE, et al. Normal serum bilirubin levels in the newborn and the effect of breast feeding. Pediatrics 1986;78:837.

breast-fed newborn. In one study, 11 of 27 breast-fed infants (41%), but none of the formula-fed infants, had bilirubin levels higher than 12 mg/dL (205 μmol/L) at 1 week of age.[188] In another study, 13 of 36 breast-fed infants (36%) had serum bilirubin levels higher than 5 mg/dL (85 μmol/L) at 16 ± 2.4 days of age.[191] Kivlahan and James used a transcutaneous jaundice meter to perform a prospective study of 140 newborns for the first 3 weeks of life (Fig. 38-12).[189] Breast-fed infants had significantly higher transcutaneous bilirubin (TcB) readings from day 6, and these were still abnormally elevated by day 21. Twenty-one percent of breast-fed infants had a TcB index higher than 20, which is about equal to a serum bilirubin level of 12.9 mg/dL, whereas none of the formula-fed infants exceeded this level.[189] In a similar study, newborns were studied for 6 weeks using the TcB meter. From weeks 1 through 6, breast-fed infants had significantly higher TcB indices than the formula-fed population.[190]

Thus, prolonged hyperbilirubinemia in breast-fed newborns is much more common than previously suggested and, depending on the age at measurement, occurs in about 20% to 30% of all breast-feeding infants. The magnitude and frequency of prolonged indirect hyperbilirubinemia in breast-feeding infants suggests a substantial overlap between the breast-milk jaundice syndrome and early-onset

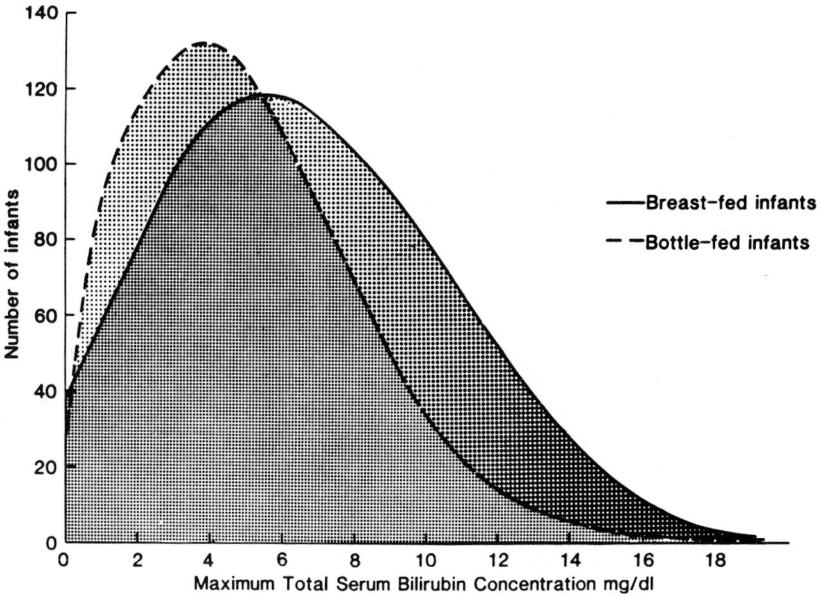

FIG. 38–11. Distribution of maximum serum bilirubin concentrations in Caucasian infants who weigh more than 2500 g. (From Maisels MJ, Gifford K, Antle CE, et al. Normal serum bilirubin levels in the newborn and the effect of breast feeding. Pediatrics 1986;78:837.)

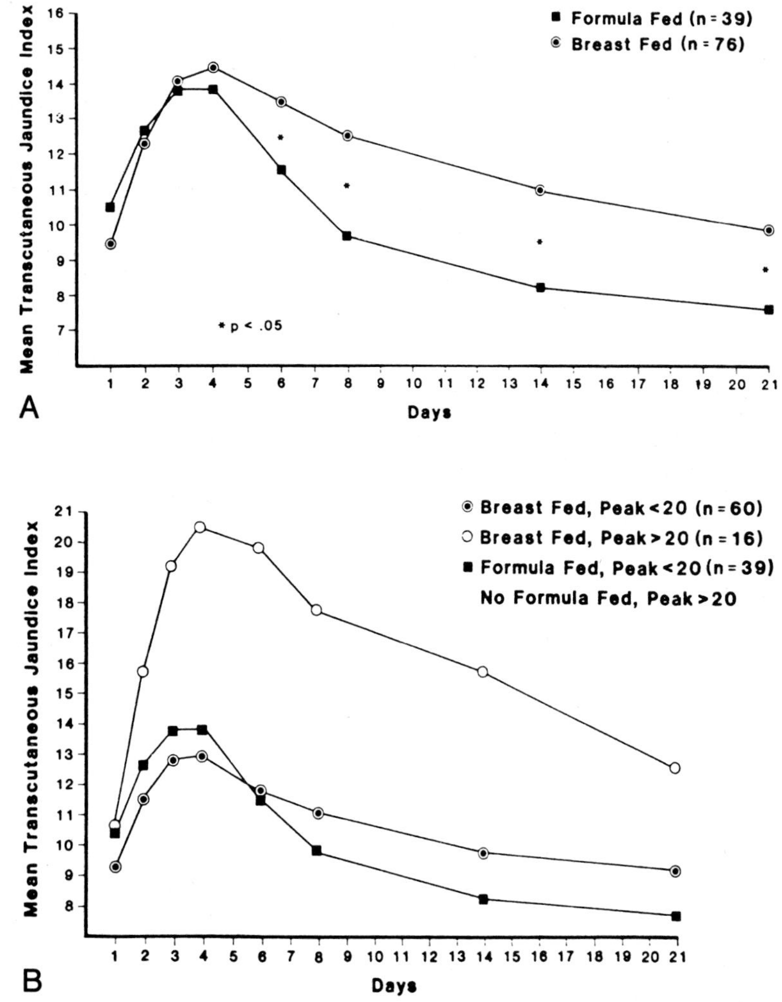

FIG. 38–12. Natural history of jaundice in Caucasian breast-fed and formula-fed infants. The transcutaneous jaundice index was measured with the Minolta Jaundice Meter. **(A)** The natural history of jaundice in the formula-fed and breast-fed infants. Significant differences in the TcB index were found from days 6 to 21. **(B)** Bimodal distribution of jaundice in the breast-fed infants. Twenty-one percent of breast-fed infants had TcB indexes greater than 20 (≅ 12.9 mg/dL), but in the remaining breast-fed infants, the bilirubin pattern was similar to that of the formula-fed infants. (From Kivlahan C, James EJP. The natural history of neonatal jaundice. Pediatrics 1984;74:364.)

breast-feeding jaundice, calling into question whether or not these are separate entities.

Jaundice associated with breast milk has also been described in premature infants. Lucas and Baker studied 186 preterm infants who weighed less than 1850 g at birth.[192] These infants were randomly assigned to receive either banked donor breast milk or a preterm infant formula. Those fed banked breast milk had significantly higher peak bilirubin concentrations and more prolonged jaundice than infants fed the preterm formula, and those fed breast milk were over four times more likely to achieve plasma bilirubin levels above 11.7 mg/dL (200 μmol/L). This effect was also seen in sick, ventilated infants who weighed less than 1500 g and whose enteral intake during the first week was only 200 mL.

The pathogenesis of breast-milk jaundice has been reviewed in detail,[186,193] and the suggested mechanisms are listed in Table 38-4.

Bilirubin Production

Breast-fed infants do not produce more bilirubin than formula-fed infants. Measurements of carbon monoxide production, an index of bilirubin production, show no differences between breast- and bottle-fed infants.[194,195]

Decreased Bilirubin Clearance by the Liver

Decreased Caloric Intake

As discussed previously, a decreased caloric intake is associated with increased serum bilirubin levels.[157,158] In the first few days after birth, breast-fed infants

TABLE 38–4
SUGGESTED PATHOPHYSIOLOGY OF JAUNDICE ASSOCIATED WITH BREAST-FEEDING

Decreased Bilirubin Clearance by the Liver
Decreased caloric intake
Inhibitory substances in breast milk
Pregnanediol
Free fatty acids
Other inhibitors
Genetic factors
Increased Intestinal Reabsorption of Bilirubin
Delayed meconium passage
Decreased formation of urobilinogen
Beta-glucuronidase
Bile acid abnormalities

consume less calories than formula-fed infants, and there is a significant association between hyperbilirubinemia and weight loss in the first few days after birth.[76,81,83,93,110,115,167] Also, during fasting, NEFA levels increase and may impede hepatic clearance of bilirubin.[172–174]

Inhibitory Substances in Breast Milk

Pregnanediol. The original observations of Arias and Gartner suggested that a progestational steroid, 3-α-20-β-pregnanediol, which is present in the milk of certain mothers, was responsible for inhibiting bilirubin conjugation *in vitro* and could also cause hyperbilirubinemia when administered to full-term infants.[182] Although others have confirmed the inhibitory properties of breast milk from certain mothers, they have not found this particular steroid to be the offending compound.[196,197]

Lipase and Free Fatty Acids. Nonesterified fatty acids inhibit bilirubin conjugation.[174,198,199,200,201] These free fatty acids may be liberated as a result of the lipolytic action of breast-milk lipase on triglycerides. Both lipoprotein lipase (LPL) and bile salt–stimulated lipase are found in human milk.[202,203,204,205] Bile salt–stimulated lipase is about 100 times more active than LPL, requires exposure to bile salts, and is important in the digestion of milk fat.[206] Lipoprotein lipase does not appear to have much activity in normal human milk, and observations regarding the role of LPL activity and NEFAs in neonatal jaundice are conflicting.[174,198,199,207,201] Some investigators have found elevated LPL activity in the milk of mothers of infants with the breast-milk jaundice syndrome,[201] but others have found no difference in LPL activity in milk samples from mothers of jaundiced and nonjaundiced infants. Alonso and colleagues found no relation between infant bilirubin levels and either NEFA levels in fresh human milk or the ability of the milk to inhibit glucuronosyl transferase activity *in vitro.*[191] Nonesterified fatty acids accumulate in stored milk, and there is a relation between free fatty acid levels and the inhibition of glucuronosyl transferase.[174,198–201] Foliot and colleagues found that milk from mothers of jaundiced infants, when stored at 4°C, strongly inhibited bilirubin conjugation, but when assayed immediately after thawing, had no inhibitory effect.[199] Breast-milk lipase activity normally increases significantly from day 3 to day 21.[208] Thus, failure to use age-matched controls produces misleading results.

Uhari and colleagues assigned 332 breast-feeding mothers to receive a diet containing a low or high polyunsaturated–saturated fatty acid ratio.[209] Although there were significant differences in breast milk and maternal and infant serum levels of oleate, linoleate, and linolenate, which was previously shown to inhibit bilirubin conjugation,[174,199] there were no significant differences in neonatal serum bilirubin levels. Intake of specific dietary fatty acids does not appear to be related to neonatal jaundice.

Other Possible Inhibitors. Many factors are involved in the control of glucuronosyl transferase activity,[210] including compounds such as metal irons,[211,212] steroids,[213] and nucleotides.[213,214] Nucleotides might inhibit bilirubin clearance and play a role in the pathogenesis of breast-milk jaundice. Genetic factors must also be considered.[47,68] Navajo infants have a high incidence of unconjugated hyperbilirubinemia, which is exaggerated in those who are breastfed. In these breast-feeding mothers, an inhibitor of glucuronosyl transferase activity was found in colostrum and breast milk in the first 3 days after birth, and the degree of inhibition observed was related to the elevation of serum bilirubin.[68]

Intestinal Reabsorption of Bilirubin

Direct and indirect evidence support the conclusion that an increase in intestinal absorption of bilirubin is the most important mechanism responsible for the jaundice associated with breast-feeding. Bilirubin is present in fetal bile as early as 14 to 15 weeks of gestation and, by 20 to 30 weeks of gestation, bilirubin conjugates appear. The cumulative excretion of bilirubin during fetal life accounts for the fact that significant quantities of bilirubin are found in meconium[54]; it has been estimated that about 100 to 200 mg of bilirubin is present in the meconium of a normal 3-kg infant. This is about 4 to 7 times more bilirubin than the infant will produce daily from the normal catabolism of heme,[52,53] and delay in meconium passage leads to higher serum bilirubin levels.[215,216] In the first few days of life, breast-fed infants pass less stool by weight, and their stools contain less bilirubin than those of formula-fed infants.[180,217] Since there is no difference in the rate of bilirubin production,[195] the implication is that breast-fed infants reabsorb more bilirubin through the gut than do formula-fed infants.

Gourley and colleagues evaluated the effect of diet on feces and jaundice during the first 3 weeks of life.[180] They found that breast-fed infants produced lower-weight individual wet and dry stools than formula-fed infants and that the cumulative wet and dry stool output was also lower in the breast-fed infants. In these infants, a decrease in serum bilirubin levels from day 3 to day 21 correlated positively with the 21-day total wet and dry cumulative stool weights. They concluded that the quantity of stool excreted is related to decreases in serum bilirubin levels in infants fed human milk. Infants fed human milk passed stool significantly less frequently than infants fed casein-predominant formulas,[217,180] while those fed casein hydrolysate formulas passed less stool, cumulatively, than those fed whey-predominant or casein-predominant formulas. There was no difference between the cumulative wet or dry stool output during the first 3 weeks of life in infants fed casein hydrolysate formulas or human milk.[180] Gartner and colleagues instilled unconjugated bilirubin into the duodenum of adult rats. When the bilirubin was given with phosphate buffer, 25% of the administered dose was absorbed and excreted in bile within 5 hours (Fig. 38-13).[218,219] When the bilirubin was administered with human milk or cow milk, absorption was less than 2%; however, when bilirubin was administered in milk from mothers of infants with the breast-milk jaundice syndrome, absorption was 25% during the first 5 hours and persisted for an additional 11 hours, leading to a total absorption of 65% of the administered dose. Thus, milk from mothers of infants with breast-milk jaundice appeared to enhance the enterohepatic circulation of bilirubin.

Alonso and colleagues[191] collected milk from unselected, normal mothers and serum from their infants at 16.3 ± 2.4 days. They labeled bilirubin with ^{14}C and studied its absorption when administered into the duodenum of adult rats. When the bilirubin was administered with a bicarbonate buffer, 25.29% ± 4% was absorbed. Absorption was 4.67% ± 2.4% when given with Similac formula and 7.7% ± 2.9% when given with fresh human milk. They also found a positive correlation between the percentage of bilirubin absorbed when administered with human milk and the serum bilirubin level in the infant being fed that milk. These data provide additional confirmation that enhanced intestinal absorption of bilirubin contributes to the jaundice associated with breast-feeding. These studies also confirm that cow milk inhibits reabsorption of bilirubin, which explains why interrupting breast-feeding or supplementing breast-feeding with formula generally lowers serum bilirubin levels.

Alonso and colleagues also analyzed the breast milk for β-glucuronidase, NEFAs, and the ability of the milk to inhibit glucuronosyl transferase activity of rat liver microsomes *in vitro*.[191] None of these measurements correlated with the infant's serum bilirubin.

Urobilinogen Formation. Once in the small intestine, conjugated bilirubin is not reabsorbed. In a healthy adult, it is largely reduced by the action of colonic bacteria, principally clostridium ramosum,[221] to a series of tetrapyrroles, collectively known as urobilinogen. As a result, in the adult, there is minimal reabsorption of bilirubin from the intestinal tract. At birth, however, the fetal gut is sterile, and although there is an increase in the bacterial content of the gut after delivery, the neonatal intestinal flora do not convert conjugated bilirubin to urobilinogen. This leaves bilirubin in the bowel and allows it to be deconjugated and become available for reabsorption. The bile pigments in newborn stool are similar to those found in duodenal bile.[193] Formula-fed infants excrete urobilin in their stools earlier than breast-fed infants,[222] perhaps due to the effect of the feeding on intestinal flora.[223] Thus, the effect of breast milk on intestinal flora, by slowing the formation of urobilin, further enhances the possibility of intestinal reabsorption of bilirubin.

Beta-Glucuronidase. Beta-glucuronidase is an enzyme that cleaves the ester-linkage of bilirubin glucuronide, producing unconjugated bilirubin, which can then be reabsorbed through the gut. Significant concentrations of β-glucuronidase are found in the neonatal intestine. Beta-glucuronidase activity is also significantly greater in human milk than in infant formulas. Gourley and Arend found a relation between serum bilirubin levels and breast-milk β-glucuronidase activity in the first 3 to 4 days after birth,[208] but others have not been able to confirm this.[191,224] Because the neonate's intestine contains large quantities of mucosal β-glucuronidase, the relatively small amounts of enzyme in milk would not be expected to add much to the overall activity. Nevertheless, Gourley and colleagues suggest that milk β-glucuronidase may be a significant additional source of fecal β-glucuronidase.[225] These investigators also found a correlation between neonatal serum bilirubin levels and β-glucuronidase activity in the first stool passed after birth.[225] Finally, Gourley and colleagues infused rat bile plus breast milk into the rat's duodenum. Rats that received this infusion with saccharolactone, a β-glucuronidase inhibitor, excreted significantly less

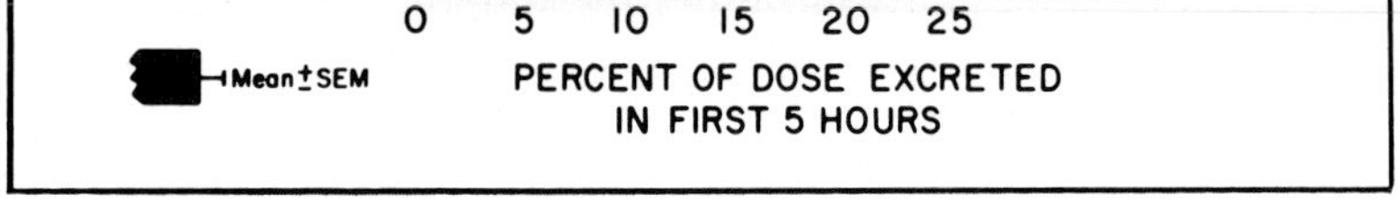

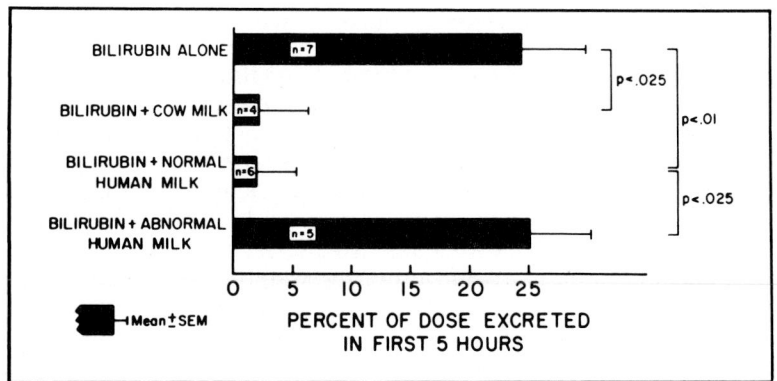

FIG. 38–13. Bilirubin excretion in the bile of adult male rats during the first 5 hours after 1 mg unconjugated bilirubin in phosphate buffer, *p*H 8.6, was introduced into the duodenum. Bilirubin was administered without milk, with a combination of fresh normal human milk and cow milk, and with milk from mothers of infants with the breast-milk jaundice syndrome (*i.e.*, abnormal human milk; n = number of animals in each group; from Gartner LM. Breast milk jaundice. In: Levine RJ, Maisels MJ, eds. Hyperbilirubinemia in the newborn: report of the 85th Ross Conference on Pediatric Research. Columbus, OH: Ross Laboratories, 1983:75.)

bilirubin in their bile than those that did not receive saccharolactone, suggesting that inhibition of β-glucuronidase decreased the intestinal absorption of bilirubin.[226]

Bile Acids. Some studies suggest that breast-fed infants with prolonged unconjugated hyperbilirubinemia may also have a mild degree of cholestasis.[227-229] Finni and colleagues found elevated serum levels of alkaline phosphatase, cholic and chenodeoxycholic acids, and α-fetoprotein in jaundiced, breast-fed infants at 1 month of age.[227] Cholic and chenodeoxycholic acids were still significantly elevated at 12 months of age, although the alkaline phosphatase and α-fetoprotein levels had returned to normal. Tazawa and colleagues did not find a significant increase in total serum bile acid levels in breast-fed infants with prolonged jaundice.[228] All breast-fed infants, regardless of the presence or absence of jaundice, had a bile acid pattern dominated by taurine conjugates, whereas in bottle-fed infants, glycine conjugates predominated. In the jaundiced breast-fed infants, however, the ratio of glycine- to taurine-conjugated bile acid was significantly lower than in nonjaundiced infants. Lipoprotein X levels were normal in breast-fed jaundiced infants. This pattern of bile acids does not suggest the usual type of cholestasis but indicates the possibility of an increased enterohepatic circulation of bile acids in breast-fed infants.[228,229] High-performance liquid chromatographic analysis of bilirubin in breast-fed and formula-fed infants revealed no differences in bilirubin monoconjugates or diconjugates on the third and fifth day of life.[230]

Meconium Passage. Because the enterohepatic circulation of bilirubin appears to be an important contributor to neonatal hyperbilirubinemia, increasing the rate of bilirubin evacuation from the bowel should decrease the incidence of neonatal jaundice. Two controlled trials tested this hypothesis. In one, infants were randomly assigned to have their temperatures taken either rectally or in the axilla directly after birth, on the assumption that the insertion of a rectal thermometer would stimulate earlier meconium evacuation, which it did.[215] Weisman and colleagues randomly assigned infants to receive one-half of an infant suppository within the first hour after birth and then every 4 hours until the appearance of the first transitional stool.[216] In both these studies, the peak serum bilirubin levels were about 1 mg/dL (17 μmol/L) lower in the treated than in the control groups, and a pooled analysis of the data indicates that the effect is significant.[105]

In summary, early and frequent feeding promotes fluid and caloric intake and minimizes weight loss. Such feeding also decreases intestinal transit time and facilitates early passage of meconium, which decreases the enterohepatic circulation of bilirubin. These measures should reduce neonatal bilirubin levels.

PHENOLIC DETERGENTS

The use of excessive concentrations of a phenolic disinfectant detergent to clean surfaces in the nursery was associated with an epidemic of neonatal hyperbilirubinemia in two hospitals.[231] There was no evidence for hemolysis, and the pathogenesis for the hyperbilirubinemia is not known. Daum and colleagues demonstrated inhibition of glucuronosyl transferase activity in liver homogenates, but they could not confirm this *in vivo* using the Gunn rat.[232] Doan and colleagues found that use of a phenolic detergent, even when used at the manufacturer's recommended concentrations, was associated with higher bilirubin levels than those found in infants in a nursery in which a nonphenolic quarternary ammonium disinfectant was used.[233] In view of these observations, it is recommended that phenolic detergents not be used in the nursery.

TRACE METALS

Plasma zinc levels were significantly lower in neonates with unexplained jaundice and their mothers than in controls.[234,235] The data on magnesium levels in these infants are conflicting—increased in one study,[235] but normal in another.[234] It is possible that zinc deficiency produces structural defects in the erythrocyte membrane and leads to hemolysis.

ALTITUDE

Moore and colleagues observed an association between hyperbilirubinemia, with serum bilirubin levels higher than 12 mg/dL (205 μmol/L), and high altitude. Infants born at 3100 meters above sea level had more than twice the incidence of hyperbilirubinemia than those born at 1600 meters (32.7% *versus* 13%) and four times the incidence reported for those born at sea level.[236] The infants born at higher altitudes had higher hematocrits, but there was no difference in hematocrits between infants with high bilirubin levels and those with low levels at each altitude. The presence of other risk factors known to affect serum bilirubin levels was similar in the different groups, but the incidence of maternal smoking was, unfortunately, not assessed. Both short- and long-term exposure to high altitudes increases bilirubin levels in adults.[237,238] Possible mechanisms for these observations include an increase in bilirubin load due to higher hematocrits,[239] impaired conjugation,[237] and impaired excretion of bilirubin.[240]

DRUGS ADMINISTERED TO THE INFANT

Large doses (up to 30 mg) of synthetic vitamin K analogs have been associated with significant increases in bilirubin levels and kernicterus.[241,242] The standard dose (1 mg) of intramuscular vitamin K_1 has no effect on neonatal bilirubin levels.

Freeman and colleagues found that infants exposed to pancuronium were at greater risk for hyperbilirubinemia (bilirubin–birth weight index > 0.5).[243] The risk was greatest among exposed infants during the 4 days after the last dose of pancuronium (relative risk, 1.4; 95% confidence interval, 1–1.8). It is possible that pancuronium alters bilirubin metabolism and increases the risk of hyperbilirubinemia in ill newborns. It is also possible that the use of pancuronium simply identifies a group of newborns who are at higher risk for this complication.[243]

Chloral hydrate, which is widely used as a sedative in neonates and infants, is associated with significant elevations in indirect and direct serum bilirubin levels (see Chap. 58).[244,245] Chloral hydrate is metabolized to trichloroacetic acid and the toxic trichloroethanol, both of which accumulate in the tissues of compromised infants. The half-life of trichloroethanol is 37 hours in the newborn, compared with 14 hours in the adult.[244] In ill preterm infants, there is indirect evidence of competition by trichloroethanol for hepatic glucuronidation of bilirubin. The administration of chloral hydrate is also associated with direct hyperbilirubinemia. Infants with direct hyperbilirubinemia had received much higher total cumulative doses of chloral hydrate than those that did not develop direct hyperbilirubinemia, and the hyperbilirubinemia resolved after chloral hydrate was discontinued.[244] Thus, chloral hydrate should be used with caution in newborns and particularly low-birth-weight, ventilator-dependent infants.

FREE-RADICAL PRODUCTION

Bilirubin appears to have an important physiologic function as an antioxidant and may play a role in the prevention of oxidative membrane damage *in vivo* (see Physiologic Effects of Bilirubin).[14] Benaron and Bowen investigated the possibility that bilirubin has a role as a free-radical scavenger.[246] Although sick newborns might be expected to have an exaggerated rise in bilirubin levels, Benaron and Bowen found that this was not the case. Infants with illnesses such as circulatory failure, proven sepsis, aspiration syndromes, and asphyxia—conditions believed to enhance free-radical production—had a significantly lower daily rise in mean serum bilirubin levels (2.1 mg/dL, or 36.1 μmol/L) than control infants (3.9 mg/dL, or 66.7 μmol/L). Control infants were initially ill but proved not to have any active medical disorder. They were selected from infants with myelomeningoceles, other surgical disorders, and suspected sepsis that was ruled out by negative studies. Neither group received enteral feedings during the study. If the conditions identified in the study infants actually enhance free-radical production, then this finding is consistent with the hypothesis that bilirubin is consumed as an antioxidant. The role of bilirubin as an antioxidant is discussed later.

JAUNDICE IN THE HEALTHY NEWBORN

NORMAL SERUM BILIRUBIN LEVELS

Mean bilirubin levels in cord blood range from 1.4 to 1.9 mg/dL (24–32 μmol/L),[152,153,155] and elevated cord bilirubin levels are associated with an increased risk of hyperbilirubinemia.[151,152,154]

In the national Collaborative Perinatal Project (CPP), conducted from 1959 to 1966, serum bilirubin concentrations were obtained prospectively on more than 35,000 infants.[74] The serum bilirubin level was measured routinely at about 48 hours of age and repeated daily if the initial level was 10 mg/dL (171 μmol/L) or greater until the value decreased below 10 mg/dL. Additional serum bilirubin determinations were obtained when clinically indicated. The maximal bilirubin levels measured are shown in Tables 38-5 and 38-6. Of infants weighing more than 2500 g at birth, 6.2% of Caucasian infants and 4.5% of black infants had serum bilirubin levels of 13 mg/dL (222 μmol/L) or greater. Although this population included sick infants and those with hemolytic disease, about 95% of all infants had serum bilirubin concentrations that did not exceed 12.9 mg/dL.

Serum bilirubin concentrations were measured in 2297 consecutive infants, who weighed more than 2500 g, admitted to a well-baby nursery between 1976 and 1980.[184] The maximal total serum bilirubin levels before hospital discharge are shown in Table 38-7. Bilirubin levels of 13 mg/dL (22 μmol/L) or greater occurred in 6%—virtually identical with the incidence (6.2%) in the CPP study. Note, however, that the data in Tables 38-5 through 38-7 were all obtained from hospitalized newborns, and although at the time of study the infants remained in hospital for at least 72 hours, when outpatient bilirubin levels are included, the values are considerably higher.[75,247] In the study by Newman and colleagues, which included outpatients, 10% of Caucasian infants, 4.4% of black infants, and 23% of East Asian infants had a serum bilirubin level of 13 mg/dL (222 μmol/L) or higher.[75] In a group of Argentinian breast-fed infants followed as inpatients and outpatients, 7.4% had a bilirubin level of 17 mg/dL (291 μmol/L) or higher.[247] Maximal bilirubin levels vary considerably depending on the racial composition of the population, the incidence of breast-feeding, and other epidemiologic factors discussed previously (see Tables 38-1 and 38-2; see Epidemiology of Neonatal Jaundice).

Normal plasma bilirubin concentrations in human adults range from 0.3 to 1 mg/dL (5–17 μmol/L).[248] In 3.3% of infants, maximal serum bilirubin levels never exceeded 1 mg/dL (5 μmol/L), and 8.2% had serum bilirubin levels that did not exceed 1.5 mg/dL (20 μmol/L).[184]

TABLE 38–5
MAXIMAL TOTAL SERUM BILIRUBIN OF NEWBORN CAUCASIAN INFANTS BY BIRTH WEIGHT

Serum Bilirubin Level (mg/dL)	<2501 g			>2500 g			Total		
	Live Births	%	Cumulative %	Live Births	%	Cumulative %	Live Births	%	Cumulative %
0–7	488	42.73	100	11908	73.73	100	12396	71.69	100
8–12	336	29.42	57.27	3243	20.08	26.27	3579	20.7	28.31
13–15	128	11.21	27.85	531	3.29	6.19	659	3.81	7.62
16–19	114	9.98	16.64	315	1.95	2.9	429	2.48	3.81
20+	76	6.65	6.65	153	0.95	0.95	229	1.32	1.32
Total	1142	100		16150	100		17292	100	
Unknown	177	13.42		1012	5.9		1189	6.43	
Grand total	1319			17162			18481		

From Hardy JB, Drage JS, Jackson EC. The first year of life: the collaborative perinatal project of The National Institutes of Neurological and Communicative Disorders and Stroke. Baltimore: Johns Hopkins University Press, 1979:104.

DIRECT BILIRUBIN LEVELS

Newman and colleagues analyzed 5255 direct bilirubin measurements performed on full-term infants born at the hospitals of the University of California, San Francisco (UCSF), and Stanford University.[249] Each institution used different methods to measure direct or conjugated bilirubin levels, which almost certainly accounts for the fact that the values for the 50th through 95th percentiles at UCSF were more than double those at Stanford (Table 38-8). The measurements of total and direct bilirubin levels are both subject to laboratory error, and it is important to recognize that direct bilirubin is not synonymous with conjugated bilirubin. Laboratory methods for estimating serum bilirubin concentrations are discussed in detail in the section on clinical management.

PHYSIOLOGIC JAUNDICE

According to the criteria for normal adult serum bilirubin concentrations, about 97% of Caucasian infants with birth weights greater than 2500 g have some degree of chemical jaundice, and about two thirds have serum bilirubin levels of 5 mg/dL (85 μmol/L) or greater (see Table 38-7). Because it is almost universal during the first week of life, this transient hyperbilirubinemia has been called physiologic jaundice. Gartner and colleagues studied the newborn rhesus monkey and found that the newborn human and monkey develop a similar biphasic pattern of physiologic jaundice. In the monkey, phase I is characterized by a rapid increase in serum bilirubin levels to 4.5 mg/dL (77 μmol/L) by 19 hours followed by a decline to 1 mg/dL (17 μmol/L) by 48 hours. In phase II, bilirubin levels remain elevated at 1 mg/dL (17

TABLE 38–6
MAXIMAL TOTAL SERUM BILIRUBIN OF NEWBORN AFRICAN-AMERICAN INFANTS BY BIRTH WEIGHT

Serum Bilirubin Level (mg/dL)	<2501 g			>2500 g			Total		
	Live Births	%	Cumulative %	Live Births	%	Cumulative %	Live Births	%	Cumulative %
0–7	1137	50.29	100	11734	74.48	100	12871	71.45	100
8–12	719	31.8	49.71	3309	21	25.52	4028	22.36	28.55
13–15	225	9.95	17.91	412	2.62	4.51	637	3.54	6.19
16–19	113	5	7.96	202	1.28	1.9	315	1.75	2.66
20+	67	2.96	2.96	97	0.62	0.62	164	0.91	0.91
Total	2261	100		15754	100		18015	100	
Unknown	356	13.6		1133	6.71		1489	7.63	
Grand total	2617			16887			19504		

From Hardy JB, Drage JS, Jackson EC. The first year of life: the collaborative perinatal project of The National Institutes of Neurological and Communicative Disorders and Stroke. Baltimore: Johns Hopkins University Press, 1979:104.

TABLE 38–7
MAXIMAL TOTAL SERUM BILIRUBIN CONCENTRATIONS BEFORE DISCHARGE IN NEWBORN CAUCASIAN INFANTS WEIGHING > 2500 g

Serum Bilirubin Levels		All Infants* (n = 2297)			Breast-Fed Infants (n = 1260)			Formula-Fed Infants (n = 1026)		
mg/dL	μmol/L	Number	Percentage	Cumulative Percentage	Number	Percentage	Cumulative Percentage	Number	Percentage	Cumulative Percentage
0–0.9	0–16	51	2.22	2.22	29	2.3	2.3	22	2.14	2.14
1–1.9	17–33	221	9.62	11.84	90	7.14	9.44	130	12.67	14.82
2–2.9	34–50	180	7.84	19.68	86	6.83	16.27	94	9.16	23.98
3–3.9	51–67	187	8.14	27.82	82	6.51	22.78	105	10.23	34.21
4–4.9	68–84	186	8.1	35.92	90	7.14	29.92	95	9.26	43.47
5–5.9	85–102	204	8.88	44.8	98	7.78	37.7	106	10.33	53.8
6–6.9	103–119	241	10.49	55.29	118	9.37	47.06	122	11.98	65.69
7–7.9	120–136	235	10.23	65.52	135	10.71	57.78	99	9.65	75.34
8–8.9	137–153	225	9.8	75.32	140	11.11	68.89	85	8.29	83.63
9–9.9	154–170	171	7.44	82.76	104	8.25	77.14	66	6.43	90.06
10–10.9	171–187	117	5.09	87.85	77	6.11	83.25	39	3.8	93.86
11–11.9	188–204	87	3.79	91.64	59	4.68	87.94	26	2.53	96.39
12–12.9	205–221	54	2.35	93.99	39	3.09	91.03	14	1.37	97.76
13–13.9	222–238	43	1.87	95.86	35	2.78	93.81	8	0.78	98.54
14–14.9	239–256	30	1.31	97.17	26	2.06	95.87	2	0.19	98.73
15–15.9	257–273	31	1.35	98.52	24	1.91	97.78	7	0.68	99.42
16–16.9	274–290	16	0.7	99.22	16	1.27	99.05	0	0	99.42
17–17.9	291–307	11	0.48	99.7	8	0.63	99.68	3	0.29	99.71
18–18.9	308–324	4	0.17	99.87	2	0.16	99.84	2	0.19	99.9
19–19.9	325–341	3	0.13	100	2	0.16	100	1	0.1	100

* Includes 11 infants who were both breast- and bottle-fed.
From Maisels MJ, Gifford KL, Antle CE, et al. Normal serum bilirubin levels in the newborn and the effect of breast feeding. Pediatrics 1986;78:837.

TABLE 38–8
MAXIMAL DIRECT BILIRUBIN LEVELS IN FULL-TERM INFANTS AT TWO HOSPITALS

	University of California, San Francisco* (n = 4948)		Stanford University† (n = 307)	
Percentile	μmol/L	mg/dL	μmol/L	mg/dL
50	19	1.1	7	0.4
75	24	1.4	10	0.6
90	32	1.9	14	0.8
95	39	2.3	17	1.0
99	63	3.7	77	4.5

* Direct bilirubin was measured either on a Dupont-automated chemical analyzer (DuPont Instruments, Wilmington, DE) or a Coulter Dacos analyzer (Coulter Electronics, Hialeah, FL).

† The Kodak Ektachem 700 (Eastman Kodak Company, Rochester, NY) was used. This instrument measures conjugated bilirubin, which is not synonymous with direct bilirubin.

From Newman TB, Hope S, Stevenson DK. Direct bilirubin measurements in jaundiced term newborns. Am J Dis Child 1991;145:1305.

μmol/L) until about 4 days of age, when they decline to normal adult values. There is a similar pattern in the full-term human neonate, but both phases last much longer and vary considerably among different racial groups. The pattern is also strongly influenced by breast- or formula-feeding (Fig. 38-14). Compared with formula-fed infants, breast-fed infants tend to have a more rapidly rising and prolonged phase I and a very prolonged phase II that, in some infants, may extend for several weeks (see Figs. 38-12 and 38-14). As can be seen from Figure 38-14, mean peak serum bilirubin levels in full-term newborns range from about 5.6 to 12.8 mg/dL (96–219 μmol/L), depending on the population and feeding method. Low-birth-weight infants, if untreated, have exaggerated and prolonged hyperbilirubinemia, with peak serum bilirubin levels of 10 to 15 mg/dL (171–257 μmol/L) on days 5 to 6 (*i.e.*, phase I), then lower concentrations, which may persist for up to 4 weeks.

Jaundice may result from an increased load of bilirubin on the liver cell, including that contributed by the enterohepatic circulation, and a decrease in the ability of the liver to clear the bilirubin from the plasma as a result of defective uptake, conjugation, or excretion, singly or in any combination. Physiologic jaundice is probably the result of the interaction of a number of these factors (Table 38-9).

CLINICAL DIAGNOSIS OF JAUNDICE

CEPHALOPEDAL PROGRESSION

In newborns, jaundice is detected by blanching the skin with digital pressure, thus revealing the underlying color of the skin and subcutaneous tissue. This dermal icterus is seen first in the face and then pro-

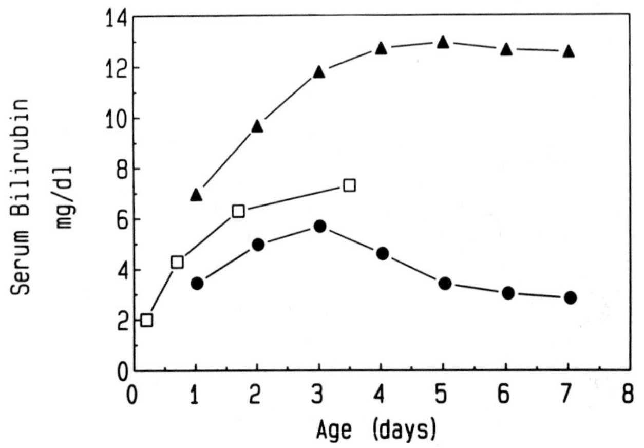

FIG. 38–14. Mean total daily bilirubin concentrations in normal full-term infants. (▲) Fifty healthy Japanese newborn infants, 37–42 weeks of gestation, all breast-fed. Excludes Rh and ABO incompatibility. (Data from Yamauchi Y, Yamanouchi I. Transcutaneous bilirubinometry in normal Japanese infants. Acta Paediatr Jpn 1989;31:65.) (□) Two hundred and seventy-five full-term Israeli infants.) 37–41 weeks of gestation, 65% breast-fed, 30% breast- and formula-fed, 5% formula-fed. Excludes infants with hemolytic disease, respiratory distress, or sepsis. Values estimated from graphic data. (Data from Frishberg Y, Zelicovic I, Merlob P, et al. Hyperbilirubinemia and influencing factors in term infants. Isr J Med Sci 1989;25:28.) (●), Twenty-nine full-term American infants, all formula-fed, about 50% African American and 50% Caucasian. Values estimated from graphic data. (Data from Gartner LM, Lee K-S, Vaisman S, et al. Development of bilirubin transport and metabolism in the newborn rhesus monkey. J Pediatr 1977;90:513.)

TABLE 38–9
POSSIBLE MECHANISMS INVOLVED IN PHYSIOLOGIC JAUNDICE

Increased Bilirubin Load on Liver Cell
Increased erythrocyte volume
Decreased erythrocyte survival
Increased early-labeled bilirubin
Increased enterohepatic circulation of bilirubin
Defective Hepatic Uptake of Bilirubin From Plasma
Decreased ligandin (*i.e.*, Y protein)
Binding of Y and Z proteins by other anions
Decreased relative hepatic uptake deficiency, phase II
Defective Bilirubin Conjugation
Decreased uridine diphosphoglucuronosyltransferase activity
Increased uridine diphosphoglucose dehydrogenase activity
Defective Bilirubin Excretion
Excretion impaired but not rate-limiting

gresses in a cordad manner to the trunk and extremities. First observed over 100 years ago, the cephalocaudal progression of dermal icterus may be a useful clinical tool (Fig. 38-15; Table 38-10). Kramer studied the relation between the progression of dermal icterus and serum indirect bilirubin levels in 103 American, full-term infants (80% Caucasian).[250] Infants whose jaundice was restricted to the face and trunk and did not extend below the umbilicus all had serum bilirubin concentrations of about 12 mg/dL (205 μmol/L) or less. Those whose hands and feet were jaundiced all had serum bilirubin levels in excess of 15 mg/dL (257 μmol/L). Ebbesen did a similar study but examined infants in daylight[251]; Kramer's observations were carried out under blue–white fluorescent light.[250] Although Ebbesen confirmed the usual cephalocaudal progression, distal icterus corresponded with much lower bilirubin levels than those found by Kramer. Ebbesen found that if dermal icterus did not progress below the knees, serum bilirubin levels never exceeded 6.4 mg/dL (μmol/L). The differences may be related to the different populations studied. Ebbesen studied a mixed Scandinavian population of full-term and premature infants. He found no effect of prematurity on dermal icterus.[251]

The cephalocaudal progression of jaundice has also been studied using transcutaneous bilirubinometry.[252–255] These measurements provide objective confirmation that, at any given bilirubin level, the skin in the face is more yellow than that in the foot. Knudsen suggested that the cephalocaudal color difference in newborns is explained by conformational changes in the bilirubin–albumin complex.[254] He hypothesizes that the yellow color of the skin in icteric newborns is made up of a contribution from natural skin color, bilirubin–albumin complexes that are located outside the vascular space, and precipitated bilirubin acid in phospholipid membranes. Bilirubin is formed in the reticuloendothelial system, primarily in the liver, spleen, and bone marrow, and once it reaches the plasma, it is bound tightly to albumin. The initial binding process is extremely rapid (*i.e.*, within 10 msec) and is followed by a train of slow relaxing changes in the conformation of the bilirubin–albumin complex. Major conformational changes in the biliru-

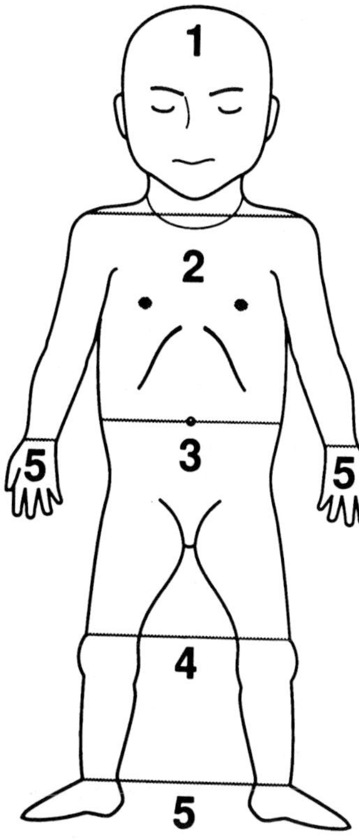

FIG. 38–15. Dermal zones of jaundice.

TABLE 38–10
INDIRECT SERUM BILIRUBIN CONCENTRATION AND ITS RELATION TO THE PROGRESSION OF DERMAL ICTERUS IN FULL-TERM INFANTS*

Dermal Zone†	Bilirubin (mg/100 mL) Mean ± SD	Range	Observations
1	5.9 ± 0.3	4.3–7.9	13
2	8.9 ± 1.7	5.4–12.2	49
3	11.8 ± 1.8	8.1–16.5	52
4	15.0 ± 1.7	11.1–18.3	45
5		>15	29

* Includes all infants whose rate of serum bilirubin rise was 0.7 mg/dL/h or less.

† See Figure 38-15.

From Kramer LI. Advancement of dermal icterus in the jaundiced newborn. Am J Dis Child 1969;118:454.

bin–albumin complex occur within 1 to 30 seconds, and a final conformation is reached 8 minutes after binding.[256] Initially, therefore, there is a lower bilirubin-binding affinity to albumin until the final stage of conformation has occurred. Thus, lower bilirubin affinity for albumin is present in the blood immediately after it has left the reticuloendothelial system, but increasing affinity is present as the blood reaches the distal portions of the body. If some of the yellow color of the skin is the result of precipitated bilirubin acid, then, in the presence of reduced bilirubin-binding affinity to albumin, there is an increase in precipitation of bilirubin acid and thus an increase in the yellow color of the skin. This is more likely to occur in the proximal parts of the body because of the conformational changes in the young bilirubin–albumin complexes. Consistent with this hypothesis, Knudsen found that there was a significant and linear correlation between the cephalocaudal color difference, the plasma bilirubin concentration, and the square of the hydrogen ion concentration.[254] The cephalocaudal color difference was inversely related to the reserve albumin concentration, thus suggesting that the conformational change in the young bilirubin–albumin complex enhances the precipitation of bilirubin acid in the skin of the proximal parts of the body. If this is the mechanism, then objective measurement of the yellow color of the skin using a transcutaneous bilirubinometer could be a better predictor of potential bilirubin encephalopathy than a serum bilirubin measurement.

EVALUATING JAUNDICED INFANTS

Because clinical jaundice becomes apparent at serum bilirubin levels of about 5 mg/dL (85 μmol/L), 65% of all normal newborns are jaundiced during the first week of life (see Table 38-7). It is therefore important for the physician caring for newborns to develop a relatively consistent approach to the investigation and management of the jaundiced newborn. Such an approach is suggested by the following questions:

Is the jaundice physiologic or nonphysiologic, and, possibly, pathologic?
If not physiologic jaundice, what are the possible causes?
Which infants require further investigation, and what investigations are needed?
Is the jaundice a threat to the infant?
  What investigations are required to assess the potential danger?
  If danger exists, what treatment is appropriate?

DIFFERENTIATING PHYSIOLOGIC FROM NONPHYSIOLOGIC JAUNDICE

The definitions of physiologic and nonphysiologic jaundice are based on the natural history of bilirubinemia and normal serum bilirubin levels in the first weeks of life. These definitions have led to the establishment of criteria for the evaluation and treatment of jaundiced infants. Some authorities advise measuring bilirubin levels in all jaundiced infants.[257,258] In those with early jaundice or bilirubin levels higher than 12 to 13 mg/dL (205–222 μmol/L), additional diagnostic evaluation is recommended.[257,259] These recommendations are likely to lead to unnecessary testing of many jaundiced full-term infants,[260] and they can do more harm than good.[261] It has also become clear that in the United States, the heterogeneity of the population no longer permits the application of standard measurements to the definition of physiologic jaundice. Tables 38-2, 38-3, and 38-5 through 38-7 and Figure 38-14 show the effect of breast-feeding, racial group, and other epidemiologic factors on bilirubin levels. An infant with many of the known nonpathologic risk factors may have a 6 to 16 times greater risk of developing a serum bilirubin level of 13 mg/dL (222 μmol/L) or greater (Table 38-11).

IDENTIFYING NONPHYSIOLOGIC JAUNDICE

In the past, whenever nonphysiologic jaundice was suspected, standard investigations included the following tests:

- serum bilirubin concentration, direct and total
- complete blood cell count, including hemoglobin, reticulocyte count, and peripheral smear for erythrocyte morphology
- blood type and Rh determination of mother and infant and direct Coombs test of infant's blood.

Problems with this approach include the following[260]:

First, the data from which definitions of physiologic and nonphysiologic jaundice are derived are based on bilirubin levels obtained during an era when about 25% of infants were breast-fed and most remained in the nursery for several days. In most nurseries in the United States today, at least 50% and sometimes more than 80% of infants are breast-fed, and all vaginally delivered infants are discharged within 48 hours, necessitating reevaluation of the infant by a health visitor, physician, or parent in the first few days after birth.

Second, with few exceptions, the recommended laboratory tests listed previously are not particularly helpful. In studies at the Hershey Medical Center[81] and UCSF,[75] almost 5000 jaundiced infants who weighed more than 2500 g were evaluated using the tests listed above. The only diagnoses made as a result of the routine investigation of jaundice were polycythemia and ABO or Rh immunization. These conditions accounted for jaundice in fewer than 20% of infants.

TABLE 38–11
PROBABILITY OF JAUNDICE IN HYPOTHETICAL INFANTS

Variable Factors	Infant A	Infant B	Infant C	Infant D	Infant E
Gestation (wk)	39	40	38	42	38
Weight loss (%)	5	7	15	10	10
East Asian	−	−	−	+	−
Oxytocin induction	−	−	−	−	+
Maternal diabetes	−	−	−	−	+
Breast-fed	−	+	+	+	+
Male gender	−	−	+	+	+
Odds	0.014	0.0626	0.720	2.032	5.335
Jaundice risk (%)	1.4	5.9	42	67	84
95% confidence limits for jaundice risk (%)	0.7–2.6	3.7–9.3	19–68.4	17.2–95.1	38.5–97.9

Odds = (probability of serum bilirubin ≤ 12.9 mg/dL)/(probability of serum bilirubin ≤ 12.9 mg/dL). Jaundice risk = probability of having serum bilirubin > 12.9 mg/dL = (odds)/(1 + odds). Example: Infant C is a breast-fed boy with a 15% weight loss. The odds of his having a serum bilirubin > 12.9 mg/dL are 0.720:1, and the risk of jaundice is 42%. Note: In our population, the prevalence of hyperbilirubinemia (*i.e.*, serum bilirubin > 12.9 mg/dL) is 6.1%. If no information is available on an infant, the odds are 0.065, and the risk of jaundice is 6.1%. Confidence limits are 5% to 7%.

+, factor present; −, factor absent.

From Maisels MJ, Gifford K, Antle CE, et al. Jaundice in the healthy newborn infant: a new approach to an old problem. Pediatrics 1988;81:505.

In most circumstances, the Rh type of the mother and her infant is known, whether or not the infant is jaundiced. Mothers who have had no antenatal care must have blood typing performed to identify the need for Rh immunoglobulin. The diagnosis of ABO isoimmunization is much more difficult (see Chap. 45).[262] Although as many as 33% of group A or B infants born to group O mothers have anti-A or anti-B antibodies attached to their erythrocytes, only a small proportion of these (perhaps 1 in 5) have hyperbilirubinemia or other evidence of hemolytic disease. ABO-incompatible Coombs-positive infants are about twice as likely as their compatible peers to have a serum bilirubin level of more than 12 mg/dL (205 μmol/L),[263] but severe jaundice in these infants is uncommon.[263–266] The presence of jaundice in an ABO-incompatible, Coombs-positive infant does not necessarily mean that the infant has ABO hemolytic disease. Because evidence from earlier studies suggests that hyperbilirubinemia is more hazardous in the presence of isoimmunization, it is probably worthwhile to identify ABO immunization in infants with severe jaundice and to treat them more aggressively than infants with nonhemolytic jaundice. The rate of rise of serum bilirubin is helpful when some form of hemolytic process is being considered, and a bilirubin level of 15 mg/dL (257 μmol/L) at 30 hours of age would raise concerns that are different from those suggested by a similar bilirubin level at 3 to 5 days of age. In certain populations, the diagnosis of G6PD deficiency or other hereditary hemolytic anemias must be considered as well as other less common causes of jaundice.[267–270]

No jaundice should be dismissed as physiologic without at least a review of the maternal and infant history, examination of the infant, and if necessary, pursuit of further laboratory investigations. On occasion, jaundice may be one sign of serious illness, and the presence of any of the associated signs listed in Table 38-12 demands evaluation and treatment as indicated. The problems are that jaundice is common, most of the diseases the tests aim to identify are rare, and the tests are neither sensitive nor specific.

Bacterial infection is a recognized cause of hyperbilirubinemia in the newborn, and some reports have suggested that unexplained indirect hyperbilirubinemia may be the only manifestation of sepsis in otherwise healthy-appearing newborns.[271–273] However, jaundice is rarely the only manifestation of bacteremia or incipient sepsis. In 306 newborns admitted to a

TABLE 38–12
DANGER SIGNS IN JAUNDICED INFANTS

Family history of significant hemolytic disease
Onset of jaundice in first 24 hours of life
Onset of jaundice after day 3 of life
Vomiting
Lethargy
Poor feeding
Fever
High-pitched cry
Dark urine
Light stools

pediatric ward within 21 days of birth with the diagnosis of indirect hyperbilirubinemia (peak serum bilirubin levels 18.5 ± 2.8; range 12.7 – 29.1 mg/dL, or 316 ± 4.8, 217–498 μmol/L), not one case of sepsis was identified (upper 95% confidence limit for the risk of sepsis = 1%).[185] If a good screening test for sepsis were available, it would be worth looking for in spite of its rarity because it is both serious and treatable. As can be seen in Table 38-13, in most full-term, jaundiced newborns, no pathologic cause of the jaundice can be identified. Jaundice is a common entity, and the finding of a positive blood or urine culture in a newborn with indirect hyperbilirubinemia does not prove that the infection is the cause of the jaundice. On the other hand, infants who exhibit other signs or symptoms (see Table 38-12) deserve more careful evaluation, particularly those who have late-onset jaundice after physiologic icterus has resolved, direct hyperbilirubinemia, or something in the history, physical examination, or laboratory investigations that is out of the ordinary.

MEASURING DIRECT BILIRUBIN CONCENTRATIONS

In many nurseries, routine determinations of direct bilirubin levels are obtained whenever the total bilirubin level exceeds a predetermined level. Measurements of direct bilirubin, however, are notoriously inaccurate (see Table 38-8; see Clinical Management),[249,274–277] and when used as a screening test in the newborn nursery, direct bilirubin measurements provide a low yield and are nonspecific if the intent is to rule out treatable causes of cholestasis, such as biliary atresia or galactosemia.[249] Biliary atresia occurs in 10 of every 100,000 births and galactosemia in about 2 in 100,000 births. In contrast, 15,000 of 100,000 infants have significant jaundice, of whom at least 750 (5%) have a direct bilirubin level above the 95th percentile. Fortunately, galactosemia can be identified by a routine metabolic screen performed in the nursery, and biliary atresia should be diagnosed by selective testing of infants with prolonged jaundice (>2 weeks), light stools, or dark urine.

Every infant who is jaundiced beyond 2 weeks of age must have a measurement of direct bilirubin performed. If this is elevated, the urine should be tested for bile and the stool color evaluated.[278] This approach is essential for the early identification of infants with biliary atresia. If these infants are to benefit from the operation of portoenterostomy, surgery must be performed before 60 days of age.[279,280] If an elevated direct bilirubin measurement is obtained while the infant is in the nursery, it must be repeated; if it remains elevated, the infant must be investigated for possible causes of cholestatic jaundice (Fig. 38-16).

PRACTICAL APPROACH TO EVALUATION

Given that jaundice in the newborn nursery is extremely common, but only rarely due to a pathologic entity, and recognizing that early neonatal discharge has rendered daily evaluation impossible, Newman and Maisels suggested two different strategies for the evaluation and follow-up of jaundiced infants.[260] Guidelines for evaluation and a diagnostic approach to the jaundiced infant are given in Figures 38-15 and 38-16 and in Tables 38-10, 38-14, and 38-15. Although most routine laboratory testing rarely reveals information of importance, jaundice should not be ignored. Particularly in association with other findings, jaundice may be a sign of serious illness. Thus, jaundice in an infant should always trigger a clinical evaluation to determine whether any danger signs are present (see Table 38-12). If they are, more aggressive evaluation and treatment are indicated.

Since a short postdelivery hospital stay is the norm for newborns and the length of stay is likely to become even shorter, it may be advantageous to try to

TABLE 38–13
DISCHARGE DIAGNOSIS IN 306 INFANTS ADMITTED WITH SEVERE HYPERBILIRUBINEMIA*

Diagnosis	Number	Percentage
Hyperbilirubinemia of unknown cause or breast-milk jaundice	290	94.8
Cephalhematoma or bruising	3	1.0
ABO hemolytic disease†	11	3.6
Anti-E hemolytic disease	1	0.3
Galactosemia	1	0.3
Sepsis	0	

* Infants were readmitted after discharge as newborns. Mean age at admission was 5 days (range, 2–17 days), and mean bilirubin level was 18.5 ± 2.8 mg/dL (range, 12.7–29.1 mg/dL).

† Mother was type O, infant was type A or B, direct Coombs test was positive.

From Maisels MJ, Kring E. Risk of sepsis in newborns with severe hyperbilirubinemia. Pediatrics 1992;90:741.

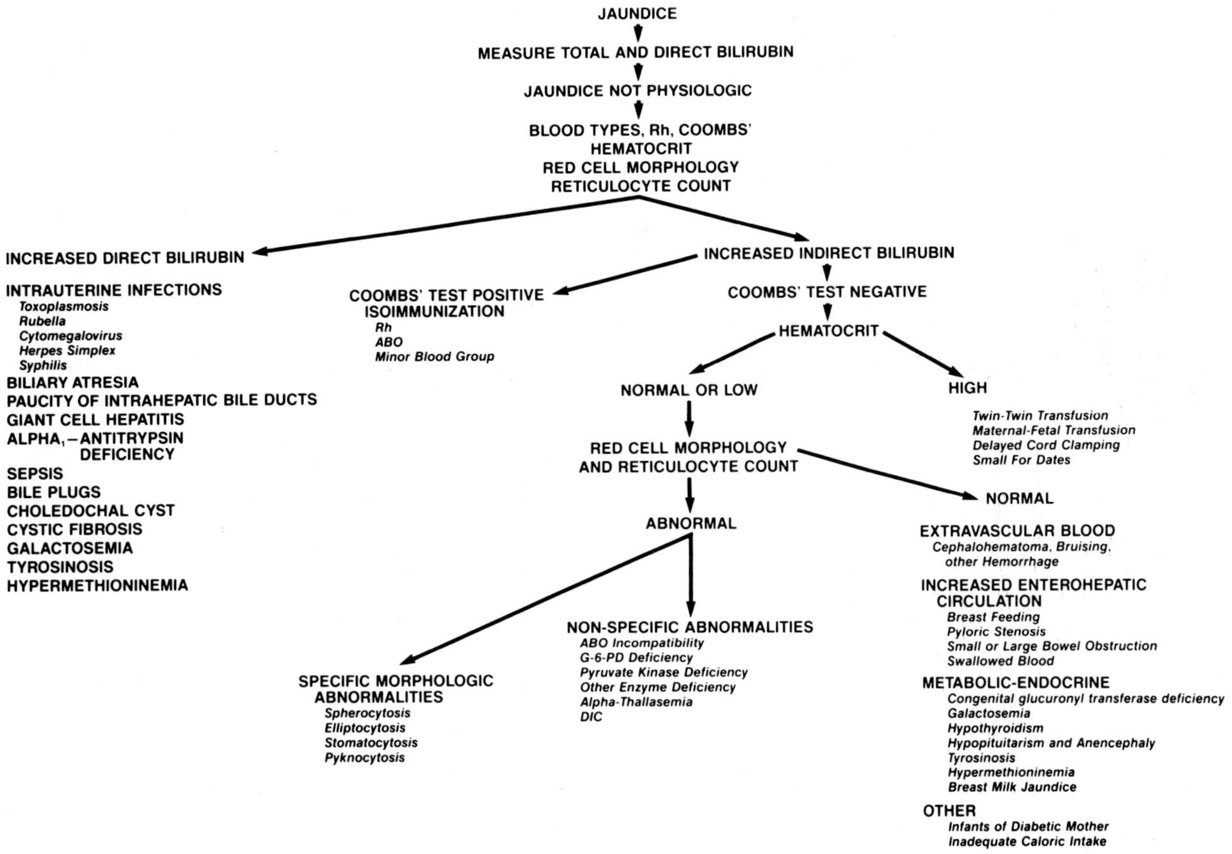

FIG. 38–16. Diagnostic approach to neonatal jaundice.

TABLE 38–14
SUGGESTED GUIDELINES FOR EVALUATION AND FOLLOW-UP OF JAUNDICE IN FULL-TERM INFANTS*

Indications	Maneuvers
Rh-negative mothers†	Blood type, group, and Coombs test, determined from cord blood
Any jaundice in first 24 hours‡	Serum bilirubin level
Jaundice after 24 hours	Observe for dermal distribution
Jaundice below umbilicus from 24–48 hours	Transcutaneous bilirubin, icterometer assessment, or serum bilirubin level
Jaundice below knee	Transcutaneous bilirubin, icterometer assessment, or serum bilirubin level
Jaundice in hands or feet	Serum bilirubin level
Infants with evidence of hemolysis	Follow bilirubin until peak

* Note that these guidelines cannot take into account all possible situations. Full-term infants are infants of at least 37 weeks of gestation.

† In some institutions, blood type, group, and Coombs tests are performed on the cord blood of infants of all group-O mothers to identify ABO incompatibility. This information could be helpful, particularly if follow-up is difficult or uncertain.

‡ This time period is not immutable. As is clear from Figure 38-14, many normal infants appear slightly jaundiced by 24 hours of age. Nevertheless, if jaundice is present well before 24 hours of age, it is almost always due to increased bilirubin production (usually hemolysis), and possible causes must be sought. Similarly, obvious jaundice appearing at 25 hours of age is more likely to be pathologic than jaundice at 48 hours of age. Hemolytic jaundice associated with glucose-6-phosphate dehydrogenase deficiency can be an exception.

TABLE 38–15
ADDITIONAL LABORATORY EVALUATION OF THE JAUNDICED FULL-TERM INFANT

Indications	Maneuvers
Suspicion of hemolytic disease or anemia (*e.g.*, pallor, early jaundice, or TB > 14 mg/dL [239 μmol/L] in first 48 hours of life)	Blood type, group, and Coombs test, if not obtained with cord blood Complete blood count and smear Reticulocyte count
Asian or Mediterranean infants, especially males, with TB > 15 mg/dL (257 μmol/L), particularly if late-onset jaundice	Glucose-6-phosphate dehydrogenase screen
Jaundice beyond 2 weeks of age	Direct bilirubin level, urine dipstick for bilirubin, inspect stools for color Check results of newborn thyroid screen, evaluate infant for signs or symptoms of hypothyroidism
Infant ill	Direct bilirubin level, check urine for reducing substances, check results of newborn screen for galactosemia, and evaluate for sepsis

TB, total bilirubin concentration.

identify isoimmunization soon after birth by performing a blood type and Coombs test on infants of group O mothers. Such testing is mandatory for all infants of Rh-negative mothers. The most frequent cause of isoimmunization is ABO incompatibility. Although the risk for severe jaundice in these infants is low,[263–266] the identification of ABO isoimmunization suggests the need for more careful surveillance, perhaps delaying discharge if outpatient follow-up cannot be ensured. A positive Coombs test is more likely to occur on cord blood than on a blood sample drawn several days later. Nevertheless, there is no good evidence that routine testing of infants of group O mothers is beneficial, and it increases costs.

Because most infants are discharged well before the peak serum bilirubin has been attained (see Fig. 38-14), it would be reassuring if these infants could be seen at about 3 to 4 days after birth. In some countries, this is achieved by a home visit from a nurse. Although nonhemolytic jaundice is usually benign, some workers in this field have encountered apparently healthy full-term, Coombs-negative infants who were discharged from the hospital only to reappear on days 4 to 7 with serum bilirubin levels of 30 mg/dL (513 μmol/L) or greater. Some of these infants developed kernicterus.[281] Unfortunately, apart from the epidemiologic and other factors already discussed, there is no easy way to identify these infants before they leave the hospital, nor is it known how often hyperbilirubinemia of this magnitude occurs. To prevent an unknown number of infants from becoming severely jaundiced, every infant would have to be seen at age 3 to 4 days, a practice that would lead to an increase in costs and other risks (*e.g.*, repeated laboratory tests, visits, and treatment in infants who would otherwise have done perfectly well).

Clinical jaundice is easy to recognize in newborns, but the ability of physicians and parents to estimate the degree of jaundice varies considerably. For this reason, the use of noninvasive methods for screening jaundiced infants should be encouraged. The Minolta Air-Shields Jaundice Meter (Air-Shields, Vickers, Hatboro, PA) and the Ingram Icterometer (Cascade Health Care Products, Salem, OR) are both effective screening tools.[282] Even the use of these simple devices, however, requires contact between the infant and a health care professional, and many infants need to be followed closely for each one that becomes significantly jaundiced. If jaundice persists beyond 2 weeks of age, a urinalysis with dipstick test for bilirubin and a direct bilirubin measurement should be performed to rule out treatable causes of cholestasis.

Some causes of jaundice, such as G6PD deficiency, are particularly problematic (see Chap. 45).[283] In contrast to the jaundice caused by blood-group incompatibilities, jaundice in infants with G6PD deficiency commonly does not appear until the second day of life and often appears much later. Furthermore, the risk for jaundice and subsequent neurologic damage probably depends on the particular isoenzyme present and on triggering environmental factors that may account for the striking differences in the incidence of neonatal hyperbilirubinemia in different populations.[284] The risk for kernicterus in G6PD-deficient infants appears to be similar to that associated with Rh disease.[268–270]

Although they usually weigh more than 2500 g and are treated as normal infants in the well-baby nursery, infants who are even slightly premature (35–37 weeks of gestation) are much more likely to develop hyperbilirubinemia. Gale and colleagues found that infants at 37 weeks of gestation were four times more likely than those at 40 weeks of gestation to have a serum bilirubin level of 13 mg/dL or higher.[76] These slightly premature infants do not feed as well as their full-term peers, particularly if they are breast-fed, and they require more careful scrutiny than full-term infants.

PATHOLOGIC JAUNDICE

INDIRECT HYPERBILIRUBINEMIA

The causes of pathologic indirect hyperbilirubinemia in the neonate are listed in Table 38-16.

INCREASED BILIRUBIN LOAD

Hemolytic Disease. Hemolytic causes of hyperbilirubinemia are discussed fully in Chapter 45. The introduction of Rh immunoglobulin has dramatically reduced the incidence of erythroblastosis fetalis, and the combination of postpartum and antepartum prophylaxis has reduced the incidence of antepartum sensitization of Rh-negative mothers to 0.17%.[285] Other hemolytic processes to be considered include spherocytosis and other morphologic abnormalities of the erythrocyte, in addition to erythrocyte enzyme deficiencies (see Fig. 38-16; see Table 38-16; see Chap. 45). Cord blood screening programs for hemoglobinopathies permit the diagnosis of sickle-cell disease in the immediate neonatal period. Although previous reports suggested an association between sickle-cell disease and jaundice in the newborn, a matched, case-control study of 68 neonates with sickle-cell disease found no increase in the rate of clinical jaundice and no increase in bilirubin levels in patients with sickle-cell disease compared with controls.[286]

Extravascular Blood. Cephalhematomas, intracranial or pulmonary hemorrhage, or any occult bleeding may lead to an elevated serum bilirubin level from breakdown of the extravascular erythrocytes.[287–289] In two reports, severe hyperbilirubinemia followed delayed absorption of intraperitoneal blood in infants who received fetal transfusions before birth.[287,289] In both reported cases, despite multiple exchange transfusions, hyperbilirubinemia was not controlled until peritoneal lavage was performed.

In the very-low-birth-weight infant, the presence of periventricular–intraventricular hemorrhage (PIVH) has been associated with an increase in serum bilirubin levels in some studies,[290,291] but not in others.[292] Amato and colleagues studied 88 infants with birth weights less than 1500 g.[292] Phototherapy was initiated only when serum bilirubin levels exceeded 12 mg/dL (205 μmol/L). The incidence of serum bilirubin levels greater than 12 mg/dL was 39% in the PIVH group and 46.8% in the infants without PIVH. There was no difference in the duration of phototherapy in the two groups. Unless phototherapy is withheld, as was done in Amato's study, it is difficult to evaluate the effect of PIVH on serum bilirubin levels, making some studies difficult to interpret.[293] In infants of less than 1250 g of birth weight, mean serum bilirubin levels on day 5 were about 8.0 mg/dL in those with PIVH, compared with levels of 6.2 mg/dL in infants with no hemorrhage.[290] Linear regression analysis showed a significant influence of PIVH on the bilirubin birth weight index (*i.e.*, the bilirubin level divided by the birth weight in kg), and the effect of PIVH was most prominent in infants with birth weights less than 1000 g.[290]

TABLE 38–16
CAUSES OF PATHOLOGIC INDIRECT HYPERBILIRUBINEMIA IN NEWBORN INFANTS

Increased Production
Fetomaternal blood group incompatibility; Rh, ABO, and others
Hereditary spherocytosis
Nonspherocytic hemolytic anemias
Glucose-6-phosphate dehydrogenase deficiency and drugs
Pyruvate kinase deficiency
Other erythrocyte enzyme deficiencies
Alpha thalassemia
Beta-γ-thalassemia
Vitamin K_3–induced hemolysis
Sepsis*†
Exravasation of blood; petechiae; hematoma; pulmonary, cerebral, or occult hemorrhage
Polycythemia
Maternofetal and fetofetal transfusion
Delayed clamping of cord
Swallowed blood
Increased enterohepatic circulation of bilirubin
Pyloric stenosis*
Small or large bowel obstruction or ileus
Infants of diabetic mothers
Decreased Clearance
Inborn errors of metabolism
Familial nonhemolytic jaundice types 1 and 2 and Gilbert syndrome
Galactosemia†
Tyrosinemia†
Hypermethioninemia†
Drugs and hormones
Hypothyroidism
Hypopituitarism†
Breast-milk jaundice
Prematurity

* Decreased clearance also part of pathogenesis.
† Elevation of direct-reacting bilirubin also occurs.

Polycythemia. The catabolism of 1 g of hemoglobin produces 35 mg of bilirubin, and it is reasonable to assume that a high hematocrit is a risk factor for neonatal jaundice. Twin-to-twin transfusion, maternofetal transfusion, or other factors that produce elevated hemoglobin levels or an increase in the erythrocyte mass should increase the bilirubin load presented to the liver. Nevertheless, mean bilirubin levels and the incidence of hyperbilirubinemia were similar in polycythemic infants randomly assigned to receive either partial exchange transfusions or symptomatic treatment (see Epidemiology).[144–146]

Increased Enterohepatic Circulation. Intestinal obstruction or a delay in bowel transit time increases the enterohepatic circulation by allowing more time for bilirubin deconjugation and reabsorption. Jaundice is common in infants with small bowel obstruction and also occurs in infants with pyloric stenosis.[294,295] Correction of the obstruction produces a prompt decline in bilirubin levels.

Infants of Diabetic Mothers. Recent studies suggest that hyperbilirubinemia is limited to macrosomic infants of mothers with insulin-dependent diabetes and is the result of increased bilirubin production (see Epidemiology of Neonatal Jaundice: Maternal Factors).

DECREASED BILIRUBIN CLEARANCE

Nonhemolytic Unconjugated Hyperbilirubinemia

Three degrees of defect are recognized:

1. Marked defect, characterized by absolute failure of bilirubin biotransformation through the normal pathway
2. Moderate defect, characterized by a marked to moderate decrease in the activity of the pathway that responds to inducing agents such as phenobarbital
3. Mild defect, characterized by a mild decrease in the activity of the pathway reaching clinical significance only under special circumstances.

The principal characteristics of these three types are listed in Table 38-17.[296–298]

Type I Glucuronosyl Transferase Deficiency. Type I glucuronosyl transferase dificiency is inherited as an autosomal recessive gene and is also known as the type I Crigler-Najjar syndrome. Infants with this condition have virtually complete absence of hepatic glucuronosyl transferase. They develop severe jaundice in the first 2 to 3 days of life, and exchange transfusion is commonly necessary in the first week of life. Subsequently, intensive home phototherapy controls bilirubin levels to some extent,[299,300] but as these children get older, increasing skin thickness and pigmentation and a decrease in the surface area–body mass ratio render phototherapy less effective.[301,302] Brain damage can occur at any time in the first two decades,[303] and plasmapheresis is used to reduce bilirubin concentrations during acute exacerbations of hyperbilirubinemia.[10,301,304] One 16-year-old boy with type I Crigler–Najjar syndrome had 72 plasma exchanges over a period of 28 months before undergoing orthotopic liver transplantation.[305] Serum bilirubin concentrations decline dramatically within hours of liver transplantation (Fig. 38-17).[300,306]

Infants who develop kernicterus generally have the classic syndrome, including choreoathetosis, hearing loss, and severe mental retardation. Labrune and colleagues described three children with Crigler–Najjar type I disease whose first manifestations of kernicterus were seen between the ages of 2.5 to 6 years.[307] All three children had the onset of acute cerebellar symptoms after an intercurrent infection or, in one case, the interruption of phototherapy. The clinical presentation was characterized by gait disturbances, ataxia, and dysmetric movements. These features have not been described in the typical syndrome of acute bilirubin encephalopathy in the neonate (see Bilirubin Toxicity), perhaps because the onset of neurologic disease in the neonate is rapid or because it is difficult to detect cerebellar symptoms in the neonatal period. Cerebellar symptoms have been described as sequelae of kernicterus in some older patients.[303,308] Gunn rats, the animal model for the Crigler–Najjar syndrome, have degenerative lesions of the brain, of which cerebellar hypoplasia is one of the most striking.[309] In children with Crigler–Najjar disease, it is important to manage intercurrent infections promptly and to follow bilirubin levels closely.

The diagnosis of Crigler–Najjar syndrome is made most readily by high-performance liquid chromatography analysis of serum and bile obtained by a duodenal tube and by evaluating the response to phenobarbital. In type I Crigler–Najjar disease, phenobarbital has little or no effect on the serum bilirubin concentrations, and bile pigments are found to contain about 90% unconjugated bilirubin, 9% monoconjugates, and 1% or less diconjugates. In children with type II disease, serum bilirubin levels decrease by 27% to 72% during phenobarbital treatment, and the bile pigment consists mainly of monoconjugates (57%), with unconjugated bilirubin and diconjugates representing 33% and 10%, respectively.

Type II Glucuronosyl Transferase Deficiency. This disease is also known as type II Crigler–Najjar disease or Arias syndrome. These infants generally manifest with less severe jaundice, although severe hyperbilirubinemia can occur, and kernicterus has been

TABLE 38–17
CONGENITAL NONHEMOLYTIC UNCONJUGATED HYPERBILIRUBINEMIA: CLINICAL SYNDROMES

Characteristics	Marked (Crigler–Najjar Syndrome; Arias Type I)	Moderate (Arias Type II)	Mild (Gilbert Syndrome)
Steady-state serum bilirubin	>20 mg/dL	<20 mg/dL	<5 mg/dL
Range of bilirubin values	14–50 mg/dL	5.3–37.6 mg/dL	0.8–10 mg/dL
Bilirubin in bile			
Total	<10 mg/dL (increased with phototherapy)	50–100 mg/dL	Normal
Conjugated	Absent	Present (only monoglucuronide)	Present (50% monoglucuronide)
Bilirubin–UDPGT activity *in vitro*	None detected	None detected	20%–30% of normal
Bilirubin clearance	Extremely decreased	Markedly decreased	20%–30% of normal
Hepatic bilirubin uptake	Normal	Normal	Reduced
Glucuronide formation with other substrates	Reduced	Reduced	Reduced?
Response to phenobarbital			
Plasma bilirubin	Unchanged	Decreased but remains above normal range	Within normal range
Bilirubin–UDPGT activity	None detected	None detected	Within normal range
Glucuronidation of other substrates	Increased from previous subnormal levels	Increased from previous subnormal levels	Increased
Smooth endoplasmic reticulum	Hypertrophy	Hypertrophy	Hypertrophy
Bilirubin encephalopathy	Usually present	Uncommon; may occur only in the neonatal period	Not present
Genetics	Autosomal recessive; parents often related; both demonstrate impairment of glucuronidation but have normal bilirubin levels	Heterogeneity of defect distinctly possible; autosomal dominant?; double heterozygotes?; no parental consanguinity; abnormal glucuronidation or Gilbert defect in one of the parents	Autosomal dominant (heterozygotes); usually one of the parents demonstrates similar abnormality

UDPGT, UDP glucuronosyltransferase.
From Valaes T. Bilirubin metabolism: review and discussion of inborn errors. Clin Perinatol 1976;3:177.

reported in some infants. Both infants and adults with type II Crigler–Najjar syndrome respond readily to phenobarbital therapy with a sharp decline in serum bilirubin levels within 7 to 10 days. This response can be used to differentiate between the two syndromes. The pattern of inheritance for Crigler–Najjar type II disease has not been clearly established.[298] Suggested inheritance patterns include an autosomal dominant disease with incomplete penetrance and varied expressivity as well as autosomal recessive inheritance. Labrune and colleagues described a brother and sister who both developed prolonged indirect hyperbilirubinemia in infancy that was responsive to phenobarbital therapy.[310] The parents were unrelated, and none of the family members had ever been jaundiced. Needle biopsy specimens of the liver obtained from both infants and parents revealed markedly reduced hepatic glucuronosyl transferase activity in both infants and both parents, suggesting autosomal recessive inheritance.

Other Inborn Errors of Metabolism

Galactosemia. Galactosemia is a rare disease (worldwide incidence, about 1 in 50,000 infants), and jaundice may be one of the presenting features; but

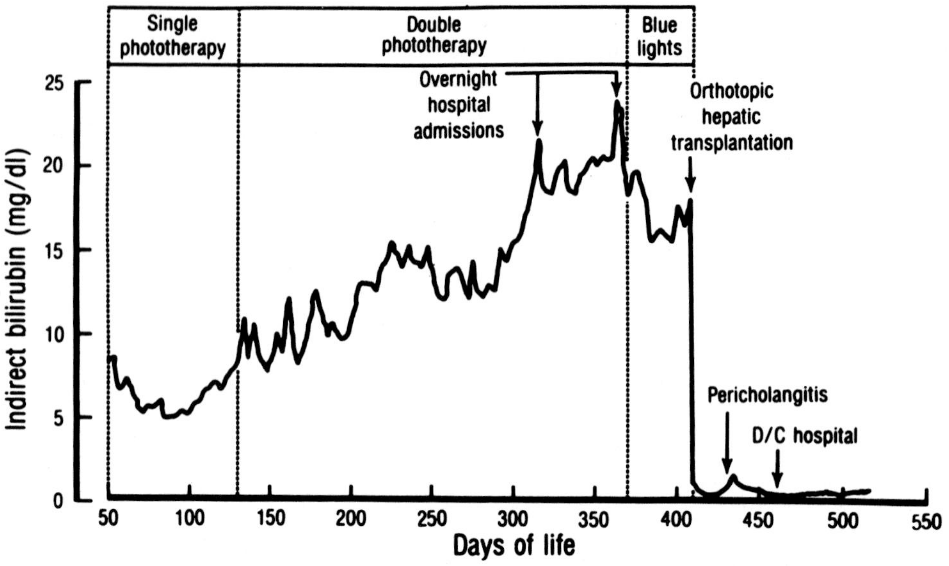

FIG. 38–17. Effect of time and various therapeutic maneuvers on indirect bilirubin concentrations in patient with Crigler–Najjar syndrome type I after discharge from neonatal intensive care unit. (From Shevell MI, Bernard B, Adelson JW, et al. Crigler-Najjar syndrome type I: treatment by home phototherapy followed by orthotopic hepatic transplantation. J Pediatr 1987;110:429.)

infants with significant hyperbilirubinemia due to galactosemia almost all have some other manifestations of the disease (*e.g.*, vomiting, excessive weight loss, hepatomegaly, splenomegaly).[185,311] Hyperbilirubinemia during the first week of life is almost exclusively unconjugated, and the conjugated fraction tends to rise during the second week, probably reflecting liver damage.[312] The presence of a positive family history, hepatomegaly, lethargy, poor feeding, or other signs of illness merit additional diagnostic evaluation, including testing the urine for reducing substances using Clinitest.

Tyrosinemia and Hypermethioninemia. The relation between these inborn errors of metabolism and jaundice is primarily due to the presence of neonatal liver disease, which may initially manifest as indirect hyperbilirubinemia but which generally is accompanied by some evidence of cholestasis (*i.e.*, direct hyperbilirubinemia).

Hypothyroidism. Prolonged indirect hyperbilirubinemia is one of the clinical features of congenital hypothyroidism, a condition that must be ruled out in any infant who has indirect hyperbilirubinemia beyond 2 to 3 weeks of age.[313–315] Although widespread availability of screening programs for congenital hypothyroidism should allow early identification of this problem as a possible cause of jaundice, screening programs do not detect every infant, and errors are more likely to occur with early discharge of infants in whom the T4 level may still be spuriously elevated. A single case of cholestasis associated with hypothyroidism has been described in a 54-year-old woman.[316]

The pathogenesis of hyperbilirubinemia associated with hypothyroidism is not clear.[317] In hypothyroid rats after thyroidectomy, the excretion rates of both unconjugated bilirubin and bilirubin monoconjugates were markedly decreased. Hypothyroidism also produced cholestasis with a 50% decrease in bile flow and bile salt excretion and an elevation in the serum conjugated bilirubin level.[317] On the other hand, there was a significant increase in hepatic bilirubin UDPGT activity. Thyroidectomized rats actually had significantly lower unconjugated bilirubin concentrations and higher concentrations of bilirubin monoconjugate and diconjugates than control rats. Thus, the mechanism for indirect hyperbilirubinemia in infants with congenital hypothyroidism is obscure.[10,307] The administration of triiodothyronine to full-term and preterm infants does not lower peak serum bilirubin levels.[318,319]

DRUGS

The use of pancuronium[243] and chloral hydrate[244,245] is associated with higher bilirubin levels in sick preterm infants, and chloral hydrate is associated with an increased risk of direct hyperbilirubinemia (see Epidemiology of Neonatal Jaundice).

BREAST-MILK JAUNDICE

See previous section on breast-feeding and jaundice.

PROLONGED INDIRECT HYPERBILIRUBINEMIA

Prolonged indirect hyperbilirubinemia is defined as indirect bilirubinemia persisting beyond 2 weeks of age in the full-term infant. The causes of prolonged indirect hyperbilirubinemia are listed in Table 38-18.

TABLE 38–18
CAUSES OF PROLONGED INDIRECT HYPERBILIRUBINEMIA

Breast-milk jaundice	Pyloric stenosis
Hemolytic disease	Crigler–Najjar syndrome
Hypothyroidism	Extravascular blood

MIXED FORMS OF JAUNDICE

SEPSIS

Jaundice is one sign of bacterial sepsis, and some reports suggest that unexplained hyperbilirubinemia may be the only manifestation of sepsis in otherwise healthy-appearing newborns.[271–273] Rooney and colleagues described a series of 22 newborns with documented bacterial infection and hyperbilirubinemia.[273] In some of these newborns, serum bilirubin levels were exceptionally high, at 28.3 to 50 mg/dL (484–855 μmol/L), and several had significant elevations of direct-reacting bilirubin. Nevertheless, nine infants were said to be "active and well throughout and jaundice was the only abnormal clinical finding."[273] In another prospective study of 69 newborn infants with unexplained hyperbilirubinemia, bacterial infection was documented in two infants, both of whom had asymptomatic gram-negative urinary tract infections.[272] Elevation of direct-reacting bilirubin has been described, particularly in infants with urinary tract infections in whom jaundice develops after the first week of life.[320–322]

Linder and colleagues identified 93 of a population of 5805 newborns who had serum bilirubin levels exceeding 10 mg/dL (171 μmol/L) in the first 48 hours after birth or 15 mg/dL (257 μmol/L) thereafter. Three had positive blood cultures; the organisms identified were *Proteus mirabilis, Bacteroides* species, and *Klebsiella pneumoniae.* Apart from the unusual nature of these organisms, all three of these infants had other signs indicating that they were not well. One had an increase in serum bilirubin of 5.4 mg/dL (92 μmol/L) over 6 hours while the infant received phototherapy; another refused feeding; and a third was vomiting.

Should newborns with unexplained hyperbilirubinemia be subjected to lumbar puncture and blood and urine cultures even if they appear otherwise well? I reviewed the charts of 306 newborns admitted to a pediatric ward within 21 days of birth with a diagnosis of indirect hyperbilirubinemia (peak serum bilirubin level 18.5 ± 2.8; range 12.7–29.1 mg/dL, or 316 ± 48, 217–498 μmol/L). Ninety percent of these infants were fully or partially breast-fed; none were septic (upper 95% confidence limit for the risk of sepsis = 1%). I concluded that if indirect hyperbilirubinemia is ever the only manifestation of bacteremia or incipient sepsis, it must be a rare occurrence. Furthermore, the finding of a positive blood or urine culture in a newborn with indirect hyperbilirubinemia does not prove that the infection is the cause of the jaundice. On the other hand, infants who appear sick or who have late-onset jaundice after physiologic icterus has resolved, direct hyperbilirubinemia, or something else in the history, physical examination, or laboratory investigations that is out of the ordinary, should be evaluated carefully for possible sepsis.

HYPOPITUITARISM

Copeland and colleagues described three full-term infants with congenital hypopituitarism and hypoglycemia who developed prolonged hyperbilirubinemia.[323] Two of the infants had evidence of significant cholestatic jaundice, but in one infant, the hyperbilirubinemia was predominantly indirect. Liver biopsies in this type of patient revealed a mixed picture, ranging from normal hepatic histology to giant-cell hepatitis and cholestatic cirrhosis with bile duct proliferation.[324–326] The pathogenesis of hyperbilirubinemia in this condition remains to be elucidated.

OTHER CAUSES

Congenital syphilis, the TORCH group of chronic intrauterine infections (*i.e.,* toxoplasmosis, rubella, cytomegalovirus, herpes simplex), and coxsackievirus B infection are the other important causes of mixed jaundice. The clinical features and diagnoses of these conditions are described in Chapter 47.

BILIRUBIN TOXICITY

PATHOLOGY OF KERNICTERUS

In 1875, Orth observed bilirubin pigment at autopsy in the brains of infants who were severely jaundiced.[327] Schmorl subsequently described two forms of "brain icterus."[328] The first was "characterized by a diffuse yellow coloration of the entire brain substance."[328] Actually, descriptions of this type of bilirubin staining of the brain had already appeared in textbooks of that era.[328] A second form had not yet "been described in detail, but has been mentioned in passing by Orth. In this form, the jaundiced coloration appears to be completely circumscribed and . . . limited to the so-called 'kern' or nuclear region of the brain."[328] Full-term infants dying from kernicterus demonstrate bilirubin staining in a characteristic distribution (Table 38-19), although a variety of patterns have been described, grossly and microscopically.[329] Kernicteric premature infants and Gunn rats with inherited glucuronosyl transferase deficiency display a similar topography of neuronal damage (see Table 38-19).[330–332] Those regions most commonly affected are the basal ganglia, particularly the subthalamic nu-

TABLE 38–19
COMPARATIVE NEUROPATHOLOGY OF KERNICTERUS

Topography of Lesions	Full-Term Infants, Hyperbilirubinemia	Homozygous Gunn Rats	Premature Infants, Low Bilirubin Levels
Globus pallidus	+	+	+
Subthalamus	+	+	+
Hypothalamus	+	−	−
Horn of Ammon	+	+	+
Reticular zone of the substantia nigra	+	+	+
Cranial nerve nuclei	+	+	+
Reticular formation	+		+
Central pontine nuclei			
Interstitial nucleus			
Locus ceruleus	−	+	+
Lateral cuneate nucleus of the medulla	+	+	+
Cerebellum			
Dentate nuclei	+	−	+
Nuclei of roof of fourth ventricle	+	+	+
Purkinje cells	−	+	+
Spinal cord	+	+	+

+, yellow pigment present; −, yellow pigment absent.
From Ahdab-Barmada M, Moossy J. The neuropathology of kernicterus in the premature neonate: diagnostic problems. J Neuropathol Exp Neurol 1984;43:45.

cleus and the globus pallidus; the hippocampus; the geniculate bodies; various brain stem nuclei, including the inferior colliculus, oculomotor, vestibular, cochlear, and inferior olivary nuclei; and the cerebellum, especially the dentate nucleus and the vermis.[329,332,333]

Neuronal necrosis is the dominant histopathologic feature after 7 to 10 days of postnatal life, and, for the most part, its distribution corresponds with the distribution of bilirubin staining, although there are some exceptions to this rule. For example, intense staining develops in the olivary and dentate nuclei, but there is little neuronal necrosis in these regions. The important areas of neuronal injury (as opposed to staining) include the basal ganglia, brain stem oculomotor nuclei, and brain stem auditory pathways, especially cochlear nuclei and inferior colliculi.[333] The involvement of these regions explains some of the clinical sequelae of bilirubin encephalopathy (see Clinical Features of Bilirubin Encephalopathy).

Originally a pathologic diagnosis, and later a well-defined acute and chronic neurologic syndrome, kernicterus or bilirubin encephalopathy appears to be a less well-circumscribed entity that includes nuclear bilirubin staining of very-low-birth-weight infants who have died from other causes and, possibly, a subtle chronic encephalopathy in which extrapyramidal motor disturbances and sensorineural hearing deficit are not the predominant features.

Full-term infants in whom the aforementioned pathologic manifestations of kernicterus are seen usually manifest the classic clinical symptomatology of this disorder, including very high serum bilirubin levels, commonly higher than 20 mg/dL (342 μmol/L). Yellow staining of the brain, however, has been observed in premature infants who manifested none of the clinical signs of kernicterus during life and in whom serum bilirubin levels remained low.[334–338] Is this yellow staining actually toxic bilirubin encephalopathy, or is it merely bilirubin staining of brain cells previously damaged by hypoxia or ischemia? Turkel and colleagues identified 32 infants with kernicterus at autopsy and compared them with 32 control infants of similar gestational ages without kernicterus.[339,340] In the kernicteric infants, although the gross pattern of staining followed that of classic kernicterus, the typical histologic changes characteristic of kernicterus were found in only three patients. These authors suggest that the bilirubin staining they observed was probably not the same clinicopathologic entity as the kernicterus of posticteric encephalopathy. Instead of the neuronal degeneration typically seen, they found spongy change and gliosis, which both imply nonspecific damage to the brain. This suggests that prior diffuse injury may predispose the brain to bilirubin deposition at relatively low levels of serum bilirubin.[339,340]

Ahdab-Barmada and Moossy found kernicterus in 97 autopsies of neonates (95 were younger than 36 weeks of gestation).[330] The neuropathology in these infants was strikingly similar to that of classic kernicterus in the full-term neonate[332] and in the Gunn rat.[331,341] In the NICHHD cooperative phototherapy study, four low-birth-weight infants had autopsy-proven kernicterus.[342] The neuropathologic findings in these infants were those of classic kernicterus.[343]

As can be seen from Table 38-20, the neuropathology of kernicterus is different from that of hypoxic ischemic encephalopathy. Even though in some low-birth-weight infants, hypoxic ischemic insults may predispose the brain to bilirubin deposition, it appears that kernicterus may occur in low-birth-weight infants in the absence of hypoxic–ischemic brain injury.

Autopsies on jaundiced infants reveal bilirubin staining of the aorta, pleural fluid, ascitic fluid, or a generalized yellow cast throughout the viscera. The staining is not usually considered a sign of tissue damage unless other cytologic changes are found.[329] Bilirubin staining can also be found in necrotic tissue anywhere in the body and has been described in the gastrointestinal tract, kidney, adrenals, and gonads. In infants with hemolytic disease, bile plugs are commonly found in the canaliculi between the hepatocytes, especially in the periportal areas. The kidneys may show bilirubin-stained tubular casts, bilirubin crystals in the small vessels or in edematous interstitium, and renal tubular necrosis. The bilirubin infarcts (*i.e.*, patches of yellow staining in the renal medulla) are probably the result of focal areas of acute tubular necrosis that have been stained by bilirubin.[329]

In infants dying from hyaline membrane disease, the lungs often appear grossly yellow or orange, and there is microscopic staining by bilirubin of the pulmonary hyaline membranes (*i.e.*, yellow hyaline membrane disease).[344,345] Hyaline membranes are formed from necrotic cellular debris and transudation of plasma proteins from the capillaries after damage to the alveolar epithelium, and it appears likely that the transudate also contains bilirubin, which is deposited in the membranes with albumin and other plasma molecules.

PATHOPHYSIOLOGY

BILIRUBIN CHEMISTRY AND NEUROTOXICITY

As already discussed in the section on the formation, structure, and properties of bilirubin, the bilirubin molecule, in its usual conformation, is stabilized by the presence of intramolecular hydrogen bonds that saturate the hydrophilic groups of the molecule, leaving no affinities for the attachment of water and rendering it nearly insoluble in water at *p*H 7.4 (see Figs. 38-4 and 38-5). In an alkaline medium, the hydrogen bonds are open to form a divalent anion that has several hydrophilic groups, resulting in a molecule with much greater solubility. Because of its pronounced tendency for aggregation, it has been suggested that bilirubin 9α (ZZ) acid is the neurotoxic form of bilirubin.[123,346] The *p*H of plasma profoundly affects the solubility of bilirubin and its binding to tissue sites.[347,348] At a *p*H of 7.4, the limit of bilirubin solubility is reached with 0.5 moles of bilirubin per

TABLE 38–20
COMPARATIVE NEUROPATHOLOGY OF KERNICTERUS AND ANOXIC–ISCHEMIC ENCEPHALOPATHY IN THE PREMATURE NEONATE

Topography of Lesions*	Kernicterus	Anoxic–Ischemic Encephalopathy
Cerebral cortex	Absent	Present
Periventricular white matter	Absent	Present
Corpus striatum	Globus pallidus	Putamen and caudate nuclei
Thalamus	Subthalamus	Anterior and lateral nuclei
Horn of Ammon	Resistant sector (H2–3)	Sommer sector (H_1)
Midbrain	Interstitial nucleus	Inferior colliculi
	Nuclei of nerve III†	Nuclei of nerve III†
	Reticular portion of substantia nigra	Compact portion of substantia nigra
Pons	Locus ceruleus	Basal pontine nuclei
	Nuclei of nerves VI, VII	Superior olivary complex
	Reticular formation†	Reticular formation†
Medulla	Vestibular and cochlear nuclei	Inferior olivary nuclei
		Superior olivary nuclei
Cerebellum	Purkinje cells†	Purkinje cells†
	Nuclei of roof of fourth ventricle	Granular cells

* Only topographic areas considered helpful for differential diagnosis were selected in this table.

† Whenever neuronal damage involved in the same structure in kernicterus and anoxic–ischemic encephalopathy, the cytopathology was different.

From Ahdab-Barmada M, Moosy J. The neuropathology of kernicterus in the premature neonate: diagnostic problems. J Neuropathol Exp Neurol 1984;43:45.

mole of albumin; at a *p*H of 7, this limit is less than 0.1 mole of bilirubin per mole of albumin.[335] Thus, when the concentration of bilirubin acid exceeds its solubility, bilirubin may gradually aggregate and come out of solution.[123] Bilirubin crystals have been found in the brain cells of infants dying from kernicterus,[349] and bilirubin in concentrations of 2 mg/dL (34 μmol/L) has been extracted from kernicteric brains.[350] It is likely that even higher concentrations of pigment exist in the presence of kernicterus.[123] Brodersen and Stern have proposed, therefore, that kernicterus occurs when aggregates of precipitated bilirubin acid are deposited in the cells of the brain.[347] Wennberg offered a different model for the development of bilirubin encephalopathy; he suggested that bilirubin monoanion and membranes form reversible complexes and that this mechanism is responsible for the development of bilirubin encephalopathy (Fig. 38-18).[351,352]

CELLULAR TOXICITY OF BILIRUBIN

Bilirubin appears to be a cell poison, but exactly how it exerts its toxic effect is not known. Cashore reviewed the evidence for bilirubin toxicity to the neuron and summarized several histologic and biophysical findings from different clinical and experimental studies.[6] These studies show a range of effects of bilirubin, including binding to cell membranes, decreased sodium–potassium exchange and increased water accumulation, axonal swelling, lowering of membrane potentials and decreased action potential, decreased activity of the auditory brain stem response, decreased phosphorylation of protein kinase and synapsone 1, decreased tyrosine uptake and dopamine synthesis, decreased methionine and thymidine uptake, and decreased mitochondrial viability.[6] Bilirubin decreases the rate of tyrosine uptake and dopamine synthesis in dopaminergic striatal synaptosomes.[353,354] These effects can be reversed by albumin. No single mechanism of bilirubin intoxication has been demonstrated in all cells, and specific studies of metabolism and toxicity have not been performed on basal ganglia cells, the cells commonly involved in kernicterus.

Other experimental data are conflicting. *In vitro*, bilirubin uncouples oxidative phosphorylation[355] and blocks the production of ATP, which is required for the energy-dependent processes in the cell,[355] but studies in guinea pigs[118] and piglets[356] infused with high concentrations of bilirubin, did not show the changes in glucose metabolism or oxygen consumption consistent with mitochondrial injury as the primary pathway of bilirubin toxicity in the intact brain. Bilirubin reduces the responsiveness of cyclic adenosine monophosphate to insulin-stimulated glucose transport,[357] but in whole-brain studies, glucose transport and glucose metabolism were unaffected.[356] Nevertheless, bilirubin infusion in the rat, after osmotic opening of the blood–brain barrier, produced a

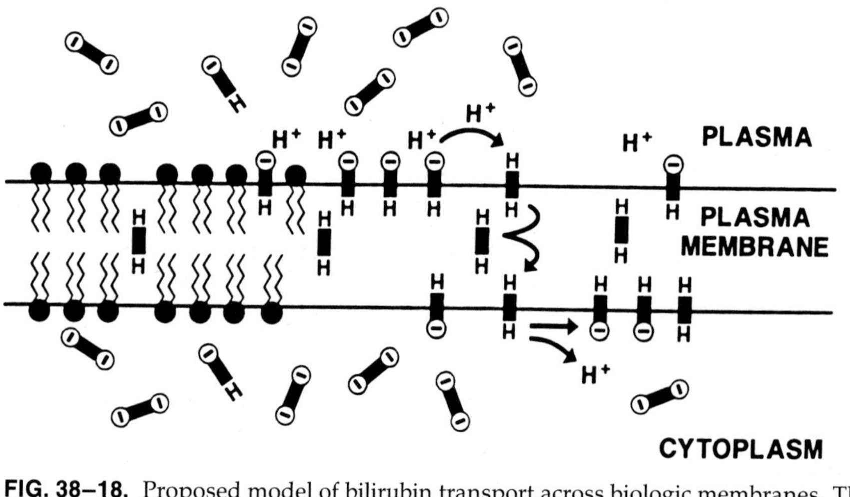

FIG. 38–18. Proposed model of bilirubin transport across biologic membranes. The relatively hydrophilic bilirubin monovalent anion H▬⊖ partitions much like a detergent from the aqueous phase to the lipid membrane surface. Addition of the second H^+ forms the bilirubin acid H ▬ H that enters the lipid phase of the membrane. The process reverses as bilirubin emerges at the cytoplasmic membrane surface. The symbol ⊖▬⊖ indicates the bilirubin dianion. The box gives typical values for unbound bilirubin concentration (UBC) and the different subfractions (molecules per liter) expected at *p*H 7.4 with a total serum bilirubin level of 15 to 20 mg/dL (250–340 μmol/L). (From Wennberg RP. Cellular basis of bilirubin toxicity. NY State J Med 1991;91:493.)

TABLE 38–21
HYPOTHETICAL MODEL OF PATHOPHYSIOLOGY OF BILIRUBIN TOXICITY

Site of Bilirubin Uptake	Effect on Neurons	Duration of Effect
Aggregation of bilirubin at nerve terminals	Lowers membrane potentials; decreases auditory brain stem conduction	Usually reversible
↓	↓	
Bilirubin binds to cell components	Impairs substrate transport, neurotransmitter synthesis, and mitochondrial functions	Prevented or reversed by equimolar albumin
↓	↓	
Retrograde uptake of bilirubin by neuronal body	Dysfunction and death of neurons in acute clinical syndrome	Irreversible
↓	↓	
Pyknosis and gliosis of neurons—bilirubin staining of affected areas	Long-term clinical sequelae	Irreversible

From Cashore WJ. The neurotoxicity of bilirubin. Clin Perinatal 1990;17:437.

marked increase in the lactate–pyruvate ratio, indicating accumulation of NADH, which reflects severe mitochondrial dysfunction.[348]

Changes in energy metabolism produced by hyperbilirubinemia have been studied using ^{31}P nuclear magnetic resonance *in vitro* and *in vivo*. Ives and colleagues studied the effects of bilirubin on brain energy metabolism in slices of adult guinea pig cortex under conditions of normoxia and hypoxia.[358] They found that hypoxia produced a steady-state reduction of $PCr–P_i$ ratio, and the addition of bilirubin lead to a further reduction in the ratio. These changes were reversible when the brain slices were exposed to a bilirubin-free medium and normoxic conditions were reestablished. These investigators also evaluated the effects of bilirubin on energy metabolism during hyperosmolar opening of the blood–brain barrier in adult rats. Hyperbilirubinemia alone caused no measurable disturbance in the energy metabolism, but after opening of the blood–brain barrier, exposure to serum bilirubin levels of about 28 mg/dL (479 μmol/L) produced a decrease in the $PCr/(PCr + P_i)$ ratio. There was a significant correlation between a reduced $PCr/(PCr + P_i)$ ratio and brain-tissue bilirubin content.[359]

When toad bladder membranes are exposed to bilirubin, there is a decrease in water and sodium transport and a decrease in the epithelial response to vasopressin[360]; and in newborn rabbits, bilirubin decreases the phosphorylation of protein kinase.[361,362] These findings illustrate the wide range of responses found when cells are directly exposed to high bilirubin concentrations.

Mayor and colleagues showed that incubation of synaptosomes with bilirubin lowers membrane potential,[363] and Hansen and colleagues also found action potentials reduced in brain slices exposed to bilirubin.[361] It is not known why bilirubin is preferentially deposited in the basal ganglia, but it is possible that it may first attach to nerve terminals, thus lowering membrane potentials and decreasing nerve conduction, and, after further exposure, may penetrate nerve terminals or axons with retrograde uptake of bilirubin in the cell body. Cashore offers a hypothetical format for the progression of bilirubin toxicity from the initial, possibly benign stage of bilirubin accumulation at the cell surface to ultimate neuronal damage and permanent sequelae (Table 38-21).[6]

ALBUMIN BINDING AND THE CONCEPT OF FREE BILIRUBIN

Bilirubin (B) is transported in the plasma as a dianion bound reversibly to serum albumin (A):

$$B^{2-} + A \leftrightarrow AB^{2-}$$

Binding of bilirubin to the high-affinity site of albumin can be expressed as follows:

$$K = \frac{AB^{2-}}{(B^{2-})(A)}.$$

The association constant (K), derived from the equilibrium concentrations of bound (AB^{2-}) and free (B^{2-}) bilirubin, is about 10^7 to 10^8 moles.[366,367] Albumin has a primary binding site with the capacity for binding up to 1 molecule of bilirubin per molecule of albumin and one or more binding sites with much lower affinities. When the bilirubin–albumin ratio exceeds 1, the concentration of free or unbound bilirubin increases, but binding at the lower-affinity sites continues up to a molar bilirubin–albumin ratio of 3:1. It has been widely accepted that bilirubin toxicity occurs when free bilirubin enters the brain and binds to cell membranes.[368,369] The presence of albumin mitigates the *in vivo* and *in vitro* toxic effects of bilirubin,[118,370] and drugs, such as sulfisoxazole, that decrease albumin binding of bilirubin also increase the risk of kernicterus.[125,371] These observations are consistent with the hypothesis that free bilirubin is able to move across the blood–brain barrier, bind to tissues, and damage the cells of the central nervous system.[346,347] They do not exclude the possibility that, under certain circumstances, albumin-bound bilirubin may do the same.

The studies of Wennberg and Hance suggest that if albumin-bound bilirubin gains access to the brain in the absence of a disrupted blood–brain barrier, it is unlikely that toxic effects will occur.[370] Disruption of the blood–brain barrier, on the other hand, permits leakage of the albumin–bilirubin complex into the interstitium of the brain. Under these circumstances, the brain cells are exposed to the same free bilirubin concentration that exists in the serum, and the bilirubin equilibrates with binding sites on albumin and cellular membranes. If the free bilirubin is sufficiently high, and the reservoirs are sufficiently large, the amount of bilirubin bound to membranes might impair neuronal function.

Measurement of Free Bilirubin

Several techniques have been developed for measuring free or loosely bound bilirubin and the binding capacity and affinity of bilirubin for albumin. Some of these tests are listed in Table 38-22, and the subject has been reviewed in detail.[372] Acute changes in free bilirubin concentrations, however, are probably transient because there is rapid equilibration and redistribution of bilirubin between the plasma (*i.e.*, albumin) and the tissues. Thus, although sulfisoxazole administration produces acute changes in binding status and an elevation in free bilirubin levels, within a few minutes, the concentration of free bilirubin returns to normal.[373] Even under experimental conditions that lead to a significant increase in brain bilirubin content, the differences in free bilirubin concentrations in the serum between control and study animals is small.[374]

Although there is a vast literature dealing with bilirubin-binding tests,[372] none is in general use in clinical decision making. Because one molecule of albumin is capable of binding one molecule of bilirubin tightly at the primary binding site, a bilirubin–albumin molar ratio of 1 represents about 8.5 mg of bilirubin per gram of albumin. Thus, a full-term infant with a serum albumin concentration of 3 to 3.5 g/dL should be able to bind about 25 to 28 mg/dL of bilirubin (428–479 μmol/L). The albumin-binding capacity of sick, low-birth-weight infants is less than that of full-term infants, and their serum albumin levels are often lower. Stevenson and Wennberg suggest using a factor of 7 times the albumin level to predict the binding capacity of bilirubin in a healthy full-term infant and a multiple of 5 to 6 times the albumin concentration in sick, low-birth-weight infants.[375]

Factors Affecting the Binding of Bilirubin to Serum Albumin

This subject has been reviewed in great detail.[346] A few of the factors are discussed here.

Fatty Acids. Free fatty acids in plasma may compete with bilirubin for its binding to albumin, but significant interference with bilirubin binding probably does not occur until molar ratios of free fatty acids to albumin exceed 4 : 1.[346,376] Brodersen has estimated that at a free fatty acid–albumin ratio of 6, the free bilirubin concentration increases by a factor of 2.6.[377] Intravenous lipid preparations do not displace bilirubin from albumin binding, but they produce an increase in free fatty acids that is potentially dangerous.

Unbound bilirubin concentrations were measured by hematofluorometry in infants receiving 1, 2, or 3 g/kg of intralipid over a 15- to 20-hour period. A linear relation was found between the serum free fatty acid–albumin (F–A) molar ratio and the concentration of unbound bilirubin, although there was considerable scatter.[378] The largest increases in unbound bilirubin were seen in infants with an F–A ratio greater than 4, and such ratios tended to occur in infants of fewer than 30 weeks of gestation. The infusion of 1 g/kg of intralipid over a 15-hour period in infants of fewer than 30 weeks of gestation produced an F–A ratio of less than 3 and minimal increases in unbound bilirubin concentrations. With doses of 2 to 3 g/kg, however, higher ratios were found. In a recent study, intravenous fat was given as a continuous infusion of 2 g/kg/day for 7 days to infants of 32 weeks or less of gestation (mean birth weight, 1200 g). This produced F–A ratios of only 0.1 to 1.8.[379] Intralipid has been administered to congenitally jaundiced (*i.e.*, Gunn) rats in which the total-body bilirubin pool was uniformly labeled with radioactive bilirubin.[380] Intralipid was found to have no effect on the kinetics of bilirubin formation, transport, tissue distribution, or clearance.

***p*H.** The binding of bilirubin to albumin is unaffected by changes in the serum *p*H.[381–383] Nevertheless, the correction of neonatal acidosis in 11 sick newborns appeared to decrease the serum free bilirubin concentration as measured by a peroxidase technique.[384] The role of *p*H, on the other hand, may be pivotal in determining the binding of bilirubin to cells and, therefore, its deposition in the central nervous system (see *p*H and Bilirubin Solubility).[351,352,385] Bilirubin interaction with rat brain synaptosomal membranes is augmented as *p*H decreases.[386] In addition, a decrease in *p*H reduces the solubility of bilirubin in plasma, encouraging precipitation of the insoluble acid form.[347] A decrease in *p*H of 0.3 produces a fourfold increase

TABLE 38–22
BILIRUBIN BINDING TESTS

Method	Measures	Reported as	Units*
Tiration with BR and:			
Sephadex column elution	Adsorption of BR on Sephadex columns	Binding capacity; loosely bound BR	mg/dL or mmol/L
Peroxidase oxidation	Enzyme-catalyzed oxidation of BR	Free bilirubin	nmol/L
		Binding capacity	mg/dL or mmol/L
		Binding affinity (association constant)	K_A
Fluorescence quenching	Fluorescence quenching of ALB by BR	Binding capacity	mol BR/mol ALB
		Binding affinity	K_A
Front-face fluorometry	Fluorescence of BR in whole blood	Total BR; bound BR	mg/dL
		Binding capacity (total bound)	mg/dL
		Saturation index	(bound/reserve) × 10
Dye binding			
HABA and related methods	Residual binding of dye, compared with a bilurubin-free standard	Reserve dye-binding capacity	Percent of dye binding compared with standard
Direct yellow 7	Fluorescence of dye and its quenching due to BR	BR-binding capacity	mol BR/mol ALB
Selective trace ligand (^{14}C-MADDS)	Dialysis rate of MADDS in serum, compared with an albumin standard	Reserve albumin	mmol/L
Electron spin resonance	Spectral emissions of bound *versus* unbound selective ligand	Binding capacity	mol BR/mol ALB
		Reserve BR-loading capacity	mol BR/mol ALB
Loosely bound or unbound BR			
Sephadex methods	As above	As above	mg/dL or mmol/L
Peroxidase oxidation	As above	As above, or apparent free BR	nmol/L or μg/dL
Erythrocyte bilirubin	Adsorption of BR onto red blood cells	Erythrocyte BR	mg/dL red blood cell
Paper chromatoelectrophoresis	Separation of bound and unbound BR on chromatography paper	Reserve binding capacity	mg/dL
		Loosely bound BR	Semiquantitative (diazo-positive)
Saturation index	Percent decrease in optical density at 460 nm caused by addition of salicylate	Saturation index	Percent decrease in optical density at 460 (maximum 14%)
Difference spectroscopy Circular dichroism	Spectral changes induced by saturation of binding sites or displacement of BR	Graphic display of spectral changes as percentage of baseline	mol BR/mol ALB, or % BR bound or displaced

* For conversion of gram or milligram concentrations to moles, molecular weight of bilirubin = 585 and of albumin = 68,000.
ALB, albumin; BR, bilirubin; HABA; hydroxybenzene azobenzoic acid; MADDS, monoacetyl diaminodiphenylsulfone.
From Cashore WJ. Bilirubin binding tests. In: Levine RJ, Maisels MJ, eds. Hyperbilirubinemia in the newborn: report of the 85th Ross Conference on Pediatric Research. Columbus. OH: Ross Laboratories, 1983:101.

in the concentration of bilirubin acid. Because the acid is insoluble in water, deposition of the substance in the tissues is likely in the presence of acidosis.[17]

Drugs. The effect of numerous drugs on bilirubin–albumin binding has been tested *in vitro* using different methods. The measured effect varies with the method used; some systems require much greater concentrations of the drug than others to demonstrate an increase in unbound bilirubin. For example, although sulfisoxazole is clearly capable of displacing bilirubin from its binding to albumin, when the serum is diluted 40-fold to perform the peroxidase assay, no displacing effect is found.[387] Drug-displacing effects are probably transient. When sulfisoxazole is administered to rats, there is a transient increase in free bilirubin concentrations, but this returns to pretreatment values despite continued infusion of the displacing drug.[373] Robertson and colleagues reviewed the bilirubin displacing effect of drugs used in neonatology.[388] They believe that every drug used in newborns should be tested for its effect on bilirubin–albumin binding before these drugs are licensed for use in the newborn, although such testing is not required by governmental authorities.

Because oral medications are rarely given to sick, preterm infants, and topical medications do not lead to concentrations that would effectively compete with bilirubin for albumin binding, they do not require testing. Other drugs can be excluded from testing either because of low albumin-binding (*e.g.*, the aminoglycosides) or low serum concentrations (*e.g.*, thyroxine, adrenal hormones, vitamins). Robertson and colleagues arbitrarily chose to consider an increase in the free bilirubin concentration of 5% as potentially dangerous, and they consider a drug to be a potential displacer if it occupies 5% or more of the available albumin. Knowledge of the usual peak serum bilirubin concentrations and the percentage of albumin-bound drug can also be used to calculate the concentration of bound drug. If the bound drug concentration is less than 15 μmol/L, it is unlikely that this drug will cause significant displacement of bilirubin.[388]

Robertson and colleagues calculated a maximal displacement factor, δ, from the K_D value, using the following equation:

$$\delta = K_D d + 1,$$

where d is the concentration of free drug in the patient's plasma and K_D is the displacement constant, which represents the competitive effect of the drug with bilirubin for albumin binding. If K_D is 0, then $\delta = 1$, and the drug does not displace bilirubin. If $\delta = 1.2$, there has been a 20% increase of free bilirubin concentration after drug administration. Although an arbitrary value of 1.2 has been suggested as the upper permissible limit for bilirubin displacement,[389] it is recommended that, as far as possible, drugs with the lowest δ values be selected. Appendix H-6 lists the effects of drugs used in neonatology on bilirubin–albumin binding. The free drug concentration is calculated from the serum concentration and the percentage of bound drug as taken from existing data in the literature.

Robertson and Brodersen have also evaluated the effect of drug combinations on bilirubin–albumin binding.[390] This is important because drug combinations are commonly administered to sick neonates, and the data show that the bilirubin-displacing effect of these combinations cannot be predicted from each drug's effect. For example, the administration of aminophylline with vancomycin increased the displacing effect when compared with either drug alone, but the overall effect was still minimal. Robertson and Brodersen recommend that, in the absence of published data, drugs should be selected in which therapeutic concentrations are much lower than the usual concentration of albumin (about 2.8 mg/dL in a very-low-birth-weight newborn infant). Drugs should be selected that are not bound to albumin, and simultaneous treatment with several drugs should be limited as far as possible.[390]

Other Competing Anions. It is possible that certain unidentified anions interfere with the albumin binding of bilirubin. Evidence for this is suggested by the failure of exchange transfusion to alter significantly the albumin binding of infants' serum[391,392] despite the fact that exchange transfusion removes bilirubin, replaces much of the infant's serum albumin with bilirubin-free albumin, and lowers the free bilirubin level. Anions that interfere with albumin binding may not be removed by exchange transfusion.

Clinical Status of the Infant. A relation may exist between bilirubin-binding capacity and the clinical condition and gestational age of the infant. In some studies, very premature infants were able to bind less bilirubin per mole of albumin than were more mature infants,[387,393] but in others studies, no relation was found between bilirubin-binding ability and gestational age.[394,395]

HYPERBILIRUBINEMIA AND BRAIN BILIRUBIN LEVELS

Under normal circumstances, there is a constant influx and efflux of bilirubin in and out of the brain, but under experimental conditions, regardless of how much bilirubin is infused, it is difficult to get it to stay in the brain of healthy animals or to produce electrical central nervous system changes.[370,396–398] Gross staining of the brain and electrophysiologic changes, however, occur readily in asphyxiated animals.[396,397,399]

Bilirubin is found in the cerebrospinal fluid at a mean concentration of 0.24 ± 0.098 mg/dL (4.1 ± 1.7 μmol/L) in normal, full-term infants and 0.61 ± 0.15 mg/dL (10.4 ± 2.6 μmol/L) in preterm infants, and there is a correlation between serum bilirubin and spinal fluid bilirubin levels.[400–402] Bilirubin is found in the brain of rats or piglets made hyperbilirubinemic by continuous intravenous infusions of bilirubin,[374,403–406] but compared with other body organs, bilirubin does not get into the brain easily—higher concentrations are found in the liver, spleen, fat, and muscle than in the brain.[407]

Genetic factors may be involved in determining the susceptibility of patients to bilirubin-induced neurotoxicity. For example, in different strains of Gunn rats exposed to similar bilirubin and albumin concentrations, there were significant differences in susceptibility to kernicterus and mortality, suggesting that genetic or other factors may be important in determining individual susceptibility to bilirubin toxicity.[408]

BLOOD–BRAIN BARRIER

A blood–brain barrier exists that limits the entry of certain substances into the central nervous system. This barrier, at the cerebral blood vessels, is due to a continuous lining of endothelial cells connected by tight junctions that restrict intercellular diffusion.[409,410] The blood–brain barrier normally excludes most water-soluble substances and proteins but is permeable to lipid-soluble substances that are not protein-bound. Large molecules, such as albumin, are excluded from the brain but may enter when the brain is made permeable by the infusion of a hypertonic solution.[411]

EXPERIMENTAL OPENING OF THE BLOOD–BRAIN BARRIER

Levine and colleagues opened the blood–brain barrier on one side of the brain in adult rats by infusing hypertonic arabinose into the internal carotid artery.[412] One minute after the arabinose was given, a bilirubin–albumin solution was infused through the femoral vein. Yellow staining of the brain occurred on the side on which the blood–brain barrier had been opened by the infusion of arabinose.[412] Clearly, the blood concentration of bilirubin, both free and bound, on both sides of the brain was identical, yet only one side was stained yellow, indicating that entry of bilirubin into the brain was determined by disruption of the blood–brain barrier, not by the level of serum free bilirubin. Bratlid and colleagues confirmed Levine's observations using a different technique.[403] They induced hyperbilirubinemia in chronically catheterized rats and produced hyperosmolality by injecting urea. A direct relation was found between serum osmolality and both brain bilirubin and albumin content.[403]

Wennberg and Hance infused bilirubin into rats whose blood–brain barriers had been opened with arabinose.[370] One group of rats received 1.5 g/kg of human serum albumin before the arabinose solution; the other group received saline only. Electroencephalogram (EEG) changes were monitored during and after these infusions. Successful opening of the blood–brain barrier was reflected by ipsilateral changes in the EEG. Bilirubin staining of the brain occurred when the blood–brain barrier was open, but the staining was most intense in the albumin-treated animals. Both the albumin-primed and control animals developed EEG changes and differential staining of the ipsilateral hemisphere. Electroencephalogram encephalopathy, however, occurred at much lower brain bilirubin concentrations in the control animals, where serum binding was poor, than in the albumin-primed rats. When free bilirubin levels were low, encephalopathy occurred only when the blood–brain barrier was open and permeable to the albumin–bilirubin complex.

Opening of the blood–brain barrier might allow albumin-bound bilirubin to bathe the neurons, but whether or not free bilirubin binds to albumin or to cellular membranes may be determined by the binding of bilirubin to albumin. At some point, sufficient tissue binding occurs to impair neuronal function. This can be documented by changes in the EEG. It is possible, therefore, that both disruption of the blood–brain barrier and the levels of free bilirubin may be important in the pathogenesis of bilirubin toxicity. This experimental model supports the proposal that yellow staining of the brain is not synonymous with bilirubin toxicity and may provide an explanation for the neuropathologic observations of Turkel and colleagues.[340] Bratlid also measured the brain uptake of bilirubin by rats after a bolus injection of sulfisoxazole.[413] A significant increase in plasma unbound bilirubin and brain bilirubin concentration occurred without any increase in brain albumin concentration.

EFFECT OF MATURITY ON BLOOD–BRAIN BARRIER PERMEABILITY

Is the blood–brain barrier of the neonate more permeable to bilirubin and albumin than in older children or adults? The immature brain demonstrates greater passive permeability between the blood and central nervous system for lipid-insoluble molecules.[414] Studies in newborn piglets have shown that the blood–brain barrier is more permeable to bilirubin in 2-day-old than in 2-week-old piglets, while the permeability to albumin does not change.[415]

LIPID SOLUBILITY

Lipid-soluble substances that are not protein-bound and gases, such as carbon dioxide and oxygen, cross the blood–brain barrier easily, by simple diffusion, while water-soluble substances, proteins, and polar compounds (*i.e.*, ions) do not. The permeability of the blood–brain barrier to different substances is proportional to the octanol–water partition coefficient, a measure of lipid solubility.[409,410] Although there has been some debate about whether bilirubin can be regarded as a lipid-soluble molecule, studies of blood–brain barrier permeability to albumin-bound and free bilirubin, show that, *in vivo*, in relation to the cerebral microvasculature, free bilirubin behaves like a lipid-soluble molecule.

MEASUREMENT OF PERMEABILITY

The permeability of the blood–brain barrier to bilirubin has only recently been quantified by Ives and Gardner.[19] Using the single-pass (*i.e.*, Oldendorf) and *in situ* perfusion (*i.e.*, Takasato) techniques in adult male rats, these investigators found that for free bilirubin, the brain uptake index was 28.5 ± 9.3 and the permeability surface area product was 54.84 ± 36.38 × 10^{-4} mL/sec/g. No permeability to albumin-bound bilirubin was demonstrated.

MECHANISMS FOR TRANSPORT ACROSS THE BLOOD–BRAIN BARRIER

Wennberg suggests a mechanism for the transport of bilirubin across membranes.[351,352] This is based on the fact that the partitioning of bilirubin between water and organic solvents, such as octanol and chloroform, is directly related to the hydrogen ion concentration.[416] Although Brodersen and Stern[347] suggest that tissue uptake of bilirubin involves the precipitation of bilirubin acid in phospholipid membranes, Wennberg suggests that bilirubin concentrates as the monovalent anion at the cell surface (see Fig. 38-18), facilitating the addition of another hydrogen ion to form bilirubin acid, which enters the lipid phase of the membrane. The process reverses as bilirubin emerges at the cytoplasmic membrane surface. Thus, although free bilirubin in plasma (*i.e.*, water) is thought to be present in the dianion form (B^{2-}), the partitioning studies indicate the existence of a bilirubin monoanion or bilirubin acid salt (BH^{-}) as well. Once it has crossed the blood–brain barrier, bilirubin probably enters the brain extracellular space and is bound by albumin or the brain cells.[385] Free bilirubin should cross the blood–brain barrier as the monovalent ion, while the entry of albumin-bound bilirubin is more restricted.

FACTORS AFFECTING BLOOD–BRAIN BARRIER PERMEABILITY

Anoxia, hypercarbia, and hyperosmolality open the blood–brain barrier and increase the deposition of bilirubin and albumin in the brain,[374,403,404,409,412] producing neurophysiologic and biochemical changes[370] as well as changes in brain physiology and energy metabolism.[348] Thus, opening of the blood–brain barrier is likely to be one important mechanism in the pathogenesis of kernicterus, although other mechanisms undoubtedly exist. For example, during hypercarbia, the increased bilirubin that is deposited in the brain is predominantly in the unbound form, although some is also albumin-bound.[374,405] Burgess and colleagues found that the regional deposition of bilirubin in the brain of piglets occurs in areas where hypercarbia produces the greatest increase in regional blood flow.[405] Respiratory acidosis increases bilirubin deposition in the brain; metabolic acidosis does not.[404,405]

REGIONAL LOCALIZATION OF BILIRUBIN WITHIN THE BRAIN

Autopsy findings in infants with erythroblastosis fetalis who died from kernicterus show that the regions of the brain most commonly affected are the basal ganglia, particularly the subthalamic nucleus and the globus pallidus; the hippocampus; the geniculate bodies; various brain stem nuclei; and the cerebellum (see Table 38-19). The distribution of brain bilirubin in animal studies has varied; some investigators found a distinct regional distribution after hyperosmolality and hypercarbia,[405,406] while others did not find a similar regional pattern.[374] Regional differences in brain bilirubin deposition may be related to blood flow differences in different areas of the brain, the binding properties of the bilirubin molecule, and the clearance of bilirubin once it has entered the brain (half-life is 1.7 hours in the rat).[417]

Mitochondria in the brain and other tissues contain a highly specific bilirubin oxidase that converts bilirubin to biliverdin and other nontoxic products.[418,419] Local breakdown of bilirubin may also have a role in determining the distribution and detoxification of bilirubin in the brain. The addition of bilirubin oxidase reversed the toxic effects of bilirubin on mouse neuroblastoma cells.[419]

CELLULAR BASIS OF BILIRUBIN TOXICITY

This subject was reviewed by Wennberg[352] and by Bratlid.[385]

*p*H AND BILIRUBIN SOLUBILITY

Brodersen demonstrated the relation between bilirubin solubility and the serum *p*H and emphasized the importance of bilirubin solubility in determining the binding of bilirubin to cells.[17,347] As discussed previously, bilirubin is reversibly bound to albumin in the form of a dianion (B^{2-}):

$$B^{2-} + A \leftrightarrow AB^{2-}.$$

This binding obeys the laws of mass action, and the concentration of bilirubin dianion can be calculated:

$$b = B/p \times 1/K,$$

where b is the concentration of free bilirubin dianion, B the concentration of bound bilirubin, p the concentration of albumin with a vacant site for high-affinity binding of bilirubin, and K the binding constant. B is measured as the concentration of unconjugated bilirubin, and p is approximated as the reserve albumin concentration for binding of monoacetyl diaminodiphenylsulfone. $K = 6.8 \times 10^7\ M^{-1}$ at 37°C. Thus, the concentration of free bilirubin in the sample can be calculated from equation 4. At a *p*H of 7.4, the solubility of bilirubin is only 7 nmol, and newborns frequently have higher concentrations of free bilirubin dianion. Thus, the plasma of newborns is supersaturated with respect to bilirubin acid, and this favors a process of precipitation of bilirubin. Using this information, an index of plasma bilirubin toxicity (I) has been derived[347,387]:

$$I = \log B/p - 2\,pH + 15.5.$$

As the toxicity index increases, bilirubin deposition in tissues is expected to occur.[387,420]

MONOVALENT ANION HYPOTHESIS

Wennberg pointed out that within the range of physiologic *p*H, the binding of bilirubin to albumin is not affected by changes in the hydrogen ion concentration,[352] and the reason for increasing tissue uptake of bilirubin with decreasing *p*H must be the result of the interaction of bilirubin with the cells,[421] rather than an effect of *p*H on albumin binding. The linear relation between hydrogen ion concentration and cell binding indicates that a single proton or hydrogen ion is added to bilirubin in the binding process.[422] Wennberg suggests that the development of bilirubin encephalopathy is the result of the formation of reversible complexes of bilirubin monoanion and cell membranes rather than the precipitation of bilirubin acid in phospholipid membranes, as proposed by Brodersen and Stern.[347] The hydrogen ion dependence of tissue binding for bilirubin can be explained, not by the effect of *p*H on bilirubin solubility, but by the conversion of the bilirubin dianion (B^{2-}) to monovalent anion (BH^-; see Fig. 38-18).

Based on this, it is possible to estimate the relative bilirubin load to tissue in equilibrium with plasma bilirubin by measuring the free bilirubin concentration and blood *p*H. Because the free bilirubin level is usually a function of the bilirubin–albumin ratio, it is possible to calculate the serum bilirubin concentrations that would yield the same tissue bilirubin load at varying *p*H and concentrations of albumin. From Figure 38-19, it can be seen that an infant with an albumin level of 2.4 g/dL and a *p*H of 7.3 has the same

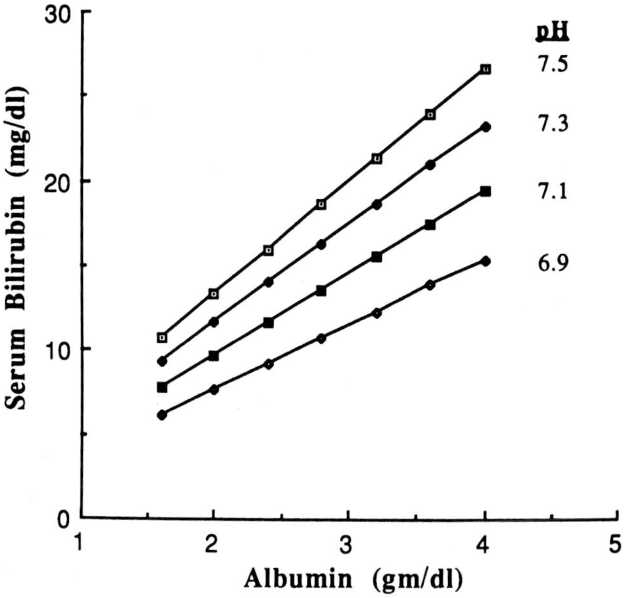

FIG. 38–19. Serum bilirubin concentrations yield the same tissue bilirubin load at varying *p*H and serum albumin concentrations. The reference exchange transfusion level of 20 mg/dL occurs with an albumin level of 3.3 g/dL and *p*H of 7.35. (From Wennberg RP. Cellular basis of bilirubin toxicity. NY State J Med 1991;91:493.)

pressure for bilirubin deposition in the brain when the serum bilirubin level is 14 mg/dL (239 μmol/L) as another infant who has a bilirubin level of 20 mg/dL (342 μmol/L) but an albumin level of 3.3 g/dL and a normal *p*H of 7.35. These calculations assume a normal albumin-binding capacity that may not be present in sick, low-birth-weight infants or in the presence of competition of drugs or endogenous anions. They also cannot take into account changes in permeability of the blood–brain barrier, variations in *p*H within the brain, and variations in the susceptibility of the brain cells. Nevertheless, these calculations suggest the importance of attempting to correct acidosis in the severely jaundiced infant, particularly, respiratory acidosis, since carbon dioxide equilibrates rapidly in the brain. Hypercapnia also increases cerebral blood flow and bilirubin delivery to the brain.[404,405]

Wennberg and colleagues also demonstrated that bilirubin toxicity can be augmented and reversed by altering cellular *p*H.[423] These investigators infused bilirubin into premature rhesus monkeys and then exposed them to carbon dioxide. At total bilirubin levels of 24 to 29 mg/dL (410–496 μmol/L; unbound bilirubin levels 2.5 − 3.8 μg/dL), the addition of carbon dioxide produced a decrease in arterial *p*H to 6.86 − 7.04 and changes in the brain stem audiometric evoked response (BAER) in 6 of 7 animals. Correction of the respiratory acidosis produced partial to complete reversal of the BAER changes within 3 to 20 minutes, and reexposure to carbon dioxide immediately reproduced the BAER abnormality. These data support the hypothesis that bilirubin toxicity can be both potentiated and reversed by modulating environmental *p*H.[423]

The monovalent anion hypothesis is consistent with the ready extraction of tissue-bound bilirubin by exchange transfusion and the reversibility of the bilirubin-induced changes in BAER.[424–427] As illustrated in Figure 38-18 and discussed previously, this hypothesis suggests that when the monoanion enters the lipid core of the membrane, it accepts a second proton, making it more lipid-soluble. This proton would be released as bilirubin emerges on the opposite surface. If the immature cell membrane has sufficient fluidity, bilirubin can pass through in its monoionic form; and if membrane fluidity is important in determining bilirubin toxicity, pharmacologic intervention can affect this.[352] For example, benzyl alcohol increases membrane fluidity,[428] and the use of benzyl alcohol appears to be strongly associated with a very high incidence of kernicterus in low-birth-weight infants.[429]

Other mechanisms have been determined by which bilirubin might alter membrane function. If tissue binding involves bilirubin acid–lipid complexes,[430] bilirubin might adversely affect membrane function by changing the lipid environment of membrane proteins.[352] Bilirubin binding to specific receptor sites on enzymes might be another mechanism for bilirubin membrane toxicity.[352]

WINDOWS OF VULNERABILITY

The permeability of the blood–brain barrier and the susceptibility of the brain to damage from bilirubin or other insults change as maturation occurs.[352] Damage to the Purkinje cells and the cerebellum of Gunn rats was significantly mitigated when these rats were exposed to phototherapy on certain days,[431] while other studies using displacing agents found that bilirubin staining of regions of the cerebellum, other than the Purkinje cells, was most intense on day 15. Although pathologic kernicterus occurs in very-low-birth-weight infants, they do not manifest the classic clinical picture; this may be due to the differences discussed previously. The distribution and type of bilirubin toxicity appear to be dependent on the maturity of the brain.[352]

MECHANISMS BY WHICH BILIRUBIN ENTERS THE BRAIN

Bratlid has provided a schematic presentation of possible mechanisms of bilirubin entry into the brain, its binding to neuronal cell membranes, and the potential clinical signs that may follow (Fig. 38-20).[385] Under normal circumstances, bilirubin enters the brain. Clinical confirmation of this fact is provided by the observation that modest elevations of serum bilirubin can produce clinical and electrophysiologic altera-

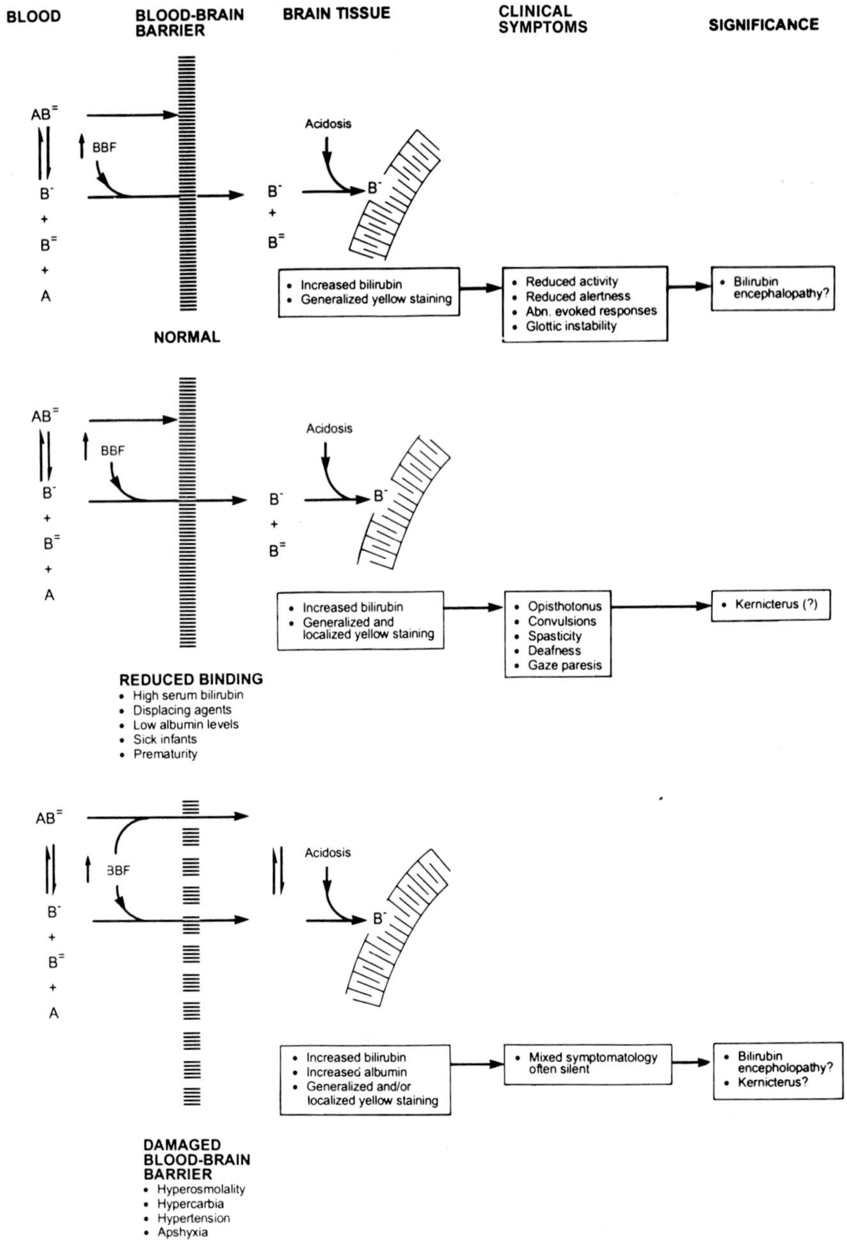

FIG. 38–20. Possible mechanisms for bilirubin entry into the brain and binding to neuronal cell membranes. The different factors affecting this process are also indicated. (A, albumin; AB^-, albumin–bilirubin complex; B^-, bilirubin monoanion; B^{2-}, bilirubin dianion; BBF, brain–blood flow; from Bratlid D. How bilirubin gets into the brain. Clin Perinatol 1990;17:449.)

tions in healthy full-term infants. Such infants demonstrate changes in behavior, characteristics of the cry, and changes in the BAER.[432] These changes reverse as the bilirubin level decreases.

The second mechanism for bilirubin entry into the brain occurs when there is a marked increase in the serum level of unbound bilirubin. In the unbound state, bilirubin readily enters the brain and has the potential for producing kernicterus. Finally, bilirubin bound to albumin can enter the brain through a disrupted blood–brain barrier. Even in the presence of a damaged blood–brain barrier, however, on a molar basis, more bilirubin than albumin is deposited in the brain.[374,403,404] In all these situations, acidosis increases deposition of bilirubin in brain cells.

CLINICAL FEATURES OF BILIRUBIN ENCEPHALOPATHY

ACUTE BILIRUBIN ENCEPHALOPATHY OR KERNICTERUS

In classic kernicterus, markedly jaundiced infants progress through three fairly distinct clinical phases.[433–435] In the first few days, the infant becomes lethargic, hypotonic, and sucks poorly. Later in the first week, the second phase evolves; the infant becomes hypertonic and frequently develops a fever and a high-pitched cry.[435] The hypertonia involves the extensor muscle groups, and most infants exhibit backward arching of the neck (*i.e.*, retrocollis) and trunk (*i.e.*, opisthotonus). The fever may be due to diencephalic involvement. In the third phase, usually after 1 week, hypertonia subsides and is replaced by hypotonia. Infants who manifest hypertonia during the second phase invariably develop the clinical features of chronic bilirubin encephalopathy.[435,436] Van Praagh found that those who were consistently neurologically normal during the first week of life never developed the features of chronic encephalopathy,[435] but other investigators found later evidence of brain damage in some infants in whom no, or equivocal, manifestations of kernicterus were apparent in the newborn.[434,436,437]

CHRONIC BILIRUBIN ENCEPHALOPATHY

Temporal Evolution

Byers and colleagues described the temporal evolution of chronic bilirubin encephalopathy after neonatal erythroblastosis fetalis.[438] In the first year, infants typically feed poorly, develop a high-pitched cry, and are hypotonic but have increased deep tendon reflexes, a persistent tonic neck reflex, and motor delay.[438] There is a delay in acquisition of motor skills, although most infants walk alone by 5 years of age. The other typical features of chronic bilirubin encephalopathy are not usually apparent before 1 year of age and often not for several years.[433] These children generally are hypotonic at rest for the first 6 or 7 years. By the time they reach their teens, hypertonia has replaced hypotonia.[439]

Clinical Features

The classic sequelae of posticteric encephalopathy constitute a tetrad consisting of extrapyramidal disturbances, auditory abnormalities, gaze palsies, and dental dysplasia.[439]

Extrapyramidal Disturbances. Athetosis (*i.e.*, involuntary, sinuous, writhing movements) may develop as early as 18 months but may be delayed as late as 8 or 9 years.[438] If sufficiently severe, athetosis may prevent useful limb function. These movements are described as "uncontrollable, purposeless, involuntary and incoordinate. They may be rapid and jerky (choreiform), slow and worm-like (orthodox athetosis) or so slowed by hypertonicity that the patient may assume momentarily fixed attitudes with stiffness of the extremities (dystonia)."[439] Occasionally, extrapyramidal rigidity may predominate, rather than involuntary motion. In Perlstein's opinion, "the absence of athetosis or of other forms of extrapyramidal dyskinesia, makes the diagnosis of post-icteric encephalopathy dubious, if not untenable."[439] Severely affected children may also have dysarthria, facial grimacing, drooling, and difficulty chewing and swallowing.

Auditory Abnormalities. Some degree of hearing loss is often found in children with chronic bilirubin encephalopathy. Pathologic studies[330,440] and studies of BAER[424,427,441–445] indicate that injury to the brain stem, specifically the cochlear nuclei, is the principal cause of hearing loss, although occasional studies suggest possible involvement of the peripheral auditory system as well.[425,426]

Hyman, Keaster, and colleagues followed 405 survivors of hemolytic disease of the newborn and compared 119 children whose maximal indirect serum bilirubin levels exceeded 20 mg/dL (342 μmol/L) with 286 who had lower bilirubin levels.[446,447] Those with higher bilirubin levels had three times the risk of neurologic abnormality (20% *versus* 6.6%) and 4.4 times the risk of sensorineural hearing loss (9.2% *versus* 2.1%). All the infants who received exchange transfusions, and 16 of the 17 later found to have hearing loss, received prophylactic streptomycin, an ototoxic antibiotic. Although infants with elevated bilirubin levels had a higher risk of hearing loss even when those not receiving streptomycin were excluded from the comparison group, it is impossible to exclude effect modification because all infants with high bilirubin levels received streptomycin.[448]

Johnston and colleagues followed 129 children who had indirect serum bilirubin levels above 20 mg/dL (342 μmol/L).[437] Ninety-two of these infants had Rh hemolytic disease, and 26 had ABO hemolytic disease. Seven children had neurologic sequelae, all of whom had sensorineural hearing impairment. All these hearing-impaired infants received exchange transfusions, and six of the seven received streptomycin. Hearing loss is generally most severe in the high frequencies, and an association between moderate hyperbilirubinemia and subsequent sensorineural hearing loss has been described in low-birth-weight infants (see Clinical Sequelae of Hyperbilirubinemia and Hearing Loss in Low-Birth-Weight Infants).

Gaze Abnormalities. Limitation of upward gaze and other gaze abnormalities occur, and the fact that full vertical eye movements during the doll's-eye maneuver are attained in most affected children suggests that the lesion is above the level of the oculomotor nuclei.[333] Some patients have paralytic gaze palsies. Supranuclear palsies can be explained by bilirubin deposition and neuronal injury in the rostral midbrain, and nuclear palsies can be explained by damage to the oculomotor nuclei.[330,449]

Dental Dysplasia. About 75% of children with posticteric encephalopathy have some degree of dental enamel hypoplasia. A smaller percentage have green discoloration of the teeth.[439]

CLINICAL SEQUELAE OF HYPERBILIRUBINEMIA

This subject remains a source of lively debate. Is there evidence for a subtle form of bilirubin encephalopathy in otherwise healthy full-term infants?[260,450–458] What about preterm infants?[459,460] What does yellow staining of the brain found at autopsy mean in some very-low-birth-weight infants?

Hsia and colleagues[461] and Mollison and Cutbush[462] first established the link between bilirubin levels and brain damage in the early 1950s, when they demonstrated that the risk of kernicterus in infants with Rh hemolytic disease increased dramatically with rising bilirubin levels and that exchange transfusion could markedly reduce the risk. It subsequently became clear that in untreated infants with severe hemolytic disease, the incidence of kernicterus (30%–50% in those with the highest bilirubin levels) was much higher than the incidence in markedly jaundiced infants without hemolytic disease.[463–468] As a result, there was considerable disagreement about how jaundice in preterm and full-term infants without Rh isoimmunization should be treated.[469,470] Some investigators described clinical and pathologic kernicterus in premature infants who did not have hemolytic disease and whose bilirubin levels were well below 20 mg/dL (342 μmol/L).[335,371,471–473] In other studies, similar infants did not appear to be at risk unless their serum bilirubin levels were well above 20 mg/dL.[468,474–476] In some small, sick infants, yellow staining of the brain was seen at autopsy, with bilirubin levels less than 10 mg/dL (171 μmol/L).[334,337,338,342,477,478]

Starting in 1967 and continuing into the late 1970s, reports from the CPP, a study of 53,000 pregnant women and their offspring, linked moderate elevations of neonatal serum bilirubin to lower developmental scores,[479,480] lower IQ scores,[481] and increased risk of neurologic abnormalities.[481,482] These findings occurred at levels of bilirubin previously presumed to be safe.

These data and the results of other studies suggested that acute bilirubin encephalopathy or classic kernicterus was the most obvious and extreme manifestation of a spectrum of bilirubin toxicity; at the other end of the spectrum were more subtle forms of neurotoxicity that occurred at much lower bilirubin levels and in the absence of any obvious abnormal clinical findings in the neonatal period.

Two subsequent studies found little association between serum bilirubin levels and bilirubin staining of the brain of very-low-birth-weight infants.[483,484] The finding that gross bilirubin staining of the brain could occur in the absence of the typical microscopic neuronal damage described with kernicterus called into question the meaning of yellow staining of the brain in some very-low-birth-weight infants.[340] This led Valaes to adopt the term neonatal intensive care unit (NICU) kernicterus. Unlike the classic form of fatal kernicterus, these very-low-birth-weight infants, although they may have had kernicterus, died from other causes.[485,486]

Rh HEMOLYTIC DISEASES OF THE NEWBORN

A lone controlled trial was done on the treatment of hemolytic disease of the newborn. In March 1952, Mollison and Walker reported the results of their prospective, randomized, controlled trial on the effect of exchange transfusion *versus* simple transfusion in infants with Rh hemolytic disease.[487] Armitage and Mollison subsequently analyzed the data in more detail.[488] They enrolled 119 infants with Rh hemolytic disease and randomly assigned them to receive an exchange transfusion or a simple transfusion within 9.5 hours of birth. Infants of fewer than 35 weeks of gestation were excluded. Thirty-two percent of the infants who received a simple transfusion died from kernicterus, compared with 10% of those who received an exchange transfusion ($p = 0.0028$). Two infants in the exchange transfusion group died after 1 week of age, but no further deaths occurred in the simple transfusion group. Survivors were followed to 6 months of age, and the incidence of brain damage was similar in both groups (7%).

No bilirubin levels were reported in these studies, therefore no conclusions can be drawn about the possible relation between serum bilirubin levels and fatal kernicterus. There is also no clear statement about how the diagnosis of kernicterus was made—clinically, by autopsy, or both. Nevertheless, the study demonstrated beyond reasonable doubt that exchange transfusion in infants improved their chance of survival and decreased the risk of fatal kernicterus. The results of these studies, combined with the uncontrolled observations of Hsai and colleagues[461] and Mollison and Cutbush,[462] established exchange transfusion as the standard treatment for preventing kernicterus in infants with erythroblastosis fetalis. These investigators found that kernicterus was unlikely to occur if serum bilirubin levels were kept below 20 mg/dL (342 μmol/L), an observation that has been amply confirmed by subsequent experience with the treatment of hemolytic disease.

As a complication of hemolytic disease, clinical kernicterus has essentially disappeared in the Western world, and since Rh disease is largely preventable, there is no reason to consider any change in this approach. It is interesting to recall, however, that these studies were performed on infants born in the late 1940s and early 1950s. These infants were commonly asphyxiated and seriously ill, and many were delivered prematurely to prevent stillbirth. Streptomycin was frequently administered to infants who received exchange transfusion.[447,465,468] Later experience with Rh hemolytic disease was far more encouraging.[437] It would be interesting to reevaluate a similar series of infants managed under contemporary conditions of high-risk obstetric and neonatal intensive care.

An 18-year follow-up of 55 boys with a history of neonatal hyperbilirubinemia (>15 mg/dL, or 257 μmol/L) was performed in Norway at the time of military draft physical examinations.[489] Compared with the total cohort of Norwegian conscripts, there were no significant differences revealed on physical examination or tests of vision, hearing, or IQ. As neonates, one-half of these boys had positive Coombs tests; and seven boys who had a history of positive Coombs tests and bilirubin in excess of 15 mg/dL (25 μmol/L) for more than 5 days had significantly lower IQ scores than the national average.

FULL-TERM INFANTS WITHOUT HEMOLYSIS

Full-term infants without hemolytic disease appear to be at significantly lower risk for bilirubin encephalopathy at bilirubin levels that are considered hazardous to infants with hemolytic disease. When the serum bilirubin level concentration reached 20 mg/dL (342 μmol/L), Killander and colleagues assigned 94 infants alternately to receive or not to receive an exchange transfusion.[349,466] None of these infants had Rh hemolytic disease; 21 were ABO incompatible, but only 6 had evidence of ABO hemolytic disease (3 in the exchange group and 3 in the nonexchange group). Forty-six infants received exchange transfusions, and 48 did not (controls). In three control and four treated infants, bilirubin levels exceeded 25 mg/dL (428 μmol/L). The infants were followed for at least 2 years and underwent detailed physical and neurologic examinations at a mean age of 27 months. No audiometry or IQ testing was done, but a detailed history was obtained with specific attention to behavioral abnormalities, hearing and vision impairment, and possible deviations in motor performance. The examiners were not blinded. With the exception of one infant in the treated group who probably had an inherited myopathy, none of the children in either of the groups showed any major neurologic abnormalities. There are no other controlled trials that address the question of whether or not serum bilirubin levels of 20 mg/dL are harmful to otherwise healthy full-term infants.

In their extensive review, Newman and Maisels could find no evidence of a clinically significant effect of bilirubin level on intelligent quotients, neurologic abnormalities, or hearing loss (Tables 38-23 through 38-25).[260,448] In a reanalysis of the data from the CPP, however, Newman and Klebanoff identified a significant association between serum bilirubin levels in excess of 15 mg/dL (257 μmol/L) and an increase in subtle neurologic abnormalities (*e.g.*, oculomotor disturbance, minor muscle and coordination problems).[490]

The CPP was a multicenter cohort study of 53,043 women who became pregnant in the years 1959 to 1965. Each infant born to these mothers and weighing more than 2500 g had a total serum bilirubin drawn at age 48 ± 12 hours. If the initial bilirubin concentration was at least 10 mg/dL (171 μmol/L), the measurement was repeated daily until the bilirubin level fell below 10 mg/dL. The predictor variable in each of the CPP studies is the highest total bilirubin value recorded. The infants in this study were followed to 8 years of age, during which time they were evaluated with full psychometric testing including IQ, formal neurologic evaluations, and evaluations of speech and hearing. Unfortunately, some important results from the CPP have been published only in monographs and are unfamiliar to many in the field because monographs are neither peer-reviewed nor listed in the *Index Medicus*.

In their analysis, Newman and Maisels restricted their attention to full-term infants without hemolysis and found that, although statistically significant, serum bilirubin levels are not associated with subsequent IQ score in any clinically important way.[260,448] They reached this conclusion by calculating the magnitude of associations (*i.e.*, the effect size) rather than relying on p values to estimate the importance of reported associations. This is necessary because some statistically significant correlations in the CPP occurred only by virtue of the enormous sample size.

To put these effect sizes into perspective and to facilitate comparisons of different studies, Newman and Maisels calculated the observed change in outcome per 5 mg/dL (85 μmol/L) of serum bilirubin. This figure was chosen because it represents the upper limit of what is usually obtained in bilirubin-lowering interventions used in clinical practice. For example, phototherapy introduced at a serum bilirubin

TABLE 38–23
ASSOCIATION BETWEEN MAXIMAL TOTAL SERUM BILIRUBIN LEVEL AND INTELLIGENCE QUOTIENT IN STUDIES PRIMARILY OF FULL-TERM INFANTS WITHOUT HEMOLYSIS

Reference	Number	Age at Follow-Up (years)	Predicted Change: Points per 85 μmol/L (5 mg/dL)	Probability
Bjure et al.[786]	181	2–3	None	
Culley et al.[787]	121	5–6	None	
Rosta et al.[788]	84	8	None	
Broman et al.[493*†]				
Caucasians	11,497	4	−0.7	<.01
African Americans	13,388		−1.4	<.01
Naeye[481*†]	29,410	4	−1.6	<0.001
Rubin et al.[789*†]	343	4, 7	None	
Valaes et al.[131†]	411	5–7	None	
Seidman et al.[496]	1,948	17	<−1	NS‡

* Study did not exclude premature or low-birth-weight infants.
† Study did not exclude infants with hemolysis.
‡ No association between mean IQ and bilirubin category, but a higher risk of IQ < 85 in full-term Coombs-negative boys with bilirubin levels > 20 mg/dL (347 μmol/L; odds ratio = 2.96; *p* = .01).
From Newman TB, Maisels MJ. Evaluation of jaundice in the term newborn: a kinder, gentler approach. Pediatrics 1992;89:809.

level of 18 mg/dL (308 μmol/L) is commonly discontinued when the bilirubin reaches 13 mg/dL (222 μmol/L). Exchange transfusion results in a drop after rebound of about 30% to 40% of the peak bilirubin level.[491] In a group of ABO incompatible infants, tin protoporphyrin (SnPP) reduced the mean serum bilirubin by 2 to 3 mg/dL (34–51 μmol/L).[492]

The association of bilirubin level with IQ in the CPP was only about one point per 5 mg/dL (85 μmol/L; see Table 38-23). This is probably a worst-case estimate because premature infants and those with hemolysis were not excluded from the study.[493] Bilirubin levels were also unrelated to subsequent school performance.[494] Finally, of nearly 15,000 subjects with complete hearing evaluations at 8 years of age, no association was found between sensorineural hearing loss and serum bilirubin levels (see Table 38-25).[495]

Thus, even if the observed associations were completely causal and interventions to reduce hyperbilirubinemia could completely eliminate the risk, the

TABLE 38–24
PROPORTION OF INFANTS WITH DEFINITE NEUROLOGIC ABNORMALITY BY MAXIMAL TOTAL SERUM BILIRUBIN LEVEL IN STUDIES PRIMARILY OF FULL-TERM INFANTS WITHOUT HEMOLYSIS

	Total Serum Bilirubin Level		
Reference	<15 mg/dL (<257 μmol/L)	≥15 mg/dL (≥257 μmol/L)	≥20 mg/dL (≥342 μmol/L)
Hardy and Peeples[482]	39/2885	1/110	0/35
Mores et al.[467]		0/54	0/54
Killander et al.[466]		1/93	1/93
Fohl and Lombos[464]	0/3	2/37	2/29
Holmes et al.[465]	0/46	0/34	
Culley et al.[787]	1/97*	1/24	
Bengtsson and Verneholt[463]	1/115	2/11	2/111
Total	41/3146	7/463	5/322
Percentage	1.3	1.5	1.6

* Includes infants with bilirubin level up to 16 mg/dL (274 μmol/L).
From Newman TB, Maisels MJ. Evaluation of jaundice in the term newborn: a kinder, gentler approach. Pediatrics 1992;89:809.

TABLE 38–25
ASSOCIATION BETWEEN SERUM BILIRUBIN LEVEL AND RISK OF SENSORINEURAL HEARING LOSS IN STUDIES PRIMARILY OF FULL-TERM INFANTS WITHOUT HEMOLYSIS

Reference	Bilirubin Level mg/dL	Bilirubin Level μmol/L	Number With Hearing Loss/Number Examined	Effect
Bjure et al.[786]	18–19.9	308–340	0/14	No hearing loss found
	≥20	≥342	0/39	
Holmes et al.[465]	≥15	≥257	0/34	No hearing loss found
Culley et al.[787]	*	*	0/230	None of 230 infants examined had sensorineural hearing loss
Bengtsson and Verneholt[463]	<20	<342	0/115	Risk ratio is undefined; p = .057 (Fisher's Exact Test)
	≥20	≥342	4/111	
Valaes et al.[131]	<12	<205	4/350	Relative risk = 8.1; 95% confidence interval = 2.3 to 28
	≥12	≥205	6/65	
Lassman et al.[495]	*	*	†	Trend toward higher risk with lower bilirubin; details not given

* Distribution not given.
† n = 14,900.
From Newman TB, Maisels MJ. Evaluation of jaundice in the term newborn: a kinder, gentler approach. Pediatrics 1992;89:809.

potential gain in IQ would be only about 0.75 to 1.5 points—an effect only about 5% to 10% as large as the effect of race or socioeconomic status.[493,494] The prediction of reduction in definite or suspected neurologic abnormality is also small; decreasing the serum bilirubin level from 18 to 13 mg/dL, for example, produces a predicted change in the incidence of definite or suspected abnormality from 14% to 13%.[448] It is unlikely that a search for new interventions directed at preventing or treating hyperbilirubinemia will be rewarding, particularly in full-term infants without hemolysis.

Seidman and colleagues evaluated a group of Israeli army draftees (n = 1948) and matched their preinduction psychologic and physical examinations at age 17 years to their neonatal records.[496] They found an association between risk of IQ below 85 and bilirubin level higher than 20 mg/dL (342 μmol/L) in full-term boys with a negative Coombs test (p = 0.01). This association was not found in girls. When adjusted for various confounders, no association was found between bilirubin levels and mean IQ score, risk of physical or neurologic abnormality, or hearing loss. Seidman and colleagues suggest that their finding of a significantly increased risk of low IQ scores in association with serum bilirubin levels higher than 20 mg/dL is consistent with the concept of a threshold level of bilirubin above which there is significant danger.[457,496] If there were no danger from bilirubin until it reached a certain threshold, however, one would expect to see an effect of bilirubin on the mean IQ of the population.

Newman and Maisels used linear regression analysis to summarize the effect of bilirubin on IQ.[448] This could be misleading if the relation between bilirubin and IQ were nonlinear.[453] Newman and Klebanoff reanalyzed the CPP data and found no association between bilirubin and IQ—adjusted for confounding variables—in either linear or nonlinear models.[490] They also found no effect of peak bilirubin on definite neurologic abnormalities. An effect was found, however, on suspected neurologic abnormalities (*e.g.*, minor muscle and coordination problems and oculomotor abnormalities) at age 7; these increased from 15% in those with a peak bilirubin level of 10 mg/dL (171 μmol/L) or higher to 22% at a bilirubin level of 20 mg/dL (342 μmol/L; $p < 0.001$). So far, there is no evidence that treating hyperbilirubinemia at these levels has reduced the incidence of these types of neurologic problems.[497]

BILIRUBIN-BINDING CAPACITY AND DEVELOPMENTAL OUTCOME

Odell and colleagues examined 32 children 4 to 7 years of age in whom bilirubin levels were measured in the neonatal period.[498] They found no relation between total serum bilirubin levels and abnormal performance, but there was a strong relation between the bilirubin saturation index, which is a measure of the saturation of serum bilirubin-binding sites by bilirubin, and subsequent abnormality. The effect size observed was remarkable: a risk difference of 58% (*i.e.*, brain damage occurred in 76% of those with high saturation, compared with 18% of those with low saturation). Sixteen of the 18 abnormal infants were either premature or had hemolytic disease. Two thirds of the infants enrolled were lost to follow-up, raising the possibility of substantial bias, and the small sample size could lead to gross overestimation of the effect simply by chance.

Johnson and Boggs reported results of detailed neurologic and psychometric examinations on 83 infants with a history of neonatal jaundice.[499] They found a relation between developmental outcome and the HBABA-binding test. Infants with binding levels of 50% or less were more likely to be considered suspect on neurologic psychometric or speech and hearing examinations.

In the NICHHD Cooperative Phototherapy Study, albumin binding of bilirubin was measured by the HBABA technique and Sephadex G-25 gel column chromatography. Three infants who died were found to have kernicterus at autopsy. Two had one or more abnormal HBABA values (<40%), whereas only one infant had positive findings on the Sephadex. No relation was found between IQ measured at age 6 years and the results of the binding tests during the neonatal period.[500]

DURATION OF HYPERBILIRUBINEMIA

Johnson and Boggs also found a relation between peak indirect bilirubin levels higher than 15 mg/dL (257 μmol/L) and the risk of neurologic and psychometric abnormalities. The strongest relation, however, was with duration of hyperbilirubinemia; the longer the hyperbilirubinemia lasted, the greater the risk.[499] Odell and colleagues found that brain-damaged infants were exposed to bilirubin levels higher than 15 mg/dL (257 μmol/L) for significantly longer than were normal infants.[498] As with Odell's study, Johnson and Boggs' data cannot be applied to healthy full-term infants because 44 (53%) of the infants had hemolytic disease and 27 (33%) were premature. In the large NICHHD collaborative phototherapy trial, a 6-year follow-up of 224 control infants who did not receive phototherapy and had birth weights lower than 2000 g showed no association between IQ and mean bilirubin level, time and duration of exposure to bilirubin, or measures of bilirubin–albumin binding.[497]

It is possible, however, that one explanation for the poor correlation between maximal serum bilirubin and outcome is that maximal serum bilirubin is only weakly associated with the true risk factor—free serum bilirubin or duration of hyperbilirubinemia. Unfortunately, it is difficult to base clinical decisions on binding tests, since they are generally unavailable, or on the duration of hyperbilirubinemia, since at the time decisions need to be made, the duration is not yet known.

HEARING LOSS AND AUDIOMETRIC EVOKED RESPONSES

The BAER test is an accurate and noninvasive means of assessing the functional status of the auditory nerve and the brain stem auditory pathway. The BAER tracing of a normal full-term infant is shown in Figure 38-21. The three positive wave forms labeled in the figure are those most easily identified in the neonate. The neural generators of the BAER include the auditory nerve (*i.e.*, wave I), the cochlear nucleus and superior olive (*i.e.*, wave III), and the inferior colliculus (*i.e.*, waves IV and V). The latency for wave I represents the peripheral conduction time. Latency of waves III and V and the interpeak latency of waves I to III, III to V, and I to V all represent measurements of central conduction time. The interpeak latency I to V is referred to as the *brainstem conduction time.* Reports also include amplitudes of the wave forms. These may decrease or be lost in response to various insults.

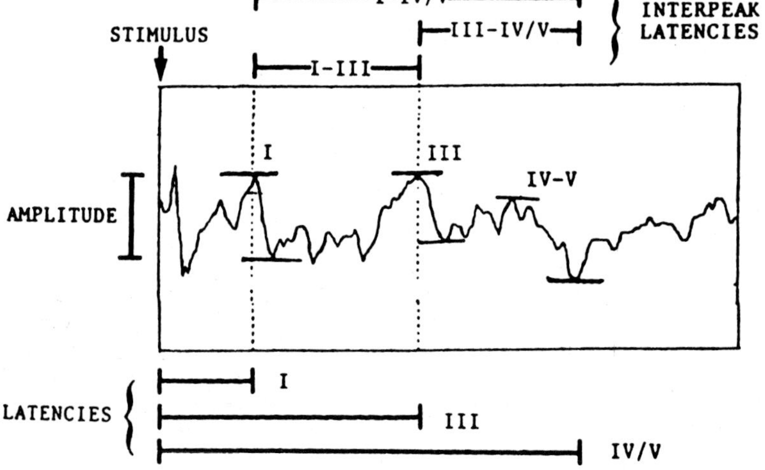

FIG. 38–21. A typical tracing of brain stem audiometric evoked response has various components. Wave I reflects the response of the peripheral auditory nerve; wave III reflects the superior olive; waves IV to V reflect the inferior colliculus with peak and trough shown. Wave I peak to waves IV to V trough (*i.e.*, interpeak latency) reflects brain stem conduction time. (From Vohr BR. New approaches to assessing the risks of hyperbilirubinemia. Clin Perinatol 1990;17:293.)

Several studies have evaluated the relation between serum bilirubin levels and the BAER. Most have identified an effect of bilirubin on central conduction time,[427,432,441–445] although some suggest an effect on the peripheral auditory nerve.[425,426,501] According to Vohr,[432] the reported differences may be due to the inclusion of both full-term and premature infants, the use of different definitions of hyperbilirubinemia, and variations in technique. Histologic studies in infants and Gunn rats suggest involvement of the brain stem auditory nuclei.[502–504]

The acute changes seen in BAER can be reversed by bilirubin-lowering interventions (*e.g.*, phototherapy, exchange transfusion).[424–427,443,505,506] Nakamura and colleagues[426] and Esbjörner and colleagues[507] found that abnormalities of the BAER were more closely related to the unbound bilirubin levels than to total bilirubin levels. In Nakamura's study, abnormalities were present in 89% of infants with unbound bilirubin levels of 1 μg/dL or higher, compared with 42% of those with levels of 0.5 to 0.99 μg/dL and 33% of those with levels of 0.5 μg/dL or lower.[426] On the other hand, Streletz and colleagues were unable to demonstrate any relation between serum bilirubin levels and prolongation of the BAER central conduction time in a NICU population.[508] Prolongation of wave I latency was found in hypoxemic infants. Streletz and colleagues also pointed out that middle ear effusion may occur in as many of one third of the NICU population and may result in transient BAER abnormalities, difficult to distinguish from the changes due to hyperbilirubinemia or hypoxemia.[508] Thoma and colleagues studied 85 children with serum bilirubin levels between 8.2 and 25 mg/dL (141–430 μmol/L).[509] About 20 infants had serum bilirubin levels that exceeded 20 mg/dL (340 μmol/L), and 72 had bilirubin levels of 17.5 mg/dL (299 μmol/L) or higher. No correlation was found between serum bilirubin concentrations and BAER.[509]

In spite of evidence for acute bilirubin toxicity on the auditory pathway in full-term and preterm infants, there is virtually no evidence for a risk of hearing loss related to hyperbilirubinemia in full-term infants who do not have hemolytic disease. In a study of almost 15,000 children who received complete hearing evaluations at 8 years of age, the incidence of sensorineural hearing loss was actually highest in the infants with the lowest bilirubin levels, as was the incidence of conductive hearing loss (see Table 38-25).[495] In their 17-year follow-up study, Seidman and colleagues found no relation between hearing loss and hyperbilirubinemia.[496] In the NICHHD controlled trial of phototherapy, the incidence of sensorineural hearing loss in children followed to age 6 years was identical in the phototherapy and control groups (1.8% *versus* 1.9%). Valaes and colleagues, however, reported a statistically significant relation between serum bilirubin levels of 12 mg/dL (205 μmol/L) or higher and the risk of sensorineural hearing loss in the children of mothers who enrolled in a prenatal phenobarbital trial (relative risk 8.1; $p < 0.001$).[131] Interpretation of this result is complicated by the lack of information on the severity of hearing loss, how it was measured, whether those measuring it were blinded to bilirubin values, and the inclusion of infants with hemolytic disease. Although most of the subjects did not have hemolytic disease, of the 45 infants with bilirubin values higher than 16 mg/dL (205 μmol/L), 13 had ABO incompatibility, 7 were premature, and 1 was G6PD-deficient.

Johnson and colleagues found that deficits in central hearing, speech, and language can occur in the absence of pure-tone hearing loss.[510] They also noted that these deficits are easier to detect at 7 years of age than at 4 years of age and that they correlate more closely with measures of bilirubin binding than with peak serum bilirubin levels. Johnson also pointed out that in their earlier study,[499] there was a high incidence of perceptual dysfunction in spite of normal IQ scores. Deficits in central processing can occur in spite of a normal hearing threshold and a normal IQ.[281]

CRY ANALYSIS

An abnormal cry is a sign of neurologic distress and has been associated with acute bilirubin encephalopathy.[511] Modest degrees of hyperbilirubinemia also affect the infant's cry.[432] Glottal instability appeared in 11 of 12 infants with serum bilirubin levels between 10 and 20 mg/dL (171–342 μmol/L).[512] Using high-speed computer technology, Vohr and colleagues found that infants with bilirubin levels of 10 to 20 mg/dL (171–342 μmol/L) had a significant increase in percentage of phonation and in the variability of first formant when compared with infants with bilirubin levels lower than 8 mg/dL (137 μmol/L).[445] They also found that the percentage of phonation correlated with the BAER interpeak latency of waves I to III and brain stem conduction time (*i.e.*, waves I to IV).

INFANT BEHAVIOR

Investigators have used the Brazelton Neonatal Behavioral Assessment Scale (BNBAS) to evaluate the effect of hyperbilirubinemia on infant behavior. Most studies show some effect, although several are confounded by the use of phototherapy. Escher-Gräub and Fricker used the BNBAS with examiners blinded to evaluate behavioral integrity in 76 infants whose serum bilirubin levels ranged from 11.7 to 14.6 mg/dL (200–250 μmol/L) and compared them with 401 infants with serum bilirubin levels below 5.8 mg/dL (100 μmol/L).[513] The jaundiced infants scored lower than the controls in habituation, orientation, motor performance, regulation of state, and autonomic stability. Paludetto and colleagues compared 31 moderately jaundiced full-term infants on days 3 and 4 (bilirubin level, 8.4 to 14.3 mg/dL, or 144–245 μmol/L) with nonjaundiced matched controls; they found no differences between the two groups.[514] Other investigators have evaluated behavior in infants undergoing phototherapy. Telzrow and colleagues[515] and Paludetto and colleagues[516] found that infants receiving phototherapy for hyperbilirubinemia scored lower on orientation items when compared with controls.

Vohr and colleagues studied 23 jaundiced full-term infants with bilirubin levels of 10 to 20 mg/dL (171–342 μmol/L) and compared them with 27 whose bilirubin levels were 8 mg/dL (137 μmol/L) or lower on days 2 to 3.[444] Infants in the jaundiced group had lower BNBAS cluster scores for orientation and state regulation. The serum bilirubin level correlates inversely with the BNBAS orientation score and state regulation score. The orientation cluster score was also inversely correlated with cry dysphonation and variability of the fundamental frequency.

These studies suggest that mild to moderate elevations of serum bilirubin have an effect on neurosensory systems that can be measured and documented. Changes in the BAER are mediated by the 8th cranial nerve pathway, and cry characteristics by the vagal complex cranial nerves. The nuclei of these cranial nerves are located close to one another in the brain stem, and bilirubin might affect both areas simultaneously.[432]

PREMATURE INFANTS

It is generally believed that premature infants are at greater risk for developing kernicterus or bilirubin encephalopathy than are full-term newborns exposed to similar bilirubin levels. The evidence for this, although suggestive, is not entirely convincing.

Watchko and Oski provide a historical review of kernicterus in prematurity from the 1950s to the present.[460] Reports during the years 1950 to 1965 suggested that kernicterus or the clinical sequelae of hyperbilirubinemia were unlikely to develop if exchange transfusions were used to maintain serum bilirubin levels below 18 to 22 mg/dL (308–376 μmol/L).[471,517–521] Killander and colleagues found that premature infants with nonhemolytic hyperbilirubinemia did not develop kernicterus or evidence of bilirubin encephalopathy if the serum bilirubin level was maintained below 20 mg/dL (342 μmol/L) using exchange transfusions.[349] Shiller and Silverman found no association between bilirubin levels and neurologic deficits or mental retardation in their study of premature infants.[476]

Wishingrad and colleagues conducted a prospective randomized study of 187 preterm infants with nonhemolytic hyperbilirubinemia, most of whom weighed more than 1500 g.[468] One-hundred infants whose serum bilirubin levels exceeded 18 mg/dL (308 μmol/L) after 36 hours of age were randomly assigned to receive or not to receive an exchange transfusion (50 in each group). An additional 87 infants whose serum bilirubin concentrations did not exceed 15 mg/dL (257 μmol/L) were selected as a control group. There were no differences in the mortality among the three groups. In the exchange transfusion group, there was no evidence of kernicterus at 1 year of age despite the fact that 7 of the 50 infants had levels of indirect bilirubin exceeding 24 mg/dL (410 μmol/L). In the no-exchange group, 10 of the infants had bilirubin levels exceeding 24 mg/dL, and one developed fatal kernicterus. This infant had respiratory distress syndrome, edema, and a peak indirect serum bilirubin concentration of 27.6 mg/dL (472 μmol/L). Lethargy and jitteriness were noted at an indirect serum bilirubin level of 17.7 mg/dL (303 μmol/L), and a seizure occurred at 22.8 mg/dL (390 μmol/L). Neurologic assessment of the remaining infants at 1 year of life revealed no evidence of kernicterus. The authors concluded that exchange transfusions in the management of nonhemolytic hyperbilirubinemia of prematurity need not be performed if indirect serum bilirubin levels are below 24 mg/dL. In the one infant who developed fatal kernicterus, however, one might question whether intervention at a bilirubin level of 17.7 mg/dL (303 μmol/L) might not have been helpful when symptoms of lethargy and jitteriness appeared.[459]

Several other studies published during this era failed to demonstrate evidence of an association between serum bilirubin levels lower than 20 mg/dL (342 μmol/L) and developmental outcome in the premature neonate.[476,520,522–524] Most of the infants reported in the studies mentioned previously were larger (1250–2500 g) and more mature (28–36 weeks of gestation) than the extremely low-birth-weight infants seen in NICUs.

LOW-BILIRUBIN KERNICTERUS

Between 1958 and 1972, a group of studies reported the occurrence of kernicterus at serum bilirubin levels well below 20 mg/dL (342 μmol/L).[335,371,473,478,525] In general, these infants were significantly more premature and of much lower birth weight than those previously observed with kernicterus, and some were exposed to sulfisoxazole,[371]—subsequently shown in a controlled trial to be a powerful displacer of bilirubin from its binding to albumin.[125] As a result of these findings, various authors suggested the use of exchange transfusions in preterm infants at serum bilirubin levels of less than 20 mg/dL (342 μmol/L).[526–528] The publication of data from the CPP that suggested an association between impaired psychomotor performance and bilirubin levels higher than 10 to 14 mg/dL (171–239 μmol/L) in low-birth-weight infants provided additional support for these recommendations.[480,481]

Similar guidelines were incorporated into the NICHHD cooperative phototherapy study. In this study, infants were randomly assigned to a control group that received no phototherapy or to a group that received phototherapy at predetermined serum bilirubin levels. The criteria for exchange transfusion for all infants mandated exchange transfusions at relatively low levels of serum bilirubin (10 mg/dL, or 171 μmol/L, in high risk newborns with birth weights less than 1250 g).[529] A total of 1339 infants entered the study—672 in the phototherapy group and 667 in the control group. Infants who weighed less than 2000 g at birth were assigned to receive phototherapy at 24 ± 12 hours of age, irrespective of their serum bilirubin levels. In this birth weight category, of 462 infants assigned to the phototherapy group, only 17.7% had serum bilirubin levels higher than 10 mg/dL (171 μmol/L), compared with 62.8% of the 460 controls. One-hundred and nineteen infants died, and 64% had autopsies performed. Kernicterus was found in four infants, all of whom weighed less than 1500 g and had a complicated neonatal course. Their peak serum bilirubin levels ranged from 6.5 to 14.2 mg/dL (111–243 μmol/L). One of these infants was in the phototherapy group, and three were in the control group ($p = 0.2$). The results were complicated by the fact that the infant in the phototherapy group who had kernicterus did not get phototherapy until 43 hours of age and received an exchange transfusion at 44 hours of age. The infant died at 7 days of age. If this infant is excluded, the p value for the Fisher exact test is .081. The four infants who had kernicterus at autopsy had birth weights ranging from 760 to 1270 g. All were asphyxiated or had hyaline membrane disease, and all had some degree of PIVH. Two had periventricular leukomalacia. Since 36% of those who died did not have autopsies, the interpretation of these results remains uncertain.

Surviving infants in the study were followed and evaluated at 1 year of age with the Bayley Scales of Mental and Psychomotor Development and at 6 years of age with the Wechsler Verbal and Performance IQ. No differences were found in the incidence of definite and suspect cerebral palsy, clumsy or abnormal movements, hypotonia, or an IQ lower than 70. There were no differences between the two groups in growth, speech, hearing loss, or evidence of hyperactivity.[497]

Scheidt and colleagues published a 6-year follow-up of 224 control children with birth weights lower than 2000 g.[500] None of these infants received phototherapy, but bilirubin levels were maintained below specified levels by the use of exchange transfusion. No relation was found between serum bilirubin levels and the incidence of cerebral palsy, nor was there any association between maximal bilirubin level and IQ. IQ was not associated with mean bilirubin level, time and duration of exposure to bilirubin, or measures of bilirubin–albumin binding.[500]

Because the predictor variable in the NICHHD phototherapy study was phototherapy *versus* no phototherapy, it provides only indirect although clinically relevant evidence regarding the question of whether bilirubin affects neurodevelopmental outcome. In fact, because in infants who weighed 2500 g or more, phototherapy was not begun until the serum bilirubin level reached an average of 15.7 mg/dL, the peak serum bilirubin levels in the two groups at this birth weight were practically identical.[529] A difference existed in the duration of hyperbilirubinemia, which can be expressed as a difference in areas under the two curves of serum bilirubin level plotted against age. This difference was about 12.5 mg/dL/day in infants who weighed more than 2500 g. In the infants who weighed 2000 to 2499 g and in those who weighed less than 2000 g, the differences in peak bilirubin levels were about 1 mg/dL and 6 mg/dL, respectively, and the areas under the curves were substantially greater in the control infants.[448]

HEARING LOSS IN LOW-BIRTH-WEIGHT INFANTS

Several epidemiologic studies have identified elevated serum bilirubin levels as a risk factor for hearing loss in low-birth-weight survivors of NICUs.[365,530–532] On the other hand, in a study of 975 infants cared for in an intensive care nursery, Halpern and colleagues identified craniofacial anomalies, congenital perinatal infections, and meconium aspiration as the strongest predictors of hearing loss, especially in full-term infants.[533] They found a negative association between hyperbilirubinemia and hearing loss. In a 5-year follow-up of 814 infants of less than 32 weeks of gestation or less than 1500 g birth weight, van de Bor and colleagues found no association between bilirubin levels and hearing loss.[534]

DeVries and colleagues found a significant increase in bilateral sensorineural deafness in infants with birth weights lower than 1500 g who were classified as high risk.[535] High-risk criteria included the following:

- Apgar score <5 at 5 minutes, or requirement for intubation lasting more than 4 minutes
- intermittent positive-pressure ventilation for more than 24 hours
- hyaline membrane disease requiring ventilation
- pneumothorax
- persistent fetal circulation severe enough to require treatment with tolazoline
- persistent patent ductus arteriosus requiring treatment
- proven infection
- hyperglycemia
- PIVH.

If serum bilirubin levels exceeded 14 mg/dL (240 μmol/L), the incidence of deafness was 36% in these high-risk infants, compared with only 4% in high-risk infants with birth weights of more than 1500 g ($p < 0.05$).[535] After more aggressive use of phototherapy and exchange transfusion, the incidence of sensorineural deafness in this population was reduced to zero.[536]

LOW-BIRTH-WEIGHT INFANTS IN THE 1980s AND 1990s

In 1980, Kim and colleagues[483] and Turkel and colleagues[484] reviewed the risk factors previously suggested to predict the development of kernicterus. They were unable to identify any risk factor or group of factors that was associated with the development of kernicterus in the premature neonate, including birth weight less than 1500 g, hypothermia, asphyxia, acidosis, hypoalbuminemia, sepsis, meningitis, drug therapy, and serum bilirubin levels.[483,484]

It is likely that there are some risk factors for the development of kernicterus that are unknown. An excellent example of this possibility is the experience reported by Jardine and Rogers.[429] They found that the proportion of premature infants with kernicterus who underwent autopsy fell abruptly from 31% to 0% when they stopped flushing intravenous catheters with bacteriostatic saline that contained benzyl alcohol. In an earlier study from their NICU, the incidence of kernicterus diagnosed postmortem among neonates of 25 to 32 weeks of gestation was a remarkably high 25%.[330] As mentioned previously, benzyl alcohol is an agent that increases membrane fluidity[352] and may thus facilitate the passage of bilirubin. At the same institution, Watchko and Claasen found only three cases of kernicterus in 72 autopsies performed from 1984 through 1991 on newborns of less than 34 weeks of gestation who lived at least 48 hours.[537] This sustained decrease in the incidence of kernicterus supports their contention, confirmed by experience in most nurseries, that kernicterus in premature newborns has disappeared almost completely from the NICU. In Watchko and Claasen's population of 69 newborns who did not have kernicterus, the peak serum bilirubin level ranged from 6.3 to 20.6 mg/dL (108–352 μmol/L), and 56% had peak serum bilirubin values higher than those suggested for exchange transfusion by the NICHHD phototherapy study guidelines.[537] Thus, kernicterus is an uncommon event, even when serum bilirubin levels are allowed to rise above those previously thought to place the premature infant at risk.

Several studies have failed to document an association between maximal serum bilirubin levels and developmental outcomes in very-low-birth-weight infants.[534,538,539] Van de Bor and colleagues found a relation between maximal serum bilirubin concentrations in the neonatal period and neurodevelopmental outcome at a corrected age of 2 years.[540] The handicaps described were not those characteristically found with kernicterus and were mainly caused by cerebral palsy. In addition, no relation was found between maximal serum bilirubin concentrations and hearing defects. In a follow-up of the same population at 5 years, in which a remarkable 98% of 831 surviving children were evaluated, no significant difference was found in mean maximal serum bilirubin concentrations between children with and without handicaps. A dose–response relation between maximal serum total bilirubin concentration and the risk of adverse outcome was again observed, but after correction for seven suspected confounding factors (*i.e.*, gestational age, birth weight, intracranial hemorrhage, ventriculomegaly, seizures, bronchopulmonary dysplasia, and socioeconomic status), the previously observed association between bilirubin levels and handicap disappeared (odds ratio, 1.2; confidence interval, 0.89 to 1.43 per 50 μmol/L increase of total bilirubin). The investigators did find, however, that children who had suffered an intracranial hemorrhage were at significantly greater risk of handicap (odds ratio, 1.84; confidence interval, 1.08 to 3.15 per 50 μmol/L increase of bilirubin). The association between maximal serum bilirubin concentration and handicap was most prominent, however, in children with grade I hemorrhage. This effect was not seen in the more severe hemorrhages, but the number of infants with severe hemorrhages was small. Furthermore, only 109 children (13.4%) had a handicap at 5 years of age; 63 (7.7%) had a minor and 46 (5.7%) had a major handicap. Failure to achieve statistical significance was probably the result of the small number of children with handicaps in the 5-year-old cohort.

Although these data are reassuring, few of these infants had markedly elevated bilirubin levels. In the study by Graziani and colleagues,[538] only 3 of 249 infants had a serum bilirubin level higher than 14.6 mg/dL (250 μmol/L). In van de Bor's study, mean maximal total serum bilirubin levels averaged 10.4 mg/dL (178 μmol/L)[534]; and in O'shea's study, median bilirubin levels were about 9 mg/dL (154 μmol/L).[539] O'shea followed a geographically based sample of 495 very-low-birth-weight infants born between January 1, 1985 and December 31, 1989 who survived to 1 year of adjusted age. Median bilirubin levels were about 9 mg/dL, and only 52 infants had a maximal serum bilirubin level above 11.6 mg/dL (22 μmol/L). Maximal neonatal serum bilirubin level was not associated with the risk of developmental problems identifiable at 1 year.[539] Although they found an increase in the odds ratio for developmental problems of 1.3 for each 50 μmol/L of bilirubin similar to that of van de Bor,[540] much of the apparent association was due to the confounding effect of neonatal intracranial abnormalities.[539] When the effect of intracranial abnormalities was controlled using stratified analyses, an association between maximal bilirubin level and developmental problems was found only among subjects with uncomplicated subependymal or intraventricular hemorrhage.[539]

CLINICAL MANAGEMENT

The clinical diagnosis of jaundice and the use of the cephalopedal progression of jaundice to evaluate the infant are discussed in the section Clinical Diagnosis of Jaundice. Guidelines for the initiation of noninvasive or invasive measurements of serum bilirubin levels are given in Tables 38-14 and 38-15.

LABORATORY MEASUREMENTS OF BILIRUBIN

METHODS BASED ON THE DIAZO REACTION

The reaction of diazotized sulfanilic acid with bilirubin, described by Ehrlich in 1883, is the basis for bilirubin measurements in most laboratories. In 1916, van den Bergh and Muller noted that this diazo reagent reacted rapidly with serum from patients with cholestatic jaundice, thus measuring the direct-reacting bilirubin, whereas serum from those with hemolytic jaundice required the addition of alcohol to obtain the red–purple derivatives (*i.e.*, azodipyrroles) of the yellow tetrapyrrole, bilirubin. This measured the total bilirubin.[541] The basic diazo reactions for total and direct bilirubin measurements are shown in Figure 38-22. The azobilirubins produced in these reactions are measured spectrophotometrically at 600 nm. The presence of accelerators, such as caffeine and methanol, break up the intramolecular hydrogen bonds of unconjugated bilirubin and the unconjugated, as well as conjugated, bilirubin reacts rapidly and completely, yielding the total diazo reaction.

Laboratory measurements of serum bilirubin concentrations can be inaccurate.[276,277,542,543] Two surveys in 1982 disclosed a high level of interlaboratory variation in the measurements of total and direct serum bilirubin concentrations in neonatal sera.[276,277] In a survey of 67 laboratories in Indiana, bilirubin values of 10.9 to 24 mg/dL (186–410 μmol/L) were reported for a serum with a mean total bilirubin concentration of 18.1 mg/dL (310 μmol/L), and a range of 1.8 to 9.2 mg/dL (31–157 μmol/L) was found for a mean direct-reacting bilirubin of 5.8 mg/dL (99 μmol/L).[276] Watkinson and colleagues also found a high interlaboratory variation in Australia and New Zealand.[277] With regard to conjugated bilirubin analyses, they concluded that "laboratories are unable to repeat accurately conjugated bilirubin results," which were, at best, "only an approximation to the true value."[277] Rather than reporting the actual value for conjugated bilirubin, they recommended that these results be reported in ranges of 25 to 50 μmol/L (1.5–3 mg/dL).[277]

When different laboratories measure total bilirubin on standard samples with identical bilirubin concentrations, the coefficient of variation (*i.e.*, the standard deviation divided by the mean) is about 10% when the total bilirubin is in the range of 5 to 20 mg/dL (85–342 μmol/L).[276,277] Coefficients of variation within the same laboratory (*i.e.*, on duplicate analyses of the same specimen) are only about one-half as large.[277] The American College of Pathologists' proficiency survey, in December 1988, found that the coefficient of variation for all methods measuring total bilirubin with a mean of 0.94 mg/dL (16 μmol/L) was 14.9%, and with a mean of 5.29 mg/dL (90 μmol/L), it was 8.1%. Unfortunately, proficiency surveys do not usually provide samples with bilirubin levels that are relevant to therapeutic decisions in the newborn. If the true serum bilirubin is 20 mg/dL (342 μmol/L), a 10% coefficient of variation between laboratories means that a repeat value could fall anywhere between 16 and 24 mg/dL (274–410 μmol/L; assuming 95% confidence limits). Within the same laboratory, however, a repeat measurement should fall between 18 and 22 mg/dL (308–376 μmol/L). These results can be improved with careful attention to standardization and other details. In William Beaumont Hospital laboratory, the coefficient of variation for a serum bilirubin level of 6.7 mg/dL (115 μmol/L) is 2%, and at 17.5 mg/dL (299 μmol/L), it is 3%.

Total Bilirubin

Conjugated Bilirubin + Unconjugated Bilirubin + Diazotized sulfanilic acid + Caffeine-benzoate

→ Azobilirubin A and B (Isomers I and II)

Direct Bilirubin

Conjugated Bilirubin + Diazotized sulfanilic acid

→ Azobilirubin B (Isomers I and II)

Indirect Bilirubin

Total Bilirubin − Direct Bilirubin = Indirect Bilirubin

FIG. 38–22. Basic diazo reactions for determination of total and direct bilirubins. Indirect bilirubin is obtained by calculation.

DIRECT SPECTROPHOTOMETRY

Direct spectrophotometry is frequently used to measure total bilirubin in the newborn. This measurement is based on the fact that bilirubin absorbs light at about 454 nm, and hemoglobin absorbs light equally at both 454 nm and 540 nm. By subtracting the 540 nm absorbance from the 454 nm absorbance, effects of hemolysis are eliminated, and only bilirubin absorbance is measured. The assay is only suitable for neonatal serum (<2–3 weeks of age) because other pigments, notably carotene, appear as infants get older and cause interference at 454 nm.[541]

HIGH-PRESSURE LIQUID CHROMATOGRAPHY

Considered the gold standard for bilirubin measurement, reverse-phase high-pressure liquid chromatography permits the measurement of all four fractions of bilirubin in a small sample (see Fig. 38-1). Unfortunately, high-pressure liquid chromatography is too elaborate, expensive, and time-consuming for the clinical laboratory.

REFLECTIVE SPECTROPHOTOMETRY

Developed by the Eastman Kodak Company, this method is available as an automated procedure using Kodak Ektachem Analizers. The method involves the use of two thin film slides, one of which directly measures conjugated and unconjugated bilirubin; the second measures total bilirubin (including δ-bilirubin; Fig. 38-23).

BILIRUBIN OXIDASE

The enzyme bilirubin oxidase oxidizes both conjugated and unconjugated bilirubin to biliverdin. The biliverdin is then oxidized to unknown purple compounds. Total bilirubin can be measured accurately by using direct spectrophotometric techniques before and after treatment of serum with bilirubin oxidase. The method can also be used to measure conjugated bilirubin. By allowing the reaction involving bilirubin oxidase to occur at *p*H 4.5, only the conjugated forms of bilirubin are measured.[541]

CONJUGATED AND DIRECT-REACTING BILIRUBIN

Although the two terms are used synonymously, direct-reacting bilirubin is not the same as conjugated bilirubin. Direct-reacting bilirubin refers to the bilirubin that reacts directly with diazotized sulfanilic acid (*i.e.*, without the addition of an accelerating agent), while conjugated bilirubin refers to bilirubin that has been made water-soluble by binding with glucuronic acid in the liver. Although measurements of total bilirubin have lacked precision and accuracy, this problem is considered more serious in the measurement of direct-reacting and conjugated bilirubin levels.[249,274,277,544–547] The measured direct-reacting bilirubin depends on the concentration of conjugated bilirubin but also on other factors, including the amount of time it is allowed to react, the concentration of various reagents, and the concentration of unconjugated bilirubin.[274] In contrast to total bilirubin, however, for which interlaboratory standardization is available through the College of American Pathologists, there is no standardization of direct-reacting bilirubin measurements from laboratory to laboratory. An example of this is the study by Newman and colleagues, in which measurements of direct-reacting bilirubin using the DuPont ACA or Coulter DACOS analyzer produced direct-reacting bilirubin levels in a population of full-term newborns at one hospital that were twice as high as those measured in a similar population at another institution, where the Kodak Ektachem 700 method was used (see Table 38-8).[249] As mentioned previously, the Ektachem method measures conjugated bilirubin, while the other methods measure direct-reacting bilirubin.

Unconjugated Bilirubin (α fraction) Conjugated Bilirubin (β and γ fractions) Total Bilirubin (α, β, γ and δ fractions)	} Direct measurement
Neonatal Bilirubin (α + β + γ fractions) Delta (δ) Bilirubin (Total−Neonatal)	} Calculations

FIG. 38–23. Bilirubin determinations performed by the Kodak Ektachem reflectance spectrophotometric method.

SITE OF BLOOD SAMPLING

Leslie and colleagues measured total serum bilirubin in paired capillary and venous samples in 118 newborns.[548] Although there was a significant correlation between the values, they found that capillary samples were lower than the venous bilirubin values when venous levels exceeded 10 mg/dL (171 μmol/L). Capillary samples were, on average, 0.9 mg/dL (15 μmol/L) lower in infants not receiving phototherapy and 0.6 mg/dL (10 μmol/L) lower in those receiving phototherapy. Eidelman and colleagues also found significant differences, but in the opposite direction.[549] Values were higher in capillary than venous samples. The reasons for these differences are obscure, but it is useful to recall that virtually all the data on bilirubin levels published in the literature were obtained from capillary samples. Some data have been derived from umbilical artery samples in very-low-birth-weight infants. Whether these are similar to capillary values is unknown, but for the purpose of making clinical decisions, capillary blood samples for measuring serum bilirubin levels remain the gold standard; and whatever the differences between capillary and venous samples may mean, there is no reason to measure the venous bilirubin level until there are data identifying the relation between venous bilirubin and the risk of kernicterus.

SAMPLING TECHNIQUE

Because of the well-known effects of light on bilirubin, laboratory manuals recommend that blood samples be protected from light until the serum is analyzed. Using serum samples with bilirubin levels of 16.0, 11.8, and 7.9 mg/dL (273, 202, and 135 μmol/L), Sykes and colleagues found that under the usual laboratory conditions, there was no measurable effect of ambient light on serum bilirubin levels for at least 8 hours.[550]

NONINVASIVE MEASUREMENTS OF BILIRUBIN

Two devices have proved useful as screening techniques for gauging the depth of jaundice in newborns.[282] The Ingram Icterometer (Cascade Health

Care Products, Salem, OR) is a piece of transparent plastic (Perspex) on which are painted five transverse stripes of graded yellow hue. The instrument is pressed against the nose, the yellow color of the blanched skin is matched with the appropriated yellow stripe, and a jaundice score is assigned. The Minolta Air Shields Jaundice Meter is a more sophisticated and much more costly device. When pressure is applied to the photoprobe of this hand-held, rechargeable instrument, a strobe light is generated by a xenon tube and passes through a fiberoptic filament, penetrating the blanched skin and entering the subcutaneous tissue. The reflected light returns through a second fiberoptic bundle to the spectrophotometric module, where the intensity of the yellow color, corrected for hemoglobin, is measured and displayed as arbitrary units—the transcutaneous bilirubin (TcB) index.

The accuracy and utility of these instruments has been reviewed in depth by Schumacher.[282] Measurements with the Minolta Air-Shields Jaundice Meter are highly reproducible and related in linear fashion to the total serum bilirubin concentration. Although there are some differences in slopes and intercepts in different populations, in full-term infants of the same racial group, the slopes of the regression lines are remarkably similar. Transcutaneous bilirubin measurements are affected by the infant's race, gestational age, and birth weight, which limits the use of the jaundice meter in heterogeneous populations. When used in selected groups, however, the jaundice meter has performed well as a screening device.[282] Because of the bleaching effect of phototherapy on cutaneous bilirubin, transcutaneous bilirubin measurements are less reliable in infants receiving phototherapy, although if an area of skin is covered with an opaque patch, the relation between the TcB index and the serum bilirubin level improves.

Schumacher used receiver-operating characteristic (ROC) curves to compare the merits of these devices. He found that the Minolta Air-Shields Jaundice Meter and the Ingram Icterometer performed equally well.[282] Receiver-operating characteristic curves of visual estimates of jaundice using the dermal zones of jaundice (see Cephalopedal Progression of Jaundice) indicate that this method is also an effective screening tool.[282] An important advantage of Minolta's jaundice meter is the virtual absence of interobserver variability. On the other hand, the jaundice meter sells for about $2500.00, while the Ingram Icterometer costs $20.00. Although none of these methods can replace serum bilirubin measurements, they can be recommended as good screening techniques. At William Beaumont Hospital, use of the Minolta Air-Shields Jaundice Meter has led to a 30% reduction in the number of serum bilirubin measurements obtained in the well-baby nursey.

Because the major concern regarding bilirubin toxicity is the amount of bilirubin in the tissue, rather than the blood, the use of transcutaneous bilirubinometry ultimately may prove to be a better predictor of the potential for brain damage than serum bilirubin concentrations.[255]

TREATMENT

MECHANISMS AND PRINCIPLES

Hyperbilirubinemia can be treated by exchange transfusion, which removes bilirubin mechanically; phototherapy, which converts bilirubin to products that can bypass the liver's conjugating system and be excreted in the bile or in the urine without further metabolism; and pharmacologic agents that interfere with heme degradation, accelerate the normal metabolic pathways for bilirubin clearance, or inhibit the enterohepatic circulation of bilirubin. Phototherapy is the most common treatment in use for hyperbilirubinemia; exchange transfusions generally are reserved for phototherapy failures. The bilirubin level at which intervention is necessary is still a contentious issue.[260,281,450–454,456–460]

The background to treatment decisions for hyperbilirubinemia has been provided (see Bilirubin Toxicity). The basic principles underlying the recommendations given in Tables 38-26 through 38-31 are as follows:

Full-term infants without hemolytic disease are at a low risk of bilirubin toxicity.
Because of the tremendous changes in obstetric and neonatal care in the past 40 years, the existing data on the use of exchange transfusion in hemolytic disease may not be applicable to infants in the 1990s.
Evidence for treatment efficacy is lacking for many infants.
Treatment is not free of risk.

There is a problem with the first principle listed. Except in the most obvious circumstances (*i.e.*, major blood group incompatibility with a rapidly rising bilirubin level), it is difficult, and sometimes impossible, to rule out an underlying hemolytic process. Stan-

TABLE 38–26
APPROACHES TO THE PREVENTION AND TREATMENT OF JAUNDICE ASSOCIATED WITH BREAST-FEEDING

Prevention
1. Encourage frequent nursing (*i.e.*, at least eight times per day)
2. Do not supplement with water or dextrose water

Treatment Options
1. Observe
2. Discontinue nursing, substitute formula
3. Alternate feedings of breast milk and formula
4. Discontinue nursing, administer phototherapy
5. Continue nursing, administer phototherapy

TABLE 38–27
APPROACHES TO THE TREATMENT OF HYPERBILIRUBINEMIA IN FULL-TERM INFANTS*

Treatment	Bilirubin Level in mg/dL (μmol/L) Total Sereum†	
	No Hemolysis‡ and Infant Well	Hemolysis Likely or Infant Sick
Phototherapy§	17–22 (290–325)	13–15 (220–255)
Interrupt or modify nursing, with or without phototherapy‖	17–22 (290–325)	Usually not indicated
Exchange transfusion#	25–29 (425–500)	17–22 (290–375)

* Refers to infants born at 37 or more weeks of gestation.
† Consider initiating therapy at these levels. Range is intended to allow discretion based on clinical conditions or other circumstances (see Table 38-30).
‡ Refers to absence of obvious hemolytic disease due to Rh or ABO incompatibility or glucose-6-phosphate dehydrogenase deficiency. It may be difficult to rule out ABO hemolytic disease as well as other, rarer, causes of hemolysis. Diagnosis of glucose-6-phosphate dehydrogenase deficiency requires an awareness of genetic background and should be considered in families from Greece, Turkey, Sardinia, China, and Nigeria and in Sephardic Jews from Kurdistan, Iraq, Iran, Syria, Turkey, and Buchara.
§ Assumes phototherapy will be used in adequate doses.
‖ Phototherapy and modification of breast-feeding are interventions that can be used separately or concurrently, depending on physician preference and parental choice.
Assumes bilirubin continues to rise or remains at these levels in spite of intensive (*i.e.*, double) phototherapy. Double phototherapy refers to light placed above and below infant.

dard diagnostic tests for hemolysis, such as the reticulocyte count, hematocrit, or examination of the peripheral smear, are neither sensitive nor specific. Nevertheless, it is reasonable to assume that most full-term infants with significant elevations of their serum bilirubin do not have hemolytic disease.[75,185,551] The possibility of G6PD deficiency must be considered in areas where this condition is prevalent and in certain ethnic groups (see Chap. 45). These infants cannot be distinguished from the normal population by measurements of hematocrit or reticulocyte count.[552]

RISKS

Phototherapy is an effective method of lowering the serum bilirubin concentration, and its use reduces the risk of exchange transfusion, but it has not been

TABLE 38–28
APPROACHES TO THE USE OF PHOTOTHERAPY AND EXCHANGE TRANSFUSION IN LOW-BIRTH-WEIGHT INFANTS*

Birth Weight (g)	Total Bilirubin Level in mg/dL (μmol/L)†	
	Phototherapy‡	Exchange Transfusion§
<1500	5–8 (85–140)	13–16 (220–275)
1500–1999	8–12 (140–200)	16–18 (275–300)
2000–2499	11–14 (190–240)	18–20 (300–340)

* Note that these guidelines reflect ranges used in neonatal intensive care units. They cannot take into account all possible situations. In some units, prophylactic phototherapy is used for all infants who weigh less than 1500 g. Higher intervention levels may be used for small-for-gestational-age infants, based on gestational age rather than birth weight.
† Consider initiating therapy at these levels.
Range allows discretion based on clinical conditions or other circumstances (see Table 38-30).
‡ Used at these levels and in therapeutic doses, phototherapy should, with few exceptions, eliminate the need for exchange transfusion. There are no data, however, to indicate that phototherapy used in this way will improve developmental outcome.
§ Levels for exchange tranfusion assume that bilirubin continues to rise or remains at these levels in spite of intensive (*i.e.*, double) phototherapy. (Double phototherapy refers to light placed above and below infant.)

TABLE 38–29
USE OF PHOTOTHERAPY IN FULL-TERM INFANTS WITH ABO HEMOLYTIC DISEASE

Age (hours)	Total Serum Bilirubin Level (mg/dL)
<12	10
12–17	12
18–23	14
≥24	15

From Osborn LM, Lenarsky C, Oakas RC, et al. Phototherapy in full-term infants with hemolytic disease secondary to ABO incompatibility. Pediatrics 1984;74:371.

shown to have any effect on neurologic or developmental outcome.[496,497] Nevertheless, it appears that liberal use of phototherapy in jaundiced premature newborns has contributed to the virtual disappearance of kernicterus and a marked reduction in the need for exchange transfusion in this population.[460]

Phototherapy is a relatively benign intervention. On the other hand, in full-term newborns, it can lead to separation of the mother and infant, increase parental concern, decrease the likelihood of successful breast-feeding, and adversely affect the mother–infant relationship.[261] At a time when pediatricians are trying to promote breast-feeding in the face of considerable odds (*e.g.*, early discharge from hospital, the rapid return of mothers to the work force, commercial marketing of formulas), attention should be given to an intervention that has a negative impact on the nursing mother. Given the low risk for adverse outcome in the nonhemolyzing full-term infant and the potentially harmful effects of bilirubin-lowering interventions (*e.g.*, phototherapy, interrupting breast-feeding) in hundreds of thousands of infants throughout the world, pediatricians must be sure that the potential benefits of interventions outweigh the risks.

TABLE 38–30
CONDITIONS THAT MAY MODIFY INTERVENTION FOR HYPERBILIRUBINEMIA

Immediate Exchange Transfusion
Clinical signs of bilirubin encephalopathy

Earlier or Prophylactic Phototherapy Due to Increased Procedural Risk of Morbidity and Mortality or Technical Difficulty in Performing Exchange Transfusion
Serious complication with previous exchange transfusions
Serious cardiovascular, coagulation, or other disease
Potential graft-*versus*-host reaction (*e.g.*, acquired or inherited immunedeficiencies, mother exposed to immunosuppressive agents)
Inability to use umbilical vessels (*e.g.*, abdominal surgery, omphalocele)

Earlier Phototherapy or Exchange Transfusion Due to Possible Increased Risk of Bilirubin Toxicity
Serum bilirubin rising more than 1 mg/dL (17 μM/L) per hour
Serum albumin < 2.5 mg/dL
Reduced bilirubin-binding capacity, if measured
Persistent, severe, metabolic or respiratory acidosis*
Persistent, severe hypercapnia*
Persistent, severe hypoxemia*
Sepsis
Very sick low-birth-weight infants

* Attempt to correct blood gas abnormality.

TABLE 38–31
SIZE OF EXCHANGE TRANSFUSION AND REPLACEMENT OF INFANT'S BLOOD

Donor Volume as Fraction* of Infant's Blood Volume	Percentage of Blood Volume Removed and Replaced by Exchange
0.5	40
1	63
2	87
3	95

* The fraction of blood removed from the infant follows the theoretical equation for the dilution of a closed volume:

$$y = 1 - e^{-x},$$

where y is the fraction of original fluid removed, x is the number of volumes exchanged, and e is 2.71828.

From Sproul A, Smith I. Bilirubin equilibration during exchange transfusion in hemolytic disease of the newborn. J Pediatr 1964;65:12.

The risk of exchange transfusion includes both risks from the transfused blood and from the procedure. Blood bank screening procedures have reduced the risk of acquired immunodeficiency syndrome and hepatitis significantly, but this risk is never zero. In experienced hands, the risk of the procedure is about 2 to 3 deaths per 1000 procedures overall, and this risk is generally restricted to sick, low-birth-weight infants.[553–555] Experience with exchange transfusion is decreasing, and with new interventions in immune hemolytic disease, it is likely to decrease even further.[556,557] It is common for a resident to complete a pediatric training program without ever having performed an exchange transfusion. Under the circumstances, the mortality and morbidity for this procedure might increase in the years ahead.

RECOMMENDATIONS

JAUNDICE ASSOCIATED WITH BREAST-FEEDING

Because of the association between breast-feeding and elevated bilirubin levels in the first week of life, attempts have been made to mitigate this effect. Observational studies suggest that increasing the frequency of breast-feeding during the first few days after birth decreases maximal serum bilirubin values.[558–560] In a controlled trial, Vain and colleagues randomly assigned mothers to one of two feeding schedules, frequent or demand.[561] The mothers in the frequent group nursed their infants on average 9.1 ± 1.4 times per day and in the demand group, 6.8 ± 1.0 times per day. Serum bilirubin levels, measured at an average age of 55 hours, were minimally lower in the frequent group (0.6 mg/dL, or 10 μmol/L); this did not achieve statistical significance. Bilirubin levels in these infants were measured between 48 and 72 hours, and it is likely that maximal bilirubin levels had not yet been achieved. Nevertheless, these data suggest that increasing the frequency of breast-feeding is unlikely to have a significant effect on serum bilirubin levels in the first three days of life.[561]

The other intervention commonly used is to provide supplemental feedings of water or dextrose water to breast-fed infants. This practice is widespread, potentially harmful, and, when studied, has consistently produced an increase in maximal serum bilirubin levels in the supplemented infants.[562–564] Kuhr and Paneth showed that dextrose water intake in the first 3 days of life was significantly and inversely related to breast-milk intake on the fourth day, and those breast-fed infants with a low breast-milk intake on the fourth day tended to have higher bilirubin levels.[565] Providing glucose water supplements to breast-fed infants not only had no effect on serum bilirubin levels but also significantly reduced the number of infants being nursed exclusively at 3 months of age.[563] If supplementation is elected as one intervention for jaundice associated with breast-feeding, formula should be chosen. Corchia and colleagues studied breast-fed infants who were assigned to be supplemented with formula or dextrose water.[566] The formula-supplemented infants were significantly less likely to reach a serum bilirubin level of 12 mg/dL (205 μmol/L).

Osborn and Bolus developed a protocol for the management of jaundiced breast-fed infants.[567] Mothers of infants whose bilirubin levels reached 14 mg/dL (239 μmol/L) were asked to discontinue breast-feeding, and the infant was fed formula every 2 hours. In 87 infants, nursing was interrupted for 24 to 48 hours, and the bilirubin declined in 81 (93%).

Amato and colleagues compared the effect of interrupting breast-feeding with phototherapy when serum bilirubin levels reached 15 mg/dL (257 μmol/L).[568] There was no difference between the groups or the amount of time needed to reduce the bilirubin to less than 12 mg/dL (205 μmol/L). They concluded that interrupting breast-feeding was a reasonable alternative to phototherapy.

In a controlled clinical trial, Martinez and colleagues compared the effect of four different interventions on hyperbilirubinemia in 125 full-term breast-fed infants.[247] When the serum bilirubin level reached 17 mg/dL (291 μmol/L), the infants were assigned at random to one of four interventions:

1. Continue breast-feeding and observe.
2. Discontinue breast-feeding and substitute formula.
3. Discontinue breast-feeding, substitute formula, and administer phototherapy.
4. Continue breast-feeding and administer phototherapy.

The serum bilirubin concentration reached 20 mg/dL (342 μmol/L) in 24% of infants in group 1, 19% in group 2, 3% in group 3, and 14% in group 4 (p = 0.0001 for groups 3 and 4 *versus* group 1). Phototherapy produced a significantly greater and more rapid decline in bilirubin than no phototherapy.

Although serum bilirubin levels reached 20 mg/dL (342 μmol/L) in 14% of the group in which phototherapy was administered and breast-feeding was continued, compared with 3% of the group in which phototherapy was administered and breast-feeding was discontinued, the decline in serum bilirubin levels over 48 hours was about the same in both groups. These data suggest that it is feasible to allow mothers to continue breast-feeding while phototherapy is being administered. When the circumstances permit, parents should be given this information and the option of making an informed decision regarding which intervention they prefer. Many mothers do not want to interrupt nursing if at all possible, and the option of doing nothing or providing phototherapy while nursing is continued should be offered. The availability of fiberoptic phototherapy systems also makes this alternative more appealing to many parents because it obviates the necessity for eye patching and permits more maternal–infant contact. If necessary, it also allows for double phototherapy, which is significantly more effective than single phototherapy (see Phototherapy).[569] Table 38-26 provides an approach to the management of breast-feeding–associated jaundice.

FULL-TERM NEWBORNS

Most infants who are treated for neonatal jaundice have no identifiable pathology and no evidence of hemolytic disease[75,184,185]; about 90% of these infants are fully or partially breast-fed.[185] Given the low risk of harm, it is reasonable to encourage individualization of treatment, taking the preferences and biases of the parent and pediatrician into account. Ranges for serum bilirubin levels are given rather than single numbers (see Table 38-27). This is a more accurate reflection of the uncertainty about when to treat jaundiced newborns. The data on which these recommendations are based are scant, however, and pediatricians are forced to compromise between a desire to avoid unnecessary and potentially harmful treatment and a reluctance to accept the possibility of some risk,[496] even if this is small.

Recommendations for treatment of full-term infants are given in Table 38-27. When phototherapy is used, it should be used in a therapeutic, not homeopathic, dose. There is a strong dose–response relation for phototherapy,[570] and a more rapid decline in serum bilirubin can be achieved by increasing the dose of light delivered. This is done by placing a standard phototherapy light closer to the infant. I do this by placing all full-term infants who receive phototherapy in bassinets, not incubators, and placing the light as close as possible to the infant. Occasionally, this produces an increase in the infant's temperature, in which case the light is elevated slightly. Exposing a greater surface area to light also lowers bilirubin levels more rapidly, and this is easily achieved by using double phototherapy (*i.e.*, placing a infant on a fiberoptic blanket with a conventional phototherapy lamp above).[569]

The recommendations for exchange transfusion assume that phototherapy has failed to keep the bilirubin below the designated levels. In some breast-fed infants, the first physician contact after discharge from the hospital occurs when the infant presents with significant jaundice. In these infants, a trial of phototherapy and interruption of nursing should be attempted even if the bilirubin level is 25 mg/dL (428 μmol/L) or higher. At these levels, I usually interrupt nursing as well, although it is by no means certain that this is necessary. Should these measures fail, exchange transfusion is an alternative.

Suggested guidelines for the management of hyperbilirubinemia in low-birth-weight infants are provided in Table 38-28. As discussed previously, there has been a remarkable decrease in the incidence of kernicterus found at autopsy in infants dying in NICUs. Some of this decrease may be due to the liberal use of phototherapy. On the scale of interventions carried out in NICUs, phototherapy is one of the most benign. There is also no question that phototherapy dramatically reduces the necessity for exchange transfusion. In a study of 1338 infants born during 1983 in the Netherlands, with a gestational age of less than 32 weeks, birth weight less than 1500 g, or both, 37 (2.8%) required at least one exchange transfusion. In a cohort of 833 infants with birth weights between 500 and 1500 g born in North Carolina in 1985 to 1989, only 2 infants (0.24%) underwent exchange transfusion.

Phototherapy is directed primarily at preventing exchange transfusion and possible developmental handicap.[534,540] The suggested association between relatively low serum bilirubin levels and cerebral palsy has been questioned,[538,539] however, and even if it were true, there is no evidence that the use of phototherapy to treat mild jaundice has prevented any form of handicap.[500] Most neonatal units apply phototherapy on a sliding scale—the lower the birth weight, the lower the bilirubin level at which phototherapy is introduced. In spite of its widespread acceptance, no data are available to support this approach. A reasonable justification is that infants weighing less than 1500 g are more likely to be sick, acidotic, hypoxic, hypercapnic, or septic, and it seems particularly pedantic to debate whether or not to introduce phototherapy at a bilirubin level of 5 or 6 mg/dL (85 or 103 μmol/L) in an infant weighing 1000 g. The use of exchange transfusion, on the other hand, merits more careful deliberation.

In the NICHHD phototherapy study, maximal bilirubin levels were established for each weight group, and exchange transfusions were performed in both phototherapy-treated and control infants when these levels were reached.[529] These criteria have been widely applied, but their validity has been questioned. Watchko and Claasen reviewed 72 postmortem examinations in infants of less than 34 weeks of gestation who were born between 1984 and 1991 and who lived at least 48 hours.[537] There were three cases of kernicterus in infants who had serum bilirubin levels of 11.3, 18.5, and 26 mg/dL, respectively (193, 316, and 452 μmol/L). All had complicated neonatal courses, including asphyxia, hyaline membrane disease, grade III–IV intraventricular hemorrhage (in two patients), and nonimmune hydrops (in one patient). Of the 69 infants who did not have kernicterus, peak bilirubin levels ranged from 6.3 to 20.6 mg/dL (108–352 μmol/L), and 56% had bilirubin levels higher than those suggested as criteria for exchange transfusion in the NICHHD study. Three infants received exchange transfusions. One infant of gestational age 28 weeks died during an exchange that was performed at a bilirubin level of 13 mg/dL (222 μmol/L).

With the introduction of more effective means of administering phototherapy to low-birth-weight infants,[571] much of the discussion regarding exchange transfusion in this population is moot. In my experience, in the very-low-birth-weight population, exchange transfusions are a rare event and are restricted to those infants who are profoundly bruised or have severe hemolytic disease. Even in these infants, the introduction of more effective phototherapy or the use of intravenous γ-globulin in hemolytic disease should reduce the need for exchange transfusion.[556] Although recommended in certain high-risk infants with bilirubin levels as low as 10 to 13 mg/dL (171–222 μmol/L), exchange transfusion at these bilirubin levels is inefficient.[572] For example, an exchange transfusion at 10 mg/dL (171 μmol/L) would probably lower the serum bilirubin level to about 5 mg/dL (85 μmol/L). With the usual rebound, however, the bilirubin would increase to about 7 mg/dL (120 μmol/L) within one-half hour of the exchange. Phototherapy is more effective than exchange transfusion in achieving prolonged reduction of bilirubin levels in infants with nonhemolytic jaundice.[572]

DIRECT-REACTING BILIRUBIN

The problem of how to deal with the occasional infant who has a high total bilirubin level as well as an elevation in direct-reacting bilirubin has never been resolved satisfactorily. Because of the evidence that indirect-, and not direct-, reacting bilirubin is toxic to the central nervous system, most texts in the 1960s and early 1970s provided guidelines for exchange transfusion based on the level of indirect serum bilirubin. More recently, most guidelines have either ignored the subject or have referred to total bilirubin levels as criteria for treatment. Kernicterus has been described in a full-term infant with the bronze-baby syndrome. The maximal total serum bilirubin in this infant was 18 mg/dL (308 μmol/L), and the direct-reacting bilirubin was 4.1 mg/dL (17 μmol/L).[573] I have had occasion to review the medical record of one full-term infant who developed clinical kernicterus when the total bilirubin level was 27.6 mg/dL (472 μmol/L), but the direct bilirubin level was 8.7 mg/dL (149 μmol/L). Others have seen similar cases. These are anecdotal observations, but they raise the question of how elevated direct bilirubin levels should be handled in assessing the risk of kernicterus. It is possible that direct-reacting bilirubin causes competitive displacement of indirect bilirubin from its binding site to albumin. Ebbesen found that infants with elevated direct bilirubin levels (6.4–9.9 mg/dL, or 109–169 μmol/L) and the bronze-baby syndrome had a decrease in reserve albumin binding.[574] Alternatively, the conditions that lead to elevation of direct-reacting bilirubin may produce changes in the ability of albumin to bind bilirubin.[575] Gartner and Lee recommend that direct bilirubin concentrations should not be subtracted from the total bilirubin level unless they amount to more than one-half of the total serum bilirubin concentration.[576] Although this is purely empiric advice, it is reasonable.

HEMOLYTIC DISEASE

In the studies of erythroblastosis fetalis done in the early 1950s, the incidence of kernicterus—30% to 50% in those with the highest bilirubin levels—was much higher than that in markedly jaundiced infants without hemolytic disease (see Clinical Sequelae of Hyperbilirubinemia).

Not all studies had such negative outcomes, however. Johnston and colleagues conducted a 5-year follow-up on 129 infants whose indirect serum bilirubin levels were higher than 20 mg/dL (342 μmol/L) in the neonatal period.[437] Ninety-two (71%) of these infants had Rh hemolytic disease and 26 (20%) ABO hemolytic disease. Forty-two infants had indirect serum bilirubin levels higher than 25 mg/dL (428 μmol/L). Only one infant developed definite kernicterus in the neonatal period, although there were 11 cases in which kernicterus was suspected because of lethargy, poor feeding, weak cry, and mild head retraction. Nine of these children were normal on follow-up examination at 5 years of age, while two had athetoid neurologic sequelae. Only seven children (5.4%) showed any sequelae at 5 years of age. All seven had sensorineural hearing impairment, but six of the seven had received streptomycin. Thus, the developmental outcome for infants with erythroblastosis may not be nearly as bleak as depicted by the earlier studies.

Why do infants with hemolytic disease appear to be at greater risk for bilirubin encephalopathy than infants with similar serum bilirubin levels who do not have hemolysis? As far as Rh disease is concerned, the infants reported in the trials of the late 1940s and early 1950s were often asphyxiated and severely ill, and many were delivered prematurely to prevent stillbirth, a practice later shown to increase the risk of kernicterus.[487] The results of subsequent studies in the 1960s were far more encouraging,[437] and given contemporary obstetric and neonatal care, it is highly unlikely that the outcome for such infants today would be nearly as gloomy. It has been suggested that one mechanism that might account for the increased risk of neurotoxicity in infants with hemolytic disease is the presence of products of erythrocyte destruction, such as hematin, which may compete with bilirubin for binding sites on albumin.[577] Studies in infants with erythroblastosis show no effect of the hemolysis or the level of bilirubin on the newborn's ability to bind hematin.[578] Catterton and colleagues could find no effect of hemolytic disease on the albumin-binding capacity,[579] but others have demonstrated a significant adverse effect of hematin on bilirubin binding.[580,581] This only occurred, however, at high hematin concentrations (*i.e.*, molar ratio of hematin to bilirubin of 0.5). The apparent unbound bilirubin concentration in control sera and sera from Coombs-positive ABO-incompatible infants was identical, suggesting that either there was no significant increase of hematin in ABO hemolytic disease or the hematin present is insufficient to alter bilirubin binding.[581] Thus, apart from the clinical condition of the infant, there is no ready explanation for the apparent increase in risk of bilirubin encephalopathy in infants with isoimmune hemolytic disease. There is also no obvious explanation for the increased risk of bilirubin encephalopathy in infants with G6PD deficiency.[268–270]

MANAGEMENT OF ABO INCOMPATIBILITY

The situation regarding ABO hemolytic disease is less clear than for Rh disease, although some studies suggest that the indications for exchange transfusion in ABO hemolytic disease could be less stringent.[349,464]

Follow-up data for infants with ABO incompatibility are not nearly as extensive as those for Rh disease. In one study by Ose and colleagues, developmental retardation or cerebral palsy occurred in 15% of 89 Japanese infants with apparent hemolytic disease whose serum bilirubin levels were between 20 and 24.9 mg/dL (342–426 μmol/L).[582] Seventy-nine percent of these infants were ABO-incompatible and 21% Rh-incompatible. Seven percent weighed less than 2500 g.

Osborn and colleagues conducted a prospective evaluation of 476 newborns admitted to their well-baby nursery.[263] Forty-seven (10%) were ABO-incompatible and had positive indirect Coombs tests measured on the cord blood. Three infants were eliminated from the study, which left 44 remaining infants. The investigators elected to use phototherapy at the bilirubin levels shown in Table 38-29. Using these criteria, two infants received phototherapy for bilirubin levels higher than 10 mg/dL (257 μmol/L) in the first 12 hours and two for levels higher than 15 mg/dL (257 μmol/L) after 24 hours. None of the infants required an exchange transfusion. Of the 40 untreated infants, 6 had bilirubin levels that exceeded 12 mg/dL (205 μmol/L). This study confirms the clinical observation that although some infants with ABO hemolytic disease have rapidly rising serum bilirubin levels in the first 12 hours of life, many do not develop significant hyperbilirubinemia subsequently. It should also be noted that about 90% of infants who have ABO incompatibility and positive Coombs tests do not have hemolytic disease.[263,264,583] Standard hematologic indices do not predict the degree of hemolysis in ABO-incompatible infants. Brouwers and colleagues found that an assay of antibody-dependent cell-mediated cytotoxicity (ADCC) in maternal serum was the most sensitive assay to predict ABO hemolytic disease.[584] Combining the ADCC assay with an assay of the antigen density of A or B antigens on the infant's erythrocytes provided the most specificity.

SEVERE HEMOLYTIC DISEASE

Exchange transfusion remains the only effective therapy in infants who have failed phototherapy or other interventions in the management of hemolytic disease. Exchange transfusions are indicated in two situations: to correct anemia rapidly in infants severely affected with erythroblastosis and to treat potential or actual hyperbilirubinemia. In hemolytic anemia, both of these conditions may exist.

In the past, various criteria for early or immediate exchange transfusion were proposed for infants with hemolytic disease based on cord blood levels of hemoglobin and bilirubin, but these measurements do not predict the severity of hyperbilirubinemia with sufficient accuracy to warrant their use as therapeutic guidelines. Early studies of the natural history of Rh and ABO hemolytic disease allowed us to predict whether or not the serum bilirubin concentration would reach 20 mg/dL (342 μmol/L), and rules of thumb were developed for exchange transfusion based on serum bilirubin levels at different ages. The use of intensive phototherapy and intravenous γ-globulin[556] has rendered such guidelines irrelevant.

If, despite intensive phototherapy, the serum bilirubin level continues to rise rapidly, an exchange transfusion is indicated (see Tables 38-27 and 38-30). The rationale for early intervention is the removal of sensitized erythrocytes from the blood, which aborts the hemolytic process. An early exchange transfusion also corrects anemia and removes some bilirubin before large amounts are distributed into the extravascular space.

REPEAT EXCHANGE TRANSFUSIONS

In general, the criteria for repeat exchange transfusions should be similar to those used for the initial exchange. The effect of exchange transfusion on unbound bilirubin levels and reserve albumin binding is variable. Some authors observed a salutary effect,[391,585] but others found no effect during or immediately after single or even multiple exchange transfusions.[392,555,586]

HYDROPS FETALIS

Obstetric management allows us to anticipate the delivery of infants with hydrops fetalis. They suffer significant hypoxia *in utero,* and women who are to deliver such infants should be managed exclusively in perinatal centers capable of the full range of obstetric and neonatal intensive care. Hydropic infants and those who are obviously pale and asphyxiated demand immediate treatment. Otherwise, therapy for jaundice is based on serial bilirubin determinations.

The pathogenesis of hydrops fetalis, with its attendant edema and serous effusions, is not clear. Hydrops commonly occurs when the fetal hemoglobin drops below 6 to 7 g/dL,[587,588] and hydrops can be reversed with intravascular intrauterine transfusions, which raise fetal hemoglobin concentrations.[587] In Rh isoimmunization, fetal edema may result from the extensive erythropoiesis in the fetal liver that disrupts the portal circulation and impairs albumin synthesis[587,589] and also from the cardiovascular adaptations that are seen in anemic fetuses.[590] Moya and colleagues found that fetuses with severe hydrops had high atrial natriuretic factor concentrations and were also significantly more anemic than fetuses with either mild or no hydrops.[591] They also found an inverse relation between the hemoglobin and atrial natriuretic factor concentrations. This may be the result of atrial natriuretic factor release induced by hypoxia. Hypoxia produces myocardial dysfunction, which increases umbilical venous pressure and leads to a release of atrial natriuretic factor.[592] After intravascular transfusion *in utero,* there was a significant decrease in plasma atrial natriuretic factor concentration.[591]

Most authors suggest that infants with hydrops due to hemolysis die from congestive heart failure secondary to the severe anemia and that the edema is secondary to the heart failure. Studies of premature infants with moderate to severe erythroblastosis, however, suggest that chronic congestive heart failure is rare at birth in hydropic infants.[593,594] Central venous pressures, measured in the thoracic inferior vena cava, reflect not only blood volume but also venous tone, pulmonary vascular resistance, and right ventricular dynamics.[595,596] Elevated pressures probably result from acute intrapartum asphyxia and may decline to normal or subnormal levels after correction of acidosis, hypoxia, hypercarbia, and anemia.[596] Severely affected infants die from progressive cardiorespiratory failure, in which asphyxia and hyaline membrane disease play a major role. Acute intrapartum asphyxia, superimposed on chronic asphyxia in a premature and anemic fetus, leads to delivery of an asphyxiated infant with hypoxemia, hypercarbia, and mixed respiratory and metabolic acidosis. A high incidence of hyaline membrane disease can be expected in such infants.

A linear relation has been found between the umbilical cord hematocrit and the erythrocyte volume in infants with erythroblastosis,[593] and in nonhemolytic infants, between the hematocrit and the blood volume.[595] No correlation was observed, however, between the severity of hydrops fetalis and the infants' blood volumes.[593] In the study by Phibbs and colleagues,[593] the blood volumes of almost all infants were within the normal range of 70 to 90 mL/kg. Only one infant, who was severely hydropic, had a significantly elevated blood volume (113 mL/kg), whereas in another infant, the blood volume was low (48 mL/kg). Not all hydropic infants are severely anemic, but most are hypoalbuminemic.[594] These data suggest that low plasma colloid osmotic pressure, as a result of hypoalbuminemia, is another important mechanism in the pathogenesis of hydrops.

The management of these infants demands a comprehensive approach that includes intensive monitoring and vigorous treatment of asphyxia, acidosis, hypoglycemia, and hypothermia. Assisted ventilation is the rule because of the frequent presence of hyaline membrane disease, pulmonary edema, and chest wall edema. Significant ascites hampers ventilatory efforts and can be relieved by paracentesis. Thrombocytopenia and coagulation disorders are common. Hydropic infants and those who are severely anemic (*i.e.*, hematocrit $< 35\%$) and asphyxiated demand immediate treatment. An exchange transfusion of about 50 mL/kg of packed cells soon after birth raises the hematocrit to about 40%. Phlebotomy should not be routinely performed on these infants because they are usually normovolemic and may be hypovolemic.[594,597,598] Furthermore, no manipulations of blood volume should be performed without appropriate measurements of central venous and arterial blood pressures. For accurate monitoring of the central venous pressure, however, the umbilical venous catheter must enter the inferior vena cava by way of the ductus venosus. If the catheter is in a portal vein or the umbilical vein, the pressures so measured are meaningless and preclude interpretation of the infant's circulatory status. The practice of measuring central venous pressure by means of an umbilical vein catheter may lead to serious therapeutic error unless the position of the catheter is confirmed radiographically or by pressure tracing. In addition, before making therapeutic decisions based on measurements of central venous pressure, the physician must also correct acidosis, hypercarbia, hypoxia, and anemia. Serum glucose levels should be monitored carefully because hypoglycemia is common.

EXCHANGE TRANSFUSION

TYPES OF BLOOD USED

Citrate phosphate dextrose (CPD) is the anticoagulant of choice for banked blood in the United States. Heparinized blood, once used exclusively in some centers, has been displaced by the use of component therapy and the need to screen all donors for human immunodeficiency virus, hepatitis, and so forth. Most blood banks reconstitute blood by adding plasma or albumin–saline solutions to stored packed erythrocytes or to previously frozen erythrocytes.[599] Some blood transfusion centers have recommended the use of preparations in which packed erythrocytes are suspended in other solutions. There are potential hazards to the use of these solutions. If additional albumin is not added, a marked depletion in albumin and other plasma proteins occurs after exchange transfusion.[600,601]

METABOLIC COMPLICATIONS

The citrate in CPD blood binds ionic calcium and magnesium and produces a significant depression in these divalent cations. The temporary hypomagnesemia has not been associated with clinically recognizable problems, but the depression of calcium ion may produce deleterious hemodynamic and cardiac effects that are not caused by toxicity of the citrate.

Some physicians administer calcium gluconate during exchange transfusions to counteract the citrate binding, but this does not appear to have any significant effect on the serum ionized calcium,[602,603] although there is a temporary increase directly after the calcium is given (Fig. 38-24). In some centers, supplemental calcium is never administered, and this has been without apparent ill effects.[553] The addition of 0.1 g calcium chloride to 1 U of heparinized CPD blood prevented a fall in ionized calcium in full-term infants, but not in preterm infants.[604] It is probably unnecessary to administer additional calcium to most infants. Clinical tetany is rarely seen during exchange transfusion, which is remarkable considering the low levels of ionized calcium that occur. Jitteriness, crying, and irritability occur but cannot be correlated with levels of ionized calcium.[602] Parathormone levels rise initially but then decline during the exchange.[603]

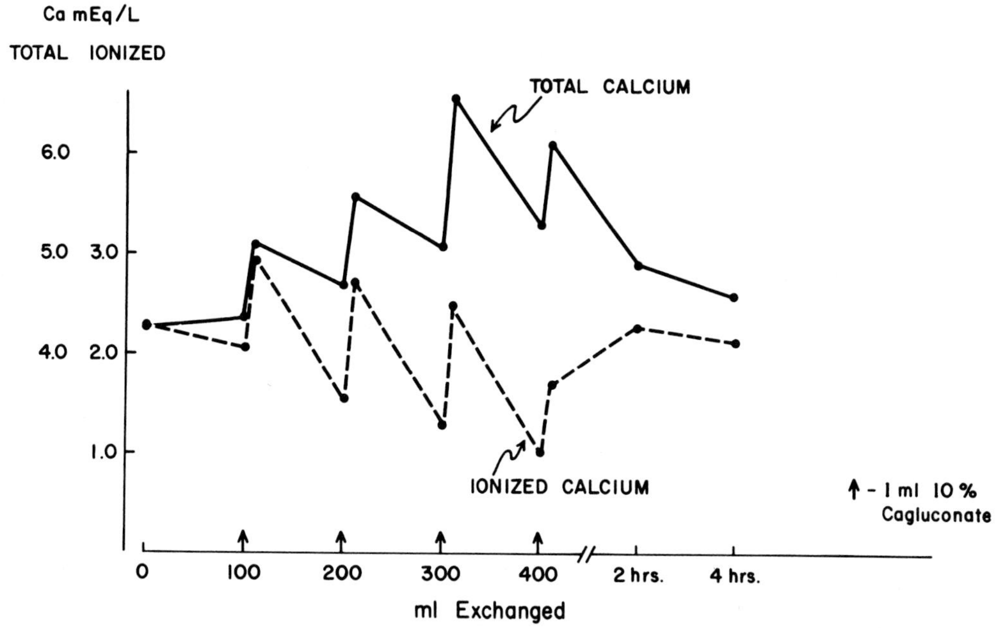

FIG. 38–24. Effect of added calcium gluconate on total ionized calcium during exchange transfusion with acid citrate dextrose (ACD) blood. (From Maisels MJ, Li TK, Piechocki JT, et al. The effect of exchange transfusion on serum ionized calcium. Pediatrics 1974;53:683.)

Citrate phosphate dextrose blood contains 300 to 350 mg/dL of glucose. This stimulates insulin secretion in the infant and may lead to rebound hypoglycemia after the exchange. Blood sugar levels should be monitored in the first few hours after the procedure.

POTASSIUM IN STORED BLOOD

Potassium levels in stored blood increase rapidly. Levels as high as 9.1 mEq/L occur after 1 day, and levels may exceed 20 mEq/L after 2 days of storage.[605] Previously, it was recommended that exchange transfusions be performed with blood no more than 4 days old. Such blood may have dramatically elevated serum potassium levels.[605–607] The blood bank can eliminate this problem by washing packed erythrocytes before reconstitution with fresh-frozen plasma. This produced a mean plasma potassium concentration of 4.4 mEq/L or less, even when 5-day-old erythrocytes were used.[606,608] Use of an IBM blood cell processor, however, produced serum potassium levels of about 2 mEq/L. Such levels could result in hypokalemia and cardiac dysrhythmia.[606]

BILIRUBIN REBOUND

During the exchange transfusion, bilirubin from the extravascular space is drawn into the plasma. Partial equilibration between extravascular and plasma bilirubin occurs almost instantaneously,[609] so that by the end of an exchange, in which only 13% of the circulating erythrocytes remain, the serum bilirubin is still 45% of the preexchange level. Immediately after the exchange, further equilibration takes place, which is complete within 30 minutes and which produces the early rebound of plasma bilirubin to 60% of the preexchange level.[491] Despite exchange transfusion, rapid heme breakdown may continue, producing a further increase in serum bilirubin that may necessitate repeat exchange transfusion. This hemolysis may result from catabolism of sensitized erythrocytes that exist as pools previously sequestered in the bone marrow or spleen and therefore not removed by exchange transfusion, from production of early-labeled bilirubin, or from the hemolysis of transfused erythrocytes.

EFFICIENCY

The mass of bilirubin removed is related to the plasma bilirubin level[610] and the size of the exchange transfusion, with the most critical factor being the amount of plasma removed (see Table 38-31). A volume of twice the infants' circulating blood volume has generally been recommended (*i.e.*, double-volume exchange transfusion). In a randomized trial, however, Amato and colleagues compared single- and double-volume exchange transfusions in full-term infants with ABO hemolytic disease and found no difference in the efficiency of the exchange.[611] Because of the rapid equilibration between extravascular and plasma bilirubin, the rate of the exchange has little effect on the amount of bilirubin removed. The extravascular bilirubin concentration decreases at the same rate as the plasma bilirubin concentration and cannot be influenced by the rate of the exchange. For practical purposes, the size of the blood aliquots exchanged also has no significant effect on the efficiency.[612] Therefore, exchanging increments of 5 or 10 mL is as efficient as using 20-mL aliquots. Withdrawal of 20 mL of blood from a 3000-g infant represents an acute depletion of total blood volume and may cause a decrease in cardiac return, cardiac output, and blood pressure, particularly if done rapidly.[613] As the cardiovascular system is adapting to these changes, an equal volume of blood is rapidly reinfused, which reverses the adaptation.[612] This could be repeated 25 to 30 times during a double-volume exchange. The use of smaller aliquots places less stress on the infants's cardiovascular adaptive mechanisms.

ALBUMIN ADMINISTRATION

The administration of albumin before or during an exchange transfusion has produced conflicting results with regard to its effect on the efficiency of the exchange. Some authors reported that 1 g/kg of 25% salt-poor albumin, given 1 hour before the exchange, increased the amount of bilirubin removed by the exchange, although others did not find this to be the case.[610]

TECHNIQUE

This is described in Allen and Diamond's classic monograph,[614] and more recent detailed descriptions also are available.[615] The most commonly used technique is the push–pull method, in which a single syringe and special four-way stopcock are used. Various other techniques have been described, which include the use of syringe pumps that mechanically infuse and withdraw blood.[616,617] Simultaneous withdrawal from the umbilical artery and gravity-assisted infusion by way of the umbilical vein has also been employed.[618] This method adds the hazard of an additional catheter but may be of considerable value when dealing with sick infants because it eliminates the swings in blood volume and pressure that occur with the push–pull method. A technique of exchange transfusion in which peripheral veins are used also has been described.[619,620]

RATE OF EXCHANGE

Rapid exchange transfusion may aggravate cardiovascular changes,[613] may affect cerebral blood flow and intracranial pressure,[621] and may not allow time for the liver to metabolize the infused acid and citrate. With adequate monitoring and good temperature control, there does not seem to be any need to hurry the procedure. Generally, an exchange of twice the blood volume should take about 1 to 1.5 hours in any infant. This means a slower rate for the smaller and sicker infants.

COMPLICATIONS

Morbidity and Mortality. In the NICHHD collaborative phototherapy study, 190 patients received a total of 331 exchange transfusions.[555] One infant died within 6 hours of the procedure. He was an 850-g infant with severe respiratory distress syndrome and thrombocytopenia. The overall mortality for the procedure was 5.3 per 1000 patients and 3 per 1000 procedures. Of 172 infants who were in good, or critical but stable, clinical condition, none died after exchange transfusion. Significant morbidity (*e.g.*, apnea, bradycardia, cyanosis, vasospasm with thrombosis) was associated with 5.2% of the exchange transfusions. Of infants in whom serious events related to the exchange transfusion occurred, all but two were critically ill before the procedure.

The results of 1472 exchange transfusions with fresh heparinized blood in 1069 newborns from 1968 to 1981 were reported by Hovi and Siimes.[554] Fourteen infants had a major complication during the procedure, including respiratory arrest, pulmonary edema, cardiac arrest, and bradycardia. The incidence of major complications was 13 in 1000 patients and 9.5 in 1000 procedures. In four infants, death was considered possibly related to the exchange transfusion (3.7 in 1000 patients or 2.7 in 1000 procedures). Remarkably, three of these infants died after developing necrotizing enterocolitis between the ages of 2 days and 3 weeks. One infant died of *Pseudomonas* septicemia at 5 days of age, after five exchange transfusions. Note that in the NICHHD collaborative phototherapy study, procedure-related mortality was defined as death occurring within 6 hours of the procedure, whereas Hovi and Siimes defined mortality as deaths possibly related to exchange transfusions.[554]

Ellis and colleagues surveyed their experience with exchange transfusion over a 27-year period (1951–1977).[553] Before 1965, 19 infants died, but death was considered inevitable. Seventeen infants had unexplained deaths. Since 1965, however, no unexplained death occurred in 1004 infants who underwent exchange transfusion.

Necrotizing Enterocolitis. Necrotizing enterocolitis with intestinal perforation has been reported following exchange transfusion.[554,622–626] This has occurred in both full-term and premature infants and after both single and multiple exchanges. The cause remains obscure, and it has been suggested that malpositioning of the umbilical venous catheter in the portal system, with its close relation to the mesenteric veins, may produce retrograde obstructive hemodynamic changes with hemorrhage and thrombosis at the microcirculatory level. Studies in piglets demonstrated a significant increase in portal venous pressure during the injection phase of the exchange.[627]

In some infants, exchange transfusion may be the primary etiologic event, whereas in others, it represents an additional insult to a bowel compromised by infection or hypoxia.[628] Black and colleagues present evidence to support this possibility.[629] In their study, infants with polycythemia and hyperviscosity were randomly assigned to receive partial plasma exchange transfusions or symptomatic care. Eight of 43 hyperviscous infants who received partial exchange transfusions developed necrotizing enterocolitis, whereas none of the symptomatically treated infants did ($p < 0.001$). Twenty-two (51%) of the infants who received partial exchange transfusions had evidence of some gastrointestinal problem, such as abdominal distention, diarrhea, blood in the stool, emesis, and signs of systemic illness. Both polycythemia and exchange transfusions have been associated with gastrointestinal injury, but the results of this study suggest that when both conditions occur in the same patient, the risk of serious gastrointestinal problems increases significantly.

Blood-Borne Infection. Exchange transfusion carries the usual risk of any blood product. With the screening techniques employed by blood banks, however, the risk of acquired immunodeficiency syndrome, hepatitis, and cytomegalovirus infection is low.[630,631]

Graft-versus-Host Disease. Graft-*versus*-host disease has occurred in infants who received intrauterine transfusions and subsequently received exchange transfusions after delivery.[632] These infants apparently did not reject the donor lymphocytes because the previous introduction of viable lymphocytes during intrauterine life had rendered them relatively immunologically tolerant. Graft-*versus*-host disease has also occurred after exchange transfusion in apparently normal, but presumably immunologically compromised, newborns.[633] Irradiation of blood before exchange transfusion is advisable for immunocompromised infants and for those who have received intrauterine transfusions.

A clinical syndrome of transient maculopapular rash with associated eosinophilia, thrombocytopenia, and mild lymphopenia was described in 21 of 35 neonates who received both intrauterine transfusions and postnatal exchange transfusions and in 6 of 17 neonates who received multiple exchange transfusions for erythroblastosis fetalis.[634] These infants did not progress to the typical syndrome of graft-*versus*-host disease and were well at follow-up. The authors suggest that extensive immunologic investigation for graft-*versus*-host disease is not necessary unless the rash fails to improve within a week or there are other indications of immunodeficiency.[634]

Other Complications. Malfunctioning blood warmers may overheat blood and produce acute hemolysis,[635,636] so it is prudent to verify the temperature of the water (37°C) directly with a mercury thermometer.[635]

The unwitting use of hemoglobin SC blood produced massive intravascular sickling and death in one infant, suggesting the advisability of screening a donor for sickle-cell trait or disease.[637]

Exchange transfusion modifies serum drug concentrations in infants who are being treated with various pharmacologic agents (see Chap. 58; see Table 38-3).[638] Unless repeated exchange transfusions are performed, the drug loss of antibiotics after exchange transfusions is clinically insignificant, and the effect on digoxin levels also is negligible. A double-volume exchange, however, is likely to decrease serum theophylline levels by 32%.[638]

Careful attention to detail helps to avoid most of the described hazards of exchange transfusions, although complications related to the placement of a catheter and to the procedure can never be eliminated completely. This is particularly so because this procedure is performed on the smallest and sickest infants and may be responsible for problems not previously considered.[621] For example, the high sodium content of CPD blood (165–170 mmol/L),[639] although of little consequence for the vigorous full-term infant, may not be benign in infants who weigh less than 1500 g.[640] In vigorous infants, exchange transfusion is usually a benign procedure, but necrotizing enterocolitis, in particular, appears to be a complication that may occur in both compromised and uncompromised infants.

PHOTOTHERAPY

In 1958, Cremer and colleagues observed that the exposure of premature infants to sunlight or blue fluorescent light produced a fall in serum bilirubin concentration.[641] Since then, visible light for the treatment of hyperbilirubinemia has been used extensively throughout the world.

TERMINOLOGY

The language of phototherapy is confusing, and interpretation of measurements quoted in the literature is difficult because different investigators use different instruments (*i.e.*, photometers) with varying spectral responses, different filters, and different units for expressing the results. The irradiance, or flux, is the radiant power incident on a surface per unit area of that surface and is expressed in watts per square centimeter (W/cm^2). Spectral irradiance is the irradiance in a narrow wavelength band centered at a specific wavelength and is expressed as watts per square centimeter nanometers ($W/cm^2/nm$). Irradiance can be converted to spectral irradiance by dividing the irradiance by the width of the interval (*e.g.*, an irradiance of 585 μW/cm² in the 425- to 475-nm range is equal to 585/50 or 11.7 μW/cm²/nm). The irradiance of various lamp combinations as measured by different commercially available meters has been studied by Hammerman and colleagues.[642] Illuminance is the photometric analog of irradiance—weighted for the visual response of the eye—and is measured in foot-candles by the familiar photographic light meter.

EFFECTIVENESS

Phototherapy is an effective means of preventing or treating hyperbilirubinemia. After random assignment in the NICHHD phototherapy study, 672 infants received phototherapy, and 667 were controls.[529] Phototherapy was effective in preventing hyperbilirubinemia. Of the 462 low-birth-weight infants treated with light, only 17.7% had bilirubin levels higher than 10 mg/dL (171 μmol/L), compared with 62.8% of the 460 controls. Furthermore, 24.4% of control infants in this weight group received exchange transfusions, compared with only 4.1% of infants in the phototherapy group. Phototherapy was also effective in controlling hyperbilirubinemia in larger infants.

In all weight groups, light treatment appeared to have its greatest impact in the first 24 to 48 hours of therapy, after which efficacy decreased. The declining efficacy of phototherapy after 48 hours is consistent with the observation that the configurational isomer, formed during light treatment, reverts to natural unconjugated bilirubin in the intestine after hepatic excretion. Natural bilirubin is then reabsorbed through the enterohepatic circulation and contributes to the bilirubin load to be cleared by the liver.[529]

Phototherapy is more effective than exchange transfusion in achieving prolonged reduction of bilirubin levels in infants with nonhemolytic jaundice,[572] and it modifies the course of hyperbilirubinemia in ABO and Rh hemolytic disease and reduces significantly the need for exchange transfusion.

Although virtually all attention has been directed toward serum bilirubin levels, the efficacy of phototherapy extends well beyond its ability to lower the plasma bilirubin concentration. Phototherapy is beneficial because it detoxifies bilirubin instantaneously and continuously, regardless of the serum bilirubin level (see Mechanism of Action).[3]

FACTORS INFLUENCING THE EFFICIENCY OF PHOTOTHERAPY

TYPES OF LIGHT

Various types of fluorescent lights have been used for phototherapy, including broad-spectrum, daylight, cool white, blue, monochromatic special blue, green, and a quartz halide white light with a tungsten filament that has a significant output in the blue spectrum. In contrast to the commonly used phototherapy units (*i.e.*, a bank of fluorescent lights), the field of irradiance produced by the quartz halide lamp is extremely heterogeneous, with a high intensity in the center and a marked decrease toward the sides that may impair the efficacy of these lamps in relation to the energy output.[643]

The first event in phototherapy is the absorption of a photon of light by a bilirubin molecule. Only light of certain colors or wavelengths can be absorbed by bilirubin. Because bilirubin is a yellow pigment, only violet, blue, and some green light can be absorbed, and when infants are treated with broad-spectrum white light, only a fraction of the light is acting on the bilirubin.[13] Bilirubin does not absorb the different colors of light equally; blue light at about 450 nm is absorbed most readily, while green light is less well absorbed. To reach the bilirubin in an infant, however, the light must penetrate the skin. The depth to which light penetrates the skin depends on the color or wavelength of light; the longer the wavelength, the deeper the penetration.[644] Green light penetrates better than blue light, which penetrates better than violet light.

The efficacy of light at different wavelengths has been studied by a number of authors, and most studies suggest that irradiance at wavelengths 425 to 475 nm is effective both *in vitro*[645,646] and *in vivo*.[646–649] Concern for potential mutagenic effects of light with wavelengths of 350 to 450 nm has resulted in the suggestion that green light (525 nm) should be used.[650–652] In clinical trials, however, the clinical efficacy of green phototherapy lamps has been equivalent[653,654] or inferior to blue or daylight phototherapy.[220,655] Since no one likes to look at green infants or work in the presence of green light, green phototherapy lamps cannot be recommended.

Hammerman and colleagues studied the efficacy of different combinations of special blue and daylight bulbs and found that a combination of four special blue lamps and four daylight lamps was effective and did not produce discomfort in the nursery staff.[642] Monochromatic blue light has been associated with discomfort and vertigo in nursery staff.[656] In jaundiced preterm infants, blue light was more effective in converting bilirubin to its isomer (4Z,15E-bilirubin) than was white light, even though the irradiance at 450 nm was the same for both light sources (12 μW/cm²/nm).[657] There was no significant difference in the percentage of lumirubin produced under white or blue light therapy.[657] Note that special blue lamps are not the same as regular blue fluorescent lamps, although some authors fail to distinguish between the two. Special blue are narrow-spectrum lamps that carry the designation F20T12/BB, while regular blue are designated F20T12/B. Special blue lamps are superior to broad-spectrum white light, but no data are available to show that regular blue lamps have any advantage.[13]

Fiberoptic light systems have been developed that deliver light from a high-intensity lamp to a fiberoptic pad or blanket. Two devices on the market are the Wallaby Phototherapy System (Fiberoptic Medical Products, Inc., Allentown, PA) and the BiliBlanket Phototherapy System (Ohmeda, Columbia, MD). In the Wallaby system, illumination is transmitted from a halogen lamp source to a bundle of fiberoptic fibers contained in a cummerbund, which can be wrapped around the infant. Alternatively, the infant can lie on the blanket. In the Ohmeda system, the infant lies on a woven fiberoptic mat. The mat may also be tucked under the shirt while the infant is held. These systems have obvious advantages over conventional phototherapy systems—eye patches are probably unnecessary, which eliminates the possibility of nasal obstruction from eye pads; the equipment is less bulky than conventional phototherapy equipment; and infants can be held and nursed while they receive phototherapy. This is also a convenient way to deliver double phototherapy when it is necessary to reduce the bilirubin level as rapidly as possible (see Exposed Body Surface Area). Only the Wallaby system has been tested in controlled trials,[571,658–660] and it appears to have an efficacy similar to conventional phototherapy. There is no reason to believe that the Ohmeda system is not similarly effective. When used at home, fiberoptic phototherapy appears to be better accepted by parents than conventional phototherapy.[661]

DOSE–RESPONSE RELATION

A clear dose–response relation can be demonstrated between irradiance and the response of the serum bilirubin concentration to phototherapy. Tan studied nine groups of full-term infants with nonhemolytic hyperbilirubinemia.[570] These infants had maximal serum bilirubin levels ranging from 15.7 to 17.8 mg/dL (269–304 μmol/L). A maximal decline in serum bilirubin level of 50% was obtained when infants were exposed to an irradiance of 34 μW/cm²/nm in the 425- to 475-nm range. This rate of decline in serum bilirubin indicates how effective phototherapy can be when given in adequate dose. Tan obtained 24-hour declines in serum bilirubin levels of 7 to 8 mg/dL (120–137 μmol/L), compared with the maximal decline of less than 2.5 mg/dL (43 μmol/L) in the first 24 hours obtained in the NICHHD phototherapy study.[529]

In the well-baby nursery at William Beaumont Hospital, I use standard fluorescent phototherapy lamps with four daylight lamps and four regular blue lamps. The measured irradiance when these lamps are placed 30 to 35 cm above the infant is about 9 μW/cm²/nm. Lowering the lamp to within 15 cm of the infant increases the irradiance to 15 μW/cm²/nm. It is my standard practice to place infants in bassinets and lower the phototherapy lamps as close as possible to the infant. Occasionally, the radiant heat produced leads to slight temperature elevations in the infant, in which case the phototherapy lamp is raised slightly. This is a simple method of achieving an increase in the dose of light.

Note, however, that as the distance between lamp and infant decreases, there is an increase in the heterogeneity of irradiation, with a much greater increase in irradiance occurring at the center than at the periphery.[643] Lining the incubator or bassinet with a reflecting white cloth produces greater homogeneity of the field of irradiance and an increase in radiant power. The lining also increases the amount of indirect reflected irradiance. Lining an incubator with a reflecting cloth may be a more effective measure for increasing the efficacy of phototherapy than moving the lamp closer to the patient.[662]

EXPOSED BODY SURFACE AREA

The efficacy of phototherapy is also influenced by the amount of body surface area exposed to the light. Phototherapy systems that simultaneously irradiate the front and the back of the infant increase the dose by delivering the same amount of irradiance per square centimeter of skin to a larger skin area. This lowers the serum bilirubin concentration more rapidly than one-sided systems,[569,663–666] but these double-surface systems are impractical. The advent of fiberoptic phototherapy systems has made it easy to use double phototherapy. Holtrop and colleagues performed a randomized trial comparing the efficacy of double phototherapy with conventional single phototherapy in infants of less than 2500-g birth weight.[569] Infants in the double phototherapy group lay on a fiberoptic phototherapy blanket with a conventional phototherapy light above. Those in the double phototherapy group had a 31% decline in bilirubin level after 18 hours of phototherapy, compared with a 16% decline in the single-phototherapy group ($p = 0.00002$).

INTERMITTENT *versus* CONTINUOUS PHOTOTHERAPY

Clinical studies comparing intermittent with continuous phototherapy have produced conflicting results. Some authors found continuous phototherapy to be more effective than the intermittent use of light,[667–669] but others did not.[670,671] Vogl and colleagues found that 15 minutes of illumination followed by 60 minutes with the lights off was found to be as effective as continuous illumination.[671] Lau and Fung found that a schedule of 1 in 4 hours of irradiation achieved the same effect as continuous phototherapy.[670] The interaction of a photon of appropriate energy with a bilirubin molecule at a skin-binding site probably occurs in nanoseconds.[672] The products of this reaction then migrate from the skin to the serum, while an unactivated bilirubin molecule assumes the skin site. The migration of bilirubin to the skin takes 1 to 3 hours and is probably the rate-limiting step.[673] Thus, intermittent light, timed to match the migration time of bilirubin, should be effective in reducing serum bilirubin while minimizing the total light dosage. The observation that intermittent phototherapy is more deleterious than continuous phototherapy to the genetic material of human cells in tissue culture has raised questions regarding intermittent phototherapy regimens,[674] although no such adverse effects have been documented in newborns, and the relevance of these *in vitro* observations to the human newborn is unknown.

CHOLESTYRAMINE AND AGAR

When it reaches the small bowel, the configurational isomer of bilirubin produced by phototherapy (4Z,15E-bilirubin) is readily converted back to ordinary unconjugated bilirubin, which can be reabsorbed through the intestinal wall. Thus, the administration of substances that bind bilirubin in the gut might decrease the enterohepatic circulation and enhance the efficacy of phototherapy. Nicolopoulos and colleagues found that administration of cholestyramine significantly reduced the duration of phototherapy.[675] Tan and colleagues assigned infants to receive phototherapy or phototherapy with cholestyramine (1.5 g/kg/day).[676] Infants entered the study when the serum bilirubin levels exceeded 15 mg/dL (257 μmol/L). There was no difference in the percentage decline in serum bilirubin levels after 24 hours of therapy, but the dose of phototherapy used by Tan was substantially higher than that used in most other studies. The side-effects of cholestyramine include hyperchloremia, hypercalcemia, acidosis, and altered stool frequency (*i.e.*, diarrhea or constipation). Exposure to higher light intensities or increasing the exposed surface area by double phototherapy are probably more effective and more tolerable methods of enhancing the efficacy of phototherapy.

Agar, like cholestyramine, can bind unconjugated bilirubin in the intestinal lumen and sequester it from the enterohepatic circulation. It has also been tested as an adjunct to phototherapy in jaundiced newborns, but its effects are slight, although the administration of Agar increased the amount of bile pigment excreted in the stool.[677,678]

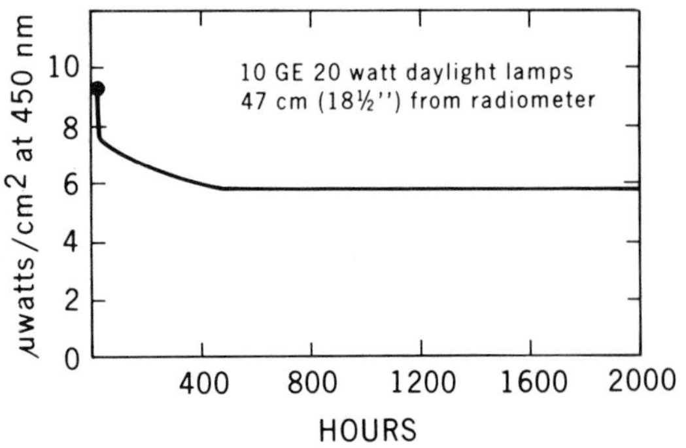

FIG. 38–25. Decay in energy output at 450 nm of phototherapy lamps.

LAMP LIFE

Wide ranges in decay of energy output have been reported with phototherapy lamps. Heat produces deterioration of the phosphors and shortens the lamp life, but with adequate cooling, effective lamp life is probably several thousand hours.[679] Figure 38-25 shows the change in blue light energy over 2000 hours with continuous use of a phototherapy lamp.

HOME PHOTOTHERAPY

Concerns about the dangers of hyperbilirubinemia and the economic and social pressures for early discharge of infants from hospital after delivery have led to the widespread use of home phototherapy. When used appropriately, phototherapy at home is as effective as that used in the hospital, is much cheaper, and poses no obvious hazards to the infant.[661,680–682] When compared with other infant therapies used in the home (*e.g.*, apnea monitors, nasal oxygen, respirators), phototherapy ranks among the more benign. The use of fiberoptic systems has also made it easier to administer phototherapy at home.[661] Home phototherapy reduces costs and avoids parent–child separation, and there is evidence that mothers of infants who receive phototherapy at home are less likely to stop breast-feeding during the period of phototherapy and, if stopped, are more likely to resume breastfeeding than women whose infants are treated in hospital.[683]

MECHANISM OF ACTION

Phototherapy is a mechanism for detoxifying bilirubin. It does this by converting bilirubin to photoproducts that are less lipophilic than bilirubin. These products partially bypass the liver's conjugating system and can be excreted without further metabolism.[3,13] Bilirubin is one of the few substances in the body that absorbs light, and when it does, one of three chemical reactions can occur: photooxidation, configurational isomerization, and structural isomerization.

PHOTOOXIDATION

If a sample of serum containing bilirubin is left exposed to sunlight, the bilirubin gradually disappears—one of the observations that led to the development of phototherapy. This bleaching phenomenon is the result of photooxidation of bilirubin to water-soluble, colorless products.[684] Because these products are small and polar, they can be excreted in the urine. Photooxidation is a slow process, however, and it is probably only a minor contributor to the elimination of bilirubin during phototherapy.

CONFIGURATIONAL ISOMERIZATION

Isomers are substances that have different physicochemical properties but the same molecular formula. Configurational, or geometric, isomerization occurs with compounds containing double bonds. Bilirubin contains two symmetrically substituted double bonds, one starting at carbon atom C4 and the other at C15 (see Figs. 38-3 and 38-5). Therefore, there are four possible geometric isomers of bilirubin: 4Z,15Z; 4Z,15E; 4E,15Z; and 4E,15E. Bilirubin bound to human serum albumin, however, shows about a 100-fold preference for configurational isomerization at the double bond between C15 and C16 over the double bond between C4 and C5.[13] Thus, in infants receiving phototherapy, the stable 4Z,15Z isomer (*i.e.*, the one produced *in vivo* by the breakdown of hemoglobin) is converted predominantly to only one of the three other isomers—the 4Z,15E isomer (Fig. 38-26). In this reaction, one of the end rings undergoes a 180° rotation around the double bond at C15. When this occurs, the polar N and O groups are exposed, making one end of the molecule polar and allowing it to be excreted in bile without conjugation. The formation of 4Z,15E-bilirubin is spontaneously reversible in the dark, unlike photooxidation or lumirubin formation (see Structural Isomerization). This reverse reaction is slow when the pigment is bound to serum albumin but occurs rapidly in bile. Thus, the 4Z,15E-bilirubin formed in the skin and excreted by the liver is readily converted back to ordinary unconjugated bilirubin. Furthermore, the photochemical conversion of the normal Z,Z isomer to the less stable 4Z,15E isomer is reversible by light, and irradiation of either isomer with visible light leads to rapid formation of the other.

In rats, the process by which bilirubin isomers are formed during phototherapy and then transported from the skin and excreted in the bile is exceptionally efficient. When Gunn rats are exposed to phototherapy, virtually instantaneous changes occur in bile composition.[685] This process is so efficient that equilibrium between configurational E isomers and the natural Z,Z isomer is not achieved, and the photoisomers accumulate in the circulation only if their excretion is blocked by ligating the bile duct.[686,687] Clearance of light-generated 4Z,15E-bilirubin isomer in jaundiced infants is slow, however, and a steady-state concentration of the two isomers is achieved (see Fig. 38-26). The absorption spectra of these isomers are similar but not identical, and different wavelengths (*i.e.*, colors) of light produce different rates of the forward and reverse reactions. The steady-state amount of the 4Z,15E isomer is dependent on the wavelength of the light used but is independent of intensity. Greater intensity leads to more rapid achievement of the steady-state concentrations but not their amounts.[13] During phototherapy, the plasma concentration of 4Z,15E isomer increases to about 20% of the total bile pigment within less than 12 hours, and this isomer may persist for hours after phototherapy is discontinued. At the same wavelength, however, the intensity of the light does not affect the steady-state concentration of the configurational isomer in serum. In the jaundiced infant, therefore, the 4Z,15E isomer behaves "as it does in other closed systems, and although it is formed fastest, it has nowhere to go."[13]

STRUCTURAL ISOMERIZATION

In this reaction, intramolecular cyclization of bilirubin occurs in the presence of light to form a substance known as lumirubin (Fig. 38-27). Lumirubin is excreted in bile, without the need for conjugation,[688] and in urine.[689] During phototherapy, the serum concentration of lumirubin is about 2% to 6% of the total serum bilirubin—considerably lower than the concentration of the configurational isomers (about 20% of the total bilirubin).[690] Lumirubin is cleared from the serum much more rapidly than the 4Z,15E isomer. The mean serum half-life for lumirubin is less than 2 hours, compared with 15 hours for the 4Z,15E isomer.[690] Thus, although the quantum yield for the configurational isomerization reaction is at least 40 times

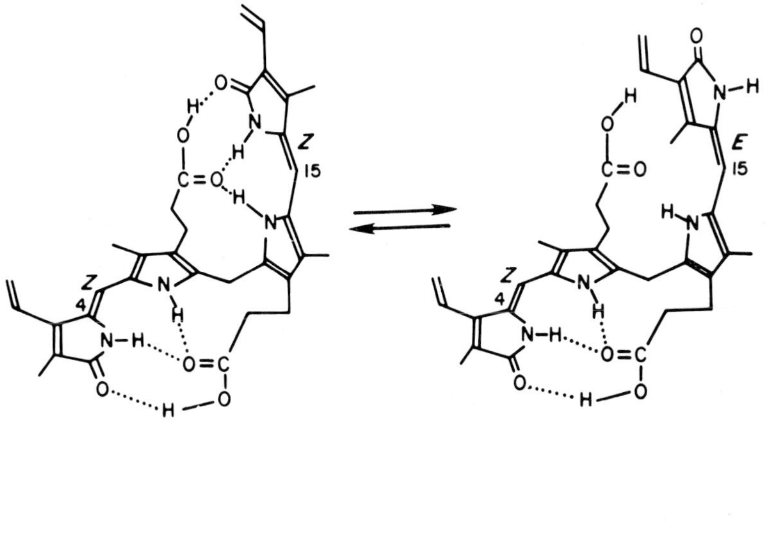

FIG. 38–26. Z–E carbon–carbon double bond configurational isomerization of bilirubin in humans. (From McDonagh AF, Lightner DA. "Like a shrivelled blood orange": bilirubin, jaundice and phototherapy. Pediatrics 1985;75:443.)

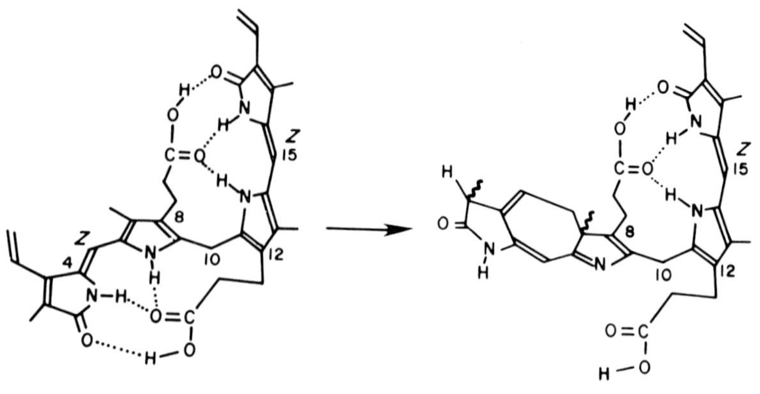

FIG. 38–27. Intramolecular cyclization of biirubin in presence of light to form lumirubin. (From McDonagh AF, Lightner DA. "Like a shrivelled blood orange": bilirubin, jaundice and phototherapy. Pediatrics 1985;75:443.)

greater than that for any other photochemical reaction of bilirubin,[691] the rate of elimination of the 4Z,15E isomer is so slow that it cannot account for the decline in serum bilirubin observed in infants treated with phototherapy.[690] Lumirubin formation is responsible for this decline. Furthermore, the formation of lumirubin is not a reversible reaction, so that once formed it is excreted unchanged in the bile and urine.

Costarino and colleagues exposed premature infants to low-dose (6 $\mu W/cm^2/nm$) *versus* high-dose (12 $\mu W/cm^2/nm$) phototherapy.[688] The lower light intensity was sufficient to drive the conversion of native 4Z,15Z-bilirubin to 4Z,15E isomer nearly to equilibrium. Doubling the irradiance produced no increase in the percentage of this configurational isomer. The proportion of lumirubin, however, increased from 0.7% to 1.3%. In a subsequent study, these investigators used high-pressure chromatography to analyze bile samples obtained from premature infants during phototherapy. They found that the major pigment and, in some infants, the only pigment present in the bile was lumirubin.[692] The serum half-life of the lumirubin was 120 ± 25 minutes. These data suggest that structural isomers (*i.e.*, lumirubin), rather than the configurational isomers (*i.e.*, E-bilirubin), are primarily responsible for the ability of phototherapy to lower serum bilirubin levels, and they account for the dose–response relation of phototherapy to the decrement in serum bilirubin.

Figure 38-28 summarizes the general mechanism of phototherapy for neonatal jaundice.

As McDonagh and Lightner point out,

> It is important to realize that formation and excretion of bilirubin photoisomers are rapid processes that begin as soon as the icteric baby is exposed to light. Thus, detoxification starts with the flick of the light switch, although it may be hours before a decline in the plasma bilirubin concentration becomes evident. Just as the tip of an iceberg represents only a small proportion of its mass, the plasma bilirubin represents only about ⅓ of the bilirubin in the body. Its disappearance in response to phototherapy is a secondary effect. Consequently, it is an insensitive, tardy, and possibly misleading parameter of the effectiveness of phototherapy. When a baby looks jaundiced, it is because pigment molecules in super-

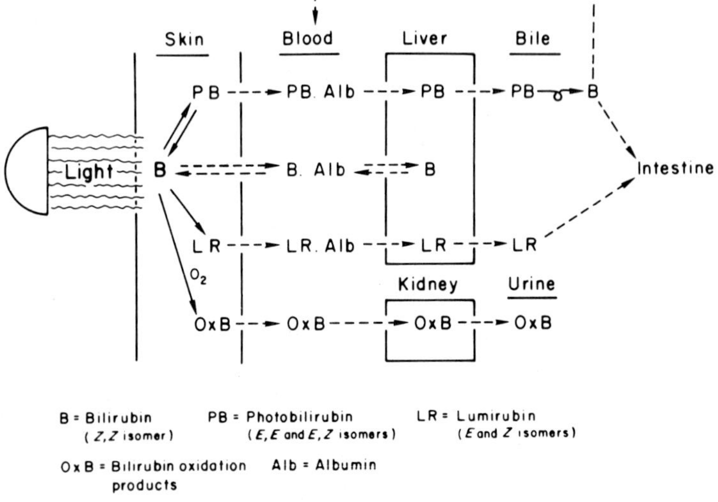

FIG. 38–28. General mechanisms of phototherapy for neonatal jaundice. Chemical reactions (*solid arrows*) and transport processes (*broken arrows*) are indicated. Pigments may be bound to proteins in compartments other than blood. Some excretion of photoisomers, particularly lumirubin, in urine also occurs. (From McDonagh AF, Lightner DA. "Like a shrivelled blood orange": bilirubin, jaundice and phototherapy. Pediatrics 1985;75:443.)

ficial tissues are absorbing blue light. What can be seen by eye is also accessible to the phototherapy lamp. . . . phototherapy is bound to accelerate the detoxification and elimination of bilirubin, irrespective of what the plasma bilirubin concentration may show.[3]

BIOLOGIC EFFECTS AND POSSIBLE COMPLICATIONS

The extensive use of light has stimulated considerable research into its possible effects on the human organism. For many years, photobiologists have been aware of the numerous effects of light on humans and other mammals. These include effects on several biologic rhythms, the pineal gland, gonadal function, and vitamin D synthesis. Nevertheless, no significant toxicity of phototherapy has been noted in over 30 years of clinical use, during which millions of infants have received this treatment.

TOXICITY OF PHOTOTHERAPY PRODUCTS

Human, animal,[693] and *in vitro* studies[694,695] suggest that the products of photodecomposition have no direct neurotoxic effects.

CELL DAMAGE

Exposure of cells to light intensities similar to those used in phototherapy can produce DNA strand breaks,[696,697] sister chromatid exchanges,[698,699] and mutations.[700] Bilirubin appears to act as a photosensitizing agent, enhancing the level of DNA damage in cells exposed to phototherapy light.[701] Intermittent illumination appears to produce more DNA damage than a similar light dosage administered continuously,[674] and illumination of sperm and oocytes in the American sea urchin produces abnormal embryos and cleavage patterns.[702] Because it is likely that light penetrates the thin scrotal skin and perhaps even reaches ovaries, it has been suggested that shielding the gonads with diapers may be indicated during phototherapy.[702] No chromosomal damage, however, was seen in lymphocyte cultures from infants receiving double phototherapy.[703]

PHOTODYNAMIC DAMAGE

Because bilirubin is a photosensitizer, it has been suggested that it may act as a photodynamic agent in the presence of light and produce damage. Bilirubin is a weak photosensitizer, however, and there is no evidence for photodynamic damage in patients receiving phototherapy. If abnormal levels of endogenous or exogenous photosensitizing pigments are present, as in some porphyrias, phototherapy is contraindicated.[704] It is also dangerous to administer known photodynamic agents to infants to improve the efficacy of phototherapy.[705,706]

INTRAVENOUS ALIMENTATION

The exposure of amino acid solutions used for intravenous alimentation to light in the blue spectrum produced a significant reduction in tryptophan. In addition, when a multivitamin solution was added to the amino acids, a significant reduction in methionine (40%) and histidine (22%) occurred. The decrease in methionine was accompanied by an increase in methionine sulfoxide.[707] Multivitamin concentrate enhanced the generation of single-strand DNA breaks in cells exposed to fluorescent light.[645]

Studies of several animal species have demonstrated the potential toxic effects of light on the retina. Most of these studies were performed in animals with pharmacologically dilated pupils and retinas that are unusually sensitive to phototoxicity. The effects of clinical levels of phototherapy (400 foot-candles) on the retinas of newborn stump-tail monkeys were studied.[708,709] These animals were maintained in standard nursery incubators and were restrained in the supine position facing the light source. No mydriatic drops were used, and the monkeys could open and close their eyes as desired. One control eye was sutured closed and covered with a patch. Exposure to the phototherapy lights for 12 hours to 7 days produced severe and progressive damage to the retina.[709] In a subsequent study, monkeys were exposed to light for 3 to 10 days, then returned to normal environments for 10 months before being sacrificed.[708] Substantial recovery in retinal cytoarchitecture was evident if the original exposure was for less than 3 days. All the exposed retinas, however, showed some loss of rod and cone cells when compared with the controls. This loss is similar to the normal attrition of photoreceptor cells that occurs in the aging process in the mammalian retina. These changes therefore represent a form of premature aging. Thus, if an infant has suffered phototoxic retinal damage (*e.g.*, as a result of a slipped eye patch), visual acuity, electroretinography, and ophthalmic examination may well be normal in childhood, despite considerable loss of tissue.

The eyes of infants receiving phototherapy should be protected with appropriate eye patches. Commercially available eye patches effectively prevent light transmission, but homemade devices are less effective.[710] Displaced eye patches not only allow the light to reach the retina but also may obstruct the nares and cause respiratory distress,[364] and the use of patches has also been associated with transient abdominal distention.[711] The choice of eye patches should therefore take into account not only their effectiveness in preventing light transmission but also the simplicity and effectiveness with which they can be secured. In follow-up studies of infants whose eyes were adequately shielded, visual function as assessed clinically and electroretinographically was normal.[712–714]

SKIN CHANGES

Because the skin becomes bleached during phototherapy, skin color cannot be used as a means of assessing serum bilirubin levels; they must be measured at regular intervals. The skin of black infants contains preformed melanin and may show a tanning effect from phototherapy.[715] Exposure to some long-wave ultraviolet and short-wave visible light (300–600 nm) produces pigmentation without an initial erythema, which is apparently caused by reoxidation of preformed melanin, a process known as immediate pigment darkening (IPD). If this light exposure continues, the initial IPD reaction fades after 1 to 24 hours and is followed within 48 to 72 hours by hyperpigmentation, secondary to increased melanosome synthesis. Plexiglas essentially eliminates the passage of short-wave (200–280 nm) and middle-wave (280–320 nm) ultraviolet light but allows a significant portion of long-wave (320–400 nm) light to pass through. Exposure to energies in the 360- to 400-nm wave band may cause an increase in peripheral blood flow and has caused erythema in adults.[716] At wavelengths greater than 650 nm, which includes infrared energy, most of this energy is absorbed by the Plexiglas.

BRONZE-BABY SYNDROME

Infants with cholestatic jaundice who are exposed to phototherapy may develop a dark grayish brown discoloration of the skin, serum, and urine.[573,717–719] Because the bronzing effect occurs exclusively in infants with some degree of cholestasis, it is reasonable to assume that the color changes are produced by the retention of some product of phototherapy. During phototherapy, the duodenal bile changes from its normal color to brownish black.[720] Onishi and colleagues identified an increase in serum concentrations of an "unknown pigment" (probably lumirubin) in infants with the bronze-baby syndrome.[718] By free-radical reaction, this pigment may be polymerized to form the brown bilifuscin.[718,721] Adults and infants with cholestasis accumulate large amounts of porphyrins and copper in their serum.[722] Further confirmation of the role of copper-bound porphyrins was presented by Jori and colleagues.[723] They produced an animal model of the bronze-baby syndrome by ligating the common bile duct in adult Wistar rats. This produced an accumulation of porphyrins and copper in the liver and a 20% conversion of protoporphyrin IX into Cu(II)-protoporphyrin IX. When exposed to phototherapy, the plasma content of Cu(II)-protoporphyrin increased by about 30%. The spectroscopic changes seen in the sera of irradiated rats whose bile ducts had been ligated were consistent with the formation of products that have the typical spectrum found in the bronze-baby syndrome. These findings provide confirmatory evidence that the brown discoloration found in the bronze-baby syndrome results from the phototransformation of copper porphyrins subsequent to an electron transfer between photoexcited bilirubin and the copper iron.[723]

Most infants with this syndrome have not suffered any deleterious consequences, although kernicterus was described in a full-term infant with the bronze-baby syndrome who died.[573] Maximal total serum bilirubin in this infant was 18 mg/dL (308 μmol/L), and the direct-reacting bilirubin was 4.1 mg/dL (17 μmol/L). A decrease in the reserve albumin binding of bilirubin has been found in infants with the bronze-baby syndrome.[574] Discontinuance of phototherapy generally results in the disappearance of the bronze pigments.

GASTROINTESTINAL TRACT DISORDERS

Phototherapy is associated with an increased incidence of watery diarrhea,[724] an increase in fecal water loss,[725,726] and a decrease in gut transit time.[727] Although suggested in one study,[728] the diarrhea is probably not the result of a phototherapy-induced lactase deficiency.[729–732] During phototherapy, unconjugated bilirubin is excreted into the gut. Unconjugated bilirubin can induce intestinal secretions, and diarrhea may be a consequence of the high concentrations of bilirubin within the intestinal lumen.[733] Increased concentrations of bile salts also have been found in the gut of neonates during phototherapy and may be a factor in the pathogenesis of phototherapy-associated diarrhea.[734]

FLUID LOSSES, THERMOREGULATION, AND BLOOD FLOW

Significant increases in insensible water loss occur during phototherapy, particularly in infants who are already under radiant warmers.[735] In full-term infants, insensible water loss increases by 40%,[725] whereas in low-birth-weight infants, insensible water loss may increase by as much as 80% to 190% in non-servocontrolled incubators.[736] This effect can be partially mitigated by the use of servocontrolled incubators. In addition to the previously noted increases in stool water loss, there is an increased fecal excretion of nitrogen, sodium, and potassium.[726]

During phototherapy, there is a marked increase in skin blood flow (228%) and, to a lesser extent, muscle blood flow.[737] When servocontrolled incubators are not used, there also is a significant increase in skin temperature from the phototherapy lamps and an increase in incubator temperature, heart rate, and respiration. The use of a servocontrolled incubator prevents a rise in skin temperature and the previously noted changes in muscle blood flow, respiration, and heart rate, although there remains a significant, but less dramatic, increase in skin blood flow (52%).[737]

GROWTH PROBLEMS

Infants receiving phototherapy gain less weight in the first week of life than those not receiving phototherapy but show catch-up growth in the next 2 weeks. In a study of 120 infants receiving phototherapy from the second to sixth days of life, 44% of those receiving continuous therapy had regained their birth weights by the seventh day, compared with 57.6% of those receiving intermittent phototherapy (12 hours on, 12 hours off) and 80% of control infants.[738] Similar but less marked changes were seen in length and head circumference. The phototherapy groups had greater increases in weight and length during the second and third postnatal weeks. These growth effects may be caused by the aforementioned increases in fluid and caloric losses. A 2-year follow-up of these infants revealed no differences in weight, length, or head circumference.[739] A 2-year follow-up of another group studied earlier, however, revealed significantly smaller head circumferences in those infants who had received phototherapy. Nevertheless, the phototherapy-treated infants showed no difference in developmental and neurologic performance when compared with the controls.[739] The difference in growth in this group of infants has not been explained. In both these studies, only one-half of the infants who entered the study were available for follow-up measurements at the age of 2 years. Other studies that have followed the growth of infants receiving phototherapy for 2 to 6 years demonstrated no effect on weight, length, or head circumference.[740–742]

GONADOTROPIN CHANGES

Changes have been observed in serum gonadotropins during and after phototherapy. Values for luteinizing hormone (LH) declined within 24 to 48 hours after phototherapy was begun but increased significantly 6 to 9 days after phototherapy was discontinued.[743] Increases in LH and follicle-stimulating hormone (FSH) were observed 3 to 4 weeks after phototherapy was administered to preterm girls. In the boys, LH increased, but FSH did not.[744] These observations suggest that light may affect pituitary-gonadal function in the human neonate, although the mechanism for these changes is not clear.

RADIANT-ENERGY EXPOSURE

Newborns are constantly exposed to the ambient nursery lighting as well as to light that passes through windows, which varies with the amount of sunlight on any particular day. An infant in an incubator near a window who is exposed to 6 hours of summer sunlight receives more radiant energy exposure in the 440- to 470-nm range than does an infant receiving 24 hours of phototherapy with daylight bulbs.[745] Thus, phototherapy may be a less important source of radiant energy than sunlight in some nurseries, and it is a minute portion of the radiant energy exposure that an infant will receive in a lifetime.[741]

ALBUMIN BINDING OF BILIRUBIN

The isomers produced during phototherapy do not compete with bilirubin for binding sites on albumin. Infants receiving phototherapy do not demonstrate any decrease in the bilirubin-binding capacity of albumin.[746–749]

INFANT BEHAVIOR

During REM sleep, infants receiving phototherapy have a slight increase in respiratory rate, whereas during non-REM sleep, the respiratory rate increases significantly. In infants who are not receiving phototherapy, respiratory rates in non-REM sleep decrease as serum bilirubin levels increase.[750] Other studies suggest changes in infant behavior and mother–infant interaction during and after phototherapy.[515,516] Because infants receiving phototherapy are more jaundiced than control infants, however, it is difficult to separate the effects of the jaundice from those of phototherapy. Phototherapy in hospital requires mother–infant separation, which may affect the infant's behavior.[515]

DEVELOPMENTAL OUTCOME

When evaluated at 6 years of age in the NICHHD cooperative phototherapy study, no differences were found between children in the phototherapy or control groups in the incidence of definite or suspect cerebral palsy, clumsy or abnormal movements, hypertonia, or IQ less than 70. There were no differences between the two groups in growth, speech, hearing loss, or evidence of hyperactivity.[497]

OTHER EFFECTS

Phototherapy has been associated with an increased incidence of hypocalcemia in preterm infants[751] and in newborn rats.[752,753] In one study, it was found that hypocalcemia in rats could be prevented by covering the entire head or by shielding the occiput with tape or India ink, and phototherapy-associated hypocalcemia persisted in blinded newborn rats but was prevented by melatonin administration.[753] On the basis of these studies, Hakanson and Bergstrom suggest an extraretinal photoreceptive mechanism involving direct transcranial photon perception by the pineal gland and a reduction of melatonin secretion.[753] The resultant low serum concentration of melatonin permits the unopposed uptake of calcium by bone. Phototherapy does not appear to stimulate the photobiosynthesis of vitamin D.[754] No effect of phototherapy was found on serum free fatty acid levels or leucine amino peptidase values.[745]

Light penetration has been measured through the newborn scalp and skull bones,[745] something that would be expected in view of the clinical experience with transillumination of the head.

PHARMACOLOGIC TREATMENT

Pharmacologic agents used in the management of hyperbilirubinemia can accelerate the normal metabolic pathways for bilirubin clearance, inhibit the enterohepatic circulation of bilirubin, and interfere with bilirubin formation by either blocking the degradation of heme or inhibiting hemolysis.

ACCELERATION OF NORMAL METABOLIC PATHWAYS FOR BILIRUBIN CLEARANCE

PHENOBARBITAL

The drug most widely tested in human studies is phenobarbital, a potent inducer of microsomal enzymes that increases bilirubin conjugation and excretion and abolishes phase I physiologic jaundice in the newborn.[56] In addition, phenobarbital enhances uptake and excretion of certain compounds and increases bile flow. Numerous studies have demonstrated that phenobarbital, when given in sufficient doses to the mother, the infant, or both, is effective in lowering serum bilirubin levels in the first week of life.[105,755] Conjugated bilirubin levels in cord blood are significantly higher in infants of mothers who receive antenatal phenobarbital compared with those who receive no therapy, demonstrating that antenatal phenobarbital enhances fetal bilirubin conjugation before delivery.[756]

The possible long-term effects of antenatal phenobarbital administration are unknown. Although a 7-year follow-up of children whose mothers received phenobarbital in the last trimester was reassuring,[131] at adolescence, the boys in the phenobarbital group were significantly taller and had a lower mean testicular volume than those in the control group.[757] These observations are significant in view of the well-documented effects, in rats, of antenatal phenobarbital on growth, sex hormones, and the onset of puberty.[757] Thus, the routine administration of phenobarbital to pregnant women does not appear justified in most Western countries, given that most infants will not develop significant hyperbilirubinemia. In the Far East and Greece, where the incidence of severe jaundice is much higher, and in developing nations, the use of antenatal phenobarbital might merit consideration.

When phenobarbital was given to mothers of erythroblastotic infants before delivery, the treated infants had a slower postnatal rise of indirect bilirubin than did nontreated controls, and significantly fewer of the phenobarbital-treated group required exchange transfusions.[758] Infants with G6PD deficiency treated from the first day of life with phenobarbital also required fewer exchange transfusions than control infants.[759] The results of the clinical trials involving the use of phenobarbital have been reviewed.[105,755]

Combining phenobarbital with phototherapy in a newborn does not reduce serum bilirubin levels more rapidly than phototherapy does alone.[760] Phenobarbital reduces serum bilirubin levels in patients with the type II Crigler–Najjar syndrome, but it has no effect on infants with the type I syndrome.

OTHER PHARMACOLOGIC AGENTS

Many chemicals are capable of inducing the enzymes in the hepatic endoplasmic reticulum and enhancing not only their own biotransformation but also that of many other substances.[755]

A number of different compounds that induce UDPGT have been tried, including clofibrate,[761,762] buculome,[762] and zixoryn.[763] Antenatal administration of ethanol[764] and antipyrine[126] has also been used with some success. Much more data are needed on the efficacy and safety of these agents before they can be considered for general clinical use.

Because of speculation that reduced synthesis of uridine diphosphate glucuronic acid, the donor substance for UDPGT, might contribute to impaired conjugation of bilirubin in the newborn, orotic and aspartic acid, precursors of uridine, have been administered without apparent effect to neonates.[765–767]

AGENTS THAT ACT ON THE ENTEROHEPATIC CIRCULATION

Pharmacologic agents have been used in an attempt to reduce the enterohepatic circulation of bilirubin. These include activated charcoal, polyvinyl pyrrolidine, and agar, which bind bilirubin in the intestinal lumen. The efficacy of agar in decreasing serum bilirubin levels has been reviewed.[755,768] A metaanalysis of five controlled studies in infants without hemolytic disease suggests a possible, but small, benefit from agar. Even if further studies produced a more significant result, the effect size appears to be too small to be clinically important. No effect was found in infants with G6PD deficiency.[769]

Cholestyramine has been used as an adjuvant to phototherapy (see Phototherapy). The results were conflicting, and the modest benefit does not outweigh the significant side-effects of this compound.

Bilirubin oxidase, an enzyme that degrades bilirubin, significantly lowers bilirubin levels when fed to Gunn rats. The presumed mechanism is its effect on decreasing the enterohepatic circulation of bilirubin.[418] Bilirubin can also be removed from the blood by passage through a filter containing bilirubin oxidase.[770]

DECREASING BILIRUBIN PRODUCTION BY INHIBITING HEME OXYGENASE

As illustrated in Figure 38-2, the enzyme microsomal heme oxygenase is necessary for the conversion of heme to biliverdin, one of the first steps in the formation of bilirubin from hemoglobin. An exciting series of observations has demonstrated that certain synthetic metalloporphyrins are powerful competitive inhibitors of heme oxygenase. Tin protoporphyrin (SnPP) and tin mesoporphyrin (SnMP), in contrast to other methods for controlling serum bilirubin levels, act by suppressing the formation of bilirubin.[755,771–775] The inhibition of heme degradation to bilirubin does not result in the accumulation of heme, which is excreted in the bile in quantities that compensate for the decreased excretion of bilirubin.[776] Thus, heme can be eliminated by pathways other than the formation of bilirubin.

Valaes and colleagues have evaluated the contribution of the classic pathway (*i.e.*, by bilirubin) and the alternative pathway of heme elimination in the bile and meconium from autopsies of stillbirths and neonatal deaths.[755] It appears that heme excreted in the bile of fetuses and neonates is either totally or partially absorbed in the bowel, either after oxidation to bilirubin by intestinal heme oxygenase or as intact heme. This suggests that this pathway predominates during fetal life and may be a mechanism for the preservation of iron in the fetus. In the absence of evacuation of bowel contents in the fetus, the enterohepatic circulation of heme may be more efficient than the standard bilirubin formation pathway.[755]

One randomized controlled trial was done on the effect of SnPP on infants with Coombs-positive ABO hemolytic disease of the newborn.[492] In the first part of the trial (*i.e.*, study I), a single dose of 0.5 μmol/kg SnPP was given at 5.5 hours after birth (range, 1–11 hours). In the second phase (*i.e.*, study II), the initial dose was increased to 0.75 μmol/kg, and a second dose was given to all infants 24 hours later. Infants whose bilirubin levels exceeded 10 mg/dL (171 μmol/L) received a third dose (9 of 24 infants). The incremental changes in plasma bilirubin level were lower in the SnPP-treated groups than in the control groups. These differences were not statistically significant in study I, but in study II, they became significant within 24 to 48 hours and remained so up to 96 hours. The investigators calculated an area under the curve for the elevation of bilirubin above the initial bilirubin value for the first 96 hours of life. This measurement was significantly lower in the SnPP-treated infants in study II. Twenty-nine percent of the SnPP-treated infants required phototherapy, compared with 46% of the control group, but these differences were not significant.

It is intriguing to contemplate the use of a drug that could eliminate the problem of hyperbilirubinemia in the newborn. To be effective, however, SnPP probably needs to be administered prophylactically to most infants. Before that is considered, excellent documentation of its lack of toxicity is needed. Transient erythema was reported in two infants in the controlled trial,[492] and other animal evidence raises concerns about possible photosensitization. In this respect, SnMP is probably as effective and less phototoxic.[777]

SnPP was used to treat three patients with the type I Crigler–Najjar syndrome. Rubaltelli and colleagues described their experience with the treatment of an infant who was 2.5 months old.[778] She received intermittent doses of SnPP (1 μmol/kg IM). They found that the duration of phototherapy necessary to maintain the serum bilirubin concentrations below 14 to 15 mg/dL (239–257 μmol/L) decreased by about 85% after SnPP administration. An injection of 1 μmol/kg given every 7 to 10 days diminished the duration of phototherapy by about 56%.[778] Galbraith and colleagues used SnMP in the treatment of two 17-year-old boys with type I Crigler–Najjar syndrome.[779] The administration of SnMP in doses of 0.5 to 1 μmol/kg achieved a temporary reduction in serum bilirubin levels and a decrease in the rebound hyperbilirubinemia that occurs after plasmapheresis. The total-body bilirubin in an adolescent with type I Crigler–Najjar syndrome is many times greater than the bilirubin contained in the intravascular space, and the initiation of heme oxygenase inhibitor therapy in an adolescent with this disease would not be expected to be as effective as earlier administration.

DECREASING BILIRUBIN PRODUCTION BY INHIBITING HEMOLYSIS

Another interesting approach to the treatment of hemolytic disease is the use of high-dose intravenous immunoglobulin therapy in infants with isoimmune hemolytic disease. Sato and colleagues administered 1 g/kg of intravenous γ-globulin over 6 to 8 hours to three infants.[557] One had Rh incompatibility due to anti-E and anti-c, and two infants had ABO incompatibility. The hyperbilirubinemia was refractory to conventional phototherapy but responded rapidly to the administration of γ-globulin. Rubo and colleagues conducted a controlled trial of 32 infants with Rh hemolytic disease.[556] They were randomly assigned to receive conventional treatment, including phototherapy with or without additional intravenous γ-globulin therapy in a dose of 500 mg/kg given over 2 hours as soon as the diagnosis was established. In the intravenous γ-globulin group, 2 of 16 children required exchange transfusions, compared with 11 of 16 in the control group ($p < 0.005$); and bilirubin levels were consistently lower in the intravenous γ-globulin group, even though they had fewer exchange transfusions. Anti-D–coated erythrocytes are removed from the circulation through antibody-dependent lysis by cells of the reticuloendothelial system. The mechanism of action of intravenous immunoglobulin is unknown, but it is possible that it might alter the course of Rh hemolytic disease by blocking Fc receptors and thus inhibiting hemolysis. Intravenous γ-globulin has been used widely in a variety of pediatric conditions, and significant complications are rare. The risks of therapy are almost certainly less than the risk of exchange transfusion.

PHYSIOLOGIC ROLE OF BILIRUBIN

This subject has been reviewed in depth by McDonagh.[14] In spite of its potential toxicity, bilirubin may have an important and positive physiologic role. Bilirubin, even when bound to human serum albumin, and at physiologic concentrations (1.1 mg/dL, or 19 μmol/L), protects linoleic acid from peroxyradical-induced oxidation *in vitro*.[780,781] It does this by efficiently scavenging peroxyradicals and intercepting the radical chain reaction that leads to the destruction of unsaturated fatty acids. At low partial pressures of oxygen, bilirubin is a better inhibitor of lipid peroxidation in liposomes than vitamin E, which is considered to be an important antioxidant in the defense against lipid peroxidation in plasma.

Unconjugated bilirubin readily diffuses through and partitions into biologic membranes, and the concentration of bilirubin in liver plasma membranes at normal adult serum bilirubin concentrations is about 0.25 mole% (mole/100 moles phospholipid).[782] The newborn has much higher concentrations of serum bilirubin, and the membrane concentration is therefore likely to be higher as well. In early neonatal life, bilirubin may play a role in preventing oxidative membrane damage. This could be important as the fetus emerges from an hypoxic environment (PO_2 of about 30 torr) into the relatively hyperoxic atmosphere. Under these circumstances, oxidative stress may occur, particularly when the levels of antioxidant enzyme systems and endogenous vitamin E may be depressed.[783,784]

Unconjugated bilirubin also reacts rapidly with another, nonradical, form of oxygen—singlet oxygen,[14] the toxic intermediate thought to be responsible for the cutaneous damage seen in patients with photosensitizing porphyric diseases. Bilirubin may have a role as a free-radical scavenger.[246] Infants with illnesses believed to enhance free-radical production (*e.g.*, circulatory failure, sepsis, asphyxia) had a significantly lower daily rise in mean serum bilirubin levels than control infants. These findings are consistent with the hypothesis that bilirubin is consumed as an antioxidant.[246]

Pauly and colleagues tested the hypothesis that bilirubin protects piglets against oxyradical-dependent pulmonary hypertension in arterial hypoxemia when they are infected with group B streptococci.[785] One group of animals was pretreated with a bolus of 50 mg/kg of bilirubin followed by a continuous infusion. There was no difference in group B streptococcus–induced increases in pulmonary arterial pressure or in the decrease in PaO_2 between control and bilirubin-treated animals. In this model, at least, bilirubin did not exhibit appreciable oxyradical-scavenging activity.[785] Bilirubin may help to keep oxyradicals and their lipid peroxide reaction products, which are essential for other reasons, under control, although the physiologic significance of bilirubin's antioxidant activity to the well-being of the neonate is unknown.

REFERENCES

1. Gautam A, Seligson A, Gordon ER, et al. Irreversible binding of conjugated bilirubin to albumin in cholestatic rats. J Clin Invest 1984;73:873.
2. Weiss JS, Gautam A, Lauff JJ, et al. The clinical importance of protein-bound fraction of serum bilirubin in patients with hyperbilirubinemia. N Engl J Med 1983;309:147.
3. McDonagh AF, Lightner DA. "Like a shrivelled blood orange": bilirubin, jaundice and phototherapy. Pediatrics 1985; 75:443.
4. Brett EM, Hicks JM, Powers DM, et al. Delta bilirubin in serum of pediatric patients: correlations with age and disease. Clin Chem 1984;30:1561.
5. Ostrea EM, Ongtengco EA, Tolia VA, Apostol E. The occurrence and significance of bilirubin species, including delta bilirubin, in jaundiced infants. J Pediatr Gastroenterol Nutr 1988;7:511.
6. Cashore WJ. The neurotoxicity of bilirubin. Clin Perinatol 1990;17:437.
7. Bernstein J, Landing BH. Extraneural lesions associated with neonatal hyperbilirubinemia and kernicterus. Am J Pathol 1962;40:371.
8. Sen Gupta PC, Ghosal SP, Mukherjee AK, Maity TR. Bilirubin crystals in neutrophils of jaundiced neonates and infants. Acta Haematol 1983;70:79.
9. Ostrow JD, Schmid R. The protein binding of C^{14}-bilirubin in human and murine serum. J Clin Invest 1963;42:1286.
10. Blaschke TF, Berke PD, Scharschmidt BT, et al. Crigler-Najjar syndrome: an unusual course with development of neurologic damage at age eighteen. Pediatr Res 1984;8:573.
11. Odell GB. The distribution and toxicity of bilirubin. Pediatrics 1970;45:16.
12. McDonagh AF, Palma LA, Schmid R. Reduction of biliverdin and placental transfer of bilirubin and biliverdin in the pregnant guinea pig. Biochem J 1981;194:273.
13. Ennever JF. Blue light, green light, white light, more light: treatment of neonatal jaundice. Clin Perinatol 1990;17:467.
14. McDonagh AF. Is bilirubin good for you? Clin Perinatol 1990;17:359.
15. Brodersen R. Bilirubin transport in the newborn period, reviewed with relation to kernicterus. J Pediatr 1980;96:348.
16. Bonnett R, Davies JE, Hursthouse MB, Sheldrick GM. The structure of bilirubin. Proc R Soc Lond 1978;202:249.
17. Brodersen R. Bilirubin solubility and interaction with albumin and phospholipid. J Biol Chem 1979;254:2364.
18. McDonagh AF. Bile pigments: bilatrienes and 5,15-biladienes. In: Dolphin D, ed. The prophyrins. New York: Academic Press, 1979:293.
19. Ives NK, Gardner RM. Blood-brain barrier permeability to bilirubin in the rat: studies using intracarotid bolus injection and *in-situ* brain perfusion techniques. Pediatr Res 1990;27: 436.
20. Deleze G, Sidiropoulos D, Baumgartner G. Determination of bile acid concentration in human amniotic fluid for prenatal diagnosis of intestinal obstruction. Pediatrics 1977;59:647.

21. Hisanaga S, Shimokawa H, Kurokawa T et al. Relation of the site of congenital upper gastrointestinal obstruction to amniotic fluid bilirubin concentration. Asia Oceania J Obstet Gynaecol 1983;9:435.
22. Wynn RJ, Schreiner RL. Spurious elevation of amniotic fluid bilirubin in acute hydramnios with fetal intestinal obstruction. Am J Obstet Gynecol 1979;134:105.
23. Goodlin R, Lloyd D. Fetal tracheal excretion of bilirubin. Biol Neonate 1968;12:1.
24. Ruoslahti E, Estes T, Seppala M. Binding of bilirubin by bovine and human alpha fetoprotein. Biochim Biophys Acta 1979;578:511.
25. Felsher BF, Maidman JE, Carpio NM, et al. Reduced hepatic bilirubin uridine diphosphate glucuronyl transferase and uridine diphosphate glucose dehydrogenase activity in the human fetus. Pediatr Res 1978;12:838.
26. Kawade N, Onishi S. The prenatal and postnatal development of UDP-glucuronyl transferase activity toward bilirubin and the effect of premature birth on this activity in the human liver. Biochem J 1981;196:257.
27. Onishi S, Kawade N, Itoh S, et al. Postnatal development of uridine diphosphate glucuronyl transferase activity towards bilirubin and O-aminophenol in human liver. Biochem J 1979;194:705.
28. Blumenthal SG, Stucker T, Rasmussen RD, et al. Changes in bilirubin in human prenatal development. Biochem J 1980; 186:693.
29. Bernstein BR, Novy MJ, Piasecki GJ, et al. Bilirubin metabolism in the fetus. J Clin Invest 1969;48:1678.
30. Lester R, Behrman RE, Lucey JF. Transfer of bilirubin-C^{14} across monkey placenta. Pediatrics 1963;32:416.
31. Rosenthal P. Human placental bilirubin metabolism. Pediatr Res 1990;27:223A.
32. Schenker S, Dawber NH, Schmid R. Bilirubin metabolism in the fetus. J Clin Invest 1964;43:32.
33. Cotton DB, Brock BD, Schifrin BS. Cirrhosis and fetal hyperbilirubinemia. Obstet Gynecol 1981;57:25S.
34. Dubey AP, Garg A, Bhatia BD. Fetal exposure to maternal hyperbilirubinemia. Indian Pediatr 1983;20:527.
35. Lipsitz PJ, Flaxman LM, Tartow LR, et al. Maternal hyperbilirubinemia and the newborn. Am J Dis Child 1973;126:525.
36. Waffarn F, Carlisle S, Pena I, et al. Fetal exposure to maternal hyperbilirubinemia: neonatal course and outcome. Am J Dis Child 1982;136:739.
37. Fort AT, Morrison JC, Ragland JV, et al. Correlation of maternal serum and amniotic fluid bilirubin in gravid patients with sickle cell anemia who were actively hemolyzing. Am J Obstet Gynecol 1972;112:227.
38. DiZoglio JD, Cardillo E. Dubin-Johnson syndrome and pregnancy. Obstet Gynecol 1973;42:560.
39. Davis DR, Yeary RA. Impaired fertility in the jaundiced female (Gunn) rat. Lab Anim Sci 1979;29:739.
40. Davis DR, Yeary RA, Lee K. Improved embryonic survival in the jaundiced female rat fed activated charcoal. Pediatr Pharmacol 1983;3:79.
41. Bissell DM. Heme catabolism and bilirubin formation. In: Ostrow JD, ed. Bile pigments in jaundice. New York: Marcel Dekker, 1986:133.
42. Brodersen R. Aqueous solubility, albumin binding, and tissue distribution of bilirubin. In: Ostrow JD, ed. Bile pigments in jaundice. New York: Marcel Dekker, 1986:157.
43. Sorrentino D, Berk PD. Mechanistic aspects of hepatic bilirubin uptake. Semin Liver Dis 1988;8:119.
44. Crawford JM, Howswer SC, Gollan JL. Formation, hepatic metabolism, and transport of bile pigments: a status report. Semin Liver Dis 1988;8:105.
45. Wolkoff AW, Ketley JN, Waggoner JG, et al. Hepatic accumulation and intracellular binding of conjugated bilirubin. J Clin Invest 1978;61:142.
46. Bock KW, Burchell B, Dutton GJ, et al. UDP-glucuronosyl transferase activities: guidelines for the consistent interim terminology and assay conditions. Biochem Pharmacol 1983;32: 953.
47. Burchell B, Coughtrie MWH. UDP-glucuronyl transferases. Pharmacol Ther 1989;43:261.
48. Rosenthal P, Blanckaert N, Cabra PM, et al. Formation of bilirubin conjugates in human newborns. Pediatr Res 1986;20: 947.
49. Balistreri WF, Hubei JE, Suchy SJ. Immaturity of the enterohepatic circulation in early life: factors predisposing to "physiologic" maldigestion and cholestasis. J Pediatr Gastroenterol Nutr 1983;2:346.
50. Jansen PLM, Mulder GJ, Burchell B, Bock KW. New developments in glucuronidation research: report of a work shop on "glucuronidation, its role in health and disease." Hepatology 1992;15:532.
51. Ostrow JA. Bile pigments and jaundice: molecular, metabolic, and medical aspects. New York: Marcel Dekker, 1986.
52. Bartoletti AL, Stevenson DK, Ostrander CR, et al. Pulmonary excretion of carbon monoxide in the human infant as an index of bilirubin production. I. Effects of gestational age and postnatal age and some common neonatal abnormalities. J Pediatr 1979;94:952.
53. Maisels MJ, Pathak A, Nelson NM, et al. Endogenous production of carbon monoxide in normal and erythroblastotic newborn infants. J Clin Invest 1971;50:1.
54. Brodersen R, Herman LS. Intestinal reabsorption of unconjugated bilirubin: a possible contributing factor in neonatal jaundice. Lancet 1963;1:1242.
55. Takimoto M, Matsuda I. β-Glucuronidase activity in the stool of a newborn infant. Biol Neonate 1971;18:66.
56. Gartner LM, Lee K-S, Vaisman S, et al. Development of bilirubin transport and metabolism in the newborn rhesus monkey. J Pediatr 1977;90:513.
57. Poland RL, Odell GB. Physiologic jaundice: the enterohepatic circulation of bilirubin. N Engl J Med 1971;284:1.
58. Levi AJ, Gatmaitan Z, Arias IM. Deficiency of hepatic organic anion-binding protein, impaired organic anion uptake by liver and "physiologic jaundice" in newborn monkeys. N Engl J Med 1970;283:1136.
59. Wolkoff AW, Goresky CA, Sellin J, et al. Role of ligandin in transfer of bilirubin from plasma into liver. Am J Physiol 1979;236:E638.
60. Brown WR, Boon WH. Ethnic group differences in plasma bilirubin levels of full-term, healthy Singapore newborns. Pediatrics 1965;65:745.
61. Drew JH, Marriage KJ, Bayle VV, et al. Phototherapy: short and long-term complications. Arch Dis Child 1976;54:454.
62. Friedman L, Lewis PJ, Clifton P, Bulpitt CJ. Factors influencing the incidence of neonatal jaundice. Br Med J 1978;1:1235.
63. Horiguchi T, Bauer C. Ethnic differences in neonatal jaundice: comparison of Japanese and Caucasian newborn infants. Am J Obstet Gynecol 1975;121:71.
64. Linn S, Schoenbaum SC, Monson RR, et al. Epidemiology of neonatal hyperbilirubinemia. Pediatrics 1985;75:770.
65. Sivasuriya M, Tan KL, Salmon YM, et al. Neonatal serum bilirubin levels in spontaneous and induced labor. Br J Obstet Gynaecol 1978;85:619.
66. Johnson JD, Angelus P, Aldrich M, et al. Exagerated jaundice in Navajo neonates: the role of bilirubin production. Am J Dis Child 1986;140:889.
67. Munroe M, Shah CP, Badgley R, et al. Birthweight, length,

head circumference and bilirubin level in Indian newborns in the Sioux Lookout Zone, Northwestern Ontario. Can Med Assoc J 1984;131:453.
68. Saland J, McNamara H, Cohen MI. Navajo jaundice: a variant of neonatal hyperbilirubinemia associated with breast feeding. J Pediatr 1974;85:271.
69. Chen S-H. Endogenous formation of carbon monoxide in Chinese newborn with hyperbilirubinemia. Journal of the Formosan Medical Association 1981;80:68.
70. Stevenson DK, Freman HJ, Fischer AF, et al. Comparison of bilirubin production in Japanese and Caucasion infants. Pediatr Res 1987;21:377A.
71. Valaes T, Petmezaki S, Doxiadis SE. Effect on neonatal hyperbilirubinemia of phenobarbital during pregnancy or after birth: practical value of the treatment in a population with high risk of unexplained severe neonatal jaundice. Birth Defects 1970;6:46.
72. Fessas PH, Doxiadis SA, Valaes T. Neonatal jaundice in glucose-6-phosphate dehydrogenase deficient infants. Br Med J 1962;11:1359.
73. Drew JH, Kitchen WH. Jaundice in infants of Greek parentage: the unknown factor may be environmental. J Pediatr 1976;89:284.
74. Hardy JB, Drage JS, Jackson EC. The first year of life: the Collaborative Perinatal Project of the National Institutes of Neurological and Communicative Disorders and Stroke. Baltimore, MD: Johns Hopkins University Press, 1979:104.
75. Newman TB, Easterling MJ, Goldman ES, et al. Laboratory evaluation of jaundiced newborns: frequency, cost and yield. Am J Dis Child 1990;144:364.
76. Gale R, Seidman DS, Dollberg S, et al. Epidemiology of neonatal jaundice in the Jerusulem population. J Pediatr Gastroenterol Nutr 1990;10:82.
77. Khoury MJ, Calle EE, Goesoef RM. Recurrence risk of neonatal hyperbilirubinemia in siblings. Am J Dis Child 1988;142: 1065.
78. Nielsen H, Haase P, Blaabjerg J, et al. Risk factors and sib correlation in physiological neonatal jaundice. Acta Paediatr Scand 1977;76:504.
79. Diwan VK, Vaughan TL, Yang CY. Maternal smoking in relation to the incidence of early neonatal jaundice. Gynecol Obstet Invest 1989;27:22.
80. Hardy JB, Mellits ED. Does maternal smoking during pregnancy have a long-term effect on the child? Lancet 1972;2: 1332.
81. Maisels MJ, Gifford KL, Antle CE, et al. Jaundice in the healthy newborn infant: a new approach to an old problem. Pediatrics 1988;81:505.
82. Nymand G. Maternal smoking and neonatal hyperbilirubinemia. Lancet 1974;2:173.
83. Tudehope D, Bayley G, Monro D, Townsend S. Breast feeding practices and severe hyperbiliurinaemia. Journal of Paediatrics and Child Health 1991;27:240.
84. Knudsen A. Maternal smoking and the bilirubin concentration in the first 3 days of life. Eur J Obstet Gynecol Reprod Biol 1991;40:123.
85. Jones JB. The smoking disease. Br Med J 1971;1:228.
86. Jährig D, Jährig K, Stiet S, et al. Neonatal jaundice in infants of diabetic mothers. Acta Paediatr Scand 1989;360:101.
87. Taylor P, Wolfson J, Bright N, et al. Hyperbilirubinemia in infants of diabetic mothers. Biol Neonate 1963;5:289.
88. Berk MA, Mimouni F, Miodovnik M, et al. Macrosomia in infants of insulin-dependent diabetic mothers. Pediatrics 1989;83:1029.
89. Peevy KJ, Landaw SA, Gross SJ. Hyperbilirubinemia in infants of diabetic mothers. Pediatrics 1980;66:417.
90. Stevenson DK, Bartoletti AL, Johnson JD. Pulmonary excretion of carbon monoxide in the human infant as an index of bilirubin production. II. Infants of diabetic mothers. J Pediatr 1979;94:956.
91. Stevenson DK, Ostrander CR, Cohen RS, et al. Pulmonary excretion of carbon monoxide in the human infant as an index of bilirubin production. II. Evidence for the possible effect of maternal prenatal glucose metabolism on postnatal bilirubin production in a mixed population of infants. Eur J Pediatr 1981;137:255.
92. Widness JA, Susa JB, Garcia JF, et al. Increased erythropoiesis and elevated erythropoietin in infants born to diabetic mothers and in hyperinsulinemic rhesus fetuses. J Clin Invest 1981; 67:637.
93. Osborn LM, Reiff MI, Bolus R. Jaundice in the full term neonate. Pediatrics 1984;73:520.
94. Buchan PC. Pathogenesis of neonatal hyperbilirubinemia after induction of labour with oxytocin. Br Med J 1979;2:1255.
95. Calder AA, Moar VA, Ounsted MK, et al. Increased bilirubin levels in neonates after induction of labor by intravenous prostaglandin E2 or oxytocin. Lancet 1974;2:1339.
96. Campbell N, Harvey D, Norman AP. Increased frequency of neonatal jaundice in a maternity hospital. Br Med J 1975;2: 548.
97. Chew EC, Swann IL. Influence of simultaneous low amniotomy and oxytocin infusion and other maternal factors on neonatal jaundice: a prospective study. Br Med J 1977;1:72.
98. Chew WC. Neonatal hyperbilirubinemia: a comparison between prostaglandin E_2 and oxytocin inductions. Br Med J 1977;3:679.
99. Davies DP, Gomersall R, Robertson R, et al. Neonatal jaundice in maternal oxytocin infusion. Br Med J 1973;3:467.
100. Jeffares MJ. A multifactorial survey of neonatal jaundice. Br J Obstet Gynaecol 1977;84:452.
101. Maisels MJ, Leib G, Gifford K, et al. The "yellow baby syndrome" (or why well babies are jaundiced). Pediatr Res 1985;19:240A.
102. Sims DG, Neligan GA. Factors affecting the increasing incidence of severe non-haemolytic neonatal jaundice. Br J Obstet Gynaecol 1975;82:863.
103. Lange AP, Secher NJ, Westergaard JG, Skovgard I. Neonatal jaundice after labour induced or stimulated by prostaglandin E_2 or oxytocin. Lancet 1982;1:991.
104. Haeri AD, Scher J, Davey DA, Leader M. Comparison of oral prostaglandin E2 and intravenous oxytocin for induction of labor. S Afr Med J 1976;50:516.
105. Maisels MJ. Neonatal jaundice. In: Sinclair JC, Bracken MB, eds. Effective care of the newborn infant. Oxford: Oxford University Press, 1992:507.
106. Singhi SC, Choo-kang E, Hall J St. E. Intrapartum infusion of oxytocin and glucose water and neonatal jaundice. Wis Med J 1984;33:80.
107. Johnson JD, Aldrich M, Angelis P, et al. Oxytocin and neonatal hyperbilirubinemia: studies of bilirubin production. Am J Dis Child 1984;138:1047.
108. Pedersen S, Moller-Petersen J, Aegidius J. Comparison of oestradiol and prostaglandin E_2 vaginal gel for ripening the unfavorable cervix at term. Br J Obstet Gynaecol 1981;282: 1395.
109. Peedicayil A, Jasper P, Balasubramanian N, et al. A randomized control trial of extra-amniotic ethinyloestradiol in ripening the cervix at term. Br J Obstet Gynaecol 1989;96:973.
110. Wood B, Culley P, Roginski C, et al. Factors affecting neonatal jaundice. Arch Dis Child 1979;54:111.
111. Jouppila R, Larva L, Jouppila P, et al. Effect of segmental epidural analgesia on neonatal serum bilirubin concentration

and incidence of neonatal hyperbilirubinemia. Acta Obstet Gynaecol Scand 1983;62:179.
112. Pedersen H, Morishima HO, Finster M. Uptake and effects of local anesthetics in mother and fetus. Int Anesthesiol Clin 1978;16:73.
113. Clark DA, Landaw SA. Bupivacaine alters red blood cell properties: a possible explanation for neonatal jaundice associated with maternal anesthesia. Pediatr Res 1985;19:341.
114. Cheek TG, Storniolo F, Banner R, et al. Is newborn jaundice associated with maternal epidural bupivacaine? Anesthesiology 1988;69:A653.
115. Johnson CA, Liese BS, Hassanein RE. Factors predictive of third-day bilirubin levels: a multiple step wise regression analysis. Fam Med 1989;21:283.
116. DeKornfeld TJ, Pearson JW, Lasagna L. Methotrimeprazine in the treatment of labor pain. N Engl J Med 1964;270:391.
117. DeLamerens S, Tuttle AH, Aballi AJ. Neonatal bilirubin levels after use of phenothiazine derivatives for obstetrical analgesia. J Pediatr 1964;65:925.
118. Diamond I, Schmid R. Experimental bilirubin encephalopathy: the mode of entry of bilirubin-^{14}C into the central nervous system. J Clin Invest 1966;45:678.
119. McDonald R, Shaw M, Craig C. Effect of phenothiazines and analgesics given during labor, on neonatal serum bilirubin. Br Med J 1964;1:677.
120. Rowley WF, Tannrikulu O, Grossman A, et al. A controlled study on effect of promethazine hydrochloride and meperidine hydrochloride upon serum bilirubin levels in the newborn infant. J Pediatr 1963;62:934.
121. Drew JH, Kitchen WH. The effect of maternally administered drugs on bilirubin concentrations in the newborn infant. J Pediatr 1976;89:657.
122. Brodersen R, Friis-Hansen B, Stern L. Drug-induced displacement of bilirubin from albumin in the newborn. Dev Pharmacol Ther 1983;6:217.
123. Brodersen R, Robertson A. Chemistry of bilirubin and its interaction with albumin. In: Levine RL, Maisels MJ, eds. Hyperbilirubinemia in the newborn: report of the 85th Ross Conference on Pediatric Research. Columbus, OH: Ross Laboratories, 1983:91.
124. Levine RL. Perinatal influence on the hyperbilirubinemia of the newborn infant. J Pediatr 1977;90:859.
125. Silverman WA, Andersen DH, Blanc WA, et al. A difference in mortality rate in incidence of kernicterus among premature infants allotted to two prophylactic antibacterial regimens. Pediatrics 1956;18:614.
126. Lewis PJ, Friedman LA. Prophylaxis of neonatal jaundice with maternal antipyrine treatment. Lancet 1979;1:300.
127. Nathenson G, Cohen MI, Litt IF, et al. The effect of maternal heroin addiction on neonatal jaundice. J Pediatr 1972;81:899.
128. Maurer HM, Wolff JA, Ginster M, et al. Reduction in concentration of total serum bilirubin in offspring of women treated with phenobarbital during pregnancy. Lancet 1968;2:122.
129. Ramboer C, Thomson RPH, William R. Controlled trials of phenobarbitone therapy in neonatal jaundice. Lancet 1969;1:966.
130. Trolle D. Decrease of total serum-bilirubin concentration in newborn infants after phenobarbital treatment. Lancet 1968;2:705.
131. Valaes T, Kipouros K, Petmezaki S, et al. Effectiveness and safety of prenatal phenobarbital for the prevention of neonatal jaundice. Pediatr Res 1980;14:947.
132. McAuley DM, Halliday HL, Johnston JR, et al. Cimetidine in labour: absence of adverse effect on the high-risk fetus. Br J Obstet Gynaecol 1985;92:350.
133. Hill RB, Kennell JH, Barnes AC. Vitamin K administration and neonatal hyperbilirubinemia of unknown etiology. Am J Obstet Gynecol 1961;82:320.
134. Liggins GC, Howie RN. A controlled trial of antepartum glucocortioid treatment for prevention of the respiratory distress syndrome in premature infants. Pediatrics 1972;50:515.
135. Nemeth I, Szeleczki T, Boda D. Hyperbilirubinemia and urinary D-glucose and excretion in premature infants following antepartum dexamethasone treatment. J Perinat Med 1981;9:35.
136. Hancock DJ, Setzer ES, Beydown SN. Physiologic and biochemical effects of ritodrine therapy on the mother and perinate. Am J Perinatol 1985;2:1.
137. Hopper AO, Cohen RS, Ostrander CR, et al. Maternal-adrenergic tocolysis and neonatal bilirubin production. Am J Dis Child 1983;137:58.
138. Ferguson JE II, Schutz TE, Stevenson DK. Neonatal bilirubin production after preterm labor tocolysis with nifedipine. Dev Pharmacol Ther 1989;12:113.
139. Caritis SN, Toig G, Heddinger LA, et al. A double-blind study comparing ritodrine and terbutaline in the treatment of preterm labor. Am J Obstet Gynecol 1984;150:7.
140. Yamauchi Y, Yamanouchi I. Difference in TcB readings between full term newborn infants born vaginally and by cesarean section. Acta Paediatr Scand 1989;79:824.
141. Wallace RL, Schifrin BS, Paul RH. The delivery route for very-low-birth-weight infants. A preliminary report of a randomized, prospective study. J Reprod Med 1984;29:736.
142. Dell DL, Sightler SE, Plauche WC. Soft cup vacuum extraction: a comparison of outlet delivery. Obstet Gynecol 1985;66:624.
143. Vacca A, Grant A, Wyatt G, et al.. Portsmouth operative delivery trial: a comparison of vacuum extraction and forceps delivery. Br J Obstet Gynaecol 1983;90:1107.
144. Black VD, Lubchenco LO, Koops BL, et al. Neonatal hyperviscosity: randomized study of effect of partial plasma exchange transfusion on long-term outcome. Pediatrics 1985;75:1048.
145. Black VD, Lubchenco LO, Luckey DW, et al. Developmental and neurologic sequela neonatal hyperviscosity syndrome. Pediatrics 1982;69:426.
146. Goldberg K, Wirth FH, Hathaway WE, et al. Neonatal hyperviscosity. II. Effect of partial plasma exchange transfusion. Pediatrics 1982;69:419.
147. Linderkamp O. Placental transfusion: determinants and effects. Clin Perinatol 1982;9:559.
148. Buckels LJ, Usher R. Cardiopulmonary effects of placental transfusion. J Pediatr 1965;67:239.
149. Philip AGS. Further observations on placental transfusion. Obstet Gynecol 1973;42:334.
150. Saigal S, O'Neill A, Surainder Y, et al. Placental transfusion and hyperbilirubinemia in the premature. Pediatrics 1972;49:406.
151. Risemberg HM, Mazzi E, MacDonald MG, et al. Correlation of cord bilirubin levels with hyperbilirubinemia in ABO incompatibility. Arch Dis Child 1977;52:219.
152. Knudsen A. Prediction of the development of neonatal jaundice by increased umbilical cord blood bilirubin. Acta Paediatr Scand 1989;78:217.
153. Knudsen A, Lebech M. Maternal bilirubin, cord bilirubin and placental function at delivery in the development of jaundice in mature newborns. Acta Obstet Gynecol Scand 1989;68:719.
154. Rosenfeld J. Umbilical cord bilirubin levels as a predictor of subsequent hyperbilirubinemia. J Fam Pract 1986;23:556.
155. Saigal S, Lunyk O, Bennett JJ, et al. Serum bilirubin levels in breast- and formula-fed infants in the first five days of life. Can Med Assoc J 1982;127:985.

156. Frishberg Y, Zelicovic I, Merlob P, et al. Hyperbilirubinemia and influencing factors in term infants. Isr J Med Sci 1989;25:28.
157. Barrett PVD. Hyperbilirubinemia of fasting. JAMA 1971;217: 1349.
158. Felsher BF, Rickard D, Redeker AG. The reciprocal relation between caloric intake and the degree of hyperbilirubinemia in Gilbert's syndrome. N Engl J Med 1970;283:170.
159. Cornblath M, Forbes AE, Pildes RS, et al. A controlled study of early fluid administration on survival of low birth weight infants. Pediatrics 1966;38:547.
160. Wennberg RP, Schwartz R, Sweet AY. Early vs. delayed feeding of low birth weight infants: effect on physiologic jaundice. J Pediatr 1966;68:860.
161. Wharton BA, Bower BD. Immediate or later feeding for premature babies? A controlled trial. Lancet 1965;2:969.
162. Wu PYK, Teilmann P, Gabler M, et al. "Early" vs. "late" feeding of low birth weight neonates: effect on serum bilirubin, blood sugar and responses to glucagon and epinephrine tolerance tests. Pediatrics 1967;39:733.
163. Weber HP, Kowalewski S, Gilje A, et al. Different caloric intake in 75 "low birth weights": effect on weight gain, blood sugar, serum protein and serum bilirubin. Eur J Pediatr 1976;122:207.
164. Bucci G, Mendicina M, Scalamandre A, et al. A control trial on therapy for newborns weighing 750–1250 gm. II. Blood chemistry and electrocardiographic observations in the newborn. Acta Paediatr Scand 1971;60:417.
165. Mamunes P, Baden M, Bass JW, et al. Early intravenous feeding of the low birth weight neonate. Pediatrics 1969;43:241.
166. Wu PYK, Hodgman JE, Kirkpatrick BV, et al. Metabolic aspects of phototherapy. Pediatrics 1985;75:427.
167. Butler DA, MacMillan JP. Relationship of breast feeding and weight loss to jaundice in the newborn period: review of the literature and results of a study. Cleveland Clinic Quarterly 1983;50:263.
168. Bloomer JR, Barrett PV, Rodkey FL, et al. Studies of the mechanisms of fasting hyperbilirubinemia. Gastroenterology 1971;61:479.
169. Bakken AF, Thaler MM, Schmid R. Metabolic regulation of heme catabolism and bilirubin production. I. Hormonal control of hepatic heme oxygenase activity. J Clin Invest 1972;51: 530.
170. Bensinger TA, Maisels MJ, Carlson DE, et al. Effect of low caloric diet on endogenous carbon monoxide production: normal adults and Gilbert's syndrome. Proc Soc Exp Biol Med 1973;144:417.
171. Stevenson DK, Bartoletti AL, Ostrander CR, et al. Effect of fasting on bilirubin production in the first postnatal week. Clin Res 1980;1:126A.
172. Bloomer JR, Berk PD, Vergalla J, et al. Influence of albumin on the hepatic uptake of unconjugated bilirubin. Clin Sci 1973;45: 505.
173. Levi AJ, Gatmaitin Z, Arias IM. Two hepatic cytoplasmic protein fractions, Y and Z, and their possible role in the hepatic uptake of bilirubin, sulfobromophthalein and other anions. J Clin Invest 1969;48:2156.
174. Bevan BR, Holten JB. Inhibition of bilirubin conjugation in rat liver slices by free fatty acids with relevance to the problem of breast-milk jaundice. Clin Chim Acta 1972;41:101.
175. Brown MR, Thunberg BJ, Golub L, et al. Decreased cholestasis with oral instead of intravenous protein in the very low birth weight infant. Pediatr Res 1986;20:236A.
176. Glass EJ, Hume R, Lang MA, et al. Parenteral nutrition compared with transpyloric feeding. Arch Dis Child 1984;59: 131.
177. Yu VYH, James E, Hendry P, et al. Total parenteral nutrition in very low birth weight infants: a control trial. Arch Dis Child 1979;54:653.
178. Vileisis RA, Inwood RJ, Hunt CE. Prospective controlled study of parenteral nutrition–associated cholestatic jaundice: effect of protein intake. J Pediatr 1980;96:893.
179. Gollan JL, Hatt KJ, Billing BH. The influence of diet on unconjugated hyperbilirubinemia in the Gunn rat. Clin Sci Mol Med 1975;49:229.
180. Gourley GR, Kreamer B, Arend R. The effect of diet on feces and jaundice during the first three weeks of life. Gastroenterology 1992;103:660.
181. Newman AJ, Gross S. Hyperbilirubinemia in breast fed infants. Pediatrics 1963;32:995.
182. Arias IM, Gartner IM, Seifter SA, et al. Prolonged neonatal unconjugated hyperbilirubinemia associated with breastfeeding and a steroid, pregnane-3-alpha 20 beta-diol in maternal milk that inhibits glucuronide formation in vitro. J Clin Invest 1964;43:2037.
183. Schneider AP. Breast milk jaundice in the newborn: a real entity. JAMA 1986;255:3270.
184. Maisels MJ, Gifford K, Antle CE, et al. Normal serum bilirubin levels in the newborn and the effect of breast feeding. Pediatrics 1986;78:837.
185. Maisels MJ, Kring E. Risk of sepsis in newborns with severe hyperbilirubinemia. Pediatrics 1992;90:741.
186. Auerbach KG, Gartner LM. Breast feeding and human milk: their association with jaundice in the neonate. Clin Perinatol 1987;14:89.
187. Lascari AD. "Early" breast-feeding jaundice: clinical significance. J Pediatr 1986;108:156.
188. Hall RT, Braun WJ, Callenbach JC, et al. Hyperbilirubinemia in breast-vs-formula-fed infants in the first six weeks of life: relationship to weight gain. Am J Perinatol 1983;1:47.
189. Kivlahan C, James EJP. The natural history of neonatal jaundice. Pediatrics 1984;74:364.
190. Maisels MJ, D'Arcangelo MR. Breast feeding and jaundice in the first six weeks of life. Pediatr Res 1983;17:324A.
191. Alonso EM, Whitington PF, Whitington SH, et al. Enterohepatic circulation of non-conjugated bilirubin in rats fed with human milk. J Pediatr 1991;118:425.
192. Lucas A, Baker BA. Breast milk jaundice in premature infants. Arch Dis Child 1986;61:1063.
193. Gourley GR. Pathophysiology of breast-milk jaundice. In: Polin RA, Fox WW, eds. Fetal and neonatal physiology. Philadelphia: WB Saunders, 1992:1173.
194. Meyers CH, Kwong LK, Vreman HJ, et al. The role of bilirubin production in breast-fed infants with elevated serum bilirubin concentrations at 2 weeks of life. Clin Pediatr 1984;23: 480.
195. Stevenson DK, Bartoletti AL, Ostrander CR, et al. Pulmonary excretion of carbon monoxide in the human infant as an index of bilirubin production. IV. Effects of breast feeding and caloric intake in the first postnatal week. Pediatrics 1980;65: 1170.
196. Murphy JF, Hughes I, Jones ERV, et al. Pregnanediols and breast milk jaundice. Arch Dis Child 1981;56:474.
197. Ramos A, Silverberg M, Stern L. Pregnanediols and neonatal hyperbilirubinemia. Am J Dis Child 1966;111:353.
198. Cole AP, Hargreaves T. Conjugation inhibitors in early neonatal hyperbilirubinemia. Arch Dis Child 1972;47:451.
199. Foliot TA, Ploussard JP, Housset E, et al. Breast milk jaundice: in vitro inhibition of rat liver bilirubinuridine diphosphate glucuronyl transferase activity and Z protein-bromusulfophthale in binding by human breast milk. Pediatr Res 1976;10:594.

200. Hargreaves T. Effect of fatty acids on bilirubin conjugation. Arch Dis Child 1973;48:446.
201. Poland RL, Schultz GE, Garg G. High milk lipase activity associated with breast milk jaundice. Pediatr Res 1980;14: 1328.
202. Blackberg L, Hernell O. The bile-salt-stimulated lipase in human milk: purification and characterization. Eur J Biochem 1981;116:221.
203. Blackberg L, Hernell O. Further characterization of the bile-salt-stimulated lipase in human milk. FEBS Lett 1983;157:337.
204. Hamosh M. Bile-salt-stimulated lipase of human milk and fat digested in the preterm infant. J Pediatr Gastroenterol Nutr 1983;2:S248.
205. Hernell O, Gebre-Medhin M, Olivecrona T. Breast milk composition in Ethiopian and Swedish mothers. IV. Milk lipases. Am J Clin Nutr 1977;30:508.
206. Hamosh M, Bitman J, Wood L, et al. Lipids in milk and the first steps in their digestion. Pediatrics 1985;75(Suppl):146.
207. Jalili F, Garza C, Huang C, et al. Free fatty acids in the development of breast-milk jaundice. J Pediatr Gastroenterol Nutr 1985;4:435.
208. Gourley GR, Anend RA. Beta-glucuronidase and hyperbilirubinemia in breast-fed and formula-fed babies. Lancet 1986;1: 644.
209. Uhari M, Aikkn A, Nikkari T, et al. Neonatal jaundice and fatty acid composition of the maternal diet. Acta Paediatr Scand 1985;74:867.
210. Dutton GJ. Control of UDP-glucuronyl transferase activity. Biochem Pharm 1975;24:1835.
211. Zakim D, Goldenberg J, Vessey DA. Effects of metals on the properties of hepatic microsomal urodine diphosphate glucuronyl transferase. Biochemistry 1973;12:4068.
212. Zakim D, Vessey DA. Regulation of micorosomal UD-glucuronyl transferase by metal irons. Eur J Biochem 1976;64:459.
213. Adlard BPF, Lathe GH. The effect of steroids and nucleotides on solublized bilirubin urodine diphosphate-glucuronyl transferase. Biochem J 1970;119:437.
214. Winsnes A. Inhibition of hepatic UDP-glucuronyl transferase by nucleotides. Biochim Biophys Acta 1972;298:88.
215. Cottrell BH, Anderson GC. Rectal or axillary temperature measurement: effect on plasma bilirubin and intestinal transit of meconium. J Pediatr Gastroenterol Nutr 1984;3:734.
216. Weisman LE, Merenstein GB, Digirol M, et al. The effect of early meconium evacuation on early-onset hyperbilirubinemia. Am J Dis Child 1983;137:666.
217. De Carvalho M, Robertson S, Klaus M. Fecal bilirubin excretion and serum bilirubin concentration in breast-fed and bottle-fed infants. J Pediatr 1985;107:786.
218. Gartner LM. Breast milk jaundice. In: Levine RL, Maisels MJ, eds. Hyperbilirubinemia in the newborn: report of the 85th Ross Conference on Pediatric Research. Columbus, OH: Ross Laboratories, 1983:75.
219. Gartner LM, Lee K-S, Moscioni AD. Effect of milk feeding on intestinal bilirubin absorption in the rat. J Pediatr 1983;103: 464.
220. Amato M, Inaebnit D. Clinical usefulness of high-intensity green phototherapy in the treatment of neonatal jaundice. Eur J Pediatr 1991;150:274.
221. Midtvedt T, Gustafsson BE. Microbial conversion of bilirubin to urobilins in vitro and in vivo. Acta Pathol Microbiol Immunol Scand (B) 1981;89:57.
222. Yoshioka H, Matsuda I, Imai K. Bilirubin and urobilin excretion into stools in infancy. Acta Paediatr Jpn 1965;7:30.
223. Yoshioka H, Iseki K, Fujita K. Development and differences of intestinal flora in the neonatal period in breast-fed and bottle-fed infants. Pediatrics 1983;72:317.
224. Wilson DC, Afrasiabi M, Reid MM. Breast-milk beta-glucuronidase and exaggerated jaundice in the early neonatal period. Biol Neonate 1992;61:232.
225. Gourley GR, Kremer B, Arend R. Is ingested milk beta glucuronidase excreted in infant stools? Pediatr Res 1989;25: 112A.
226. Gourley GR, Gourley MF, Arend R, et al. The effect of saccharolactone on rat intestinal absorption of bilirubin in the presence of human breast milk. Pediatr Res 1989;25: 234.
227. Finni K, Similä S, Koivisto M, et al. Colic acid, chenodeoxycholic acid, alpha-1-fetoprotein and alpha-1-antitrypsin serum concentrations in breast-fed infants with prolonged jaundice. Eur J Pediatr 1982;138:53.
228. Tazawa Y, Yamada M, Nakagawa M, et al. Serum bile acids and their conjugates in breast-fed infants with prolonged jaundice. Eur J Pediatr 1985;144:37.
229. Yamada M, Tazawa Y, Nakagawa M, et al. Alterations of serum bile acid profile in breast-fed infants with prolonged jaundice. J Pediatr Gastroenterol Nutr 1985;4:741.
230. Rubaltelli FF, Muraca M, Vilei MT, et al. Unconjugated and conjugated bilirubin pigments during prenatal development. III. Studies on serum of breast-fed and formula-fed neonates. Biol Neonate 1991;60:144.
231. Wysowski DK, Flynt JW, Goldfield M, et al. Epidemic neonatal hyperbilirubinemia and use of a phenolic disinfectant detergent. Pediatrics 1978;61:165.
232. Daum F, Cohen MI, McNamara H. Experimental toxicologic studies on a phenol detergent associated with neonatal hyperbilirubinemia. J Pediatr 1976;89:853.
233. Doan H McK, Keith L, Shennan AT. Phenol and neonatal jaundice. Pediatrics 1979;64:324.
234. Misra PK, Kapoor RK, Dixit S, et al. Trace metals in neonatal hyperbilirubinemia. Indian Pediatr 1988;25:761.
235. Tuncer M, Demirsoy S, Ozsoylu S, et al. The significance of zinc, copper and magnesium levels of maternal, cord and newborns' sera in hyperbilirubinemia of unknown etiology. Turk J Pediatr 1982;24:227.
236. Moore LG, Newberry MA, Freeby GM, et al. Increased incidence of neonatal hyperbilirubinemia at 3,100 m in Colorado. Am J Dis Child 1984;138:157.
237. Berendsohn S. Hepatic function at high altitudes. Arch Intern Med 1962;109:256.
238. Ramsoe K, Jarjarnum S, Preisig R, et al. Liver function and blood flow at high altitudes. J Appl Physiol 1970;28:725.
239. Atland PD, Parker MG. Bilirubinemia and intravascular hemolysis during acclimatization to high altitude. Int J Biometeorol 1977;21:165.
240. Barron ESG. Bilirubinemia. Medicine 1931;10:114.
241. Bound JP, Telfar TP. Effective vitamin-K dosage on plasma-bilirubin levels in premature infants. Lancet 1956;1:720.
242. Mayer TC, Angus J. The effect of large doses of "synkavit" in the newborn. Arch Dis Child 1956;31:212.
243. Freeman J, Lesko S, Mitchell AA, et al. Hyperbilirubinemia following exposure to pancuronium bromide in newborns. Dev Pharmacol Ther 1990;14:209.
244. Lambert GH, Muraskas J, Anderson CL, et al. Direct hyperbilirubinemia associated with chloral hydrate administration in the newborn. Pediatrics 1990;86:277.
245. Reimche LD, Sankaran K, Hindmarsh KW, et al. Chloral hydrate sedation in neonates and infants: clinical and pharmacologic consideration. Dev Pharmacol Ther 1989;12:57.
246. Benaron DA, Bowen FW. Variation of initial serum bilirubin rise in newborn infants with type of illness. Lancet 1991;338:78.
247. Martinez JC, Maisels MJ, Otheguy L, et al. Hyperbilirubine-

mia in the breast-fed newborn: a controlled trial of four interventions. Pediatrics 1993;91:470.
248. Gollan JL, Knapp AB. Bilirubin metabolism and congenital jaundice. Hosp Pract 1985;(February 15):83.
249. Newman TB, Hope S, Stevenson DK. Direct bilirubin measurements in jaundiced term newborns. Am J Dis Child 1991;145:1305.
250. Kramer LI. Advancement of dermal icterus in the jaundiced newborn. Am J Dis Child 1969;118:454.
251. Ebbesen F. The relationship between the cephalo-pedal progress of clinical icterus and the serum bilirubin concentration in newborn infants without blood type sensitization. Acta Obstet Gynecol Scand 1975;54:329.
252. Hegyi T, Hiatt M, Gertner I, et al. Transcutaneous bilirubinometry: the cephalocaudal progression of dermal icterus. Am J Dis Child 1981;135:547.
253. Knudsen A. The cephalocaudal progression of jaundice in newborns in relation to the transfer of bilirubin from plasma to skin. Early Hum Dev 1990;22:23.
254. Knudsen A. The incidence of the reserve albumin concentration and pH on the cephalocaudal progression of jaundice in newborns. Early Hum Dev 1991;25:37.
255. Knudsen A, Brodersen R. Skin colour and bilirubin in neonates. Arch Dis Child 1989;64:605.
256. Jacobsen J, Brodersen R. Albumin-bilirubin binding mechanism: kynetic and spectroscopic studies of binding of albumin and zanthobilirubic acid to human serum albumin. J Biol Chem 1983;10:6319.
257. Behrman RE, Vaughan VC. Nelson textbook of pediatrics. Philadelphia: WB Saunders, 1987:406.
258. Rosenthal P, Sinatra F. Jaundice in infancy. Pediatr Rev 1989; 11:79.
259. Poland RL, Ostrea EM Jr. Neonatal hyperbilirubinemia. In: Klaus MS, Fanaroff AA, eds. Care of the high risk neonate. Philadelphia: WB Saunders, 1986:239.
260. Newman TB, Maisels MJ. Evaluation of jaundice in the term newborn: a kinder, gentler approach. Pediatrics 1992;89:809.
261. Kemper K, Forsyth B, McCarthy P. Jaundice, terminating breast-feeding, and the vulnerable child. Pediatrics 1989;84: 773.
262. Zipursky A. Isoimmune hemolytic disease. In: Nathan DG, Oske FA, eds. Hematology of infancy and childhood. Philadelphia: WB Saunders, 1987:44.
263. Osborn LM, Lenarsky C, Oakes RC, et al. Phototherapy in full-term infants with hemolytic disease secondary to ABO incompatibility. Pediatrics 1984;74:371.
264. Kanto WP, Marino B, Godwin AS, et al. ABO hemolytic disease: a comparative study of clinical severity and delayed anemia. Am J Dis Child 1978;62:365.
265. Quinn MW, Weindling AM, Davidson DC. Does ABO incompatibility matter? Arch Dis Child 1988;63:1258.
266. Serrao PA, Modanlou HD. Significance of anti-A and anti-B isohemagglutinins in cord blood of ABO incompatible newborn infants: correlation with hyperbilirubinemia. J Perinatol 1989;9:154.
267. Beutler E. Glucose-6-phosphate dehydrogenase deficiency. N Engl J Med 1991;324:169.
268. Brown WR, Boon WH. Hyperbilirubinemia and kernicterus in glucose-6-phosphate dehydrogenase deficient infants in Singapore. Pediatrics 1968;41:1055.
269. Gibbs WN, Gray R, Lowry M. G6PD deficiency and neonatal jaundice in Jamaica. Br J Haematol 1979;43:263.
270. Singh H. G-6-PD deficiency: a preventable cause of mental retardation. Br Med J 1986;292:397.
271. Chavalitdhamrong P-O, Escobedo MB, Barton LL, et al. Hyperbilirubinemia and bacterial infection in the newborn. Arch Dis Child 1975;50:652.
272. Linder N, Yatsiv I, Tsur M, et al. Unexplained neonatal jaundice as an early diagnostic sign of septicemia in the newborn. J Perinatol 1988;8:325.
273. Rooney JC, Hill DJ, Danks DM. Jaundice associated with bacterial infection in the newborn. Am J Dis Child 1971;122:39.
274. Chan KM, Scott MG, Wu TW, et al. Inaccurate values for direct bilirubin with some commonly used direct bilirubin procedures. Clin Chem 1985;31:1560.
275. Rosenthal P. The laboratory method as a variable in the diagnosis of hyperbilirubinemia. Am J Dis Child 1987;141:1066.
276. Schreiner RL, Glick MR. Interlaboratory bilirubin variability. Pediatrics 1982;69:277.
277. Watkinson LR, St John A, Penberthy LA. Investigation into paediatric bilirubin analyses in Australia and New Zealand. J Clin Pathol 1982;35:52.
278. Hussein M, Howard ER, Mieli-Vergani G, et al. Jaundice at 14 days of age: exclude biliary atresia. Arch Dis Child 1991;66: 1177.
279. Mieli-Vergani G, Howard ER, Portman B, et al. Late referral for biliary atresia: missed opportunities for surgical intervention. Lancet 1986;1:421.
280. Ohi R, Nio M, Chiba T, et al. Long-term follow-up after surgery for patients with biliary atresia. J Pediatr Surg 1990;25:442.
281. Johnson L. Hyperbilirubinemia in the term infant: when to worry, when to treat. NY State J Med 1991;91:483.
282. Schumacher RE. Non-invasive measurements of bilirubin in the newborn. Clin Perinatol 1990;17:417.
283. Oski FA, Naiman JL. Hematologic problems in the newborn. 3rd ed. Philadelphia, WB Saunders, 1982:115.
284. Piomelli S. G-6-PD deficiency and related disorders of the pentose pathway. In: Nathan DG, Oski FA, eds. Hematology of infancy and childhood. Philadelphia: WB Saunders, 1987:583.
285. Davey MG, Zipursky A. McMaster conference on prevention of Rh immunization. Vox Sang 1979;36:50.
286. Bainbridge R, Khoury J, Mimouni F. Jaundice in neonatal sickle cell disease: a case controlled study. Am J Dis Child 1988;148:569.
287. Rajagopalan I, Katz BZ. Hyperbilirubinemia secondary to hemolysis of intrauterine intraperitoneal blood transfusion. Clin Pediatr 1984;23:511.
288. Rose J, Berdon WE, Sullivan T, Baker DH. Prolonged jaundice as presenting sign of massive adrenal hemorrhage in newborn. Radiology 1971;98:263.
289. Wright K, Tarr PI, Hickman RO, Guthrie RD. Hyperbilirubinemia secondary to delayed absorption of intraperitoneal blood following intrauterine transfusion. J Pediatr 1982;100: 302.
290. Epstein MF, Leviton A, Quban KCK, et al. Bilirubin interventricular hemorrhage and phenobarbital in very low birth weight babies. Pediatrics 1988;82:350.
291. Pasnick M, Lucey JF. Serum bilirubin in preterm infants following intracranial hemorrhage. Pediatr Res 1983;17:329A.
292. Amato M, Fouchere JC, von Muralt G. Relationship between peri-interventricular hemorrhage and neonatal hyperbilirubinemia in very low birth weight infants. Am J Perinatol 1987;4:275.
293. Valaes T. Bilirubin, interventricular hemorrhage, and phenobarbital. Pediatrics 1989;83:648.
294. Bleicher MA, Reiner MA, Rapaport SA, et al. Extraordinary hyperbilirubinemia in a neonate with idiopathic hypertrophic pyloric stenosis. J Pediatr Surg 1979;14:527.

295. Wooley MM, Felsher BF, Asch MJ, et al. Jaundice, hypertrophic pyloric stenosis, and glucuronyl transferase. J Pediatr Surg 1974;9:359.
296. Jansen PLM, Oude Elferink RPJ. Hereditary hyperbilirubinemias: a molecular and mechanistic approach. Semin Liver Dis 1988;8:168.
297. Reichen J. Familial unconjugated hyperbilirubinemia syndromes. Semin Liver Dis 1983;3:24.
298. Valaes T. Bilirubin metabolism: review and discussion of inborn errors. Clin Perinatol 1976;3:177.
299. O'Reilly C, Dixon R. Crigler-Najjar syndrome: treatment at home with phototherapy. Scott Med J 1988;33:335.
300. Shevell MI, Bernard B, Adelson JW, et al. Crigler-Najjar syndrome type I: treatment by home phototherapy followed by orthotopic hepatic transplantation. J Pediatr 1987;110:429.
301. Wolkoff AW, Chowdhury JR, Gartner LA, et al. Crigler-Najjar (type I) syndrome in an adult male. Gastroenterology 1979;76:840.
302. Yohannen MD, Terry HJ, Littlewood JM. Long-term phototherapy in Crigler-Najjar syndrome. Arch Dis Child 1983;58: 460.
303. Blumenschein SD, Kallen RJ, Storey P, et al. Familial nonhemolytic jaundice with late onset of neurological damage. Pediatrics 1968;42:786.
304. Mooney RA, Smith CH, Zarkowski HS. Free bilirubin measurements in a patient with Crigler-Najjar syndrome after crush injury. J Pediatr 1983;103:262.
305. Ahmad P, Pratt A, Land VJ, et al. Multiple plasma exchanges successfully maintain a young adult patient with Crigler-Najjar syndrome type I. J Clin Apheresis 1989;5:17.
306. Kaufman SS, Wood RP, Shaw BW Jr, et al. Orthotopic liver transplantation for type I Crigler-Najjar syndrome. Hepatology 1986;6:1259.
307. Labrune PH, Myara A, Francoual J, et al. Cerebellar symptoms as the presenting manifestations of bilirubin encephalopathy in children with Crigler-Najjar type I disease. Pediatrics 1992;88:768.
308. Solomon G, Labar D, Galbreath RA, et al. Neurophysiological abnormalities and adolescence of type I Crigler-Najjar syndrome. Electroencephalogr Clin Neurophysiol 1990;76:473.
309. Keino H, Sato H, Semba R, et al. Mode of prevention by phototherapy of cerebellar hypoplasia in a new Sprague-Dawley strain of jaundiced Gunn rats. Pediatr Neurosci 1985–86;12:145.
310. Labrune PH, Myara A, Hennion C, et al. Crigler-Najjar type II disease inheritance: a family study. J Inherited Metab Dis 1989;12:303.
311. Levy HL. Inborn errors of metabolism. In: Taeusch HW, Ballard RA, Avery ME, eds. Diseases of the newborn. Philadelphia: WB Saunders, 1991:120.
312. Korsin M, Irons M, Levy HL. The neonatal phenotype of galactosemia. Pediatr Res 1987;21:343A.
313. Akerren Y. Prolonged jaundice in newborn associated with congenital myxedema. Acta Paediatr Scand 1954;43:411.
314. Christenson JF. Prolonged icterus neonatorum and congenital myxedema. Acta Paediatr Scand 1956;45:367.
315. Weldon AP, Danks DM. Congenital hypothyroidism and neonatal jaundice. Arch Dis Child 1972;47:469.
316. Ariza CR, Frati AC, Sierra I. Hypothyroidism-associated cholestasis. JAMA 1984;252:2392.
317. Van Steenbergen W, Fevery J, DeVos R, et al. Thyroid hormones and the hepatic handling of bilirubin. I. Effects of hypothyroidism and hyperthyroidism on the hepatic transport of bilirubin mono- and diconjugates in the Wistar rat. Hepatology 1989;9:314.
318. Lees MH, Ruthven CRJ. The effects of triiodothyronine on neonatal hyperbilirubinemia. Lancet 1959;2:371.
319. Shrand H, Ruthven CRJ. Effect of triiodothyronine on serum bilirubin level in neonatal development of the premature infant. Lancet 1960;2:1274.
320. Bernstein J, Brown SK. Sepsis and jaundice in early infancy. Pediatrics 1962;29:873.
321. Hamilton JR, Sass-Kortsak A. Jaundice associated with severe bacterial infection in young infants. J Pediatr 1963;63:121.
322. Seeler RA, Hahn K. Jaundice and urinary tract infection in infancy. Am J Dis Child 1969;118:553.
323. Copeland KC, Franks RC, Ramamurthy R. Neonatal hyperbilirubinemia and hypoglycemia in congenital hypopituitarism. Clin Pediatr 1981;20:523.
324. Herman SP, Baggenstoss AH, Cloutier MD. Liver dysfunction and histologic abnormalities in neonatal hypopituitarism. J Pediatr 1975;87:892.
325. Johnson JD, Hansen RC, Albritton WL, et al. Hypoplasia of the anterior pituitary in neonatal hypoglycemia. J Pediatr 1973;82:634.
326. Lanes R, Bancheette V, Edwin C, et al. Congenital hypopituitarism and conjugated hyperbilirubinemia in two infants. Am J Dis Child 1978;132:926.
327. Orth J. Ueber das vorkommen von bilirubinkrystallen bei neugebornen kindern. Virchows Arch [A] 1875;63:447.
328. Schmorl G. Zur kenntnis des ikterus neonatorum, Insbesondere der dabei auftretenden gehirnveranderungen. Verh Dtsch Ges Pathol 1904;15:109.
329. Turkel SB. Autopsy findings associated with neonatal hyperbilirubinemia. Clin Perinatol 1990;17:381.
330. Ahdab-Barmada M, Moossy J. The neuropathology of kernicterus in the premature neonate: diagnostic problems. J Neuropathol Exp Neurol 1984;43:45.
331. Blanc WA, Johnson L. Studies on kernicterus. J Neuropathol Exp Neurol 1959;18:165.
332. Haymaker W, Margoles C, Pentschew A, et al. Pathology of kernicterus and posticteric encephalopathy. Springfield, IL: Charles C Thomas, 1961.
333. Volpe JJ. Neurology of the newborn. 2nd ed. Philadelphia: WB Saunders, 1987:386.
334. Cashore WJ, Oh W. Unbound bilirubin and kernicterus in low birthweight infants. Pediatrics 1982;69:481.
335. Gartner LM, Snyder RN, Chabon RS, et al. Kernicterus: high incidence in premature infants with low serum bilirubin concentration. Pediatrics 1970;45:906.
336. Maisels MJ. Clinical studies of the sequelae of hyperbilirubinemia. In: Levine RL, Maisels MJ, ed. Hyperbilirubinemia in the newborn: report of the 85th Ross Conference on Pediatric Research. Columbus, OH: Ross Laboratories, 1983:26.
337. Pledger DR, Scott JM, Belfield A. Kernicterus at low levels of serum bilirubin: the impact of bilirubin albumin-binding capacity. Biol Neonate 1982;41:38.
338. Ritter DA, Kenny JD, Norton HJ, et al. A prospective study of free bilirubin and other high-risk factors in the development of kernicterus in premature infants. Pediatrics 1982;69:260.
339. Turkel SB. Clinical and pathologic correlations with kernicterus and yellow pulmonary hyaline membranes. In: Levine RL, Maisels MJ, ed. Hyperbilirubinemia in the newborn: report of the 85th Ross Conference on Pediatric Research. Columbus, OH: Ross Laboratories, 1983:11.
340. Turkel SB, Miller CA, Guttenberg ME, et al. A clinical pathologic reappraisal of kernicterus. Pediatrics 1982;69:267.
341. Johnson L, Sarmiento F, Blanc WA, et al. Kernicterus in rats with an inherited deficiency of glucouronyl transferase. Am J Dis Child 1960;97:591.

342. Lipsitz PJ, Gartner LM, Bryla DA. Neonatal and infant mortality in relation to phototherapy. Pediatrics 1985;75(Suppl): 422.
343. Brown AK, Kim MH, Bryla D. Report on the NIH Cooperative Study of Phototherapy: efficacy of phototherapy in controlling hyperbilirubinemia and preventing kernicterus. In: Levin RL, Maisels MJ, eds. Hyperbilirubinemia in the newborn: report of the 85th Ross Conference on Pediatric Research. Columbus, OH: Ross Laboratories, 1983:55.
344. Doshi N, Klionsky B, Fujikura TEA. Pulmonary yellow hyaline membranes in neonates. Hum Pathol 1980;11:520.
345. Valdes-Dapena MA, Nissim JE, Arey JB, et al. Yellow pulmonary hyaline membranes. J Pediatr 1976;89:128.
346. Brodersen R. Binding of bilirubin to albumin. CRC Crit Rev Clin Lab Sci 1980;11:305.
347. Brodersen R, Stern L. Deposition of bilirubin acid in the central nervous system: a hypothesis for the development of kernicterus. Acta Paediatr Scand 1990;79:12.
348. Wennberg RP, Johansson BB, Folbergrova J, et al. Bilirubin-induced changes in brain energy metabolism after osmotic opening of the blood brain barrier. Pediatr Res 1991;30:473.
349. Killander A, Mueller-Eberhard U, Sjolin S. Indications for exchange transfusion in newborn infants with hyperbilirubinemia not due to Rh immunization. Acta Paediatr Scand 1960;49:477.
350. Claireaux A. Icterus of the brain in the newborn. Lancet 1953;2:1226.
351. Wennberg RP. Experimental bilirubin encephalopathy: role of the blood-brain barrier. In: Johansson BB, Owman C, Widner H, eds. Pathophysiology of the blood brain barrier: long-term consequences of barrier dysfunction for the brain. Fernstrom Foundation series. vol. 14. Amsterdam, Elsevier Science Publishers, 1990:269.
352. Wennberg RP. Cellular basis of bilirubin toxicity. NY State J Med 1991;91:493.
353. Cashore WJ, Kilguss NV. Inhibition of synaptosomal tyrosine uptake by bilirubin. Pediatr Res 1989;25:209A.
354. Cashore WJ, Kilguss NV, Chung CE. Effects of bilirubin and albumin on dopamine synthesis in striatal synaptosomes. Pediatr Res 1989;25:210A.
355. Zetterstrom R, Ernster L. Bilirubin, an uncoupler of oxidative phosphorylation in isolated mitochondria. Nature 1956;178: 1335.
356. Brann BS, Stonestreet BS, Ohw Wea. The in-vivo effect of bilirubin and sulfisoxazole on cerebral oxygen, glucose, and lactate metabolism in newborn piglets. Pediatr Res 1987;22: 135.
357. Shepherd RE, Moreno P, Cashore WJ, et al. Effects of bilirubin on fat cell metabolism and lipolysis. Am J Physiol 1980;37: E505.
358. Ives NK, Cox DWG, Gardner RM, et al. The effects of bilirubin on brain energy metabolism during normoxia and hypoxia: an in-vitro study using ^{31}P nuclear magnetic resonance spectroscopy. Pediatr Res 1988;23:569.
359. Ives NK, Bolas NM, Gardner RM. The effects of bilirubin on brain energy metabolism during hyperosmolar opening of the blood brain barrier: an in-vivo study using ^{31}P nuclear magnetic resonance spectroscopy. Pediatr Res 1989; 26:356.
360. Brem AS, Cashore WJ, Pacholski, et al. Effects of bilirubin on transepithelial transport of sodium, water and urea. Kidney Int 1985;27:51.
361. Hansen TWR, Paulsen O, Gjerstad Lea. Short-term exposure to bilirubin reduces synaptic activation in rat transverse hipocanthus slices. Pediatr Res 1988;23:453.
362. Morphis L, Constantopoulos A, Matsaniotos N. Bilirubin-induced modulation of cerebral protein phosphorylation in neonate rabbits in-vivo. Science 1982;218:156.
363. Mayor F Jr, Diez-Guerra J, Valdivieso Fea. Effect of bilirubin on the membrane potential of rat synaptosomes. J Neurochem 1986;47:363.
364. Al-Salihi FL, Curran JP. Airway obstruction by displaced eye mask during phototherapy. Am J Dis Child 1975;129:1362.
365. Abramovich SJ, Gregory S, Slemick M, et al. Hearing loss in very low birth weight infants treated with neonatal intensive care. Arch Dis Child 1979;54:421.
366. Jacobsen J. Binding of bilirubin to human serum albumin: determination of the dissociation constants. FEBS Lett 1969;5: 112.
367. Jacobsen J, Wennberg RP. Determination of unbound bilirubin in the serum of newborns. Clin Chem 1974;20:783.
368. Odell GB. The influence of pH on distribution of bilirubin between albumin and mitochondria. Proc Soc Exp Biol Med 1965;120:352.
369. Wennberg RP, Ahlfors CE, Rasmussen LF. The pathochemistry of kernicterus. Early Hum Dev 1979;31:353.
370. Wennberg RP, Hance AJ. Experimental encephalopathy: importance of total bilirubin, protein binding and blood brain barrier. Pediatr Res 1986;20:789.
371. Harris RC, Lucey JF, MacLean JR. Kernicterus in premature infants associated with low concentrations of bilirubin in the plasma. Pediatrics 1958;21:875.
372. Cashore WJ. Bilirubin binding tests. In: Levine RL, Maisels MJ, eds. Hyperbilirubinemia in the newborn: report of the 85th Ross Conference on Pediatric Research. Columbus, OH: Ross Laboratories, 1983:101.
373. Oie S, Levy G. Effect of sulfisoxazole on pharmacokinetics of free and plasma protein-bound bilirubin in experimental unconjugated hyperbilirubinemia. J Pharm Sci 1979;68:6.
374. Hansen TWR, ϕyasÆter S, Stiris T, et al. Effects of sulfisoxazole, hypercarbia, and hyperosmolality on entry of bilirubin and albumin into brain regions in young rats. Biol Neonate 1989;56:22.
375. Stevenson DK, Wennberg RP. Predictors of a new therapy for jaundice. West J Med 1990;153:648.
376. Whitington PF, Burchart GJ, Gross SR, et al. Alterations in reserve bilirubin binding capacity of albumin by free fatty acids. II. In-vitro and in-vivo studies using difference spectroscopy. J Pediatr Gastroenterol Nutr 1982;1:495.
377. Brodersen R. Prevention of kernicterus based on recent progress in bilirubin chemistry. Acta Paediatr Scand 1977;66:625.
378. Spear ML, Stahl GE, Paul MH, et al. The effect of 15-hour fat infusions of varying dosage on bilirubin binding to albumin. JPEN 1985;9:144.
379. Nizar L, Vyhmeister N, Ross R, et al. A jaundiced look at intravenous fat administration and the risk factor for kernicterus. Clin Res 1990;38:197A.
380. Thaler MM, Pelger A. Influence of intravenous nutrients on bilirubin transport. III. Emulsified fat infusion. Pediatr Res 1977;11:171.
381. Jacobsen J, Brodersen R. The effects of pH on the albumin bilirubin binding affinity. Birth Defects 1976;12:175.
382. Levine RL. Fluorescence quenching studies of the binding of bilirubin to albumin. Clin Chem 1972;23:2292.
383. Nelson P, Jacobsen J, Wennberg RP. Effect of pH on the interaction of bilirubin with albumin and tissue culture cells. Pediatr Res 1974;8:963.
384. Kozuki K, Oh W, Widness J, Cashore W. Increase in bilirubin binding to albumin with correction of neonatal acidosis. Acta Paediatr Scand 1979;68:213.
385. Bratlid D. How bilirubin gets into the brain. Clin Perinatol 1990;17:449.

386. Mayor F Jr, Pages M, Diez-Guerra J, et al. Effect of postnatal anoxia on bilirubin levels in rat brain. Pediatr Res 1985;19:231.
387. Cashore WJ, Oh W, Brodersen R. Reserve albumin and bilirubin toxicity index in infant serum. Acta Paediatr Scand 1983; 72:415.
388. Robertson A, Carp W, Brodersen R. Bilirubin displacing effect of drugs used in neonatology. Acta Paediatr Scand 1991;80: 1119.
389. Brodersen R. Free bilirubin in blood plasma of the newborn: effects of albumin, fatty acids, pH, displacing drugs, and phototherapy. In: Stern L, Oh W, Friis-Hansen B, eds. Intensive care of the newborn. New York: Masson, 1978:331.
390. Robertson A, Brodersen R. Effect of drug combinations on bilirubin-albumin binding. Dev Pharmacol Ther 1991;17:95.
391. Arkans HD, Cassady G. Estimation of unbound serum bilirubin by the peroxidase assay method: effect of exchange transfusion on unbound bilirubin and serum binding. J Pediatr 1978;92:1001.
392. Valaes T, Hyte M. Effect of exchange transfusion on bilirubin binding. Pediatrics 1977;59:881.
393. Cashore WJ, Horwich A, Karotkin EH, et al. Influence of gestational age and clinical status on bilirubin-binding capacity in newborn infants. Am J Dis Child 1977;131:898.
394. Ritter DA, Kenny JD. Influence of gestational age on cord serum bilirubin binding studies. J Pediatr 1985;106:118.
395. Robertson A, Sharp C, Karp W. The relationship of gestational age to reserve albumin concentration for binding of bilirubin. J Perinatol 1988;8:17.
396. Chen H-C, Lien I-N, Lu T-C. Kernicterus in newborn rabbits. Am J Pathol 1965;46:331.
397. Jirka JH, Duckrow B, Kendig JW, et al. Effect of bilirubin on brainstem auditory evoked potentials in the asphyxiated rat. Pediatr Res 1985;19:556.
398. Rozdilsky B, Olszewski J. Experimental study of the toxicity of bilirubin in newborn animals. J Neuropathol Exp Neurol 1961;20:193.
399. Lucey JF, Hibbard E, Behrman RE, et al. Kernicterus in asphyxiated newborn rhesus monkeys. Exp Neurol 1964;9:43.
400. Kulkarni SV, Merchant RH, Gupte SC, et al. Clinical significance of serum and cerebrospinal fluid bilirubin indices in neonatal jaundice. Indian Pediatr 1989;26:1202.
401. Meisel P, Jahrig D, Weinkie I, et al. Distribution of bilirubin between serum and cerebral spinal fluid in newborn infants. In: Rubaltelli FF, Jori G, eds. Neonatal jaundice: new trends in phototherapy. New York: Plenum, 1984:45.
402. Nasralla M, Gawronska E, Hsia D-Y. Studies on the relation between serum and spinal fluid bilirubin during early infancy. J Clin Invest 1958;37:703.
403. Bratlid D, Cashore WJ, Oh W. Effect of serum hyperosmolality on opening of blood brain barrier for bilirubin in rat brain. Pediatrics 1983;71:909.
404. Bratlid D, Cashore WJ, Oh W. Effects of acidosis on bilirubin deposition in rat brain. Pediatrics 1984;73:431.
405. Burgess GH, Oh W, Bratlid D, et al. The effects of brain blood flow on brain bilirubin deposition in newborn piglets. Pediatr Res 1985;19:691.
406. Burgess GH, Stonestreet BS, Cashore WJ, Oh W. Brain bilirubin deposition and brain blood flow during acute urea-induced hyperosmolality in newborn piglets. Pediatr Res 1985; 19:537.
407. Bowen WR, Porter E, Waters WJ. The protective effect of albumin in bilirubin toxicity in newborn puppies. Am J Dis Child 1959;48:568.
408. Stobie PE, Hansen CT, Hailey JR, et al. A difference in mortality between two strains of jaundiced rats. Pediatrics 1991;87: 88.
409. Rapoport SI. Blood-brain barrier in physiology and medicine. New York: Raven, 1976.
410. Rapoport SI. Reversible osmotic opening of the blood-brain barrier for experimental and therapeutic purposes. In: Levine RL, Maisels MJ, eds. Hyperbilirubinemia in the newborn: report of the 85th Ross Conference on Pediatric Research. Columbus, OH: Ross Laboratories, 1983:116.
411. Chiueh CC, Sun CL, Kopin IJ, et al. Entry of [^{3}H]norepinephrine, [^{125}I]albumin and Evans blue from blood into brain following unilateral osmotic opening of the blood-brain barrier. Brain Res 1978;145:291.
412. Levine RL, Fredericks WR, Rapoport SI. Entry of bilirubin into the brain due to opening of the blood brain barrier. Pediatrics 1982;69:255.
413. Bratlid D. Mechanism of bilirubin entry into the brain in an animal model. In: Rubaltelli FF, Jori G, eds. Neonatal jaundice: new trends in phototherapy. New York: Plenum, 1984:23.
414. Saunders NR, Møllgård K. Development of the blood-brain barrier. J Dev Physiol 1984;6:45.
415. Lee C, Oh W, Stonestreet BS, et al. Permeability of the blood-brain barrier for ^{125}I-albumin-bound bilirubin in newborn piglets. Pediatr Res 1989;25:452.
416. Wennberg RP, Ahlfors CE, Wieth JO. Interaction of bilirubin with tissue. Clin Res 1983;31:139A.
417. Levine RL, Fredericks WR, Rapoport SI. Clearance of bilirubin from rat brain after reversible osmotic opening of the blood brain barrier. Pediatr Res 1985;19:1040.
418. Johnson L, Dworanczyk R, Abbasi M, et al. Bilirubin oxidase (BOX) feeding significantly decrease serum bilirubin levels in jaundiced infant Gunn rats. Pediatr Res 1988;23:412A.
419. Kimura M, Matsumura Y, Konno T, et al. Enzymatic removal of bilirubin toxicity by bilirubin oxidase *in-vitro* and excretion of degredation products *in-vivo*. Proc Soc Exp Biol Med 1990; 195:64.
420. Ebbesen F, Brodersen R. Risk of bilirubin acid precipitation in preterm infants with respiratory distress syndrome: considerations of blood/brain bilirubin transfer equilibrium. Early Hum Dev 1982;6:341.
421. Bratlid D. The effect of pH on bilirubin binding to human erythrocytes. Scand J Clin Lab Invest 1972;29:453.
422. Wennberg RP. The importance of bilirubin acid salt in bilirubin uptake by erythrocytes and mitochondria. Pediatr Res 1988;23:443.
423. Wennberg R, Rhine W, Gospe S, et al. Brainstem bilirubin toxicity may be potentiated and reversed by modulating PCO_2. Pediatr Res 1992;31:229A.
424. Chin KC, Taylor MJ, Perlman M. Improvement in auditory and visually evoked potentials in jaundiced preterm infants after exchange transfusion. Arch Dis Child 1985;60:714.
425. Kuriyama H, Tomiwa K, Konishi Yea. Improvement in auditory brain stem response of hyperbilirubinemic infants after exchange transfusion. Pediatr Neurol 1986;2:127.
426. Nakamura H, Takada S, Shimabuku R, et al. Auditory and brainstem responses in newborn infants with hyperbilirubinemia. Pediatrics 1985;75:703.
427. Perlman M, Fainmesser P, Sohmer H, et al. Auditory nerve-brainstem evoked responses in hyperbilirubinemic neonates. Pediatrics 1983;72:658.
428. Friedlander G, Le Grimellec C, Giocondi MC. Benzyl alcohol increases membrane fluidity and modulates cyclic AMP synthesis in intact renal epithelial cells. Biochem Biophys Acta 1987;903:341.
429. Jardine DS, Rogers K. Relationship of benzyl alcohol to kernicterus, intraventricular hemorrhage, and mortality in preterm infants. Pediatrics 1989;83:153.

430. Ostrow JD, Celic L, Mukerje P. Molecular and micellar associations in the pH-dependent stable and metastable dissolution of unconjugated bilirubin by bile salts. J Lipid Res 1988;29: 335.
431. Keino H, Kashiwamata S. Critical period of bilirubin-induced cerebellar hypoplasia in a new Sprague-Dawley strain of jaundiced Gunn rats. Neurosci Res 1989;6:209.
432. Vohr BR. New approaches to assessing the risks of hyperbilirubinemia. Clin Perinatol 1990;17:293.
433. Connolly AM, Volpe JJ. Clinical features of bilirubin encephalopathy. Clin Perinatol 1990;17:371.
434. Gerrard J. Kernicterus. Brain 1952;75:526.
435. Van Praagh R. Diagnosis of kernicterus in the neonatal period. Pediatrics 1961;28:870.
436. Jones MH, Sands R, Hyman CB, et al. Longitudinal study of incidence of central nervous system damage following erythroblastosis fetalis. Pediatrics 1954;14:346.
437. Johnston WH, Angara V, Baumal R, et al. Erythroblastosis fetalis and hyperbilirubinemia: a five-year follow-up with neurological, physiological and audiological evaluation. Pediatrics 1967;39:88.
438. Byers RK, Paine RS, Crothers V. Extrapyramidal cerebral palsy with hearing loss following erythroblastosis. Pediatrics 1955;15:248.
439. Perlstein MA. The late clinical syndrome of post-icteric encephalopathy. Pediatr Clin North Am 1960;7:665.
440. Gerrard J. Nuclear jaundice and deafness. J Laryngol Otol 1952;66:39.
441. Kaga K, Kitazume E, Dodama K. Auditory brain stem response of kernicterus infants. Int J Pediatr Otorhinolaryngol 1979;1:255.
442. Lenhardt M, McArtor R, Bryant B. Effects of neonatal hyperbilirubinemia on the brain stem electric response. J Pediatr 1984;104:184.
443. Nwaesei CG, Van Aerde J, Boyden M, et al. Changes in auditory brainstem responses in hyperbilirubinemic infants before and after exchange transfusion. Pediatrics 1984;74:800.
444. Vohr BR, Carp D, O'Dea C, et al. Behavioral changes correlated with brain-stem auditory evoked responses in term infants with moderate hyperbilirubinemia. J Pediatr 1990;117: 288.
445. Vohr BR, Lester B, Rapisardi G, et al. Abnormal brain-stem function (brain-stem auditory evoked response) correlates with acoustic cry features in term infants with hyperbilirubinemia. J Pediatr 1989;115:303.
446. Hyman CB, Keaster J, Hanson V, et al. CNS abnormalities after neonatal hemolytic disease or hyperbilirubinemia. Am J Dis Child 1969;117:395.
447. Keaster J, Hyman DB, Harris I. Hearing problems subsequent to neonatal hemolytic disease of hyperbilirubinemia. Am J Dis Child 1969;117:406.
448. Newman TB, Maisels MJ. Does hyperbilirubinemia damage the brain of healthy full-term infants? Clin Perinatol 1990;17: 331.
449. Hoyt C, Billson FA, Alpins M. The supranuclear disturbances of gaze in kernicterus. Ann Ophthalmol 1978;10:1487.
450. Brown AK, Seidman DS, Stevenson DK. Jaundice in healthy, term neonates: do we need new action levels or new approaches? Pediatrics 1992;89:827.
451. Cashore WJ. Hyperbilirubinemia: should we adopt a new standard of care? Pediatrics 1992;89:824.
452. Gartner LM. Management of jaundice in the well baby. Pediatrics 1992;89:826.
453. Johnson L. Yet another expert opinion of bilirubin toxicity! Pediatrics 1992;89:829.
454. Merenstein GB. "New" bilirubin recommendations questioned. Pediatrics 1992;89:822.
455. Newman TP, Maisels MJ. Response to commentaries re: evaluation and treatment of jaundice in the term newborn: a kinder, gentler approach. Pediatrics 1992;89:831.
456. Poland RL. In search of a "gold standard" for bilirubin toxicity. Pediatrics 1992;89:823.
457. Valaes T. Bilirubin toxicity: the problem was solved a generation ago. Pediatrics 1992;89:819.
458. Wennberg RP. Bilirubin recommendations present problems: new guidelines simplistic and untested. Pediatrics 1992;89: 821.
459. Ives NK. Kernicterus in preterm infants: lest we forget (to turn on the lights). Pediatrics 1992;90:757.
460. Watchko JF, Oski FA. Kernicterus in preterm newborns: past, present and future. Pediatrics 1992;90:707.
461. Hsia DY-Y, Allen FH, Diamond LK, et al. Serum bilirubin levels in the newborn infant. J Pediatr 1953;42:277.
462. Mollison PL, Cutbush M. Haemolytic disease of the newborn. In: Gairdner D, ed. Recent advances in pediatrics. New York: P Blakiston & Son, 1954:110.
463. Bengtsson B, Verneholt J. A follow-up study of hyperbilirubinemia in healthy, full term infants without isoimmunization. Acta Paediatr Scand 1974;63:70.
464. Fohl E, Lombos O. The prognosis of neonatal hemolysis due to A-B-O incompatibility, without exchange transfusion. Ann Paediatr 1964;203:279.
465. Holmes GE, Miller JB, Smith EE. Neonatal bilirubinemia in production of long-term neurological deficits. Am J Dis Child 1968;116:37.
466. Killander A, Michaelsson M, Muller-Eberhard U, et al. Hyperbilirubinemia in full term newborn infants: a follow-up study. Acta Paediatr Scand 1963;52:481.
467. Mores A, Fargasova I, Minarikova E. The relation of hyperbilirubinemia in newborns without isoimmunization to kernicterus. Acta Paediatr Scand 1959;48:490.
468. Wishingrad L, Cornblath M, Takakuwa P, et al. Studies of non-hemolytic hyperbilirubinemia in premature infants: prospective randomized selection for exchange transfusion with observations on the levels of serum bilirubin with and without exchange transfusion and neurologic evaluations one year after birth. Pediatrics 1965;36:162.
469. McKay RJ. Current status of use of exchange transfusion in newborn infants. Pediatrics 1964;33:763.
470. Smith CH. The magic numbers: "20 mg of bilirubin." Pediatrics 1960;36:712.
471. Crosse VM, Meyer TC, Gerrard JW. Kernicterus and prematurity. Arch Dis Child 1955;30:501.
472. Govan ADT, Scott JM. Kernicterus and prematurity. Lancet 1953;1:611.
473. Stern L, Denton RL. Kernicterus in small, premature infants. Pediatrics 1965;35:486.
474. Newns GH, Norton KR. Hyperbilirubinemia in prematurity. Lancet 1958;2:1138.
475. Rapmund G, Bowman JM, Harris RC. Bilirubinemia in non-erythroblastotic premature infants. Am J Dis Child 1960;99: 604.
476. Shiller JG, Silverman WA. "Uncomplicated" hyperbilirubinemia of prematurity. Am J Dis Child 1961;101:587.
477. Cashore WJ. Free bilirubin concentrations and bilirubin-binding affinity in term and preterm infants. J Pediatr 1980;96:521.
478. Keenan WJ, Perlstein PH, Light IJ, et al. Kernicterus in small, sick, premature infants receiving phototherapy. Pediatrics 1972;49:652.
479. Boggs T, Hardy J, Frazier T. Correlation of neonatal serum

total bilirubin concentration and developmental status at age eight months. J Pediatr 1967;71:553.

480. Scheidt PC, Mellits ED, Hardy JB, et al. Toxicity to bilirubin in neonates: infant development during first year in relation to maximum neonatal serum bilirubin concentration. J Pediatr 1977;91:292.
481. Naeye RL. Amniotic fluid infections, neonatal hyperbilirubinemia, and psychomotor impairment. Pediatrics 1978;62:497.
482. Hardy JB, Peeples MO. Serum bilirubin levels in newborn infants: distributions and associations with neurological abnormalities during the first year of life. Johns Hopkins Med J 1971;128:265.
483. Kim MH, Yoon JJ, Sher J, et al. Lack of predictive indices in kernicterus: a comparison of clinical and pathologic factors in infants with or without kernicterus. Pediatrics 1980;66:852.
484. Turkel SB, Guttenberg ME, Moynes DR, et al. Lack of identifiable risk factors for kernicterus. Pediatrics 1980;66:502.
485. Valaes T. Estimation and clinical significance of bilirubin binding status. In: Rubaltelli FF, Jori G, eds. Neonatal jaundice: new trends in phototherapy. New York: Plenum, 1984:79.
486. Valaes T, Gellis SS. Is kernicterus always the definitive evidence of bilirubin toxicity? Pediatrics 1981;67:940.
487. Mollison PL, Walker W. Controlled trials of the treatment of haemolytic disease of the newborn. Lancet 1952;1:429.
488. Armitage P, Mollison PL. Further analysis of controlled trials of treatment of haemolytic disease of the newborn. J Obstet Gynaecol British Empire 1953;60:602.
489. Nilsen ST, Finne PH, Bergsjo P, et al. Males with neonatal hyperbilirubinemia examined at 18 years of age. Acta Paediatr Scand 1984;73:176.
490. Newman TB, Klebanoff M. Peak serum bilirubin in normal-sized infants and neurodevelopmental outcome at age 7: a closer look at the Collaborative Perinatal Study. Am J Dis Child 1992;146:493.
491. Valaes T. Bilirubin distribution and dynamics of bilirubin removal by exchange transfusion. Acta Paediatr Scand 1963; 52(Suppl):149.
492. Kappas A, Drummond GS, Manola T, et al. Sn-protoporphyrin use in the management of hyperbilirubinemia in term newborns with direct Coombs'-positive ABO incompatibility. Pediatrics 1988;81:485.
493. Broman SH, Nichols PL, Kennedy WA. Preschool IQ: prenatal and early developmental correlates. Hillsdale, NJ: Lawrence Erlbaum Associates, 1975:123.
494. Broman SH, Bien E, Shaughanessy P. Low achieving children: the first seven years. Hillsdale, NJ: Lawrence Erlbaum Associates, 1985:132.
495. Lassman FM, Fisch RO, Vetter DK, et al. Early correlates of speech, language and hearing. Littleton, MA: PSG, 1980:366.
496. Seidman DS, Paz I, Stevenson DK, et al. Neonatal hyperbilirubinema and physical and cognitive performance at age 17 years. Pediatrics 1991;88:828.
497. Scheidt PC, Bryla DA, Nelson KB, et al. Phototherapy for neonatal hyperbilirubinemia: six year follow-up of the NICHD clinical trial. Pediatrics 1990;85:455.
498. Odell GB, Storey GNB, Rosenberg LA. Studies in kernicterus. III. The saturation of serum proteins with bilirubin during neonatal life and its relationship to brain damage at five years. J Pediatr 1970;76:12.
499. Johnson L, Boggs TR. Bilirubin-dependent birth damage: incidence and indications for treatment. In: Odell GB, Schaffer R, Simopoulous AP, eds. Phototherapy in the newborn: an overview. Washington, DC: National Academy of Sciences, 1974:122.
500. Scheidt PC, Graubard BI, Nelson KB, et al. Intelligence at six years in relation to neonatal bilirubin level: follow-up of the National Institute of Child Health and Human Development Clinical Trial of Phototherapy. Pediatrics 1991;87:797.
501. Chisin R, Perlman M, Sohmer H. Cochlear and brainstem responses in hearing loss following neonatal hyperbilirubinemia. Ann Otol Rhinol Laryngol 1979;88:352.
502. Belal A Jr. Effects of hyperbilirubinemia on the inner ear in Gunn rats. J Laryngol Otol 1975;89:259.
503. Crabtree N, Gerrard J. Perceptive deafness associated with severe neonatal jaundice. J Laryngol Otol 1950;64:482.
504. Dublin WB. Neurologic lesions of erythroblastosis in relation to nuclear deafness. Am J Clin Pathol 1951;21:935.
505. Tan KL, Skurr BA, Yip YY. Phototherapy in the brain-stem auditory evoked response in neonatal hyperbilirubinemia. J Pediatr 1992;120:306.
506. Wennberg RP, Ahlfors CE, Bickers R, et al. Abnormal auditory brainstem response in a newborn infant with hyperbilirubinemia: improvement with exchange transfusion. J Pediatr 1982;100:624.
507. Esbjörner E, Larsson P, Leissner P, et al. The serum reserve albumin concentration for monoacetyldiaminodiphenyl sulphone and auditory evoked responses during neonatal hyperbilirubinemia. Acta Paediatr Scand 1991;80:406.
508. Streletz LJ, Graziani LJ, Branca PA, et al. Brainstem auditory evoked potentials in full-term and preterm newborns with hyperbilirubinemia and hypoxemia. Neuropediatrics 1986; 17:66.
509. Thoma J, Gerull G, Mrowinski D. A long-term study of hearing in children following neonatal hyperbilirubinemia. Arch Otorhinolaryngol 1986;243:133.
510. Johnson L, Winchester R, Atkins T. Central hearing and communication disorders in hyperbilirubinemia. Pediatr Res 1990; 27:210A.
511. Zimmerman HM, Yannet H. Cerebral sequelae of icterus gravis neonatorum and their relation to kernicterus. Am J Dis Child 1935;49:418.
512. Golub HL, Corwin MJ. Infant cry: a clue to diagnosis. Pediatrics 1982;69:197.
513. Escher-Gräub DC, Fricker HS. Jaundice and behavioral organization in the full-term neonate. Helv Paediatr Acta 1986;41:425.
514. Paludetto R, Mansi G, Rinaldi P, et al. Moderate hyperbilirubinemia does not influence the behavior of jaundiced infants. Biol Neonate 1986;50:43.
515. Telzrow RW, Snyder DM, Tronick E, et al. The behavior of jaundiced infants undergoing phototherapy. Dev Med Child Neurol 1980;22:317.
516. Paludetto R, Mansi G, Rinaldi P, et al. The behavior of jaundiced infants treated with phototherapy. Early Hum Dev 1983;8:259.
517. Crosse VM, Obst D. The incidence of kernicterus (not due to haemolytic disease) among premature babies. In: Sass-Kortsak A, ed. Kernicterus. Toronto: University of Toronto Press, 1961:4.
518. Crosse VM, Wallis PG, Walsh AM. Replacement transfusion of preventing kernicterus of prematurity. Arch Dis Child 1958;33:403.
519. Hugh-Jones K, Slack J, Simpson K, et al. Clinical course of hyperbilirubinemia in premature infants. N Engl J Med 1960; 263:1223.
520. Koch CA, Jones DV, Dine MS, et al. Hyperbilirubinemia in preterm infants: a follow up study. J Pediatr 1959;55:23.
521. Meyer TC. A study of serum bilirubin levels in relation to kernicterus and prematurity. Arch Dis Child 1956;31:75.

522. Grewar DAI. Experiences with kernicterus in premature infants. In: Sas-Kortsak A, ed. Kernicterus. Toronto: University of Toronto Press, 1961:13.
523. Koch CA. Hyperbilirubinemia in premature infants: a follow-up study. J Pediatr 1964;65:1.
524. Vuchovich DM, Haimowitz N, Bowers ND, et al. The incidence of serum bilirubin levels upon the ultimate development of low birth weight infants. J Ment Defic Res 1965; 9:51.
525. Ackerman BD, Dyer GY, Leydorf MM. Hyperbilirubinemia and kernicterus in small premature infants. Pediatrics 1970; 45:918.
526. American Academy of Pediatrics. Standards and recommendations for hospital care of newborn infants. 6th ed. Evanston, IL: American Academy of Pediatrics, 1977.
527. Cashore WJ, Stern L. The jaundiced newborn. In: Warshaw JB, Hobbins JC, eds. The principles and practices of perinatal medicine. Menlo Park, CA: Addison-Wesley, 1982:342.
528. Lee K-S, Gartner LM, Eidelman AI, et al. Unconjugated hyperbilirubinemia in very low birth weight infants. Clin Perinatol 1977;4:305.
529. Brown AK, Kim MH, Wu PYK, et al. Efficacy of phototherapy in prevention and management of neonatal hyperbilirubinemia. Pediatrics 1985;75(Suppl):393.
530. Anagnostakis D, Petmezakis J, Papzissis J, et al. Hearing loss in low-birth-weight infants. Am J Dis Child 1982;136:602.
531. Bergman I, Hirsch RP, Fria TJ, et al. Cause of hearing loss in the high-risk premature infant. J Pediatr 1985;106:95.
532. Salamy A, Eldredge L, Tooley WH. Neonatal status and hearing loss in high risk infants. J Pediatr 1989;114:847.
533. Halpern J, Hosford-Dunn H, Malachowski N. Four factors that actually predict hearing loss in "high risk" neonates. Ear Hear 1987;8:21.
534. Van de Bor M, Ens-Dokkum M, Schreuder AM, et al. Hyperbilirubinemia in low birth weight infants and outcome at 5 years of age. Pediatrics 1992;89:359.
535. DeVries KL, Lary S, Dubowitz LMS. Relationship of serum bilirubin levels to ototoxicity and deafness in high-risk low-birth-weight infants. Pediatrics 1985;76:351.
536. DeVries LS, Lary S, Whitelaw AG, et al. Relationship of serum bilirubin levels and hearing impairment in newborn infants. Early Hum Dev 1987;15:269.
537. Watchko JF, Claasen T. Kernicterus in premature infants: is it gone but not forgotten? Pediatr Res 1992;31:229A.
538. Graziani LJ, Mitchell DG, Kornhauser M, et al. Neurodevelopment of preterm infants: neonatal neurosonographic and serum bilirubin studies. Pediatrics 1992;89:229.
539. O'Shea TM, Dillard RG, Klinepeter KL, et al. Serum bilirubin levels, intracranial hemorrhage, and the risk of developmental problems in very low birth weight infants. Pediatrics 1992;90:888.
540. Van de Bor M, van Zeben-van der Aa TM, Verloove-Vanhorick SP, et al. Hyperbilirubinemia in very preterm infants and neurodevelopmental outcome at two years of age: results of a national collaborative survey. Pediatrics 1989;83: 915.
541. Sykes E, Epstein E. Laboratory measurement of bilirubin. Clin Perinatol 1990;17:397.
542. Mather A. Reliability of bilirubin determinations in icterus of the newborn infant. Pediatrics 1960;26:350.
543. Westphal M, Viergiver E, Roth R. Analysis of a bilirubin survey. Pediatrics 1962;30:12.
544. Maier B, Klempner LB. Abnormally high values for direct bilirubin in the serum of newborns as measured with the DuPont ACA. Am J Clin Pathol 1987;87:642.
545. Ou C-N, Buffone GJ, Herr-Calomeni PJ, et al. Unconjugated hyperbilirubinemia is over-estimated in neonates with cholestasis. Am J Clin Pathol 1985;84:752.
546. Pleasure JR. Bilirubin measurement problems. Pediatrics 1988;82:808.
547. Rutledge JC, Ou C-N. Bilirubin and the laboratory: advances in the 1980's, considerations for the 1990's. Pediatr Clin North Am 1989;36:189.
548. Leslie GI, Philips JB, Cassady G. Capillary and venous bilirubin values: are they really different? Am J Dis Child 1987;141: 1199.
549. Eidelman AI, Schimmel, Algur N, et al. Capillary and venous bilirubin values: they are different—and how! Am J Dis Child 1989;143:642.
550. Sykes E, Maisels MJ, Kusack S. The effect of ambient light on serum bilirubin levels. Pediatr Res 1991;29:236A.
551. Maisels MJ, Gifford K. Neonatal jaundice in full-term infants: role of breastfeeding and other causes. Am J Dis Child 1983; 137:561.
552. Kaplan K, Abramov A. Neonatal hyperbilirubinemia associated with glucose-6-phosphate-dehydrogenase deficiency in Sephardic-Jewish neonates: incidence, severity, and the effect of phototherapy. Pediatrics 1992;90:401.
553. Ellis MI, Hey EN, Walker W. Neonatal death in babies with rhesus isoimmunization. Q J Med 1979;48:211.
554. Hovi L, Siimes MA. Exchange transfusion with fresh heparinized blood is a safe procedure: experiences from 1069 newborns. Acta Paediatr Scand 1985;74:360.
555. Keenan WJ, Novak KK, Sutherland JM, et al. Morbidity and mortality associated with exchange transfusion. Pediatrics 1985;75(Suppl):417.
556. Rubo J, Albrecht K, Lasch P, et al. High-dose intravenous immune globulin therapy for hyperbilirubinemia caused by Rh hemolytic disease. J Pediatr 1992;121:93.
557. Sato K, Hara T, Kondo T, et al. High-dose intravenous gammaglobulin therapy for neonatal immune haemolytic jaundice due to blood group incompatibility. Acta Paediatr Scand 1991;80:163.
558. De Carvalho M, Klaus MH, Merkatz RB. Frequency of breastfeeding and serum bilirubin concentration. Am J Dis Child 1982;136:737.
559. Varimo P, Simili S, Wendt L, et al. Frequency of breast feeding and hyperbilirubinemia. Clin Pediatr 1986;25:112.
560. Yamauchi Y, Yamanouchi I. Breast-feeding frequency during the first 24 hours after birth in full-term neonates. Pediatrics 1990;86:171.
561. Vain N, Acquavita AM, Maisels MJ, et al. The effect of breast feeding frequency on serum bilirubin levels. Pediatr Res 1990; 27:259A.
562. De Carvalho M, Holl M, Harvey D. Effects of water supplementation on physiological jaundice in breast fed babies. Arch Dis Child 1981;56:568.
563. Herrera AJ. Supplemented versus unsupplemented breast feeding. Perinatol Neonatol 1984;:70.
564. Nicoll A, Ginsburg R, Tripp JH. Supplementary feeding and jaundice in newborns. Acta Paediatr Scand 1982;71:759.
565. Kuhr M, Paneth N. Feeding practices and early neonatal jaundice. J Pediatr Gastroenterol Nutr 1982;1:485.
566. Corchia C, Ruiu M, Orzalesi M. Breast feeding and hyperbilirubinemia in full-term newborn infants. Pediatrics 1985;75: 617.
567. Osborn LM, Bolus R. Breast feeding and jaundice in the first week of life. J Fam Pract 1985;20:475.
568. Amato M, Howald H, von Muralt G. Interruption of breast feeding versus phototherapy as treatment of hyperbilirubinemia in full term infants. Helv Paediatr Acta 1985;40:127.
569. Holtrop PC, Ruedisueli K, Maisels MJ. Double versus single

phototherapy in low birthweight infants. Pediatrics 1992;90: 674.

570. Tan KL. The pattern of bilirubin response of phototherapy for neonatal hyperbilirubinemia. Pediatr Res 1982;16:670.
571. Holtrop PC, Madison K, Maisels MJ. A clinical trial of fiberoptic phototherapy versus conventional phototherapy. Am J Dis Child 1992;146:235.
572. Tan KL. Comparison of the effectiveness of phototherapy and exchange transfusion in the management of nonhemolytic neonatal hyperbilirubinemia. J Pediatr 1975;87:609.
573. Clark CF, Torii S, Hamamoto Y, et al. The "bronze" baby syndrome: post mortem data. J Pediatr 1976;88:461.
574. Ebbesen F. Low reserve albumin for binding of bilirubin in neonates with deficiency of bilirubin excretion and bronze baby syndrome. Acta Paediatr Scand 1982;71:415.
575. Ebbesen F, Foged N, Brodersen R. Reduced albumin binding of MADDS—a measure for bilirubin binding—in sick children. Acta Paediatr Scand 1986;75:550.
576. Gartner LM, Lee K-S. Jaundice and liver disease. In: Fanaroff AA, Martin RJ, eds. Neonatal-perinatal medicine. St Louis: CV Mosby, 1992:1075.
577. Odell GB. The dissociation of bilirubin from albumin and its clinical implications. J Pediatr 1959;55:268.
578. Dossett J, Bentley HP Jr. Protein binding of hematin in the newborn. Am J Dis Child 1963;105:27.
579. Catterton Z, Carp W, Bunyaten C, et al. Bilirubin binding capacity in ABO hemolytic disease of the newborn. Clin Res 1979;27:817A.
580. Dawodu AH, Sutherland JN, Becker LE, et al. Influence of heme on the kynetics of bilirubin binding. Pediatr Res 1977; 11:532.
581. Kirk JJ, Ritter DA, Kenny JD. The effect of hematin on bilirubin binding in bilirubin-enriched neonatal cord serum. Biol Neonate 1984;54:53.
582. Ose T, Tsuruhara T, Araki M, et al. Follow-up study of exchange transfusion for hyperbilirubinemia in infants in Japan. Pediatrics 1967;74:371.
583. Desjardins L, Blajchman MA, Chintu C, et al. The spectrum of ABO hemolytic disease of the newborn infant. J Pediatr 1979;95:447.
584. Brouwers HAA, Overbeeke MAM, van Ertbruggen I, et al. What is the best preditor of the severity of ABO-haemolytic disease of the newborn? Lancet 1988;2:641.
585. Ebbesen F. Effect of exchange on serum reserve albumin for binding of bilirubin and index of bilirubin toxicity. Acta Paediatr Scand 1981;70:643.
586. Cepeda EE, Shankaran S. The effect of multiple exchange transfusions on bilirubin binding. Acta Paediatr Scand 1985; 74:545.
587. Grannum P, Kopel J, Moya F, et al. The reversal of hydrops fetalis by intravascular intrauterine transfusion in severe isoimmune fetal anemia. Am J Obstet Gynecol 1988;158: 914.
588. Nicolaides K, Thilaganathan B, Rodeck C, et al. Erythroblastosis and reticulocytosis in anemic fetuses. Am J Obstet Gynecol 1988;159:1063.
589. Nicolaides K, Warensky J, Rodeck C. The relationship of fetal plasma protein concentration and hemoglobin level to the development of hydrops in Rhesus isoimmunization. Am J Obstet Gynecol 1985;152:341.
590. Rightmire D, Nicolaides K, Rodeck C, et al. Mid-trimester fetal blood flow velocities in Rhesus isoimmunization. Obstet Gynecol 1986;68:233.
591. Moya FR, Granham PAT, Riddick L, et al. Atrial natriuretic factor in hydrops fetalis caused by Rh isoimmunization. Arch Dis Child 1990;65:683.
592. Weiner C. Non-hematologic effects of intravascular transfusion on the human fetus. Semin Perinatol 1989;13:338.
593. Phibbs RH, Johnson P, Kitterman JA, et al. Cardiorespiratory status of erythroblastotic infants. I. Relationship of gestational age, severity of hemolytic disease and birth asphyxia to idiopathic respiratory distress syndrome and survival. Pediatrics 1972;49:5.
594. Phibbs RH, Johnson P, Tooley WH. Cardiorespiratory status of erythroblastotic newborn infants. II. Blood volume, hematocrit, and serum albumin concentration in relation to hydrops fetalis. Pediatrics 1974;53:13.
595. Brans YW, Milstead RR, Bailey PE, et al. Blood volume estimates in Coombs'-test-positive infants. N Engl J Med 1974; 290:1450.
596. Phibbs RH, Johnson P, Kitterman JA, et al. Cardiorespiratory status of erythroblastotic newborn infants. III. Intravascular pressures during the first hours of life. Pediatrics 1976;58:484.
597. Barss V, Doubilet P, John-Sutton M, et al. Cardiac output in a fetus with erythroblastosis fetalis: assessment using pulse Doppler. Obstet Gynecol 1987;70:442.
598. Nicolaides K, Clewell W, Rodeck C. Measurement of human fetoplacental blood volume in erythroblastosis fetalis. Am J Obstet Gynecol 1987;157:50.
599. Grawjer LA, Pildes R, Zarif M, et al. Exchange transfusion in the neonate: a controlled study using frozen-stored erythrocytes resuspended in plasma. Am J Clin Pathol 1976;66:117.
600. Ryan SW, Bhaduri B, Harran MJ. Concern over safety of SAGM blood. Arch Dis Child 1988;63:104.
601. Tuchsmid P, Mieth D, Burger R, et al. Potential hazard of hypoalbuminemia in newborn babies after exchange transfusions with adzol red blood cell concentrates. Pediatrics 1990; 85:234.
602. Maisels MJ, Li TK, Piechocki JT, et al. The effect of exchange transfusion on serum ionized calcium. Pediatrics 1974;53:683.
603. Wieland P, Duc G, Binswanger U, et al. Parathyroid hormone response in newborn infants during exchange transfusion with blood supplemented with citrate and phosphate: effects of IV calcium. Pediatr Res 1979;13:963.
604. Maisels MJ, Friedman Z, Marks KH, et al. Calcium homeostasis in exchange transfusion. Pediatr Res 1977;11:537.
605. Batton DG, Maisels MJ, Schulman G. Serum potassium changes following packed red cell transfusions in newborn infants. Transfusion 1983;23:163.
606. Blanchette VS, Gray E, Hardie MJ, et al. Hyperkalemia after neonatal exchange transfusion: risk eliminated by washing red cell concentrates. J Pediatr 1984;105:321.
607. Scanlon JW, Krakaur R. Hyperkalemia following exchange transfusion. J Pediatr 1980;96:108.
608. Thompson S, Inwood MJ, Ferries P, et al. Hyperkalemia in the neonate: a method to provide acceptable donor blood for exchange transfusion. Can J Med Tech 1982;44:31.
609. Sproul A, Smith L. Bilirubin equilibration during exchange transfusion in hemolytic disease of the newborn. J Pediatr 1964;65:12.
610. Chan G, Schiff D. Variance in albumin loading in exchange transfusions. J Pediatr 1976;88:609.
611. Amato M, Blumberg A, Hermann U Jr, et al. The effectiveness of single vs. double volume exchange transfusion in newborn infants with ABO hemolytic disease. Helv Paediatr Acta 1988;43:177.
612. Phibbs RH. Advances in the theory and practice of exchange transfusions. California Medicine 1966;105:442.
613. Aranda JV, Sweet AY. Alterations in blood pressure during exchange transfusion. Arch Dis Child 1977;52:545.
614. Allen FH, Diamond LK. Erythroblastosis fetalis including exchange transfusion technique. Boston: Little, Brown, 1958.

615. Edwards MC, Fletcher MA. Exchange transfusions. In: Fletcher MA, MacDonald MG, eds. Atlas of procedures in neonatology. 2nd ed. Philadelphia: JB Lippincott, 1993.
616. Funato M, Shimada S, Tamai H, et al. Automated exchange transfusion and exchange rate. Acta Paediatr Jpn 1989;31:572.
617. Goldman SL, Tu HC. Automated method for exchange transfusion: a new modification. J Pediatr 1983;102:115.
618. Martin JR. A double catheter technique for exchange transfusion in the newborn infant. N Z Med J 1973;77:167.
619. Campbell N, Stewart I. Exchange transfusion in ill newborn infants using peripheral arteries and veins. J Pediatr 1979; 94:820.
620. Srinivasan G, Shankar AG, Yeh TF, et al. A critical care problem in neonates: exchange transfusion through peripheral artery. Crit Care Med 1980;8:338.
621. Bada HS, Chua C, Salmon JH, et al. Changes in intracranial pressure during exchange transfusion. J Pediatr 1979;94:129.
622. Castor WR. Spontaneous perforation of bowel in newborn following exchange transfusion. Can Med Assoc J 1968;99: 934.
623. Corkery JJ, Dubowitz V, Lister J, et al. Colonic perforation after exchange transfusion. Br Med J 1968;4:345.
624. Hilgartner MW, Lanzkowsky P, Lipsitz P. Perforation of small and large intestine following exchange transfusion. Am J Dis Child 1970;120:70.
625. Livaditis A, Wallgren G, Faxelieus G. Necrotizing enterocolitis after catheterization of the umbilical vessels. Acta Paediatr Scand 1974;63:277.
626. Orme RL, Eades SM. Perforation of the bowel in the newborn as a complication of exchange transfusion. Br Med J 1968;4: 349.
627. Touloukian RJ, Kadar A, Spencer RP. The gastrointestinal complications of neonatal umbilical venous exchange transfusion: a clinical and experimental study. Pediatrics 1973;51:36.
628. Shapiro N, Stein H, Olinsky A. Necrotizing enterocolitis and exchange transfusion. S Afr Med J 1973;47:1236.
629. Black VD, Rumack CM, Lubochenco LO, et al. Gastrointestinal injury in polycythemic term infants. Pediatrics 1985;75: 225.
630. Dodd RY. The risk of transfusion-transmitted infection. N Engl J Med 1992;327:419.
631. Walker RH. Special report: transfusion risks. Am J Clin Pathol 1987;88:374.
632. Parkman R, Mosier D, Umanski I, et al. Graft versus host disease after intrauterine and exchange transfusions for hemolytic disease of the newborn. N Engl J Med 1974;290:359.
633. Lauer BA, Githens JH, Hayward AR, et al. Probable graft-versus-graft reaction in an infant after exchange transfusion and marrow transplantation. Pediatrics 1982;70:43.
634. Chudwin DS, Ammann AJ, Wara DW, et al. Post-transfusion syndrome: rash, eosinophilia, and thrombocytopenia following intrauterine and exchange transfusions. Am J Dis Child 1982;136:612.
635. Seshadri RS, Blake GP. Disseminated intravascular coagulation due to an exchange transfusion with over-heated blood. Aust Paediatr J 1979;15:33.
636. Vaughn RL. Morbidity due to exchange transfusion with heat-hemolyzed blood. Am J Dis Child 1982;136:646.
637. Murphy RJC, Malhotra C, Sweet AY. Death following an exchange transfusion with hemoglobin SC blood. J Pediatr 1980; 96:110.
638. Lackner TE. Drug replacement following exchange transfusion. J Pediatr 1982;100:811.
639. Bailey DN, Bove JR. Chemical and hematological changes in stored CPD blood. Transfusion 1975;15:244.
640. Doyle PE, Eidelman AI, Lee K-S, et al. Exchange transfusion and hypernatremia: possible role in intracranial hemorrhage in very-low birthweight infants. J Pediatr 1978;92:848.
641. Cremer RJ, Perryman PW, Richards DH. Influence of light on the hyperbilirubinemia of infants. Lancet 1958;1:1094.
642. Hammerman C, Eidelman A, Lee K-S, et al. Comparative measurements of phototherapy: a practical guide. Pediatrics 1981;67:368.
643. Eggert P, Stick C. The distribution of radiant power in a phototherapy unit equipped with a metal halide lamp. Eur J Pediatr 1985;143:224.
644. Anderson RR, Parrish JA. The optics of human skin. J Invest Dermatol 1981;77:13.
645. Ennever JF, Carr HS, Speck WT. Potential for genetic damage from multivitamin solutions exposed to phototherapy illumination. Pediatr Res 1983;17:192.
646. Gutcher GR, Yen WM, Odell GB. The *in vitro* and *in vivo* photoreactivity of bilirubin. I. Laser-defined wave length dependence. Pediatr Res 1983;17:120.
647. Gaethel HA. Wavelengths of light producing photodecomposition of bilirubin in serum from a neonate with hyperbilirubinemia. J Pediatr 1975;87:110.
648. Ostrow JD. Photocatabolism of labeled bilirubin in the congenitally jaundiced (Gunn) rat. J Clin Invest 1971;50:707.
649. Sisson TR, Kendall N, Shaw E, et al. Phototherapy of jaundice in the newborn infant. II. Effect of various light intensities. J Pediatr 1972;81:35.
650. Bradley MO, Sharkey NA. Mutagenicity and toxicity of visible fluorescent light to cultured mamalian cells. Nature 1977;266: 724.
651. Speck MT, Rosenkranz PG, Behrman M, Rosenkranz HS. The embryotoxic effects of phototherapy: separation of therapeutic and gametotoxic activities. Photochem Photobiol 1981;33: 121.
652. Speck WT, Rosenkranz HS. Phototherapy for neonatal hyperbilirubinemia: a potential environmental health hazard to newborn infants. Environmental Mutagenesis 1979;1:321.
653. Ayyash H, Hadjigorgiou E, Sofatzis I, et al. Green or blue light phototherapy for neonates with hyperbilirubinemia. Arch Dis Child 1987;82:843.
654. Ayyash H, Hadjigorgiou E, Sofatzis J, et al. Green light phototherapy in newborn infants with ABO hemolytic disease. J Pediatr 1987;111:882.
655. Tan KL. Efficacy of fluorescent daylight, blue, and green lamps in the management of non-hemolytic hyperbilirubinemia. J Pediatr 1989;114:132.
656. Wanamaker WL, Van Gils JF, TerVrugt JW. New blue lamp for phototherapy of hyperbilirubinemia. Lighting, Research, and Technology 1975;7:19.
657. Costarino AT, Ennever JF, Baumgart S, et al. Effect of spectral distribution on isomerization of bilirubin in vivo. J Pediatr 1985;107:125.
658. Gale R, Dranitzki Z, Dohlberg S, Stevenson DK. A randomized, controlled application of the Wallaby Phototherapy System compared with standard phototherapy. J Perinatol 1990; 10:239.
659. Rosenfeld W, Twist D, Concepcion L. A new device for phototherapy treatment of jaundiced infants. J Perinatol 1990;10: 243.
660. Woodall D, Karas JG. A new light on jaundice. Clin Pediatr 1992;31:353.
661. Schuman AJ, Karush G. Fiberoptic vs. conventional home phototherapy for neonatal hyperbilirubinemia. Clin Pediatr 1992;31:345.
662. Eggert P, Stick C, Schroder H. On the distribution of irradiation intensity in phototherapy: measurements of effective irradiance in an incubator. Eur J Pediatr 1985;142:58.

663. Ebbesen F, Moller J. Blue double light: improved method of phototherapy. Arch Dis Child 1976;51:476.
664. Sharma SK, Sood SC, Sharma A, et al. Double vs. single surface phototherapy in neonatal hyperbilirubinemia. Indian Pediatr 1985;2:235.
665. Srivastava KS, Misra PK, Kaul R, et al. Double surface phototherapy vs. single surface phototherapy in neonatal jaundice. Indian J Med Res 1980;71:746.
666. Tan KL. The nature of the dose-response relationship of phototherapy for neonatal hyperbilirubinemia. J Pediatr 1977;90: 446.
667. Maurer HM, Shumway CN, Draper DA, et al. Controlled trial comparing agar, intermittent phototherapy, and continuous phototherapy for reducing neonatal hyperbilirubinemia. J Pediatr 1973;82:73.
668. Rubaltelli FF, Zanardo V, Granati B. Effect of various phototherapy regimens on bilirubin decrement. Pediatrics 1978;61: 838.
669. Wu PYK, Lim RC, Hodgman JE, et al. Effect of phototherapy in preterm infants on growth in the neonatal period. J Pediatr 1974;85:563.
670. Lau SP, Fung KP. Serum bilirubin kinetics in intermittent phototherapy of physiological jaundice. Arch Dis Child 1984;59:892.
671. Vogl TP, Heggy IT, Hiatt IM, et al. Intermittent phototherapy in the treatment of jaundice in the premature infant. J Pediatr 1978;92:627.
672. Indyk L. Physical aspects of phototherapy. In: Bergsma D, Blondheim SH, eds. Bilirubin metabolism in the newborn. New York: American Elsevier, 1976:23.
673. Vogl TP. Phototherapy of neonatal hyperbilirubinemia: bilirubin in unexposed areas of the skin. J Pediatr 1974;85:707.
674. Santella RG, Rosenkranz HS, Speck WT. Intracellular deoxyribonucleic acid-modifying activity of intermittent phototherapy. J Pediatr 1978;93:106.
675. Nicolopoulos D, Hadjigeorgiou E, Malamitsi A, et al. Combined treatment of neonatal jaundice with cholestyramine and phototherapy. J Pediatr 1978;93:684.
676. Tan KL, Jacob E, Liew DSM, et al. Cholestyramine and phototherapy for neonatal jaundice. J Pediatr 1984;104:284.
677. Ebbesen F, Moller J. Agar ingestion combined with phototherapy in jaundiced newborn infants. Biol Neonate 1977; 31:7.
678. Odell GB, Gutcher GR, Whitington PF, et al. Enteral administration of agar as an effective adjunct to phototherapy of neonatal hyperbilirubinemia. Pediatr Res 1983;17:810.
679. Ente G, Lanning EW, Cukor P, et al. Chemical variables and new lamps in phototherapy. Pediatr Res 1972;6:246.
680. Eggert LD, Pollary RA, Folland DS, et al. Home phototherapy treatment of neonatal jaundice. Pediatrics 1985;76:579.
681. Grabert BE, Wardwell C, Harburg SK. Home phototherapy: an alternative to prolonged hospitalization of a full-term, well newborn. Clin Pediatr 1986;25:291.
682. Slater L, Brewer MF. Home versus hospital phototherapy for term infants with hyperbilirubinemia: a comparative study. Pediatrics 1984;73:515.
683. James J, Williams SD, Osborn LM. Home phototherapy for treatment of exaggerated neonatal jaundice enhances breast feeding. Am J Dis Child 1990;144:431.
684. Lightner DA, Linnane WP III, Ahlfors CE. Bilirubin oxidation products in the urine of jaundiced neonates receiving phototherapy. Pediatr Res 1984;18:696.
685. McDonagh AF, Ramonas LM. Jaundice phototherapy: microflow cell photometry reveals rapid billiary response of Gunn rats to light. Science 1978;20:829.
686. Ballowitz L, Muller H-W, Wiese G. Phototherapy in bile duct ligated Gunn rats. Biol Res Pregnancy Perinatol 1984;5: 36.
687. Davis DR, Yeary RA, Lee K. The failure of phototherapy to reduce plasma bilirubin levels in the bile duct-ligated rat. J Pediatr 1981;99:956.
688. Costarino AT, Ennever JF, Baumgart S, et al. Bilirubin photoisomerization in premature neonates under low- and high-dose phototherapy. Pediatrics 1985;75:519.
689. Knox I, Ennever JF, Speck WT. Urinary excretion of an isomer of bilirubin during phototherapy. Pediatr Res 1985;19:198.
690. Ennever JF, Knox I, Denne SC, et al. Phototherapy for neonatal jaundice, in vivo clearance of bilirubin photoproducts. Pediatr Res 1985;19:205.
691. Lamola AA, Flores J, Doleiden FH. Quantum yield and equilibrium position of the configurational photoisomerization of bilirubin bound to human serum albumin. Photochem Photobiol 1982;35:649.
692. Ennever JF, Costarino AT, Knox I, et al. Where does bilirubin go when you turn on the lights? Pediatr Res 1985;19:218A.
693. Diamond I, Schmid R. Neonatal hyperbilirubinemia and kernicterus: experimental support for treatment by exposure to visible light. Arch Neurol 1968;18:699.
694. Haddock JH, Nadler HL. Bilirubin toxicity in human cultivated fibroblasts and its modification by light treatment (34724). Proc Soc Exp Biol Med 1970;134:45.
695. Silberberg DH, Johnson L, Schutta H, et al. Effects of photodegradation products of bilirubin on myelinating cerebellum cultures. J Pediatr 1970;77:613.
696. Bradley MO, Erickson LC, Cohn KW. Non-enzymatic DNA strand breaks induced in mammalian cells by fluorescent lights. Biochim Biophys Acta 1978;520:11.
697. Speck WT, Rosenkranz HS. Intracellular deoxyribonucleic acid-modifying activity of phototherapy lights. Pediatr Res 1976;10:553.
698. Montichone RE, Schneider EL. Induction of sister chromatid exchanges in human cells by fluorescent light. Mutat Res 1979;59:215.
699. Sideris EG, Papageorgiou GC, Charalampous SC, et al. A spectrum response study on single strand DNA breaks, sister chromatid exchanges and lethality induced by phototherapy lights. Pediatr Res 1981;15:1019.
700. McGinty LD, Faller RG. Visible light mutogenesis in *Escherichia coli*. Mutat Res 1982;95:171.
701. Rosenstein BS, Ducore JM. Enhancement by bilirubin of DNA damage induced in human cells exposed to phototherapy light. Pediatr Res 1984;18:3.
702. Speck WT. Effect of phototherapy on fertilization and embryonic development. Pediatr Res 1979;13:506.
703. Amato M, von Muralt G, Auf der Maur P. Double direction phototherapy and light-induced genetic abnormalities in human lymphocytes. Helv Pediatr Acta 1985;40:285.
704. Brown AK, McDonagh AF. Phototherapy for neonatal hyperbilirubinemia: efficacy, mechanism and toxicity. In: Barness LA, ed. Advances in pediatrics. Chicago: Year Book, 1980:341.
705. Maisel P, Jahrig D, Jahrig K. Photodegradation of bilirubin is enhanced by photosensitizers in vitro. Acta Biologica et Medica Germanica 1978;37:1229.
706. Pascale JA, Mims LC, Greenberg MH, et al. Riboflavin and bilirubin response during phototherapy. Pediatr Res 1976;10: 854.
707. Bhatia J, Mims LC, Roesel RA. The effect of phototherapy on amino acid solutions containing multivitamins. J Pediatr 1980; 96:284.
708. Messner KH. Light toxicity to newborn retina. Pediatr Res 1978;12:530.

709. Messner KH, Maisels MJ, Leure duPree AE. Phototoxicity to the newborn primate retina. Invest Ophthalmol 1978;17:178.
710. Robinson J, Moseley MJ, Fielder AR, et al. Light transmission measurements in phototherapy eye patches. Arch Dis Child 1991;66:59.
711. Preis I, Rudolph N. Abdominal distention in newborn infants on phototherapy: the role of eye occlusion. J Pediatr 1979;94:816.
712. Bhupathy K, Sethupathy R, Pildes RS, et al. Electroretinography in neonates treated with phototherapy. Pediatrics 1978;61:189.
713. Dobson V, Corvett RM, Riggs LA. Long-term effect of phototherapy on visual function. J Pediatr 1975;86:555.
714. Dobson V, Riggs LA, Signeland FR. Electroretinographic determination of dark adaptation functions of children exposed to phototherapy as infants. J Pediatr 1974;85:25.
715. Woody NC, Brodkey MJ. Tanning from phototherapy for neonatal jaundice. J Pediatr 1973;82:1042.
716. Gartner LM, Lee K-S. The bronze baby syndrome. J Pediatr 1976;88:465.
717. Kopelman AE, Brown RS, Odell GB. The "bronze" baby syndrome: a complication of phototherapy. J Pediatr 1972;81:466.
718. Onishi I, Itoh S, Isobe K, et al. Mechanism of development of bronze baby syndrome in neonates treated with phototherapy. Pediatrics 1982;69:273.
719. Rubaltelli FF, Jori G, Reddi E. Bronze baby syndrome: a new porphyrin-related disorder. Pediatr Res 1983;17:327.
720. Lund HT, Jacobsen J. Influence of phototherapy on the biliary bilirubin excretion pattern in newborn infants with hyperbilirubinemia. J Pediatr 1974;85:262.
721. Onishi S, Fujikake M, Ogawa Y, et al. Photodegradation products of bilirubin studied by high-pressure liquid chromatography, gel permeation chromatography, nuclear magnetic resonance and mass spectrometry. Birth Defects 1976;12:41.
722. Rubaltelli FF, Jori G, Rossi E, et al. Bronze baby syndrome: new insights on bilirubin-photosensitization of copper-porphyrins. In: Rubaltelli FR, Jori G, eds. Neonatal jaundice: new trends in phototherapy. New York: Plenum, 1984:265.
723. Jori G, Reddi E, Rubaltelli FF. Bronze-baby syndrome: an animal model. Pediatr Res 1990;27:22.
724. Brown RJK, Valman HB, Daganah EG. Diarrhea and light therapy in neonates. Lancet 1970;1:498.
725. Oh W, Karecki H. Phototherapy and insensible water loss in the newborn infant. Am J Dis Child 1972;124:230.
726. Wu PYK, Moosa A. Effect of phototherapy on nitrogen and electrolyte levels and water balance in jaundiced preterm infants. Pediatrics 1978;61:193.
727. Rubaltelli FF, Largajolli G. Effect of light exposure on gut transit time in jaundiced newborns. Acta Paediatr Scand 1973;62:146.
728. Bakken AF. Temporary intestinal lactase deficiency in light-treated jaundiced infants. Acta Paediatr Scand 1977;1977:91.
729. Bujanover Y, Schwartz G, Milbauer B, et al. Lactose malabsorption is not a cause of diarrhea during phototherapy. J Pediatr Gastroenterol Nutr 1985;4:196.
730. Ebbesen F, Edelstein D, Hurtel J. Gut transit time and lactose malabsorption during phototherapy. I. A study using lactose-free human mature milk. Acta Paediatr Scand 1980;69:65.
731. Ebbesen F, Edelsten D, Hurtel J. Gut transit time and lactose malabsorption during phototherapy. II. A study using raw milk from the mothers of infants. Acta Paediatr Scand 1980;69:69.
732. Whitington PF. Effect of jaundice phototherapy on intestinal mucosal bilirubin concentration and lactase activity in the congenitally jaundiced Gunn rat. Pediatr Res 1981;15:345.
733. Whitington PF, Olsen WA, Odell GB. The effect of bilirubin on the function of hamster small intestine. Pediatr Res 1981;15:1009.
734. Berant M, Diamond E, Brick R, et al. Phototherapy-associated diarrhea. Acta Paediatr Scand 1983;72:853.
735. Bell EF, Neidich GA, Cashore WJ, et al. Combined effect of radiant warmer and phototherapy on insensible water loss in low birth weight infants. J Pediatr 1979;94:810.
736. Wu PYK, Hodgman JE. Insensible water loss in preterm infants: changes with post-natal development and non-ionizing radiant energy. Pediatrics 1974;54:704.
737. Wu PYK, Wong WH, Hodgman JE, et al. Changes in blood flow in the skin and muscle with phototherapy. Pediatr Res 1974;8:257.
738. Yeung CY, Tam LS, Chan A, et al. Phenobarbitone prophylaxis for neonatal hyperbilirubinemia. Pediatrics 1971;48:372.
739. Teberg AJ, Hodgman JE, Wu PYK. Effect of phototherapy on growth of low birth weight infant: two year follow up. J Pediatr 1977;91:92.
740. Drew JH, Marriage KJ, Bayle VV, et al. Phototherapy: short and long-term complications. Arch Dis Child 1976;54:454.
741. Lucey JF. Another view of phototherapy. J Pediatr 1974;84:145.
742. Ogawa J, Ogawa Y, Onishi S, et al. Five years' experience in phototherapy. In: Brown AK, Showacre J, ed. Phototherapy for neonatal hyperbilirubinemia: long term implications. Washington, DC: US Department of Health, Education and Welfare, 1977.
743. Dacou-Voutetakis C, Anagnostakis D, Matsaniotis N. Effect of prolonged illumination (phototherapy) on concentrations of luteinizing hormone in human infants. Science 1978;199:1229.
744. Lemaitre B, Toubas PL, Guillo TM, et al. Changes of serum gonadotropin concentrations in premature babies submitted to phototherapy. Biol Neonate 1977;32:113.
745. Lucey JF, Hewitt J. Recent observations on light in neonatal jaundice. Washington, DC: US Department of Health, Education and Welfare, 1977:123.
746. Ahlfors CE, Shwer ML. Absence of bilirubin binding competitors during phototherapy for neonatal jaundice. Early Hum Dev 1982;6:125.
747. Cashore WJ, Karotkin EH, Stern L, et al. The lack of effect of phototherapy on serum bilirubin binding capacity in newborn infants. J Pediatr 1975;87:977.
748. Gartner LM, Lee K-S, Keenan WJ, et al. Effect of phototherapy on albumin-binding of bilirubin. Pediatrics 1985;75:401.
749. Porto SO, Pildes RS, Goodman H. Studies on the effect of phototherapy on neonatal hyperbilirubinemia among low birth weight infants. 2. Protein binding capacity. J Pediatr 1969;75:1048.
750. Korinthenberg R, Schaten TH, Palm D. Sleep state and respiration in newborn infants undergoing phototherapy. Neuropediatrics 1983;14:155.
751. Ramagnoli G, Polidori G, Catalbi L, et al. Phototherapy-induced hypocalcemia. J Pediatr 1979;94:815.
752. Gutcher GR, Odell GB. Hypocalcemia associated with phototherapy in newborn rats: light source dependence. Photochem Photobiol 1983;37:177.
753. Hakanson DO, Bergstrom WH. Phototherapy-induced hypocalcemia in newborn rats: prevention by melatonin. Science 1981;214:807.
754. Gillies DRN, Hay A, Sheltaway MJ, et al. Effect of phototherapy on plasma 25 (OH)-vitamin D in neonates. Biol Neonate 1984;45:225.
755. Valaes T, Harvey-Wilkes K. Pharmacologic approaches to the prevention and treatment of neonatal hyperbilirubinemia. Clin Perinatol 1990;17:245.

756. Rayburn W, Donn S, Piehl E, et al. Antenatal phenobarbital and bilirubin metabolism in the very low birth weight infant. Am J Obstet Gynecol 1988;159:1491.
757. Yaffe SJ, Dorn LD. Effects of prenatal treatment with phenobarbital. Dev Pharmacol Ther 1990;15:215.
758. Wennberg RP, Depp R, Heinrichs WL. Indications for early exchange transfusion in patients with erythroblastosis fetalis. J Pediatr 1978;92:789.
759. Meloni T, Cagnazzo G, Dore A, et al. Phenobarbital for prevention of hyperbilirubinemia in glucose-6-phosphate dehydrogenase-deficient newborn infants. J Pediatr 1973;82:1048.
760. Valdes OS, Maurer HM, Shumway CN, et al. Controlled clinical trial of phenobarbital and/or light in reducing neonatal hyperbilirubinemia in a predominantly Negro population. J Pediatr 1971;79:1015.
761. Lindenbaum L, Hernandorena X, Vial M, et al. Traitement curatif de l'ictère du nouveau-né a terme par le clofibrate: essai therapeutique contrôlé en double aveugle. Arch Fr Pediatr 1981;38:867.
762. Segni G, Polidori G, Romagnoli C. Buculome in prevention of hyperbilirubinaemia in preterm infants. Arch Dis Child 1977; 52:549.
763. Koranyi G, Boriss G. Enzyme inducing action of zixoryn (3-trifluoromethyl-alphaethyl-benzhydrole) in the treatment of neonatal jaundice. Monatsschr Kinderheilkd 1985;133:99.
764. Waltman R, Bonura F, Nigren G, et al. Ethanol in prevention of hyperbilirubinemia in the newborn. Lancet 1969;2:1265.
765. Cutillo S, Meloni T, Dore A. Effect of orotic acid upon serum bilirubin in newborn infants with erythrocyte G-6-PD deficiency. Acta Paediatr Scand 1974;63:143.
766. Gray DWG, Mowart AP. Effects of aspartic acid, orotic acid and glucose on serum bilirubin concentrations in infants born before term. Arch Dis Child 1971;45:123.
767. Kintzel H, Hinkel GK, Schwarze R. The decrease in the serum bilirubin level in premature infants by orotic acid. Acta Paediatr Scand 1971;60:1.
768. Kemper K, Horowitz RI, McCarthy P. Decreased neonatal serum bilirubin with plain agar: a meta-analysis. Pediatrics 1988;82:631.
769. Meloni T, Costa S, Corti R, et al. Agar in control of hyperbilirubinemia in mature newborn infants with erythrocyte G-6-PD deficiency. Biol Neonate 1978;34:295.
770. Lavin A, Sung C, Klibanov AM, et al. Enzymatic removal of bilirubin from blood: a potential treatment for neonatal jaundice. Science 1985;230:543.
771. Cornelius CE, Rogers PA. Prevention of neonatal hyperbilirubinemia in rhesus monkeys by tin-protoporphyrin. Pediatr Res 1984;18:728.
772. Drummond GS, Kappas A. Prevention of neonatal hyperbilirubinemia by tin-protoporphyrin IX, a potent competitive inhibitor of heme oxidation. Proc Natl Acad Sci 1981;78:6466.
773. Drummond GS, Kappas A. Chemoprevention of neonatal jaundice: potency of tin-protoporphyrin in an animal model. Science 1982;217:1250.
774. Kappas A, Drummond GS, Simionatto CS, et al. Control of heme-oxygenase and plasma levels of bilirubin by a synthetic heme analogue, tin-protoprophyrin. Hepatology 1984;4:336.
775. Maines MD. Zinc protoprophyrin is a selective inhibitor of heme oxygenase activity in the neonatal rat. Biochim Biophys Acta 1981;673:339.
776. Berglund L, Angelin B, Blomstrand R, et al. Sn-protoporphyrin lowers serum bilirubin levels, decreases bilirubin output, enhances biliary heme excretion and potently inhibits microsomal heme oxygenase activity in normal human subjects. Hepatology 1988;8:625.
777. Fort FL, Gold J. Phototoxicity of tin-protoporphyrin, tin-mesoporphyrin, and tin-diiododeuteroporphyrin under neonatal phototherapy conditions. Pediatrics 1989;84:1031.
778. Rubaltelli FF, Guerrini P, Reddi E, et al. Tin-protoporphyrin in the management of children with Crigler-Najjar disease. Pediatrics 1989;84:728.
779. Galbraith RA, Drummond GS, Kappas A. Suppression of bilirubin production in the Crigler-Najjar type I syndrome: studies with the heme oxygenate inhibitor tin-mesoporphyrin. Pediatrics 1992;89:175.
780. Stocker R, Glazer AN, Ames BN. Antioxidant activity of albumin-bound bilirubin. Proc Natl Acad Sci USA 1987;84:5918.
781. Stocker R, Yamamoto Y, McDonagh AF, et al. Bilirubin as an antioxidant of possible physiological importance. Science 1987;235:1043.
782. Leonard M, Noy N, Zakim D. The interactions of bilirubin with model and biological membranes. J Biol Chem 1989;264: 5648.
783. Lindeman JH, von Zoeren-Grobben D, Schrijver J, et al. The total free radical trapping ability of cord blood plasma in preterm and term babies. Pediatr Res 1989;26:20.
784. Phelps DL. The role of vitamin E therapy in high-risk neonates. Clin Perinatol 1988;15:955.
785. Pauly TH, Smith M, Gillespie M. Bilirubin as an anti-oxidant: effect on group B streptococci-induced pulmonary hypertension in infant piglets. Biol Neonate 1991;60:320.
786. Bjure J, Liden G, Reinard T, et al. A follow-up study of hyperbilirubinemia in full term infants without isoimmunization. Acta Paediatr Scand 1961;50:437.
787. Culley P, Powell J, Waterhouse J, et al. Sequelae of neonatal jaundice. Br Med J 1970;3:383.
788. Rosta ZM, Bekefi D, Popper P, et al. Neonatal pathological jaundice: seven to nine years follow-up. Acta Paediatr Acad Sci Hung 1971;12:317.
789. Rubin RA, Balow B, Fisch RO. Neonatal serum bilirubin levels related to cognitive development at ages 4 through 7 years. J Pediatr 1979;94:601.

Neonatology: Pathophysiology and Management of the Newborn, Fourth Edition,
edited by Gordon B. Avery, Mary Ann Fletcher, and Mhairi G. MacDonald.
J.B. Lippincott Company, Philadelphia © 1994.

chapter 39

Inherited Metabolic Disorders

BARBARA K. BURTON

Major advances in the recognition and treatment of inborn errors of metabolism have made it more essential than ever that the neonatologist be familiar with the clinical presentation of these disorders. Many of the diseases in this group are associated with symptoms in the neonatal period, and many affected infants find their way into neonatal intensive care units. The likelihood of establishing a diagnosis is often directly related to the awareness of the neonatologist responsible for the neonate's care. Although many of the individual inborn errors of metabolism occur infrequently, collectively, they are not rare. With current diagnostic methods and mass screening programs operating in several states, many of these disorders have been found to be significantly more common than previously believed. There is no doubt that a significant number of children with these disorders are undiagnosed. Every geneticist has had the experience of diagnosing an inborn error of metabolism in a child and discovering that the parents have had one or more other children who died in early infancy of vague or undetermined causes. The other children were probably similarly affected but undiagnosed. Autopsy findings in such cases are often nonspecific and unrevealing unless special biochemical studies are done. Infection is often suspected as the cause of death, and sepsis is a common accompaniment of inherited metabolic disorders.

The significance of the precise diagnosis of metabolic disease cannot be overemphasized. Increasingly, these disorders are lending themselves to successful medical management, and if treatment means the prevention of significant mental retardation or death, even when the numbers are small, the diagnosis is clearly worth pursuing. However, the success of most treatment regimens depends on the earliest possible institution of therapy, stressing the importance of early clinical diagnosis. Even in cases for which no effective therapy exists or if an infant cannot be salvaged, diagnosis is critical for purposes of genetic counseling.

Inborn errors of metabolism are all genetically transmitted, usually in an autosomal recessive or X-linked recessive fashion, and there is usually a substantial risk of recurrence. Prenatal diagnosis is available for many conditions in this group. Awareness of the diagnosis before birth of an at-risk infant can lead to earlier therapy and improved prognosis.

This chapter defines the constellation of findings in the newborn that should alert the clinician to the possibility of inherited metabolic disease. The discussion is confined to the disorders for which manifestations are observed in the first few months of life and does not include the many disorders (*e.g.*, most lysosomal storage diseases) that typically present in later infancy or childhood. The laboratory tools used for infants suspected of having metabolic disease are discussed. Treatment of important groups of metabolic disorders are addressed, focusing on the stabilization and acute management of patients with these conditions.

MANIFESTATIONS OF INBORN ERRORS OF METABOLISM

A list of the inborn errors of metabolism that have been described clinically in early infancy is found in Table 39-1. This table cannot be considered complete because it includes only the disorders for which manifestations in the first few months of life have been documented in the literature. It is likely that disorders typically occurring later in childhood may occasionally present as early as the first month of life. New disorders causing neonatal disease will undoubtedly continue to be described. A single literature reference is listed for each disorder in the table, and detailed information about most of the disorders listed can be found in recent editions of reference textbooks.[79,80]

Table 39-2 is a summary of the major clinical findings seen in infants with inborn errors of metabolism and the disorders with which they have been associated. Table 39-3 serves as a guideline for abnormal laboratory findings seen in these disorders.

ACUTE LIFE-THREATENING SYMPTOMS

Several inherited metabolic disorders, most notably the organic acidemias, urea cycle defects, and certain disorders of amino acid metabolism, typically present with acute life-threatening symptoms in the neonatal period. Because they are associated with protein intolerance, symptoms usually begin after feedings have been instituted. Affected infants are typically full term and usually appear normal at birth. The interval between the first protein feeding and clinical symptoms ranges from hours to weeks. The initial findings are usually those of lethargy and poor feeding, as seen in almost any sick infant. Although sepsis is often the first consideration in infants who present in this way, these symptoms in a full-term infant with no specific risk factors strongly suggest a metabolic disorder. Infants with inborn errors of metabolism may rather quickly become debilitated and septic, and it is therefore important that the presence of sepsis not exclude consideration of other possibilities. The lethargy associated with these conditions is an early symptom of a metabolic encephalopathy that may progress to coma. Other signs of central nervous system (CNS) dysfunction, such as seizures and abnormal muscle tone, may exist. Evidence of cerebral edema may be observed, and intracranial hemorrhage occasionally occurs.[81]

An infant with an inborn error of metabolism who presents more abruptly or in whom the lethargy and poor feeding go unnoticed may first come to attention because of apnea or respiratory distress. The apnea is typically central in origin and a symptom of the metabolic encephalopathy, but tachypnea may be a symptom of an underlying metabolic acidosis, as occurs in the organic acidemias. Infants with urea cycle defects and evolving hyperammonemic coma initially exhibit hyperventilation, which leads to respiratory alkalosis.

Vomiting is a striking feature of many of the inborn errors of metabolism associated with protein intolerance, although somewhat less common in the newborn than in the older infant. If persistent vomiting occurs in the neonatal period, it usually signals significant underlying disease. Inborn errors of metabolism should always be considered in the differential diagnosis. It is common for an infant to be diagnosed as having a metabolic disorder after having undergone surgery for suspected pyloric stenosis.[82] Formula intolerance is frequently suspected, and many affected infants have numerous formula changes before a diagnosis is finally established.

The basic laboratory studies that should be obtained for an infant who has acute life-threatening symptoms consistent with an inborn error of metabolism are listed in Table 39-4.

HYPERAMMONEMIA

Among the most important laboratory findings associated with inborn errors of metabolism presenting with acute overwhelming symptoms is hyperammonemia. A plasma ammonia level should be obtained for any infant with unexplained vomiting, lethargy, or other evidence of an encephalopathy. Significant hyperammonemia is observed in a limited number of conditions. Inborn errors of metabolism, including urea cycle defects and many of the organic acidemias, are at the top of the list. Also in the differential diagnosis is a condition referred to as transient hyperammonemia of the newborn (THAN).[83] Ammonia levels in these conditions frequently exceed 1000 μmol/L. The finding of marked hyperammonemia provides an important clue to diagnosis and indicates the need for urgent treatment to reduce the ammonia level. The degree of neurologic impairment and developmental delay subsequently observed in infants with urea cycle defects depends on the duration of the neonatal hyperammonemic coma.[84]

A flow chart for the differentiation of conditions producing significant hyperammonemia in the newborn is provided in Figure 39-1. The timing of the onset of symptoms may provide an important clue. Infants with urea cycle defects typically do not become symptomatic until after 24 hours of age. Patients with some of the organic acidemias, such as glutaric acidemia type II, or with pyruvate carboxylase deficiency may exhibit symptomatic hyperammonemia during the first 24 hours. Symptoms in the first 24 hours are characteristic of THAN, a condition that is poorly understood but apparently not genetically determined. The typical patient with this disorder is a large premature infant (mean gestational age, 36 weeks) who has symptomatic pulmonary disease, often from birth, and severe hyperammonemia. Survivors do not have recurrent episodes of hyperam-

Text continued on page 730

TABLE 39–1
INBORN ERRORS OF METABOLISM THAT PRESENT IN EARLY INFANCY

Disorder	Reference
Disorders of Carbohydrate Metabolism	
1. Galactosemia (*i.e.*, galactose-1-phosphate uridyl transferase deficiency)	1
2. Hereditary fructose intolerance (*i.e.*, fructose-1-phosphate aldolase deficiency)	2
3. Fructose-1,6-diphosphatase deficiency	3
4. Glycogen storage disease type I (*i.e.*, von Gierke disease, glucose-6-phosphatase deficiency)	4
5. Glycogen storage disease type II (*i.e.*, Pompe disease, α-glucosidase deficiency)	5
6. Glycogen storage disease type III (*i.e.*, limit dextrinosis, debrancher deficiency)	4
7. Glycogen storage disease type IV (*i.e.*, amylopectinosis, brancher deficiency)	6
8. Phosphoenolpyruvate carboxykinase deficiency	7
Disorders of Amino Acid Metabolism	
9. Maple syrup urine disease	8
10. Hypervalinemia	9
11. Hyper-β-alaninemia	10
12. Nonketotic hyperglycinemia	11
13. Phenylketonuria	12
14. Hereditary tyrosinemia	13
15. Hyperornithinemia-hyperammonemia-homocitrullinuria syndrome	14
16. Lysinuric protein intolerance	15
17. Methylene tetrahydrofolate reductase deficiency	16
18. Pyridoxine dependency with seizures (*i.e.*, presumed glutamic acid decarboxylase deficiency)	17
Organic Acidemias	
19. Methylmalonic acidemia	18
20. Methylmalonic acidemia with homocystinuria	19
21. Propionic acidemia	20
22. Isovaleric acidemia	21
23. 3-Methyl crotonyl CoA carboxylase deficiency	22
24. Holocarboxylase synthetase deficiency (*i.e.*, early-onset multiple carboxylase deficiency)	23
25. Biotinidase deficiency (*i.e.*, late-onset multiple carboxylase deficiency)	24
26. Glutaric acidemia type I	25
27. Glutaric acidemia type II (*i.e.*, multiple acyl CoA dehydrogenase deficiency, severe)	26
28. Ethylmalonic-adipic aciduria (*i.e.*, later-onset glutaric acidemia type II, multiple acyl CoA dehydrogenase deficiencies, mild)	27
29. 3-Hydroxy-3-methylglutaric acidemia	28
30. 2-Methylacetoacetyl-CoA thiolase deficiency	29
31. D-Glyceric acidemia with hyperglycinemia	30
32. 3-Hydroxyisbutyryl-CoA deacylase deficiency	31
33. Mevalonic aciduria	32
34. Glutathione synthetase deficiency	33
35. 3-Hydroxyisobutyric aciduria	34
36. 3-Methylglutaconic aciduria	35
Urea Cycle Disorders	
37. Carbamyl phosphate synthetase deficiency	36
38. Ornithine transcarbamylase deficiency	36
39. Citrullinemia	36
40. Arginosuccinic aciduria	36
41. Arginase deficiency	37
42. *N*-Acetylglutamate synthetase deficiency	38

(*continued*)

TABLE 39–1
INBORN ERRORS OF METABOLISM THAT PRESENT IN EARLY INFANCY (*continued*)

Disorder	Reference
Fatty Acid Oxidation Defects	
43. Short-chain acyl CoA dehydrogenase deficiency	39
44. Medium-chain acyl CoA dehydrogenase deficiency	40
45. Long-chain acyl CoA dehydrogenase deficiency	41
46. Primary systemic carnitine deficiency	42
47. Long-chain 3-hydroxyacyl-CoA dehydrogenase deficiency	43
Lactic Acidemias	
48. Pyruvate dehydrogenase deficiency	44
49. Pyruvate carboxylase deficiency	45
50. Fumaric aciduria	46
51. NADH-CoQ reductase (*i.e.*, complex I) deficiency	47
52. Cytochrome oxidase (*i.e.*, complex IV) deficiency	48
Transport Disorders	
53. Cystic fibrosis	49
54. Infantile free sialic acid storage disease	50
55. Hartnup disease	51
Lysosomal Storage Disorders	
56. GM_1 gangliosidosis type I (*i.e.*, generalized gangliosidosis, β-galactosidase deficiency)	52
57. Gaucher disease type II (*i.e.*, glucocerebrosidase deficiency)	53
58. Niemann–Pick disease types A and B (*i.e.*, sphingomyelinase deficiency)	54
59. Mannosidosis (*i.e.*, α-mannosidase deficiency)	55
60. Fucosidosis (*i.e.*, α-fucosidase deficiency)	56
61. Farber disease (*i.e.*, acid ceramidase deficiency)	57
62. Wolman disease (*i.e.*, acid lipase deficiency)	58
63. Krabbe disease (*i.e.*, galactocerebrosidase deficiency)	59
64. Mucopolysaccharidosis type VI (*i.e.*, Maroteaux–Lamy syndrome, arylsulfatase B deficiency)	60
65. Mucopolysaccharidosis type VII (*i.e.*, β-glucuronidase deficiency)	61
66. Mucolipidosis type II (*i.e.*, I-cell disease)	62
67. Mucolipidosis type IV	63
68. Multiple sulfatase deficiency	64
69. Sialidosis type II (*i.e.*, neuraminidase deficiency)	65
Peroxisomal Disorders	
70. Zellweger syndrome	66
71. Neonatal adrenoleukodystrophy	66
72. Hyperpipecolic acidemia	66
73. Rhizomelic chondrodysplasia punctata	66
Other Disorders	
74. Congenital adrenal hyperplasia	67
75. Lysosomal acid phosphatase deficiency	68
76. Menke kinky-hair syndrome	69
77. Hereditary orotic aciduria	70
78. Hypophosphatasia	71
79. Molybdenum cofactor deficiency	72
80. Sulfite oxidase deficiency	73
81. Crigler–Najjar syndrome	74
82. $Alpha_1$-antitrypsin deficiency	75
83. Canavan disease (*i.e.*, aspartoacylase deficiency)	76
84. Steroid sulfatase deficiency	77
85. Senger syndrome	78

TABLE 39–2
MAJOR CLINICAL MANIFESTATIONS OF INBORN ERRORS OF METABOLISM IN EARLY INFANCY

Clinical Findings	Associated Disorders*
Failure to thrive, poor feeding	Essentially all
Vomiting	1–3, 9, 10, 13–16, 19–24, 26–30, 35, 37–47, 61, 62, 74, 75
Diarrhea	1–4, 14, 16, 30, 33, 53, 54, 58, 62
Lethargy or coma	1, 3, 9–12, 15, 16, 19–26, 29, 30, 33–35, 43–50
Abnormal muscle tone	1, 5–12, 16, 19–27, 29, 31–34, 37–41, 43–47, 50–52, 54, 56–58, 61, 63, 65, 66, 70–72, 76–80, 83
Seizures	1–4, 6, 8, 9, 11, 12, 15–22, 24–27, 29–31, 33, 35, 37–40, 43–51, 54, 56, 57, 60, 61, 63, 70, 71, 74, 76, 78, 79, 83
Respiratory distress, apnea, or both	3–6, 8, 9, 12, 17, 19–22, 24, 25, 27, 35, 37–45, 47–52, 56, 57, 61, 78–80
Hepatomegaly	1–8, 15, 16, 19, 26, 27, 29, 33, 38, 40, 41, 43–47, 49, 54, 56–62, 64–66, 68–70, 72, 82
Abnormal eye findings (*e.g.*, cataract, lens dislocation, retinopathy)	1, 16, 33, 46, 55, 57, 58, 60, 64–72, 75, 78, 79, 82–84
Dysmorphic features	27, 32, 33, 35, 48, 70–73, 79
Cardiomyopathy	5–7, 30, 36, 45–47, 85
Abnormal skin (*i.e.*, ichthyosis or rashes)	13, 24, 25, 55, 68, 73, 84
Coarse facial features	54, 56, 59, 60, 64–66, 68, 69
Macroglossia	5, 56, 61, 66
Macrocephaly	26, 56, 63, 64, 83
Abnormal odor	9, 13, 14, 22–24, 27
Abnormal hair	16, 40, 76

* Numbers in this column refer to the numbered disorders in Table 39-1.

monemia and may or may not exhibit neurologic sequelae, depending on the extent of the neonatal insult. There are some affected infants who survive with normal intelligence despite extraordinarily high ammonia levels.[83]

Infants who develop severe hyperammonemia after 24 hours of age usually have a urea cycle defect or an organic acidemia; the infants with organic acidemias usually have a metabolic acidosis and ketonuria. Urine organic acids should always be obtained, regardless of whether or not acidosis is present. Metabolic acidosis is not a feature of the urea cycle defects. Plasma amino acid analysis is helpful in the differentiation of the specific defects in this group. Characteristic amino acid abnormalities provide a definitive diagnosis of citrullinemia and argininosuccinic aciduria. Although no diagnostic amino acid elevations are observed in carbamyl phosphate synthetase deficiency or ornithine transcarbamylase deficiency, a low or undetectable level of plasma citrulline is observed in both of these conditions. This finding is helpful in differentiating these two conditions from THAN, in which the plasma citrulline level is normal. However, plasma citrulline is not accurately measured in all laboratories performing amino acid analysis, probably because it is important in few other clinical settings, and in clinical situations in which this is a critical diagnostic test, samples should be sent to laboratories with expertise in the differentiation of urea cycle defects. Carbamyl phosphate synthetase deficiency and ornithine transcarbamylase deficiency may be differentiated by measuring urine orotic acid,

TABLE 39–3
COMMON LABORATORY FINDINGS ASSOCIATED WITH INBORN ERRORS OF METABOLISM IN EARLY INFANCY

Laboratory Findings	Associated Disorders*
Metabolic acidosis	1–4, 6, 8, 9, 19–30, 34, 35, 43–52, 85
Hyperammonemia	15, 16, 19, 21, 22, 24–26, 28–30, 37–47
Hypoglycemia	1–4, 6, 8, 14, 19, 23, 26–29, 36, 43–47, 49, 75
Elevated lactate	3, 4, 8, 19, 21, 24, 25, 28, 29, 35, 36, 43–52, 85
Direct hyperbilirubinemia, elevated transaminases, or both	1, 2, 6–8, 14, 16, 26, 33, 38, 40, 41, 43–47, 58, 62, 70, 72, 82
Non-glucose reducing substance in urine	1, 2, 14
Positive urine ferric chloride test	9, 13, 14
Ketonuria	3, 9, 19, 21–26, 30, 35, 49
Neutropenia	12, 16, 19, 21, 22, 34, 36, 37, 77
Thrombocytopenia	16, 19–23, 25, 43
Anemia	14, 16, 19, 20, 22, 33, 34, 36, 54, 62, 77, 78
Vacuolated lymphocytes on peripheral smear	4, 56–60, 62, 64–66, 69

* Numbers in this column refer to the numbered disorders in Table 39-1.

which is low in the former and elevated in the latter. The pattern of inheritance of the two may help to differentiate them; ornithine transcarbamylase deficiency, an X-linked disorder, rarely produces severe hyperammonemia in a female infant, and carbamyl phosphate synthetase deficiency, an autosomal recessive disorder, occurs with equal frequency in the two genders.

Although the clinical and laboratory evaluation outlined should lead to a specific tentative diagnosis for virtually all patients, liver biopsy may be indicated for enzymatic confirmation of the diagnoses of carbamyl phosphate synthetase and ornithine transcarbamylase deficiencies, because these diagnoses dictate rigid lifelong therapy. Acute treatment should be based on the presumptive diagnosis, with biopsy considered only after the infant is stabilized.

Less significant elevations of plasma ammonia than those associated with inborn errors of metabolism and THAN can be observed in a variety of other conditions associated with liver dysfunction, including sepsis, generalized herpes infection, and perinatal asphyxia. Liver function studies should be obtained in evaluating the significance of moderate elevations of plasma ammonia. However, even in cases of severe hepatic necrosis, it is rare for ammonia levels to exceed 500 μmol/L or 900 μg/100 mL.[85] Mild transient hyperammonemia with ammonia levels as high as twice normal is relatively common in the newborn, especially in the premature infant, and is usually asymptomatic. It appears to be of no clinical significance, and there are no long-term neurologic sequelae.[86]

TABLE 39–4
LABORATORY STUDIES FOR AN INFANT SUSPECTED OF HAVING AN INBORN ERROR OF METABOLISM

Complete blood count with differential
Urinalysis
Blood gases
Electrolytes
Blood glucose
Plasma ammonia
Urine reducing substances
Urine ketones if acidosis or hypoglycemia present
Urine ferric chloride dinitrophenylhydrazine test
Plasma and urine amino acids, quantitative
Urine organic acids
Lactate and pyruvate, if acidosis present

METABOLIC ACIDOSIS

The second important laboratory feature of many of the inborn errors of metabolism during acute episodes of illness is metabolic acidosis with an in-

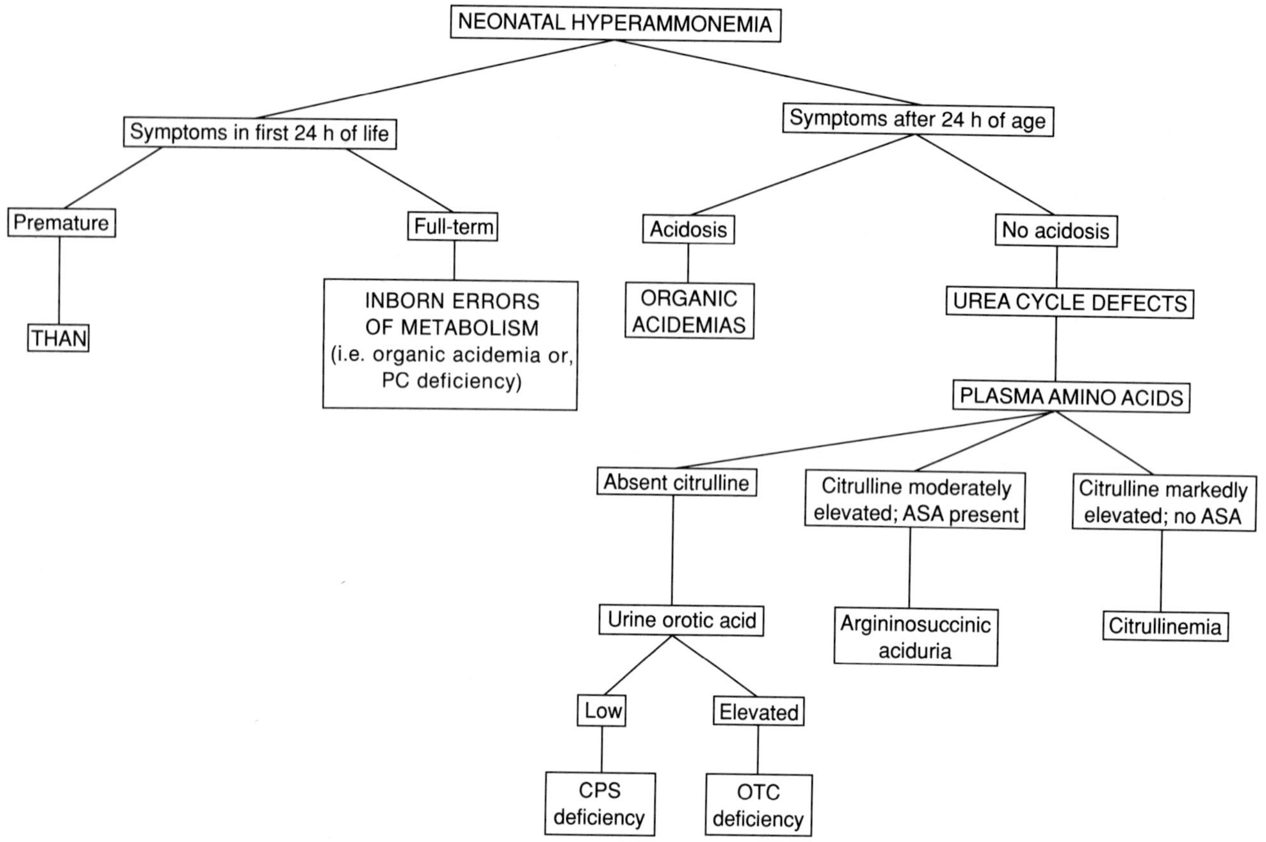

FIG. 39–1. Differentiating between conditions that produce severe neonatal hyperammonemia. (ASA, argininosuccinic acid; CPS, carbamyl phosphate synthetase; OTC, ornithine transcarbamylase; PC, pyruvate carboxylase; THAN, transient hyperammonemia of the newborn.)

creased anion gap, readily demonstrable by measurement of arterial blood gases or serum electrolytes and bicarbonate. A flow chart for the evaluation of infants with this finding is provided in Figure 39-2. An increased anion gap (> 16) is observed in many inborn errors of metabolism and in most other conditions producing metabolic acidosis in the neonate. The differential diagnosis of metabolic acidosis with a normal anion gap is essentially limited to two conditions, diarrhea and renal tubular acidosis. Among the inborn errors, the largest group typically associated with overwhelming metabolic acidosis in infancy is the group of organic acidemias, including methylmalonic acidemia, propionic acidemia, and isovaleric acidemia. The list of disorders in this group has expanded dramatically as new disorders have been defined through the use of organic acid analysis.

In addition to specific organic acid intermediates, plasma lactate is often elevated in organic acidemias as a result of secondary interference with coenzyme A (CoA) metabolism. Neutropenia and thrombocytopenia are commonly observed and further underscore the clinical similarity of these disorders to neonatal sepsis. Hyperammonemia, sometimes as dramatic as that associated with urea cycle defects, is commonly but not uniformly seen in critically ill neonates with organic acidemias.

The metabolic acidosis associated with organic acidemias and certain other inborn errors of metabolism may have significant adverse impact on many different organ systems, which may lead to the erroneous diagnosis of a wide variety of seemingly unrelated disorders. I had the experience of caring for an infant with isovaleric acidemia who presented at 10 days of age with respiratory distress, severe metabolic acidosis, a dilated heart, and poor cardiac output. The infant was suspected of having the hypoplastic left heart syndrome or other severe congenital heart disease, and cardiac catheterization was performed, even though members of the nursing staff had observed that the infant had a strong unpleasant odor, reminiscent of sweaty feet. Personnel in the catheterization laboratory also noticed that the blood had a strong peculiar odor, but it was not until 18 hours later, long after significant heart disease had been ruled out, that the diagnosis of metabolic disease was first considered. Despite attempts at therapy with dialysis and other measures, the child succumbed to the disease. In this case, the metabolic acidosis led to poor function of the cardiac muscle and not the reverse.

Another child subsequently found to have methylmalonic acidemia was admitted through the emergency room with severe metabolic acidosis and a tight, distended abdomen with evidence of multiple air–fluid levels on x-ray films. The history revealed that the child had fed poorly since birth and had repeated episodes of vomiting despite several formula changes. Intestinal obstruction was suspected, and the child was taken to the operating room, where most of the small intestine was found to be infarcted, presumably secondary to the acidosis and poor tissue perfusion. No anatomic abnormalities were found. Postoperatively, metabolic disease was considered, and the diagnosis of a vitamin B_{12}–responsive form of methylmalonic acidemia was made. The infant died of complications of the disease despite the fact that early diagnosis and treatment of this disorder, before the terminal episode, should have been associated with a good prognosis.

Defects in pyruvate metabolism or in the respiratory chain may lead to primary lactic acidosis presenting as severe metabolic acidosis in infancy.[87,88] Unlike most of the other conditions presenting acutely in the newborn, the clinical features of these disorders are unrelated to protein intake. Disorders in this group should be considered in patients with lactic acidosis who have normal urine organic acids. Differentiation of the various disorders in this group can be facilitated by measuring plasma pyruvate and calculating the lactate/pyruvate ratio. A normal ratio (<25) suggests a defect in pyruvate dehydrogenase (PDH) or in gluconeogenesis, and an elevated ratio (>35) suggests pyruvate carboxylase deficiency, a respiratory chain defect, or a mitochondrial myopathy.

Disorders of protein intolerance and certain other inborn errors of metabolism should be seriously considered in any infant who presents with symptoms of acute overwhelming illness or who has a history of poor feeding or vomiting. The finding of metabolic acidosis or hyperammonemia, with or without other supportive findings, should lead to a strong suspicion of metabolic disease, prompting immediate diagnostic evaluation and treatment.

Not all infants with life-threatening metabolic disease have metabolic acidosis or hyperammonemia. For example, patients with nonketotic hyperglycinemia typically present in the neonatal period with evidence of severe and progressive CNS dysfunction, including obtundation, seizures, and altered muscle tone, but exhibit neither metabolic acidosis nor hyperammonemia.[89] Even patients with galactosemia may rarely present with symptoms of acute CNS toxicity, which may progress to cerebral edema, when galactose-1-phosphate levels rise precipitously. A series of laboratory studies designed to screen for inborn errors of metabolism should be obtained for any infant with clinical findings suggesting an inborn error of metabolism, even if metabolic acidosis and hyperammonemia are not present. These studies are listed in Table 39-4. Most are self-explanatory. Although not available in many hospital laboratories,

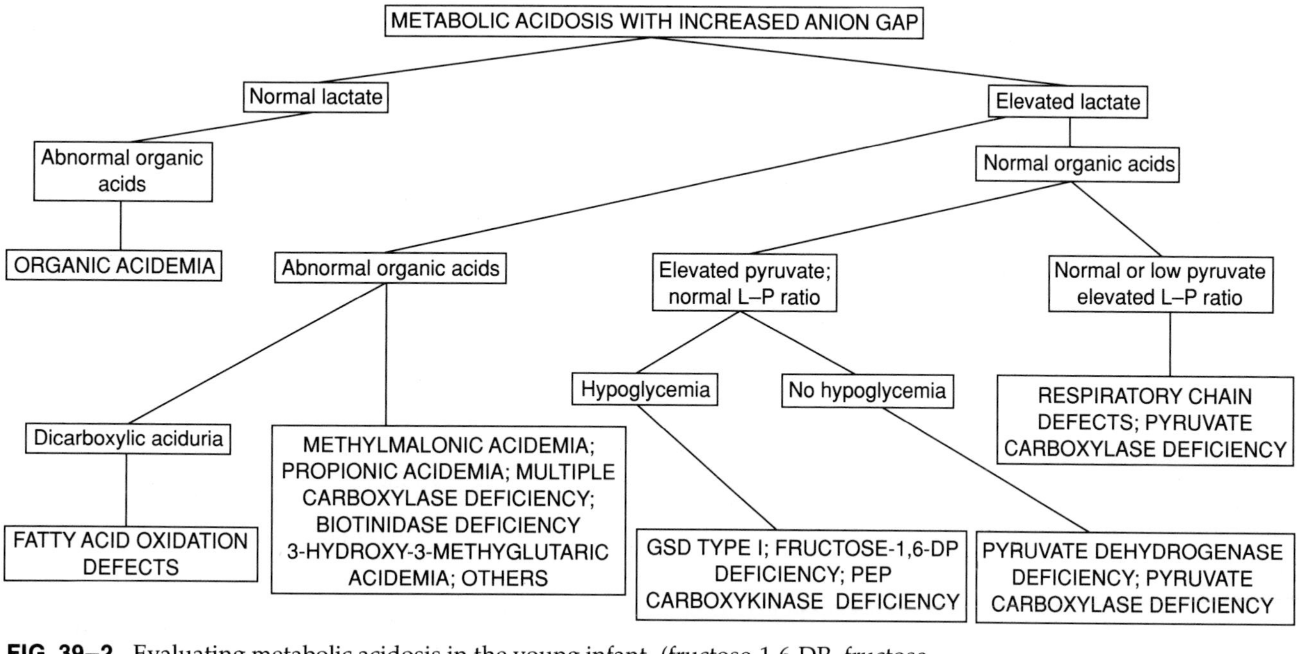

FIG. 39–2. Evaluating metabolic acidosis in the young infant. (fructose-1,6-DP, fructose-1,6-diphosphatase; GSD, glycogen storage disease; L/P; lactate/pyruvate.)

TABLE 39–5
DISORDERS ASSOCIATED WITH NON-GLUCOSE REDUCING SUBSTANCES IN URINE

Disorder	Compound
Galactosemia	Galactose
Hereditary fructose intolerance	Fructose
Hereditary tyrosinemia	*p*-Hydroxy-phenylpyruvic acid
Galactokinase deficiency	Galactose
Essential fructosuria	Fructose
Pentosuria	Xylulose
Severe liver disease with secondary galactose intolerance	Galactose

amino acid and organic acid analysis can be obtained in any part of the country through reference laboratories or through referral of samples to medical center genetics units. It is important to insist that any reference laboratory used for this purpose provide prompt test results and reference ranges and provide interpretation of abnormal results.

Urine testing for reducing substances should be performed using Benedict reagent (Clinitest tablets, Miles, Elkhart, IN). If positive, the urine should be tested for glucose by dipstick. A non-glucose reducing substance in the urine is probably galactose, but there are other possibilities (Table 39-5). The urine ferric chloride test is a simple and rapid test that can lead to the early recognition of maple syrup urine disease, before results of amino acid analysis are available. In addition to the branched chain ketoacids, there are several other substances and disorders that produce a color change with ferric chloride. These are shown in Table 39-6. The dinitrophenylhydrazine screening test is useful in screening for maple syrup urine disease. All of these tests are simple and straightforward and can be performed at the bedside. Reagents should be available in any hospital chemistry laboratory.

TREATMENT

When an inborn error of metabolism, such as an organic acidemia or urea cycle defect, is suspected in a critically ill infant, immediate treatment should be initiated even if a definitive diagnosis may not yet be established. Within 48 to 72 hours, the results of amino acid and organic acid analyses should be available, allowing diagnostic confirmation in most cases. Appropriate and aggressive treatment before the confirmation of a diagnosis may be lifesaving and may avert or reduce the neurologic sequelae of some of these disorders. The immediate treatment of infants with disorders in this group has two primary goals. The first is the removal of accumulated metabolites, such as organic acid intermediates or ammonia. At the first suspicion of a disorder associated with protein intolerance, protein intake in the form of breast milk, infant formula, or hyperalimentation should immediately be discontinued. In critically ill infants, accumulated metabolites should be removed by hemodialysis or peritoneal dialysis. Although either can be used, hemodialysis is a much more expeditious method of reducing the plasma ammonia level.[91] Exchange transfusions have been used in the past but are substantially less effective than dialysis. In infants who are comatose, ventilator dependent, or exhibit evidence of cerebral edema, dialysis should be instituted immediately without waiting to see if there is a response to dietary manipulation, bicarbonate infusion, medication, or other less aggressive therapy. Maximal supportive care should be provided simultaneously.

TABLE 39–6
DISORDERS ASSOCIATED WITH A POSITIVE FERRIC CHLORIDE REACTION

	Urine	
Disorder	Major Compound	Color
Phenylketonuria	Phenylpyruvic acid	Green
Hereditary tyrosinemia	*p*-Hydroxyphenylpyruvic acid	Green, fading rapidly
Maple syrup urine disease	Branched-chain ketoacids	Gray-green
Histidinemia	Imidazolepyruvic acid	Blue-green
Alkaptonuria	Homogentisic acid	Dark brown
Diabetic ketoacidosis	Acetoacetic acid	Cherry red
Melanoma	Melanin	Black
Pheochromocytoma	Catecholamines	Blue-green
Formimino-transferase deficiency	Imidazolcarboxamide	Gray-green
Drug intoxication	Salicylates	Purple
	Phenothiazines	Purple
	p-Aminosalicylic acid	Red-brown
	Lysol	Green
Conjugated hyperbilirubinemia	Bilirubin	Green

If an organic acidemia is suspected, vitamin B_{12} (1 mg) should be given intramuscularly in case the patient turns out to have a B_{12}-responsive form of methylmalonic acidemia. Biotin (10 mg) should be given orally or by nasogastric tube, because some patients with multiple carboxylase deficiency are biotin responsive. If acidosis exists, intravenous bicarbonate should be liberally administered. Calculations of bicarbonate requirements appropriate for the treatment of other conditions are rarely adequate because of ongoing production of organic acids or lactate. The acid–base status should be monitored frequently, with therapy adjusted accordingly.

After removing toxic metabolites, the second major goal of therapy in infants with inborn errors of metabolism should be to prevent catabolism. Ten percent glucose should be liberally administered intravenously, because it is important to provide as many calories as possible. Intralipids can be given to infants with urea cycle defects and other disorders in which dietary fat plays no role. Protein should not be withheld indefinitely. If clinical improvement is observed and a final diagnosis has not been established, some amino acid intake should be provided after 2 to 3 days of complete protein restriction. Essential amino acids or total protein can be provided orally or intravenously at an initial dose of 0.5 g protein/kg body weight/24 hours. This should be increased incrementally to 1.0 g/kg/24 hours and held at that level until the diagnostic evaluation is complete and plans can be made for definitive long-term therapy. Therapy should be planned in conjunction with a geneticist or specialist in metabolic disease. Until then, supplemental calories and nutrients can be provided orally using protein-free diet powder (Product 80056, Mead Johnson, Evansville, IN).

The chronic therapy of urea cycle defects and most of the organic acidemias involves restriction of dietary protein. Depending on the specific diagnosis, this may be accomplished by simple restriction of total protein intake in breast milk or standard infant formula or by use of special formulas designed for individual inborn errors of metabolism. Formulas have been developed for many of the more common metabolic disorders and are commercially available. These specialized formulas are typically deficient in one or several specific amino acids. Dietary treatment alone may be effective in management of some patients with organic acidemias and in several disorders of amino acid metabolism, such as maple syrup urine disease.

In several of the vitamin-responsive disorders, such as methylmalonic acidemia, multiple carboxylase deficiency and homocystinuria, dietary protein restriction may be combined with specific cofactor therapy. In the organic acidemias and certain other disorders, L-carnitine, usually beginning with a dose of 100 mg/kg/day, may be given. Acyl CoAs accumulating in these disorders combine with carnitine to produce acylcarnitines that are water soluble and excreted in the urine. Without treatment, many patients with these disorders develop a secondary carnitine deficiency. Treatment with exogenous carnitine prevents the development of symptoms of carnitine deficiency and provides a measure of protection against recurrent episodes of metabolic decompensation by providing an augmented mechanism for excretion of accumulated metabolites.

Patients with urea cycle defects require supplementation with oral arginine or, in some cases, citrulline, which is converted to arginine. In normal persons, adequate amounts of arginine are synthesized via the urea cycle. Patients with a defect in urea synthesis have deficient arginine production and must depend on dietary supplementation. In the case of carbamylphosphate synthetase and ornithine transcarbamylase deficiencies, the most severe of the urea cycle defects, drug therapy is also required. These disorders were formerly almost uniformly lethal in the neonatal period. The development of novel drugs that provide an alternate pathway for waste nitrogen excretion has allowed survival of many affected infants.[91] Sodium benzoate and sodium phenylacetate were the agents originally used, but these have been replaced in clinical trials by sodium phenylbutyrate.

Despite rigorous therapy and intensive surveillance, patients with urea cycle defects remain at risk for intercurrent episodes of hyperammonemia which may result in death. The risk appears to be greatest for patients with ornithine transcarbamylase deficiency. Liver transplantation should be seriously considered for patients with this disorder if they can be stabilized, survive the neonatal period, and appear to have a reasonable developmental prognosis.

No clearly effective therapy has been developed for some of the inborn errors of metabolism presenting with acute overwhelming symptoms in the newborn. An example of a disorder in this group is nonketotic hyperglycinemia. Although therapy has been attempted with dietary protein restriction, sodium benzoate, and a variety of other drugs, the results have been disappointing. Most infants with this disorder die or exhibit significant neurologic impairment.

HYPOGLYCEMIA

Hypoglycemia and its associated symptoms may occasionally be seen in infants with disorders of protein intolerance, but it is more commonly seen in disorders of carbohydrate metabolism or of fatty acid oxidation. Among the best known inborn errors of metabolism associated with hypoglycemia are the glycogen storage diseases, of which types I (*i.e.*, von Gierke disease or glucose-6-phosphatase deficiency) and III (*i.e.*, limit dextrinosis or debrancher deficiency) are the most likely to be associated with manifestations in the neonatal period. The hypoglycemia in these disorders is related to the inability of the liver to release glucose from glycogen, and it is most profound during periods of fasting. Hypoglycemia, hepatomegaly, and lactic acidosis are prominent features of these disorders. Hypoglycemia is not a feature of glycogen storage disease type II (*i.e.*, Pompe disease), because cytoplasmic glycogen metabolism and release is normal in this disorder in which glycogen accumulates within lysosomes as a result of the deficiency of the lysosomal enzyme α-1,4-glucosidase. The clinical manifestations of this disorder include macroglossia, hypotonia, cardiomegaly with congestive heart failure, and hepatomegaly. Cardiomegaly is the most striking and may be apparent in the neonatal period. Congestive heart failure is the cause of death in most cases.

A disorder that presents clinically with findings virtually indistinguishable from the hepatic glycogen storage diseases types I and III is fructose-1,6-diphosphatase deficiency, a disorder of gluconeogenesis. Several other disorders of gluconeogenesis have been described. The basic immediate treatment of all of these disorders is frequent feedings and glucose administration, and the definitive diagnosis is made by liver biopsy and assay of appropriate hepatic enzymes. In some cases, enzymatic assays can be performed using lymphocytes or cultured skin fibroblasts.

Several inherited defects in fatty acid oxidation have been identified in infants presenting with hypoglycemia. Although most of the disorders in this group typically present after 2 months of age, neonatal manifestations may be observed. These disorders are important because of their apparent frequency and because of the variability of the initial presentation. Affected infants have an impaired capacity to use stored fat for fuel during periods of fasting and readily deplete their glycogen stores. Despite the development of hypoglycemia, acetyl CoA production is diminished, and ketone production is impaired. The hypoglycemia occurring in these conditions is typically characterized as nonketotic, although small amounts of ketones may be produced. Hypoglycemia may occur as an isolated finding or may be accompanied by many of the other biochemical derangements typically associated with Reye syndrome, such as hyperammonemia, metabolic acidosis, and elevated transaminases. Hepatomegaly may or may not be present. Any infant presenting with findings suggesting Reye syndrome should be evaluated for fatty acid oxidation defects. As the incidence of true Reye syndrome has decreased, most children presenting at any age with this constellation of findings have an inherited metabolic disorder.

The most common of the fatty acid oxidation defects is medium-chain acyl CoA dehydrogenase deficiency, which is estimated to occur in 1 of 15,000 births, an incidence similar to that observed for phenylketonuria (PKU).[92] It is among the most common inborn errors of metabolism. In addition to presenting as nonketotic hypoglycemia or a Reyelike syndrome, it may present as sudden infant death syndrome (SIDS) or a near-miss event. Many infants diagnosed as having medium-chain acyl CoA dehydrogenase deficiency have a history of a sibling who died of SIDS.[93] Microvascular fat accumulation in the liver in any infant dying of SIDS should strongly suggest the possibility of this or a related disorder. Long-chain fatty acyl CoA dehydrogenase deficiency is associated with similar clinical findings, although there may be evidence of a significant cardiomyopathy. Infants with this defect may present with cardiac arrhythmias or unexplained cardiac arrest. Several less common fatty acid oxidation defects present in a similar, although variable, fashion.

The accumulation of fatty acyl CoAs in patients with fatty acid oxidation defects leads to a secondary carnitine deficiency, probably as a result of excretion of excess acylcarnitines in the urine.[94,95] There is a rare syndrome of primary systemic carnitine deficiency with similar symptoms, although many of the original patients reported as having this condition were later shown to have medium-chain acyl CoA dehydrogenase deficiency.[95] In other cases, the various disorders that may result in secondary carnitine deficiency were not completely ruled out.

Urine organic acid analyses and measurements of serum carnitine are most helpful in the initial screening for defects in fatty acid oxidation. If the serum free carnitine level is low and the urine organic acids are normal or nondiagnostic, oral L-carnitine should be given in a single dose of 100 mg/kg. A urine specimen should be collected 6 to 8 hours later for an acylcarnitine profile, which should be adequate to establish the diagnosis of medium-chain acyl CoA dehydrogenase deficiency, the most common of the fatty acid oxidation defects. This disorder is confirmed by the demonstration of the characteristic metabolite, octanoylcarnitine. Alternatively, chronic carnitine therapy can be initiated at a dosage of 100 mg/kg/day divided in three or four equal doses, with a urine sample collected for acylcarnitine analysis after 3 days of treatment. Enzymatic assays may be necessary for the diagnosis of some of the fatty acid oxidation defects. As is true for the defects in carbohydrate metabolism leading to hypoglycemia, treatment of the fatty acid oxidation defects involves avoidance of fasting and provision of adequate glucose. Restriction of dietary fat intake and supplemental L-carnitine therapy are recommended. With appropriate therapy, patients with medium-chain acyl CoA dehydrogenase deficiency appear to have an excellent prognosis. The prognosis for the other fatty acid oxidation defects is more variable.

LIVER DYSFUNCTION

JAUNDICE AND OTHER BIOCHEMICAL DISORDERS

Jaundice or other evidence of liver dysfunction may be the presenting finding in several inherited metabolic disorders in the neonatal period. For most of the inborn errors of metabolism associated with jaundice, the elevated serum bilirubin is of the direct-reacting type. This generalization does not include those inborn errors of erythrocyte metabolism, such as glucose-6-phosphate dehydrogenase deficiency or pyruvate kinase deficiency, that are occasionally responsible for hemolytic disease in the newborn. The best-known metabolic disease associated with jaundice is galactosemia, in which the deficiency of the enzyme galactose-1-phosphate uridyltransferase results in an accumulation of galactose-1-phosphate and other metabolites, such as galactitol, which are thought to have a direct toxic effect on the liver and on other organs. Jaundice and liver dysfunction in this disorder are progressive and usually appear at the end of the first or during the second week of life with vomiting, diarrhea, poor weight gain, and eventual cataract formation if the infant is receiving breast milk or a galactose-containing formula. Hypoglycemia may be observed. The disease may present initially with indirect hyperbilirubinemia resulting from hemolysis secondary to high levels of galactose-1-phosphate in erythrocytes. Alternatively, the effects of acute galactose toxicity on the brain may rarely cause the CNS symptoms to predominate.

If galactosemia is suspected, the urine should be tested simultaneously with Benedict reagent and with a glucose oxidase method. The glucose oxidase method is specific for glucose, and Benedict reagent can detect any reducing substance. A negative dipstick for glucose with a positive Benedict reaction means that a non-glucose reducing substance is present. With appropriate clinical findings, this is most likely to be galactose. Paper or thin-layer chromatography can be used to positively identify the reducing substance. If a child has been on intravenous fluids and has not recently been receiving galactose in the diet, galactose may not be present in the urine.

If the diagnosis of galactosemia is suspected, whether or not reducing substances are found in the urine, galactose-containing feedings should immediately be discontinued and replaced by soy formula or other lactose-free formula pending the results of appropriate enzyme assays on erythrocytes to confirm the diagnosis. Untreated galactosemics, if they survive the neonatal period, have persistent liver disease, cataracts, and severe mental retardation. Many affected infants die of *E. coli* sepsis in the neonatal period, and the early onset of sepsis may alter the presentation of the disorder.[96]

Treatment of the disorder by maintenance of strict dietary restriction of galactose, if started early, results in complete reversal of the physical manifestations of the disorder and enables many affected persons to develop normal or near-normal intelligence. Unfortunately, there continues to be an increased incidence of mental retardation even among treated patients. There are some late sequelae of the disorder that appear to be unaffected by current therapy. These include premature ovarian failure in females and a late-onset neurologic syndrome involving ataxia and tremors in both genders.[97,98] Many states have newborn screening programs for galactosemia, but clinical manifestations of the disorder often appear before the results of screening studies are available, and it is therefore critical that the physicians remain alert to this possibility.

Another inborn error of metabolism that occasionally presents in the newborn period with jaundice, hepatomegaly, and the presence of reducing substances in the urine is hereditary fructose intolerance, which is characterized by episodes of profound hypoglycemia, vomiting, and metabolic acidosis. This disorder is uncommonly seen in the neonate, because most newborns are not immediately exposed to a fructose-containing diet unless they have been given a soy formula with sucrose as the carbohydrate source. In the uncommon event that an infant who has been receiving fructose should present with these findings, this diagnosis should be considered. Analysis of the urine reveals the presence of a non-glucose reducing substance that by chromatography can be demonstrated to be fructose. Treatment involves elimination of fructose from the diet and results in a complete resolution of all clinical signs and symptoms. Confirmation of the diagnosis is by assay of the deficient enzyme fructose-1-phosphate aldolase in liver tissue, but this is rarely necessary.

Another disorder that may be associated with neonatal jaundice is α_1-antitrypsin deficiency, a puzzling disorder that is among the most common of all inherited metabolic diseases.[99] The clinical manifestations of this disorder may be identical to those of traditional neonatal or giant cell hepatitis, and a determination of serum α_1-antitrypsin should be a part of the initial evaluation of all children presenting with this syndrome. Infants with deficient levels of α_1-antitrypsin on quantitative analysis should have protease inhibitor typing performed to confirm the diagnosis. There is no specific treatment for the liver disease associated with α_1-antitrypsin deficiency, but approximately one-half of all affected infants eventually exhibit complete resolution of the liver dysfunction. Others may progress to end-stage disease and require liver transplantation.

Another disorder that presents with liver disease in early infancy is hereditary tyrosinemia. The biochemical hallmarks of this disorder include marked elevations of plasma tyrosine and methionine and generalized aminoaciduria with a disproportionate increase in the excretion of tyrosine. However, these findings are relatively nonspecific and may be observed as a secondary phenomenon in other forms of liver disease. Hereditary tyrosinemia was once among the most difficult of inborn errors of metabolism to diagnose clinically. The finding of succinylacetone in the urine of patients with this disease has led to a helpful diagnostic test for the disorder.[100] It has become possible to establish the diagnosis definitively by demonstration of a deficiency of the enzyme fumarylacetoacetate fumarylhydrolase in lymphocytes and cultured skin fibroblasts of affected individuals.[101]

In contrast to disorders in which there is an elevation of the direct-reacting bilirubin, a persistent elevation of indirect bilirubin beyond the limits of physiologic jaundice, without evidence of hemolysis, suggests the diagnosis of the Crigler-Najjar syndrome. The hyperbilirubinemia in this disorder is related to a partial or complete deficiency of glucuronyl transferase, the liver enzyme responsible for the normal conjugation of bilirubin to bilirubin diglucuronide. There is no effective long-term therapy for all patients with this disorder, but the standard modalities of phototherapy and exchange transfusion may prevent the development of kernicterus in the neonatal period.[102,103] Hepatic transplantation has been performed successfully for patients with this disorder. Patients with a partial deficiency of the enzyme may respond to phenobarbital therapy.[103]

HEPATOMEGALY

The disorders associated with hepatomegaly in the neonatal period fall into two general categories: the storage diseases and disorders associated with liver damage or dysfunction. The latter have been previously discussed. Many of the well-known lipid storage diseases do not typically present in the neonatal period. Among those that may occasionally be associated with hepatomegaly in the neonatal period are GM_1-gangliosidosis type I, Gaucher disease, Niemann–Pick disease, and Wolman disease, all of which are associated with splenomegaly. The glycogen storage diseases that are associated with hepatomegaly in the newborn have previously been discussed and are listed in Table 39-2. Infants with the most common mucopolysaccharidoses, such as the Hurler and Hunter syndromes, uncommonly exhibit clinical abnormalities in the first month of life. Newborns with the typical features of these syndromes, such as coarse facial features, hepatosplenomegaly, skeletal abnormalities, and hernias, are more likely to have GM_1-gangliosidosis or a mucolipidosis, such as I-cell disease. Beta-glucuronidase deficiency, also classified as mucopolysaccharidosis type VII, may present in the neonatal period with features virtually indistinguishable clinically from those seen later in the Hurler and Hunter syndromes. An infantile form of sialidosis (*i.e.*, neuraminidase deficiency) is typically associated with findings at birth. The clinical manifestations of several of these conditions may be so severe *in utero* that fetal hydrops develops.

If one of these disorders is suspected, urine screening tests for mucopolysaccharides and oligosaccharides should be performed. These can be helpful diagnostically, but negative results do not rule out the possibility of a storage disorder. False-positive mucopolysaccharide spot tests are not uncommonly observed in neonates. The definitive diagnosis of most disorders of lipid or mucopolysaccharide metabolism is made by appropriate biochemical studies on leukocytes or cultured skin fibroblasts.

COARSE FACIAL FEATURES

Coarse facial features, a classical finding in older infants with mucopolysaccharidoses and oligosaccharide storage diseases, are observed occasionally in neonates with GM_1-gangliosidosis, β-glucuronidase deficiency, I-cell disease, and infantile sialidosis.

MACROGLOSSIA

Macroglossia is a typical finding in Pompe disease, or glycogen storage disease type II. It has been described in neonates with GM_1-gangliosidosis.

DIARRHEA

Diarrhea is described in relatively few of the inborn errors of metabolism, unlike vomiting, which is seen in so many of them. Notable exceptions to this are galactosemia, certain cases of cystic fibrosis, and less familiar disorders, such as Wolman disease (*i.e.*, acid lipase deficiency) and hereditary tyrosinemia.

ABNORMAL ODOR

Abnormal body or urinary odor, probably observed by nurses or mothers rather than physicians, is an important but often overlooked clue to the diagnosis of several of the inborn errors of metabolism and may be the most specific clinical finding in these patients. It is best described for PKU, for which the urine was found to have a peculiar musty odor years before the biochemical basis of the disease was understood. In the acutely ill neonate with an abnormal odor, isovaleric acidemia, glutaric acidemia type II, and maple syrup urine disease are the most likely entities to be encountered. In maple syrup urine disease, the urine has a distinctive sweet odor, reminiscent of maple syrup or burnt sugar. The odor associated with isovaleric acidemia and glutaric acidemia type II is pungent and similar to that of sweaty feet.

DYSMORPHIC FEATURES

There formerly appeared to be a clear distinction between inborn errors of metabolism and dysmorphic syndromes, both of which may be inherited in a similar fashion. Infants with inherited metabolic disease were thought to be phenotypically normal at birth with no evidence of major or minor structural anomalies. It is becoming increasingly apparent that inherited metabolic disorders may be associated with consistent patterns of birth defects, suggesting that metabolic derangements *in utero* may disrupt the normal process of fetal development.

This phenomenon is best illustrated by the group of disorders associated with multiple defects in peroxisomal enzymes, including those involved in fatty acid oxidation and plasmalogen synthesis.[104,105] These include Zellweger syndrome (*i.e.*, cerebrohepatorenal syndrome), neonatal adrenoleukodystrophy, and several variant conditions, all of which are associated with congenital hypotonia and dysmorphic features, such as epicanthal folds, Brushfield spots, large fontanels, simian creases, and renal cysts. Patients with glutaric acidemia type II, one of the organic acidemias, have a characteristic phenotype including a high forehead, hypertelorism, low-set ears, abdominal wall defects, palpably enlarged kidneys, hypospadias, and rocker bottom feet.[106,107] An energy-deficient mechanism (*i.e.*, fuel-mediated teratogenesis), similar to that postulated for maternal diabetes mellitus, has been suggested to explain these findings. Several of the other organic acidemias, such as mevalonic aciduria, 3-hydroxyisobutyryl CoA deacylase deficiency, and 3-hydroxyisobutyric aciduria have been associated with multiple dysmorphic features.

Some infants with PDH deficiency have dysmorphic facial features resembling those observed in the fetal alcohol syndrome (FAS).[44] The specific findings observed include a narrow forehead with frontal bossing, a broad nasal bridge, short nose with anteverted nostrils, and a long philtrum. The resemblance to FAS has been explained by suggesting that there is a common mechanism in the two disorders, involving a deficiency of PDH activity. It has been postulated that, in FAS, acetaldehyde from the maternal circulation inhibits fetal PDH, which leads to malformations.

Isolated malformations may be more commonly associated with inherited metabolic disorders. Patients with nonketotic hyperglycinemia frequently have agenesis of the corpus callosum and may have gyral malformations related to defects in neuronal migration as well.[108] Patients with PDH deficiency may exhibit agenesis of the corpus callosum.[109] It is not uncommon for patients with almost any of the inborn errors of metabolism to exhibit one or more dysmorphic features or anomalies that are nonspecific. The observation of dysmorphic features in an infant should in no way preclude consideration of an inherited metabolic disorder. In selected circumstances, it may heighten the clinical suspicion.

ABNORMAL EYE FINDINGS

Abnormal eye findings are typically associated with many of the inborn errors of metabolism, although they are not always found at the time of initial presentation. Cataracts are classically associated with galactosemia and other disorders of galactose metabolism, but may be observed in disorders such as Zellweger syndrome. Dislocated lenses, seen in homocystinuria, molybdenum cofactor deficiency, and sulfite oxidase deficiency, may be found as early as the first month of life and are an important clue to diagnosis. Retinal degenerative changes are typical of the peroxisomal disorders, including Zellweger syndrome and neonatal adrenoleukodystrophy, and are observed in several other conditions. Other abnormalities that may be associated with inborn errors of metabolism include corneal clouding and congenital glaucoma. A careful eye examination, preferably by an ophthalmologist, should be performed whenever an inherited metabolic disorder is suspected.

SAMPLES TO OBTAIN FROM A DYING CHILD WITH A SUSPECTED INBORN ERROR OF METABOLISM

If death appears imminent in a child suspected of having an inborn error of metabolism, it is important to obtain the appropriate samples for postmortem analysis. This is critical for resolution of the cause of death and is essential for subsequent genetic counseling and prenatal diagnosis. The following samples should be collected and stored: urine, frozen; plasma, separated from whole blood and frozen; and a small snip of skin obtained using sterile technique and stored at room temperature or 37°C in tissue culture medium, if available, or sterile saline. The latter sample can be obtained by slipping a 25-gauge needle under the skin, lifting the skin and snipping a 2- to 3-mm ellipse with a sterile scissors, which can often be found in a suture removal tray. The skin should be cleansed with alcohol. If an autopsy is performed, a sample of unfixed liver tissue should be obtained as soon as possible after death and frozen at −20°C for subsequent biochemical studies. Additional tissue should be preserved for electron microscopy. If consent for autopsy is denied, consent for a postmortem needle biopsy of the liver should be requested. The liver tissue should be frozen in total or in part if histologic studies appear to be indicated. As soon as possible after death, the case should be reviewed with a metabolic specialist and plans made for the transport of samples to the appropriate laboratory.

NEWBORN SCREENING FOR INHERITED METABOLIC DISORDERS

All 50 states and the District of Columbia in the United States and many other countries have newborn screening programs in place for genetic disorders. In the United States, there are significant state-to-state differences in the disorders that are included and in the methods of screening and in follow-up.

The only two disorders for which screening is routine in all 50 states and the District of Columbia are PKU and hypothyroidism. Because neonates with PKU are usually asymptomatic, neonatologists rarely encounter this condition except in the context of following abnormal screening test results. Because phenylalanine levels are normal in the cord blood of infants with this condition and rise only after milk feedings have been initiated, newborn screening samples should be obtained after 24 hours of age. In the case of infants discharged before 24 hours, most states recommend that a sample be obtained at discharge and subsequently repeated. In the case of sick infants who are not being fed, the initial newborn screening sample should not be withheld indefinitely but should be submitted at the recommended time (often 7 days), because screening for some other disorders, such as hypothyroidism, is not affected by the feeding history. For PKU screening, however, another specimen should be submitted after feedings are instituted. If the phenylalanine level is elevated on the first sample, a repeat specimen may be requested. If it is elevated again, referral for definitive diagnosis should be made immediately. This includes quantitative plasma amino acids and analysis of urinary pterins to rule out disorders of biopterin metabolism, which result in hyperphenylalaninemia. Newborn screening and early dietary treatment of PKU have completely altered the natural history of this disorder, which once accounted for 1% of all institutionalized mentally retarded persons. Children whose disorder is maintained under strict dietary control can now be expected to exhibit normal growth and intellectual development.

Several other inherited metabolic disorders are included in the newborn screening programs of selected states. The specific disorders and the number of states engaged in newborn screening for each are as follows: galactosemia, 37; maple syrup urine disease, 20; homocystinuria, 19; biotinidase deficiency, 12; hereditary tyrosinemia, 7; congenital adrenal hyperplasia, 5; and cystic fibrosis, 3. A likely candidate for the future may be medium-chain acyl CoA dehydrogenase deficiency. Although there is no simple screening test for the abnormal metabolites in this disorder, a single DNA mutation has been identified that accounts for approximately 90% of the defective genes.[92] It may be possible to implement newborn screening by direct DNA analysis, and a pilot screening program is underway in North Carolina to test this approach. This disorder appears to be an excellent candidate for newborn screening, because it is estimated to be among the most common of the inborn errors of metabolism with an incidence of approximately 1 in 15,000 and is associated with an excellent prognosis if recognized and treated.

Neonatologists should attempt to be actively involved in the evaluation of disorders considered for inclusion in newborn screening programs. Several criteria should be met before screening is considered on other than a research basis. The disorder should be sufficiently common to justify screening. A relatively simple, accurate and inexpensive screening test should be available. Treatment for the disorder should be available, and there should be some demonstrable benefit to starting treatment before clinical symptoms appear and the diagnosis is made on clinical grounds. It is on the basis of the last criterion that newborn screening for cystic fibrosis has often been criticized. Newborn screening for purposes of genetic counseling alone, when there is no clear benefit to the affected infant, is generally not viewed as appropriate. It is a inefficient method of identifying couples at risk of having a child with a recessively inherited disorder, because it identifies such couples only after the birth of an affected child. Carrier testing in the child-bearing age group is a far more appropriate approach to the identification of at-risk couples.

MATERNAL METABOLIC DISORDERS

With advances in therapy for inborn errors of metabolism, it is now common for patients with many of these disorders to reach adult life with normal or near-normal intelligence and the desire to have families of their own. This has led to serious concerns about the potential adverse effects of maternal metabolic derangements on fetal growth and development. The real potential for adverse consequences is illustrated by the experience that has accumulated with maternal PKU. In the past, patients with PKU were severely retarded and did not reproduce. This changed completely with the initiation of newborn screening programs and early dietary management. Dietary therapy was once maintained until 5 to 6 years of age and then discontinued. Treatment is now continued indefinitely in most cases, because it was later demonstrated that some patients exhibited neurologic deterioration and loss of IQ points after discontinuation of the diet. Nonetheless, most patients with PKU who are now adults have been off the diet for years and have high phenylalanine levels. After women with PKU began reproducing, it became clear that the maternal metabolic environment in this condition had extremely harmful effects on fetal development. A spectrum of findings referred to as "maternal PKU syndrome" is observed in a large percentage of exposed infants, most of whom do not themselves have PKU.[110,111] Over 90% of exposed infants exhibit mental retardation, and microcephaly occurs in 72%, growth retardation in 40%, and congenital heart disease in 12%. Altered facial features, similar to those observed in FAS, may be observed. Mothers with "benign" hyperphenylalaninemia, a condition that is associated with lower phenylalanine levels than classical PKU and does not require treatment, may be at increased risk for fetal abnormalities.

There is some suggestion that dietary treatment of pregnant women before conception and throughout pregnancy, with careful control of phenylalanine levels, may reduce the risk.[112] This is a difficult goal to achieve, because the phenylalanine-restricted diet is a onerous one to patients who have ever been on a normal diet, and some adult patients, despite early therapy, may have borderline intellectual functioning. A national collaborative study is in progress to address many of the issues related to the identification and treatment of maternal PKU. There has been no evidence for an increased risk of birth defects or any other problems in infants born to fathers with PKU.

Pregnancies have been reported in mothers with a variety of other inherited metabolic disorders, including several forms of glycogen storage disease, isovaleric acidemia, homocystinuria, hereditary orotic aciduria and several others, with no adverse outcomes clearly attributable to the maternal disorder. The collaborative experience with many disorders, however, is limited to single cases or small numbers of patients. It is probable that other maternal metabolic disorders will be identified that adversely affect fetal development.

REFERENCES

1. Fishler K, Koch R, Donnell GN, Wenz E. Developmental aspects of galactosemia from infancy to childhood. Clin Pediatr 1980;19:38.
2. Baerlocher K, Gitzelmann R, Steinmann B, Gitzelmann-Cumara-Samy N. Hereditary fructose intolerance in early childhood: a major diagnostic challenge. Survey of 20 symptomatic cases. Helv Paediatr Acta 1978;33:465.
3. Pagliara AS, Karl IE, Keating JP, et al. Hepatic fructose-1,6-diphosphatase deficiency. A cause of lactic acidosis and hypoglycemia in infancy. J Clin Invest 1972;51:2115.
4. Moses SW, Gutman A. Inborn errors of glycogen metabolism. Adv Pediatr 1972;19:95.
5. Huijing F, van Creveld S, Losekoot G. Diagnosis of generalized glycogen storage disease (Pompe's disease). J Pediatr 1963;63:984.
6. Levin B, Burgess EA, Mortimer PE. Glycogen storage disease type IV: amylopectinosis. Arch Dis Child 1968;43:548.
7. Clayton PT, Hyland K, Brand M, Leonard JV. Mitochondrial phosphoenolpyruvate carboxykinase deficiency. Eur J Pediatr 1986;145:46.
8. Clow CL, Reade TM, Scriver CR. Outcome of early and long-term management of classical maple syrup urine disease. Pediatrics 1981;68:856.
9. Tada K, Wada Y, Arakawa T. Hypervalinemia. Am J Dis Child 1967;113:64.
10. Scriver CR, Pueschel S, Davies E. Hyper-β-alaninemia associated with β-amnioaciduria and -aminobutyricaciduria, somnolence and seizures. N Engl J Med 1966;274:636.
11. Baumgartner R, Ando T, Nyhan WL. Nonketotic hyperglycinemia. J Pediatr 1969;75:1022.
12. Smith I, Wolff OH. Natural history of phenyketonuria and influence of early treatment. Lancet 1974;2:540.
13. Kvittingen EA. Hereditary tyrosinemia type I—an overview. Scand J Clin Lab Invest 1986;46:27.
14. Fell V, Pollitt RJ, Sampson GA, Wright T. Ornithinemia, hyperammonemia and homocitrullinuria. A disease associated with mental retardation and possibly caused by defective mitochondrial transport. Am J Dis Child 1974;127:752.
15. Simell O, Perheentupa J, Rapola J, Visakorpi JK, Eskelin L-E. Lysinuric protein intolerance. Am J Med 1975;59:229.
16. Allen RJ, Wong PWK, Rothenberg SP, et al. Progressive neonatal leukoencephalomyopathy due to absent methylenetetrahydrofolate reductase, responsive to treatment. Ann Neurol 1980;8:211.
17. Scriver CR, Whelan DT. Glutamic acid decarboxylase (GAD) in mammalian tissue outside the central nervous system, and its possible relevance to hereditary B_6 dependency with seizures. Ann N Y Acad Sci 1969;166:83.
18. Matsui SM, Mahoney MJ, Rosenberg LE. The natural history of the inherited methylmalonic acidemias. N Engl J Med 1983; 308:857.
19. Mitchell GA, Watkins D, Melancon SB, et al. Clinical heterogeneity in cobalamin C variant of combined homocystinuria and methylmalonic aciduria. J Pediatr 1986;108:410.
20. Wolf B, Hsia YE, Sweetman L, et al. Propionic acidemia: a clinical update. J Pediatr 1981;99:835.
21. Newman CGH, Wilson BDR, Callaghan P, Young L. Neonatal death associated with isovaleric acidemia. Lancet 1967; 2:439.
22. Finnie MDA, Cottrall K, Seakins JWT, Snedden W. Massive excretion of 2-oxoglutaric acid and 3-hydroxyisovaleric acid in a patient with a deficiency of 3-methylcrotonyl-CoA carboxylase. Clin Chim Acta 1976;73:513.
23. Burri BJ, Sweetman L, Nyhan WL. Heterogeneity of holocarboxylase synthetase in patients with biotin-responsive multiple carboxylase deficiency. Am J Hum Genet 1985;37:426.
24. Wolf B, Heard GS, Weissbecker KA, et al. Biotinidase deficiency; initial clinical features and rapid diagnosis. Ann Neurol 1985;18:614.
25. Leibel RL, Shih VE, Goodman SI, et al. Glutaric acidemia: a metabolic disorder causing progressive choreoathetosis. Neurology 1980;30:1163.
26. Goodman SI, Stene DO, McCabe ERB, et al. Glutaric acidemia type II: clinical, biochemical and morphologic considerations. J Pediatr 1982;100:946.
27. Mantagos S, Genel M, Tanaka K. Ethylmalonic-adipic aciduria: in vivo and in vitro studies indicating deficiency of activities of multiple acyl-CoA dehydrogenases. J Clin Invest 1979;64:1580.
28. Wysocki SJ, Hahnel R. 3-Hydroxy-3-methylglutaryl-CoA lyase deficiency: a review. J Inherited Metab Dis 1986;9:225.
29. Robinson BH, Sherwood WG, Taylor J, et al. Acetoacetyl CoA thiolase deficiency: a cause of severe ketoacidosis in infancy simulating salicylism. J Pediatr 1979;95:228.
30. Brandt NJ, Rasmussen K, Brandt S, et al. D-Glyceric-acidaemia and non-ketotic hyperglycinaemia. Acta Paediatr Scand 1976;65:17.
31. Brown GK, Hunt SM, Scholem R, et al. Beta-hydroxyisobutyryl coenzyme A deacylase deficiency: a defect in valine metabolism associated with physical malformations. Pediatrics 1982;70:532.
32. Hoffmann G, Gibson KM, Brandt IK, et al. Mevalonic aciduria—an inborn error of cholesterol and nonsterol isoprene biosynthesis. N Engl J Med 1986;314:1610.
33. Hagenfeldt L, Larsson A, Zetterstrom R. Pyroglutamic aciduria. Studies of an infant with chronic metabolic acidosis. Acta Paediatr Scand 1974;63:1.
34. Fang-Jong D, Nyhan WL, Wolff J, et al. 3-Hydroxyisobutyric aciduria: an inborn error of valine metabolism. Pediatr Res 1991;30:322.
35. Kelley RI, Cheatham JP, Clark BJ, et al. X-linked dilated cardiomyopathy with neutropenia, growth retardation, and 3-methylglutaconic aciduria. J Pediatr 1991;119:738.
36. Hudak ML, Jones MD Jr, Brusilow SW. Differentiation of transient hyperammonemia of the newborn and urea cycle enzyme defects by clinical presentation. J Pediatr 1985;107: 712.
37. Cederbaum SD, Shaw KNF, Valente M. Hyperargininemia. J Pediatr 1977;90:569.
38. Bachmann C, Krahenbiihl S, Colombo JP, et al. *N*-acetylgluta-

mate synthetase deficiency: a disorder of ammonia detoxification. N Engl J Med 1981;304:543.
39. Amendt BA, Greene C, Sweetman L, et al. Short chain acyl-CoA dehydrogenase deficiency: clinical and biochemical studies in two patients. J Clin Invest 1987;79:1303.
40. Stanley CA. New genetic defects in mitochondrial fatty acid oxidation and carnitine deficiency. Adv Pediatr 1987;34:59.
41. Hale DE, Batshaw ML, Coates PM, et al. Long chain acyl coenzyme A dehydrogenase deficiency: an inherited cause of nonketotic hypoglycemia. Pediatr Res 1985;19:666.
42. Waber LJ, Valle D, Neill C, et al. Carnitine deficiency presenting as familial cardiomyopathy: a treatable defect in carnitine transport. J Pediatr 1982;101:700.
43. Przyrembel H, Jakobs C, Ijlot L, et al. Long-chain 3-hydroxyacyl-CoA dehydrogenase deficiency. J Inherited Metab Dis 1991;14:674.
44. Robinson BH, McMillan H, Petrova-Benedict R, Sherwood WG. Variable clinical presentation in patients with deficiency of pyruvate dehydrogenase complex. A review of 30 cases with a defect in the E component of the complex. J Pediatr 1987;111:525.
45. Robinson BH, Oei J, Sherwood WG, et al. The molecular basis for the two different clinical presentations of classical pyruvate carboxylase deficiency. Am J Hum Genet 1984;36:283.
46. Zinn AB, Kerr DS, Hoppel CL. Fumarase deficiency: a new cause of mitochondrial encephalomyopathy. N Engl J Med 1986;315:469.
47. Robinson BH, DeMeirleir L, Glerum M, et al. Clinical presentation of patients with mitochondrial respiratory chain defects in NADH-coenzyme Q reductase and cytochrome oxidase: clues to the pathogenesis of Leigh disease. J Pediatr 1987;110:216.
48. Dimauro S, Mendell JR, Sahenk Z, et al. Fatal infantile mitochondrial myopathy and renal dysfunction due to cytochrome-C oxidase deficiency. Neurology 1980;30:795.
49. Taussig LM, ed. Cystic fibrosis. New York: Thieme-Stratton, 1984.
50. Stevenson RE, Lubinsky M, Taylor HA, et al. Sialic acid storage disease with sialuria: clinical and biochemical features in the severe infantile type. Pediatrics 1983;72:441.
51. Scriver CR, Mahon B, Levy HL, et al. The Hartnup phenotype: mendelian transport disorder, multifactorial disease. Am J Hum Genet 1987;40:401.
52. O'Brien JS, Stern MB, Landing BH, et al. Generalized gangliosidosis. Am J Dis Child 1965;109:338.
53. Barranger JA, Murray GJ, Ginns EI. Genetic heterogeneity of Gaucher's disease. In Barranger JA, Brady RO, eds. Molecular basis of lysosomal storage disorders. New York: Academic, 1984:311.
54. Besley GT, Elleder M. Enzyme activities and phospholipid storage patterns in brain and spleen samples from Niemann-Pick disease variants: a comparison of neuropathic and non-neuropathic forms. J Inherited Metab Dis 1986;9:59.
55. Autio S, Louhimo T, Helenius M. The clinical course of mannosidosis. Ann Clin Res 1982;14:93.
56. Dawson G, Spranger JW. Fucosidosis: a glycosphingolipidosis. N Engl J Med 1971;285:122.
57. Antonarakis SE, Valle D, Moser HW, et al. Phenotypic variability in siblings with Farber disease. J Pediatr 1984;104:409.
58. Young LW, Sty JR, Babbitt JP. Wolman's disease. Am J Dis Child 1979;133:959.
59. Clarke JTR, Ozere RL, Krause VW. Early infantile variant of Krabbe globoid cell leukodystrophy with lung involvement. Arch Dis Child 1981;8:640.
60. Spranger JW, Koch F, Mekusick VA, et al. Mucopolysaccharidosis VI (Maroteaux-Lamy's disease). Helv Paediatr Acta 1970;25:337.
61. Nelson A, Peterson L, Frampton B, Sly WS. Mucopolysaccharidosis VII (β-glucuronidase deficiency) presenting as nonimmune hydrops fetalis. J Pediatr 1982;101:574.
62. Leroy JG, Spranger JW, Feingold M, Dopitz JM. I-cell disease: a clinical picture. J Pediatr 1971;79:360.
63. Amir N, Zlotogora J, Bach G. Mucolipidosis type IV: clinical spectrum and natural history. Pediatrics 1987;79:953.
64. Burk RD, Valle D, Thomas GH, et al. Early manifestations of multiple sulfatase deficiency. J Pediatr 1984;104:574.
65. Aylsworth AS, Thomas GH, Hood JL, et al. A severe infantile sialidosis: clinical, biochemical and microscopic features. J Pediatr 1980;96:662.
66. Wilson GN, Holmes RD, Hajra AK. Peroxisomal disorders: clinical commentary and future prospects. Am J Med Genet 1988;30:771.
67. White PC, New MI, Dupont B. Congenital adrenal hyperplasia. N Engl J Med 1987;316:1519, 1580.
68. Nadler HL, Egan TJ. Deficiency of lysosomal acid phosphatase. A new familial metabolic disorder. N Engl J Med 1970; 282:303.
69. Danks DM, Campbell PE, Stevens BJ, et al. Menkes kinky hair syndrome: an inherited defect in copper absorption with widespread effects. Pediatrics 1972;50:188.
70. McClard RW, Black MJ, Jones ME, et al. Neonatal diagnosis of orotic aciduria: an experience with one family. J Pediatr 1983;102:85.
71. Kozlowski K, Sutcliffe J, Barylak A, et al. Hypophosphatasia: review of 24 cases. Pediatr Radiol 1976;5:103.
72. Wadman SK, Duran M, Beemer FA, et al. Absence of hepatic molybdenum cofactor: an inborn error of metabolism leading to a combined deficiency of sulphite oxidase and xanthine dehydrogenase. J Inherited Metab Dis 1983;1(Suppl 6):78.
73. Mudd SH, Irreverre F, Laster L. Sulfite oxidase deficiency in man: demonstration of the enzymatic defect. Science 1967;156:1599.
74. Berk PD, Jones EA, Howe RB, Berlin NI. Disorders of bilirubin metabolism in Bondy, PK, Rosenberg LE, eds. Metabolic control and disease. 8th ed. Philadelphia: WB Saunders, 1980:1009.
75. Sveger T. Liver disease in alpha$_1$-antitrypsin deficiency detected by screening of 200,000 infants. N Engl J Med 1976;294:1316.
76. Matalon R, Michals K, Sebesta D, et al. Aspartoacylase deficiency and *N*-acetylaspartic aciduria in patients with Canavan disease. Am J Med Genet 1988;29:463.
77. Shapiro LJ, Buxman MM, Weiss R, et al. Enzymatic basis of typical X-linked ichthyosis. Lancet 1978;2:756.
78. Cruysberg JRM, Sengers RCA, Pinckers A, et al. Features of a syndrome with congenital cataracts and hypertrophic cardiomyopathy. Am J Ophthalmol 1986;102:740.
79. Scriver CR, Beaudet AL, Sly WS, Valle D, eds. The Metabolic Basis of Inherited Disease. 6th ed. New York: McGraw-Hill, 1989.
80. Emery AEH, Rimoin DL, eds. Principles and practice of medical genetics. New York: Churchill Livingstone, 1983.
81. Fischer AQ, Challa VR, Burton BK, McLean WT. Cerebellar hemorrhage complicating isovaleric acidemia: a case report. Neurology 1981;31:746.
82. Nyhan WL. Patterns of clinical expression and genetic variation in the inborn errors of metabolism. In: Nyhan WL, ed. Heritable disorders of amino acid metabolism. New York: John Wiley & Sons, 1974;3.
83. Ballard RA, Vinocur B, Reynolds JW, et al. Transient hy-

perammonemia of the preterm infant. N Engl J Med 1978; 299:920.

84. Msall M, Batshaw ML, Suss R, et al. Neurologic outcome in children with inborn errors of urea synthesis. N Engl J Med 1984;310:1500.
85. Goldberg RN, Cabal LA, Sinatra FR, et al. Hyperammonemia associated with perinatal asphyxia. Pediatrics 1979;64: 336.
86. Batshaw ML, Wachtel RC, Cohen L, et al. Neurologic outcome in premature infants with transient asymptomatic hyperammonemia. J Pediatr 1986;108:27.
87. Robinson BH, Taylor J, Sherwood WG. The genetic heterogeneity of lactic acidosis: occurrence of recognizable inborn errors of metabolism in a pediatric population with lactic acidosis. Pediatr Res 1980;14:956.
88. Robinson BH, Glerum DM, Chow W, et al. The use of skin fibroblast cultures in the detection of respiratory chain defects in patients with lacticacidemia. Pediatr Res 1990;28:549.
89. Carson NAJ. Non-ketotic hyperglycinemia—a review of 70 patients. J Inherited Metab Dis 1982;2(Suppl 5):126.
90. Wiegand C, Thompson T, Bock GH, et al. The management of life-threatening hyperammonemia: a comparison of several therapeutic modalities. J Pediatr 1980;96:142.
91. Batshaw ML, Brusilow SW, Waber L, et al. Treatment of inborn errors of urea synthesis: activation of alternative pathways of waste nitrogen synthesis and excretion. N Engl J Med 1982;306:1387.
92. Matsubara Y, Narisawa K, Tada K, et al. Prevalence of K329E mutation in medium-chain acyl-CoA dehydrogenase gene determined from Guthrie cards. Lancet 1991;1:552.
93. Duran M, Hofkamp M, Rhead WJ, et al. Sudden death and "healthy" affected family members with medium-chain acyl coenzymes A dehydrogenase deficiency. Pediatrics 1986;78: 1052.
94. Stanley CA, Hale DE, Coates PM, et al. Medium chain acyl-CoA dehydrogenase deficiency in children with non-ketotic hypoglycemia and low carnitine levels. Pediatr Res 1983; 17:877.
95. Engel AG, Rebouche CJ. Carnitine metabolism and inborn errors. J Inherited Metab Dis 1984;1(Suppl 7):38.
96. Levy HL, Sepe SJ, Shih VE, et al. Sepsis due to Escherichia coli in neonates with galactosemia. N Engl J Med 1977;297: 823.
97. Kaufman FR, Kogut MD, Donnell GN, et al. Hypergonadotropic hypogonadism in female patients with galactosemia. N Engl J Med 1981;304:994.
98. Friedman JH, Levy HL, Boustany RM. Late onset of distinct neurologic syndromes in galactosemic siblings. Neurology 1989;39:741.
99. Cutz E, Cox DW. Alpha$_1$-antitrypsin deficiency: the spectrum of pathology and pathophysiology. Perspect Pediatr Pathol 1979;5:1.
100. Lindbland B, Lindstedt S, Stein G. On the enzymic defects in hereditary tyrosinemia. Proc Natl Acad Sci USA 1977;74: 4641.
101. Kvittingen EA, Halvorsen S, Jellum E. Deficient acetoacetate fumarylhydrolase activity in lymphocytes and fibroblasts from patients with hereditary tyrosinemia. Pediatr Res 1983;14:541.
102. Karon M, Imach D, Schwartz A. Phototherapy in congenital non-obstructive non-hemolytic jaundice. N Engl J Med 1970;282:377.
103. Garodischer R, Levy G, Krasner J, Yaffe SJ. Congenital non-obstructive non-hemolytic jaundice: effect of phototherapy. N Engl J Med 1970;282:375.
104. Schutgens RBH, Heymans HSA, Wanders RJA, et al. Peroxisomal disorders: a newly recognized group of genetic diseases. Eur J Pediatr 1986;144:430.
105. Wilson GN, Holmes RD, Hajra AK. Peroxisomal disorders: clinical commentary and future prospects. Am J Med Genet 1988;30:771.
106. Sweetman L, Nyhan WL, Trauner DA, et al. Glutaric acidemia type II. J Pediatr 1980;96:1020.
107. Chalmers RA, Tracy BM, King GS, et al. The prenatal diagnosis of glutaric acidemia type II using quantitative gas chromatography–mass spectroscopy. J Inherited Metab Dis 1980;3:67.
108. Dobyns WB. Agenesis of the corpus callosum and gyral malformations are frequent manifestations of nonketotic hyperglycinemia. Neurology 1989;39:817.
109. Wick H, Schweizer KK, Baumgartner R. Thiamine dependency in a patient with congenital lactic acidemia due to pyruvate dehydrogenase deficiency. Agents Actions 1977;7: 405.
110. Lenke RR, Levy HL. Maternal phenylketonuria and hyperphenylkalaninemia. An international survey of untreated and treated pregnancies. N Engl J Med 1980;303:1202.
111. Levy HL, Waisbren SE. Effects of untreated maternal phenylketonuria and hyperphenylalaninemia on the fetus. N Engl J Med 1983;309:1269.
112. Rohr FJ, Doherty LB, Waisbren SE, et al. Benacerraf B, Levy HL. New England Maternal PKU project. Prospective study of untreated and treated pregnancies and their outcomes. J Pediatr 1987;11:391.

Neonatology: Pathophysiology and Management of the Newborn, Fourth Edition,
edited by Gordon B. Avery, Mary Ann Fletcher, and Mhairi G. MacDonald.
J.B. Lippincott Company, Philadelphia © 1994.

chapter 40

Congenital Malformations

MURRAY FEINGOLD

Birth defects are being diagnosed in an increasing number of infants during the prenatal and neonatal period because of improved diagnostic technology, especially ultrasonography (see Chaps. 12 and 13). Because of this, it is even more important for the neonatolgist to be knowledgeable about congenital malformations. There are various causes of birth defects, including genetic abnormalities, dysmorphogenesis, and environmental affects on the fetus.

TYPES OF INHERITANCE

AUTOSOMAL DOMINANT INHERITANCE

If a dominant gene is present in a person, the patient will be affected. The manifestations, however, vary depending on the expressivity and penetrance of the gene. Therefore, in some affected newborns the diagnosis will be very obvious, whereas in others it will be much more difficult to make. A person inherits one gene for a specific trait from the mother, and another gene from the father. If one of these genes is abnormal, and it is a dominant gene, the child has a one-in-two chance of inheriting the gene from the affected parent (Fig. 40-1).

It is important to remember that this 50% chance occurs with each pregnancy. Also, if the infant does not inherit the affected gene, then it will not be passed on to his or her children.

There are many autosomal dominant syndromes, such as achondroplasia and tuberous sclerosis, in which neither parent is affected. In these situations, the inherited disease is most likely to be due to a mutation. Because of expressivity and penetrance of the gene, it is important that both parents be examined to make certain that they do not have the disease in a mild or undetected form. From a genetic counseling point of view, if the syndrome is secondary to a mutation, it is unlikely that the parents will have a second affected child. As a general rule, autosomal dominant diseases tend to be less severe than those inherited in an autosomal recessive manner.

AUTOSOMAL RECESSIVE INHERITANCE

In this type of inheritance, neither parent is affected, but both are carriers of the abnormal gene. The chance of the couple having a child with an autosomal recessive disease such as cystic fibrosis, is one in four with each pregnancy (Fig. 40-2). A child who does not have cystic fibrosis, but whose sibling does—indicating the parents are obligate carriers—has a two-in-three chance of being a carrier of the disease. For his or her children to be affected, however, it is necessary for the mate to be a carrier. In an increasing number of genetic diseases, newer DNA probe techniques make it possible to determine whether or not a person has the affected gene. By knowing this information, the physician can then provide very specific genetic counseling. For example, if it is known that one mate has the gene and the other does not, then none of their children will be affected but 50% will be carriers. If the patient has a genetic disease in the family in which the carrier state can not be determined, then it is necessary to know

	A	a
a	Aa	aa
a	Aa	aa

FIG. 40–1. In autosomal dominant inheritance, a person with the Aa phenotype inherits the disease, while a person with the aa genotype does not have the disease and is not a carrier. The chance of recurrence of the disease is 1 in 2.

	X	X•
X	XX	XX•
Y	XY	X•Y

FIG. 40–3. In X-linked inheritance, a person with the XX genotype may be either a normal girl or a female carrier, whereas a person with the XY genotype may be either a normal boy or a boy with the disease. The chance of recurrence of the disease is 1 in 4.

the gene frequency of the disease to ascertain the chance of having an affected child. If it is a very common gene, such as the gene for cystic fibrosis, then chances of one carrier marrying another are greater than when it is a rare gene.

X-LINKED INHERITANCE

X-linked recessive conditions occur more frequently than do X-linked dominant ones. Examples of X-linked recessive syndromes are hemophilia A and B, Duchenne muscular dystrophy, hypohydrotic ectodermal dysplasia, mucopolysaccharidosis II (*i.e.*, Hunter syndrome), and Lesch–Nyhan syndrome.

In this type of inheritance, the abnormal gene is present on one of the two X chromosomes of the female. When the affected gene is recessive, the normal gene on the other X chromosome prevents the expression of the abnormal gene. Because the Y chromosome contains much less genetic material than the X chromosome, if a male inherits the mother's X chromosome with the abnormal gene he will be affected. Parents of a child with an X-linked disease have a one-in-four chance of having an affected child with each pregnancy (Fig 40-3). None of the females will be affected, but one-half will be carriers. In providing genetic counseling for a normal sister of a male with an X-linked disease, it must be determined whether she is a carrier. The normal male sibling of a child with an X-linked disease did not inherit the X chromosome containing the gene for the disease and, therefore, will not only be normal but will not be a carrier. If the disease is X-linked dominant, then both males and females can be affected, as demonstrated by vitamin D–resistant rickets. In this type of inheritance, the chance of an affected person having an affected child is 50%.

MULTIFACTORIAL INHERITANCE

This type of inheritance is associated with many genetic conditions, including cleft lip and palate and meningomyelocele. In autosomal dominant and X-linked recessive inheritance, only one abnormal gene is needed to have an affected child; in autosomal recessive inheritance, two abnormal genes are necessary. In multifactorial inheritance, however, many genes from both parents are necessary before the child will be affected. Because of this, the chances of recurrence are much less than in the other forms of inheritance. For example, parents who have a child with an isolated cleft lip with or without a cleft palate have a 3% to 4% statistical chance of reoccurrence.

CHROMOSOMAL ABNORMALITIES

An infant born with some type of chromosomal abnormality occurs in approximately 1 of every 200 deliveries, although many of these patients are phenotypically normal. It is important to realize that approximately 50% of all spontaneous abortions involve a chromosomal abnormality.

NONDISJUNCTION

Nondisjunction is the most common cause of chromosomal syndromes. As a result of nondisjunction, an extra chromosome usually is present, as in Down

	B	b
B	BB	Bb
b	Bb	bb

FIG. 40–2. In autosomal recessive inheritance, a person with the BB genotype is normal, a person with the Bb genotype is normal but a carrier, and a person with the bb genotype has the disease. The chance of recurrence of the disease and the chance of being normal are each 1 in 4; the chance of being a carrier is 2 in 4.

syndrome (*i.e.*, trisomy 21). Chromosomes undergo reduction during meiosis, at which time the total number of chromosomes decreases from 46 to 23. They then divide, producing daughter cells that also have 23 chromosomes. At fertilization, the egg and sperm each contain 23 chromosomes, and this results in the fetus having the normal number of 46 chromosomes; one-half come from the mother and one-half from the father. In nondisjunction Down syndrome, during meiosis in one mate, the two 21 chromosomes do not separate. At fertilization, these two chromosomes join with the single chromosome 21 of the other mate, resulting in three 21 chromosomes, or trisomy 21. Maternal age is a risk factor for nondisjunction to occur (Table 40-1). Studies using DNA probes, show that the extra 21 chromosome comes from the father approximately 5% to 10% of the time. The most common types of nondisjunction abnormalities associated with autosomes in live-born babies are trisomies 21, 18, and 13.

TRANSLOCATION

Chromosomal material may break off from one chromosome and translocate on to another. It is important to determine whether a translocated chromosome is present, because the chromosome can be passed on from parent to child and, in certain situations, can result in an abnormal child. Translocation of part of a chromosome 21 to another chromosome—usually chromosomes 14, 22, or 21—is responsible for approximately 3% of Down syndrome cases. If the mother is the carrier of the translocated chromosome, there is about a 10% chance that her next child will have Down syndrome. If the father is the carrier, however, the chance is approximately 2%. Many translocation syndromes do not have classic clinical findings, and therefore may be difficult to diagnose. Manifestations usually are present when the translocation is unbalanced, resulting in extra or missing chromosomal material. In the carrier state (*i.e.*, balanced translocation), manifestations usually are not present.

TABLE 40–1
INCIDENCE OF DOWN SYNDROME ACCORDING TO MATERNAL AGE

Maternal Age (y)	Incidence
20	1:1667
25	1:1250
30	1:952
35	1:385
36	1:295
37	1:227
38	1:175
39	1:137
40	1:106
41	1:82
42	1:64
43	1:50
44	1:38
45	1:30
46	1:23
47	1:18
48	1:14
49	1:11

From D'Alton ME, DeCherney AH. Prenatal diagnosis. N Engl J Med 1993;328:114.

DELETION

A deletion occurs when chromosomal material is missing from either the upper (p) or lower (q) arms of a chromosome. An example of a deletion is the cri du chat syndrome, in which material is missing from the upper or short arm of chromosome 5 (5p−).

PARTIAL TRISOMY

Partial trisomy, which occurs when there is duplication of the long or short arm of a chromosome, is associated with various manifestations, some more severe than others. The facial features of these patients may or may not be typical enough to make the diagnosis on physical examination. Partial trisomies have been described, involving the short or long arms of at least ten different chromosomes.

ABNORMAL NUMBERS OF X AND Y CHROMOSOMES

An abnormal number of X and Y chromosomes, such as in Turner or Klinefelter syndromes, is a common type of chromosomal abnormality (see Chap. 41). The most common chromosomal abnormality in Turner syndrome is the absence of one of the X chromosomes; thus, there are only 45 chromosomes. Although patients with only one X chromosome have a greater chance of surviving than patients who are missing one of their autosomes (*i.e.*, monosomy), spontaneous abortions do occur quite frequently when the fetus has an XO karyotype. Isochromosome X is another chromosomal abnormality associated with Turner syndrome. In this situation, the centromere (*i.e.*, the center of the chromosome) divides transversally instead of longitudinally, resulting in duplication of the long arm of the X chromosome and lack of the short arm. Isochromosome X occurs in approximately 15% to 20% of all patients with Turner syndrome. A less common type of Turner syndrome is Turner mosaic. Mosaicism occurs when there is more than one cell line (*e.g.*, some cells containing a XO line and other cells containing a XX line). There are various types of Turner mosaics including XO/XX, XO,i(Xq) (*i.e.*, isochromosome of the long arm of the X chromosome), and XO/XX/XY. Patients with classic XO Turner syndrome cannot reproduce, although this is not always true in patients with mosaic Turner syndrome. Klinefelter syndrome is one of the more common chromosomal aberrations in males and usually is characterized by the presence of an extra X chromosome (*i.e.*, 47XXY). Although it may be difficult to make this diagnosis during the newborn period, two helpful clues are radioulnar synostosis and abnormal genitalia such as small penis and cryptorchidism. There are numerous other abnormalities involving the X and Y chromosomes, including the XYY karyotype, which occurs in 1 in 1000 male births.

The fragile X syndrome is the most common genetic cause of mental retardation in males. Cytogenetically, there is a gap or fragile site located near the distal end of the long arm of the X chromosome. For the fragile site to be seen, a special culture medium must be used to grow the cells, one that is low in folic acid and thymidine. The gene for the fragile X syndrome is located near the fragile site. The inheritance of the fragile X syndrome is complicated. One reason for this is that approximately 20% of males who have the fragile X gene do not exhibit any manifestations; these are called normal transmitting males. Also, not all patients who are affected with fragile X syndrome show the fragile site on cytogenetic examination. Using techniques involving DNA probes, the diagnosis of fragile X can be made with greater accuracy prenatally and postnatally. The facial features of patients with fragile X are characteristic and include large, simple ears, prominent forehead, broad nose, and a wide mouth. The prominent mandible usually is not present in a neonate. Although macroorchidism has been reported during infancy, it usually occurs later in life. Most carrier females are normal, especially if they inherited their abnormal X chromosome from the normal transmitting father, although some of them may have learning difficulties or retardation.

To provide optimal genetic counseling to parents, chromosomal analyses should be done on stillbirths or newborns who have multiple congenital anomalies of unknown etiology, or to confirm a suspected chromosomal diagnosis. When obtaining chromosomes, blood or skin are adequate, but it is important to make certain that there is no bacterial contamination. Because this probably is the only opportunity to obtain chromosomes on the patient, getting more than one specimen is advisable. Other tissues also can be used. Numerous syndromes are associated with neonatal death. Some of them are listed in Table 40-2. It is very important that necessary studies be done before or immediately after death because this may be the only time that pertinent specimens are available. In addition to obtaining chromosomes, other studies should include radiographic examination, especially if there are skeletal abnormalities, a postmortem examination that includes preservation of various tissues for future studies, and photographs.

TABLE 40–2
SYNDROMES ASSOCIATED WITH NEONATAL DEATH

Achondrogenesis
Camptomelic dysplasia
Holoprosencephaly
Hypophosphatasia
Jarcho–Levin
Jeune thoracic dystrophy
Lethal multiple pterygia
Osteogenesis imperfecta
Meckel–Gruber
Neu–Laxova
Pena–Shokeir
Rhizomelic chondrodysplasia punctata
Trisomy 18
Trisomy 13
Trisomy 9 mosaicism

EVALUATING THE MALFORMED INFANT

Before examining the infant, all pertinent historic data must be obtained. Pregnancy history provides valuable information, especially if there is a history of frequent spontaneous abortions or exposure to infections, medications, alcohol, or radiographic examinations. Details concerning labor, delivery, birth weight, Apgar score, placenta, and number of umbilical vessels also are helpful. Family history, especially regarding mental retardation, presence of birth defects, chromosomal abnormalities, and skeletal dysplasias, help to make a diagnosis. A family pedigree should be obtained routinely.

FACIES

It is important to get an overall impression of the facies. Is the face normal in configuration? Is it triangular, as seen in patients with marked loss of subcutaneous fat? The triangular facies of patients with progeria and diencephalic syndrome are not apparent in the newborn period. A rounded facies may be present in patients with the Prader–Willi, Laurence–Moon–Biedl, and cri du chat syndromes. In myotonic dystrophy, the face is expressionless, and, in the newborn period, drooling frequently occurs. Other terms used to describe the face include birdlike (Seckel dwarf and Hallermann–Streiff syndromes), elfin (Williams syndrome and leprechaunism), flattened (Potter syndrome and congenital syphilis), coarse (congenital hypothyroidism, GM_1 gangliosidosis, and mucolipidosis II), and abnormally shaped skull (Apert, Crouzon, and Saethre–Chotzen syndromes). Patients with various types of mucopolysaccharidoses are not included because they generally do not have coarse facial features in the newborn period. The diagnosis of some type of storage disease should be strongly considered in infants with a coarse facies and an enlarged liver or spleen.

HEAD

The size and shape of the head should be noted. If the head size is significantly small (*i.e.*, microcephaly), de Lange syndrome, intrauterine infections (*e.g.*, rubella, toxoplasmosis, cytomegalovirus), cebocephaly, and various syndromes associated with chromosomal abnormalities should be considered. The most common cause of an enlarged head is hydrocephalus, which may or may not be associated with a meningomyelocele. Hydrocephalus also may be found in achondroplasia, cerebral gigantism, hydrancephaly, and congenital toxoplasmosis. Another cause of an enlarged head is macrocephaly, which is present in achondroplasia, cerebral gigantism, osteopetrosis, Conradi–Hünermann syndrome, and pyknodysostosis. An enlarged anterior fontanelle is present in a variety of syndromes, including osteogenesis imperfecta, Conradi–Hünermann syndrome, pyknodysostosis, cleidocranial dysplasia, congenital hypothyroidism, congenital syphilis, and various skeletal dysplasias such as achondroplasia. Other abnormalities of the head, including a prominent frontal bone, flattened occiput, prominent occiput, and premature closure of sutures, should be noted. The latter is found in Apert and Saethre–Chotzen syndromes and Crouzon disease, but also may be an isolated finding.

The size and shape of the infant's skull are helpful in determining the correct diagnosis in a patient suspected of having a skeletal dysplasia. For example, in achondroplasia, thanatophoric dwarfism, cleidocranial dysplasia, and achondrogenesis, a large head is present. In spondyloepiphyseal dysplasia, however, a fairly common type of dwarfism, the head size is normal, as it is in the Ellis–van Creveld syndrome.

An ultrasound examination of the brain, through the open fontanelle, frequently provides useful information when performed on an infant whose head is abnormal in size or shape.

EYES

The eye examination can be divided into an external and internal examination. It is difficult, and frequently not practical, for the physician to do a complete ophthalmologic examination on all newborn infants. It should be thorough enough, however, to alert the physician to the possibility of any ocular abnormalities so that a more extensive evaluation can be done by an ophthalmologist.

On external examination, the presence of colobomas of the iris and lid should be noted. A coloboma of the upper lid (*i.e.*, interruption of the normal curvature of the lid) raises the question of the Goldenhar syndrome, whereas in the Treacher Collins syndrome the lower lid is involved. Cataracts may be the result of an intrauterine infection or an inherited biochemical defect. Cataracts may not be present in the newborn period, but occur later (*e.g.*, galactosemia). Long eyelashes are unusual in the newborn but are present in patients with de Lange syndrome, which also includes synophrys (*i.e.*, eyebrows that meet in the middle). Structural abnormalities of the iris may be found at birth in Rieger syndrome, but heterochromia or iris bicolor associated with the Waardenburg syndrome does not occur until the infant is at least 3 months of age. The size of the eyes should be noted; if they are small, trisomy 13, Hallermann–Streiff syndrome, and congenital toxoplasmosis should be considered. Some external abnormalities that may occur include nystagmus, ptosis of the lids, megalocornea, Brushfield spots, and dermoids. The presence of epicanthal folds may be difficult to interpret because the newborn usually has a broad nasal bridge, giving the appearance of an epicanthal fold. Epicanthal folds frequently are associated with Down, cri du chat, Noonan, and Smith–Lemli–Opitz syndromes.

An important factor to consider in the eye examination is whether the eyes are too far apart (*i.e.*, ocular hypertelorism) or too close together (*i.e.*, ocular hypotelorism). These findings have important clinical significance not only because there are numerous syndromes associated with both but also because there is a significant incidence of mental retardation associated with hypotelorism. Some of the syndromes that manifest hypertelorism and hypotelorism are listed in Table 40-3.

The slant of the palpebral fissures should be observed to determine whether they go in an upward and outward direction (*i.e.*, mongoloid slant) or downward and outward (*i.e.*, antimongoloid slant). Because it is difficult to quantitate the slant of the eyes, it is mainly a clinical impression. Some of the

TABLE 40–3
SYNDROMES ASSOCIATED WITH OCULAR HYPERTELORISM AND HYPOTELORISM

Ocular Hypertelorism
Aarskog
Apert
Cerebrohepatorenal
Chromosome 4p−
Cleidocranial dysplasia
Coffin–Lowry
Craniometaphyseal dysplasia
Cri du chat (*i.e.*, cat-cry; 5p−)
Crouzon
Fetal hydantoin
Fetal warfarin
Larsen
Leprechaunism
Multiple lentigens (LEOPARD)
Median cleft face
Neu–Laxova
Otopalatodigital
Robinow
Turner
Williams
Ocular Hypotelorism
Cebocephaly
Ethmocephaly
Oculodentodigital
Trisomy 13
Holoprosencephaly

conditions associated with downward and outward slants are the Rubinstein–Taybi, Treacher Collins, Noonan, otopalatodigital, and ring chromosome 18 syndromes.

Abnormalities on internal (*i.e.*, funduscopic) examination of the eye also may lead the examiner to suspect a diagnosis. For example, the finding of chorioretinitis suggests the possibility of an intrauterine infection, and, if microcephaly and a skin rash also are present, the possibility becomes even stronger. Other findings such as a cherry-red spot, corneal opacities, iritis, macular degeneration, optic atrophy, and retinitis pigmentosa should be looked for.

EARS

A variety of ear abnormalities are associated with syndromes, and it is important to note whether they are unilateral or bilateral. For example, patients with Goldenhar syndrome and hemifacial microsomia usually have unilateral ear involvement, whereas patients with Treacher Collins syndrome have bilateral abnormalities. There also is a higher incidence of renal anomalies present in patients with unilateral ear and facial bone abnormalities. Other abnormalities include those affecting the length of the ear (increased in cerebral gigantism and decreased in Down syndrome), prominent anthelix (deletion of chromosome 18), absence of ear lobes (Seckel dwarf syndrome), and square ears (Down syndrome). Low-set ears are found in numerous genetic syndromes, including Apert, Crouzon, Turner, Noonan, and Rubinstein–Taybi syndromes, and trisomies 13 and 18. There are various methods used to determine whether the ears are low-set. One method consists of extending a line from both medial canthi to the ear and determining the percentage of the ear above this line. A graph can then be used to determine whether the ear is low-set (see Figs. 40-26 and 40-27).

NOSE

There are numerous terms used to describe the shape of the nose, including "beaked" (Apert, Crouzon, Hallermann–Streiff, achondroplasia, de Lange, and Smith–Lemli–Opitz syndromes), "bulbous" (trisomy 13), and "pinched" (oculodentodigital syndrome). The nasolabial distance (*i.e.*, philtrum) varies greatly in the neonate. Prominence of the philtrum is characteristic of various conditions, including the de Lange and Smith–Lemli–Opitz syndromes. A broad bridge of the nose is a common finding and occurs in Down, Williams, and Conradi syndromes and in achondroplasia.

ORAL REGION

The most obvious abnormalities involving the oral region are cleft lip and cleft palate, which usually are inherited in a multifactorial manner. It is important to examine such patients for the presence of lip pits, which are indentations or depressions located on the lower lip. When present and associated with a cleft lip or cleft palate, the chance for recurrence of the cleft lip, cleft palate, or both changes from approximately 4% to 50% because it is then inherited in an autosomal dominant fashion. Other oral abnormalities include natal teeth (pyknodysostosis), serrated gingivae (Ellis–van Creveld) and high-arched palate (Treacher Collins, Apert, Crouzon, Smith–Lemli–Opitz, Marfan, Turner, and Noonan syndromes, and familial microcephaly). The tongue also provides clues to diagnoses. An absent or very small tongue may be noted in the hypoglossia and hypodactyly syndrome. A large tongue is found in Beckwith syndrome, gangliosidosis, congenital hypothyroidism, isolated macroglossia, and angiomas and hamartomas of the tongue. In dysautonomia, there is absence of the fungiform papillae. Clefts of the tongue are seen in the orofaciodigital, Meckel, and glossopalatine ankylosis syndromes.

Various terms are used to describe the shape of the mouth, including "broad" (Williams syndrome), "fishlike" (Treacher Collins, Prader–Willi, and Silver syndromes), "open" (Down syndrome, Apert syndrome, and myotonic dystrophy), and "small" (Schwartz–Jampel syndrome, Hallermann–Streiff syndrome, and craniocarpotarsal dystrophy). Micrognathia occurs in many conditions, including the Pierre Robin, Treacher Collins, and Hallermann–Streiff syndromes and trisomies 13 and 18. Prognathism (*i.e.*, prominence of the mandible) frequently is seen in Crouzon, Apert, and Rieger syndromes and in cerebral gigantism.

NECK

On examination of the neck, note should be made as to whether it is short (Turner, Noonan, and Klippel–Feil syndromes, spondyloepiphyseal dysplasia, and trisomy 13) or webbed (Turner, Noonan, and Down syndromes, and trisomy 18), or both. Deafness should be suspected in patients with preauricular pits and branchial cleft sinuses located along the anterior border of the sternocleidomastoid muscle, associated with cup-shaped ears.

SKELETON

There is a large number of skeletal abnormalities secondary to birth defects or genetic syndromes. They may be isolated (*e.g.*, polydactyly) or part of a syndrome (*e.g.*, polydactyly associated with trisomy 13). The most common type of polydactyly is postaxial (*i.e.*, the extra digit or digits are on the ulnar or fibular side of the middle finger or toe). Syndactyly, which also occurs in many syndromes, most frequently is an isolated finding involving the second and third toes and can be inherited in an autosomal dominant manner. The hand is very accessible for examination and frequently provides clues to syndrome diagnoses (Table 40-4). Other hand abnormalities that should be looked for include clinodactyly, broad hands, camptodactyly (*i.e.*, bent fingers), tapered fingers, and abnormal dermatoglyphics. Nails also should be observed for abnormal findings (*e.g.*, dysplasia associated with Ellis–van Creveld syndrome, ectodermal dysplasia, hereditary osteoonychodysplasia, fetal hydantoin syndrome, and focal dermal hypoplasia).

Most skeletal dysplasias can be suspected in the newborn period. It is very difficult to keep abreast of the changing classifications of the skeletal dysplasias, but the pediatrician should have a general approach to these problems to raise the possibility of such a diagnosis.

The most common and also the most overdiagnosed skeletal dysplasia is achondroplasia. An infant who dies in the newborn period and resembles an achondroplastic dwarf is most likely to have thanatophoric dwarfism or achondrogenesis, and not achondroplasia. Radiographic findings and microscopic examination of the cartilage differ in each syn-

TABLE 40–4
HAND ABNORMALITIES PRESENT IN THE NEWBORN PERIOD

Abnormality	Syndrome	Abnormality	Syndrome
Arachnodactyly	Contractual arachnodactyly	Abnormal thumbs	
	Homocystinuria	Broad	Apert
	Marfan		Larsen
Brachydactyly	Achondroplasia		Pfeiffer
	Coffin–Lowry		Otopalatodigital
	Congenital hypothyroidism		Rubinstein–Taybi
	de Lange	Proximally placed	de Lange
	Diastrophic dwarfism		Diastrophic dwarf
	Down		Trisomy 13
	Ellis–van Creveld	Fingerlike and triphalangeal	Fetal hydantoin
	Hypochondroplasia		Heart–hand
	Laurence–Moon–Biedl		Holt–Oram
	Multiple epiphyseal dysplasia		Hypoplastic congenital anemia
	Orofaciodigital		VATER association
	Pseudoachondroplasia	Stub thumb	Isolated, autosomal dominant
	Robinow	Thumb sign*	Ehlers–Danlos
	Silver–Russell		Marfan
	Turner	Dorsal swelling	Congenital hypothyroidism
Polydactyly	Achondrogenesis		Noonan
	Cerebrohepatorenal		Thrombocytopenia–absent radius
	de Lange		
	Ellis–van Creveld		Turner
	Fetal alcohol	Shortened metacarpals	Albright hereditary osteodystrophy
	Focal–dermal hypoplasia		
	Jeune thoracic dysplasia		Basal cell nevus syndrome
	Laurence–Moon–Biedl		Cri du chat
	Meckel		Otopalatodigital
	Short-rib polydactyly		Short-rib polydactyly
	Smith–Lemli–Opitz		Sjögren–Larsson
	Trisomy 13		
	Trisomy 18		
Syndactyly	Apert		
	de Lange		
	Fetal hydantoin		
	Goltz		
	Holt-Oram		
	Meckel		
	Orofaciodigital		
	Otopalatodigital		
	Poland		
	Russell–Silver		
	Saethre–Chotzen		
	Short–rib polydactyly		
	Smith–Lemli–Opitz		

* Extension of the flexed thumb beyond the ulnar border when the fingers are flexed over the thumb.

TABLE 40-5
SKELETAL DYSPLASIAS PRESENT IN THE NEWBORN PERIOD

Syndrome	Large Head	Narrow Chest	Inheritance
Achondrogenesis	+	+	AR, −
Achondroplasia	+	+	AD
Camptomelic dysplasia	−	++	AR
Cleidocranial dysplasia	+	−	AD
Chondrodysplasia punctata, rhizomelic type	±	−	AR
Chondrodysplasia punctata, Conradi-Hünermann type	±	−	AD
Diastrophic dwarfism	−	−	AR
Ellis–van Creveld	−	++	AR
Hypophosphatasia	−	+	AR
Jeune thoracic dystrophy	−	++	AR
Kniest dysplasia	−	−	AD
Metatropic	−	+	AD/AR
Osteogenesis imperfecta congenita	+	−	AR
Pyknodysostosis	+	−	AR
Robinow	+	−	AD/AR
Short-rib polydactyly	−	++	AR
Spondylocostal dysplasia	−	±	AD
Spondyloepiphyseal dysplasia congenita	−	−	AD
Spondylothoracic dysplasia	−	++	AR
Thanatophoric dwarfism	+	++	?

++, present to a severe degree; +, present; − absent; ±, may or may not be present; AD, autosomal dominant; AR, autosomal recessive.

drome. Some of the bone dysplasias that have manifestations at birth associated with dwarfism are listed in Table 40-5. Patients with thanatophoric dwarfism and achondrogenesis do not survive the newborn period. In asphyxiating thoracic dysplasia and the camptomelic syndrome, respiratory distress is present. It is important to note whether the long bones are shorter proximally, as in achondroplasia, or distally, as in Ellis–van Creveld syndrome, and whether the chest is narrow. Radiographic examination will confirm the diagnosis.

For a compilation of inherited disorders in humans, see McKusick's text on mendelian inheritance.[1] Malformations of particular organs are described in their related chapters.

COMMON MALFORMATION SYNDROMES

ACHONDROPLASIA

Major manifestations of achondroplasia (Fig. 40-4) include short stature, with the proximal segments of the limbs being more involved than the distal segments. The hands are short and stubby. There is enlargement of the head, which may be secondary to macrocephaly or hydrocephalus or both, and the forehead is prominent. There is a depressed nasal bridge with an upturned nose. The chest cavity appears small. As the child grows older, there is lordosis, and the abdomen protrudes. Motor development, such as sitting and standing, may be delayed, but intelligence usually is normal. Radiographic examination substantiates the diagnosis. The ilia are square, the sacrosciatic notch is small, the pubic and ischial bones are short, and there is a lack of the normal increase in the interpediculate distance from L1 to L5.

Achondroplasia is inherited as an autosomal dominant trait, although approximately 80% of the cases are secondary to a new mutation.

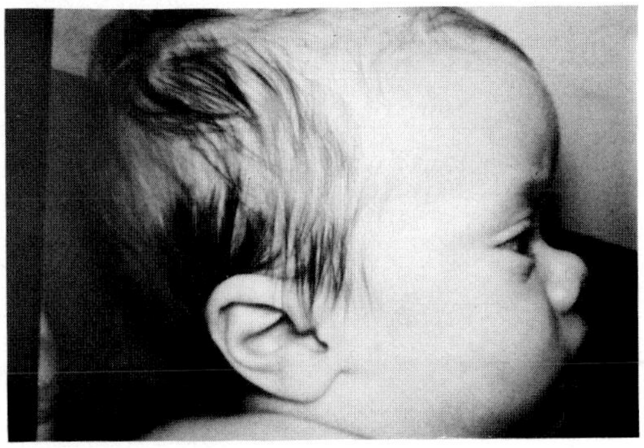

FIG. 40–4. Achondroplasia.

APERT SYNDROME

Major manifestations of Apert syndrome (*i.e.*, acrocephalosyndactyly; Fig. 40-5) include craniosynostosis, mainly of the coronal sutures; depressed broad bridge of the nose, which is beaked; hypoplasia of the maxilla; apparent ocular hypertelorism; downward and outward slant of the palpebral fissures; and a high-arched, narrow palate. Skeletal abnormalities consist mainly of syndactyly of the hands and feet, usually including the second to fifth digits.

Mental retardation has been reported, although many children have normal intelligence. Most of the cases are sporadic, but autosomal dominant inheritance has been reported.

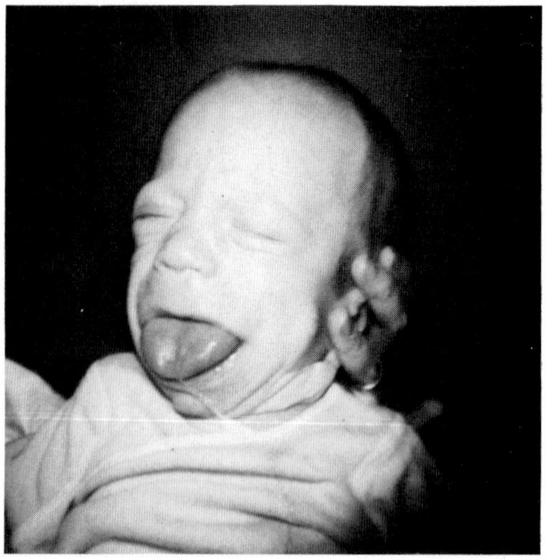

FIG. 40–6. Beckwith syndrome.

BECKWITH–WIEDEMANN SYNDROME

Major manifestations of Beckwith–Wiedemann syndrome (Fig. 40-6) include birth weight over 3200 g, large tongue and viscera, neonatal hypoglycemia, usually after the first day of life, leucine sensitivity, strabismus, and an omphalocele, or large umbilical hernia. After an initial weight loss, there is an increase in both height and weight. The hypoglycemia may be severe enough to cause death or slow development. Other findings include microcephaly, indentation or notching of the ear lobes, facial nevus flammeus, diaphragmatic eventration, visceromegaly, cliteromegaly, cryptorchidism, and asymmetry. The type of inheritance is uncertain, but polygenic, autosomal recessive, and autosomal dominant inheritance have been reported.

CHONDRODYSPLASIA PUNCTATA, RHIZOMELIC TYPE

In the newborn period, chondrodysplasia punctata, rhizomelic type (Fig. 40-7) is characterized by dwarfism, microcephaly, flat bridge of a hypoplastic nose, puffy cheeks, cataracts, contractures, club feet, dyskeratotic skin lesions, respiratory distress, and congenital heart disease. The limbs may be quite short, causing some confusion with achondroplasia or osteogenesis imperfecta. Death may occur within the first year of life. Radiographic examination reveals a characteristic deformity of vertebral bodies. The spine has vertical radiolucent bars of cartilage that separate the anterior and posterior ossification centers; shortened femora or humeri or both; metaphyseal irregularities; and symmetric stippling.

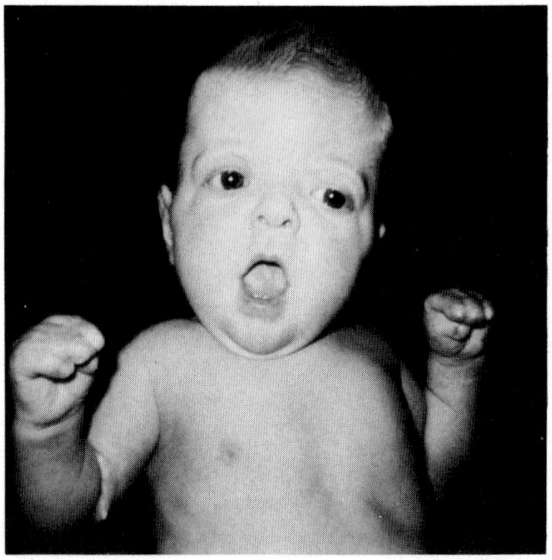

FIG. 40–5. Apert syndrome.

Chondrodysplasia punctata, Conradi–Hunermann type, is more benign and is inherited in an autosomal dominant manner.

CRI DU CHAT SYNDROME

Major manifestations of cri du chat syndrome (Fig. 40-8) are a high-pitched, catlike cry present during infancy, microcephaly, ocular hypertelorism, rounded face, mental retardation, and deletion of the short arm of chromosome 5. The infant with cri du chat syndrome is small for dates and has low-set ears, short metacarpals or metatarsals, and epicanthal folds.

The partial deletion of the short arm of chromosome 5 usually is a sporadic occurrence, although occasionally one of the parents may be a balanced translocation carrier.

DE LANGE SYNDROME

Manifestations of de Lange syndrome (Fig. 40-9) include short stature, hirsutism, synophrys, long eyelashes, upturned nose with anteverted nares, prominent philtrum, thin lips, congenital heart disease, and a variety of skeletal abnormalities, including limb abnormalities. Mental retardation almost always is present, as is microcephaly. A growling cry frequent-

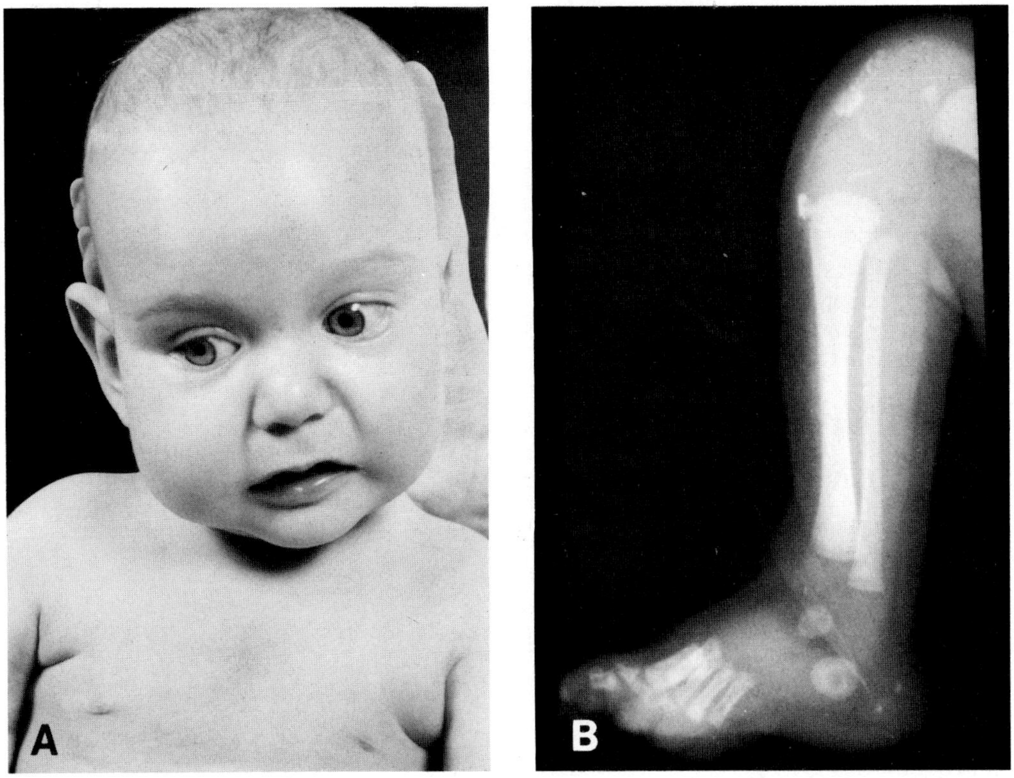

FIG. 40–7. (A, B) Chrondrodysplasia punctata.

ly is heard. Neonatal respiratory and feeding problems are common.

The cause is unknown, and recurrence is unlikely. There have been rare reports of familial translocation abnormalities.

DOWN SYNDROME

Clinical findings in Down syndrome (*i.e.*, trisomy 21; Fig. 40-10) include brachycephaly, broad-bridged nose, speckled iris, upward slant of the palpebral fissures, epicanthal folds, flattened facies, high-arched, narrow palate, protruding tongue, small, square ears, short, broad hands, simian line, short or missing fifth middle phalanx, congenital heart disease, webbing of the neck, hypotonia, and mental retardation. Trisomy 21 is present in approximately 95% of the patients, and a translocation abnormality is seen in 2% to 3%. See Table 40-1 for frequency according to maternal age.

This syndrome is so familiar that a lengthy description is not included here. There are varying degrees of mental retardation.

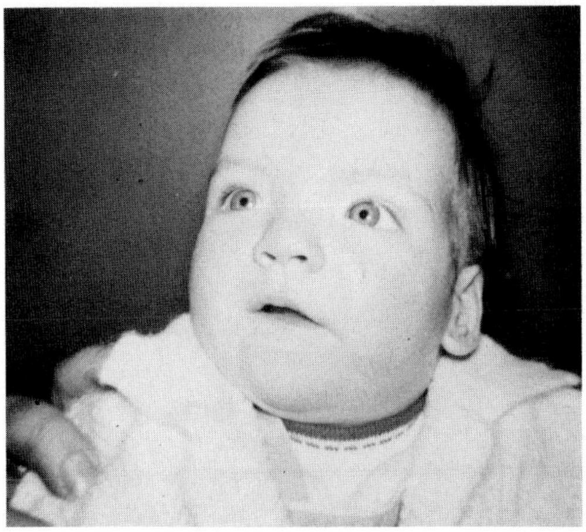

FIG. 40–8. Cri du chat syndrome.

MANDIBULOFACIAL DYSOSTOSIS

Major manifestations of mandibulofacial dysostosis (*i.e.*, Treacher Collins Syndrome; Fig. 40-11) include an abnormal facial appearance manifested by a downward slant of the palpebral fissures, beaklike nose, coloboma of the lower lid, hypoplasia of the supraorbital ridges, facial bone dysostosis, micrognathia, dysplastic ears, conductive hearing loss, defects of the auditory ossicles, preauricular tags, flame-shaped projections of hair extending from the ear onto the cheek, and micrognathia. Mental retardation usually is not present.

The syndrome is inherited as an autosomal dominant trait with a varying degree of expressivity.

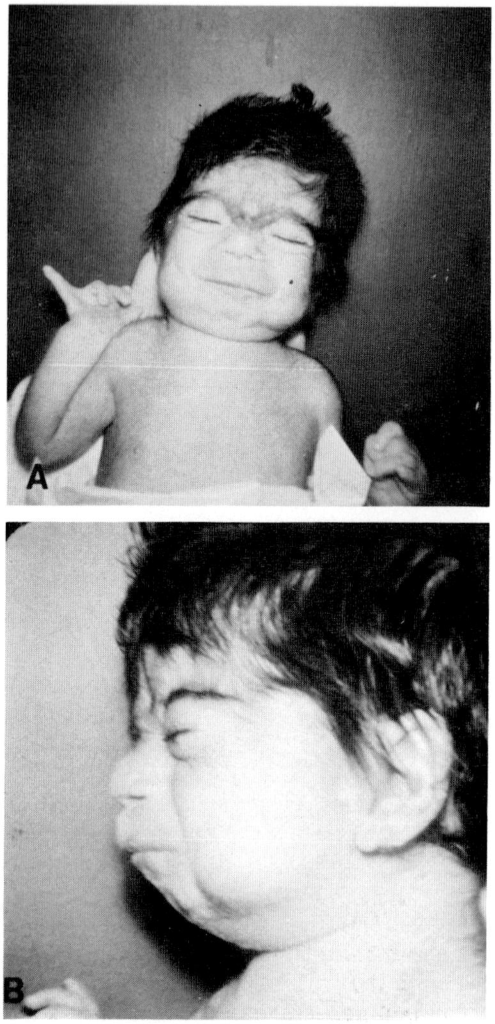

FIG. 40–9. (A, B) de Lange syndrome.

OSTEOGENESIS IMPERFECTA CONGENITA

At birth, multiple fractures and skeletal deformities characterize osteogenesis imperfecta congenita (Fig. 40-12). The skull is soft, and there is a ping-pong sensation on palpation of the enlarged skull, which has wide-open fontanelles. In very severe cases, the face may be birdlike. The limbs usually are very small and bowed, with multiple deformities and hyperextensibility of the joints. Blue sclerae occasionally may be present. Hydrocephalus and intracranial hemorrhage are frequent findings. Radiographs show multiple wormian bones and fractures, especially of the long bones and ribs.

The mode of inheritance in the neonatal type usually is autosomal recessive, but in the lethal type a new dominant mutation may occur. Osteogenesis imperfecta tarda is inherited in an autosomal dominant manner, and manifestations generally are not present in the neonatal period.

POTTER SYNDROME

Major manifestations of Potter syndrome (Fig. 40-13) include typical facial appearance, absent or dysplastic kidneys, pulmonary hypoplasia, and neonatal death. The facies appear flattened with micrognathia, low-set and abnormally shaped ears, flattened, beaked nose, apparent ocular hypertelorism, and a skin fold below the eye. Other malformations include arthrogryposis, abnormal genitalia, lower limb abnormalities, and gastrointestinal malformations. Oligohydramnios and amnion nodosum (*i.e.*, nodular plaques of debris and cells on the fetal surface of the placenta) are associated with this syndrome.

The etiology is not certain, and there does not appear to be an inherited pattern, although one report has indicated a 3% recurrence risk.

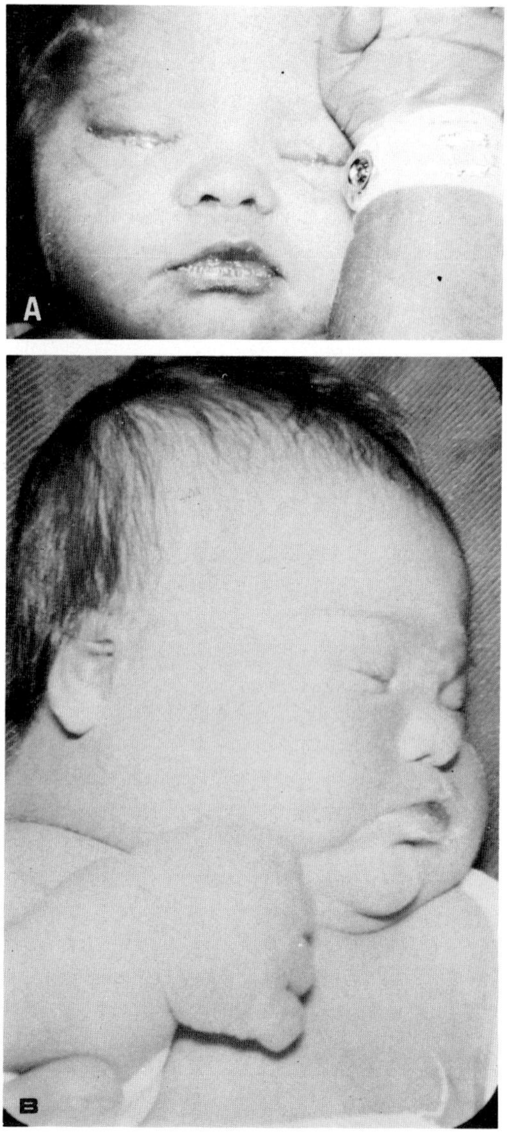

FIG. 40–10. (A, B) Down syndrome.

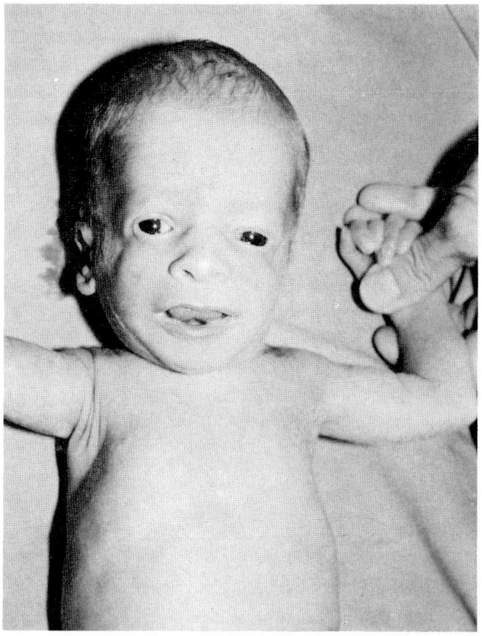

FIG. 40–11. Treacher Collins syndrome (mandibulofacial dysostosis).

SMITH–LEMLI–OPITZ SYNDROME

Major manifestations of Smith–Lemli–Opitz syndrome (Fig. 40-14) include marked failure to thrive, mental and motor retardation, a classic facial appearance, vomiting and pyloric stenosis, microcephaly, a shrill cry, cryptorchidism, hypospadias, small penis, simian line, syndactyly of the second and third toes, and abnormal dermatoglyphics. The facial appearance includes ptosis of the eyelids, strabismus, anteverted nostrils, prominent philtrum, and broad maxillary alveolar ridge. There are other, less frequently found congenital birth defects, including a clenched hand with the index finger over the middle finger. Many of these children die within the first year of life; Smith–Lemli–Opitz type II produces more major malformation and almost always results in a neonatal death. The syndrome is inherited in an autosomal recessive manner, and the carrier state is not detectable.

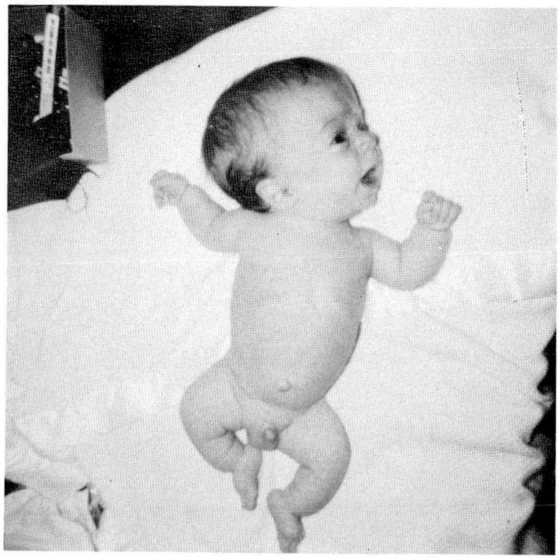

FIG. 40–12. Osteogenesis imperfecta congenita.

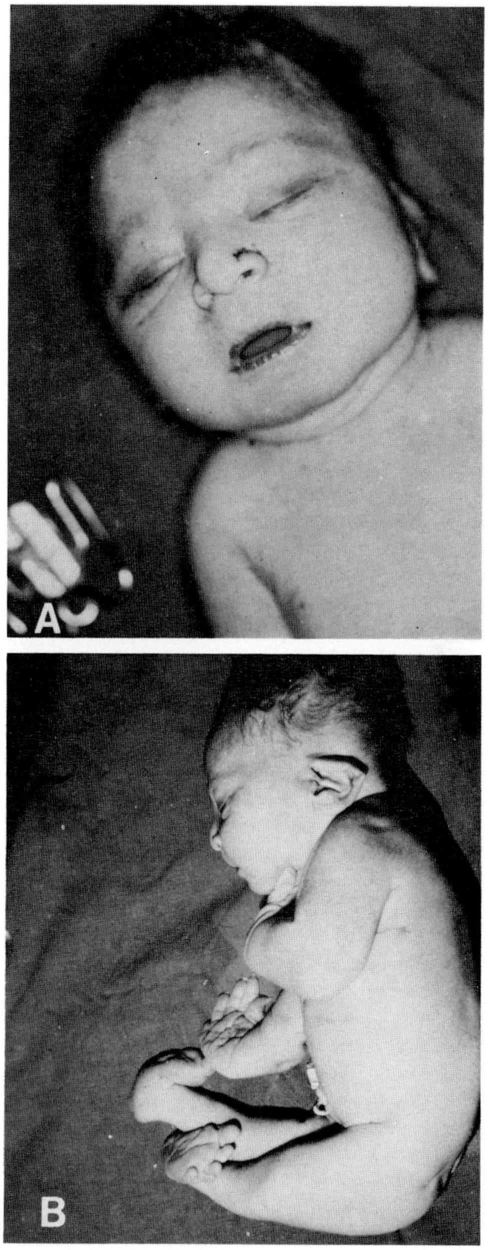

FIG. 40–13. (A, B) Potter syndrome.

STURGE–WEBER SYNDROME

The major manifestation of Sturge–Weber syndrome (Fig. 40-15) is a port-wine vascular malformation involving the distribution of the fifth cranial nerve. A

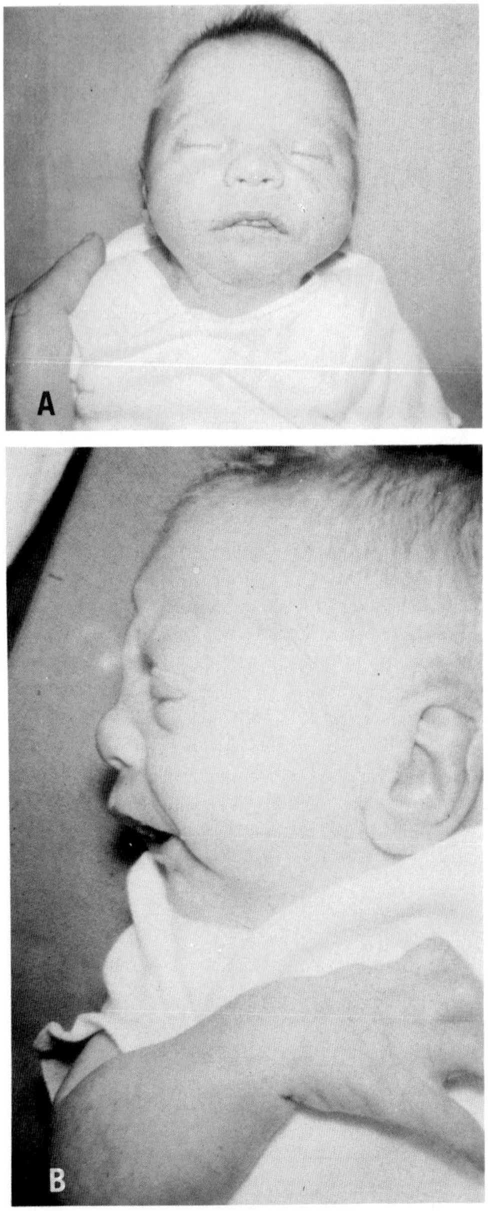

FIG. 40–14. **(A, B)** Smith–Lemli–Opitz syndrome.

vascular malformation also may affect the brain, resulting in seizures and intracerebral calcifications that usually are not present in the neonatal period. Glaucoma also may be present on the side of the malformation. Hemianopia and hemiplegia frequently are present.

The etiology is unknown, and there does not appear to be an inherited pattern.

TRISOMY 13

Major manifestations of trisomy 13 (Fig. 40-16) include marked mental and motor retardation, microcephaly, ocular hypotelorism, microphthalmos, low-

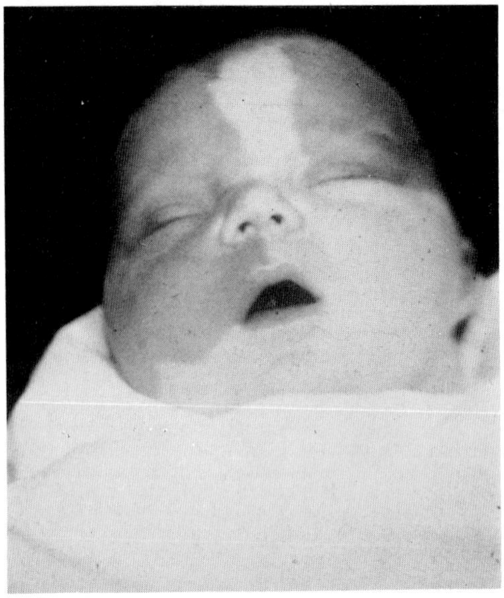

FIG. 40–15. Sturge–Weber syndrome.

set, malformed ears, cleft lip, palate, or both, micrognathia, webbing of the neck, undescended testicles, congenital heart disease, hand abnormalities, capillary hemangioma, and scalp defects. Postmortem examination reveals various renal and gastrointestinal abnormalities, holoprosencephaly, and a

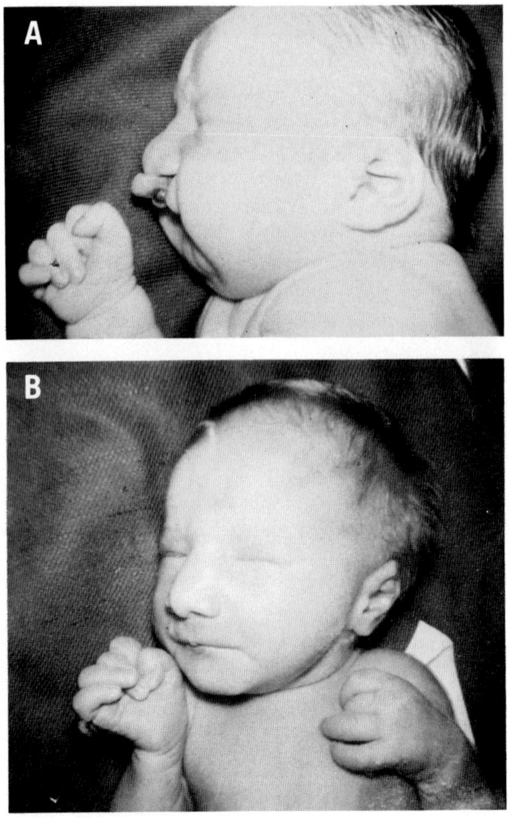

FIG. 40–16. **(A, B)** Trisomy 13.

bicornuate uterus. Most patients die by 1 year of age. There are 47 chromosomes; chromosome 13 is the extra one.

TRISOMY 18

Common manifestations of trisomy 18 (Fig. 40-17) include prominent occiput, low-set, malformed ears, ptosis of the eyelids, small palpebral fissures, Grecian or upturned nose, narrow palate or clefting of the palate, congenital heart disease, and renal abnormalities. Skeletal anomalies include overlapping of the second over the third fingers, retroflexed or distally placed thumb, rocker-bottom feet, syndactyly, short sternum, and small pelvis. Other findings include failure to thrive, poor suck, abnormal cry, pyloric stenosis, Meckel diverticulum, webbing of the neck, and meningomyelocele. Mental retardation and early death are constant findings. The chromosomal abnormality consists of an extra chromosome 18.

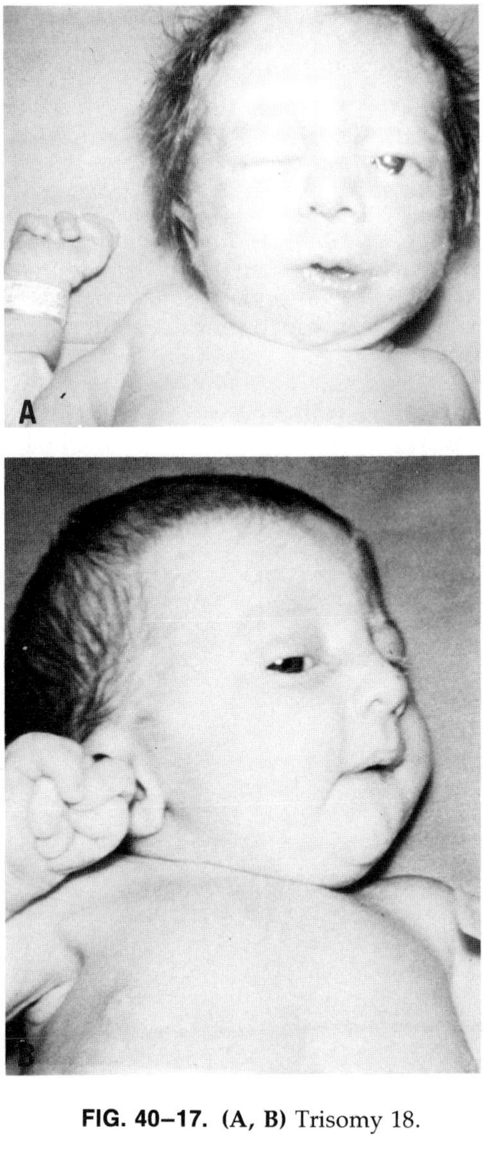

FIG. 40–17. (A, B) Trisomy 18.

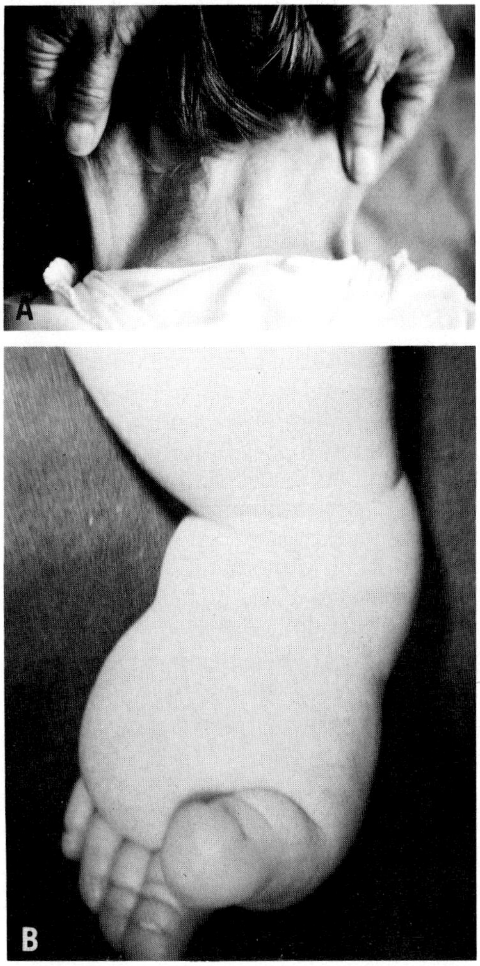

FIG. 40–18. (A, B) Turner syndrome.

TURNER SYNDROME

Major manifestations of Turner syndrome (Fig. 40-18) include short stature; broad nasal bridge; low-set ears; ptosis of the eyelids; epicanthal folds; webbing of the neck; low posterior hairline; narrow palate; lymphedema on the dorsa of the hands and feet; hypoplastic or inverted nipples; congenital heart disease, usually coarctation of the aorta; abnormal dermatoglyphics; increased number of pigmented moles; dysplastic or hyperconvex fingernails; gonadal dysplasia or streak gonads; lack of secondary sexual characteristics; horseshoe kidneys; and unilateral renal agenesis. Intelligence is normal. Classically, an X chromosome is missing, but isochromosome X and a variety of mosaic forms may be present. Recurrence in the same family is unusual.

FETAL ALCOHOL SYNDROME

Major manifestations of fetal alcohol syndrome include slow prenatal and postnatal growth, mental retardation, microcephaly, characteristic facial appearance (*i.e.*, broad nasal bridge, short palpebral fissures, ptosis, and prominent philtrum), congenital heart defects, congenital dislocated hip and other joint abnormalities, poor motor coordination, and tremulousness during the newborn period. Manifestations also can occur in offspring born to mothers who were moderate drinkers, but the symptoms usually are not as marked (Fig. 40-19).

FETAL HYDANTOIN SYNDROME

Major manifestations of fetal hydantoin syndrome include slow prenatal and postnatal growth, microcephaly, mental retardation, and a characteristic facial appearance, including epicanthal folds, ptosis of the eyelids, broad nasal bridge, small, upturned nose, apparent ocular hypertelorism, and prominent philtrum. Various types of congenital heart disease are present. Limb abnormalities include fingerlike thumbs, hypoplasia of the distal phalanges, and nail dysplasia. Frequently, only a few of these findings are present (Fig. 40-20).

POLAND MALFORMATION SEQUENCE

Major manifestations of Poland malformation sequence (Fig. 40-21) include symbrachydactyly (*i.e.*, syndactyly and short digits) and a defect of the pectoralis muscle. All variations of syndactyly and brachydactyly can occur, but the thumb usually is not as severely affected. The sternal head of the pectoralis muscle on the same side as the hand anomaly is abnormal, whereas the clavicular head always is present. Other findings include asymmetric breast development, absent breast on same side, ipsilateral webbing of the axilla, rib abnormalities, shortening of the arm and forearm, and Sprengel deformity (*i.e*,. congenital high scapula).

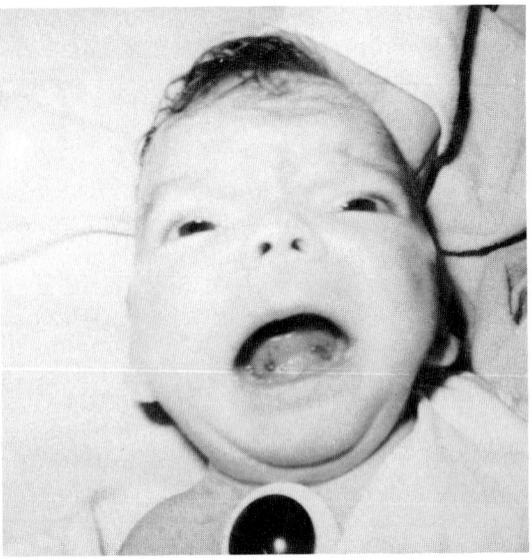

FIG. 40–20. Fetal hydantoin syndrome.

PRUNE-BELLY SYNDROME

The major manifestation of prune-belly syndrome is aplasia or hypoplasia of the abdominal wall muscles. This results in wrinkling and redundant skin over the abdominal wall and protrusion of the abdominal organs (Fig. 40-22). A variety of urinary tract abnormalities may be present, including megaureter and hydronephrosis. If renal involvement is significant, the facies may appear flat, as in Potter syndrome. Gastrointestinal and skeletal abnormalities are not uncommon. Most reported cases have been sporadic.

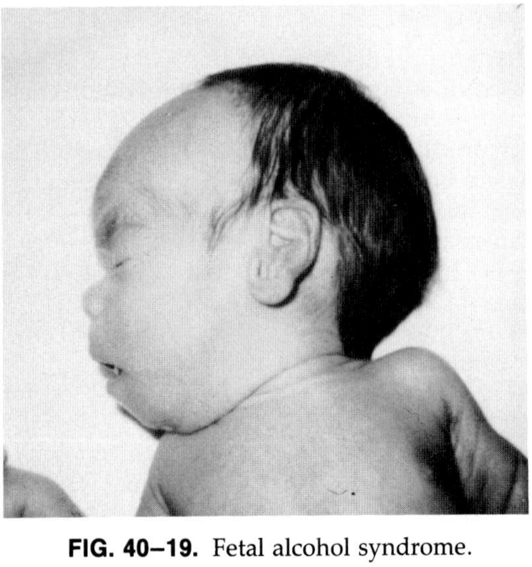

FIG. 40–19. Fetal alcohol syndrome.

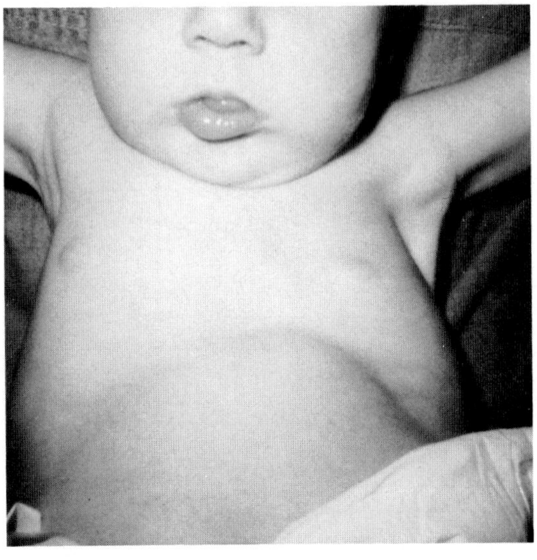

FIG. 40–21. Poland malformation sequence.

THROMBOCYTOPENIA–ABSENT RADIUS SYNDROME

Major manifestations of thrombocytopenia–absent radius syndrome (Fig. 40-23) are absence of the radius with the thumb present and thrombocytopenia. Both radii usually are missing or hypoplastic, and other limb abnormalities such as club hand, syndactyly, missing bones of the limbs, and dislocated hips may be present. The thrombocytopenia usually persists for the first few months of life and may require platelet transfusions. A leukemoid reaction often is present. Other findings include a triangular facial shape and micrognathia, congenital heart disease, diarrhea, swelling on the dorsal aspects of the feet, and bleeding episodes secondary to the thrombocytopenia. The syndrome is inherited in an autosomal recessive manner.

VATER ASSOCIATION OR SEQUENCE

VATER stands for vertebral abnormalities, anal atresia, tracheoesophageal fistula, usually with esophageal atresia, and renal or radial limb abnormalities. The acronym VACTERL also has been used, in which the C stands for cardiac abnormalities, and the L for limb anomalies. Less frequently found manifestations include abnormalities of the brain, respiratory tract, and ribs. The diagnosis usually is made if three or more of the major manifestations are present. Nearly all the cases have been sporadic.

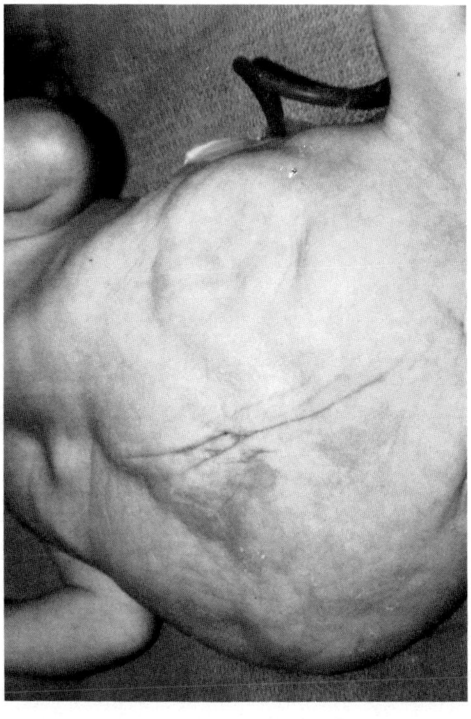

FIG. 40–22. An infant with prune-belly syndrome shows redundant abdominal skin and lax abdominal muscles.

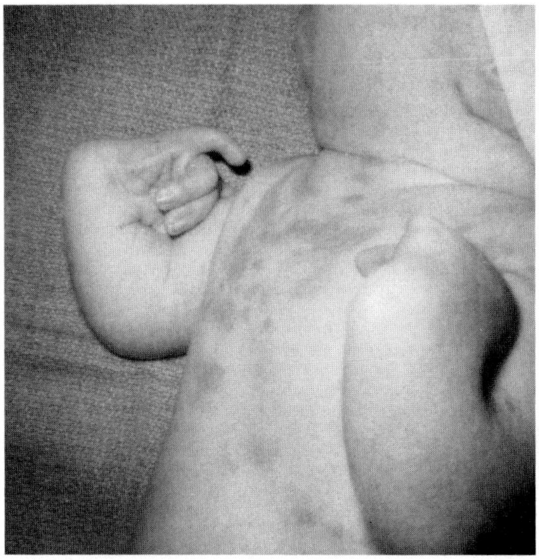

FIG. 40–23. An infant with thrombocytopenia–absent radius syndrome has thrombocytopenia, absent radius, and associated deformities.

PHYSICAL NORMS FOR SYNDROMES

One of the difficulties in syndrome identification is the lack of specific descriptive measurements (Fig. 40-24). For example, the definition of low-set ears varies from observer to observer. The same is true in defining other facial features. Various physical parameters have been studied in a normal population to provide standards.[2]

EYE MEASUREMENTS

Although the presence of ocular hypertelorism or hypotelorism is extremely important in syndrome diagnosis, direct interpupillary measurements are difficult to obtain and therefore are unreliable in infants and children.

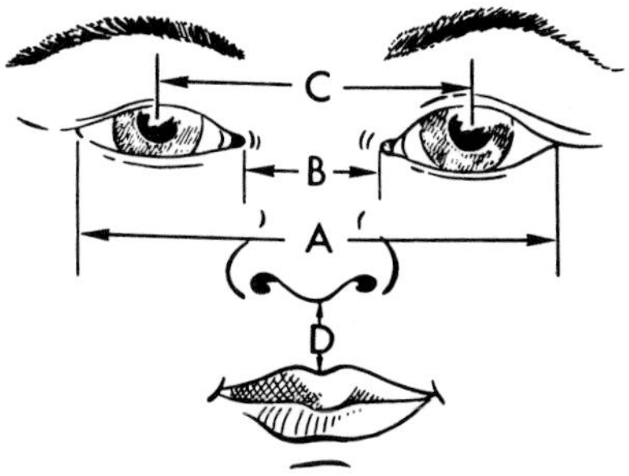

FIG. 40–24. A, outer canthal distance; B, inner canthal distance; C, interpupillary distance; D, nasolabial distance.

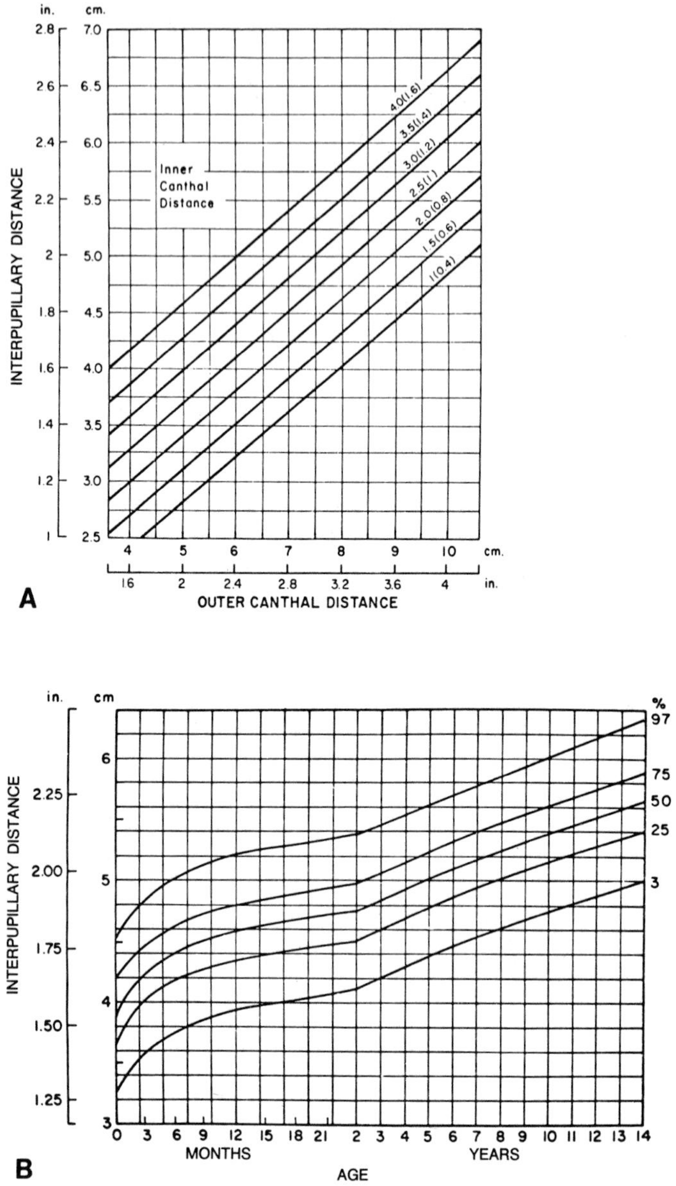

FIG. 40–25. **(A)** Nomogram for computing interpupillary distance from inner and outer canthal distance. **(B)** Age-specific norms for interpupillary distance. Key percentiles are designated.

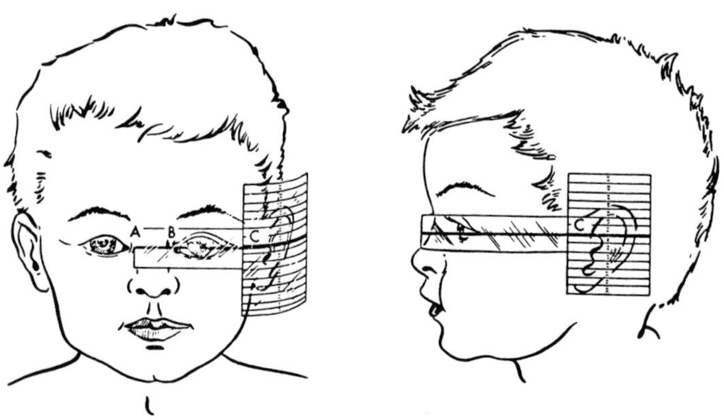

FIG. 40–26. An x-ray film device can be used to measure ear length and compute the percentage of the ear above and below the inner canthal eyeline.

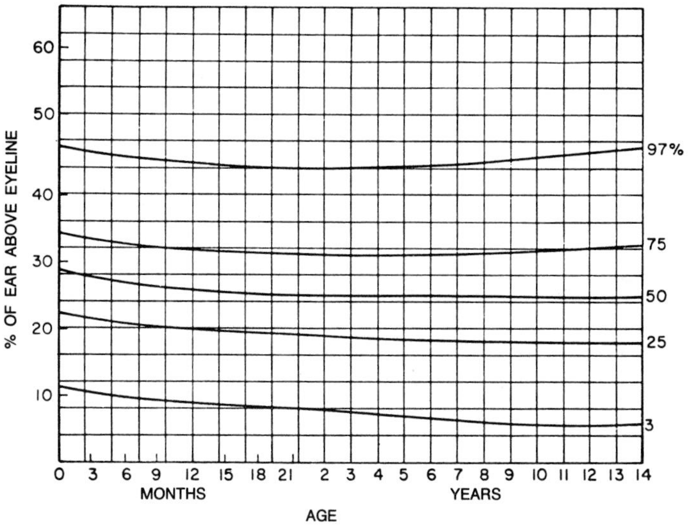

FIG. 40–27. Age-specific norms for the percentage of the ear above the eyeline.

A graph was prepared that allows the determination of interpupillary distance (Fig. 40-25*A*). By plotting the inner and outer canthal distances, one can obtain the interpupillary distance, plot it against the patient's age (Fig. 40-25*B*), and determine the percentile.

EAR MEASUREMENTS

Figure 40-26 depicts a measuring instrument made from x-ray film and its application.[2] Both sides of the instrument are divided into millimeters, allowing the right and left ears to be measured by the same instrument. A central horizontal line is drawn on the instrument, and the length of the ear above or below this line is determined. The medial canthi (see Fig. 40-26) were used as landmarks, rather than the lateral canthi, because an upward or downward slant of the palpebral fissures can provide incorrect landmarks. The central horizontal line is placed over both inner canthi, and point C is found by extending this center line to the side of the face. The measuring part of the instrument covers the ear, and the length of the ear above or below the center line is determined. The percentage of the ear above the line is determined, and this percentage is then related to age, with Figure 40-27 used to ascertain the percentile. Because this measurement is more difficult to obtain than the others, at least two measurements should be done so that reliability is improved.

HAND MEASUREMENTS

The hands were measured according to the landmarks depicted in Figure 40-28. The length of the middle finger, as a percentage of the total hand size (Fig. 40-29*A*), remained fairly constant from the newborn period to 14 years of age (42%–43%). This measurement helps to determine whether the fingers are longer or shorter than normal. The total length of the hand was plotted against age (Fig. 40-29*B*).

INTERNIPPLE DISTANCE

The internipple distance as a percentage of the chest circumference is plotted in Figure 40-30. This percentage was highest during the newborn period and then remained fairly constant. When this measurement is obtained for patients with Turner syndrome, an increased internipple distance is not documented.

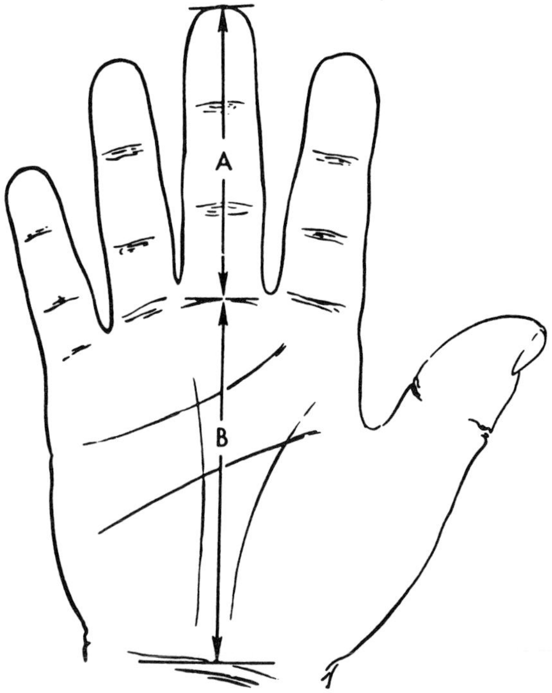

FIG. 40–28. Landmarks are used in measuring palm and finger length.

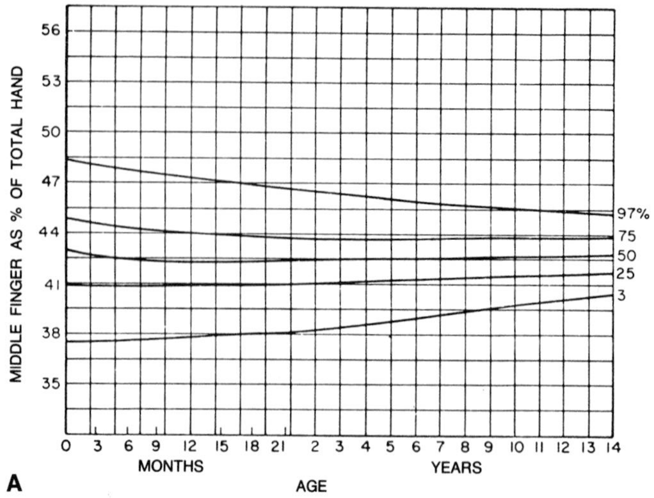

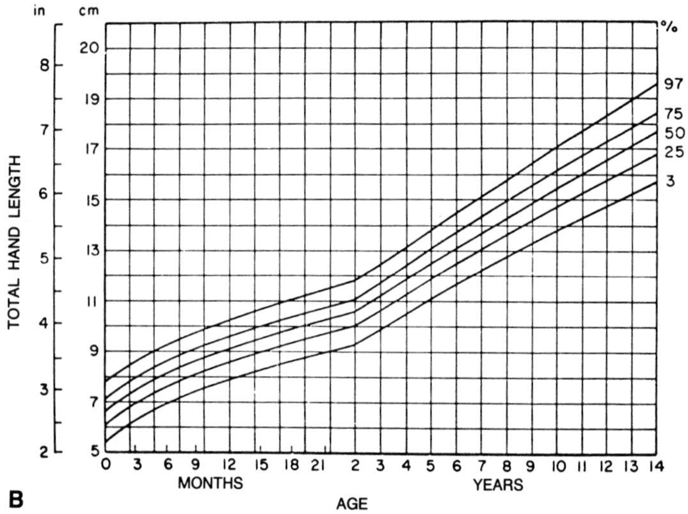

FIG. 40–29. **(A)** Age-specific norms for middle finger length as a percentage of total hand length. **(B)** Age-specific norms for total hand length.

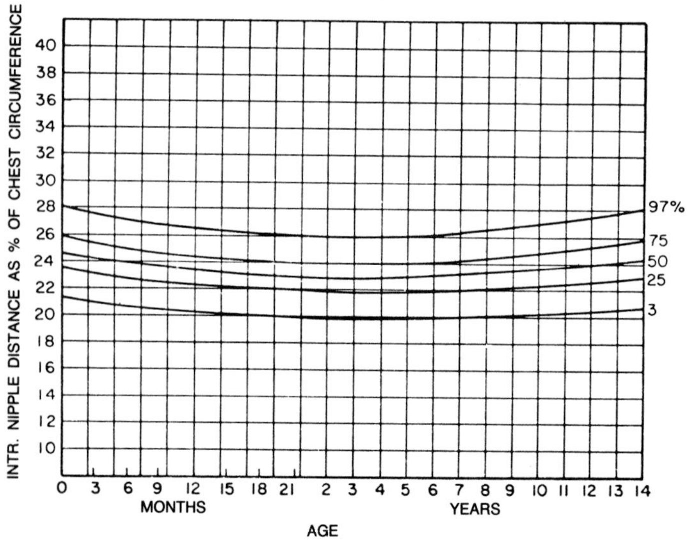

FIG. 40–30. The internipple distance as a percentage of chest circumference.

REFERENCES

1. McKusick VA. Mendelian inheritance in man. 9th ed. Baltimore: Johns Hopkins Press, 1990.
2. Feingold M, Bossert WH. Normal values for selected physical parameters. Birth Defects 1974;10(13).

BIBLIOGRAPHY

Aase JM. Diagnostic dysmorphology. New York: Plenum Medical Book Company, 1990.

Buyse ML. Birth defects encyclopedia. Cambridge, MA: Blackwell Scientific Publications, 1990.

Emery AEH, Rimoin DL. Principles and practice of medical genetics. New York: Churchill-Livingston, 1990.

Feingold M, Pashayan J. Genetics and birth defects in clinical practice. Boston: Little, Brown & Co., 1983.

Goldberg MJ. The dysmorphic child: an orthopedic perspective. New York: Raven Press, 1987.

Jones KL. Smith's recognizable patterns of human malformation. 4th ed. Philadelphia: WB Saunders, 1988.

Thompson JS, Thompson MW. Genetics in medicine. Philadelphia: WB Saunders, 1986.

Neonatology: Pathophysiology and Management of the Newborn, Fourth Edition,
edited by Gordon B. Avery, Mary Ann Fletcher, and Mhairi G. MacDonald.
J.B. Lippincott Company, Philadelphia © 1994.

chapter 41

Endocrine Disorders

THOMAS MOSHANG, JR.
PAUL S. THORNTON

Almost from the moment of conception, endocrine physiologic processes are actively involved in the growth and development of the human fetus. Disturbances of the interplay of these complex hormonal processes can cause somatic or biochemical alterations in the fetus and newborn infant. Therefore, the clinical disorders of endocrine function in the newborn are reflections of altered physiologic function, in either the fetus or the mother, during intrauterine life. Moreover, the disturbances of endocrine physiologic function can occur during different stages of fetal development, resulting in different clinical situations. Knowledge about the physiologic fetomaternal hormonal processes and the ontogeny of the fetal endocrine glands makes the clinical disorders of endocrine function in the newborn more readily understandable.

NORMAL SEXUAL DIFFERENTIATION

A schematic representation of the controls of sexual development is depicted in Figure 41-1. The gonadal anlagen are recognized as genital ridges by the fifth or sixth week of gestation. These primitive gonads are bipotential, consisting of cortical (*i.e.*, ovarian) and medullary (*i.e.*, testicular) components. The differentiation of the gonadal anlage into either a testis or an ovary is directed by the genetic information contained within the sex chromosomes.

In 1959, Ford and colleagues determined that the Y chromosome was necessary for male development,[1] which was further localized to the short arm of the Y chromosome in 1966.[2] H-Y antigen, which is located on the short arm of Y, was subsequently thought to represent the testis-determining factor (TDF).[3] In 1986, Page and associates postulated that a gene coding for a zinc finger protein in region one (*i.e.*, Yp1A2) on the short arm of the Y chromosome was the TDF.[4] Most recently, however, Sinclair and colleagues have localized a gene in the Yp1A1 region of the short arm of the Y chromosome that is present in all 46XY males, all 46XX males, and not found in any 46XY females. This gene is now referred to as the SRY gene (*i.e.*, the sex-determining region of the Y chromosome).[5] This complex story certainly is not complete, however, since the SRY gene has not been found in most 46XX true hermaphrodites in which testicular tissue is present. The current concept is that the SRY gene is the primary TDF, but more than one factor downstream of the SRY gene is involved in testicular determination.

In males, under the influence of TDF, the primary sex chords, which are the bipotential gonads, develop to form the testes. Testicular development is complete by 6 to 7 weeks of gestation. In the absence of a Y chromosome or the SRY gene and in the presence of two X chromosomes, the primary sex chords become follicles and the ovaries are formed by 10 weeks of gestation.

The differentiated gonads, in turn, play a critical role in directing the differentiation of the internal

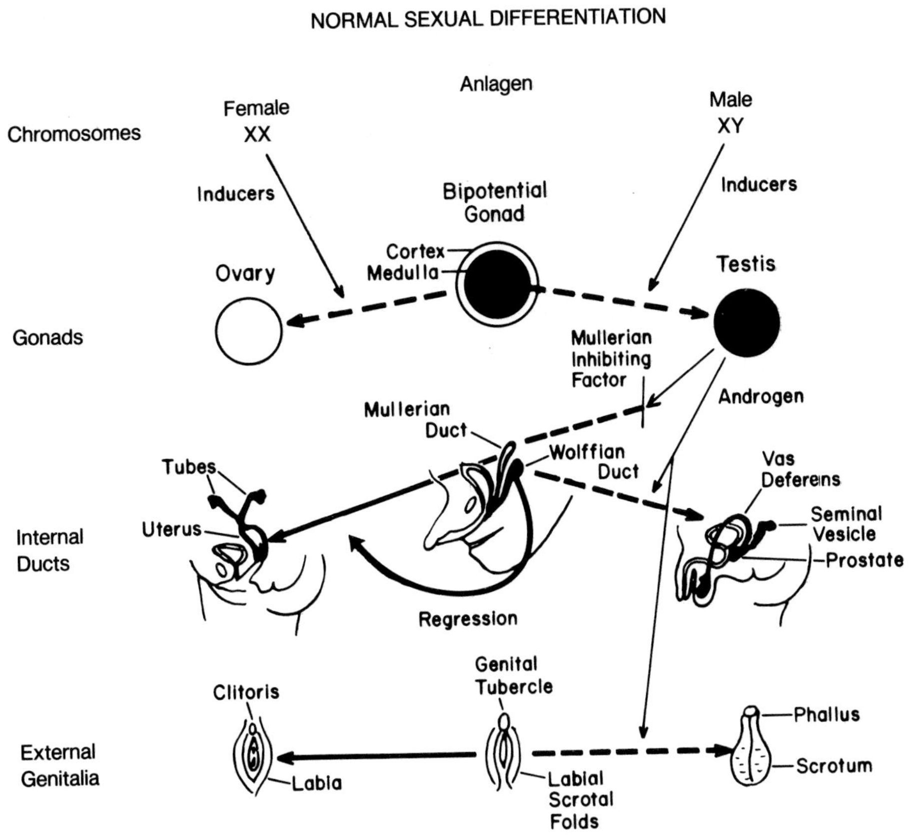

FIG. 41–1. Various inducers (*thin arrows*) are necessary for differentiation of the gonads and masculine development (*dashed arrows*). In the absence of these inducers, the differentiation is female (*thick arrows*).

genital ducts, as well as the external genitalia. In males, at 7 to 8 weeks of gestation, Sertoli cells in the seminiferous tubules secrete a 140-kd glycoprotein now referred to as anti-müllerian hormone or müllerian-inhibiting substance (MIS), previously referred to as müllerian inhibiting factor. Müllerian-inhibiting substance causes degeneration of the müllerian duct with resultant absence of the uterus, fallopian tubes, and proximal two thirds of the vagina. Leydig cells in the testes, stimulated by human chorionic gonadotropin (hCG), secrete testosterone, which locally stimulates the wolffian ducts to proliferate into the vas deferens, seminal vesicle, and epididymis. Testosterone is converted locally, by 5α-reductase, to dihydrotestosterone (DHT), which causes fusion of the urogenital slit and genital tubercle and development of the scrotum and penis. Male genital development is completed by 12 weeks of gestation. In the second trimester, abdominal descent of the testes is stimulated by MIS. Further descent of the testes into the scrotum and penile growth in the second and third trimester of gestation is in response to increasing testosterone production. This increase in testosterone production is stimulated by pituitary gonadotropins.

In the absence of the SRY gene and the presence of two X chromosomes, the primary sex chords develop into follicles and form the ovaries. The fetal ovaries, in the absence of androgens and MIS, do not descend. The müllerian ducts persist with resultant formation of the uterus, fallopian tubes, and vagina. There is no stimulus to the wolffian duct. The development of female external genitalia does not depend on hormone action or on the presence of functioning gonads.

SEXUAL AMBIGUITY AND GONADAL DISORDERS

The first thought for most parents of a newborn infant is the gender of the child. Even when many parents today are aware of the probable gender of a fetus because of prenatal ultrasonography or amniocentesis, the declaration of gender at birth is necessary. In those situations when gender is unclear or is discordant from prenatal chromosomal findings, the situation is truly a medical emergency. It is important for those attending at the birth of such infants to be extremely cautious but simultaneously reassuring to parents that the gender of their child will be discerned in a short period of time.

DISORDERS OF CHROMOSOMAL SEX

The normal complement of sex chromosomes directs the bipotential gonad to differentiate into either ovary or testicle. Many varieties of sex chromosome aberrations have been reported (see Chap. 40). Some of these are lethal to the fetus (*e.g.*, YO), and some probably cause very few somatic or biochemical abnormalities in terms of sexual differentiation (*e.g.*, XXX). It is clear that aberrations of sex chromosomes influence gonadal differentiation. In contrast to the autosomal chromosomes (*e.g.*, trisomy 21), extra genetic material from the X chromosome (*e.g.*, 47XXX) can be tolerated with minor untoward effects. This is because, both in normal 46XX females and in patients with an extra X chromosome (*e.g.*, 47XXX), the second and subsequent X chromosomes are inactivated and do not contribute to the pool of genetic information. Studies of natural chromosomal disorders indicate that at least two X chromosomes are required for complete ovarian development. Although more than two X chromosomes do not interfere with gonadal differentiation, a percentage of the reported patients with X polyploidy have manifested early menopause.[6,7] It generally is true that a Y chromosome is necessary for testicular development; however, case reports of true hermaphrodites and normal male phenotypes with only XX chromosomes are well documented.[8,9] The presence of testicular tissue in the absence of a Y chromosome previously was difficult to explain. The discovery of the SRY gene and the knowledge that translocations of small amounts of genetic material may occur, make this possibility more easily understood. The etiology of the 46XX true hermaphrodite, however, still is not fully explained.

The classic sex chromosomal aberrations occur relatively frequently as determined by newborn screening. In the New Haven Study, XXY occurred once in 545 males, XYY occurred once in 728 males, XXX occurred once in 727 females, and only one case of 45 XO occurred in 2181 female newborns.[10] The diagnosis of Turner syndrome, however, is made with greater frequency than the other sex chromosomal aberrations because of the associated somatic abnormalities. Various combinations and deletions of sex chromosomal material have been reported, which cause a range of abnormalities of gonadal and sexual differentiation. The interested reader is referred to the discussion by Morishima and Grumbach concerning the interrelationship of various sex chromosome aberrations and phenotype.[11] Common sex chromosome abnormalities other than Turner syndrome (*e.g.*, XXX, XXY, XYY) do not present with problems during the neonatal period.

TURNER SYNDROME

Turner syndrome is preferred to other eponyms and descriptive terms (*e.g.*, Bonnevie–Ullrich Syndrome, gonadal dysgenesis) because of the linking of this eponym with the somatic characteristics of the 45XO chromosomal karyotype. The terms "gonadal dysgenesis" and "ovarian dysgenesis" can be confused with those embryologic situations designated "pure gonadal dysgenesis" (see Disorders of Gonadal Sex). The classic chromosomal abnormality is total loss of an X chromosome. Other chromosomal abnormalities have been reported, however, such as mosaicism of cells with an XO cell line with normal 46XX cells, or 46XY and deletion of part of an X chromosome (*e.g.*, 46X isochromosome X). Chromosomal analysis of girls with Turner syndrome suggests that over 50% are 45XO, 17% are isochromosome mosaic 46X,i(Xq), 8% are 45XO/46XX, and all of the other mosaics comprise the remainder.[12] It is estimated that 99.9% of concepta that are 45XO abort before week 28 of gestation,[13] and that 1 in 15 spontaneous abortions are 45XO.

The loss of some of the genetic information in the X chromosomes results in varying degrees of the somatic abnormalities of Turner syndrome. The presence of a 46XX cell line in mosaicism does not modify the short stature or somatic abnormalities to a great degree, but does seem to influence gonadal development. In the study by Goldberg and associates, spontaneous female sexual development occurred in 3 of 25 patients with mosaic karyotypes but in none of the XO group.[14]

In 1930, Ullrich described an 8-year-old girl with what are now accepted as the classic features of Turner syndrome.[15] Bonnevie described a collection of anomalies consisting of distention of the neck (pterygium colli), malformations of the ears and face, and swelling of the limb buds in a strain of mice.[16] He ascribed these features to distention of the tissues by fluid. Ullrich suggested that this effect was the cause of the phenotype of Turner syndrome. It is known that this swelling is caused by lymphangiectasia and lymphedema. It was not until 1938 that Henry Turner described seven females with the uniform appearance that now bears his name. In 1949, Ullrich confirmed what most endocrinologists now believe, that Bonnevie–Ullrich syndrome is a description of Turner syndrome in the neonate. The pterygium colli most often is seen as redundant folds about the posterior neck. The lymphedema involves the dorsa of the hands and feet. A host of associated somatic defects have been described in this syndrome,[17] most of which become more readily identifiable with age and growth of the child. The most common defects include triangular facies with low-set ears, high-arched palate, low hairline, shieldlike chest with widespread and hypoplastic areolas, and cubitus valgus. Coarctation of the aorta is a common cardiovascular abnormality; however, the more benign condition of bicuspid aortic valves is more common. Skin manifestations include hemangiomas, cutis laxa, pigmented nevi, dysplastic nails, and tendency to keloid formation. Skeletal abnormalities such as "beaking" of the medial tibial condyle, drumstick-shaped distal phalanges, and vertebral anomalies have been described.[18] Short metacarpals, resulting in the knuckle sign, may be detected clinically or radiologically. Palmar simian creases, distal axial triradius, and increased number of digital ulnar whorls are documented as dermatoglyphic abnormalities. The most consistent characteristics are seen in the older child, and these are short stature and sexual infantilism.

The diagnosis should be suspected in female neonates of low birth weight with lymphedema, pterygium colli, or coarctation of the aorta, and confirmed by chromosomal analyses. There is no specific therapy for this syndrome in the newborn period unless the developmental anomalies, such as coarctation of the aorta, create a clinical problem. These children have a high incidence of recurrent otitis media, chronic lymphocytic thyroiditis, and idiopathic hypertension. There is an increased incidence of mental retardation, but many Turner syndrome children are intellectually normal or even bright. Hormonal therapy at the appropriate age is indicated for the treatment of sexual infantilism.

Because one of the major psychological problems for girls with Turner syndrome is short stature, efforts to increase the final height in these children have been attempted by the use of low-dose estrogens, low-dose androgens, and human growth hormone. One retrospective study indicated that low-dose androgens did not enhance final height in Turner syndrome patients.[19] The availability of recombinant growth hormone has led to a large, multicenter trial, preliminary results of which indicate that final height is improved by growth hormone treatment of Turner syndrome patients.[20]

The question of fertility in later life might arise even in the newborn period. Studies have indicated that women with Turner syndrome can achieve pregnancy, with successful outcome, using *in vitro* fertilization of donor oocytes and hormonal therapy, at a rate similar to couples with infertility for other reasons.[21]

In Turner syndrome with XO/XY or XX/XY mosaicism or variations, the gonadal elements frequently will contain testicular components. In these situations, the presence of both medullary and cortical elements in gonadal remnants is referred to as mixed gonadal dysgenesis. Various external genitalia phenotypes have been documented in the mosaic variant of Turner syndrome, including normal female, normal male, intersex female with clitoromegaly, and male with hypospadias and unilateral cryptorchidism. The most frequent phenotype is female, although occasionally with clitoromegaly. In nine cases of XO/XY chromosome mosaicism described by Morishima and Grumbach, only one had male genital development.[11] These patients may have many of the somatic abnormalities typical of classic XO Turner syndrome. In mixed gonadal dysgenesis, however, especially in the presence of a Y chromosome, the likelihood of malignant degeneration of the gonadal tissues is markedly increased. Because any gonadal hormonal function in this disorder is more likely to be androgenic in nature and inappropriate for the usual phenotype, early gonadectomy is recommended for this specific variant of Turner syndrome.[22]

DISORDERS OF GONADAL SEX

A number of conditions have been documented in which there is gonadal failure of one degree or another. The etiologies of these disorders may include sex chromosome aberrations, but in many reported conditions no chromosome aberrations have been noted. Certainly, various teratogens, including radiation, viruses, and drugs might cause *in utero* gonaditis and damage to the developing gonad. The degree and timing of the damage to the developing testis will cause varying levels of failure of development of the internal ducts and external genitalia.

PURE GONADAL DYSGENESIS

Complete dysgenesis of the genital ridges results in normal phenotypic females. Affected girls tend to be tall and eunuchoid and have primary amenorrhea and sexual infantilism. The chromosomal karyotype may be either 46XX or 46XY. In the 46XX females, the condition can be inherited in an autosomal recessive manner and is associated with sensory neural deafness.[23] In the 46XY females, the condition also is inherited in an autosomal recessive fashion but also may be transmitted as an X-linked mutation.[24] Such patients have no gonads (*i.e.*, gonadal dysgenesis), in contrast to the 46XY females with deletion of the SRY gene, where a gonad is present. Teratogenic factors may also cause gonadal dysgenesis. A high incidence of neoplasia has been reported in pure gonadal dysgenesis. Most infants with 46XY gonadal dysgenesis will be detected in the neonatal period only if chromosome studies are done for other reasons, because they are phenotypically normal females.

PARTIAL GONADAL DYSGENESIS

Teratogenic factors that damage the testis at later stages of fetal development cause varying clinical situations. Destruction of the testis from between weeks 9 and 12 of gestation will not prevent involution of the müllerian structures since MIS will have been secreted, but will result in failure of fusion and development of the external genitalia, which is dependent on testosterone production by the testes. Thus, the external genitalia will be phenotypically female but there will be no gonads, no uterus or fallopian tubes. If the testes disappear late in the second trimester (*i.e.*, vanishing testes syndrome), the infant will have congenital anorchia with otherwise normal male external and internal genitalia. Lesser damage occurring between these times in gestation may cause micropenis or cryptorchidism.

TRUE HERMAPHRODITISM

In true hermaphroditism, both ovarian and testicular elements are present. Findings may consist of an ovary on one side and a testis on the contralateral side, an ovary or a testis and a contralateral ovotestis, or two ovotestes. Therefore, this terminology also includes those patients with mixed gonadal dysgenesis associated with sex chromosome aberrations (*e.g.*, 45XO/46XY). In those patients without chromosome aberrations, two thirds have a 46XX karyotype, and one third have a 46XY karyotype. It is interesting to note that of the true hermaphrodite patients with 46XX karyotype, very few have the SRY gene, yet 50% express the H-Y antigen. This contrasts with the 46XX males, of whom 90% carry the SRY gene. It has been suggested that the 46XX true hermaphrodite has an autosomal or X-linked mutation of a gene downstream of the SRY gene that plays a role in gonadal differentiation.

The development and differentiation of the internal duct structures and external genitalia in the true hermaphrodite depend on the degree of functioning testicular tissue. The sex differentiation of the gonaduct corresponds to the gonad on the same side, because it is apparent that MIS acts locally. Most true hermaphrodites have ambiguous external genitalia.

DISORDERS OF PHENOTYPIC SEX

Disorders of phenotypic sex result when the anatomic development of the external genitalia does not correspond to the chromosomal or gonadal sex. This condition is called pseudohermaphroditism, and may either be male (*i.e.*, inadequate virilization of the male) or female (*i.e.*, a virilized female). These conditions usually occur in the presence of normal gonads and sex chromosomes. Such derangements may be secondary to teratogens causing defective embryogenesis, genetic defects causing abnormal and inappropriate hormonal changes, or receptor abnormalities.

The external genitalia may be truly ambiguous—that is, the sex of the infant cannot be ascertained by physical examination. Alternatively, the phenotype may be completely normal but inappropriate for the genotype and detected only because the genotype was known for other reasons.

FEMALE PSEUDOHERMAPHRODITISM

Masculinization of the female fetus is caused by androgens, either produced by the fetus or transferred across the placenta from the mother. Exposure to androgens prior to week 12 of gestation results in fusion of the urogenital sinus and genital folds. Labial scrotal fusion may occur at the same time. With exposure to androgens from week 12 of gestation onward, however, pure clitoral enlargement may occur. Clitoral enlargement also may occur with postnatal androgen exposure.

Congenital Adrenal Hyperplasia. This condition is the most common cause of virilization in the female. The more common inherited enzymatic deficiencies of adrenal biosynthesis (*i.e.*, 21-hydroxylase, 11-hydroxylase, and 3β-hydroxysteroid dehydrogenase defects) all cause virilization of the female. The gonaducts remain normal, with persistence and development of the müllerian ducts. This is as expected, because these patients are true females without testes, and therefore do not have MIS to suppress müllerian duct development. The excess adrenal androgens, however, cause fusion of the labia, fusion of the urogenital sinus with the genital fold, and clitoral enlargement. In the 21-hydroxylase and 3β-hydroxysteroid dehydrogenase defects, the virilization often is associated with salt-losing crises presenting in the first week of life. The various enzymatic defects of this disorder and the methods of diagnosis and treatment are more fully discussed in the section on adrenal disorders.

Drug-Induced Female Pseudohermaphroditism. A number of female newborns have been virilized by progestational agents or androgens used during the first trimester of pregnancy. The incidence of drug-induced female pseudohermaphroditism has decreased because, with recognition of this iatrogenic cause of virilization of the fetus, there has been a decreased use of the incriminated drugs. Such drugs were used most commonly during the first trimester of gestation, for prevention of spontaneous abortion or maintenance of pregnancy in patients with habitual abortion. When these drugs are used during the first trimester of gestation, the anatomic changes are similar to those found in congenital adrenal hyperplasia. There will be fusion of the labioscrotal folds with formation of a urogenital sinus and clitoromegaly.[25] Rarely, virilization can be so extreme as to cause complete external masculinization. When used after the first trimester, these drugs will cause only phallic enlargement, without fusion of the labioscrotal folds. The bone age often is advanced at birth. Unlike congenital adrenal hyperplasia, however, there is neither progressive virilization nor progressive acceleration of growth, bone age, or sexual development postnatally. The androgens are not elevated. These children will feminize normally at puberty and are quite capable of bearing children. The only therapy necessary is surgical correction of the labioscrotal fusion and clitoromegaly, when these findings are present.

The drugs that have been incriminated include testosterone, 17-methyltestosterone, 17α-ethinyl-19-nortestosterone (Norlutin), 17α-ethyl-19-nortestosterone (Nilevar), 17α-ethinyltestosterone (Pranone), progesterone, diethylstilbestrol, 17α-hydroxyprogesterone, 17-methylandrostenediol, and the combination of ethinyl estradiol 3-methylester and 17α-ethinyl-19-nortestosterone (Ortho-Novum).

Virilizing Disorders in the Mother. The virilization of a female fetus as the result of an androgen-producing tumor of the mother is a relatively rare condition. These tumors almost always are caused by an ovarian lesion, although in one report the lesion was a benign adrenal adenoma.[26] The reported tumors have included arrhenoblastomas, Krukenberg tumors, luteomas, a lipoid tumor of the ovary, and a stromal cell tumor. Haymond and Weldon reviewed the reported cases and noted that maternal virilization has been characterized by clitoromegaly, acne, deepening of the voice, decreased lactation, hirsutism, and elevated excretion of urinary 17-ketosteroids.[27] The offspring tend to have a low birth weight as well as virilization. The degree of virilization of the fetus is variable.

More mothers who themselves have congenital adrenal hyperplasia have come of childbearing age. It is very important that control of their disease is good, to minimize the effects of excess androgens on the fetus.

Idiopathic Female Pseudohermaphroditism. There are two forms of idiopathic female pseudohermaphroditism. There is a small group of genotypically normal females in whom virilization of the external genitalia is seen in association with congenital anomalies of the gastrointestinal and urinary tracts. The reported anomalies include imperforate anus, renal agenesis, urinary tract obstructions, urethrovaginal fistulas, and defective formation of the müllerian ducts. The masculinization of these infants cannot be explained on the basis of androgens, and is thought to be caused by nonhormonal factors. There is another group of female pseudohermaphrodites in whom there are no associated anomalies and no history of maternal exposure to androgens. It is possible that, in this last form, there is an as yet unknown disturbance of steroid metabolism in either the mother or the placenta.

MALE PSEUDOHERMAPHRODITISM

Incomplete masculinization of the male fetus may be secondary to an enzymatic deficiency of testosterone synthesis, unresponsiveness to testosterone action (*i.e.*, androgen-resistance syndromes), or teratogenic damage to either the gonad or the genital anlagen (see Disorders of Gonadal Sex).

Congenital Adrenal Hyperplasia. This disorder can cause incomplete masculinization of the male fetus when the enzyme deficient in the adrenal also is deficient in the testes and is necessary for testosterone synthesis. Deficiency of the 3β-hydroxysteroid dehydrogenase enzyme causes a block early in the biosynthetic pathway of cortisol and aldosterone synthesis, resulting in a severe salt-losing syndrome.[28] The inability to form testosterone indicates that the enzymatic defect also affects both testicular and adrenal steroid biosynthesis.[29] This results in a variable degree of ambiguity of the external genitalia, because the high levels of dehydroepiandrosterone (DHA) have mild androgenic effects, ranging from mild coronal hypospadias to severe perineoscrotal hypospadias and micropenis. The testes usually are within the scrotum. Other, and more rare, defects of adrenal steroid biosynthesis affecting testicular synthesis of testosterone include deficiencies of 17α-hydroxylase, 17-ketosteroid reductase, 17,20-lyase, and the 20,22-desmolase enzymes. In the latter two disorders, there may be a normal female phenotype due to the complete absence of any androgens, and absence of both müllerian and wolffian structures. The full details of these disorders, including diagnosis and treatment, are outlined in the section on adrenal hyperplasia.

Syndromes of Androgen Resistance. This is a group of disorders characterized by normal regression of the müllerian duct structures and normal synthesis of testosterone. The syndrome of androgen resistance occurs when there is either a defect in the conversion of testosterone to DHT caused by deficiency of 5α-reductase, or abnormalities of the androgen receptor or in translation of the message, post androgen receptor.

In the 5α-reductase deficiency, the testis produces both MIS and testosterone. Thus, there is regression of müllerian structures and normal development of the wolffian structures; however, because external genitalia fuse and develop secondary to the local action of DHT, which is absent in this syndrome, these patients may have a blind vaginal pouch, a small phallic structure with chordee and a hooded prepuce, and severe hypospadias. At puberty, these patients will masculinize under the influence of testosterone, and develop pubic hair, penile enlargement, and descent of the testes. The diagnosis is suspected by demonstrating that the patients have 46XY chromosomes and an elevated testosterone–DHT ratio, both basally (>35) and following hCG stimulation (>74). The diagnosis is confirmed by finding reduced 5α-reductase activity in fibroblasts from genital skin.

The classic androgen resistance syndrome is the testicular feminization syndrome. Affected patients are XY male pseudohermaphrodites with normal female external genitalia, absent wolffian and müllerian structures, but with testes that may be located in the abdomen, inguinal canal, or in inguinal hernias. There is a blind vaginal pouch. Unlike patients with 5α-reductase deficiency, they do not virilize at puberty, and breasts do in fact develop secondary to the peripheral conversion of the high levels of testosterone to estradiol. There also is normal estrogenization of the labia minora and the vagina. Most affected patients, however, have very little pubic hair and approximately one third have total absence of sexual hair. In all other respects, including height, habitus, voice, and breast development, these individuals are completely feminine. They frequently marry and have normal sexual relations. When the diagnosis is made during childhood, it usually is because of testicular masses or discovery of testicular tissue during a herniorrhaphy. Because of the lack of formation of a uterus, these patients also frequently will come to attention because of primary amenorrhea. These patients may be either androgen receptor–negative or androgen receptor–positive. Molecular studies have demonstrated mutations in the androgen receptor gene, accounting for the variations in receptor binding of androgens.[30] Testosterone levels in both plasma and urine are in the normal to high male range after puberty. This syndrome is inherited as an X-linked disorder.

There are incomplete forms of androgen resistance, including Reifenstein syndrome, where qualitatively abnormal or reduced binding to the androgen receptor results in defective virilization of the fetus and subsequent feminization at puberty. These abnormalities were previously referred to as partial testicular feminization syndromes. They present with either phenotypic female genitalia and 46XY chromosomes or variable degrees of sexual ambiguity.

PHENOTYPE INCONSISTENT WITH CHROMOSOMAL SEX

Chorionic villus sampling or amniocentesis is being performed more routinely for a variety of reasons. Chromosomal sex generally is determined during such procedures. A problem ensues at birth when the phenotype, with completely normal external genitalia, is inconsistent with the chromosomal sex determined during amniocentesis or chorionic villus sampling. One possible explanation is that there was an error in the initial karyotyping. There are, however, a number of conditions that present at birth with normal external genitalia that are discordant with chromosomal sex. Table 41-1 lists these conditions. These children always should be raised according to the phenotypic sex.

HYPOSPADIAS AND CRYPTORCHIDISM

Twenty-five percent of infants born with undescended testes and hypospadias have a disorder of intersex. This incidence of intersex increases with severity of the hypospadias and bilateral undescended testes. The incidence of isolated hypospadias is 8 in 1000 newborn males, and most cases have no associated endocrine abnormality.

MICROPENIS

Isolated micropenis generally is not considered as ambiguous genitalia, and is dealt with in the section on hypopituitarism.

EVALUATION OF SEXUAL AMBIGUITY

The evaluation of a newborn with ambiguous genitalia should be treated as an emergency, for several reasons. First, life-threatening illness can occur in several of the types of congenital adrenal hyperplasia. Second, the uncertainty of a child's gender, if handled poorly, can cause parents to have long-term psychological concerns which may in turn affect the child's own perception of body image.

Parents should be informed immediately that, although gender can not be determined at that moment by physical examination, a definitive gender will be determined within several days. This allows enough time—generally 72 hours—for most experienced cytogenetic laboratories to provide sex chromosome determination. The parents should be reassured that appropriate gender will be established in their child. It is our general philosophy not to discuss the pending studies in detail because there are occasions for gender assignment that are not consistent with either chromosomal or gonadal sex. It is recommended not to use such terms as penis and clitoris or testis and ovary, when talking to the parents, but rather to say the baby has unfinished external genitalia or underdeveloped gonads. Some parents find it useful not to announce the birth of their child, and to remain in seclusion for a few days, until the gender of their child is known. This will minimize the need for long explanations to relatives and friends. It is advisable to suggest to the parents not to name the child until the

TABLE 41–1
ETIOLOGY OF NORMAL PHENOTYPE INAPPROPRIATE FOR THE GENOTYPE

Disorder	Genotype	Phenotype	Etiology
Pure gonadal dysgenesis	XY	Female	AR, XLR
46XX Males	XX	Male	SRY translocation
46XY Females	XY	Female	SRY deletion
20,22-Desmolase	XY	Female	CAH
17,20-Lyase deficiency	XY	Female	CAH
17-Hydroxylase deficiency	XY	Female	CAH
Androgen resistance syndrome	XY	Female	XLR/AD

AD, autosomal dominant; AR, autosomal recessive; CAH, congenital adrenal hyperplasia; SRY, testicular determining gene; XLR, X-linked recessive; XLR/AD, may be either X-linked recessive or autosomal dominant.

child's gender is known and, in particular, not to use ambiguous names.

As in any diagnostic problem, the approach to the child with ambiguous genitalia should begin with a thorough history, a careful physical examination, and then laboratory and radiologic testing. Table 41-2 outlines the different causes of sexual ambiguity.

The history may provide some clues. It is important to ask about drug ingestion during the pregnancy, particularly in the first trimester, and to inquire about the possibility of any recent androgenic changes in the mother that might suggest the cause for female pseudohermaphroditism. A history of infection or exposure to teratogens in the first trimester might suggest partial gonadal dysgenesis. The family history of a previous sibling who died in the first 10 days of life, or siblings who are overvirilized or had precocious puberty, might suggest the possibility of congenital adrenal hyperplasia.

Physical examination may be of some value, but on no account should a diagnosis be made purely on the grounds of physical examination. The presence or absence of palpable gonads is very important and can direct appropriate laboratory and radiologic investigations. The measurement of the length and diameter of the penis is important both for prognostic information and also as a baseline if treatment is given in an attempt to enlarge the penis. Severe micropenis or agenesis, despite the presence of testes or a normal 46XY karyotype, may necessitate a gender reassignment to female gender. The urethral opening should be identified and the existence or absence of a vagina should be determined. The degree of fusion of the labia should be assessed. Finally, the presence of any abnormalities involving the urinary tract or anal region and any of the other organ systems should be evaluated.

TABLE 41–2
ETIOLOGY OF AMBIGUOUS GENITALIA

Virilization of Females
Congenital adrenal hyperplasia
21-Hydroxylase deficiency
11-Hydroxylase deficiency
3β-Hydroxysteroid dehydrogenase deficiency
Chromosomal aberrations
XO/XY
XX/XY
Variants
Maternal virilization
Drug-induced
Excess androgen production by mother
True hermaphroditism
Idiopathic
Isolated
Associated with midline congenital anomalies
Inadequate Masculinization of Males
Congenital adrenal hyperplasia
3β-Hydroxysteroid dehydrogenase deficiency
Partial androgen resistance syndromes
5α-Reductase deficiency
Partial androgen receptor defects
Testicular dysgenesis
True hermaphroditism
Idiopathic
Isolated
Associated with midline congenital anomalies

TABLE 41–3
STUDIES TO EVALUATE AMBIGUOUS GENITALIA

Immediate Studies
Chromosomal analysis
Bone marrow
Blood
Pelvic ultrasonography
Serum
17-Hydroxyprogesterone
17-OH pregnenolone
Testosterone
11-Deoxycortisol
Dihydrotestosterone
Later Studies
Vaginogram
Exploratory laparotomy and gonadal biopsy
Radiologic studies, intravenous pyelography, barium enema
Skin biopsy to evaluate testosterone metabolism

Certain tests should be obtained as soon as it is apparent that there is sexual ambiguity, to determine the appropriate gender of the infant (Table 41-3). Other tests may be required at a later time to make an accurate diagnosis. It should be stressed, however, that gender determination does not require that all studies leading to a final diagnosis be completed (*e.g.*, the exact type of congenital adrenal hyperplasia may be important for genetic counseling and future prenatal diagnosis, but not for gender assignment).

Some laboratories can use bone marrow for chromosomal estimation and have a karyotype result available in 6 hours; however, this should be used as an adjunct to standard chromosomal analysis because bone marrow karyotyping may miss mosaicism. Chromosomal results enable mosaicism to be determined whether the infant is a virilized female or an inadequately virilized male. Karyotype, however, should not be used *per se* as the major factor in gender determination because gonadal function and future sexual function are more important.

Pelvic ultrasound should be undertaken by an experienced radiologist as soon as possible, to determine the presence or absence of uterus and gonads. The presence of a uterus indicates the absence of any functioning testicular tissue early on in gestation, and almost certainly indicates that the child, no matter what the karyotype, should be raised as a female. Conversely, the absence of müllerian structures implies the presence of functioning testicular tissue at 7 to 9 weeks of gestation and secretion of MIS. Their absence also almost certainly indicates the presence of the SRY gene and probably an XY karyotype. This finding alone should not determine a male gender assignment. Karyotype, phallic size, degree of hypospadias, and the continued presence of testicular tissue, as suggested by testosterone concentrations, should be considered. Ultrasonography may identify gonads previously nonpalpable, and may even define them as either ovarian or testicular tissue, depending on the echogenic pattern.[31]

The results of chromosomal analysis, ultrasound, and steroid determinations should be available within 48 to 72 hours. Gender assignment should be made by this time.

To evaluate further the possible cause of sexual ambiguity, secondary studies may be necessary. The algorithms in Figures 41-2 and 41-3, which are based on the initial ultrasound findings, delineate the steps that may be necessary to make a definitive diagnosis. These algorithms do not include those patients with a normal phenotype that is inappropriate for the genotype. In cases of androgen resistance, some time will be required to evaluate the skin biopsy. Surgical exploration frequently will be required in cases of true hermaphroditism; this also may be done at a later time. It should be stressed that the final diagnosis is not necessary for gender assignment.

When the baby has been fully evaluated, including consultations from an endocrinologist, a urologist,

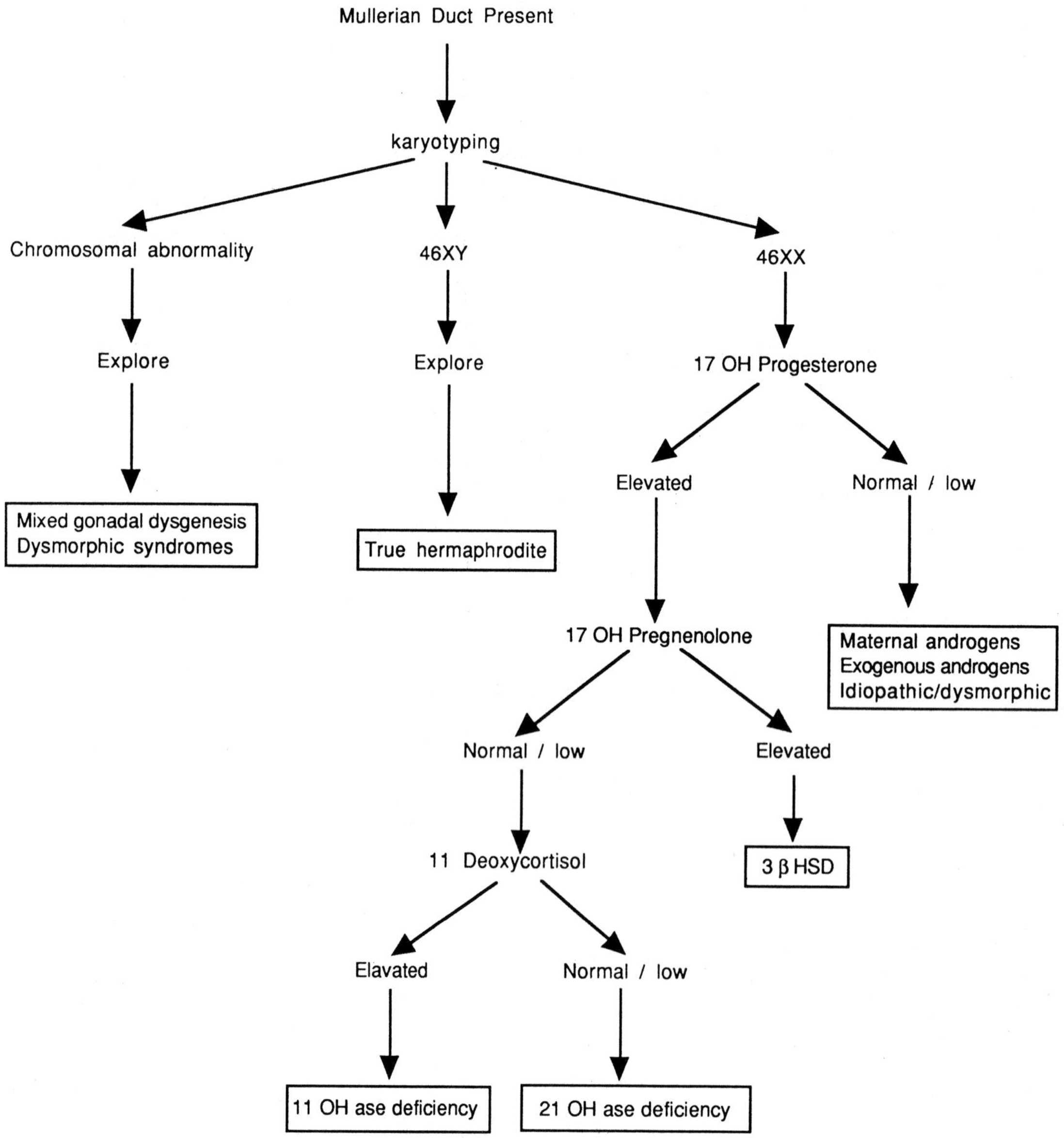

FIG. 41–2. An algorithm for evaluating sexual ambiguity in infants with müllerian structures.

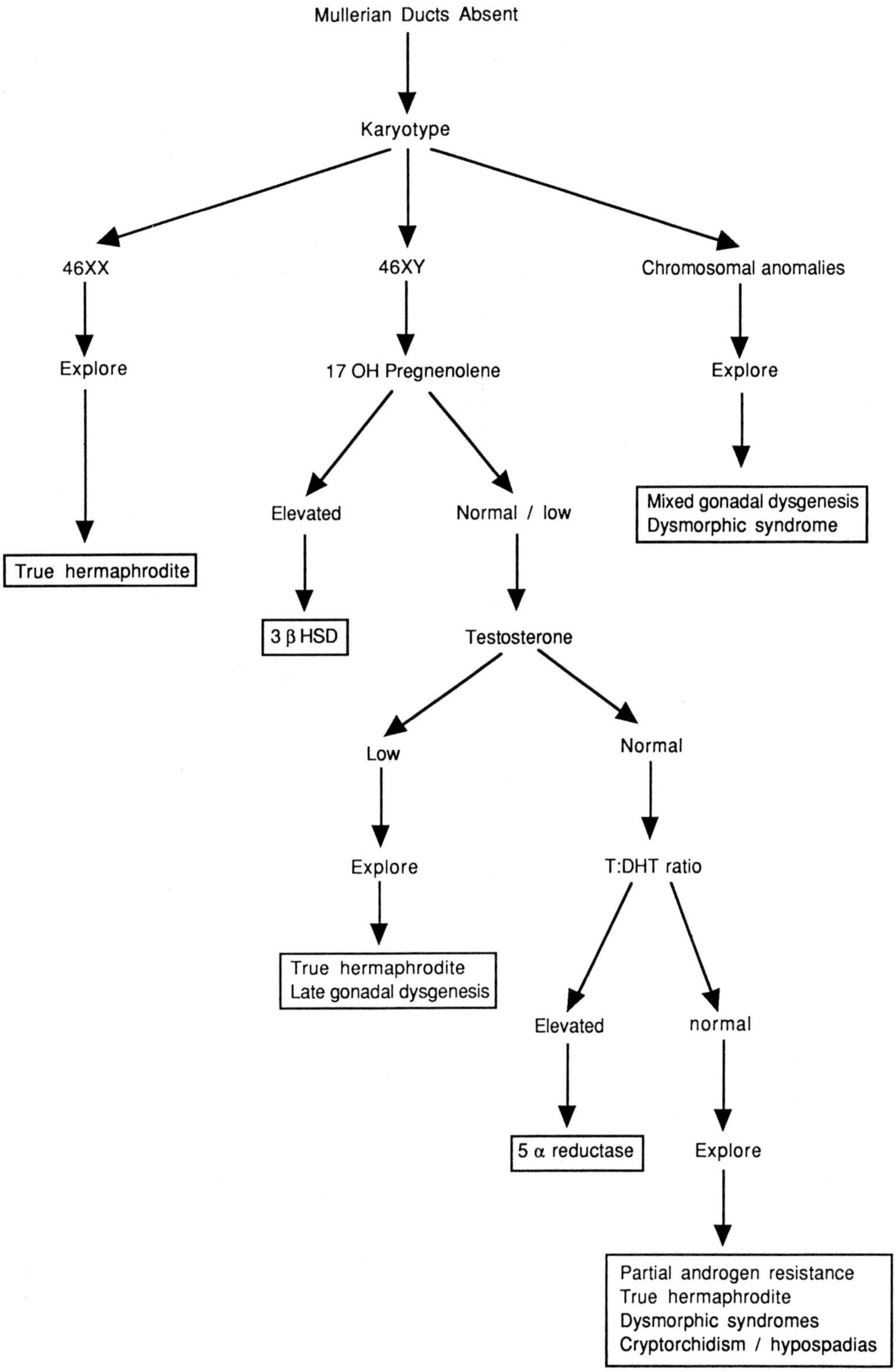

FIG. 41–3. An algorithm for evaluating sexual ambiguity in infants without müllerian structures.

and possibly a psychiatrist, there must be a consensus of agreement as to the appropriate gender, with future heterosexual function and fertility as major determining factors, before discussion with the parents. The attending physician should then discuss the condition fully with the parents, including expectations for future sexual function and fertility and whether any hormonal medications or surgery will be needed.

Gender assignment for most infants with ambiguous genitalia is not difficult, because chromosomal sex and gonadal sex will correlate with the internal structures. The external genitalia will, in general, require minor to moderate surgery to improve function and cosmetic appearance. In some cases, hormonal therapy may be required later on in life, but not during the neonatal period. Rarely, as in cases of incomplete androgen resistance syndromes or in true hermaphroditism or mixed gonadal dysgenesis, gender assignment contrary to chromosomal or gonadal sex must be considered. In this case, careful consideration must be given to the likelihood of adequate normal sexual function as an adult. If it is thought that the penis will be very small and nonfunctional as an adult (<4 cm), it often is more considerate to raise the child as a female.

DISORDERS OF THE ENDOCRINE HYPOTHALAMUS AND PITUITARY

Development of the Hypothalamic–Pituitary Axis

The hypothalamus and pituitary glands regulate the fetal endocrine system after week 12 of gestation. In general terms, the hypothalamus regulates the anterior pituitary by secreting stimulatory hormones and inhibiting hormones. The stimulatory hormones identified include growth hormone-releasing hormone, thyrotropin-releasing hormone (TRH), corticotropin-releasing hormone, and gonadotropin-releasing hormone (GnRH). Somatostatin inhibits pituitary growth hormone release and prolactin inhibitory factor inhibits prolactin release. In response to these hypothalamic controlling hormones, the anterior pituitary secretes growth hormone, thyroid-stimulating hormone (TSH), adrenocorticotropic hormone (ACTH), prolactin, luteinizing hormone (LH), and follicle-stimulating hormone (FSH). The posterior pituitary secretes vasopressin and oxytocin.

The pituitary gland is formed of two distinct parts. The anterior pituitary, or adenohypophysis, arises embryonically from an invagination of the oral ectodermal cavity called the Rathke pouch. This diverticulum arises at 3 weeks of gestation, and by 5 weeks has migrated to its final position and separates completely from the oral cavity. At approximately the same time in gestation, the posterior pituitary, or neurohypophysis, is formed from an invagination of the floor of the diencephalon. This invagination grows downward and joins up with the Rathke pouch, to form the posterior portion of the pituitary gland. Neural fibers migrate from the hypothalamus down to the posterior pituitary to form the neurohypophyseal tract. The hypothalamus itself arises by proliferation of neuroblasts in the intermediate zone of the diencephalic wall. The supraoptic and periventricular nuclei of the hypothalamus are formed. By 12 weeks of gestation, both the hypothalamus and pituitary gland are functioning.

Most disorders of the hypothalamic–pituitary axis in the newborn period, except for the syndrome of inappropriate secretion of antidiuretic hormone (SIADH), are those of insufficiency. In the newborn, most hypothalamic and pituitary problems are related to malformations, unlike in older children and adults, where tumors may both secrete hormones and disrupt hormone function. Causes of disorders of the hypothalamic–pituitary axis in the newborn child are outlined in Table 41-4.

DISORDERS OF THE ANTERIOR PITUITARY

Disorders of anterior pituitary function often are difficult to detect in the newborn; however, there is a series of characteristic findings that may occur. The predominant symptoms of anterior pituitary insufficiency are hypoglycemia, micropenis and, rarely, cholestatic jaundice. There may be combined deficiency of multiple hormones of the anterior pituitary or isolated deficiency of a single hormone.

Growth Hormone Deficiency. Deficiency of growth hormone does not present as intrauterine growth retardation, but may present as hypoglyce-

TABLE 41–4
ETIOLOGY OF DISORDERS OF THE HYPOTHALAMIC–PITUITARY AXIS

Malformations
Cleft lip and palate
Optic nerve atrophy
Septooptic dysplasia
Transphenoidal encephalocele
Holoprosencephaly
Anencephaly
Trauma associated with breech delivery
Congenital infection
Rubella
Toxoplasmosis
Tumor
Hypothalamic hamartoblastoma (*i.e.*, Pallister Hall syndrome)
Rathke pouch cyst
Craniopharyngioma
Isolated or combined familial or idiopathic pituitary hormone deficiency
Autosomal recessive or X-linked recessive familial panhypopituitarism

mia, micropenis, or both in the newborn period. Intrauterine growth is determined by maternal factors, including nutritional status, placental function, and gestational infection or drugs. During early postnatal life, thyroid hormone, insulin, and nutrition are more important growth determinants than growth hormone. The effect of growth hormone deficiency on linear growth often is not discerned until 6 to 9 months of age.

Gonadotropin Deficiency. Micropenis most often is secondary to gonadotropin deficiency, which can occur as either isolated hypogonadotropic hypogonadism or combined multiple pituitary hormone deficiency. Micropenis is defined as penile size less than 2.5 cm stretched length. In female infants, there are no clinical signs of hypogonadotropic hypogonadism at birth.

Adrenocorticotropic Hormone Deficiency. Adrenocorticotropic hormone deficiency rarely presents as adrenal crisis; it is more likely to result only in cortisol insufficiency and to present as hypoglycemia or hyponatremia without hyperkalemia. Occasionally, cholestatic jaundice (*i.e.*, conjugated hyperbilirubinemia) is associated with ACTH deficiency in the newborn. Newborn patients with prolonged direct hyperbilirubinemia should be evaluated for pituitary insufficiency.[32] Isolated ACTH deficiency is extremely rare. The combination of both growth hormone and ACTH deficiency may cause hypoglycemia of such severity that it is difficult to differentiate from congenital hyperinsulinism.

Thyroid-Stimulating Hormone Deficiency. Thyroid-stimulating hormone deficiency results in secondary hypothyroidism in the newborn. This generally is not detected clinically, and more often is detected by the newborn screening tests as a low thyroxine (T_4) level but a normal TSH level. This finding may be misinterpreted as the euthyroid sick syndrome (see Disorders of the Thyroid) in a stressed neonate. Furthermore, secondary hypothyroidism may be missed in those countries using only TSH determinations for thyroid screening. Isolated TSH deficiency, like ACTH deficiency, is extremely rare, and TSH deficiency usually is seen only in panhypopituitarism. Thus, in an infant with any of the abnormalities outlined in Table 41-4, the routine newborn screening procedures should not be relied on to detect secondary hypothyroidism.

Diagnosis. The diagnosis of hypothalamic and pituitary deficiency may be made by stimulation tests, as well as by determination of random hormone levels. Growth hormone levels are tonically elevated in the first few days of life, and thus, as a screening test, a random growth hormone level greater than 10 ng/mL suggests adequate growth hormone function. A random low growth hormone level requires provocative growth hormone testing to confirm growth hormone deficiency. Provocative growth hormone testing in normal newborn infants often results in growth hormone levels of 25 ng/mL or higher, whereas growth hormone–deficient infants will not respond to provocative testing. Adrenocorticotropic hormone deficiency and adrenal insufficiency are unlikely if a random cortisol level is greater than 20 μg/dL, because newborns normally have very low cortisol levels, without diurnal variation. In general, ACTH stimulation testing is necessary to test the hypothalamic–pituitary–adrenal axis. Gonadotropin-releasing hormone will stimulate pituitary secretion of LH and FSH during the first few months of life but, subsequently, normal children will not respond to GnRH. Therefore, to assess gonadotropin function, GnRH testing should be performed in the first 2 to 3 months of life.

In those infants suspected of anterior pituitary deficiency, ultrasonography through the open fontanelle may discern malformations of the brain, including the defects seen in septooptic dysplasia. To evaluate further the possibility of septooptic dysplasia in suspected infants, ophthalmologic examination also should be performed. In those infants in whom malformation is strongly suspected, magnetic resonance imaging or computed tomography scanning may be useful in delineating the abnormality.

Treatment. Anterior pituitary deficiency often is not detected clinically during the neonatal period because the hypoglycemia may be very modest, micropenis—obviously not a clinical feature in hypopituitary females—is marginal, and jaundice is not severe. Treatment considerations, therefore, are based on the severity of symptoms. The child who is severely hypoglycemic will require growth hormone and glucocorticoid replacement. The dose of these hormones for replacement therapy can be relatively modest. Recombinant growth hormone is injected subcutaneously, at a dose of 0.04 mg/kg daily. Data indicate that the production rate of cortisol is less than previously believed, and, based on this information, replacement of glucocorticoid insufficiency requires 8 to 10 mg/m^2 of oral hydrocortisone per day.[33] If the newborn is ill, it is recommended that initially the child be treated with at least three times the replacement dose. In male infants with micropenis, a short trial of hCG, testosterone, or both, is recommended to stimulate the penis to grow. Not only will this improve penile size, but such treatment provides an opportunity to evaluate testicular response to hCG and penile response to testosterone. Testosterone can be administered by injecting testosterone enanthate, 25 mg intramuscularly every month, for a total of three injections. Penile response to this treatment can be assessed at the end of 3 months. Some authors have recommended a prolonged course of hCG, which will test both testicular response and penile growth in response to endogenous testosterone production.

DISORDERS OF THE POSTERIOR PITUITARY

There are two hormones secreted from the posterior pituitary, vasopressin or antidiuretic hormone (ADH) and oxytocin. Oxytocin has no known function in the neonate. Antidiuretic hormone is manufactured in the supraoptic and periventricular nuclei of the hypothalamus. It is bound to neurophysin and is transported by axonal transport along the neurons of the neurohypophyseal tract to the posterior pituitary, where it is stored and released as necessary. Antidiuretic hormone can be found in the fetus after 12 weeks of gestation; ADH secretion is stimulated by hyperosmolar states and volume depletion. Antidiuretic hormone release is inhibited predominantly by volume overload. It acts on the collecting tubules of the kidney by increasing the permeability to water and urea. There are two main disorders of ADH secretion, diabetes insipidus (DI) and SIADH.

Diabetes Insipidus. Diabetes insipidus in the newborn may be due to central ADH insufficiency or renal unresponsiveness to ADH (*i.e.*, nephrogenic DI). This section will deal only with central DI.

Diabetes insipidus in the neonate may present with failure to thrive, irritability, fever, vomiting, and hypernatremia. There may be a history of polyhydramnios in the mother. Polyuria is difficult to detect in newborn infants because normal newborn infants will void up to 20 times a day.[34] Diabetes insipidus should be suspected, however, in symptomatic, cachectic-appearing, hypernatremic infants. Sustained urine output greater than 60% of fluid input is unusual, and single-void volumes of greater than 6 mL/kg suggest DI. The diagnosis is confirmed by demonstrating inappropriately dilute urine in the presence of a hyperosmolar serum, and by demonstrating an appropriate concentration of the urine after administration of vasopressin. Unresponsiveness to vasopressin indicates renal problems rather than central DI. Water deprivation tests should not be done in newborn infants, since acute dehydration and hypernatremia may cause permanent brain damage.

A list of causes of central DI is given in Table 41-5. Secondary DI is more common than primary in the neonatal period. Diabetes insipidus should be strongly suspected in infants with the listed malformations.

TABLE 41–5
ETIOLOGY OF CENTRAL DIABETES INSIPIDUS

Primary
Familial
X-linked recessive
Autosomal dominant
Idiopathic
Secondary
Malformation sequences
Optic atrophy
Septooptic dysplasia
Holoprosencephaly
Birth trauma
Periventricular hemorrhage
Infection
Meningitis
Encephalitis

Treatment. Treatment of DI requires strict management of fluid balance. These infants require enormous quantities of free water; it is not unusual to provide several times usual maintenance quantities of water as 5% glucose intravenously, while providing nutrition and electrolytes by the oral route. Desmopressin is a long-acting analogue of vasopressin, and can be given intranasally or sublingually. Intranasal administration is the best and most consistent route of administration; however, sublingual administration can be helpful in patients with cleft lip and palate. The dose and dose interval must be carefully evaluated, by trial and error, in each child individually. The usual intranasal dose is 5 μg once or twice daily. Rapid shifts in the serum sodium, caused by excessive fluid input or urine output, should be avoided.

Syndrome of Inappropriate Antidiuretic Hormone Secretion. In the premature infant, from 26 weeks of gestation onward, elevated levels of ADH have been clearly documented.[35] Increased ADH secretion occurs for many reasons in sick premature infants, and these are outlined in Table 41-6. A common mechanism for the elevated ADH levels in many of these pathologic cases is intravascular volume depletion. This is detected by stretch receptors in the left atrium, which are either compressed by increased air trapping and artificial positive pressure in the lungs or stimulated by true volume depletion. Thus, in these circumstances, the elevated ADH levels are appropriate for the volume status, but inappropriate for the osmolar status. True SIADH is uncommon in

TABLE 41–6
CAUSES OF ELEVATED LEVELS OF ANTIDIURETIC HORMONE IN THE NEWBORN

Birth asphyxia
Acute deterioration of hyaline membrane disease and bronchopulmonary dysplasia
Respiratory syncytial virus infection
Pneumothorax
Pulmonary interstitial emphysema
Artificial ventilation
Acute blood loss
Periventricular hemorrhage
Surgery
Pain
Syndrome of inappropriate ADH secretion

ADH, antidiuretic hormone.

neonates,[36] and this condition should be differentiated from appropriately elevated ADH levels because not only is it vitally important to control water and sodium intake and prevent hyponatremia, but it is equally important to treat the volume depletion states causing the appropriate ADH secretion.

The SIADH, by definition, occurs when there is hyponatremia associated with a urine osmolarity that is less than maximally diluted, and continued sodium loss in the urine (*i.e.*, urine sodium > 10 mEq/L) in the absence of volume depletion, renal failure, or adrenal insufficiency. Hyponatremia occurs commonly in newborn premature infants, with the most common cause being renal sodium wasting due to diuretics. The differential diagnosis of hyponatremia in the newborn also must include prerenal failure, renal failure, adrenal insufficiency and SIADH. The SIADH, if it occurs, is associated more commonly with sepsis and central nervous system infection in older infants, but perhaps in critically ill neonates as well. Unlike volume depletion states, SIADH is treated by fluid restriction.

DISORDERS OF THE ADRENAL GLAND

DEVELOPMENT AND FUNCTION OF THE ADRENAL GLAND

The adrenal gland is two separate glands, the adrenal cortex and the adrenal medulla. The fetal adrenal cortex is of mesodermal origin, whereas the chromaffin cells of the adrenal medulla are of neuroectodermal origin. The classes of hormones secreted by these two glands differ and are independent of each other, although Wurtman and Axelrod have suggested that the intraadrenal level of glucocorticoids may influence the level of the enzyme, phenylethanolamine-*N*-methyl transferase, necessary for the conversion of norepinephrine to epinephrine.[37] It certainly is possible that the influence of these two glands on each other may be greater than appreciated currently. In as much as diseases of the adrenal medulla during the neonatal period are extremely rare, this section will focus on the adrenal cortex.

The anlage of the adrenal cortex arises as two large masses on either side of the aorta, at about the level of the first thoracic nerve. Immediately adjacent are the medullary cells that have migrated from the neural crest. Fetal adrenal cortical cells can be identified by 4 weeks of gestation. By 7 weeks of gestation, the medullary cells begin to migrate to the interior of the adrenal cortex. These original adrenal cortical cells make up the fetal zone of the adrenal cortex. There is a second downgrowth of coelomic epithelium that envelops the original cortical cells and remains as an outer shell. The fetal adrenal gland is extremely large during gestation, but involutes during the last one-half of pregnancy and especially after birth. The adult adrenal cortex slowly develops from the outer shell, with involution of the fetal zone. The fetal zone is active in steroid metabolism, and the rapid involution after birth suggests a role in the maintenance of pregnancy.

The trophic hormonal control of the fetal adrenal is not clear. In anencephalic fetuses, the fetal adrenal appears to be normal during the first 12 weeks of gestation, with subsequent involution of the gland. In patients with enzymatic defects of cortisol biosynthesis, however, the excessive androgen production in association with hyperplasia of the adrenal glands during the first 12 weeks of gestation suggests that ACTH must play some role during that time.

The adrenal cortex secretes three main groups of steroid hormones, glucocorticoids, mineralocorticoids, and androgens. The glucocorticoids, of which cortisol (*i.e.*, hydrocortisone) is the most important, exert their major physiologic effects on carbohydrate, protein, and fat metabolism. The mineralocorticoids, desoxycorticosterone and aldosterone, maintain salt and water balance by promoting sodium retention in exchange for hydrogen and potassium in the distal convoluted tubules of the kidney. The adrenal androgens, DHA, Δ^4-androstenedione, and 11β-hydroxyandrostenedione, are protein anabolic and responsible for the development of sexual hair in girls at puberty. Adrenal androgens are not secreted in appreciable amounts until puberty, except during the neonatal period. The slightly higher levels of adrenal androgens during the neonatal period may be secondary to the relative deficiency of 3β-hydroxysteroid dehydrogenase in the fetal zone of the fetal adrenal cortex, which is reflected in the higher concentrations of Δ^5 steroids (*e.g.*, DHA, 17-OH pregnenolone) noted especially in premature infants.

The production of adrenocortical steroids is controlled by a hypothalamic–pituitary–adrenal homeostatic mechanism. The hypothalamic ACTH-releasing factor, corticotropin-releasing hormone (CRH), provokes release of pituitary ACTH. The hypothalamic CRH center is sensitive both to tissue levels of cortisol and to stress. Adrenocorticotropic hormone, in turn, stimulates adrenocortical steroid biosynthesis—mainly cortisol. Increased levels of cortisol inhibit the production of ACTH, probably acting at the level of the hypothalamus.

The regulation of aldosterone, however, is influenced by many factors. The main regulatory homeostatic mechanism controlling aldosterone secretion is the renin–angiotensin system. Acute changes in pressure receptors control the release of renin from the juxtaglomerular cells of the kidney. Increased levels of circulating renin, in turn, increase angiotensin II. Angiotensin II acts on the zona glomerulosa of the adrenal cortex to increase aldosterone secretion and directly to cause vascular contractility. Increased pressure within the arterial receptors, secondary to the contracted vessels and the increased blood volume produced by elevated aldosterone, operates a negative-feedback inhibition of the renin–angiotensin system.

Other mechanisms are involved in a secondary fashion in the control of aldosterone secretion. A low sodium or high potassium intake will increase aldosterone excretion. It has been demonstrated that the sodium or potassium concentration in the blood perfusing the adrenals has a direct effect on aldosterone secretion.[38] Adrenocorticotropic hormone also will cause a transient, albeit unsustained, increase in aldosterone excretion,[39] and aldosterone secretion will be diminished in the absence of ACTH.[40] Finally, cortisol itself may have a permissive role in aldosterone action at the tissue level.[41]

ADRENAL INSUFFICIENCY

The disorders of the adrenal cortex during the neonatal period consist almost entirely of those conditions that cause adrenal insufficiency. The inborn errors of steroid biosynthesis (*i.e.*, congenital adrenal hyperplasia) can cause excessive production of various steroids, but Cushing syndrome or cortisol excess rarely occurs during the neonatal period. Cushing syndrome may occur secondary to exposure to exogenous steroids such as dexamethasone. Adrenal cortical tumors resulting in Cushing syndrome can present very early in life (*i.e.*, several months of age) but not in the neonate. Cushing disease has not been described in the very young infant. Adrenal insufficiency can result from lack of trophic hormone stimulation, ACTH receptor abnormalities, damage to fetal adrenal gland, inherited degenerative disorders, or inborn errors of steroid biosynthesis.

ADRENOCORTICOTROPIC HORMONE INSUFFICIENCY

There have been a number of neonatal deaths, after shock and peripheral vascular collapse associated with severe hyponatremia and hyperkalemia, in which the adrenal glands were noted to be hypoplastic at autopsy. Some of these cases of failure of development of the adrenal cortex after involution of the fetal zone have been reported in infants with anencephaly and in patients with partial or total pituitary aplasia. The probable basis of the developmental failure in these cases is the lack of ACTH. The possibility, however, that the lack of another central nervous system factor also might be involved in these cases is suggested in the patients with congenital hypopituitarism. In the latter group of patients, the adrenal insufficiency produces decreased cortisol production, but mineralocorticoid function remains normal.[42] Such patients tend to have hypoglycemia, poor feeding, and failure to thrive. These patients can, in general, maintain water and electrolyte balance and can respond to sodium deprivation with increase in aldosterone excretion; however, hyponatremia with normokalemia has been noted in hypopituitarism and isolated glucocorticoid insufficiency. The limitation, with ACTH deficiency, of the developmental failure to the zona fasciculata and reticularis can be explained by the fact that the trophic hormone for zona glomerulosa function is angiotensin II and not ACTH.

ADRENOCORTICOTROPIC HORMONE UNRESPONSIVENESS

Migeon and associates have postulated that the dichotomy of control of the various zones of the adrenal cortex may be the explanation for a familial syndrome of isolated glucocorticoid deficiency. This syndrome was reported initially by Shepard and associates in 1959.[43] It presents in early childhood with hyperpigmentation, hypoglycemia, failure to thrive, and poor feeding. These patients have cortisol insufficiency and cannot increase 17-hydroxysteroid excretion in response to ACTH stimulation. These patients can, however, respond to sodium deprivation with increased aldosterone excretion and decreased sodium excretion. Migeon and associates, based on *in vitro* experiments, have suggested that this syndrome is the result of an inherited defect in the ACTH receptor system.[44] This syndrome has since been referred to as the syndrome of ACTH unresponsiveness. A family with this syndrome has been reported, however, in whom the pathogenesis of the disorder appears to be more compatible with a degenerative process (see Familial Isolated Glucocorticoid Insufficiency).[45] It is probable that this familial syndrome is caused by a variety of defects, including ACTH unresponsiveness.

DAMAGE

Adrenal insufficiency can occur during the newborn period as a result of damage to the relatively large and hyperemic adrenal glands. Trauma in association with a difficult delivery, particularly breech delivery; hemorrhagic diseases; or infectious processes can damage the adrenal glands. Minor hemorrhage or unilateral damage may not cause adrenal insufficiency, and may present subsequently as calcification of the adrenal glands detected on an abdominal radiograph obtained for other purposes. All patients with shock symptoms in association with hyponatremia should be suspect for adrenal insufficiency. Newer, highly sensitive ACTH determinations using monoclonal antibodies and immunoradiometric assays can detect elevated plasma ACTH, diagnostic of primary adrenal insufficiency.

DEGENERATIVE DISORDERS

The most common cause of chronic adrenal insufficiency is idiopathic atrophy, or degeneration of the adrenal glands. Chronic adrenal insufficiency (*i.e.*, Addison disease), however, is extremely uncommon in childhood and unheard of during the newborn period, if the cases of congenital hypoplasia of the adrenal glands are excluded. It is possible that some of the cases of congenital hypoplasia of the adrenals are caused by a degenerative process, especially when the central nervous system, including the pituitary gland, is intact.

FAMILIAL ISOLATED GLUCOCORTICOID INSUFFICIENCY

This disorder can occur during the neonatal period. Affected infants present during the neonatal period with shock, hyperpigmentation, and hypoglycemia. Some of the families with this syndrome probably have a defect in ACTH responsiveness; however, there is a substantial number of case histories with a clinical course suggestive of an inherited degenerative process.

A family was studied, of which five siblings had hyperpigmentation, hypoglycemia, convulsions, and deficient glucocorticoid production.[45] Mineralocorticoid function was normal. Of these five children, two were studied during early infancy, and glucocorticoid function initially was normal. The development of deficient glucocorticoid production at a later age in these two patients suggests an inherited degenerative process of the adrenal glands as the pathogenetic basis for this syndrome in this family.

CONGENITAL ADRENAL HYPERPLASIA

This is a genetic disorder involving deficiency of one of several enzymatic systems required for normal steroid biosynthesis. The various clinical manifestations of this syndrome can be correlated with the different defects of cortisol synthesis. The biochemical basis of this syndrome has been extensively reviewed.[46] The principal biochemical reactions in the conversion of cholesterol into active adrenocortical steroids require a series of hydroxylations (Fig. 41-4). These hydroxylations actually are mediated by cytochrome P450 oxidases. The side chain cleavage of cholesterol is mediated by P450scc. The most common disorder is lack of 21-hydroxylation. Hydroxylation of both progesterone and 17-hydroxyprogesterone is mediated by a single enzyme, P450c21. A single enzyme, P450c11, mediates 11β-hydroxylase, 18-hydroxylase,

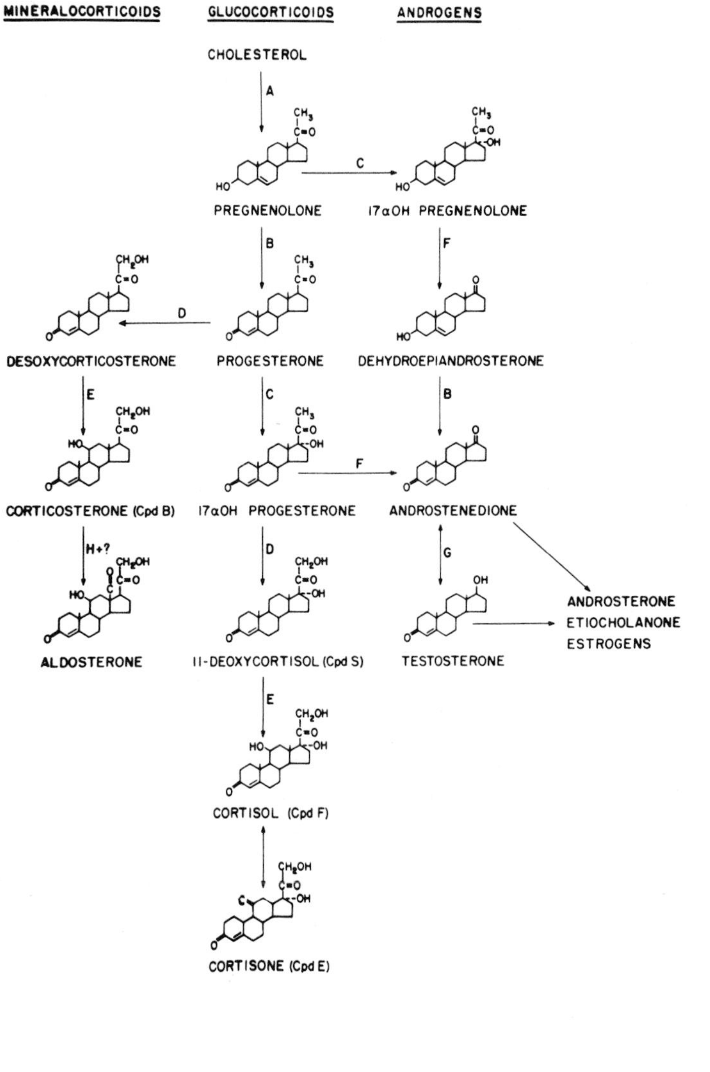

FIG. 41–4. The biosynthetic pathway of adrenal steroid biosynthesis. The classic enzyme terminology is represented by the alphabetical letters with the appropriate cytochrome P450 oxidases in parentheses. A, 20,22-desmolase (P450scc); B, 3β-hydroxysteroid dehydrogenase; C, 17α-hydroxylase (P450c17); D, 21-hydroxylase (P450c21); E, 11-hydroxylase (P450c11); F, 17,20-lyase (P450c17); G, 17-keto reductase; H+, 18-hydroxylase + 18-oxidase (P450c11).

and aldehyde synthase activities. Similarly, a single enzyme, P450c17, mediates 17α-hydroxylase and 17,20-lyase activities. There probably are several 3β-hydroxysteroid dehydrogenase enzymes, which are not P450 enzymes. The gene for one of these enzymes, located on chromosome 1, has been cloned and has been identified to be responsible for the disease, 3β-hydroxysteroid dehydrogenase deficiency.

The three synthetic pathways produce mineralocorticoids, glucocorticoids, and androgens. Both steroidogenesis and adrenocortical growth are stimulated by the trophic influence of ACTH. Deficient cortisol synthesis secondary to an enzymatic deficiency causes increased ACTH production. Increased ACTH production, in turn, causes a compensatory hypertrophy of the adrenal cortex, and in this manner the block in the biosynthetic pathway may be partially overcome. This increased production of ACTH, however, also leads to an increased production and accumulation of precursor steroids. The clinical findings and the steroidal patterns of the individual defects are summarized in Table 41-7.

Virilization. Virilization of the female is secondary to the elevation of adrenal androgens caused by those enzymatic defects subsequent to 17-hydroxylation. In most cases, there is some fusion of the labioscrotal folds with clitoral enlargement, which may be bound down by chordee. Occasionally, virilization may be so severe that a phallic urethra develops. Virilization of the male generally is not noted during the neonatal period, and, in the non–salt-losing forms of this disorder, the male often will be undetected until age 5 or 6 years. At this time, he may be noted to be large for his age, and muscular, demonstrating secondary sexual changes. The classic virilizing form of congenital adrenal hyperplasia is the result of a deficiency of the cytochrome P450c21 (*i.e.*, 21-hydroxylase deficiency). This defect also is the most common, accounting for almost 90% of recognized cases. As discussed later, elevation of 17-hydroxyprogesterone is not diagnostic of 21-hydroxylase deficiency. A mistaken diagnosis of 21-hydroxylase deficiency can result in errors in genetic counseling and prenatal treatment.

Incomplete Masculinization. Failure of complete masculine development occurs in those forms of adrenal hypoplasia in which synthesis of testosterone is blocked. The incomplete masculinization in the male, which is under fetal testicular control, suggests that the enzymatic deficiency in these defects occurs in both the adrenal gland and the testis. The lack of 3β-hydroxysteroid dehydrogenase activity occurring in both the adrenal gland and the testis has been demonstrated.[28] In the 3β-hydroxysteroid dehydrogenase defect, the block results in secretion of steroids that consist almost entirely of compounds with Δ^5-3β-hydroxy configuration. The lack of the enzyme in the fetal testis causes incomplete masculinization in the male by interfering with testosterone synthesis.[29] The marked elevation of Δ^5-3β-hydroxyadrenal androgens, especially DHA, however, accounts for the vir-

TABLE 41–7
CLINICAL AND BIOCHEMICAL FINDINGS OF THE COMMON VARIANTS OF CONGENITAL ADRENAL HYPERPLASIA

Enzyme Deficiency (Classic)	Phenotype 46XX	Phenotype 46XY	Other Clinical Manifestations	Predominant Steroids
Cholesterol side-change cleavage deficiency ("desmolase")	Female	Female	Salt-wasting crisis	Low level—all steroids No response to ACTH
3β-Hydroxysteroid dehydrogenase deficiency	Virilized	Hypospadias	Salt-wasting crisis	Dehydroepiandrosterone 17-OH pregnenolone Increased Δ^5–Δ^4 ratio of steroids
21-Hydroxylase deficiency	Virilized	Male	Pseudoprecocious puberty in male Late virilization in female Salt-wasting crisis	17-OH progesterone Androstenedione Testosterone
11α-Hydroxylase deficiency	Virilized	Male	Pseudoprecocious puberty in male Hypertension	11-Deoxycortisol 11-Deoxycorticosterone Androstenedione Low renin
17α-Hydroxylase deficiency	Female	Female	Sexual infantilism Hypertension	Corticosterone 11-Deoxycorticosterone (Low renin)

ACTH, adrenocorticotrophic hormone.

ilization of the female infant. The elevation of serum 17-hydroxypregnenolone is diagnostic of 3β-hydroxysteroid dehydrogenase deficiency. In 3β-hydroxysteroid dehydrogenase deficiency, however, 17-hydroxyprogesterone concentrations also are markedly elevated.[47] Therefore, the finding of elevations of 17-hydroxyprogesterone requires further studies to delineate the exact enzymatic defect. The reported cases of genetic males with both the 20,22-desmolase defect and the 17α-hydroxylase defect support the hypothesis that the adrenal and testicular enzymatic mechanisms for testosterone biosynthesis share common genetic controls.

Hypertension. Hypertension has been associated with enzymatic blocks resulting in excessive secretion of mineralocorticoids. A defect of cytochrome P450c11 (*i.e.*, 11-hydroxylase deficiency) causes an accumulation of desoxycorticosterone, a potent mineralocorticoid, as well as 11-deoxycortisol.[48] The 17α-hydroxylase defect (*i.e.*, P450c17) blocks 17-hydroxylation of progesterone, interfering with cortisol and androgen biosynthesis, and the mineralocorticoid excess results in hypertension.[49] Hypertension in these forms of congenital adrenal hyperplasia, however, is an inconstant feature. Whether the hypertension is related to the duration of excessive secretion of mineralocorticoid, the degree of the defect (*i.e.*, variations of the genetic mutation), or variations in sodium intake is not clear. It is not known whether hypertension occurs during the newborn period in infants with these forms of the congenital adrenal hyperplasia syndrome.

Salt Loss. The salt-losing form of the 21-hydroxylase defect, the 3β-hydroxysteroid dehydrogenase defect, and the 20,22-desmolase defect block steroid synthesis early in the biosynthetic pathway, resulting in mineralocorticoid insufficiency and severe sodium loss. The electrolytes initially are normal, but, within a week of life, serum sodium concentration will slowly decrease with a concomitant increase in serum potassium concentration. These infants may manifest acute adrenal crisis with shock, peripheral collapse, and dehydration, by 10 to 14 days of age.

The underlying metabolic defects for two varieties of the 21-hydroxylase enzyme defect are not clearly understood. Bongiovanni and Eberlein postulated that both varieties are the result of the same hydroxylase deficiency.[50] In the salt-loser, there is almost complete 21-hydroxylase deficiency, whereas in the compensated patient there is sufficient 21-hydroxylase to permit aldosterone synthesis. Childs and associates and Prader found that each form (*i.e.*, salt-loser or non–salt-loser) occurred consistently within individual families and proposed separate genotypes.[51,52] Rosenbloom and Smith, however, described salt-losers and non–salt-losers within the same sibship.[53] Bartter favored the hypothesis that there are two 21-hydroxylase enzymes, and that the compensated form is caused by a genetic error in which only the 21-hydroxylase enzyme specific for 17-hydroxyprogesterone is deficient, whereas the salt-losing form is the result of a second 21-hydroxylase specific for progesterone as well. Aldosterone hypersecretion in the compensated form has been reported by Bartter and associates.[54] Their very high values for aldosterone secretion, however, have not been generally confirmed, although there are reports of modest elevations. The dual enzyme hypothesis is no longer viewed as likely, since it is clear that a single gene mediates the hydroxylation of both progesterone and 17-hydroxyprogesterone. It is likely that variations in the mutation of the P450c21 gene account for the heterogeneity of 21-hydroxylase deficiency disorders, including the nonclassic late-onset variant.

A few instances of aldosterone deficiency caused by a specific defect of 18-dehydrogenase, the last enzymatic transaction toward aldosterone, have been described.[55,56] There is salt and water loss, without the other clinical consequences of congenital adrenal hyperplasia. It is possible that some of the infants reported by Jaudon to have transient adrenal insufficiency of the newborn had the same defect.[57] These disorders probably are secondary to point mutations of the P450c11 enzyme that mediates these activities.

Prenatal Diagnosis and Treatment. It is possible, using molecular and genetic techniques, to diagnosis 21-hydroxylase deficiency in the fetus prenatally. It should be stressed, however, that these techniques should be considered experimental, and such diagnosis and treatment should be performed in major medical centers well versed in performing them. It is equally important to stress that only 21-hydroxylase deficiency can be diagnosed prenatally with any degree of confidence. A proband diagnosed to have 21-hydroxylase deficiency on the basis of elevated 17-hydroxyprogesterone levels, without confirmation by measurement of other steroids, can lead to a mistaken diagnosis.[47]

The gene regulating P450c21 is closely linked to the human leukocyte antigen (HLA) locus on chromosome 6. Once the diagnosis of 21-hydroxylase deficiency has been established in a propositus, HLA typing should be done in the propositus and the parents. The parents should be tested with ACTH, to confirm biochemically that they are genetic heterozygotes for 21-hydroxylase deficiency. The management of the pregnancy, the techniques used for diagnosis, the treatment of the female fetus with 21-hydroxylase deficiency, and the problems with these techniques have been reviewed.[58,59] In brief, the mother is started on dexamethasone early in the first trimester and, subsequently, chorionic villus sampling or amniocentesis is performed to determine the sex and the HLA type of the fetus. DNA is extracted from cultured tissue and analyzed using appropriate cDNA probes. If molecular and genetic techniques confirm the diagnosis and the fetus is female, dexamethasone treatment is continued to term.

DIAGNOSIS

It is difficult to make the diagnosis of acute adrenal insufficiency in the newborn. There must be a high index of suspicion in any acutely ill infant with shock, peripheral collapse, and a rapid and weak pulse, and in any infant with poor feeding, failure to thrive, intermittent pyrexia, or even hypoglycemia and convulsions. A subtle sign of congenital adrenal hypoplasia is hyperpigmentation, especially in the extensor creases and genitalia; however, this sign is recognized most often after the diagnosis has been made. Decreased serum sodium and chloride and increased serum potassium levels are suggestive of mineralocorticoid deficiency. Isolated hyponatremia does not exclude glucocorticoid insufficiency, and should be viewed as a possible sign of adrenal insufficiency. Certainly, ambiguous external genitalia at birth always should suggest the possibility of congenital adrenal hyperplasia.

The serum cortisol levels are low in all newborns, and especially in premature infants. There is no diurnal variation of cortisol levels, and therefore cortisol determinations without stimulation testing are not useful. In clinical situations highly suggestive of adrenal insufficiency, it is recommended that a rapid, 1-hour ACTH stimulation test be performed and that pharmacologic doses of glucocorticoids be administered, along with fluid and mineral resuscitation, after testing. Plasma concentrations of ACTH are elevated in those infants with primary adrenal insufficiency, including congenital adrenal hyperplasia. A plasma sample for ACTH determination should be obtained before ACTH testing.

Delineation of the specific enzyme defect in congenital adrenal hyperplasia can be determined by measuring serum concentrations of the various steroidal precursors to cortisol synthesis (see Table 41-7). The serum concentration of 17-hydroxyprogesterone is elevated in the affected newborn, and may serve as a screening device using a filter paper technique.[60] Normal newborn levels are less than 100 ng/dL,[61] and may increase to levels as high as 200 ng/dL in the male infant at 1 to 2 months of age. Stressed newborns may have higher levels, but these are significantly less than the values noted in patients with 21-hydroxylase deficiency. This is especially true in the preterm sick newborn, whose 17-hydroxyprogesterone values can be above 600 ng/dL. Affected infants with 21-hydroxylase deficiency often have serum levels markedly above 2000 ng/dL. Serum levels of 17-hydroxyprogesterone normally are elevated in cord blood with levels ranging between 900 and 5000 ng/dL. The serum levels rapidly decrease by the second or third day of life, and values above 1000 ng/dL are suspect. Moreover, elevated serum concentrations of 17-hydroxyprogesterone are not diagnostic of the 21-hydroxylase defect. Serum levels of 17-hydroxyprogesterone can be mildly elevated in the 11-hydroxylase defect and can be markedly elevated in the 3β-hydroxysteroid dehydrogenase defect secondary to peripheral conversion of 17-hydroxypregnenolone to 17-hydroxyprogesterone.[47] Serum levels of 17-hydroxypregnenolone are especially elevated in the premature infant, and levels up to 2000 ng/dL are normal.[62]

TREATMENT

The immediate need of the critically ill infant in adrenal crisis is for cortisol. If possible, cortisol should be withheld until the diagnosis can be established, either by ACTH testing or by obtaining serum and plasma assay for determination of the appropriate steroids and ACTH. If a newborn infant is in shock and *in extremis*, however, the use of glucocorticoids as a lifesaving measure is justified, whatever the diagnosis. In the usual situation, salt and water alone will relieve the clinical crisis. Intravenous isotonic saline in 5% glucose water should be infused at a rate of 100 to 120 mL/kg during the first 24 hours. If the infant is in severe shock, the use of plasma or 5% albumin, 10 to 20 mL/kg, as well as cortisol, often is necessary. Hydrocortisone hemisuccinate or phosphate, 1.5 to 2 mg/kg, should be given intravenously immediately. Constant infusion of hydrocortisone hemisuccinate or phosphate (30 mg/m^2/day) should be continued. Hydrocortisone hemisuccinate, 2 mg/kg, can be given intramuscularly if intravenous access is a problem. Desoxycorticosterone acetate was used in the past to aid electrolyte control, but this drug is no longer available commercially. The infant with severe shock may at times require a vasopressor. In severe adrenal cortical insufficiency, vasopressor drugs may be without effect until after the administration of hydrocortisone.

Hydrocortisone or cortisone acetate, 7 to 15 mg/m^2/day, is the mainstay for long-term treatment of patients with adrenal insufficiency. The newer steroid analogues, especially in the patient with mineralocorticoid deficiency, should be avoided. Many of these analogues were synthesized with the express aim of eliminating the sodium-retaining property of hydrocortisone. In fact, some of these drugs, such as dexamethasone, promote sodium excretion. Cortisone acetate also can be given intramuscularly every 3 days for long-term replacement therapy, but this regimen seldom is necessary. During severe stress, such as pernicious vomiting or surgery, cortisone acetate (30 mg/m^2) should be given parenterally on a daily basis.

A mineralocorticoid often is a necessary adjunct for the chronic treatment of adrenal insufficiency. The oral mineralocorticoid, 9α-hydrocortisone (Florinef), has supplanted the use of desoxycorticosterone acetate. The dose of 9α-hydrocortisone is 0.05 to 0.1 mg/day, which is sufficient for most forms of adrenal insufficiency. In the salt-losing forms of congenital adrenal hyperplasia, higher doses of 9α-hydrocortisone occasionally are required for control of electrolyte balance. It has been recognized that even the compensated (*i.e.*, non–salt-losing) form of the 21-hydroxylase defect may be treated better when a small amount of mineralocorticoid is added to the therapeutic regimen.

IATROGENIC ADRENAL INSUFFICIENCY

It often is necessary during the neonatal period to use pharmacologic doses of glucocorticoids for adjunctive treatment of a number of diseases, such as bronchopulmonary dysplasia. There are no good studies, especially in newborn infants, as to the dose and duration of glucocorticoid therapy that will result in adrenal insufficiency. It is probable, however, that high-dose glucocorticoid therapy for a very brief duration (<1 week) will not cause adrenal insufficiency, and treatment longer than 30 days will result in at least transient adrenal insufficiency. Therefore, after a very short course of treatment, tapering glucocorticoids in decreasing increments is not necessary in terms of adrenal function, although the clinical course of the primary condition may worsen with rapid discontinuation of glucocorticoids. After prolonged glucocorticoid therapy, the dose of glucocorticoids can be decreased by one-half every several days until a physiologic replacement dose (10 mg of hydrocortisone/m^2/day orally) is achieved. The dose can then be lowered more gradually, by 20% increments every 4 or 5 days.

It is likely that adrenal function will be suppressed for some time after prolonged pharmacologic glucocorticoid therapy. Again, there are no studies correlating dose, duration of pharmacologic treatment, and time needed for recovery of adrenal function after high-dose glucocorticoid therapy. There have been anecdotal reports of adrenal crisis occurring during stress 6 months and longer after discontinuation of pharmacologic glucocorticoid therapy. It is possible to evaluate periodically the adrenal response to exogenous ACTH to determine when iatrogenic adrenal insufficiency has resolved. Alternatively, the empiric use of pharmacologic doses of glucocorticoids during situations of stress, for at least a year after discontinuation of prolonged high-dose glucocorticoid therapy, is not inappropriate. A minimal dose of glucocorticoid to be used during stress situations is 30 mg of hydrocortisone/m^2/day, orally.

DISORDERS OF THE THYROID

DEVELOPMENT AND FUNCTION OF THE THYROID

The fetal thyroid begins as a thickening of epithelium at the base of the tongue. The thyroid anlage subsequently migrates down the trachea, leaving the thyroglossal duct as an embryonic remnant. During its caudal migration, the thyroid anlage assumes a more bilobate shape. Thyroid function is apparent by 12 weeks of gestation, with the ability to accumulate and concentrate iodide present. Organification of iodine, with synthesis of T_4 and triiodothyronine (T_3), occurs by 14 weeks of gestation. The fetal hypothalamic–pituitary feedback mechanisms are operative by the latter part of gestation, and the fetal thyroid is responsive to TSH. There is no placental transfer of maternal or fetal TSH, although thyroid-stimulating immunoglobulins (TSI) will cross the placenta. Free T_4 and, more so, T_3 are capable, to a small degree, of crossing the placenta in either direction.[63,64]

The biosynthesis of thyroid hormones is illustrated in Figure 41-5. Circulating plasma iodide is concen-

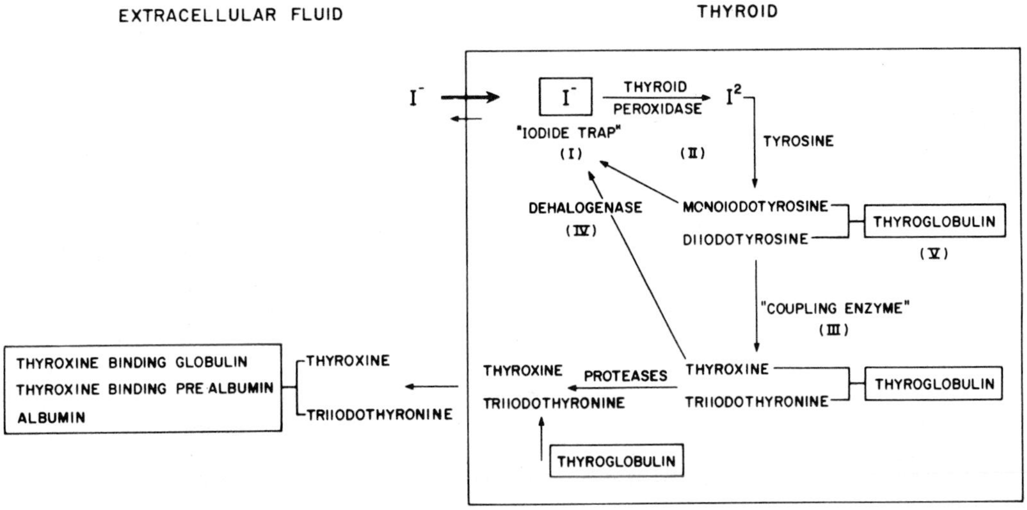

FIG. 41–5. Thyroid hormone synthesis. The roman numerals represent described enzymatic defects of thyroxine synthesis.

TABLE 41–8
RANGE OF MEAN VALUES FOR THYROID AND THYROID-STIMULATING HORMONES DURING THE NEONATAL PERIOD IN FULL-TERM INFANTS

	T_4 (μg/dL)	T_3 (ng/dL)	TBG (mg/dL)	TSH (μU/mL)
Cord blood	10.9 (7–13)	48 (12–90)	5.4 (1.2–9.6)	9.5 (2.4–20)
2 hours of age	22.1	217		86
24–72 hours of age	17.2 (12.4–21.9)	125 (89–256)	5.4	7.3 (< 2.5–16.3)
2 weeks of age	12.9 (8.2–16.6)	250	5 (1–9)	
6 weeks of age	10.3 (7.9–14.4)	163 (114–189)	4.8 (2–7.6)	2.5 (< 2.5–6.3)

T_3, triiodothyronine; T_4, thyroxine; TBG, thyroxine-binding globulin; TSH, thyroid-stimulating hormone.

trated by the thyroid gland. The concentrated iodide is then oxidized by a thyroid peroxidase and bound to tyrosine to form monoiodotyrosine (MIT) and diiodotyrosine (DIT). The iodotyrosines are held in peptide linkage to thyroglobulin. These iodotyrosines are then coupled to form T_3 and T_4, still linked to thyroglobulin. The thyroid hormones are cleaved from thyroglobulin by thyroid proteases, and T_3 and T_4 are secreted into the circulatory system. Intrathyroidal iodotyrosines and iodothyronines are deiodinated by dehalogenase enzymes and remain within the intrathyroidal iodide pool to be reused. The thyroid gland secretes both T_3 and T_4; however, a large percentage of the circulating T_3 is secondary to deiodination of T_4 by the peripheral tissues.[65] The iodide released from the peripheral metabolism of iodothyronines enters the circulatory system to be reconcentrated by the thyroid gland or excreted by the kidneys. The iodothyronines are transported in the plasma by proteins. Thyroxine-binding globulin (TBG), an α-globulin, is the major carrier of T_4, but TBG also will bind T_3 to a lesser extent. Thyroxine also is bound by T_4-binding prealbumin and by albumin. At the cellular level, free T_3 and T_4 are active. Disorders, either genetic or acquired, that quantitatively change the concentration of TBG will alter the level of total T_4 in serum without altering biologic thyroid status.

The secretion of the thyroid hormones is under hypothalamic–pituitary control. The hypothalamus secretes a tripeptide, TRH, which stimulates release of TSH from the pituitary.[66,67] Thyroid-stimulating hormone, in turn, stimulates the production of thyroid hormones. Every step of thyroid hormone biosynthesis and release, from iodide accumulation to proteolysis of thyroglobulin, is under TSH stimulation. The thyroid hormones, in turn, exercise negative feedback control of TSH response to TRH at the pituitary level.

THYROID FUNCTION TESTS

Thyroid function tests in the newborn are elevated compared to values obtained for older children. This is secondary to the surge of TSH that occurs in the immediate postnatal period. The total T_4 ranges from 7.3 to 22.9 μg/dL during the first month of life, with mean values greater than 10 μg/dL (Tables 41-8 and 41-9). The thyroid function tests remain elevated compared to the values found in older children, for the first several months of life. The TBG levels are elevated, secondary to maternal estrogen effect, causing the increased T_4 levels. Thyroid function tests normally are lower in premature and sick newborns than in healthy term newborn infants (Table 41-10). This also is an effect of TBG levels, which are decreased in the premature infant.

CONGENITAL HYPOTHYROIDISM

The causes of congenital hypothyroidism are many and include disorganized embryogenesis, genetic disorders, including errors of T_4 biosynthesis, and environmental factors. It is useful to classify congenital hypothyroidism into the following subgroups:

- agenesis of the thyroid gland (*e.g.*, athyrotic cretinism) or dysgenesis of the thyroid gland (*e.g.*, thyroid hypoplasia, thyroid ectopia)
- endemic goitrous hypothyroidism
- inborn errors of T_4 synthesis (*e.g.*, familial goitrous cretinism)
- drug-induced hypothyroidism
- end-organ unresponsiveness to thyroid hormone
- thyroid unresponsiveness to thyrotropin
- secondary hypothyroidism (*e.g.*, pituitary hypothyroidism)
- tertiary hypothyroidism (*e.g.*, hypothalamic hypothyroidism).

TABLE 41–9
THE UPPER LIMIT OF NORMAL FOR MEASUREMENTS OF THYROID-STIMULATING HORMONE IN THE FIRST 5 DAYS OF LIFE

Age at Collection (d)	Standard TSH Cutoff		Age-Adjusted TSH Cutoff	
	Number of Infants	TSH Value (mU/L)	Number of Infants	TSH Value (mU/L)
0–1	19	> 20	8	> 30
2	54	> 20	26	> 25
3	136	> 20	45	> 25
4	30	> 20	30	> 20
5	34	> 20	34	> 20
Total	273		143	

Retrospective study of 37,927 infants with definite abnormal results during a 6-month period (1988–1989).
TSH, thyroid-stimulating hormone.
From Allen DB, Sieger JE, Litsheim T, Duck SC. Age-adjusted thyrotropin criteria for neonatal screening of hypothyroidism. J Pediatr 1990;117:310.

AGENESIS OR DYSGENESIS OF THE THYROID GLAND

Disorganization of embryogenesis of the thyroid gland is the most frequent cause of congenital hypothyroidism in the United States. Although congenital endemic goitrous hypothyroidism may have been more prevalent throughout the world at one time, the frequency of this disorder has declined with the introduction of iodine into endemic areas.

Little is known of the causes of defective fetal thyroid development. There may be genetic factors. Athyrotic congenital hypothyroidism has been documented in siblings[68,69] and in identical twins.[70] Nonetheless, athyrosis generally is a sporadic disorder. Thyroid antibodies have been detected with increased incidence among mothers of children with hypothyroidism.[71] Most mothers with thyroid antibodies have normal children, however, and, conversely, most mothers who deliver children with congenital hypothyroidism do not have thyroid antibodies. Thyroid hypoplasia has been reported in children with congenital toxoplasmosis, but *in utero* infectious disorders have not been implicated commonly as a cause of thyroid dysgenesis.

TABLE 41–10
MEAN VALUES FOR THYROID AND THYROID-STIMULATING HORMONES IN CORD BLOOD OF FULL-TERM AND PREMATURE INFANTS

	T_4 (μg/dL)	T_3 (ng/dL)	TSH (μU/mL)
Term	10.9	48	9.5
35 weeks of gestation	9.5	29	12.7
32 weeks of gestation	7.6	15	

T_3, triiodothyronine; T_4, thyroxine; TSH, thyroid-stimulating hormone.

ENDEMIC GOITROUS HYPOTHYROIDISM

Although endemic goiter still remains one of the most widespread nutritional diseases in the world, the introduction of iodine into various foods, including infant formulas, has markedly decreased the incidence of endemic goitrous hypothyroidism. The dietary requirements for iodine vary, but 40 to 100 μg/day is sufficient for most children. In areas with endemic goiters, it is probable that factors other than iodine (*e.g.*, enzymatic defects, other genetic factors, other dietary factors such as goitrogens) contribute to goiter formation. The contributory factors are suggested by the evidence that females are more commonly afflicted than males, many of the population within the endemic area may not be afflicted, and the incidence of endemic cretinism varies in different areas. In the Alps, deaf–mutism is a common finding in association with endemic cretinism, suggesting possibly an associated enzymatic defect of organification of iodide. When cretinism occurs in conjunction with an endemic goiter, the signs and symptoms are similar to the dysgenetic form of cretinism except for the presence of a goiter and an elevated radioactive iodine uptake.

INBORN ERRORS OF THYROXINE SYNTHESIS

The inherited disorders of T_4 synthesis involve deficiencies in one or more of the enzymes necessary for hormonogenesis or release of thyroid hormones, resulting in hypothyroidism. A compensatory increase in TSH production produces hyperplasia and enlargement of the thyroid gland, creating the clinical picture of familial goitrous cretinism. These defects of T_4 biosynthesis have been reviewed by Dumont and colleagues.[72]

Iodide Trap Defect. The thyroid gland has the ability to concentrate iodide, so that the intrathyroidal iodide concentration may be 40-fold greater than the serum concentration. In this rare inherited defect of T_4 synthesis, this ability is lost. As would be anticipated, the 24-hour radioactive iodine uptake is negligible. Thyroid scans do not demonstrate the presence of thyroid tissue, although there may be some uptake, but the gland is detected by ultrasonography. Several other organs, including the salivary glands, share the ability to concentrate iodide, and this defect can be distinguished from athyrosis because the salivary iodide concentration also is low and there usually is a goiter. The serum T_4 is low in this defect, but the TSH is elevated. In a manner of speaking, this defect represents iodine deficiency, and high dosages of iodide can overcome this defect to some degree.

Organification or Peroxidase Defect. A defect in the organification of iodide is one of the most frequent defects of T_4 synthesis. In this defect, the thyroid has an increased uptake for iodide but is unable to oxidize it and cannot combine it with tyrosine. This leads to the accumulation of free iodide in the gland, and the administration of anions such as perchlorate or thiocyanate will cause a discharge or release of the unbound iodide. Iodine that is bound to tyrosine or thyronines cannot be discharged. These findings have led to a simple test for the organification defect. The patient is given a tracer amount of radioactive iodine, and the radioactivity over the thyroid gland is noted. In a patient with the organification defect, the radioactive iodine is rapidly concentrated into the gland. When the radioactivity over the gland has leveled off, a dose of potassium perchlorate or thiocyanate given orally (0.5–1 g) will displace the unorganified iodine, causing a rapid discharge of the radioactive iodine from the thyroid gland. The measurement of T_4 usually is low or low normal, but the TSH is elevated.

A variant of this form of familial goiter secondary to a defect in organification is associated with deaf–mutism (*i.e.*, Pendred syndrome). The clinical pattern differs slightly from the full organification defect, in that patients with the Pendred syndrome often have only small goiters and the perchlorate discharge is not as complete. The hearing loss in this variant is neurosensory. Intelligence usually is normal.

Coupling Defect. The failure of coupling of MIT and DIT into T_4 and T_3 has been identified as a cause of goitrous hypothyroidism. The coupling of the iodotyrosines into the final product of the thyroid hormones probably is a complex intermediate step involving many processes, and the block should not be thought of as a defined enzymatic deficiency. The inability of the thyroid gland to couple MIT and DIT into T_4 and T_3 leads to the accumulation of large amounts of MIT and DIT in the gland, with the small amounts of T_4 and T_3 synthesized being immediately released into the circulation. Thus, when extracts of the thyroid gland are subjected to chromatographic analysis after radioactive iodine labeling, large amounts of MIT and DIT are detected with only trace quantities of T_4 and T_3. The TSH is elevated. The radioactive iodine uptake by the thyroid gland is rapid and high. Definitive diagnosis requires thyroid biopsy and chromatographic analysis of the iodotyrosines and iodothyronines.

Dehalogenase Defect. The deiodination of the iodotyrosines and iodothyronines occurs in the thyroid as well as in the liver, kidneys, and other organs. The inherited inability of the thyroid to deiodinate MIT and DIT causes leakage of these precursors from the gland and depletion of iodide stores. This loss of iodide causes decreased hormone synthesis, resulting in compensatory TSH release, thyroid hyperplasia, and increased synthesis of MIT, DIT, and the iodothyronines. The loss of iodide is compounded by further intermediate formation and their increased loss. The goitrous hypothyroidism in this defect is not caused by a biosynthetic block but, in a sense, by iodine deficiency. Radioactive iodine is rapidly accumulated and turned over. Large amounts of iodine can permit adequate hormone synthesis. The T_4 is low or low normal, and the TSH is elevated. When the protein-bound iodine (PBI) was used as a determinant of thyroid hormone levels in the past, the increased circulating levels of MIT and DIT often caused the PBI determination to be normal. Because this defect is extrathyroidal as well as intrathyroidal, administered radioactive MIT and DIT appears unchanged in the urine.

Abnormal Thyroglobulin. Thyroglobulin is synthesized exclusively within the thyroid. The iodination of the tyrosyl residues with the thyroglobulin complex leads to the formation of MIT and DIT, and coupling of these iodinated tyrosyl residues leads to formation of T_4 and T_3. A defect of thyroglobulin formation incorporates a group of disorders. Errors of thyroglobulin synthesis, as well as decreased synthesis, are possible. Deficient protease activity for thyroglobulin degradation also has been postulated to result in deficiency of thyroid hormone release.

These disorders are characterized by abnormal, non–butanol-extractable iodoproteins in the thyroid and the serum. These peptides sometimes have been described as albuminlike, and have been identified by

Savoie and associates as the iodoalbumin thyroalbumin, in which the major iodinated compounds appear to be monoiodohistadines and diiodohistadines.[73,74] These investigators concluded that the abnormality of thyroglobulin causes iodination of inappropriate proteins, mainly albumin, with a subsequent low yield of T_4. A compensatory increase in TSH secretion causes thyroid hyperplasia and a rapid turnover of T_4 or albumin. Proteolysis of the iodohistadinethyroalbumin results in a high secretion of iodohistadine, which can be detected in the urine.

DRUG-INDUCED NEONATAL GOITER

Many agents (*e.g.*, paraaminosalicylic acid, cobalt, iodides, thiourea drugs) as well as foods (*e.g.*, cabbage, turnips, rutabaga) have been demonstrated to be goitrogenic. In the newborn infant, the most commonly implicated drugs are iodides and thiourea derivatives used for treatment of maternal thyrotoxicosis. The use of these drugs not only has caused goiter in the newborn but also has been associated with scattered reports of hypothyroidism.[75] Although the correlation between the dose of the drug and the occurrence of goiter is poor, prolonged administration of thiourea drugs to the mother increases the risk of fetal goiter. Herbst and Selenkow suggest lowering the dose of thiourea drugs during the last trimester and concurrent use of thyroid hormone, in the treatment of a thyrotoxic pregnant woman.[76] In the infants of these women, it is necessary to distinguish the drug-induced goiter from the long-acting TSI-induced goiter. A low T_4 suggests that the goiter is secondary to the drug, whereas a high T_4 is more compatible with a TSI-induced goiter and possible neonatal hyperthyroidism. Treatment usually is not necessary for the infant with a drug-induced goiter unless the goiter is asphyxiating or, more rarely, the infant is hypothyroid. Thyroid hormone will cause the goiter to subside. If the goiter is suffocating, however, subtotal thyroidectomy may be necessary.[77]

UNRESPONSIVENESS TO THYROID HORMONES

Refetoff and associates reported a family with deaf–mutism, stippled epiphyses, delayed bone age, goiter, and an elevated serum T_4.[78] The children appeared to be euthyroid. The serum thyroid hormone-binding proteins and hormone biosynthesis appeared to be normal. This family has been postulated to represent tissue unresponsiveness to thyroid hormone.

It now is clear that there are several expressions of this syndrome. Refetoff's patients probably represent a variant that is totally resistant to thyroid hormones and, despite elevated T_4 levels, is basically hypothyroid. There are patients with isolated central resistance to thyroid hormone who usually are clinically hyperthyroid in infancy and childhood.[79]

UNRESPONSIVENESS TO THYROID-STIMULATING HORMONE

Stanbury and associates reported a severely retarded 8-year-old boy with a normal thyroid gland, a low PBI, normal radioactive iodine uptake, and high endogenous levels of biologically active TSH.[80] Exogenous TSH neither stimulated the thyroid gland *in vivo* nor increased glucose metabolism by thyroid slices *in vitro*. Thyroid-stimulating hormone unresponsiveness of the thyroid gland was postulated by these investigators as an explanation for this clinical syndrome.

SECONDARY AND TERTIARY HYPOTHYROIDISM

These conditions are due to failure of secretion of TSH and TRH from the pituitary and hypothalamus, respectively. Newborn infants with these disorders may be missed in some of the newborn screening programs because they rely on both low T_4 and elevated TSH levels. All patients with the midline abnormalities outlined in Table 41-4 should be suspected of having secondary and tertiary hypothyroidism. Therefore, they should have more complete thyroid studies (*e.g.*, T_4, TSH, T_3 uptake) performed because of the risk that they might be missed by the newborn screening test.

SYMPTOMS

Symptoms of agenesis of the thyroid gland are detectable by 6 weeks of age; however, a number of infants will have clinical manifestations at birth or during the immediate neonatal period. The signs during the early neonatal period are subtle and include prolonged neonatal jaundice, poor suck, poor feeding, lethargy (*i.e.*, the quiet baby), respiratory difficulties, bradycardia, constipation, and intermittent cyanosis. Later, the more classic symptoms of cretinism appear. The progressive myxedema causes coarsening of the facies, with puffy eyelids, flattened nasal bridge, and enlarged tongue. The cry is hoarse secondary to myxedema of the larynx and epiglottis. The infant is extremely lethargic and hypotonic. Constipation, poor feeding, poor weight gain, dry hair, umbilical hernia, and pallor become more notable with time.

There is considerable evidence for the essential role of the thyroid hormones in the growth and development of the central nervous system.[81] The final outcome of mental development in children with congenital hypothyroidism depends on the severity, the time of onset, and duration of thyroid insufficiency. By the time the above clinical symptoms are clinically evident, it is likely that brain injury has occurred.

Infants with ectopic or residual thyroid tissue (*i.e.*, dysgenetic cretinism) or inborn errors of T_4 synthesis often will produce enough thyroid hormone to delay the onset of clinical symptoms. Although the signs and symptoms are similar to those for the athyrotic cretin, the prognosis for mental function is greatly improved.

DIAGNOSIS

The incidence of congenital hypothyroidism has been estimated to be 1 in 4000 births. In view of the desirability of early diagnosis and treatment, screening of newborn infants, using filter paper spots, as for phenylketonuria testing, is now standard in the United States. Some 34% of low T_4 values detected by this method are not the result of true hypothyroidism, but represent diminished levels of TBG. If the initial T_4 is in the lowest 10% of the samples being tested, a repeat T_4 and a TSH are determined on the same sample. If the repeat T_4 is still low ($<6\ \mu g/dL$) or the TSH is elevated, confirmatory tests are requested. A serum sample should be obtained and studied in detail. A low T_4 and a normal TSH may represent secondary or tertiary hypothyroidism or TBG deficiency. Low T_4 levels also are found normally in premature infants and severely ill newborn infants, and are not necessarily indicative of hypothyroidism (see Euthyroid Sick Syndrome). If the T_4 is greater than 7 $\mu g/dL$, it is regarded as normal in premature or sick infants.[82] Note the need to avoid using specimens obtained in the early hours after birth because of the normal surge of TSH (see Tables 41-8 and 41-9).

The diagnosis should be confirmed by serum T_4 and TSH levels, as well as some determination of T_4 binding (*e.g.*, T_3 resin uptake). In those cases suggestive of deficient thyroid hormone binding, a direct measurement of TBG should be determined. Thyroxine-binding globulin deficiency is an X-linked disorder and occurs in 1 in 2000 screening studies of boys. The initial confirmatory serologic studies should not include TBG measurements, because the test is more expensive than a T_3 resin uptake and also will miss binding abnormalities involving other proteins. Radiographic skeletal age often is useful, because one-half of full-term infants with congenital hypothyroidism will not have the osseous centers normally present at birth. It is important to perform a thyroid scan on all patients with congenital hypothyroidism to identify those patients with inborn errors of T_4 synthesis so that appropriate genetic counseling may be given.

The incidence figures for various forms of congenital hypothyroidism, as determined by the newborn screening studies, are listed in Table 41-11. It is probable that the hypothalamic–hypopituitary forms of hypothyroidism have been underestimated by the newborn screening studies, because many of the TSH-deficient patients have normal serum T_4 concentrations at birth. Also, the syndromes of T_4 resistance and thyroid resistance to TSH can be missed by the newborn screening method. Probably the most common cause of undetected congenital hypothyroidism is omitting the screening study. This is more likely to occur in intensive care situations, because of the magnitude of other ongoing problems. The problems with newborn screening for congenital hypothyroidism have been reviewed.[83]

TABLE 41–11
INCIDENCE OF VARIOUS FORMS OF CONGENITAL HYPOTHYROIDISM

Disorder	Incidence
Congenital thyroid agenesis or dysgenesis	1:4000
Inborn errors of thyroxine synthesis	1:30,000
Hypothalamic–hypopituitary hypothyroidism	1:66,000*

* Hypothalamic–hypopituitary hypothyroidism incidence is based on newborn screening studies.

TREATMENT AND PROGNOSIS

It is possible to treat some of the inborn errors of T_4 synthesis with iodide, but T_4 therapy is inexpensive and effective for all of the disorders causing congenital hypothyroidism. The dose of thyroid hormone prescribed should be sufficient to achieve high euthyroid levels of serum T_4 within 2 weeks of starting therapy. This usually is achieved with a starting dose of L-thyroxine, during the newborn period, of 10 $\mu g/kg/day$, with 37.5 $\mu g/day$ being a fairly convenient dose for most full-term infants, since the smallest tablet size is 25 μg. Once treated, the serum T_4 returns to normal before the serum TSH. It is recommended that, to avoid overdosing with L-thyroxine during the first 4 weeks, the serum concentration of T_4 should be used as the laboratory guide for adequate treatment. After 4 to 6 weeks of therapy, however, the TSH level is the best monitor of treatment, and if the TSH remains elevated, the dose of L-thyroxine should be increased.

The prognosis for mental development has been correlated with time of onset of therapy. Klein and associates studied 31 patients and, in 9 patients treated before the age of 3 months, the mean IQ was significantly greater than that of the children treated after 3 months of age.[84] The prognosis for mental development in children with congenital hypothyroidism who have treatment started within 1 month of life is good. There is some evidence that there may be an increase in learning disabilities even in those infants treated within 1 month of age.[85] Another survey, however, indicated no differences in IQ testing or other psychometric parameters studied when children with congenital hypothyroidism treated within 1 month of age were compared to matched normal controls.[86] In the latter survey, the only factor that correlated with poor IQ levels was inadequate treatment.

EUTHYROID SICK SYDNROME

The euthyroid sick syndrome is a reflection of adaptive physiologic processes that occur during acute and chronic illness. Thyroid hormones increase basal metabolism, cardiac output, and oxygen consumption. Reduced production of thyroid hormones, especially T_3, which reduces oxygen consumption and basal metabolic rate, is beneficial for certain illnesses (*e.g.*, catabolic or hypoxic conditions). In animal studies, hypophysectomized rats survive longer during oxygen deprivation than intact animals. The euthyroid sick syndrome has been noted in both premature and full-term sick newborn infants.

The euthyroid sick syndrome is characterized by a low normal T_4 concentration, an extraordinarily low T_3 concentration, and a normal TSH level. The latter two findings distinguish the euthyroid sick syndrome from primary and secondary hypothyroidism. Triiodothyronine levels generally are in the low normal range in both primary and secondary hypothyroidism, with TSH levels markedly elevated in primary hypothyroidism. In those cases difficult to distinguish from secondary hypothyroidism, administration of TRH to a patient with the euthyroid sick syndrome results in a normal rise and prompt decline of TSH. In patients with hypothalamic hypothyroidism, however, there will be a marked and prolonged increase in TSH, and in patients with pituitary hypothyroidism, there will not be any increase in TSH, after TRH administration. Unlike older infants and children, reverse T_3 is not useful in the diagnosis of euthyroid sick syndrome, because it is elevated normally in the newborn infant. Euthyroid sick syndrome does not require any treatment other than correction of the primary disease.

CONGENITAL THYROTOXICOSIS

Thyrotoxicosis in the neonatal period is relatively rare. Affected infants almost always are born of mothers who have either active Graves disease or who have a history of previous Graves disease and are now euthyroid. Neonatal thyrotoxicosis also may present in infants born to mothers with Hashimoto thyroiditis. Fewer than 5% of infants born to mothers with Graves disease will have thyrotoxicosis in the newborn period. It is thought that the etiologic factor for neonatal thyrotoxicosis is the placental transfer of maternal TSI. Thyroid-stimulating immunoglobulins have been demonstrated in over 90% of studied cases.[87]

Neonatal thyrotoxicosis is manifested by poor weight gain or excessive weight loss, goiter, irritability, tachycardia, flushing, and exophthalmos. A number of these infants tend to be small for gestational age. In an infant of a thyrotoxic mother, a high normal T_4 should be viewed with suspicion and the child followed closely. A low or suppressed TSH is further suggestive of neonatal thyrotoxicosis. Onset of symptoms usually occurs within the first week of life, but may be delayed until the second week. Arrhythmias, such as paroxysmal atrial tachycardia,[88] cardiac failure, and death may occur if thyrotoxicity is especially severe. The prognosis generally is good, however, because the thyrotoxic state is transient. Most cases will have resolved by 9 months of age, when maternal antibodies have disappeared from the infant. In several reported cases, there has been a rapid advance in skeletal maturation, with advanced bone age and premature closure of the cranial sutures.[89,90]

Major therapeutic concerns in neonatal thyrotoxicosis are tracheal obstruction secondary to goitrous encroachment, and cardiac failure. Subtotal thyroidectomy rarely is required to relieve tracheal obstruction. In non-neonatal thyrotoxicosis, iodide usually is reserved for preoperative management of thyrotoxicosis, because the duration of its therapeutic effects is limited. Because neonatal thyrotoxicosis is a self-limiting disorder, however, iodide (1 drop every 8 hours of Lugol iodide), along with a β-adrenergic blocking agent such as propranolol hydrochloride, often is used. Iodide has the advantage of interfering not only with T_4 synthesis but also with release of thyroid hormones. In the most severe cases, digitalis, sedation, or glucocorticoids may be necessary to prevent cardiovascular collapse.

REFERENCES

1. Ford CE, Jones KW, Polani PE, et al. A sex-chromosome anomaly in a case of gonadal dysgenesis. Lancet 1959;1:711.
2. Jacobs PA, Ross A. Structural abnormalities of the Y chromosome in man. Nature 1966;210:352.
3. Wachtell SS, Ono S, Koo GC, et al. Possible role for H-Y antigen in the primary determination of sex. Nature 1975;257:235.
4. Page DC, Mosher R, Simpson EM, et al. The sex-determining region of the human Y chromosome encodes a finger protein. Cell 1987;51:1091.
5. Sinclair AH, Berta P, Palmer MS, et al. A gene from the human sex determining region encodes a protein with homology to a conserved DNS binding motif. Nature 1990;346:240.
6. Jacobs PA, Baikie AG, Court Brown WM, et al. Evidence for the existence of the human "super-female." Lancet 1959;2:423.
7. Johnston AW, Ferguson-Smith MA, Handmaker SD Jr, et al. The triple-X syndrome: clinical, pathological and chromosomal studies in three mentally retarded cases. Br Med J 1961;2:1047.
8. Anderson M, Page DC, de la Chapelle A. Chromosome Y-specific DNA is transferred to the short arm of X chromosome in human XX males. Science 1986:233;786.
9. Winters SJ, Wachtel SS, White BJ, et al. H-Y antigen mosaicism in the gonad of a 46XX true hermaphrodite. N Engl J Med 1979;300:745.
10. Lus HA, Rudd FH. Chromosomal abnormalities in the human population: estimation of rates based on New Haven Newborn Study. Science 1970;169:496.
11. Morishima A, Grumbach M. The interrelationship of sex chromosome constitution and phenotype in the syndrome of gonadal dysgenesis and its variants. Ann NY Acad Sci 1968; 155:695.

12. Lippe BM. Primary ovarian failure. In: Kaplan SA, ed. Clinical pediatric endocrinology. Philadelphia: WB Saunders, 1990:325.
13. Carr DH, Gedeon M. Population cytogenetics in human abortuses. In: Hook EB, Porter IH, eds. Population cytogenetics. New York: Academic Press, 1977:1.
14. Goldberg MD, Scully AL, Solomon IL, et al. Gonadal dysgenesis in phenotypic female subjects. Am J Med 1968;45:529.
15. Ullrich O. Uber typische kombinations bilder multipler abartunigen. Z. Kinder Klinik 1930;49:271.
16. Bonnevie K. Embryological analysis of gene manifestation in Little and Bagg's abnormal mouse tribe. J Exp Zool 1934;67:443.
17. Haddad HM, Wilkins L. Congenital anomalies associated with gonadal aplasia. Pediatrics 1959;23:885.
18. Preger L, Steinbach HL, Moskowitz P. Roentgenographic abnormalities in phenotypic females with gonadal dysgenesis. AJR 1968;104:899.
19. Sybert VP. Adult height in Turner syndrome with and without androgen treatment. J Pediatr 1984;104:365.
20. Rosenfeld RG, Hintz RL, Johanson AJ, et al. Three year results of a randomized prospective trial of methinyl human growth hormone and oxandrolone in Turner syndrome. J Pediatr 1988;113:393.
21. Serhal PF, Craft IL. Oocyte donation in 61 patients. Lancet 1989;1:1185.
22. Moshang T, Vallet HL, Cintron C, et al. Gonadal function in XO/XY or XX/XY Turner's syndrome. J Pediatr 1972;80:460.
23. Pallister PD, Opitz JM. The Perrault syndrome: autosomal recessive ovarian dysgenesis with facultative, non-sex-limited sensorineural deafness. Am J Med Genet 1979;4:239.
24. Sternberg WH, Barclay DL, Kloepfer HW. Familial XY gonadal dysgenesis. N Engl J Med 1968;278:695.
25. Grumbach MM, Ducharme J, Moloshok RE. On the fetal masculinizing action of certain oral progestins. J Clin Endocrinol Metab 1959;19:1369.
26. Murset G, Zachman M, Prader A, et al. Male external genitalia of a girl caused by virilizing adrenal tumor in the mother. Acta Endocrinol 1970;65:627.
27. Haymond MW, Weldon VV. Female pseudohermaphroditism secondary to a maternal virilizing tumor. J Pediatr 1973;82:682.
28. Bongiovanni AM. Adrenogenital syndrome with deficiency of 3 β-hydroxysteroid dehydrogenase. J Clin Invest 1962;41:2086.
29. Bongiovanni AM, Eberlein WR, Goldman AS, et al. Disorders of adrenal steroid biogenesis. Recent Prog Horm Res 1967; 23:375.
30. Griffen JE, Wilson JD. Syndromes of androgen resistance. Hosp Pract 1987;22:159.
31. Eberenz W, Rosenberg HK, Moshang T, et al. True hermaphroditism: sonographic determination of ovotestes. Radiology 1991;179:429.
32. Fitzgerald JF. Cholestatic disorders of infancy. Pediatr Clin North Am 1989;35:357.
33. Linder BL, Esteban NV, Yergey AL, et al. Cortisol production rate in childhood and adolescence. J Pediatr 1990;117:892.
34. Goellner MH, Ziegler EE, Fomon SI. Urination during the first three years of life. Nephron 1981;28:174.
35. Rees L, Brook CGD, Shaw JCL, et al. Hyponatremia in the first week of life in preterm infants: parts I and II. Arch Dis Child 1984;59:414.
36. Judd BA, Haycock GB, Dalton N, et al. Hyponatremia in premature babies and following surgery in older children. Acta Paediatr Scand 1987;76:385.
37. Wurtman RJ, Axelrod J. Adrenaline synthesis: control by the pituitary gland and adrenal glucocorticoids. Science 1956; 150:1464.
38. Denton DA, Goding JR, Wright RD. Control of adrenal secretion of electrolyte-active steroids: adrenal stimulation by cross-circulation experiments in conscious sheep. Br Med J 1959; 2:522.
39. Newton MA, Laragh JH. Effect of corticotropin on aldosterone excretion and plasma renin in normal subjects, in essential hypertension and in primary aldosteronism. J Clin Endocrinol Metab 1968;28:1006.
40. David JO, Yankopoulos NA, Lieberman F, et al. Role of the anterior pituitary in the control of aldosterone secretion in experimental secondary hyperaldosteronism. J Clin Invest 1960; 39:765.
41. Eberlein WR, Bongiovanni AM. Steroid metabolism in the "salt-losing" form of congenital adrenal hyperplasia. J Clin Invest 1958;37:889.
42. Peters JP, German WI, Man EB, et al. Functions of gonads, thyroid and adrenals in hypopituitarism. Metabolism 1954; 3:118.
43. Shepard TH, Landing BH, Mason DG. Familial Addison's disease. Am J Dis Child 1959;97:154.
44. Migeon CJ, Kenny EM, Kowarski A, et al. The syndrome of congenital adrenocortical unresponsiveness to ACTH. Pediatr Res 1968;2:501.
45. Moshang T Jr, Rosenfield RL, Bongiovanni Am, et al. Familial glucocorticoid insufficiency. J Pediatr 1973;82:821.
46. Miller WL, Levine LS. Molecular and clinical advances in congenital adrenal hyperplasia. J Pediatr 1987;111:1.
47. Cara J, Moshang T, Bongiovanni AM. Elevated 17 hydroxyprogesterone and testosterone in a newborn male with 3 β-hydroxysteroid dehydrogenase deficiency. N Engl J Med 1985;313:618.
48. Eberlein WR, Bongiovanni AM. Plasma and urinary corticosteroids in hypertensive form of congenital adrenal hyperplasia. J Biol Chem 1956;223:85.
49. Goldsmith O, Solomon DH, Horton R. Hypogonadism and mineralocorticoid excess: the 17-hydroxylase deficiency syndrome. N Engl J Med 1967;277:673.
50. Eberlein WR, Bongiovanni AM. Defective steroidal biogenesis in congenital adrenal hyperplasia. Pediatrics 1958;21:661.
51. Childs B, Grumbach MM, Van Wyk JJ. Virilizing adrenal hyperplasia: a genetic and hormonal study. J Clin Invest 1956; 35:213.
52. Prader A. Die Hanfigkeit des kongenitalen adrenogenitalen Syndromes. Helv Paediatr Acta 1958;13:426.
53. Rosenbloom AL, Smith DW. Varying expression for salt losing in related patients with congenital adrenal hyperplasia. Pediatrics 1966;38:215.
54. Bartter FC, Henkin RI, Bryan CT. Aldosterone hypersecretion in "non-salt-losing" congenital adrenal hyperplasia. J Clin Invest 1968;47:1747.
55. Ulick S, Gautier E, Vetterik K, et al. An aldosterone biosynthetic defect in a salt-losing disorder. J Clin Endocrinol Metab 1964;24:669.
56. Visser HK, Cost WS. A new hereditary defect in the biosynthesis of aldosterone: urinary C 21-corticosteroid pattern in three related patients with a salt-losing syndrome, suggesting an 18-oxidation defect. Acta Endocrinol 1964;47:589.
57. Jaudon JC. Addison's disease in children. Pediatrics 1946;28: 737.
58. Pang S, Pollack MS, Marshall RN, et al. Prenatal treatment of congenital adrenal hyperplasia due to 21-hydroxylase deficiency. N Engl J Med 1990;322:111.
59. Speiser PW, Laforgia N, Kato K, et al. First trimester prenatal treatment and molecular genetic diagnosis of congenital adrenal hyperplasia (21-hydroxylase deficiency). J Clin Endocrinol Metab 1990;70:838.

60. Pang S, Hotchkiss J, Drash AL, et al. Microfilter paper method for 17-hydroxyprogesterone RIA: screen for congenital adrenal hyperplasia. J Clin Endocrinol Metab 1977;45:1003.
61. Weiner D, Smith J, Dahlem S, et al. Serum adrenal steroid levels in full term infants. J Pediatr 1987;110:122.
62. Lee MM, Rajagopalen L, Berg GJ, et al. Serum adrenal steroid concentrations in premature infants. J Clin Endocrinol Metab 1989;69:1133.
63. Fisher DA, Hobel CJ, Garza R, et al. Thyroid function in the preterm fetus. Pediatrics 1970;46:208.
64. Dussault J, Row VV, Lickrish G, et al. Studies of serum triiodothyronine concentration in maternal and cord blood: transfer of triiodothyronine across the human placenta. J Clin Endocrinol Metab 1969;29:595.
65. Pittman CS, Chambers JB Jr, Read VH. The extrathyroidal conversion rate of thyroxine to triiodothyronine in normal man. J Clin Invest 1971;50:1187.
66. Burgus R, Dunn TF, Desiderio DM, et al. Characterization of ovine hypothalamic hypophysiotropic TSH-releasing factor. Nature 1970;226:321.
67. Nair RMG, Barret JF, Bowers CX, et al. Structure of porcine thyrotropin releasing hormone. Biochemistry 1970;9:1103.
68. Lowrey GH, Aster RH, Carr EA, et al. Early diagnostic criteria of congenital hypothyroidism. Am J Dis Child 1958;96:131.
69. Childs B, Gardner LI. Etiologic factors in sporadic cretinism. Ann Hum Genet 1954;19:90.
70. Greig WR, Henderson AS, Boyle JA, et al. Thyroid dysgenesis in two pairs of monozygotic twins and in a mother and child. J Clin Endocrinol Metab 1966;26:1309.
71. Blizzard RM, Chandler RW, Landing BH, et al. Maternal autoimmunization to thyroid as a probable cause of athyrotic cretinism. N Engl J Med 1960;262:327.
72. Dumont JE, Vassart G, Refetoff S. Thyroid disorders. In: Scriver CR, Beaudet AC, Sly WS, et al, eds. The metabolic basis of inherited disease. 6th ed. New York: McGraw-Hill, 1989: 1843.
73. Savoie JC, Thompoulos P, Savoie F. Studies on mono and diiodohistidine: I. The identification of histadines from thyroidal iodoproteins and their peripheral metabolism in the normal man and rat. J Clin Invest 1973;52:106.
74. Savoie JC, Massin JP, Savoie F. Studies on mono and di-iodohistidine: II. Congenital goitrous hypothyroidism with thyroglobulin defect and iodohistidine-rich iodoalbumin production. J Clin Invest 1973;52:116.
75. Burrow GN. Neonatal goiter after maternal propylthiouracil therapy. J Clin Endocrinol Metab 1965;5:403.
76. Herbst AL, Selenkow JA. Hyperthyroidism during pregnancy. N Engl J Med 1965;273:627.
77. Bongiovanni AM, Eberlein WR, Jones IT. Sporadic goiter of the newborn infant. Dallas Medical Journal 1957;43:167.
78. Refetoff S, DeWind LT, DeGroot LJ. Familial syndrome combining deaf-mutism, stippled epiphyses, goiter, and abnormally high PBI: possible target organ refractoriness to thyroid hormone. J Clin Endocrinol Metab 1967;27:279.
79. Bode HH, Danon M, Weintraub BD, et al. Partial target organ resistance to thyroid hormone. J Clin Invest 1973;52:776.
80. Stanbury JB, Rocmans P, Butler UK, et al. Congenital hypothyroidism with impaired thyroid response to thyrotropin. N Engl J Med 1968;279:1132.
81. French FS, Van Wyk JJ. Fetal hypothyroidism: I. Effects of thyroxine on neural development. II. Fetal versus maternal contributions to fetal thyroxine requirements. III. Clinical implications. J Pediatr 1964;64:589.
82. Committee on Genetics, American Academy of Pediatrics. Screening for congenital deficiency of thyroid hormone. Pediatrics 1977;60:389.
83. Willi SM, Moshang T Jr. Diagnostic dilemmas: results of screening tests for congenital hypothyroidism. Pediatr Clin North Am 1991:38;555.
84. Klein AH, Meltzer S, Kenny FM. Improved prognosis in congenital hypothyroidism treated before age 3 months. J Pediatr 1972;81:912.
85. Glorieux J, Dussault J, Letarte J, et al. Preliminary results on the mental development of hypothyroid infants detected by the Quebec screening program. J Pediatr 1983;102:19.
86. New England Congenital Hypothyroidism Collaborative. Characteristics of infantile hypothyroidism discovered on neonatal screening. J Pediatr 1984;102:539.
87. Foley TP Jr, White C, New A. Juvenile Graves' disease: usefulness and limitations of thyrotropin receptor antibody determinations. J Pediatr 1989;110:378.
88. Riopel DA, Mullins CE. Congenital thyrotoxicosis with paroxysmal atrial tachycardia. Pediatrics 1972;50:140.
89. Farrehi C. Accelerated maturity in fetal thyrotoxicosis. Clin Pediatr 1968;7:134.
90. Hollingsworth DR, Mabry CC, Eckard JM. Hereditary aspects of Grave's disease in infancy and childhood. J Pediatr 1972; 81:446.

Neonatology: Pathophysiology and Management of the Newborn, Fourth Edition,
edited by Gordon B. Avery, Mary Ann Fletcher, and Mhairi G. MacDonald.
J.B. Lippincott Company, Philadelphia © 1994.

chapter 42

Renal Disease

LUC P. BRION
LISA M. SATLIN
CHESTER M. EDELMANN, JR.

DEVELOPMENTAL PHYSIOLOGY

The kidney plays a central role in the physiologic transition from fetal to postnatal life. Although the neonatal kidney traditionally has been characterized as dysfunctional, closer analysis indicates that the kidney functions at a level that is appropriate to the growing infant's physiologic needs, except in very-low-birth-weight (VLBW) infants.

EMBRYOLOGY

Embryologic development of the mammalian kidney proceeds through three sequential stages: the rudimentary pronephros, which appears at about week 3 of fetal life, the mesonephros, which degenerates by week 12, and the definitive kidney, the metanephros.[1] The ureteral bud, an offshoot of the mesonephros, ultimately forms the ureter, pelvis, calyces, and collecting ducts and induces formation of nephrons within the metanephric blastema. The nephroblastic cells of the blastema, on contact with the ureteric bud, differentiate into the glomerulus, proximal convoluted tubule, loop of Henle, and distal convoluted tubule.

Nephronogenesis proceeds in a centrifugal pattern. Thus, the first nephrons to develop are those residing in the juxtamedullary region, whereas the youngest are located in the superficial cortex. In the 22-week-old human fetus, all glomeruli present belong to juxtamedullary nephrons. At a conceptional age of 40 to 42 weeks, the juxtamedullary glomeruli are about twice the size of the outer cortical glomeruli. By 1 year of age, the juxtaglomerular glomeruli are only about 20% larger than cortical glomeruli, similar to the relationship observed in the adult.

The full complement of approximately 1 million nephrons per kidney in the human is achieved at a body weight of about 2300 g or 36 weeks of gestational age (GA).[2] When birth occurs before 36 weeks of conceptional age, nephron formation continues until a full complement is achieved. Once complete, nephronogenesis never is resumed, even after extensive loss of renal tissue. Thus, the full-term newborn is born with as many nephrons as he or she will have for the duration of life.

Physiologic, biochemical, and enzymatic maturation of newly formed nephrons may lag behind anatomic maturation by weeks or months. Thus, the immature kidney is characterized by structural and functional heterogeneity arising from the concurrent presence of nephrons in diverse stages of differentiation.

RENAL PHYSIOLOGY

Urine produced by the metanephric kidneys of 12- to 16-week-old fetuses contributes to the formation of amniotic fluid.[3] Although renal function is not necessary for long-term regulation of fetal water and electrolyte homeostasis, a process assumed by the placenta, evidence indicates its importance in normal growth,[4] lung development,[5] and protection from acute changes in fetal vascular volume.[6] The rate of urine production in normal fetuses is about 10 mL/hour at 30 weeks, increasing to 28 mL/hour at 40 weeks.[7]

RENAL BLOOD FLOW

The effective renal plasma flow (ERPF) traditionally has been measured from the renal clearance of the organic acid paraaminohippurate (PAH), corrected for the fraction of PAH extracted by the kidney[8]; the value for ERPF divided by (100 − hematocrit [%])/100 provides an estimate of renal blood flow (RBF). The ERPF increases from 20 mL/minute/1.73 m^2 at 30 weeks of GA to 45 mL/minute/1.73 m^2 by 35 weeks, and 83 mL/minute/1.73 m^2 at term.[8] During the first 3 months of postnatal life, ERPF increases rapidly to 300 mL/minute/1.73 m^2; by 24 months of age, ERPF averages 650 mL/minute/1.73 m^2.[8]

Because the renal extraction ratio for PAH varies with age, measurements of ERPF must be interpreted with caution in the fetus and neonate. Indeed, the rate of extraction of PAH in the full-term newborn at 1 week of age is only about 60%, reaching 90%, the adult value, by 5 months.[9] Paraaminohippurate clearance averages 148 mL/minute/1.73 m^2 in full-term infants at 2 weeks of life, increasing to 200 mL/minute/1.73 m^2 by 2 to 3 months.[10] Paraaminohippurate clearance, corrected for body surface area (BSA), reaches adult levels sometime between 1 and 2 years of age.[8] The incomplete PAH extraction early in life appears to arise from the relatively greater blood flow to juxtamedullary nephrons and efferent arteriovenous shunting in cortical nephrons (see following), thereby allowing blood to bypass PAH-transporting segments of the nephron. In addition, the organic acid secretory pathways in the proximal tubule are immature early in development.[11] Thus, RBF and renal plasma flow (RPF) will be underestimated by PAH clearance alone in neonates, particularly in premature infants, in the absence of determination of the PAH extraction ratio.

The rate of RBF is determined by the cardiac output and the ratio of renal to systemic vascular resistance. Developmental changes in both determinants contribute to the postnatal increase in RBF.

The two kidneys of the adult, which comprise 0.5% of the total body mass, receive approximately 20% of the total cardiac output,[12] corresponding to a RBF of 4 mL/minute/g kidney weight. In contrast, the previable fetus receives only about 5% of the cardiac output.[13]

Although it has been proposed that imposition of functional demand at birth causes a dramatic increase in RBF, experimental evidence suggests that clamping of the umbilical cord does not in itself result in a sudden increase in RBF.[14] Indeed, RBF has been shown to increase progressively to 6% of cardiac output by the end of the first week, reaching 15% to 18% by the end of the first month of life.[15] Because further increases in the percentage of cardiac output received by the kidneys occur in parallel with increases in renal mass, the rate of RBF per unit kidney weight thereafter remains relatively constant.

The intrarenal distribution of RBF in the newborn differs from that reported in the adult, reflecting the relative size and number of glomeruli present in the different regions of the kidney at that stage of development. The newborn kidney has a greater percentage of blood flow to the inner cortical and medullary areas compared to the adult (Fig. 42-1).[16,17] Maturation is accompanied by a redistribution of blood flow toward the superficial cortex, so that the ratio of inner cortical to outer cortical blood flow becomes progressively less than in the fetus.[15,16–18] At maturity, about 93% of RBF goes to the cortex, which constitutes about 75% of the renal mass, whereas only 7% is distributed to the renal medulla and perirenal fat.

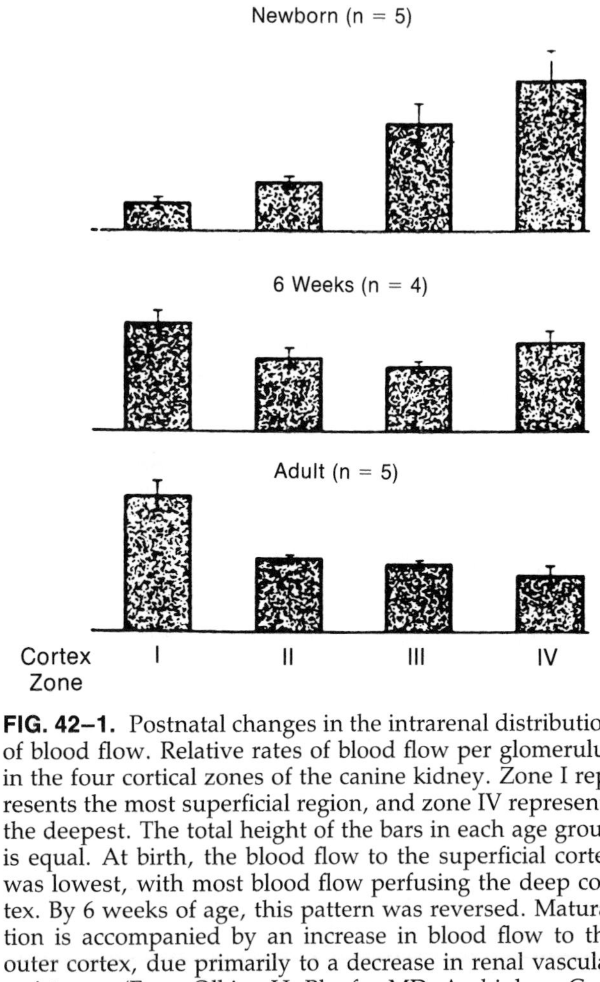

FIG. 42–1. Postnatal changes in the intrarenal distribution of blood flow. Relative rates of blood flow per glomerulus in the four cortical zones of the canine kidney. Zone I represents the most superficial region, and zone IV represents the deepest. The total height of the bars in each age group is equal. At birth, the blood flow to the superficial cortex was lowest, with most blood flow perfusing the deep cortex. By 6 weeks of age, this pattern was reversed. Maturation is accompanied by an increase in blood flow to the outer cortex, due primarily to a decrease in renal vascular resistance. (From Olbing H, Blaufox MD, Aschinberg C, et al. Postnatal changes in renal glomerular blood flow distribution in puppies. J Clin Invest 1973;52:2891.)

The primary factor responsible for the maturational increase in RBF and change in intrarenal distribution is a decrease in renal vascular resistance,[19] the rise in cardiac output and mean arterial blood pressure (MAP) accounting only partially for postnatal changes in renal hemodynamics.[19,20] Indeed, the intrarenal vascular resistance, localized both at the afferent and efferent arterioles,[21] is much higher in the newborn than in the adult.[19,22] The maturational decrease in vascular resistance in the kidney is of greater magnitude than in other organs.

A major contribution to the evolution of the kidney from a high-resistance, low-flow organ, with most of the blood supplying the inner cortex, into a low-resistance, high-flow organ, with most of the blood supplying the outer cortex, is provided by anatomic changes in the renal vasculature.[21] Because RBF increases during the neonatal period after volume expansion,[23,24] however, anatomic immaturity cannot be solely responsible for the low perfusion rate of the newborn kidney; a functional constraint also must exist.

Several vasoactive substances suggested to have a role in the regulation of RBF include the renin–angiotensin system, the kallikrein–kinin system, prostaglandins (PG), vasopressin, and atrial natriuretic peptides. The renal nerves and adrenergic nervous system also may play important roles in regulating renal vascular resistance in the neonate. These factors are considered in subsequent sections.

Anatomic Maturation of Vascular Structures. Experimental evidence indicates that the postnatal increase in RBF may be due in part to glomerulogenesis or structural changes in the vascular bed, or both. Although development and formation of new glomeruli may continue after birth in premature infants of less than 34 to 36 weeks of conceptional age, the increase in RBF continues long after nephronogenesis is complete,[25,26] suggesting that other factors are involved.

The intrarenal vascular system distal to the afferent arteriole in the neonate differs from that in the adult. Variability in the complexity of the glomerular capillary network exists early in postnatal life, with some glomeruli in the nephrogenic zone possessing only a single capillary loop.[27] Inner cortical glomeruli at this age generally have a smaller number of capillaries than the adult, although they appear similar in overall structure.

Efferent arterioles in the outer cortex of the neonatal kidney join the venous system by way of venous channels or sinusoids.[28] Few of the efferent arterioles descend into the medulla to divide to form the vasa recta and peritubular capillaries. Thus, the renal vasculature of the neonatal kidney is characterized by fewer vessels and by efferent arterioles that connect directly to the venous system, thereby bypassing the proximal tubules.[21]

Renin–Angiotensin System. The renin–angiotensin system is very active in the fetus and newborn. The fetus produces renin as early as 17 weeks of GA.[29] Plasma renin activity (PRA) is inversely related to GA, decreasing from 60 ng/mL/hour at 30 weeks to about 10 to 20 ng/mL/hour at term.[30] Plasma renin activity in the newborn may be 20-fold greater than in the adult.[31] It increases gradually to a maximum by 3 to 6 days, then falls by 3 to 6 weeks to a level that still exceeds normal adult levels.[31]

The high levels of PRA in the neonate may be due to increased secretion, decreased clearance, or smaller volume of distribution.[32] Plasma renin activity increases as expected in response to changes in position from recumbent to upright, volume depletion (*e.g.*, hemorrhage, administration of furosemide), and hypoxia.[24,32–37] Plasma renin activity levels decrease after volume expansion with isotonic saline and administration of substances such as the β-adrenergic antagonist propranolol, the PG synthetase inhibitor (PGSI) indomethacin, or vasopressin.[32,38–40] The administration of saralasin, a competitive antagonist of angiotensin II (AII), results in an increase in PRA, indicating a functional short-loop feedback mechanism in the newborn.[41]

The high levels of PRA in the neonate are associated in general with levels of AII and aldosterone[42] that exceed those in the adult. Despite this, in contrast to the adult, systemic blood pressure is low and systemic vascular resistance is very low. Circulating levels of plasma AII decrease during postnatal life in parallel with PRA.[43]

Although the renin–angiotensin system does not appear to play a major role in the control of basal blood flow in the fetus and newborn, the system may be important under conditions of stress. An acute reduction in fetal blood volume or onset of fetal hypoxia results in significant increases in renin and AII levels.[7,44,45]

Kinins. Bradykinins are potent vasodilator peptides generated from the protein precursor kininogen by the proteolytic enzyme kallikrein. The kinins are inactivated by two kininases, kininase I, which is a carboxypeptidase, and kininase II, which is a peptidyl dipeptide hydrolase and is also known as angiotensin-converting enzyme (ACE). Thus, inhibition of ACE not only decreases AII production but also prevents breakdown of kinins.

Premature infants have undetectable levels of urinary kinins[46]; urinary excretion of kallikreins and kinins is lower in newborns than older children.[47] The role of these substances in modulating the function of the immature kidney remains unclear.

Prostaglandins. Complex interactions between PGs and the renin–angiotensin and kinin systems have been described, making it difficult to identify the specific effects of PGs on regulation of blood pressure, RBF, and electrolyte and water homeostasis.

Prostaglandins E_2, D_2, and I_2 (PGE_2, PGD_2, PGI_2) have been shown to reduce renal vascular resistance and increase RBF[48,49]; prostaglandin $F_{2\alpha}$ ($PGF_{2\alpha}$) and thromboxane A_2 (TXA_2) contribute to the vasoconstrictor tone.[48,50] The urinary excretion of PGs, including PGE_2, $PGF_{2\alpha}$, and metabolites of PGI_2 and TXA_2, is high in the fetus,[51,52] presumably reflecting a high rate of renal synthesis. Urinary excretion of PGE_2 and prostacyclin metabolites in the premature infant is 5 times that noted at term and 20 times that measured in older children.[53] Although rates of excretion decrease after birth, urinary PG excretion remains significantly higher in neonates, especially premature infants, than in children or adults.[54,55]

Evidence suggests that PGs produced by the fetal kidney are involved in the regulation of RBF.[56] Inhibition of PG synthesis results in reduction in RBF in the fetus,[56,57] presumably mediated by an increase in renal vascular resistance. In contrast, administration of indomethacin to the unstressed adult causes little change in RBF.

Urinary excretion of these substances decreases in parallel with changes in PRA; however, it remains unclear whether the effects on RBF are mediated by PGs or through their effects on the renin–angiotensin system. Thus, in the newborn, as in the adult, PGs probably play little or no role in control of RBF in the normal subject at rest. Prostaglandins may, however, attenuate renal vasoconstriction in pathologic conditions.

Renal Nerves and the Adrenergic System. Circulating catecholamine levels, particularly norepinephrine, are very high just before and immediately after birth.[58] The abrupt decrease in catecholamine release postnatally is not associated with any change in renal vascular resistance. It has been suggested that the high vascular resistance of the maturing kidney is due to a high sensitivity of the neonatal renal vasculature to circulating catecholamines, acting directly on α-adrenergic receptors or indirectly on β-adrenergic receptors by means of renin–angiotensin release.[59]

In general, the renal vascular bed of the newborn seems to be more sensitive, but less reactive, than that of the adult in response to renal nerve stimulation. The sensitivity of the newborn renal vasculature to the effects of the adrenergic nervous system may be related in part to differences in adrenergic receptor density compared to the adult. Innervation of the developing kidney is incomplete at birth,[60] and most of the adrenergic receptors in the fetal and neonatal kidney are α-type.[61] Alpha-adrenergic–mediated vasoconstrictor effects are enhanced, whereas β-adrenergic and dopaminergic vasodilatory responses are decreased in the newborn compared to those in the adult.[62–64] The gradual appearance of β-adrenergic receptors in the developing kidney may account for some vasodilation of the renal circulation.[65]

Dopamine and Dopamine Receptors. Exogenous administration of dopamine, which results in an increase in RBF in the adult, has no effect in the young animal unless there also is an increase in systemic blood pressure and cardiac output.[66–68] Renal cortical dopamine 1 receptor density does not appear to change with age, whereas that of dopamine 2 receptors decreases.[69]

Arginine Vasopressin. The plasma concentration of arginine vasopressin (AVP) in neonates increases abruptly after birth and is highest in infants whose mothers labored before vaginal delivery.[70] Although AVP has the potential to contribute to the increased renal vascular resistance characteristic of the neonate through its action on vascular and glomerular V_1 receptors, its role in regulating basal renal hemodynamics remains to be defined. Infusion of synthetic AVP does not alter RBF and renal vascular resistance in fetal sheep[40]; however, AVP may play a role in certain stress-induced reductions in renal hemodynamics. For example, during hemorrhage, but not during hypoxemia, the marked decrease in RBF and increase in renal vascular resistance have been correlated closely with the rise in plasma AVP.[7,44,71]

Atrial Natriuretic Factor. Atrial natriuretic peptides and messenger ribonucleic acids (mRNA) are present in both atria and ventricles of the fetus in several species, and circulating levels of these peptides are significantly elevated compared to those of the adult,[72–74] due in part to decreased renal clearance. Although the plasma levels of atrial natriuretic factor (ANF) fall to adult levels within the first few weeks of life,[74] ANF release appears to respond to various stimuli that are associated with volume overload.

The role of ANF in volume and sodium homeostasis early in life remains uncertain. Infusion of ANF into the renal artery of sheep results in renal vasodilation and an increase in RBF in fetal and newborn animals[75]; systemic infusion causes a decline in MAP and thereby reduces RBF.[76]

Autoregulation of Renal Blood Flow. Autoregulation in the mature kidney allows for constancy of RBF as renal perfusion pressure varies over a wide range, from about 80 to 150 torr. Although systemic blood pressure in the fetus (*i.e.*, 40–60 torr) and neonate (see Clinical Evaluation) is less than the lower limit of autoregulatory range defined for adults, experimental evidence suggests that the fetus and newborn are able efficiently to autoregulate RBF at their prevailing low arterial pressure.[77–79] The autoregulatory response probably is mediated in part by a myogenic response of the renal afferent arteriole,[80] which dilates in response to a decrease in renal perfusion pressure, as well as by hormonal factors.

GLOMERULAR FILTRATION

Initiation of glomerular filtration in the human fetus occurs between weeks 9 and 12 of GA.[81,82] It has been suggested that the functional demand placed on the neonatal kidney by cessation of placental function at birth stimulates glomerular filtration rate (GFR) to increase. However, accurate estimates of GFR, assessed by inulin clearance (C_{in}) or true creatinine methodology, indicate a developmental pattern of change in GFR that occurs whether the fetus remains *in utero* or is born prematurely.[83–86] Specifically, GFR averages approximately 8 to 10 mL/minute/1.73 m^2 at 28 weeks of GA, and increases only slightly before 34 weeks of conceptional age, although body size and kidney weight increase appreciably during this time. After about 34 weeks of conceptional age, at which time GFR averages 25 mL/minute/1.73 m^2, regardless of postnatal age, GFR increases rapidly, often by threefold to fivefold within 1 week,[83,85,87] coincident with completion of nephronogenesis (Fig. 42-2). Thus, an infant born prematurely at 28 weeks of GA shows little increase in GFR until the infant is about 6 weeks old (*i.e.*, until a conceptional age of 34 weeks is attained). On the other hand, GFR increases from birth in infants born at 34 weeks or beyond as it does in full-term infants. The GFR of neonates who are small for GA (SGA) is similar to that of infants whose body weight is appropriate for the same GA.[87]

Changes in GFR immediately after birth are variable. In the human, however, the general pattern is one of an increase in GFR in the first 2 hours, followed by a decrease to lower values at 4 hours.[88]

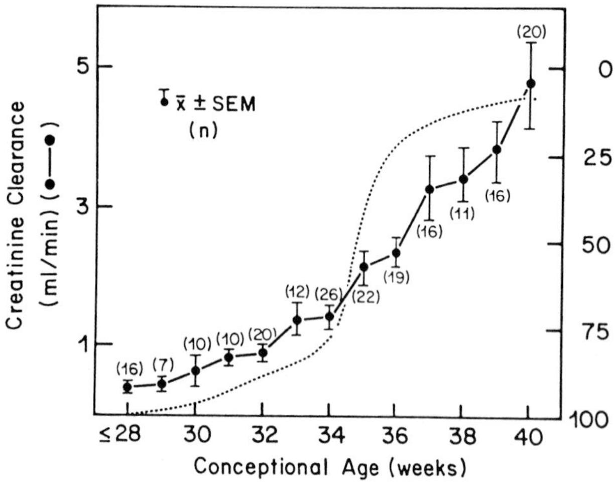

FIG. 42–2. Changes in glomerular filtration rate (GFR; mL/minute), estimated by creatinine clearance, and nephrogenic activity in the kidney cortex (%) are plotted as a function of postconceptional age in the human infant. There is a temporal relationship between the accelerated rate of increase in GFR and completion of nephrogenesis after 34 weeks of gestation. (From Arant BS. Neonatal adjustments to extrauterine life. In: Edelmann CM Jr, ed. Pediatric kidney disease. Boston: Little, Brown & Co, 1992:1021.)

During the first 4 months of life, GFR increases rapidly relative to body size, kidney weight, and surface area.[8] Thereafter, a slower rise is noted until adult values, determined on the basis of BSA, are reached by 2 years of age.[8,89,90] Overall, the increase in absolute GFR (in mL/minute) observed during development is about 25-fold in a number of species.

Total-kidney GFR (TKGFR) is determined by the number of functional nephrons and the rate of filtration per nephron. Increases in either one or both of these factors can account for the postnatal increase in GFR.

Analysis of the similar developmental pattern of change in GFR for several mammalian species indicates that the accelerated rate of increase in GFR is observed around the time nephronogenesis is complete. Thus, those species that complete nephronogenesis *in utero*, including the full-term human neonate,[2] sheep,[15] and guinea pig,[91] show a rapid increase in GFR after birth.[83,91] In contrast, premature infants continue to produce new nephrons after birth[2,92]; GFR increases rapidly only after nephronogenesis has been completed.[93]

Glomeruli are formed in the nephrogenic zone of the kidney, that area of the renal cortex directly under the renal capsule. With maturation, those glomeruli migrate to deeper zones of the renal cortex. At birth, the more mature glomeruli in the juxtamedullary cortex, nearly as large as glomeruli in the adult kidney, will have higher filtration rates than the most recently formed glomeruli in the superficial cortex, some of which may not begin filtration for some time. Thus, GFR matures centrifugally. As nephrons enlarge and forces that regulate filtration permit, GFR increases, with most of the surge due to enhanced perfusion of superficial nephrons,[15,20,25,91,94] related temporally to the increase in total RBF and its centrifugal redistribution within the renal cortex.

The addition of newly functioning nephrons is insufficient, however, to account for the large increases in GFR observed during maturation. A substantial rise in rate of filtration per nephron also must occur. Measurements of single-nephron GFR (SNGFR) and TKGFR by micropuncture techniques in superficial nephrons of the guinea pig show little increase in SNGFR in the first 2 weeks of life, followed by a surge thereafter that continues until the SNGFR of the adult, about 20 nL/minute, is reached by 4 to 5 weeks.[91] During this time period, TKGFR increases at a constant rate. These data indicate that the increase in TKGFR arises initially from an increase in SNGFR of deep nephrons; superficial nephrons appear to contribute to TKGFR later.

The process of urine formation starts with ultrafiltration of plasma through the glomerular capillary membrane. The rate of filtration depends on filtration characteristics of the membrane and on the net ultrafiltration pressure, represented by the difference between hydrostatic pressure (*i.e.*, glomerular capillary hydraulic pressure minus the Bowman space pressure) and colloid osmotic pressure within the capillary loop. The capillary hydrostatic pressure promotes filtration, whereas the colloid osmotic pressure of the blood and the hydrostatic pressure in the Bowman space oppose it.

The postnatal increase in GFR may result from changes in all of these variables, including surface area available for filtration, permeability of the filtering membrane, and effective filtration pressure. The variables that must be considered in describing changes in GFR are described by the following formula:

$$\text{SNGFR} = P_{uf} \times k \times S,$$

where P_{uf} is the net ultrafiltration pressure, k is the hydraulic conductivity of the glomerular capillary per unit surface area (*i.e.*, index of membrane permeability), and S is the surface area for filtration. The product of k times S is indicated by K_f.

Net Ultrafiltration Pressure. The low systemic blood pressure in the immediate postnatal period, substantially less than in the adult in many mammalian species, suggests that glomerular capillary pressure might be low as well. In fact, measurements of glomerular capillary pressure performed in newborn guinea pigs indicate an increase from 18 to 38 torr between day 1 and 30 of life. During this same period, MAP increases from 40 to 60 torr.[21] Concomitantly, plasma oncotic pressure rises, as does proximal tubular pressure, an index of the pressure in the Bowman space. The net effect of these changes is a 2.5-fold increase in net ultrafiltration pressure between birth and 50 days of life, an increase accounting for only about 10% of the 25-fold increase in GFR observed with maturation.[21]

K_f. K_f, the product of the total surface area available for filtration and the hydraulic conductivity of the capillary, provides an index of the net permeability property of the glomerular capillary. An increase in K_f appears to be necessary for the increases in glomerular plasma flow and SNGFR observed during the later stages of maturation.

Measurements of hydraulic conductivity, or water permeability per unit surface area, have not been performed during development. Analysis of the clearance of macromolecules in dogs suggests that changes in the permeability characteristics of the glomerular capillary membrane play only a small role in the increase in GFR with development.[95]

Glomerular capillary surface area increases during development by an average of fourfold in the juxtamedullary glomeruli and by tenfold in the superficial glomeruli, providing a combined increase in capillary surface area of approximately eightfold during the first 6 weeks of life,[96–98] indicating that the maturational increase in GFR is caused primarily by an increase in glomerular surface area.

Many of the vasoactive substances known to affect RBF also influence GFR. Cortisone and growth hormone have been reported to increase GFR concomitant with an increase in RBF.[99,100] Angiotensin II, a powerful vasoconstrictor of both afferent and efferent arterioles, present in high circulating levels in the infant, is known to reduce RBF and constrict the glomerular mesangium, thereby reducing the surface area available for filtration[101]; thus, it may determine glomerular blood flow and hydrostatic pressure within glomerular capillaries. A role for PGs in regulation of GFR has been suggested by the observation that administration of PGSI to newborn babies results in a transient decrease of GFR.[102,103]

Autoregulation of Glomerular Filtration Rate. In the adult, RBF and GFR are maintained over a wide range of MAPs (*i.e.*, 60–150 torr). This autoregulation is accomplished primarily by changes in renal vascular resistance at the afferent and efferent arteriolar level. As MAP falls, efferent arteriolar resistance increases, resulting in maintenance of glomerular capillary pressure and preservation of filtration rate. If MAP falls below a critical lower value, renal perfusion pressure and GFR decrease and prerenal azotemia ensues. On the other hand, as MAP increases, afferent arteriolar resistance increases to limit a rise in glomerular hydrostatic pressure and thus protect the glomeruli from the effects of systemic hypertension. Experimental evidence indicates that the full-term newborn also can autoregulate, albeit at a lower range of MAP.[77,104] The autoregulatory range, however, has not been established.

Filtration Fraction. The normal balance between GFR and RBF is calculated as the filtration fraction (GFR/RPF), and averages 0.2 in the adult kidney. Evidence indicates that the developmental increase in filtration fraction appears to be determined mainly by changes in GFR. Renal blood flow increases in a linear fashion that parallels renal growth, whereas GFR increases in a nonlinear pattern until nephronogenesis is complete.

Tubuloglomerular Feedback. Maturational relationships between tubular flow and GFR (*i.e.*, tubuloglomerular feedback) also occur with growth; this mechanism is thought to contribute to the autoregulatory maintenance of RBF and GFR. A stimulus (*e.g.*, tubular flow rate, ion concentration) at the macula densa is transmitted to the vascular structures of the nephron that control GFR. The feedback system aims at maintaining a constant rate of water and salt delivery to distal segments of the nephron in which reabsorption is regulated to maintain fluid balance. The tubuloglomerular feedback mechanism (*i.e.*, change of SNGFR induced by a given change in tubular flow rate) is maximally sensitive in a range that corresponds to the values of SNGFR and tubular flow rate under normal conditions. As GFR increases with maturation, the maximal response and flow range of maximum sensitivity also increase, so that the relative sensitivity of the tubuloglomerular feedback mechanism is unaltered during growth.[105,106]

TUBULAR FUNCTION

Sodium, bicarbonate, phosphate, amino acids, and glucose are reabsorbed primarily by the proximal tubule. Although most filtered potassium also is reabsorbed proximally, net urinary potassium secretion occurs in the distal tubule, primarily in the cortical collecting duct. Tubular secretion of organic acids occurs in the proximal tubule. Hydrogen ion secretion occurs in both the proximal and distal tubules.

Sodium. Term infants are in a state of positive sodium balance, a requisite for growth, particularly of bone. Healthy infants fed a variety of formulas retain approximately 30% of ingested dietary sodium. The magnitude of this positive balance remains relatively constant within a wide range of sodium intakes.[107,108]

The fractional excretion of sodium (FENa), which may be as high as 20% during fetal life,[109] decreases progressively during gestation,[110,111] so that the FENa in the full-term newborn generally averages about 0.2%.[112,113] Premature infants of less than 30 weeks of GA continue to show elevated values of FENa, similar to those observed in the fetus, which may exceed 5% during the first few days of life.[112,114] In these infants, excessive urinary sodium losses exceeding dietary sodium intake (*e.g.*, breast milk, low-salt formula), often create a state of negative sodium balance and loss of body weight during the first 2 weeks of life (*i.e.*, hyponatremia of prematurity).[115] It has been estimated that these infants require at least 2 mEq/kg/day of supplemental sodium to maintain a normal sodium concentration and remain in positive balance.[116,117]

Postnatal changes in renal sodium excretion proceed in two phases, at least in the sheep. The first phase, which occurs within 2 hours of birth, is characterized by a transient increase in FENa and urinary sodium excretion to levels exceeding those observed during fetal life.[110] This phenomenon may be related to changes in the distribution of intrarenal blood flow, changes in secretion of natriuretic substances and hormones that regulate sodium balance, or both. After the first few hours of postnatal life, in the second phase, the FENa and urinary sodium excretion decline rapidly, possibly related to contraction of the extracellular fluid (ECF) volume.[110]

Studies of full-term human infants and other newborn animals demonstrate parallel and proportionate increases in GFR and the reabsorptive capacity of the proximal tubule, thereby maintaining glomerulotubular balance. Thus, the fractional reabsorption of sodium in the proximal tubule remains constant at about 70% in euvolemic animals.[25,91] A functional glomerulotubular imbalance may exist in the premature infant whereby the reabsorptive capacity of the proximal tubule lags behind the capacity for glomerular filtration.[118]

Clearance studies in premature infants indicate low rates of proximal tubular reabsorption of sodium, resulting in increased delivery to the distal tubule.[119] Because the increased distal delivery is not compensated for by increased distal reabsorption, despite very high circulating aldosterone levels, increased sodium excretion occurs. Explanations for this distal tubular limitation include a relative tubular insensitivity to aldosterone in the premature infant,[120] and the presence of maximal aldosterone stimulation without possibility of additional effect.[42,121,122] Conditions that may augment the FENa include hypoxia, respiratory distress, hyperbilirubinemia, acute tubular necrosis (ATN), administration of theophylline or diuretics, polycythemia, and increased fluid and salt intake.[53,123–125]

Although both term and preterm newborns can tolerate a wide range of salt intake, the newborn kidney is characterized by a limited capacity to excrete a sodium load compared to its mature counterpart. Exogenous administration of a sodium load to an adult is followed by immediate expansion of the extracellular fluid space. This signals the kidney to decrease tubular sodium reabsorption, resulting in increased excretion of sodium and a relatively rapid return of the ECF space to the baseline condition. When full-term newborn infants are given a sodium load in excess of 12 mEq/kg/day, however, they experience a rise in serum sodium levels, abnormal increase in weight, and generalized edema.[126] This blunted natriuresis of the newborn kidney appears to be due more to enhanced sodium reabsorption by the distal nephron than to the low GFR.[127]

The ability to excrete a sodium load increases with age over the first year of life, due to increases in filtered sodium with increased GFR and FENa.[128] Paradoxically, preterm infants of 34 to 36 weeks of GA excrete a sodium load more efficiently than do term newborns, but not as efficiently as adults.[85,114,129] In these subjects with decreased proximal reabsorption under basal conditions, the further depression in proximal reabsorption during saline loading increases distal delivery even further, presumably exceeding the reabsorptive capacity of this segment.

The observation that the fractional reabsorption of sodium in the proximal tubule of the full-term newborn is similar to that observed in the adult indicates that sodium retention in the infant must arise from enhanced reabsorption in more distal segments of the nephron.[130] The avidity of the distal nephron for sodium reabsorption, which increases with GA,[119] may be related to the high levels of stimulation of the renin–angiotensin–aldosterone system. Sulyok and colleagues showed that infants born between 30 and 32 weeks of gestation and studied at 1 week of age, while receiving 1.5 to 2.0 mEq/kg/day of sodium, generally were in negative sodium balance with high urinary sodium excretion rates.[42] Plasma renin activity was directly related to urinary sodium loss but was inversely related to plasma aldosterone concentration and sodium balance. There was a positive correlation between plasma aldosterone concentration and sodium balance, however, suggesting that premature infants can augment their PRA in response to salt wasting, but that their adrenals initially fail to respond adequately to this stimulation. The relative hypoaldosteronism results in an inability to conserve sodium, manifested clinically by weight loss and hyponatremia.

In addition to the renin–angiotensin–aldosterone system, regulation of sodium excretion during maturation is by circulating catecholamines, renal sympathetic innervation, ANF, and glucocorticoids. Studies in newborns indicate a relatively poor natriuretic response to ANF compared to their adult counterparts.[72,131,132] Renal PGE_2 and PGI_2 are natriuretic in the adult. Thus, administration of indomethacin to the adult reduces sodium excretion; in contrast, however, this inhibitor causes a natriuresis when administered to fetal sheep, despite a decrease in fetal RBF.[56] Administration of cortisol to fetal sheep is associated with depression of proximal sodium reabsorption.[99,133]

Potassium. Potassium is transported actively across the placenta from mother to fetus.[134] Indeed, fetal potassium is maintained at levels exceeding 5 mEq/L even in the face of maternal potassium deficiency.[134,135]

Unlike adults who are in zero balance, growing infants maintain a state of positive potassium balance.[42,137] The relative conservation of potassium early in life generally is associated with higher plasma potassium values than in the adult[119,136–138]; plasma potassium levels average 5.2 mEq/L from birth to age 4 months, decreasing to 4.3 mEq/L by 1 year of age.[138] The renal clearance of potassium in the infant is less than in the older child, even when corrected for GFR.[138] Children and adults ingesting a regular diet containing sodium in excess of potassium excrete urine with a sodium–potassium ratio greater than one, as expected. Although the sodium–potassium ratio of breast milk and commercial infant formulas averages 0.5, the urinary sodium–potassium ratio of the newborn also is greater than one, consistent with significant potassium retention.

Infants, like adults, can excrete potassium at a rate that exceeds its glomerular filtration when given a potassium load, indicating the capacity for net tubular secretion[139]; however, the rate of potassium excretion per unit body weight in response to exogenous potassium loading is less in newborn than older animals.[140] Clearance studies in saline-expanded dogs also provide indirect evidence for a diminished secretory and enhanced reabsorptive capacity of the immature distal nephron to potassium.[141]

Filtered potassium is reabsorbed almost entirely in proximal segments of the nephron, urinary potassium being derived predominantly from distal potassium secretion. Therefore, potassium balance, at least in the adult, is maintained by renal secretion rather than reabsorption. Approximately 50% of the filtered load of potassium is reabsorbed along the proximal tubule in both newborns and adults.[136] Up to 40% of the filtered load of potassium reaches the superficial distal tubule of the newborn, in contrast to about 10% in mature animals, providing evidence for functional immaturity of the loop of Henle.[136,142]

The capacity of the immature distal tubule and collecting duct for potassium transport has not been well defined. Micropuncture data indicate that the mass flow of potassium entering the tubular fluid between the late distal tubule and final urine in the newborn is less than that in the adult.[136] Examination of single-nephron segments during postnatal development indicates that the rate of potassium secretion in the cortical collecting duct, that segment responsible for potassium secretion in the adult, is low early in life.[143] Na–K–ATPase activity in neonatal segments has been reported to be only 50% of that measured in the mature nephron.[144] Because the cell potassium content is similar in neonatal and mature collecting ducts,[145] the limitation in potassium secretion at this site probably derives from an unfavorable electrical gradient opposing secretion or reduced apical membrane permeability of this segment to potassium.

Additional factors that may limit potassium secretion early in life include the low distal flow rates characteristic of the newborn,[127] and the unresponsiveness of the immature nephron to mineralocorticoid stimulation.[146] Plasma aldosterone concentrations in the fetus and newborn are high compared to the adult's; yet, clearance studies demonstrate a relative insensitivity of the immature kidney to this hormone.[146] Distal tubular flow rates are low in newborn animals, even when appropriate correction is made for the small tubular size.[127] Low flow rates in the cortical collecting duct may lead to higher concentrations of potassium in the tubular fluid, creating a less favorable cell-to-lumen concentration gradient, thereby limiting potassium secretion. The postnatal surge in superficial SNGFR that occurs in maturing animals at about 3 to 4 weeks of postnatal life should increase fluid delivery into the cortical collecting duct and promote potassium secretion.[91]

Acid–Base. The acid–base status of the fetus is maintained by placental function and maternal mechanisms. The fetal kidney in the second one-half of pregnancy, however, is able to acidify the urine.[147,148] The bicarbonate threshold, low in the fetus, increases with GA.[149]

Immediately after birth, the acid–base state of the full-term newborn is characterized by a metabolic acidosis.[150] Recovery occurs within 24 hours in the full-term infant, an increase accomplished in large measure through pulmonary excretion of CO_2.

The normal range for serum bicarbonate is lower

for preterm infants (16–20 mmol/L) and full-term infants (19–21 mEq/L) than for children and adults (24–28 mmol/L),[151,152] presumably due to a low renal tubular bicarbonate threshold.[153] The low threshold may arise from a relatively expanded extracellular fluid compartment in the neonate or immaturity of the renal tubular reabsorptive capacity for bicarbonate reabsorption.[149,154,155] Experimental evidence suggests that renal tubular carbonic anhydrase activity, present in the human fetal kidney in late gestation,[156] does not limit the capacity of the fetal kidney for bicarbonate reabsorption.

The capacity of the neonatal kidney for renal acidification is limited, due in part to decreased excretion of urinary buffers, including phosphate and ammonium ions. Phosphate loading, administration of cow milk that is rich in protein and phosphate instead of breast milk, or high protein feeding enhances the ability of the newborn to excrete titratable acids and ammonia.[157] Before feeding, newborns excrete 10% to 25% of H^+ as titratable acid. In 1-week-old babies fed cow milk, net acid excretion per kilogram body weight is high and 60% of urinary acid is in the form of titratable acid.[158] In contrast, 1-week-old breast-fed babies, who ingest a milk low in phosphate and protein, excrete 60% less net acid than cow-milk–fed infants, and only 20% of this is titratable acid.[158]

Term newborns generally are able to excrete a maximal acid load within the first 2 months of life.[159] Premature infants born at 34 to 35 weeks of GA and studied 1 to 3 weeks after birth exhibit rates of excretion of net acid, titratable acid, and ammonium that are about 50% lower than term babies of similar postnatal age; net acid excretion increases to levels observed in term newborns only after 3 weeks of age.[159,160] In response to acid loading with ammonium chloride, urinary *p*H of premature infants rarely decreases below 5.9 until the second month of life.[161] In contrast, by the end of the second postnatal week, urine *p*H values of 5.0 or lower, comparable to those in the adult, can be consistently achieved in term infants.[152,157]

The final site of urinary acidification is the renal collecting duct. Functional immaturity of this segment and the acid–base transporting intercalated cells therein may further limit the ability of the neonate to eliminate an acid load.[162,163]

Low rates of ammonia synthesis and excretion may contribute to the inability of the immature kidney to excrete acid.[164] The rate of ammonia excretion in response to acid loading in human infants does not reach mature values until 2 months of age.[152,165]

Up to 10% of preterm infants develop a partially compensated hyperchloremic metabolic acidosis during weeks 1 to 3 of life (*i.e.*, late metabolic acidosis),[153] despite an otherwise healthy appearance. Typically, spontaneous remission occurs in the subsequent 2 weeks. These infants are characterized further by an apparent delay in postnatal weight gain despite ample dietary intake, suggesting a high rate of endogenous acid formation in infants whose dietary intake exceeds their anabolic capacity.[166] Although infants provided supplemental sodium bicarbonate to maintain acid–base homeostasis showed greater increases in length than controls, there were no differences in weight gain between the two groups.[151,167] Because supplementation with sodium results in an increase in serum bicarbonate, it has been suggested that the late metabolic acidosis and low bicarbonate threshold results in part from large urinary sodium losses.

Calcium. Urinary excretion of calcium varies inversely with GA in the first week of life and varies directly with urine flow and sodium excretion (see Chap. 36).[168] Increased calcium excretion may contribute in part to early neonatal hypocalcemia, which occurs in the first 24 to 48 hours of life.[169] The urinary calcium–creatinine ratio in full-term infants ranges from 0.05 to 1.2 during the first week of life, but may exceed 2 in premature neonates.[168,170] In children over 1 year of age, the ratio is approximately 0.2, and in adults, less than 0.11.[171] Urinary calcium excretion from 1 to 15 years of age averages 2.4 mg/kg/day, with an upper limit of 4 mg/kg/day.[171]

The high fractional excretion of calcium in preterm infants may be related to maturational changes in the tubular handling of calcium. Approximately 50% of filtered calcium is reabsorbed along the superficial proximal tubule in mature rats, yet only 1% of filtered calcium is excreted.[136] Thus, in the adult, almost one-half of the filtered calcium is reabsorbed at a site beyond the proximal tubule or in deep nephrons.[136] The fractional reabsorption of calcium in the neonate has been shown to be decreased in the loop of Henle, as is the case for sodium, potassium, and chloride.[136]

The roles of parathyroid hormone (PTH) and calcitonin in the regulation of renal calcium excretion in the neonatal period are unclear. In mature animals and in adults, PTH decreases the urinary excretion of calcium,[172] whereas calcitonin at high doses increases calciuria.[173] Parathyroid hormone–responsive adenylate cyclase has been found in renal cortical homogenates from preterm rabbits[174] and in the thick ascending loop of Henle in 2-day-old puppies.[175] It has been suggested that neonatal hypocalcemia may be due to end organ unresponsiveness to PTH. In premature and full-term newborns, however, the administration of exogenous PTH increases urinary excretion of cyclic adenosine monophosphate (cAMP),[176,177] results in a calcemic response but affects calciuria and phosphaturia only minimally.[178] The response of the thick ascending limb to PTH is decreased at birth and increases with age; similar maturational increases are seen with calcitonin.[175]

Magnesium. Ninety-seven percent of the filtered magnesium is reabsorbed by the mature nephron, largely in the loop of Henle.[179] Although tubular reabsorption of magnesium is almost complete in the case of hypomagnesemia, it decreases in the case of hypermagnesemia.[179] The administration of PTH results in an increase in serum concentration of magnesium (see Chap. 36).[180]

Only limited data are available on the maturation of renal magnesium transport during postnatal life. Micropuncture analysis of magnesium transport in developing rats showed a decrease in the fractional reabsorption of magnesium in the proximal tubule during maturation.[136] In contrast, the fractional reabsorption of magnesium in the loop of Henle had already reached mature values of about 60% in the youngest animals.[136,181]

Phosphate. In contrast to most other transport processes, the capacity of the immature kidney to reabsorb phosphate is greater than in the adult (see Chap. 36).[182–184] The tubular reabsorption of phosphate increases from 85% of the filtered load at 28 weeks of GA to 99% at term and decreases thereafter to about 85% between 3 and 20 months of age. An increase in phosphate load, provided by a change in formula from breast milk to cow milk, results in doubling in the renal clearance of phosphate and a decrease in fractional reabsorption from 95% to 80%.[185]

Clearance studies performed in infants and children suggest that phosphate retention in the young is due in large part to the low GFR.[184,185] Studies in experimental animals, however, demonstrate enhanced tubular reabsorption early in life.[186,187] Younger subjects have a higher maximal net reabsorption (Tm) of phosphate per unit glomerular filtrate (Tm/GFR) than adults.[187–189] Micropuncture analysis of newborn and adult guinea pigs confirm a higher fractional reabsorption of phosphate in the newborn proximal tubule (75%) compared to the adult (65%); distal phosphate reabsorption also is higher in younger than older animals.[190]

The high reabsorptive capacity of the immature kidney for phosphate is thought not to be related to PTH levels. Serum levels of PTH are low immediately after birth, increasing substantially thereafter to levels in infancy exceeding those observed in later childhood.[191,192] Exogenous administration of PTH to humans or experimental animals results in a blunted phosphaturic effect in immature kidneys.[177,186] The lack of effect may be related to poorly developed proximal tubular segments responsive to PTH or a low intracellular phosphate concentration.[193] By the end of the first week of life, however, full-term infants exhibit a prompt phosphaturic response and an increase in urinary cAMP excretion after PTH administration. The mechanisms responsible for the high reabsorptive capacity of the kidney for phosphate early in life include developmental differences in the intrinsic properties of sodium phosphate cotransport in the luminal membrane of the tubule or hormonal regulation of phosphate transport between the neonate and adult.

Glucose. Premature infants of less than 34 weeks of GA have a higher urinary glucose concentration, higher fractional glucose excretion, and lower fractional reabsorption of filtered glucose than full-term infants and older children. The tubular reabsorptive capacity for glucose appears to increase with increasing GA[83]; however, the maximal reabsorption of glucose factored by GFR, the fractional reabsorption of glucose, is similar in full-term newborn infants and adults.[83] Similar observations have been made in experimental animals.[93,194] These results provide additional evidence for preservation of glomerulotubular balance, at least in term infants. The renal threshold for glucose, however, is lower in newborns than in older animals,[93] suggesting a greater degree of nephron heterogeneity early in life.

Studies in the rat and guinea pig indicate that the neonatal renal tubule possesses two distinct membrane transport systems for glucose, whereas only one, the low-affinity system, is present in adults.[195,196] It is not clear when the high-affinity system disappears during maturation, but its presence early in life may enable the anatomically immature kidney to reabsorb sugar more efficiently from the glomerular filtrate. The single glucose transport system in the fetus is qualitatively similar to that of the adult; specifically, it is sodium dependent, electrogenic, and *p*H sensitive.[197]

Organic Acids. Organic acids, including PAH (see Renal Blood Flow) and endogenously produced uric acid, are eliminated by filtration and proximal tubular secretion. Organic acids are transported from the peritubular circulation across the basolateral surface of the proximal tubule to the tubular fluid. The renal clearance of organic acids is low in the neonate, even when corrected for body size, and increases gradually with age.[14,198,199] As discussed previously, the limitation in tubular excretion of weak acids may be due in part to the preponderance of blood flow to the juxtamedullary region, bypassing tubular secretory sites. Additional variables that may account for the low clearance of organic acids include the low GFR, reduced numbers of transporter sites, and limited energy for transport.

Amino Acids. The renal reabsorption of many amino acids in newborn animals and humans is low compared to that of adults, often resulting in aminoaciduria.[200,201] This does not appear to be a generalized defect in amino acid reabsorption because other amino acids (*e.g.*, methionine, isoleucine, leucine, tyrosine) are reabsorbed more completely. Specific amino acid transport systems have been identified in newborn kidneys.[202–205] Experimental evidence suggests that the limitation in luminal reabsorption arises from a lower rate of efflux out of the cell into the peritubular circulation compared to the adult, a mechanism that also would account for the high intracellular concentrations of amino acids observed early in life.[202]

Urinary Concentration. In mammals, fetal urine is hypotonic with respect to fetal plasma.[109] This observation may reflect a limited medullary osmotic gradient, arising either from structural immaturity of the medulla or a relatively high blood flow through the vasa recta, which disperses the intrarenal solute gradient normally found in the medulla of more mature animals. Another possibility is reduced sensitivity of the fetal nephron to vasopressin due to reduced numbers of AVP receptors or poor coupling between AVP receptor binding and cAMP generation. The fetal kidney is able both to concentrate and to dilute urine, depending on the hydration state of the fetus and thus the mother. Maternal water deprivation[206] or infusion of AVP into the fetus[207] leads to a fall in fetal urine flow rate and a decrease in free water clearance.

Urine voided at or shortly after birth generally is hypotonic with respect to plasma.[88,208] Maximal urinary concentrating ability in the neonate has been shown to be less than that of children and adults. After fluid deprivation for 12 to 24 hours, the maximal urine osmolality achieved in both premature infants and full-term newborns averages about 500 mOsm/kg,[209–212] a value roughly 60% that observed in older children and adults. A few 1- to 2-month-old infants may be able to achieve a urine osmolality as high as 1000 mOsm/kg, a maximal value generally not seen before 12 months of age.[210,212]

The limited ability of infant kidneys to concentrate urine may be related to several factors, including low GFR (see Glomerular Filtration), immaturity of the countercurrent multiplication and exchange system thereby preventing buildup of a medullary gradient, and diminished responsiveness of the distal nephron to antidiuretic hormone (ADH).

Medullary Gradient. A direct relationship has been demonstrated in the rat between elongation of the loops of Henle, their penetration into the medulla, and the capacity to concentrate the urine.[213] The inner medulla and renal papillae are poorly developed in the immature kidney. In the rat, the 1.6-fold increase in length of the renal medulla correlates well with the 1.5-fold increase in urine osmolality observed between 10 and 20 days of age.[213]

Associated with this anatomic maturation is the buildup of a high interstitial solute concentration gradient in the medulla. This buildup occurs mostly through development of two aspects of the urinary concentrating mechanism: the ability of the thick ascending limb of the loop of Henle to reabsorb sodium and the ability of this segment to sequester urea.[214–216]

Antidiuretic Hormone. The decreased ability of the immature kidney to concentrate urine is not due to an inability of the fetus or neonate to synthesize ADH. Circulating levels of ADH are elevated in preterm and term infants and decrease rapidly in term infants within 24 hours of birth.[217,218] Studies in fetal and newborn animals,[44,219,220] as well as human infants,[218,221] indicate an appropriate response to osmolar or volume stimuli known to affect ADH release, similar to that observed in their mature counterparts. Thus, it is likely that diminished end organ responsiveness to ADH in the young contributes to the low concentrating ability of the newborn.

Exogenous administration of AVP or 1-des-amino-8-D-AVP (DDAVP) to healthy 1- to 3-week-old newborns leads to a response of shorter duration and reduced magnitude than that observed at 4 to 6 weeks.[221a] The diminished sensitivity of the newborn kidney to AVP may be due to a paucity of vasopressin receptors,[222] limited activation of adenylate cyclase and therefore cAMP generation by AVP, or both.[175,223]

Prostaglandin E_2 inhibits the action of AVP on the hydraulic permeability of the collecting duct.[224] Although infants excrete more PGE_2 per unit BSA than do older children (see Prostaglandins), inhibition of PG synthesis in fetal lambs has no effect on urinary concentrating ability.[56]

Thus, the limited ability of the neonatal kidney to concentrate the urine is due to both structural and functional constraints that together prevent generation of the requisite corticopapillary osmotic gradient.

Urinary Dilution. Premature infants (<35 weeks of GA) studied under conditions of maximal water diuresis decrease urine osmolality to 70 mOsm/kg, whereas infants over 35 weeks of GA are able to reduce urine osmolality to 50 mOsm/kg.[119] This is associated with a significantly greater osmolar clearance in the premature infants, indicating that they cannot dilute their urine as well as term infants or adults. Although there is greater proximal sodium rejection in preterm than term infants, the high avidity of the distal nephron for sodium reabsorption allows the neonate, especially the preterm infant, to generate a free water clearance greater than that in adults.[127,130,141] Despite the greater capacity for free water clearance, the ability of the neonate to excrete a hypotonic load is limited, presumably due to the low GFR.

CLINICAL EVALUATION OF FUNCTION AND DISEASE

A newborn infant presenting with oligoanuria or with Potter syndrome, in the absence of prolonged rupture of the membranes, obviously has a renal problem. On the other hand, renal anomalies or malfunction can remain unnoticed until routine observations reveal abnormalities such as a mass, hypertension, an unexpectedly high gentamicin level, or a high serum or plasma creatinine concentration (P_{cr}). Temperature instability or unexpected jaundice may lead to the diagnosis of urinary tract infection (UTI). If an early diagnosis of a renal anomaly is made, several complications may be prevented, including those related to the kidney itself (*e.g.*, progressive loss of renal function due to systemic hypertension, obstructive or reflux uropathy, or infection) and those related to other organs (*e.g.*, cerebral hemorrhage, seizures or congestive heart failure [CHF] secondary to hypertension, ventricular arrhythmia secondary to hyperkalemia).

In this section, clinical and laboratory features that should raise suspicion of a renal problem are reviewed, and an approach to establish the correct diagnosis is presented. Factors that increase the risk for renal or urinary tract malformations are analyzed.

INCIDENCE OF RENAL AND URINARY TRACT MALFORMATIONS

The exact incidence of major renal and urinary tract malformations in newborn infants can only be estimated, since a large prospective population-based study using ultrasonography (US) has not been reported (Table 42-1). Early studies using neonatal abdominal palpation as the screening method showed an incidence of 0.2% to 0.6%,[225-227] whereas neonatal autopsy series had an incidence of 7% to 9%.[228,229] Series using routine prenatal US have detected anomalies in 0.1% to 0.7% of fetuses.[230,231] In two prospective studies that used routine US screening in a cohort of newborn infants, 1.0% of infants were found to have renal anomalies.[232,233] However, in one of these studies,[232] this figure may be an underestimation of the true incidence in a neonatal population, since only those infants not requiring intensive care were included. A small study done in a predominantly Caucasian population, using a perinatal approach that combined family history, prenatal US, physical examination, and case-oriented neonatal imaging showed an incidence of 1.3%.[234] A similar incidence (1.4%) was found in 2- to 10-month-old infants by routine US.[235] The incidence of urinary tract anomalies in males in all large series is approximately twice that in females. Whether the incidence varies with geography or race remains to be determined.

HISTORY

FAMILY HISTORY

Positive family history should be sought for hereditary disease, including renal cystic disease, tubular disorders, and nephrotic syndrome. There is a 9% incidence of asymptomatic renal malformations—most often unilateral renal agenesis—in the first-degree relatives of infants with agenesis or dysgenesis of both kidneys or agenesis of one kidney and dysgenesis of the other.[236] A study using US has confirmed that in some families, bilateral agenesis or dysplasia is inherited as an autosomal dominant trait.[237] The clinician should be cautious not to immediately exclude a diagnosis of an autosomal dominant disease, since there may be variable penetrance or time of presentation (*e.g.*, adult-type polycystic disease) and because of the possibility of a new mutation. In addition, the history for prior fetal loss should be carefully reviewed, with autopsy review if possible.

TERATOLOGY

The risk of renal or urinary tract malformations is increased by maternal diabetes and by certain medications or drugs, including alcohol, trimethadione, thalidomide, and cocaine (see Appendix I-1). Maternal diabetes, at least in the absence of tight diabetic control initiated before conception, is associated with urogenital malformations, with an incidence of 2.6%, compared to an incidence of 1.2% in controls,[238] as well as with neonatal renal venous thrombosis. The risk for renal or urinary tract malformations is high when an infant of diabetic mother has either a caudal regression syndrome or a femoral hypoplasia–unusual facies syndrome (see Appendix I-1). Fetal alcohol syndrome is associated with various types of renal malformations, including unilateral renal agenesis, renal hypoplasia, ureteral duplication, and hydronephrosis.[239] The effect of maternal cocaine abuse on fetal malformations is controversial. In a recent metaanalysis of cocaine abuse in pregnancy based on 20 case–control or cohort studies and at least one control group, the odds ratio of genitourinary malformations comparing pregnancies exposed to cocaine to drug-free controls was 5.0 (95% confidence interval 1.1–23.6).[240] The odds ratio was 6.1 (95% confidence interval 1.2–31.3) in studies comparing cocaine–polydrug users to polydrug users without cocaine.[240]

PREGNANCY

Oligohydramnios should lead to the suspicion of oligoanuria, unless the amniotic sac has ruptured or has been leaking. Fetal oligoanuria can result from congenital malformations of the genitourinary tract, such as bilateral renal agenesis, bilateral or lower urinary tract obstruction, bilateral cystic kidneys, or renal hypoplasia–dysplasia, or from acquired fetal renal disease, such as that due to administration of indomethacin to the mother for the treatment of premature labor.

Although polyhydramnios is due most commonly to other causes, it may be the first clue to the diagnosis of a nephrogenic defect of urinary concentration. Similarly, fetal hydrops may be the first sign of congenital nephrotic syndrome. The diagnosis of a urologic problem may have been obtained by US performed as a routine examination or as a part of the work up for another anomaly.

Prenatal urinary indices (*e.g.*, urinary osmolality, electrolyte concentration, response of fetal urinary

TABLE 42–1
INCIDENCE OF RENAL AND URINARY TRACT MALFORMATIONS IN INFANCY AND CHILDHOOD

Author	Number of Subjects	Selection Criteria	Method of Screening	Most Common Anomalies (Final Diagnosis)	Number of Subjects With Anomalies (% of Total)
Sherwood, 1956	12,160	Consecutive newborn infants	Palpation Confirmation by IVU	Ectopia (7), horseshoe/fused kidneys (5), obstruction (6), Wilms (1)	22 (0.2%)
Museles, 1971	12,150	Consecutive newborn infants	Palpation Confirmation by IVU	Ectopia (7), horseshoe (4), agenesis (3)	22 (0.2%)
Rubenstein, 1961	2153	<12-year-old autopsies	Autopsy	Agenesis (11), hypoplasia/dysplasia (89), ectopia (31), duplication (14)	181 (8.4%)
Brion, 1984	1200	Consecutive newborn infants	Prenatal US (2/3), physical examination, US screening for various indications	Hypoplasia/agenesis (4), obstructive uropathy (8), reflux (1)	15 (1.3%)
Helin, 1986	11,986	Consecutive pregnancies	Prenatal US	Hydronephrosis (9), VUR (3), mild dilatation (10), cystic disease (3)	33 (0.3%)
Steinhart, 1988	437	Healthy infants	US	VUR (3), obstructive uropathy (3)	6 (1.4%)
Gillerot, 1988	900	Newborn infant autopsies	Autopsy	Dysplasia/agenesis (30), polycystic kidneys (18), obstructive uropathy (11), cloacal exstrophy (4)	63 (7%)
Scott, 1991	1061	Newborn infants in well-baby nursery	Postnatal US, followed by appropriate workup	Duplex kidney (1), solitary kidney (2), hydronephrosis	11 (1.0%)
Mihara, 1992	2351	Asymptomatic 3-year-old children	US	Pelvic dilation (6), solitary kidney (3), hypoplasia (2)	11 (0.5%)

IVU, intravenous urography; US, ultrasonography; VUR, vesicoureteral reflux.

output to the maternal administration of furosemide), which are obtained from amniotic fluid or, better, from aspiration of urine from the fetal bladder, are not specific and sensitive enough to predict outcome in individual cases. A high maternal serum or amniotic α-fetoprotein concentration is associated with several anomalies, including bladder exstrophy or myelodysplasia, which are associated with urinary tract malformations (see Appendix I-1). Increased maternal serum α-fetoprotein concentration is associated with pyelectasis and thick-walled bladder.[241]

Maternal treatment with indomethacin or with ACE inhibitors has been associated with prenatal renal damage leading to early-onset neonatal renal failure with nephron dysgenesis and cystic dilatations (see Acute Renal Failure).[242–244] Severe perinatal asphyxia frequently is associated with oligoanuria or acute renal failure (ARF).

DYSMORPHISM

RENAL AND URINARY TRACT ANOMALIES ASSOCIATED WITH MULTIPLE CONGENITAL ANOMALIES

Any dysmorphic feature (*e.g.*, abnormal ears) should lead the clinician to look for the other anomalies and structural defects. Appendix I-1 lists the major signs of multiple congenital anomalies (MCA) associated with renal and urinary tract anomalies (see Chap. 40). The most typical sequence related to kidney disease is the oligohydramnios sequence, described in the next section.

OLIGOHYDRAMNIOS SEQUENCE

The oligohydramnios sequence (*i.e.*, Potter syndrome) can be due either to prolonged leakage of amniotic fluid or to intrauterine oligoanuria secondary to bilateral renal agenesis, lower urinary tract obstruction, polycystic kidneys, or renal hypoplasia–dysplasia–aplasia–dysgenesis. Severe oligohydramnios results in facial deformation (*e.g.*, Potter facies characterized by a redundant skin, flat nose, low-set ears, bilateral skinfolds arising at the inner canthus and receding chin), wrinkled skin, and malposition of the hands and feet, which are attributed to *in utero* compression, on the basis of animal studies and observations in twins discordant for renal or urinary tract malformations.[245] On the other hand, lung hypoplasia may be due to several factors, including fetal compression caused by oligohydramnios, abnormal composition of the urine that possibly includes a decrease in proline,[246,247] and, in some cases, massive abdominal distention. The risk for lung hypoplasia is high during the pseudoglandular period (12–16 weeks of GA) and the canalicular period (17–28 weeks of GA) of lung development.[247] Animal data suggest that the lung is more severely damaged during the latter period.[246,248] Even a short duration of oligohydramnios (1 week) at a critical period can induce pulmonary hypoplasia.[245,248,249] Thus, the severity of the lung hypoplasia seems to depend more on the time of onset of the oligohydramnios than on its duration.

ASSOCIATIONS OF RENAL AND URINARY TRACT ANOMALIES WITH SINGLE SIGNS

Although several associations have been described between upper urinary tract anomalies and isolated anomalies of other body systems, such as abnormal vertebrae, anorectal malformations, congenital diaphragmatic hernia, hypospadias, lung hypoplasia, spontaneous air leak syndrome, single umbilical artery (UA), and supernumerary nipples, some of these associations are controversial (see Appendix I-2).[250–255]

Urinary tract malformations may be present in infants with a single UA but an otherwise normal physical examination.[251] Based on 35 published series (see Appendix I-2), the minimum incidence of renal and urinary tract malformations, excluding hypospadias, in patients with a single UA is estimated to be 6.5% (89 of 1375). In clinical studies, the incidence of renal and urinary tract malformation in series using a high percentage of intravenous urography (IVU) is twice that in the other series (9 of 72, or 12.5%, *versus* 63 of 1256, or 5.0%). In approximately 8% of those patients with a urinary tract malformation (3 of 40), the latter is isolated. The incidence of malformations in newborn infants with a single UA is approximately seven times that seen in control infants in prospective series (26.4% *versus* 3.7%), and twice that seen in controls in autopsy series (68.3% *versus* 31.4%).[253] The distribution of malformations in infants with a single UA is skewed toward a higher incidence of polymalformations and of isolated malformations pertaining to the gastrointestinal tract.[254] In patients with polymalformations, the presence of a single UA does not increase the risk of finding renal or urinary tract malformations as compared to other malformed patients.[252]

The presence of any of the index signs shown in Appendix I-2 should raise the suspicion of a known MCA; the presence of vertebral or anorectal anomalies can suggest a possible VATER syndrome (*i.e.*, vertebral defects, anal atresia, tracheoesophageal fistula with esophageal atresia, and radial and renal defects). The risk of finding renal or urinary tract anomalies increases if additional anomalies are present. This is well shown by the study by Khuri and colleagues, in which the incidence of urinary tract anomalies was 7.7% in those with one additional system anomaly, 13% in those with two additional system anomalies, and 37% in those with three or more additional system anomalies.[250] The presence of other anomalies in patients with hypospadias depends on its severity; the incidence of urinary tract malformations was found to be 1.3% in first-degree hypospadias, 2.2% in second-degree hypospadias, and 5.3%

in third-degree hypospadias.[250] Some signs may be an indication for performance of US only in some families (*e.g.*, preauricular pits).[255] Thus, it appears justified to obtain an US but not an IVU in newborn infants who are suspected clinically of having a recognized MCA, as well as in those with several anomalies. In the absence of rigorous large-scale studies, decisions must be made on an individual basis.

PHYSICAL EXAMINATION

VITAL SIGNS AND GENERAL EXAMINATION

Severe cyanosis or apneic events can lead to prerenal or functional failure. Tachycardia, peripheral vasoconstriction, hypotension, or narrowing of the pulse pressure may suggest prerenal failure due to hypovolemia or low-output cardiac failure. Tachyarrhythmia, premature ventricular contractions, or abnormal QRS complexes on the electrocardiographic monitoring may be the first sign of hyperkalemia, often due to or at least related to renal immaturity or renal failure. Seizures or coma may be due to hypertension or complications of renal failure.

MEASUREMENT AND EVOLUTION OF BLOOD PRESSURE IN THE NEONATAL PERIOD

Although a direct technique is the ideal method for the measurement of blood pressure, the transducer must be calibrated regularly and the tubing and the transducer dome checked for the presence of air bubbles or blood clots, which may result in damping of the pulse wave and falsely low measurements of systolic blood pressure.[256] On the other hand, overestimation of systolic blood pressure may result from a low resonant frequency system, which should not be used in newborn infants (see Appendices C-1a through C-1d).

Blood pressure in normal newborn infants is obtained by the computerized oscillometric or Doppler technique; either of these methods provides an accurate assessment of the systolic and mean blood pressure compared to direct measured values, unless the patient is in shock.[257] Differences between direct and indirect measurements of systolic and mean blood pressure can be minimized by selecting an appropriate cuff size. The American Heart Association has recommended that the ratio between the width of the inflatable part (*i.e.*, bladder) of the cuff and the arm circumference be 0.40 for adults and children.[258] A larger ratio has been found to be more accurate using the Doppler technique in newborn infants (0.4–0.6).[259] Similarly, the most appropriate ratio between the cuff width, rather than the bladder width, and the arm circumference for measurement of blood pressure using the oscillometric technique in newborn infants was found to be 0.45–0.70.[257] The length of the bladder should be 80% of the arm circumference.[258] Although measurements of diastolic blood pressure by indirect techniques, especially the Doppler technique, usually are not as accurate as systolic or mean pressure, excellent results may be obtained by some oscillometric devices.[260]

The average difference between arm systolic blood pressure and thigh systolic blood pressure obtained by oscillometry using appropriate cuff sizes was found to be 0.9 ± 5.3 torr (mean ± SD) in normal full-term infants.[261] The average difference in systolic blood pressure between arm and calf was 1.1 ± 7.7 torr; the same cuff size was adequate for both limbs.[262] Thus, statistically, when the systolic blood pressure in the upper limbs is more than 10 torr higher than that in the thigh or 15 torr higher than in the calf, coarctation of the aorta should be suspected.

After variable trends during the first hour of life, arterial blood pressure in normal newborn infants at any GA increases by approximately 1 torr per day during the first week of life and then by 1 torr per week until 5 to 6 weeks of life (see Appendices C-1a through C-1d). It is unclear why some studies[263] report higher blood pressure values than most of the other ones. The upper limit of normal systolic blood pressure in infancy reported in a large-scale prospective study was 113 torr.[264] Interindividual differences in blood pressure are related mostly to GA, weight, and ponderal index.[265,266] Even when considering infants of similar GA, size, and postnatal age, there is a wide range of normal values. Blood pressure increases with awake state (see Appendix C-1d), knee–chest position, crying, pain, physical examination, and performance of procedures.[267,268] In addition, a circadian blood pressure pattern was described in some, but not all, full-term infants.[269] There is significant tracking (*i.e.*, a trend for the same individual) of blood pressure during the first months of age.[266]

CHEST

A small chest suggests hypoplastic lungs, which can be associated with renal and urinary tract malformations. Congestive heart failure, patent ductus arteriosus, and severe respiratory distress all can cause prerenal failure.

ABDOMEN

The physical examination of a normal newborn infant should include bimanual palpation of the abdomen for the presence of a normal kidney in each flank.[225,226,234] The examination is easiest in the delivery room, before the bowel is filled with gas; later on, it is facilitated by relaxation of the abdominal wall musculature obtained, for instance, by eliciting the sucking reflex. Several characteristics of the kidneys should be evaluated, including their location (normally in the flank; an ectopic kidney may be located in the pelvis), size (the normal size in a full-term infant is 4–5 cm × 2–3 cm),[270] long axis (normally cephalocaudal; a horseshoe kidney may be suspected if the lower pole is closer to the midline than the upper pole), consistency (normally firm, as opposed to a cyst or a hydronephrotic kidney, which may be depressible), and surface (normally smooth, as opposed to large cysts in multicystic or autosomal dominant polycystic kidneys). A careful examination may raise the suspicion of ectopia, agenesis, hypoplasia, cystic dysplasia, polycystic kidney, hydronephrosis, or a horseshoe kidney. Abdominal masses most often are of renal or urologic origin,[271] and may correspond to polycystic or multicystic kidney, renal vein thrombosis, renal tumor, congenital hydronephrosis, or acquired hydronephrosis (*e.g.*, fungus ball, papillary necrosis); a suprapubic mass suggests bladder distention. In some patients, one or both kidneys cannot be palpated: this may be due to a less than optimal examination (*e.g.*, absence of patient relaxation, bowel distention); unilateral renal agenesis; renal malposition, in which case the kidney may be felt at another place in the abdomen; or renal hypoplasia or aplasia. Some abnormalities of the abdominal wall, such as bladder exstrophy, cloacal exstrophy, and prune-belly syndrome, are associated with renal anomalies. The umbilical cord should be examined for the number of umbilical arteries. Anorectal anomalies or ambiguous genitalia, including severe hypospadias,[250] should raise the suspicion of renal or urologic malformations.

The physical examination of the abdomen also should include percussion for detecting ascites or a large bladder. In the absence of hydrops fetalis, neonatal ascites commonly is due to the rupture of an obstructed urinary tract (7 of 27 patients, or 26%).[272] Sphincter dysfunction may suggest an occult spinal dysraphism.

LIMBS

Motor and sensory dysfunction of the lower limbs suggests an occult spinal dysraphism. Several limb anomalies are part of syndromes or sequences associated with renal or urinary tract malformations, such as skeletal dysplasia, radial aplasia, femoral hypoplasia, rocker bottom feet, compression deformation, polydactyly, syndactyly, and hemihypertrophy.

HYDRATION

Body weight should be obtained on a daily basis and the net weight (*i.e.*, without equipment such as arm boards, endotracheal tube, chest tubes) compared to the normal postnatal weight evolution.[273] Edema may be a sign of renal disease, including renal failure or nephrotic syndrome, or be secondary to a wide variety of generalized or local problems. In newborn infants in a prone or supine position, generalized edema starts around the eyes, at the perineum, and on the lateral sides of the trunk. Dehydration may be evident on the basis of weight loss, dry skin and mucosae, sunken fontanelle, sometimes with the signs of hypovolemia mentioned previously. Because edema fluid and third-space fluid do not participate in the effective ECF volume, hydration status should not be based upon weight alone. A comprehensive evaluation of hydration status should include a complete history and physical examination, as well as assessment of urine output, and serum and urine biochemical analysis (see Chap. 23).

CLINICAL OBSERVATIONS

TIME OF THE FIRST POSTNATAL VOIDING

The time of first voiding after birth has been analyzed by several researchers (Table 42-2).[274–278] The selection criteria were mentioned in only one study.[277] Between 4% and 22% of infants were reported to void in the delivery room. The cumulative percentage of infants who void within 24 hours after birth has increased from 92% before 1960 to 97% after 1970; this most probably results from an increase in total fluid intake during the first day of life. Thus, according to the more recent studies, delayed voiding indicates that first voiding occurred later than 24 hours after birth. Nevertheless, the significance of delayed voiding, as defined above, is unclear. The most recent study failed to detect any difference in gender, weight, type of delivery, 5-minute Apgar score, time to first feeding, or incidence of respiratory distress syndrome (RDS), compared to infants voiding for the first time before 24 hours.[278] In addition, whether urine passed in the delivery room should be included to assess postnatal urine output is questionable, because it is virtually impossible to exclude urination during labor. Although observation of urination in the delivery room is reassuring, because it demonstrates the presence of functional kidneys and urinary tract, it is not associated with an earlier second urination.[277] Urine produced *in utero* normally is very dilute, with an average osmolality less than 200 mOsm/kg.[109] Higher osmolality may result from obstructive urinary tract disease caused by poor tubular reabsorption of sodium, from administration of oxytocin or indomethacin to the mother, or from acute or subacute intrauterine asphyxia. On the other hand, urine produced after birth usually is isotonic or hypertonic, probably as a result of increased release of oxytocin and ADH.

URINE OUTPUT

The urine output depends on GFR and tubular reabsorption of water. In full-term infants, the urine output is low during the first day of life and increases progressively in parallel with daily intake. On the other hand, in LBW and VLBW infants, Bidiwala and associates have described three phases in the early postnatal period: an oliguric phase, during which the urine output is always lower than the intake; a polyuric phase starting between 24 and 72 hours of age,

TABLE 42–2
TIME OF FIRST POSTNATAL VOIDING

			Cumulative Percentage of Infants at First Postnatal Voiding				
Author	**Criteria**	**Number**	Delivery Room	≤20 h	≤24 h	≤30 h	≤48 h
Sherry, 1955	>2500 g	500	17.0%		92.4%		99.8%
Kramer, 1957	<2500 g	200	21.5%		90.5%		100.0%
Pynnönen, 1972*	Boys	155	16.1%	94.2%		97.4%	
	Girls	164	4.3%	92.1%		98.8%	
Clark, 1977	Full-term	395	12.9%		100.0%		
	Premature	80	21.1%		100.0%		
	Postterm	25	12.0%		100.0%		
Chih, 1991	>2500 g	920	18.5%		96.0%		100.0%
	<2500 g	80	20.0%		96.2%		100.0%
Total before 1970		700	18.3%		92%†		
Total after 1970‡		1819	15.9%		97%§		

* Physical examination did not show any overt abnormalities, significant for this study.
† Significantly different from the percentage before 1970, $p < 0.001$, chi-square analysis.
‡ Early feedings used as current practice.
§ The exact value may range between 96.6% and 97.6%. Pynnönen's study did not report the percentage at 24 h.

during which the output is always greater than the intake; and an adaptive phase, during which the kidney adjusts to the rate of fluid intake.[279] A diuretic phase was observed in most infants, whether or not the course was complicated by respiratory distress syndrome. Whether this triphasic pattern is present in most infants remains to be validated in prospective randomized studies using various predetermined amounts of fluid intake. The diagnosis and treatment of oligoanuria and polyuria are discussed elsewhere in this chapter (see Acute Renal Failure; Tubular Dysfunction).

CHARACTERISTICS OF URINATION

The baby should be observed for dribbling, urination through an abnormal location, or persistence of a large bladder after urination. Additional discussion can be found in Chapter 43.

URINALYSIS

Urinalysis at the bedside includes the dipstick, which can help diagnose proteinuria, hematuria–hemoglobinuria–myoglobinuria, glucosuria and leukocyturia, and the measurement of urine specific gravity (SG) by refractometry. Normal newborn infants have a physiologic proteinuria, the amount of which changes with GA and postnatal age (Table 42-3). The first step in the assessment of hemoprotein in the urine is a microscopic examination (see Hematuria and Proteinuria). Glucosuria usually is absent until the glycemia is greater than 150 mg/dL, although mild glucosuria is common in VLBW infants even when glycemia is normal. Urine SG is inversely proportional to urine output. The relationship between SG and osmolarity in newborn infants is different from that in older patients.[279a] This may result from frequent proteinuria and glucosuria, as well as differences in major solutes with increasing maturity (*e.g.*, decrease in sodium concentration, increase in urea concentration).

Pink urine may correspond to the presence of heme compounds or uric acid–urate; the latter may be seen in some normal infants. If a dipstick is positive for heme compounds, the clinician first should differentiate hemoglobinuria, myoglobinuria, and hematuria. This can be done by examining the urine under the microscope for the presence of erythrocytes, and the color of the plasma, which should be pink in the case of significant hemoglobinuria. Definitive differentiation of hemoglobinuria and myoglobinuria can be obtained by electrophoresis of urinary proteins. Hemoglobinuria is diagnostic of a significant intravascular hemolytic process, whereas myoglobinuria has been observed in severely asphyxiated newborn infants, particularly those with birth trauma.

TABLE 42–3
PROTEINURIA DURING THE FIRST DAYS OF LIFE

Gestational Age (wk)	Number of Infants	Mean and Range ($mg/m^2/h$)
≤ 28	5	0.86 (0.2–1.33)
30	12	2.08 (0–9.4)
32	15	2.32 (0–5.22)
34	15	2.48 (0–13.07)
36	17	1.27 (0–4.60)
40	26	1.29 (0–6.14)

Arant BS Jr. Developmental patterns of renal functional maturation compared in the human neonate. J Pediatr 1978;92:705.

LABORATORY EVALUATION

MEASUREMENT OF GLOMERULAR FILTRATION RATE USING EXOGENOUS SUBSTANCES

To be an adequate marker for GFR, a substance must not be metabolized, must be completely filtered through the glomerulus, must not be secreted by the tubule, and must be eliminated from the body only by the kidney, unless GFR is determined by classic clearance method.[280] Adequate markers include inulin, polyfructosan, and radionuclides such as ^{99m}Tc-diethylenetriaminepentacetic acid (DTPA). Renal clearance can be measured by classic clearance techniques with collection of samples of blood and urine, by the rate of constant infusion that is associated with a steady-state plasma concentration, or by a noncompartmental analysis or a double-slope analysis of the plasma concentration after a single injection.[281] Coulthard and colleagues showed in 1983 that an infusion duration for constant infusion technique or a sampling time for single injection technique prolonged as long as 24 to 72 hours is required to measure GFR.[282]

ASSESSMENT OF GLOMERULAR FILTRATION RATE USING CREATININE CLEARANCE

In the clinical setting, GFR often is estimated by creatinine clearance (C_{cr}). Comparisons of C_{cr} with C_{in} have shown reasonable agreement, but the $C_{cr}:C_{in}$ ratio tends to increase in parallel with a decrease in C_{in}.[283,284] Limitations of C_{cr} as an assessment of GFR have been attributed to inaccurate determination of P_{cr}, effect of maternal or diet creatinine load on creatinine concentration, tubular secretion of creatinine, and difficulty in obtaining complete urine collections in newborn infants, especially in girls.

One of the major limitations of C_{cr} for assessing renal function is the difficulty of accurately measuring P_{cr}. The gold standard technique is isotope dilution mass spectrometry, and various high-performance liquid chromatography (HPLC) techniques have been proposed as reference techniques.[285,286] The clinician should know which technique is used in the laboratory, its accuracy and precision, as well as possible sources of interference.[287]

The value of P_{cr} during the first days of life depends both on maternal creatinine load and on neonatal GFR. Cord blood creatinine concentration is almost equivalent to the maternal level, and the serum concentration decreases exponentially during the first few days of life, with a half-life of 2.1 days in normal full-term infants.[288] Because of this maternal load, the rate of decrease of P_{cr} may be a better indicator than its absolute concentration in full-term infants during the first days of life, especially when the mother is in renal failure.[288] The agreement between C_{cr} and C_{in} in LBW infants during the first days of life suggests that creatinine secretion is minimal in immature tubules.[289]

Obtaining an adequate urine collection is a difficult task, especially in girls. This often can be resolved by using either an adhesive plastic collection bag on the perineum, by bladder catheterization if hourly urine output measurement or bladder decompression is necessary, by using a modified metabolic bed or by collecting urine samples from diapers, taking care to limit evaporation, and correcting for diaper weight.

Several units have been used for expressing GFR (*e.g.*, mL/minute; mL/minute/1.73 m^2 of BSA; mL/minute/kg of weight; mL/minute/kg of lean body mass). Which of these units should be used in infants is controversial. Indeed, the normal values of GFR corrected for 1.73 m^2, which are stable throughout childhood and midadulthood, increase significantly with age until 2 years of age; thus, there is no obvious advantage to correcting GFR for body surface area in infancy. Although correcting GFR for body weight (mL/minute/kg) results in more homogenization of the normal values of GFR with maturation in newborn infants,[290] it also results in apparent changes in GFR due to day-to-day weight changes. It may be best to express GFR both in absolute units (*i.e.*, mL/minute) and with correction for body size, to facilitate comparison between various studies.

ESTIMATION OF GLOMERULAR FILTRATION RATE USING PLASMA CREATININE CONCENTRATION

The most commonly obtained laboratory test used routinely to monitor renal function is P_{cr}. The value should be compared to normal values for GA and postnatal age using the same technique of measurement. Figure 42-3 shows the normal evolution of P_{cr} in mg/dL during the first month of life.[291] In addition to the limitations of C_{cr} for assessing GFR, another limitation is relevant to the use of P_{cr} for this purpose. The relationship between P_{cr} and GFR results from the formula for creatinine clearance:

$$C_{cr} = V \times U_{cr}/P_{cr},$$

where C_{cr} is C_{cr} in mL/minute, V is urinary volume in mL/minute, U_{cr} is the urinary creatinine concentration in mg/dL, and P_{cr} is P_{cr} in mg/dL. It is obvious from this formula that the relationship depends on the amount of creatinine excreted per unit of time into the urine; this amount depends on the rate of biotransformation of creatinine in striated muscle, and thus on the amount of muscle.[292] Identical values of P_{cr} represent lower values of GFR for patients with less muscle per unit of body size, such as in SGA or large for GA (LGA) infants. As a result, a seemingly normal P_{cr} for age may be obtained in an infant with severe intrauterine growth retardation (IUGR) and renal failure, because of the loss in muscle mass.

To take this into account, Schwartz and colleagues have developed a formula designed to estimate GFR corrected for BSA:

$$GFR = kL/P_{cr},$$

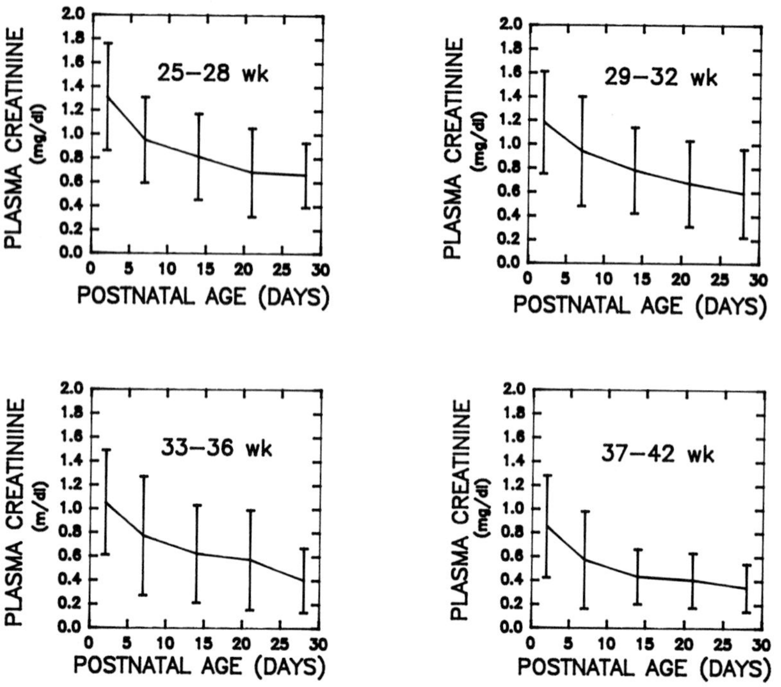

FIG. 42–3. The normal values of plasma creatinine concentration (mean ± 2 SD) during the first month of life are shown at four gestational age ranges. Infants were excluded from this study if they had congenital heart disease, heart failure with patent ductus arteriosus, indomethacin therapy within 48 hours, postasphyxic oligoanuria, renal anomalies, or muscle disease. These values were obtained using a kinetic Jaffé technique with a Beckman Creatinine Analyzer 2. This method reportedly had no interference with bilirubin up to 400 μmol/L (23 mg/dL); the addition of 0.1 mmol/L of pyruvate produced a rise of 5 μmol/L (0.06 mg/dL) in the creatinine value. (Adapted from Rudd PT, Hughes EA, Placzek MM, et al. Reference ranges for plasma creatinine during the first month of life. Arch Dis Child 1983;58:212, using a conversion factor of 1 IU = 0.0113 mg/100 mL.)

where GFR is in mL/minute/1.73 m^2, the constant k is a factor corresponding to the rate of urinary creatinine excretion per unit of body size for a group of similar body habitus (mg/100 minute/cm/1.73 m^2), L is body length (cm), and P_{cr} is in mg/dL.[293] The value of k was found to be 0.45 in appropriate for GA (AGA) full-term infants, 0.33 in LBW infants, 0.33 in SGA full-term infants, and 0.31 in LGA full-term infants.[289,292,293] During the first week of life in LBW infants, the formula kL/P_{cr} gave values similar to those obtained by C_{in}.[289] The low value of the constant k in LBW, SGA, and LGA infants is related to the lower amount of muscle mass per unit of body size compared to full-term AGA infants. Within each group, the coefficient of variation of the value of k was 30% to 35%; for LBW infants, 77% of the values of k were found to be within a range of 0.20 to 0.50, whereas in full-term infants, 79% of the values were within a range of 0.30 to 0.70.

Despite all the criticisms over the use of P_{cr} to estimate GFR in newborn infants, several researchers have found a significant correlation between P_{cr} and the half-life of several medications eliminated by the kidney.[294–297] Thus, if a reliable technique of creatinine measurement is available, the clinician can use P_{cr} for routine, sequential evaluation of glomerular filtration in most newborn infants. Formal repeated measurements of C_{cr} or GFR are recommended for those patients in renal failure.

BLOOD UREA NITROGEN

The blood urea nitrogen (BUN) can increase as a result of catabolism, dehydration, high protein load (*e.g.*, oral, intravenous, gastrointestinal bleeding), or renal failure. On the other hand, a low value of BUN can be observed in association with either ECF expansion or decreased production of urea. The latter may result from anabolism, low protein intake, urea cycle disorder, liver failure, or liver immaturity.

URIC ACID

The concentration of uric acid is higher in cord blood than in maternal blood. Renal handling of uric acid along the nephron includes glomerular filtration, tubular reabsorption, tubular secretion, and further reabsorption distal to the secretory site. Fractional excretion of uric acid during the first 24 hours decreases from about 70% at 29 to 31 weeks of GA to 39% ± 14% (mean ± SD) at 38 to 40 weeks of GA,[299] and decreases with postconceptional age, to reach less than 20% at 1 year of age and less than 10% in adults. This results from progressive tubular maturation.[300] An abnormally high serum level of uric acid may result from a wide range of disorders associated with decreased renal excretion of uric acid, including maternal toxemia, ECF contraction, renal failure, hypertension, medications (*e.g.*, diuretics), and lead intoxication. Rarely, elevated levels of uric acid result from increased production (*e.g.*, leukemia). A very low serum level of uric acid suggests a tubular disorder.

PLASMA RENIN ACTIVITY

The most common indication for the measurement of PRA is the evaluation of hypertension. Normal levels of PRA are higher in the newborn infant than in older children or adults. This is discussed further in the section on Hypertension.

GENETIC DIAGNOSIS

Chromosome analysis is indicated if a hereditary syndrome is suspected. Molecular diagnosis using recombinant technology is available for an increasing number of renal diseases. For most cases with a family history of autosomal dominant polycystic kidney disease (ADPKD), a correct diagnosis can be made in the infant if there are restriction length polymorphisms close to the relevant gene, which is usually, but not always, on chromosome 16.[301,302]

URINARY ACIDIFICATION

Immaturity of renal tubular acidification results in a significantly lower value of serum bicarbonate concentration in VLBW infants than in full-term infants. In parallel, the serum base deficit is often between −5 and 10 mEq/L in VLBW infants, compared with 0 to 5 mEq/L in full-term infants, and the anion gap, obtained by the difference between sodium concentration and the sum of chloride and bicarbonate concentrations, is normally 15 to 22 mEq/L in premature infants, compared to 12 ± 2 mEq/L (<15 mEq/L) in full-term infants. In newborn infants, metabolic acidosis often is secondary to asphyxia, hypoxia, shock, or erythrocyte transfusion. If metabolic acidosis is persistent, a defect in tubular acidification, among other diagnoses, should be suspected, whether urine *p*H is low or high; a low urine *p*H suggests but does not assure that distal tubular acidification is normal (see Tubular Function).

MICROSCOPIC EXAMINATION OF URINE

The shape of erythrocytes in freshly voided urine should be observed under the microscope. The presence of deformed cells suggests a hematuria from glomerular origin, whereas undeformed cells predominate in either massive hematuria, or in cases of lower urinary tract disease. Leukocyturia is common in normal infants during the first few days of life.[303] On the other hand, leukocyturia may be lacking in a newborn infant with a positive urine culture, in contrast to older children. The presence of bacteria on a Gram stain may be a better predictor of UTI. The presence of erythrocyte casts in the urine suggests the diagnosis of glomerulopathy, whereas leukocyte casts can be observed during UTI.

URINE ELECTROLYTES AND OSMOLALITY

The measurement of urinary and blood osmolality, urea, creatinine, and electrolytes is indicated for the differential diagnosis of polyuria and for the early diagnosis of oliguria.

PROTEINURIA AND β_2-MICROGLOBULINURIA

Maturation of the infant is associated not only with a decrease in the daily amount of proteinuria (see Table 42-3), but also with qualitative changes that can be demonstrated by two-dimensional gel electrophoresis.[304] The first voided urine in 22- to 28-week-old infants contains many serum proteins and peptides, whereas urine in full-term infants contains much less polypeptides. One of the identified proteins is called Tamm–Horsfall glycoprotein, which is derived from the tubule.

Beta$_2$-microglobulin is a low-molecular-weight protein (11,800 kd), which in the normal adult is filtered through the glomerulus and almost entirely reabsorbed and catabolized by the tubule. Because the tubular reabsorption of β_2-microglobulin increases with maturation, its fractional excretion decreases until 2 years of age.[305] Several studies have shown that the urinary concentration of this and other proteins is a more sensitive indicator for renal damage due to asphyxia or medications, than the measurement or the estimation of GFR (see Acute Renal Failure).

IMAGING OF THE KIDNEY AND THE URINARY TRACT

ULTRASONOGRAPHY

This technique is performed to screen for renal and urologic malformations or as one of the first steps in the workup of renal failure, oligoanuria, hypertension, UTI, and hematuria.[306] Suggested indications for the performance of neonatal US are shown in Table 42-4. In a series using similar indications, 71 of 1500 newborns had neonatal US performed, and 15 (21%) were found to have a congenital renal or urinary tract malformation.[234] The size of the kidneys should be compared to normal for size, GA, and gender.[270] The examiner should assess not only the kidneys but also the adrenal glands, the aorta, the renal arteries, the renal veins, the inferior vena cava, the ureters, and the bladder. The differential diagnosis of US anomalies is presented in Table 42-5.[307–313]

Blood flow through renal vessels can be assessed by Doppler US, which is indicated for the evaluation of hematuria, hypertension, and ARF, especially in a patient with UA catheterization. Pulsed Doppler flow analysis (*i.e.*, duplex scanning) allows the calculation of the ratio of end-diastolic minimum velocity to systolic peak velocity (*i.e.*, diastolic–systolic ratio), which gives an assessment of renal artery vascular resistance.[314,315]

VOIDING CYSTOURETHROGRAM

Vesicoureteral reflux (VUR) and bladder obstruction should be ruled out in patients with hydronephrosis, trabeculated bladder, bladder distention, or myelomeningocele.[316] In patients with UTI, the voiding cystourethrogram (VCUG) best is delayed, because VUR, often present during a UTI, may disappear within 4 to 6 weeks. Sterile technique is imperative to prevent iatrogenic infection; the role of prophylactic antibiotic therapy has not been evaluated.

TABLE 42–4
INDICATIONS FOR ULTRASONOGRAPHY TO RULE OUT RENAL–URINARY TRACT MALFORMATIONS AND ACQUIRED RENAL DISEASE IN NEWBORN INFANTS

History*

Family history
- First-degree relative with Potter syndrome (bilateral renal agenesis/dysgenesis), autosomal dominant polycystic kidney disease
- Sibling with autosomal recessive polycystic kidney disease

Abnormal prenatal ultrasonography (*e.g.*, kidney, bladder, ascites)

Oligohydramnios, unless normal posnatal renal function and oligohydramnios attributed to:
- Prolonged rupture of the membranes
- Postdate delivery, subacute fetal distress

Physical Examination or Evidence for Other Congenital Anomalies

Syndrome, sequence, or field defect described in Appendix I-1†

Any part of a possible VATER syndrome (*i.e.*, vertebral anomalies, anorectal anomalies, tracheoesophageal fistula)

Preauricular pits, if family history

Supernumerary nipples, if associated anomalies or according to ethnic or geographic background

Congenital diaphragmatic hernia with additional anomalies

Lung hypoplasia, symptomatic spontaneous pneumothorax

Abnormal abdominal examination:
- Abnormal kidney palpation
- Abdominal mass
- Bruit‡

Ascites

Single umbilical artery

Second- or third-degree hypospadias

Ambiguous genitalia

Evidence for Renal Disease

Renal failure, oligoanuria‡

Systemic hypertension‡

Urinary tract infection

Hematuria‡

Significant proteinuria

Nephrotic syndrome

* The best timing of ultrasonography remains to be determined: a negative test immediately after birth does not rule out hydronephrosis or vesicoureteral reflux; a repeat test should be obtained within a few weeks or earlier if clinically indicated.

† The frequency of urinary tract anomalies in many of these entities has not been determined. Since a cost–benefit analysis has not been performed, the indication for neonatal ultrasonographic (US) screening should be decided on an individual basis. The frequency of fetal urinary tract anomalies in association with maternal diabetes or cocaine use probably is too low to justify neonatal US in asymptomatic infants.

‡ These patients also should have a Doppler ultrasonography.

RENAL RADIONUCLIDE SCAN

The most commonly used radionuclides in the study of newborn infants include ^{99m}Tc, which is preferred because it is a pure γ-ray emitter and has a half-life of only 6 hours, and ^{123}I, which also emits x-rays and has a half-life of 13 hours. ^{131}I should be avoided in infants because of its long half-life. ^{99m}Tc-DTPA is eliminated mostly by glomerular filtration and very little by tubular secretion; analysis of the radioactivity due to that compound can be used for assessing renal perfusion if measurements are taken immediately after the injection, renal mass if measurements are taken within 1 to 3 minutes after the injection, and GFR if using a double-compartment analysis of radioactivity in sequential blood measurements or convolution analysis after a single injection, as well as for visualizing the urinary tract.[317] In normal newborn infants, however, routinely measuring GFR using radionuclides is not ethically justifiable, even though the amount of radioactivity is minimal. Therefore, normal values for age are not available. On the other hand, ^{99m}Tc-dimercaptosuccinic acid (DMSA) binds to the tubules and is only minimally excreted into the urine; it is preferred for the analysis of renal morphology and differential function. Typical indications for radionuclide studies include renovascular hypertension, lack of visualization of a kidney by US, preoperative evaluation of the severity of urinary tract obstruction, and evaluation of differential renal function. Chapter 43 provides details on anatomic diagnoses.

INTRAVENOUS UROGRAPHY

In newborn infants, IVU largely has been replaced by US, because of the improved resolution of the new generations of US probes, increased recognition of the nephrotoxicity of standard radiopaque products, and the poor contrast obtained, which is due to the low GFR during the first weeks of life. If needed, a

TABLE 42–5
RENAL ULTRASONOGRAPHIC PATTERNS IN NEWBORN INFANTS

Normal Appearance
Prerenal failure
Renal artery thrombosis
Congenital renal disease (*e.g.*, renal tubular acidosis)
Renal cystic disease, in which cysts develop late
Developing hydronephrosis or vesicoureteral reflux
Increased Cortical Echogenicity
With increased corticomedullary differentiation in large kidneys
Beckwith–Wiedemann syndrome
With normal corticomedullary differentiation
Prerenal failure
Renal ischemia
Mild renal dysplasia
Congenital nephrotic syndrome, Finnish type
With loss of corticomedullary differentiation in normal-to-small kidneys*
Severe renal dysplasia
Pyelonephritis, including renal candidiasis, which often is heterogeneous
Renal tubular dysgenesis or glomerular dysgenesis†
With loss of corticomedullary differentiation in large kidneys*
Renal vein thrombosis
Edema results in decreased echoes
Hemorrhage results in increased echoes
Corticomedullary necrosis‡
Autosomal recessive polycystic kidney disease
Renal glomerular dysgenesis or tubular dysgenesis
Benign transient nephromegaly
Contrast nephropathy
Lymphangioma
Mesoblastic nephroma§
Cysts‖
See Appendix I-3
Increased Medullary Echogenicity
Nephrocalcinosis
Medullary cystic disease
Tamm–Horsfall proteinuria, acute tubular necrosis
Medullary sponge kidney
Intrapyelic Echogenicity
Renal candidiasis (*i.e.*, fungus ball)
Lithiasis
Hydronephrosis

This list does not include findings shown by Doppler ultrasonography.
* Diffuse or heterogeneous hyperechogenicity of cortex or whole kidney.
† The kidney may be enlarged.
‡ The kidney may be normal or enlarged.
§ A solid mass that causes distorsion of the intrarenal collecting system, with occasional cystic areas corresponding to necrosis or hemorrhage.
‖ The absence of cysts visualized at ultrasound does not rule out a renal cystic disease in a newborn infant. Some entities result in development of cysts later in life, while others (*e.g.*, autosomal recessive polycystic kidney disease) result in hyperechogenicity.

low-osmolality contrast material is preferred (see Nephrotoxicity). Optimally, the procedure is delayed a few weeks, at which time improved renal function usually results in better visualization.

PERCUTANEOUS ANTEGRADE PYELOGRAPHY

This technique may be diagnostic in some cases of cystic disease or urinary tract obstruction.[318]

ANGIOGRAM

The frequency of this procedure, mostly used during cardiac catheterization, has decreased dramatically since the development of two-dimensional echocardiography. The anatomy of the kidneys always should be examined during cardiac catheterization. Angiography may be indicated in case of an abdominal tumor, renovascular hypertension, or an aortic thrombus.

COMPUTED TOMOGRAPHY AND MAGNETIC RESONANCE IMAGING

Computed tomography (CT) and magnetic resonance imaging (MRI) are indicated in case of an abdominal tumor. In addition, MRI may be a useful technique to exclude a spina bifida occulta. Using MRI, we have diagnosed a tethered cord in a patient with bladder distention who had a normal US and neither VUR nor urethral stenosis with VCUG.

RENAL PATHOLOGY

Renal biopsy is indicated in cases of nephrotic syndrome and may be indicated in polycystic kidney disease, hematuria, or persistent severe renal failure when the workup has failed to lead to a definitive diagnosis. Major contraindications to renal biopsy include bleeding diathesis, anticoagulant therapy, moderate or severe hypertension, solitary kidney, and intrarenal tumor.[319] The technique includes visualization of the kidney using US, radioisotope, or radiopaque contrast. The most common complication is macroscopic hematuria, which occurs in 5% to 7% of biopsies.

ACUTE RENAL FAILURE AND OLIGOANURIA

Acute renal failure, usually defined as an acute deterioration in the ability of the kidneys to maintain the homeostasis of body fluids,[320] is associated with an acute decrease in the rate of glomerular filtration, as opposed to isolated acute tubular dysfunction. Since the placenta fulfills that role *in utero*, congenital malformations associated with limitation of renal function will not lead to renal failure until birth.

INCIDENCE

The incidence of intrinsic oliguric ARF in newborn infants admitted to the neonatal intensive care unit (NICU) ranges between 1% and 6% in retrospective studies,[321–323] and between 6% and 8% in prospective studies.[322,323] In a prospective study on 314 NICU admissions, Norman and Assadi found 72 infants (23%) with azotemia (*i.e.*, BUN $\geq$ 20 mg/dL) and urine output equal to or less than 25 mL/kg/day for at least 24 hours.[322] Administration of a fluid and diuretic challenge resulted in normalization of the urine output in 52 of 72 patients (72%). Thus, in that series, the incidence of prerenal failure was 17%, whereas that of intrinsic renal failure was 6%. Stapleton and colleagues found an incidence of oliguric renal failure (*i.e.*, urine output $<$ 1 mL/kg/hour unresponsive to fluid challenge, accompanied by a P_{cr} greater than 1.5 mg/dL) of 8% in NICU patients.[323] In a subsequent prospective study on 186 patients including systematic determinations of P_{cr}, these researchers found an incidence of 8% (14 of 186); during the same study period, only one patient had a nonoliguric renal failure. In other series, 30% to 50% of newborn infants with renal failure were not oliguric.[321,324]

DIAGNOSIS

Intrauterine oligoanuria can be suspected when oligohydramnios develops in the absence of rupture of the amniotic membranes; it can be due to a congenital urinary tract anomaly (*e.g.*, urinary tract obstruction, renal agenesis, dysgenesis), to toxins (*e.g.*, ACE inhibitors, indomethacin), or to intrauterine asphyxia.[325,326] If urine output alone is used to assess renal function, ARF often will be both overlooked and overdiagnosed. Indeed, normal urine output is found in approximately one third of neonates with ARF,[321,327] and anuria may occur as a result of the syndrome of inappropriate antidiuretic hormone secretion (SIADHS), in the absence of ARF. Renal function should be evaluated, for possible ARF, in infants who have been subjected to perinatal asphyxia, shock, hypoxemia, and various nephrotoxins (Fig. 42-4). Clinical signs of ARF include syndromes or signs suggestive of renal or urogenital malformations, oligoanuria, polyuria, hematuria, proteinuria, fluid overload, dehydration, cardiac arrhythmia, and systemic hypertension. Other signs include decreased activity, seizures, anemia, vomiting, and anorexia. Sometimes ARF is suspected on the basis of electrolyte abnormalities or elevated plasma levels of medications (*e.g.*, aminoglycosides).

Acute renal failure is characterized by decreased GFR and renal tubular function compared to normal values for either postconceptional age or GA and postnatal age. Although the diagnosis of ARF is strongly suggested by a P_{cr} that is above the upper limit of normal, during the first days of life such an elevation also may result from abnormal maternal re-

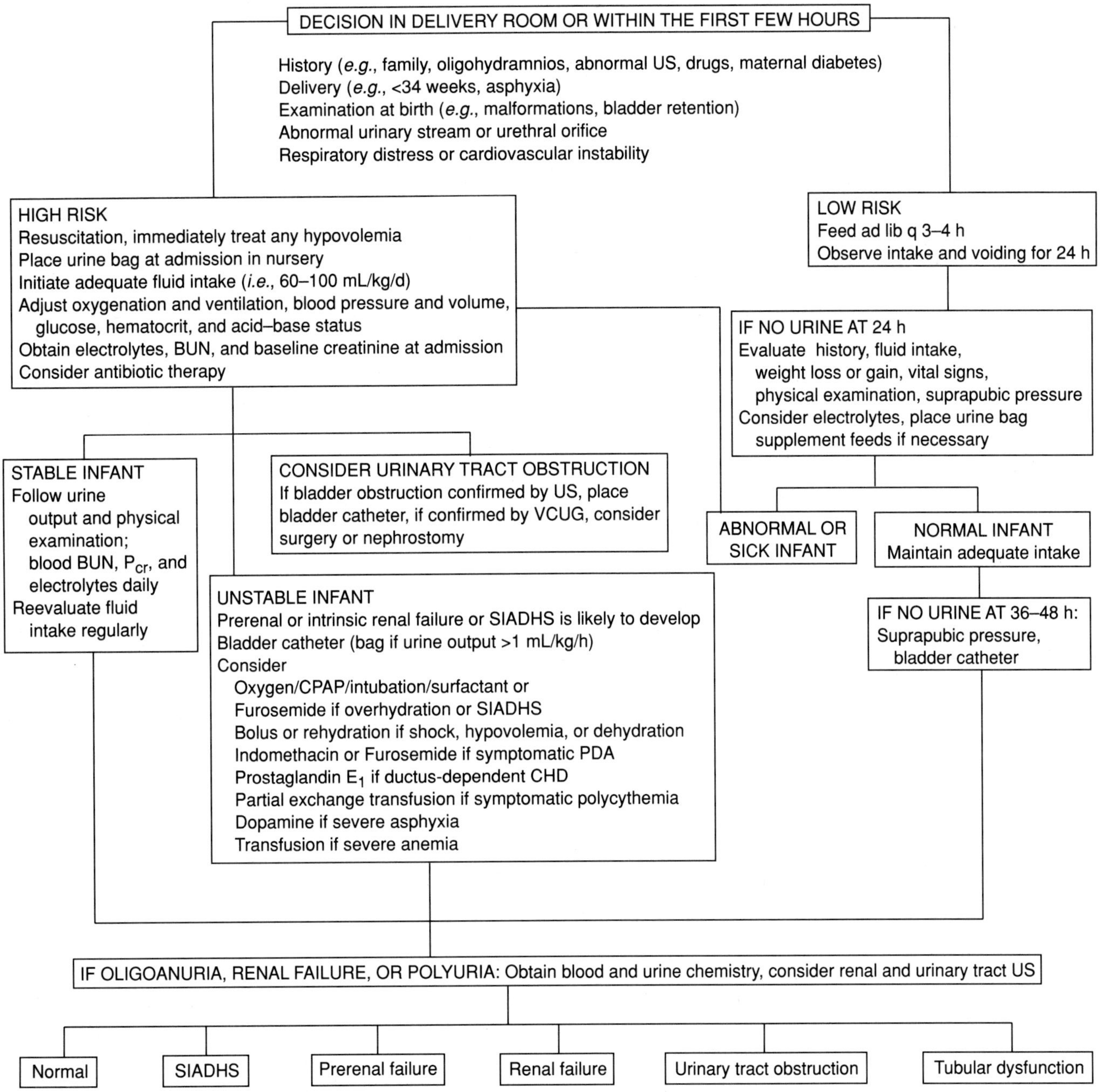

FIG. 42–4. Proposed approach for monitoring urinary output and preventing prerenal failure. (ad lib, *ad libitum;* BUN, blood area nitrogen; CHD, congenital heart disease; CPAP, continuous positive airway pressure; P_{cr}, plasma creatinine concentration; PDA, patent ductus arterosus; q, every; SIADHS, syndrome of inappropriate antidiuretic hormone secretion; US, ultrasonography; VCUG, voiding cystourethrogram.)

nal function. Thus, measuring GFR or following P_{cr} over time is required to diagnose ARF in a newborn infant during the first days of life. Because renal tubular function changes with maturation, it is important to use criteria appropriate for age; indices developed for more mature subjects are not indicative of intrinsic renal failure in VLBW infants.

ETIOLOGY

A wide variety of malformations and prenatal, perinatal, and postnatal events may cause neonatal renal failure (Table 42-6).[323,328–333] The most common type of acute intrinsic renal failure is ATN, which is discussed in the next section.

TABLE 42–6
ETIOLOGIC CLASSIFICATION OF ACUTE NEONATAL RENAL FAILURE

Parenchymal Malformation*

- Renal agenesis
- Renal hypoplasia
  - Simple hypoplasia
  - Oligonephronic hypoplasia
- Renal dysplasia
  - Multicystic
  - Hypoplastic
  - Aplastic
  - Associated with urinary tract obstruction or VUR
- Nephron dysgenesis
  - Tubular dysgenesis: congenital hypernephronic nephromegaly with tubular dysgenesis = congenital tubular dysgenesis = isolated congenital renal tubular immaturity
  - Glomerular dysgenesis:
    - Idiopathic
    - Secondary to maternal administration of indomethacin or angiotensin-converting enzyme inhibitors
- Polycystic kidney disease
  - Adult type (*i.e.,* autosomal dominant)
  - Infant type (*i.e.,* autosomal recessive)
  - Others

Acquired Renal Dysfunction or Lesion†

- Asphyxia/hypoxia/ischemia
  - Functional (may lead to prerenal or intrinsic renal failure):
    - Prenatal, perinatal, or postnatal asphyxia
    - Respiratory distress, hypoxemia
    - Sepsis
    - Surgery (*e.g.,* cardiopulmonary bypass, shock)
    - Heart failure
    - Patent ductus arteriosus
    - Hypovolemia, shock, and severe dehydration
    - Hyperviscosity, polycythemia
    - Severe anemia
  - Vascular
    - Arterial or arteriolar thrombosis, embolism, stenosis
    - Cortical or medullary necrosis, renal infarction
    - Venous thrombosis
- Urinary tract obstruction, massive VUR
- Urinary tract infection
- Disseminated intravascular coagulation
- Drugs
  - Antibiotics (*e.g.,* aminoglycosides, amphotericin, acyclovir)
  - Indomethacin
  - Tolazoline
  - α-Adrenergic agents
  - Angiotensin converting enzyme inhibitors
  - Radiocontrast agents
  - Cyclosporine
- Toxins
  - Hemoglobinuria
  - Myoglobinuria
  - Hyperoxaluria
  - Benzyl alcohol
  - Intravenous tocopherol (polysorbate probably responsible)
  - Uric acid nephropathy
- Glomerular disease
  - Membranous glomerulonephritis (IgG-mediated)
  - Congenital syphilis
  - Diffuse mesangial sclerosis

* May not cause acute renal failure until after the neonatal period.
† May occur *in utero.*
VUR, vesicoureteral reflex.

PATHOPHYSIOLOGY OF ACUTE TUBULAR NECROSIS

The evolution of ATN, the most common cause of ARF, is characterized by three successive phases: initiation, maintenance, and recovery. Although ATN may be precipitated by a single event, its development is multifactorial and involves vascular (*i.e.*, hemodynamic), nephronal, and cellular (*i.e.*, metabolic) factors.[320] The relative importance of these various factors may vary according to the etiology; specific aspects of toxic ATN are described in the section on Nephrotoxicity.

VASCULAR FACTORS

Vascular changes, characterized by vasoconstriction of the afferent arterioles, play a major role in the initiation phase of ATN,[334] even in the absence of shock. The kidney can be protected before the initiating event by the administration of vasodilator compounds.[335] Tubular damage due to any factor will result in increased amounts of solutes in the tubule; this stimulates the release of vasoactive compounds by the juxtaglomerular apparatus. Despite high PRA, the stimulation of the renin–angiotensin system alone cannot explain all the findings at this stage.[320] Renal vasoconstriction may result from systemic or local changes in the relative concentrations of vasoconstrictive agents such as PRA, adenosine, thromboxane (TX), and platelet activating factor, and vasodilator agents such as PGs and prostacyclin.

NEPHRONAL FACTORS

Nephronal factors play a major role during the maintenance phase of ARF. A decrease in GFR and in tubular flow may result from obstruction of the tubule by cellular debris, and from backleak of fluid and solutes secondary to loss of integrity of the tubule. Although an increase in proximal tubule pressure has been demonstrated only in animals,[336] tubular cell casts also are evident in humans with ARF. Backleak has been demonstrated in humans,[337] and its localization has been shown in animal data to be the proximal tubule.[320] In addition, glomerular membrane permeability may decrease during ARF.

CELLULAR FACTORS

During both the initiation and the maintenance phase of ARF, several disturbances may occur in tubular cells.[320] They can be classified into four groups, the respective importance of which, however, is unclear: cessation of oxidative phosphorylation, which results in depletion of adenosine triphosphate (ATP) and diphosphate; disruption of several major cellular functions, including Na^+/K^+-ATPase and cell swelling; formation of free radicals, lipid alterations, and membrane damage; and calcium influx.

During the recovery phase, GFR initially increases in parallel with a decrease in intratubular pressure and in intratubular casts; GFR then increases in parallel with PRF and urine output.[336] Slowing of the recovery or even secondary deterioration of renal function may occur if hypovolemia results from lack of replacement of the large amounts of urine lost during the polyuric phase.

PREVENTION OF PRERENAL FAILURE AND EARLY DIAGNOSIS OF ACUTE RENAL FAILURE

The first step in prevention is to identify infants at high risk for renal failure or oligoanuria immediately after birth (see Fig. 42-4). In these infants, careful observation of urine output using a urine collection bag should be initiated immediately after delivery, and serial assessment of vital signs, electrolytes, and renal function should be initiated as indicated. If urinary tract anomalies are suspected on the basis of prenatal diagnosis, associated risk factors (see Appendices I-1 and I-2), or other clinical evidence (see Clinical Evaluation of Function and Disease), a complete urologic workup should be considered (see Chap. 43). Decompression of the urinary tract by bladder catheterization, surgical intervention, or both is indicated if obstruction or massive VUR is demonstrated.

Prevention of prerenal failure includes correction of any abnormality in and maintenance of adequate oxygenation, ventilation, blood pressure, blood glucose, and hematocrit. Fluid intake should be initiated immediately, 60 to 120 mL/kg/day, according to size, maturity, and environment (see Chap. 23). Assessment of hydration status and renal function should be made on a routine schedule (*i.e.*, every shift or every day) according to the status of the infant, and the intake of fluid and electrolytes should be adjusted. An increase of plasma sodium concentration within the first 8 to 12 hours, assuming that no sodium has been administered, may be the first sign of progressive dehydration in a VLBW infant; it most often indicates that the fluid intake should be increased. Prevention and rapid correction of respiratory failure, cyanosis, hypotension, poor cardiac output, dehydration, peritonitis, hypoglycemia, symptomatic hypocalcemia, symptomatic polycythemia, and sepsis are essential.

URINE OUTPUT

In stable, low-risk, full-term infants, low or even absent urine output during the first 24 hours of life is a normal event and does not by itself require any workup. These infants should be evaluated carefully for significant history or physical signs such as bladder distention, dehydration (*e.g.*, excessive weight loss, dry mucosae), hypotension, excessive weight gain, or heart failure. If any of these conditions is present, further workup and treatment should be initiated. In other cases, intake and urine output should be monitored, and breast-feeding should be supplemented if necessary, but invasive and other therapeutic procedures may be avoided. If spontaneous urination is not observed within an additional 12 to 24 hours (*i.e.*, at 36–48 hours of life), suprapubic pressure (*i.e.*, Credé maneuver) should be performed, to assess the possibility of bladder distention or of oligoanuria. If bladder distention is suspected, bladder and renal US should be performed. If no urine is obtained by suprapubic pressure, the bladder should be catheterized. If little or no urine is obtained by catheterization, oligoanuria is suspected, and further workup should be initiated (see Oligoanuria).

In contrast, in high-risk infants, urine output should be followed carefully from birth. If possible, a urine dipstick test should be obtained before catheterization; this may provide the first evidence for hematuria or myoglobinuria.[338] If urine output is less than 1 mL/kg/hour and is not increased by suprapubic pressure, bladder catheterization should be performed and a full evaluation should be obtained (see Fig. 42-4).

If polyuria develops during the first day, possible diagnoses include hypervolemia, tubular dysfunction, diabetes insipidus, glucose overload, polyuric phase of ATN, and polyuric phase of postrenal failure (*e.g.*, after decompression of the bladder by catheterization).

PERINATAL ASPHYXIA

Early diagnosis of ARF secondary to perinatal asphyxia is suggested by the finding of increased tubular proteinuria (see Hematuria and Proteinuria) immediately after birth, specifically β_2-microglobulin, retinol-binding protein (>27,000 μg/mmol creatinine) or myoglobin (>1500 μg/mmol creatinine).[339–341] Asphyxiated infants with a urine output less than 1 mL/kg/hour for 36 hours usually have high urinary concentration of β_2-microglobulin as well as clinical signs of hypoxic–ischemic encephalopathy and often have long-term neurologic deficits. Oligoanuria in infants with hypoxic–ischemic encephalopathy may result from prerenal (*i.e.*, functional) failure, intrinsic renal failure, and SIADHS. One additional factor that may contribute to ARF in some neonates with severe asphyxia and birth trauma is rhabdomyolysis, which may result in significant myoglobinemia and oliguric ARF.[338] Myoglobinuria may result both from increased filtered load and decreased tubular reabsorption. This is discussed further elsewhere in the chapter (see Nephrotoxicity).

One prospective randomized study showed that infusion of dopamine at low dose (2–5 μg/kg/minute) in severely asphyxiated newborn infants increased systolic blood pressure and urine output, and decreased the incidence of abnormal P_{cr}.[342] In premature hypotensive infants (29–34 weeks of GA) with RDS, the infusion of dopamine at a rate of 0.5–2 μg/kg/minute resulted in a transient elevation in blood pressure compared to controls, followed by an increase in urine output, creatinine clearance, and natriuresis.[343,344] In another series, the administration of low-dose dopamine to premature infants with RDS increased blood pressure and natriuresis, but the increase in GFR and urine output did not reach significance.[345] Low-dose dopamine may stimulate PRA in the absence of any change in blood pressure.[346]

INDOMETHACIN

Renal side-effects of the administration of indomethacin to premature infants with patent ductus arteriosus (PDA) can be prevented by the simultaneous administration of furosemide.[347] Other specific preventive measures are discussed elsewhere in the chapter (see Nephrotoxicity).

GENERAL APPROACH IN OLIGOANURIA

The diagnosis of oligoanuria (*i.e.*, urinary output < 0.5–1.0 mL/kg/hour) should be confirmed by reviewing the chart and demonstrating absence of urine by suprapubic pressure (*i.e.*, Credé maneuver) and by bladder catheterization performed under sterile conditions, using a 3.5- or 5-Fr lubricated feeding tube, which then is left in place and connected to a sterile system for accurate measurement of the hourly urine output. Delayed micturition has been described in association with transient bladder distention attributed to severe perinatal asphyxia.[348] Bladder puncture should be avoided, because of the high likelihood of causing trauma.

Once oligoanuria is confirmed, the history should be reviewed for severe asphyxia, respiratory failure, hypotension, shock, and renal toxins. Intake and output over the last few days should be reviewed. The patient should be evaluated for possible central nervous system disease, such as meningitis, which may be associated with SIADHS. The physical examination should seek evidence of weight loss, dehydration, malformations, respiratory failure, CHF, shock, hypotension, and central nervous system disease. General care should be optimized, including ventilation using artificial means if required, oxygenation, cardiac output, functional circulatory volume, and extracellular volume.

URINE AND BLOOD ANALYSIS

The differential diagnosis of oligoanuria includes not only renal failure but also SIADHS and decreased urine production secondary to the administration of ADH or its analogues (Table 42-7). The differentiation between prerenal and true renal ARF is presented in Table 42-8.

Urine should be examined promptly for protein, cellular elements, electrolytes, creatinine, and SG or osmolality. A blood sample should be obtained for

TABLE 42–7
DIFFERENTIAL DIAGNOSIS OF OLIGOANURIA

Renal Failure
Prerenal: see Table 42-6
Intrinsic: see Table 42-6
Postrenal
- Bladder retention
  - Urethral valves
  - Meningomyelocele, tethered cord
- Massive vesicoureteral reflux
- Bilateral ureteral obstruction
  - Ureteropelvic junction obstruction
  - Ureterovesical junction obstruction, ureterocele
  - Lithiasis
  - Fungus ball
- Extrinsic compression
- Uroascites (*i.e.*, ruptured urinary tract)
  - Secondary to urinary tract obstruction
  - Bladder perforation due to umbilical artery catheterization or direct bladder trauma

Syndrome of Inappropriate Secretion of Antidiuretic Hormone
Exogenous administration to mother or newborn infant
- Antidiuretic hormone, desmopressin
- Oxytocin
- Indomethacin

Acute Bladder Distension Without Renal Failure
Curarization
Neurogenic bladder
Hematoma of the anterior wall of the bladder (*i.e.*, traumatic suprapubic aspiration)

hematocrit, electrolytes, creatinine, BUN, and glucose. Plasma osmolality can be either measured, or calculated from the following formula:

$$\text{Posm(mOsm/kg)} = 2 \times \text{Na(mEq/L)} + \text{glucose(mg/dL)}/18 + \text{BUN(mg/dL)}/2.8.$$

Use of this formula is not recommended for infants with a birth weight less than 1000 g, in whom it may substantially underestimate true osmolality.[349]

While waiting for the results of these tests and ordering a renal US, and in some instances a renal scan, an initial therapeutic decision often can be made on the basis of the history and physical examination. This is especially important in patients in whom no urine can be obtained for analysis. Prerenal failure is a reasonable presumptive diagnosis in the presence of respiratory failure, CHF, dehydration, or shock, if osmolality or SG is high in the absence of casts in the urine. Rapid correction of the problem may be the only therapeutic intervention needed. The syndrome of inappropriate antidiuretic hormone secretion can be suspected on the basis of severe neurologic dysfunction, pneumothorax, or pleural effusion, with weight gain, oligoanuria, and high urinary SG.

The urine obtained initially (*i.e.*, before any diuretic or fluid challenge) should be sent for urinalysis and urine chemistry for the assessment of tubular function. Various indices and tests have been proposed to differentiate ATN from prerenal or functional failure, by the presence of tubular dysfunction in ATN.[350,351] Fractional excretion of sodium is the preferred index; it is obtained from the following formula:

$$\text{FeNa} = \frac{100 \times U_{Na}/U_{cr}}{P_{Na}/P_{cr}},$$

where U_{Na} is the urinary concentration of sodium (mEq/L), U_{cr} is the urinary concentration of creatinine (mg/dL), P_{Na} is the plasma sodium concentration (mEq/L), and P_{cr} is the plasma creatinine concentration (mg/dL). The FENa is the ratio of the sodium clearance to the creatinine clearance, expressed as a percent. A FENa greater than 3%, low urinary osmolality, or low SG, suggests a diagnosis of intrinsic or postrenal failure (*i.e.*, obstruction), but also can be observed in prerenal failure in patients younger than 28 weeks of GA or postconceptional age with adrenal insufficiency, or after the administration of diuretics, volume expansion, or an episode of osmotic diuresis.

Asphyxiated newborn infants may manifest transient tubular dysfunction associated with a normal or mildly decreased GFR and a normal or decreased urine output. Their tubular dysfunction is characterized by a positive dipstick test for blood, moderate tubular proteinuria (*i.e.*, β_2-microglobulin, myoglobin, retinol-binding globulin, and N-acetyl-β-D-glucos-

TABLE 42–8
DIFFERENTIAL DIAGNOSIS: PRERENAL *versus* INTRINSIC OLIGURIC RENAL FAILURE*

	Prerenal	Intrinsic
FeNa	≤2.5%	>3%
U_{Na}	≤20	>50
Uosm	≥350	≤300
U/P osm†	≥1.2	0.8–1.2
U_{SG}	>1012	<1014
Urine retinol binding protein‡	<20 mg/mmol creatinine	>27 mg/mmol creatinine
Urine myoglobin‡	<0.5 mg/mmol creatinine	>1.5 mg/mmol creatinine
Ultrasonography	Normal	May be abnormal§
BUN/P_{cr}	>30	<20
Response to challenge‖	UO > 2mL/kg/h	No increase in UO

* Indices using urine sodium, osmolality, and specific gravity are not useful for the differential diagnosis between prerenal and intrinsic renal failure (falsely suggesting an intrinsic renal failure) after diuretic administration or volume expansion, or in case of glycosuria, adrenal insufficiency, or gestational age less than 28 weeks. In case of urinary tract obstruction, indices most oten are similar to intrinsic renal failure.

† Although plasma osmolality can be estimated using the formula Posm: $2 \times P_{Na}$ (mEq/L) + gl (mg/dL)/18 + BUN (mg/dL)/2.8, the measured value of Posm is preferable, especially in critically ill patients, because of large differences in the case of sick cell syndrome (*i.e.*, leaking cellular membranes), and in infants with a birth weight less than 1000 g.[349]

‡ Transient tubular dysfunction secondary to neonatal asphyxia is characterized by moderate proteinuria with normal or mildly decreased GFR and normal or mildly increased FeNa; it is shown here in the prerenal category. Very high urine levels of myoglobin or retinol-binding protein may in some cases precede the increase in FeNa of intrinsic renal failure.[341]

§ Ultrasonography in intrinsic renal failure may show increased echogenicity of the pyramids, which probably corresponds to precipitation of Tamm–Horsfall protein, signs of renal vein thrombosis, renal artery thrombosis, adrenal hemorrhage, hydronephrosis, cystic kidney disease, renal dysplasia or hypoplasia, or other pathology (see Table 42–5).

‖ The challenge corresponds to the administration of 20 mL/kg of crystalloid (more should be given if there is evidence of hypovolemia) and/or 1 mg/kg of furosemide. Normalization of the urine output after such a challenge may correspond to a prerenal failure or to the polyuric phase following an oliguric renal failure.

BUN/P_{cr}, ratio of blood urea nitrogen to plasma creatinine concentration; FeNa, fractional excretion of sodium; P_{Na}, plasma sodium concentration GFR, glomerular filtration rate; gl, glycemia; U_{Na}, urinary sodium concentration; UO, urine output; Uosm, urine osmolality; U/P osm, ratio of urine to plasma osmolality; U_{SG}, urine specific gravity.

aminidase [NAG]), and a FENa that is either normal or mildly increased.[339,340,352–354] On the other hand, ATN is associated with marked proteinuria, markedly decreased GFR, and often oligoanuria. Urinary concentration of myoglobin and retinol-binding protein, but not NAG, can be used to differentiate between normal, transient tubular dysfunction and ATN[339,340]; β_2-microglobulin has not been assessed for that purpose.[340] Emergency renal and bladder US may establish a diagnosis of urinary tract obstruction, uroascites, renal cystic disease (see Appendix I-3), suggest renal vein or artery thrombosis, adrenal hemorrhage, or show abnormal cortical, medullary, or pyelocalicial echogenicity (see Table 42-5).[307–313,355–357] One common finding is increased echogenicity of the pyramids,[355,356] which may correspond to the precipitation of Tamm–Horsfall protein in patients with ATN.

The diagnosis of SIADHS can be suspected on the basis of plasma osmolality less than 280 mOsm/kg, a ratio of urinary to plasma osmolality that is greater than 1, high urine SG, and an inappropriate increase in weight. It is important to note that the strict criteria used for the diagnosis of SIADHS in adults rarely are met in newborn infants. In most instances, inappropriate levels of ADH are found in patients with abnormal renal function, because asphyxia is a common cause of both problems. The treatment of SIADHS usually includes severe fluid restriction, with a normal sodium intake. In some cases, more rapid correction is necessary because of either severe CHF secondary to fluid overload, severe hypoglycemia secondary to drastic fluid restriction during treatment of SIADHS, or central nervous system signs (*e.g.*, seizures, coma) associated with severe hyponatremia. In these cases, the treatment includes the administration of furosemide, followed by careful replacement of the sodium lost in the urine.

CHALLENGE TEST

A challenge test is indicated only if the etiology of the renal failure is not evident from the assessment of risk factors, clinical signs, US, and urine indices (see

Table 42-8). This can be a fluid challenge (20 mL/kg of crystalloid solution, such as 5% glucose, isotonic saline, or any combination of the two) or a diuretic challenge (usually furosemide 1 mg/kg intravenously). Although patients who fail to respond to furosemide may respond to bumetanide (5 μg/kg/dose intravenously), a more potent loop diuretic, this medication has not been evaluated prospectively in acute neonatal oligoanuria. Whereas the use of mannitol (1 g/kg) has been recommended,[358] its administration has resulted in ARF in adult patients,[359] and may enhance the risk for intraventricular hemorrhage in VLBW infants through an acute increase in serum osmolality. Thus, mannitol cannot be recommended for routine use in newborn infants with oligoanuria and is contraindicated in premature infants.

Which challenge test (*i.e.*, diuretic administration *versus* fluid challenge) to be used depends first on the best judgment of the probability of hypovolemia *versus* hypervolemia. If no satisfactory response, defined by a normal urine output, is obtained after the first challenge test, the other test should be considered. Although normalization of the urine output in response to a fluid challenge is most commonly observed in prerenal failure, it also is compatible with the beginning of the polyuric phase after oliguric intrinsic renal failure, and with transformation of an incipient oliguric renal failure into nonoliguric renal failure.[360] Although the FENa often is not useful in clarifying this differential diagnosis because either ECF expansion secondary to fluid challenge or diuretic administration may cause a high FENa, US and the subsequent development of polyuria may suggest the correct diagnosis. In any of these situations, renal function is expected to improve, and the prognosis usually is good. In contrast, if anuria persists despite optimization of general care and double-challenge test, the diagnosis of intrinsic renal failure is likely, severe fluid restriction is indicated, and the prognosis is guarded.

Nonrandomized studies in adult patients with oliguria and azotemia suggest that the administration of low-dose dopamine may result in the improvement of urine output and creatinine clearance, even in patients who failed to respond to furosemide.[361–364] A prospective study is required to evaluate the possible role of dopamine in the early management of diuretic-resistant oliguria in newborn infants.

DIAGNOSIS OF NONOLIGURIC RENAL FAILURE

Nonoliguric renal failure is characterized by a sudden decrease in GFR and tubular function in the absence of oligoanuria. It may be overlooked in the absence of routine measurement of blood chemistries and urinalysis.[321,323] As mentioned previously, it may be confused initially with the polyuric phase of an intrinsic or postrenal renal failure, especially after an undiagnosed oligoanuric episode, or with prerenal failure that has been treated by the administration of fluids or low-dose dopamine for shock or hypovolemia.[360] Although the evolution of nonoliguric renal failure usually is better than oliguric renal failure,[327] it can be complicated by symptomatic hyperkalemia.[365]

TREATMENT OF ACUTE RENAL FAILURE

In our experience, prevention of ARF and of its complications avoids the need for renal replacement therapy (*e.g.*, dialysis, hemo[dia]filtration) in most patients. Some researchers argue that early institution of replacement therapy may result in improvement in mortality and morbidity.

SUPPORTIVE TREATMENT AND PREVENTION OF COMPLICATIONS

Supportive treatment of infants with ARF, whether oliguric or nonoliguric, includes the establishment and maintenance of adequate fluid and electrolyte balance, as well as the adjustment of the dosage of medications that are eliminated by the kidney.[321,366–370]

Many complications of ARF, such as water or medication intoxication and hyperkalemia, may be prevented by early suspicion of ARF and by careful monitoring of intake and output and appropriate adjustment of therapy to renal function and to serum levels. The prognosis of ARF depends not only on the severity and the duration of the renal injury, but also, and perhaps mainly, on the overall status of the patient.

Fluid and Electrolytes

Water and Sodium. In the presence of oligoanuria refractory to the initial fluid and diuretic challenge, fluid restriction is indicated. Fluid intake is limited to ongoing losses (*e.g.*, gastrointestinal losses, urinary output, third-space losses, drainage), plus 25 mL/kg/24 hours in a full-term infant, and 50 to 75 mL/kg/24 hours in a LBW or VLBW infant. If fluid restriction is not initiated early in the course of ARF, fluid overload will result, with potential CHF, pulmonary edema, and pulmonary hemorrhage. If massive fluid overload leads to severe CHF, hemo(dia)filtration may be indicated. Neither sodium nor potassium should be administered routinely during this phase. On the other hand, high doses of calcium may be required to treat hypocalcemia or for the electrocardiographic consequences of hyperkalemia.

Hyperkalemia

Diagnosis. The most common electrolyte abnormality observed in patients with acute renal failure is hyperkalemia, which can be defined either as a plasma potassium concentration greater than 7 mEq/L or on the basis of electrocardiographic abnormalities.[371] True hyperkalemia can be diagnosed only on a nonhemolyzed plasma sample that is not obtained from a heparin-coated umbilical catheter. Factitious hyperkalemia can result from hemolysis or clot formation during sampling (*i.e.*, release of potassium from erythrocytes or platelets) or interference with the measurement of potassium concentration by benzalkonium released from a heparin-coated umbilical catheter.[372]

Treatment. The treatment of hyperkalemia includes discontinuing potassium intake from sources such as unwashed erythrocytes, antibiotics, and intravenous solutions; discontinuing any medication that could cause hyperkalemia (*e.g.*, indomethacin, ACE inhibitors, potassium-sparing diuretics); and correcting hypovolemia using isotonic saline to promote tubular secretion of potassium. Several modalities are available to treat hyperkalemia (Table 42-9)[365,371,373–379]; each has potential side-effects that may limit or preclude its repetitive administration. Simultaneous administration of several forms of therapy often is required for the acute treatment of life-threatening hyperkalemia.

If electrocardiographic changes are associated with hyperkalemia, administration of calcium chloride or calcium gluconate is indicated; this will rapidly, but only transiently, decrease myocardial cell excitability, and will not decrease potassium concentration (see Table 42-9).[374] Thus, the administration of calcium should be followed immediately by at least one other method to decrease the potassium concentration.

Cellular uptake of potassium can be induced by an infusion of sodium bicarbonate, the combination of glucose and insulin, or salbutamol. Because their mechanisms are different, more than one method may be used; none has been shown to be superior to the others. If glucose and insulin are infused, the initial ratio for VLBW infants (500–1000 g) should be approximately 2.2 g/unit;[375] the ratio should be adjusted (range, 1–3 g/unit) according to the evolution of the glycemia. European data have shown that salbutamol infusion also is effective in treating hyperkalemia[376]; its action is mediated by an induction

TABLE 42–9
TREATMENT OF HYPERKALEMIA IN RENAL FAILURE

Medication	Dose (Intravenous Unless Otherwise Specified)	Mechanism	Onset of Action	Duration
Calcium chloride	0.25–0.5 mEq/kg over 5–10 min	Modifies myocardial excitability	1–3 min	30–60 min
Calcium gluconate	0.5–1 mEq/kg over 5–10 min			
Sodium bicarbonate	1 mEq/kg over 10–30 min	Intracellular uptake of K	5–10 min	2 h
Glucose and insulin	0.5 g/kg/h 1 U/2.2 g glucose (1–3)*	Intracellular uptake of K	30 min	4–6 h
Salbutamol (albuterol)	4 μg/kg over 20 minutes†	Intracellular uptake of K	40 min	>120 min
Cation-exchange resin (Na/Ca polystyrene sulfonate)	1 g/kg intrarectally q 6 hr‡	Exchange of K for Na or Ca	1–2 h	6 h
Exchange transfusion	⅔ washed erythrocytes reconstituted with 5% albumin	Uptake of K by erythrocytes	Minutes§	>12 h
Peritoneal dialysis	Use a dialysate with low K concentration	Dialysis	Minutes§	No limit
Hemofiltration and hemodialysis		Filtration, dialysis	Minutes§	Days

* The preparation of an insulin drip requires saturating the plastic tubing with the insulin solution before infusing to the patient. The average ratio of glucose to insulin associated with maintenance of normal glycemia in VLBW infants is 2.2 ± 0.6 g/unit (mean ± SD).[375]

† The intravenous preparation is not available in the United States. Salbutamol also is efficient by aerosol, but no experience is available in newborn infants.

‡ Oral administration of polystyrene resin should be avoided in VLBW infants and those with poor peristalsis because they may be at risk for concretions.[378] Substantial load of calcium or sodium may result from the respective resin. The effect on potassium concentration is slower than glucose insulin combination.[377]

§ These techniques are both rapid and extremely effective in correcting potassium levels. The time to set them up may be the limiting factor; other techniques may be used to stabilize the infant initially.

VLBW, very low birth weight.

Adapted from Smith JD, Bia MJ, DeFronzo RA. Clinical disorders of potassium metabolism. In: Arieff AI, DeFronzo RA, eds. Fluid, electrolyte, and acid–base disorders. Vol. 1. New York: Chuchill-Livingstone, 1985:413.

of Na^+/K^+-ATPase through cAMP and is independent of insulin or aldosterone.

Although an enema with cation-exchange resin offers the potential advantage of removing potassium from the body rather than moving potassium from the extracellular into the intracellular compartment, resin used alone has a much slower effect than infusion of glucose and insulin. One prospective randomized study showed that using a cation-exchange resin alone for the treatment of hyperkalemia resulted in greater mortality than using glucose–insulin.[377] One potential problem associated with the use of cation-exchange resin is excessive sodium load; this complication may be avoided by using a resin with calcium instead of sodium. Oral administration of cation-exchange resins is not recommended.[378]

If these techniques fail to correct hyperkalemia, exchange transfusion with washed, packed erythrocytes reconstituted with plasma or albumin is extremely efficient in normalizing potassium concentration for as long as 12 hours[379]; it is the treatment of choice in those patients in whom renal replacement therapy is contraindicated by peritonitis or cardiovascular instability. Renal replacement therapy, especially hemo(dia)filtration, is the procedure of choice for the infant with severe oliguric ARF.

If hyperkalemia is associated with hyponatremia, hypoglycemia, and hypotension, a diagnosis of adrenal insufficiency should be considered. This most often results either from congenital adrenal hyperplasia or from bilateral adrenal hemorrhage, which may be suspected on the basis of anemia with thrombocytopenia, jaundice, and bilateral abdominal masses.

Acid–Base and Mineral Disturbances

Metabolic acidosis develops rapidly in most infants with ARF. It may require the administration of large doses of sodium bicarbonate, which may aggravate fluid overload.

Hypocalcemia will develop rapidly in almost all patients with ARF. It may result from hyperphosphatemia and increased deposition of calcium in injured tissues, especially in rhabdomyolysis; skeletal resistance to PTH, which results from decreased production of 25-hydroxyvitamin D and 1,25-dihydroxyvitamin D (1,25[OH]$_2$D)[380]; and, in aminoglycoside-induced ARF, parathyroid dysfunction secondary to hypomagnesemia, which is due to increased tubular loss.[381] Hypercalcemia may occur as a late complication of rhabdomyolysis, as a result of reabsorption of calcium deposited in necrotic tissues. Hyperphosphatemia is due to tissue damage (*e.g.*, severe asphyxia, shock, rhabdomyolysis)[380] and decreased urine excretion. In addition, ARF usually causes hypermagnesemia,[382] which may result from decreased excretion and from shift from the intracellular space. The polyuric phase of ATN is associated with increased urinary excretion of phosphate and magnesium.

Hypocalcemia should be prevented or treated with early intravenous administration of calcium gluconate or chloride. During the oliguric phase, no intake of magnesium (*e.g.*, antacids) or phosphate should be provided, to limit both hypermagnesemia and hyperphosphatemia.

Polyuric Phase

The oliguric phase of ARF is followed by a polyuric phase, during which continuous replacement of ongoing losses is essential. Because of individual variability and the change over time in electrolyte content of the urine, serial measurements of urine electrolytes and hourly monitoring of the urine output are imperative. This will permit accurate replacement of urinary losses and prevent dehydration, hyponatremia, and hypokalemia. In some cases, bicarbonate, phosphate, and magnesium need to be given to replace urinary losses. When GFR approaches normal levels, fluid intake should be decreased gradually and carefully, while following weight, serum chemistries, and urine output. Replacing the urine output volume for volume for an indefinite duration would cause an adaptive persistence of the polyuria. In contrast, some patients may not recover a normal urinary concentrating ability despite normalization of GFR; these patients need to continue to receive higher fluid intake.[383]

Nutrition. If fluid restriction is required, glucose intake often is minimal, and severe hypoglycemia may develop, unless a hypertonic solution of glucose is infused through a central venous catheter. If refractory hypoglycemia occurs despite an adequate glucose intake per kilogram and per minute (see Chap. 35), the infant should be evaluated for possible hormonal anomalies, and specific treatment should be initiated, if indicated. Otherwise, steroids or an infusion of glucagon[384] can be given. If this is unsuccessful, hemofiltration should be considered. This technique will allow increased fluid and glucose intake while rapidly correcting the hypervolemia.

The importance of adequate nutrition results from the fact that renal load decreases with anabolism.[385] Breast milk or low-protein formula should be initiated as soon as possible; if the infant cannot be fed, total parenteral nutrition (TPN) should be initiated. If the ARF is severe, the usual amino acid solution should be replaced by essential L-amino acids supplemented with L-histidine (Levamin Essential; Leiras, Turku, Finland), initially given at a dose of 0.5 to 1 g/kg/day.[385]

Hematologic Disturbances. Anemia associated with ARF may result from several factors, including decreased erythropoietin production, abnormal or ineffective erythropoiesis, impaired iron use, and shortened erythrocyte survival. Transfusion of packed erythrocytes may be necessary. Bleeding tendency may result from abnormal platelet function and, in some patients (*e.g.*, those with renal venous thrombosis), from thrombocytopenia.

Adjustment of Medication Dosage. Adjustment of the dosage of medications with renal elimination must be done to avoid toxic levels. The interval of administration should be prolonged, unless renal replacement therapy that removes the particular drug is initiated. Toxic levels of some drugs may in turn increase the severity of the renal failure (*e.g.*, aminoglycosides, acyclovir, amphotericin B, cyclosporine; see Nephrotoxicity). In newborn infants, the commonly used drugs of concern include antibiotics (*e.g.*, aminoglycosides, vancomycin, penicillins, cephalosporins, amphotericin B, acyclovir), paralyzing agents (*e.g.*, vecuronium), tolazoline, theophylline, antiepileptic drugs, and digoxin. Although there are insufficient data to calculate adjustment of dosage in newborn infants, predictions can be made from the relationship between serum creatinine concentration and the half-life of serum concentration of a particular drug.[294–297] Further adjustments can be made by monitoring drug levels. When possible, medications with minimal or no renal toxicity should be chosen.

RENAL REPLACEMENT THERAPY

Renal replacement therapy is indicated only if aggressive symptomatic treatment fails to manage life-threatening complications due to massive fluid overload, hyperkalemia, or hypertension. Hemodialysis has been replaced largely by peritoneal dialysis, hemofiltration, and hemodiafiltration.[386–390] Availability of large-bore intravascular catheters in a patient on extracorporeal membrane oxygenation (ECMO) makes the latter two techniques particularly easy to initiate. Hemo(dia)filtration is the technique of choice for the treatment of massive fluid overload. Although these techniques offer excellent potential renal replacement in newborn infants, their use has remained limited for several reasons.

Peritoneal dialysis is contraindicated in patients with respiratory failure, shock, peritonitis, or necrotizing enterocolitis, although it can be used in some cases after abdominal surgery. In patients with liver failure, lactate contained in standard dialysis solution may result in the accumulation of lactic acid; a dialysis solution containing bicarbonate should then be used.[387] The other techniques usually require heparinization, which is contraindicated in premature infants because of the risk of intraventricular hemorrhage. Nevertheless, efficient continuous arteriovenous hemofiltration has been performed in premature infants with ARF and fluid overload, using prostacyclin instead of heparin to prevent hemofilter clotting.[389] If MAP is less than 40 torr, or if arterial access is impossible, hemo(dia)filtration requires a pump to be efficient. Renal transplantation is not an available option; this is discussed in greater detail elsewhere in the chapter (see Chronic Renal Failure).

Before renal replacement therapy is initiated, serious consideration should be given to the possibility that the patient has a dysmorphic syndrome consistent with a fatal disease or one associated with a very poor future quality of life, or the possibility that the patient is suffering from severe, irreversible multiorgan failure, secondary to profound immaturity or asphyxia, including irreversible neurologic damage or severe lung compromise (Table 42-10).

PROGNOSIS

SHORT-TERM

The short-term prognosis for neonatal ARF depends on the general condition of the infant and the status of all major organs and systems (see Table 42-10). It is essential to assess the whole patient, not only the renal condition.

Immediate mortality of infants with congenital urinary tract malformations depends primarily on the presence of respiratory failure associated with pulmonary hypoplasia and oligohydramnios.[391] Infants with severe pulmonary hypoplasia, often associated with typical Potter syndrome, die within the first postnatal hours or days; after certainty of the diagnosis, resuscitation or active intervention appears futile and therefore inappropriate. In patients with prenatal diagnosis of urinary tract anomalies, satisfactory renal function is observed more frequently in association with a normal volume of amniotic fluid, absence of cortical cysts, fetal urinary sodium concentration less than 100 mEq/L, Cl^- less than 90 mEq/L, osmolality less than 210 mOsm/kg, and urine output greater than 2 mL/hour.[392] The reliability of these indicators to prognosticate in individual cases, however, has not been established.[393]

In one series, the mortality rate in patients with oliguric ARF was 60% in ARF due to acquired conditions (*i.e.*, asphyxia and sepsis) and even higher in those with congenital heart disease.[323] A similar mortality rate (61%) was observed in a series of infants requiring peritoneal dialysis in the first 60 days of life.[388] For newborn infants in whom ARF develops while on ECMO, the prognosis is grim. In contrast, the prognosis for nonoliguric renal failure or for prerenal failure is excellent, unless major arrhythmia secondary to hyperkalemia develops or multiorgan failure develops.

LONG-TERM

A team approach to management is crucial and should include a neonatologist, nephrologist, urologist, geneticist, and radiologist.

Long-term abnormalities in GFR and in tubular function are common in acquired as well as congenital causes of ARF. In one series, limited urinary con-

TABLE 42–10
PROGNOSTIC FACTORS IN RENAL–URINARY TRACT MALFORMATIONS

Poor Prognosis for Survival or for Future Quality of Life

- General condition
  - Dysmorphic syndrome associated with poor prognosis (*e.g.*, trisomy 13, severe oligohydramnios or Potter sequence)
  - Severe immaturity
  - Multiorgan failure (*e.g.*, asphyxia, ARF in a patient on ECMO, overwhelming sepsis)
- Other major organs and systems
  - Severe pulmonary hypoplasia or oligohydramnios
  - Severe, irreversible neurologic damage
  - Refractory cardiac output failure, major arrhythmia
  - Sepsis
- Renal function*
  - Oligoanuria unresponsive to general treatment and to fluid and diuretic challenge

Poor Prognosis for Renal Function

- Severe bilateral renal parenchymal disease (*e.g.*, agenesis, hypoplasia, aplasia, dysplasia, severe PKD)
- Late diagnosis of obstruction, reflux, or infection

* Although fetal urinary Na concentration < 100 mEq/L, Cl concentration < 90 mEq/L, osmolality < 210 mOsm/kg, and urinary output > 2 mL/kg/h all are statistically associated with good prognosis, none of these tests is reliable in individual cases.[393]

ARF, acute renal failure; ECMO, extracorporeal membrane oxygenation; PKD, polycystic kidney disease.

centrating ability tested using DDAVP was observed at 1 to 36 months of age in 11% of patients who had a neonatal P_{cr} greater or equal to 1.5 mg/dL.[383] Fanconi syndrome has been reported as a sequela of renovascular accident in the neonatal period.[394] The presence of bilateral renal parenchymal disease is the major factor predicting poor renal function in cases with congenital renal or urinary tract malformations. Chronic renal failure (CRF) may develop despite early surgical intervention for urinary tract obstruction or reflux (*i.e.*, *in utero* or immediately after birth).[395]

SPECIAL CONSIDERATIONS

NEPHRON DYSGENESIS: TUBULAR OR GLOMERULAR IMMATURITY

Several cases of perinatal ARF have been described in association with immature nephrons, either predominantly with glomerular lesions or predominantly with tubular lesions. Oligohydramnios developed in most patients during the second trimester, and they died *in utero* or soon after birth. Whether these cases represent a spectrum of presentations due to the same pathophysiology or several different entities has not been determined. In any case, we propose to call this syndrome nephron dysgenesis and its two main subtypes tubular dysgenesis and glomerular dysgenesis.

Congenital Tubular Dysgenesis. Congenital tubular dysgenesis (*i.e.*, congenital oligomeganephronic nephromegaly with tubular dysgenesis, congenital renal tubular immaturity) has been described in 1% of 500 consecutive perinatal autopsies.[396] This syndrome, probably autosomal recessive, is characterized by short and undifferentiated tubules and lack of identifiable proximal tubules by lectin staining, contrasting to the presence of numerous glomeruli.[397–401] The size of the kidneys usually is normal or slightly enlarged, but in some instances the kidneys are hypoplastic. Renal US shows normal or increased cortical echogenicity and decreased corticomedullary differentiation.[311,397] Oligohydramnios develops during the second trimester, usually after 20 weeks of gestation, and results in Potter sequence and perinatal death. Some cases have been described in association with twin-to-twin transfusion or polymalformations.

Glomerular Dysgenesis. Glomerular dysgenesis is characterized by immature glomeruli, often with dilation of the Bowman space. It has been reported mostly in association with prenatal administration of indomethacin or ACE inhibitors, but also in the absence of prenatal therapy.[401] In contrast to tubular dysgenesis, glomerular dysgenesis may be associated with hematuria and casts.[309,401]

Administration of indomethacin for the prevention of premature labor can result in fetal oligoanuria and oligohydramnios; this effect of indomethacin on fetal urine output has been used for the treatment of polyhydramnios.[309] Six infants have been reported who presented with persistent oligoanuria after prenatal administration of indomethacin[244]; these infants eventually died and had either massive cortical necrosis (1 patient) or ischemic changes in the cortex associated with cystic dilation of the superficial nephrons and increased intrarenal renin.[244] Indomethacin also may cause milder forms of nephron dysgenesis, as suggested by one case report of a monozygotic twin pregnancy with polyhydramnios in which prolonged indomethacin administration resulted in severe oligohydramnios in one of the twins.[309]

The administration of ACE inhibitors during pregnancy can result in oligohydramnios, lung hypoplasia, neonatal renal failure with oligoanuria for 3 to 9 days, hypotension, hypoplasia of the calvaria, and, in many cases, perinatal death.[242,243,326] Pathologic examination may show nephron dysgenesis with immature glomeruli and dilation of glomerular spaces, convoluted tubules, and collecting ducts.[242,243]

RENAL ARTERY THROMBOSIS

The clinical presentation of renal artery thrombosis may include systemic hypertension, high PRA, and hematuria, as well as severe oligoanuric ARF if the lesion is bilateral. In some patients, the presence of a major aortic thrombus may be suspected from loss of femoral pulses and of blood flow to the lower extremities. The diagnosis of renal artery thrombosis should be suspected, especially in a newborn infant who has or has had a UA catheter.[402–405] The incidence of thrombi in infants with a UA catheter in place ranges between 24% and 95%.[406–410] These thrombi may become symptomatic when massive or when embolism occurs. Whether the incidence of UA line complications, including hypertension, can be minimized by specific position in the aorta or by continuous heparinization remains controversial.[409,410] Renal thromboembolism may occur in the absence of UA catheterization.[411]

Renal US may be normal or show increased cortical echogenicity or nephromegaly. Real-time US may show a blood clot in the aorta or a renal artery, and Doppler flow studies may show decreased renal arterial flow. Isotopic renogram may show absence of renal blood flow or a localized defect. If the UA catheter is still in place, angiography may be performed, preferably using a low-osmolality radiocontrast agent (see Nephrotoxicity).

Acute renal failure associated with bilateral renal artery thrombosis may require prolonged replacement therapy (*e.g.*, peritoneal dialysis).[403] The indications for surgical treatment of aortic or renal thromboembolism are not clear. Whereas at one time nephrectomy or thrombectomy was recommended, success has been reported by several researchers using a selective approach.[403,412–414] Thrombolysis and, if it fails, thrombectomy, should be considered for patients with refractory hypertension and those with massive aortic thrombus resulting in major complications (*e.g.*, compromised limb perfusion or anuria).[403,412–414] The other patients usually can be treated with antihypertensive agents and symptomatic management of the complications of ARF; heparinization may help to limit further extension of the thrombus. The therapeutic decision should take into account the risk of disseminated bleeding and of intraventricular hemorrhage, especially in premature infants.

Although renal artery thrombosis often results in localized or diffuse renal hypotrophy, renal function often improves to a level that is close to normal, and hypertension resolves in most patients within a few months.[415,416] Fanconi syndrome may occur in rare patients.[416]

RENAL VENOUS THROMBOSIS

Neonatal renal venous thrombosis is an uncommon condition. It may be associated with polycythemia; severe perinatal asphyxia; severe dehydration, sometimes with shock; maternal diabetes; angiography for congenital cyanotic heart disease; and adrenal hemorrhage.[417–421] Suboptimal fibrinolysis in stressed newborn infants may be an important factor.[422] Renal venous thrombosis presents clinically as the association of a unilateral or bilateral palpable flank mass with hematuria, proteinuria, and, in some cases, oligoanuria. Ultrasonography and Doppler studies show whether the renal venous thrombosis extends to the inferior vena cava. Ultrasonography of the kidney shows a typical image, characterized by enlargement of the kidney, loss of definition of the corticomedullary junction, abnormal focal or generalized increase in echo amplitude of the renal parenchyma, and some diminution of the size and echo amplitude of the central echo complex.[420] The acute complications of renal venous thrombosis include ARF, systemic hypertension, and disseminated intravascular coagulation (DIC); it ultimately may result in renal atrophy.[423,424]

Whereas nephrectomy used to be recommended in all cases, some series report good results using a conservative approach, except in the most severe cases. In the presence of consumption coagulopathy, administration of heparin may be considered. In cases associated with bilateral renal venous thrombosis or inferior vena cava thrombosis, similar results have been reported using either thrombectomy or thrombolysis.[425,426]

CORTICAL NECROSIS AND MEDULLARY NECROSIS

Renal cortical or medullary necrosis is the most severe type of ARF. The most common causes of renal necrosis include severe asphyxia and shock.[427–429] A rare cause of renal infarction is idiopathic arterial calcification.[430] The symptomatology is not specific and includes oligoanuric ARF, proteinuria, and hematuria that is often grossly apparent. The kidneys often are enlarged; renal US shows homogeneously hyperechoic kidneys, with loss of sharp corticomedullary definition.[312] The renal scan either will show very poor renal function or will not visualize the kidneys. Calcifications may become visible both on the US and the abdominal radiography. The treatment is similar to that described previously for ATN. The prognosis of bilateral global cortical necrosis is dismal; the diagnosis has been made most often at autopsy. Patients with focal or unilateral necrosis may recover, but often have chronic hypertension and CRF. Infants with medullary necrosis typically have persistent limitations in urinary concentrating ability.

POSTRENAL FAILURE

The medical treatment of postrenal failure is similar to that of intrinsic renal failure. Decompression of the urinary tract often results in an increase in GFR as well as a polyuric phase that usually is transient. During the polyuric phase, severe dehydration, hyponatremia, and hyperkalemia may develop despite adequate increase of serum aldosterone levels.[431] Careful sequential assessment of fluid balance and serum electrolytes is imperative to prevent or limit such complications, some of which may result from ECF contraction due to insufficient replacement of urine losses. As mentioned previously (see Fluid and Electrolyte Balance), when GFR comes to baseline within 1 week after surgery, fluid intake should be reduced slowly and carefully, taking into account the fact that limited urine-concentrating ability is expected in association with dysplastic kidneys. The evolution of renal function depends on the degree of renal dysplasia, which is very common in congenital urinary tract obstruction, and the frequency of UTI, which is related to VUR, urinary stasis, and the presence of an indwelling catheter. Surgical treatment is described in Chapter 43.

NEPHROTOXICITY: DRUGS AND TOXINS

PATHOPHYSIOLOGY

Several drugs that cross the placenta (see Chap. 16) can damage the fetal kidney, including aminoglycosides, heavy metals, alcohol,[432] and organic solvents (Table 42-11).[433] Chapters 16 and 56 provide a discus-

TABLE 42–11
NEPHROTOXIC EFFECTS OF VARIOUS DRUGS AND TOXINS

Substance	Renal Side-Effects
Drugs	
Aminoglycosides	Proteinuria, increased urinary excretion of Na, K, Mg, and glucose, Fanconi syndrome, myelin figures, decreased concentrating ability, decreased RBF, polyuric ARF, ATN, interstitial nephritis
Methicillin	Interstitial nephritis
Amphotericin B	Hyperkaliuria, hyposthenuria, NDI, hypernatriuria, ATN, oliguria, RTA, nephrocalcinosis
Acyclovir	Crystalluria, obstructive nephropathy
Indomethacin	Decreased RBF, ATN, oligoanuria, hyponatremia, hyperkalemia, *in utero* nephron dysgenesis, oligohydramnios
Tolazoline	Hypotension and hypoxemia resulting in decreased GFR, ATN, oliguria, hematuria
α-Adrenergic agents	Decreased RBF, ATN
ACE inhibitors	Hypotension, decreased RBF, ATN, *in utero* nephron dysgenesis
Radiocontrast agents	Decreased RBF, oliguric ATN, Tamm–Horsfall proteinuria, nephromegaly with US similar to ARPKD, increased urinary excretion of uric acid
Cyclosporine	Renal vasoconstriction, decreased RBF and GFR, interstitial nephritis
Loop diuretics	Nephrocalcinosis, nephrolithiasis
Toxins	
Hemoglobin	ATN
Myoglobin	ATN
Oxalate	Nephrocalcinosis, nephrolithiasis, oxalosis with ARF
Benzyl alcohol	Cardiovascular collapse, ATN
Polysorbate in intravenous tocopherol	ATN
Uric acid	Crystalluria, ATN
Organic solvents (*e.g.*, toluene)	Fanconi syndrome, aminoaciduria, hyperchloremic acidosis
Alcohol (*in utero*)	Distal RTA

ACE, angiotensin-converting enzyme; ARF, acute renal failure; ARPKD, autosomal recessive polycystic kidney disease; ATN, acute tubular necrosis; GFR, glomerular filtration rate; NDI, nephrogenic diabetes insipidus; RBF, renal blood flow; RTA, renal tubular acidosis; US, ultrasound.

sion of the relevant pharmacokinetics. Although high doses often are required to produce toxicity in animal models, once the threshold is reached, the pathologic and pathophysiologic processes often are similar to those observed in human toxicology.

Depending on the compound and its dose, nephrotoxicity may result either from direct cytotoxicity or from renal ischemia; the latter mechanism may be especially important during the initial phase. Direct cytotoxicity is related to the concentration of drug or metabolite in renal tubular cells, which depends on the concentration of free drug in the plasma, GFR, and the characteristics of tubular transport.

CLINICAL PRESENTATION AND DIAGNOSIS

Nephrotoxicity may present as oligoanuria, ARF, drug toxicity caused by decreased clearance of a medication with renal excretion, hypotension, hematuria, proteinuria, renal tubular acidosis (RTA), nephrocalcinosis or nephrolithiasis, polyuria, abnormal plasma electrolyte concentrations, or cardiac arrhythmia (see Table 42-11). Methods of screening for nephrotoxicity depend on the drug or toxin and may include urinalysis, measurement of urinary concentration of low-molecular-weight proteins, sequential measurements of P_{cr}, GFR, or serum drug levels, urine output, or renal US. Since most NICU patients also are exposed to multiple drugs as well to episodes of hypoxemia and ischemia, it often is very difficult to determine whether a particular drug is the major renal offender.

PREVENTION AND TREATMENT

Prevention of nephrotoxicity includes avoiding teratogens (*e.g.*, ACE inhibitors), adjusting the interval of administration of nephrotoxic agents (*e.g.*, aminoglycosides, acyclovir) according to measured or predicted GFR, avoiding known toxins (*e.g.*, methicillin, benzyl alcohol,[434,435] polysorbate[329]), selecting drugs with the best risk–benefit ratio (*e.g.*, choosing a thiazide rather than furosemide for chronic oral therapy of bronchopulmonary dysplasia [BPD] except in refractory patients), and avoiding, if possible, synergistic nephrotoxic combinations. In addition, the dosage of all these medications should be adjusted to renal function, which is predicted from GA during the first day of life and estimated from P_{cr} afterward.

Treatment of nephrotoxicity is symptomatic; the dosage of all medications with renal elimination should be adjusted to renal function and to drug levels, fluid and electrolyte disturbances should be corrected, and, if appropriate, the toxic medication should be replaced by a less toxic one.

SPECIFIC CONSIDERATIONS

AMINOGLYCOSIDES

Pathophysiology. Aminoglycoside nephrotoxicity results from renal vasoconstriction and from direct cellular toxicity, especially in the proximal tubule. Within the same species, there is a dose–effect relationship and a characteristic time course. In the dog, low doses of gentamicin induce successively an increase in urinary excretion of PGE_2, a decrease in urinary osmolality, a rise in PRA, and finally, after 2 weeks or more, a sudden decrease in PGE_2 followed immediately by polyuric ARF with high FENa and tubulointerstitial nephritis[436,437]; higher doses result in hypokalemia, hypocalcemia, and a more prominent decrease in GFR.[437] Continuous exposure to gentamicin after tubular necrosis and regeneration is associated with aminoglycoside insensitivity, which is characterized by normalization of GFR, but only partial recovery of renal concentrating ability. At that stage, pathologic examination discloses chronic tubulointerstitial changes in the medulla.[438]

Renal vasoconstriction associated with aminoglycoside administration may be mediated by an increase in TX synthesis.[439] Indeed, inhibition of TX synthesis or volume expansion with isotonic saline diminishes aminoglycoside-induced nephrotoxicity; furthermore, the enhanced nephrotoxicity of the association of gentamicin, captopril, and potassium depletion is dependent largely on an increase in TXB_2 synthesis.[439] Prostaglandins may limit that vasoconstriction, as suggested by the natural history of gentamicin nephrotoxicity in the dog,[436] and by enhanced nephrotoxicity resulting from the association of indomethacin with gentamicin.[440]

Aminoglycoside nephrotoxicity is predominantly a proximal tubular disease. Histopathologic features include a loss of brush border, an increase in number and size of lysosomes, and formation of myeloid bodies.[441] In the proximal tubule, the aminoglycoside is absorbed by pinocytosis and stored in lysosomes. Cellular uptake of aminoglycoside results in inhibition of lysosomal enzymes, including cathepsins and phospholipase A_1, which leads to the development of myeloid figures; inhibition of endocytosis, mitochondrial Ca^{2+} uptake, and Na^+/K^+-ATPase; and alterations of membrane phospholipids. Cellular uptake may explain two pharmacologic findings, the presence of a "tissue compartment" and the fact that plasma clearance of gentamicin is greater than its urinary clearance.[294,442]

Functional tubular changes include decreased glucose, electrolyte, and fluid absorption in the proximal tubule, decreased maximum PAH secretion, decreased urea and sodium concentration in the papillary tip, and decreased fluid absorption in the papillary duct.[437,443] Proteinuria is mediated by two mechanisms: decreased tubular reabsorption, which results in urinary excretion of low-molecular-weight proteins, and loss of integrity and desquamation of cells, which results in urinary excretion of cytoplasmic enzymes (*e.g.*, lactate dehydrogenase, alanine aminopeptidase) and lysosomal enzymes (*e.g.*, NAG).[444] Eventually, tubular necrosis, tubular atrophy, intratubular myeloid bodies, and interstitial nephritis may be apparent.[437,445]

Several mechanisms are involved in the decrease in GFR associated with aminoglycoside use. In rats, low doses of gentamicin may induce a mild reduction in GFR secondary to a decrease in ultrafiltration coefficient, whereas high doses induce a severe reduction in GFR secondary to a decrease in RBF, ultrafiltration coefficient, and transglomerular hydraulic pressure; the latter is associated with tubular lesions.[446] High doses of gentamicin also may induce a reduction in the number and size of the glomerular endothelial fenestrae, which may further decrease the ultrafiltration coefficient.[445,446]

Risk Factors. Gentamicin, kanamycin, and tobramycin are more nephrotoxic than amikacin or netilmicin.[445,447] Several factors may enhance aminoglycoside nephrotoxicity under experimental conditions. In subtotally nephrectomized dogs, morphologic and functional (*i.e.*, GFR) measures of nephrotoxicity are less severe when the interval of administration is adjusted with a fixed dose than when the dose is adjusted with a fixed administration interval.[448] Nephrotoxic effects of aminoglycosides may be enhanced by reduced renal mass; ischemia; metabolic acidosis; sodium or potassium depletion; pyelonephritis; endotoxemia; indomethacin; ACE inhibition, especially in association with potassium depletion; and furosemide. Although vancomycin has been reported to increase aminoglycoside-induced nephrotoxicity in adult patients,[449] several studies in newborn rats, infants, and children have failed to confirm an additive toxicity.[450–454] Renal susceptibility to aminoglycosides also depends on renal maturity. In mongrel dogs, newborn puppies are less susceptible to gentamicin nephrotoxicity than older puppies or adult animals.[455]

Clinical Presentation and Diagnosis. Aminoglycoside nephrotoxicity most commonly presents either as isolated proteinuria or polyuric ARF with a high FENa.[441] Laboratory findings may include proteinuria, decreased GFR, decreased urine-concentrating ability, glucosuria, increased natriuresis and kaliuresis, and alterations in tubular transport of organic acids[441,456]; hypomagnesemia secondary to increased urinary excretion has been reported.[382] A reversible Fanconi syndrome has developed rarely in children receiving gentamicin, either within a few days or after prolonged therapy.[457,458]

The diagnosis of aminoglycoside toxicity should be suspected if tubular or glomerular damage disappears after the medication is stopped. During the first days of therapy, the most sensitive indicator of nephrotoxicity is an increase in urinary excretion of low-molecular-weight proteins (*i.e.*, β_2-microglobulin, retinol-binding protein, lysozyme), whereas after 1 week of therapy, the most common indicator is an increase in urinary excretion of NAG.[447,459] Neither low-molecular-weight proteinuria nor NAG enzymuria is specific.[460,461] On the other hand, the presence of myelin figures in the urinary sediment is associated with nephrotoxicity related to cationic amphophilic compounds (*e.g.*, aminoglycosides) but not with ischemic nephropathy[462,463]; however, their detection requires electron microscopy.

Prevention and Treatment. Serum aminoglycoside levels should be obtained at least weekly. Plasma creatinine concentration, serum electrolytes, urinalysis, and urine output should be followed serially in high-risk patients. The interval of administration of medications such as digoxin, indomethacin, and the aminoglycoside itself may have to be adjusted according to P_{cr} and to respective plasma levels, which should be kept within the therapeutic range (for gentamicin: peak level, 4–10 μg/mL; trough level, 1–2 μg/mL).[464] Sodium and potassium intake should be adequate to prevent depletion of either electrolyte. If severe Fanconi syndrome or polyuric ARF develops, the aminoglycoside should be replaced by another antibiotic, and nonspecific treatment should be given (see Acute Renal Failure; Fanconi Syndrome).

INDOMETHACIN

Pathophysiology. Because the half-life of indomethacin depends on GA, similar doses result in higher levels for longer duration in more immature patients.[465] Indomethacin, which is a cyclooxygenase inhibitor, blocks the synthesis of PG. Since renal synthesis of PGs already occurs in fetuses who are 22 weeks of GA, it is not surprising that indomethacin may cause renal side-effects at all ages.

Indomethacin administration acutely decreases RBF.[315,466] Although in premature infants with symptomatic PDA, RBF decreases only transiently after each dose of indomethacin (0.2 mg/kg),[315] in some patients it may result in transient renal dysfunction.[467] The latter is associated with suppression of PG synthesis, a fall of PRA from the high levels that are attributed to renal hypoperfusion before closure of the PDA, and a transient rise in the plasma level of AVP.[467] During prolonged administration of indomethacin (*i.e.*, up to 1 week), hormonal levels normalize, and renal function tends to improve.[467,468]

Indomethacin and its glucuronide are excreted into the urine almost entirely through the organic secretory pathway of the proximal tubule, involving active transport at the basolateral surface.[469] Indomethacin induces a marked reduction in microsomal enzymes (*e.g.*, cytochrome P450), increased reabsorption of solutes in the proximal part of the nephron, increased corticomedullary gradient, and enhanced hydroosmotic effect of antidiuretic hormone. The latter two changes result in an increased ratio of urine to plasma osmolality and decreased free water clearance; water retention and dilutional hyponatremia develop in some patients.[470] The effect of indomethacin administration on urinary electrolyte excretion is variable; in some premature infants it may result in decreased natriuresis. Indomethacin-mediated hyperkalemia is due to decreased renal K^+ excretion, which may result from hyporeninemic hypoaldosteronism, decreased Na^+ delivery to the distal tubule, or ARF, but is not due to alteration of the extrarenal handling of K^+.[471] Simultaneous administration of PG prevents all renal side-effects of indomethacin, except for NAG enzymuria.

An indomethacin-mediated decrease in RBF may result in ARF in some patients. Papillary necrosis, nephrotic syndrome, and interstitial nephritis have been described in animals and adult humans treated with nonsteroidal antiinflammatory agents, such as indomethacin, but not in newborn infants.

Risk Factors. The risk of nephrotoxicity is increased by the combination of indomethacin with other nephrotoxins, such as aminoglycosides[440] or cyclosporine.[460]

Clinical Presentation. Maternal administration of indomethacin, which has been used for the prevention of premature labor and for the treatment of polyhydramnios, results in equivalent plasma indomethacin concentrations in fetal and maternal circulations. Maternal indomethacin administration may induce nephron dysgenesis (see Acute Renal Failure),[309,402] oligohydramnios, and neonatal renal failure.[470]

Renal side-effects of postnatal administration of indomethacin include decreased free water clearance[472] and oligoanuria, which can cause dilutional hyponatremia; hyperkalemia; ARF; and decreased digoxin clearance.[473,474]

Prevention and Treatment. Indomethacin is contraindicated if P_{cr} is elevated (*i.e.*, usual criterion is $P_{cr} > 1.8$ mg/dL) and in the presence of oligoanuria or hyperkalemia. The incidence of indomethacin-related nephrotoxicity can be decreased by volume expansion for a few hours before its administration,[475] or by simultaneous administration of furosemide.[347]

Because GFR decreases frequently in association with indomethacin administration, P_{cr}, serum electrolyte concentrations, and urine output should be monitored. In addition, the interval of drug administration should be adjusted according to P_{cr} or GFR. The digoxin administration interval should be increased preventively.[473] Treatment of indomethacin-induced ARF or hyperkalemia is symptomatic (see Acute Renal Failure). Dilutional hyponatremia can be prevented by adjusting fluid intake to urine output. If oligoanuria develops, a challenge dose of furosemide should be given; fluid restriction should be initiated if oligoanuria persists.

TOLAZOLINE

Pathophysiology and Risk Factors. Administration of tolazoline (see Chaps. 29, 31, and 56) to hypoxic animals induces systemic hypotension and a more severe decrease in RBF and GFR and increase in FENa than hypoxia alone.[476] In newborn infants with pulmonary hypertension, tolazoline has predominantly a nonspecific vasodilator effect (*i.e.*, acting on both the pulmonary and the systemic vasculature, presumably as an α-antagonist). Whether tolazoline has a specific action on the renal vasculature or renal function in newborn infants has not been investigated; it may be that the renal side-effects of tolazoline are mediated through ischemia caused by tolazoline-induced systemic hypotension.

Because tolazoline is excreted unchanged into the urine, both by glomerular filtration and by tubular secretion,[477] its half-life is expected to increase in parallel with decreasing renal function. Very little information is available about the pharmacokinetics of tolazoline in the newborn infant. In one study, a 2 mg/kg loading dose given in 3 minutes followed by a maintenance dose of 2 mg/kg/hour resulted in plasma levels of 5 to 20 μg/mL at a GA of 27 to 41 weeks.[478] The data suggested that these levels were higher than optimal (<14 μg/mL). The half-life of tolazoline ranged between 3 and 10 hours in all patients, with the exception of one who was hypotensive and in whom the half-life was 33 hours.

Clinical Presentation. Renal complications, including oliguria, transient oliguric ARF, and hematuria, are common in newborn infants with pulmonary hypertension in whom systemic hypotension and persistent hypoxemia develop after tolazoline administration.[479–481]

Prevention and Treatment. Tolazoline administration is contraindicated in patients with ARF, intravascular volume depletion, or low systemic blood pressure. We never administer tolazoline unless systolic blood pressure has been at least 60 torr for a few hours in a full-term infant. In addition, we always expand the intravascular volume and initiate a low-dose dopamine infusion just before and during the administration of tolazoline.

AMPHOTERICIN B

Pathophysiology. Administration of amphotericin B produces immediate nephrotoxicity, which is mediated by renal vasoconstriction[482] and by the affinity of amphotericin B to sterols, which are important components of cellular and lysosomal membranes. Functional tubular alterations include an increase in urinary *p*H, in fractional excretion of Na^+, K^+, and phosphate, and in NAG enzymuria.[483] Histopathologic features after prolonged amphotericin administration in adults include glomerular changes (*e.g.*, subcortical atrophy, juxtamedullary hypertrophy), interstitial edema, focal tubular atrophy, and nephrocalcinosis.[484]

Risk Factors. Glomerular and tubular toxicity of a 5-hour infusion of amphotericin is lower than that of a rapid intravenous injection.[485] The degree of damage to renal tubular cell membranes is directly related to the cholesterol content of the membrane.[486,487] The toxicity of amphotericin to proximal tubular cells in culture is decreased by its inclusion into liposomes. Preliminary data in adults using a liposomal formulation of amphotericin B appear promising.[488]

Clinical Presentation. In adults, the incidence of renal damage is 40% after a total dose of more than 4 g and 90% after a dose of more than 5 g[489]; permanent renal damage may result from even higher total doses.[484] Acute signs may include decreased RBF and GFR, azotemia, oligoanuria, increased urinary excretion of Na^+, K^+, phosphate, and bicarbonate, and hyposthenuria; later complications include nephrogenic diabetes insipidus (NDI), distal RTA, and nephrocalcinosis.[484,489]

In newborn infants receiving amphotericin B at doses adjusted to serum levels, the most frequent signs of nephrotoxicity include increased P_{cr} and BUN, and transient hypokalemia, which responds readily to additional K^+ intake.[490] Inadvertent administration of an amphotericin overdose has been reported in a handful of newborn infants,[490–492] who were treated with various modalities, including exchange transfusion. Acute nephrotoxicity in these patients was limited; distal RTA developed in one patient who received a 50-fold overdose of amphotericin.[491] The most adequate therapy of amphotericin overdose remains to be determined.

Prevention and Treatment. If TPN is used, the dose of lipid administration should be adjusted to prevent hypercholesterolemia. The interval of administration of amphotericin B should be adjusted to GFR during therapy. Serum levels may need to be monitored in VLBW infants, and compared to the minimum inhibitory concentration (0.2–25 μg/mL in one study)[493] and the minimum fungicidal concentration (0.2–0.4 μg/mL).[493] Supplementary K^+ intake may help prevent hypokalemia. If oligoanuric ARF develops during amphotericin administration, amphotericin should be withheld temporarily and restarted later at a lower dose.[490]

ACYCLOVIR

Pathophysiology. Acyclovir administration may result in an increase in urine β_2-microglobulin and an obstructive nephropathy mediated by crystalluria.[494]

Risk Factors. The incidence of acyclovir-related nephropathy increases with rapid intravenous injections and fluid restriction.[494]

Clinical Presentation. In children, acyclovir-related nephrotoxicity is associated with crystalluria and increased P_{cr}.[494] Acyclovir overdose in two well-hydrated newborn infants did not result in nephrotoxicity. Neither exchange transfusion nor administration of activated charcoal appeared significantly to enhance the elimination of acyclovir.[495]

Prevention and Treatment. Because acyclovir is excreted in the urine, the interval of administration should be adjusted for GA and renal function to prevent neurologic toxicity.[496] If acyclovir is administered at a correct dose and interval[496] in a slow infusion, and if sufficient fluid intake is provided to maintain adequate urinary output, the risk of clinical nephrotoxicity is negligible. If acyclovir is considered in a patient who also needs fluid restriction, the urine should be checked regularly for crystalluria and increased P_{cr}; if renal dysfunction is observed, the dose of acyclovir should be withheld or decreased, and fluid intake increased temporarily.

RADIOCONTRAST AGENTS

Pathophysiology. The pathophysiologic presentation of radiocontrast nephropathy includes a combination of ischemia, direct toxicity, and tubular obstruction by Tamm–Horsfall protein[497] or by uric acid crystals resulting from increased uricosuria.[498] Histopathologic features include vacuolization of proximal tubular cells, mild dilation of proximal tubules, areas of luminal inspissation by waxy debris, and interstitial edema.[499]

Risk Factors. In adult patients, risk factors for radiocontrast-induced increase in P_{cr} include a high baseline P_{cr} and diabetes mellitus.[500] Whether the incidence of radiocontrast nephropathy in adults is lower with low-osmolality contrast agents than with conventional high-osmolality products is controversial; no significant difference was observed in two prospective studies on stable patients with rigorous selection criteria and adequate fluid intake.[501,502] Although there is no study comparing low- and high-osmolality products in infants, only the latter cause a decrease in GFR in immature rabbits.[503]

Clinical Presentation. The signs of radiocontrast nephrotoxicity may include poor visualization or a prolonged nephrogram, proteinuria with casts, and oliguric ARF.[497] One premature infant, who had no visualization after injection of an iodinated product, had a transient oligoanuric ARF with a specific gravity of 1.020, low FENa, and nephromegaly[499]; US suggested the diagnosis of autosomal recessive polycystic kidney disease (ARPKD).

Prevention and Treatment. Intravenous urography best is avoided in the neonatal period, especially during the first days of life. In newborn infants who need angiography or CT with contrast, a low-osmolality agent is preferred; adequate hydration should be provided before the procedure.

ANGIOTENSIN-CONVERTING ENZYME INHIBITORS

Pathophysiology. Especially in association with hypovolemia, ACE inhibition may cause hypotension, decreased RBF, and oliguric ARF.

Risk Factors. The combination of ACE inhibitors and diuretics may lead to severe refractory hypotension, profound decrease in RBF, oligoanuria, and ARF. Angiotensin-converting enzyme inhibition enhances the renal toxicity of aminoglycosides.[439]

Clinical Presentation. Maternal administration of ACE inhibitors has been associated with glomerular dysgenesis, oliguric ARF, hypotension, hypoplasia of the calvaria, and perinatal death (see Acute Renal Failure).[242,243,326] Neonatal administration of ACE inhibitors has resulted in reversible oliguric ARF,[504] which may occur at the time of initiation of therapy or much later, without any precipitating event.[505] The neurologic complications are of greater concern than the renal side-effects.[505]

Prevention and Treatment. Angiotensin-converting enzyme inhibitors never should be used during pregnancy. Because of the neurologic complications associated with chronic ACE inhibition in newborn infants,[505] ACE inhibitors should be used only for life-threatening refractory hypertension, with continuous measurement of systemic blood pressure and central venous pressure. Hypotension caused by ACE inhibition often responds only to massive amounts of crystalloids and colloids, and then sometimes poorly.[505]

CYCLOSPORINE A

Cyclosporine is used infrequently in newborn infants; however, its use is expected to increase in parallel with the increasing frequency of cardiac transplantation.

Pathophysiology. Cyclosporine induces reversible renal vasoconstriction, apparently through stimulation of α_1-receptors.[506]

Risk Factors. Cyclosporine toxicity is enhanced by high serum levels of the drug, ischemia, concomitant administration of nephrotoxic drugs (*e.g.*, indomethacin), and reduced renal function.[460] Cyclosporine toxicity is decreased by cotreatment with α-antagonists or spironolactone.[506]

Clinical Presentation. Cyclosporine nephrotoxicity develops in approximately two thirds of patients receiving cyclosporine after liver transplantation.[507] It may present as an increase in P_{cr} and BUN and NAG enzymuria, associated with a normal renal US and Doppler flow analysis and a ^{99m}Tc-DTPA scan that shows normal perfusion with loss of tubular function. The incidence of systemic hypertension with moderately decreased GFR and proteinuria also is very high.[507] Acute renal failure is a less common complication.

Prevention and Treatment. The incidence and severity of cyclosporine nephrotoxicity may be decreased by monitoring the blood levels of cyclosporine and avoiding the use of other nephrotoxic drugs. Cyclosporine-induced nephrotoxicity, with or without hypertension, usually is easily controlled medically; other immunosuppressive drugs should be considered if severe nephrotoxicity has appeared during cyclosporine therapy.

MYOGLOBINURIA–HEMOGLOBINURIA

Pathophysiology. Myolysis results in increased intercompartmental exchanges, including influx into the intracellular compartment of water, sodium, chloride, and calcium, which result in shock and hypocalcemia, and efflux of potassium, phosphate, purines, lactic acid, myoglobin, thromboplastin, creatine kinase, and creatinine into the ECF compartment.

The renal damage associated with rhabdomyolysis is mediated by factors observed in other types of ATN (*i.e.*, vasomotor, obstructive, and nephrotoxic), as well as metabolic factors resulting from the myolysis (*i.e.*, hyperphosphatemia, hyperuricemia, and the formation of thrombi in the glomerular capillary tufts due to DIC).[508] The formation of intratubular hemoprotein casts is favored by oligoanuria and low *p*H. Hemoprotein catabolism liberates iron pigments, which may catalyze the formation of free radicals[509] and peroxidation of lipids, and inhibit the vasodilation mediated by endothelium-derived relaxing factors in the kidney.[510]

Risk Factors. In contrast to the adult literature, only rare reports of neonatal rhabdomyolysis have been published.[338,511,512] This low incidence may result from the low myoglobin content of immature muscle, especially in premature infants.[513]

Clinical Presentation. Adult patients with traumatic rhabdomyolysis manifest the so-called crush syndrome, characterized by shock, high serum concentration of creatinine phosphokinase, high P_{cr}–BUN ratio, hyperkalemia, metabolic acidosis, hyperphosphatemia, hypocalcemia, hyperuricemia, DIC, and oligoanuric ATN.[508] In severely asphyxiated infants, a strongly positive reaction for heme in the absence of microscopic hematuria suggests a serum myoglobin concentration greater than 200 ng/mL.[338]

Prevention and Treatment. In adults with crush syndrome, immediate initiation of forced alkaline diuresis, with mannitol for patients in whom oligoanuria develops, results in dramatic improvement in outcome; this treatment prevents hypovolemia and intratubular hemoprotein casts.[514] In contrast, in newborn infants with profound perinatal asphyxia or massive hemolysis, a similar approach cannot be recommended, because the potential benefit to the kidney may be outweighed by an increased risk for brain edema, pulmonary edema, and PDA. The treatment of established myoglobinuric or hemoglobinuric ATN is nonspecific.

CHRONIC RENAL FAILURE

The definition of chronic renal insufficiency is a reduction in GFR to a level between 25% and 50% of normal, whereas that of CRF is a reduction in GFR to less than 25% of normal for at least 3 months.[515] End-stage renal disease (ESRD) is the stage of CRF at which the patient requires chronic dialysis or renal transplantation for survival.

INCIDENCE

The incidence of ESRD in children (age range, 0–16 years) is three to eight cases per one million children.[515–517] Only 6% of children with ESRD are under 3 years of age.[515] In 1989, of the 754 children (age range, 0–18 years) who received 761 renal transplants in the United States, less than 7% were under 2 years of age, and less than 2% were under 1 year of age.[518] Infants rarely survive the neonatal period and either have CRF or ESRD in infancy; the exact incidence is not known.

ETIOLOGY

Most reports of CRF in children combine patients who developed CRF as neonates with those in whom CRF develops as a result of a later insult to the kidney (Table 42-12).[519] The underlying disease in recipients of renal transplants changes with age. Among patients under 24 months of age there is a high percentage of aplastic–hypoplastic–dysplastic kidneys (34%, *versus* ≤ 23% in patients 2 years or older) and obstructive uropathy (21%, *versus* ≤ 16% in patients 6 years or older).[518] By far the most common (29%) underlying disease during the first 2 years of age is renal dysplasia.[520] Focal segmental glomerulosclerosis is not observed, in contrast to the experience in older age groups. Typically, the course in infants is characterized by slow, progressive deterioration of renal function.

DIAGNOSIS

History, physical examination, US, measurement of GFR using a radionuclide for the estimation of the functional level of each kidney, urinalysis, and urine culture should be obtained initially. In patients with hydronephrosis, meningomyelocele, or UTI, a VCUG is indicated, and a furosemide radionuclide scan should be considered. In certain patients, an IVU, a percutaneous antegrade pyelography, or a renal biopsy may be indicated (see Clinical Evaluation of Renal Function and Disease).

The signs and symptoms suggestive of CRF are nonspecific, especially in infants, and include growth failure, anorexia, vomiting, pallor, edema, seizures, dehydration, heart failure, hypertension, polyuria,

TABLE 42–12
ETIOLOGY OF CHRONIC RENAL FAILURE IN 75 PATIENTS YOUNGER THAN 2 YEARS OF AGE

Diagnosis	Number of Patients	Percentage
Hypoplasia	24	32
Obstructive uropathy	15	20
Oxalosis	8	11
Congenital nephrotic syndrome	6	8
Hemolytic uremic syndrome*	4	5
Cortical necrosis	3	4
Infantile polycystic kidney disease	3	4
Glomerulonephritis*	3	4
Steroid-resistant nephrotic syndrome	2	3
Birth hypoxia with renal failure	2	3
Jeune syndrome	1	1
Drash syndrome	1	1
Anatomical problems	1	1
Unknown	2	3

* These diagnoses virtually are not seen during the neonatal period.
From Najarian JS, Frey DJ, Matas AJ, et al. Renal transplantation in infants. Ann Surg 1990; 212:353.

fever, hematuria, proteinuria, and pyuria. In children, symptoms such as lassitude, fatigue, headache, and nausea can be present. The diagnosis of CRF is confirmed by a persistently low GFR corrected for postconceptional age.

PATHOPHYSIOLOGY AND TREATMENT

Any patient with chronic renal insufficiency should have periodic physical examinations, including measurement of blood pressure, regular monitoring of growth rate and GFR, and not only serial measurements of plasma or serum creatinine concentration, acid–base status, serum electrolytes, mineral metabolism (*i.e.*, serum concentrations of calcium, phosphate, alkaline phosphatase, and PTH), hemoglobin, and hematocrit. Urinalysis, including dipstick, urinary electrolytes, *p*H, and calcium, should be done serially, and UTI should be excluded on a regular basis. The treatment of CRF ideally should make it possible to achieve normal growth rate, hematocrit, and fluid and electrolyte homeostasis, while limiting the rate of progression of the renal disease toward ESRD. Provision is made for limitations in renal function, while allowing an acceptable quality of life.[515,521,522] Although the cost–benefit ratio of many aspects of treatment has not been determined, therapeutic outcome has improved, in parallel with changes in both maintenance therapy (*e.g.*, maintenance of growth) and replacement therapy (*i.e.*, early renal transplantation).

GROWTH

One major problem of CRF in childhood, especially in infancy, is severe growth failure, which is multifactorial in etiology. Known causes include acidosis, reduced caloric intake, anemia, hypertension, renal osteodystrophy, aluminum intoxication, abnormalities of growth hormone and somatomedin, recurrent episodes of fluid and electrolyte disturbances, recurrent infections, and administration of steroids. Ten years ago, ESRD due to congenital renal disease was associated with profound growth failure.[523] Until very recently, only limited catch-up growth was observed, despite increased caloric intake, administration of vitamin D and phosphate-binding gels, and renal transplantation.

Every effort should be made to limit growth failure at the beginning of CRF; this is most critical in infants, who normally grow much faster than children. Assessment of growth is made by serially plotting the height standard deviation score (SDS) against age.[524] Height SDS is the number of standard deviations below the mean height for age. Because bone maturation is delayed in CRF, height SDS corrected for bone age is preferred.[521] Normal growth rate corresponds to a height SDS that is constant with age, whereas catch-up growth is associated with a progressive improvement in the height SDS. The advantages of improving the rate of growth include a reduction in the renal load of potassium and phosphate, accelerated weight gain, which allows a renal transplant at an earlier age, and achievement of improved adult height. Improved growth has been obtained, at least in some patients, by provision of additional caloric intake using nasogastric feeding or TPN,[524] treatment and prevention of renal osteodystrophy,[525,526] elimination of aluminum intake,[525] limitation of steroid dosage made possible by the use of cyclosporine, prevention, early diagnosis, and treatment of complications such as UTI, administration of erythropoietin, administration of growth hormone, and early transplantation.

NUTRITION

Protein restriction is recommended in adults with CRF to prevent glomerular capillary hyperfiltration, which has been implicated in the development of focal segmental glomerulosclerosis.[527] Hyperfiltration corresponds to the increase in GFR observed after a high-protein diet in normal people and in those with chronic renal disease. Dietary protein restriction slows down the progression of renal disease in several animal models and, perhaps, in adult patients.[528] Postulated mechanisms include not only a reduction in hyperfiltration but also a reduction in glomerular prostanoid production, in glomerular hypertrophy, in insulinlike growth factor type 1 (IGF-1), in glomerular eicosanoid production, and in glomerular selectivity.[529]

The diet should provide sufficient calories and individual nutrients for a normal rate of growth. The ideal amount of protein intake in infants with CRF has not been established. It seems prudent to follow the recommended dietary allowance (RDA) for normal infants (*i.e.*, 2.2 g/kg body weight at 0–2 months of age, 2.0 g/kg at 2–6 months of age, and 1.8 g/kg at 6–12 months of age), corresponding to 8% of the RDA of calories.[530–532] Breast milk, SMA (Wyeth Ayerst, Radnor, PA), and Similac PM 60/40 (Ross, Columbus, OH), provide adequate high-quality protein and minerals with limited phosphate and sodium content for most infants with CRF. To maintain adequate growth despite decreased appetite, the caloric content of the formula often needs to be supplemented with carbohydrates and with medium-chain triglycerides to reach 120% to 180% of the RDA, and continuous nocturnal feeding through a nasogastric tube or a gastrostomy tube may be required.[531] In the few patients who cannot tolerate enough enteral feeding (*e.g.*, most infants with congenital nephrotic syndrome of the Finnish type [CNF]), TPN should be initiated; in patients with severe CRF, only essential amino acids should be provided (*e.g.*, Nephramine; American McGaw, Santa Ana, CA).[532]

As the degree of renal failure increases (*i.e.*, GFR $<$ 25% of normal), protein intake should be decreased to maintain a BUN below 100 mg/dL, using milk with high-quality proteins that are at least 35% essential amino acids, such as breast milk, SMA, Similac PM 60/40, or Special Formula S-29 (Wyeth Ayerst). Patients with severe renal failure may require special diets that contain limited amounts of protein and are supplemented with essential amino acids or their corresponding keto acids.

MAINTENANCE OF ADEQUATE FLUID AND ELECTROLYTE AND ACID–BASE BALANCE

Because the ability of the failing kidney to concentrate urine is limited, additional water may be required to compensate for polyuria. On the other hand, the failing kidney usually is able to maintain normal serum levels of sodium, potassium, and bicarbonate until GFR falls below 25% of normal. As stated previously, the electrolyte requirements should be assessed for every patient from the measurement of serum and urinary electrolytes. Sodium intake should be normal, except in patients with salt-losing nephropathy, such as obstructive uropathy, primary tubulointerstitial disease, and dysplastic kidneys, who may need sodium supplements, and those with hypertension or edema, who may need sodium restriction. Metabolic acidosis is commonplace in patients with CRF. Administration of bicarbonate usually is initiated when the serum bicarbonate concentration falls below normal. An initial dose of 3 mEq/kg/day is used and increased as needed to achieve a serum level of 22 to 24 mEq/L. Citrate can be given instead of bicarbonate, unless aluminum intoxication is suspected (see Aluminum Intoxication). Hyperkalemia usually develops only when GFR is less than 25% of normal, but it may appear earlier in patients with interstitial disease or secondary to exogenous potassium intake, hemolysis, or acidosis.

Acute episodes of fluid or electrolyte imbalance, characterized by hyponatremia, hyperkalemia, azotemia, hypocalcemia or hypercalcemia, metabolic acidosis, and hyperphosphatemia can be precipitated by diarrhea, UTI, sepsis, or increased catabolism associated with poor nutritional intake. Rapid diagnosis and correction of the imbalance are critical. The treatment of dehydration, hyperkalemia, hyponatremia, hypernatremia, and acidosis is similar to that described for ARF. Peritoneal dialysis may be needed. Hyperkalemia in adults with terminal renal failure requiring chronic dialysis responds poorly to the administration of bicarbonate infusion.[533]

ADJUSTMENT OF MEDICATION DOSAGE

The interval of administration of medications excreted by the kidney needs to be modified, based on the level of renal function or their removal by means of dialysis. Recommendations are given in the section on Acute Renal Failure.

CARDIOVASCULAR SYSTEM

Rigorous control of hypertension is important to avoid its complications and its known effect in accelerating progression of renal failure. A detailed discussion is presented elsewhere in the chapter (see Hypertension).

MINERAL METABOLISM AND RENAL OSTEODYSTROPHY

Vitamin D and Parathyroid Hormone. The two major disturbances of mineral metabolism associated with chronic loss of renal function are decreased 1-α-hydroxylation of vitamin D as a result of loss of kidney tissue, and an increased secretion of PTH (Table 42-13).[525] Initially, the latter is an appropriate response to low serum ionized calcium, but in CRF the set point for the inhibition of PTH secretion by extracellular calcium is raised, which corresponds to secondary hyperparathyroidism.

Mild decrease in GFR is associated with a decrease in ionized calcium concentration, which induces the secretion of PTH (see Table 42-13). Higher levels of PTH result in phosphaturia and low levels of fasting phosphatemia; daytime phosphatemia may be normal.[525] At that point, the lack of increase in serum level of $1,25(OH)_2D_3$, despite hyperparathyroidism, is evidence for lack of response of renal 1-α-hydroxylase to the hypocalcemia. When GFR decreases further (*i.e.*, GFR $<$ one-half of normal), the serum concentration of $1,25(OH)_2D_3$ decreases.[534] If phosphate intake is restricted, 1-α-hydroxylase is stimulated and PTH decreases. The decrease in PTH might be mediated by an increase in ionized calcium secondary to the increase in $1,25(OH)_2D_3$. When GFR decreases further to below 25% of normal, hyperphosphatemia develops, except in patients with a proximal tubular defect.

The radiographic signs of renal osteodystrophy include ricketslike lesions (*i.e.*, radiolucent bands), as well as signs of osteitis fibrosa related to increased PTH secretion (*i.e.*, subperiosteal resorption zones and metaphyseal changes); the latter may result in slipped epiphyses.[535] Histologic examination of the metaphysis in renal osteodystrophy shows accumulation of woven bone, fibrous tissue, or both, rather than the accumulation of cartilage and chondro-osteoid seen in rickets.[535] Although severe renal osteodystrophy, associated with GFR less than 30 mL/minute/1.73 m^2, is related to poor growth, the effect of mild renal osteodystrophy on growth is unclear; histologic bone disease can be observed at the same frequency regardless of growth status.

Aluminum Intoxication. Some of the bone changes seen in renal osteodystrophy are related to aluminum intoxication, resulting from aluminum-containing phosphate-binding gels or aluminum-containing dialysis water. In adults, a syndrome charac-

TABLE 42–13
DISTURBANCES IN MINERAL METABOLISM ASSOCIATED WITH CHRONIC LOSS OF RENAL FUNCTION IN CHILDREN

Stage	Ionized Calcium	Phosphate	$1,25(OH)_2D_3$	iPTH	Alkaline Phosphatase
Early (*i.e.*, GFR 70%–80%)	Low	Low when fasting Normal during the daytime	Normal but inadequate for low Ca	High	Normal–high
Moderate (*i.e.*, GFR < 50%)					
Normal P intake	Low	Normal	Low	High	High
Restricted P intake	Normal (low)	Low	Normal	Normal	
Advanced (*i.e.*, GFR <25%)	Low	High	Low	High	High
Aluminum intoxication	High while on vitamin D, otherwise normal	Normal–high	Normal	Normal (high)	Normal (high)

Pathophysiology in Patients With Moderate Loss of Renal Function

Normal phosphate intake:

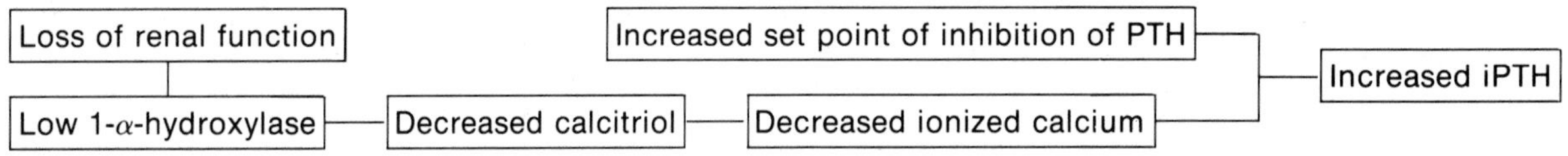

Effect of reduction in phosphate intake:

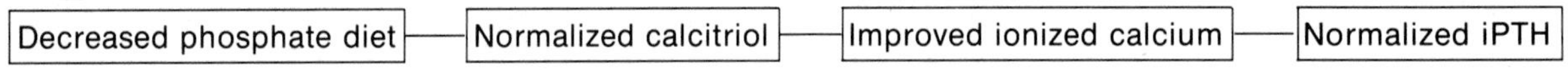

$1,25(OH)_2D_3$, serum concentration of 1,25-dihydroxyvitamin D_3 or calcitriol; Ca, calcium; GFR, glomerular filtration rate expressed in % of normal; iPTH, serum level of immunoreactive parathyroid hormone; P, phosphate.

terized by bone pain, proximal myopathy, fractures, and encephalopathy was shown to be associated with high tissue levels of aluminum.[536] Radiographs show growth zone abnormalities and metaphyseal solid bands, and accumulation of aluminum in bone can be demonstrated in biopsy specimens. Similar changes are observed in rats injected with aluminum. Aluminum-related bone disease increases in conditions associated with decreased PTH secretion, such as parathyroidectomy and administration of vitamin D.

Aluminum was removed from dialysis fluids around 1980, and aluminum-containing phosphate-binding agents were replaced by calcium carbonate in 1984.[537] Because some preparations of parenteral medications (*e.g.*, calcium gluconate, potassium and sodium phosphate, 5% albumin, heparin) may contain substantial amounts of aluminum despite lack of evidence on the package label,[538] VLBW infants on TPN may accumulate aluminum even in the absence of CRF, probably because of their limited GFR.[539–541] The Food and Drug Administration intends to set upper limits on the aluminum content of intravenous preparations.[538]

Aluminum intoxication in a patient with renal osteodystrophy may be suggested by hypercalcemia, which may occur spontaneously but most often happens during vitamin D administration. Hypercalcemia is associated with a normal alkaline phosphatase level, normal PTH levels, and metaphyseal solid bands, but any of these signs can be absent (see Table 42-12).[525] Confirmation of aluminum intoxication requires the demonstration of increased aluminum stores, which are not evaluated reliably by serum aluminum concentration, unless serum aluminum level is greater than 100 μg/L.[542] Aluminum stores are evaluated best by the increase in serum level after an intravenous desferrioxamine test, or by a bone biopsy using flameless atomic absorption spectrophotometry.

Treatment of Renal Osteodystrophy. Treatment includes removal of all sources of aluminum intake. Citrate should be used with caution in aluminum-intoxicated patients. Indeed, it has two opposite effects on aluminum balance; although it has been used as an aluminum chelator in aluminum-intoxicated mice, it also increases aluminum absorption by the gastrointestinal tract in several species as well as in patients with CRF.[543,544] The only medication that has been shown to result in efficient elimination of aluminum is desferrioxamine, which can be given intravenously during hemodialysis, or intraperitoneally.[545] Lowering calcium concentration in the dialysis fluid enhances the efficacy of desferrioxamine by stimulating PTH secretion.

Early detection of renal osteodystrophy requires sequential measurements of serum PTH level and urinary cAMP excretion; photon absorptiometry is much more sensitive than bone radiography for the detection of mild demineralization (*e.g.*, in osteopenia of prematurity), but no series have been published about its use in infants with CRF.

The treatment of renal osteodystrophy includes the administration of vitamin D analogues, which raises serum calcium, decreases PTH, improves bone changes, and may accelerate growth (Table 42-14).[546,547] The preferred forms of vitamin D are $1{,}25(OH)_2D_3$, dihydrotachysterol, and $1\text{-}\alpha\text{-}OHD_3$ because of their potency, lack of need for 1-α-hydroxylation, and short half-life, which limits the duration of hypercalcemia, should it occur. The initial doses are increased progressively until PTH reaches a normal level or serum or urinary calcium reaches the upper limit of normal. Preliminary data suggest that early administration of 10 to 15 ng/kg/day of $1{,}25(OH)_2D_3$ may efficiently prevent renal osteodystrophy, probably by inhibiting the development of hyperparathyroidism; growth in a small group of patients appeared better when the administration of $1{,}25(OH)_2D_3$ was initiated before 12 months than in patients in whom it was started after 21 months of age.[526]

An additional aspect of treatment is the administration of calcium supplements and the limitation of phosphate intake. Restriction of phosphate intake early in the course results in increased serum levels of $1{,}25(OH)_2D_3$ and limits the degree of hyperparathyroidism. This requires avoidance of cow milk and dairy products and using breast milk or formulas for premature infants, such as PM 60/40, which has a high calcium–phosphorus ratio and limited phosphate content. Calcium carbonate not only provides calcium (40% on a weight basis), but also is an efficient phosphate-binding agent, which reduces intestinal absorption of phosphate. It should be given with meals, to increase the inhibition of phosphate absorption and to decrease the absorption of calcium and limit the risk for hypercalcemia.

HEMATOLOGIC DISTURBANCE

Chronic renal failure is associated with a normochromic, normocytic, hypoproliferative anemia, resulting from many factors, including low erythropoietin (Epo) levels, shortened erythrocyte survival, iron and folate deficiency, and aluminum intoxication. Although steady-state levels of Epo are low relative to the degree of anemia, levels do increase in response to hypoxemic stress.[548]

Erythropoietin is a glycoprotein that is synthesized, under hypoxic conditions, by endothelial cells of the peritubular capillary in the renal cortex and the outer medulla.[549] Even after bilateral nephrectomy, serum levels of Epo increase progressively, which demonstrates that extrarenal sites take over that role of the kidney.[550] Children with ESRD at one time required many transfusions, which resulted in severe iron overload. Extensive experience in adults has proven that recombinant human Epo administration can correct the anemia of ESRD and eliminate the need for transfusion in almost all patients.[551] Failure to respond to Epo has been attributed to several causes, including iron deficiency, underlying inflammatory disease, aluminum intoxication, and poorly controlled hyperparathyroidism.[552] The most common side-effects are an increase in blood pressure in one third of the patients and seizures in 3%; seizures most often are associated with a sudden increase in blood pressure and hematocrit at the initiation of therapy.

The experience with the administration of Epo to children is growing rapidly. Epo administered subcutaneously or intravenously in children with ESRD resulted in an increase in hematocrit, an improvement in symptomatology, and a reduction in iron overload. The response is dose dependent. One fourth of patients responded to the administration of 25 U/kg of

TABLE 42–14
INITIAL DOSES AND SIDE-EFFECTS OF MEDICATIONS COMMONLY USED IN CHRONIC RENAL FAILURE

Medication	Initial Dose	Mineral Metabolism and Growth	Kidney	Other
Vitamin D		Hypercalcemia	Renal failure due to metastatic calcifications	Metastatic calcifications
$1{,}25(OH)_2D_3$	20–60 ng/kg/d			
DHT	15–40 μg/kg/d			
$1\text{-}\alpha\text{-}OHD_3$	1–2 μg/kg/d			
$CaCO_3$	10–20 mg/kg/d of elemental Ca	Hypercalcemia	Hypercalciuria	
Erythropoietin	25–50 U/kg 3 times/wk		Hypertension	Seizures due to hypertension

Epo two to three times a week, whereas two thirds responded to 50 U/kg.[553] Side-effects included hypertension and thromboocclusion of vascular access. Seizures and increase in liver enzymes occurred in only a minimal number of patients. Although there is no controlled study on the administration of Epo in children and infants with CRF, the administration of Epo (see Table 42-14) should be strongly considered for infants in CRF with a hematocrit below 30%. Because Epo results in increased use of iron stores[554] and decreased need for transfusions, iron supplementation should be added. During the duration of the Epo administration, hemoglobin, hematocrit and reticulocyte count, and ferritin levels should be monitored.

GROWTH HORMONE

Growth failure in CRF occurs in the absence of low levels of growth hormone or of total serum concentration of IGF-1, but with an increased concentration of the high-molecular-weight IGF-1 binding protein.[555–557] The administration of supraphysiologic doses of recombinant human growth hormone resulted in an improvement of the ratio of IGF-1 to its binding protein.[557] Administration of growth hormone for up to 4 years accelerated growth in growth-retarded children with ESRD,[557–559] without acceleration of bone maturity or other side-effects. It may be that the administration of growth hormone could prevent growth failure in infants with CRF. This hypothesis remains to be investigated.

SURGICAL TREATMENT

Surgical treatment of urinary tract obstruction and of severe VUR has an important role but may not prevent progressive loss of renal function.[560] In addition, bilateral nephrectomy is commonly performed in patients with CNF, and allows the preparation of the infant for the renal transplantation.

INFECTION

Infants with CRF are at risk for infections because of urinary stasis, malnutrition, peritoneal dialysis, and immunosuppression at the time of transplantation. Chemoprophylaxis for UTI is indicated in infants at increased risk because of VUR, ADPKD, or urinary tract obstruction, and at the time of invasive procedures. The incidence of peritonitis in children receiving either continuous ambulatory peritoneal dialysis (CAPD) or continuous cyclic peritoneal dialysis (CCPD) is similar, and ranges between one episode every 5 months and one every 12 months.[561,562] The most common agents include *Staphylococcus* sp, gram-negative organisms, and *Candida* sp.[561]

CENTRAL NERVOUS SYSTEM

The complications of CRF include polyneuropathy and encephalopathy, which can result from aluminum intoxication, hypertension, and electrolyte imbalance related to uremia. In the 1970s, a dialysis encephalopathy syndrome was described in adults receiving hemodialysis and was shown to be associated with high aluminum content in the gray matter of the brain.[542] A similar encephalopathy, characterized by regression of developmental milestones, ataxia, seizures, myoclonus, dementia, loss of bulbar function, and severe renal osteodystrophy was described in children with CRF,[563] and subsequently was associated with aluminum intoxication.[564] Since it became standard practice to remove aluminum from all dialysis fluid and to avoid aluminum hydroxide as phosphate-binding therapy, most acute CNS complications have been limited by careful monitoring of renal function; careful monitoring of blood pressure, especially during Epo administration; and early initiation of dialysis. Nevertheless, some motor and mental delay commonly is observed in children with ESRD, and electroencephalogram abnormalities are frequent in those with significant mental delay.[565,566] Successful transplantation may be associated with a significant improvement in mental performance and in an acceleration in head growth.[566]

DIALYSIS

Two modalities are available, hemodialysis and peritoneal dialysis. Since the description of CAPD in 1976, this technique rapidly has become the procedure of choice for infants, in whom the large peritoneal surface makes it more efficient than in adults. Usually, four to five exchanges are performed per day, using a Silastic Tenckhoff catheter.[522] The peritoneal dialysis fluid should have a low concentration of calcium, to avoid hypercalcemia. It should not contain aluminum; it should not contain citrate if any aluminum ingestion is possible. The advantages of CAPD over hemodialysis include better hemodynamic stability, increased serum bicarbonate concentration, decreased transfusion requirements, augmented caloric intake, and increased freedom for the patient and the family. The side-effects of CAPD are the burden to the family, the risk of peritonitis, and chronic loss of protein, calcium, and phosphate. Another technique now available is CCPD, in which five to eight 2-hour exchanges are performed automatically at night.[567] Data of the North American Pediatric Renal Transplant Cooperative Study suggest that early initiation of peritoneal dialysis, in association with nasogastric feeding to augment caloric intake, is the treatment of choice of ESRD in infants.[568]

TRANSPLANTATION

Benefits and Complications of Renal Transplantation. Although no randomized study is available, renal transplantation in children younger than 5 years of age with ESRD offers a potential of improving growth and development that is not observed in patients on long-term dialysis.[566,569,570] The success of renal transplantation in young children has improved progressively during the last two decades. This improvement has been attributed to several factors, including improvement of the patient's preoperative condition, with nutritional support and dialysis, and bilateral nephrectomy in patients with CNF; improvement in graft survival by multiple preoperative transfusions[571]; improvement in the quality of human leukocyte antigen matching, made possible both by the availability of large multicenter organizations and by the increased use of grafts from living related donors, which offer the best success rates; improvement of the surgical technique, including shortened cold storage time of the graft; improvement of anesthetic and postoperative therapy[572]; and introduction of various immunosuppressive drugs to prevent and to treat graft rejection. Available drugs include cyclosporine, azathioprine, steroids, antithymocyte globulin, antilymphocyte globulin, and monoclonal antibody against OKT_3, an antigen of T lymphocytes.[572–575]

The complications of renal transplantation include postoperative renal failure, fluid and electrolyte disturbances, hypertension, hypotension, infection, and the side-effects of the various immunosuppressive medications. Difficult problems include the early detection of rejection and differentiating renal failure due to cyclosporine from rejection or other complications of the transplant.

Controversy Over Renal Transplantation Before 1 Year of Age. The issue of undertaking renal transplantation in infancy before or after the age of 1 year is controversial. Because the best results are obtained using grafts from living related donors, determining the best time for transplantation is critical for the family.

The results of the North American Pediatric Renal Transplant Cooperative Study show that the most important factor for graft survival for cadaveric transplants is a recipient age greater than 24 months (relative risk 2.8, 95% confidence interval of (1.6–4.7), although the prognosis for living donor transplants improves as early as age 12 months with a weight of approximately 8 kg.[520,575]

In contrast, a few centers have reported excellent results using living related donor kidneys in recipients as young as 6 to 7 months or weighing 5 to 7 kg, and cadaveric transplants during the second year of life.[569,570] In such centers, the size of the donor is a more important factor for deciding the time of transplantation: an average-sized adult kidney (*i.e.*, 12–13 cm) is tolerated by the abdominal cavity of an infant with a length of 65 cm.[576] The wide differences in reported success in infants cannot be explained. Sequential administration of several immunosuppressive medications, prophylactic suppression of T-lymphocyte–related immunity for cadaveric transplants, and aggressive intraoperative administration of colloids are potential factors. At the University of Minneapolis, the 1-year and 5-year related living graft survival rates in 18 recipients less than 12 months were, respectively, 100% and 83%, with a patient survival rate of 94% and 71%, whereas the graft and patient survival rates for cadaveric transplant were 25% both at 1 year and 5 years.[519] The actuarial allograft survival was similar in infants and in 1- to 5-year-old children.[576] A more recent report from the same institution showed that infants (age range, 6 weeks–12 months) who received a graft from a living related donor, as well as cyclosporine A, had a 100% 1-year survival and improved growth.[570] It is not clear what are the critical factors associated with the good results of renal transplants in these centers. It is likely that the prognosis for renal transplantation in young infants will improve over the next few years in other institutions as well, in parallel with further improvements in immunosuppressive therapy.

PROGNOSIS

The prognosis for several types of diseases that cause CRF in infancy has improved considerably over the last two decades. The improvement in prognosis may have resulted in part from a change in the percentage of patients diagnosed during the neonatal period, due to prenatal and postnatal ultrasonography, but also from aggressive management, as described previously. The literature contains only limited data on the long-term prognosis for infants born with or rapidly developing renal failure during the neonatal period. Considerable variability in outcome remains, which depends in part on the severity of the renal dysfunction (*e.g.*, the presence of renal dysplasia in obstructive disease). Early neonatal death is related most often to respiratory failure due to pulmonary hypoplasia associated with severe cases of polycystic kidney disease (PKD) or renal dysplasia, whereas later death is related to renal failure or other complications.

The prognosis depends also on the diagnosis and the severity of the renal disease (Table 42-15). For obstructive urinary tract disease, the presence of associated renal dysplasia–hypoplasia is the main prognostic factor.[577–579] Despite early intervention and intact renal function for many years during childhood, progression to ESRD may occur. Isolated posterior urethral valves are associated with a low mortality rate and a low risk of ESRD.[577] Infants with prune-belly syndrome can be divided into three groups, according to the severity of renal dysplasia.[578] Most deaths occur in the first group, during the neonatal period, and are due to respiratory failure caused by pulmonary hypoplasia; the autopsy most often shows severe renal dysplasia involving an average of 70% of the parenchyma in most cases. Patients in the second group have mild impairment of renal function and may develop progressive CRF. Since pathologic examination of nephrectomy specimens in this second group shows evidence of pyelonephritis and obstructive or reflux nephropathy, but only mild renal dysplasia involving an average of 25% of the paren-

TABLE 42–15
PROGNOSIS OF VARIOUS CONGENITAL DISEASES AT RISK FOR END-STAGE RENAL DISEASE

Diagnosis	Transplant Offered	n	Percentage that Survive the Neonatal Period (Causes of Death)	Percentage Survival at 1 Year	Percentage of Those Surviving the Neonatal Period in Whom ESRD Develops; (Age)	Long-Term Survival	Reference
Posterior urethral valves	Yes	50	98% (UTI and sepsis)	98%	8%	96% at 2–12 y (6.8)	Connor, 1990[577]
Prune-belly syndrome	No	50	72% (respiratory failure, renal failure, or both)	68%	6%	68% at ? y (≤35)	Burbige, 1987[579]
	Yes	32	72% (respiratory failure)	66%	48%	63% at ? y	Reinberg, 1991[578]
	Yes	7	57% (CHF, stillborn,	57%	50% (13–14 y)	57% at 3–14 y	Reinberg, 1991[578]
			bronchopneumonia)		23% (1 mo–>10 y)	46% at 15 y (actuarial)	Kaplan, 1989[580]
ARPKD	No	46*	NA	79% (from birth)	41% (8 mo–16 y)	88% at 6.1 ± 4.3 y	Cole, 1987[581]
	Yes		17 (sample)	88% (from 1 mo)	100%	0% at 4 y	Mahan, 1984[582]
Nephrotic		14	100%	NA	100% (8–90 mo)	75% until transplant;	Mahan, 1984[582]
syndrome	No	27	100%	NA		82% at 2 y after transplant	
	Yes						

* This series involved 23 cases of neonatal PKD, 23 cases of infantile PKD, and 7 patients diagnosed after 1 year of age. Seven patients were lost to follow-up.

ARPKD, autosomal recessive polycystic kidney disease; CHF, congestive heart failure; ESRD, end-stage renal disease; NA, not available; PKD, polycystic kidney disease; UTI, urinary tract infection.

chyma, it appears that aggressive prevention of these complications using surgery and antibiotic therapy may decrease the incidence of ESRD in some.[578] Finally, patients in the third group, the least severe, do not have CRF and have a normal life expectancy.

Infants with ARPKD diagnosed at birth have a 46% survival rate at 15 years.[580] Those who survive the neonatal period have a high potential for survival, although portal hypertension eventually develops in one-third to one-half of them, which may require a portocaval shunt.[580,581] Other common complications include hyponatremia and systemic hypertension. Although only limited data are available on ADPKD, the prognosis for renal function seems better than in ARPKD. Of five infants who survived the neonatal period and were followed until the age of 3.5 ± 3.4 (mean ± SD) years, ESRD developed only in one.[581]

Congenital nephrotic syndrome of the Finnish type, which used to be a fatal disease, now has a much better prognosis, using bilateral nephrectomy for recovery from the nephrotic syndrome, followed by renal transplantation. Two-year patient and graft survival rates of 82% and 71%, respectively, have been reported.[582]

Obtaining an accurate diagnosis of the etiology of the CRF is as important for predicting later complications and for genetic counseling as for the management of the CRF *per se*. Assessment of renal function and anatomy in the family may clarify the type of genetic transmission and hence the probable diagnosis and prognosis in the infant. In addition, assessment of the family may result in early diagnosis of hereditary conditions, either in the parents or the siblings, and lead to genetic counseling.

HYPERTENSION

Systemic hypertension is defined by a blood pressure that persistently exceeds the mean + 2 SD for normal subjects of similar GA, size, and postnatal age (see Appendices C-1a through C-1d). Hypertension is very likely if the blood pressure consistently exceeds 90/60 torr in a full-term infant or 80/50 torr in a premature infant,[583] and is likely in an infant after the neonatal period if systolic blood pressure is higher than 113 torr.[264] The measurement of diastolic blood pressure by indirect techniques, especially the Doppler method, is only approximate.

INCIDENCE

The reported incidence of neonatal hypertension ranges between 0.2%[584] and 43%.[585] This variability may in part result from the following factors:

- The sample studied. Groups at high risk include infants who had a UA catheter (3%)[412] and those in whom BPD developed (as much as 43%).[585] Hypertension may develop in some patients only after discharge from the nursery.[586]
- The percentage of infants screened and the frequency of measurement of blood pressure in the nursery.
- The care taken in measuring blood pressure accurately at rest, not during feeding or during various examinations (see Clinical Evaluation).
- The normative values used.

ETIOLOGY AND PATHOPHYSIOLOGY

An etiology can be determined only in approximately one third of hypertensive newborn infants (see Appendices C-1e and C-1f).[587,588] Although there is a weak correlation between neonatal blood pressure and maternal blood pressure, there is no convincing evidence that essential hypertension as seen in older children and adults starts in the neonatal period. The most common mechanisms of neonatal hypertension include iatrogenic disease, renovascular hypertension, and renal disease.[587]

IATROGENIC HYPERTENSION

Direct or indirect iatrogenic causes of neonatal hypertension are shown in Appendix C-1e. Hypertension induced by pancuronium probably is mediated by release of catecholamines, the mechanism of which is unknown.[589–591] As many as 30% of infants receiving dexamethasone for BPD manifest hypertension, defined as a systolic blood pressure greater than 90 torr.[592]

Hypertension develops in 11% to 92% of newborns placed on ECMO, either immediately or at variable times after initiation of the procedure.[593] Because hypertension in these infants is more common when accompanied by high fluid intake, and it responds well to diuretic administration, fluid overload may be an important mechanism.[593] This hypothesis remains to be demonstrated by prospective studies.

Another common cause of hypertension is BPD.[585,586] Umbilical artery catheterization and the administration of corticosteroids are contributing factors in some infants, but the etiology in many remains unknown. Because hypertension often develops after discharge from the NICU, frequent monitoring of blood pressure during follow-up is important.[586,588]

Hypertension may develop after surgical repair of abdominal wall defects. Three of four patients in one series had edema of the lower extremities and normal PRA, and one had evidence for ureteropelvic obstruction and high PRA.[594] The duration of hypertension in these patients ranged from 12 days to 6 months.

RENOVASCULAR HYPERTENSION

Hyperreninemia is present in most infants with renovascular hypertension. The most common cause of neonatal renovascular hypertension is aortic or renal thromboembolism related to UA catheterization.[412] Hypertension develops in approximately 3% of infants with UA catheterization.[408,412] Hypertension may develop either while the catheter is in place or long after its removal,[595] and may be associated with a history of renal failure or hematuria. Associated signs may include hematuria, ARF in patients with bilateral renal thromboembolism, and loss of femoral pulses and of blood flow to the lower extremities in patients with extensive aortic thrombosis.

Congenital vascular anomalies responsible for renovascular hypertension in newborn infants include stenosis or hypoplasia of the renal artery,[596,597] segmental intimal hyperplasia,[598] and idiopathic arterial calcification of infancy[430]; all these anomalies may involve the aorta as well as the renal arteries. Idiopathic arterial calcification of infancy is a rare disorder for which there have been approximately 90 reported cases. It is characterized by the presence of calcium deposits in all layers of the arteries, including the aorta and the coronary arteries, as well as in the heart valves.[430,599–601] Some of these deposits may be visible on a plain radiogram. Most cases have been diagnosed at autopsy.[601]

Other causes of renovascular hypertension include neonatal renal arterial embolism in the absence of UA catheterization,[411] intramural hematoma of the renal artery,[602] renal vein thrombosis,[423] and external compression of the renal artery by hydronephrosis,[603] adrenal hemorrhage,[604] or urinoma.[605]

RENAL CAUSES OF HYPERTENSION

Hypertension is a common complication of renal anomalies and diseases such as PKD[581]; renal dysplasia[606]; tumors, of which mesoblastic nephroma is the most common in newborn infants[607,608]; hydronephrosis[609]; and interstitial nephritis.[587] Hypertension may develop in patients with ATN as a result of fluid and sodium overload. Hypertension may be associated with hyperreninemia in some cases,[610,611] especially when it occurs with renal tumors. Hyperreninemia can be either primary (*i.e.*, renin within the tumor itself), or secondary (*i.e.*, increased renin in hypertrophied juxtaglomerular cells adjacent to residual glomeruli entrapped in the tumor).[611]

COARCTATION OF THE AORTA

Coarctation of the aorta (see Chaps. 33 and 34) produces hypertension limited to the upper extremities or to the right arm, with hypotension and decreased pulse volume in lower extremities and normal PRA.

NEUROLOGIC HYPERTENSION

Neurologic causes of hypertension include intracranial hypertension, drug withdrawal, seizures, and familial dysautonomia. Although seizures are common complications of severe hypertension, blood pressure may increase transiently during seizure episodes.[612]

ENDOCRINE HYPERTENSION

Several adrenal disturbances can induce hypertension directly. Hyperthyroidism is associated with systolic hypertension and sustained tachycardia and, sometimes, with episodes of supraventricular tachycardia.[613] Neural crest tumors are uncommon in newborn infants.[614]

CLINICAL FEATURES

Mild to moderate hypertension may be asymptomatic.[615–617] The symptoms associated with hypertension are nonspecific (Table 42-16), and may be due to the underlying disease, to the hypertension itself, or to its complications (*e.g.*, neurologic, cardiovascular).[618,619] The infant's chart should be reviewed carefully for the administration of excessive fluids or of medications causative of hypertension. Infants with a UA catheter may have had transient episodes of blood pressure elevation associated with an increase in P_{cr} and hematuria, all suggestive of renal artery thromboembolism.

Pertinent points of the physical examination are listed in Table 42-16. Indirect ophthalmoscopy may reveal abnormalities similar to those observed in older patients with hypertension. Skalina and associates observed significant retinal changes in 11 of 21 newborn infants with a mean blood pressure greater than 70 torr, including increased ratio of venous to arterial caliber, vascular tortuosity including arteriovenous crossing changes, superficial and deep hemorrhages, and exudates.[620] These anomalies appeared to resolve after control of the hypertension.

INVESTIGATION

The first step is to determine whether the infant is indeed hypertensive, or if the blood pressure rises only during periods of agitation, pain (*e.g.*, even an infiltrated intravenous line may cause an increase in blood pressure), crying, feeding, or performance of procedures. All newborn infants with hypertension should have a urinalysis and routine blood chemistry tests (see Appendix C-1f). If it appears that the hypertension is iatrogenic or secondary to drug withdrawal, specific therapy can be tried before additional investigations are performed.

A thorough workup should be initiated in every patient with persistent or severe hypertension (see Appendix C-1f), both to rule out cardiovascular complications and to reach a specific diagnosis (see Appendix C-1e). If myocardial dysfunction, cardiomegaly, or heart failure is secondary to hypertension, the blood pressure should be reduced rapidly. The presence of metabolic alkalosis in a hypertensive neonate suggests the diagnosis of congenital adrenal hyperplasia (CAH) or primary hyperaldosteronism. Ambiguous genitalia in a hypertensive infant should raise the suspicion of CAH. If the maternal history is

TABLE 42–16
SIGNS AND SYMPTOMS ASSOCIATED WITH NEONATAL HYPERTENSION

	History and Observation	Physical Examination
Growth	Failure to thrive	Weight and length may be small for age
Vital signs	Tachypnea, fever	Tachypnea, tachycardia, fever
Respiratory system	Apnea, cyanosis, tachypnea	Apnea, central cyanosis, tachypnea, rales
Cardiovascular system	Sweating	Hyperdynamic precordium, heart murmur, congestive heart failure, tachyarrhythmia, mottling, peripheral cyanosis, poor perfusion, abdominal bruit, increased pulse, differential pulse in upper *versus* lower extremities, ischemia of the lower extremities with absent pulse
Fluids and renal system	Edema, hematuria	Edema
	Weight loss, polyuria	Abdominal mass
Gastrointestinal system and liver	Anorexia, abdominal distention	Hepatomegaly
Neurologic system	Irritability, lethargy, seizures	Irritability; tremors; seizures; lethargy; coma; bulging fontanelle; increased, decreased, or asymmetrical tone; facial palsy; abnormal reflexes; abnormal optic fundus
Genitalia		Hypogonadism (*i.e.*, congenital adrenal hyperplasia)

Some of these findings are directly related to hypertension, whereas other signs are related to the primary cause.

positive for Graves disease, and the infant has a goiter or is constantly tachycardic with systolic hypertension, thyroid studies should be ordered urgently.

If no cause is evident, or if a renal or renovascular etiology is suspected, the workup usually will include a US of the kidneys, adrenals, aorta, and bladder, with a flow study (*i.e.*, Doppler US with duplex scan) of the aorta and the renal arteries, as well as a renal scan and PRA[621]; IVU, angiography, MRI, or CT may be indicated in specific patients. If there is any suspicion of hydronephrosis or reflux, urine obtained by suprapubic aspiration or bladder catheterization should be sent for both bacterial and fungal culture. Of 17 patients with fungal uropathy, hypertension was one of the presenting signs in 7.[622]

If PRA is elevated compared to age-appropriate normal values for the same laboratory, a perfusion renal scan should be obtained in addition to the renal US and Doppler, since the scan is more sensitive for the detection of small defects. Renal microemboli from an umbilical artery catheter, however, can elude detection by any of the above means. High PRA may be secondary to the administration of diuretics or adrenergic medications or to severe respiratory disease, and mild elevations of PRA may be seen in normal infants. In addition, one normal value of PRA does not exclude hyperreninemic hypertension.[583]

TREATMENT

Various modalities of treatment for neonatal hypertension have been recommended. Because no prospective comparative study has been performed, knowledge is based on published case reports and series. Although malignant hypertension should be corrected immediately and vigorously to prevent central nervous system hemorrhage, the treatment of chronic or subacute hypertension usually is aimed at a rapid decrease of blood pressure to a level that is not less than approximately three-fourths of the initial value, followed by progressive normalization. A rapid decrease of blood pressure to a normal level, which is easily obtained by using the combination of a diuretic and a potent vasodilator, might place the infant at risk for both cerebral ischemia and renal failure,[505] secondary to compromised central nervous system and renal blood flow, respectively.

NONSPECIFIC TREATMENT

In many patients antihypertensive medications may not be required (see Specific Treatment). In patients with sodium or volume overload, sodium restriction with or without diuretics may control mild hypertension (see Diuretics). Many newborn infants in whom hypertension develops already are receiving diuretics, however, and more intensive diuretic therapy may cause dehydration and a further increase in PRA. In more severe cases, the treatment may consist of hydralazine, α-methyldopa, or a β-blocker. Hydralazine is used frequently as the first-line antihypertensive medication in newborn infants. Because its side-effects include fluid retention and tachycardia, it often is used in combination with a diuretic or a β-blocker or both, which also increases its efficacy.

Acute, severe hypertension probably is treated best

with the combination of sodium and fluid restriction and a potent diuretic (*e.g.*, furosemide, bumetanide), plus a potent short-term vasodilator such as diazoxide, which is an arteriolar vasodilator,[623] or sodium nitroprusside, which is both an arteriolar and venous vasodilator.[624] Although the effect of diazoxide on blood pressure is difficult to predict, the rate of administration of a nitroprusside drip can be titrated, with rapid and excellent control of severe hypertension. The major side-effect of nitroprusside is the production of cyanide and thiocyanate toxicity, suggested by the development of metabolic acidosis and increased mixed venous oxygen content secondary to decreased tissue oxygen extraction. These side-effects are uncommon with short-duration infusions of up to 4 days.[624]

Labetolol has been used successfully in a limited number of neonates with severe hypertension; its effect was reported to be more gradual than that of nitroprusside or diazoxide.[617] It is effective even in patients with renal failure.[625]

Angiotensin-converting–enzyme inhibitors (*e.g.*, enalapril, captopril) are extremely potent and have been used successfully in newborn infants[626–630]; however, they may result in prolonged and profound hypotension that requires massive doses of crystalloids and colloids and is refractory to inotropes. Such hypotensive episodes often develop at the initiation of treatment if the patient is relatively hypovolemic after diuretic administration and if inappropriately high doses are being used; correct doses in newborn infants are much lower than those in children. The most serious reservation with the use of ACE inhibitors is the risk of late-onset hypotensive episodes, even after weeks of apparently successful and well tolerated therapy. These episodes may be associated with decreased cerebral blood flow and significant central nervous system dysfunction or even cerebral infarction.[505] Although additional knowledge of ACE pharmacokinetics may lead to safer use in the future,[631] ACE inhibitors seem to be indicated only for patients with refractory hypertension.

SPECIFIC TREATMENTS

Iatrogenic Hypertension. If the infant is hypervolemic secondary to excessive administration of sodium or fluids, intake should be restricted and a diuretic—usually furosemide—administered. It is imperative to eliminate hidden sources of sodium, such as isotonic saline used to flush an arterial line and sodium-containing medications (*e.g.*, antibiotics). If fluid restriction is not possible, and severe hypertension with CHF is present, hemofiltration should be strongly considered.

If one or more medications is responsible for the hypertension, several choices are possible. In some cases, the medication can be replaced by another (*e.g.*, pancuronium can be replaced by vecuronium). In some cases, withholding the medication, decreasing the dose, or using an infusion instead of a repeated bolus may result in the resolution of the high blood pressure. On the other hand, the neonatologist may choose to use steroids in VLBW infants with severe BPD, even at the risk of mild hypertension that can be controlled by a diuretic, sodium restriction, and hydralazine. If severe hypertension develops, however, the risk of IVH, CHF, and renal failure may outweigh the possible beneficial effects on the lung disease. If hypertension develops in an infant on ECMO, the first step is to induce diuresis vigorously.[593] There is no specific treatment for hypertension that develops after closure of abdominal wall defects.[594]

Renovascular Hypertension. The choice of antihypertensive medications is controversial. Whereas ACE inhibitors are considered the drugs of choice for adults and children with renovascular hypertension, and some centers have had good success in neonates as well, many neonatologists have serious concerns about the potential major side-effects mentioned previously. Other medications, such as a β-blocker or, in the case of a hypertensive crisis, a potent vasodilator, should be tried first. The advantage of a β-blocker such as propranolol is that it reduces the secretion of renin and the release of norepinephrine. Several side-effects of propranolol (*e.g.*, bronchoconstriction, hypoglycemia) are related to absence of specificity. A more specific β_1-blocker, metoprolol, has been used in infants.

Although the treatment of aortic or renal thrombosis remains controversial, a selective approach seems justified (see Acute Renal Failure). A thrombus that compromises only renal perfusion usually can be treated using antihypertensive agents; heparinization should be considered. If hypertension cannot be controlled despite aggressive medical therapy, or if massive aortic thrombosis results in other major complications, thrombolysis should be considered, using urokinase, streptokinase, or thromboplastin antecedent.[412–414] If severe hypertension persists despite antihypertensive treatment and thrombolysis, thrombectomy or nephrectomy should be considered. Although hypertension resolves within a few months in most patients, refractory hypertension may develop in rare patients, and nephrectomy ultimately may be necessary.

Patients with renovascular hypertension due to a congenital vascular anomaly or to external compression of the renal artery should be treated surgically. Infants with unilateral renal artery disease not infrequently can be managed only with unilateral nephrectomy.[597] Hypertension due to idiopathic arterial calcification typically fails to respond to standard antihypertensive medication and to nephrectomy.[599,600]

Renal Causes of Hypertension. Surgical correction of hydronephrosis, VUR, or renal compression (see Chap. 43) usually results in cure of the hypertension, unless there is postoperative edema with postrenal failure or renal dysplasia.[632] If hydronephrosis is present, antibiotic therapy should be initiated immediately, pending results of the culture. The presence of yeast in the urine should lead to immediate initiation of systemic amphotericin therapy; if hydronephrosis is secondary to a fungus ball, surgical relief of the obstruction should be followed by local irrigation with amphotericin. Hypertension due to PKD sometimes is severe; if medical therapy fails, nephrectomy may have to be performed.

Coarctation of the Aorta. For a discussion of treatment of coarctation of the aorta, see Chapter 34.

Neurologic Hypertension. Narcotic withdrawal should be treated as described in Chapter 57. Appropriate pain relief should be given before undertaking procedures such as placement of a chest tube or performance of a cut-down and after major surgical procedures (see Chap. 58). A discussion of treatment of intracranial hypertension is presented elsewhere (see Chaps. 49 and 50).

Endocrine Hypertension. For a discussion of treatment of endocrine hypertension, see Chapter 41.

PROGNOSIS

The prognosis depends mainly on etiology, although timing of the diagnosis, presence of neurologic complications, and response to therapy are important factors. Until devices became available for routine and reliable monitoring of blood pressure in neonates, hypertension was detected early only in patients with a UA line in place. Patients in whom hypertension is diagnosed on the basis of either neurologic, cardiovascular, or renal decompensation have a high mortality rate. Nevertheless, the use of routine monitoring should allow early detection of most infants with mild to moderate hypertension, even after discharge from the nursery.

The mortality rate of patients with idiopathic calcification of the arteries or with massive aortic thrombosis remains high despite aggressive therapy. The long-term prognosis for newborn infants with thromboembolism of the renal artery or the aorta is good, often with progressive resolution of the hypertension within a year and only mild to moderate decrease in renal function.[413,415] Most hypertensive neonates with PKD or dysplastic kidney sooner or later will require nephrectomy.

DIURETICS

This section reviews the major characteristics of the various types of diuretics, classified according to their major site of action along the nephron, from proximal to distal (Table 42-17).[633]

TYPES OF DIURETICS

CARBONIC ANHYDRASE INHIBITORS

Carbonic anhydrase is present in a wide range of cell types. It is an important enzyme for the secretion of cerebrospinal fluid and for acid–base transport. Carbonic anhydrase inhibition reduces bicarbonate reabsorption by the proximal tubule; it increases the urinary excretion of Na^+, K^+, bicarbonate, and phosphate. The diuretic action of carbonic anhydrase inhibitors is limited by the presence of carbonic anhydrase–independent Na^+ reabsorption in the proximal tubule, compensatory mechanisms for Na^+ reabsorption in distal segments of the tubule, and the development of metabolic acidosis, which results from carbonic anhydrase inhibition.

Some infants with hydrocephalus respond favorably to the combination of acetazolamide and furosemide.[634] This treatment may be indicated in VLBW infants with posthemorrhagic hydrocephalus, who are too small to tolerate a ventriculoperitoneal shunt (see Chap. 50). In our experience, the side-effects of acetazolamide may be minimized by increasing the dose of acetazolamide gradually over the course of 2 weeks while carefully monitoring serum chemistries and titrating the amounts of supplementary sodium bicarbonate and potassium acetate that are needed.

OSMOTIC DIURETICS

The administration of hypertonic mannitol causes a shift of water from the intracellular fluid (ICF) to the ECF, which results in dilutional hyponatremia and hypochloremia, and increased total and medullary renal blood flow. Mannitol is filtered freely by the glomerulus. Because it is not reabsorbed in the tubule, its luminal concentration increases progressively along the nephron, which decreases tubular fluid reabsorption. This increases the backflux of Na^+ into the lumen, thereby decreasing net Na^+ reabsorption. In addition, the decreased medullary solute gradient leads to decreased urinary concentration.

Although mannitol has been reported to decrease the incidence of ARF in certain surgical situations (*e.g.*, cardiopulmonary bypass, aneurysm of the aorta, obstructive jaundice), in myoglobinuria–hemoglobinuria with shock, and in the use of radiocontrast agents in patients with CRF, and it may convert oliguric to nonoliguric ARF, it has been associated with the development of renal failure in some patients.[359] Mannitol-induced water shifts may induce hyperkalemic metabolic acidosis and, if no diuresis occurs, it may precipitate CHF by acute expansion of the ECF. On the other hand, brisk diuresis may be followed by hypernatremic dehydration unless free water is provided.

Although mannitol has been used in newborn infants, its risk–benefit ratio has not been assessed.[358,635] It is contraindicated in premature infants because of the risk of inducing an intraventricular

TABLE 42–17
EFFECTS OF VARIOUS TYPES OF DIURETICS ON URINARY OUTPUT

			Urine Characteristics								
Type of Diuretic	**Site of Major Action**	**Elimination**	FENa (%)	Volume	CH_2O	K^+	Ca^{2+}	Mg^{2+}	$H_2PO_4^-$	Cl^-	HCO_3^-
CA inhibitors	PCT	Secretion	3–6	+	+	+++	0,+	0,+	++	0	+++
Osmotic	Loop	Filtration	>10	+++	+	+	+	++	+	+	+
Loop	TAL > PCT*	Secretion	15–30	+++	+,−†	++	+++	++	++	+++	+,−‡
Thiazides	DCT > PCT	Secretion	5–10	++	0	++	−,+§	++	++	+++	+,−‡
Metolazone	DCT > PCT	Secretion	4–7	+++	0,−	0	+	+	+	+++	0
Spironolactone	CD	Metabolization	2–3	+	0	−−	+	+	+	+	0
Other K-sparing	CD > DCT‖	Variable¶	2–3	+	0	−−	−	−	+	+	+

Most of these studies were obtained in adults.

* Ethacrynic acid at usual doses does not have any significant effect on PCT reabsorption. Ethacrynic acid is not recommended because of its ototoxicity.

† CH_2O decreases during water loading and increases during dehydration.

‡ Despite decreased reabsorption of bicarbonate related to the inhibition of carbonic anhydrase, the acute result is a contraction alkalosis; chronic administration results in increased urine acidification in the distal part of the nephron.

§ Thiazides may be associated with hypercalciuria after salt-loading.

‖ Amiloride causes mild metabolic acidosis by decreasing Na^+–H^+ exchange, especially in the DCT.

¶ Amiloride is not metabolized, and acts on the luminal side. Triamterene is hydroxylated in the liver; it acts on the basolateral side.

+, increase; 0, no change; −, decrease; CA, carbonic anhydrase; CD, connecting tubule and collecting duct; CH_2O, free water clearance; DCT, distal convoluted tubule; FENa, fractional excretion of sodium; loop, thin loop of Henle; PCT, proximal convoluted tubule; TAL, thick ascending loop of Henle.

Adapted from Chemtob S, Kaplan BS, Sherbotie JR, et al. Pharmacology of diuretics in the newborn. Pediatr Clin North Am 1989;36:1231.

hemorrhage. The efficacy of mannitol in the treatment of cerebral edema in newborn infants is controversial; no benefit was observed in a randomized study (see Chaps. 49 and 50).[636,637] Thus, the use of mannitol in neonates is of questionable benefit.

LOOP DIURETICS

Loop diuretics—diuretics with a site of action in the loop of Henle—include furosemide, ethacrynic acid, bumetanide, and several other drugs. They have multiple actions that can affect blood pressure and fluid and electrolyte balance. First, they are vasodilators. They decrease peripheral vascular resistance in patients with CHF. They increase RBF and redistribute renal cortical and pulmonary blood flow. The vasodilator action, observed before any diuretic effect, is responsible for the rapid improvement of blood gas exchange and pulmonary compliance in patients with pulmonary edema (*e.g.*, in CHF, in BPD).[638]

Loop diuretics reach their site of action in the tubular lumen by secretion by the organic transport system of the proximal tubule, which is inhibited by probenecid. The major diuretic effect on the tubule results from the inhibition of chloride reabsorption at the cortical thick ascending loop of Henle, by blocking Na^+–K^+–$2Cl^-$ cotransport.[639] The increase in CH_2O induced by loop diuretics may be useful for the treatment of situations associated with fluid retention and hyponatremia.[640]

A less important potential effect is a decrease in proximal tubular fluid reabsorption, which results in part from the weak ability to inhibit carbonic anhydrase activity, due to the sulfamoylbenzoic structure. In contrast to other loop diuretics, ethacrynic acid does not have any effect on the proximal tubule at doses used clinically.

Loop diuretics decrease the reabsorption of calcium, first by decreasing the lumen-positive transepithelial potential that favors the reabsorption of calcium, and, second, by blocking active reabsorption of calcium at the cortical thick ascending limb.

Finally, loop diuretics stimulate renin secretion and PG synthesis.[641] Increased PG synthesis may be an important mediator of the effects of these diuretics; indomethacin prevents or limits all the effects of furosemide.[642]

Indications for loop diuretics include oligoanuria, prevention of oligoanuria due to indomethacin administration,[347] and fluid retention with hyponatremia (*e.g.*, SIADHS, CHF, nephrotic syndrome, liver failure). The most commonly used loop diuretic is furosemide. Bumetanide is much more potent than furosemide on a weight basis;[639] pharmacologic data are becoming available in neonates.[642a]

In newborn infants, a single dose of intravenous furosemide has an onset of action within 1 hour and a duration of approximately 6 hours (see Chap. 56). In infants with a postconceptional age of fewer than 31 weeks, the secretory clearance of furosemide is very low, suggesting that the amount of diuretic reaching the site of action is entirely dependent on GFR.

BENZOTHIAZIDES OR THIAZIDES

Similarly to loop diuretics, the benzothiazides (*i.e.*, thiazides) are secreted into the tubule to reach their site of action. Their primary action is an inhibition of the reabsorption of Cl^-, coupled with that of Na^+, at the early distal convoluted tubule. A second effect of thiazides is the inhibition of proximal reabsorption of chloride, which may be mediated in part through the inhibition of carbonic anhydrase activity secondary to the sulfonamide moiety of the benzothiazides. Finally, thiazides decrease NaCl and fluid reabsorption at the inner medullary collecting duct. In contrast to loop diuretics, they are not vasodilators.

Thiazides may decrease calciuria by enhancing reabsorption of calcium at the level of the proximal convoluted tubule in response to ECF contraction, as well as at the level of the distal convoluted tubule. A positive calcium balance as a result of hypocalciuria is noted during chronic thiazide administration, except after salt loading or during sodium replacement.[643] Thiazide administration may result in a prolonged increase in total and ionized serum calcium concentration.[644]

Thiazides generally are ineffective in patients with renal failure. There is good evidence to show that the association of a thiazide and a potassium-sparing diuretic is effective in the treatment of VLBW infants with BPD.[645] In addition, because of their hypocalciuric effect, they are indicated for the prevention and the treatment of nephrocalcinosis in patients with hypercalciuria (see Hypercalciuria). Finally, they are used for the treatment of NDI in association with a PGSI (see Tubular Dysfunction).

QUINAZOLINE

Like the thiazides, metolazone, a quinazoline, is an inhibitor of the reabsorption of sodium and chloride at the diluting segment, but its action is more complete and more prolonged. In contrast to thiazides, metolazone causes little or no increase in urinary potassium excretion, and its diuretic action on the proximal tubule is independent of carbonic anhydrase, which is not blocked by metolazone. It also has an antihypertensive action.

Metolazone is efficient even in patients with CRF, if higher dosage is used.[646] It has been used successfully in adults and children with edema refractory to furosemide and thiazides,[647] as well as in VLBW infants with BPD in whom tolerance to furosemide develops.[648]

POTASSIUM-SPARING DIURETICS

Potassium-sparing diuretics, including spironolactone, triamterene, and amiloride, inhibit sodium reabsorption by the principal cells of the connecting tubule and the cortical collecting duct and thereby decrease potassium secretion. Spironolactone is a steroid analogue and competes with aldosterone for binding to intracellular receptor proteins. Metabolites of spironolactone, including canrenone, also have antimineralocorticoid activity. In contrast to spironolactone, the effect of the two other potassium-sparing diuretics is independent of aldosterone. Triamterene is hydroxylated in the liver and exerts its action on the basolateral side of the tubule. Amiloride is not metabolized; its major effect is the blockade of an electrogenic Na^+ channel on the luminal membrane of the collecting duct, thereby reducing K^+ secretion. In addition, usual doses of amiloride decrease Na^+ reabsorption and completely block K^+ secretion at the distal convoluted tubule, causing a mild metabolic acidosis by decreasing Na^+–H^+ exchange in this segment.

In newborn infants, the most commonly used potassium-sparing diuretic is spironolactone. Potassium-sparing diuretics are used most often in addition to a thiazide. They are especially useful in situations associated with primary hyperaldosteronism (see Hypertension) or hyperaldosteronism secondary to CHF, nephrotic syndrome, or liver failure.[649] They also may be used for the treatment of Bartter syndrome and, in association with a PGSI, for the treatment of NDI (see Tubular Dysfunction).[650]

STRATEGY IN USING DIURETICS

The choice of diuretic depends on the acuity of hypertension or fluid overload, on the adequacy of renal function, and on the expected side-effects. For emergencies (*e.g.*, cardiovascular or respiratory failure as a result of fluid overload), loop diuretics are the best choice because of their rapidity of action and their potency. In most patients with lung edema, fluid restriction should be initiated along with diuretic therapy. Since the goal of the administration of diuretics is a decrease in ECF and a decrease in body sodium content, mild hyponatremia (130–135 mEq/L) should be expected. The clinician should avoid the vicious cycle of diuretic–low serum sodium concentration–increased sodium intake–more hypertension or lung edema–more diuretic; however, potassium and chloride depletion should be prevented.

Both hypokalemia and hypochloremic metabolic alkalosis[651] are common complications of thiazide or loop diuretic administration, unless the patient has renal failure or appropriate preventive therapy is initiated. Despite decreased reabsorption of bicarbonate related to the inhibition of carbonic anhydrase, acute thiazide or loop diuretic administration results in a "contraction" alkalosis because of a reduction of the ECF volume and a relatively low bicarbonate concentration in the urine.[652,653] During chronic diuretic administration, metabolic alkalosis results from increased distal urine acidification, which may be due to hypokalemia, mineralocorticoid excess, and increased delivery of Na^+ to the distal convoluted tubule, where protons are secreted in exchange for Na^+. There is serious concern about the effects of metabolic alkalosis associated with diuretic therapy both in adults with chronic obstructive pulmonary disease and in infants with BPD.[652] Thus, both potassium depletion and metabolic alkalosis should be treated or, better, prevented by adding KCl or a potassium-sparing diuretic as soon as diuretic therapy is initiated, except in the presence of renal failure.

Resolution of peripheral edema is neither an emergency nor a priority. An effective circulatory volume and normal blood pressure should be maintained carefully at all times; this is especially critical when a potent vasodilator is administered to a patient with marginal circulatory volume (*e.g.*, during administration of tolazoline, antihypertensive medications, general anesthesia). In a patient with low circulatory volume and abnormally low serum protein concentration (*e.g.*, postoperative phase, third space losses, nephrotic syndrome, hydrops fetalis) with visceral (*e.g.*, pleural, peritoneal, pericardiac) fluid accumulation, the circulatory volume should be expanded with colloids before administration of diuretics.

During chronic diuretic therapy, the sensitivity to a single diuretic decreases progressively, as a result of compensatory mechanisms for solute reabsorption at other sites of the nephron.[648,654] Thus, the combination of two diuretics from different groups often is required. To minimize bone calcium loss and prevent nephrocalcinosis and nephrolithiasis (see Nephrotoxicity), thiazides should be used as first choice for chronic diuretic therapy, rather than loop diuretics. The association of a thiazide and spironolactone is efficient in premature infants with BPD[645]; intermittent doses of furosemide can be added to this regimen when necessary. In refractory patients, the association of metolazone and furosemide should be considered.[648]

BACTERIURIA AND URINARY TRACT INFECTIONS

Until the early 1970s, significant bacteriuria was defined as a colony count of 10^5/mL or greater in specimens obtained either by bag or by clean catch. It was shown subsequently that such samples frequently are contaminated by perineal flora. There is general agreement that in infants, bacteriuria can be diagnosed with certainty only by culturing samples obtained by invasive techniques (*i.e.*, bladder catheterization, suprapubic aspiration). There is no consensus, however, about the magnitude of bacteriuria required to reach significance (Table 42-18).

In this review, only those series in which bacteriuria or candiduria was established by invasive technique will be considered. Bacteriuria in newborn infants can be either asymptomatic or an indication of

TABLE 42–18
METHODS OF DIAGNOSIS OF BACTERIURIA OR URINARY TRACT INFECTIONS IN NEWBORN INFANTS

	Suprapubic Aspiration	Bladder Catheterization
Contraindications	No clinical or US evidence for presence of urine in the bladder Abdominal distension, peritonitis, organomegaly Hemorrhagic tendency, thrombocytopenia Local skin infection	Hypospadias, phimosis, local skin infection
Complications*	Microscopic hematuria (common); gross hematuria, hypovolemia requiring transfusion; bladder wall hematoma, urinary tract obstruction; aspiration of bowel content; bowel perforation, peritonitis; perforation of abdominal organ; abdominal wall abscess; sepsis, death	Microscopic hematuria (common), gross hematuria (rare), UTI
Positive culture	$\geq 10^2$ or 10^5 organisms/mL†	$\geq 10^4$ or 10^5 organisms/mL†
Indeterminate culture	$<10^2$ or 10^5 organisms/mL	$<10^4$ or 10^5 organisms/mL

* Except for hematuria, most complications are very rare.
† Some authors define UTI as a count $\geq 10^5$/mL of a single bacterial species.[669,687,720]
US, ultrasound; UTI, urinary tract infection.

pyelonephritis, which is characterized by local and systemic inflammatory response. Lower UTI (*i.e.*, cystitis) usually cannot be diagnosed on clinical grounds in newborn infants, except when associated with hematuria.

FREQUENCY IN NEWBORN INFANTS

The frequency of bacteriuria demonstrated by suprapubic aspiration or bladder catheterization ranges between 0% and 2.0% in an unselected neonatal population and between 0.6% and 10% in a NICU population.[655–668] Risk factors include prematurity (frequency of bacteriuria is 0%–10%),[660,663,666,667] male gender (male–female ratio ranges from 1:1 to 9:1 in newborn infants),[655,656,661,663–667] and absence of circumcision (relative risk of UTI during the first month of life is ten times as high in uncircumcised as in circumcised males).[664–668] The frequency of UTI in uncircumcised male newborn infants was found to be similar to that in females.[664] The frequency of UTI also is increased in infants with urinary tract anomalies and after invasive procedures.

PATHOPHYSIOLOGY

The risk of UTI depends on bacteriologic factors (see Chap. 48), including the size of the inoculum and the virulence of the organism, as well as host characteristics. Periurethral cultures obtained in uncircumcised infants show higher total bacterial counts, as well as a higher prevalence of *Escherichia coli* than cultures obtained in circumcised infants.[669] Virulence factors include the ability of bacteria to adhere to uroepithelial cells, the presence of specific antigen combinations, hemolysin, endotoxin, or colicin, and resistance to the bactericidal effect of the serum. The normal defense against UTI includes maintenance of an adequate flow of urine and complete emptying of the bladder. Either may be compromised by urinary tract obstruction or bladder dysfunction (*e.g.*, neurogenic bladder).[670,671] The relationship between UTI and VUR is discussed elsewhere in this chapter (see Underlying Abnormalities) and in Chapter 43. In addition, the normal anatomic barrier (*i.e.*, the bladder outlet) may be compromised by urinary tract malformation or manipulation (*e.g.*, prolonged or repeated bladder catheterization). Immune defenses in general are described in Chapter 46. In the case of pyelonephritis, endocytosis of bacteria is performed not only by inflammatory cells but also by proximal tubular cells; in parallel, an increase in cellular superoxide dismutase is observed.[672]

PATHOLOGY

Acute pyelonephritis commonly is associated with nephromegaly. It is characterized by the presence of polymorphonuclear leukocytes in the glomeruli, tubules, and interstitium.[673,674] Some glomeruli are completely destroyed, whereas others are infiltrated with leukocytes and surrounded by fibrin. The tubules are necrotic, dilated, and their lumens are filled with polymorphonuclear cells and bacteria. Suppuration may develop in the kidney, often with multiple abscesses at autopsy, as well as other parts of the genitourinary tract. Chronic or recurrent pyelonephritis is characterized by infiltration of chronic inflammatory cells, loss or hyalinization of glomeruli, and atrophy of tubules, with obstruction of the lumen with colloid casts. The development of renal scars may not occur until after 1 year of life.

CLINICAL PRESENTATION

The percentage of infections that are asymptomatic is high in some series,[657,659,660] and low in others.[663] The clinical presentation of UTI in newborn infants may include one or more of the following signs[662]:

Growth failure and gastrointestinal symptoms. Failure to thrive, excessive weight loss, poor feeding, diarrhea, and vomiting are the most common clinical features of neonatal UTI.

Jaundice. The hyperbilirubinemia observed in newborn infants with UTI may be either direct or indirect and sometimes is associated with hemolytic anemia. It is commonly the main clinical feature at presentation and may be the only sign of UTI in some infants.[662,675–677]

Temperature instability or fever (temperature ≥ 38°C). Urinary tract infection has been reported in 7.5% to 11% of febrile infants presenting to the emergency room during the first 8 to 12 weeks of life.[668,678]

Irritability, lethargy.

Abnormal urination. This includes poor urinary stream, malodorous urine, and polyuria, which may lead to severe dehydration.

Signs associated with bacteremia (*e.g.*, respiratory distress) or with focal infection (*e.g.*, mucocutaneous candidiasis, omphalitis).

Hypertension. This may develop as a result of hydronephrosis associated with the UTI (see Complications).[679]

LABORATORY FEATURES

URINALYSIS

Based on specimens obtained by bladder catheterization or suprapubic aspiration, only one-half of febrile outpatients with documented UTI during the first 3 months of life had an abnormal urinalysis defined either by the presence of more than five leukocytes per high power field or by the presence of any bacteria.[668] The positive predictive value of pyuria on samples obtained by suprapubic aspiration ranges between 71% (pyuria > 10 leukocytes/mm^3)[658] and 96% (pyuria ≥ 20 leukocytes/mm^3).[666] Thus, although the presence of pyuria, at least on a sample obtained by suprapubic aspiration, is suggestive of UTI, its absence is insufficient to rule out UTI.[667,680,681] Microscopic demonstration of yeast cells in urine obtained by suprapubic aspiration or bladder catheterization is very suggestive of candiduria.

URINE CULTURE

Clean voided urine or urine collected by a bag, even after cleansing the perineum, often yields a false-positive culture, when a simultaneous culture of urine obtained by suprapubic aspiration or bladder catheterization is negative. On the other hand, a negative culture of urine obtained by a noninvasive technique is sufficient to rule out bacteriuria; this may avoid the need for invasive collection of urine in a substantial number of patients.[660] The validity of suprapubic aspiration and bladder catheterization for detecting significant bacteriuria in newborn infants was demonstrated by the fact that both techniques only rarely yield equivocal bacterial counts, in contrast to bag-collected samples (*i.e.*, bacterial counts most often are either > 10^5/mL or < 10^3/mL; see Table 42-18).[655,682]

The incidence of UTI during the first 3 days of life is very low among infants suspected of sepsis.[683,684] Thus, urine culture usually is part of a sepsis workup only if the infant is more than 3 days of age. If antibiotic therapy is to be started immediately because of suspicion of sepsis, urine should be obtained by suprapubic aspiration or by bladder catheterization. In other cases, these invasive procedures can be delayed until the result of a culture obtained from a bag-collected specimen is positive.

COMPLICATIONS

Acute complications of UTI in newborn infants include bacteremia; suppuration; VUR; urinary tract obstruction, sometimes associated with hypertension or acute renal failure; severe hydromineral imbalance;[685] methemoglobinemia;[686] and ARF, which may be associated with urinary tract obstruction or massive VUR.

The incidence of bacteremia in association with UTI in infants depends on the population studied. Crain and colleagues[668] and Krober and associates[678] reported an incidence of 6% in infants under 2 months of age and in infants under 3 months of age who presented with fever in the emergency room. On the other hand, the incidence of bacteremia in patients with UTI was found to be 29% in infants under 1 month of age and 31% to 36% in neonates.[665,687]

Suppurative complications of UTI are extremely rare in newborn infants. Only one case of renal abscess in the neonatal period has been reported; the predisposing factor was congenital nephrotic syndrome.[688] Other sites of abscess include the perirenal area, where abscess can be caused by group B streptococci;[689] the prostate; and other genitourinary organs.

Vesicoureteral reflux is observed commonly during the acute stage of UTI; it often decreases or disappears after treatment and may reappear at the time of recurrent infections.[690,691] Intraparenchymal reflux is associated with a high risk of renal scarring (see Chap. 43).

Bacterial UTI can be associated with the development of hypertension in infants with hydronephrosis.[609] Mycotic UTI can lead to the development of fungus balls, which may cause obstruction in the renal pelvis or the bladder[622,679,692–694]; this may lead to the development of an abdominal mass, systemic hypertension, and anuria.

INVESTIGATION

PYELONEPHRITIS *versus* BACTERIURIA

Once bacteriuria is documented, the clinician should differentiate between pyelonephritis, which presents a high risk for renal scarring, and asymptomatic bacteriuria, which presents a low risk for renal scarring. Clinical and laboratory features suggesting the diagnosis of pyelonephritis include fever, an increase in leukocyte count with a left shift, an elevated sedimentation rate, an increase in the serum concentration of C-reactive protein, and renal tubular dysfunction.[695–697] Unfortunately, none of these tests, alone or in combination, can reliably establish the diagnosis or predict the development of renal scars.[695] Although bacterial or fungal pyelonephritis may cause parenchymal hyperechogenicity,[312,694] the sensitivity and the specificity of US to diagnose pyelonephritis have not been evaluated.

Since ^{99m}Tc-DMSA binds to the proximal tubules and is excreted only minimally into the urine, it yields excellent visualization of the functioning parenchyma, and is therefore ideal for the detection of cortical defects.[317] The presence of focal, multifocal, or diffuse areas of decreased cortical uptake was shown reliably to detect pathologic inflammatory changes in a piglet model of acute pyelonephritis.[698] Thus, the ^{99m}Tc-DMSA scan may be the most reliable indicator of acute pyelonephritis. In addition, the DMSA scan has a very good predictive value (80%) for the development of renal scars.[699] One study included newborn as well as older infants with UTI, in whom the DMSA scan was performed after resolution of the infection, which was always after 1 month of age; defects detected by the DMSA scan were associated with VUR and with the development of renal scars.[700]

SEPSIS

On diagnosing UTI, a systemic infection must be ruled out. Most often a full sepsis workup is performed.[683]

RENAL FUNCTION

Renal glomerular and tubular function should be assessed at the time of the diagnosis and during treatment and follow-up. Urinary tract infection can be associated with transient or permanent decrease in GFR, RTA, decreased urine concentrating ability, or other tubular damage demonstrated by increased NAG enzymuria.[696]

UNDERLYING ABNORMALITIES

Although US of the entire urinary tract should be obtained immediately, further evaluation for the presence of a congenital or acquired urinary tract anomaly should be performed after the infection has resolved. The recommended approach has changed considerably over the last decade.[701–704] Although previously used routinely, IVU is almost never performed in the neonatal period because of poor visualization as a result of limited renal function during the first weeks of life and the risk of nephrotoxicity inherent to radiopaque contrast products. Ultrasonography and VCUG have become the procedures of choice. Because VUR associated with UTI often decreases after resolution of infection, the VCUG most often is delayed by approximately 1 month,[705] unless the US demonstrates an abnormality that requires further investigation or surgical intervention.

During the last few years, the DMSA scan has become routine for the workup of acute UTI in infants, children, and adults.[703,706] It may be reasonable to perform VCUG only in children with abnormal US or DMSA scan,[706] but this needs further confirmation before being accepted as the standard approach.

TREATMENT

The treatment of UTI is discussed in Chapter 48. The interval of administration of the antibiotics may have to be adjusted during the course of therapy, since renal function may be compromised both by aminoglycoside or amphotericin nephrotoxicity and by pyelonephritis. The interval of gentamicin administration can be modified according to P_{cr}.[294] A cephalosporin can be substituted, if renal failure develops. Third-generation cephalosporins, piperacillin, and aztreonam[707] are alternatives to the ampicillin–gentamicin combination and are chosen according to local epidemiology. A repeat urine culture should be obtained during treatment and after completion of the antibiotic therapy. In the case of failure to respond to treatment, US should be repeated, antibiotic therapy may have to be adjusted, and a systemic infection or other foci should be ruled out. Low-dose antibiotic therapy may be indicated after the initial 10-day course until the VCUG or the DMSA scan is performed, at least in those patients with abnormal US.[705]

Therapy for asymptomatic bacteriuria in the absence of bacteremia can be given orally after the first few days. It is possible that shorter courses for the treatment of asymptomatic bacteriuria may be adequate,[705] but this has not been evaluated in newborn infants. Although most neonatologists recommend treating bacteriuria in any infant during or after the neonatal period regardless of the presence or absence of symptoms,[708,709] growing evidence supports simple observation of infants and children with asymptomatic bacteriuria.[705,710] Additional experience in newborn infants must be obtained before withholding of therapy for asymptomatic bacteriuria can be recommended.

Surgical intervention may be required for patients with severe VUR and those with urinary tract obstruction (see Chap. 43).[711] If a fungus ball is associated with urinary tract obstruction or does not disappear during systemic treatment, daily washings with amphotericin B through a bladder catheter or a nephrostomy tube usually are a necessary addition to systemic therapy.[712–714]

LONG-TERM COMPLICATIONS AND FOLLOW-UP

In patients with pyelonephritis or urinary tract anomalies, GFR, urinary concentrating ability, and tubular acidification should be assessed serially. The development of renal failure, once a common complication of UTI in small children, is observed only rarely, except in patients with major urinary tract malformations and renal dysplasia.

Although the association between segmental hypoplasia of the kidney (*i.e.,* Ask–Upmark kidney), VUR, and UTI has been known for more than a decade,[715,716] the development of renal scars remains a serious potential complication.[717] In patients in whom UTI develops before 1 year of age, approximately one-half of the kidneys with VUR will develop renal scars, and 70% of the kidneys that eventually develop scars have VUR.[706] Several risk factors for formation of renal scars can be identified early, including UTI associated with specific strains of *E. coli*[718]; grades III to IV VUR, especially if complicated by recurrent infections[668,717,718]; and abnormal DMSA scan at the time of the UTI.[699] In the piglet model, the DMSA scan was shown to have a sensitivity of 85% and a specificity of 97% for detection of scars caused by VUR and UTI.[719] Infants at risk for chronic renal scarring need long-term follow-up by a nephrologist and a urologist, including repeat urine cultures and sequential isotopic scans, and should be considered for prophylactic antibiotic therapy.[691]

PREVENTION

Several epidemiologic studies have shown an association between circumcision and a higher frequency of UTI in the neonatal period and early infancy. It is possible, however, that other, unassessed factors may explain these differences, at least in part. In one of the studies, a high incidence of urinary tract malformations (26%) was found in uncircumcised boys.[720]

Intermittent bladder catheterization with anticholinergic medication is performed more and more frequently in infants with neurogenic bladder associated with myelodysplasia; this method has been shown to result in a lower frequency of long-term deterioration of the radiologic appearance of the kidney, despite a relatively high incidence (19%–42%) of bacteriuria–UTI.[721,722] It appears that prophylactic antibiotic administration may reduce the risk for UTI, but this has not been evaluated prospectively.[722]

Chemoprophylaxis usually is recommended after a first UTI for infants with VUR or other urinary tract anomalies.[723] The role of chemoprophylaxis in newborn infants with prenatally diagnosed urinary tract malformations has not been established. In one series of 25 infants, prenatal dilation of the urinary tract led to early diagnosis of VUR in the neonatal period.[724] Chemoprophylaxis was associated with absence of infection in 17 infants, a single infection in 3, and 2 or more infections in only 5.

TUBULAR DYSFUNCTION

In this section, tubular disorders that present commonly in the neonatal period are discussed, in addition to those for which early onset of treatment during the neonatal period may modify or delay the evolution toward renal failure. The reader is referred to other sources for discussion of uncommon disorders not included here.[319,725]

HYPERCALCIURIA, NEPHROCALCINOSIS, AND NEPHROLITHIASIS

There are many causes of hypercalciuria, with or without hypercalcemia (Table 42-19). Congenital disorders associated with decreased renal tubular reabsorption of calcium include distal RTA,[726] X-linked hypophosphatemic rickets during vitamin D and phosphate therapy,[727,728] arthrogryposis multiplex congenita with renal and hepatic anomalies (see Appendix I-1), Bartter syndrome, and hyperprostaglandinuric tubular syndrome.[729] Prenatal development of nephrocalcinosis has been observed in neonatal familial hyperparathyroidism associated with hypercalciuria and distal RTA, partly associated with proximal RTA.[726]

In the absence of hypercalciuria, nephrocalcinosis may develop in infants with cystinosis (see Fanconi Syndrome) or with primary hyperoxaluria (see Primary Oxalosis and Hyperoxaluria). Hypercalciuria and nephrocalcinosis, however, are associated most commonly with prematurity, which is the subject of this section.

NEPHROCALCINOSIS AND NEPHROLITHIASIS IN PREMATURE INFANTS

Incidence. In 1982, ten premature infants 28 to 34 weeks of GA with birth weights from 700 to 1950 g were described with abdominal calcifications visible on plain radiography; renal localization of the calcification was demonstrated by ultrasonography. Their calciuria was ten times greater than that of control infants of similar GA who had no calcification and had not received furosemide.[730] In eight of these ten patients, urinalysis showed calcium oxalate crystals. All ten infants had been receiving furosemide (≥2 mg/kg/day) for respiratory distress for at least 12 days. Administration of chlorothiazide resulted in a fourfold to fivefold decrease in calciuria and disappearance of radiologically detectable calcification. Urinary tract infection developed in six of the ten

TABLE 42–19
MECHANISMS OF NEPHROCALCINOSIS AND NEPHROLITHIASIS IN INFANCY

Hypercalciuria
Increased calcium intake with or without hypercalcemia
Excessive calcium intake orally or intravenously
Rapid calcium infusion
Hypervitaminosis D
Low phosphate intake
Decreased renal tubular reabsorption
Furosemide, ethacrynic acid, aldactone
Extracellular volume expansion
Osmotic diuresis
Phosphate depletion syndrome
Distal renal tubular acidosis, type I
Arthrogryposis multiplex congenita with renal and hepatic anomalies
Bartter syndrome
Hyperprostaglandinuric tubular syndrome with hypercalciuria and hypokalemia
Increased bone reabsorption
Primary hyperparathyroidism, including neonatal familial hyperparathyroidism
Secondary hyperparathyroidism
Acidosis
Hyperthyroidism
Chronic corticosteroid therapy
Hypophosphatasia
Other Mechanisms
Factors facilitating precipitation of calcium phosphate and oxalate
Low urine output
Alkaline urine
Absence of inhibitors (*e.g.*, citrate, inorganic phosphate, magnesium)
X-linked hypophosphatemic rickets during phosphate and vitamin D administration
Other causes of nephrolithiasis
Primary oxaluria
Cystinosis

infants, including three with recurrent UTI-related sepsis. Autopsy performed in four of seven infants who died of respiratory failure showed nephrolithiasis and calcium deposits in the interstitium of the renal papillae as large as 0.5 mm and composed of calcium oxalate and calcium phosphate, but autopsy did not show tubular calcifications, such as those seen in nephrocalcinosis in other age groups, or hydronephrosis.

Since that first report, US has become more sensitive than plain radiography in detection of nephrocalcinosis, and furosemide has become widely used for the treatment of BPD. The incidence of nephrocalcinosis or nephrolithiasis in premature infants (<32 weeks of GA) is 25% to 60%.[731–734]

Definition. Hypercalciuria was defined in 1- to 15-year-old children either as urinary calcium excretion greater than 6 mg/kg/day (0.15 mmol/kg/day),[735] or as a urinary calcium–creatinine ratio greater than 0.4 ± 0.06 mg/mg (mean ± SD; 2 mmol/mmol).[735] Although factoring urinary calcium excretion for creatininuria allows the use of spot urine rather than timed collections, values established in children may not be adequate for LBW infants, because the low muscle mass in LBW infants is associated with a 40% lower rate of creatinine excretion than in children (see Clinical Evaluation). Normal values of calcium–creatinine ratio in full-term infants during the first 9 days of life were found by Goldsmith and associates to be a maximum of 0.15 mg/mg.[736]

Pathophysiology. The mechanisms responsible for hypercalciuria include increased calcium intake or gastrointestinal absorption, decreased renal tubular calcium reabsorption, and abnormal regulation of bone mineral content.[737] Chronic use of discontinuous daily calcium infusions is associated with recurrent periods of hypercalcemia and hypercalciuria.[736] High enteral calcium intake from using a formula associated with high calcium and phosphate retention may be associated with hypercalciuria in the absence of hypercalcemia.[738] Chronic phosphate depletion due to insufficient phosphate intake may result in hypophosphatemia, hypercalcemia, hypercalciuria, and osteopenia of prematurity.[739] Increased phosphate intake results in a decrease in calcemia and reduces calciuria.[740]

Although infants at highest risk for nephrocalcinosis and nephrolithiasis are those receiving prolonged furosemide therapy for chronic lung disease,[733] not all affected infants have received furosemide.[731,741] Acute administration of furosemide induces a tenfold increase in calciuria in premature infants[742]; this effect is related to the inhibition of calcium reabsorption at the level of the ascending limb of the loop of Henle. Chronic administration of furosemide is associated with a mild increase in calciuria,[731] which leads to a negative calcium balance.[743] Furosemide-induced hypercalciuria may lead to secondary hyperparathyroidism and demineralization in some infants.[744]

Hypercalciuria also is associated with administration of ethacrynic acid—another loop diuretic—and spironolactone.[745,746] Thiazides usually increase tubular reabsorption of calcium, both directly and by decreasing extracellular volume (see Diuretics).[643,644,737] In some patients, however, thiazide administration induces an increase in calciuria, attributed in premature infants to increased sodium intake and natriuresis.[745] Hypercalciuria associated with TPN in adults has been attributed to excessive calcium intake[747]; high protein intake, which increases not only GFR but also fractional excretion of calcium[748]; and the acid load.[749] Addition of acetate to the TPN resulted in a significant decrease in calciuria in the absence of any change in serum levels of calcium, PTH, or vitamin D.[749] Acute as well as chronic acid loading induces bone calcium reabsorption and hypercalciuria.

Because neither the level of calciuria[731] nor the total

dose of furosemide[741] separates LBW infants with nephrocalcinosis or nephrolithiasis from other LBW infants, the development of nephrocalcinosis in an individual infant appears to be multifactorial. Factors in addition to those mentioned include low urine output and the oxalaturia that is associated with the use of TPN.

Treatment and Prognosis. Although nephrocalcinosis and nephrolithiasis are not associated with any specific signs or symptoms and tend to decrease during the first year of life, in some patients they are associated with compromised renal function.[733,741] Follow-up to 1 to 2 years of age has shown signs of tubular dysfunction in patients with persistent calcifications, including decrease in tubular reabsorption of phosphate, increase in FENa, and limitation of distal renal tubular acidification.[750]

Low-birth-weight infants with BPD should be screened by ultrasonography for nephrolithiasis and for hyperechogenicity of the renal pyramids; those with abnormal ultrasonography should have a measurement of calciuria, which is the first step in the differential diagnosis (see Table 42-19).[313] Prevention of hypercalciuria includes administering enough phosphate and avoiding chronic administration of calcium boluses and of furosemide; the latter should be used only when other diuretics are ineffective or contraindicated. To the extent possible, thiazides should be used in place of furosemide to limit both the development of chronic renal compromise and of severe bone demineralization.

PRIMARY HYPEROXALURIA AND OXALOSIS

Pathophysiology. Primary hyperoxaluria is a rare disorder, two types of which have been described. Type I (*i.e.*, glycolic aciduria) is an autosomal recessive disorder, due to a functional deficiency in the hepatic peroxisomal enzyme alanine glyoxylate aminotransferase, for which pyridoxine is a cofactor.[725] This defect results in excessive production of oxalate, glyoxylic acid, and glycolic acid. The severity of type I is related to the progressive accumulation of calcium oxalate in various tissues, a condition called oxalosis. Type II hyperoxaluria (*i.e.*, L-glyceric aciduria) is a very rare disorder that probably is transmitted as an autosomal recessive trait, and does not cause oxalosis.[725]

Clinical Presentation and Diagnosis. Approximately 12% of patients with primary hyperoxaluria present in infancy, with anorexia, failure to thrive, vomiting, dehydration and fever; presentation in the neonatal period is rare.[751–753]

Treatment. In patients with type I hyperoxaluria, early administration of high doses of pyridoxine should be tried in an attempt to limit the development of oxalosis.[754] Therapy includes pyridoxine, inhibitors of calcium oxalate precipitation, and a large fluid intake (2 L/m^2/day). Aggressive therapy, including dialysis, of hyperoxaluria type I does not prevent oxalosis and ESRD. The most severely affected infants (*i.e.*, those with the neonatal form with oxalosis) usually die before the age of 1 year. Although renal transplantation initially may be successful,[755] it usually is disappointing because of rapid accumulation of oxalate in the graft, leading to recurrent renal failure. Combined liver–kidney transplantation has been performed successfully in at least 22 patients.[756,757] Early liver transplantation before ESRD appears to be a promising approach.[758]

FANCONI SYNDROME

PATHOPHYSIOLOGY

Fanconi syndrome is characterized by a generalized dysfunction of the proximal tubule. The cardinal signs are renal glucosuria, renal phosphaturia, and generalized aminoaciduria; other features, present inconsistently, include RTA (see Renal Tubular Acidosis), tubular proteinuria, increased urinary excretion of urate, sodium, potassium, and calcium, and decreased ability to concentrate the urine and to secrete PAH.[759] In some cases, distal tubular dysfunction is present, and the disease evolves toward renal failure, with less evidence of tubular dysfunction.

Because several transport systems are deficient in this syndrome, the pathophysiologic process presumably involves a global disturbance such as an alteration of the integrity of the tubular membranes or of sulfhydryl-requiring enzymes.[759]

ETIOLOGY

Idiopathic cases of Fanconi syndrome most often are sporadic, although autosomal recessive, autosomal dominant, and X-linked recessive transmission have been described.[760] Fanconi syndrome occurs in association with a variety of acquired and congenital disorders (Table 42-20), the most common of which is cystinosis.[761] Disorders associated with late onset renal dysfunction, such as glycogenosis type I and Wilson disease, will not be reviewed here. General discussions of galactosemia, fructose intolerance, tyrosinemia, and vitamin D–deficient rickets can be found in Chapters 36 and 39.

CLINICAL FEATURES AND DIAGNOSIS

The clinical presentation of Fanconi syndrome includes polyuria, polydipsia, dehydration, and failure to thrive. Signs include acidosis, hypophosphatemia, and rickets. The diagnosis is confirmed by the demonstration of glucosuria in the presence of a normal glycemia (<120–150 mg/dL), decreased tubular reabsorption of phosphate, and generalized hyperaminoaciduria. The prognosis of Fanconi syndrome depends on the underlying disorder.

TABLE 42–20
CAUSES OF FANCONI SYNDROME IN INFANCY

	Secondary	
Idiopathic	Inherited (AR Unless Specified)	Acquired
Isolated	Cystinosis	Renovascular accident in neonatal period
Deal syndrome (AR)	Fructose 1,6-diphosphatase deficiency	Interstitial nephritis
	Hepatorenal tyrosinemia	Medications (*e.g.*, valproate, aminoglycosides)*
	Galactosemia	Nephrotic syndrome
	Glycogenosis with Fanconi syndrome (*i.e.*, Fanconi–Bickel syndrome)	Renal transplantation
	Oculocerebrorenal (Lowe) syndrome (X-linked)	Toluene; heavy metal poisoning
	Vitamin D–dependent rickets	Vitamin D–deficiency rickets
		Dysproteinemia

* Fanconi syndrome also has been reported after administration of other medications in older patients.
AR, autosomal recessive.

TREATMENT

The treatment includes replacement therapy, usually of sodium phosphate, sodium citrate, and potassium citrate and, if rickets has developed, vitamin D administration. Indomethacin has been given successfully in some patients. Specific diet therapy for fructose intolerance, galactosemia, or tyrosinemia results in disappearance of the Fanconi syndrome. In many other diseases, treatment serves only to slow the deterioration of renal function.

SPECIAL CONSIDERATIONS

Cystinosis. The reported incidence of cystinosis ranges between 1:20,000 and 1:326,000.[319] It is an autosomal recessive lysosomal storage disease, due to a defect in the carrier-mediated transport of cystine from the lysosomes to the cytosol.[762] The infantile (*i.e.*, nephropathic) type of cystinosis is the most severe form.[319,759]

At birth, patients with cystinosis appear normal except for lighter skin and hair pigmentation than in siblings. Signs of Fanconi syndrome appear by 3 to 12 months of age. In some patients, the initial presentation may suggest a diagnosis of Bartter syndrome or of NDI.[763] Patients also have photophobia, which is secondary to retinopathy; the latter is characterized by generalized, often patchy, depigmentation of the peripheral retina and pigment clumps, and may be detected within the first weeks of life.[764] In contrast, characteristic corneal opacities appear only after 1 year.

Laboratory findings include urinary excretion of typical cystine crystals, generalized hyperaminoaciduria, mild to moderate glucosuria, severe phosphaturia, RTA, marked increase in urinary excretion of nonaminated organic acids, and tubular or mixed glomerular and tubular proteinuria.[761] Progressive deterioration of the GFR leads to ESRD at a median age of 9.2 years.[765]

The treatment of cystinosis in infancy includes the nonspecific treatment of Fanconi syndrome and the administration of cysteamine (*i.e.*, β-mercaptoethylamine) hydrochloride.[766] Cysteamine administration to children with cystinosis results in improvement of growth and delay in progression of the renal failure.[766] The administration before 2 weeks of age has been shown in a limited number of patients to delay the progression of the renal disease.[767] Tolerance of cysteamine is limited by its foul taste and odor; this may result in suboptimal intake of the medication and early development of ESRD. Phosphocysteamine, which lacks the taste and odor of cysteamine, may replace it in the future if collaborative trials show equivalent efficacy.

Deal Syndrome. Deal and colleagues described a new, probably autosomal recessive, syndrome, characterized by ichthyosis, jaundice, musculoskeletal deformities, diarrhea, failure to thrive, and early onset Fanconi syndrome; all six patients with this syndrome have died within the first 6 months of life.[768]

Glycogenosis With Fanconi Syndrome. More than 20 patients have been described with Fanconi–Bickel syndrome (*i.e.*, glycogenosis with Fanconi syndrome), an autosomal recessive disorder characterized by impaired use of galactose and glucose and hepatorenal glycogenosis.[760] In the kidney, glycogen accumulation is limited to the proximal tubule, with maximal levels in the straight part. The etiology is unknown. This syndrome should be differentiated from glycogenosis type I, which is due to glucose-6-phosphatase or glucose-6-phosphate translocase deficiency and is associated with late onset of proximal tubular dysfunction in approximately 15% of the cases.[769]

Fever, vomiting, growth failure, and rickets develop in the patients within 6 weeks to 10 months of birth, followed by hepatomegaly, protuberant abdomen, moon-shaped face, and fat deposition around the shoulder and the abdomen.[760,770] Laboratory findings include glucosuria on the first day of life, galactosemia on the fourth day, and hypophosphatemia by the eighth week. The Fanconi syndrome is severe. Over time, GFR does not decrease and the tubular defects improve. Hepatic glycogenosis causes a tendency toward hypoglycemia, ketonuria, hypercholesterolemia, and hypertriglyceridemia, but no lactic acidosis. The diagnosis of Fanconi–Bickel syndrome is confirmed by normal enzyme activity in liver or kidney biopsy.

Particular attention should be given to treating possible acute decompensations at the time of surgery or infections. Hypoglycemia can be prevented by frequent protein-enriched feedings. The treatment of the nephropathy is nonspecific.

Galactose-1-Phosphate Uridyl Transferase Deficiency. Galactosemia (see Chap. 39) is an autosomal recessive disorder that results in intracellular accumulation of galactose-1-phosphate in various tissues, including the kidney. Symptoms often develop in the neonatal period, soon after initiating lactose intake (*i.e.*, milk), and include hypoglycemia, anorexia, vomiting, diarrhea, hepatomegaly, jaundice, and hypoprothrombinemia.[771] Renal dysfunction develops within 2 weeks after initiation of galactose intake; it is characterized by severe proteinuria, generalized aminoaciduria, and a significant defect in transport of phosphate, bicarbonate, and PAH.[771–773] Lactose intake leads to galactosuria, which produces a positive test for reducing substances but no glucosuria. Removing lactose and galactose from the diet results in rapid resolution.[771]

Hereditary Fructose Intolerance. Hereditary fructose intolerance is an autosomal recessive disorder due to deficiency in fructose-1-phosphate aldolase which normally is present in the liver, small intestine, and renal cortex (see Chap. 39). In patients with fructose intolerance, ingestion of fructose results in the accumulation of fructose-1-phosphate in these tissues. Other tissues either possess another isoenzyme of the aldolase (*e.g.*, muscle, brain) or lack the enzymes required to metabolize fructose (*e.g.*, renal medulla) and therefore are not involved. Although fructose is not part of the normal diet in the neonatal period, the routine use of sucrose has been recommended for sedation during neonatal procedures such as circumcision.[774,775]

A single dose of fructose immediately will induce hypophosphatemia, generalized hyperaminoaciduria, RTA, proteinuria, and phosphaturia; mild glucosuria may be present.[776,777] Liver failure may result in high plasma concentrations of tyrosine and methionine, and thereby in a pattern of aminoaciduria similar to that seen in tyrosinemia. Removal of fructose and sucrose from the diet results in normalization of tubular function within 2 weeks.

Hepatorenal Tyrosinemia. Hereditary tyrosinemia type I (*i.e.*, hepatorenal tyrosinemia, tyrosinosis) is an autosomal recessive disorder due to a deficiency in fumarylacetoacetate hydrolyase (*i.e.*, fumarylacetoacetase); maleylacetoacetate hydrolyase may be decreased as well (see Chap. 39).[725] More than 100 cases have been reported. Accumulation of succinylacetoacetate and succinylacetone results in renal tubular dysfunction and inhibition of hepatic metabolism of tyrosine and of porphobilinogen synthase.

Clinical presentation includes failure to thrive, a cabbagelike odor, vomiting, diarrhea, severe metabolic acidosis, hepatomegaly, jaundice, melena, ascites, edema, fever, and tubular dysfunction.[778,779] Renal dysfunction includes hyperaminoaciduria, severe phosphaturia, and mild proteinuria, but no glucosuria.[778,779] The acute form of tyrosinemia type I is associated with liver failure and death by the age of 1 year in most untreated patients. Removal of phenylalanine, tyrosine, and methionine from the diet results in normalization of tubular function but does not prevent liver failure.

Oculocerebrorenal Dystrophy. More than 100 cases of Lowe syndrome (*i.e.*, oculocerebrorenal dystrophy) have been reported (see Chap. 39). Fanconi syndrome appears in infancy, includes proteinuria, generalized aminoaciduria, phosphaturia, intermittent glucosuria, RTA, and carnitine wasting, and causes rickets and failure to thrive.[780] Glomerular involvement develops progressively in childhood and eventually leads to renal failure.[781,782] The treatment includes alkalinization therapy and supplements of potassium, phosphate, calcium, and carnitine.

NEPHROGENIC DIABETES INSIPIDUS

The differential diagnosis of polyuria in infancy includes central diabetes insipidus (see Chap. 41) and nephrogenic defects in urinary concentration. The latter defects can result either from a decreased effect of ADH on tubular permeability to water or from a decreased corticomedullary osmotic gradient (Table 42-21). Several entities, congenital[783] or acquired, may result in impaired urinary concentration. Many of these disorders are discussed in other sections of this chapter or in Chapter 41; therefore, only NDI is reviewed here.

PATHOPHYSIOLOGY

Nephrogenic diabetes insipidus is characterized by lack of V_2 receptor-mediated response to arginine vasopressin.[784] This disorder usually is transmitted as

TABLE 42–21
ETIOLOGY OF NEPHROGENIC DEFECT IN URINARY CONCENTRATION

Decreased Effect of Antidiuretic Hormone on Tubular Permeability to Water Gradient	Decreased Corticomedullary Concentration
Congenital	
Nephrogenic diabetes insipidus	Medullary cystic disease, polycystic kidney disease
Hypokalemia	Bilateral dysplastic kidneys
Bartter syndrome	Urinary tract obstruction
Hyperprostaglandinuric tubular syndrome	
Pseudohypoaldosteronism	
Proximal renal tubular acidosis	
Duplication of the mitochondrial genome	
Acquired	
Drugs (*e.g.*, PGE_2, PGE_1, amphotericin, lithium)	Polyuria (*i.e.*, water/osmotic diuresis)
Hypokalemia	Obstructive disease before and after treatment
Hypercalcemia	Chronic or acute renal failure
	Pyelonephritis
	Nephrocalcinosis
	Medullary necrosis
	Malnutrition

PG, prostaglandin.

an X-linked recessive trait, but other modes of transmission have been proposed. The NDI gene has been mapped to the distal long arm of chromosome X by linkage analysis of affected kindreds with restriction fragment length polymorphism.[785] The molecular basis for the disease has not been determined.

CLINICAL PRESENTATION AND DIAGNOSIS

Most patients with congenital NDI present with polyuria, dehydration, fever, and constipation. If untreated, mental retardation may develop. Pertinent laboratory findings include a persistently low urine osmolality, even if there is evidence for dehydration, and hypernatremia. There is no other evidence of tubular dysfunction.

The diagnosis of NDI is confirmed by the failure to respond to intranasal administration of DDAVP, in contrast to patients with central diabetes insipidus (*i.e.*, ADH deficiency). The response of urinary cAMP can be compared to that seen in vasopressin-sensitive diabetes insipidus (*i.e.*, 200%–250% increase).[786] Diagnosis *in utero* can be made by linkage analysis if other family members have the disease.[785] Female carriers do not present with any symptomatology, but they may have mild impairment of urine-concentrating ability.

TREATMENT

Thiazide diuretics result in a decrease in urine output.[787] Prostaglandin synthesis inhibitors, especially indomethacin, additionally reduce urine output; successful long-term results are obtained in most patients, in association with a decrease in urinary PGE_2 excretion. The most common therapeutic regimen is the combination of chlorothiazide, indomethacin, and potassium supplements.[787,788] Preliminary data suggest that an alternative may be the use of amiloride and hydrochlorothiazide, without potassium supplements.[785]

HYPOKALEMIC ALKALOSIS

The differential diagnosis of hypokalemic alkalosis in infancy is given in Table 42-22. The discussion in this section is limited to the renal causes.

BARTTER SYNDROME

Bartter syndrome is a sporadic or familial disorder, characterized by hypokalemic alkalosis, impaired urinary-concentrating ability, hyperaldosteronism, hyperreninemia, hyperplasia of the juxtaglomerular apparatus, and normal blood pressure.[789] The etiology presumably is a PG-independent defect of chloride transport at the level of the thick ascending loop of Henle.[790] Hyperkaliuria may result from the primary defect itself, from increased distal flow, or from secondary hyperaldosteronism. Hypokalemia stimulates PGE_2 and prostacyclin synthesis; the latter, together with increased serum bradykinin concentration, leads to generalized vasodilation. High PRA and sympathoadrenal activity are critical in maintaining a normal blood pressure, whereas hypersecretion of PGE_2 and bradykinin results in pressor resistance to angiotensin II and norepinephrine. Decreased urinary diluting ability results from the defect in chloride reabsorption, whereas decreased urinary concentrating ability results from the combination of

TABLE 42–22
DIFFERENTIAL DIAGNOSIS OF HYPOKALEMIC ALKALOSIS

Inadequate intake
Cl^--deficient diet
Insufficient K and Cl intravenously
Gastrointestinal losses
Vomiting, pyloric stenosis
Gastric suction
Cl^- diarrhea
Kidney
Diuretics (*e.g.*, loop diuretics, thiazides)
Hypovolemia and other cause for hypokalemia (*e.g.*, proximal RTA, cystinosis)
Bartter syndrome
Gitelman syndrome
Hypercalciuria syndrome with hyperprostaglandinuria
Endocrine
Primary hyperaldosteronism
Cushing syndrome
Congenital adrenal hyperplasia with hypertension
11β-Hydroxylase deficiency
17α-Hydroxylase deficiency
11β-Hydroxysteroid dehydrogenase deficiency
Cystic fibrosis

RTA, renal tubular acidosis.

hypokalemia, increased PGE_2, and a decreased corticomedullary gradient. The defect in chloride reabsorption in the thick ascending loop of Henle could be the cause of decreased magnesium reabsorption in that segment. In addition, patients with Bartter syndrome have a circulating inhibitor of platelet aggregation, which results from PG metabolism disturbance.[791]

Patients with Bartter syndrome typically present with failure to thrive, polyuria, polydipsia, and a tendency to dehydration. Bartter syndrome may present rarely in the neonatal period.[792] In contrast to adults, nephrocalcinosis secondary to hypercalciuria develops in children with Bartter syndrome.[793]

Laboratory abnormalities include hypokalemic, hypochloremic alkalosis, elevated PRA, a high serum aldosterone, creatinine, and uric acid, and low magnesium concentration. Renal abnormalities include hyperkaliuria, hypercalciuria, high excretion of PGE_2 and 6-keto-prostaglandin-$I_{1\alpha}$ (6-keto-$PGI_{1\alpha}$), decreased fractional water clearance, decreased concentrating ability and, in some patients, high excretion of magnesium.

The treatment includes supplementation with KCl and, if necessary, $MgCl_2$. If this is insufficient, either a potassium-sparing diuretic or a PGSI is indicated. The administration of indomethacin decreases PG, bradykinin, PRA, and sympathoadrenal activity, but fails to correct the hyperkaliuria and the chloride reabsorption defect, as shown by persistence of impaired concentration and dilution ability.[790]

HYPERPROSTAGLANDINURIC TUBULAR SYNDROME

This syndrome has also been called calcium-losing tubulopathy, hypercalciuric Bartter syndrome, and congenital hypokalemia with hypercalciuria.[729] Although it was thought initially to be a neonatal variant of Bartter syndrome with enhanced renal and systemic formation of PGE_2, the primary cause probably is a defect in tubular calcium reabsorption, rather than high secretion of PGE_2 or a defect in tubular chloride reabsorption.[794] Although the disorder shares several features with Bartter syndrome, hyperkaliuria is not as severe, and spironolactone administration results in normalization of the urinary excretion of potassium. In addition, the fractional excretion of water is normal. Prostaglandin E_2 hypersecretion contributes to increased bone resorption, increased renal 1-α-hydroxylase, decreased tubular reabsorption of calcium, and decreased urinary concentration ability.[795–797]

Clinical features include polyhydramnios, premature labor, failure to thrive, and episodes of fever, vomiting, diarrhea, renal electrolyte and water wastage, and hypercalciuria with nephrocalcinosis and osteopenia.[729]

Laboratory abnormalities are similar to those seen in Bartter syndrome, except that there is no increase in prostacyclin, hypokalemia may be mild or intermittent, and fractional water excretion is normal.[729,794]

Prolonged treatment with indomethacin results in substantial improvement of clinical and most biochemical features, although some degree of hypercalciuria persists. The response to indomethacin is much better than in Bartter syndrome.

GITELMAN SYNDROME

Gitelman syndrome or magnesium-losing nephropathy (*i.e.*, primary renal tubular hypokalemic metabolic alkalosis with hypocalciuria and magnesium deficiency) is a benign autosomal recessive disorder that frequently is complicated by febrile seizures and tetanic episodes. It is not associated with polyhydramnios, prematurity, defect in urinary concentration, or hypercalciuria.[793,798]

RENAL TUBULAR ACIDOSIS

Metabolic acidosis in newborn infants usually is normochloremic with an increased serum anion gap. The most common cause is lactic acidosis resulting from asphyxia, ischemia, hypoxemia, or local tissue damage. Less commonly, it is due to a congenital metabolic disorder (see Chap. 39) or to renal failure.

Hyperchloremic metabolic acidosis results from bicarbonate losses through the gastrointestinal tract or the urinary tract. Increased bicarbonaturia may result from either renal tubular acidosis (RTA) or a defect in urinary acidification attributed to a deficit in distal sodium delivery; the latter commonly is observed in association with diarrhea.[799,800] In contrast to adults, the urinary anion gap is not a valid measurement in newborn infants.[801]

Clinical presentation of RTA includes polyhydramnios, polyuria with episodes of dehydration, failure to thrive, vomiting, and serum biochemical disturbances. Failure to thrive appears to be a direct consequence of acidosis; correction of acidosis often results in catch-up growth, unless other complications (*e.g.*, rickets, renal failure) have developed.

DIFFERENTIAL DIAGNOSIS

Four types of RTA have been described: classical distal (*i.e.*, type I), proximal RTA (*i.e.*, type II), hyperkalemic distal (*i.e.*, type IV), which is the most common type of RTA, and mixed proximal and distal (*i.e.*, type III; Table 42-23).[319,802–804] The differential diagnosis depends on the findings of hypertension, hyponatremia and salt wasting, hyperkalemia, generalized proximal tubular dysfunction, decreased ability to acidify the urine, UTI, nephrocalcinosis, or urinary tract malformation. Further workup (*e.g.*, measurement of urinary ammonium, titratable acid, or PCO_2; ammonium chloride, sodium sulfate, or bicarbonate loading) may be required in specific cases, in consultation with a nephrologist.[801–805]

PROXIMAL RENAL TUBULAR ACIDOSIS

Proximal RTA or type II may be caused by a defect of one of the mechanisms involved in bicarbonate absorption in the proximal tubule or occur in association with other signs of proximal tubular dysfunction (*e.g.*, Fanconi syndrome). Although it may be a primary defect, it is associated most often with other entities. The diagnosis is suspected when the serum bicarbonate concentration is low for age and urinary *p*H is adequately low in the presence of mild to moderate acidosis. The diagnosis is confirmed either by the presence of a Fanconi syndrome, or by measuring the urinary concentration of bicarbonate at various serum levels during a bicarbonate infusion.

Treatment consists in the administration of sodium bicarbonate or citrate (initially at 5–10 mEq/kg/day) and potassium citrate. In some patients, acidosis will persist despite administration of high doses of alkali; hydrochlorothiazide or PGSI may be beneficial. Patients with Fanconi syndrome require additional therapy (see Fanconi Syndrome).

DISTAL RENAL TUBULAR ACIDOSIS

Several criteria have been proposed for the diagnosis of defects in distal RTA,[806–808] including the inability to decrease urinary *p*H during metabolic acidosis, limited urinary ammonium concentration, limited urinary PCO_2, and decreased difference between urinary and arterial blood PCO_2.

Hyperkalemic Distal Renal Tubular Acidosis. Hyperkalemic distal RTA or type IV is the most common type of distal RTA. It results from the association of defects in K^+ and H^+ secretion at the level of the collecting duct.

Primary type IV RTA or early-childhood hyperkalemic RTA has been described in some infants and children who presented with failure to thrive and frequent vomiting.[803] These patients had isolated signs of distal RTA with hyperkalemia, without nephrocalcinosis, and responded very well to alkali therapy.

Type IV RTA can be associated with a variety of disorders. These secondary cases of type IV RTA can be divided into five groups (see Table 42-23).[803] Subtype 1 is caused by primary aldosterone deficiency or adrenal insufficiency in the absence of intrinsic renal disease. Subtypes 2 and 3 are caused by hyporeninemic hypoaldosteronism secondary to advanced renal disease, and are very rare in infancy. Subtypes 4 and 5 are caused by unresponsiveness to aldosterone.

The treatment of type IV RTA includes correction of the metabolic acidosis, limitation of potassium intake, and specific therapy for each specific disorder.

Classic Distal Renal Tubular Acidosis. In classic or type I RTA, there is no defect of potassium secretion; nephrocalcinosis and nephrolithiasis are common.[809] The development of nephrocalcinosis is attributed to the association of hypercalciuria, high urine *p*H, and low citraturia.[810]

Idiopathic RTA type I in infants can be associated with bicarbonate wastage. It can be hereditary, and may be associated with several other conditions (see Table 42-23).

The treatment includes the administration of sodium bicarbonate or citrate and potassium citrate. Administration of citrate is important for the prevention of nephrolithiasis.

Mixed Renal Tubular Acidosis. In some disorders, both proximal and distal RTA are present; this is known as mixed RTA or type III (see Table 42-23). Very-low-birth-weight infants during the first days or weeks of life have a mild degree of mixed tubular acidosis, with lower normal values of serum bicarbonate concentration and higher urine *p*H despite metabolic acidosis (see Renal Physiology).

HYPERPHOSPHATURIC SYNDROMES

Hyperphosphaturia results from decreased proximal tubular reabsorption. Whereas severe hypophosphaturia may result from hyperparathyroidism or Fanconi syndrome, mild hyperphosphaturia occurs in association with the administration of diuretics (*e.g.*, loop diuretics, carbonic anhydrase inhibitors, thiazides) or proximal tubular toxicity from drugs or toxins. Other causes of hypophosphatemia such as vitamin D–deficiency rickets and hypophosphatemia of

TABLE 42–23
ETIOLOGY OF RENAL TUBULAR ACIDOSIS IN INFANCY

Proximal RTA (Type 2)	Hyperkalemic RTA (Type 4)*	Distal RTA (Type 1)	Mixed (Type 3)
Primary			
AR, AD Sporadic transient	Early childhood hyperkalemic RTA	With bicarbonate wasting in infancy and early childhood AR with sensorineural deafness AD, sporadic With cystic fibrosis	Familial hyperparathyroidism with hypercalciuria and RTA (Nishiyama[726]) VLBW infant
Secondary			
Fanconi syndrome Metachromatic leukodystrophy† Mitochondrial diseases Hereditary nephritis Tetralogy of Fallot† Vitamin D deficiency Vascular accident in neonatal period Hereditary nephritis Carbonic anhydrase inhibition Carbonic anhydrase II deficiency with osteopetrosis (AR) Drugs and toxins (*e.g.*, valproic acid, heavy metals)	1: Primary hypoaldosteronism, adrenal insufficiency 2–3: Hyporeninemic hypoaldosteronism with chronic renal disease‡ 4: Pseudohypoaldosteronism with or without salt wasting 5: Partial unresponsiveness to aldosterone Toxins, drugs, K-sparing diuretics Tubulointerstitial disease Urinary tract obstruction, UTI Unilateral dysplastic kidney or RVT Drugs (*e.g.*, KCl, K-sparing diuretics, heparin, ACE inhibitors, PGSI, cyclosporine)	Hypergammaglobulinemia (*i.e.*, maternal Sjögren syndrome) Fetal alcohol syndrome Toluene, amphotericin B, lithium Hypercalcemic hyperthyroidism Vitamin D intoxication Nephrocalcinosis Medullary sponge kidney Urinary tract obstruction Carnitine palmitoyltransferase type I deficiency† Carbonic anhydrase II deficiency with osteopetrosis (AR)	Carbonic anhydrase II deficiency with osteopetrosis (AR) Hyperparathyroidism Nephrocalcinosis and Fanconi syndrome Renal transplantation

Renal tubular acidification may also be deficient in the case of renal failure (*i.e.*, normochloremic metabolic acidosis) or of acute diarrhea (*i.e.*, hypochloremic metabolic acidosis).

* Numbers represent subtypes.

† The only patients with this type of RTA were diagnosed after more than 12 months of age.[119]

‡ Subtypes 2 and 3, associated with hyporeninemic hypoaldosteronism, are mostly seen in adults.

ACE, angiotensin-converting enzyme; AD, autosomal dominant; AR, autosomal recessive; PGSI, prostaglandin synthetase inhibitor; RTA, renal tubular acidosis; RVT, renal venous thrombosis; UTI, urinary tract infection; VLBW, very low birth weight.

the premature infant caused by insufficient phosphate intake are discussed in Chapter 36.

FAMILIAL HYPOPHOSPHATEMIC RICKETS OR VITAMIN D–RESISTANT RICKETS

This is the most common disease associated with hyperphosphaturia in infancy. It is transmitted most often as an X-linked disorder. Low tubular reabsorption of phosphate is due to a mutation at a locus in region Xp22.31-p21.3.[811]

Clinical signs, including bone deformations, usually appear after the first year of life. Hypophosphatemia and low tubular reabsorption of phosphate can be detected during the first month of life when family cases are known.[812]

The treatment includes oral supplementation with sodium and potassium phosphate and $1,25(OH)_2D_3$.

VITAMIN D–DEPENDENT RICKETS OR PSEUDOVITAMIN D–RESISTANT RICKETS

In this disorder, increased phosphaturia is due to hyperparathyroidism. In type 1, which is the most frequent and is transmitted as an autosomal trait, hyperparathyroidism results from a defect of renal synthesis of $1,25(OH)_2D_3$ due to a defect of 1-α-hydroxylation in the proximal tubule.[813] In type 2, there is a lack of sensitivity of target organs to $1,25(OH)_2D_3$,[814–816] which, at least in some patients, is due to defective nuclear uptake of the hormone.[815]

This disorder presents during infancy with typical signs of rickets including hypotonia, tetany, irritability, motor retardation, deformations and growth failure. Some patients with type 2 have alopecia.[816] Serum levels of $1,25(OH)_2D_3$ are lower than normal in type 1 and very high in type 2. At birth, serum calcium and phosphate levels are normal, but gastrointestinal absorption of calcium is decreased.

Patients with type 1 respond to the administration of physiologic doses of 1-α-OHD_3 or $1,25(OH)_2D_3$.[813] In type 2, a response is observed only when extremely high doses are used.[816]

GLUCOSURIA

Several disorders are associated with renal glucosuria: an isolated defect, or primary glucosuria, which is a benign condition; congenital glucose–galactose malabsorption; Fanconi syndrome; and other rare entities. They all are associated with mild to moderate glucosuria, which does not require specific therapy.[817,818]

In VLBW infants, the incidence of glucosuria is increased because of two factors: decreased tubular reabsorption of glucose (see Renal Physiology) and instability of glycemia.[819] At a mean GA of 29 weeks, glucosuria appears when glycemia exceeds 152 ± 8 mg/dL.[819] This may lead to osmotic diuresis, which is associated with loss of several electrolytes, especially sodium and potassium, and may cause severe dehydration. The treatment includes careful replacement of the urinary losses. Prevention of hyperglycemia is a much better approach. Glycemia should be kept at a maximum of 120 to 150 mg/dL, using insulin if required in specific patients (see Chap. 35).

URIC ACID

INCREASED SERUM URIC ACID CONCENTRATION

Because the risk of uric acid precipitation is favored by a high urinary concentration and a low urine *p*H, the newborn infant is at relatively low risk for tubular obstruction by uric acid crystalluria, despite low ability of the immature renal tubule to reabsorb uric acid. Drug-induced decrease in uric acid excretion (*e.g.*, secondary to diazoxide, diuretics, dopamine, ethambutol) may result in higher serum levels but not in renal toxicity. Uric acid crystalluria with tubular obstruction has been described rarely in newborn infants with ARF secondary to perinatal asphyxia[820]; the treatment is nonspecific. The prevention of uric acid nephropathy in patients at high risk includes maintaining a high tubular flow rate by the administration of high volumes of alkaline fluids.[821] Allopurinol is indicated for infants with hyperuricemia secondary to neoplasia.[822]

DEFECTS OF TUBULAR HANDLING OF URIC ACID

Increased urinary excretion of uric acid may result from various medications (*e.g.*, ascorbic acid, glycine, citrate, and iodinated radiocontrast agents) and rare defects of tubular handling of uric acid. These disorders may be suspected on the basis of family history, low serum concentration of uric acid, or crystalluria. Early diagnosis may allow specific therapy and prevention of urolithiasis, which may develop in childhood.

CONGENITAL NEPHROTIC SYNDROME

Nephrotic syndrome is defined by the association of marked proteinuria (>1 g/m^2/day) with hypoalbuminemia (<2.5 g/dL). A nephrotic syndrome is called congenital if it presents within the first 3 months of life; this definition is based on the natural history of the Finnish type, the most common type of nephrotic syndrome in newborn infants.

FINNISH TYPE

CLINICAL PRESENTATION AND LABORATORY FINDINGS

The incidence of CNF is estimated to be 1.2 per 10,000 births in Finland[823]; CNF should be suspected if there is a history of CNF in a sibling, hydrops fetalis or edema of the placenta (*i.e.*, placental weight > 25% of birth weight), or an elevated α-fetoprotein or total protein concentration in the amniotic fluid. Since the disease begins *in utero* in all patients, an increased α-fetoprotein (>10 SD above the mean amniotic fluid concentration during the second trimester) is a reliable indicator of the disease.[823]

The natural history of the disease is based on experience before the availability of renal transplantation in young patients.[582,823–825] The mean GA was 36.6 ± 1.8 weeks (mean ± SD), and 42% of the infants were premature (<37 weeks of GA). Many infants were SGA, especially those with a GA at or above 37 weeks. In some patients, the typical signs of nephrotic syndrome (*i.e.*, edema, proteinuria, hypoalbuminemia) did not develop until the third month of life. The evolution of the disease was not affected by the administration of steroids or cytotoxic medications.[582] Complications included severe failure to thrive and ascites in all patients, severe bacterial infections in 85%, pyloric stenosis in 12%, and thrombotic events in 10%.[582] An increase in P_{cr} or BUN was observed in approximately 20% of the patients, but none had frank uremia. One-half of the patients died by 6 months of life, and all of them by 4 years. The immediate cause of death appeared to be infection in one third. Autopsy showed thrombi in large vessels in 19%. Since this early report, aggressive management has considerably improved the survival rate (see Treatment and Prognosis).

The proteinuria, initially very selective (*i.e.*, almost entirely albumin as a result of increased permeability of the glomerulus only for small proteins), increases progressively and becomes nonselective, corresponding to increased sieving coefficient and to tubular damage.[825] Blood chemistry is significant for low serum albumin concentration and total thyroxine concentration as a result of low thyroxine-binding globulin, a normal or mildly elevated P_{cr}, and hyperlipidemia. Ultrasonography shows enlarged kidneys, increased echogenicity of the renal cortex compared to the liver and the spleen, decreased differentiation between cortex and medulla, and poor visualization of the pyramids.[826] Tubular dilations may be misinterpreted as other causes of cystic disease, including ARPKD.[827] The diagnosis is confirmed by renal biopsy (see Histopathology).

HISTOPATHOLOGY

Although the basic defect in CNF is unknown, the pathologic findings are characteristic. Glomerular changes are seen by scanning electron microscopy in human fetuses at 13 to 24 weeks of GA.[828] Renal biopsy in infancy shows irregularities of the glomerular basement membrane and thinning of the lamina densa,[828] followed by fusion of the epithelial cell foot processes, all of which are similar to the findings in minimal-change, steroid-sensitive nephrotic syndrome. On light microscopy, the mature glomeruli initially typically show only minimal abnormalities, including mild mesangial hypercellularity and an increase in mesangial matrix. Immature-appearing glomeruli show a dilated urinary space surrounding a small glomerular tuft. Progressive changes include obliteration of capillary loops and glomerular hyalinization. Immune deposits become visible by electron microscopy within the mesangium only at late stages of the disease.

Except in the early stages, the biopsy frequently shows dilated tubules from both proximal and distal origin (*e.g.*, microcystic disease). Although these tubular changes have been used by some neonatologists as a diagnostic criterion, they are not pathognomonic and have caused some confusion in the differential diagnosis. Although the etiology of the tubular dilation is unknown, it has been attributed to the heavy proteinuria.[829] Progressive interstitial fibrosis and tubular atrophy develop; the latter is well correlated with increasing proteinuria.[823]

TREATMENT AND PROGNOSIS

Infants with CNF require intensive management, which includes repetitive administration of albumin and diuretics for ascites, oral and parenteral hyperalimentation, and the treatment of multiple complications.[582] Chronic renal insufficiency develops between 6 and 23 months of age. As a consequence, most patients eventually receive dialysis while waiting for transplantation. All reported infants treated before the availability of renal transplantation died, mostly of infection. In one report, of the 17 patients who received renal transplantation, the 2-year patient and graft survival rates were 82% and 71%, respectively.[582] Recurrence of nephrotic syndrome was not observed after transplantation. Most infants had a normal or accelerated growth, although the mean height remained significantly lower than normal. Although 16 of 17 had delayed psychomotor development at the time of transplantation, marked improvement was evident 1 year later, and 12 of 15 surviving children had normal school and social performance (range, 2.5–17 years).

OTHER CAUSES

DIFFERENTIAL DIAGNOSIS

Several entities are associated with congenital nephrotic syndrome. An increase in α-fetoprotein in the amniotic fluid may be observed, but this is far less consistent than in CNF. Although therapy with corticosteroids and cytotoxic agents invariably has proven ineffective, specific therapy may be available for some patients (*e.g.*, those with congenital infection). Classification of a patient into one of the major entities may not be possible.[824]

DIFFUSE MESANGIAL SCLEROSIS

The second most common cause of congenital nephrotic syndrome is diffuse mesangial sclerosis, which appears to be a heterogenous group.[824] The onset may be as late as 1 year of life. In contrast to CNF, CRF develops rapidly in these patients, and is the major cause of death in the absence of dialysis and renal transplantation. Renal venous thrombosis is a frequent complication. In most families, diffuse mesangial sclerosis is transmitted as an autosomal recessive trait. Histologic examination of the glomeruli shows mesangial cells embedded in a periodic acid-Schiff–positive and silver-positive fibrillar network occluding the capillaries. Tubular changes are similar to those seen in CNF, and interstitial fibrosis is more pronounced than in CNF.

In some infants, diffuse mesangial sclerosis is part of a Drash syndrome, which also includes ambiguous genitalia—most often male pseudohermaphroditism (*i.e.*, 46XY karyotype)—and Wilms tumor.[830] Patients present between 2 weeks and 33 months of age with proteinuria, with or without nephrotic syndrome, sometimes hematuria, often arterial hypertension, and progressive CRF leading to ESRD within a few months to 2 years from the onset. Several patients have presented with incomplete forms of Drash syndrome (*i.e.*, only two of the three signs of the triad).[830]

CONGENITAL INFECTION

Nephrotic syndrome due to congenital infection is seen most commonly in congenital syphilis,[831,832] in which case the lesion is characterized by epimembranous or proliferative glomerulopathy, with diffuse deposits of γ-immunoglobulin and treponemal antigen along the glomerular capillaries and subepithelial electron-dense deposits.[831] The condition responds very well to the administration of penicillin. The nephrotic syndrome associated with congenital toxoplasmosis is less common[833,834]; the lesion is characterized by the deposition in the glomeruli of immunoglobulins, complement, and *Toxoplasma* antigen and antibody. It may respond to administration of pyrimethamine, sulfadiazine, and steroid. Only one case of congenital nephrotic syndrome has been reported in association with congenital cytomegalovirus infection[835]; whether or not the nephrotic syndrome was mediated by the infection was uncertain.

OTHER CAUSES

Even though some infants with congenital nephrotic syndrome have been found to have minimal change disease on biopsy, corticosteroid and cyclophosphamide therapy has not proven useful. Some cases of congenital nephrotic syndrome are associated with dysmorphic features, such as pachygyria, microcephaly, buphthalmos, or disturbances of neuronal migration.[836–838]

Transient cases of congenital nephrotic syndrome have been described due to maternal transmission,[839] intoxication with mercury, or nail patella syndrome.[840] One 3-month-old infant with infantile systemic lupus erythematosus reportedly had steroid-responsive membranous glomerulopathy.[841]

HEMATURIA AND PROTEINURIA

DIFFERENTIAL DIAGNOSIS OF HEMATURIA

Pink or red urine or coloration of the diaper may result from hematuria, hemoglobinuria, myoglobinuria, uric acid, or bile pigments. The presence of blood on the diaper may also result from rectal bleeding or vaginal mucoid sanguinous discharge caused by maternal hormone withdrawal. On a dipstick test, the reagent strip based on the orthotolidine peroxidase reaction will give a positive reaction with hemoglobinuria, myoglobinuria, hematuria, or other oxidants, such as hydrogen peroxide and ascorbic acid. A dipstick can detect 5 to 20 intact erythrocytes per microliter of urine, and 0.05 to 0.3 mg of free hemoglobin/100 mL urine, which corresponds to 2–10 lysed erythrocytes per microliter. The diagnosis of hematuria requires the visualization of an excessive number of erythrocytes in an uncontaminated specimen of urine.

Significant hematuria in childhood has been defined as at least 5 erythrocytes per high-power field in the sediment of freshly centrifuged urine, at least 6 erythrocytes per 0.9 μL of unspun urine, or an Addis count of at least 129,000 to 800,000 erythrocytes per 12 hours. During the first week of life, Addis counts in normal full-term newborn infants do not appear to be different from those reported in older children and range between 0 and 630,000 erythrocytes per 12 hours (mean, 90,219).[303] Erythrocytes are most abundant during the first few days of life. Although most urine samples during the first week of life contain zero to four erythrocytes per microliter, more than one-half of the samples do not contain any erythrocytes. After the first week of life, erythrocytes are sparse. The presence of erythrocyte casts always is abnormal.[303,842]

INCIDENCE

Gross hematuria during the first month of life occurred in 35 of 132,050 admissions (0.21/1000) to a major tertiary center between 1950 and 1967.[843] In a more recent series, the incidence of hematuria during the first 48 hours of life was much lower in normal full-term infants (0/63) than in patients admitted to the NICU (48/78); none of these patients, however, had abnormalities on physical examination or had

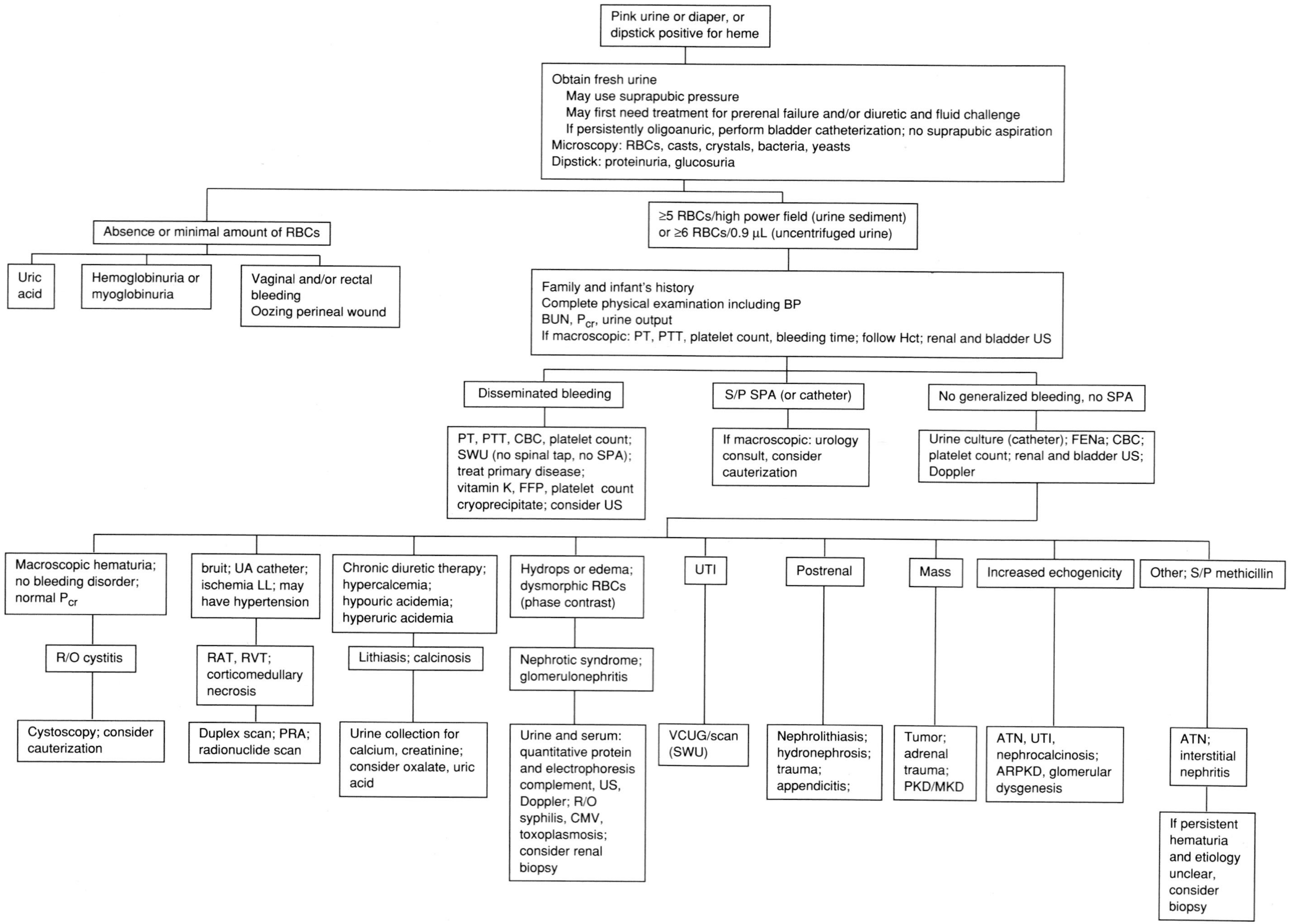

Pink urine or diaper, or dipstick positive for heme
Obtain fresh urine
May use suprapubic pressure
May first need treatment for prerenal failure and/or diuretic and fluid challenge
If persistently oligoanuric, perform bladder catheterization; no suprapubic aspiration
Microscopy: RBCs, casts, crystals, bacteria, yeasts
Dipstick: proteinuria, glucosuria
Absence or minimal amount of RBCs
Uric acid
Hemoglobinuria or myoglobinuria
Vaginal and/or rectal bleeding
Oozing perineal wound
≥5 RBCs/high power field (urine sediment) or ≥6 RBCs/0.9 μL (uncentrifuged urine)
Family and infant's history
Complete physical examination including BP
BUN, P_{cr}, urine output
If macroscopic: PT, PTT, platelet count, bleeding time; follow Hct; renal and bladder US
Disseminated bleeding
PT, PTT, CBC, platelet count; SWU (no spinal tap, no SPA); treat primary disease; vitamin K, FFP, platelet count cryoprecipitate; consider US
S/P SPA (or catheter)
If macroscopic: urology consult, consider cauterization
No generalized bleeding, no SPA
Urine culture (catheter); FENa; CBC; platelet count; renal and bladder US; Doppler
Macroscopic hematuria; no bleeding disorder; normal P_{cr}
R/O cystitis
Cystoscopy; consider cauterization
bruit; UA catheter; ischemia LL; may have hypertension
RAT, RVT; corticomedullary necrosis
Duplex scan; PRA; radionuclide scan
Chronic diuretic therapy; hypercalcemia; hypouric acidemia; hyperuric acidemia
Lithiasis; calcinosis
Urine collection for calcium, creatinine; consider oxalate, uric acid
Hydrops or edema; dysmorphic RBCs (phase contrast)
Nephrotic syndrome; glomerulonephritis
Urine and serum: quantitative protein and electrophoresis complement, US, Doppler; R/O syphilis, CMV, toxoplasmosis; consider renal biopsy
UTI
VCUG/scan (SWU)
Postrenal
Nephrolithiasis; hydronephrosis; trauma; appendicitis;
Mass
Tumor; adrenal trauma; PKD/MKD
Increased echogenicity
ATN, UTI, nephrocalcinosis; ARPKD, glomerular dysgenesis
Other; S/P methicillin
ATN; interstitial nephritis
If persistent hematuria and etiology unclear, consider biopsy

proteinuria, hypertension, or abnormal values of P_{cr} or BUN.[844] Transient hematuria was found in 76% of asphyxiated newborns.[845] In another series, hematuria was estimated to occur in 62% of newborn infants with UA catheter in place and US evidence of an arterial clot, and in 25% in those without evidence for a clot.[846] Hematuria was present in one-half of infants with ARF secondary to cardiac surgery, and in two thirds of newborn infants with irreversible ARF.[847,848]

ETIOLOGY

Hematuria may occur in a wide variety of diseases, including bleeding diathesis and renal and postrenal disorders. Prostaglandin synthesis inhibitor–mediated hematuria may be due to platelet dysfunction, ATN, or tubular dysfunction. Congenital infections (*e.g.*, syphilis, toxoplasmosis, cytomegalovirus) may cause thrombocytopenia or, rarely, glomerulonephritis. Common congenital causes of hematuria include hydronephrosis, PKD, tumors, and sponge kidneys. Although before 1967 the only commonly recognized acquired etiology of hematuria in the newborn infant was renal venous thrombosis,[843] neonatal hematuria is known to be secondary often to asphyxia, coagulation abnormalities, infectious and vascular disorders, and nephrotoxicity.

EVALUATION

The first step is to confirm the diagnosis of hematuria by the demonstration of erythrocytes in fresh urine voided spontaneously or after suprapubic pressure (Fig. 42-5). Suprapubic aspiration is contraindicated, because it can cause microscopic or macroscopic hematuria. If the patient is anuric, despite treating any condition associated with prerenal failure and despite a diuretic challenge and a fluid challenge (see Acute Renal Failure), the bladder should be catheterized using a lubricated 3.5- to 5-Fr catheter.

The history may disclose familial nephritis, and maternal history may be positive for diabetes (suggesting renal venous thrombosis, infection, thrombocytopenia, glomerulonephritis), and autoimmune disease, or recent use of PGSI. The patient's history should be reviewed, especially for asphyxia, sepsis, shock, hypertension, renal failure, medications, and placement of a UA line. Pertinent points in the physical examination include hypertension; bruising; edema suggesting ARF or glomerulonephritis; an abdominal mass that may indicate hydronephrosis, cystic disease, adrenal hemorrhage, and, rarely, renal trauma; and bruit (suggesting renovascular disease). In some patients, the presumptive etiology is obvious (*e.g.*, bleeding disorder, bladder trauma, severe asphyxia, ATN, renovascular disease, glomerulonephritis, nephrotic syndrome).

The initial workup should include a microscopic examination of the urine, dipstick test, and measurement of urine output, BUN, and P_{cr} (see Fig. 42-5). In addition, most patients should have a bladder and renal US and a urine culture. Microscopic examination of the urine may show dysmorphic erythrocytes or erythrocyte casts indicating glomerulonephritis, crystalluria as a result of rapid administration of acyclovir to a dehydrated patient, bacteriuria, or yeast forms, and the dipstick may show glucosuria or proteinuria. If any of these is present, further, specific investigations should be obtained. If a glomerular disease is suspected, fresh urine should be examined using phase contrast microscopy, which is the method of choice for identifying the presence of dysmorphic erythrocytes. The origin of the hematuria cannot be assessed by microscopic analysis when the hematuria is massive.

Transient microscopic hematuria during the first 48 hours of life may be insignificant,[844] as long as the infant is asymptomatic (*i.e.*, has no bleeding diathesis) and does not exhibit other evidence of a renal lesion (*e.g.*, no familial renal disease; normal physical examination, blood pressure, P_{cr}, US and BUN; no erythrocyte casts in the urine).

In patients with macroscopic hematuria, the first diagnoses to exclude are bleeding disorder, trauma, and cystitis. In those patients, coagulation tests, platelet count, and bleeding time should be assessed, and a renal and bladder US should be obtained. Purpura, excessive bleeding after venipuncture, or thrombocytopenia suggests that hematuria is due to a bleeding disorder. Specific treatment for sepsis or endocarditis and the bleeding disorder should be initiated. If renal function and urine output are normal, and hematuria disappears after resolution of the bleeding diathesis, no additional renal workup is required. It should be remembered, however, that thrombocytopenia with hematuria may occur in association with renal diseases, such as renal venous thrombosis and UTI with sepsis. Macroscopic hema-

◄ **FIG. 42–5.** Differential diagnosis of hematuria. (ARF, acute renal failure; ARPKD, autosomal recessive polycystic kidney disease; ATN, acute tubular necrosis; BP, blood pressure; BUN, blood urea nitrogen; CBC, complete blood count; CMV, cytomegalovirus; FeNa, fractional excretion of sodium; Hct, hematocrit; LL, lower limbs; MKD/PKD, multicystic/polycystic kidney disease; P_{cr}, plasma creatinine concentration; PRA, plasma renin activity; PT, prothrombin time; PTT, partial thromboplastin time; RAT, renal artery thrombosis; RBC, erythrocyte; R/O, rule out; RVT, renal venous thrombosis; S/P, status post; SPA, suprapubic aspiration; SWU, sepsis workup; UA, umbilical artery; UO, urine output; US, ultrasonography; UTI, urinary tract infection; VCUG, voiding cystourethrogram).

turia also may occur after suprapubic aspiration or catheterization of the bladder; if hematuria disappears rapidly, US is normal, and urine output, BUN and P_{cr} remain normal, no additional investigations are required. In patients with massive hematuria in whom a bleeding disorder has been excluded, cystoscopy should be performed, unless the presumptive etiology is renal.

All other patients should have a urine culture, as well as a renal and bladder US, which may disclose an intravascular thrombus, renal venous or arterial thrombosis, cystic kidney disease, lithiasis or nephrocalcinosis, hydronephrosis, adrenal hemorrhage, or other anomalies. The association of hematuria with UA catheterization, an abdominal bruit, or blanching of the lower extremities, especially with hypertension, strongly suggests the diagnosis of a renovascular etiology.[846,849] Hematuria is an unusual complication of nephrolithiasis or nephrocalcinosis during the neonatal period; it has been reported in one 10-week-old patient with familial hypercalciuria.[850]

Glomerulonephritis is a rare occurrence in newborn infants. It should be suspected if the patient has either hydrops or generalized edema with massive proteinuria or erythrocyte casts or dysmorphic erythrocytes. Although hematuria of glomerular origin is suggested by the presence of erythrocyte casts, severe proteinuria, or dysmorphic erythrocytes, it is not excluded by their absence. These patients should be assessed for possible congenital syphilis, toxoplasmosis, cytomegalovirus infection, various causes of nephrotic syndrome, familial nephritis, and immune-mediated glomerulonephritis. A decrease in the serum concentration of the third fraction of complement has been described in glomerulonephritis due to congenital syphilis and in one mother–infant pair with a benign glomerulonephritis with isolated hematuria.[851] Consultation with a pediatric nephrologist should be obtained, and a renal biopsy should be considered.

For the other patients, the differential diagnosis includes a wide range of diseases; US is the most important initial investigation. Further workup depends on the clinical presentation (*e.g.*, hypertension, ARF) or presumed etiology (*e.g.*, ATN, cystic disease, tumor). If hematuria persists without obvious etiology, a renal biopsy should be considered.

DIFFERENTIAL DIAGNOSIS OF PROTEINURIA

Proteinuria may be suggested by a strongly positive dipstick test. Significant proteinuria is diagnosed by a timed collection for quantitative proteinuria. Abnormal proteinuria is defined according to normal values for age (see Table 42-3).

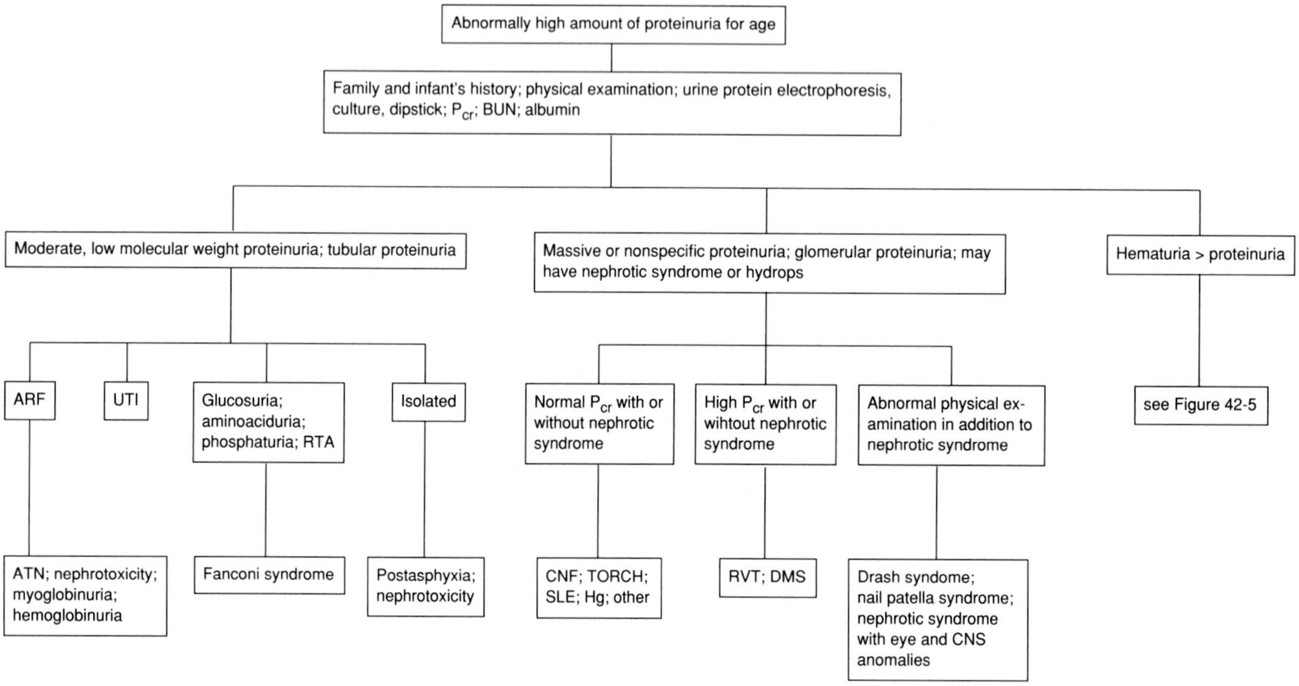

FIG. 42–6. Differential diagnosis of proteinuria. (AFR, acute renal failure; ATN, acute tubular necrosis; BUN, blood urea nitrogen; CNF, congenital nephrotic syndrome (Finnish type); DMS, diffuse mesangial sclerosis; Hg, mercury intoxication; P_{cr}, plasma creatinine concentration; RTA, renal tubular acidosis; RVT, renal venous thrombosis; SLE, systemic lupus erythematosus; UTI, urinary tract infection.)

FREQUENCY

Increased proteinuria occurs frequently in newborn infants admitted to the NICU; it is associated with various types of renal injury. The detection of increased tubular proteinuria is a sensitive screening test for renal damage after perinatal asphyxia,[852] as well as for tubular damage due to nephrotoxicity (see Acute Renal Failure and Nephrotoxicity).

ETIOLOGY

The most common type of proteinuria is tubular proteinuria, which never is massive. It includes low-molecular-weight proteins (*i.e.*, <60,000 kd), which, as in the normal situation, are freely filtered through the glomerulus. These include β_2-microglobulin, retinol-binding protein, and myoglobin. In addition, in some patients, lysosomal proteins such as NAG can be found in the urine. Although tubular proteinuria can be isolated, it is associated most often with perinatal asphyxia or renal ischemia, UTI, ARF, Fanconi syndrome, or nephrotoxicity (see Acute Renal Failure; Tubular Dysfunction).

In contrast, proteinuria of glomerular origin includes proteins with higher molecular weight such as albumin. In addition, it may become massive and lead to nephrotic syndrome (see Nephrotic Syndrome).

EVALUATION

Because proteinuria occurs frequently, an extensive workup is not indicated unless there is evidence for renal disease. Apart from history and physical examination, a major step in the differential diagnosis is the differentiation between tubular and glomerular proteinuria. This can be obtained by an electrophoresis of urinary proteins or by quantitative measurement of specific low-molecular-weight proteins and albumin (Fig. 42-6). In addition, there may be evidence of tubular damage (*e.g.*, glucosuria, RTA). Discussions of specific disorders are provided elsewhere in this chapter.

REFERENCES

DEVELOPMENTAL PHYSIOLOGY

1. Saxen L. Organogenesis of the kidney. Cambridge, MA: Harvard University Press, 1987.
2. Potter EL, Thierstein ST. Glomerular development in the kidney as an index of foetal maturity. J Pediatr 1943;22:695.
3. Lumbers ER. A brief review of fetal renal function. J Dev Physiol 1984;6:1.
4. Thorburn GD. The role of the thyroid gland and kidneys in fetal growth. Ciba Found Symp 1974;27:185.
5. Perlman M, Levin M. Fetal pulmonary hypoplasia, anuria, and oligohydramnios: clinicopathologic observations and review of the literature. Am J Obstet Gynecol 1974;118:1119.
6. Gomez RA, Meernick JG, Kuehl WD, et al. Developmental aspects of the renal response to hemorrhage during fetal life. Pediatr Res 1984;18:40.
7. Wladimiroff JW, Campbell S. Fetal urine production rates in normal and complicated pregnancy. Lancet 1974;1:151.
8. Rubin MI, Bruck E, Rapoport MJ. Maturation of renal function in childhood: clearance studies. J Clin Invest 1949;28:1144.
9. Calcagno PL, Rubin MI. Renal extraction of para-amino-hippurate in infants and children. J Clin Invest 1963;42:1632.
10. Barnett HL, Hare WK, McNamara H, et al. Influence of postnatal age on kidney function of premature infants. Proc Soc Exp Biol Med 1948;69:55.
11. Schwartz GJ, Goldsmith DI, Fine LG. p-Aminohippurate transport in the proximal straight tubule: development and substrate stimulation. Pediatr Res 1978;12:793.
12. Pitts RF. Physiology of the kidney. Chicago: Year Book, 1974:158.
13. Rudolph AM, Heymann MA, Teramo KAW, et al. Studies on the circulation of the previable human fetus. Pediatr Res 1971;5:452.
14. Aperia A, Broberger O, Herin P, et al. Renal hemodynamics in the perinatal period: a study in lambs. Acta Physiol Scand 1977;99:261.
15. Robillard JE, Weismann DN, Herin P. Ontogeny of single glomerular perfusion rate in fetal and newborn lambs. Pediatr Res 1981;15:1248.
16. Kleinman LI, Reuter JH. Maturation of glomerular blood flow distribution in the newborn dog. J Physiol (Lond) 1973;228:91.
17. Olbing H, Blaufox MD, Aschinberg LC, et al. Postnatal changes in renal glomerular blood flow distribution in puppies. J Clin Invest 1973;52:2885.
18. Aschinburg LC, Goldsmith DI, Olbing H, et al. Neonatal changes in renal blood flow distribution in puppies. Am J Physiol 1975;228:1453.
19. Gruskin AB, Edelmann CM Jr, Yuan S. Maturational changes in renal blood flow in piglets. Pediatr Res 1970;4:7.
20. Aperia A, Broberger O, Herin P. Maturational changes in glomerular perfusion rate and glomerular filtration rate in lambs. Pediatr Res 1974;8:758.
21. Spitzer A, Schwartz GJ. The kidney during development. In: Windhagen E, ed. The handbook of physiology. Bethesda, MD: American Physiology Society, 1992:475.
22. Ichikawa I, Maddox DA, Brenner BM. Maturational development of glomerular ultrafiltration in the rat. Am J Physiol 1979;236:F465.
23. Elinder G, Aperia A, Herin P, et al. Effect of isotonic volume expansion on glomerular filtration rate and renal hemodynamics in the developing rat kidney. Acta Physiol Scand 1980;108:411.
24. Drukker A, Goldsmith DI, Spitzer A, et al. The renin angiotensin system in newborn dogs: developmental patterns and response to acute saline loading. Pediatr Res 1980;14:304.
25. Horster M, Valtin H. Postnatal development of renal function: micropuncture and clearance studies in the dog. J Clin Invest 1971;50:779.
26. Jose PA, Logan AG, Slotkoff LM, et al. Intrarenal blood flow distribution in canine puppies. Pediatr Res 1971;5:335.
27. Vernier RL, Birch-Andersen A. Studies of the human fetal kidney: I. Development of the glomerulus. J Pediatr 1962;60:754.
28. Evan AP, Stoeckel JA, Loemker V, et al. Development of the intrarenal vascular system of the puppy. Anat Rec 1979;194:187.
29. Ljungqvist A, Wagermark J. Renal juxtaglomerular granula-

tion in the human foetus and infant. Acta Pathol Microbiol Scand 1966;67:257.

30. Richer C, Hornych H, Amiel-Tison C, et al. Plasma renin activity and its postnatal development in preterm infants. Biol Neonate 1977;31:301.
31. Kotchen TA, Strickland AL, Rice TW, et al. A study of the renin–angiotensin system in newborn infants. J Pediatr 1972; 80:938.
32. Pelayo JC, Eisner GM, Jose PA. The ontogeny of the renin–angiotensin system. Clin Perinatol 1981;8:347.
33. Van Acker KJ, Scharpe SL, Deprettere AJR, et al. Renin–angiotensin–aldosterone system in the healthy infant and child. Kidney Int 1979;16:196.
34. Smith FG, Lupu AN, Barajas L, et al. The renin–angiotensin system in the fetal lamb. Pediatr Res 1974;8:611.
35. Mott JC. The place of the renin angiotensin system before and after birth. Br Med Bull 1975;31:64.
36. Siegel SR, Fisher DA. The renin angiotensin–aldosterone system in the newborn lamb: response to furosemide. Pediatr Res 1977;11:837.
37. Lumberg ER, Reid GC. Effects of vaginal delivery and caesarian section on plasma renin activity and angiotensin II levels in human umbilical cord blood. Biol Neonate 1977;31:127.
38. John EG, Zeis PM, Samayo C. Renin–aldosterone system response to chronic salt loading and volume contraction in puppies. Int J Pediatr Nephrol 1981;2:9.
39. Sulyok E, Varga F, Nemeth M, et al. Furosemide-induced alterations in the electrolyte status, the function of renin angiotensin–aldosterone system and the urinary excretion of prostaglandins in newborn infants. Pediatr Res 1980;14:765.
40. Robillard JE, Weitzman RE. Developmental aspects of the fetal response to exogenous arginine vasopressin. Am J Physiol 1980;238:F407.
41. Fiselier R, Monnens L, Lameire N, et al. Effects of angiotensin II blockade in the canine puppy under different salt-intake. Kidney Int 1984;26:823.
42. Sulyok E, Nemeth M, Tenyi I, et al. Relationship between maturity, electrolyte balance and the function of the renin–angiotensin–aldosterone system in newborn infants. Biol Neonate 1979;35:60.
43. Arant BS Jr, Stephenson WH. Developmental change in systemic vascular resistance compared with prostaglandins and angiotensin II concentration in arterial plasma of conscious dogs. Pediatr Res 1982;16:120A.
44. Robillard JE, Weitzman RE, Fisher DA, et al. The dynamics of vasopressin release: blood volume regulation during fetal hemorrhage in the lamb fetus. Pediatr Res 1979;13:606.
45. Nakamura KT, Ayres NA, Gomez RA, et al. Renal responses to hypoxemia during renin–angiotensin system inhibition in fetal lambs. Am J Physiol 1985;249:R116.
46. Tortorolo G, Porcelli G, Cuatalo P. Urinary kallikreins in premature, small at term and normal newborns and in children. In: Pisano JJ, Austen KF, eds. Chemistry and biology of kallikrein: kinin system in health and disease. Washington, DC: PHEW (National Institutes of Health) 1974:76.
47. Godard C, Vallotton MB, Favre L. Urinary prostaglandins, vasopressin, and kallikrein excretion in healthy children from birth to adolescence. J Pediatr 1982;100:898.
48. Gerber JG, Nies AS. The hemodynamic effects of prostaglandins in the rat: evidence for important species variation in renovascular responses. Circ Res 1979;44:406.
49. Lifschitz MD. Prostaglandins and renal blood flow: in vivo studies. Kidney Int 1981;19:781.
50. Moncada S, Vane JR. Pharmacology and endogenous roles of prostaglandin endoperoxides, thromboxane A_2 and prostacyclin. Pharmacol Rev 1979;30:293.
51. Walker DW, Mitchell MD. Prostaglandins in urine of foetal lambs. Nature 1978;271:161.
52. Walker DW, Mitchell MD. Presence of thromboxane B_2 and 6-keto-prostaglandin F1-α in the urine of fetal sheep. Prostaglandins Med 1979;3:249.
53. Arant BS Jr. Renal disorders of the newborn infant. Pediatr Nephrology 1984;12:111.
54. Robillard JE, Weismann DN, Gomez RA, et al. Renal and adrenal responses to converting-enzyme inhibition in fetal and newborn life. Am J Physiol 1983;244:R249.
55. Benzoni D, Vincent M, Betend B, et al. Urinary excretion of prostaglandins and electrolytes in developing children. Kidney Int 1981;20:386.
56. Matson JR, Stokes JB, Robillard JE. Effects of inhibition of prostaglandin synthesis on fetal renal function. Kidney Int 1981;20:621.
57. Millard RW, Baig H, Vatner SF. Prostaglandin control of the renal circulation in response to hypoxemia in the fetal lamb in utero. Circ Res 1979;45:172.
58. Lagercrantz H, Bistoletti P. Catecholamine release in the newborn infant at birth. Pediatr Res 1973;11:889.
59. Jose PA, Slotkoff LM, Lilienfield LS, et al. Sensitivity of neonatal renal vasculature to epinephrine. Am J Physiol 1974; 226:796.
60. McKenna OC, Angelakos ET. Adrenergic innervation of the canine kidney. Circ Res 1968;22:345.
61. Felder RA, Pelayo JC, Calcagno PL, et al. Alpha adrenoceptors in the developing kidney. Pediatr Res 1983;17:177.
62. Buckley NM, Brazeau P, Fraiser ID. Cardiovascular effects of dopamine in developing swine. Biol Neonate 1983;43:50.
63. Buckley NM, Brazeau P, Charney AN, et al. Cardiovascular and renal effects of isoproterenol infusions in young swine. Biol Neonate 1984;45:69.
64. Fildes RD, Eisner GM, Calcagno PL, et al. Renal α-adrenoceptors and sodium excretion in the dog. Am J Physiol 1985; 248:F128.
65. Felder CC, Piccio MM, Mckelvey AM, et al. Ontogeny of renal beta-adrenoceptors in the sheep. Pediatr Nephrol 1990;4:635.
66. Nakamura KT, Matherne GP, Jose PA, et al. Ontogeny of renal β-adrenoceptor mediated vasodilation in sheep: comparison between endogenous catecholamines. Pediatr Res 1987;22:465.
67. Feltes TF, Hansen TN, Martin CG, et al. The effects of dopamine infusion on regional blood flow in newborn lambs. Pediatr Res 1987;21:131.
68. Driscoll DJ, Gillette PC, Lewis RM, et al. Comparative hemodynamic effects of isoproterenol, dopamine, and dobutamine in the newborn dog. Pediatr Res 1979;13:1006.
69. Felder RA, Nakamura KT, Robillard JE, et al. Dopamine receptors in the developing kidney. Pediatr Nephrol 1988;2: 156.
70. Pohjavuori M, Fyhrquist F. Hemodynamic significance of vasopressin in the newborn infant. J Pediatr 1980;97:462.
71. Weismann DN, Robillard JE. Renal hemodynamic responses to hypoxemia during development: relationship to circulatory vasoactive substances. Pediatr Res 1988;23:155.
72. Chevalier RL, Gomez RA, Carey RM, et al. Renal effects of atrial natriuretic peptide infusion in young and adult rats. Pediatr Res 1988;24:333.
73. Tulassay T, Rascher W, Seyberth HW, et al. Role of atrial natriuretic peptide in sodium homeostasis in premature infants. J Pediatr 1986;109:1023.
74. Wei Y, Rodi CP, Day ML, et al. Developmental changes in the rat atriopeptin hormonal system. J Clin Invest 1987;79:1325.
75. Varille VA, Nakamura KT, McWeeny OJ, et al. Renal hemo-

dynamic response to atrial natriuretic factor in fetal and newborn sheep. Pediatr Res 1989;25:291.
76. Robillard JE, Nakamura KT, Varille VA, et al. Ontogeny of the renal response to natriuretic peptide in sheep. Am J Physiol 1988;254:F634.
77. Chevalier RL, Kaiser DL. Autoregulation of renal blood flow in the rat: effect of growth and uninephrectomy. Am J Physiol 1983;244:F483.
78. Jose PA, Slotkoft LM, Montgomery S, et al. Autoregulation of renal blood flow in the puppy. Am J Physiol 1975;229:983.
79. Buckley NM, Brazeau P, Frasier ID. Renal blood flow autoregulation in developing swine. Am J Physiol 1983;245:H1.
80. Semple SJG, deWardener HE. Effect of increased venous pressure on circulatory "autoregulation" of isolated dog kidneys. Circ Res 1959;7:643.
81. Altschule MD. The changes in the mesonephric tubules of human embryos seven to twelve weeks old. Anat Rec 1930;46:81.
82. Gersh I. The correlation of structure and function in the developing mesonephros and metanephros. Contributions to Embryology 1937;153:35.
83. Arant BS Jr. Developmental patterns of renal functional maturation compared in the human neonate. J Pediatr 1978;92:705.
84. Coulthard MG. Maturation of glomerular filtration in preterm and mature babies. Early Hum Dev 1985;11:281.
85. Aperia A, Broberger O, Elinder G, et al. Postnatal development of renal function in pre-term and full-term infants. Acta Paediatr Scand 1981;70:183.
86. Leake RD, Trygstad CW, Oh W. Inulin clearance in the newborn infant. Relationship to gestational and postnatal age. Pediatr Res 1976;10:759.
87. Oh W, Arcilla RA, Oh MA, et al. Renal and cardiovascular effects of body tilting in the newbcrn infant: a comparative study of infants born with early and late cord clamping. Biol Neonate 1966;10:76.
88. Strauss J, Daniel SS, James LS. Postnatal adjustment in renal function. Pediatrics 1981;68:802.
89. Barnett HL. Renal physiology in infants and children: I. Method for estimation of glomerular filtration rate. Proc Soc Exp Biol Med 1940;44:654.
90. Arant BS Jr. Postnatal development of renal function during the first year of life. Pediatr Nephrol 1987;1:308.
91. Spitzer A, Brandis M. Functional and morphologic maturation of the superficial nephrons: relationship to total kidney function. J Clin Invest 1974;53:279.
92. MacDonald MS, Emery JL. The late intrauterine and postnatal development of human renal glomeruli. J Anat 1959;93:331.
93. Arant BS Jr, Edelmann CM Jr, Nash MA. The renal reabsorption of glucose in the developing canine kidney: a study of glomerulo-tubular balance. Pediatr Res 1974;8:638.
94. Aperia A, Herin P. Development of glomerular perfusion rate and nephron filtration rate in rats 17–60 days old. Am J Physiol 1975;228:1319.
95. Goldsmith DI, Jodorkovsky RA, Sherwinter J, et al. Glomerular capillary permeability in developing canines. Am J Physiol 1986;251:F528.
96. John E, Goldsmith DI, Spitzer A. Quantitative changes in the canine glomerular vasculature during development: physiologic implications. Kidney Int 1981;20:223.
97. Fetterman GH, Sheeplock NA, Philipp FJ, et al. The growth and maturation of human glomeruli and proximal convolutions from term to adulthood: studies by microdissection. Pediatrics 1965;35:601.
98. Knutson DW, Chieu F, Bennett CM, et al. Estimation of relative glomerular capillary surface area in normal and hypertrophic rat kidneys. Kidney Int 1978;14:437.
99. Hill KJ, Lumbers ER, Elbourne I. The actions of cortisol on fetal renal function. J Dev Physiol 1988;10:85.
100. Corvilain J, Abramow M. Effect of growth hormone on tubular transport of phosphate in normal and parathyroidectomized dogs. J Clin Invest 1964;43:1608.
101. Ausiello DA, Kreisberg JI, Roy C, et al. Contraction of cultured rat glomerular cells of apparent mesangial origin after stimulation with angiotensin II and arginine vasopressin. J Clin Invest 1980;65:754.
102. Friedman Z, Demers LM, Marks KH, et al. Urinary excretion of prostaglandin E following the administration of furosemide and indomethacin to sick low-birth-weight infants. J Pediatr 1978;93:512.
103. Cifuentes RF, Olley PM, Balfe JW, et al. Indomethacin and renal function in premature infants with persistent ductus arteriosus. J Pediatr 1979;95:583.
104. Aperia A, Herin P. Effect of arterial blood pressure reduction on renal hemodynamics in the developing lamb. Acta Physiol Scand 1976;98:387.
105. Briggs JP, Schubert G, Schnermann J. Quantitative characterization of the tubuloglomerular feedback response: effect of growth. Am J Physiol 1984;247:F808.
106. Muller-Suur R, Ulfendahl HR, Persson AEG. Evidence for tubuloglomerular feedback in juxtamedullary nephrons of young rats. Am J Physiol 1983;244:F425.
107. Gordon HH, Levine SZ, Marples E, et al. Water exchange of premature infants: comparison of metabolic (organic) and electrolyte (inorganic) methods of measurement. J Clin Invest 1939;18:187.
108. McCance RA, Widdowson EM. The response of the newborn puppy to water, salt and food. J Physiol (Lond) 1958;141:81.
109. Houston IB, Zeis PM. Intrauterine renal function and the amniotic fluid. J Physiol 1976;257:20P.
110. Nakamura KT, Matherne GP, McWeeny OJ, et al. Renal hemodynamics and functional changes during the transition from fetal to newborn life in sheep. Pediatr Res 1987;21:229.
111. Robillard JE, Sessions C, Kennedey RL, et al. Interrelationship between glomerular filtration rate and renal transport of sodium and chloride during fetal life. Am J Obstet Gynecol 1977;128:727.
112. Siegel SR, Oh W. Renal function as a marker of human fetal maturation. Acta Paediatr Scand 1976;65:481.
113. Engelke SC, Shah BL, Vasan U, et al. Sodium balance in very low birth-weight infants. J Pediatr 1978;93:837.
114. Aperia A, Broberger O, Thodenius K, et al. Developmental study of the renal response to an oral salt load in preterm infants. Acta Paediatr Scand 1974;63:517.
115. Ross B, Cowett RM, Oh W. Renal functions of low birth weight infant during the first two months of life. Pediatr Res 1977;11:1162.
116. Lorenz JM, Kleinman LI, Kotagal UR, et al. Water balance in very low-birth-weight infants: relationship to water and sodium intake and effect on outcome. J Pediatr 1982;101:423.
117. Al-Dahhan J, Haycock GB, Nichol B, et al. Sodium homeostasis in term and preterm neonates: III. The effect of salt supplementation. Arch Dis Child 1984;59:945.
118. Merlet-Benichou C, de Rouffignac C. Renal clearance studies in fetal and young guinea pigs: effect of salt loading. Am J Physiol 1977;232:F178.
119. Rodriguez-Soriano J, Vallo A, Oliveros R, et al. Renal handling of sodium in premature and full-term neonates: a study using clearance methods during water diuresis. Pediatr Res 1983;17:1013.
120. Robillard JE, Smith FG, Segar JL, et al. Mechanisms regulating renal sodium excretion during development. Pediatr Nephrol 1992;6:205.

121. Ito Y, Goldsmith DI, Spitzer A. The role of aldosterone in renal electrolyte transport during development. [Abstract] Pediatr Res 1984;18:370A.
122. Stephenson G, Hammet M, Hadaway G, et al. Ontogeny of renal mineralocorticoid receptors and urinary electrolyte responses in the rat. Am J Physiol 1984;247:F665.
123. Broberger U, Aperia A, Thodenius K, et al. Renal function in infants with hyperbiliremia. Acta Paediatr Scand 1979;68:75.
124. Aperia A, Bergqvist G, Brogerger O, et al. Renal function in newborn infants with high hematocrit values before and after isovolemic haemodilution. Acta Paediatr Scand 1974;63:878.
125. Harkavy KL, Scanlon JW, Jose P. The effects of theophylline on renal function in the premature newborn. Biol Neonate 1979;35:126.
126. Aperia A, Broberger O, Thodenius K, et al. Renal response to an oral sodium load in newborn full-term infants. Acta Paediatr Scand 1972;61:670.
127. Aperia A, Elinder G. Distal tubular sodium reabsorption in the developing rat kidney. Am J Physiol 1981;240:F487.
128. Dean RFA, McCance RA. The renal responses of infants and adults to the administration of hypertonic solutions of sodium chloride and urea. J Physiol 1949;109:81.
129. Aperia A, Broberger O, Herin P, et al. Sodium excretion in relation to sodium intake and aldosterone excretion in newborn preterm and full term infants. Acta Paediatr Scand 1979;68:813.
130. Kleinman LI. Renal sodium reabsorption during saline loading and distal blockade in newborn dogs. Am J Physiol 1975;228:1403.
131. Brace RA, Bayer LA, Cheung CY. Fetal cardiovascular, endocrine, and fluid responses to atrial natriuretic factor infusion. Am J Physiol 1989;257:R580.
132. Semmekrot BA, Wiesel PH, Monnens LAH, et al. Age differences in renal response to atrial natriuretic peptide in rabbits. Life Sci 1990;46:849.
133. Wintour EM, Coghlan JP, Towstoless MK. Cortisol is natriuretic in the immature ovine fetus. J Endocrinol 1985; 106:1213.
134. Serrano CV, Talbert LM, Welt LG. Potassium deficiency in the pregnant dog. J Clin Invest 1964;43:27.
135. Dancis J, Springer D. Fetal homeostasis in maternal malnutrition: potassium and sodium deficiency in rats. Pediatr Res 1970;4:345.
136. Lelievre-Pegorier M, Merlet-Benichou C, Roinel N, et al. Developmental pattern of water and electrolyte transport in rat superficial nephrons. Am J Physiol 1983;245:F15.
137. Sulyok E. The relationship between electrolyte and acid–base balance in the premature infant during early postnatal life. Biol Neonate 1971;17:227.
138. Satlin LM. Maturation of renal potassium transport. Pediatr Nephrol 1991;5:260.
139. Tuvdad F, McNamara H, Barnett HL. Renal response of premature infants to administration of bicarbonate and potassium. Pediatrics 1954;13:4.
140. McCance RA, Widdowson EM. The response of the new-born piglet to an excess of potassium. J Physiol 1958;141:88.
141. Kleinman LI, Banks RO. Segmental nephron sodium and potassium reabsorption in newborn and adult dogs during saline expansion. Proc Soc Exp Biol Med 1983;173:231.
142. Zink H, Horster M. Maturation of diluting capacity in loop of Henle of rat superficial nephrons. Am J Physiol 1977;-233:F519.
143. Satlin LM. Postnatal maturation of potassium (K) secretion in the rabbit cortical collecting duct (CCD). [Abstract] Pediatr Res 1992;31:342A.
144. Schmidt U, Horster M. Na-K-activated ATPase: activity maturation in rabbit nephron segments dissected in vitro. Am J Physiol 1977;233:F55.
145. Satlin LM, Evan AP, Gattone V III, et al. Postnatal maturation of the rabbit cortical collecting duct. Pediatr Nephrol 1988; 2:135.
146. Robillard JE, Nakamura KT, Lawton WJ. Effects of aldosterone on urinary kallikrein and sodium excretion during fetal life. Pediatr Res 1985;190:1048.
147. Vaughn D, Kirschbaum TH, Bersentes T, et al. Fetal and neonatal response to acid loading in the sheep. J Appl Physiol 1968;24:135.
148. Smith FG Jr, Schwartz A. Response of the intact lamb fetus to acidosis. Am J Obstet Gynecol 1970;106:52.
149. Robillard JE, Sessions C, Burmeister L, et al. Influence of fetal extracellular volume contraction on renal reabsorption of bicarbonate in fetal lambs. Pediatr Res 1977;11:649.
150. Weisbrot IM, James LS, Prince CE, et al. Acid–base homeostasis of the new-born infant during the first 24 hrs of life. J Pediatr 1958;52:395.
151. Schwartz GJ, Haycock GB, Edelmann CM Jr, et al. Late metabolic acidosis: a reassessment of the definition. J Pediatr 1979;95:102.
152. Ranlov P, Siggaard-Andersen O. Late metabolic acidosis in premature infants. Acta Paediatr Scand 1965;54:531.
153. Edelmann CM Jr, Rodriguez-Soriano J, Boichis H, et al. Renal bicarbonate reabsorption and hydrogen ion excretion in normal infants. J Clin Invest 1967;46:1309.
154. Schwartz GJ, Evan AP. Development of solute transport in rabbit proximal tubule: I. HCO_3 and glucose absorption. Am J Physiol 1983;245:F382.
155. Moore ES, Fine BP, Satrasook SS, et al. Renal reabsorption of bicarbonate in puppies: effect of extracellular volume contraction on the renal threshold for bicarbonate. Pediatr Res 1972;-6:859.
156. Lonnerholm G, Wistrand PJ. Carbonic anhydrase in the human fetal kidney. Pediatr Res 1983;17:390.
157. Svenningsen NW, Lindquist B. Postnatal development of renal hydrogen ion excretion capacity in relation to age and protein intake. Acta Paediatr Scand 1974;63:721.
158. McCance RA, Widdowson EM. Renal aspects of acid–base control in the newly born: I. Natural development. Acta Paediatr Scand 1960;49:409.
159. Svenningsen NW. Renal acid–base titration studies in infants with and without metabolic acidosis in the postneonatal period. Pediatr Res 1974;8:659.
160. Kerpel-Fronius E, Heim T, Sulyok E. The development of the renal acidifying processes and their relation to acidosis in low-birth-weight infants. Biol Neonate 1970;15:156.
161. Sulyok E, Heim T. Assessment of maximal urinary acidification in premature infants. Biol Neonate 1971;19:200.
162. Satlin LM, Schwartz GJ. Postnatal maturation of rabbit renal collecting duct: intercalated cell function. Am J Physiol 1987;253:F622.
163. Mehrgut FM, Satlin LM, Schwartz GJ. Maturation of HCO_3 transport in rabbit collecting duct. Am J Physiol 1990; 259:F801.
164. Goldstein L. Ammonia metabolism in kidneys of suckling rats. Am J Physiol 1971;220:213.
165. Peonides A, Levin B, Young WF. The renal excretion of hydrogen ions in infants and children. Arch Dis Child 1965; 40:33.
166. Kildeberg P, Engel K, Winters RW. Balance of net acid in growing infants: endogenous and transintestinal aspects. Acta Paediatr Scand 1969;58:321.
167. Radde IC, Chance GW, Bailey K. Growth and mineral metabolism in very low birth-weight infants: I. Comparison of the

effects of two modes of $NaHCO_3$ treatment of late metabolic acidosis. Pediatr Res 1975;9:564.
168. Arant BS Jr. Renal handling of calcium and phosphorus in normal human neonates. Semin Nephrol 1983;2:94.
169. Brown DR, Steranka BH. Renal cation excretion in the hypocalcemic premature human neonate. Pediatr Res 1981; 15:1100.
170. Karlen J, Aperia A, Zetterstrom R. Renal excretion of calcium and phosphate in preterm and term infants. J Pediatr 1985; 106:814.
171. Ghazali S, Barratt TM. Urinary excretion of calcium and magnesium in children. Arch Dis Child 1974;49:97.
172. Jahan I, Pitts RF. Effect of parathyroid on renal tubular reabsorption of phosphate and calcium. Am J Physiol 1948;155:42.
173. Ardaillou R. Kidney and calcitonin. Nephron 1975;15:250.
174. Linarelli LG, Bobick J, Bobick C. The effect of parathyroid hormone on rabbit renal cortex adenyl cyclase during development. Pediatr Res 1973;7:878.
175. Imbert-Teboul M, Chabardes D, Clique A, et al. Ontogenesis of hormone-dependent adenylate cyclase in isolated rat nephron segments. Am J Physiol 1984;247:F316.
176. Mallet E, Basuyau J-P, Brunelle P, et al. Neonatal parathyroid secretion and renal receptor maturation in premature infants. Biol Neonate 1978;33:304.
177. Linarelli LG. Nephron urinary cyclic AMP and developmental renal responsiveness to parathyroid hormone. Pediatrics 1972;50:14.
178. Tsang RC, Light IJ, Sutherland JM, et al. Possible pathogenetic factors in neonatal hypocalcemia of prematurity. J Pediatr 1973;82:423.
179. Quamme GA, Dirks JH. Intraluminal and contraluminal magnesium on magnesium and calcium transfer in the rat nephron. Am J Physiol 1980;238:F187.
180. Bethune JE, Turpin RA, Inoue H. Effect of parathyroid hormone extract on divalent ion excretion in man. J Clin Endocrinol Metab 1968;28:673.
181. Brunette MG, Vigneault N, Carriere S. Micropuncture study of magnesium transport along the nephron in the young rat. Am J Physiol 1974;227:891.
182. Smith FG Jr, Adams FH, Borden N, et al. Studies of renal function in the intact fetal lamb. Am J Obstet Gynecol 1966;96:240.
183. Richmond JB, Kravitz H, Segar W, et al. Renal clearance of endogenous phosphate in infants and children. Proc Soc Exp Biol Med 1951;77:83.
184. Brodehl J, Gellison K, Weber HP. Postnatal development of tubular phosphate reabsorption. Clin Nephrol 1982;17:163.
185. McCrory WW, Forman CW, McNamara H, et al. Renal excretion of inorganic phosphate in newborn infants. J Clin Invest 1952;31:357.
186. Johnson V, Spitzer A. Renal reabsorption of phosphate during development: whole kidney events. Am J Physiol 1986; 251:F251.
187. Caversazio J, Bonjour JP. Fleisch H. Tubular handling of Pi in young growing and adult rats. Am J Physiol 1982;242:F705.
188. Senterre J, Salle B. Renal aspects of calcium and phosphorus metabolism in preterm infants. Biol Neonate 1988;53:220.
189. Haramati A, Mulroney SE, Webster SK. Developmental changes in the tubular capacity for phosphate reabsorption in the rat. Am J Physiol 1988;255:F287.
190. Kaskel FJ, Kumar AM, Feld LG, et al. Renal reabsorption of phosphate during development: tubular events. Pediatr Nephrol 1988;2:129.
191. Arnaud SB, Goldsmith RS, Stickler GB, et al. Serum parathyroid hormone and blood minerals: interrelationships in normal children. Pediatr Res 1973;7:485.
192. David L, Anast CS. Calcium metabolism in newborn infant: the interrelationship of parathyroid function and calcium, magnesium, and phosphorus metabolism in normal sick and hypocalcemic newborns. J Clin Invest 1974;54:287.
193. Barac-Nieto M, Dowd TL, Gupta RK, et al. Changes in NMR-visible kidney cell phosphate with age and diet: relationship to phosphate transport. Am J Physiol 1991;261:F153.
194. Robillard JE, Sessions C, Kennedy RL, et al. Maturation of the glucose transport process by the fetal kidney. Pediatr Res 1978;12:680.
195. Roth KS, Hwang SM, Yudkoff M, et al. The ontogeny of sugar transport in kidney. Pediatr Res 1978;12:1127.
196. Seigle R, Kinne R, Spitzer A. Glucose transport in newborn guinea pig brush border membrane fragments. [Abstract] Kidney Int 1982;21:287A
197. Beck JC, Lipkowitz MS, Abramson RG. Characterization of the fetal glucose transporter in rabbit kidney: comparison with the adult brush border electrogenic Na^+-glucose symporter. J Clin Invest 1988;82:379.
198. Horster M, Lewy JE. Filtration fraction and extraction of PAH during neonatal period in the rat. Am J Physiol 1970;219: 1061.
199. Friis C. Postnatal development of renal function in piglets: glomerular filtration rate, clearance of PAH and PAH extraction. Biol Neonate 1979;35:180.
200. Brodehl J, Gellissen K. Endogenous renal transport of free amino acid in infancy and childhood. Pediatrics 1968;42:395.
201. Webber WA, Cairns JA. A comparison of the amino acid concentrating ability of the kidney cortex of newborn and mature rats. Can J Physiol Pharmacol 1968;46:165.
202. Chesney RW, Jax DK. Developmental aspects of renal β-amino acid transport: II. Ontogeny of uptake and efflux processes and effect of anoxia. Pediatr Res 1979;13:861.
203. Roth KS, Hwang SM, London JW, et al. Ontogeny of glycine transport in isolated rat renal tubules. Am J Physiol 1977; 233:F241.
204. Hwang SM, Serabian MA, Roth KS, et al. L-proline transport by isolated renal tubules from newborn and adult rats. Pediatr Res 1983;17:42.
205. Segal S, Smith I. Delineation of separate transport systems in rat kidney cortex for L-lysine and L-cystine by developmental patterns. Biochem Biophys Res Comm 1969;35:771.
206. Ross MG, Sherman DJ, Ervin MG, et al. Maternal dehydration-rehydration: fetal plasma and urinary responses. Am J Physiol 1988;255:E674.
207. Woods LL, Cheung CY, Power GG, et al. Role of arginine vasopressin in fetal renal response to hypertonicity. Am J Physiol 1986;251:F156.
208. McCance RA, Widdowson EM. Renal function before birth. Proc R Soc Lond (Biol) 1953;141:488.
209. Hansen JDL, Smith CA. Effects of withholding fluid in the immediate postnatal period. Pediatrics 1953;12:99.
210. Edelmann CM Jr, Barnett HL, Troupkou V. Renal concentrating mechanisms in newborn infants: effect of dietary protein, and water content, role of urea and responsiveness to antidiuretic hormone. J Clin Invest 1960;39:1062.
211. Calcagno PL, Rubin MI, Weintraub DH. Studies on the renal concentrating and diluting mechanisms in the premature infant. J Clin Invest 1954;33:91.
212. Polacek E, Vocel J, Neugebauerova L, et al. The osmotic concentrating ability in healthy infants and children. Arch Dis Child 1965;40:291.
213. Trimble ME. Renal response to solute loading in infant rats: relation to anatomical development. Am J Physiol 1970; 219:1089.
214. Horster MF, Gilg A, Lory P. Determinants of axial osmotic

gradients in the differentiating counter-current system. Am J Physiol 1984;246:F124.
215. Edwards BR, Mendel DB, LaRochelle FT Jr, et al. Postnatal development of urinary concentrating ability in rats: changes in renal anatomy and neurohypophysial hormones In: Spitzer A, ed. The kidney during development: morphology and function. New York: Masson, 1982:233.
216. Edelmann CM Jr, Barnett HL, Stark H. Effect of urea on concentration of urinary nonurea solute in premature infants. J Appl Physiol 1966;21:1021.
217. Hadeed AJ, Leake RD, Weitzman RE, et al. Possible mechanisms of high blood levels of vasopressin during the neonatal period. J Pediatr 1979;94:805.
218. Rees L, Forsling ML, Brook CGD. Vasopressin concentrations in the neonatal period. Clin Endocrinol 1980;12:357.
219. Leake RD, Weitzman RE, Weinberg JA, et al. Control of vasopressin secretion in the new-born lamb. Pediatr Res 1979;13:257.
220. Weitzman RE, Fisher DA, Robillard JE, et al. Arginine vasopressin response to an osmotic stimulus in the fetal sheep. Pediatr Res 1978;12:35.
221. DeVane GW, Porter JC. An apparent stress-induced release of arginine vasopressin by human neonates. J Clin Endocrinol Metab 1980;51:1412.
221a. Svenningsen NW, Aronson AS. Postnatal development of renal concentration capacity as estimated by DDAVP-test in normal and asphyxiated neonates. Biol Neonate 1974;25:230.
222. Rajerison RM, Butlen D, Jard S. Ontogenic development of kidney and liver vasopressin receptors. In: Spitzer A, ed. The kidney during development: morphology and function. New York: Masson, 1982:249.
223. Schlondorff D, Weber H, Trizna W, et al. Vasopressin responsiveness of renal adenylate cyclase in newborn rats and rabbits. Am J Physiol 1978;234:F16.
224. Anderson RJ, Berl T, McDonald KM, et al. Evidence for an in vivo antagonism between vasopressin and prostaglandin in the mammalian kidney. J Clin Invest 1975;56:420.

CLINICAL EVALUATION OF FUNCTION AND DISEASE

225. Museles M, Gaudry CC Jr, Bason WM. Renal anomalies in the newborn found by deep palpation. Pediatrics 1971;47:97.
226. Sherwood DW, Smith RC, Lemmon RH, et al. Abnormalities of the genitourinary tract discovered by palpation of the abdomen of the newborn. Pediatrics 1956;36:127.
227. Perlman M, Williams J. Detection of renal anomalies by abdominal palpation in newborn infants. Br Med J 1976;2:347.
228. Gillerot Y, Koulischer L. Major malformations of the urinary tract: anatomic and genetic aspects. Biol Neonate 1988;53:186.
229. Rubenstein M, Meyer R, Bernstein J. Congenital abnormalities of the urinary system: I. A postmortem survey of developmental anomalies and acquired congenital lesions in a children's hospital. J Pediatr 1961;58:356.
230. Helin I, Persson PH. Prenatal diagnosis of urinary tract abnormalities by ultrasound. Pediatrics 1986;78:879.
231. Livera LN, Brookfield DSK, Egginton JA, et al. Antenatal ultrasonography to detect fetal renal abnormalities: a prospective screening programme. Br Med J 1989;298:1421.
232. Scott JES, Lee REJ, Hunter EW, et al. Ultrasound screening of newborn urinary tract. Lancet 1991;2:338:1571.
233. Rubecz I, Kodela I, Gasztonyi V, et al. Postnatal screening examination of renal developmental anomalies: classical diagnosis, screening of risk group and routine screening. Orv Hetil 1991;132:585.
234. Brion L, Rondia G, Avni FE, et al. Importance of deep abdominal palpation in the perinatal diagnosis of urologic malformations. Biol Neonate 1984;46:215.
235. Steinhart JM, Kuhn JP, Eisenberg B, et al. Ultrasound screening of healthy infants for urinary tract abnormalities. Pediatrics 1988;82:609.
236. Roodhooft AM, Birnholz JC, Holmes LB. Familial nature of congenital absence and severe dysgenesis of both kidneys. N Engl J Med 1984;310:1341.
237. McPherson E, Carey J, Kramer A, et al. Dominantly inherited renal adysplasia. Am J Med Genet 1987;26:863.
238. Neave C. Congenital malformation in offspring of diabetics. Perspect Pediatr Pathol 1984;8:213.
239. Havers W, Majewski F, Olbing H, et al. Anomalies of the kidneys and genitourinary tract in alcohol embryopathy. J Urol 1980;124:108.
240. Lutiger B, Graham K, Einarson TR, et al. Relationship between gestational cocaine use and pregnancy outcome: a meta-analysis. Teratology 1991;44:405.
241. Petrikovsky BM, Nardi DA, Rodis JF, et al. Elevated maternal serum alpha-fetoprotein and mild fetal uropathy. Obstet Gynecol 1991;78:262.
242. Barr M Jr, Cohen MM Jr. ACE inhibitor fetopathy and hypocalvaria: the kidney–skull connection. Teratology 1991;44:485.
243. Cunniff C, Jones KL, Phillipson J, et al. Oligohydramnios sequence and renal tubular malformation associated with maternal enalapril use. Am J Obstet Gynecol 1990;162:187.
244. Gubler MC, vd Heijden AJ, Carlus C, et al. Persistent anuria in 6 neonates exposed to indomethacin (ID) during pregnancy (Abstract). J Am Soc Nephrol 1991;2:307.
245. Thomas IT, Smith DW. Oligohydramnios, cause of the nonrenal features of Potter's syndrome, including pulmonary hypoplasia. J Pediatr 1974;84:811.
246. Hislop A, Hey E, Reid L. The lungs in congenital bilateral renal agenesis and dysplasia. Arch Dis Child 1979;54:32.
247. Nimrod C, Varela-Gittings F, Machin G, et al. The effect of very prolonged membrane rupture on fetal development. Am J Obstet Gynecol 1984;148:540.
248. Moessinger AC, Collins MH, Blanc WA, et al. Oligohydramnios-induced lung hypoplasia: the influence of timing and duration in gestation. Pediatr Res 1986;20:951.
249. Thibeault DW, Beatty EC Jr, Hall RT, et al. Neonatal pulmonary hypoplasia with premature rupture of fetal membranes and oligohydramnios. J Pediatr 1985;107:273.
250. Khuri FJ, Hardy BE, Churchill BM. Urologic anomalies associated with hypospadias. Urol Clin North Am 1981;8:565.
251. Faierman E. The significance of one umbilical artery. Arch Dis Child 1960;35:285.
252. Froehlich LA, Fujikura T. Significance of a single umbilical artery. Am J Obstet Gynecol 1966:94:274.
253. Heifetz SA. Single umbilical artery: a statistical analysis of 237 autopsy cases and review of the literature. Perspect Pediatr Pathol 1984;8:345.
254. Ainsworth P, Davies PA. The single umbilical artery: a five-year survey. Dev Med Child Neurol 1969;11:297.
255. Lachiewicz AM, Sibley R, Michael AF. Hereditary renal disease and preauricular pits: report of a kindred. J Pediatr 1985;106:948.
256. Rothe CF, Kim KC. Measuring systolic arterial blood pressure: possible errors from extension tubes or disposable transducer domes. Crit Care Med 1980;8:683.
257. Kimble KJ, Darnall RA Jr, Yelderman M, et al. An automated oscillometric technique for estimating mean arterial pressure in critically ill newborns. Anesthesiology 1981;54:423.
258. Kirkendall WM, Feinleib M, Freis ED, et al. Recommendations for human blood pressure determination by sphygmo-

manometers: Subcommittee on the AHA Postgraduate Education Committee. Circulation 1980;62:1146A.
259. Lum LG, Jones MD Jr. The effect of cuff width on systolic blood pressure measurements in neonates. J Pediatr 1977; 91:963.
260. Baker DM, Maisels MJ, Marks KH. Indirect BP monitoring in the newborn: evaluation of a new oscillometer and comparison of upper- and lower-limb measurements. Am J Dis Child 1984;138:775.
261. Piazza SF, Chandra M, Harper RG, et al. Upper- vs lower-limb systolic blood pressure in full-term normal newborns. Am J Dis Child 1985;139:797.
262. Park MK, Lee DH. Normative arm and calf blood pressure values in the newborn. Pediatrics 1989;83:240.
263. Tan KL. Blood pressure in very low birth weight infants in the first 70 days of life. J Pediatr 1988;112:266.
264. de Swiet M, Fayers P, Shinebourne EA. Systolic blood pressure in a population of infants in the first year of life: the Brompton Study. Pediatrics 1980;65:1028.
265. Versmold HT, Kitterman JA, Phibbs RH, et al. Aortic blood pressure during the first 12 hours of life in infants with birth weight 610 to 4,220 grams. Pediatrics 1981;67:607.
266. Zinner SH, Lee YH, Rosner B, et al. Factors affecting blood pressures in newborn infants. Hypertension 1980;2(Suppl 1):I-99.
267. Spahr RC, MacDonald HM, Mueller-Heubach E. Knee–chest position and neonatal oxygenation and blood pressure. Am J Dis Child 1981;135:79.
268. Sinkin RA, Philips BL, Adelman RD. Elevation in systemic blood pressure in the neonate during abdominal examination. Pediatrics 1985;76:970.
269. Gemelli M, Manganaro R, Mami C, et al. Circadian blood pressure pattern in full-term newborn infants. Biol Neonate 1989;56:315.
270. Scott JES, Hunter EW, Lee REJ, et al. Ultrasound measurement of renal size in newborn infants. Arch Dis Child 1990; 65:361.
271. Longino LA, Martin LW. Abdominal masses in the newborn infant. Pediatrics 1958;596.
272. Griscom NT, Colodny AH, Rosenberg HK, et al. Diagnostic aspects of neonatal ascites: report of 27 cases. AJR 1977; 128:961.
273. Shaffer SG, Quimiro CL, Anderson JV, et al. Postnatal weight changes in low birth weight infants. Pediatrics 1987;79:702.
274. Sherry SN, Kramer I. The time of passage of the first stool and first urine by the newborn infant. J Pediatr 1955;46: 158.
275. Kramer I, Sherry SN. The time of passage of the first stool and urine by the premature infant. J Pediatr 1957;51:373.
276. Clark DA. Time of first void and first stool in 500 newborns. Pediatrics 1977;60:457.
277. Pynnönen AL, Kouvalainen K, Jäykkä S. Time of the first urinations in male and female newborns. Acta Paediatr Scand 1972;61:303.
278. Chih TW, Teng RJ, Wang CS, et al. Time of the first urine and the first stool in Chinese newborns. Acta Paediatr Sin 1991;32:17.
279. Bidiwala KS, Lorenz JM, Kleinman LI. Renal function correlates of postnatal diuresis in preterm infants. Pediatrics 1988;82:50.
279a. Benitez OA, Benitez M, Slynen T, et al. Inaccuracy in neonatal measurement of urine concentration with a refractometer. J Pediatr 1986;108:613.
280. Coulthard MG, Ruddock V. Validation of inulin as a marker for glomerular filtration in preterm babies. Kidney Int 1983; 23:407.
281. Summerville DA, Potter CS, Treves ST. The use of radiopharmaceuticals in the measurement of glomerular filtration rate: a review. In: Freeman LM, ed. Nuclear medicine annual 1990. New York: Raven Press, 1990:191.
282. Coulthard MG. Comparison of methods of measuring renal function in preterm babies using inulin. J Pediatr 1983; 102:923.
283. Arant BS Jr, Edelmann CM Jr, Spitzer A. The congruence of creatinine and inulin clearances in children: use of the Technicon autoanalyzer. J Pediatr 1972;84:559.
284. Bauer JH, Brooks CS, Burch RN. Clinical appraisal of creatinine clearance as a measurement of glomerular filtration rate. Am J Kidney Dis 1982;2:337.
285. Welch MJ, Cohen A, Hertz HS, et al. Determination of serum creatinine by isotope dilution mass spectrometry as a candidate definitive method. Anal Chem 1986;58:1681.
286. Rosano TG, Ambrose RT, Wu AHB, et al. Candidate reference method for determining creatinine in serum: method development and interlaboratory validation. Clin Chem 1990;36:1951.
287. Weber JA, van Zanten AP. Interferences in current methods for measurements of creatinine. Clin Chem 1991;37:695.
288. Schwartz GJ, Feld LG, Langford DJ. A simple estimate of glomerular filtration rate in full term infants during the first year of life. J Pediatr 1984;104:849.
289. Brion L, Fleischman AR, McCarton C, et al. A simple estimate of glomerular filtration rate in low birth weight infants during the first year of life: non invasive assessment of body composition and growth. J Pediatr 1986;109:698.
290. Coulthard MG, Hey EN. Weight as the best standard for glomerular filtration in the newborn. Arch Dis Child 1984;59:373.
291. Rudd PT, Hughes EA, Placzek MM, et al. Reference ranges for plasma creatinine during the first month of life. Arch Dis Child 1983;58:212.
292. Schwartz GJ, Brion L, Spitzer A. The use of plasma creatinine concentration for estimating glomerular filtration rate in infants, children and adolescents. Pediatr Clin North Am 1987;34:579
293. Schwartz GJ, Haycock G, Edelmann CM Jr, et al. A simple estimate of glomerular filtration rate in children derived from body length and plasma creatinine. Pediatrics 1976;58:259
294. Brion LP, Fleischman AR, Schwartz GJ. Gentamicin interval in newborn infants determined by renal function and postconceptional age. Pediatric Nephrology 1991;5:675.
295. McCracken GH, Chrane DF, Thomas ML. Pharmacologic evaluation of gentamicin in newborn infants. J Infect Dis 1971;124:S214.
296. Koren G, James A, Perlman M. A simple method for the estimation of glomerular filtration rate by gentamicin pharmacokinetics during routine monitoring in the newborn. Clin Pharmacol Therap 1985;38:680.
297. Kildoo CW, Lin LM, Gabriel MH, et al. Vancomycin pharmacokinetics in infants: relationship to postconceptional age and serum creatinine. Dev Pharmacol Ther 1990;14:77.
298. Oyanagi K, Nakamura K, Sogawa H, et al. A study of urea-synthesizing enzymes in prenatal and postnatal human liver. Pediatr Res 1980;14:236.
299. Stapleton FB. Renal uric acid clearance in human neonates. J Pediatr 1983;103:290.
300. Stapleton FB, Arant BS Jr. Ontogeny of renal uric acid excretion in the mongrel puppy. Pediatr Res 1981;15:1513.
301. Germino GG, Barton NJ, Lamb J, et al. Identification of a locus which shows no genetic recombination with the autosomal dominant polycystic kidney disease gene on chromosome 16. Am J Hum Genet 1990;46:925.
302. Saris JJ, Breuning MH, Dauwerse HG, et al. Rapid detection

of polymorphism near gene for adult polycystic kidney disease. Lancet 1 1990;335:1102.
303. Aas K. The cellular excretion in the urine of normal newborn infants. Acta Paediatrica 1961;50:361.
304. Kronquist KE, Crandall BF, Tabsh KM. Characterization of fetal urinary proteins at midgestation and term. Biol Neonate 1984;46:267.
305. Van Oort A, Monnens L, van Munster P. Beta-2-microglobulin clearance, an indicator of renal tubular maturation. Int J Pediatr Nephrol 1980;1:80.
306. Gordon I, Barratt TM. Imaging the kidneys and urinary tract in the neonate with acute renal failure. Pediatr Nephrol 1987;1:321.
307. Slovis TL. Pediatric renal anomalies and infections. Clinics in Diagnostic Ultrasound 1989;24:157.
308. McCarten KM, Cleveland RH, Simeone JF, et al. Renal ultrasonography in Beckwith-Wiedemann syndrome. Pediatr Radiol 1981;11:46.
309. Restaino I, Kaplan BS, Kaplan P, et al. Renal dysgenesis in a monozygotic twin: association with in utero exposure to indomethacin. Am J Med Genet 1991;39:252.
310. Stapleton FB, Hilton S, Wilcox J, et al. Transient nephromegaly simulating infantile polycystic disease of the kidneys. Pediatrics 1981;67:554.
311. Lusiri A, Salinas-Madrigal L, Noguchi A, et al. Renal tubular dysgenesis. AJR 1991;157:383.
312. Shackelford GD, Kees-Folts D, Cole BR. Imaging the urinary tract. Clin Perinatol 1992;19:85.
313. Shultz PK, Strife JL, Strife CF, et al. Hyperechoic renal medullary pyramids in infants and children. Radiology 1991; 181:163.
314. Glickstein J, Friedman D, Schacht R, et al. Renal artery Doppler waveforms in neonates with umbilical artery catheters. Clin Res 1991;39:669A
315. Van Bel F, Guit GL, Schipper J, et al. Indomethacin-induced changes in renal blood flow velocity waveform in premature infants investigated with color Doppler imaging. J Pediatr 1991;118:621
316. Gaum LD, Wese FX, Alton DJ, et al. Radiologic investigation of the urinary tract in the neonate with myelomeningocele. J Urol 1982;127:510.
317. Ash JM, Antico VF, Gilday DL, et al. Special considerations in the pediatric use of radionuclides for kidney studies. Semin Nucl Med 1982;12:345.
318. Kullendorf CM, Salmonson EC, Laurin S. Diagnostic cyst puncture of multicystic kidney in neonates. Acta Radiol 1990;31:287.
319. Edelmann CM Jr, ed. Pediatric kidney disease. 2nd ed. Boston: Little, Brown & Co, 1992:499.

ACUTE RENAL FAILURE AND OLIGOANURIA

320. Gaudio KM, Siegel NJ. Pathogenesis and treatment of acute renal failure. Pediatr Clin North Am 1987;34:771.
321. Chevalier RL, Campbell F, Norman A, Brenbridge AG. Prognostic factors in neonatal acute renal failure. Pediatrics 1984;74:265.
322. Norman ME, Asadi FK. A prospective study of acute renal failure in the newborn infant. Pediatrics 1979;63:475.
323. Stapleton FB, Jones DP, Green RS. Acute renal failure in neonates: incidence, etiology and outcome. Pediatr Nephrol 1987;1:314.
324. Medani CR, Davitt MK, Huntington DF, et al. Acute renal failure in the newborn. Contrib Nephrol 1979;15:47.
325. Hanssens M, Keirse MJNC, Vankelecom F, et al. Fetal and neonatal effects of treatment with angiotensin-converting enzyme inhibitors in pregnancy. Obstet Gynecol 1991;78: 128.
326. Rosa FW, Bosco LA, Graham CF, et al. Neonatal anuria with maternal angiotensin-converting enzyme inhibition. Obstet Gynecol 1989;74:371.
327. Grylack L, Medani C, Hultzen C, et al. Non oliguric acute renal failure in the newborn: a prospective evaluation of diagnostic indexes. Am J Dis Child 1982;136:518.
328. McCroy WW. Congenital malformations causing renal failure in the neonatal period. Contrib Nephrol 1979;15:55.
329. Arrowsmith JB, Faich GA, Tomita DK, et al. Morbidity and mortality among low birth weight infants exposed to an intravenous vitamin E product, E-Ferol. Pediatrics 1989;83:244.
330. Tack ED, Perlman JM. Renal failure in sick hypertensive premature infants receiving captopril therapy. J Pediatr 1988; 112:805.
331. Parchoux B, Bourgeois J, Gilly J, et al. Hypertrophic kidneys in utero and neonatal renal failure by diffuse mesangial sclerosis. Pédiatrie 1988;43:219.
332. Nauta J, de Heer E, Baldwin III WM, et al. Transplantal induction of membranous nephropathy in a neonate. Pediatr Nephrol 1990;4:111.
333. Ridgen SPA, Barratt TM, Dillon MJ, et al. Acute renal failure complicating cardiopulmonary bypass surgery. Arch Dis Child 1982;57:425.
334. Hollenberg NK, Epstein M, Rosen SM, et al. Acute oliguric renal failure in man: evidence for preferential renal cortical ischemia. Medicine (Baltimore) 1968;47:455.
335. Isenberg G, Racelis D, Oh J, et al. Prevention of ischemic renal damage with prostacyclin. Mt Sinai J Med (NY) 1982; 49:415.
336. Finn WF, Chevalier RL. Recovery from postischemic acute renal failure in the rat. Kidney Int 1979;16:113.
337. Myers BD, Chui F, Hilberman M, et al. Transtubular leakage of glomerular filtrate in human acute renal failure. Am J Physiol 1979;237:F319.
338. Kasik JW, Leuschen MP, Bolam DL, et al. Rhabdomyolysis and myoglobinemia in neonates. Pediatrics 1985;76:255.
339. Perlman JM, Tack ED. Renal injury in the asphyxiated newborn infant: relationship to neurologic outcome. J Pediatr 1988;113:875.
340. Roberts DS, Haycock GB, Dalton RN, et al. Prediction of acute renal failure after birth asphyxia. Arch Dis Child 1990;65: 1021.
341. Kojima T, Kobayashi T, Matsuzaki S, et al. Effects of perinatal asphyxia and myoglobinuria on development of acute, neonatal renal failure. Arch Dis Child 1985;60:908.
342. DiSessa TG, Leitner M, Ti CC, et al. The cardiovascular effects of dopamine in the severely asphyxiated neonate. J Pediatr 1981;99:772.
343. Seri I, Tulassay T, Kiszel J, et al. Cardiovascular response to dopamine in hypotensive preterm neonates with severe hyaline membrane disease. Eur J Pediatr 1984;142:3.
344. Tulassay T, Seri I, Machay T, et al. Effects of dopamine on renal functions in premature neonates with respiratory distress syndrome. Int J Pediatr Nephrol 1983;4:19.
345. Cuevas L, Yeh TF, John EG, et al. The effect of low-dose dopamine infusion on cardiopulmonary and renal status in premature newborns with respiratory distress syndrome. Am J Dis Child 1991;145:799.
346. Sulyok E, Seri I, Tulassay T, et al. The effect of dopamine administration on the activity of the renin–angiotensin–aldosterone system in sick preterm infants. Eur J Pediatr 1985; 143:191.
347. Yeh TF, Wilks A, Singh J, et al. Furosemide prevents the renal

side effects of indomethacin in premature infants with patent ductus arteriosus. J Pediatr 1982;101:433.
348. Ivey HH. The asphyxiated bladder as a cause of delayed micturition in the newborn. J Urol 1978;120:498
349. Giacoia GP, Miranda R, West KI. Measured vs calculated plasma osmolality in infants with very low birth weights. Am J Dis Child 1992;146:712.
350. Ellis EN, Arnold WC. Use of urinary indexes in renal failure in the newborn. Am J Dis Child 1982;136:615.
351. Matthew OP, Jones AS, James E, et al. Neonatal renal failure: usefulness of diagnostic indices. Pediatrics 1980;65:57.
352. Tack ED, Perlman JM, Robson AM. Renal injury in sick newborn infants: a prospective evaluation using urinary β_2-microglobulin concentrations. Pediatrics 1988;81:432.
353. Cole JW, Portman RJ, Lim Y, et al. Urinary β_2-microglobulin in full-term newborns: evidence for proximal tubular dysfunction in infants with meconium-stained amniotic fluid. Pediatrics 1985;76:958.
354. Tsukahara H, Yoshimoto M, Saito M, et al. Assessment of tubular function in neonates using urinary β_2-microglobulin. Pediatr Nephrol 1990;4:512.
355. Chiara A, Chirico G, Comelli L, et al. Increased renal echogenicity in the neonate. Early Hum Dev 1990;22:29.
356. Avni EF, Spehl-Robberecht M, Lebrun D, et al. Transient acute tubular disease in the newborn: characteristic ultrasound pattern. Ann Radiol (Paris) 1983;26:175.
357. Dmochowski RR, Crandell SS, Corriere JN Jr. Bladder injury and uroascites from umbilical artery catheterization. Pediatrics 1986;77:421.
358. Gouyon JB, Guignard JP. Drugs and acute renal insufficiency in the neonate. Biol Neonate 1986;50:177.
359. Dorman HR, Sondheimer JH, Cadnapaphornchai P. Mannitol-induced acute renal failure. Medicine (Baltimore) 1990; 69:153.
360. Myers BD, Moran SM. Hemodynamically mediated acute renal failure. N Engl J Med 1986;314:97.
361. Davis RF, Lappas DG, Kirklin JK, et al. Acute oliguria after cardiopulmonary bypass: renal functional improvement with low-dose dopamine infusion. Crit Care Med 1982;10: 852.
362. Henderson IS, Beattie TK, Kennedy AC. Dopamine hydrochloride in oliguric states. Lancet 1980;1:827.
363. Lindner A. Synergism of dopamine and furosemide in diuretic-resistant, oliguric acute renal failure. Nephron 1983; 33:121.
364. Parker S, Carlon GC, Isaacs M, et al. Dopamine administration in oliguria and oliguric renal failure. Crit Care Med 1981; 9:630.
365. Brion LP, Schwartz GJ, Campbell D, et al. Early hyperkalemia in very low birthweight infants in the absence of oliguria. Arch Dis Child 1989;64:270.
366. Meeks ACG, Sims DG. Treatment of acute renal failure in neonates. Arch Dis Child 1988;63:1372.
367. Finn WF. Diagnosis and management of acute tubular necrosis. Med Clin North Am 1990;74:873.
368. Shaffer SE, Norman ME. Renal function and renal failure in the newborn. Clin Perinatol 1989;16:199.
369. Engle WD. Evaluation of renal function and acute renal failure in the neonate. Pediatr Clin North Am 1986;33:129.
370. Karlowicz MG, Adelman RD. Acute renal failure in the neonate. Clin Perinatol 1992;19:139.
371. Usher R. The respiratory distress syndrome of prematurity: I. Changes in potassium in the serum and the electrocardiogram and effects of therapy. Pediatrics 1959;25:562.
372. Gaylord MS, Pittman PA, Bartness J, et al. Release of benzalkonium chloride from a heparin-bonded umbilical catheter with resultant factitious hypernatremia and hyperkalemia. Pediatrics 1991;87:631.
373. Gruskay J, Costarino AT, Polin RA, et al. Nonoliguric hyperkalemia in the premature infant weighing less than 1000 grams. J Pediatr 1988;113:381.
374. Smith JD, Bia MJ, DeFronzo RA. Clinical disorders of potassium metabolism. In: Arieff AI, DeFronzo RA, eds. Fluid, electrolyte, and acid–base disorders. vol. 1. New York: Churchill-Livingstone, 1985:413.
375. Lui K, Thungappa U, Nair A, et al. Treatment with hypertonic dextrose and insulin in severe hyperkalaemia of immature infants. Acta Paediatr 1992;81:213.
376. Murdoch IA, Dos Anjos R, Haycock GB. Treatment of hyperkalemia with intravenous salbutamol. Arch Dis Child 1991;66:527.
377. Malone TA. Glucose and insulin versus cation-exchange resin for the treatment of hyperkalemia in very low birth weight infants. J Pediatr 1991;118:121.
378. Ohlsson A, Hosking M. Complications following oral administration of exchange resins in extremely low-birth-weight infants. Eur J Pediatr 1987;146:571.
379. Setzer ES, Ahmed F, Goldberg RN, et al. Exchange transfusion using washed red blood cells reconstituted with fresh-frozen plasma for treatment of severe hyperkalemia in the neonate. J Pediatr 1984;104:443.
380. Llach F, Felsenfeld AJ, Haussler MR. The pathophysiology of altered calcium metabolism in rhabdomyolysis-induced acute renal failure: interactions of parathyroid hormone, 25-hydroxy-cholecalciferol and 1,25-dihydroxycholecalciferol. N Engl J Med 1981;305:117.
381. Patel V, Savage A. Symptomatic hypomagnesemia associated with gentamicin therapy. Nephron 1979;23:50.
382. Arieff AI, Massry SG. Effects of uremia, hemodialysis, and parathyroid hormone. J Clin Invest 1974;53:837.
383. Zamarella P, Zorzi C, Pavanello L, et al. The prognostic significance of acute neonatal renal failure. Child Nephrol Urol 1991;11:15.
384. Carter PE, Lloyd DJ, Duffty P. Glucagon for hypoglycemia in infants small for gestational age. Arch Dis Child 1988;63: 1264.
385. Kekömaki M. Uremic catabolism in a neonate: reversal by parenteral nutrition. J Pediatr Surg 1981;16:35.
386. Matthews DE, West KW, Rescorla FJ, et al. Peritoneal dialysis in the first 60 days of life. J Pediatr Surg 1990;25:110.
387. Nash MA, Russo JC. Neonatal lactic acidosis and renal failure: the role of peritoneal dialysis. J Pediatr 1977;91:101.
388. Bishof NA, Welch TR, Strife CF, et al. Continuous hemodiafiltration in children. Pediatrics 1990;85:819.
389. Zobel G, Ring E, Müller W. Continuous arteriovenous hemofiltration in premature infants. Crit Care Med 1989;17:534.
390. Ronco C, Brendolan A, Bragantini L, et al. Treatment of acute renal failure in newborns by continuous arterio-venous hemofiltration. Kidney Int 1986;29:908.
391. Callan NA, Blakemore K, Park J, et al. Fetal genitourinary tract anomalies: evaluation, operative correction, and follow-up. Obstet Gynecol 1990;75:67.
392. Glick PL, Harrison MR, Golbus MS, et al. Management of the fetus with congenital hydronephrosis: II. Prognostic criteria and selection for treatment. J Pediatr Surg 1985;20:376.
393. Elder JS, O'Grady JP, Ashmead G, et al. Evaluation of fetal renal function: unreliability of fetal urinary electrolytes. J Urol 1990 (Part 2);144:574.
394. Stark H, Geiger R. Renal tubular dysfunction following vascular accidents of the kidney in the newborn period. J Pediatr 1973;83:933.
395. Bensman A, Baudon JJ, Jablonski JP, et al. Uropathies diag-

nosed in the neonatal period: symptomatology and course. Acta Paediatr Scand 1980;69:499.
396. Genest DR, Lage JM. Absence of normal-appearing proximal tubules in the fetal and neonatal kidney: prevalence and significance. Hum Pathol 1991;22:147.
397. Swinford AE, Bernstein J, Toriello HV, et al. Renal tubular dysgenesis: delayed onset of oligohydramnios. Am J Med Genet 1989;32:127.
398. Schwartz BR, Lage JM, Pober BR, et al. Isolated congenital renal tubular immaturity in siblings. Hum Pathol 1986; 17:1259.
399. Allanson JE, Pantzar JT, Mac Leod PM. Possible new autosomal recessive syndrome with unusual renal histopathological changes. Am J Med Genet 1983;16:57.
400. Voland JR, Hawkins EP, Wells TR, et al. Congenital hypernephronic nephromegaly with tubular dysgenesis: a distinctive inherited renal anomaly. Pediatr Pathol 1985;4:231.
401. Lorentz WB, Trillo AA. Neonatal renal failure and glomerular immaturity. Clin Nephrol 1983;19:154.
402. Malin SW, Baumgart S, Rosenberg HK, et al. Nonsurgical management of obstructive aortic thrombosis complicated by renovascular hypertension in the neonate. J Pediatr 1985; 106:630.
403. Payne RM, Martin TC, Bower RJ, et al. Management and follow-up of arterial thrombosis in the neonatal period. J Pediatr 1989;114:853.
404. Kennedy LA, Drummond WH, Knight ME, et al. Successful treatment of neonatal aortic thrombosis with tissue plasminogen activator. J Pediatr 1990;116:798.
405. Seibert JJ, Northington FJ, Miers JF, et al. Aortic thrombosis after umbilical artery catheterization in neonates: prevalence of complications on long-term follow-up. AJR 1991; 156:567.
406. Neal WA, Reynolds JW, Jarvis CW, et al. Umbilical artery catheterization: demonstration of arterial thrombosis by arteriography. Pediatrics 1972;50:16.
407. Mokrohisky ST, Levine RL, Blumhagen JD, et al. Low positioning of umbililical-artery catheters increases associated complications in newborn infants. N Engl J Med 1978;299:561.
408. Goetzman BW, Stadalnik RC, Bogren HG, et al. Thrombotic complications of umbilical artery catheters: a clinical and radiologic study. Pediatrics 1975;56:374.
409. Umbilical Artery Catheter Trial Study Group. Relationship of intraventricular hemorrhage or death with the level of umbilical artery catheter placement: a multicenter randomized clinical trial. Pediatr 1992;90:881.
410. Schmidt B, Andrew M. Neonatal thrombotic disease: prevention, diagnosis and management. J Pediatr 1988;113:407.
411. Durante D, Jones D, Spitzer R. Neonatal renal arterial embolism syndrome. J Pediatr 1976;89:978.
412. Adelman RD, Merten D, Vogel J, et al. Nonsurgical management of renovascular hypertension in the neonate. Pediatrics 1978;62:71.
413. Caplan MS, Cohn RA, Langman CB, et al. Favorable outcome of neonatal aortic thrombosis and renovascular hypertension. J Pediatr 1989;115:291.
414. Vailas GN, Brouillette RT, Scott JP, et al. Neonatal aortic thrombosis: recent experience. J Pediatr 1986;109:101.
415. Seibert JJ, Northington FJ, Miers JF, et al. Aortic thrombosis after umbilical artery catheterization in neonates: prevalence of complications on long-term follow-up. AJR 1991;156:567.
416. Adelman RD. Long-term follow-up of neonatal renovascular hypertension. Pediatr Nephrol 1987;1:35.
417. Olson D. Renal vein thrombosis in infants. In: Lieberman E, ed. Clinical pediatric nephrology. 1st ed. Philadelphia: JB Lippincott, 1976:372.
418. Takeuchi A, Benirschke K. Renal venous thrombosis of the newborn and its relation to maternal diabetes: report of 16 cases. Biol Neonate 1961;3:237.
419. Rasoulpour M, McLean RH. Renal venous thrombosis in neonates. Initial and follow-up abnormalities. Am J Dis Child 1980;134:276.
420. Lam AH, Warren PS. Ultrasonographic diagnosis of neonatal renal venous thrombosis. Ann Radiol 1981;24:7.
421. Lebowitz JM, Belman AB. Simultaneous idiopathic adrenal hemorrhage and renal vein thrombosis in the newborn. J Urol 1983;129:574.
422. Corrigan JJ Jr, Jeter MA. Tissue-type plasminogen activator, plasminogen activator inhibitor, and histidine-rich glycoproteins in stressed human newborns. Pediatrics 1992;89:43.
423. Evans DJ, Silverman M, Bowley NB. Congenital hypertension due to unilateral renal vein thrombosis. Arch Dis Child 1981;56:306.
424. Mocan H, Beattie TJ, Murphy AV. Renal venous thrombosis in infancy: long-term follow-up. Pediatr Nephrol 1991;5:45.
425. Clark AGB, Saunders A, Bewick M, et al. Neonatal inferior vena cava and renal venous thrombosis treated by thrombectomy and nephrectomy. Arch Dis Child 1985;60:1076.
426. Bromberg WD, Firlit CF. Fibrinolytic therapy for renal vein thrombosis in the child. J Urol 1990;143:86.
427. Leonidas JC, Berdon WE, Gribetz D. Bilateral renal cortical necrosis in the newborn infant: roentgenographic diagnosis. J Pediatr 1971;79:623.
428. Kurnetz R, Bernstein J. Neonatal blood loss and hematuria. J Pediatr 1974;84:452.
429. Anand K, Northway JD, Smith JA. Neonatal renal papillary and cortical necrosis. Am J Dis Child 1977;131:773.
430. Van Reempts PJ, Boven KJ, Spitaels SE, et al. Idiopathic arterial calcification of infancy. Calcif Tissue Int 1991;48:1.
431. Terzi F, Assael BM, Claris-Appiani A, et al. Increased sodium requirement following early postnatal surgical correction of congenital uropathies in infants. Pediatr Nephrol 1990;4:581

NEPHROTOXICITY: DRUGS AND TOXINS

432. Assadi FK. Renal tubular dysfunction in fetal alcohol syndrome. Pediatr Nephrol 1990;4:48.
433. Lindemann R. Congenital renal tubular dysfunction associated with maternal sniffing of organic solvents. Acta Paediatr Scand 1991;80:882.
434. Brown WJ, Buist NR, Gipson HT, et al. Fatal benzyl alcohol poisoning in a neonatal intensive care unit. Lancet 1982; 1:1250.
435. Gershanik J, Boeckler B, Enlsey H, et al. The gasping syndrome and benzyl alcohol poisoning. N Engl J Med 1982; 307:1384.
436. McNeil JS, Jackson B, Nelson L, et al. The role of prostaglandins in gentamicin-induced nephrotoxicity in the dog. Nephron 1983;33:202.
437. Cronin RE, Bulger RE, Southern P, et al. Natural history of aminoglycoside nephrotoxicity in the dog. J Lab Clin Med 1980;95:463.
438. Elliott WC, Houghton DC, Gilbert DN, et al. Gentamicin nephrotoxicity: II. Definition of conditions necessary to induce acquired insensitivity. J Lab Clin Med 1982;100:513.
439. Klotman PE, Boatman JE, Volpp BD, et al. Captopril enhances aminoglycoside nephrotoxicity in potassium-depleted rats. Kidney Int 1985;28:118.
440. Higa EMS, Schor N, Boim MA, et al. Role of the prostaglandin and kallikrein-kinin systems in aminoglycoside-induced acute renal failure. Braz J Med Biol Res 1981;18:355.
441. Cojocel C, Hook JB. Aminoglycoside nephrotoxicity. Trends Pharmacol Sci 1983;4:174.

442. Riviere JE. Limitations on the physiologic interpretation of aminoglycoside body clearance derived from pharmacokinetic studies. Res Commun Chem Pathol Pharmacol 1982; 38:31.
443. Safirstein R, Miller P, Kahn T. Cortical and papillary absorptive defects in gentamicin nephrotoxicity. Kidney Int 1983; 24:526.
444. Chahwala SB, Harpur ES. Gentamicin-induced hypercalciuria in the rat. Acta Pharmacol Toxicol 1983;53:358.
445. Cojocel C, Dociu N, Ceacmacudis E, et al. Nephrotoxic effects of aminoglycoside treatment on renal protein reabsorption and accumulation. Nephron 1984;37:113.
446. Baylis C, Rennke HE, Brenner BM. Mechanisms of the defect in glomerular ultrafiltration associated with gentamicin administration. Kidney Int 1977;12:344.
447. Rajchgot P, Prober CG, Soldin S, et al. Aminoglycoside-related nephrotoxicity in the premature newborn. Clin Pharmacol Ther 1984;35:394.
448. Riviere JE, Carver MP, Coppoc GL, et al. Pharmacokinetics and comparative nephrotoxicity of fixed-dose versus fixed-interval reduction of gentamicin dosage in subtotal nephrectomized dogs. Toxicol Appl Pharmacol 1984;75:496.
449. Rybak MJ, Frankowski JJ, Ewards DJ, et al. Alanine aminopeptidase and beta-2-microglobulin excretion in patients receiving vancomycin and gentamicin. Antimicrob Agents Chemother 1987;31:1461.
450. Kacew S, Bergeron MG. Pathogenic factors in aminoglycoside-induced nephrotoxicity. Toxicol Lett 1990;51:241.
451. Nahata MC. Lack of nephrotoxicity in pediatric patients receiving concurrent vancomycin and aminoglycoside therapy. Chemotherapy 1987;33:302.
452. Swinney VR, Rudd CC. Nephrotoxicity of vancomycin-gentamicin therapy in pediatric patients. J Pediatr 1987;110:497.
453. Goren MP, Baker DK Jr, Shenep JL. Vancomycin does not enhance amikacin-induced tubular nephrotoxicity in children. Pediatr Infect Dis J 1989;8:278.
454. Kacew S, Hewitt WR, Hook JB. Gentamicin-induced renal metabolic alterations in newborn rat kidney: lack of potentiation by vancomycin. Toxicol Appl Pharmacol 1989;99:61.
455. Cowan RH, Jukkola AF, Arant BS Jr. Pathophysiologic evidence of gentamicin nephrotoxicity in neonatal puppies. Pediatr Res 1980;14:1204.
456. Heimann G. Renal toxicity of aminoglycosides in the neonatal period. Pediatr Pharmacol 1983;3:251.
457. Russo JC, Adelman RD. Gentamicin-induced Fanconi syndrome. J Pediatr 1980;96:151.
458. Casteels-Van Daele M, Corbeel L, Van de Casseye W, et al. Gentamicin-induced Fanconi syndrome. J Pediatr 1980;97: 507.
459. Ylitalo P, Mörsky P, Parviainen MT, et al. Nephrotoxicity of tobramycin: value of examining various protein and enzyme markers. Methods Find Exp Clin Pharmacol 1991;13:281.
460. Williamson HE. Interaction of cyclosporine and indomethacin in the rat. Res Commun Chem Pathol Pharmacol 1988;61: 141.
461. Falzon M, Whiting PH, Ewen SWB, et al. Comparative effects of indomethacin on hepatic enzymes and histology and on serum indices of liver and kidney function in the rat. Br J Exp Pathol 1985;66:527.
462. Katz SM, Sufian S, Matsumoto T. Urinary myelin figures in gentamicin nephrotoxicity. Am J Clin Pathol 1979;72:621.
463. Sufian S, Katz SM. Urinary myelin figures in gentamicin treated vs. ischemic kidneys. Am Surg 1983;49:254.
464. Sande MA, Mandell GL. Antimicrobial agents (continued): the aminoglycosides. Gilman AG, Goodman LS, Rall TW, et al, eds. In: Goodman and Gilman's the pharmacological basis of therapeutics. New York: MacMillan, 1985:1150.
465. Bhat R, Vidyasagar D, Vadapalli M, et al. Disposition of indomethacin in preterm infants. J Pediatr 1979;95:313.
466. Bergamo RR, Cominelli F, Kopple JD, et al. Comparative acute effects of aspirin, diflunisal, ibuprofen and indomethacin on renal function in healthy man. Am J Nephrol 1989; 9:460.
467. Seyberth HW, Rascher W, Hackenthal R, et al. Effect of prolonged indomethacin therapy on renal function and selected vasoactive hormones in very-low-birth-weight infants with symptomatic patent ductus arteriosus. J Pediatr 1983;103: 979.
468. Hammerman C, Aramburo MJ. Prolonged indomethacin therapy for the prevention of recurrences of patent ductus arteriosus. J Pediatr 1990;117:771.
469. Jansen HML, Russel FGM, Wouterse AC, et al. Renal handling of indomethacin: isolated membrane vesicles of proximal tubular cells as an in vitro model system for transport. Neth J Med 1989;35:134.
470. vd Heijden AJ, Provoost AP, Grose W, et al. Renal functional impairment in preterm neonates related to intrauterine indomethacin exposure. Pediatr Res 1988;24:644.
471. Spital A, Akrawi A. Indomethacin does not impair cellular potassium uptake in the rat. Am J Kidney Dis 1990;15:316.
472. John EG, Vasan U, Hastreiter AR, et al. Intravenous indomethacin and changes of renal function in premature infants with patent ductus arteriosus. Pediatr Pharmacol 1984;4:11.
473. Koren G, Zarfin Y, Perlman M, et al. Effects of indomethacin on digoxin pharmacokinetics in preterm infants. Pediatr Pharmacol 1984;4:25.
474. Hammerman C, Zaia W, Wu HH. Severe hyponatremia with indomethacin: a more serious toxicity than previously realized? Dev Pharmacol Ther 1985;8:260.
475. Leititis JU, Burghard R, Gordjani N, et al. Effect of a modified fluid therapy on renal function during indomethacin therapy for persistent ductus arteriosus. Acta Paediatr Scand 1987; 76:789.
476. John EG, Bhat R, Vidyasagar D. Renal response to tolazoline in normal and hypoxemic newborn puppies. [Abstract] Pediatr Res 1979;14:514.
477. Brodie BB, Aronow L, Axelrod J. The fate of benzazoline (Priscoline) in dog and man and a method for its estimation in biological material. J Exp Pharmacol Ther 1952;106:200.
478. Monin P, Vert P, Morselli PL. A pharmacodynamic and pharmacokinetic study of tolazoline in the neonate. Dev Pharmacol Ther 1982;4(Suppl 1):124.
479. Trompeter RS, Chantler C, Haycock GB. Tolazoline and acute renal failure in the newborn. Lancet 1981;1:1219.
480. Bhat R, Gupta M, John E, et al. Acute renal failure (ARF) in the newborn due to priscoline (prisc). [Abstract] Pediatr Res 1978;12:519.
481. Goetzman BW, Sunshine P, Johnson JD, et al. Neonatal hypoxia and pulmonary vasospasm: response to tolazoline. J Pediatr 1976;89:617.
482. Heyman SN, Clark BA, Kaiser N, et al. In-vivo and in-vitro studies on the effect of amphotericin B on endothelin release. J Antimicrob Chemother 1992;29:69.
483. Joly V, Dromer F, Barge J, et al. Incorporation of amphotericin B (AMB) into liposomes alters AMB-induced acute nephrotoxicity in rabbits. J Pharmacol Exp Ther 1989;251:311.
484. Reynolds ES, Tomkiewicz ZM, Dammin GJ. The renal lesion related to amphotericin B treatment for coccidioidomycosis. Med Clin North Am 1963;47:1149.
485. Rubin SI, Krawiec DR, Gelberg H, et al. Nephrotoxicity of amphotericin B in dogs: a comparison of two methods of administration. Can J Vet Res 1989;53:23.
486. Joly V, Saint-Pierre-Chazalet M, Saint-Julien L, et al. Inhibiting cholesterol synthesis reduces the binding and toxicity of

amphotericin B against rabbit renal tubular cells in primary culture. J Infect Dis 1992;165:337.
487. Vadiei K, Lopez-Berestein G, Luke DR. Disposition and toxicity of amphotericin-B in the hyperlipidemic Zucker rat model. Int J Obes 1990;14:465.
488. Lopez-Berenstein G, Bodey GP, Frankel LS, et al. Treatment of hepatosplenic candidiasis with liposomal-amphotericin B. J Clin Oncol 1987;5:310.
489. McCurdy DK, Frederic M, Elkinton JR. Renal tubular acidosis due to amphotericin B. N Engl J Med 1968;278:124.
490. Baley JE, Meyers C, Kliegman RM, et al. Pharmacokinetics, outcome of treatment, and toxic effects of amphotericin B and 5-fluorocytosine in neonates. J Pediatr 1990;116:791.
491. Koren G, Lau A, Kenyon CF, et al. Clinical course and pharmacokinetics following a massive overdose of amphotericin B in a neonate. Clin Toxicol 1990;28:371.
492. Brent J, Hunt M, Kulig K, et al. Amphotericin B overdoses in infants: is there a role for exchange transfusion? Vet Hum Toxicol 1989;31:347.
493. Baley JE, Kliegman RM, Fanaroff AA. Disseminated fungal infections in very-low-birth-weight infants: therapeutic toxicity. Pediatrics 1984;73:153.
494. Bianchetti MG, Roduit C, Oetliker OH. Acyclovir-induced renal failure: course and risk factors. Pediatr Nephrol 1991; 5:238.
495. McDonald LK, Tartaglione TA, Mendelman PM, et al. Lack of toxicity in two cases of neonatal acyclovir overdose. Pediatr Infect Dis J 1989;8:529.
496. Englund JA, Fletcher CV, Balfour HH. Acyclovir therapy in neonates. J Pediatr 1991;119:129.
497. Berdon WE, Schwartz RH, Becker J, et al. Tamm-Horsfall proteinuria: its relationship to prolonged nephrogram in infants and children and to renal failure following intravenous urography in adults with multiple myeloma. Radiology 1969;92:714.
498. Sleasman JE, Stapleton FB, Tonkin II. Marked uricosuric effect of contrast media during cardiac catheterization in children. [Abstract] Pediatr Res 1986;17:219A.
499. Avner ED, Ellis D, Jaffe R, et al. Neonatal radiocontrast nephropathy simulating infantile polycystic kidney disease. J Pediatr 1982;100:85.
500. Lautin EM, Freeman NJ, Schoenfeld AH, et al. Radiocontrast-associated renal dysfunction: incidence and risk factors. AJR 1991;157:49.
501. Moore RD, Steinberg EP, Powe NR, et al. Nephrotoxicity of high-osmolality versus low-osmolality contrast media: randomized clinical trial. Radiology 1992;182:649.
502. Deray G, Bellin MF, Boulechfar H, et al. Nephrotoxicity of contrast media in high-risk patients with renal insufficiency: comparison of low- and high-osmolar contrast agents. Am J Nephrol 1991;11:309.
503. Harvey LA, Caldicott WJH, Kuruc A. The effect of contrast media on immature renal function: comparison of agents with high and low osmolality. Radiology 1983;148:429.
504. Wood EG, Bunchman TE, Lynch RE. Captopril-induced reversible acute renal failure in an infant with coarctation of the aorta. Pediatrics 1991;88:816.
505. Perlman JM, Volpe JJ. Neurologic complications of Captopril treatment of neonatal hypertension. Pediatrics 1989;83:47.
506. Mehring N, Neumann KH, Rahn KH, et al. Mechanisms of ciclosporin A-induced vasoconstriction in the isolated perfused rat kidney. Nephron 1992;60:477.
507. Eid A, Steffen R, Porayko MK, et al. Beyond 1 year after liver transplantation. Mayo Clin Proc 1989;64:446.
508. Ward MM. Factors predictive of acute renal failure in rhabdomyolysis. Arch Intern Med 1988;148:1553.
509. Shah SV, Walker PD. Evidence suggesting a role for hydroxyl radical in glycerol-induced acute renal failure. Am J Physiol 1988;255:F438.
510. Martin W, Villani GM, Jothianandan D, et al. Selective blockade of endothelium-dependent and glyceryl trinitrate-induced relaxation by hemoglobin and by methylene blue in the rabbit aorta. J Pharmacol Exp Ther 1985;232:708.
511. Haftel AJ, Eichner J, Haling J, et al. Myoglobinuric renal failure in a newborn infant. J Pediatr 1978;93:1015.
512. Turner MC, Naumburg EG. Acute renal failure in the neonate: two fatal cases due to group B streptococci with rhabdomyolysis. Clin Pediatr 1987;26:189.
513. Kagen LJ, Christian CL. Immunologic measurements of myoglobin in human adult and fetal skeletal muscle. Am J Physiol 1966;211:656.
514. Better OS, Stein JH. Early management of shock and prophylaxis of acute renal failure in traumatic rhabdomyolysis. N Engl J Med 1990;322:825.

CHRONIC RENAL FAILURE

515. Foreman JW, Chan JCM. Chronic renal failure in infants and children. J Pediatr 1988;113:793.
516. Potter DE, Holliday MA, Piel CF, Feduska NJ, Belzer FO, Salvatierra O, Jr. Treatment of end stage renal disease in children: a 15-year experience. Kidney Int 1980;18:103.
517. Pistor K, Olbing H, Schärer K. Children with chronic renal failure in the Federal Republic of Germany: I. Epidemiology, modes of treatment, survival. Clin Nephrol 1985;23:272.
518. Alexander SR, Arbus GS, Butt KMH, et al. The 1989 report of the North American Pediatric Renal Transplant cooperative study. Pediatr Nephrol 1990;4:542.
519. Najarian JS, Frey DJ, Matas AJ, et al. Renal transplantation in infants. Ann Surg 1990;212:353.
520. McEnery PT, Stablein DM, Arbus G, et al. Renal transplantation in children: a report of the North American Pediatric Renal Transplant Cooperative Study. N Engl J Med 1992; 326:1727.
521. Hanna JD, Foreman JW, Chan JCM. Chronic renal insufficiency in infants and children. Clin Pediatr 1991;30:365.
522. Tapper D, Watkins S, Burns M, et al. Comprehensive management of renal failure in infants. Arch Surg 1990;125:1276.
523. Miller LC, Bock GH, Lum CT, et al. Transplantation of the adult kidney into the very small child: long-term outcome. J Pediatr 1982;100:675.
524. Rees L, Rigden SPA, Ward GM. Chronic renal failure and growth. Arch Dis Child 1989;64:573.
525. Mehls O, Salusky IB. Recent advances and controversies in childhood renal osteodystrophy. Pediatr Nephrol 1987;1: 212.
526. Chesney RW, Dabbagh S, Uehling DT, et al. The importance of early treatment of renal bone disease in children. Kidney Int 1985;28(Suppl 17):S75.
527. Hostetter TH, Olson JL, Rennnke HT, et al. Hyperfiltration in remnant nephrons: a potentially adverse response to renal ablation. Am J Physiol 1981;241:F85.
528. Rosman JB, Meijer S, Sluiter WJ, et al. Prospective randomised trial of early dietary protein restriction in chronic renal failure. Lancet 1984;2:1291.
529. Diamond JR. Brief review: effects of dietary interventions on glomerular pathophysiology. Am J Physiol 1990;258:F1.
530. Wassner SJ, Abitbol S, Alexander S, et al. Nutritional requirements for infants with renal failure. Am J Kidney Dis 1986; 7:300.
531. Brewer ED. Growth of small children managed with chronic

peritoneal dialysis and nasogastric tube feedings: 203-month experience in 14 patients. Adv Perit Dial 1990;6:269.
532. Feld LG. Total parenteral nutrition in children with renal insufficiency. In: Lebenthal E, ed. Total parenteral nutrition: indications, utilization, complications and pathophysiological considerations. New York: Raven Press, 1986:385.
533. Blumberg A, Weidmann P, Ferrari P. Effect of prolonged bicarbonate administration on plasma potassium in terminal renal failure. Kidney Int 1992;41:369.
534. Portale AA, Booth BE, Tsai HC, et al. Reduced plasma concentration of 1,25-dihydroxy-vitamin-D in children with moderate renal insufficiency. Kidney Int 1982;21:627.
535. Mehls O, Ritz E, Krempien B, et al. Slipped epiphyses in renal osteodystrophy. Arch Dis Child 1975;50:545.
536. Alfrey AC, LeGendre GR, Kaehny WD. The dialysis encephalopathy syndrome: possible aluminum intoxication. N Engl J Med 1976;294:184.
537. Polinsky MS, Gruskin AB. Aluminum toxicity in children with chronic renal failure. J Pediatr 1984;105:758.
538. ASCN/ASPEN Working Group on Standards for Aluminum Content of Parenteral Nutrition Solutions. Parenteral drug products containing aluminum as an ingredient or a contaminant: response to Food and Drug Administration notice of intent and request for information. JPEN J Parenter Enteral Nutr 1991;15:194.
539. Sedman AB, Klein GL, Merritt RJ, et al. Evidence of aluminum loading in infants receiving intravenous therapy. N Engl J Med 1985;312:1337.
540. Bozynski MEA, Sedman AB, Naglie RA, et al. Serial plasma and urinary aluminum levels and tissue loading in preterm twins. JPEN J Parenter Enteral Nutr 1989;13:428.
541. Koo WWK, Kaplan LA, Krug-Wispe SK, et al. Response of preterm infants to aluminum in parenteral nutrition. JPEN J Parenter Enteral Nutr 1989;13:516.
542. Alfrey AC. Aluminum intoxication. N Engl J Med 1984; 310:1113.
543. Weberg R, Berstad A. Gastrointestinal absorption of aluminium from single doses of aluminium containing antacids in man. Eur J Clin Invest 1986;16:428.
544. Nordal KP, Dahl E, Srhus K, et al. Gastrointestinal absorption and urinary excretion of aluminium in patients with predialysis chronic renal failure. Pharmacol Toxicol 1988;63:351.
545. Freundlich M, Zilleruelo G, Faugere MC, et al. Treatment of aluminum toxicity in infantile uremia with deferoxamine. J Pediatr 1986;109:140.
546. Chesney RW, Moorthy AV, Eisman JA, et al. Increased growth after long-term oral 1-α-25-vitamin-D_3 in childhood renal osteodystrophy. N Engl J Med 1978;298:238.
547. Chan JCM, Kodroff MB, Landwehr DM. Effects of 1,25-dihyroxyvitamin-D_3 on renal function, mineral balance and growth in children with severe chronic renal failure. Pediatrics 1981;68:559.
548. Chandra M, Clemons GK, McVicar MI. Relation of serum erythropoietin levels to renal excretory function: evidence for lowered set point for erythropoietin production in chronic renal failure. J Pediatr 1988;113:1015.
549. Lacombe C, Da Silva J-L, Bruneval P, et al. Peritubular cells are the site of erythropoietin synthesis in the murine hypoxic kidney. J Clin Invest 1988;81:620.
550. Beckman BS, Brookins JW, Garcia MM, et al. Measurement of erythropoietin in anephric children: a report of the Southwest Pediatric Nephrology Study Group. Pediatr Nephrol 1989; 3:75.
551. Eschbach JW, Adamson JW. Guidelines for recombinant human erythropoietin therapy. Am J Kidney Dis 1989;14:2.
552. Stivelman JC. Resistance to recombinant human erythropoietin therapy: a real clinical entity? Semin Nephrol 1989; 9:Suppl 2:8.
553. Kitagawa T, Ito K, Komatsu Y, et al. The clinical studies of recombinant human erythropoietin (Epoetin) in children with renal anemia. Japanese Journal of Pediatrics 1988;41:3251.
554. Sinai-Trieman L, Salusky IB, Fine RN. Use of subcutaneous recombinant human erythropoietin in children undergoing continuous cycling peritoneal dialysis. J Pediatr 1989;114:550.
555. Bercu BB, Corden BJ, Schulman JD, et al. Circulating somatomedin C levels in nephropathic cystinosis. Isr J Med Sci 1984;20:236.
556. El-Bishti MM, Counahan R, Bloom S, et al. Hormonal and metabolic responses to intravenous glucose in children on regular hemodialysis. Am J Clin Nutr 1978;31:1865.
557. Tönshoff B, Mehls O, Heinrich U, et al. Growth-stimulating effects of recombinant human growth hormone in children with end-stage renal disease. J Pediatr 1990;116:561.
558. Koch VH, Lippe BM, Nelson PA, et al. Accelerated growth after recombinant human growth hormone treatment of children with chronic renal failure. J Pediatr 1989;115:365.
559. Fine RN, Yadin O, Moulton L, et al. Recombinant human growth hormone (rhGH) long term treatment of growth retarded children with chronic renal failure (CRF). [Abstract] J Am Soc Nephrol 1991;2:235.
560. Warshaw BL, Edelbrock HH, Ettenger RB, et al. Progression to end-stage renal disease in children with obstructive uropathy. J Pediatr 1982;100:183.
561. Hogg RJ. Continuous ambulatory and continuous cycling peritoneal dialysis in children: a report of the Southwestern Pediatric Nephrology Study Group. Kidney Intern 1985; 27:558.
562. Fennell RS, Orak JK, Garin EH, et al. Continuous ambulatory peritoneal dialysis in a pediatric population. Am J Dis Child 1983 137:388.
563. Baluarte HJ, Gruskin AB, Hiner LB, et al. Encephalopathy in children with chronic renal failure. Proc Dial Transpl Forum 1977;7:95.
564. Sedman AB, Wilkening GN, Warady BA, et al. Encephalopathy in childhood secondary to aluminum toxicity. J Pediatr 1984;105:836.
565. Bock GH, Conners CK, Ruley J, et al. Disturbances of brain maturation and neurodevelopment during chronic renal failure in infancy. J Pediatr 1989;114:231.
566. Davis ID, Pi-Nian C, Nevins TE. Successful renal transplantation accelerates development in young uremic infants. Pediatrics 1990;86:594.
567. Offner G, Latta K, Hoyer PF. CAPD in children with special aspects of renal transplantation. Contrib Nephrol 1991;89:243.
568. Alexander SR. CAPD in infants less than one year of age. In: Fine RN, Gruskin AB, eds. End stage renal disease in children. Philadelphia: WB Saunders, 1984:149.
569. So SK, Chang PN, Najarian JS, et al. Growth and development in infants after renal transplantation. J Pediatr 1986; 110:343.
570. Najarian JS, Almond PS, Mauer M, et al. Renal transplantation in the first year of life: the treatment of choice for infants with end-stage renal disease. J Am Soc Nephrol 1992;2:S228.
571. Opelz G, Graver B, Terasaki PI. Induction of high kidney graft survival rate by multiple transfusions. Lancet 1981; 1:1223.
572. Beebe DS, Belani KG, Mergens P, et al. Anesthetic management of infants receiving an adult kidney transplant. Anesth Analg 1991;73:725.
573. Almond PS, Matas AJ, Gillingham K, et al. Pediatric renal transplants: results with sequential immunosuppression. Transplantation 1992;53:46.

574. So SK, Gillingham K, Cook M, et al. The use of cadaver kidneys for transplantation in young children. Transplantation 1990;50:979.
575. North American Pediatric Renal Transplant Cooperative Study. Annual Report. 1991.
576. Nevins T. Treatment of very young infants with ESRD: renal transplantation as soon as possible (less than 1 yr of age): controversy. Adv Perit Dial 1990;6:283.
577. Connor JP, Burbige KA. Long-term urinary continence and renal function in neonates with posterior urethral valves. J Urol 1990;144:1209.
578. Reinberg Y, Manivel JC, Pettinato G, et al. Development of renal failure in children with the prune belly syndrome. J Urol 1991;145:1017.
579. Burbige KA, Amodio J, Berdon WE, et al. Prune belly syndrome: 35 years of experience. J Urol 1987;137:86.
580. Kaplan BS, Fay J, Shah V, et al. Autosomal recessive polycystic kidney disease. Pediatr Nephrol 1989;3:43.
581. Cole BR, Conley SB, Stapleton FB. Polycystic kidney disease in the first year of life. J Pediatr 1987;111:693.
582. Mahan JD, Mauer SM, Sibley RK, et al. Congenital nephrotic syndrome: evolution of medical management and results of renal transplantation. J Pediatr 1984;105:549.

HYPERTENSION

583. Adelman RD. The hypertensive neonate. Clin Perinatol 1988;15:567.
584. Ingelfinger J. Hypertension in the first year of life. In: Ingelfinger J, ed. Pediatric hypertension. Philadelphia: WB Saunders, 1982:229.
585. Abman SH, Warady BA, Lum GM, et al. Systemic hypertension in infants with bronchopulmonary dysplasia. J Pediatr 1984;104:928.
586. Sheftel DN, Hustead V, Friedman A. Hypertension screening in the follow-up of premature infants. Pediatrics 1983;71:763.
587. Buchi KF, Siegler RL. Hypertension in the first month of life. J Hypertens 1986;4:525.
588. Friedman AL, Hustead VA. Hypertension in babies following discharge from a neonatal intensive care unit: a 3-year follow-up. Pediatr Nephrol 1987;1:30.
589. Bancalari E, Gerhardt T, Feller R, et al. Muscle relaxation during IPPV in prematures with RDS. Pediatr Res 1980; 14:590.
590. Greenough A, Gamsu HR, Greenall F. Investigation of the effects of paralysis by pancuronium on heart rate variability, blood pressure and fluid balance. Acta Paediatr Scand 1989; 78:829.
591. Cabal LA, Siassi B, Artal R, et al. Cardiovascular and catecholamine changes after administration of pancuronium in distressed neonates. Pediatrics 1985;75:284.
592. Ferrara TB, Couser RJ, Hoekstra RE. Side effects and long-term follow-up of corticosteroid therapy in very low birthweight infants with bronchopulmonary dysplasia. J Perinatol 1990;10:137.
593. Sell LL, Cullen ML, Lerner GR, et al. Hypertension during extra-corporeal membrane oxygenation: cause, effect, and management. Surgery 1987;102:724.
594. Adelman RD, Sherman MP. Hypertension in the neonate following closure of abdominal wall defects. J Pediatr 1980; 97:642.
595. Merten DF, Vogel JM, Adelman RD, et al. Renovascular hypertension as a complication of umbilical arterial catheterization. Radiology 1978;126:751.
596. Angella JJ, Sommer LS, Poole C, et al. Neonatal hypertension associated with renal artery hypoplasia. Pediatrics 41:524.
597. Wilson DI, Appleton RE, Coulthard MG, et al. Fetal and infantile hypertension caused by unilateral renal arterial disease. Arch Dis Child 1990;65:881.
598. Schmidt DM, Rambo ON Jr. Segmental intimal hyperplasia of the abdominal aorta and renal arteries producing hypertension in an infant. Am J Clin Pathol 1965;44:546.
599. Milner LS, Heitner R, Thomson PD, et al. Hypertension as the major problem of idiopathic arterial calcification of infancy. J Pediatr 1984;105:934.
600. Van Dyck M, Proesmans W, Van Hollebeke E, et al. Idiopathic infantile arterial calcification with cardiac, renal and central nervous system involvement. Eur J Pediatr 1989; 148:374.
601. Meradji M, de Villeneuve VH, Huber J, et al. Idiopathic infantile arterial calcification in siblings: radiologic diagnosis and successful treatment. J Pediatr 1978;92:401.
602. Takahashi G, Nakano H, Ueda K, et al. Neonatal renovascular hypertension: haematoma within the renal arterial wall: a case report. Z Kinderchir 1984;39:341.
603. Davis RS, Manning JA, Branch GL, et al. Renovascular hypertension secondary to hydronephrosis in a solitary kidney. J Urol 1973;110:724.
604. Bensman A, Neuenschwander S, Lavollay B, et al. Hypertension artérielle et compression du pédicule vasculaire rénal par un hématome de la surrénale chez un nouveau-né. Ann Pediatr (Paris) 1982;29:670.
605. Patel MR, Mooppan MMU, Kim H. Subcapsular urinoma: unusual form of "page kidney" in newborn. Urology 1984; 23:585.
606. Tokunaka S, Takamura T, Osanai H, et al. Severe hypertension in an infant with unilateral hypoplastic kidney. Urology 1987;29:618.
607. Chan HSL, Cheng MY, Mance K, et al. Congenital mesoblastic nephroma: a clinicoradiologic study of 17 cases representing the pathologic spectrum of the disease. J Pediatr 1987; 111:64.
608. Malone PS, Duffy PG, Ransley PG, et al. Congenital mesoblastic nephroma, renin production and hypertension. J Pediatr Surg 1989;24:599.
609. Munoz AI, Baralt JF, Melendez MT. Arterial hypertension in infants with hydronephrosis: report of six cases. Am J Dis Child 1977;131:38.
610. Roth A. An unusual renal tumor, associating a nephroblastoma, nephroblastomatosis, a teratoma, cystic dysplasia, hypertension and the secretion of α-foetoprotein. J Urol (Paris) 1984;90:7.
611. Yokomori K, Hori T, Takemura T, et al. Demonstration of both primary and secondary reninism in renal tumors in children. J Pediatr Surg 1988;23:403.
612. Perlman JM, Volpe JJ. Seizures in the premature infant: effects on cerebral blood flow velocity, intracranial pressure and arterial blood pressure. J Pediatr 1983;102:288.
613. Schoenwetter BS, Libber SM, Jones D, et al. Hypertension in neonatal hyperthyroidism. Am J Dis Child 1983;137:854.
614. Kaufman BH, Telander RL, Van Heerden JA, et al. Pheochromocytoma in the pediatric age group: current status. J Pediatr Surg 1983;18:879.
615. Guignard JP, Gouyon JB, Adelman RD. Arterial hypertension in the newborn infant. Biol Neonate 1989;55:77.
616. Goble MM, Rocchini AP. Neonatal hypertension: why it happens, what to do about it. Contemporary Pediatrics 1990;7:89.
617. Rasoulpour M, Marinelli KA. Systemic hypertension. Clin Perinatol 1992;19:121.
618. Miall-Allen VM, deVries LS, Whitelaw AGL. Mean arterial blood pressure and neonatal cerebral lesions. Arch Dis Child 1987;62:1068.
619. Moore P, Fiddler GI. Facial palsy in an infant with coarcta-

tion of the aorta and hypertension. Arch Dis Child 1980;55:315.
620. Skalina MEL, Annable WL, Kliegman RM, et al. Hypertensive retinopathy in the newborn infant. J Pediatr 1983;103:781.
621. Stringer DA, de Bruyn R, Dillon MJ. Comparison of aortography, renal vein renin sampling, radionuclide scans, ultrasound and IVU in the investigation of childhood renovascular hypertension. Br J Radiol 1984;57:111.
622. Baetz-Greenwalt B, Debaz B, Kumar ML. Bladder fungus ball: a reversible cause of neonatal obstructive uropathy. Pediatrics 1988;81:826.
623. McLaine PN, Drummond KN. Intravenous diazoxide for severe hypertension in childhood. J Pediatr 1971;79:829.
624. Benitz WE, Malachowski N, Cohen RS, et al. Use of sodium nitroprusside in neonates: efficacy and safety. J Pediatr 1985;106:102.
625. Bunchman TE, Lynch RE, Wood EG. Intravenously administered labetolol for treatment of hypertension in children. J Pediatr 1992;120:140.
626. Wells TG, Bunchman TE, Kearns GL. Treatment of neonatal hypertension with enalaprilat. J Pediatr 1990;117:664.
627. Bifano E, Post EM, Springer J, et al. Treatment of neonatal hypertension with captopril. J Pediatr 1982;100:143.
628. Hymes LC, Warshaw BL. Captopril: long-term treatment of hypertension in a preterm infant and older children. Am J Dis Child 1983;137:263.
629. O'Dea RF, Mirkin BL, Alward CT, et al. Treatment of neonatal hypertension with captopril. J Pediatr 1988;113:403.
630. Marcadis ML, Kraus DM, Hatzopoulos FK, et al. Use of enalaprilat for neonatal hypertension. [Letter] J Pediatr 1991;119:505.
631. Sfakianakis GN, Sfakianaki E, Paredes A, et al. Single-dose captopril scintigraphy in the neonate with renovascular hypertension: prediction of renal failure, a side effect of captopril therapy. Biol Neonate 1988;54:246.
632. Hendren WH, Kim SH, Herrin JT, et al. Surgically correctable hypertension of renal origin in childhood. Am J Surg 1982;143:432.

DIURETICS

633. Chemtob S, Kaplan BS, Sherbotie JR, et al. Pharmacology of diuretics in the newborn. Pediatr Clin North Am 1989;36:1231.
634. Shinnar S, Gammon K, Bergman EW, et al. Management of hydrocephalus in infancy: use of acetazolamide and furosemide to avoid cerebrospinal fluid shunts. J Pediatr 1985;107:31.
635. Velasquez Jones L, Rivera Acosta F, Gordillo Paniagua G. Evaluation of the urinary and plasma urea ratio and osmolarity in newborn infants and malnourished children with pathological and normal renal function. Bol Med Hosp Infant Mex 1976;33:651.
636. Adhikari M, Moodley M, Desai PK. Mannitol in neonatal cerebral oedema. Brain Dev 1990;12:349.
637. Levene MI, Evans DH. Medical management of raised intracranial pressure after severe birth asphyxia. Arch Dis Child 1985;60:12.
638. Najak ZD, Harris EM, Lazzara A, et al. Pulmonary effects of furosemide in preterm infants with lung disease. J Pediatr 1983;102:758.
639. Imai M. Effect of bumetanide and furosemide on the thick ascending limb of Henle's loop of rabbits and rats perfused in vitro. Eur J Pharmacol 1977;41:409.
640. Schrier RW, Lehman D, Zacherle B, et al. Effect of furosemide on free water excretion in edematous patients with hyponatremia. Kidney Int 1973;3:30.
641. Sulyok E, Varga F, Nèmeth F, et al. Furosemide-induced alterations in the electrolyte status, the function of renin–angiotensin–aldosterone system, and the urinary excretion of prostaglandins in newborn infants. Pediatr Res 1980;14:765.
642. Friedman Z, Demers LM, Marks KH, et al. Urinary excretion of prostaglandin E following the administration of furosemide and indomethacin to sick low-birth-weight infants. J Pediatr 1978;93:512.
642a. Wells TG, Fasules JW, Taylor BJ, et al. Pharmacokinetics and pharmacodynamics of bumetanide in neonates treated with extracorporeal membrane oxygenation. J Pediatr 1992;121:974.
643. Brickman AS, Massry SG, Coburn JW. Changes in serum and urinary calcium during treatment with hydrochlorothiazide: studies on mechanisms. J Clin Invest 1972;51:945.
644. Costanzo LS, Windhager EE. Calcium and sodium transport by the distal convoluted tubule of the rat. Am J Physiol 1978;235:F492.
645. Albersheim SG, Solimano AJ, Sharma AK, et al. Randomized, double-blind, controlled trial of long-term diuretic therapy for bronchopulmonary dysplasia. J Pediatr 1989;115:615.
646. Dargie HJ, Allison MEM, Kennedy AC, et al. High dosage metolazone in chronic renal failure. Br Med J 1972;4:196.
647. Arnold WC. Efficacy of metolazone and furosemide in children with furosemide resistant edema. Pediatrics 1984;74:872.
648. Segar JL, Robillard JE, Johnson KJ, et al. Addition of metolazone to overcome tolerance to furosemide in infants with bronchopulmonary dysplasia. J Pediatr 1992;120:966.
649. Bull MB, Laragh JH. Amiloride: a potassium-sparing natriuretic agent. Circulation 1968;37:45.
650. Knoers N, Monnens LAH. Amiloride-hydrochlorothiazide versus indomethacin-hydrochlorothiazide in the treatment of nephrogenic diabetes insipidus. J Pediatr 1990;117:499.
651. Perlman JM, Moore V, Siegel MJ, et al. Is chloride depletion an important contributing cause of death in infants with bronchopulmonary dysplasia? Pediatrics 1986;77:212.
652. Cannon PJ, Heinemann HO, Albert MS, et al. "Contraction" alkalosis after diuresis of edematous patients with ethacrynic acid. Ann Intern Med 1965;62:979.
653. Loon NR, Wilcox CS, Kanthanatana S, et al. Metabolic alkalosis during furosemide infusion in man: roles of volume contraction and acid excretion. [Abstract] Kidney Int 1987;31:208.
654. Mirochnick MH, Miceli JJ, Kramer PA, et al. Renal response to furosemide in very low birth weight infants during chronic administration. Dev Pharmacol Ther 1990;15:1.

BACTERIURIA AND URINARY TRACT INFECTIONS

655. McCarthy J, Pryles CV. Clean voided and catheter neonatal urine specimens: bacteriology in the male and female neonate. Am J Dis Child 1963;106:473.
656. O'Doherty NJ. Urinary tract infection in the neonatal period and later infancy. In: O'Grady F, Brumfitt W, eds. Urinary tract infection: proceedings of the First National Symposium. London: Oxford University Press, 1968:113.
657. Zies L, Ramirez J, Jannach JR. Incidence of bacteriuria in the premature infant as determined by suprapubic aspiration. J Fla Med Assoc 1968;55:452.
658. Gower PE, Husband P, Coleman JC, et al. Urinary infection in two selected neonatal populations. Arch Dis Child 1970;45:259.

659. Pendarvis BC Jr, Chitwood LA, Wenzl JE. Bacteriuria in the premature infant. American Society of Microbiology Pediatric News 1970;4:33.
660. Edelmann CM Jr, Ogwo JE, Fine BP, et al. The prevalence of bacteriuria in full-term and premature newborn infants. J Pediatr 1973;82:125.
661. Winberg J, Andersen HJ, Bergström T, et al. Epidemiology of symptomatic urinary tract infection. Acta Paediatr Scand Suppl 1974;252:1.
662. Drew JH, Acton CM. Radiological findings in newborn infants with urinary infection. Arch Dis Child 1976;51:628.
663. Maherzi M, Guignard JP, Torrado A. Urinary tract infection in high-risk newborn infants. Pediatrics 1978;62:521.
664. Wiswell TE, Roscelli JD. Corroborative evidence for the decreased incidence of urinary tract infections in circumcised male infants. Pediatrics 1986;78:96.
665. Wiswell TE, Geschke DW. Risks from circumcision during the first month of life compared with those for uncircumcised boys. Pediatrics 1989;83:1011.
666. Olusanya O, Owa JA, Olusanya OI. The prevalence of bacteriuria among high risk neonates in Nigeria. Acta Paediatr Scand 1989;78:94.
667. Vilanova Juanola JM, Canos Molinos J, Rosell Arnold E, et al. Urinary tract infection in the newborn infant. An Esp Pediatr 1989;31:105.
668. Crain EF, Gershel JC. Urinary tract infections in febrile infants younger than 8 weeks of age. Pediatrics 1990;86:363.
669. Wiswell TE, Miller GM, Gelston HM, et al. Effect of circumcision status on periurethral bacterial flora during the first year of life. J Pediatr 1988;113:442.
670. Fernandez Escribano A, Garcia Meseguer C, Pastor Abascal I, et al. Neonatal pelvic ectasia. An Esp Pediatr 1989;31:570.
671. Ehrlich O, Brem AS. A prospective comparison of urinary tract infections in patients treated with either clean intermittent catheterization or urinary diversion. Pediatrics 1982; 70:665.
672. Strand WR, Sesterhenn I, Rushton HG. Role of superoxide dismutase in the pathogenesis of pyelonephritis: immunological localization of superoxide dismutase in human renal tissues. J Urol 1989 (Part 2);142:616.
673. Neumann CG, Pryles CV. Pyelonephritis in infants and children. Am J Dis Child 1962;104:215.
674. Porter KA, Giles HM. A pathological study of live cases of pyelonephritis in the newborn. Arch Dis Child 1956;31:303.
675. Rooney JC, Hill DJ, Danks DM. Jaundice associated with bacterial infection in the newborn. Am J Dis Child 1971;122: 39.
676. Moraga Llop FA, del Alcázar Muñoz R, Casado Toda M, et al. Jaundice associated with urinary infection in the first three months of life: study of 66 cases. An Esp Pediatr 1980;13:5.
677. Ng SH, Rawstron JR. Urinary tract infections presenting with jaundice. Arch Dis Child 1971;46:173.
678. Krober MS, Bass JW, Powell JM, et al. Bacterial and viral pathogens causing fever in infants less than 3 months old. Am J Dis Child 1985;139:889.
679. Pappu LD, Purohit DM, Bradford BF, et al. Primary renal candidiasis in two preterm neonates: report of cases and review of the literature on renal candidiasis in infancy. Am J Dis Child 1984;138:923.
680. Newman CGH, O'Neill P, Parker A. Pyuria in infancy, and the role of suprapubic aspiration of urine in diagnosis of infection of urinary tract. Br Med J 1967;2:277.
681. Bonadio WA. Urine culturing technique in febrile infants. Pediatr Emerg Care 1987;3:75.
682. Nelson JD, Peters PC. Suprapubic aspiration of urine in premature and term infants. Pediatrics 1965;36:132.
683. Visser VE, Hall RT. Urine culture in the evaluation of suspected neonatal sepsis. J Pediatr 1979;94:635.
684. DiGeronimo RJ. Lack of efficacy of the urine culture as part of the initial sepsis workup of suspected neonatal sepsis. Pediatr Infect Dis J 1992;11:764.
685. Vaid YN, Lebowitz RL. Urosepsis in infants with vesicoureteral reflux masquerading as the salt-losing type of congenital adrenal hyperplasia. Pediatr Radiol 1989;19:548.
686. Luk G, Riggs D, Luque M. Severe methemoglobinemia in a 3-week-old infant with a urinary tract infection. Crit Care Med 1991;19:1325.
687. Ginsburg CM, McCracken GH, Jr. Urinary tract infections in young infants. Pediatrics 1982;69:409.
688. Crawford DB, Rasoulpour M, Dhawan VM, et al. Renal carbuncle in a neonate with congenital nephrotic syndrome. J Pediatr 1978;93:78.
689. Walker KM. Suprarenal abscess due to group B streptococcus. J Pediatr 1979;94:970.
690. Pais VM, Retik AB. Reversible hydronephrosis in the neonate with urinary sepsis. N Engl J Med 1975;465.
691. Edwards D, Normand ICS, Prescod N, et al. Disappearance of vesicoureteral reflux during long-term prophylaxis of urinary tract infection in children. Br Med J 1977;2:285.
692. Yadin O, Ben-Ezer DG, Golan A, et al. Survival of a premature neonate with obstructive anuria due to *Candida*: the role of early sonographic diagnosis and antimycotic treatment. Eur J Pediatr 1988;147:653.
693. Patriquin H, Lebowitz R, Perreault G, et al. Neonatal candidiasis: renal and pulmonary manifestations. AJR 1980;135:1205.
694. Tung KT, MacDonald LM, Smith JC. Neonatal systemic candidiasis diagnosed by ultrasound. Acta Radiol 1990;31:293.
695. Hellerstein S, Duggan E, Welchert E, et al. Serum C-reactive protein and the site of urinary tract infections. J Pediatr 1982;100:21.
696. Johnson CE, Shurin PA, Marchant CD, et al. Identification of children requiring radiologic evaluation for urinary tract infection. Pediatr Infect Dis 1985;4:656.
697. Pylkkänen J, Vilska J, Koskimies O. The value of level diagnosis of childhood urinary tract infection in predicting renal injury. Acta Paediatr Scand 1981;70:879.
698. Rushton HG, Majd M, Chandra R, Yim D. Evaluation of ^{99m}technetium-dimercapto-succinic acid renal scans in experimental acute pyelonephritis in piglets. J Urol 1988 (Part 2); 140:1169.
699. Verber IG, Meller ST. Serial ^{99m}Tc dimercaptosuccinic acid (DMSA) scans after urinary infections presenting before the age of 5 years. Arch Dis Child 1989;64:1533.
700. Rossleigh MA, Wilson MJ, Rosenberg AR, et al. DMSA studies in infants under one year of age. Contrib Nephrol 1990; 79:166.
701. Leonidas JC, McCauley RGK, Klauber GC, et al. Sonography as a substitute for excretory urography in children with urinary tract infection. AJR 1985;144:815.
702. Mage K, Zoppardo P, Cohen R, et al. Imaging of the first urinary infection in children: respective role of each examination technique in the initial assessment: a report on 122 observations. J Radiol 1989;70:279.
703. Rickwood AMK, McKendrick T, Williams MPL, et al. Current imaging of childhood urinary tract infections: prospective survey. Br Med J 1992;304:663.
704. Bourchier D, Abbott GD, Maling TMJ. Radiologic abnormalities in infants with urinary tract infections. Arch Dis Child 1984;59:620.
705. Feld LG. Urinary tract infections in childhood: definition, pathogenesis, diagnosis, and management. Pharmacotherapy 1991;11:326.

706. Gleeson FV, Gordon I. Imaging in urinary tract infection. Arch Dis Child 1991;66:1282.
707. Constantopoulos A, Thomaidou L, Loupa H, et al. Successful response of severe neonatal gram-negative infection to treatment with aztreonam. Chemotherapy 1989;35(Suppl 1):101.
708. Zhanel GG, Harding GKM, Guay DRP. Asymptomatic bacteriuria: which patients should be treated? Arch Intern Med 1990;150:1389.
709. Leung AKC, Robson WLM. Urinary tract infection in infancy and childhood. Adv Pediatr 1991;38:257.
710. Wettergreen B, Hellstrom M, Stockland E, et al. Six year follow up of infants with bacteriuria on screening. Br Med J 1990;13:845.
711. Dore B, Irani J, Istin A, et al. Vesicorenal reflux in children under age 2: indications and results of surgery. J Urol (Paris) 1990;96:365.
712. Rehan VK, Davidson DC. Neonatal renal candidal bezoar. Arch Dis Child 1992;67:63.
713. Bartone FF, Hurwitz RS, Rojas EL, et al. The role of percutaneous nephrostomy in the management of obstructing candidiasis of the urinary tract in infants. J Urol 1988;140:338.
714. Matsumoto AH, Dejter SW Jr, Barth KH, et al. Percutaneous nephrostomy drainage in the management of neonatal anuria secondary to renal candidiasis. J Pediatr Surg 1990;25:1295.
715. Arant BS Jr, Sotelo-Avila C, Bernstein J. Segmental "hypoplasia" of the kidney (Ask-Upmark). J Pediatr 1979;95:931.
716. Welch TR, Nogrady MB, Outerbridge EW. Roentgenologic sequelae of neonatal septicemia and urinary tract infection. American Journal of Roentgenology, Radium Therapy, and Nuclear Medicine 1973;118:28.
717. Holland NH, Jackson EC, Kazee M, et al. Relation of urinary tract infection and vesicoureteral reflux to scars: follow-up of thirty-eight patients. J Pediatr 1990;116:S65.
718. Majd M, Rushton HG, Jantausch BG, et al. Relationship among vesicoureteral reflux, P-fimbriated *Escherichia coli*, and acute pyelonephritis in children with febrile urinary tract infection. J Pediatr 1991;119:578.
719. Arnold AJ, Brownless SM, Carty HM, et al. Detection of renal scarring by DMSA scanning-an experimental study. J Pediatr Surg 1990;25:391.
720. Herzog LW. A case-control study: urinary tract infections and circumcision. Am J Dis Child 1989;143:348.
721. Joseph DB, Bauer SB, Colodney AH, et al. Clean, intermittent catheterization of infants with neurogenic bladder. Pediatrics 1989;84:74.
722. Kasabian NG, Bauer SB, Dyro FM, et al. The prophylactic value of clean intermittent catheterization and anticholinergic medication in newborns and infants with myelodysplasia at risk of developing urinary tract deterioration. Am J Dis Child 1992;146:840.
723. Anderson PAM, Rickwood AMK. Features of primary vesicoureteric reflux detected by prenatal sonography. Br J Urol 1991;67:267.
724. Gordon AC, Thomas DFM, Arthur RJ, et al. Prenatally diagnosed reflux: a follow-up study. Br J Urol 1990;65:407.

TUBULAR DYSFUNCTION

725. Scriver CR, Beaudet AL, Sly WS, et al, eds. The metabolic basis of inherited disease. 6th ed. New York: McGraw-Hill, 1989.
726. Nishiyama S, Tomoeda S, Inoue F, et al. Self-limited neonatal familial hyperparathyroidism associated with hypercalciuria and renal tubular acidosis in three siblings. J Pediatr 1990; 86:421.
727. Reusz GS, Latta K, Hoyer PF, et al. Evidence suggesting hyperoxaluria as a cause of nephrocalcinosis in phosphate-treated hypophosphataemic rickets. Lancet 1 1990;335: 1240.
728. Alon U, Donaldson DI, Hellerstein S, et al. Metabolic and histologic investigation of the nature of nephrocalcinosis in children with hypophosphatemic rickets and in the Hyp mouse. J Pediatr 1992;120:899.
729. Seyberth HW, Rascher W, Schweer H, et al. Congenital hypokalemia with hypercalciuria in preterm infants: a hyperprostaglandinuric tubular syndrome different from Bartter syndrome. J Pediatr 1985;107:694.
730. Hufnagle KG, Khan SN, Penn D, et al. Renal calcifications: a complication of long-term furosemide therapy in preterm infants. Pediatrics 1982;70:360.
731. Jacinto JS, Modanlou HD, Crade M, et al. Renal calcification incidence in very low birth weight infants. Pediatrics 1988; 88:31.
732. Noe HN, Bryant JF, Roy S III, et al. Urolithiasis in pre-term neonates associated with furosemide therapy. J Urol 1984; 132:93.
733. Short A, Cooke RWI. The incidence of renal calcification in preterm infants. Arch Dis Child 1991;66:412.
734. Woolfield N, Haslam R, Le Quesne G, et al. Ultrasound diagnosis of nephrocalcinosis in preterm infants. Arch Dis Child 1988;63:86.
735. Ghazali S, Barratt TM, Williams DI. Childhood urolithiasis in Britain. Arch Dis Child 1973;48:291.
736. Goldsmith MA, Bhatia SS, Kanto WP, et al. Gluconate calcium therapy and neonatal hypercalciuria. Am J Dis Child 1981;135:538.
737. Coe FL, Bushinsky DA. Pathophysiology of hypercalciuria. Am J Physiol 1984;16:F1.
738. Rowe JC, Goetz CA, Carey DE, et al. Achievement of in utero retention of calcium and phosphorus accompanied by high calcium excretion in very low birth weight infants fed a fortified formula. J Pediatr 1987;110:581.
739. Senterre J, Salle B. Renal aspects of calcium and phosphorus metabolism in preterm infants. Biol Neonate 1988;53:220.
740. Chessex P, Pineault M, Zebiche H, et al. Calciuria in parenterally fed preterm infants: role of phosphorus intake. J Pediatr 1985;107:794.
741. Ezzedeen F, Adelman RD, Ahifors CE. Renal calcification in preterm infants: pathophysiology and long-term sequelae. J Pediatr 1988;113:532.
742. Savage MO, Wilkinson AR, Baum JD, et al. Furosemide in respiratory distress syndrome. Arch Dis Child 1975;50:709.
743. Warshaw BL, Anand SK, Kerian A, et al. The effect of chronic furosemide administration on urinary calcium excretion and calcium balance in growing rats. Pediatr Res 1980;14:1118.
744. Venkatarman PS, Han BK, Tsang RC, et al. Secondary hyperparathyroidism and bone disease in infants receiving long term furosemide therapy. Am J Dis Child 1983;137:1157.
745. Atkinson SA, Shah JK, McGee C, et al. Mineral excretion in premature infants receiving various diuretic therapies. J Pediatr 1988:113:540.
746. Fischer AF, Parker BR, Stevenson DK. Nephrolithiasis following in utero diuretic exposure: an unusual case. Pediatrics 1988;81:712.
747. Adelman RD, Abern SB, Merten D, et al. Hypercalciuria with nephrolithiasis: a complication of total parenteral nutrition. Pediatrics 1977;59:473.
748. Bengoa JM, Sitrin MD, Wood RJ, et al. Amino acid-induced hypercalciuria in patients on total parenteral nutrition. Am J Clin Nutr 1983;38:264.
749. Berkelhammer CH, Wood RJ, Sitrin MD. Acetate and hyper-

calciuria during total parenteral nutrition. Am J Clin Nutr 1988;48:1482.
750. Downing GJ, Egelhoff JC, Daily DK, et al. Kidney function in very low birth weight infants with furosemide-related renal calcifications at ages 1 to 2 years. J Pediatr 1992;120:599.
751. De Zegher FE, Wolff ED, vd Heijden AJ, et al. Oxalosis in infancy. Clin Nephrol 1984;22:114.
752. Morris MC, Chambers TL, Evans PWG, et al. Oxalosis in infancy. Arch Dis Child 1982;57:224.
753. Furuta M, Torii S. Congenital oxalosis: first report of two neonatal cases. Annales Paediatrici Japonica 1967;13:42.
754. Rose GA, Arthur LJH, Chambers TL, et al. Successful treatment of primary hyperoxaluria in a neonate. Lancet 1982; 1:1298.
755. Leumann EP, Wegmann W, Largiadèr F. Prolonged survival after renal transplantation in primary hyperoxaluria of childhood. Lancet 1986;2:340.
756. Watts RWE, Calne RY, Rolles K, et al. Successful treatment of primary hyperoxaluria type I by combined hepatic and renal transplantation. Lancet 1987;2:474.
757. Jouvet P, Hubert P, Jan D, et al. Combined hepatic and renal transplantation for primary hyperoxaluria type I. Arch Fr Pediatr 1991;48:637.
758. Watts RWE, Danpure CJ, De Pauw L, et al. Combined liver–kidney and isolated liver transplantations for primary hyperoxaluria type I: The European experience. Nephrol Dial Transplant 1991;6:502.
759. Roth KS, Foreman JW, Segal S. The Fanconi syndrome and mechanisms of tubular transport dysfunction. Kidney Int 1981;20:705.
760. Manz F, Bickel H, Brodehl J, et al. Fanconi-Bickel syndrome. Pediatr Nephrol 1987;1:509.
761. Worthen HG, Good RA. The de Toni-Fanconi syndrome with cystinosis. Am J Dis Child 1958;95:653.
762. Gahl WA, Tietze F, Bashan N, et al. Defective cystine exodus from isolated lysosome-rich fractions of cystinotic leucocytes. J Biol Chem 1982;257:9570.
763. Lemire J, Kaplan BS. The various renal manifestations of the nephropathic form of cystinosis. Am J Nephrol 1984;4:81.
764. Wong VG, Lietman PS, Seegmiller JE. Alterations of pigment epithelium in cystinosis. Arch Ophthalmol 1967;77:361.
765. Gretz N, Man F, Augustin R, et al. Survival time in cystinosis: a collaborative study. Proceedings of the European Dialysis and Transplant Association 1982;19:582.
766. Schneider JA, Schulman JD, Theone JG. Cysteamine therapy in cystinosis. N Engl J Med 1981;290:878.
767. Reznik VM, Adamson M, Bernardini, et al. Failure of cysteamine to prevent renal Fanconi syndrome in nephropathic cystinosis. [Abstract] Clin Res 1989;39:218A.
768. Deal JE, Barratt M, Dillon MJ. Fanconi syndrome, ichthyosis, dysmorphism, jaundice and diarrhoea: a new syndrome. Pediatr Nephrol 1990;4:308.
769. Chen YT, Scheinman JI, Park HK, et al. Amelioration of proximal renal tubular dysfunction in type I glycogen storage disease with dietary therapy. N Engl J Med 1990;323;590.
770. Garty R, Cooper M, Tabachnik E. The Fanconi syndrome associated with hepatic glycogenosis and abnormal metabolism of galactose. J Pediatr 1974;85:821.
771. Komrower GM, Schwarz V, Holzel A, et al. A clinical and biochemical study of galactosemia: a possible explanation of the nature of the biochemical lesion. Arch Dis Child 1956; 31:254.
772. Hsia DY-Y, Hsia H-H, Green S, et al. Amino-aciduria in galactosemia. Am J Dis Child 1954;88:458.
773. Darling S, Mortensen O. Aminoaciduria in galactosaemia. Acta Paediatrica 1954;43:337.
774. Editorial. Pacifiers, passive behaviour, and pain. Lancet 1992; 1:275.
775. Blass EM, Hoffmeyer LB. Sucrose as an analgesic for newborn infants. Pediatrics 1991;87:215.
776. Levin B, Snodgrass GJAI, Oberholzer VG, et al. Fructosaemia. Arch Dis Child 1968;45:826.
777. Mass RE, Smith WR, Walsh JR. The association of hereditary fructose intolerance and renal tubular acidosis. Am J Med Sci 1966;251:516.
778. Halvorsen S, Pande H, Løken AC, et al. Tyrosinosis: a study of 6 cases. Arch Dis Child 1966;41:238.
779. Gentz J, Jagenburg R, Zetterström R. Tyrosinemia: an inborn error of tyrosine metabolism with cirrhosis of the liver and multiple renal tubular defects (de Toni-Debré-Fanconi syndrome). J Pediatr 1965;66:670.
780. Charnas LR, Bernardini I, Rader D, et al. Clinical and laboratory findings in the oculocerebrorenal syndrome of Lowe, with special reference to growth and renal function. N Engl J Med 1991;324:1318.
781. Van Acker KJ, Roels H, Beelaerts W, et al. The histologic lesions of the kidney in the oculo-cerebro-renal syndrome of Lowe. Nephron 1967;4:193.
782. Witzleben CL, Schoen EJ, Tu WH, et al. Progressive morphologic renal changes in the oculo-cerebro-renal syndrome of Lowe. Am J Med 1968;44:319.
783. Rötig A, Bessis JL, Romero N, et al. Maternally inherited duplication of the mitochondrial genome in a syndrome of proximal tubulopathy, diabetes mellitus, and cerebellar ataxia. Am J Hum Genet 1992;50:364.
784. Anderson JG, Notmann DD, Springer J. Studies in nephrogenic diabetes insipidus. Clin Res 1969;27:477A.
785. Knoers NV, van der Heyden H, van Oost BA, et al. Linkage of X-linked nephrogenic diabetes insipidus with DXS52, a polymorphic DNA marker. Nephron 1988;50:187.
786. Ohzeki T. Urinary adenosine 3′5′-monophosphate (cAMP): response to antidiuretic hormone in diabetes insipidus (DI): comparison between congenital nephrogenic DI type 1 and 2, and vasopressin sensitive DI. Acta Endocrinol 1985;108:485.
787. Libber S, Harrison H, Spector D. Treatment of nephrogenic diabetes insipidus with prostaglandin synthesis inhibitors. J Pediatr 1986;108:305.
788. Rasher W, Rosendahl W, Hendrichs IA, et al. Congenital nephrogenic diabetes insipidus-vasopressin and prostaglandins in response to treatment with hydrochlorothiazide and indomethacin. Pediatr Nephrol 1987;1:485.
789. Bartter FC, Pronove P, Gill JR Jr, et al. Hyperplasia of the juxtaglomerular complex with hyperaldosteronism and hypokalemic alkalosis: a new syndrome. Am J Med 1962;33:811.
790. Gill JR Jr, Bartter JC. Evidence for a prostaglandin-independent defect in chloride reabsorption in the loop of Henle as a proximal cause of Bartter's syndrome. Am J Med 1978;65: 766.
791. O'Regan S, Rivard GE, Mongeau J-G, et al. A circulating inhibitor of platelet aggregation in Bartter's syndrome. Pediatrics 1979;64:939.
792. Moorthy MB, Cade MSJ. Bartter's syndrome: a rare cause of a severe metabolic abnormality in a pre-term neonate. J R Army Med Corps 1992;138:46.
793. Bettinelli A, Blanchetti MG, Girardin E, et al. Use of calcium excretion values to distinguish two forms of primary renal tubular hypokalemic alkalosis: Bartter and Gitelman syndromes. J Pediatr 1992;120:38.
794. Houser M, Zimmerman B, Davidman M, et al. Idiopathic hypercalciuria associated with hyperreninemia and high urinary prostaglandin E. Kidney Int 1984;26:176.
795. Roman RJ, Skelton M, Lechene C. Prostaglandin–vasopressin

interactions on the renal handling of calcium and magnesium. J Pharmacol Exp Ther 1984;230:295.
796. Yamada M, Matsumoto T, Takahashi N, et al. Stimulatory effect of prostaglandin E_2 on 1α,25-dihydroxyvitamin D_3 synthesis in rats. Biochemistry 1983;216:237.
797. Raisz LG, Dietrich JW, Simmons HA, et al. Effect of prostaglandin endoperoxides and metabolites on bone resorption in vitro. Nature 1977;267:532.
798. Gitelman HJ. Hypokalemia, hypomagnesemia, and alkalosis: a rose is a rose—or is it? J Pediatr 1992;120:79.
799. Batlle DC, Hizon M, Cohen E, et al. The use of the urinary anion gap in the diagnosis of hyperchloremic metabolic acidosis. N Engl J Med 1988;318:594.
800. Izraeli S, Rachmel A, Frishberg Y, et al. Transient renal acidification defect during acute infantile diarrhea: the role of urinary sodium. J Pediatr 1990;117:711.
801. Sulyok E, Guignard JP. Relationship of urinary anion gap to urinary ammonium excretion in the neonate. Biol Neonate 1990;57:98.
802. Carlisle EJF, Donnelly SM, Halperin ML. Renal tubular acidosis (RTA): recognize the ammonium defect and pHorget the urine pH. Pediatr Nephrol 1991;5:242.
803. McSherry E. Renal tubular acidosis in childhood. Kidney Int 1981;20:799.
804. Sebastian A, Morris RC Jr. Renal tubular acidosis. Clin Nephrol 1977;7:216.
805. Svenningsen NW. Renal acid-base titration studies in infants with and without metabolic acidosis in the postneonatal period. Pediatr Res 1974;8:659.
806. Dubose TD Jr, Pucacco LR, Green JM. Hydrogen ion secretion by the collecting duct as a determinant of the urine to PCO_2 gradient in alkaline urine. J Clin Invest 1982;69:145.
807. Wrong O. Distal tubular acidosis: the value of urinary pH, pCO_2 and NH_4^+ measurements. Pediatr Nephrol 1991;5:249.
808. Alon U, Hellerstein S, Warady BA. Oral acetazolamide in the assessment of (urine-blood) PCO_2. Pediatr Nephrol 1991;5:307.
809. Brenner RJ, Spring DB, Sebastian A, et al. Incidence of radiographically evident bone disease, nephrocalcinosis, and nephrolithiasis in various types of renal tubular acidosis. N Engl J Med 1982;307:217.
810. Norman ME, Feldman NI, Cohn RM, et al. Urinary citrate excretion in the diagnosis of distal renal tubular acidosis. J Pediatr 1978;92:394.
811. Tennenhouse HS, Scriver CR. X-linked hypophosphatemia: a phenotype in search of a cause. Int J Biochem 1992;24:685.
812. Chan JCM, Alon U, Hirschman GM. Renal hypophosphatemic rickets. J Pediatr 1985;106:533.
813. Delvin EE, Glorieux FH, Marie PJ, et al. Vitamin D dependency: replacement therapy with calcitriol. J Pediatr 1981;99:26.
814. Brooks MH, Bell NH, Love L, et al. Vitamin-D-dependent rickets type II: resistance of target organs to 1,25-dihydroxyvitamin D. N Engl J Med 1978;298:996.
815. Eil C, Liberman UA, Rosen JF, et al. A cellular defect in hereditary vitamin D-dependent rickets type II: defective nuclear uptake of 1,25-dihydroxyvitamin D in cultured skin fibroblasts. N Engl J Med 1981;304:1588.
816. Balsan S, Garabedian M, Liberman UA, et al. Rickets and alopecia with resistance to 1,25-dihydroxyvitamin D: two different clinical courses with two different cellular defects. J Clin Endocrinol Metab 1983;57:803.
817. Elsas LJ, Hillman RE, Patterson JH, et al. Renal and intestinal hexose transport in familial glucose–galactose malabsorption. J Clin Invest 1970;49:576.
818. Horowitz L, Schwarzer S. Renal glycosuria: occurrence in two siblings and a review of the literature. J Pediatr 1955;47:634.
819. Stonestreet BS, Rubin L, Pollak A, et al. Renal functions of low birth weight infants with hyperglycemia and glucosuria produced by glucose infusions. Pediatrics 1980;66:561.
820. Ahmadian Y, Lewy PR. Possible urate nephropathy of the newborn infant as a cause of transient renal insufficiency. J Pediatr 1977;91:96.
821. Conger JD, Falk SA. Intrarenal dynamics in the pathogenesis and prevention of acute urate nephropathy. J Clin Invest 1977;59:786.
822. Krakoff IH, Murphy ML. Hyperuricemia in neoplastic disease in children: prevention with allopurinol, a xanthine oxidase inhibitor. Pediatrics 1968;41:52.

CONGENITAL NEPHROTIC SYNDROME

823. Huttunen NP. Congenital nephrotic syndrome of Finnish type: study of 75 patients. Arch Dis Child 1976;51:344.
824. Norio R, Rapola J. Congenital and infantile nephrotic syndromes. In: Bartsocas CS, ed. Genetics of kidney disorders. New York: Alan R Liss, 1989:179.
825. Huttunen NP, Vehaskari M, Vihikari M, et al. Proteinuria in congenital nephrotic syndrome of the Finnish type. Clin Nephrol 1980;13:12.
826. Lanning P, Uhari P, Koulavainen K, et al. Ultrasonic features of the congenital nephrotic syndrome of the Finnish type. Acta Paediatr Scand 1989;78:717.
827. Bratton VS, Ellis EN, Seibert JT. Ultrasonographic findings in congenital nephrotic syndrome. Pediatr Nephrol 1990;4:515.
828. Autio-Harmainen H, Rapola J. The thickness of the glomerular basement membrane in congenital nephrotic syndrome of the Finnish type. Nephron 1983;34:48.
829. Rapola J, Sariola H, Ekblom P. Pathology of fetal congenital nephrosis: immunohistochemical and ultrastructural studies. Kidney Int 1984;25:701.
830. Habib R, Loirat C, Gubler MC, et al. The nephropathy associated with male pseudohermaphroditism and Wilms' tumor (Drash syndrome): a distinctive glomerular lesion—report of 10 cases. Clin Nephrol 1985;24:269.
831. Wiggelinkhuizen J, Kaschula ROC, Uys CJ, et al. Congenital syphilis and glomerulonephritis with evidence for immune pathogenesis. Arch Dis Child 1973;48:375.
832. Papaioannou AC, Asrow GG, Schuckmell NH. Nephrotic syndrome in early infancy as a manifestation of congenital syphilis. Pediatrics 1961;27:636.
833. Shahin B, Papadopoupou ZL, Jenis EH. Congenital nephrotic syndrome associated with congenital toxoplasmosis. J Pediatr 1974;85:366.
834. Couvreur J, Alison F, Coccon-Gibod L, et al. Rein et toxoplasmose. Ann Pediatr (Paris) 1984;31:847.
835. Amir G, Hurvitz H, Neeman Z, et al. Neonatal cytomegalovirus infection with pancreatic cystadenoma and nephrotic syndrome. Pediatr Pathol 1986;6:393.
836. Shapiro LR, Duncan PA, Farnsworth PB, et al. Congenital microcephaly, hiatus hernia and nephrotic syndrome: an autosomal recessive syndrome. Birth Defects 1976;12:275.
837. Robain O, Deonna T. Pachygyria and congenital nephrosis disorder of migration and neuronal orientation. Acta Neuropathol 1983;60:137.
838. Palm L, Hägerstrand I, Kristofferssen U, et al. Nephrogenesis and disturbances of neuronal migration in male siblings: a new hereditary disorder? Arch Dis Child 1986;61:545.
839. Lagrue G, Branellec A, Niaudet P, et al. Transmission of ne-

phrotic syndrome to two neonates: spontaneous regression. Presse Med 1991;20:255.
840. Similä S, Vesa L, Wasz-Höckert O. Hereditary onycho-osteodysplasis (the nail-patella syndrome) with nephrosis-like renal disease in a newborn boy. Pediatrics 1970;46:61.
841. Ty A, Fine B. Membranous nephritis in infantile systemic lupus erythematosus associated with chromosomal abnormalities. Clin Nephrol 1979;12:137.

HEMATURIA AND PROTEINURIA

842. Halvorsen S, Aas K. Observation on the urine of asphyxiated and dysmature newborn infants. Acta Paediatrica 1962; 51:417.
843. Emmanuel B, Aronson N. Neonatal hematuria. Am J Dis Child 1974;208:204.
844. Cramer A, Steele A, Wishne P, et al. Transient hematuria in premature and sick neonates. Pediatr Res 1981;15:692.
845. Thullen JD, Fanaroff AA, Makker SP. Renal manifestations of perinatal asphyxia. Pediatr Res 1979;13:380.
846. Seibert JJ, Taylor BJ, Williamson SL, et al. Sonographic detection of neonatal umbilical-artery thrombosis: clinical correlation. AJR 1987;148:965.
847. Chesney RW, Kaplan BS, Freedom RM, et al. Acute renal failure: an important complication of cardiac surgery in infants. J Pediatr 1975;87:381.
848. Pillion G, Sonsino E, Beaufils F. Insuffisance rénale aiguë du nouveau-né. In: Journées annuelles de pédiatrie. Paris: Flammarion, 1982:29.
849. Willis J, Duncan C, Gottschalk S. Paraplegia due to peripheral venous air embolus in a neonate: a case report. Pediatrics 1981;67:472.
850. Kalia A, Travis LB, Brouhard BH. The association of idiopathic hypercalciuria and asymptomatic gross hematuria in children. J Pediatr 1981;99:716.
851. Linshaw MA, Stapleton FB, Cuppage FE, et al. Hypocomplementemic glomerulonephritis in an infant and mother: evidence for an abnormal form of C_3. Am J Nephrol 1987;7: 470.
852. Miltényi M, Pohlandt F, Boka G, et al. Tubular proteinuria after perinatal hypoxia. Acta Paediatr Scand 1981;70:399.

Neonatology: Pathophysiology and Management of the Newborn, Fourth Edition,
edited by Gordon B. Avery, Mary Ann Fletcher, and Mhairi G. MacDonald.
J.B. Lippincott Company, Philadelphia © 1994.

chapter 43

Structural Abnormalities of the Genitourinary System

GEORGE W. KAPLAN

A discussion of neonatal pediatric urology in essence encompasses most of pediatric urology. Admittedly, there are age-specific problems that do not present in early infancy, but there are many more problems that present primarily or specifically in the neonatal months. It is these latter lesions on which this discussion will focus. The development of antenatal ultrasonography over the past two decades has had a profound effect on detection, management, and understanding of many lesions of the urinary tract.

To understand properly and interpret the symptoms and findings that are seen in most urologic problems, an understanding of the significant events of embryogenesis of the lesions seen is essential. Because normal embryology is discussed elsewhere in this text (see Chap. 42), abnormalities of embryogenesis will be addressed as the resulting lesions are covered.

The ureteral bud arises from the mesonephric duct at 4 to 5 weeks of gestation, the kidney begins to form at 6 weeks, and the bladder develops during the sixth to seventh week. The wolffian duct is then incorporated into the bladder (Fig. 43-1). It is not until week 10 of gestation that urine production begins, and usually not until 14 to 16 weeks of gestation that the urinary tract is evident on antenatal ultrasonography.[1] A number of anomalies may result from disordered embryogenesis of the ureter or kidney. Although some of the abnormalities are familial and others are related to chromosomal abnormalities, most seem to be sporadic in occurrence.

IMAGING

Urologic diagnostic imaging in the newborn, and to some extent in the infant, is limited by the level of renal function. Even though renal functional parameters may be sufficient to maintain homeostasis, they may not suffice to produce the accuracy of diagnosis that would be expected from some imaging examinations when used in older children and adults.

Ultrasonography and voiding cystourethrography are not dependent on renal function, and hence assume even greater diagnostic import than in other age groups. Intravenous urography, and to a lesser extent, renal scintigraphy, depend on renal function to produce images and may be less reliable than in the adult (Fig. 43-2).

ANOMALIES OF THE KIDNEY

With normal embryogenesis as background, the anomalies and problems that are likely to be encountered can be anticipated, because most have an embryologic basis. Some are incompatible with life, some may lead to an early demise, some are of no clinical significance, but most are potential, yet correctable, sources of morbidity that can be minimized if the children are treated at an early age.

Renal anomalies include the cystic diseases as well as abnormalities of number, position, and rotation. If the pronephros fails to develop, the mesonephros

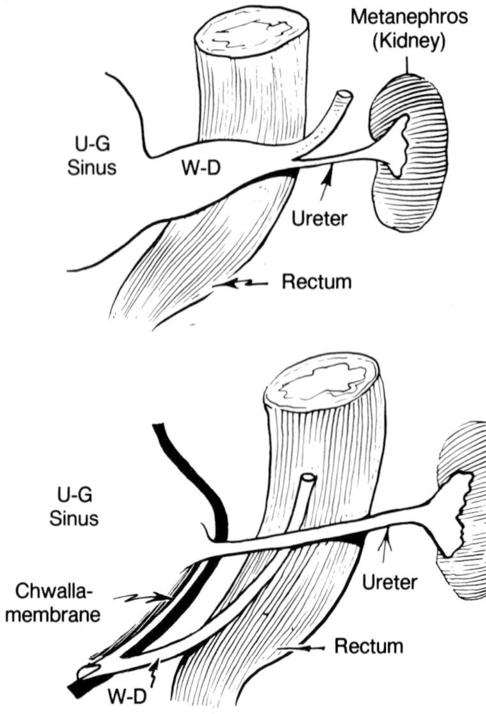

FIG. 43–1. Incorporation of the wolffian (*i.e.*, mesonephric) duct (W-D) into the urogenital sinus (U-G). (From Kelalis PP, King LR, Belman AB, eds. Clinical pediatric urology. vol. 1. Philadelphia: WB Saunders, 1976:504.)

will not develop, resulting in renal and ureteral agenesis and absence of the ipsilateral genital ducts in the male. If the mesonephric duct develops but the metanephros does not, there will be renal agenesis but the genital ducts will be present and there might be a blind-ending ureter.

Because nephrogenesis is induced by the ureter, normal nephrogenesis depends on the ureteral bud meeting normal metanephrogenic blastema.[2] Should the ureter fail to do so, a blind-ending ureter might result. If the ureter meets a degenerating portion of the metanephrogenic blastema (*i.e.*, the cephalic or caudal end of the blastema), renal dysplasia might result.[2]

RENAL AGENESIS

Renal agenesis can be unilateral or bilateral. Bilateral renal agenesis obviously is incompatible with extrauterine life. In cases of bilateral renal agenesis, there is no *in utero* urine production, and thus there is marked oligohydramnios and the affected fetus may exhibit the deformational changes of Potter syndrome.[3] Because adequate amniotic fluid is required for normal lung development, the lungs may be hypoplastic. The incidence of bilateral renal agenesis is roughly 1 in 5000 births.[3] Renal agenesis sometimes may be associated with sirenomelus.[3] Bilateral renal agenesis can be diagnosed antenatally by a combination of sonographic findings that include lack of identifiable renal masses, absent bladder, and severe oligohydramnios.[1] Renal agenesis must be considered postnatally when Potter facies are noted, when there is no urinary output within 24 to 48 hours, or when there is evidence of ventilatory failure with small lungs on chest radiograph. The postnatal diagnosis can be confirmed ultrasonographically by the absence of identifiable kidneys as well as the absence of urine in the bladder. When the postnatal diagnosis of bilateral renal agenesis is made and confirmed, attempts at life support, which may have been initiated because of respiratory distress, should, in my opinion, be abandoned.

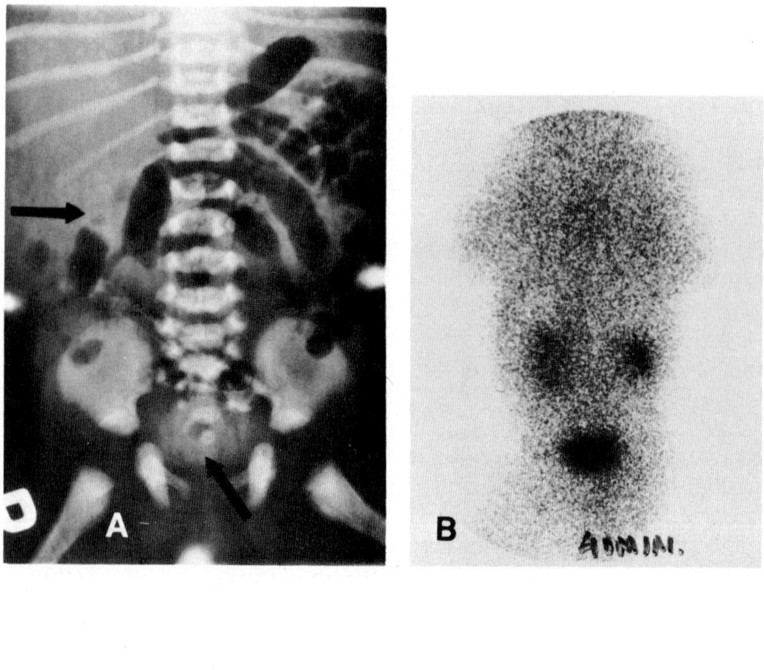

FIG. 43–2. (A) In an excretory urogram in a newborn infant. The right kidney barely concentrates contrast (*arrow*); there is no evidence of the left kidney. Contrast is apparent in the bladder (*arrow*). **(B)** An isotope renal scan the next day demonstrates the presence and function of two kidneys. The child was normal.

Unilateral renal agenesis previously was not thought to affect longevity or health, as long as the contralateral kidney was normal. Recent experimental studies have suggested that renal injury may be produced in the solitary kidney by hyperfiltration, and that a reduced protein diet may be somewhat protective. Clinical studies of patients with a solitary kidney (*e.g.*, transplant donors, trauma victims), however, have failed to confirm this.[4] The incidence of unilateral renal agenesis is roughly 1 in 500.[3] There is a higher incidence of contralateral renal abnormality in patients with unilateral renal agenesis, when compared to the general population, and many of these may be obstructive in nature. One-third of the patients with a solitary kidney in one series required some form of surgical procedure on the solitary unit.[5] Unilateral renal agenesis also is associated with congenital scoliosis as well as with vaginal and uterine agenesis.[6,7] It is the most common nonskeletal anomaly seen with imperforate anus.[8]

RENAL ECTOPIA AND FUSION

Failure of renal ascent will result in a pelvic kidney, and may be associated with vaginal or vertebral anomalies.[6] If the two metanephrogenic masses come into contact with each other in the pelvis, they may fuse and form a pancake or a horseshoe kidney.[7] The embryogenesis of crossed ectopia, with or without fusion, is harder to explain but might result from lateral bending and rotation of the tail bud of the embryo, thereby altering the course of ascent.[7]

Renal malrotation occurs when the kidney, as it ascends, maintains its early fetal orientation in which the renal pelvis is directed anteriorly. Malrotation is present routinely in fusion anomalies and in pelvic and crossed ectopias, and occasionally is seen in kidneys located in the renal fossa. It is of no clinical significance, but does introduce difficulties in interpretation of some imaging studies, and occasionally is of surgical import in planning reconstructive procedures.

Abnormalities of renal position (*i.e.*, ectopia) are interesting anomalies that are in themselves of no clinical import but may become apparent because of trauma (*i.e.*, hematuria), a palpable mass, or associated urologic abnormality. The ectopic kidney may be located in the chest or the pelvis. Thoracic kidneys usually are associated with eventration of the diaphragm, and are of no clinical significance except as a finding on a chest radiograph.[9] Pelvic ectopia is the most common of the abnormalities of position and often is associated with vesicoureteral reflux or ureteropelvic junction obstruction.[10] In addition, girls with müllerian anomalies have an increased incidence of pelvic kidney compared to the general population; hence, the finding of a pelvic kidney in a girl warrants investigation of the genital tract to uncover associated anomalies.[11]

Fusion anomalies, such as horseshoe or pancake kidneys, may present in the same way that anomalies of position present. Horseshoe kidneys are found with increased frequency in girls with Turner syndrome.[12] There is an increased incidence of ureteropelvic junction obstruction in horseshoe kidneys.[10] Crossed ectopia with or without fusion (*i.e.*, one kidney is found on the opposite side of the body) is uncommon. When crossed ectopia occurs, the left kidney more commonly crosses to the right side than *vice versa*.[13] By definition, the ipsilateral ureteral orifice is located on the correct side of the body (*i.e.*, the left ureter is on the left side of the trigone and the right ureter is on the right side of the trigone). There is an increased incidence of vesicoureteral reflux and of ureteropelvic junction obstruction in crossed ectopic kidneys.[10] Patients with crossed ectopia have an increased incidence of skeletal and cardiac abnormalities.[7]

SUPERNUMERARY KIDNEY

The presence of a supernumerary (*i.e.*, third) renal mass is a very rare anomaly, the clinical significance of which is determined by any associated pathologic condition.[14] The supernumerary kidney usually is small, and more often caudal than cranial to the normally placed kidney. Many patients and some physicians confuse a supernumerary kidney with a duplication of the collecting system and commonly, but incorrectly, refer to a duplication as a third kidney.

TABLE 43–1
CLASSIFICATION OF RENAL CYSTIC DISEASE

Polycystic Disease
Autosomal recessive
Autosomal dominant
Renal Cortical Cysts in Hereditary Syndromes
Tuberous sclerosis
von Hippel–Lindau disease
Meckel syndrome
Zellweger cerebrohepatorenal syndrome
Jeune asphyxiating thoracic dysplasia
Syndromes of multiple malformations that include cortical cysts
Renal Medullary Cysts
Familial juvenile nephronophthisis
Medullary cystic disease
Renal retinal dysplasia
Medullary sponge disease
Renal Dysplasia
Multicystic kidney disease
Other cystic dysplasias
Multilocular mesoblastic nephroma
Other Cystic Diseases
Simple cysts, single or multiple
Unilateral segmental cystic disease

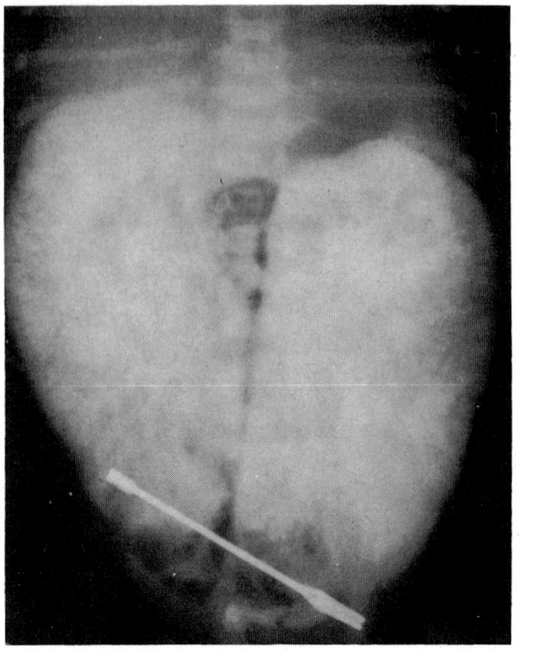

FIG. 43–3. An excretory urogram in a 2-day-old girl with infantile polycystic kidney disease shows the sunray appearance of the contrast material and the enormous renal size. (From Kelalis PP, King LR, Belman AB, eds. Clinical pediatric urology. vol. 2. Philadelphia: WB Saunders, 1976:686.)

CYSTIC DISEASE

Renal cystic diseases are a group of disorders seen in pediatric urologic practice that sometimes will present in the neonatal period. Because there is no agreed-on uniform system of classification, there can be difficulty in communication between disciplines. An accurate diagnosis is needed for prognosis and for genetic counseling. It is for this reason that communication must be clear. Table 43-1 is a classification scheme that has been of some clinical utility in my practice.

Autosomal recessive polycystic kidney disease, as the name implies, is an inherited disorder whose mode of transmission follows a mendelian recessive pattern. In this disorder, formerly known as infantile polycystic disease, the kidneys are very large and often occupy the entire retroperitoneum (Fig. 43-3). The cysts in this disorder are small, and are in reality enlargements of the collecting ducts.[15] The liver almost always is abnormal. At times there will be periportal hepatic fibrosis as a significant part of this complex. Death in the neonatal period is secondary to either renal or pulmonary failure. Those who survive the neonatal period usually will exhibit decreased renal function and hypertension, but at times liver failure due to hepatic fibrosis may be the most prominent part of the clinical picture.[16] Imaging studies such as antenatal or postnatal ultrasonography and intravenous urography usually are diagnostic.

Autosomal dominant polycystic kidney disease is inherited in a mendelian dominant fashion and is more common than the recessive form. It usually does not present until adult life, however—hence its former name, adult polycystic disease. These patients usually present with hypertension, hematuria, urinary tract infection, or renal failure. When this problem presents in childhood, it may do so as an abdominal mass. Imaging studies will prove diagnostic, because multiple large cysts that splay and distort the collecting system will be present. Although there often are associated hepatic cysts, liver failure is not usually a clinical feature of this disorder. Microdissection studies have shown that the cysts are due to abnormal branching of the collecting tubules and cystic dilations of portions of the nephron.[17] Detectable cysts may not develop in affected people until middle to late adult life, however, and the disease is undetectable clinically until they appear.

Tuberous sclerosis can mimic both autosomal recessive and autosomal dominant polycystic disease, in that lesions grossly similar to both forms of polycystic disease can be found in the tuberous sclerosis complex.[18] Microscopically, lesions characteristic of tuberous sclerosis will be seen on biopsy of the affected kidneys. Angiomyolipomas (*i.e.*, renal hamartomas), however, are the more usual renal lesion in patients with tuberous sclerosis.

Multicystic kidney disease is the most common form of cystic disease seen in neonates. As originally defined by Spence and colleagues, this is a unilateral lesion in which the entire kidney is replaced by cysts of varying sizes.[19] Grossly, there is no recognizable renal tissue present, but microscopically there may be dysplastic renal elements in the septa between the cysts (Fig. 43-4). Bilateral multicystic kidney disease is incompatible with life. Multicystic kidney disease is sporadic and is not inherited. Some multicystic kidneys involute, probably by absorption of the cyst fluid. This can occur antenatally or in the first few months of life. It is likely that many cases of presumed renal agenesis are multicystic kidneys that have undergone involution. Multicystic kidneys usually are detectable as palpable masses. Ultrasonography should demonstrate multiple cysts in a random pattern (Fig. 43-5), and there usually is no function on renal scan or intravenous urography. There is a great deal of controversy surrounding the management of these lesions; traditional therapy had been nephrectomy, but many pediatric urologists advocate observation because the incidence of sequelae such as infection, pain, hypertension, or malignancy is very low. Nephrectomy seems a reasonable alternative to lifelong follow-up, however, and is my current recommendation if the kidney does not completely involute within 6 to 12 months. Roughly 25% of the patients with multicystic kidney disease have an obstructive lesion such as ureteropelvic junction obstruction on the contralateral side, and it is this fact that will determine the patient's ultimate prognosis.

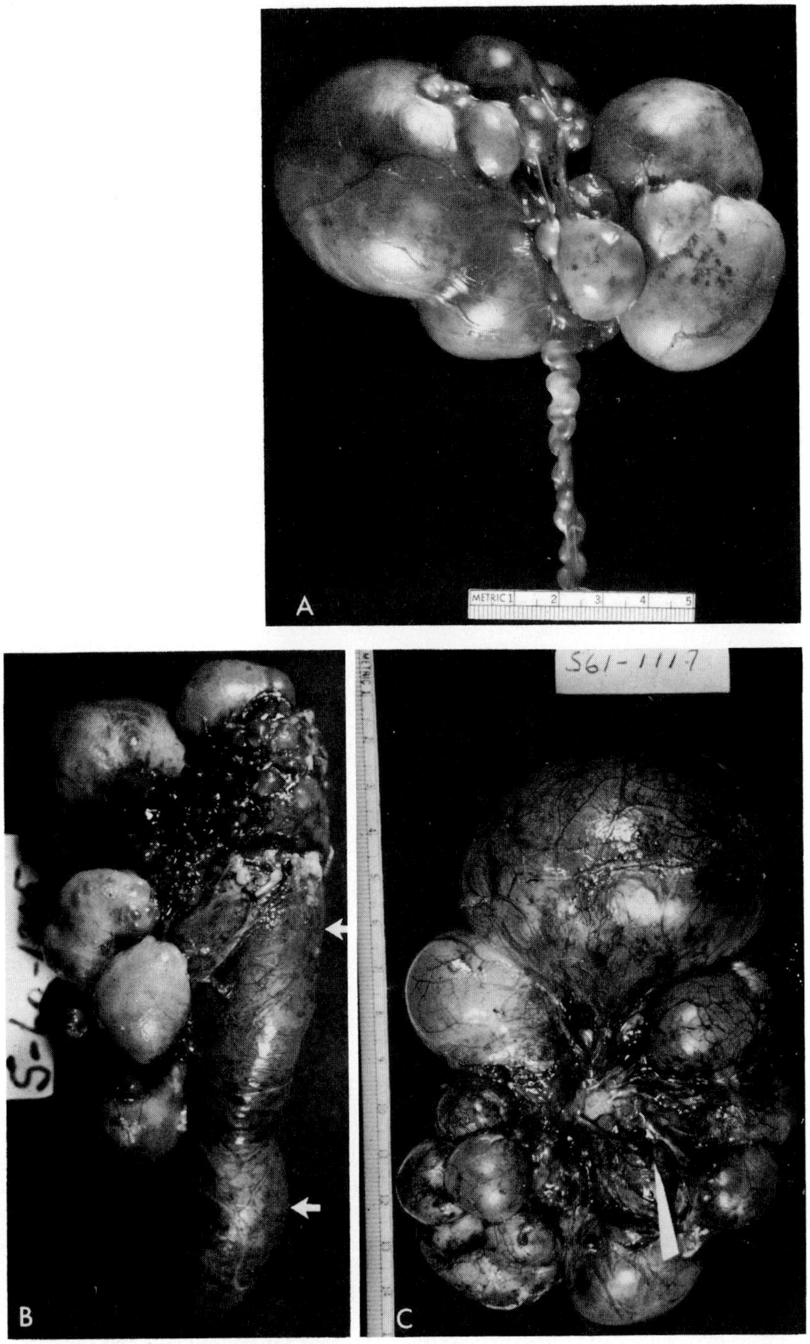

FIG. 43–4. Three examples of the variety of multicystic diseases. **(A)** Multicystic kidney with a torturous atretic ureter. The cysts vary in size and appear to be held together by fibrous tissue. **(B)** Multicystic kidney in a 1-month-old girl. The dilated pelvis and proximal ureter are indicated (*arrows*). **(C)** Multicystic kidney in a 4-day-old girl. No ureter was found during the nephrectomy. (From Kelalis PP, King LR, Belman AB, eds. Clinical pediatric urology. vol. 2. Philadelphia: WB Saunders, 1976: 210.)

ANOMALIES OF THE URETERS AND BLADDER

DUPLICATION AND TRIPLICATION OF THE URETERS

Multiple ureteral buds or premature division of the ureteral bud could produce ureteral duplication or triplication.[20] If there are multiple ureteral buds, one bud is likely to meet degenerating rather than normal nephrogenic tissue. This could account for the increased incidence of renal dysplasia in the upper pole of a duplicated system.[2] Duplication of the urinary collecting system is one of the more common abnormalities seen in the urinary tract. Duplication can be either complete or incomplete. Incomplete duplication usually is of no clinical significance, although, rarely, there can be ureteroureteral reflux between the two limbs of the partial duplication that can result in dilation of one of the moieties, usually the lower one. Complete duplication occurs once in every 500 cases.[20] Complete duplication by itself is of no clinical significance, but it is associated with a higher incidence of other abnormalities in the urinary system.

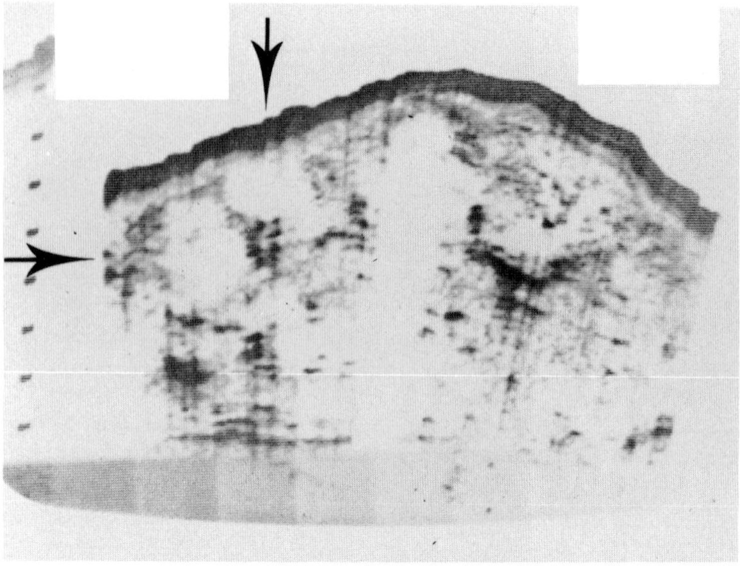

FIG. 43–5. A transverse abdominal ultrasonographic study carried out in prone position 3 cm above the iliac crest in an infant with left multicystic (*i.e.*, cystic dysplastic) kidney. Note the multiple echo-free areas (*arrows*).

These abnormalities include both vesicoureteral reflux and obstructions.

Vesicoureteral reflux probably is the more common of these associated anomalies and usually occurs into the lower moiety of a duplicated system (Fig. 43-6). Duplication is seen in approximately one in five people with vesicoureteral reflux, which is much higher than its incidence in the general population.[21] The grade of reflux associated with a complete duplication usually is greater than that seen with a single system. When the upper moiety of a complete duplication is abnormal, obstruction is the more common abnormality. Both obstruction and vesicoureteral reflux associated with duplications may present as either mass lesions or urosepsis.

If the ureteral bud arises from a locus that is more cranial or caudad than normal, ureteral ectopia, vesicoureteral reflux, or paraureteral diverticula might be produced.[22] Ectopic ureteroceles probably result from abnormalities of the ureteral bud as well as ureteral ectopia.[23] Simple ureteroceles are thought to be produced by persistence of the Chwalla membrane (*i.e.*, the membrane covering the distal end of the ureter during development).[24]

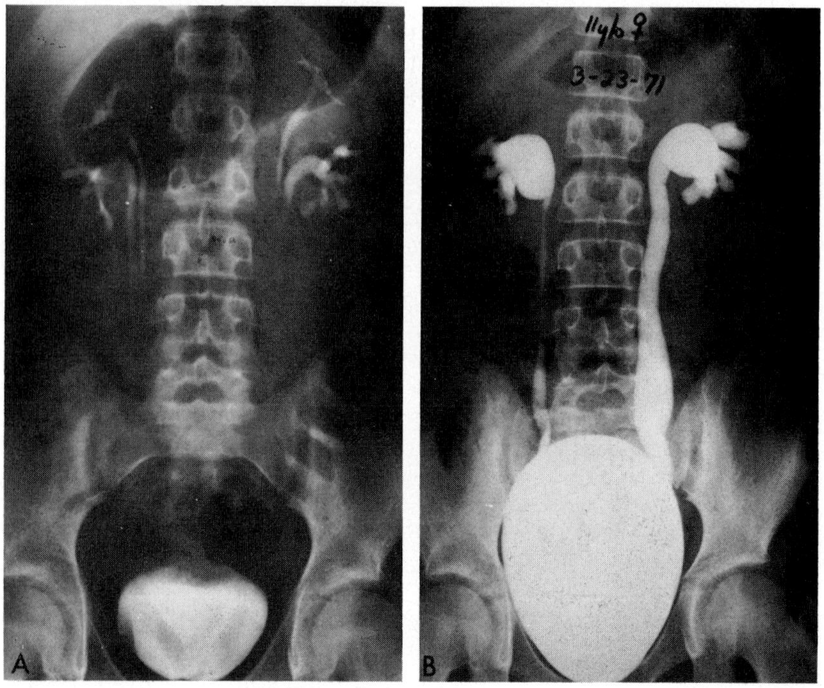

FIG. 43–6. (A) An intravenous urogram in a girl with complete, bilateral duplication of the collecting system. Note the blunting of the lower calyces. **(B)** A cystogram in the same child demonstrates reflux into both lower collecting systems only. (From Belman AB. The clinical significance of vesicoureteral reflux. Pediatr Clin North Am 1976;23:707.)

Ureteral obstructions occur primarily at the ureteropelvic and ureterovesical junctions. These obstructions usually are intrinsic in nature, and the ureter may be of normal or reduced caliber externally.[25,26] Multicystic kidney disease has been said to result from ureteral obstruction early in gestation but, in my opinion, is more likely to be secondary to disordered induction of the metanephrogenic mass by a faulty ureteral bud.[27]

BLADDER ANOMALIES

Agenesis of the bladder could result if the allantoic stalk failed to develop.[28] It could also occur if there were bilateral failure of ureteral migration with bilateral ureteral ectopia, because migration of the ureters is necessary for formation of the trigone, which, in turn, might be necessary for enlargement of the allantoic stalk.[29] Urachal anomalies occur because of a general mesodermal failure, as in the prune-belly syndrome, or because of delayed closure of the urachus.[30] Duplications of the bladder and urethra often are associated with duplications of the hindgut and lower spinal cord. Hence, it would seem that splitting of the hind end of the embryo might be responsible for this type of anomaly.[31]

Posterior urethral valves probably result from abnormal insertion and persistence of the mesonephric ducts distal to the Müller tubercle (type I), or from persistence of the cloacal membrane (type III).[32] Type II valves probably do not exist (see Fig. 43-17).

URETERAL ECTOPIA

Ureteral ectopia exists when the ureter opens in a position other than its normal location at the corner of the trigone. Ectopia may occur in ureters of single or duplex kidneys (Fig. 43-7). The most common form of ureteral ectopia is lateral ureteral ectopia, in which the ureteral orifice lies within the bladder lateral to its normal position. This is the etiologic mechanism for primary vesicoureteral reflux (see Vesicoureteral Reflux). Significant medial or distal ureteral ectopia is less common than lateral ureteral ectopia, and causes clinical pathologic conditions that vary depending on the location of the ureteral orifice and the gender of the patient. An abnormal proximal budding locus on the mesonephric duct allows the ureteral bud to remain in prolonged contact with the wolffian duct, so that the medially ectopic ureteral orifice may open anywhere along the course of the wolffian duct (Fig. 43-8). In males, this includes the posterior urethra, seminal vesicles, vas deferens, or epididymis.[33] In females, the ectopic ureter may open into the urethra, the uterus, or proximal vagina or anywhere along the course of the Gartner duct in the anterolateral wall of the vagina. If a medially ectopic ureter opens within the confines of the bladder, no clinical abnormality

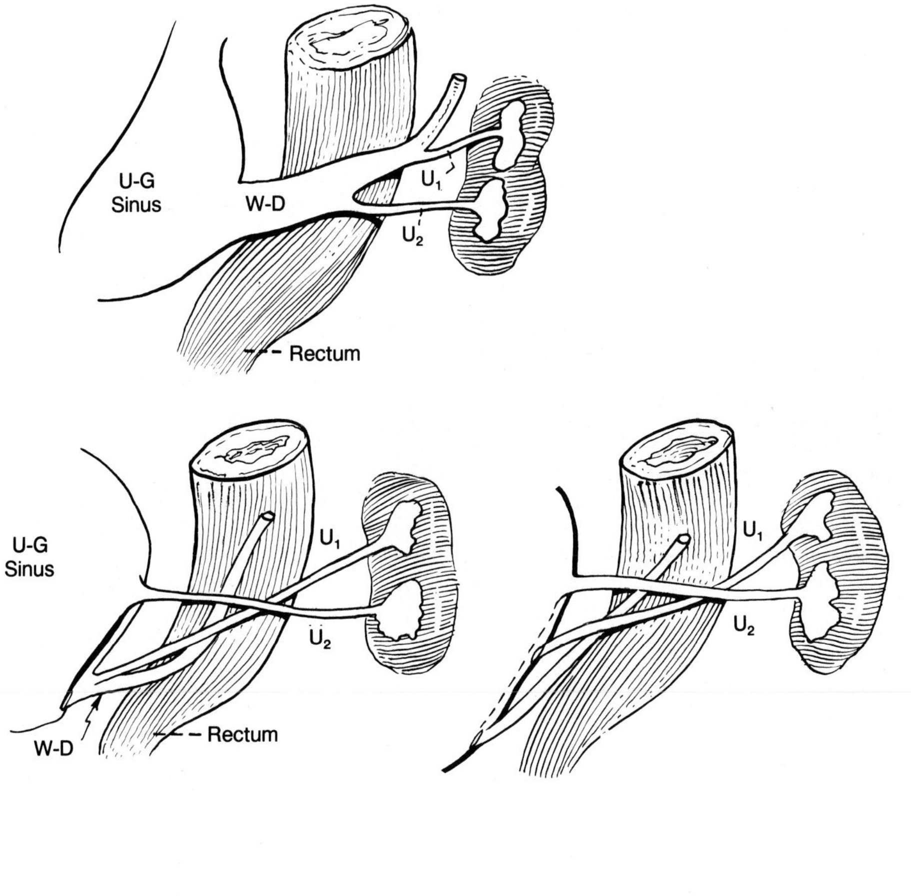

FIG. 43–7. Development of ectopic ureter. (U, ureter; U-G, urogenital; W-D, wolffian duct; (from Kelalis PP, King LR, Belman AB, eds. Clinical pediatric urology. vol. 1. Philadelphia: WB Saunders, 1976:510.)

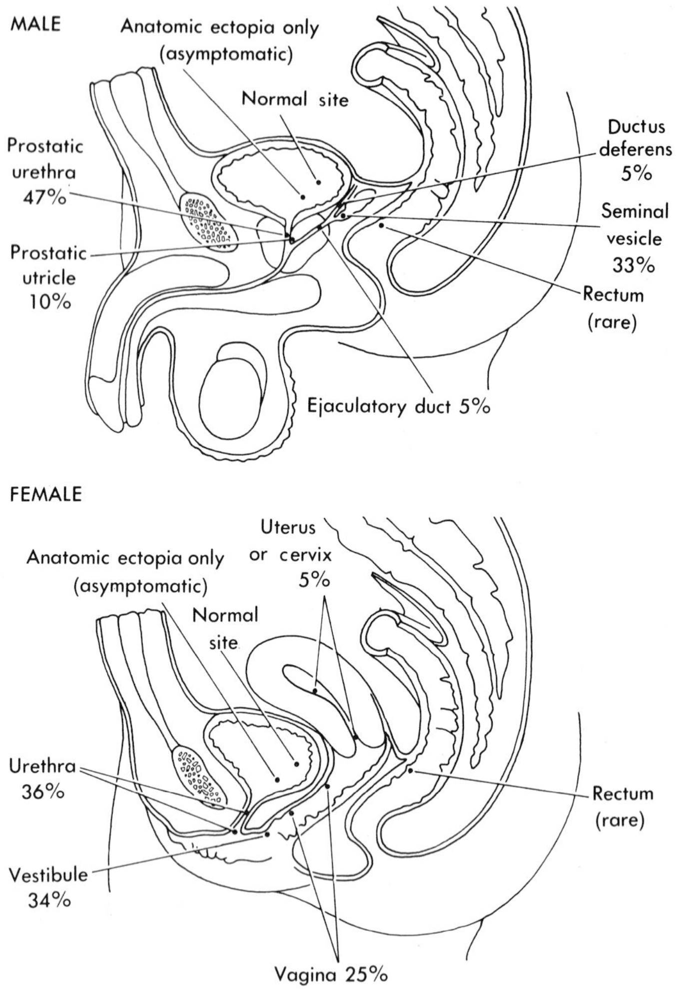

FIG. 43–8. Sites of ectopic ureteral orifices and their relative frequencies of occurrence in men and women. (From Gray, SW, Skandalakis JE Embryology for surgeons. Philadelphia: WB Saunders, 1972:536.)

occurs. If, however, the ureter opens within the confines of the bladder neck mechanism, obstruction of the involved renal unit or urethroureteral reflux may occur.

In females, ectopic ureteral orifices that lie distal to the internal sphincter mechanism of the bladder neck can cause incontinence.[34] Older girls usually present with constant dampness that is associated with an otherwise symptom-free, normal voiding pattern. Infant girls may be constantly wet or have a purulent discharge if the system is infected. Physical examination suggests the diagnosis if urine can be seen to well up in the vagina, or if a spurt of urine is seen coming from the perineal ectopic ureteral orifice. Eighty percent of these ectopic ureters arise from the upper pole segment of a total ureteral duplication, and an intravenous urogram often will suggest the diagnosis.[34] Because the ectopic segment in these patients frequently functions poorly, it may not be visible on excretory urography despite the use of delayed radiographs. A high index of suspicion and an awareness of the radiographic clues to a nonvisible duplication (*i.e.*, the drooping lily sign) often will lead to the diagnosis (Fig. 43-9). Since an ectopic vaginal ureter may drain a poorly functioning, and thus nonvisualizable single renal unit, congenital absence of one kidney in a girl with incontinence must not be accepted as a diagnosis without a thorough investigation that should include abdominal sonography, nuclear renal scan, and occasionally computed tomography scan.[35]

Treatment of the ectopic ureter depends on the presence or absence of significant function in the involved renal unit. If the ureter drains an otherwise healthy system, ureteral reimplantation into the bladder will correct the problem and preserve maximal renal function. If the ureteral anomaly is associated with a duplex kidney, ipsilateral ureteroureterostomy is indicated. In the more usual case, in which the involved renal unit functions poorly, excision of the involved segment is indicated. The distal ureteral stump is left undisturbed to avoid compromise of the normal sphincter mechanisms. The male infant with an ectopic ureter more frequently presents with a mass, urinary tract infection, or epididymitis.[33] In boys, an ectopic ureter will arise more frequently from a nonduplicated kidney and can drain into the male genital tract anywhere from the prostatic ure-

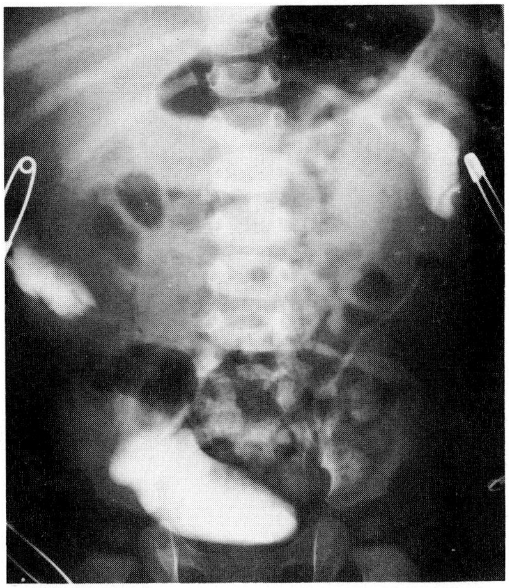

FIG. 43–9. Excretory urogram in an infant with ureteral duplication. Ectopic ureters from upper segments produced massive displacement of lower segments, leading to a misdiagnosis of abdominal mass and neuroblastoma. (From Kelalis PP, King LR, Belman AB, eds. Clinical pediatric urology. vol. 1. Philadelphia: WB Saunders, 1976:518.)

thra to the epididymis. Treatment is similar to that in females.

URETEROCELE

A ureterocele is a cystic dilation of the distal submucosal or intravesical portion of a ureter. Ureteroceles account for a broad spectrum of associated or secondary pathologic conditions, and constitute one of the more complex and confusing groups of anomalies of the lower urinary tract.[36]

Ureteroceles in children most commonly involve the end of the upper pole ureter of a duplex kidney (*i.e.*, ectopic ureterocele), but may less commonly involve a single-system ureter (*i.e.*, simple ureterocele).[37] The etiology of ureteroceles is uncertain. Failure of reabsorption of the Chwalla membrane from over the ureteral orifice has been proposed as an obstructive etiology.[24] It seems more likely that ureteroceles result from an intrinsic defect in the ureteral bud itself, and from faulty or delayed incorporation of the ureteral bud into the urethra and bladder base.[34]

Ureteroceles associated with a single-system ureter (*i.e.*, simple ureteroceles) tend to be intravesical and in the normal position. Intravesical ureteroceles in children often are associated with hydronephrosis of varying degrees.[38]

Ureteroceles may be associated with significant derangement of the upper and lower urinary tract. Since the ureterocele most commonly associated with secondary pathology originates from the upper pole ureter of a duplex kidney the most frequently noted associated pathologic condition is hydronephrosis and impaired function of the upper pole system and obstruction or reflux in the ipsilateral lower pole system (Fig. 43-10). Contralateral reflux or obstruction also may occur. The pathophysiology of the associated findings is understood easily when it is recognized that a ureterocele may dissect under the trigonal epithelium and cause deformity of the ipsilateral or contralateral ureterovesical junction, causing various combinations of vesicoureteral reflux or obstruction in any or all of the ureters.[39] Ten percent of ureteroceles occur bilaterally.[36] If the ureterocele prolapses into or otherwise occludes the bladder outlet, bilateral hydronephrosis may occur. The upper pole system associated with a ureterocele frequently is minimally functional, and may show evidence of dysplasia on microscopic evaluation.

Ureteroceles occur more commonly in females and usually manifest in early childhood.[36] One-third of my patients have presented during the first year of life. The most common presentation is that of a febrile infant with a urinary tract infection. If the ureterocele prolapses into the urethra, difficult voiding or azotemia may prompt evaluation. Ureterocele is the most common cause of urinary retention in the female infant. Rarely, a ureterocele will prolapse through the external urethral meatus in a female, and present as an introital mass.

In the classic situation, the diagnosis of a ureterocele should be fairly straightforward. Renal and bladder ultrasonography will reveal the upper tract dilation and the wall of the ureterocele in the bladder.[40]

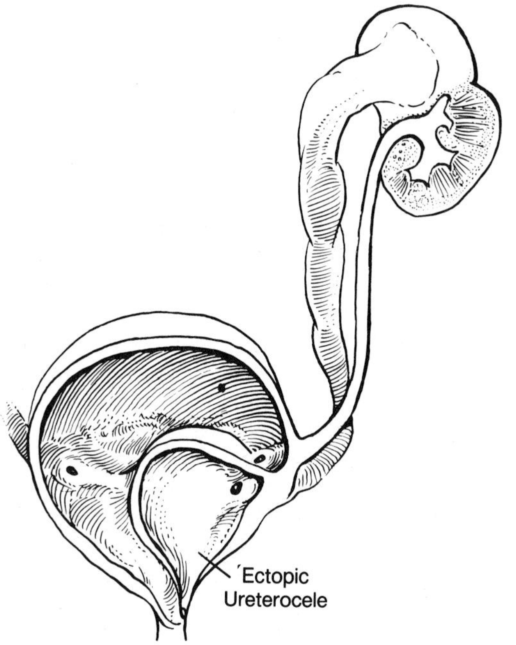

FIG. 43–10. Ectopic ureterocele. (From Malek RS, Kelalis PP, Burke EC, et al. Simple and ectopic ureterocele in infancy and childhood. Surg Gynecol Obstet 1972;134:611.)

This can be seen antenatally. The intravenous urogram most commonly reveals an ipsilateral complete ureteral duplication and upper pole hydronephrosis, coupled with the characteristic lucency of the ureterocele in the bladder. Cystography is necessary to establish the presence or absence of associated vesicoureteral reflux and to assess the integrity of the detrusor muscle backing the ureterocele.

The choice of treatment of a ureterocele depends on several factors. The age and clinical condition of the patient, the presence or absence of significant function in the involved renoureteral unit, and the presence of reflux or obstruction in the ipsilateral or contralateral uninvolved ureters all influence the choice of therapy. In the critically ill, septic infant transurethral or transvesical unroofing of the ureterocele may provide decompression and allow stabilization of the child until his or her clinical condition allows definitive treatment. Alternatively, placement of a temporary percutaneous nephrostomy into the involved renal unit often can be done without the need for general anesthesia. The best form of definitive treatment has been debated over the years. If an intravesical ureterocele is associated with a single kidney and minimal hydronephrosis, simple excision of the ureterocele and reimplantation of the involved ureter may suffice. Even if the system is duplex, an *en bloc* ureteral reimplantation can be performed if the ureters are not too dilated.[36]

There is general agreement as to the best form of management of the hydronephrotic upper tract associated with a ureterocele. If sufficient function exists in the involved unit, pyeloureterostomy or ureteroureterostomy to the ipsilateral uninvolved unit is appropriate.[36] In the most common situation, however, function usually is so poor that removal of the involved upper pole unit is necessary.[36] Debate centers over the management of the distal ureter and ureterocele itself. Once upper pole nephrectomy has been accomplished, the distal ureter and ureterocele may collapse, alleviating any associated pathologic condition caused by the mass effect of the ureterocele. If there is significant reflux into the ureter associated with the ureterocele, which is uncommon, or if the ureterocele tends to evert because of poor detrusor muscle backing, upper pole nephroureterectomy, excision of the involved ureter and ureterocele, and reconstruction of the bladder base is preferred. This obviates the need for a secondary, delayed surgical excision of the ureterocele because of recurrent urinary tract infections or persistent reflux.[39] At times, preliminary cutaneous diversion of the involved ureter with delayed reconstruction is warranted, to allow maximal recovery of function before deciding on the need for nephrectomy *versus* reconstruction.[36]

URETEROPELVIC JUNCTION OBSTRUCTION

Obstruction at the ureteropelvic junction probably is the most common cause of a palpable abdominal mass in the newborn, and is a frequent cause of antenatal hydronephrosis. This lesion usually is the result of narrowing of the ureter at the junction of the renal pelvis with the ureter. Because the renal pelvis is compliant, there can be a great deal of renal preservation despite massive dilation of the kidney behind the obstruction (Fig. 43-11).[41]

The diagnosis of ureteropelvic junction obstruction can be made sonographically because there is a sonolucent central mass within the renal area, surrounded by thin renal parenchyma (Fig. 43-12*A*). Vesicoureteral reflux must be excluded from the differential diagnosis, and this is done by cystography. The function of the obstructed kidney can be determined by intravenous urography or radionuclide scanning (Fig. 43-12*B*). One of the advantages of radionuclide scanning is that the physiologic significance of dilation can be determined by administering furosemide.[42] If the dilation that is present is of significance, there will be retention of the radionuclide behind the obstruction, whereas if there is no physiologic significance to the hydronephrosis, the administered diuretic will cause the radionuclide to wash out rapidly from the dilated system. It is becoming apparent that some instances of what was formerly thought to be significant hydronephrosis in the newborn are physiologically insignificant, and with time stabilize or improve and require no treatment. In instances that are physiologically significant, repair, usually consisting of a dismembered pyeloplasty, results in improvement in drainage and renal function in most instances.[41]

URETEROVESICAL OBSTRUCTION

Obstruction at the ureterovesical junction is not nearly so common as obstruction at the ureteropelvic

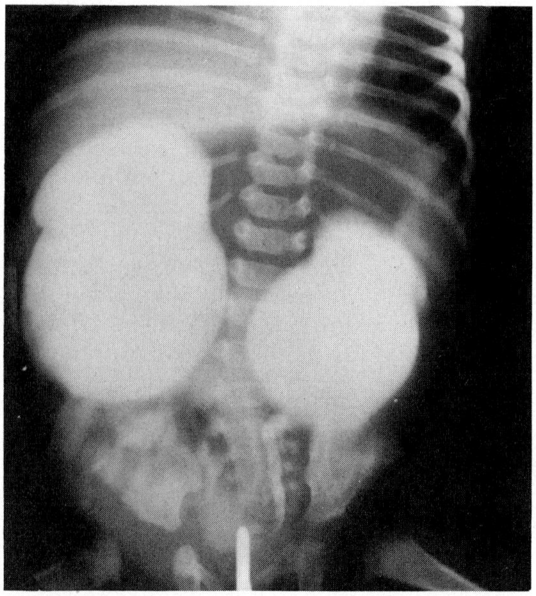

FIG. 43–11. Severe bilateral hydronephrosis secondary to ureteropelvic junction obstructions.

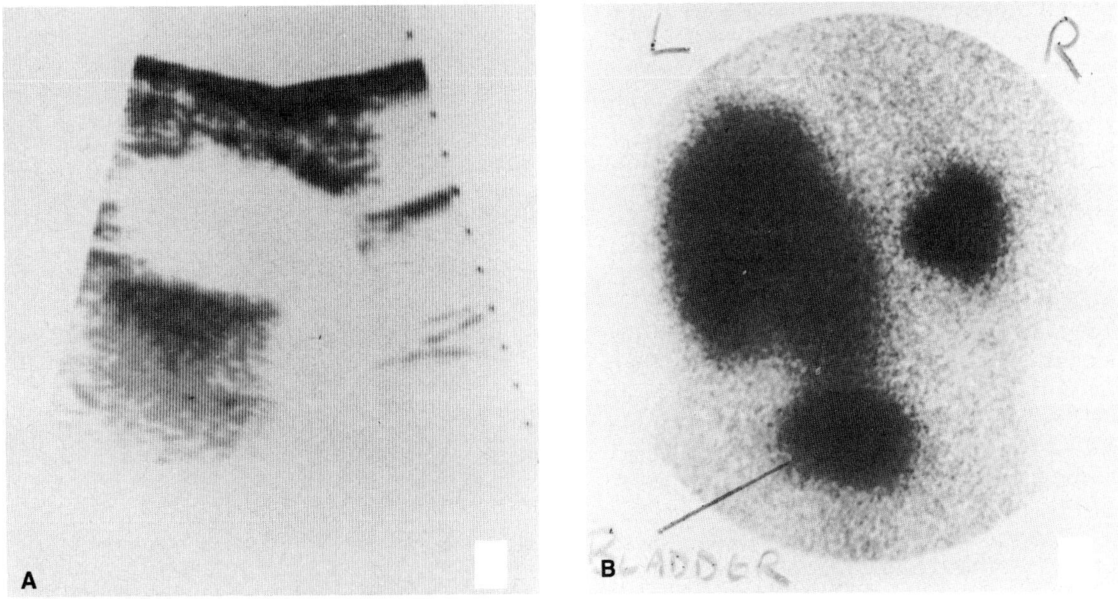

FIG. 43–12. **(A)** A longitudinal abdominal ultrasonogram in a newborn infant demonstrates a single, large echo-free region consistent with hydronephrosis. **(B)** A delayed renal scan in a newborn infant with massive left hydronephrosis secondary to ureteropelvic junction obstruction demonstrates that the renal pelvis extends all the way to the child's true pelvis.

junction, but it is far from rare.[26] Lower ureteral obstruction may present as marked hydroureteronephrosis (*i.e.*, a mass), but also sometimes presents as urinary infection (Fig. 43-13). Just as with ureteropelvic obstruction, it has become apparent with experience that not all ureterovesical obstructions are physiologically significant; therefore, some may require no treatment. Radionuclide scanning with diuretics is helpful in making the diagnosis of a physiologic obstruction.[42] At times, however, an antegrade pyelogram with pressure perfusion studies is necessary to determine the significance or lack of significance of an apparent narrowing at the ureterovesical junction.[43] These lesions, when identified to be obstructive, are treated by excision of the obstructing segment, tailoring or tapering of the dilated ureter, and reimplantation of the ureter into the bladder.[44]

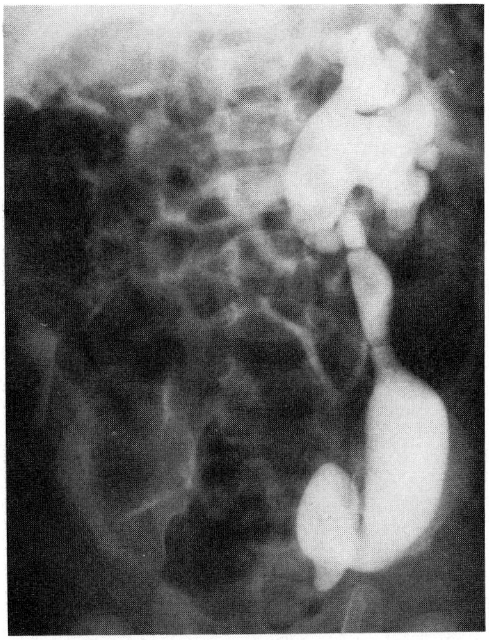

FIG. 43–13. Left ureterovesical obstruction in a 3-month-old boy who presented with unresponsive diarrhea. Urine culture was positive, and radiographic evaluation demonstrated significant pathology, as is evident in this illustration. The diarrhea resolved with treatment of the urinary infection. The ureterovesical obstruction was treated surgically. (From Kelalis PP, King LR, Belman AB, eds. Clinical pediatric urology. vol. 1. Philadelphia: WB Saunders, 1976:276.)

VESICOURETERAL REFLUX

Vesicoureteral reflux is the most common abnormality of the urinary system seen in children. The actual incidence is unknown, but there is no question that it is at least as common as cryptorchidism or hypospadias.

Vesicoureteral reflux is known to be a familial problem. When one child in a family is identified as having reflux, up to 30% of the siblings of that child may have vesicoureteral reflux. For that reason, it is thought that all younger siblings of any proband identified to have reflux should be screened.[45] The normal ureterovesical junction is a relatively efficient mechanism that allows egress of urine into the lumen of the bladder, but, because of its oblique course through the ureteral wall, prevents the bladder urine from reentering the ureter (Fig. 43-14).[46] It is obvious that there is maturation of the ureterovesical junction with both time and growth because infants have a much higher incidence of vesicoureteral reflux than do older children.[47]

Reflux is graded on a scale of 1 to 5.[48] The major significance of this grading system is that the higher the grade of reflux, the more likely it is that reflux will persist despite somatic growth, and that there is associated or eventual reflux nephropathy. Conversely, the lower the grade of reflux, the more likely there will be spontaneous resolution of the vesicoureteral reflux without reflux nephropathy.[49]

Although the presence of hydronephrosis suggests an abnormality in the urinary tract, the radiologic confirmation of vesicoureteral reflux is accomplished by voiding cystourethrography. Generally, this should not be performed while the child is actively infected, but, in those in whom infection has been the presenting sign, once the urine is sterile and the patient afebrile, there is no need to delay investigation. Because renal scarring is produced easily in the neonate, it is especially important to establish the presence or absence of vesicoureteral reflux before discontinuing antibiotics in patients who have presented with urinary infection.

Once reflux is demonstrated, especially in the infant, the patient should be maintained on low-dose antibacterial therapy in hopes of preventing urinary infection. The choices of agents are limited in the newborn, but amoxicillin is a reasonable alternative until hepatobiliary maturation is sufficient to allow the use of sulfa or nitrofurantoin. Breakthrough infection, especially while the patient is on antibacterial suppression or due to poor parental compliance, suggests the need for surgical repair.

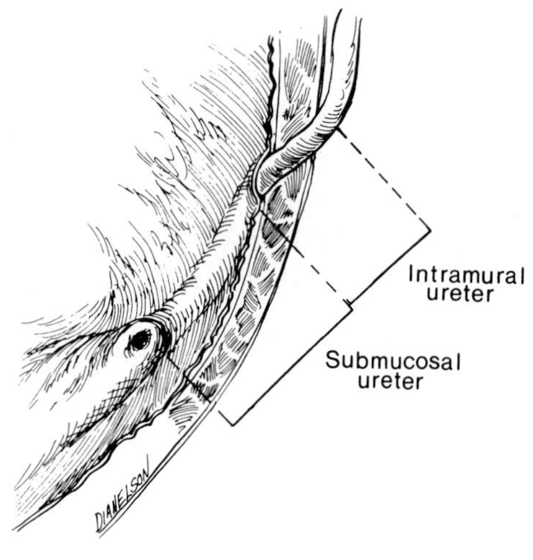

FIG. 43–14. Normal ureterovesical junction. (From Harrison JH, et al, eds. Campbell's urology. 4th ed. Philadelphia: WB Saunders, 1979:1597.)

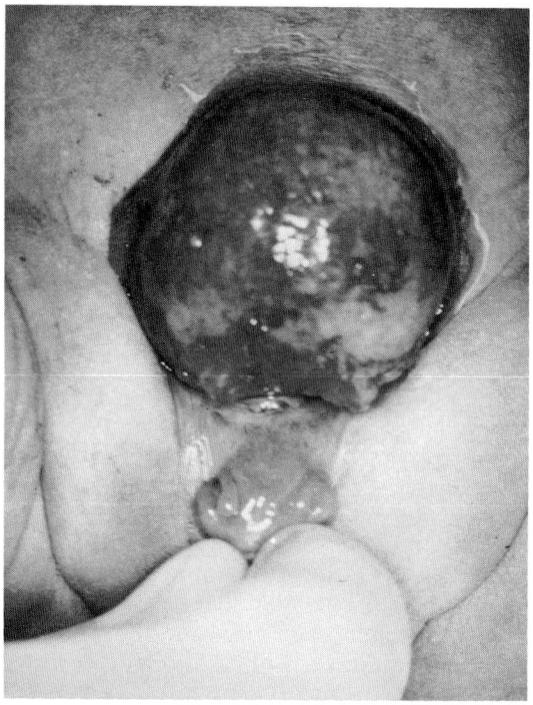

FIG. 43–15. Complete bladder exstrophy in a male child. Note that the penis is epispadiac, short, and stubby.

EXSTROPHY

Exstrophy of the bladder is a rare, but extremely significant, abnormality (Fig. 43-15). It affects roughly 1 child in every 25,000 live births. Exstrophy is not commonly associated with abnormalities in other organ systems, and the remainder of the urinary tract usually is normal in these children. Functional reconstruction of the exstrophic bladder, although a formidable surgical undertaking, in experienced hands can result in a continent child with a relatively normal upper urinary tract.[50] The major factor affecting the success of closure in terms of continence seems to be the size of the exstrophic bladder at presentation.

The epithelium of the exstrophic bladder is grossly normal at birth, but becomes hyperplastic very shortly thereafter if the bladder is not closed. It is preferable, if possible, that the exstrophic bladder be left uncovered and kept moist pending closure, assuming that closure can be accomplished in the newborn period.

Functional closure of exstrophy usually is a staged procedure. In the first stage, iliac osteotomies are performed to facilitate closure. Even though osteotomy can be omitted, especially in newborns, success rates are higher when osteotomy is used.[51] The exstrophic bladder is then dissected free from the anterior abdominal wall, closed into a sphere, and dropped back into the pelvis. The abdominal wall is then closed over the bladder. There is no attempt at the first stage to produce urinary continence. A second-stage procedure, performed after 2 to 3 years of life, is then performed in an attempt to produce urinary control. In the past, ureterosigmoidostomy was used as an alternative to functional closure. In this operation, the ureters were anastomosed to the colon and the patient voided a mixture of urine and stool. There are metabolic abnormalities (*e.g.*, hyperchloremic acidosis) associated with this form of diversion, and it has become apparent that patients who have been treated by ureterosigmoidostomy have an increased risk for development of adenocarcinoma of the colon at some time after their diversion.[52] Similarly, the unclosed exstrophic bladder is at high risk for development of adenocarcinoma of the bladder in the second or third decade of life.[53] Functional closure seems to obviate this latter risk.

Exstrophy of the cloaca is a severe anomaly, once thought incompatible with long-term survival. In this anomaly, two halves of an exstrophic bladder are separated by a midline strip of exteriorized cecum (Fig. 43-16).[54] The ileum may prolapse through the bowel plate. In addition, the child has an imperforate anus with almost no colon present distal to the exstrophic bowel plate. The small intestine often is short, and there may be a malrotation anomaly. The genital tubercle is split and widely separated. Hence, it is almost impossible to produce a functional penis in boys with this anomaly and genetic males so affected are best raised as females.[55] These children often have spinal dysraphism and a neurogenic bladder and bowel. For this reason, as well as the very short colon, a functional anus is almost impossible to produce and permanent colostomy, incorporating the exstrophic bowel, is the bowel diversion of choice. Even though the colon is short, it is best to preserve as much of it as possible to improve water reabsorption. Permanent ileostomy, although used in the past, may lead to problems with dehydration and short gut syndrome. The bladder in these children can be closed and reconstructed using iliac osteotomy and then uniting the two halves of the exstrophic bladder before anterior closure. Although normal urinary control usually is not possible, dryness provided by clean intermittent catheterization is a reasonable goal.

PATENT URACHUS

The urachus is a tube that connects the urogenital sinus and the allantois between months 3 and 5 of intrauterine life. The urachus normally regresses first to a small-caliber, epithelialized tube and then into a sealed, obliterated cord by term or during the neonatal period; it may remain patent up to the infraumbilical area in the premature infant.[56] Thirty-two percent of all bladders have tubular remnants of the urachus noted at necropsy.[57] Significant urachal anomalies are rare; they occur twice as often in males as females.[57]

Complete failure of obliteration results in a persistent communication between the bladder and the umbilicus that leaks urine; it is the most common urachal anomaly encountered. The etiology of this condition is unknown. It has been suggested that bladder outlet obstruction may be a contributing factor, although the chronology of embryologic events suggests that the urachal lumen obliterates before urethral tubularization. The diagnosis may be confirmed by retrograde fistulography, instillation of methylene blue into the tract or intravesically, or injection of indigo carmine intravenously. A voiding cystourethrogram

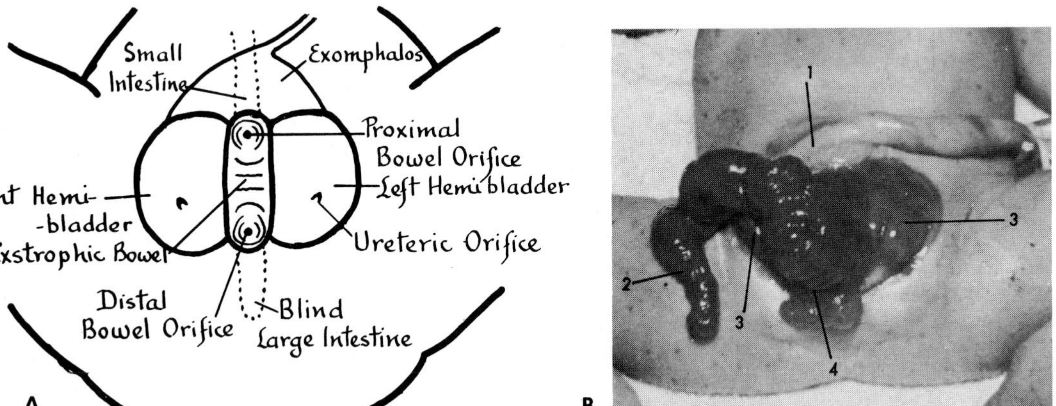

FIG. 43–16. Exstrophy of the cloaca. **(A)** Diagram of the external anatomy. **(B)** In a patient with exstrophy of the cloaca, the anatomic features as numbered include exomphalos (1), ileum that has prolapsed through the proximal bowel orifice (2), and the hemibladders lying on either side of the exstrophic bowel (3). Note the absence of an anus (4) and of definable external genitalia. (From Johnston JH, Penn IA. Exstrophy of the cloaca. Br J Urol 1966:38:302.)

occasionally will demonstrate the communication, but this study is more useful in ruling out other associated lower urinary tract anomalies such as obstruction or vesicoureteral reflux. A persistent omphalomesenteric duct must be considered in the differential diagnosis. In infants with minimal umbilical drainage that causes a small stain on the diaper, an umbilical granuloma or a patch of gastric mucosa may be at fault.[58] Iatrogenic creation of a vesicoumbilical fistula, during an umbilical artery cutdown, has been reported.[56] Treatment of a patent urachus consists of complete extraperitoneal excision of the urachus with an attached cuff of bladder.

MEGALOCYSTIS MICROCOLON INTESTINAL HYPOPERISTALSIS SYNDROME

Megalocystis microcolon intestinal hypoperistalsis syndrome was first described in 1976, and is considered rare.[59] The disorder primarily affects full-term female neonates and generally is fatal within the first year of life. Presentation includes abdominal distention, an abdominal mass (*i.e.*, a distended bladder), and functional intestinal obstruction characterized by bilious vomiting and absent or decreased bowel sounds. The small bowel is short, dilated, and hypoactive, with an accompanying microcolon but no anatomic obstruction.

The etiology is unknown, but the dilated bladder may be seen on antenatal ultrasound. Treatment consists of parenteral alimentation and urinary diversion by means of a cutaneous vesicostomy. Patients with Ochoa urofacial syndrome also may present with megalocystis in infancy.[60]

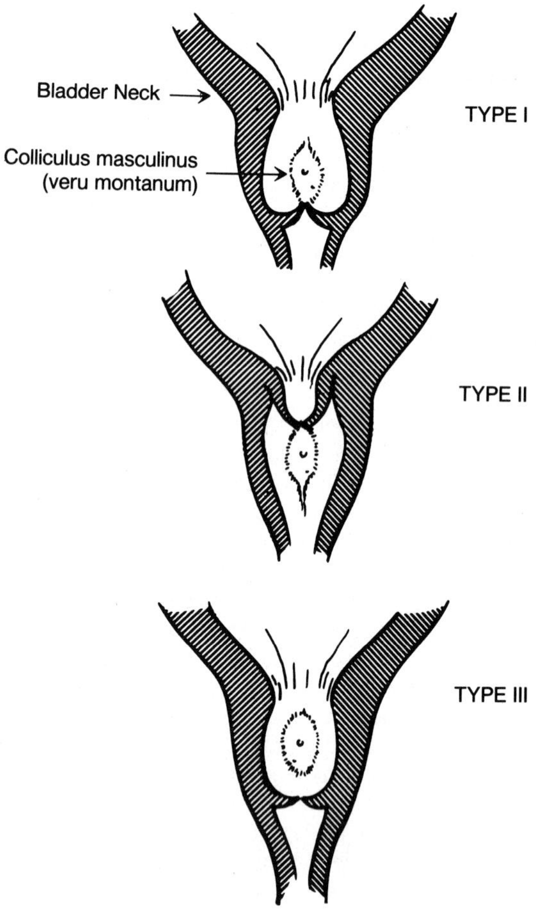

FIG. 43–17. Young classified valves into three types. The type II valve probably does not exist. (From Kelalis PP, King LR, Belman AB, eds. Clinical pediatric urology. vol. 1. Philadelphia: WB Saunders, 1976:306.)

POSTERIOR URETHRAL VALVES

The most commonly seen obstructing lesion of the lower urinary tract in a boy is the lesion termed posterior urethral valves (Fig. 43-17). The name really is a misnomer, because the valves are really a diaphragm that traverses the urethra from a point just distal to the verumontanum to the proximal limit of the membranous urethra.[61] Embryologically, these occur because there is an abnormal anterior insertion and persistence of the distal extent of the wolffian duct.[32] To understand the clinical picture of urethral valves, one must consider the dynamics and pathophysiologic consequences of the obstruction itself. The valves are best considered a rigid band or membrane, despite their frequently flimsy nature. The vesical neck also is a relatively rigid area. With antegrade flow of fluid, this membrane obstructs. When obstruction is present, the urethra dilates proximally and elongates. The detrusor hypertrophies in response to the extra work involved in voiding, with resultant trabeculation and sacculation. Detrusor hypertrophy also produces relative hypertrophy of the vesical neck.

The prostatic urethra becomes dilated in a fusiform manner between two relatively rigid points, creating a subvesical chamber. If there is a primary abnormality of the ureterovesical junction or if a paraureteral saccule develops, vesicoureteral reflux may result. Hydroureteronephrosis may develop, with or without reflux. Renal parenchymal damage in the form of renal dysplasia or interstitial nephritis, with or without superimposed pyelonephritis, often is concomitant or a result of valvular obstruction. Renal dysplasia often is present at birth in infants with posterior urethral valves and has been found at as early as 15 weeks of gestational age in the fetus.[62]

Osathanondh and Potter state that dysplasia is a consequence of intrauterine urinary obstruction.[63] In experimental animals, intrauterine urethral obstruction early in gestation usually has led to a patent urachus, without hydronephrosis or dysplasia—a situation that does not correspond to the clinical sequence in humans.[64] Later in gestation, experimental intrauterine urethral obstruction results in hydronephrosis without dysplasia.[65]

Clinically, dysplasia is found more often in association with severe vesicoureteral reflux.[66] In addition, dysplasia often is unilateral and not bilateral, as one would expect if it resulted from intrauterine urethral obstruction. Maizels and Simpson, using chick embryos, have shown that dysplasia results from problems associated with the renal blastema and not from obstruction of the ureter.[67] It seems that dysplasia, when present, represents a primary abnormality of the ureterorenal unit and has no direct causal relationship to the presence of intrauterine urethral obstruction.

The clinical presentation of the infant with posterior urethral valves often is related to the severity of the obstruction. Virtually all of the signs and symptoms seen in the boy with posterior urethral valves are secondary to the obstructive nature of the valves, the effect of intrauterine oligohydramnios, or the presence of superimposed urinary infection or azotemia.

Twenty-five to 50% of boys with posterior urethral valves present during the neonatal period.[68] The nonrenal features of Potter syndrome may be seen in newborns with posterior urethral valves, including intrauterine growth deficiency, pulmonary hypoplasia, limb positioning defects (*e.g.*, talipes equinovarus), and the characteristic Potter facies. All are thought to be due to a deficiency of amniotic fluid and subsequent fetal compression. The incidence of anomalies in other organ systems not directly attributable to urethral obstruction is low.[69] A palpably enlarged bladder, urinary tract infection, failure to thrive, or gastrointestinal disturbances may lead to investigation. A strong urinary stream does not preclude the diagnosis of posterior urethral obstruction.[70] Pulmonary hypoplasia will present with respiratory distress, especially with spontaneous pneumothorax or pneumomediastinum. This is an unusual but important symptom of valves in newborns. Any full-term boy with respiratory distress should be suspect for a renal problem. Hydronephrosis is present in 90% of infants with valves.[70]

Paradoxically, boys who present with posterior urethral valves very early in infancy carry a poorer prognosis than children who present at an older age. Presumably, this is because there is a high incidence of renal dysplasia associated with early presentation.

Urinary ascites is one of the rarer forms of presentation of children with posterior urethral valves.[71] The presence of ascitic fluid in a newborn infant should prompt investigation of the urinary tract, because urinary ascites is responsible for one-third of all cases of neonatal ascites.[72] Although the ascites rarely may be secondary to frank perforation of the urinary tract,[73] most often it is due to leakage of urine through the renal fornices and transudation of fluid across the peritoneal membrane into the peritoneal cavity.[74] The ascitic fluid usually has a chemical content equivalent to that of serum, because the high urea and creatinine content of urine has dialyzed passively across the peritoneal membrane and into the vascular system. These children may not have marked hydronephrosis because the urinary tract has been decompressed by leakage of urine.[74] These boys often present as extremely ill infants, but occasionally may appear initially healthy except for abdominal distention. Their prognosis with regard to renal preservation often is better than that of a child who does not present with urinary ascites, presumably because the leakage of urine from the distended system protects the upper urinary tract from the ravages of high intraluminal pressure.[74] Occasionally, a localized retroperitoneal urinoma will form. The diagnosis of urinary ascites usually is made clinically, and confirmed by ultrasound examination or a plain radiograph of the abdomen demonstrating bowel displaced to the central abdomen and a ground-glass appearance of the remainder of the abdomen.

Twenty-five percent of patients with posterior urethral valves have vesicoureteral reflux at presentation.[75] In one-half of cases, the reflux is bilateral. When there is massive unilateral vesicoureteral reflux associated with posterior urethral valves, the kidney on the refluxing side often is dysplastic and does not function at presentation or subsequently. Hence, marked hydronephrosis without vesicoureteral reflux usually carries a better prognosis for long-term renal function than does the presence of vesicoureteral reflux. In patients with posterior urethral valves, reflux, when present, will resolve with relief of obstruction in one-third to one-half of cases.[75]

Obstructive uropathy will be suggested on ultrasonography by findings such as bilateral hydronephrosis or by a distended, thick-walled bladder. Patients with posterior urethral valves often have a dilated and elongated posterior urethra that can be imaged sonographically. Perirenal urinoma or ascites also can be detected.

The single most important study in the diagnosis of infravesical obstruction is the voiding cystourethrogram. An adequate study requires complete visualization of the urethra from the bladder neck to the meatus and oblique and lateral projections of the urethra during voiding without a catheter in the urethra, because an indwelling catheter may obscure the lesion.

Posterior urethral valves appear as a sharply defined transverse or oblique lucency, with proximal urethral elongation and distention and diminution of flow distal to the valve. The bladder neck in valve cases may be secondarily thickened and collarlike. The bladder usually is trabeculated with saccules or diverticula, especially paraurethral diverticula (Fig 43-18). Vesicoureteral reflux often is present at diagnosis, and the refluxing ureters frequently are grossly dilated and tortuous.

Functional imaging studies of the upper urinary tracts will determine the degree of upper tract damage produced by lower tract obstruction. Historically, intravenous urography has been used routinely in upper tract imaging but may be inconclusive, especially if renal function is poor. If function is sufficient

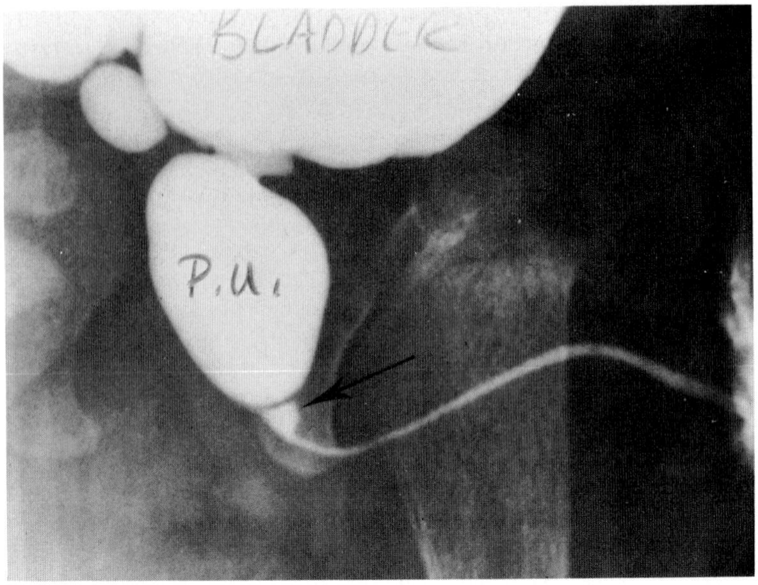

FIG. 43–18. Voiding cystourethrogram in a newborn boy with posterior urethral value (*arrow*). The prostatic urethra (PU) is dilated, and the bladder is trabeculated with multiple diverticula (*upper left*).

for radiographic visualization, and if delayed radiographs are obtained, marked hydroureteronephrosis should be evident. Delayed filling, visualizing a poorly functioning renal unit, may be secondary to vesicoureteral reflux rather than evidence of renal function. In the newborn or azotemic infant in whom obstruction is suspected, a radionuclide renal scan usually provides more information than excretory urography. A scan allows estimation of differential renal function. Scintigraphy also may be safer than excretory urography because it eliminates the need for iodinated contrast agents that have a small risk of associated morbidity.

When these infants first present, resuscitative measures often are necessary to treat associated urinary infection, to replace fluid and electrolytes, and, most important, to drain the urinary tract. A small intraurethral catheter (*e.g.*, a feeding tube) often will suffice to drain the urinary tract for a few days. Once the child is stable, the valves must be either transurethrally resected primarily or the urinary tract should be drained for a prolonged period using a cutaneous vesicostomy.

The long-term outlook for infants who present with posterior urethral valves is only fair, because approximately 50% of boys who present with posterior urethral valves eventually will progress to renal failure and transplantation despite treatment.[76] This does not mean that a fatalistic attitude must be adopted, but, nonetheless, expectations must be realistic. If the serum creatinine is normal at 2 years of age, the prognosis for long-term normal renal function is good but not perfect.[77]

RENAL TUMORS

Fortunately, tumors of the urinary tract are rare in infancy and those that do occur tend to exhibit a benign behavior. Variants of Wilms tumor can be seen in the neonatal period and include mesoblastic nephroma,[78] nephroblastomatosis,[79] and benign cystic nephroma.[80] These lesions usually will present as a palpable flank mass and occasionally can produce hypertension.[81]

Mesoblastic nephroma is the most frequent of these tumors. This recognized variant of Wilms tumor behaves in an almost uniformly benign manner.[78] Histologically, mesoblastic nephroma is composed largely of mesenchymal stroma with spindle-shaped fibrous or leiomyomatous cells. Ultrasonography will demonstrate a solid intrarenal mass. Radionuclide scans will show the mass to be nonfunctioning tissue. Intravenous urography will reveal distortion of the calyceal architecture by the tumor. Nephrectomy is curative, but there have been a few reports of local recurrence and rare reports of distant metastasis.[78] Chemotherapy and radiation therapy are not necessary adjuncts to therapy.

Nephroblastomatosis can be diffuse or nodular.[79] Diffuse nephroblastomatosis usually presents as marked enlargement of both kidneys. The kidneys are grossly enlarged and have a whitish hue. Biopsy reveals primitive metanephric epithelium resembling that seen in Wilms tumor. This lesion usually responds to chemotherapy (*i.e.*, actinomycin D). Nodular renal blastoma consists of microscopic foci of primitive metanephric epithelium and often is an incidental autopsy finding in infants. It is thought that Wilms tumor may in some instances arise from foci of nodular renal blastema.

Benign cystic nephroma occasionally is classified with the cystic diseases, but more properly belongs with the renal tumors because elements of Wilms tumor may be found in the septa between the cysts.[82] As with the other tumors, patients with cystic nephroma present with a palpable mass. Ultrasonography will identify the mass as multiple cysts or as complex (*i.e.,* mixed cystic and solid). Although enucleation of the mass is a theoretical therapeutic option, nephrectomy usually is the treatment of choice. Despite the presence of Wilms tumor elements in the septa, chemotherapy is not necessary for cure.

RENAL VEIN THROMBOSIS

Another renal lesion that has a definite predilection for the neonatal period is renal vein thrombosis.[83] This problem usually results from hemoconcentration secondary to dehydration, and also is seen in infants of diabetic mothers. Sludging in the intrarenal venules occurs, with subsequent thrombosis. The thrombus then tends to propagate centrally. The infants present with a palpable mass, hematuria, albuminuria, and thrombocytopenia. If both kidneys are involved, the infant will become uremic. Treatment is supportive and involves correction of the underlying problems. Surgery (*i.e.,* nephrectomy) was once thought essential to survival; however, it is recognized that nephrectomy is unnecessary and that, if collateral circulation is present, there may be renal recovery. Thrombectomy is of no help because the problem is in the peripheral rather than the central veins.

ADRENAL HEMORRHAGE

At times, either spontaneously or in association with renal vein thrombosis, there may be hemorrhage into the adrenal gland.[84] The infant may present with icterus from absorption of hemoglobin and an abdominal mass. Ultrasonography will demonstrate a sonolucent or solid mass above the kidney. Over the course of a few weeks, the mass will be reabsorbed or, rarely, will form an adrenal pseudocyst.[85] If the latter occurs, percutaneous drainage is the preferred mode of therapy. Otherwise, no therapy is necessary. Adrenal calcification often is seen several weeks after an adrenal hemorrhage.

PRENATAL ULTRASONOGRAPHY

The advent of high-resolution, real-time ultrasonography has allowed the antenatal diagnosis of many anomalies of the urinary tract. It has become apparent with time, however, that diagnostic accuracy *in utero* is not complete and that the natural history of some lesions is not as clear-cut as once thought.[86] The hope that antenatal intervention might result in improvement in outcome has proven ill-founded.[87] The maternal risk of morbidity with intervention has been reported to be as high as 4% to 5%,[89] and there are no clear-cut examples of improvement in fetal outcome as a result of such interventions.[88] Studies of the results of postnatal treatment after antenatal identification of lesions have, however, clearly demonstrated improved outcome.[89] There seems to be no advantage to early delivery, and thus the timing of delivery in fetuses with hydronephrosis is in my opinion dictated best by obstetric factors rather than fetal concerns.[90]

As stated earlier, the fetal kidneys can be identified in the early part of the second trimester of pregnancy. Dilation of the renal pelvis and calices in a nonduplex system, without identification of a dilated ureter, suggests the presence of ureteropelvic obstruction. It has become apparent that some instances of hydronephrosis resolve spontaneously and completely *in utero,* whereas others that are present at birth may stabilize or improve with time. Conversely, some seem to dilate progressively with time. Hence, not all dilations of the upper urinary tract are obstructive in nature.[86] Most of those that are of significance prove to be secondary to narrowing at the ureteropelvic junction.

In a duplicated system, there can be dilation of either the lower pole system or the upper pole system. Dilations of the lower pole system usually are due to ureteropelvic junction obstruction or to vesicoureteral reflux. Obstructions of the upper pole system usually are associated with hydroureter and often are accompanied by a ureterocele. Solid intrarenal lesions are most commonly mesoblastic nephromas, with neuroblastoma occurring infrequently.

Ureteral dilation can at times be massive, and may be confused with bowel on sonography; however, following the ureter from a dilated upper system down to the bladder usually will distinguish the dilated ureter from bowel because dilated ureters often do not demonstrate peristalsis. Bilateral hydroureter, although it may be associated with bilateral ureterovesical obstruction, is more commonly due to either high-grade vesicoureteral reflux, posterior urethral valves, or the prune-belly syndrome.

An enlarged bladder, when thick-walled and in a male fetus, often is secondary to posterior urethral valves or the prune-belly syndrome, and in females might be due to the megalocystis microcolon syndrome. If sought, ureteroceles can be reliably identified by sonography in the bladder. If no bladder is identified on ultrasonography, this suggests bilateral renal agenesis, in which case oligohydramnios also should be present; bilateral single ureteral ectopy; or exstrophy of the bladder.

Lesions associated with hydronephrosis and normal amounts of amniotic fluid generally carry a good prognosis, whereas those associated with increased renal echogenicity and decreased amounts of amniotic fluid generally carry a poor prognosis for pulmonary maturation as well as renal function.[91]

ABDOMINAL MASSES

The finding of an abdominal mass is not infrequent in the newborn nursery. An unselected series of infants in the newborn nursery revealed abdominal masses arising from the genitourinary tract in approximately

TABLE 43–2
ABDOMINAL MASSES OF RENAL ORIGIN

Mass	Texture	Renal Scan or Excretory Urogram	Ultrasonogram
Hydronephrosis	Smooth	Delayed drainage	Sonolucent
Multicystic kidney (*i.e.*, cystic dysplasia)	Irregular	Nonfunction	Multiple large and small cysts
Polycystic kidney	Smooth (recessive); irregular or smooth (dominant)	Delayed function; distortion of collecting system	Diffuse small cysts (recessive) Multiple large and small cysts (dominant)
Tumor	Smooth	Distortion of collecting system	Solid
Renal vein thrombosis	Smooth	Poor function to nonfunction	Relatively normal renal architecture; enlarged kidney

1 in every 500 admissions.[92] It is quite clear from multiple reports that the urinary tract often is the source of any palpable abdominal mass in infants.[93,94] In most reported series, approximately two thirds of the infants presenting with an abdominal mass eventually are found to have lesions in the urinary tract to account for the presenting mass. In infancy, hydronephrosis and cystic kidneys are the most common lesions producing abdominal masses, whereas in older children tumors are more common.[95] The obvious inference from these data is that ultrasonography, because the urinary tract is easily visualized, is the study most likely to identify the source of a palpable abdominal mass. The physical, sonographic, and urographic or renographic characteristics of the common abdominal masses of renal origin are listed in Table 43-2.

HEMATURIA

Hematuria in the infant can be a sign of renal vein thrombosis, urinary infection, or urinary tract obstruction.[96] The presence of hematuria must be confirmed by examination of the urine, both chemically and microscopically. A positive chemical test may reflect hemoglobinuria, rather than hematuria, which implies the presence of cellular elements in the urine. Even more common than the presence of hematuria or hemoglobinuria, however, is concern about a red diaper in an infant. Two relatively common causes for red diapers are the presence of urates in the urine, which can give a pink hue to the urine, especially in the diaper, and, if cloth diapers are used, the growth of *Serratia* sp. on urine-soaked diapers left standing in the diaper pail. Obviously, these latter two situations are of no clinical consequence but must be separated from true hematuria or hemoglobinuria in diagnostic considerations.

GENITAL ABNORMALITIES

CRYPTORCHIDISM

Undescended testes are a very common finding in the newborn period, affecting perhaps as many as 1 in every 50 newborn males.[97] Most testes that are undescended at birth, however, will descend during the first 6 to 9 months of life, so that the incidence of cryptorchidism at 1 year of age is approximately 0.7%, which is exactly the same incidence that has been found in postpubertal males.[97] The newborn examination is important in determining testicular position because the cremasteric reflex at that time is weak to absent.[98] If the testis is well descended in a newborn, it is unlikely that there will be problems with true cryptorchidism later in life. Because it is thought that optimal results from treatment of cryptorchidism are produced by interventions after the possibility of testicular descent has passed (*i.e.*, beyond 9 months of age) and before adverse effects of testicular nondescent are seen histologically (*i.e.*, approximately 1.5–2 years of age), the optimal time for treatment of cryptorchidism would seem to be approximately 1 year of age.[99]

PENILE AGENESIS

Although many of the penile anomalies are common, some, such as agenesis of the penis, are rare (Fig. 43-19). Penile agenesis suggests an early embryologic failure in the development of the genital tubercle and occurs once in every 10 to 30 million live births. The urethra usually exits on the perineum or near the anal verge. It is believed that these children are best raised as females and that castration and reconstruction of the external genitalia should be performed at an early age.[100]

PENILE DUPLICATION

Penile duplication (*i.e.*, true diphallia) is a rare anomaly that also may involve duplications of the urethra and bladder (Fig. 43-20).[101] Reconstruction of these anomalies involves complex decisions about functional capability of the urinary, genital, and gastrointestinal tracts, as well as appearance.

MICROPHALLUS

The boy born with an abnormally small phallus presents a true therapeutic dilemma. Most cases of microphallus are due to hypogonadism,[102] and will respond to testosterone, but an occasional patient with microphallus has end organ failure and will not respond to exogenous testosterone. It is notable that, despite the relatively common finding of microphallus in the newborn nursery, it is an extremely rare event to find an adult with a phallus so small that it is incapable of sexual function.

The normal full-term newborn phallus measures approximately 3 to 3.5 cm in stretched length; the definition of microphallus requires a phallus that is less than 2.5 cm in stretched length.[102] To determine whether or not microphallus will respond to hormonal stimulation, 25 mg of testosterone enanthate is administered intramuscularly every 4 weeks for a total of 75 mg (see Chap. 41).[103] Some element of response usually is evident after the first dose, and, in most instances, after the course is completed the child has a relatively normal phallus. If there is no response to testosterone, gender reassignment should be strongly considered.[104]

HYPOSPADIAS

The term hypospadias, by definition, refers to the abnormal location of the urethral meatus somewhere ventral to the normal glanular tip (Fig. 43-21); however, the term actually encompasses a complex that includes chordee (*i.e.*, a ventral curvature of the penis on erection) as well as an abnormality of the prepuce. Although it is traditional in some circles to categorize hypospadias by degrees (*i.e.*, first, second, and third), I find it more helpful, because there is no gen-

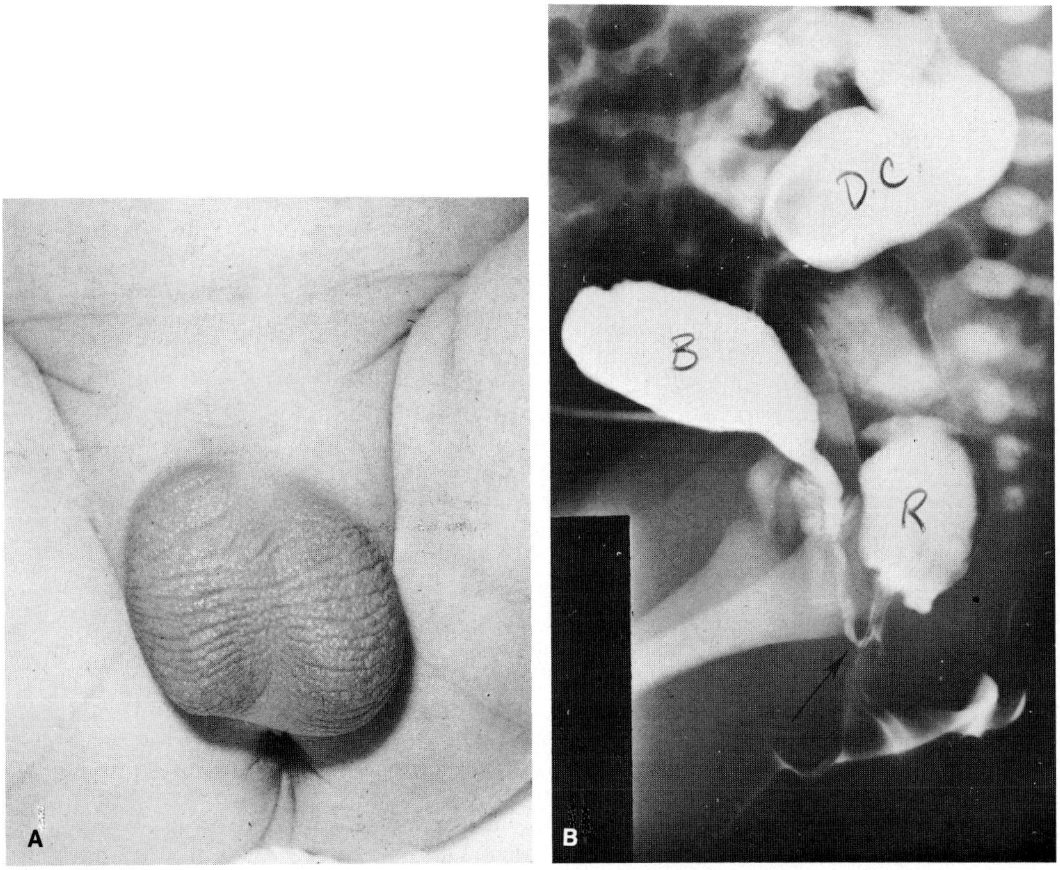

FIG. 43–19. (A) Genetic boy born with complete penile agenesis. **(B)** An antegrade cystourethrogram in a genetic boy with penile agenesis. The bladder is full (B), and there is communication between the urethra and rectum (*arrow*). The rectum (R) and descending colon (DC) are filled with voided contrast material.

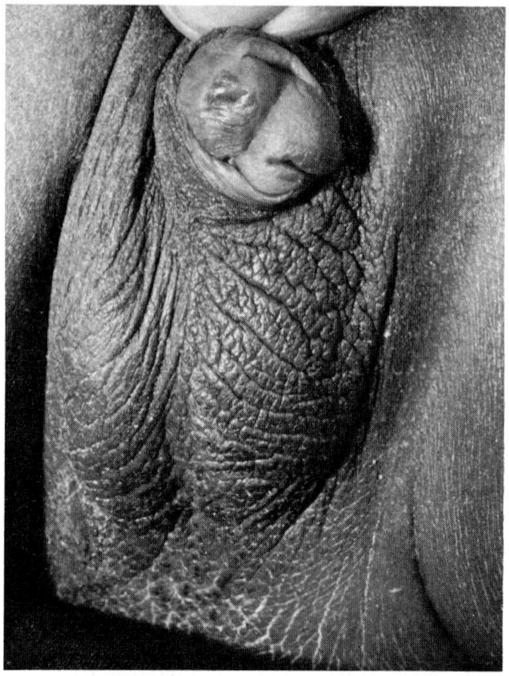

FIG. 43–20. Duplication of the glans in a 2-year-old boy. (From Kossow JH, Morales PA. Duplication of bladder and urethra and associated anomalies. Urology 1973;1:71.)

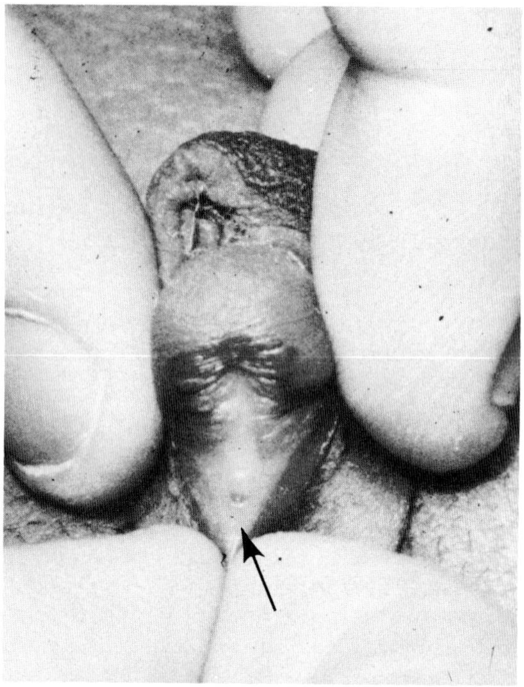

FIG. 43–21. The hypospadiac meatal position (*arrow*) is demonstrated by pulling the ventral shaft of skin away from the penis.

eral agreement on the meaning of these terms, to describe hypospadias by the location of the meatus and the presence or absence of chordee (Fig. 43-22). At times, the meatus is quite stenotic and can be very difficult to see, especially in the newborn.

It has become obvious that the sibling of a child with hypospadias has an increased (14%) chance of having hypospadias.[105] It is thought that hypospadias is inherited as a multifactorial problem. It once was thought that there might be associated abnormalities of the upper urinary tract in children with hypospadias, but critical analysis of series of children with hypospadias who have been investigated uniformly reveals that there is no increased incidence of upper tract abnormalities when children with hypospadias are compared to those of the general population.[106]

Most forms of hypospadias can be surgically corrected and, although there is no ideal age for genital surgery, it is thought preferable to perform this surgery late in the first year of life. The presence of the foreskin greatly facilitates the repair of these problems and it is for this reason that circumcision should be delayed in children with hypospadias. One of the primary clinical clues that hypospadias may be present is an abnormality of the foreskin, and whenever such abnormality is noted, circumcision should be avoided until the surgeon who will be involved in the repair can assess the child and determine whether it will be necessary to repair the foreskin.

EPISPADIAS

Epispadias usually is associated with exstrophy, but occasionally appears as an isolated defect (Fig. 43-23). The incidence of isolated epispadias is 1 in 100,000 live births. The repair of this lesion is moderately difficult. The more severe degrees of epispadias usually are associated with urinary incontinence and are more common than those associated with continence. In incontinent cases, the bladder neck must be reconstructed. Children with epispadias tend to have a relatively short phallus and, although attempts at lengthening the phallus are somewhat helpful, this aspect of the problem sometimes defies correction.

URETHRAL DUPLICATION

Urethral duplication is an uncommon anomaly that can present either as a partial or complete duplication. The more ventral urethra usually is the functional urethra, and the dorsal urethra often is stenotic and unusable.[107] Repair of these anomalies must be tailored to the individual situation.

AMBIGUOUS GENITALIA

Ambiguity of the external genitalia is a quandary encountered with some regularity in the newborn nursery (see Chap. 41). These patients often pose difficult diagnostic and therapeutic challenges. It is

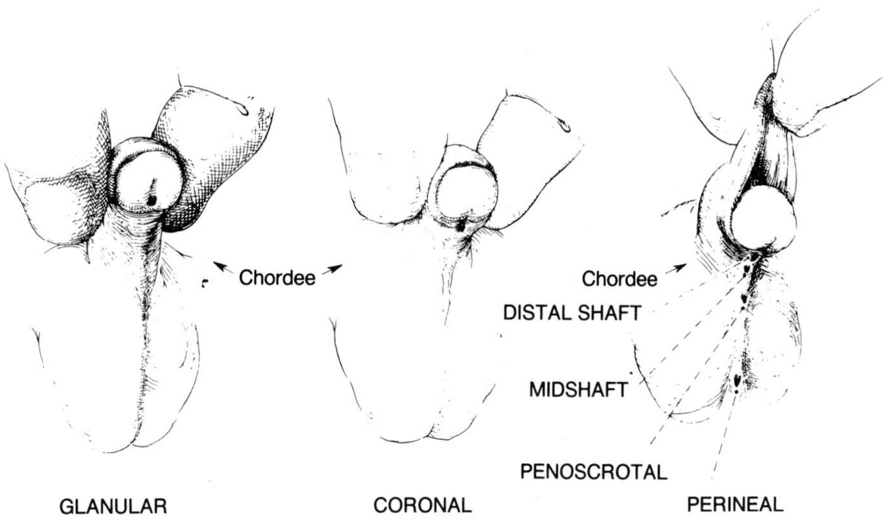

FIG. 43–22. Classification of hypospadias is based on anatomic location of the urethral meatus. The associated chordee is best described in terms of its severity (mild, moderate, or severe). (From Kelalis PP, King LR, Belman AB, eds. Clinical pediatric urology. vol. 1. Philadelphia: WB Saunders, 1976:577.)

important to establish a diagnosis rapidly. On physical examination, the presence or absence of palpable gonads is very helpful. If a gonad is palpably present, it almost certainly is a testis. Hence, bilaterally palpable gonads suggest very strongly that the patient is a genetic male. If a gonad is palpable only unilaterally, there probably is a testis on that side. There could conceivably be a normal testis, a streak, or an ovary on the other side. If no testes are palpable, the patient could be an XX female, an XY male with abdominal testes and mixed gonadal dysgenesis, or a true hermaphrodite.

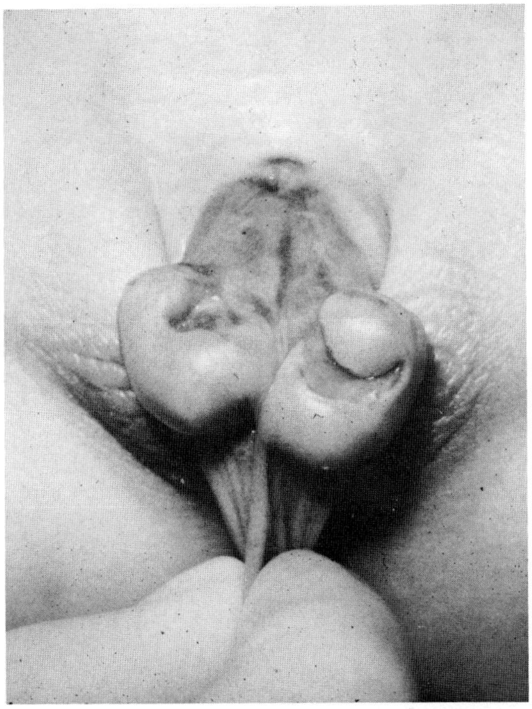

FIG. 43–23. Isolated epispadias without exstrophy. The bladder neck is intact in this child, who has good but not excellent urinary continence. Note also the incomplete duplication of glans.

Chromosomal gender is established by karyotype. An XY male who is undervirilized could have Klinefelter syndrome, true hermaphroditism, 5α-reductase deficiency, hypopituitarism, 17-hydroxylase deficiency, or 3β-O6 deficiency.

If the patient is an XX female, ambiguity could be produced by excessive maternal androgens or the adrenogenital syndrome, which is most commonly caused by a 21-hydroxylase deficiency. This latter must be considered in any patient with nonpalpable gonads if the genitalia appear masculinized, to avoid an Addisonian crisis in a patient with a salt-losing adrenogenital syndrome (Fig. 43-24).

Gender assignment (*i.e.*, gender of rearing) should be accomplished with some dispatch, to avoid excessive parental anxiety; however, assignment should not be made in a cavalier manner. Anxiety produced by indecision over gender assignment is exponentially increased by changes in gender assignment. The elements that should be considered are potential fertility, capacity for sexual function, and the possibility for satisfactory reconstruction. This last factor mandates, in my opinion, that an experienced surgeon participate in the decision regarding gender of rearing.

DEVELOPMENT OF THE PREPUCE AND CIRCUMCISION

The prepuce forms as a roll of epithelium that fuses ventrally at the frenulum. If there is failure of urethral development, this will interfere with development of the prepuce so that abnormalities of the prepuce are very suggestive of other penile abnormalities (*e.g.*, hypospadias, chordee, epispadias). Once the prepuce has covered the glans, its inner epithelial surface fuses with the epithelium of the glans and does

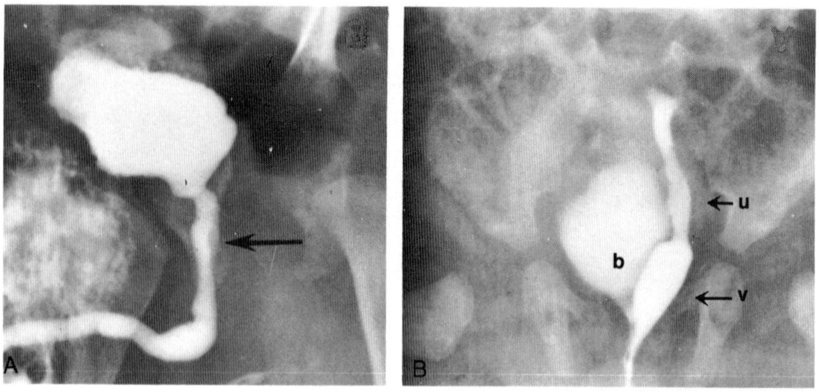

FIG. 43–24. Voiding cystourethrogram in a genetic girl who was totally masculinized by adrenal hyperplasia. **(A)** Utriculus masculinus (*arrow*), as would normally be expected in a male. **(B)** Retrograde vaginohistogram reveals a normal vagina (v) and uterus (u), as well as an overflow of contrast into the urinary bladder (b).

not separate from it until some time in childhood.[108] It is unusual for a male to have a completely retractable foreskin at birth. In the process of separation of the inner epithelial layer from the glans, cystic spaces form between the two layers and are sometimes filled with desquamated epithelial cells that form white, pearl-like beads that can be seen through the overlying skin. These areas resemble sebaceous cysts and occasionally become inflamed or infected.

Because circumcision is so common in the United States, the natural history of preputial development has been lost and one must depend upon observations made in countries where circumcision usually is not practiced. The foreskin in the newborn normally is not retractable. In a large series from Denmark, the foreskin was not completely retractable in most boys until puberty.[109] Phimosis is defined as the inability to retract the foreskin. In early childhood, this is the normal physiologic state. Although by definition this may be phimosis, there is every anticipation that the child will develop normally and will not have problems as a result of the temporary inability to retract the foreskin. Forcible retraction of the prepuce tends to produce tears in the preputial orifice, with resulting scarring that may lead to pathologic phimosis.

Circumcision is performed for a multitude of reasons. Medically, it is true that carcinoma of the penis, pathologic phimosis, paraphimosis, some sexually transmitted diseases, and some urinary infections in infancy may be prevented by circumcision.[110] If the overall population is considered from a public health and economic basis, however, the advantages to the

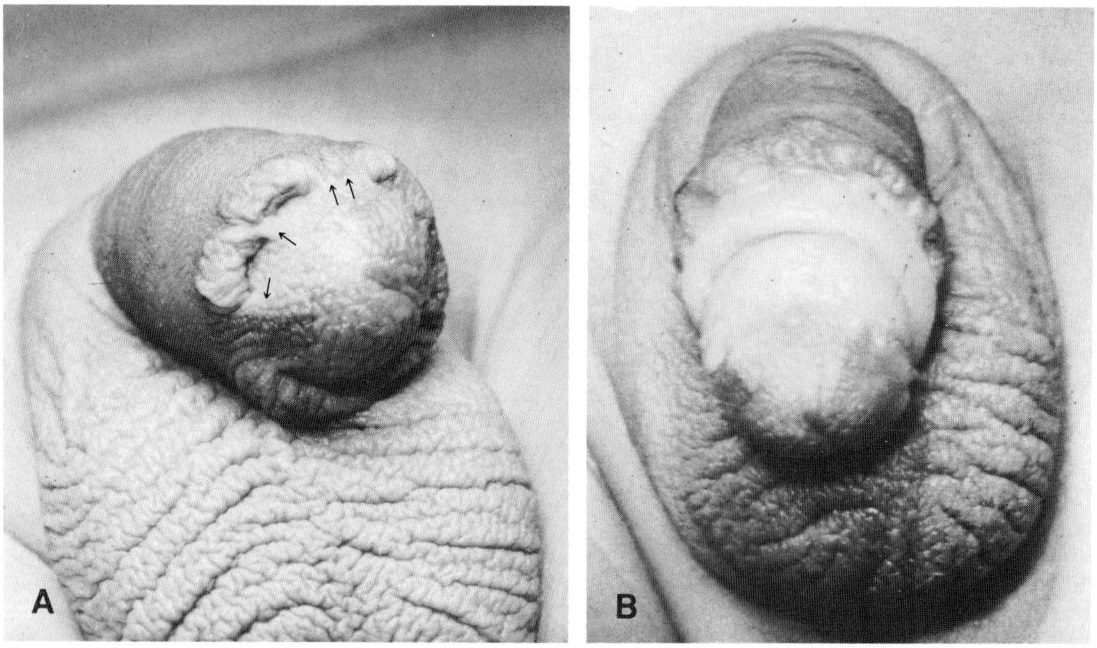

FIG. 43–25. Adhesions (*arrows*) between the distal foreskin and glans penis **(A)** before and **(B)** after surgical transection.

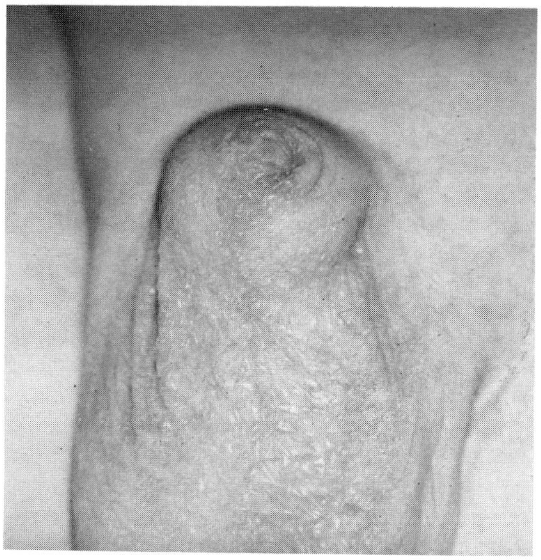

FIG. 43–26. In this patient with circumcision injury, excessive skin of the shaft healed over the retracted glans, obscuring the glans. The appearance is that of amputation of the glans. (From Belman AB. The penis. Urol Clin North Am 1978;5:17.)

individual patient may perhaps be mitigated by the cost of circumcising the entire male population to prevent problems in a minority.

At times, the benefits of circumcision are offset by the complications that may arise from this surgical procedure, because complications occur after circumcision just as after any surgical procedure.[111] The most common complications seen are hemorrhage and wound infection. Both of these usually prove to be easily treated, minor annoyances. Serious complications do occur rarely. These include sepsis, amputation of part of the glans, loss of the entire penis, urethrocutaneous fistulas, bands of scar between the shaft and the glans (Fig. 43-25), denudation of the skin of the entire shaft of the penis, recurrent phimosis (Fig. 43-26), and urethral fistulas (Fig. 43-27).[112] At times, parents are very unhappy with the cosmetic appearance of the penis if an inadequate amount of skin has been excised, even though the functional result is good.

TESTICULAR TORSION

Torsion of the testis in the newborn usually presents as a firm, slightly enlarged testis. There rarely is much abnormality of the overlying skin. Neonatal torsion seems to be painless, and actually may be an antenatal event.[113] Exploration of the testis that has undergone torsion in the newborn period probably is of extremely limited value because it is too late for testicular salvage.[114] Ten percent of neonatal torsions are bilateral; some are asynchronous, and some are of the intravaginal rather than the extravaginal type. Therefore, contralateral exploration when the infant is stable may prevent contralateral torsion.[115]

TESTICULAR TUMORS

Tumors of the testis occasionally present at birth or in early infancy.[116] Teratomas of the testis are benign and are treated by excision. On some occasions, this can be excision of the tumor only, leaving the remainder of the testis *in situ*. On other occasions, because the entire testis has been destroyed, orchiectomy is necessary. The most common type of tumor presenting in the newborn testis is one of the gonadal stromal tumors[117]; Sertoli cell tumors are the most common of these. Although these tumors histologically may appear malignant, in infancy they invariably exhibit a benign behavior, and, for this reason, orchiectomy is curative. This is in contradistinction to gonadal stromal tumors appearing in later childhood, where malignant behavior has been documented.

Yolk sac tumors, which are malignant tumors of the testis, do present in infancy and rarely present at birth. These tumors are best treated by radical orchiectomy. As long as there is no evidence of metastatic

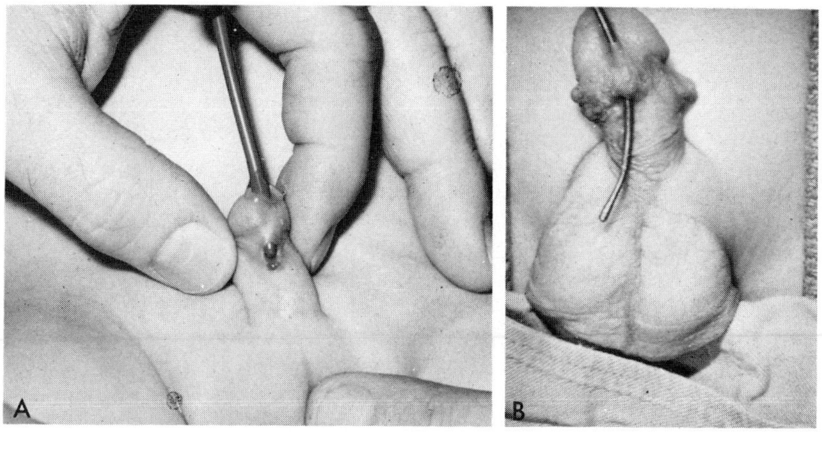

FIG. 43–27. Two examples of circumcision injuries with secondary coronal fistulas. (From Belman AB. The penis. Urol Clin North Am 1978;5:17.)

disease, adjunctive chemotherapy, node dissection, or radiation therapy are thought to be unwarranted.[118]

URINARY TRACT INFECTION

Infancy is one period of life at which there is reversal in the gender incidence of bacteriuria. The overall incidence of neonatal urinary tract infections is somewhere between 1.5 to 5 cases per 1000 live births. The male–female ratio is somewhere between 3:1 and 5:1,[119] whereas later in childhood and until later adult life, there is a female preponderance of patients with urinary infections. It has been documented that uncircumcised males are ten times more likely to have urinary infections than are circumcised males.[120] The incidence of urinary infection in uncircumcised males approximates 1 per 100. At times, the source of the urinary infection is hematogenous rather than ascending.[121]

It is imperative that there be radiographic evaluation of any newborn with culture documented bacteriuria. Vesicoureteral reflux is present in approximately one half of those evaluated, and obstructive uropathy is not an unusual finding.[122] Therefore, at a minimum, the avoidance of cystourethrography and ultrasonography is indicated.

UROLOGIC ASPECTS OF MYELODYSPLASIA

Almost any child with myelodysplasia will have involvement of the urinary tract. This may be of little consequence in the newborn period, but it is essential that the patient be appropriately evaluated shortly after birth, and that a surveillance program be instituted. It was thought that hydronephrosis was found at birth in roughly 10% of children with myelodysplasia, but studies have suggested that the hydronephrosis formerly detected actually was a result of spinal shock after closure of the neurologic lesion, and in many children resolved spontaneously.[123] Although manual expression of the bladder has been used to empty the bladders of children with myelodysplasia, it is not recommended because the intravesical pressures that are produced can be quite high and this can lead to upper tract deterioration, especially in patients with associated vesicoureteral reflux.[124] Intermittent catheterization can be used successfully in both male and female infants if needed, and, where these procedures are not successful or acceptable and bladder emptying is thought to be necessary, temporary cutaneous vesicostomy is a proven management modality.[125] Children with myelodysplasia, if at all possible, should be managed by a multidisciplinary team that includes neurosurgeons, urologists, and orthopaedic surgeons. With this approach, these children have an excellent chance of survival and development as productive citizens in modern society.

PRUNE-BELLY SYNDROME

This lesion is a spectrum of abnormalities characterized by the triad of abdominal wall deficiency, hydronephrosis, and cryptorchidism. It is the abdominal wall defect that gives the characteristic appearance leading to its name. The incidence of this lesion has been estimated to be 1 per 50,000 live births.[126] Males are affected ten times more frequently than females.[127] There is no clear-cut evidence that this is an inherited disorder. Theories of embryogenesis include obstructive uropathy and mesenchymal dysplasia.[128]

There can be massive hydroureteronephrosis and the bladder often is very dilated. There is prostatic hypoplasia with dilation of the prostatic urethra; thus, antenatal studies may not differentiate these patients from boys with posterior urethral valves.

The kidneys often are dysplastic, and it is the renal dysplasia that will determine prognosis.[129] Although some affected children die in infancy, many today will survive. Reconstruction of the urinary tract, orchiopexy, and repair of the abdominal wall defect often are helpful in altering the outlook for these children.[130]

UROLOGIC IMPLICATIONS OF IMPERFORATE ANUS

Because of the intimate relationships of the lower urinary and gastrointestinal tract in their respective development, it is not at all surprising that the urinary tract will be affected in a high proportion of children with imperforate anus; the higher the lesion, the greater the chance of urinary involvement.[131] It is for this reason that all newborns with imperforate anus should, in my opinion, be screened for urinary tract abnormalities. There often are other associated anomalies, and the constellation has come to be known as the VACTERRL association. This acronym stands for Vertebral, Anorectal, Cardiac, Tracheoesophageal, Renal, Radial, and Limb. When two elements are present, the others should be sought, because three elements qualify as the association. This is a nongenetic, sporadically occurring lesion.

ACKNOWLEDGMENT

I thank A. Barry Belman M.D., M.S. for his generosity in allowing the republication of illustrations from his chapter in the third edition of this book.

REFERENCES

1. Townsend RR, Manlo-Johnson M. Prenatal diagnosis of urinary tract abnormalities with ultrasound: a review. Scand J Urol Nephrol [Suppl] 1991;138:13.

2. Mackie GG, Stephens FD. Duplex kidneys: a correlation of renal dysplasia with position of the ureteral orifice. J Urol 1979;114:274.
3. Potter EL. Normal and abnormal development of the kidney. Chicago: Year Book, 1972:86.
4. Brenner B, Meyer TW, Hostetter TH. Dietary protein intake and the progressive nature of kidney disease: role of hemodynamically mediated glomerular injury in the pathogenesis of progressive glomerular sclerosis in aging, renal ablation and intrinsic renal disease. N Engl J Med 1983;307:652.
5. Emanuel B, Nachman R, Aronson N, et al. Congenital solitary kidney: a review of 74 cases. Am J Dis Child 1974;127:17.
6. McGee MD, Lucey DT, Fried FA. A new embryologic classification for urogynecological malformations: the syndrome of mesonephric duct induced müllerian deformities. J Urol 1979;121:265.
7. Cook WA, Stephens FD. Fused kidneys: morphologic study and theory of embryogenesis. In: Bergsma D, Duckett JW, eds. Urinary system malformations in children. Birth Defects: Original Article Series. New York: March of Dimes, 1977: 327.
8. Belman AB, King LR. Urinary tract abnormalities associated with imperforate anus. J Urol 1972;108:823.
9. Burke EC, Wenzel JE, Utz DC. The intrathoracic kidney: report of a case. Am J Dis Child 1967;113:487.
10. Kelalis PP, Malek RS, Segura JW. Observations on renal ectopia and fusion in children. J Urol 1973;110:588.
11. Leduc B, Van Campenhout J, Simaro R. Congenital absence of the vagina: observations on 25 cases. Am J Obstet Gynecol 1968;100:512.
12. Elli F, Stalder G. Malformations of kidney and urinary tract in common chromosomal aberrations. Hum Genet 1973;18:1.
13. McDonald JH, McClellan DS. Crossed renal ectopia. Am J Urol 1957;93:995.
14. N'Guessan G, Stephens FD. Supernumerary kidney. J Urol 1983;130:649.
15. Osathanondh V, Potter EL. Pathogenesis of polycystic kidneys: type I due to hyperplasia of interstitial portions of collecting tubules. Arch Pathol 1964;77:466.
16. Blythe H, Ockenden BG. Polycystic disease of kidneys and liver presenting in childhood. J Med Genet 1971;8:257.
17. Osathanondh V, Potter EL. Pathogenesis of polycystic kidneys: type 3 due to multiple abnormalities of development. Arch Pathol 1964;77:485.
18. Stapleton FB, Johnson DL, Kaplan GW, et al. The cystic renal lesion in tuberous sclerosis. J Pediatr 1980;97:574.
19. Spence HM, Baird SS, Ware EW Jr. Cystic disorders of the kidney: classification, diagnosis, treatment. JAMA 1957; 163:1466.
20. Campbell MF. Embryology and anomalies of the urogenital tract. In: Clinical pediatric urology. Philadelphia: WB Saunders, 1951:198.
21. Ambrose SS, Nicholson WP. Ureteral reflux into duplicated ureters. J Urol 1964;92:439.
22. Stephens FD, Lenaghan D. The anatomical basis and dynamics of vesicoureteral reflux. J Urol 1962;87:669.
23. Stephens FD. Caecoureterocele and concepts of the embryology and aetiology of ureteroceles. Aust N Z J Surg 1971; 40:239.
24. Chwalla R. The process of formation of cystic dictations of the vesical end of the ureter and of diverticula at the ureteral ostium. Urologic Cutaneous Review 1927;31:499.
25. Johnston JH. The pathogenesis of hydronephrosis in children. Br J Urol 1969;41:724.
26. McLaughlin AP III, Pfister RC, Leadbetter WF, et al. Pathophysiology of primary megaureter. J Urol 1973;109:805.
27. Osathanondh V, Potter EL. Pathogenesis of polycystic kidneys: type 2 due to inhibition of ampullary activity. Arch Pathol 1964;77:459.
28. Glenn JF. Agenesis of the bladder. JAMA 1959;169:2016.
29. Williams DI. The development of the trigone of the bladder. Br J Urol 1951;23:123.
30. Bauer SB, Retik AB. Urachal and related umbilical disorders. Urol Clin North Am 1978;5:195.
31. Satler EJ, Mossman HW. A case of double bladder and double urethra in the female child. J Urol 1968;79:274.
32. Stephens FD. Congenital malformations of the urinary tract. New York: Praeger, 1983.
33. Das S, Amar AD. Extravesical ureteral ectopia in male patients. J Urol 1981;125:842.
34. Brock WA, Kaplan GW. Voiding dysfunction in children. Curr Probl Pediatr 1980;10.
35. Weiss JP, Duckett JW, Snyder HM. Single unilateral vaginal ectopic ureter: is it really a rarity? J Urol 1984;132:1177.
36. Brock WA, Kaplan GW. Ectopic ureteroceles in children. J Urol 1978;119:800.
37. Mandel J, Colodny AH, Lebowitz R, et al. Ureteroceles in infants and children. J Urol 1980;123:921.
38. Snyder HM, Johnston JH. Orthotopic ureteroceles in children. J Urol 1978;119:543.
39. Scherz HC, Kaplan GW, Packer MG, et al. Ectopic ureteroceles: surgical management with preservation of continence: review of 60 cases. J Urol 1989;142:538.
40. Somner TE, Crowe JE, Resnick MI. Diagnosis of ectopic ureterocele using ultrasound. Urology 1980;15:82.
41. White JM, Kaplan GW, Brock WA. Ureteropelvic junction obstruction in children. Am Fam Physician 1984;29:211.
42. Koff SA, Thrall JH, Keyes JW Jr. Assessment of hydroureteronephrosis in children using diuretic radionuclide urographs. J Urol 1980;132:531.
43. Whitaker RH. Methods of assessing obstruction in the dilated ureter. Br J Urol 1973;45:15.
44. Johnston JH. Reconstructive surgery of megaureter in childhood. Br J Urol 1967;39:17.
45. Dwoskin JY. Sibling uropathology. J Urol 1976;115:726.
46. Paquin AJ. Ureterovesical anastomosis: the description and evaluation of a technique. J Urol 1954;82:573.
47. Baker R, Maxted W, Maylith J, et al. Relation of age, sex, and infection to reflux: data indicating high spontaneous cure rate in pediatric patients. J Urol 1966;95:27.
48. Levitt SA, Duckett J. Spitzer A, et al. Medical versus surgical treatment of primary vesicoureteral reflux: report of the International Reflux Study Committee. Pediatrics 1981;67: 392.
49. Dwoskin JY, Perlmutter AD. Vesicoureteral reflux in children: a computerized review. J Urol 1973;109:888.
50. Jeffs RD. Exstrophy and cloacal exstrophy. Urol Clin North Am 1978;5:127.
51. Scherz HC, Kaplan GW, Sutherland DH, et al. Fascia lata and early spica casting as adjuncts in closure of bladder exstrophy. J Urol 1990;144:550.
52. Eraklis A, Folkman J. Adenocarcinoma at the site of ureterosigmoidostomies for exstrophy of the bladder. J Pediatr Surg 1978;13:730.
53. McIntosh JF, Worley G Jr. Adenocarcinoma arising in exstrophy of the bladder: report of two cases and review of the literature. J Urol 1955;73:820.
54. Johnston JH, Penn IA. Exstrophy of the cloaca. Br J Urol 1966;38:302.
55. Tank ES, Lindenauer SM. Principles of management of exstrophy of the cloaca. Am J Surg 1970;119:95.
56. Waffarn F, Devasker UP, Hodgman JE. Vesico-umbilical fis-

tula: a complication of umbilical artery cutdown. J Pediatr Surg 1980;15:211.
57. Walden TB, Karafin L, Kendall AR. Urachal diverticulum in a 3 year old boy. J Urol 1979;122:554.
58. Bambirra EA, Miranda D. Gastric polyp of the umbilicus in an 8 year old boy. Clin Pediatr 1980;19:430.
59. Berdon WE, Baker DH, Becker JA, et al. Megacystis—microcolon intestinal hypoperistalsis syndrome: a new cause of intestinal obstruction: report of radiologic findings in five newborn girls. AJR 1976;126:957.
60. Ochoa B, Curlin RJ. Urofacial (Ochoa) syndrome. Am J Med Genet 1987;27:661.
61. Robertston WB, Hayes JA. Congenital diaphragmatic obstruction of the male posterior urethra. Br J Urol 1969;41:592.
62. Rattner WH, Meyer R, Bernstein J. Congenital abnormalities of the urinary system: IV. Valvular obstruction of the posterior urethra. J Pediatr 1963;63:94.
63. Osathanondh V, Potter EG. Pathogenesis of polycystic kidneys: type 4 due to urethral obstruction. Arch Pathol 1964;77:502.
64. Javadpour N, Graziano MF, Terrill R. Experimental induction of patent allantoic duct by intrauterine bladder outlet obstruction. J Surg Res 1974;17:341.
65. Tanagho EA. Surgically induced partial urinary obstruction in the fetal lamb: II. Urethral obstruction. Invest Urol 1972;10:25.
66. Johnston JH. Vesicoureteral reflux with urethral valves. Br J Urol 1979;51:100.
67. Maizels M, Simpson SB Jr. Primitive ducts of renal dysplasia induced by cultured ureteral buds and condensed renal mesenchyme. Science 1983;219:509.
68. Cass AS, Stephens FD. Posterior urethral valves: diagnosis and management. J Urol 1974;112:519.
69. Sheldon CH, Gonzales R, Bauer MS, et al. Obstructive uropathy, renal failure, and sepsis in the neonate: a surgical emergency. Urology 1980;16:457.
70. Egami K, Smith ED. A study of the sequelae of posterior urethral valves. J Urol 1982;127:84.
71. Scott TW. Urinary ascites secondary to posterior urethral valves. J Urol 1976;116:87.
72. Tank ES, Carey TC, Seifert NL. Management of neonatal urinary ascites. Urology 1980;16:270.
73. Weller MH, Miller KE. Unusual aspects of urine ascites. Radiology 1973;129:665.
74. Parker RM. Neonatal urinary ascites: a potentially favorable sign in bladder outlet obstruction. Urology 1974;3:589.
75. Johnston JH. Vesicoureteral reflux with urethral valves. Br J Urol 1979;51:100.
76. Johnston JH, Kulatilake AE. The sequelae of posterior urethral valves. Br J Urol 1971;43:743.
77. Mayor G, Genton N, Tobrado A, et al. Renal function in obstructive uropathy: long-term effect of reconstructive surgery. Pediatrics 1975;56:740.
78. Howell CG, Othersen HB Jr, Kiviat NE, et al. Therapy and outcome in 51 children with mesoblastic nephroma: a report of the National Wilms' Tumor Study. J Pediatr Surg 1982; 6:826.
79. Machin GA. Persistent renal blastema (nephroblastomatosis) as a frequent precursor of Wilms' tumor: a pathological and clinical review: 2. significance of nephroblastomatosis in the genesis of Wilms' tumor. Am J Pediatr Hematol Oncol 1980;2:253.
80. Gonzalez-Cirraso F, Kidd JM, Hernandez RJ. Cystic nephroma: morphologic spectrum and implications. Urology 1982;20:88.
81. Ganguly A, Gribble J, Tune B, et al. Renin-secreting Wilms' tumor with severe hypertension: report of a case and brief review of renin-secreting tumors. Ann Intern Med 1973; 79:835.
82. Joshi VV, Banarsee AK, Yadak K, et al. Cystic partially differentiated nephroblastoma: a clinicopathologic entity in the spectrum of infantile renal neoplasia. Cancer 1977;40:789.
83. Belman AB, King LR. The pathology and treatment of renal vein thrombosis in the newborn. J Urol 1972;107:852.
84. Khuri FJ, Alton DJ, Hardy BE, et al. Adrenal hemorrhage in neonates: report of 5 cases and review of the literature. J Urol 1980;124:684.
85. Levin S, Collins D, Kaplan GW, et al. Neonatal adrenal pseudocyst mimicking metastatic disease. Ann Surg 1974; 174:186.
86. Blane CE, Koff SA, Bowerman RA, et al. Non-obstructive fetal hydronephrosis: sonographic recognition and therapeutic implications. Radiology 1983;147:95.
87. Elder JS, Duckett JW Jr, Snyder HM. Intervention for fetal obstructive uropathy: has it been effective? Lancet 1987;2: 1007.
88. Manning FA, Harrison MR, Rodeck C, et al. Catheter shunts for fetal hydronephrosis: report of the International Fetal Surgery Registry. N Engl J Med 1985;315:336.
89. Murphy JL, Kaplan GW, Packer MG, et al. Prenatal diagnosis of severe urinary tract anomalies improves renal function and growth. Child Nephrol Urol 1988–89;9:290.
90. Montana MA, Cyr DR, Lenke RR, et al. Sonographic detection of fetal ureteral obstruction. AJR 1985;145:595.
91. Glick PL, Harrison MR, Golbus MS, et al. Management of the fetus with congenital hydronephrosis: II. Prognostic criteria and selection for treatment. J Pediatr Surg 1985;20:376.
92. Sherwood DW, Smith RC, Lemmon RH, et al. Abnormalities of the genitourinary tract discovered by palpation of the abdomen of the newborn. Pediatrics 1956;18:782.
93. Wedge JJ, Grosfeld JL, Smith JP. Abdominal masses in the newborn: 63 cases. J Urol 1971;106:770.
94. Raffensberger J, Abdusleiman A. Abdominal masses in children under one year of age. Surgery 1968;63:514.
95. Melicow MM, Uson AC. Palpable abdominal masses in infants and children: a report based on a review of 653 cases. J Urol 1959;81:705.
96. Emanuel B, Nachman R, Aronson N, et al. Congenital solitary kidney. Am J Dis Child 1974;127:17.
97. Scorer CG. The descent of the testicle. Arch Dis Child 1964;39:605.
98. Scorer CG, Farrington GH. Congenital deformities of the testis and epididymis. London: Butterworths, 1971.
99. Kogan JJ, Tennenbaum SY, Gill B, et al. Efficacy of orchiopexy by patient age 1 year for cryptorchidism. J Urol 1990;144: 508.
100. Kessler WO, McLaughlin AP. Agenesis of the penis: embryology and management. Urology 1973;1:226.
101. Rodriguez C. Report of a case of diphallus. J Urol 1965;94:436.
102. Lee PA, Mazur T, Danish R, et al. Micropenis: criteria, etiologies, and classification. Johns Hopkins Medical Journal 1980;146:156.
103. Burstein S, Grumbach MM, Kaplan SL. Early determination of androgen responsiveness is important in the management of microphallus. Lancet 1979;2:983.
104. Money J, Potter R, Stall CS. Sex reannouncement in hereditary sex deformity: psychology and sociology of habilitation. Soc Sci Med 1969;3:207.
105. Bauer SB, Retik AB, Colodny AH. Genetic aspects of hypospadias. Urol Clin North Am 1981;8:559.
106. Cerasaro TS, Brock WA, Kaplan GW. Upper urinary tract

anomalies associated with congenital hypospadias: is screening necessary? J Urol 1986;135:537.
107. Williams DI, Kenawi MM. Urethral duplications in the male. Eur Urol 1975;1:209.
108. Gairdner D. The fate of the foreskin: a study of circumcision. Br Med J 1949;2:1433.
109. Oster J. Further fate of the foreskin. Arch Dis Child 1968; 43:200.
110. Wiswell TE. Routine neonatal circumcision: a reappraisal. Am Fam Physician 1990;41:859.
111. MacDonald MG. Circumcision. In: Fletcher MA, MacDonald MG, eds. Atlas of procedures in neonatology. 2nd ed. Philadelphia: JB Lippincott, 1993:378.
112. Kaplan GW. Complications of circumcision. Urol Clin North Am 1983;10:543.
113. Burge DM. Neonatal testicular torsion and infarction: etiology and management. Br J Urol 1987;59:70.
114. Jerkins GR, Noe HN, Hollabauch RS, et al. Spermatic cord torsion in the neonate. J Urol 1983;129:121.
115. Kaplan GW, Silber I. Neonatal torsion: to pex or not? In: King LR, ed. Neonatal problems in urology. Philadelphia: JB Lippincott, 1988:386.
116. Kaplan GW. Prepubertal testicular tumors. World J Urol 1984;2:238.
117. Kaplan GW, Chromie WJ, Kelalis PP, et al. Gonadal stromal tumors: a report of the Prepubertal Testicular Tumor Registry. J Urol 1986;136:300.
118. Kaplan GW, Chromie WJ, Kelalis PP, et al. Prepubertal yolk sac testicular tumors: report of the Testicular Tumor Registry. J Urol 1988;140:1109.
119. Drew JH, Acton CK. Radiologic findings in newborn infants with urinary infection. Arch Dis Child 1976;51:628.
120. Wiswell TE, Smith FR, Bass JW. Decreased incidence of urinary tract infections in circumcised male infants. Pediatrics 1985;75:401.
121. Stamey TA. Urinary infections. Baltimore: Williams & Wilkins, 1972.
122. Bergstrom T, Larson H, Lincoln K, et al. Studies of urinary tract infections in infancy and childhood: XII. Eighty consecutive patients with neonatal infection. J Pediatr 1972;80: 858.
123. Chiaramonte RM, Horowitz EM, Kaplan GW, et al. Implications of hydronephrosis in the newborn with myelodysplasia. J Urol 1986;136:147.
124. Barbalias GA, Klauber GT, Blaivas JG. Critical evaluation of the Credé maneuver: a urodynamic study of 207 patients. J Urol 1983;130:720.
125. Cohen JS, Harbach LS, Kaplan GW. Cutaneous vesicostomy for temporary diversion in infants with neurogenic bladder dysfunction. J Urol 1978;119:120.
126. Garlinger P, Ott J. Prune belly syndrome: possible genetic implications. Birth Defects 1974;10:173.
127. Rabinowitz R, Schillinger JF. Prune belly syndrome in the female subject. J Urol 1977;118:454.
128. Silverman FM, Huang N. Congenital absence of the abdominal muscle associated with malformation of the genitourinary and alimentary tracts: report of cases and review of literature. Am J Dis Child 1950;80:9.
129. Williams DI, Parker RM. The role of surgery in the prune belly syndrome. In: Johnston JH, Goodwin WF, eds. Review of pediatric urology. Amsterdam: Excerpta Medica, 1974:315.
130. Woodard JR, Parrott TS. Reconstruction of the urinary tract in prune belly syndrome. J Urol 1978;119:824.
131. Fleisher MH, McLorie GA, Churchhill BM, et al. The yield of investigation of the urinary tract in imperforate anus. J Urol 1985;133:142.

Neonatology: Pathophysiology and Management of the Newborn, Fourth Edition,
edited by Gordon B. Avery, Mary Ann Fletcher, and Mhairi G. MacDonald.
J.B. Lippincott Company, Philadelphia © 1994.

chapter 44

General Surgery

PHILIP C. GUZZETTA
KATHRYN D. ANDERSON
MARTIN R. EICHELBERGER
KURT D. NEWMAN
THOMAS M. ROUSE
JAY J. SCHNITZER
MICHAEL BOYAJIAN
SHARON M. TOMASKI

Cooperation between the neonatologist and the pediatric surgeon is essential to the success of any major neonatal surgical procedure. Together they can assure comprehensive care throughout the preoperative and postoperative phase. In the immediate postoperative period, the regulation of parenteral fluid and electrolytes, antibiotics, and other supportive drugs is best directed by the surgeon. For respiratory support and for the special metabolic considerations in the premature, optimal care is provided when the neonatologist and surgeon work in close cooperation.

When an infant is being prepared for an operation, a fasting period of 6 hours is adequate to ensure an empty stomach. For longer periods without oral fluids, maintenance intravenous fluids should be started. Fluid administration during major surgery requires an intravenous catheter of adequate size. In babies weighing more than 1000 g, a 22-gauge catheter can usually be placed percutaneously. Central venous pressure lines can be placed percutaneously or by cutdown. Arterial lines are preferentially placed in the right radial artery to reflect preductal arterial blood gases, but if an umbilical artery line is in place when the child goes to surgery, that line is usually maintained to monitor arterial blood gases.

Severe hypothermia is a significant problem in the premature infant undergoing a lengthy operation. A heat-conserving covering of the extremities and head is helpful in maintaining the neonate's temperature, as is using surface-warming lights, a heating blanket, and draping materials that are impervious to fluids. The anesthesiologist can prevent hypothermia by warming the blood that is to be transfused and by warming and humidifying the inhaled gas mixture. The infant's temperature is constantly monitored by the anesthesiologist by means of a rectal or esophageal temperature probe. The surgical team must strive for maximal efficiency, especially when the bowel or thoracic contents are exposed. Irrigating solutions should be warmed to body temperature. Cold stress is a potentially lethal problem in neonatal surgery, and the importance of maintaining the infant's thermal environment near normal cannot be overemphasized.[1]

Throughout the surgical procedure, blood must be replaced with precision. Sponges are weighed or carefully estimated, with the understanding that the amount of blood absorbed in one or two sponges can account for profound hypovolemia in a neonate.

Careful selection of anesthetic technique is important for preterm infants, and if feasible, regional anesthesia is preferred over general anesthesia.[2] Proper postoperative management includes adequate analgesic medication to keep the neonate comfortable and minimize the stressful physiologic responses to pain.[3]

Postoperative monitoring implies meticulous attention to fluid balance, including losses caused by creation of enterostomies. Serial measurements of the baby's weight, hematocrit, electrolytes, urine volume, and urine specific gravity serve as a guide for fluid replacement in the postoperative phase.[4]

Postoperative fluid therapy includes maintenance requirements and replacement of losses. Gastrostomy and ileostomy drainages are measured, their electrolyte content is determined, and replacement is tailored to individual needs. The infant's losses are replaced at 8-hour intervals, because the deficits incurred in 24 hours can be excessive.

The successful management of many of these fragile patients depends on strict adherence to these principles of management.

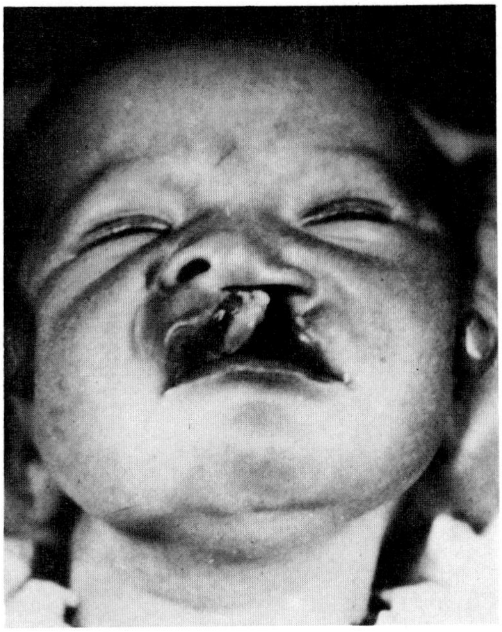

FIG. 44–1. Complete congenital cleft of the lip with associated cleft of the palate that extends forward through the alveolar ridge.

LESIONS OF THE HEAD AND NECK

Congenital abnormalities of the head and neck occur commonly in the newborn. Because of the short, fat neck of the baby, some of these lesions are not immediately apparent, and the examiner must be alert to their possibility to detect them.

CLEFT LIP

Clefts of the lip or palate occur in approximately 1 of every 600 to 700 Caucasian newborns. The frequency is doubled in Asians and halved in African Americans. Cleft lip occurs somewhat more often in male patients and on the left side. The defect probably results from lack of the mesodermal reinforcement of the junction of the nasomedial and lateral facial processes that normally takes place in the sixth to seventh week of gestation. Multiple genetic influences seem to be more important than environmental factors. The cleft deformity ranges from minor notching to complete separation of the entire lip and nasal floor (Fig. 44-1). The defect may involve the lip, the lip and palate, or only the palate, and it may be unilateral or bilateral. Median cleft lip is rare and is usually associated with hypotelorism, microcephaly, and early death.

Airway obstruction is not typically a consequence of isolated cleft lip or palate. Initial care focuses on feeding the infant and counseling the parents. Swallowing and airway protection should be normal, but the negative pressure of the normal suck is vented through the cleft, resulting in inadequate inflow. Fatigue during feeding is common and may mimic satiation. Although suckling is not altogether discouraged, a baby with a complete cleft lip or any degree of cleft palate should be expected to suffer mechanical feeding difficulty. The solution may be to rely on an enlarged nipple aperture, a compressible bottle, or a syringe feeder. With the use of a positive-pressure delivery system, the feeding schedule should be normal.

Lip closure is usually carried out at around 3 months of age. The major goals are muscle continuity, balanced lip height, the normal Cupid's-bow lip shape, a smooth and pout-free lip margin, a good nasal sill, adequate sulcus lining, and a minimal, well-placed scar. The wide, complete unilateral and the complete bilateral clefts present greater challenges. Preliminary lip adhesion for the unilateral case or presurgical orthodontics can improve anatomic associations and facilitate the definitive surgery. Residual nasal deformity is often a stubborn problem and may require secondary surgery.

CLEFT PALATE

The embryologic palatal shelves initially hang vertically, and then rise to meet and fuse from front to back between weeks 7 and 12 of gestation. Interference with this process may result in complete, incomplete, or submucous cleft of the palate. Initial care is discussed in the section on cleft lip.

The major significance of this defect is the effect on speech. Normal modulation of speech requires reliable, dynamic palatal separation of the mouth from the nose. This requires a palate of adequate length, suppleness, and muscle power. Velopharyngeal incompetence or incomplete nasal closure results in hypernasal speech and significant communication disability.

Chronic or recurrent effusion and infection in an otherwise normal ear is common in the child with a cleft palate because eustachian tube function is compromised. This child usually needs myringotomies and ventilation tubes.

Early surgery seems to have a negative effect on facial growth, but the trend is toward closure during infancy because of the improved speech results. Most American surgeons choose 9 to 12 months of age as optimal timing for a single-stage closure.

Palatal closure is accomplished with local soft tissue. Mucoperiosteal flaps are mobilized and closed in the midline, with oral and nasal lining, effecting muscle apposition and retroposition. No bone reconstruction is involved. The goal is normal speech, and this is achieved in approximately 85% of patients. A second operation produces good results for almost all the remaining infants.

An essential concept in the treatment of these children is a multidisciplinary approach. The patient should be followed through adolescence by a team consisting of a plastic surgeon, otolaryngologist, audiologist, pedodontist, orthodontist, speech pathologist, geneticist, pediatrician, and social worker.

PIERRE–ROBIN SEQUENCE

The Pierre–Robin sequence is characterized by retrognathia or microgenia (*i.e.*, small or recessed jaw or chin), glossoptosis, airway obstruction, and cleft palate. The lack of forward support of the tongue allows it to fall back and compromise the airway. The basic defect may result from intrauterine restriction of mandibular growth.

Intensive monitoring, including a home apnea monitor, is necessary for many patients. The airway can usually be maintained by conservative measures. Prone positioning allows the tongue to fall forward. An appropriately apertured board may facilitate this positioning, and a nasal airway may be useful. Early gavage feedings may obviate hazardous oral feedings. A lip–tongue adhesion may be performed in more difficult cases, but its effectiveness varies. Tracheostomy should be avoided, but it is sometimes the only safe choice. Management should be as conservative as the clinical situation permits. The airway problem is typically self-limited, resolving as the child grows.

MASSES IN THE NECK

Masses in the neck are common in children and may be congenital, infectious, or neoplastic. Thyroglossal duct remnants, branchial apparatus anomalies, and lymphangiomas (*i.e.*, cystic hygromas) are the most common congenital pediatric lesions in the neck.

THYROGLOSSAL DUCT REMNANTS

Thyroid tissue left behind in an abnormal location during normal developmental descent can result in a thyroglossal duct cyst, which presents in the midline of the neck. Infection may lead to a cutaneous salivary fistula. After appropriate therapy for infection, treatment consists of resection of the cyst, the central portion of the hyoid bone, and dissection of the tract up to its origin at the foramen cecum (*i.e.*, Sistrunk operation).[5–7]

BRANCHIAL CLEFT ANOMALIES

Branchial clefts with their corresponding arches and pouches are embryologic structures that give rise to many of the components of the lower face and neck. Abnormal persistence of any portion of the branchial apparatus leads to specific anomalies about the face and neck.[8,9]

Preauricular Tabs and Sinuses. These lesions are not true branchial cleft remnants because they originate from an abnormal formation of the ear, rather than a branchial cleft component. The preauricular sinus almost always ends blindly, and excision is indicated to prevent recurrent infection in later years.

Cervical Fistulas. Fistulas that originate from the first branchial arch present in the neck just below the ear and communicate with the external auditory canal. A fistula originating from the second branchial arch is the most common branchial cleft remnant. The fistula usually extends from the skin of the lower neck upward along the sternocleidomastoid muscle and then passes inward between the internal and external carotid arteries to attach to the posterolateral pharynx just below the tonsillar fossa (Fig. 44-2). The presenting complaint is usually related to persistent or intermittent drainage onto the neck. Complete surgical extirpation is necessary for cure. A large incision in the neck can be avoided by the use of two or three small, neat, transverse stair-step incisions.

Branchial Cyst. Approximately 10% of persistent branchial deformities are cystic. These invariably arise low in the anterior triangle of the neck and present as smooth cysts anterior to the sternocleidomastoid muscle. Dissection with excision is curative.

Cervical Cutaneous Tabs. Occasionally, a baby presents with a cutaneous tab in the skin of the anterior aspect of the neck. A small, irregular mass of cartilage may be contained in the skin tab. The cartilage is never associated with a fistula, and removal of this small appendage is not urgent.

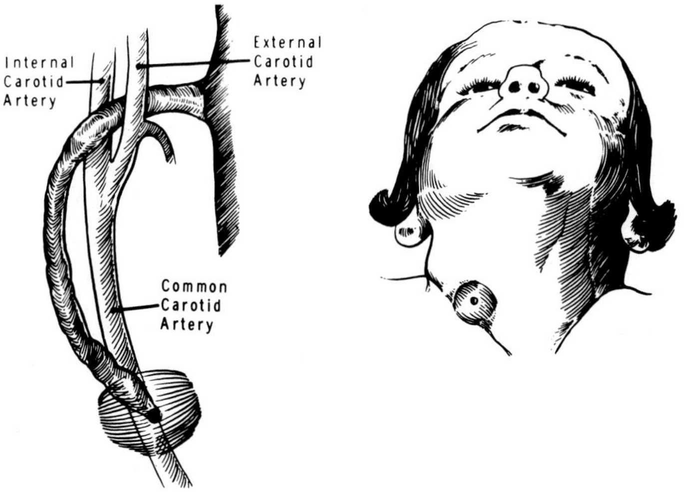

FIG. 44–2. Brachial cleft cyst, which presents low in the neck as a mass or an opening in the skin, extends upward and laterally in the neck, passing between the branches of the carotid artery to connect with the pharynx below the tonsillar facia. (From Nardi GL, Zuidema GD. Surgery. 3rd ed. Boston: Little, Brown, 1972.)

CYSTIC HYGROMA

Cystic hygroma (*i.e.*, lymphangioma) arises as a result of congenital deformity of development of lymphatic channels (Fig. 44-3).[10] About 80% of these watery cysts occur in the neck, and most are located posterior to the sternocleidomastoid muscle. Other sites of occurrence are the groin, the axilla, and the mediastinum. The term "hygroma" suggests the watery fluid contained in the endothelium-lined spaces. The cyst may be unilocular, but more often there are numerous cysts of various sizes that permeate the surrounding structures and distort the local anatomy. Supporting connective tissue often shows extensive lymphocytic infiltration. Except in the case of a single large cyst, no definite cleavage plane is found between hygroma and normal tissue.

The lesion is usually evident at birth. Occasionally, the mass occupies the entire submandibular region, distorting the subglottic area and compromising the airway. A supraclavicular mass may become prominent with the Valsalva maneuver. This form of cystic hygroma is usually associated with a mediastinal component. Some cystic hygromas contain nests of poorly supported vascular channels that are prone to bleeding and may produce sudden enlargement and discoloration of the lesion.

Symptoms are related entirely to the location and size of the mass. Disfigurement is often severe. Infection in the mass may lead to dangerous regional cellulitis, but after the infection subsides, the resultant intracystic fibrosis and scar may significantly reduce the size of the tumor mass. Prenatal ultrasonography has been used to diagnose cystic hygroma.[11] This modality has demonstrated a hidden mortality with a high incidence of associated anomalies, including abnormal karyotypes and hydrops fetalis, when lymphangiomas are detected before 30 weeks of gestation.

Repeated aspiration of the cyst with injection of sclerosing agents is not recommended, because any surgical excision that is subsequently required is rendered significantly more difficult by the sclerosing procedure. Elective surgical excision between 4 and

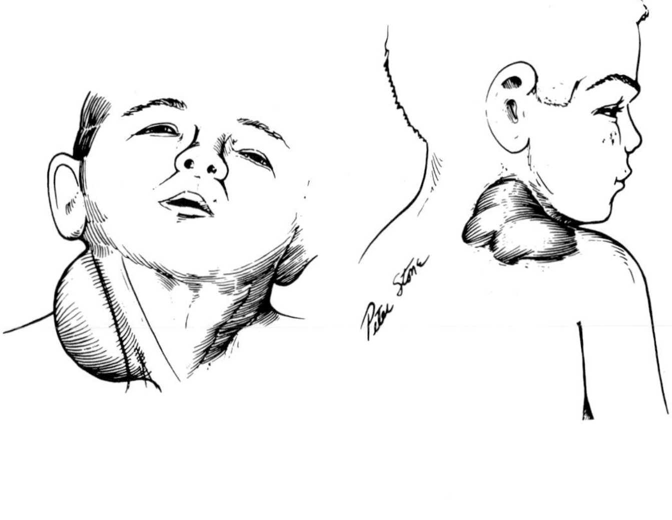

FIG. 44–3. The typical cystic hygroma occurs in the lateral neck. The mass may extend into the scapular, axillary, or thoracic compartments, or the hygroma may present separately in any of these locations. Although depicted here as a single cyst, the hygroma is often a multiloculated, ill-defined mass. (From Nardi GL, Zuidema GD. Surgery. 3rd ed. Boston: Little, Brown, 1972.)

12 months of age is indicated for asymptomatic patients. Airway compression or recurrent infections may necessitate removal at an earlier age.[12] Total excision is often impractical because of the extent of the hygroma and its proximity to vital structures. Important nerves and vascular structures must not be sacrificed in an attempt to achieve total excision of this benign lesion; multiple excisions of the residual hygroma are preferable. Postoperative wound drainage using closed-suction drains may reduce recurrence.

UPPER AIRWAY OBSTRUCTION CAUSING RESPIRATORY DISTRESS

Neonatal respiratory distress from partial obstruction in the larynx or trachea may arise suddenly and threaten the life of the infant or may be subtle, mild, or intermittent and require special techniques to define its cause. Inspiratory stridor, although an alarming symptom in the newborn, is often self-limited and requires no specific therapy. Before this reassurance can be given, however, an orderly evaluation is required to exclude mechanical causes that may present a threat to the infant.

The newborn infant has several inherent disadvantages in respiratory mechanics. The diameters of the trachea and bronchi are small, and the risk of major obstruction from a mucous plug is increased. The musculature of the chest wall is relatively weak, and coughing is less efficient than in older patients.

Most neonates are obligatory nose breathers, and patency of the nares must be established by catheter if airway obstruction is suspected. Obstruction of the upper airway may be caused by laryngomalacia, vocal cord paralysis, subglottic stenosis, laryngeal webs, or subglottic hemangioma. Diagnosis is made by direct laryngoscopy.[13]

Unilateral cord paralysis is associated with cardiac, pulmonary, or esophageal lesions. Bilateral paralysis is associated with lesions of the central nervous system. Birth trauma has been implicated in vocal cord paralysis. Laryngeal webs are rare, and the diagnosis suggested by airway compromise and a weak cry. Treatment varies with the thickness of the web. Thin webs are incised with a knife or laser, and thick webs require tracheostomy and definitive surgery at a later time.

Hemangiomas involving the vocal cords or trachea can compromise the airway. Surgical excision of these hemangiomas is often impossible. If obstructive symptoms are severe, a course of parenteral steroids is tried to accelerate involution of the vascular anomalies. Some hemangiomas may be amenable to excision with the surgical laser.

An overpenetrated chest radiograph is useful in defining the location and patency of the trachea and its major divisions. An extrinsic pressure defect or major displacement of the trachea is readily appreciated on this study. All infants with respiratory distress should have a barium swallow in the lateral projection, which demonstrates compression by vascular structures within the mediastinum (*i.e.*, vascular ring). Most symptoms of vascular entrapment of the trachea and esophagus are referable to swallowing, but the airway can be compromised and ventilation impaired. Because of the interference with swallowing, aspiration with pneumonia is commonly seen as a cause of respiratory distress in this group of infants.

NASAL OBSTRUCTION

Choanal atresia was first described by Roederer in 1755. The incidence of choanal atresia is reported to be 1 in 5000 to 7000 live births. Unilateral atresia is much more common than bilateral atresia, and the female-to-male ratio is 2:1.[14] Ninety percent of atresias are bony, and 10% are membranous.

Twenty percent to 50% of patients with choanal atresia have associated anomalies. The most common are of the CHARGE (*i.e.*, colobomata of the eyes, heart defects, renal anomaly, growth and mental retardation, ear deficits, and gastroesophageal reflux) association.[15] A genetic consultation is recommended for all patients diagnosed with choanal atresia, and a thorough search for additional anomalies should be made.

The most widely held hypothesis about the pathogenesis of choanal atresia is based on the failure of the bucconasal membrane to rupture during the seventh week of gestation.[16] Hengere and Oas postulated that misdirection of mesodermal flow due to local factors results in alteration of opening of the choana.[17]

The neonatologist should have intimate knowledge of the presenting signs and symptoms of choanal atresia. Because infants are obligate nasal breathers for the first 6 to 8 weeks of life, newborns with bilateral choanal atresia can present with immediate respiratory distress and cyanosis. This distress is relieved by crying and is known as cyclic dyspnea or cyanosis while suckling. Unilateral choanal atresia is commonly not diagnosed until the patient's nostril becomes occluded with secretions. The differential diagnosis includes congenital or traumatic deviation of the nasal septum and stuffy nose syndrome, which is usually a self-limited condition that is treated medically.

A dislocated nasal septum can occur as a result of a traumatic delivery. Radiographs are of little value in demonstrating cartilaginous injury alone. A thorough examination of the nose is needed to rule out a septal hematoma. A hematoma should be evacuated by an otolaryngologist. An uncomplicated septal dislocation can be reduced by gentle traction on the nose to effect realignment. Despite reduction of nasal fractures and cartilaginous dislocations, a subsequent nasal growth disturbance may occur. The parents should be counseled about the possibility of future rhinologic surgery.

The diagnosis and workup of choanal atresia begins in the delivery room. A catheter is passed through each nostril into the nasopharynx as part of the routine newborn physical examination. A 6-Fr (2-mm) catheter should pass into the nasopharynx in full-term infants. Care must be taken that the catheter does not coil in the anterior nares and obscure the diagnosis. If doubt persists, a firm, curved, metal dilator can be used to palpate and verify an atretic plate. At birth, the posterior aspect of the bony septum is approximately 3 cm from the nostril entrance in full-term infants.[16] A flexible nasopharyngoscope can be used to view the region. High-resolution computed tomography (CT) is the gold standard for documenting the exact location and extent of the atresia. Just before the CT scan, intranasal vasoconstriction and thorough, gentle suctioning must be performed. If this is not done, the scans will be suboptimal and perhaps misleading (*e.g.*, indicating stenosis instead of atresia). Thin-section axial and coronal CT scans should be requested.[18]

Emergent management of bilateral atresia necessitates an artificial airway. An oral anesthesia airway usually suffices, unless there are other airway anomalies. A McGovern nipple (*i.e.*, large rubber nipple with an enlarged hole) can be used in the neonatal period until oral breathing occurs. These children are not usually able to feed normally until oral breathing begins.

A pediatric otolaryngologist usually undertakes surgical correction of bilateral atresia in the neonatal period for patients who cannot be managed with conservative measures. If a unilateral atresia is not causing any respiratory embarrassment, definitive surgical correction is generally carried out before school entry to abate the chronic unilateral nasal discharge. Several techniques for correction have been described: transnasal, transpalatal, and endoscopic.[16,19] Although transpalatal is accepted as the preferred method for all age groups, concerns about possible stunting of palatal growth and subsequent orthodontic problems remain.[16] Some surgeons elect to perform an initial transnasal repair in the neonate, with a planned definitive transpalatal procedure performed when the child is larger and anatomic visualization is better. After the transnasal procedure, a stent is left in place in the nostrils for several weeks. The surgical approach is decided on an individual basis.[20]

LARYNGOMALACIA

Laryngomalacia is the most common obstructing lesion of the larynx. The lack of firm cartilaginous support permits compromise of the lumen with each inspiration. Collapse of the larynx and cervical trachea results in a characteristic stridor, which is accentuated when respiratory efforts are most vigorous, such as when the infant is crying. Although alarming, the stridor associated with laryngomalacia is usually self-limited, requiring no specific treatment. It generally resolves by 6 to 12 months of age as the cross-sectional diameter of the tracheal lumen increases and the supporting cartilage matures.

Laryngoscopy is performed so that the motions of the larynx can be observed during inspiration. This is best done with the infant awake. The flexible bronchoscope can be introduced through the infant's nose with minimal discomfort. Laryngomalacia is a diagnosis that is made only after obstructing tracheal lesions are ruled out.

Parents of infants with laryngomalacia are advised that respiratory infections, with resultant edema of the mucous lining of the larynx and trachea, may accentuate the symptoms. A humidified environment and antibiotics are key factors in therapy when these babies contract respiratory infections.

Although spontaneous resolution of laryngomalacia is the rule, some infants expend an inordinate amount of energy in the work of breathing. This caloric loss occurs at the expense of growth. Infrequently, the amount of inspiratory obstruction is so severe that cyanosis and cardiac instability result. In these rare instances, tracheostomy may be required as a life-saving procedure.

TRACHEOMALACIA

Tracheomalacia results from abnormal softness of the cartilaginous rings of the trachea and causes collapse of the intrathoracic airway during expiration. It may be localized to a few tracheal rings or involve the entire trachea. It may be congenital, with no associated anomalies. Tracheomalacia also occurs secondary to abnormalities of esophageal and aortic arch development. In cases of esophageal atresia, the dilated upper esophageal pouch compresses the adjacent tracheal cartilage during development.[21] Aortic arch anomalies, including vascular rings and an anomalous innominate artery, may result in a softening of the tracheal cartilage by compressing the fetal airway.[22]

A barking, seal-like cough is characteristic in the postoperative period. Some infants with repaired esophageal atresia have apneic episodes during feedings that may be caused by a transient distention of the upper esophagus, with compression of the trachea between the innominate artery anteriorly and the esophagus posteriorly. Rarely, infants fail extubation because, without the support of the endotracheal tube, the airway collapses during expiration. Ventilation is impaired by air trapping and overdistention of the lungs.

Standard anteroposterior and lateral radiographs may show airway narrowing. Cinefluoroscopy, with a small amount of contrast in the upper esophagus, more precisely defines the dynamic airway collapse during swallowing. Rigid laryngotracheobronchoscopy, with the infant anesthetized but spontaneously breathing, is essential for diagnosis. Under direct vision, the tracheal lumen is elliptical rather than C-shaped, and it collapses or becomes occluded with coughing or deep inspiration. The transmitted pulsation of the aortic arch may be observed anteriorly. As with laryngomalacia, most infants recover spontaneously as the tracheal wall stabilizes with growth. Children with life-threatening airway compromise due to vascular compression require aortopexy. In a procedure originally described by Gross, the aortic arch and innominate artery are elevated away from the trachea and sutured to the sternum.[22] The anterior elevation of the wall of the trachea results in a larger intratracheal lumen, but the attachments between the vascular structures and the trachea are not disturbed. Rarely, external splinting or tracheostomy is required.[23]

TRACHEOSTOMY

Acute respiratory emergencies in infants can usually be managed by temporary placement of endotracheal tubes. An endotracheal tube is surprisingly well tolerated by the infant, even for extended periods. Rarely is emergency tracheostomy necessary in the newborn period. Only if the respiratory crisis extends beyond 3 to 4 weeks is the infant considered for tracheostomy. The operation is always undertaken in the operating room. An endotracheal tube or bronchoscope is put in place so that stabilization of the delicate trachea is ensured and good control of the infant's airway is provided until the trachea can be identified and opened.

Proper placement of the tracheostomy is essential. The tracheostomy should be placed at the level of the second or third tracheal ring, avoiding the cricoid, but not so low that the tube enters the right main stem bronchus when the neck is flexed. The incision is made transversely between the second and third tracheal cartilages. Alternatively, a vertical incision may be made through two cartilages. Tracheal substance is never resected. Stay sutures are placed on the incised margins of the trachea to facilitate insertion of the tracheostomy tube and to serve as traction sutures if the tube becomes dislodged in the early postoperative period. With the development of the new Silastic tracheostomy tubes, problems relating to erosion and postoperative stenosis have been minimized.

Before tracheostomy is begun, the care team and the parents must understand that decannulization may be difficult. When tracheostomy becomes necessary in an infant, it may be many months or even years before the tube can be removed safely. Complications can be minimized if postoperative surgical care is meticulous and Silastic tubes are used.

THORACIC LESIONS CAUSING RESPIRATORY DISTRESS

CONGENITAL LOBAR EMPHYSEMA

Congenital lobar emphysema can be severe or life threatening as a result of hyperexpansion of a single lobe of the lung. Air is permitted into the involved lobe but denied egress. The lobe becomes emphysematous, resulting in compression of adjacent pulmonary parenchyma and mediastinal displacement. Symptoms may appear shortly after birth and invariably develop before 4 months of age.[24] The cause is unknown. An inherent, cartilaginous defect in the bronchus has been postulated, but the bronchial abnormality is not always recognizable in the resected specimen.

A chest radiograph is characteristic, showing hyperaeration of the involved lobe with mediastinal shift away from the affected side. The lobar distribution of the hyperaeration can be appreciated, and adjacent pulmonary parenchyma is compressed. The upper lobes are most frequently involved, but the condition may be seen in the middle lobe. Rarely, the lesion is bilateral.[25]

Treatment is surgical, and prompt thoracotomy and lobectomy are undertaken after the diagnosis is made. An infant may remain compensated for some weeks and then deteriorate rapidly from acute hyperinflation of the involved lobe. There is no place for expectant management of congenital lobar emphysema.

An identical clinical picture may be seen in the neonate who has been ventilated for a prolonged time and develops a large pneumatocele as a result of respiratory tract barotrauma. It is often difficult for the physician to determine whether respiratory distress is due to the pneumatocele or generalized pulmonary parenchymal disease. Surgical excision of the pneumatocele is indicated if the lesion is enlarging and the respiratory status is worsening without another apparent cause.

CYSTIC ADENOMATOID MALFORMATION

Cystic adenomatoid malformation (CAM) is a pulmonary maldevelopment that presents with cystic replacement of pulmonary parenchyma. If the cysts are small (*i.e.*, microcystic CAM) and constitute a small portion of one lung, the child may be asymptomatic. If the lesion is microcystic and replaces a large portion of the lung, the fetus may develop hydrops, and the prognosis is poor.[26] If the cysts are macroscopic and the child is in respiratory distress at birth, the problem may be misdiagnosed as congenital diaphragmatic hernia. Appropriate therapy for the symptomatic neonate with CAM is thoracotomy and resection of the involved lung. Postoperative support with extracorporeal membrane oxygenation (ECMO) has been necessary for infants developing severe persistent pulmonary hypertension after CAM excision.[27]

BRONCHOGENIC CYST

Bronchogenic cyst is another lung bud anomaly in which the normal bronchiole-to-bronchiole communication is absent or atretic, resulting in a mucus-producing cyst that may obstruct the trachea, bronchus, or esophagus. This seldom causes severe problems in the neonate, but it must be considered if a space-occupying lesion is detected on a chest x-ray film obtained for investigation of respiratory distress. Excision of the bronchogenic cyst is the preferred treatment.

IATROGENIC AIRWAY INJURY

As aggressive management of the pulmonary disease of newborns has developed, there has been a concurrent increase in injury to the airway or pulmonary parenchyma. Long-term intubation and high peak inspiratory pressure settings on the ventilator place these children at an increased risk of airway injury. It has been known since 1976 that perforation of bronchi, particularly the bronchus of the right lower lobe, can be prevented by careful measurement of suction catheters so that they do not extend more than 1 cm beyond the carina.[28] The development of a bronchopulmonary fistula after chest tube evacuation of a pneumothorax can be life threatening and may require surgical closure of the fistula, although some children have been successfully treated nonoperatively.[29]

Complications of high-pressure ventilation include development of interstitial emphysema and bronchopulmonary dysplasia. The interstitial emphysema is usually self-limited, although some infants may benefit from a surgical approach to the problem.[30] Surgery can be curative for granulomas within the airway of chronically intubated neonates, particularly if the lesions contribute to air trapping or stenosis. The best management for iatrogenic airway injury is prevention, and although not totally avoidable, careful attention to ventilator management and suction techniques should reduce the incidence and severity of these problems.

DIAPHRAGMATIC HERNIA

Failure of the development of the posterolateral portion of the diaphragm results in persistence of the pleuroperitoneal canal or foramen of Bochdalek. By week 12 of gestation, the bowel has returned to the abdominal cavity. The incomplete formation of the posterior diaphragm allows the viscera to occupy the chest cavity, and the abdomen is undeveloped and scaphoid after birth. Both lungs are hypoplastic, more so on the side of the hernia. Bronchial branching, lung weight, and lung volume are decreased. The pulmonary arteries are hypoplastic.[31,32] The lesion occurs in 1 of every 3000 live births, with equal frequency in male and female infants. Sporadic occurrence is the rule, but a familial pattern has been reported.[33]

The prenatal diagnosis of congenital diaphragmatic hernia (CDH) can be made using fetal sonography by as early as 15 weeks of gestation.[34] Sonographic findings include herniated abdominal viscera, abnormal anatomy of the upper abdomen, and mediastinal shift away from the herniated viscera.[35] The high-risk fetus is identified by a diagnosis early in gestation, a dilated stomach in the chest, low lung–thorax ratio, and polyhydramnios. Amniocentesis with a fetal karyotype identifies chromosomal defects; trisomy 18 and 21 are most common. More than 40% of newborns with CDH have associated anomalies of the heart, brain, limbs, genitourinary system, or craniofacial region.[36]

Typically, babies with congenital Bochdalek hernia present dramatically with cyanosis and severe respiratory distress immediately after birth. Because the abdominal viscera are dislocated through the defect into the chest, the abdominal contour is scaphoid. Breath sounds are diminished or absent, and because the mediastinal structures have been displaced, the heart sounds are heard in the right chest. As the bowel fills with gas, respiration and cardiac action are further compromised, hypoxia and respiratory acidosis are increased, and death is inevitable unless surgical intervention is undertaken. In some instances, the infants remain relatively asymptomatic in the early hours and days of life, and rarely, a diaphragmatic hernia is an incidental finding in an older child. The respiratory symptoms demand an immediate x-ray film, which is diagnostic. The hernia is on the left side in 90% of these infants, and the air-filled bowel is seen occupying the left hemithorax, with resultant displacement of the mediastinum to the right (Fig. 44-4). The abdomen is airless. Additional x-ray films are unnecessary, and contrast studies for additional confirmation are contraindicated.

Many newborns with CDH have respiratory failure within minutes of birth and urgent stabilization is mandatory to reverse hypoxia, hypercarbia, and metabolic acidosis. No longer is CDH considered to be an operative emergency; instead, rather prompt and aggressive preoperative care is essential.[37] This includes mechanical ventilation with 100% oxygen, sedation with narcotics, muscle paralysis, controlled alkalosis with hyperventilation and intravenous sodium bicarbonate, and vasopressors. The goal is to reverse the baby's persistent fetal circulation with right-to-left shunting of oxygen-poor blood across the open foramen ovale and the ductus arteriosus.

Some infants do not improve despite aggressive therapy, and many centers use ECMO before hernia repair to stabilize these desperately ill infants.[38,39] Venovenous or venoarterial bypass is used, depending on the infant's hemodynamic stability. Bypass is continued until the pulmonary hypertension is reversed and lung function is improved. Most infants respond within 7 to 10 days, but some require 3 weeks of support. Newborns who have not improved after this time probably have such severe pulmonary hypoplasia that further extracorporeal life support is futile.

There are no absolute respiratory criteria that exclude newborns with CDH from consideration for

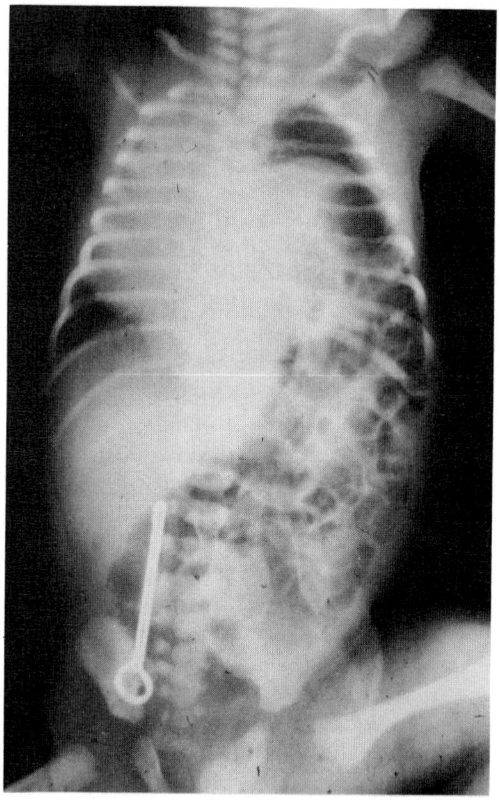

FIG. 44–4. X-ray film of left diaphragmatic hernia with loops of bowel well up into the chest. Although most diaphragmatic hernias do not have a sac, the smooth curve of the sac in this instance is visible. Notice the heart is displaced to the border of the right chest.

ECMO support.[40,41] More than 70% of infants with CDH who are supported by ECMO are expected to survive (see Chap. 32).

The surgical findings are usually those of a posterolateral defect in the left diaphragm, with most or all of the abdominal viscera in the chest. The surgeon reduces the hernia gently by withdrawing the viscera from the chest. If a sac is present, it is delivered and excised. There may be adequate diaphragmatic tissue to accomplish direct suture repair. If a significant portion of the diaphragm is lacking, prosthetic material is used to close the defect. Before completion of the repair, a small chest tube is placed in the left hemithorax and brought out through an intercostal space.

The temptation to expand the compressed lung at the time of initial surgery must be resisted. Aggressive attempts at expansion can result in pneumothorax on the contralateral side, which, if unrecognized, is a disastrous complication.

The abdominal viscera have been located in the thorax throughout most of the developmental period of the fetus, and there is insufficient room within the abdomen to accommodate the intestine without increasing dangerously the intraabdominal pressure, compressing the vena cava, and compromising respirations by elevating the diaphragm. To avoid these potential problems, the surgeon may omit anatomic closure of the abdominal wall. Skin flaps are quickly mobilized and only the skin is closed. The ventral pouch created accommodates the intraabdominal organs; diaphragmatic action and venous return are unimpeded. The ventral hernia is repaired after the infant has been weaned off the ventilator and is in stable clinical condition.

Ten percent of infants with Bochdalek hernias present with the defect on the right side. The difference in incidence on the two sides is probably explained by the presence of the liver, which partially blocks the pleuroperitoneal canal and limits the amount of bowel that can herniate into the chest. Symptoms in babies with right-sided hernias may be less severe, but when a right diaphragmatic hernia of Bochdalek presents as an emergency, it is managed as already described.

After CDH repair and removal from ECMO, ventilation is continued with ventilation rates and oxygen concentrations necessary to maintain adequate oxygenation. Continuous transcutaneous oxygen monitoring of upper and lower body areas is useful. To avoid relapse into pulmonary hypertension, weaning from the ventilator should be achieved by making small incremental changes in the inspired oxygen and ventilator rate.

New modalities being investigated may offer an increased chance of survival for infants with CDH. These include surfactant replacement therapy, intratracheal pulmonary ventilation, and pulmonary lobar transplantation.[42,43] Prenatal repair of CDH has been performed in selected fetuses, but many issues need further evaluation before *in utero* correction of CDH can become a widely accepted treatment.[44]

Babies who present after the first day of life with signs and symptoms prompting a diagnosis of diaphragmatic hernia are almost always hardier patients and have greater pulmonary reserve, and they can be expected to make a satisfactory recovery.

The anterior retrosternal hernia of Morgagni is rarely encountered in the newborn. The diagnosis is confirmed by chest radiograph in the lateral projection. The standard treatment is surgical reconstruction, beginning with an abdominal approach through a thoracoabdominal incision. The prognosis is usually favorable, and these lesions are not associated with the severe cardiopulmonary complications seen with Bochdalek hernias in the neonatal period.

EVENTRATION OF THE DIAPHRAGM

Eventration of the diaphragm may be congenital or acquired. The congenital presentation may mimic that of a congenital diaphragmatic hernia with a sac. The acquired lesion is due to paralysis of the diaphragm, most commonly caused by operative trauma or birth injury.[45]

Large eventrations and diaphragmatic paralysis are poorly tolerated by infants.[46] Paradoxic cephalad motion of the diaphragm on inspiration produces a shift of the mobile, neonatal mediastinum that limits the function of the contralateral lung. Moderate or severe respiratory distress is evident; many newborns with eventration require ventilatory support.

Diagnosis is suggested by a marked elevation of a hemidiaphragm on a chest radiograph. Fluoroscopic examination identifies paradoxic movement of the diaphragm. Treatment is plication of the diaphragm with nonabsorbable sutures that reef up or overlap the diaphragm. The taut diaphragm results in less abnormal motion and improved ventilation.

LESIONS OF THE ESOPHAGUS

ESOPHAGEAL ATRESIA AND ASSOCIATED ANOMALIES

The success story of the management of infants born with esophageal atresia and tracheoesophageal fistula is one of the most dramatic and satisfying that the surgeon, the neonatologist, and the pediatrician can point to. In the early 1900s, virtually all babies born with esophageal atresia and tracheoesophageal fistula died. In 1941, Haight and Towsley were the first to bring an infant with esophageal atresia and tracheoesophageal fistula successfully through the rigors of primary transthoracic reconstruction.[47] This landmark accomplishment occurred before antibiotics, respiratory support, or sophisticated intravenous nutrition were available. This surgical approach formed the basis of modern operative and postoperative care of infants born with this anomaly. Fifty years after the first survivor was announced, every baby born with atresia of the esophagus who is spared coexisting fatal abnormalities and is offered appropriate care has an excellent chance of leading a normal life.

EMBRYOLOGIC AND GENETIC CONSIDERATIONS

The cause of esophageal atresia is unknown, but it is related to the common origin of the esophagus and trachea.[48] The embryonic trachea and esophagus are first recognized as a ventral diverticulum of the foregut approximately 22 or 23 days after fertilization.[49] As the diverticulum elongates, a proliferation of endodermal cells appears on the lateral walls. These cell masses become ridges of tissue that ultimately divide the foregut into tracheal and esophageal channels. The division into separate tubes is completed between 34 and 36 days after fertilization. Many embryologic studies indicate that interruption in the fourth fetal week allows persistence of fistulas and clefts between the esophagus and trachea and permits incomplete development of the esophagus.

There have been several reports of a mother and her child having esophageal atresia, which raises the possibility of a heritable genetic factor, but it is not yet possible to verify this statistically. Numerous accounts of siblings with esophageal atresia have been reported.[50] Conversely, certain commonly coexistent anomalies, such as the VACTERL (*i.e.*, vertebral, anal, cardiac, tracheal, esophageal, renal, and limb anomalies) association (see Chap. 40) and other malformations, strongly suggest that a teratogen may influence the developing fetus at a certain time.[51] Most evidence points to environmental agents or events that exert a more substantial effect on the developing esophagus than genetic factors.

In many babies with esophageal atresia, it is the associated anomalies that alter treatment and affect survival. Congenital heart defects and chromosomal abnormalities are the most worrisome. Major anomalies that may seriously affect the infant, but that are not usually fatal, include imperforate anus and other congenital obstructions of the gut. Grosfeld and Ballantine found that 31 (37%) of 84 infants had cardiac anomalies; 18 (21.4%) had gastrointestinal malformations, of whom 11 (13%) had imperforate anus; and 6 (7%) had the VACTERL association.[52] A ventricular septal defect is the most common cardiac lesion, followed in frequency by patent ductus arteriosus and tetralogy of Fallot. Piekarski and Stephens suggest that the high incidence of coexisting anomalies is a reflection of generalized damage to the mesenchymal tissue in the fourth week of gestation.[53]

ESOPHAGEAL ATRESIA WITH TRACHEOESOPHAGEAL FISTULA

Esophageal atresia occurs approximately in 1 of 3000 to 4500 births. In the most common form of esophageal anomaly (86% of patients), the blind-ending upper esophageal segment usually extends into the upper portion of the thorax, and the lower portion of the esophagus is connected to the trachea at or just above the tracheal carina (Fig. 44-5).[54] This connection is 3 to 5 mm in diameter and easily admits inspired air or, in a retrograde fashion, acidic gastric secretions. The earliest clinical sign of esophageal atresia is excessive oral secretions or regurgitation of saliva. The saliva pools in the blind-ending esophagus and then accumulates until it is apparent around the lips as excessive mucus. The first feeding is followed by choking, coughing, and regurgitation. Abdominal distention is a prominent feature, occurring as inspired air is transmitted through the fistula and distal esophagus into the stomach. Gastric juice may pass upward in the distal esophagus, traversing the tracheoesophageal fistula and spilling into the trachea and lungs, leading to chemical pneumonia. Pulmonary difficulties are compounded by atelectasis and diaphragmatic elevation secondary to gastric distention.

Diagnosis. Attentive members of the nursing staff who are feeding the baby are often the first to suspect

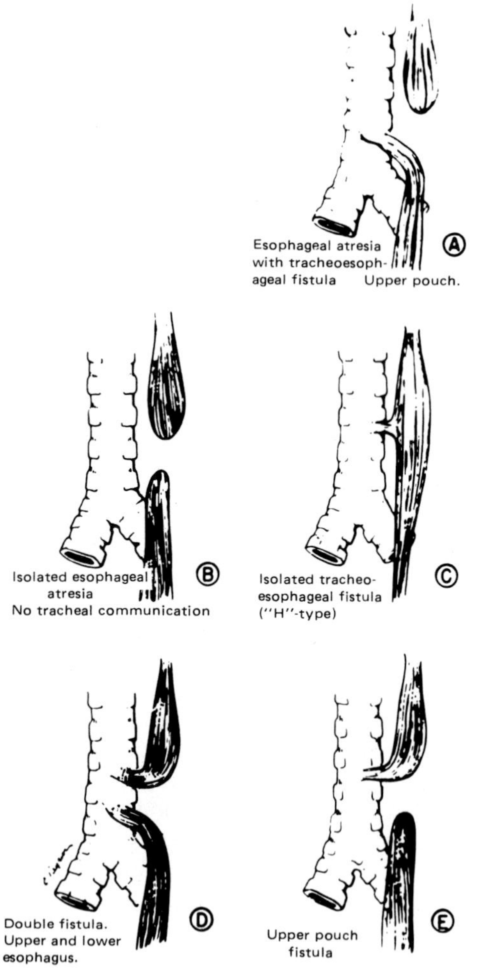

FIG. 44–5. The various forms of esophageal malformations are shown in the order of the frequency in which they occur. (From Nardi GL, Zuidema GD. Surgery. 3rd ed. Boston: Little, Brown, 1972.)

the esophageal blockage. Esophageal atresia may not be obvious on the initial newborn examination, unless an attempt is made to pass a tube into the stomach. Thin, flexible feeding catheters should be avoided, because they may coil up in the esophagus and give the misleading impression that they have passed into the stomach. A larger, stiffer catheter carefully advanced will meet the obstruction. Occasionally, a tube dissects into the wall of a normal esophagus leading to a misdiagnosis of esophageal atresia, particularly in a premature infant. A contrast x-ray film rules this out and confirms the diagnosis of atresia; a lateral projection with 1 mL of dilute barium or an isoosmolar contrast agent (*e.g.*, metrizamide) shows the length of the upper pouch, defines its precise extension into the chest, and demonstrates the rare upper pouch fistula (Fig. 44-6*A,B*). Air seen in the bowel confirms the presence of a tracheoesophageal fistula. The existence of pneumonia or atelectasis also can be demonstrated on the initial radiographs.

Evaluation of the heart and great vessels with echocardiography is important to identify potential cardiac anomalies and verify the aortic arch position. A right-sided arch may alter the surgical approach and exposure. Bronchoscopy is useful for identifying the level of the fistula and exclusion of upper pouch fistulas and laryngotracheoesophageal clefts.

Esophageal atresia has become more frequently recognized during maternal ultrasonography. Failure to visualize a fetal stomach in a mother who has polyhydramnios suggests esophageal atresia. Prenatal diagnosis permits a search for associated problems and allows a comprehensive, coordinated approach to the family and infant in the perinatal period.

Management. After the diagnosis is secure, the following measures should be instituted promptly:

Use an infant warmer.
Place the infant in a 30° to 40° head-up position.
Give nothing orally.
Provide antibiotic treatment for possible aspiration.
Place a sump suction catheter in the upper pouch to remove the excess secretions (Fig. 44-7).
Consult with the appropriate pediatric surgical service.

A classification developed by Waterston and colleagues in 1962 was useful in the stratification of patients for different management plans and the comparison of outcomes.[55] This system was based on low birth weight and the presence of pneumonia as significant risk categories for infants with esophageal atresia and tracheoesophageal fistula. The infants were classified as follows:

Category A: birth weight over 2.5 kg (5.5 lb) and otherwise well
Category B: birth weight of 1.8 to 2.5 kg and well, or higher birth weight but moderate pneumonia and other congenital anomalies
Category C: birth weight under 1.8 kg, or higher birth weight but severe pneumonia and severe congenital anomaly.

Neonatal care has evolved to the point that neither low birth weight nor the presence of pneumonia are risk factors for poor survival. Severe anomalies and their consequences are now the crucial determinants of survival.

At Children's National Medical Center (CNMC), each baby admitted with esophageal atresia is managed according to his or her physiologic status alone.[56] If the infant is stable, immediate primary repair is undertaken. If unstable, surgery is delayed until the clinical status is stabilized, the impact of associated anomalies is determined, and the infant can be anesthetized and operated on safely.

Immediate Operative Repair. A thoracic incision provides exposure of the upper pouch and tracheoesophageal fistula. A right thoracotomy is stan-

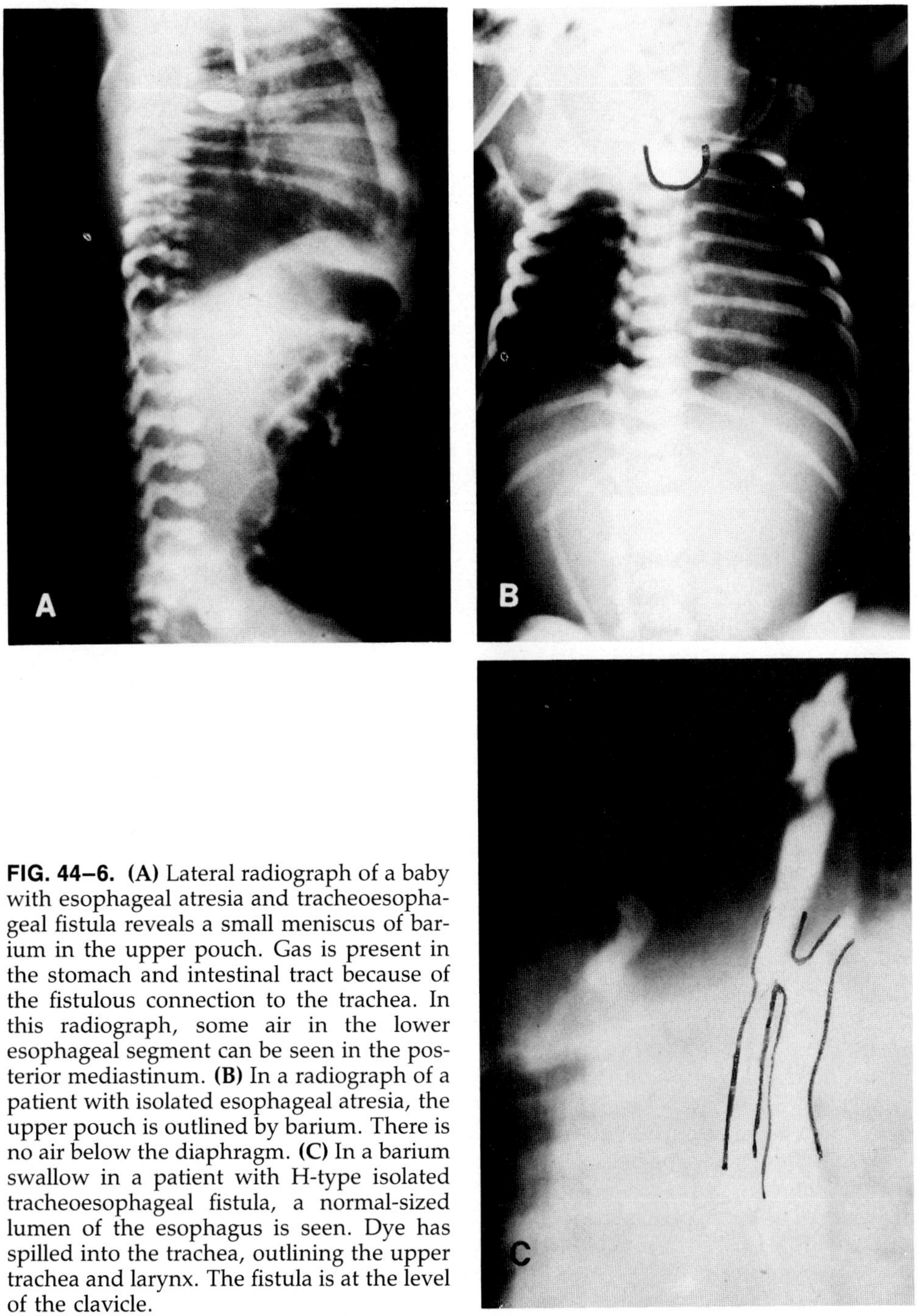

FIG. 44–6. **(A)** Lateral radiograph of a baby with esophageal atresia and tracheoesophageal fistula reveals a small meniscus of barium in the upper pouch. Gas is present in the stomach and intestinal tract because of the fistulous connection to the trachea. In this radiograph, some air in the lower esophageal segment can be seen in the posterior mediastinum. **(B)** In a radiograph of a patient with isolated esophageal atresia, the upper pouch is outlined by barium. There is no air below the diaphragm. **(C)** In a barium swallow in a patient with H-type isolated tracheoesophageal fistula, a normal-sized lumen of the esophagus is seen. Dye has spilled into the trachea, outlining the upper trachea and larynx. The fistula is at the level of the clavicle.

dard unless the aortic arch is on the right, which would interfere with the dissection. A retropleural approach affords protection of the lung by maintaining its pleural envelope. If an anastomotic leak occurs, it will not communicate with the pleural cavity but can be drained posteriorly from the mediastinum with less morbidity.

The fistula is identified and carefully divided from the trachea. The tracheal opening is closed with several sutures, with care to avoid narrowing the tracheal lumen. Although some centers have advocated simple ligation of the fistula, this procedure is associated with an unacceptably high rate of recurrence.[57]

The circumference of the lower esophageal fistula is usually small and is enlarged by trimming and spatulating its open end. The tip of the upper pouch is mobilized extensively and cut across to expose the lumen. Most surgeons employ a single-layer circumferential anastomosis to approximate the two ends, instead of the classic two-layer Haight anastomosis.[58]

Avoiding undue tension on the repair and averting compromise of the blood supply to the two ends are

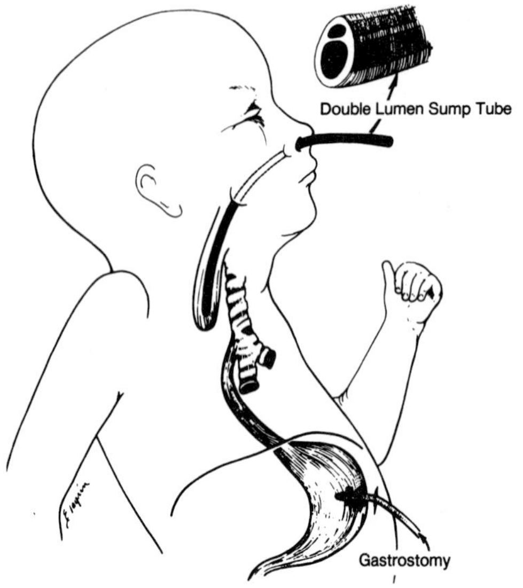

FIG. 44–7. Temporary care of a patient with esophageal atresia and tracheoesophageal fistula is performed with the patient in the upright position. A gastrostomy is in the stomach, and a double-lumen sump tube is in the upper pouch to clear secretions and saliva.

key factors in obtaining good results. The upper pouch is more amenable to mobilization than the fistula because the blood supply comes submucosally from the neck. The blood supply to the fistula is more easily compromised because it derives from tiny branches off the aorta. If the ends do not come together easily, there are surgical techniques available for extending the length of the upper pouch.[59]

Although once routine, gastrostomy is now rarely used in stable infants. Postoperatively, infants are maintained on intravenous nutrition. A chest tube is placed to drain the mediastinum and pleural space if necessary. The chest tube is connected to suction and monitored for evidence of air leak, blood loss, or saliva indicating an anastomotic leak. Postoperative management requires meticulous care to avoid disruption of the tracheal suture line if suctioning or reintubation is required. A contrast swallow is usually obtained on the fifth or sixth postoperative day. If all looks well, and there is no leak, feedings are begun and quickly advanced. Some surgeons routinely dilate the esophagus of all infants before discharge to prevent potential stricture formation. We have not found this approach helpful.

Delayed Primary Repair and Staged Repair. If the infant is unstable, an intermediate plan allows correction of minor difficulties before repair. This plan involves delay of the surgical repair for several days. Management of these babies includes upper pouch suction with a Replogle tube, head-up position, antibiotics, and parenteral nutrition. These maneuvers provide for stabilization, improvement of pulmonary status, and diagnosis and management of certain higher priority malformations, particularly cardiac lesions. Primary retropleural repair, as described previously, is undertaken when the infant's condition is stable and the risk of surgery reduced.

Unstable infants with serious coexisting anomalies or severe prematurity have diminished chances for survival. For these infants, a gastrostomy is placed, and repair is postponed. This approach uses early retropleural fistula division without anastomosis, gastrostomy feedings, and continuous sump suction of the upper pouch. Division of the fistula is important to prevent reflux of gastric contents. In some premature infants with noncompliant lungs, division of the fistula is required to allow adequate ventilation, in essence closing off the lower resistance pathway through the fistula and stomach. Immediate closure of the fistula may be lifesaving in these instances.

This clinical arrangement of gastrostomy and fistula division without anastomosis requires constant, intensive nursing care, but it can be safely maintained for many weeks. Coupled with the holding pattern provided by suction of the upper pouch and gastrostomy drainage, infants with esophageal atresia and tracheoesophageal fistula can be maintained indefinitely by intravenous nutrition while weight and pulmonary status are improved and other congenital anomalies are studied and corrected. Later, the definitive transthoracic operation is performed and the esophageal anastomosis accomplished electively.

Results. At the Children's National Medical Center in Washington, D.C., 118 patients with a blind upper esophageal pouch and a fistula arising from the bifurcation of the trachea were treated between 1966 and 1989. Eighty-eight percent of these patients survived. Since 1982, the physiologic status of the infant has been the sole guide to therapy. The survival for infants who were classified as stable and had primary repair is 100%. Survival in the unstable group who had staged repair is 57%. The deaths were due to associated anomalies, including congenital diaphragmatic hernia and hypoplastic left heart. As a result of this experience with high-risk infants, we concluded that a staged procedure, even one that abandons the esophagus, is preferable to primary repair for selected infants in the highest-risk group. This decision is controversial. Most pediatric surgeons eschew the staged approach, preferring primary repair in most infants with esophageal atresia and tracheoesophageal fistula.[60]

Complications. Complications are not uncommon and require scrupulous diagnostic evaluation. Strictures, gastroesophageal reflux, poor motility, recurrent fistula, and tracheomalacia produce similar respiratory symptoms and may be difficult to differentiate.

Gastroesophageal reflux after repair of esophageal

atresia has become increasingly recognized as a clinical problem because of more alert physicians and more sensitive diagnostic tools, such as 24-hour *p*H monitoring. Werlin and coworkers showed that all of the 14 postoperative esophageal atresia patients they studied exhibited severe esophageal motor dysfunction. Only 5 of the 14 complained of a swallowing problem.[61] In 1980, Jolley and others studied 25 young patients between 3 and 83 months after repair of esophageal atresia and tracheoesophageal fistula. Seventeen of 25 had significant gastroesophageal reflux demonstrated by prolonged *p*H monitoring, and 12 of these patients had significant symptoms in the form of vomiting, respiratory difficulty, or esophagitis.[62] Fonkaslrud concluded that esophageal dysmotility and gastroesophageal reflux were serious problems in combination and recommended fundoplication in selected patients.[63]

Esophageal stricture is a common complication (*i.e.*, 31% in our series) after the anastomosis of the esophagus. Stricture may present early with an inability to swallow, choking, or failure to thrive but may show up later, particularly at the time of transition to solid foods. In most infants esophageal dilation is successful, but some require repetitive dilations as often as every 2 weeks for 1 year. Occasionally, a recalcitrant stricture requires operative resection.

Anastomotic disruption with leakage of saliva, gastric juice, and swallowed liquid into the mediastinum or thoracic space was once a dreaded complication after surgery. It is no longer universally fatal, due to improvements in nutrition and antibiotics. The leak may be identified on a contrast study obtained before feeding or by an increase in the output from the chest tube or the drainage of saliva through the chest tube. If the operative repair has been accomplished with a retropleural approach and the pleura remains intact, external drainage posteriorly from the mediastinum is a relatively simple matter. If transthoracic repair is followed by esophageal disruption, the leak is best treated by extensive drainage, parenteral nutrition, and delayed repair. If the baby is deteriorating, it may be wise to abandon the esophagus and create a diverting cervical esophagostomy.

Recurrent fistulas may develop in a few infants.[64] Usually, there is a history of a perioperative leak. The symptoms are often those of recurrent respiratory problems, such as bronchitis or pneumonia related to silent aspiration. Reoperation is required to divide the fistula.

Tracheomalacia is an uncommon complication, but it is difficult to manage. It may be related to a congenital weakness of the trachea or operative injury. The spectrum of presentation ranges from complete collapse of the airway, with an inability to ventilate without positive pressure, to mild tracheal compromise. Bronchoscopy reveals the level and degree of collapse. In severe cases, operative suspension of the aorta and trachea is curative.

ESOPHAGEAL ATRESIA WITHOUT FISTULA

Esophageal atresia may occur without a fistulous connection to the respiratory tract. This variant accounts for approximately 8% of esophageal malformations. As with other forms of esophageal atresia, these babies cannot swallow food or saliva. Because there is no tracheoesophageal fistula, air is absent from the gastrointestinal tract, and the abdomen is noticeably scaphoid. The radiologic findings of a blind upper pouch coupled with the absence of air below the diaphragm are pathognomonic of isolated esophageal atresia.

For many years, the standard treatment of isolated esophageal atresia included cervical esophagostomy and gastrostomy. At a later time, a feeding pathway would be created with a segment of small bowel or colon or with construction of a reversed gastric tube. This time-proven practice still has a place in the treatment of pure esophageal atresia. Since the mid-1970s, new methods for bridging the gap between the disparate esophageal segments have evolved. Howard and Myers reported a technique for elongating the blind upper pouch using daily stretching by bougie dilators, allowing the two esophageal ends to be successfully united after several months.[65] Mechanical stretching of the pouches may not be necessary. Natural growth in the first months of life produces impressive elongation of the esophageal pouches.[66] During the interval, meticulous nursing care is required to prevent aspiration of saliva and ensure adequate nutrition. In many infants, the wisest course may still be cervical esophagostomy and gastrostomy, with later esophageal replacement. This course is even more appropriate for the premature infant, especially if respiratory distress proves troublesome.

The decision to preserve or abandon the esophagus rests on the patient's weight, pulmonary status, presence of other serious anomalies, and general hardiness during the early diagnostic and sustaining maneuvers. Our experience has led us to treat the last 15 consecutive infants that presented with isolated atresia of the esophagus by cervical esophagostomy and gastrostomy, reconstructing the esophagus at 1 year of age using a reversed gastric tube. The latter is a tube created from the greater curve of the stomach, brought up through the chest, and anastomosed to the upper esophageal segment. Fourteen of the 15 infants survived and are growing well.

ISOLATED TRACHEOESOPHAGEAL FISTULA

Isolated (*i.e.*, H-type) tracheoesophageal fistula is a rare lesion, representing approximately 4% of esophageal anomalies. Although congenital tracheoesophageal communication without atresia may be found at any level, most of these fistulas occur in the upper portion of the trachea and the esophagus, at or above the level of the second thoracic vertebra.[67] Larger fistulas and communications extending throughout the length of the trachea have been seen, defects appropriately called laryngotracheoesophageal clefts.

The infant suffering from congenital tracheoesophageal fistula usually chokes and coughs with feeding. Prompt relief may be achieved by gavage feeding. Frequently the diagnosis is not made in infancy, because the symptoms can be subtle. Pneumonitis often develops in the early days of life and recurs frequently as patchy bronchopneumonia. With continued aspiration through the fistula, a constant state of bronchopneumonia supervenes, attended by all of the manifestations of chronic infection. For any child with recurrent pneumonia, a wide variety of disease entities must be considered, but the list should include H-type tracheoesophageal fistula.

A contrast esophageal swallow with a dilute or isoosmolar medium may reveal the fistula (see Fig. 44-6C). Tracheobronchoscopy is usually successful in demonstrating this anomaly, but simultaneous esophagoscopy may be required. The fistula can be exposed through a cervical collar incision in most instances. A thoracic approach is necessary in 10% to 15% of patients. Surgery produces complete cures for most patients.

Although once uniformly fatal, laryngotracheoesophageal clefts can now be repaired with good results. Early diagnosis is essential to prevent repeated aspiration through the communication between the trachea and esophagus below the vocal cords. Bronchoscopy allows identification of the cleft and its severity. Defects range from those involving only the upper trachea to those extending the entire length and beyond the carina. Management involves tracheostomy and an antireflux procedure to prevent aspiration, with later repair of the defect.[68]

GASTROESOPHAGEAL REFLUX

In 1947, Berenberg and Neuhauser defined a condition they called "chalasia," or abnormal relaxation of the gastroesophageal junction.[69] The affected babies manifest relentless regurgitation that may present as spitting, mild vomiting, or vigorous vomiting after every feeding. The deleterious effects of gastroesophageal reflux in infants have been recognized with increasing frequency.[70–72] The spectrum of symptoms caused by gastroesophageal reflux in the infant is distinctly different from that seen in the adult. In infants, the main symptoms of gastroesophageal reflux are regurgitation, significant growth retardation, aspiration pneumonia, apneic spells, stridor, and esophagitis.[63,64,73,74] The abnormality is the absence of a normal valvular mechanism at the gastroesophageal junction that allows unimpeded reflux of gastric content. Associated medical conditions affect many infants. Congenital or acquired central nervous system disorders are most frequent, including severe asphyxia, cerebral palsy, chromosomal anomalies, and microcephaly.

Infants with repaired esophageal atresia and tracheoesophageal fistula may have reflux that leads to anastomotic strictures, poor weight gain, or aspiration pneumonias.

Most infants with gastroesophageal reflux have some form of vomiting from birth. In some babies, the vomiting suggests the diagnosis of pyloric stenosis. Retardation of growth and development is the second most common presenting symptom, occurring in approximately 50% of our patients. These babies rank below the tenth percentile on their growth chart or show a marked falling off of growth progression. Recurrent aspiration with pneumonia occurs in approximately one-third of infants with pernicious gastroesophageal reflux. Reflux may also be the underlying cause of severe apnea in some infants.[72]

A barium swallow demonstrates reflux in about 75% of symptomatic patients. However, reflux can also be shown in many otherwise normal, healthy infants, and radiologists have understandable difficulty in defining gastroesophageal reflux that is pathologic. Gastroesophageal reflux can be documented and quantitated with radionuclide material. This examination permits an accurate appraisal of the pathophysiologic effects of reflux in most patients. It has proved adaptable to infants, and when serial observations are extended over several hours, normal reflux can usually be differentiated from pathologic reflux. Gastric emptying is also measured by this scan.

Monitoring of *p*H at different levels of the esophagus can demonstrate gastric acid reflux. With timed studies, physicians can now chart reflux in relation to sleeping, various body positions, and during eating, documenting episodes that lead to characteristic symptoms or life-threatening incidents.[75] Esophagoscopy helps physicians to document the presence of esophagitis in selected infants.

Every effort should be made to reverse the consequences of pernicious gastroesophageal reflux by conservative therapy. Medical therapy of symptomatic infants with gastroesophageal reflux consists of maintaining a semiupright posture and small frequent feedings of thickened material. Bethanechol has yielded little or no benefit, but metaclopramide, which increases the tone and amplitude of gastric contraction, relaxes the pyloric sphincter, and accelerates gastric emptying, has proved more helpful.

In rare instances, the extent of a baby's nutritional depletion or chronic pneumonitis may demand hospitalization. In infants sick enough to be hospitalized, 3 weeks is an ample period to determine whether their symptoms can be controlled by intensive medical measures. Infants less severely affected should be evaluated in an outpatient setting over 2 to 4 months. If symptoms are controlled by medical means, reflux usually disappears by 15 months, coincident with the development of upright posture. In our experience, medical therapy fails for approximately 15% of the patients.

With worsening or protraction of symptoms despite adherence to conservative treatment, surgical

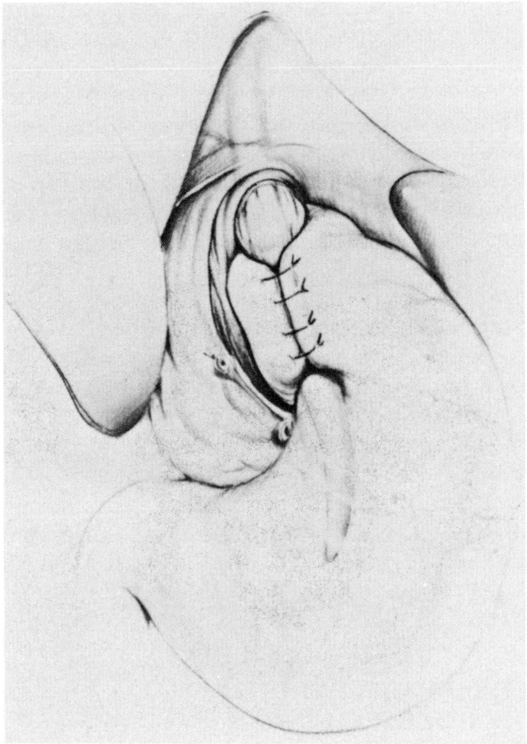

FIG. 44–8. A successful method for the surgical correction of gastroesophageal reflux employs gastric fundoplication as described by Nissen.

correction is recommended if the infant fails to gain weight and grow adequately, has recurrent pneumonitis, has life-threatening apnea spells, or has esophagitis. Prompt operative correction is thought appropriate without medical trial for those patients with thoracic translocation of a significant portion of the stomach and esophageal stricture.

Surgical intervention is undertaken to place the gastroesophageal junction well below the diaphragm (*i.e.*, lengthen the intraabdominal esophagus), recreate an acute angle of His, and create a valvelike mechanism to force the fundus of the stomach against the esophagus. The Nissen fundoplication involves wrapping the fundus of the stomach completely around the esophagogastric junction (Fig. 44-8). In the Thal procedure, the wrap is partial (*i.e.*, 210°–270°). Postoperative problems, such as dysphagia and inability to burp and vomit (*i.e.*, gas-bloat syndrome) appear less likely with the Thai procedure.[74] Gastroesophageal reflux is discussed in more detail in Chapter 37.

ABDOMINAL SURGERY

The indications for abdominal surgery are distention and bilious vomiting. To these should be added the scaphoid contour seen if there is high intestinal obstruction or the abdominal viscera are in an ectopic location, as in infants with congenital diaphragmatic hernia. Extreme degrees of abdominal distention are associated with intestinal and gastric perforation. Tenderness signifying peritoneal irritation can be elicited by careful examination. A tender, erythematous abdominal wall is a reliable sign of an intraabdominal catastrophe with resultant peritonitis and ischemic intestine. Reliance on bowel sounds can be misleading. Peristalsis can exist despite peritonitis or be absent when intestinal distention is caused by mechanical obstruction.

Pertinent radiologic studies to be obtained in all cases of suspected intraabdominal surgical lesions are the flat and upright views of the abdomen. The left lateral decubitus radiograph may be substituted for the upright radiograph if pneumoperitoneum is suspected. Intestinal obstruction can be diagnosed and the level of obstruction determined by the configuration of the air–fluid levels. Pneumoperitoneum is usually readily appreciated on abdominal x-ray films. Supine radiographs may show the football sign produced by superimposition of the falciform ligament on a large bubble of free air (Fig. 44–9). The bowel wall may be outlined by air outside and inside the bowel lumen. The left lateral decubitis radiograph may show air around the liver. Not infrequently, the findings on radiographs may be subtle, requiring an alert physician to make the diagnosis. Distended bowel and the absence of air fluid levels in intestinal loops of various sizes suggest obstruction secondary to meconium ileus. Calcifications scattered within the abdomen indicate intrauterine perforation with meconium peritonitis.

Unless precluded by a deteriorating clinical condition, a contrast enema, usually of isoosmotic Gastrografin initially, requires only a short delay that is usually justified by the information obtained. The enema need not be an elaborate study in these precarious subjects.

The diagnosis of malrotation is most accurately made with a small amount of contrast placed into the stomach to confirm the position of the ligament of Treitz. Incomplete obstructions of the gastrointestinal tract, such as those caused by congenital stenosis or intraluminal web, are often the most difficult congenital lesions to diagnose and require contrast studies of the upper gastrointestinal (UGI) tract, with careful attention to every centimeter of intestine on fluoroscopy.

PNEUMOPERITONEUM: GASTRIC PERFORATION

Spontaneous perforation of a hollow viscus is most frequently seen in distressed neonates who have undergone resuscitation immediately after birth. The presence of free air in the peritoneal cavity may be secondary to perforation anywhere in the gastrointestinal tract and is a surgical emergency. The surgeon

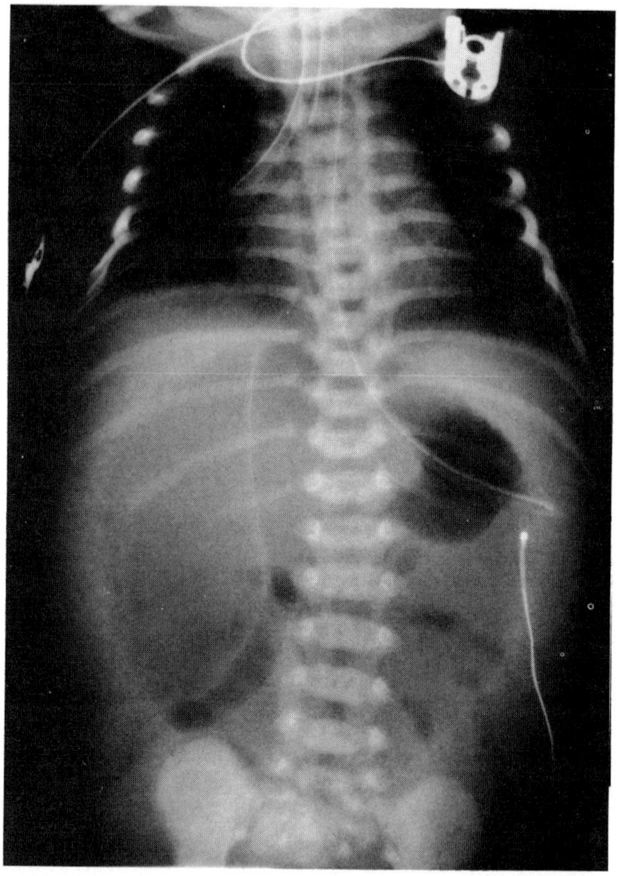

FIG. 44–9. Supine abdominal x-ray film demonstrates a massive intraperitoneal air collection. The air is seen as a large central bubble upon which is superimposed a dense linear opacity produced by the falciform ligament (*arrow*). The falciform ligament forms the lace for the football sign.

approaching the infant with pneumoperitoneum must be prepared to investigate systematically the entire gastrointestinal tract and anticipate problems such as gastric perforation, necrotizing enterocolitis (NEC), Hirschsprung disease, or other ischemic insults to the intestine resulting in perforation.[76–78]

After perforation, egress of air into the free peritoneal cavity usually leads to impressive abdominal distention. Elevation of the diaphragm occurs with considerable embarrassment of the infant's respiratory dynamics. A temporary but lifesaving maneuver is needle aspiration of the peritoneal cavity, which diminishes air under pressure, allowing the diaphragm to return to a more normal position. There is usually dramatic relief of abdominal distention and respiratory distress. It is not hazardous to insert a needle adapted to a 50-mL syringe through the anterior abdominal wall. The bowel is usually compressed against the posterior parietes and is not likely to be injured by this maneuver.

Surgical intervention must be prompt. When massive distention of the abdomen occurs, a gastric perforation can be anticipated. Typically, the rent occurs high on the greater curvature of the stomach. Because the perforation may be located on the posterior wall, thorough exploration of the relatively inaccessible areas of the stomach must be carried out. Although it has been suggested that perforation of the stomach results from congenital deficiency of musculature in the gastric wall, this explanation is questionable. The apparent absence of musculature at the margin of the perforation probably represents retraction of the muscles of an overdistended stomach, with a ballooning of mucosa between the muscle fibers.

Repair is accomplished by primary closure in two layers after debridement of the margins of the perforation. A gastrostomy tube, inserted through a noninvolved area of the stomach, is advisable to ensure postoperative decompression. The subsequent course of the infant is usually uncomplicated if the underlying problem for which resuscitation was required is controlled. Cautious feedings can be started within a few days of surgical repair. For diagnosis and management of perforations occurring elsewhere in the gastrointestinal tract, see Meconium Peritonitis and Necrotizing Enterocolitis.

TEMPORARY DIVERSION OF THE INTESTINAL TRACT

Newborn intestinal emergencies often demand a temporary vent or enterostomy. Although not as desirable as an end-to-end union of the bowel, these measures may be lifesaving in fragile infants who are critically ill as the result of intestinal obstruction or peritonitis or who are threatened by serious congenital defects. An abdominal stoma in the infant does not carry the same implications as in the adult; the physician must stress this fact to allay the fears and doubts of a worried parent. Most enterostomies are temporary, and the outlook for restoration of complete intestinal continuity is good.

GASTROSTOMY

The stomach requires venting for two reasons. First, decompression of the gastrointestinal tract is necessary in the face of any abdominal catastrophe. Placement of the gastrostomy obviates the need for a nasogastric tube. It is more efficient and eliminates the danger of pressure necrosis of the alar cartilage of the infant's nose and the respiratory hazards that attend nasogastric tubes. Second, the gastrostomy tube provides access for feeding a depleted neonate.

Gastrostomy can be performed under local anesthesia, although it is usually done under general anesthesia. Frequently, the procedure complements a primary abdominal operation. A simple Stamm gastrostomy is preferred, and it is not difficult to remove or replace the tube as an office procedure. If the gastrostomy tube is to be maintained for a long time, it may be replaced after 1 month with a gastrostomy button, which is easier for the parents to care for at home.[79]

ILEOSTOMY

Temporary ileostomy is less desirable than primary union of the bowel, but there are clinical circumstances for which its creation as a temporary diverting procedure is prudent, including inflammatory necrosis of the distal small bowel with intraperitoneal soiling and peritonitis, ischemic insult with marginal viability of the bowel, and marked disparity in lumen size, as in intestinal atresia or meconium ileus.

A properly performed ileostomy is usually well tolerated and rarely causes skin breakdown. With appropriate supportive care, weight gain and healing proceed, and intestinal reconstruction can be carried out electively with greater safety for the infant. We recommend closure of the ileostomy when the infants weigh 2.5 to 3.0 kg to minimize fluid and electrolyte imbalances that these babies may develop.[80]

In very sick infants or in babies with other underlying conditions such as meconium ileus, the double-barrel enterostomy of Mikulicz has proved valuable. The common wall that has been created is gradually crushed with a special clamp, partly reestablishing intestinal continuity. Complete closure of the bowel can be achieved without reentering the peritoneal cavity. Another effective technique of intestinal venting that permits access to the distal gastrointestinal tract is the end-to-side enteroenterostomy described by Bishop and Koop.[81] This technique has particular application for lesions in the proximal gastrointestinal tract, such as jejunal and high ileal atresia.

COLOSTOMY

The four usual indications for colostomy in the neonate are impending or actual perforation of the colon, colonic atresia with huge disparity of the bowel lumen, Hirschsprung disease, and high imperforate anus. The loop colostomy has the advantage of simplicity and speed in critically ill babies. An end-colostomy is mechanically sound, easily managed, and avoids spillage into the distal loop, which is an advantage in treating Hirschsprung disease and imperforate anus. A diaper neatly covers the colostomy during the early months of life, until definitive surgical correction of the primary problem is accomplished and the colostomy closed (see Chap. 37).

ROTATIONAL ABNORMALITIES

MALROTATION

In the developing embryo, the elongating intestine must undergo rotation as it returns to the celomic cavity so that it can be accommodated within the confines of the abdominal cavity. The proximal small intestine assumes the characteristic C-shaped contour, and the duodenum is fixed to the left of the midline at the ligament of Treitz. The cecum takes a counterclockwise rotation, reaching its final location in the right lower abdomen.[82] Incomplete intestinal rotation, with consequent inadequate fixation of the intestinal mesentery, may be an asymptomatic occurrence, may give rise to subtle symptoms difficult to diagnose, or may present as a life-threatening intraabdominal catastrophe. An understanding of the mechanism by which the lesion becomes symptomatic is necessary if the physician is to recognize and prevent the devastating complications that can accompany midgut volvulus.

If rotation is abnormal, bands are formed between the ectopic cecum, located in the right upper quadrant, and the right lateral abdominal wall. As these bands course from the cecum to the abdominal wall, they traverse the duodenum and can cause intermittent, incomplete duodenal obstruction. Symptoms of partial duodenal obstruction are often baffling. The infant may experience intervals of a normal feeding pattern that are interspersed with exasperating episodes of vomiting. Because the obstruction is high in the gastrointestinal tract, abdominal distention does not occur. The telltale sign of an underlying mechanical problem is bile in the vomitus. This lesion, more than any other, supports the contention that bile-stained vomitus in an infant necessitates a thorough diagnostic workup to detect a malrotation and subsequent midgut volvulus. More than 50% of babies present with symptoms before 1 week of age, but 10% remain asymptomatic until after 1 year of age.[83]

The most reliable diagnostic study is a UGI series for localization of the ligament of Treitz. Surgical correction of malrotation of the colon prevents a future volvulus of the midgut and relieves the partial duodenal obstruction. The bands binding the cecum to the right abdominal wall are lysed, and the large bowel is freed and transposed to the left side of the abdomen. The duodenum is mobilized on its medial aspect, where the narrow mesentery is intimately associated with the superior mesenteric artery. As the mesentery of the small bowel is freed medially, it assumes a broad position over the posterior abdominal wall. With the mesentery splayed, the potential for torsion is eliminated. It is unnecessary to fix the intestine in its new position with sutures.[84] The appendix, because it now lies on the left side of the abdomen, is usually removed or inverted. Operative correction of malrotation in this manner is known as the Ladd procedure.

MALROTATION WITH MIDGUT VOLVULUS

If fixation of the mesentery of the small bowel has not occurred normally, the intestine is subject to torsion on the axis of the superior mesenteric artery. This mechanism of obstruction must be considered for an infant with bile-stained vomiting, especially if there is no abdominal distention. Abdominal tenderness is an ominous finding.

Roentgenographic abnormalities are often characteristic, with evidence of duodenal obstruction and scanty gas distributed through the remainder of the bowel. The air–fluid levels typical of intestinal obstruction elsewhere in the gastrointestinal tract are not usually associated with this malrotation. An airless abdomen is an ominous sign and usually indicates that infarction of the intestine has already taken place. Bloody stools imply that significant compromise to the intestinal vasculature has occurred. A UGI series shows a corkscrewlike constriction of the third portion of the duodenum.

If midgut volvulus is diagnosed or suspected as the underlying mechanism for the infant's illness, emergency surgical exploration is undertaken. If the findings are favorable and the bowel is viable, the torsion is reduced by counterclockwise rotation, and a Ladd procedure, is carried out as described for the treatment of malrotation without volvulus. The prognosis is favorable as long as the viability of the intestine is not in question. However, if the diagnosis has been delayed or the volvulus has been an intrauterine event, intestinal ischemia, infarction, or both may be encountered in the distribution of the superior mesenteric artery. Initial judgments regarding the viability of the intestine are not easy; intestinal resection at the time of initial exploration is contraindicated. The ischemic intestine must be given every opportunity to recover after the torsion has been reduced. The first operation consists of untwisting the small bowel and establishing a gastrostomy.

Reexploration is undertaken 24 to 36 hours later, and areas of obvious infarction are identified. These are resected, and appropriate enterostomies are brought out to the abdominal wall; anastomosis is contraindicated. Any intestine of marginal viability is retained in hope that it will recover. Reexploration to determine recovery or further loss of small bowel is repeated after another interval of 36 to 48 hours. After the full extent of intestinal loss has been established and the margins of viable bowel exteriorized, the surgeon is faced with the management of a desperately ill infant at risk from sepsis, disseminated intravascular coagulation, and the inevitable nutritional crisis attending a short bowel syndrome.

A central venous catheter for total parenteral alimentation is established, and nourishment is provided by this technique throughout the early postoperative weeks. After the infant has achieved positive nitrogen balance and the reestablishment of intestinal continuity is complete, there is then a difficult period of weaning from parenteral onto oral feedings. About 40 cm of residual small intestine seems to be required for successful adaptation of the intestine in full-term infants, although adaptation has been reported for children with considerably less than 40 cm of intestine.[85] If the distal ileum and ileocecal valve are intact, slightly less bowel may be tolerated. Infant formulas that are fat free and contain monosaccharides and hydrolyzed protein should be used to feed these babies, because these formulas require only a minimal absorptive surface and little enzyme activity for assimilation. Gradually, the volume and concentration of these substances may be increased, until all calories are taken orally. The process of weaning the infant from total intravenous to total oral alimentation may take months. This underscores the devastating complications of a midgut volvulus and indicates the need for vigilance by pediatrician and surgeon in the pursuit of the diagnosis of malrotation.

HYPERTROPHIC PYLORIC STENOSIS

Pyloric stenosis occurs in approximately 1 of 300 to 1000 live births. Its cause is obscure. Male infants are affected about four times as frequently as females, and the disease seems to have a predilection for the first-born child. There is a familial tendency, with a 2.5% to 20% incidence of pyloric stenosis in children of affected parents; the variation in incidence depends on the gender of the affected parent and child.[86] It has been speculated that hypertrophy of the circular muscles of the pylorus results from propulsion of milk curds against the spastic pyloric canal, producing edema, additional spasm, and subsequent hypertrophy of the musculature, leading to complete obstruction. Some researchers have postulated that the muscle hypertrophy is a response to vagal stimulation. This is somewhat substantiated by the observation that infants undergoing surgery for esophageal atresia and tracheoesophageal fistula seem to have a higher incidence of pyloric stenosis, a result perhaps of vagal nerve irritation in the operative field. No infectious agent has been isolated despite the apparent seasonal incidence of the disease. The clinical onset of bile-free projectile vomiting at 2 to 8 weeks of age in a first-born male strongly suggests the diagnosis of congenital hypertrophic pyloric stenosis. Occasionally, the onset is insidious and these babies can present to the pediatrician as perplexing feeding problems. A typical history reveals intermittent vomiting that gradually increases in frequency and intensity over a week, until the baby vomits most ingested feedings with impressive force.

Abdominal examination is carried out with the stomach empty. If the infant has not just vomited, the physician may need to use a nasogastric tube to ensure an adequate examination. The baby can be given a pacifier for relaxation. Visible peristalsis may be observed moving across the upper abdomen. The examiner stands to the left, elevating the baby's feet with his left hand to relax the abdominal muscles and then palpates gently in the right upper quadrant. The pyloric olive is palpable to the experienced examiner in 90% of patients, and radiographic studies are usually not needed. If pyloric stenosis is suspected but the olive cannot be palpated, the diagnostic procedure of choice is abdominal ultrasonography, which is more than 90% accurate in centers experienced with this technique.[87] A UGI series is usually reserved for those patients with vomiting but a normal ultrasonographic examination, in whom another cause of obstruction is suspected. Hyperbilirubinemia is seen in

8% of babies with pyloric stenosis. Almost all the bilirubin is of an indirect type and may be related to a decreased level of hepatic glycuronyl transferase.[88] Jaundice clears after pyloromyotomy.

Infants with pyloric stenosis are conveniently grouped according to their clinical condition at the time they are seen by the surgeon. About one-half are well hydrated and in a satisfactory nutritional state. Serum electrolytes are normal, and the urine, although concentrated, is of adequate volume. These babies can undergo surgical correction without preoperative preparation. For the remaining infants, preparation before surgery is necessary. The typical pattern of electrolyte disturbance is that of mild or moderate metabolic alkalosis. The hypokalemia may not be reflected in the serum electrolytes, but potassium supplements must be provided before the alkalosis can be corrected. Salt-losing adrenogenital syndrome can present with symptoms identical to pyloric stenosis. However, this condition is characterized by an elevated serum potassium and metabolic acidosis.

These moderately dehydrated infants usually can be corrected within 12 hours with 5% Dextrose–half-normal saline solution at a rate of 0.5 to 2 times that of maintenance. After urine production is certain, potassium should be replaced at 2 mEq/kg for the 12-hour period of therapy.

A few infants present with severe dehydration and malnutrition and are often well below their birth weight. In this group, extensive rehydration is mandatory before surgery. The infants are profoundly alkalotic and potassium deficient. Their protein stores are depleted, urine is scanty, and they may be anemic. Intensive therapy for 2 to 3 days is required to bring these infants into metabolic balance. Fluids, electrolytes, colloid, and even blood may be necessary. Fortunately, it is rare to see such children today.

A Ramstedt–Fredet pyloromyotomy is best performed through a transverse skin incision placed in the right upper quadrant of the abdomen. This short, safe, surgical procedure accomplishes division of the hypertrophic circular muscles of the gastric outlet and reestablishes patency of the pyloric channel (Fig. 44-10). In most cases, glucose water feedings can be reinstituted 6 to 8 hours postoperatively. If the child tolerates the first feeding, slow advancement of the volume of his regular formula is encouraged. The infant commonly vomits a few times postoperatively, but this should not alter his feeding advancement. Explanation to the parents that this vomiting is common can allay their anxiety. The child is generally ready for discharge on the second or third postoperative day, when he attains adequate oral intake. Typically, the babies enjoy a growth spurt in the immediate postoperative weeks, much to the satisfaction of the parents.

DUODENAL ATRESIA, STENOSIS, AND ANNULAR PANCREAS

Duodenal obstruction may be complete or partial and results from intrinsic causes or external compression.[89] An intraluminal diaphragm can cause partial, intermittent obstruction, which is difficult to recognize. Only a carefully performed UGI series outlines an intraluminal web and determines the site of obstruction. Annular pancreas, duodenal stenosis, and congenital bands are other causes of partial duodenal obstruction in which the need for early surgical intervention is more apparent.

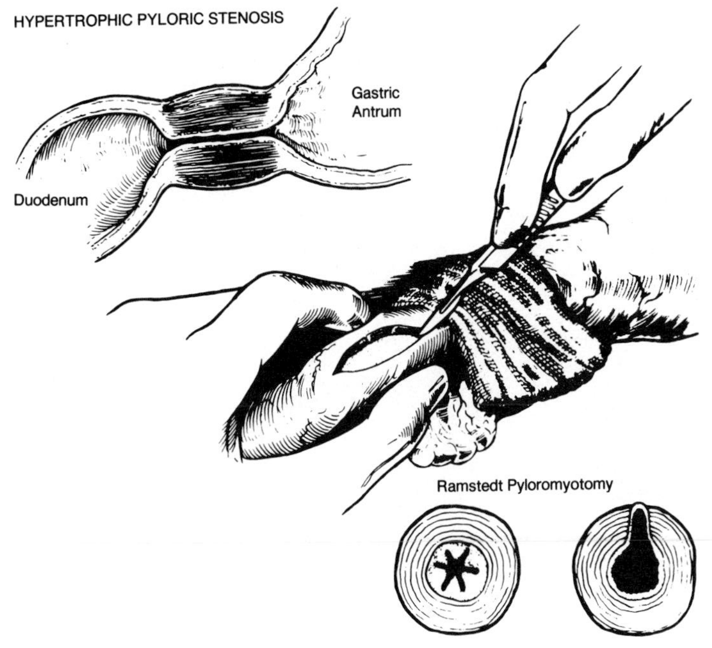

FIG. 44–10. A Ramstedt pyloromyotomy is made through all layers of the pylorus except the mucosa. The cross section demonstrates how the mucosa of the pylorus expands into the defect created, enlarging the cross-sectional diameter of the pyloric channel.

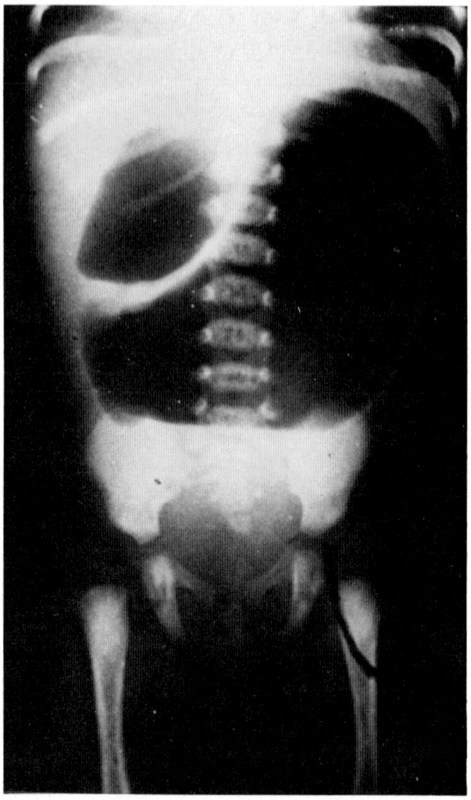

FIG. 44–11. Characteristic double bubble of congenital duodenal obstruction.

Duodenal atresia results in complete obstruction. In instances of complete duodenal obstruction, swallowed air is prevented from passing beyond the duodenum, and the middle and lower abdomen are scaphoid. The characteristic x-ray finding is that of a double bubble of ingested air filling the stomach and blind-ending duodenum (Fig. 44-11). Duodenal atresia is often associated with trisomy 21.

Unless the underlying cause of obstruction is related to malrotation, an initial period of nasogastric drainage and resuscitation with intravenous fluids and electrolytes is appropriate before duodenal obstruction is surgically corrected. Surgical therapy is tailored to the particular lesion encountered. The intraluminal web can be resected through a transduodenal approach. It may be necessary for the surgeon to perform a gastrotomy or duodenotomy, through which a Foley catheter with the balloon minimally inflated is passed, to identify the site at which the web is attached.

Some stenotic lesions can be managed by local duodenoplasty, but obstruction from duodenal atresia requires bypass for relief. Obstruction secondary to duodenal atresia or annular pancreas is best treated by creating a duodenoduodenostomy.[90] A duodenojejunostomy is an alternative method to establish intestinal continuity.

JEJUNOILEAL ATRESIA

Atresia of the bowel probably results from an ischemic insult to the intestine during its development.[91] The atresia may be discrete, involving only a short segment of jejunum or ileum (Fig. 44-12), or it may involve the intestine over many centimeters.[92] Atretic areas are sometimes multiple, and although the intervening bowel is normal, considerable length may be missing. Abdominal distention and bile-stained vomitus are the usual presenting symptoms. Radiographs show air–fluid levels distributed throughout the abdomen (Fig. 44-13). In cases of distal ileal obstruction, the contrast enema adds confirmation, showing the typical microcolon.

A short period of restoration with fluids, electrolytes, and colloid may be necessary, but this should never exceed a few hours. The method of surgical correction depends on the intraoperative findings. If the intestinal length is normal, the dilated proximal end is excised back to near-normal-caliber bowel, and an end-to-back anastomosis is performed. In the infant with a large gap atresia, the proximal end is ta-

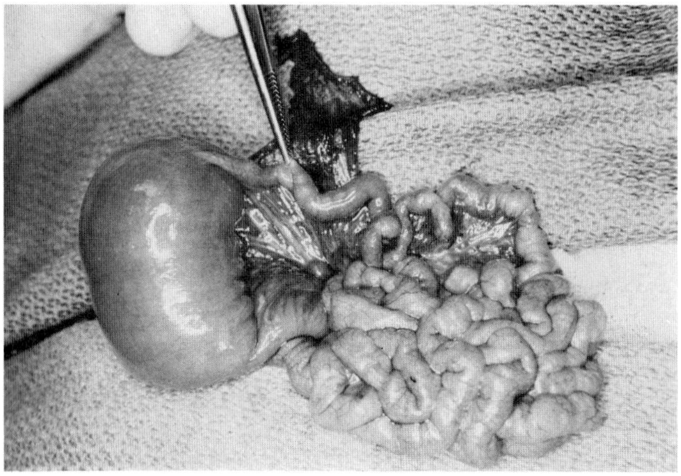

FIG. 44–12. In this patient with jejunal atresia, a dilated proximal segment and a narrow distal jejunum are evident.

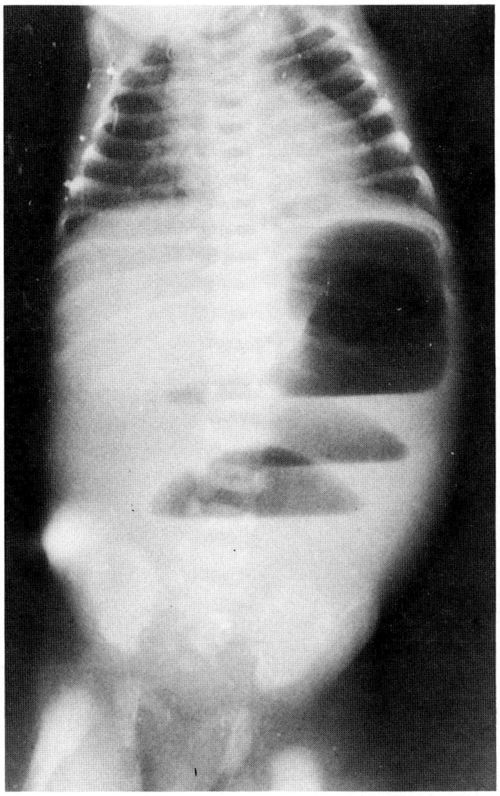

FIG. 44–13. An upright, abdominal x-ray film of a patient with jejunal atresia shows gastric distention and approximately three loops of bowel with no gas beyond the obstruction.

pered and anastomosis accomplished.[93,94] The end-to-side reconstruction, described by Bishop and Koop, has proved safe and effective and has the added advantage of providing access to the gastrointestinal tract for irrigations postoperatively.[81] This type of repair is particularly helpful if there is a major disparity in the size of the ends of the intestine. A Mikulicz enterostomy or simple end-enterostomy may be lifesaving in critically ill, depleted newborns with distal bowel obstruction.

Incomplete obstruction resulting from stenosis of the bowel can be puzzling and hazardous because there is a confusing clinical picture. The infants feed poorly, occasionally vomit, or become distended without pattern. These symptoms continue despite changes in the formula. The pediatrician may consider food allergies, nonspecific failure to thrive, and even a nervous mother as underlying causes. The obstruction finally becomes complete or the bowel perforates. Surgical exploration may be needed to confirm a diagnosis of ileal stenosis, and this approach is considered even if x-ray examinations of the intestine have been normal when the clinical course of the infant suggests this diagnosis. Cure is achieved by appropriate intestinal tailoring procedures such as a Y–V plasty or longitudinal incision and transverse closure (*i.e.*, Heineke–Mikulicz principle).

MECONIUM PLUG SYNDROME

The meconium plug syndrome is a benign form of colon obstruction in the neonate caused by a firm white plug of mucus. These babies usually present with abdominal distention. Abdominal x-ray films reveal distended loops of bowel. A barium enema shows a long radiolucency within the descending colon. The plug is passed after the barium enema or a saline rectal irrigation. Although meconium plug syndrome is found in otherwise completely normal infants, because it can be difficult to differentiate from Hirschsprung disease and to rule out cystic fibrosis, many surgeons routinely perform a rectal biopsy and obtain a sweat chloride test in infants with meconium plug syndrome.

MECONIUM PERITONITIS

Meconium peritonitis usually follows antenatal intestinal obstruction and perforation of the bowel above the obstruction in conditions such as bowel atresia, volvulus, meconium ileus, and neonatal Hirschsprung disease. If it occurs early in gestation, the perforation may have sealed off, but the chemical peritonitis gives rise to tiny scattered foreign-body reactions that may become calcified and be visible radiographically. If the perforation occurs closer to birth, calcifications are usually not seen on radiographs, and chemical peritonitis may be followed by bacterial peritonitis. More frequently, the presenting signs are those of intestinal obstruction.

MECONIUM ILEUS

Intestinal obstruction resulting from viscid meconium impacted in the terminal ileum is seen as the earliest manifestation of cystic fibrosis. This problem affects about 10% of the cystic fibrosis population. Infants with meconium ileus subsequently develop other complications of their underlying disease, but the later respiratory sequelae are not necessarily more severe.[95]

The clinical presentation of meconium ileus is not unlike that seen with other forms of distal intestinal obstruction. Abdominal distention and bile-stained vomitus are characteristic. The upright radiograph of the abdomen is especially helpful in this form of intestinal obstruction in the newborn. The characteristic soap bubble mass in the right lower abdomen and a paucity of air–fluid levels despite the presence of many gas-filled loops of intestine is pathognomonic (Fig. 44-14). The air–fluid levels characteristic of obstruction do not develop because air is trapped by the tenacious meconium and a clear interface is not produced. The contrast enema shows a microcolon, unused because of the distal ileal obstruction. Concretions of meconium in the terminal ileum immediately proximal to the ileocecal valve are often seen.

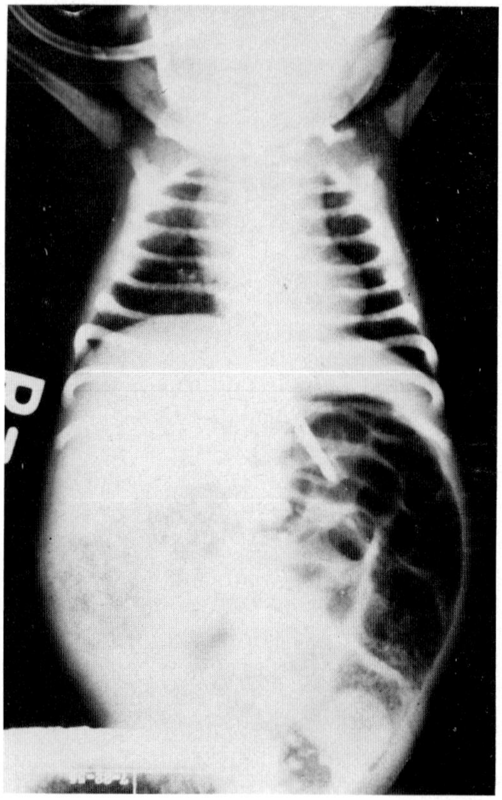

FIG. 44–14. An x-ray film of a newborn infant with meconium ileus reveals many gas-filled loops, but little fluid is seen. The right lower quadrant is filled with a large loop of intestine distended by meconium. Gas trapped in the meconium gives the typical ground-glass appearance.

Surgical intervention may be required for relief of obstruction, but enemas of Gastrografin often eliminate the obstructing mass of meconium.[96] At our institution, the Gastrografin is diluted 1:4 with saline so that the complications of a hyperosmolar fluid enema are avoided. This radiopaque contrast material contains a wetting agent (*i.e.,* Tween 80) in which the thick meconium is soluble. If the Gastrografin can be successfully advanced through the microcolon and into the obstructed distal ileum, there is reasonable expectation that meconium will be passed spontaneously with relief of obstruction.[97] When the first attempt moves some meconium out, but the infant's obstruction is not completely relieved, a second enema is justified several hours later. Complete removal of the meconium may take several Gastrografin enemas over a few days. If these maneuvers fail to relieve the obstruction or if meconium peritonitis is present, surgical exploration is the only acceptable treatment.

If surgical correction is necessary, technical problems associated with evacuating the tarlike meconium from the distended ileum and establishing intestinal continuity between the dilated proximal intestine and the distal microcolon have been solved in various ways. Irrigation through an ileostomy with dilute acetylcysteine has proved effective in some infants. A rapid and safe anastomosis involving the Bishop–Koop technique is well suited for this problem.[81] A Mikulicz enterostomy has the virtue of speed, while providing decompression and establishment of continuity. These techniques allow access to the distal intestine for postoperative irrigations with acetylcysteine. With use, the colon has the potential to function normally, and the vent established by the Mikulicz or Bishop–Koop procedure is closed surgically. In selected infants, resection and primary anastomosis can be performed at the first operation. In the postoperative period, the infant is subject to respiratory difficulty secondary to impacted secretions. These may require tracheal suctioning or bronchoscopy for relief. When oral feedings are instituted, exogenous pancreatic supplements are provided so that digestion and use of calories are ensured.

DUPLICATIONS

An uncommon cause of intestinal obstruction in the newborn is that arising secondary to duplications of the bowel. These can exist at any level of the intestine and may cause obstruction when the lumen is compromised by the gradually expanding duplication or by the duplication acting as a focus for segmental intestinal volvulus. Because they occur on the mesenteric aspect of the bowel, duplications are intimately involved with the blood supply to the normal intestine. Small, cystic duplications are easily resected with a segment of the adjacent bowel.[98] However, extensive fusiform or intramural duplications may tax the surgeon's ingenuity. In these instances, resection of the common wall, with creation of a single conduit, may enable the surgeon to preserve an extensive segment of normal intestine.[99] Gastric mucosa can exist within a duplication and result in gastrointestinal hemorrhage.[100] This cause of gastrointestinal bleeding is considered in the evaluation of a baby with melena.

HIRSCHSPRUNG DISEASE

The clinical presentation of Hirschsprung disease (*i.e.,* aganglionic megacolon) may be subtle and go unrecognized for months or years until the classic symptoms of constipation and abdominal distention are unmistakable. However, the history of constipation goes back to the early days of life in most patients with Hirschsprung disease. The consequences of aganglionosis can be life threatening in the newborn period.[101] The absence of ganglion cells modifies neuromuscular conduction and prevents proper evacuation of the bowel. Abdominal distention or debilitating enterocolitis brings the infant to the surgeon's attention.

Failure of an infant to pass meconium in the first 36 hours of life should alert the pediatrician to the possibility of Hirschsprung disease. Retention of a meconium plug, requiring mechanical assistance for its evacuation, is another presumptive sign that the colon may be aganglionic. A positive barium enema, even in a newborn, can be a reliable indication of Hirschsprung disease.[102] The characteristic terminal narrow segment, with transition to dilated bowel in the area of the rectosigmoid, is a classic finding in older children but may not be present in neonates. Anal dilation produced by a rectal examination may confuse the findings. A normal barium enema in the neonate does not exclude the diagnosis of aganglionosis, and confirmatory evidence must be obtained by rectal biopsy.

Several techniques of biopsy have been described, but any one that provides an adequate specimen of the rectal wall can establish the diagnosis. The absence of ganglion cells in the submucosal or muscular plexus confirms the diagnosis. Experienced pathologists can interpret the more superficial biopsies, which include only the submucosal tissue. The advantage of partial-thickness biopsy is that there is less intramural scarring to complicate the definitive surgical procedure for correction of Hirschsprung disease. A suction biopsy technique is available that is readily adapted for use in infants.[103] This bedside procedure provides adequate submucosal tissue for interpretation by an experienced pediatric pathologist. A histochemical technique estimating acetylcholinesterase activity has been helpful in establishing the diagnosis in some centers and has the added advantage of requiring only tiny fragments of bowel tissue.[104]

The clinical presentation of Hirschsprung disease varies. Intestinal obstruction is not always typical. Enterocolitis is often the presenting complaint in a newborn, and this may be confused with NEC, seen primarily in premature infants with respiratory distress. The effects of enterocolitis associated with Hirschsprung disease can be devastating unless recognized and treated appropriately.[105] Enterocolitis often presents with diarrhea and signs of collapse. Sepsis may be fatal if not promptly recognized and treated. The enterocolitis can sometimes be controlled by careful rectal lavage with quarter-normal solutions of saline. It is vital that the volume of solutions instilled be recovered during the lavage.

Whether the symptoms are those of obstruction or enterocolitis, after resuscitating the infant, the safest course of action is the performance of a colostomy in an area of bowel containing ganglion cells. Most babies have a transition somewhere in the rectosigmoid, and a high sigmoid colostomy usually ensures normal innervation.[106] The presence of ganglion cells at the site of the colostomy should be verified by biopsy at the time of colostomy formation. In desperately ill infants, the condition may preclude a controlled laparotomy with frozen-section confirmation of the transition area. In these babies, a right transverse colostomy ensures that ganglionic bowel has been exteriorized in 98%. The few remaining infants have total colonic aganglionosis or aganglionic small bowel and present special problems in management. In these infants, barium enema is helpful, showing marked foreshortening of the entire colon. The basic surgical principle is to achieve exteriorization of the most distal normally innervated bowel.

Definitive surgical therapy is deferred until the infants are managed through the initial crisis and have achieved a weight of about 7 to 9 kg. At that time, the ganglionic intestine is transposed to the anus by one of the several pull-through techniques now available. These include the classic operation described by Swenson[107] and the modification popularized by Duhamel.[108] Many centers favor the endorectal pull-through procedure of Soave.[109] Several centers have advocated surgery in the newborn period with a pull-through operation and no colostomy.[110] The early results are promising, but the follow-up period has been too short to allow proper scrutiny.

If the physician suspects Hirschsprung disease, the diagnosis is made early. The outlook for these infants is favorable because currently available operations have now become standardized.[111] Minor constipation is the most frequent sequela of surgery. Most babies with congenital megacolon achieve excellent functional results.[112]

NECROTIZING ENTEROCOLITIS

Necrotizing enterocolitis is a condition predominantly seen in premature infants, which is characterized by partial- or full-thickness intestinal ischemia, usually involving the terminal ileum. The cause is unknown, but the common pathway appears to be a combination of factors that leads to intestinal ischemia.[113] Studies suggest that the combination of ischemia and reperfusion injury may be a factor in the development of NEC.[114] Known risk factors include prematurity, neonatal stress, formula feedings, and surgery in the newborn period. Other factors considered to increase the risk of NEC are umbilical artery catheterization, infection with certain types of bacteria, and hypoalbuminemia.[115]

Although the cause is uncertain, the histopathology is well established. Initially, the disease begins as mucosal ischemia, with resultant sloughing of this layer. As the disease progresses, gas develops within the muscular layers (Fig. 44-15) and may be seen on x-ray films as pneumatosis cystoides intestinalis. If full-thickness necrosis occurs, perforation and peritonitis develop. The rapidity of disease progression differs in each patient, but those who perforate usually do so within the first few days of the disease.

The diagnosis of NEC is based on clinical assessment and x-ray studies. The earliest signs are often an intolerance of feedings with vomiting. The vomitus of about one-half of the patients is bile stained. Abdominal distention is a common early finding. Hematest-positive stools help confirm the diagnosis, but blood may be absent or a late finding. Abdominal wall erythema and a palpable abdominal mass are commonly

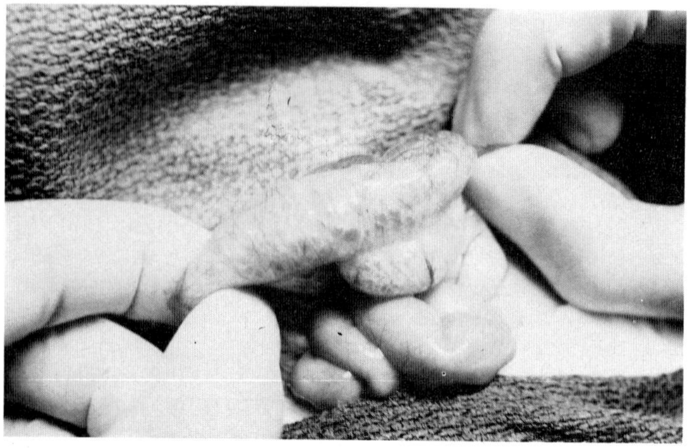

FIG. 44–15. Operative photograph of a loop of intestine affected by necrotizing enterocolitis. The gas in the seromuscular layer distorts the segment of intestine. Normal loops of uninvolved intestine also are evident.

late findings and signify more extensive disease. The use of paracentesis to choose surgical candidates has been advocated by Kosloske[116] and Ricketts.[117]

Radiographic findings in early NEC may show only separated loops of distended intestine, suggesting bowel wall thickening. Pneumatosis cystoides intestinalis is pathognomonic for NEC and may be present early in the disease process. A persistent large loop of intestine seen on a series of x-ray films has been used by some as an indication for surgery, but in our experience, many children with persistent loops have been successfully treated medically.

Hepatic portal venous gas usually implies a particularly severe or extensive form of the disease, and more than 80% of children with this finding required surgery. Free intraperitoneal air is an absolute indication for surgery, although pneumoperitoneum from air dissecting down from the chest in the ventilator-dependent child must be ruled out so that an unnecessary laparotomy is not performed (dissecting air − PO_2 of air in abdomen ≈ FiO_2 provided to infant by the ventilator; pneumoperitoneum peritoneum − PO_2 of air in peritoneum = 21 torr).

Initial management of the child with NEC without pneumoperitoneum is standardized. The child receives nothing orally, the stomach is decompressed with a gastric sump tube, and intravenous antibiotics are begun. Antibiotics must cover gram-negative and gram-positive aerobic organisms, but anaerobic bacteria coverage is less necessary.[118] Fungal infection is common after surgical treatment of NEC, and oral Mycostatin should be given postoperatively.[119] The best method of determining which babies require surgery consists of repeated physical examinations by the same examiner; flat and left lateral decubitus abdominal radiographs every 4 to 6 hours for detection of pneumoperitoneum; careful monitoring of the respiratory status and acid–base balance; and monitoring of the leukocyte and platelet counts for signs of sepsis.

In our experience, indications for surgery include pneumoperitoneum, persistent acidosis (*i.e.*, *p*H less than 7.2), rapidly worsening pulmonary status, and unremitting neutropenia or thrombocytopenia.[120] Because many of our patients with hepatoportal venous gas come to surgery, we operate on these children if they do not improve promptly on medical therapy. Our experience is similar to that of others in that mortality is higher in patients who have perforated before surgery, and it is therefore better to operate before perforation has occurred.

Surgery in these infants should be expeditious and conservative. The frankly necrotic or perforated intestine should be removed and ileostomies formed. Although routine primary anastomosis in NEC has been advocated by some, most surgeons prefer ileostomy formation in almost all patients.[121] When massive resection is necessary, the chance for the child's survival is limited, but the premature infant's intestine still has potential for growth and adaptation, and rarely is the entire intestine involved in the disease. Drainage of the peritoneum under local anesthesia in the infant weighing under 1500 g has been advocated for perforated NEC by Ein and colleagues, although most babies managed by this method eventually require formal laparotomy.[122]

If ileostomy is performed, the mucous fistula should be exteriorized close to the functioning ileostomy, and closure should be planned when the child is large enough (*i.e.*, approximately 2 kg) and at a sufficient time after the event (*i.e.*, at least 4 to 6 weeks) to minimize the possibility of recurrence.[123] Because of a 20% incidence of stricture after medical or surgical treatment of NEC in our patients, barium enema is performed in all our surgical patients before ileostomy closure and any medical patients with feeding difficulties. Other physicians have advocated a UGI study for all babies with medically treated NEC before feeding.[124]

The children are not fed orally for at least 2 to 3 weeks after the onset of NEC, and it frequently takes more than 1 month for those patients successfully treated medically to attain adequate oral caloric intake. Hyperalimentation is mandatory in these children as soon as NEC is diagnosed, and we prefer central intravenous alimentation for most children with NEC.

The long-term success rate for treatment for NEC has been good, despite long hospitalization for gastrointestinal adaptation when massive resection is necessary. The quoted survival rate for children with medically treated NEC is now more than 80%, and the survival rate for those requiring surgery is approximately 50%. At CNMC, the survival rate for NEC has steadily increased since 1980 and is 80% for the surgical and medical groups combined.[120] Successful medical treatment may be followed by late-onset intestinal obstruction due to scarring, and an interesting long-term complication of ileocolic anastomosis in infancy is the development of anastomotic ulcers. These ulcers present as painless rectal bleeding or melena years after the NEC surgery.[125] Necrotizing enterocolitis is discussed in more detail in Chapter 37.

IMPERFORATE ANUS

Imperforate anus affects male and female infants with equal frequency and occurs in approximately 1 of every 20,000 live births. The lesion results from a failure of differentiation of the urogenital sinus and cloaca. Associated anomalies include urogenital, cardiac, spinal cord, and esophageal malformations, especially esophageal atresia and tracheoesophageal fistula. The latter lesion occurs in 10% of patients with imperforate anus.[126]

Imperforate anus can be broadly classified as high or low, depending on the relation of the distal rectal pouch to the levator complex. High imperforate anus in either gender implies that the rectal pouch is above the sphincter muscle complex. Low imperforate anus implies that the rectum has descended past this level, with an abnormal location in the perineum. Because the levator musculature is actually funnel shaped, these associations are somewhat approximate and should be considered as guidelines. Infants with low imperforate anus can be expected to have rectal continence after repair. The sphincter muscle complex must be precisely located and preserved in infants with high imperforate anus and a normal relation to the rectum established surgically for continence to be achieved.

Eighty percent of girls have imperforate anus of the low type. Usually, the rectum terminates by means of a fistula anterior to the normal location of the anus on the perineum (Fig. 44-16*A*), on the vaginal fourchette (Fig 44-16*B*), or low in the vagina. Because the termination of the colon is accessible and colostomy is not

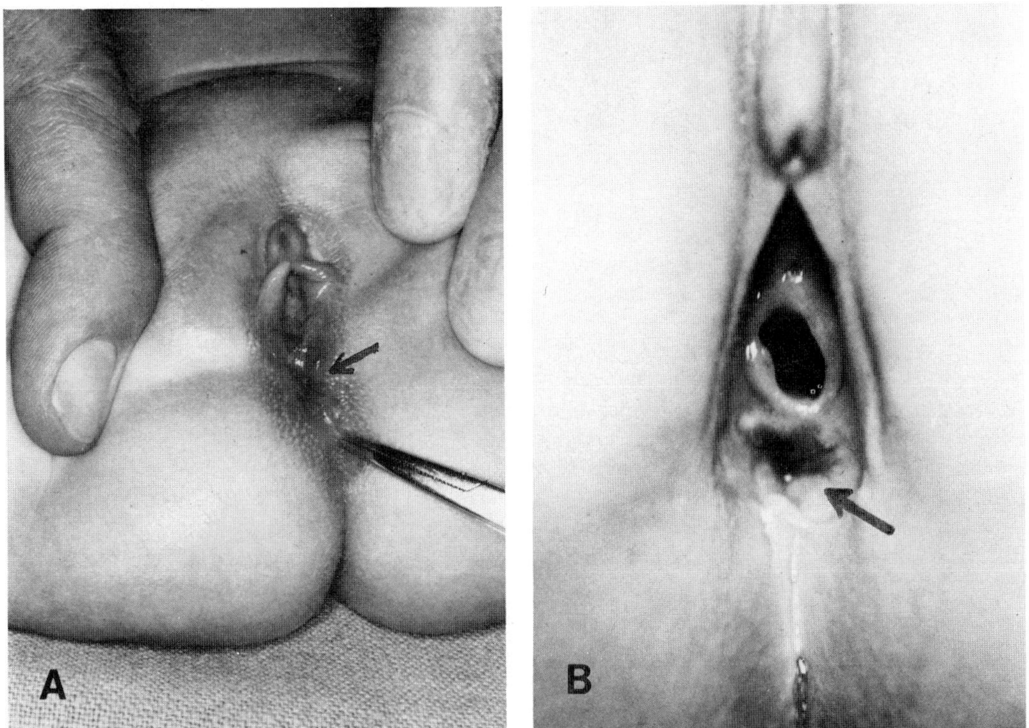

FIG. 44–16. (A) Female infant with an imperforate anus. The *arrow* demonstrates the opening of the perineal fistula. The clamp is at the point where a normal anus would open. **(B)** Close-up photograph of imperforate anus and an introital fistula just inside the labia minora and immediately beneath the hymenal ring. This is the most common form of fistulous opening in a female imperforate anus.

necessary, early therapy can be directed at decompression of the bowel by catheter irrigation and dilation of the fistula.

It is possible to transpose the anus from the posterior vagina or perineum to its normal position in the newborn period. This is not always necessary if the bowel is easily decompressed or the baby can stool spontaneously through the fistula. A judicious interval is appropriate to allow the baby to grow before surgery is carried out. Definitive repair usually can be accomplished by means of perineal operation, because the rectum is properly related to the muscles of continence. In instances in which the fistula cannot be identified, it is usually high in the vagina and not accessible to dilation or surgical revision in the newborn period. In this 20% of female infants, a colostomy is necessary. Definitive therapy for high imperforate anus in the female is deferred until the baby weighs 7 to 9 kg.

In boys, the incidences of high and low imperforate anus are equal. Approximately one-half of the babies present with a fistula placed ectopically on the perineum, anterior to the normal location of the anus. The fistula can terminate as far forward as the penoscrotal junction. At birth, the opening of the fistula is not always apparent, and an interval of 12 to 24 hours may be required until the bowel fills with air or meconium reaches the most distal point in the gastrointestinal tract (Fig. 44-17*A*). When a spot of meconium or beads of mucus can be identified on the perineum, there is assurance that the rectal pouch is low, implying that the rectum has traversed the sphincter muscle complex and continence is expected after repair. In babies with these findings, a perineal anoplasty in the newborn period accomplishes decompression of the bowel and no colostomy is needed.

If no fistula is visible on the perineum, the male infant can be presumed to have a high imperforate anus. The fistula usually communicates with the posterior urethra. A colostomy is needed for decompression, and the definitive pull-through operation is generally deferred until the baby is about 1 year of age. Improved results in children with high imperforate anus are being reported with the use of the posterior sagittal anoplasty, described by Pena and DeVries, at approximately 1 year of age.[127]

The use of an x-ray film with the infant in the upside-down position (*i.e.*, Wangensteen–Rice position) is limited in the diagnosis of the level of imperforate anus (Fig. 44-17*B*) and is primarily of historic inter-

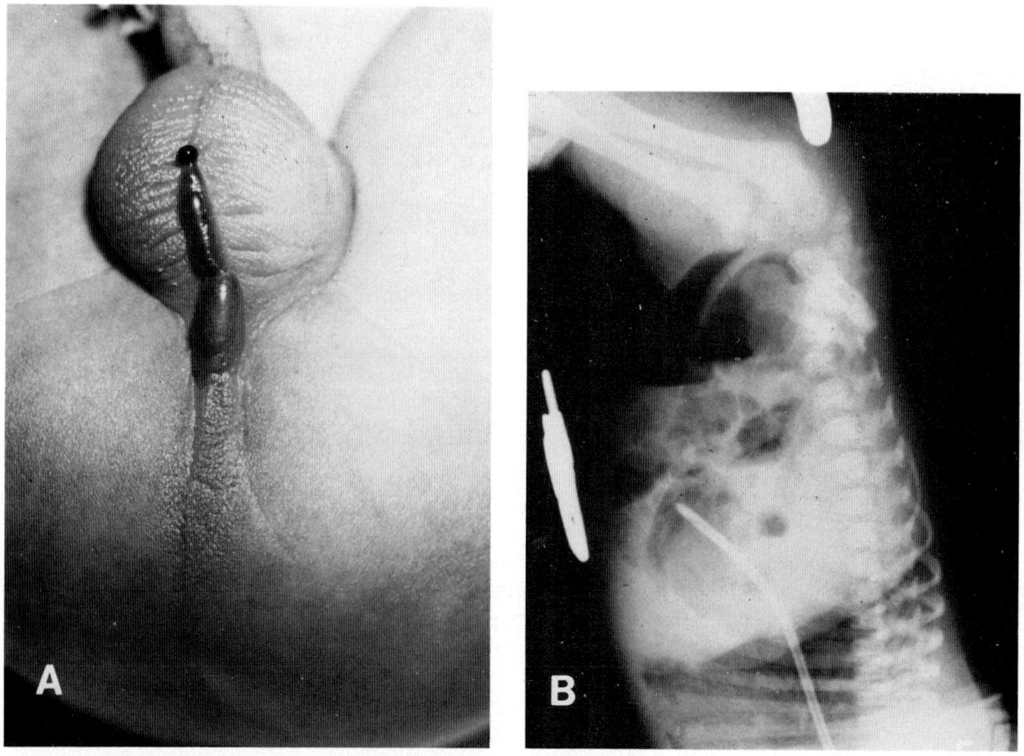

FIG. 44–17. (A) Imperforate anus and partly covered perineal fistula that opens on the scrotum always occurs with a low pouch. The rectum has traversed the levator sling musculature properly. **(B)** Upside-down radiographic technique of Wangensteen–Rice using a metal marker at the anus shows the distance between the rectal pouch and the anal skin. It is clearly above a line drawn between the pubis and lower border of the sacrum. There is a second gas-containing space anterior to the rectum. This indicates the presence of a rectourethral fistula with air trapped in the bladder.

est.[128] Although it may help when it shows the rectal pouch at or near the perineum, it can also be misleading if the distal rectum is filled with meconium that prevents air from reaching the most distal aspect of this pouch, and complete reliance on this view for the selection of therapy is ill advised. Ultrasonography may be helpful in locating the rectal pouch.

Needle aspiration for detecting meconium in the blind perineum, with or without injection of contrast material, has been advocated by some physicians but should be performed only by the pediatric surgeon responsible for the child's care.[129] If there is no fistula and a low imperforate anus cannot be diagnosed with certainty, a colostomy is advised. Risk of a colostomy performed for a low imperforate anus is preferable to prejudicing the chances of a successful pull-through procedure by an ill-advised perineal exploration in the newborn period. With realization of the importance of the accurate transposition of the rectal pouch to the perineum, successful functional restoration has become the rule.

IMPERFORATE HYMEN AND VAGINAL ATRESIA

Errors in the development of the vagina range from simple defects (*e.g.*, imperforate hymen) to complex anomalies, including distal, proximal, and complete vaginal atresia.[130] These anomalies may result from abnormal development of the Müllerian ducts or the urogenital sinus. Most often, the diagnosis is apparent on physical examination of the perineum. The hymen is visibly bulging in babies with imperforate hymen. Accumulated secretions in an obstructed reproductive tract create hydrocolpos, which can be appreciated as a pelvic or abdominal mass by ultrasonography. The surgical approach depends on the severity of the defect. Simple excision by a perineal approach suffices for imperforate hymen and low transverse septum. More severe forms of vaginal atresia mandate complex reconstructive surgery, which may include mobilizing vaginal remnants down to the perineum, creation of skin flaps, or forming a neovagina from a bowel segment.

OVARIAN CYSTS AND MASSES

The increased frequency of prenatal ultrasound has lead to increased detection of ovarian cysts.[131,132] Surgical excision was previously recommended for all cysts larger than 5 cm in diameter because of the perceived risk of ovarian torsion. On the basis of serial ultrasound examinations, it has become evident that many of these lesions resolve spontaneously without apparent sequelae. However, complex cysts of any size mandate prompt surgical intervention.[133] Surgeons have four options for managing simple ovarian cysts:

1. Follow the lesion sonographically, and operate if it fails to disappear after several months.
2. Drain the cyst percutaneously by ultrasound-guided needle aspiration, and periodically check on it sonographically.
3. Drain the cyst by laparoscopic-guided needle aspiration and periodically check on it by using ultrasound.
4. Excise the cyst by conventional surgery.

AMBIGUOUS GENITALIA

Normal sexual differentiation occurs in the sixth fetal week (see Chap. 41). Any disruption of the orderly steps in sexual differentiation may be reflected clinically as variants of the intergender syndromes. These may be classified as true hermaphroditism with ovarian and testicular gonadal tissue, male pseudohermaphroditism with testicles only, female pseudohermaphroditism with ovarian tissue only, and mixed gonadal dysgenesis with usually undeveloped or imperfectly formed gonads. Most of these clinical forms present with ambiguous external genitalia, which may or may not be obvious at birth.[134]

When the physician is confronted with a newborn infant with ambiguous genitalia, the following diagnostic steps should be initiated within the first 24 hours of life:

1. Review the genetic background and family history.
2. Delineate the anatomic structures by physical examination and x-ray studies.
3. Perform chromosome studies.
4. Determine biochemical factors in serum and urine.
5. When necessary, perform laparotomy and gonadal biopsy.

By employing the two criteria of gonadal symmetry and cytologic analysis, most infants can be assigned to one of the four categories accurately within the first day of life, avoiding errors in gender assignment. Genetic females should be assigned the female gender, regardless of the degree of virilization. For genetic males, the gender assignment depends on the size of the phallus, because satisfactory surgical techniques do not exist to reconstruct an inadequate phallus.

Certain plastic surgical procedures are required to harmonize the external genitalia with the gender of rearing. Operations to reduce the size of the enlarged clitoris preserve the sensation and function of the clitoris. Plastic procedures to exteriorize the vagina or separate it from the urethra are necessary in patients born with a urogenital sinus. If the male assignment is appropriate for an infant with ambiguous genitalia, hypospadias repair will be necessary. When contradictory gonads or ovotestes are present, removal of these structures prevents the possibility of hormone secretion or malignant degeneration. For some teenage male patients with inadequate or absent gonads, the insertion of testicular prostheses may be psychologically beneficial. Children with endocrine insufficiency may require lifetime exogenous supplementation. Prompt recognition of infants with intersexual anomalies, followed by appropriate gender assignment and proper treatment, prevents the social and psychologic derangements that have occurred in the past because of delayed diagnosis or inappropriate gender assignment.

OBSTRUCTIVE JAUNDICE

A variety of neonatal cholestatic syndromes overlap in presentation with obstructive jaundice from biliary atresia. Many conditions causing direct hyperbilirubinemia have been grouped under the term "neonatal hepatitis." To some extent, this is misleading because hepatitis implies an inflammatory process within the liver. It is preferable to separate the infants into one group with cholestatic syndromes and another group with extrahepatic obstruction, such as biliary atresia. In the former group, specific disease entities are further identified by serologic testing or metabolic screening (see Chap. 37). A common metabolic condition that causes neonatal jaundice is α_1-antitrypsin deficiency. Screening for this inherited disorder is recommended for all infants with conjugated hyperbilirubinemia. Infants with cystic fibrosis may present with obstructive jaundice that mimics biliary atresia, and infants receiving intravenous hyperalimentation for weeks or months may develop cholestatic jaundice.

Advances in hepatobiliary imaging using ^{99m}Tc scans have made it possible to differentiate cholestatic from obstructive jaundice with a high degree of accuracy, particularly after administration of phenobarbital for 5 days before the scan.[135] Numerous diagnostic blood tests have been recommended, but none is completely reliable and most represent unnecessary procrastination. The infant who has an obstructive profile on liver function tests and hepatic scan, with a negative evaluation for cystic fibrosis and α_1-antitrypsin deficiency, should be evaluated with an abdominal ultrasound to identify the gallbladder and extrahepatic biliary ducts and should have a percutaneous liver biopsy. Absence of the extrahepatic duct on ultrasound and the finding of extrahepatic cholestasis on biopsy mandate surgical exploration.

An initial exploration is made through a limited right subcostal incision. If a normal gallbladder is seen, a transcholecystic cholangiogram is obtained. If the extrahepatic biliary tree appears normal, a liver biopsy is obtained, and the incision is closed.

If the gallbladder is atretic or the liver is obviously cirrhotic, suggesting an obstructive process, the incision is enlarged so that the extrahepatic biliary system can be formally explored. Any remnant of the gallbladder or extrahepatic biliary duct through which a cholangiogram can be performed is used. In the infant with extrahepatic biliary atresia, only threadlike remnants of the biliary tree are identified. The atretic ducts are transected at their confluence, deep into the porta hepatis, and an anastomosis is created to a segment of the small intestine. This procedure is called a portoenterostomy (*i.e.*, Kasai procedure). When the operation is performed in infants younger than 3 months of age, there is reasonable expectation that bile will drain into the intestine.[136] Children who fail to drain bile after the portoenterostomy may be rescued by liver transplantation before 1 year of age, although the complication rate in these infants is higher than in older children with liver transplants.[137]

Other causes of jaundice that can be relieved surgically are choledochal cysts, common duct stones, and inspissated sludge in the bile ducts. True choledochal cysts are rarely encountered in the newborn period but should be treated by cyst excision and intestinal drainage of the hepatic duct, using a technique similar to the Kasai procedure. Bile peritonitis after spontaneous rupture of the bile duct may resemble a choledochal cyst to the unwary surgeon. These babies require only drainage of the area, with anticipation that the perforation will heal spontaneously while the infant is maintained on antibiotics.[138,139]

Biliary hypoplasia, is a descriptive term for the radiologic finding of a diminutive extrahepatic ductal system. This may be a secondary condition resulting from intrahepatic cholestasis. Biliary hypoplasia has been associated with intrahepatic disease conditions, such as the cholestasis seen in α_1-antitrypsin deficiency.[140] A cholangiogram confirms the patency of these structures and their narrow caliber. Liver biopsy invariably shows cholestasis, and there is often a paucity of intrahepatic bile ducts. Speculation that there is an inflammatory component associated with biliary hypoplasia and that it represents a phase of a dynamic process, leading perhaps to total biliary obstruction, has prompted the use of corticosteroids for treatment. In some instances of steroid therapy, the jaundice resolved and subsequent biopsies reverted to normal.

With the increased use of abdominal ultrasonography, cholelithiasis has been diagnosed in infants with increasing frequency, particularly in infants with ileal resection or long-term intravenous hyperalimentation.[141] In the asymptomatic baby, observation often is rewarded with spontaneous disappearance of the gallstones, although symptomatic cholelithiasis should be managed by cholecystectomy.[142] Obstructive jaundice is discussed in more detail in Chapters 37 and 38.

HERNIA AND HYDROCELE

Inguinal hernia and hydrocele occur commonly, especially in male infants. They result from the persistence of a patent processus vaginalis, a fingerlike projection of the peritoneum accompanying the testicle as it descends into the scrotum. In the female infant, the peritoneal extension accompanies the round ligament and can remain patent, becoming a potential hernia sac. A hydrocele is often associated with an inguinal hernia, or it may be an isolated finding. The fluid may be in communication with the peritoneal cavity, and the hydrocele may therefore wax and wane in size, or it may be separated and completely isolated in the scrotum, in the inguinal canal, or, in female infants, the canal of Nuck. A hydrocele presents a smooth, cylindric contour, with the superior margin generally distinct. It is not tender and is often asymptomatic. The hernia is often large enough that it is easily appreciated as a swelling in the groin or scrotum. The mass can usually be reduced back into the abdominal cavity.

The special anatomic associations of infants puts them at particular risk for incarceration of a hernia. The internal inguinal ring is narrow, and an intestine finding its way into the hernia sac in the inguinal canal can become trapped and is reduced only with great difficulty. The incidence of inguinal hernia is dramatically increased in children born earlier than 36 weeks of gestation, with as many as 35% of them developing hernias.

In premature infants in our neonatal unit, we repair the hernias before discharge. If the premature infant has a hernia that freely moves in and out of the inguinal canal, has no history of incarceration, and is first seen as an outpatient, we prefer to delay elective repair until the baby is at least 46 weeks of gestation to minimize postoperative apnea,[2] especially in the anemic child.[143] If a troublesome hernia in a premature infant must be repaired earlier than the elective 46 weeks of gestational age, we prefer to use spinal anesthesia rather than general anesthesia to minimize the risk of postoperative apnea.[2]

If there is diagnostic confusion between an incarcerated hernia and a hydrocele, a rectal examination with bimanual palpation of the internal inguinal ring delineates the structures passing through the ring into the inguinal canal. The vas deferens is a constant reference point, and the intestine adjacent to the vas and between the examining fingers confirms the diagnosis of a hernia. Surgical repair is indicated in all cases of inguinal hernia.

If incarceration of a hernia occurs, moderate, bimanual pressure, applied by compressing the sac from below while providing a gentle downward counterforce with the hand above the inguinal ring, usually achieves reduction. Occasionally, these hernias reduce spontaneously after sedation is given and struggling and crying are terminated. If the hernia fails to reduce or if there is obvious intestinal obstruction and systemic toxicity, emergency surgical reduction and repair are necessary.

An inguinal hernia in a female infant is often diagnosed by palpation of a nontender ovoid mass in the groin. The mass represents an ovary herniated into the open sac. Although the gonad can usually be reduced back into the abdomen, it often prolapses in and out until surgical repair is carried out. If the inguinal hernia is apparent unilaterally, the opposite side is routinely explored in all children younger than 1 year of age, because the incidence of bilateral hernias in these children is approximately 50%.

ABNORMALITIES OF THE UMBILICUS AND ABDOMINAL WALL

UMBILICAL HERNIA

Umbilical hernia is a common condition of the newborn, presenting as a central fascial defect beneath the umbilicus. Incarceration is a rare complication in patients with umbilical hernia, but it occurs more commonly in patients with smaller defects of the fascia, such as those seen in the neonate. Umbilical hernias are more common in African Americans, in premature infants, and in patients with congenital deficiencies of thyroid hormone.

Most babies with umbilical hernia require no surgical treatment, because the hernia disappears spontaneously by 2 or 3 years of age. With persistence of the hernia until 3 years of age, repair is indicated. In a few patients, there is progressive enlargement of the skin of the umbilicus until a prominent proboscis is produced. Surgical repair is indicated early. A simple repair suffices for all these patients and can be accomplished through a small semilunar incision made in the curve of the umbilicus. Complicated fascial flap repairs, such as may be required in adults, are unnecessary and contraindicated in young patients. The umbilicus is never excised.

Adhesive dressings with coins and metallic or plastic objects have no place in the management of umbilical hernia, because they are ineffective and merely cover the defect at the expense of irritating the surrounding skin.

PRIMARY INFECTION OF THE UMBILICUS

With the advent of sound prenatal care, the incidence of infection around the umbilicus (*i.e.*, omphalitis) has been markedly reduced. Potentially serious complications can result from infections in this area. Cellulitis of the abdominal wall, with direct spread into the peritoneal cavity and resultant peritonitis of the newborn, has been recorded. The most serious consequence is ascending infection along the umbilical vein to the portal system and liver. Before antibiotics, the resultant multiple hepatic abscesses were often fatal. A more common sequela is portal vein thrombosis, which is a major cause of portal hypertension in children. In the past, this was a significant cause of esophageal varices in young patients, and although this condition now occurs less often, it must be assiduously avoided by prompt local and systemic antibiotic treatment of suspected infections in and around the umbilicus.

UMBILICAL GRANULOMA

The formation of weeping granulation tissue at the umbilicus is not unusual in the newborn. Failure of the umbilical epithelium to grow over the severed stump of the umbilicus results in a persistent crusting mass of granulomatous tissue. Cauterization with silver nitrate is diagnostic and therapeutic. Applications of silver nitrate twice weekly for 1 month clear most umbilical granulations. With persistence of fluid at the umbilicus, a patent omphalomesenteric duct or patent urachus should be considered.

PATENT OMPHALOMESENTERIC DUCT

During fetal development, the omphalomesenteric duct forms a connection from the intestinal tract to the placenta. If this duct fails to involute, a tubular attachment persists between the ileum and the abdominal wall (Fig. 44-18). Liquid ileal content refluxes out of this duct.

Diagnosis of a congenital fistula at the umbilicus is made by inspection and probing of the tract. The introduction of radiopaque material into the ostium at the umbilicus demonstrates a connection to the intestinal lumen on lateral x-ray films of the abdomen.

Treatment for patent omphalomesenteric duct is elective abdominal exploration with division and closure of the fistula at its origin in the ileum and total excision of the fistula, including its attachment to the undersurface of the umbilicus. This procedure must not be postponed, because there is a potential for intestinal volvulus to occur around the postlike attachment between the umbilicus and the ileum.

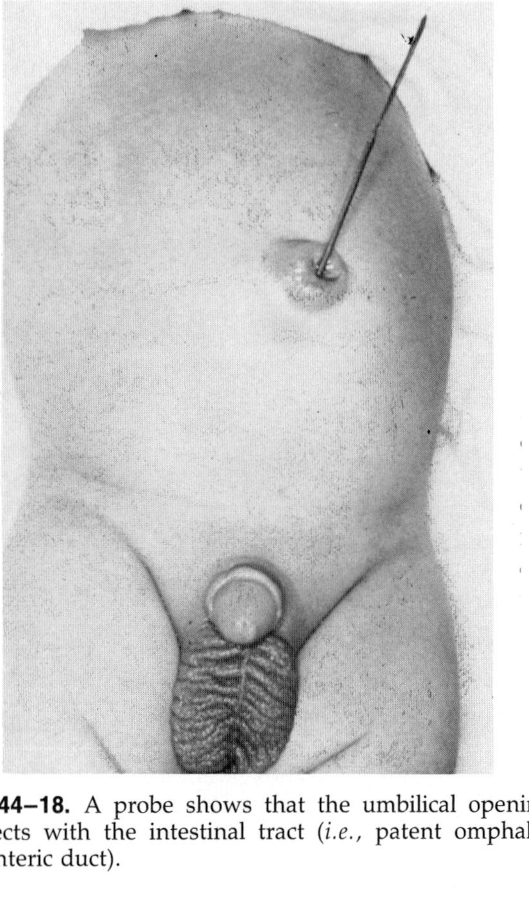

FIG. 44–18. A probe shows that the umbilical opening connects with the intestinal tract (*i.e.*, patent omphalomesenteric duct).

In rare instances, if the patent omphalomesenteric duct opening is large, the peristaltic activity of the bowel can result in eversion of proximal intestine, as in intussusception, through the opening onto the abdominal wall. Clinically, this appears as a mucosa-covered extrusion, and the resulting mass is easily confused with a small ruptured omphalocele. Careful inspection of the neck of the defect at the border of the abdominal skin discloses the true nature of the lesion. The bowel has in effect turned inside out and prolapsed through the patent omphalomesenteric duct. Immediate operation, with reduction and repair, is indicated.

PATENT URACHUS

During embryologic development, there is free communication between the urinary bladder and the abdominal wall. Persistence of this tract establishes a communication between the urinary bladder and the umbilicus, through which urine may pass. Although this passage is small, the umbilicus is constantly wet. The first sign of a patent urachus may be urinary infection. In some patients, a portion of the urachus has obliterated with only a partially patent remnant or cyst remaining beneath the umbilicus. Urachal cysts may present after the newborn period as an infected infraumbilical mass caused by colonization with skin organisms from the umbilicus.

In the diagnostic workup of a newborn suspected of having a patent urachus, the cystogram in lateral projection demonstrates the abnormal tract. Another diagnostic technique is the introduction of a colored dye into the bladder through the urethral catheter. The appearance of dye on the abdominal wall confirms the connection between the umbilicus and the bladder. Extraperitoneal surgical exploration of the infraumbilical area allows complete excision of the urachal tract and closure of the bladder. Partial urachal remnants, sinus tracts, and cysts are easily excised.

OMPHALOCELE

Developmental arrest of those somites that form the peritoneal, muscular, and ectodermal layers of the abdominal wall results in a central defect called an omphalocele. The defect is covered by a translucent membrane overlying the bowel and solid viscera and may vary in size from a small hernia of the cord that is 1 or 2 cm in diameter to a huge mass containing essentially all the abdominal viscera (Fig. 44-19). Usually, the sac remains intact, but it is occasionally ruptured during delivery.

The diagnosis of this lesion is made entirely by inspection, because it is readily apparent immediately

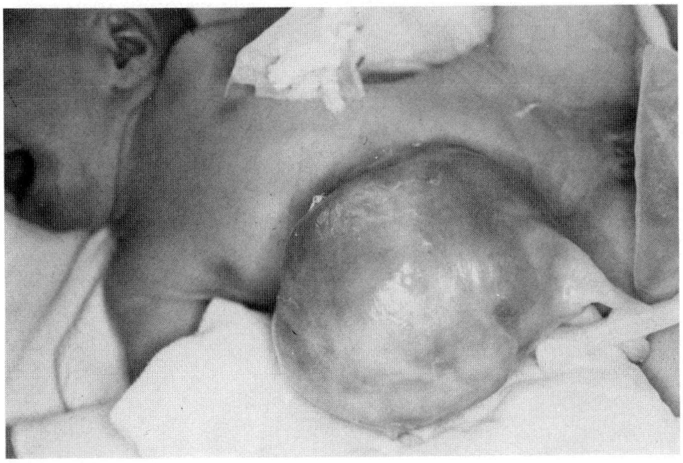

FIG. 44–19. Large omphalocele. Notice the covering of the sac and its relation to the umbilicus, which protrudes from the lower portion.

after delivery of the baby. The abdomen is wrapped carefully with well-padded, saline-soaked gauze and an outer dry layer in preparation for transport. No pressure is placed on the omphalocele in an attempt to reduce it. This is hazardous to the integrity of the sac, may interfere with venous return, and may impede the infant's respiratory efforts.

Small omphaloceles are usually amenable to complete one-stage surgical repair. For larger omphaloceles (>6 cm), a sheet of Silastic with interwoven Marlex can be sewn around the edge of the defect to envelop the omphalocele.[144,145] Steady pressure on the prosthesis and a reduction in size over several days brings about gradual reduction of the omphalocele so that surgical closure can be accomplished. Irrigation with povidone–iodine (Betadine) solution or coverage with a layer of silver sulfadiazine (Silvadene) has been effective in reducing surface contamination throughout the time for which the prosthesis is required.

Coexisting anomalies, such as exstrophy of the cloaca or congenital heart disease, may make surgical closure inappropriate. Painting the omphalocele sac with 4% mercurochrome promotes a firm, strong crust to cover the defect. This protection serves until the natural process of epithelialization occurs. Although success with a plastic prosthesis has obviated the need for the painting method, it is still a useful treatment in certain instances.

Congenital malrotation of the colon usually occurs in patients born with omphalocele. Although it is in itself not a serious defect, the anomaly can lead to midgut volvulus, and the symptoms of intestinal obstruction in a baby who has previously recovered from treatment of omphalocele must be considered a dire emergency.

GASTROSCHISIS

Originally confused as a type of omphalocele, gastroschisis is now recognized as a separate entity. It differs embryologically in that the abdominal wall has completed its development but a defect remains at the base of the umbilical stalk, through which a portion of the intestinal tract has escaped. Gastroschisis always occurs as a defect lateral to the base of the umbilicus, and the defect may represent an isolated congenital defect in the abdominal wall. An alternate theory of the embryogenesis of gastroschisis holds that closure of the celomic cavity has been completed while a portion of the intestinal tract remained trapped outside the abdomen in the base of the umbilical cord. It is postulated that this hernia of the cord then ruptures, allowing the intestine to float freely in the amnion while the umbilical arteries and vein remain attached to the baby.

The escape of the intestine into the amniotic cavity apparently can occur at different times in fetal development. This conclusion follows the observation that in some infants the intestines are glistening and normal looking, as if they had escaped a celomic envelope just before birth. Many infants with gastroschisis, however, are born with edematous and matted intestinal loops that appear to have been exposed to the amniotic fluid for many weeks (Fig. 44-20).

Immediate treatment in the delivery room consists of wrapping the baby and the exteriorized intestine in saline-soaked gauze and dry sterile dressings. Prompt surgical repair is undertaken. In about one-half of the patients, the viscera can be returned to the abdomen and secure closure obtained. In favorable cases, peristalsis returns in a few days, and normal bowel function can be expected. If the bowel is matted and edematous, it may take many weeks before intestinal function recovers. Nutrition can be successfully supported during this interval by intravenous hyperalimentation. Previously, many of these babies died of malnutrition before intestinal function returned.

If the abdominal wall cannot be closed without undue tension, which interferes with respiration and venous return, an extraabdominal prosthetic compartment must be fashioned. As in staged omphalocele repair, Silastic-covered Marlex is well suited for this purpose because its surface is inert and does not adhere to the bowel. After the prosthesis is fastened

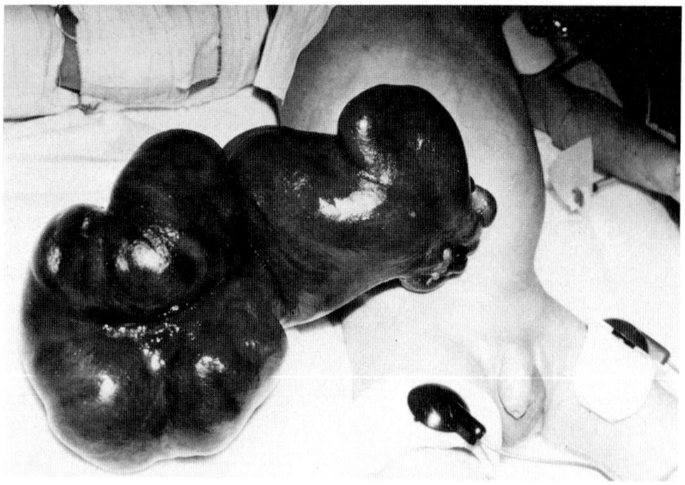

FIG. 44–20. Patient with gastroschisis. The edematous, matted bowel is the result of the intestines floating freely in the amniotic fluid. Remarkably, these distorted viscera ultimately fit back into the abdominal cavity and assume a normal appearance and function.

to the fascial margins, the capacity of the plastic compartment is gradually reduced until complete surgical closure is possible, usually within 7 to 10 days. This staged maneuver, coupled with intravenous alimentation, has resulted in an increased percentage of survivors from a previously hopeless anomaly.[146] Intestinal atresia occurs in about 10% of patients with gastroschisis. In these babies, the clinical course is one of early complete obstruction, which requires abdominal exploration if the lesion has been inadvertently overlooked at the time of initial repair of the gastroschisis.

CONGENITAL DEFICIENCY OF THE ABDOMINAL MUSCLE

The prune-belly syndrome consists of three major anomalies:

1. Deficiency of the abdominal musculature
2. Dilation of the urinary collecting system
3. Bilateral cryptorchidism.

By definition, all patients with this syndrome are male, but a similar condition has been reported in female patients. In severely affected infants, there is marked wrinkling of the skin of the abdomen and no muscular substance beneath (Fig. 44-21). Lower abdominal musculature is most frequently and severely involved.

The bladder is characteristically large, and the ureters are dilated and tortuous. The kidneys may be hypoplastic, but usually there is enough renal parenchyma for adequate function from at least one side. There is an increased incidence of patent urachus, particularly if the renal function is poor.

The cause of the condition is unknown. It has been proposed that all these infants have some degree of urethral obstruction, with resultant overdistention of the bladder and abnormal pressure on the developing muscular somites.[147] Others have suggested that the primary deficiency is in the abdominal musculature, allowing overdistention of the bladder with secondary changes in the urinary collecting system. It is probable that neither of these explanations is com-

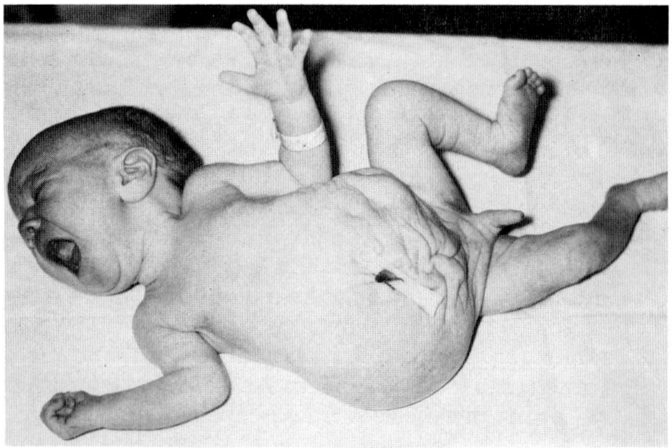

FIG. 44–21. An infant with congenital deficiency of the abdominal musculature shows the typical prune-belly appearance.

pletely valid, and that some more comprehensive explanation exists for the coexistence of the unusual abdominal deficiency and the distortion of the collecting system.

The treatment of these infants is conservative and nonoperative if their renal function is good.[148] If the renal function is poor, urinary diversion may be necessary in the neonatal period to eliminate pressure in the collecting system. Abdominal wall reconstruction and bilateral orchiopexy can be performed between 1 and 2 years of age, if the renal function is stable. Reconstruction of the abdominal wall is best performed through a low transverse incision, so that the use of normal upper abdominal musculature is maximized.[149]

SACROCOCCYGEAL TERATOMA

A sacrococcygeal teratoma is an unusual tumor that frequently comes to attention in the fetus or newborn infant.[150] It is usually a large mass arising from the coccyx. The mass is made of mature and immature elements of different cell types. The mass may be several centimeters in diameter, or it may rival the size of the newborn infant.[151] In the newborn period, the tumor is usually benign; however, when discovered later, the incidence of malignancy rises.[152]

The diagnosis is frequently made at the time of prenatal ultrasound.[153] A large solid or cystic mass is observed in the sacral region. The maternal serum α-fetoprotein level may be elevated. Occasionally, the blood flow through the tumor is large enough to produce heart failure and hydrops in the fetus.[154] Langer and colleagues proposed using a large mass and heart failure as an indication for fetal surgery to arrest the tumor growth.[155] If a sacrococcygeal teratoma is diagnosed prenatally, a multidisciplinary approach to the pregnancy and delivery is indicated.[156]

The key to the management of an infant born with a sacrococcygeal teratoma is an expeditious surgical resection. The infant is stabilized, with careful attention to high-output cardiac failure. Hypothermia can be a major problem in the nursery and the operating room because of the large surface area of the mass. After a search for coexisting anomalies and after appropriate resuscitation, the mass is resected. Complete resection is usually possible without long-term sequelae, although bowel continence can be a problem if the sphincter mechanism is disturbed by the tumor or the surgery. It is important to remove the coccyx to prevent recurrence. The tumors are rarely malignant in the newborn period, and complete surgical resection is curative.

VASCULAR ACCESS

An excellent text, *Atlas of Procedures in the Newborn*, is recommended for an in-depth review of vascular access techniques in the infant.[157] The traditional method of maintaining vascular access in the neonate for blood sampling, medications, and parenteral nutrition has been to use an umbilical artery catheter. When the umbilical artery catheter must be maintained for an extended period of time, the risk of complications, such as arterial emboli, aortic thrombosis, and infections, becomes prohibitive, and the line must be removed. The use of transcutaneous pulse oximetry has greatly reduced the need for arterial lines in neonates with pulmonary problems, but when arterial access is required, the right radial artery is preferred because its preductal location accurately reflects intracerebral blood oxygenation.

Even in the smallest babies, a radial artery line can be placed by cutdown with optical magnification. Placing an arterial line percutaneously is preferable to the cutdown technique, with the aim of maintaining future arterial patency. However, multiple attempts to access the radial artery percutaneously should be discouraged to avoid damage to the artery, preventing access by cutdown. The posterior tibial artery is an alternate site for arterial lines in neonates. More proximal arterial lines in the brachial or femoral arteries have been used in selected patients, although the risk of extremity ischemia is substantial with these locations.

Establishing reliable venous access in the preterm infant has become one of the most common procedures done by pediatric surgeons. The placement of a catheter into the central venous circulation allows the use of more concentrated intravenous solutions and eliminates the risk of subcutaneous infiltration of solutions and resultant skin sloughs. In the past, central venous catheters were placed predominantly by a percutaneous approach; this is now restricted to larger neonates, using a Seldinger technique. In preterm infants, a Silastic catheter is placed by cutdown, with a Dacron cuff attached to the catheter placed beneath the skin to prevent catheter infection and accidental removal. A percutaneous ultrathin Silastic catheter that can be threaded from a peripheral vein to the central venous system is used with increasing frequency at the CNMC, but many children continue to require the cutdown technique.

The site of venous catheter placement depends on patient anatomy, disease, location of previous catheters, and surgeon preference. The sites of choice are the external jugular or facial vein to avoid damage to the internal jugular vein. In the infant weighing less than 1000 g, the internal jugular vein may be the only one of adequate size, and its use unilaterally should not cause serious problems. When the line is placed in the neck, the tip of the catheter should be in the superior vena cava just cephalad to the right atrium. Silastic catheters within the atrium may cause atrial thrombus formation, atrial perforation, or dysrythmias.

If the superior vena caval system cannot be used, the saphenous vein, at its junction with the femoral vein, can usually be cannulated, even in infants weighing less than 1000 g. If the saphenous vein is used, it is best to keep the catheter tip caudad to the renal veins, approximately at the level of T12.

Central venous catheters in neonates are plagued with complications. Infection remains the most common complication, occurring in approximately 10% of infants. Although catheter infection can be successfully treated with intravenous antibiotics, it is better to remove the catheter, give intravenous medications and nutrition temporarily through a peripheral intravenous line, and replace the central line, if still needed, after all cultures are free of infection. Most of the organisms that contaminate central venous lines originate from the infant's skin or from careless decontamination of the connecting tubing before line changes or the administration of medication.

Central vein thrombosis is a serious problem that may lead to superior vena caval syndrome, which includes head and arm swelling and pleural effusions due to obstruction of the thoracic duct drainage. Babies weighing less than 1000 g are at particularly high risk of developing thrombus.[158] Management of vena caval thrombosis with thrombolytic agents, such as urokinase, may be beneficial, but the risk of systemic anticoagulation must always be considered. Some reduction in the risk of thrombosis may be achieved by the use of 1 U of heparin per 1 mL of intravenous solution.

REFERENCES

1. Roe CF, Santulli RV, Blair CS. Heat loss in infants during general anesthesia and operations. J Pediatr Surg 1966;1:266.
2. Welborn LG, Rice LJ, Hannallah RS, et al. Postoperative apnea in former preterm infants: prospective comparison of spinal and general anesthesia. Anesthesiology 1990;72:838.
3. Anand KJS, Hickey PR. Pain and its effects in the human neonate and fetus. N Engl J Med 1987;317:1321.
4. Rowe MI, Lloyd DA, Lee M. Is the refractometer specific gravity a reliable index for pediatric fluid management? J Pediatr Surg 1986;21:580.
5. Gross RE, Connerly JL. Thyroglossal cysts and sinuses. N Engl J Med 1940;223:616.
6. Brown PM, Judd ES. Thyroglossal cysts and sinuses: results of radical (Sistrunk) operation. Am J Surg 1961;102:494.
7. Athow AC, Fagg NL, Drake DP. Management of thyroglossal cysts in children. Br J Surg 1989;76:811.
8. Gray SW, Skandalakis JE. The pharynx and its derivatives. In: Gray SW, Skandalakis JE, eds. Embryology for surgeons: the embryologic basis for the treatment of congenital defects. Philadelphia: WB Saunders, 1972.
9. Bill AH Jr, Vadheim JL. Cysts, sinuses, and fistulas of the neck arising from the first and second branchial clefts. Ann Surg 1955;142:904.
10. Gray SW, Skandalakis JE. The lymphatic system. In: Gray SW, Skandalakis JE, eds. Embryology for surgeons: the embryologic basis for the treatment of congenital defects. Philadelphia: WB Saunders, 1972.
11. Langer JC, Fitzgerald PG, Desa D, et al. Cervical cystic hygroma in the fetus: clinical spectrum and outcome. J Pediatr Surg 1990;25:58.
12. Grosfeld JL, Weber TR, Vane DW. One stage resection for massive cervicomediastinal hygroma. Surgery 1982;92:693.
13. Richardson MA, Cotton RT. Anatomic abnormalities of the pediatric airway. Pediatr Clin North Am 1984;31:821.
14. Hengerer A, Newburg J. Congenital malformations of the nose and paranasal sinuses. In: Bluestone CD, Stool SE, eds. Pediatric otolaryngology. 2nd ed. Philadelphia: WB Saunders, 1990:718.
15. Coniglio J, Manzione J, Hengerer A. Anatomic findings and management of choanal atresia and the CHARGE association. Ann Otol Rhinol Laryngol 1988;97:448.
16. Stankiewicz J. The endoscopic repair of choanal atresia. Otolaryngol Head Neck Surg 1990;102:931.
17. Hengerer A, Oas R. Congenital anomalies of the nose: their embrology, diagnosis and management. Washington, DC: The American Academy of Otolaryngology Head and Neck Surgery Foundation, 1987.
18. Kearns D, Wickstead M, Choa D, et al. Computed tomography in choanal atresia. Laryngol Otol 1988;102:414.
19. Richardson M, Osguthorpe J. Surgical management of choanal atresia. Laryngoscope 1988;98:915.
20. Grundfast KM, Thomsen J, Barber C. An improved stent method for choanal atresia repair. Laryngoscope 1990; 100:1132.
21. Messineo A, Filler RM, Vinograd I. Severe tracheomalacia associated with esophageal atresia: short and long term results of surgical treatment. J Pediatr Surg 1992;27:1136..
22. Gross RE. Surgical relief for tracheal obstruction from a vascular ring. N Engl J Med 1945;233:586.
23. Blair GK, Cohen R, Filler RM. Treatment of tracheomalacia: eight years' experience. J Pediatr Surg 1986;21:781.
24. Murray GF. Congenital lobar emphysema. Surg Gynecol Obstet 1967;124:611.
25. Ekkelkamp S, Vos A. Successful surgical treatment of a newborn with bilateral congenital lobar emphysema. J Pediatr Surg 1987;22:1001.
26. Adzick NS, Harrison MR, Glick PL, et al. Fetal cystic adenomatoid malformation: prenatal diagnosis and natural history. J Pediatr Surg 1985;20:483.
27. Atkinson JB, Ford EG, Kitagawa H, et al. Persistant pulmonary hypertension complicating cystic adenomatoid malformation in neonates. J Pediatr Surg 1992;27:54.
28. Anderson KD, Chandra R. Pneumothorax secondary to perforation of sequential bronchi by suction catheters. J Pediatr Surg 1976;11:687.
29. Gangitano ES, Pomerance JJ, Gans SL. Successful surgical repair of iatrogenic lung perforation in a neonate. J Pediatr Surg 1981;16:70.
30. Zerella JT, Trump DS. Surgical management of neonatal interstitial emphysema. J Pediatr Surg 1987;22:34.
31. Geggel RL, Murphy JD, Langleben D. Congenital diaphragmatic hernia: arterial structural changes and persistent pulmonary hypertension after surgical repair. J Pediatr Surg 1985;92:805.
32. Levin DL. Morphologic analysis of the pulmonary vascular bed in congenital left-sided diaphragmatic hernia. J Pediatr Surg 1978;92:805.
33. Crane JP. Familial congenital diaphragmatic hernia: prenatal diagnostic approach and analysis of twelve families. Clin Genet 1979;16:244.
34. Adzick NS, Vacanti JP, Lillehei CW. Fetal diaphragmatic hernia: ultrasound diagnosis and clinical outcome in 38 cases. J Pediatr Surg 1989;24:654.
35. Adzick NS, Harrison MR, Glick PL. Diaphragmatic hernia in the fetus: prenatal diagnosis and outcome in 94 cases. J Pediatr Surg 1985;20:357.

36. Benjamin DR, Juul S, Siebert JR. Congenital posterolateral diaphragmatic hernia: associated malformations. J Pediatr Surg 1988;23:899.
37. Nakayama DK, Motoyama EK, Tagge EM. Effect of preoperative stabilization on respiratory system compliance and outcome in newborn infants with congenital diaphragmatic hernia. J Pediatr Surg 1991;118:793.
38. Breaux CW, Rouse TM, Cain WS, et al. Improvement in survival of patients with congenital diaphragmatic hernia utilizing a strategy of delayed repair after medical and/or extracorporeal membrane oxygenation stabilization. J Pediatr Surg 1991;26:333.
39. Connors RH, Tracy T, Bailey PV, et al. Congenital diaphragmatic hernia repair on ECMO. J Pediatr Surg 1990;25:1043.
40. Van Meurs KP, Newman KD, Anderson KD, et al. Effect of extracorporal membrane oxygenation on survival of infants with congenital diaphragmatic hernia. J Pediatr Surg 1990; 117:954.
41. Newman KD, Anderson KD, Van Meurs K, et al. Extracorporeal membrane oxygenation and congenital diaphragmatic hernia: should any infant be excluded? J Pediatr Surg 1990; 25:1048.
42. Wilson JM, Thompson JR, Schnitzer JJ, et al. Intratracheal pulmonary ventilation and congenital diaphragmatic hernia: a report of two human cases. J Pediatr Surg 1993;28:484..
43. Crombleholme TM, Adzick NS, Hardy K, et al. Pulmonary lobar transplantation in neonatal swine: a model for treatment of congenital diaphragmatic hernia. J Pediatr Surg 1990; 25:11.
44. Harrison MR, Langer JC, Adzick NS. Correction of congenital diaphragmatic hernia *in utero*: initial clinical experience. J Pediatr Surg 1990;25:47.
45. Haller JA, Pickard LR, Tepas JJ, et al. Management of diaphragmatic paralysis in infants with special emphasis on selection of patients for operative plication. J Pediatr Surg 1979; 14:779.
46. Langer JC, Filler RM, Coles J, et al. Plication of the diaphragm for infants and young children with phrenic nerve palsy. J Pediatr Surg 1988;23:749.
47. Haight C, Towsley HA. Congenital atresia of the esophagus with tracheoesophageal fistula. Extrapleural ligation of fistula and end to end anastomosis of esophageal segments. Surg Gynecol Obstet 1943;76:672.
48. Smith EI. The early development of trachea and esophagus in relation to atresia of the esophagus and tracheoesophageal fistula. Contributors to Embryology #245 Carnegie Institute of Washington Publication #611 1957;36:41.
49. Hopkins WA. The esophagus. In: Gray SW, Skandalakis JE, eds. Embryology for surgeons, 63. Philadelphia: WB Saunders, 1972.
50. Chen J, Goei GS, Hertzler JH. Family studies on congenital esophageal atresia with or without tracheoesophageal fistula. Birth Defects 1979;15:117.
51. Berry JE, Auldist AW. The VATER association: one end of a spectrum of anomalies. Am J Dis Child 1984;128:769.
52. Grosfeld JL, Ballantine TDN. Esophageal atresia and tracheoesophageal fistula: effect of delayed thoracotomy on survival. Surgery 1978;84:394.
53. Piekarski DH, Stevens FD. The association and embryogenesis of tracheoesophageal and anorectal anomalies. Prog Pediatr Surg 1976;9:63.
54. Holder TM, Cloud DT, Lewis JE Jr, et al. Esophageal atresia and tracheoesophageal fistula. A survey of its members by the Surgical Section of the American Academy Pediatrics. Pediatrics 1961;34:542.
55. Waterston DJ, Bonham-Carter RE, Aberdeen E. Oesophageal atresia: tracheoesophageal fistula—a study of survival in 218 infants. Lancet 1962;1:819.
56. Randolph JG, Newman K, Anderson KD. Current results and repair of esophageal atresia with tracheoesophageal fistula using physiologic status as a guide to therapy. Ann Surg 1989;209:525.
57. Spitz L, Keily E, Brereton RJ. Esophageal atresia: a five year experience with 148 cases. J Pediatr Surg 1987;22:103.
58. Pohlson EC, Schaller R, Tapper D. Improved survival with primary anastomosis in the low birth weight neonate with esophageal atresia and tracheoesophageal fistula. J Pediatr Surg 1988;23:418.
59. Livaditas A. Esophageal atresia, a method of overbridging large segmental gaps. Z Kinderchir 1973;13:298.
60. Manning P, Morgan RA, Coran A, et al. 50 years' experience with esophageal atresia in tracheoesophageal fistula. Ann Surg 1987;204:446.
61. Werlin SC, Dodds WJ, Hogan WJ, et al. Esophageal function in esophageal atresia. Dig Dis Sci 1981;26:796.
62. Jolley SJ, Johnson DG, Roberts CC, et al. Patterns of gastroesophageal reflux in children following repair of esophageal atresia and distal tracheoesophageal fistula. J Pediatric Surg 1980;15:857.
63. Fonkalsrud EW. Gastroesophageal fundoplication for reflux following repair of esophageal atresia. Arch Surg 1979;114: 48.
64. Ghandour KE, Spitz L, Brereton RJ, et al. Recurrent tracheoesophageal fistula: experience with 24 patients. J Paediatr Child Health 1990;26:89.
65. Howard R, Myers NA. Esophageal atresia: a technique for elongating the upper pouch. Surgery 1965;58:725.
66. Puri T, Blake N, O'Donnell B, et al. Delayed primary anastomosis following spontaneous growth of esophageal segments in esophageal atresia. J Pediatr Surg 1981;16:180.
67. Schneider JM, Becker JM. The H-type tracheoesophageal fistula in infants and children. Surgery 1962;51:677.
68. Dubois JJ, Pokorny W, Harberg FJ. Current management of laryngeal and laryngotracheoesophageal clefts. J Pediatr Surg 1990;25:855.
69. Neuhauser EBD, Berenberg W. Cardioesophageal relaxation as cause of vomiting in infants. Radiology 1947;48:480.
70. Randolph JG, Lilly JR, Anderson KD. Surgical treatment of gastroesophageal reflux in infants. Ann Surg 1974;180:479.
71. Foglia RM, Fonkalsrud EW, Ament ME, et al. Gastroesophageal fundoplication for management of chronic pulmonary disease in children. Am J Surg 1980;140:72.
72. Leape LL, Holder TM, Franklin JD, et al. Respiratory arrest in infants secondary to gastroesophageal reflux. Pediatrics 1977;50:924.
73. Nielson DW, Heldt GP, Tooley WH. Stridor and gastroesophageal reflux in infants. Pediatrics 1990;85:1034.
74. Randolph JG. Experience with the Nissen fundoplication for correction of gastroesophageal reflux in infants. Ann Surg 1983;198:579.
75. Halpern LM, Jolley SG, Tunell WP, et al. The mean duration of gastroesophageal reflux during sleep as an indicator of respiratory symptoms from gastroesophageal reflux in children. J Pediatr Surg 1991;26:686.
76. Holgersen LO. The etiology of spontaneous gastric perforation of the newborn: a reevaluation. J Pediatr Surg 1981; 16:608.
77. Bell MJ. Perforation of the gastrointestinal tract and peritonitis in the neonate. Surg Gynecol Obstet 1985;160:20.
78. Tan CE, Krily EM, Agrawal M, et al. Neonatal gastrointestinal perforation. J Pediatr Surg 1989;24:888.
79. Gauderer MWL, Olsen MM, Stellato TA, et al. Feeding gas-

trostomy "button"—experience and recommendations. J Pediatr Surg 1988;23:24.
80. Gertler JP, Seashore JH, Touloukian RJ. Early ileostomy closure in necrotizing enterocolitis. J Pediatr Surg 1987;22:140.
81. Bishop HC, Koop CE. Management of meconium ileus: resection, Roux-en-Y anastomosis and ileostomy irrigation with pancreatic enzymes. Ann Surg 1957;145:410.
82. Moore K. The developing human. 3rd ed. Philadelphia: WB Saunders, 1981.
83. Ford EG, Senac MO, Srikanth MS, et al. Malrotation of the intestine in children. Ann Surg 1992;215:172.
84. Stauffer UG, Herrmann P. Comparison of late results in patients with corrected intestinal malrotation with and without fixation of the mesentery. J Pediatr Surg 1980;15:9.
85. Cooper A, Floyd TF, Ross AJ, et al. Morbidity and mortality of short-bowel syndrome acquired in infancy: an update. J Pediatr Surg 1984;19:711.
86. Carter CO, Evans KA. Inheritance of congenital pyloric stenosis. J Med Genet 1969;6:233.
87. Tunell WP, Wilson PA. Pyloric stenosis: diagnosis by real time sonography, the pyloric muscle length method. J Pediatr Surg 1984;19:795.
88. Woolley MM, Feesher BF, Asch MJ, et al. Jaundice, hypertrophic pyloric stenosis and hepatic glucuronyl transferase. J Pediatr Surg 1974;9:359.
89. Fonkalsrud EW, deLorimier AA, Hays DM. Congenital atresia and stenosis of the duodenum—a review compiled from the members of the surgical section of the American Academy of Surgery. Pediatrics 1969;43:79.
90. Merrill JR, Raffensperger JG. Pediatric annular pancreas: twenty year experience. J Pediatr Surg 1976;11:921.
91. Louw JH, Barnard CN. Congenital intestinal atresia: observations on its origin. Lancet 1955;1:1065.
92. de Lorimier AA, Fonkalsrud EW, Hays DM. Congenital atresia and stenosis of the jejunum and ileum. Surgery 1969;65:819.
93. Thomas CG. Jejunoplasty for the correction of jejunal atresia. Surg Gynecol Obstet 1969;129:545.
94. Weber TR, Vane DW, Grosfeld JL. Tapering enteroplasty in infants with bowel atresia and short gut. Arch Surg 1982;17:684.
95. LoPresti JM, Altman RP, Kulczychi L. Meconium ileus: operative therapy and pulmonary complications in the newborn. Clinical Proceedings of the Children's Hospital of the District of Columbia 1972;28:221.
96. Noblett HR. Treatment of uncomplicated meconium ileus by Gastrografin enema: a preliminary report. J Pediatr Surg 1969;4:190.
97. Mabogunje OA, Wang CI, Mahour H. Improved survival of neonates with meconium ileus. Arch Surg 1982;117:37.
98. Bishop HC, Koop CE. Surgical management of duplication of the alimentary tract. Am J Surg 1964;107:434.
99. Wrenn EL. Tubular duplication of the small intestine. Surgery 1962;52:494.
100. Leape LL. Case records of the Massachusetts General Hospital: duplication of the ileum. N Engl J Med 1980;302:958.
101. Fraser GC, Berry C. Mortality of neonatal Hirschsprung's disease: with particular reference to enterocolitis. J Pediatr Surg 1967;2:205.
102. Taxman TL, Ulish BS, Rothstein FC. How useful is the barium enema in the diagnosis of infantile Hirschsprung's disease? Am J Dis Child 1986;140:881.
103. Campbell PE, Noblett HR. Experience with rectal suction biopsy in the diagnosis of Hirschsprung's Disease. J Pediatr Surg 1969;4:410.
104. Huntley CC, Shaffner L deS, Challa VR, et al. Histochemical diagnosis of Hirschsprung's disease. Pediatrics 1982;69:755.
105. Teich S, Schisgall RM, Anderson KD, et al. Ischemic enterocolitis as a complication of Hirschsprung's disease. J Pediatr Surg 1986;21:143.
106. Harrison MW, Dytes DM, Campbell JR, et al. Diagnosis and management of Hirschsprung's disease. Am J Surg 1986;152:49.
107. Swenson O, Bill AH Jr. Resection of rectum and rectosigmoid with preservation of the sphincter for benign spastic lesions producing megacolon. An experimental study. Surgery 1948;24:212.
108. Duhamel B. Retrorectal and transanal pullthrough procedure for the treatment of Hirschsprung's disease. Dis Colon Rectum 1964;7:455.
109. Soave F. Hirschsprung's disease: a new surgical technique. Arch Dis Child 1964;39:116.
110. Carcassonne N, Guys J, Morisson-Lacombe G, et al. Management of Hirschsprung's disease: curative surgery before 3 months of age. J Pediatr Surg 1989;24:1032.
111. Foster P, Cowan G, Wrenn EL, et al. 25 years' experience with Hirschsprung's disease. J Pediatr Surg 1990;25:531.
112. Sherman JO, Snyder ME, et al. A 40-year multi-national retrospective study of 880 Swenson procedures. J Pediatr Surg 1989;24:833.
113. Touloukian RJ, Posch JN, Spencer R. The pathogenesis of ischemic gastroenterocolitis of the neonate: selective gut mucosal ischemia in asphyxiated neonatal piglets. J Pediatr Surg 1972;7:194.
114. Czyrko C, Steigman C, Turley DL, et al. The role of reperfusion injury in occlusive intestinal ischemia of the neonate: malonaldehyde-derived fluorescent products and correlation of histology. J Surg Res 1991;51:1.
115. Atkinson SD, Tuggle DW, Tunell WP. Hypoalbuminemia may predispose infants to necrotizing enterocolitis. J Pediatr Surg 1989;24:674.
116. Kosloske AM, Lilly JR. Paracentesis and lavage for diagnosis of intestinal gangrene in neonatal necrotizing enterocolitis. J Pediatr Surg 1978;13:315.
117. Ricketts RR. The role of paracentesis in the management of infants with necrotizing enterocolitis. Am Surg 1986;52:61.
118. Mollitt DL, Tepas JJ, Talbert JL. The microbiology of neonatal peritonitis. Arch Surg 1988;123:176.
119. Smith SD, Tagge EP, Miller J, et al. The hidden mortality in surgically treated necrotizing enterocolitis: fungal sepsis. J Pediatr Surg 1990;25:1030.
120. Buras R, Guzzetta P, Avery GB, et al. Acidosis and hepatic portal venous gas: indications for surgery in necrotizing enterocolitis. Pediatrics 1986;78:273.
121. Harberg FJ, McGill CW, Saleem MM, et al. Resection with primary anastomosis for necrotizing enterocolitis. J Pediatr Surg 1983;18:743.
122. Ein SH, Shandling B, Wesson D, et al. A 13-year experience with peritoneal drainage under local anesthesia for necrotizing enterocolitis perforation. J Pediatr Surg 1990;25:1034.
123. Musemeche CA, Kosloske AM, Ricketts RR. Enterostomy in necrotizing enterocolitis: an analysis of techniques and timing of closure. J Pediatr Surg 1987;22:479.
124. Radhakrishnan J, Blechman G, Shrader C, et al. Colonic strictures following successful medical management of necrotizing enterocolitis: a prospective study evaluating early gastrointestinal contrast studies. J Pediatr Surg 1991;26:1043.
125. Parashar K, Kyawhla S, Booth IW, et al. Ileocolic ulceration: a long term complication following ileocolic anastomosis. J Pediatr Surg 1988;23:226.
126. Kiesewetter WB. Rectum and anus. In: Ravitch MM, Welch

KJ, Benson CD, et al, eds. Pediatric surgery, vol 2. Chicago: Year Book, 1979:1059.
127. Pena A, DeVries PA. Posterior sagittal anoplasty: important technical considerations and new applications. J Pediatr Surg 1982;17:796.
128. Wangensteen OH, Rice CO. Imperforate anus: a method of determining the surgical approach. Ann Surg 1930;92:77.
129. Danis RK, Graviss ER. Imperforate anus: avoiding a colostomy. J Pediatr Surg 1978;13:759.
130. Hendren WH, Donahoe PK. Correction of congenital abnormalities of the vagina and perineum. J Pediatr Surg 1980; 15:751.
131. Brandl ML, Luks FI, Filiatrault D, et al. Surgical indications in antenatally diagnosed ovarian cysts. J Pediatr Surg 1991; 26:276.
132. Sakala EP, Leon ZA, Rouse GA. Management of antenatally diagnosed fetal ovarian cysts. Obstet Gynecol Surg 1991; 46:407.
133. Croitoru DP, Aaron LE, Laberge JM, et al. Management of complex ovarian cysts presenting in the first year of life. J Pediatr Surg 1991;26:1366.
134. Donahoe PK, Crawford JD. Ambiguous genitalia in the newborn. In: Welch KJ, Randolph JG, Ravitch MM, O'Neill JA Jr, Rowe MI, eds. Pediatric surgery. 4th ed. Chicago: Year Book, 1986.
135. Majd M, Reba RC, Altman RP. Effect of phenobarbital on ^{99m}Tc-IDA scintigraphy in the evaluation of neonatal jaundice. Semin Nucl Med 1981;11:194.
136. Karrer FM, Lilly JR, Stewart BA, et al. Biliary atresia registry, 1976 to 1989. J Pediatr Surg 1990;25:1076.
137. Stevens LH, Emond JC, Piper JB, et al. Hepatic artery thrombosis in infants: a comparison of whole livers, reduced-size grafts, and grafts from living-related donors. Transplantation 1992;53:396.
138. Lilly JR, Weintraub WW, Altman RP. Spontaneous perforation of the extrahepatic bile ducts and bile peritonitis in infancy. Surgery 1974;75:664.
139. Megison SM, Votteler TP. Management of common bile duct obstruction associated with spontaneous perforation of the biliary tree. Surgery 1992;111:237.
140. Altman RP, Chandra R. Biliary hypoplasia consequent to alpha-1-antitrypsin deficiency. Surg Forum 1976;37:377.
141. King DR, Ginn-Pease ME, Lloyd TV, et al. Parenteral nutrition with associated cholelithiasis: another iatrogenic disease of infants and children. J Pediatr Surg 1987;22:593.
142. Jacir NN, Anderson KD, Eichelberger MR, et al. Cholelithiasis in infancy: resolution of gallstones in three of four infants. J Pediatr Surg 1986;21:567.
143. Welborn LG, Hannallah RS, Luban NLC, et al. Anemia and postoperative apnea in former preterm infants. Anesthesiology 1991;74:1003.
144. Schuster SR. A new method for the staged repair of large omphaloceles. Surg Gynecol Obstet 1967;125:837.
145. Yazbeck S, Ndoye M, Khan AH. Omphalocele: a 25-year experience. J Pediatr Surg 1986;21:761.
146. Caniano DA, Brokaw B, Ginn-Pease ME. An individualized approach to the management of gastroschisis. J Pediatr Surg 1990;25:297.
147. Moerman P, Fryns JP, Goddeeris P, et al. Pathogenesis of the prune-belly syndrome: a functional urethral obstruction caused by prostatic hypoplasia. Pediatrics 1984;73:470.
148. Tank ES, McCoy G. Limited surgical intervention in the prune-belly syndrome. J Pediatr Surg 1983;18:688.
149. Randolph J, Cavett C, Eng G. Surgical correction and rehabilitation for children with "prune-belly" syndrome. Ann Surg 1981;193:757.
150. Tapper D, Lack EE. Teratoma in infancy in childhood: a 54-year experience at the Children's Hospital Medical Center. Ann Surg 1983;198:389.
151. Altman RP, Randolph JG, Lilly, JR. Sacrococcygeal teratoma: American Academy of Pediatric Surgical Section Survey. J Pediatr Surg 1974;9:389.
152. Billmire DF, Grosfeld JL. Teratomas in childhood: analysis of 142 cases. J Pediatr Surg 1986;21:548.
153. Sepulveda WH. Prenatal sonographic diagnosis of congenital sacrococcygeal teratoma and management. J Perinat Med 1989;17:93.
154. Smith KG, Silverman NH, Harrison MR, et al. High output cardiac failure in fetuses with large sacrococcygeal teratoma: diagnosis by echocardiography and Doppler ultrasounds. J Pediatr 1989;114:1023.
155. Langer JC, Harrison MR, Schmidt KG, et al. Fetal hydrops and deaths from sacrococcygeal teratoma: rational for fetal surgery. Am J Obstet Gynecol 1990;163:682.
156. Nakayama DK, Killian A, Hill LM, et al. The newborn with hydrops and sacrococcygeal teratoma. J Pediatr Surg 1991; 26:1435.
157. Fletcher MA, MacDonald MG, eds. Atlas of procedures in neonatology. 2nd ed. Philadelphia: JB Lippincott, 1993.
158. Mehta S, Connors AF, Danish EH, et al. Incidence of thrombosis during central venous catheterization of newborns: a prospective study. J Pediatr Surg 1992;27:18.

Neonatology: Pathophysiology and Management of the Newborn, Fourth Edition,
edited by Gordon B. Avery, Mary Ann Fletcher, and Mhairi G. MacDonald.
J.B. Lippincott Company, Philadelphia © 1994.

chapter 45

Hematology

VICTOR BLANCHETTE
JOHN DOYLE
BARBARA SCHMIDT
ALVIN ZIPURSKY

During the neonatal period, the clinician is confronted with a variety of life-threatening hematologic problems. Some of these disturbances are primary, and some merely reflect the presence of other diseases. The interpretation of laboratory findings and institution of appropriate therapy require an understanding of basic hematologic principles and an appreciation of normal physiologic variations in the formed blood elements and coagulation factors in the newborn.

ANEMIAS

ERYTHROCYTE PRODUCTION

The explosion of information on early hematopoiesis and hematopoietic growth factors has expanded the understanding of the fetal and neonatal erythron. As growth factors, particularly erythropoietin (EPO), enter into clinical use in this population, it becomes important to understand the physiology behind their application.

Early hematopoietic cells originate in the yolk sac. By the eighth week of gestation, more definitive fetal erythropoiesis is taking place in the liver. The liver remains the primary site of erythroid production throughout the early fetal period. By 6 months of gestation, the bone marrow becomes the principal site of erythroid cell development. Later during gestation, a switch occurs in the type of hemoglobin being formed, with adult hemoglobin (HbA) replacing fetal hemoglobin (HbF). The site of production of EPO switches from the less sensitive hepatic to the more sensitive renal site.[1]

The earliest characterized erythroid precursor is the burst-forming unit (BFU-E), which gives rise to colony-forming units (CFU-E). These are identified by their growth characteristics in culture. Neonatal BFU-E and CFU-E are as sensitive as their adult counterparts to EPO stimulation.[2,3] Earlier development is a function of other factors, including interleukins and burst-promoting activity. The numbers of BFU-E progressively decline along the series of fetal blood, cord blood, adult bone marrow, and adult blood. More than 40 times the number of BFU-E can be cultured from fetal blood compared with adult blood.[1] Measurement of the peripheral blood pool does not indicate the size of the total body pool, so that it cannot be inferred that the fetus has a markedly greater erythropoietic potential than an adult.[4] It is probably at least comparable.

The major difference between fetal and adult erythropoiesis is in the EPO response. Erythropoiesis is controlled by a feedback loop involving EPO. A decrease in erythrocyte mass is reflected by an increase in EPO, which drives erythropoiesis to increase erythrocyte mass and diminish EPO production. The expected correlations between EPO and measures of oxygen delivery (*e.g.*, hemoglobin, mixed venous oxygen tension, available oxygen) can be detected in premature neonates, providing evidence that the same feedback loop exists.[5–7] The measured levels of EPO are much lower than those of older children and adults with corresponding degrees of anemia. Brown and colleagues presented evidence that the magnitude of the EPO response was lowest in the least mature infant (*i.e.*, 27–31 weeks of gestation).[7] Forestier and associates found low EPO values in cordocentesis samples from infants between 18 and 37 weeks of gestation.[8] Surprisingly, there was no correlation between gestational age and EPO level. This poor EPO response persists through the neonatal period and is one of the reasons for the physiologic anemia of prematurity.

NORMAL HEMOGLOBIN LEVELS

The first requirement in any study of anemia is a clear definition of the normal hemoglobin range for the population under study. At no other time is this principle more important than in the newborn period, when the hemoglobin concentration is undergoing constant physiologic change.

Normal hemoglobin values at birth have been determined through measurement of levels in cord blood of newborn infants. In a review of normal blood values in the newborn, Oski and Naiman cite a range of 13.7 to 20.1 g/dL, with a mean of 16.8 g/dL.[9] Blanchette and Zipursky obtained similar results in studies of healthy newborns yielding cord hemoglobin values (mean ± 1 SD) of 16.9 ± 1.6 g/dL in full-term infants and 15.9 ± 2.4 g/dL in premature infants.[10] Definitive values for premature infants are known as a result of cordocentesis sampling. Data from Forestier and colleagues for 18 to 29 weeks of fetal life and our own data for fetuses older than 36 weeks of gestation are given in Table 45-1.[8] Based on these data, cord hemoglobin levels of less than 13.0 g/dL should be considered abnormal in term and premature (<36 weeks of gestation) neonates. In the very premature infant (<26 weeks of gestation), values as low as 12.0 g/dL may be acceptable. If anemia is confirmed, a prompt and careful search for the cause should be initiated.

One factor that can significantly influence the hemoglobin level in newborn infants is the amount of placental transfusion. At birth, blood is rapidly transferred from the placenta to the infant, with one-fourth of the placental transfusion occurring within 15 seconds of birth and one-half by the end of the first minute.[11] The placental vessels contain 75 to 125 mL of blood at birth.[12] Usher and associates demonstrated that the blood volume of an infant can be increased by as much as 61% by delayed cord clamping.[13] In that study, the average erythrocyte mass in a group of infants with delayed cord clamping was 49 mL/kg at 72 hours of age compared with 31 mL/kg in a group in whom the cord was clamped immediately after birth. Although infants delivered after delayed cord clamping have higher hemoglobin values, it should be recognized that the placental transfusion may be markedly reduced or prevented if the infant is held above the level of the placenta at the time of delivery; in this situation, it is possible for an infant to lose blood into the placenta and be born anemic.[14]

PHYSIOLOGIC ANEMIA AND THE ANEMIA OF PREMATURITY

The hemoglobin concentration of healthy full-term and premature infants undergoes typical changes during the first weeks of life.[15–18] After birth, there is a transient increase in hemoglobin concentration (Fig. 45-1) as plasma moves extravascularly to compensate for the placental transfusion and increase in circulating erythrocyte volume that occurs at the time of delivery.[19] Thereafter, the hemoglobin concentration gradually falls, to reach minimal levels of 11.4 ± 0.9 g/dL in term infants by 8 to 12 weeks of age and 7.0 to 10.0 g/dL in premature infants by 6 weeks of age (see Fig. 45-1).[18]

There are several reasons for the fall in hemoglobin. The first is the decline in erythrocyte production, which occurs in the first few days of life and is evidenced by a fall in reticulocyte counts during that time (Fig. 45-2; see Fig. 45-1). Normally, reticulocyte counts may be elevated during the first 1 or 2 days of life (20–30 × 10^9/dL) but then fall to low levels (5 × 10^9/dL) through the remainder of the neonatal period. This diminution of erythropoiesis is probably due to decreased EPO production. The reduced EPO re-

TABLE 45–1
NORMAL ERYTHROCYTE VALUES DURING GESTATION*

Weeks of Gestation	Erythrocytes (× 10^{12}/L)	Hemoglobin (g/dL)	Hematocrit (%)	Mean Corpuscular Volume (fl)
18–21	2.85 ± 0.36	11.7 ± 1.3	37.3 ± 4.3	131.11 ± 10.97
22–25	3.09 ± 0.34	12.2 ± 1.6	38.6 ± 3.9	125.1 ± 7.84
26–29	3.46 ± 0.41	12.9 ± 1.4	40.9 ± 4.4	118.5 ± 7.96
>36	4.7 ± 0.4	16.5 ± 1.5	51.0 ± 4.5	108 ± 5

* Values are given ±1 standard deviation.

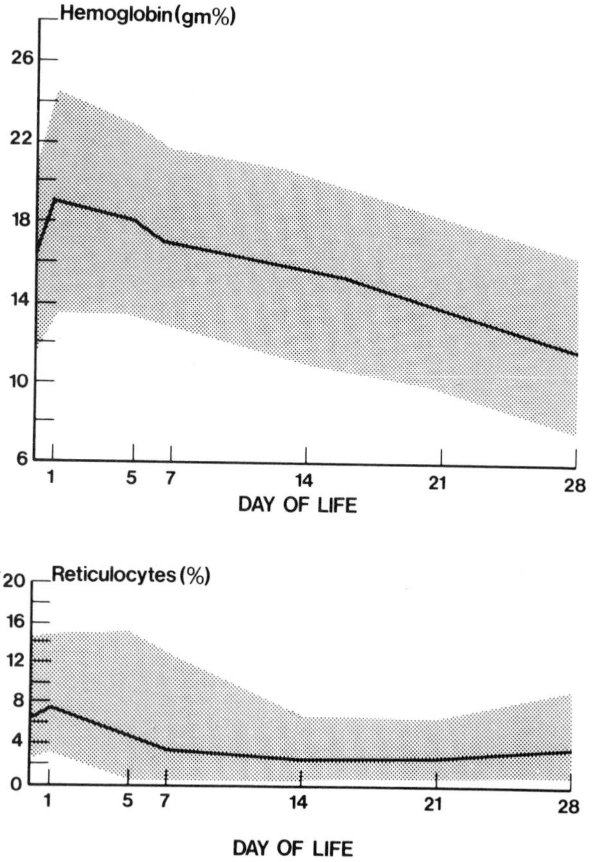

FIG. 45–1. Hemoglobin values of 178 normal premature infants ≤36 weeks of gestation. Data at the first point, day 0, are cord blood values. Subsequent points represent data from capillary blood samples on 1, 5, 7, 14, and 28 days of life. The dark line represents the mean value, and the shaded area includes 95% of all values.

sponse persists until approximately 6 weeks of age, at which time erythrocyte production increases, as evidenced by a sharp rise in reticulocyte numbers in the blood and an increase in total-body hemoglobin (see Fig. 45-2). Other factors that contribute to the physiologic anemia in newborns, particularly the more profound anemia in premature infants, are the shortened survival of neonatal erythrocytes and rapid body growth (see Fig. 45-2).[20,21]

There is considerable controversy about whether the anemia of prematurity is physiologic. Low hemoglobin levels in the newborn have been associated with apneic spells, bradycardia, and failure to thrive.[22] Other studies have not confirmed the relation between hemoglobin levels and clinical signs.[23,24]

Trials of transfusion therapy at certain values have not demonstrated clear benefit and may expose these infants to infection (*e.g.*, cytomegalovirus [CMV], hepatitis, human immunodeficiency virus [HIV]).[25,26] The signs and symptoms of anemia in premature infants are nonspecific and reflect changes in metabolic rate or cardiorespiratory function and perfusion. Controversy exists about whether tachycardia, tachypnea, periodic breathing, and apnea are reliable indicators of anemia.[27–30] Stockman and Clark demonstrated an improvement in weight gain in premature infants with poor weight gain after transfusion.[31] Trials of transfusion therapy for anemia in premature infants require a better defined end point before they can yield a definitive result. Prevention of anemia would be a better intervention. Trials of folate, iron, and vitamin E have not shown any evidence of benefit in preventing the physiologic anemia of infancy.[32] Protein supplementation may be of some value and requires further study.[33] Iron supplementation is im-

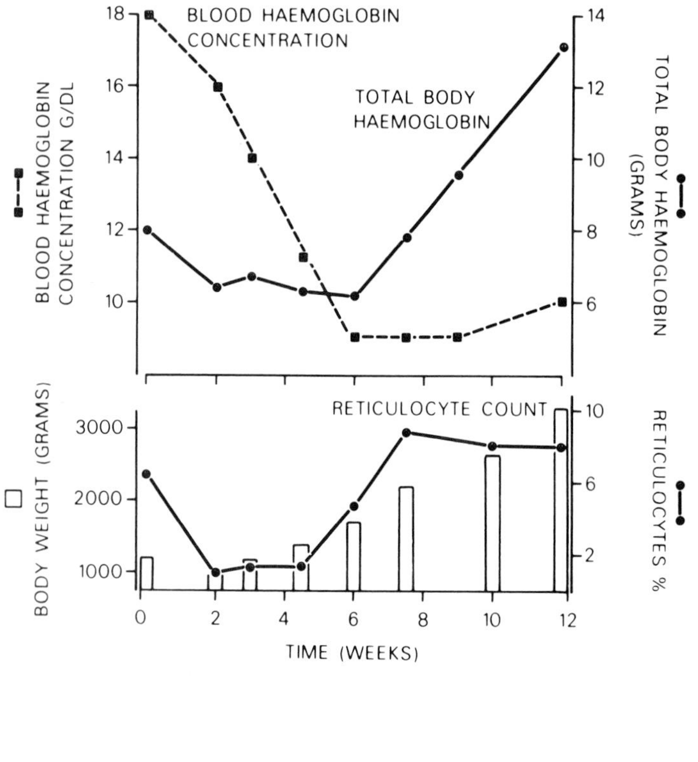

FIG. 45–2. Changes in total body hemoglobin, blood hemoglobin concentration, reticulocyte count, and body weight in a representative premature infant. The vertical bars represent the infant's body weight. During the first 6 weeks of life, the blood hemoglobin concentration and total body hemoglobin fall as a result of decreased erythrocyte production, as evidenced by the low reticulocyte count. The more rapid decline in blood hemoglobin concentration from the third to the sixth week is the result of the increasing body size and "dilution" of the hemoglobin mass. After 6 weeks of age, hemoglobin production increases, as evidenced by the increased reticulocyte count and the rapid increase in total body hemoglobin. The blood hemoglobin concentration during that period may rise slightly, or not at all, because the totaly body size increases at approximately the same rate as the total hemoglobin mass.

portant for the prevention of the anemia seen at about 6 months of age in premature infants.[34–36]

Several groups have begun to examine the use of EPO administration to prevent the physiologic anemia of prematurity.[37–39] There is no convincing evidence of benefit, and the possible side-effects of neutropenia and poor weight gain have been observed. A large multicenter trial is underway to address the possible benefits and risks of EPO in this population. Until the results of that trial are known, the use of EPO must be considered experimental.

EVALUATION

Anemia is a disorder characterized by an abnormally low erythrocyte mass; in clinical practice the hemoglobin concentration is assumed to reflect the circulating erythrocyte mass, and an abnormally low hemoglobin concentration defines the anemic state. After diagnosis, causes of anemia are traditionally considered under the pathophysiologic categories of decreased erythrocyte production, increased destruction (*i.e.*, hemolysis), and blood loss. In newborn infants, this classic approach to anemia is complicated by a hemoglobin concentration that undergoes constant physiologic change during the first few weeks of life. The site of blood sampling, quantity of blood sampled for laboratory monitoring, and the effect of rapid growth can significantly influence the hemoglobin values observed in newborn infants. Failure to consider these factors may lead to errors in diagnosis and result in unnecessary investigation and therapy. A practical approach to the assessment of anemia in newborn infants is the classic pathophysiologic method, with special emphasis on factors such as growth and blood sampling, which must be considered for an accurate assessment of anemia in this age group.

ACCURACY OF CAPILLARY HEMOGLOBIN LEVELS

Blanchette and Zipursky compared capillary hemoglobin values obtained by duplicate puncture of the right and left heels of 35 healthy full-term infants.[40] The standard deviation of the difference in hemoglobin concentration of the duplicate samples was 0.8 g/dL; in an infant with a hemoglobin concentration of 17.0 g/dL, 95% of hemoglobin values obtained fall between 15.4 and 18.6 g/dL. It is evident that a difference as large as 1.5 g/dL of hemoglobin in consecutive laboratory reports may reflect the error inherent in the technique of capillary blood sampling in the newborn infant.

EFFECT OF THE SAMPLING SITE ON HEMOGLOBIN LEVELS

In newborn infants, hemoglobin levels measured in capillary blood samples may be significantly higher than values obtained from simultaneously collected venous blood samples. Oettinger found an average difference of 3.6 g/dL between simultaneous capillary and venous hemoglobin determinations in 24 infants studied on the first day of life.[41] Similar differences have been reported by other investigators (Fig. 45-3).[40,42,43] These differences have been found in term and premature infants, and they persist through the first 6 weeks to 3 months of life.[40,44] The difference in capillary and venous hemoglobin levels is most marked in the more premature infants.[44] Linderkamp and colleagues suggested that warming of the heel reverses the poor circulation and stasis in peripheral

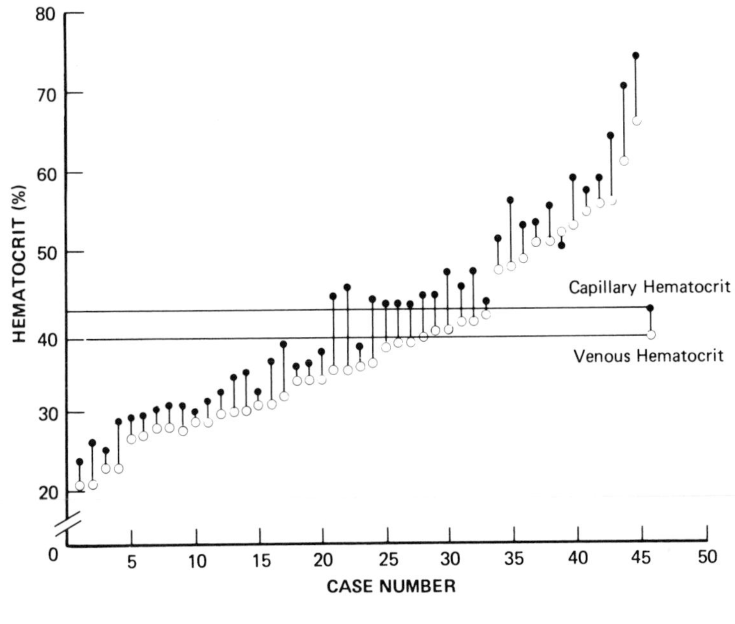

FIG. 45–3. Simultaneous capillary (*dark circles*) and venous (*open circles*) hematocrit levels in 45 premature infants studied during the first 6 weeks of life. Each vertical line represents values for 1 infant, and the horizontal solid line represent mean capillary and venous hematocrit levels for the whole group. Data are not shown for 5 infants in whom capillary and venous hematocrit levels were identical.

vessels that is largely responsible for capillary and venous differences.[42] If the heel is prewarmed before collection of a capillary sample, the difference in capillary and venous hemoglobin values decreases significantly.[40,43]

CORRELATION OF CAPILLARY HEMATOCRIT LEVELS AND TOTAL ERYTHROCYTE MASS

Erythrocyte mass is probably the best measurement of anemia. In adults, it correlates directly with hemoglobin values, which can be used as a valid means of determining anemia. In infants, the correlation between erythrocyte mass and hemoglobin values, although statistically significant, is poor.[40,45] Figures 45-4 and 45-5 show the results of measurements made using a microtechnique using ^{51}Cr to measure erythrocyte mass in premature infants in the first and sixth weeks of life.[40] Extremely wide variations in erythrocyte mass occur for any given hematocrit value. The capillary hematocrit is often a poor reflection of the circulating erythrocyte mass in newborn infants. This is particularly true for ill infants, in whom a poor peripheral circulation may exaggerate capillary and venous hematocrit differences, and for premature infants during periods of rapid body growth, when increases in the total circulating blood volume may influence hemoglobin levels through hemodilution.[42]

Of the many techniques available for measuring erythrocyte mass, the use of chromium-labeled erythrocytes (^{51}Cr) remains the gold standard.[46] This technique allows a direct measurement of erythrocyte mass and does not depend on approximations involving the use of measured plasma volumes, body

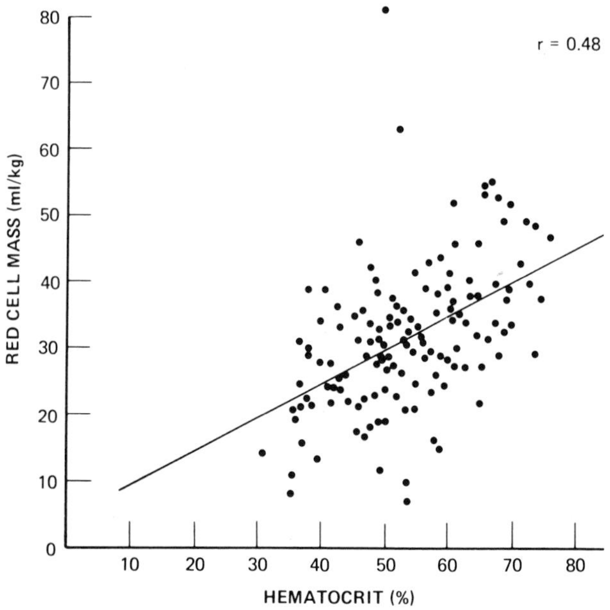

FIG. 45–4. Simultaneous capillary hematocrit and circulating erythrocyte mass levels in 135 premature infants who had birth weights less than 1500 g and were studied during the first week of life. (r, correlation coefficient.)

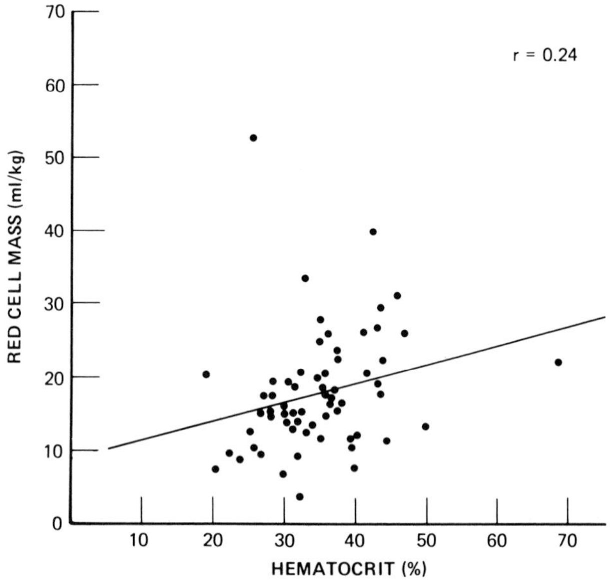

FIG. 45–5. Simultaneous capillary hematocrit and circulating erythrocyte mass levels in 63 premature infants who had birth weights less than 1500 g and were studied at 6 weeks of age. (r, correlation coefficient.)

weights, hematocrit values, or dilution of fetal hemoglobin after transfusion. The values shown in Figure 45-4 agree with those obtained by other researchers.[47–51] Another technique involving the use of biotinylated erythrocytes has been applied in neonates and yields values similar to those obtained by previous researchers using ^{51}Cr.[52,53] The newer, nonradioactive technique will lead to more accurate study of anemia in premature newborns.

EFFECT OF GROWTH ON HEMOGLOBIN LEVELS

Healthy premature infants are in a phase of rapid growth when active erythropoiesis, as evidenced by a mild reticulocytosis, resumes at 6 to 8 weeks of age. Associated with this rapid gain in body weight is an obligatory increase in the total circulating blood volume. The resultant hemodilution may cause a peripheral hemoglobin concentration that is static or even falling slightly. The apparent paradox of a stable or falling hemoglobin concentration despite active erythropoiesis (*i.e.*, mild reticulocytosis and an increasing erythrocyte mass) gradually corrects, and the peripheral hemoglobin concentration increases (see Fig. 45-2). Failure to recognize the important effect of rapid body growth on the peripheral hemoglobin concentration may lead to erroneous investigation and treatment of apparent anemia.[16,54]

IMPACT OF BLOOD SAMPLING ON HEMOGLOBIN LEVELS

Despite the adoption of micromethods using small volumes of blood by most laboratories servicing neonatal units (Table 45-2), cumulative blood losses

TABLE 45–2
VOLUME OF WHOLE BLOOD REQUIRED FOR COMMON LABORATORY TESTS

Test	Volume (mL)
Hemoglobin, total leukocytes, platelets	0.11
Blood gases	0.44
Electrolytes	0.21
Bilirubin	0.14
Calcium	0.14
Protein (total), albumin	0.21
PT, PTT, TCT fibrinogen	0.9

PT, prothrombin time; PTT, partial thromboplastin time; TCT, thrombin clotting time.

through sampling for laboratory monitoring are often surprisingly large in small infants. Blanchette and Zipursky measured an average blood loss of 22.9 mL of packed cells from 59 premature infants studied through the first 6 weeks of life.[40] Forty-six percent (26 of 57) of the infants studied had cumulative losses that exceeded their circulating erythrocyte mass at birth (Fig. 45-6); in a few cases, losses were amazingly large and were equivalent to two or three times the infants' initial circulating erythrocyte masses. Because these losses must be replaced, at least in part, by erythrocyte transfusions, some infants had the equivalent of a double- or triple-volume exchange transfusion, simply as a result of blood sampling for laboratory tests. Approximately 10% of all blood loss during sampling for laboratory monitoring was hidden and represented blood on cotton swabs or in the dead space of syringes or tubing of butterfly sets used to collect blood samples.[55]

There is a correlation between the volume of blood sampled and transfused (Fig. 45-7), suggesting that much of the erythrocyte transfusion requirement of ill, premature infants is a direct consequence of blood loss for essential laboratory monitoring.[40] In the study of Blanchette and Zipursky, significantly more blood was sampled from infants judged to be clinically ill than from healthy premature infants.[40] Iatrogenic blood loss through sampling was significant in both groups (mean ± 1 SD = 26.9 ± 9 and 14.6 ± 5 mL, respectively). These comparative volumes may not appear large, particularly to those who regularly deal with older children or adults, but the actual values must be compared with a total erythrocyte mass that varies between 32.3 and 45.5 mL/kg.[47–51] In practical terms, the removal of 1 mL of blood from a 1-kg infant is equivalent to removing 70 mL of blood from an average adult, and it is therefore not surprising that repeated blood sampling, even with capillary samples, can have a profound effect on the hemoglobin concentration of small, premature infants. Ballin and colleagues, demonstrated in animals that, if the erythrocytes that were discarded from samples drawn in which only the plasma was used were instead reinfused, the fall in hemoglobin concentration was substantially reduced.[56]

CLASSIFICATION

Anemia at birth or appearing during the first few weeks of life can be broadly categorized into three major groups. The anemia may be the result of blood loss, hemolysis, or underproduction of erythrocytes.

ANEMIA CAUSED BY BLOOD LOSS

Blood loss resulting in anemia may occur prenatally, at the time of delivery, or postnatally. Blood loss may be a result of occult hemorrhage before birth, obstetric accidents, internal hemorrhages, or excessive blood sampling for diagnostic studies (Table 45-3). Faxelius and colleagues associated a low erythrocyte volume with a maternal history of bleeding in the late

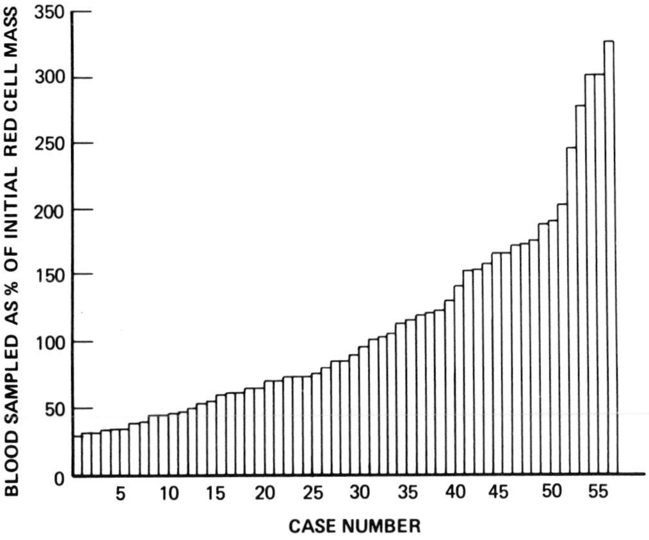

FIG. 45–6. Cumulative blood losses through sampling in premature infants, expressed as a percentage of their erythrocyte mass at birth. Infants were studied during the first 6 weeks of life, and each vertical bar represents a single infant.

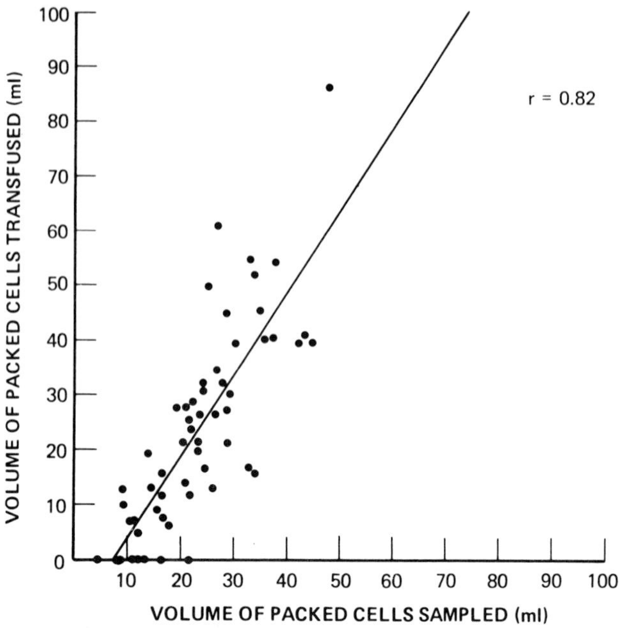

FIG. 45–7. Relation during the first 6 weeks of life between the cumulative volumes of blood sampled from and transfused into 57 premature infants who had birth weights less than 1500 g. Volumes represent milliliters of packed erythrocytes. (r, correlation coefficient.)

third trimester, placenta previa, abruptio placentae, nonelective cesarean section, deliveries associated with cord compression, Apgar scores of less than 6, an early central venous hematocrit of less than 45%, and a mean arterial pressure of less than 30 torr.[45]

Occult Hemorrhage Before Birth

Occult hemorrhage before birth may be caused by bleeding of the fetus into the maternal circulation or by bleeding of one fetus into another in multiple pregnancies. In approximately 50% of all pregnancies, some fetal cells can be demonstrated in the maternal circulation.[57] In about 8% of pregnancies, from 0.5 to 40.0 mL of blood is transferred from the fetus to the mother at birth, and in 1% of pregnancies, the blood loss exceeds 40 mL. Fetomaternal hemorrhages are more common after traumatic diagnostic amniocentesis or external cephalic version.

Fetomaternal Hemorrhage. The clinical manifestations of a fetomaternal hemorrhage depend on the volume of the hemorrhage and the rapidity with which it has occurred. If the hemorrhage has been prolonged or repeated during the course of the pregnancy, anemia develops slowly, giving the fetus an opportunity to develop hemodynamic compensation. These infants may manifest only pallor at birth. After acute hemorrhage just before delivery, the infant may be pale and sluggish, with gasping respirations and signs of circulatory shock.

The degree of anemia varies. Usually, the hemoglobin is less than 12.0 g/dL before signs and symptoms of anemia are recognized by the physician. Hemoglobin values as low as 3.0 to 4.0 g/dL have been recorded in infants who were born alive and survived. If the hemorrhage has been acute, and particularly in hypovolemic shock, the hemoglobin value may not reflect the magnitude of the blood loss. Several hours may elapse before hemodilution occurs and the magnitude of the hemorrhage is appreciated. In general, a loss of 20% of the blood volume acutely is sufficient to produce signs of shock and is reflected in a fall in hemoglobin concentration within 3 hours of the event.

In acute and chronic hemorrhage, the erythrocytes usually appear normochromic and normocytic. Rarely in chronic hemorrhage, the cells appear hypochromic and microcytic, indicating fetal iron deficiency anemia.[58]

If anemia is a direct result of a fetal-to-maternal hemorrhage, the Coombs test is negative, and the infant is not jaundiced. Infants with anemia secondary to blood loss generally have lower than average bilirubin values throughout the neonatal period as a consequence of their reduced erythrocyte mass.

The diagnosis of a fetomaternal hemorrhage great enough to result in anemia at birth can be made with certainty only by the demonstration of fetal cells in the maternal circulation. The Kleihauer technique of

TABLE 45–3
TYPES OF HEMORRHAGE IN THE NEONATE

Occult Hemorrhage Before Birth
Fetomaternal
Traumatic amniocentesis
Spontaneous
After external cephalic version
Twin-to-twin
Obstetric Accidents, Malformations of the Placenta and Cord
Rupture of a normal umbilical cord
Precipitous delivery
Entanglement
Hematoma of the cord or placenta
Rupture of an abnormal umbilical cord
Varices
Aneurysm
Rupture of anomalous vessels
Aberrant vessel
Velamentous insertion
Communicating vessels in multilobed placenta
Incision of placenta during cesarean section
Placenta previa
Abruptio placentae
Internal Hemorrhage
Intracranial
Giant cephalohematomas
Subgaleal
Retroperitoneal
Laceration of the liver
Ruptured spleen

acid elution is the simplest and most commonly employed method for the detection of fetal cells.[59] The test is based on the property of HbF to resist elution from the cell in an acid medium. The acid elution technique can be relied on with certainty for diagnosis only when other conditions capable of producing elevations in maternal HbF levels are absent. These include maternal thalassemia minor, sickle-cell anemia, hereditary persistence of HbF, and in some normal women, a pregnancy-induced rise in HbF production.[60] In these conditions, the appearance of the Kleihauer test, with many cells containing variable amounts of HbF, is easily differentiated from that of a true transplacental hemorrhage, in which the fetal cells containing high concentrations of HbF are readily differentiated from the maternal cells containing no HbF.

Diagnosis of a fetomaternal hemorrhage may be missed in situations in which the mother and infant are incompatible in the ABO blood group system. In such instances, the infant's A or B cells are rapidly cleared from the maternal circulation by the maternal anti-A or anti-B and may not be seen in the Kleihauer preparation.

Twin-to-Twin Transfusion. Twin-to-twin transfusion is observed in 13% to 33% of monozygotic multiple births with monochorial placentas.[61] In approximately 70% of monozygotic twin pregnancies, a monochorial placenta exists. Blood exchange between twins may produce anemia in the donor and polycythemia in the recipient. If a significant hemorrhage has occurred, the difference in hemoglobin between the twins exceeds 5.0 g/dL. There is a maximal discrepancy of 3.3 g/dL in cord blood hemoglobin concentration in dizygotic twins. The anemic twin may develop congestive heart failure, and the plethoric twin may manifest symptoms and signs of the hyperviscosity syndrome, disseminated intravascular coagulation (DIC) and hyperbilirubinemia.

The hemorrhage may be acute or chronic. Tan and associates, on the basis of a review of 482 twin pairs in which 35 were found to have the transfusion syndrome, pointed out how the difference in weight of the twins could be used to establish the timing of the hemorrhage.[61] If the weight difference exceeded 20% of the weight of the larger twin, the transfusion was chronic, and the smaller infant was invariably the donor. The anemic, smaller twin displayed reticulocytosis. If the difference in the weight of the twins did not exceed 20% of the weight of the larger twin, the larger twin was the donor in almost 50% of cases. In these presumably acute transfusions around the time of birth, significant reticulocytosis was not observed in the anemic donor.

If twin-to-twin transfusion is suspected, attempts to confirm it by placental examination should be made. The placentas of all multiple pregnancies should be routinely examined for purposes of genetic counselling. If hematologic evidence has not been obtained and the infants have died, other findings may suggest the diagnosis, including polyhydramnios of one of the recipient's amniotic sac and oligohydramnios of the donor and marked differences in the size and organ weights of the twins.

Obstetric Accidents and Complications

Obstetric accidents and malformations of the placenta and cord may be responsible for major blood loss at the time of delivery. These accidents may be unreported to the pediatrician and may result in diagnostic confusion about the cause of shock in the early hours of life or the presence of pallor and unexplained anemia during the second or third day of life.

The obstetric conditions that can produce neonatal hemorrhage are listed in Table 45-3. Severe and often fatal fetal hemorrhage may accompany placenta previa, abruptio placentae, or accidental incision of the placenta or umbilical cord during a cesarean section.

In women with late-third-trimester bleeding, Clayton and associates were able to anticipate the birth of a possible anemic infant by examining the vaginal blood for the presence of fetal erythrocytes, employing the acid elution technique of Kleihauer.[59,62]

It is good pediatric practice to obtain a hemoglobin measurement routinely at the time of delivery of all babies born of women with late-third-trimester bleeding and of those born by cesarean section. This determination should be repeated in 6 to 12 hours to observe the expected fall in hemoglobin due to the hemodilution that follows recent blood loss.

Severe bleeding as a result of an obstetric accident or complication of delivery often results in the birth of a pale, limp infant. Respirations, which usually commence spontaneously, are often irregular and gasping. They are not associated with retraction, as in conditions accompanied by primary pulmonary disease. Cyanosis is minimal, and the infant's pale color is not improved by oxygen administration. The peripheral pulses are weak or absent, and the blood pressure is reduced. The venous pressure measured after the insertion of an umbilical catheter is found to be extremely low.

Internal Hemorrhage

Anemia that appears in the first 24 to 72 hours of life and is not associated with jaundice is commonly caused by hemorrhage at the time of birth or by a postnatal internal hemorrhage. Traumatic deliveries may result in subdural or subarachnoid hemorrhages or cephalohematomas of sufficient magnitude to produce anemia.

Breech deliveries may be associated with hemorrhage into the adrenals, kidney, spleen, or retroperitoneal area. Rupture of the liver or subcapsular hemorrhage into the liver may occur more commonly than is clinically recognized.[63–65] An infant with a ruptured liver may appear well for the first 24 to 48 hours of life and then suddenly go into shock. The abdomen may appear distended, and a mass contiguous with the liver is often palpable. Shifting dullness on abdominal percussion can often be demonstrated, and an elevation of the right hemidiaphragm may be seen on the radiograph.

Splenic rupture may occur after a difficult delivery or as a result of the extreme distension of the spleen that is often seen in babies with severe erythroblastosis fetalis. The physician should always suspect a rupture of the spleen when an anemic, and often hydropic, infant with erythroblastosis is found to have a low initial venous pressure at the time of exchange transfusion.

Bleeding into the ventricles and subarachnoid space can also produce significant decreases in hemoglobin concentration. This is more common in infants with birth weights of less than 1500 g.

Iatrogenic Anemia

Anemia appearing during the first week of life is often caused by blood removal for diagnostic studies required for the frequent monitoring of critically ill infants. Removal of more than 20% of a subject's blood volume produces anemia. In an infant of 1500 g, this represents a blood loss of only 25 mL. If frequent blood sampling is necessary, a flow sheet should be attached to the infant's incubator, and the amount removed at any given time should be recorded. This simple technique often converts a diagnosis of idiopathic anemia to one of iatrogenic anemia.

Treatment

The treatment of anemia due to blood loss depends on the degree of anemia and the acuteness of the hemorrhage. For acute hemorrhage, the following measures must be employed:

1. If the infant is pale and limp at birth, clear the airway, administer oxygen, and intubate if necessary.
2. Obtain venous access immediately. In some circumstances, this may be through the insertion of an umbilical venous line. Blood specimens for hematologic determinations and crossmatching should be drawn. If an umbilical line is placed, it may be possible to measure a central venous pressure.
3. As soon as it is apparent that pallor is a result of hypovolemic shock or profound anemia and not a consequence of asphyxia, administer 20 mL/kg of the available solution. In order of preference, these are group O Rh-negative blood, plasma, 5% albumin, and isotonic saline. Infants with acute external blood loss usually demonstrate dramatic improvement after such a procedure. Infants with massive internal hemorrhages show less evidence of response.
4. A repeat injection of 10 to 20 mL/kg of whole blood may be given after the first transfusion, particularly if whole blood was not administered initially and the venous pressure and arterial pressure have not returned to normal.

After resuscitating the infant, make efforts to determine the cause of blood loss. Examine the placenta and cord for evidence of abnormalities. Obtain a blood sample from the mother for the detection of a fetomaternal hemorrhage. The infant who is mildly anemic at birth as a consequence of chronic blood loss and who is in no distress may not require transfusion.

For anemic infants still requiring intensive supports, especially mechanical ventilation, it is probably appropriate to treat anemia with blood transfusion. The decision to transfuse must be based on the hemoglobin level and on the clinical condition of the baby. The exact guidelines are not determined. Infants requiring multiple blood tests should receive transfusions after 10% of the calculated blood volume has been removed.

HEMOLYTIC ANEMIA

Anemia as a consequence of a hemolytic process is common in the newborn period and has multiple causes. Hemolytic anemia in the newborn period is almost always associated with elevation of the serum bilirubin value to 170 μmol/L (10 mg/dL) or greater. In general, a hemolytic process is first detected during the investigation of jaundice occurring during the first week of life.

Diagnosis of Hemolytic Disease

Detection and diagnosis of hemolytic disease in newborn infants are difficult, because many of the tests used in older children and in adults are of little value during the first days of life. Hemolytic disease in adults is diagnosed if there is evidence of a rapidly falling hemoglobin concentration, increased erythrocyte production in the absence of hemorrhage, abnormal erythrocyte morphology, and increased erythrocyte destruction within the blood stream with the release of free hemoglobin or within the reticuloendothelial system with production of bilirubin. In the newborn infant, these signs of a hemolytic process are of limited value and require additional interpretation.

Rapidly Falling Hemoglobin Concentration. The assessment of anemia in newborn infants was described previously. Hemolytic disease may be suspected if there is anemia or if hemoglobin levels fall rapidly in the absence of hemorrhage, significant removal of blood for testing, or fluid shifts.

Evidence of Increased Erythrocyte Production. In adults, an increased reticulocyte count with a stable or falling hemoglobin concentration is evidence of increased erythrocyte production and, in the absence of hemorrhage, is diagnostic of a hemolytic process. Growth of the newborn must also be considered.

The reticulocyte count is an inaccurate measure of erythrocyte production, particularly in the newborn, in whom other causes of reticulocytosis may complicate the issue. The reticulocyte count in normal newborns has a wide range, further limiting its value except in severe hemolytic disease. A valuable test for erythrocyte production is the determination of erythrocyte creatine levels.[66,67] The concentration of erythrocyte creatine is high in young erythrocytes and decreases as the cell ages. Erythrocyte creatine is a measure of mean erythrocyte age and is valuable in the study of hemolytic disease in newborn infants.

Erythrocyte Morphology. The shape of erythrocytes in newborns differs from that in adults. Abnormally shaped cells are frequent in newborn infants, particularly in premature infants. Quantitative assessment of the three-dimensional shape of the erythrocyte is of considerable value in the diagnosis of hemolytic disease in newborns.[68] Erythrocyte morphology found in newborn infants is shown in Figure 45-8, and the percentage of these cells found in full-term and premature infants is shown in Table 45-4.

Evidence of Intravascular Erythrocyte Destruction. In adults and children, intravascular hemolysis is evidenced by increased levels of hemoglobin in the plasma (*i.e.*, hemoglobinemia), a fall in serum haptoglobin, and the appearance of hemoglobinuria and methemalbuminemia. In the normal newborn, haptoglobin levels may be zero, and plasma hemoglobin levels are above those found in adults. Gross elevations in plasma hemoglobin and hemoglobinuria are evidence of intravascular hemolysis in newborns, but the value of these tests in detecting mild hemolysis is limited.

Evidence of Extravascular Erythrocyte Destruction. When erythrocytes are destroyed in the reticuloendothelial system, bilirubin is produced, with elevation of indirect bilirubin in the blood. In the newborn, there are many other causes of hyperbilirubinemia (see Chap. 38). In newborns, unlike adults, indirect hyperbilirubinemia is not a specific or helpful sign of hemolytic disease. Unusually rapid appearance of jaundice, particularly in the first 24 hours, suggests hemolytic disease. Because there are many causes of indirect hyperbilirubinemia, all newborns with abnormally high indirect bilirubin levels must be studied for evidence of hemolytic disease.

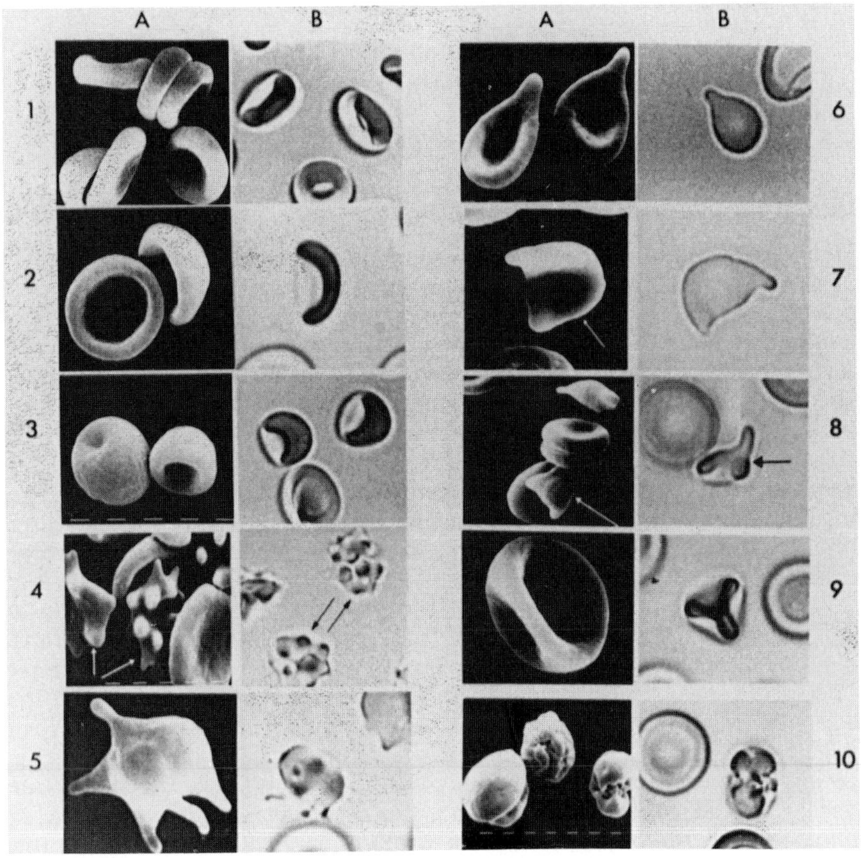

FIG. 45–8. The three-dimensional appearance of erythrocytes as seen by **(A)** scanning electron microscopy and **(B)** by light microscopy of glutaraldehyde-fixed cells. The terminology used to describe the cells is that of Bessis,[69] with the exception of images 2 and 10. (1, discocytes; 2, bowls; 3, spherocytes; 4, echinocytes; 5, acanthocytes; 6, dacrocytes; 7, keratocytes; 8, schizocytes; 9, knizocytes; 10, immature erythrocytes.)

TABLE 45–4
ERYTHROCYTE DIFFERENTIAL COUNTS IN ADULTS AND NEONATES

	Median (5%–95%)*		
Erythrocytes	Adults	Full-Term Infants†	Premature Infants‡
Number studied	53	31	52
Disks	78 (42–94)	43 (18–62)	39.5 (18–57)
Bowls	18 (4–50)	40 (14–58)	29 (13–53)
Ratio of disks to bowls	2 (0–4)	2 (0–5)	3 (0–10)
Spherocytes	0 (0–0)	0 (0–1)	0 (0–3)
Echinocytes	0 (0–3)	1 (0–4)	5.5 (1–23)
Acanthocytes	0 (0–1)	1 (0–2)	0 (0–2)
Dacrocytes	0 (0–1)	1 (0–3)	1 (0–5)
Keratocytes	0 (0–1)	2 (0–5)	3 (0–7)
Schizocytes	0 (0–1)	0 (0–2)	2 (0–5)
Knizocytes	1 (0–4)	3 (0–8)	1 (0–6)
Others	1 (0–4)	3 (0–7)	4 (1–11)

* All values are expressed as a median plus the 5% to 95% range, because the distribution of most values was nongaussian.
† Of the sample, 29 were ABO compatible, 1 was AB with an A mother, and 1 was AB with a B mother.
‡ Includes ABO-compatible and ABO-incompatible infants.

There are several signs of hemolytic disease in newborn infants:

- rapid fall in hemoglobin concentration in the absence of hemorrhage
- increased erythrocyte production (*i.e.*, reticulocytosis or elevated erythrocyte creatine) with a stable or falling hemoglobin concentration
- abnormal erythrocyte morphology
- hemoglobinuria
- jaundice during the first 24 hours of life.

Isoimmune Hemolytic Disease

Hemolytic disease in the newborn as a consequence of isoimmunization of the mother is caused by the passage of fetal erythrocytes into the maternal circulation, where they stimulate the production of antibody. Antibodies of the IgG class return to the fetal circulation, attach to antigenic sites on the surface of the erythrocyte, and cause its rapid removal and destruction. The incidence and clinical manifestations of isoimmunization depend on the type of blood group incompatibility between the mother and fetus. This topic has been the subject of many comprehensive reviews.[70–73]

Rhesus Hemolytic Disease

The incidence of Rh incompatibility in a population depends, in large part, on the prevalence of the Rh-negative antigens. The prevalence of the Rh-negative genotype ranges from approximately zero in Japanese, Chinese, and North American Indian populations to 5.5% among African Americans and 15% among American Caucasians. Among Caucasian women, it has been estimated that in approximately 9% of all pregnancies an Rh-negative woman carries an Rh-positive fetus. In 6% (1 of 15) of pregnancies at risk, isoimmunization of the mother occurs if there is no immunoprophylaxis.

The severity of Rh hemolytic disease varies greatly from infant to infant. It is estimated that, without antenatal diagnosis and treatment, the perinatal mortality in this disease would be approximately 17.5%, with stillbirths accounting for about 14% of deaths.[72] Although hemolytic disease tends to be more severe in a second pregnancy than in a first one in which sensitization has occurred, the severity of disease in subsequent pregnancies tends to be uniform.

Pathogenesis. The entry of fetal cells into the maternal circulation is the cause of Rh isoimmunization. As few as 0.05 to 0.1 mL of cells, particularly if transferred repeatedly, are sufficient to produce immunization. Rh immunization tends to occur more frequently in pregnancies that have been complicated by toxemia, cesarean section, or manual removal of the placenta, because transplacental hemorrhages occur with greater frequency and in greater volume under these circumstances. It is estimated that 1% of Rh-negative women develop antibodies as a consequence of these transplacental hemorrhages before the delivery of their first child. An additional 7.5% manifest evidence of sensitization within 6 months of the delivery of their first child, and another 7.5% show no evidence of immunization 6 months after delivery but develop antibodies during their next pregnancy if their fetus is Rh-positive, presumably as a consequence of a sensitization during the first pregnancy.

Destruction of Fetal Erythrocytes by Anti-D. The transfer of antibody from the mother into the fetal circulation is responsible for the clinical manifestations of the hemolytic process. The erythrocyte, coated with an antibody of the IgG class, is removed primarily in the spleen of the fetus. The rate of destruction is proportional to the amount of antibody on the cell. At very high levels of antibody, the cell may be destroyed by intravascular hemolysis and splenic sequestration.

Before birth, the chief danger of excess erythrocyte destruction is profound anemia. After birth, the infant is primarily at risk from the toxic products of erythrocyte breakdown, such as bilirubin. *In utero*, the infant responds to the increased breakdown of cells by increasing the rate of erythrocyte production. This is reflected by an elevation of reticulocyte count and the presence of nucleated erythrocytes in the peripheral circulation. This accelerated demand for erythrocytes results in active erythropoiesis in nonmarrow sites such as the liver, spleen, and lung. A major portion of the hepatosplenomegaly observed in infants with hemolytic disease is a result of this extramedullary erythropoiesis.

In infants with severe Rh incompatibility, the liver and pancreas exhibit pathologic changes. Islet cell hyperplasia can be observed in the pancreas, and focal cellular necrosis with cholestasis may be seen in the liver.

The most severely affected infants manifest hydrops fetalis. This massive edema with pleural effusions and ascites is not strictly related to the hemoglobin level of the infant. Other factors play a role in the development of hydrops, including intrauterine hypoxia, hypoproteinemia, and a lowering of the nonprotein oncotic pressure of the plasma. Hydrops fetalis has been observed in a variety of other conditions (Table 45-5).

TABLE 45-5
CAUSES OF HYDROPS FETALIS

Severe Chronic Anemia *In Utero*
Erythroblastosis fetalis
Homozygous alpha-thalassemia
Chronic fetomaternal transfusion or twin-to-twin transfusion
Glucose-6-phosphate dehydrogenase deficiency (rare)
Cardiac Failure
Severe congenital heart disease
Premature closure of foramen ovale
Large arteriovenous malformation (*e.g.*, hemangioma)
Intrauterine arrhythmias
Hypoproteinemia
Renal disease
Congenital nephrosis
Renal vein thrombosis
Congenital hepatitis
Intrauterine Infections
Syphilis
Toxoplasmosis
Cytomegalovirus
Miscellaneous
Maternal diabetes mellitus
Parabiotic syndrome in multiple pregnancies
Sublethal umbilical or chorionic vein thrombosis
Fetal neuroblastomatosis
Cystic adenomatoid malformation of the lung
Pulmonary lymphangiectasia
Chorioangioma of the placenta[74]
Transient leukemia of Down syndrome[75]

Clinical Manifestations. The main signs of hemolytic disease in the newborn are jaundice, pallor, and enlargement of the liver and spleen. Jaundice usually becomes evident during the first 24 hours of life, frequently within the first 4 to 5 hours of life, and becomes maximal by the third or fourth day. Jaundice and the metabolism of bilirubin are extensively discussed in Chapter 38.

The degree of anemia reflects the severity of the hemolytic process and the infant's capacity to respond to it with increased erythrocyte production. Late anemia may develop in infants with Rh isoimmunization. This is observed in two clinical settings. In one, the infant does not become sufficiently jaundiced in the initial newborn period to require exchange transfusion. This is more common since the advent of light therapy, which may control the jaundice even though the hemolytic process continues. Continued erythrocyte destruction occurs, and the infant can develop severe or fatal anemia between 7 and 21 days of life. The other, more common situation occurs in infants who have had exchange transfusions. In these infants, a gradual fall in hemoglobin may be observed, with hemoglobin values of 5 to 6 g/dL being reached by 4 to 6 weeks of life. This results from continued destruction of residual and newly formed Rh-positive cells. Spontaneous correction can expected by 6 to 8 weeks of age.

Petechiae and purpura may be observed in infants with severe anemia as a result of thrombocytopenia and a disturbance in the intrinsic system of coagulation. This disturbance may result from DIC or from hepatic dysfunction with consequent inability to synthesize the vitamin K-dependent factors.[76,77]

Laboratory Findings. Decreased hemoglobin concentration, increased reticulocyte count, and increased numbers of nucleated erythrocytes in the peripheral blood reflect the presence of the hemolytic process. Hemoglobin determinations performed on venous samples most accurately reflect the severity of the hemolytic process. Values of less than 13 g/dL in the cord blood should be regarded as abnormal. The reticulocyte count is usually greater than 6% and may reach 30% to 40%. In the peripheral blood, nucleated erythrocytes may be observed in addition to some degree of polychromasia and anisocytosis. Spherocytes are not found in patients with Rh hemolytic disease.

The erythrocytes of infants with Rh hemolytic disease test positive on direct Coombs testing, indicating the presence of maternal IgG on the erythrocyte surface.

Prevention. The management of Rh hemolytic disease focuses primarily on prevention of the disease by the administration of anti-Rh immunoglobulin to the mother after the delivery or abortion of an Rh-positive infant and on the prevention of the intrauterine death of the infant at risk.

The early proposals for the use of anti-Rh immunoglobulin were based on the observation that ABO incompatibility offered protection against the development of Rh sensitization, probably by allowing destruction of the fetal erythrocytes in the mother before they could stimulate Rh antibody formation. Because most major transfers of fetal erythrocytes occur at the time of delivery, efforts were undertaken to destroy such cells soon after delivery. The development of a human γ-globulin concentrate of anti-D (RhoGAM) greatly facilitated application of this means of prevention. Prevention of Rh sensitization is now about 90% effective with the use of anti-D immune globulin at the time of delivery. Failures appear to be caused by hemorrhages that occur before term or by massive hemorrhages that occur at the time of delivery in which the amount of anti-D immunoglobulin administered is inadequate to destroy the large numbers of cells that have entered the circulation. The physician can detect massive hemorrhages at delivery by examining maternal blood for fetal erythrocytes by the Kleihauer technique. It has been estimated that approximately 1 in 250 deliveries involve a transplacental hemorrhage of more than 30 mL.[72] In such instances, a larger dose of anti-D γ-globulin should be given.

Immunization before delivery occurs in approximately 1% of women at risk.[72] The Rh immunization can be prevented by administration of anti-D γ-globulin at week 28 of gestation. It has been suggested that this may not be cost-effective therapy; however, this matter has been discussed in detail elsewhere, and it is the researchers' recommendation that all Rh-negative women with Rh-positive partners should be treated at week 28 of gestation with anti-D γ-globulin to prevent Rh immunization.[78]

Stillbirths are prevented by intrauterine transfusions or by the early termination of pregnancy. The pregnant woman at risk is one who is Rh (D)-negative, has an Rh (D)-positive husband, and has anti-D antibodies in her serum. All such women must be followed carefully during pregnancy.[71,79]

Intrauterine Diagnosis and Treatment. The most accurate assessment of severity of disease in the fetus is the estimation of amniotic fluid bilirubin levels. Amniotic fluid is normally clear and colorless. It acquires a yellow pigmentation in cases of severe hemolytic disease because of the passage of bilirubin into it. The amount of bile pigment in the amniotic fluid more accurately reflects the degree of fetal involvement than does the maternal antibody titer. The concentration of bilirubin pigments, usually measured by spectrophotometry of amniotic fluid, is approximately 350 to 700 nm. Normal amniotic fluid, when plotted on a logarithmic scale, describes a straight line, but when a pigment is present, a bulge appears at approximately 450 nm. This can be measured, and the change in optical density (OD) as a function of gestational age can be employed to gauge the severity of the hemolytic process.[79,80] Women who should have amniocentesis are those with a history of hemolytic disease in previous infants and those whose anti-D titers are greater than 0.125 by the indirect Coombs test, remembering that titers may vary from laboratory to laboratory.

Analysis of the amniotic fluid indicates whether the infant is suffering from severe disease, and this is used as a guide to therapy, which may include continued observation with amniocentesis at 2-week intervals, premature induction after 33 weeks of gestation, or intrauterine blood transfusion.

In severe cases, in which the amniotic OD is high, it is recommended that fetal blood be sampled from the umbilical vein to determine directly the hemoglobin level in the fetal blood and the severity of the hemolytic disease.

The treatment of severe hemolytic disease *in utero* has been by intrauterine transfusions into the peritoneum of the fetus. The preferred method is direct intrauterine transfusion through the umbilical vein. Using intrauterine diagnosis (*e.g.*, amniotic fluid or fetal blood analyses), most fetuses with severe Rh disease can be salvaged. Those who reach 33 weeks of gestation can be induced prematurely, and the survival rate is expected to be the same as for a full-term infant with Rh disease. For those with more severe disease who would not survive to 33 weeks of gestation, intrauterine transfusion beginning at 20 to 22 weeks of gestation results in salvage of as many as 87% of patients.[81]

Management. Newborns with Rh hemolytic disease are at risk of death or damage, primarily from anemia or hyperbilirubinemia. As soon as the infant has been delivered and respirations have been established, the infant should be evaluated in an attempt to judge the severity of the hemolytic process. Assess pallor, organomegaly, petechiae, edema, ascites, respiratory rate, pulse, and blood pressure. Cord blood samples should be analyzed for hemoglobin concentration, reticulocyte count, nucleated erythrocyte count, blood type, direct Coombs reaction, and serum bilirubin concentration, direct-reacting and total.

In the infant with a positive-reacting Coombs test, the major initial decision is whether to perform an immediate exchange transfusion or to observe the infant's clinical status. In many instances, the outcome of previous pregnancies and the result of amniocentesis during the current pregnancy provide valuable information about what to anticipate in the way of severity. Except for the obviously pale or edematous child, the decision to perform an immediate exchange transfusion is based on laboratory findings.

It has been suggested that a cord hemoglobin of less than 11.0 g/dL or a cord bilirubin of more than 4.5 mg/dL are indications for immediate exchange transfusion.[79] The value of immediate transfusion is that it is more efficient to remove "potential bilirubin" (*i.e.*, antibody-coated erythrocytes) than to allow hemolysis to occur, with distribution of bilirubin throughout the tissues, from which it is removed with greater difficulty by exchange transfusion.

For less severely affected infants, exchange transfusion is indicated if it becomes apparent that the rate of bilirubin rise is such that total indirect bilirubin will exceed 20 mg/dL (330 nmol/L) in otherwise healthy full-term infants. The physician needs to use lower maximal bilirubin levels in sick or premature infants (see Chap. 38).

ABO Hemolytic Disease

ABO hemolytic disease results from the action of maternal anti-A or anti-B antibodies on fetal erythrocytes of the corresponding blood group. Although approximately 20% of all pregnancies are associated with ABO incompatibility between the mother and fetus, the incidence of severe hemolytic disease is low. Anti-A and anti-B antibodies are found in the IgA, IgM, and IgG fractions of plasma. Only the IgG antibodies cross the placenta and are responsible for the production of disease. These naturally occurring antibodies result from continuous immune stimulation by A and B substances that exist in foods and gram-negative bacteria. It is not understood why some women develop high anti-A or anti-B titers. They may be the result of repeated, asymptomatic bacterial infections. ABO hemolytic disease tends to occur in the newborns of mothers with high levels of IgG anti-A or anti-B titers.

Fewer A or B antigenic sites are present on the erythrocytes of the newborn, which is responsible for the weakly reactive Coombs test in infants with ABO hemolytic disease. The sparse distribution of A and B sites on the erythrocytes of the newborn also explains why the erythrocyte life span in ABO hemolytic disease is only slightly shortened. This phenomenon is caused by the fetal erythrocyte, which is supported by the fact that adult group A erythrocytes transfused into a baby with maternally acquired anti-A antibody are rapidly destroyed and may produce severe intravascular hemolysis.

The diagnosis of ABO hemolytic disease is often difficult and may first require the exclusion of other causes of hyperbilirubinemia. Usually, the diagnosis is suspected when hyperbilirubinemia appears in the A or B baby of a blood group O mother. The disease is more common and more severe in black infants. Jaundice appearing in the first 24 hours (*i.e.*, icterus praecox) is particularly characteristic of ABO hemolytic disease. Anemia may be mild or not exist. Evidence of isoimmunization is difficult to interpret because the Coombs test may be negative or only weakly positive. A positive Coombs test in ABO incompatible infants does not necessary indicate disease; it has been observed that one-third of all A or B babies of O mothers have a positive direct Coombs test.[82] In approximately two-thirds of these babies, an elution test demonstrated anti-A or anti-B on the surfaces of their erythrocytes.[82] The Coombs test and elution test are not specific for ABO hemolytic disease because these tests are frequently positive in infants who are not affected with disease.

The diagnosis of ABO hemolytic disease is supported by the finding of increased numbers of spherocytes; these are best detected by evaluating the three-dimensional shape of the erythrocyte (Fig. 45-9). Increased erythrocyte production is also demonstrated by an increased reticulocyte count or increased erythrocyte creatine. The diagnosis of ABO hemolytic disease is supported by the following tests and findings:

- indirect hyperbilirubinemia
- jaundice during the first 24 hours
- an A or B baby of an O mother
- increased numbers of spherocytes in the blood

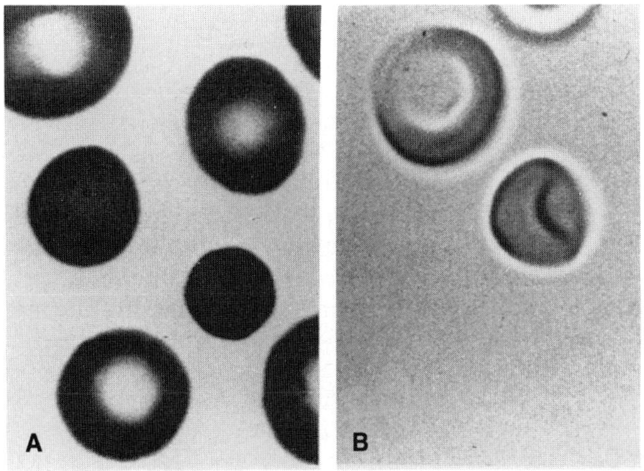

FIG. 45–9. The erythrocytes of a patient with hereditary spherocytosis, as seen **(A)** on a stained blood smear and **(B)** by three-dimensional viewing of glutaraldehyde-fixed cells.

- increased erythrocyte production evidenced by reticulocytosis or an elevated erythrocyte creatine concentration.

The levels of IgG, anti-A, or anti-B in the mothers of babies with ABO hemolytic disease are significantly higher than in mothers whose infants do not have the disease. These tests are often not available and, unfortunately, are of neither high specificity nor sensitivity in the diagnosis of ABO hemolytic disease.

Treatment of this disease is primarily directed toward the prevention of hyperbilirubinemia. Phototherapy reduces the need for exchange transfusion.[83]

Hemolytic Disease Resulting From Minor Blood Group Incompatibility

Hemolytic disease due to maternal erythrocyte antibodies other than anti-D, anti-A, or anti-B is relatively uncommon. In one study, minor group antibodies were found in 121 (0.08%) of 142,800 pregnant women.[84] The principal antibodies found were anti-E, anti-c, and anti-Kell. Anti-Kell antibodies may cause severe hemolytic disease in newborn infants, including hydrops and neonatal death.[85] In a report of 30 cases of hemolytic disease of the newborn, the following antibodies were responsible: 14 anti-c, 9 anti-E, 2 anti-Ce, 2 anti-Kell, 1 anti-Fy^a, 1 anti-JK^a, and 1 anti-U.[86] It is recommended that all pregnant women should have their blood screened for antibodies at least once during pregnancy before week 34 of gestation.

Congenital Defects of the Erythrocyte

Inherited defects of erythrocyte metabolism, membrane function, and hemoglobin synthesis all may manifest themselves in the newborn period. Defects of erythrocyte metabolism include glucose-6-phosphate dehydrogenase (G6PD) deficiency and less common disorders such as pyruvate kinase deficiency.

Glucose-6-Phosphate Dehydrogenase Deficiency

The major function of the erythrocyte is the delivery of oxygen to the tissues. The cell is constantly exposed to oxygen, and the erythrocyte membrane and cytoplasm are subjected to oxidative damage. Oxidation causes the formation of precipitates of denatured hemoglobin (*i.e.*, Heinz bodies), which appear to be associated with a shortened erythrocyte life span *in vivo* (Fig. 45-10). The erythrocyte has a metabolic system that can prevent oxidative damage (Fig. 45-11). Glucose-6-phosphate dehydrogenase is an enzyme in this system; if it is absent, there is a risk of oxidative damage to the erythrocyte, particularly if the cell is stressed by chemicals or drugs capable of oxidative damage (Table 45-6).

Glucose-6-phosphate dehydrogenase deficiency is a common genetic disorder affecting millions of people in the world. There are three major types of deficiency, all of which are inherited as a gender-linked recessive disorder. The most severe deficiency occurs rarely and is associated with a chronic hemolytic anemia. With this type of deficiency, the person has a mild or moderate anemia throughout life and may have severe hemolytic disease as a newborn. The second type affects Asians (*e.g.*, 5.5% of Chinese) and many populations in the Middle East and Mediterranean region (*e.g.*, 0.7% to 3% of Greeks, with the highest incidence of 53% among Kurds). These persons are healthy but are at risk of developing hemolytic anemia when exposed to oxidative drugs or chemicals (*e.g.*, sulpha drugs, fava beans). The anemia may be of sudden onset and may be severe. In the absence of drug exposure, hemoglobin levels are normal, although there is evidence that the erythrocyte life span is slightly shorter than normal.

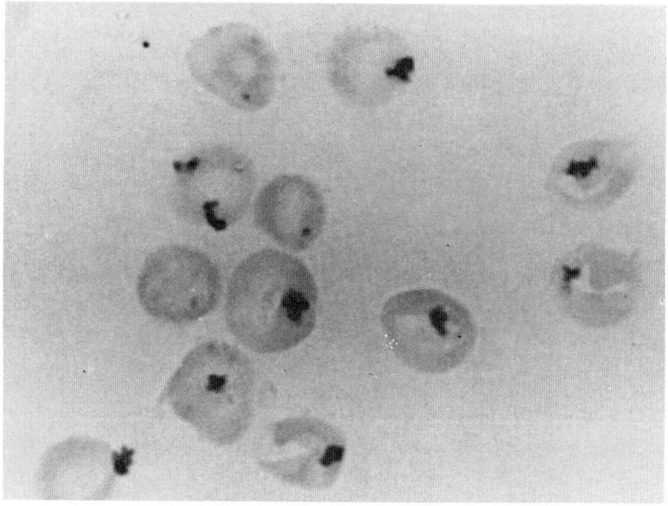

FIG. 45–10. Heinz bodies in a newborn who developed hemolytic anemia after exposure to naphthalene in mothballs.

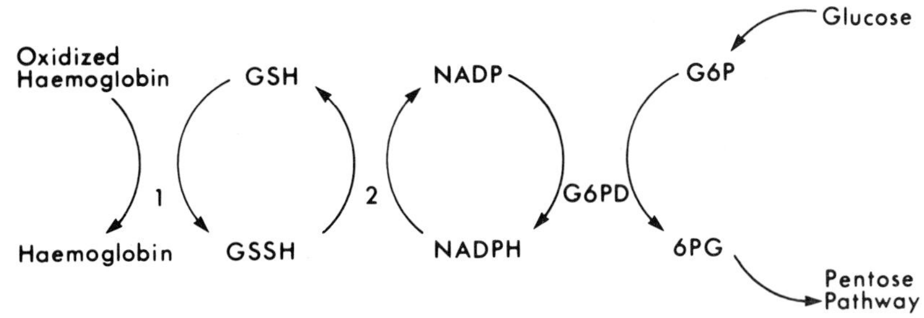

FIG. 45–11. Protection against oxidative stress in erythrocytes. The erythrocyte is constantly exposed to oxygen; as a result, there is formation of hydrogen peroxide (H_2O_2), lipid peroxides in the membrane, and oxidized products of hemoglobin such as methemoglobin and Heinz bodies. To prevent the formation of and to reduce the levels of these oxidized products, the erythrocyte has a system by which a series of enzyme steps link the metabolism of glucose through the pentose pathway to the reduction of oxidized products. (1, glutathione peroxidase; 2, glutathione reductase; G6PD, glucose-6-phosphate dehydrogenase; 6PG, 6-phosphogluconate; G6P, glucose-6-phosphate; GSH, reduced glutathione; GSSH, oxidized glutathione; NADP, nicotinamide-adenine dinucleotide phosphate; NADPH, nicotinamide-adenine dinucleotide phosphate, reduced.)

The third type of deficiency affects blacks (*e.g.*, 10%–14% of African Americans), in whom the severity of the defect is not as great as in those with the other two types. Anemia appears only with drug exposure, is less severe than that of the Asian–Mediterranean type, and tends to be self-limited.

Glucose-6-Phosphate Dehydrogenase Deficiency and Neonatal Jaundice. Because their erythrocytes have a diminished capacity to deal with oxidative stress as a result of lower levels of glutathione peroxidase and catalase and a relative deficiency of vitamin E, newborn infants with G6PD deficiency are at greater risk of developing hemolytic anemia than are adults (see Fig. 45-10). It appears that G6PD deficiency is associated with an increased incidence of neonatal hyperbilirubinemia, especially in the more severe type affecting the Asian and Mediterranean groups. Hyperbilirubinemia in G6PD-deficient boys has been reported in newborns in Greece, Italy, Singapore, and Thailand.[87,88] Although the hyperbilirubinemia is largely the result of G6PD deficiency,

TABLE 45–6
DRUGS, CHEMICALS, AND OTHER FACTORS THAT CAUSE GLUCOSE-6-PHOSPHATE DEHYDROGENASE DEFICIENCY HEMOLYTIC DISEASE

Antimalarials	**Sulfonamides**
Primaquine	Sulfanilamide
Pamaquine	N^2-Acetylsulfanilamide
Pentaquine	Sulfacetamide (Sulamyd)
Antipyretics and Analgesics	Sulfamethoxazole (Gantanol)
Aspirin*	Salicylazosulfapyridine (Azulfidine)
Acetanilid	**Sulfones**
Acetophenetidin (phenacetin)*	Thiazolesulfone
Acetaminophin*	**Others**
Diabetic Acidosis	Methylene blue
Vitamin K analogs	Toluidine blue
Infections	Naphthalene
Respiratory viruses	Phenylhydrazine
Infectious hepatitis	Acetylphenylhydrazine
Infectious mononucleosis	Fava beans
Bacterial pneumonia	Nalidixic acid (Neggram)
Nitrofurans	Niridazole (Ambilhar)
Nitrofuranto (Furadantin)	Chloramphenicol
Furazolidone (Furoxone)	
Furaltadone (Altafur)	
Nitrofurazone (Furacin)	

* Of doubtful significance.

there is a tendency for the jaundice to occur more frequently in particular families and communities, indicating that genetic and environmental factors must influence the incidence of the disease. In this group of patients, jaundice may be severe and may lead to kernicterus.[89–91] In most cases, however, hemoglobin and reticulocyte counts are normal, although in some affected infants the cord blood contains increased bilirubin and decreased hemoglobin levels, suggesting the presence of a mild hemolytic process *in utero.* There is no evidence of intravascular hemolysis in most of these patients. Full-term African-American infants with G6PD deficiency do not develop hyperbilirubinemia more frequently than normal infants do, although the incidence in premature infants may be slightly higher.[92] It has been reported from Africa, however, that black male infants with G6PD deficiency have a significantly higher incidence of hyperbilirubinemia than do controls.[93]

Clinical Manifestations. The jaundice that occurs in these infants appears to be an accentuation of the physiologic jaundice of newborns, although jaundice may appear in some during the first 24 hours of life. There is seldom evidence of a hemolytic process. Abnormal erythrocyte morphology has been documented during hemolytic episodes in adults, but this is seldom described in newborns. However, a more severe hemolytic anemia may appear, with evidence of abnormal erythrocyte morphology, Heinz bodies in the peripheral blood, and intravascular hemolysis. This may be the result of exposure to drugs or chemicals (*e.g.*, naphthalene in mothballs).[94]

Diagnosis. The presence of unexplained hyperbilirubinemia in an infant of a high-risk population may suggest G6PD deficiency. The enzyme defect can be detected by one of the many screening tests.[95,96] The finding of G6PD deficiency in a jaundiced infant does not in itself prove that the jaundice was due to the enzyme defect. All other causes of jaundice must be excluded first. Glucose-6-phosphate dehydrogenase deficiency is most severe and frequent in male infants, because it is a recessive gender-linked disorder. However, female infants may be affected because they have two populations of erythrocytes, one with normal and one with low levels of G6PD, in keeping with the Lyon hypothesis. Given the high gene frequency, it is also possible for a female infant to be homozygous for the deficiency.

Treatment. Treatment is the same as that for hyperbilirubinemia described in Chapter 38. Drugs and chemicals likely to produce hemolytic anemia (see Table 45-6) should be avoided by these patients.

Other Metabolic Abnormalities of the Erythrocyte

Other abnormalities are far less common than G6PD deficiency and are unusual causes of a hemolytic process during the newborn period. Virtually all the recognized defects have been associated with jaundice and anemia during the first week of life. Of this group, erythrocyte pyruvate kinase deficiency appears to be most commonly responsible for a severe hemolytic process during the first week of life. These disorders are usually characterized by the presence of a normal osmotic fragility of unincubated blood, few or no spherocytes in the peripheral blood smear, and failure of splenectomy in later life to correct the hemolytic process. It is practical to defer diagnosis of these infants until approximately 3 months of life, after it has been established that the hemolytic process observed in the neonatal period is chronic and that the more common reasons for it have been excluded.

Abnormalities of the Erythrocyte Membrane: Hereditary Spherocytosis and Elliptocytosis

In approximately 50% of patients with hereditary spherocytosis, a history of neonatal jaundice can be obtained. Hyperbilirubinemia may require exchange transfusions. Untreated hyperbilirubinemia has resulted in kernicterus in infants with hereditary spherocytosis.

Although most patients with hereditary spherocytosis are anemic, the degree of anemia, reticulocytosis, and hyperbilirubinemia is quite variable. The hemoglobin may fall rapidly during the first several weeks of life, reaching values of 5.0 to 7.0 g/dL by 1 month of age. Neither the hematologic values observed during the immediate newborn period nor the values observed during the first several months of life are reliable indicators of the eventual severity of the disease. It has been my experience that hemoglobin levels in many infants of 4.0 to 7.0 g/dL during the first several months of life subsequently stabilize in the range of 7.0 to 10.0 g/dL. Repeated transfusions are rarely needed, except during the course of infections or aplastic crises. Splenectomy, if indicated, should be deferred until 3 or 4 years of age, so that the risk of postsplenectomy infections is minimized.

Hereditary spherocytosis can be diagnosed during the newborn period. Examination of the peripheral blood reveals characteristic microspherocytes, and the osmotic fragility of erythrocytes is increased. The osmotic fragility of the erythrocytes of normal newborn infants is lower than that of adults' erythrocytes, and if an infant is suspected of having spherocytosis, the osmotic fragility should be compared with normal newborn standards. Family studies are extremely useful in confirming the diagnosis, although an affected parent is identified in only approximately 70% of cases.

Hereditary elliptocytosis may manifest in the newborn period as a hemolytic anemia. Only 12% to 15% of newborns with this morphologic abnormality have a shortened erythrocyte survival in later life, but many more appear to have a hemolytic anemia during the first several weeks or months of life. In the newborn period, hereditary elliptocytosis may manifest as hyperbilirubinemia and anemia associated with the presence of fragmented and deformed erythrocytes in the circulation. This is referred to as neonatal poikilocytosis. The erythrocytes of these infants are unusually susceptible to fragmentation after heating. This defect disappears within the first few months of life, and the erythrocytes assume an elliptic appearance, usually with no or minimal evidence of hemolytic disease. As in hereditary spherocytosis, demonstration of an affected parent or sibling helps to establish the diagnosis.

Most patients do not require treatment, although an exchange transfusion may be required for infants with hyperbilirubinemia. For patients with persistent hemolytic anemia, splenectomy has proved beneficial, but as in hereditary spherocytosis, it should be deferred until the patient is 3 or 4 years of age.

Disorders of Hemoglobin Synthesis

The predominant hemoglobin in the newborn infant is HbF ($\alpha_2\gamma_2$); therefore, it is not surprising that abnormalities in β-chain production (*e.g.*, sickle-cell disease, β-thalassemia) do not manifest during the first month of life. Thalassemia has been diagnosed as early as the second month of life.[97] Patients with sickle-cell disease are usually found to be anemic by 3 months of age, but cases of jaundice and systemic signs during the neonatal period have been reported.[98]

Abnormalities in γ-chain production have been described during the first month of life, although most of these are not clinically significant. One case of Heinz body hemolytic anemia with an unstable γ-chain abnormality has been reported.[99] Cases of microcytic anemia in newborns with reduced γ-chain synthesis have been described as part of a γ-β-thalassemia syndrome.[100–103]

Alpha-chain disorders occur frequently in the newborn period. Although there are many structural defects of the α-chain that have been reported in the newborn, these are rarely of clinical significance. Alpha-thalassemia manifests clinically in newborn infants and can be serious. The α-thalassemia group of diseases represents abnormalities in the synthesis of the α-chains of hemoglobin. Synthesis of these chains is determined by two pairs of α genes. A deletion of one or more of these four α genes results in one of the α-thalassemia disorders. The severity of the disease in the newborn and in the adult depends on the number of genes deleted. If one gene is lacking, the patient is hematologically normal, unless he or she is a newborn, in which case there is a slight elevation of Bart hemoglobin (γ_4). If two genes are absent (*i.e.*, two missing from one chromosome or one missing from each of the two chromosomes), the patient has α-thalassemia, which manifests as microcytosis in the newborn (mean corpuscular volume $< 95\ \mu m^3$/cell) and elevation of Bart hemoglobin. If three genes are deleted, the patient has hemoglobin H (HbH; β_4) disease, a lifelong hemolytic anemia that manifests in the newborn as jaundice and anemia. If all four genes are absent, the patient can form no α-chains and cannot form HbA or HbF. As a result, the infant is born dead or severely hydropic, with death occurring several hours after birth. The hemoglobin of these infants is predominantly Bart hemoglobin.

In patients with HbH disease, one parent is lacking one α gene (*i.e.*, a silent carrier), and the other is lacking two α genes on one chromosome (*i.e.*, α-thalassemia trait). In the patient with homozygous α-thalassemia, each parent is lacking two genes on one chromosome. It is now thought that the α-thalassemia trait that is found in 2% to 10% of blacks is in the *trans* form in which one abnormal gene is present on each of the two chromosomes (*i.e.*, -1α, -1α), and that the *cis* form ($--,\alpha\alpha$) does not occur in blacks but does occur with various frequencies in populations in Southeast Asia and the Mediterranean region. Homozygous α-thalassemia and HbH disease are not found in blacks.

The incidence of α-thalassemia can be determined through measurement of levels of Bart hemoglobin in newborns. Silent carriers (*i.e.*, $-\alpha,\alpha\alpha$) have as much as 2% of Bart hemoglobin. Those with α-thalassemia trait ($--,\alpha\alpha$ or $-\alpha,-\alpha$) have 2% to 9% Bart hemoglobin. Those with HbH disease ($-\alpha,--$) have up to 20% of Bart hemoglobin.

Acquired Defects of the Erythrocyte

Infections and drugs can produce a hemolytic anemia in the newborn infant who has no underlying inherited defect of erythrocyte metabolism. It is frequently suggested that neonatal sepsis causes a hemolytic process. Certain infections in the newborn are associated with hyperbilirubinemia, which initially may be indirect and subsequently include direct hyperbilirubinemia. Hemolytic anemia infrequently complicates sepsis. One exception is *Clostridium welchii* sepsis, in which severe hemolytic anemia associated with microspherocytosis occurs.

Congenital syphilis, toxoplasmosis, cytomegalic inclusion disease, rubella, generalized coxsackie B infections, and *Escherichia coli* septicemia are examples of infections in which anemia and jaundice are common. Some of the nonhematologic manifestations of these diseases (*e.g.*, rash, chorioretinitis, purpura, hepatosplenomegaly) are useful in differentiating these disorders from isoimmunization or other primary erythrocyte abnormalities.

The erythrocytes of the newborn infant are particularly sensitive to the toxic effects of oxidant drugs. The erythrocytes of infants, particularly those of premature babies, demonstrate increased numbers of Heinz bodies, marked glutathione instability, and an increased tendency to develop methemoglobinemia when incubated with acetylphenylhydrazine or menadione. In many respects, the cells of these infants mimic the metabolic abnormalities observed in cells from patients with G6PD deficiency. Severe Heinz body hemolytic anemia (see Fig. 45-10) occurs in infants with severe G6PD deficiency and in normal newborns who are exposed to oxidant drugs. The best and most frequent example of this is naphthalene-induced hemolytic anemia caused by exposure to mothballs. This disease is associated with a severe hemolytic anemia, hemoglobinuria, and the presence of fragmented erythrocytes and spherocytes in the circulation. If these are detected, a careful search for exposure to naphthalene or other oxidant drugs (see Table 45-6) should be carried out. This increased susceptibility to oxidative damage may be related to the low levels of antioxidants, including glutathione peroxidase, catalase, and vitamin E, in the newborn infant. Idiopathic Heinz body hemolytic anemia probably reflects a similar mechanism, resulting in hyperbilirubinemia and anemia with Heinz bodies present, but the infant has normal G6PD levels, a normal hemoglobin electrophoresis, and a negative heat test for the presence of unstable hemoglobins.[104] Evaluation of the family yields no evidence of an inherited disorder, and in the affected neonate, the disorder appears to be self-limited, disappearing within the first several months of life. The role of previously unsuspected agents capable of causing oxidative damage to hemoglobin, such as vitamin C, is being investigated.[105]

ANEMIA CAUSED BY IMPAIRED ERYTHROCYTE PRODUCTION

Diamond–Blackfan Syndrome. Impaired erythrocyte production appears to be an unusual cause for anemia in the newborn. The most common cause is the Diamond–Blackfan syndrome, also known as congenital hypoplastic anemia or pure erythrocyte aplasia. In approximately one-third of infants with this abnormality, anemia exists at birth.[106] The leukocyte count and platelet count are normal. Diagnosis may be established by demonstrating anemia, reticulocytopenia, and a marked decrease in the bone marrow erythroid–myeloid ratio in an otherwise healthy newborn. Erythroid–myeloid ratios range from 1:6 to more than 1:200. Low birth weight affects about 10% of these patients, with about one-half being small for gestational age. Physical anomalies are found in about 30% of patients. Anomalies apparent at birth include microcephaly, cleft palate, eye defects, web neck, and abnormalities of the thumb. A trial of prednisone is recommended, and a response, reflected by a reticulocytosis and a rise in the hemoglobin level, often occurs within 2 weeks. After the hemoglobin has returned to normal, the medication is reduced to the lowest dose necessary to maintain a hemoglobin in the acceptable range. Most patients become refractory to steroid therapy and require a lifelong transfusion program or bone marrow transplantation. Pure erythrocyte aplasia has also been associated with triphalangeal thumbs.[107]

Vitamin Deficiencies. Specific vitamin deficiencies may cause anemia in newborn infants because of decreased erythrocyte production, increased erythrocyte destruction, or a combination of these two mechanisms.

Nutritional anemia secondary to iron or folate deficiency is uncommon in neonates.[108] Studies by Siep and Halvorsen indicate that stainable iron disappears from bone marrow aspirates by 12 weeks of age in premature infants and by 20 to 24 weeks in term infants, and it is only after this period that iron deficiency manifests in infants who do not receive supplemental iron.[109] To prevent the development of iron deficiency, premature infants should receive supplemental iron from no later than 2 months of age. Although most premature infants have low serum folate levels by 1 to 3 months of age, they rarely manifest evidence of a megaloblastic anemia. Cases of megaloblastic anemia due to folate deficiency typically involve newborn infants receiving goat's milk or phenytoin therapy and infants with chronic diarrhea or infection. Folic acid and vitamin B_{12} deficiency are rare disorders of the neonatal period and have been reviewed by Shojania.[110]

The syndrome of vitamin E deficiency anemia in newborn infants, first described by Hassan and colleagues in 1966, typically occurs in premature infants (birth weight < 1500 g) at 6 weeks of age.[111] Characteristic features include anemia, reticulocytosis, thrombocytosis, decreased serum vitamin E levels (<0.5 mg/dL), increased fragility of erythrocytes in the presence of dilute solutions of hydrogen peroxide, and shortened erythrocyte survival.[112] Damage to the erythrocyte membrane by lipid peroxides, formed naturally during peroxidation of polyunsaturated fatty acids (PUFA) in the erythrocyte membrane, is thought to be the mechanism of the anemia; vitamin E, a biologic antioxidant, inactivates lipid peroxides and protects against erythrocyte damage. The anemia may be exaggerated by increasing the PUFA content of the diet, particularly if infants are also given supplemental iron, a catalyst in the autooxidation of PUFA to free radicals and lipid peroxides.[113] After the association of the PUFA content of the diet, iron supplementation, and the vitamin E requirement of premature infants was recognized, the PUFA content of infant formulas was reduced. Vitamin E deficiency is now rare in premature infants, and there is no evidence that routine vitamin E supplementation is of benefit in preventing the anemia of prematurity.[114]

DIAGNOSIS

At no other time does such a variety of disorders result in anemia as in the first week of life. The need for rapid treatment often adds to the diagnostic confusion. It is because of the multiple causes and the need for prompt therapy that the fundamentals of diagnosis should be appreciated and practiced without delay. Attempts at diagnosis begin with a history if the cause is not immediately apparent. In the family history, attention should be paid to anemia in other members of the family or to unexplained episodes of jaundice or cholelithiasis. A positive family history is frequently obtained in cases of infants with hereditary spherocytosis, but a history of affected siblings may be encountered in cases of patients with enzymatic defects of the erythrocyte.

In the maternal history, information should be obtained concerning drug ingestion near term. Information about drugs known to initiate hemolysis in cases of G6PD deficiency should especially be sought with any history of recent exposure to mothballs containing naphthalene.

The obstetric history should provide information about vaginal bleeding during pregnancy, placenta previa, abruptio placentae, vasa previa, and cesarean section. Additional questions should be answered. Was the birth traumatic? Did the cord rupture? Was it a multiple birth?

The age at which anemia is first noticed is also of diagnostic value. Marked anemia at birth is usually the result of hemorrhage or severe isoimmunization. Anemia manifesting itself during the first 2 days of life is frequently caused by external or internal hemorrhages, but anemia appearing after the first 48 hours of life is most commonly hemolytic and is usually associated with jaundice.

One approach to the differential diagnosis of anemia in the newborn period is presented in Figure 45-12. The physician should first decide whether the low hemoglobin level can be explained by blood loss from sampling. Cumulative losses, particularly in ill premature infants, may be extremely large, and correct interpretation of rapid changes in hemoglobin level can be made only if careful attention is paid to exact volumes of blood sampled and transfused. If the cause of anemia remains unknown, several laboratory tests may aid in diagnosis: reticulocyte count, a direct antiglobulin test (*i.e.*, Coombs test) of the infant's blood, examination of a peripheral blood smear, and examination of the maternal blood smear for fetal erythrocytes. From these studies and the history, a diagnosis often can be made, or at least the list of diagnostic possibilities can be greatly shortened.

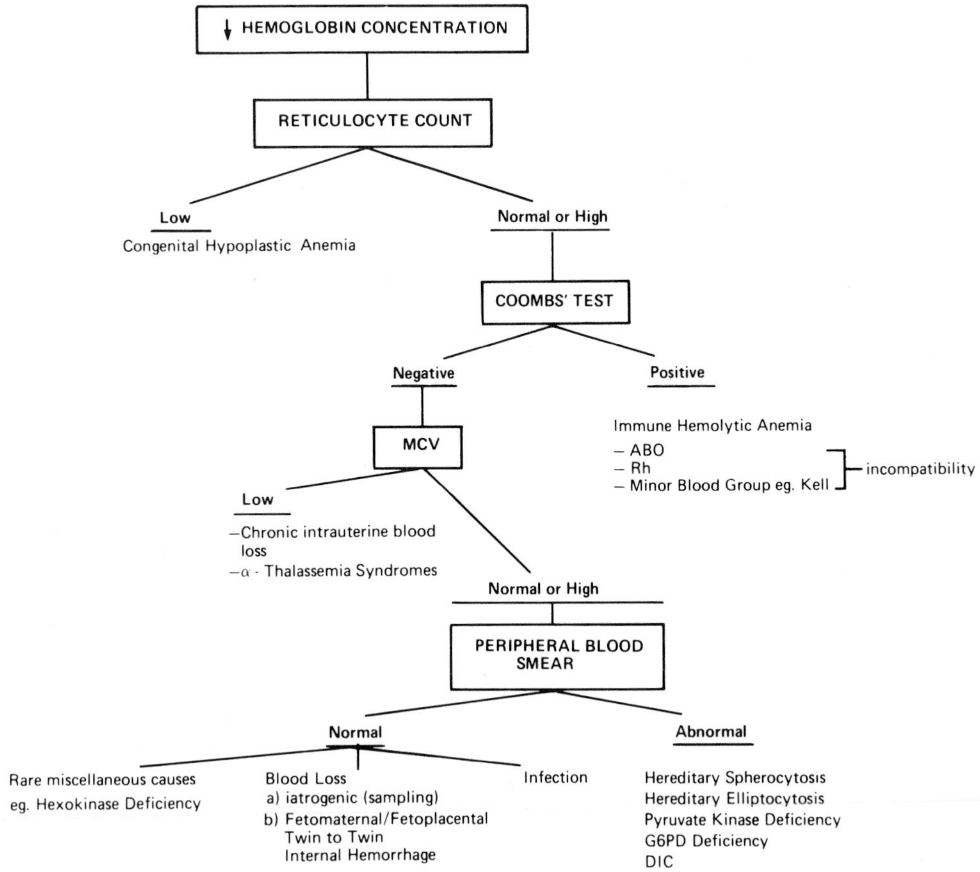

FIG. 45–12. Diagnostic approach to anemia in the newborn infant.

TABLE 45–7
NEONATAL POLYCYTHEMIA

Possible Causes by Placental Hypertransfusion
Twin-to-twin transfusion
Maternofetal transfusion
Delayed cord clamping
Intentional
Unassisted home delivery
Possible Associations
Placental insufficiency
Small-for-gestational-age infants
Postmaturity birth
Toxemia of pregnancy
Placental previa
Endocrine and metabolic disorders
Congenital adrenal hyperplasia
Neonatal thyrotoxicosis
Maternal diabetes
Miscellaneous
Trisomies 21, 13, and 19
Hyperplastic visceromegaly (*i.e.*, Beckwith syndrome)
Erythroderma icthyosiforme congenita

POLYCYTHEMIA

A venous hemoglobin of more than 22.0 g/dL or a venous hematocrit of more than 65% during the first week of life should be regarded as polycythemia. Although neonatal polycythemia may be the result of fetal disorders such as twin-to-twin transfusion, placental insufficiency, and certain metabolic disorders (Table 45-7), most cases occur in otherwise normal infants. Most of these infants have been full term, appropriate for gestational age, and without asphyxia at birth. Polycythemia occurs in 1.5% to 4% of newborn infants.[115–117]

The symptoms observed in the polycythemic infant appear to be primarily a consequence of hypervolemia and an increase in blood viscosity. After the central venous hematocrit reaches 60% to 65%, the increase in blood viscosity becomes much greater as a result of the exponential relation between hematocrit and viscosity.[118] Plasma and erythrocyte factors also affect the viscosity of neonatal blood.[119–121]

Respiratory distress, cyanosis, congestive heart failure, convulsions, priapism, jaundice, renal vein thrombosis, hypoglycemia, and hypocalcemia appear to be more common in infants with polycythemia.[117] Many infants with polycythemia are asymptomatic.

In addition to supportive care, partial exchange transfusion with 5% albumin has been used for the treatment of polycythemia. Reduction of the venous hematocrit to less than 60% may improve symptoms, but it has not been shown to improve long-term neurologic outcome.[122–124]

FETAL HEMOGLOBIN, NEONATAL ERYTHROCYTES, AND 2,3-DIPHOSPHOGLYCERATE

Human tissue metabolism critically depends on an adequate supply of oxygen. The oxygen transport system in humans is the erythrocyte, which contains the iron–protein conjugate, hemoglobin. The erythrocyte's primary function is to bring oxygen to the tissues in adequate quantities at a partial pressure sufficient to permit its rapid diffusion from the blood. The ultimate supply of oxygen to the cell is determined by a number of factors, including the content of oxygen in the inspired air, the pulmonary and alveolar ventilation, the diffusion of oxygen from the alveolar air to the capillary bed, the cardiac output, the blood volume, the hemoglobin concentration, and the passive diffusion of oxygen from the capillaries to the cells. The initial passive diffusion of oxygen from the lungs and its final release to the tissues is largely determined by the affinity of hemoglobin for oxygen.

The oxygen–hemoglobin equilibrium curve reflects the affinity of hemoglobin for oxygen (Fig. 45-13). As blood circulates in the normal lung, arterial oxygen tension rises from 40 torr and reaches approximately 110 torr, sufficient to ensure at least 95% saturation of the arterial blood. The shape of the curve is such that a further increase in the oxygen tension in the lung results in only a small increase in the degree of satu-

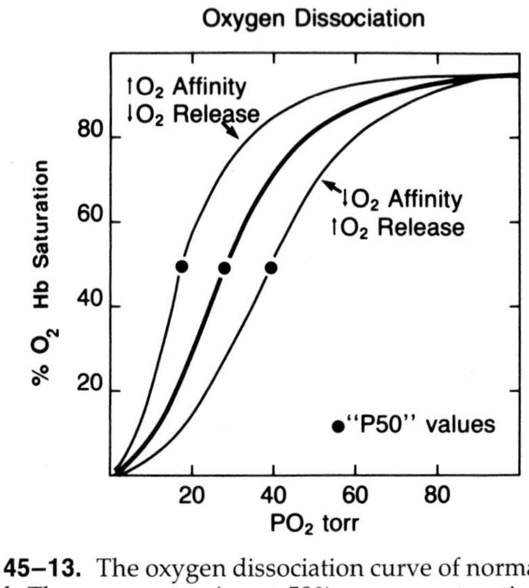

FIG. 45–13. The oxygen dissociation curve of normal adult blood. The oxygen tension at 50% oxygen saturation (P50) is approximately 27 torr. As the curve shifts to the right, the oxygen affinity of hemoglobin decreases, and more oxygen is released at a given oxygen tension. With a shift to the left, the opposite effects are observed. A decrease in *p*H or an increase in temperature decreases the affinity of hemoglobin for oxygen.

ration of the blood. As blood travels from the lung, the oxygen tension falls as oxygen is released to the tissues from hemoglobin. In the normal adult, when the oxygen tension has fallen to approximately 27 torr, at a *p*H of 7.4 and a temperature of 37°C, 50% of the oxygen bound to hemoglobin has been released. The P_{50}, the whole blood oxygen tension at 50% oxygen saturation, is 27 torr. If the affinity of hemoglobin for oxygen is reduced, more oxygen is released to the tissues at a given oxygen tension. In such situations, the oxygen–hemoglobin equilibrium curve is shifted to the right of normal. It has long been recognized that increases in blood acidity, carbon dioxide content, ionic concentration, and temperature are capable of decreasing the affinity of hemoglobin for oxygen and shifting the curve to the right. If the affinity of hemoglobin for oxygen is increased, as occurs with alkalosis or a decrease in temperature, the equilibrium curve appears shifted to the left, and the tension must drop lower than normal before the hemoglobin releases an equivalent amount of oxygen.

The oxygen dissociation curve of the erythrocytes of newborn infants is shifted to the left, reflecting an increase in the affinity of the hemoglobin for oxygen compared with the blood of adults (see Fig. 45-13). This shift is due primarily to less binding of 2,3-diphosphoglycerate to HbF than to HbA.[125] As a result, the unloading of oxygen in the tissues requires a greater fall of oxygen tension in the newborn than in adults. Conversely, the uptake of oxygen in the lung is enhanced in newborns. It is not clear whether this phenomenon is a benefit or handicap to newborns; presumably, its role in intrauterine life was to permit greater movement of oxygen from the mother to the fetus. There is no evidence that provision of blood containing HbA improves tissue oxygenation in the newborn.

BLEEDING DISORDERS

The hemostatic system is not completely developed at birth, and this may affect the appearance and interpretation of bleeding disorders. There is little evidence to suggest that this incomplete development places neonates at increased risk of hemorrhage, although they may be more prone to thrombosis. However, in the neonatal period many hemorrhagic problems appear as a result of the diseases and disorders that occur at that time of life. The study of hemorrhagic disorders in the newborn period demands an understanding of the development of the hemostatic system, of congenital and acquired factors that can affect it, and appreciation of the role of disease in producing disturbances in the system.

Because of the incomplete development of the hemostatic system, interpretation of laboratory tests requires knowledge of normal values for infants of similar gestational and postnatal age, as shown in Table 45-8. The complexity of hemorrhagic disorders in the neonatal period demand that laboratory testing be as complete as possible. This requires the use of microtechnology for the assessment of the hemostatic system in the newborn. A complete assessment can be done with as little as 0.2 mL of plasma.

There are several important features of the coagulation system in the newborn (see Table 45-8). The prothrombin time of full-term and premature infants is

TABLE 45–8
SCREENING TESTS FOR BLEEDING DISORDERS*

Test	Adults	Full-Term Infants	Disease-Free Premature Infants†
Prothrombin time (seconds)	12 ± 1	14 ± 1.3	14 ± 1.3
Partial thromboplastin time (seconds)	42 ± 4	51 ± 10	57 ± 10.5
Thrombin clotting time (2 U)	25 ± 2	23 ± 2.9	23 ± 2.4
Factor II (%)	81 ± 17‡	50 ± 14.5	31 ± 8.6
Factor V (%)	90 ± 19	79 ± 17	70 ± 22
Factor VII–X (%)	93 ± 20	54 ± 12.2	37 ± 11
Factor VIII (%)	87 ± 27	126 ± 56	116 ± 73
Factor IX (%)	99 ± 23	35 ± 12.6	28 ± 11
Factor X (%)	89 ± 23	45 ± 12	31 ± 9.0
Antithrombin III (%)	99 ± 10	58 ± 9.6	33 ± 9.0
Fibrinogen (mg/dL)§	315 ± 60	215 ± 35	256 ± 20

* All results are expressed as means ± SD.
† Infants of birth weight less than 1500 g who were free of any clinical disease.
‡ Data from Johnston M, Zipursky A. Microtechnology for the study of the blood coagulation system in newborn infants. Can J Med Technol 1980;42:133.
§ Data from Hathaway WE, Bonnar J. Perinatal coagulation. New York: Grune and Stratton, 1978:56.

only slightly outside the adult range of 10 to 12 seconds. The partial thromboplastin time (PTT), which is a frequently used screening test in adults, is much longer in newborn infants, particularly premature infants. It is my impression that children with a long PTT may not be prone to hemorrhagic phenomena. It is likely that the prolongation of the PTT is due to relatively reduced levels of contact factors, which should not cause a significant hemorrhagic disorder. The PTT is of little value in the newborn. The two-unit thrombin time is a valuable screening test, because it can detect heparin contamination and fibrinogen deficiency. Bleeding disorders in newborn infants are best separated into local bleeding problems and generalized hemorrhagic diatheses.

LOCAL BLEEDING PROBLEMS

Bleeding in newborn infants can occur from the cord, into the scalp, into the gastrointestinal tract, into the abdomen (*e.g.*, liver, adrenal glands), and into the lung. There is little evidence to suggest that the physiologically low levels of coagulation factors in the newborn play any role in the genesis of these disorders.

Intraventricular hemorrhage (IVH) is a major problem of premature infants (see Chap. 49). There is little evidence to suggest that a hemorrhagic diathesis underlies this disorder. Therapeutic trials of infusing plasma or coagulation factor concentrates have been equivocal or unsuccessful. Although it is likely that IVH occurs as a result of local phenomena related to hypoxia, hemodynamic changes, and prematurity, it is possible that a deficiency of hemostasis may contribute to the continuation of the hemorrhage. Supportive evidence for this is found in the preliminary trials of ethamsylate, an agent that appears to affect the platelet capillary component of hemostasis and that was found in one study to prevent or diminish the severity of IVH.[126]

ACQUIRED HEMORRHAGIC DIATHESIS

I believe that there are only two major causes of generalized acquired hemorrhagic diathesis due to blood coagulation factor deficiency that occur in the newborn period. These are vitamin K deficiency hemorrhagic disease of the newborn and DIC.

VITAMIN K DEFICIENCY

Newborn infants have a tendency to spontaneously hemorrhage in the first days of life. This has been referred to as hemorrhagic disease of the newborn. It was shown many years ago that the administration of vitamin K at birth prevented hemorrhagic disease of the newborn, the classic form of which occurs in the first week of life. It has become an accepted procedure to administer 1 mg of vitamin K_1 oxide intramuscularly at birth, and as a result, hemorrhagic disease in the newborn has virtually disappeared. However, there has been controversy about the question of vitamin K deficiency in newborns and the need for prophylactic treatment. Vitamin K is a cofactor necessary for the γ-carboxylation of a prothrombin precursor to active prothrombin. In the absence of vitamin K, this precursor (proteins induced by vitamin K absence [PIVKA]) can be detected in the plasma.[127] Because PIVKA was found in only one-third of term infants, it has been suggested that not all infants are vitamin K–deficient and not all need to receive prophylactic vitamin K.[128] Some studies have shown that, unlike adults, normal newborns demonstrate no vitamin K in their serum, and therefore, relative to adults, they are vitamin K deficient.[129] In several cases of hemorrhagic disease of the newborn, Dreyfus and colleagues observed low levels of vitamin K–dependent factors and high levels of PIVKA and a response to vitamin K.[129] Current evidence suggests that many newborn infants are vitamin K deficient, even though elevated PIVKA levels are not found in all of them. Because it is not possible to select babies who are likely to bleed, it is recommended that all babies receive 1 mg of vitamin K_1 at birth.

Babies born to mothers who are on anticonvulsant medication are at particularly high risk of having vitamin K deficiency (*e.g.*, early hemorrhagic disease of the newborn), and these mothers should receive vitamin K before delivery.[130] Late hemorrhagic disease of newborns (*i.e.*, vitamin K deficiency hemorrhagic disease) manifests at 4 to 6 weeks of age. Infants with this disease characteristically have not received vitamin K prophylaxis at birth; have been maintained on breast milk, which is low in vitamin K; and may have suffered from diarrhea.[131] This disorder continues to be reported from areas in which routine prophylaxis is not given.[132] It is recommended that vitamin K be given intramuscularly to prevent hemorrhagic disease of the newborn.[133] Oral vitamin K is effective in raising vitamin K levels, but there is evidence that it is not as effective in preventing late hemorrhagic disease of the newborn.[134–136]

DISSEMINATED INTRAVASCULAR COAGULATION

There have been many reports of DIC in newborn infants associated with a variety of diseases. Some reports suggest that most cases of DIC in neonates are caused by cardiovascular collapse.[137] This refers to those infants who have had an episode of cardiac arrest, an Apgar score of 0 to 1, or an episode of profound hypotension.

The infant is found to have a generalized hemorrhagic diathesis with bleeding from venipuncture sites, bruising, and widespread internal hemorrhage. Blood studies reveal prolongation of screening tests (*e.g.*, prothrombin time, PTT, thrombin time), elevated fibrin split products, depressed factor V levels, and hypofibrinogenemia. Platelet counts may be normal or only slightly depressed. The findings in this syndrome should be differentiated from those observed in sepsis or necrotizing enterocolitis, in which thrombocytopenia is severe, coagulation factors may be normal or slightly reduced, and bleeding is minimal.[137]

Disseminated intravascular coagulation in newborns is treated first by the correction of cardiovascular collapse. If the circulation is restored to normal, the coagulopathy will correct itself spontaneously. If bleeding is a problem, replacement therapy with cryoprecipitate 0.5 U/kg (10 mL/kg), and if necessary, platelet concentrate should be given. After correction of the coagulopathy, patients should be monitored at 4-hour intervals with prothrombin time and fibrinogen levels. If fibrinogen falls, the DIC is continuing.

The syndrome of DIC is typically a difficult problem, complicating a serious illness in an infant. Diagnosis and treatment of the hemorrhagic diathesis are relatively straightforward. Unfortunately, the underlying disease and the ischemic damage due to the cardiovascular collapse and the DIC result in high mortality rates.[137]

OTHER CAUSES OF ACQUIRED BLEEDING DISORDERS

Profound liver disease can produce a hemorrhagic diathesis as a result of vitamin K deficiency or a primary failure of production of coagulation factors.

Despite the use of small doses of heparin to maintain intravenous lines, a hemorrhagic diathesis due to heparin therapy is unusual. However, it is not uncommon in studies of newborn infants for blood samples to be contaminated with heparin. All laboratories studying blood coagulation in newborns should be able to detect heparin contamination.

CONGENITAL HEMORRHAGIC DISORDERS IN THE NEONATAL PERIOD

Hemophilia A (*i.e.*, factor VIII deficiency) and hemophilia B (*i.e.*, factor IX deficiency) may present with bleeding symptoms in the newborn period.[138] Because of gender-linked inheritance, male infants are affected. All cases of hemophilia A can be diagnosed at birth, because the lower limit of the reference range for factor VIII (>50% or 0–0.05 U/mL) is similar to the adult value. Although the severe (<1%) and moderate (1%–5%) forms of hemophilia B can be confidently diagnosed in the neonatal period, children with the mild forms may require investigation in later infancy because their levels of factor IX may fall within the lower limit of the reference range for full-term and premature infants at birth (see Table 45-8).[139] The delay in confirming the diagnosis is usually of no consequence, because children with mild deficiencies of factor IX are not at risk for spontaneous bleeding.

The bleeding manifestations of neonatal hemophilia include scalp hematomas, prolonged bleeding from venipuncture sites or from surgical procedures such as circumcision, and intracranial hemorrhage. Management of bleeding involves the infusion of factor VIII or IX to restore hemostasis; the replacement product of choice is a factor concentrate treated during preparation to inactivate the acquired immunodeficiency syndrome (AIDS) and hepatitis viruses.[140] Factor IX concentrates should not be used in the newborn, because of the risk of inducing thrombosis secondary to low antithrombin III levels.

Deficiencies of factors II, V, VII, VIII, and X and of fibrinogen are inherited in an autosomal manner. The homozygous forms of the disorders may present with bleeding in the newborn period. Delayed bleeding from the umbilical stump is characteristic of homozygous factor XIII deficiency or of a severe quantitative or qualitative abnormality of fibrinogen.[141] Screening coagulation tests (*e.g.*, prothrombin time, PTT, thrombin time) are normal in patients with factor XIII deficiency, and the diagnosis should be confirmed by specific factor assay. Treatment of the coagulation factor deficiencies involves infusion of stored plasma (except for factor V), fresh-frozen plasma, or specific factor concentrates (*e.g.*, factor XIII).

Bleeding is uncommon in newborns with von Willebrand disease.[142] The diagnosis of von Willebrand disease cannot be made with confidence in the newborn period because levels of von Willebrand factor are elevated at birth, masking the presence of most forms of von Willebrand disease.[143]

PLATELET DISORDERS

A platelet count of less than 150×10^9/L is abnormal in term and premature infants.[144] The level of platelets in the blood reflects a balance between their production and destruction. Thrombocytopenia may result from decreased production, increased destruction, or a combination of both. Examination of a well-stained smear of peripheral blood to assess platelet morphology and number and of bone marrow to assess megakaryocyte morphology and number has traditionally yielded important information concerning the mechanism of thrombocytopenia. Decreased numbers of platelets and megakaryocytes indicate a production defect, and megakaryocytic hyperplasia and the presence of megathrombocytes (*i.e.*, young large platelets) in a peripheral blood smear are characteristic of thrombocytopenic states in which there is increased peripheral destruction of platelets. Unfortunately, these indices are not as useful in newborn infants as in older children or adults because the number of megakaryocytes in bone marrow aspirates obtained even from healthy newborn infants often appears reduced. In my experience, aspirates obtained from the iliac crest are more satisfactory than those obtained from the tibia.

There are many causes of thrombocytopenia in the newborn. The most common of these disorders appear in Table 45-9 and have been reviewed elsewhere.[144,145]

NEONATAL IMMUNE THROMBOCYTOPENIA

Immune thrombocytopenia occurs when antibody-sensitized platelets are prematurely destroyed in the reticuloendothelial system, particularly the spleen. Characteristic laboratory features include isolated thrombocytopenia and an increased number of immature megakaryocytes in a bone marrow aspirate. Elevated levels of platelet-bound IgG can be demonstrated in many cases.

A variety of conditions are associated with the transplacental passage of antibody, resulting in immunologic destruction of the infant's platelets. The antibody may be formed against an antigen on the platelets of the infant (*i.e.*, if isoimmune or alloimmune, mother's platelet count is normal) or an antigen present on the platelets of the mother (*i.e.*, if autoimmune, mother has immune thrombocytopenic purpura [ITP] or thrombocytopenia associated with a collagen vascular disorder such as systemic lupus erythematosus).

Neonatal Isoimmune Thrombocytopenia. In neonatal isoimmune or alloimmune thrombocytopenia, the infant possesses a platelet antigen of paternal origin that is lacking in the mother. Typically, the infant's platelets cross the placenta into the maternal circulation during pregnancy or at the time of delivery and cause immunization of the mother, with the formation of antibodies against the foreign platelet antigen. Less frequently, the cause of immunization is exposure of an antigen negative mother to antigen positive platelets during transfusion. During pregnancy, transplacental passage of the maternal IgG antibodies leads to sensitization of fetal platelets. Sensitized platelets are rapidly destroyed in the fetal reticuloendothelial system, particularly the spleen, and the result may be thrombocytopenia *in utero* and in the infant at the time of delivery. This mechanism is analogous to that causing hemolytic disease of the newborn.

The platelet-specific antigen system most often involved in cases of neonatal alloimmune thrombocytopenia is Pl^{A1}.[146,147] Other platelet-specific antigens are involved less frequently.[148–154] In the largest series of cases of suspected neonatal alloimmune thrombocytopenia, 91% (120 of 132) of serologically proven cases were due to Pl^{A1} alloantibodies.[147] Of the remaining 12 cases, the pathologic alloantibodies were anti-Br^a-9; anti-Pl^{A2}-1; anti-Bak^a with HLA antibody-1; and blood group B isoagglutinins-1. Although HLA alloantibodies often develop as a result of pregnancy, they rarely are the cause of severe neonatal thrombocytopenia.

The incidence of neonatal alloimmune thrombocytopenia is estimated to be 1 per 5000 live births or less.[155] In my opinion, the incidence of platelet alloimmunization is higher, probably on the order of 1 in 1000 to 2000 pregnancies in a Caucasian population. This opinion is based on the finding of three cases of Pl^{A1} alloimmunization in a prospective study of 5000 pregnant women.[156]

The typical infant with neonatal alloimmune thrombocytopenia is term, and thrombocytopenia is unexpected. Cutaneous manifestations of severe thrombocytopenia (*e.g.*, bruising, petechial rash) are often the only abnormalities found on physical examination. A complete blood count shows severe isolated thrombocytopenia, with a normal hemoglobin and leukocyte count.

Affected infants are at risk for serious hemorrhage, particularly into the central nervous system (CNS). In a review by Pearson and colleagues, the incidence of fatal hemorrhage was 10% to 15%.[155] In some cases, CNS hemorrhage occurs *in utero* before delivery.[157–161] Bussell and colleagues estimated that as many as 25% of CNS hemorrhage cases associated with neonatal alloimmune thrombocytopenia occur antenatally.[162]

Early diagnosis and effective therapy of infants with neonatal alloimmune thrombocytopenia is important. The disorder should be suspected in all infants with severe, isolated thrombocytopenia in whom a specific cause for the thrombocytopenic state cannot be identified (*e.g.*, sepsis, DIC, and skeletal anomalies such as absent radii) and if the maternal platelet count is normal. These infants should receive antigen-negative, compatible platelets, harvested from the mother or a phenotyped blood donor. If maternal platelets are used, supernatant plasma with pathologic antibody should be removed by centrifu-

TABLE 45–9
CAUSES OF NEONATAL THROMBOCYTOPENIA

Decreased Production of Platelets
Congenital megakaryocytic hypoplasia
Thrombocytopenia–absent radius syndrome
Megakaryocytic hypoplasia without anomalies
Congenital leukemias and histiocytoses
Inherited thrombocytopenias
Wiskott–Aldrich syndrome
Other X-linked or recessively transmitted thrombocytopenias
Increased Destruction of Platelets
Immune thrombocytopenias
Neonatal alloimmune thrombocytopenia
Neonatal autoimmune thrombocytopenia
Drug-induced thrombocytopenia
Giant hemangioma syndrome
Other states with disseminated intravascular coagulation
Both Decreased Production and Increased Destruction of Platelets
Infections
Congenital, usually viral
Acquired, usually bacterial
Osteopetrosis

gation or washing and the compatible maternal platelets infused after irradiation. In clinical practice, severely thrombocytopenic infants (*i.e.*, platelet counts $< 30 \times 10^9$/L) are often initially transfused with a unit of random donor platelets; in such cases, the platelet response is of diagnostic value.[163,164] Because most persons type positively for the Pl^{A1} and Bak^a antigens (98% and 88%, respectively), most random donor platelets are incompatible in cases of neonatal alloimmune thrombocytopenia due to these alloantigens, and their infusion fails to produce a satisfactory posttransfusion platelet increment. In situations in which alloimmune thrombocytopenia is clinically suspected, this pattern of response provides additional evidence for the diagnosis, and it is then most important that severely affected infants receive compatible antigen-negative platelets collected from the mother or blood donors of known antigen type. Regional blood centers serving large neonatal intensive care units should be encouraged to develop a small bank of blood donors phenotyped for common platelet antigens who are readily available for donation. In selected cases, it may be useful to harvest and store in the frozen state the platelets from mothers or antigen-negative donors for immediate use if an affected infant is anticipated.[165]

Other therapeutic interventions for neonatal alloimmune thrombocytopenia include exchange transfusion to remove pathologic antibody and intravenous administration of large doses of immunoglobulin G. This latter strategy is of proven benefit in children with ITP and has been used with variable success in infants with alloimmune thrombocytopenia.[166–171] However, if compatible platelets can be quickly obtained, these additional therapeutic interventions are rarely indicated. If compatible platelets cannot be obtained or if a significant delay can be anticipated before this ideal product will be available, the therapy of choice is a trial of high-dose intravenous IgG. Our current practice is to administer a total dose of 2 g per 1 kg of body weight, given as 1 g/kg over 6 to 8 hours on each of 2 consecutive days. Corticosteroid therapy (*e.g.*, prednisone) is of no proven benefit used in the traditional dose of 1 to 2 mg/kg/day.

The risk of the disorder recurring in subsequent pregnancies is high; approximately 75% of the offspring of a sensitized Pl^{A1}-negative woman manifest thrombocytopenia. Because of the significant risk of CNS hemorrhage *in utero*, especially in cases of $P1^{A1}$ alloimmunization with a history of a previously severely affected infant, most experts involved with management of these high-risk pregnancies advocate determination of the fetal platelet count by percutaneous umbilical vessel sampling (PUBS) at 18 to 20 weeks of gestation. If the fetus is determined to have severe thrombocytopenia, weekly administration of intravenous IgG to the mother is started and continued until delivery.[162,172] Although the benefit of *in utero* transfusion of compatible platelets has been reported, the relatively short half-life of even compatible donor platelets makes this approach impractical.[172] The route of delivery is determined by the fetal platelet count obtained by PUBS or scalp vein sampling before delivery; of these two methods, PUBS is preferred because of its higher accuracy. If the fetal platelet count is less than 50×10^9/L, delivery by cesarean section is recommended. At the time of delivery, a cord blood platelet count should be obtained, and thrombocytopenia should be verified in a peripheral blood sample obtained shortly after delivery. If the infant is severely thrombocytopenic, compatible platelets should be infused immediately. These high-risk pregnancies should be managed by a team of obstetricians, neonatologists, and hematologists.

Neonatal Autoimmune Thrombocytopenia. Clinical and laboratory features of neonatal autoimmune thrombocytopenia parallel those of the alloimmune state. In both disorders, the observation of ecchymoses, a petechial rash, or both in an otherwise well infant may be the first clue to the disorder. Measurement of a maternal platelet count and examination of a peripheral blood smear obtained from the mother can help to differentiate autoimmune from alloimmune neonatal thrombocytopenia. In neonatal alloimmune thrombocytopenia, the maternal peripheral blood smear and platelet count are normal, but in the autoimmune condition (*i.e.*, mothers with ITP), the platelet count is reduced, and the existing platelets are often large (*i.e.*, megathrombocytes). Occasionally, the finding of unexpected thrombocytopenia in an infant may lead to the diagnosis of previously unrecognized ITP in the mother. Autoimmune thrombocytopenia may occur in infants of mothers with ITP who have normal platelet counts after splenectomy. Occasionally in mothers with ITP, increased bone marrow activity can compensate for accelerated destruction of antibody-sensitized platelets. These women may have normal platelet counts, but their infants are at risk of developing acquired thrombocytopenia.

Management of infants with autoimmune neonatal thrombocytopenia differs from that of those with the alloimmune form of the disease. Compatible platelets cannot be found, because platelet autoantibodies react with all donor platelets. Therapeutic options include exchange transfusion to remove passively acquired maternal autoantibodies, corticosteroids, and high-dose intravenous immunoglobulin G. In infants with significant thrombocytopenia (*i.e.*, platelet counts $< 50 \times 10^9$/L) or clinical bleeding, we favor administration of immunoglobulin G in a dose of 1 g/kg daily for 2 consecutive days. A marked increment in platelet count can be anticipated within 24 to 48 hours in 75% of patients.[173,174] If this response is not observed, exchange transfusion should be considered and oral corticosteroids started (*e.g.*, prednisone or an equivalent corticosteroid at a dose of 3–4 mg/kg/day initially, with rapid tapering once the platelet count increases above 50 × 10^9/L). Splenectomy should not be considered in newborn infants unless there is a real clinical emergency with life-threatening bleeding into the CNS and no effective alternative.

The same considerations apply to the route of delivery as have been outlined in the discussion of neonatal alloimmune thrombocytopenia. The maternal platelet count and levels of platelet-bound IgG and serum platelet antibody do not predict with certainty which infants will be thrombocytopenic.[175–177] In some high-risk obstetric units, PUBS or fetal scalp vein sampling during labor is used to determine the fetal platelet count and allow a decision about cesarean section (*i.e.*, recommended if the fetal platelet count is < 50 × 10^9/L). Another approach to the antenatal management of women with ITP is the use of oral steroids administered to the mother before delivery. In an uncontrolled study of 17 pregnant women with ITP, Karpatkin and colleagues found that the mean platelet count in infants after delivery was 151 ± 25,000/μL in the group whose mothers were given steroids before delivery, compared with 42 ± 12,000/μL in the group of 7 infants whose mothers did not receive steroids antenatally.[178] This observation was not confirmed in a prospective study in which mothers with ITP were randomized to receive low-dose corticosteroids (*e.g.*, betamethasone, 1.5 mg/day) or a placebo antenatally.[179] The role of therapy, corticosteroids, or high-dose intravenous IgG administered antenatally to mothers with ITP for the sole benefit of their offspring is unclear.

OTHER FORMS OF THROMBOCYTOPENIA

A variety of other disorders may produce a reduction in platelet count. Thrombocytopenia is particularly common in ill infants admitted to neonatal intensive care units. In a prospective study of 807 consecutive infants admitted to a regional intensive care neonatal center, Castle and colleagues reported a 22% incidence of thrombocytopenia, defined as a platelet count of less than 50 × 10^9/L.[180] In 38% of thrombocytopenic infants, the platelet count was 50 to 100 × 10^9/L, and in 20%, the platelet count was less than 50 × 10^9/L. Thrombocytopenia was associated with laboratory evidence of increased platelet destruction or DIC in 52% and 21% of patients, respectively. There was an association of thrombocytopenia with birth asphyxia. Although only 7% of the thrombocytopenic infants had positive blood cultures, sepsis is an important cause of neonatal thrombocytopenia, and a low platelet count may be an early clue to infection in this patient population.[171] Inherited defects in platelet production or platelet function also manifest themselves during this period of life.

An approach to the multiple diagnostic possibilities is outlined in Figure 45-14. In this scheme, it is as important to study the mother as it is to study the infant. Points requiring specific inquiry include a history of previous bleeding in the form of purpura, bruising, or nosebleeds that might suggest a diagnosis of maternal ITP at some time in the past; ingestion of drugs that may cause thrombocytopenia in the

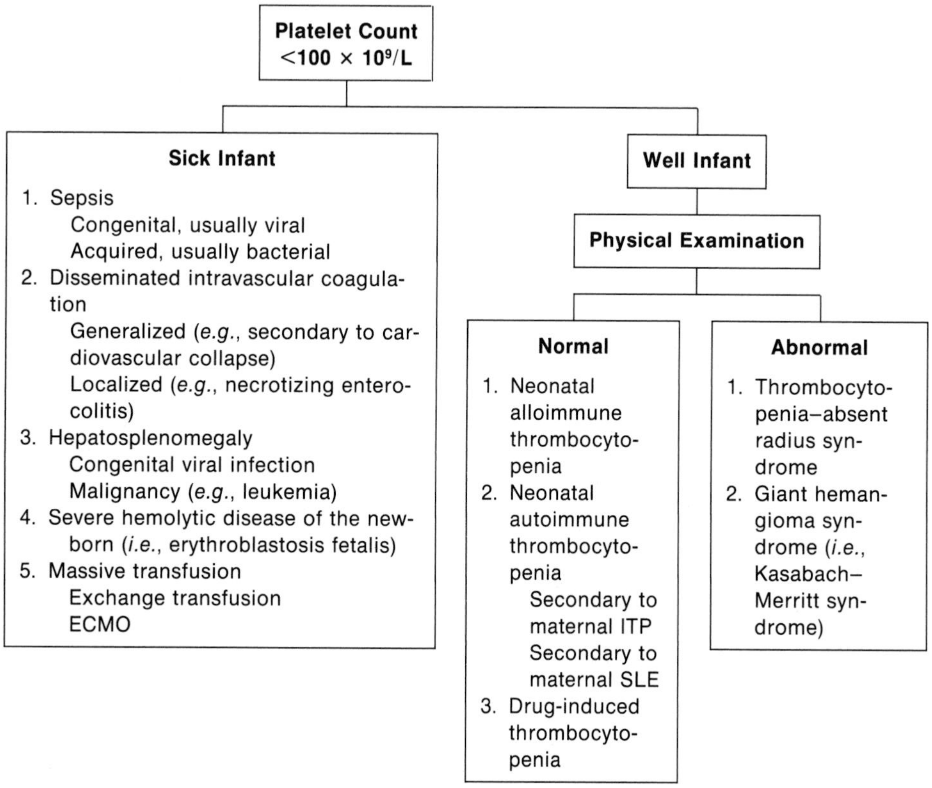

FIG. 45–14. Approach to the diagnosis of the thrombocytopenic newborn. (ECMO, extracorporeal membrane oxygenation; ITP, immune thrombocytopenic purpura; SLE, systemic lupus erythematosus.)

mother and infant (*e.g.*, quinidine, quinine); previous siblings affected with purpura, suggesting one of the immune or inherited thrombocytopenias; and skin rash or exposure to rubella in the first 8 weeks of pregnancy. Serologic evidence of congenital infections (*e.g.*, syphilis, CMV, herpesvirus, toxoplasmosis) should be sought and recorded. An accurate maternal platelet count should be performed as soon as possible after delivery, so that immune neonatal thrombocytopenia caused by maternal ITP can be differentiated from that due to platelet isoimmunization, in which case the mother's platelet count is normal.

Physical findings of importance in differential diagnosis of the affected newborn include hepatosplenomegaly and congenital anomalies. Hepatosplenomegaly is often accompanied by jaundice and suggests an infectious process as the most likely cause of thrombocytopenia. In some cases, congenital leukemia may have to be considered. Among the congenital anomalies associated with neonatal thrombocytopenia, the commonest group recognizable at birth is that occurring in the rubella syndrome (*i.e.*, congenital heart defects, cataracts, and microcephaly). Deformity and shortening of the forearms should suggest bilateral absence of the radii, with associated amegakaryocytic thrombocytopenia. A single large hemangioma or multiple smaller hemangiomas point to possible platelet trapping.

A complete blood count on the infant should include hemoglobin determination, leukocyte count, platelet count, and a smear. Associated anemia may be due to blood loss, concurrent hemolysis (*e.g.*, in an infectious processes), or marrow infiltration caused by congenital leukemia. Leukocytosis of a mild degree may accompany infection or blood loss, but if this exceeds 40,000 to 50,000/μL, it may point to congenital leukemia. Bone marrow examination should be considered if thrombocytopenia is persistent and a specific cause cannot be identified. Serologic tests for platelet antibodies and platelet antigen typing are available in reference laboratories. If isoimmune thrombocytopenia is suspected by the finding of an otherwise normal newborn with thrombocytopenia and a healthy mother with a normal platelet count, blood should be drawn from the parents soon after delivery for serologic testing. Characteristically, the maternal serum contains an antibody reactive against paternal platelets. Platelet antigen typing should be performed on both parents, if available; in cases of neonatal alloimmune thrombocytopenia, the mother will type negative and the father positive for the pathologic platelet-specific antigen. In this situation, the infant's platelet type is assumed to be identical to that of the father, because it is usually not possible to obtain sufficient blood from severely thrombocytopenic newborn infants for extensive serologic testing. Results of platelet studies may not be available for some time, and therapy should not be delayed pending their results.

LEUKOCYTE DISORDERS

A diverse group of leukocyte disorders is encountered in newborn infants. Different blood cells are involved (*e.g.*, neutrophils, lymphocytes, eosinophils), and the disorders may be quantitative or qualitative in nature. This section focuses on abnormalities that are particularly relevant to newborn infants because of the frequency with which they are encountered (*e.g.*, neutrophil changes associated with bacterial infections) or because they are unique to this age group (*e.g.*, congenital leukemia, neonatal alloimmune neutropenia).

NEUTROPHIL DISORDERS

NORMAL LEUKOCYTE COUNT IN THE NEONATAL PERIOD

Counts of segmented and band (*i.e.*, nonsegmented, young) neutrophils of healthy full-term infants studied by us during the first 5 days of life are illustrated in Figure 45-15.[181]

In premature infants, neutrophil counts during the first 5 days of life are similar to or slightly lower than those in full-term infants (see Fig. 45-15). In a series of 180 premature infants, mean values were found at 0, 24, and 120 hours to be 4000, 7500, and 3500/mm^3, respectively (Fig. 45-16).[182] Similar values have been found by others.[173–185] Peak values excluding the top 2.5% were 8000, 15,500, and 8500/mm^3, which is significantly lower than the values for full-term infants (see Fig. 45-16).

The lower limit for a normal neutrophil count in full-term and premature infants is not clearly established. In a series of 180 infants, some of the infants were found to have values of 0 without a cause.[182] Xanthou,[183] Coulombel,[184] and Lloyd and Oto[185] reported smaller series that indicated a neutrophil count of less than 1000/mm^3 would be considered abnormal. A helpful rule of thumb is to consider a neutrophil count of less than 1000/mm^3 to be abnormal in full-term and premature infants.

During the first month of life, the neutrophil count in premature infants falls slowly, so that at 30 days the mean value is approximately 2000/mm^3, with a range of 1000 to 6000/mm^3.[183,184]

For my studies, a cell was considered to be a segmented neutrophil if its nucleus was distinctly segmented into two or more lobes connected by a thin filament. Cells with no lobulation and those in which the width of the narrowest segment of the nucleus was greater than one-third the width of the broadest segment were referred to as nonsegmented neutrophils or bands (Fig. 45-17). During the first 2 weeks of life for full-term and premature infants, a band–segmented neutrophil ratio of greater than 0.3 was considered to be abnormal.[171] Other investigators have reported reference ranges for total neutrophil and immature neutrophil counts in newborn infants

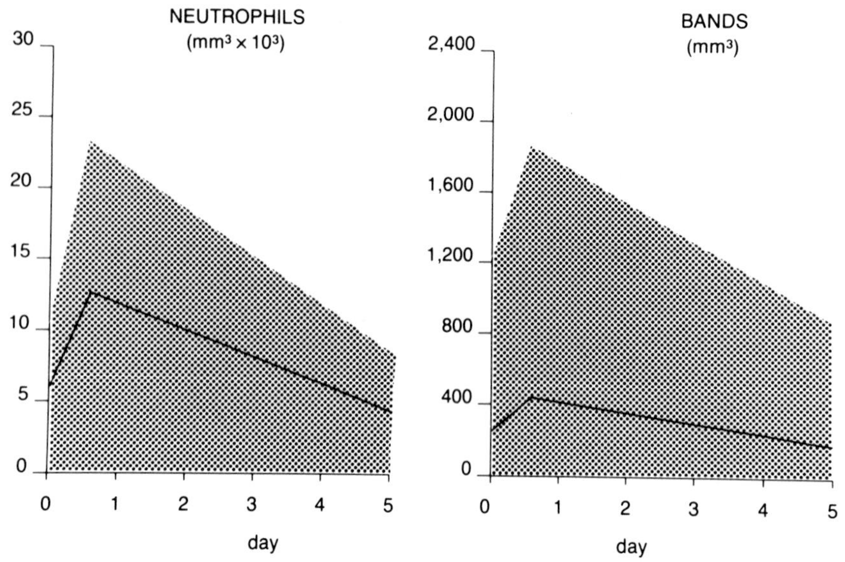

FIG. 45–15. Neutrophil and band counts of 169 normal full-term infants. Data at the first point, day 0, are cord blood values. Subsequent points represent data from capillary blood samples on 1 and 5 days of life. The heavy line represents the mean at each point. The shaded area includes 95% of the patients, excluding the top and bottom 2.5% of the group. The mean of all values on blood collected from 4 to 24 hours of age is plotted at 14 hours.

throughout the first 28 days of life.[186–188] Examination of a peripheral blood smear during the first few days of life characteristically reveals an excess of polymorphonuclear neutrophils. Particularly in premature infants, some immature forms (*e.g.*, promyelocytes, myelocytes) may be seen. Sometime between the fourth and seventh days of life, the lymphocyte becomes the predominant cell and remains so until the fourth year of life.

CHANGES IN BLOOD NEUTROPHILS DURING BACTERIAL INFECTION

In newborn infants, clinical signs of infection may be minimal, and the speed of evolution of disease may be rapid. Changes in neutrophil number and appearance are often helpful in the diagnosis of bacterial infections in this age group.

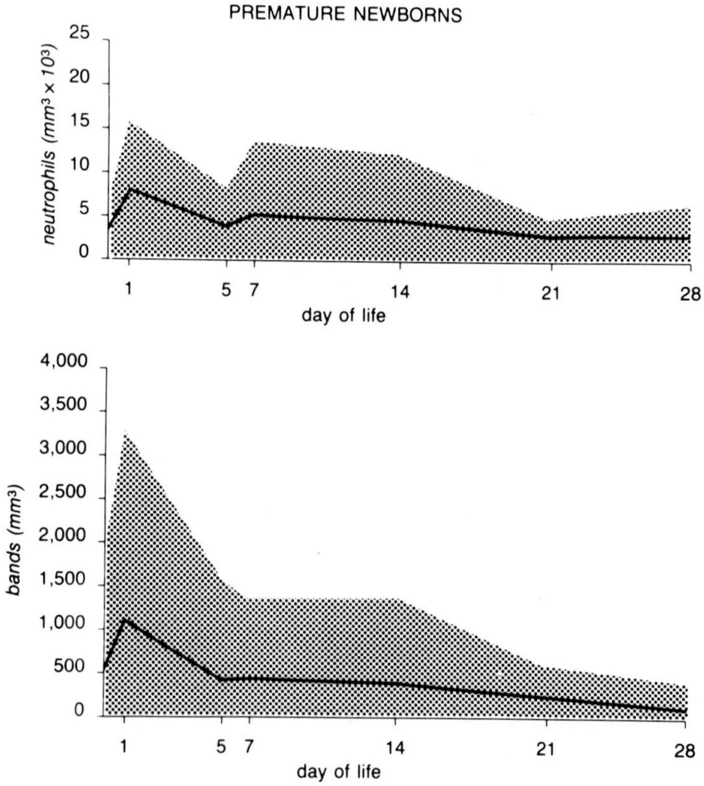

FIG. 45–16. Neutrophil and band counts of 180 premature infants. Data at the first point, day 0, are cord blood values. Subsequent points represent data from capillary blood samples on 1, 5, 7, 14, 21, and 28 days of life. The heavy line represents the mean at each point. The shaded area includes 95% of the subjects, excluding the top and bottom 2.5% of the group.

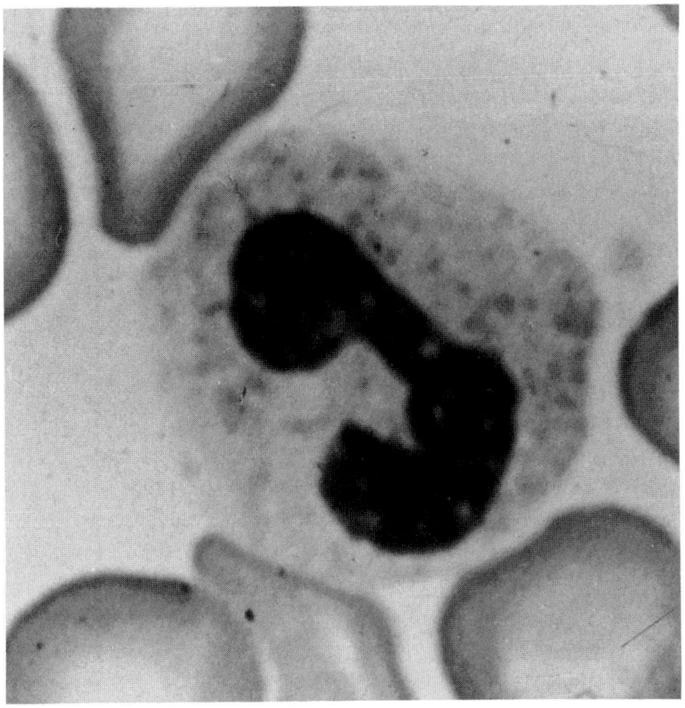

FIG. 45–17. A band neutrophil.

Changes in Neutrophil Numbers. In infants with systemic bacterial infection, the total neutrophil count may be increased (*i.e.*, neutrophilia), decreased (*i.e.*, neutropenia), or fall within normal limits. In a study of 24 newborn infants with proven bacterial sepsis (*e.g.*, positive bacterial cultures from the blood, cerebrospinal fluid, bladder-tap urine, or peritoneal fluid), neutropenia was observed in 5, neutrophilia was seen in 3, and normal neutrophil counts were observed in the remaining 16.[181] Although neutrophilia is a relatively nonspecific finding and may occur in conditions other than sepsis, the finding of neutropenia is highly significant in newborn infants and may be the first clue to bacterial infection. In the study of Manroe and colleagues, neutropenia was observed in 77% of counts associated with confirmed or suspected bacterial disease; neutrophilia was absent almost as often in infected infants (42%) as it was present (58%).[188] In addition to neutropenia, increased numbers of immature neutrophils (*i.e.*, band forms) and an elevated band–segmented neutrophil ratio are of considerable value in the diagnosis of bacterial infection. In a study of premature infants with proven bacterial infection, 73% (11 of 15) of the infants had elevated band counts and a reversed band–segmented neutrophil ratio.[182]

Changes in Neutrophil Morphology. During infection, the neutrophils of newborn infants have increased numbers of Döhle bodies (*i.e.*, aggregates of rough endoplasmic reticulum), vacuoles, and toxic granules.[182]

Neutrophil Response to Bacterial Infection. There is a characteristic pattern of neutrophil response that can assist greatly in the diagnosis of infection in newborn infants. When bacterial infection occurs, neutrophils migrate from the circulating pool to the walls of blood vessels. Massive infection may produce neutropenia by causing complement-dependent neutrophil aggregation, with disappearance from the circulation. If the demand is sufficient, neutropenia occurs. The baby's response is a release of its marrow storage pool, which consists mostly of young or band neutrophils. This is evidenced by an increase in the band–segmented neutrophil ratio and slowly thereafter by an increase in the absolute band count. The body continues to produce neutrophils, and the resulting neutrophil count is then a balance between demand and production. In the newborn infant, there is evidence that marrow reserves are relatively limited compared with those of the adult; neutrophilia may not occur, or if it does, it may be seen only late in the disease. With increased production under the stress of infection, abnormal neutrophils (*i.e.*, those containing vacuoles, Döhle bodies, toxic granulations) are produced, providing further evidence of bacterial infection. As a myeloid response continues, it is not unusual to find in the blood stream early myeloid precursors such as promyelocytes or even myeloblasts.

Neutrophil response to infection is also of importance in terms of understanding the susceptibility of newborns to infection. Neutrophil function, particularly chemotaxis and phagocytosis, is reduced in newborns and may contribute to their susceptibility to infection.[189] The neutrophil storage pool is lower in newborns, accounting for the neutropenia frequently seen in association with neonatal infections and contributing to the relative inability of the newborn to fight infections.[190]

There is evidence that the reduced function of the neutrophils may be secondary to relatively low levels of humoral factors (*i.e.*, antibody, complement) in the plasma of newborns. The low neutrophil counts during infection may be reversed by administration of γ-globulin.[191]

Because of the occurrence of neutropenia, the reduced marrow storage pools, and decreased neutrophil function, it has been suggested that leukocyte transfusions may be valuable in the treatment of neonatal sepsis. There have been several contradictory reports regarding the benefit of such transfusions.[189] Because of the risks of leukocyte transfusions and the difficulty in obtaining leukocyte concentrates, this therapy is rarely used.

NEUTROPENIA

Causes of neutropenia include decreased production of neutrophils, increased destruction, or a combination of both mechanisms (Table 45-10).

Decreased Production of Neutrophils

Impaired granulopoiesis and neutropenia are features of a number of inherited disorders. In Kostmann syndrome and reticular dysgenesis, severe neutropenia from birth leads to early diagnosis. In the other syndromes described in this section, persistent or periodic neutropenia does not typically present a problem in the neonatal period, and these disorders are usually diagnosed later in life.

TABLE 45–10
CAUSES OF NEONATAL NEUTROPENIA

Decreased Production of Neutrophils
Kostmann syndrome
Reticular dysgenesia
Shwachman–Diamond syndrome
Neutropenia associated with cartilage–hair hypoplasia
Neutropenia associated with immunodeficiency syndromes
Cyclic neutropenia
Increased Destruction of Neutrophils
Neonatal alloimmune neutropenia
Neonatal autoimmune neutropenia
Drug-induced neutropenia
Decreased Production and Increased Destruction of Neutrophils
Infections
Congenital, usually viral
Acquired, usually bacterial
Drug-induced neutropenia

Kostmann Syndrome. Congenital neutropenia is severe in patients with Kostmann syndrome; cases are reported in which there was striking neutropenia from the first day of life.[192] Bone marrow smears typically reveal normal cellularity, with a maturation arrest at the promyelocyte–myelocyte level. Serious bacterial infections occur early in life, and the disorder is usually fatal. However, infusions of the cytokine granulocyte colony-stimulating factor have proven to be successful therapy for this disease.[193] Inheritance is autosomal recessive in most cases.

Reticular Dysgenesia. In their original report, deVaal and Seynhaeve described premature monozygotic twins in whom recognizable leukocytes were absent from the peripheral blood.[194] Both infants died of infection within the first 2 weeks of life. At autopsy, thymic tissue and lymph node tissue were absent. Smears of aspirated marrow showed normal erythroid and megakaryocytic development, with absent myeloid and lymphocytic cells.

Shwachman–Diamond Syndrome. In 1964, Shwachman and colleagues described 5 children with evidence of pancreatic insufficiency and neutropenia.[195] Growth retardation, normal sweat electrolytes, and absence of pulmonary disease ordinarily characteristic of cystic fibrosis were other features of the disorder. Bone marrow findings include hypocellularity with maturation arrest of myeloid elements. Inheritance appears to be autosomal recessive.

Neutropenia Associated With Immunodeficiency Syndromes. Approximately one-third of boys with X-linked agammaglobulinemia are neutropenic at some time.[196] Neutropenia may also be associated with deficiencies of IgG and IgA.[197]

Cyclic Neutropenia. Cyclic neutropenia is a sporadic or familial disorder characterized by a regular, repetitive decrease in peripheral blood neutrophils at approximately 21-day intervals.[198,199] The disorder reflects a regulatory abnormality of the stem cell pool and is rarely diagnosed in the neonatal period.

Increased Destruction of Neutrophils

Neonatal Alloimmune Neutropenia. Neonatal alloimmune neutropenia is the neutrophil counterpart of the erythrocyte disorder of hemolytic disease of the newborn. The incidence of alloimmune neutropenia is reported to be in the range of 1 in 500 to 2000 newborn infants.[200,201] Alloimmune neutropenia occurs when a mother becomes sensitized to a foreign antigen present on the neutrophils of her infant and is then stimulated to form specific IgG antibody directed against this fetal antigen. Transplacental passage of IgG antibody into the fetal circulation results in neutropenia. Because neutropenia is the direct consequence of transplacentally acquired maternal IgG, the condition is self-limiting, and neutropenia persists for only a few weeks or months. The severity of neutropenia is influenced by the titer and subclass of the maternal IgG neutrophil antibody, the phagocytic activity of the infant's reticuloendothelial system, and the capacity of the infant's marrow to compensate for the shortened survival of antibody-sensitized neutrophils.

Investigation of infants with neonatal alloimmune neutropenia has contributed much to current knowledge of neutrophil-specific antigens, and the antigen systems most often involved are NA1, NA2, and NB1.[202] The neutrophil-specific antigens NA1 and NA2 are located on the neutrophil Fc-gamma receptor III (FcRIII), and antibodies to this neutrophil membrane glycoprotein have caused neonatal neutropenia.[203,204] Although HLA antigens are present on granulocytes, and alloimmunization to these antigens is common in pregnancy, HLA antibodies are not thought to be a significant cause of neutropenia in newborn infants. It appears that maternal HLA antibodies are effectively absorbed by HLA antigens placental tissue; the antibodies that reach the fetus are neutralized by soluble antigens or weakened by having to react with antigens on various cells distributed in the blood and other tissues. In contrast, neutrophil-specific antibodies cross the placenta without any obstacle and concentrate on the target antigen, which occurs only on the relatively small mass of mature neutrophils.

The clinical course of infants with alloimmune neutropenia is of interest. Neutropenia is usually severe. In a review of 19 affected infants reported before 1974, Lalezari found that 12 infants had total absence of circulating neutrophils for at least part of their course.[202] The duration of neutropenia ranged from 2 to 17 weeks, with a mean of 7 weeks. Infections were common, and most were due to *Staphylococcus aureus*. Two infants died, one with staphylococcal septicemia and the other with pneumonia and possible meningitis. Alloimmune neutropenia is not a benign disorder. Affected infants with severe neutropenia are at risk for serious bacterial infections, and therapeutic intervention may be necessary. In addition to intravenous antibiotic therapy for infants with suspected or proven infection, possible therapies include exchange transfusion to remove passively acquired maternal neutrophil antibodies, transfusion with compatible antigen-negative granulocytes harvested from the mother or known antigen-negative blood donors, corticosteroids; and high-dose intravenous IgG.

There is little evidence that steroids are of value in this condition. The response to high-dose intravenous γ-globulin therapy varies.[205–207] My experience is limited to therapy of twins with severe neutropenia due to maternally derived anti-NA1 antibody; both infants failed to respond to 2 g/kg of intravenous IgG. It is possible that higher doses of IgG may be required in the therapy of immune neutropenia. The use of exchange transfusion or transfusion with compatible antigen-negative neutrophils should be reserved for infected infants who have failed an adequate trial of high-dose intravenous IgG (2–5 g/kg administered as 1 g/kg/day for 2–5 days) and who are not responding to broad-spectrum intravenous antibiotic therapy.

Neonatal Autoimmune Neutropenia. Transient neutropenia in the neonatal period may reflect transfer of IgG neutrophil antibodies from mother to fetus during pregnancy. In these cases, the maternal serum contains the pathologic neutrophil antibodies, and the mother may be neutropenic and may have a history of an autoimmune disorder, such as systemic lupus erythematosus. Therapy of the affected neonate, if clinically indicated, is high-dose intravenous IgG (2–5 g/kg administered as 1 g/kg/day for 2–5 days). Such therapy produces dramatic, albeit transient, increases in absolute neutrophil counts in older children with autoimmune neutropenia.[208]

Evaluation of the Infant With Neutropenia. The unexpected finding of neutropenia in a newborn infant should prompt consideration of bacterial infection. A peripheral blood smear should be carefully examined for Döhle bodies, vacuolization, and toxic granulation, and the band–segmented neutrophil ratio should be determined. In infants with some combination of neutropenia, an increased band–segmented neutrophil ratio, and morphologic features suggestive of bacterial infection, empiric broad-spectrum antibiotic therapy should be started until the results of cultures are known. If there is no clinical or laboratory evidence of infection, other causes of neutropenia must be considered. A maternal history, including a drug history, and a maternal neutrophil count should be obtained to exclude maternal illness (*e.g.*, systemic lupus erythematosus) as a cause of neutropenia. The physician should obtain a careful family history, asking specifically about family members with documented neutropenia or a history of severe or unusual infections. This information may provide an important clue to the possibility of an inherited neutropenic syndrome (*e.g.*, Kostmann syndrome). Physical examination of affected infants suggests or excludes hypersplenism and congenital viral infections as likely causes of neutropenia. In well infants with no apparent cause for the neutropenic state, neonatal alloimmune neutropenia should be considered. In such cases, a search should be made for neutrophil antibodies in a sample of maternal serum; these antibodies are typically reactive against paternal neutrophils. In some infants, a bone marrow aspirate may be necessary to exclude the possibility of an intrinsic marrow disorder, such as congenital leukemia.

Congenital Leukemia and Leukemoid Reactions

Congenital leukemia is an extremely rare disorder. The predominant form of congenital leukemia is acute myeloblastic leukemia; in older children, acute leukemia is typically lymphoblastic. In all forms of congenital leukemia, the prognosis is poor. Approximately 50% of infants with congenital leukemia manifest skin nodules. The nodules are bluish and feel like fibromatous tumors deep within the skin. Other presenting features include hepatosplenomegaly, poor weight gain, fever, diarrhea, pallor, and petechiae. There are a number of disorders that can appear similar to acute leukemia in the newborn. Congenital infections such as CMV disease, toxoplasmosis, and syphilis may manifest as hepatosplenomegaly with a pronounced leukemoid response in the peripheral blood. Severe bacterial infections also may be associated with a leukemoid blood picture.

Special mention should be made of the transient leukemia seen in patients with Down syndrome. Although the incidence of acute and congenital leukemia is higher in Down syndrome, there is also an unusual syndrome in which a picture of acute megakaryoblastic leukemia appears and then, during the subsequent weeks, regresses and disappears.[199,209]

Some cases of transient leukemia are severe, with evidence of hydrops fetalis, hepatosplenomegaly, liver disease or congestive failure.[75,210,211] Most cases of transient leukemia recover completely without antileukemic therapy. However, approximately 20% of these patients subsequently develop acute megakaryoblastic leukemia during the first 4 years of life, a disease that is fatal unless treated.

Lymphopenia

In the newborn infant, an absolute lymphocyte count consistently less than 1500/μL is abnormal and requires evaluation. During this period, lymphopenia is most often associated with immunodeficiency disorders, including reticular dysgenesia, Swiss-type agammaglobulinemia, agammaglobulinemia associated with short-limb dwarfism, X-linked recessive agammaglobulinemia, and lymphopenia with dysgammaglobulinemia (*e.g.*, Nezelof syndrome). Affected infants should be promptly investigated for defects of cellular and humoral immune function. If they require blood transfusions, they should be given only irradiated blood products so that graft-*versus*-host disease does not develop.

Eosinophilia

An elevated eosinophil count is common in premature infants. Normal values for a group of healthy premature infants studied by us are illustrated in Figure 45-18. The upper limit of normal (95th percentile) for absolute eosinophil counts in a group of 167 full-term infants was 1016/μL, 1323/μL, and 1372/μL at 0, 1, and 5 days, respectively. The corresponding mean values were 475/μL, 496/μL, and 540/μL. In a prospective study of 45 premature infants, Bhat and colleagues found the incidence of eosinophilia to be 75.5%.[212] Similar results have been reported by other investigators.[213–215] In Bhat's study, an absolute eosinophil count of more than 700/μL was considered to be abnormal. The frequency and severity of eosinophilia were greatest in the subgroup of infants younger than 30 weeks of gestational age. There was a significant association between the development of eosinophilia and number of blood transfusions administered, use of parenteral nutrition, and duration of intubation. The causative nature of these associations is uncertain because these features are common in ill, premature infants. Prolonged processing of antigens at the cellular level is required for the development of eosinophilia, and the investigators suggest that eosinophilia in the premature infant may be a physiologic process needed to handle foreign antigens. The fact that eosinophilia is more frequent in premature infants than in term infants may reflect immaturity of barrier mechanisms in the gastrointestinal tract, respiratory tract, or both.

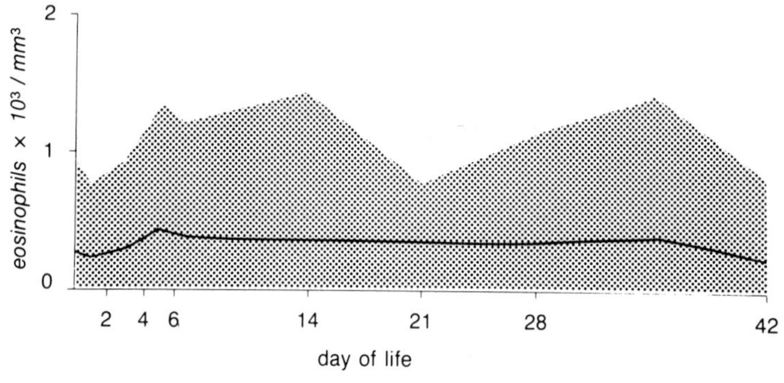

FIG. 45–18. Eosinophil counts in 142 healthy, premature infants. Data at the first point, day 0, are cord blood values. Subsequent points represent data from capillary blood samples on 1, 5, 7, 14, 28, 35, and 42 days of life. The heavy line represents the mean of each point. The shaded area includes 95% of the infants studied, excluding the top and bottom 2.5% of the group.

TRANSFUSION OF BLOOD AND BLOOD PRODUCTS

Transfusions of blood products to newborn infants are essential in many clinical situations, and guidelines for transfusion practice in this patient population have been published.[216] However, guidelines simply provide a list of acceptable clinical situations in which transfusions may be given, and they should not serve as absolute indications for transfusion therapy. In all cases, the responsible physician should take into account the general condition of the infant. The decision to transfuse blood products should reflect careful consideration of the risk–benefit ratio for the individual patient.

ERYTHROCYTE TRANSFUSIONS

Transfusion of erythrocytes in newborn infants, particularly in premature newborns, is a common practice. The indications are those that hold for any other time of life: hypovolemia and anemia. Transfusion for anemia has created much controversy. Anemia is defined as a hemoglobin concentration lower than that which is normal for the given patient. This concept of normality is difficult to apply to the premature infant, who as part of his normal course may require respiratory assistance, may have apneic spells, and may have much blood sampled for laboratory tests. There is significant controversy about whether a low hemoglobin concentration is harmful to the infants or whether transfusions to maintain an arbitrary hemoglobin concentration improve their clinical condition. The following guidelines for administering a blood transfusion, although lacking definitive proof, include the caution that is necessary in view of the risks of this procedure:

- Shock due to blood loss
- Venous hemoglobin level less than 13 g/dL in neonates younger than 24 hours of age
- Removal of blood for diagnostic purposes when the volume removed exceeds 10% of the infant's blood volume and significant continuing iatrogenic losses are anticipated
- Hemoglobin less than 13.0 g/dL in newborn infants with severe pulmonary disease, cyanotic heart disease, or heart failure
- Hemoglobin less than 8 g/dL in stable newborn infants; transfusion may be considered if the infant has symptoms (*e.g.*, tachycardia, tachypnea, recurrent apnea, decreased vigor, poor weight gain unexplained by other causes) that can be improved by blood transfusion.

The decision for transfusion should be made by the physician caring for the infant after considering the relative risks and benefits of the procedure.

PREPARATION OF BLOOD FOR TRANSFUSION AND CROSSMATCHING

There are several principles of blood transfusion and crossmatching that should be understood by those caring for neonates. First, omission of the major antiglobulin crossmatch for initial and subsequent transfusions of neonates is recommended, if the initial antibody screen does not demonstrate unexpected antibodies and the erythrocytes transfused are type O and of an Rh type that is compatible with the baby and mother. This recommendation reflects the fact that newborn infants appear unable to form alloantibodies to erythrocyte antigens.[217,218] Repeated blood sampling for pretransfusion testing only contributes to phlebotomy losses from small newborn infants. Second, the practice of using fresh-frozen plasma to adjust erythrocyte preparations to a predetermined hematocrit value for small-volume transfusions (*i.e.*, not exchange transfusion) may lead to exposure of newborn infants to two different donors per transfusion. This practice should be discouraged.[219] If necessary, isotonic saline or albumin should be used to adjust hematocrit.

EXCHANGE TRANSFUSIONS

It is generally recommended that blood for exchange transfusion be as fresh as possible and less than 5 days old. Because extracellular potassium increases rapidly during storage of erythrocyte concentrates at 4°C, I recommend that erythrocyte units for exchange transfusion of ill, premature infants be saline washed before reconstitution with fresh-frozen plasma. Manual and automated saline wash processes are effective.[220] This maneuver effectively eliminates any chance of iatrogenic hyperkalemia, a complication reported in ill premature infants after exchange transfusion.[221]

EFFICIENT USE OF BLOOD

Because newborn babies require only small volumes of blood for transfusion (approximately 10 mL/kg), there can be a great waste from a unit of blood, which usually contains 250 mL of packed erythrocytes. As a result, a number of methods of efficient use of blood have been employed; for example, a single unit may be collected into a quadruple pack. These individual bags may be used for transfusion of as many as 4 infants. Use may be improved by subsampling from a single erythrocyte unit through a sterile docking system, which means that one bag of blood may provide transfusion for 10 or more infants. The problem with this technique is that, although it provides for efficient use of blood, the small infant who requires several transfusions during his hospital stay may receive blood from many donors, with the increasing risks associated with each donation.

The ideal system of transfusion of blood would be one that uses only one donor for each patient. One way in which this can be achieved is by the use of a walking blood donor system, in which one adult provides blood for a single infant. The blood, when required, is simply taken into a heparinized syringe and administered directly to the patient. Although such donors are regularly tested to ascertain that they are free of disease, loss of routine blood bank collection techniques, record keeping, and laboratory testing of the blood collected are potential disadvantages. Care must be taken that the heparin used in the blood collection (*i.e.*, 250 U/50 mL of whole blood) does not lead to inadvertent anticoagulation of the neonate. For these reasons, a walking donor program is not advocated. Another way in which donor exposure can be kept to a minimum is by designating for use by a single baby 1 unit of blood divided into a quadruple pack. Because blood can remain in storage for up to 35 days—up to 42 days for erythrocytes preserved in extended storage media such as Adsol—this is a feasible method, although there is a moderate amount of wastage.

PLATELET TRANSFUSIONS

A platelet count of less than 150×10^9/L in a newborn infant is abnormal and requires investigation. In older children and adults, the risk of serious internal hemorrhage, particularly intracranial hemorrhage, increases significantly when the platelet count falls below 20,000/μL. Donor platelets are usually infused prophylactically when this degree of thrombocytopenia occurs. The situation in newborn infants is less clear. Particularly in ill premature infants, in whom the risk of hemorrhage into the CNS is high, factors other than the absolute platelet count may play a role. Many of these infants are on medications, such as antibiotics, that may impair platelet function. Immaturity of blood vessels in the periventricular area and changes in cerebral blood flow and pressure associated with fluid and ventilation therapy may play a role. Alternatively, IVH may be the final result of cerebral infarction, perhaps related to asphyxia, with hemorrhage into the infarcted area. The clinical impact of significant neonatal thrombocytopenia (*i.e.*, platelet counts $< 100 \times 10^9$/L) in infants weighing less than 1500 g at birth has been studied prospectively by Andrew and associates.[222] The incidence of IVH in 97 thrombocytopenic infants was 78%, compared with 48% in nonthrombocytopenic control infants. The more severe grades of IVH (*i.e.*, grades III or IV) were more frequent in the thrombocytopenic infants. These observations provide a rationale for the guidelines for transfusion of platelet concentrates outlined in Table 45-11.

The standard platelet product available from blood banks is harvested from a single whole blood donation of approximately 450 mL. After centrifugation of this whole blood unit, platelet-rich plasma (PRP) is separated from the erythrocyte fraction, and the PRP is further centrifuged to yield 1 unit of fresh-frozen plasma and 1 unit of random donor platelets. Each platelet concentrate contains approximately 0.7×10^{11} platelets in a volume of 50 mL; this product can be stored for as long as 5 days at 22°C. The objective of most platelet transfusions is to increase the infant's platelet count to more than 100×10^9/L. This can be achieved by the infusion of 10 mL of a standard platelet concentrate per kilogram of body weight. Generally, this volume is not excessive, providing intake of other fluids is monitored and adjusted as needed.

TABLE 45–11
GUIDELINES FOR TRANSFUSION OF PLATELET CONCENTRATES IN NEONATES

Premature Infants (Gestational Age <37 wk)
Blood platelets $< 30 \times 10^9$/L in a stable infant
Blood platelets $< 50 \times 10^9$/L in a sick infant
All Other Infants
Blood platelet count $< 20 \times 10^9$/L
Blood platelet count $< 50 \times 10^9$/L with active bleeding or the need for an invasive procedure
Blood platelet count $< 100 \times 10^9$/L with active bleeding plus disseminated intravascular coagulation or other coagulation abnormalities*
Bleeding with qualitative platelet defect and marked prolongation of bleeding time, regardless of the platelet count
Cardiovascular bypass surgery with unexplained excessive bleeding, regardless of the platelet count

* Statements that are underlined require additional definition by a local transfusion committee.

Adapted from Blanchette VS, Hume HA, Levy GJ, et al. Guidelines for auditing pediatric blood transfusion practices. Am J Dis Child 1991;145:787.

Although methods exist to reduce the volume of platelet concentrates, additional processing should be performed with care because of possible platelet loss, clumping, and dysfunction caused by the additional handling.[223] Platelets should be administered through a standard 170-μ blood filter as rapidly as the infant's overall condition permits and certainly within 2 hours. A microaggregate filter should not be used because it will trap a large number of platelets.

GRANULOCYTE TRANSFUSIONS

The neutrophil has a critical role in the body's defense against bacterial infections. When the absolute neutrophil count falls below 1×10^9/L, the risk of bacterial infection increases and becomes substantial with counts less than 0.5×10^9/L. In the newborn infant, profound neutropenia may be the result rather than the cause of sepsis. The outlook for infants with infection-related neutropenia is poor, even if intensive antibiotic therapy is administered early in the course of the illness. This is particularly true if the marrow neutrophil storage pool is decreased.[224] During the first week of life, in the setting of an ill newborn infant with sepsis, a blood neutrophil count of less than 3×10^9/L and evidence of a depleted marrow neutrophil storage pool (*i.e.*, <10% of nucleated marrow cells are polymorphonuclear neutrophil leukocytes), granulocyte transfusion therapy appears to be beneficial, as reviewed by Blanchette and colleagues.[212]

Granulocyte concentrates may be prepared from units of fresh (<24 hours old) whole blood or harvested by apheresis of blood donors.[225,226] The product of choice is a granulocyte concentrate prepared by automated leukapheresis. The donor should be seronegative for hepatitis, CMV, HIV, human T-cell leukemia virus, and syphilis. There should be erythrocyte compatibility between donor and neonate. The concentrates should be irradiated (1500–5000 cGy) before use and infused intravenously over 45 minutes through a standard 170-μ blood filter after the results of predonation testing are available and certainly within several hours of product collection because granulocyte concentrates should be as fresh as possible. Neonates should receive 1 to 2×10^9/L neutrophils per kilogram per infusion, and transfusions should be given daily until there is clinical improvement and the neutrophil plus band count is greater than 3×10^9/L. However, the use of leukocyte transfusions in the neutropenia of sepsis is controversial and is rare in most centers.

Like alloimmune thrombocytopenia, the clinical disorder alloimmune neutropenia requires special consideration. Granulocytes harvested from random blood donors are unlikely to be effective, because the incidence of compatible antigen-negative donors in the general population is low: 46% for NA1, 7% for NA2, and 8% for NB1. Compatible granulocytes may be harvested from the mother or from blood donors of known granulocyte antigen types. If maternal granulocytes are used, they should be washed to remove pathologic antibody and irradiated before transfusion. I do not recommend granulocyte transfusion therapy unless the infant has a systemic infection, is not responding to intravenous broad-spectrum antibiotic therapy, and has failed a trial of high-dose intravenous IgG therapy.

RISKS

Potential complications of blood transfusion have been reviewed by Mollison.[227] For newborn infants, post-transfusion hepatitis, CMV infection, HIV infection, and graft-*versus*-host disease are of particular concern. Because of these potential complications, it is important that physicians order blood or blood product support for newborns only in situations in which the infant will clearly benefit from such therapy.

HEPATITIS

Transfusion-associated hepatitis may be caused by the hepatitis A or B viruses or more commonly by the hepatitis C virus (HCV).[228,229] Cases of HCV were previously classified as non-A, non-B hepatitis. Unfortunately, little information is available concerning HCV infection in newborn infants. In adults, the incidence of hepatitis C was previously reported to be 5% to 15% among persons who received 1 to 5 units of blood.[230] More than 90% of these cases have now been confirmed to be caused by HCV infection. Approximately 50% of all patients with HCV develop chronic persistent or chronic active hepatitis. A subgroup of those with chronic hepatitis ultimately develop cirrhosis or hepatocellular carcinoma. These data are derived from studies of adults; the natural history of transfusion-acquired hepatitis in newborn infants is unknown.

CYTOMEGALOVIRUS INFECTION

Transfusion-acquired CMV infection can occur when at-risk CMV antibody-negative infants are infused with CMV antibody-positive blood products.[217] In the study of Yeager and colleagues, 13.5% (10 of 74) of seronegative infants who received CMV antibody-positive erythrocytes developed CMV infection.[231] Infection did not occur in 90 seronegative infants who received only CMV antibody-negative blood. Two of the 10 infected infants in this series died, and 3 others developed serious symptoms including pneumonia, hepatitis, hemolytic anemia, and thrombocytopenia. All of the fatal or other serious infections occurred in infants with a birth weight of less than 1200 g; infection was more common in infants who received 50 mL or more of blood. Similar data have been reported by Adler and colleagues, and other reports have stressed the morbidity and mortality that may be associated with transfusion-acquired CMV infection in neonates.[232–234]

Based on these studies, it has been recommended that CMV antibody-negative blood products be made available to preterm infants of birth weight 1250 g or less who are CMV antibody negative. A study of Preiksaitis and colleagues challenges this recommendation for all neonates.[235] In this prospective study of 120 seronegative infants, only one case of acquired CMV infection was observed. Because no mortality and little morbidity could be attributed to transfusion-acquired CMV, the investigators did not recommend that all neonatal units provide specialized blood components for the prevention of CMV infection. The indications for use of CMV seronegative blood products in newborn infants have been comprehensively reviewed by Preiksaitis and associates.[236] They include low-birth-weight (LBW) neonates (*i.e.*, birth weight < 1500 g) born to seronegative mothers in centers that have documented a high incidence of transfusion-acquired CMV infection in neonates; LBW neonates born to seronegative or seropositive mothers and who require granulocyte transfusions; and neonates receiving extracorporeal membrane oxygenation (ECMO).

The importance of breast milk as a source of CMV infection in newborn infants has also been stressed.[237,238] In future studies of transfusion-acquired CMV infection in newborn infants, it will be important to control for this variable, particularly in nurseries in which pooled breast milk is used. If a decision to transfuse CMV low-risk blood products to selected LBW infants is made and CMV seronegative erythrocytes are not available, products that are associated with a low-risk of transmitting CMV infection include frozen, deglycerolized erythrocytes; washed erythrocytes; and filtered erythrocytes.[239–241]

ACQUIRED IMMUNODEFICIENCY SYNDROME

Since the first report of AIDS in 1981, much has been learned about the disorder.[242] The causative agent of the syndrome is now known to be the HIV-1 virus. The virus can be grown in culture, and antibody to the virus can be detected with immunologic techniques, such as an enzyme-linked immunosorbent assay. Blood donations are routinely screened for evidence of antibodies to the HIV-1 virus, and the risk of HIV-1 transmission by blood products is extremely small. However, HIV-1 transmission has occurred in newborn infants, and this potentially fatal complication demands that blood or blood component therapy be restricted to situations in which therapy is clinically indicated and is likely to be of benefit to the newborn infant.[243–245] The potential complication of HIV infection is a major reason to limit the number of blood donors to whom a given newborn infant is exposed.

GRAFT-*versus*-HOST DISEASE

Graft-*versus*-host disease has been reported in congenitally immunodeficient infants, after blood transfusion in premature infants, after ECMO, and in apparently normal infants with Rh isoimmunization who have received intrauterine transfusions followed by exchange transfusion.[246–250] Features of transfusion associated graft-*versus*-host disease, usually a fatal disorder, include fever, generalized rash, diarrhea, hepatitis, and pancytopenia. Irradiation of blood products to prevent graft-*versus*-host disease is recommended for the following groups:

- neonates with known or suspected congenital immunodeficiency disorders
- neonates requiring intrauterine transfusions
- neonates who received intrauterine transfusions and who require transfusion postnatally
- recipients of cellular blood products from first-degree blood relatives
- premature infants weighing less than 1500 g at birth.

Data supporting the last recommendation are not available. However, very low birth weight infants (<1500 g) may have an associated immunodeficiency, and it is reasonable to offer protection to this group of infants.[251] The dose of irradiation used varies among centers, ranging from 1500 to 5000 cGy; a dose of 1500 cGy is most frequently used.[252]

PLASMA DERIVATIVES

ALBUMIN

Albumin is available in 5% and 25% solutions. Although albumin infusion has been recommended as a means of drawing more bilirubin into the intravascular space before exchange transfusion, convincing data in support of such a practice is lacking.

FRESH-FROZEN PLASMA

Centrifugation of whole blood within 6 hours of collection yields a concentrate of erythrocytes and 1 unit of fresh-frozen plasma. If stored at −30°C, the plasma product has a shelf life of 12 months and contains all coagulation factors.

CRYOPRECIPITATE

Cryoprecipitate is prepared from fresh-frozen plasma by slow thawing at 2°C to 4°C. Each unit of cryoprecipitate contains approximately 80 units of factor VIII and 250 mg of fibrinogen in 5 to 10 mL of plasma. If stored at −30°C, the product has a shelf life of 12 months. Cryoprecipitate also contains various amounts of factor XIII.

FACTOR VIII AND IX CONCENTRATES

Concentrates of factor VIII and IX are commercially manufactured from large pools (2000–20,000 donors) of plasma. Each concentrate lot is assayed for coagulation factor activity, and this value is stated in units on each vial. Traditionally, concentrates of factors VIII and IX have not been used in newborn infants or young children because of the increased risk of hepatitis associated with infusion of factor VIII and IX concentrates and of DIC and thrombotic complications associated with infusion of factor IX concentrates because of thrombogenic materials in such concentrates and low antithrombin III levels in newborns. Disseminated intravascular coagulation is particularly likely if liver dysfunction occurs. The introduction of high-purity virus-inactivated factor concentrates appears to have eliminated the risk of HIV-1 infection and to have significantly reduced the incidence of hepatitis. altering the previous general recommendations. However, factor IX concentrates are not recommended for use in newborns. Most North American hemophilia centers now recommend that infants with newly diagnosed, severe hemophilia immediately receive hepatitis B immunization, and then they can be started on virus-inactivated factor replacement therapy, as clinically indicated for prevention or control of bleeding.[140]

HYPERIMMUNE SERUM GLOBULIN

PREVENTION OF HEPATITIS B VIRUS INFECTIONS

Infants of mothers who are positive for hepatitis B surface antigen (HBsAg) are frequently infected with hepatitis B virus. Infection is most likely to occur if mothers are also positive for hepatitis Be antigen. Approximately 90% of infants whose mothers are positive for both markers will become infected, and most of these infants will be permanent carriers of the hepatitis B virus. It is estimated that 1 in 4 infants who are chronic carriers after perinatal infection will later develop cirrhosis or hepatocellular carcinoma.[253]

Infants receive greatest protection from a combination of active immunization with three doses of hepatitis B vaccine, together with passive immunization using hepatitis B immune globulin (HBIG). The following schedule is recommended: at birth, 0.5 mL of HBIG and 10 μg of hepatitis B vaccine.[241] Both the vaccine and immunoglobulin are given intramuscularly and can be administered at the same time if separate sites are used. At 1 and 6 months, 10 μg of hepatitis B vaccine is given. Infants should be tested for presence of anti-HBsAg at 9 months. If they are found to be negative (<10% of all cases), a repeat dose of the vaccine should be given.

PREVENTION OF CYTOMEGALOVIRUS INFECTIONS

The administration of CMV hyperimmune globulin to CMV antibody-negative patients who undergo bone marrow transplantation decreases the incidence of transfusion-acquired CMV infection. Whether a similar approach may be beneficial for the CMV antibody-negative premature infant exposed to multiple blood products is unknown.

NEONATAL THROMBOSIS AND EMBOLISM

In childhood, the incidence of thrombotic disease is highest in the newborn period and in early infancy.[254] Spontaneous and catheter-induced thromboses appear to be more common in early life than in later childhood.[254] Thromboembolic vascular obstruction may result in death or severe morbidity due to irreversible organ damage.

The vessels affected include renal, adrenal, portal, and hepatic veins; peripheral, cerebral, pulmonary, coronary, renal, and mesenteric arteries; and the aorta, vena cava, and right atrium.[254] Clinical presentation may be dramatic and fairly specific, as in the case of peripheral arterial obstruction; it can be nonspecific, such as disseminated pulmonary emboli presenting as persistent pulmonary hypertension of the newborn.[255] Occasionally, clinical signs of neonatal thrombosis are too subtle to be recognized in the acute stage of the disease, and thrombosis is suspected only retrospectively, after sequelae of vessel occlusion become apparent (*e.g.*, portal hypertension as a consequence of portal vein thrombosis). Table 45-12 summarizes the major sites of thrombotic vessel obstruction and their clinical signs in the newborn infant.

RISK FACTORS AND PATHOGENESIS

Three major factors contribute to the formation of thrombi: abnormalities of the vessel wall, disturbances of blood flow, and changes in blood coagulation and fibrinolysis.[256]

ABNORMAL VESSEL WALL

Intravascular Catheters. Abnormalities of the vessel wall are most frequently caused by intravascular catheters that damage or abrade the vessel wall endothelium, in addition to introducing a foreign surface with thrombogenic properties. The placement of vascular catheters carries a potential risk of thrombosis, regardless of which vessel is used; however, because of their widespread use, umbilical catheters are responsible for most published catheter-related thromboses in newborn infants.

TABLE 45–12
CLINICAL PRESENTATION OF THROMBOEMBOLIC DISEASE IN NEONATES

Vessel Obstruction	Clinical Signs and Symptoms
Venous Sites	
Vena cava inferior	May be associated with renal venous thrombosis; edema and cyanosis of legs
Vena cava superior	Soft tissue edema of head, neck, and chest; chylothorax
Cerebral	Seizures
Renal	Enlarged kidney(s); hematuria
Adrenal	Often associated with adrenal hemorrhagic necrosis
Portal and hepatic	Clinically silent during acute phase
Arterial Sites	
Aorta	Congestive heart failure; systolic gradient between upper and lower limbs; decreased femoral pulses; renal failure
Peripheral	Pulselessness; fall in skin temperature; discoloration
Cerebral	Prolonged apnea; seizures
Pulmonary	Respiratory distress; pulmonary hypertension
Coronary	Congestive heart failure, cardiac shock
Renal	Systemic hypertension; congestive heart failure
Mesenteric	Signs of necrotizing enterocolitis

Umbilical Artery Catheters. In a retrospective review of 4000 infants who underwent umbilical artery catheterization in the 1970s, severe symptomatic vessel obstruction was observed in approximately 1% of patients.[257] Clinically silent thromboses have been detected more often at autopsy or during contrast angiography in asymptomatic infants with an umbilical artery catheter in place. Between 3% and 59% of cases had postmortem evidence of catheter-related thrombosis.[257–267] In six prospective angiographic studies of infants who had had umbilical artery catheter in place, thrombosis was demonstrated in 10% to 95% of patients.[268–275]

Umbilical Vein Catheters. During a time when many umbilical vein catheters were malpositioned in the portal or hepatic veins and hyperosmolar solutions were injected rapidly through those catheters, thrombi were found in 20% to 61% of autopsies.[263,274] The incidence of thrombosis associated with an umbilical venous catheter that is correctly positioned in the inferior vena cava above the diaphragm and properly managed is unknown.

Abnormal Chorionic Vessels. Abnormal chorionic vessels occur in a wide range of maternal disorders, such as hypertension, and predispose to the development of chorionic thrombi, which can embolize into the fetal circulation, mainly into the pulmonary arteries and portal veins.[275]

Abnormal Closure of the Ductus Arteriosus. During abnormal closure of the ductus arteriosus, thrombi may form within the vessel and provide a source of emboli to the pulmonary circulation and the systemic circulation.[276]

ABNORMAL BLOOD FLOW

Blood flow is a critical determinant of thrombus formation, site, location, and structure. Increased blood viscosity as a consequence of polycythemia or dehydration has been implicated in cases of neonatal thrombotic disease.[277] Hyperviscosity due to polycythemia is also thought to contribute to the alleged thrombotic tendency in infants with diabetic mothers.[254]

Shock is another example of a severe disturbance of blood flow, predisposing to thrombosis and necrosis.

ABNORMAL HEMOSTASIS AND FIBRINOLYSIS

Congenital Deficiencies. Homozygous protein C and protein S deficiency are the only well-documented, congenital prethrombotic abnormalities of the clotting profile in the neonatal period. Affected infants present with purpura fulminans or massive large vein thrombosis.[278,279] Complete neonatal deficiency of antithrombin III, the main inhibitor of thrombin, has not been reported. Heterozygous antithrombin III deficiency has been implicated in neonatal thrombotic disease, but the magnitude of the risk remains uncertain.[280,281] I am not aware of any reported associations between dysfibrinogemia or dysplasminogenemia and neonatal thrombotic disease.

Acquired Deficiencies. It is not known whether and to what degree any of the special features of neonatal coagulation and fibrinolysis account for thrombotic complications in sick neonates. Research is particularly required to assess whether the low levels of antithrombin III, protein C, protein S, or plasminogen increase the risk of thrombosis in early life.

MANAGEMENT

Clinical investigators of adult cardiovascular diseases have made considerable progress through a series of well designed studies, which enabled them to make firm recommendations regarding the diagnosis and treatment of deep vein thrombosis and pulmonary embolism.[282] In contrast, the literature on neonatal thrombotic disease consists almost entirely of case reports and case series.[283] Such anecdotal observations are poor guides to management, because they are uncontrolled and fraught with bias.[283] Extrapolation of findings in adult patients to newborn infants may be inappropriate, because the cause and localization of thrombi and the coagulation system and its response to antithrombotic and fibrinolytic agents differ markedly between the two age groups. The following recommendations are in keeping with those endorsed by the Scientific and Standardization Subcommittee on Neonatal Hemostasis of the International Society on Thrombosis and Hemostasis.[284] Current approaches to the management of neonatal thrombosis require validation in future clinical trials.

DIAGNOSIS

Whenever thrombotic disease is suspected in the newborn (see Table 45-12), every effort should be made to confirm or refute the diagnosis. Contrast angiography with the use of nonionic contrast media is the best imaging technique for the confirmation of thrombosis before embarking on thrombolytic or surgical therapy. Other, less invasive tests, such as real-time ultrasonography, Doppler flow studies, or radioisotope scans, may be helpful adjunctive measures, but their precision and accuracy in neonatal thrombotic disease are still uncertain.[283]

Predisposing factors should be sought and eliminated. In the absence of obvious risk factors, such as vessel catheterization or shock, a family history looking for of thrombotic disease should be taken. Patient and parents should be tested for hereditary deficiencies of protein C, protein S, and antithrombin III and for dysfibrinogenemia or dysplasminogenemia.[284] Maternal lupus anticoagulant has been associated with severe thrombosis in a liveborn infant.[285]

TREATMENT

Organ or limb dysfunction as a result of thrombosis is the most compelling indication for active intervention. The lack of strong evidence for the benefits of antithrombotic therapy and the propensity of neonatal thrombi to resolve spontaneously do not usually justify aggressive therapy for asymptomatic thrombosis or thrombosis with minor symptoms.[283,286]

Intracranial hemorrhage or hemorrhagic infarction should be ruled out by suitable imaging techniques before prescribing anticoagulant or fibrinolytic drugs.[273] In all infants who receive antithrombotic therapy, the platelet count should be maintained above 50×10^9/L, and the fibrinogen concentration at greater than 1 g/L.

HEPARIN

Standard heparin is the most commonly used anticoagulant in infants with thrombotic disease, despite the observation that the low neonatal antithrombin III levels decrease the recovery and antithrombotic properties of heparin *in vitro* and in animal studies.[287,288] Thrombin inhibitors that do not depend on antithrombin III may prove to be preferable to standard heparin for the treatment of neonatal thrombosis in the future.

Heparin has been used in neonates at an initial loading dose of 50 U per 1 kg of body weight by intravenous injection, followed by approximately 20 U/kg/hour by continuous intravenous infusion.[289] Laboratory monitoring should be performed, to avoid excessive heparinization as indicated by plasma levels of heparin that are considered unsafe in adult patients (>0.5 μ/mL).

There is no validated therapeutic range for heparin therapy in newborn infants, and the optimal heparin assay for neonatal plasma has yet to be found. In adults, the PTT is widely used to monitor heparin therapy, but the use of the PTT in heparinized newborn infants has been less successful, because the PTT may become unmeasurably prolonged even in the presence of low concentrations of heparin.[290] Chromogenic antifactor-Xa assays may be preferable in the neonatal period.

THROMBOLYTIC AGENTS

The experience with thrombolytic agents (*e.g.*, streptokinase, urokinase, tissue plasminogen activator) is limited in newborns.[291] Successes and failures have been reported.[291] Urokinase appears to have been used most commonly. Dosages are derived from the adult literature. A loading dose of 4400 U/kg over 20 minutes has been recommended, followed by a maintenance regimen of 4400 U/kg/hour for up to 48 hours.[284] Local continuous perfusion of the affected vessel with lower doses of urokinase may also be beneficial if appropriate catheter placement is possible.[291] *In vitro* neonatal fibrin clots are more resistant to lysis by any of the three thrombolytic agents, possibly because of lack of functional plasminogen.[292] Whether this observation translates into higher neonatal drug requirements *in vivo* is unknown.

It is recommended that thrombolytic treatment be adjusted based on clinical and laboratory response. The latter includes a decrease in plasma fibrinogen concentration and an increase in fibrinogen–fibrin degradation products.[293] If such a lytic state cannot be induced, supplementation of plasminogen, such as through infusion of fresh-frozen adult plasma, may be considered.[292]

Any clinician who is contemplating the institution of thrombolytic therapy in sick neonates must weigh the risk of prolonged vessel occlusion and the uncertain drug benefits against the infant's risk of suffering from bleeding complications.

SURGERY

The main objectives of surgical intervention in neonatal large vessel thrombosis have been to remove the occluding clot and to resect a supposedly nonviable product of the vessel obstruction (*e.g.*, amputation for limb gangrene, resection of necrotic bowel). Thrombectomy may be used in selected cases, particularly if the thrombus obstructs a major artery.

Because of the devastating functional loss, with all ensuing problems, amputation in peripheral arterial occlusion should be postponed as long as possible. The main aim is to prevent superimposed secondary infection. Ideally, surgical intervention should be delayed until the necrotic parts are well demarcated. In some cases, surgery is not necessary because autoamputation occurs, which results in the least possible loss of tissue.

PROGNOSIS

Data on long-term follow-up of neonatal thrombosis is limited. Two of the relatively better studied conditions are renal venous thrombosis and aortic thrombosis.

A total of 58 neonates with renal venous thrombosis have been followed for 0.1 to 17 years by four investigator teams.[293] Persistent hypertension was found in 28% of all children, and 21% had residual renal tubular defects.[293]

The available follow-up data on survivors of aortic thrombosis suggest that blood pressure and renal function are likely to normalize during early childhood, but persistent hypertension, leg-growth discrepancies, and abnormalities in renal size and function have been described.[294–297]

PROPHYLAXIS

To reduce the risk of thromboembolic disease in the newborn, intravascular monitoring devices should be used judiciously, and blood flow should be optimized at all times.

Heparin has been advocated as a possible means of preventing catheter-related thrombosis. Heparin is added to the infusate of umbilical artery catheters in 74% of 117 American nurseries.[299] There is good evidence from controlled clinical trials that the continuous infusion of low doses of heparin (<200 U/kg/day) prolongs the patency of umbilical artery catheters.[299–302] Unfortunately, none of the published trials had sufficient power to conclusively answer the question of whether low doses of heparin reduce catheter-associated thrombus formation.[303]

The safety of heparin prophylaxis in LBW infants has been questioned by Lesko and colleagues, who implicated heparin as a risk factor for intracranial hemorrhage.[304] Although the evidence provided in their retrospective case-control study is not strong, the researchers' hypothesis is plausible and awaits testing in a future controlled clinical trial.

REFERENCES

1. Brown MS. Fetal and neonatal erythropoiesis. In: Stockman JA, Pochedly C, eds. Developmental and neonatal hematology. New York: Raven Press, 1988:39.
2. Shannon KM, Naylor GS, Torkildson JC, et al. Circulating erythroid progenitors in the anemia of prematurity. N Engl J Med 1987;317:728.
3. Rhondeau SM, Christensen RD, Ross MP, et al. Responsiveness to recombinant human erythropoietin of marrow erythroid progenitors from infants with the "anemia of prematurity." J Pediatr 1988;112:935.
4. Christensen RD. Hematopoiesis in the fetus and neonate. Pediatr Res 1989;26:531.
5. Stockman JA III, Garcia JF, Oski FA. The anemia of prematurity. Factors governing the erythropoietin response. N Engl J Med 1977;296:647.
6. Stockman JA III, Graeber JE, Clark DA, et al. Anemia of prematurity: determinants of the erythropoietin response. J Pediatr 1984;105:786.
7. Brown MS, Garcia JF, Phibbs RH, Dallman PR. Decreased response of plasma immunoreactive erythropoietin to "available oxygen" in anemia of prematurity. J Pediatr 1984;105:793.
8. Forestier F, Daffos F, Catherine N, et al. Developmental hematopoiesis in normal human fetal blood. Blood 1991;77:2360.
9. Oski FA, Naiman JL. Normal blood values in the newborn period. In: Oski FA, Naiman JL, eds. Hematologic problems in the newborn. 3rd ed. Philadelphia: WB Saunders, 1982:11.
10. Blanchette V, Zipursky A. Neonatal hematology. In: Avery GB, ed. Neonatology: pathophysiology and management. 3rd ed. Philadelphia: JB Lippincott, 1987:639.
11. Yao AC, Moinian M, Lind J. Distribution of blood between infant and placenta after birth. Lancet 1969;2:871.
12. Colozzi AE. Clamping of the umbilical cord: its effect on the placental transfusion. N Engl J Med 1954;250:629.
13. Usher R, Shephard M, Lind J. The blood volume of the newborn infant and placental transfusion. Acta Pediatr 1963;52:497.
14. Gunther M. The transfer of blood between baby and placenta in the minutes after birth. Lancet 1957;1:1277.
15. O'Brien RT, Pearson HA. Physiologic anemia of the newborn infant. J Pediatr 1971;79:132.
16. Schulman I, Smith CH, Stern GS. Studies on the anemia of prematurity. Am J Dis Child 1954;88:567.
17. Stockman JA III. Anemia of prematurity. Clin Perinatol 1977;4:239.
18. Stockman JA III, Oski FA. Physiological anemia of infancy and the anemia of prematurity. Clin Hematol 1978;7:3.
19. Gairdner D, Marks J, Roscoe JD. Blood formation in infancy. Part II. Normal erythropoiesis. Arch Dis Child 1952;27:214.
20. Bratteby LE, Garby L, Groth T, et al. Studies on erythrokinetics in infancy. XIII. The mean life span and life span frequency function of red blood cells formed during foetal life. Acta Pediatr Scand 1968;57:311.
21. Pearson HA. Life-span of the fetal red blood cell. J Pediatr 1967;70:166.

22. Wardrop CAJ, Holland BM, Veale KEA, et al. Non-physiologic anemia of prematurity. Arch Dis Child 1978;53:855.
23. Keyes WG, Donohue PK, Spivak JL, et al. Assessing the need for transfusion of premature infants and role of hematocrit, clinical signs and erythropoietin level. Pediatrics 1989;84:412.
24. Stevens D. Available oxygen in pre-term babies. Lancet 1979;1:877.
25. Blank JP, Sheagren TG, Vajaria J, et al. The role of RBC transfusion in the premature infant. Am J Dis Child 1984;138:831.
26. Ross MP, Christensen RD, Rothstein G, et al. A randomized trial to develop criteria for administering erythrocyte transfusions to anemic preterm infants 1 to 3 months of age. J Perinatol 1989;9:246.
27. Bifano E, Smith F, Borer J, Goldwasser E. Oxygen supply and demand in infants with anemia of prematurity with and without apnea. Pediatr Res 1988;23:461A.
28. Sasidharan P, Heimler R, Pelegano J. Effect of transfusion on the control of breathing in preterm anemic infants. Pediatr Res 1988;23:523A.
29. Bifano E, Borer J, Smith F, et al. Effect of transfusion on apnea of prematurity: red cells or volume? Pediatr Res 1988;23:402A.
30. Ross MP, Christensen RD, Koenig JM, et al. The "anemia of prematurity" in unwell infants: is it physiologic or pathologic, is transfusion beneficial, is erythropoietin administration an alternative? Pediatr Res 1988;23:467A.
31. Stockman JA, Clark DA. Weight gain: a response to transfusion in selected preterm infants. Am J Dis Child 1984;138:828.
32. Doyle JJ, Zipursky A. Neonatal blood disorders. In: Sinclair JC, Bracken MB, eds. Effective care of the newborn infant. Oxford: Oxford University Press, 1992;425.
33. Rönnholm KAR, Siimes MA. Hemoglobin concentration depends on protein intake in small preterm infants fed human milk. Arch Dis Child 1985;60:99.
34. James JA, Combes M. Iron deficiency in the premature infant: significance and prevention by the intramuscular administration of iron dextran. Pediatrics 1960;26:368.
35. Gorten MK, Cross ER. Iron absorption in premature infants. II. Prevention of iron deficiency. J Pediatr 1964;64:509.
36. Hammond D, Murphy A. The influence of exogenous iron on formation of hemoglobin in the premature infant. Pediatrics 1960;25:362.
37. Halprin DS, Wacker P, Lacourt G, et al. Effects of recombinant human erythropoietin in infants with the anemia of prematurity: a pilot study. J Pediatr 1990;116:779.
38. Shannon KM. Anemia of prematurity: progress and prospects. Am J Pediatr Hematol Oncol 1990;12:14.
39. Shannon KM, Mentzer WC, Abels RI, et al. Recombinant human erythropoietin in the anemia of prematurity: results of a placebo-controlled pilot study. J Pediatr 1991;118:949.
40. Blanchette VS, Zipursky A. Assessment of anemia in newborn infants. Clin Perinatol 1984;11:489.
41. Oettinger L Jr, Mills WB. Simultaneous capillary and venous hemoglobin determinations in the newborn infant. J Pediatr 1949;35:362.
42. Linderkamp O, Versmold HT, Strohhacker I, et al. Capillary-venous hematocrit differences in newborn infants. I. Relationship to blood volume, peripheral blood flow, and acid-base parameters. Eur J Pediatr 1977;127:9.
43. Oh W, Lind J. Venous and capillary hematocrit in newborn infants and placental transfusion. Acta Pediatr Scand 1966;55:38.
44. Rivera LM, Rudolph N. Postnatal persistence of capillary-venous differences in hematocrit and hemoglobin values in low-birth-weight and term infants. Pediatrics 1982;70:956.
45. Faxelius G, Raye J, Gutberlet R, et al. Red cell volume measurements and acute blood loss in high-risk newborn infants. J Pediatr 1977;90:273.
46. International Committee for Standardization in Haematology. Recommended methods for measurement of red-cell and plasma volume. J Nucl Med 1980;21:793.
47. Mollison PL, Veall N, Cutbush M. Red cell and plasma volume in newborn infants. Arch Dis Child 1950;25:242.
48. Bratteby LE. Studies on erythro-kinetics in infancy. XI. The change in circulating red-cell volume during the first five months of life. Acta Pediatr Scand 1968;57:215.
49. Bratteby LE. Studies on erythro-kinetics in infancy. X. Red-cell volume of newborn infants in relation to gestational age. Acta Pediatr Scand 1968;57:132.
50. Dyer NC, Brill AB, Faxelius G, et al. Blood volume and hemorrhage timing in newborn infants with respiratory distress using the stable tracer ^{50}Cr. Proceed Am Nucl Soc 1971;5:46.
51. Francoual C, Relier J-P, Thérain F. Interet de la mesure du volume globulaire total chez le nouveau-ne en distresse respiratoire. Arch Fr Pediatr 1977;34:83.
52. Cavill I, Trevett D, Fisher J, Hoy T. The measurement of the total volume of red cells in man: a non-radioactive approach using biotin. Br J Haematol 1988;70:491.
53. Hudson IRB, Cavill IAJ, Cooke A, et al. Biotin labelling of red cells in the measurement of red cell volume in preterm infants. Pediatr Res 1990;28:199.
54. Schulman I. The anemia of prematurity. J Pediatr 1959;54:663.
55. Bell EF, Nahmias C, Sinclair JC, et al. The assessment of anemia in small premature infants. [Abstract] Pediatr Res 1977;11:467.
56. Ballin A, Koren G, Hasu M, Zipursky A. Evaluation of a new method for the prevention of neonatal anemia. Pediatr Res 1989;25:274.
57. Zipursky A, Hull A, White FD, Israels LG. Foetal erythrocytes in the maternal circulation. Lancet 1959;1:451.
58. Pai MKR, Bedritis I, Zipursky A. Massive transplacental hemorrhage: clinical manifestations in the newborn. Can Med Assoc J 1975;112:585.
59. Kleihauer E, Hildegard B, Betke K. Demonstration von fetalem Hamoglobin in den Erythrocyten eines Blutausstrichs. Klin Wochenschr 1957;35:637.
60. Pembrey ME, Weatherall DJ, Clegg JB. Maternal synthesis of hemoglobin F in pregnancy. Lancet 1973;1:1350.
61. Tan KL, Tan R, Tan SH, Tan AM. The twin transfusion syndrome. Clinical observations on 35 affected pairs. Clin Pediatr 1979;18:111.
62. Clayton EM, Pryor JA, Wierdsma JG, Whitacre FE. Fetal and maternal components in third-trimester obstetric hemorrhage. Obstet Gynecol 1964;24:56.
63. Potter EL. Fetal and neonatal deaths: a statistical analysis of 2000 autopsies. JAMA 1940;115:996.
64. Holmberg E. Rupture of liver in newborn observed at General Lying-In Hospital in Helsingfors from 1924 to 1932. Finska Lak-Sallsk Handl 1933;75:1067.
65. Henderson JL. Hepatic haemorrhage in stillborn and newborn infants; clinical and pathologic study of 47 cases. J Obstet Gynaecol Br Commw 1941;48:377.
66. Paes B, Andrew M, Milner R, et al. Developmental changes in red cell creatine and free erythrocyte protoporphyrin in healthy full-term infants during the first six months of life. J Pediatr 1986;108:732.
67. Paes B, Andrew M, Milner R, et al. Developmental changes in red cell creatine and free erythrocyte protoporphyrin in healthy premature infants during the first six months of life. J Pediatr 1987;111:745.
68. Zipursky A, Brown E, Palko J, Brown EJ. The erythrocyte

differential count in newborn infants. Am J Pediatr Hematol Oncol 1983;5:45.
69. Bessis M. Red cell shapes. In: Bessis M, Weed RI, LeBlond PF, eds. An illustrated classification and its rationale—red cell shape, physiology, pathology, ultrastructure. New York: Springer-Verlag, 1973:1.
70. Naiman JL. Current management of hemolytic disease of the newborn infant. J Pediatr 1972;80:1049.
71. Queenan JT. Modern management of the Rh problem. New York: Harper & Row, 1967.
72. Zipursky A. Erythroblastosis fetalis. In: Nathan DG, Oski FA, eds. Hematology of infancy and childhood. Philadelphia: WB Saunders, 1974:46.
73. Liley AW. Diagnosis and treatment of erythroblastosis in the fetus. Adv Pediatr 1968;15:29.
74. Cassady G, Daniel SJ. Non-immunologic hydrops fetalis associated with large hemangioendothelioma. Pediatrics 1968; 42:828.
75. Doyle J, Poon A, Zipursky A. Transient leukemia and Down syndrome. Blood 1991;78:41A.
76. Chessells JM, Wigglesworth JS. Haemostatic failure in babies with rhesus isoimmunization. Arch Dis Child 1971;46:38.
77. Hathaway WE. Coagulation problems in the newborn infant. Pediatr Clin North Am 1970;17:929.
78. Torrance GW, Zipursky A. Cost-effectiveness of antepartum prevention of Rh immunization. Clin Perinatol 1984;11:267.
79. Bowman JM, Friesen RF. Hemolytic disease of the newborn. In: Gellis SS, Kogan BM, eds. Current pediatric therapy, vol 4. Philadelphia: WB Saunders, 1970:405.
80. Bowman JM, Pollack JM. Amniotic fluid spectrophotometry and early delivery in the management of erythroblastosis fetalis. Pediatrics 1965;35:815.
81. Zipursky A, Bowman JM. Erythroblastosis fetalis. In: Nathan DG, Oski FA, eds. Hematology of infancy and childhood. vol. 4. Philadelphia: WB Saunders, 1993:44.
82. Desjardins L, Blajchman MA, Chintu C, et al. The spectrum of ABO hemolytic disease of the newborn infant. J Pediatr 1979;95:447.
83. Kaplan E, Herz F, Scheye E, Robinson L Jr. Phototherapy in ABO hemolytic disease of the newborn. J Pediatr 1971;79:911.
84. Kornstad L. New cases of irregular blood group antibodies other than anti-D in pregnancy. Acta Obstet Gynecol Scand 1983;62:431.
85. Pepperell RJ, Barrie JU, Fliegner JR. Significance of red cell irregular antibodies in the obstetric patient. Med J Aust 1977; 2:453.
86. Giblett ER. Blood group antibodies causing hemolytic disease of the newborn. Clin Obstet Gynecol 1964;7:1044.
87. Doxiadis SA, Valaes T, Karaklis A, Stavrakakis D. Risk of severe jaundice in glucose-6-phosphate dehydrogenase deficiency of the newborn. Lancet 1964;2:1210.
88. Lu TC, Wei H, Blackwell RQ. Increased incidence of severe hyperbilirubinemia among Chinese infants with G6PD deficiency. Pediatrics 1966;37:994.
89. Fessas P, Doxiadis S, Valaes T. Neonatal jaundice in glucose-6-phosphate dehydrogenase-deficient infants. Br Med J 1962; 2:1359.
90. Olowe SA, Ransome-Kuti O. The risk of jaundice in glucose-6-phosphate deficient babies exposed to menthol. Acta Pediatr Scand 1980;69:341.
91. Necheles T, Rai US, Valaes T. The role of hemolysis in neonatal hyperbilirubinemia as reflected in carboxyhemoglobin levels. Acta Pediatr Scand 1976;65:361.
92. Eshaghpour E, Oski FA, Williams M. The relationship of glucose-6-phosphate dehydrogenase deficiency to hyperbilirubinemia in Negro premature infants. J Pediatr 1967;70:595.
93. Bienzle U, Effiong C, Luzatto L. Erythrocyte glucose-6-phosphate dehydrogenase deficiency (G6PD type A) and neonatal jaundice. Acta Pediatr Scand 1976;65:701.
94. Valaes T, Doxiadis SA, Fessas P. Acute hemolysis due to naphthalene inhalation. J Pediatr 1963;63:904.
95. Motulsky AG, Campbell-Kraut JM. Population genetics of glucose-6-phosphate dehydrogenase deficiency of the red cell. In: Blumber BS, ed. Proceedings of the conference on genetic polymorphisms and geographic variations in disease. New York: Grune & Stratton, 1961:159.
96. Beutler E, Mitchell M. Special modifications of the fluorescent screening method for glucose-6-phosphate dehydrogenase deficiency. Blood 1968;32:816.
97. Erlandson ME, Hilgartner M. Hemolytic disease in the newborn period. J Pediatr 1959;54:566.
98. Hegye T, Delphin ES, Bank A, et al. Sickle cell anemia in the newborn. Pediatrics 1977;60:213.
99. Lee-Potter JP, Deacon-Smith RA, Simpkiss AJ, et al. A new cause of hemolytic anemia in the newborn. A description of an unstable fetal hemoglobin: F Poole, $\alpha 2G\gamma 2$ 130 tryptophan—glycine. J Clin Pathol 1975;28:317.
100. Oort M, Roos HD, Flavell RA, Bernini LF. Haemolytic disease of the newborn and chronic anemia induced by gamma-beta thalassemia in a Dutch family. Br J Haematol 1981;48:251.
101. Kan YW, Forget BG, Nathan DG. Gamma-beta thalassemia: a cause of hemolytic disease of the newborn. N Engl J Med 1972;286:129.
102. Fearon ER, Kazazian HH, Waber PG, et al. The entire beta-globin gene cluster is deleted in a form of delta-beta-gamma thalassemia. Blood 1983;61:1273.
103. Piratsu M, Kan YW, Lin CC, et al. Hemolytic disease of the newborn caused by a new deletion of the entire beta-globin cluster. J Clin Invest 1989;72:602.
104. Ballin A, Brown EJ, Zipursky A. Idiopathic Heinz body hemolytic anemia in newborn infants. Am J Pediatr Hematol Oncol 1989;11:3.
105. Ballin A, Brown EJ, Koren G, Zipursky A. Vitamin C induced erythrocyte damage in premature infants. J Pediatr 1988; 113:114.
106. Diamond LK, Wang WC, Alter BP. Congenital hypoplastic anemia. Adv Pediatr 1976;22:349.
107. Aase JM, Smith DW. Congenital anemia and triphalangeal thumbs. A new syndrome. J Pediatr 1969;74:471.
108. Dallman PR. Iron, vitamin E and folate in the preterm infant. J Pediatr 1974;85:742.
109. Seip M, Halvorsen S. Erythrocyte production and iron stores in premature infants during the first months of life. The anemia of prematurity—aetiology, pathogenesis, iron requirement. Acta Pediatr 1956;45:600.
110. Shojania AM. Folic acid and vitamin B_{12} deficiency in pregnancy and in the neonatal period. Clin Perinatol 1984;11:433.
111. Hassan H, Hashim SA, Van Itallie TB, et al. Syndrome in premature infants associated with low plasma vitamin E levels and high polyunsaturated fatty acid diet. Am J Clin Nutr 1966;19:147.
112. Oski FA, Barness LA. Vitamin E deficiency: a previously unrecognized cause of hemolytic anemia in the premature infant. J Pediatr 1967;70:211.
113. Williams ML, Shott R, O'Neal PL, Oski FA. Role of dietary iron and fat on vitamin E deficiency anemia of infancy. N Engl J Med 1975;292:887.
114. Zipursky A, Brown EJ, Watts J, et al. Oral vitamin E supplementation for the prevention of anemia in premature infants: a controlled trial. Pediatrics 1987;79:61.
115. Wirth FH, Goldberg KE, Lubchenco LO. Neonatal hyperviscosity: I. Incidence. Pediatrics 1979;63:833.

116. Stevens K, Wirth FH. Incidence of neonatal hyperviscosity at sea level. J Pediatr 1980;97:118.
117. Wiswell TE, Cornish JD, Northam RS. Neonatal polycythemia: frequency of clinical manifestation and other associated findings. Pediatrics 1986;78:26.
118. Shohat M, Reisner SH, Mimouni F, Merlob P. Neonatal polycythemia: II. Definition related to time of sampling. Pediatrics 1984;73:11.
119. Linderkamp O, Wu PYK, Meiselman HJ. Deformability of density separated red blood cells in normal newborn infants and adults. Pediatr Res 1982;16:964.
120. Riopel L, Fouron J, Bard H. Blood viscosity during the neonatal period: the role of plasma and red blood cell type. J Pediatr 1982;100:449.
121. Linderkamp O, Versmold HT, Riegel KP, Betke K. Contributions of red cells and plasma to blood viscosity in preterm and full term infants and adults. Pediatrics 1984;74:45.
122. Black VD, Lubchenco LO, Koops BL, et al. Neonatal hyperviscosity: randomized study of effect of partial plasma exchange transfusion on long-term outcome. Pediatrics 1985; 75:1048.
123. Black V, Camp BW, Roberts L, et al. Neonatal hyperviscosity: outcome at school age following a randomized trial of partial plasma exchange. J Dev Behav Pediatr 1986;7:202.
124. Black VD, Camp BW, Lubchenco LO, et al. Neonatal hyperviscosity is associated with lower achievement and IQ scores at school age. Pediatr Res 1988;23:442A.
125. Bauer C, Ludwig I, Ludwig M. Different effects of 2,3-diphosphoglycerate and adenosine triphosphate on the oxygen affinity of adult and foetal human hemoglobin. Life Sci 1968; 7:1339.
126. Morgan MEI, Benson JWT, Cooke RWI. Ethamyslate reduces the incidence of periventricular hemorrhage in very low birth weight infants. Lancet 1981;2:830.
127. Bloch CA, Rothberg AD, Bradlow BA. Mother-infant prothrombin status at birth. J Pediatr Gastroenterol Nutr 1984; 3:101.
128. Shearer MJ, Rahin S, Barkhan P, Stimmlier L. Plasma vitamin K in mothers and their newborn babies. Lancet 1982;2:460.
129. Dreyfus M, Lelong-Tissier MC, Lombard C, Tchernia G. Vitamin K deficiency in the newborn. Lancet 1979;1:1351.
130. Blayer WA, Skinner AL. Fetal neonatal hemorrhage after maternal anticonvulsant therapy. JAMA 1976;235:626.
131. Goldman HI, Desposito F. Hypoprothrombinemic bleeding in young infants. Am J Dis Child 1966;111:430.
132. Minford AMB, Eden OB. Hemorrhage responsive to vitamin K in a 6-week-old infant. Arch Dis Child 1979;54:310.
133. Committee on Nutrition, American Academy of Pediatrics. Vitamin K compounds and the water-soluble analogs: use in therapy and prophylaxis in pediatrics. Pediatrics 1961;28:501.
134. Sann L, Leclerq BSC, Guillaumont BS, et al. Serum vitamin K, concentration after oral administration of vitamin K_1, in low birth weight infants. J Pediatr 1985;107:608.
135. Hathaway WE, Isarangkura PB, Mahasandana C, et al. Comparison of oral and parenteral vitamin K prophylaxis for prevention of late hemorrhage disease of the newborn. J Pediatr 1991;119:461.
136. von Kries R. Neonatal vitamin K. Br Med J 1991;303:1083.
137. Zipursky A, deSa D, Hsu E, et al. Clinical and laboratory diagnosis of hemostatic disorders in newborn infants. Am J Pediatr Hematol Oncol 1979;1:217.
138. Baehner RL, Straus HS. Hemophilia in the first year of life. N Engl J Med 1966;275:524.
139. Andrew M, Paes B, Milner R, et al. Development of the human coagulation system in the full-term infant. Blood 1987; 70:165.
140. Brellter DB, Levine PH. Factor concentrates for treatment of hemophilia: which one to choose? Blood 1989;73:2067.
141. Lorand L, Losowsky MS, Miloszewski KJN. Human factor XIII fibrin stabilizing factor. Prog Hemost Thromb 1980;5:245.
142. Croizat P, Revol L, Favre-Gilly J, et al. Les Hémorrhagies néonatales dans les diethesis hemorrhagiques congénital. Nouv Rev Franc Hematol 1964;4:181.
143. Katz JA, Moake JL, McPherson PD, et al. Relationship between human development and disappearance of unusually large von Willebrand factor multimers from plasma. Blood 1989;73:1851.
144. Andrew M, Kelton J. Neonatal thrombocytopenia. Clin Perinatol 1984;1:359.
145. Pearson HA, McIntosh S. Neonatal thrombocytopenia. Clin Haematol 1978;7:111.
146. von dem Borne AEGKr, van Leeuwen EF, von Riesz LE, et al. Neonatal alloimmune thrombocytopenia: detection and characterization of the responsible antibodies by the platelet immunofluorescence test. Blood 1981;57:649.
147. Mueller-Eckhardt C, Kiefel V, Grubert A, et al. 348 cases of suspected neonatal alloimmune thrombocytopenia. Lancet 1989;1:363.
148. von dem Borne AEGK, von Riesz E, Verheugt FWA, et al. Bak^a a new platelet-specific antigen involved in neonatal alloimmune thrombocytopenia. Vox Sang 1980;39:113.
149. Friedman JM, Aster RW. Neonatal alloimmune thrombocytopenic purpura and congenital porencephaly in two siblings associated with a "new" maternal antiplatelet antibody. Blood 1985;65:1412.
150. Mueller-Eckhardt C, Becker T, Weisheit M, et al. Neonatal alloimmune thrombocytopenia due to fetomaternal Zw^b incompatability. Vox Sang 1986;50:94.
151. Shibata Y, Miyaji T, Ichikawa Y, Matsuda I. A new platelet system, Yuk^a/Yuk^b. Vox Sang 1986;51:334.
152. Kiefel V, Santoso S, Katzmann B, Mueller-Eckhardt C. A new platelet-specific alloantigen Br^a. Report of 4 cases with neonatal alloimmune thrombocytopenia. Vox Sang 1988;54:101.
153. Kroll H, Kiefel V, Santoso S, Mueller-Eckhardt C. Sr^a, a private platelet antigen on glycoprotein IIIa associated with neonatal alloimmune thrombocytopenia. Blood 1990;76:2296.
154. Kaplan C, Morel-Kopp MC, Kroll H, et al. HPA-5b (Br(a)) neonatal alloimmune thrombocytopenia: clinical and immunological analysis of 39 cases. Br J Haematol 1991;78:425.
155. Pearson HA, Shulman NR, Marder VJ, Cone TE Jr. Isoimmune neonatal thrombocytopenic purpura; clinical and therapeutic considerations. Blood 1964;23:154.
156. Blanchette VS, Chen L, de Friedberg ZS, et al. Alloimmunization to the $P1^{A1}$ platelet antigen: results of a prospective study. Br J Haematol 1990;74:209.
157. Herman JH, Jumbelic MI, Ancona RJ, Kickler TS. *In utero* cerebral hemorrhage in alloimmune thrombocytopenia. Am J Pediatr Hematol Oncol 1986;8:312.
158. Lester RB, Sty JR. Prenatal diagnosis of cystic CNS lesions in neonatal isoimmune thrombocytopenia. J Ultrasound Med 1987;6:479.
159. Burrows RF, Caco CC, Kelton JF. Neonatal alloimmune thrombocytopenia: spontaneous *in utero* intracranial hemorrhage. Am J Hematol 1988;28:98.
160. Manson J, Speed I, Abbott K, Crompton J. Congenital blindness, porencephaly, and neonatal thrombocytopenia: a report of four cases. J Child Neurol 1988;3:120.
161. de Vries LS, Connell J, Bydder GM, et al. Recurrent intracranial hemorrhages *in utero* in an infant with alloimmune thrombocytopenia. Case report. Br J Obstet Gynecol 1988; 95:299.
162. Bussel JB, Berkowitz RL, McFarland JG, et al. Antenatal treat-

ment of neonatal alloimmune thrombocytopenia. N Engl J Med 1988;319:1374.

163. Gill FM, Schwartz E. Platelet transfusion as a diagnostic and therapeutic aid in the newborn. Pediatr Res 1971;5:409.
164. McIntosh S, O'Brien RT, Schwartz AD, Pearson HA. Neonatal isoimmune purpura: response to platelet infusions. J Pediatr 1973;82:1020.
165. McGill M, Mayhaus C, Hoff R, Carey P. Frozen maternal platelets for neonatal thrombocytopenia. Transfusion 1987; 27:347.
166. Massey GV, McWilliams NB, Mueller DG, et al. Intravenous immunoglobulin in treatment of neonatal isoimmune thrombocytopenia. J Pediatr 1987;111:133.
167. Suarez CR, Anderson C. High-dose intravenous gammaglobulin (IVG) in neonatal immune thrombocytopenia. Am J Hematol 1987;26:247.
168. Beck R, Reid DM, Lazarte R. Intravenous gammaglobulin therapy for neonatal alloimmune thrombocytopenia. Am J Perinatol 1988;5:79.
169. Kaplan M, Abramov A, Goren A. Repeated single-dose intravenous immunoglobulin therapy for neonatal passive immune thrombocytopenia. Isr J Med Sci 1987;23:844.
170. Mueller-Eckhardt C, Kiefel V, Grubert A. High-dose IgG treatment for neonatal alloimmune thrombocytopenia. Blut 1989;59:145.
171. Pietz J, Kiefel V, Sontheimer D, et al. High-dose intravenous gammaglobulin for neonatal alloimmune thrombocytopenia in twins. Acta Paediatr Scand 1991;80:129.
172. Bussel J, Kaplan C, McFarland J, and The Working Party on Neonatal Immune Thrombocytopenia of the Neonatal Hemostasis Subcommittee of the Scientific and Standardization Committee of the ISTH. Recommendations for the evaluation and treatment of neonatal autoimmune and alloimmune thrombocytopenia. Thromb Haemost 1991;65:631.
173. Ballin A, Andrew M, Ling E, et al. High-dose intravenous gammaglobulin therapy for neonatal autoimmune thrombcytopenia. J Pediatr 1988;112:789.
174. Hanada T, Saito K, Nagasawa T, et al. Intravenous gammaglobulin therapy for thromboneutropenic neonates of mothers with systemic lupus erythematosus. Eur J Hematol 1987;38:400.
175. Kelton JG, Inwood MJ, Barr RM, et al. The prenatal prediction of thrombocytopenia in infants of mothers with clinically diagnosed immune thrombocytopenia. Am J Obstet Gynecol 1982;144:449.
176. Cines DB, Dusak B, Tomaski A, et al. Immune thrombocytopenic purpura and pregnancy. N Engl J Med 1982;306: 826.
177. Kelton JG. Management of the pregnant patient with idiopathic thrombocytopenic purpura. Ann Intern Med 1983; 99:796.
178. Karpatkin M, Porges RF, Karpatkin S. Platelet counts in infants of women with autoimmune thrombocytopenia: effects of steroid administration to the mother. N Engl J Med 1981;305:936.
179. Christiaens GC, Nieuwenhuis HK, von dem Borne AE, et al. Idiopathic thrombocytopenic purpura in pregnancy: a randomized trial on the effect of antenatal low dose corticosteroids on neonatal platelet count. Br J Obstet Gynaecol 1990;97:893.
180. Castle V, Andrew M, Kelton J, et al. Frequency and mechanism of neonatal thrombocytopenia. J Pediatr 1986;108:749.
181. Akenzua GI, Hui YT, Milner R, et al. Neutrophil and band counts in the diagnosis of neonatal infection. Pediatrics 1974; 54:38.
182. Zipursky A, Palko J, Milner R, Akenzua GI. The hematology of bacterial infections in premature infants. Pediatrics 1976; 57:839.
183. Xanthou M. Leukocyte blood picture in healthy full-term and premature babies during neonatal period. Arch Dis Child 1970;45:242.
184. Coulombel L, Dehan M, Tchernia G, et al. The number of polymorphonuclear leukocytes in relation to gestational age in the newborn. Acta Pediatr Scand 1979;68:709.
185. Lloyd BW, Oto A. Normal values from mature and immature neutrophils in very preterm babies. Arch Dis Child 1982; 57:233.
186. Zipursky A, Jaber HM. The hematology of bacterial infection in newborn infants. Clin Hematol 1978;7:175.
187. Gregory J, Hey E. Blood neutrophil response to bacterial infection in the first month of life. Arch Dis Child 1972;47:747.
188. Manroe BL, Weinberg AG, Rosenfeld CR, Browne R. The neonatal blood count in health and disease. I. Reference values for neutrophilic cells. J Pediatr 1979;95:89.
189. Berger M. Complement deficiency and neutrophil dysfunction as risk factors for bacterial infection in newborns and the role of granulocyte transfusion in therapy. Rev Infect Dis Suppl 1990;4:S401.
190. Christensen RD, Rothstein G. Exhaustion of mature marrow neutrophils in neonates with sepsis. J Pediatr 1980;96:316.
191. Christensen RD, Brown MS, Hall DC, et al. Effect on neutrophil kinetics and serum opsonic capacity of intravenous administration of immune globulin to neonates with clinical signs of early-onset sepsis. J Pediatr 1991;118:606.
192. Kostmann R. Infantile genetic agranulocytosis. Acta Paediatr Scand 1975;64:362.
193. Boxer L, Hutchinson R, Emerson S. Recombinant human granulocyte colony-stimulating factor in the treatment of patients with neutropenia. Clin Immunol Immunopathol 1992;62:539.
194. DeVaal OM, Seynhaeve V. Reticular dysgenesia. Lancet 1959; 2:1123.
195. Shwachman H, Diamond LK, Oski FA, et al. The syndrome of pancreatic insufficiency and bone marrow dysfunction. J Pediatr 1964;65:645.
196. Buckley RH, Rowlands DT Jr. Agammaglobulinemia, neutropenia, fever and abdominal pain. J Allergy Clin Immunol 1973;51:308.
197. Rosen FS. The dysgammaglobulinemias and X linked thymic dysplasias. In: Bergsma D, ed. Immunologic deficiency diseases in man. New York: National Foundation March of Dimes, 1968:67.
198. Page AR, Good RA. Studies on cyclic neutropenia. Am J Dis Child 1957;94:623.
199. Guerry DIV, Dale DC, Omine M, et al. Periodic hematopoiesis in human cyclic neutropenia. J Clin Invest 1973;52:3220.
200. Levine DH, Madyastha PR. Isoimmune neonatal neutropenia. Am J Perinatol 1986;3:231.
201. Minchinton RM, McGrath KM. Alloimmune neonatal neutropenia—a neglected diagnosis? Med J Aust 1987;147:139.
202. Lalezari P, Radel E. Neutrophil-specific antigens: immunology and clinical significance. Semin Hematol 1974;11:281.
203. Huizinga TW, Kuijpers RW, Kleijer M, et al. Maternal genomic neutrophil FcRIII deficiency leading to neonatal isoimmune neutropenia. Blood 1990;76:1927.
204. Stroncek DF, Skubitz KM, Plachta LB, et al. Alloimmune neonatal neutropenia due to an antibody to the neutrophil Fc-gamma receptor III with maternal deficiency of CD16 antigen. Blood 1991;77:1572.
205. Hanada T, Shin R, Hosoi M, et al. Intravenous gammaglobulin in treatment of isoimmune neonatal neutropenia. Eur J Pediatr 1988;148:218.

206. Jarvenpa AL, Koskimies S, Rajantie J. Alloimmune granulocytopenia in three newborn infants of two families. Acta Paediatr Scand 1990;79:1244.
207. Cartron J, Tchernia G, Celton JL, et al. Alloimmune neonatal neutropenia. Am J Pediatr Hematol Oncol 1991;13:21.
208. Bussel J, Lalezari P, Fikrig S. Intravenous treatment with gammaglobulin of autoimmune neutropenia of infancy. J Pediatr 1988;112:298.
209. Zipursky A, Peeters M, Poon A. Megakaryoblastic leukemia and Down's syndrome. Pediatr Hematol Oncol 1987;4:211.
210. Miyauchi J, Ito Y, Kawaivo T, et al. Diffuse liver fibrosis accompanying transient abnormal myelopoiesis in Down's syndrome. Blood 1991;78:40A.
211. Ruchelli ED, Uri A, Dimmick JE, et al. Severe perinatal liver disease and Down syndrome: an apparent relationship. Hum Pathol 1991;22:1274.
212. Bhat AM, Scanlon JW. The pattern of eosinophilia in premature infants. J Pediatr 1981;98:612.
213. Gibson EL, Vaucher Y, Corrigan JJ Jr. Eosinophilia in premature infants: relationship to weight gain. J Pediatr 1979;95:99.
214. Lawrence R Jr, Church JA, Richards W, Lipsey AI. Eosinophilia in the hospitalized neonate. Ann Allergy 1980;44:349.
215. Rothberg AD, Cohn RJ, Argent AC, et al. Eosinophilia in premature neonates. Phase 2 of a biphasic granulopoietic response. South Afr Med J 1983;64:539.
216. Blanchette VS, Hume HA, Levy GJ, et al. Guidelines for auditing pediatric blood transfusion practices. Am J Dis Child 1991;145:787.
217. Floss AM, Strauss RG, Goeken N, Kox L. Multiple transfusions fail to provoke antibodies against blood cell antigens in human infants. Transfusion 1986;26:419.
218. Ludvigsen CW Jr, Swanson JL, Thompson TR, McCullough J. The failure of neonates to form red cell alloantibodies in response to multiple transfusions. Am J Clin Pathol 1987;87:250.
219. Sacher RA, Strauss RG, Luban NLC, et al. Blood component therapy during the neonatal period: a national survey of red cell transfusion practice, 1985. Transfusion 1990;30:271.
220. Blanchette VS, Gray E, Hardie MJ, et al. Hyperkalemia after neonatal exchange transfusion: risk eliminated by washing red cell concentrates. J Pediatr 1984;105:321.
221. Scanlon JW, Krakaur R. Hyperkalemia following exchange transfusion. J Pediatr 1980;96:108.
222. Andrew M, Castle V, Saigal S, et al. Clinical impact of neonatal thrombocytopenia. J Pediatr 1987;110:457.
223. Moroff G, Friedman A, Robkin-Kline L, et al. Reduction of the volume of stored platelet concentrates for use in neonatal patients. Transfusion 1984;24:144.
224. Christensen RD, Rothstein G, Anstall HB, et al. Granulocyte transfusions in neonates with bacterial infection, neutropenia, and depletion of mature marrow neutrophils. Pediatrics 1982;70:1.
225. Poon A, Wilson S. Simple manual method of harvesting granulocytes. Transfusion 1980;20:71.
226. Rock G, Zurakowski S, Baxter A, et al. Simple and rapid preparation of granulocytes for the treatment of neonatal septicemia. Transfusion 1984;24:510.
227. Mollison PL. Blood transfusion in clinical medicine. 6th ed. London: Blackwell Scientific Publications, 1979:617.
228. Giacoia GP, Kasprisin DO. Transfusion in acquired hepatitis A. South Med J 1989;82:1357.
229. Azimi PH, Roberto RR, Guralnik J, et al. Transfusion in acquired hepatitis A in a premature infant with secondary nosocomial spread in an intensive care nursery. Am J Dis Child 1986;140:23.
230. Dienstag JL, Alter HJ. Non-A, non-B hepatitis: evolving epidemiologic and clinical perspective. Semin Liver Dis 1986;6:67.
231. Yeager AS, Grumet FC, Hafleigh EB, et al. Prevention of transfusion-acquired cytomegalovirus infections in newborn infants. J Pediatr 1981;98:281.
232. Adler SP, Chandrika T, Lawrence L, Baggett J. Cytomegalovirus infections in neonates acquired by blood transfusions. Pediatr Infect Dis 1983;2:114.
233. de Cates CR, Roberton NR, Walker JR. Fatal acquired cytomegalovirus infection in a neonate with maternal antibody. J Infect 1988;17:235.
234. Weston PJ, Farmer K, Croxson MC, Ramirez AM. Morbidity from acquired cytomegalovirus infection in a neonatal intensive care unit. Aust Paediatr J 1989;25:138.
235. Preiksaitis JK, Brown L, McKenzie M. Transfusion-acquired cytomegalovirus infection in neonates. A prospective study. Transfusion 1988;28:205.
236. Preiksaitis JK. Indications for the use of cytomegalovirus-seronegative blood products. Trans Med Rev 1991;5:1.
237. Rawls WE, Wong CL, Blajchman M, et al. Neonatal cytomegalovirus infections: the relative role of neonatal blood transfusion and maternal exposure. Clin Invest Med 1984;7:13.
238. Wu J, Tang ZY, Wu YX, Li WR. Acquired cytomegalovirus infection of breast milk in infancy. Chin Med J 1989;102:124.
239. Taylor BJ, Jacobs RF, Baker RL, et al. Frozen deglycerolyzed blood prevents transfusion-acquired cytomegalovirus infections in neonates. Pediatr Infect Dis 1986;5:188.
240. Luban NLC, Williams AE, MacDonald MG, et al. Low incidence of acquired cytomegalovirus infection in neonates transfused with washed red blood cells. Am J Dis Child 1987;141:416.
241. Gilbert GL, Hayes K, Hudson IL, James J. Prevention of transfusion-acquired cytomegalovirus infection in infants by blood filtration to remove leukocytes. Neonatal Cytomegalovirus Infection Study Group. Lancet 1989;1:1228.
242. Shannon KM, Ammann AJ. Acquired immune deficiency syndrome in childhood. J Pediatr 1985;106:332.
243. Ammann AJ, Cowan MJ, Wara DW, et al. Acquired immunodeficiency in an infant: possible transfusion by means of blood products. Lancet 1983;1:956.
244. Shannon K, Ball E, Wasserman RL, et al. Transfusion-associated cytomegalovirus infection and acquired immune deficiency syndrome in an infant. J Pediatr 1983;103:859.
245. McCarthy VP, Charles DL, Unger JL. Transfusion-associated HIV infection in a neonate from a seronegative donor. Am J Dis Child 1987;141:1145.
246. Seemayer TA, Bolande RP. Thymic involution mimicking thymic dysplasia: a consequence of transfusion-induced graft-versus-host disease in a premature infant. Arch Pathol Lab Med 1980;104:141.
247. Berger RS, Dixon SL. Fulminant transfusion-associated graft-versus-host disease in a premature infant. J Am Acad Dermatol 1989;20:945.
248. Funkhouser AW, Vogelsang G, Zehnbauer B, et al. Graft versus host disease after blood transfusions in a premature infant. Pediatrics 1991;87:247.
249. Hatley RM, Reynolds M, Paller AS, et al. Graft-versus-host disease following ECMO. J Pediatr Surg 1991;26:317.
250. Bastian JF, Williams RA, Ornelas W, et al. Maternal isoimmunisation resulting in combined immunodeficiency and fatal graft-versus-host disease in an infant. Lancet 1984;1:1435.
251. Luban NLC, Ness PM. Irradiation of blood products: indications and guidelines and comment. Transfusion 1985;25:301.
252. Leitman SF, Holland PV. Irradiation of blood products: indications and guidelines. Transfusion 1985;25:293.

253. Committee on Infectious Diseases. Prevention of hepatitis B virus infections. Pediatrics 1985;75:362.
254. Schmidt B, Zipursky A. Thrombotic disease in newborn infants. Clin Perinatol 1984;11:461.
255. Levin DL, Weinberg AG, Perken RM. Pulmonary microthrombi syndrome in newborn infants with unresponsive persistent pulmonary hypertension. J Pediatr 1983;102:299.
256. Freiman DG. The structure of thrombi. In: Colman RW, Hirsh J, Marder VJ, Salzman EW, eds. Hemostasis and thrombosis. Philadelphia: JB Lippincott, 1982:766.
257. O'Neill JA Jr, Neblett WW III, Born ML. Management of major thromboembolic complications of umbilical artery catheters. J Pediatr Surg 1981;16:972.
258. Cochran WD, Davis HT, Smith CA. Advantages and complications of umbilical artery catheterization in the newborn. Pediatrics 1968;42:769.
259. Gupta JM, Roberton NRC, Wigglesworth JS. Umbilical artery catheterization in the newborn. Arch Dis Child 1968;43:382.
260. Larroche JC. Umbilical catheterization: its complications. Biol Neonate 1970;16:101.
261. Wigger JH, Bransilver BR, Blanc WA. Thrombosis due to catheterization in infants and children. J Pediatr 1970;76:1.
262. Egan EA, Eitzman DV. Umbilical vessel catheterization. Am J Dis Child 1971;121:213.
263. Symansky MR, Fox HA. Umbilical vessel catheterization: indications, management and evaluation of the technique. J Pediatr 1972;80:820.
264. Tooley WH. What is the risk of an umbilical artery catheter? Pediatrics 1972;50:1.
265. Marsh JL, King W, Barrett C, et al. Serious complications after umbilical artery catheterization for neonatal monitoring. Arch Surg 1975;110:1203.
266. Tyson JE, deSa DJ, Moore S. Thromboatheromatous complications of umbilical arterial catheterization in the newborn period. Clinicopathological study. Arch Dis Child 1976;51:744.
267. MacDonald MG. Umbilical artery catheterization. In: Fletcher MA, MacDonald MG, eds. Atlas of procedures in neonatology. Philadelphia: JB Lippincott, 1993.
268. Neal WA, Reynolds JW, Jarvis CW, et al. Umbilical artery catheterization: demonstration of arterial thrombosis by aortography. Pediatrics 1972;50:6.
269. Goetzman BW, Stadalnik RC, Bogren HG, et al. Thrombotic complications of umbilical artery catheters: a clinical and radiographic study. Pediatrics 1975;56:374.
270. Olinsky A, Aitken FG, Isdale JM. Thrombus formation after umbilical arterial catheterization. An angiographic study. S Afr Med J 1975;49:1467.
271. Mokrohisky ST, Levine R, Blumhagen JD, et al. Low positioning of umbilical artery catheters increases associated complications in newborn infants. N Engl J Med 1978;299:561.
272. Saia OS, Rubaltelli FF, D'Elia RD, et al. Clinical and aortographic assessment of the complications of arterial catheterization. Eur J Pediatr 1978;128:169.
273. Wesstrom G, Finnstrom O, Stenport G. Umbilical artery catheterization in newborns. I. Thrombosis in relation to catheter type and position. Acta Paediatr Scand 1979;68:575.
274. Scott JM. Iatrogenic lesions in babies following umbilical vein catheterization. Arch Dis Child 1965;40:426.
275. DeSa DJ. Intimal cusions in foetal placental veins. J Pathol 1973;110:347.
276. Morisot C, Dubos JP, Kacet N, et al. Neonatal hypertension and thrombosis of the ductus arteriosus. Am J Perinatol 1991;8:77.
277. Amit M, Camfield PR. Neonatal polycythemia causing multiple cerebral infarcts. Arch Neurol 1980;37:109.
278. Marlar RA, Montgomery RR, Broekmans AW, and the Working Party. Diagnosis and treatment of homozygous protein C deficiency: report of the working party on homozygous protein C deficiency of the subcommittee on protein C and protein S, International Committee on Thrombosis and Haemostasis. J Pediatr 1989;114:528.
279. Mahasandana C, Suvatte V, Marlar RA, et al. Neonatal purpura fulminans associated with homozygous protein S deficiency. Lancet 1990;335:61.
280. De Stefano V, Leone G, De Carolis MP, et al. Antithrombin III in full-term and pre-term newborn infants: three cases of neonatal diagnosis of AT III congenital defect. Thromb Haemostas 1987;57:329.
281. Brenner B, Fishman A, Goldsher D, et al. Cerebral thrombosis in a newborn with a congenital deficiency of antithrombin III. Am J Hematol 1988;27:209.
282. Hyers TM, Hull RD, Weg JG. Antithrombotic therapy for venous thromboembolic disease. Summary and recommendations. Arch Intern Med 1986;146:467.
283. Schmidt B, Andrew M. Neonatal thrombotic disease: prevention, diagnosis, and treatment. J Pediatr 1988;113:407.
284. Schmidt B, Andrew M. Report of Scientific and Standardization Subcommittee on Neonatal Hemostasis. Diagnosis and treatment of neonatal thromboses. Thromb Haemostas 1992;67:381.
285. Finazzi G, Cortelazzo S, Viero P, et al. Maternal lupus anticoagulant and fetal neonatal thrombosis. Thromb Haemostas 1987;57:238.
286. Seibert JJ, Taylor BJ, Williamson SL, et al. Sonographic detection of neonatal umbilical-artery thrombosis: clinical correlation. Am J Roentgenol 1987;148:965.
287. Schmidt B, Ofosu FA, Mitchell L, et al. Anticoagulant effects of heparin in neonatal plasma. Pediatr Res 1989;25:405.
288. Schmidt B, Buchanan MR, Ofosu F, et al. Antithrombotic properties of heparin in a neonatal piglet model of thrombin induced thrombosis. Thromb Haemostas 1988;60:289.
289. McDonald MM, Hathaway WE. Anticoagulant therapy by continuous heparinization in newborn and older infants. J Pediatr 1982;101:451.
290. Barnard D, Hathaway WE. Neonatal thrombosis. Am J Pediatr Hematol Oncol 1979;1:235.
291. Corrigan JJ. Neonatal thrombosis and the thrombolytic system: pathophysiology and therapy. Am J Pediatr Hematol Oncol 1988;10:83.
292. Andrew M, Brooker L, Leaker M, et al. Fibrin clot lysis by thrombolytic agents is impaired in newborns due to a low plasminogen concentration. Thromb Haemostas 1992;68:325.
293. Mocan H, Beattie TJ, Murphy AV. Renal venous thrombosis in infancy: long-term follow up. Pediatr Nephrol 1991;5:45.
294. Adelman R. Long-term follow-up of neonatal renovascular hypertension. Pediatr Nephrol 1987;1:35.
295. Caplan MS, Cohn RA, Langman CB, et al. Favorable outcome of neonatal aortic thrombosis and renovascular hypertension. J Pediatr 1989;115:291.
296. Payne RM, Martin TC, Bower RJ, et al. Management and follow-up of arterial thrombosis in the neonatal period. J Pediatr 1989;114:853.
297. Seibert JJ, Northington FJ, Miers JF, et al. Aortic thrombosis after umbilical artery catheterization in neonates: prevalence of complications on long-term follow-up. Am J Roentgenol 1991;156:567.
298. Gilhooly J, Lindenberg J, Reynolds JW. Survey of umbilical artery catheter practices. Crit Care Med 1990;18:247.
299. Rajani K, Goetzman BW, Wennberg RP, et al. Effect of heparinization of fluids infused through an umbilical artery cathe-

ter on catheter patency and frequency of complications. Pediatrics 1979;63:552.

300. David RJ, Merten DF, Anderson JC, et al. Prevention of umbilical artery catheter clots with heparinized infusates. Dev Pharmacol Ther 1981;2:117.
301. Bosque E, Weaver L. Continuous versus intermittent heparin infusion of umbilical artery catheters in the newborn infant. J Pediatr 1986;108:141.
302. Horgan MJ, Bartoletti A, Polansky S, et al. Effect of heparin infusates in umbilical artery catheters on frequency of thrombotic complications. J Pediatr 1987;111:774.
303. Detsky AS, Sackett D. When was a "negative" trial big enough? Arch Intern Med 1985;145:709.
304. Lesko SM, Mitchell AA, Epstein MF, et al. Heparin use as a risk factor for intraventricular hemorrhage in low birth weight infants. N Engl J Med 1986;314:1156.

Neonatology: Pathophysiology and Management of the Newborn, Fourth Edition,
edited by Gordon B. Avery, Mary Ann Fletcher, and Mhairi G. MacDonald.
J.B. Lippincott Company, Philadelphia © 1994.

chapter 46

Immunology

JOSEPH A. BELLANTI
YUNG-HAO PUNG
BARBARA J. ZELIGS

Immunology has come a long way since 1905, when the Russian biologist Eli Metchnikoff prophetically wrote:

> Within a very short period, immunity has been placed in possession not only of a host of medical ideas of the highest importance, but also of effective means of combating a whole series of maladies of the most formidable nature in man and the domestic animals. Science is far from having said its last word, but the advances already made are amply sufficient to dispel pessimism in so far as this has been suggested by the feat of diseases and the feeling that we are powerless to struggle against them.[1]

Once the branch of medicine that dealt exclusively with the study of protection of the host against microorganisms, immunology now enjoys a much broader biologic scope and is concerned with the host processes that recognize and eliminate foreignness. Immunologic responses serve three functions: defense (*i.e.*, resistance to infection by microorganisms), homeostasis (*i.e.*, removal of worn-out host cells), and surveillance (*i.e.*, perception and destruction of mutant cells).[2]

Although not fully developed, the cells of the immunologic system of the fetus and neonate manifest a striking capacity for response to the environment. However, the fetus and newborn appear to be particularly vulnerable to injury caused directly by immunologic mechanisms or inflicted by infectious agents that take advantage of the relatively immature and inexperienced immune system. Immaturity refers to the genetically programmed low response or lack of response of the fetal and newborn immune system. Inexperience refers to the fact that the newborn immune system has not yet had its first immunologic encounter. Those who care for newborns must understand these processes because they form the basis for the prevention, diagnosis, and treatment of many diseases that afflict these patients (Table 46-1).

DEVELOPMENT OF THE IMMUNE SYSTEM

ROLE OF THE ENVIRONMENT

The development of the immune response may be visualized as a series of adaptive cellular responses to an ever-changing and potentially hostile environment. Development can be considered at several levels: the species, the individual, or the cell (Table 46-2).

From an evolutionary standpoint, the effect of a hostile macroenvironment provided the selective pressures leading to the survival of those life forms within the species that were best adapted to that environment (*i.e.*, phylogeny). Within the developing fetus, the microenvironment in which undifferentiated progenitor cells exist (*e.g.*, thymus, bursa of Fabricius) provides yet another type of inductive environment, permitting the full expression of immunity

TABLE 46–1
APPLICATIONS OF IMMUNOLOGY FOR THE NEONATOLOGIST

Type	Example of Immunologic Procedure	Disease
Prevention	Rhogam	Hemolytic disease of the newborn
Diagnosis	Elevated IgM globulins in cord serum	Intrauterine infections
Therapy	Fresh blood transfusions	Acute sepsis of the newborn

within the developing infant. The immunologically mature person may be considered as the best-selected form resulting from this type of development (*i.e.*, ontogeny). The molecular environment (*i.e.*, antigen) in which immunologically reactive cells exist provides the best-studied inductive stimulus leading to the proliferative and differentiating events commonly associated with cellular immune responses. The establishment of memory cells may be considered the best-adapted form for this environment.

Fetal and neonatal development of the immunologic system is best understood in terms of the developing host responding to his environment.

The cells and functions that constitute the immune system appear early in fetal life, but at least some of them are fully activated only after birth, after interaction of the neonate with his environment. Under certain circumstances (*e.g.*, intrauterine infections), the environment of the developing fetus may be so altered that it begins activation *in utero*.

The neonatologist and those entrusted with the care of the newborn must be concerned with the deleterious effect of factors introduced to the fetus from the ever-changing and complex external environment. Threatening agents that may gain access to the fetus during prenatal development include maternal drugs, infecting organisms, and antibiotics. The obstetrician and the neonatologist, who have already made significant contributions to the understanding of teratogenic effects of these agents, must be made aware of their effects on the developing immunologic system.

DEVELOPMENT OF COMPONENTS

For ease of discussion, the immunologic system may be considered under two major headings. The nonspecific immune system, which functions primarily during inflammatory responses, includes the phagocytic cell system (*i.e.*, polymorphonuclear leukocytes [PMNs]), mononuclear phagocytes (*i.e.*, monocytes and macrophages), and several amplification systems, including complement, coagulation, and kinin systems. The specific immune system consists of cell-mediated (*i.e.*, T-cell) and humoral (*i.e.*, B-cell) systems.

It is important to stress that the nonspecific and specific systems are intimately interrelated and interdependent. For example, the activation of the complement system by immunoglobulins (*i.e.*, IgM and IgG) or the production of chemotactic factors and other cytokines plays a significant role in the whole inflammatory response. The monocyte or macrophage may function in inflammatory responses and play a significant role in the processing of antigen—steps that are essential to the induction of the specific immune response. The macrophage forms part of the nonspecific and specific immune systems and is important to the afferent and efferent limbs of the immune response. The cytokines are other products secreted by cells that play a role in nonspecific and specific immune mechanisms.

Several abnormalities of nonspecific immunity may affect the newborn infant, including abnormalities of quantitative and qualitative factors of cellular function (*e.g.*, neutrophils, mononuclear phagocytes) and humoral factors (*e.g.*, specific antibody, complement, fibronectin).[3,4] The quantitative cellular abnormalities are related to size and ability to regenerate mature cells for the storage pools of phagocytic cells in the fetal liver, neonatal spleen, bone marrow, and local sites such as lung and skin. The qualitative cellular abnormalities are related to the adherence and directed migration (*i.e.*, chemotaxis) of phagocytic cells in response to and toward a chemoattractant that is exogenous (*e.g.*, bacterial proteins) or endogenous (*e.g.*, cellular or plasma products), the attachment

TABLE 46–2
EFFECT OF ENVIRONMENT ON THE DEVELOPMENT OF THE IMMUNE RESPONSE

Target	Inductive Environment	Process	Selected Form
Species	Macroenvironment	Phylogeny	Existing life forms
Individual	Microenvironment	Ontogeny	Immunologically mature individual
Cell	Molecular environment (*i.e.*, antigen)	Induction of immune response	Memory cells

TABLE 46–3
DEFICIENCIES IN NEONATAL HOST DEFENSES THAT PREDISPOSE TO INFECTION

Anatomic Barriers
Injuries during delivery (*e.g.*, skin abrasions)
Invasive procedures in the nursery (*e.g.*, umbilical artery catheters, endotracheal tubes)
Phagocytic Cells
Small polymorphonuclear leukocytes storage pool
Decreased polymorphonuclear leukocytes adherence
Decreased polymorphonuclear leukocytes and monocyte chemotaxis
Decreased polymorphonuclear leukocytes intracellular killing in stressed neonates
Decreased phagocytosis in stressed neonates
Complement
Decreased levels of complement
Decreased expression of complement receptors
Cellular Immunity
Possible defects in T-cell immunoregulation
Humoral Immunity
Decreased IgA, IgM
Decreased IgG in premature neonates
Impaired antibody function
Decreased levels of fibronectin
Decreased levels of cytokine (*e.g.*, interferon-γ, tumor necrosis factor)

and internalization (*i.e.*, phagocytosis) of the source of the inflammation after its precoating (*i.e.*, opsonization) by specific plasma factors such as antibody or complement, and the inactivation (*i.e.*, microbicidal activity) and digestion (*i.e.*, antigen processing) of the phagocytosed material. The deficiencies in the neonatal phagocytic cell system that may predispose to infection are summarized in Table 46-3.

INFLAMMATORY RESPONSE

After tissue injury or invasion by microorganisms, a cascade of systemic and local events is triggered. This generalized response to injury is referred to as an inflammatory response.

The febrile response is believed to reflect enhanced metabolic activity and to be related to the release of endogenous pyrogens (*i.e.*, cytokines interleukin-1 [IL-1] and tumor necrosis factor [TNF]) from the host's leukocytes, which then trigger a hypothalamic response.[5] Because these pathways are not particularly well developed in the neonate, fever is not a valuable sign of infection in this age group. Similarly, leukocytosis and an increased rate of sedimentation, commonly associated with bacterial infections in the older infant and child, are not particularly useful predictive markers of inflammation in neonates. However, other parameters in the inflammatory response, such as the increase in α- and β-globulins with the elevation of C-reactive protein, occur in the neonatal period and are commonly used in the diagnosis of infectious diseases in the neonate. An elevation in total neutrophil count is an inconsistent and unreliable index of neonatal sepsis; neutropenia during sepsis is more common in the neonate. If neutropenia reflects storage pool exhaustion, it is a poor prognostic sign, even with appropriate antibiotic therapy.[6–8]

An important event accompanying nonspecific immune responses in the newborn is the activation of the coagulation system, with disseminated intravascular coagulation, as seen in bacterial sepsis. The measurement of clotting factors and fibrin split products may provide another marker for infection.

CELLULAR COMPONENTS

The cellular responses are carried out primarily by phagocytic cells, such as PMNs, monocytes, and macrophages, and secondarily by eosinophils and lymphocytes. The storage pool size and the function of PMNs play a critical role in the inflammatory response.

POLYMORPHONUCLEAR LEUKOCYTES

Polymorphonuclear Leukocyte Storage Pools. Leukocytes are first produced in the liver at about 2 months of gestation. By 5 months of gestation, the bone marrow has become the primary hematopoietic center, and liver production has diminished.[9] Polymorphonuclear leukocyte (PMN) storage pools are considerably smaller per kilogram of body weight in the premature and full-term newborn than in adults.[10,11] Neonates are less capable of increasing their PMN numbers because the proliferative rate of their progenitor cells is already near maximum compared with adults.[12]

Polymorphonuclear Leukocyte Adherence, Mobility, and Chemotaxis. The skin of the newborn is relatively deficient in expressions of nonspecific immunity. After introduction of a foreign substance into the skin, several inflammatory cells begin to adhere to the wall of vessels near the substance and move in a directed fashion toward it in response to a chemical released from the foreign material or surrounding tissue. In the adult, a prominent PMN infiltration occurs during the first 4 to 12 hours, followed by a predominant mononuclear response consisting of macrophages and lymphocytes. In the newborn, the shift from a PMN response to a mononuclear cell response is slower and less intense than in the adult, reflecting maturational deficiency. In some studies, a curiously high percentage of eosinophils is observed in the 2- and 4-hour exudate of newborns older than 24 hours but not in those younger than 24 hours. Although the precise mechanisms for this eosinophilic response are unknown, it is of interest that the lesions of erythema toxicum, well known to neonatologists, consist primarily of eosinophilic leukocytes.

Mobility or movement encompasses a series of cellular events that are decreased in the neonate and include cell responsiveness to chemoattractants.[13–17] The latter reflects expression of cell surface receptors (particularly complement receptor [CR] 3), adherence, deformability, and aggregation, all of which are necessary for normal chemotaxis.[18–26] Chemotaxis does not appear to reach adult levels until 16 years of age.[27]

Neonatal PMNs exhibit less chemotactic activity than do adult cells because of deficiencies of intrinsic cellular factors and extrinsic humoral factors. The primary deficient humoral factors are complement components C3 and C5.[28]

PHAGOCYTOSIS

Once mobilized, the phagocytic cells mount an attack on their target by a process of phagocytosis. In the adult, many foreign substances, such as damaged tissue or nonvirulent organisms, may be ingested by phagocytic cells through unenhanced processes involving cell receptors (*e.g.*, integrins, fibronectin), nonspecific plasma, and tissue factors. More virulent organisms require opsonization by a specific antibody or complement. The newborn may have compromised cellular and humoral factors involved in phagocytosis. Of the immunoglobulins, only the IgG globulins are transmitted across the placenta. The complement factors do not cross the placenta.[29] Complement and fibronectin levels are deficient in the neonate.[30,31]

Several investigations of phagocytosis in the neonate have had conflicting results. In some studies, phagocytosis by neonatal leukocytes is abnormal when suspended in neonatal serum. Normal activity is restored when the same cells are resuspended in adult serum. However, under certain *in vitro* and *in vivo* conditions, neonatal PMNs are deficient in phagocytic capacity compared with the adult PMN.[32] For example, if the concentration of adult serum is varied or if phagocytes are taken from sick full-term infants, phagocytic activity is deficient relative to that in normal full-term neonates. The decreased phagocytic activity may be related to the decreased expression of the complement receptor CR3 in the newborn, which is reported to reach only 60% to 70% of adult levels during stimulation.[29] This receptor is important for complement-dependent adherence, surface adherence with albumin and fibronectin, and penetration of PMN into tissues.[29] Decreased expression of C3 may contribute to the relatively poor adherence and chemotaxis of neonatal cells.

Microbicidal and Metabolic Activity

After particle uptake by phagocytes, there is an increase in oxygen consumption and in glucose use by the hexose monophosphate pathway (HMP), events that are collectively referred to as the "respiratory burst."[2] The formation of hydrogen peroxide, the result of increased HMP activity, is considered to be of major importance in the killing of many bacteria by the oxygen-dependent antimicrobial system. A second antimicrobial system, which is oxygen-independent and granule associated, plays an important role in phagocytic cell function.

Oxygen-Dependent Systems. Phagocytic leukocytes, such as PMNs, respond to a particulate or soluble stimulus with a respiratory burst of increased oxygen consumption and the production of toxic microbicidal oxygen radicals, including superoxide (O_2^-), hydrogen peroxide (H_2O_2), and hydroxyl radicals. When the cell membrane is stimulated, NADPH oxidase (*i.e.*, membrane-associated oxidative enzymatic system), which consists of the oxidase and nonmitochondrial flavoprotein and cytochrome components, is activated and transfers electrons to molecular oxygen, reducing it to the free-radical superoxide anion.[17,33]

Chronic granulomatous disease (CGD) is a genetic disorder in which the PMNs and monocytes are incapable of generating the oxidative burst necessary to produce the antimicrobial oxygen metabolites (*i.e.*, hydrogen peroxide and related compounds). This is the result of a deficiency of one of the components of the NADPH oxidase complex.[17,33] The consequent loss of the important antibacterial mechanisms of the human host defense is the basis for recurrent bacterial and fungal infections in these children. There has been marked clinical improvement in CGD patients treated with interferon-γ (IFN-γ).[17,33]

The production of high-energy oxygen radicals and

superoxide by the newborn's PMNs is evaluated differently by various researchers. The O_2^- generation system seems to be efficient in the normal newborn and human fetus.[34,35] There is some evidence that the NADPH oxidase system in granulocytes generating O_2^- is completely developed during fetal life, but triggering mechanisms are probably deficient. The release by fetal and newborn bone marrow of many immature phagocytic cells with significantly reduced phagocytic function into the peripheral blood and the relatively rapid exhaustion of this cell reservoir may explain the defect in granulocyte function observed in stressed and infected newborns.[36]

Oxygen-Independent Systems. The oxygen-independent microbicidal system is demonstrated by the ability of phagocytic cells to kill organisms in anaerobic conditions and by non–O_2-dependent microbicidal activity of the cells from patients with CGD.

The active components of the O_2-independent system reside in the phagocytic cell granules. In the PMN, the primary (*i.e.*, azurophilic) granules contain acid hydrolases, neutral proteases, lysozyme, bactericidal cationic protein, and myeloperoxidase, a critical component in the O_2-dependent system, which catalyses the generation of toxic oxyhalide ($HOCl^-$) from H_2O_2. The specific granules contain vitamin B_{12}-binding protein, phospholipase-A_2, collagenase, more lysozyme, and lactoferrin, which has an important role in OH generation by the O_2-dependent system. The secondary granules contain stores of cell receptors for complement components (*e.g.*, CR3) and chemoattractant. It is clear from the contents of the granules that degranulation plays a key role in both microbicidal systems and that deficiencies in granule population could result in a poor inflammatory response. This is particularly demonstrated by the role that the first granules to be released play in the amplification of the complement cascade, generation of chemoattractant C5a, release of a monocyte chemoattractant, and promotion of PMN adherence to endothelial cells.[37] The granule complement is established early in cell differentiation. Primary granules appear in the promyelocyte stage and secondary granules in the myelocyte stage. Except under extreme conditions, when very immature cells are released from the bone marrow (*e.g.*, severe neonatal sepsis), the granule content of neonatal phagocytes is similar to that of the adult.

The results obtained in studies of bactericidal activity of neonatal PMNs are similar to those found in studies of phagocytosis; results obtained under apparently normal conditions differ from those obtained under stress. A deficient bactericidal activity has been shown in PMNs from neonates with a variety of clinical abnormalities, including sepsis, meconium aspiration, respiratory distress syndrome, hyperbilirubinemia, and premature rupture of the membranes.[38] When subjected to the demands of adjustment to extrauterine life, relative deficiencies of the bactericidal activities of PMNs contribute significantly to the compromised host defense mechanisms of the neonate.

MONOCYTES AND MACROPHAGES

The other major phagocyte system involved in immunologic processes is the mononuclear phagocyte system, which consists of circulatory monocytes and tissue macrophages. Tissue macrophages comprise a wide network of phagocytic cells, including alveolar and gastrointestinal tract macrophages important for initial defense at major portals of entry and dendritic cells important in antigen processing and presentation of antigen at local sites (*i.e.*, Langerhans cells in the skin). Liver (*i.e.*, Kupffer cells) and spleen macrophages are vital for the systemic clearance of microorganisms, cellular debris, and immunocomplexes.

Monocytes–macrophages perform a variety of functions, from microbicidal activity to secreting over 100 molecules important in inflammatory regulation.[39] These secretory products include cytokines, growth factors, eicosanoids, enzymes, enzyme inhibitors, clotting factors, complement components, plasma-binding proteins, and low-molecular-weight reactive oxygen and nitrogen products. Macrophages play a vital role in angiogenesis and wound healing.

Inflammation, which is a vital part of the immune defense, is marked by the rapid movement of monocytes out of the circulation in response to several factors, including bacterial protein, complement components, fibrinopeptides, and several cytokines (*e.g.*, transforming growth factor [TGF], platelet-derived growth factor [PDGF], IL-1, TNF, IL-2). During this inflammatory response, the monocytes may be further primed by cytokines (*e.g.*, interferon-γ [IFN-γ], IL-2, granulocyte–macrophage colony-stimulating factor [GM-CSF]). Interferon-γ activated macrophages are more bactericidal, tumoricidal, and express more major histocompatibility complex class II (MHC II) molecules on their surface. They are enabled to present antigens to lymphocytes and are primed to release cytokines (*e.g.*, TNF-α).[39] Monocytes–macrophages can express several plasma membrane receptors, such as those for immunoglobulin (*i.e.*, FcR) and complement components (*i.e.*, CR1 and CR3), that enhance their function, and carbohydrate receptors (*e.g.*, MMR on resident macrophages only). Although studies of Fc and C3b receptors on newborn monocytes reflect the level similar to those in adult cells, cord blood monocytes are less efficient in the phagocytosis of group B streptococci and intracellular killing of *Staphylococcus aureus* and group B streptococci.[40] The reason for this defective intracellular killing is unknown, but the characteristic susceptibility of the newborn to group B streptococcal (GBS) infections may depend, in part, on the immunologic immaturity of the mononuclear phagocyte system.

Monocytes, particularly cytokine-activated macrophages, are the first and the most important defense against many intracellular microorganisms (*e.g.*, *Toxoplasma gondii*). Although the antibacterial activity of the newborn's monocytes is comparable to that of the adult, these cells probably have only an initial role in limiting infection. The high incidence (65%) of congenital toxoplasmosis after maternal infection during the third trimester and the significant incidence of serious tissue damage in the fetus may result from a deficient activation of the fetal tissue macrophages. Decreased generation by neonatal lymphocytes of IFN-γ, which is necessary for killing of intracellular pathogens, for the increased expression of MHC II and cytokine production, and for normal inflammatory response and antigen presentation, may facilitate the survival and replication of *T. gondii* in fetal tissues.[41,42]

Macrophage function is deficient in the neonate.[43] This may be related to decreased cytokine production. Investigation has focused on the functional capabilities of monocytes in neonates, including chemotaxis, phagocytosis, microbial killing, and antibody-dependent cellular cytotoxicity (ADCC). Only chemotaxis has been shown to be primarily deficient, although the total number and the function of alveolar macrophages has been reported to be deficient in the neonatal period.[44,45] This observation may partially explain the newborn's susceptibility to GBS pneumonia.

HUMORAL COMPONENT

COMPLEMENT SYSTEM

The complement system is a key component in the production of innate or natural resistance to infection in vertebrates. Deficiencies of complement components can contribute to the susceptibility of the neonatal host to infection.

Despite its significant biologic role, relatively little is known about the complement system in the neonate, except that it is deficient in this period and the components do not cross the placenta from mother to fetus.[29] The third component of complement, C3, can be synthesized in different tissues in the human conceptus, beginning as early as 290 days of gestation.[46] The sites of synthesis for C3 appear to be the fibroblast, the lymphoid cell, and the macrophage. There is some evidence that the liver is the major producer of C3 in adults. Serum concentration of C3 in the fetus rises almost exponentially, from 1.9 mg/dL at 5.5 weeks of gestation to between 52 and 167 mg/dL at 28 to 41 weeks.[46] The mean level in cord blood is ± 90 mg/dL, approximately one-half the maternal levels. Studies of C3 phenotypes indicate that C3 is synthesized *in utero*. The concentration of complement in the newborn falls slightly after birth and recovers before the infant is 3 weeks of age. By 6 months of age, C3 reaches adult levels. Phagocytosis of bacterial products enhances production of complement components. It can be deduced that antigen stimulation after birth may play a role in the induction of complement synthesis.

Complement components C3, C4, and C5 are deficient in premature and full-term infants compared with maternal and adult standards. Propp and colleagues found that C1q, C3, C4, and C5 in cord blood from full-term neonates were approximately 50% of the respective maternal levels.[47] Low levels of properdin, factor B(C3PA), C1, C2, C3, and C4 also have been reported in cord blood.

Levels of C1q, C2, C3, C4, C5, factor B(C3PA), properdin, and total hemolytic complement are lower in the neonatal period. Most of the biologic effects of complement, including opsonization, immune adherence, complement-dependent viral neutralization, generation of anaphylactic and chemotactic factors, and production of cell membrane lesions, require only the first five complement components. Because the fetus can synthesize each of these components in biologically active form within the first trimester of development—however, in smaller quantities than the adult—all these immunologic functions could be affected to some degree by complement levels. There is a decreased expression of CR3, the receptor for the complement component C3bi on neonatal PMN, which is important in a variety of adhesion reactions, such as cell adherence, mobility, and phagocytosis.[29]

FIBRONECTIN AND ADHESION MOLECULES

Fibronectin is a nonimmune opsonin that exists in an insoluble form on most cells and in a soluble form in plasma and interstitial fluid.[31] Newborn infants have fibronectin levels in the plasma that are one-third to one-half those found in the adult. These levels are further reduced in premature infants and under various pathologic conditions in the newborn (*e.g.*, sepsis, malnutrition, respiratory distress syndrome, asphyxia).[30,31,48] Fibronectin is a glycoprotein with a molecular weight of 450,000 that promotes the clearance by phagocytic cells of fibrin, platelets, immune complexes, and collagenous debris. Fibronectin is also an important opsonic factor for numerous pathogenic microorganisms, including *Staphylococcus aureus*, *Streptococcus* sp., and some gram-negative bacteria. It functions as a chemoattractant for phagocytic cells alone, as for macrophages, or by increasing the response in PMNs. Fibronectin induces the expression of the complement receptors (*i.e.*, CR1 and CR3), amplifying functions of the phagocytic cell system.[29] Low levels of fibronectin may contribute to hypofunction of the neonatal phagocytic cell system, predisposing to the development of sepsis.

Adhesion molecules are a group of glycoproteins on cells that mediate cell-to-cell or cell-to-matrix (*e.g.*, fibronectin, basement membrane) attachments. This attachment occurs through ligand–receptor interaction, as with ICAM-1, VCAM-1, and ELAM-1 on endothelial cells with the ligands LFA-1 (CD11a/CD18), VLA-4, and slex integrin–selectin molecules on pha-

TABLE 46–4
CHARACTERISTICS OF MAJOR CYTOKINES

Cytokine	Molecular Weight	Primary Cell Sources	Activity	Principal Effects
IL-1	17,500	Macrophages, NK and B cells	Immunoaugmentation	Inflammatory and hematopoietic
IL-2	15,500	T lymphocytes and LGL	T- and B-cell growth factor	Activates T and NK cells
IL-3	28,000	T lymphocytes	Hematopoietic growth factor	Promotes growth of early myeloid progenitor cells
IL-4	20,000	TH cells	T- and B-cell growth factor; promotes IgE reactions	Promotes IgE switch and mast cell growth
IL-5	50,000–60,000	TH cells	Stimulates B cells and eosinophils	Promotes IgA switch and eosinophilia
IL-6	25,000	Fibroblasts and others	Hybridoma growth factor; augments inflammation	Growth factor for B cells and polyclonal immunoglobulin production
IL-7	25,000	Stromal cells	Lymphopoietin	Generates pre-B and pre-T cells and is lymphocyte growth factor
IL-8	8,800	Macrophages and others	Chemoattracts, neutrophils, and T lymphocytes	Regulates lymphocyte homing and neutrophil infiltration
IL-9	30,000–40,000	Activated T lymphocytes	T-cell growth factor; stimulation of hematopoiesis	Together with IL-2 increases fetal thymocyte proliferation; stimulates erythroid precursor cell proliferation
IL-10	18,000	B and T lymphocytes (TH2) and thymocytes	Effects on T cells, B cells, and mast cells; inhibition of cytokine synthesis by TH1 cells; IL-10 shows homology with EBV proteins.	Proliferation of mature and immature thymocytes in presence of IL-2 and IL-4; stimulates mast cells only when combined with IL-3 or IL-4; interference with antigen presentation
IL-11	23,000	Bone marrow stroma cells	Functions as cofactor in hematopoiesis; B-cell growth factor; regulator of stem cell cycle	Stimulates megakaryocyte colony forming units; stimulates Ig synthesis in the presence of T cells
G-CSF	18,000–22,000	Monocytes and others	Myeloid growth factor	Generates neutrophils
M-CSF	18,000–26,000	Monocytes and others	Macrophage growth factor	Generates macrophages
GM-CSF	14,000–38,000	T cells and others	Monomyelocytic growth factor	Myelopoiesis
IFN-α	18,000	Leukocytes	Antiviral, antiproliferative, and immunomodulating	Stimulates NK and phagocytic cells
IFN-β	20,000	Fibroblasts		Induce cell membrane antigens (*e.g.*, MHC)
IFN-γ	20,000–25,000	TH lymphocytes and NK cells	Inflammatory, immunoenhancing, and tumoricidal	Vascular thromboses, tumor necrosis and enhances phagocytic cell function
TNF-α	17,000	Macrophages and others		
LT-TNF-β	25,000	T lymphocytes		
TGF-β	25,000	Platelets, bone, and others	Fibroplasia and immunosuppression	Wound healing and bone remodeling

B, bursal dependent; EBV, Epstein-Barr virus; G-CSF, granulocyte-colony–stimulating factor; GM-CSF, granulocyte–macrophage-colony–stimulating factor; IL, interleukin; INF, interferon; LGL, large granular lymphocytes; M-CSF, macrophage–colony stimulating factor; MHC, major histocompatibility complex; NK, natural killer; T, thymus derived; TGF, tumor growth factor; TH, thymic; TNF, tumor necrosis factor.

gocytic cell plasma membranes.[39,48] This binding facilities recruitment of these cells into inflammatory sites. Activation of phagocytic cells by a variety of events, including adherence and by cytokines such as TNF and IL-1, induces the expression of the adhesion molecules. If the cytokine production is deficient, the adhesion molecule expression may also be reduced. Deficient cytokine production may be responsible for the decreased inflammatory response seen in newborns.[42]

CYTOKINES

There are a group of hormonelike proteins, or glycoproteins, secreted primarily by lymphocytes and macrophages and a variety of other cells, that act as mediators of systemic inflammatory and immune responses by being molecular messengers between participating cells. Some of these were previously referred to as lymphokines or monokines, based on their cellular origin, but they are all generically referred to as cytokines. A summary of the major cytokines appears in Table 46-4, listing their primary cell sources and principal functions. In the neonatal period, there are deficiencies in two very important cytokines that may be key in the age-dependent susceptibility of the infant to viral and bacterial infections.

The primary deficiency appears to result from an immaturity in T-cell function, particularly in the production of IFN-γ in the neonate, which is reported to be 10-fold less than in the adult.[42] Interferon-γ has antiviral effects and is an important immune cell modulator. It increases MHC expression and the cell functions, particularly microbicidal activity, of natural killer (NK) cells, PMNs, and macrophages. It induces T-cell differentiation and IgG and TNF production, which augments antimicrobial activity of phagocytic cells. In the neonate, the T-cell production of TNF is 50% less than in the adult, and IFN-γ–enhanced mononuclear phagocyte production of TNF is 7% less than adult levels. Tumor necrosis factor plays a major role in enhancing phagocytic cell function and inducing a variety of other antimicrobial, inflammatory, and immune functions, such as the expression of adhesion molecules (*i.e.*, integrins ICAM-1, VCAM-1, ELAM-1 on endothelial cells and phagocytic cells) alone or by inducing the production of other cytokines.[48] Deficiencies in TFN and IFN-γ may play a major role in the increased susceptibility to infections of neonates.

ANTIBODIES

Antibodies react with antigens, and they appear to play a significant role in events mediating inflammatory responses, such as phagocytosis, chemotaxis, and the release of mediators. The extent to which the antibodies affect these functions in the fetus and newborn depends on the permeability of the placenta to a given antibody and maturation of the antibody-producing system.

Silverstein and colleagues studied the maturation of immunologic capability and lymphoid tissues in the normal fetal lamb *in utero* (Fig. 46-1).[49] They established the sequence of the antibody response to different antigens. Bacteriophage OX174 given on day 37 elicited the earliest antibody response, at 41 days of gestation. This is a remarkable observation, because the fetal sheep has little organized lymphoid tissue at this stage. At approximately 66 days of gestation, the fetus becomes able to respond to the protein ferritin, but not until 125 days of gestation can it respond to egg albumin. Antibodies against *Salmonella typhi* or bacillus Calmette–Guérin appear only after birth. The researchers were unable to induce tolerance until the lamb reached the age at which it was able to recognize the antigen and produce antibody. It is possible to draw an analogy between this phenomenon and the poor response of human newborn infants to the polysaccharide antigens. These phenomena must be understood in the human if adequate immunization techniques are to be developed and allergic diseases are to be prevented (Table 46-5).

OPSONIC CAPACITY

The opsonic capacity of blood refers to the enhancement of phagocytosis and includes the activities of antibodies, complement, and other proteins that are not well defined. IgM appears to have the greatest opsonic activity. Full-term and premature human newborns appear to be relatively deficient in opsonic

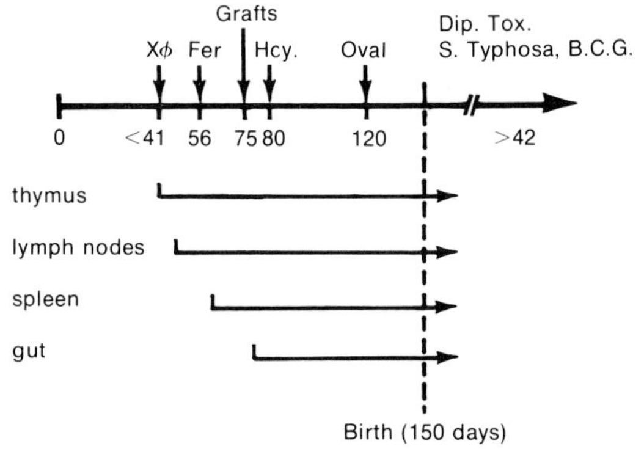

FIG. 46–1. Comparison of immunologic and lymphoid development in the fetal lamb. Numbers on the upper horizontal axis show the earliest times at which antibody responses and graft rejection could be detected. The order in which lymphocytes appear in different tissues is as follows. bacteriophage (Xϕ), horse ferritin (Fer); snail hemocyanin (Hcy); hen albumin (Oval); diptheria toxoid (Dip Tox). (Adapted from Silverstein A, Prendergast R. The maturation of lymphoid tissue structure and function in ontogeny. In: Lindahl-Kiessling K, Alm G, Hanna MG Jr, eds. Morphological and functional aspects of immunity. New York, Plenum Press, 1971.)

TABLE 46–5
DEVELOPMENT OF THE IMMUNE SYSTEM IN THE FETUS

Gestation (wk)	Findings
4	First blood centers appear in yolk sac
5.5	Synthesis of complement is detected
7	Lymphocytes appear in peripheral blood, about 1000/mm^3
7–9	Lymphocytes appear in the thymus
11	CD_2 receptors (*i.e.*, E rosette) develop in thymus lymphocytes; B-cell maturation occurs in liver and spleen, with IgG, IgA, IgM, and IgD surface markers; serum IgM levels can be detected
12	Antigen recognition is demonstrable
13	Graft-versus-host reactivity is present
14	Phytohemagglutinin response by thymus lymphocyte occurs
17	Serum IgM levels can be detected
20	Secondary lymphoid complex is present
20–25	Lymphocytes in blood number about 10000/mm^3
22	Complement levels detectable in serum
30	IgA level detectable in serum

Adapted from Cauchi MN. Immunological aspects of pregnancy and the newborn. In: Cauchi MN, Gilbert GL, Brown JB, eds. The clinical pathology of pregnancy and the newborn infant. London: Edward Arnold Publishers, 1984:325.

activity toward a variety of agents. The degree of deficiency varies with different agents and probably particularly involves antibodies of the IgM type. This deficiency of antibodies may account for the susceptibility of the newborn to gram-negative infections, because IgM antibodies do not traverse the placenta. However, Miller observed that addition of purified IgM to neonatal sera does not enhance opsonization of yeast particles.[32] Complement and other heat-labile factors amplify the opsonic activity of IgM to a much greater extent than they amplify IgG opsonic activity. The deficit in opsonic activity derives from deficiencies of complement, particularly of components C3, C5, and C3PA. In the premature infant, lowered levels of IgG may play a role in the opsonic deficiency.[50] Rigorously controlled studies of the opsonic capacity of the fetus and newborn are needed so that the usefulness of potentially harmful treatments, such as fresh plasma transfusion in the septicemic neonate, can be determined.

One of the important clinical sequelae of deficient antimicrobial antibody is seen in GBS infection of the newborn. The increased susceptibility of newborns to GBS infection has been correlated with deficiency of maternal antibody directed against the type-specific polysaccharides of the organism.

SPECIFIC IMMUNE MECHANISMS

The maturation of specific immune responses in the human begins *in utero* between 8 and 12 weeks of gestation. The differentiation of cells destined to perform these functions appears to arise from a population of progenitor cells, referred to as stem cells, that are located within the yolk sac, fetal liver, and bone marrow of the developing embryo (Fig. 46-2). Depending on the type of microchemical environment surrounding these cells, differentiation occurs along at least two avenues: hematopoietic and lymphopoietic.

HEMATOPOIETIC DIFFERENTIATION

One type of microchemical environment leads to the proliferation and differentiation of stem cells into myeloid, erythroid, and megakaryocyte precursors. The products of these cell lines are the monocytes, granulocytes, erythrocytes, and platelets of the circulation. In the human, granulocytic cells are first observed in the liver of the fetus in the second month of gestation. Leukocyte production by the fetal liver declines at about the fifth month of gestation, when the bone marrow activity increases.

LYMPHOPOIETIC DIFFERENTIATION

Classically, the lymphoid system develops along two independent pathways leading to morphologically and functionally distinct populations of immune lymphocytes: the thymus-derived system of cell-mediated immunity (CMI), whose principal effector cells are the T lymphocytes, and the bursal-dependent system of antibody-mediated immunity, which is effected by the B lymphocytes.

The T lymphocyte is commonly identified by the T-cell receptor–CD3 (TCR–CD3) complex or CD2 surface marker (*i.e.*, binding site for sheep erythrocytes). The B lymphocyte is recognized primarily by its surface CD19 or CD20 markers or immunoglobulin.

T-CELL SYSTEM

The basic cell type differentiates into lymphoid cells when the progenitor cells are influenced by certain microchemical environments. The first is the thymus, which leads to the differentiation of T cells.[51,52] The thymus gland is derived from the epithelium of the third and fourth pharyngeal pouches at about the sixth week of fetal life. The parathyroid glands also begin their development at about this time from the same pouches. With further differentiation, a caudal migration of epithelium occurs, and beginning in the eighth week, blood-borne stem cells enter the gland and begin lymphoid differentiation. With further development, the thymus is infiltrated with lymphocytes and is differentiated into a dense cortex contain-

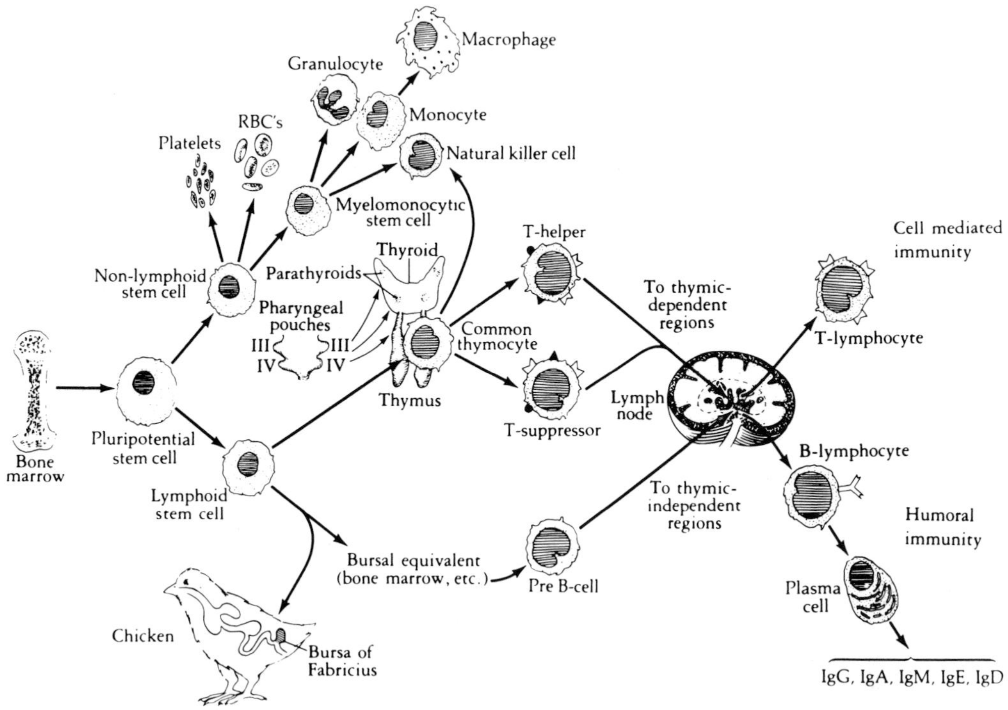

FIG. 46–2. Ontogeny of immune response, showing differentiation of progenitor cells into hematopoietic and immunocompetent cells. (From Bellanti JA. Immunology III. Philadelphia, WB Saunders, 1985:48.)

ing many small lymphocytes and a less dense, central medulla with relatively more epithelial elements.

Thymocyte precursors are probably derived from multipotential hematopoietic precursors in the fetal liver and later in the bone marrow.[53–55] Under the influence of thymic epithelium-derived chemoattractants, pro-T cells initially localize to the thymic corticomedullary junction. These CD4-negative, CD8-negative T-cell precursors undergo extensive gene rearrangement, phenotypic alteration, and biochemical modification to yield the population of thymocytes that undergoes intrathymic selection. First, precursor T cells with affinity for self MHC (*i.e.*, usually CD4-positive and CD8-positive) are positively selected in the cortex of the thymus. Subsequently, in the medulla, they undergo negative selection, and those that recognize self-antigens are deleted. More than 95% of the thymocytes, which includes cells that have not been positively selected and those that have been negatively selected, proceed to programmed cell death, a process called apoptosis. The selected mature thymocyte, usually bearing mature TCRs with CD8 or CD4 molecules (*i.e.*, single positive), seed the peripheral lymphoid tissue.

In the developing thymus, there exists a dynamic interplay of cytokines that act in a coordinated and temporal manner to control the passage of the precursor cell through different stages of development in the thymus (Fig. 46-3). In particular, IL-1, IL-2, IL-4, and IL-7 may play central roles in precursor proliferation and differentiation.[56]

T-cell differentiation within the thymus appears to be regulated by several factors synthesized by the thymic epithelial cells. Several peptides have been described, and they share several properties that may result from their relative impurity.[57] One of the best characterized of these thymic hormones is thymopoietin (molecular weight, 5562), which promotes prothymocyte to thymocyte differentiation, as demonstrated in the appearance of typical T-cell surface markers.[58] Some synthetic polypeptide molecules that seem to have all the differentiation-inducing properties of the original molecule are being evaluated. Although the characterization of hormones is preliminary, the use of thymosin has intriguing applications in clinical medicine as a replacement therapy for immunoincompetence.

The clinical importance of the simultaneous embryogenesis of the parathyroid and thymus is seen in one of the immunologic deficiency disorders of infancy, the DiGeorge anomaly. The DiGeorge anomaly is a developmental field defect in which derivatives of pharyngeal pouches III and IV do not arise, usually because of inadequate neural crest contributions. The conditions in which this occurs include exposure to teratogens, cytogenetic abnormalities, and mendelian disorders. The facies and cardiovascular defects that occur are very characteristic. There is

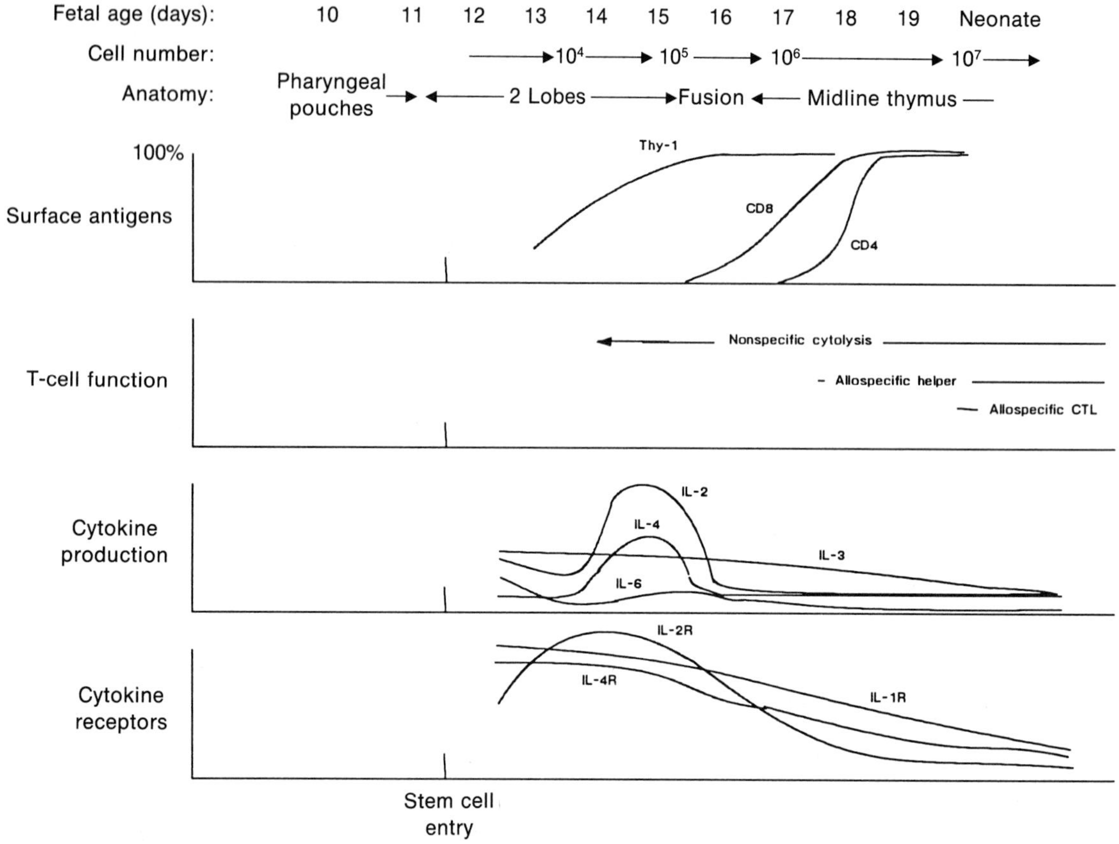

FIG. 46–3. Temporal relations among the production of cytokines, expression of cytokine receptors, and the differentiating events occurring in precursor cells in the murine fetal thymus during T-cell ontogeny. (CTL, cytotoxic T lymphocytes; adapted from Carding SR, Haydan AC, Bottomly K, et al. Cytokines in T-cell development. Immunol Today 1991;12:240.)

no known feature that uniformly occurs, and the diagnosis of DiGeorge anomaly is usually based on two or more of the following:

- typical facies (*e.g.*, hypoplastic mandible, short philtrum, hypertelorism, ears low set or malformed or both)
- characteristic heart lesion (*e.g.*, conotruncal malformation, usually interrupted aortic arch [IAA] type B)
- persistent hypocalcemia with onset in the first month of life
- documented inability to identify the thymus at surgery or autopsy
- decrease in T-cell response to mitogens
- decrease in T-cell number.[59,60]

Two rare conotrucal anomalies, type B IAA and truncus arteriosus, account for over one-half of the cardiac lesions seen in DiGeorge anomaly. Of all patients with IAA type B, 68% had DiGeorge anomaly; of all patients with truncus arteriosus, 33% had DiGeorge anomaly.

Failure of descent of the thymus is extremely common in DiGeorge anomaly, but immunodeficiency that requires correction occurs in only approximately 25% of the patients. The term, complete DiGeorge anomaly, should be reserved for patients in need of reconstitution of the immune system. The physician can identify patients requiring treatment of the thymic defect by T-cell enumeration and *in vitro* proliferation assays. Two alternatives for therapy are thymus transplantation and bone marrow transplantation from a HLA-matched sibling.

After emigration of the T cells from the thymus, they circulate through the lymphatic and vascular systems as the long-lived lymphocytes (*i.e.*, the recirculating pool), which then populate certain restricted regions of the lymph nodes, the thymic-dependent subcortical areas, and the periarteriolar regions of the spleen. Removal of the thymus in neonatal mice renders them deficient in the number of circulating T cells and leads to depletion of the thymic-dependent areas in lymphoid tissue. The long-lived nature of these lymphocytes and the degree of competence in the human may explain in part why, after thymectomy, immediate deficits are not usually seen in the newborn period, although they may become apparent later in life.

After birth, the thymus plays a continually changing role in relation to body size. It is largest compared with body size during fetal life, and at birth, it weighs 10 to 15 g.[2] The gland continues to increase in size, reaching a maximum of 30 to 40 g at puberty, after which involution occurs. The increased incidence of autoimmunity and malignancy with aging have associated with senescence of thymic function.

T CELLS

The stages in the life history of T cells are marked by the gradual appearance of a variety of membrane-bound glycoproteins (Fig. 46-4). Many of them have been identified by employing monoclonal antibodies. Immature thymocytes are characterized by the expression of some surface markers acquired during intrathymic development, such as transferrin receptor (CD71), CD1, CD2, CD4, CD8, and the CD3–TCR complex. After the T cells enter the circulation, they lose the transferrin receptor and CD1 molecule.

In the peripheral blood, approximately 70% of T cells express the CD4 marker, and CD8 is found on approximately 30%. T cells that acquire helper activity characteristically express CD4, and suppressor T cells have CD8 but not CD4 on their surface. The CD4 receptor with antigen-specific TCR–CD3 complex allows the helper T cell to recognize antigens combined with antigen-presenting cell surface MHC II molecules. Helper T cells are induced to undergo blast transformation and cell division after interaction with antigen and MHC II molecules on the macrophage and other antigen-presenting cells. T-cell activation leads to the production of a variety of cytokines (*e.g.*, IL-2, IL-3, IL-4, IL-5, IL-6, GM-CSF, IFN-γ, TNF), cell proliferation, and increased cell surface receptor expression (*e.g.*, CD71, IL-2 receptor).

Significantly decreased production of IL-4 and IFN-γ by neonatal T cells has been observed after activation.[61] T-cell helper function in newborns is quite low, but it develops almost to adult levels by 6 months of age. T-cell–mediated suppression of immune responsiveness is somewhat higher in the infant than in the adult. The percentage of putative suppressors with the CD8 phenotype is lower in cord blood than in adult blood.[62] However, in functional assays, neonatal T cells elicit increased spontaneous suppressor activity compared with adult T cells. Moreover, suppressor T cells exert a strong cytostatic effect on adult B- and T-cell proliferation, probably to prevent graft-*versus*-host (GVH) reaction by maternal cells transferred to the fetus. Natural killer CD3-negative CD56-positive cell activity is extremely low in the neonatal period, and it reaches the adult level by be-

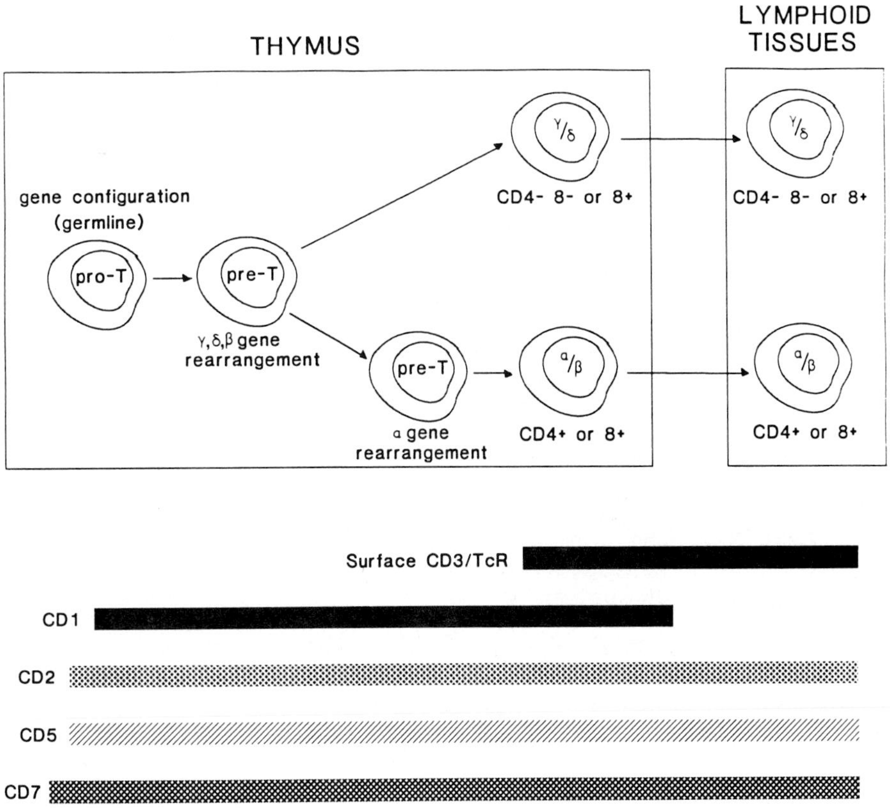

FIG. 46–4. Temporal relation among T-cell maturation, differentiation, and cell surface antigen expression.

tween 1 to 5 months of age. Although the percentage of NK cells in the peripheral mononuclear cell population is decreased in neonates, the absolute number of these cytotoxic NK cells is high in infancy and even higher from 1 month to 4 years of age compared with that in adults.[63] The increased number of NK cells with adequate cytotoxic abilities present from 1 month to 4 years of age indicates the predominance of NK immunity during infancy to early childhood, in the presence of immaturity in other aspects of immunologic system. In the neonatal period, the decreased NK cell activity predisposes to increased severity of viral infections.

As a general rule, T cells acquire immunocompetence (*i.e.*, strong proliferation in mixed lymphocyte culture and antigen binding) early during fetal life, even though their functional capacities are not always comparable to those of the adult.

Newborns, particularly premature infants, have a significantly lower rate and degree of skin sensitization to dinitrochlorobenzene (DCNB), and rejection of skin allografts is slower in newborns than in normal adults. Delayed hypersensitivity can be induced in newborns during the first month of life. The newborn's inconsistency in this capacity appears to be caused more by a decreased inflammatory response and macrophage function than by depressed T-cell activity. A depressed T-cell function may be a consequence of neonatal viral infection, hyperbilirubinemia, corticosteroid therapy, or maternal medications taken late during pregnancy. Specific T-cell immunity can result from antigenic exposure *in utero* to certain antigens such as penicillin, mumps virus, *Escherichia coli,* diphtheria and tetanus toxoid, and dental plaque in the mother. There are some suggestions that specific CMI can be acquired from the ingestion of T cells contained in colostrum or breast milk or transferred through the placenta. The proliferative capabilities of immature lymphocytes are well developed early in gestation and, at the time of birth, are equal to or may exceed those of adult lymphocytes; the inflammatory response and macrophage functions, however, appear to be impaired in the newborn period.

B-CELL SYSTEM

If the progenitor cells fall under the influence of a second type of microchemical environment, differentiation produces a population of lymphocytes and plasma cells concerned with humoral immunity or antibody synthesis (see Fig. 46-2). This B-cells population comes under the influence of the bursa of Fabricius in birds.[64] In humans, bone marrow constitutes one of the equivalents of the bursa, but all available evidence indicates that the human fetal liver is the analog of the bursa of Fabricius in humans.

The process of B-cell differentiation from a multipotent stem cell begins in fetal liver between 8 and 9 weeks of gestation, with the appearance of pre-B cells. Pre-B cells have MHC II antigens on their surface and the CD19 receptors (*i.e.*, pan-B cell marker) shown in Figure 46-5. These cells begin to synthesize the cytoplasmic μ, the heavy chain of IgM, that later becomes the surface IgM that appears on "baby" or immature B cells. CD21, which is the receptor for complement C3d and Epstein–Barr virus (EBV), also begins to appear on the immature B-cell surface. Although these cells continue to express surface IgM, they begin to express one of the surface immunoglobulins (*i.e.*, IgA, IgG, IgD) shown in Figure 46-6. After stimulation by antigen, mitogen, and helper T cells, the immature cells become mature plasma cells or memory cells. As in T-cell development, the B-cell development involves several cytokines, such as IL-3, IL-4, IL-5, IL-6, and IL-7. These cytokines influence the B-cell growth and differentiation and regulate the immunoglobulin class switch and secretion. For instance, IL-4 and IL-5 induce B-cell immunoglobulin class switch to IgE and IgA committed B cells, respectively. IL-6 induces the committed B cells to become immunoglobulin-secreting plasma cells.

The first surface immunoglobulin expressed by a B cell is an IgM; at 13 weeks of fetal life, most B cells express IgM and IgD. In the next differentiation step, B-cell clones start to express IgG (*i.e.*, subclasses 1, 2, 3, 4), IgA (*i.e.*, subclasses 1, 2), or IgE. Full-term babies probably have a complete repertoire of B-cell

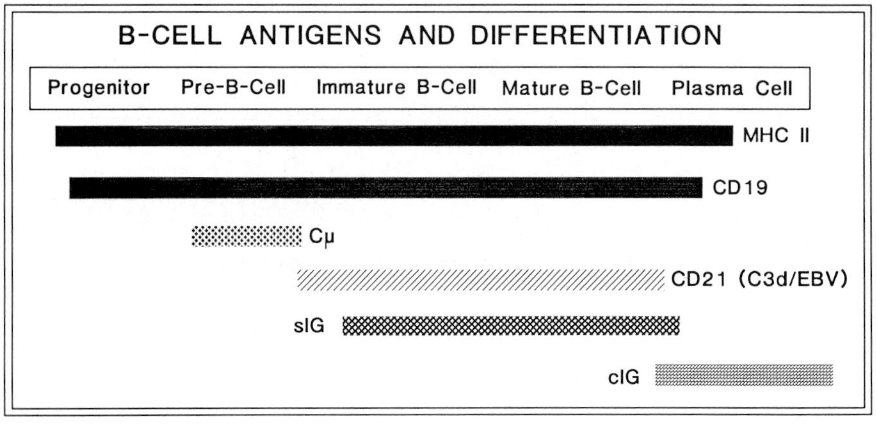

FIG. 46–5. Temporal relation among B-cell maturation, differentiation, and cell surface marker or antigen expression.

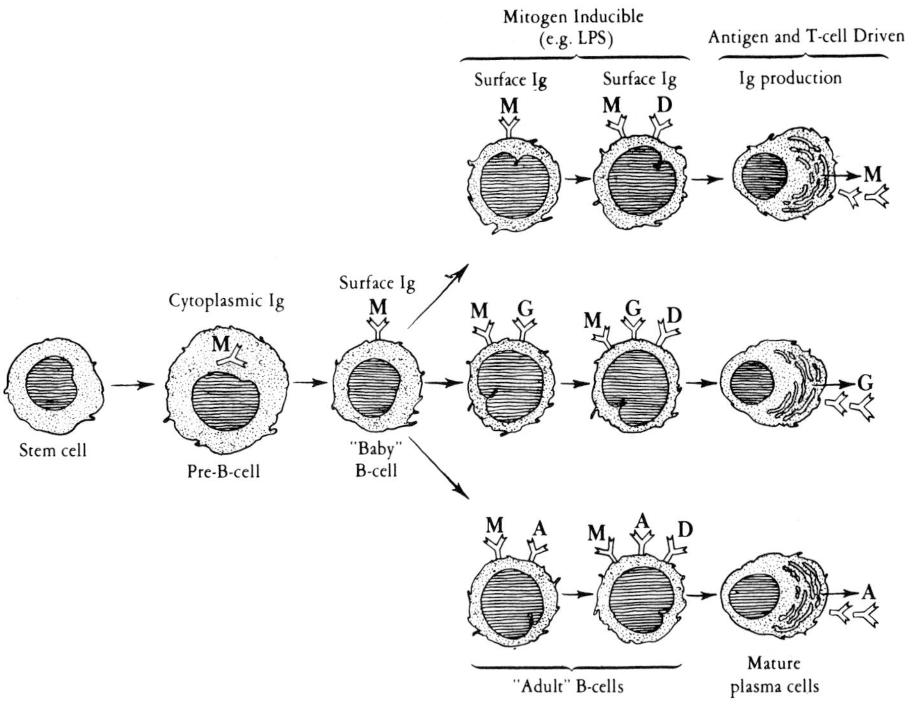

FIG. 46–6. Mammalian B-cell differentiation model. B cells differentiate from a stem cell to a rapidly dividing pre-B cell lacking functional antibody receptors. These cells initially synthesize cytoplasmic IgM that later becomes surface IgM (*i.e.*, baby B cells). These baby B cells can easily be made tolerant and are pivotal for further differentiation of immunoglobulin-producing cells. While they continue to express surface IgM, they begin to express one of the surface IgG subclasses or IgA, followed later by the appearance of surface IgD. When these double or triple cells are triggered by antigen, helper T cells, or B-cell mitogens, they become mature plasma cells or memory cells (not illustrated in this figure). The antigen-dependent T-cell–driven stage requires the presence of surface IgD that is lost after antigenic stimulation. (LPS, lipopolysaccharide; adapted from Cooper MD, Seligmann M. In: Bellanti JA, ed. Immunology III. Philadelphia: WB Saunders, 1985.)

clones, and they can theoretically synthesize each type of immunoglobulin. However, human newborns fail to respond efficiently to all antigens; for example, they are unable to mount an antibody response to polysaccharide antigens.

Infants respond to protein antigens (*i.e.*, T-dependent antigens), mainly with IgM production and a slow progression compared with that of the adult to IgG response. Children younger than 18 months fail to respond with an IgG2 production to *Hemophilus influenzae* type B capsular antigen; this deficient synthesis of IgG2, which is the predominant subclass of antibody against *H. influenzae*, may explain the frequent appearance of *H. influenzae* infections in young children. The acquisition of adult levels of immunoglobulins is achieved by approximately 1 year of age for IgM, at 5 to 7 years for IgG, and at 10 to 14 years for IgA.[65] The reasons for this defective antibody response are under investigation. Excessive suppressor T-cell activity in newborn blood, defective regulatory cytokine production, and a partial immaturity of the B cell have been suggested as limiting factors in the perinatal response.[61,66,67]

The fetal liver occupies the central role in B-cell development, as it probably does in T-cell development. The B cells constitute a much smaller part of the recirculating pool of lymphocytes than the T cells and populate the thymic-independent regions of the lymphoid tissue, including the germinal centers of lymph nodes. Removal of the bursa or its mammalian equivalent leads to a profound deficiency of γ-globulin with little or no effect on CMI.[68]

Antibody provides a major defense against encapsulated high-grade pyogenic pathogens including *Streptococcus pneumoniae*, *H. influenzae*, and *Neisseria meningitidis*. The development of immunity in the fetus and the newborn must not be considered separate from maternal influences.

MATERNAL, FETAL, AND NEONATAL INTERACTIONS

In the human, the predominant transfer of antibody occurs by way of the passage of the IgG immunoglobulins from the maternal circulation to that of the fetus. This is accomplished by means of an active transport of this immunoglobulin by virtue of a receptor located on one portion of the molecule. In this manner, the fetus receives a library of preformed antibody from his or her mother, reflecting most of her experiences with infectious agents. The secretory IgA immunoglobulins found in breast milk also provide local protection on the mucous membranes of the gastrointestinal tract. Although these antibodies are not absorbed, their unique structure renders them more effective in these sites and may explain the lower incidence of enteric infections seen in breast-fed infants. It has been shown that as much as 11 g of IgA may be delivered initially to the newborn infant in 24 hours, based on total output in the early colostrum. Subsequently, total IgA output appears to decrease significantly, and between 3 and 50 days postpartum, as much as 3 g of IgA may be delivered to the breast-fed infant.[69] The fate of ingested IgA has not been clearly defined. A small amount may be absorbed from the intestine and appear in the circulation within the first 24 hours of life.[70]

Significant numbers of granulocytes, macrophages, and B and T lymphocytes appear in breast milk.[71] The B lymphocytes in human milk can produce IgA antibodies.[71] Secretory antibodies in milk are directed against antigens occurring in the gastrointestinal tract: *Escherichia coli* O and K antigens, *Shigella* O antigen, *Vibrio cholerae* O antigen, *E. coli* and *V. cholerae* enterotoxins, poliovirus, and rotavirus. There appears to be a direct relation between the extent of intestinal antigenic exposure and the level of specific secretory antibodies in milk. It is possible that, after antigenic stimulation, the lymphoid cells from the Peyer patches of the gastrointestinal tract home by way of the mesenteric lymph nodes and the blood to the mammary gland tissue and appear in the milk. As a result of this homing mechanism, human milk contains secretory IgA antibodies against many microorganisms harbored in the maternal intestine at the time of lactation (*i.e.*, microorganisms that the baby is most likely to be exposed to after birth). Because of the same homing mechanism, human milk contains IgA antibodies to many food protein antigens (*e.g.*, cow-milk proteins). It is possible, particularly in infants with atopic predisposition, that the frequency and magnitude of food allergy may be decreased by a prolonged period of breast-feeding.[72] In the early period of life, when the infant's own secretory IgA system is maturationally deficient, breast-feeding may provide the infant with antibodies that support the local immune defense system. Decreasing the antigenic exposure or influencing the infant immune response by prolonged breast-feeding may prevent or delay the development of atopic disease. Other protective factors are present in human milk, such as lactoferrin, lactoperoxidase, *Lactobacillus bifidus* factor, complement components, and leukocytes.

Necrotizing enterocolitis, a disease seen primarily in premature infants who have suffered severe perinatal stress, affects predominantly formula-fed infants. Neonatal rats subjected daily to a short period of hypoxia developed a reproducible model of the disease. All animals died as a result of necrotizing enterocolitis if they were formula-fed but not if breast-fed. The viable macrophages in their breast-feedings appears to have afforded the survivors protection and to have prevented the mortality seen in control animals. However, studies carried out after naturally acquired maternal cytomegalovirus infection or other viral and bacterial infections have demonstrated acquisition of neonatal infections in breast-feeding babies of infected mothers.[73]

Occasionally, fetal cells or other proteins may gain access to the maternal circulation and actively immunize the mother to the paternal allotypes found on these substances. This process, referred to as isoimmunization, may lead to serious disease in the infant, such as hemolytic disease of the newborn, thrombocytopenia, and leukopenia.

The development of serum immunoglobulins during intrauterine life and postnatally is shown in Figure 46-7. The amount and type of γ-globulin found in the blood of the newborn at birth is higher than those of the mother and are made up almost exclusively of the IgG immunoglobulins. There are few or no IgA and IgM globulins in cord sera because the fetus is usually protected *in utero* from antigenic stimuli. If challenged *in utero* as a consequence of immunization of the mother with *Salmonella* vaccine or infection (*e.g.*, congenital rubella, cytomegalic inclusion disease, toxoplasmosis), the fetus responds with antibody production, largely of the IgM variety. The exclusion of other classes of antibody is beneficial to the fetus in many cases. For example, the exclusion of the IgM isohemagglutinins, leukoagglutinins, or the IgE antibodies of allergy prevents disease that may be produced by these antibodies. However, it also prevents the passage of other maternal antibodies that would be beneficial to the newborn, such as the IgM antibodies important in bacterial defense (*e.g.*, opsonins, agglutinins, bactericidal antibodies) against gram-negative bacteria. This may explain the increased susceptibility of the newborn to infection with gram-negative organisms such as *E. coli.*

There is great variability in the types of antibodies that are obtained transplacentally by the fetus (Table 46-6). This reflects the quantity of antibodies in the maternal circulation and of their molecular sizes. For example, low-molecular-weight IgG antibodies (*e.g.*, rubeola antibody), present in high concentrations in maternal serum, are readily transferred. IgG antibodies in lower concentrations (*e.g.*, *Bordetella pertussis*) are poorly transferred, and macroglobulin antibodies

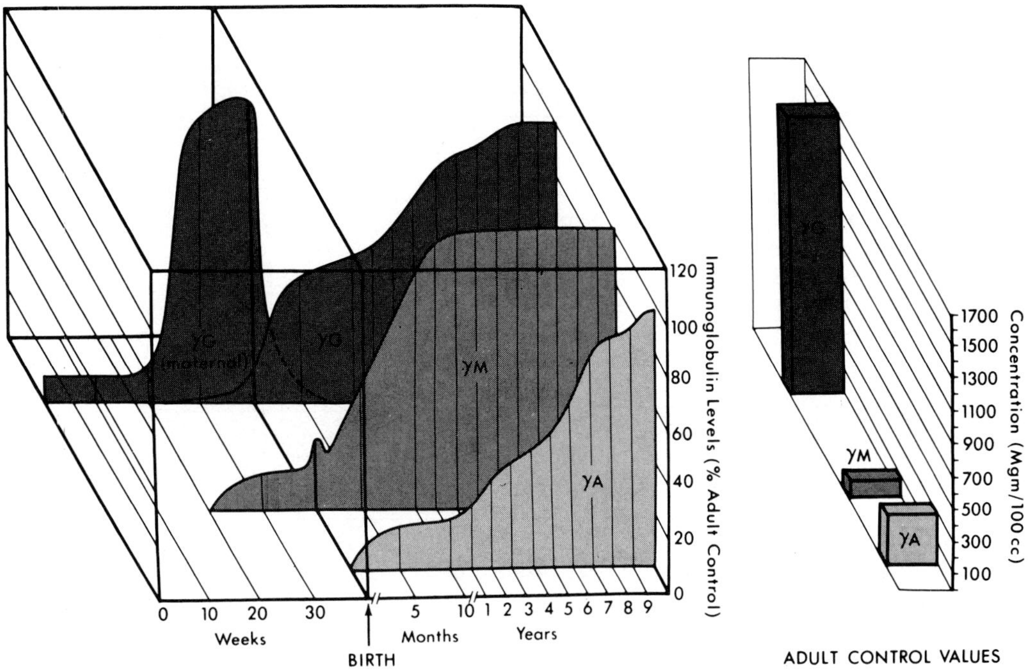

FIG. 46–7. Development of serum immunoglobulins in the human during maturation. (From Bellanti JA. Immunology III. Philadelphia: WB Saunders, 1985:49.)

(*e.g.*, Wassermann antibody) are completely excluded.

Because the IgG immunoglobulins are passively transferred, they have a finite half-life, between 20 and 30 days, and their concentration in serum falls rapidly within the first few months of life, reaching its lowest level between the second and fourth months. This period is referred to as physiologic hypogammaglobulinemia. During the course of the first few years, the levels of γ-globulin increase because of exposure of the maturing infant to antigens in the environment. There appears to be a sequential development in the γ-globulins at different rates. The IgM globulins attain adult levels by 1 year of age. Under physiologic conditions, little or no IgA synthesis is observed *in utero*. Plasma cells appear in the intestinal lamina propria of the neonate shortly after birth. IgA is not detectable in the serum or in the secretions during the first 2 to 3 days of life, although IgA is frequently present in the secretions after the fourth day of life. The secretory IgA concentration matures rapidly, reaching adult levels by 4 to 6 weeks of life. Serum IgA levels rise more slowly, and adult levels are observed after 10 to 14 years. This pattern of appearance of immunoglobulins recapitulates that seen in phylogeny and appears to parallel that seen after

TABLE 46–6
RELATION OF ANTIBODY TYPE AND TRANSPLACENTAL TRANSFER

Good Passive Transfer	Poor Passive Transfer	No Passive Transfer
Diphtheria antitoxin	*Hemophilus influenzae*	Enteric somatic (*i.e.*, O) antibodies (*Salmonella* sp., *Shigella* sp., *Escherichia coli*)
Tetanus antitoxin	*Bacillus pertussis*	Skin-sensitizing antibody
Antierythrogenic toxin	Dysentery	Heterophile antibody
Antistaphylococcal antibody	Streptococcus MG	Wasserman antibody
Salmonella flagella (H) antibody		
Antistreptolysin		
All the antiviral antibodies present in maternal circulation (*e.g.*, rubeola, rubella, mumps, poliovirus)		
VDRL antibodies		

VDRL, veneral disease research laboratory.

TABLE 46–7
MATERNAL ANTIBODIES THAT CAN PRODUCE HARMFUL EFFECTS IN THE INFANT

Maternal Disease	Antibodies	Effect on Infant
Hyperthyroidism	LATS	Transient hyperthyroidism (*i.e.*, exophthalmos)
Idiopathic thrombocytopenia	Platelet antibodies	Transient thrombocytopenia
Isoimmunization (*e.g.*, platelets, neutrophils, red blood cells)	Platelet, neutrophil, isohemagglutinins, $Rh_o(D)$ antibodies	Transient thrombocytopenia, neutropenia, anemia
Lupus erythematosus	Autoantibodies to blood elements (*e.g.*, LE-cell factor, Coombs test, platelets)	Transient LE-cell phenomenon, neutropenia, thrombocytopenia, congenital heart disease (*i.e.*, AV block)
Myasthenia gravis	Cholinergic receptor antibody	Transient neonatal myasthenia gravis

AV, arteriovenous; LATS, long-acting thyroid stimulation; LE, lupus erythematosus.
Adapted from Bellanti JA, ed. Immunology III. Philadelphia: WB Saunders, 1985:579.

antigenic exposure during the primary immune response.

In addition to providing protection to the newborn, passively acquired IgG antibodies may interfere with active antibody synthesis after immunization procedures. Several studies have confirmed that passively acquired antibody to diphtheria and to pertussis may actually inhibit active antibody formation after active immunization. This occurs in the case of killed vaccines, appears to be dose related, and can be overcome by increasing the inoculum size. In the case of immunization with live virus vaccines, the effect of passively acquired antibody is to neutralize the vaccine virus, inhibiting successful immunization with parenteral live vaccines. Immunization at 2 to 3 months of age with killed vaccines (*e.g.*, diphtheria, pertussis, tetanus) does not appear to be appreciably inhibited by this passive antibody. Live virus immunization procedures are usually delayed until the end of the first year of life because of the inhibitory effect of the passive antibody.

Another situation in which passive acquired antibody may interfere with active antibody synthesis is the natural immunity acquired by the newborn infant from breast milk. IgA in breast milk may interfere with successful immunization with live poliovirus vaccines by neutralizing virus in the gastrointestinal tract. Poliovirus immunizations are not usually delayed, even in breast-fed infants, because active immunization follows sequential poliovirus administration according to recommended immunization schedules for infants and children. Maternal antibodies can have harmful effects, as shown in Table 46-7.

IMMUNOLOGIC CONSEQUENCES OF INTRAUTERINE INFECTIONS

The possibility of intrauterine infection should be suspected in a newborn infant if there is a known exposure of the mother to an infectious disease during pregnancy or if the infant is small for gestational age or fails to thrive. Manifestations of intrauterine infection include petechiae, hepatosplenomegaly, congenital malformation, inguinal hernia, thrombocytopenia, and unusual skin rash (see Chap. 47).

An IgM concentration greater than 20 mg/dL in the cord blood or in the infant serum is considered abnormal. It should be pointed out that an elevated IgM level may be the result of leakage of maternal blood into the fetus; under these circumstances, the infant's IgA level usually exceeds the IgM level, reflecting the IgA–IgM ratio in maternal blood. IgM concentration test repeated after 3 to 4 days disclose a significant fall in the case of maternal transfusion, but the amount of IgM actively synthesized by the newborn will have increased.

Congenital infections frequently become chronic and persist for weeks or years with signs and symptoms that are not seen in children or adults with the same infection. The agents that produce persistent infection of the human fetus exhibit a predilection for the reticuloendothelial system. Impaired function of reticuloendothelial cells may be associated with the development of immunodeficiency.

In the congenital rubella syndrome, infection results from transmission of the virus from the pregnant mother to the fetus in the first 5 months of gestation. The infection of the child continues after birth for 6 months to 3 years, despite passive antibody acquired from the mother and active antibody synthesis by the infant. After birth, the child may continue to shed virus while making antibody. A variety of abnormal antibody responses have been reported in children with congenital rubella, including increased levels of IgM with low IgG and absent IgA and low levels of IgM with low levels of IgG and absent IgA.[74,75] Reports have appeared of poor antibody responses in patients with congenital rubella as determined by delayed appearance of isohemagglutinins, suboptimal vaccine responses, immune paresis with no response to tetanus or *Salmonella typhi* vaccines, and impaired CMI as demonstrated by impaired lymphoproliferative responses to phytohemagglutinin and decreased lymphocytotoxicity.[76–78] These abnormal responses have been associated with an increased frequency of infections. Many of the alterations reverted to normal responses later, when the child was no longer excreting virus.[79] This could represent a form of immunologic blockade while the child is shedding virus, reversal of which may be linked to the maturity of the immunologic systems.

Cytomegalovirus and herpesviruses produce infections that persist for years or throughout life when infection is acquired *in utero*. Cell-mediated immunity appears to be particularly important in these infections. In one study, eight infants with congenital cytomegalovirus infection and six of their mothers showed decreased specific CMI.[80] The decreased CMI in the mothers may have contributed to the transmission of the infection to the infant. The earlier the infection, the more devastating is the effect on the ontogeny of the immune system. If an insult occurs to the thymus in the first trimester, the normal development of T-cell function is affected; if the insult occurs in the third trimester, no resulting damage should be expected.

Viral infection of the fetus may be limited by the degree of cellular immune competence, as exemplified by the infants with proven congenital infection and intact cellular responses who are no longer shedding virus at birth. The cellular competence of the fetus may also modulate the manifestations of intrauterine infection. Intrauterine syphilis, for example, presents in late pregnancy, at which time the body mounts a brisk cellular immune response to the spirochete. Infection occurring early in gestation may go unnoticed because the spirochete has neither a toxic nor a teratogenic effect on the fetus. The spirochete is teratogenic only when the immune response to the organism is activated. In contrast, rubella in very early gestation has primarily teratogenic effects (*e.g.*, congenital defects). In later pregnancy (2–4 months), a primarily inflammatory effect is seen (*e.g.*, hepatitis, iridocyclitis, meningitis). These differences may result from an intact cellular immune response characteristic of the older fetus, but in some cases, the immune response of the child may fail to limit or clear these infections.

IMMUNOLOGIC EVALUATION

The functional significance of the two-compartment system is important in clinical medicine. It provides a useful basis on which understanding of the primary immunodeficiency disorders rests and a framework for a more logical approach to the management of maturational deficiencies in the newborn period. Selective deficiencies of the thymic-independent B system (*i.e.*, agammaglobulinemias) present with recurrent bacterial infections. Selective deficiencies of the thymic-dependent tissues are associated with fungal and viral infections. Patients with combined B- and T-cell defects have the most serious of all the immunodeficiency syndromes, with profound deficiencies in cell-mediated and antibody-mediated functions; they present with a diversity of infections.

Evaluation of the immune system during the perinatal period is not an easy task. The evaluator must take into consideration the dynamic, rapidly growing, and adaptive parameters of the immune function in response to a changing internal and external environment. Table 46-8 shows some of the major classes of immunodeficiencies that can be diagnosed in the newborn period, with their time of onset and associated infections. A detailed history, with emphasis on family background and a careful physical examination, should offer a solid foundation for interpretation of clinical and research laboratory data. Table 46-9 presents some suggestions for the clinical evaluation of the newborn. Table 46-10 lists some of the pertinent clinical and historic information that could be useful in the diagnosis of immunodeficiency disorders in the newborn period. Although most immunologic defects are not clinically apparent until postnatal life, it is not unlikely that in certain instances the result of immunologic deficiency may be intrauterine infection with a resultant damaged baby at birth or an aborted conceptus.

Cohen and Zuelzer and others have shown maternal blood-formed elements in fetal circulation.[81] Theoretically, early passage of immunologically active mononuclear cells from the mother to the fetus could be responsible for GVH reaction. Although direct proof of GVH reactions in the fetus is lacking, several clinical situations suggest that such processes may occur in the newborn and fetus. Among these can be cited the report of an XX/XY chimerism in a 12-week-old abortus of a mother who had several repeated spontaneous abortions.[82] A case was reported by Naiman and colleagues, in which, after three exchange transfusions, the infant developed jaundice, aplastic anemia, and marked histiocytosis.[83] This infant also showed chimerism of the mononuclear cells, with one line representing donor cells.

EVALUATION OF THE HUMORAL IMMUNE SYSTEM

Table 46-11 summarizes the evaluation of the humoral immune system. Pure humoral immunodeficiency syndromes are not clinically manifested in the prenatal period because of the protective effect of maternal IgG. However, very premature infants, particularly those born at less than 32 weeks of gestation, may have IgG serum levels below 400 mg/dL. Small-for-gestational-age infants also have decreased IgG, some impairment of specific antibody responses (*e.g.*, to attenuated polio virus), reduction in specific IgG secretory antibody responses, and an increased incidence of antibodies to food.[84] Another factor to

TABLE 46–8
IMMUNODEFICIENCY DISORDERS THAT CAN BE DIAGNOSED IN THE NEONATAL PERIOD

Disorder	Example	Genetics	Time of Onset	Type of Infection
Phagocytic disorders				
Quantitative	Neutropenia	Variable	At birth	Virulent bacteria
	Congenital asplenia	Variable	At birth or later	Gram-negative
Qualitative	Chronic granulomatous disease	X-linked, autosomal recessive	At birth	Less virulent bacteria
Disorders of antibody-forming cells	Agammaglobulinemia	Variable	>6 months of age, earlier if infant is premature or small for dates	Virulent bacteria
T-cell immunodeficiency (*i.e.*, cell-mediated or delayed hypersensitivity)	Congenital aplasia of thymus (*i.e.*, DiGeorge syndrome)	Variable	At birth	Fungal, viral
	Chronic mucocutaneous candidiasis	Sporadic forms, autosomal recessive		Fungal
	Pediatric acquired immunodeficiency syndrome	None	At birth or later	Bacterial, fungal, protozoal, viral, *Pneumocystis carinii*
Combined B- and T-cell immunodeficiency	Severe combined immunodeficiency	X-linked recessive, autosomal recessive, sporadic forms	6 months	Bacterial, fungal, viral, *Pneumocystis carinii*
	Cellular immunodeficiency with abnormal immunoglobulins (*i.e.*, Nezelof syndrome)	Variable	Variable	Bacterial, viral, fungal
Complex (*i.e.*, multisystem) immunodeficiencies	Immunodeficiency with ataxia and telangiectasia	Autosomal recessive	>6 months	Bacterial, viral, fungal
	Immunodeficiency with eczema and thrombocytopenia (*i.e.*, Wiskott–Aldrich syndrome)	X-linked recessive	>6 months	Bacterial, viral, fungal, *Pneumocystis carinii*
Disorders of early and late components of complements	Deficiency of C1, C2, C4, and later components of complement have been described	Variable	At birth	Gram-negative

be considered is hypogammaglobulinemia in the mother, which, although rare, can lead to inadequate levels of IgG in the newborn.

NEONATAL IMMUNE RESPONSE TO HUMAN IMMUNODEFICIENCY VIRUS

The immune response to human immunodeficiency virus (HIV) infection in neonates is described in greater detail in Chapter 47.

The complexity of the immune response to HIV infection seen in the adult is equal or greater in the newborn. Human immunodeficiency virus has a tropism for human CD4-positive T cells and bone-marrow-derived dendritic cells, megakaryocytes, cells of monocyte–macrophage lineage, and the macrophage–microglial and endothelial cells of the central nervous system. A characteristic depletion of CD4-positive cell numbers is seen in HIV infections, after which there is a continuous but variable rate of decline of CD4 cells. In adults there is acute loss of CD4-positive T cells around the time of seroconversion and in the late symptomatic phase of disease.

There are several proposed mechanisms to explain the depletion of CD4 cells, because infection of the cell is not necessarily cytopathic. One possible mech-

TABLE 46–9
CLINICAL EVALUATION OF THE IMMUNE SYSTEM IN NEONATES

History
Previous newborn deaths in the family; history of immune diseases
Previous isoimmunization in mother (*e.g.,* due to pregnancy or transfusions (Rh, ABO) or to γ-globulin administration
Previous diseases in the mother (*e.g.,* autoimmune diseases: SLE, thyroiditis, myasthenia gravis, idiopathic thrombocytopenic purpura)
History of medications in mother (*e.g.,* quinine, guinidine, Sedormid, chlorpromazine)
History of infections during pregnancy (*e.g.,* rubella, cytomegalic inclusion disease, toxoplasmosis, syphilis, herpes simplex, UTI, vaginal infections, TB)
Physical Examination
General appearance (*i.e.,* assess degree of activity: if there is hyperactivity, consider hyperthyroidism, passive transfer of LATS; if there is hypoactivity or muscle weakness, consider myasthenia gravis with transfer of antibodies to muscle; if there is purpura, consider thrombocytopenia due to the passive transfer of antibodies to platelets)
Skin (*e.g.,* jaundice in first 24 hours of life, petechiae are characteristic of isoimmunization such as erythroblastosis fetalis)
Eyes (*e.g.,* exophthalmos due to LATS)
Chest (*e.g.,* pneumonitis seen in many intrauterine infections)
Cardiovascular (*e.g.,* evaluate for congenital heart disease, congenital heart block in infants of mothers with SLE)
Abdomen (*e.g.,* hepatosplenomegaly seen in severe erythroblastosis fetalis, in congenital intrauterine infections, in GVH reactions, and in absence of spleen)
Extremities (*e.g.,* deformities, and other birth defects)
Neurologic (*e.g.,* convulsions, weakness)

GVH, graft-versus-host; LATS, long-acting thyroid stimulation; SLE, systemic lupus erythematosus; TB, tuberculosis; UTI, urinary tract infection.
From Bellanti JA, ed. Immunology III. Philadelphia: WB Saunders, 1985:578.

TABLE 46–10
DIAGNOSTIC CLUES FOR IMMUNODEFICIENCY DISORDERS IN NEONATES

Findings	Comments
Hypocalcemic tetany Absence of thymic shadow Moniliasis	DiGeorge syndrome—characteristic features are *in vitro* lymphocyte stimulation with phytohemagglutinin and MLR
History of immunodeficiency in other family members	Most immunologic defects genetically determined; gender-linked most common
Agammaglobulinemia	Quantitative immunoglobulins not useful because of passive transfer of IgG; determination after 2 to 4 months helpful in establishing diagnosis; allotypes helpful; B-cell (CD19) enumeration
Chronic granulomatous disease	NBT helpful as screening test only because there may be nonspecific elevation; tests of bactericidal function fail to reach normal values in presence of adult sera
Poor growth, splenomegaly, hepatomegaly, diffuse dermatitis, diarrhea	GVH—laboratory findings include anemia, decrease in serum complement, histiocytic infiltration of bone marrow, and erythrophagocytosis; skin biopsy shows mummified cells
Howell–Jolly bodies in peripheral smear, absence of spleen, shadow in x-ray film	Congenital absence of spleen and other associated malformations
Seborrheic dermatitis	C5 deficiency (*i.e.,* Leiner disease)
Chronic diarrhea	Defect in phagocytosis of baker's yeast particles secondary to failure of sera to opsonize yeast

GVH, graft-versus-host; MLR, mixed lymphocyte reaction; NBT, nitroblue tetrazine.

TABLE 46–11
DIAGNOSTIC TESTS FOR EVALUATION OF THE HUMORAL IMMUNOFUNCTION IN NEONATES

Test	Comment
Practical	
Quantitative measurement of immunoglobulins	May reveal elevated IgM or IgA; does not differentiate maternal from fetally produced IgG
B-cell mitogen stimulation (*e.g.*, pokeweed)	As with PHA (routine test), Ig synthesis determined in supernatant or cells stained with intracytoplasmic immunofluorescence techniques
IgG subclass determination	IgG3 increases in prenatal period and reaches adult levels after 3 months; IgG1, IgG2, IgG4 close to adult levels years later
Determination of total number B cells by CD19 or CD20 markers	Does not necessarily correlate with decreased Ig synthesis; helpful to elucidate level of B-cell defect
Specialized	
Specific antibody responses to *de novo* sensitization (*e.g.*, *Salmonella sp.*)	O antigen induces IgM; H antigen induces IgG
Regional lymph node biopsy after immunization	Helpful for humoral and cell-mediated immunity

PHA, phytohemagglutinin.

anism is that discharge of virions may be vigorous enough to disrupt the cell and cause death, depleting cell numbers. Alternatively, expression of viral antigens on the cell surface can result in CMI cytotoxicity. These losses may be compounded by the inability of the bone marrow to respond appropriately to replenish CD4 cells. Because CD4 cells play a pivotal role in many immunoregulatory functions, the loss in these cells is responsible for a reduction in their helper-inducer function and a decrease in other T-cell, B-cell, and monocyte activities, resulting in wide-ranging functional defects in cellular and humoral immunity.

Immune dysregulation and nonspecific immune activation are features of HIV disease. Generalized immune activation evidenced by polyclonal hypergammaglobulinemia and elevated activation markers (*e.g.*, β_2-microglobulin, neopterin) is recognized, and the levels of these activation markers are used to predict disease progression. Human immunodeficiency virus encoding a superantigen has been suggested; this may play a role in the generalized polyclonal activation and subsequent clonal deletion of T cells.

One of the most perplexing clinical problems for the pediatrician and neonatologist is the diagnosis of acquired immunodeficiency syndrome in children younger than 15 months of age, because maternal IgG antibody to HIV is passively transferred across the placenta and may persist until 15 to 18 months of age in uninfected infants. Detection of HIV antibody is therefore not reliable for infants younger than 15 months of age. Moreover, viral culture and P24 antigen assays have a low sensitivity (*i.e.*, viral culture detects approximately 50% of infected neonates). Although potentially useful, polymerase chain reaction (PCR) assay is limited by the high false positives due to contamination or carryover during testing, the complexity of the test and required laboratory facilities, and the cost. With improved quality control, PCR can identify as many as 50% of asymptomatic perinatally infected infants at birth. Viral-specific IgA antibody (*i.e.*, HIV-IgA) immunoblot assay has a high sensitivity (99.4%) and high specificity (99.7%) for children older than 3 months of age but a much lower sensitivity in neonates. As a practical approach, identification of the infected infant relies on identification of the infected mother, followed by careful clinical and laboratory monitoring of the infant throughout the first year of life. Suggested laboratory tests include serial HIV antibody testing (*i.e.*, ELISA and immunoblot); serial P24 antigen testing; HIV culture; immunoglobulin levels; T-cell numbers and subsets, remembering that neonates have significantly higher T-cell numbers than older children; and one or more other diagnostic techniques (*e.g.*, PCR, HIV-IgA, immunoblot assay). The aim is to diagnose HIV infection before the onset of severe opportunistic infection, especially *Pneumocystis carinii* pneumonia.

EVALUATION OF THE CELL-MEDIATED IMMUNE SYSTEM

Table 46-12 summarizes the evaluation of the CMI system of the newborn. Evaluation of the CMI system begins with a total and differential leukocyte count. Lymphopenia is seen in most of the CMI deficiencies, but the lymphocyte count may be normal in some patients. The number of T cells, B cells, CD4 helper cells, and CD8 suppressor cells can be ascertained by flow cytometry, using specific monoclonal antibody for individual cell markers (*e.g.*, CD3 for T cells, CD19 or CD20 for B cells). *In vitro* lymphoblastogenic responses of T cells to specific antigens also are informative for host CMI, provided the antigens have been encountered previously (*e.g.*, *Candida* for a baby with history of thrush).

Tests of lymphoproliferative responses should be performed with different concentrations of T-cell mitogens, such as concanavalin A and phytohemagglutinin. Newborn lymphocytes seem to respond better than those of adults at low dosages of mitogens; at higher concentrations, they are less responsive than adult lymphocytes.[85] Mixed lymphocyte culture reactions may be helpful in diagnosing CMI deficiencies. A dissociation of low phytohemagglutinin, with normal MLC, can be seen in some patients with CMI deficiency. On the basis of phylogeny and ontogeny, it can be speculated that such a defect originates at a higher level of T-cell differentiation. Lack of MLC responses suggests a defect occurring earlier in ontogenic development. Determinations of enzymes, such as adenine deaminase and nucleoside phosphorylase, may help clarify some of the cases of severe combined immunodeficiency and motivate the clinician to investigate enzyme replacement therapy or possible gene therapy.

Skin testing with fungal, bacterial, and viral antigens for delayed hypersensitivity has not proved useful in the newborn. Skin testing with PHA is claimed to be somewhat more sensitive.[86] Contact sensitization to DNCB offers advantages over intradermal testing. Dinitrochlorobenzene is positive in 90% of normal persons. Viral infections sometimes depress CMI, and some of the patients who are referred to us may show anergy because of persistent viral infections. In these cases, sound medical judgment, patience, and repeated studies are necessary. Fetal growth retardation and malnutrition also depress CMI and humoral responses for several months after birth.[84]

Evaluation of the nonspecific immune responses in the newborn is almost limited to testing PMN function with the Rebuck skin-window technique (Table 46-13), which has not yet been standardized for the newborn. The nitroblue tetrazine test may be used as a screening test for CGD; the results should be confirmed by bactericidal assay. Lowered numbers of complement components have been described in the prenatal and cord blood. The extent to which these reflect actual functional abnormalities of complements is uncertain. Phagocytic tests should include evaluation of influences of C3 and C5. Separate evaluation of the complement effects on phagocytosis, chemotaxis, and bactericidal activities must be made. A functional deficiency of C5 activity has been described in Leiner disease. Monocyte function, although important, is not usually clinically evaluated because of a lack of adequate methods. Poplack and colleagues have shown that in humans, ADCC activity against erythrocytes depends only on the monocyte.[87] It is hoped that this test will prove significant in the evaluation of the monocyte in the fetus and newborn infant.

TABLE 46–12
DIAGNOSTIC TESTS FOR EVALUATION OF CELL-MEDIATED IMMUNITY IN NEONATES

Test	Comment
Practical	
Leukocyte and differential counts	Normal lymphocyte count does not rule out CMI deficiency; low count compatible but not diagnostic
Determination of absolute number of T cells by CD2/CD3 marker; T-cell subsets by CD4 and CD8 markers	No functional test, but correlates well with CMI status
Mitogen stimulation of lymphocytes (*e.g.*, PHA)	Optimal, suboptimal, and overoptimal concentrations of PHA should be used
Specific antigen stimulation of lymphocytes	Previously known exposure required (*e.g.*, *Candida*)
Specialized	
Skin testing with DNCB	Positive result practically rules out CMI deficiency
MLR	Could be positive in absence of responses to PHA
Lymph node biopsy after stimulation with *de novo* organism	To determine whether dependent areas are normal
Biopsy of thymus	To be performed in patients with obvious CMI; helps elucidate different types of CMI deficiencies that could orient new therapeutic measures
MHC I and MHC II antigen expression	Such as bare lymphocyte syndrome (*i.e.*, MHC II deficiency)

CMI, cell-mediated immunity; DNCB, dinitrochlorobenzene; MHC, major histocompatibility complex; MLR, mixed lymphocyte reaction; PHA, phytohemagglutinin.

TABLE 46–13
DIAGNOSTIC TESTS FOR POLYMORPHONUCLEAR LYMPHOCYTE FUNCTION IN NEONATES

Test	Comment
Peripheral blood count and differential	Often of help, count important (*e.g.*, neutropenia); morphology of cells important (*e.g.*, Chediak–Higashi syndrome)
Rebuck skin window	May give general clue to defect of inflammatory function, particularly ability to marshal leukocytes to site of infection
Phagocytosis	Results vary with assay used; particle being phagocytized critical; assay used must distinguish humoral and cellular components of process
Chemotaxis	Decreased in cellular and humoral activity during neonatal period
Quantitative NBT	Screening test; if normal or high, does not rule out CGD
Bactericidal activity	Measured by direct killing assay; CGD can be diagnosed during neonatal period
Measurement of specific leukocyte enzymes	Not done routinely

GD, chronic granulomatous disease; NBT, nitroblue tetrazine.

IMMUNOLOGIC THERAPY

Because newborn infants are less immunologically competent than adults and premature infants are even more susceptible to serious infections than full-term infants, several replacement therapies have been tried with variable results.

PREVENTION OF INFECTION IN LOW-BIRTH-WEIGHT INFANTS

There is little transport of maternal IgG to the fetus before 32 weeks of gestation, and endogenous synthesis does not begin until about 24 weeks after birth.[88–91] In low-birth-weight infants, serum IgG levels by 3 months of age are only 60 to 150 mg/dL, compared with 100 to 350 mg/dL for infants born at term.[91–94] It is reasonable to consider intravenous immunoglobulin (IVIG) prophylaxis in premature infants. Some pilot studies indicated a lower rate of severe infection in IVIG-treated low birth weight infants compared with placebo-treated patients.[95–98] In a randomized, double-blind, placebo-controlled trial involving 588 infants with birth weights of 500 to 1750 g, mortality was not significantly reduced among IVIG recipients.[99] However, the number of infections was significantly reduced among IVIG recipients. There was some evidence that the beneficial effect may vary by birth-weight category, and significantly more placebo patients were small for gestational age. Information about long-term results (>56 days) is not available from this trial. Preliminary analysis of other trials indicates no significant differences in infection rates between IVIG recipients and placebo recipients.[100–101] Another multicenter, randomized, controlled trial, involving more than 2000 neonates with birth weights between 500 and 1500 g, has been completed.[102] Intravenous immunoglobulin was initiated at less than 72 hours of age, and continued every 2 weeks until hospital discharge or a weight of 1.8 kg. No significant difference was seen in the rate of nosocomial infection or in the mortality rate between control and treated groups.

The disparity in these results may be due to several variables. For instance, these studies are complicated by the fact that multiple factors contribute to the predisposition to infection in premature neonates and that different predominant pathogens occur in different nurseries. There are differences in the titers of antibodies to various pathogens, especially GBS infection, in different lots of IVIG preparations. Moreover, differences in the study design and IVIG dosage and schedule make direct comparison of the various trials difficult. At this time, IVIG cannot be recommended as standard prophylaxis for low-birth-weight infants.

TREATMENT OF PRESUMED NEONATAL INFECTION

Small trials using primarily historic controls have yielded mixed results. Questions remain concerning dose, schedule, and patient selection. Sidiropoulos and colleagues treated successively admitted infants suspected of neonatal sepsis with antibiotics or antibiotics plus IVIG (0.5–1.0 g/day for 6 days).[103] A reduction of mortality was found. Two of 20 infants treated with antibiotics plus IVIG died, compared with 4 of 15 infants treated with antibiotics alone (10% *versus* 26%; $p = 0.16$). Among premature infants weighing less than 2500 g, IVIG made a significant difference. Four (44%) of 9 patients who received antibiotics alone died, compared with 1 (9%) of the 11 who received antibiotics plus IVIG ($p < 0.05$).

Haque and associates studied 60 preterm infants of 28–37 weeks of gestation who were suspected of having bacterial sepsis.[104] One-half of the group was treated with antibiotics alone and one-half was treated with antibiotics plus IgM-enriched IVIG. The doses were 190 mg/kg/day of IgG and 30 mg/kg/day of IgM for 4 days. Six (20%) of the 30 infants who received antibiotics alone died, compared with 1 (3.3%)

of the 30 who received antibiotics plus IVIG, a statistically significant difference. Christensen and associates used IVIG plus antibiotics in neonates with clinical signs of sepsis. They found IVIG recipients to have a more rapid correction of neutropenia, a more rapid appearance of immature neutrophils in the peripheral circulation suggesting release of neutrophils from marrow storage pools, and an increase in arterial oxygen tension compared with control infants receiving albumin.[105] There were no deaths in either group, and no difference in mortality rates were observed.

These studies suggest, but do not prove, that IVIG is a valuable form of therapy in septic premature newborns.

GROUP B STREPTOCOCCAL INFECTION

Group B streptococcal infection is one of the serious diseases in the newborn period. The use of IVIG in this condition has been addressed by Fischer[106–108] and Santos.[109] Some of these preparations are opsonic for multiple strains of group B streptococci *in vitro* and protect animals against experimental GBS disease. Such passively administered IgG could ensure that premature infants who are at high risk of infection or already ill are protected by antibody to group B streptococci, even if little of it has been obtained transplacentally. However, not all GBS strains are uniformly susceptible to opsonization by antibody to group B streptococci. Lot-to-lot variation in antibody activity to group B streptococci has been observed. To ensure that an appropriate quantity of antibody is administered, screening of immunoglobulin lots for functional activity and pharmacokinetic studies in neonates are necessary.

Studies by Hill and colleagues indicated that administration of IVIG in neonatal rats improved the outcome of GBS pneumonia and sepsis by increasing opsonization and by enhancing PMN migration.[110] The mechanisms of these actions are unclear, but antibody may prevent neutrophil depletion by localizing bacteria to the lung where they can be phagocytized by pulmonary leukocytes and may generate inflammatory mediators, causing the release of PMNs from the marrow.[110–112] Combined use of other plasma factors may provide even better protection against bacterial pathogens. Neonatal rats with GBS infection had significantly lower mortality rates if given IVIG and fibronectin than if given fibronectin alone.[110] If IVIG is used, it seems reasonable to normalize the IgG level to between 700 and 1000 mg/dL, using frequent infusions and determination of IgG levels. A dose of 100 mg/kg usually raises serum IgG by about 100 mg/dL.

SPECIFIC ANTIBODY REPLACEMENT THERAPY

Variability in IVIG preparations and lots creates several difficulties in predicting results of treatment for specific organisms. There is a potential role for directed preparations containing specific antibodies. Intravenous immunoglobulin apparently has minimal short-term side effects or complications.[99–102] Nevertheless, large, multicenter studies must be completed before possible long-term problems such as hepatitis or inhibition of subsequent antibody synthesis can be identified or ruled out.

The fact that IVIG has known immunomodulating properties should be kept in mind when one is considering its use in persons without antibody deficiency.[113] Passively administered antibodies are potent antigen-specific immunosuppressive agents, as illustrated by the high degree of efficacy of $Rh_o(D)$ immune globulin (RhoGAM) in preventing sensitization of Rh-negative women to the Rh-D antigen on the erythrocytes of their Rh-positive fetuses. Recent studies in patients with systemic vasculitis demonstrated a 51% decrease in antineutrophil cytoplasm antibodies after high-dose therapy with IVIG, and this decrease was maintained during follow-up.[114]

Although there are no controlled clinical studies of the suppression of immune responses to other antigens by passively administered antibody, there is no reason to believe that antibodies to the Rh-D and neutrophil cytoplasm antigens are unique in this regard. There is evidence from animal and *in vitro* studies that IVIG can suppress antibody formation, T-cell proliferation and the activity of NK cells.[115–119] In addition to the masking of antigens, IVIG has many potential mechanisms for suppressing the immune response, including interaction with Fc receptors on the membranes of various cells of the immune system and the combination of antiidiotypic antibodies with antibody-producing cells or secreted antibodies.[114,120] Antiidiotypic antibodies in IVIG could impair the capacity of B cells from even immune hosts to secrete antibody. Blockade of the Fc receptor by high doses of IVIG, as in the treatment of idiopathic thrombocytopenic purpura, or by the formation of immune complexes of IVIG with antigens could also impair the normal clearance of opsonized infectious agents and lead to overwhelming infection.[120]

There are many reasons not to administer IVIG unless there is a demonstrated broad antibody-deficiency state or other accepted clinical indications. Furthermore, studies in neonatal animals have shown that, in some situations, survival rates are reduced with high concentrations of IVIG plus antibiotic compared with antibiotic alone. The routine use of IVIG as adjuvant therapy of neonatal infections cannot be recommended at this time.[121]

ACTIVE IMMUNIZATION OF PREGNANT WOMEN

Although the results of specific antibody replacement therapies seems promising, the availability and delay of the initiation of therapy (*i.e.,* using it only when the condition is clinically suspected) are of concern. If pregnant women could be safely immunized at the beginning of the third trimester, producing high levels of protective antibody which then cross the placental barrier, this would probably give protection to neonates early enough to significantly decrease the incidence of the infection.

Group B streptococcal sepsis develops in approximately 3 neonates per 1000 live births, resulting in approximately 11,000 cases annually in the United States. Mortality and morbidity from these infections continue to be substantial.[122–125]

Because human immunity to group B streptococci correlates with type-specific anticapsular antibodies and low levels of these antibodies predict susceptibility to invasive disease, to actively immunize women with capsular polysaccharide antigens of group B streptococci to stimulate production of type-specific, IgG antibody for transplacental protection of the fetus might be a valuable therapeutic or prophylactic approach.[126–129]

Baker and associates immunized 40 pregnant women, at a mean gestation of 31 weeks, with a single 50-μg dose of the type III capsular polysaccharide of group B streptococci.[130] Twenty-five women (63%) responded to the vaccine. Of the infants born to these women, 80% continued to have protective levels of antibody (*e.g.*, IgG-specific antibody $\geq 2\ \mu$g/mL) at 1 month of age, and 64% had protective levels at 3 months. Serum samples from infants with $\geq 2\ \mu$g of antibody to type III group B streptococci per milliliter uniformly promoted efficient opsonization, phagocytosis, and bacterial killing *in vitro* of type III strains. This effect may be mediated exclusively by the alternative complement pathway.

Although this vaccine, with an overall response rate of 63%, is not optimally immunogenic, this study suggests that maternal immunization is feasible and can provide passive immunity against systemic infection with type III group B streptococci in most newborns. Larger trials with better vaccines are required to evaluate the safety and clinical effectiveness of this strategy.

PLASMA COMPONENT TRANSFUSION

Neonates have significant impairment in humoral and cellular immune factors. Augmentation of deficient humoral factors by transfusion of transfer factor, fresh frozen plasma, antibody, or whole blood has been protective in humans or neonatal animals with infection.[108,112,131–140] Because of the extensive interaction between cellular and humoral factors, the positive effect of these therapies is thought to be produced, at least partially, by their improvement of neonatal neutrophil function. One study showed that replacement of humoral factors and PMNs is superior to replacement of humoral factors alone.[134]

Transfer factor is a dialyzable extract from human leukocytes with chemoattractant activity. The results of its use in patients with chemotactic defects vary. Some investigators found that transfer factor corrected the PMN chemotactic defect in patients with candidiasis and the hyper-IgE syndrome, but others found that it suppressed PMN function in several patients with the hyper-IgE syndrome.[131,132]

Fresh frozen plasma contains antibody, complement, fibronectin, and other proteins that help protect against infection and have been found to be deficient in the neonate, especially the premature infant.[141–143] Fresh frozen plasma infusions are commonly given to neonates with hypotension and are well tolerated. A preliminary study suggests that fresh frozen plasma transfusions improve PMN chemotaxis in newborn infants.[133] Whether this improvement results in decreased morbidity or mortality from infection is unknown.

NEUTROPHIL TRANSFUSION THERAPY

Bone marrow reserve for PMN in neonates is limited, and bone marrow pool exhaustion during neonatal infection is common. The most direct way to correct the impairment in neonatal PMN function and reserve is to transfuse adult PMNs into newborn infants. Several studies of transfusion of adult PMNs in human neonates with sepsis have produced mixed results.[144–150] The first clinical trial of PMN transfusion in human neonates was carried out by Laurenti and associates.[145] In this nonrandomized study, the mortality rate was 10% in the transfused group and 72% in the nontransfused group. No untoward effects of the transfusions were observed. The striking improvement in morbidity and mortality rates in the transfused group suggested that PMN transfusions could benefit septic newborns. Christensen and colleagues carried out a prospective trial of adult PMN transfusion in 26 septic neutropenic neonates.[144] Ten neonates with moderate or no depletion of their marrow PMN reserve did not receive PMN transfusion, and none died. Eight (89%) of 9 neonates with severe depletion of marrow PMN reserve who did not receive PMN transfusion died. These data indicate that septic neutropenic neonates with normal marrow PMN reserve who are given standard antibiotic and supportive care are likely to survive without PMN transfusion. In contrast, septic neutropenic neonates with severe marrow PMN depletion have a high mortality rate despite antibiotics and supportive care and can probably benefit from adult PMN transfusions. Two studies of the use of transfusion of PMNs from whole blood buffy coat layers failed to demonstrate a beneficial effect in septic neonates.[149,150] Baley and associates conducted a prospective, randomized, controlled trial of PMN transfusions for septic neonates that failed to demonstrate any improvement in survival.[150]

Several researchers have recommended bone marrow examination before neonatal PMN transfusion to detect bone marrow exhaustion. Neonates with marrow exhaustion have a poor prognosis and may benefit most from PMN transfusion. Because this procedure is invasive and delays delivery of PMNs to neonates with fulminant infection, a rapid, accurate, and easily performed test to document marrow exhaustion would be useful.

There are several potential problems associated with PMN transfusion. Polymorphonuclear leukocyte sequestration in the lung, resulting in pulmonary decompensation (*e.g.*, decreased PaO_2), occurs in adults and children.[151,152] Graft-*versus*-host disease has been reported after PMN transfusion in the immunocompromised host.[153] Irradiation of leukocytes with minimum of 3000 cGy should be sufficient to impair lymphocyte function and prevent GVH disease without altering PMN number and function. Human immunodeficiency virus transmission from PMN transfusion is another potential concern. Although minimized with current antibody screening programs, an estimated 1 in 100,000 to 1,000,000 units of antibody-negative blood may contain transmissible virus as a result of recent HIV infection in the donor.[154] Whether the risk of HIV transmission is greater with PMN transfusion than with whole blood or packed cell transfusions is unknown. Cytomegalovirus, EBV, and hepatitis virus are other infectious agents that may be transmitted by PMN transfusion. Use of one of the recipient's parents, preferably the mother, as the PMN donor minimizes the risk of viral transmission.

Although the results of studies of PMN transfusion in neonates appear promising, large prospective randomized trials must be carried out before it can be concluded that the potential benefits of PMN transfusion outweigh the risks. Polymorphonuclear leukocyte transfusion cannot be recommended for routine adjunctive therapy of neonatal sepsis at this time.[8,155] Polymorphonuclear leukocyte transfusion can be considered for the subgroup of septic neonates with neutrophil storage pool depletion, because this group of high-risk infants appear to be the most likely to benefit.

REFERENCES

1. Metchnikoff E. Immunity in Infective Diseases. London: Cambridge University Press, 1905.
2. Bellanti JA. Immunology III. Philadelphia: WB Saunders, 1985.
3. Baker CJ. Group B streptococcal infections in newborns. Pediatr Rev 1979;64:5.
4. McCracken GH, Mize SG. A controlled study of intrathecal antibiotic therapy in gram-negative enteric meningitis of infancy. J Pediatr 1976;89:66.
5. Vogel SN, Nogan MM. Role of cytokines in endotoxin-mediated host responses. In: Opperheim JJ, Shevach EM, eds. Immunophysiology. The role of cells and cytokines in immunity and inflammation. New York: Oxford, University Press, 1990:238.
6. Christensen RD, Rothstein G, Anstall HB, et al. Granulocyte transfusions in neonates with bacterial infection, neutropenia, and depletion of mature marrow neutrophils. Pediatrics 1982;70:1.
7. Christensen RD, Bradley PP, Rothstein G. The leukocyte left shift in clinical and experimental neonatal sepsis. J Pediatr 1981;98:101.
8. Krause PJ, Herson VC, Eisenfeld L, Johnson GM. Enhancement of neutrophil function for treatment of neonatal infections. Pediatr Infect Dis J 1989;8:362.
9. Playfair JHL, Wolfendale MR, Kay HEM. The leukocytes of peripheral blood in the human foetus. Br J Haematol 1963; 9:336.
10. Cartwright GE, Athens JW, Wintrobe MM. The kinetics of granulopoiesis in normal man. Blood 1964;24:780.
11. Erdman SH, Cristensen RD, Bradley PP, et al. The supply and release of storage neutrophils: a developmental study. Biol Neonate 1982;41:132.
12. Christensen RD, Hill HR, Rothstein G. Granulocyte stem cell (CFU_c) proliferation in experimental group B streptococcal sepsis. Pediatr Res 1983;17:278.
13. Miller ME. Phagocytic function in the neonate: selected aspects. Pediatrics 1979;64(Suppl):709.
14. Mohandes AE, Touraine JL, Osman M, et al. Neutrophil chemotaxis in infants of diabetic mothers and in preterms at birth. J Clin Lab Immunol 1982;8:117.
15. Sacchi F, Rondini G, Mingrat G, et al. Different maturation of neutrophil chemotaxis in term and preterm newborn infants. J Pediatr 1982;101:273.
16. Anderson DC, Hughes BJ, Edwards E, et al. Impaired chemotaxigenesis by type III group B streptococci in neonatal sera: relationship to diminished concentration of specific anticapsular antibody and abnormalities of serum complement. Pediatr Res 1983;17:496.
17. Abramson JS, Wheeler JG, Quie PG. The polymorphonuclear phagocytic system. In: Stiehm ER, ed. Immunologic disorders in infants and children. Philadelphia: WB Saunders, 1989:68.
18. Nunoi H, Endo F, Chikazawa S, et al. Chemotactic receptor of cord blood granulocytes to the synthesized chemotactic peptide N-formyl-methionyl-leucyl-phenylalanine. Pediatr Res 1983;17:57.
19. Bruce MC, Baley JE, Medvik K, et al. Impaired surface membrane expression of C3bi but not C3b receptors on neonatal neutrophils. Pediatr Res 1987;21:306.
20. Anderson DC, Hughes BJ, Smith CW. Abnormal mobility of neonatal polymorphonuclear leukocytes. J Clin Invest 1981; 68:683.
21. Krause PJ, Maderazo EG, Scroggs M. Abnormalities of neutrophil adherence in newborns. Pediatrics 1982;69:184.
22. Anderson DC, Becker, Freeman KL, et al. Abnormal stimulated adherence of neonatal granulocytes: impaired induction of surface MAC-1 by chemotactic factors or secretagogue. Blood 1987;70:740.
23. Miller MH. Cell elastimetry in the study of normal and abnormal movement of human neutrophils. Clin Immunol Immunopathol 1979;14:502.
24. Yasui K, Masuda M, Matsuooka T, et al. Abnormal membrane fluidity as a cause of impaired functional dynamics of chemoattractant receptors on neonatal polymorphonuclear leukocytes: lack of modulation of the receptors by a membrane fluidizer. Pediatr Res 1988;24:442.
25. Krause PJ, Maderazo EG, Scroggs M. Abnormalities of neutrophil adherence in newborns. Pediatrics 1982;69:184.
26. Olson TA, Ruymann FB, Cook BA, et al. Newborn polymorphonuclear leukocyte aggregation: a study of physical properties and ultrastructure using chemotactic peptides. Pediatr Res 1983;17:993.
27. Klein RB, Fischer TJ, Gard SE, et al. Decreased mononuclear and polymorphonuclear chemotaxis in human newborns, infants and young children. Pediatrics 1977;60:467.

28. Miller ME. Chemotactic function in the human neonate: humoral and cellular function. Pediatr Res 1971;5:487.
29. Berger M. Complement deficiency and neutrophil dysfunction as risk factors for bacterial infection in newborns and the role of granulocyte transfusion in therapy. Rev Infect Dis 1990;12:S401.
30. Roth P, Polin RA. Adherence of human newborn infants' monocytes to matrix-bound fibronectin. J Pediatr 1992;121:285.
31. Polin RA. Role of fibronectin in diseases of newborn infants and children. Rev Infect Dis 1990;12:5428.
32. Miller ME. Phagocytosis in the newborn infant: humoral and cellular factors. J Pediatr 1969;74:255.
33. Gallin JI. Interferon-γ in the management of chronic granulomatous disease. Rev Inf Dis 1971;13:973.
34. Ambruso DR, Altenburger KM, Johnston RB Jr. Defective oxidative metabolism in newborn neutrophils: discrepancy between superoxide anion and hydroxyl radical generation. Pediatrics 1979;64:722.
35. Newburger PE. Superoxide generation by human fetal granulocytes. Pediatr Res 1982;16:373.
36. Shigeoka AO, Charette RP, Wyman ML, Hill HR. Defective oxidative metabolic responses of neutrophils from stressed neonates. J Pediatr 1981;98:392.
37. Falloon J, Gallin JI. Neutrophil granules in health and disease. J Allergy Clin Immunol 1986;77:653.
38. Wright WC Jr, Ank BJ, Herbert J, et al. Decreased bactericidal activity of leukocytes of stressed newborn infants. Pediatrics 1975;56:578.
39. Stein M, Keshav S. The versatility of macrophage. Clin Exp Allergy 1992;22:19.
40. Marodi L, Leijh PCJ, Van Furth R. Characteristics and functional capacities of human cord blood granulocytes and monocytes. Pediatr Res 1984;18:1127.
41. Wilson CB, Haas JE. Cellular defenses against Toxoplasma gondii in newborns. J Clin Invest 1984;73:1606.
42. Wilson CB, Lewis DB. Basis and implications of selectively diminished cytokine production in neonatal susceptibility to infection. Rev Infect Dis 1990;12:5410.
43. Blaese RM. Macrophages and the development of immunocompetence. In: Bellanti JA, Dayton DH, eds. The phagocytic cell in host resistance. New York: Raven Press, 1975:309.
44. Klein RB, Fisher TJ, Gard SE, et al. Decreased mononuclear and polymorphonuclear chemotaxis in human newborns, infants, and young children. Pediatrics 1977;60:467.
45. Weston WL, Carson BS, Barkin RM, et al. Monocyte—macrophage function in the newborn. Am J Dis Child 1977;131:1291.
46. Gitlin D, Biasucci A. Development of gamma G, gamma M, beta 1_c, beta 1_a, C'1 esterase inhibitor, ceruloplasmin, transferrin, hemopexin, haptoglobin, fibrinogen, plasminogen, alpha-1-antitrypsin, orosomucoid, beta-lipoprotein, α_2-macroglobin and pre-albumin in the human conceptus. J Clin Invest 1969;48:1433.
47. Propp RP, Alper CA. C'3 synthesis in the human fetus and lack of transplacental passage. Science 1968;162:672.
48. Zimmerman GA, Prescott SM, McIntyre TM. Endothelial cell interactions with granulocytes: tethering and signaling molecules. Immunol Today 1992;13:93.
49. Silverstein A, Uhr J, Kramer K, et al. Fetal response to antigenic stimulus: II. Antibody production by the fetal lamb. J Exp Med 1963;117:799.
50. Froman ML, Stiehm ER. Impaired opsonic activity but normal phagocytosis in low birth-weight infants. N Engl J Med 1969;281:926.
51. August CS, Berkel AJ, Driscoll B, et al. Onset of lymphocyte function in the human fetus. Pediatr Res 1971;5:539.
52. Stites DP, Carr MC, Fudenberg HH. Development of cellular immunity in the human fetus: dichotomy of proliferative and cytotoxic responses of lymphoid cells to phytohemagglutinin. Proc Natl Acad Sci USA 1972;69:1440.
53. Boyd RL, Hugo P. Towards an integrated view of thymopoiesis. Immunol Today 1991;12:71.
54. Finkel TH, Kubo RT, Cambier JC. T-cell development and transmembrane signaling: changing biological responses through an unchanging receptor. Immunol Today 1991;12:79.
55. Nikolic-Zugic J. Phenotypic and functional stages in the intrathymic development of αβ T cells. Immunol Today 1991;12:65.
56. Carding SR, Hayday AC, Bottomly K. Cytokines in T-cell development. Immunol Today 1991;12:239.
57. Low TL, Goldstein AL. Thymic hormones: an overview. Methods Enzymol 1985;116:213.
58. Goldstein G, Scheid M, Boyse EA, et al. Thymopoietin and bursopoietin: induction signals regulating early lymphocyte differentiation. Cold Spring Harbor Symp Quant Biol 1977;41:5.
59. Hong R. The DiGeorge Anomaly. Immunodef Rev 1991;3:1.
60. Bastian J, Law S, Vogler L, et al. Prediction of persistent immunodeficiency in the DiGeorge anomaly. J Pediatr 1989;115:391.
61. Lew DB, Yu CC, Meyer J, et al. Cellular and molecular mechanisms for reduced interleukin 4 and interferon-γ production by neonatal T cells. J Clin Invest 1991;87:194.
62. Haywood AR, Loyword L, Lyslyard PM, et al. Fc receptor heterogeneity of human suppressor T cells. J Immunol 1978;121:1.
63. Yabuhara A, Kawai H, Komiyama A. Development of natural killer cytotoxicity during childhood: marked increases in number of natural killer cells with adequate cytotoxic abilities during infancy to early childhood. Pediatr Res 1990;28:316.
64. Cooper MD, Lawton AR. The mammalian "bursa equivalent": does lymphoid differential along plasma cell lines begin in the gut-associated lymphoepithelial tissues (GALT) of mammals? In: Hanne MG, ed. Contemporary topics in immunobiology. New York: Plenum Press, 1972:49.
65. Rosen FS, Cooper MD, Wedgewood RJP. The primary immunodeficiencies. N Engl J Med 1984;311:235.
66. Andersson U, Bird G, Britton S. Cellular mechanisms of restricted immunoglobulin formation in the human neonate. Eur J Immunol 1980;10:888.
67. Gathings WE, Kubagawa H, Cooper MD. A distinctive pattern of B cell immaturity in perinatal human. Immunol Rev 1981;57:107.
68. Cooper MD, Lawton AR, Kincade PW. A two stage model for development of antibody producing cells. Clin Exp Immunol 1972;2:143.
69. Losonsky GA, Ogra PL. Development of immunocompetence in the products of lactation. In: Ogra PL, ed. Monograph on neonatal infections: nutritional and immunologic interactions. New York: Grune & Stratton, 1983.
70. Ogra SS, Weintraub D, Ogra PL. Immunologic aspects of human colostrum and milk. III. Fate and absorption of cellular and soluble components in the gastrointestinal tract of newborns. J Immunol 1977;119:245.
71. Smith EV, Goldman AS. The cell of human colostrum: I. In vitro studies of morphology and functions. Pediatr Res 1968;2:103.
72. Hanson LA, Ahlstedt S, Carlsson B, Fallstrom SP. Secretory IgA antibodies against cow's milk proteins in human milk and their possible effect in mixed feeding. Int Arch Allergy Appl Immunol 1977;54:457.

73. Ogra PL, Greene HL. Human milk and breast feeding: an update on the state of the art. Pediatr Res 1982;16:266.
74. Bellanti JA, Artenstein MS, Olson LC, et al. Congenital rubella: clinicopathologic, virologic, and immunologic studies. Am J Dis Child 1965;110:464.
75. Alford CA Jr. Studies on antibody in congenital rubella infections. Am J Dis Child 1965;110:455.
76. South MA, Montgomery JR, Rowls WE. Immune deficiency in congenital rubella and other viral infections. Birth Defects 1975;9:234.
77. Michaels RH. Suspension of antibody response in congenital rubella. J Pediatr 1972;80:583.
78. Fuccillo DA, Steele RW, Henson SA, et al. Impaired cellular immunity to rubella virus in congenital rubella. Infect Immun 1974;9:81.
79. Stern LM, Forbes IJ. Dysgammaglobulinemia and temporary immune paresis in case of congenital rubella. Aust Paediatr J 1975;77:38.
80. Rola-Pleszczynski M, Frenkel LD, Fuccillo DA, et al. Specific impairment of cell-mediated immunity in mothers and infants with congenital infection due to cytomegalovirus. J Infect Dis 1977;135:386.
81. Cohen F, Zuelzer WW. Mechanism of isoimmunization. II. Transplacental passage and postnatal survival of fetal erythrocytes in heterospecific pregnancy. Blood 1967;30:796.
82. Taylor AI, Polani PE. XX/XY mosaicism in man. Lancet 1965; 1:1226.
83. Naiman TL, Punnet HH, Lischner HW, et al. Possible graft-versus-host-reaction after intrauterine transfusion for Rh erythroblastosis fetalis. N Engl J Med 1969;281:697.
84. Chandra RH. Fetal malnutrition and postnatal immunocompetence. Am J Dis Child 1975;129:450.
85. Stites DP, Wybran J, Carr MC, et al. Development of cellular immunocompetence in man. In: Porter R, Knight J, eds. Ontogeny of acquired immunity: Ciba Foundation symposium. Amsterdam: Elsevier/North Holland, 1972:113.
86. Bonforte RJ, Topilsky M, Siltzbach LE, et al. Phytohemagglutinin skin test: a possible in vivo measure of cell-mediated immunity. J Pediatr 1972;81:775.
87. Poplack DG, Bonnard GD, Holiman BJ, et al. Monocyte-mediated antibody-dependent cellular cytotoxicity: a clinical test of monocyte function. Blood 1976;48:809.
88. Yoder MC, Polin RA. Immunotherapy of neonatal septicemia. Pediatr Clin North Am 1990;33:481.
89. Stiehm ER. Role of immunoglobulin therapy in neonatal infections: where we stand today. Rev Infect Dis 1990;12 (Suppl):439.
90. Hobbs JR, Davis JA. Serum γ-globulin levels and gestational age in premature babies. Lancet 1967;1:757.
91. Ballow M, Cates KL, Rowe JC, et al. Development of the immune system in very low birth weight (less than 1500 g) premature infants: concentrations of plasma immunoglobulins and patterns of infections. Pediatr Res 1986;20:899.
92. Noya FJD, Rench MA, Garcia-Prats JA, et al. Disposition of an immunoglobulin intravenous preparation in very low birth weight neonates. J Pediatr 1988;112:278.
93. Noya FJD, Rench MA, Courtney JT, et al. Pharmacokinetics of intravenous immunoglobulin in very low birth weight neonates. Pediatr Infect Dis J 1989;8:759.
94. Sasidharan P. Postnatal IgG levels in very-low-birth weight infants: preliminary observations. Clin Pediatr 1988;27:271.
95. Buaael JB. Intravenous gammaglobulin in the prophylaxis of late sepsis in very-low-birth weight infants: preliminary results of a randomized, double-blind, placebo-controlled trial. Rev Infect Dis 1990;12:2457S.
96. Chiricl G, Rondini G, Plebani A, et al. Intravenous gammaglobulin therapy for prophylaxis of infection in high-risk neonates. J Pediatr 1987;110:437.
97. Clapp DW, Kliegman RM, Baley JE, et al. Use of intravenously administered immune globulin to prevent nosocomial sepsis in low birth weight infants: report of a pilot study. J Pediatr 1989;115:973.
98. Haque KN, Zaidi MH, Haque SK, et al. Intravenous immunoglobulin for prevention of sepsis in preterm and low birth weight infants. Pediatr Infect Dis 1986;5:622.
99. Baker CJ, Melish ME, Hall RT, et al. Intravenous immune globulin for the prevention of nosocomial infection in low-birth-weight neonates. N Engl J Med 1992;327:213.
100. Stabile A, Sopo SM, Romanelli V, et al. Intravenous immunoglobulin for prophylaxis of neonatal sepsis in premature infants. Arch Dis Child 1988;63:441.
101. Magny J-F, Bremard-Oury C, Brault D, et al. Intravenous immunoglobulin therapy for prevention of infection in high-risk premature infants: report of a multicenter, double-blind study. Pediatr 1991;88:437.
102. Fanaroff A, Wright E, Korones S, et al. A controlled trial of prophylactic intravenous immunoglobulin (IVIG) to reduce nosocomial infection (NI) in VLBW infants. [Abstract] Pediatr Res 1992;33:202A.
103. Sidiropoulos D, Boehme U, Von Muralt G, et al. Immunoglobulin supplementation in prevention or treatment of neonatal sepsis. Pediatr Infect Dis 1986;5:193S.
104. Haque KN, Zaidi MH, Bahakim H. IgM-enriched intravenous immunoglobulin therapy in neonatal sepsis. A J Dis Child 1988;142:1293.
105. Christensen RD, Brown MS, Hall DC, et al. Effect on neutrophil kinetics and serum opsonic capacity of intravenous administration of immune globulin to neonates with clinical signs of early-onset sepsis. J Pediatr 1991;118:606.
106. Fisher GW, Hunter KW, Wilson SR, Hensen SA. The role of antibody in group B streptococcal disease. In: Alving BM, Finlayson JS, eds. Immunoglobulins: characteristics and uses of intravenous preparations, vol 1. Washington DC: US Government Printing Office, 1980:81.
107. Fisher GW, Hunter KW, Wilson SR. Modified human immune serum globulin for intravenous administration: in vitro opsonic activity and in vivo protection against group B streptococcal disease in suckling rats. Acta Paediatr Scand 1982; 71:639.
108. Fischer GW, Hemming VG, Hunter KW, et al. Intravenous immunoglobulin in the treatment of neonatal sepsis: therapeutic strategies and laboratory studies. Pediatr Infect Dis 1986;5:S171.
109. Santos JI, Shigeoka AO, Rote NS, Hill HR. Protective efficacy of a modified immune serum globulin in experimental group B streptococcal infections. J Pediatr 1981;99:873.
110. Hill HR, Shigeoka AO, Pineus S, Christensen RD. Intravenous IgG in combination with other modalities in the treatment of neonatal infection. Pediatr Infect Dis 1986;5: S180.
111. Stiehm ER. Intravenous immunoglobulins in neonates and infants: an overview. Pediatr Infect Dis 1986;5:S217.
112. Hall RT, Shigeoka AO, Hill HR. Serum opsonic activity and peripheral neutrophil counts before and after exchange transfusion in infants with early onset group B streptococcal septicemia. Pediatr Infect Dis 1983;2:356.
113. Dwyer JM. Intravenous therapy with gamma globulin. Adv Intern Med 1987;32:111.
114. Jayne DRW, Davies MJ, Fox CJV, et al. Treatment of systemic vasculitis with pooled intravenous immunoglobulin. Lancet 1991;337:1137.
115. Stohl W. Cellular mechanisms in the in vitro inhibition of

pokeweed mitogen-induced B cell differentiation by immunoglobulin for intravenous use. J Immunol 1986;136:4407.
116. Hashimoto F, Sakiyama Y, Matsumoto S. The suppressive effect of gammaglobulin preparations on in vitro pokeweed mitogen-induced immunoglobulin production. Clin Exp Immunol 1986;65:409.
117. Bussel J, Pahwa S, Porges A, et al. Correlation of in vitro antibody synthesis with the outcome of intravenous γ-globulin treatment of chronic idiopathic thrombocytopenic purpura. J Clin Immunol 1986;6:50.
118. Kawada K, Terasaki PI. Evidence of immunosuppression by high-dose gammaglobulin. Exp Hematol 1987;15:133.
119. Engelhard D, Waner JL, Kapoor N, Good RA. Effect of intravenous immune globulin on natural killer cell activity: possible association with autoimmune neutropenia and idiopathic thrombocytopenia. J Pediatr 1986;108:77.
120. Bussel JB. Intravenous immunoglobulin therapy for the treatment of idiopathic thrombocytopenic purpura. Prog Hemost Thromb 1986;8:103.
121. NIH Consensus Conference. Intravenous immunoglobulin. JAMA 1990;264:3189.
122. Baker CJ, Edwards MS. Group B streptococcal infections. In: Remington JS, Klein JO, eds. Infectious diseases of the fetus and newborn infant. 2nd ed. Philadelphia: WB Saunders, 1983:820.
123. Dillon HC Jr, Khare S, Gray BM. Group B streptococcal carriage and disease: a 6-year prospective study. J Pediatr 1987;110:31.
124. Institute of Medicine, National Academy of Sciences. New vaccine development: establishing priorities. In: Diseases of importance in the United States. vol 1. Washington, DC: National Academy Press, 1985:424.
125. Wald ER, Bergman I, Taylor HG, et al. Long-term outcome of group B streptococcal meningitis. Pediatrics 1986;77:217.
126. Boyer KM, Gotoff SP. Prevention of early-onset neonatal group B streptococcal disease with selective intrapartum chemoprophylaxis. N Engl J Med 1986;314:1665.
127. Baker CJ, Kasper DL. Correlation of maternal antibody deficiency with susceptibility to neonatal group B streptococcal infection. N Engl J Med 1976;294:753.
128. Baker CJ, Kasper DL, Tager IB, et al. Quantitative determination of antibody to capsular polysaccharide in infection with type III strains of group B Streptococcus. J Clin Invest 1977;59:810.
129. Stewardson-Kreiger PB, Albrandt K, Nevin T, et al. Perinatal immunity to group B beta-hemolytic Streptococcus type Ia. J Infect Dis 1977;136:619.
130. Baker CJ, Rench MA, Edwards MS, et al. Immunization of pregnant women with a polysaccharide vaccine of group B streptococcus. N Engl J Med 1988;319:1180.
131. Friendenberg WR, Marx JJ Jr, Hensen RL, et al. Hyperimmunoglobulin E syndrome: response to transfer factor and ascorbic acid therapy. Clin Immunol Immunopathol 1979;12:132.
132. Snyderman R, Altman LC, Frankel A. Defective mononuclear leukocyte chemotaxis: a previously unrecognized immune dysfunction. Studies in a patient with chronic mucocutaneous candidiasis. Ann Intern Med 1973;78:509.
133. Eisenfeld L, Krause PJ, Herson VC, et al. Enhancement of neonatal polymorphonuclear leukocyte (PMN) motility with adult fresh frozen plasma (FFP). [Abstract 1409] Washington, DC: The Society for Pediatric Research, 1986.
134. Santos JI, Shigeoka AO, Hill HR. Functional leukocyte administration protection against experimental neonatal infection. Pediatr Res 1980;14:1408.
135. Santos JI, Shigeoka AO, Rote NS, et al. Protective efficacy of a modified immune serum globulin in experimental group B streptococcal infection. J Pediatr 1981;99:873.
136. Harper TE, Christensen RD, Rothstein G, et al. Effect of intravenous immunoglobulin G on neutrophil kinetics during experimental group B streptococcal infection in neonatal rats. Rev Infect Dis 1986;8:S401.
137. Bortulussi R, Fischer GW. Opsonic and protective activity of immunoglobulin, modified immunoglobulin and serum against neonatal E. coli K1 infection. Pediatr Res 1986;20:175.
138. Givner LB, Edwards MS, Baker CJ. A polyclonal Ig preparation hyperimmune for type III Group B Streptococcus: in vitro opsonophagolytic activity and efficacy in experimental models. J Infect Dis 1988;158:724.
139. Shigeoka AD, Gobel RJ, Janatova J, et al. Neutrophil mobilization induced by complement fragments during experimental group B streptococcal (GBS) infection. Am J Pathol 1988;133:623.
140. Shigeoka AO, Hall RT, Hill HR. Blood transfusion in group B streptococcal sepsis. Lancet 1978;1:636.
141. Miller ME, Stiehm ER. Immunology and resistance to infection. In: Remington JS, Klein JO, eds. Infectious diseases of the fetus and newborn infant. Philadelphia: WB Saunders, 1983:27.
142. Cates KL, Rowe JC, Ballow M. The premature infant as a compromised host. Curr Probl Pediatr 1983;13:63.
143. Gerdes JS, Yoder MC, Douglas SD, et al. Decreased plasma fibronectin in neonatal sepsis. Pediatrics 1983;72:877.
144. Christensen RD, Rothstein G, Anstall HB, et al. Granulocyte transfusions in neonates with bacterial infection, neutropenia, and depletion of mature marrow neutrophils. Pediatrics 1982;70:1.
145. Laurenti F, Ferro R, Giancarlo I, et al. Polymorphonuclear leukocyte transfusion for the treatment of sepsis in the newborn infant. J Pediatr 1981;98:118.
146. Cairo MS, Rucker R, Bennetts GA, et al. Improved survival of newborns receiving leukocyte transfusions for sepsis. Pediatrics 1984;74:887.
147. Laing IA, Boulton FE, Hume R. Polymorphonuclear leukocyte transfusion in neonatal septicaemia. Arch Dis Child 1983;58:1003.
148. Cairo MS, Worcester C, Rucker R, et al. Role of circulating complement and polymorphonuclear leukocyte transfusion in treatment and outcome in critically ill neonates with sepsis. J Pediatr 1987;110:935.
149. Wheeler JG, Chauvenet AR, Johnson CA, et al. Buffy coat transfusion in neonates with sepsis and neutrophil storage depletion. Pediatr 1987;79:411.
150. Baley JE, Stork EK, Warentin PI, et al. Buffy coat transfusions in neutropenic neonates with presumed sepsis, a prospective radomized trial. Pediatrics 1987;80:712.
151. Wright DG, Robichaud KJ, Pizzo PA, et al. Lethal pulmonary reactions associated with the combined use of amphotericin B and leukocyte transfusions. N Engl J Med 1981;304:1185.
152. Strauss RG, Connett JE, Gale RP, et al. A controlled trial of prophylactic granulocyte transfusion during induction chemotherapy for acute myelogenous leukemia. N Engl J Med 1981;305:597.
153. Rosen RC, Huestis DW, Corrigan JJ. Acute leukemia and granulocyte transfusion: fatal graft-versus-host reaction following transfusion of cells obtained from normal donors. J Pediatr 1978;93:268.
154. Friedland GH, Klein RS. Transmission of the human immunodeficiency virus. N Engl J Med 1987;317:1125.
155. Hill HR. Phagocyte transfusion: ultimate therapy of neonatal disease? J Pediatr 1981;98:59.

Neonatology: Pathophysiology and Management of the Newborn, Fourth Edition,
edited by Gordon B. Avery, Mary Ann Fletcher, and Mhairi G. MacDonald.
J.B. Lippincott Company, Philadelphia © 1994.

chapter 47

Chronic Infections

BISHARA J. FREIJ
JOHN L. SEVER

Maternal infections acquired shortly before conception or during gestation can adversely affect pregnancy outcome indirectly through nonspecific effects of severe maternal illness (*e.g.*, increased rates of spontaneous abortions, stillbirths, premature births associated with measles infection during pregnancy) or directly through microbial invasion of the fetus or neonate.[1] Pathogens can be transmitted from mothers to their infants through hematogenous spread across the placenta (*e.g.*, cytomegalovirus [CMV], *Toxoplasma gondii*), ascension from an infected cervix (*e.g.*, herpes simplex virus [HSV]), or intimate contact between a fetus and infected genital secretions during vaginal delivery (*e.g.*, HSV, hepatitis B virus [HBV], probably human immunodeficiency virus type 1 [HIV-1]).[2] Iatrogenic fetal infections can occur after invasive procedures such as fetal scalp monitoring or intrauterine transfusions.

The outcome of a fetal or neonatal infection depends on the stage of pregnancy during which infection occurs, virulence of the pathogen, preexisting maternal immunity to the infecting agent, and efficacy of drug therapy for maternal or neonatal disease. Intrauterine infections may lead to resorption of the embryo, to fetal demise resulting in a spontaneous abortion or a stillbirth, or to the delivery of an infected neonate. Infected infants who are asymptomatic at birth may develop chronic problems in late infancy or early childhood (*e.g.*, HIV, CMV), or during adulthood (*e.g.*, rubella, HBV).[3–6] Others suffer from severe acute neonatal disease such as pneumonia or hepatitis (*e.g.*, HSV, syphilis), congenital malformations (*e.g.*, CMV, rubella), intrauterine growth retardation, or prematurity.[5,7,8] The number of infants born each year with these conditions is substantial (Table 47-1),[9–15] and the lifetime expenditures for their medical and educational needs are considerable. Compounding the problem is a resurgence in the incidence of congenital syphilis and congenital rubella after years of steady decline.[8,14]

The acronym TORCH (*T. gondii*, "other", rubella virus, CMV, HSV) has long been used as a reminder that a number of pathogens can cause clinically indistinguishable illnesses in the neonate. These agents were originally grouped together because of shared clinical features (*e.g.*, microcephaly, hepatosplenomegaly, petechiae, ocular abnormalities), their ability to cause asymptomatic infections in the mother and newborn, and their propensity for causing long-term sequelae that are inapparent at birth.[16] Because many other agents (*e.g.*, HIV, *Treponema pallidum*, varicella-zoster virus [VZV], coxsackievirus, human parvovirus B19, *Mycobacterium tuberculosis*) are capable of causing similar illnesses, the diagnostic workup of infants suspected of having a TORCH infection should not be restricted to the original four agents, as is common in medical practice.[17] The clinical utility of this mnemonic is limited, and its use should be minimized or abandoned altogether.

The epidemiology, clinical manifestations, diagnosis, and treatment of maternal and fetal infections caused by *Treponema pallidum* subsp. *pallidum*, *T. gon-*

TABLE 47–1
ESTIMATED NUMBER OF INFANTS WITH SELECTED CHRONIC CONGENITAL OR PERINATAL INFECTIONS BORN ANNUALLY IN THE UNITED STATES

Infection	Number of Infants	Year of Estimate
Congenital cytomegalovirus[9]	40,000	1992
Hepatitis B virus[6]		
Exposed	22,113	1988
Chronic carriers*	6,012	1988
Congenital toxoplasmosis[10]	3,700	1990
Congenital syphilis[11]	4,322	1991
Perinatal human immunodeficiency virus type 1[12]	1,800	1989
Neonatal herpes[13]	700–1,000	1990
Congenital rubella syndrome[11]†	47	1991

* If not given hepatitis B immune globulin and hepatitis B recombinant vaccine at birth.
† Due to the passive nature of the reporting system and to missed diagnoses of less severe cases, this figure probably only represents 20% to 30% of the actual cases.[14,15]

dii, rubella virus, HIV-1, CMV, HSV, VZV, human parvovirus B19, and hepatitis B are summarized in this chapter. Strategies for the prevention of maternal infection by these organisms or their vertical spread to the fetus or newborn infant are emphasized.

SYPHILIS

T. pallidum subsp. *pallidum*, the causative agent of syphilis, is a motile, nonculturable, gram-negative, microaerophilic spirochete that is too slender to be observed by light microscopy. The laboratory differentiation of *T. pallidum* from the other pathogenic treponemes that cause yaws (*e.g.*, *Treponema pallidum* subsp. *pertenue*), endemic syphilis (*e.g.*, *Treponema pallidum* subsp. *endemicum*), or pinta (*e.g.*, *Treponema carateum*) is difficult. Ultrastructurally, *T. pallidum* has an outer cell membrane (*i.e.*, envelope), periplasmic flagella that arise at each end of the cell, cell wall, and a multilayer cytoplasmic membrane; a capsulelike amorphous layer coats the organism.[18]

Person-to-person transmission of *T. pallidum* occurs primarily through contact with infectious lesions during sexual activity. The organism enters the body through sites of minor trauma that disrupt mucosal or epithelial barriers.[19] Fibronectin receptors appear to mediate the attachment of *T. pallidum* to epithelial or mucosal cells.[20] Parenteral transmission of this spirochete through transfusions is rare because of routine serologic screening of blood or blood products, but intravenous drug users occasionally acquire syphilis by sharing needles contaminated with *T. pallidum*–infected blood.[21] Intrauterine transmission from an infected mother to her developing fetus accounts for most congenitally infected infants; rarely, infection is acquired at birth through contact with a genital lesion.[8] *In utero* transmission can occur as early as 9 to 10 weeks of gestation. The most important determinant for the risk of fetal infection is the maternal stage of syphilis. Mothers with primary, secondary, early latent, or late latent stages of syphilis have at least a 50%, 50%, 40%, or 10% risk, respectively, of delivering an infant with congenital syphilis.[8] Concomitant maternal infection with *T. pallidum* and HIV may enhance the transplacental spread of either pathogen to the fetus.[8]

Natural and experimental *T. pallidum* infections elicit complex cellular and humoral immune responses. Most antitreponemal antibodies produced during the course of a syphilitic infection cross-react with antigens from nonpathogenic treponemes (*i.e.*, culturable treponemes that are part of the normal oral, intestinal, or genital flora) and are not pathogen specific.[22,23] Antibodies directed against integral membrane lipoproteins with molecular masses of 47, 17, and 15 kd appear to be *T. pallidum* specific; their detection on Western immunoblot assays indicates syphilitic infection.[24–26] A variety of other host immunologic defenses are activated after *T. pallidum* infection, including infiltration of inoculation sites with polymorphonuclear leukocytes that contain treponemicidal peptides (*i.e.*, defensins), T-lymphocyte activation and proliferation with interferon-γ production, cytokine secretion, macrophage-mediated phagocytosis and intracellular killing of opsonized *T. pallidum*, and complement activation.[27–30] A few treponemes manage to evade these clearance mechanisms during the acute phase of untreated infection, and this allows them to disseminate and establish a chronic infection.[29]

MATERNAL SYPHILIS

EPIDEMIOLOGY

The number of primary and secondary syphilis cases in the United States increased steadily between 1985 and 1990, with 50,223 cases reported for 1990 alone (*i.e.*, 20.1 cases per 100,000 persons); the rates increased most dramatically among African-American women (231%) and African-American men (126%) during this period.[31] The number of cases reported during 1991 declined for the first time in several years to 42,935 (*i.e.*, 17.3 cases per 100,000 persons).[11] Although the highest syphilis rates are encountered in urban areas, increased *T. pallidum* transmission has occurred in rural areas as well.[32] Nationally, adolescents 15 to 19 years of age experienced a 40% increase in the incidence of primary and secondary syphilis from 1987 through 1991.[32] Factors contributing to the increase in syphilis cases include cocaine use (especially crack cocaine) and exchange of drugs for sex, frequently with multiple, anonymous sex partners.[33] Partner notification for diagnosis and treatment purposes is especially difficult under these circumstances.[34] Declines in resources for syphilis control programs and in the socioeconomic and educational levels of certain populations have promoted the spread of syphilis.[8,32]

Pregnant women with syphilis are usually in their twenties (60%–80%), unmarried (65%–90%), and African American (45%–70%) or Hispanic (25%–55%). They usually receive no prenatal care (45%–65%) and are likely to be substance abusers (55%–70%).[35–37]

CLINICAL MANIFESTATIONS

Approximately 10 to 90 days (mean, 21 days) after sexual contact with an infected person, a painless chancre with regional lymphadenopathy develops (*i.e.*, primary syphilis).[19] Chancres heal within 3 to 6 weeks, even without specific therapy.

Secondary syphilis develops after hematogenous spread of *T. pallidum*. Its most recognizable manifestations include widely distributed rashes (*e.g.*, macular, maculopapular, pustular, follicular) that typically involve the palms and soles, alopecia, condyloma lata (*i.e.*, broad, flat, painless, highly infectious papules found in moist areas such as the vulva or anus), oropharyngeal lesions (*e.g.*, mucous patches, erosions, ulcers), constitutional symptoms (*e.g.*, low-grade fever, myalgias, sore throat, malaise, weight loss), and generalized painless lymphadenopathy. Asymptomatic central nervous system (CNS) involvement is found in 8% to 40%; headache or meningismus occurs in 1% to 2%. Hepatitis, glomerulonephritis, nephrotic syndrome, osteitis, bursitis, and arthritis are uncommon.

Secondary syphilis can resolve spontaneously without specific treatment. Untreated patients enter a latent phase of their illness, which is subdivided into an early stage, defined as 1 year of disease duration by the Centers for Disease Control and Prevention (CDC) and as 2 years by the World Health Organization, and a late stage. About 25% of patients in this phase experience relapses of secondary syphilis within 4 years, with approximately 75% of these relapses occurring during the first year.[8,19]

Tertiary syphilis is a slowly progressive inflammatory process that develops after several years in about one-third of untreated patients. Manifestations include the invasion of various organs with gumma formation (*i.e.*, late benign tertiary syphilis) or cardiovascular and CNS disease. Infection does not spread to the fetus during this stage.

The natural history of syphilis may be altered in patients co-infected with HIV. Support for this concept stems from several case reports describing unusual or florid symptoms and signs of disease, atypical skin rashes, and uveitis.[19] Delayed healing of primary lesions and impaired immune responses to syphilis have been observed in HIV-infected rabbits and simian immunodeficiency virus–infected rhesus macaques.[38,39]

Women with untreated gestational syphilis are at increased risk of spontaneous abortion, stillbirth, premature delivery, or neonatal death.[40] Congenitally infected infants who are asymptomatic at birth subsequently develop clinical manifestations if left untreated.

LABORATORY DIAGNOSIS

Several methods are currently available for the direct detection of *T. pallidum* in suspicious lesions (*e.g.*, chancre, condyloma lata, mucous patch), body fluids (*e.g.*, nasal discharge, amniotic fluid), placentas, umbilical cords, and tissue biopsy or autopsy specimens. The organism can be visualized using darkfield microscopy, and it can be differentiated from nonpathogenic treponemes by its corkscrew appearance, characteristic 90° flexion centrally, and motility.[19] A practical alternative to darkfield examination is the direct fluorescent antibody test for *T. pallidum* (DFA-TP). The DFA-TP uses pathogen-specific monoclonal antibodies as reagents.[41,42] Another method involves the inoculation of animals with cerebrospinal fluid (CSF) or other clinical specimens (*i.e.*, rabbit infectivity test) and examining the animals for evidence of a syphilitic infection over several weeks; this method is impractical for clinical purposes.[43,44] An innovation uses the polymerase chain reaction (PCR) for the detection of minuscule amounts of *T. pallidum* DNA in CSF, amniotic fluid, lesion exudate, serum, or biopsy specimens.[45–47] Polymerase chain reaction methodologies for syphilis diagnosis are not yet commercially available.

Serologic methods, despite their limitations, are the most popular and practical means of diagnosing syphilis. Two different types of antibodies are measured: nonspecific, nontreponemal reaginic (*i.e.*, Wassermann) antibodies and specific, antitreponemal antibodies.[48]

Nontreponemal tests detect IgG and IgM antibodies directed against cardiolipin–lecithin–cholesterol antigens.[19] The Venereal Disease Research Laboratory (VDRL) test and the rapid plasma reagin (RPR) 18-mm-circle card test are the two most popular tests in use. These flocculation tests are inexpensive and simple to perform, making them suitable for screening purposes. Quantitative results can be obtained, and the measured titers are helpful in monitoring the response to therapy and in detecting reinfections.[19] These antibodies are detectable in 70% to 80% of patients with primary syphilis and in almost 100% of those with secondary syphilis. They may disappear even without specific therapy in 25% of patients with latent disease. The RPR or VDRL tests may become nonreactive within 1 or 2 years of adequate treatment of patients with primary or secondary syphilis, respectively. The length of time needed to serorevert depends on pretreatment titers.[49]

False-positive VDRL or RPR test results occur for 1% to 2% of the general population and for about 10% of intravenous drug users. Many infectious conditions (*e.g.*, hepatitis, leptospirosis, HIV infection, infectious mononucleosis, bacterial endocarditis, chancroid, tuberculosis, *Mycoplasma* pneumonia, Lyme disease) and noninfectious conditions (*e.g.*, pregnancy, chronic liver disease, connective tissue disease, multiple blood transfusions) are associated with false-positive test results, and specific treponemal tests are required for confirmation of the diagnosis. The titers in false-positive reactions are usually low (<1:8).[19,50] Prozone (*i.e.*, false-negative) reactions occur in 1% to 2% of patients with secondary syphilis because of the excess reaginic antibodies that prevent flocculation; diluting the serum and retesting yield high RPR or VDRL titers.[51]

Specific treponemal tests include fluorescent treponemal antibody-absorption (FTA-ABS), *T. pallidum* immobilization, microhemagglutination assay for antibody to *T. pallidum* (MHA-TP), and the hemagglutination treponemal tests for syphilis.[19,48] These tests are expensive and cumbersome to perform and are not suitable for screening purposes. Reactive test results are obtained in 65% (by MHA-TP) to 85% (by FTA-ABS) of women with primary syphilis, in 100% with secondary syphilis, and in 95% to 98% with later stages of disease. Because these tests remain positive indefinitely in most patients, they are not helpful in detecting reinfections. However, the FTA-ABS and MHA-TP tests have been shown to serorevert in 24% and 13%, respectively, of patients with primary or secondary syphilis within 36 months of adequate treatment.[49] The specific treponemal tests are most useful in differentiating a syphilitic infection from a false-positive reaction on the VDRL or RPR tests. False-positive treponemal test reactions occur in about 1% of the general population; these are usually transient. Conditions associated with false-positive reactions include infectious mononucleosis, leprosy, leptospirosis, Lyme disease, and systemic, discoid, or drug-induced lupus erythematosus.[19]

Newer serologic techniques under evaluation include enzyme immunoassays and Western blots for the detection of IgG and IgM antibodies to *T. pallidum* and antigen-capture enzyme immunoassays.[24,26,48,52] In the future, these tests may help differentiate active from previously treated syphilis and aid in the accurate diagnosis of congenital infection.[19]

TREATMENT

Penicillin remains the drug of first choice for the treatment of maternal syphilis and for the prevention of fetal infection.[53] The dosage of the drug and the duration of treatment varies with the stage of the disease. Early syphilis (*i.e.*, primary, secondary, early latent) is treated with 2.4 million units of benzathine penicillin G given once intramuscularly. The cure rate with this regimen is about 95%. For syphilis of longer than a 1-year duration (*i.e.*, late syphilis), 2.4 million units of benzathine penicillin G are given intramuscularly once weekly for 3 consecutive weeks. A variety of regimens are used for neurosyphilis. About 45% of treated pregnant women have Jarisch–Herxheimer reactions during the first 24 hours after benzathine penicillin therapy.[54] This reaction consists of fever, myalgias, headache, tachycardia, and mild hypotension. Uterine contractions and decreased fetal movements are observed in two-thirds of pregnant women.[54] The reaction is usually at its peak at 6 to 12 hours after therapy.

Formal recommendations for syphilis therapy are the same for HIV-positive and HIV-negative patients; however, many reports have documented the failure of standard penicillin therapy in curing early syphilis in HIV-infected patients.[19] Consequently, most experts in the field now use higher doses of penicillin for the HIV-positive patient.[55]

The failure of maternal penicillin treatment to prevent congenital syphilis in some infants is well documented.[56] Most of these failures occur when treatment is given during the last 4 weeks of pregnancy.

Antimicrobials other than penicillin are probably effective in the treatment of syphilis. Tetracyclines can be used in the penicillin-allergic patient, but their use during pregnancy is contraindicated. Erythromycin has a lower cure rate in early syphilis compared with penicillin.[53] It is not well tolerated because of gastrointestinal adverse effects, and its transplacental transfer is unpredictable. Congenital syphilis after maternal erythromycin therapy has been observed repeatedly.[53,57] Limited data on the use of first-generation cephalosporins (*e.g.*, cephalothin, cephalexin), ceftriaxone, nafcillin, amoxicillin, and chloramphenicol suggest that they may be acceptable alternatives to penicillin in adults with early syphilis; information on their use during pregnancy is minimal.[19,53,58,59] Aminoglycosides, clindamycin, and rifampin are considered ineffective.[58]

Penicillin-allergic pregnant women should be skin tested for reactions to major and minor penicillin determinants.[60] If the skin tests are negative, penicillin can be used for the treatment of syphilis. If the skin test is positive, desensitization with oral penicillin over 3 to 4 hours should be attempted and the patient subsequently treated with standard doses of the drug.[61]

Follow-up of treated pregnant women is essential. Monthly nontreponemal serologic tests should be performed. A fourfold decline in titer should be observed within 3 months after therapy. If the decline in titer does not occur or if the titer rises, retreatment is recommended.[60]

PREVENTION

Pregnant women should be tested for syphilis on their first antenatal visit and again at the time of delivery. For high-risk women, an additional test around 28 weeks of gestation is advisable. Screening is performed with quantitative nontreponemal tests, and positive results are confirmed with treponemal tests to exclude biologic false-positive reactions. Women who test positive for syphilis should be investigated for other sexually transmitted pathogens, especially HIV.[60,62–64]

CONGENITAL SYPHILIS

EPIDEMIOLOGY

The number of cases of congenital syphilis reported to the CDC increased steadily between 1980 and 1991, reflecting a true increase in the number of primary and secondary maternal syphilis cases and a change since 1989 in the surveillance case definition for congenital syphilis.[65] The new surveillance case definition (Table 47-2) was implemented to provide guidelines for reporting but not for making a clinical diagnosis of congenital syphilis.[66] In essence, the change involved considering stillbirths and infants born to women with untreated syphilis as presumptively infected, regardless of symptoms or results of subsequent follow-up evaluations. Because vertical transmission of *T. pallidum* does not occur in all instances, the new definition leads to the inclusion of a number of uninfected infants in the "presumptive case" category.[66] The older surveillance case definition led to underestimates of the true incidence of congenital syphilis. Many infants in whom the diagnosis could not be made at birth were presumptively treated but not reported because the diagnosis could not be confirmed; others were inconsistently reported or lost to follow-up. The new case definition improves sensitivity at the expense of specificity.[67] Compared with traditional criteria for diagnosis, the new definition results in about a fivefold increase in the reported number of congenital syphilis cases.[8,68]

CLINICAL MANIFESTATIONS

The pathologic and morphologic alterations of congenital syphilis are due to host immune and inflammatory responses to spirochetal fetal invasion.[69–71]

TABLE 47–2
CENTERS FOR DISEASE CONTROL SURVEILLANCE CASE DEFINITION FOR CONGENITAL SYPHILIS

Confirmed Case
An infant in whom *Treponema pallidum* is identified by darkfield microscopy, fluorescent antibody, or other specific stains in specimens from lesions, placenta, umbilical cord, or autopsy material
Presumptive Case
Any infant whose mother had untreated or inadequately treated syphilis at delivery, regardless of findings in the infant*
Any infant or child who has a reactive treponemal test for syphilis and any one of the following:
Any evidence of congenital syphilis on physical examination
Any evidence of congenital syphilis on long-bone radiograph
Reactive cerebrospinal fluid Venereal Disease Research Laboratory test
Elevated cerebrospinal fluid cell count or protein without other cause
Quantitative nontreponemal serologic titers which are fourfold higher than the mother's when both are drawn at birth
Reactive test for FTA-ABS-19S-IgM antibody
Syphilitic Stillbirth
Fetal death in which the mother had untreated or inadequately treated syphilis at delivery of a fetus of more than 20 weeks of gestation or of a fetus weighing more than 500 g *

* Inadequate treatment consists of any nonpenicillin therapy, or penicillin given <30 days prior to delivery.

From Center for Disease Control. Congenital syphilis—New York City, 1986–1988. MMWR 1989;38:825.

The most prominent histopathologic abnormalities are vasculitis with resultant necrosis and fibrosis.[40] Syphilitic stillbirths are usually macerated with *T. pallidum*–rich vesiculobullous cutaneous lesions, hepatosplenomegaly, and protuberant abdomen.

Most infants with congenital syphilis are asymptomatic at birth. Infants who develop clinical manifestations during the first 2 years of life are considered to have early congenital syphilis, while features that appear later, usually near puberty, comprise late congenital syphilis.[40]

The placenta may be larger than normal.[72] The main histopathologic abnormalities are a focal, proliferative villitis with necrosis and focal mononuclear cell infiltration; endovascular and perivascular proliferation in villous vessels, leading to vascular obliteration; and focal or diffuse villous immaturity.[73,74] *T. pallidum* is demonstrable in the placenta using immunohistochemical stains; silver staining methods are difficult to perform and easy to misinterpret.[73] The focal placental villitis and obliterative arteritis is associated with increased resistance to placental perfusion; antenatal measurements of uterine and umbilical systolic–diastolic ratios using Doppler velocity waveform analysis reveal higher mean ratios in pregnancies complicated by syphilis compared with noninfected controls.[75] Necrotizing funisitis, a deep inflammatory process involving the matrix of the umbilical cord and accompanied by phlebitis and thrombosis, is common in syphilitic stillbirths and infants symptomatic at birth.[76]

Clinical signs of congenital syphilis appear in approximately two-thirds of affected infants during the third to eighth week of life and in most by 3 months of age.[40] Symptoms may be generalized and nonspecific (*e.g.*, fever, lymphadenopathy, irritability, failure to thrive); alternatively, the highly suggestive triad of snuffles, palmar and plantar bullae, and splenomegaly may be apparent.[40] The severity of the clinical illness can vary from mild to fulminant, life-threatening disease.[77–81]

Congenitally infected infants may be small for their gestational ages.[40,80] However, a carefully conducted study by Naeye of 36 stillborn and newborn infants with congenital syphilis revealed that fetal growth was almost normal despite widespread evidence of tissue destruction.[82] The observed growth retardation in some reports may be related to confounding factors such as maternal intravenous drug use or coinfection with other pathogens.

Hepatosplenomegaly occurs in 50% to 90% of infants with early congenital syphilis.[8,40] The enlargement is caused mainly by abundant extramedullary hematopoiesis and by subacute hepatic and splenic inflammation. Jaundice, with direct and indirect hyperbilirubinemia, occurs in about a third of infants and may be contributed to by hepatitis or hemolysis.[8] Syphilitic hepatitis is common and may worsen with penicillin therapy.[79,83,84] Alkaline phosphatase elevation is a frequent biochemical abnormality.[79] Transaminase and γ-glutamyltransferase concentrations may be high at presentation and increase with antimicrobial therapy to levels approaching 150 times normal.[83] Fulminant syphilitic hepatitis can manifest with hypoglycemia, lactic acidosis, encephalopathy, disseminated intravascular coagulation, and shock, mimicking metabolic or other infectious causes of acute liver failure.[81,85] Hepatic and splenic abnormalities may persist for as long as 1 year after treatment.[40] Liver cirrhosis is uncommon.[8]

Generalized lymphadenopathy is found in 20% to 50% of infants with congenital syphilis.[40] The enlarged nodes are firm and nontender.

The mucocutaneous lesions of congenital syphilis are varied and occur in 30% to 60% of infants.[40] The most characteristic are vesiculobullous eruptions that are most pronounced on the palms and soles; the blister fluid abounds with active spirochetes and is highly infectious.[40] When a blister ruptures, it leaves behind a macerated red surface that rapidly dries and crusts. The most commonly encountered rash consists of oval, red, maculopapular lesions that are most prominent on the buttocks, back, thighs, and soles; they later change to a copper–brown color with superficial desquamation. Other lesions may be annular, circinate, petechial, purpuric, or have a blueberry-muffin appearance.[40] Mucous patches involving the nares, palate, tongue, lips, and anus can occur; these lesions become deeply fissured and hemorrhagic and subsequently result in rhagades (*i.e.*, Parrot radial scars of late congenital syphilis).[40] Condyloma lata are usually encountered later in infancy in untreated patients. These raised, flat, moist, and wartlike lesions most commonly affect perioral (*e.g.*, nares, angles of mouth) and perianal areas.[8]

Rhinitis (*i.e.*, snuffles) is encountered in 10% to 50% of infected infants and usually precedes the appearance of cutaneous eruptions by 1 to 2 weeks.[40,77,79,86,87] The extremely contagious discharge is initially watery, but it later becomes thicker, purulent, and even hemorrhagic.[40] Without treatment, the nasal cartilage ulcerates with ensuing chondritis, necrosis, and septal perforation (*i.e.*, saddle nose deformity of late congenital syphilis).[8] Throat involvement can produce hoarseness or aphonia.[40]

Roentgenographic abnormalities are detected in 20% to more than 95% of infants with early congenital syphilis.[86–92] The lower rates are usually seen in asymptomatic infants.[90] Multiple, symmetric bony lesions are common. The metaphyses and diaphyses of long bones, particularly those of the lower extremities, are most commonly affected. Radiologic changes include osteochondritis, periostitis, and osteitis.[8] The earliest changes occur in the metaphysis and consist of transverse, serrated radiopaque bands (*i.e.*, Wegner sign) alternating with zones of radiolucent osteoporotic bone.[40,89] Osteochondritis becomes evident radiographically 5 weeks after fetal infection.[40] The metaphysis may become fragmented; focal erosions involving the proximal medial tibia are referred to as the Wimberger sign (Fig. 47-1). Periosteal reactions may consist of a single layer of new bone formation, of multiple layers (*i.e.*, "onion peel periosteum"), or of a severe lamellar form (*i.e.*, periostitis of Pehu).[89] Periostitis is radiologically apparent after at least 16 weeks of fetal infection.[40] Osteitis can give rise to a celery-stick appearance of longitudinal translucent lines that extend into the diaphysis or lead to a diffuse moth-eaten rarefaction of the shaft. Dactylitis, absence of lower extremity ossification centers, cranial nodules, and pathologic fractures or joint involvement leading to immobility of the affected limb (*i.e.*, pseudoparalysis of Parrot) are occasionally seen.[40,89,91]

Hematologic abnormalities are common and include anemia, leukocytosis, leukopenia, and thrombocytopenia.[87] Anemia may be due to Coombs-negative hemolysis, to replacement of bone marrow by syphilitic granulation tissue, or to a maturation arrest in the erythroblastoid cell line.[8] Thrombocytopenia is due to shortened peripheral platelet survival.

Clinically silent CNS involvement occurs in as many as 60% of infants with congenital syphilis.[8]

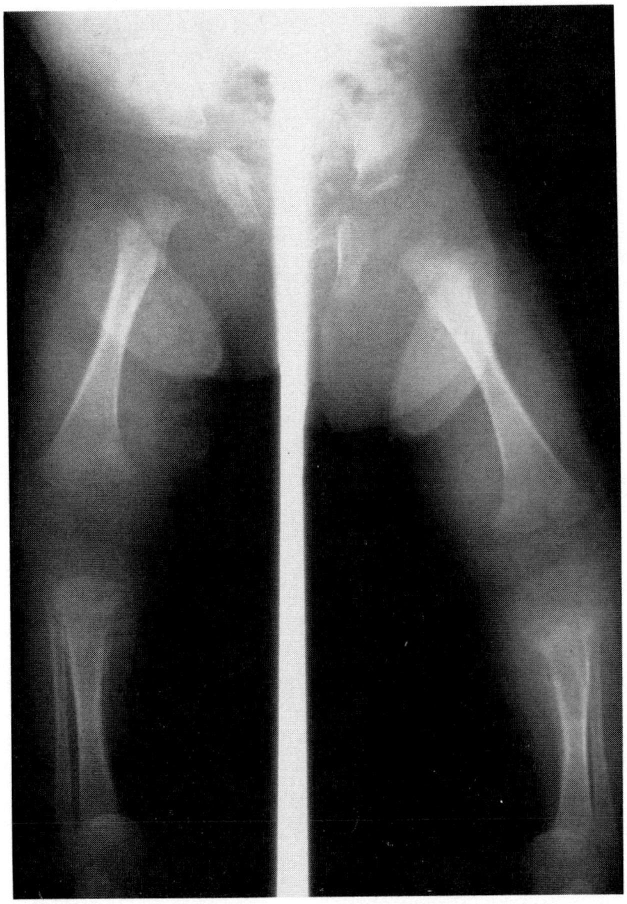

FIG. 47–1. Bone abnormalities in an infant with early congenital syphilis. Findings include bilateral, symmetric tibial periosteal new bone formation, and bilateral bony erosions involving the proximal tibial metaphysis medially (*i.e.*, Wimberger sign).

Acute syphilitic meningitis may present with neck stiffness, vomiting, bulging anterior fontanelle, and a positive Kernig sign. Cerebrospinal fluid examination reveals a normal glucose concentration, modestly elevated protein content, and mononuclear pleocytosis (usually <200 cells/μL), a pattern consistent with aseptic meningitis. Chronic meningovascular syphilis develops in untreated infants and manifests in late infancy with progressive, communicating hydrocephalus, cranial nerve palsies, optic atrophy, and cerebral infarctions leading to hemiplegia or seizure disorders.[40]

Other less common pathologic changes of early congenital syphilis involve the eyes (*e.g.*, salt and pepper chorioretinitis, glaucoma, chancres of eyelids, uveitis), lungs (*e.g.*, pneumonia alba, interstitial scarring, extramedullary hematopoiesis), and kidneys (*e.g.*, nephrotic syndrome, glomerulonephritis).[40,93,94] Nonimmune hydrops is found in a sixth of liveborn infants with congenital syphilis.[36] Myocarditis, pancreatitis, diarrhea, and malabsorption also occur.[40]

The clinical manifestations of late congenital syphilis represent residual scars after therapy of early congenital infection or persistent inflammation in untreated persons. Abnormalities of dentition are secondary to early damage incurred by developing tooth buds and are preventable by penicillin treatment during the neonatal period or in early infancy. Unilateral or bilateral interstitial keratitis occurs in about 10% of patients and is usually diagnosed between 5 and 20 years of age. Saddle nose deformity, high-arched palate, and poor maxillary growth are late consequences of syphilitic rhinitis. Eighth nerve deafness occurs infrequently (3% of patients) and is due to osteochondritis of the otic capsule and resulting cochlear degeneration. Rhagades are linear scars that radiate from sites of earlier mucocutaneous lesions of the mouth, nares, and anus. Skeletal manifestations are caused by persistent or recurrent periostitis and its associated bone thickening.[40,95,96]

DIAGNOSIS

Antenatal sonography may reveal placental thickening or fetal abnormalities such as hydrops, hepatomegaly, ascites, or dilated small bowel loops.[97–100] Spirochetes can be visualized in amniotic fluid samples using darkfield microscopy or indirect immunofluorescent staining.[97,99,101] The presence of *T. pallidum* or its DNA in amniotic fluid can be demonstrated by rabbit infectivity tests or PCR techniques, respectively.[102] With the availability of umbilical blood sampling, intrauterine infection has been confirmed as early as 24 weeks of gestation by detecting the spirochete or its DNA in fetal blood and by measuring specific IgM antibodies directed against the 47-kd antigen of *T. pallidum* in fetal serum.[97,100,102]

At birth, the diagnosis of congenital syphilis is best established by demonstrating the spirochete or its DNA in tissues or body fluids as previously alluded to. Serologic data obtained from cord blood or neonatal sera are helpful if interpreted with their limitations in mind.

Rapid plasma reagin measurements on cord blood samples yield false-positive and false-negative results in 10% and 5% of cases, respectively.[103] If an infant's RPR or VDRL titer is at least fourfold higher than a concomitantly obtained maternal titer, the diagnosis of congenital syphilis is likely. The RPR may be negative in infants whose mothers had acquired syphilis shortly before delivery.[79] The FTA-ABS-IgM test yields false-positive and false-negative results in 35% and 10% of cases, respectively.[8] This is due to interference with test performance by rheumatoid factor (*i.e.*, fetal IgM antibodies directed against maternal IgG). This problem can be overcome by separating the IgG and IgM fractions of the serum and then testing the IgG-depleted fraction with FTA-ABS-IgM. This assay is known as FTA-ABS-19S-IgM, and it is available through a few reference laboratories and the CDC.[48] The detection of IgM antibodies against specific *T. pallidum* antigens, especially the 47-kd outer membrane protein antigen, by Western immunoblot assays is diagnostically helpful.[8]

In addition to serologic tests for syphilis, the complete diagnostic evaluation of an infant with congenital syphilis should include bone radiography, CSF examination, complete blood count, platelet count, liver function tests, and HIV antibody determination.

The diagnosis of congenital neurosyphilis is difficult to ascertain. Cerebrospinal fluid abnormalities such as mononuclear pleocytosis ($\geq$25 cells/μL), elevated protein concentration (>170 mg/dL), and reactive CSF VDRL are widely used criteria.[8] However, the CSF VDRL can be positive in the absence of neurosyphilis because of passive diffusion of nontreponemal IgG antibodies from serum to CSF and in infants with traumatic lumbar punctures.[8] A specific IgM response to the *T. pallidum* 47-kd antigen has been detected in the CSF of some infants with congenial syphilis, and this may prove helpful for the diagnosis of neurosyphilis.[104] Cerebrospinal fluid IgM reactivity can be present in infants with negative CSF VDRL test results.[48] The presence of *T. pallidum* in the CSF of some infants with normal CSF cell counts, protein concentrations, and VDRL test results has been demonstrated using sensitive rabbit infectivity tests or PCR methods.[8,102]

TREATMENT

Infants should be treated at birth if they are symptomatic, if maternal therapy was inadequate or unknown, or if follow-up cannot be ensured. Adequate maternal therapy is defined as penicillin treatment at a dose appropriate for the stage of syphilis and started at least 30 days before delivery.[65]

One of two dosage regimens can be used for confirmed or presumptive congenital syphilis:

1. Crystalline penicillin G at a dose of 100,000 to 150,000 U/kg/day administered intravenously in divided doses every 8 to 12 hours for 10 to 14 days
2. Procaine penicillin G at a dose of 50,000 U/kg/day given intramuscularly once daily for 10 to 14 days.

Because congenital neurosyphilis cannot be reliably excluded in many infants, benzathine penicillin G given as a single intramuscular dose of 50,000 U/kg is recommended only for infants at low risk for congenital infection who were born to HIV-negative mothers adequately treated for syphilis but in whom close follow-up cannot be guaranteed. The 10- to 14-day regimens of crystalline or procaine penicillin G should be used if the mother is HIV positive.[62] The Jarisch–Herxheimer reaction occurs in some infants within hours of initiation of penicillin therapy.

The VDRL titers should be monitored at 1, 2, 4, 6, and 12 months of age until they become nonreactive. Untreated infants should have FTA-ABS tests. Passively acquired maternal antibodies usually disappear by 6 to 12 months of age in uninfected infants. If the VDRL titers are stable or rising or if the FTA-ABS test result remains positive beyond 1 year of age, the infant should be thoroughly reexamined and treated. The VDRL titers of adequately treated infants with congenital syphilis gradually decline, but FTA-ABS reactivities persist. Infants with CSF abnormalities should be retested at 6 months of age. If the CSF VDRL is positive at that time, a second course of penicillin is indicated. Follow-up examinations should emphasize developmental assessment and a careful search for stigmata of congenital syphilis.

TOXOPLASMOSIS

Toxoplasmosis is a common zoonosis, afflicting approximately 1 in 3 people worldwide. Infections of immunocompetent hosts are typically asymptomatic or benign, but intrauterine infections and illnesses in immunosuppressed patients can be severe or fatal. The causative organism, *T. gondii,* is an obligate intracellular protozoan that can be encountered in the form of a tachyzoite, tissue cyst, or oocyst. In addition to humans, *T. gondii* can infect other warm-blooded animals such as cats, dogs, sheep, swine, and some birds; cats and other felines are the only known complete hosts for this parasite.[10]

The life cycle of *T. gondii* is usually divided into an enteroepithelial, sexual phase that occurs only in felines and an extraintestinal, asexual phase that takes place in definitive (*e.g.*, cats) and intermediate (*e.g.*, humans) hosts.[105] Susceptible cats can acquire *Toxoplasma* infection by ingesting oocysts or parasite-harboring tissues of other animals. Some of the organisms released in cat intestines invade gut epithelial cells and undergo sexual differentiation into microgametes and macrogametes; the gametocytes later fuse to produce a zygote. After a rigid wall forms around the zygote, it is excreted in feces as an oocyst. Acutely infected cats generally shed millions of oocysts in their feces daily for periods of 1 to 3 weeks. Parasites that do not undergo sexual differentiation may instead penetrate the gut wall and spread to other tissues by way of the blood and lymphatics; this extraintestinal or asexual stage can occur in humans and other susceptible animals as well.

The tachyzoite is the actively proliferating form that is encountered in organs during the acute stage of infection. Tachyzoites gain entry into the cytoplasm of host cells and multiply rapidly. Infected cells subsequently burst and release progeny parasites that go on to attack neighboring host cells; this leads to the formation of necrotic areas that are surrounded by an inflammatory cellular reaction. This process is eventually curtailed by specific cellular and humoral host immune responses. In immunodeficient persons, the acute infection can continue relentlessly and cause serious illnesses.

After the host develops specific immunity against *T. gondii,* the organism can remain in organs in a viable, clinically inapparent tissue cyst form. *T. gondii* tissue cysts are most commonly found in the brain, eyes, myocardium, and skeletal muscles. Each cyst contains a number of slowly propagating or dormant parasites. Encysted organisms can reactivate and cause serious illnesses such as encephalitis and pneumonia in patients who become immunodeficient later in life because of malignancy, acquired immunodeficiency syndrome (AIDS), or immune suppressant therapy (*e.g.*, organ transplants).

T. gondii is transmitted to humans primarily through the ingestion of oocyst-contaminated water or food or the consumption of cyst-containing raw or undercooked beef, pork, mutton, or chicken. Unwashed hands can serve as vehicles for the transport of contaminating oocysts from the soil, dust, or cat litter box material into the mouth. Transmission can occasionally occur by eating raw infected eggs, by transfusion of infected blood or blood products, by heart or kidney transplants from seropositive donors to seronegative recipients, or by accidental self-inoculation of laboratory workers who are in contact with infected animals, needles, or glassware. Direct human-to-human transmission occurs only in the context of transplacental spread of the parasite to a developing fetus.[106]

MATERNAL TOXOPLASMOSIS

EPIDEMIOLOGY

The prevalence of anti-*Toxoplasma* antibodies among women of childbearing age varies geographically, ranging from none to more than 90%. A seroprevalence of 39% was found in a large study of 22,845 pregnancies from diverse parts of the United States conducted between 1959 and 1966.[107] More recent surveys demonstrate the divergence of seroprevalence figures by region: Denver, CO, 3.3%; Palo Alto, CA, 10%; Boston, MA, 14%; and Birmingham, AL, 30%. Seroprevalence figures for women of childbearing age from other countries include Australia with a rate of 4%; Finland, 20%; Poland, 36%; Ethiopia, 48%; Belgium, 53%; Panama, 63%; France, 71%; and El Salvador, 75%.[10,106,108,109]

The incidence of acute *T. gondii* infection during pregnancy varies by locale. Reported frequencies per 1000 pregnancies include Alabama with 0.6; Finland with 2.4; Australia with 5; Germany with 7.5; and Belgium with 14.3.[10,109] The risk of infection is greatest for pregnant women leaving a region with a low incidence of toxoplasmosis to reside in an area where the infection is prevalent.[108]

CLINICAL MANIFESTATIONS

Acute toxoplasmosis is asymptomatic in 80% to 90% of pregnant women. Those with clinically evident illnesses most commonly present with lymphadenopathy, primarily of the head and neck region; a single node is involved in about two-thirds of patients.[110] *T. gondii* causes about 1% to 5% of infectious mononucleosis cases and should be considered a likely etiologic agent in patients with negative heterophile antibody test results.[111] Complications such as hepatitis, pneumonia, myocarditis, encephalitis, and deafness are rare in immunocompetent women.[106,112,113] Fulminating illnesses are common in immunosuppressed patients.[113–115]

T. gondii spreads transplacentally to involve the developing fetus in 25%, 54%, or 65% of pregnant women with untreated primary toxoplasmosis during the first, second, or third trimesters, respectively.[106] Proper maternal therapy reduces the overall incidence of fetal infection by more than 50%, and fewer infected infants manifest with severe congenital toxoplasmosis.[116,117] These data underscore the importance of an accurate and timely diagnosis of acute toxoplasmosis in pregnant women.

DIAGNOSTIC TESTS

A clinical diagnosis of toxoplasmosis should be considered dubious unless supported by appropriate laboratory test results. *T. gondii* can be isolated from infected blood, CSF, aqueous humor, amniotic fluid, or homogenized tissues (*e.g.*, placenta, brain, muscle) by inoculating these specimens into the peritoneal cavities of mice or onto tissue cultures. Tissue culture techniques are faster (≈1 week) but less sensitive than intraperitoneal inoculation methods (≤6 weeks); both methods are impractical for clinical purposes. Tachyzoites can be visualized in tissue sections or smears of body fluids, especially if labeled specific anti-*Toxoplasma* antibodies are used for staining; their presence denotes acute infection. The demonstration of tissue cysts on histopathology can be consistent with an acute or a chronic *Toxoplasma* infection.[106]

Other immunologic techniques that have been used for the diagnosis of toxoplasmosis include intradermal skin tests and transformation of lymphocytes on exposure to *Toxoplasma* antigens, both of which connote chronic infection.[106] *Toxoplasma* antigens can be detected in CSF, urine, serum, or amniotic fluid using enzyme-linked immunosorbent assays (ELISA) or immunoblotting methods. A positive antigen test result indicates that the infection is recent. This is particularly helpful in newborns and immunodeficient persons, in whom antibody responses to infection may be absent or unpredictable.[10] The antigen test is not available commercially. The PCR has been successfully used for the direct detection of *T. gondii* DNA in clinical samples by amplification of the *P30* or *B1* genes of the parasite.[118–120]

The diagnosis of toxoplasmosis most often rests on serologic confirmation. The Sabin–Feldman dye test, traditionally the reference test against which newer methods are compared, requires the use of live parasites. Positive titers are usually in the 1:256 to 1:128,000 range. Most laboratories have abandoned the dye test in favor of simpler techniques that use killed antigens, such as the indirect fluorescent antibody (IFA), ELISA, agglutination, and indirect hemagglutination (IHA) tests.

Toxoplasma-specific IgM antibodies can be measured by IFA, ELISA, or IgM-immunosorbent agglutination assay (IgM-ISAGA). False-positive IgM-IFA or IgM-ELISA are encountered in sera containing rheumatoid factor; this problem is circumvented if a double-sandwich IgM-ELISA (DS-IgM-ELISA) is performed.[106] Specific IgM antibodies usually become positive within 1 to 2 weeks of infection and continue to be detectable for months or years, especially when measured by very sensitive assays such as DS-IgM-ELISA or IgM-ISAGA. The detection of specific IgM antibodies should not be considered proof that an infection is acute. High specific IgM titers suggest acute infection, especially if accompanied by high specific IgG titers of about 1:1000 or greater as measured by IFA or the Sabin–Feldman dye test. Low specific IgM titers measured by DS-IgM-ELISA or IgM-ISAGA are generally encountered in patients whose infections occurred several months earlier. IgM-IFA tests are considerably less sensitive than DS-IgM-ELISA or IgM-ISAGA and are positive in only 60% to 70% of patients with acute infections and 25% to 50% of infants with congenital toxoplasmosis.[10,121,122] Fewer than 25% of patients are still positive by the IgM-IFA assay 9 months after an acute infection.[122] It is important to know the type of assay used to measure specific IgM antibodies in pregnant women to correctly interpret the significance of positive and negative results.

Anti-*Toxoplasma* IgG antibodies usually appear early during an infection. IgG titers peak at about 2 months, gradually drop thereafter, but remain detectable for years. The predominant IgG antibody response is of the IgG1 subclass.[123] A single high specific IgG titer is considered only suggestive of an acute infection.

Anti-*Toxoplasma* IgA antibodies directed against the major surface protein of tachyzoites (P30) are present in over 95% of patients with acute infections.[124–126] These antibodies are detected at the end of the first month of infection and usually disappear within 4 to 7 months.[126,127] Specific IgA antibodies are rarely found in patients with chronic infections.[126–128]

Specific serum IgE antibodies are present in about 86% of women who seroconvert during pregnancy.[129] They appear shortly before or concomitantly with specific IgA antibodies, and they persist for less than 4 months.

Antibodies detected by IHA are different from those measured by the dye test, ELISA, or IFA. The titers take several weeks before becoming positive, making the test unsuitable for the diagnosis of acute toxoplasmosis during pregnancy.[10]

SEROLOGIC DIAGNOSIS OF MATERNAL INFECTION

Acute infection in immunologically normal women can be diagnosed if seroconversion or a fourfold or greater rise in antibody titers occurs when serum samples are collected 3 to 6 weeks apart.[106] The absence of *Toxoplasma*-specific IgM antibodies as measured by the DS-IgM-ELISA or IgM-ISAGA essentially excludes the diagnosis of acute toxoplasmosis; elevated titers obtained by these assays are considered suggestive of the diagnosis, especially if specific IgG titers are high as well. Positive IgM-IFA results are more likely to represent recent infection. Specific antibodies detected by IgM-ISAGA or DS-IgM-ELISA usually persist at low levels for months or years after infection; high levels measured many years after the acute infection are rare.[130] The detection of *Toxoplasma*-specific serum IgA or IgE antibodies indicates a recent infection; conversely, absence of these antibodies in a seropositive woman suggests that the infection is old.[126–129]

Immunodeficient women with acute *T. gondii* are frequently unable to mount a specific IgM response, and their IgG responses may be absent or low. Use of the more sensitive antibody assays may be helpful, but direct detection of the parasite or its components (*e.g.*, antigen, DNA) in body fluids or tissues is sometimes the only means of establishing the diagnosis of acute toxoplasmosis.[106]

DIAGNOSIS OF INTRAUTERINE INFECTION

Estimation of the duration of maternal *T. gondii* infection is usually difficult, and consequently, assessment of the true risk to the fetus is often fraught with uncertainties. The parasite can be transmitted to the developing fetus at any stage of pregnancy and, in some cases, at or shortly before conception.[10,131] This creates considerable anxiety for parents, who may choose an unwarranted end to the pregnancy or unnecessary maternal chemotherapy with potentially toxic drugs.

Prenatal diagnosis of fetal toxoplasmosis can be achieved safely and reliably. Pregnant women shown to have acquired acute *Toxoplasma* infections during the course of their pregnancies can undergo amniocentesis and ultrasound-guided cordocentesis. Parasite isolation studies, if available, include inoculation of these clinical samples into mice or onto tissue cultures. Fetal blood should be shown to be free of maternal blood contamination, using the Kleihauer–Betke stain or hemoglobin electrophoresis, before it is assayed for *Toxoplasma*-specific IgM antibodies or other nonspecific indicators of fetal infection (*e.g.*, leukocyte and differential cell counts, platelet count, total IgM content, lactic dehydrogenase level, γ-glutamyltransferase concentration). Serial ultrasound examinations should be done at 2-week intervals to detect ventricular dilation, cerebral or hepatic calcifications, ascites, hydrops, or other fetal abnormalities.

Daffos and colleagues applied this approach to prenatal diagnosis to 746 women with gestational toxoplasmosis occurring within the first 25 weeks of pregnancy.[132] All mothers were treated with spiramycin. Fetal infection occurred in 42 pregnancies, of which 39 (93%) were successfully identified prenatally. The most sensitive test in this study proved to be parasite isolation from amniotic fluid or fetal blood (81%). Despite the use of the sensitive IgM-ISAGA assay, only 21% of infected fetuses tested positive. Serial ultrasound examinations showed abnormalities in 45% of fetuses. Among nonspecific tests, γ-glutamyltransferase or total IgM contents of fetal blood were elevated in more than one-half of the patients. Results of prenatal testing led to pregnancy terminations in 62% of cases; the diagnosis was confirmed postnatally in the remainder. No false-positive diagnoses of fetal toxoplasmosis were made in this study, although other investigators have encountered this problem.[133]

Because maternal IgA and IgE antibodies do not cross the placenta, fetal serum IgA and IgE have been explored as possible markers for intrauterine *T. gondii* infection. Decoster and colleagues were able to detect specific IgA antibodies in fetal blood as early as 23 weeks of gestation.[134] The sensitivity of the assay was only 50%, slightly higher than that for *Toxoplasma*-specific IgM. No false-positive results were obtained. Pinon and colleagues were unable to detect specific anti-*Toxoplasma* IgE antibodies in fetal blood.[129]

Polymerase chain reaction methods have been employed in prenatal diagnosis of fetal toxoplasmosis.[135,136] Cazenave and colleagues studied 80 women with documented acute toxoplasmosis during pregnancy.[136] Polymerase chain reaction analysis (*i.e.*, *P30* gene amplification) of the amniotic fluid was negative in 70 cases without intrauterine infection and positive for all 10 with fetal toxoplasmosis. In this study, the PCR was considerably more sensitive than recovering the parasite from amniotic fluid using culture methods (40%) or detection of specific fetal IgM (40%).[136] Similarly, Grover and associates amplified the *B1* gene and found the PCR method to be more sensitive than the traditional techniques used for the prenatal diagnosis of toxoplasmosis.[135] The PCR can provide results within hours, compared with tissue cultures which require a minimum of 4 days or animal inoculation techniques, which take at least 5 weeks to complete.[136] The sensitivity of PCR analysis, coupled with its rapidity, makes it promising as a diagnostic tool because it can minimize the rate of late pregnancy terminations with their relatively increased risk.

TREATMENT

Acute toxoplasmosis in the healthy, nonpregnant woman usually requires no specific therapy because of its benign, self-limited nature. Drugs used to treat toxoplasmosis are active against tachyzoites, but they generally have no effect on the encysted form of the parasite.

Pregnancy termination should be confined to women who become infected during the first one-half of their pregnancy. Although the risk of transmission of the parasite to the fetus is at its lowest during this stage, the severity of fetal disease is usually at its greatest. Acutely infected women who elect to proceed with their pregnancies should be treated with spiramycin as soon after diagnosis as possible.[106] Spiramycin is a macrolide antibiotic that is active against *T. gondii* and can cross the placenta to enter the cord blood and amniotic fluid.[137] It achieves high tissue levels, especially in the placenta. The main adverse effects of spiramycin are nausea, vomiting, and diarrhea. The drug reduces the risk of intrauterine transmission of the parasite, but it does not alter fetal pathology after infection has developed. Spiramycin is only available by request from the Food and Drug Administration; the adult dose is 2 to 4 g daily, given orally in two to four divided doses.[106]

If prenatal diagnosis is attempted and a fetus is shown to be infected, drugs such as pyrimethamine and sulfadiazine are added. Pyrimethamine, an antimalarial drug, is a folic acid antagonist. Its half-life in adults is about 100 hours, and it achieves tissue concentrations (*e.g.*, brain) that are higher than in serum.[138] The drug causes bone marrow suppression with resultant anemia, granulocytopenia, and thrombocytopenia; severe pancytopenia occasionally occurs.[139] Other side-effects include a bad taste in the mouth, headache, and gastrointestinal discomfort. Pyrimethamine has been shown to be teratogenic in animals receiving massive doses of the drug early in organogenesis, and it should not be used before the fifth month of pregnancy.[106] Sulfadiazine or the trisulfapyrimidines act synergistically with pyrimethamine against *Toxoplasma* tachyzoites; other sulfonamides show less synergy and are not used. These drugs are folic acid antagonists. Side-effects include bone marrow suppression, rashes, crystalluria, hematuria, and reversible acute renal failure.[138] One regimen used to treat pregnant women with an infected fetus incorporates 3-week courses of a combination of pyrimethamine (50 mg/day), sulfadiazine (3 g/day), and leucovorin supplements (10 mg/day), alternating with 3 weeks of spiramycin (3 g/day).[116] Leucovorin (folinic acid) is used to counteract the bone marrow suppressive effects of pyrimethamine and sulfadiazine. This treatment regimen is thought to reduce the occurrence of severe congenital infection and increase the proportion of infants born with asymptomatic toxoplasmosis. For ethical reasons, the study inferring that the drugs were efficacious did not include a control group of patients and relied on historic comparisons for its conclusions.[116]

PREVENTION

A vaccine against *T. gondii* is not yet available. Primary prevention rests on educating susceptible pregnant women on how to avoid becoming infected with this parasite. Cats that are kept indoors and only eat dried, cooked, or canned food are unlikely to get infected and shed oocysts. Contact with cat feces should be avoided; disposable gloves should be worn when handling cat litter boxes or while gardening. Cat litter boxes should be emptied of cat feces daily and disinfected by adding boiling water to the empty box for 5 minutes. Covering children's sandboxes decreases the risk of contamination. Meat should be cooked at 66°C or higher temperatures, smoked, or cured in brine. Hands should not touch the eyes or mouth when handling raw meat, and they must be washed thoroughly afterward. Kitchen surfaces should be cleaned carefully. Fruits and vegetables may have oocysts on their surfaces and should be washed or peeled before being eaten.[140–142]

Prenatal education programs can bring about changes in personal behavior that reduce a susceptible woman's risk of acquiring toxoplasmosis.[143] Although it is generally believed that health education reduces the occurrence of gestational toxoplasmosis, the extent of this benefit is uncertain.[144–146] Foulon and colleagues found that when a group of susceptible pregnant women in Belgium implemented these suggestions, the predicted seroconversion rates decreased by only 34%.[144] This is possibly a reflection of how difficult it is to consistently follow the instructions.

Secondary prevention entails the identification and treatment of pregnant women who are acutely infected. Because about 90% of patients with acute toxoplasmosis have minimal or no symptoms, a systematic serologic screening program would be needed. A national prevention program for congenital toxoplasmosis that mandates monthly serologic screening of all seronegative pregnant women has been in place since 1976 in France.[142] A comparable policy for routine screening does not exist for the United States.

Women found to be seronegative early in pregnancy should be advised to follow the hygienic measures outlined earlier. Retesting at 18 to 22 weeks of gestation can identify women who seroconverted during the first one-half of their pregnancy, affording them the opportunity to consider options such as maternal chemotherapy, prenatal diagnostic procedures, or elective pregnancy termination. Seronegative women gain from testing at the end of pregnancy; this helps to identify asymptomatic newborns with toxoplasmosis who may derive benefit from treatment during the first year of life.

Women found to be seropositive early in gestation should be evaluated further to exclude a recent *Toxoplasma* infection. As a group, infants born to seropositive pregnant women with IHA titers of 1:256 to 1:512 have double the predicted frequency of deafness, a 60% increase in microcephaly, and a 30% increase in the occurrence of intelligence quotients less than 70.[107]

CONGENITAL TOXOPLASMOSIS

EPIDEMIOLOGY

The true incidence of congenital toxoplasmosis is unknown. Reported figures underestimate its occurrence. Published rates vary by locale, but they range from 0 to 10 per 1000 live births. Representative incidence estimates per 1000 live births include New York City with 0.7, Birmingham, AL, with 0.12, Mexico City with 2, Paris with 3, and Austria with 8.3.[106]

As treatment of acutely infected pregnant women becomes more commonplace, the occurrence of congenital toxoplasmosis should decline. Trimester-specific *T. gondii* transmission rates have been shown to decrease with proper maternal chemotherapy from 25% to 8% for the first trimester, from 54% to 19% for the second trimester, and from 65% to 44% for the third trimester.[106]

CLINICAL MANIFESTATIONS

About two-thirds of infants with congenital toxoplasmosis have inapparent disease at birth; however, a third of all asymptomatic neonates who undergo detailed examinations are found to have abnormalities such as CSF pleocytosis or elevated protein content (20%), chorioretinitis (15%), or intracranial calcifications (10%).[106] Several weeks or months later, untreated infants develop signs or symptoms of disease.

Symptomatic *Toxoplasma* infection of the newborn can be mild, moderate, or severe. It can involve multiple organ systems or present as isolated abnormalities such as hydrocephalus, hepatosplenomegaly, or prolonged hyperbilirubinemia. Approximately 25% to 50% of symptomatic infants are delivered prematurely. Only 10% of infected infants have severe disease at birth. Systemic manifestations such as fever, jaundice, anemia, hepatomegaly, splenomegaly, or chorioretinitis may predominate in some infants, and neurologic abnormalities such as encephalitis, seizures, hydrocephalus, or intracranial calcifications may be prominent in others. About 10% of congenitally infected infants who have severe disease die, and most surviving infants are left with major neurologic sequelae, such as mental retardation, seizures, spasticity, or visual deficits.[10]

Central nervous system involvement is common. Parenchymal lesions may extend to surrounding blood vessels, leading to vasculitis with thrombosis and infarction. Substantial destruction of brain parenchyma can lead to obstruction of the aqueduct of Sylvius with resultant secondary enlargements of the third and lateral ventricles and, ultimately, hydrocephalus. Hydrocephalus can be the sole manifestation of congenital toxoplasmosis. It may be present at birth or develop later in infancy, and it may be static or gradually worsen to the point of requiring shunt placement. Diffuse intracranial calcifications occur in 10% to 15% of infants with congenital toxoplasmosis, but they can be found in 30% to 65% of those with symptomatic disease at birth (Fig. 47-2).[106] They may increase in number and size over time. Other neurologic findings encountered in this infection include bulging anterior fontanelle, encephalitis, hydranencephaly, hypotonia or paralysis, spasticity, microcephaly, opisthotonus, swallowing difficulties, and CSF pleocytosis. Radiologic CNS findings may be consistent with an old insult (*e.g.*, hydrocephalus, porencephaly, encephalomalacia, cortical atrophy) or, less commonly, with an acute process (*e.g.*, single or multiple hypodense lesions with contrast ring enhancement).[147]

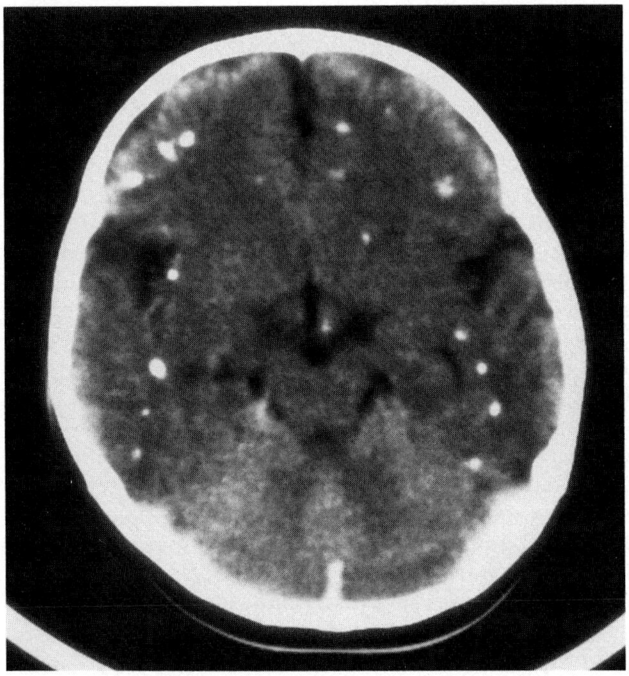

FIG. 47–2. Computerized axial head tomogram of a 5-month-old girl with congenital toxoplasmosis. Notice the diffuse parenchymal calcifications and the prominent subarachnoid space bilaterally.

Manifestations of active congenital ocular toxoplasmosis may include chorioretinal scars, chorioretinitis, iritis, leukocoria, microphthalmia. nystagmus, optic atrophy, optic coloboma, retinal folds and traction detachments, granulomas in the posterior pole, strabismus, small cornea, or cataracts.[10,148] On ophthalmoscopy, the typical findings are single or multiple yellow–white, fluffy necrotic lesions with indistinct margins that arise at the borders of preexisting, healed, hyperpigmented retinochoroidal scars. Macular involvement is common; other findings may include retinal hemorrhages, iridocyclitis, vitreous haziness, papillitis, and papilledema. Untreated infants who were asymptomatic at birth are at great risk of subsequent development of chorioretinitis (about 50% for patients older than 10 years).[10]

Sensorineural hearing loss may occur in 15% to 25% of congenitally infected infants, and educationally significant hearing loss afflicts 10% to 15% of infected infants.[149] *T. gondii* has been found in the mastoid and middle ear at autopsy of some infants. Gastrointestinal disturbances such as feeding difficulties, diarrhea, and vomiting are common. The liver and spleen may be enlarged, and hepatic calcifications may be found. Conjugated hyperbilirubinemia sometimes takes months to subside. Biliary atresia associated with congenital toxoplasmosis has been reported in 1 infant.[150] Myocarditis, nephrotic syndrome, hydrops fetalis, interstitial pneumonia, and skeletal metaphyseal lucencies occur infrequently. Cutaneous lesions include ecchymoses, petechiae, purpura, or maculopapular rashes.

Hematologic abnormalities include anemia, eosinophilia, and thrombocytopenia.[106] Transient quantitative (*e.g.*, neutropenia) and qualitative (*e.g.*, enlarged, vacuolated lymphocytes) changes in the leukocytes are common.[151] Total CD4 lymphocyte counts and CD4 : CD8 ratios are usually depressed.[152] Compared with adults, infants with congenital toxoplasmosis have no or reduced lymphocyte blastogenic responses on exposure to *Toxoplasma* lysate antigens, with failure to produce interferon-γ or interleukin-2; however, they do respond normally to nonspecific stimulators such as concanavalin A.[153] The severe organ damage seen in congenital toxoplasmosis may be due to specific deficits in cell-mediated immune responses to *Toxoplasma* antigens.

DIAGNOSIS

Congenital toxoplasmosis is diagnosed if the parasite is recovered from the placenta. *T. gondii* can be isolated from the blood of asymptomatic or symptomatic infants; isolation rates peak at 71% during the first week of life and then decline to 33% at 2 to 4 weeks of age. Attempts at recovering the parasite from the blood of older infants are generally fruitless. The detection of *Toxoplasma* antigens or DNA in body fluids such as urine, CSF, or serum is considered diagnostic.[10,154]

Specific IgM antibodies can be detected in the serum of 25% of congenitally infected infants with the IFA method and in as many as 75% with the DS-IgM-ELISA technique.[106] The sensitivity of the IgM-ISAGA test is probably even greater.[155] Passively transferred maternal anti-*Toxoplasma* IgG antibodies can suppress an infant's specific IgM response. Gross and colleagues have shown that about 5% of sera have strain-specific immune responses.[127,154] Unless antigens from more than one *T. gondii* strain are used in the assay, the sera would have no detectable specific antibodies in one test but be positive in another.[127] IgM antibodies can persist for over 1 year when measured by very sensitive assays.[155] Rarely, intrathecal production of anti-*Toxoplasma* IgM is demonstrable despite the absence of specific antibodies in the serum of congenitally infected infants with CNS involvement.[154]

Levels of anti-*Toxoplasma* IgG antibodies of maternal origin typically drop at a rate of 50% per month in the infant's serum, but they may continue to be detectable for about 1 year. Active congenital infection should be suspected if specific IgG titers do not show the anticipated decline or if they increase. Untreated infants begin synthesizing their own anti-*Toxoplasma* IgG antibodies by 3 months of age. The intrathecal production of specific IgG is demonstrable in about 2% of infants with CNS involvement.[106]

Toxoplasma-specific serum IgA antibodies are detectable in most congenitally infected infants, significantly more often than IgM antibodies.[126,128,134,156] Specific IgA antibodies were found in the CSF of the few infants in whom it had been measured.[128] Specific serum IgE antibodies can be measured from birth in some patients, especially infants with complications such as hydrocephalus or chorioretinitis.[129]

Transformation of lymphocytes on exposure to *Toxoplasma* antigens is a sensitive and specific indicator of congenital infection if performed on symptomatic or asymptomatic infants 3 months of age or older.[10,157] The observed blastogenic response is lower in infants than in infected adults.[153]

TREATMENT

Controlled trials examining the benefits of various treatment protocols are lacking. Drug regimens have been arrived at empirically, and conclusions about their efficacies are based on comparisons with historic data. A randomized, prospective study by the Toxoplasmosis Study Group aiming at addressing these deficiencies is under way.

The treatment of symptomatic infants during the first 6 months of life usually consists of a combination of pyrimethamine, sulfadiazine, and leucovorin supplements. Pyrimethamine (1 mg/kg orally; maximum, 25 mg) in one or two divided doses is given daily or every other day. A 75 mg/kg/day loading dose of sulfadiazine (maximum, 4 g/day) in two divided oral doses is given for the first 2 days, followed by 100 mg/kg/day (maximum, 8 g/day) in two divided oral doses administered daily thereafter. Leucovorin (5 mg) is injected intramuscularly every 3 days; the dose can be increased to 10 mg every 3 days in infants with bone marrow toxicities.[106] After the first 6 months of treatment are completed, the regimen is modified to include 1-month courses of spiramycin alternating with 1-month courses of pyrimethamine, sulfadiazine, and leucovorin supplements for an additional 6 months. Spiramycin is given daily at a dose of 100 mg/kg/day (maximum, 2–4 g/day) in two to four divided oral doses.

Corticosteroids such as prednisone or methylprednisolone (1.5 mg/kg/day orally in two divided doses) are used in infants with chorioretinitis or CSF protein elevations to reduce the inflammatory response.[106,158] They should be used concurrently with anti-*Toxoplasma* drugs.

Infants with asymptomatic congenital toxoplasmosis are treated for 1 year. They receive an initial 6-week course of pyrimethamine, sulfadiazine, and leucovorin supplements, followed by alternating courses of spiramycin for 6 weeks and the pyrimethamine, sulfadiazine, and leucovorin combination for 4 weeks.

Healthy infants born to mothers with gestational toxoplasmosis can be treated with a 3-week course of pyrimethamine, sulfadiazine, and leucovorin followed by 4 to 6 weeks of spiramycin. If the diagnosis of congenital toxoplasmosis is later established, chemotherapy is continued as delineated earlier for infants with subclinical *T. gondii* infection. For healthy infants born to mothers with high Sabin–Feldman dye test titers and undetermined timing of maternal infection, a 1-month course of spiramycin is usually prescribed. Therapy is extended if clinical or laboratory evidence of congenital toxoplasmosis is uncovered.

Pyrimethamine serum levels do not vary significantly with age during infancy; they are comparable for infants receiving the drug daily or every other day. Pyrimethamine serum concentrations and half-life may be reduced in infants concomitantly treated with phenobarbital. The drug achieves CSF concentrations that are 10% to 25% of concurrently measured serum levels. Seizures have been observed in patients with pyrimethamine overdosage.[159]

Clindamycin has been used effectively for the treatment of ocular toxoplasmosis in older patients because of its tendency to concentrate in the choroid.[158] There are no data on its efficacy in congenital infection. Photocoagulation of active lesions and of normal retinal tissues immediately bordering chorioretinal scars may be helpful in reducing recurrences.[160]

Infants treated with pyrimethamine and sulfadiazine should be closely monitored. Weekly blood counts, platelet counts, and urine microscopic analysis are suggested for the early detection of adverse drug effects.

PROGNOSIS

Most infants with severe symptomatic congenital toxoplasmosis who survive beyond the neonatal period suffer from serious long-term residual problems, such as mental retardation and blindness.[108] This grim outlook does not apply to all infants with congenital infection. Short-term follow-up studies indicate that maternal therapy during gestation, followed postnatally by treatment of all congenitally infected infants, improves prognosis by reducing the frequency and severity of late-appearing disease sequelae. In the study by Hohlfeld and colleagues, congenital infection remained subclinical in 76%. Almost all treated infants developed normally and were neurologically normal.[116] Peripheral chorioretinitis that did not impair vision developed in about 10% between 5 and 17 months of age. In another study, early institution of anti-*Toxoplasma* therapy may have prevented the occurrence of sensorineural hearing loss in congenitally infected infants.[149] Preliminary data by Guerina and colleagues after only 2 years of follow-up suggest that progression of congenital toxoplasmosis can be halted for most infants by beginning specific therapy early in infancy.[161]

Long-term follow-up of infants with symptomatic or subclinical congenital toxoplasmosis suggest that most patients develop chorioretinitis or chorioretinal scars by 10 to 20 years of age, but treatment may reduce the frequency and severity of adverse sequelae.[162–164] The rates at which other residual abnormalities, such as mental retardation or neurologic dysfunction, occur are unknown.

RUBELLA

Rubella (*i.e.*, German measles, third disease) typically is a subclinical or mild exanthematous infection of children and adults. Gestational rubella can have deleterious effects on the fetus. The infant may have physical and mental abnormalities, such as cataracts, congenital heart disease, deafness, microcephaly, or psychomotor retardation, or present with severe neonatal diseases that include thrombocytopenia, bleeding, hepatosplenomegaly, pneumonia, and myocarditis. Some manifestations of congenital rubella infection may not appear until years or decades later, even among patients asymptomatic at birth.[5]

The rubella virus is an enveloped, single-stranded RNA virus that is spherical and has spikelike projections containing hemagglutinin. Only one antigenic type of the virus is known, and man is its only natural host. It has three structural polypeptides; two are envelope glycoproteins (*i.e.*, E1 and E2), and one is a nonglycosylated RNA-associated capsid protein (*i.e.*, C). Different epitopes of E1 are responsible for viral hemagglutination and neutralization, and E2 accounts for the minor differences among rubella strains.[165]

Person-to-person transmission usually occurs by airborne spread of infected respiratory secretions, and direct contact with virus-containing urine or feces is a less likely route of infection. Although rubella virus can be recovered from the genital tract of infected women, vertical transmission during pregnancy is believed to occur almost exclusively through the placenta.[166,167]

On entry into the body in cases of postnatal infection, the rubella virus multiplies in nasopharyngeal epithelial cells and in local lymph nodes. This is followed by a period of viremia and shedding from the throat. It is during this maternal viremic phase that placental and fetal infection occurs. The frequency and nature of fetal involvement depends on the mother's immune status against the virus and the timing during gestation of maternal rubella.[5]

The mechanisms by which the virus ravages the fetus are not clearly understood. Necrotic placental vascular endothelial cells can serve as a source of virus-infected emboli. Damage to endothelial cells can lead to thrombosis of small blood vessels, resulting in hypoxic tissue damage.[168,169] Rubella-infected cells have diminished mitotic activity due to chromosomal breaks, the production of a mitosis-inhibiting protein, or damaging effects of the virus on actin-containing cytoskeletal filaments.[170–173] Focal lysis of infected cells can be seen in some organs, but inflammation is not a salient feature of congenital rubella.[168] Growth-retarded infants have reduced cell numbers on histopathologic examination.[174] Moreover, the virus can modify cell receptors for specific growth factors.[175] Late-onset manifestations of congenital rubella may be due to viral persistence with ongoing cell destruction or to organ damage by means of a number of immune mechanisms such as circulating rubella-specific immune complexes, defective cytotoxic effector cell function, or the development of autoimmunity.[176–179] Rubella virus E1 and E2 structural proteins, but not the C nucleoprotein, appear to be responsible for autoantibody induction.[180]

Long-lasting immunity normally develops after recovery from postnatal rubella. Reinfections can occur in persons with low antibody titers, but these are usually asymptomatic.[167] Persons with low antibody levels after rubella vaccination are more prone to reinfections than persons with similarly low titers after natural infection.[167]

Circulating antibodies and cell-mediated immune responses are generated after rubella infection. Rubella-specific IgM, IgG, IgA, IgD, and IgE antibodies are induced in response to postnatal infection.[181] IgM antibodies appear early and are short lived, and they usually disappear 5 to 8 weeks after onset of illness, although rubella-specific IgM antibodies rarely persist for months or years.[182,183] The IgM response after rubella vaccination or natural reinfection is generally weak and of brief duration.[184–186] Specific IgD and IgE antibodies appear early and then decline more slowly than specific IgM antibodies.[181] Specific IgA antibodies generally emerge within the first 10 days of illness, and they may continue to be measurable for periods ranging from 3 weeks to several years.[181,187] Rubella-specific IgG antibodies increase rapidly and persist throughout life; rubella-specific IgG1 has been shown to be the principal IgG subclass.[167,188] The most vigorous antibody and lymphocyte proliferative responses in postnatal rubella are directed against glycoprotein E1.[189,190] Men and women appear to differ in the nature and magnitude of their antibody responses to rubella virus structural proteins.[191] Men never produce anti-E2 IgA and generate significantly lower levels of IgG antibodies directed against E2 than women. Anti-E1 IgM and IgG antibodies appear earlier in male patients, but female patients have higher levels of rubella-specific IgG antibodies after recovery from the illness. The observed gender differences in antibody responses to viral proteins may be under genetic or hormonal influences and may be related to the increased susceptibility of women to the joint complications of rubella.[191]

Immune responses in congenitally infected infants differ from those observed in adults with rubella. Fetal IgM production usually begins after 16 weeks of gestation. Rubella-specific IgM antibodies are detectable until 6 to 12 months of age. Specific IgG antibody levels decrease over time; as many as 20% of affected children have no measurable antibody titers by 5 years of age.[167] Circulating antirubella antibodies in infants with intrauterine infection have lower affinities to rubella antigen than antibodies from adults with natural infection.[192] Serum antibodies to the E2 glycoprotein are quantitatively more abundant than those directed against E1 in some patients with congenital rubella, particularly among older infants; antibody reactivities against the C protein are poor.[189,193] Infants with congenital rubella have diminished cell-mediated immune responses on exposure to rubella antigens compared with children or adults with postnatal infection, and the responses are weakest for infants infected earlier during gestation.[194]

MATERNAL RUBELLA

EPIDEMIOLOGY

Epidemics of rubella formerly occurred at 6- to 9-year intervals in the United States. The last major pandemic took place between 1964 and 1965, during which time 20,000 cases of congenital rubella occurred. Rubella did not become a notifiable disease in the United States until 1966. From 1966 through 1971, between 45,000 and 58,000 cases of postnatal rubella were reported to the CDC each year.[11] Since licensure of the rubella vaccine in 1969, the number of rubella cases declined by more than 99%, and from 1980 to 1988, the number of cases decreased from 3904 to 225.[11] However, a resurgence of rubella was found for 1989 through 1991, and 1401 cases were reported for 1991 alone. Outbreaks of infection occur mostly in unimmunized populations such as inner city children and adults, illegal aliens, prison inmates, and religious groups that refuse vaccination (*e.g.*, Amish communities).[14,195–198] Medical students and other health professionals serve as vectors for rubella infection, placing susceptible pregnant women to whom they are exposed in a medical setting at significant risk.[199]

Approximately 10% to 20% of women of childbearing age (≥15 years of age) are susceptible to rubella, and more than 70% of cases occur among persons in this age group.[200] Women delivering infants with the congenital rubella syndrome (CRS) tend to be younger than the national average for mothers giving birth in the United States; a disproportionate number of these mothers are African-American or Hispanic.[195] Rubella susceptibility rates for women of childbearing age in European countries are generally comparable to those found in the United States, but lower seropositivity rates are encountered among island populations such as in Hawaii and Jamaica and in certain tropical African countries.[167,201–204] Significant regional differences have been found in large countries, such as India and China.[205,206]

CLINICAL MANIFESTATIONS

Over 30% of postnatal rubella infections are subclinical.[200] Illness occurs 14 to 21 days (mean, 18 days) after exposure. A prodrome consisting of malaise, low-grade fever that rarely lasts beyond the first day of the exanthem, headache, and conjunctivitis precede the rash by 1 to 5 days. The exanthem consists of discrete macules or papules that initially appear on the face and behind the ears, spread downward over 1 to 2 days, and usually disappear over 3 to 5 days; rubella virus can be isolated from these skin lesions.[207] Postauricular, suboccipital, and posterior cervical lymphadenopathy is common and may persist for several weeks. Complications of rubella develop more frequently in adults. Transient arthralgias may occur in as many as one-third of infected women, but arthritis is uncommon.[5] Other complications are rare and include thrombocytopenic purpura, hemolytic anemia, hepatitis, Guillain–Barré syndrome, encephalitis, progressive panencephalitis, myelitis, peripheral neuritis, myocarditis, and pericarditis.[5,208–210]

Pregnancy has no effect on the natural course of rubella infection. However, rubella is associated with an increased risk of miscarriages, spontaneous abortions, and stillbirths.[5]

LABORATORY DIAGNOSIS

The diagnosis of rubella on clinical grounds alone is unreliable because similar illnesses may be produced by enteroviruses, measles virus, or parvovirus B19. Laboratory confirmation by virus isolation or serologic testing is thus essential in pregnant women, for whom an accurate diagnosis of gestational rubella is critical. Shirley and colleagues investigated 627 patients clinically suspected of having rubella, but they could confirm this diagnosis in only 229 (37%).[211] Human parvovirus B19 infection accounted for 7%, measles for 1%, and other infectious agents for 1%; the causes for the remainder (54%) remained unknown.

Rubella virus is shed from the nasopharynx for 1 week before and 1 week after onset of the rash. The virus is present in blood and urine during the week preceding the exanthem but disappears thereafter. Rubella virus isolation is impractical for diagnostic purposes because it is expensive, labor intensive, and frequently unavailable to the clinician.

Serologic techniques are the most useful methods for diagnosing rubella infection. Available tests include hemagglutination inhibition (HI), ELISA, immunofluorescence, radioimmunoassay (RIA), hemolysis in gel, complement fixation, passive hemagglutination, and latex agglutination tests.[186,212] Serum specimens obtained as soon as feasible after the appearance of the exanthem and again 2 weeks later can prove the diagnosis if seroconversion or a fourfold or greater rise in rubella-specific antibody titers can be documented. Paired sera are best tested in unison because of the variability in results of assays done on separate days or by different personnel. If measured by ELISA, HI, or RIA, rubella-specific IgG antibodies can be found as early as 1 to 2 days before the emergence of the rash; if assayed by the less readily available passive hemagglutination method, these antibodies are not detected until 15 to 50 days after onset of the exanthem, and peak approximately 6 to 7 months later. The detection of rubella-specific IgM antibodies within 28 days of the appearance of the rash is also diagnostic.[213] Newer tests that can be used for the diagnosis of acute postnatal rubella include avidity-ELISA, in which acutely infected persons have low IgG avidity compared with persons previously immune to rubella who exhibit greater IgG avidity.[214] IgG produced in response to rubella vaccination shows low avidity to rubella antigens during the first 2 months after immunization, but this increases significantly over the ensuing months and remains at high levels thereafter.[215] Immunoblot techniques have been developed for the sensitive detection of rubella-specific IgG, IgM, and IgA antibodies.[216]

Rubella reinfections are confirmed by a fourfold or greater rise in the titer of preexisting rubella-specific IgG antibodies. The specific IgM response is absent or weak, but it is sometimes high enough to be within the range deemed sufficient for the diagnosis of primary rubella.[186]

False-positive IgM reactions can occur in sera containing rheumatoid factor, although the IgM capture assay appears to be unaffected by its presence.[186] Cross-reactions between rubella and human parvovirus B19 infections in specific IgM tests necessitate caution in interpreting low or equivocal levels of rubella-specific IgM antibodies.[217]

TREATMENT

Therapy of postnatal rubella is symptomatic. Patients with rubella shed the virus from the nasopharynx for 1 week after appearance of the rash, and they should therefore avoid contact with susceptible persons until the exanthem has vanished.

PREVENTION

The principal goal of rubella immunization programs is the elimination of CRS. The vaccine used in the United States is the RA 27/3 attenuated live rubella virus vaccine.[200] It is available in a monovalent form (*i.e.*, rubella only) and in combinations with measles, mumps, or both (*i.e.*, MMR). The vaccine induces antirubella antibodies in more than 95% of recipients 12 months of age or older, and its protective efficacy is greater than 90% for at least 15 years.[200] Immunizing children whose pregnant mothers are susceptible to rubella does not pose a threat to the mother or her fetus. The vaccine is recommended for all susceptible persons 12 months of age or older and is usually given at 15 months of age; a second booster dose is given to children at the time of school entry.

A clinical diagnosis of rubella is considered unreliable and cannot be considered proof of immunity. Persons are deemed protected if they have serologic evidence of immunity or had previously been vaccinated on or after their first birthday.

Pregnant women whose rubella-immune status is not known should be tested for the presence of antirubella antibodies during their first prenatal visit. If a previously unimmunized pregnant woman with unknown antibody status is exposed to rubella, a blood sample should be immediately obtained for rubella antibody testing. If antibody to rubella is found, the woman is considered immune. The risk of rubella reinfection after natural disease or vaccination is small, but it is more likely to occur in women with low specific IgG titers. Significant fetal pathology after reinfection occurs infrequently, despite rubella virus transmission to the fetus.[218–228]

Susceptible women exposed to rubella should be informed of the risks to the fetus if maternal infection occurs. If the woman develops fever, lymphadenopathy, or a rash within the expected incubation period, serum for rubella-specific IgM assay should be obtained. If a clinical illness does not occur, serum should be obtained 6 to 8 weeks after exposure to exclude a subclinical infection. For women who seroconvert or become positive for rubella-specific IgM, the rate of fetal infection is 81% after maternal rubella during the first 12 weeks of gestation, 54% at 13 to 16 weeks, 36% at 17 to 22 weeks, 30% at 23 to 30 weeks, 60% at 31 to 36 weeks, and 100% at more than 36 weeks of pregnancy.[229] Infants infected before 11 weeks of gestation usually develop congenital defects, most often cardiac anomalies and deafness, but only 35% of infants infected at 13 to 16 weeks of gestation have abnormalities at birth, usually deafness.[229] In a study of 106 infants with confirmed CRS in whom the timing of maternal infection was known with reasonable accuracy, Munro and colleagues found deafness in 58% of patients, and it was the sole abnormality in 40% of all infants; infants with congenital cardiac, ocular, or CNS defects were almost always deaf as well.[230] The risk of deafness is small if maternal infection occurs at 17 weeks of gestation or later.[229,230] Other investigators have confirmed that rubella virus can be transmitted to the fetus at any stage of pregnancy, and that the earlier the maternal infection during pregnancy, the greater is the severity of congenital defects.[231–233]

If maternal rubella occurs during the first 5 months of pregnancy, the option of therapeutic pregnancy termination can be considered. Infections occurring after this time do not produce congenital defects. If available, an attempt at prenatal diagnosis can be made, because fetal involvement after maternal rubella is not universal. The virus has been isolated from amniotic fluid by culture or directly visualized using electron microscopy in a few cases.[234,235] The low sensitivities of these methods limits their usefulness. Daffos and colleagues studied 18 pregnancies complicated by maternal rubella; fetal blood was obtained at 20 to 26 weeks of gestation, and rubella-specific IgM was detected in 12 fetuses.[236] Contamination of fetal blood specimens by maternal blood was excluded. Of the 6 fetuses without detectable rubella-specific IgM antibodies, 1 was found to be infected at birth.[236] In another study, investigators were able to detect rubella-specific IgM and IgA as early as 22 weeks of pregnancy.[187] The drawbacks of this method are that the fetus does not synthesize IgM until the fifth month of gestation, and the quantity produced initially may be meager and below the limits of detection of the assay. Despite these disadvantages, the technique has been found to be helpful in the management of pregnancies complicated by maternal rubella.[237]

Terry and associates detected rubella antigens and RNA sequences in a chorionic villus biopsy specimen obtained at 11 weeks of gestation from a woman with rubella in early pregnancy, and this led to pregnancy termination at week 13 of gestation; infection was verified in the aborted fetus and placenta by virus isolation, immunoblotting, and hybridization methods.[238] Hybridization techniques appear to be more sensitive than viral isolation methods, and the PCR has been used successfully to enhance the yield from infected fetal and placental tissues.[235,239,240] Molecular biologic techniques for the prenatal diagnosis of rubella are research tools and are not readily available for clinical use.

The administration of immunoglobulin to susceptible pregnant women who are exposed to rubella does not prevent maternal or fetal infection. Its use is confined to women who would not contemplate pregnancy termination under any circumstances.[200]

Pregnant women who do not have rubella antibody are usually immunized in the immediate postpartum period. However, reports by a group of investigators from Canada have shown that acute arthritis occurs in as many as 8% of women receiving the rubella RA 27/3 vaccine in the postpartum period, and that some subsequently develop chronic arthropathy, neurologic abnormalities such as the carpal tunnel syndrome or paresthesias, and chronic rubella viremia.[241] These women tend to transmit rubella virus to some of their infants through breast-feeding, and a few infected infants develop chronic rubella viremia.[241,242] Data from the United States and elsewhere indicate that such complications are rare with the RA 27/3 live rubella vaccine.[200] The mechanisms of rubella vaccine-induced joint disease are poorly understood, but they may include infection of the synovial membrane by vaccine virus or the deposition of rubella antigen-containing immune complexes in the synovium.[243] It is advised that all susceptible pregnant women be vaccinated against rubella before hospital discharge.[200] It is estimated that 40% to 55% of CRS cases could have been prevented had the opportunity to implement postpartum rubella immunization of susceptible women not been missed.[195,197] Although rubella vaccine virus can be shed in breast milk, breastfeeding is not a contraindication to maternal immunization.[200,244]

The rubella vaccine should not be knowingly administered during pregnancy because of its small risk of teratogenicity. Data for the 1979 to 1988 period from the CDC indicate that none of 562 infants born to 683 women inadvertently immunized with the RA 27/3 vaccine within 3 months of conception in the United States had malformations compatible with CRS.[245] Between January 1971 and April 1989, 321 known rubella-susceptible women who had been immunized against rubella within 3 months before or after their estimated date of conception with the RA 27/3 or earlier vaccines (Cendehill, HPV-77) were followed by the CDC; none of the 324 infants born to these women had defects consistent with the CRS.[200] The RA 27/3 rubella vaccine virus, however, does cross the placenta and produces a subclinical infection in about 3% of infants; the rate of fetal infection was considerably higher (20%) for the earlier rubella vaccines.[245] The possible risk of serious congenital defects after accidental rubella vaccination has been calculated by the CDC to be 0% to 1.6%; the observed risk has been zero.[200] This risk is considerably lower than the 20% or greater risk of CRS after maternal gestational infection, and it is comparable to the 2% to 3% rate of major birth defects observed in the absence of rubella vaccine exposure.[245]

CONGENITAL RUBELLA

EPIDEMIOLOGY

The incidence of congenital rubella has shown a consistent decline since the introduction of rubella vaccination programs in the United States. From 1980 to 1989, the incidence of CRS decreased from 0.39 per 100,000 live births to 0.05 per 100,000 live births.[14] However, the number of indigenous and imported CRS cases for 1989, 1990, and 1991 were 3, 11, and 47, respectively.[11] The observed increase was largely due to a cluster of cases from southern California.[197] About one-half of the cases could have been prevented by postpartum immunization of susceptible mothers after earlier pregnancies. Maternal risk factors for CRS include young age, African-American race, and Hispanic ethnicity.[14] In the southern California cluster, approximately 40% of the mothers were never married and about 60% were primigravidas.[197] Because of the passive nature of the CRS reporting system, it is estimated that the reported number of infants with CRS represents only 20% to 30% of actual cases.[15]

Congenital rubella syndrome continues to be a problem in other parts of the world.[201,246] However, rubella immunization programs have been successful in reducing the occurrence of CRS wherever implemented.[247,248] As an example, the incidence of CRS declined from 3.5 per 100,000 live births in 1980 to 0.41 per 100,000 live births in 1986 in 19 European birth defects registries.[248]

CLINICAL MANIFESTATIONS

More than one-half of all newborns with congenital rubella are asymptomatic at birth, but most later manifest with one or more signs and symptoms of disease. The most common abnormalities encountered in CRS listed in order of decreasing frequency are sensorineural hearing loss, mental retardation, cardiac malformations, and ocular defects.[249] Clinical abnormalities encountered in congenital rubella are summarized in Table 47-3.[5,174,177,178,208,230,250–280]

If the findings of mental retardation and infection of neurosensory organs such as the eyes or ears are combined, then CNS involvement occurs in more than 80% of CRS patients.[208] Vascular abnormalities, a prominent pathologic characteristic of congenital rubella, contributes to the neuropathology by causing ischemic necrosis of adjacent tissues. Microcephaly may be due to the generalized organ hypocellularity seen with rubella infection.[174]

The development of late-onset CRS manifestations that were inapparent in early infancy may be related to persistence or reactivation of rubella virus infection, to the body's immune responses to the infection, or to vascular damage. Insulin-dependent diabetes mellitus occurs in about 20% of patients by 35 years of age.[280] Rubella virus can infect human fetal pancreatic islet cells and can reduce secretion of insulin.[281] About 20% of CRS patients and 50% to 80% of those with glucose intolerance have circulating pancreatic islet cell cytotoxic or surface antibodies.[282] These autoantibodies are triggered by rubella virus and cause destruction of pancreatic β cells, unmasking the person with a genetic susceptibility to diabetes mellitus.[283] Thyroid abnormalities develop in about 5%; thyroid microsomal or thyroglobulin antibodies are found more frequently in deaf CRS patients than in those who are hearing impaired from other causes.[178] Rare cases of growth hormone deficiency of hypothalamic origin have been described.[284] About 10% of CRS patients incur additional forms of late-appearing ocular insults such as glaucoma, keratoconus, corneal hydrops, and spontaneous lens absorption. Permanent damage to the vascular endothelium can induce the formation of obstructive lesions of major vessels such as the pulmonary and renal arteries. Choroidal neovascularization with significant visual loss can complicate CRS retinopathy. Autism and behavioral problems are usually delayed in appearance, and can be progressive. Progressive rubella panencephalitis is a rare but ultimately fatal CNS manifestation of CRS that appears late, usually in the second decade of life.[280]

DIAGNOSIS

The CDC has established clinical and laboratory criteria for the classification of CRS cases to allow better CRS surveillance (Table 47-4).[285]

The diagnosis of CRS usually is suspected on the basis of the maternal history and the clinical findings. A definitive diagnosis can be achieved by isolating the virus from pharyngeal washings or, less commonly, from urine, CSF, conjunctivae, or available organs such as the lens at surgery or autopsy. Although nasopharyngeal shedding of rubella virus may continue for 6 to 12 months, the frequency of its isolation declines from about 85% during the first month of life to approximately 10% at 9 to 12 months of age.[286] In children with congenital rubella encephalitis, the virus can be isolated from the CSF for months or even years.[262] However, viral isolation is seldom employed in clinical practice because of its difficulty, expense, and limited availability.

Rubella-specific IgM is usually present in congenitally infected infants and may persist for 6 to 12 months. It can be used to make a definitive diagnosis of congenital rubella infection; false-positive results may be encountered in sera containing rheumatoid factor. Delays in obtaining serum for IgM measurements can introduce interpretation difficulties be-

Text continued on page 1050

TABLE 47–3
CLINICAL ABNORMALITIES IN INFANTS WITH SYMPTOMATIC CONGENITAL RUBELLA

Clinical Abnormality	Remarks
General	
Intrauterine growth retardation	Common (50%–85%); usually have other manifestations of congenital infection; may be due to reduced number of body cells[174]
Postnatal growth retardation	Retarded growth is most severe in infants with multiple congenital defects; long-term follow-up studies indicate that most will have subnormal growth[250,251]
Cardiovascular system	
Patent ductus arteriosus	Most frequently encountered structural defect (30%); may occur with other heart lesions, especially pulmonary valvular or artery stenosis[230]
Pulmonary artery stenosis	Second most common heart defect; results from intimal proliferation[252]
Miscellaneous defects	Individually uncommon; include coarctation of the aorta, atrial and ventricular septal defects, myocarditis, tetralogy of Fallot, and ventricular aneurysm
Hearing loss	The most common congenital defect; almost always present in infants with other malformations; uncommon if maternal rubella occurs at ≥17 weeks of gestation; usually bilateral; may be present at birth or develop later; can be progressive[5,253]
Ocular abnormalities	
Cataract	Found in about 35% of infants; can be unilateral or bilateral; noted at birth or early infancy; virus can be isolated from lens; spontaneous reabsorption of cataracts has been described in rare cases[254–257]
Retinopathy	Common (35%); may be present at birth or appear later in life; often unilateral; salt-and-pepper appearance; does not affect visual acuity[258–260]
Cloudy cornea	Rare; usually present at birth; may coexist with glaucoma; resolves spontaneously; rarely persists[261]
Glaucoma	Occurs in ≤5%; may be bilateral; can be found at birth or appear later in life; leads to blindness if not treated[5]
Microphthalmia	Common in infants with unilateral cataract[5]
Miscellaneous abnormalities	Uncommon; includes iris hypoplasia, strabismus, and iridocyclitis
Interstitial pneumonia	Occurs in about 5%; probably immunologically mediated; may be acute, subacute, or chronic[177]
Central nervous system	
Meningoencephalitis	Occurs in as many as 20%; manifests with bulging anterior fontanelle, hypotonia, irritability, and seizures; cerebrospinal fluid findings include elevated protein concentration, mononuclear pleocytosis, and rubella virus isolation in 30%; transient; most infants have neurodevelopmental deficits[208,262,263]
Microcephaly	Uncommon; may be associated with normal intelligence
Intracranial calcifications	Rare[264,265]
Electroencephalographic abnormalities	Occurs in 36%; usually resolves by 1 year of age[208]
Mental retardation	Occurs in 10%–20%; associated with other stigmata of congenital rubella
Speech defects	Uncommon in absence of hearing impairment
Behavioral disorders	Common; occurs primarily in deaf patients[262]
Miscellaneous problems	Autism; central language disorders; spastic quadriparesis; hydrocephalus; cerebral arterial stenosis
Skin	
Blueberry-muffin spots	Transient; infrequent (5%); represents dermal erythropoiesis[266]
Chronic rashes	Generalized; persists for weeks; appears in infancy; virus can be isolated from skin[267]
Dermatoglyphic abnormalities	May serve as marker for viral teratogenicity[268]
Genitourinary system	Cryptorchidism; testicular agenesis; polycystic kidneys; renal agenesis; renal artery stenosis with hypertension; hypospadias; hydroureter; hydronephrosis; ureteral duplication[269–272]

(continued)

TABLE 47–3
CLINICAL ABNORMALITIES IN INFANTS WITH SYMPTOMATIC CONGENITAL RUBELLA (*continued*)

Clinical Abnormality	Remarks
Skeletal system	
Metaphyseal radiolucencies	Occurs in 10%–20%; most common in distal femur and proximal tibia; usually normalizes by 3 months of age; due to a direct inhibitory effect of rubella virus on bone and cartilage cells[273–277]
Large anterior fontanelle	Found in the most severely affected infants[273]
Miscellaneous problems	Micrognathia; pathologic fractures; myositis
Gastrointestinal system	
Hepatosplenomegaly	Common (>50%); transient
Hepatitis	Occurs in 5%–10%; may not be associated with jaundice
Obstructive jaundice	Infrequent (5%)
Miscellaneous problems	Esophageal, jejunal, or rectal atresia; pancreatitis; chronic diarrhea
Blood	
Thrombocytopenic purpura	Occurs in 5%–10%; associated with severe disease; transient[273,278]
Anemia	Transient[278]
Miscellaneous abnormalities	Hemolytic anemia; altered blood group expression[279]
Immune system	
Hypogammaglobulinemia	Rare; transient
Thymic hypoplasia	Rare; fatal
Endocrine glands	Diabetes mellitus; hypothyroidism; hyperthyroidism; thyroiditis; growth hormone deficiency; precocious puberty[5,178,280]

TABLE 47–4
OUTLINE OF THE CENTERS FOR DISEASE CONTROL CRITERIA FOR THE CLASSIFICATION OF CONGENITAL RUBELLA SYNDROME CASES

I. Congenital Rubella Syndrome Confirmed

Defects present and at least one of the following:
- Isolation of rubella virus
- Detection of rubella-specific IgM antibodies
- Persistence of rubella-specific hemagglutination inhibition (HI) titer beyond the period expected from that of passively transferred maternal antibodies

II. Congenital Rubella Syndrome Compatible

Incomplete laboratory data for confirmation of diagnosis and any two complications from A or one from A and one from B:
- A. Cataracts or congenital glaucoma, congenital heart disease, hearing loss, pigmentary retinopathy
- B. Purpura, splenomegaly, jaundice, bone radiolucencies, meningoencephalitis, microcephaly, mental retardation

III. Congenital Rubella Syndrome Possible

Some compatible clinical findings but insufficient criteria for the confirmed or compatible categories

IV. Congenital Rubella Infection Only

No defects, but laboratory evidence of infection is found

V. Stillbirths

Stillbirths believed to be a consequence of maternal rubella infection

VI. Congenital Rubella Syndrome Excluded

At least one of the following inconsistent laboratory findings in a child without evidence of an immunodeficiency disease:
- Absence of rubella-specific HI titer in a child ≤24 months of age
- Absence of rubella-specific HI titer in the mother
- Decrease of rubella-specific HI titer in an infant in a manner consistent with that expected from passively transferred maternal antibodies (*i.e.*, a twofold dilution drop per month)

HI, hemagglutination inhibition.
Adapted from Centers for Disease Control. Rubella and congenital rubella syndrome—New York City. MMWR 1986;35:770.

cause of the possibility that the infant may have acquired rubella infection postnatally. Persistence of rubella-specific IgG antibodies at 6 to 12 months of age, especially in high titers, provides presumptive evidence of congenital or early postnatal infection.

Other techniques for establishing the diagnosis of congenital rubella include negative virus-specific lymphocyte transformation responses in seropositive children younger than 3 years of age, detection of rubella-specific IgM in CSF, or demonstration of low avidity rubella-specific IgG in seropositive infants.[192,287,288]

TREATMENT

There is no specific therapy for CRS. A few patients have been treated with amantadine or interferon-α with minimal or no clinical improvement.[179,289–291] Susceptible pregnant women should avoid contact with CRS patients during their first year of life. The appearance of delayed manifestations of CRS that were not present early in life underscores the importance of close follow-up. Congential rubella syndrome patients often require surgical correction of heart or genitourinary defects, removal of dense cataracts, hearing aids, and special schooling.

HEPATITIS B

Hepatitis B virus afflicts nearly 200,000 to 300,000 persons in the United States each year, 6% to 10% of whom become chronic HBV carriers. Estimates from the CDC place the number of chronic, infectious HBV carriers in the United States at about 1 to 1.25 million people.[292] Globally, the number of chronic carriers is approximately 300 million, and more than 250,000 persons die each year from HBV-related acute and chronic hepatic disease.[293] More than a fourth of all carriers develop HBV-related chronic active hepatitis, liver cirrhosis, or hepatocellular carcinoma.[292] Chronic carriers of this virus can transmit HBV to their offspring during pregnancy; as many as 70% to 90% of perinatally infected infants become chronic carriers themselves.[294]

The complete HBV is known as the Dane particle and consists of an outer lipid-containing envelope and an inner core or nucleocapsid. On the surface of the outer coat is the hepatitis B surface antigen (HBsAg), an antigenically complex glycoprotein. HBsAg has many antigenic epitopes that permit the identification of several HBV subtypes; the subtyping scheme is valuable as an epidemiologic tool, but it has no correlation with disease severity. The surface envelope contains three proteins (*i.e.*, major, middle, and large S proteins) coded for by the HBV DNA genome. Variations in the major protein account for the subtype determinants, and the middle and large proteins are implicated in receptor-mediated virus uptake by hepatocytes.[295]

The virus inner core consists of hepatitis B core antigen (HBcAg), hepatitis B e antigen (HBeAg), hepatitis B x antigen (HBxAg), a partially double-stranded DNA molecule, DNA-dependent DNA polymerase enzyme with reverse transcription activity, and a protein kinase. HBcAg is found primarily in the nuclei of infected hepatocytes. In serum, HBcAg is found only as a component of circulating Dane particles, but it is never found in free form. HBeAg is a prematurely terminated polypeptide product of the same gene that codes for HBcAg; its presence in serum indicates infectivity. HBxAg is probably an independent marker of infectivity. Hepatitis B virus DNA is a partially double-stranded DNA, and HBV DNA polymerase repairs the single-stranded HBV DNA region to form a complete double-stranded molecule.[295]

With very sensitive assays, HBsAg can be detected in the blood within 1 to 2 weeks of exposure to HBV. However, clinical disease usually occurs 1 to 3 months, and occasionally 6 months, after exposure. HBeAg can be detected late in the incubation period, usually coinciding with or within days of HBsAg appearance. Hepatitis B virus DNA polymerase and HBV DNA are measurable at this stage and generally peak by the latter part of the incubation period. Their concentrations fall with onset of liver disease. In patients who recover, HBsAg usually can no longer be detected at about the time of clinical resolution.[296]

The earliest antibodies to appear are those directed against HBcAg (anti-HBc), typically 2 to 4 weeks after HBsAg is first detected. Anti-HBc titers increase during the acute stage of infection and persist for many years. Antibodies to HBeAg (anti-HBe) appear immediately after or within several weeks of HBeAg clearance and usually while HBsAg is still present. A window period that occasionally can be as long as 20 weeks follows HBsAg clearance from the circulation, during which neither HBsAg nor anti-HBs are detectable. However, specific IgM and IgG anti-HBc antibodies are usually present, and they may be the only laboratory indicators of an acute HBV infection. The patient is contagious during this period. After anti-HBs antibodies become measurable, their titers continue to increase for approximately 6 to 12 months.[295,296] About 18% of patients have detectable HBV DNA in their serum for 3 to 6 months after first appearance of anti-HBs antibodies.[297] Anti-HBs antibodies persist for life and protect against future HBV reinfections. Antibodies to HBxAg (anti-HBx) can be detected in only 17% of patients with acute HBV infection and usually appear 3 to 4 weeks after onset of clinical symptoms; their clinical significance is not yet defined.[298]

Patients who continue to have detectable serum HBsAg for 20 weeks or longer, HBeAg for 10 weeks or longer, or HBV DNA for 4 weeks or longer are likely to become chronic HBsAg carriers; their serum anti-HBc titers are usually high, and IgM anti-HBc tends to persist for a long time. Approximately 25% to 50% of chronic carriers are HBeAg positive, and the remainder have anti-HBe. Persons who are positive for HBeAg, HBV DNA polymerase, or HBV DNA are highly contagious. Most chronic carriers remain HBV-infected for life, but 1.5% to 2% of carriers spontaneously lose their HBsAg each year. About 25% of chronic carriers whose HBsAg resolves spontaneously have HBV DNA in their serum that can be detected by PCR and are potentially infectious to others; HBV DNA ultimately clears from serum.[295]

Young age is an important risk factor for developing the chronic carrier state; 70% to 90% of infected newborns become carriers, compared with 25% to 50% of children infected before their fifth birthday, and 6% to 10% of adults. Other risk factors include a positive HIV-1 antibody status, hemodialysis, immunodeficiency, Down syndrome, and male gender.[6,295,299] Reactivation of chronic HBV infection can occur during pregnancy, but this is rare.[300]

CLINICAL MANIFESTATIONS

Most HBV infections are subclinical, particularly in children. Symptomatic infections can be mild and anicteric or be severe enough to produce encephalopathy, coagulopathy, and death. Fulminant hepatitis is more common in adults than in children and in those infected with certain mutant HBV strains or co-infected with the hepatitis delta virus.[295,301,302] Extrahepatic disease may include a serum sickness–type illness in 10% to 20% of patients with acute infections, polyarteritis nodosa, membranous glomerulonephritis, cryoglobulinemia, and infantile papular acrodermatitis.[303,304]

Approximately two-thirds of chronic HBsAg carriers develop chronic persistent hepatitis. They are usually healthy but have persistent or recurrent serum transaminase elevations. The remaining third eventually develop chronic active hepatitis, a progressive disorder that ultimately results in postnecrotic liver cirrhosis. Primary hepatocellular carcinoma, a common malignant tumor in certain parts of the world such as Southeast Asia, Japan, Greece, and Italy, may be as much as 300 times more common in HBsAg-positive men than in their HBsAg-negative counterparts. Primary hepatocellular carcinoma develops after an average of 35 years of HBsAg carriage; coexisting cirrhosis is found in 60% to 90%.[295]

Most neonates and infants who acquire HBV from their mothers remain asymptomatic; those with symptoms typically have benign illnesses. Fulminant disease is rare. Most infected infants become chronic carriers and have a 25% or greater life-time chance of dying of primary hepatocellular carcinoma or liver cirrhosis.

MODES OF TRANSMISSION

HBsAg has been found in blood, blood products, urine, feces, bile, saliva, tears, sweat, semen, vaginal secretions, gastric contents of newborns, breast milk, cord blood, CSF, synovial fluid, and wound exudate.[6] Many routes for HBV spread are possible, but the most significant ones are percutaneous or permucosal exposure to infected blood or body fluids during birth or sexual intercourse or by contaminated needles.[295]

Hepatitis B virus–infected blood can enter the body through contaminated needles shared by drug users, if health care providers mistakenly puncture themselves, or if other persons reuse unsterilized devices in medical or dental offices, acupuncture clinics, or tattooing parlors. Contaminated blood can be introduced through mucous membranes, open wounds, and abrasions.

Screening of blood and blood products for HBsAg has almost eradicated transfusion-acquired HBV infection. Nonetheless, blood that is nonreactive to HBsAg may still be infectious. In Taiwan, a region where 15% to 20% of adults are chronic HBsAg carriers, a study of 206 volunteer blood donors who were HBsAg-negative and had normal serum transaminase activities revealed that about 4% were positive for HBV DNA in plasma by using the PCR; their blood was possibly infectious to susceptible recipients.[305] The frequency of HBsAg-negative, HBV DNA-positive blood in the donor pool of areas of low HBV endemicity is probably substantially less.

Hepatitis B virus can spread to sexual partners of chronic HBsAg carriers or patients with acute hepatitis B. Hepatitis B virus infection is more likely in persons with multiple sex partners, more years of sexual activity, and histories of other sexually transmitted diseases. Heterosexual transmission now accounts for 25% of new HBV cases in the United States, a 38% increase from the early 1980s. It is the most important risk factor for women, with parenteral drug abuse in second place.[306] Close, long-term contact with chronic carriers, as happens in households or institutions for the developmentally disabled, is a risk factor. Intrafamilial nonsexual transmission accounts for 2% of new HBV infections in the United States each year. Transplanted organs are uncommon vehicles of HBV spread to susceptible recipients. About 30% to 40% of all patients have no identifiable risk factors.[306]

PERINATAL EPIDEMIOLOGY

About 0.2% of American Caucasians and 0.9% of African Americans are HBsAg positive. The prevalence is notably higher in certain high-risk groups, such as immigrants from areas of high HBV endemicity (13%), Alaskan natives or Pacific islanders (5%–15%), clients in institutions for the developmentally disabled (10%–20%), users of illicit parenteral drugs (7%), household contacts of an HBV carrier (3%–6%), health care workers with frequent blood contact (1%–2%), and heterosexuals with multiple partners (0.5%).[307]

Perinatal HBV transmission accounts for 35% to 50% of all chronic carriers of this virus in high-incidence areas, such as Taiwan, and for about 15% of those in intermediate-incidence areas, such as certain

African countries. Vertical transmission accounts for a small fraction of cases of chronic infection in areas of low endemicity, such as the United States, where most HBV infections are acquired in adulthood.

The rate of vertical transmission from mother to infant hinges on several factors. For women with acute HBV infection, the risk is about 76% if infection occurs during the third trimester or shortly after delivery, but it is only about 10% if it takes place during the first or second trimesters. For HBsAg carrier mothers, the risk of mother-to-infant transmission depends on their HBeAg/anti-HBe status. The rate is estimated to be 70% to 90% for those who are HBeAg positive, 31% for those who are negative for HBeAg and anti-HBe, and 10% or less for those who are positive for anti-HBe. About a third of HBsAg-positive pregnant women in the United States are also HBeAg positive. Other variables that enhance vertical transmission are high maternal HBsAg and anti-HBc titers and a high HBV DNA concentration.[6] Carrier mothers can transmit HBV to infants born after sequential pregnancies.

Mother-to-infant transmission occurs during delivery in most cases through transplacental microhemorrhages or from ingestion of contaminated maternal secretions. Intrauterine infection is uncommon but may account for 5% to 15% of cases for HBeAg-positive mothers.[294] HBsAg is found in about 71% of breast milk samples from carrier mothers, but no differences in antigenemia rates have been found between breast-fed and bottle-fed infants born to infected mothers.

Unimmunized infants who acquire HBV infection from their mothers usually have no detectable serum HBsAg until 1 to 4 months later. Passively acquired low levels of HBsAg may be detected in the peripheral blood of some neonates, and they do not necessarily imply HBV infection. Cord blood should not be used for HBsAg testing because it can be contaminated with maternal blood.

IMMUNOPROPHYLAXIS

Two preparations have been employed for passive immunization against HBV: immune serum globulin and hepatitis B immunoglobulin (HBIG). Immune serum globulin has anti-HBs titers of 1:16 to 1:1,000. Hepatitis B immunoglobulin, a hyperimmunoglobulin product, has anti-HBs titers of 1:100,000 to 1:250,000. Hepatitis B immunoglobulin is prepared from plasma obtained from HIV antibody-negative donors with a high anti-HBs titer, and its administration does not interfere with the host's immune response to hepatitis B vaccines.

Plasma-derived and recombinant hepatitis B vaccines are used for active immunization. The plasma-derived vaccine, Heptavax-B, is no longer manufactured in the United States. Two recombinant hepatitis B vaccines are available: Recombivax HB and Engerix-B. These vaccines are prepared by insertion of a plasmid containing the HBsAg gene into common bakers' yeast, followed by lysis of yeast cells after the intracellular production, assembly, and accumulation of HBsAg polypeptides. HBsAg is later separated from disrupted yeast cell components; less than 5% of the final product is yeast-derived protein. Recombivax HB contains 10 μg of HBsAg protein/mL, and Engerix-B contains 20 μg/mL.[308]

The CDC's recommended regimen for primary hepatitis B vaccination consists of three intramuscular doses given at 0, 1, and 6 months; an alternative schedule of four doses given at 0, 1, 2, and 12 months has been approved for Engerix-B only. The three-dose schedule induces a good antibody response in more than 90% of healthy adults and more than 95% of pediatric patients (*i.e.*, newborn through 19 years of age). Hepatitis B vaccines have a protective efficacy of 80% to 95% when given to susceptible recipients. About 30% to 50% of vaccinees have no detectable anti-HBs titer after 7 years.[308] The optimal schedule for booster doses has not been defined.

Children younger than 11 years of age can be immunized with 0.5 mL per dose of the Engerix-B vaccine, and adolescents and adults need 1.0 mL per dose. The regimen for Recombivax HB consists of 0.5 mL per dose for infants of HBV-carrier mothers, 0.25 mL per dose for other infants and children younger than 11 years of age, 0.5 mL per dose for adolescents 11 to 19 years of age, and 1.0 mL per dose for adults.

Susceptible pregnant women with accidental percutaneous or permucosal exposure to HBV-infected blood or who have had sexual contact with a chronic HBV carrier or an acutely infected man should receive immunoprophylaxis. Regimens using multiple HBIG doses or vaccine alone are only 70% to 85% effective in preventing HBV infection if used for postexposure prophylaxis of otherwise healthy persons.[308]

Pregnancy is not a contraindication to hepatitis B vaccination. However, vaccine manufacturers advise against their use during pregnancy for liability reasons. Avoidance of vaccination in early pregnancy (*i.e.*, period of embryogenesis) is recommended by some experts. No fetal or maternal risks from hepatitis B vaccination are known, and the limited available data suggest that its use in early or late pregnancy is safe.[309]

Immunoprophylaxis after exposure to HBV-contaminated blood should consist of two doses of HBIG (0.06 mL/kg given intramuscularly; maximum, 5 mL). The first dose of HBIG should be given as soon as possible or within 24 hours of exposure; its effectiveness when given after 7 days of exposure is unknown. The second dose is given 1 month later. This regimen has not been specifically evaluated in pregnant women, but it is about 75% effective in preventing infection in healthy persons. If the physician decides to use the hepatitis B vaccine, which is the preferred approach, only one HBIG dose needs to be given; the vaccine should be administered intramuscularly at a site different from that used for HBIG, and the first dose can be given concomitantly with HBIG or within 7 days of exposure. For sexual HBV exposure, the prophylactic regimen is similar, except that immunization can begin within 14 days of the last sexual encounter.

PREVENTION OF PERINATAL HEPATITIS B VIRUS TRANSMISSION

The CDC estimates that 22,000 births per year occur to HBsAg-positive women in the United States and, unless immunoprophylaxis is given at birth, about 6000 of these newborns become chronic HBV carriers.[6] The administration of HBIG and the initiation of hepatitis B vaccination is 85% to 95% effective in preventing the development of the chronic carrier state in these infants.[294]

The CDC initially recommended that all high-risk women be screened for HBsAg during pregnancy. However, targeting women in high-risk groups identifies only about 35% to 65% of HBsAg carriers. The guidelines were later revised, and universal prenatal screening for HBsAg is now recommended.[310] All pregnant women should be routinely screened for HBsAg during an early prenatal visit. HBsAg-negative women at high risk for infection (*e.g.*, those with other sexually transmitted diseases, illicit drug users) should be retested late in pregnancy. Opinions are divided regarding the cost-effectiveness of this approach when applied to low-risk prenatal populations.[311,312]

Infants born to HBsAg-positive mothers should be bathed as soon as possible to remove HBV-infected blood and other secretions. Suctioning of the stomach contents, if needed, should be performed gently to avoid mucosal trauma that could promote HBV entry into the blood. Delivery by elective cesarean section has been advocated by some as a way of reducing maternal-infant HBV transmission; this approach is not recommended because of the lack of evidence to support the practice and because of the efficacy of immunoprophylaxis.

Hepatitis B immunoglobulin at a dose of 0.5 mL intramuscularly should be given as soon as possible after birth and no later than 12 hours of life. An HBIG dose given at 12 to 48 hours of life is probably effective, but this has not been proved. The first vaccine dose should be given within the first week of life, preferably within the first 12 hours. The intramuscular dose is 0.5 mL, regardless of the vaccine product used. Later doses are given at 1 and 6 months of age. Breast-feeding should be allowed for infants who have started immunoprophylaxis.

The CDC and the American Academy of Pediatrics recommend universal hepatitis B vaccination of all infants, regardless of the maternal HBsAg status.[292,313] Infants born to HBsAg-positive women are given HBIG and the vaccine as outlined earlier. Infants born to women admitted in labor and whose HBsAg status is unknown should receive the first dose of the vaccine within 12 hours of birth in the dosage used for those born to HBsAg-positive mothers (*i.e.*, 0.5 mL of either vaccine type); maternal HBsAg testing should be immediately performed, and if positive, the infant should receive HBIG (0.5 mL) as soon as feasible after birth and no later than 7 days of age. The second and third vaccine doses are given at 1 to 2 months and at 6 months of age, respectively. Household contacts and sex partners of HBsAg-positive women should be vaccinated against hepatitis B; prevaccination susceptibility testing should be done in adults whenever possible but is not required in children because of low rates of HBV infection in that age group and the lower costs of smaller individual vaccine doses.

The recommendations for infants born to HBsAg-*negative* mothers are different. These infants do not need HBIG administration. The vaccine dose depends on the product used. Recombivax HB is given in a dose of 0.25 mL, and the Engerix-B dose is 0.5 mL. Two schedules for vaccine delivery are acceptable, but the preferred one involves giving the first vaccine dose to newborns before hospital discharge, the second dose 1 to 2 months later, and the third dose at 6 to 18 months of age. An alternative schedule for those not immunized at birth is to give the three vaccine doses at 2, 4, and 6 to 18 months of age. Hepatitis B virus vaccines can be given concurrently but in different syringes with poliomyelitis, diphtheria–tetanus–pertussis, measles–mumps–rubella, or *Haemophilus influenzae* type b conjugate vaccines.

Massive newborn immunization programs are already in place in at least 20 countries. In the United States, such programs have been successfully implemented in high-incidence areas, such as Alaska and American Samoa.

Infants who become infected despite immunoprophylaxis may have been infected *in utero*, or their mothers may have had a high virus load. Infants who fail immunoprophylaxis do not become HBsAg positive until 6 to 9 months of age. Immunized infants born to HBsAg-positive mothers should be tested at the age of 9 months or later for HBsAg and anti-HBs; those negative for both should receive a fourth vaccine dose and be tested again 1 month later, and infants found to be HBsAg positive should be monitored closely to determine whether a chronic carrier state has developed.[294]

HERPES SIMPLEX VIRUS INFECTIONS

Infections caused by HSV are common. Conservative estimates indicate that in the United States each year almost 500,000 people have their first episode of genital herpes, and another 10 million have recurring genital lesions.[314] Neonatal HSV infection occurs in at least 700 to 1000 newborns, and approximately 720,000 cesarean sections are performed annually for the purpose of preventing neonatal herpetic infection.[13,314] The optimal management of women with active or suspected genital HSV infections during pregnancy or at labor is not well-defined.[315]

Herpes simplex virus is a double-stranded DNA virus that can infect a broad range of hosts.[316] The virus enters the body through mucosal surfaces or abraded skin, and it multiplies in cells of the epidermis or dermis. Sensory or autonomic nerve endings in its vicinity become infected, and the virus travels intraaxonally in a retrograde fashion to the ganglia. Herpes simplex virus can then continue its multiplication in the ganglia and later spread to other skin and mucous membrane areas through anterograde travel along peripheral sensory nerves, or it can enter a phase of latency in the ganglia. The virus intermittently reactivates and travels to the body surface, where it can produce clinical disease. Exposure to ultraviolet light, trauma to skin, or immunosuppression can provoke HSV reactivation.[316,317] Antibody- and cell-mediated immune reactions are generated in response to HSV, both of which are important for control of the infection.[316,318–320]

The various HSV strains found in the general population can be grouped into two serologic subtypes, HSV-1 and HSV-2. The two subtypes can be differentiated on the basis of their cell culture range, restriction endonuclease analysis, or by monoclonal antibody-based serologic assays.[321]

Seven HSV glycoproteins (g) have been characterized; three (*i.e.*, B, D, H) are essential for HSV replication, and four (*i.e.*, C, E, G, I) are not essential for viral multiplication but may play a role in the pathogenesis and spread of HSV.[322] One of the glycoproteins, gG-2, is a highly type-specific antigen and has been found to be helpful in differentiating HSV-1 from HSV-2 antibody responses.

MATERNAL INFECTION

EPIDEMIOLOGY

Serologic surveys conducted in the United States reveal that the prevalence of antibodies to HSV increases with age, and it is higher in persons from lower socioeconomic strata and in groups with greater levels of sexual activity. Antibodies to HSV-1 may be present in 90% or more of adults from lower socioeconomic groups but only about 30% of college students. Antibodies to HSV-2 are present in approximately 16.4% of the United States population 15 to 74 years of age and in 20.2% of the group 30 to 44 years old. African-Americans are more likely to have antibodies against HSV-2 than American Caucasians. Among African Americans, women are twice as likely as men to be seropositive for this virus.[323] Higher seropositivity rates (17%–32%) have been documented when populations of pregnant women were studied, and this appeared to be independent of socioeconomic status.[315] A recent survey that focused on adults in an inner-city community found that 62% and 33% had antibodies against HSV-1 and HSV-2, respectively.[324] Herpes simplex virus type 1 seropositivity was significantly correlated with being Hispanic or African American, and HSV-2 seropositivity significantly correlated with being female or African American or Hispanic and with low educational level and the number of lifetime sexual partners.[324]

By measuring type-specific antibodies against HSV-2 gG in a group of 190 pregnant women and their husbands, Kulhanjian and colleagues found that 73% of the couples were concordant with respect to their HSV-2 serologies (*i.e.*, both partners were seronegative or seropositive).[325] However, about 9.5% of the pregnant women were seronegative but had seropositive spouses, and they were therefore at risk for gestational primary HSV-2 infection; 56% of these husbands had no history of previous genital HSV infection. Approximately 5% of pregnant women in this particular study were susceptible to HSV-2 infection but were unaware of their risk for acquiring the virus from their seropositive spouses who gave no history of prior genital herpes.[325]

Asymptomatic shedding of HSV occurs in 0.2% to 7.4% of pregnant women and in 0.2% to 4% of those at or near term. Most HSV infections during pregnancy represent recurrent disease. The frequency of asymptomatic shedding increases as pregnancy advances.[7]

CLINICAL MANIFESTATIONS

Many primary HSV infections are subclinical. Symptomatic primary HSV disease can include gingivostomatitis, genital herpes, herpetic whitlow, keratitis, chorioretinitis, encephalitis, esophagitis, pneumonia, and hepatitis.[7]

The most common manifestations of primary HSV-1 infections are gingivostomatitis and pharyngitis.[326,327] Herpes simplex virus type 1 causes 7% to 50% of primary genital herpes infections.[328] Recurrent episodes of herpes labialis are common, and HSV-1 may be recovered from the pharynx of as many as 5% of asymptomatic healthy persons.[7]

The most common clinical illness caused by HSV-2 is genital herpes. Most initial HSV-2 infections are subclinical or mild. Symptomatic patients can have extensive, painful, vesicular or ulcerative genital lesions with or without associated systemic manifestations.[329,330] Women with recurrent disease typically have mild or subclinical infections. Serious complications of HSV infections include pneumonia, hepatitis, and encephalitis.[331,332] The likelihood of reactivation of HSV infection is greater for genital than oral–labial disease and for HSV-2 than for HSV-1.[333,334] Asymptomatic HSV-2 shedding occurs more often during the first 3 months after the primary genital HSV-2 infection than during subsequent periods.[334]

Genital herpes infections are categorized according to HSV subtype, serologic evidence of past HSV-1 or HSV-2 infection, and the presence or absence of symptoms. This classification scheme is useful when examining the impact of gestational HSV infection on pregnancy outcome according to the type of maternal genital infection. First episode, primary HSV-1 or HSV-2 infection is considered if the virus is isolated from the genital tract of a symptomatic or asymptomatic woman who has no serologic evidence of prior infection with HSV-1 or HSV-2 in the acute phase serum, but she subsequently has antibodies to the same HSV subtype when convalescent serum is tested. If the acute-phase serum contains antibodies to the other HSV subtype (*e.g.*, HSV-1 antibodies in a woman with an HSV-2 genital isolate), first episode, nonprimary genital infection is considered present. Recurrent HSV-1 or HSV-2 infection is diagnosed if the patient has antibodies to the same HSV subtype isolated from the genital tract in the acute- and convalescent-phase sera.[315]

DIAGNOSIS

The diagnosis can be made by isolating the virus from tissue cultures of clinical specimens. The best specimen is usually vesicle fluid obtained within 3 days of its appearance.[321] Positive culture results may be obtained within 16 hours to 7 days, depending on the viral load in the clinical specimen. Shell vial cultures may become positive within 16 to 48 hours.[321] Direct detection of HSV antigens in exfoliated cells using a DFA stain can yield a positive result within 45 minutes. The Tzanck smear is a rapid and inexpensive method, but it is only 60% sensitive for HSV infections.[335] It involves scraping the base of a fresh vesicle with a scalpel and spreading the cells and debris on a glass slide. The adherent cells are stained with Giemsa, Sedi, or Wright stain. The slide is examined for the presence of virus-induced cytopathic abnormalities such as multinucleated giant cells, atypical keratinocytes with large nuclei, and ground-glass cytoplasm.[335] A positive Tzanck smear cannot differentiate between VZV and HSV lesions.

Serologic diagnosis is infrequently used for the diagnosis of acute HSV infections. Herpes simples virus–specific IgM may be detected within 3 to 10 days of onset of infection, and it persists for 6 to 8 weeks.[321] Demonstration of seroconversion or a fourfold rise in HSV-specific IgG titers is significant.

Molecular biologic techniques have been applied for the diagnosis of HSV infection through the detection of viral DNA in clinical specimens.[335–337] The PCR continues to detect HSV DNA in clinical specimens for several days after the culture becomes negative; the test is relatively rapid and can be completed within a few hours. The clinical relevance of culture-negative, PCR-positive results from genital specimens remains to be elucidated. Polymerase chain reaction detection of HSV DNA in CSF specimens helps in the diagnosis of herpes encephalitis.[338] Because the PCR technique is sensitive to even minuscule amounts of HSV, contamination from external sources, such as laboratory personnel, physicians, or nurses who may be shedding the virus, can yield false-positive results.[339] Extreme care should be taken while handling the CSF specimen to avoid making an erroneous diagnosis of herpes encephalitis and possibly missing the true culprit.[340]

TREATMENT

Acyclovir is the drug of choice for primary and symptomatic recurrent genital HSV infection.[341] The drug inhibits the replication of HSV-1, HSV-2, and VZV. Acyclovir is converted in the body to its active triphosphate form, initially through the action of viral thymidine kinase to the monophosphate form and later by cellular enzymes to the diphosphate and triphosphate forms. Acyclovir triphosphate concentrations are 40 to 100 times higher in HSV-infected cells than in uninfected cells. The active form of the drug competes with deoxyguanosine triphosphate as a substrate for viral DNA polymerase and, once incorporated into viral DNA, leads to termination of HSV DNA synthesis.[341]

The use of acyclovir during pregnancy is not approved and is generally reserved for life-threatening or severe HSV infections such as pneumonia. Maternal antiviral therapy may fail to prevent fetal infection with HSV.[342] Acyclovir is teratogenic in rats.[343] It can cross the placenta, becomes concentrated in amniotic fluid, and can accumulate in human breast milk.[344,345]

A registry of acyclovir use in pregnancy was established in June 1984. As of June 30, 1990, 312 acyclovir-exposed pregnancies had been reported and followed.[346] Of 239 exposures that took place during the first trimester, outcomes included 24 spontaneous fetal losses, 47 induced abortions, 159 live births without congenital malformations, and 9 with congenital anomalies. Among 73 second- and third-trimester exposures, 1 infant only was born with an anomaly. These findings were not different from what was expected for the general population of pregnant women. Although the size of the cohort is relatively small, the data provide some reassurance for women who are inadvertently treated with acyclovir during pregnancy or have major HSV-related diseases such as pneumonia or encephalitis.[346]

Acyclovir-resistant HSV strains are uncommon, except in patients with AIDS. The mechanism of resistance appears to be a mutation that renders the virus thymidine kinase deficient.[341] Infections caused by these acyclovir-resistant HSV strains can be treated with foscarnet or vidarabine; neither drug is approved by the Food and Drug Administration for use during pregnancy.[347]

FETAL AND NEONATAL INFECTION

EPIDEMIOLOGY

Most neonatal HSV infections are acquired during passage through an infected birth canal. Transplacental spread occurs occasionally, with major deleterious fetal effects. Primary HSV infections during the first one-half of gestation are associated with significantly greater frequencies of spontaneous abortions and stillbirths.[7] About 40% of newborns with herpes are delivered before week 36 of pregnancy.

Intrapartum transmission is more likely to occur with primary maternal HSV genital infection. Other risk factors for HSV acquisition by the infant are cervical HSV infection, multiple genital lesions, prematurity, prolonged rupture of maternal membranes, intrauterine instrumentation (*e.g.*, scalp electrodes), and absent or low titers of transplacentally acquired neutralizing anti-HSV antibodies. The risk of vertical transmission is about 40% to 50% for mothers with primary herpes and about 5% for those with recurrent infections.[7] Postpartum HSV spread to newborns occurs infrequently.[13]

CLINICAL MANIFESTATIONS

Asymptomatic HSV infections are rare in the newborn. Disease manifestations may be localized or widely disseminated. About 60% to 80% of infants with HSV infections are born to women who are asymptomatic at the time of delivery and who have no history of genital herpes.[348] Infants born to asymptomatic women shedding HSV in early labor are 10 times more likely to develop neonatal HSV infection if the mother has recently experienced a first episode genital herpes than neonates born to women whose HSV shedding is secondary to reactivated infection.[349] Serious perinatal morbidity is encountered in 40% of infants born to women who acquire primary genital herpes during pregnancy.[350]

Intrauterine HSV infection is uncommon.[351,352] Its hallmarks are a vesicular rash that is present at birth or appears shortly thereafter; associated abnormalities include microcephaly (60%), chorioretinitis (40%–50%), and microphthalmia (25%). The rash is more likely to be generalized than localized. Other skin lesions include bullae and cutaneous scars in 10% to 15% of patients. The intracranial calcifications seen in 15% may be present at birth or evolve later in infancy. Lesions indicative of brain damage, such as hydranencephaly, cerebral necrosis, and brain atrophy, can be seen on computed tomography (CT) scans of the head. Other findings can include radiographic bone lucencies, intrauterine growth retardation, hepatosplenomegaly, cloudy corneas, and cataracts. About 30% have seizures during the neonatal period. The mortality rate is 40%, and about one-half of the survivors are expected to have significant long-term residual problems such as psychomotor retardation, seizure disorders, spasticity, blindness, or deafness.[352] Most cases have been caused by HSV-2.

About a fourth of infants with neonatal HSV infection become sick within the first day of life, and about two-thirds are ill by the end of the first week.[320] Infections resulting from the intrapartum acquisition of HSV may not manifest until about 10 to 11 days of age with disease localized to the skin, eyes, or oral cavity.[7] Cutaneous lesions include discrete vesicles, large bullae, or denuded skin (Fig. 47-3). Recurrent mucocutaneous herpes develops in some of these infants. Ulcerative mouth lesions without skin disease may sometimes occur. Eye disease includes keratoconjunctivitis and chorioretinitis. Neurologic abnormalities eventually develop in 25% of these infants, despite the fact that CNS involvement may not have been evident during the acute illness.

A second group of infants may present at 15 to 17 days of age with localized CNS involvement, with or without skin, mouth, or ocular lesions. The mortality rate for this group is about 17%, and 40% of survivors suffer long-term sequelae.

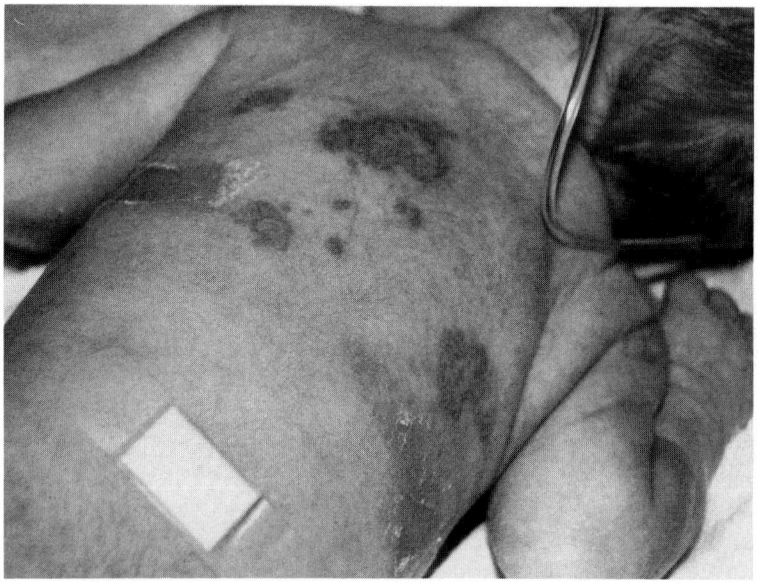

FIG. 47–3. Localized cutaneous herpes simplex virus type 2 infection in a neonate. Notice the coalescing vesicular lesions on the back and right arm. The vesicles are surrounded by an erythematous border.

A third group presents at 9 to 11 days of age with disseminated disease. CNS involvement is found in about two-thirds of these infants; other organs that are severely affected are the adrenal glands, gastrointestinal tract, liver, heart, pancreas, and kidneys. Without appropriate therapy, about 80% die. With acyclovir therapy, the mortality rate is 15% to 20%, but 40% to 55% of the survivors have severe neurologic impairments.

The National Institute of Allergy and Infectious Diseases Collaborative Antiviral Study Group (NIAID CASG) recently published their findings on 210 infants younger than 1 month of age with HSV infection.[353,354] About 4% of infants had congenital HSV infection, and 40% had disease confined to the skin, eyes, or mouth. Central nervous system disease occurred in 34%, and 22% had disseminated infections. Two-thirds of the isolates were HSV-2.

The clinical manifestations of herpes encephalitis in the newborn includes focal or generalized seizures, lethargy, apnea, and pyramidal tract signs.[13] Eventual loss of gag and suck reflexes is common.[320] Involvement of other organs is frequent. Skin vesicles may be absent in about 40% of infants, mandating a high index of suspicion for the diagnosis.[13] Cerebrospinal fluid analysis reveals mononuclear pleocytosis and elevated protein concentrations (as high as 1000 mg/dL).[13] Rarely, the CSF may show a predominance of neutrophils or be completely normal.[13,355] Focal or generalized electroencephalographic abnormalities are common.[356] About 8% of surviving infants have CNS relapse within 1 month of completing therapy.[353]

Ocular herpetic infection may be an isolated problem, but it is more likely to occur in infants with CNS disease. Eye abnormalities include keratitis, conjunctivitis, chorioretinitis, optic atrophy, and cataracts. Long-term follow-up studies of survivors of neonatal HSV infection indicate that 40% (94% in patients with neurologic impairment; 20% in patients who are neurologically normal) have persistent abnormalities, such as cataracts, corneal scars, optic atrophy, and chorioretinal scars; about 44% have disturbed oculomotor control.[357]

Herpes simplex virus pneumonia usually presents between days 3 and 14 of life with gradually worsening respiratory distress.[358–360] Chest roentgenograms reveal perihilar infiltrates that gradually progress into severe diffuse interstitial and alveolar disease (*i.e.*, "white-out" lungs).[361] Other findings include thrombocytopenia, neutropenia, jaundice, and hyperammonemia.[362] The mortality rate of neonatal HSV pneumonia is about 80%, and almost 100% in infants with pneumonia and disseminated intravascular coagulopathy.[354]

DIAGNOSIS

Neonatal HSV infections are best diagnosed by isolating the virus from a vesicular lesion. The virus can be recovered from 25% to 40% of CSF specimens obtained from infants with CNS disease. Cultures of urine, feces, nasopharyngeal secretions, and conjunctivae may yield the virus in some patients. Serology is not useful in neonatal HSV infections. Direct fluorescent antibody staining of scrapings from the base of fresh vesicles may reveal HSV antigens. In culture-negative infants, the use of molecular techniques such as the PCR may establish the diagnosis.[363]

TREATMENT

Antiviral therapy with acyclovir or vidarabine is the mainstay of treatment. In the NIAID CASG reports, infants treated with acyclovir or vidarabine had comparable morbidity and mortality rates.[353] No deaths occurred among 85 infants with localized skin, eyes, or mouth disease; about 94% seemed developmentally normal after 1 year. The mortality rates for the encephalitis and the disseminated HSV groups were 14% and 54%, respectively, and 40% to 70% of the survivors were neurologically impaired. Factors influencing mortality included level of consciousness at the start of treatment, prematurity, disease classification, pneumonia, and disseminated intravascular coagulopathy.[354] Cutaneous HSV recurrences occurred in 46% of survivors by 6 months after the end of therapy, and the rates were similar for infants treated with acyclovir or vidarabine. Seventy-five percent of survivors with disease caused by HSV-2 were impaired, compared with 27% of infants with HSV-1 infection. This is explained partially by the greater *in vitro* susceptibility of HSV-1 to acyclovir.[341]

Infants receiving acyclovir shed lower virus titers than those on vidarabine. Given the ease of administration of acyclovir compared with vidarabine, its fairly benign toxicity profile, and its efficacy against HSV, acyclovir (10 mg/kg/dose given every 8 hours intravenously) is preferred as initial therapy of suspected or proven neonatal HSV infections. Dosage reductions are needed in infants with renal or hepatic dysfunction.[364] The optimal duration of therapy is unknown, but it appears that 14 days to 21 days may be preferable to the 10-day course; higher dosage regimens (about 60 mg/kg/day) are being evaluated, but no data are available yet.[320] Topical antiviral agents such as the ophthalmic preparations of trifluorothymidine, vidarabine, or iododeoxyuridine should be used in newborns with ocular involvement.[320] The use of commercial intravenous γ-globulin preparations for HSV postexposure prophylaxis or treatment of neonates is not recommended.[365]

PREVENTION

Because of the enormous morbidity and mortality rates of neonatal HSV infections despite the early initiation of antiviral therapy, the focus of many research groups has been the development of effective prevention strategies. In a detailed decision analysis study, Libman and colleagues used published data to theoretically evaluate nine different obstetric approaches for the prevention of neonatal HSV disease.[366] The investigators concluded that, given the state of technology, physical examination at the time of labor was the most reasonable strategy. This tactic would be expected to reduce the number of neonatal HSV cases by 36% while increasing the rate of cesarean sections by only 3%. The strategy of obtaining genital HSV cultures at weekly intervals from women with a history of recurrent genital herpes and then delivering by cesarean section those whose most recent culture results were positive by onset of labor would result in 547 additional cesarean sections performed to prevent less than one case of neonatal HSV infection (rates per 100,000 deliveries).[366] Studies on women with histories of recurrent genital herpes have demonstrated that weekly antepartum cultures fail to predict the risks to their infants of HSV exposure at delivery and that most infants exposed to asymptomatic HSV shedding at delivery are born to women without a history of recurrent genital herpes infection.[367,368] Use of rapid antigen detection methods on all women in labor would be the most effective approach in terms of preventing neonatal disease, but this would come at the cost of a 10-fold increase in the number of cesarean sections.[366]

Cesarean section should be performed on women with signs and symptoms suggesting genital HSV infection at the onset of labor. Infants delivered through an infected birth canal should be isolated to protect other infants in the nursery. The risk of invasive HSV infection is small for infants delivered vaginally to women with recurrent genital herpes who are asymptomatic but shedding the virus at the time of labor.[369,370] Cultures of exposed mucous membranes (*e.g.*, eyes, nasopharynx) should be obtained at 24 to 48 hours of life. Earlier positive cultures may reflect transient contamination and not true infection. If the cultures are positive for HSV, antiviral therapy should be started, even if the infant is asymptomatic.

Numerous HSV candidate vaccines are currently in various stages of development.[371,372] Although animal protection studies have provided encouraging results, clinical trials with one vaccine type have been disappointing.[373] None of the HSV vaccines are available commercially.

CYTOMEGALOVIRUS INFECTIONS

Cytomegalovirus is the most common congenital viral infection of humans in the United States.[374] It is one of the most important opportunistic pathogens causing serious illness and death in immunocompromised patients.[375] Cytomegalovirus infections are benign for most adults. However, when CMV infection occurs during pregnancy, the virus can be transmitted to the fetus and result in symptomatic neonatal disease or subclinical congenital infection that may later manifest with hearing loss or learning disabilities.

Cytomegalovirus is an enveloped, double-stranded DNA virus that belongs to the herpes family of viruses.[375] Cytomegalovirus is not eradicated after resolution of the primary infection. It persists in the body in a low-grade chronic infection form or in a latent state with periodic reactivations.[376] Cytomegalovirus transmission occurs primarily by direct or indirect person-to-person spread of infected oropharyngeal secretions, sexual intercourse, blood transfusions, or transplacental spread from mother to fetus.

MATERNAL INFECTION

Serologic surveys in the United States and Great Britain have shown that about 40% to 60% of adults of middle or upper socioeconomic status have antibodies to CMV; the seropositivity rate is about 80% for adults of lower socioeconomic status.[377] The higher the prevalence of maternal CMV antibody in a population, the greater is the rate of congenital CMV infection.[377] Factors correlating with CMV seropositivity in pregnant women include non-Caucasian race, unmarried status, lower educational and income levels, and increasing parity.[378,379] Sexual activity is an important risk factor for CMV infection in adolescent girls, and co-infection with bacterial vaginosis, trichomoniasis, or gonorrhea increases the odds of intrauterine CMV transmission.[380,381]

Intrafamilial CMV transmission from young children to their seronegative pregnant mothers can occur. The risk of CMV seroconversion for a seronegative mother with an infected child is estimated at 10% to 30% per year and is even higher if the child is younger than 20 months of age.[377,382] Annual seroconversion rates for seronegative day-care providers is about 8%.[383] Health care workers with CMV-infected patient contact do not appear to be at increased risk for CMV acquisition compared with persons without patient contact.[384]

About 2% to 2.5% of susceptible women acquire primary CMV infection during pregnancy, a risk comparable to that of nonpregnant women.[7] Seropositive women can reactivate their latent CMV infection during pregnancy or, less commonly, become reinfected by an exogenous CMV strain. Pregnant women may shed CMV from the cervix (8%), urinary tract (4%), throat (2%), and breast milk in the postpartum period (14%).[7]

Primary and recurrent maternal CMV infection can result in transmission of the virus to the fetus. This occurs in about 40% of pregnancies complicated by primary CMV infection.[7] The presence of maternal antibodies to CMV in women with recurrent infection does not prevent viral transmission to the fetus, but it does protect against major fetal damage by CMV.[385]

Most women (90%) with primary CMV infection are asymptomatic. The remainder usually have illnesses resembling infectious mononucleosis. Other manifestations are rare but include interstitial pneumonia, myocarditis, aseptic meningitis, hepatitis, colitis, thrombocytopenia, and hemolytic anemia. Primary CMV infection during the first trimester of pregnancy does not cause fetal loss.[386]

Infection can be documented by isolating the virus from urine, saliva, buffy coat, or cervical secretions. Viral isolation, however, does not differentiate between primary and recurrent CMV infections. Measurement of CMV-specific IgM antibodies is useful for the diagnosis of primary infection, but this antibody can persist in serum for 4 to 8 months.[387] Cytomegalovirus-specific IgG antibody levels are helpful if seroconversion or a fourfold titer rise can be demonstrated. The IFA and ELISA are the most practical and reliable methods for detecting CMV antibodies. Rapid diagnosis of CMV infection is possible using newly developed antigen assays or molecular biologic techniques such as the PCR.[388–390]

Ganciclovir, an acyclic nucleoside analog of acyclovir, has excellent inhibitory activity against CMV.[391] It has been extensively evaluated in immunocompromised patients (*e.g.*, AIDS, organ transplant recipients) with serious CMV infections such as pneumonia or retinitis, but its use in immunocompetent persons has not been examined. Foscarnet (phosphonoformate), another anti-CMV drug, inhibits the DNA polymerase of CMV. Like ganciclovir, foscarnet is used only in the immunosuppressed patient with CMV disease.[392]

CONGENITAL INFECTION

Congenital infection with CMV occurs in 0.4% to 2.3% of all live births.[377] About 10% are symptomatic, and the rest have subclinical infections. Infants with symptomatic congenital CMV have a mortality rate of 15% to 30%, and most survivors have long-term sequelae.[7,393–396] Petechiae, jaundice, and hepatosplenomegaly are found in two-thirds of patients; conjugated hyperbilirubinemia and thrombocytopenia are found in about 80% of cases.[385,393] Neurologic abnormalities such as seizures and hypotonia are common, and microcephaly occurs in about 50% to 75% of infants. Intracranial calcifications are seen on one-half of the patients' CT scans. At autopsy, evidence of multiorgan involvement is apparent.[393] Neuropathologic findings include periventricular necrosis, calcifications, cerebellar hypoplasia, periventricular leukomalacia, hydrocephalus, and porencephalic cyst.[396] Hearing loss and neurologic impairment (*e.g.*, psychomotor and mental retardation) develop in one-half of the survivors.[394,395]

Chorioretinitis is the most frequent eye abnormality, followed by optic atrophy. Microphthalmia, cloudy cornea, optic nerve hypoplasia, nystagmus, and strabismus also occur. Eye abnormalities are common in infants with intracranial calcifications.[7]

Unilateral or bilateral sensorineural hearing loss that can vary from mild to profound develops in about 30% of infants with symptoms at birth, and in 8% to 13% of those with subclinical infections. Hearing loss may be present at birth in otherwise asymptomatic infants, and it subsequently deteriorates in more than one-half of the patients.[397,398] Some patients have normal hearing for the first several years of life, but they then develop sudden hearing loss.

Intellectual deficits are common, particularly in infants with symptomatic congenital CMV. Many infants with subclinical disease may develop mental or behavioral problems.

Dental defects can be found in 40% of the survivors of symptomatic neonatal disease but in only 5% of asymptomatic cases.[399] A variety of congenital anomalies have been described in infants with congenital CMV infection, but these probably reflect coincidental associations rather than true cause-and-effect associations.[400] Reported associations include atrial and ventricular septal defects, tetralogy of Fallot, congenital mitral stenosis, inguinal hernia, hip dislocation, clubfoot, esophageal atresia, megacolon, and extrahepatic biliary atresia.[7,401]

Maternal anti-CMV antibody protects the fetus against major CMV pathology. Fowler and colleagues found that 18% of 125 infants born to women with primary CMV during pregnancy had symptomatic neonatal disease, compared with none of 64 infants born to women with reactivated CMV infection.[385] After a 5-year follow-up period, 13% of infants born to mothers with primary infection had mental impairment (*i.e.*, intelligence quotient ≤ 70) compared with none in the recurrent infection group. Sensorineural hearing loss was found in 15% and 5% of infants born to mothers with primary and recurrent CMV infections, respectively.[385] Bilateral hearing loss occurred only in the primary infection group.

Congenital infection can be diagnosed by isolation of CMV from the urine or saliva within the first 2 weeks of life. Positive cultures from specimens obtained at 3 weeks or later may reflect perinatal CMV acquisition. Congenitally infected infants shed CMV in their urine for many years. The use of shell vial cultures hastens viral isolation. Cytomegalovirus can be detected in the urine by electron microscopy or ELISA. Cytomegalovirus DNA can be detected in a variety of clinical specimens using sensitive hybridization or PCR methods. Cytomegalovirus-specific IgM antibody is detected in many of the infected newborns. IgM detection by RIA or ELISA is superior to immunofluorescence.[377,402–406]

Ganciclovir is being evaluated as treatment for congenital CMV disease. Ganciclovir suppresses viral replication in immunocompromised patients with serious CMV infections. Several problems are associated with ganciclovir use, including the resumption of viral replication on discontinuation of therapy, emergence of ganciclovir-resistant CMV strains after prolonged use in immunosuppressed patients, and drug toxicity (*e.g.*, neutropenia, thrombocytopenia).[407] Demmler reported preliminary data on 25 babies with symptomatic congenital CMV infections who were treated with ganciclovir.[377] Urinary shedding of CMV lessened during therapy but increased again after stopping the drug. More detailed descriptions appear in reports of 2 neonates with severe CMV pneumonia and 1 infant with CNS involvement.[408–410] All 3 infants exhibited modest improvements during ganciclovir therapy, but 1 infant developed significant bone marrow depression and a diffuse bullous rash.[409] The 2 infants with pneumonia died a few months later of long-standing pulmonary problems. Cytomegalovirus hyperimmunoglobulin used in conjunction with ganciclovir has improved the survival of bone marrow transplant recipients with CMV pneumonia. The combination was not beneficial in the 1 infant in whom it was tried.[409] The need for more effective anti-CMV chemotherapeutic agents is evident. Foscarnet has not been tried in congenitally infected infants.

PERINATAL INFECTION

Infants can acquire CMV during passage through an infected birth canal or by ingestion of CMV-positive breast milk.[411] In contrast to congenital disease, perinatally acquired CMV infection is usually benign. Most infections are subclinical. A self-limited, infantile pneumonitis is the most commonly encountered clinical abnormality among symptomatic term infants. Premature infants may have severe illness, including pneumonia, hepatitis, anemia, thrombocytopenia, and neutropenia. The long-term prognosis for intellectual abilities and intact hearing for patients with perinatal CMV infection is excellent.[412]

PREVENTION

Termination of the pregnancy can be considered for women who develop a primary CMV infection during gestation. With primary infection, the overall risk of delivering an infant with symptomatic congenital infection is only about 5%. Prenatal diagnosis of fetal CMV infection is feasible but usually requires a battery of tests. Fourteen of 30 infants born to women with primary CMV infection during pregnancy were infected *in utero*.[413–415] The amniotic fluid cultures were positive for all 14 infected fetuses and negative for the remaining 16 who had escaped infection. Fetal blood samples obtained between weeks 21 to 28 of gestation revealed the presence of CMV-specific IgM antibodies in 9 (64%) of 14 infected fetuses. Cytomegalovirus was isolated from the fetal blood of only 1 (11%) of 9 shown to be infected using other tests. Abnormalities of fetal hematologic indices, liver function tests, and total IgM concentrations were observed in some; the prognostic significance of these abnormalities is uncertain. One report describes the detection of CMV DNA in the amniotic fluid of a woman who later delivered an infant with asymptomatic congenital CMV.[416] Isolation of CMV from the amniotic fluid implies intrauterine infection but does not provide information regarding the severity of fetal disease. A false-positive amniotic fluid culture or PCR result is possible if contamination with maternal blood occurs.

Failure to isolate the virus does not rule out fetal infection with certainty.[377] Fetal abnormalities detected by ultrasonography in women with gestational primary or recurrent CMV infection generally indicate more severe fetal disease. A variety of sonographic findings have been reported, including microcephaly, ventricular dilation, ascites, hydrops, pericardial effusions, oligohydramnios, and intracranial and abdominal calcifications.[413,417,418]

Cytomegalovirus vaccines are not yet available in the United States, but they are being tested in special populations. Routine CMV serologic screening of pregnant women is not cost effective.

Because blood from seropositive donors contains leukocytes that are latently infected with CMV, many blood banks now screen the blood for CMV antibodies (68%), use leukocyte filters, or use washed erythrocytes. The practice of giving only CMV-negative blood or blood products to ill neonates has greatly reduced or eliminated the occurrence of transfusion-acquired CMV infections in many nurseries. Disseminated CMV infection after extracorporeal membrane oxygenation has been described, and CMV screening of blood had not been done.[419]

VARICELLA

Varicella (*i.e.*, chickenpox) and herpes zoster (*i.e.*, shingles) are caused by VZV. Varicella-zoster virus is an enveloped, double-stranded DNA virus. Only one serotype is known.

MATERNAL INFECTION

In the United States, about 95% of women of childbearing age have serologic evidence of past VZV infection. The proportion of seropositive women is smaller in those from tropical or semitropical countries.[420]

Varicella is a highly communicable and usually benign disease of childhood. Children younger than 15 years of age account for more than 90% of cases. Fewer than 2% of reported cases occur in persons 20 years of age or older.[421] The estimated incidence of gestational varicella is 1 to 7 per 10,000 pregnancies.[422,423] Zoster results from reactivation of latent VZV and is more frequently encountered in elderly or immunosuppressed patients. Its incidence in pregnancy is unknown, but it is probably lower than that of varicella. One estimate places the incidence at about 0.5 per 10,000 pregnancies.[422]

Less than 5% of primary VZV infections are subclinical.[424] Varicella usually becomes clinically evident

10 to 20 days after exposure of susceptible persons to VZV. The typical illness consists of fever, malaise, and a pruritic rash. The exanthem is mostly truncal in distribution and is characterized by crops of maculopapules that rapidly evolve into vesicles. The vesicles gradually crust over. New lesions continue to appear for 3 to 5 days, producing the distinctive finding of cutaneous lesions in various stages of evolution. Complications of varicella include pneumonia, encephalitis, arthritis, bacterial cellulitis, and bleeding diathesis. The risk of incurring complications from varicella in otherwise normal adults may be up to 25-fold greater than that for normal children.[421] Pregnancy is not a risk factor for maternal complications. Immunity after varicella is usually long lasting. Recurrent VZV infections can occur in immunocompetent persons who respond appropriately to the virus in terms of mounting seemingly adequate VZV-specific humoral and cellular immune responses.[425]

Zoster is characterized by pain localized to the area of distribution of one or more sensory nerve roots. The rash is unilateral in most patients and follows the same evolutionary pattern seen in varicella except for its restricted distribution.

Varicella and herpes zoster are usually diagnosed clinically, and laboratory confirmation is infrequently needed. The virus can be isolated from vesicular fluid by inoculating freshly collected specimens onto human diploid cell lines. The VZV-specific antigens can be detected in vesicular fluid by immunofluorescence staining of smears of cell scrapings collected from the base of fresh vesicles.[426] Varicella-zoster virus DNA can be detected in vesicle samples, including most crusted lesions, by PCR methodologies.[427,428]

Several serologic assays are available for the detection of antibodies to VZV. These include complement fixation, neutralization, IHA, immune adherence hemagglutination, fluorescent antibody against membrane antigen (FAMA), IFA, and ELISA. These tests can be used to diagnose VZV infections or to ascertain the susceptibility status of an individual.[321]

Complement fixation antibodies develop within 10 days of onset of varicella and peak at 2 to 3 weeks. These antibodies appear earlier in herpes zoster. Complement fixation antibodies tend to disappear with time. By 1 year after infection, about two-thirds of persons do not have detectable complement fixation antibody titers. The complement fixation test is relatively insensitive compared with FAMA or ELISA, and it is now rarely used in clinical laboratories. The FAMA test is very sensitive and is considered to be the gold standard for VZV antibody measurements. However, FAMA is arduous to perform and is not readily available. The ELISA test is being increasingly used for VZV antibody measurements. The IFA methods have been shown to be as sensitive as FAMA.[321]

Two serum samples collected 1 to 2 weeks apart can provide a retrospective diagnosis of VZV infection if a fourfold or greater rise in antibody titer is demonstrated. If the first sample is collected late in the course of the illness, a single high titer indicates a recent primary or a reactivated VZV infection.

Measurement of VZV-specific IgM antibodies is useful for documenting a recent infection with this virus. The VZV-specific IgM antibodies can be detected in serum for several weeks after varicella and may be transiently found after herpes zoster.

For uncomplicated varicella, symptomatic treatment with antipruritics and cleansing of lesions is adequate. Analgesics are needed for pain control in herpes zoster. Early therapy of varicella within the first day of illness with oral acyclovir (800 mg given orally five times per day for 7 days) hastens resolution of fever and shortens the time period to complete crusting of the lesions.[429–431] Acyclovir is not recommended for use during pregnancy, but it can be given for the treatment of severe or life-threatening VZV complications such as pneumonia.

There have been several reports of pregnant women with varicella pneumonia treated with acyclovir.[432–436] The drug was used at doses ranging from 5 to 18 mg/kg every 8 hours, and the treatment results have generally been favorable.[432] At least 312 women have been treated with acyclovir during pregnancy, and there has been no evidence of a teratogenic effect.[346]

TRANSMISSION TO THE FETUS

Varicella-zoster virus transmission to the fetus occurs primarily through the transplacental route. Congenital malformations after maternal infection during the first one-half of pregnancy occur infrequently. This, however, provides support for the notion of transplacental fetal VZV acquisition and infection, even though attempts at isolating the virus from these infants have been largely unsuccessful.[437]

About one-fourth of newborns delivered to mothers who contract varicella during the last 3 weeks of pregnancy develop clinical infection.[438] Paryani and Arvin used several clinical and immunologic criteria to document intrauterine transmission of VZV in 43 pregnancies complicated by varicella and 14 others complicated by herpes zoster.[439] These criteria included malformations consistent with the congenital varicella syndrome, acute varicella of the newborn, detection of VZV-specific IgM in the neonatal period, specific lymphocyte transformation to VZV antigen, persistence of anti-VZV IgG antibodies, and the occurrence of herpes zoster in infancy. The rate of intrauterine transmission was 24% after maternal varicella and 0% after maternal herpes zoster.[439]

FETAL INFECTION

Varicella during pregnancy is not associated with an increased incidence of prematurity or fetal death.[439–441] Chromosomal abnormalities have occurred after VZV infections in experimentally infected human diploid fibroblasts and in the peripheral leukocytes of patients with acute varicella.[442,443] Leukocyte chromosomal breaks were described in 1 child whose mother had gestational varicella.[444] An increased risk for leukemia in the offspring of women with gestational varicella has been found by some investigators, but the numbers are too small to confirm the association.[445]

Several case reports published over the past 45 years have described the occurrence of congenital malformations in the progeny of women who acquire chickenpox during pregnancy.[437,440,446–476] With the exception of 2 infants with congenital anomalies (*e.g.*, skin ulcers, microcephaly, cataracts, intracranial calcifications) after maternal varicella at 25.5 to 28 weeks of gestation, these infections usually occurred between weeks 8 and 20 of pregnancy.[477,478] Abnormalities are primarily cutaneous, musculoskeletal, neurologic, and ocular (Table 47-5).

Cicatricial lesions are the most common skin abnormalities (Fig. 47-4). Cutaneous scars usually occur on hypoplastic extremities, but they can extend to the trunk or opposite extremity. Limb hypoplasia is usually unilateral and most commonly involves the leg. The arm, mandible, or hemithorax can be affected. Rudimentary digits are common on hypoplastic extremities. Detailed clinical and histopathologic studies of some patients suggest that limb abnormalities after intrauterine VZV infection are probably due to a neuropathy resulting from damage to dorsal ganglia and anterior columns of the spinal cord.[464,466]

Central nervous system pathology is common and includes microcephaly, cortical and cerebellar atrophy, psychomotor retardation, seizures, and focal brain calcifications. Autonomic dysfunction, manifested by loss of bowel and urinary sphincter control, dysphagia, intestinal obstruction, and Horner syndrome, is observed in some patients. Unilateral or bilateral ocular anomalies are common; the eye may be the only organ affected in fetal VZV infection.

The literature contains references to a few infants born with congenital malformations after maternal herpes zoster during pregnancy.[479–482] Reported birth defects include microcephaly, microphthalmia, cataracts, and talipes equinovarus. These rare cases probably represent chance occurrences rather than true associations. Paryani and Arvin prospectively followed 14 pregnancies complicated by herpes zoster and were unable to uncover any clinical or immunologic evidence of intrauterine VZV infection.[439]

NEONATAL INFECTION

About 25% of newborns become infected when maternal varicella occurs during the last 3 weeks of pregnancy.[438] The most important determinant of the severity of neonatal disease is the time of onset of maternal varicella relative to delivery. If maternal infection occurs within 5 days before and 2 days after delivery, varicella lesions in neonates usually appear at 5 to 10 days of age. The illness may be mild with only a few cutaneous lesions or may become severe with fever, hemorrhagic rash, and generalized visceral involvement (see Table 47-5). The mortality rate is about 30%, and death usually is caused by severe pulmonary disease. If maternal varicella occurs 5 to 21 days before delivery, lesions in newborns typically appear in the first 4 days of life and the prognosis is good, with no associated mortality. The mild course is probably due to the production and transplacental passage of maternal antibodies, which modify the course of the illness in newborns. Passive transfer of maternal VZV antibodies across the placenta at titers considered to be protective can occur as early as 24 to 28 weeks of gestation.[483]

The diagnosis can be confirmed by viral isolation or VZV antigen detection. Infected newborns may have VZV-specific IgM antibodies, but these usually disappear shortly after birth. Newborns with varicella should be kept in strict isolation if they require hospi-

TABLE 47–5
ABNORMALITIES IN NEWBORNS AFTER MATERNAL GESTATIONAL VARICELLA

Timing of Maternal Varicella	Neonatal Clinical Abnormalities
0–20 weeks of pregnancy	Cicatricial skin lesions, denuded skin, herpes zoster, limb hypoplasia, rudimentary digits, muscle atrophy, intrauterine growth retardation, psychomotor retardation, microcephaly, cerebellar and cortical atrophy, seizures, intracranial calcifications, sensory deficits, Horner syndrome, anal sphincter dysfunction, dysphagia, recurrent aspiration pneumonia, clubfoot, microphthalmia, optic atrophy, hypoplasia of optic disc, chorioretinitis, chorioretinal scars, cataract, nystagmus
Last 5 days of pregnancy–2 days postpartum	Fever, vesicular exanthem, hemorrhagic rash, respiratory distress, cyanosis, pneumonia, widespread necrotic lesions of the viscera (in fatal cases)

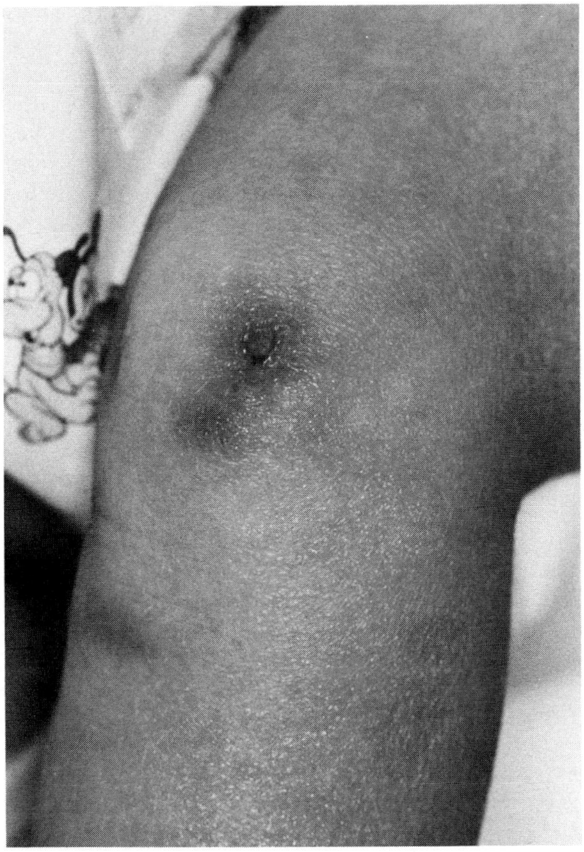

FIG. 47–4. Newborn with congenital varicella after maternal infection at about week 13 of pregnancy. Notice the ulcerated area with surrounding scars over the knee; a second scar is visible distally, over the tibia. Despite an otherwise normal physical examination, computerized tomography of the head revealed multiple areas of cerebral infarction and diffuse intracranial calcifications.

talization. Vidarabine or acyclovir can be used for infants with severe disease.[341,484] If started early in the illness, acyclovir usually leads to more rapid resolution of disease symptoms and signs. Varicella-zoster immunoglobulin (VZIG) is not beneficial after clinical disease has developed.

PREVENTION

Management of persons exposed to VZV is critical because varicella is a highly communicable infection that can adversely affect pregnant women and their offspring. Exposed susceptible persons can be protected by passive immunization with VZIG. Varicella-zoster immunoglobulin is prepared from plasma of normal blood donors found to have high IgG antibody titers to VZV. Varicella-zoster immunoglobulin can prevent or modify clinical varicella in susceptible persons if given shortly after exposure.

A live, attenuated varicella vaccine is available but awaits licensing in the United States. Extensive trials have shown it to be effective and safe.[485–488] There are no formal guidelines for its use, but adults susceptible to varicella are likely to benefit from the vaccine.

Pregnant women exposed to varicella who have negative or uncertain prior histories of this infection should be tested for VZV susceptibility if sensitive assays are available and the results can be rapidly obtained. About 80% to 95% of these women are immune to varicella, as indicated by positive FAMA, IFA, or ELISA test results.[421,489]

If a pregnant woman has significant exposure to varicella and is susceptible or if the laboratory test result cannot be obtained in a timely fashion, VZIG should be administered for the purpose of preventing or modifying the infection in the mother to avoid complications. It is not known whether passive maternal immunization can prevent fetal VZV infection.[421] Varicella-zoster immunoglobulin is most efficacious when given as soon after exposure as is feasible, but not later than 96 hours.

Congenital malformations after first-trimester maternal varicella are estimated to occur at a rate of 5%.[439] Balducci and colleagues found no cases of congenital varicella among 35 term pregnancies complicated by first-trimester maternal varicella.[490] Borzyskowski and collaborators reported a set of female identical twins sharing a single placenta whose mother developed varicella at 10 weeks of gestation.[449] The first twin was normal, and the second had congenital defects consistent with intrauterine VZV infection.

Prenatal diagnosis by detection of VZV-specific IgM in fetal blood has been successful in 1 fetus evaluated at about 32 weeks of gestation, approximately 12 weeks after his mother developed chickenpox.[453] Isada and colleagues attempted to diagnose intrauterine VZV infection in 2 patients by chorionic villus sampling and PCR.[491] Tissues from both mothers were PCR positive but culture negative. One mother elected to terminate her pregnancy at 23 weeks; examination of the fetal brain by Southern blot hybridization was negative. The second woman continued her pregnancy to term, and her newborn infant was clinically normal. Tests for VZV-specific IgM antibody in cord blood and viral placental cultures were negative. The detection of VZV DNA sequences in chorionic villus samples does not equate with fetal infection.[491]

Children born to mothers who develop varicella within 5 days before and 2 days after delivery should receive 125 U of VZIG as soon as possible. Varicella-zoster immunoglobulin does not reduce the clinical attack rate in treated newborns, but these infants generally contract milder infections than untreated neonates.[421,492] Because severe varicella can develop in newborns despite timely administration of VZIG, some clinicians have advocated the use of acyclovir prophylaxis in these infants.[493,494]

Although a few cases of severe neonatal varicella after exposure to mothers who developed the infection more than 2 days after delivery have been described, routine VZIG administration is not recommended, because this group of infants is not regarded to be at increased risk of varicella complications.[421,495]

Pregnant women with varicella at the time of delivery should be isolated from their newborns until all vesicles have crusted. Neonates with varicella lesions should be isolated from other infants but not from their mothers.

PARVOVIRUS B19 INFECTIONS

Human parvovirus B19 was discovered fortuitously in 1975 by British scientists who had been evaluating new laboratory methods for the improved detection of HBsAg in blood donor sera.[496] Since then, B19 has been etiologically linked to a variety of conditions, including erythema infectiosum (*i.e.*, fifth disease), aplastic crises in sickle-cell anemia and other hemolytic diseases, chronic anemia in immunocompromised patients, acute arthritis, and fetal hydrops.[497,498]

B19 is a small, nonenveloped, single-stranded DNA virus. Despite its many genotypes, only one B19 antigenic type is recognized at present.[497] The virus does not grow in conventional cell lines, but it can be propagated in erythropoietin-stimulated bone marrow explant cultures, fetal liver cells of erythroid lineage, a novel cell line with megakaryocytic phenotype, and in erythroid progenitor cells generated *in vitro* from peripheral human blood in the presence of recombinant erythropoietin and interleukin-3.[499–501]

B19 causes a lytic infection of human erythroid progenitor cells. Cessation of erythrocyte production, manifesting as reticulocytopenia, does not cause symptomatic anemia in otherwise healthy persons. However, patients who have reduced erythrocyte life spans (*e.g.*, sickle-cell anemia, thalassemia major) may develop transient aplastic crises. Patients with congenital or acquired immunodeficiency disorders may fail to clear the acute B19 infection, and a persistent B19 infection ensues, resulting in chronic anemia.[502] The rash and arthropathy seen in B19 infections are immune-mediated phenomena and are not directly related to the lytic infection of erythrocyte progenitor cells.

MATERNAL INFECTION

Serologic surveys have found 30% to 60% of adults to have serum antibodies against B19, indicating prior infection.[503] The virus is transmitted primarily by means of B19-infected respiratory secretions. Transmission through transfusions of blood or blood products is uncommon. The incubation period is 4 to 14 days, but it can be as long as 20 days.

About 1% of susceptible pregnant women without known exposure to B19-infected persons seroconvert each year in the United States.[504] During a large erythema infectiosum outbreak in Connecticut, pregnant women were tested for serologic evidence of recent B19 infection. The highest infection rates among exposed susceptible pregnant women were for schoolteachers (16%), day care workers (9%), and homemakers (9%).[505] Attack rates of 36% to 38% have been documented among susceptible nursing staff who were exposed to patients with sickle-cell anemia and aplastic crisis at a children's hospital.[506]

About 20% of acute B19 infections are subclinical. Erythema infectiosum is the most commonly identified B19-related condition. This illness is seen primarily in children, and its most characteristic feature is a facial exanthem (*i.e.*, slapped-cheek appearance). The rash is lacy or reticulated, spreads to the trunk and extremities, and fades within 2 weeks. Recrudescence of the rash is observed with stimuli such as temperature changes, sunlight, or emotional stress. Pruritic, petechial, purpuric, vesicular, or erythema multiforme types of rashes are possible with acute B19 infection.[497,507,508]

In addition to erythema infectiosum, acute B19 infections in otherwise healthy adults can manifest with influenza-type illnesses and symmetric polyarthropathies (*e.g.*, polyarthralgias, polyarthritis); B19-associated joint disease is more common in women.[509] Rheumatoid factor may be positive transiently, and the illness could therefore be misdiagnosed as early rheumatoid arthritis.[510] B19 infections in compromised patients can result in transient aplastic crises, chronic anemia, and viral-induced hemophagocytic syndrome.[497,511,512]

A diagnosis of acute or recent B19 infection can be made by detecting B19-specific IgM using enzyme immunoassays. These antibodies are present in the serum of over 90% of patients by the third day of illness. B19-specific IgM antibodies can persist for 4 months or longer in more than 75% of patients, rendering the distinction between acute or recent B19 infection on serologic grounds alone difficult.[513] B19-specific IgG antibodies are usually formed by the end of the first week of the illness, and they persist for life. The detection of B19-specific antibodies of the IgG class with negative IgM test results is considered evidence of past infection and, probably, immunity to B19 reinfections.

B19 DNA can be detected in serum and tissues by nucleic acid hybridization techniques and the PCR.[497] B19 DNA can be found in serum for as long as 2 months after the onset of illness.[513] B19 antigens can be detected by immunofluorescence or enzyme immunoassays, but these methods are not widely available.

There is no specific treatment for B19-associated illnesses. Immunosuppressed patients with chronic anemia secondary to persistent B19 infections have benefited from intravenous immunoglobulin (IVIG) administration.[497] Patients with erythema infectiosum are not contagious to others after the rash is evident, and those with aplastic crises continue shedding their viruses during the first few days of their hospitalization and require contact isolation.

FETAL INFECTION

Maternal B19 infection during pregnancy can adversely affect pregnancy outcome, but most fetuses escape infection. Fetal infection can lead to hydrops fetalis or death. B19 is responsible for about 8% of nonimmune hydrops cases.[503] The histopathology of fetal B19 infection consists principally of infected erythroblasts with intranuclear inclusions, which are found mostly in the liver, spleen, and bone marrow.[514]

Gestational B19 infections are associated with a less than 10% risk of pregnancy loss from spontaneous abortion, stillbirth, or the delivery of a hydropic infant. In a British prospective study of 190 pregnant women found to be positive for B19-specific IgM, the B19-related fetal death rate was estimated at 9%.[515] In a case–control study conducted in the United States, it was shown that B19 was not a common cause of fetal death in the general population.[516]

B19 suppresses fetal bone marrow erythrocyte production, leading to a chronic anemia. This is not well tolerated by the fetus because of its rapidly expanding cell volume and its immature immune system, which fails to rapidly contain the B19 infection. Congestive heart failure ensues, usually secondary to the severe anemia. Direct infection of cardiac muscles by B19 can occur and may contribute to cardiac dysfunction.[517]

Congenital malformations after intrauterine B19 infections have rarely been described, and they may represent chance occurrences rather than a true teratogenic effect of B19. Hartwig and colleagues described a 9-week-old embryo whose tissues were positive for B19 DNA and who had abnormalities of the eyes and damage to skeletal and smooth muscles.[518] Rodis and associates described an electively terminated pregnancy in which the B19-infected fetus had anencephaly.[519] If B19 is a true teratogen, the associated risk must be small.

The diagnosis of intrauterine B19 infection in a newly born infant is difficult and rests on detection of B19-specific IgM in serum or B19 DNA in the fetal blood or tissues. Parvovirus particles can be observed in tissues by electron microscopy.[520,521]

Management of hydropic newborns is supportive and almost invariably includes packed erythrocyte transfusions. There are no recognized long-term sequelae for healthy infants born to mothers with gestational B19 infection.

PREVENTION

Pregnant women who sustain a significant exposure to a B19-associated illness at home (*e.g.*, erythema infectiosum in a child) and whose B19 antibody status is unknown can be informed that their overall risk of fetal death is at most 2.5%. This figure can be arrived at by multiplying the rate of susceptibility (about 50%), the rate at which exposed susceptible persons acquire B19 infection (maximum of 50%), and the estimated rate of death in documented infection (9%). Had the exposure taken place in a school or day care setting, the risk would decline to less than 1.5%.

Some investigators have suggested the use of IVIG for postexposure prophylaxis of B19-susceptible pregnant women.[522] Commercial IVIG preparations contain anti-B19 IgG antibodies, and they have been shown to be helpful in the treatment of immunosuppressed patients with B19-induced chronic anemia. There are no data to support or refute the use of IVIG for the prevention or amelioration of B19 infection.

If acute or recent B19 infection is confirmed in the pregnant woman by means of a positive B19-specific IgM assay, serial ultrasound examinations should be performed for the detection of early signs indicative of fetal hydrops. Ultrasound examination was instrumental in diagnosing meconium peritonitis at 25 weeks of gestation in an infant with intrauterine B19 infection.[523] Maternal serum α-fetoprotein elevations have been observed in pregnancies with B19-related adverse fetal outcomes such as hydrops.[524]

Limited published experience suggests that the prenatal diagnosis of fetal B19 infection is possible and accurate.[525–528] B19 can be demonstrated in fetal blood by electron microscopy, molecular biologic techniques, or detection of B19-specific IgM antibodies. Török and colleagues used the sensitive PCR assay to detect B19 DNA in amniotic fluid and fetal blood.[528] Fifteen mothers who were positive for B19-specific serum IgM antibodies were evaluated. Eight of 15 fetuses were positive for B19 DNA only, and the other 7 were positive for B19 DNA and B19-specific IgM. Nine (60%) fetuses had hydrops. Ten infants were born healthy, including 4 found to have hydrops at 17 to 23 weeks of gestation, which resolved without specific intervention. Polymerase chain reaction detected B19 DNA in the sera of 20% of mothers with negative B19-specific IgM assay results, with or without B19-specific IgG; one-half of the fetal specimens corresponding to this group of mothers were B19 DNA positive by PCR.[528]

Some B19-infected pregnant women may remain negative for B19-specific IgM and IgG antibodies, despite the detection of B19 particles in serum and saliva using electron microscopy or the detection of B19 DNA with PCR or other techniques.[528,529] B19 infection of their newborns may or may not be symptomatic.

Fetal therapy with intrauterine blood transfusions or digitalization has been attempted in some infants.[503,525–527] The indications for intrauterine transfusion are not well defined. Fetal hydrops has been shown to resolve spontaneously before birth in several patients without specific intervention. All of these infants remained well after birth and during several months of follow-up.[528,530] This indicates that fetal hydrops is not uniformly fatal if not treated and that some fetuses are capable of eventually resolving their B19 infection and reversing the observed pathophysiologic abnormalities.

HUMAN IMMUNODEFICIENCY VIRUS TYPE 1 INFECTION

Acquired immunodeficiency syndrome accounted for 49% of deaths due to infectious diseases and 1.1% of deaths from all causes in the United States during 1991; mortality rates were much higher for African Americans than for Caucasians (31.2 *versus* 8.8 per 100,000, respectively).[531] The HIV-related mortality rates for all races increased between 1989 and 1991 (8.7 *versus* 11.2 per 100,000, respectively).[531] The infant mortality rate per 100,000 live births due to HIV infection was 3.0 in 1989 (10.1 for African-American children; 1.6 for Caucasian children); the provisional HIV-related infant mortality rate for 1991 is estimated at 2.0 per 100,000 live births.[531]

Acquired immunodeficiency syndrome in children younger than 13 years of age (*i.e.*, 4051 cases through September 1992) accounts for 1.7% of all AIDS cases in the United States.[532] Approximately 86% of these children have acquired their HIV infections from their mothers.[532] The situation is worse in Africa, where 80% of the global pool of HIV-infected women live; pediatric patients account for 20% of all AIDS cases in these regions.[533]

Approximately 3 million women worldwide are believed to be HIV-infected.[534] In the United States, women account for 10.7% of all AIDS cases.[532] The proportion of AIDS cases involving female patients continues to increase.[535] As HIV continues to spread among women of childbearing age, a parallel rise in the number of infants born with this infection is expected.

MATERNAL INFECTION

Approximately 12% of the 242,146 AIDS cases reported to the CDC between 1981 and September 1992 were in female patients.[532] African-Americans and Hispanics accounted for 74% of AIDS cases among women; only 19% of all U.S. women belong to these two minorities.[532,536] About 85% of women with AIDS are of reproductive age (*i.e.*, 15 to 44 years). The most important sources of infection are intravenous drug use (50%), heterosexual contact (36%), and transfusions (7%); about 7% of affected women do not belong to any of the recognized risk groups.[532,536]

The prevalence of HIV-1 infection among women is not known with certainty and shows significant geographic and racial variations.[537–544] Rates can be less than 0.2% in a cross-sectional population of pregnant women seeking care at an army base to as high as 8.3% among pregnant African-American women in a rural Florida community.[539,544] The odds of infection within a given group depend on the high-risk behaviors practiced: use of crack cocaine, multiple sexual partners, sexual intercourse with a high-risk partner, and presence of other sexually transmitted diseases.[544] Another factor is low levels of condom use among heterosexual partners. Nationally, only 17% of people with multiple sexual partners use condoms; 12.6% of persons with risky sexual partners use condoms.[545]

To obtain more representative figures for the prevalence of HIV-1 among pregnant women in the United States, Gwinn and associates exploited the fact that maternal IgG antibodies against HIV-1 can passively cross the placenta.[12] This group was able to calculate that 1.5 per 1000 women giving birth in the United States were seropositive for this virus; the rates were highest in large metropolitan areas along the Atlantic coast (*e.g.*, New York, New Jersey, District of Columbia, Florida). This national, population-based survey in childbearing women used residual dried-blood specimens on filter paper that had been collected from newborns for the mandatory metabolic disease screening; anti-HIV-1 antibodies were detected by enzyme immunoassays and Western blots. The detection of these antibodies in newborn blood signifies maternal infection. Gwinn and associates estimated that 6079 births occurred to HIV-infected women in the United States during 1989 and that 1800 infants were infected perinatally during that year.[12]

Human immunodeficiency virus screening programs targeted at patients who acknowledge high-risk behavior generally fail to identify most HIV-infected pregnant women. At Grady Memorial Hospital in Atlanta, Georgia, a program for routine voluntary HIV screening has been in place for several years. The hospital provides care for a predominantly African-American inner-city population. About 95% of pregnant women consented to voluntary HIV screening after pretest counseling. The rate of seropositivity increased from 3.5 per 1000 in 1987 to 5.3 per 1000 in 1990; the increase was significantly associated with history of crack cocaine use. Only 30% of seropositive women had acknowledged high-risk behavior before being tested, but an additional 26% admitted such activities after learning their test results. Targeting only women with self-acknowledged high-risk behavior for HIV testing would have missed 70% of infected women.[546] With nondirective counseling about options for terminating or continuing pregnancy, 85% of HIV-infected women elect to continue their pregnancies.[546,547]

MOTHER-TO-INFANT TRANSMISSION

Vertical transmission of HIV can occur *in utero*, intrapartum, or postpartum. Although most investigators think that vertical HIV-1 transmission in the United States occurs chiefly through intrauterine, transplacental spread of the virus, a growing body of evidence indicates that intrapartum transmission may be a major mode of fetal infection.[548–552]

Laboratory investigations of second trimester abortuses from HIV-infected mothers have shown that about 30% of the fetuses were infected.[553] On this basis, *in utero* transmission could account for most perinatal infections in the United States. Another group of investigators examined 13 second-trimester pregnancies of HIV-positive women that were scheduled for elective pregnancy termination.[554] Maternal serum, amniotic fluid, and fetal blood samples were obtained on all patients. Although HIV antibody patterns were similar in maternal and fetal sera, the P24 antigen was detected in serum and amniotic fluid samples of 38% of the women and from the sera of 23% of the fetuses. These results confirm the importance of the intrauterine route of HIV transmission.[554]

The importance of resolving the controversy surrounding the major mode of spread cannot be overemphasized. If intrapartum transmission proves to be the major route of spread, as for HBV, preventive approaches aiming at interrupting HIV transmission can be more vigorously pursued. These might include the administration at birth of zidovudine or recombinant soluble CD4, the administration of an HIV-hyperimmunoglobulin, or cesarean deliveries.

Consistent, universally applied definitions would be helpful in resolving this issue. Data collected by different investigators from around the world can then be compared directly and conclusions can be reached. The Pediatric Virology Committee of the AIDS Clinical Trials Group published a consensus working definition. An infant is considered to have early (*i.e., in utero*) infection if the HIV-1 genome was detected by PCR or if HIV-1 was isolated from blood within 48 hours of birth; positive results should be confirmed with at least one sample obtained after the neonatal period. An infant is considered to have late (*i.e.,* intrapartum) infection if diagnostic studies (*e.g.,* HIV-1 isolation, PCR, serum P24 antigen assays) were negative in blood samples obtained during the first week of life but became positive during the period from day 7 to day 90, and the infant has not been breast fed. Care should be exercised to avoid contaminating cord blood with maternal blood.[555]

In the United States, breast-feeding of infants by infected mothers is not recommended.[556,557] Postnatal HIV transmission by breast-feeding was examined prospectively in a cohort of 219 infants born to 217 seronegative women at the Centre Hospitalier de Kigali, Rwanda.[558] Among 212 mother–infant pairs who were seronegative, 16 mothers seroconverted within 24 months of delivery. Nine infants born to the 16 mothers became HIV-positive by Western blot analysis, PCR, or both before the age of 18 months; all were breast-fed. Five of the infants seroconverted by the age of 3 months and were more likely to have acquired the virus late in gestation or during delivery. Four infants became HIV-positive at 6 to 18 months of age and were presumably infected postnatally through breast milk. Case reports describing the postnatal acquisition of HIV through breast-feeding have appeared from the United States, France, Zaire, and Australia.[559]

Vertical HIV transmission has been reported to occur at various rates in different areas throughout the world. A report by the 19-center European Collaborative Study provided a rate of 14.4% among a cohort of 721 children followed for 18 months or longer; a similar rate of 14% to 20% was observed in a nationwide study of a cohort of 286 children born to HIV-positive mothers in Switzerland.[560,561] The rate is about 30% in the United States.[562] Rates as high as 50% have been reported from African countries such as Zaire and Kenya.[558] The reason for these geographic differences are unknown, but they may be related to the duration and severity of maternal disease, the frequency of cofactors for HIV activation such as other sexually transmitted diseases, viral strain differences, or host genetic factors.

Maternal factors enhancing the rate at which HIV is transmitted to their infants may include advanced disease, low CD4-positive lymphocyte percentage, low absolute CD4-positive counts, higher plasma virus titers, P24 antigenemia, coexisting infections, viral strain differences, premature delivery, and obstetric factors such as prolonged rupture of maternal membranes or chorioamnionitis. In the report of the European Collaborative Study, infants born at 33 weeks of gestation or earlier were about fourfold more likely to become HIV-1 infected than those born closer to term.[560] For twins born to HIV-infected mothers, the first infant delivered, whether vaginally or by cesarean section, is at least twice as likely to be infected as the second-born twin.[563] This may be due to more intense exposure of the first born to HIV-infected genital secretions. De Martino and associates could not confirm these observations in their studies of twins born to HIV-infected mothers.[564] They did observe that, if the first-born twin became infected, only 42% of their second-born siblings were infected. If the first-born escaped HIV infection, only 13% of their second-born siblings were infected.[564]

Multiple HIV variants exist in infected persons. These variants arise during retroviral replication through errors in reverse transcription, perhaps as a result of immunologic pressure, alterations in cell tropism or replication efficiency. Wolinsky and colleagues studied 3 mother–infant pairs and found that only a small subset of maternal HIV variants is transmitted to infants.[565] A proviral form that was infrequently found in 2 mothers predominated in their infants. Other variants present in the 3 mothers were absent from all infants.

TREATMENT

The safety and efficacy of zidovudine as a chemoprophylactic agent against the vertical transmission of

HIV is under investigation. Zidovudine crosses the placenta, and its concentration in umbilical cord blood may be higher than maternal levels.[566–569] Sperling and colleagues described a retrospective survey of 43 women who had received zidovudine (300–1200 mg/day) during pregnancy.[569] Their report is flawed by missing data and errors of definition. These investigators found no increased risk for premature birth, intrauterine growth retardation, or neonatal asphyxia. There were no malformations in the 12 newborns exposed to zidovudine during the first trimester. Birth defects observed in 5 newborns showed no consistent pattern and included one each of the following: ventricular septal defect, albinism, polydactyly, clitoral enlargement, and ureteropelvic junction obstruction. At least 7 newborns had hemoglobin concentrations below the lowest limit of normal for term infants; 3 were born prematurely. This finding is potentially of concern because zidovudine crosses the placental barrier and may suppress the bone marrow of a developing fetus. Data from larger, prospective studies are urgently required.

Zidovudine has a direct embryotoxic effect on pregnant mice, resulting in fewer fetuses and more resorptions.[570] Zidovudine's mouse embryotoxicity is dose-dependent and can be reduced by concomitant treatment of the animals with erythropoietin, vitamin E, or interleukin-3; the relevance of these animal findings to the human fetus has not been examined.[571]

FETAL AND NEONATAL INFECTION

Congenitally infected infants are usually asymptomatic during the neonatal period, although detectable subtle signs such as lymphadenopathy and hepatosplenomegaly have been observed in approximately 5% of cases, and some infants have been born with evidence of cerebral atrophy. The latency period to development of symptoms is considerably shorter than that for adults, with a median age at onset of 8 months. The shorter latency does not appear to be caused by higher titers of replicating virus in the blood of vertically infected infants compared with HIV-infected adults.[550]

The diagnosis of HIV infection during the neonatal period or early infancy is difficult.[572,573] Measurement of the anti-HIV-1 IgG is not useful because of passive transplacental passage of this antibody and its persistence for several months. A few infants who serorevert to an HIV-seronegative status in early infancy may actually be HIV-infected, and close follow-up is required.[574,575] Human immunodeficiency virus cultures, P24 antigen detection, and HIV-specific IgM and IgA measurements are all hampered by low sensitivities in the first weeks of life.[576–579] Human immunodeficiency virus cultures and P24 antigen measurements are about 50% sensitive in the early neonatal period. This apparently high false-negative rate may due to poor sensitivity of the technique itself, tropism of the virus for organs such as the lymph nodes and thymus, which allows it to evade detection in blood, or to the possibility that many infants acquire HIV late in pregnancy or at delivery and are truly negative when tested at birth. A technique that dissociates HIV antibodies from their bound antigens can provide a rapid and sensitive means of detecting HIV antigens in cord sera of infected infants by disrupting HIV antigen–containing immune complexes.[580] Assays for anti-HIV IgA antibodies during the first month of life detect fewer than 10% of HIV-infected infants, but their sensitivities increase to 60% for patients at 3 months of age and to 77% to 100% at 6 months of age or older.[578,579] The PCR method detects HIV proviral sequences in the blood of more than one-half of the infected newborns.[574,581] Like all the other tests, the sensitivity of the PCR improves as infants become older.[572] The PCR can be falsely positive if contamination with maternal blood occurs.

More than 50% of perinatally infected children become symptomatic by 2 years of age. The most common AIDS-defining conditions in pediatric patients are *Pneumocystis carinii* pneumonia, lymphoid interstitial hyperplasia, recurrent bacterial infections, HIV wasting syndrome, candidiasis, and HIV encephalopathy. *P. carinii* prophylaxis with trimethoprim-sulfamethoxazole is usually started in asymptomatic HIV-infected infants when the CD4-positive lymphocyte count is less than 1500 cells/μL during the first year of life.[582] *Mycobacterium avium-intracellulare* has emerged as a common opportunistic pathogen in AIDS patients.[583] *M. tuberculosis,* including strains with multidrug resistance patterns, has increased in prevalence among AIDS patients.[584,585] Infusions of IVIG at 2- to 4-week intervals and initiation of antiretroviral agents such as zidovudine and 2′,3′-dideoxyinosine reduce the frequency and severity of various complications. However, reports of HIV-1 resistance to zidovudine are rapidly increasing for adults and children.

REFERENCES

1. Atmar RL, Englund JA, Hammill H. Complications of measles during pregnancy. Clin Infect Dis 1992;14:217.
2. Zeichner SL, Plotkin SA. Mechanisms and pathways of congenital infections. Clin Perinatol 1988;15:163.
3. Kline MW, Shearer WT. Impact of human immunodeficiency virus infection on women and infants. Infect Dis Clin North Am 1992;6:1.
4. Freij BJ, Sever JL. Congenital viral infections. Curr Opin Infect Dis 1992;5:558.
5. Freij BJ, South MA, Sever JL. Maternal rubella and the congenital rubella syndrome. Clin Perinatol 1988;15:247.
6. Shapiro CN, Margolis HS. Impact of hepatitis B virus infection on women and children. Infect Dis Clin North Am 1992;6:75.
7. Freij BJ, Sever JL. Herpesvirus infections in pregnancy: risks to embryo, fetus, and neonate. Clin Perinatol 1988;15:203.
8. Sánchez PJ. Congenital syphilis. Adv Pediatr Infect Dis 1992;7:161.

9. Dobbins JG, Stewart JA, Demmler GJ, and the Collaborating Registry Group. Surveillance of congenital cytomegalovirus disease, 1990–1991. MMWR 1992;41(SS-2):35.
10. Remington JS, Desmonts G. Toxoplasmosis. In: Remington JS, Klein JO, eds. Infectious diseases of the fetus and newborn infant. 3rd ed. Philadelphia: WB Saunders, 1990:89.
11. Centers for Disease Control. Summary of notifiable diseases, United States, 1991. MMWR 1991;40(53):1.
12. Gwinn M, Pappaioanou M, George JR, et al. Prevalence of HIV infection in childbearing women in the United States: surveillance using newborn blood samples. JAMA 1991; 265:1704.
13. Whitley RJ. Herpes simplex virus infections. In: Remington JS, Klein JO, eds. Infectious diseases of the fetus and newborn infant. 3rd ed. Philadelphia: WB Saunders, 1990:282.
14. Lindegren ML, Fehrs LJ, Hadler SC, Hinman AR. Update: rubella and congenital rubella syndrome, 1980–1990. Epidemiol Rev 1991;13:341.
15. Cochi SL, Edmonds LE, Dyer K, et al. Congenital rubella syndrome in the United States, 1970–1985: on the verge of elimination. Am J Epidemiol 1989;129:349.
16. Kinney JS, Kumar ML. Should we expand the TORCH complex? A description of clinical and diagnostic aspects of selected old and new agents. Clin Perinatol 1988;15:727.
17. Alpert G, Plotkin SA. A practical guide to the diagnosis of congenital infections in the newborn infant. Pediatr Clin North Am 1986;33:465.
18. Gutman LT. The spirochetes. In: Joklik WK, Willett HP, Amos DB, Wilfert CM, eds. Zinsser microbiology. 20th ed. Norwalk: Appleton & Lange, 1992:657.
19. Hook EW III, Marra CM. Acquired syphilis in adults. N Engl J Med 1992;326:1060.
20. Baughn RE. Role of fibronectin in the pathogenesis of syphilis. Rev Infect Dis 1987;9:S372.
21. Nelson KE, Vlahov D, Cohn S, et al. Sexually transmitted diseases in a population of intravenous drug users: association with seropositivity to the human immunodeficiency virus (HIV). J Infect Dis 1991;164:457.
22. Dobson SRM, Taber LH, Baughn RE. Recognition of Treponema pallidum antigens by IgM and IgG antibodies in congenitally infected newborns and their mothers. J Infect Dis 1988;157:903.
23. Wicher V, Zabek J, Wicher K. Pathogen-specific humoral response in Treponema pallidum-infected humans, rabbits, and guinea pigs. J Infect Dis 1991;163:830.
24. Sànchez PJ, McCracken GH Jr, Wendel GD, et al. Molecular analysis of the fetal IgM response to Treponema pallidum antigens: implications for improved serodiagnosis of congenital syphilis. J Infect Dis 1989;159:508.
25. Lewis LL, Taber LH, Baughn RE. Evaluation of immunoglobulin M Western blot analysis in the diagnosis of congenital syphilis. J Clin Microbiol 1990;28:296.
26. Byrne RE, Laska S, Bell M, et al. Evaluation of a Treponema pallidum Western immunoblot assay as a confirmatory test for syphilis. J Clin Microbiol 1992;30:115.
27. Borenstein LA, Selsted ME, Lehrer RI, Miller JN. Antimicrobial activity of rabbit leukocyte defensins against Treponema pallidum subsp. pallidum. Infect Immun 1991;59:1359.
28. Borenstein LA, Ganz T, Sell S, et al. Contribution of rabbit leukocyte defensins to the host response in experimental syphilis. Infect Immun 1991;59:1368.
29. Fitzgerald TJ. The Th_1/Th_2-like switch in syphilitic infection: is it detrimental? Infect Immun 1992;60:3475.
30. Baker-Zander SA, Lukehart SA. Macrophage-mediated killing of opsonized Treponema pallidum. J Infect Dis 1992; 165:69.
31. Centers for Disease Control. Primary and secondary syphilis—United States, 1981–1990. MMWR 1991;40:314.
32. Centers for Disease Control. Syphilis—Ford County, Kansas, 1992. MMWR 1992;41:644.
33. Rolfs RT, Goldberg M, Sharrar RG. Risk factors for syphilis: cocaine use and prostitution. Am J Public Health 1990;80:853.
34. Andrus JK, Fleming DW, Harger DR, et al. Partner notification: can it control epidemic syphilis? Ann Intern Med 1990;112:539.
35. Mascola L, Pelosi R, Blount JH, et al. Congenital syphilis: why is it still occurring? JAMA 1984;252:1719.
36. Ricci JM, Fojaco RM, O'Sullivan MJ. Congenital syphilis: the University of Miami/Jackson Memorial Medical Center experience, 1986–1988. Obstet Gynecol 1989;74:687.
37. Ong KR, Rubin S, Brome-Bunting M, Labes K. Congenital syphilis in New York City: 1985–1990. N Y State J Med 1991; 91:531.
38. Tseng CK, Hughes MA, Hsu P-L, et al. Syphilis superinfection activates expression of human immunodeficiency virus 1 in latently infected rabbits. Am J Pathol 1991;138:1149.
39. Marra CM, Handsfield HH, Kuller L, et al. Alterations in the course of experimental syphilis associated with concurrent simian immunodeficiency virus infection. J Infect Dis 1992;165:1020.
40. Schulz KF, Murphy FK, Patamasucon P, Meheus AZ. Congenital syphilis. In: Holmes KK, Mårdh P-A, Sparling PF, Wiesner PJ, Cates W Jr, Lemon SM, Stamm WE, eds. Sexually transmitted diseases. 2nd ed. New York: McGraw-Hill, 1990:821.
41. Hook EW III, Roddy RE, Lukehart SA, et al. Detection of Treponema pallidum in lesion exudate with a pathogen-specific monoclonal antibody. J Clin Microbiol 1985;22:241.
42. Ito F, Hunter EF, George RW, et al. Specific immunofluorescent staining of pathogenic treponemes with a monoclonal antibody. J Clin Microbiol 1992;30:831.
43. Lukehart SA, Hook EW III, Baker-Zander SA, et al. Invasion of the central nervous system by Treponema pallidum: implications for diagnosis and treatment. Ann Intern Med 1988;109:855.
44. Penn CW. Pathogenicity and molecular biology of treponemes. Rev Med Microbiol 1991;2:68.
45. Burstain JM, Grimprel E, Lukehart SA, et al. Sensitive detection of Treponema pallidum by using the polymerase chain reaction. J Clin Microbiol 1991;29:62.
46. Noordhoek GT, Wolters EC, De Jonge MEJ, Van Embden JDA. Detection by polymerase chain reaction of Treponema pallidum DNA in cerebrospinal fluid from neurosyphilis patients before and after antibiotic treatment. J Clin Microbiol 1991;29:1976.
47. Wicher K, Noordhoek GT, Abbruscato F, Wicher V. Detection of Treponema pallidum in early syphilis by DNA amplification. J Clin Microbiol 1992;30:497.
48. Lewis LL. Congenital syphilis: serologic diagnosis in the young infant. Infect Dis Clin North Am 1992;6:31.
49. Romanowski B, Sutherland R, Fick GH, et al. Serologic response to treatment of infectious syphilis. Ann Intern Med 1991;114:1005.
50. Rompalo AM, Cannon RO, Quinn TC, Hook EW III. Association of biologic false-positive reactions for syphilis with human immunodeficiency virus infection. J Infect Dis 1992; 165:1124.
51. Berkowitz K, Baxi L, Fox HE. False-negative syphilis screening: the prozone phenomenon, nonimmune hydrops, and diagnosis of syphilis during pregnancy. Am J Obstet Gynecol 1990;163:975.
52. Young H, Moyes A, McMillan A, Patterson J. Enzyme immu-

noassay for anti-treponemal IgG: screening or confirmatory test? J Clin Pathol 1992;45:37.
53. Wendel GD. Gestational and congenital syphilis. Clin Perinatol 1988;15:287.
54. Klein VR, Cox SM, Mitchell MD, Wendel GD Jr. The Jarisch-Herxheimer reaction complicating syphilotherapy in pregnancy. Obstet Gynecol 1990;75:375.
55. Musher DM. Syphilis, neurosyphilis, penicillin, and AIDS. J Infect Dis 1991;163:1201.
56. Rawstron SA, Bromberg K. Failure of recommended maternal therapy to prevent congenital syphilis. Sex Transm Dis 1991; 18:102.
57. Fenton LJ, Light IJ. Congenital syphilis after maternal treatment with erythromycin. Obstet Gynecol 1976;47:492.
58. Rein MF. Biopharmacology of syphilotherapy. J Am Vener Dis Assoc 1976;3:109.
59. Marra CM, Slatter V, Tartaglione TA, et al. Evaluation of aqueous penicillin G and ceftriaxone for experimental neurosyphilis. J Infect Dis 1992;165:396.
60. Centers for Disease Control. Guidelines for the prevention and control of congenital syphilis. MMWR 1988;37(Suppl 1):1.
61. Wendel GD Jr, Stark BJ, Jamison RB, et al. Penicillin allergy and desensitization in serious infections during pregnancy. N Engl J Med 1985;312:1229.
62. Ikeda MK, Jenson HB. Evaluation and treatment of congenital syphilis. J Pediatr 1990;117:843.
63. Quinn TC, Cannon RO, Glasser D, et al. The association of syphilis with risk of human immunodeficiency virus infection in patients attending sexually transmitted disease clinics. Arch Intern Med 1990;150:1297.
64. Temmerman M, Ali FM, Ndinya-Achola J, et al. Rapid increase of both HIV-1 infection and syphilis among pregnant women in Nairobi, Kenya. AIDS 1992;6:1181.
65. Zenker PN, Berman SM. Congenital syphilis: trends and recommendations for evaluation and management. Pediatr Infect Dis J 1991;10:516.
66. Centers for Disease Control. Congenital syphilis—New York City, 1986–1988. MMWR 1989;38:825.
67. Zenker PN, Berman SM. Congenital syphilis: reporting and reality. Am J Public Health 1990;80:271.
68. Cohen DA, Boyd D, Prabhudas I, Mascola L. The effects of case definition in maternal screening and reporting criteria on rates of congenital syphilis. Am J Public Health 1990;80: 316.
69. Baughn RE. Congenital syphilis: immunologic challenges. Pathol Immunopathol Res 1989;8:161.
70. Fitzgerald TJ, Froberg MK. Congenital syphilis in newborn rabbits: immune functions and susceptibility to challenge infection at 2 and 5 weeks of age. Infect Immun 1991;59:1869.
71. Wicher K, Baughn RE, Wicher V, Nakeeb S. Experimental congenital syphilis: guinea pig model. Infect Immun 1992; 60:271.
72. Benirschke K. Syphilis—the placenta and the fetus. Am J Dis Child 1974;128:142.
73. Russell P, Altshuler G. Placental abnormalities of congenital syphilis: a neglected aid to diagnosis. Am J Dis Child 1974; 128:160.
74. Ohyama M, Itani Y, Tanaka Y, et al. Syphilitic placentitis: demonstration of Treponema pallidum by immunoperoxidase staining. Virchows Arch A Pathol Anat Histopathol 1990; 417:343.
75. Lucas MJ, Theriot SK, Wendel GD Jr. Doppler systolic-diastolic ratios in pregnancies complicated by syphilis. Obstet Gynecol 1991;77:217.
76. Fojaco RM, Hensley GT, Moskowitz L. Congenital syphilis and necrotizing funisitis. JAMA 1989;261:1788.
77. Ewing CI, Roberts C, Davidson DC, Arya OP. Early congenital syphilis still occurs. Arch Dis Child 1985;60:1128.
78. Boot JM, Oranje AP, Menke HE, et al. Congenital syphilis in The Netherlands: diagnosis and clinical features. Genitourin Med 1989;65:300.
79. Dorfman DH, Glaser JH. Congenital syphilis presenting in infants after the newborn period. N Engl J Med 1990;323:1299.
80. Rosenberg NM. Congenital syphilis: an emerging emergency. Pediatr Emerg Care 1991;7:171.
81. Wright MS, Tecklenburg FW. Critical illness in congenital syphilis after the newborn period. Clin Pediatr (Phila) 1992; 31:247.
82. Naeye RL. Fetal growth with congenital syphilis: a quantitative study. Am J Clin Pathol 1971;55:228.
83. Long WA, Ulshen MH, Lawson EE. Clinical manifestations of congenital syphilitic hepatitis: implications for pathogenesis. J Pediatr Gastroenterol Nutr 1984;3:551.
84. Venter A, Pettifor JM, Duursma J, et al. Liver function in early congenital syphilis: does penicillin cause a deterioration? J Pediatr Gastroenterol Nutr 1991;12:310.
85. Noseda G, Roy C, Phan P, et al. Acute hepatic failure in an infant with congenital syphilis. Arch Fr Pediatr 1990;47:445.
86. Mascola L, Pelosi R, Blount JH, et al. Congenital syphilis revisited. Am J Dis Child 1985;139:575.
87. Berry MC, Dajani AS. Resurgence of congenital syphilis. Infect Dis Clin North Am 1992;6:19.
88. Hira SK, Bhat GJ, Patel JB, et al. Early congenital syphilis: clinico-radiologic features in 202 patients. Sex Transm Dis 1985;12:177.
89. Rasool MN, Govender S. The skeletal manifestations of congenital syphilis: a review of 197 cases. J Bone Joint Surg [Br] 1989;71:752.
90. Brion LP, Manuli M, Rai B, et al. Long-bone radiographic abnormalities as a sign of active congenital syphilis in asymptomatic newborns. Pediatrics 1991;88:1037.
91. Schulman M, Levin T, Zieba P, Goldman HS. Absence of lower extremity ossification centers in term infants with congenital syphilis [abstract]. Clin Res 1992;40:661A.
92. Greenberg SB, Bernal DV. Are long bone radiographs necessary in neonates suspected of having congenital syphilis? Radiology 1992;182:637.
93. Austin R, Melhem RE. Pulmonary changes in congenital syphilis. Pediatr Radiol 1991;21:404.
94. Hill LL, Singer DB, Falletta J, Stasney R. The nephrotic syndrome in congenital syphilis: an immunopathy. Pediatrics 1972;49:260.
95. Fiumara NJ, Lessell S. Manifestations of late congenital syphilis: an analysis of 271 patients. Arch Dermatol 1970;102:78.
96. Hendershot EL. Luetic deafness. Otolaryngol Clin North Am 1978;11:43.
97. Wendel GD Jr, Sánchez PJ, Peters MT, et al. Identification of Treponema pallidum in amniotic fluid and fetal blood from pregnancies complicated by congenital syphilis. Obstet Gynecol 1991;78:890.
98. Hill LM, Maloney JB. An unusual constellation of sonographic findings associated with congenital syphilis. Obstet Gynecol 1991;78:895.
99. Satin AJ, Twickler DM, Wendel GD Jr. Congenital syphilis associated with dilation of fetal small bowel: a case report. J Ultrasound Med 1992;11:49.
100. Hallak M, Peipert JF, Ludomirsky A, Byers J. Nonimmune hydrops fetalis and fetal congenital syphilis: a case report. J Reprod Med 1992;37:173.
101. Glover DD, Winter CA, Charles D, Larsen B. Diagnostic considerations in intra-amniotic syphilis. Sex Transm Dis 1985; 12:145.

102. Grimprel E, Sanchez PJ, Wendel GD, et al. Use of polymerase chain reaction and rabbit infectivity testing to detect Treponema pallidum in amniotic fluid, fetal and neonatal sera, and cerebrospinal fluid. J Clin Microbiol 1991;29:1711.
103. Rawstron SA, Bromberg K. Comparison of maternal and newborn serologic tests for syphilis. Am J Dis Child 1991; 145:1383.
104. Sánchez PJ, Wendel GD, Norgard MV. IgM antibody to Treponema pallidum in cerebrospinal fluid of infants with congenital syphilis. Am J Dis Child 1992;146:1171.
105. Jackson MH, Hutchison WM. The prevalence and source of Toxoplasma infection in the environment. Adv Parasitol 1989; 28:55.
106. Freij BJ, Sever JL. Toxoplasmosis. Pediatr Rev 1991;12:227.
107. Sever JL, Ellenberg JH, Ley AC, et al. Toxoplasmosis: maternal and pediatric findings in 23,000 pregnancies. Pediatrics 1988;82:181.
108. Couvreur J, Desmonts G. Toxoplasmosis. In: MacLeod CL, ed. Parasitic infections in pregnancy and the newborn. Oxford: Oxford University Press, 1988:112.
109. Lappalainen M, Koskela P, Hedman K, et al. Incidence of primary Toxoplasma infections during pregnancy in Southern Finland: a prospective cohort study. Scand J Infect Dis 1992; 24:97.
110. McCabe RE, Brooks RG, Dorfman RF, Remington JS. Clinical spectrum in 107 cases of toxoplasmic lymphadenopathy. Rev Infect Dis 1987;9:754.
111. Sayre MR, Jehle D. Elevated Toxoplasma IgG antibody in patients tested for infectious mononucleosis in an urban emergency department. Ann Emerg Med 1989;18:383.
112. Katholm M, Johnsen NJ, Siim C, Willumsen L. Bilateral sudden deafness and acute acquired toxoplasmosis. J Laryngol Otol 1991;105:115.
113. Evans TG, Schwartzman JD. Pulmonary toxoplasmosis. Semin Respir Infect 1991;6:51.
114. Holland GN. Ocular toxoplasmosis in the immunocompromised host. Int Ophthalmol 1989;13:399.
115. Luft BJ, Remington JS. Toxoplasmic encephalitis in AIDS. Clin Infect Dis 1992;15:211.
116. Hohlfeld P, Daffos F, Thulliez P, et al. Fetal toxoplasmosis: outcome of pregnancy and infant follow-up after in utero treatment. J Pediatr 1989;115:765.
117. Ghidini A, Sirtori M, Spelta A, Vergani P. Results of a preventive program for congenital toxoplasmosis. J Reprod Med 1991;36:270.
118. Burg JL, Grover CM, Pouletty P, Boothroyd JC. Direct and sensitive detection of a pathogenic protozoan, Toxoplasma gondii, by polymerase chain reaction. J Clin Microbiol 1989; 27:1787.
119. Savva D, Morris JC, Johnson JD, Holliman RE. Polymerase chain reaction for detection of Toxoplasma gondii. J Med Microbiol 1990;32:25.
120. van de Ven E, Melchers W, Galama J, et al. Identification of Toxoplasma gondii infections by BI gene amplification. J Clin Microbiol 1991;29:2120.
121. van Loon AM. Laboratory diagnosis of toxoplasmosis. Int Ophthalmol 1989;13:377.
122. Del Bono V, Canessa A, Bruzzi P, et al. Significance of specific immunoglobulin M in the chronological diagnosis of 38 cases of toxoplasmic lymphadenopathy. J Clin Microbiol 1989; 27:2133.
123. Huskinson J, Stepick-Biek PN, Araujo FG, et al. Toxoplasma antigens recognized by immunoglobulin G subclasses during acute and chronic infection. J Clin Microbiol 1989;27: 2031.
124. Decoster A, Caron A, Darcy F, Capron A. IgA antibodies against P30 as markers of congenital and acute toxoplasmosis. Lancet 1988;2:1104.
125. Huskinson J, Thulliez P, Remington JS. Toxoplasma antigens recognized by human immunoglobulin A antibodies. J Clin Microbiol 1990;28:2632.
126. Bessières MH, Roques C, Berrebi A, et al. IgA antibody response during acquired and congenital toxoplasmosis. J Clin Pathol 1992;45:605.
127. Gross U, Roos T, Appoldt D, Heesemann J. Improved serological diagnosis of Toxoplasma gondii infection by detection of immunoglobulin A (IgA) and IgM antibodies against P30 by using the immunoblot technique. J Clin Microbiol 1992; 30:1436.
128. Stepick-Biek P, Thulliez P, Araujo FG, Remington JS. IgA antibodies for diagnosis of acute congenital and acquired toxoplasmosis. J Infect Dis 1990;162:270.
129. Pinon JM, Toubas D, Marx C, et al. Detection of specific immunoglobulin E in patients with toxoplasmosis. J Clin Microbiol 1990;28:1739.
130. Bobić B, Šibalić D, Djurković-Djaković O. High levels of IgM antibodies specific for Toxoplasma gondii in pregnancy 12 years after primary Toxoplasma infection: case report. Gynecol Obstet Invest 1991;31:182.
131. Haentjens M, Sacré L, Demeuter F. Congenital toxoplasmosis after maternal infection before or slightly after conception. Acta Paediatr Scand 1986;75:343.
132. Daffos F, Forestier F, Capella-Pavlovsky M, et al. Prenatal management of 746 pregnancies at risk for congenital toxoplasmosis. N Engl J Med 1988;318:271.
133. Holliman RE, Johnson JD, Constantine G, et al. Difficulties in the diagnosis of congenital toxoplasmosis by cordocentesis: case report. Br J Obstet Gynaecol 1991;98:832.
134. Decoster A, Darcy F, Caron A, et al. Anti-P30 IgA antibodies as prenatal markers for congenital Toxoplasma infection. Clin Exp Immunol 1992;87:310.
135. Grover CM, Thulliez P, Remington JS, Boothroyd JC. Rapid prenatal diagnosis of congenital Toxoplasma infection by using polymerase chain reaction and amniotic fluid. J Clin Microbiol 1990;28:2297.
136. Cazenave J, Forestier F, Bessieres MH, et al. Contribution of a new PCR assay to the prenatal diagnosis of congenital toxoplasmosis. Prenat Diagn 1992;12:119.
137. Couvreur J, Desmonts G, Thulliez P. Prophylaxis of congenital toxoplasmosis: effects of spiramycin on placental infection. J Antimicrob Chemother 1988;22(Suppl B):193.
138. McCabe RE, Oster S. Current recommendations and future prospects in the treatment of toxoplasmosis. Drugs 1989; 38:973.
139. Pajor A. Pancytopenia in a patient given pyrimethamine and sulphamethoxidiazine during pregnancy. Arch Gynecol Obstet 1990;247:215.
140. Wilson CB, Remington JS. What can be done to prevent congenital toxoplasmosis? Am J Obstet Gynecol 1980;138:357.
141. Koskiniemi M, Lappalainen M, Hedman K. Toxoplasmosis needs evaluation: an overview and proposals. Am J Dis Child 1989;143:724.
142. Jeannel D, Costagliola D, Niel G, et al. What is known about the prevention of congenital toxoplasmosis? Lancet 1990; 336:359.
143. Carter AO, Gelmon SB, Wells GA, Toepell AP. The effectiveness of a prenatal education programme for the prevention of congenital toxoplasmosis. Epidemiol Infect 1989;103:539.
144. Foulon W, Naessens A, Lauwers S, et al. Impact of primary prevention on the incidence of toxoplasmosis during pregnancy. Obstet Gynecol 1988;72:363.
145. Conyn-van Spaendonck MAE. Prevention of congenital toxo-

plasmosis: experience in the Netherlands. Int Ophthalmol 1989;13:403.
146. Forsgren M, Gille E, Ljungström I, Nokes DJ. Toxoplasma gondii antibodies in pregnant women in Stockholm in 1969, 1979, and 1987. Lancet 1991;337:1413.
147. Taccone A, Fondelli MP, Ferrea G, Marzoli A. An unusual CT presentation of congenital cerebral toxoplasmosis in an 8-month-old boy with AIDS. Pediatr Radiol 1992;22:68.
148. de Jong PTVM. Ocular toxoplasmosis; common and rare symptoms and signs. Int Ophthalmol 1989;13:391.
149. McGee T, Wolters C, Stein L, et al. Absence of sensorineural hearing loss in treated infants and children with congenital toxoplasmosis. Otolaryngol Head Neck Surg 1992;106:75.
150. Glassman MS, Dellalzedah S, Beneck D, Seashore JH. Coincidence of congenital toxoplasmosis and biliary atresia in an infant. J Pediatr Gastroenterol Nutr 1991;13:298.
151. Rajantie J, Siimes MA, Taskinen E, et al. White blood cells in infants with congenital toxoplasmosis: transient appearance of cALL antigen on reactive marrow lymphocytes. Scand J Infect Dis 1992;24:227.
152. Hohlfeld P, Forestier F, Marion S, et al. Toxoplasma gondii infection during pregnancy: T lymphocyte subpopulations in mothers and fetuses. Pediatr Infect Dis J 1990;9:878.
153. McLeod R, Mack DG, Boyer K, et al. Phenotypes and functions of lymphocytes in congenital toxoplasmosis. J Lab Clin Med 1990;116:623.
154. Gross U, Müller J, Roos T, et al. Possible reasons for failure of conventional tests for diagnosis of fatal congenital toxoplasmosis: report of a case diagnosed by PCR and immunoblot. Infection 1992;20:149.
155. Skinner LJ, Chatterton JMW, Joss AWL, et al. The use of an IgM immunosorbent agglutination assay to diagnose congenital toxoplasmosis. J Med Microbiol 1989;28:125.
156. Decoster A, Slizewicz B, Simon J, et al. Platelia-Toxo IgA, a new kit for early diagnosis of congenital toxoplasmosis by detection of anti-P30 immunoglobulin A antibodies. J Clin Microbiol 1991;29:2291.
157. Wilson CB, Desmonts G, Couvreur J, Remington JS. Lymphocyte transformation in the diagnosis of congenital Toxoplasma infection. N Engl J Med 1980;302:785.
158. Wilson CB. Treatment of congenital toxoplasmosis. Pediatr Infect Dis J 1990;9:682.
159. McLeod R, Mack D, Foss R, et al. Levels of pyrimethamine in sera and cerebrospinal and ventricular fluids from infants treated for congenital toxoplasmosis. Antimicrob Agents Chemother 1992;36:1040.
160. Dutton GN. Recent developments in the prevention and treatment of congenital toxoplasmosis. Int Ophthalmol 1989; 13:407.
161. Guerina N, Meissner HC, Maguire J, et al. Prospective newborn screening and treatment program for congenital Toxoplasma infection. [Abstract 80] In: Program and abstracts of the 32nd Interscience Conference on Antimicrobial Agents and Chemotherapy. Washington, DC: American Society for Microbiology, 1992:124.
162. Wilson CB, Remington JS, Stagno S, Reynolds DW. Development of adverse sequelae in children born with subclinical congenital Toxoplasma infection. Pediatrics 1980;66:767.
163. Koppe JG, Loewer-Sieger DH, de Roever-Bonnet H. Results of 20-year follow-up of congenital toxoplasmosis. Lancet 1986; 1:254.
164. Koppe JG, Rothova A. Congenital toxoplasmosis: a long-term follow-up of 20 years. Int Ophthalmol 1989;13:387.
165. Lamprecht CL. Rubella virus. In: Belshe RB, ed. Textbook of human virology. 2nd ed. St. Louis: Mosby Year Book, 1991:675.
166. Seppälä M, Vaheri A. Natural rubella infection of the female genital tract. Lancet 1974;1:46.
167. Horstmann DM. Rubella. In: Evans AS, ed. Viral infections of humans: epidemiology and control. 3rd ed. New York: Plenum Publishing, 1989:617.
168. Töndury G, Smith DW. Fetal rubella pathology. J Pediatr 1966;68:867.
169. Garcia AGP, Marques RLS, Lobato YY, et al. Placental pathology in congenital rubella. Placenta 1985;6:281.
170. Chang TH, Moorhead PS, Boué JG, et al. Chromosome studies of human cells infected in utero and in vitro with rubella virus. Proc Soc Exp Biol Med 1966;122:236.
171. Ansari BM, Mason MK. Chromosomal abnormality in congenital rubella. Pediatrics 1977;59:13.
172. Plotkin SA, Vaheri A. Human fibroblasts infected with rubella virus produce a growth inhibitor. Science 1967;156:659.
173. Bowden DS, Pedersen JS, Toh BH, Westaway EG. Distribution by immunofluorescence of viral products and actin-containing cytoskeletal filaments in rubella virus-infected cells. Arch Virol 1987;92:211.
174. Naeye RL, Blanc W. Pathogenesis of congenital rubella. JAMA 1965;194:1277.
175. Yoneda T, Urade M, Sakuda M, Miyazaki T. Altered growth, differentiation, and responsiveness to epidermal growth factor of human embryonic mesenchymal cells of palate by persistent rubella virus infection. J Clin Invest 1986;77: 1613.
176. Coyle PK, Wolinsky JS, Buimovici-Klein E, et al. Rubella-specific immune complexes after congenital infection and vaccination. Infect Immun 1982;36:498.
177. Boner A, Wilmott RW, Dinwiddie R, et al. Desquamative interstitial pneumonia and antigen-antibody complexes in two infants with congenital rubella. Pediatrics 1983;72:835.
178. Clarke WL, Shaver KA, Bright GM, et al. Autoimmunity in congenital rubella syndrome. J Pediatr 1984;104:370.
179. Verder H, Dickmeiss E, Haahr S, et al. Late-onset rubella syndrome: coexistence of immune complex disease and defective cytotoxic effector cell function. Clin Exp Immunol 1986;63:367.
180. Yoon J-W, Choi D-S, Liang H-C, et al. Induction of an organ-specific autoimmune disease, lymphocytic hypophysitis, in hamsters by recombinant rubella virus glycoprotein and prevention of disease by neonatal thymectomy. J Virol 1992; 66:1210.
181. Salonen E-M, Hovi T, Meurman O, et al. Kinetics of specific IgA, IgD, IgE, IgG, and IgM antibody responses in rubella. J Med Virol 1985;16:1.
182. Al-Nakib W, Best JM, Banatvala JE. Rubella-specific serum and nasopharyngeal immunoglobulin responses following naturally acquired and vaccine-induced infection: prolonged persistence of virus-specific IgM. Lancet 1975;1:182.
183. Herrmann KL. Available rubella serologic tests. Rev Infect Dis 1985;7:S108.
184. Banatvala JE, Best JM, O'Shea S, Dudgeon JA. Persistence of rubella antibodies after vaccination: detection after experimental challenge. Rev Infect Dis 1985;7:S86.
185. Zolti M, Ben-Rafael Z, Bider D, et al. Rubella-specific IgM in reinfection and risk to the fetus. Gynecol Obstet Invest 1990;30:184.
186. Cradock-Watson JE. Laboratory diagnosis of rubella: past, present and future. Epidemiol Infect 1991;107:1.
187. Grangeot-Keros L, Pillot J, Daffos F, Forestier F. Prenatal and postnatal production of IgM and IgA antibodies to rubella virus studied by antibody capture immunoassay. J Infect Dis 1988;158:138.
188. Stokes A, Mims CA, Grahame R. Subclass distribution of IgG

and IgA responses to rubella virus in man. J Med Microbiol 1986;21:283.
189. Katow S, Sugiura A. Antibody response to individual rubella virus proteins in congenital and other rubella virus infections. J Clin Microbiol 1985;21:449.
190. Chaye HH, Mauracher CA, Tingle A, Gillam S. Cellular and humoral immune responses to rubella virus structural proteins E1, E2, and C. J Clin Microbiol 1992;30:2323.
191. Mitchell LA, Zhang T, Tingle AJ. Differential antibody responses to rubella virus infection in males and females. J Infect Dis 1992;166:1258.
192. Fitzgerald MG, Pullen GR, Hosking CS. Low affinity antibody to rubella antigen in patients after rubella infection in utero. Pediatrics 1988;81:812.
193. de Mazancourt A, Waxham MN, Nicolas JC, Wolinsky JS. Antibody response to the rubella virus structural proteins in infants with the congenital rubella syndrome. J Med Virol 1986;19:111.
194. Buimovici-Klein E, Cooper LZ. Cell-mediated immune response in rubella infections. Rev Infect Dis 1985;7:S123.
195. Kaplan KM, Cochi SL, Edmonds LD, et al. A profile of mothers giving birth to infants with congenital rubella syndrome: an assessment of risk factors. Am J Dis Child 1990;144:118.
196. Centers for Disease Control. Outbreaks of rubella among the Amish—United States, 1991. MMWR 1991;40:264.
197. Lee SH, Ewert DP, Frederick PD, Mascola L. Resurgence of congenital rubella syndrome in the 1990s: report on missed opportunities and failed prevention policies among women of childbearing age. JAMA 1992;267:2616.
198. Briss PA, Fehrs LJ, Hutcheson RH, Schaffner W. Rubella among the Amish: resurgent disease in a highly susceptible community. Pediatr Infect Dis J 1992;11:955.
199. Poland GA, Nichol KL. Medical students as sources of rubella and measles outbreaks. Arch Intern Med 1990;150:44.
200. Centers for Disease Control. Rubella prevention: recommendations of the Immunization Practices Advisory Committee (ACIP). MMWR 1990;39(RR-15):1.
201. Assaad F, Ljungars-Esteves K. Rubella—world impact. Rev Infect Dis 1985;7:S29.
202. Lever AML, Ross MGR, Baboonian C, Griffiths PD. Immunity to rubella among women of child-bearing age. Br J Obstet Gynaecol 1987;94:208.
203. Mingle JAA. Frequency of rubella antibodies in the population of some tropical African countries. Rev Infect Dis 1985;7:S68.
204. Prabhakar P, Bailey A, Smikle MF, et al. Seroprevalence of Toxoplasma gondii, rubella virus, cytomegalovirus, herpes simplex virus (TORCH) and syphilis in Jamaican pregnant women. West Indian Med J 1991;40:166.
205. Seth P, Manjunath N, Balaya S. Rubella infection: the Indian scene. Rev Infect Dis 1985;7:S64.
206. Wannian S. Rubella in the People's Republic of China. Rev Infect Dis 1985;7:S72.
207. Heggie AD. Pathogenesis of the rubella exanthem: isolation of rubella virus from the skin. N Engl J Med 1971;285:664.
208. Waxham MN, Wolinsky JS. Rubella virus and its effects on the central nervous system. Neurol Clin 1984;2:367.
209. Onji M, Kumon I, Kanaoka M, et al. Intrahepatic lymphocyte subpopulations in acute hepatitis in an adult with rubella. Am J Gastroenterol 1988;83:320.
210. Thanopoulos BD, Rokas S, Frimas CA, et al. Cardiac involvement in postnatal rubella. Acta Paediatr Scand 1989;78:141.
211. Shirley JA, Revill S, Cohen BJ, Buckley MM. Serological study of rubella-like illnesses. J Med Virol 1987;21:369.
212. Mahony JB, Chernesky MA. Rubella virus. In: Rose NR, de Macario EC, Fahey JL, Friedman H, Penn GM, eds. Manual of clinical laboratory immunology. 4th ed. Washington, DC: American Society for Microbiology, 1992:600.
213. Katow S, Sugiura A, Janejai N. Single-serum diagnosis of recent rubella infection with the use of hemagglutination inhibition test and enzyme-linked immunosorbent assays. Microbiol Immunol 1989;33:141.
214. Hedman K, Rousseau SA. Measurement of avidity of specific IgG for verification of recent primary rubella. J Med Virol 1989;27:288.
215. Hedman K, Hietala J, Tiilikainen A, et al. Maturation of immunoglobulin G avidity after rubella vaccination studied by an enzyme linked immunosorbent assay (avidity-ELISA) and by haemolysis typing. J Med Virol 1989;27:293.
216. Zhang T, Mauracher CA, Mitchell LA, Tingle AJ. Detection of rubella virus-specific immunoglobulin G (IgG), IgM, and IgA antibodies by immunoblot assays. J Clin Microbiol 1992; 30:824.
217. Kurtz JB, Anderson MJ. Cross-reactions in rubella and parvovirus specific IgM tests. Lancet 1985;2:1356.
218. Forsgren M, Carlström G, Strangert K. Congenital rubella after maternal reinfection. Scand J Infect Dis 1979;11:81.
219. Levine JB, Berkowitz CD, St Geme JW Jr. Rubella virus reinfection during pregnancy leading to late-onset congenital rubella syndrome. J Pediatr 1982;100:589.
220. Enders G, Calm A, Schaub J. Rubella embryopathy after previous maternal rubella vaccination. Infection 1984;12:96.
221. Forsgren M, Sörén L. Subclinical rubella reinfection in vaccinated women with rubella-specific IgM response during pregnancy and transmission of virus to the fetus. Scand J Infect Dis 1985;17:337.
222. Grangeot-Keros L, Nicolas JC, Bricout F, Pillot J. Rubella reinfection and the fetus. N Engl J Med 1985;313:1547.
223. Hornstein L, Levy U, Fogel A. Clinical rubella with virus transmission to the fetus in a pregnant woman considered to be immune. N Engl J Med 1988;319:1415.
224. Best JM, Banatvala JE, Morgan-Capner P, Miller E. Fetal infection after maternal reinfection with rubella: criteria for defining reinfection. BMJ 1989;299:773.
225. Gilbert J, Kudesia G. Fetal infection after maternal reinfection with rubella. BMJ 1989;299:1217.
226. Das BD, Lakhani P, Kurtz JB, et al. Congenital rubella after previous maternal immunity. Arch Dis Child 1990;65:545.
227. Keith CG. Congenital rubella infection from reinfection of previously immunised mothers. Aust N Z J Ophthalmol 1991; 19:291.
228. Condon R, Bower C. Congenital rubella after previous maternal vaccination. Med J Aust 1992;156:882.
229. Miller E, Cradock-Watson JE, Pollock TM. Consequences of confirmed maternal rubella at successive stages of pregnancy. Lancet 1982;2:781.
230. Munro ND, Sheppard S, Smithells RW, et al. Temporal relations between maternal rubella and congenital defects. Lancet 1987;2:201.
231. Grillner L, Forsgren M, Barr B, et al. Outcome of rubella during pregnancy with special reference to the 17th–24th weeks of gestation. Scand J Infect Dis 1983;15:321.
232. Bitsch M. Rubella in pregnant Danish women 1975–1984. Dan Med Bull 1987;34:46.
233. Enders G, Nickerl-Pacher U, Miller E, Cradock-Watson JE. Outcome of confirmed periconceptional maternal rubella. Lancet 1988;1:1445.
234. Segondy M, Boulot J, N'Dakortamanda N, et al. Detection of rubella virus in amniotic fluid by electron microscopy. Eur J Obstet Gynecol Reprod Biol 1990;37:77.
235. Sandow D, Rosmus K, Karnahl K, et al. Ein Beitrag zur pränatalen Rötelndiagnostik. Z Geburtshilfe Perinatol 1991;195:95.

236. Daffos F, Forestier F, Grangeot-Keros L, et al. Prenatal diagnosis of congenital rubella. Lancet 1984;2:1.
237. Enders G, Jonatha W. Prenatal diagnosis of intrauterine rubella. Infection 1987;15:162.
238. Terry GM, Ho-Terry L, Warren RC, et al. First trimester prenatal diagnosis of congenital rubella: a laboratory investigation. BMJ 1986;292:930.
239. Cradock-Watson JE, Miller E, Ridehalgh MKS, et al. Detection of rubella virus in fetal and placental tissues and in the throats of neonates after serologically confirmed rubella in pregnancy. Prenat Diagn 1989;9:91.
240. Ho-Terry L, Terry GM, Londesborough P. Diagnosis of foetal rubella virus infection by polymerase chain reaction. J Gen Virol 1990;71:1607.
241. Tingle AJ, Chantler JK, Pot KH, et al. Postpartum rubella immunization: association with development of prolonged arthritis, neurological sequelae, and chronic rubella viremia. J Infect Dis 1985;152:606.
242. Losonsky GA, Fishaut JM, Strussenberg J, Ogra PL. Effect of immunization against rubella on lactation products. II. Maternal-neonatal interactions. J Infect Dis 1982;145:661.
243. Howson CP, Katz M, Johnston RB Jr, Fineberg HV. Chronic arthritis after rubella vaccination. Clin Infect Dis 1992;15:307.
244. Landes RD, Bass JW, Millunchick EW, Oetgen WJ. Neonatal rubella following postpartum maternal immunization. J Pediatr 1980;97:465.
245. Centers for Disease Control. Rubella vaccination during pregnancy—United States, 1971–1988. MMWR 1989;38:289.
246. De Owens CS, De Espino RT. Rubella in Panama: still a problem. Pediatr Infect Dis J 1989;8:110.
247. Menser MA, Hudson JR, Murphy AM, Upfold LJ. Epidemiology of congenital rubella and results of rubella vaccination in Australia. Rev Infect Dis 1985;7:S37.
248. De la Mata I, De Wals P, Dolk H, et al. Incidence of congenital rubella syndrome in 19 regions of Europe in 1980–1986. Eur J Epidemiol 1989;5:106.
249. South MA, Sever JL. Teratogen update: the congenital rubella syndrome. Teratology 1985;31:297.
250. Tokugawa K, Ueda K, Fukushige J, et al. Congenital rubella syndrome and physical growth: a 17-year, prospective, longitudinal follow-up in the Ryukyu Islands. Rev Infect Dis 1986;8:874.
251. Chiriboga-Klein S, Oberfield SE, Casullo AM, et al. Growth in congenital rubella syndrome and correlation with clinical manifestations. J Pediatr 1989;115:251.
252. Campbell PE. Vascular abnormalities following maternal rubella. Br Heart J 1965;27:134.
253. Peckham CS. Clinical and laboratory study of children exposed in utero to maternal rubella. Arch Dis Child 1972; 47:571.
254. Gregg NM. Congenital cataract following German measles in the mother. Trans Ophthalmol Soc Aust 1941;3:35.
255. Romano A, Weinberg M, Bar-Izhak R, et al. Rate and various aspects of eye infection resulting from congenital rubella. J Pediatr Ophthalmol Strabismus 1979;16:26.
256. Kanra G, Firat T. Isolation of rubella virus from lens material in cases of congenital cataracts. J Pediatr Ophthalmol Strabismus 1979;16:31.
257. Smith GTH, Shun-Shin GA, Bron AJ. Spontaneous reabsorption of a rubella cataract. Br J Ophthalmol 1990;74:564.
258. Kresky B, Nauheim JS. Rubella retinitis. Am J Dis Child 1967; 113:305.
259. Geltzer AI, Guber D, Sears ML. Ocular manifestations of the 1964–65 rubella epidemic. Am J Ophthalmol 1967;63:221.
260. Collis WJ, Cohen DN. Rubella retinopathy: a progressive disorder. Arch Ophthalmol 1970;84:33.
261. Deluise VP, Cobo LM, Chandler D. Persistent corneal edema in the congenital rubella syndrome. Ophthalmology 1983; 90:835.
262. Desmond MM, Fisher ES, Vorderman AL, et al. The longitudinal course of congenital rubella encephalitis in nonretarded children. J Pediatr 1978;93:584.
263. Carey BM, Arthur RJ, Houlsby WT. Ventriculitis in congenital rubella: ultrasound demonstration. Pediatr Radiol 1987; 17:415.
264. Parisot S, Droulle P, Feldmann M, et al. Unusual encephaloclastic lesions with paraventricular calcification in congenital rubella. Pediatr Radiol 1991;21:229.
265. Yamashita Y, Matsuishi T, Murakami Y, et al. Neuroimaging findings (ultrasonography, CT, MRI) in 3 infants with congenital rubella syndrome. Pediatr Radiol 1991;21:547.
266. Hendricks WM, Hu C-H. Blueberry muffin syndrome: cutaneous erythropoiesis and possible intrauterine viral infection. Cutis 1984;34:549.
267. Marshall WC, Trompeter RS, Risdon RA. Chronic rashes in congenital rubella: isolation of virus from skin. Lancet 1975; 1:1349.
268. Alter M, Schulenberg R. Dermatoglyphics in the rubella syndrome. JAMA 1966;197:685.
269. Menser MA, Dorman DC, Reye RDK, Reid RR. Renal-artery stenosis in the rubella syndrome. Lancet 1966;1:790.
270. Menser MA, Robertson SEJ, Dorman DC, et al. Renal lesions in congenital rubella. Pediatrics 1967;40:901.
271. Forrest JM, Menser MA. Congenital rubella in schoolchildren and adolescents. Arch Dis Child 1970;45:63.
272. Kaplan GW, McLaughlin AP III. Urogenital anomalies and congenital rubella syndrome. Urology 1973;2:148.
273. Rudolph AJ, Singleton EB, Rosenberg HS, et al. Osseous manifestations of the congenital rubella syndrome. Am J Dis Child 1965;110:428.
274. Reed GB Jr. Rubella bone lesions. J Pediatr 1969;74:208.
275. London WT, Fuccillo DA, Anderson B, Sever JL. Concentration of rubella virus antigen in chondrocytes of congenitally infected rabbits. Nature 1970;226:172.
276. Sekeles E, Ornoy A. Osseous manifestations of gestational rubella in young human fetuses. Am J Obstet Gynecol 1975;122:307.
277. Heggie AD. Growth inhibition of human embryonic and fetal rat bones in organ culture by rubella virus. Teratology 1977; 15:47.
278. Zinkham WH, Medearis DN Jr, Osborn JE. Blood and bone-marrow findings in congenital rubella. J Pediatr 1967;71: 512.
279. Sherman LA, Silberstein LE, Berkman EM. Altered blood group expression in a patient with congenital rubella infection. Transfusion 1984;24:267.
280. Sever JL, South MA, Shaver KA. Delayed manifestations of congenital rubella. Rev Infect Dis 1985;7:S164.
281. Numazaki K, Goldman H, Wong I, Wainberg MA. Infection of cultured human fetal pancreatic islet cells by rubella virus. Am J Clin Pathol 1989;91:446.
282. Ginsberg-Fellner F, Witt ME, Fedun B, et al. Diabetes mellitus and autoimmunity in patients with the congenital rubella syndrome. Rev Infect Dis 1985;7:S170.
283. McEvoy RC, Fedun B, Cooper LZ, et al. Children at high risk of diabetes mellitus: New York studies of families with diabetes and of children with congenital rubella syndrome. Adv Exp Med Biol 1988;246:221.
284. Preece MA, Kearney PJ, Marshall WC. Growth-hormone deficiency in congenital rubella. Lancet 1977;2:842.
285. Centers for Disease Control. Rubella and congenital rubella syndrome—New York City. MMWR 1986;35:770.

286. Cooper LZ, Krugman S. Clinical manifestations of postnatal and congenital rubella. Arch Ophthalmol 1967;77:434.
287. O'Shea S, Best J, Banatvala JE. A lymphocyte transformation assay for the diagnosis of congenital rubella. J Virol Methods 1992;37:139.
288. Vesikari T, Meurman OH, Mäki R. Persistent rubella-specific IgM-antibody in the cerebrospinal fluid of a child with congenital rubella. Arch Dis Child 1980;55:46.
289. Plotkin SA, Klaus RM, Whitely JP. Hypogammaglobulinemia in an infant with congenital rubella syndrome; failure of 1-adamantanamine to stop virus excretion. J Pediatr 1966; 69:1085.
290. Larsson A, Forsgren M, Hård af Segerstad S, et al. Administration of interferon to an infant with congenital rubella syndrome involving persistent viremia and cutaneous vasculitis. Acta Paediatr Scand 1976;65:105.
291. Arvin AM, Schmidt NJ, Cantell K, Merigan TC. Alpha interferon administration to infants with congenital rubella. Antimicrob Agents Chemother 1982;21:259.
292. Centers for Disease Control. Hepatitis B virus: a comprehensive strategy for eliminating transmission in the United States through universal childhood vaccination. Recommendations of the Immunization Practices Advisory Committee (ACIP). MMWR 1991;40(RR-13):1.
293. Margolis HS, Alter MJ, Hadler SC. Hepatitis B: evolving epidemiology and implications for control. Semin Liver Dis 1991;11:84.
294. Stevens CE. Immunoprophylaxis of hepatitis B virus infection. Semin Pediatr Infect Dis 1991;2:135.
295. Lutwick LI. Hepatitis B virus. In: Belshe RB, ed. Textbook of human virology. 2nd ed. St. Louis: Mosby Year Book, 1991:719.
296. Hoofnagle JH, Di Bisceglie AM. Serologic diagnosis of acute and chronic viral hepatitis. Semin Liver Dis 1991;11:73.
297. Baker BL, Di Bisceglie AM, Kaneko S, et al. Determination of hepatitis B virus DNA in serum using the polymerase chain reaction: clinical significance and correlation with serological and biochemical markers. Hepatology 1991;13:632.
298. Levrero M, Stemler M, Pasquinelli C, et al. Significance of anti-HBx antibodies in hepatitis B virus infection. Hepatology 1991;13:143.
299. Bodsworth NJ, Cooper DA, Donovan B. The influence of human immunodeficiency virus type 1 infection on the development of the hepatitis B virus carrier state. J Infect Dis 1991;163:1138.
300. Rawal BK, Parida S, Watkins RPF, et al. Symptomatic reactivation of hepatitis B in pregnancy. Lancet 1991;337:364.
301. Omata M, Ehata T, Yokosuka O, et al. Mutations in the precore region of hepatitis B virus DNA in patients with fulminant and severe hepatitis. N Engl J Med 1991;324:1699.
302. Liang TJ, Hasegawa K, Rimon N, et al. A hepatitis B virus mutant associated with an epidemic of fulminant hepatitis. N Engl J Med 1991;324:1705.
303. Aach RD. Viral hepatitis. In: Feigin RD, Cherry JD, eds. Textbook of pediatric infectious diseases. 3rd ed. Philadelphia: WB Saunders, 1992:677.
304. Jonas MM, Ragin L, Silva MO. Membranous glomerulonephritis and chronic persistent hepatitis B in a child: treatment with recombinant interferon alfa. J Pediatr 1991;119:818.
305. Wang J-T, Wang T-H, Sheu J-C, et al. Detection of hepatitis B virus DNA by polymerase chain reaction in plasma of volunteer blood donors negative for hepatitis B surface antigen. J Infect Dis 1991;163:397.
306. Alter MJ, Hadler SC, Margolis HS, et al. The changing epidemiology of hepatitis B in the United States: need for alternative vaccination strategies. JAMA 1990;263:1218.
307. Centers for Disease Control. Protection against viral hepatitis: recommendations of the Immunization Practices Advisory Committee (ACIP). MMWR 1990;39(S-2):1.
308. Hadler SC, Margolis HS. Hepatitis B immunization: vaccine types, efficacy, and indications for immunization. In: Remington JS, Swartz MN, eds. Current clinical topics in infectious diseases, vol 12. Boston: Blackwell Scientific Publications, 1992:282.
309. Levy M, Koren G. Hepatitis B vaccine in pregnancy: maternal and fetal safety. Am J Perinatol 1991;8:227.
310. Centers for Disease Control. Prevention of perinatal transmission of hepatitis B virus: prenatal screening of all pregnant women for hepatitis B surface antigen. MMWR 1988;37:341.
311. Koretz RL. Universal prenatal hepatitis B testing: is it cost-effective? Obstet Gynecol 1989;74:808.
312. Okun NB, Bryce Larke RP, Waters JR, Joffres MR. Success of a program of routine prenatal screening for hepatitis B surface antigen: the first 2 years. Can Med Assoc J 1990;143:1317.
313. Committee on Infectious Diseases. Universal hepatitis B immunization. Pediatrics 1992;89:795.
314. Roizman B. Introduction: objectives of herpes simplex virus vaccines seen from a historical perspective. Rev Infect Dis 1991;13:S892.
315. Prober CG, Corey L, Brown ZA, et al. The management of pregnancies complicated by genital infections with herpes simplex virus. Clin Infect Dis 1992;15:1031.
316. Corey L, Spear PG. Infections with herpes simplex virus (first of two parts). N Engl J Med 1986;314:686.
317. Stevens JG. Human herpesviruses: a consideration of the latent state. Microbiol Rev 1989;53:318.
318. Kohl S. Role of antibody-dependent cellular cytotoxicity in defense against herpes simplex virus infections. Rev Infect Dis 1991;13:108.
319. Eriksen NL, Gonik B, Loo LS. Natural killer cell cytotoxicity to herpes simplex virus-1-infected cells is not altered by pregnancy. Am J Obstet Gynecol 1991;165:965.
320. Jenkins M, Kohl S. New aspects of neonatal herpes. Infect Dis Clin North Am 1992;6:57.
321. Wiedbrauk DL, Johnston SL. Manual of clinical virology. New York: Raven Press, 1993.
322. Courtney RJ. Membrane-associated antigens of herpes simplex virus. Rev Infect Dis 1991;13:S917.
323. Johnson RE, Nahmias AJ, Magder LS, et al. A seroepidemiologic survey of the prevalence of herpes simplex virus type 2 infection in the United States. N Engl J Med 1989;321:7.
324. Siegel D, Golden E, Washington AE, et al. Prevalence and correlates of herpes simplex infections: the population-based AIDS in Multiethnic Neighborhoods Study. JAMA 1992; 268:1702.
325. Kulhanjian JA, Soroush V, Au DS, et al. Identification of women at unsuspected risk of primary infection with herpes simplex virus type 2 during pregnancy. N Engl J Med 1992; 326:916.
326. Taieb A, Body S, Astar I, et al. Clinical epidemiology of symptomatic primary herpetic infection in children: a study of 50 cases. Acta Paediatr Scand 1987;76:128.
327. Kuzushima K, Kimura H, Kino Y, et al. Clinical manifestations of primary herpes simplex virus type 1 infection in a closed community. Pediatrics 1991;87:152.
328. Straus SE, Rooney JF, Sever JL, et al. Herpes simplex virus infection: biology, treatment, and prevention. Ann Intern Med 1985;103:404.
329. Breinig MK, Kingsley LA, Armstrong JA, et al. Epidemiology of genital herpes in Pittsburgh: serologic, sexual, and racial correlates of apparent and inapparent herpes simplex infections. J Infect Dis 1990;162:299.

330. Koutsky LA, Stevens CE, Holmes KK, et al. Underdiagnosis of genital herpes by current clinical and viral-isolation procedures. N Engl J Med 1992;326:1533.
331. Whitley RJ. Herpes simplex virus infections of the central nervous system: encephalitis and neonatal herpes. Drugs 1991;42:406.
332. Jacques SM, Qureshi F. Herpes simplex virus hepatitis in pregnancy: a clinicopathologic study of three cases. Human Pathol 1992;23:183.
333. Lafferty WE, Coombs RW, Benedetti J, et al. Recurrences after oral and genital herpes simplex virus infection: influence of site of infection and viral type. N Engl J Med 1987;316:1444.
334. Koelle DM, Benedetti J, Langenberg A, Corey L. Asymptomatic reactivation of herpes simplex virus in women after the first episode of genital herpes. Ann Intern Med 1992;116:433.
335. Nahass GT, Goldstein BA, Zhu WY, et al. Comparison of Tzanck smear, viral culture, and DNA diagnostic methods in detection of herpes simplex and varicella-zoster infection. JAMA 1992;268:2541.
336. Cone RW, Hobson AC, Palmer J, et al. Extended duration of herpes simplex virus DNA in genital lesions detected by the polymerase chain reaction. J Infect Dis 1991;164:757.
337. Rogers BB, Josephson SL, Mak SK, Sweeney PJ. Polymerase chain reaction amplification of herpes simplex virus DNA from clinical samples. Obstet Gynecol 1992;79:464.
338. Aurelius E, Johansson B, Sköldenberg B, et al. Rapid diagnosis of herpes simplex encephalitis by nested polymerase chain reaction assay of cerebrospinal fluid. Lancet 1991;337:189.
339. Editorial. Acute diagnosis of herpes simplex encephalitis. Lancet 1991;337:205.
340. Whitley RJ, Cobbs CG, Alford CA Jr, et al. Diseases that mimic herpes simplex encephalitis: diagnosis, presentation, and outcome. JAMA 1989;262:234.
341. Whitley RJ, Gnann JW Jr. Acyclovir: a decade later. N Engl J Med 1992;327:782.
342. Berger SA, Weinberg M, Treves T, et al. Herpes encephalitis during pregnancy: failure of acyclovir and adenine arabinoside to prevent neonatal herpes. Isr J Med Sci 1986;22:41.
343. Stahlmann R, Klug S, Lewandowski C, et al. Teratogenicity of acyclovir in rats. Infection 1987;15:261.
344. Frenkel LM, Brown ZA, Bryson YJ, et al. Pharmacokinetics of acyclovir in the term human pregnancy and neonate. Am J Obstet Gynecol 1991;164:569.
345. Lau RJ, Emery MG, Galinsky RE. Unexpected accumulation of acyclovir in breast milk with estimation of infant exposure. Obstet Gynecol 1987;69:468.
346. Andrews EB, Yankaskas BC, Cordero JF, et al. Acyclovir in pregnancy registry: six years' experience. Obstet Gynecol 1992;79:7.
347. Safrin S, Crumpacker C, Chatis P, et al. A controlled trial comparing foscarnet with vidarabine for acyclovir-resistant mucocutaneous herpes simplex in the acquired immunodeficiency syndrome. N Engl J Med 1991;325:551.
348. Stone KM, Brooks CA, Guinan ME, Alexander ER. National surveillance for neonatal herpes simplex virus infections. Sex Transm Dis 1989;16:152.
349. Brown ZA, Benedetti J, Ashley R, et al. Neonatal herpes simplex virus infection in relation to asymptomatic maternal infection at the time of labor. N Engl J Med 1991;324:1247.
350. Brown ZA, Vontver LA, Benedetti J, et al. Effects on infants of a first episode of genital herpes during pregnancy. N Engl J Med 1987;317:1246.
351. Baldwin S, Whitley RJ. Teratogen update: intrauterine herpes simplex virus infection. Teratology 1989;39:1.
352. Freij BJ, Sever JL. Fetal herpes simplex virus infection. In: Buyse ML, ed. Birth defects encyclopedia. Boston: Blackwell Scientific Publications, 1990:713.
353. Whitley R, Arvin A, Prober C, et al. A controlled trial comparing vidarabine with acyclovir in neonatal herpes simplex virus infection. N Engl J Med 1991;324:444.
354. Whitley R, Arvin A, Prober C, et al. Predictors of morbidity and mortality in neonates with herpes simplex virus infections. N Engl J Med 1991;324:450.
355. Silverman MS, Gartner JG, Halliday WC, et al. Persistent cerebrospinal fluid neutrophilia in delayed-onset neonatal encephalitis caused by herpes simplex virus type 2. J Pediatr 1992;120:567.
356. Cameron PD, Wallace SJ, Munro J. Herpes simplex virus encephalitis: problems in diagnosis. Dev Med Child Neurol 1992;34:134.
357. el-Azazi M, Malm G, Forsgren M. Late ophthalmologic manifestations of neonatal herpes simplex virus infection. Am J Ophthalmol 1990;109:1.
358. Andersen RD. Herpes simplex virus infection of the neonatal respiratory tract. Am J Dis Child 1987;141:274.
359. Hubbell C, Dominguez R, Kohl S. Neonatal herpes simplex pneumonitis. Rev Infect Dis 1988;10:431.
360. Barker JA, McLean SD, Jordan GD, et al. Primary neonatal herpes simplex virus pneumonia. Pediatr Infect Dis J 1990;9:285.
361. Dominguez R, Rivero H, Gaisie G, et al. Neonatal herpes simplex pneumonia: radiographic findings. Radiology 1984;153:395.
362. Schutze GE, Edwards MS, Adham BI, Belmont JW. Hyperammonemia and neonatal herpes simplex pneumonitis. Pediatr Infect Dis J 1990;9:749.
363. Kimura H, Futamura M, Kito H, et al. Detection of viral DNA in neonatal herpes simplex virus infections: frequent and prolonged presence in serum and cerebrospinal fluid. J Infect Dis 1991;164:289.
364. Englund JA, Fletcher CV, Balfour HH Jr. Acyclovir therapy in neonates. J Pediatr 1991;119:129.
365. Toltzis P. Current issues in neonatal herpes simplex virus infection. Clin Perinatol 1991;18:193.
366. Libman MD, Dascal A, Kramer MS, Mendelson J. Strategies for the prevention of neonatal infection with herpes simplex virus: a decision analysis. Rev Infect Dis 1991;13:1093.
367. Arvin AM, Hensleigh PA, Prober CG, et al. Failure of antepartum maternal cultures to predict the infant's risk of exposure to herpes simplex virus at delivery. N Engl J Med 1986;315:796.
368. Prober CG, Hensleigh PA, Boucher FD, et al. Use of routine viral cultures at delivery to identify neonates exposed to herpes simplex virus. N Engl J Med 1988;318:887.
369. Prober CG, Sullender WM, Yasukawa LL, et al. Low risk of herpes simplex virus infections in neonates exposed to the virus at the time of vaginal delivery to mothers with recurrent genital herpes simplex virus infections. N Engl J Med 1987;316:240.
370. Arvin AM. Relationships between maternal immunity to herpes simplex virus and the risk of neonatal herpesvirus infection. Rev Infect Dis 1991;13:S953.
371. Burke RL. Development of a herpes simplex virus subunit glycoprotein vaccine for prophylactic and therapeutic use. Rev Infect Dis 1991;13:S906.
372. Stanberry LR. Evaluation of herpes simplex virus vaccines in animals: the guinea pig vaginal model. Rev Infect Dis 1991;13:S920.
373. Corey L. Clinical studies with herpes simplex virus type 2 Curtis strain vaccine. Rev Infect Dis 1991;13:S904.

374. Alford CA, Stagno S, Pass RF, Britt WJ. Congenital and perinatal cytomegalovirus infections. Rev Infect Dis 1990;12:S745.
375. Gehrz RC. Human cytomegalovirus: biology and clinical perspectives. Adv Pediatr 1991;38:203.
376. Grundy JE. Virologic and pathogenetic aspects of cytomegalovirus infection. Rev Infect Dis 1990;12:S711.
377. Demmler GJ. Summary of a workshop on surveillance for congenital cytomegalovirus disease. Rev Infect Dis 1991; 13:315.
378. Walmus BF, Yow MD, Lester JW, et al. Factors predictive of cytomegalovirus immune status in pregnant women. J Infect Dis 1988;157:172.
379. Tookey PA, Ades AE, Peckham CS. Cytomegalovirus prevalence in pregnant women: the influence of parity. Arch Dis Child 1992;67:779.
380. Sohn YM, Oh MK, Balcarek KB, et al. Cytomegalovirus infection in sexually active adolescents. J Infect Dis 1991;163:460.
381. Fowler KB, Pass RF. Sexually transmitted diseases in mothers of neonates with congenital cytomegalovirus infection. J Infect Dis 1991;164:259.
382. Adler SP. Cytomegalovirus and child day care: risk factors for maternal infection. Pediatr Infect Dis J 1991;10:590.
383. Murph JR, Baron JC, Brown CK, et al. The occupational risk of cytomegalovirus infection among day-care providers. JAMA 1991;265:603.
384. Balfour CL, Balfour HH Jr. Cytomegalovirus is not an occupational risk for nurses in renal transplant and neonatal units: results of a prospective surveillance study. JAMA 1986; 256:1909.
385. Fowler KB, Stagno S, Pass RF, et al. The outcome of congenital cytomegalovirus infection in relation to maternal antibody status. N Engl J Med 1992;326:663.
386. Putland RA, Ford J, Korban G, et al. Investigation of spontaneously aborted concepti for microbial DNA: investigation for cytomegalovirus DNA using polymerase chain reaction. Aust N Z J Obstet Gynaecol 1990;30:248.
387. Griffiths PD, Stagno S, Pass RF, et al. Infection with cytomegalovirus during pregnancy: specific IgM antibodies as a marker of recent primary infection. J Infect Dis 1982;145:647.
388. Einsele H, Ehninger G, Steidle M, et al. Polymerase chain reaction to evaluate antiviral therapy for cytomegalovirus disease. Lancet 1991;338:1170.
389. Brytting M, Xu W, Wahren B, Sundqvist V-A. Cytomegalovirus DNA detection in sera from patients with active cytomegalovirus infections. J Clin Microbiol 1992;30:1937.
390. Erice A, Holm MA, Gill PC, et al. Cytomegalovirus (CMV) antigenemia assay is more sensitive than shell vial cultures for rapid detection of CMV in polymorphonuclear blood leukocytes. J Clin Microbiol 1992;30:2822.
391. Fan-Havard P, Nahata MC, Brady MT. Ganciclovir—a review of pharmacology, therapeutic efficacy and potential use for treatment of congenital cytomegalovirus infections. J Clin Pharmacol Ther 1989;14:329.
392. Drew WL. Cytomegalovirus infection in patients with AIDS. Clin Infect Dis 1992;14:608.
393. Boppana SB, Pass RF, Britt WJ, et al. Symptomatic congenital cytomegalovirus infection: neonatal morbidity and mortality. Pediatr Infect Dis J 1992;11:93.
394. Bale JF Jr, Blackman JA, Sato Y. Outcome in children with symptomatic congenital cytomegalovirus infection. J Child Neurol 1990;5:131.
395. Ramsay MEB, Miller E, Peckham CS. Outcome of confirmed symptomatic congenital cytomegalovirus infection. Arch Dis Child 1991;66:1068.
396. Perlman JM, Argyle C. Lethal cytomegalovirus infection in preterm infants: clinical, radiological, and neuropathological findings. Ann Neurol 1992;31:64.
397. Williamson WD, Demmler GJ, Percy AK, Catlin FI. Progressive hearing loss in infants with asymptomatic congenital cytomegalovirus infection. Pediatrics 1992;90:862.
398. Fowler K, McCollister F, Pass R, et al. Childhood deafness: the importance of congenital cytomegalovirus screening. [Abstract] Am J Epidemiol 1992;136:954.
399. Stagno S, Pass RF, Thomas JP, et al. Defects of tooth structure in congenital cytomegalovirus infection. Pediatrics 1982; 69:646.
400. Morris DJ. Epidemiological evidence is crucial as proof of causation in cytomegalovirus disease. J Infect 1991;23:233.
401. Hart MH, Kaufman SS, Vanderhoof JA, et al. Neonatal hepatitis and extrahepatic biliary atresia associated with cytomegalovirus infection in twins. Am J Dis Child 1991;145:302.
402. Jenson HB, Robert MF. Congenital cytomegalovirus infection with osteolytic lesions: use of DNA hybridization in diagnosis. Clin Pediatr (Phila) 1987;26:448.
403. Warren WP, Balcarek K, Smith R, Pass RF. Comparison of rapid methods of detection of cytomegalovirus in saliva with virus isolation in tissue culture. J Clin Microbiol 1992;30:786.
404. Dankner WM, Pass RF, Stagno S, et al. Polymerase chain reaction (PCR) for the detection of cytomegalovirus (CMV) in placentas from congenitally infected infants. [Abstract 943] Pediatr Res 1992;31:160A.
405. Balcarek KB, Lyon MD, Smith RJ, et al. Neonatal screening for congenital cytomegalovirus (CMV) infection by detection of virus in saliva. [Abstract 1627] Pediatr Res 1992;31:274A.
406. Chang M-H, Huang H-H, Huang E-S, et al. Polymerase chain reaction to detect human cytomegalovirus in livers of infants with neonatal hepatitis. Gastroenterology 1992;103:1022.
407. Drew WL, Miner RC, Busch DF, et al. Prevalence of resistance in patients receiving ganciclovir for serious cytomegalovirus infection. J Infect Dis 1991;163:716.
408. Hocker JR, Cook LN, Adams G, Rabalais GP. Ganciclovir therapy of congenital cytomegalovirus pneumonia. Pediatr Infect Dis J 1990;9:743.
409. Evans DGR, Lyon AJ. Fatal congenital cytomegalovirus infection acquired by an intra-uterine transfusion. Eur J Pediatr 1991;150:780.
410. Reigstad H, Bjerknes R, Markestad T, Myrmel H. Ganciclovir therapy of congenital cytomegalovirus disease. Acta Paediatr 1992;81:707.
411. Alford C. Breast milk transmission of cytomegalovirus (CMV) infection. Adv Exp Med Biol 1991;310:293.
412. Gentile MA, Boll TJ, Stagno S, Pass RF. Intellectual ability of children after perinatal cytomegalovirus infection. Dev Med Child Neurol 1989;31:782.
413. Lynch L, Daffos F, Emanuel D, et al. Prenatal diagnosis of fetal cytomegalovirus infection. Am J Obstet Gynecol 1991; 165:714.
414. Hohlfeld P, Vial Y, Maillard-Brignon C, et al. Cytomegalovirus fetal infection: prenatal diagnosis. Obstet Gynecol 1991;78:615.
415. Lamy ME, Mulongo KN, Gadisseux J-F, et al. Prenatal diagnosis of fetal cytomegalovirus infection. Am J Obstet Gynecol 1992;166:91.
416. Weber B, Opp M, Born HJ, et al. Laboratory diagnosis of congenital human cytomegalovirus infection using polymerase chain reaction and shell vial culture. Infection 1992; 20:155.
417. Pletcher BA, Williams MK, Mulivor RA, et al. Intrauterine cytomegalovirus infection presenting as fetal meconium peritonitis. Obstet Gynecol 1991;78:903.

418. Grose C, Meehan T, Weiner CP. Prenatal diagnosis of congenital cytomegalovirus infection by virus isolation after amniocentesis. Pediatr Infect Dis J 1992;11:605.
419. Tierney AJ, Higa TE, Finer NN. Disseminated cytomegalovirus infection after extracorporeal membrane oxygenation. Pediatr Infect Dis J 1992;11:241.
420. Weller TH. Varicella and herpes zoster: changing concepts of the natural history, control, and importance of a not-so-benign virus (first of two parts). N Engl J Med 1983;309:1362.
421. Centers for Disease Control. Varicella-zoster immune globulin for the prevention of chickenpox. MMWR 1984;33:84.
422. Sever JL, Ellenberg JH, Ley A, Edmonds D. Incidence of clinical infections in a defined population of pregnant women. In: Marois M, ed. Prevention of physical and mental congenital defects. Part B: epidemiology, early detection and therapy, and environmental factors. New York: Alan R Liss, 1985:317.
423. Stagno S, Whitley RJ. Herpesvirus infections of pregnancy. Part II: herpes simplex virus and varicella-zoster virus infections. N Engl J Med 1985;313:1327.
424. Ross AH. Modification of chicken pox in family contacts by administration of gamma globulin. N Engl J Med 1962; 267:369.
425. Junker AK, Angus E, Thomas EE. Recurrent varicella-zoster virus infections in apparently immunocompetent children. Pediatr Infect Dis J 1991;10:569.
426. Enders G. Varicella-zoster virus infection in pregnancy. Prog Med Virol 1984;29:166.
427. Kido S, Ozaki T, Asada H, et al. Detection of varicella-zoster virus (VZV) DNA in clinical samples from patients with VZV by the polymerase chain reaction. J Clin Microbiol 1991;29:76.
428. Koropchak CM, Graham G, Palmer J, et al. Investigation of varicella-zoster virus infection by polymerase chain reaction in the immunocompetent host with acute varicella. J Infect Dis 1991;163:1016.
429. Feder HM Jr. Treatment of adult chickenpox with oral acyclovir. Arch Intern Med 1990;150:2061.
430. Rothe MJ, Feder HM Jr, Grant-Kels JM. Oral acyclovir therapy for varicella and zoster infections in pediatric and pregnant patients: a brief review. Pediatr Dermatol 1991;8:236.
431. Wallace MR, Bowler WA, Murray NB, et al. Treatment of adult varicella with oral acyclovir: a randomized, placebo-controlled trial. Ann Intern Med 1992;117:358.
432. Broussard RC, Payne DK, George RB. Treatment with acyclovir of varicella pneumonia in pregnancy. Chest 1991;99: 1045.
433. Esmonde TF, Herdman G, Anderson G. Chickenpox pneumonia: an association with pregnancy. Thorax 1989;44:812.
434. Cox SM, Cunningham FG, Luby J. Management of varicella pneumonia complicating pregnancy. Am J Perinatol 1990; 7:300.
435. Lotshaw RR, Keegan JM, Gordon HR. Parenteral and oral acyclovir for management of varicella pneumonia in pregnancy: a case report with review of literature. W V Med J 1991;87:204.
436. Smego RA Jr, Asperilla MO. Use of acyclovir for varicella pneumonia during pregnancy. Obstet Gynecol 1991;78:1112.
437. Brunell PA. Fetal and neonatal varicella-zoster infections. Semin Perinatol 1983;7:47.
438. Meyers JD. Congenital varicella in term infants: risk reconsidered. J Infect Dis 1974;129:215.
439. Paryani SG, Arvin AM. Intrauterine infection with varicella-zoster virus after maternal varicella. N Engl J Med 1986; 314:1542.
440. Siegel M, Fuerst HT. Low birth weight and maternal virus diseases: a prospective study of rubella, measles, mumps, chickenpox, and hepatitis. JAMA 1966;197:680.
441. Siegel M, Fuerst HT, Peress NS. Comparative fetal mortality in maternal virus diseases: a prospective study on rubella, measles, mumps, chicken pox and hepatitis. N Engl J Med 1966;274:768.
442. Benyesh-Melnick M, Stich HF, Rapp F, Hsu TC. Viruses and mammalian chromosomes. III. Effect of herpes zoster virus on human embryonal lung cultures. Proc Soc Exp Biol Med 1964;117:546.
443. Aula P. Chromosomes and viral infections. Lancet 1964;1: 720.
444. Massimo L, Vianello MG, Dagna-Bricarelli F, Tortorolo G. Chicken-pox and chromosome aberrations. BMJ 1965;2:172.
445. Muñoz N. Perinatal viral infections and the risk of certain cancers. Prog Biochem Pharmacol 1978;14:104.
446. Alexander I. Congenital varicella. BMJ 1979;2:1074.
447. Alkalay AL, Pomerance JJ, Rimoin DL. Fetal varicella syndrome. J Pediatr 1987;111:320.
448. Bennet R, Forsgren M, Herin P. Herpes zoster in a 2-week-old premature infant with possible congenital varicella encephalitis. Acta Paediatr Scand 1985;74:979.
449. Borzyskowski M, Harris RF, Jones RWA. The congenital varicella syndrome. Eur J Pediatr 1981;137:335.
450. Brice JEH. Congenital varicella resulting from infection during second trimester of pregnancy. Arch Dis Child 1976; 51:474.
451. Charles NC, Bennett TW, Margolis S. Ocular pathology of the congenital varicella syndrome. Arch Ophthalmol 1977;95: 2034.
452. Cotlier E. Congenital varicella cataract. Am J Ophthalmol 1978;86:627.
453. Cuthbertson G, Weiner CP, Giller RH, Grose C. Prenatal diagnosis of second-trimester congenital varicella syndrome by virus-specific immunoglobulin M. J Pediatr 1987;111:592.
454. Dodion-Fransen J, Dekegel D, Thiry L. Congenital varicella-zoster infection related to maternal disease in early pregnancy. Scand J Infect Dis 1973;5:149.
455. Essex-Cater A, Heggarty H. Fatal congenital varicella syndrome. J Infect 1983;7:77.
456. Frey HM, Bialkin G, Gershon AA. Congenital varicella: case report of a serologically proved long-term survivor. Pediatrics 1977;59:110.
457. Hajdi G, Mészner Z, Nyerges G, et al. Congenital varicella syndrome. Infection 1986;14:177.
458. Higa K, Dan K, Manabe H. Varicella-zoster virus infections during pregnancy: hypothesis concerning the mechanisms of congenital malformations. Obstet Gynecol 1987;69:214.
459. König R, Gutjahr P, Kruel R, et al. Konnatale Varizellen-Embryo-Fetopathie. Helv Paediatr Acta 1985;40:391.
460. Kotchmar GS Jr, Grose C, Brunell PA. Complete spectrum of the varicella congenital defects syndrome in 5-year-old child. Pediatr Infect Dis 1984;3:142.
461. LaForet EG, Lynch CL Jr. Multiple congenital defects following maternal varicella: report of a case. N Engl J Med 1947; 236:534.
462. McKendry JBJ, Bailey JD. Congenital varicella associated with multiple defects. Can Med Assoc J 1973;108:66.
463. Rinvik R. Congenital varicella encephalomyelitis in surviving newborn. Am J Dis Child 1969;117:231.
464. Savage MO, Moosa A, Gordon RR. Maternal varicella infection as a cause of fetal malformations. Lancet 1973;1:352.
465. Siegel M. Congenital malformations following chickenpox, measles, mumps, and hepatitis: results of a cohort study. JAMA 1973;226:1521.
466. Srabstein JC, Morris N, Bryce Larke RP, et al. Is there a congenital varicella syndrome? J Pediatr 1974;84:239.
467. Taranger J, Blomberg J, Strannegård Ö. Intrauterine varicella:

a report of two cases associated with hyper-A-immunoglobulinemia. Scand J Infect Dis 1981;13:297.
468. Trlifajová J, Benda R, Beně Č. Effect of maternal varicella-zoster virus infection on the outcome of pregnancy and the analysis of transplacental virus transmission. Acta Virol (Praha) 1986;30:249.
469. Unger-Köppel J, Kilcher P, Tönz O. Varizellenfetopathie. Helv Paediatr Acta 1985;40:399.
470. Williamson AP. The varicella-zoster virus in the etiology of severe congenital defects: a survey of eleven reported instances. Clin Pediatr (Phila) 1975;14:553.
471. Lambert SR, Taylor D, Kriss A, et al. Ocular manifestations of the congenital varicella syndrome. Arch Ophthalmol 1989; 107:52.
472. Lloyd KM, Dunne JL. Skin lesions as the sole manifestation of the fetal varicella syndrome. Arch Dermatol 1990;126:546.
473. Scharf A, Scherr O, Enders G, Helftenbein E. Virus detection in the fetal tissue of a premature delivery with a congenital varicella syndrome. A case report. J Perinat Med 1990;18:317.
474. Da Silva O, Hammerberg O, Chance GW. Fetal varicella syndrome. Pediatr Infect Dis J 1990;9:854.
475. Scheffer IE, Baraitser M, Brett EM. Severe microcephaly associated with congenital varicella infection. Dev Med Child Neurol 1991;33:916.
476. Magliocco AM, Demetrick DJ, Sarnat HB, Hwang WS. Varicella embryopathy. Arch Pathol Lab Med 1992;116:181.
477. Asha Bai PV, John TJ. Congenital skin ulcers following varicella in late pregnancy. J Pediatr 1979;94:65.
478. Salzman MB, Sood SK. Congenital anomalies resulting from maternal varicella at 25 ½ weeks of gestation. Pediatr Infect Dis J 1992;11:504.
479. Brazin SA, Simkovich JW, Johnson WT. Herpes zoster during pregnancy. Obstet Gynecol 1979;53:175.
480. Duehr PA. Herpes zoster as a cause of congenital cataract. Am J Ophthalmol 1955;39:157.
481. Klauber GT, Flynn FJ Jr, Altman BD. Congenital varicella syndrome with genitourinary anomalies. Urology 1976;8:153.
482. Webster MH, Smith CS. Congenital abnormalities and maternal herpes zoster. BMJ 1977;2:1193.
483. Mendez DB, Sinclair MB, Garcia S, et al. Transplacental immunity to varicella-zoster virus in extremely low birthweight infants. Am J Perinatol 1992;9:236.
484. Williams H, Latif A, Morgan J, Ansari BM. Acyclovir in the treatment of neonatal varicella. J Infect 1987;15:65.
485. Gershon AA. Varicella vaccine: still at the crossroads. Pediatrics 1992;90:144.
486. Weller TH. Varicella and herpes zoster: changing concepts of the natural history, control, and importance of a not-so-benign virus (second of two parts). N Engl J Med 1983;309:1434.
487. Brunell PA. Varicella in pregnancy, the fetus, and the newborn: problems in management. J Infect Dis 1992;166:S42.
488. Gershon AA, LaRussa P, Hardy I, et al. Varicella vaccine: the American experience. J Infect Dis 1992;166:S63.
489. McGregor JA, Mark S, Crawford GP, Levin MJ. Varicella zoster antibody testing in the care of pregnant women exposed to varicella. Am J Obstet Gynecol 1987;157:281.
490. Balducci J, Rodis JF, Rosengren S, et al. Pregnancy outcome following first-trimester varicella infection. Obstet Gynecol 1992;79:5.
491. Isada NB, Paar DP, Johnson MP, et al. In utero diagnosis of congenital varicella zoster virus infection by chorionic villus sampling and polymerase chain reaction. Am J Obstet Gynecol 1991;165:1727.
492. Hanngren KAJ, Grandien M, Granström G. Effect of zoster immunoglobulin for varicella prophylaxis in the newborn. Scand J Infect Dis 1985;17:343.
493. Bakshi SS, Miller TC, Kaplan M, et al. Failure of varicella-zoster immunoglobulin in modification of severe congenital varicella. Pediatr Infect Dis 1986;5:699.
494. Haddad J, Simeoni U, Messer J, Willard D. Acyclovir in prophylaxis and perinatal varicella. Lancet 1987;1:161.
495. Rubin L, Leggiadro R, Elie MT, Lipsitz P. Disseminated varicella in a neonate: implications for immunoprophylaxis of neonates postnatally exposed to varicella. Pediatr Infect Dis 1986;5:100.
496. Cossart YE, Field AM, Cant B, Widdows D. Parvovirus-like particles in human sera. Lancet 1975;1:72.
497. Anderson LJ, Török TJ. The clinical spectrum of human parvovirus B19 infections. In: Remington JS, Swartz MN, eds. Current clinical topics in infectious diseases, vol 11. Boston: Blackwell Scientific Publications, 1991:267.
498. Kumar ML. Human parvovirus B19 and its associated diseases. Clin Perinatol 1991;18:209.
499. Takahashi T, Ozawa K, Takahashi K, et al. Susceptibility of human erythropoietic cells to B19 parvovirus in vitro increases with differentiation. Blood 1990;75:603.
500. Shimomura S, Komatsu N, Frickhofen N, et al. First continuous propagation of B19 parvovirus in a cell line. Blood 1992;79:18.
501. Schwarz TF, Serke S, Hottenträger B, et al. Replication of parvovirus B19 in hematopoietic progenitor cells generated in vitro from normal human peripheral blood. J Virol 1992; 66:1273.
502. Frickhofen N, Young NS. Persistent parvovirus B19 infections in humans. Microb Pathog 1989;7:319.
503. Centers for Disease Control. Risks associated with human parvovirus B19 infection. MMWR 1989;38:81.
504. Koch WC, Adler SP. Human parvovirus B19 infections in women of childbearing age and within families. Pediatr Infect Dis J 1989;8:83.
505. Cartter ML, Farley TA, Rosengren S, et al. Occupational risk factors for infection with parvovirus B19 among pregnant women. J Infect Dis 1991;163:282.
506. Bell LM, Naides SJ, Stoffman P, et al. Human parvovirus B19 infection among hospital staff members after contact with infected patients. N Engl J Med 1989;321:485.
507. Lobkowicz F, Ring J, Schwarz TF, Roggendorf M. Erythema multiforme in a patient with acute human parvovirus B19 infection. J Am Acad Dermatol 1989;20:849.
508. Zerbini M, Musiani M, Venturoli S, et al. Different syndromes associated with B19 parvovirus viraemia in paediatric patients: report of four cases. Eur J Pediatr 1992;151:815.
509. Woolf AD, Campion GV, Chishick A, et al. Clinical manifestations of human parvovirus B19 in adults. Arch Intern Med 1989;149:1153.
510. Naides SJ, Field EH. Transient rheumatoid factor positivity in acute human parvovirus B19 infection. Arch Intern Med 1988;148:2587.
511. Frickhofen N, Abkowitz JL, Safford M, et al. Persistent B19 parvovirus infection in patients infected with human immunodeficiency virus type 1 (HIV-1): a treatable cause of anemia in AIDS. Ann Intern Med 1990;113:926.
512. Muir K, Todd WTA, Watson WH, Fitzsimons E. Viral-associated haemophagocytosis with parvovirus-B19-related pancytopenia. Lancet 1992;339:1139.
513. Erdman DD, Usher MJ, Tsou C, et al. Human parvovirus B19 specific IgG, IgA, and IgM antibodies and DNA in serum specimens from persons with erythema infectiosum. J Med Virol 1991;35:110.
514. Schwarz TF, Nerlich A, Hottenträger B, et al. Parvovirus B19 infection of the fetus: histology and in situ hybridization. Am J Clin Pathol 1991;96:121.

515. Public Health Laboratory Service Working Party on Fifth Disease. Prospective study of human parvovirus (B19) infection in pregnancy. BMJ 1990;300:1166.
516. Kinney JS, Anderson LJ, Farrar J, et al. Risk of adverse outcomes of pregnancy after human parvovirus B19 infection. J Infect Dis 1988;157:663.
517. Porter HJ, Quantrill AM, Fleming KA. B19 parvovirus infection of myocardial cells. Lancet 1988;1:535.
518. Hartwig NG, Vermeij-Keers C, van Elsacker-Niele AMW, Fleuren GJ. Embryonic malformations in a case of intrauterine parvovirus B19 infection. Teratology 1989;39:295.
519. Rodis JF, Hovick TJ Jr, Quinn DL, et al. Human parvovirus infection in pregnancy. Obstet Gynecol 1988;72:733.
520. Clewley JP, Cohen BJ, Field AM. Detection of parvovirus B19 DNA, antigen, and particles in the human fetus. J Med Virol 1987;23:367.
521. Field AM, Cohen BJ, Brown KE, et al. Detection of B19 parvovirus in human fetal tissues by electron microscopy. J Med Virol 1991;35:85.
522. Schwarz TF, Roggendorf M, Hottenträger B, et al. Immunoglobulins in the prophylaxis of parvovirus B19 infection. J Infect Dis 1990;162:1214.
523. Bloom MC, Rolland M, Bernard JD, et al. Materno-fetal infection by parvovirus associated with antenatal meconium peritonitis. Arch Fr Pediatr 1990;47:437.
524. Carrington D, Gilmore DH, Whittle MJ, et al. Maternal serum α-fetoprotein—a marker of fetal aplastic crisis during intrauterine human parvovirus infection. Lancet 1987;1:433.
525. Naides SJ, Weiner CP. Antenatal diagnosis and palliative treatment of non-immune hydrops fetalis secondary to fetal parvovirus B19 infection. Prenat Diagn 1989;9:105.
526. Peters MT, Nicolaides KH. Cordocentesis for the diagnosis and treatment of human fetal parvovirus infection. Obstet Gynecol 1990;75:501.
527. Sahakian V, Weiner CP, Naides SJ, et al. Intrauterine transfusion treatment of nonimmune hydrops fetalis secondary to human parvovirus B19 infection. Am J Obstet Gynecol 1991; 164:1090.
528. Török TJ, Wang Q-Y, Gary GW Jr, et al. Prenatal diagnosis of intrauterine infection with parvovirus B19 by the polymerase chain reaction technique. Clin Infect Dis 1992;14:149.
529. Weiner CP, Naides SJ. Fetal survival after human parvovirus B19 infection: spectrum of intrauterine response in a twin gestation. Am J Perinatol 1992;9:66.
530. Morey AL, Nicolini U, Welch CR, et al. Parvovirus B19 infection and transient fetal hydrops. Lancet 1991;337:496.
531. Wegman ME. Annual summary of vital statistics—1991. Pediatrics 1992;90:835.
532. Centers for Disease Control and Prevention. Statistics from the Centers for Disease Control. AIDS 1993;7:145.
533. Goldfarb J. The acquired immunodeficiency syndrome (AIDS) in African children. Adv Pediatr Infect Dis 1993;8:145.
534. Hankins CA, Handley MA. HIV disease and AIDS in women: current knowledge and a research agenda. J Acquir Immune Defic Syndr 1992;5:957.
535. Allen MH, Marte C. HIV infection in women: presentations and protocols. Hosp Pract (Off Ed) 1992;27(3):113.
536. Ellerbrock TV, Bush TJ, Chamberland ME, Oxtoby MJ. Epidemiology of women with AIDS in the United States, 1981 through 1990: a comparison with heterosexual men with AIDS. JAMA 1991;265:2971.
537. Hoff R, Berardi VP, Weiblen BJ, et al. Seroprevalence of human immunodeficiency virus among childbearing women: estimation by testing samples of blood from newborns. N Engl J Med 1988;318:525.
538. Sperling RS, Friedman F Jr, Joyner M, et al. Seroprevalence of human immunodeficiency virus in women admitted to the hospital with pelvic inflammatory disease. J Reprod Med 1991;36:122.
539. Horowitz GM, Scott RT, Hankins GDV. Results of a prenatal screening program for the human immunodeficiency virus in a cross-sectional population. J Reprod Med 1991;36:773.
540. Repke JT, Townsend TR, Coberly JS, et al. Seroprevalence of human immunodeficiency virus type 1 among pregnant women. Am J Perinatol 1992;9:293.
541. Tabet SR, Palmer DL, Wiese WH, et al. Seroprevalence of HIV-1 and hepatitis B and C in prostitutes in Albuquerque, New Mexico. Am J Public Health 1992;82:1151.
542. Donegan SP, Steger KA, Recla L, et al. Seroprevalence of human immunodeficiency virus in parturients at Boston City Hospital: implications for public health and obstetric practice. Am J Obstet Gynecol 1992;167:622.
543. Lindsay MK, Johnson N, Peterson HB, et al. Human immunodeficiency virus infection among inner-city adolescent parturients undergoing routine voluntary screening, July 1987 to March 1991. Am J Obstet Gynecol 1992;167:1096.
544. Ellerbrock TV, Lieb S, Harrington PE, et al. Heterosexually transmitted human immunodeficiency virus infection among pregnant women in a rural Florida community. N Engl J Med 1992;327:1704.
545. Catania JA, Coates TJ, Stall R, et al. Prevalence of AIDS-related risk factors and condom use in the United States. Science 1992;258:1101.
546. Lindsay MK, Peterson HB, Willis S, et al. Incidence and prevalence of human immunodeficiency virus infection in a prenatal population undergoing routine voluntary human immunodeficiency virus screening, July 1987 to June 1990. Am J Obstet Gynecol 1991;165:961.
547. Stratton P, Mofenson LM, Willoughby AD. Human immunodeficiency virus infection in pregnant women under care at AIDS clinical trials centers in the United States. Obstet Gynecol 1992;79:364.
548. Douglas GC, King BF. Maternal-fetal transmission of human immunodeficiency virus: a review of possible routes and cellular mechanisms of infection. Clin Infect Dis 1992;15:678.
549. Ehrnst A, Lindgren S, Dictor M, et al. HIV in pregnant women and their offspring: evidence for late transmission. Lancet 1991;338:203.
550. Alimenti A, Luzuriaga K, Stechenberg B, Sullivan JL. Quantitation of human immunodeficiency virus in vertically infected infants and children. J Pediatr 1991;119:225.
551. Luzuriaga K, McQuilkin P, Alimenti A, Sullivan JL. Vertical HIV-1 infection: intrauterine vs. intrapartum transmission. [Abstract 1000] Pediatr Res 1992;31:169A.
552. Krivine A, Firtion G, Cao L, et al. HIV replication during the first weeks of life. Lancet 1992;339:1187.
553. Soeiro R, Rubinstein A, Rashbaum WK, Lyman WD. Maternofetal transmission of AIDS: frequency of human immunodeficiency virus type 1 nucleic acid sequences in human fetal DNA. J Infect Dis 1992;166:699.
554. Viscarello RR, Cullen MT, DeGennaro NJ, Hobbins JC. Fetal blood sampling in human immunodeficiency virus-seropositive women before elective midtrimester termination of pregnancy. Am J Obstet Gynecol 1992;167:1075.
555. Bryson YJ, Luzuriaga K, Sullivan JL, Wara DW. Proposed definitions for in utero versus intrapartum transmission of HIV-1. N Engl J Med 1992;327:1246.
556. Dunn DT, Newell ML, Ades AE, Peckham CS. Risk of human immunodeficiency virus type 1 transmission through breastfeeding. Lancet 1992;340:585.
557. Van de Perre P, Lepage P, Homsy J, Dabis F. Mother-to-infant transmission of human immunodeficiency virus by breast

milk: presumed innocent or presumed guilty? Clin Infect Dis 1992;15:502.
558. Van de Perre P, Simonon A, Msellati P, et al. Postnatal transmission of human immunodeficiency virus type 1 from mother to infant: a prospective cohort study in Kigali, Rwanda. N Engl J Med 1991;325:593.
559. Lederman SA. Estimating infant mortality from human immunodeficiency virus and other causes in breast-feeding and bottle-feeding populations. Pediatrics 1992;89:290.
560. European Collaborative Study. Risk factors for mother-to-child transmission of HIV-1. Lancet 1992;339:1007.
561. Kind C, Brändle B, Wyler C-A, et al. Epidemiology of vertically transmitted HIV-1 infection in Switzerland: results of a nationwide prospective study. Eur J Pediatr 1992;151:442.
562. Hutto C, Parks WP, Lai S, et al. A hospital-based prospective study of perinatal infection with human immunodeficiency virus type 1. J Pediatr 1991;118:347.
563. Goedert JJ, Duliège A-M, Amos CI, et al. High risk of HIV-1 infection for first-born twins. Lancet 1991;338:1471.
564. de Martino M, Tovo P-A, Galli L, et al. HIV-I infection in perinatally exposed siblings and twins. Arch Dis Child 1991; 66:1235.
565. Wolinsky SM, Wike CM, Korber BTM, et al. Selective transmission of human immunodeficiency virus type-1 variants from mothers to infants. Science 1992;255:1134.
566. Watts DH, Brown ZA, Tartaglione T, et al. Pharmacokinetic disposition of zidovudine during pregnancy. J Infect Dis 1991; 163:226.
567. Pons JC, Taburet AM, Singlas E, et al. Placental passage of azathiothymidine (AZT) during the second trimester of pregnancy: study by direct fetal blood sampling under ultrasound. Eur J Obstet Gynecol Reprod Biol 1991;40:229.
568. Sperling RS, Roboz J, Dische R, et al. Zidovudine pharmacokinetics during pregnancy. Am J Perinatol 1992;9:247.
569. Sperling RS, Stratton P, O'Sullivan MJ, et al. A survey of zidovudine use in pregnant women with human immunodeficiency virus infection. N Engl J Med 1992;326:857.
570. Toltzis P, Marx CM, Kleinman N, et al. Zidovudine-associated embryonic toxicity in mice. J Infect Dis 1991;163:1212.
571. Gogu SR, Beckman BS, Agrawal KC. Amelioration of zidovudine-induced fetal toxicity in pregnant mice. Antimicrob Agents Chemother 1992;36:2370.
572. Sison AV, Campos JM. Laboratory methods for early detection of human immunodeficiency virus type 1 in newborns and infants. Clin Microbiol Rev 1992;5:238.
573. Phair JP, Wolinsky S. Diagnosis of infection with the human immunodeficiency virus. Clin Infect Dis 1992;15:13.
574. Borkowsky W, Krasinski K, Pollack H, et al. Early diagnosis of human immunodeficiency virus infection in children < 6 months of age: comparison of polymerase chain reaction, culture, and plasma antigen capture techniques. J Infect Dis 1992;166:616.
575. Lepage P, Van de Perre P, Simonon A, et al. Transient seroreversion in children born to human immunodeficiency virus 1-infected mothers. Pediatr Infect Dis J 1992;11:892.
576. Burgard M, Mayaux M-J, Blanche S, et al. The use of viral culture and p24 antigen testing to diagnose human immunodeficiency virus infection in neonates. N Engl J Med 1992; 327:1192.
577. Palomba E, Gay V, de Martino M, et al. Early diagnosis of human immunodeficiency virus infection in infants by detection of free and complexed p24 antigen. J Infect Dis 1992; 165:394.
578. Landesman S, Weiblen B, Mendez H, et al. Clinical utility of HIV-IgA immunoblot assay in the early diagnosis of perinatal HIV infection. JAMA 1991;266:3443.
579. Quinn TC, Kline RL, Halsey N, et al. Early diagnosis of perinatal HIV infection by detection of viral-specific IgA antibodies. JAMA 1991;266:2439.
580. Miles SA, Balden E, Magpantay L, et al. Rapid serologic testing with immune-complex-dissociated HIV p24 antigen for early detection of HIV infection in neonates. N Engl J Med 1993;328:297.
581. Rogers MF, Ou C-Y, Rayfield M, et al. Use of the polymerase chain reaction for early detection of the proviral sequences of human immunodeficiency virus in infants born to seropositive mothers. N Engl J Med 1989;320:1649.
582. Hughes WT. Pneumocystis carinii pneumonia: new approaches to diagnosis, treatment and prevention. Pediatr Infect Dis J 1991;10:391.
583. Hoyt L, Oleske J, Holland B, Connor E. Nontuberculous mycobacteria in children with acquired immunodeficiency syndrome. Pediatr Infect Dis J 1992;11:354.
584. Braun MM, Cauthen G. Relationship of the human immunodeficiency virus epidemic to pediatric tuberculosis and Bacillus Calmette-Guérin immunization. Pediatr Infect Dis J 1992;11:220.
585. Khouri YF, Mastrucci MT, Hutto C, et al. Mycobacterium tuberculosis in children with human immunodeficiency virus type 1 infection. Pediatr Infect Dis J 1992;11:950.

Neonatology: Pathophysiology and Management of the Newborn, Fourth Edition,
edited by Gordon B. Avery, Mary Ann Fletcher, and Mhairi G. MacDonald.
J.B. Lippincott Company, Philadelphia © 1994.

chapter 48

Acute Infections

BISHARA J. FREIJ
GEORGE H. McCRACKEN, JR.

Infections are significant causes of mortality and long-term morbidity in neonates, especially for premature infants of very low birth weight.[1–3] Temporal and geographic differences in the relative frequencies of various neonatal pathogens are well recognized.[4,5] In North America in the 1930s and 1940s, gram-positive cocci such as group A β-hemolytic streptococci and *Staphylococcus aureus* were the most common bacterial isolates from neonates with sepsis, with *Escherichia coli* accounting for most of the remaining cases. *S. aureus* and *E. coli* became the major pathogens in the 1950s, but since the late 1960s, group B β-hemolytic streptococci and *E. coli* have predominated. Coagulase-negative staphylococci emerged in the 1980s and have surpassed *S. aureus* and gram-negative enteric bacilli as the bacteria most frequently associated with nosocomial infections in many neonatal intensive care units; this has largely been a result of the survival of very-low-birth-weight infants who require lengthy hospitalizations and considerable mechanical and nutritional support.[6,7]

The outcome of neonatal infections can be improved if illness is recognized early and appropriate antimicrobial agents are promptly administered. This chapter presents pertinent epidemiologic and pathogenetic concepts of specific infections, clinical manifestations, and diagnostic evaluations of patients with these diseases with a rational approach to therapy and control of neonatal infections.

PHARMACOLOGIC BASIS OF ANTIMICROBIAL THERAPY

Selection of antimicrobial therapy for neonatal infections must be based on pharmacokinetic properties of antibiotics in newborn infants of different gestational and postnatal ages, antimicrobial susceptibilities of commonly encountered pathogens within each nursery, and the natural history of the infectious disease being treated.[8]

Combining two or more antibiotics is the usual clinical practice when initiating therapy for presumed systemic bacterial disease (*e.g.*, ampicillin and an aminoglycoside are combined to treat suspected early-onset septicemia or meningitis before identification of the pathogen). After a bacterium has been identified and its susceptibility to various antimicrobials is determined, a single appropriate antibiotic is usually satisfactory for treating most infections.

Although antibiotics are commonly used to prevent infection, they are effective prophylactically only if directed against a single pathogen. For example, a single dose of penicillin G given intramuscularly at birth reduces the colonization rate and incidence of early-onset group B streptococcal (GBS) disease, except in infants who acquire the infection *in utero*.[9] However, if antibiotics are used as broad-spectrum coverage against many potential pathogens, they are rarely effective. This umbrella method of chemoprophylaxis encourages the emergence of resistant strains among previously susceptible bacteria and alters the normal flora of the gastrointestinal and respiratory tracts with overgrowth of potentially virulent organisms. Broad-coverage prophylaxis may partially suppress a bacterium, masking the development of clinical disease and causing neglect of important surgical measures or serious delay in administering more effective therapy.

EPIDEMIOLOGY

The two principal sources of newborn infection are the mother and the nursery environment. Infection is acquired from the mother transplacentally at the time of delivery or in the postnatal period. The infant may acquire infection postnatally from environmental sources, such as nursery personnel, respiratory equipment, sinks, and incubators. Infections manifesting within the first week of life are usually the result of exposure to microorganisms of maternal origin, but infections presenting later can have a maternal or environmental source.

Myriad aerobic and anaerobic bacteria, mycoplasmas, chlamydiae, fungi, viruses, and protozoa can be found in the maternal genital tract. Some of these organisms pose little threat to the newborn infant (*e.g.*, *Lactobacillus*, α-hemolytic streptococci, *Veillonella*), and others are infrequent causes of neonatal disease (*e.g.*, *Haemophilus influenzae*, *Streptococcus pneumoniae*, *Neisseria meningitidis*).[10–16] More commonly, organisms such as groups A and B β-hemolytic streptococci, *E. coli*, *Listeria monocytogenes*, *Neisseria gonorrhoeae*, cytomegalovirus, and herpes simplex virus are responsible for serious neonatal infections.

Within a few days after birth, α-hemolytic streptococci, *Staphylococcus epidermidis*, and gram-negative enteric bacilli colonize the throat, nose, umbilicus, and stool.[17] The gastrointestinal tract of newborns becomes heavily colonized by lactobacilli. Infants in neonatal intensive care units tend to have delayed colonization, which is probably related to early antimicrobial therapy for possible sepsis, and are more likely to acquire nosocomial strains of gram-negative bacilli such as *Klebsiella*, *Enterobacter*, *Citrobacter*, and *E. coli*.[17–19] Colonization of the scalp, axilla, and groin by coagulase-negative staphylococci is universal by 48 hours of age.[7] In a prospective study of 18 premature infants admitted to a neonatal intensive care unit, *S. epidermidis* as the only coagulase-negative staphylococcal species isolated from the axilla, ear, nasopharynx, and rectum was found in about 11% of infants during their first day of life; this increased to 100% by 4 weeks of age. None of these infants had a predominant *S. epidermidis* biotype on the first day, compared with 89% by 4 weeks of age. The prevalence of slime production and multidrug resistance among isolates rose from 68% to 95% and from 32% to 82%, respectively, during the 4-week study period.[20]

Postnatal fungal colonization is more likely to occur in low-birth-weight infants. An estimated 10% of term infants have gastrointestinal *Candida* colonization within the first 5 days of life; infants weighing less than 1500 g have colonization rates of about 25%. Early colonization (<2 weeks of age) is more common, involves the gastrointestinal and respiratory tracts, and is with *Candida albicans* or *Candida tropicalis*, unlike late colonization (>2 weeks of age), which usually involves the skin and is more likely to be *Candida parapsilosis*.[21] Cutaneous colonization with *Malassezia (Pityrosporum) furfur*, a lipophilic yeast best known as the cause of tinea versicolor, is common and is found in as many as two-thirds of all critically ill newborns; fewer than 3% of healthy newborns and young infants have skin colonization by this fungus.[22,23]

The vagina or cervix of asymptomatic, sexually active women is colonized by *Ureaplasma urealyticum* in 40% to 80% and by *Mycoplasma hominis* in 21% to 53%.[24] Vertical transmission rates of from 45% to 66% for preterm and term neonates have been reported for *U. urealyticum*.[24] By 3 months of age, about 33% to 68% of these infants continue to have detectable pharyngeal, ocular, or vaginal colonization.[25] Vertical transmission rates for infants born to women with cervical *Chlamydia trachomatis* infections have been estimated at 40% to 70%; about 35% of untreated infants continue to be infected at one or more sites (*e.g.*, conjunctiva, nasopharynx, oropharynx, rectum, vagina) at 12 months of age.[26–28]

The incidence of neonatal sepsis is from 1 to 10 cases per 1000 live births and 1 per 250 live premature births; the incidence is higher (1%–5%) for infants born to mothers with chorioamnionitis.[4] The average national incidence rate for nursery-acquired infections is about 1.4%, but figures reported for neonatal intensive care units are considerably higher and range from 5% to 30%.[6,29,30] The most important risk factor for acquiring a nosocomial infection is low birth weight; others include prolonged hospitalization, invasive procedures, placement of indwelling devices such as central venous catheters or ventriculoperitoneal shunts, bacterial or fungal colonization, and overcrowded nurseries.

INFECTION CONTROL IN THE NURSERY

Microorganisms can be transmitted to infants through direct contact with infected or colonized persons (*e.g.*, mother, hospital personnel), indirect contact with a contaminated object (*e.g.*, resuscitation equipment, pressure monitoring transducers), droplet contact (*e.g.*, coughing or sneezing by infected caretakers), and contaminated products (*e.g.*, milk, lipid emulsions, blood). Transmission of bacteria by the hands of hospital personnel is the most important mode of transmission within nurseries.[29]

Prevention of nosocomial infection depends on recognizing and correcting environmental risk factors. Personnel should wash their hands thoroughly with a scrub brush and an antibacterial cleaning agent before and between the handling of patients. Overcrowding in nurseries and a high infant–nurse ratio have increased the risk of nosocomial infections by 5- to 15-fold.[29] Continuous surveillance through review of patient and microbiologic records helps to identify changing colonization patterns, to detect newly introduced virulent organisms in the nursery environment, and to recognize changes in the antibiotic susceptibility patterns of the predominant pathogens. Repeated treatment with broad-spectrum antimicrobials encourages colonization of infants by *Candida* and multiresistant bacteria. Routine neonatal surveillance cultures are usually inadequate predictors of future infection of newborns by their colonizing microorganisms, but they are useful during outbreaks because they allow cohorting of infants within the nursery to minimize spread of an epidemic viral or bacterial strain to uninfected patients. Invasive procedures, such as endotracheal intubation, placement of fetal scalp electrodes, and insertion of ventriculoperitoneal shunts, are well-recognized risk factors for hospital-acquired infections.

Umbilical and peripheral arterial and venous indwelling catheters are important sources of nosocomial bacteremia.[31,32] As many as 60% of umbilical catheters become colonized by bacteria, but the prevalence of umbilical catheter–related sepsis has been estimated at 3% to 16%. The most common causative agents are coagulase-negative staphylococci, followed by *S. aureus;* gram-negative bacilli and fungi account for about a third of all cases. Risk factors for umbilical arterial catheter–related sepsis include very low birth weight and duration of antibiotic therapy. Umbilical venous catheter–related sepsis occurs most often in larger infants receiving infusions of hyperalimentation solutions.[32]

There is increasing use of central venous catheters in seriously ill infants for providing prolonged, dependable vascular access for the administration of intravenous fluids, hyperalimentation solutions, and drugs. About 30% of critically ill infants with central venous catheters develop catheter-related sepsis.[33] Central venous catheter infections can be caused by contaminated infusates, hematogenous seeding from distant sites of infection, or contamination of the catheter hub. The most important source appears to be organisms found on an infant's skin, such as coagulase-negative staphylococci, that travel along the central venous catheter track to the catheter tip, where colonization takes place.[34]

Preventive measures designed to reduce the incidence of central venous catheter–related infections generally aim at decreasing the number of organisms at catheter exit sites. Disinfection of central venous catheter insertion sites by repeatedly applying topical antiseptics is viewed as one of the most important ways of reducing the frequency of catheter-related sepsis. Two percent aqueous chlorhexidine has been more efficacious than 10% povidone–iodine or 70% alcohol for this purpose when used in adults.[35] Chlorhexidine is nontoxic to newborns, and its absorption through neonatal skin is minimal.[36–38] The popular semipermeable transparent dressings that are applied to central venous catheter exit sites produce significantly heavier bacterial growth on the underlying skin compared with gauze dressings and result in a higher incidence of central venous catheter contamination.[34,39] The use of silver-impregnated collagen cuffs that can be attached to central venous catheters has reduced the incidence of catheter-related sepsis in adults, but this approach has not been studied in neonates.[40,41]

NOSOCOMIAL BACTERIAL OUTBREAKS

When an infectious disease caused by the same organism appears in several infants from the same nursery in a short period, a nosocomial outbreak should be suspected. The sick infants should be isolated and cultured to identify the pathogen. If a specific pathogen is responsible for the outbreak, epidemiologic investigations to determine the source of infection must be initiated, and measures should be taken to prevent further colonization and disease. Specific typing of organisms, using techniques such as phage typing for *S. aureus*, determination of antibiotic susceptibility and biochemical profiles for *S. epidermidis*, and pyocin typing for *Pseudomonas* are being replaced by the more powerful tools of molecular biology. Plasmid fingerprinting, restriction endonuclease analysis of plasmid and genomic DNA, DNA hybridization, immunoblotting, ribosomal RNA typing, multilocus enzyme electrophoresis, and polymerase chain reactions are increasingly used in the analysis of nosocomial epidemics.[42]

Staphylococcus aureus INFECTION

In the late 1950s and early 1960s, phage group I *S. aureus* (*i.e.*, phage types 29, 52, 52A, 79, 80, and 81) caused significant hospital disease, ranging from pustules and cellulitis to pneumonia, septicemia, and meningitis. Although most infants are colonized with the epidemic strain during outbreaks, staphylococcal disease occurs in only a small fraction of those infants. Disease caused by phage group I staphylococci has diminished in the past decade. Theories to explain this decline are unsatisfactory but include changes in the virulence of the organism, implementation of infection control techniques in nurseries, and introduction of the semisynthetic β-lactamase–resistant penicillins.

Disease caused by phage group II *S. aureus* (*i.e.*, phage types 3A, 3B, 3C, 55, and 71) in newborn and young infants has been encountered. Clinical manifestations caused by this organism have been broadly classified as the expanded scalded skin syndrome.[43,44] Nursery epidemics of bullous impetigo, toxic epidermal necrolysis, or both caused by group II staphylococci have been reported.[45] Outbreaks are usually a result of lapses in infection control techniques and spread of the organism to other infants through hand carriage by nursery personnel; a staphylococcal nasal carrier among the nursery staff is only rarely the source.

Methicillin-resistant *S. aureus* (MRSA) strains have become important nosocomial pathogens in the United States since 1975.[46] The major route by which MRSA is spread is through hand carriage by transiently colonized personnel.[47] Nasal MRSA carriage rates for hospital personnel caring for colonized patients are from 1% to 6%.[46] Outbreaks of disease caused by multiresistant *S. aureus* strains have been reported from several nurseries in North America.[48,49] These organisms are resistant to the antistaphylococcal penicillins, cephalosporins, lincomycin, and aminoglycosides but are susceptible to vancomycin, rifampin, and trimethoprim–sulfamethoxazole. Vancomycin is the preferred therapy.

When staphylococcal disease occurs in a nursery, the extent of infection must be determined. Cultures are obtained from all infants and personnel associated with the index patient and a random sampling of the other infants. Culture sites include the nasopharynx and umbilicus for infants and the anterior nares and hands for personnel. Several measures are commonly employed to control a nursery epidemic:

Increase emphasis on hand washing by all personnel.

Isolate all symptomatic and asymptomatic infants colonized with the virulent staphylococcal strain, with cohorting of all exposed but not colonized infants and all new admissions to the nursery and cohorting of caretakers. Maintain infant cohorts until discharge from the nursery.

Use parenteral antistaphylococcal therapy to treat systemic disease, with application of topical agents such as triple dye (*i.e.*, mixture of brilliant green, crystal violet, and proflavine hemisulfate), bacitracin ointment, sulfadiazine cream, isopropyl alcohol, iodophor, chlorhexidine, or mupirocin to the umbilical stump of infants to delay or reduce colonization.[50–52]

Initiate routine bathing with antistaphylococcal cleansing agents such as chlorhexidine. Iodophor detergents are not recommended because of cutaneous staining and the potential for transdermal absorption of iodine, with resultant suppression of neonatal thyroid function.[29] Hexachlorophene is neurotoxic and should not be routinely used. This agent remains an option for difficult-to-contain epidemics, but it should be used in a 1 : 4 or 1 : 5 dilution in water and only in full-term infants.[50]

Colonize the umbilical stump of infants with a less virulent *Staphylococcus* species such as the 502A strain of *S. aureus* (*i.e.*, bacterial interference).[50] Although associated with low risk if properly performed, this procedure is rarely used and should be undertaken only after other control techniques have failed.

Close the nursery to new admissions if an outbreak is difficult to control.

ENTEROPATHOGENIC *Escherichia coli*

Because diarrhea caused by enteropathogenic strains of *E. coli* occurs rarely during the first week of life, nosocomial disease is usually confined to intensive and special care nurseries. The mother is frequently the source of infection for the index case; subsequent cases are usually transmitted from infant to infant by nursery personnel. The epidemiology, symptoms, treatment, and control measures for enteropathogenic *E. coli* diarrhea are considered later.

GROUP A STREPTOCOCCAL INFECTION

Group A β-hemolytic streptococci were a common cause of puerperal and neonatal sepsis in the 1930s and early 1940s. With the advent of penicillin and its frequent use in maternity and nursery units, neonatal infections caused by this organism have become relatively uncommon.[53,54] However, the resurgence of serious, invasive group A streptococcal disease among children and adults may herald an increase in the incidence of neonatal infections by this organism.[55–58] The primary source of group A streptococci in nursery outbreaks is a nurse or physician working in the unit or the mother. After group A streptococci are introduced into a nursery, many infants become colonized, but few develop clinical disease. The most common clinical manifestation is a low-grade granulating omphalitis that fails to heal despite local measures. However, more significant disease may occur, including extensive cellulitis, pneumonia, septicemia, and meningitis.

One neonate with group A streptococcal colonization is enough to warrant investigation of the nursery for a potential source of disease. All infants in close contact with the index case, a random sampling of other infants, and nursery personnel should be cultured. Nasopharyngeal and umbilical cultures from infants and nasopharyngeal, skin, and rectal cultures from personnel should be obtained. The epidemiologic workup should be coordinated with the obstetric service of the hospital.

Infants with streptococcal disease should be treated with aqueous penicillin G. During nosocomial outbreaks, all asymptomatic infants colonized with group A streptococci should receive penicillin. The prophylactic use of penicillin for new admissions to the nursery may be indicated. Benzathine penicillin G has been used effectively as prophylaxis against group A streptococcal infection in one nursery outbreak.

GRAM-NEGATIVE BACILLARY INFECTIONS

Routine nasopharyngeal and rectal cultures from normal newborn infants usually reveal one or several coliform organisms. These bacteria and others represent the normal flora of the neonate's gastrointestinal tract. It is likely that the gastrointestinal tract is a source of systemic neonatal infections caused by coliform and other gram-negative bacteria.[17,59]

Several nursery outbreaks caused by specific gram-negative bacteria have been described.[60–72] Among the organisms incriminated were *Klebsiella pneumoniae, Flavobacterium meningosepticum, Serratia marcescens, Pseudomonas aeruginosa, Proteus mirabilis, Citrobacter diversus, Enterobacter* spp., *Salmonella* spp., and *E. coli.* A common feature of these outbreaks was that most colonized infants were asymptomatic, and those who developed disease usually had pneumonia, septicemia, or meningitis.

Infected fomites represent the single most common source of nursery outbreaks caused by gram-negative bacteria. Contaminated faucet aerators, sink traps, drains, suction equipment, bottles containing distilled water, cleansing solutions, humidification apparatus, and incubators have been incriminated. Contaminated formula and breast milk are infrequent sources.[73] Colonized infants may act as a source of infection, and the organism is transmitted from infant to infant by way of the hands or gowns of personnel. During epidemics, the rate of asymptomatic colonization of infants with the specific pathogen ranges from 0% to 90%.

The general approach to nursery outbreaks caused by gram-negative organisms is similar to that for outbreaks caused by *S. aureus.* Identification of an infant in a nursery or intensive care unit with a potentially virulent pathogen such as *P. aeruginosa* should serve as a warning. This infant should be segregated, preferably outside the nursery, from the other infants and managed appropriately. All infants in the same unit should be cultured. If additional infants are discovered to be asymptomatic carriers of the organism, they should be segregated from other infants in the nursery, and an epidemiologic investigation should be initiated. Resuscitation and inhalation equipment, cleansing solutions, washing facilities, and other objects in the patient's environment are cultured so that the source of nosocomial infection can be identified. It may become necessary to close the nursery to new admissions until the source of infection is identified and appropriate measures have been taken to prevent new cases.

NOSOCOMIAL VIRAL OUTBREAKS

Several viral agents have been incriminated in nursery outbreaks of infection.[74,75] Most viral nosocomial outbreaks tend to parallel the activity of the agent in the community. The original source of infection is frequently the mother, who transmits the viral agent transplacentally or by direct contact postnatally. A second common source of nosocomial viral disease is infected nursery personnel. Although the mechanisms accounting for spread of virus from infant to infant are not well defined, it appears likely that respiratory viruses such as influenza and parainfluenza are spread by the airborne route, while respiratory syncytial virus (RSV) is spread primarily by infected hands of personnel. Viruses causing diarrhea may be transferred from infant to infant by the hand-to-mouth route through intermediary nursery personnel. Viruses excreted in the urine in high concentrations may be aerosolized when diapers or sheets are changed.

During a nursery outbreak of viral infection, most infected infants are asymptomatic and serve as reservoirs for perpetuation of infection. Even more important, infants with minimal symptoms and signs of disease such as sneezing, stuffy nose, or several loose stools may contribute significantly to transmission of virus by way of the airborne or fecal–oral routes.

COXSACKIEVIRUSES

Coxsackievirus A is rarely incriminated in nursery epidemics. In one outbreak at a regular nursery in Bangkok, 48 of 598 infants developed herpangina in the first week of life.[76] Several infants had coxsackievirus A5 isolated from their throat or rectum or developed rising antibody titers to the virus.

There have been several well-documented nursery outbreaks of the encephalomyocarditis syndrome associated with coxsackieviruses of the B group.[77,78] Coxsackieviruses B1 through B5 have been etiologically associated with this illness, and the virus has been isolated from multiple organs, including the myocardium, lung, brain, blood, kidney, and liver. The severe involvement found in many infants explains the relatively high mortality rate of this condition. The clinical picture is one of abrupt onset of fever, listlessness, and feeding difficulty. Respiratory distress and cyanosis are found frequently, and cardiac signs such as tachycardia, cardiomegaly, murmurs, and gallop rhythm are present in most patients.[79] Hepatosplenomegaly is common, and signs and symptoms referable to central nervous system involvement affect one-third of patients. The newborn can apparently acquire coxsackievirus infection *in utero* or after birth. The postnatally acquired disease has been traced to direct contact with the mother or an infected attendant.

ECHOVIRUSES

Several echovirus types cause illness in premature and term infants.[79–88] Although echovirus 9 is the most prevalent type, it is echovirus 11 that has been responsible for most nursery outbreaks caused by this group of viruses.[74] Reported neonatal secondary attack rates during hospital outbreaks have been as high as 50%.[75]

Mother-to-infant vertical transmission appears to be the major route of infection. The virus spreads to other newborns through the contaminated hands of nursery personnel, especially to infants requiring mouth care and gavage feeding.[87] Echovirus infections acquired from the mother tend to be more serious than those acquired through secondary nosocomial spread; this may be because of the lack of passively transferred protective maternal neutralizing antibodies against the offending agent in infants born to women infected at or near the time of delivery.[86,89]

The clinical manifestations of echovirus infection range from mild diarrhea to overwhelming hepatic necrosis. Separate nursery outbreaks caused by the same echovirus type may produce different clinical diseases. For example, in a premature nursery outbreak, echovirus type 19 produced respiratory illness associated with roentgenographic findings of cystic emphysema.[80] In a separate outbreak of echovirus type 19, the initial clinical picture was strikingly similar to that of sepsis neonatorum and was characterized by overwhelming infection and hepatic necrosis.[83] This disparity in the clinical diseases that characterize individual nosocomial outbreaks has also been observed for echovirus type 11.[85]

During nursery outbreaks, infection control measures should include cohorting of cases and increased emphasis on hand washing.[75,90] The use of gloves and gowns is helpful, especially when handling secretions and feces.[75] Closure of the nursery to new admissions is sometimes needed. The administration of immune serum globulin to uninfected newborns has been tried, but its benefits are unproved.[87,91]

HEPATITIS A

There have been several reported outbreaks of hepatitis A in neonatal intensive care units.[92–96] The virus is transmitted primarily by person-to-person contact through fecal contamination and oral ingestion.[97] Approximately 16% to 30% of an inoculum of hepatitis A virus can be recovered from infected hands after 4 hours.[98] Indirect person-to-person transmission of infectious virus can also occur through contact with inanimate objects, such as hard surfaces.[98] In some of the nursery outbreaks, the initial infection occurred through transfusion of neonates with blood or fresh frozen plasma from donors with hepatitis A viremia during the prodromal phase of their illness.[92,94–96]

Hepatitis A virus is highly communicable; in one nursery outbreak, 20% of infants, 24% of nurses, and several non-nursing staff and household contacts were affected.[95] Fecal excretion of hepatitis A virus may persist for 4 to 5 months.[95] Risk factors for spread of hepatitis A to other infants and nursery personnel include asymptomatic infection, prolonged fecal shedding of the virus, frequent contact with soiled diapers, and breaks in infection control measures. One study found that having long fingernails, not wearing gloves for certain procedures, smoking, and drinking beverages in the nursery facilitated direct hand-to-mouth contact.[95] The use of intramuscular immune serum globulin for postexposure prophylaxis may be helpful in controlling hospital outbreaks. To be most effective, immune globulins in a dosage of 0.02 mL per 1 kg of body weight should be given as soon as possible after the last exposure and within a period not exceeding 2 weeks.

ADENOVIRUSES

Neonatal adenoviral infections are infrequent but can be severe.[99,100] Nursery outbreaks have been caused by adenovirus serotypes 1, 2, 3, 7, 7a, 8, and 21.[101–104] Manifestations of nosocomial adenovirus infection can include pseudomembranous conjunctivitis, apnea, bradycardia, tachypnea, wheezing, coryza, fever, hypothermia, feeding intolerance, and diarrhea. Deaths during nosocomial outbreaks have been described.[102] Adenoviruses can spread by means of contaminated hands and fomites; fecal–oral and small-particle aerosol spread is also possible.[75] Conjunctival shedding of the virus persists for 7 to 10 days; rectal shedding is intermittent and more prolonged.[102] Adenoviruses remain stable on environmental surfaces for long periods; this property enhances their ability to spread to susceptible infants and personnel.

Outbreak control can be achieved through cohorting of infected infants, exclusion of ill personnel from the workplace, hand washing, and wearing of gloves and masks; the use of goggles is advocated by some investigators. The use of immune serum globulins was ineffective in preventing or modifying adenoviral infection in one nursery outbreak, and the administered preparation had minimal neutralizing activity against the specific serotype responsible for that outbreak.[103]

RESPIRATORY SYNCYTIAL VIRUS

Community outbreaks of RSV infection occur in winter and early spring. The virus is highly contagious; as many as 50% of personnel on pediatric wards become infected during nosocomial RSV outbreaks. Shedding of RSV in respiratory secretions of infants usually lasts from 1 to 21 days (mean, 7 days) but can continue for 6 or more weeks in immunosuppressed patients.[75]

Respiratory syncytial virus has caused nursery outbreaks of bronchiolitis and pneumonia.[105–109] Infants initially demonstrated coryza and cough lasting several days, followed by the acute onset of dyspnea associated with roentgenographic evidence of pneumonia in most patients.[105] During a community outbreak in Rochester, New York, 35% of infants in a nursery acquired RSV infection.[106] Illness was often atypical, especially in infants younger than 3 weeks of age, in whom lower respiratory tract involvement was less common. Four infants died; 2 infants died unexpectedly after the acute illness had subsided. Infection was acquired by 34% of the nursery staff, who appeared to be important in the spread of RSV within the nursery. Infected infants are at risk of respiratory arrest due to RSV-related apnea.[110] Patients with pulmonary disease, congenital heart disease, or immunodeficiency are at highest risk for severe and potentially fatal RSV infections.[111] Simultaneous outbreaks of viral respiratory disease caused by RSV and rhinovirus or parainfluenza virus type 3 have been described in newborn nurseries.[107,108]

Control of nosocomial RSV infection should emphasize diligent hand washing before and after handling infants, cohorting of RSV-infected neonates, and not allowing nursery personnel to care for infected and uninfected infants at the same time. Gowns and masks are generally ineffective in reducing nosocomial RSV spread.[75] The use of eye–nose goggles has reduced the rates of nosocomial RSV infections among infants and personnel.[112,113] It is occasionally necessary to close the nursery to admissions if new cases of disease continue to occur despite the strict infection control measures.

The use of aerosolized ribavirin for the treatment of RSV infection in high-risk infants should be considered.[114] When given early in the course of an RSV infection, ribavirin can reduce the amount and duration of viral shedding, lead to a more rapid resolution of the illness, and lower mortality rates. Ribavirin can be administered safely to mechanically ventilated infants if careful attention is paid to correcting problems resulting from drug precipitation in the respirator tubing and around the expiratory valves of ventilators.[115]

INFLUENZA

Epidemics of usually mild respiratory illness caused by influenza A virus have been described in newborn infants.[116,117] Clinical findings are nonspecific and can be indistinguishable from bacterial sepsis. Apnea, lethargy, nasal congestion, and poor feeding have been observed. Interstitial pneumonia may be seen on chest radiographs.[117]

SEPSIS NEONATORUM

The term sepsis neonatorum is used to describe a disease of infants who are younger than 1 month of age, are clinically ill, and have positive blood cultures. The presence of clinical manifestations differentiates this condition from the transient bacteremia observed in some healthy neonates.

The incidence of sepsis neonatorum is from 1 to 10 cases per 1000 live births and 1 per 250 live premature births.[4,118] These incidence rates vary from nursery to nursery and depend on conditions predisposing to infection.

PATHOGENESIS

Maternal, environmental, and host factors determine which infants exposed to a potentially pathogenic organism will develop sepsis, meningitis, or other serious invasive infections.

Many prepartum and intrapartum obstetric complications have been associated with increased risk of infection in the newborn, the most significant of which are premature onset of labor, prolonged rupture of fetal membranes, chorioamnionitis, and maternal fever. In one study of 963 pregnancies complicated by premature rupture of membranes, the incidence of clinical sepsis increased from 2% among infants born within 23 hours of membrane rupture to 7% and 11% among those delivered 24 to 47 hours and 48 to 71 hours after rupture, respectively; the risk was highest for the premature, low-birth-weight infants.[119] The incidence of infection has been estimated at 8.7% for infants born to mothers with prolonged rupture of membranes (≥24 hours) and clinical chorioamnionitis.[120] Intraamniotic infection is associated with a higher incidence of sepsis among infants weighing less than 2500 g at birth compared with those weighing 2500 g or more (16% and 4%, respectively); death from sepsis is greater in the low-birth-weight group (11% and 0%, respectively).[121] Isolation of bacteria from the chorioamnion has been associated with an increased risk for neonatal death among preterm infants.[122] Maternal urinary tract infections, coitus near the time of delivery, and the use of internal monitoring devices are risk factors for chorioamnionitis.[118] Concurrent maternal and neonatal bacteremia has been documented for many microorganisms.[123–125]

With improved supportive care of the sick neonate has come increased opportunity for microorganisms of relatively low virulence to cause systemic disease. The use of arterial and venous umbilical catheters, central venous catheters, and endotracheal tubes provides access to the debilitated infant for organisms in the respiratory or gastrointestinal tract, on the skin, or in respiratory support equipment.[4]

Bacterial colonization of the skin and mucosal surfaces precedes invasive disease in most infants with sepsis. Type III strains of GBS, the ones most commonly associated with early-onset septicemia and with meningitis at any age in early infancy, adhere better to vaginal and neonatal buccal epithelial cells *in vitro* than do other GBS strains.[126,127] Bloodstream invasion generally follows local multiplication of the organism at sites of colonization. Aspiration of infected amniotic fluid is another proposed route for fetal infection among infants born to mothers with chorioamnionitis.

Animals have been used to define the host–bacteria interactions that determine pathogenesis of disease. Bloodstream infection in infant rats or mice caused by *E. coli* K1 or any of the GBS serotypes can be prevented by pretreatment with type-specific capsular polysaccharide antibody.[128,129] The orogastric route for *E. coli* K1 in the infant rat and the intratracheal installation of GBS in the rhesus monkey or rat produce illnesses that closely parallel the human syndromes.[130–132]

Several investigations of the host–parasite association of humans with group B streptococci have focused on measurement of specific antibody in the serum of infected and colonized persons. Protective concentrations of antibody to GBS serotype III were found in 73% of women whose newborn infants were well but in only 17% of women whose neonates developed sepsis or meningitis caused by this organism.[133] The amount of antibody to GBS serotype III was considerably lower in ill infants than in healthy neonates born to mothers with vaginal colonization.[133] Levels of GBS serotype III antibodies correlate with *in vitro* opsonic activity and *in vivo* protection of animals experimentally infected with these strains.[134,135] The administration of standard intravenous immunoglobulin preparations with activities against GBS, of human GBS monoclonal antibodies, or of GBS hyperimmune polyclonal antibodies provides significant protection to animals experimentally infected with this pathogen.[136,137] Asymptomatic colonization is also associated with antibody formation.[138,139] Although less extensively studied, similar observations have been made for other GBS serotypes.[137,140–143]

Evidence suggests that antibodies to the K1 *E. coli* antigen are protective against infection by this organism, but this is not firmly established.[144] Neonatal serum has been shown to be inefficient in killing *E. coli* because of a deficiency of non-IgG serum components, such as complement factor 9.[145,146]

Physiologic deficiencies of the classic and alternative pathways of complement activation in neonates contribute to inefficient bacterial opsonization.[147,148] Organisms such as GBS and *E. coli* with a high capsular sialic acid content tend to be poor activators of the alternative complement pathway.[149]

Fibronectin is a multifunctional glycoprotein found in the plasma and on the surface of certain epithelial cells, basement membranes, and connective tissues. In plasma, fibronectin acts as a nonspecific opsonin that enhances clearance of invading bacteria.[150] Fibronectin is deficient in neonatal plasma, and its concentration varies inversely with gestational age.[150,151] Septic infants have been shown to have significantly lower plasma concentrations of this glycoprotein than healthy, age-matched controls.[152] The soluble form of fibronectin binds poorly to GBS.[153] Fibronectin enhances phagocyte function *in vitro* and *in vivo*.[150]

Quantitative and qualitative deficiencies in neonatal neutrophils contribute to the immaturity of the immune system of newborns.[118,154] The abnormalities become most pronounced at times of stress or during infections and include impaired chemotaxis, decreased deformability, reduced C3bi receptor expression, depressed bacterial killing by phagocytes, and oxidative metabolic abnormalities. The neutrophil storage pool of neonates is markedly depleted compared with that of adults. Stem cell proliferative rates are near maximal capacity and cannot increase appreciably in response to infection.[154]

CLINICAL MANIFESTATIONS

Most infants with septicemia present with nonspecific signs and symptoms that are usually first observed by the nurse or mother rather than by the physician. The most common of these vague signs are temperature instability, lethargy, apnea, and poor feeding.[155] Although hypothermia is more common, a temperature elevation above 37.8°C is significant in the neonate and frequently associated with bacterial infections, especially with temperatures above 39°C.[156] The signs and symptoms in some infants may suggest respiratory or gastrointestinal disease (*e.g.*, tachypnea and cyanosis or vomiting, diarrhea, abdominal distention). Septicemia must always be included in the differential diagnosis when evaluating an infant with these findings.[155]

Although it is tempting to recommend a workup for septicemia in all infants with nonspecific clinical manifestations, this is impractical and unnecessary in many cases. A complete history and physical examination, coupled with clinical experience, are the best guides in determining the extent of the workup. If doubt exists, a blood culture should be obtained. Hepatosplenomegaly, jaundice, and petechiae are classic signs of neonatal infection but represent late manifestations.

STREPTOCOCCAL DISEASE

Group B β-hemolytic streptococcus is the most common gram-positive bacterium isolated from blood of infants with septicemia in North America.[157] The epidemiology, pathogenesis, and clinical features of GBS disease have been defined.[158] The organism is a common inhabitant of the female genital tract and can be isolated from vaginal and anorectal cultures of as many as 35% of asymptomatic pregnant women.[159–161] Risk factors for maternal GBS colonization include lower parity, higher frequency of intercourse, multiple sexual partners, and concurrent colonization with *Candida* spp.[161] Peripartum GBS colonization of the lower urogenital tract has been associated with several maternal complications including preterm labor, premature rupture of membranes, endometritis, chorioamnionitis, urinary tract infection, intrapartum or postpartum fever, late abortions, and invasive infections, such as bacteremia or meningitis.[125,162–166] The identical serotype can be isolated frequently from urethral cultures of the sexual partners of these culture-positive women.[167] Although most infected pregnant women have normal, healthy infants, 1% to 2% of pregnancies involving maternal infection result in stillbirths or infants with neonatal disease. Vertical transmission of group B organisms occurs in approximately 50% to 70% of mother–infant pairs, resulting in neonatal colonization rates of from 8% to 25%; transmission is most likely to occur among infants born to heavily colonized mothers.[168]

The early-onset GBS syndrome occurs within the first 72 hours of life (mean age of onset, 20 hours), and 65% of reported cases involve premature infants. There is often a history of other maternal obstetric complications. Onset is sudden and follows a fulminant course with the primary focus of inflammation in the lungs, although meningitis can develop. Respiratory distress is the most common initial sign among infants with early-onset meningitis.[169] Apnea, hypotension, and disseminated intravascular coagulation cause rapid deterioration and often lead to the patient's demise within 24 hours. It is difficult to identify the infant with respiratory distress caused by GBS infection, because in 60% of infected patients, the chest radiograph shows a reticulogranular pattern with air bronchograms indistinguishable from that seen with uncomplicated hyaline membrane disease. The mortality rate is approximately 20% and is inversely correlated with birth weight.[158,170] All five GBS serotypes have been incriminated in early-onset disease in roughly similar proportions. A similar syndrome has been associated with groups D and G streptococci.[171,172]

A late-onset syndrome caused by GBS or *L. monocytogenes* occurs most frequently at 2 to 4 weeks of age, but it may be seen as late as 16 weeks. The onset is insidious; poor feeding and fever are the most frequent presenting symptoms. A fulminant illness with rapid onset and progressive deterioration is occasionally encountered.[173] Meningitis is seen in approximately 60% of infants with the late-onset syndrome, and GBS serotype III accounts for 93% of these cases.[158] Rarely, infants with late-onset meningitis caused by group B streptococci present with hydrocephalus. These infants may appear to have uncomplicated hydrocephalus with normal lumbar cerebrospinal fluid (CSF). Examination of ventricular fluid reveals pleocytosis, and the organism is recovered on culture. Spinal fluid cultures of infants with meningitis caused by gram-positive organisms are usually sterile within 24 to 36 hours of therapy, and the mortality rate is 10% to 15%.

Approximately 20% of neonatal infections caused by GBS do not fit into the early- or late-onset syndromes and extend over a broad clinical spectrum involving many different organ systems. Several manifestations have been observed:[158,174,175]

- cellulitis
- scalp abscess
- impetigo
- breast abscess
- adenitis
- supraglottitis
- conjunctivitis
- orbital cellulitis
- ethmoiditis
- otitis media
- pneumonia complicated by empyema
- endocarditis
- hepatitis
- septic arthritis
- osteomyelitis
- urinary tract infection
- omphalitis
- asymptomatic transient bacteremia

The transient bacteremia is remarkable because these infants appear clinically well and are cultured because of a history of maternal obstetric complications. A repeat blood culture before the institution of antibiotic therapy is frequently sterile.

COAGULASE-POSITIVE STAPHYLOCOCCAL DISEASE

The phage group I *S. aureus,* which was common in the late 1950s, still exists in some nurseries and occasionally causes serious systemic neonatal disease. The pathogenicity of this organism is based on its ability to invade the skin and musculoskeletal system, producing furuncles, breast abscesses, adenitis, and osteomyelitis. Septicemia is usually secondary to local invasion. After *S. aureus* is recovered from blood cultures of neonates, a careful search should be made for a primary focus. Some group I *S. aureus* strains produce toxic shock syndrome toxin-1, formerly known as enterotoxin F or pyrogenic toxin C, and have caused toxic shock syndrome in older neonates.[176,177] Clinical characteristics of this disease include the sudden onset of fever, diarrhea, shock, mucous membrane hyperemia, and a diffuse erythematous macular rash with subsequent desquamation of the hands and feet, commencing on about the fifth or sixth day of illness.

In the early 1970s, phage group II coagulase-positive staphylococci emerged as a common cause of neonatal infection. Although this organism may be invasive, pathogenicity depends principally on production of an exotoxin (*i.e.,* exfolatin or epidermolytic toxin). Common areas of primary infection include the umbilical stump, conjunctiva, and throat. Clinical disease may take one of several forms, including bullous impetigo, toxic epidermal necrolysis (*i.e.*, Ritter disease), and nonstreptococcal scarlatina. Collectively, these diseases have been referred to as the expanded scalded skin syndrome.[43]

The initial finding in Ritter disease is generalized erythema associated with edema and tenderness on palpation, usually noticed between days 3 to 16 of life.[178] After several days, a distinctive desquamation of large sheets of epidermis occurs, which is different from the fine desquamation observed in the second and third weeks of streptococcal scarlet fever. Large flaccid bullae are commonly observed in Ritter disease that, on rupture, leave a tender, weeping erythematous base. Some infants may appear quite toxic with the generalized form of disease. A rare, congenital form of staphylococcal scalded skin syndrome has been described.[179]

Umbilical venous or arterial catheters and central venous lines are well-recognized risk factors for staphylococcal bacteremia. *S. aureus* is second only to coagulase-negative staphylococci as a cause of catheter-related infections.[32]

The mortality rate for neonates with *S. aureus* bacteremia is about 20%. Low-birth-weight infants are at highest risk for death from this infection.[180]

COAGULASE-NEGATIVE STAPHYLOCOCCAL DISEASE

The isolation of coagulase-negative staphylococci from blood, CSF, or urine of newborns with signs and symptoms of sepsis can be significant, and these bacteria should not be dismissed as contaminants. Of the 21 recognized coagulase-negative staphylococcal species, *S. epidermidis* is clinically the most significant for neonates.[181,182] Experience indicates that these bacteria are responsible for about 10% of cases of sepsis in neonatal intensive care units.[157,183] Coagulase-negative staphylococcal infections are nosocomial in origin and result in substantially longer hospitalizations for affected infants.[184,185] Risk of infection with these organisms increases with decreasing gestational age and birth weight.[186–189]

Clinical manifestations of coagulase-negative staphylococcal infections are similar to those caused by other pathogens and include apnea, bradycardia, temperature instability (*e.g.*, hypothermia, hyperthermia), respiratory distress (*e.g.*, tachypnea, retractions, cyanosis), gastrointestinal manifestations (*e.g.*, poor feeding, abdominal distention, bloody stools), lethargy, and metabolic acidosis.[7,182] Clinical illnesses include septicemia, meningitis with or without CSF abnormalities, necrotizing enterocolitis, pneumonia, omphalitis, soft tissue abscesses associated with persistent bacteremia, endocarditis, and scalp abscesses and osteomyelitis at insertion sites of fetal monitoring electrodes.[186–196]

Risk factors for coagulase-negative staphylococcal infections include the presence of foreign bodies, such as central venous lines, ventriculoperitoneal shunts, or peritoneal dialysis catheters, and prior antibiotic therapy and the intravenous infusion of lipid emulsions for nutritional support.[182,197] The organisms travel along catheter tracks from colonization sites. They eventually adhere to and proliferate on certain biosynthetic materials and later cause local or systemic reactions. The mechanism by which adherence occurs appears to initially involve hydrophobic and electrostatic interactions between the bacteria and the biopolymers.[182] Once attached, a viscous exopolysaccharide referred to as slime is formed. Slime covers the bacteria to form a surface biofilm that protects them from such environmental factors as antibiotics and host defenses while allowing continued access to nutrition.[182] The density of the biofilm may be increased if the organisms are exposed to subinhibitory concentrations of antibiotics to which they are susceptible (*e.g.*, vancomycin).[198] Slime appears to inhibit neutrophil chemotaxis and phagocytosis and the lymphoproliferative responses of mononuclear cells to mitogens.[199,200] Slime-producing strains account for most coagulase-negative staphylococci isolated from infants with invasive infections.[189] Ineffective opsonophagocytosis due to intrinsic deficiencies in neonatal host defenses contributes to the increased susceptibility of low-birth-weight infants to infection with these organisms.[201,202]

Coagulase-negative staphylococci produce a variety of toxins that may serve as virulence factors, including hemolysins, proteases, urease, and fibrinolysin.[7] Most fecal isolates produce a hemolysin that is functionally and immunologically identical to the delta toxin produced by *S. aureus*.[203] This toxin causes severe mucosal necrosis and hemorrhage when injected into ligated infant rat bowel loops and may play a role in the pathogenesis of neonatal necrotizing enterocolitis.[204,205]

Listeria monocytogenes DISEASE

The pathogenesis of clinical diseases caused by *L. monocytogenes* are similar to those caused by GBS. A fulminant, disseminated disease (*i.e.*, granulomatosis infantiseptica) may occur during the first several days of life. The pathogen is acquired transplacentally or by aspiration at the time of vaginal delivery, and multiple organ systems are involved.[206] The infant frequently presents with hypothermia, lethargy, and poor feeding. Early passage of meconium in a premature infant suggests *Listeria* infection.[207] A characteristic rash consisting of small, salmon-colored papules scattered primarily on the trunk can be observed in some infants. The chest roentgenogram shows parenchymal infiltrates suggestive of aspiration pneumonitis in most infants. A miliary-type of bronchopneumonia can be seen in some cases. *Listeria* serotypes Ia, Ib, and IVb produce the early-onset disease, whereas serotype IVb is the predominant type in late-onset meningitic disease.[208]

A delayed form of neonatal listeriosis occurs during

the second through fifth weeks of life and primarily involves the meninges.[208,209] The infected infant usually is the full-term product of an uncomplicated labor and delivery. Onset of symptoms and signs is relatively insidious and indistinguishable from those observed with meningitis caused by other pathogens. The source of the organism in late-onset disease is unclear. Although acquisition of *Listeria* may occur during passage through an infected birth canal, it appears that most cases result from postpartum horizontal spread. In favor of the latter route of infection are several reported clusters of neonatal listeriosis and the demonstration of cross-infections between newborns using enzyme electrophoretic typing and DNA fingerprinting.[206,210–212] The bacteriology laboratory should be forewarned of the clinical suspicion of listerial meningitis, because these microorganisms are occasionally discarded as contaminants because of their tinctorial and morphologic similarities with diphtheroids. Overnight refrigeration of spinal fluid specimens frequently enhance growth of this organism.

The peripheral leukocyte count usually shows a brisk leukocytosis, with a predominance of polymorphonuclear leukocytes in the differential count.[213] A significant elevation in the number of monocytes, to 7% to 21% of the total leukocyte count, has been documented on admission laboratory evaluation of infected infants. A monocytosis of this magnitude can be demonstrated in most remaining infants on repetitive testing of the peripheral leukocyte count, but monocytes are not typically found in the spinal fluid of infants infected with *L. monocytogenes.* Polymorphonuclear leukocytes predominate in about 75% of cases, with a relative lymphocytosis in the remaining 25%. As with other pyogenic meningitides, hypoglycorrhachia and elevated protein concentrations are frequent findings. Examination of the stained smear of spinal fluid has not been rewarding in more than 50% of cases. This is a reflection of the relatively low concentrations of organisms in the fluid.

ENTEROCOCCAL INFECTION

Group D streptococci are divided into enterococcal and nonenterococcal types. The enterococci are now included in the new genus *Enterococcus;* most neonatal infections are caused by *Enterococcus faecalis* and, to a lesser extent, by *E. faecium.*[214–216]

Early-onset enterococcal disease (<7 days of age) is relatively mild and presents clinically with respiratory distress or diarrhea; no associations with underlying conditions, invasive procedures, or maternal obstetric complications have been observed.[217] Late-onset disease (≥7 days of age) most commonly afflicts low-birth-weight infants with complicated clinical problems that often require surgical procedures (*e.g.,* bowel resection), central venous catheters, or prior treatment with antimicrobials. Clinical manifestations of late-onset disease include apnea, bradycardia, circulatory failure, meningitis, pneumonia, scalp abscesses, catheter-related bacteremia, and necrotizing enterocolitis-associated septicemia.[217] About 20% of enterococcal blood isolates represent skin contamination; clinical correlation is needed to differentiate contamination from true infection.[215]

Enterococci can spread rapidly within a nursery.[218] Nosocomial outbreaks of enterococcal septicemia in neonatal intensive care units are well documented.[216,219] The mortality rate is estimated at 6% to 11%, but it can be as high as 17% in infants with necrotizing enterocolitis-associated septicemia.[215,217]

The importance of identifying *Enterococcus* as the etiologic agent in septicemia primarily relates to selection of proper antimicrobial agents. The group D enterococci are moderately resistant to penicillin alone, due to certain properties of their penicillin-binding proteins.[215,220] Some enterococcal strains have acquired new mechanisms of antibiotic resistance that include β-lactamase production and high-level aminoglycoside resistance (*i.e.,* minimal inhibitory concentrations $\geq$ 2000 μg/mL).[218,221,222] Strains resistant to vancomycin have been encountered.[223] Nonenterococcal group D streptococci continue to be highly susceptible to penicillin.[215]

GRAM-NEGATIVE INFECTION

In North America, *E. coli* is the most common gram-negative organism causing septicemia during the neonatal period. *Klebsiella* and *Enterobacter* strains are second.[157] In Dallas, annual incidence rates have remained reasonably constant at 0.5 to 1 case per 1000 live births since 1970. In contradistinction to illness caused by GBS and *L. monocytogenes, E. coli* infections do not fit into distinct clinical syndromes of early- and late-onset disease. Approximately 40% of *E. coli* strains causing septicemia possess K1 capsular antigen, and strains identical with those isolated from blood cultures can usually be identified in the patient's nasopharynx or rectal cultures. The clinical features of *E. coli* sepsis are generally similar to those observed in infants with disease caused by other pathogens. Localized *E. coli* infections have included breast abscess, cellulitis, pneumonia, lung abscess, empyema, osteomyelitis, septic arthritis, urinary tract infection, ascending cholangitis, and otitis media.

Pseudomonas septicemia may present with a characteristic violaceous papular lesion or lesions that, after several days, develop central necrosis. Although these skin lesions are most commonly seen in *Pseudomonas* infection, they may be associated with other organisms.[224]

ANAEROBIC INFECTIONS

Anaerobes have accounted for 1% to 25% of all bacteria isolated from blood cultures of neonates with suspected septicemia in various studies.[225–228] *Bacteroides* spp., primarily *Bacteroides fragilis,* and clostridia are most commonly recovered.[228] *Peptostreptococcus* spp., *Veillonella* spp., *Propionibacterium acnes, Eubacterium* spp., and *Fusobacterium* spp. occur relatively infrequently. Anaerobes are found mixed in cultures with aerobic bacteria in about a third of cases. Clinical illnesses include transient bacteremia, fulminant septicemia, postoperative infections, and intrauterine death associated with septic abortion.[225] Localized diseases such as omphalitis, cellulitis, and necrotizing fasciitis are commonly seen with clostridia.[229] Conditions predisposing to anaerobic septicemia include prolonged rupture of membranes, chorioamnionitis, prematurity, and gastrointestinal disease.

Anaerobes isolated from blood within the first 2 days of life are usually gram positive and penicillin G susceptible, but those isolated from older newborns tend to be gram negative and penicillin G resistant.[227] Gram-positive anaerobes are more likely to be recovered from blood of infants with sepsis associated with chorioamnionitis, whereas gram-negative anaerobes predominate in necrotizing enterocolitis-associated bacteremia.[227] The mortality rates for reported cases of anaerobic septicemia are about 35% for illnesses caused by *Bacteroides* spp., and 12% for other anaerobes.[228]

GENITAL MYCOPLASMAS

M. hominis and *U. urealyticum* are occasionally isolated from the blood of neonates with sepsis.[24] Cassell and colleagues observed concomitant bacteremia in 40% and 26% of preterm infants with positive endotracheal cultures for *M. hominis* and *U. urealyticum,* respectively.[24] Other investigators have been unable to recover genital mycoplasmas from the blood or CSF of neonates with suspected sepsis.[230,231] An association between persistent pulmonary hypertension and *U. urealyticum* sepsis and pneumonia has been observed.[232]

FUNGAL INFECTIONS

Fungal infections occur in as many as 5% of low-birth-weight infants.[233] Most cases are due to *Candida* spp., particularly *C. albicans.*[233–235] *C. tropicalis, C. parapsilosis, Candida lusitaniae,* and *Candida glabrata* also cause systemic candidiasis.[233] Congenital candidiasis is uncommon and results from ascending infection through intact membranes; it usually manifests with early skin lesions (*e.g.,* maculopapular rash, pustules, vesicles, desquamation, skin abscesses) but disseminated and life-threatening infections can occur.[236,237]

Risk factors for late-onset systemic candidiasis include prematurity, low birth weight, use of broad-spectrum antimicrobial agents, central vascular catheters, parenteral hyperalimentation, intralipid infusions, prolonged endotracheal intubation, necrotizing enterocolitis, and immunologic immaturity.[234] The most important of these factors appears to be the number of prior antibiotics and the duration of therapy.[238,239] Low-birth-weight infants in whom mucocutaneous candidiasis develops are at considerable risk for subsequent invasive disease.[238] Infants with invasive candidiasis caused by *C. albicans* are more likely to have antecedent candidal thrush or perineal dermatitis and to die of their infection than neonates with severe *C. parapsilosis* infections.[240] Clinical manifestations vary and are indistinguishable from those caused by other pathogens. A fungal cause for sepsis should be strongly considered in an infant weighing less than 1500 g who has been hospitalized for a prolonged period, is receiving parenteral hyperalimentation through a central vascular catheter, and has previously been treated with multiple antibiotics; a history of gastrointestinal disease or surgery adds to the clinical suspicion. Diseases caused by *Candida* spp. include but are not limited to pneumonia, endocarditis, endophthalmitis, meningitis, cerebral abscesses, pyelonephritis, fungal balls in the kidney and bladder, peritonitis, hepatosplenic abscesses, arthritis, and osteomyelitis.[234,241–248]

M. furfur causes invasive neonatal fungal disease. Most infections involve chronically ill premature infants who are receiving lipid emulsions through a central venous catheter.[249] The most commonly reported presenting symptoms and signs include fever (50%) and respiratory distress (50%).[249] Pathologic analysis reveals mycotic thrombi around catheter tips, endocardial vegetations, and lung lesions that include mycotic emboli with occlusion of pulmonary arteries, septic thrombi, pulmonary vasculitis, and alveolitis.[249] Involvement of other organs is uncommon. Systemic infections due to other fungi such as *Hansenula anomala, Aspergillus* spp., *Cryptococcus neoformans, Coccidioides immitis, Blastomyces* spp., and *Trichosporon beigelii* are rare.[233,250]

LABORATORY TESTS AND FINDINGS

Since the early 1970s, several screening tests and scoring systems have been described that are purported to aid the physician in making the diagnosis of neonatal infection. Although a few are helpful in identifying the infant at high risk of developing infection, the diagnosis of septicemia can be made only by recovery of the organism from blood cultures or other normally sterile body fluids.[118,251] It is imperative that these cultures be obtained by strict aseptic technique. Blood should be obtained from a peripheral vein rather than from the umbilical vessels, the outer several millimeters of which are frequently contaminated with bacteria. Femoral vein aspiration may result in cultures contaminated with coliform organisms from the perineum. Heel stick samples have low sensitivities. The skin above the vein to be punctured should be cleansed with an antiseptic solution, such as an iodophor, and allowed to dry for maximal antiseptic effect. The amount of blood drawn is critical; 0.5 to 1 mL of blood is required for optimal results. The sensitivity of a single blood culture in identifying septicemia is only 80%.[251] Obtaining blood cultures from multiple sites may enhance the yield and aid in identifying false-positive results.[252] Quantitative blood cultures, if available, are helpful in differentiating true pathogens from culture contaminants.[253,254]

It is frequently helpful to obtain cultures of other sites before initiating antimicrobial therapy. For example, percutaneous bladder aspiration of urine for culture can be helpful in identifying the urinary tract as the focus of infection. This is particularly true for illness occurring after the third day of life.[118] Nasopharyngeal, skin, umbilical cord, gastric, and rectal cultures are frequently positive in the early septicemic form of listeriosis and GBS disease. However, these colonization sites are not predictive of the cause of bloodstream infection and should not be used to guide antimicrobial therapy.[255] All clinically stable infants with suspected septicemia should have CSF obtained for examination and culture before therapy.[256] This practice has been challenged for infants younger than 7 days of age because of its low yield; the yield from a lumbar puncture is much higher when performed on infants older than 1 week of age.[257–259]

The peripheral leukocyte count is the most useful of the indirect indicators of bacterial infection. After correction for the nucleated erythrocyte count, the total absolute neutrophil count and the ratio of immature to total neutrophilic forms are compared with normal standard values for age. In the absence of maternal hypertension, severe asphyxia, periventricular hemorrhage, maternal fever, or hemolytic disease, absolute total neutropenia and an elevated ratio of immature to total neutrophilic forms strongly suggest bacterial infection.[260,261] Infants born in high-altitude areas have higher total and immature neutrophil counts.[262] Repeating complete blood counts within 24 hours of birth has been shown to enhance the value of the test as a screen for sepsis.[263] Gastric aspirate stains and culture, erythrocyte sedimentation rate, C-reactive protein, and the nitroblue tetrazolium test have not proved useful as indicators of bacterial infection, although in combination these tests may offer some guidance.[118] C-reactive protein values appear not to be influenced by perinatal asphyxia, hyperbilirubinemia, periventricular hemorrhage, or respiratory distress syndrome and may prove to be a useful marker for bacterial infection.[264]

Detection of the soluble antigens of *E. coli* K1, GBS, *H. influenzae* type b, *N. meningitidis*, and *S. pneumoniae* by counterimmunoelectrophoresis and agglutination procedures is useful for identifying the infant infected with these pathogens. The absence of antigen does not rule out infection by these organisms. Substantial sensitivity differences have been found among the commercially available latex particle agglutination (LPA) assays for GBS antigen.[265] False-positive LPA test results for GBS in urine specimens can result from contamination of bag specimens with these bacteria from perineal and rectal colonization, cross-reacting antigens, or absorption of antigen from the gastrointestinal tract.[266,267] Similar false-positive test results may be obtained for the other bacteria. Rapid diagnosis of invasive *Candida* infection by detection of its circulating cell-wall (*e.g.*, mannan) or cytoplasmic (*e.g.*, enolase) antigens is possible, although the reliability of these tests is yet to be proved.[268–270]

THERAPY

After septicemia is suspected, suitable cultures should be obtained and therapy with ampicillin and an aminoglycoside started immediately. If meningitis has been excluded, ampicillin is administered intravenously or intramuscularly in a dosage of 50 mg/kg/day divided in two doses for infants younger than 1 week of age and 100 to 150 mg/kg/day divided in three or four doses for infants 1 to 4 weeks of age. The selection of the aminoglycoside antibiotic should be based on antimicrobial susceptibilities of enteric organisms isolated from infants in each nursery. Gentamicin is the drug of choice for treatment of infections caused by susceptible gram-negative organisms and is administered intravenously or intramuscularly in a dosage of 5 to 7.5 mg/kg/day divided in two or three doses, depending on infant's age.

Aminoglycoside-resistant *E. coli* have been encountered in some nurseries in North America.[271] In these nurseries or in an infant from whom an isolate is shown to be resistant to kanamycin or gentamicin, amikacin or cefotaxime should be used. Studies have demonstrated no significant ototoxicity in infants and children who were treated in the neonatal period with kanamycin or gentamicin.[8] However, in premature infants and in those receiving these drugs for prolonged periods, brain stem evoked response audiometry should be performed whenever possible. Serum concentrations of the aminoglycosides should be monitored in the low-birth-weight premature infants because of erratic absorption and elimination of the drugs in these infants. Although cefotaxime should not be routinely used for initial empiric therapy of neonatal sepsis, it is an effective agent alone or combined with an aminoglycoside for infections caused by coliform bacilli.

When the type of skin lesions or historic experience suggests the possibility of *Pseudomonas* infection, ceftazidime or ticarcillin with or without an aminoglycoside is the therapy of choice. Although not approved for use in neonates by the Food and Drug Administration, we have successfully used Timentin (ticarcillin and clavulanate) for treatment of sepsis caused by multiresistant gram-negative enteric bacilli, *Pseudomonas*, or anaerobic bacteria.

If staphylococcal sepsis is suspected but not proved, parenteral methicillin or nafcillin should be substituted for penicillin or ampicillin, because approximately 80% of staphylococci encountered in neonates are penicillin-resistant. Although gentamicin and kanamycin possess activity against most staphylococci, these agents cannot be recommended because there are no studies of their efficacy in neonatal staphylococcal disease. For disease caused by coagulase-negative staphylococci or multiresistant *S. aureus* strains, vancomycin is the preferred therapy. Peak and trough serum vancomycin concentrations should be monitored because of the drug's narrow therapeutic index.

After the pathogen is identified and its antimicrobial susceptibilities are known, the most appropriate drug or drugs should be selected. As a general rule, gentamicin alone or in combination with ampicillin, or cefotaxime alone or in combination with an aminoglycoside should be used for susceptible *E. coli*, *Klebsiella* spp., and *Enterobacter* spp.; amikacin alone or in combination with cefotaxime for gentamicin-resistant coliform bacteria; ceftazidime, ticarcillin, or Timentin, with or without an aminoglycoside, for *Pseudomonas;* ampicillin alone or in combination with an aminoglycoside for *P. mirabilis,* enterococci, and *L. monocytogenes;* and penicillin for other gram-positive organisms, except for penicillin-resistant *S. aureus,* for which methicillin or nafcillin is the drug of choice. Vancomycin is used for coagulase-negative staphylococci and MRSA. Rarely, coagulase-negative staphylococcal strains that are resistant to vancomycin can emerge during treatment with this agent.[272] The minimal inhibitory concentration (MIC) and minimal bactericidal concentration (MBC) of penicillin and ampicillin should be determined for GBS because a small percentage of these organisms are tolerant (*i.e.,* has an MBC : MIC ratio > 32) to these antibiotics.[273,274] These strains are best treated with a penicillin–aminoglycoside combination. *U. urealyticum* infections are treated with erythromycin.[275]

The drug of choice for systemic fungal infections is amphotericin B, with or without flucytosine.[234] The half-life and serum concentrations of amphotericin B are highly variable during the neonatal period.[276] The drug appears to be better tolerated by infants than older children and adults, but renal and hepatic functions should be carefully monitored.[234,277] The optimal daily dosage of amphotericin B is not universally agreed on. The most commonly employed dosage regimen is to begin with 0.5 mg/kg of the drug on the first day and, if tolerated, to increase the daily dosage to 1.0 mg/kg by the second or third day of treatment. The cumulative dosage of amphotericin B needed for the adequate treatment of systemic *Candida* infection is not well defined, but it is estimated to be 20 to 30 mg/kg.[234] Resistance to amphotericin B among *Candida* species is not a major clinical problem.[278] Amphotericin B is frequently combined with flucytosine for the treatment of central nervous system fungal infection because of flucytosine's excellent CSF penetration and the *in vitro* synergy of this drug combination against *Candida.* Gastrointestinal intolerance, myelosuppression, and hepatotoxicity are common side-effects of flucytosine.[234] Experience with the use of liposomal amphotericin B, miconazole, or fluconazole in newborns is limited.[234,279,280]

Guidelines for determining duration of therapy in the neonatal period are often lacking, because objective evidence of illness may be minimal. Culture of the blood should be repeated 24 to 48 hours after initiation of therapy; if positive, alteration of therapy may be necessary. In the absence of deep tissue involvement or abscess formation, treatment is usually continued 5 to 7 days after clinical improvement. If multiple organs are involved or clinical response is slow, treatment may need to be continued for 2 to 3 weeks.

Suspected central venous catheter–related bacterial sepsis can be initially managed with the intraluminal infusion of vancomycin combined with ceftazidime or an aminoglycoside. After infection is confirmed and the pathogen identified, single-drug therapy is usually sufficient. Reported cure rates with antibiotics alone without catheter removal have ranged from 50% to more than 90% for pediatric patients. Persistently positive blood cultures after 2 to 4 days of appropriate antimicrobial therapy warrants catheter removal. A continuous infusion of a low dose of urokinase for 24 hours may help in clearing catheter-related infections in some infants who fail conventional antibiotic therapy.[281] Patients responding to antibiotic therapy should be treated for 2 to 3 weeks or at least for 10 days from the time of the first negative blood culture. Catheter-related fungal infections are rarely cured without catheter removal.

Immunotherapy of neonatal sepsis is discussed in in Chapter 46. Extracorporeal membrane oxygenation for newborns with persistent pulmonary hypertension due to overwhelming early-onset GBS sepsis may improve their survival.[282]

PREVENTION

The identification of high-risk GBS-carrier mothers and the subsequent interruption of vertical transmission by intrapartum maternal chemotherapy can prevent many cases of early-onset neonatal GBS disease.[283] If this approach is used, pregnant women should be screened for anogenital GBS carriage at 26 to 28 weeks of gestation. Latex agglutination tests can be used at the time of delivery for women with no prenatal care. Culture-positive women with onset of labor or rupture of membranes before 37 weeks of gestation, fever during labor, rupture of membranes for more than 12 hours, a history of GBS bacteriuria during pregnancy, or a history of having previously delivered an infant with GBS disease should be treated intravenously with ampicillin until delivery. The management of infants born to women given intrapartum antimicrobial prophylaxis depends on their clinical status and culture results; most premature infants are treated with ampicillin and an aminoglycoside for 36 to 72 hours unless sepsis becomes evident.[283] Immunologic approaches to prevention include passive or active immunization of mothers, with transplacental passage of protective antibodies to the fetus, but immunoprophylaxis is not a clinically available option.

MENINGITIS

BACTERIAL MENINGITIS

The incidence of bacterial meningitis is 0.4 per 1000 live births, but rates as high as 1 per 1000 live births have been reported in a few nurseries.[155] The disease is seen more commonly in premature infants, male infants, and infants born to mothers with complicated pregnancies or deliveries.

ETIOLOGY

The bacteria causing neonatal meningitis are similar to those causing sepsis neonatorum. Group B β-hemolytic streptococci and *E. coli* presently account for approximately 75% of all cases. The next most common etiologic agent is *L. monocytogenes*.[284]

PATHOLOGY

The pathologic findings in cases of neonatal meningitis are similar, regardless of the bacterial agent. The most consistent finding at necropsy is a purulent exudate coating the meninges and ependymal surfaces of the ventricles.[285] Perivascular inflammation is observed. The inflammatory response of neonates is similar to that in adults with meningitis, with the exception that babies show a relative sparsity of plasma cells and lymphocytes during the subacute stage of meningeal reactions. Hydrocephalus and a noninfectious encephalopathy can be demonstrated in approximately 50% of infants dying of meningitis. Subdural effusions occur rarely in neonates. Various degrees of phlebitis and arteritis of intracranial vessels can be found in all infants. Thrombophlebitis with occlusions of veins may occur in the subependymal zone. Ventriculitis can be demonstrated in virtually all infants dying of meningitis and in approximately 75% of infants at the time of diagnosis.

CLINICAL MANIFESTATIONS

The signs and symptoms of central nervous system infection are frequently indistinguishable from those associated with neonatal septicemia. Lethargy, feeding problems, and altered temperature are the most frequent presenting complaints, and respiratory distress, vomiting, diarrhea, and abdominal distention are common findings. Seizures are observed frequently and may be caused by direct central nervous system inflammation or may be associated with hypoglycemia or hypocalcemia. Signs suggesting meningeal involvement, such as a bulging anterior fontanelle, neck stiffness, or opisthotonus, are uncommon.

PATHOGENESIS

Most cases of meningitis result from bacteremia and spread from a contiguous infected focus is rare. Although there are more than 100 K types of *E. coli*, *E. coli* K1 accounts for more than 70% of meningitis cases.[128] The extracellular polysaccharide capsule allows the organism to avoid host clearance mechanisms. The outer membrane lipopolysaccharide (*i.e.*, endotoxin) is released from dying bacteria and initiates an intense inflammatory reaction. Endotoxin stimulates the production of tumor necrosis factor, interleukin-1β (IL-1β), and other mediators by monocyte–macrophage cells. Tumor necrosis factor and IL-1β induce phospholipase A_2 activity, production of other mediators and receptor–ligand interactions between leukocytes and endothelia. Phospholipase A_2 then acts on membrane phospholipids to produce a variety of lipid proinflammatory substances such as platelet-activating factor, leukotrienes, prostaglandins, and thromboxanes. The inflammatory changes result in vascular injury and alterations in the permeability of the blood–brain barrier, with resultant vasogenic edema. The cytokines activate adhesion-promoting receptors on cerebral vascular endothelial cells which leads to recruitment of leukocytes to sites of stimulation. These polymorphonuclear leukocytes subsequently enter the subarachnoid space, release toxic substances, and cause cytotoxic edema.[286] The net pathophysiologic effect is the development of increased intracranial pressure and severe brain edema. Cerebral edema, increased intracranial pressure, systemic hypotension, decreased cerebral perfusion pressure, and a variety of vascular changes result in global or regional reductions of cerebral blood flow and can lead to brain ischemia.[287] The pathophysiologic aberrations ultimately cause focal or diffuse neuronal injury, which may be irreversible.

Among the five GBS serotypes, the BIII organisms account for more than 80% of cases of neonatal GBS meningitis. The presence of type-specific antibodies enhances opsonization of the organism in the presence of complement. Cell wall components of the organism can stimulate the inflammatory cascade in a manner similar to that described for endotoxins.

LABORATORY FINDINGS

Interpretation of CSF values in newborn infants may be difficult. Any one or a combination of the following CSF values should alert the pediatrician to the possibility of meningeal infection:

More than 32 leukocytes/mm^3, of which more than 60% are polymorphonuclear cells

CSF glucose less than 50% to 75% of a simultaneous serum glucose
Protein greater than 150 mg/dL
Microorganisms on gram-stained smears of CSF.[288]

The upper limits of "normal" for infants with birth weights of 1500 g or less are even higher.[289]

It is important to carefully examine a stained smear of the CSF of every infant with suspected meningitis. In babies with meningitis caused by GBS or coliform bacteria, each oil-immersion field usually contains several to many bacteria. This is because there are 10^4 to 10^8 bacteria per 1 mL of spinal fluid (average, 10^7/mL) present at the time of diagnosis. *Listeria* organisms are often difficult to identify on stained smears because the bacterial counts are frequently on the order of 10^3/mL.

Blood and urine cultures should be obtained from every infant suspected of meningitis. As many as 15% of infants with positive CSF cultures have sterile blood cultures.[256]

TREATMENT

Considerable data have been gathered on the pharmacokinetic properties of antibiotics in neonates with meningitis.[290,291] After an intramuscular dose of 2.5 mg/kg of gentamicin, peak levels in lumbar CSF and ventricular fluid are approximately 1 to 2 μg/mL. If lumbar intrathecal gentamicin is added to this regimen, values of 20 to 40 μg/mL or greater several hours after instillation may be observed in the lumbar area. Intraventricular administration of 2.5 mg results in ventricular fluid levels of 20 to 80 μg/mL and in lumbar spinal fluid values of 10 to 50 μg/mL 1 to 4 hours later. With kanamycin, peak CSF values of 6 to 10 μg/mL are observed 4 to 6 hours after an intramuscular dose of 7.5 mg/kg. However, peak values of 10 to 30 μg/mL are demonstrated in CSF approximately 2 to 4 hours after a 50 to 70 mg/kg/dose of ampicillin.

For the aminoglycosides, the MIC values for the common pathogens are frequently greater than the antibiotic levels achieved in CSF. For example, an *E. coli* with a gentamicin MIC value of 2.5 or 5 μg/mL is considered susceptible when bloodstream infection is being treated but may be resistant when meningitis is being treated. This is because peak cerebrospinal and ventricular fluid gentamicin levels after parenteral therapy are usually lower than this MIC value. Alternative therapeutic regimens must be considered, such as adding a second antibiotic, selecting a different antibiotic class, or changing the route of administration.

Ampicillin and gentamicin or ampicillin and cefotaxime are recommended for initial empiric therapy of neonatal meningitis. The dosage of ampicillin or cefotaxime is 100 mg/kg/day in two divided doses during the first week of life and 200 mg/kg/day in three or four divided doses thereafter. The gentamicin dosage is the same as that used for septicemia. All infants should have repeat spinal fluid examinations and cultures at 48 hours after initiation of therapy. If organisms are seen on methylene blue or Gram stain of the fluid, the patient should be completely reevaluated with regard to making alterations in antimicrobial therapy and to obtaining computerized tomography of the head. The radiologic procedures may demonstrate the presence of a subdural empyema, brain abscess, or ventriculitis that requires neurosurgical intervention.

Cefotaxime, with or without an aminoglycoside, can be used for therapy of neonatal meningitis due to susceptible gram-negative enteric organisms.[292] Although there are no large controlled trials of cefotaxime in neonates, accumulated experience from open studies indicates that this cephalosporin is effective for therapy of neonatal sepsis and meningitis.

The Neonatal Meningitis Cooperative Study group reported that there is no beneficial effect of lumbar intrathecal or of intraventricular instillation of gentamicin in the therapy of meningitis caused by gram-negative organism.[291] The mortality rate in infants given intraventricular gentamicin was threefold greater than that in infants treated with systemic therapy only. The mean and peak ventricular CSF concentrations of endotoxin and IL-1β were significantly higher for infants treated with intraventricular gentamicin than those receiving intravenous antibiotics alone.[293] This difference may have resulted from the enhanced bacterial killing achieved through higher ventricular CSF gentamicin concentrations, with the consequent increased release of damaging inflammatory mediators, which resulted in greater periventricular inflammation.

Therapy for meningitis is continued for a minimum of 2 weeks after sterilization of CSF cultures. This equates to 14 days of therapy for meningitis caused by gram-positive organisms and a minimum of 21 days of therapy for meningitis caused by gram-negative pathogens.

Attention to general supportive therapy is essential in caring for infants with meningitis and is the single most important factor that accounts for the improved outcome during recent years. Disturbances of fluid and electrolyte balance are common, particularly in the first several days of illness when inappropriate antidiuretic hormone secretion may lead to fluid retention and hyponatremia. Hypoglycemia, hypocalcemia, and hyperbilirubinemia are frequent complications. Ventilatory assistance is frequently necessary, and blood pressure should be carefully monitored. During the course of illness, hemoglobin and hematocrit values should be checked frequently because infection may exaggerate and prolong the anemias of infancy, particularly in premature infants. Because of the frequent occurrence of bleeding diathesis, platelet counts, prothrombin time, and partial thromboplastin time should be followed.

PROGNOSIS

The mortality from neonatal meningitis is considerable. The overall mortality rate is approximately 10% to 30%, but this varies with etiologic agent, infant population, and the nursery or intensive care unit.

Short- and long-term sequelae of neonatal meningitis are frequent. The acute complications include communicating or noncommunicating hydrocephalus, subdural effusions, ventriculitis, and blindness. In 70% of infants with *Citrobacter diversus* meningitis, there is associated brain abscess.[290,291,294,295] With computed tomography scanning of the head, abnormalities can be identified in approximately 70% of neonates with coliform meningitis. Gross retardation may be obvious immediately, but many infants appear relatively normal at the time of discharge. It is only after prolonged and careful follow-up that perceptual difficulties, reading problems, or minimal brain damage is apparent. It is estimated that 30% to 50% of survivors have some evidence of neurologic damage.[169,296–298]

ASEPTIC MENINGITIS

Aseptic meningitis is an acute nonbacterial inflammatory disease of the meninges that is caused principally by viral agents. The illness occurs frequently in older infants and children and is uncommon in newborn infants. Disease in young infants is sporadic or occurs in sharply defined epidemics. It is important to differentiate aseptic from bacterial meningitis of infancy, because the therapy and prognosis are different in the two conditions.

It is frequently difficult to make a clinical distinction between aseptic meningitis and encephalitis in young infants. The cause of viral central nervous system disease depends in part on seasonal variation, age, and immune status of the host. In older infants and children, the enteroviruses (*e.g.*, coxsackievirus B, echoviruses) account for most cases of aseptic meningitis during the summer months, and mumps, lymphocytic choriomeningitis, and other viruses are more common during the other seasons. During epidemics of encephalitis, such as those caused by St. Louis encephalitis virus, a mild aseptic meningitis may be seen in young infants and occasionally in neonates. The mild nature of the disease in early life may be due in part to passively transferred antibodies from immune mothers and the relatively isolated status of young infants during community outbreaks.

Certain viruses appear to cause significant disease in the very young, such as encephalomyocarditis caused by type B coxsackieviruses. In this disease, brain, myocardium, blood, kidney, and liver are involved. In one nursery outbreak, coxsackievirus type B5 caused aseptic meningitis only.[299] Echovirus type II has been etiologically associated with a nursery epidemic of aseptic meningitis, and sporadic cases have been caused by echoviruses 1, 2, 3, 5, 9, 11, 14, 16, 17, 18, 19, 24, 25, 30, 31, and 71.[300]

Encephalitis, with or without involvement of the meninges, may occur in young infants and is caused by the aforementioned viral agents and by other arboviruses, principally Eastern equine encephalomyelitis virus and Western equine encephalomyelitis virus. St. Louis encephalomyelitis is rare in newborn infants. Congenital cytomegalovirus, herpes simplex virus types 1 and 2, rubella, and varicella-zoster viruses produce encephalitis in some infants.

SYMPTOMS

Poor temperature control, lethargy, irritability, loose stools, vomiting, diminished appetite, and "failure to thrive" are the most common symptoms.[301] In some infants, a shocklike syndrome occurs associated with seizures. It may be difficult to differentiate this clinical illness from that of bacterial meningitis. In a few patients, an erythematous maculopapular eruption, with or without petechiae, may suggest a viral cause.

DIAGNOSIS

Aseptic meningitis should be suspected if several infants in a nursery develop illness over a short period or if illness is detected in an infant during a community outbreak of aseptic meningitis. Although the outbreak is caused by a single etiologic agent, the clinical manifestations may differ among infected infants. Although one infant manifests respiratory symptoms primarily, another may have gastrointestinal illness, and all may have findings indicating involvement of the meninges. Aseptic meningitis is diagnosed in these infants by failure to demonstrate bacteria on stained smears and cultures of CSF. Although the CSF leukocyte count is usually lower than that observed in bacterial meningitis, high counts with predominance of polymorphonuclear cells may be observed early in aseptic meningitis. The CSF protein and sugar content are usually within normal limits. A definitive diagnosis is made by isolation of a viral agent from cultures of CSF or from the throat or rectum, accompanied by a significant rise in serum antibody titer to the specific agent.

With the exception of meningoencephalitis caused by herpes simplex, there is no specific antiviral therapy for postnatally acquired viral aseptic meningitis. Acyclovir is the preferred drug for herpes CNS infections.[302] Intensive supportive care is frequently necessary, with particular attention to maintenance of *p*H and electrolyte balance, respiratory assistance, and adequate nutrition. It is possible, although unproved, that intravenous immunoglobulins may be beneficial in some infants with persistent viral CNS disease, especially that caused by the enteroviruses. If an infant develops illness in a newborn nursery, every effort should be made to define the cause and source of infection. The affected infants should be isolated and treated as cohorts until discharge. Survivors may be at risk for development of significant neurologic sequelae, especially if they had seizures during their illness.[303,304]

OSTEOMYELITIS AND SEPTIC ARTHRITIS

Because of the unique nature of the vascular supply of the neonatal skeletal system, osteomyelitis and septic arthritis frequently occur concomitantly. During the first 12 months of life, capillaries perforate the epiphyseal plate of long bones and provide a communication between the metaphysis and the joint space.[305] Infections originating in one anatomic location easily spread to the other. This is not true after approximately 1 year of age, when the perforating capillaries disappear.

The capsules of the hip and shoulder attach below the metaphysis of the femur and humerus, respectively. Infection of the epiphyseal cartilage may rupture through the periosteum and enter the joint space, producing purulent arthritis. Because of the capsular articulation of the hip and shoulder, osteomyelitis and septic arthritis may coexist, making the origin of infection difficult to determine.

Infections of the musculoskeletal system are uncommon in the neonate, but incidence figures are not available.

ETIOLOGY AND PATHOGENESIS

The infecting organisms in osteomyelitis and septic arthritis vary, but the predominant ones are group B streptococci, *S. aureus*, and gram-negative enteric organisms such as *Klebsiella* spp., *Proteus* spp., and *E. coli.* Although gonococcal arthritis and tenosynovitis were commonly encountered in previous decades, they are seen only occasionally today. Other etiologic agents associated with newborn bone and joint infection are *Salmonella* spp., *Pseudomonas* spp., and *C. albicans.*[306] Hospital-acquired MRSA osteomyelitis and septic arthritis can develop in sick premature infants after catheter-associated septicemia.[307]

Osteomyelitis and arthritis have been reported after several invasive procedures in newborns, including heel puncture, femoral venipuncture, exchange transfusions, fetal monitoring electrode placement, and umbilical artery catheterization.[196,306] Osteomyelitis of cranial bones has complicated infected cephalhematomas. In most cases, the origin is unknown and is presumed to be hematogenous.

CLINICAL PRESENTATION

Nonspecific symptoms of infection, such as lethargy, irritability and poor feeding, may be the initial manifestations of neonatal musculoskeletal infection. Diminished movement of the affected limb, unrelated temporally to birth trauma, is a common clinical sign.[308] Heat, erythema, and swelling are late manifestations. The long bones are most commonly affected. Occasionally, the diagnosis is made unsuspectingly when purulent material is obtained on attempted aspiration of the femoral vein and the needle enters the swollen hip capsule. Group B streptococcal osteomyelitis is indolent and usually involves a single bone, most commonly the proximal humerus.[305]

Although blood cultures are frequently positive, the infants are usually not clinically toxic. The exception is group A β-hemolytic streptococcal infection, in which the infant may appear gravely ill.

LABORATORY TESTS AND FINDINGS

Blood cultures should be obtained from all infants with suspected infection of the musculoskeletal system. A diagnostic aspiration of the joint or subperiosteal space should be attempted in all patients, and the material obtained should be treated with Gram stain and cultured. The identification of the organism is particularly important, because it may be necessary to treat with more than one potentially nephrotoxic drug until the causative bacterium has been isolated.

The peripheral leukocyte count is frequently elevated, and juvenile forms may be seen. There is little information regarding the erythrocyte sedimentation rate during the neonatal period. In older infants and children, the sedimentation rate is accelerated in osteomyelitis; its return toward normal is a rough indicator of therapeutic success.

Radiographs of the affected bone or joint taken early in illness may be normal or show widening of the articular space. Later in the course of disease, subluxation and destruction of the joint are common. If osteomyelitis is present, the normal fat markings on roentgenograms of the deep tissues may be obliterated, indicating inflammation. Lifting of the periosteum from the bone may be observed, but cortical destruction is unusual before the second week of illness. A complete skeletal survey should be performed because of frequent involvement of multiple sites.[308,309] Resolution of bone changes is considerably slower than clinical improvement. Although radioisotope scans (*e.g.*, technetium, gallium) of bone are useful in early diagnosis of osteomyelitis in older infants and children, they may be normal in newborns with proven infection.[306]

THERAPY

Selection of initial antimicrobial therapy should be based on results of Gram and methylene blue stains of aspirated purulent material and associated clinical findings, such as furuncles or cellulitis. If gram-positive cocci are observed on stained smears, methicillin or nafcillin should be started. Vancomycin may be preferable in nurseries with multiresistant *S. aureus* strains. Cefotaxime or gentamicin is indicated if gram-negative organisms are observed. If no organisms are identified on stained smears, a combination of an antistaphylococcal drug and an aminoglycoside is used. After the organism has been identified and susceptibility studies are available, the most appropriate antibiotic or combination of antibiotics should be used. Direct instillation of an antimicrobial agent into the joint space is unnecessary because most antibiotics penetrate the inflamed synovium, and adequate concentrations are achieved in purulent material.[310] This also applies to treatment of osteomyelitis; direct instillation of antibiotics into infected bone is unwarranted.

As a general rule, infection of the joint space and bone should be drained by repeated aspiration or by surgery. Suppurative arthritis of the hip and shoulder is best treated with incision and drainage to prevent vascular compromise or extension of infection into the metaphysis. Orthopaedic consultation must be obtained for all patients.

Antimicrobial therapy of neonatal musculoskeletal infections caused by *Staphylococcus* or coliform organisms should be continued for approximately 3 weeks and, in some patients, for a longer period. For gonococcal or streptococcal infections, 10 days of therapy are generally sufficient with adequate surgical drainage. The duration of therapy must be individualized. In general, systemic symptoms disappear within several days of initiation of therapy and drainage, but local signs such as heat, erythema and swelling may persist for 4 to 7 days. Full range of motion of the involved limb may not return for several months, and physical therapy should be instituted early to prevent contractures. Complete resolution of roentgenographic changes may take several months. The use of large oral dosages of antibiotics for outpatient therapy of neonatal musculoskeletal infections has not been studied systematically and should be undertaken with caution.[311]

PROGNOSIS

Death from these diseases is unusual. However, morbidity may be considerable, particularly if weight-bearing joints such as the hip are involved. Contractures and muscle damage can be permanent.[306,312]

CUTANEOUS INFECTIONS

Most infections of the skin and subcutaneous tissues in neonates are caused by *S. aureus.* There are three major presentations of superficial staphylococcal disease. The first and most common are pustules and furuncles, which may be solitary or appear in clusters during the neonatal period. Pustules are frequently in the periumbilical and diaper areas, and they may coalesce gradually and spread to other areas of the body. Bloodstream or organ invasion is unusual unless the cutaneous infection involves extensive areas. Omphalitis is usually caused by staphylococci or streptococci, and infected circumcisions are usually caused by *S. aureus.*

The occurrence of staphylococcal skin infections in several infants from the same nursery should alert the physician to the possibility of nosocomial infection caused by a single, virulent strain of *S. aureus.* If infections are caused by the same strain of *Staphylococcus*, prompt measures should be instituted so that the source of infection can be determined and further colonization and disease can be prevented.

Therapy of cutaneous staphylococcal disease depends on the extent of the lesions and the general condition of the infant. Small, isolated pustules can be managed by local care with a mild cleansing agent or an antiseptic agent such as hexachlorophene or povidone–iodine. Infants with more extensive cutaneous involvement, systemic signs and symptoms of infection, or both should be treated with parenteral antimicrobial agents. The selection of the proper penicillin is based on historic experience and antimicrobial susceptibility studies of staphylococci isolated from the nursery unit.

The second form of neonatal staphylococcal disease has been described as the expanded scalded skin syndrome.[43] This group of illnesses includes bullous impetigo, toxic epidermal necrolysis (*i.e.,* Ritter disease), and nonstreptococcal scarlatina, usually caused by phage group II staphylococci. The pathogenesis of these entities appears to be related to release of an exotoxin (*i.e.,* exfolatin) that acts primarily on the stratum granulosa of the epidermis, causing a generalized erythema, edema, and tenderness, frequently progressing to desquamation and formation of flaccid bullae. The usual sites of staphylococcal infection are conjunctivae, throat, and umbilicus. Infants are usually afebrile. Cultures of blood, nasopharynx, eyes, and other areas should be obtained before therapy. Because phage group II staphylococci are frequently resistant to penicillin, methicillin is the initial drug of choice. Vancomycin should be used for multiresistant strains.

The third form of staphylococcal disease is necrotizing fasciitis, which also can be caused by streptococci or *E. coli.*[313–315] Necrotizing fasciitis, an unusual disease of newborns, is associated with surgical procedures, birth trauma, or cutaneous infections. In this condition, subcutaneous tissues, including muscle layers, are invaded, and the organism spreads along the fascial planes. Overlying skin may appear violaceous, and the borders of the lesion are usually indistinct. Extensive surgery to resect the destroyed tissue is imperative in treating necrotizing fasciitis. Blood and tissue cultures should be obtained, and the patient started on methicillin or nafcillin. The necrotic fatty tissue may combine with calcium, resulting in tetany and convulsions.

Breast abscesses are most commonly caused by *S. aureus*, but gram-negative enteric organisms can be causative.[316] Anaerobes can be recovered from as many as 40% of samples, one-half of which are in mixed cultures with aerobic bacteria.[317] Bacteremia is rare. The physician should attempt to establish an etiologic diagnosis by expressing fluid from the nipple after thorough cleaning. Treatment is with methicillin or an aminoglycoside, depending on the results of the Gram stain and culture, and it should be continued for 5 to 7 days. For mild infections, antibiotic therapy is adequate; with more severe inflammation, incision and drainage of the abscess are required.

Scalp abscesses occur most commonly as a complication of fetal monitoring in which scalp electrodes are used and may occur as localized manifestations of systemic disease (*e.g.*, enterococcal sepsis).[217,318] Etiologic agents include staphylococci, enterococci, gram-negative enteric bacteria, and gonococci.[217,318,319] Treatment consists of incision and drainage. If there is an associated cellulitis, antibiotics are given and continued for 5 to 7 days.

URINARY TRACT INFECTION

Improved methods for obtaining sterile specimens have made it possible for investigators to define more accurately the incidence of neonatal urinary tract infection. Bacteriuria may be demonstrated in 0.5% to 1.0% of full-term infants and as many as 3% of premature infants in studies using bladder aspiration technique.[320] Urinary tract infections are more common in babies born to bacteriuric mothers and in male neonates, in contrast to the predominance of female infants beyond this period of life.

ETIOLOGY

E. coli is the most common etiologic agent of urinary tract infection, as found in older patients. Approximately 50% of causative *E. coli* strains belong to one of eight common O antigen groups. Several polysaccharide capsular antigens (*e.g.*, K1, K2, K12, K13) are found more often in infants with upper tract disease. This particularly pertains to the K1 antigen.[321] Fimbriated *E. coli* can attach to specific receptors on uroepithelial cells. Glycolipids of the P blood group constitute a specific receptor that is believed to be associated with pyelonephritis in patients who do not have reflux. *Klebsiella* and *Pseudomonas* species are encountered less frequently. Gram-positive bacteria, with the exception of enterococci, are rare causes of urinary tract infections. Fungal cystitis and pyelonephritis are encountered in chronically ill premature infants previously treated with multiple broad-spectrum antibiotics and are associated with mucocutaneous candidiasis or invasive disease.[234]

CLINICAL MANIFESTATIONS

Many infants with significant bacteriuria are asymptomatic.[322] If clinical signs are present, they are usually nonspecific and consist of poor weight gain, altered temperature, cyanosis or gray skin color, abdominal distention, malodorous urine, and poor feeding. In a few patients, jaundice and hepatomegaly may be the presenting features of urinary tract infection.[323,324] Thrombocytopenic purpura is found in some of these infants. Localizing signs suggesting urinary tract involvement are unusual; they usually consist of a weak urinary stream or an abdominal tumor from bladder distention or hydronephrosis.[324] The most important predisposing factor is vesicoureteral reflux, which allows easy access for bacteria to ascend to the kidneys and leads to residual urine in the bladder.[324,325]

DIAGNOSIS

The diagnosis of urinary tract infection is confirmed by examination and culture of urine. The result of these tests depends largely on the method of urine collection. Most pediatricians obtain urine with a sterile, plastic receptacle applied to the cleansed perineum. However, urine obtained by this method may have an elevated cell count because of recent circumcision, vaginal reflux of urine, or contamination from the perineum. Neonatal asphyxia may increase the urinary cell count. Leukocytes must be differentiated from round epithelial cells that appear in the urine in appreciable numbers during the early days of life. Although pyuria commonly accompanies significant bacteriuria, cells can be few or absent in the presence of bacteriuria in as many as one-half of the patients.[326] Direct microscopic examination of uncentrifuged, fresh urine is useful. If bacteria are readily seen in each oil-immersion field, there are generally more than 10^5 bacteria per 1 mL. Glitter cells are felt by many to be diagnostic of urinary tract infections.

Quantitative urine cultures from infants with documented disease contain more than 50,000 colonies per 1 mL (usually ≥100,000/mL), but a small number of organisms can be found. Any number of bacteria in a urine specimen obtained by percutaneous needle puncture of the bladder should be considered significant. This latter procedure is the single best source of urine for culture and is safe in most newborn infants; its primary complication is transient gross hematuria lasting less than 24 hours in 0.6% of patients.[324]

TREATMENT

There are several approaches to the treatment of neonatal urinary tract infections. Antimicrobial agents should initially be administered parenterally, because septicemia is found in 15% to 30% of infants, and absorption after oral administration may be erratic in neonates.[327] The physician must assume that there is infection of renal parenchyma resulting from hematogenous spread.

Antibiotic selection should be based on results of antimicrobial susceptibility studies. Gentamicin is effective against the commonly encountered coliform bacteria. Because urinary concentrations of these drugs are considerably higher than those seen in serum, the usual dosages may be halved; for gentamicin, 2 to 3 mg/kg/day is satisfactory, provided the initial blood cultures are sterile. Ampicillin and gentamicin should be administered to symptomatic infants with pyuria before results of culture and susceptibility tests. Renal candidiasis should be treated systemically with amphotericin B. Bladder irrigation with amphotericin B for infants with uncomplicated *Candida* cystitis has not been properly evaluated, and its use cannot be recommended.[328]

A repeat urine culture should be sterile 36 to 48 hours after initiation of appropriate therapy. Infants with persistent bacteriuria must be evaluated for possible abscess formation, with or without urinary obstruction. In the uncomplicated patient, therapy is usually continued for a period of approximately 10 days. Blood urea nitrogen and serum creatinine levels should be determined at the initiation of therapy. If there is evidence of renal compromise, dosage and frequency of administration of the drugs, particularly the aminoglycosides, may need to be reduced. Approximately 1 week after therapy is discontinued, a repeat urine culture is obtained. If the culture is positive, therapy is reinstituted and a thorough investigation of the urinary tract is made to rule out obstruction or abscess formation.

All infants with documented urinary tract infections should have radiologic evaluation of the urinary tract. A renal scan or ultrasound examination is obtained sometime during therapy so that the possibility of gross congenital abnormalities of the urinary system can be excluded. If obstruction is demonstrated, urologic procedures to ensure proper drainage are mandatory if therapy is to be successful. A voiding cystourethrogram is usually obtained several weeks after therapy has been completed. Radiologic abnormalities, such as vesicoureteral reflux, obstructive uropathy, and renal scars, are found in approximately 45% of infants, especially in girls.[324,327,329]

PROGNOSIS

It is the physician's responsibility to be certain that neonates with documented urinary tract infections do not have congenital abnormalities of the urinary system. In such patients, recurrent urinary tract infections are common, and physical growth may be retarded until definitive surgery for stage IV or V vesicoureteral reflux has been performed.[330] Renal growth retardation is common after neonatal urinary tract infections, even in patients without reflux.[331] Every patient must have careful long-term follow-up studies to detect recurrent infections, many of which are asymptomatic. Prophylactic antibiotics should be provided for infants with clinically significant reflux to avoid new scar formation and to ensure normal renal growth.

NEONATAL OPHTHALMIA

Infections of the eye of the newborn may be caused by a variety of microorganisms, including *N. gonorrhoeae, C. trachomatis, S. aureus,* and *P. aeruginosa.* From a review of more than 300 cases of eye infections in newborns at Grady Memorial Hospital in Atlanta, it was determined that 29% were caused by chlamydiae, 14% by gonococci, 10% by staphylococci, 2% by chemical reactions, and 1% by mixed gonococcal and chlamydial infections.[332] The causes of the remaining 44% were uncertain. This frequency distribution of etiologic agents is typical of the experience at large urban general hospitals.

The incidence of ophthalmia neonatorum has not paralleled the significant increase in gonococcal disease rates among adolescents and young adults. This is almost certainly a result of universal neonatal gonococcal prophylaxis. The invasive, destructive ophthalmitis described so vividly in old literature is rarely seen today. Several agents have been effective prophylactically against gonococci: 1% silver nitrate, erythromycin or tetracycline ophthalmic ointments, and one dose of ceftriaxone administered intramuscularly.[333]

CLINICAL MANIFESTATIONS

Gonococcal ophthalmia usually becomes apparent within the first 5 days of life and is characterized initially by a clear, watery discharge. Conjunctival hyperemia and chemosis are associated with a copious discharge of thick, white, purulent material. Both eyes are usually involved but not necessarily to the same degree. Untreated gonococcal ophthalmia may extend to involve the cornea (*i.e.,* keratitis) and the anterior chamber of the eye. Corneal perforation and blindness may occur. Before the introduction of adequate prophylactic measures, ophthalmia neonatorum was the most frequent cause of acquired blindness in the United States.

DIFFERENTIAL DIAGNOSIS

Any infant presenting with a conjunctival discharge should be evaluated carefully to determine the cause. Three tests should be performed:

1. Gram stain of the exudate
2. Culture of the exudate
3. Direct immunofluorescent chlamydial stain of scrapings made from the lower palpebral conjunctiva after exudate has been wiped away.[334]

Appropriate therapy should be instituted on the basis of the results of the stained smears.

Conjunctivitis occurring in the first days of life can be chemical or bacterial. Chemical irritants, such as silver nitrate, cause transient conjunctival hyperemia and a watery discharge that rarely turns purulent.

If gram-negative rods are seen in the stained exudate, the greatest concern is *P. aeruginosa* because of the virulent, necrotizing endophthalmitis that can result. In this condition, a relatively mild conjunctivitis can progress to infection of the entire globe within 12 to 24 hours. Prompt diagnosis and immediate institution of appropriate antimicrobial therapy are mandatory.[335]

Conjunctivitis during the second or third week of life may be caused by viral, bacterial, or chlamydial agents. Viral conjunctivitis is frequently associated with other symptoms of respiratory tract disease, such as rhinorrhea, cough, and rash, and several persons in the family or nursery may simultaneously have the disease. The discharge in viral conjunctivitis is watery or mucopurulent but rarely purulent. Preauricular adenopathy is common. Staphylococci, streptococci, and occasionally gonococci cause conjunctivitis in this age group. A smear of purulent material helps differentiate these bacterial agents. However, the presence of bacteria on a gram-stained smear of exudate is not necessarily related etiologically to the conjunctivitis. Normal inhabitants of the skin and mucous membranes such as *Staphylococcus,* diphtheroids, and *Neisseria* may be observed.

Chlamydial eye infection may begin in the first days of life, but it usually does not come to the attention of the physician until the second or third week.[336] Clinical manifestations of chlamydial infection vary from mild conjunctivitis to intense inflammation and swelling of the lids, associated with copious purulent discharge. Pseudomembrane formation and a diffuse injection of the tarsal conjunctiva are common. The cornea is rarely affected, and preauricular adenopathy is unusual. In the early stages of disease, one eye may appear more swollen and infected than the other, but both eyes are usually involved. The physician establishes the diagnosis by scraping the tarsal conjunctiva and looking for typical cytoplasmic inclusions within epithelial cells or by direct immunofluorescent staining for chlamydial antigens.

THERAPY

Initial therapy is based on the results of stained smears of exudate and epithelial cells. If gonococci are seen, parenteral ceftriaxone is employed. Penicillin can be used in areas with a low prevalence of penicillinase-producing *N. gonorrhoeae* strains.[337] If staphylococci are seen, methicillin or another penicillinase-resistant penicillin analog is used. Topical antibiotics are unnecessary, because ample antibiotic to inhibit bacteria exists in the eye secretions.

Pseudomonas eye infection should always be treated with parenteral therapy consisting of ceftazidime and gentamicin. Gentamicin ophthalmic drops are used for simple *Pseudomonas* conjunctivitis, and subconjunctival or sub-Tenon space injections of gentamicin are given daily for endophthalmitis.[338]

Ophthalmic solutions containing 1% tetracycline, erythromycin, or sulfacetamide may be used in the treatment of chlamydial conjunctivitis. These are applied four times daily for 2 weeks. Topical and oral erythromycin regimens are equally effective in treating this condition, but oral therapy has the advantage of eradicating nasopharyngeal carriage of *Chlamydia* spp.[339]

Patients with gonococcal ophthalmia should be segregated, and strict hand-washing techniques should be employed because of the highly contagious nature of the exudate. The eyes should be irrigated with saline to remove the purulent material. Follow-up examination of infants treated for gonococcal ophthalmia is important to treat subsequent *C. trachomatis* ophthalmia, which can manifest after completion of therapy for gonococcal infection.

DIARRHEAL DISEASE

Although diarrheal disease during the neonatal period is usually brief and self-limited, it can cause significant morbidity in some infants and represents a potential danger to other infants in the nursery unit.

ETIOLOGY AND PATHOGENESIS

The most common cause of diarrhea in young infants is alteration of diet and feeding practices, rather than specific bacterial or viral pathogens. Of the infectious causes of diarrhea, rotaviruses are important agents.[340] Their significance in the neonatal period has not been determined except in several isolated outbreaks. A study from France indicates that 32% of neonates shed rotavirus in their stools. However, of the neonates shedding the virus, 71% in this study had no associated diarrhea.[341] The finding of rotavirus in the stools of a neonate with diarrhea may be coincidental and not represent the true etiologic agent.

Enteropathogenic *E. coli* serotypes were once considered the most common bacterial agents responsible for diarrhea in young infants.[342] These strains are referred to as enteroadherent or enteroaggregate on the basis of the purported mechanism by which they cause diarrhea. Failure to demonstrate enteropathogenic serotypes of *E. coli* in rectal cultures does not rule out coliform disease. Enterotoxigenic strains of *E. coli* with nonenteropathogenic serotypes have been identified in nursery outbreaks of diarrheal disease.[343] These organisms inhabit the small bowel, where they attach to—but do not invade—the intestinal mucosa. The enterotoxin produced by these organisms stimulates cyclic AMP, which inhibits Na and Cl transport across the intestinal wall. These salts are lost into the lumen of the upper bowel, followed passively by water, causing a net loss of stools high in electrolyte content. *Vibrio cholerae,* some *E. coli* serotypes (*i.e.,* almost exclusively nonenteropathogenic strains), and *Vibrio parahaemolyticus* are examples of bacteria that cause diarrhea by this mechanism.

Toxigenic and nontoxigenic *Clostridium difficile* strains are commonly recovered from stool cultures of newborn infants.[344] Their significance, however, is unknown because most culture-positive or toxin-positive infants are asymptomatic.

A second mechanism for bacterial diarrhea involves invasion of the intestinal mucosa. *Shigella* dysentery is the classic example of this disease. Colonic invasion, with subsequent destruction of the mucosa, causes an outpouring of polymorphonuclear cells and mucus. The resultant diarrhea is usually bloody and contains mucus and pus.[345] Other organisms causing bloody diarrhea are *Campylobacter, Yersinia,* and *Aeromonas* species.[346–349] *Salmonella* species also invade the intestinal mucosa, but extensive destruction does not occur. The epithelial lining is left intact and the organisms reach the lamina propria, where an inflammatory response is elicited.

EPIDEMIOLOGIC CONTROL

Serotyping of *E. coli* for identification of the traditional enteropathogenic strains is no longer practiced in most hospitals. After an index case of enteropathogenic *E. coli* diarrhea is recognized in a nursery, secondary cases are likely to ensue. This applies to the other etiologic agents of diarrhea in neonates. Any nursery infant with diarrhea should be suspected of having a potentially communicable disease. All infants in proximity of the index case should have rectal swabs tested by culture or by fluorescent antibody technique, which is more sensitive for identifying asymptomatic carriers of enteropathogenic *E. coli.* Ill and healthy colonized infants should be segregated and treated with orally administered neomycin (100 mg/kg/day in four divided doses) or with colistin sulfate (15 mg/kg/day in three divided doses) for 5 days. Neomycin causes rapid disappearance of the organism and abbreviates the period of diarrhea, but approximately 20% of infants revert to the asymptomatic carrier state after treatment.[350] Repeated surveillance of infants is necessary until the pathogenic strain has been eliminated from the nursery.

CLINICAL MANIFESTATIONS

The cause of diarrhea cannot be differentiated on clinical grounds in newborn infants. Diarrhea caused by enteropathogenic strains of *E. coli* is insidious in onset, is associated with seven to ten green, watery stools daily, and is usually without blood or mucus. The infants do not appear acutely ill. Complications are rare and are related primarily to dehydration and electrolyte disturbances. *Shigella* infection is uncommon, usually episodic in neonates, and does not spread within nurseries. Shigellosis in the newborn may present as a diarrheic or dysenteric syndrome or may be evidenced only by a septic or toxic infant.[345] Suppurative complications are rare, but dehydration and electrolyte disturbances are common and need immediate and constant attention. *Campylobacter* species can cause bloody diarrhea in an otherwise asymptomatic infant.[351]

Rotavirus infection has been described in newborn infants as a sporadic disease or as part of a nursery outbreak. Infection may be asymptomatic or associated with vomiting and diarrhea. The infants are usually afebrile, but temperature elevation as high as 39°C can occur. Most patients vomit, and the diarrhea is characterized by watery stools containing mucus and no blood. Moderate or severe dehydration may occur, which results in significant electrolyte disturbance in some infants. Fatal disease has been described in a small number of infants. In one report, an outbreak of necrotizing enterocolitis was associated with rotavirus infection.[352]

THERAPY

The most important aspect of therapy for diarrheal disease of newborn infants is maintenance of hydration and electrolyte balance. Parenteral solutions containing appropriate electrolytes should be administered during the time of active diarrhea, and the infant should be examined and weighed frequently so that proper rehydration and prevention of complications are ensured. Estimation of fluid loss from diarrhea and vomiting should be carefully recorded and used as a basis for replacement therapy.

Selection of appropriate antimicrobial therapy depends in part on the mechanism of diarrhea. An absorbable antibiotic, such as ampicillin or trimethoprim–sulfamethoxazole, is indicated for disease caused by invasive bacteria (*i.e.,* shigellosis), but orally administered, nonabsorbable drugs, such as neomycin or colistin sulfate, are used for noninvasive organisms that produce enterotoxin (*e.g.,* strains of *E. coli*).

Antimicrobial therapy for *Salmonella* gastroenteritis is controversial. Antibiotics do not alter the course of illness and usually prolong intestinal carriage of the organism. Clinical relapse is more common in antibiotic-treated infants. We do not recommend antibiotic therapy for uncomplicated *Salmonella* gastroenteritis if it occurs in older infants and children. Therapy is probably indicated for those with prolonged illness or evidence of colitis, for all neonates, and for infants with systemic symptoms suggesting bloodstream invasion. Ampicillin or amoxicillin is usually satisfactory, as are trimethoprim–sulfamethoxazole, cefotaxime, or ceftriaxone.

Ampicillin was formerly the antibiotic of choice for

shigellosis, but in recent years, significant resistance to this agent has been observed in many areas of the country. Most strains are susceptible *in vitro* to trimethoprim–sulfamethoxazole, and infants respond clinically and bacteriologically to a regimen of 10 mg trimethoprim with 50 mg sulfamethoxazole/kg/day in two divided doses given for 5 days. However, we have limited experience with this agent in newborn infants, and the drug should not be used in those with jaundice.

Any infant with diarrhea must be isolated from other babies in the nursery. Surveillance of all infants in contact with the index case and adoption of strict infection control measures are mandatory.

LOWER RESPIRATORY TRACT INFECTION

Lower respiratory tract infection is an important cause of morbidity in the neonate and is demonstrable on postmortem examination in approximately 20% of neonatal deaths.

Pneumonias can be divided into three categories on the basis of route of acquisition and age at presentation. The first is transplacental pneumonitis, which is acquired *in utero* and presents clinically in the early hours of life. Pneumonia may be part of a generalized congenital infection caused by cytomegalovirus, herpesvirus, rubella virus, *Toxoplasma* spp., or *L. monocytogenes*. *Treponema pallidum* produces a severe, usually fatal pneumonitis (*i.e.*, pneumonia alba), and mycoplasma can cause congenital pneumonia. These infants usually have many organ systems involved, and the pneumonitis may be obscured. Clinical findings may include hepatosplenomegaly, cutaneous manifestations such as rash or petechiae, neurologic abnormalities, and teratogenic effects.

The second category, aspiration pneumonia, is acquired in the immediate perinatal period, and onset of illness occurs within the first hours to days of life. Pathogenesis is by way of aspiration of amniotic fluid or material from the maternal cervix during the period immediately before or during delivery. Most infants with roentgenographic evidence of aspiration have not swallowed infected material and do not require antimicrobial therapy. This is also true of meconium aspiration, in which the pneumonitis is chemical. The bacterial pathogens most commonly encountered are the group B β-hemolytic streptococci, group D streptococci, pneumococci, and coliform organisms. Infants with these infections may present in the first 12 hours of life with acute respiratory distress, with or without shock. The mortality is considerable in this condition, even if appropriate antimicrobial therapy is instituted early.

The third category of pneumonias are acquired during delivery or in the postpartum period, usually beyond the first week of life. Acquired pneumonitis may be caused by viral, chlamydial, or bacterial agents and is most frequently bronchopneumonic or interstitial. The respiratory syncytial virus is the most important pathogen causing lower respiratory tract disease in young infants.[353] The parainfluenza viruses, enteroviruses, rhinoviruses, and adenoviruses cause bronchiolitis and pneumonia during early infancy. Herpes simplex virus infection can be acquired at the time of delivery and present in the first week of life. Bronchiolitis, pneumonia, or both usually occur in epidemics among premature and full-term nursery infants or in the community.

Documented nursery outbreaks of lower respiratory tract disease have been associated with RSV, adenovirus, echovirus type 22, influenza A and B viruses, and parainfluenza virus infections. During these outbreaks, many infants are colonized with the epidemic virus strains, but only a few manifest clinical disease.

S. aureus and coliform organisms are the most common bacterial pathogens causing postnatally acquired pneumonia. Disease caused by *S. aureus* and *K. pneumoniae* may occur sporadically or in epidemic fashion during the neonatal period. Pyogenic complications, such as septicemia, osteomyelitis and meningitis, are frequently associated with the epidemic form of these infections.

Acquisition of *C. trachomatis* in the intrapartum period may result in conjunctivitis (*i.e.*, inclusion blennorrhea) or in pneumonia that usually presents between the fourth and twelfth weeks of life. The pneumonia is associated with a staccato cough, often terminating in vomiting or cyanosis, and with tachypnea; the infants are usually afebrile.[354] Rales are heard, and there may be a history of the infant having conjunctivitis in the newborn period. Eosinophilia affects approximately one-half of the patients. *C. trachomatis* can cause severe and chronic pneumonia in low-birth-weight infants.[355,356] *C. trachomatis* pneumonia in otherwise healthy infants has been associated with long-term pulmonary function abnormalities.[357]

Considerable data indicates that *U. urealyticum* colonization of low-birth-weight infants is associated with the subsequent development of chronic lung disease.[358–360] *Pneumocystis carinii* is an uncommon cause of pneumonia in the neonatal period; susceptible infants include malnourished premature newborns living in endemic geographic areas, infants with congenital immunodeficiencies (*e.g.*, severe combined immunodeficiency), and neonates infected with the human immunodeficiency virus type 1.[361,362]

CLINICAL MANIFESTATIONS

The early signs of lower respiratory tract disease in the neonate and young infant are frequently nonspecific and include change in feeding status, listlessness or irritability, and poor color. More specific findings that may not be present at the onset of illness are tachypnea, dyspnea, cyanosis, hypothermia, cough, and grunting. Accentuation of the normal irregularity of breathing is a common finding in neonates.

The physical findings of pneumonia vary. Flaring of the alae nasi, rapid respirations, and sternal and subcostal retractions are frequently observed. A cough is indicative of lower respiratory tract involvement; a brassy cough is frequently found in viral disease. Percussion dullness is difficult to demonstrate, but it is indicative of consolidation, effusion, or both. Auscultation may reveal diminished breath sounds over the affected area. Rales, wheezes, or both can usually be heard on deep inspiration or when the baby is crying, but may be absent early in the illness. The clinician is frequently surprised by the meager clinical signs in the face of clearly demonstrable and sometimes extensive roentgenographic findings of pneumonia.

DIAGNOSIS

The leukocyte count can sometimes help to differentiate viral from bacterial pneumonia. Infants with early-onset bacterial pneumonia with sepsis may have leukopenia with an increased number of band forms. Chorioamnionitis has been demonstrated in the mothers of some infants with congenital pneumonia.

Cultures of blood and material from the trachea frequently help to define the etiologic agent of neonatal pneumonia. However, results of cultures from the ear canal, throat, and other external sites are not helpful and may be misleading in newborn and young infants. Lung puncture should be considered in infants with consolidated pneumonia if the cause is unknown or the infant fails to respond to conventional antimicrobial therapy. Material obtained at puncture should be Gram stained for direct visualization of bacteria and cultured. Chlamydial pneumonia is best diagnosed by direct immunofluorescent staining and culture of nasopharyngeal secretions.[363]

A chest radiograph is indicated in all infants with nonspecific signs of infection. There may be roentgenographic evidence of pneumonia despite the absence of physical findings. Although it is not usually possible to determine the cause of neonatal pneumonia from chest radiographs, certain roentgenographic patterns may be associated with specific diseases. A consolidating bronchopneumonia with pneumatoceles, with or without empyema, suggests staphylococcal disease. This is particularly true when the radiologic findings advance markedly in a few hours. If a lobar infiltrate is associated with bulging fissures on the radiograph, *K. pneumoniae* infection should be considered. A miliary-type of bronchopneumonia in a septic neonate is characteristic of listeriosis. Group B streptococcal pneumonia is frequently indistinguishable radiographically from hyaline membrane disease.

A bronchopneumonic infiltrate is most commonly encountered in the first month of life.[364] This can be caused by aspiration of sterile or infected amniotic fluid or by viral, chlamydial, or bacterial pathogens, or it can represent patchy atelectasis.

Staphylococcal pneumonia is found most commonly in young infants—30% of patients are younger than 3 months of age, and 70% are younger than 1 year of age. Epidemics of staphylococcal disease caused by phage group I organisms are encountered infrequently.

Staphylococci cause a confluent bronchopneumonia, characterized by extensive areas of hemorrhagic necrosis and irregular areas of cavitation. The pleural surface is usually covered by a thick layer of fibrinopurulent exudate. Multiple small abscesses are scattered throughout the lungs. Rupture of a small subpleural abscess may result in a pyopneumothorax, which may erode into a bronchus, producing a bronchopleural fistula.

The onset of illness in staphylococcal pneumonia is abrupt, with fever, cough, and respiratory distress as the major manifestations. Tachypnea, grunting respirations, retractions, cyanosis, and anxiety are usually observed. Severe dyspnea and a shocklike state may occur. Rapid progression of symptoms is characteristic. Moist, scattered rales, diminished breath sounds, and rhonchi may be heard early in the illness. With the development of pleural effusion, dullness on percussion is associated with diminished breath sounds.

Most patients with staphylococcal pneumonia have roentgenographic evidence of bronchopneumonia early in the illness. The infiltrate may be patchy and limited in extent or be dense and homogeneous, involving an entire lobe or hemithorax. Pleural effusion or empyema are found in most infants.[365] Pneumatoceles of various sizes are common. Although no radiographic change can be considered diagnostic, progression over a few hours from bronchopneumonia to effusion or pyopneumothorax with or without pneumatoceles is highly suggestive of staphylococcal pneumonia.

TREATMENT

All diagnostic procedures and cultures should be obtained before initiation of therapy. Methicillin is the initial drug of choice for staphylococcal pneumonia and should be administered parenterally in a dosage of 75 mg/kg/day, divided in two or three doses for infants younger than 1 week of age and in a dosage of 100 mg/kg/day divided in four doses for older infants.

If infection extends to the pleural surfaces, surgical intervention usually becomes necessary. With small amounts of effusion, repeated pleural taps may be successful in removing fluid, but empyema is best treated by closed drainage with a chest tube of the largest possible caliber.

Vancomycin is preferred for disease due to MRSA. For pneumonia caused by *K. pneumoniae* or other coliforms, kanamycin or gentamicin should be used in a total dosage of 15 mg/kg/day or 5 to 7.5 mg/kg/day, respectively. Alternatively, a third-generation cephalosporin, such as cefotaxime, can be used. Treatment for *Listeria* pneumonia is parenteral ampicillin in a dosage of 50 to 100 mg/kg/day, divided in two doses for infants younger than 1 week of age and 100 to 150 mg/kg/day divided in three doses for older neonates. Infants with GBS septicemia and pneumonia should be given penicillin in a dosage of 50,000 U/kg/day divided in two doses for infants younger than 1 week of age and 75,000 to 100,000 U/kg/day divided in three or four doses for older infants. Larger doses are required for meningitis. Ampicillin or cefotaxime may be used in place of penicillin.

Chlamydial and ureaplasmal pneumonias are probably best treated with orally or intravenously administered erythromycin, depending on the infant's clinical status. This agent has been shown to shorten the course of illness and to eradicate shedding of the organisms from the nasopharynx. Trimethoprim–sulfamethoxazole is the initial drug of choice for *P. carinii* pneumonia; pentamidine is reserved for treatment failures.

Pneumonia may be one manifestation of generalized congenital viral infections. It is important to differentiate these infections from congenital syphilis and bacterial pneumonias resulting from aspiration. There is no convincing evidence that antiviral chemotherapy is effective in infants with congenital cytomegalovirus infection. Vidarabine or acyclovir are effective if given early in disease caused by herpes simplex virus.

Most infants with aspiration pneumonia do not require antimicrobial therapy. It is frequently difficult to differentiate infants with aspiration of sterile amniotic fluid from those aspirating infected materials. If doubt exists, therapy with penicillin and kanamycin or gentamicin should be initiated and continued until results of cultures are available.

OTITIS MEDIA

Otitis media is a frequent finding in premature infants receiving intensive care and an almost universal finding in autopsy studies of infants who died after a period of intensive care.[366,367] A principal predisposing factor for otitis media in the newborn is nasotracheal intubation that results in ipsilateral obstruction of the eustachian tube, establishing the conditions eventuating in middle ear infection. The diagnosis is frequently missed because pneumatic otoscopy is not routinely performed in neonates.

The exact incidence of this condition is unknown. In one prospective study of 70 infants followed from birth, 34% developed their first episode of otitis media before 2 months of age.[368] Symptoms are nonspecific and include irritability, lethargy, fever, cough, diarrhea, vomiting, tachypnea, and anorexia.[369] An associated conjunctivitis, pneumonia, or meningitis may be found in one-half of the patients. The diagnosis is usually made by pneumatic otoscopy. Tympanometry is unreliable in neonates.

Pathogenic organisms include *S. pneumoniae, H. influenzae, S. aureus, Moraxella catarrhalis,* and coliforms. The predominant isolates vary in different study populations.[366,369–371]

Tympanocentesis should be performed on all newborns with otitis media who develop illness while in the nursery or intensive care unit.[372] This may yield an etiologic agent when cultures of other sites are sterile. Some infants have positive blood cultures. The choice of antibiotic therapy can be based on the results of the Gram stain and culture of the aspirated middle ear effusion. If no organisms are seen on the smear, treatment should be with methicillin and an aminoglycoside until additional information is available. Infants with otitis media who are seen in the clinic or office do not usually require tympanocentesis for etiologic diagnosis if the illness is mild and can be managed at home. In these infants, cefaclor or Augmentin (amoxicillin and clavulanate) is preferred for therapy, and the patients should be reexamined 2 or 3 days after initiation of therapy to ascertain improvement. Infants with onset of otitis media before 2 months of age need as long as 3 months to clear the effusion, and 33% of them develop chronic otitis media.[368]

PERITONITIS

Spontaneous bacterial (*i.e.*, primary) peritonitis without an evident intraabdominal source is rare during the neonatal period.[373] It is postulated that bacteria can reach the peritoneal cavity by means of hematogenous, lymphatic, genital, or transmural (*i.e.*, across the gut wall) routes of spread.[374] A concurrent omphalitis is common.[375] Gram-positive bacteria (*e.g.*, *S. pneumoniae,* groups A and B streptococci) are the predominant pathogens, but gram-negative bacilli such as *Pseudomonas* or *Klebsiella* are responsible for some cases.

Most infants develop peritonitis after perforation of an abdominal viscus, usually as a complication of necrotizing enterocolitis. Other predisposing conditions include spontaneous focal gastrointestinal perforations, wound infections after abdominal surgery, traumatic perforations (*e.g.*, feeding tube, rectal thermometer), ruptured omphalocele, and meconium peritonitis with subsequent bacterial contamination. Organisms isolated from peritoneal fluid cultures generally mirror the infant's gut flora and include *E. coli, Klebsiella* spp., *Enterobacter* spp., *Pseudomonas,* coagulase-positive and coagulase-negative staphylococci, streptococci, enterococci, anaerobic bacteria (*e.g.*, clostridia, *Bacteroides* spp.), and *Candida.*[376–379]

Clinical signs of peritonitis include vomiting, abdominal distention, abdominal wall edema or discoloration, constipation, diarrhea, grunting, temperature instability (*i.e.*, usually hypothermia), shock, and scrotal or vulvar swelling.[380] Abdominal radiographs may reveal free air in the peritoneal cavity, indicating intestinal perforation, or patterns suggesting necrotizing enterocolitis (*e.g.*, pneumatosis intestinalis) or intestinal obstruction. Abdominal ultrasound is helpful in visualizing peritoneal fluid. An abdominal paracentesis may yield pus or reveal a different cause for the illness (*e.g.*, hemoperitoneum, bile peritonitis). Aerobic and anaerobic cultures of the peritoneal fluid and of the blood should be obtained in all cases.

The management of peritonitis consists of supportive measures aimed at reversing hypovolemia, shock, and electrolyte imbalances; of surgical correction of underlying conditions; and of the administration of broad-spectrum antimicrobial agents. Acceptable initial antibiotic regimens include ampicillin, gentamicin and clindamycin, Timentin and an aminoglycoside, or vancomycin, ceftazidime, and metronidazole. The broadest antibacterial coverage is attained by the vancomycin, ceftazidime, and metronidazole combination. Treatment can be simplified after the blood and peritoneal fluid culture results become available. Antibiotics are usually continued for 10 days. The prognosis depends on several factors, including birth weight and precipitating conditions, and fatality rates range from 10% to 50%.[373]

REFERENCES

1. Jason JM. Infectious disease-related deaths of low birth weight infants, United States, 1968 to 1982. Pediatrics 1989; 84:296.
2. Bennet R, Bergdahl S, Eriksson M, Zetterström R. The outcome of neonatal septicemia during fifteen years. Acta Paediatr Scand 1989;78:40.
3. Msall ME, Buck GM, Rogers BT, et al. Risk factors for major neurodevelopmental impairments and need for special education resources in extremely premature infants. J Pediatr 1991;119:606.
4. Siegel JD, McCracken GH Jr. Sepsis neonatorum. N Engl J Med 1981;304:642.
5. Freedman RM, Ingram DL, Gross I, et al. A half century of neonatal sepsis at Yale: 1928 to 1978. Am J Dis Child 1981; 135:140.
6. Jarvis WR. Epidemiology of nosocomial infections in pediatric patients. Pediatr Infect Dis J 1987;6:344.
7. St Geme JW III, Harris MC. Coagulase-negative staphylococcal infection in the neonate. Clin Perinatol 1991;18:281.
8. McCracken GH Jr, Freij BJ. Clinical pharmacology of antimicrobial agents. In: Remington JS, Klein JO, eds. Infectious diseases of the fetus and newborn infant. 3rd ed. Philadelphia: WB Saunders, 1990:1020.
9. Boyer KM, Gotoff SP. Antimicrobial prophylaxis of neonatal group B streptococcal sepsis. Clin Perinatol 1988;15:831.
10. Khuri-Bulos N, McIntosh K. Neonatal Haemophilus influenzae infection: report of eight cases and review of the literature. Am J Dis Child 1975;129:57.
11. Campognone P, Singer DB. Neonatal sepsis due to nontypable Haemophilus influenzae. Am J Dis Child 1986;140:117.
12. Abdul-Rauf A, Schreiber JR. Neonatal Haemophilus influenzae type b sepsis. Pediatr Infect Dis J 1990;9:918.
13. Takala AK, Pekkanen E, Eskola J. Neonatal Haemophilus influenzae infections. Arch Dis Child 1991;66:437.
14. Cox RA. Neonatal septicaemia due to non-capsulate Haemophilus influenzae in three siblings. J Infect 1991;23:317.
15. Bortolussi R, Thompson TR, Ferrieri P. Early-onset pneumococcal sepsis in newborn infants. Pediatrics 1977;60:352.
16. Chugh K, Bhalla CK, Joshi KK. Meningococcal brain abscess and meningitis in a neonate. Pediatr Infect Dis J 1988;7:136.
17. Goldmann DA. Bacterial colonization and infection in the neonate. Am J Med 1981;70:417.
18. Fryklund B, Tullus K, Burman LG. Epidemiology of enteric bacteria in neonatal units—influence of procedures and patient variables. J Hosp Infect 1991;18:15.
19. Goering RV, Ehrenkranz NJ, Sanders CC, Sanders WE Jr. Long term epidemiological analysis of Citrobacter diversus in a neonatal intensive care unit. Pediatr Infect Dis J 1992;11:99.
20. D'Angio CT, McGowan KL, Baumgart S, et al. Surface colonization with coagulase-negative staphylococci in premature neonates. J Pediatr 1989;114:1029.
21. Baley JE, Kliegman RM, Boxerbaum B, Fanaroff AA. Fungal colonization in the very low birth weight infant. Pediatrics 1986;78:225.
22. Aschner JL, Punsalang A Jr, Maniscalco WM, Menegus MA. Percutaneous central venous catheter colonization with Malassezia furfur: incidence and clinical significance. Pediatrics 1987;80:535.
23. Bell LM, Alpert G, Slight PH, Campos JM. Malassezia furfur skin colonization in infancy. Infect Control Hosp Epidemiol 1988;9:151.
24. Cassell GH, Waites KB, Crouse DT. Perinatal mycoplasmal infections. Clin Perinatol 1991;18:241.
25. Syrogiannopoulos GA, Kapatais-Zoumbos K, Decavalas GO, et al. Ureaplasma urealyticum colonization of full term infants: perinatal acquisition and persistence during early infancy. Pediatr Infect Dis J 1990;9:236.
26. Hammerschlag MR, Anderka M, Semine DZ, et al. Prospective study of maternal and infantile infection with Chlamydia trachomatis. Pediatrics 1979;64:142.
27. Schachter J, Grossman M, Sweet RL, et al. Prospective study of perinatal transmission of Chlamydia trachomatis. JAMA 1986;255:3374.
28. Bell TA, Stamm WE, Wang SP, et al. Chronic Chlamydia trachomatis infections in infants. JAMA 1992;267:400.
29. Peter G, Cashore WJ. Infections acquired in the nursery: epidemiology and control. In: Remington JS, Klein JO, eds. Infectious diseases of the fetus and newborn infant. 3rd ed. Philadelphia: WB Saunders, 1990:1000.
30. Thompson PJ, Greenough A, Hird MF, et al. Nosocomial bacterial infections in very low birth weight infants. Eur J Pediatr 1992;151:451.
31. Adams JM, Speer ME, Rudolph AJ. Bacterial colonization of radial artery catheters. Pediatrics 1980;65:94.
32. Landers S, Moise AA, Fraley JK, et al. Factors associated with umbilical catheter-related sepsis in neonates. Am J Dis Child 1991;145:675.
33. Hruszkewycz V, Holtrop PC, Batton DG, et al. Complications associated with central venous catheters inserted in critically ill neonates. Infect Control Hosp Epidemiol 1991;12:544.
34. Toltzis P, Goldmann DA. Current issues in central venous catheter infection. Annu Rev Med 1990;41:169.
35. Maki DG, Ringer M, Alvarado CJ. Prospective randomised trial of povidone-iodine, alcohol, and chlorhexidine for prevention of infection associated with central venous and arterial catheters. Lancet 1991;338:339.

36. Cowen J, Ellis SH, McAinsh J. Absorption of chlorhexidine from the intact skin of newborn infants. Arch Dis Child 1979; 54:379.
37. Alder VG, Burman D, Simpson RA, et al. Comparison of hexachlorophane and chlorhexidine powders in prevention of neonatal infection. Arch Dis Child 1980;55:277.
38. Meberg A, Schøyen R. Bacterial colonization and neonatal infections: effects of skin and umbilical disinfection in the nursery. Acta Paediatr Scand 1985;74:366.
39. Hoffmann KK, Weber DJ, Samsa GP, Rutala WA. Transparent polyurethane film as an intravenous catheter dressing: a meta-analysis of the infection risks. JAMA 1992;267:2072.
40. Maki DG, Cobb L, Garman JK, et al. An attachable silver-impregnated cuff for prevention of infection with central venous catheters: a prospective randomized multicenter trial. Am J Med 1988;85:307.
41. Flowers RH III, Schwenzer KJ, Kopel RF, et al. Efficacy of an attachable subcutaneous cuff for the prevention of intravascular catheter-related infection: a randomized, controlled trial. JAMA 1989;261:878.
42. John JF Jr. Molecular analysis of nosocomial epidemics. Infect Dis Clin North Am 1989;3:683.
43. Melish ME, Glasgow LA, Turner MD. The staphylococcal scalded-skin syndrome: isolation and partial characterization of the exfoliative toxin. J Infect Dis 1972;125:129.
44. Curran JP, Al-Salihi FL. Neonatal staphylococcal scalded skin syndrome: massive outbreak due to an unusual phage type. Pediatrics 1980;66:285.
45. Albert S, Baldwin R, Czekajewski S, et al. Bullous impetigo due to group II Staphylococcus aureus: an epidemic in a normal newborn nursery. Am J Dis Child 1970;120:10.
46. Boyce JM. Methicillin-resistant Staphylococcus aureus: detection, epidemiology, and control measures. Infect Dis Clin North Am 1989;3:901.
47. Boyce JM. Should we vigorously try to contain and control methicillin-resistant Staphylococcus aureus? Infect Control Hosp Epidemiol 1991;12:46.
48. Graham DR, Correa-Villasenor A, Anderson RL, et al. Epidemic neonatal gentamicin-methicillin-resistant Staphylococcus aureus infection associated with nonspecific topical use of gentamicin. J Pediatr 1980;97:972.
49. Dunkle LM, Naqvi SH, McCallum R, Lofgren JP. Eradication of epidemic methicillin-gentamicin-resistant Staphylococcus aureus in an intensive care nursery. Am J Med 1981;70:455.
50. Goldmann DA. Prevention and management of neonatal infections. Infect Dis Clin North Am 1989;3:779.
51. Rosenfeld CR, Laptook AR, Jeffery J. Limited effectiveness of triple dye in preventing colonization with methicillin-resistant Staphylococcus aureus in a special care nursery. Pediatr Infect Dis J 1990;9:290.
52. Davies EA, Emmerson AM, Hogg GM, et al. An outbreak of infection with a methicillin-resistant Staphylococcus aureus in a special care baby unit: value of topical mupirocin and of traditional methods of infection control. J Hosp Infect 1987; 10:120.
53. Dillon HC Jr. Group A type 12 streptococcal infection in a newborn nursery: successfully treated neonatal meningitis. Am J Dis Child 1966;112:177.
54. Geil CC, Castle WK, Mortimer EA Jr. Group A streptococcal infections in newborn nurseries. Pediatrics 1970;46:849.
55. Givner LB, Abramson JS, Wasilauskas B. Apparent increase in the incidence of invasive group A beta-hemolytic streptococcal disease in children. J Pediatr 1991;118:341.
56. Wheeler MC, Roe MH, Kaplan EL, et al. Outbreak of group A streptococcus septicemia in children: clinical, epidemiologic, and microbiological correlates. JAMA 1991;266:533.
57. Jackson MA, Burry VF, Olson LC. Multisystem group A β-hemolytic streptococcal disease in children. Rev Infect Dis 1991;13:783.
58. Stevens DL. Invasive group A streptococcus infections. Clin Infect Dis 1992;14:2.
59. Lambert-Zechovsky N, Bingen E, Denamur E, et al. Molecular analysis provides evidence for the endogenous origin of bacteremia and meningitis due to Enterobacter cloacae in an infant. Clin Infect Dis 1992;15:30.
60. Hill HR, Hunt CE, Matsen JM. Nosocomial colonization with Klebsiella, type 26, in a neonatal intensive-care unit associated with an outbreak of sepsis, meningitis, and necrotizing enterocolitis. J Pediatr 1974;85:415.
61. Eidelman AI, Reynolds J. Gentamicin-resistant Klebsiella infections in a neonatal intensive care unit. Am J Dis Child 1978;132:421.
62. Plotkin SA, McKitrick JC. Nosocomial meningitis of the newborn caused by a flavobacterium. JAMA 1966;198:662.
63. Abrahamsen TG, Finne PH, Lingaas E. Flavobacterium meningosepticum infections in a neonatal intensive care unit. Acta Paediatr Scand 1989;78:51.
64. Smith PJ, Brookfield DSK, Shaw DA, Gray J. An outbreak of Serratia marcescens infection in a neonatal unit. Lancet 1984;1:151.
65. Duggan TG, Leng RA, Hancock BM, Cursons RT. Serratia marcescens in a newborn unit—microbiological features. Pathology 1984;16:189.
66. Bobo RA, Newton EJ, Jones LF, et al. Nursery outbreak of Pseudomonas aeruginosa: epidemiological conclusions from five different typing methods. Appl Microbiol 1973;25:414.
67. Burke JP, Ingall D, Klein JO, et al. Proteus mirabilis infections in a hospital nursery traced to a human carrier. N Engl J Med 1971;284:115.
68. Parry MF, Hutchinson JH, Brown NA, et al. Gram-negative sepsis in neonates: a nursery outbreak due to hand carriage of Citrobacter diversus. Pediatrics 1980;65:1105.
69. Modi N, Damjanovic V, Cooke RWI. Outbreak of cephalosporin resistant Enterobacter cloacae infection in a neonatal intensive care unit. Arch Dis Child 1987;62:148.
70. Simmons BP, Gelfand MS, Haas M, et al. Enterobacter sakazakii infections in neonates associated with intrinsic contamination of a powdered infant formula. Infect Control Hosp Epidemiol 1989;10:398.
71. Khan MA, Abdur-Rab M, Israr N, et al. Transmission of Salmonella worthington by oropharyngeal suction in hospital neonatal unit. Pediatr Infect Dis J 1991;10:668.
72. Cook LN, Davis RS, Stover BH. Outbreak of amikacin-resistant Enterobacteriaceae in an intensive care nursery. Pediatrics 1980;65:264.
73. Biering G, Karlsson S, Clark NC, et al. Three cases of neonatal meningitis caused by Enterobacter sakazakii in powdered milk. J Clin Microbiol 1989;27:2054.
74. Modlin JF. Perinatal echovirus and group B coxsackievirus infections. Clin Perinatol 1988;15:233.
75. Graman PS, Hall CB. Epidemiology and control of nosocomial viral infections. Infect Dis Clin North Am 1989;3:815.
76. Chawareewong S, Kiangsiri S, Lokaphadhana K, et al. Neonatal herpangina caused by coxsackie A-5 virus. J Pediatr 1978;93:492.
77. Javett SN, Heymann S, Mundel B, et al. Myocarditis in the newborn infant: a study of an outbreak associated with coxsackie group B virus infection in a maternity home in Johannesburg. J Pediatr 1956;48:1.
78. Swender PT, Shott RJ, Williams ML. A community and intensive care nursery outbreak of coxsackievirus B5 meningitis. Am J Dis Child 1974;127:42.

79. Krajden S, Middleton PJ. Enterovirus infections in the neonate. Clin Pediatr (Phila) 1983;22:87.
80. Butterfield J, Moscovici C, Berry C, Kempe CH. Cystic emphysema in premature infants: a report of an outbreak with the isolation of type 19 ECHO virus in one case. N Engl J Med 1963;268:18.
81. McDonald LL, St Geme JW Jr, Arnold BH. Nosocomial infection with ECHO virus type 31 in a neonatal intensive care unit. Pediatrics 1971;47:995.
82. Lapinleimu K, Hakulinen A. A hospital outbreak caused by ECHO virus type 11 among newborn infants. Ann Clin Res 1972;4:183.
83. Philip AGS, Larson EJ. Overwhelming neonatal infection with ECHO 19 virus. J Pediatr 1973;82:391.
84. Purdham DR, Purdham PA, Wood BSB, et al. Severe echo 19 virus infection in a neonatal unit. Arch Dis Child 1976;51:634.
85. Davies DP, Hughes CA, MacVicar J, et al. Echovirus-11 infection in a special-care baby unit. Lancet 1979;1:96.
86. Modlin JF, Polk BF, Horton P, et al. Perinatal echovirus infection: risk of transmission during a community outbreak. N Engl J Med 1981;305:368.
87. Kinney JS, McCray E, Kaplan JE, et al. Risk factors associated with echovirus 11′ infection in a hospital nursery. Pediatr Infect Dis 1986;5:192.
88. Rabkin CS, Telzak EE, Ho M-S, et al. Outbreak of echovirus 11 infection in hospitalized neonates. Pediatr Infect Dis J 1988; 7:186.
89. Reyes MP, Ostrea EM Jr, Roskamp J, Lerner AM. Disseminated neonatal echovirus 11 disease following antenatal maternal infection with a virus-positive cervix and virus-negative gastrointestinal tract. J Med Virol 1983;12:155.
90. Larson E. A causal link between handwashing and risk of infection? Examination of the evidence. Infect Control Hosp Epidemiol 1988;9:28.
91. Nagington J. Echovirus 11 infection and prophylactic antiserum. Lancet 1982;1:446.
92. Noble RC, Kane MA, Reeves SA, Roeckel I. Posttransfusion hepatitis A in a neonatal intensive care unit. JAMA 1984; 252:2711.
93. Klein BS, Michaels JA, Rytel MW, et al. Nosocomial hepatitis A: a multinursery outbreak in Wisconsin. JAMA 1984; 252:2716.
94. Azimi PH, Roberto RR, Guralnik J, et al. Transfusion-acquired hepatitis A in a premature infant with secondary nosocomial spread in an intensive care nursery. Am J Dis Child 1986;140:23.
95. Rosenblum LS, Villarino ME, Nainan OV, et al. Hepatitis A outbreak in a neonatal intensive care unit: risk factors for transmission and evidence of prolonged viral excretion among preterm infants. J Infect Dis 1991;164:476.
96. Lee KK, Vargo LR, Lê CT, Fernando L. Transfusion-acquired hepatitis A outbreak from fresh frozen plasma in a neonatal intensive care unit. Pediatr Infect Dis J 1992;11:122.
97. Centers for Disease Control. Protection against viral hepatitis: recommendations of the Immunization Practices Advisory Committee (ACIP). MMWR 1990;39(S-2):1.
98. Mbithi JN, Springthorpe VS, Boulet JR, Sattar SA. Survival of hepatitis A virus on human hands and its transfer on contact with animate and inanimate surfaces. J Clin Microbiol 1992; 30:757.
99. Abzug MJ, Levin MJ. Neonatal adenovirus infection: four patients and review of the literature. Pediatrics 1991;87:890.
100. Brown M, Rossier E, Carpenter B, Anand CM. Fatal adenovirus type 35 infection in newborns. Pediatr Infect Dis J 1991;10:955.
101. Eichenwald HF, Kotsevalov O. Immunologic responses of premature and full-term infants to infection with certain viruses. Pediatrics 1960;25:829.
102. Finn A, Anday E, Talbot GH. An epidemic of adenovirus 7a infection in a neonatal nursery: course, morbidity, and management. Infect Control Hosp Epidemiol 1988;9:398.
103. Piedra PA, Kasel JA, Norton HJ, et al. Evaluation of an intravenous immunoglobulin preparation for the prevention of viral infection among hospitalized low birth weight infants. Pediatr Infect Dis J 1990;9:470.
104. Piedra PA, Kasel JA, Norton HJ, et al. Description of an adenovirus type 8 outbreak in hospitalized neonates born prematurely. Pediatr Infect Dis J 1992;11:460.
105. Berkovich S. Acute respiratory illness in the premature nursery associated with respiratory syncytial virus infections. Pediatrics 1964;34:753.
106. Hall CB, Kopelman AE, Douglas RG Jr, et al. Neonatal respiratory syncytial virus infection. N Engl J Med 1979; 300:393.
107. Valenti WM, Clarke TA, Hall CB, et al. Concurrent outbreaks of rhinovirus and respiratory syncytial virus in an intensive care nursery: epidemiology and associated risk factors. J Pediatr 1982;100:722.
108. Meissner HC, Murray SA, Kiernan MA, et al. A simultaneous outbreak of respiratory syncytial virus and parainfluenza virus type 3 in a newborn nursery. J Pediatr 1984;104:680.
109. Snydman DR, Greer C, Meissner HC, McIntosh K. Prevention of nosocomial transmission of respiratory syncytial virus in a newborn nursery. Infect Control Hosp Epidemiol 1988;9:105.
110. Church NR, Anas NG, Hall CB, Brooks JG. Respiratory syncytial virus-related apnea in infants: demographics and outcome. Am J Dis Child 1984;138:247.
111. MacDonald NE, Hall CB, Suffin SC, et al. Respiratory syncytial viral infection in infants with congenital heart disease. N Engl J Med 1982;307:397.
112. Gala CL, Hall CB, Schnabel KC, et al. The use of eye-nose goggles to control nosocomial respiratory syncytial virus infection. JAMA 1986;256:2706.
113. Agah R, Cherry JD, Garakian AJ, Chapin M. Respiratory syncytial virus (RSV) infection rate in personnel caring for children with RSV infections: routine isolation procedure vs routine procedure supplemented by use of masks and goggles. Am J Dis Child 1987;141:695.
114. Lau YR, Whitley RJ. Evaluation of ribavirin for treatment of respiratory syncytial virus. Semin Pediatr Infect Dis 1991; 2:279.
115. Smith DW, Frankel LR, Mathers LH, et al. A controlled trial of aerosolized ribavirin in infants receiving mechanical ventilation for severe respiratory syncytial virus infection. N Engl J Med 1991;325:24.
116. Bauer CR, Elie K, Spence L, Stern L. Hong Kong influenza in a neonatal unit. JAMA 1973;223:1233.
117. Meibalane R, Sedmak GV, Sasidharan P, et al. Outbreak of influenza in a neonatal intensive care unit. J Pediatr 1977; 91:974.
118. Polin RA, St Geme JW III. Neonatal sepsis. Adv Pediatr Infect Dis 1992;7:25.
119. Bada HS, Alojipan LC, Andrews BF. Premature rupture of membranes and its effect on the newborn. Pediatr Clin North Am 1977;24:491.
120. St Geme JW Jr, Murray DL, Carter JA, et al. Perinatal bacterial infection after prolonged rupture of amniotic membranes: an analysis of risk and management. J Pediatr 1984;104:608.
121. Sperling RS, Newton E, Gibbs RS. Intraamniotic infection in low-birth-weight infants. J Infect Dis 1988;157:113.
122. Hillier SL, Krohn MA, Kiviat NB, et al. Microbiologic causes

and neonatal outcomes associated with chorioamnion infection. Am J Obstet Gynecol 1991;165:955.
123. Marston G, Wald ER. Hemophilus influenzae type b sepsis in infant and mother. Pediatrics 1976;58:863.
124. Tarpay MM, Turbeville DF, Krous HF. Fatal streptococcus pneumoniae type III sepsis in mother and infant. Am J Obstet Gynecol 1980;136:257.
125. Grossman J, Tompkins RL. Group B beta-hemolytic streptococcal meningitis in mother and infant. N Engl J Med 1974; 290:387.
126. Botta GA. Hormonal and type-dependent adhesion of group B streptococci to human vaginal cells. Infect Immun 1979; 25:1084.
127. Broughton RA, Baker CJ. Role of adherence in the pathogenesis of neonatal group B streptococcal infection. Infect Immun 1983;39:837.
128. Robbins JB, McCracken GH Jr, Gotschlich EC, et al. Escherichia coli K1 capsular polysaccharide associated with neonatal meningitis. N Engl J Med 1974;290:1216.
129. Givner LB, Baker CJ. Pooled human IgG hyperimmune for type III group B streptococci: evaluation against multiple strains in vitro and in experimental disease. J Infect Dis 1991; 163:1141.
130. Glode MP, Sutton A, Moxon ER, Robbins JB. Pathogenesis of neonatal Escherichia coli meningitis: induction of bacteremia and meningitis in infant rats fed E. coli K1. Infect Immun 1977;16:75.
131. Larsen JW Jr, London WT, Palmer AE, et al. Experimental group B streptococcal infection in the rhesus monkey. I. Disease production in the neonate. Am J Obstet Gynecol 1978; 132:686.
132. Martin TR, Ruzinski JT, Rubens CE, et al. The effect of type-specific polysaccharide capsule on the clearance of group B streptococci from the lungs of infant and adult rats. J Infect Dis 1992;165:306.
133. Baker CJ, Edwards MS, Kasper DL. Role of antibody to native type III polysaccharide of group B streptococcus in infant protection. Pediatrics 1981;68:544.
134. Anderson DC, Edwards MS, Baker CJ. Luminol-enhanced chemiluminescence for evaluation of type III group B streptococcal opsonins in human sera. J Infect Dis 1980;141:370.
135. Vogel LC, Kretschmer RR, Boyer KM, et al. Human immunity to group B streptococci measured by indirect immunofluorescence: correlation with protection in chick embryos. J Infect Dis 1979;140:682.
136. Fischer GW, Hemming VG, Hunter KW Jr, et al. Intravenous immunoglobulin in the treatment of neonatal sepsis: therapeutic strategies and laboratory studies. Pediatr Infect Dis 1986;5:S171.
137. Hill HR, Gonzales LA, Knappe WA, et al. Comparative protective activity of human monoclonal and hyperimmune polyclonal antibody against group B streptococci. J Infect Dis 1991; 163:792.
138. Baker CJ, Webb BJ, Kasper DL, et al. The natural history of group B streptococcal colonization in the pregnant woman and her offspring. II. Determination of serum antibody to capsular polysaccharide from type III, group B streptococcus. Am J Obstet Gynecol 1980;137:39.
139. Anthony BF, Concepcion NF, Concepcion KF. Human antibody to the group-specific polysaccharide of group B streptococcus. J Infect Dis 1985;151:221.
140. Klegerman ME, Boyer KM, Papierniak CK, Gotoff SP. Estimation of the protective level of human IgG antibody to the type-specific polysaccharide of group B streptococcus type Ia. J Infect Dis 1983;148:648.
141. Boyer KM, Kendall LS, Papierniak CK, et al. Protective levels of human immunoglobulin G antibody to group B streptococcus type Ib. Infect Immun 1984;45:618.
142. Gotoff SP, Papierniak CK, Klegerman ME, Boyer KM. Quantitation of IgG antibody to the type-specific polysaccharide of group B streptococcus type 1b in pregnant women and infected infants. J Pediatr 1984;105:628.
143. Gray BM, Pritchard DG, Dillon HC Jr. Seroepidemiological studies of group B streptococcus type II. J Infect Dis 1985;151: 1073.
144. Anthony BF. The role of specific antibody in neonatal bacterial infections: an overview. Pediatr Infect Dis 1986;5:S164.
145. Lassiter HA, Tanner JE, Miller RD. Inefficient bacteriolysis of Escherichia coli by serum from human neonates. J Infect Dis 1992;165:290.
146. Lassiter HA, Watson SW, Seifring ML, Tanner JE. Complement factor 9 deficiency in serum of human neonates. J Infect Dis 1992;166:53.
147. Edwards MS, Buffone GJ, Fuselier PA, et al. Deficient classical complement pathway activity in newborn sera. Pediatr Res 1983;17:685.
148. Máródi L, Leijh PCJ, Braat A, et al. Opsonic activity of cord blood sera against various species of microorganism. Pediatr Res 1985;19:433.
149. Edwards MS, Kasper DL, Jennings HJ, et al. Capsular sialic acid prevents activation of the alternative complement pathway by type III, group B streptococci. J Immunol 1982; 128:1278.
150. Yoder MC. Therapeutic administration of fibronectin: current uses and potential applications. Clin Perinatol 1991;18:325.
151. Gerdes JS, Yoder MC, Douglas SD, Polin RA. Decreased plasma fibronectin in neonatal sepsis. Pediatrics 1983;72:877.
152. Domula M, Bykowska K, Wegrzynowicz Z, et al. Plasma fibronectin concentrations in healthy and septic infants. Eur J Pediatr 1985;144:49.
153. Butler KM, Baker CJ, Edwards MS. Interaction of soluble fibronectin with group B streptococci. Infect Immun 1987; 55:2404.
154. Cairo MS. Neonatal neutrophil host defense: prospects for immunologic enhancement during neonatal sepsis. Am J Dis Child 1989;143:40.
155. Klein JO, Marcy SM. Bacterial sepsis and meningitis. In: Remington JS, Klein JO, eds. Infectious diseases of the fetus and newborn infant. 3rd ed. Philadelphia: WB Saunders, 1990:601.
156. Voora S, Srinivasan G, Lilien LD, et al. Fever in full-term newborns in the first four days of life. Pediatrics 1982;69:40.
157. Gladstone IM, Ehrenkranz RA, Edberg SC, Baltimore RS. A ten-year review of neonatal sepsis and comparison with the previous fifty-year experience. Pediatr Infect Dis J 1990;9:819.
158. Baker CJ, Edwards MS. Group B streptococcal infections. In: Remington JS, Klein JO, eds. Infectious diseases of the fetus and newborn infant. 3rd ed. Philadelphia: WB Saunders, 1990:742.
159. Easmon CSF, Hastings MJG. GBS colonisation in mothers and babies. Antibiot Chemother 1985;35:28.
160. Dillon HC Jr, Khare S, Gray BM. Group B streptococcal carriage and disease: a 6-year prospective study. J Pediatr 1987;110:31.
161. Regan JA, Klebanoff MA, Nugent RP, for the Vaginal Infections and Prematurity Study Group. The epidemiology of group B streptococcal colonization in pregnancy. Obstet Gynecol 1991;77:604.
162. Bobitt JR, Damato JD, Sakakini J Jr. Perinatal complications in group B streptococcal carriers: a longitudinal study of prenatal patients. Am J Obstet Gynecol 1985;151:711.
163. Daugaard HO, Thomsen AC, Henriques U, Østergaard A.

Group B streptococci in the lower urogenital tract and late abortions. Am J Obstet Gynecol 1988;158:28.
164. Newton ER, Clark M. Group B streptococcus and preterm rupture of membranes. Obstet Gynecol 1988;71:198.
165. Schwartz B, Schuchat A, Oxtoby MJ, et al. Invasive group B streptococcal disease in adults: a population-based study in metropolitan Atlanta. JAMA 1991;266:1112.
166. Haft RF, Kasper DL. Group B streptococcus infection in mother and child. Hosp Pract 1991;26(12):75.
167. Gardner SE, Yow MD, Leeds LJ, et al. Failure of penicillin to eradicate group B streptococcal colonization in the pregnant woman: a couple study. Am J Obstet Gynecol 1979; 135:1062.
168. Jones DE, Kanarek KS, Lim DV. Group B streptococcal colonization patterns in mothers and their infants. J Clin Microbiol 1984;20:438.
169. Chin KC, Fitzhardinge PM. Sequelae of early-onset group B hemolytic streptococcal neonatal meningitis. J Pediatr 1985; 106:819.
170. Pyati SP, Pildes RS, Ramamurthy RS, Jacobs N. Decreasing mortality in neonates with early-onset group B streptococcal infection: reality or artifact. J Pediatr 1981;98:625.
171. Siegel JD, McCracken GH Jr. Group D streptococcal infections. J Pediatr 1978;93:542.
172. Dyson AE, Read SE. Group G streptococcal colonization and sepsis in neonates. J Pediatr 1981;99:944.
173. Isaacman SH, Heroman WM, Lightsey AL. Purpura fulminans following late-onset group B β-hemolytic streptococcal sepsis. Am J Dis Child 1984;138:915.
174. Howard JB, McCracken GH Jr. The spectrum of group B streptococcal infections in infancy. Am J Dis Child 1974; 128:815.
175. Yagupsky P, Menegus MA, Powell KR. The changing spectrum of group B streptococcal disease in infants: an eleven-year experience in a tertiary care hospital. Pediatr Infect Dis J 1991;10:801.
176. Whitley CB, Thompson LR, Osterholm MT, et al. Toxic shock syndrome in a newborn infant. [Abstract 1053] Pediatr Res 1982;16:254A.
177. Chesney PJ, Jaucian RC, McDonald RA, et al. Exfoliative dermatitis in an infant: association with enterotoxin F-producing staphylococci. Am J Dis Child 1983;137:899.
178. Dancer SJ, Simmons NA, Poston SM, Noble WC. Outbreak of staphylococcal scalded skin syndrome among neonates. J Infect 1988;16:87.
179. Loughead JL. Congenital staphylococcal scalded skin syndrome: report of a case. Pediatr Infect Dis J 1992;11:413.
180. Espersen F, Frimodt-Møller N, Rosdahl VT, Jessen O. Staphylococcus aureus bacteraemia in children below the age of one year: a review of 407 cases. Acta Paediatr Scand 1989;78:56.
181. Pfaller MA, Herwaldt LA. Laboratory, clinical, and epidemiological aspects of coagulase-negative staphylococci. Clin Microbiol Rev 1988;1:281.
182. Patrick CC. Coagulase-negative staphylococci: pathogens with increasing clinical significance. J Pediatr 1990;116:497.
183. Vesikari T, Isolauri E, Tuppurainen N, et al. Neonatal septicaemia in Finland 1981–85: predominance of group B streptococcal infections with very early onset. Acta Paediatr Scand 1989;78:44.
184. Sidebottom DG, Freeman J, Platt R, et al. Fifteen-year experience with bloodstream isolates of coagulase-negative staphylococci in neonatal intensive care. J Clin Microbiol 1988; 26:713.
185. Freeman J, Epstein MF, Smith NE, et al. Extra hospital stay and antibiotic usage with nosocomial coagulase-negative staphylococcal bacteremia in two neonatal intensive care unit populations. Am J Dis Child 1990;144:324.
186. Munson DP, Thompson TR, Johnson DE, et al. Coagulase-negative staphylococcal septicemia: experience in a newborn intensive care unit. J Pediatr 1982;101:602.
187. Baumgart S, Hall SE, Campos JM, Polin RA. Sepsis with coagulase-negative staphylococci in critically ill newborns. Am J Dis Child 1983;137:461.
188. Noel GJ, Edelson PJ. Staphylococcus epidermidis bacteremia in neonates: further observations and the occurrence of focal infection. Pediatrics 1984;74:832.
189. Hall RT, Hall SL, Barnes WG, et al. Characteristics of coagulase-negative staphylococci from infants with bacteremia. Pediatr Infect Dis J 1987;6:377.
190. Gruskay J, Harris MC, Costarino AT, et al. Neonatal Staphylococcus epidermidis meningitis with unremarkable CSF examination results. Am J Dis Child 1989;143:580.
191. Gruskay JA, Abbasi S, Anday E, et al. Staphylococcus epidermidis-associated enterocolitis. J Pediatr 1986;109:520.
192. Mollitt DL, Tepas JJ, Talbert JL. The role of coagulase-negative Staphylococcus in neonatal necrotizing enterocolitis. J Pediatr Surg 1988;23:60.
193. Patrick CC, Kaplan SL, Baker CJ, et al. Persistent bacteremia due to coagulase-negative staphylococci in low birth weight neonates. Pediatrics 1989;84:977.
194. Noel GJ, O'Loughlin JE, Edelson PJ. Neonatal Staphylococcus epidermidis right-sided endocarditis: description of five catheterized infants. Pediatrics 1988;82:234.
195. Wagener MM, Rycheck RR, Yee RB, et al. Septic dermatitis of the neonatal scalp and maternal endomyometritis with intrapartum internal fetal monitoring. Pediatrics 1984;74:81.
196. Overturf GD, Balfour G. Osteomyelitis and sepsis: severe complications of fetal monitoring. Pediatrics 1975;55:244.
197. Freeman J, Goldmann DA, Smith NE, et al. Association of intravenous lipid emulsion and coagulase-negative staphylococcal bacteremia in neonatal intensive care units. N Engl J Med 1990;323:301.
198. Dunne WM Jr. Effects of subinhibitory concentrations of vancomycin or cefamandole on biofilm production by coagulase-negative staphylococci. Antimicrob Agents Chemother 1990;34:390.
199. Gray ED, Peters G, Verstegen M, Regelmann WE. Effect of extracellular slime substance from Staphylococcus epidermidis on the human cellular immune response. Lancet 1984; 1:365.
200. Johnson GM, Lee DA, Regelmann WE, et al. Interference with granulocyte function by Staphylococcus epidermidis slime. Infect Immun 1986;54:13.
201. Fleer A, Gerards LJ, Aerts P, et al. Opsonic defense to Staphylococcus epidermidis in the premature neonate. J Infect Dis 1985;152:930.
202. Schutze GE, Hall MA, Baker CJ, Edwards MS. Role of neutrophil receptors in opsonophagocytosis of coagulase-negative staphylococci. Infect Immun 1991;59:2573.
203. Scheifele DW, Bjornson GL. Delta toxin activity in coagulase-negative staphylococci from the bowels of neonates. J Clin Microbiol 1988;26:279.
204. Scheifele DW, Bjornson GL, Dyer RA, Dimmick JE. Delta-like toxin produced by coagulase-negative staphylococci is associated with neonatal necrotizing enterocolitis. Infect Immun 1987;55:2268.
205. Scheifele DW. Role of bacterial toxins in neonatal necrotizing enterocolitis. J Pediatr 1990;117:S44.
206. Gellin BG, Broome CV. Listeriosis. JAMA 1989;261:1313.
207. Becroft DMO, Farmer K, Seddon RJ, et al. Epidemic listeriosis in the newborn. BMJ 1971;3:747.

208. Mulder CJJ, Zanen HC. Listeria monocytogenes neonatal meningitis in The Netherlands. Eur J Pediatr 1986;145:60.
209. Kessler SL, Dajani AS. Listeria meningitis in infants and children. Pediatr Infect Dis J 1990;9:61.
210. Schuchat A, Lizano C, Broome CV, et al. Outbreak of neonatal listeriosis associated with mineral oil. Pediatr Infect Dis J 1991;10:183.
211. Facinelli B, Varaldo PE, Casolari C, Fabio U. Cross-infection with Listeria monocytogenes confirmed by DNA fingerprinting. Lancet 1988;2:1247.
212. Farber JM, Peterkin PI, Carter AO, et al. Neonatal listeriosis due to cross-infection confirmed by isoenzyme typing and DNA fingerprinting. J Infect Dis 1991;163:927.
213. Visintine AM, Oleske JM, Nahmias AJ. Listeria monocytogenes infection in infants and children. Am J Dis Child 1977;131:393.
214. Bavikatte K, Schreiner RL, Lemons JA, Gresham EL. Group D streptococcal septicemia in the neonate. Am J Dis Child 1979;133:493.
215. Boulanger JM, Ford-Jones EL, Matlow AG. Enterococcal bacteremia in a pediatric institution: a four-year review. Rev Infect Dis 1991;13:847.
216. Coudron PE, Mayhall CG, Facklam RR, et al. Streptococcus faecium outbreak in a neonatal intensive care unit. J Clin Microbiol 1984;20:1044.
217. Dobson SRM, Baker CJ. Enterococcal sepsis in neonates: features by age at onset and occurrence of focal infection. Pediatrics 1990;85:165.
218. Rhinehart E, Smith NE, Wennersten C, et al. Rapid dissemination of β-lactamase-producing, aminoglycoside-resistant Enterococcus faecalis among patients and staff on an infant-toddler surgical ward. N Engl J Med 1990;323:1814.
219. Luginbuhl LM, Rotbart HA, Facklam RR, et al. Neonatal enterococcal sepsis: case-control study and description of an outbreak. Pediatr Infect Dis J 1987;6:1022.
220. Klare I, Rodloff AC, Wagner J, et al. Overproduction of a penicillin-binding protein is not the only mechanism of penicillin resistance in Enterococcus faecium. Antimicrob Agents Chemother 1992;36:783.
221. Patterson JE, Singh KV, Murray BE. Epidemiology of an endemic strain of β-lactamase-producing Enterococcus faecalis. J Clin Microbiol 1991;29:2513.
222. Sahm DF, Boonlayangoor S, Schulz JE. Detection of high-level aminoglycoside resistance in enterococci other than Enterococcus faecalis. J Clin Microbiol 1991;29:2595.
223. Kaplan AH, Gilligan PH, Facklam RR. Recovery of resistant enterococci during vancomycin prophylaxis. J Clin Microbiol 1988;26:1216.
224. Ghosal SP, Gupta PCS, Mukherjee AK, et al. Noma neonatorum: its aetiopathogenesis. Lancet 1978;2:289.
225. Chow AW, Leake RD, Yamauchi T, et al. The significance of anaerobes in neonatal bacteremia: analysis of 23 cases and review of the literature. Pediatrics 1974;54:736.
226. Dunkle LM, Brotherton TJ, Feigin RD. Anaerobic infections in children: a prospective study. Pediatrics 1976;57:311.
227. Noel GJ, Laufer DA, Edelson PJ. Anaerobic bacteremia in a neonatal intensive care unit: an eighteen-year experience. Pediatr Infect Dis J 1988;7:858.
228. Brook I. Pediatric anaerobic infection: diagnosis and management. 2nd ed. St. Louis: CV Mosby, 1989:65.
229. Spark RP, Wike DA. Nontetanus clostridal neonatal fatality after home delivery. Arizona Med 1983;40:697.
230. Likitnukul S, Kusmiesz H, Nelson JD, McCracken GH Jr. Role of genital mycoplasmas in young infants with suspected sepsis. J Pediatr 1986;109:971.
231. Izraeli S, Samra Z, Sirota L, et al. Genital mycoplasmas in preterm infants: prevalence and clinical significance. Eur J Pediatr 1991;150:804.
232. Waites KB, Crouse DT, Philips JB III, et al. Ureaplasmal pneumonia and sepsis associated with persistent pulmonary hypertension of the newborn. Pediatrics 1989;83:79.
233. Phillips G, Golledge C. Fungal infection in neonates. J Antimicrob Chemother 1991;28:159.
234. Baley JE. Neonatal candidiasis: the current challenge. Clin Perinatol 1991;18:263.
235. Sharp AM, Odds FC, Evans EGV. Candida strains from neonates in a special care baby unit. Arch Dis Child 1992;67:48.
236. Schwartz DA, Reef S. Candida albicans placentitis and funisitis: early diagnosis of congenital candidemia by histopathologic examination of umbilical cord vessels. Pediatr Infect Dis J 1990;9:661.
237. Santos LA, Beceiro J, Hernandez R, et al. Congenital cutaneous candidiasis: report of four cases and review of the literature. Eur J Pediatr 1991;150:336.
238. Faix RG, Kovarik SM, Shaw TR, Johnson RV. Mucocutaneous and invasive candidiasis among very low birth weight (< 1,500 grams) infants in intensive care nurseries: a prospective study. Pediatrics 1989;83:101.
239. Wey SB, Mori M, Pfaller MA, et al. Risk factors for hospital-acquired candidemia: a matched case-control study. Arch Intern Med 1989;149:2349.
240. Faix RG. Invasive neonatal candidiasis: comparison of albicans and parapsilosis infection. Pediatr Infect Dis J 1992; 11:88.
241. Sánchez PJ, Siegel JD, Fishbein J. Candida endocarditis: successful medical management in three preterm infants and review of the literature. Pediatr Infect Dis J 1991;10:239.
242. Zenker PN, Rosenberg EM, Van Dyke RB, et al. Successful medical treatment of presumed Candida endocarditis in critically ill infants. J Pediatr 1991;119:472.
243. Annable WL, Kachmer ML, DiMarco M, DeSantis D. Long-term follow-up of Candida endophthalmitis in the premature infant. J Pediatr Ophthalmol Strabismus 1990;27:103.
244. Goldsmith LS, Rubenstein SD, Wolfson BJ, et al. Cerebral calcifications in a neonate with candidiasis. Pediatr Infect Dis J 1990;9:451.
245. Baetz-Greenwalt B, Debaz B, Kumar ML. Bladder fungus ball: a reversible cause of neonatal obstructive uropathy. Pediatrics 1988;81:826.
246. Rehan VK, Davidson DC. Neonatal renal candidal bezoar. Arch Dis Child 1992;67:63.
247. Butler KM, Rench MA, Baker CJ. Amphotericin B as a single agent in the treatment of systemic candidiasis in neonates. Pediatr Infect Dis J 1990;9:51.
248. Ward RM, Sattler FR, Dalton AS Jr. Assessment of antifungal therapy in an 800-gram infant with candidal arthritis and osteomyelitis. Pediatrics 1983;72:234.
249. Marcon MJ, Powell DA. Human infections due to Malassezia spp. Clin Microbiol Rev 1992;5:101.
250. Henwick S, Henrickson K, Storgion SA, Leggiadro RJ. Disseminated neonatal Trichosporon beigelii. Pediatr Infect Dis J 1992;11:50.
251. Gerdes JS. Clinicopathologic approach to the diagnosis of neonatal sepsis. Clin Perinatol 1991;18:361.
252. Wiswell TE, Hachey WE. Multiple site blood cultures in the initial evaluation for neonatal sepsis during the first week of life. Pediatr Infect Dis J 1991;10:365.
253. Phillips SE, Bradley JS. Bacteremia detected by lysis direct plating in a neonatal intensive care unit. J Clin Microbiol 1990;28:1.
254. St Geme JW III, Bell LM, Baumgart S, et al. Distinguishing sepsis from blood culture contamination in young infants

with blood cultures growing coagulase-negative staphylococci. Pediatrics 1990;86:157.
255. Evans ME, Schaffner W, Federspiel CF, et al. Sensitivity, specificity, and predictive value of body surface cultures in a neonatal intensive care unit. JAMA 1988;259:248.
256. Visser VE, Hall RT. Lumbar puncture in the evaluation of suspected neonatal sepsis. J Pediatr 1980;96:1063.
257. Fielkow S, Reuter S, Gotoff SP. Cerebrospinal fluid examination in symptom-free infants with risk factors for infection. J Pediatr 1991;119:971.
258. Weiss MG, Ionides SP, Anderson CL. Meningitis in premature infants with respiratory distress: role of admission lumbar puncture. J Pediatr 1991;119:973.
259. Schwersenski J, McIntyre L, Bauer CR. Lumbar puncture frequency and cerebrospinal fluid analysis in the neonate. Am J Dis Child 1991;145:54.
260. Manroe BL, Weinberg AG, Rosenfeld CR, Browne R. The neonatal blood count in health and disease. I. Reference values for neutrophilic cells. J Pediatr 1979;95:89.
261. Benuck I, David RJ. Sensitivity of published neutrophil indexes in identifying newborn infants with sepsis. J Pediatr 1983;103:961.
262. Carballo C, Foucar K, Swanson P, et al. Effect of high altitude on neutrophil counts in newborn infants. J Pediatr 1991; 119:464.
263. Greenberg DN, Yoder BA. Changes in the differential white blood cell count in screening for group B streptococcal sepsis. Pediatr Infect Dis J 1990;9:886.
264. Schouten-Van Meeteren NYN, Rietveld A, Moolenaar AJ, Van Bel F. Influence of perinatal conditions on C-reactive protein production. J Pediatr 1992;120:621.
265. Ascher DP, Wilson S, Fischer GW. Comparison of commercially available group B streptococcal latex agglutination assays. J Clin Microbiol 1991;29:2895.
266. Sánchez PJ, Siegel JD, Cushion NB, Threlkeld N. Significance of a positive urine group B streptococcal latex agglutination test in neonates. J Pediatr 1990;116:601.
267. Ascher DP, Wilson S, Mendiola J, Fischer GW. Group B streptococcal latex agglutination testing in neonates. J Pediatr 1991; 119:458.
268. Schreiber JR, Maynard E, Lew MA. Candida antigen detection in two premature neonates with disseminated candidiasis. Pediatrics 1984;74:838.
269. Kahn FW, Jones JM. Latex agglutination tests for detection of Candida antigens in sera of patients with invasive candidiasis. J Infect Dis 1986;153:579.
270. Walsh TJ, Hathorn JW, Sobel JD, et al. Detection of circulating Candida enolase by immunoassay in patients with cancer and invasive candidiasis. N Engl J Med 1991;324:1026.
271. Howard JB, McCracken GH Jr. Reappraisal of kanamycin usage in neonates. J Pediatr 1975;86:949.
272. Schwalbe RS, Stapleton JT, Gilligan PH. Emergence of vancomycin resistance in coagulase-negative staphylococci. N Engl J Med 1987;316:927.
273. Kim KS, Anthony BF. Penicillin tolerance in group B streptococci isolated from infected neonates. J Infect Dis 1981; 144:411.
274. Siegel JD, Shannon KM, DePasse BM. Recurrent infection associated with penicillin-tolerant group B streptococci: a report of two cases. J Pediatr 1981;99:920.
275. Waites KB, Crouse DT, Cassell GH. Antibiotic susceptibilities and therapeutic options for Ureaplasma urealyticum infections in neonates. Pediatr Infect Dis J 1992;11:23.
276. Baley JE, Meyers C, Kliegman RM, et al. Pharmacokinetics, outcome of treatment, and toxic effects of amphotericin B and 5-fluorocytosine in neonates. J Pediatr 1990;116:791.
277. Koren G, Lau A, Klein J, et al. Pharmacokinetics and adverse effects of amphotericin B in infants and children. J Pediatr 1988;113:559.
278. Conly J, Rennie R, Johnson J, et al. Disseminated candidiasis due to amphotericin B-resistant Candida albicans. J Infect Dis 1992;165:761.
279. Lackner H, Schwinger W, Urban C, et al. Liposomal amphotericin-B (AmBisome) for treatment of disseminated fungal infections in two infants of very low birth weight. Pediatrics 1992;89:1259.
280. Wiest DB, Fowler SL, Garner SS, Simons DR. Fluconazole in neonatal disseminated candidiasis. Arch Dis Child 1991; 66:1002.
281. Fishbein JD, Friedman HS, Bennett BB, Falletta JM. Catheter-related sepsis refractory to antibiotics treated successfully with adjunctive urokinase infusion. Pediatr Infect Dis J 1990; 9:676.
282. Hocker JR, Simpson PM, Rabalais GP, et al. Extracorporeal membrane oxygenation and early-onset group B streptococcal sepsis. Pediatrics 1992;89:1.
283. Noya FJD, Baker CJ. Prevention of group B streptococcal infection. Infect Dis Clin North Am 1992;6:41.
284. Smith AL, Haas J. Neonatal bacterial meningitis. In: Scheld WM, Whitley RJ, Durack DT, eds. Infections of the central nervous system. New York: Raven Press, 1991:313.
285. Bell WE, McGuinness GA. Suppurative central nervous system infections in the neonate. Semin Perinatol 1982;6:1.
286. Sáez-Llorens X, Ramilo O, Mustafa MM, et al. Molecular pathophysiology of bacterial meningitis: current concepts and therapeutic implications. J Pediatr 1990;116:671.
287. Ashwal S, Tomasi L, Schneider S, et al. Bacterial meningitis in children: pathophysiology and treatment. Neurology 1992; 42:739.
288. Sarff LD, Platt LH, McCracken GH Jr. Cerebrospinal fluid evaluation in neonates: comparison of high-risk infants with and without meningitis. J Pediatr 1976;88:473.
289. Rodriguez AF, Kaplan SL, Mason EO Jr. Cerebrospinal fluid values in the very low birth weight infant. J Pediatr 1990; 116:971.
290. McCracken GH Jr, Mize SG. A controlled study of intrathecal antibiotic therapy in gram-negative enteric meningitis of infancy: report of the Neonatal Meningitis Cooperative Study Group. J Pediatr 1976;89:66.
291. McCracken GH Jr, Mize SG, Threlkeld N. Intraventricular gentamicin therapy in gram-negative bacillary meningitis of infancy: report of the Second Neonatal Meningitis Cooperative Study Group. Lancet 1980;1:787.
292. Kaplan SL, Patrick CC. Cefotaxime and aminoglycoside treatment of meningitis caused by gram-negative enteric organisms. Pediatr Infect Dis J 1990;9:810.
293. Mustafa MM, Mertsola J, Ramilo O, et al. Increased endotoxin and interleukin-1β concentrations in cerebrospinal fluid of infants with coliform meningitis and ventriculitis associated with intraventricular gentamicin therapy. J Infect Dis 1989; 160:891.
294. Graham DR, Anderson RL, Ariel FE, et al. Epidemic nosocomial meningitis due to Citrobacter diversus in neonates. J Infect Dis 1981;144:203.
295. Foreman SD, Smith EE, Ryan NJ, Hogan GR. Neonatal Citrobacter meningitis: pathogenesis of cerebral abscess formation. Ann Neurol 1984;16:655.
296. Edwards MS, Rench MA, Haffar AAM, et al. Long-term sequelae of group B streptococcal meningitis in infants. J Pediatr 1985;106:717.
297. Wald ER, Bergman I, Taylor HG, et al. Long-term outcome of group B streptococcal meningitis. Pediatrics 1986;77:217.

298. Franco SM, Cornelius VE, Andrews BF. Long-term outcome of neonatal meningitis. Am J Dis Child 1992;146:567.
299. Brightman VJ, McNair Scott TF, Westphal M, Boggs TR. An outbreak of coxsackie B-5 virus infection in a newborn nursery. J Pediatr 1966;69:179.
300. Miller DG, Gabrielson MO, Bart KJ, et al. An epidemic of aseptic meningitis, primarily among infants, caused by echovirus 11-prime. Pediatrics 1968;41:77.
301. Dagan R, Jenista JA, Menegus MA. Association of clinical presentation, laboratory findings, and virus serotypes with the presence of meningitis in hospitalized infants with enterovirus infection. J Pediatr 1988;113:975.
302. Whitley R, Arvin A, Prober C, et al. A controlled trial comparing vidarabine with acyclovir in neonatal herpes simplex virus infection. N Engl J Med 1991;324:444.
303. Sells CJ, Carpenter RL, Ray CG. Sequelae of central-nervous-system enterovirus infections. N Engl J Med 1975;293:1.
304. Wilfert CM, Thompson RJ Jr, Sunder TR, et al. Longitudinal assessment of children with enteroviral meningitis during the first three months of life. Pediatrics 1981;67:811.
305. Ogden JA. Pathophysiology of neonatal osteomyelitis and septic arthritis. In: Polin RA, Fox WM, eds. Fetal and neonatal physiology. Philadelphia: WB Saunders, 1992:1679.
306. Asmar BI. Osteomyelitis in the neonate. Infect Dis Clin North Am 1992;6:117.
307. Ish-Horowicz MR, McIntyre P, Nade S. Bone and joint infections caused by multiply resistant Staphylococcus aureus in a neonatal intensive care unit. Pediatr Infect Dis J 1992;11:82.
308. Fox L, Sprunt K. Neonatal osteomyelitis. Pediatrics 1978; 62:535.
309. Mok PM, Reilly BJ, Ash JM. Osteomyelitis in the neonate. Radiology 1982;145:677.
310. Nelson JD. Antibiotic concentrations in septic joint effusions. N Engl J Med 1971;284:349.
311. Perkins MD, Edwards KM, Heller RM, Green NE. Neonatal group B streptococcal osteomyelitis and suppurative arthritis: outpatient therapy. Clin Pediatr (Phila) 1989;28:229.
312. Wopperer JM, White JJ, Gillespie R, Obletz BE. Long-term follow-up of infantile hip sepsis. J Pediatr Orthop 1988;8:322.
313. Weinberger M, Haynes RE, Morse TS. Necrotizing fasciitis in a neonate. Am J Dis Child 1972;123:591.
314. Ramamurthy RS, Srinivasan G, Jacobs NM. Necrotizing fasciitis and necrotizing cellulitis due to group B streptococcus. Am J Dis Child 1977;131:1169.
315. Wilson HD, Haltalin KC. Acute necrotizing fasciitis in childhood: report of 11 cases. Am J Dis Child 1973;125:591.
316. Rudoy RC, Nelson JD. Breast abscess during the neonatal period: a review. Am J Dis Child 1975;129:1031.
317. Brook I. The aerobic and anaerobic microbiology of neonatal breast abscess. Pediatr Infect Dis J 1991;10:785.
318. Plavidal FJ, Werch A. Fetal scalp abscess secondary to intrauterine monitoring. Am J Obstet Gynecol 1976;125:65.
319. Plavidal FJ, Werch A. Gonococcal fetal scalp abscess: a case report. Am J Obstet Gynecol 1977;127:437.
320. Nelson JD, Peters PC. Suprapubic aspiration of urine in premature and term infants. Pediatrics 1965;36:132.
321. Israele V, Darabi A, McCracken GH Jr. The role of bacterial virulence factors and Tamm-Horsfall protein in the pathogenesis of Escherichia coli urinary tract infection in infants. Am J Dis Child 1987;141:1230.
322. Nebigil I, Tümer N. Asymptomatic urinary tract infection in childhood. Eur J Pediatr 1992;151:308.
323. Bergström T, Larson H, Lincoln K, Winberg J. Studies of urinary tract infections in infancy and childhood. XII. Eighty consecutive patients with neonatal infection. J Pediatr 1972; 80:858.
324. Leung AKC, Robson WLM. Urinary tract infection in infancy and childhood. Adv Pediatr 1991;38:257.
325. Anderson PAM, Rickwood AMK. Features of primary vesicoureteric reflux detected by prenatal sonography. Br J Urol 1991;67:267.
326. Crain EF, Gershel JC. Urinary tract infections in febrile infants younger than 8 weeks of age. Pediatrics 1990;86:363.
327. Ginsburg CM, McCracken GH Jr. Urinary tract infections in young infants. Pediatrics 1982;69:409.
328. Wong-Beringer A, Jacobs RA, Guglielmo J. Treatment of funguria. JAMA 1992;267:2780.
329. Bourchier D, Abbott GD, Maling TMJ. Radiological abnormalities in infants with urinary tract infections. Arch Dis Child 1984;59:620.
330. Feld LG, Greenfield SP, Ogra PL. Urinary tract infections in infants and children. Pediatr Rev 1989;11:71.
331. Hellström M, Jacobsson B, Jodal U, et al. Renal growth after neonatal urinary tract infection. Pediatr Nephrol 1987;1:269.
332. Armstrong JH, Zacarias F, Rein MF. Ophthalmia neonatorum: a chart review. Pediatrics 1976;57:884.
333. Laga M, Naamara W, Brunham RC, et al. Single-dose therapy of gonococcal ophthalmia neonatorum with ceftriaxone. N Engl J Med 1986;315:1382.
334. Rapoza PA, Quinn TC, Kiessling LA, et al. Assessment of neonatal conjunctivitis with a direct immunofluorescent monoclonal antibody stain for Chlamydia. JAMA 1986; 255:3369.
335. Burns RP, Rhodes DH Jr. Pseudomonas eye infection as a cause of death in premature infants. Arch Ophthalmol 1961;65:517.
336. Rowe DS, Aicardi EZ, Dawson CR, Schachter J. Purulent ocular discharge in neonates: significance of Chlamydia trachomatis. Pediatrics 1979;63:628.
337. Centers for Disease Control. Plasmid-mediated antimicrobial resistance in Neisseria gonorrhoeae—United States, 1988 and 1989. MMWR 1990;39:284.
338. Golden B. SubTenon injection of gentamicin for bacterial infections of the eye. J Infect Dis 1971;124:S271.
339. Patamasucon P, Rettig PJ, Faust KL, et al. Oral v topical erythromycin therapies for chlamydial conjunctivitis. Am J Dis Child 1982;136:817.
340. Haffejee IE. Neonatal rotavirus infections. Rev Infect Dis 1991;13:957.
341. Champsaur H, Questiaux E, Prevot J, et al. Rotavirus carriage, asymptomatic infection, and disease in the first two years of life. I. Virus shedding. J Infect Dis 1984;149:667.
342. Moffet HL, Shulenberger HK, Burkholder ER. Epidemiology and etiology of severe infantile diarrhea. J Pediatr 1968;72:1.
343. Boyer KM, Petersen NJ, Farzaneh I, et al. An outbreak of gastroenteritis due to E. coli 0142 in a neonatal nursery. J Pediatr 1975;86:919.
344. Lyerly DM, Krivan HC, Wilkins TD. Clostridium difficile: its disease and toxins. Clin Microbiol Rev 1988;1:1.
345. Haltalin KC. Neonatal shigellosis: report of 16 cases and review of the literature. Am J Dis Child 1967;114:603.
346. Wong S-N, Tam AY-C, Yuen K-Y. Campylobacter infection in the neonate: case report and review of the literature. Pediatr Infect Dis J 1990;9:665.
347. Reina J, Borrell N, Fiol M. Rectal bleeding caused by Campylobacter jejuni in a neonate. Pediatr Infect Dis J 1992; 11:500.
348. Paisley JW, Lauer BA. Neonatal Yersinia enterocolitica enteritis. Pediatr Infect Dis J 1992;11:331.
349. Freij BJ. Aeromonas: biology of the organism and diseases in children. Pediatr Infect Dis 1984;3:164.
350. Nelson JD. Duration of neomycin therapy for enteropatho-

genic Escherichia coli diarrheal disease: a comparative study of 113 cases. Pediatrics 1971;48:248.
351. DiNicola AF. Campylobacter jejuni diarrhea in a 3-day-old male neonate. Am J Dis Child 1986;140:191.
352. Rotbart HA, Levin MJ, Yolken RH, et al. An outbreak of rotavirus-associated neonatal necrotizing enterocolitis. J Pediatr 1983;103:454.
353. Abzug MJ, Beam AC, Gyorkos EA, Levin MJ. Viral pneumonia in the first month of life. Pediatr Infect Dis J 1990;9:881.
354. Tipple MA, Beem MO, Saxon EM. Clinical characteristics of the afebrile pneumonia associated with Chlamydia trachomatis infection in infants less than 6 months of age. Pediatrics 1979;63:192.
355. Attenburrow AA, Barker CM. Chlamydial pneumonia in the low birthweight neonate. Arch Dis Child 1985;60:1169.
356. Numazaki K, Chiba S, Kogawa K, et al. Chronic respiratory disease in premature infants caused by Chlamydia trachomatis. J Clin Pathol 1986;39:84.
357. Weiss SG, Newcomb RW, Beem MO. Pulmonary assessment of children after chlamydial pneumonia of infancy. J Pediatr 1986;108:659.
358. Sánchez PJ, Regan JA. Ureaplasma urealyticum colonization and chronic lung disease in low birth weight infants. Pediatr Infect Dis J 1988;7:542.
359. Walsh WF, Stanley S, Lally KP, et al. Ureaplasma urealyticum demonstrated by open lung biopsy in newborns with chronic lung disease. Pediatr Infect Dis J 1991;10:823.
360. Wang EEL, Frayha H, Watts J, et al. Role of Ureaplasma urealyticum and other pathogens in the development of chronic lung disease of prematurity. Pediatr Infect Dis J 1988;7:547.
361. Gajdusek DC. Pneumocystis carinii—etiologic agent of interstitial plasma cell pneumonia of premature and young infants. Pediatrics 1957;19:543.
362. Beach RS, Garcia ER, Sosa R, Good RA. Pneumocystis carinii pneumonia in a human immunodeficiency virus 1-infected neonate with meconium aspiration. Pediatr Infect Dis J 1991;10:953.
363. Paisley JW, Lauer BA, Melinkovich P, et al. Rapid diagnosis of Chlamydia trachomatis pneumonia in infants by direct immunofluorescence microscopy of nasopharyngeal secretions. J Pediatr 1986;109:653.
364. Haney PJ, Bohlman M, Sun C-CJ. Radiographic findings in neonatal pneumonia. AJR 1984;143:23.
365. Freij BJ, Kusmiesz H, Nelson JD, McCracken GH Jr. Parapneumonic effusions and empyema in hospitalized children: a retrospective review of 227 cases. Pediatr Infect Dis 1984;3:578.
366. Berman SA, Balkany TJ, Simmons MA. Otitis media in the neonatal intensive care unit. Pediatrics 1978;62:198.
367. deSa DJ. Mucosal metaplasia and chronic inflammation in the middle ear of infants receiving intensive care in the neonatal period. Arch Dis Child 1983;58:24.
368. Marchant CD, Shurin PA, Turczyk VA, et al. Course and outcome of otitis media in early infancy: a prospective study. J Pediatr 1984;104:826.
369. Tetzlaff TR, Ashworth C, Nelson JD. Otitis media in children less than 12 weeks of age. Pediatrics 1977;59:827.
370. Bland RD. Otitis media in the first six weeks of life: diagnosis, bacteriology, and management. Pediatrics 1972;49:187.
371. Shurin PA, Howie VM, Pelton SI, et al. Bacterial etiology of otitis media during the first six weeks of life. J Pediatr 1978;92:893.
372. Arriaga MA, Bluestone CD, Stool SE. The role of tympanocentesis in the management of infants with sepsis. Laryngoscope 1989;99:1048.
373. Bell MJ. Peritonitis in the newborn—current concepts. Pediatr Clin North Am 1985;32:1181.
374. Freij BJ, Votteler TP, McCracken GH Jr. Primary peritonitis in previously healthy children. Am J Dis Child 1984;138:1058.
375. Duggan MB, Khwaja MS. Neonatal primary peritonitis in Nigeria. Arch Dis Child 1975;50:130.
376. Genta VM, Gilligan PH, McCarthy LR. Clostridium difficile peritonitis in a neonate: a case report. Arch Pathol Lab Med 1984;108:82.
377. Aronoff SC, Olson MM, Gauderer MWL, et al. Pseudomonas aeruginosa as a primary pathogen in children with bacterial peritonitis. J Pediatr Surg 1987;22:861.
378. Mollitt DL, Tepas JJ III, Talbert JL. The microbiology of neonatal peritonitis. Arch Surg 1988;123:176.
379. Kaplan M, Eidelman AI, Dollberg L, Abu-Dalu K. Necrotizing bowel disease with Candida peritonitis following severe neonatal hypothermia. Acta Paediatr Scand 1990;79:876.
380. Fonkalsrud EW, Ellis DG, Clatworthy HW Jr. Neonatal peritonitis. J Pediatr Surg 1966;1:227.

Neonatology: Pathophysiology and Management of the Newborn, Fourth Edition,
edited by Gordon B. Avery, Mary Ann Fletcher, and Mhairi G. MacDonald.
J.B. Lippincott Company, Philadelphia © 1994.

chapter 49

Neurologic Disorders

ALAN HILL
JOSEPH J. VOLPE

Neurologic problems are a major cause of morbidity and mortality in neonatal medicine. Improvements in obstetric care, treatment of respiratory disease, and control of infection have dramatically increased the survival of premature infants. Detailed fetal assessment, especially the use of antenatal real-time ultrasonography, revealed that many abnormalities presenting during the neonatal period actually originate antenatally. Extensive discussions of the advances in fetal assessment are reviewed elsewhere.[1,2]

Advanced methods of neurologic assessment of the fetus allow limited intrauterine intervention for prevention of cerebral injury. Management of neurologic problems in the newborn are based on the scientific principles of neuroanatomy, physiology, and biochemical mechanisms.[1] In many instances, the most effective management of complex neurologic problems involves a team approach, which draws expertise from obstetrics, neonatology, genetics, neurology, and neurosurgery.

In this chapter, an approach to the neurologic assessment of the newborn is outlined, and the practical aspects of diagnosis and management of the most common neurologic problems of the newborn (*e.g.*, seizures, hypoxic–ischemic cerebral injury, intracranial hemorrhage, traumatic birth injury) are reviewed. The major bacterial and viral infections, major metabolic derangements, and cerebral dysgenesis that affect the central nervous system are discussed in Chapters 40, 47, 48, and 50.

NEUROLOGIC EVALUATION OF THE NEWBORN

HISTORY AND PHYSICAL EXAMINATION

The importance of a detailed history and neurologic examination in assessing the newborn with neurologic problems cannot be overemphasized.[1] The history must include details of the family history and complications encountered during pregnancy, delivery, and the neonatal period that may indicate an increased risk for neurologic problems.

The format of the neurologic examination in the newborn is similar to that used in older patients, but neurologic observations must be interpreted in the context of the level of cerebral maturation at different gestational ages. Physical examination should not be prolonged unnecessarily to avoid hypoxemia and fluctuations in arterial blood pressure that may be associated with routine handling, especially in premature newborns.

Neurologic observations are influenced by the level of alertness of the infant. After 28 weeks of gestation, infants are able to awaken spontaneously or may be roused for several minutes by stimulation. Distinct sleep–wake patterns may be recognized by 40 weeks of gestation. In an examination of the cranial nerves, pupillary constriction to light and the blink reflex may be elicited as early as 28 weeks of gestation. Pupillary responsiveness is consistent by 31 to 32 weeks. Definite visual following of a bright light and opticokinetic nystagmus can be elicited consistently in the awake infant at term. Fundoscopy may reveal retinal hemorrhages in 20% to 50% of newborn infants. Such hemorrhages rarely indicate significant injury to the central nervous system. Dysconjugate and jerky eye movements are common in premature infants and may persist to some degree for several months after term. Full extraocular eye movements to doll's-head maneuver or to caloric stimulation may be elicited after 32 weeks of gestation.

Observation of facial movement and symmetry must be evaluated to identify the dysfunction as peripheral or central in origin. Hearing may be difficult to assess, although infants startle to loud noises as early as 28 weeks of gestation. The act of feeding requires integrated action of breathing, sucking, and swallowing, which involve the cranial nerves V, VII, IX, X, and XII. The major features of the motor examination include posture of limbs, motility, muscle power, tendon reflexes, and primary neonatal reflexes. Muscle tone can be assessed by careful observation of the infant's resting posture during various maneuvers of passive manipulation. With increasing gestational age, there is increasing flexor tone, which predominates in all limbs by term. Asymmetry of muscle tone and spontaneous limb movements may indicate focal cerebral lesions. Brachial plexus injury may result in asymmetric paralysis of the upper limbs. Tendon reflexes are elicited readily in the newborn. Undue emphasis should not be placed on brisk responses, ankle clonus, or crossed adductor responses without other corroborative abnormal neurologic signs.

Careful evaluation of sensory function is particularly important in the evaluation of spinal cord or peripheral nerve injury. Sensory evaluation is useful for determining habituation, such as the normal dampening of responses to multiple (*i.e.*, 5–10) stimulations. Habituation indicates a high level of response that appears to require input from cerebral hemispheres. It is characteristically absent in anencephalic infants.

TABLE 49–1
DIAGNOSTIC TECHNIQUES FOR NEUROLOGICAL ASSESSMENT

Structural Cerebral Imaging
Ultrasonography
Computed tomography
Magnetic resonance imaging
Technetium brain scanning
Physiological Brain Imaging
Single photon emission computed tomography
Positron emission tomography
Neurophysiological Techniques
Electroencephalography
Brain stem auditory evoked responses
Visual evoked responses
Somatosensory evoked responses
Peripheral nerve conduction/electromyography
Other
Cerebrospinal fluid examination
Noninvasive measurement of intracranial pressure by Ladd monitor
Cerebral blood flow velocity by Doppler ultrasound
Cerebral magnetic resonance spectroscopy
Cerebral hemodynamics and oxygenation by near-infrared resonance spectroscopy

NEURODIAGNOSTIC TECHNIQUES

Because the neurologic examination is often limited by associated systemic illness and the use of complex life support systems, especially in premature infants, a variety of noninvasive neurodiagnostic techniques have been used as adjunctive methods for the assessment of neurologic problems in the newborn. The major neurodiagnostic techniques that have clinical application in the newborn are summarized in Table 49-1. The usefulness of individual techniques is discussed in the context of individual neurologic conditions.

NEONATAL SEIZURES

Seizures are the most frequent manifestation of serious neurologic disease in premature and term newborns. Immediate diagnosis and intervention are indicated because seizures indicate serious underlying disease and may interfere with supportive care (*e.g.*, ventilation, alimentation).[3,4] Experimental data suggest that neonatal seizures may have a deleterious effect on the developing brain, depleting cerebral glucose, which may interfere with DNA synthesis, glial proliferation and differentiation, and myelination.[5–7] Although the relevance of the animal study data to the human newborn is not entirely clear, their potential importance is suggested by *in vivo* studies performed with magnetic resonance (MR) spectroscopy.[8]

CLINICAL FEATURES

Seizures observed in newborns differ significantly from seizures observed in older children, principally because the immature newborn brain is less capable of propagating generalized or organized electrical discharges. The principal types of neonatal seizures are summarized in Table 49-2.[9] Although individual seizure types are not indicative of specific varieties of brain injury, certain types are associated more commonly with some conditions. For example, generalized tonic seizures, which may represent brain stem release phenomena, have been observed with severe intraventricular hemorrhage (IVH).[10,11] Focal clonic seizures may be associated with focal cerebral infarc-

TABLE 49–2
CLINICAL FEATURES OF NEONATAL SEIZURES

Seizure Type	Major Clinical Manifestations
Subtle	Repetitive blinking, eye deviation, staring Repetitive mouth or tongue movements Apnea Bicycling movements
Tonic (*i.e.*, generalized or focal)	Tonic extension of limb or limbs Tonic flexion of upper limbs, extension of lower limbs
Clonic (*i.e.*, multifocal or focal)	Multifocal, synchronous or asynchronous limb movements Repetitive, jerky limb movements Nonordered progression Localized repetitive clonic limb movements with preservation of consciousness
Myoclonic (*i.e.*, generalized, focal, multifocal)	Single or several flexion jerks of upper limbs (common) and lower limbs (rare)

tion or traumatic cerebral contusion. Differentiation of seizures from nonconvulsive movements may be difficult in the newborn. Clonic seizures may be difficult to differentiate clinically from jitteriness, particularly because both conditions often occur in identical clinical contexts, such as hypoxic–ischemic encephalopathy, metabolic derangements, and drug withdrawal. However, jitteriness is a movement disorder often associated with a good outcome. The distinction between jitteriness and seizures can be made clinically.

Jitteriness is not accompanied by abnormalities of eye movements.
Jitteriness is exquisitely stimulus sensitive.
The predominant movement of jitteriness is tremor (*i.e.*, alternating movements are of equal rate and amplitude), but the clonic movements of seizures typically have fast and slow components.
The repetitive movements of limbs affected by jitteriness may be stopped by passive flexion of the affected limb.

Simultaneous video and electroencephalographic (EEG) monitoring has raised questions about the incidence, classification, pathophysiology, and management of neonatal seizures. Some stereotypic, paroxysmal clinical phenomena, such as subtle seizures, generalized tonic, and extensor posturing, are not associated consistently with cortical electrographic seizure activity based on EEG recordings from surface electrodes.[10–15] Subtle clinical phenomena correlate more frequently with simultaneous abnormal EEG discharges in premature than in term newborns.[13,14,16–18]. Myoclonic seizures that are rare but associated with a grave prognosis and must be differentiated from benign neonatal sleep myoclonus, which may occur in healthy newborns.[19,20]

ETIOLOGY

Although neonatal seizures may be due to numerous underlying disorders, most result from a relatively few causes. Seizures are commonly the result of a combination of factors, such as hypoxic–ischemic cerebral injury, intracranial hemorrhage, and metabolic derangements. Determination of the cause permits specific treatment and allows meaningful prediction of outcome. The most important causes of seizures in the newborn are listed in order of relative frequency in Table 49-3.

Several less common causes of seizures are worthy of mention. Hyperbilirubinemia *per se* is a rare cause of seizures, but approximately 50% of infants with kernicterus exhibit seizures.[21]

Intoxication with local anesthetic occurs rarely after inadvertent injection into the infant's scalp during placement of pudendal, paracervical, or epidural blocks.[22] Severe tonic seizures begin during the first hours of life and are associated with low Apgar scores, bradycardia, apnea, severe hypoventilation, hypotonia, fixed and dilated pupils, and absence of extraocular movements in response to the doll's-head maneuver. The latter two features are often useful in differentiating anesthetic intoxication from hypoxic–ischemic encephalopathy. Seizures are usually self-limited. Evaluation includes inspection of the scalp for evidence of injection, and management consists of vigorous support and removal of the drug by diuresis.

Seizures are a relatively uncommon manifestation of withdrawal from passive addiction to narcotics, such as heroin, methadone, or barbiturates.[23] Cocaine, which has become the most common illicit drug abused in North America, has caused epileptiform EEG abnormalities, although not clinical sei-

TABLE 49–3
ETIOLOGY AND PROGNOSIS OF NEONATAL SEIZURES

Etiology	Gestational Age: Premature	Gestational Age: Term	Time of Onset (days of age): 0–3	Time of Onset (days of age): 4–10	Outcome Normal (%)
Hypoxic–ischemic encephalopathy	+	+	+		50
Intracranial hemorrhage					
Intraventricular hemorrhage	+	−	+		<10
Subarachnoid hemorrhage	−	+	+		90
Hypoglycemia	+	+	+		50
Infection	+	+		+	<50
Developmental Anomalies	+	+		+	0
Hypocalcemia					
Early onset	+	+	+		50
Late onset	−	+		+	100

+, common; −, rare.
Adapted from Volpe JJ. Neurology of the newborn. Philadelphia: WB Saunders, 1987:136.

zures, in approximately 50% of infants exposed *in utero* and through breast-feeding.[24–27]

A benign, autosomal dominant form of neonatal seizures has been described that begins dramatically on the second or third day of life, with more than 10 or 20 seizures per day.[28] Affected infants appear remarkably well interictally, and long-term neurologic outcome is normal. The gene for this transient form of epilepsy has been located on chromosome 20q.[29,30]

DIAGNOSIS

Diagnostic evaluation must begin with a careful history and physical examination. The maternal history is critical and should be obtained directly from the mother if possible. It is important for determining the possibility of drug abuse, intrauterine infection, and genetic or metabolic disorders. Laboratory investigations should focus initially on treatable causes, such as metabolic disorders (*e.g.*, hypoglycemia, hypocalcemia, hypomagnesemia) and infection. Lumbar puncture or treatment with meningitic doses of antibiotics and acyclovir may be indicated.

Although the EEG may be useful for establishing prognosis, it is rarely of help in determining the cause. Continuous EEG monitoring may be of value for the diagnosis of seizures in newborns who are treated with muscular paralysis to improve assisted ventilation.[31] The major EEG correlates of neonatal seizures include focal or multifocal spikes or sharp waves and focal monorhythmic discharges. Care must be taken not to confuse epileptiform activity and normal sharp transients in recordings of premature newborns or the trace alternant pattern of quiet sleep in term newborns with seizures.

Clinical observation and EEG recording may underestimate the true incidence or duration of seizures.[12] In newborns with frequent EEG seizures, the sensitivity of clinical observation has been as low as 21%.[32,33] Abnormal motor activity is associated with EEG abnormalities on routine surface recordings in only approximately one-third of of the recordings.[12] If initial screening investigations fail to identify a specific cause, additional neuroimaging or metabolic studies should be considered.

MANAGEMENT

Infants who exhibit clinical seizures require urgent intervention that includes maintenance of adequate ventilation and perfusion. Correction of even moderate hypoglycemia is of paramount importance, because studies indicate an association with adverse neurologic outcome.[34] Hypoglycemia should be corrected with intravenous administration of dextrose. Hypocalcemia may be corrected by intravenous administration of 5% calcium gluconate.

Seizures related to hypocalcemia may be controlled by phenobarbital, but correction of the underlying derangement of calcium homeostasis is still necessary. In the absence of hypoglycemia, phenobarbital should be administered intravenously in a single loading dose of 20 mg/kg administered over 5 to 10 minutes with concomitant surveillance of cardiorespiratory status. If seizures persist, an additional 20 mg/kg of phenobarbital administered in aliquots of 5 mg/kg as required to a maximum of 40 mg/kg have controlled seizures in 85% of patients without significant side-effects.[35–37] If seizures persist despite the previous measures, a loading dose of 20 mg/kg of phenytoin (5- to 10-mg/kg aliquots) may be administered slowly intravenously, at a rate of 0.5 to 1.0 mg/kg/minute, because of potential cardiac toxicity. Limited experience demonstrates that prolonged status epilepticus or refractory seizures may respond to other anticonvulsants (*e.g.*, lorazepam, paraldehyde, primidone, thiopental).[38–44]

PROGNOSIS

The mortality rate for neonatal seizures has improved during the past 20 years.[1] The most important determinant of prognosis is the underlying cause of the seizure, as outlined in Table 49-3. Mental retardation and motor deficits (*e.g.*, cerebral palsy) are more common long-term sequelae than epilepsy. The mortality rate for premature infants with seizures is increased as much as fourfold compared with term newborns. Early onset of seizures, more frequent or prolonged seizures, and seizures refractory to multiple anticonvulsants are associated with poor prognoses.[45] These features probably reflect the severity of the underlying cerebral injury. The characteristics observed on the interictal EEG are prognostically valuable. A normal interictal EEG has been associated with normal development in more than 85% of the patients, but interictal EEGs with a flat, periodic, or multifocal pattern have an approximately 8% probability of normal outcome.[46,47] In 25% to 35% of newborns with seizures, the EEG is borderline, equivocal, or contains less marked abnormalities and is associated with an uncertain prognosis.

HYPOXIC–ISCHEMIC CEREBRAL INJURY

Hypoxic–ischemic cerebral injury results from a combination of hypoxemia and ischemia often associated with impaired cerebrovascular autoregulation and possibly exacerbated by diminished glucose supply to the brain, lactic acidosis, accumulation of free radicals and excitotoxic amino acids, and other metabolic derangements. The extent and distribution of hypoxic–ischemic cerebral injury is determined principally by the maturity of the brain at the time of insult and the severity and duration of the insult.[1,48,49]

Although the importance of antepartum and intrapartum factors have been recognized since 1862, when Little initially described a relation between perinatal complications and cerebral palsy, data from large epidemiologic studies, such as the National Collaborative Perinatal Project and the Western Australian Cerebral Palsy Register, suggest that the etiologic role of antepartum factors may have been markedly underestimated previously.[50,51] Review of these large populations of children with cerebral palsy have revealed evidence of severe, hypoxic–ischemic cerebral insult in only 10% to 15% of them. Approximately one third of these patients had at least one congenital anomaly unrelated to the central nervous system. This observation raises the possibility that an insult that originated much earlier during gestation may have predisposed these infants to subsequent hypoxic–ischemic cerebral injury at the time of delivery. Advances in the monitoring of fetal heart rate, fetal scalp blood gas sampling, and biophysical profile may improve the accuracy of diagnosing the timing of antepartum insult.[1,2]

DIAGNOSIS

Infants who sustain hypoxic–ischemic cerebral injury earlier in gestation and before delivery may be asymptomatic during the neonatal period. However, term newborns who sustain sufficient intrapartum insult that results in long-term sequelae invariably demonstrate clinical evidence of acute encephalopathy during the first days of life. The clinical features of hypoxic–ischemic encephalopathy are nonspecific, and similar clinical abnormalities may occur in the context of other types of brain injury, such as metabolic derangements, cerebral dysgenesis, and infection. It is important to establish that the insult is due to hypoxia–ischemia based on assessment of factors such as complications of pregnancy, labor, and delivery that support the occurrence of asphyxia, including prolonged fetal bradycardia or late decelerations of fetal heart rate, acidosis of scalp blood gas samples or cord *p*H, presence of thick meconium, or low Apgar scores beyond 5 minutes of age. There are no single factors that predict accurately the severity or duration of hypoxic–ischemic insult or long-term sequelae.[52,53] However, the clinical features and patterns of cerebral injury as determined by imaging techniques, EEG, and biochemical markers may permit determination of prognosis with a reasonable degree of accuracy.[54,55]

Although there is a spectrum of hypoxic–ischemic encephalopathy, classification of severity as mild, moderate, or severe has prognostic value (Table 49-4).[54,55] Mild encephalopathy is characterized by hyperalertness, jitteriness, exaggerated tendon reflexes, and Moro responses that do not last longer than 24 hours and are not associated with long-term neurologic sequelae. Moderate encephalopathy is associated with lethargy and stupor, hypotonia, and suppressed tendon reflexes. Seizures may occur. Abnormal long-term outcome has been reported in 20% to 40% of affected infants. Severe encephalopathy is associated invariably with coma, seizures, and brain stem and autonomic dysfunction. Elevated intracranial pressure occurs in a minority of cases, and it is associated invariably with severe encephalopathy.[56–58] All infants with severe encephalopathy die or develop major neurologic sequelae, such as microcephaly, spastic quadriplegia, and seizures. In severe encephalopathy, the clinical features characteristically worsen during the first 3 days of life. Death occurs most commonly between 24 and 72 hours of life. Maximal elevation of intracranial pressure occurs during this time. Autopsy studies of patients who had elevated intracranial pressures demonstrated extensive cerebral necrosis. It appears that elevated intracranial pressure is a consequence rather than a cause of extensive brain injury, and intervention with antiedema agents may reduce the intracranial pressure but probably could not be expected to improve the ultimate neurologic outcome.

Seizures occur in approximately 50% of asphyxi-

TABLE 49–4
SEVERITY AND OUTCOME OF HYPOXIC–ISCHEMIC ENCEPHALOPATHY IN THE FULL-TERM NEONATE

Severity	Level of Consciousness	Seizures	Primitive Reflexes	Brain Stem Dysfunction	Elevated Intracranial Pressure	Duration	Poor Outcome* (%)
Mild	Increased irritability, hyperalertness	−, Jitteriness	Exaggerated	−	−	<24	0
Moderate	Lethargy	Variable	Suppressed	−	−	>24 h (variable)	20–40
Severe	Stupor or coma	+	Absent	+	Variable	>5 d	100

* Poor outcome was defined as the pressure of mental retardation, cerebral palsy, or seizures.
+, present; −, absent.

ated infants and usually begin during the first 24 hours of life. The seizures are often prolonged and may be resistant to anticonvulsants. Infants who survive beyond 72 hours of age usually demonstrate an improving level of consciousness, although with persistent impairment of feeding, abnormal muscle tone, and developmental delay.

In addition to clinical examination, neuroimaging techniques enable assessment of the extent of cerebral injury. In the term newborn, computed tomography (CT) scanning during the newborn period has excellent prognostic value and may demonstrate diffuse or focal cerebral injury. Optimal timing of CT scans is between 2 and 4 days of age to demonstrate maximal extent of decreased tissue attenuation, which is presumed to correspond to irreversible cerebral necrosis and associated edema (Fig. 49-1*A*).[56] Accurate interpretation of tissue attenuation on CT scans requires careful attention to scanning technique; scans should be photographed using a narrow window width of 60 to 80 Hounsfield units and window level between 25 and 30 Hounsfield units. Computed tomography scans performed later in childhood may demonstrate generalized or focal cerebral atrophy, often with multicystic encephalomalacia (Fig. 49-1*B*). Visualization of a brain stem injury or documentation of the extent of injury in the premature infant is limited using CT because of the normally low attenuation of the premature brain.

Cranial ultrasonography may identify periventricular leukomalacia in the premature infant. Increased periventricular echoes in the early days of life may herald development of cystic changes in these regions during the ensuing weeks. However, these areas of increased echogenicity are often transient, and the absence of such changes does not preclude the existence of hypoxic–ischemic injury to periventricular white matter. In the term newborn, cerebral necrosis may be suspected on the basis of diffuse increased echogenicity on cranial ultrasonography.[59,60] Problems with this technique are caused by limited visualization of the cerebral cortex and posterior fossa, the subjectivity of interpretation of increased echogenicity, and the inability to differentiate between ischemic and hemorrhagic cerebral injury.

Magnetic resonance scans may produce more detailed images of the injury to the posterior fossa structures and brain stem. Preliminary investigations using MR imaging suggest that it may be of value for documenting delayed myelination and cerebral atrophy.[61–65]

Radionuclide scanning can document various patterns of injury. O'Brien and associates and Pasternak and colleagues demonstrated the value of technetium scanning.[66,67] The development of new radionuclides with the capacity to cross the intact blood–brain barrier should provide new insights into abnormalities in regional cerebral blood flow, as in single photon emission CT and positron emission tomography.[68,69] Other noninvasive techniques, such as MR spectroscopy and near-infrared spectroscopy, permit detailed evaluation of cerebral metabolism in this context.[70–72] Infants whose MR spectra remain normal, with normal levels of high-energy phosphate compounds have normal outcomes.[71] Infants with abnormally decreased ratios of phosphocreatine to phosphorus compounds have extensive cerebral injuries and poor outcomes. Near-infrared spectroscopy permits regional quantification of oxyhemoglobin, deoxyhemoglobin, and oxidized cytochromes, which provides information on cerebral oxygen saturation, cerebral blood volume, cerebral blood flow, and tissue oxygen delivery.[72]

In addition to neuroimaging techniques and studies for evaluation of cerebral blood flow, electrodiagnostic techniques have been used in the evaluation of asphyxiated newborns. Electroencephalographic recordings that demonstrate a discontinuous pattern with voltage suppression and rapid bursts of sharp activity and slow waves indicate a poor outcome. Rapid resolution of EEG abnormalities and a normal interictal EEG pattern are associated

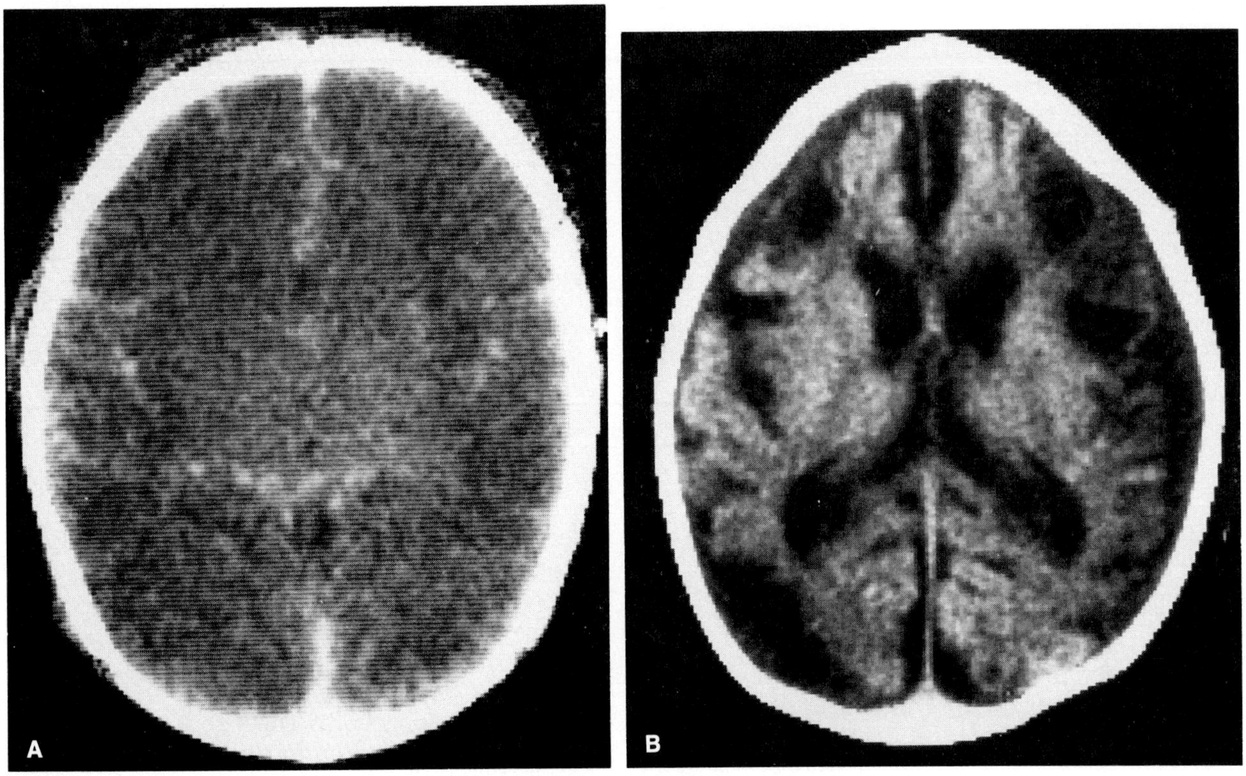

FIG. 49–1. **(A)** Computed tomography scan of a full-term newborn with severe, acute hypoxic–ischemic encephalopathy shows generalized, decreased tissue attenuation throughout both cerebral hemispheres. **(B)** Computed tomography scan performed at 4 months of age after hypoxic–ischemic cerebral injury at term demonstrates multicystic encephalomalacia and cerebral atrophy.

with a good outcome.[55] Evoked responses, including brain stem evoked responses, visual evoked responses, and somatosensory evoked responses, have some prognostic value.[73,74] However, their routine clinical application has been limited by technical constraints.

Several enzymes and metabolites (*e.g.*, creatine kinase BB, hypoxanthine, vasopressin) in blood or cerebrospinal fluid (CSF) are being studied as possible indicators of perinatal hypoxic–ischemic cerebral injury.[1] Other metabolic derangements, such as hypoglycemia and hyponatremia due to inappropriate secretion of antidiuretic hormone and acidosis, may contribute to the cerebral injury.

PATHOGENESIS AND NEUROPATHOLOGY

The neuropathologic lesions associated with perinatal hypoxic–ischemic insult result usually from a combination of hypoxemia and ischemia. These basic pathogenetic mechanisms have been refined to the extent that the major neuropathologic patterns of hypoxic–ischemic cerebral injury can be explained satisfactorily on the basis of a combination of regional circulatory and metabolic factors combined with the regional distribution of excitatory amino acid synapses, principally glutamate receptors.[49] The major neuropathologic patterns of hypoxic–ischemic cerebral injury are listed in Table 49-5.

CIRCULATORY FACTORS

The initial circulatory response to perinatal asphyxia involves redistribution of cardiac output, with increased perfusion of vital organs, such as the brain, heart, and adrenals, and concomitant decreased blood flow to other organs, such as the lungs, kidneys, and gastrointestinal tract. Prolonged hypoxic–ischemic insult results in systemic hypotension. The potential significance of hypotension is potentiated by impairment of cerebrovascular autoregulation, which has been reported even after relatively moderate hypoxic–ischemic insult.[75–77] Cerebrovascular autoregulation is a homeostatic mechanism that maintains relatively constant cerebral perfusion over a wide range of systemic arterial blood pressures by means of cerebral arteriolar constriction or dilation. Due to a deficiency in the muscular lining of cerebral arterioles in the immature brain, the frequent association of hypercarbia or hypoxemia, the fact that the normal blood pressure of the newborn is close to the down slope of the normal autoregulatory curve, or a combination of these factors, this protective mechanism may be disrupted. Impaired cerebrovascular

TABLE 49–5
MAJOR NEUROPATHOLOGIC PATTERNS

Pattern of Injury	Gestational Age: Full-Term	Gestational Age: Premature	Anatomic Distribution
Selective neuronal necrosis	+	+	Cerebral cerebellar cortex, thalamus, brain stem
Parasagittal neuropathy	+	−	Parasagittal cortex, subcortical white matter
Status marmoratus of basal ganglia or thalamus	+	−	Thalamus, basal ganglia, cerebral cortex
Focal or multifocal necrosis	+	+	Unilateral or bilateral cerebral cortex
Periventricular leukomalacia	−	+	Periventricular white matter

+, present; −, absent.

autoregulation results in a linear relation between cerebral perfusion and systemic blood pressure.

Systemic hypotension associated with moderate decreases in cerebral perfusion may result in injury that is confined principally to watershed zones of arterial supply. In the term newborn, the watershed zones among the anterior, middle, and posterior cerebral arteries are located in the parasagittal regions of cerebral cortex, but in the premature newborn, the most vulnerable watershed zone is located in periventricular white matter.

METABOLIC FACTORS

Regional differences in the rate of energy metabolism, energy requirements, lactate accumulation, calcium influx, and free-radical formation may partially explain the increased susceptibility of the thalamus and brain stem to hypoxic–ischemic injury under certain circumstances.[78,79] Selective vulnerability may relate to active myelination in these regions during the neonatal period.

There is increasing evidence for the fact that excitatory amino acids, particularly glutamate, play a critical role in the expression of hypoxic–ischemic neuronal injury. For example, hippocampal neurons in tissue culture are able to survive prolonged oxygen and glucose deprivation in the absence of glutamatergic synapses or after the addition of glutamate receptor blockers, such as magnesium, dextromethorphan, or ketamine. In experimental models, there is a dramatic increase in the concentration of extracellular glutamate within minutes after oxygen deprivation because of excessive release of glutamate from neurons and impaired energy-dependent glutamate uptake by presynaptic nerve terminals and astrocytes.[80–83] There appears to be a relation between the distribution of glutamatergic synapses in the mammalian brain and the common neuropathologic patterns of hypoxic–ischemic cerebral injury.[84] The potential clinical applications of glutamate antagonists are being explored.

MAJOR NEUROPATHOLOGIC PATTERNS OF INJURY

Selective Neuronal Necrosis. Selective necrosis of neurons, which is recognized principally in the term newborn, involves specific regions of the cortex, such as the Sommer sector of the hippocampus and thalamus, brain stem, cerebellum, and anterior horn cells of the spinal cord. The extent of injury relates to the severity and duration of the insult (*i.e.*, acute, total *versus* prolonged, partial asphyxia). Although circulatory factors may be involved, the major pathogenetic mechanisms appear to relate to relative rates of metabolism and state of maturation, including anatomic distribution of glutamatergic synapses. The late

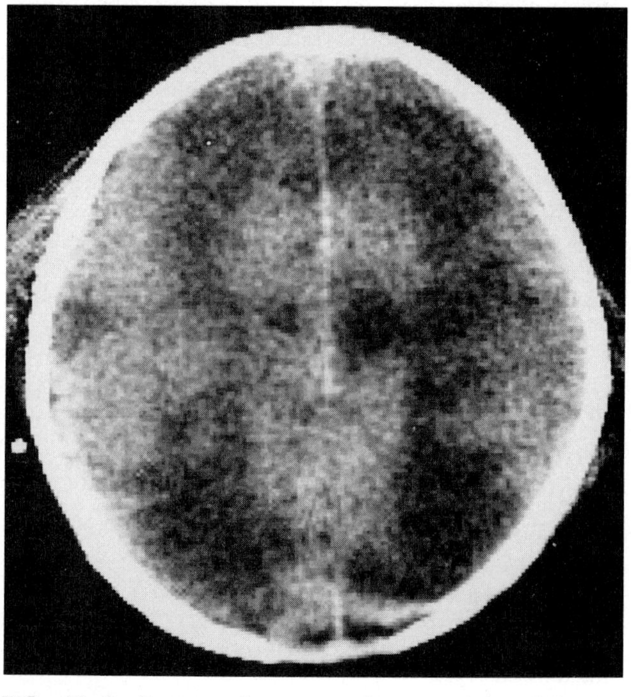

FIG. 49–2. Computed tomography scan of a full-term newborn demonstrates decreased tissue attenuation in the parasagittal watershed zones.

neuropathologic sequelae of selective neuronal necrosis are cerebral atrophy and multicystic encephalomalacia. Affected children develop various degrees of spastic quadriplegia, microcephaly, mental retardation, and seizures.

Parasagittal Cerebral Injury. In the term newborn, the parasagittal cortex represents the watershed area of arterial supply among the anterior, middle, and posterior cerebral arteries, which may sustain injury from systemic hypotension (Fig. 49-2). Clinical features of this pattern during the newborn period include hypotonia and weakness, which are more prominent in the proximal upper extremities than the lower extremities.

Status Marmoratus of Basal Ganglia and Thalamus. Neuronal necrosis, gliosis, and hypermyelination of astrocytes in basal ganglia, thalamus, and cerebral cortex may result in a striking marbled appearance of these structures (Fig. 49-3). This neuropathologic pattern reflects the transient, dense glutamatergic innervation of basal ganglia during the newborn period and the increased metabolic demands of actively differentiating neurons in these regions.[85–87] The clinical neurologic abnormalities during the newborn period that are associated with this pattern of injury are not known. Late sequelae include choreoathetotic cerebral palsy.

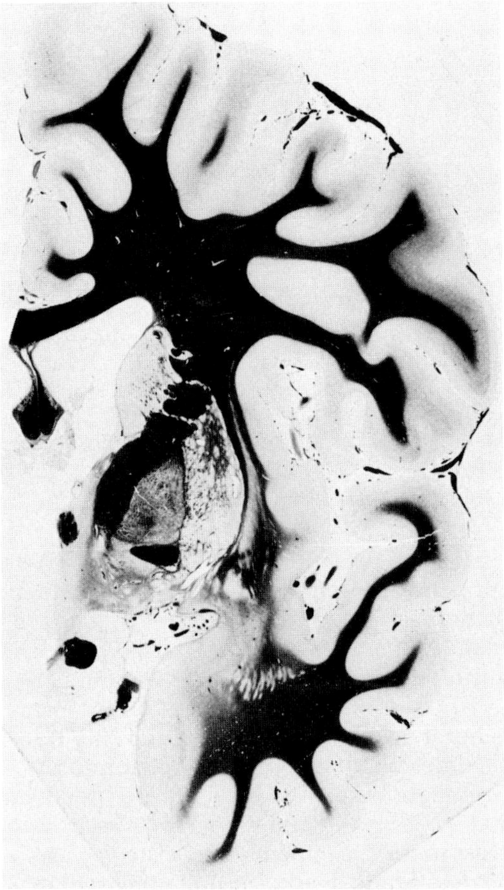

FIG. 49–3. Status marmoratus of basal ganglia is demonstrated in a coronal section of cerebral hemisphere, stained for myelin, from a patient who died years after the insult. The marbled appearance is especially striking in the putamen. (Courtesy of Dr. E.P. Richardson, Jr.)

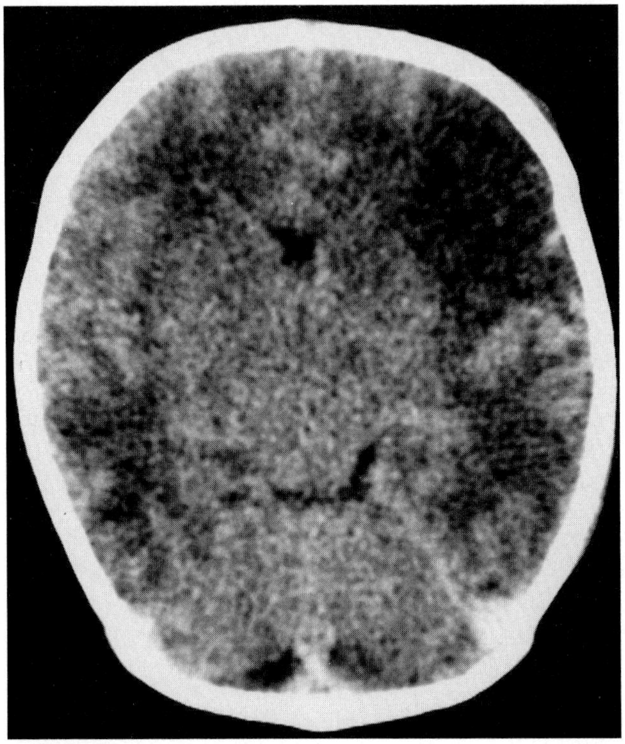

FIG. 49–4. Computed tomography scan of a full-term newborn with acute, focal infarction involving the territory of the middle cerebral artery.

Focal and Multifocal Cerebral Necrosis. Focal arterial occlusion by embolus or thrombus is well recognized in the newborn period (Fig. 49-4). There is evidence of cortical venous thrombosis.[88] Conditions predisposing to focal ischemic necrosis include polycythemia, disseminated intravascular coagulation, protein C deficiency, intrauterine cocaine exposure, isoimmune thrombocytopenia, vascular maldevelopment, and emboli from punctured or catheterized vessels or involuting fetal vessels. It is usually impossible to document the specific vascular lesion. In premature newborns, infarction is often multifocal.

Newborn infants who develop focal cerebral infarction may be asymptomatic or may have asymmetric motor function and focal or multifocal seizures. Long-term sequelae may include cerebral palsy (often hemiparesis), seizures, and intellectual impairment.

Periventricular Leukomalacia. This hypoxic–ischemic lesion involves the arterial end zones within periventricular white matter in the premature newborn.[89–91] A similar neuropathologic lesion called "telencephalic leukoencephalopathy" has been studied by Gilles, Leviton, and colleagues.[92–94] Secondary hemorrhage has been reported in 25% of patients with periventricular leukomalacia.[95] Periventricular hemorrhagic infarction is often unilateral (Fig. 49-5), and if associated with severe germinal matrix hemorrhage (GMH) or IVH, it is considered to result from obstruction of the terminal vein by a large subependymal GMH.[96] The severity of periventricular leukomalacia ranges from small areas of gliosis to larger areas of necrosis that may exhibit various degrees of cavitation (Fig. 49-6). These neuropathologic lesions may be seen by cerebral ultrasonography as areas of increased echogenicity in periventricular white matter during the first days of life that subsequently evolve into cystic lesions after 2 to 3 weeks.[97,98]

The clinical features of periventricular leukomalacia in the premature newborn may be subtle and include weakness or altered muscle tone involving predominantly the lower extremities. Long-term sequelae include spastic diplegia and occasional visual impairment related to involvement of the optic radiations.[99]

MANAGEMENT

There is no consensus about the optimal management of hypoxic–ischemic cerebral injury in the newborn.[100,101] Awareness of the events during the intrauterine period has promoted prevention of cerebral injury by early diagnosis and close monitoring of the high-risk fetus and consideration of rapid delivery in the event of persistent fetal distress. An asphyxiated newborn requires immediate and close surveillance to minimize postnatal injury. Provision of adequate ventilation and perfusion, maintenance of normal blood pressure and normoglycemia, and control of seizures are essential. There is a high incidence of dysfunction of other organ systems, such as the heart, kidneys, and gastrointestinal tract, which must be monitored carefully.

Avoidance of hypoxemia and hypercapnia has been simplified by the use of continuous transcutaneous oximetry and carbon dioxide monitoring. Adequate ventilation and the avoidance of postnatal hypoxemia may be difficult to achieve because of the cardiorespiratory problems associated with severe hyaline membrane disease in the premature newborn and persistent fetal circulation and pulmonary hypertension in the term newborn. Administration of artificial surfactant and extracorporeal membrane oxygenation are newer treatment modalities. Because hypoxemic episodes in the premature newborn may

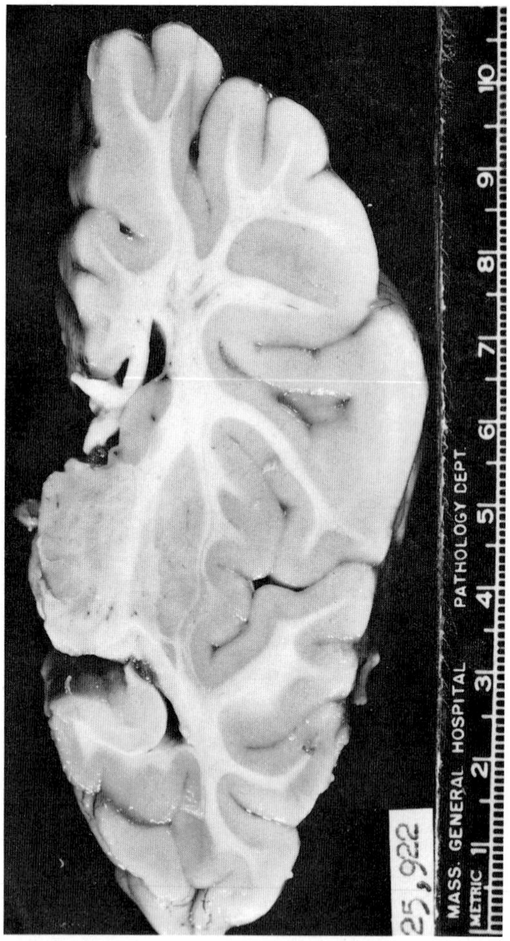

FIG. 49–6. Periventricular leukomalacia is demonstrated in the coronal section of cerebral hemisphere from a 20-month-old child who was the product of a 35-week pregnancy and experienced cardiorespiratory difficulties in the neonatal period. Small, cavitated lesions can be seen approximately 5 mm from the external angle of the lateral ventricle of the parietal lobe. (From DeReuck J, Chattha AS, Richardson EP Jr. Pathogenesis and evolution of periventricular leukomalacia in infancy. Arch Neurol 1972;27:229.)

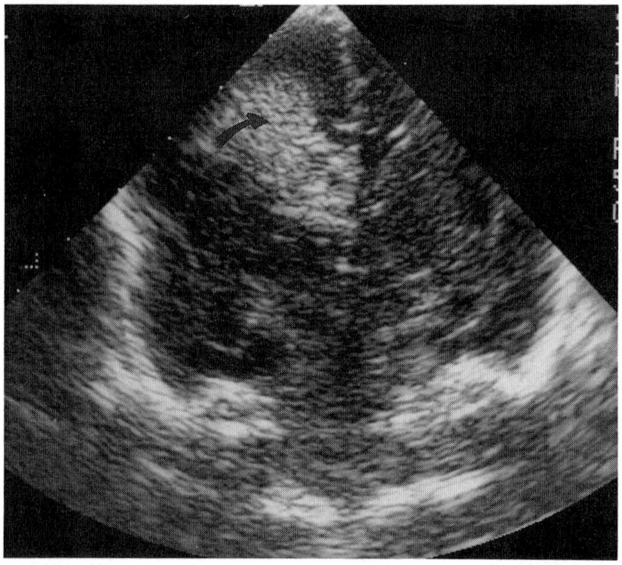

FIG. 49–5. Coronal ultrasound scan delineates the periventricular hemorrhagic infarction (*arrow*) in a premature newborn with intraventricular hemorrhage.

be associated with routine care such as suctioning or spontaneous crying, minimal handling is recommended for these infants. However, hyperoxia must be avoided because of the possibility of pontosubicular necrosis and retrolental fibroplasia.[102] Theoretically, hypercapnia may result in worsening of the intracellular acidosis and impairment of cerebrovascular autoregulation, but there are no conclusive data to support the routine use of hyperventilation in asphyxiated newborns.

The maintenance of normal systemic arterial blood pressure and adequate cerebral perfusion may require volume replacement and the use of inotropic agents (*e.g.*, dopamine) if there is evidence of myocardial dysfunction. In the premature newborn, systemic hypotension may occur in the context of patent ductus arteriosus and recurrent apnea with bradycardia. However, systemic hypertension must be avoided, especially in the premature newborn, because it may predispose the infant to hemorrhage originating within the fragile vasculature of the germinal matrix.

Seizures that occur in the context of hypoxic–ischemic encephalopathy may be refractory to anticonvulsant intervention. Nevertheless, treatment is indicated to minimize associated apnea, hypertension, and metabolic derangements, such as depletion of brain glucose and high-energy phosphate compounds.

The optimal levels of blood glucose after asphyxia have not been established clearly. Maintenance of normoglycemia is recommended, and fluid overload should be avoided. Inappropriate antidiuretic hormone secretion after major hypoxic–ischemic cerebral injury may result in hyponatremia and decreased osmolality, with a consequent increase in cerebral edema and seizures.

Data from human and animal studies suggest that elevated intracranial pressure associated with hypoxic–ischemic encephalopathy in the term newborn reflects extensive cerebral necrosis, which represents a consequence rather than a cause of hypoxic–ischemic brain injury. Maximal elevations of intracranial pressure are observed between 36 and 72 hours after the initial insult and are associated with a poor outcome.[54] Although it is possible to reduce elevated intracranial pressure by antiedema agents (*e.g.*, mannitol, diuretics) and hyperventilation, there is no evidence to indicate that such intervention improves long-term neurologic outcome.[53]

Several management strategies are under investigation. Data on asphyxiated animals suggest that pretreatment with barbiturates before the onset of metabolic stress may improve survival and reduce the severity of brain injury.[100] There is compelling evidence that pretreatment and treatment after the hypoxic–ischemic event with glutamate receptor antagonists (*e.g.*, phencyclidine, dextromethorphan, ketamine, MK-801) appear to reduce neuronal injury. Calcium channel blockers (*e.g.*, flunarizine, nimodipine) may prevent intracellular calcium accumulation, cell membrane disintegration, and neuronal death.[103–107] Toxic free-radical scavengers and inhibitors (*e.g.*, indomethacin, allopurinol) are being investigated.[108,109]

PROGNOSIS

The major factors associated with poor outcome in the term newborn are summarized in Table 49-6. In our experience with full-term newborns, the severity and duration of clinical hypoxic–ischemic encephalopathy, combined with the extent of decreased tissue attenuation seen on CT scans performed between 2 and 5 days after the original insult, can provide the most accurate combination of prognostic factors. The prediction of outcome in the premature newborn who sustains hypoxic–ischemic insult may be more difficult.

INTRACRANIAL HEMORRHAGE

The incidence of GMH/IVH in premature newborns is 25% to 40%. Although there has been a reduction in incidence during the past decade, GMH/IVH remains a major concern, principally because of the improved survival rates of very-low-birth-weight infants (<1000 g), who are at highest risk for the development of GMH/IVH. In the premature newborn, GMH/IVH originates from the rupture of fragile vessels in the subependymal germinal matrix (Fig. 49-7). In approximately 80% of patients, there is associated IVH, and in approximately 10% to 15%, there is cerebral infarction involving the periventricular tissues. Serial cranial ultrasonography has demonstrated that in 50% of the patients, GMH/IVH originates during the first day of life. In 90%, hemorrhage originates before 4 days of age. In 20% to 40%, the hemorrhage progresses during the first week of life.

TABLE 49–6
MAJOR PROGNOSTIC FACTORS FOR HYPOXIC–ISCHEMIC BRAIN INJURY IN FULL-TERM NEWBORNS

Fetal factors: congenital anomalies, abnormal fetal heart rate, acid–base disturbances during scalp blood sampling
Extended poor Apgar scores ≥ 5 minutes of age
Neonatal encephalopathy: severity, duration, occurrence of seizures
Neuroimaging data: cranial ultrasonography, computed tomography, radionuclide scans, magnetic resonance imaging
Electrophysiologic data: electroencephalography, evoked responses, magnetic resonance spectroscopy
Biochemical markers

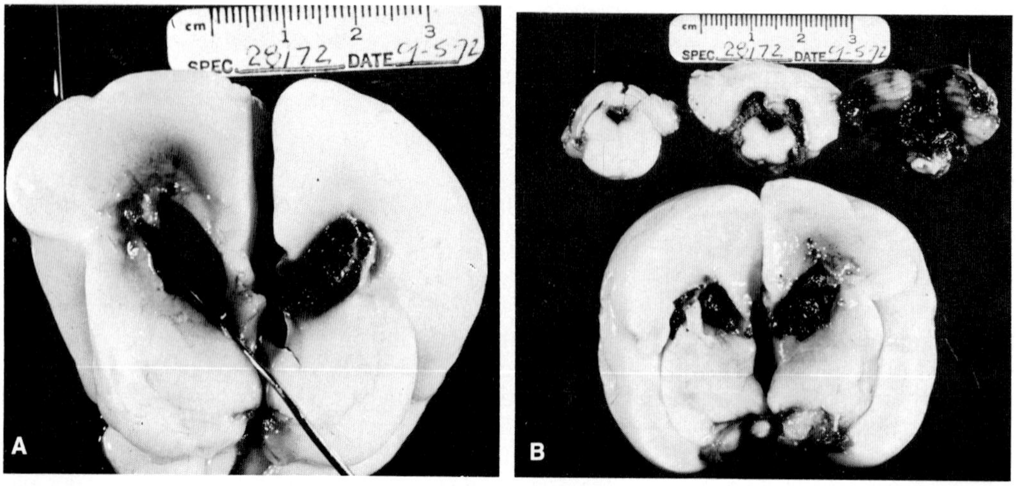

FIG. 49–7. **(A)** Periventricular hemorrhage with intraventricular rupture at the level of the foramen of Monro; blood fills both lateral ventricles. The site of rupture of the hemorrhage from the right subependymal region can be seen. **(B)** Extension of intraventricular hemorrhage, same case as shown in Fig. 49–7. Hemorrhage can be seen in the lateral ventricles, the aqueduct of Sylvius, the fourth ventricle, and the subarachnoid space around the cerebellum and base of the brain. (Courtesy of Dr. John Axley.)

DIAGNOSIS

Although CT and cranial ultrasonography have the capability for diagnosis of the spectrum of GMH/IVH, ultrasonography is considered the technique of choice because of its portability, high resolution, and lack of ionizing radiation. Nevertheless, CT scanning remains superior for the diagnosis of other varieties of intracranial hemorrhage, including primary subarachnoid, convexity, and posterior fossa subdural and epidural hematomas and for differentiating hemorrhagic and ischemic parenchymal infarctions. Figure 49-8 illustrates the appearance of IVH on CT scan.

Because of the high risk of GMH/IVH, routine cranial ultrasonography is recommended at 4 days of age for high-risk infants younger than than 32 weeks of gestation. Ultrasound scanning should be performed sooner if there are clinical concerns. Because there may be progression in the size of the hemorrhage in 20% to 40% of patients with GMH/IVH, the ultrasound scans should be repeated after the first week of life to establish the maximal extent of the hemorrhage. After major GMH/IVH, serial scans should be performed on a weekly basis for surveillance of ventricular size and possible development of post-hemorrhagic hydrocephalus (Fig. 49-9). This is particularly important because of the high degree of compliance of the premature brain and cranium and the relatively large subarachnoid space that permits considerable increase in ventricular size before excessive increase in head growth occurs.

The diagnosis of GMH/IVH may be suspected on the basis of clinical signs alone in approximately 50% of patients.[110] The severity of clinical features ranges from an asymptomatic state through a saltatory neurologic deterioration over several days to a catastrophic presentation with coma, apnea, tonic extensor posturing, brain stem dysfunction, and flaccid quadriparesis. Associated systemic abnormalities may include hypotension, metabolic acidosis, bradycardia, serum glucose, and electrolyte disturbances. Bloody or xanthochromic CSF supports a diagnosis of intracranial hemorrhage.

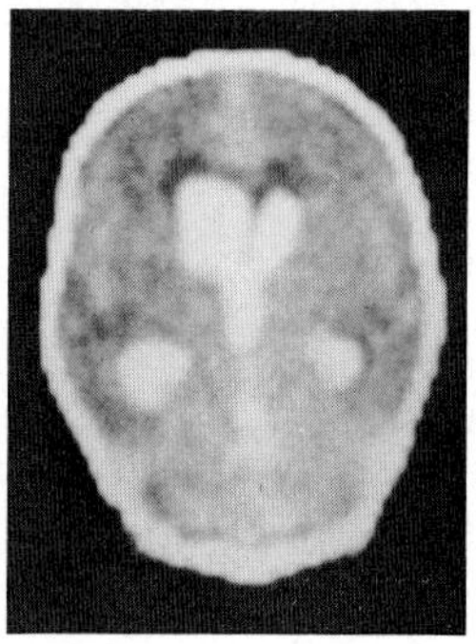

FIG. 49–8. Computed tomography scan of marked intraventricular hemorrhage demonstrates blood in the frontal horns, third ventricle, and occipital horns.

PATHOGENESIS

The pathogenesis of GMH/IVH is multifactorial and consists of a combination of intravascular, vascular, and extravascular factors (Table 49-7). The importance of individual factors may vary in different situations. Consideration of these major pathogenetic mechanisms provides a framework for the selection of appropriate interventional strategies.

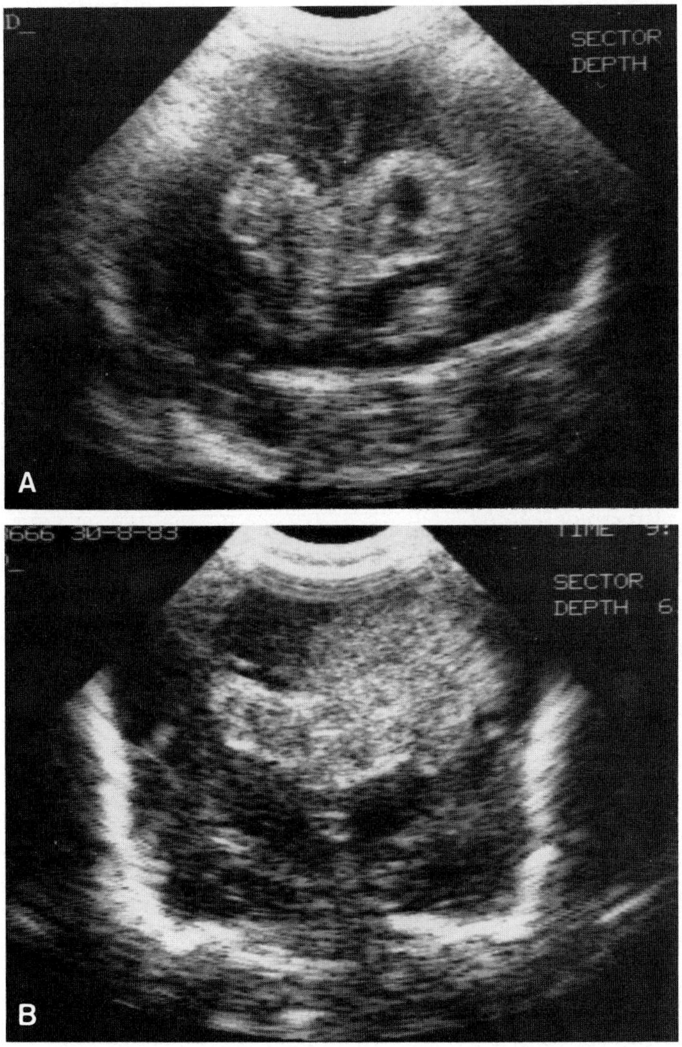

FIG. 49–9. **(A)** Ultrasonographic scan in the coronal plane of marked intraventricular hemorrhage delineates blood in the dilated frontal horns of the lateral ventricles and central clearing of the hematoma (*left*). **(B)** Ultrasonographic scan in the coronal plane of marked intraventricular hemorrhage shows blood in the dilated frontal horns of lateral ventricles and intraparenchymal hematoma (*left*).

Intravascular factors involve principally the regulation of cerebral perfusion (*i.e.*, cerebral blood flow and pressure) within the fragile vasculature of the germinal matrix and platelet–capillary interactions and coagulation disturbances. Vascular pathogenetic factors include the fragility of vessels in the germinal matrix and their vulnerability to hypoxic–ischemic insult. Extravascular factors are the characteristics of the supporting tissues, excessive fibrinolytic activity, and the decrease in tissue pressure postnatally.

Post-hemorrhagic hydrocephalus and periventricular hemorrhagic infarction are the major mechanisms of cerebral injury observed after GMH/IVH. Other mechanisms involved in cerebral injury associated with GMH/IVH include concomitant or preceding hypoxic–ischemic cerebral injury (*e.g.*, periventricular leukomalacia, neuronal necrosis of the brain stem); acute increase in intracranial pressure associated with major hemorrhage; destruction of the germinal matrix with its glial precursors; and focal ischemia, possibly secondary to vasospasm.

Ventriculomegaly and hydrocephalus occur commonly after major GMH/IVH (Table 49-8). Communicating hydrocephalus is related to impaired CSF reabsorption secondary to an obliterative arachnoiditis in the posterior fossa. A second potential mechanism involves the blockage of CSF resorption at the small arachnoid villi by particulate debris floating in CSF after GMH/IVH.[111] Obstructive hydrocephalus may occur secondary to blockage of the flow of CSF at the level of the aqueduct of Sylvius by a blood clot or other intraventricular debris.[112] Although the accumulation of excessive quantities of blood within the ventricular system may produce ventricular dilation at the time of the initial GMH/IVH, it usually does not become progressive until several weeks after the hemorrhage.[1]

The characteristic clinical signs of hydrocephalus (*e.g.*, abnormally rapid increase in head circumference, bulging anterior fontanel, suture diastasis) may be delayed for days or weeks after the onset of ventricular dilation is seen on serial ultrasound scans.[1]

TABLE 49–7
PATHOGENESIS AND MANAGEMENT OF GERMINAL MATRIX–INTRAVENTRICULAR HEMORRHAGE

Pathogenic Factor	Management
Intravascular	
Alterations in cerebral blood flow	Avoidance of systemic hypertension or hypotension; paralysis of ventilated infants
Alterations in cerebral venous pressure	Avoidance of prolonged labor and difficult vaginal delivery Avoidance of pneumothorax, minimal handling
Coagulation disturbances	Avoidance of hypoxic-ischemic insult; prophylactic infusion of fresh-frozen plasma (?); platelet infusion (?)
Vascular	
Fragility of vessels in subependymal germinal matrix	Ethamsylate (?), vitamin E (?)
Extravascular	
Poor vascular support of germinal matrix	Tranexamic acid (?)
Decrease in tissue pressure (?)	

Delayed clinical manifestations of progressive ventriculomegaly are related to the high compliance of periventricular tissue in the immature brain, especially after hypoxic–ischemic injury, the relatively generous subarachnoid space in the premature infant, and the distensible cranium, all of which allow increase in ventricular size without expansion of head circumference.

Ventriculomegaly after GMH/IVH may become static or resolve spontaneously after days or months in approximately 50% of the patients. In the remainder, temporary amelioration of increased intracranial pressure by serial lumbar punctures or more permanent surgical drainage are required.

Hemorrhagic necrosis of periventricular white matter occurs in approximately 15% of infants, usually those with severe GMH/IVH. These parenchymal lesions may be the single most important determinant of major long-term neurologic sequelae. The lesion is usually unilateral or asymmetric, located in regions that are dorsal and lateral to the external angle of the lateral ventricle on the side of the more extensive IVH (see Fig. 49-5).[95] Neuropathologic studies suggest that the pathogenesis of this type of hemorrhagic necrosis differs from that of hemorrhagic periventricular leukomalacia, which represents an arterial ischemic lesion with secondary hemorrhage. Periventricular hemorrhagic necrosis with IVH probably represents venous infarction. The fan-shaped parenchymal hemorrhage associated with IVH is located near the external angle of the lateral ventricle, where the medullary veins of the periventricular white matter become confluent to form the terminal vein in the subependymal region. Hemorrhagic necrosis probably represents venous infarction with obstruction of medullary and terminal veins by intraventricular and germinal matrix blood clots.[112–116]

The intraventricular blood may contribute to periventricular necrosis through the release of injurious or vasoactive substances, such as lactic acid or potassium from hemolyzed erythrocytes.[117,118]

TABLE 49–8
MAJOR COMPLICATIONS OF GERMINAL MATRIX–INTRAVENTRICULAR HEMORRHAGE

Ventriculomegaly or post-hemorrhagic hydrocephalus
Periventricular hemorrhagic cerebral infarction
Acute increased intracranial pressure with major intraventricular hemorrhage
Destruction of germinal matrix glial precursors
Focal ischemia (?)
Concomitant hypoxic–ischemic cerebral injury (*i.e.*, periventricular leukomalacia)

MANAGEMENT

Management strategies should address the major pathogenetic mechanisms as outlined previously. The primary goal is prevention of GMH/IVH. Prevention of premature labor and delivery are the most direct means of accomplishing this goal. Transportation of the infants *in utero* to a perinatal center specializing in high-risk deliveries results in fewer cases of IVH than for infants transported postnatally.[115,117]

Correction or prevention of major hemodynamic disturbances, including fluctuating cerebral blood flow, systemic hypotension and hypertension, and increases in cerebral venous pressure, can reduce the incidence of GMH/IVH and major degrees of hemorrhage. Because of the impaired cerebrovascular autoregulation in the sick premature newborn, alterations in systemic blood pressure are reflected directly in changes in cerebral blood flow. Care must be taken to prevent the hypertension associated with excessive handling, suctioning, and rapid infusions of blood or other colloid, and adequate ventilation must be maintained to avoid apnea, pneumothorax, and hypercapnia.[117,119,120]

In mechanically ventilated infants, muscle paralysis with pancuronium bromide is highly effective for regulating a fluctuating pattern of cerebral blood flow into a stable pattern, resulting in an impressive decrease in all grades of IVH.[117,119,120] Muscle paralysis is effective for preventing increases in venous pressure associated with tracheal suctioning.[120,121]

Two pharmacologic agents, phenobarbital and indomethacin, may influence intravascular factors associated with GMH/IVH. Administration of phenobarbital prenatally and postnatally may dampen the rises in arterial blood pressure associated with motor activity and handling. Although the incidence of IVH was decreased in infants of mothers who received antenatal phenobarbital, the interpretation of these studies is hampered by methodologic problems.[122,123] Results of several controlled studies involving postnatal phenobarbital administration are inconsistent, although the largest study suggests a possible deleterious effect of phenobarbital.[124–129]

Indomethacin, an agent that inhibits prostaglandin synthesis, blunts vasodilatory responses, prevents increases in cerebral blood flow, and inhibits formation of free radicals, may decrease the likelihood of GMH/IVH.[130,131] Other studies suggest no prophylactic value.[132,133]

Abnormalities of coagulation or platelet–capillary interactions may play a role in the pathogenesis of IVH in some patients. Prenatal administration of vitamin K has been reported to be beneficial, but the data are inconclusive.[134] Administration of fresh-frozen plasma reduced the overall incidence of IVH without affecting the incidence of severe IVH or had no effect.[135,136]

Two pharmacologic agents, ethamsylate and vitamin E, are theoretically valuable for the stabilization of the fragile germinal matrix vessels. Ethamsylate has been evaluated in at least three controlled trials, two of which demonstrated a reduction in the overall incidence of IVH as well as a reduction of severe hemorrhage.[137,138] This agent is not available in the United States.

Vitamin E has antioxidant properties and may function as a free-radical scavenger to protect endothelial cells of germinal matrix from hypoxic injury. There are conflicting data about the use of vitamin E for prevention of IVH. Several studies reported a reduction of all grades of IVH, but Phelps and associates observed a higher incidence of IVH in treated infants than in controls.[139–142] Additional data are required.

Because the magnitude of the pressure gradient across the capillary walls in the germinal matrix may influence the likelihood of GMH/IVH and because there is evidence for postnatal loss of extracellular fluid in studied animals, prolactin, a hormone involved in water homeostasis, has been proposed as a potential preventive measure for IVH. Preliminary data demonstrated a significant reduction in the incidence of GMH/IVH in newborn beagles who were treated with prolactin.[143] The significance of these observations for the management of high-risk human newborns is unknown.

In approximately 50% of patients with post-hemorrhagic hydrocephalus drainage of CSF by serial lumbar punctures, with or without administration of acetalomide or furosemide to decrease CSF production, or ventricular drainage (*e.g.*, ventriculoperitoneal shunt), ventriculostomy with or without a subcutaneous reservoir is required.[1] The optimal timing for intervention has not been identified because the role of ventriculomegaly in the genesis of brain injury is unknown. Although it is assumed that hydrocephalus with raised intracranial pressure is deleterious, the significance of slowly progressive ventricular dilation without raised intracranial pressure is unknown. Data suggest that ventricular dilation may cause periventricular edema, axonal stretching, or axonal loss with astrocytosis and alteration in the lipid and protein content of the periventricular white matter.[144,145] Alterations in the caliber and number of periventricular vessels may occur.[140] Studies of human infants have demonstrated decreased blood flow velocity in the anterior cerebral arteries of infants with ventriculomegaly that was reversible after drainage of CSF.[147] Impairment of cerebral perfusion and correction by CSF removal has been demonstrated by positron emission tomography.[148] Similarly, reversal of increased latency of visual evoked responses has been demonstrated in affected infants; the latency was presumably related to disturbed axonal function in the optic radiations by the dilation of the occipital horns of the lateral ventricles.[149]

A randomized trial of 157 infants in 15 centers attempted to compare the value of early drainage of CSF by repeated lumbar punctures and observation alone without intervention.[150] Of the survivors, 62% in the treated and untreated groups ultimately required permanent surgical ventricular drainage. Data on neurologic outcome at 12 months of age demonstrated a high overall incidence of neurologic abnormalities (85%). There was no apparent benefit for early treatment in children who did not have parenchymal lesions at the time of entry into the study. Although the period of follow-up was relatively brief, there was some indication that neurologic sequelae, except motor impairment, may be reduced in infants with parenchymal lesions who are treated early.[150]

PROGNOSIS

The short-term outcome of GMH/IVH is related principally to the size of the hemorrhage and may be considered in terms of mortality or hydrocephalus among survivors. The short-term outcome of the infant with GMH/IVH appears to have improved because of detection by routine cranial ultrasonography of small lesions that are silent clinically and of little practical consequence. Improvements in neonatal intensive care have contributed to a decrease in mortality rate during the newborn period for infants with larger lesions. For infants with small hemorrhages, survival without ventricular dilation is the rule. With moderate-sized hemorrhages, mortality is low (approximately 10%), and progressive hydrocephalus occurs in fewer than 20%. However, large hemorrhages have a high mortality rate (50%–60%), and post-hemorrhagic hydrocephalus often develops (65%–100%).[1,151,152] The most critical determinant of long-term outcome is the extent of parenchymal involvement. Major GMH/IVH occurs frequently in the context of hypoxic–ischemic cerebral insult, and long-term neurologic outcome depends on concomitant or preceding hemorrhagic or nonhemorrhagic hypoxic–ischemic cerebral injury.

SUBDURAL HEMORRHAGE

Improvements in obstetric practice and a decrease in mechanical birth trauma have reduced considerably the incidence of severe subdural hemorrhage. This type of hemorrhage accounts for less than 5% to 10% of intracranial hemorrhage in the newborn.[153] However, the data must be interpreted with the recognition that mild subdural hemorrhage may have few associated clinical abnormalities and may remain undiagnosed.

Subdural hemorrhage occurs in premature and term infants and results from laceration of the major veins and sinuses, usually associated with a tear of the dura or dural reflections (*e.g.*, falx, tentorium) overlying the cerebral hemispheres or cerebellum. Excessive molding of the head may play a role in the genesis of subdural hemorrhage. Clinical features include a decreased level of consciousness, seizures, or asymmetry of motor function. Clinical outcome is determined in large part by the extent of associated hypoxic–ischemic injury.

DIAGNOSIS

Computed tomography is the technique of choice for the identification of subdural hemorrhage. Differentiating subdural from intracerebellar hemorrhage may be difficult in infants who have evidence of hemorrhage in the posterior fossa on CT scans. Intracerebellar hemorrhage appears to be more common in premature infants, and posterior fossa subdural hemorrhage is more common in term newborns.[1]

The diagnosis of posterior fossa hemorrhage and small lesions located over the cerebral convexities may be difficult using cranial ultrasonography alone. However, large convexity subdural hemorrhage, especially if associated with lateral displacement of midline structures, can be detected by this technique.

Occipital diastasis and skull fractures are demonstrated best by skull radiographs.

MANAGEMENT

Convexity subdural hemorrhage, particularly if associated with displacement of the midline, should be evacuated by subdural tap or craniotomy, especially if there is clinical deterioration with signs of transtentorial herniation. Massive subdural hemorrhage located in the posterior fossa may require surgical evacuation. Surgical intervention may not significantly improve the long-term outcome if there are no major neurologic signs.[1]

PROGNOSIS

The prognosis for infants with major lacerations of the tentorium or falx is poor. The mortality rate is approximately 45%, and survivors frequently develop hydrocephalus and other sequelae. More than 50% of survivors who sustain lesser degrees of hemorrhage are neurologically normal at follow-up. Concomitant hypoxic–ischemic cerebral injury is often the critical factor in determining outcome.

PRIMARY SUBARACHNOID HEMORRHAGE

Primary subarachnoid hemorrhage, which is located most prominently in the subarachnoid space over the cerebral convexities and in the posterior fossa refers to hemorrhage within the subarachnoid space that is not secondary to extension of subdural hemorrhage, IVH, or cerebellar hemorrhage. Unlike the dramatic arterial hemorrhage in adults, subarachnoid hemorrhage in the newborn is usually self-limited and of venous origin, originating from small vessels in the leptomeningeal plexus or in bridging veins within the subarachnoid space.[1] Trauma or hypoxic events may be important antecedents of major degrees of primary subarachnoid hemorrhage, although the pathogenesis is usually uncertain. Long-term sequelae are uncommon. Rarely, hydrocephalus may develop secondary to adhesions at the outflow of the fourth ventricle or over the cerebral convexities.

CLINICAL FEATURES

Definition of the clinical features related solely to primary subarachnoid hemorrhage has been made difficult by its association with trauma, hypoxia, and other forms of intracerebral hemorrhage that produce abnormal neurologic signs. Nevertheless, three syndromes of primary subarachnoid hemorrhage are recognized.[1] The first syndrome of minimal or no clinical features is the most common. In the second syndrome, seizures occur most commonly on the second day of life, and the infant is usually well between seizures. The third syndrome, associated with massive subarachnoid hemorrhage, consists of rapid neurologic deterioration and is rare. The infant has usually sustained severe hypoxic–ischemic cerebral injury, with or without trauma, or has a major vascular abnormality, such as arteriovenous malformation or aneurysm.

DIAGNOSIS

The diagnosis of primary subarachnoid hemorrhage is based on the finding of uniformly blood-stained CSF on lumbar puncture in an infant in whom other forms of intracranial hemorrhage have been excluded by CT scans. With primary subarachnoid hemorrhage, the CT scans usually demonstrate blood in the superior longitudinal fissure and in sulci.

MANAGEMENT

Seizures are treated with anticonvulsant medication. Hydrocephalus is managed as described earlier in this chapter.

PROGNOSIS

In the absence of preceding severe trauma, hypoxic–ischemic cerebral injury, or ruptured vascular lesion, the outcome is favorable. Outcome correlates well with the neonatal clinical syndrome. In infants with minimal or no clinical signs, prognosis is excellent. In term infants with seizures, 90% are normal at follow-up. In the rare instance of massive subarachnoid hemorrhage with catastrophic deterioration, death and hydrocephalus are common.

INTRACEREBELLAR HEMORRHAGE

Postmortem studies suggested that primary hemorrhage into the cerebellum is a relatively common lesion, reported in 15% to 25% of infants younger than 32 weeks of gestation or with birth weights less than 1500 g.[154,155] The routine use of ultrasonographic study of premature infants has confirmed that this lesion is much less common in surviving infants than was once the case. Cerebellar hemorrhage has been reported in full-term infants.[156,157]

NEUROPATHOLOGY

The several causes of cerebellar hemorrhage include traumatic laceration of the cerebellum, major veins, or sinuses secondary to occipital diastasis, venous infarction, or extension of IVH or massive subarachnoid hemorrhage into the cerebellum. Pathogenetic factors include tenuous vascular integrity, skull deformation, occipital diastasis, impaired cerebrovascular autoregulation with hypoxic–ischemic insult, and bleeding from fragile vessels of the germinal external granule cell layer of the cerebellum.[1,158] Cerebellar hemorrhage was reported by Pape and colleagues in infants who received ventilation by face masks that were held in place by a Velcro strap around the infants' heads.[158]

CLINICAL FEATURES

Most reports of intracerebellar hemorrhage in premature infants are based on autopsy studies. Clinical details are based on retrospective analyses. There was usually a history of perinatal asphyxia or an association with severe respiratory distress syndrome. In most instances, there was a catastrophic deterioration with apnea, bradycardia, and a fall in hematocrit. The signs appeared in the first 3 weeks of life, with most beginning within the first 2 days of life. For term infants, there were usually histories of difficult breech deliveries with subsequent development of neurologic signs referable to brain stem compression, such as stupor or coma, cranial nerve abnormalities, apnea, bradycardia, and opisthotonus.

DIAGNOSIS

The lesion is suspected on the basis of the history and physical features described previously. Definitive diagnosis can be made by CT or MR scans.[156] In some instances, ultrasound scanning can demonstrate intracerebellar hemorrhage.[4]

MANAGEMENT

Early detection by CT, MR, or ultrasound scans is essential. Decisions concerning surgical or conservative management are based on the size of the lesion and the clinical state of the infant. Recovery without surgical intervention has been reported. Fishman and colleagues reported successful conservative management of four full-term infants with intracerebellar hemorrhage and concluded that, if the clinical picture is stable and there is no increase in intracranial pressure, supportive care and serial CT examinations may be all that is necessary.[157] Our experience with nonsurgical management of selected cases supports this notion.

PROGNOSIS

Most reports of intracerebellar hemorrhage in the premature infant are based on autopsy studies. For the infant with severe intracerebellar hemorrhage, the prognosis is poor. Scotti and associates, in a study of 700 newborns diagnosed using CT scans, observed eight cases of intracerebellar hemorrhage.[156] Four premature infants had concomitant IVH and died. In the four term infants, the intracerebellar hemorrhages were evacuated. All these infants survived but with neurologic handicap; two had quadriplegia and mental retardation, one had mental retardation, and one had hemiparesis.

EXAMPLES OF INTRACRANIAL HEMORRHAGE IN THE NEWBORN

Intracranial hemorrhage in the newborn may be associated uncommonly with trauma, hemorrhagic infarction, coagulation defects, vascular abnormalities, and tumors.

TRAUMA

Perinatal trauma usually results in subdural or primary subarachnoid hemorrhage. Occasionally, epidural or intracerebral hemorrhages occur, usually associated with other evidence of cranial injury, such as cephalhematoma or subgaleal hematoma. The extent and precise location of traumatic intracranial hemorrhage may be established with CT scans. Ultrasound scanning may be of value in detecting intracerebral hemorrhage.

VASCULAR ABNORMALITIES

Congenital arterial aneurysm and arteriovenous malformation are uncommon causes of intracranial hemorrhage in the newborn. Rupture of congenital aneurysms in the newborn has been reported.[159,160] The most common arteriovenous malformation encountered in this age group involves the vein of Galen.[161,162] High-output cardiac failure is the usual mode of presentation. Hydrocephalus occurs occasionally secondary to obstruction of the aqueduct by the dilated vein of Galen. Intracranial hemorrhage is more likely to occur later in childhood than in early infancy.

CEREBRAL TUMOR

Brain tumors in the newborn rarely present with intracranial hemorrhage. The most common presenting features are increased intracranial pressure and hydrocephalus.[163,164] However, intracranial hemorrhage has been the presenting feature in isolated cases.[164,165]

UNKNOWN CAUSE

Investigation of infants with neonatal seizures rarely reveals an intracerebral hemorrhage without an obvious cause.[166–168] In many of these cases, the outcome is favorable, although hydrocephalus may occur.

MANAGEMENT

General management of these miscellaneous varieties of intracranial hemorrhage should include provision of appropriate supportive care and control of seizures. The precise location and extent of the hemorrhage may be established by CT or ultrasound scanning. Treatment of underlying problems that may be responsible for the hemorrhage (*e.g.*, polycythemia, meningitis, disseminated intravascular coagulation, deficiency of clotting factors) should be undertaken as rapidly as possible. Surgical drainage of the hematoma may be indicated.

In infants with arterial aneurysms, surgical clipping has been successful in two cases. In infants with arteriovenous malformations, attention to cardiac failure is necessary. Although most of these infants die before surgery, approximately 30% have survived surgery.[162] In infants with cerebral tumors, surgical intervention may be required for removal of the tumor and for shunting the hydrocephalus.

REFERENCES

1. Volpe JJ. Neurology of the newborn. Philadelphia: WB Saunders, 1987.
2. Hill A, Volpe JJ, eds. Fetal neurology. International review of child neurology series. New York: Raven Press, 1989.
3. Lou HC, Friis-Hansen B. Arterial blood pressure elevations during motor activity and epileptic seizures in the newborn. Acta Pediatr Scand 1979;68:803.
4. Perlman JM, Volpe JJ. Seizures in the preterm infant: effects on cerebral blood flow velocity, intracranial pressure and arterial blood pressure. J Pediatr 1983;102:288.
5. Vannucci RC, Vasta F. Energy state of the brain in experimental neonatal status epilepticus. Pediatr Res 1985;19:396.
6. Wasterlain CG, Dwyer B. Brain metabolism during prolonged seizures in neonates. Adv Neurol 1983;34:241.
7. Wasterlain CG, Vert P, eds. Neonatal seizures. New York: Raven Press, 1990.
8. Younkin DP, Delivoria-Papadopoulos M, Maris J, Donlon E, Clancy R, Chance B. Cerebral metabolic effects of neonatal seizures measured with in vivo ^{31}P NMR spectroscopy. Ann Neurol 1986;20:513.
9. Volpe JJ. Neonatal seizures: current concepts and revised classification. Pediatrics 1989;84:422.
10. Sarnat HG. Pathogenesis of decerebrate seizures in the premature infant with intraventricular hemorrhage. J Pediatr 1975;87:154.
11. Mizrahi EM, Kellaway P. Characterization of seizures in neonates and young infants by time-synchronized electroencephalographic/polygraphic video monitoring. Ann Neurol 1984; 16:383.
12. Legido A, Clancy RR, Berman PH. Recent advances in the diagnosis, treatment and prognosis of neonatal seizures. Pediatr Neurol 1988;4:79.
13. Mizrahi EM, Kellaway P. Characterization and classification of neonatal seizures. Neurology 1987;37:1837.
14. Mizrahi EM. Neonatal seizures: problems in diagnosis and classification. Epilepsia 1987;28:546.
15. Sher MS, Painter MJ. Controversies concerning neonatal seizures. Pediatr Clin N Am 1989;2:281.
16. Radvanji-Bouvet MF, Vallecalle MH, Morel-Kaln F, et al. Seizures and electrical discharges in premature infants. Neuropediatrics 1985;43:266.
17. Dreyfus-Brisac C. The electroencephalogram of the premature and full-term infant. In: Kellaway P, Peterson I, eds.

Neurological and electroencephalographic correlative studies in infancy. New York: Grune & Stratton, 1964:186.
18. Kellaway P, Mizrahi EM. Neonatal seizures. In: Lueders H, Lesser RP, eds. Epilepsy: electroclinical syndromes. London: Springer-Verlag, 1987:13.
19. Blennow G. Benign infantile nocturnal myoclonus. Acta Paediatr Scand 1985;74:505.
20. Coulter DL, Allen RJ. Benign neonatal sleep myoclonus. Arch Neurol 1982;39:191.
21. Craig WS. Convulsive movements in the first ten days of life. Arch Dis Child 1960;35:336.
22. Hillman L, Hillman R, Dodson WE. Diagnosis, treatment and follow-up of neonatal mepivacaine intoxication secondary to paracervical and pudendal blocks during labor. J Pediatr 1979;95:472.
23. Herzlinger RA, Kandall SR, Vaughan HG. Neonatal seizures associated with narcotic withdrawal. J Pediatr 1977;91:638.
24. Doberczak T, Shanzer S, Senie R, Kendall S. Neurological and electroencephalographic effects of intrauterine cocaine exposure. J Pediatr 1988;113:354.
25. Roland EH, Volpe JJ. Effect of maternal cocaine use on the fetus and newborn: review of the literature. Pediatr Neurosci 1989;15:88.
26. Chaney N, Franke J, Wodlingten W. Cocaine convulsions in a breast-feeding baby. J Pediatr 1988;112:134.
27. Chasnoff I, Lewis D, Squires L. Cocaine intoxication in a breastfed infant. Pediatrics 1987;80:836.
28. Zonana J, Silvey K, Strimling B. Familial neonatal and infantile seizures: an autosomal dominant disorder. Am J Med Genet 1984;18:455.
29. Leppert M, Anderson VE, Quattlebaum T, et al. Benign familial neonatal convulsions linked to genetic markers on chromosome 20. Nature 1989;337:647.
30. Ryan SG, Wiznitzer M, Hollman C, Torres CM, Szekerosova M, Schneider SI. Benign familial neonatal convulsions: evidence for clinical and genetic heterogeneity. Ann Neurol 1991;29:469.
31. Eyre JA, Oozeer RC, Wilkingson AR. Diagnosis of neonatal seizures by continuous recording and rapid analysis of the electroencephalogram. Arch Dis Child 1983;58:785.
32. Clancy RR, Legido A, Lewis D. The effects of mental status and ictal duration on the clinical visibility of EEG-proven neonatal seizures. Ann Neurol 1986;20:411.
33. Clancy RR, Legido A, Lewis D. Occult neonatal seizures. Epilepsia 1988;29:256.
34. Lucas A, Morley R, Cole TJ. Adverse neurodevelopmental outcome of moderate hypoglycemia. Br Med J 1988;297:1304.
35. Donn SM, Grasela TH, Goldstein GW. Safety of higher loading doses of phenobarbital in the term newborn. Pediatrics 1985;75:1061.
36. Gal P, Toback J, Boer HR, et al. Efficacy of phenobarbital monotherapy for control of neonatal seizures. Neurology 1982;32:1401.
37. Gilman JT, Duchowny MS, Gal P, Weaver R. Phenobarbital serum concentration and response in neonatal seizures. Ann Neurol 1987;22:417.
38. Crawford TO, Mitchell WG, Snodgrass SR. Lorazepam in childhood status epilepticus and serial seizures: effectiveness and tachyphylaxis. Neurology 1987;37:190.
39. Deshmuch A, Witter W, Schnitzler E, Mangurten HH. Lorazepam in the treatment of refractory neonatal seizures. Am J Dis Child 1986;140:1042.
40. Roddy SM, McBride MC, Torres CT. Treatment of neonatal seizures with lorazepam. Ann Neurol 1987;22:412.
41. McDermott CA, Kowalczyk AL, Schmitzler ER, et al. Pharmacokinetics of lorazepam in critically ill neonates with seizures. J Pediatr 1992;120:479.
42. Koren G, Butt W, Rajchgot P, et al. Intravenous paraldehyde for seizure control in newborn infants. Neurology 1986;36:108.
43. Powell G, Painter MJ, Pippenger CE. Primidone therapy in refractory neonatal seizures. J Pediatr 1984;105:651.
44. Cloyd JC, Wright BD, Perrier D. Pharmacokinetics of thiopental in two patients treated for uncontrollable seizures. Epilepsia 1979;20:31.
45. Bergman I, Painter MJ, Hirsch RP, et al. Outcome in neonates with convulsions treated in an intensive care unit. Ann Neurol 1983;14:642.
46. Rose AL, Lombroso CT. Neonatal seizure states. A study of clinical, pathological and electroencephalographic features in 137 full-term babies with a long-term follow-up. Pediatrics 1972;45:404.
47. Tibbles JAR, Pritchard JS. The prognostic value of the electroencephalogram in neonatal convulsions. Pediatrics 1965;35:778.
48. Hill A. Current concepts of hypoxic-ischemic cerebral injury in the term newborn. Pediatr Neurol 1991;7:317.
49. Volpe JJ. Pathophysiology of perinatal hypoxic-ischemic brain injury. Can Med Assoc J 1989;(Suppl):38.
50. Nelson KB, Ellenberg JH. Antecedents of cerebral palsy: multivariate analysis of risk. N Engl J Med 1986;315:82.
51. Blair E, Stanley FJ. Intrapartum asphyxia: a rare cause of cerebral palsy. J Pediatr 1988;112:515.
52. Freeman JM, Nelson KB. Intrapartum asphyxia and cerebral palsy. Pediatrics 1988;82:240.
53. Grant A. The relationship between obstetrically preventable intrapartum asphyxia, abnormal neonatal neurologic signs and subsequent motor impairment in babies born at or after term. In: Kubli F, ed. Perinatal events and brain damage in surviving children. Berlin: Springer-Verlag, 1988:149–159.
54. Finer NN, Robertson CN, Richards RT, Pinnell LE, Peters KL. Hypoxic-ischemic encephalopathy in term neonates: perinatal factors and outcome. J Pediatr 1981;98:112.
55. Sarnat HB, Sarnat MS. Neonatal encephalopathy following fetal distress. Arch Dis Child 1976;33:696.
56. Lupton BA, Hill A, Roland EH, Whitfield MF, Flodmark O. Brain swelling in the asphyxiated term newborn: pathogenesis and outcome. Pediatrics 1988;82:139.
57. Levene MI, Evans DH. Medical management of raised intracranial pressure after severe birth asphyxia. Arch Dis Child 1985;60:12.
58. Levene MI, Evans DH, Forde A, et al. Value of intracranial pressure monitoring of asphyxiated newborn infants. Dev Med Child Neurol 1987;29:311.
59. Siegel MJ, Shackelford GD, Perlman JM, et al. Hypoxic-ischemic cerebral injury in the neonatal brain: a report of sonographic features with computed tomographic correlation. J Pediatr Radiol 1983;13:307.
60. Martin DJ, Hill A, Daneman AR, et al. Hypoxic-ischemic cerebral injury in the neonatal brain: a report of sonographic features with computed tomographic correlation. J Pediatr Radiol 1983;13:307.
61. McArdle CB, Richardson CJ, Hayden CK, et al. Abnormalities of the neonatal brain in MR imaging, part II. Hypoxic-ischemic brain injury. Radiology 1987;163:395.
62. Johnson MA, Pennock JM, Bydder GM, Dubowitz LMS, Thomas DJ, Young IR. Serial MR imaging in neonatal cerebral injury. AJNR 1987;8:89.
63. Van de Bor M, Guit GL, Schreuder AM, et al. Early detection of delayed myelination in preterm infants. Pediatrics 1989;84:407.
64. Flodmark O, Lupton BA, Li D, et al. Magnetic resonance imaging of periventricular leukomalacia (PVL) in childhood. Am J Neuroradiol 1989;10:110.

65. Keeney SE, Adcock EW, McArdle CB. Prospective observations of 100 high-risk neonates by high-field (1.5 Tesla) magnetic resonance imaging of the central nervous system. II. Lesions associated with hypoxic-ischemic encephalopathy. Pediatrics 1991;87:431.
66. O'Brien MJ, Ash JM, Gilday DL. Radionuclide brain scanning in perinatal hypoxia-ischemia. Dev Med Child Neurol 1979; 21:161.
67. Volpe JJ, Pasternak JF. Parasagittal cerebral injury in neonatal hypoxic-ischemic encephalopathy: clinical and neuroradiologic features. J Pediatr 1977;91:472.
68. Denays R, Pachterbeke TV, Tondeur M, et al. Brain single photon emission computed tomography in neonates. J Nucl Med 1989;30:1337.
69. Volpe JJ, Herscovitch P, Perlman JM, et al. Positron emission tomography in the asphyxiated term newborn: parasagittal impairment of cerebral blood flow. Ann Neurol 1985;17:287.
70. Hope PL, Reynolds EOR. Investigation of cerebral energy metabolism in newborn infants by phosphorus nuclear magnetic resonance spectroscopy. Clin Perinatal 1985;12:261.
71. Hope PL, Cady EB, Tofts PS, et al. Cerebral energy metabolism studied with phosphorus NMR spectroscopy in normal and birth asphyxiated infants. Lancet 1984;2:366.
72. Wyatt JS, Cope M, Delpy DT, Wray S, Richardson C, Reynolds EOR. Responses of cerebral vasculature to changes in arterial carbon dioxide measured by near infrared spectroscopy in newborn infants. Pediatr Res 1987;22:230.
73. Whyte HE, Taylor MJ, Menzies R, Chin KC, MacMillan LJ. Prognostic utility of visual evoked potentials in term asphyxiated neonates. Pediatr Neurol 1986;2:220.
74. Stockard JE, Stockard JJ, Kleinberg F, Westmoreland BF. Prognostic value of brain stem auditory evoked potentials in neonates. Arch Neurol 1983;40:360.
75. Lou HC, Lassen NA, Friis-Hansen B. Impaired autoregulation of cerebral blood flow in the distressed newborn. J Pediatr 1979;94:119.
76. Lou HC, Lassen NA, Tweed WA, et al. Pressure-passive cerebral blood flow and breakdown of the blood-brain barrier in experimental fetal asphyxia. Acta Pediatr Scan 1979;68:35.
77. Pryds O, Greisen G, Lou H, et al. Vasoparalysis associated with brain damage in asphyxiated term infants. J Pediatr 1990;119.
78. Roland EH, Hill A, Norman MG, Flodmark O, MacNab AJ. Selective brain stem injury in an asphyxiated newborn. Ann Neurol 1988;23:89.
79. Duffy TE, Cavazzuti M, Cruz NF, Sokoloff L. Local cerebral glucose metabolism in newborn dogs: effects of hypoxia and halothane anesthesia. Ann Neurol 1982;11:233.
80. Clark GD, Rothmann SM. Blockade of excitatory amino acid receptors protects anoxic hippocampal slices. Neuroscience 1987;21:665.
81. Choi DW, Koh J-Y, Peters S. Pharmacology of glutamate neurotoxicity in cortical cell culture: attenuation by NMDA antagonists. J Neurosci 1988;8:185.
82. Choi DW. Dextrorphan and dextromethorphan attenuate glutamate neurotoxicity. Brain Res 1987;403:333.
83. Benveniste H, Drejer J, Schousboe A, et al. Elevation of the extracellular concentrations of glutamate and aspartate in rat hippocampus during transient cerebral ischemia monitored by intracerebral microdialysis. J Neurochem 1984;43:1369.
84. Engelsen B. Neurotransmitter glutamate: its clinical importance. Acta Neurol Scand 1986;74:337.
85. Greenamyre JT, Penney JB, Young AB, et al. Evidence for transient perinatal glutamatergic innervation of globus pallidum. J Neurosci 1987;7:1022.
86. Barks JD, Silverstein FS, Sims K, et al. Glutamate recognition sites in human fetal brain. Neurosci Lett 1988;84:131.
87. Johnston MV, Coyle JT. Development of central neurotransmitter systems. In: Elliot K, Whelan J, eds. The fetus and independent life. Ciba symposium 86. London: Pitman, 1981;251–270.
88. Roland E, Flodmark O, Hill A. Thalamic hemorrhage with intraventricular hemorrhage in the full-term newborn. Pediatrics 1990;85:737.
89. DeReuck J, Chattha AS, Richardson EP Jr. Pathogenesis and evolution of periventricular leukomalacia in infancy. Arch Neurol 1972;27:229.
90. DeReuck JL. Cerebral angioarchitecture and perinatal brain lesions in premature and full-term infants. Acta Neurol Scand 1984;70:391.
91. Van den Bergh R, van der Eeken H. Anatomy and embryology of the cerebral circulation. Prog Brain Res 1968;30:1.
92. Leviton A, Gilles FH, Neff R, Yaney P. Multivariate analysis of risk of perinatal telencephalic leukoencephalopathy. Am J Epidemiol 1976;104:621.
93. Gilles FH, Averill DR Jr, Kerr CS. Neonatal endotoxin encephalopathy. Ann Neurol 1977;2:49.
94. Leviton A, Gilles FH. Acquired perinatal leukoencephalopathy. Ann Neurol 1984;16:1.
95. Armstrong D, Norman MG. Periventricular leukomalacia in neonates: complications and sequelae. Arch Dis Child 1974; 99:367.
96. Guzzetta F, Shackelford GD, Volpe S, et al. Periventricular intraparenchymal echodensities in the premature newborn: critical determinant of neurological status. Pediatrics 1986; 78:995.
97. Dolfin T, Skidmore MB, Fong KW, et al. Diagnosis and evolution of periventricular leukomalacia: a study with real-time ultrasound. Early Hum Dev 1984;9:105.
98. Dubowitz LMS, Bydder GM, Mushin J. Developmental sequence of periventricular leukomalacia. Arch Dis Child 1985; 60:349.
99. Roland EH, Jan JE, Hill A, et al. Cortical visual impairment following birth asphyxia. Pediatr Neurol 1986;2:133.
100. Vannucci RC. Current and potentially new management strategies for perinatal hypoxic-ischemic encephalopathy. Pediatrics 1990;85:961.
101. Donn SM, Goldstein GW, Schork A. Asphyxia neonatorum: a national survey of management practices. [Abstract] Pediatr Res 1986;20:461.
102. Barmada MA, Moosy J, Painter M. Pontosubicular necrosis and hyperoxemia. Pediatrics 1980;68:840.
103. McDonald JW, Silverstein FS, Johnston MW. MK-801 protects the neonatal brain from hypoxic-ischemic damage in the neonatal rat. Neurology 1989;39:713.
104. Hattori H, Morin AM, Schwartz PH, et al. Posthypoxic treatment with MK-801 reduces hypoxic-ischemic damage in the neonatal rat. Neurology 1989;39:713.
105. Germano IM, Bartkowski HM, Cassel MF, et al. The therapeutic value of nimodipine in experimental focal cerebral ischemia. J Neurosurg 1987;67:81.
106. Silverstein FS, Buchanan K, Hudson C, et al. Flunarizine limits hypoxia-ischemia induced morphologic injury in immature rat brain. Stroke 1986;17:477.
107. Gunn AJ, Mydlar T, Bennet L, et al. The neuroprotective actions of a calcium channel antagonist, flunarizine in the infant rat. Pediatr Res 1989;25:573.
108. Rosenberg AA, Murdaugh E, White CW. The role of oxygen free radicals in postasphyxia cerebral hypoperfusion in newborn lambs. Pediatr Res 1989;26:215.
109. Sasaki T, Nakagomi T, Kirino T, et al. Indomethacin ameliorates ischemic neuronal damage in the gerbil hippocampal CA1 sector. Stroke 1988;19:1399.
110. Lazzara A, Ahmann P, Dykes F, Brann AW, Schwartz J. Clini-

cal predictability of intraventricular hemorrhage in preterm infants. Pediatrics 1980;65:30.
111. Hill A, Shackelford GD, Volpe JJ. A potential mechanism for the pathogenesis of post-hemorrhagic hydrocephalus. Pediatrics 1984;73:1123.
112. Larroche JD. Developmental pathology of the neonate. Amsterdam: Elsevier/North Holland 1977:380.
113. Takashima S, Mito T, Ando Y. Pathogenesis of periventricular white matter hemorrhages in preterm infants. Brain Dev 1986;8:25.
114. Takashima S, Mito T, Houdou S, Ando Y. Relationship between periventricular hemorrhage, leukomalacia and brain stem lesions in prematurely born infants. Brain Dev 1989; 11:121.
115. Volpe JJ. Intraventricular hemorrhage and brain injury in the premature infant: neuropathology and pathogenesis. Clin Perinatol 1989;16:361.
116. Volpe JJ. Intraventricular hemorrhage in the premature infant—current concepts. Part I. Ann Neurol 1989;25:3.
117. Volpe JJ. Intraventricular hemorrhage in the premature infant—Current concepts. Part II. Ann Neurol 1989;35:109.
118. Pranzatelli MR, Stumpf DA. The metabolic consequences of experimental intraventricular hemorrhage. Neurology 1985; 35:1299.
119. Perlman JM, Goodman S, Kreusser KL, Volpe JJ. Reduction in intraventricular hemorrhage by elimination of fluctuating cerebral blood-flow velocity in preterm infants with respiratory distress syndrome. N Engl J Med 1985;313:1353.
120. Perlman JM, Volpe JJ. Are venous circulatory abnormalities important in the pathogenesis of hemorrhagic and/or ischemic cerebral injury? Pediatrics 1987;80:705.
121. Fanconi S, Duc G. Intratracheal suctioning in sick preterm infants: prevention of intracranial hypertension and cerebral hypoperfusion by muscle paralysis. Pediatrics 1987;79:538.
122. Morales WJ, Koerten J. Prevention of intraventricular hemorrhage in very low birthweight infants by maternally administered phenobarbital. Obstet Gynecol 1986;68:295.
123. Shankaran S, Cepeda EE, Ilagan N, et al. Antenatal phenobarbital for the prevention of neonatal intracerebral hemorrhage. Am J Obstet Gynecol 1986;154:53.
124. Donn SM, Roloff DW, Goldstein GW. Prevention of intraventricular hemorrhage in preterm infants by phenobarbitone: a controlled trial. Lancet 1981;2:215.
125. Morgan MEI, Massey RF, Cooke RWI. Does phenobarbitone prevent periventricular hemorrhage in very low-birth-weight infants: a controlled trial. Pediatrics 1982;70:186.
126. Whitelaw A, Placzek M, Dubowitz L, et al. Phenobarbitone for prevention of periventricular hemorrhage in very low-birth-weight infants: a randomized double-blind trial. Lancet 1983;2:1168-1170.
127. Bedard MP, Shankaran S, Slovis TL, et al. Effect of prophylactic phenobarbital on intraventricular hemorrhage in high-risk infants. Pediatrics 1984;73:435.
128. Kuban KC, Leviton A, Krishnamoorthy KS, et al. Neonatal intracranial hemorrhage and phenobarbital. Pediatrics 1986; 77:443.
129. Kuban KC, Skouteli H, Cherer A, et al. Hemorrhage, phenobarbital and fluctuating cerebral blood flow velocity in the neonate. Pediatrics 1988;82:548.
130. Ment LR, Duncan CC, Ehrenkranz RA, et al. Randomized low-dose indomethacin trial for the prevention of intraventricular hemorrhage in very low birth weight neonates. Ann Neurol 1987;22:406.
131. Ment LR, Duncan CC, Ehrenkranz RA, et al. Randomized low-dose indomethacin trial for prevention of intraventricular hemorrhage in very low-birth-weight neonates. J Pediatr 1988;112:948.
132. Hanigan WC, Kennedy G, Roemisch F, Anderson R, Cusack T, Powers W. Administration of indomethacin for the prevention of periventricular-intraventricular hemorrhage in high-risk neonates. J Pediatrics 1988;112:941.
133. Bandstra ES, Bauer CR, Duenas ML, et al. Prophylactic indomethacin for prevention of intraventricular hemorrhage: neurodevelopmental follow-up. [Abstract] Ann Neurol 1987; 22:427.
134. Pomerance JJ, Teal JG, Gogolok JF, et al. Maternally administered antenatal vitamin K_1: effect on neonatal prothrombin activity, partial thromboplastin time and intraventricular hemorrhage. Obstet Gynecol 1987;70:235.
135. Beverley DW, Pitts-Tucker TJ, Congdon PJ, et al. Prevention of intraventricular hemorrhage by fresh frozen plasma. Arch Dis Child 1985;60:710.
136. Van De Bor M, Briet E, Van Bel F, et al. Hemostasis and periventricular-intraventricular hemorrhage of the newborn. Am J Dis Child 1986;140:1131.
137. Cooke RWI, Morgan MEI. Prophylactic ethamsylate for periventricular hemorrhage. Arch Dis Child 1984;59:82.
138. Benson JWT, Hayward C, Osborne JP, et al. Multicentre trial of ethamsylate for prevention of periventricular hemorrhage in very low birthweight infants. Lancet 1986;1:1297.
138a. Morgan MEI, Benson JWT, Cooke RWI. Ethamsylate reduces the incidence of periventricular hemorrhage in very low birthweight babies. Lancet 1981;2:830.
139. Chiswick ML, Johnson M, Woodhall C, et al. Protective effect of vitamin E (D,L-alpha-tocopherol) against intraventricular hemorrhage in premature babies. Br Med J 1983;287;81.
140. Sinha S, Davies J, Toner N, et al. Vitamin E supplementation reduces frequency of periventricular hemorrhage in very preterm babies. Lancet 1987;1:466.
141. Speer ME, Blifeld C, Rudolph AJ, et al. Intraventricular hemorrhage and vitamin E in the very low-birth-weight infant: evidence for efficacy of early intramuscular vitamin E administration. Pediatrics 1984;74:1107.
142. Phelps DL, Rosenbaum AL, Isenberg SJ, et al. Tocopherol efficacy and safety for preventing retinopathy of prematurity: a randomized, controlled, double-masked trial. Pediatrics 1987;79:489.
143. Coulter DM, LaPine TR, Gooch WM III. Treatment to prevent postnatal loss of brain water reduces the risk of intracranial hemorrhage in the beagle puppy. Pediatr Res 1985;19:1322.
144. Rubin RC, Hochwald GM, Tiell M, Mizutani H, Ghatak N. Hydrocephalus and ultrastructural changes in the preshunted cortical mantel. Surgical Neurology 1976;5:109.
145. Fishman RA, Greer M. Experimental obstructive hydrocephalus. Arch Neurol 1963;8:156.
146. Wozniak M, MacLean DE, Raymondi AJ. Micro- and macrovascular changes as the direct cause of congenital murine hydrocephalus. J Neurosurg 1975;43:535.
147. Hill A, Volpe JJ. Decrease in pulsatile flow in the anterior cerebral arteries in infantile hydrocephalus. Pediatrics 1982; 67:4.
148. Volpe JJ, Herscovitch P, Perlman JM, et al. Positron emission tomography in the newborn: extensive impairment of regional cerebral blood flow with intraventricular hemorrhage and hemorrhagic intracerebral involvement. Pediatrics 1983; 72:589.
149. Ehle A, Sklar F. Visual evoked potentials in infants with hydrocephalus. Neurology 1979;29:1541.
150. Ventriculomegaly Trial Group. Randomised trial of early tapping in neonatal posthemorrhagic ventricular dilation. Arch Dis Child 1990;65:3.
151. Krishnamoorthy KS, Shannon DC, Deloong GR, Todres ID, Davis KR. Neurological sequelae in the survivors of neonatal intraventricular hemorrhage. Pediatrics 1979;64:233.

152. Papile L-A, Burstein J, Burstein R, Koffler H. Incidence and evolution of subependymal and intraventricular hemorrhage. J Pediatr 1978;92:529.
153. Bergman I, Bauer RE, Barmada MA, et al. Intracerebral hemorrhage in the full-term neonatal infant. Pediatrics 1985; 74:488.
154. Grunnet ML, Shields WO. Cerebellar hemorrhage in the premature infant. J Pediatr 1975;88:605.
155. Martin R, Roesmann U, Fanaroff A. Massive intracerebellar hemorrhage in low birth weight infants. J Pediatr 1976;89:290.
156. Scotti G, Flodmark O, Harwood-Nash DC, Humphries RP. Posterior fossa hemorrhages in the newborn. J Comput Assist Tomogr 1981;5:68.
157. Fishman MA, Percy AK, Cheek WR, Speer ME. Successful conservative management of cerebellar hematomas in term neonates. J Pediatr 1981;98:466.
158. Pape KE, Wigglesworth JS. Hemorrhage, ischemia and the perinatal brain. Clinics in developmental medicine, 1969–70. London: Spastics International Medical Publications, 1979: 26.
159. Grode ML, Saunders M, Carton CA. Subarachnoid hemorrhage secondary to ruptured aneurysms in infants. J Neurosurg 1978;49:898.
160. Lee YJ, Kandall SR, Ghali VS. Intracerebral arterial aneurysm in the newborn. Arch Neurol 1978;35:171.
161. Iannucci AM, Buonanno F, Rizzuto N, Mazza C, Vivenza C, Maschio A. Arteriovenous aneurysm of the vein of Galen. J Neurosci 1979;40:29.
162. Watson DG, Smith RR, Brann AW. Arteriovenous malformation of the vein of Galen. Am J Dis Child 1976;130:520.
163. Jellinger K, Sunder-Plassman M. Connatal intracranial tumours. Neuropadiatrie 1973;4:46.
164. Sandbank R. Congenital astrocytoma. J Pathol Bacteriol 1962; 84:226.
165. Rothman SM, Nelson JS, DeVivo DC, Coxe WS. Congenital astrocytoma presenting with intracerebral hematoma. J Neurosurg 1979;51:237.
166. Aggett PJA, Harvey DR, Till K. Intracerebral hematoma with communicating hydrocephalus in a neonate. Proc R Soc Med 1976;69:877.
167. Cartwright GW, Culbertson K, Schreiner RL, Garg BP. Changes in clinical presentation of term infants with intracranial hemorrhage. Dev Med Child Neurol 1979;21:730.
168. Chaplin ER Jr, Goldstein GW, Norman D. Neonatal seizures, intracerebral hematoma, and subarachnoid hemorrhage in full-term infants. Pediatrics 1979;63:812.

Neonatology: Pathophysiology and Management of the Newborn, Fourth Edition,
edited by Gordon B. Avery, Mary Ann Fletcher, and Mhairi G. MacDonald.
J.B. Lippincott Company, Philadelphia © 1994.

chapter 50

Neurosurgery

THOMAS H. MILHORAT
JOHN I. MILLER

The surgical treatment of disorders affecting the newborn nervous system has advanced significantly. Contributing to this advance have been an improved understanding of the developing nervous system, improved methods of neurologic diagnosis, and improvements in surgical technique and supportive management. In some centers, the establishment of specialized units for the care of newborn patients has greatly enhanced the quality of preoperative and postoperative care.

EXCESSIVE CRANIAL ENLARGEMENT

Of the various neurologic disorders requiring surgical attention in the neonatal period, a significant number are associated with increased intracranial pressure. In this age group, owing to the patency of the cranial sutures, the most prominent clinical finding is usually an excessive rate of cranial enlargement. Because expansion of the cranial cavity tends to neutralize a rise in intracranial pressure, this may delay the onset of more obvious signs such as vomiting, papilledema, and cranial nerve palsies. For practical purposes, therefore, the differential diagnosis of an abnormally enlarged head in the neonatal period can be regarded as equivalent to the differential diagnosis of increased intracranial pressure.

In the evaluation of patients with excessive cranial enlargement, a systematic approach is desirable. A complete history and physical examination are required, and the diagnosis should be confirmed by plotting the patient's head circumference on a standard chart according to age and gender. More important than any single measurement indicating abnormal enlargement of the head are serial measurements demonstrating an excessive rate of growth. Examination of the head should include percussion, auscultation, and transillumination. Each patient deserves a thorough neurologic examination, and special attention should be given to the following signs of increased intracranial pressure:

- distention of the scalp veins
- palpable separation of the cranial sutures
- enlargement and distention of the fontanelles
- unilateral or bilateral sixth nerve palsies
- setting-sun eye sign.

In some cases, it is desirable to obtain routine skull radiographs at the time of the initial evaluation so that fractures can be excluded and the pattern of sutural separation can be defined.

The diagnostic procedure of choice for evaluating infants with presumed disorders of the nervous system is magnetic resonance imaging (MRI). This remarkable technique avoids the hazards of x-ray exposure and is an imaging breakthrough of the highest order that can be expected to supplant computed tomography (CT) scanning for all but a few diagnostic problems. Structural MRI uses magnet gantries in the range of 0.3 to 1.5 Tesla units and images anatomic slices of the brain in a detail comparable to that obtained with the prosector's knife (Fig. 50-1). One feature of MR images is their ability to distinguish subtle differences between gray and white matter density, thus allowing the display of certain lesions revealed heretofore only at the time of surgery or autopsy. Such lesions include degenerative and demyelinating diseases, polymicrogyria, hemangiomas, gray matter ectopias, diffuse granulomas, and low-grade gliomas (Fig. 50-2). To distinguish properly white matter atrophy, brain edema, and gliosis during the early months of infancy, it is necessary to appreciate the MRI correlates of normal myelinization.[1] Lesions that alter the blood–brain barrier often are brilliantly enhanced by the use of a paramagnetic contrast agent such as gadolinium,[2] which is indicated in the evaluation of tumors and inflammations.

Magnetic resonance techniques have been applied successfully to angiographic imaging.[3] Magnetic resonance angiography is noninvasive and provides detailed information concerning normal arterial and venous anatomy (Fig. 50-3), although it has not replaced conventional angiography in the conduct of surgical procedures. Magnetic resonance angiography is perhaps the ideal method for screening infants and children with presumed arteriovenous malformations, cerebral arterial occlusions, dural sinus thrombosis, and vascular tumors.

With larger-magnet gantries, in the range of 2.5 to 5 Tesla units, ionic MRI is possible, providing functional scans of brain chemistry and metabolism. This information doubtless will contribute much to the understanding of the pathophysiology of nervous system diseases and promises to shed new light on normal and abnormal developmental processes.

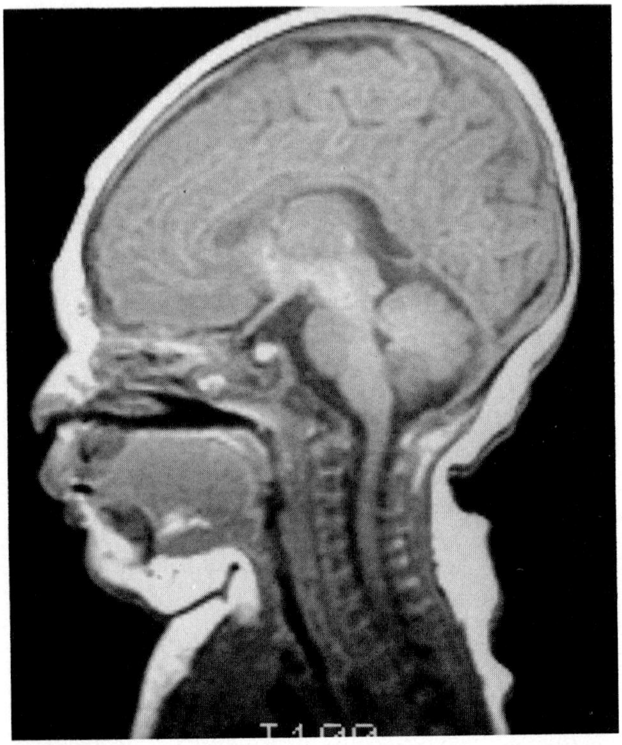

FIG. 50–1. Sagittal magnetic resonance imaging scan of a normal 4-month-old infant.

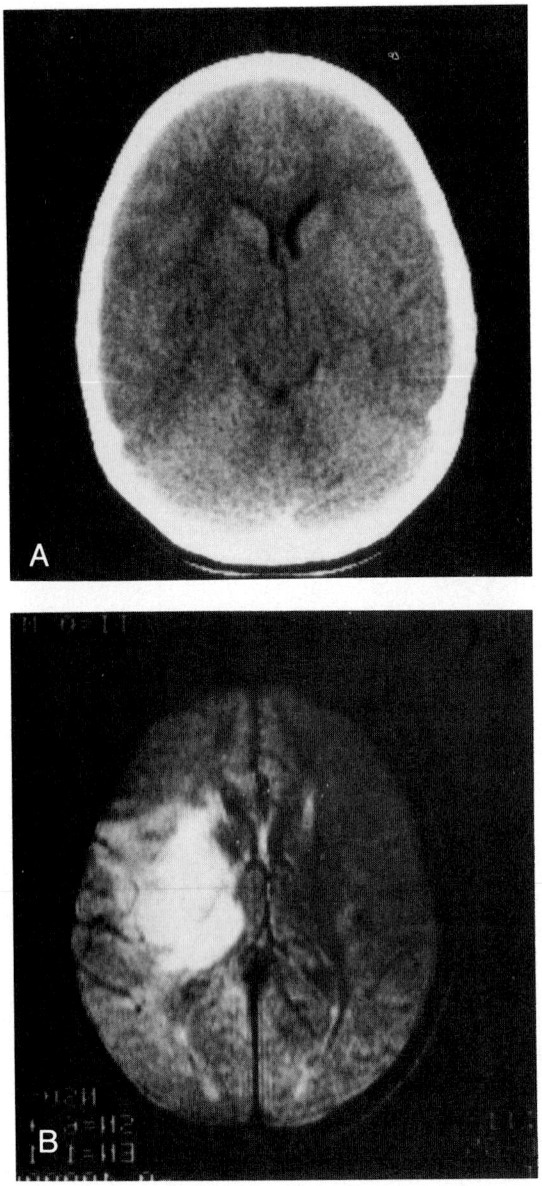

FIG. 50–2. Comparison of **(A)** computed tomography (CT) and **(B)** magnetic resonance imaging (MRI) scans depicting diffuse grade I astrocytoma of the left hemisphere. The CT scan shows slight hypodensity of left insular area with compression of left frontal horn. The MRI scan demonstrates the precise outline of the tumor.

Until MRI scans become widely available, the pediatrician must continue to rely on cranial CT. This is a noninvasive procedure and carries with it an x-ray exposure risk no greater than that for a standard skull series.[4] For screening purposes, eight cuts of a noncontrast scan with a standard axial plane usually is adequate. Contrast scans should be performed in any

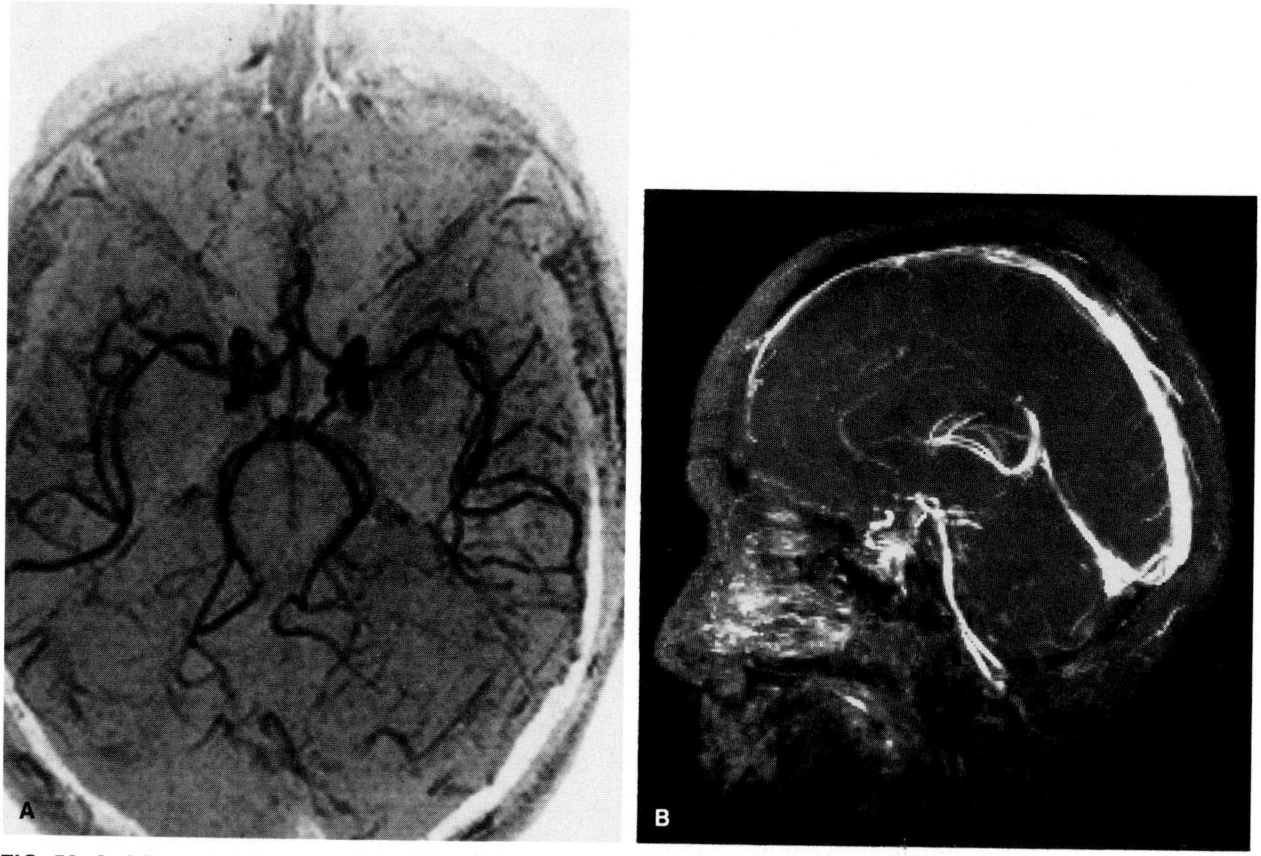

FIG. 50–3. Magnetic resonance angiography using the three-dimensional time-of-flight technique. **(A)** A horizontal section shows the intracranial arteries. **(B)** A sagittal section shows the dural sinuses and deep cerebral veins. (From Link KM. Magnetic resonance angiography. MRI Decisions 1991;5:11.)

questionable case and are especially helpful for enhancing vascular lesions such as tumors, subdural hematomas, and arteriovenous malformations.

Computed tomography scanning may be regarded as highly reliable for the diagnosis of hydrocephalus, intracranial hemorrhage, and congenital cysts and tumors. The procedure is somewhat less reliable in the assessment of subdural effusions and occasionally will miss isodense collections. Computed tomography scanning cannot be expected to provide complete or even adequate information in all cases, and the physician must decide on the basis of available clinical evidence whether or not additional studies are necessary.

Ultrasonography, much in vogue in recent years, provides crude neurodiagnostic information but is helpful in the management of very young infants. In particular, a portable sonogram is perhaps the most practical means for screening premature infants in the neonatal intensive care unit for disorders such as intraventricular hemorrhage and hydrocephalus. The anterior fontanelle is used as an ultrasonic window through which imaging of the intracranial cavity is performed. Ultrasonography can be obtained repeatedly at the bedside and involves no risk to the patient whatsoever. It is sufficient to say that a precise definition of intracranial pathology is not possible with ultrasonography and is achieved best by MRI or CT scanning.

BENIGN ENLARGEMENTS

Benign cranial enlargement may be caused by a number of easily recognizable conditions, including cephalohematoma, subgaleal effusion, and edema of the scalp. These disorders usually are the result of birth or neonatal trauma and tend to resolve spontaneously over a matter of days or weeks. Skull radiographs should be obtained to rule out fractures, and the hematocrit should be followed, since occult blood loss frequently exceeds that evidenced by the visible lesion. Surgery rarely is indicated unless the fracture is depressed.

Constitutional macrocephaly is the most important benign condition that can be confused with pathologic enlargement of the head. The diagnosis requires a convincing family history, and, if growth charts, photographs, and skull radiographs of other members of the family are available, these should be examined for comparisons. In patients with true constitutional macrocephaly, the absolute circumference of the head is large, but serial measurements demonstrate a proportional rather than an excessive rate of growth. The neurologic examination is negative, and signs of increased intracranial pressure are absent. An MRI or CT scan is most reassuring in such cases and reveals normal-sized ventricles without displacement or deformity. If continued follow-up confirms the findings of proportionate head growth and normal development, further diagnostic tests probably are unnecessary.

PATHOLOGIC ENLARGEMENTS

Pathologic cranial enlargement may be caused by such neonatal disorders as congenital and acquired hydrocephalus, subdural collections, intracranial hemorrhage, intracranial cysts and tumors, and various disorders causing brain swelling or encephalopathy.

CONGENITAL AND ACQUIRED HYDROCEPHALUS

Taken as a group, hydrocephalus constitutes the ranking cause of pathologic cranial enlargement. Congenital and acquired forms are recognized, and examples of the former are more common, in an approximate incidence of 3:1. Table 50-1 indicates the wide spectrum of congenital and acquired lesions that can cause hydrocephalus.

Etiology and Pathology. Etiologic factors responsible for congenital hydrocephalus are for the most part obscure. In a small number of cases, teratogenesis (*e.g.*, exposure to radiation), intrauterine infection (*e.g.*, toxoplasmosis, cytomegalic inclusion disease), maternal malnutrition, and genetic factors (*e.g.*, X-linked hydrocephalus) can be shown to play a role. In patients with acquired neonatal hydrocephalus, the most important etiologic factors include meningitis, trauma, and subarachnoid hemorrhage.[4]

Knowledge about the pathology of hydrocephalus was put on firm ground in 1949 with the publication of *Observations on the Pathology of Hydrocephalus* by Dorothy Russell.[5] One of the most important contributions of this monograph, and one that has been upheld to date, is the observation that in almost every case of hydrocephalus there is a pathologic obstruction at some point along the pathway of cerebrospinal fluid (CSF) circulation.[6,7] In congenital hydrocephalus, the pathologic obstruction usually is within the ventricular system proximal to the subarachnoid space (*i.e.*, noncommunicating hydrocephalus). Lesions of the aqueduct of Sylvius predominate, and in some cases there are multiple anomalies of the nervous system. In acquired hydrocephalus, the pathologic obstruction usually is in the subarachnoid space distal to the ventricular system (*i.e.*, communicating hydrocephalus). In these cases, chronic inflammation or fibrosis of the leptomeninges, or both, is the typical histologic finding.

The secondary pathologic effects of prolonged ventricular enlargement have been extensively summarized by Russell and Milhorat.[5–7] The most important findings include diffuse atrophy of the white matter, spongy edema of the brain surrounding the ventricles, and fibrosis of the choroid plexuses. As noted by Penfield and Elvidge,[8] the atrophic process in hydrocephalus involves a sequential destruction of glial cells, myelin, and axonal collaterals. Neurons are se-

TABLE 50–1
CLASSIFICATION OF HYDROCEPHALUS

Noncommunicating Hydrocephalus	Communicating Hydrocephalus
I. Congenital lesions A. Aqueductal obstruction (*i.e.*, stenosis) 1. Gliosis 2. Forking 3. True narrowing 4. Septum B. Atresia of the foramina of Luschka and Magendie (*i.e.*, Dandy–Walker cyst) C. Masses 1. Benign intracranial cysts 2. Vascular malformations 3. Tumors II. Acquired lesions A. Aqueductal stenosis (*i.e.*, gliosis) B. Ventricular inflammation and scars C. Masses 1. Tumors 2. Nonneoplastic masses	I. Congenital lesions A. Arnold–Chiari malformation B. Encephalocele C. Leptomeningeal inflammations D. Lissencephaly E. Congenital absence of arachnoid granulations II. Acquired lesions A. Leptomeningeal inflammations 1. Infections 2. Hemorrhage 3. Particulate matter B. Masses 1. Tumors 2. Nonneoplastic masses C. Platybasia III. Oversecretion of CSF caused by choroid plexus papilloma

CSF, cerebrospinal fluid.
From Milhorat TH. Pediatric neurosurgery. Philadelphia: FA Davis, 1978:96.

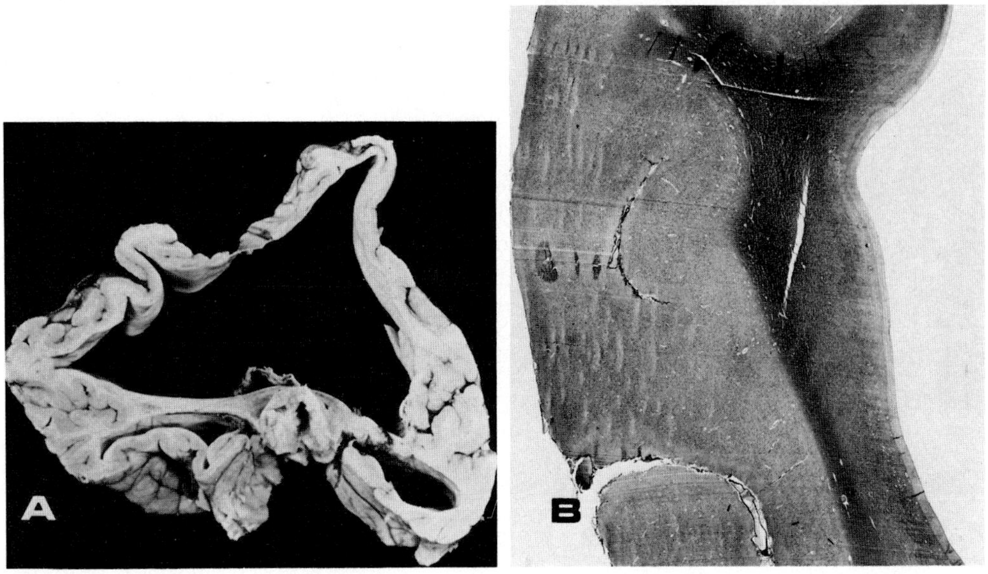

FIG. 50–4. **(A)** Severe hydrocephalus secondary to aqueductal stenosis. The cerebral mantle has been reduced to a thin ribbon and the lateral ventricles resemble a huge monolocular chamber as a result of rupture of the septum pellucidum. **(B)** Microscopic section shows relative sparing of the cortical gray matter and marked atrophy of the white matter. (Luxol blue stain; from Milhorat TH. Hydrocephalus and the cerebrospinal fluid. Baltimore: Williams & Wilkins, 1972:63.)

lectively spared (Fig. 50-4), and this may explain why the thickness of the cerebral mantle is not a reliable prognostic criterion in patients with neonatal hydrocephalus.[9]

Diagnosis. The diagnosis of congenital hydrocephalus is sometimes obvious at birth on the basis of gross cranial enlargement. In less extreme examples and in cases of acquired hydrocephalus, the head size at birth is normal and there is gradual cranial enlargement. Whereas early symptoms may be minimal, anorexia, vomiting, and lethargy or hyperirritability are common as the condition advances. The general physical examination may demonstrate any or all these nonspecific signs of increased intracranial pressure. If there is significant ventricular dilation, percussion of the head produces a hollow or cracked-pot sound over the dilated segments of the ventricular system (*i.e.*, Macewen sign). Transillumination of the head usually is negative unless the cerebral mantle is 1 cm or less in thickness. The configuration of the head and the pattern of sutural diastasis may suggest the type of hydrocephalus. In patients with aqueductal stenosis, for example, the cranial vault is expansive, and the posterior fossa is small. This is in contrast to patients with communicating hydrocephalus in whom the head is symmetrically enlarged with splitting of all of the major sutures above and below the tentorium. In patients with congenital atresia of the foramina of Luschka and Magendie, there is selective enlargement of the posterior fossa.

Ultimately, the definitive diagnosis of hydrocephalus requires special tests. This can be achieved most accurately by an MRI scan, which provides exquisite anatomic images and avoids the hazards of x-ray exposure (Fig. 50-5). Until MRI scanning becomes widely available, CT scanning remains a simple and reliable means of evaluating infants with suspected hydrocephalus (Fig. 50-6). In the initial evaluation of new patients, it generally is advisable to obtain both contrast and noncontrast CT scans so that congenital mass lesions, such as tumors and vascular malformations, can be ruled out. If these lesions are suggested by CT or MRI scanning, cerebral angiography is indicated to provide detailed information on vascular anatomy.

Under special circumstances, CT metrizamide cisternography or ventriculography may be helpful in defining CSF flow and dynamics. Such information may be necessary to distinguish certain types of communicating and noncommunicating hydrocephalus and also is useful in the assessment of shunt patency, intraventricular loculations, and the communicating nature of intracranial cysts and fluid collections. There appears to be little indication for the time-honored procedures of air ventriculography and pneumoencephalography.

Antenatal Diagnosis. Severe hydrocephalus or hydranencephaly usually can be diagnosed by week 28 of gestation, using pelvic ultrasonography. In such cases, it is advisable to consider the option of cesar-

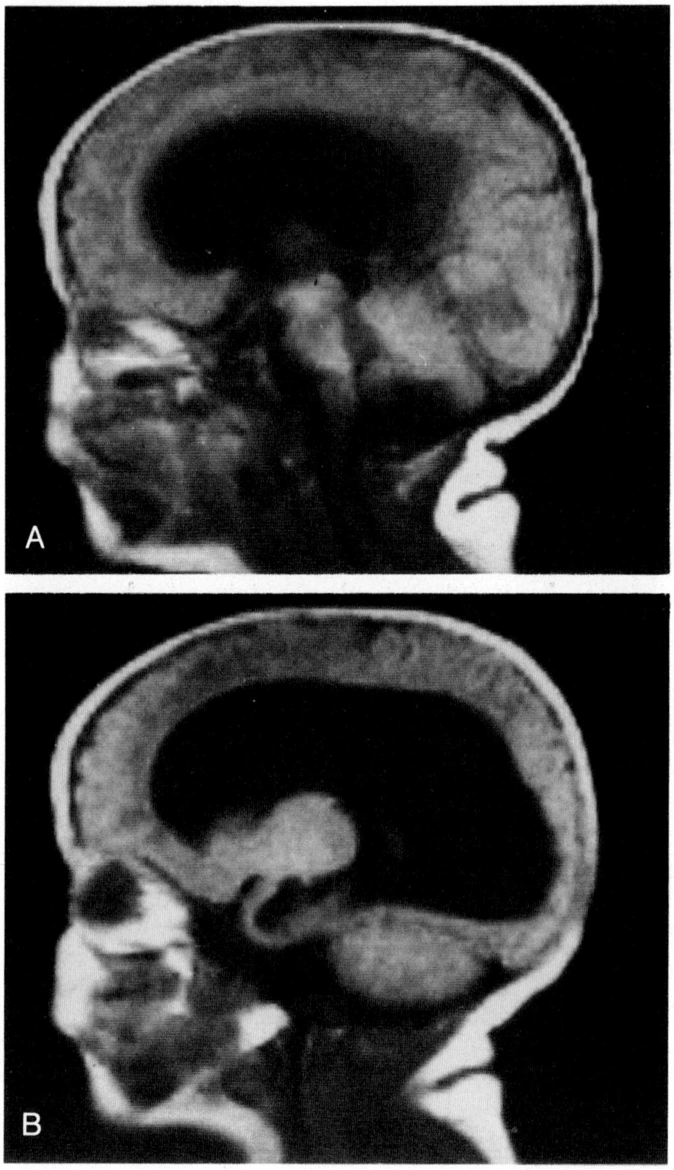

FIG. 50–5. Magnetic resonance imaging scans of congenital hydrocephalus demonstrate marked ventriculomegaly and stenosis of the aqueduct of Sylvius. **(A)** Sagittal section. **(B)** Parasagittal section.

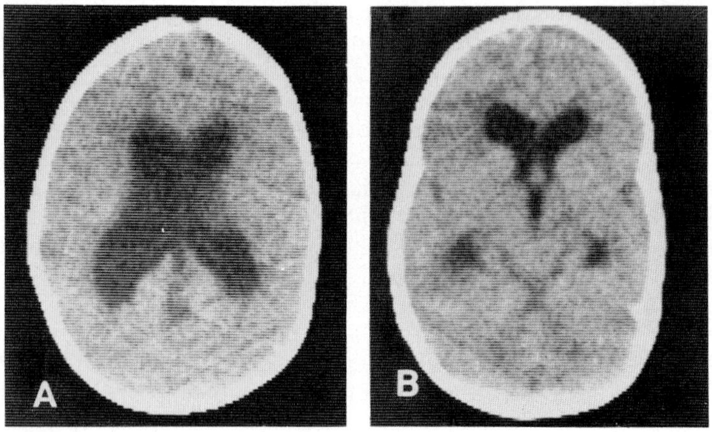

FIG. 50–6. Computed tomography scans of an infant with congenital aqueductal stenosis. The lateral and third ventricles are enlarged and the fourth ventricle is small or absent.

ean section for purposes of early shunting any time after week 34. Delivery before this time is associated with many risks, including hyaline membrane disease, and there is no convincing evidence that the pathologic effects of ventricular enlargement are sufficiently pronounced or irreversible to mandate delivery before viability of the infant is predictable. Techniques for intrauterine shunting have not been perfected and must be regarded as being of investigational interest only.

Treatment. Since the introduction of valve-regulated shunts in the 1950s, the outlook for patients with neonatal hydrocephalus has improved steadily. As experience has grown, the morbidity and mortality of these operations have been greatly reduced and the 5-year survival rate in an unselected series approaches 90%.[4,10,11] Two operations can be recommended for widespread use (Fig. 50-7): the ventriculoperitoneal shunt and the ventriculoatrial shunt. The former, because it is easier to implant, somewhat easier to revise, and much easier to lengthen electively in growing children, has become the most popular shunting procedure. It is the preferred shunt for infants and young children, and is undoubtedly safer than the ventriculoatrial shunt in patients in whom the CSF has been recently infected.

Unfortunately, for most patients with infantile hydrocephalus, a single operation is rarely curative, and multiple revisions are required to accommodate growth. In practical terms, this means that for full-term infants, a shunt performed in the neonatal period usually will require at least one elective revision before somatic growth is completed. For premature infants, the number of elective revisions is greater, and it usually is necessary to lengthen the original shunt by the end of the first year of life. It is important to point out that these elective revisions do not include revisions for shunt malfunctioning, which may be many. Obstruction and infection are the most common complications of ventriculoperitoneal shunts, and septicemia, thromboembolism, and shunt nephritis are of additional concern in patients with ventriculoatrial shunts.[4,6,12]

Despite the popularity of ventricular shunting operations, the treatment of neonatal hydrocephalus is not limited to these procedures. In a small number of cases, direct operations such as the removal of congenital cysts and tumors, suboccipital craniectomy for lesions of the craniospinal junction, and fenestration procedures for Dandy–Walker cysts and septa occluding the aqueduct of Sylvius may be effective in reestablishing the normal flow of CSF. Choroid plexectomy, however, has no place in the treatment of hydrocephalus, and there is no evidence that commercially available drugs such as acetazolamide (Diamox; Lederle Laboratories, Pearl River, NY) are of more than temporizing value in the treatment of this disorder.[4,6,7,13]

Prognosis. The prognosis of patients with neonatal hydrocephalus is uncertain owing to the lack of long-term follow-up. In most operative series, late complications occur with discouraging frequency, and it is evident that a steady decrease in the survival rate occurs the longer a series is followed.[4,6] For the purposes of short-term prognosis, it is useful to divide patients into three groups:

1. Patients with progressive hydrocephalus and evidence of irreversible damage of the brain or other major organs (*e.g.*, multiple congenital anomalies and cerebral atrophy secondary to meningitis). In this group, prognosis is uniformly poor, and shunting operations have little to offer.

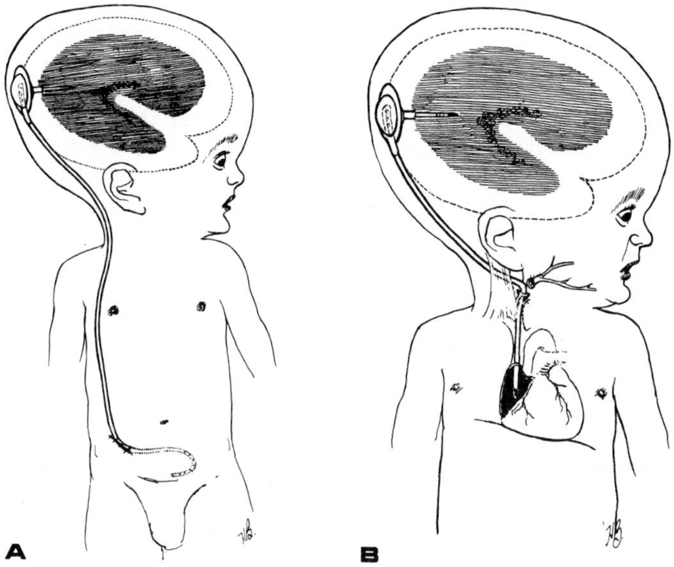

FIG. 50–7. **(A)** Ventriculoperitoneal shunt. **(B)** Ventriculoatrial shunt. (From Milhorat TH. Hydrocephalus and the cerebrospinal fluid. Baltimore: Williams & Wilkins, 1972:197.)

2. Patients with progressive hydrocephalus and little or no evidence of irreversible brain damage. In this group, prompt treatment is indicated, and the prognosis varies according to the severity of hydrocephalus and the success or failure of treatment. Although there is no definite correlation between the thickness of the cerebral mantle and the eventual development of mental and motor skills,[9] a cerebral mantle of 2 cm or more usually is associated with a good prognosis (*i.e.*, the patient is capable of functioning at a competitive level), and a cerebral mantle of 1 cm or less usually is associated with a poor prognosis.[14] The most optimistic results of 5-year follow-up in an unselected series indicate a survival rate of 90%, with approximately two thirds of the surviving patients having an intelligence quotient of 75 or above.[4,6] Detailed information on intellectual impairment occurring with hydrocephalus has been provided by Young and colleagues.[11]
3. Patients with arrested hydrocephalus. This diagnosis requires evidence of stable head size if the head is already enlarged and continuing psychomotor development with increasing age. If neurologic deficits are present, these remain stable or gradually improve. Patients in this group must be carefully followed so that slowly progressive, or "normal-pressure," hydrocephalus can be ruled out.[4,6,7]

SUBDURAL COLLECTIONS

Of the various causes of pathologic cranial enlargement in the neonatal period, the incidence of subdural collections ranks second only to hydrocephalus. Hematoma, hygroma, and effusion are the three main pathologic types, and the clinical management of these lesions is sufficiently similar to allow them to be considered a single diagnostic entity.

Etiology and Pathology. Bleeding into the subdural space is almost always of venous origin and results from the tearing of bridging veins that run from the cerebral surface to the major dural sinuses. Trauma at delivery and postnatal injuries to the head account for most cases. Less commonly, subdural hemorrhage may occur as a consequence of bleeding dyscrasias, immunization reactions, dehydration, and prolonged illnesses associated with cachexia. In neurosurgical practice, subdural collections are seen as an occasional complication of overshunting for hydrocephalus, and result from too rapid decompression of the cerebral ventricles. Hygromatous collections are thought to arise from traumatic laceration of the pia-arachnoid, and subdural effusions almost always are the result of meningeal infection.

In contrast to fluid collections in other parts of the body, accumulations in the subdural space are poorly tolerated. In many instances, the subdural fluid prompts a foreign body response that is characterized by a proliferation of fibroblasts from the dural and pia-arachnoidal surfaces. In time, a thick outer membrane contributed by the dura and a thin inner membrane contributed by the pia-arachnoid may completely envelop the lesion. In cases of acute hematoma, lysis of the clot may produce an osmotic gradient that draws additional fluid into the subdural space, and there is accumulating evidence that an important cause of persistent or enlarging lesions is spontaneous rebleeding from the neovascular membranes.[15] Because subdural hygromas generally have less vascular membranes and contain fluid not unlike CSF, they rarely undergo progressive expansion. In cases of meningitic subdural effusion, the accumulation may resolve spontaneously once the active infection subsides. Chapter 49 provides further discussion of the etiology and pathology of subdural collections.

Diagnosis. A history of trauma or infection is obtained in most patients with chronic subdural accumulations. In patients with subdural empyema, there often is a history of persistent or recurrent fever after an adequate course of treatment for meningitis. On physical examination, the following findings may be helpful in distinguishing subdural collections from hydrocephalus:

- The configuration of the head appears square rather than rounded.
- The transillumination test is positive unless the lesion consists of frank blood or pus.
- In cases of acute subdural hematoma, funduscopic examination may reveal subhyaloid hemorrhages as a consequence of blood dissecting through the dural sheaths surrounding the optic nerves.

The procedure of choice for screening patients with suspected subdural collections is CT or MRI (Fig. 50-8). This usually avoids the need for cerebral angiography and provides much useful information concerning the size and location of the collections, the presence of associated cerebral lesions such as contusions, and the size of the cerebral ventricles. In infants, chronic subdural collections occur bilaterally in approximately 80% to 85% of the cases.[4] Computed tomography typically reveals an area of decreased density between the brain and inner table of the skull, whereas acute clots invariably are dense, and liquefying lesions often are isodense (see Fig. 50-8).

Conventional radiographs of the skull rarely are helpful in the diagnostic evaluation of subdural collections but should be obtained along with radiographs of the long bones in infants who are suspected victims of criminal battering. Isotopic brain scanning is positive in only 40% to 60% of patients with this lesion,[4] and electroencephalography (EEG) is abnormal in less than 50% of the cases.

The definitive diagnosis of acute subdural hematoma requires direct surgical exploration through a burr hole or craniotomy. Negative subdural taps do not exclude this diagnosis because clotted blood may

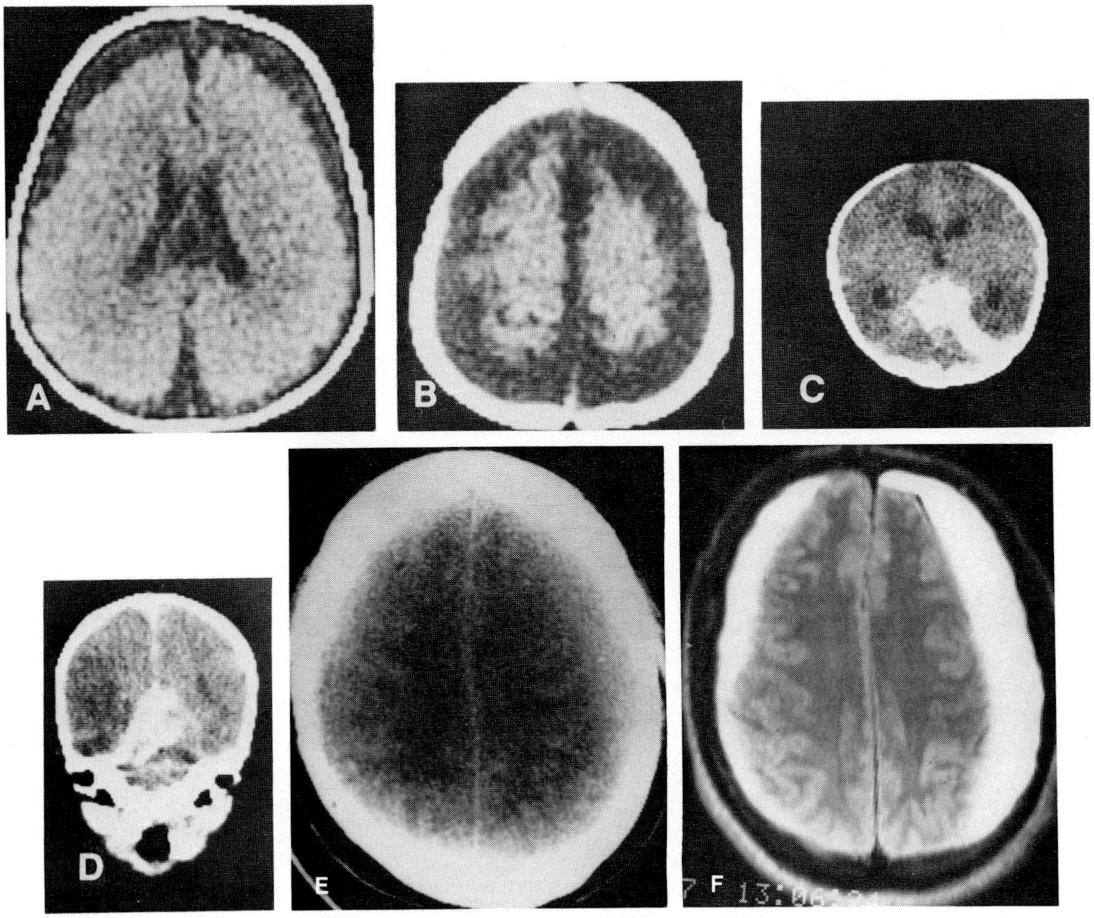

FIG. 50–8. **(A, B)** Computed tomography (CT) scans demonstrate hypodense extraaxial collections indicative of chronic, bilateral subdural hematomas. **(C, D)** Acute subdural hematoma appears as a dense clot above and below the tentorium in CT scans of a 1-day-old infant after traumatic forceps delivery. **(E)** CT scan in a patient with isodense bilateral subdural hematomas. **(F)** T2-weighted MRI scan in the same patient as shown in **(E)** demonstrates well defined subdural collections.

not be recoverable through the needle. In contrast, the definitive diagnosis of chronic subdural collections is made by subdural taps. This is most safely carried out in the hospital rather than in the office or outpatient department and should be preceded in most cases by a hematocrit to rule out anemia.

Treatment. The surgical treatment of neonatal subdural collections has not been fully standardized. In cases of acute hematoma, the lesion is evacuated through multiple burr holes or a craniotomy. In chronic accumulations, serial taps through the anterior fontanelle may be curative and can be repeated on a daily basis for 3 or 4 weeks. If, at the end of this time, there is no evidence that the lesion is resolving, surgical treatment is indicated. Of the many available operations, a subdural shunt to the peritoneal cavity is usually the safest and most effective procedure, unless the lesion is infected or contains more than 500 mg/dL protein. In such cases, the subdural space is drained externally using a closed sterile system until the fluid is suitable for shunting. Subdural peritoneal shunts usually are left in place for 2 to 3 months, at which time they can be removed if the CT or MRI scan is negative.

Prognosis. The prognosis for patients with chronic subdural collections depends on the nature and severity of the precipitating illness; the size, location, and duration of the lesion; and the success or failure of treatment. In a small number of cases, communicating hydrocephalus will develop as a late complication. This should be kept in mind in any case in which the expected results of treatment are not achieved.

INTRAVENTRICULAR HEMORRHAGE OF THE NEWBORN

Intraventricular hemorrhage of the newborn (see Chap. 49) is a distinctive disorder that occurs in premature or low-weight, term infants with respiratory

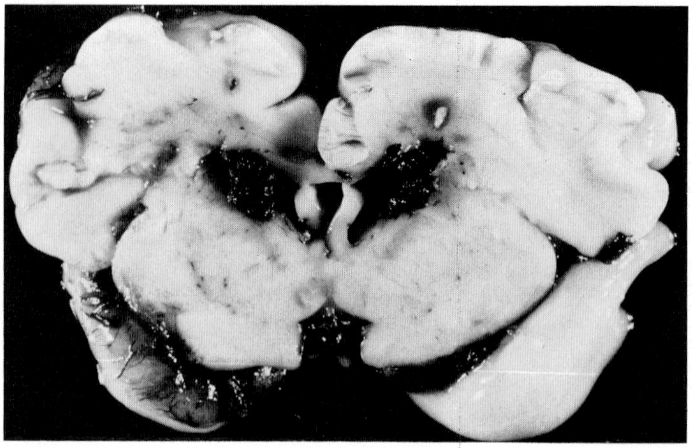

FIG. 50–9. Intraventricular and subarachnoid hemorrhage in hyaline membrane disease. (From Milhorat TH. Pediatric neurosurgery. Philadelphia: FA Davis, 1978.)

distress syndrome, and it is characterized by intraventricular bleeding within the first 24 to 48 hours of life. Although generally referred to as intraventricular hemorrhage of the newborn, the initial lesion actually is a hemorrhagic infarct of the periventricular white matter that secondarily ruptures into the cerebral ventricles. The bleeding originates from small veins in the subependymal germinal matrix,[16–19] and the hemorrhage frequently extends into the thalamus and white matter of the centrum semiovale, eventually bursting through the ependyma to fill the ventricular system and subarachnoid space (Fig. 50-9). In approximately 40% of the cases, the hemorrhage remains confined to the subependymal white matter and does not enter the ventricular system.

Pathogenesis. The pathogenesis of this condition has not been fully elucidated. Because the strongest association is with events causing hypoxia, it is likely that the combination of increased cerebral venous pressure attendant to respiratory distress and the vasodilation that occurs with hypercapnia results in the rupture of fragile veins surrounding the cerebral ventricles. These vessels reside in a germinal matrix that is almost devoid of supporting connective tissue until term, possibly explaining the almost exclusive occurrence of this condition in premature or low-weight infants.

Clinical Aspects. The diagnosis of intraventricular hemorrhage of the newborn should be considered in any premature or low-weight infant with hyaline membrane disease, pneumonia, or other syndromes of respiratory distress. That the condition is common is suggested by its presence in approximately 70% of infants with hyaline membrane disease coming to autopsy,[4] and by the surprisingly high incidence of intraventricular hemorrhage in apparently healthy premature infants. In a study of infants under 34 months of gestational age and weighing less than 1500 g, routine ultrasonography demonstrated evidence of periventricular or intraventricular hemorrhages in an incidence approaching 50%.[20] This finding has mandated a policy of routine scans on all premature patients in this weight or age category.

The clinical findings in intraventricular hemorrhage of the newborn are variable and depend on the magnitude of bleeding. Small, periventricular hemorrhages frequently produce no clinical signs at all, but massive bleeds are associated with stupor, tonic or generalized convulsions, bulging of the anterior fontanelle, and rapidly progressive anemia. If the bleeding is less pronounced, the clinical picture may be characterized by fever, generalized tremulousness, increased muscle tone, and an excessive rate of cranial enlargement.

The definitive diagnosis of intraventricular hemorrhage is made by MRI or CT scanning. In very sick infants, however, an ultrasonogram obtained at the bedside usually is a reliable means for demonstrating large bleeds (Fig. 50-10). This procedure is not definitive for small or petechial hemorrhages, but the rapid diagnosis provided by a portable sonogram and the ability to repeat the study as often as desirable to follow the progress of the patient are definite advantages. For purposes of clinical assessment, it is useful to grade hemorrhages by MRI or CT scanning in the following manner:

Grade 1: petechial bleeding, which is limited to the subependymal periventricular white matter
Grade 2: intraventricular hemorrhage without ventriculomegaly
Grade 3: intraventricular hemorrhage with ventriculomegaly
Grade 4: intracerebral hematoma with intraventricular hemorrhage and ventriculomegaly (Fig. 50-11).

Treatment and Prognosis. The management of intraventricular hemorrhage of the newborn has been significantly modified by the availability of noninvasive scanning, but it is fair to say that the indications for and the types of treatment have not been fully standardized. It is generally agreed that, unless there

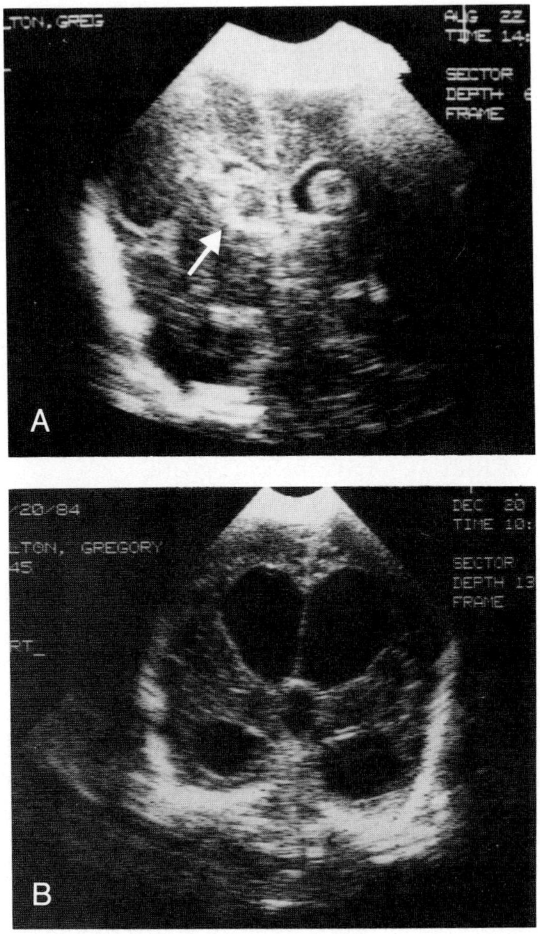

FIG. 50–10. Intraventricular hemorrhage of the newborn. **(A)** An ultrasonogram of a 1-day-old premature infant demonstrates hemorrhage into right basal ganglia (*arrow*) and subependymal zone. **(B)** An ultrasonogram in the same patient 3 months later demonstrates severe hydrocephalus.

are extenuating circumstances, it is unwise to recommend surgical treatment for infants with large grade 4 hemorrhages. Bleeding of this magnitude is associated with a mortality rate approaching 90%, and even those infants who are sustained by ventricular drainage and heroic medical management often are severely affected with varying degrees of mental retardation, spastic diplegia, and blindness. In such cases, it usually is advisable to do nothing other than to provide good nursing care and supportive management.

In the less severe examples of intraventricular hemorrhage, CSF drainage may provide lifesaving decompression and probably reduces the incidence of communicating hydrocephalus in surviving patients. Assisted ventilation often is essential in the early stages of management, and frequent transfusions may be required until hemorrhaging ceases. Anticonvulsants, antibiotics, and parenteral feedings are administered routinely. With grade 3 hemorrhages, we prefer external ventricular drainage to repeated lumbar punctures; drainage can be maintained for days or even weeks until the CSF has been cleared of gross blood. After removal of the drain, MRI or CT scanning will identify those patients who will eventually need a ventricular shunt, although in many cases chronic hydrocephalus seems to be avoided by the early institution of an effective, continuous, external drain.

In patients with grades 1 or 2 hemorrhages, because of the small risk of hydrocephalus, there is a consensus in many institutions that CSF drainage is not indicated. The long-term outcome for such patients has not been ascertained, but it is our opinion that serial lumbar punctures, carried out until the CSF is clear or only faintly xanthochromic, probably constitute optimal treatment. This takes advantage of

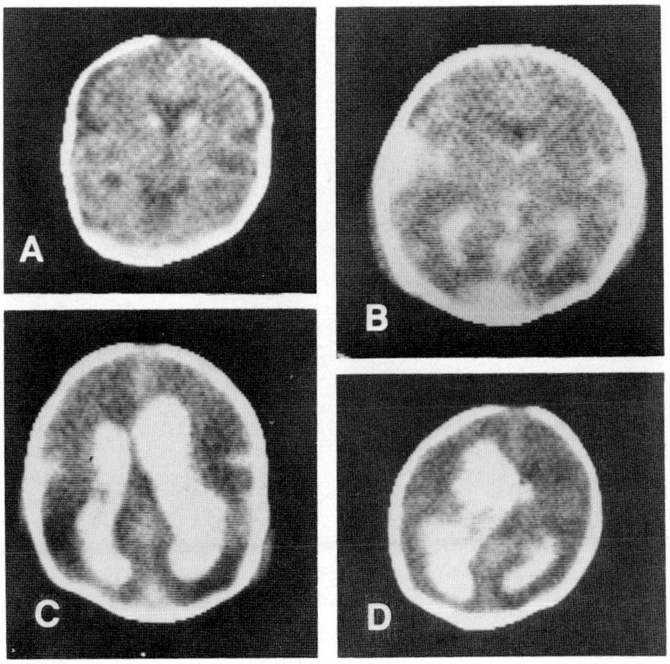

FIG. 50–11. Computed tomography scans demonstrate four grades of intraventricular hemorrhage of the newborn. **(A)** Grade 1: petechial hemorrhages in subependymal white matter lateral to frontal horns. **(B)** Grade 2: intraventricular hemorrhage without ventriculomegaly. **(C)** Grade 3: intraventricular hemorrhage with ventriculomegaly. **(D)** Grade 4: intracerebral hematoma, intraventricular hemorrhage, and ventriculomegaly.

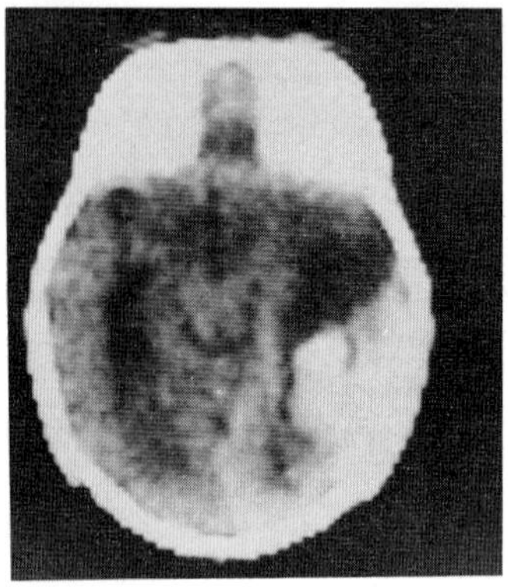

FIG. 50–12. Computed tomography scan demonstrates right temporal lobe hematoma in a 1-day-old infant after traumatic delivery.

the sink function of the CSF and helps not only to drain blood out of the ventricles but also to mobilize and remove blood pigments from the periventricular areas of the brain. The long-term benefits of such treatment, with particular reference to mental, motor, and psychological development, obviously will take many years to assess.

TEMPORAL LOBE HEMATOMA OF THE NEWBORN

This is a rare but important complication of birth trauma that results from excessive compression of the temporal or lateral surface of the head during delivery. With few exceptions, the injury is caused by the use of obstetric forceps, although it also can result from forceful uterine contractions that crush the head against the pelvic outlet. The clinical picture is characterized by irritability, anemia, hemiparesis, focal or generalized seizures, and episodic apnea. Contusions of the scalp often are evident in the temporal area, but radiographs of the skull are negative in most cases. The definitive diagnosis can be made by CT or MRI scanning (Fig. 50-12). Treatment consists of evacuation of the hematoma through a subtemporal craniectomy or osteoplastic craniotomy. The prognosis for survival is good, but seizures, hemiparesis, and mental retardation are common sequelae.

INTRACRANIAL CYSTS AND TUMORS

These lesions, although relatively rare, should not be overlooked. Intracranial tumors are exceptional in the neonatal period, but medulloblastoma, teratoma, ependymoma, choroid plexus papilloma, cerebellar astrocytoma, and craniopharyngioma all are known to occur (Fig. 50-13). Porencephalic cysts may attain sufficient size to produce abnormal cranial enlargement, and arachnoid cysts of the posterior fossa are a relatively common cause of hydrocephalus (Fig. 50-14).

In general, the diagnostic evaluation of patients with intracranial cysts and tumors is the same as that outlined for hydrocephalus. Treatment is aimed at complete surgical removal, although this is not always possible. In patients with malignant tumors of the brain, radiotherapy or chemotherapy or both may

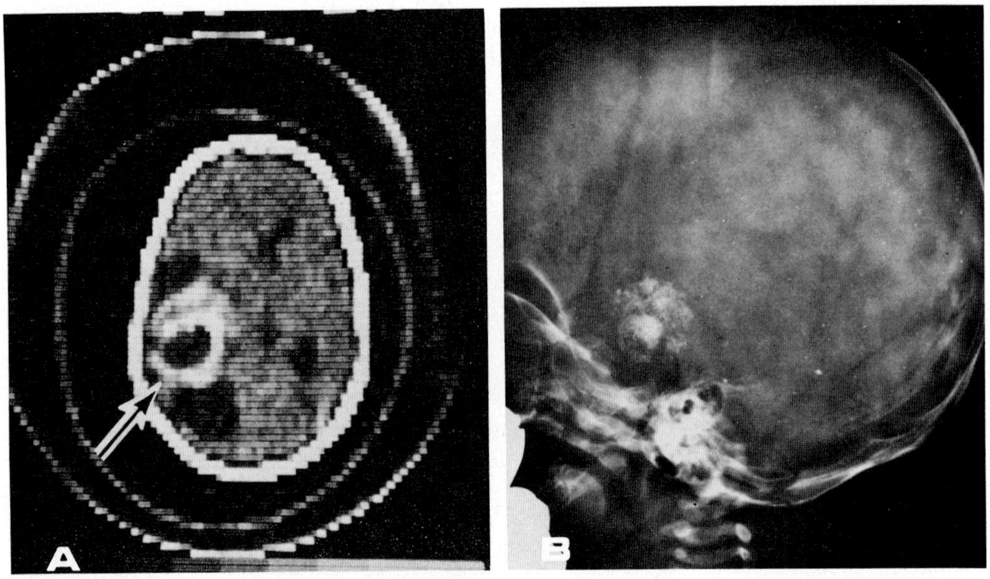

FIG. 50–13. (A) Computed tomography scan demonstrates a large cystic ependymoma situated within the left lateral ventricle of an infant who presented with cranial enlargement. (From Milhorat TH. Pediatric neurosurgery. Philadelphia: FA Davis, 1978.) (B) Lateral radiograph demonstrates calcification in a craniopharyngioma in a 1-day-old infant. (From Milhorat TH. Hydrocephalus and the cerebrospinal fluid. Baltimore: Williams & Wilkins, 1972:86.)

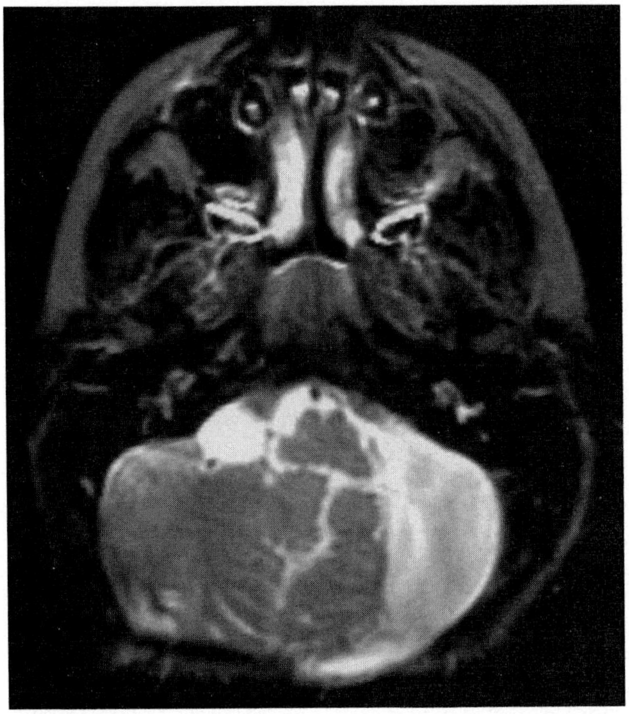

FIG. 50–14. A T2-weighted magnetic resonance imaging scan in the horizontal plain through the posterior fossa demonstrates an arachnoid cyst. The cyst is hyperintense and displaces the cerebellum laterally.

have something to offer. Ventricular shunting procedures will be required if the lesion produces an obstruction of the CSF pathways that cannot be relieved by direct operation.

DISORDERS CAUSING BRAIN SWELLING OR ENCEPHALOPATHY

Encephalopathy is a relatively common cause of pathologic cranial enlargement and is excluded best by a careful history and physical examination. Toxic, metabolic, anoxic, traumatic, and infectious causes are recognized, and of these lead poisoning is the most important consideration in some regions of the country. Vitamin A deficiency may occur in infants on a milk-substitute diet to which inadequate vitamin supplements have been added. The diagnosis is suggested by the finding of abnormal cranial enlargement in association with xerophthalmia, gynecomastia, and epithelial metaplasia. Hypervitaminosis A may occur after the administration of large amounts of vitamin A—usually 50,000 U/day for several months—and produces signs of increased intracranial pressure in association with cheilosis.

Cranial enlargement of a mild order may occur in the early stages of degenerative brain diseases such as gargoylism, metachromatic leukodystrophy, Tay–Sachs disease, and Canavan spongy cerebral sclerosis. Such enlargements are the result of an increased cerebral mass (*i.e.*, megalocephaly) and not ventricular dilation. The history and physical examination are usually sufficient to distinguish these diseases from hydrocephalus and subdural collections.

An unusual rate of cranial enlargement has been reported in otherwise normal infants recovering from severe malnutrition.[21] In extreme examples, there may be roentgenographic evidence of sutural diastasis and other signs of increased intracranial pressure. Although the explanation for this phenomenon is unknown, there probably is a preferential nutrition and growth of the brain during periods of relative deprivation. If adequate nutrition is maintained, the rate of cranial growth and the head–body proportions return to normal in a matter of months.

ABNORMAL CRANIAL CONFIGURATION

An alteration in normal cranial configuration without measurable enlargement of the head is a common clinical problem in the neonatal period. From a diagnostic standpoint, it is important to distinguish examples of benign cranial molding from conditions associated with premature closure of the cranial sutures (*i.e.*, craniosynostosis).

BENIGN CRANIAL MOLDING

As a consequence of normal delivery, the fetal head undergoes considerable molding as it passes through the birth canal. The skull, dura, and brain participate in the molding process, and compartmental shifts of the CSF probably occur to some extent. At birth, the grossly molded head is lengthened in the occipitofrontal diameter. Flattening of the forehead, narrowing of the biparietal diameter, and protuberance of the occiput are characteristic findings (Fig. 50-15). Examination of the head reveals a palpable patency of the cranial sutures, and this can be confirmed in

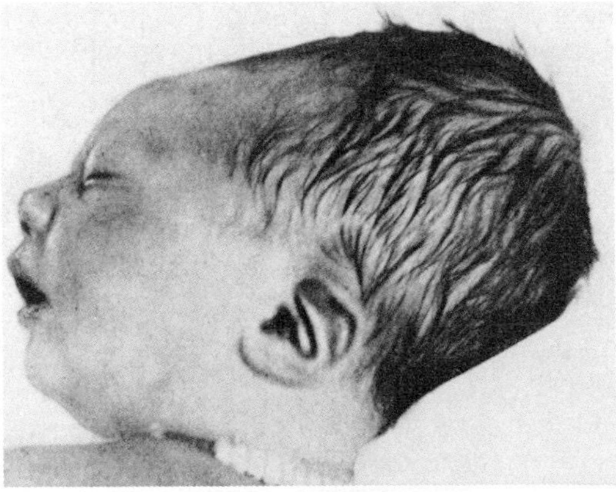

FIG. 50–15. Infant with molded head. (From William's obstetrics. 11th ed. New York: Appleton-Century-Crofts, 1956.)

doubtful cases with skull radiographs. With few exceptions, the configuration of the molded head improves steadily over a period of days and weeks.

Passive molding of the head also may occur in severely ill or brain-damaged infants on a positional basis. The most common abnormality is bilateral occipital flattening, although asymmetric deformities may occur if the infant has a preference for lying on one side. Radiographs of the skull should be obtained so that premature stenosis of the lambdoid sutures can be ruled out. If the abnormal cranial configuration is of positional origin only, there will be roentgenographic evidence of suture patency.

CRANIOSYNOSTOSIS

Craniosynostosis may be regarded as a pathologic condition encompassing a wide spectrum of disorders ranging from premature stenosis of a single cranial suture to complex syndromes in which there is generalized stenosis of the cranial vault, midface hypoplasia, and associated systemic anomalies. It is important to distinguish between the primary and secondary types. In primary craniosynostosis, the deformity is present at birth, and the premature fusion of the sutures can lead to a restriction of brain growth. In secondary craniosynostosis, the sutures close and the skull fails to grow as a consequence of brain atrophy or agenesis. This is a common occurrence in patients with microcephaly and may develop in patients with treated hydrocephalus if there is marked overlapping of the cranial sutures.

The configuration of the head in patients with primary craniosynostosis depends on the suture or sutures involved. In general, the deformity is greatest in the axial direction of the affected suture. In cases of premature closure of the sagittal suture, the lateral growth of the head is limited, and the growth of the brain causes the head to expand in the occipitofrontal diameter (*i.e.*, scaphocephaly, dolichocephaly, or boat-shaped head; Fig. 50-16). In contrast, with premature closure of the coronal sutures, the growth of the head is limited in the occipitofrontal diameter, and there is marked expansion of the vertex and lateral aspects of the skull (*i.e.*, brachycephaly; Fig. 50-17). Premature fusion of the metopic suture causes the forehead to assume a bullet-shaped configuration (*i.e.*, trigonocephaly). Fusion of the squamosal suture or of the squamosal and coronal suture on one side produces a striking deformity with flattening of the ipsilateral forehead (*i.e.*, plagiocephaly) and elevation and retraction of the lateral orbital wall (*i.e.*, Harlequin eye sign). If there is premature fusion of all the cranial sutures, the skull expands toward the vertex. This is the direction of least resistance and results in a pointed, tower-shaped head (*i.e.*, oxycephaly).

The etiology of primary craniosynostosis, like that of the other birth defects, is obscure. In occasional patients with coronal synostosis, the disorder will appear in siblings of successive generations, suggesting that genetic factors are important. This is certainly the case when coronal synostosis occurs in association with Apert syndrome, Carpenter syndrome, or Crouzon syndrome, because these conditions follow precise patterns of mendelian transmission. With other types of craniosynostosis (*e.g.*, sagittal, metopic, lambdoid), however, no familial incidence is recognized. There is no evidence that intrauterine infections or disturbances in calcium metabolism are important etiologic factors, but craniosynostosis and accelerated skeletal maturation have been reported in patients with neonatal hyperthyroidism.[4] In a few cases of single-suture stenosis, there is a history of twin birth, difficult lie, or cephalopelvic disproportion, raising the possibility that compression of the fetal head may play a causal role.

The most common type of craniosynostosis is premature stenosis of the sagittal suture. This accounts for approximately 50% of all cases coming to clinical attention and is followed in frequency by coronal synostosis, lambdoid synostosis, and metopic synostosis, in that order. Sagittal synostosis occurs about four times as frequently in boys as in girls, but coronal synostosis exhibits a slight female preponderance.

The clinical features of primary craniosynostosis are related to the cranial deformity, the effects of cerebral compression, and the presence or absence of associated congenital anomalies. In general, when there is premature closure of only one cranial suture,

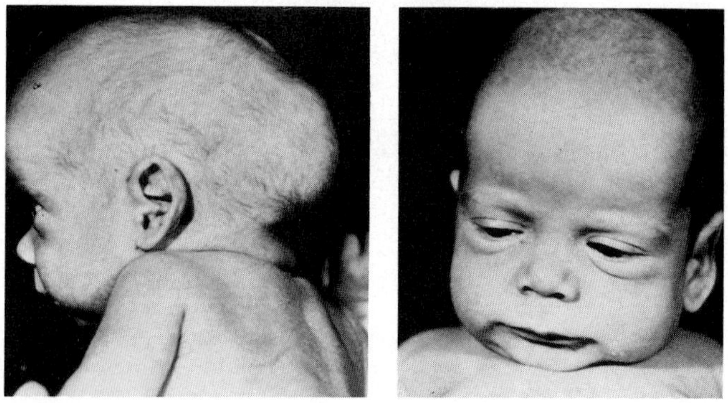

FIG. 50–16. Scaphocephaly secondary to premature stenosis of the sagittal suture. (From Milhorat TH. Pediatric neurosurgery. Philadelphia: FA Davis, 1978:173.)

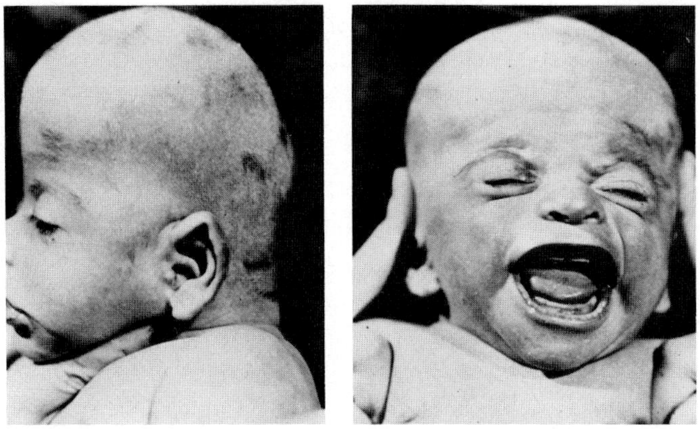

FIG. 50–17. Brachycephaly secondary to premature fusion of both coronal sutures. (From Milhorat TH. Pediatric neurosurgery. Philadelphia: FA Davis, 1978:175.)

the consequences are mainly cosmetic. When two or more sutures unite before birth, the hazards of restricted brain growth and increased intracranial pressure increase proportionately.

DIAGNOSIS

The diagnostic evaluation of patients with craniosynostosis rarely requires elaborate tests. The configuration of the head usually suggests the diagnosis, and, in most cases, the affected suture can be palpated as an elevated, hyperostotic ridge. Signs of increased intracranial pressure should be sought and a careful funduscopic examination performed so that papilledema and optic atrophy can be ruled out.

Three syndromes of craniofacial dysostosis commonly are associated with premature fusion of the coronal sutures. These include Crouzon syndrome, Apert syndrome, and Carpenter syndrome. In most cases, there is evidence of midface hypoplasia characterized by shallow orbits, exophthalmos, high arched palate, depression of the nasal and malar bones, and choanal atresia (Fig. 50-18). The latter deformity may lead to severe obstruction of the nasopharyngeal airway and frequently is a cause of persistent mucoid drainage from the nose and mouth.

The definitive diagnosis of craniosynostosis is made by radiographic examination of the skull. This readily confirms the configuration of the skull and will adequately demonstrate which sutures are fused (Figs. 50-19 and 50-20). In patients who exhibit signs of neurologic involvement, EEG and CT or MRI scanning may be appropriate.

TREATMENT

There are two principal rationales for operative treatment of primary craniosynostosis: to correct the cranial deformity and to relieve or prevent the effects of cranial or orbital compression. In patients with premature closure of one cranial suture, the considerations are mainly cosmetic; however, when there is involvement of two or more cranial sutures, surgery can be strongly recommended because of the definite risk of progressive visual and neurologic complications. Funduscopic evidence of papilledema or optic atrophy, roentgenographic signs of increased intracranial pressure, and severe exophthalmos with exposure keratitis are clear-cut indications for operative intervention.

There are few indications for operative treatment of secondary craniosynostosis. Surgical procedures should of course be avoided in patients with microcephaly, but in occasional patients with marked overlapping of the cranial sutures after a craniotomy or ventricular shunting procedure, there is evidence of

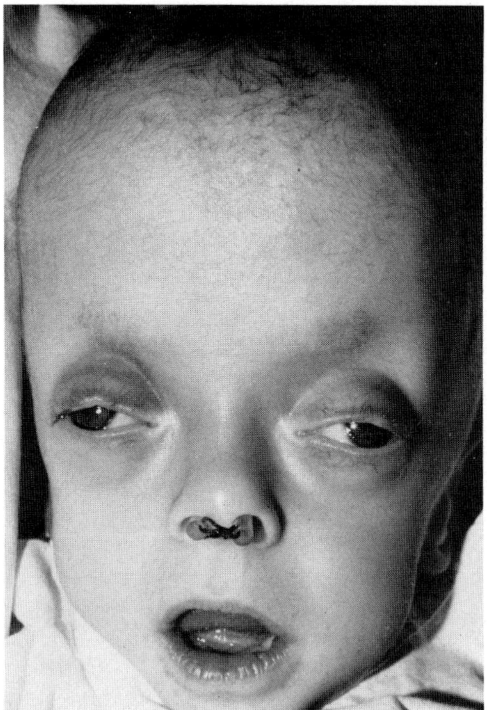

FIG. 50–18. Crouzon syndrome (*i.e.*, craniofacial dysostosis) with midface hypoplasia characterized by small orbits, exophthalmos, hypoplasia of the facial bones, and choanal atresia.

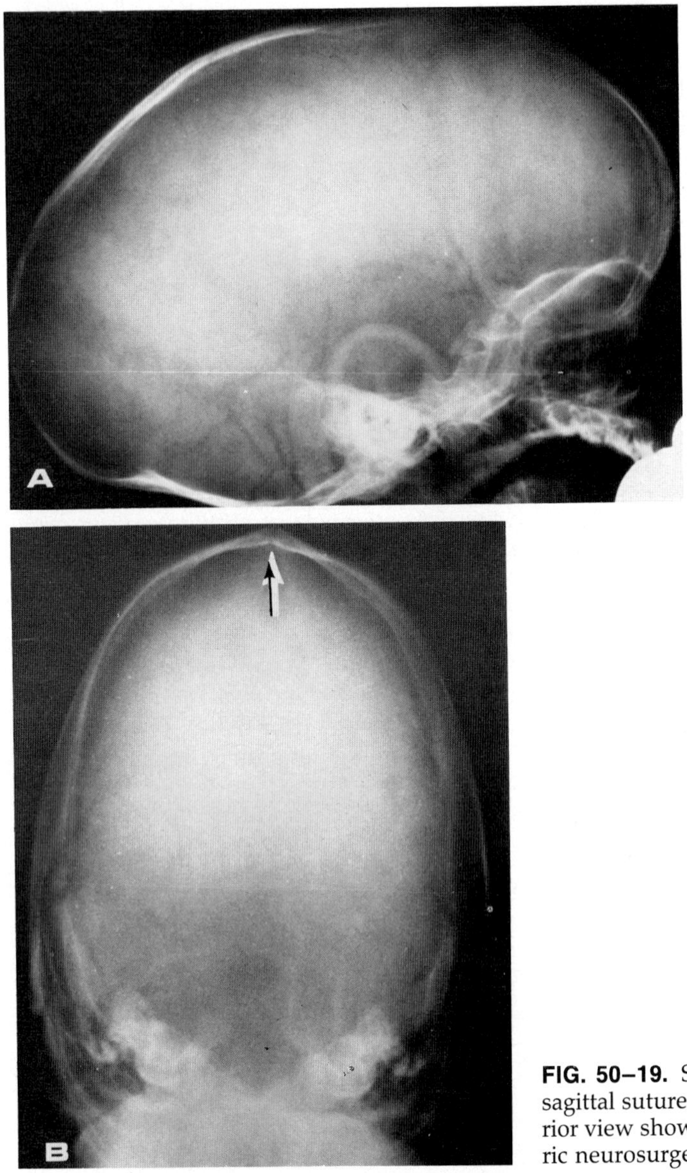

FIG. 50–19. Skull radiographs demonstrate premature stenosis of the sagittal suture. **(A)** Lateral view shows scaphocephaly. **(B)** Anteroposterior view shows hyperostotic sagittal suture. (From Milhorat TH. Pediatric neurosurgery. Philadelphia: FA Davis, 1978:174.)

restricted brain growth. In such cases, treatment usually consists of a sizeable cranial decompression followed by a cranioplasty at some later date.

Patients with stenosis of two or more cranial sutures should be operated on as soon as possible after birth. This is indicated to minimize the effects of cerebral compression during the period of rapid brain growth and is preferable to postponing surgery until symptoms develop. In patients with severe choanal atresia, surgical relief of the airway obstruction often is required before decompression of the cranial vault can be considered.

Operations for stenosis of one cranial suture are performed electively at 6 weeks of life or once the period of physiologic anemia has passed. It is advisable not to delay surgery unnecessarily because the rapid growth of the brain during the first 6 months of life is the predominant factor in achieving satisfactory remodeling of the skull and its integuments. Synectectomies performed after 9 months of age usually do not restore normal cranial configuration, and after 2 years of age more complex techniques for cranial remodelling are required.

Optimal surgical treatment for single-suture stenosis consists of resecting the affected suture, elevating the opposing cranial bones, and manually shaping any associated deformities or depressions.[4] With few exceptions, brain growth between the second and sixth months of life will spontaneously remodel the cranial vault and even will correct compensatory deformities such as hypertelorism, the Harlequin eye sign, and protrusion of the forehead or occiput. In patients with multiple-suture synostosis, staged operations, with or without orbital decompression, may be required. The treatment of midface hypoplasia must be postponed until the emergence of secondary

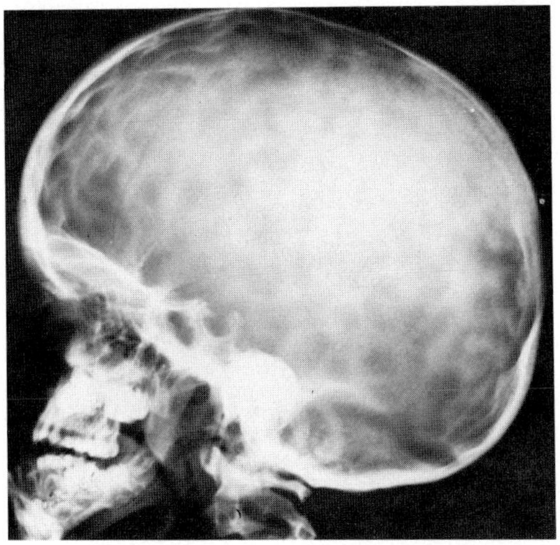

FIG. 50–20. Skull radiograph in a 2-year-old child with untreated Crouzon syndrome shows oxycephaly, increased digital markings, and hypoplasia of facial bones.

dentition at 6 to 10 years of age, when a radical craniofacial correction can be carried out. Excellent techniques have been developed for orbital advancement,[22] delayed cranial remodeling,[23] and the treatment of complex midface deformities.[24] It is important that patients awaiting such cosmetic procedures have adequate cranial decompressions to prevent neurologic and visual complications. Psychological counseling before and after surgery is strongly recommended.

MENINGOMYELOCELE AND RELATED DISORDERS

Disturbances of fetal development can produce a variety of serious and closely related anomalies. The crucial time for the development of the human nervous system is between the third and fifth weeks of gestation.[25] During this interval, the neural groove closes and the resulting neural tube separates from the overlying ectoderm to become surrounded ventrally, laterally, and dorsally by mesodermal elements (*i.e.*, the somites) that later form the vertebral column and supporting soft tissue structures. Any disturbance of this sequence of development, depending on the extent of the disturbance, can result in incomplete closure of the dorsal midline (*i.e.*, dysraphism). Less severe developmental errors produce deformities limited to the supporting structures. Of these, the best-known examples are spina bifida, spinal meningocele, cranium bifidum, and cranial meningocele. More severe errors in development produce deformities that include nervous tissue as well as supporting structures (*e.g.*, meningomyelocele, encephalocele). Perhaps the most dramatic example of craniospinal dysraphism is anencephaly (Fig. 50-21). In this condition, the brain and spinal cord are exposed, and there is complete failure of the ectodermal and mesodermal layers to close dorsally. In some cases, the exposed nervous tissue contains a persistent neural groove that is mute testimony to the severe and early arrest in development. It is important to emphasize that all the foregoing dysraphic anomalies are closely related and that they differ more in degree than in origin.

MENINGOMYELOCELE

Meningomyelocele is the most common dysraphic disorder referred to the neurosurgeon during the neonatal period. By definition, the lesion contains both meningeal and neural components and thus is distinguished from simple meningocele, which does not contain neural tissue.

ETIOLOGY AND PATHOLOGY

The etiology of meningomyelocele, like that of other congenital anomalies, is poorly understood. The disorder is common, occurring in approximately 1 of 500 live births.[26] Although statistics vary, a familial incidence is recognized, and in families in which one member is affected, the risk that subsequent offspring will be similarly affected approaches 5%.[26] If two or more members are affected, the risk factor increases to 10%.[27] Although this pattern of inheritance is too low to indicate direct, single-gene transmission, it suggests a genetic susceptibility in some families. Meningomyelocele and related disorders occur with greater frequency in Caucasians than in African Americans, and the gender ratio favors girls slightly.[26] In some instances, seasonal outbreaks or waves of meningomyelocele appear to correlate with virus epidemics having occurred 8 to 9 months before.[28]

An understanding of the pathology of meningomyelocele is fundamental to medical and surgical management. Regardless of the location of the lesion, the spinal cord and nerve roots are displaced dorsally, owing to a lack of posterior supporting structures. Lateral to the lesion, masses of muscle and bone, representing the spina bifida defect, are present. In some cases, the defect is so wide as to accommodate an orange; in other cases, only a dime-sized defect of the posterior elements is present. Overlying the lesion, meninges and skin are present to a variable extent. If the ectodermal covering is complete, the lesion can be confused with a simple meningocele. In most cases, however, the neural elements are incompletely covered, and a flattened plaque of nervous tissue (*i.e.*, the neuropore) is easily recognizable in the center of the lesion (Fig. 50-22). If the lesion is exposed or if the meninges are ruptured at the time of delivery, the lesion will exude CSF. Meningomyelocele may arise at any point along the vertebral column from C1 to the coccyx but is most common in the lumbar, lumbosacral, and sacral segments.

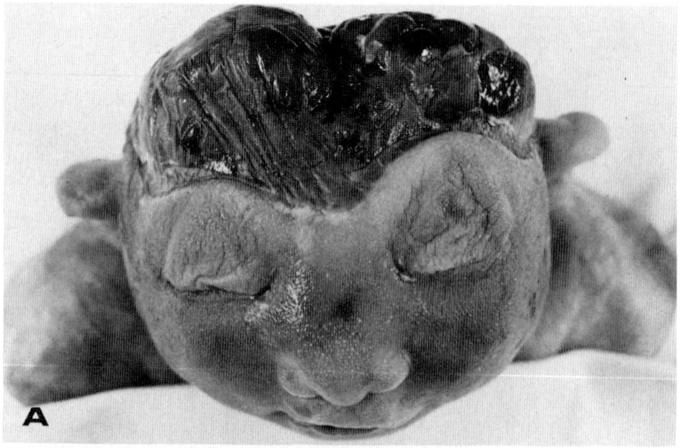

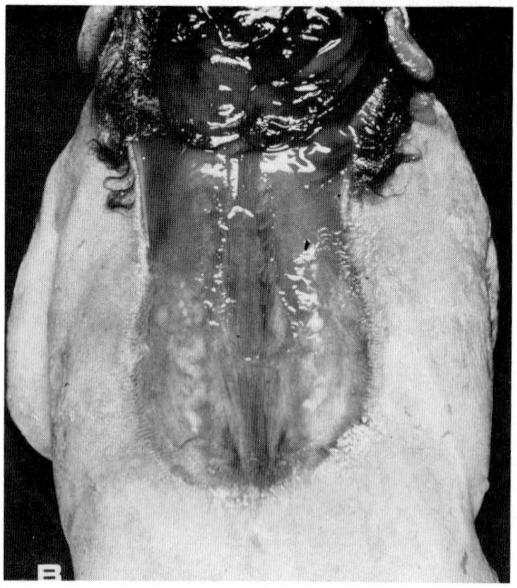

FIG. 50–21. **(A)** Anencephaly. **(B)** Craniospinal rachischisis and persistent neural groove. (From Milhorat TH. Pediatric neurosurgery. Philadelphia: FA Davis, 1978:138.)

Associated congenital anomalies are encountered in all but a few cases of meningomyelocele. Except when the lesion is small or sacral in location, an associated Arnold–Chiari malformation (*i.e.,* Chiari type II) will be present (Fig. 50-23). This is a complex hindbrain deformity and is characterized by a small posterior fossa and impaction of the posterior cerebellar vermis through the foramen magnum. Frequently, the cerebellum extends as a tonguelike prolongation to the level of the second to fifth cervical segments. The cisterna magna is obliterated, and the fourth ventricle is carried down through the cervical canal as a long, slitlike cavity. The herniated cerebellum usually is firmly attached to the back and sides of the cervical canal by arachnoidal adhesions. Frequently, there is an elongation and thinning of the lower pons and upper medulla, and, in severe cases, the lower medulla is dorsally buckled and folded back on itself at the level of the gracile and cuneate tubercles. The lower cranial nerves are greatly elongated and run upward toward the foramen magnum with the upper cervical nerve roots.

The next most common anomaly associated with meningomyelocele is aqueductal forking. This occurs in approximately 80% of all cases and produces a noncommunicating type of hydrocephalus.[6] Other congenital anomalies that may be associated with meningomyelocele include hydromyelia, syringomyelia, double spinal cord, polymicrogyria, craniolacunia, heterotopias of gray matter, beaklike deformity of the quadrigeminal plate, basilar impression, platybasia, Klippel–Feil deformity, congenital heart disease, and intestinal anomalies such as duodenal atresia or pyloric stenosis (Fig. 50-24). Although it has been argued that the Arnold–Chiari malformation may arise as a consequence of traction or tethering of the spinal cord, it is likely in view of the multiple associated anomalies that occur in this disorder that the hindbrain deformity is but one of many closely related maldevelopments.[4–6]

DIAGNOSIS

The diagnosis of meningomyelocele usually is apparent at birth. The head should be carefully examined for signs of hydrocephalus, and serial circumferential measurements are required to rule out an abnormal rate of cranial enlargement. In most cases, CT or MRI is performed so that the size of the ventricular system can be determined and so that aqueductal stenosis and the Arnold–Chiari malformation can be ruled out. MRI scanning provides superior information about associated anomalies such as polymicrogyria, heterotopias of gray matter, and deformities of the hindbrain. Electromyography is useful in assessing motor function in the lower extremities, and an abdominal sonography or intravenous pyelogram may be indicated so that hydronephrosis can be excluded.

ANTENATAL DIAGNOSIS

The measure of α-fetoprotein (AFP) in amniotic fluid has established itself as a reliable means for detecting dysraphic disorders *in utero*, and can be carried out early enough to permit safe termination of the pregnancy.[29] Except when the defect is closed, false-negative results are unusual, and the finding of an extremely high level of AFP usually is indicative of a large open anomaly. The value of this simple test in counseling women who have previously given birth to a defective infant is obvious. Somewhat less reliable is the maternal serum AFP test, which will detect 50% to 90% of open dysraphic anomalies and is falsely positive in 5%.[29]

TREATMENT AND PROGNOSIS

Until 1960, most infants with meningomyelocele and hydrocephalus were managed conservatively at home. Without surgical treatment, less than 20% survived for as long as 2 years. In patients with large meningomyeloceles and a severe degree of hydrocephalus, the natural mortality was even higher. In this group, approximately 50% of the patients died within the first month of life, and the remainder were dead within 6 months.[30,31]

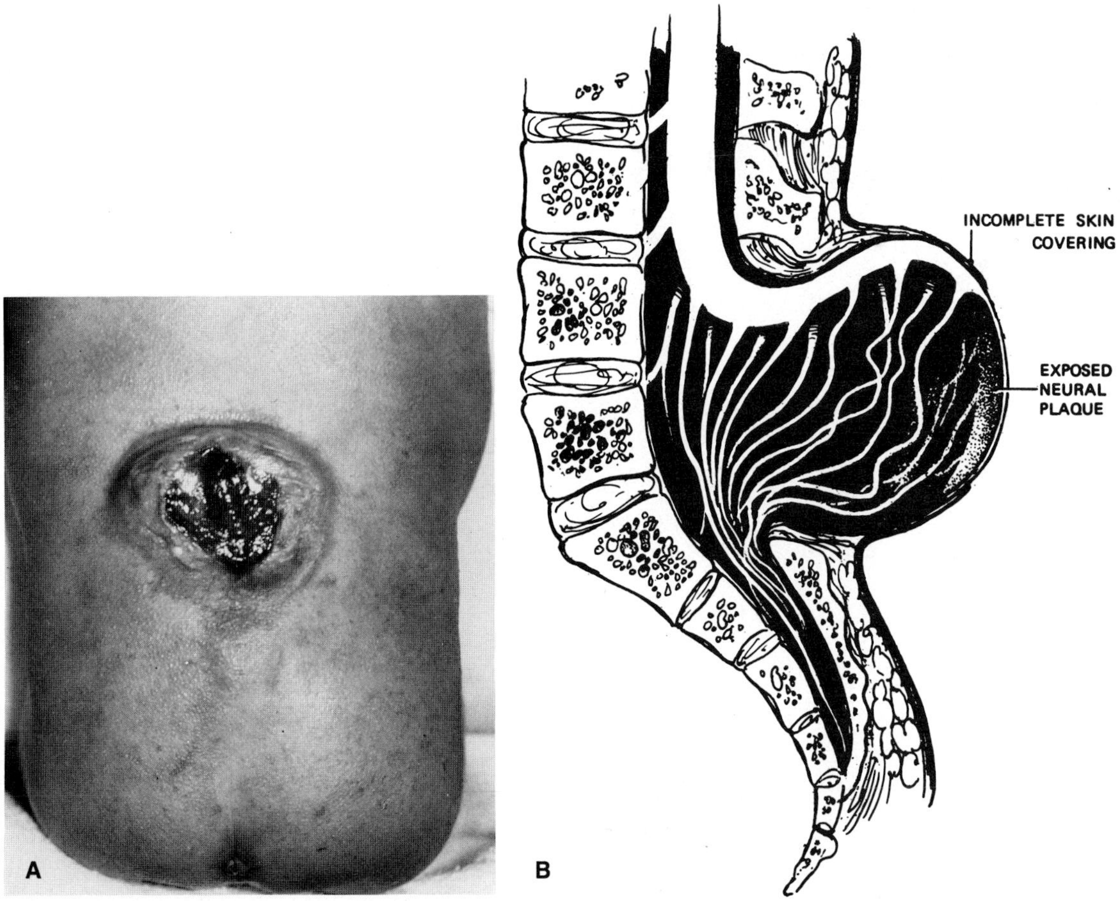

FIG. 50–22. **(A)** Thoracolumbar meningomyelocele with central neuropore and incomplete covering of meninges and skin. **(B)** Lumbosacral meningomyelocele. (From Milhorat TH. Pediatric neurosurgery. Philadelphia: FA Davis, 1978:139.)

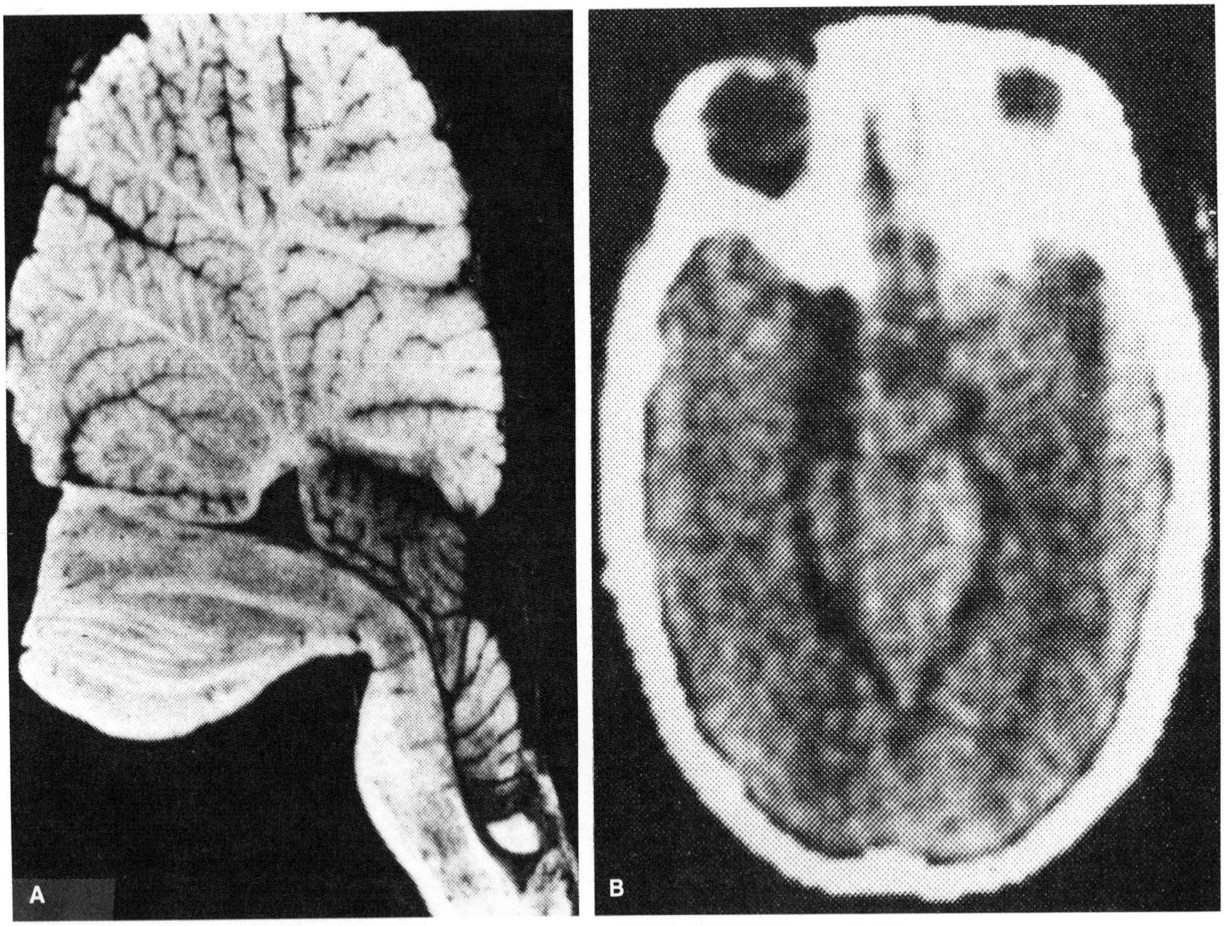

FIG. 50–23. Arnold–Chiari malformation. **(A)** Sagittal section through the cerebellum and lower brain stem. **(B)** Computed tomography scan of a newborn infant demonstrates beaklike deformity of the quadrigeminal plate. (From Milhorat TH. Pediatric neurosurgery. Philadelphia: FA Davis, 1978:140.)

In 1959, a comprehensive plan of treatment was evolved at the University of Sheffield, England.[32] The Sheffield plan, as it came to be known, consisted of repairing all meningomyeloceles within the first few hours of life. Hydrocephalus was treated with a ventriculoatrial shunt, and all patients were evaluated and followed by a team of surgeons, physicians, physiotherapists, and social workers. Shunt revisions were performed periodically, and many of the patients underwent multiple orthopaedic and urologic procedures. This multidisciplinary approach, which was widely adopted, increased the survival rate of all patients with meningomyelocele and hydrocephalus to between 60% and 70% at 2 years. As experience grew, however, it became clear that a large number of patients had been sustained who had little or no chance of ever achieving a competitive place in life.[33] Many of the surviving patients had severe handicaps and various degrees of bladder, bowel, and lower extremity paralysis; 30% to 50% were totally paraplegic, and the average patient required seven orthopaedic operations on the lower extremities. It was estimated, furthermore, that only 20% of patients with severe meningomyelocele and hydrocephalus had a normal intellect at 2 to 4 years. These dour statistics, of course, did not include the hardships imposed by multiple operations, the psychological burdens on the patient and his or her family, or the financial cost of such a comprehensive program.

In view of the foregoing, it is obvious that the management of meningomyelocele is a complicated matter for which there are no easy answers. Arbitrary rules cannot be applied, and each case must be judged on an individual basis. After considering all the clinical, prognostic, and ethical factors, however, an attempt should be made to arrive at a clear-cut decision. It rarely is possible for parents to evaluate a long list of choices and possibilities objectively, and it is therefore desirable that the physician offer advice and guidance. In many clinics, it is believed that operative procedures on totally paraplegic patients are unjustified.[33,34] Similarly, patients with severe hydrocephalus or multiple anomalies involving the major organ systems, or both, rarely are operated on. In such cases, conservative management is advised, and treatment other than that necessary to assure the comfort of the infant is avoided.

In patients who are candidates for surgical treatment, the following plan is appropriate:

1. Whenever possible, the spinal lesion should be closed within the first few hours of life. Prompt surgery cannot be expected to improve neurologic deficits, but it is performed so that infection is prevented and the progressive loss of existing neurologic function is halted. If the lesion is completely epithelialized, elective closure may be performed at some later date. If the lesion is open and the patient is not seen within the first 24 hours of life, surgery should be delayed until superficial contamination of the lesion has been controlled by moist dressings and systemic antibiotics.
2. Computed tomography or MRI scanning should be performed within the first week of life. Every effort should be made to define the type as well as the severity of hydrocephalus. In patients with moderate to severe ventriculomegaly, and in those with aqueductal stenosis, a shunt is performed between 5 and 15 days. Of the available operations, the ventriculoperitoneal shunt is preferred.
3. After surgery, the patient should be fully evaluated and followed in a multidisciplinary clinic. Repeated urinary tract infections can be avoided in most children by adopting clean techniques of straight catheterization.[35] A number of orthopaedic deformities can be modified or avoided by vigorous physical therapy, but operative procedures frequently are required during the first decade of life, including heel cord lengthening, tendon releases, and spinal instrumentation for scoliosis.[36] Parents should be instructed in the symptoms and signs of increased intracranial pressure and shunt failure should be managed as a surgical emergency. A potential delayed

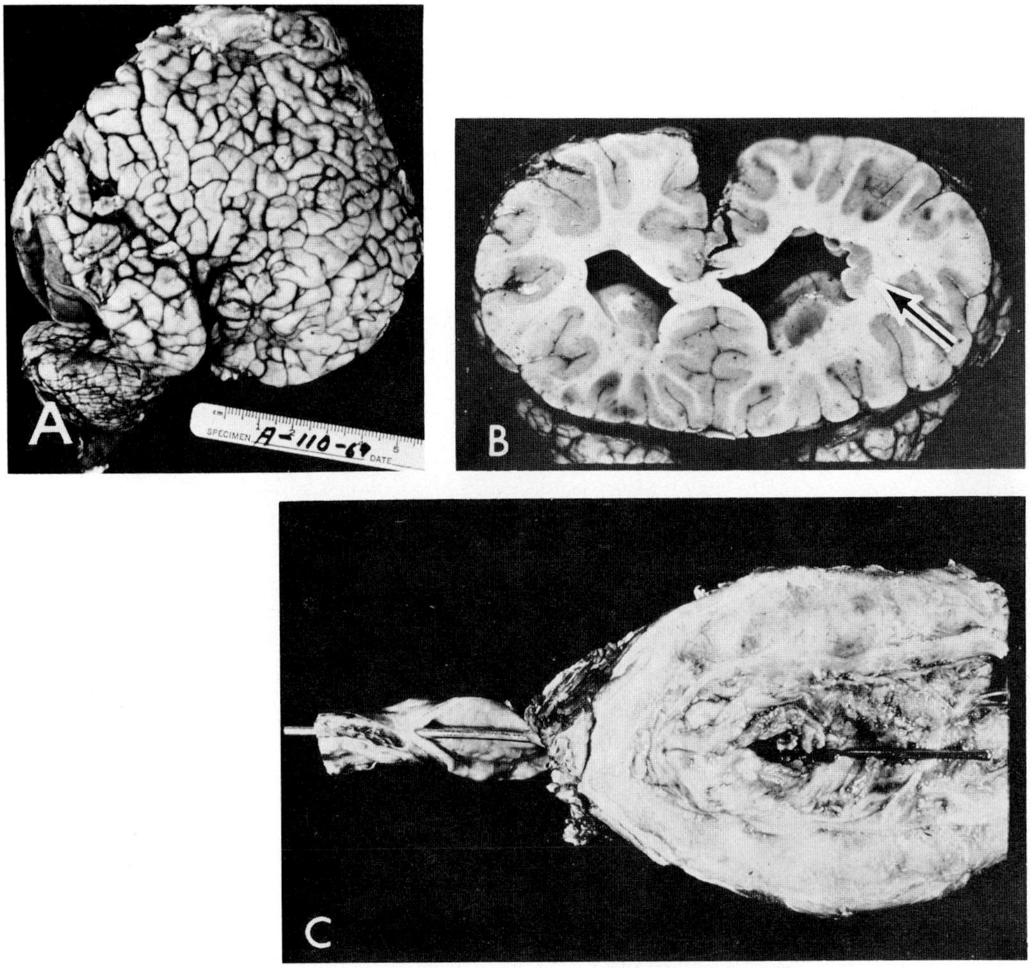

FIG. 50–24. Common anomalies associated with meningomyelocele. **(A)** Polymicrogyria. **(B)** Heterotopias of gray matter. **(C)** Meningomyelocele and hydromyelia. A probe has been passed through the central canal. (From Milhorat TH. Hydrocephalus and the cerebrospinal fluid. Baltimore: Williams & Wilkins, 1972:98.)

complication of myelomeningocele repair is spinal cord tethering. This usually occurs after the fifth year of life as a consequence of somatic growth and is characterized by increasing weakness and spasticity of the lower extremities, progressive orthopaedic deformities, and neurogenic bladder.

ENCEPHALOCELE

Cranium bifidum and encephalocele are much less common than their spinal counterparts. Although these lesions occur in a variety of locations, they are found most frequently in the posterior midline (Fig. 50-25). Occipital and suboccipital encephaloceles show a considerable variation in morbid anatomy. Deformities of the tentorium and hindbrain are common, and the external sac may contain a knuckle of occipital lobe or cerebellum or both. Owing to the distorted anatomy of the posterior fossa in some cases, hydrocephalus may be present or may develop as a delayed complication.[6] Frontal encephaloceles frequently occur in the midline just above the nasion and produce wide lateral displacement of the orbits (*i.e.*, hypertelorism). Orbital encephaloceles tend to present with unilateral exophthalmos, and nasal and nasopharyngeal lesions occasionally are mistaken for nasal polyps.

Although some encephaloceles reach gigantic proportions, the size of the external lesion gives little indication of its contents.[34] It should be emphasized that occipital encephaloceles sometimes communicate with the occipital horn of one or both lateral ventricles, and lesions in the suboccipital area almost invariably communicate with the cisterna magna or upper cervical theca. If the encephalocele is open and draining at birth, it should be repaired immediately. In cases in which the lesion is completely covered by thick skin, it usually is preferable to delay surgery until a complete diagnostic workup, including skull radiographs, CT or MRI scans, and EEGs, has been performed. If hydrocephalus is present, a ventricular shunting procedure usually is performed 7 to 10 days after the encephalocele has been repaired.

CRANIAL AND SPINAL MENINGOCELES

These lesions are similar to encephaloceles and meningomyeloceles except that they do not contain nervous tissue. Associated congenital anomalies occur with much less frequency, and, unless the lesions are open and draining at birth, surgical repair can be delayed for several weeks.

DERMAL SINUS TRACTS

By definition, these lesions consist of a tract of stratified squamous epithelium that extends inward from the skin surface. Like other dysraphic disorders, they presumably arise between the third to fifth weeks of gestation as a consequence of imperfect separation of the neuroectoderm and epithelial ectoderm. Dermal

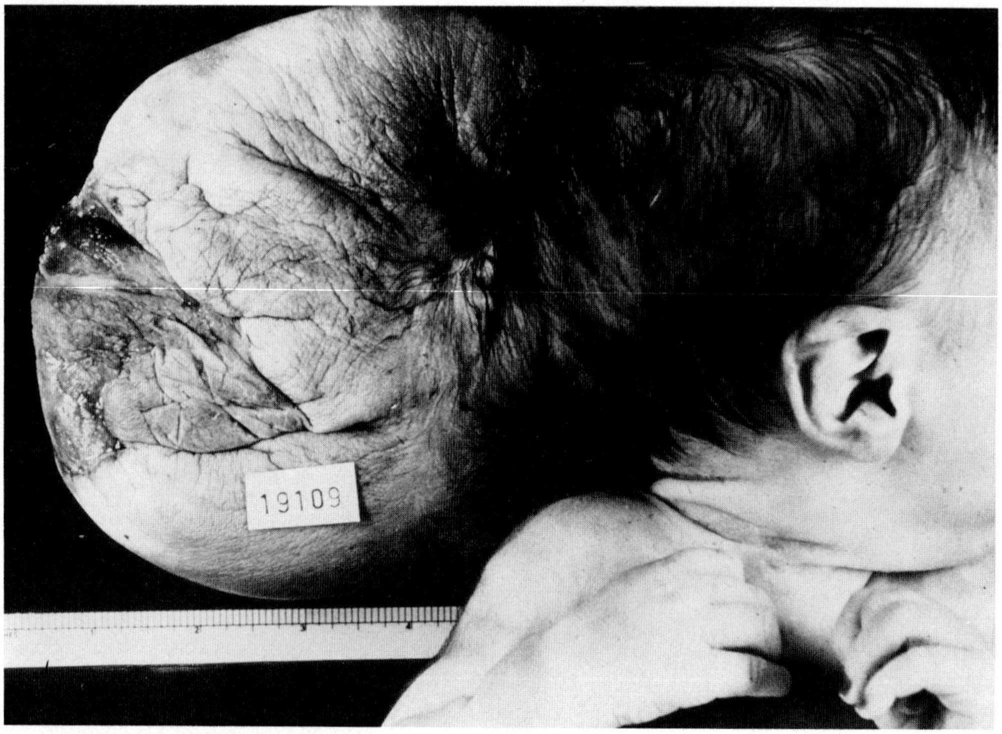

FIG. 50–25. Occipital encephalocele.

sinus tracts therefore characteristically occur in the dorsal midline. The most common sites include the sacrum, the lumbar area, and the suboccipital area, in that order. Embryologically, these sites correspond to the location of the posterior neuropore in the lumbosacral region and the anterior neuropore in the suboccipital area.

The morbid anatomy of congenital dermal sinus tracts varies considerably. In some cases, the epithelial tube ends blindly just dorsal to the vertebral column or skull. In other instances, the tract extends through a small bony defect to terminate as a large mass (*i.e.*, dermoid tumor or lipoma) that may be situated either extradurally or intradurally. In lumbosacral lesions, the intradural component may extend cephalad over many segments (Fig. 50-26). Such lesions are capable of producing an intramedullary mass that is embedded in the conus medullaris. In suboccipital lesions, the sinus tract may extend through the cerebellar vermis to terminate as a dermoid or teratomatous tumor within the fourth ventricle.

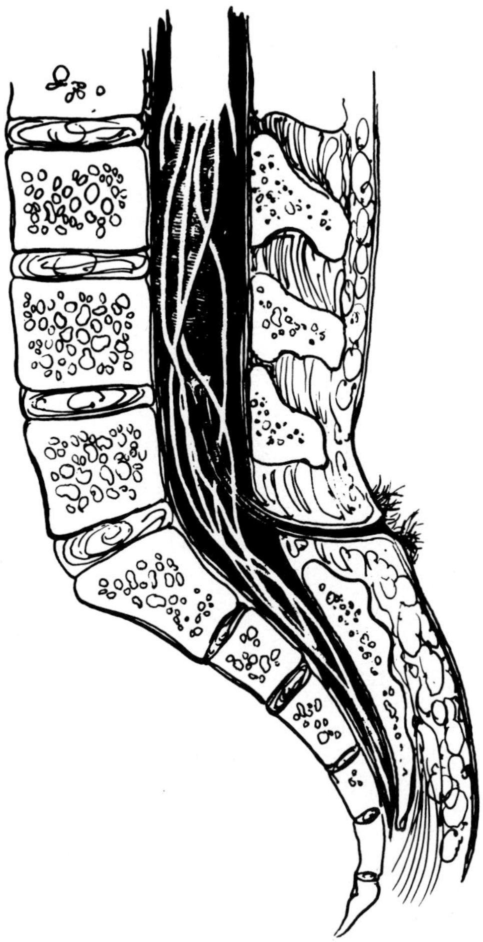

FIG. 50–26. Dermal sinus tract enters the spinal canal and extends cephalad to a dermoid tumor at embryologic point of origin. (From Milhorat TH. Pediatric neurosurgery. Philadelphia: FA Davis, 1978:160.)

The diagnosis of a congenital dermal sinus tract occasionally is made at birth. It is sufficient to say that any skin dimple or depression overlying the dorsal midline should be carefully examined by the attending physician. Computed tomography of the skull or spine occasionally may demonstrate a small bony defect, but the absence of such a finding never excludes this lesion. Unfortunately, in many cases, the disorder comes to attention only after the patient has experienced several bouts of unexplained meningitis. The responsible organism is almost always a strain of *Staphylococcus* or *Escherichia coli*. Less commonly, the patient may present with symptoms referable to an expanding intracranial or intraspinal mass.

To evaluate fully the extent of a dermal sinus tract, special diagnostic tests are required. Dermal sinography is to be condemned because it can precipitate or exacerbate a meningeal infection. In patients with sacral or lumbosacral lesions, MRI is indicated and myelography is sometimes performed to rule out an intraspinal mass. To evaluate the extent of a sinus tract in the suboccipital area, a CT or MRI scan is indicated.

The surgical treatment of dermal sinus tracts is performed with least risk and fewest complications when there are no signs of active meningeal infection. In patients who present with recurring bouts of meningitis, it usually is best to treat the infection with systemic antibiotics before proceeding with surgery. If persistent fever and meningeal signs suggest the formation of a chronic abscess, however, prolonged medical therapy is unwise. The goal of surgical treatment is complete removal of the sinus tract and its intraspinal or intracranial extensions. This usually is achieved, except when past inflammation or infection causes the lesion to adhere intimately to vital structures. In patients in whom hydrocephalus develops secondary to meningitis, a ventricular shunting procedure may be required.

LIPOMYELOMENINGOCELE

This is a relatively uncommon lesion that generally arises in the lumbar or lumbosacral area and frequently reaches the size of a grapefruit. The mass may be central or paracentral in location and usually is well covered by skin. In typical cases, the lipomatous tissue extends intradurally and is continuous with the conus medullaris, which is fixed caudally at the level of L5 or S1 (Fig. 50-27).

Lipomyelomeningocele, in contrast to ordinary myelomeningocele, rarely is associated with hydrocephalus, hydromyelia, or other congenital anomalies. With few exceptions, the neurologic examination at birth is negative. For these reasons, some physicians have regarded the lesion as a deformity for which surgical treatment is mainly cosmetic and only occasionally indicated.[34] On the basis of accumulated clinical experience, however, it is evident that progressive neurologic deficits occur in most patients as

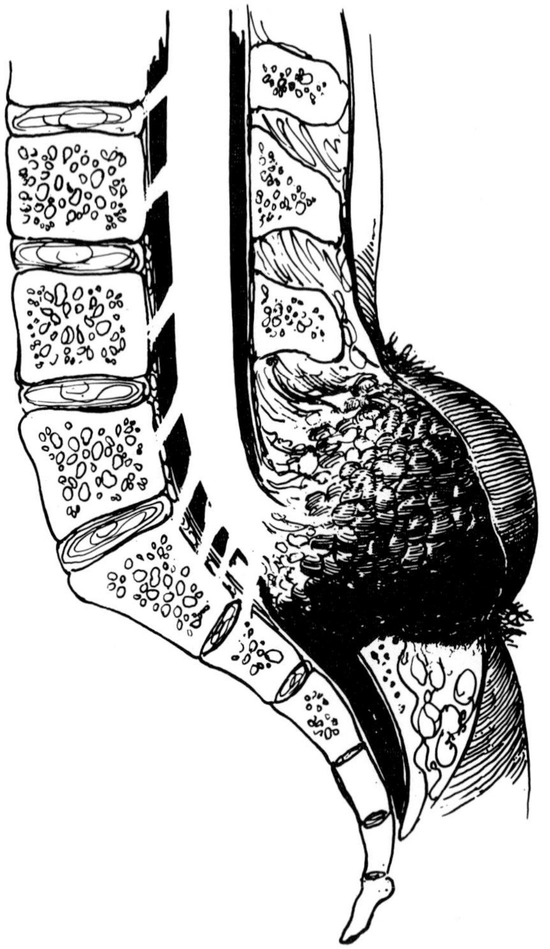

FIG. 50–27. Lipomyelomeningocele. The fatty tissue extends intradurally and is continuous with the conus medullaris, which is tethered at the level of L5. (From Milhorat TH. Pediatric neurosurgery. Philadelphia: FA Davis, 1978:151.)

a consequence of somatic growth and tethering of the spinal cord.[4] These deficits may occur at any time and are especially difficult to recognize during infancy. In older children, the most common symptoms include bladder and bowel disturbances, foot deformities, back pain, weakness in one or both legs, and dysesthesias in the lower extremities.

It is the consensus at the University Hospital of Brooklyn that lipomyelomeningoceles should be repaired on an elective basis as soon as the 2- to 3-month period of physiologic anemia has passed. The principal aim of surgery is to relieve tethering of the spinal cord before neurologic deficits supervene. Excellent surgical techniques using the operating microscope[4] and spinal evoked potential monitoring are available.

REFERENCES

1. Barkovitch AJ, Kjos BO, Jackson DE, et al. Normal maturation of the neonatal infant brain: MR imaging at 1.5 T. Radiology 1988;166:173.
2. Runge VM, Schaible TF, Goldstein HR, et al. Gd-DTPA clinical efficacy. Radiographics 1988;8:147.
3. Masaryk TJ, Modic MT, Ross JS, et al. Intracranial circulation: preliminary clinical results with three-dimensional (volume) MR angiography. Radiology 1989;171:793.
4. Milhorat TH. Pediatric neurosurgery. Philadelphia: FA Davis, 1978.
5. Russel DS. Observations on the pathology of hydrocephalus. London: His Majesty's Stationery Office, 1949.
6. Milhorat TH. Hydrocephalus and the cerebrospinal fluid. Baltimore: Williams & Wilkins, 1972.
7. Milhorat TH. Cerebrospinal fluid and the brain edemas. New York: Neuroscience Society of New York, 1987.
8. Penfield W, Elvidge AR. Hydrocephalus and the atrophy of cerebral compression. In: Penfield W, ed. Cytology and cellular pathology of the nervous system. vol 3. New York: Hafner, 1932:1208.
9. Foltz EL, Shurtleff DB. Five-year comparative study of hydrocephalus in children with and without operation (113 cases). J Neurosurg 1963;20:1064.
10. Amacher AL, Wellington J. Infantile hydrocephalus: long-term results of surgical therapy. Child's Brain 1984;11:217.
11. Young HF, Nulsen FE, Weiss MH, et al. The relationship of intelligence and cerebral mantle in treated infantile hydrocephalus. Pediatrics 1973;52:38.
12. Wald SL, McLaurin RL. Shunt-associated glomerulonephritis. Neurosurgery 1978;3:146.
13. Milhorat TH. Failure of choroid plexectomy as treatment for hydrocephalus. Surg Gynecol Obstet 1974;139:505.
14. Paine RS: Hydrocephalus. Pediatr Clin North Am 1967;14:779.
15. Rabe EF, Flynn RE, Dodge PR. Subdural collections of fluid in infants and children: a study of 62 patients with special reference to factors influencing prognosis and the efficacy of various forms of therapy. Neurology 1968;18:559.
16. Towbin A. Cerebral intraventricular hemorrhage and subependymal matrix infarction in the fetus and premature newborn. Am J Pathol 1968;52:121.
17. Larroche JC. Hémorragies cérébrales intraventriculaires chez le prematuré: I. Anatomie et physiopathologie. Biol Neonate 1964;7:26.
18. Schwartz P. Birth injuries of the newborn. New York: Hafner, 1961.
19. Towbin A. Cerebral hypoxic damage in fetus and newborn: basic patterns and their clinical significance. Arch Neurol 1969;20:35.
20. Ment LR, Ehrenkranz RA, Duncan CC. Intraventricular hemorrhage of the preterm neonate: prevention studies. Semin Perinatol 1988;12:359.
21. DeLevie M, Nogrady MB. Rapid brain growth upon restoration of adequate nutrition causing false radiographic evidence of increased intracranial pressure. J Pediatr 1970;76:523.
22. Whitaker LA, Schut L, Kerr LP. Early surgery for isolated craniofacial dysostosis. Plast Reconstr Surg 1977;60:575.
23. Persing JA, Edgerton MT, Jane JA. Scientific foundations and surgical treatment of craniosynostosis. Baltimore: Williams & Wilkins, 1989.
24. Goodrich JT, Post KD, Argamaso RV. Plastic techniques in neurosurgery. New York: Thieme, 1991.
25. Arey LB. Developmental anatomy: a textbook and laboratory manual of embryology. 7th ed. Philadelphia: WB Saunders, 1965.
26. Myrianthopoulous NC, Kurland LT. Present concepts of the epidemiology and genetics of hydrocephalus. In: Fields WS, Desmond MM, eds. Disorders of the developing nervous system. Springfield, IL: Charles C Thomas, 1961:187.

27. Carter CO, Roberts JAF. The risk of recurrence after 2 affected children with central nervous system malformations. Lancet 1967;1:306.
28. Milhorat TH. Congenital hydrocephalus. In: Sano K, Ishii S, LeVay S, eds. Recent progress in neurological surgery. Amsterdam: Excerpta Medica, 1974:68.
29. Brock JD. Alpha-fetoprotein and the prenatal diagnosis of central nervous system disorders. Child's Brain 1976;2:1.
30. Laurence KM. The natural history of spina bifida cystica. Arch Dis Child 1964;39:41.
31. Rickham PP, Mawdsley T. The effect of early operation on the survival of spina bifida cystica. Dev Med Child Neurol [Suppl] 1966;11:20.
32. Sharrard WJ, Zachary RB, Lorber J, et al. A controlled trial of immediate and delayed closure of spina bifida cystica. Arch Dis Child 1963;38:18.
33. Lorber J. Results of treatment of meningomyelocele: an analysis of 524 unselected cases, with special reference to possible selection for treatment. Dev Med Child Neurol 1971;13:279.
34. Matson DD. Neurosurgery of infancy and childhood. Springfield, IL: Charles C Thomas, 1969.
35. Action Committee of Myelodysplasia, Section of Urology. Current approaches to evaluation and management of children with myelomeningocele. Pediatrics 1979;63:663.
36. Bunch WH, Cassl AS, Bernsman AS, et al. Modern management of myelomeningocele. St. Louis: WH Green, 1972.

Neonatology: Pathophysiology and Management of the Newborn, Fourth Edition,
edited by Gordon B. Avery, Mary Ann Fletcher, and Mhairi G. MacDonald.
J.B. Lippincott Company, Philadelphia © 1994.

chapter 51

Neuromuscular Disease

GLORIA D. ENG

The principles of rehabilitation medicine are important in the evaluation and treatment of infants who present with nerve or muscle problems that affect tone, posture, and movement. They may be congenital or traumatic in origin. These principles include making an accurate diagnosis and recognizing its impact on the functional capacity of the infant; minimizing deformity that can become exaggerated with growth; and, if there is permanent disability, giving training in compensatory movements to optimize function.

Parents should be integrally involved, supported, and counseled on the nature of their child's disability. They should develop a reasonable level of comfort and be taught basic handling techniques that they can apply regularly to their infant. The rest of this chapter details the more common clinical disorders that come under the purview of rehabilitation medicine.

TRAUMATIC PERIPHERAL NERVE PALSIES AND SPINAL CORD INJURIES

Traumatic peripheral palsies as well as spinal cord injuries in the newborn usually are associated with difficult deliveries. The infant's head and face may be subject to prolonged pressure; because of their width, the baby may have difficulty slipping the shoulders through the birth canal or, if presenting in a breech position, too much traction may be exerted on the legs and lower spine. There may be vigorous distraction and hyperextension of the aftercoming head. The bony spinal column may distract and not fracture, but the spinal cord is vulnerable to injury from traction.

FACIAL PALSY

Facial palsy may occur in association with a complicated delivery, particularly when there is extended impingement of the baby's head against the maternal sacrum, prolonged application of forceps, or intracranial bleeding with or without skull fracture. The infant is unable to wrinkle the forehead, close the eyes, or suck a nipple without dribbling the milk on the affected side (Fig. 51-1). The incidence varies from 0.05% to 1.8%.[1,2]

This condition must be differentiated from congenital maldevelopment of the seventh nerve nucleus itself, which is frequently bilateral and associated with abducens palsy, as seen in the Möbius syndrome. It should not be confused with persistent partial congenital palsies seen with chondrocardiac anomalies (*e.g.*, Klippel–Feil syndrome, Sprengel deformity), some phocomelias, and cardiac malformations reflecting maldevelopment of the visceral arches. Central facial palsy involves the lower portion of the face and is characterized by flattening of the nasolabial fold, a droop of the involved corner of the mouth, and sparing of the muscles of the forehead and eye. It can be associated with intracranial hemorrhage or infarcts. To be distinguished from all others is a benign condition, described by Nelson and Eng[3]—congenital absence or hypoplasia of the depressor anguli oris

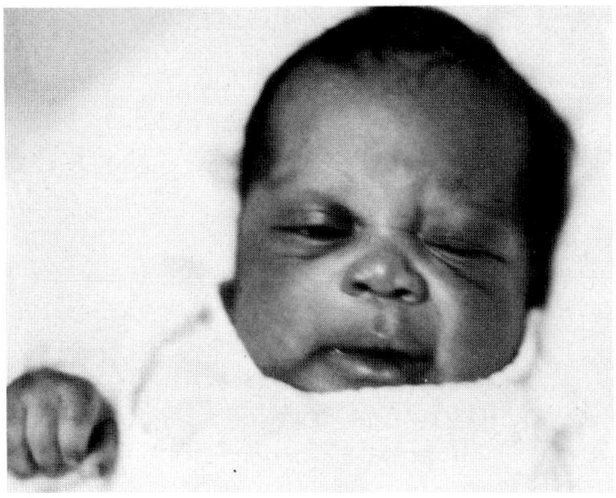

FIG. 51–1. Right facial palsy in a 2-week-old infant.

(*i.e.*, triangularis) muscle (Fig. 51-2). In this condition, one corner of the mouth does not move downward and outward with the other when the baby is crying. The rest of the facial muscles are intact, allowing the baby to frown, close the eyes, wrinkle the nose, and suck without dribbling because, despite palpable thinning of the lateral portion of the lower lip, the orbicularis oris functions normally. It may represent the least remnant of a first visceral arch syndrome. Therefore, associated congenital cardiac lesions must be considered. As the child grows and increasingly uses the smiling muscles (*i.e.*, the risorius and zygomaticus), the oral asymmetry will become less prominent.

In birth palsy of the facial nerve, the asymmetry of facial movements may be profound and may not reflect the true integrity of the nerve. Clinical criteria that may predict prognosis (*e.g.*, pain about the ear, associated symptoms such as hyperacusis and loss of taste) cannot be evaluated in an infant. Fortunately, there are simple electrodiagnostic tests that can provide valuable information on the state of the nerve.

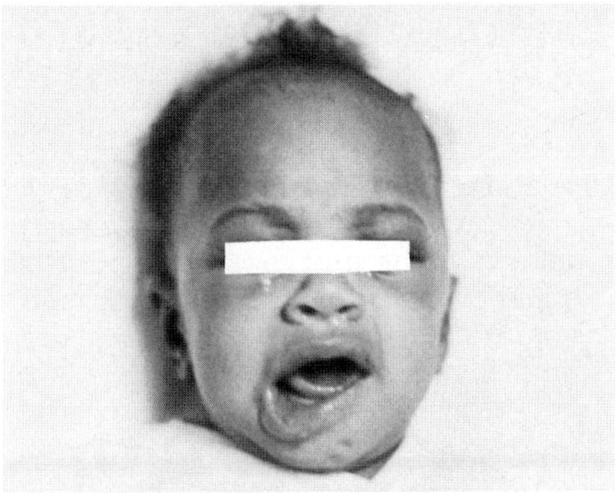

FIG. 51–2. Hypoplasia of the left depressor anguli oris muscle in a 2-month-old infant.

NERVE EXCITABILITY TEST

This can be performed 72 hours after onset. The facial nerve is stimulated in front of the ear with surface electrodes using a square wave pulse 0.1 to 0.2 milliseconds in duration. Visual observation of the muscle contraction in response to the stimulus intensity in milliamperes is compared between the normal side and the affected side. If the threshold currents are the same, then neurapraxia (*i.e.*, block of nerve impulse secondary to edema) exists, and recovery should occur in several days or weeks. Late degeneration of the nerve can occur; therefore, repeated testing is indicated at 3- to 5-day intervals until stabilization or gradual recovery becomes evident.

NERVE CONDUCTION LATENCY

The facial nerve is stimulated in front of the ear, and the impulse is recorded from the frontalis or levator anguli nasi muscles (Fig. 51-3). If the nerve loses all response to electrical stimulation, the prognosis is guarded. This test may be done 7 to 10 days after onset.

The amplitude and duration of the evoked compound motor action potential compared between the

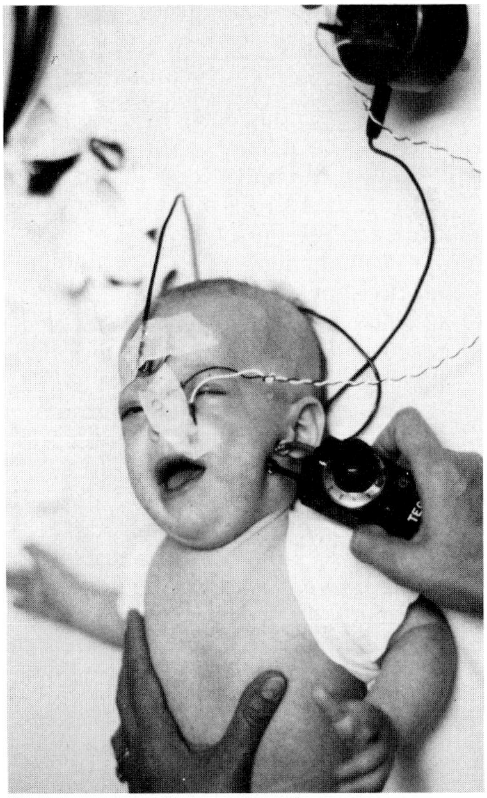

FIG. 51–3. Nerve conduction latency determination in a 6-week-old infant with hypoplasia of the left depressor anguli oris muscle. The recording electrode is on the levator nasalis, the reference electrode is on the bridge of the nose, and the ground is on the forehead.

normal and the affected side may indicate the extent of the pathologic condition and prognosis. Eliciting the blink reflex can give information on the more proximal portion of the facial nerve. The stimulus is applied to the supraorbital nerve and two responses are elicited, R_1, which represents a pontine pathway, and R_2, which is relayed presumably through the pons and medulla. R_2 may be elicited in only two thirds of neonates, according to Kimura,[4] and mostly on the side of the stimulus, rarely on the contralateral side.

ELECTROMYOGRAM

This may be done 14 to 21 days after onset. Absence of motor unit activity, and presence of fibrillation potentials and sharp waves depict a state of denervation. Sequential studies are useful for evaluation of reinnervation leading to gradual improvement.

Because many infants with facial palsy recover spontaneously within several days to 3 weeks after delivery, the pathophysiologic process in these infants is undoubtedly one of mild neurapraxia. The infants who are referred for consultation usually are more seriously involved, yet their numbers are not large in the total spectrum of facial palsies affecting children. Twenty-eight patients with facial palsy were studied over a 1-year period.[5] Only 11 were seen in the newborn period; 6 had traumatic palsies, and 5 had congenital palsies associated with other anomalies. All but one infant of the six with traumatic palsies recovered spontaneously by 5 months of age. If there was evidence of denervation on initial electrodiagnostic studies, the nerve regenerated at approximately 2.5 cm (1 inch) each month. The congenital group did not change on follow-up because, in this group, there was agenesis of a lower branch or the entire lower division of the facial nerve.

General principles of management have been formulated based on experience with this problem. If the clinical picture and electrodiagnosis suggest mild involvement or neurapraxia, no treatment is required. If partial denervation exists, physical therapy, including massage and later active exercises, is prescribed. The use of corticosteroids to suppress edema and inflammation seems to hold no justification in birth palsy. Methylcellulose drops and taping of the involved eye to prevent excoriation of the cornea are the only treatments indicated. The complications of synkinesis and contracture rarely are seen in infants.

BRACHIAL PLEXUS PALSY

The brachial plexus may be injured during delivery when the infant's head has been delivered and the shoulders are trapped in the birth canal. Hyperextension of the head may exert traction of the cervical roots and plexus.

Erb palsy is paralysis of the muscles of the arm supplied by components of C5 and C6 nerve roots. It is the most common form of paralysis and is clinically obvious in an infant who has a one-sided Moro reflex, and whose affected arm hangs limply adducted and internally rotated at the shoulder, extended and pronated at the elbow, and with flexed wrist in the typical waiter's-tip posture (Fig. 51-4). Deep tendon reflexes are diminished or absent in the paralyzed arm.

Klumpke paralysis affects only the muscles of the hand supplied by C8 to T1 nerve roots. It is seen rarely in infancy as an isolated entity after birth trauma. It has been associated with thoracic outlet tumors, cystic hygromas, cardiac surgery, and spinal cord injury. Total plexus involvement affects all the muscles in the arm because the entire plexus from C5 to T1 has been damaged (Fig. 51-5). The arm lies motionless, usually devoid of sweat and sensation, and the hand becomes small, dry, and atrophic. The deep tendon reflexes are absent in the affected arm.

Intrauterine brachial plexus palsy has been described by Koenigsberger[6] and Dunn and colleagues,[7] and I have seen a case on one occasion. Abnormal intrauterine position of the fetus's arm—usually in abduction and external rotation at the shoulder, hand impinged behind infant's head—can result in chronic traction of the plexus. The infant's hand is usually small and atrophic with very simple palmar creases. Electrodiagnostic studies are abnormal right from birth rather than 2 to 3 weeks after delivery.

In an early report of 135 infants from the Children's National Medical Center, the obstetric histories were universally complicated.[8] Long, difficult labors and the use of general anesthesia were the rule. The babies, with the exception of one, weighed between 3600 and 7000 g. The incidence of abnormal presentation was high. Associated defects included torticollis, facial palsies, subluxations of the shoulder, fracture of the clavicle and humerus, slippage of the capital

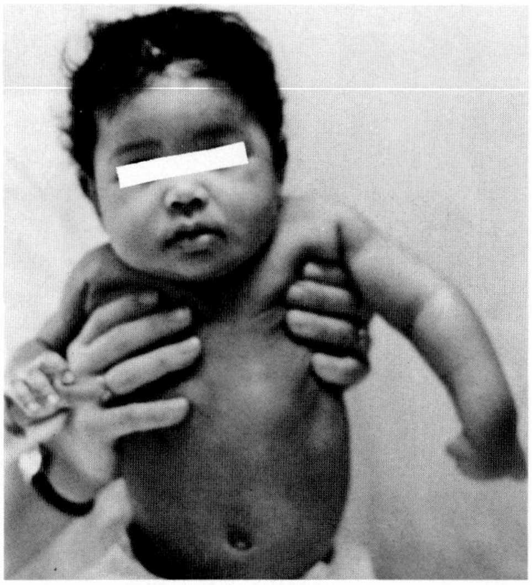

FIG. 51–4. A 2-month-old girl with a left Erb palsy.

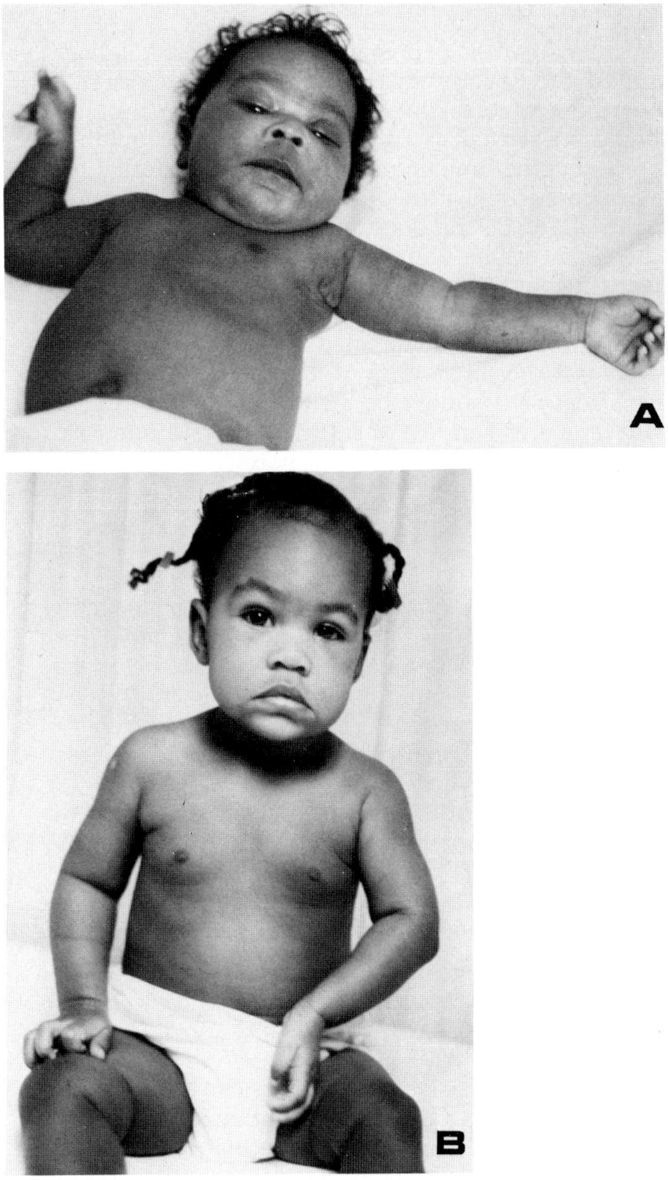

FIG. 51–5. **(A)** Newborn girl with complete brachial plexus palsy involving the left arm. Atrophy of the pectoralis major muscle and also the Horner syndrome (*i.e.*, ptosis of the left lid) are present. **(B)** At 1 year of age, return of the function of the C5- and C6-supplied muscles has occurred, but no return of function of the C7-, C8-, and T1-supplied muscles has taken place. The hand is atrophic and devoid of sensation. Note the persistent Horner syndrome.

head of the radius, subluxation of the cervical spine with evidence of traction injury of the cervical cord, ipsilateral diaphragmatic paralysis, and even periadrenal hemorrhage; all suggest the traumatic nature of these deliveries. Horner syndrome associated with complete plexus palsy was seen in eight infants. Phrenic nerve paralysis may account for acute respiratory compromise in some affected infants. The integrity of the nerve can be assessed within the first 10 to 15 days of life. Since the initial study, over 500 patients with plexopathy have been seen and treated, which suggests that the relative incidence remains the same.

Conduction latencies of the axillary, musculocutaneous, median, and ulnar nerves, as well as ulnar and median H reflexes, and electromyography (EMG) are extremely useful in accurate delineation of the extent of the pathologic condition. The first examination can be done 2.5 to 3 weeks after birth. The second study should be done at 3 months of age. This second study is critical in assessing the integrity of the C5- and C6-supplied muscles. If there is no reinnervation by 3 months into the biceps, then further radiographic studies are indicated. These include computed tomography myelography or magnetic resonance imaging of the cervical spine, and decision for surgical nerve grafting or neurotization, especially if there is disruption of the nerves. Rupture of the nerve roots as evidenced by pseudomeningocele may not mean complete root avulsion, however. Even in these infants, reinnervation may still occur, as evidenced by improvement on EMG studies. Therefore, early surgical intervention remains a controversial subject.[9–13]

CONSERVATIVE MANAGEMENT

The initial neuritic pain may preclude immediate vigorous intervention; however, gentle and meticulous movement of the joints of the paralyzed extremity should be started as soon as tolerated. Scapulohumeral winging, limitation of internal and external rotation, abduction of the shoulder, loss of supination of the elbow, flexion deformity of the wrist, and tight adduction of the thumb quickly develop without treatment. Supportive splints to hold the wrist and hand in good alignment may be indicated. Electrical stimulation of the denervated muscle to prevent fibrosis is a debatable form of treatment. To be effective, treatment should be started early, be applied with regularity, and be of sufficient current intensity to cause maximal muscle contraction. As recovery ensues, active exercises for strengthening the proximal shoulder girdle and arm muscles are included. The infant must be made aware of that extremity as a part of himself.

Sequelae, even in the mildest paralysis, include scapular winging (Fig. 51-6) and loss of shoulder abduction and elbow supination. More serious complications include loss of bone growth (Fig. 51-7), persistent loss of sensation, and total lack of awareness of the arm by the infant, even with good neuromotor and sensory recovery.

The differential diagnosis of brachial plexus palsy includes pseudoparalysis from fracture or osteomyelitis of the scapula, humerus, or other bones of the extremity, and hemiplegia of central origin. None of these entities usually is apparent at birth, and the deep tendon reflexes are preserved.

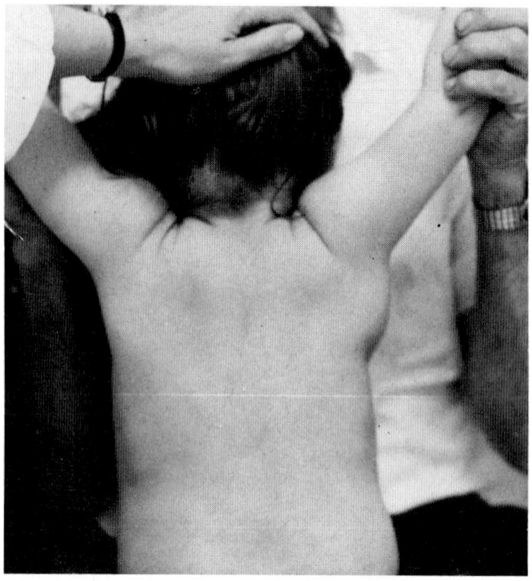

FIG. 51–6. Winging of the scapula occurred in an 18-month-old girl with a C5, C6, C7 brachial plexus palsy.

SPINAL CORD INJURY

In this era of intensive resuscitative care of asphyxiated neonates, those born with evidence of severe hypoxic ischemia may not only have encephalopathy secondary to cortical neuronal necrosis and subcortical white matter injury, but also may have ischemic necrosis of spinal cord gray matter. According to Clancy and associates,[14] depressed tone and hyporeflexia should alert the clinician that spinal cord involvement can coexist with cerebral insult. Survivors showed evidence of acute denervation on EMG in muscles supplied at or below the level of injury.

Spinal cord injury can occur after difficult breech extraction. Persistent intrauterine hyperextension of the head can result in chronic impingement of the cervical and upper thoracic spine.[15] Infants delivered by cesarean section also can sustain injury to the spinal cord, as evidenced by a case described by Hernandez-Marti and colleagues,[16] and two infants that I have seen. These latter two infants presented with bilateral plexus injury predominantly affecting C8- and T1-supplied muscles, resulting in partial paralysis of the trunk and lower extremities in one child, and complete cervicothoracic paralysis in the other. Umbilical artery catheterization has caused spinal cord as well as other major organ infarctions.[17] In such cases described in the literature, the tips of the catheters were located high in relation to the thoracic spinal cord, and thrombotic or embolic occlusion of the arterial supply to the anterior spinal cord presumably occurred. It has been recommended that the catheter be inserted to the level of the tenth thoracic vertebra or below the third lumbar vertebra, recognizing that major vessel branches arise one vertebral body higher in infants than they do in adults.[17]

In those infants suspected of spinal cord injury, routine radiographic studies are of limited value because vertebral fractures and subluxations rarely are seen. Somatosensory evoked potentials can be useful in cases affecting the midthoracic level of the cord, but upper thoracic and cervical recordings frequently are difficult to obtain even in normal infants,[18] and scalp potentials overlying the somatosensory cortex may be absent in one third of newborns.[19] Magnetic resonance imaging is considered superior to myelography in its ability to define spinal cord pathology, and provides direct visualization of the spinal cord.[20]

Management of the newborn with a spinal cord lesion requires an interdisciplinary approach. The physicians must attend to the problem of spinal cord stability and to pulmonary, urologic, and gastrointestinal complications. The physical and occupational therapists prevent contractures and malalignment, and provide appropriate developmental stimulation to the affected infant. The nurse tends to temperature stability, feeding, suctioning, prevention of skin breakdown, and instruction of parents on proper handling techniques. A lightweight polypropylene body orthosis or a canvas jacket with flexible metal stays allow support of the trunk. Hand and foot

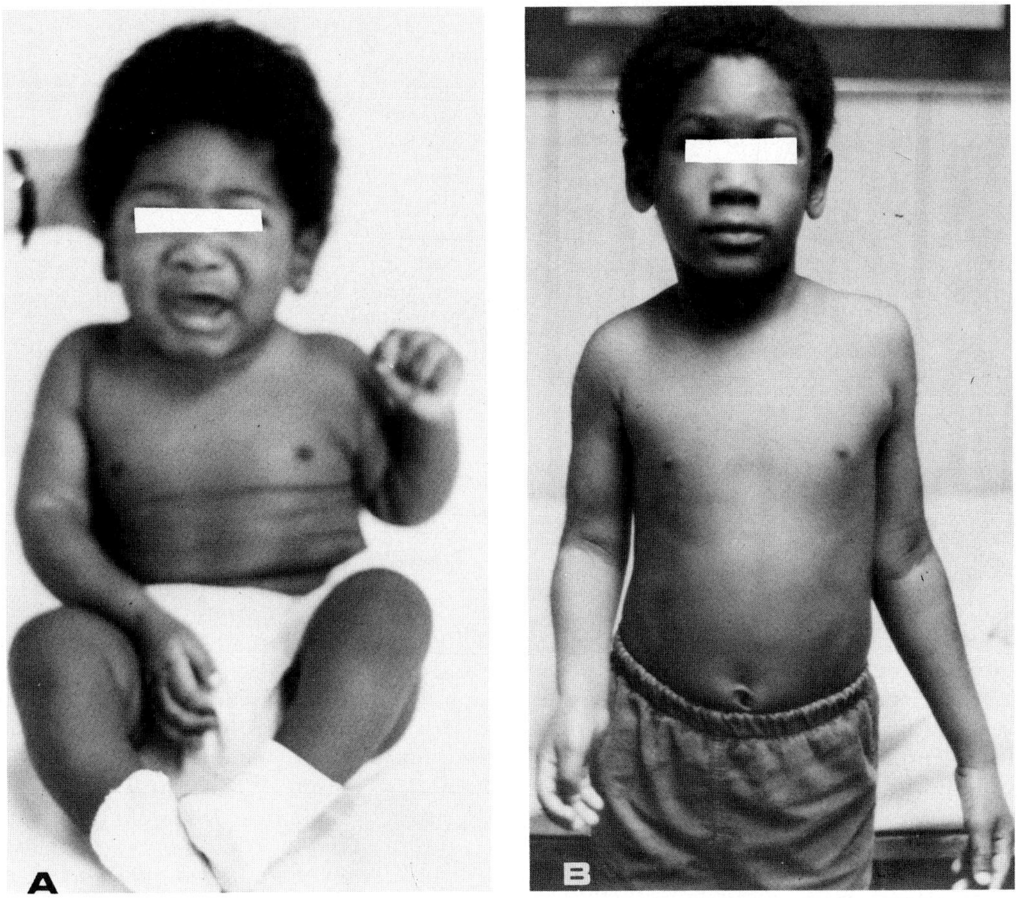

FIG. 51–7. **(A)** A 4-week-old boy with complete brachial plexus palsy involving the right arm. **(A)** The same patient at 3 years of age shows length discrepancy and loss of growth of the right arm. The hand intrinsic muscles are weak, and sensation is not intact.

splints to prevent deformity also are prescribed. An infant seat that provides well contoured support of the infant also is a necessity.

Successful rehabilitation must include the parents' understanding and care of their disabled child. Therefore, the social service personnel should play an integral role in meeting parental needs and facilitating long-term rehabilitation options.

CONGENITAL TORTICOLLIS

Torticollis, or wry neck, is recognized in an infant who persists in tilting the head to one side because of tightness of the sternocleidomastoid muscle or the trapezius and scalene muscles. There is asymmetry of the infant's face, with flattening of the cheek and temporal region, narrowing of the palpebral fissure, compression of the ear, and elevation of the shoulder on the side of the tight muscles, as well as flattening of the contralateral occiput (Fig. 51-8). By the second to fourth week of life, a hard fusiform mass (*i.e.*, an olive) is palpable in the belly of the muscle. It may increase in size, then gradually disappear when the infant is between 4 and 7 months of age, occasionally leaving a thick, fibrotic, noncontractile muscle.

The birth history in an infant with torticollis is remarkable in that it is usually difficult, is frequently a breech presentation, and occasionally even necessitates a cesarean section. Despite speculation on the pathogenesis of this problem,[21] the reason for the torticollis probably lies in the fact that the sternocleidomastoid pathologic condition exists *in utero*, precluding engagement of the infant's head in the birth canal. The concept that there is a hereditary defect in the anlage of the muscle is derived from the discovery of anomalous muscles in relatives or of the association of ipsilateral hip dislocation or clubfoot in the affected infants.[22] Intrauterine denervation and infection have not been substantiated by pathologic dissections of the involved muscle, which usually consists of glistening white fibrous tissue engulfing muscle fibers, without evidence of hemorrhage.[23]

Congenital torticollis must be differentiated from bony anomalies of the cervical spine and shoulder

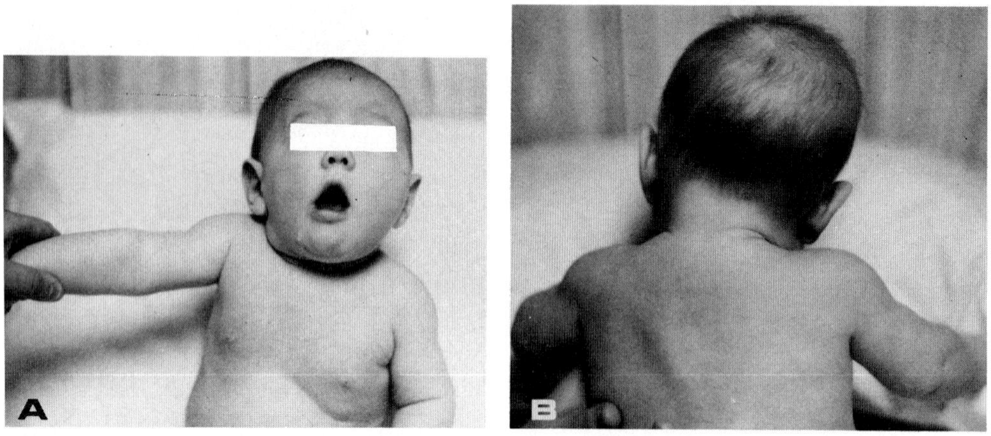

FIG. 51–8. **(A)** Congenial torticollis affecting the right sternocleidomastoid muscle in a 3-month-old infant. **(B)** Note the flattening of the left occiput and right head tilt.

girdle (*i.e.*, Klippel–Feil syndrome with or without Sprengel deformity) and acquired wry neck associated with acute trauma, pharyngotonsillitis, adenitis, cerebral irritation secondary to meningitis, posterior fossa tumors, visual and labyrinthine disorders, and postshunting for hydrocephalus. A mass in the neck may represent adenoma, cystic hygroma, dermoid, or rhabdomyoma.

In a review of 277 patients seen between 1970 and 1982, with a 2- to 13-year follow-up, 70% of the infants had resolution of the problem by 12 months of age. Tenotomies were required in ten children, eight having been first evaluated after 1 year of age.[24] In a young baby, physical therapy is eminently successful in stretching the contracted muscle. The parents are taught two basic exercises: stretching of the clavicular portion by lateral flexion of the head to the opposite side (Fig. 51-9*A*), and stretching of the sternal portion by rotation of the chin to the affected side (Fig. 51-9*B*). Occasionally, the trapezius and the muscles over the ipsilateral pelvic brim also must be stretched, because the baby tends to assume a long C-scoliotic curve. A soft, or a firmer, plasticized collar can be made readily to hold the head in good alignment (Fig. 51-10). Hanging toy mobiles above the baby's head on the affected side and placing the crib so that the baby has to turn the head to the affected side to see what is happening in the room are recommended for active stretching on the infant's part. Later, strengthening exercises will provide balanced flexion of the head. With early treatment, the asymmetry lessens as the skull and facial bones are permitted to remold. At 2 years of age, the entire contour is appreciably improved.

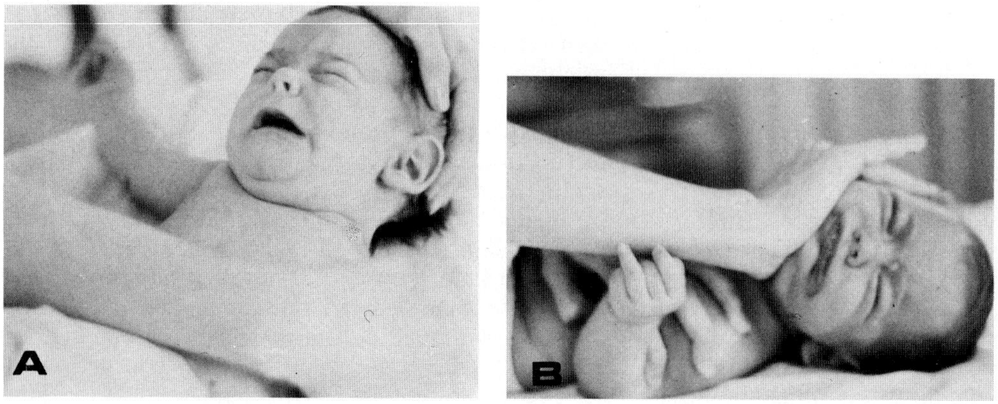

FIG. 51–9. **(A)** Stretching of the clavical portion of the contracted sternocleidomastoid muscle. **(B)** Stretching of the sternal portion of the contracted sternocleidomastoid muscle.

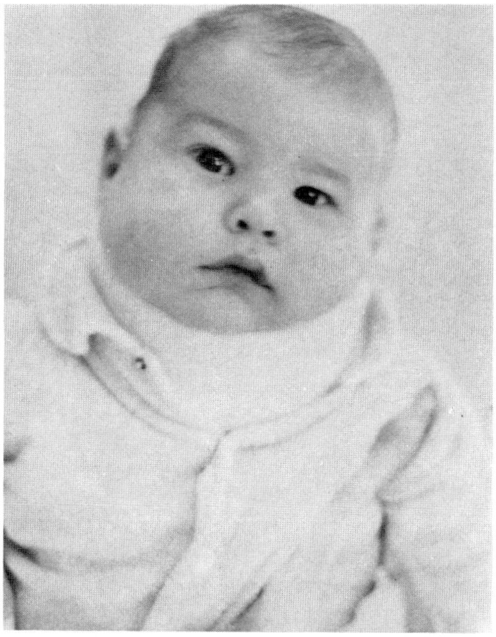

FIG. 51–10. A soft collar is used to keep the head in good alignment in a baby with a left torticollis.

TONE

Infants frequently are examined because of problems in tone. To separate tonal changes caused by upper motor neuron disorders from peripheral neuromuscular weakness, the concept of tone must be considered.

Tone is that quality in muscle that resists movement. The French call it *extensibilité,* and relate it to slow stretch while moving the muscle through a range of motion.[25] It also can be described as a recoil phenomenon. When the muscle is stretched passively and released, it springs back to its original position. When there is stretch and no rebound, allowing for limpness, this is hypotonia. When there is a constant resistance to stretch associated with a lead-pipe delay in relaxation, this is rigidity. Further, if there is stretch with too rapid rebound and too much recoil, this is spasticity.

MECHANISM

Neurophysiologists long have attempted to unravel the nervous control of posture and movement. It now appears that the γ nervous system, with its muscle spindles, the primary and secondary endings in the spindles, the afferent γ pathways, the γ motor neurons in the ventral horn of the spinal cord, and the efferent γ fibers back to the spindles, assumes important roles in the mechanism of tone. The monosynaptic connection between the group Ia γ afferent fibers and the α motor neurons, which send axons to the extrafusal fibers, constitutes the important stretch reflex. Inhibitory potentials from antagonistic muscles, as well as cutaneous and visceral afferents, affect the motor neuronal pathway. Supraspinal centers, through the corticospinal or lateral vestibulospinal tracts and reticulospinal pathways, send modifying influences to both the α motor and γ motor neurons (Fig. 51-11).

More specifically, the muscle spindles are sensory structures. They are small and fusiform in shape, lying parallel to skeletal muscle fibers. There are two types of intrafusal fibers in the muscle spindles, a nuclear bag fiber and a nuclear chain fiber. Each nuclear bag and nuclear chain fiber has a sensory ending that unites to form the group Ia sensory afferent nerve. The secondary endings come from nuclear chain fibers and form the group II afferent nerve fibers. Presumably, the primary ending from the nuclear bag intrafusals is sensitive to the rate of change of muscle length in stretch, and the secondary endings are sensitive to change in length. According to Rushworth, group Ia afferent fibers not only have monosynaptic connections with the α motor neurons in the spinal cord of the same muscle but also end in motor neurons of the synergistic and antagonistic muscles.[26] The exact function of the secondary endings is not clear, but they conduct more slowly, are polysynaptic, and are thought to facilitate flexor and inhibit extensor α motor neurons in the regulation of posture.

In the ventral horn of the spinal cord, the α motor neurons send axons back to the extrafusal muscle fibers. Gamma I and γ II motor neurons in turn send fibers that terminate in the intrafusal muscles fibers as trail endings and plate endings.[27]

The γ system modulates voluntary movement. According to Matthews, the γ afferents connect with the α motor neuron by way of the spindle loop as a "closed-loop servomechanism" controlling the length of the muscle, whereas the γ efferents control the "damping" of this loop and its controlled position.[26]

Although Rushworth believed that overactivity of the γ system resulted in spasticity and rigidity, it is known that the cortex, basal ganglia, and cerebellum modulate brain stem structures to affect motor control. Interruption of the extrapyramidal fibers results in spasticity, and selective destruction of corticospinal tracts can result in hypotonia.[28,29]

CHANGES IN TONE IN THE BRAIN-INJURED INFANT

A cerebrally damaged infant's tone may remain flaccid for days or weeks after delivery. The infant then progressively assumes abnormal postures and increasing stretch reflex. Tone can be modified by changing the infant's position. Hypotonia in prone may be hypertonia in supine and exaggerated hypertonicity in vertical suspension. The release of descending vestibulospinal impulses from higher cortical control probably is responsible for these shifts in

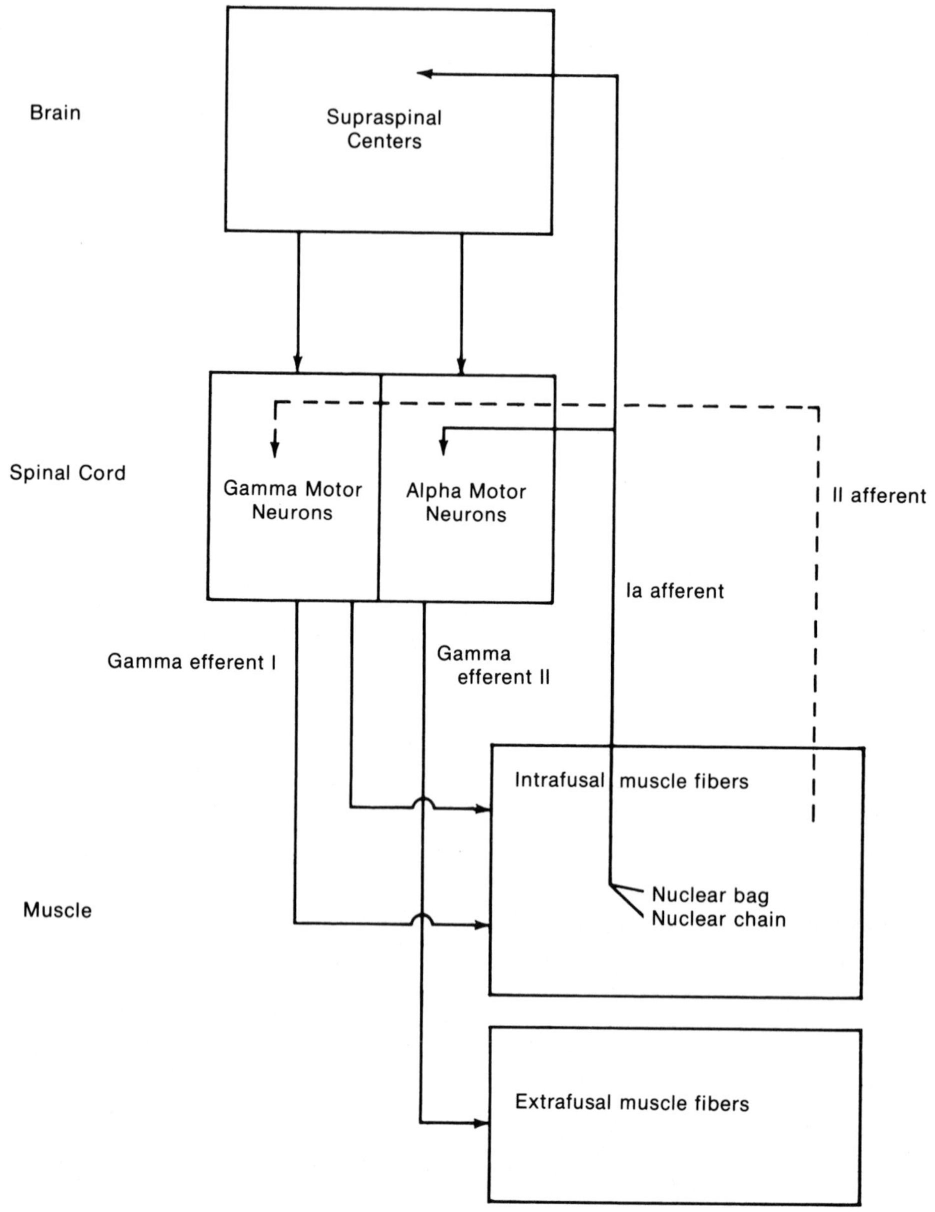

FIG. 51–11. Supraspinal, spinal, and muscle spindle pathways in muscle control.

tone. Changing the position of the infant's head will evoke the labyrinthine reflexes that also affect tone. Hyperextension of the head will elicit hyperextension of the trunk and facilitate hypertonicity of the limbs. Flexion of the head will relieve the hypertonus and relax the limbs. Imposing the tonic neck reflex increases the extensor tone in the limbs on the face side of the infant and the flexor tone on the occipital side. There may exist a discrepancy between hypotonicity affecting neck and trunk muscles and hypertonicity of the limb muscles. Deep tendon reflexes and infantile automatisms, although important in the early assessment of the infant, frequently are unreliable because they again are subservient to tone.

The problem in discrimination between brain and peripheral neuromuscular disease lies not in the overtly cerebrally damaged infant with changing tone but in the infant with persistently depressed tone. It may be hard to determine whether an infant has peripheral neuromuscular disease or brain damage because both conditions have a similar history:

- varying degrees of intrauterine immobility
- difficult labor
- slow engagement and descent in the birth canal
- a flaccid, immobile infant with weak cry and a low Apgar score at birth.

Prolonged hypotonia may be seen in the kernicteric infant after the initial rigid, opisthotonic state; athetosis may appear at the end of the first year of life.

Severe anoxia can produce a depressed baby for several months who then becomes increasingly choreoathetoid. My experience bears out Paine and Oppe's statement that "persistent and permanent hypotonicity of the body as a whole is also occasionally seen with chronic brain syndrome and may include hypo- or areflexia (and usually severe mental deficiency as well)."[30]

THE HYPERTONIC INFANT

Occasionally, an infant may present with too much tone. Such an infant tends to be stiff in the limbs, head control is too good, and on the Landau maneuver shows too much extension of the head and legs. When placed on the feet, the infant jerks into full vertical extension, rearing into almost an opisthotonic posture. Increased jitteriness, regurgitant feeding patterns, brisk jaw jerks, and deep tendon reflexes may be observed. The infant usually has a complicated gestational history that may include maternal drug abuse, may be premature, or may be small for dates. As the infant grows, the rigidity may diminish and milestones begin to be attained readily; the infant gradually evolves into a perfectly normal baby by 14 to 18 months of age. On the other hand, the infant may become overtly spastic with delayed development and varying degrees of psychomotor retardation. Drillien, in a prospective study of 300 children of low birth weights, described "transient dystonia" in some of the babies in the first year of life. Mental impairment and hyperactivity were noted in these babies by 2 to 3 years of age compared to the children who did not show abnormal neurologic signs. Those same children show deficits in language skills, motor perception, behavior, and learning when they reach school age.[31]

THE HYPOTONIC, PERIPHERAL NEUROMUSCULAR-DISEASED INFANT

The hypotonic infant with lower motor neuron involvement usually assumes very typical postures without changes in tone when his posture in space is altered. When lying supine, the arms rest slightly abducted and internally or externally rotated at the

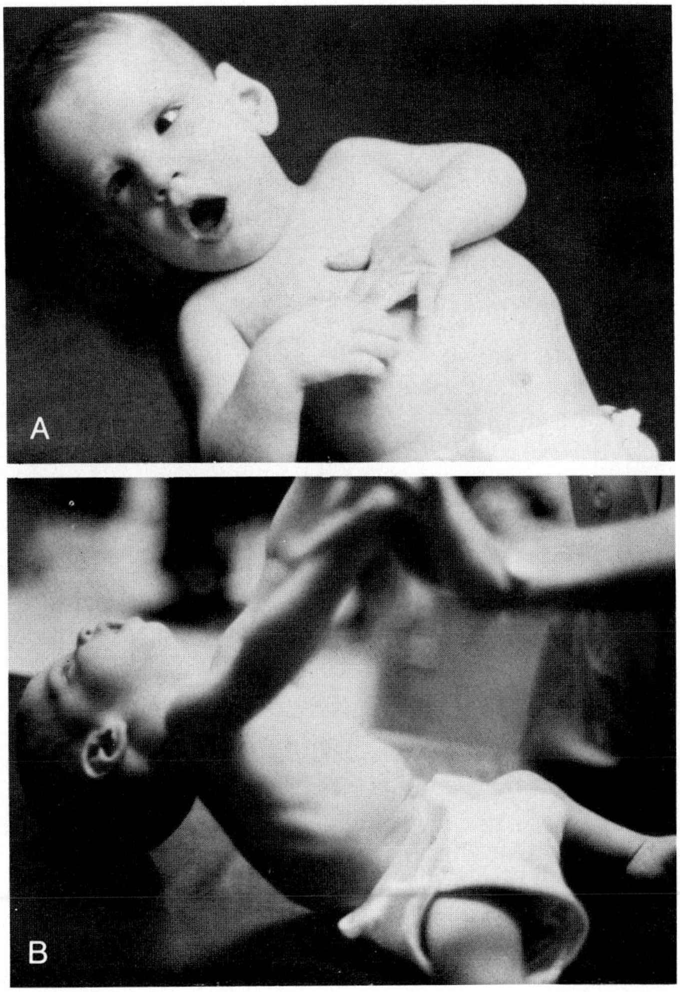

FIG. 51–12. A hypotonic 4-month-old infant with **(A)** myopathic facies and **(B)** extreme head lag during traction of the arms was diagnosed as having myotonic atrophy.

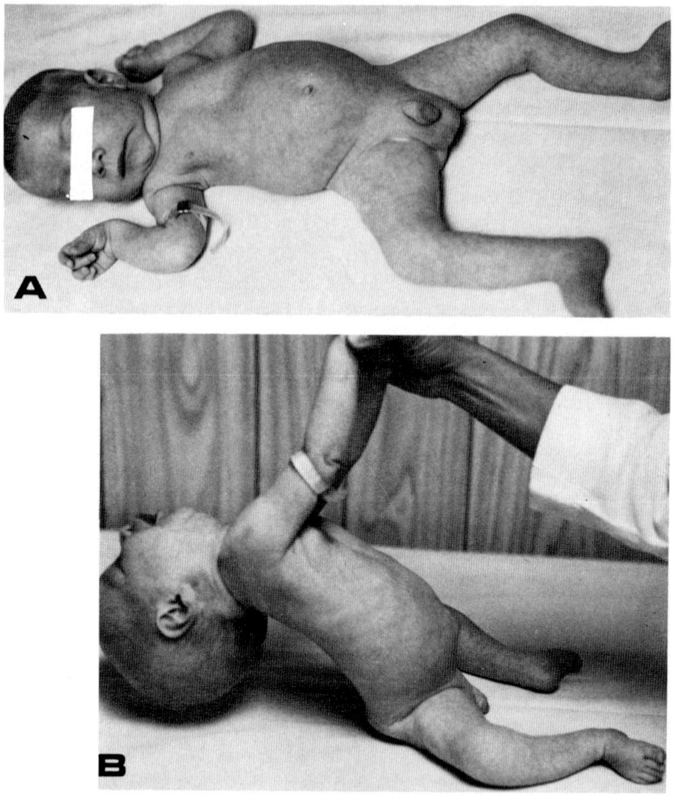

FIG. 51–13. (A) A hypotonic 3-month-old infant with Werdnig–Hoffman disease lies in a typical immobile posture. He appears alert despite profound weakness and paradoxical respirations. (B) Severe head lag is noted when traction is exerted on the infant's arms.

shoulder, with elbows flexed and pronated and fingers clenched in slight ulnar drift. The hips are maintained in an abducted externally rotated position in the pithed-frog posture. The cry is weak, breathing may be paradoxic with asynchronous expansion of the chest cage and the abdomen, and the only spontaneous movements involve small excursions of the fingers and toes. Deep tendon reflexes are depressed and frequently absent. The Moro reflex, tonic neck reflexes, and crossed adductor responses usually are not elicitable. The infant may have an expressionless facies (Fig. 51-12), but alternatively may appear vitally alert despite profound weakness (Fig. 51-13).

THE CHRONICALLY ILL INFANT

Not to be forgotten among the hypotonic babies is the chronically ill infant who has cardiac, renal, adrenal, metabolic, or nutritional problems. Such an infant may be severely hypotonic but usually maintains deep tendon reflexes and will move the extremities on stimulus. Moreover, the infant will look sick.

RESULTS IN A SERIES OF INFANTS WITH TONE PROBLEMS

Over a 3-year period, I studied 335 infants who presented with problems in tone. They ranged from birth to 3 years of age (Table 51-1). Of these, nine infants developed normally or even acquired milestones in an accelerated manner. Two hundred and seventy-five infants were categorized as infants with cerebral dysfunction (*i.e.*, 241 with cerebral palsy, 26 with nonspecific psychomotor retardation, and 8 with various degenerating or demyelinating disorders). Involvement of the spinal cord to include the anterior horn cells, the peripheral nerves, neuromuscular junction, and muscles affected 51 infants. Thus, peripheral neuromuscular diseases comprised only 15% of the total group of hypotonic–hypertonic infants that I examined.

The most common lower motor neuron disorder in the series was spinal muscular atrophy (*i.e.*, Werdnig–Hoffman disease). This is a disorder with a wide spectrum of manifestations. It may occur *in utero*, resulting in diminution of fetal movements. The baby may then be born with arthrogrypotic changes. A baby may appear normal at birth and suddenly develop extreme weakness with severe head lag, proximal limb girdle muscle paralysis, absent deep tendon reflexes, and increasing respiratory problems because of bulbar and respiratory muscle involvement. Despite severe flaccidity, the facial muscles are spared and the baby usually appears alert, wide-eyed, and intelligent. The earlier the onset of the disease, the worse the prognosis becomes. Of babies who were diagnosed under 5 months of age, 90% were dead before 1 year of age. Some infants with spinal muscular atrophy who are not diagnosed until the end of the first year or during the second year of life have a more benign variant of this disease. They may survive infancy and with good care grow into adulthood. Their disease appears to be nonprogressive or very slowly progressive, and they blend into the adult group of benign limb girdle atrophies.[32]

TABLE 51–1
TONE PROBLEMS IN 332 INFANTS FROM BIRTH TO 3 YEARS OF AGE WHO WERE HYPOTONIC–HYPERTONIC ON INITIAL EVALUATION

Site and Type of Problem	Number
Normal-to-accelerated development	9
Brain	372
Cerebral palsy	247
Psychomotor retardation	23
Degenerating–demyelinating disease	5
Krabbe syndrome	1
Tay–Sachs disease	2
Metachromatic leukodystrophy	1
Adrenoleukodystrophy	1
Cord	27
Infantile spinal muscular atrophy (*i.e.*, Werdnig–Hoffman syndrome)	15
Juvenile spinal muscular atrophy	4
Arthrogryposis secondary to neurogenic atrophy	4
Traction injury	1
Infantile poliomyelitis	1
Multiple anomalies with upper cord lesion	1
Multiple anomalies with diffuse neurogenic atrophy	1
Roots and nerves	3
Polyneuropathy	3
Neuromuscular junction	2
Congenital myasthenia gravis	2
Muscle	14
Muscular dystrophy	1
Myopathy—type I hypotrophy and central nuclei	4
Inflammatory myopathy	2
Polymyositis	1
Myotonic atrophy	5
Pompe glycogen storage disease	1
Metabolic and chronic diseases	5
Hyperthyroidism—myositis	1
Hypothyroidism—neuropathy	3
Congenital renal anomaly	1

The infantile form of spinal muscular atrophy usually is inherited as an autosomal recessive disorder and the genetic marker presumably is on chromosome 5. Prenatal diagnosis is in the investigative phase.

The fetal form of myotonic dystrophy deserves attention because of the neonatal difficulties of sucking, swallowing associated with apnea, and bradycardia. At birth, the infant is hypotonic with slack facies and a tented mouth, occasionally showing cryptorchidism and equinovarus deformities of the feet. Particular scrutiny of the mother may reveal her to be the unsuspected carrier and confirm the diagnosis.[33–35]

Since the initial survey, recognizable syndromes affecting infants that result in hypotonia and delay in development have increased in number and complexity as knowledge and diagnostic acumen in their identification increase. These include various genetic syndromes such as Prader–Willi syndrome,[36] specific lysosomal enzyme as well as peroxisomal metabolic abnormalities,[37] amino and organic acid metabolic dysfunction, as well as urea cycle defects.[38,39]

Lower motor neuron disorders include not only the spinal muscular atrophies, but peripheral neuropathies:

- hereditary motor sensory neuropathy type I (*i.e.*, Charcot–Marie–Tooth disease)
- hereditary motor sensory neuropathy type II (*i.e.*, distal spinal muscular atrophy)
- hereditary motor sensory neuropathy type IV (*i.e.*, Refsum disease)
- pure sensory neuropathies.[40]

Various lesions of the neuromuscular junction, including myasthenia gravis[41,42] and infantile botulism,[43,44] have been verified on neuromuscular transmission studies accompanied by facilitation techniques.

Congenital muscular dystrophies are relatively rare, but should be considered in the infant with a myopathic facies and extreme hypotonia.[45] A fetal form of fascioscapulohumeral dystrophy with particular weakness of the face, neck, and proximal shoulder girdle muscles accompanied by deafness, with autosomal dominant transmission, has been identified by us and others.[46] Ophthalmoplegia and generalized muscle weakness have been noted in infants who have myotubular myopathy,[47] and mitochondrial myopathies.[48,49] Nemaline myopathy,[50,51] associated with sudden respiratory compromise in a mildly hypotonic infant, also has been seen. Glycogen storage disorders,[52] such as Pompe disease with a fatal outcome, have been diagnosed. Many of the neuromuscular disorders have identifiable genetic markers, and in certain instances prenatal diagnosis is available. The reader is referred to the many articles and monographs on neuromuscular disorders.[53–55]

The physician is responsible for informing the parents of the diagnosis and to offer them the opportunity for genetic counseling. He or she needs to prescribe appropriate physical therapy intervention to maintain the infant in as optimal a state as possible. Special requirements include feeding techniques, postural drainage and suctioning, seating in well supported postural alignment, prevention of joint contractures that can add to the child's discomfort, and appropriate developmental stimulation to offset the child's relative immobility.[55–57]

LABORATORY AIDS IN PERIPHERAL NEUROMUSCULAR DISORDERS

The laboratory becomes of inestimable value in the detailed study of infants with hypotonia. Muscle enzymes, EMG, and muscle biopsy are important in laboratory confirmation of the clinical impression.

MUSCLE ENZYMES

Elevated serum enzyme levels of creatine phosphokinase, aldolase, and transaminases reflect muscle breakdown. They are normal in the cerebrally damaged infant, may be slightly elevated in neurogenic disease and some myopathies, and markedly elevated in muscular dystrophies. Creatine kinase levels are particularly specific for intrinsic muscle disease; however, they may be considerably elevated in normal infants during the first 24 hours of life, gradually tapering to near normal levels by 5 days of age, but may persist in slight elevation throughout the first year of life.[58,59] Cautious interpretation of the enzyme levels is therefore necessary, especially when a baby with possible congenital Duchenne dystrophy is being considered. The enzymes should therefore be drawn after the end of the first week of life. It also is preferable to request enzymes before EMG because trauma caused by needle exploration may elevate the creatine kinase for 72 hours. Intramuscular injection also will cause a rise in creatine kinase levels.

ELECTRODIAGNOSIS

The development of electrodiagnosis has proven a valuable adjunct to the neurologic differentiation of hypotonic infants.[5,60,61] The electrical studies are well tolerated by neonates. They include study of neuromuscular transmission, nerve conduction velocity determinations, and EMG. Their application is based on knowledge of maturation of the infant's peripheral nervous system. In this regard, even the gestational age of infants can be estimated by conduction velocities of their peripheral nerves.[62] Full-term infants' nerve conduction velocities are approximately one-half those of adults and mature to adult levels by 3 to 5 years of age. These nerve conduction velocity studies provide information relevant to the integrity of the peripheral nerve, particularly in suspected polyneuropathies.

Neuromuscular transmission likewise improves with maturation and deteriorates when disease states such as myasthenia gravis or botulism and other poisonous agents intervene.[4]

The EMG has proven especially excellent in providing information regarding the muscle. The size and duration of the motor unit action potentials, the aggregation of these potentials and firing rate to form an interference pattern, the tracing when the muscle is at rest—whether it is silent or shows fibrillation potentials and sharp waves—may reflect the presence or absence of a pathologic condition. Irritability of the muscles on needle exploration may signify sick muscles. The presence of runs of positive potentials (*i.e.*, iterative discharges) may suggest myotonia and is evidence of instability of the muscle membrane.

MUSCLE BIOPSY

The enzyme and electrodiagnostic data lead to necessary confirmation of suspected muscle disease by muscle biopsy. The importance of meticulous handling of the biopsy specimen cannot be overemphasized, especially when the possible diagnosis of a rather obscure myopathy is involved. The selection of the biopsy site is important. It should reflect disease that is active but not so advanced pathologically that all landmarks are destroyed. A muscle that has been recently studied by EMG or that has received intramuscular injections should be avoided. The biopsy then may show inflammatory reaction and frequently identifiable needle tracks. A full complement of histochemical staining, electron microscopy, dystrophin assay, and interpretation by a physician experienced in muscle disorders should be available before a biopsy is attempted.[63]

REFERENCES

1. Falco NA, Eriksson E. Facial nerve palsy in the newborn: incidence and outcome. Plast Reconstr Surg 1990;00:1.
2. Harris JP, Davidson TM, May M, et al. Evaluation and treatment of congenital facial paralysis. Arch Otolaryngol 1983;109:145.
3. Nelson K, Eng G. Congenital hypoplasia of the depressor anguli oris muscle: differentiation from congenital facial palsy. J Pediatr 1972;18:16.

4. Kimura J. Electrodiagnosis in diseases of nerve and muscle: principles and practice. 2nd ed. Philadelphia: FA Davis, 1989.
5. Eng GD. Electrodiagnosis. In: Molnar GE, ed. Pediatric rehabilitation. 2nd ed. Baltimore: Williams & Wilkins, 1992:143.
6. Koenigsberger MR. Brachial plexus palsy at birth: intrauterine or due to delivery trauma? Ann Neurol 1980;8:228.
7. Dunn DW, Engle WA. Brachial plexus palsy: intrauterine onset. Pediatr Neurol 1985;1:367.
8. Eng GD, Koch B, Smokvina MD. Brachial plexus palsy in neonates and children. Arch Phys Med Rehabil 1978;59:458.
9. Kawabata H, Masada K, Tsuyuguchi Y, et al. Early microsurgical reconstruction in birth palsy. Clin Orthop 1987;215:233.
10. Boome RS, Kaye JC. Obstetric traction injuries of the brachial plexus: natural history, indication for surgical repair and results. J Bone Joint Surg [Br] 1988;70:571.
11. Piatt JH, Hudson AR, Hoffman HJ. Preliminary experience with brachial plexus exploration in children: birth injury and vehicular trauma. Neurosurgery 1988;22:715.
12. Kline DG. "Comments," in Piatt JH Jr, Hudson AR, Hoffman JH. Preliminary experiences with brachial plexus exploration in children: birth injury and vehicular trauma. Neurosurgery 1988;22:722
13. Gilbert A, Brockman R, Carlioz H. Surgical treatment of brachial plexus palsy. Clin Orthop 1991;264:39.
14. Clancy RR, Sladkey JT, Rorke LB. Hypoxic-ischemic spinal cord injury following perinatal asphyxia. Ann Neurol 1989; 25:185.
15. Koch BM, Eng GD. Neonatal spinal cord injury. Arch Phys Med Rehabil 1979;60:378.
16. Hernandez-Marti M, DalCanto MC, Kidd JM. Evidence of spinal cord injury in an infant delivered by Cesarean section: a case report. Child's Brain 1984;11:197.
17. Brown MS, Phibbs RH. Spinal cord injury in newborns from use of umbilical artery catheters: report of two cases and review of the literature. J Perinatol 1988;8:105.
18. Bell HJ, Dykstra DD. Somatosensory evoked potentials as an adjunct to diagnosis of neonatal spinal cord injury. J Pediatr 1985;106:298.
19. Gilmore R, Brock J, Hermansen MC, et al. Development of lumbar spinal cord and cortical evoked potentials after tibial nerve stimulation in the pre-term newborns: effect of gestational age and other factors. Electroencephalogr Clin Neurophysiol 1987;68:28.
20. Lanska MJ, Roessman U, Wiznitzer M. Magnetic resonance imaging in cervical cord birth injury. Pediatrics 1990;85:760.
21. Suzuki S, Yamamuro T, Fugita A. The aetiological relationship between congenital torticollis and obstetrical paralysis. Int Orthop 1984;8:175.
22. Hara I, Ikeda T. On the ipsilateral involvement of congenital muscular torticollis and congenital dislocation of the hip. J Jpn Orthop Assoc 1962;35:1221.
23. Garceau G. Congenital muscular torticollis hematoma: fact or myth. Medical Journal of Rhode Island 1962;45:401.
24. Binder J, Eng GD, Gaiser JF, et al. Congenital muscular torticollis: results of conservative management with long-term follow-up in 85 cases. Arch Phys Med Rehabil 1987;68:222
25. Andre-Thomas CY, Saint-Anne Daigassis S. The neurological examination of the infant. Little Club Clinic, No. 1. London: National Spastics Society, 1960.
26. Boyd IA, Eyzaguirre C, Matthews P, et al. The role of the gamma system in movement and posture. New York: New York Association for the Aid of Crippled Children, 1964.
27. Dubo H, Darling R. Gamma nervous system and muscle spindles. In: Downey J, Darling R, eds. Physiological basis of rehabilitation medicine. Philadelphia: WB Saunders, 1971:49.
28. Katz RT, Rymer WZ. Spastic hypertonia: mechanisms and measurement. Arch Phys Med Rehabil 1989;70:144.
29. Meinck HM, Benecke R, Conrad B. Spasticity and flexor reflex. In: Delwaide PJ, Young RR, eds. Clinical neurophysiology in spasticity: contribution to assessment and pathophysiology. Amsterdam: Elsevier, 1985:41.
30. Paine R, Oppe T. Neurological examination of children. Clinic in Developmental Medicine. London: Heineman Medical, 1966.
31. Drillien C. Abnormal neurologic signs in the first year of life in low-birthweight infants: possible prognostic significance. Dev Med Child Neurol 1972;14:575.
32. Eng GD, Binder H, Koch B. Spinal muscular atrophy: experience in diagnosis and rehabilitation management of 60 patients. Arch Phys Med Rehabil 1984;65:549.
33. Dyken PR, Harper PS. Congenital dystrophic myotonica. Neurology 1973;23:465.
34. Harper PS, Dyken PR. Early onset dystrophia myotonica: evidence supporting a maternal environment factor. Lancet 1972;2:53.
35. Wesström G, Bensch J, Schollin J. Congenital myotonic dystrophy: incidence, clinical aspects and early prognosis. Acta Paediatr Scand 1986;75:849.
36. Cassidy SB. Prader-Willi syndrome. Curr Probl Pediatr 1984; 14:5.
37. Naidu S, Moser HW. Peroxisomal disorders. Neurol Clin 1990; 8:507.
38. Volpe JJ. Disorders of organic acid metabolism. In: Volpe JJ, ed. Neurology of the newborn. Philadelphia: WB Saunders, 1987:434.
39. Volpe JJ. Hyperammonemia and other disorders of amino acid metabolism. In: Volpe JJ, ed. Neurology of the newborn. Philadelphia: WB Saunders, 1987:434.
40. Dyck PJ, Thomas PK, Lambert EH, et al, eds. Peripheral neuropathy. Philadelphia: WB Saunders, 1984.
41. Engel AG. Congenital myasthenic syndromes. J Child Neurol 1988;3:233.
42. Gay CT, Bodensteiner JB. The floppy infant: recent advances in the understanding of disorders affecting the neuromuscular junction. Neurol Clin 1991;8:715.
43. Midura TF, Arnone SS. Infant botulism. Lancet 1976;2:934.
44. Fakadej AV, Gutman L. Prolongation of post-tetanic facilitation in infant botulism. Muscle Nerve 1982;5:727.
45. Fenichel GM. Congenital muscular dystrophies. Neurol Clin 1988;6:519.
46. Korf BR, Bresman MJ, Shapiro F, et al. Facioscapulohumeral dystrophy presenting in infancy with facial diplegia and sensorineural deafness. Ann Neurol 1985;17:513.
47. Collins JE, Collins A, Radford MR, et al. Perinatal diagnosis of myotubular (centronuclear) myopathy: a case report. Clin Neuropathol 1983;2(2):79.
48. Morgan-Hughes JA. The mitochondrial myopathies. In: Engel AG, Banker BQ, eds. Myology. New York: McGraw-Hill, 1986: 1709.
49. Zeviani M, Bonilla E, Devivo DC, et al. Mitochondrial diseases. Neurol Clin 1989;7:123.
50. Tsujihata M, Shimomura C, Yoshimura T, et al. Fatal neonatal nemaline myopathy: a case report. J Neuro Neurosurg Psychiatr 1983;46:856.
51. Martinex A, Lake BD. Childhood nemaline myopathy: a review of clinical presentations in relationship to prognosis. Dev Med Child Neurol 1987;29:815.
52. Servidei S, DiMauro S. Disorders of glycogen metabolism of muscle. Neruol Clin 1989;7:159.
53. Dubowitz V. The floppy infant. Philadelphia: JB Lippincott, 1980.
54. Dubowitz V. Color atlas of muscle disorders in childhood. Chicago: Year Book, 1989.
55. Eng GD. Rehabilitation of children with neuromuscular dis-

eases. In: Molnar GE, ed. Pediatric rehabilitation. 2nd ed. Baltimore: Williams & Wilkins, 1992:336.
56. End GD, Binder H. Rehabilitation of infants and children with neuromuscular disorders. Pediatr Ann 1988;12:745.
57. Eng GD. Rehabilitation of the child with a severe form of spinal muscular atrophy. In: Merlini L, Granata C, Dubowitz V, eds. Current Concepts in Childhood Spinal Muscluar Atrophy. New York: Springer-Verlag, 1989.
58. Wharton B, Bassie U, Gough G, Williams A. Clinical value of plasma creatine kinase and uric acid levels during the first week of life. Arch Dis Child 1971;46:356.
59. Bodensteiner J, Zellweger H. Creatine phosphokinase in normal neonates and young infants. J Lab Clin Med 1971;77:853.
60. Jones HR Jr. EMG evaluation of the floppy infant: differential diagnosis and technical aspects. Muscle Nerve 1990;13:338.
61. Jablecki CK. Pediatric electrodiagnosis. Clinics of North America—Physical Medicine and Rehabilitation 1991;2:917.
62. Bryant PR, Eng GD. Normal values for the soleus H-reflex in newborn infants 31-45 weeks post-conceptional age. Arch Phys Med Rehabil 1991;72:28.
63. Engel AG. The muscle biopsy: part 2. In: Engel AG, Banker BQ, eds. Myology. New York: McGraw-Hill, 1986:833.

Neonatology: Pathophysiology and Management of the Newborn, Fourth Edition,
edited by Gordon B. Avery, Mary Ann Fletcher, and Mhairi G. MacDonald.
J.B. Lippincott Company, Philadelphia © 1994.

chapter 52

Orthopaedics

PAUL P. GRIFFIN

The orthopaedic or musculoskeletal examination of the newborn is a significant part of the evaluation of the neonate. Normal variations in contour, size, relationships, and range of motion of joints are influenced by genetic factors and by position *in utero.* These normal variations must be distinguished from congenital anomalies and traumatic lesions. The basic principle, that the earlier appropriate treatment is started, the better the correction, makes it incumbent on those caring for the neonate to make a diagnosis early and to obtain appropriate consultation promptly.

PHYSICAL EXAMINATION

The clinician examines the musculoskeletal system first by inspection, looking for anomalies in contour and position and observing the spontaneous and reflex movements of the infant, and second by palpation and manipulation to determine whether there are abnormalities of passive motion. This is followed by stimulation, where indicated, so that active motion can be noted.

A routine for examining a newborn should be developed so that each examination will be complete. This routine may vary among physicians, but each part of the musculoskeletal system should be examined systematically.

HEAD AND NECK

The neck is examined passively for rotation, lateral flexion, anterior flexion, and extension. Rotation of 80° and lateral flexion of 40° should be present. Both these motions are normally symmetric to the right and left. Extension and flexion are difficult to measure, but in flexion the chin should touch or nearly touch the chest wall. Extension should be at least 45° from neutral. When rotation or lateral flexion is asymmetrical or when motion is limited, radiographs of the neck should be made.

UPPER EXTREMITIES

The clavicle and shoulder girdle, including the scapula and proximal humerus, elbow, forearm, and hand are inspected and palpated, with any anomalies in contour and postural attitudes noted. Range of motion of the shoulder girdle is evaluated. Flexion and abduction of the shoulder are 175° to 180°. Extension, internal rotation, and external rotation of the shoulder should be at least 25°, 80°, and 45°, respectively.

The elbow is next inspected, and its motion is evaluated. Normally, the newborn's elbow lacks 10° to 15° from going to full extension and flexes 145°. The forearm should pronate and supinate at least 80°. Limitation of these two motions can be easily missed. Supination and pronation are tested by holding the humerus at the side of the trunk with the elbow held flexed 90° with one hand while checking supination and pronation with the other. The wrist flexes 75° to 80° and extends 65° to 75°. The normally clenched fist of the newborn should have full passive extension of the thumb and all fingers. Active finger extension may be elicited if necessary by a pinprick to the palm. Extension should be to 0° at the metacarpophalangeal joint, but active extension of the interphalangeal joint usually lacks 5° to 15° from going to 0°.

SPINE

In the newborn, congenital anomalies of the spine are not readily detectable on physical examination; however, gross anomalies frequently can be recognized by inspection of the spine. Passive flexion and extension and lateral bending of the spine should show smooth contours. Lateral flexion may be slightly asymmetric secondary to position *in utero*. A hairy patch, cutaneous vascular pattern, and lipomatous mass are frequent telltale signs of underlying axial anomalies.

LOWER EXTREMITIES

The lower extremity is observed for symmetry, variations in contour, position, and size. The hips of a newborn will flex 145° and generally have a flexion contracture as shown by the Thomas test. This test is performed by flexing both the infant's hips fully, then extending the hip to be tested while the opposite hip is held in flexion to lock the pelvis. The number of degrees that the extended thigh lacks from going to 0° extension is the degree of flexion contracture present. It is normal for the newborn to have a 25° to 30° flexion contracture. The hip flexion contracture gradually diminishes during the first 12 weeks or so of life but occasionally will be present longer than 3 months. When hip extension is asymmetrical, the more extended hip may be unstable. The stability of the hip always must be evaluated by an Ortolani test (Fig. 52-1). When there is a difference in the extension of the hips or a positive Ortolani test, further evaluation of the hip by radiographs or, preferably, by sonography should be done. Internal and external rotation of the hip in general will range between 40° and 80°, abduction is between 45° and 75°, and normal abduction is between 10° and 20°. Any asymmetry of motion should be investigated to determine the cause.

Infants who have not been in the frank breech position generally will have a knee flexion contracture of 10° to 25° with additional ability to flex to 120° to 145°. In those positioned in frank breech, the knees usually will hyperextend 10° to 15° and have limitation of flexion.

Examination of the ankles and feet should include observation of the resting position and stimulation for active motion, which is accomplished by stroking the sole and the dorsal, medial, and lateral sides of the foot to observe the range of active motion. Passive motion of the ankle in both dorsiflexion and plantarflexion varies depending on the *in utero* position, but dorsiflexion to above neutral always should be present and plantarflexion of less than 10° below neutral generally would be abnormal. Abduction and adduction of the forefoot is at least 10° to 15°, and the hindfoot has 5° to 10° or more of motion in both varus and valgus.

MUSCULOSKELETAL ANOMALIES

It is not within the scope of this text to discuss all the congenital and acquired abnormalities of the musculoskeletal system seen in the neonate; this chapter does, however, cover most of the more common abnormalities.

NECK

Klippel–Feil syndrome is a defect in segmentation of the cervical vertebrae. There is both a decrease in the number of vertebrae and fusion of two or more verte-

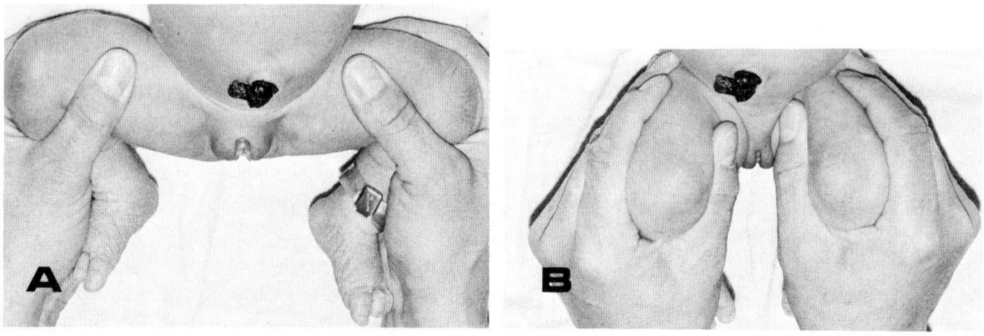

FIG. 52–1. **(A)** Ortolani sign. The fingers are on the trochanter and the thumbs grip the femurs as shown. The femurs are lifted forward as the thighs are abducted. If the head was dislocated, it can be felt to reduce. **(B)** The thighs are adducted. If the head dislocates, it will be both felt and seen as it suddenly jerks over the acetabulum.

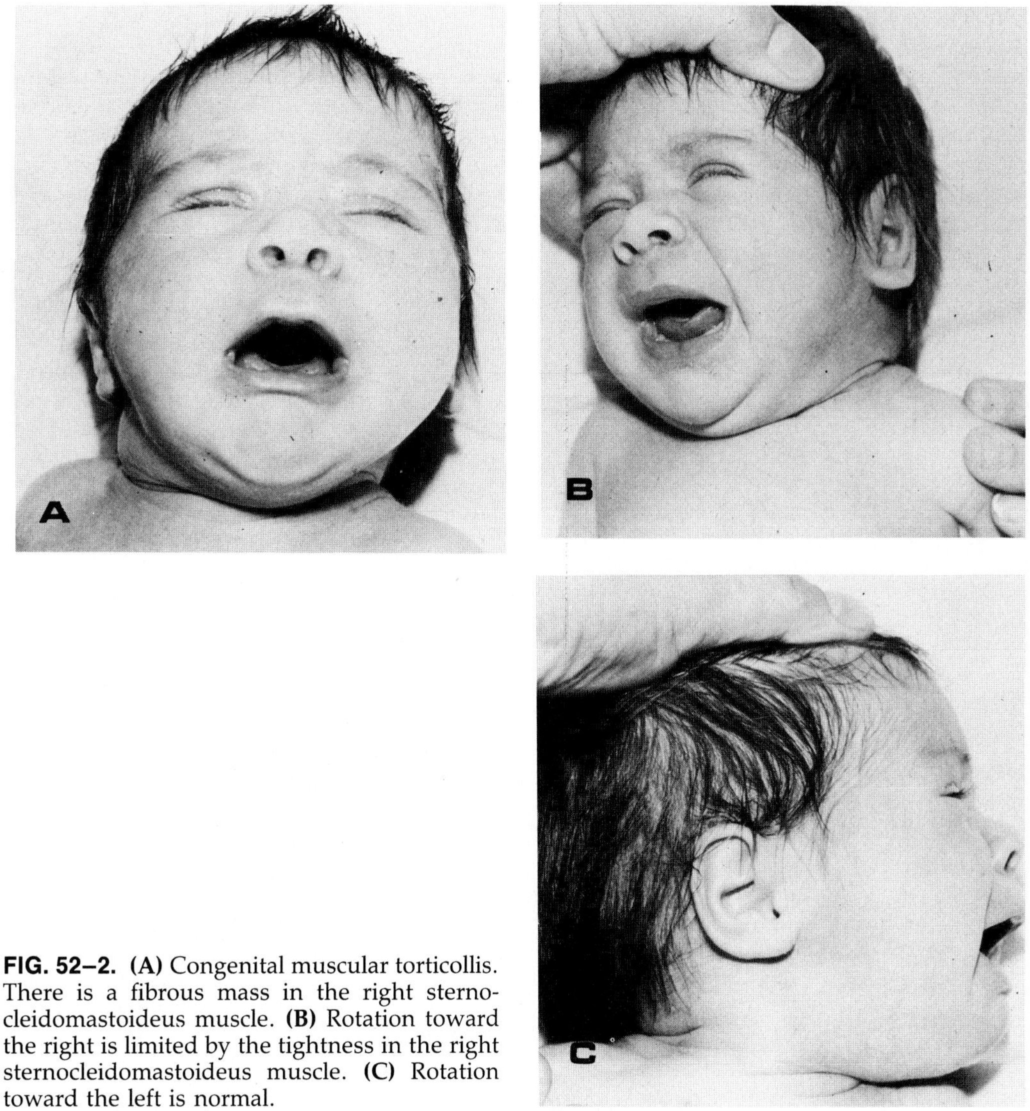

FIG. 52–2. **(A)** Congenital muscular torticollis. There is a fibrous mass in the right sternocleidomastoideus muscle. **(B)** Rotation toward the right is limited by the tightness in the right sternocleidomastoideus muscle. **(C)** Rotation toward the left is normal.

brae. The neck appears shorter than normal, and motion is limited in all directions. The limitation of motion depends on the number of fused segments and frequently is asymmetric in both rotation and lateral flexion. The asymmetric motion may simulate muscular torticollis, but radiographic examination of the neck can confirm the presence of the Klippel–Feil deformity. Treatment started early, done several times a day, and consisting of passive stretching of the neck to improve rotation, lateral bending, and flexion–extension may improve the range of motion of the neck.

Torticollis of the neonate may be one of several types. The typical muscular torticollis (Fig. 52-2*A*) involves a mass from a muscular hematoma that appears in the sternocleidomastoideus at 2 weeks of age and gradually disappears during the next 8 to 10 weeks. This mass may go unnoticed, and the torticollis unrecognized until there is facial asymmetry and limited motion of the neck. The physical findings of muscular torticollis are limited rotation of the neck toward the side of the lesion (Fig. 52-2*B,C*) and limited lateral flexion away from the lesion. In well established, persistent torticollis, there is flattening of the maxillary and frontal bones on the side of the lesion and of the occiput on the opposite side. The asymmetry is not present in the newborn but may become apparent as early as 2 or 3 weeks and is progressive until the tightness is corrected. Torticollis associated with interuterine deformation may be apparent at birth.

Initial treatment of muscular torticollis is by passive exercise and appropriate positioning of the infant in bed. The neck should be gently but firmly stretched, four or five times each day, toward the direction of limited rotation and lateral flexion. Sandbags or some similar objects may be used to position the baby's head to prevent it from assuming the position that the tight muscle encourages.

There is a type of congenital torticollis that is associated with neither a mass in the sternocleidomastoideus nor cervical spine abnormalities. In these infants, there is a myostatic contracture of the sternocleidomastoideus, probably secondary to *in utero* position. This type of torticollis often is associated with scoliosis, and abductor contracture of one hip and adductor tightness of the opposite hip, and there may be acetabular dysplasia opposite to the hip with abductor tightness (Fig. 52-3). The abductor contracture may not be detectable until the hip flexor tightness has spontaneously diminished so that the hip can be extended.

Whereas the torticollis usually will correct with little or no treatment, the tight hip adductor and, particularly, the abductor should be treated by passive stretching plus use of multiple diapers or some other abduction device. Rarely, the associated dysplasia progresses to dislocation.

SPINE

Congenital scoliosis may be difficult to recognize at birth unless there is asymmetrical motion, a cutaneous lesion (*e.g.*, aplasia, flat hemangioma, hairy patch), or a lipomatous mass. The scoliosis is caused by an isolated defect in vertebral body formation or by failure of segmentation. There is little evidence that it is an inherited anomaly. Except when associated with a genetically transmitted condition, there is no reason to expect a future sibling to have a similar problem. Treatment of congenital scoliosis is initially by observation, because spinal orthoses seldom are of benefit. When the curve is progressive, spinal fusion will be needed and should be done before the curve becomes cosmetically or functionally significant. Fusion of a short segment may be done as early as necessary. Because congenital scoliosis is associated with a high incidence of related genitourinary anomalies,

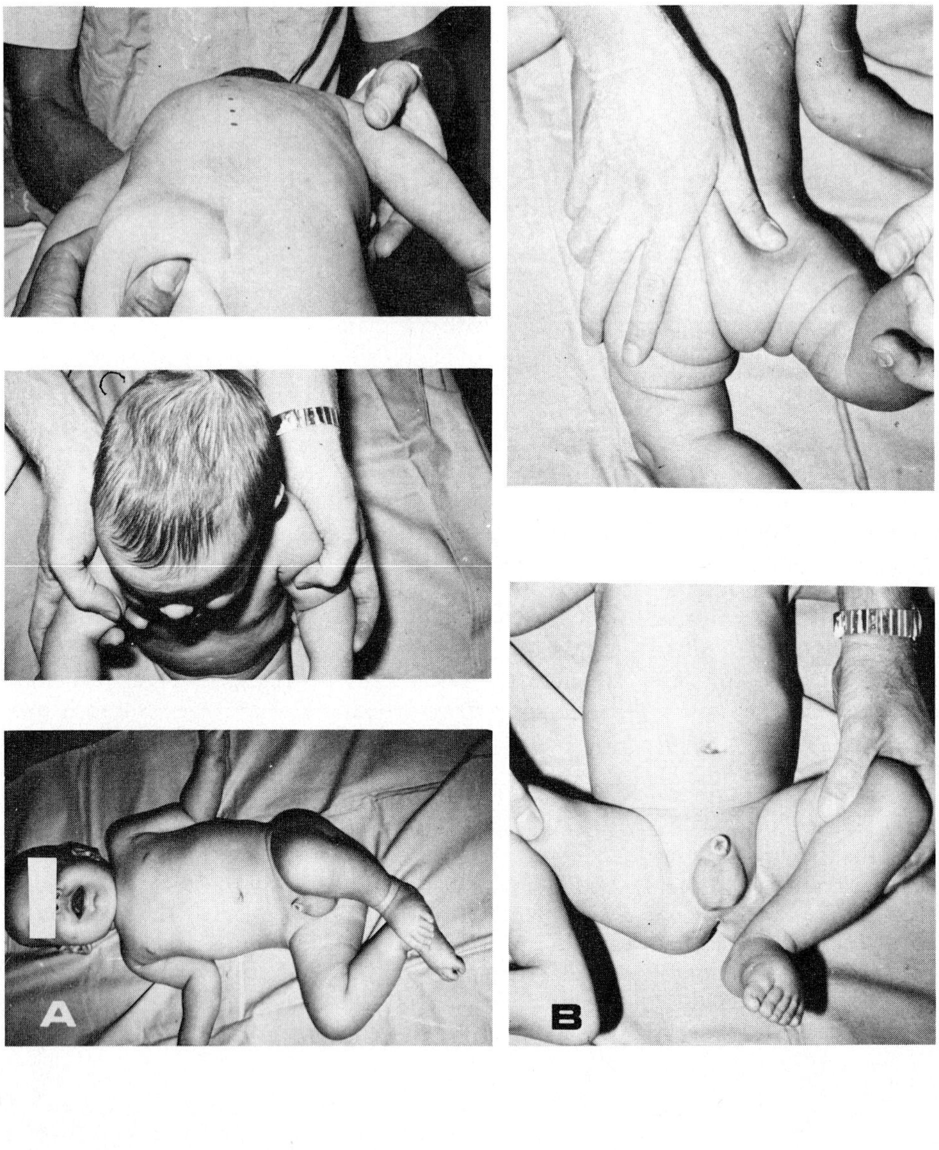

FIG. 52–3. A 6-month-old infant with left torticollis, left scoliosis, right abductor contracture, and left adductor tightness. **(B)** The right abductor and left adductor are tight.

the function and anatomy of the genitourinary system should be evaluated.

Diagnosis of a myelomeningocele generally poses little problem when there is a skin defect. Because the skin over myelomeningoceles is not always defective, any soft mass in or off the midline must be examined closely to determine its composition. Lipomas always have good skin coverage and may be off the midline.

The care of an infant born with myelomeningocele is complex and requires input from several specialties (see Chap. 50). It is important to determine immediately after birth the level of involvement by inspection of the back, careful examination of the muscle function of the lower extremities, and radiographic examination before surgical closure.

The most common abnormalities of the lower extremities associated with myelomeningocele are deformations of the feet, indicating lack of normal muscle activity *in utero*. Initial treatment of the deformed foot is with plaster cast correction followed by surgical releases if necessary. Transfer of muscle insertions frequently are needed for maintenance of the correction after release. These surgeries may be done at almost any age.

Flexion or extension deformities of the knee are treated by splinting and gentle passive exercising. New splints need to be made frequently as the deformity improves.

Treatment of a dislocated hip in the patient with a defect above L4 is controversial. Usually the dislocated hip in the newborn reduces easily in flexion and abduction. I believe the hips of a newborn with a myelomeningocele should be splinted in abduction in an effort to develop a more stable hip. The flexed, abducted, externally rotated position should not be used in treating dislocated hips in the infant with lesions above L2 because this position frequently leads to the development of fixed contractures that prevent the hips from extending and adducting.

Infants with high lumbar–low thoracic myelomeningoceles have very high early mortality, lowered significantly by early surgical closure of the lesions. The degree of disability and mental retardation can be correlated very well with the level of defect, the presence and degree of hydrocephalus, and the presence of a bony kyphosis. A lesion above L1 with hydrocephalus and kyphosis will indicate, almost without exception, significant mental and motor disability.

UPPER EXTREMITIES

DUPLICATION AND REDUCTION

Supernumerary parts, absence or reduction anomalies of the extremities, and segmentation defects of the limb should offer no problem in diagnosis. These orthopaedic anomalies seldom need immediate attention but should be seen early by the orthopaedist to plan appropriate therapy and discuss prognosis with the family. This is true for anomalies of both the upper and lower extremities.

Syndactylism, or fusion of any portion of two or more digits, is a common anomaly. It is genetically transmitted through an autosomal dominant gene with varying expressivity. Surgical treatment should be done within the first year with the timing dependent on the completeness of the syndactyly and the fingers involved. The thumb and index finger should be separated at 6 months of age, the little and ring finger separated at 1 year. It is important to determine by radiographs if there is a synostosis between fingers because this should be corrected by 1 year of age. A delay in surgical separation in synostosis will result in a bowing of the longer finger due to differential growth.

Polydactyly is correctable by surgery with timing dependent on the extent of duplication. When the duplication does not contain bone or cartilage, it should be removed in infancy. When there is a question of function, surgical correction should be delayed until the degree of function present in each of the duplicated digits can be ascertained.

Absence of the radius, commonly called radial clubhand, is easily recognized (Fig. 52-4). The wrist and hand are deviated 90° or more. Absence of the radius may be bilateral or unilateral and the thumb may be present, absent, or hypoplastic. The clubhand is caused by damage to the apical ectoderm or to the deeper mesenchymal tissue of the limb bud.[2] It is not genetically transmitted in the otherwise normal child but is associated with some genetically transmitted syndromes and frequently is associated with aplastic anemia. Early treatment by corrective splints may be sufficient to correct the radial deviation and prepare the extremity for surgery at a later date.

Congenital absence of the thumb occurs as an isolated anomaly or may be associated with a radial club-

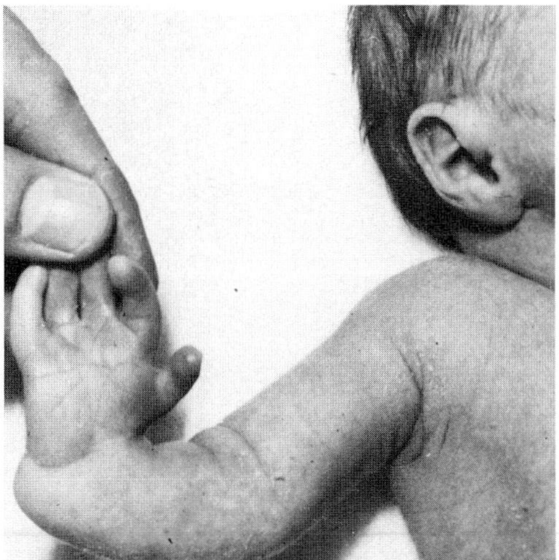

FIG. 52–4. Congenital absence of the radius.

hand. When unilateral, little or no treatment is needed, but when the absence is bilateral, pollicization of the dominant hand will improve function. When the thumb is rudimentary and nonfunctional, treatment is controversial.

SHOULDER GIRDLE

Sprengel deformity (*i.e.*, congenital elevated scapula) is one of the more common congenital anomalies of the shoulder girdle. The deformity may be bilateral or unilateral and usually is associated with other abnormalities such as Klippel–Feil syndrome, congenital anomalies of the upper thoracic vertebrae, or anomalies of the ribs. Asymmetry of the shoulders in unilateral involvement makes recognition easier. On palpation, the affected scapula is high and rotated outward and downward so that its vertebral border lies superiorly and more horizontally than normal. Shoulder abduction and flexion usually but not always are limited. The early conservative treatment is passive range-of-motion exercises. Surgical correction at 3 or 4 years or up to 16 years of age generally improves appearance and function, with the overall improvement from surgery better in the younger child.

The clavicle has two congenital malformations: congenital pseudarthrosis and congenital absence of part or all of the clavicle. The physical signs on palpation of congenital pseudarthrosis are angulation of the clavicle and a painless, bulbar mass in the midclavicular area (Fig. 52-5). The shoulder girdle is hypermobile, with motion in the clavicle at the pseudarthrosis. Early treatment is not needed. Surgical correction by grafting of the defect at 3 or 4 years of age usually is successful, but the need for such treatment is controversial, so therapy needs to be individualized.

Partial or complete absence of the clavicle may be recognized by palpation and by the presence of excessive scapulothoracic motion (Fig. 52-6). The completely absent clavicle usually is associated with cranial dysostosis or with a widened pubic symphysis. There are no symptoms, so no treatment is needed in complete absence. With partial absence, the end of the clavicle may irritate the brachial plexus, necessitating incision of the fragment. Whereas congenital pseudarthrosis usually is an isolated anomaly, partial absence of the clavicle almost always is associated with an axial or appendageal skeletal anomaly.

DEFECTS OF LIMB SEGMENTATION

Synostosis of the elbow and synostosis of the radius and ulna are two of the more common skeletal anomalies of limb segmentation. Elbow synostosis is easily recognized by the lack of motion, and, almost always, the significantly smaller size of the affected extremity. Synostosis of the radius and ulna seldom is diagnosed in the nursery, and, commonly, not for several years. This is particularly true if the defect is bilateral because the child himself will not appreciate a difference in his arms. Supinating and pronating the forearm in the initial examination of the newborn should demonstrate this anomaly by lack of range of motion.

LOWER EXTREMITIES

Variations in contours and postural attitudes of the lower extremities in general and the feet in particular are frequent causes of concern. *In utero*, the feet seldom rest at a neutral position, being either dorsiflexed, plantarflexed, inverted, or everted, or in a combination of these positions. At times, it may be difficult to determine whether there is a structural

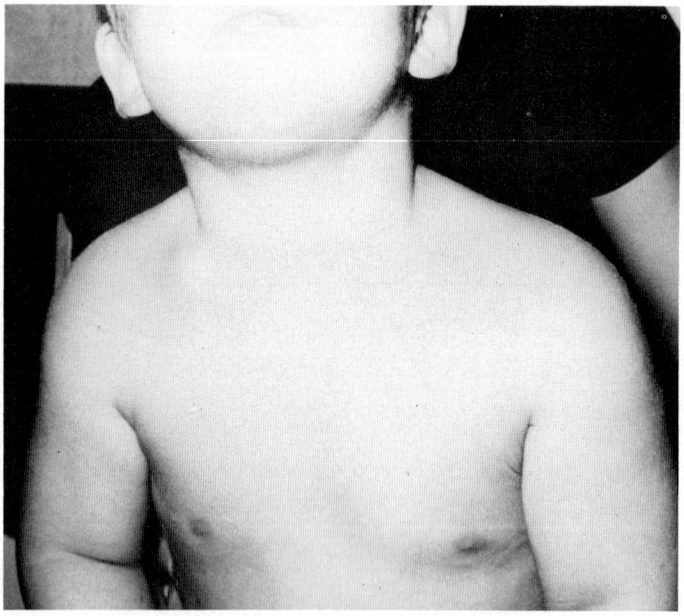

FIG. 52–5. A 2-year-old child with pseudarthrosis of the right clavicle.

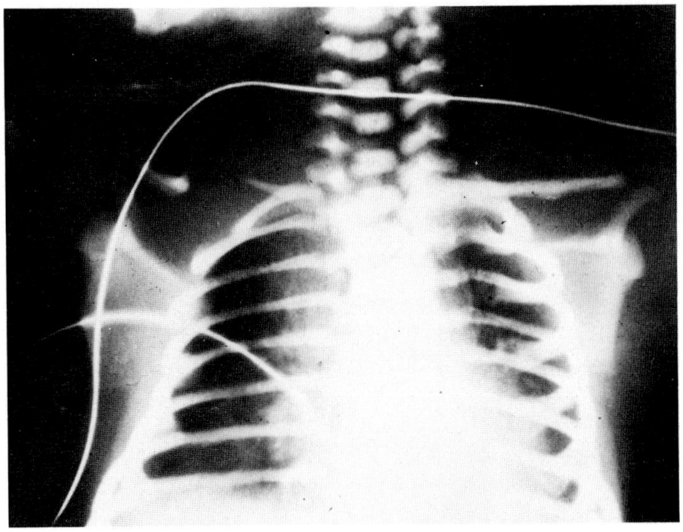

FIG. 52–6. Partial absence of the right clavicle.

abnormality, or only a temporary positional deformation.

FEET

Metatarsus adductus (Fig. 52-7) may be either a positional deformity with no bony abnormality or a structural defect, and it is not always easy to distinguish between the two. The distinction becomes easier with time because a positional metatarsus adductus corrects fairly rapidly by passive exercises or even without treatment. A structural deformity does not spontaneously correct completely, becoming more rigid with time.

The differentiation between postural and structural metatarsus adductus is made mostly by physical examination. In structural metatarsus adductus (see Fig. 52-7*A*), the base of the fifth metatarsus and the cuboid are prominent, creating an impressive, well defined skin crease on the medial side of the foot at the first metatarsal–cuneiform joint. In a positional metatarsus adductus, the lateral and medial borders of the foot are curved more gently than in the structural deformity. The most significant physical finding, however, is the presence or absence of rigidity of the forefoot as determined by its resistance to abduction. In the structural deformity, the forefoot usually cannot be abducted beyond the midline (see Fig. 52-7*B*), whereas in the positional deformity the forefoot is more flexible and can be abducted (see Fig. 52-7*C*). The heel of the structural metatarsus adductus foot usually is in valgus, and in the positional deformity it is likely to be in varus or at neutral. The valgus position of the hindfoot can be seen on clinical evaluation and, if necessary, confirmed by radiographic studies.

Treatment of the positional flexible deformity is either observation for spontaneous resolution or passive stretching of the forefoot into abduction with the foot held as in Figure 52-7*B*. Structural metatarsus adductus generally needs treatment with repeated cast changes.

Talipes calcaneovalgus is not a structural deformity but rather a reflection of the foot's position *in utero* (Fig. 52-8). The sole lies against the uterine wall, and the foot is dorsiflexed so that its dorsal skin lies against the anterior surface of the tibia. The fibula is prominent and appears to be dislocated posteriorly, being pushed backward by the excessive dorsiflexion. There is a depression over the sinus tarsus. The calcaneovalgus foot is flexible and passively plantarflexes at least to neutral and, in most instances, to 5° to 10° beyond neutral.

Treatment of the calcaneovalgus foot is by either passive exercises or corrective plaster cast, according to the severity of the deformity. Mild cases are treated with exercises that stretch the foot into equinus and varus 15 to 20 times at 4 to 5 sessions daily.

The more severely resistant deformities, those that flex only to neutral plantarflexion, are treated by repeated applications of plaster casts for 8 weeks. Casts are changed as needed with growth, and, at each change, the foot is placed in equinus and varus with a mold placed in the arch to relax the plantar ligaments and posterior tibialis muscle. The goal of treatment is to obtain a plantarflexed, varus position to allow the plantar ligaments and posterior tibialis tendon that have been stretched *in utero* to shorten. Early plaster treatment appears to give these children a better chance of having strong feet.

It is important that the positional calcaneovalgus foot not be confused with congenital vertical talus, a rare but serious anomaly. In congenital vertical talus, the forefoot is dorsiflexed, and the hindfoot is in equinus (Fig. 52-9). The talus is rigidly fixed in plantarflexion, and if the examiner places one thumb on the talus, and with the other hand dorsiflexes and plantarflexes the foot, the talus will remain almost stationary as the forefoot moves around it. The fore-

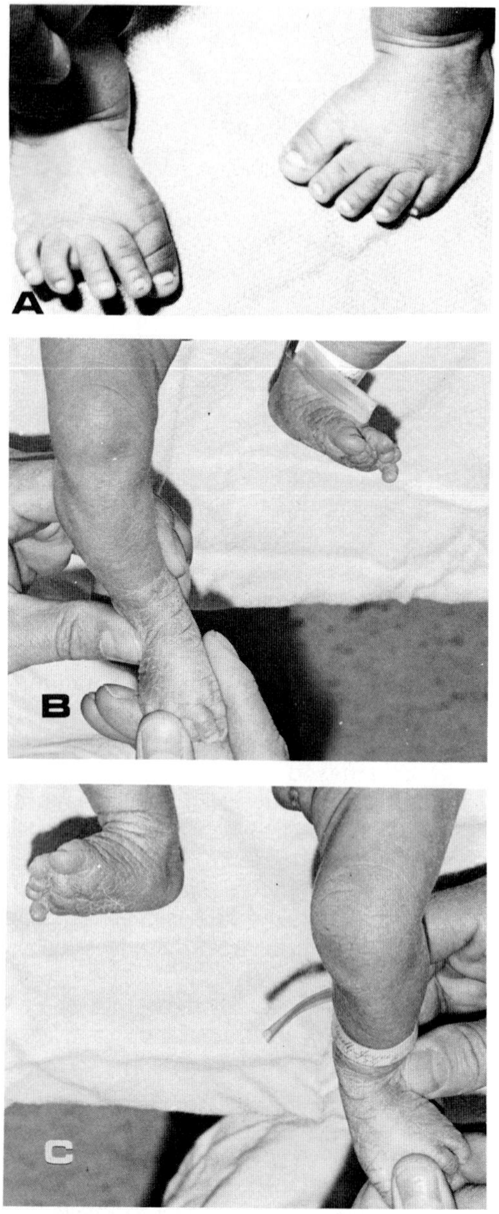

FIG. 52–7. **(A)** Structural metatarsus adductus. **(B)** Structural metatarsus adductus. The forefoot does not abduct beyond neutral. **(C)** Positional metatarsus. The forefoot abducts beyond the midline.

foot cannot be plantarflexed as much as the calcaneovalgus foot, and seldom can it be plantarflexed more than 5° beyond neutral. A radiographic examination of the foot will demonstrate the hindfoot equinus and forefoot dorsiflexion plus the other radiographic characteristics of this anomaly. Although treatment will not create a normal foot, the results are far better with early treatment.

The classic clubfoot is a developmental anomaly of the entire foot (Fig. 52-10). There is varus of the hindfoot, varus and adduction of the forefoot, and equinus that is not apparent until the varus and ad-

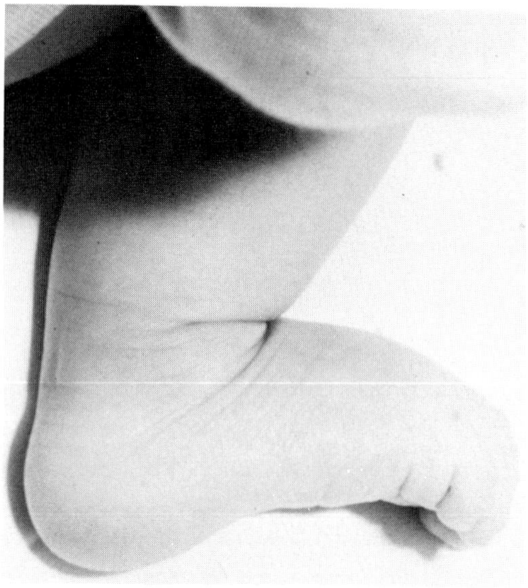

FIG. 52–8. Talipes calcaneovalgus.

duction are corrected to neutral. This is a structural deformity, and resists correction; it is easily recognized by its rigidity. There is a positional equinovarus foot that may resemble the true clubfoot, but it is flexible and can be corrected beyond neutral with little difficulty. Treatment of the structural clubfoot is by repeated manipulation and strapping or by manipulation and application of a cast. Treatment should start on the day of birth if the infant is otherwise stable. When conservative measures are unsuccessful in correcting the foot, surgical correction is necessary.

TIBIA AND FIBULA

Significant deformities of the tibia and fibula occur infrequently and are not difficult to detect. Congenital absence of the tibia or fibula, congenital amputation, and congenital bowing all are easily recognized. When the tibia is absent, the foot is in varus; when the fibula is absent, the foot has an equinovalgus deformity. These deformities should be seen early by the orthopaedist, because in some of these children

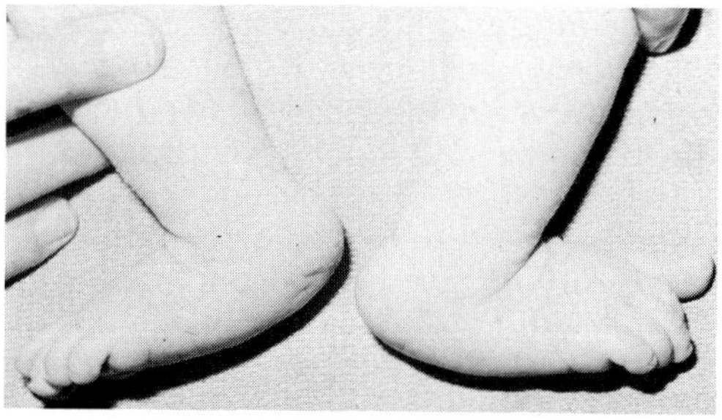

FIG. 52–9. Congenital vertical talus.

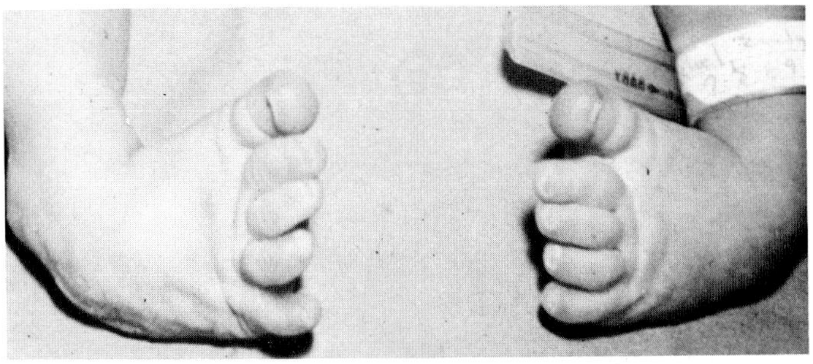

FIG. 52–10. Talipes equinocavovarus foot (*i.e.*, clubfoot).

conservative and supervised treatment of the foot deformities is indicated, whereas in others early amputation is the treatment of choice.[3–5] With newer techniques and knowledge of the biology of bone elongation, more of these limbs are being salvaged.

Anterior bowing of the tibia is a serious deformity (Fig. 52-11). The bone of the tibia is of poor quality, and in most cases it either is sclerotic with partial or complete obliteration of the intermedullary space or has cystic areas that contain material similar to that in fibrous dysplasia. Pseudarthrosis may be present at birth, or always following a fracture, which is likely within the first 2 years of life. Protection of the tibia by casts and braces is important and may be sufficient to prevent a fracture. Although the case shown in Figure 52-11 is mild, there is a narrow intramedullary canal, and the bone needs protection, for it is unlikely to heal should it fracture. There is no tendency for these cases of anterior bowing to improve spontaneously.

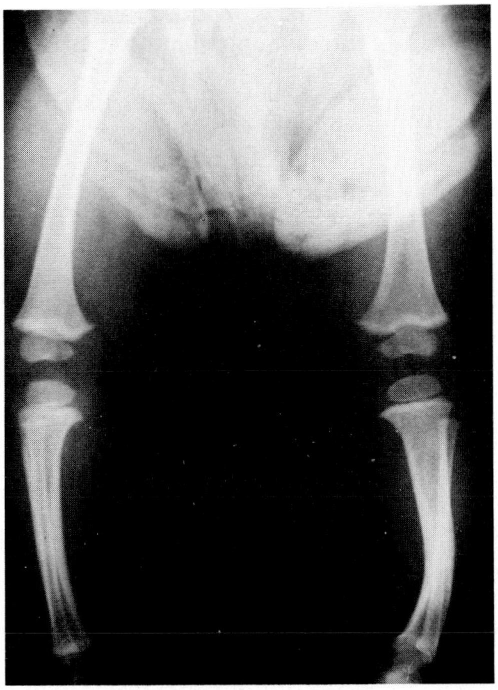

FIG. 52–11. Anterior bowed tibia.

Conversely, a tibia that is posteriorly bowed corrects spontaneously, and seldom fractures, but if it does, it usually heals. The posteriorly bowed tibia needs only to be observed.

Most neonates have an inward or medial torsion of the leg distal to the knee and outward rotation above the knee. The medial torsion below the knee may occur in the knee, tibia, ankle, or a combination of these, and, except in extreme cases, no treatment is necessary because alignment will improve progressively. The exception to this may be in relatively immobile, premature infants who lie in the same position most of the time.

KNEE

Significant deformities of the knee are very rare. Genu recurvatum, a frequent positional deformity associated with a frank breech position, is not serious and will respond to gentle exercising. The positional recurvatum must be differentiated from the more serious subluxation or dislocation. When there is doubt as to whether or not a recurvatum represents a subluxation or a dislocation, a radiograph should be made; in subluxation, the tibia is forward on the femur but not completely dislocated, whereas in dislocation, the tibia will be completely anterior to the femur. In congenital dislocation, the knee can be hyperextended but not flexed beyond neutral and the tibia is anteriorly displaced on palpation. The subluxed knee reduces with traction but the dislocated knee frequently requires open reduction.

Congenital fibrosis of part of the quadriceps is an anomaly that prevents knee flexion, causing a more extended posture than normal in neonates. Active and passive flexion is limited and seldom is more than 40°. Treatment is by surgical excision of the fibrous mass.

HIP

There are two basic types of congenital hip dislocation. The more common of the two is the developmental dislocation that is embryologically normal

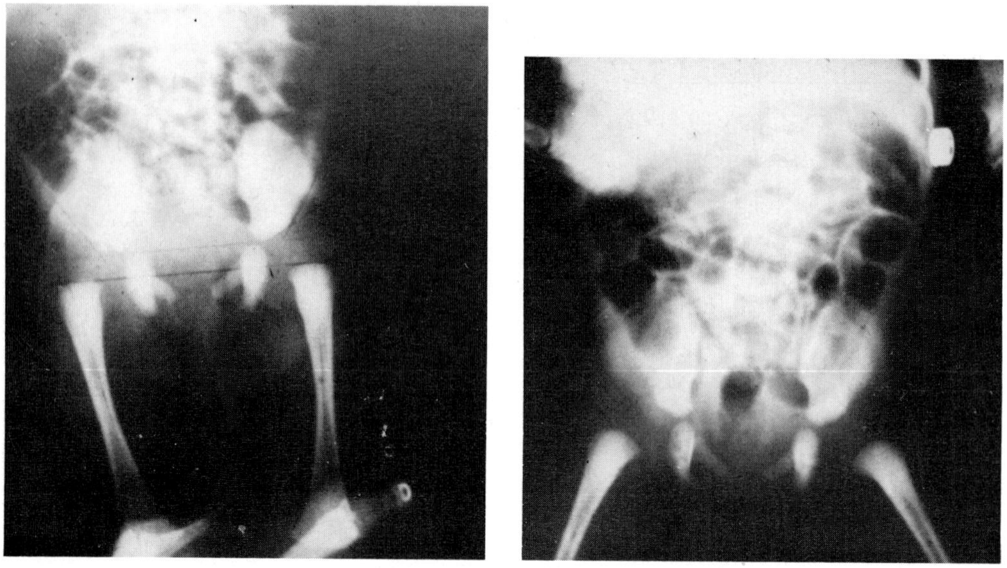

FIG. 52–12. Bilateral congenital dislocation of the hip. The metaphyseal–acetabulum distance is wide.

but, as a result of mechanical forces *in utero* and maternal hormones that relax tissues in preparation for parturition, the hip is dislocated or dislocatable in the perinatal period. The less common type is a teratogenic hip that dislocates probably in the embryologic period of gestation and is associated with malformation of the pelvis and femur.

Developmental dislocation of the hips occurs more frequently in girls, presenting in breech position at term gestation and with a positive family history. The dislocation usually is unilateral with the left hip more frequently affected, but it may be bilateral. The dislocation almost always is reduced in flexion and abduction and usually but not always is stable if held flexed 90° or above and then abducted. In the newborn, radiographs of the hip are not necessarily diagnostic, although in some, the hip appears laterally displaced in the anteroposterior projection (Fig. 52-12).

In the newborn, the typical dislocated hip may not have the classically described signs of dislocation, such as symmetric skin folds, limited abduction, and shorter-appearing femur (*i.e.*, Galeazzi sign). These signs are secondary and develop by the end of 6 weeks of life as the hip migrates laterally and superiorly. The clinician diagnoses this condition in the newborn by demonstrating that the femoral head can be lifted into the acetabulum as the thigh is abducted in flexion (*i.e.*, Ortolani maneuver; see Fig. 52-1*A*) and that it dislocates as the hip is adducted (*i.e.*, Barlow maneuver; see Fig. 52-1*B*). The Ortolani test is positive in the dislocated hip until 6 to 8 weeks of age, sometimes longer. In addition to feeling the dislocation as the thigh is adducted, the examiner should reduce the hip by abduction in flexion and, while maintaining the same degree of abduction, extend the thigh to dislocate the hip. In each instance, whether dislocation is obtained by adducting or by extending the thigh, the examiner not only can feel the hip dislocate but also see the sudden jerk that occurs as the femoral head rides out of the acetabulum.

Developmental hip dislocation usually can be recognized in the first few days of life. Opinion is that treatment should be started as soon as possible after diagnosis. Most hips that are unstable at birth become stable by the fifth day, however, so I prefer to wait until the fifth day to start treatment of only those hips that remain unstable. Early treatment is easier on the family and child, with results that are far better than when treatment is started several months or years later.

The Pavlik harness is the splint of choice from birth to 6 months of age. It must be applied properly. Excessive abduction from tight posterior straps can cause avascular necrosis.[6] Sonography, if well done, is the method of choice in the neonate both to confirm the diagnosis of hip dysplasia and to follow the progress of acetabular development during treatment. When sonograms are not available, hip radiographs in both the anteroposterior and horizontal planes should be taken with the child in the splint to determine that the hip is held reduced. Rarely, the hip dislocates posteriorly in the splint but appears to be reduced in the anteroposterior view; only the horizontal view will show the dislocation in this instance.

All infants should have follow-up hip examinations at well baby checks the first 3 months. The Ortolani test may still be positive for 6 to 12 weeks, but more commonly, the late physical signs of dislocation are the following:

- asymmetric folds in unilateral dislocation
- an apparent discrepancy of leg length caused by pelvic obliquity and a high-riding femoral head

- a high trochanter
- limited abduction
- a palpable defect in the anterior groin where the femoral head normally should be
- a piston or telescoping motion.

These signs are sufficient to make the diagnosis, but radiographs or sonography should be obtained to confirm the diagnosis.

The developmental hip dislocation is probably the most important condition in the musculoskeletal system in which a delay in diagnosis and treatment has a profound affect on the outcome. The results of treatment in the neonate are far superior to those in any other time, so special care in diagnosing this condition is warranted.

The teratogenic hip dislocation presents with different findings. The hip, which has dislocated early in fetal life, ordinarily will not reduce by flexion and abduction because the femoral head is displaced proximally. Therefore, the Ortolani sign is not present in the teratogenic dislocation. If the dislocation is unilateral, there is asymmetry of abduction of the hips. The dislocated hip will have more extension than the opposite hip, and may have limited rotation. When the dislocation is bilateral, the diagnosis is more difficult because there is no asymmetry. Abduction of both hips is limited, the thighs appear short in relation to the lower legs, and the perineum appears wider than normal. The diagnosis usually is made by radiographic examination, which in the teratogenic dislocation is always abnormal.

Proximal femoral focal deficiency is an anomaly of serious magnitude that may be either unilateral or bilateral. The degree of deficiency is variable and ranges from absence of the diaphysis, upper metaphysis, and femoral head to a very short femur with coxa vara of the neck and head. It is not uncommon as well for the fibula to be absent and the foot deformed in the more severely affected infant with proximal femoral focal deficiency. The shortness of the femur is obvious on inspection. Motion of the hip may be limited. Early referral to the orthopaedist, who will give the definitive treatment, is important. Initial treatment may include stretching exercises or traction or both for correction of contractures about the hip, although these have proven to be of limited value. Definitive surgical management depends on the potential for function in the extremity and ranges from measures to correct leg length discrepancy to fusion of the knee and amputation of the foot to create a stump for an above-knee prosthesis.

GENERALIZED MUSCULOSKELETAL ANOMALIES

The many syndromes that primarily involve the epiphysis, epiphyseal plate, metaphysis, or diaphysis are, with few exceptions, easily recognized by their phenotypes. There are similarities in all of the chondrodystrophies, but there are important differences in prognoses. Because classification of the various types generally is made by the radiographic appearance of the skeleton, radiographs of the spine, skull, and extremities should be examined before a diagnosis is made and the prognosis is discussed with the parent.[7] There is little to be done for most of these syndromes, but, when there is a deformity, treatment should be initiated early.

Achondroplasia, chondroectodermal dysplasia (*i.e.*, Ellis–van Creveld disease), and epiphyseal dysostosis (*i.e.*, diastrophic dwarfism) are three of the more common congenital, generalized skeletal affectations recognizable at birth that are associated with dwarfism. Children with large heads, short extremities, excessive or restricted motion of joints, unusual-appearing faces, and short, stubby phalanges suggest that a skeletal dysplasia is present that usually can be identified by radiographs of the skull, spine, and extremities.[8] Infants affected by certain skeletal dysplasias or by metabolic skeletal abnormalities, however, appear normal at birth, with the skeletal anomalies appearing later in infancy and childhood.

Osteogenesis imperfecta is a generalized disturbance of the skeleton manifested by soft, fragile bone. If severe, it is very obvious at birth, but it may be mild enough to go undiagnosed until the child is several years old. Osteogenesis imperfecta involves primarily the skeleton but also affects the skin, ligaments, tendons, sclera, nose, ear, platelet function, and probably other systems.[9–11]

The diagnosis of osteogenesis imperfecta is not difficult when there are multiple fractures, a very soft skull, paradoxic respirations indicating rib fractures, and bluish gray sclera. For those who survive the delivery, gentle handling to prevent further injuries and skin traction to align the extremities are important considerations. It is possible to align all four extremities simultaneously with traction. The fractures heal rapidly, and by 9 or 10 days the traction usually can be discontinued.[12] There are several classifications of osteogenesis imperfecta according to severity of involvement. The classification of Sillence appears to be the most helpful in prognosis and genetic counseling.[11]

Arthrogryposis multiplex congenita (Fig. 52-13) is an uncommon but easily recognizable syndrome of the musculoskeletal system. All four extremities and the trunk may be affected, or the abnormalities may be limited to the arms or legs. The hallmark of this entity is the lack of active and passive motion in the affected extremities.

The microscopic picture of the muscle in arthrogryposis shows changes of denervation and fibrofatty replacement. Secondary to the muscle weakness and dysfunction, there is distortion of the joints, as well as limitation of motion. Frequently, these infants have dislocation of the hips, knees, or radial heads or combinations of the three. In addition, they may have either clubfeet or vertical talus, both of which are more resistant to treatment than those not associated

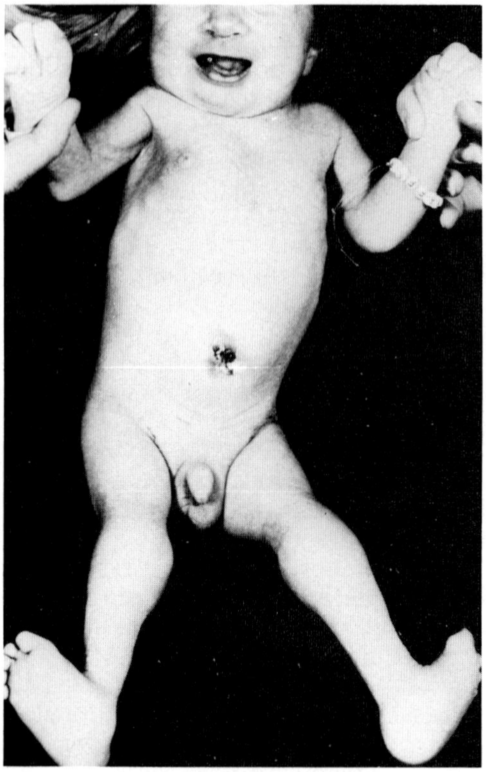

FIG. 52–13. Arthrogryposis multiplex congenita.

with arthrogryposis. Treatment should begin in the nursery and is directed at increasing the motion of all affected joints by passive exercises done six to eight times each day. Joint dislocation and the hand and foot deformities should be treated early with appropriate plaster splints or casts or with traction.

BIRTH FRACTURES

Long, difficult labor—particularly with the breech position, a large infant, or fetal distress requiring rapid extraction—makes birth injuries more likely. Birth fractures almost always involve clavicle, humerus, or femur. It is rare for birth fractures in a normal infant to occur below the elbow or below the knee. The fracture is more likely to be through either the diaphysis or the epiphyseal plate, so that the epiphysis and epiphyseal plate are separated from the metaphysis. At times, the fractures are not noted because pain may be minimal and a deformity may not be apparent. Diagnosis in such cases is made incidental to a radiograph taken for unrelated indications. In others, the fracture is painful and is a cause of pseudoparalysis, with the limb lying limp and not moving on stimulation.

DIAPHYSEAL FRACTURES

Fractures of the diaphysis of the humerus generally are diagnosed by the obstetrician, who hears and feels the snap when the humerus fractures as the baby is being extracted. The same can be said about fractures of the femoral shaft and clavicle. A radiograph confirms the fracture.

A fracture of the shaft of the humerus is treated by immobilization of the arm by the side. Soft padding is placed between the arm and the chest, and the elbow is held at 90° flexion.

Fractures of the femoral shaft can be held with a posterior splint that extends from below the knee to over the buttock and is held in place with an elastic bandage for 10 to 14 days.

Fractures of the clavicle may be asymptomatic if undisplaced and need no treatment except care in handling the infant. If the fracture is displaced, it usually is painful. The fracture can be treated either by strapping the arms to the chest with padding placed in the axilla and the elbow flexed 90° or by using a figure-of-eight bandage made of stockinette to immobilize the fracture. In 8 to 10 days, the callus is sufficient for immobilization to be discontinued.

EPIPHYSEAL INJURIES

The epiphyseal separation or fracture occurs through the hypertrophied layer of cartilage cells in the epiphysis. A fracture through the proximal epiphyseal plate of the humerus is one of the more common skeletal injuries associated with a difficult delivery. The diagnosis has to be made primarily on the clinical findings of swelling about the shoulder and crepitus and pain when the shoulder is moved. Motion is painful, and the arm lies limp by the side. The proximal humeral epiphysis is not ossified at birth and therefore is not visible on radiographs. This makes diagnosis by radiograph very difficult. If there is complete or almost complete separation of the epiphysis, the metaphysis appears displaced in relation to the glenoid of the scapula, but usually the separation is minimal and there are no radiographic changes except soft tissue swelling. After 8 to 10 days, callus appears and is visible on radiographs.

The treatment for a fracture of the proximal epiphysis of the humerus is immobilization of the arm by the side with soft padding in the axilla for 8 to 10 days. Healing is rapid, and remodeling is such that even a striking angulation will improve progressively to where the contour appears normal. If a complete separation is present, reduction by gentle traction probably should be attempted.

A fracture separation of the distal humeral epiphysis is very rare. It is difficult to diagnose radiographically because this epiphysis, like the proximal epiphysis, is completely cartilaginous. When an injury is present, there will be swelling about the elbow with pain and crepitus on passive motion. If the epiphysis is displaced, the anteroposterior radiograph will show that the olecranon is placed medially or laterally in its relationship with the long axis of the humerus. A fracture of the distal epiphysis is more likely to have a significant residual deformity than is a fracture of the proximal humeral epiphysis. I prefer traction on the forearm for 9 to 10 days to treat this injury.

Fracture of the proximal femoral epiphysis is an uncommon problem but one that can cause confusion if it is not recognized. It often is confused with a congenital dislocation or with acute pyarthrosis. The epiphyseal plate of the proximal femur is a crescent-shaped line extending from the greater to the lesser trochanter and includes the cartilaginous epiphysis of the trochanter, neck, and femoral head. Swelling about the hip is difficult to appreciate, and suspicion of the presence of this injury should be aroused when the baby does not move the extremity on stimulation. This is confirmed by the presence of pain and crepitus when the hip is moved passively. The radiograph of the hip will show the upper end of the femoral metaphysis to be displaced laterally, and, if the separation is complete, the metaphysis is likely to be displaced above the center of the acetabulum as well as displaced laterally. After several days of incomplete separation, the hip will no longer be painful, and, in my experience, most of these have been recognized only after callus formation is seen on an incidental radiograph or after a large callus presents as a firm mass in the groin or upper thigh (Fig. 52-14). If the diagnosis is recognized before healing is underway, the hip should be manipulated gently and immobilized in flexion and abduction for 10 to 14 days. When the diagnosis is uncertain, aspiration of the joint will help differentiate a fracture from congenital dislocation and acute pyarthrosis. If the fracture is present, blood should be found in the joint.

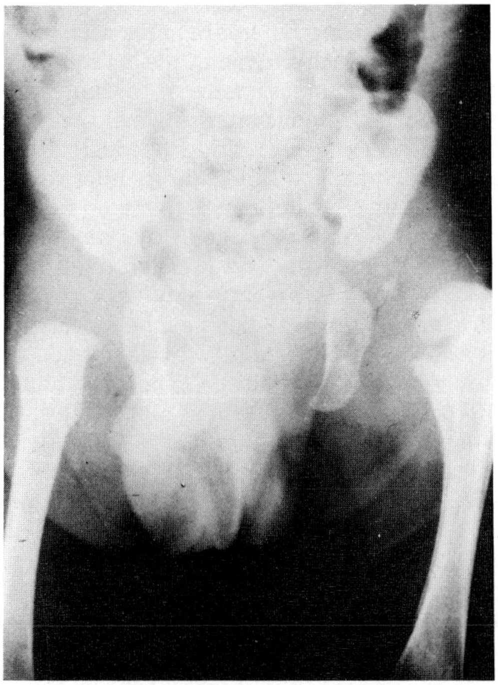

FIG. 52–14. A 3-week-old infant with a birth fracture of the proximal epiphysis of the femur.

The diagnosis of a fracture separation of the distal femoral epiphysis can be made by radiographic studies. Ossification of the distal femoral epiphysis is present at birth, and even slight displacement and angulation can be recognized. If there is swelling around the knee and pain on passive motion, a radiograph will confirm the diagnosis. Treatment is by immobilization in plaster for 10 to 14 days if displacement is not severe. When displacement or angulation is excessive, reduction by manipulation should be done and the extremity immobilized in plaster for 14 days.

OBSTETRIC PALSY

Traumatic neuropathy of the brachial plexus is one of the more common birth injuries. It is caused most usually by traction and lateral flexion of the neck. In vertex presentations, it occurs by traction and lateral flexion applied to deliver the shoulder in large babies, and in breech presentations by traction and lateral flexion to deliver the head.

The clinical picture is easily recognized by the absence of active motion of the involved extremity in the Moro reflex. There may be supraclavicular swelling, and an associated fractured clavicle.

There are three types of obstetric palsy, and the clinical findings are different in each. The upper plexus type is called Erb–Duchenne (Fig. 52-15), and in this the C5 and C6 nerve roots are affected, with C7 roots less involved. In the lower plexus type, known as Klumpke palsy, the C8 and T1 roots are involved. The third type is a total involvement of all roots that make up the plexus. If the C5 and C6 roots are affected, the shoulder is held internally rotated with the forearm supinated and the elbow extended and the wrist and fingers flexed. A grasp may be present, whereas traction will be absent. When the lower roots, C8 and T1, are involved, the hand is flaccid with little or no control. When the entire plexus is affected, the total extremity is flaccid.

The early treatment of obstetric palsy is conservative. Myelography and surgical exploration have little to offer initially in the management of this problem. Recovery of function depends, of course, on the degree of injury. When the injury is a neurapraxia, complete recovery over several weeks usually takes place. When there is a neurotmesis or complete avulsion, no recovery takes place. Loss of sensory function suggests a more severe involvement. Because it is not possible to say which degree of injury is present, all should be treated by prevention of further injury to the plexus by gentle handling. The arm needs protection for the first 4 or 5 days until swelling has subsided. After this period, the joints of the arm may be carried through a passive range of motion several times each day for maintenance of flexibility. The paralyzed muscles should be supported in a position of relaxation for part of each day, with care being taken that a contraction of the protected muscles does not

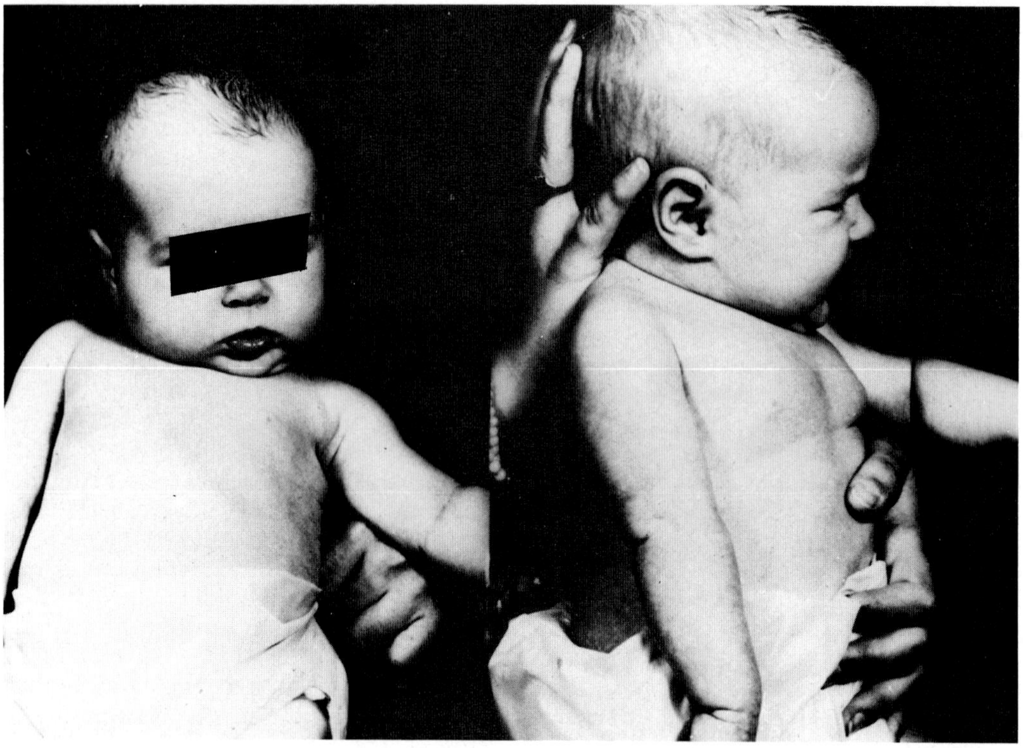

FIG. 52–15. An Erb–Duchenne type of brachial plexus injury.

occur. Denervated muscles undergo fibrosis, which can become contracted, producing a fixed deformity. Most obstetric plexus palsy patients recover within 3 months.[13] The return of function of the deltoid and biceps are the best clinical parameters to follow recovery. If these have not shown some recovery by 3 months, return of function is unlikely. When the lesion is limited to the C5 and C6 nerve roots without recovery at 3 months, surgical intervention should be considered.[14]

In those patients with residual paralysis, passive exercises and progressive active exercises should be continued for months and years, as long as there is some progressive improvement. At 3 to 5 years, certain residual deformities can be improved surgically. Brachial plexus injuries are discussed further in Chapter 51.

BONE AND JOINT INFECTIONS

Osteomyelitis and acute septic arthritis occur in the neonate, although not as frequently as in older infants. Additionally, changes in obstetric and neonatal practices have contributed to a decreased incidence of bony infections in the neonatal period. Infants with altered immune function or the presence of indwelling vascular lines remain at particular risk for these unusual infections. The priorities of treatment are different in osteomyelitis and septic arthritis, and the differences are of paramount importance.

Osteomyelitis occurs almost always by hematogenous spread, from either a cutaneous or oral lesion, or from other sources such as omphalitis or an indwelling arterial line. *Staphylococcus* and *Streptococcus* species are the most frequent causative organisms, with group B β-hemolytic streptococcus increasing in frequency most recently.

Osteomyelitis begins in the metaphyses of long bones. Bacteria reach the metaphysis through the nutrient artery, which terminates in the sinusoids adjacent to the epiphyseal plate.[15,16] The rate of flow in the sinusoid is slower, creating an ideal situation for bacterial stasis and multiplication. Edema, vascular engorgement, and cellulitis are followed by thrombosis and abscess formation, with destruction and absorption of trabeculae. The purulent exudate in the metaphysis spreads by way of Volkmann canals to the periosteal space and elevates the loosely attached periosteum, which responds by laying down new bone over the original cortex. The new bone is the involucrum. In infants, unlike in older children, the exudate perforates the cortex of the metaphysis early and does not spread down the diaphysis, sparing the endosteal and haversian vessels, and therefore does not cause massive sequestrum in infants as readily as in older children.

In children beyond infancy, the epiphyseal plate acts as a barrier against spread to the epiphysis. In the infant, Trueta has shown that vessels cross the epiphyseal plate, so that infection of the metaphysis may spread to the epiphysis and cause irreparable damage to the secondary center of the ossification and the epiphyseal plate.[15] For this reason, early diagnosis and treatment are very important to prevent destruction of the metaphysis and epiphysis.

The neonate with hematogenous osteomyelitis presents with varied complaints and findings. Movement of the affected part may provoke crying. There may be loss of active motion of the affected extremity (*i.e.*, pseudoparalysis), or the baby may have unexplained fever. Palpable swelling of the extremity appears early after the onset of bone infection and is visible in a soft tissue radiograph. In the newborn, this swelling may be massive, including the entire extremity, before visual changes in the bone are apparent on radiographic evaluation. In a newborn with extensive swelling of an extremity, osteomyelitis must be strongly considered as the diagnosis until proven otherwise. Alternatively, the infant may be so overwhelmed by infection that he or she responds very little to stimulation and may even be afebrile. In any infant who is seriously ill or who is failing to thrive, careful examination of the extremities should be done, with observation for any evidence of tenderness, pain, and swelling that may indicate the presence of osteomyelitis.

The symptoms of osteomyelitis due to group B β-hemolytic streptococcus are unusual. There may be minimal systemic response and little or no local swelling, with a pseudoparalysis or pain on motion as the only symptom of osteomyelitis. When the proximal humerus is involved, the infant holds the affected arm in the same position as does the infant with an obstetric palsy.

Early treatment with appropriate antibiotics and immobilization usually will control the osteomyelitis. If treatment is started too late, abscesses may form that will require surgical drainage.

Acute septic arthritis has even greater urgency of treatment than osteomyelitis in the neonate, although delay in either may cause irreparable damage to the secondary centers of ossification. Joint infection is primarily by hematogenous spread, although the hip may be infected by needle inoculation during attempted femoral vein puncture.

The neonate with septic arthritis generally is very ill but may be so overwhelmed that there are few specific signs. Failure to thrive, as in osteomyelitis, may be the reason for admission. Pseudoparalysis, pain on passive motion, and swelling and increased warmth are the usual physical findings. Diagnosis is difficult when the hip is affected because visible swelling and palpable warmth are minimal except when there is osteomyelitis associated with the arthritis. Radiographic examination will show a joint effusion and distention with widening of the joint space. The hip frequently will be subluxated, and, if diagnosis is delayed several days, the intraarticular pressure will cause dislocation of the hip. When dislocation occurs secondary to pyarthrosis, the joint usually is severely and permanently damaged.

Treatment of an infected joint in an infant generally should be by joint cleaning to remove debris as soon as the diagnosis is confirmed. If the hip is infected, there is no acceptable alternative to arthrotomy for decompression and debridement. A delay in surgical decompression may cause the hip to dislocate by the increasing accumulation of joint fluid. The blood supply to the femoral head is vulnerable both to the increased pressure and to the products of the infection, and delay in adequate debridement may cause occlusion of the vessels, which will result in further deterioration of the femoral head. Both these complications can be prevented by early diagnosis and surgical decompression. In other joints, repeated needle aspiration and irrigation may sufficiently debride, but the clinician never knows whether there is pannus covering the joint surface that must be removed to prevent further destruction of the articular cartilage. Because of this, open surgical decompression with debridement is a more reliable method than needle aspiration.[17] If the hip is affected, traction should pull the thigh into abduction, and moderate flexion should be applied with the traction force just sufficient to overcome muscle spasm. Great care should be taken not to overpull the hip so as to cause further distraction. If the hip joint is tending to dislocate, immobilization in abduction and flexion in a spica cast may be needed to maintain reduction of the hip.

REFERENCES

1. McMaster MJ, Ohtsuka K. The natural history of congenital scoliosis: a study of two hundred and fifty-one patients. J Bone Joint Surg [Am] 1982;64:1128.
2. Lamb DW. Radial clubhand, a continuing study of sixty-eight patients with one hundred and seventeen clubhands. J Bone Joint Surg [Am] 1977;59:1.
3. Brown FW. Construction of a knee joint in congenital total absence of the tibia. J Bone Joint Surg [Am] 1965;47:695.
4. Farmer AW, Laurin CA. Congenital absence of the fibula. J Bone Joint Surg [Am] 1960;42:1.
5. Wood WL, Zlolsky N, Westin GW. Congenital absence of the fibula: treatment by Syme amputation-indications and technique. J Bone Joint Surg [Am] 1965;47:1159.
6. Mubarak S, Garfins S, Vance R, et al. Pitfalls in the use of the Pavlik harness for treatment of congenital dysplasia, subluxation and dislocation of the hip. J Bone Joint Surg [Am] 1981;63:1239.
7. Ruben P. Dynamic classification of bone dysplasia. Chicago: Year Book, 1964.
8. Fairbank HAT. An atlas of general affectation of the skeleton. Edinburgh: E & S Livingstone, 1951.
9. McKusick VA. Heritable disorders of the connective tissue. 3rd ed. St. Louis: CV Mosby, 1966.
10. Weber M. Osteogenesis imperfecta congenita: a study of its histopathogenesis. Arch Pathol 1930;9:984.
11. Sillence D, Danks D. The differentiation of genetically distinct varieties of osteogenesis imperfecta in the newborn period. Clin Res 1978;26:178A.
12. Sofield HA, Miller EA. Fragmentation, realignment and intramedullary rod fixation of deformities of long bones of children. J Bone Joint Surg [Am] 1959;41:1371.

13. Jackson ST, Hoffer MM, Parrish N. Brachial plexus palsy in the newborn. J Bone Joint Surg [Am] 1988;70:1217.
14. Gilbert A, Razaboni R, Amar-Khodja S. Indications and results of brachial plexus surgery in obstetrical palsy. Orthop Clin North Am 1988;19:91.
15. Trueta J. The three types of acute hematogenous osteomyelitis: a clinical and vascular study. J Bone Joint Surg [Br] 1959; 41:671.
16. Trueta J. The normal vascular anatomy of the human femoral head during growth. J Bone Joint Surg [Br] 1972;39:358.
17. Griffin PP. Bone and joint infections in children. Pediatr Clin North Am 1967;3:533.

Neonatology: Pathophysiology and Management of the Newborn, Fourth Edition,
edited by Gordon B. Avery, Mary Ann Fletcher, and Mhairi G. MacDonald.
J.B. Lippincott Company, Philadelphia © 1994.

chapter 53

Eye Disorders

DAVID S. FRIENDLY

A thorough discussion of the multitudinous ocular abnormalities that appear during the first 4 weeks of life is beyond the scope and purpose of this chapter. Rather, I have elected to concentrate on those disorders that have particular importance because of high incidence, impairment of vision, and bearing on general health.

HISTORY AND EXAMINATION TECHNIQUES

The history obtained from parents may be of considerable importance when the physician is confronted with an infant with eye abnormalities. The existence of hereditary ocular disease should be explored in depth and, when indicated, should include examination of the parents and siblings. A prenatal history of maternal drug ingestion and of rubella or other illnesses may be highly significant. Whenever relevant, questions should be asked about the possibility of parental veneral disease. The birth history should include specifics pertaining to the likelihood of perinatal anoxia. The Apgar score as well as details concerning the administration of supplemental oxygen should be noted. The birth weight and gestational age of the patient may provide evidence of prematurity.

Helpful information on visual behavior often can be obtained from attendants in the nursery. The training, experience, and relative objectivity of nurses generally make their observations more reliable than those of family members.

The general medical findings may be essential to the determination of a specific and comprehensive diagnosis. Particular attention should be directed to the central nervous system. Because the optic vesicle and cup develop from the embryologic forebrain, malformations of the globe are associated with developmental defects of the brain.

Examination of the eyes of newborns may be divided conveniently into structural and functional components. Structural aspects of importance include the size of the eye, the size and clarity of the cornea, the transparency of the lens, and abnormalities of the uveal tract (*i.e.*, iris, ciliary body, and choroid), vitreous, retina, and optic disk.

The size of the eye can be estimated grossly by inspection alone or by inspection coupled with palpation. There is a tendency to equate corneal diameter and eyeball diameter. This tendency should be consciously resisted because, although these two determinations generally correlate, they do not always have the same significance. Eyeball diameter may be precisely, simply, and safely measured ultrasonographically. This technique also is useful for exploring the interior of the eye in the presence of corneal and lenticular opacities as well as other conditions that interfere with visualization of the posterior segment of the eye.

Corneal diameter generally is measured with ruled calipers. The axial diameter of the human eye at term is about 17 mm; the corneal diameter usually is between 9.5 and 10.5 mm.

Functional ophthalmologic aspects of importance

that can be tested during the newborn period include pupillary light responses, induced eye movements, ocular fixation, and tracking or following eye movements.

Pupillary responses to light normally are present even in premature infants after 32 weeks of gestation. They should be elicited before mydriasis. A strong light—preferably that of the indirect ophthalmoscope—should be used, although a conventional flashlight usually is adequate. Pocket flashlights generally are not sufficiently powerful. Pupillary responses should be demonstrated several times so that reflex responses to light can be differentiated conclusively from random changes in pupillary size. The presence of pupillary responses to light demonstrates intactness of pupillary afferent and efferent pathways, and, by inference, intactness of subcortical visual pathways. Blink responses to light in newborns likewise are indicative of subcortical visual function. Supranuclearly induced horizontal ocular rotations can be stimulated by manual rotation of the head about the longitudinal axis of the body or by rotational stimulation with the infant held facing the examiner. The former will produce doll's-head movements; the latter will produce deviation of the eyes toward the direction of rotation. Such simple maneuvers are helpful in identifying paretic ocular muscles early in life.

Ocular fixation of stationary objects and eye tracking of moving objects are present in some term newborns but generally are not well developed until 4 to 6 weeks. The absence of fixation or following at birth need not cause concern, but their presence is reassuring. With forced-choice, optokinetic stimulation and electrooculographic recordings, visual acuities of 20/400 have been demonstrated during the first few days of life. For clinical purposes, a bright light or a human face are optimal test objects for eliciting fixation and following movements.

Examination of the lens, vitreous, and fundus best is deferred until after pupillary mydriasis has been obtained. Optimal mydriasis requires both anticholinergic and sympathetic drugs. Recommended agents are 0.2% cyclopentolate (Cyclogyl, Alcon Laboratories, Inc., Fort Worth, TX) and 1.0% phenylephrine (Neo-Synephrine, Winthrop Consumer Products, New York, NY). These two drugs are combined in appropriate concentrations in Cyclomydril (Alcon), a commercially available product. One drop of Cyclomydril should be instilled in each eye. Because the conjunctival recesses of the newborn can accommodate far less than a single drop of fluid, most of the medication will flow out of the eye. Excess fluid should be absorbed with tissues. If pupillary dilation is inadequate after 45 minutes, the aforementioned medications may be repeated. Bauer and coworkers report paralytic ileus and necrotizing enterocolitis after topical installation of six drops of cyclopentolate in the eyes of newborns.[1] One death occurred. I recommend not using more than two drops in each eye of the 0.5% solution. Darkly pigmented irides (*e.g.*, those of most African Americans) require a second instillation of drops. Caution should be observed in repeating anticholinergic drops in lightly pigmented individuals because erythema, hyperthermia, and tachycardia are more likely to develop in such patients. Ten-percent phenylephrine should not be instilled in the eyes of premature infants. Its use in such infants has been reported to produce transient systemic hypertension.[2] The possibility of inducing angle-closure glaucoma in infants is so remote that it does not constitute a realistic danger. Atropine drops or ointment should never be used in infants for routine diagnostic purposes because of possible adverse reactions.

Opacities of the lens are visualized best by slit-lamp examination. Hand-held slit lamps that can be brought readily to the patient are commercially available. A bright light and plus lens magnification—such as is obtained with the indirect ophthalmoscope without the hand-held condensing lens—is a convenient but less precise diagnostic instrument. Another useful technique is to retroilluminate lenticular opacities by means of a retinoscope. The latter instrument is a readily available diagnostic device generally used for objective estimation of refractive error.

Much information on the anterior segment of the eye may be obtained by simple inspection. There are four important principles to consider:

1. To obtain maximal magnification, the examiner should reduce the distance between his or her eyes and the eyes of the patient as much as possible. If the examiner is presbyopic, reading glasses should be worn.
2. The object must be well illuminated. A conventional flashlight, such as is used for transillumination of the head, is adequate.
3. The object must be well exposed. This can be accomplished best by means of a small, self-retaining speculum (Fig. 53-1), specifically de-

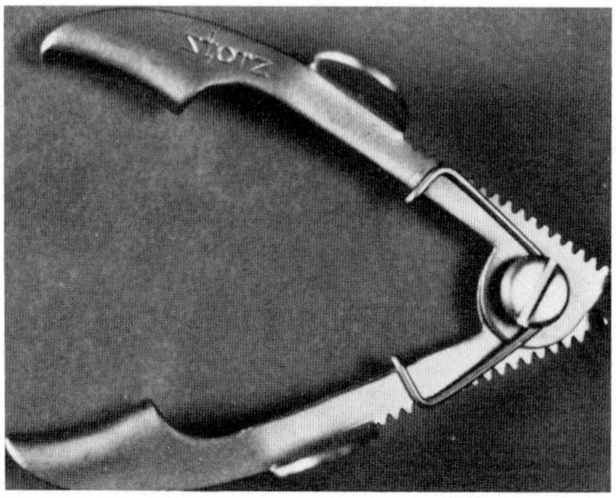

FIG. 53–1. Spring-action, self-retaining infant eyelid speculum.

signed to separate the eyelids of infants. The examiner should instill a topical anesthetic such as 0.5% proparacaine hydrochloride (Ophthaine HCl, Squibb Mark, Princeton, NJ) to anesthetize the cornea and dull conjunctival sensitivity before insertion of the speculum. If a speculum is used, normal saline should be dropped on the cornea from time to time to maintain corneal transparency. If a speculum is not available, an assistant should be asked to separate the lids. A tissue placed between the fingers and the lid surfaces will ensure dryness and reduce slippage. To obtain maximal exposure, the lids should be grasped as close as possible to their margins. The assistant's fingers actually should touch the cilia of both the upper and lower lids. Gentle pressure must be applied to the globe so that adequate exposure is obtained. This pressure may blanch the optic disk by interfering with its circulation. The unwary may misinterpret this induced blanching as optic atrophy. Slight pallor of the disks is a normal finding in about one-third of newborns.[3]

4. The patient's eye must be centered and more or less immobile. Correct positioning may at times be difficult to attain, particularly in the presence of an active Bell phenomenon (*i.e.*, the tendency of the anterior portion of the eye to roll upward toward the brow as the lids are forcibly separated against the contracting orbicularis oculi). It frequently is helpful to feed the baby during this and other portions of the examination or to place a pacifier in the baby's mouth.

The fundi are visualized best after mydriasis by indirect ophthalmoscopy (Fig. 53-2). Familiarity with the indirect ophthalmoscope unfortunately is not widespread outside the specialty of ophthalmology. The instrument has the disadvantage of producing an inverted as well as a reversed image. For screening purposes, however, this inconvenient feature is of little importance. The instrument is far superior to the conventional direct ophthalmoscope because it provides a panoramic stereoscopic view. Opacities of the media do not significantly interfere with fundus visualization unless they are dense and extensive. As with any other unfamiliar instrument, a certain amount of practice is required until proficiency is obtained. The effort is well worth making.

The infant's eyes are closed much of the time after birth. When open, a moderate divergence generally is noted. The eyes do not move together in a smooth, well coordinated (*i.e.*, conjugate) manner immediately after birth. In this sense, all newborns may be thought of as having strabismus during the first several weeks of life.[4] Definitive diagnosis of nonparalytic (*i.e.*, concomitant) strabismus rarely is possible before the third month. For this reason, this subject has little importance in neonatal pediatric ophthalmology.

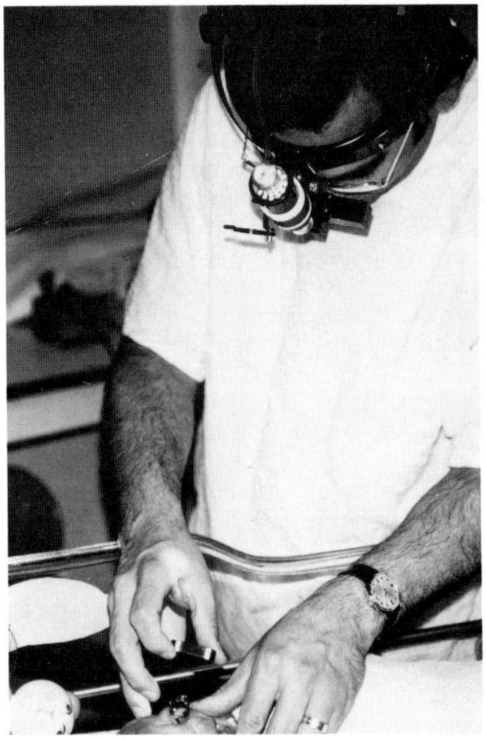

FIG. 53–2. Indirect ophthalmoscopy in the nursery.

OPHTHALMIA NEONATORUM

Although numerous infectious agents are capable of producing conjunctival inflammation in newborns,[5–7] the more common etiologies consist of silver nitrate chemical conjunctivitis and chlamydial, staphylococcal, and gonococcal infections. Herpetic infections and nasolacrimal duct obstruction also must be considered. Chlamydial, gonococcal, and herpes simplex infections can cause permanent ocular damage and can produce serious systemic complications. Because these various etiologies cannot be distinguished on clinical grounds, laboratory investigations are essential to correct diagnoses. Rational therapy requires knowledge of the cause of the ocular inflammation.

SILVER NITRATE CONJUNCTIVITIS

Conjunctival edema, hyperemia, and watery discharge occur frequently after the use of 1% silver nitrate drops. This irritative reaction occurs in about 90% of infants and begins within hours after drop instillation. It usually subsides within 48 hours. Thus, ocular inflammation developing more than 24 hours after silver nitrate prophylaxis is not likely to be due to this cause. This is perhaps the one instance in which knowledge of the time of onset of the ocular inflammation is truly useful in differential diagnosis.

CHLAMYDIAL EYE INFECTION

The incubation period for chlamydial eye infection is said to be approximately 5 to 13 days, but cases have been reported to start both earlier and later. Gonococcal and staphylococcal neonatal ophthalmitis frequently are stated to become clinically apparent 3 to 5 days and 5 to 7 days, respectively, after birth, but both earlier and later onsets are not uncommon. Incubation periods, except in silver nitrate inflammation, are notoriously unreliable and therefore do not help in determining an etiologic diagnosis. The clinical characteristics of neonatal conjunctivitis are not sufficiently distinctive to enable even the most experienced clinician to establish the precise etiology.

Chlamydia species are a common cause of ophthalmia neonatorum and indeed are possibly the most common identifiable infectious cause.[8] The reported rate of transmission of chlamydial infection from infected mothers to infants varies from 23% to 70%,[9] with conjunctivitis being the most common clinical manifestation of acquired disease.

Ocular infection has not been known to result in visual loss, but conjunctival sheet scarring and micropannus—especially of the superior limbus—have been reported. Of greater significance is the possibility that the eye may be the portal through which colonization of the respiratory tract occurs via the nasolacrimal ducts.

Cultures from the nasopharynx have been positive in a high percentage of infants exposed to infected cervices during delivery. Of particular importance is the observation of chlamydial pneumonia in some such infected neonates.[10–16] This particular form of pneumonia presents at 3 to 13 weeks of age and is characterized by a dry cough, congestion, tachypnea, and rales. It may or may not be preceded by clinically evident conjunctivitis. Affected infants are characteristically afebrile. Chest radiographs reveal areas of hyperinflation and interstitial infiltrates. IgG and IgM levels are elevated, and there is occasional eosinophilia. *Chlamydia trachomatis* is considered the etiologic agent of an appreciable proportion of cases of pneumonia in infants.[13]

The laboratory diagnosis of chlamydial conjunctivitis can be determined most simply by scraping the palpebral conjunctiva of the lower lid with a platinum spatula and spreading the contents on a clean glass slide for Giemsa staining. Infected epithelial cells reveal a basophilic paranuclear cytoplasmic inclusion (*i.e.*, Halberstaedter–Prowazek inclusion bodies). Tissue cell culture techniques using McCoy cells are becoming increasingly available and useful for recovery of *C. trachomatis*. The primary methods for demonstrating inclusions in infected cells are iodine staining, Giemsa staining, and immunofluorescent techniques.[17] Direct smear using fluorescent antibody is the most thoroughly evaluated diagnostic method second to culture.[18]

Systemic therapy of patients with chlamydial conjunctivitis is essential. Topical therapy consisting of 10% sulfacetamide drops or 1% tetracycline ointment or drops every 6 hours for 3 weeks is inadequate to eradicate the organism from the upper respiratory tract.[14,19] Erythromycin (12.5 mg/kg orally or intravenously four times a day for 14 days) should be given to affected infants.[18] Parents likewise should be treated with erythromycin for lactating women or tetracycline for 2 or 3 weeks.[19]

STAPHYLOCOCCAL INFECTION

Infection may be acquired during the birth process or postnatally by contact with the mother or nursery personnel. Infection usually is mild, with catarrhal discharge. Rare complications include corneal ulcers, corneal infiltrates, hypopyon, endophthalmitis, and a generalized exfoliative dermatitis.[20]

Recovery of staphylococci from cultures should be interpreted with caution because these organisms may be found in the conjunctival sacs of healthy neonates without conjunctivitis.

GONORRHEAL INFECTION

In the United States and elsewhere, there is an epidemic of gonorrhea. Indeed, it has been said to be the most common contagious disease next to the common cold. An upsurge in the incidence of gonorrheal ophthalmia neonatorum is therefore to be expected and actually appears to be occurring.[21]

Antibiotics have radically altered the prognosis in the presence of established disease. The rarity of serious complications in proven cases of gonococcal conjunctivitis in newborn infants has been documented.[22] In view of the rising incidence of the venereal form of the disease and the development of penicillin resistance, however, complacency toward this potentially blinding disease must not be allowed to develop.

Gonococcal ophthalmia neonatorum classically presents as a purulent conjunctivitis, usually bilateral (Fig. 53-3); however, this textbook picture often is not present. The discharge may be mild and mucoid. Ocular complications are due to corneal involvement, which may progress to endophthalmitis.

Infants with gonococcal ophthalmia may have other forms of localized disease, including rhinitis, anorectal infection, and funisitis. Dissemination of infection with development of arthritis and meningitis is a possible complication. Premature rupture of the membranes may lead to the gonococcal amniotic infection syndrome characterized by pneumonia, meningitis, sepsis, chorioamnionitis, funisitis, and recovery of organisms from orogastric aspirates.[23]

Infants with ophthalmia neonatorum routinely should have Gram stains and blood agar and chocolate agar cultures, in addition to the aforementioned conjunctival scrapings. The organisms are fastidious in their environmental and nutritional requirements.

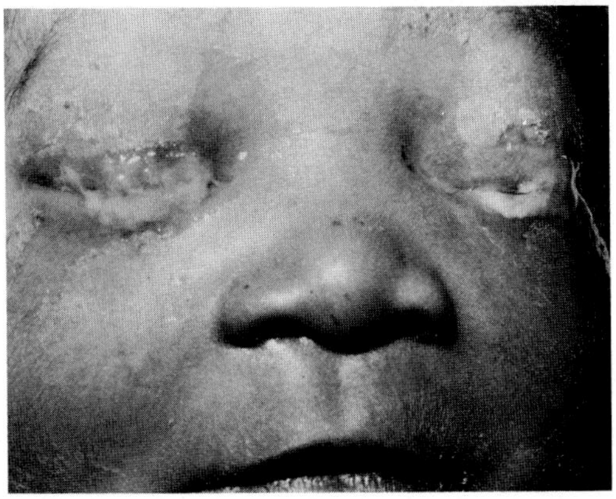

FIG. 53–3. Gonococcal ophthalmia neonatorum.

Growth occurs best in the presence of moisture, in an atmosphere containing increased concentrations of carbon dioxide, and in temperatures of 35°C to 36°C. Because organisms die rapidly at room temperature, inoculated material should be brought to the laboratory as soon as possible.

If the Gram stains suggest the possibility of the presence of *Neisseria* species organisms, which are gram-negative intracellular diplococci, the infant should be admitted to the hospital, and isolation precautions should be observed. Beta-lactamase–producing strains of gonococci have been reported, so that conventional doses of penicillin may not be adequate in all cases. Sensitivities to penicillin should be determined *in vitro*.

Recommended treatment of uncomplicated cases consists of aqueous crystalline penicillin G, 100,000 units/kg/day intravenously in four divided doses for 7 days.[18] The eyes should be irrigated with saline. Topical antibiotics are not essential. Systemic therapy is necessary, particularly in view of the possibility of localized infection in remote locations as well as the possibility of hematogenous dissemination. Ophthalmologic consultation is advisable. All cases should be reported to local health departments so that epidemiologic concerns can be addressed and so that adequate treatment of the mother and her sexual contacts can be ensured.

PREVENTION

There is good evidence that Credé prophylaxis has significantly reduced the incidence of gonorrheal ophthalmia neonatorum.[24] Silver nitrate is not effective against *C. trachomatis*, however, and for that reason as well as for the associated chemical conjunctivitis, some authorities advocate the routine use of tetracycline or erythromycin ointment[25] after birth. Both agents are effective against *Neisseria gonorrhoeae*.

The Centers for Disease Control,[18] the American Academy of Pediatrics,[26] and the National Society to Prevent Blindness[27] agree that 1% silver nitrate solution and ophthalmic ointment containing 1% tetracycline or 0.5% erythromycin are acceptable and effective choices for prophylaxis of ophthalmia neonatorum. Many institutions are reviewing their current policies pertaining to prophylaxis; however, local laws and health department regulations of many jurisdictions mandate which particular agents may or may not be used. Therefore, current local regulations must be investigated before changes are made in institutional practices.

HERPES SIMPLEX INFECTION

Nahmias and colleagues have described three forms of neonatal herpes simplex infection: disseminated, localized, and asymptomatic.[28] The last is apparently extremely rare. Infants with disseminated disease also may have localized organ involvement. Disseminated forms of infection involve the liver, adrenal glands, and lungs, thus resembling bacterial sepsis. The localized forms involve the central nervous system, skin, oral cavity, and eye. Eye involvement includes optic neuritis, chorioretinitis, cataracts, conjunctivitis, and keratitis. The eyes become involved in about 15% to 20% of infected neonates.

Most infants with herpes simplex infection acquire the disease during the birth process. Ascending infection and transplacental transmission are thought to be relatively uncommon. Genital (*i.e.*, type II) maternal infection usually is asymptomatic. When active genital disease is recognized at term—preferably by the morphologic characteristics of infected cervical cells or by tissue virus isolation techniques—cesarean section usually is considered, provided the fetal membranes have been ruptured for less than 4 to 6 hours.

Neonatal herpes simplex infection is a very serious disease. Many affected infants are born prematurely. An 85% mortality is associated with disseminated disease, and a 50% mortality is associated with untreated localized central nervous system disease.[29] There also is a high morbidity, primarily due to central nervous system sequelae.

Neonatal herpes simplex occasionally may present first as a conjunctivitis.[30] The onset generally is between 2 and 14 days after birth. The characteristics of neonatal herpetic simplex conjunctivitis are not clinically distinctive. The diagnosis is likely to be suspected only if there is a history of maternal or paternal genital herpes or if there are other manifestations of the disease in the neonate, including keratitis.

Several types of unilateral and bilateral corneal involvement have been reported, including the virtually diagnostic epithelial dendrite. A diffuse punctate keratitis, stromal keratitis, and perhaps most frequently a geographic or ameboid epithelial form have been described.

Epithelial defects can be visualized best by staining the corneal surface with a dilute solution of fluorescein dye and then examining the cornea with a portable slit lamp under blue light. Lid retractors are essential to adequate exposure of the cornea. Two assistants in addition to the physician are needed for proper immobilization and exposure.

The consulting ophthalmologist also should examine the fundus by indirect ophthalmoscopy to evaluate for possible chorioretinitis. Cataracts also have been reported. Slit-lamp biomicroscopy and fundal examinations should be repeated periodically on all children with neonatal herpes simplex infection.[31]

Herpetic neonatal conjunctivitis may be diagnosed most simply by examination of conjunctival epithelial scrapings for multinucleated giant cells and intranuclear inclusions. Papanicolaou-stained preparations should be read by a trained cytologist.

Herpes simplex virus may be isolated from the conjunctiva by means of cotton swabs that subsequently are placed in transport media. Cytopathic effects are observed in tissue culture within 1 to 3 days.

Other methods of diagnosis include identification of virus particles by electron microscopy and fluorescent antibody techniques.

After the diagnosis has been made, the infant should be placed in a special care or, preferably, a tertiary care nursery unit. Isolation precautions should be observed.[32] Topical antivirals should be administered. The most effective available drug is trifluorothymidine. One drop is instilled every 2 hours for a maximum daily dose of nine drops.

Systemic treatment with adenine arabinoside (*i.e.*, ara-A or vidarabine) has been shown to reduce the mortality in both the disseminated and localized central nervous system forms of the disease.[29]

Acyclovir is an antiviral compound with effectiveness similar to that of vidapline. Because the eyes occasionally may be the portal of entry of the virus to the body, exposed neonates may be given topical antivirals prophylactically.

Although the eye may be the only affected organ, disseminated and localized forms of the disease may precede or follow eye involvement. In an individual case, it is impossible to predict whether the disease will remain localized or disseminate. Therefore, it seems reasonable to advise systemic therapy for an infant with only corneal epithelial or conjunctival involvement. In such cases, systemic antiviral therapy should be instituted as early as possible so that morbidity and mortality are minimized.

Recurrences of keratitis are common; affected individuals should be reevaluated periodically throughout childhood. Parents should be made aware of the need for immediate ophthalmologic consultation if symptoms or signs suggestive of keratitis recur.

Further discussion of herpes simplex infections can be found in Chapter 47.

OBSTRUCTED NASOLACRIMAL DUCTS

A history of recurrent unilateral or bilateral ocular infections during the first few months of life should suggest the possibility of congenital nasolacrimal duct obstruction. Affected infants have pooling of tears in the lacrimal lake and epiphora (*i.e.*, overflow of tears onto the lower lid and cheek). The lids frequently are excoriated and the lid margins matted. Patients give a history of recurrent mucopurulent conjunctival discharge.

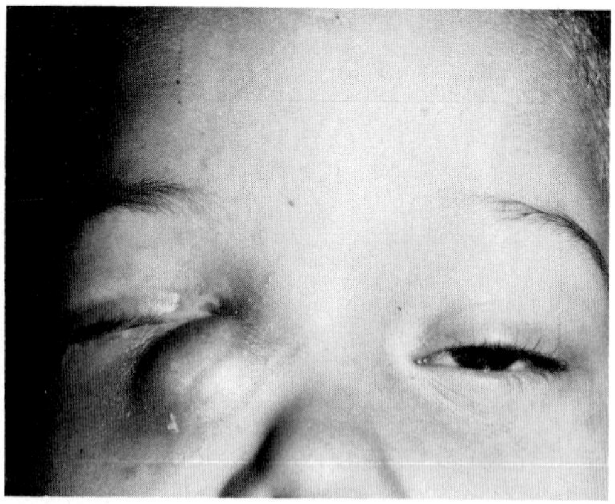

FIG. 53–4. Acute dacryocystitis with enlargement of the right nasolacrimal sac.

Pressure on the lacrimal sac may cause a reflux of mucus or pus through the puncta. When the infant cries, tears do not appear at the external nares.

The most important defect to differentiate from this entity is congenital glaucoma. In this condition, light sensitivity, blepharospasm, corneal enlargement, and opacification are common. Tears do appear at the external nares when the infant cries.

Conservative treatment of nasolacrimal duct obstruction consists of massage of the lacrimal sac and suppression of the infection with topical antibiotic drops and ointments. The eyes should be cleaned with moist compresses, and secretions should be removed mechanically.

Some ophthalmologists recommend office probing of the nasolacrimal system at approximately 3 months. Others favor postponing surgery until 8 or 9 months[33] because of the possibility of spontaneous opening of the duct. The only conditions that require prompt probing are mucoceles and acute dacryocystitis. The former are mucus collections in distended lacrimal sacs obstructed at both the proximal and distal openings; the latter are obstructed sacs distended by purulent material (Fig. 53-4).

CATARACTS

The causes of cataracts in infants and children are legion. A tabulation in 1969 listed 50 known causes and associations.[34] A survey of 386 cases reported finding "etiologic factors" in about two thirds of all cases.[35] Details are given in Table 53-1. It is significant that the birth weight was below 2500 g in 52% of the patients with central nervous system damage and in 22% of the cases for which a cause could not be estab-

TABLE 53–1
ETIOLOGY OF INFANTILE CATARACTS IN 386 CASES

	Number	Percent
Hereditary (*i.e.*, other family members affected)	32	8.3
Congenital rubella syndrome	74	19.1
Systemic disease (*e.g.*, Down syndrome, multiple congenital malformations, Lowe syndrome, galactosemia)	46	11.9
Other ocular disease, excluding microphthalmos	23	6.0
Central nervous system disorders (*e.g.*, mental retardation, convulsions, paraplegia, hemiplegia, cerebral palsy)	88	22.8
Unknown	123	31.9

Adapted from Merin S, Crawford JS. The etiology of congenital cataracts. Can J Ophthalmol 1971;6:178.

lished. The mechanisms whereby perinatal hypoxia and low birth weight contribute to the incidence of infantile cataracts are unknown. Hypoglycemia may play a role in some cases. It is of interest that cataracts associated with neurologic abnormalities and prematurity, as well as rubella cataracts, may develop postnatally.

In galactosemia, cataracts may appear as early as 7 days after birth. The most characteristic type of lens opacity resembles an oil droplet. These cataracts always are bilateral and are observed in approximately 75% of affected patients. The classic disease is caused by deficiency of the transferase enzyme that, in the presence of uridine diphosphoglucose, converts galactose-1-phosphate to glucose-1-phosphate. Cataracts of a similar type may occur within 5 months of birth in galactokinase deficiency. Galactokinase deficiency results in an inability to phosphorylate galactose. This disorder, like galactose transferase deficiency, is inherited as an autosomal recessive trait. Urinary reducing substances detectable by Clinitest (Ames Company, Elkhart, IN) but not with glucose-oxidase testing strips are present in both disorders. Systemic abnormalities are present in transferase deficiency but, with the possible exception of mental retardation, not in galactokinase deficiency. Prompt diagnosis is of the utmost importance, because in both disorders, early dietary restriction of galactose—the major source of which is the lactose of milk—can prevent cataracts from developing and also can cause regression of established cataracts.

Transient bilateral cataracts of obscure etiology have been described in premature infants.[36] Of 513 prematures examined for possible retrolental fibroplasia (RLF), transient cataracts were noted in 19.[37] These cataracts clearly were related only to gestational age and birth weight. The cataracts were not invariably present at the time of initial examination. Symmetric fluid vacuoles were noted in the region of the posterior lens sutures. At times, these cataracts were sufficiently dense to obscure fundal details. Complete spontaneous clearing invariably occurred over a period of several weeks.

The principal difficulty in rehabilitating eyes with severe congenital monocular cataracts is the presence of a particularly pernicious form of amblyopia. Experimental work in monocularly deprived kittens suggests that irreversible anatomic changes at the level of the lateral geniculate body and neurophysiologic alterations in striate cortical synapses occur very early in life and are responsible for the poor posttreatment prognoses of individuals with congenital monocular cataracts.[38,39] Patients with congenital bilateral symmetrical cataracts may fare better, presumably because of less severe or absent competitive interaction between the neural pathways from the two eyes, resulting in less severe amblyopia.

One report indicates that surgical removal of unilateral congenital cataracts performed within the first 2 months of life, followed by intense medical treatment consisting of contact lens wear to correct the aphakic refractive error and occlusion of the sound eye to eliminate amblyopia in the surgically treated eye, may result in good central vision in both eyes.[40] Because of the amblyopia-imposed requirement to operate very early in life, dense, extensive, unilateral, congenital cataracts have been termed surgical emergencies.

INFANTILE GLAUCOMA

Glaucoma in infants may be primary or secondary. The primary, or idiopathic, variety generally has been thought to be caused by autosomal recessive inheritance with incomplete penetrance. This time-honored concept has been challenged,[41] and a multifactorial genetic basis has been proposed. The secondary forms of infantile glaucoma are associated with other anomalies and disorders of the eye and of the body generally and, with a single exception, will not be considered in this discussion.

The incidence of primary infantile or, less accurately, congenital glaucoma is said to be approximately 1 in 12,500 births. The low incidence of the disease, combined with the high incidence of obstructed nasolacrimal ducts in the same age group, accounts for a high proportion of misdiagnoses and late referrals. In both conditions, tearing may be the chief complaint. Neonates with glaucoma, however, have light sensitivity and blepharospasm in addition to tearing. All infants with tearing should have careful corneal examinations. The hallmark of infantile glaucoma is corneal cloudiness (Fig. 53-5), occurring as a result of the passage of intraocular fluid, which is under abnormally high pressure, into the corneal stroma. Breaks in the Descemet membrane occur as the cornea stretches and increases in size in response to the raised intraocular pressure. The entire eye eventually may share in the enlargement, producing buphthalmos.

Approximately 70% of the optic disks of normal newborns show some degree of cupping.[3] This nearly always is symmetric. Asymmetric, extensive cupping of the optic disks is a relatively early sign of infantile glaucoma. Such findings should suggest the possibility of this diagnosis.

There is a slight but definite tendency for the disorder to occur preferentially in boys. For reasons equally obscure, approximately 25% of cases are monocular.

Immediate recognition and early referral are critically important. In late cases, irreversible damage to the angle region where aqueous humor egresses from the eye makes control of pressure difficult. Corneal scarring and retinal and optic nerve damage are largely preventable by prompt surgery.

The prognosis is related to the patient's age at the onset of corneal opacification. The earlier the corneal edema becomes apparent, the poorer the prognosis is for vision.

The treatment of infantile glaucoma is surgical. Attempts at long-term control by medications are inadvisable, except in instances in which surgery cannot be performed or is only partially successful. Although new operations have been introduced (*e.g.*, trabeculotomy), goniotomy generally still is recognized as the operation of choice. The raised intraocular pressure can be brought under control by this procedure in approximately 80% of cases. The success rate in terms of vision, however, is not nearly as favorable, primarily because of unrecognized or treatment-resistant amblyopia secondary to unequal refractive errors. Poor vision also can result from corneal scarring and irregular astigmatism.[42]

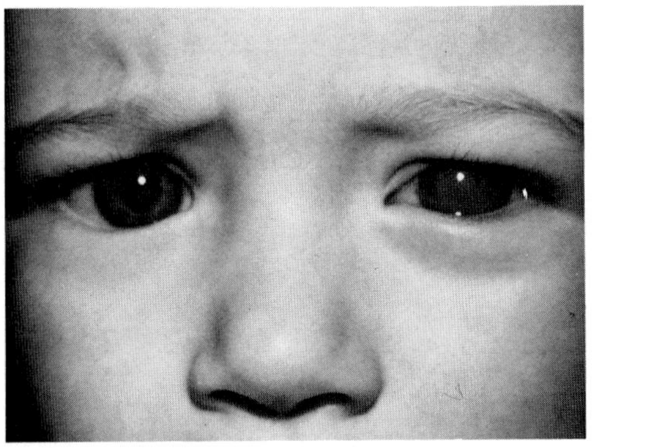

FIG. 53–5. Unilateral congenital glaucoma in an 11-month-old infant. Note the enlargement and the cloudiness of the left cornea.

The glaucoma that occasionally is seen in infants with the rubella syndrome is an exact phenocopy of primary infantile glaucoma. The diagnosis may be made on the basis of associated findings and serologic tests. Only very rarely do patients with the rubella syndrome have both cataracts and glaucoma.

Megalocornea is an inherited binocular condition largely confined to boys. Affected eyes are asymptomatic and normal except for an enlarged anterior segment. The corneas, although enlarged, are clear and do not have breaks in the Descemet membrane.

Prolonged labor, anatomic crowding during delivery, and, in particular, the application of obstetric forceps to an eye during birth may cause ruptures of the Descemet membrane and corneal edema. The intraocular pressure of such traumatized eyes is low and there is no corneal enlargement. Myopia, amblyopia, and strabismus may develop in patients with perinatal corneal injuries. Bullous keratopathy develops in some of these patients in adult life.[43]

RETINOPATHY OF PREMATURITY OR RETROLENTAL FIBROPLASIA

The term RLF was introduced in 1942 by Terry, who first described the condition.[44] He believed that the essential disturbance was an overgrowth of embryonic connective tissue behind the lens. Heath in 1951 introduced the term "retinopathy of prematurity" (ROP).[45] This term more accurately identifies the site of the initial pathologic processes.

HISTORICAL ASPECTS AND INCIDENCE

In the early 1950s, a number of investigators suggested that excess oxygen was causally associated with ROP. Three controlled nursery studies published in 1951, 1954, and 1955 convincingly demonstrated the toxic effects of excess oxygen on the retinal vessels of premature infants.[46–48] Production of the condition in experimental newborn animals raised with supplemental oxygen provided further confirmation of the detrimental effect of hyperoxia on growing retinal vessels.

The epidemic of ROP that occurred in the 1940s and early 1950s in association with the unrestricted use of oxygen was followed by a period of low incidence during which supplemented oxygen was markedly curtailed. More recent studies have shown that the restricted use of oxygen resulted in an increase in mortality,[49] and in cerebral palsy.[50] As a result, oxygen is used more liberally, but unlike the practice during the period after World War II, it is being used more selectively. An upsurge in the incidence of ROP nevertheless may occur as a result of this most recent swing of the therapeutic pendulum plus the survival of more very small prematures.

The incidence of ROP is inversely proportional to birth weight. In one study, retinal vessel changes in premature infants receiving oxygen occurred in 6 of 17 infants (35%) under 1500 g, whereas such changes occurred in only 10 of 58 infants (17%) over 1500 g.[51] In a retrospective survey, Silverman found that 82% of all cases of ROP occurred in infants under 1500 g birth weight.[52] For reasons unknown, infants of multiple births are more likely to have cicatricial ROP than are singleton infants of the same gestational age and weight.[48]

In 1970, Tasman found the overall incidence of cicatricial ROP to be 0.9% in 995 live births.[53] This investigator showed, by citing his own experience as well as the recorded experience of others, that very few cases of ROP develop in infants over 2268 g at birth but that "all gradations of severity . . . may be found no matter what the premature weighs at birth and no matter what the gestational age."[53]

In 1981, Phelps estimated the number of infants affected by cicatricial ROP in the United States.[54] She stated that there are 2100 cases annually, 550 of whom will be blind. The predominant factor leading to the increase in ROP is the enhanced survival of infants under 1 kg. The history of oxygen therapy and RLF has been reviewed by James and Lanman.[55] Current theory emphasizes multiple causal factors associated with the disease.[56,57]

PATHOPHYSIOLOGY

In a series of animal experiments, Ashton and coworkers have shown that excess oxygen produces a vasoconstriction of immature retinal vessels.[58–61] This vasoconstriction, which is reversible in its early stages, occurs first in the terminal arterioles and in the arteriolar side of the capillary tree. It is followed by an irreversible vasoobliteration, at which stage the vessel walls are adherent and show degenerative changes. Cytopathic effects are noted first in the endothelium of immature retinal capillaries. Vasoproliferation typically occurs after normalization of oxygen tension. The severity of the vasoobliteration is directly proportional to the duration and concentration of excess oxygen and to the degree of immaturity of the retinal vascular system. The toxic effects of oxygen can be prevented in kittens by intermittent air breathing. Thus, kittens alternately receiving 1-hour periods of 80% to 90% ambient oxygen and normal air showed no evidence of vasoobliteration.

Completely vascularized retinas of animals and humans are immune to the toxic effects of oxygen. The occasional case of ROP in a full-term infant probably best is explained by the fact that the human retina is incompletely vascularized at term.[62] Intrauterine hypoxia may be the basis for the rare development of ROP in infants who do not receive supplemental oxygen. It is hypothesized that, in such infants, the abnormally great postnatal increase in blood oxygen tension is sufficient to produce vasoobliteration. This theory is, however, entirely speculative and it should be recognized that there are important unknown factors in the development of proliferative retinopathy in newborns.[63,64]

The disorder usually makes its appearance between 10 days and 1 month after birth. Bilateral involvement is nearly invariable, but pathologic changes frequently are asymmetric. The active phase generally subsides in a few months and in mild cases frequently is followed by spontaneous regression. The completeness of the regression varies indirectly with the severity of the morphologic derangement during the active stages.

Flynn and coworkers have identified, by means of fluorescein angiography, a functioning arteriovenous shunt located between avascular and vascularized retina.[65] The shunt virtually always is present in the temporal fundus but, in severe cases, may extend circumferentially. Neovascularization develops from vessels posterior to the shunt. In mild cases of ROP, vasoproliferation occurs only in the retinal periphery, but in severe cases, the entire retina will undergo neovascularization. Early changes occur predominantly in the temporal periphery, presumably because this area is the last to become vascularized.

The outcome is affected by the extent of the abnormalities (*i.e.*, hours of retinal involvement) as well as by the location of the abnormalities. The more posterior the arteriovenous shunt or ridge, the worse the prognosis. Dilation and tortuosity of posterior retinal vessels are unfavorable signs. An international classification of proliferative ROP[66] and the Reese classification of cicatricial RLF[67] are given in Table 53-2.

Newly formed vessels are strikingly abnormal. They tend to leak blood and plasma. Organization of hemorrhages and exudates leads to the formation of retinal and vitreous membranes and retinal detachments. Cicatricial changes start to develop at approximately 6 months after birth. Temporal traction of the vessels as they leave the disk is noted commonly (Fig. 53-6). The proliferation of retrolental fibrous tissue produces leukocoria (*i.e.*, abnormal pupillary reflex; Fig. 53-7) and visible ciliary processes that become elongated by traction.

In more severe cases, peripheral anterior synechiae and angle closure by forward movement of the lens iris diaphragm result in glaucoma. Such eyes usually are blind but may be preserved by lens aspiration and iridectomy. The most severely affected eyes become microphthalmic, soft, atrophic, and eventually phthisical.

LONG-TERM EFFECTS

Myopia is present in a great preponderance of eyes with cicatricial ROP. At times, corrected central acu-

TABLE 53–2
CLASSIFICATION OF RETINOPATHY OF PREMATURITY*

Stage	Proliferative-Phase Fundus Changes
I	Demarcation line (*i.e.*, thin, nonelevated white line at junction between vascularized and avascular retina)
II	Ridge (*i.e.*, elevated demarcation line)
III	Ridge with extraretinal fibrovascular proliferation
IV	Retinal detachment
Grade	**Cicatricial-Phase Fundus Changes**
I	Small areas of retinal pigment irregularities; small peripheral retinal scars
II	Disk distortion
III	Retinal fold
IV	Incomplete retrolental mass; partial retinal detachment
V	Complete retrolental mass; total retinal detachment

Plus disease indicates dilation of posterior veins and tortuosity of posterior arterioles. Three zones of retinal involvement centered on the optic disk are recognized. They are consecutively numbered from posterior to anterior. Zone I includes the area circumscribed by a circle with a radius twice the distance between disk and fovea. Zone II is situated peripheral to zone I and is limited by a circle that passes through the nasal ora serrata. Zone III is peripheral to zone II.

* International classification of proliferative retinopathy of prematurity[63] and Reese classification of cicatricial retrolental fibroplasia.[64]

ity may be poor because of foveal damage that may not always be readily apparent on ophthalmoscopy. Temporal displacement of the macula in cicatricial ROP may give the false impression of exotropia (*i.e.*, pseudoexotropia).

All eyes with cicatricial ROP are susceptible to late retinal detachment. Detachments are discovered most frequently in the first and second decades of life but may occur at any age. There is a direct relationship between the degree of myopia and the incidence of retinal detachment.

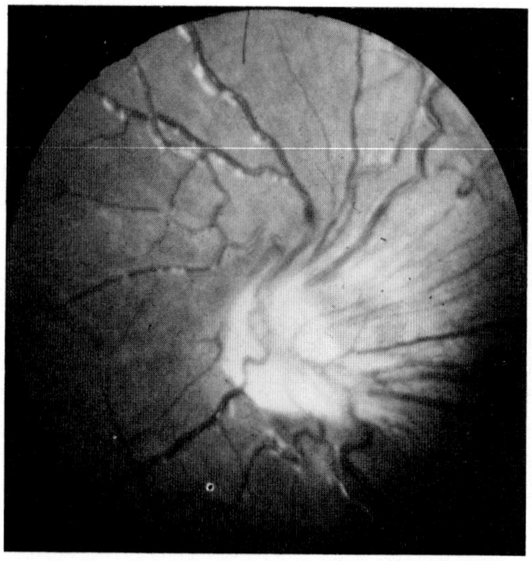

FIG. 53–6. Temporal traction of vessels from the optic disk in the left eye of an 8-month-old infant with grade II cicatricial retrolental fibroplasia.

DETECTION AND PREVENTION

Although vasoconstriction is the earliest adverse effect of oxygen on developing retinal vessels, attempts to detect this narrowing ophthalmoscopically have been unrewarding.[68] The presence of vitreous haziness in low-birth-weight infants may interfere with visualization of the retinal vessels even when the indirect ophthalmoscope is used. Persistence of the hyaloid system and the tunica vasculosa lentis may be the cause of this vitreous haze. The degree of opacifi-

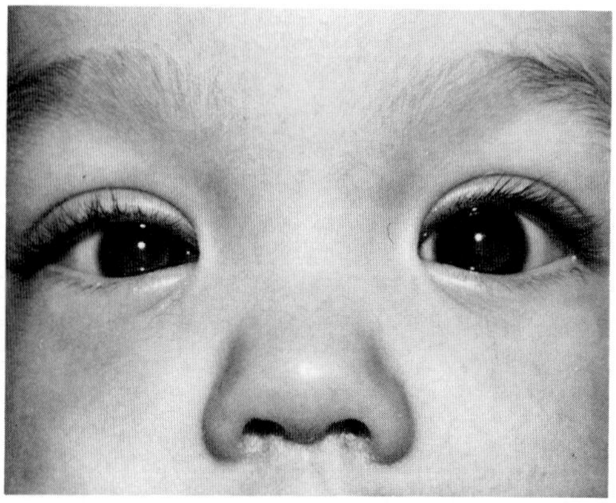

FIG. 53–7. Grade V retrolental fibroplasia in both eyes of a 7-month-old infant.

cation varies inversely with the birth weight. There also is a poor correlation between arterial PO_2 levels and retinal vessel caliber. Therefore, daily monitoring of the fundi would seem to have little practical value in assessment of the oxygen tension of arterial blood.

Retinopathy of prematurity is quite rare although not unknown in the presence of cyanosis[69]; however, the risk cannot be estimated by inspection alone once the skin color has become pink. At normal hemoglobin levels, cyanosis is observed when hemoglobin is between 75% and 85% saturated with oxygen, which for fetal hemoglobin corresponds to oxygen tensions of 32 to 42 torr. This does not mean that supplemental oxygen should be withheld until cyanosis appears. The respiratory distress syndrome is by far the most common condition for which supplemental oxygen is given to newborns. It is highly desirable to monitor the arterial PO_2 levels of such infants. This is particularly important after the infant's cardiopulmonary system has begun to improve. It is after recovery from the respiratory distress syndrome that arterial PO_2 levels are likely to reach retinotoxic levels if supplemental oxygen is not curtailed.

The safe upper level of retinal artery PO_2 is unknown. When possible, however, it is desirable to keep umbilical artery PO_2 levels below 100 torr. Unfortunately, maintenance below this level will not invariably prevent development of ROP. Susceptibility to oxygen is known to depend on multiplicity of birth, degree of immaturity, duration of oxygen exposure, and many other factors in addition to the level of arterial oxygen tension.

Low-birth-weight newborns and newborns receiving supplemental oxygen should have ophthalmologic examinations before discharge from the nursery or at approximately 4 to 6 weeks after birth, whichever comes first. A satisfactory negative examination practically eliminates the presence of the disease or the possibility of its future development. If abnormalities are noted at any age, subsequent ophthalmologic examinations must be planned according to the extent and severity of the changes and the rate of progression.

TREATMENT

There has been renewed interest in the antioxidant, vitamin E. Protective and therapeutic roles have been claimed, but not all clinical studies are in agreement. Large doses of vitamin E may have detrimental side effects (*e.g.*, sepsis, necrotizing enterocolitis). Controlled studies suggest that supplemental vitamin E does not have a favorable cost–benefit ratio. Until more definitive information is available, it probably is wise to maintain vitamin E levels within a physiologic range (*i.e.*, between 1.5 and 2 mg/dL). Blood levels should be determined periodically.

Indications for treatment during the active stages are influenced by the multicenter trial of cryotherapy for ROP,[70] which found a 50% reduction in unfavorable retinal outcomes in patients receiving cryotherapy according to protocol criteria. The criteria for cryotherapy in the study were at least five contiguous or eight cumulative clock hours of stage 3 ROP in zone 1 or 2 in the presence of plus disease. The treatment rationale for cryotherapy to the retina peripheral to the ridge or shunt is the same as for diabetic retinopathy. Ablation of this nonvascularized tissue is presumed to reduce production of a hypothetical vasoproliferative factor.

Retinal detachment surgery is possible during the cicatricial phase of the disease. Anatomic reattachment may be obtained but the functional results in terms of vision usually are poor.

It is essential that patients with significant cicatricial disease receive periodic fundus evaluations by ophthalmologists because of the possibility of late retinal detachment. This recommendation is particularly important in view of the favorable results of surgery for late retinal detachments associated with ROP.

RETINOBLASTOMA

The incidence of retinoblastoma is approximately 1 in 20,000 births. The diagnosis is made only rarely in the neonatal period except during examinations of siblings and progeny of affected individuals. The condition generally becomes manifest during infancy and is recognized most frequently between 17 and 18 months of life.[71] The mortality in the United States is about 10%. Among untreated patients, it is nearly 100%.

The presenting signs are leukocoria (*i.e.*, abnormal pupillary reflex) in about 60% (Fig. 53-8) and strabismus in about 20% of cases. About 33% of patients have bilateral involvement.

The disease occurs in both familial and sporadic forms. The familial form, defined as such whenever

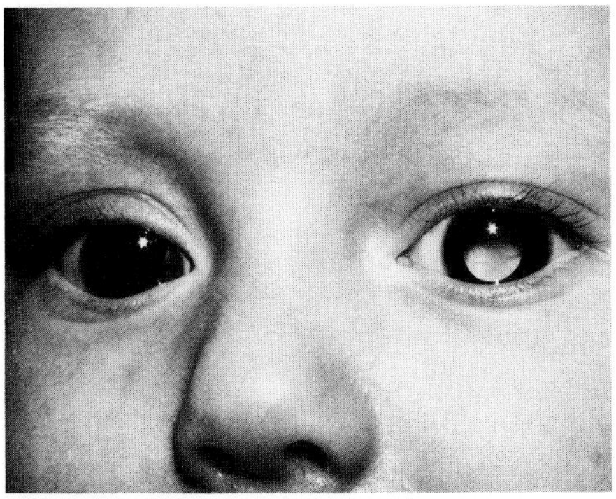

FIG. 53–8. This 2-month-old infant presented with leukocoria caused by retinoblastoma of the left eye but had bilateral disease. The left eye was more severely involved and was enucleated. The right eye was successfully treated with radiation.

there is at least one other affected family member, is only one-tenth as common as the sporadic form. The familial form is dominantly inherited and is more likely to be bilateral.

According to Knudson and associates, retinoblastoma requires two mutational events (*i.e.*, two-hit theory).[72] In the dominantly inherited form, one mutation is inherited (*i.e.*, prezygotic), whereas the second occurs in the somatic cells (*i.e.*, postzygotic). In the sporadic form of the disease, both events occur postzygotically. Tumors arising from multiple origins (*e.g.*, bilateral disease) signify the presence of the hereditary form.

In a relatively small proportion of retinoblastoma patients, a deletion on the long arm of chromosome 13 has been found by chromosomal banding techniques.[73] Clinical findings in these 13q-patients have included mental retardation, microcephaly, hypertelorism, absence or hypoplasia of the thumb, short fingers, pelvic girdle anomalies, and anogenital malformations. Eye findings have included microphthalmos and colobomata.

Patients with the hereditary form of the disease, including all bilaterally affected patients, have a tendency toward development of other malignancies later in life,[74,75] the most common of which is osteogenic sarcoma.

A likely explanation for this predisposition is offered by the Knudson hypothesis, according to which familial cases have an inherited genetic abnormality that affects all body cells. The retinoblastoma gene appears to have a suppressor function. Experimental evidence suggests the possibility that all three forms of retinoblastoma (*i.e.*, familial, sporadic, and deletion) are due to faulty genetic material in the 13q14 region. Neoplasms occur when the suppressor protein for which the gene codes is totally absent within a developing neuronal retinal cell.[76] It is vital that all patients with a history or physical findings indicating an abnormal pupillary reflex (*i.e.*, cat's-eye reflex) be referred to competent specialists as early in life as possible. In favorable cases, survival rates approach 100%. X-ray therapy, cryotherapy, and light coagulation are the mainstays of conservative management. In advanced unilateral cases, enucleation generally is performed.

Because progeny and siblings of retinoblastoma patients may be affected, it is most important to examine thoroughly the retinas of all such people shortly after birth. Thorough examination of suspected and high-risk cases requires indirect ophthalmoscopy with careful visualization of the entire retina of both eyes. Such examinations frequently require general anesthesia.

ANIRIDIA

In 1964, Miller and associates found in a retrospective study that of 440 children with Wilms tumor, 6 had aniridia (Fig. 53-9).[77] This rate of 1 in 73 is much higher than the expected rate of aniridia in the general population, which is about 1 in 50,000 births. Mental retardation, hypospadias, undescended testicles, and congenital hemihypertrophy also were found to have a higher than expected incidence in patients with Wilms tumor. In 1968, Fraumeni and Glass found 7 cases of Wilms tumor among 28 children hospitalized with aniridia.[78] In several patients with the triad of aniridia, ambiguous genitalia, and mental retardation, an interstitial deletion of the short arm of chromosome 11 has been reported.[79] Thus, patients with aniridia and other congenital abnormalities should receive high-quality chromosomal banding analysis.

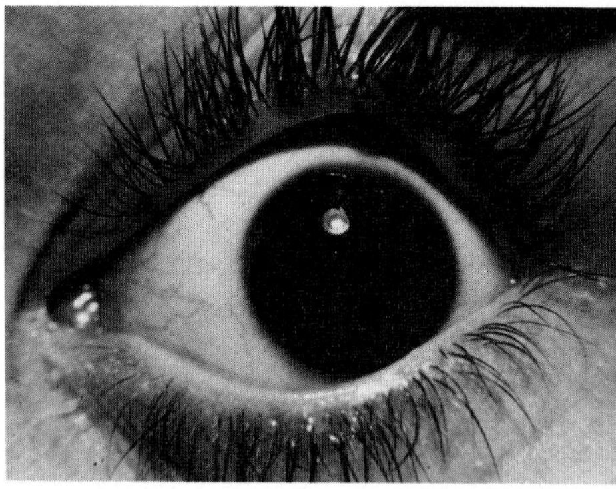

FIG. 53–9. Aniridia in the left eye of a child. Note that iris tissue is visible only in the superior nasal quadrant.

Aniridia occurs in both familial and sporadic forms. The familial form is somewhat more common. With a single possible exception, all cases of patients with both Wilms tumor and aniridia reported to date have been sporadic.

The implication of the association of Wilms tumor with aniridia is obvious. All infants with rudimentary or apparently absent irides without a positive family history of aniridia should be followed with periodic physical examinations, urinalyses, renal scans, and ultrasonograms until at least 3 years of age.

TOXOPLASMOSIS

Human toxoplasmosis (see Chap. 47) is acquired primarily by the handling and consumption of raw and undercooked meat and by contact with feces from infected cats. Desmonts and Couvreur found that of infants born to mothers who acquired the disease during pregnancy, only 11% were overtly affected.[80]

The clinical manifestations of congenital toxoplasmosis vary widely. In severely affected infants, chorioretinitis, microphthalmos, hydrocephalus, jaundice, hepatosplenomegaly, anemia, fever, and failure to thrive may be observed. As in other congenital infections, low birth weight and prematurity are common. Occasionally, microcephaly, meningoencephalitis, convulsions, and a maculopapular rash are present. In some cases, only the retinas are affected.

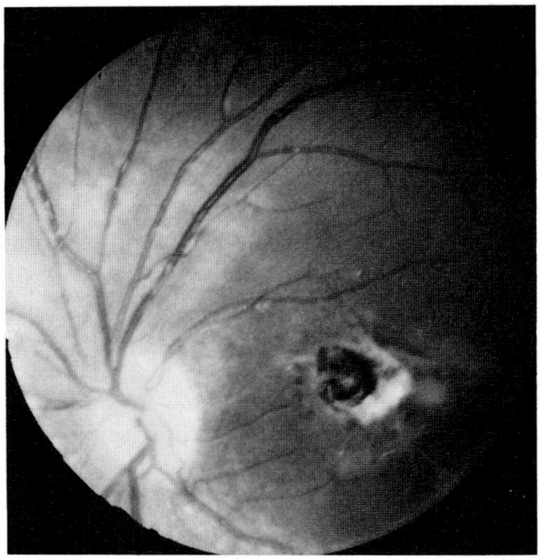

FIG. 53–10. Congenital toxoplasmosis in the macular region of the left eye of a child.

Retinal lesions may not appear, however, for days or even weeks after birth.

The most constant feature is a chorioretinitis or more properly a retinochoroiditis because the organisms lodge in the retina, producing a primary necrotizing retinitis with secondary choroidal involvement. The foveas are a favored location. There may be one or multiple foci in each fundus. The retinal lesions, when first observed, usually are bilateral and sharply outlined. They generally are quiescent, consisting of flat scars with pigmented borders (Fig. 53-10). The vitreous usually is clear. Radiographs may show diffuse intracranial calcifications. Specific hemagglutination antibody titers and Sabin and Feldman dye titers will be raised in both mother and infant. Elevated assays for IgM antibodies in the infant are particularly significant because maternal IgM does not cross the normal placenta.

Treatment of active toxoplasmosis is not very satisfactory. Administration of pyrimethamine (Daraprim; Burroughs Wellcome Co., Research Triangle Park, NC), sulfadiazine, steroids, and folinic acid does not result in dramatic improvement. Furthermore, steroids to a moderate extent and pyrimethamine to a marked extent are dangerous drugs with serious side effects.

Reactivation of congenital lesions may occur at any time throughout life. Late rupture of cysts situated at the pigmented margins of the retinal scars liberates viable organisms that produce characteristic satellite lesions. It is probable that most adult cases of ocular toxoplasmosis infection represent relapses of congenital disease.

CYTOMEGALOVIRUS DISEASE

Transplacental infection of the fetus with cytomegalovirus (CMV; see Chap. 47) results in clinical manifestations that vary from death to asymptomatic involvement. Hepatosplenomegaly is the most common physical finding. The lung, hematopoietic system, and the brain may be affected, producing pneumonitis, thrombocytopenia, and encephalitis with calcifications that are characteristically but not invariably periventricular in distribution. Approximately 25% of infants with severe neonatal CMV infection have retinochoroiditis.[81,82] Most infected infants are asymptomatic.[83]

The retinal lesions usually are described as similar to those of toxoplasmosis but tend to be less pigmented and more peripheral in location. They may not become manifest until some time after birth.

Diagnosis can be made on the basis of serologic tests, including elevated IgM levels, and virus culture from freshly obtained urine specimens.

There is no established treatment for the disease in neonates; however, ganciclovir is effective in immunodeficient adults with CMV retinopathy.

RUBELLA SYNDROME

Sir Norman Gregg in 1941 first described the rubella syndrome.[84] The virus was not isolated, however, until 1962. Today, congenital rubella is recognized as a major cause of serious eye malformations including retinopathy, glaucoma, cataract, microphthalmos, and anterior uveitis (see Chap. 47).

The classic syndrome, as originally described, consists of the triad of eye, ear, and heart defects. Involvement of other organ systems is now recognized. Microcephaly, encephalitis, hepatosplenomegaly, jaundice, anemia, thrombocytopenia, and skin and bone abnormalities are not uncommon manifestations of congenital infection. Infants with the syndrome tend to have low birth weights, fail to thrive, and have a high incidence of mental retardation.

An atypical retinitis pigmentosa–like retinopathy frequently is noted. Diffuse or localized pigment epithelium hypertrophy and atrophy are present, giving rise to a salt-and-pepper configuration. The retinopathy is not progressive and is not associated with significant visual loss. It may be either unilateral or bilateral.

The glaucoma that occurs in the rubella syndrome has been discussed previously.

Cataracts, the most common clinical ocular finding in the rubella syndrome, usually, but not invariably, are bilateral and have a characteristic morphology. A dense, white, opaque nucleus is seen centrally with gradually decreasing opacification toward the periphery of the lens (Fig. 53-11). Involved eyes usually are microphthalmic and have an anterior uveitis that results in variable degrees of iris atrophy and poor pupillary dilation with topical medications.

Treatment of rubella cataracts is similar to treatment of other types of congenital cataracts. Surgical discission and aspiration of the lens is the procedure of choice. An iridectomy should be done at the time of cataract surgery so that postoperative glaucoma

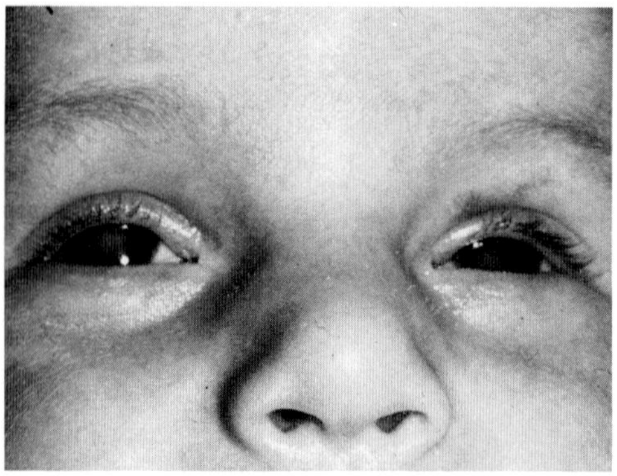

FIG. 53–11. Rubella cataracts in a 7-week-old infant.

from pupillary blockage of aqueous humor flow is prevented. It is important that pupillary dilation be obtained and retained for several months after surgery by means of topical medications. Surgery for rubella cataracts can be performed safely in early infancy.[85] Delay for ocular reasons beyond 6 months is unnecessary according to most authorities, despite the fact that virus has been isolated from lenses of congenital rubella patients up to 35 months old. For functional visual results, it is essential that surgery be performed as promptly as possible and that contact lenses be fitted early in the postoperative period.

RETINAL DANGERS ASSOCIATED WITH PHOTOTHERAPY FOR HYPERBILIRUBINEMIA

Phototherapy for hyperbilirubinemia has become increasingly popular since it was introduced in England in 1958 by Cremer and coworkers.[86] Light, obtained from ordinary fluorescent bulbs, is used to photooxidize bilirubin in the skin and subcutaneous tissues, thereby reducing the required number of exchange transfusions.

Noell and coworkers in 1966 and Kuwabara and Gorn in 1968 exposed rats to 750 foot-candles of illumination from ordinary fluorescent lights for periods of time ranging from 1 hour to several weeks.[87,88] Damage to the outer retinal layers was observed. Sisson and colleagues in 1970 exposed newborn piglets to 300 foot-candles of illumination for periods of time ranging from 12 to 72 hours.[89] Irreversible changes in the outer retinal layers were demonstrated.

Commercial phototherapy units for hyperbilirubinemia produce approximately 300 foot-candles of illumination in the incubator.[90] In view of the aforementioned animal experiments, it would appear to be necessary to shield the eyes of infants receiving phototherapy. This may be accomplished by an opaque mask secured by an elastic strap or by eye pads held in place by adhesive tape. Both eyes should be completely occluded. Incomplete occlusion of one eye is undesirable not only because of the retinotoxic effects of intense light but also for reasons related to animal experiments. Hubel and Wiesel have shown in kittens that monocular occlusion for merely a few days during the fourth or fifth weeks of life—the period of maximal sensitivity to unilateral occlusion in kittens—results in permanent amblyopia.[91]

The effects of monocular occlusion observed in kittens also potentially are applicable to newborns with unilateral cataracts, ptosis, or lid tumors that are sufficiently severe to occlude the pupillary aperture. Strenuous efforts should be made to eliminate the monocular occlusion at a very early age in such cases.

Bright, continuous nursery illumination may be a risk factor for ROP, and some attention to providing an appropriate visual environment to the premature infant may prove important.[64]

REFERENCES

1. Bauer CR, Trottier MC, Stern L. Systemic cyclopentolate (Cyclogyl) toxicity in the newborn infant. J Pediatr 1973;82:501.
2. Borromeo-McGrail V, Bordiuk JM, Keitel H. Systemic hypertension following ocular administration of 10% phenylephrine in the neonate. Pediatrics 1973;51:1032.
3. Khodadoust AA, Ziai M, Briggs SI. Optic disc in normal newborns. Am J Ophthalmol 1968;66:502.
4. Dayton GO, Jones MH, Aiu P, et al. Developmental study of coordinated eye movement in the human infant. Arch Ophthalmol 1964;71:865.
5. Armstrong JH, Zacarias F, Rein MF. Ophthalmia neonatorum: a chart review. Pediatrics 1976;57:884.
6. Pierce JM, Ward ME, Seal DV. Ophthalmia neonatorum in the 1980s: incidence, aetiology and treatment. Br J Ophthalmol 1982;66:728.
7. Stenson S, Newman R, Fedukowicz H. Conjunctivitis in the newborn: observations on the incidence, cause, and prophylaxis. Ann Ophthalmol 1981;13:329.
8. Thygeson P. Historical review of oculogenital disease. Am J Ophthalmol 1971;71:975.
9. Heggie AD, Lumicao GG, Stuart LA, et al. Chlamydia trachomatis infection in mothers and infants. A prospective study. Am J Dis Child 1981;135:507.
10. Beem MO, Saxon EM. Respiratory tract colonization and a distinctive pneumonia syndrome in infants infected with Chlamydia trachomatis. N Engl J Med 1977;296:306.
11. Frommel GT, Bruhn FW, Schwartzman JD. Isolation of Chlamydia trachomatis from infant lung tissue. N Engl J Med 1977;296:1150.
12. Frommel GT, Rothenberg R, Wang S-P, et al. Chlamydial infection of mothers and their infants. J Pediatr 1979;95:28.
13. Harrison HR, English MG, Lee CK, et al. Chlamydia trachomatis infant pneumonitis: comparison with matched controls and other infant pneumonitis. N Engl J Med 1978;298:702.
14. Rees E, Tait IA, Hobson D, et al. Persistence of chlamydial infection after treatment for neonatal conjunctivitis. Arch Dis Child 1981;56:193.
15. Schachter J, Grossman M, Holt J, et al. Prospective study of chlamydial infection in neonates. Lancet 1979;2:377.
16. Schachter J, Lunn L, Gooding CA, et al. Pneumonitis following inclusion blennorrhoea. J Pediatr 1975;87:779.
17. Schachter J. Chlamydial infections (third of three parts). N Engl J Med 1978;298:540.

18. Center for Disease Control. 1985 standard treatment guidelines. MMWR 1985;34(Suppl):53.
19. Patamasucon P, Rettig PJ, Faust KL, et al. Oral v. topical erythromycin therapies for chlamydial conjunctivitis. Am J Dis Child 1982;136:817.
20. Fox KR, Golomb HS. Staphylococcal ophthalmia neonatorum and the staphylococcal scalded skin syndrome. Am J Ophthalmol 1979;88:1052.
21. Lossick JG. Prevention and management of neonatal gonorrhea. Sex Transm Dis 1979;6:192.
22. Friendly DS. Gonorrheal ophthalmia, reappearance of an old problem. Transactions of the American Academy of Ophthalmology and Otolaryngology 1970;74:975.
23. Handsfield HH, Hodson WA, Holmes KK. Neonatal gonococcal infection: orogastric contamination with Neisseria gonorrhoeae. JAMA 1973;225:697.
24. Rothenberg R. Ophthalmia neonatorum due to Neisseria gonorrhoeae: prevention and treatment. Sex Transm Dis 1979;6:187.
25. Hammerschlag MR, Chandler JW, Alexander ER, et al. Erythromycin ointment for ocular prophylaxis of neonatal chlamydial infection. JAMA 1980;244:2291.
26. American Academy of Pediatrics Committee on Drugs, Committee on Fetus and Newborn and Committee on Infectious Diseases. Prophylaxis and treatment of neonatal gonococcal infections. Pediatrics 1980;65:1047.
27. National Society to Prevent Blindness Committee on Ophthalmia Neonatorum. Prevention and treatment of ophthalmia neonatorum, September, 1981. New York: National Society to Prevent Blindness, 1981.
28. Nahmias AJ, Alford CA, Korones SB. Infection of the newborn with herpes virus hominis. Adv Pediatr 1970;17:185.
29. Whitley RJ, Nahmias AJ, Soong SJ, et al. Vidarabine therapy of neonatal herpes simplex virus infection. Pediatrics 1980;66:495.
30. Nahmias AJ, Hagler WS. Ocular manifestations of herpes simplex in the newborn (neonatal ocular herpes). Int Ophthalmol Clin 1972;12:191.
31. Tarkkanen A, Laatikainen L. Late ocular manifestations in neonatal herpes simplex infection. Br J Ophthalmol 1977;61:608.
32. Kibrick S. Herpes simplex infection at term: what to do with mother, newborn, and nursery personnel. JAMA 1980;243:157.
33. Petersen RA, Robb RM. The natural course of congenital obstruction of the nasolacrimal duct. J Pediatr Ophthalmol Strabismus 1978;15:246.
34. Scheie HG, Albert DM. Adler's textbook of ophthalmology. 8th ed. Philadelphia: WB Saunders, 1969:123.
35. Merin S, Crawford JS. The etiology of congenital cataracts. Can J Ophthalmol 1971;6:178.
36. McCormick AQ. Transient cataracts in premature infants: a new clinical entity. Can J Ophthalmol 1968;3:202.
37. Alden ER, Kalina RE, Hodson A. Transient cataracts in low-birth-weight infants. J Pediatr 1973;82:314.
38. Wiesel TN, Hubel DH. Effects of visual deprivation on morphology and physiology of cells in the cat's lateral geniculate body. J Neurophysiol 1963;26:978.
39. Wiesel TM, Hubel DH. Single-cell responses in striate cortex of kittens deprived of vision in one eye. J Neurophysiol 1963;26:1003.
40. Beller RA, Hoyt CS, Marg E, et al. Good visual function after neonatal surgery for congenital monocular cataracts. Am J Ophthalmol 1981;91:559.
41. Merin S, Morin D. Heredity of congenital glaucoma. Br J Ophthalmol 1972;56:414.
42. Shaffer RN, Weiss DI. Congenital and pediatric glaucomas. St. Louis: CV Mosby, 1970.
43. Sugar HS, Airala MA. Birth injuries of the cornea. J Pediatr Ophthalmol 1971;8:26.
44. Terry TL. Extreme prematurity and fibroblastic overgrowth of persistent vascular sheath behind each crystalline lens: I. Preliminary report. Am J Ophthalmol 1942;25:203.
45. Heath P. Pathology of the retinopathy of prematurity; retrolental fibroplasia. Am J Ophthalmol 1951;34:1249.
46. Patz A, Hoeck LE, DeLaCruz E. Studies on the effect of high oxygen administration in retrolental fibroplasia: I. Nursery observations. Am J Ophthalmol 1952;35:1248.
47. Lanman JT, Guy LP, Dancis J. Retrolental fibroplasia and oxygen therapy. JAMA 1954;155:223.
48. Kinsey VE, Hemphill FM. Etiology of retrolental fibroplasia, and preliminary report of a cooperative study of retrolental fibroplasia. Transactions of the American Academy of Ophthalmology and Otolaryngology 1955;59:15.
49. Avery ME, Oppenheimer EH. Recent increase in mortality from hyaline membrane disease. J Pediatr 1960;57:553.
50. McDonald AD. Cerebral palsy in children of very low birth weight. Arch Dis Child 1963;38:579.
51. Aranda JV, Saheb N, Stern L, et al. Arterial oxygen tension and retinal vasoconstriction in newborn infants. Am J Dis Child 1971;122:189.
52. Silverman WA. Prematurity and retrolental fibroplasia. Sight Sav Rev 1969;39:42.
53. Tasman W. Vitreoretinal changes in cicatricial retrolental fibroplasia. Trans Am Ophthalmol Soc 1970;68:548.
54. Phelps DL. Vision loss due to retinopathy of prematurity. Letter. Lancet 1981;1:606.
55. James LS, Lanman JT. History of oxygen therapy and retrolental fibroplasia. Pediatrics 1976;57(Suppl):591.
56. Silverman WA, Flynn RT, eds. Retinopathy of prematurity. Boston: Blackwell Scientific Publications, 1986.
57. McPherson AR, Hittner HM, Kretzer FL, eds. Retinopathy of prematurity: current concepts and controversies. Burlington, Ontario: BC Decker, 1986.
58. Ashton N, Ward B, Serpel G. Role of oxygen in the genesis of retrolental fibroplasia: preliminary report. Br J Ophthalmol 1953;37:513.
59. Ashton N, Ward B, Serpell G. Effect of oxygen on developing retinal vessels with particular reference to the problem of retrolental fibroplasia. Br J Ophthalmol 1954;38:397.
60. Ashton N, Pedler C. Studies on developing retinal vessels: IX. Reaction of endothelial cells to oxygen. Br J Ophthalmol 1962;46:257.
61. Ashton N, Garner A, Knight G. Intermittent oxygen in retrolental fibroplasia. Am J Ophthalmol 1971;71:153.
62. Cogan D. Development and senescence of the human retinal vasculature. Transactions of the Ophthalmological Society of the United Kingdom 1963;83:465.
63. Karlsberg RC, Green R, Patz A. Congenital retrolental fibroplasia. Arch Ophthalmol 1973;89:122.
64. Glass PG, Avery GB, Siva Subramarian KN, et al. Effect of bright light in the hospital nursery on the incidence of retinopathy of prematurity. N Engl J Med 1985;313:401.
65. Flynn JT, O'Grady GF, Herrera J, et al. Retrolental fibroplasia: I. Clinical observations. Arch Ophthalmol 1977;95:217.
66. Committee members. An international classification of retinopathy of prematurity. Pediatrics 1984;74:127.
67. Reese AB, King MJ, Owens WC. A classification of retrolental fibroplasia. Am J Ophthalmol 1953;36:1333.
68. Cantolino SJ, O'Grady GE, Herrera JA, et al. Ophthalmoscopic monitoring of oxygen therapy in premature infants. Am J Ophthalmol 1971;72:322.
69. Kalina R, Hodson WA, Morgan BC. Retrolental fibroplasia in a cyanotic infant. Pediatrics 1972;50:765.

70. Multicenter trial of cryotherapy for retinopathy of prematurity: preliminary results. Arch Ophthalmol 1988;106:471.
71. Ellsworth R. Tumors of the retina. In: Tasman W, ed. Retinal diseases of children. New York: Harper & Row, 1971:000.
72. Knudson AG, Hethcote HW, Brown BW. Mutation and childhood cancer: a probabilistic model for the incidence of retinoblastoma. Proc Natl Acad Sci USA 1975;72:5116.
73. Knudson AG, Meadows AT, Nichols WW, et al. Chromosomal deletion and retinoblastoma. N Engl J Med 1976;295:1120.
74. Abramson DH, Ellsworth RM, Zimmerman LE. Nonocular cancer in retinoblastoma survivors. Transactions of the American Academy of Ophthalmology and Otolaryngology 1976; 81:454.
75. Roarty JD, McLean IW, Zimmerman LE. Incidence of second neoplasms in patients with bilateral retinoblastoma. Ophthalmology 1988;95:1583.
76. Burde RM. Esterase D and hereditary retinoblastoma. Am J Ophthalmol 1984;97:779.
77. Miller RW, Fraumeni JF Jr, Manning MD. Association of Wilms' tumor and aniridia, hemihypertrophy and other congenital malformations. N Engl J Med 1964;270:922.
78. Fraumeni JF Jr, Glass AG. Wilms' tumor and congenital aniridia. JAMA 1968;206:825.
79. Riccardi VM, Sujansky E, Smith AC, et al. Chromosomal imbalance in the aniridia-Wilms' tumor association: 11p interstitial deletion. Pediatrics 1978;61:604.
80. Desmonts G, Couvreur J. Congenital toxoplasmosis: a prospective study of 378 pregnancies. N Engl J Med 1974;290: 1110.
81. Eichenwald HF, Shinefeld HR. Viral infections of the fetus and of the premature and newborn infant. Adv Pediatr 1962;12:249.
82. Weller TH, Hanshaw JB. Virologic and clinical observations on cytomegalic inclusion disease. N Engl J Med 1962;266:1233.
83. Lonn LI. Neonatal cytomegalic inclusion disease chorioretinitis. Arch Ophthalmol 1972;88:434.
84. Gregg NM. Congenital cataract following German measles in the mother. Transactions of the Ophthalmological Society of Australia 1941;3:35.
85. Boniuk V, Boniuk M. The incidence of phthisis bulbi as a complication of cataract surgery in the congenital rubella syndrome. Int Ophthalmol Clin 1972;12:000.
86. Cremer RJ, Perryman PW, Richards DH. Influence of light on the hyperbilirubinemia of infants. Lancet 1958;1:1094.
87. Noell WK, Walker VS, Kang BS, et al. Retinal damage by light in rats. Invest Ophthalmol 1966;5:450.
88. Kuwabara T, Gorn RA. Retinal damage by visible light, an electron microscopic study. Arch Ophthalmol 1968;79:69.
89. Sisson TRC, Glauser SC, Glauser EM, et al. Retinal changes produced by phototherapy. J Pediatr 1970;77:221.
90. Kalina RE, Forrest GL. Ocular hazards of phototherapy for hyperbilirubinemia. J Pediatr Ophthalmol 1971;8:116.
91. Hubel DH, Wiesel TN. The period of susceptibility to the physiological effects of unilateral eye closure in kittens. J Physiol 1970;206:419.

Neonatology: Pathophysiology and Management of the Newborn, Fourth Edition,
edited by Gordon B. Avery, Mary Ann Fletcher, and Mhairi G. MacDonald.
J.B. Lippincott Company, Philadelphia © 1994.

chapter 54

Neoplasia

ROBERT J. ARCECI
HOWARD J. WEINSTEIN

Although neoplasia in infancy is quite rare, it presents important and unique biologic, diagnostic, and therapeutic problems. Such neoplasms show peculiarities that distinguish them from those occurring later. Many tumors in early life are composed of persistent embryonal or fetal tissues, suggesting a failure of proper maturation or cytodifferentiation during intrauterine or postnatal life. Indeed, the failure of proper maturation of fetal tissue may be difficult to distinguish from neoplasia. In addition, an unexpectedly large number of neoplasms of early life are associated with growth disturbances and congenital anomalies. Spontaneous regression and cytodifferentiation also occur most frequently in tumors of early life. Finally, the unique physiology of the still-developing neonate provides the clinician with special problems in terms of therapeutic interventions and their long-term sequelae.

EPIDEMIOLOGY

From the data in The Third National Cancer Survey (1969–1971), Bader and Miller reported that in the United States the annual incidence of malignant neoplasms in infants younger than 1 year of age was 183.4 per 1 million live births and within the first 28 days of life was 36.5 per 1 million live births.[1] They further estimated that approximately 653 infants a year in the United States are diagnosed with cancer and that about 130 (20%) of these patients are neonates. Approximately one-half of the neonatal malignancies are noted on the first day of life.

When incidence for all malignancies is compared with mortality as determined from death certificates, the incidence in patients younger than 1 year is 3.5 times greater than mortality, whereas the incidence in patients younger than 29 days old is 4.8 times greater than mortality.[1,2] These figures offer an interesting comparison to those reported in children up to 15 years of age, among whom the incidence of malignancy is only about 1.3 to 1.8 times greater than mortality. When individual diseases are considered, there are marked differences in incidence versus mortality. For example, in neonates, the incidence of neuroblastoma is 10 times greater than the mortality, whereas the incidence of leukemia is only 1.8 times the mortality.

The distribution of the types of malignancies found in infants younger than 1 year of age differs from that found in later childhood. In infants younger than 1 year of age, neuroblastoma is the most common malignancy and accounts for about 50% of malignancies in the neonatal period; it is followed by leukemia, renal tumors, sarcomas, central nervous system (CNS) tumors, and hepatic malignancy. In older children younger than 15 years of age, leukemia is the most common malignancy (about 30%), followed by CNS tumors, lymphoma, neuroblastoma, sarcoma, and renal tumors.

GROWTH DISTURBANCES, GENETIC ABERRATIONS, AND CANCER PATHOGENESIS

Primary, inherited, cytogenetic syndromes usually occur as a result of chromosomal aneuploidy, deletions, translocations, or increased fragility that represent the end result of germline chromosomal defects. An example of aneuploidy is Down syndrome (*i.e.*, trisomy 21), in which the frequency of acute leukemia is approximately 15 times the normal. Deletion of part of the long arm of chromosome 13 is associated with psychomotor retardation, microcephaly, cardiac and skeletal defects, and the early development of retinoblastoma. The deletion of the short arm of chromosome 11 results in mental retardation, microcephaly, aniridia, ear and genital anomalies, and an increased incidence of Wilms tumor (*i.e.*, aniridia–Wilms tumor syndrome). These syndromes provided support for the assignment of a retinoblastoma locus to chromosome 13q14 and a Wilms tumor locus to 11p14. These mutant alleles (*i.e.*, loci) are heterozygous in constitutional cells and homozygous in retinoblastoma and Wilms tumor cells. The actual development of the tumor appears to require that the mutant alleles on both chromosomes be affected. Homozygosity for the "Wilms tumor locus" has been found in embryonal rhabdomyosarcomas and hepatoblastomas, suggesting a common pathogenesis for these embryonal tumors.[3] The specific loss of constitutional heterozygosity and its relationship to oncogenesis has been confirmed in studies of transgenic mice that lack a functional tumor suppressor gene, *p53;* these animals are predisposed to development of malignancies early in life.[4]

Bloom syndrome, Fanconi syndrome, and ataxia–telangiectasia are disorders characterized by increased chromosomal fragility. All three appear to be autosomal recessive in inheritance, involving abnormal amounts or function of various DNA repair enzymes. Each syndrome is, in addition, associated with an increased incidence of various malignancies.

Malformation syndromes without obvious cytogenetic abnormalities include hemihypertrophy and Beckwith–Wiedemann syndrome, which consists of mental retardation, gigantism, macroglossia, omphalocele, and organomegaly; both of these disorders are associated with the development of Wilms tumor, hepatoblastoma, and adrenocortical carcinoma. Sacrococcygeal teratomas and teratocarcinomas are associated with anomalies of the lower spine and urogenital region.

Hamartomas are benign proliferations of cells in their normal anatomic location. Hamartomas in which malignant neoplasms arise include congenital melanotic nevi, which can progress to melanoma, and familial polyposis, which may evolve into colonic carcinoma. Finally, examples of malignancies developing from persistent fetal rests include craniopharyngioma arising from tissue derived embryologically from the Rathke pouch, and persistent neuroblastic cellularity leading to adrenal neuroblastoma.

Such predisposing conditions share at least one common element: an inherited or developmental disturbance of cellular growth.

EXPOSURE TO MATERNAL MALIGNANCY

In addition to the susceptibility of the fetus to adverse effects of chemotherapy during pregnancy, there also is the possibility that the maternal cancer will metastasize to the placenta and fetus. Although many anecdotal reports have documented such involvement, it occurs only very rarely. The types of tumors shown to be transmitted from the mother to the placenta or fetus are quite varied, with melanoma most commonly cited.[5] Although lymphoma and leukemia may involve the placenta, they have not been found transmitted to the fetus.

GENES, NEOPLASIA, AND TERATOGENESIS

Viruses, particularly the RNA retroviruses, contain genes responsible for transforming cells to a malignant phenotype.[6,7] Such genetic sequences have been termed viral oncogenes. Naturally occurring DNA sequences homologous to these viral oncogenes exist in normal, untransformed cells of all metazoa along the evolutionary ladder. Such DNA sequences are called cellular oncogenes and are used in normal cells during growth, development, and differentiation in precise temporal and tissue-specific patterns.[8–10] Some of their products function as potent growth regulators. The protein products of some cellular oncogenes are quite similar to the products from the homologous viral oncogenes.

Because of their expression during normal development, inherited or acquired mutations affecting cellular oncogene expression might lead to a variety of developmental abnormalities and congenital defects, such as hemihypertrophy syndromes and hamartomas. In addition, the persistent expression beyond birth of certain growth-related oncogenes may play a role in such proliferative states as the transient myeloproliferative disorder associated with Down syndrome and the so called stage IV-S neuroblastoma found in infants, with both conditions characterized by subsequent regression. In addition, recessive oncogenes or tumor suppressor genes are normal constituents of the genome that appear to be involved in regulating cell division and differentiation.[8–12] When the function of both alleles encoding a tumor suppressor gene is disrupted by mutation with loss of heterozygosity, the control over normal cell division is lost and tumorigenesis may ensue.[13,14] Examples of such genes include the Wilms tumor gene (*wt1*), the retinoblastoma gene (*rb*), and *p53*, which appears to be the most frequently mutated gene in human malignancies.[13,14] The finding of these genes defines a molecular link between conditions of abnormal development (*i.e.*, teratogenesis) and neoplastic transformation.[7,11,12]

TUMORS OF NEUROEPITHELIAL ORIGIN

Neuroectodermal cells of the neural tube differentiate to neuroblasts, which become nervous system tissue and melanocytes; free spongioblasts, which become either astrocytes or oligodendroglia cells; and ependymal spongioblasts, which become ependymal cells. These primitive neuroectodermal cells may be the target for neoplasia, giving rise to a group of morphologically similar tumors in central and peripheral sites of the nervous system. Neonatal tumors originating from neuroectodermal cells include neuroblastoma, retinoblastoma, peripheral nerve tumors (*i.e.*, neuroepithelioma), medulloblastoma, choroid plexus papilloma, ependymoblastoma, and melanotic neuroectodermal tumors. These tumors show varying degrees of cellular differentiation, have similar histologic features (*e.g.*, small, primitive cells with rosettes or pseudorosettes), and tend to spread along cerebrospinal fluid pathways.

NEUROBLASTOMA

Neuroblastoma is the most common malignant tumor in neonates. It originates from neural crest cells that normally give rise to the adrenal medulla and sympathetic ganglia. Its reported occurrence in siblings and other family members suggests that some cases are hereditary.[15] An interesting syndrome has been reported in several women who delivered infants diagnosed as having neuroblastoma during the first few months of life.[16] The mothers had sweating, pallor, headaches, palpitations, hypertension, and tingling in their hands and feet during the last trimester of pregnancy. The authors of that study postulated that this symptom complex is caused by the introduction of fetal tumor catecholamines into the maternal circulation.

Neuroblastoma may present as a tumor mass anywhere that sympathetic neural tissue normally occurs.[17] Most tumors arise in the adrenal medulla or retroperitoneal sympathetic ganglia. An abdominal sonogram or computed tomography (CT) scan would demonstrate displacement of the kidney without distortion of the calyceal system. The neoplasm also may originate in the posterior mediastinum, neck, or pelvis. Cervical sympathetic ganglion involvement in the neck may result in Horner syndrome; posterior mediastinal tumors may cause respiratory distress; paravertebral tumors tend to grow through the intervertebral foramina and cause symptoms of spinal cord compression; and presacral neuroblastomas may mimic presacral teratomas. Neuroblastoma also has been detected prenatally by ultrasonography, showing a solid and sometimes cystic suprarenal mass.[18,19]

Two unusual presentations of neuroblastoma are intractable diarrhea secondary to release of vasoactive intestinal peptide; and the syndrome of opsoclonus, myoclonus, and truncal ataxia,[20,21] the etiology of which remains an enigma. The diarrhea secondary to vasoactive intestinal peptide abates after removal of the neuroblastoma. In contrast is the unpredictable improvement after the removal or treatment of neuroblastoma associated with opsoclonus–myoclonus. Nevertheless, survival for children with this syndrome is excellent.

Metastatic lesions are common presenting findings of neuroblastoma, especially in the neonate.[22] The primary tumor often cannot be found in infants younger than 6 months of age. These infants present with bluish subcutaneous nodules and extensive hepatomegaly. The liver may be studded with tumor nodules and be so large that it causes respiratory distress secondary to abdominal distention. Clumps of tumor cells often are found in the bone marrow aspirates. Metastases to bones, skull, and orbit, which present as periorbital ecchymoses, are rare in the neonate. The unique metastatic pattern to liver, bone marrow, and skin in infants is classified as stage IV-S neuroblastoma.[23]

The differential diagnosis for neuroblastoma is limited. The subcutaneous nodules appear similar to those found in congenital leukemia cutis and several congenital infections. The leukoerythroblastosis secondary to bone marrow metastases from neuroblastoma also is observed with congenital infection, severe hemolytic disease, and leukemia. Over 90% of children with neuroblastoma will have elevated urinary excretion of catecholamine metabolites, vanillylmandelic acid (VMA) or homovanillic acid (HVA), or both.[24] The diagnosis of neuroblastoma is made by biopsy of the primary tumor or metastatic lesions. The most histologically primitive lesion is neuroblastoma without differentiation and is composed of small, round cells with scant cytoplasm. The ganglioneuroma, its benign counterpart, is composed of large, mature ganglion cells. The ganglioneuroblastoma is intermediate in its degree of cellular differentiation. In the absence of a tissue specimen, the findings of elevated urinary catecholamines and tumor pseudorosettes in a bone marrow specimen usually are sufficient to make a definitive diagnosis.

The prognosis for children with neuroblastoma is inversely correlated to the age of the child at diagnosis. The infant with stage IV-S disease has a better chance of survival than does the older child with less advanced disease.[17] Evans and coworkers proposed a clinical staging system for children with neuroblastoma that is prognostically useful[23]:

Stage I: tumor limited to the organ of involvement
Stage II: regional tumor spread that does not cross

the midline; includes many of the posterovertebral primaries

Stage III: tumors that extend and infiltrate across the midline

Stage IV: distant metastases to lymph nodes, bone, bone marrow, etc.

Stage IV-S: stage I or stage II primary tumor with distant metastases involving liver, skin, or bone marrow but not bone; usually observed in infants under the age of 1 year.

Infants with stage IV-S have had spontaneous regression of disease, and in other patients malignant neuroblastomas apparently have undergone maturation into mature ganglioneuromas.[25] The incidence of spontaneous regression of neuroblastoma may be more common than is clinically evident. Primitive sympathetic neuroblasts, which are derived from neural crest ectoderm, migrate in early embryonic life into the adrenal primordium, where they arrange themselves in nodules before differentiation into adrenomedullary tissue. These nodules are present in all fetal adrenal glands at 14 to 18 weeks of gestation.[26] Beckwith and Perrin detected the presence of microscopic clusters of neuroblastoma cells (*i.e.*, neuroblastoma *in situ*) in the adrenal glands in a number of autopsies from infants younger than age 3 months who had no clinical evidence of tumor.[27] They estimated that neuroblastoma *in situ* occurs in 1 of 250 stillborn infants and infants younger than 3 months of age. Clinically detectable neuroblastoma is noted in only 1 of 10,000 live births.

These observations raise the interesting question as to whether stage IV-S neuroblastoma is not a true malignancy. If stage IV-S neuroblastoma is a classic malignant neoplasm, it should be clonally derived. One such example of clonality in stage IV-S neuroblastoma tumor specimens has been demonstrated by cytogenetic analysis. Although no consistent and specific chromosomal alteration has been found in all stage IV-S specimens, there are increasing numbers of examples of cytogenetic clonality. In addition, it is becoming clear that stage IV-S neuroblastoma, unlike tumors representing stages I to IV, usually are hyperdiploid and lack the 1p deletion and double minute chromosomes (*i.e.*, N-*myc* amplification).[28*] The reason for spontaneous regression of stage IV-S disease remains a mystery.

Complete surgical removal of neuroblastoma usually is accomplished in infants with stage I or II disease. Postoperative treatment generally is not indicated for these patients, and their long-term survival is excellent.[29] It has been suggested that the infant with the special pattern of metastases (*i.e.*, stage IV-S) be observed for a period of weeks to months before treatment is initiated because of the reasonable likelihood of spontaneous regression.[30] If disease progresses, combination chemotherapy should be initiated. Respiratory difficulties and vascular compression because of hepatomegaly develop in some infants with massive hepatic involvement. Small doses of radiation therapy or cyclophosphamide usually will cause enough tumor regression to relieve these symptoms. For infants with stage III disease in whom gross residual tumor remains after surgery, postoperative chemotherapy or radiotherapy or both are indicated. Chemotherapy is the treatment of choice for infants with stage IV disease.[31] The active chemotherapeutic agents against neuroblastoma include alkylating compounds (*e.g.*, *cis*-platinum, cyclophosphamide, dacarbazine, nitrogen mustard), vincristine, and doxorubicin. Combinations of several of these agents administered for 6 months to 1 year have resulted in greater than 50% long-term survival for children younger than 1 year of age with stage IV neuroblastoma. This is in contrast to the dismal prognosis for similarly staged children who are older than 1 year of age at diagnosis and in whom bone marrow transplantation trials are being tried.

* Fletcher J, personal communication, September 1992.

RETINOBLASTOMA

Retinoblastoma is a congenital malignant tumor arising from the nuclear layer of the retina. Although an extremely rare tumor, it is the most common ocular tumor of childhood. The median age at presentation is 18 months, or 14 months for bilateral cases, but a small percentage of infants are diagnosed during the first few months of life.[32]

Approximately 10% of children with retinoblastoma have a family history of the disease. Approximately 30% with bilateral or multifocal unilateral tumors have a negative family history.[33,34] These two groups are capable of transmitting the disease to their offspring in an autosomal dominant fashion. This hereditary tendency is governed by a genetic locus on the long arm of chromosome 13 (*i.e.*, band 13q14). If there is a family history of retinoblastoma, an experienced ophthalmologist should examine the eyes of unaffected future siblings regularly while they are under general anesthesia to detect cases early.

The most common initial sign of retinoblastoma is an abnormal white pupil (*i.e.*, leukocoria), known as a cat's-eye reflex. The second most common presenting sign is a squint, or strabismus. A clinical picture resembling retinoblastoma may result from granulomatosis uveitis, congenital defects, and severe retrolental fibroplasia.

Once the diagnosis of retinoblastoma is suspected, both eyes should be examined with the infant under general anesthesia. A bone marrow aspiration and spinal tap for malignant cells should be performed for staging. A staging system for retinoblastoma is based on the size, location, number of tumors in each eye, and distant hematogenous metastases. Vitreous seeding, tumors extending anteriorly to the ora serrata, tumors invading over one-half of the retina, residual orbital disease, and optic nerve or distant metastases are adverse prognostic features.

Retinoblastoma usually is curable when diagnosed early; vision often need not be sacrificed even when bilateral disease is present. Radiotherapy always should be considered if the eye has a chance for useful vision. It usually is the infant diagnosed early with a positive family history who is an appropriate candidate for radiation. Patients with adverse prognosis features should have prompt enucleation. Chemotherapy is recommended only for children with very advanced local or metastatic disease.[32]

BRAIN TUMORS AND OTHER NEUROECTODERMAL TUMORS

Intracranial tumors presenting in the first year of life are uncommon. In a review from the Hospital for Sick Children in London,[35] 107 of 1296 children with brain tumors had symptoms before the age of 1 year; 17 were symptomatic within 2 months of birth. Brain tumors in this age group tend to be supratentorial, in contrast to those in older children, which tend to be infratentorial. In infants the most common presenting symptom is macrocrania with a bulging fontanelle secondary either to hydrocephalus or tumor volume. Seizures, vomiting, abnormal eye movement, and irritability also are frequent. Most brain tumors reported in neonates are teratomas.[36] The histologic diagnoses of the neuroectodermal tumors are similar to those of tumors in later childhood, with gliomas accounting for most. There is, however, a high frequency of choroid plexus papillomas in this age group.[37] An association of choroid plexus papillomas and the presence of SV40 viral DNA has been reported.[38]

Treatment has included surgical removal or biopsy and radiotherapy. Operative mortality has been high, and few infants have survived for longer than 1 year. In these few, brain radiotherapy has resulted in severe intellectual and psychomotor retardation. Combined surgical and experimental preradiation chemotherapeutic approaches are being evaluated.[39]

Primitive neuroectodermal tumors of peripheral nerve represent a group of soft tissue tumors known as neuroepitheliomas, medulloepitheliomas, and peripheral neuroblastomas.[40,41] They are associated with major branches of peripheral nerves (*i.e.*, tumor of the chest wall arising from intercostal nerve). These are extremely rare tumors but quite aggressive in their biologic behavior, with frequently occurring distant metastases, including to the CNS. Treatment approaches include wide excision, if possible, and chemotherapy modeled after either neuroblastoma or brain tumor protocols.

The melanotic neuroectodermal tumor of infancy has its origin in the neural crest population. Most of these tumors are diagnosed between 1 and 8 months of age and occur in the maxilla.[42] They are considered a benign neoplasm, with a local recurrence rate of about 15%. These tumors originate from pluripotential neural crest cells that give rise to both melanoblasts and neuroblasts. The rate of malignancy for this tumor is reported to be approximately 5%. Recommended treatment is wide local excision.

CONGENITAL LEUKEMIA

Leukemia in the newborn is extremely rare.[43,44] It has been customary to categorize leukemia as congenital when it is diagnosed within a few days after birth and as neonatal when it manifests itself during the first 4 to 6 weeks of life. The kinetics of leukemic cell growth and the estimated leukemic cell burden at the time of diagnosis make it reasonable to assume that clinically detectable leukemia during the first 4 weeks of life originated *in utero*. In the following discussion, congenital leukemia is considered as leukemia diagnosed from birth to 4 weeks of age.

The etiology and pathogenesis of congenital leukemia, as well as other leukemias, are unknown. The strongest evidence for a genetic predisposition to acute leukemia is its occurrence in identical twins.[45] If leukemia develops in one of identical twins before 6 years of age, the risk of disease in the other twin is 20%. Leukemia usually develops in a co-twin within months of the first case. For fraternal twins and siblings, the risk of development of leukemia is two and four times higher, respectively, than in the general population. Congenital leukemia has been associated with trisomy 9, trisomy 13, Turner syndrome, and Down syndrome.[46–49]

Over 95% of the childhood leukemias, including congenital leukemia, are classified as acute because they are characterized by a predominance of immature myeloid or lymphoid precursors. In children, the proportion of cases of acute lymphoblastic leukemia (ALL) to acute myelogenous leukemia (AML) is approximately 4:1, but this ratio is reversed in the congenital leukemias.[43] Most children with ALL have neither cell surface immunoglobulin nor T-cell–associated surface antigens that would clearly identify the disease as having B-cell or T-cell lineage.[50,51] Whereas lymphoblasts from most children with ALL express the common acute lymphoblastic leukemia antigen (CALLA) on the cell surface and also express markers of early B-cell differentiation (*e.g.*, cytoplasmic immunoglobulin, or Ig gene rearrangement), the lymphoblasts of congenital and infant ALL often are pre-B but CALLA-negative.[52,53] These infants have a higher incidence of CNS leukemia at diagnosis, a higher leukocyte count, increased frequency of hepatosplenomegaly, and a poorer prognosis than older children with ALL. A translocation involving the long arms of chromosomes 4 and 11, t(4;11), also has been associated with ALL presenting during infancy.[54]

The most common subtype of AML in the neonate is acute monocytic leukemia, which accounts for only 20% of AML in older children.[55] It is associated with a high incidence of extramedullary leukemia, especially in the CNS. Structural abnormalities of the long arm of chromosome 11 have been closely linked to this subtype of AML.[56]

Cutaneous manifestations are the most frequent clinical findings noted at birth. In addition to petechiae and purpura, leukemic skin nodules (*i.e.*, leukemia cutis) have been observed in approximately 50% of cases.[57] These skin nodules may vary in size from a few millimeters to a few centimeters, are bluish to slate gray in color, may appear in all sites, and are palpated as fibromalike tumors of the deep skin (Fig. 54-1). Neonatal leukemia cutis may undergo a spontaneous, temporary regression, but tends to recur in a more generalized form within a few weeks to months.[55] Transient spontaneous hematologic remissions are rare in the congenital leukemias.[58]

Hepatosplenomegaly is common, but lymphadenopathy is not. Respiratory distress, secondary to leukostasis within the pulmonary vasculature, may complicate the clinical course. Other nonspecific symptoms of neonatal leukemia include lethargy, pallor, poor feeding, and umbilical, gastrointestinal, or genitourinary bleeding.

In Pierce's report of congenital leukemia,[43] the mean hemoglobin concentration at birth was normal, with a wide range of values (7–20 g/dL); the mean leukocyte counts were 150,000/mm^3 (range, 2000–850,000); and mean platelet counts were 70,000/mm^3 (range, 6000–300,000). The diagnosis of leukemia is confirmed by examination of a bone marrow aspirate obtained from the posterior iliac crest.

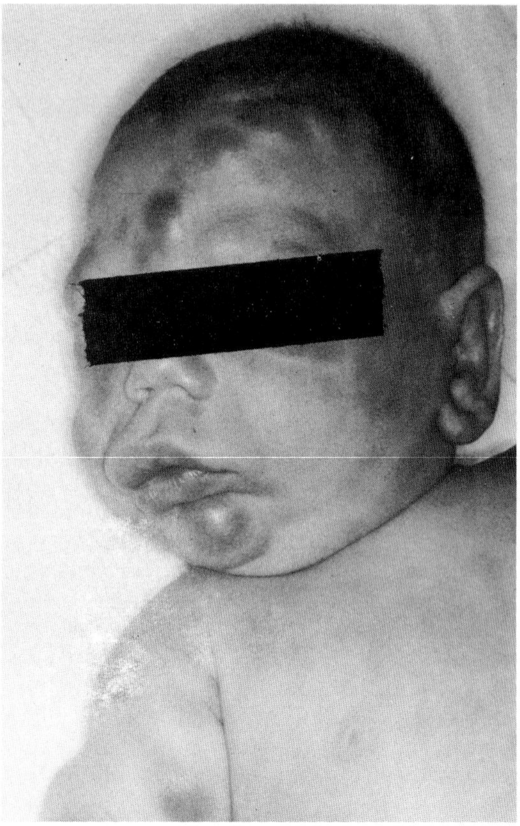

FIG. 54–1. Congenital acute monocytic leukemia with skin nodules.

A variety of disorders in the newborn imitate leukemia. The newborn bone marrow response to infection, hypoxemia, or severe hemolysis commonly is a leukemoid reaction and an increase in circulating nucleated erythrocytes. This frequently has been confused with congenital leukemia.

An enigmatic myeloproliferative disorder described as transient acute leukemia, or ineffective regulation of granulopoiesis masquerading as congenital leukemia, has been reported in infants with Down syndrome.[46,59] This syndrome, noted during the first few days of life, mimics AML. Peripheral leukocyte counts can range from 25,000 to several hundred thousand; bone marrow aspirates reveal 30% to 70% blasts. Hepatosplenomegaly and thrombocytopenia also are common findings. The hematologic status of these neonates returns to normal in 1 to 4 months with only supportive therapy. Several of these children who subsequently died of cardiac or pulmonary disease years after the resolution of their transient myeloproliferative syndrome showed no evidence of leukemia at autopsy. There are a few case reports in which a fatal leukemia developed after spontaneous regression of this myeloproliferative syndrome. This syndrome has been observed both in neonates with stigmata of Down syndrome and in phenotypically normal infants who have trisomy 21 mosaicism in their hematopoietic cells or skin fibroblasts.[60]

An infant with Down syndrome has an equal likelihood of having either a transient myeloproliferative syndrome or congenital leukemia.[46] Although time is still the most definitive indicator of transiency, serial cytogenetic studies may be of value. If there is a chromosome marker in addition to trisomy 21 in spontaneously dividing bone marrow cells, a true leukemic clone is more likely.

Congenital ALL is fatal if untreated and should be managed with chemotherapy programs used in treating childhood ALL. Cranial irradiation should not be used as part of CNS prophylaxis because of the severe morbidity associated with radiation to the developing brain; intrathecal chemotherapy should be used instead. Age has been an important prognostic variable in childhood ALL, with the most favorable prognosis for patients between 2 and 9 years of age. Prognosis for young infants with ALL remains poor.[53]

Because untreated congenital AML also is fatal, aggressive combination chemotherapy in an institution with maximal supportive services is mandatory. One report has described the successful treatment of several neonates with acute monocytic leukemia with either VP-16 or VM-26, but this experience has not been confirmed.[55] Aggressive AML treatment regimens have met with some success in achieving long remissions in neonates with AML.[61]

NEOPLASMS OF THE KIDNEY

MESOBLASTIC NEPHROMA

Most abdominal masses presenting in infancy are renal in origin, and most of these can be accounted for by cystic disease and congenital malformations of the urinary tract leading to hydronephrosis. Although neoplasms of the kidney are rare in infancy, that they do occur and have important prognostic implications makes it mandatory that they be included in the evaluation of abdominal masses.

The most common renal tumor found in infants is the mesoblastic nephroma,[62] also called fetal renal hamartoma, mesenchymal hamartoma of infancy, and leiomyomatous hamartoma. Mesoblastic nephroma commonly presents as an asymptomatic, enlarging abdominal mass during the first few months of life. It is not associated with congenital anomalies and has no race predilection. Of note is the more frequent occurrence of polyhydramnios and premature labor in women whose infants have mesoblastic nephroma.[63] The differential diagnosis includes renal cystic disease, congenital malformations of the urinary tract resulting in hydronephrosis, and Wilms tumor.

Most patients with mesoblastic nephroma are cured by surgical excision without adjuvant chemotherapy or radiotherapy.[64] The addition of chemotherapy has resulted in increased morbidity and, in some instances, fatal complications. In rare cases, such as older infants presenting with metastatic disease or when there is tumor rupture and spillage, chemotherapeutic intervention with regimens containing actinomycin D, vincristine, cyclophosphamide, and doxorubicin have been effectively used. Similar regimens have been used in the rare recurrences.[65–68] Radiotherapy also has shown efficacy in patients with local recurrence.

PERSISTENT RENAL BLASTEMA, NEPHROBLASTOMATOSIS, AND WILMS TUMOR

The adult or metanephric kidney arises from a complex, inductive interaction between the evaginating uteric bud and its bifurcations with the metanephric, mesodermally derived blastema. By 36 weeks of gestation, normal nephrogenesis is complete with no residual metanephric blastema. When these metanephric blastemal elements persist, they usually are characterized by microscopic clusters of primitive blastema and occasionally some tubular differentiation (*i.e.*, persistent metanephric blastema). If these fetal rests proliferate, they may develop along several different histologic pathways, each of which has particular relevance to the evolution of Wilms tumor.[65–67,69–71] Nephroblastomatosis represents the persistence and cellular expansion of metanephric blastema beyond the cessation of nephrogenesis. The proliferation may occur in characteristic patterns, either multifocal or diffuse.

Multifocal nephroblastomatosis refers to the widespread proliferation of blastemal cells, most prominently in the subcapsular cortex as well as along the penetrating columns of Bertin. Nephromegaly is not always evident. Unlike mesoblastic nephroma, multifocal nephroblastomatosis is associated with congenital malformation syndromes and chromosomal abnormalities.

Within the category of multifocal nephroblastomatosis there are several characteristic lesions. When persistent blastema proliferate in small 100- to 300-μm foci separated by normal renal parenchyma, they are referred to as nodular renal blastema. Nodular renal blastema may regress or evolve into what has been called sclerosing metanephric hamartoma as well as into Wilms tumorlets, which are 0.3 to 3.5 cm in diameter, noninfiltrating, often multiple, neoplastic tumors separated by normal renal parenchyma. They usually consist of blastema with a monomorphous epithelial pattern of differentiation. Although they resemble true Wilms tumor, they are distinguishable by their smaller size and their noninfiltrating behavior.

A second type of nephroblastomatosis, which is quite rare but found more commonly in infants and young children, is diffuse nephroblastomatosis. The blastemal proliferation may be pannephric or superficial, with the latter lesion encasing a normal cortex and medulla. Diffuse nephroblastomatosis presents as bilateral, palpable nephromegaly in association with congenital malformations. Radiographic examination by intravenous pyelogram reveals distortion and elongation of the pelvicalyceal system without obstruction. On gross inspection, there is an exaggerated pattern of fetal lobulation of the enlarged kidneys.

That these various histologic lesions are related to one another and to the evolution of frank Wilms tumor has been strongly suggested by case studies as well as by epidemiologic and pathologic correlations.[72–74] In about one third of cases of Wilms tumor, there is suggestive pathologic evidence for the association of nodular renal blastema, nephroblastomatosis, Wilms tumorlets, and Wilms tumor; in bilateral Wilms tumor, this association is nearly always present.[75]

Management of nephroblastomatosis involves surgery and sometimes chemotherapy, depending on the extent of disease. Radiation therapy is not very effective. If only one kidney is involved, surgical resection is sufficient, but exploration and biopsy of the contralateral kidney are critical. When both kidneys are extensively involved, nephroblastomatosis usually will respond to the combination chemotherapy used in Wilms tumor (*i.e.*, vincristine and actinomycin). The goal of such treatment is to cause regression of the nephroblastomatosis or cause its evolution to an end-stage hamartoma. The duration of treatment is based on clinical response. Close follow-up with both radiographic and second-look operations is important in that patients still may progress to the development of true Wilms tumor despite therapy.

True Wilms tumor rarely is seen in the neonatal period.[76] It generally presents as an asymptomatic abdominal mass that does not cross the midline but, occasionally, the mass is large enough to cause dystocia at the time of delivery. Rarely is it associated with gross hematuria, hypertension, or polycythemia secondary to increased erythropoietin levels. The most common congenital abnormalities associated with Wilms tumor are genitourinary and musculoskeletal anomalies, hemihypertrophy, aniridia, and hamartomas (*e.g.*, hemangiomas, nevi, café-au-lait spots). In addition, there is the Wilms tumor–aniridia syndrome with its associated deletion of part of the short arm of chromosome 11. Computed tomography, renal isotope scanning, and renal ultrasonography help define the extent of the tumor.

Pathologically, classic Wilms tumor consists of neoplastic blastemal elements with epithelial and stromal components. In the neonate, Wilms tumor is predominantly epithelial and localized, displaying little invasiveness or metastatic potential. The primary prognostic variables include histology, extent of disease, and age.[66,77,78]

The management of a patient with Wilms tumor depends primarily on staging. In the neonate, most patients will be classified as stage I in that the tumors usually are relatively small, localized, noninvasive, and resectable; show favorable histology; and appear to metastasize infrequently. At the time of surgery, a frozen section diagnosis is important in ascertaining whether or not nephroblastomatosis also is present. If it is present, wedge biopsy of the contralateral kidney is indicated, even if it is grossly normal. In cases of bilateral Wilms tumor, the more affected kidney is removed and the less involved kidney partially resected.

For all patients with stage I disease, the National Wilms' Tumor Study group has recommended 6 months of combination chemotherapy with vincristine and actinomycin; radiation therapy is not given. Disease-free, long-term survival has been greater than 90%. There is some indication, however, that in infants with localized, noninvasive, nonmetastatic, histologically favorable tumors weighing less than 550 g, reduced courses of chemotherapy or even no further therapy apart from radical nephrectomy is all that is required.[79,80] For advanced stages and for tumors with unfavorable histology, more aggressive therapy, including radiation and intensive chemotherapy, is used.

RENAL NEOPLASMS NOT ASSOCIATED WITH WILMS TUMOR

Malignant rhabdoid tumor of the kidney, which represents about 2% of primary renal malignancies in childhood and for which the mean age at diagnosis is 13 months, was first described as a rhabdomyosarcomatoid variant of Wilms tumor. Subsequent studies have suggested that this tumor is neuroepithelial in origin, possibly from neural crest, and therefore is unrelated to Wilms tumor.[81–84] This tumor also may be primary in the liver, chest wall, or paravertebral area. There is an association with posterior fossa brain tumors and a predilection for metastasizing to the brain.[85] Despite aggressive therapy, this tumor is associated with a 90% mortality.

The clear cell sarcoma of the kidney, also originally described as a Wilms tumor variant, is now considered a separate entity.[86,87] It represents about 2% to 5% of all childhood malignant tumors of the kidney. Age at presentation is similar to that in Wilms tumor. Clear cell renal sarcoma demonstrates a predilection to metastasize to bone.[88] It carries a poor prognosis, with at least a 50% mortality.

TUMORS OF GERM CELL ORIGIN

Germ cell tumors are derived from the stem cells of the embryo that ultimately are determined to differentiate into spermatocytes or ova. Such cells are totipotent and therefore are capable of giving rise to tumors containing any fetal, embryonal, or adult tissue. In addition, their spatial distribution and migration pattern during embryogenesis helps explain the various anatomic sites in which such tumors may develop. For example, human primordial germ cells can be recognized first in the 4-week embryo as large cells embedded in a restricted area of the yolk sac. During the fifth week of gestation, the germ cells migrate from the yolk sac to the hindgut wall and along the mesentery to the gonadal ridge, where they encounter the gonadal anlage. From there they descend into the pelvis or scrotal sac. During their migration from the yolk sac to the definitive gonad, germ cells may be left behind or they may migrate too far along the dorsal wall of the embryo near the midline. Thus, aside from the gonads, germ cell-derived tumors quite commonly arise in locations at or near the midline, anywhere from the sacrum to the head. Depending on their viability, embryonic stage, and anatomic location, they may differentiate along a variety of different cell lineages.

For example, germinomas arise from primitive but developmentally restricted germ cells. When they occur in the testis, they are referred to as seminomas; when they are found in the ovary, they are called dysgerminomas. These neoplasms also may be found outside the gonads, particularly in the mediastinal and pineal regions, and in such cases are referred to as extragonadal germinomas. Germinomas occur only rarely during infancy and develop almost exclusively in older children and adults.

Embryonal carcinoma, which occurs most commonly in individuals from 4 to 28 years of age (median age, 15 years), represents a highly malignant tumor of the multipotential germ cells that has the capacity to differentiate further into either extraembryonal or embryonal tissue lineages. Because of this capacity, embryonal carcinoma is considered to arise in the stem cells that can give rise to endodermal sinus (*i.e.*, yolk sac) tumor or choriocarcinoma, both of which are extraembryonal in origin, as well as to teratomas, which are embryonal in origin.

ENDODERMAL SINUS OR YOLK SAC TUMORS

The endodermal sinus, or yolk sac, tumor represents the most common testicular malignancy occurring under the age of 4 years. This tumor also has been called embryonal adenocarcinoma, mesoblastoma, orchioblastoma, and choroid teratoma, and at times it has been confused with embryonal carcinoma. These tumors characteristically form a histologic picture reminiscent of the yolk sac. They may metastasize to the retroperitoneal lymph nodes, which constitute the drainage pathway from the testis, to the liver, to the lung, and to bone, although metastatic disease in the infant is unusual.[89,90] Biochemically, yolk sac tumors usually are associated with elevated levels of α-fetoprotein, which serves as a useful marker in diagnosis, assessment of treatment response, or of relapse.

The assessment of a patient with the possibility of a germ cell tumor of the testis should include an assay for both α-fetoprotein and human chorionic gonadotropin levels; the latter, if positive, suggests a mixed tumor with choriocarcinomatous elements. Radiographic workup should include a chest radiograph, a chest CT scan, an abdominal CT scan, and, if the abdominal CT scan is not informative for bone, liver, and spleen, a radionuclide scan of those organs.

After the workup, the operation of choice is a radical orchiectomy with high ligation of the spermatic cord at the level of the internal inguinal ring. A transscrotal approach is contraindicated because of the risk of seeding the scrotal sac with tumor cells. Whether or not all children with testicular yolk sac tumors should undergo retroperitoneal dissection as part of further staging remains controversial. Some studies suggest that in the infant younger than 12 months of age, only orchiectomy is needed with close follow-up including radiographic studies, monitoring of α-fetoprotein levels, and physical examination.[90–92] In other studies, however, approximately 40% of children younger than age 2 years treated with orchiectomy only die from metastatic disease, compared to only 12% treated with retroperitoneal node dissection and radiation therapy with or without chemotherapy.[93,94] These reports suggest that management should include orchiectomy, lymph node dissection, combination chemotherapy, and radiation therapy for those patients with retroperitoneal nodes positive for metastatic disease. Endodermal sinus tumors also may arise in the ovary, usually at a median age of 19 years, as well as in extragonadal sites such as the pineal body, mediastinum, sacrococcyx, and the infant vagina.

In addition to resulting in endodermal sinus tumors, the extraembryonal pathway may lead to a trophoblastic-derived tumor called choriocarcinoma. Although this neoplasm is extremely rare, when it occurs in infants younger than 12 months of age, it usually is a result of transmission of a placental choriocarcinoma. Such a patient presents with pallor, hepatomegaly, and a history of gastrointestinal bleeding with hemoptysis or hematuria. There may be endocrinologic manifestations with breast enlargement and pubic hair. Chest radiographs may reveal pulmonary metastases; human chorionic gonadotropin levels most often are elevated. Such gestationally related choriocarcinomas are particularly responsive to treatment with methotrexate.[95]

TERATOMAS

When germ cell tumors arise from the embryonal compartment, they form teratomas. These are neoplasms that contain cellular or tissue derivatives of more than one of the three primary embryonal germ layers and that are foreign to the anatomic region in which they arise. The name teratoma is derived from the Greek *teratos,* which literally means monster, plus the ending "-oma," which is used to denote a neoplasm. This name derived from cases in which these tumors contained tissue elements so well organized as to resemble a deformed fetus.

In early childhood, teratomas primarily occur as extragonadal masses located along the midline axis; about 40% to 50% occur in the sacrococcygeal region with head and neck, brain, mediastinum, retroperitoneum, abdomen, spinal cord, and other soft tissue locations accounting for 1% to 5% each.[96] Gonadal teratomas occur more frequently after puberty, particularly in the ovary. About 80% to 90% of early childhood teratomas are benign; malignant teratomas usually are characterized histologically by areas containing embryonal carcinoma or endodermal sinus tumor. Such malignant lesions most often arise in the sacrococcygeal region.

Sacrococcygeal teratoma is the most common teratoma in infancy, with about 67% diagnosed by the age of 1 year. These tumors occur at a rate of 1 in 25,000 to 1 in 40,000 live births and display a significant gender predilection, with girls being affected over 75% of the time.[97,98]

Clinically, these tumors present as a mass protruding between the coccyx and the rectum (Fig. 54-2). They nearly always arise from the tip of the coccyx and vary greatly in the amount of their internal *versus*

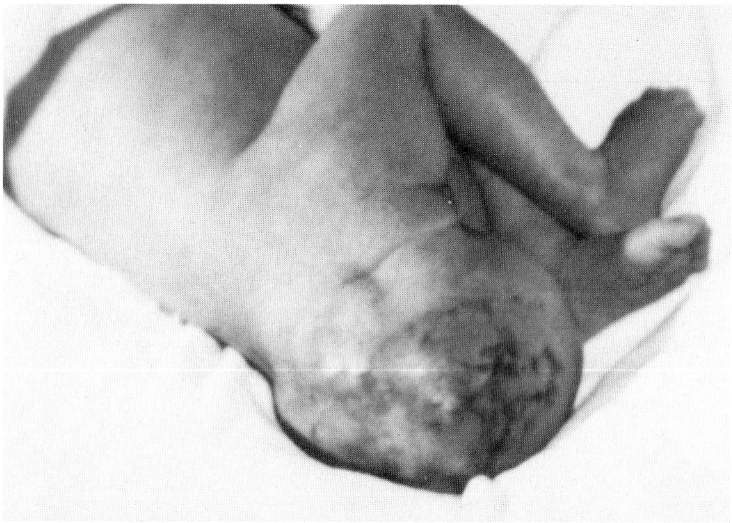

FIG. 54–2. Large sacrococcygeal teratoma in a newborn infant.

external tissue extensions.[97] Some lesions can be diagnosed only by rectal examination; however, this examination should be done with extreme care in the neonate to avoid any traumatic damage. The differential diagnosis of a sacrococcygeal teratoma includes meningomyelocele, rectal abscess, pilonidal cyst, bladder neck obstruction, rectal prolapse, duplications of the rectum, imperforate anus, dermoid cyst, angioma, lymphangioma, lipoma, neurogenic tumors of the pelvis and perineum, giant cell tumor of the sacrum, and soft tissue sarcoma.

Benign teratomas usually will produce no functional problems other than obstruction, whereas the presence of bowel or bladder dysfunction suggests a malignant lesion. Evidence for venous or lymphatic obstruction or lower leg paralysis is found more commonly in malignant tumors. Pressure applied to a meningomyelocele often will be transmitted noticeably to the anterior fontanelle. Approximately 15% of patients with sacrococcygeal teratomas have associated congenital anomalies, including imperforate anus, sacral bone defects, genitourinary abnormalities such as duplication of the uterus or vagina, and occasionally spina bifida and meningomyelocele.[99] Radiographic evaluation of the spine can be informative in that meningomyeloceles are associated with characteristic vertebral abnormalities. Abdominal and pelvic ultrasonography along with CT scanning are useful in assessing the internal extension of the mass. Barium enema may distinguish between a bowel duplication and displacement caused by a tumor mass. Chest radiographs and liver–spleen scans may indicate evidence of metastatic disease. Serum α-fetoprotein and human chorionic gonadotropin levels may be elevated in those teratomas with mixed cellular elements.

The prognosis for a patient with a sacrococcygeal teratoma depends primarily on whether the lesion is benign or malignant. For benign lesions, disease-free survival is greater than 90%, whereas for malignant components, associated mortality secondary to tumor may be greater than 90%. The age of the patient at diagnosis appears to be extremely important in determining the likelihood of malignancy. For example, the incidence of malignancy is only 7% to 10% for tumors diagnosed at younger than 2 months of age, whereas this figure increases to about 37% at age 1 year and to 50% by age 2 years. In addition, there is a significantly higher incidence of malignancy in lesions that show mostly internal tissue extension.[97]

The management of a patient with a benign sacrococcygeal teratoma is primarily surgical and includes removal of the coccyx, the site where the tumor arises. Leaving the coccyx is associated with a 30% to 40% incidence of recurrence, many of which are malignant.[100] Patients with malignant teratomas are managed after surgery with irradiation, if residual disease is present, and always with combination chemotherapy. Some regimens include vincristine, actinomycin D, and cyclophosphamide; others use vinblastine, bleomycin, and *cis*-platinum.[101,102] Regardless of intensive therapy, the prognosis in such patients is poor. The average interval between diagnosis and death usually is less than 10 months, with metastatic disease occurring in lungs, bone, liver, lymph nodes, and peritoneum.[96,103,104] Not surprisingly, there have been no survivors among patients who presented with metastatic disease.

PRIMARY HEPATIC NEOPLASMS

The differential diagnosis of a right upper quadrant mass with hepatomegaly in infants is extensive and includes nonneoplastic lesions as well as a variety of benign and malignant tumors.[105] Hepatomegaly associated with malignant disease in the infant is secondary much more commonly to leukemia or disseminated neuroblastoma than to a primary hepatic cancer.

Hepatocellular carcinoma, often associated with chronic underlying liver disease, rarely occurs in infancy. This tumor usually is massive, multifocal, and rapidly growing—all contributing factors to its frequent unresectability. In spite of aggressive combined modality treatment, such patients have a poor prognosis, with up to 90% mortality.[106,107]

Hepatoblastoma occurs primarily but not exclusively in children younger than age 3 years, with a mean age of 18 months; it also has been reported in neonates.[108–110] There have been anecdotal reports of patients with hepatoblastoma associated with the maternal use of oral contraceptives or with the fetal alcohol syndrome.[111,112] Familial cases of hepatoblastoma have been documented, suggesting an environmental or genetic contribution in some instances.[113,114] Hepatoblastoma also has been associated with a variety of congenital anomalies, most notably hemihypertrophy and renal abnormalities, but also with macroglossia, Meckel diverticulum, tetralogy of Fallot, diaphragmatic hernia, talipes equinovarus, and digital clubbing.[115] Wilms tumor and adrenal cortical neoplasms also have been found in patients with hepatoblastoma.[2]

Hepatoblastoma presents in most cases with abdominal enlargement and hepatomegaly. In approximately 25% of patients, there also will be associated anorexia, weight loss, pallor, and pain. Less common are vomiting and jaundice; diarrhea, fever, and precocious puberty are rare. Laboratory studies reveal a mild anemia and a thrombocytosis with bone marrow megakaryocytosis and, occasionally, thrombocytopenia secondary to platelet trapping.[116] Increased levels of liver enzyme transaminases and alkaline phosphatase are variable, but mild elevation of bilirubin may be present in up to 15% of cases with hepatoblastoma. Alpha-fetoprotein is elevated many-fold in nearly 70% of patients with hepatoblastoma.[117] Although not specific for hepatoblastoma, this protein marker, with a half-life of 4 to 6 days, is useful in the assessment of the response to therapy and of tumor recurrence. It should be noted, however, that not all recurring metastatic lesions are positive for α-fetoprotein, even though the primary tumor was.[118] All values for α-fetoprotein should be compared to age-matched values, because levels normally are elevated in the neonatal period. Another potential biochemical marker of hepatoblastoma is urinary cystathionine, although elevations also occur frequently in patients with neuroblastoma.[119]

Abdominal radiographs show enlargement of the liver, with the right lobe more commonly involved; areas of calcification occur in up to 20% of cases. Chest radiographs may reveal pulmonary metastases, present in about 10% of cases at diagnosis. Both abdominal CT scanning and hepatic angiography are extremely useful in determining tumor size and surgical resectability. Radioisotopic liver scans demonstrate the tumor by its decreased ability to take up the isotope; it appears as a cold lesion when compared with the surrounding, normal hepatic tissue.

The prognosis for patients with hepatoblastoma appears to depend primarily on the lesion's surgical resectability and on histology. Complete surgical excision is possible in 40% to 75% of patients, although perioperative mortality may be as high as 10% to 25%. Local and metastatic recurrences after surgical resection appear within 36 months, although there have been recurrences as late as 8 years after surgery.[109,120]

The histopathology of hepatoblastoma can be viewed as occurring in two major patterns. The first is the pure fetal epithelial type. Several studies have strongly suggested that this type of tumor is associated with a better outcome.[107,121–123] The second type, composed of both epithelial and mesenchymal elements, usually is referred to as a mixed hepatoblastoma and has been associated with a poorer prognosis. In addition, some hepatoblastomas may have anaplastic or sarcomatous elements that portend a poor prognosis.

Although some reports have demonstrated that approximately 30% to 60% of patients can be cured with complete surgical resection alone, others have shown that adjuvant chemotherapy after tumor resection significantly reduces the risk of development of distant metastases. Chemotherapy should begin about 4 weeks after resection to allow for the adequate regeneration of normal hepatic tissue. For those children with unresectable primary tumors, preoperative irradiation or combination chemotherapy or both may reduce tumor size to allow resection.[124,125] Radiation therapy has a limited role, in part because normal liver has a relatively low tolerance to irradiation. The response of both the primary tumor and metastatic disease to chemotherapeutic agents has been best when such agents have been used in combination; they include vincristine, actinomycin D, cyclophosphamide, 5-fluorouracil, doxorubicin, *cis*-platinum, and methotrexate.[126,127] Chemotherapy not only has caused regression of primary tumors but also has been associated with a few long-term remissions of pulmonary metastases. There is no precedent for survival unless the primary tumor can be fully resected.

SOFT TISSUE SARCOMAS

Soft tissue tumors represent a diverse group of neoplasms, all of which share a common cellular origin from mesenchymal elements. In the infant, the spectrum of soft tissue tumor types includes rhabdomyosarcoma, fibrosarcoma, and fibrous proliferative neoplasms as well as the rhabdoid tumor (see Neoplasms of the Kidney).

Rhabdomyosarcoma accounts for about one-half of soft tissue sarcomas but is extraordinarily rare in the neonate.[128] It may present as an orbital, nasopharyngeal, or sinus tumor; as a truncal or extremity lesion; as a genitourinary tract tumor, usually arising from bladder, prostate, or vagina; or as a paratesticular mass. At the time of diagnosis, about 20% to 40% of patients have evident metastatic disease, usually to lung, lymph nodes, liver, bone marrow, bone, and brain.[129,130]

After appropriate assessment of the primary tumor and possible metastatic sites, complete surgical resection with clean margins should be attempted. Adjuvant chemotherapy with vincristine, actinomycin D, and cyclophosphamide significantly prolongs disease-free survival. If there is residual microscopic disease as evidenced by involved surgical margins, irradiation usually is used in older children but should be modified for the neonate or infant because of long-term toxicities.

The prognosis for patients with rhabdomyosarcoma depends on stage at presentation and histology. In children with the embryonal subtype and early-stage tumors, disease-free survival is greater than 80%, whereas in those with more extensive disease or alveolar histology, prognosis remains poor.[129–131]

Fibrosarcoma represents about 10% of soft tissue sarcomas in patients younger than age 15 years, and over one-half occur in children younger than age 5 years, with about one third of these appearing at or shortly after birth.[132,133] Fibrosarcoma most commonly arises in the extremities, with the remaining cases involving the back, retroperitoneum, sacrococcyx, and the head and neck.

For extremity lesions, complete surgical resection is curative in over 90% of cases, even though local recurrences are common, appearing about 20% to 40% of the time. Occasionally, amputation may be required. Metastatic disease occurs only rarely. For tumors that are not amenable to surgical resection because of size or location or both, there is some evidence that combination chemotherapy may be quite effective.[133–136] Results with radiation therapy have been poor.[132,133]

Possibly related to fibrosarcoma, but nevertheless distinguishable pathologically, is a group of fibroblastic proliferative disorders that may be seen in the infant and newborn. The digital fibroma usually is found as a soft tissue mass on the medial side of digits, with the exclusion of the thumbs and great toes. As with fibrosarcoma, surgical resection is curative, although recurrence rates may be as high as 75% to 90%. Congenital (*i.e.*, infantile) fibromatosis may occur as solitary or multiple soft tissue lesions. The solitary lesions occur nearly anywhere on the body. When present as multiple lesions, they involve subcutaneous tissue, muscle, and bones; in some cases, the lesions may become more generalized, producing significant morbidity and mortality from visceral organ involvement.[137,138] These tumors are pathologically benign in appearance, and the solitary and multiple lesions are histologically similar.

Treatment of solitary lesions is surgical and curative. There have been several reports of patients with multiple congenital fibromatosis in which spontaneous regression has occurred.[139–141] After a diagnosis is made, treatment primarily has been supportive, with an excellent prognosis for multiple lesions involving subcutaneous tissue, muscle, and bone and a poor prognosis when visceral organ involvement is extensive.[137,138] There is little proven benefit from the use of chemotherapy in cases of fibromatosis, although a report of use of a combination of vincristine, actinomycin D, and cyclophosphamide in an infant with unresectable neck fibromatosis showed an apparently good response.[142]

VASCULAR NEOPLASMS AND MALFORMATIONS

Hemangiomas are the most common tumors found in infancy and childhood.[143] They usually appear during late fetal or early neonatal life and affect girls more commonly than boys. Skin is the most frequent site of involvement, although they may arise in any organ and often occur in multiple locations. They are soft, compressible, bright red to blue lesions found on a level with or slightly above the surface of the skin. They range in size from a few millimeters to quite massive, occupying large areas of the skin or internal organs.

Their natural course is characterized by rapid growth for the first 4 to 6 months of life followed by stabilization then gradual involution over several years. They may be considered true neoplasms in that during the proliferative phase they show greatly increased endothelial cell proliferation. They should be distinguished from vascular malformations such as arteriovenous fistulas, which represent anomalous vascular development and do not demonstrate endothelial cell proliferation. Such lesions nearly always are present at birth and increase in size along with the patient without the usual phase of involution. Lymphatic lesions, such as lymphangioma, are best considered malformations rather than neoplastic growths.[144–146]

The clinical complications that arise from hemangiomas are secondary to their size, site of origin, and physiology. They may compromise vision by encroaching on the eye; cause respiratory distress by impinging on the trachea; cause severe and even fatal congestive heart failure when they are very large, as in some liver lesions; cause gastrointestinal or CNS hemorrhage; or cause a consumptive coagulopathy from platelet and fibrinogen trapping, as in Kasabach–Merritt syndrome.

The first principle of treatment should be to do no harm, because most of these lesions eventually will regress on their own. Nevertheless, when they are the cause of significant morbidity, intervention may be necessary. Corticosteroids probably are the most useful first-line treatment and may accelerate regression.[147–149] Radiotherapy may cause undesirable side effects, such as cutaneous scarring, dermatitis, growth disturbances, and possible second tumors.[150–152] Surgery may be difficult for large lesions and may result in unsightly scarring.[153] For large lesions of the liver, hepatic artery ligation or embolization occasionally has been successful in controlling high-output cardiac failure, but liver necrosis, renal failure, and other embolic complications may result.[154,155] In cases of Kasabach–Merritt syndrome, heparin or aspirin plus dipyridamole, pentoxifylline, and steroids plus ε-aminocaproic acid have proved useful in treating the associated consumptive coagulopathy.[156–159] Laser therapy also has been used effectively.[160] The use of α-interferon has demonstrated promising results.[161]

Malignant tumors arising from vascular endothelium such as hemangioendothelioma, hemangiopericytoma, and angiosarcoma are extremely rare but reported in infants.[162,163] More information on vascular neoplasms and malformations is given in Chapter 55.

HISTIOCYTOSES

The histiocytoses represent a group of rare disorders characterized by reactive infiltrates that usually are composed of varying proportions of histiocytes, lymphocytes, plasma cells, eosinophils, and neutrophils. These infiltrates lack the usual cellular atypia characteristic of malignancies. Their benign nature is underscored further by the high frequency of spontaneous remissions. Whether these cellular infiltrates are a reaction to an infectious agent, an exaggerated response to a subtle immune system defect, or a primary proliferation disorder is unclear.[164]

The nonmalignant, proliferative histiocytoses have been grouped or classified depending on the type of histiocyte presumed to be involved primarily. Class I includes the Langerhans cell histiocytoses, which include disorders referred to as eosinophilic granuloma, Hand–Christian–Schuller disease, and Letterer–Siwe disease. Class II represents the non-Langerhans cell histiocytoses and includes familial erythrophagocytic lymphohistiocytosis (FEL), infection-associated hemophagocytic syndrome (IAHS), and congenital self-healing histiocytosis. Class III includes malignant disorders of the histiocyte, such as malignant histiocytosis and histiocytic sarcoma, neither of which occurs in the neonatal period.

Eosinophilic granuloma is found predominantly in older children, usually presenting as solitary or multiple lytic lesions of bone. Surgical curretage alone usually is curative, and low-dosage radiation also is effective. The prognosis is excellent.

Hand–Schuller–Christian disease occurs in younger children from ages 2 to 5 years and often presents with multifocal, lytic bone lesions, particularly of the skull; exophthalmia; oral soft tissue involvement; eczematoid rash; and, sometimes, diabetes insipidus secondary to hypothalamic infiltration. The clinical course is chronic with multiple recurrences over several years. For disease that is symptomatic, potentially disfiguring, or resulting in loss of function, therapeutic interventions are indicated. For localized lesions, surgical curettage or low-dose radiation therapy is very effective.[165] When there are multifocal bone lesions or multisystem disease, chemotherapy is quite effective, using vinblastine with or without prednisone. More intensive, combination chemotherapy is not indicated because it causes increased morbidity.[166,167]

Letterer–Siwe disease is the most severe form of histiocytosis. It most commonly presents within the first year of life and, occasionally, in neonates. Cases have been reported among siblings as well as in twins.[168,169]

Infants present with scaly, seborrheic, eczematoid, and sometimes purpuric rashes involving the scalp, face, ear canals, abdomen, and intertriginous areas. Hepatosplenomegaly is common, and there may be signs of hepatic dysfunction with hypoproteinemia and coagulopathy. Draining ears, lymphadenopathy, cough, and tachypnea are common. These infants are irritable and fail to thrive, secondary either to chronic disease and liver dysfunction, or to malabsorption due to gastrointestinal infiltration. Lesions in bones are not uniformly present.

The prognosis for severe Letterer–Siwe disease with liver, lung, or hematopoietic organ dysfunction is poor despite intensive combination chemotherapy, with mortality greater than 65%.[166,170–172] Hematologic studies reveal anemia, a variable leukocytosis, and thrombocytopenia, with the latter finding frequently predicting a fatal outcome. As for Hand–Schuller–Christian disease, vinblastine with prednisone often is used initially, but if there is no significant response or the disease progresses, treatment with VP-16 and steroids has been used effectively.[173,174] Anecdotal cases in which cyclosporine A has been used successfully have been reported.[175] In refractory cases, allogeneic bone marrow transplantation has been effective.[176,177] Low-dose hemi-body or whole-body radiation therapy has been used but without prolonged efficacy.[178] This severe form of histiocytosis is unresponsive to treatment with thymic extract.[179]

The diagnosis of the class I histiocytoses is made by biopsy showing characteristic pathologic changes, which include a histologically mixed, reactive infiltrate, multinucleated giant cells and proliferation of Langerhans cell histiocytes, identified by their expression of S-100 and CD1 surface antigens and the presence of cytoplasmic Birbeck granules. Birbeck granules most probably represent internalized membrane components and have a characteristic racquet appearance in the electron microscope. Therefore, biopsy specimens should be processed for immunocytochemistry and electron microscopy in addition to routine paraffin embedding.

Included in class II histiocytoses is FEL, which presents in early infancy and is presumed to be inherited as an autosomal recessive condition.[180,181] The infant presents with failure to thrive, anorexia, fever, and irritability. Seizures and spastic weakness of the limbs may occur secondary to CNS involvement.[182,183] Hepatosplenomegaly usually is prominent. Skin, bones, and lymph nodes, although often affected, are less involved than in Letterer–Siwe disease. Laboratory data characteristically show a hypofibrinogenemia as well as a distinctive hyperlipidemia with increased triglycerides and decreased high-density lipoproteins.[184] Pancytopenia often develops, as do problems with bleeding. Pathologically, there is extensive lymphohistiocytic infiltration associated with erythrophagocytosis in the visceral organs and leptomeninges, thymic involution, and depletion of lymphoid tissue.

Prognosis is poor, and most infants will die within weeks of diagnosis from sepsis or hemorrhage or both. Plasmapheresis or repeated blood exchange has been reported to produce temporary remissions.[185] Treatment with epipodophyllotoxin VP-16 along with intrathecal methotrexate has produced complete remissions in a few cases.[186–189] In addition, allogeneic bone marrow transplantation has been used successfully.[190] It frequently is difficult to clinically distinguish FEL from IAHS. A positive family history would support the diagnosis of FEL, whereas the identification of an inciting, infectious organism would suggest IAHS. There is no effective therapy. Last, some infants may present with a picture of histiocytosis localized primarily to the skin and occasionally bone. They usually have a rash that shows hard, red to dark blue nodules, which occasionally may crust over. This disorder, which undergoes spontaneous resolution within weeks to months, requires no therapy. It is referred to as congenital self-healing histiocytosis, or self-healing reticulohistiocytosis.[191,192]

THERAPEUTIC ISSUES AND LATE EFFECTS OF THERAPY

The issues surrounding the treatment of cancer in infants and young children are unique. Because of their very young age, the balance between therapy and long-term side effects becomes especially important. A close collaboration and coordination by subspecialists is critical.

Surgical management must consider the distinctive aspects of neonatal biology.[193] Some tumors, such as hemangiomas and stage IV-S neuroblastoma, frequently involute or regress on their own, obviating surgical intervention. With other tumors, such as localized neuroblastomas, a complete resection may be unnecessary, whereas in cases of hepatoblastoma an incomplete resection may portend a fatal outcome.

The detrimental effects of irradiation to infants are profoundly demonstrated in the treatment of brain tumors, resulting in a high incidence and degree of mental retardation. Skeletal growth also may be severely affected, with deformities of limbs and scoliosis. Liver, lung, and kidney are major organs whose short- and long-term function can be compromised.[194] In addition, the late appearance of second tumors may be significantly increased as a result of the mutagenic effects of irradiation.[195]

For many solid tumors, chemotherapy has been effective in the treatment of micrometastatic disease as well as residual disease after incomplete resection. In cases of disease that is disseminated at the time of diagnosis, such as in leukemia or advanced neuroblastoma, systemic chemotherapy is imperative. The use of chemotherapy in the newborn is complicated by unique differences in absorption, distribution, metabolism, and excretion of such drugs.[196] Some of the signs and symptoms of drug toxicity may be subtle and must be related to the behavioral repertoire of the infant. Survivors of the successful treatment of malignancy in infancy should be followed closely for long-term sequelae.[197,198]

REFERENCES

1. Bader JL, Miller RW. U.S. cancer incidence and mortality in the first year of life. Am J Dis Child 1979;133:157.
2. Fraumeni JF Jr, Miller RW. Adrenocortical neoplasms with hemihypertrophy, brain tumors, and other disorders. J Pediatr 1967;70:129.
3. Koufos A, Hansen M, Coperland N, et al. Loss of heterozygosity in three embryonal tumors suggests a common pathogenetic mechanism. Nature 1985;316:330.
4. Donehower LA, Harvey M, Slagle BL, et al. Mice deficient for p53 are developmentally normal but susceptible to spontaneous tumours. Nature 1992;356:215.
5. Donegan WL. Cancer and pregnancy. CA 1983;33:194.
6. Bishop JM. Viruses, genes and cancer: II. Retroviruses and cancer genes. Cancer 1985;55:2329.
7. Auersperg NaRC. Retroviral oncogenes: interrelationships between neoplastic transformation and cell differentiation. Critical Reviews in Oncogenesis 1991;2:125.
8. Slamon DJ, Cline MJ. Expression of cellular oncogenes during embryonic and fetal development of the mouse. Proc Natl Acad Sci USA 1984;81:7141.
9. Forrester LM, Brunkow M, Bernstein A. Proto-oncogenes in mammalian development. Current Opinion in Genetics and Development 1992;2:38.
10. Pavelic K, Slaus NP, Spaventi R. Growth factors and proto-oncogenes in early mouse embryogenesis and tumorigenesis. Int J Dev Biol 1991;35:209.
11. Myers C. Peptide growth factors: the parallel between fetal development and malignant transformation. Am J Reprod Immunol 1991;25:133.
12. Torry DS, Cooper GM. Proto-oncogenes in development and cancer. Am J Reprod Immunol 1991;25:129.
13. Weinberg RA. Tumor suppressor genes. Science 1991;254:1138.
14. Mitchell CD. Recessive oncogenes, antioncogens and tumor suppression. Br Med Bull 1991;47:136.
15. Chatten J, Voorhess M. Familial neuroblastoma: report of a

kindred with multiple disorders, including neuroblastomas in four siblings. N Engl J Med 1967;277:1230.
16. Voute P, Wadman S, van Putten W. Congenital neuroblastoma: symptoms in the mother during pregnancy. Clin Pediatr 1970;9:206.
17. Jaffe N. Neuroblastoma: review of the literature and an examination of the factors contributing to its enigmatic character. Cancer Treat Rev 1976;3:61.
18. Giulian BB, Chang CCN, Yoss BS. Prenatal ultrasonographic diagnosis of fetal adrenal neuroblastoma. J Clin Ultrasound 1986;14:225.
19. Forman HP, Leonidas JC, Berdon WE, et al. Congenital neuroblastoma: evaluation with multimodality imaging. Radiology 1990;175:365.
20. Iida Y, Nose O, Kai H. Watery diarrhea with vasoactive intestinal peptide-producing ganglioneuroblastoma. Arch Dis Child 1980;55:929.
21. Delalieux C, Ebinger G, Maurus R, et al. Myoclonic encephalopathy and neuroblastoma. N Engl J Med 1975;292:46.
22. D'Angio G, Evans A, Koop C. Special pattern of widespread neuroblastoma with a favorable prognosis. Lancet 1971;1:1046.
23. Evans A, D'Angio G, Randolph J. A proposed staging for children with neuroblastoma. Cancer 1971;27:374.
24. Laug W, Seigel S, Shaw K, et al. Initial urinary catecholamine metabolite concentrations and prognosis in neuroblastoma. Pediatrics 1978;62:77.
25. Schwartz A, Dadash-Zadeh M, Lee H, et al. Spontaneous regression of disseminated neuroblastoma. J Pediatr 1974;85:760.
26. Ikeda Y, Lister J, Bouton J, et al. Congenital neuroblastoma *in situ* and the normal fetal development of the adrenal. J Pediatr Surg 1981;16:636.
27. Beckwith J, Perrin E. In situ neuroblastomas: a contribution to the natural history of neural crest tumors. Am J Pathol 1963;43:1089.
28. Brodeur GM. Neuroblastoma: clinical significance of genetic abnormalities. Cancer Surv 1990;9:673.
29. Hosoda Y, Miyano T, Kimura K, et al. Characteristics and management of patients with fetal neuroblastoma. J Pediatr Surg 1992;27:623.
30. Evans A, Chatten J, D'Angio G, et al. A review of 17 IV-S neuroblastoma patients at Children's Hospital of Philadelphia. Cancer 1980;45:833.
31. Kretschmar C, Frantz C, Rosen E, et al. Improved prognosis for infants with stage IV neuroblastoma. J Clin Oncol 1984;2:799.
32. Ellsworth RM. Current concepts in the treatment of retinoblastoma. In: Peyman GA, Apple DJ, Sanders DR, eds. Intraocular tumors. New York: Appleton-Century-Crofts, 1977:335.
33. Murphree A, Benedict W. Retinoblastoma: clues to human oncogenes. Science 1984;223:1028.
34. Knudson A. Retinoblastoma: a prototypic hereditary neoplasm. Semin Oncol 1978;5:57.
35. Jooma R, Kendall BE. Intracranial tumours in the first year of life. Neuroradiology 1982;23:267.
36. Takaku A, Kodama N, Ohara H, et al. Brain tumor in newborn babies. Childs Brain 1978;4:365.
37. Matson DD. Hydrocephalus in a premature infant caused by papilloma of the choroid plexus. J Neurosurg 1953;10:416.
38. Bergsagel DJ, Finegold MJ, Butel JS, et al. DNA sequences similar to those of simian virus 40 in ependymomas and choroid plexus tumors of childhood. N Engl J Med 1992;326:988.
39. van Eys J, Cangir A, Coody D, et al. MOPP regimen as primary chemotherapy for brain tumors in infants. J Neurol Oncol 1985;3:237.
40. Das L, Chang C, Cushing B, et al. Congenital primitive neuroectodermal tumor (neuroepithelioma) of the chest wall. Med Pediatr Oncol 1982;10:349.
41. Seemayer T, Themo W, Bolande R, et al. Peripheral neuroectodermal tumors. Perspect Pediatr Pathol 1975;2:151.
42. Cutler L, Chaudhry A, Topazian R. Melanotic neuroectodermal tumor of infancy: an ultrastructural study, literature reviews, and re-evaluation. Cancer 1981;48:257.
43. Pierce MI. Leukemia in the newborn infant. J Pediatr 1959;54:691.
44. Weinstein HJ. Congenital leukemia and the neonatal myeloproliferative disorders associated with Down's syndrome. Clin Haematol 1978;7:147.
45. MacMachon B, Levy MA. Prenatal origin of childhood leukemia: evidence from twins. N Engl J Med 1964;270:1082.
46. Rosner F, Lee SL. Down's syndrome and acute leukemia: myeloblastic or lymphoblastic? Report of forty-three cases and review of the literature. Am J Med 1972;53:203.
47. Krivit W, Good RA. Simultaneous occurrence of leukemia and mongolism: report of a nationwide survey. Am J Dis Child 1957;94:289.
48. Djernes BW, Soukup SW, Bove KE, et al. Congenital leukemia associated with mosaic trisomy 9. J Pediatr 1976;88:596.
49. Miller RW. Persons with exceptionally high risk of leukemia. Cancer Res 1967;27:2420.
50. Greaves MF, Janossy G, Peto J, et al. Immunologically defined subclasses of acute lymphoblastoma leukemia in children: their relationship to presentation features and prognosis. Br J Haematol 1981;48:179.
51. Korsmezer SJ, Arnold A, Babhshi A. Immunoglobulin gene rearrangement and cell surface antigen expression in acute lymphocytic leukemias of T-cell and B-cell precursor origins. J Clin Invest 1983;71:301.
52. Spier C, Kjeldsberg G, O'Brien R, et al. Pre-B cell acute lymphoblastic leukemia in the newborn. Blood 1984;64:1064.
53. Crist W, Puller J, Boyett J. Clinical and biologic features predict a poor prognosis in acute lymphoid leukemias in infants: a pediatric oncology groups study. Blood 1986;67:135.
54. Abe R, Ryan D, Cecalupo A, et al. Cytogenetic findings in congenital leukemia: case report and review of the literature. Cancer Genet Cytogenet 1983;9:139.
55. Odom L, Gordon E. Acute monoblastic leukemia in infancy and early childhood: successful treatment with an epipodophyllotoxin. Blood 1984;4:876.
56. Berger R, Bernheim A, Weh H. Cytogenetic studies on acute monocytic leukemia. Leuk Res 1980;4:119.
57. Reimann D, Clemmens R, Pillsbury W. Congenital leukemia: skin nodules a first sign. J Pediatr 1955;46:415.
58. Chu J, O'Connor D, Gale G, et al. Congenital leukemia: two transient regressions without treatment in one patient. Pediatrics 1983;71:277.
59. Engel RR, Hammond D, Eitzman D, et al. Transient congenital leukemia in 7 infants with mongolism. J Pediatr 1964;65:303.
60. Brodeur G, Dahl G, Williams D, et al. Transient leukemoid reaction and trisomy 21 mosaicism in a phenotypically normal newborn. Blood 1980;55:691.
61. Grier H, Weinstein H. Acute nonlymphocytic leukemia. Pediatr Clin North Am 1985;32:653.
62. Bolande RP, Brough AJ, Izant RJ. Congenital mesoblastic nephroma of infancy: a report of eight cases and the relationship to Wilms' tumor. Pediatrics 1967;40:272.
63. Blank E, Nerhout RC, Burry RA. Congenital mesoblastic nephroma and polyhydramnios. JAMA 1978;240:1504.

64. Howell CG, Othersen HB, Kiviat NE. Therapy and outcome in 51 children with mesoblastic nephroma: a report of the National Wilms' Tumor Study. J Pediatr Surg 1982;17:826.
65. Steinfeld AD, Crowley CA, O'Shea PA, et al. Recurrent and metastatic mesoblastic nephroma in infancy. J Clin Oncol 1984;2:956.
66. D'Angio GJ, Evans A, Breslow N. The treatment of Wilms' tumor: results of the second National Wilms' Tumor Study. Cancer 1981;47:2302.
67. Gonzales-Crussi F, Sotelo-Avila C, Kidd JM. Malignant mesenchymal nephroma of infancy: a report of a case with pulmonary metastases. Am J Surg Pathol 1980;4:185.
68. Varsa EW, McConnell TS, Dressler LG, et al. Atypical congenital mesoblastic nephroma: report of a case with karyotypic and flow cytometric analysis. Arch Pathol Lab Med 1989;113:1078.
69. Machin GA. Persistent renal blastema (nephroblastomatosis) as a frequent precursor of Wilms' tumor: a pathological and clinical review: part I. Nephroblastomatosis in the context of embryology and genetics. Am J Pediatr Hematol Oncol 1980; 2:165.
70. Machin GA. Part II: significance of nephroblastomatosis in the genesis of Wilms' tumor. Am J Pediatr Hematol Oncol 1980;2:253.
71. Machin GA. Part III: clinical aspects of nephroblastomatosis. Am J Pediatr Hematol Oncol 1980;2:353.
72. Kulkarni R, Bailie MD, Bernsetin J, et al. Progression of nephroblastomatosis to Wilms' tumor. J Pediatr 1980;96: 178.
73. Bennington JL, Beckwith JB. Tumors of the kidney renal pelvis and ureter. In: Atlas of tumor pathology. 2nd series. fasc. 12. Washington, DC: Armed Forces Institute of Pathology, 1975:32.
74. Bove DE, McAdams AJ. The nephroblastomatosis complex and its relationship to Wilms' tumor: a clinicopathologic treatise. In: Rosenberg HS, Bolande RP, eds. Perspectives in pediatric pathology. Chicago: Year Book, 1976:185.
75. Dimmick JE, Johnson HW, Coleman GU, et al. Wilms tumorlet, nodular renal blastema and multicystic renal dysplasia. J Urol 1989;142:484.
76. Hrabovsky EE, Othersen HB Jr, deLorimier A, et al. Wilms' tumor in the neonate: a report from the National Wilms' Tumor Study. J Pediatric Surg 1986;21:385.
77. Beckwith JB. Wilms' tumor and other renal tumors of childhood. Hum Pathol 1983;14:481.
78. Cassady JR, Tefft M, Filler RM. Considerations in the radiation therapy of Wilms' tumor. Cancer 1973;32:298.
79. Corn BW, Goldwein JW, Evans I, et al. Outcomes in low-risk babies treated with half-dose chemotherapy according to the Third National Wilms' Tumor Study. J Clin Oncol 1992;10: 1305.
80. Larsen E, Perez-Atayde A, Green DM, et al. Surgery only for the treatment of patients with stage I (Cassady) Wilms' tumor. Cancer 1990;66:264.
81. Beckwith JB, Palmer NF. Histopathology and prognosis of Wilms' tumor: results from the First National Wilms' Tumor Study. Cancer 1978;41:1937.
82. Haas JE, Palmer NF, Weinberg AG, et al. Ultrastructure of the rhabdoid tumor of kidney: a distinctive renal tumor of children. Hum Pathol 1981;12:646.
83. Palmer NF, Sutlow W. Clinical aspects of the rhabdoid tumor of the kidney: a report of The National Wilms' Tumor Study Group. Med Pediatr Oncol 1983;11:242.
84. Lynch HT, Shwim SB, Dahms BB. Paravertebral malignant rhabdoid tumor in infancy. Cancer 1983;52:290.
85. Bonnin JM, Rubinstein LJ, Palmer NF, et al. The association of embryonal tumors originating in the kidney and in the brain. Cancer 1984;54:2137.
86. Gonzalez-Crussi F, Baum ES. Renal sarcomas of childhood: a clinicopathologic and ultrastructural study. Cancer 1983;51: 898.
87. Carcassonne C, Raybaud C, Lebreuil G. Clear cell sarcoma of the kidney in children: a distinct entity. J Pediatr Surg 1983;16: 645.
88. Marsden HB, Lawler W, Kumar PM. Bone metastasizing renal tumor of childhood: morphologic and clinical features and differences from Wilms' tumor. Cancer 1978;42:1922.
89. Ise T, Ohtsuki H, Matsumoto K, et al. Management of malignant testicular tumors in children. Cancer 1976;37:1539.
90. Exelby PR. Testis cancer in children. Semin Oncol 1979;6: 116.
91. Jeffs RD. Management of embryonal adenocarcinoma of the testis in childhood: an analysis of 164 cases. In: Gooden JA, ed. Cancer in childhood. New York: Plenum Press 1973:68.
92. Brosman SA. Testicular tumors in prepubertal children. Urology 1979;13:581.
93. Drago JR, Nelson RP, Palmer JM. Childhood embryonal carcinoma of testes. Urology 1978;12:499.
94. Colodny A, Hopkins TB. Testicular tumors in infants and children. Urol Clin North Am 1977;4:347.
95. Witzleben CH, Bruninga G. Infantile choriocarcinoma: a characteristic syndrome. J Pediatr 1968;73:374.
96. Tapper D, Lack E. Teratomas in infancy and childhood: a 54 year experience at The Children's Hospital Medical Center. Ann Surg 1983;198:398.
97. Altman RP, Randolph JG, Lilly JR. Sacrococcygeal teratoma: American Academy of Pediatrics Surgical Section Survey. J Pediatr Surg 1974;9:389.
98. Damjanov II, Knowles BB, Solter D, eds. The human teratomas: experimental and clinical biology. Clifton, NJ: Humana Press, 1983.
99. Fraumeni JF, Li FP, Dalager S. Teratomas in children: epidemiologic features. JNCI 1973;51:1425.
100. Donnellan WA, Swenson O. Benign and malignant sacrococcygeal teratomas. Surgery 1968;64:834.
101. Raney RB Jr, Chatten J, Littman P. Treatment strategies for infants with malignant sacrococcygeal teratoma. J Pediatr Surg 1981;16:573.
102. Einhorn H, Donohue J. *Cis*-diaminedichloroplatinum vinblastine, bleomycin combination chemotherapy in disseminated testicular cancer. Ann Intern Med 1977;87:293.
103. Noseworthy J, Lack EE, Kozakewich HPW. Sacrococcygeal germ cell tumors in childhood: an updated experience with 118 patients. J Pediatr Surg 1981;16:258.
104. Valdiserri RO, Yunis EJ. Sacrococcygeal teratomas: a review of 68 cases. Cancer 1981;48:217.
105. Edmondson HA. Differential diagnosis of tumors and tumor-like lesions of liver in infancy and childhood. Am J Dis Child 1956;91:168.
106. Lack EE, Neave C, Vawter GF. Hepatocellular carcinoma: review of 32 cases in childhood and adolescence. Cancer 1983; 52:1510.
107. Weinberg AG, Finegold MJ. Primary hepatic tumors of childhood. Hum Pathol 1983;14:512.
108. Randolph JG, Altman RP, Arensman RM. Liver resection in children with hepatic neoplasms. Ann Surg 1978;187:599.
109. Ein SH, Stephens CA. Malignant liver tumors in children. J Pediatr Surg 1974;9:491.
110. Clatworthy HW, Schiller M, Grosfeld JL. Primary liver tumors in infancy and childhood: 41 cases variously treated. Arch Surg 1974;109:143.
111. Otten J, Smets R, de Jager R, et al. Hepatoblastoma in an

infant after contraceptive intake during pregnancy. N Engl J Med 1977;297:222.
112. Khan A, Bader JL, Hoy GR, et al. Hepatoblastoma in child with fetal alcohol syndrome. Lancet 1979;1:1403.
113. Fraumeni JF Jr, Rosen PJ, Hull EW. Hepatoblastoma in infant sisters. Cancer 1969;24:2647.
114. Napoli V, Campbell W Jr. Hepatoblastoma in infant sister and brother. Cancer 1977;39:2647.
115. Berry CL, Keeling J, Hilton C. Coincidence of congenital malformation and embryonic tumors in childhood. Arch Dis Child 1970;45:229.
116. Nickerson HJ, Silberman TL, McDonald TP. Hepatoblastoma, thrombocytosis and increased thrombopoietin. Cancer 1980; 45:315.
117. Exelby PR, Filler RM, Grosfeld JL. Liver tumors in children in particular reference to hepatoblastoma and hepatocellular carcinoma: American Academy of Pediatrics Surgical Section Survey. J Pediatr Surg 1975;10:329.
118. Pritchard J, daCunha A, Cornbleet MA, et al. Alpha-fetoprotein monitoring of response to adriamycin in hepatoblastoma. J Pediatr Surg 1982;17:429.
119. Geiser CG, Baez A, Schindler AM, et al. Epithelial hepatoblastoma associated with congenital hemihypertrophy and cystathioninuria: presentation of a case. Pediatrics 1970;46:66.
120. Moazam F, Talbert JL, Rodgers BM. Primary tumors of the liver in infancy and childhood. J Fla Med Assoc 1982;69:991.
121. Lack EE, Neave C, Vawter FG. Hepatoblastoma: a clinical and pathologic study of 54 cases. Am J Surg Pathol 1982;6:693.
122. Kasai M, Watanabe I. Histologic classification of liver cell carcinoma in infancy and childhood and its clinical evaluation: a study of 70 cases collected in Japan. Cancer 1970;25:551.
123. Gonzalez-Crussi F, Upton PM, Macurer SH. Hepatoblastoma: attempt at characterization of histologic subtypes. Am J Surg Pathol 1982;6:599.
124. Weinblatt ME, Siegel SE, Siegal MM. Preoperative chemotherapy for unresectable primary hepatic malignancies in childhood. Cancer 1982;50:1061.
125. Forouhar FA, Quinn JJ, Cooke R, et al. The effect of chemotherapy on hepatoblastoma. Arch Pathol Lab Med 1984; 108:311.
126. Holton CP, Burrington JD, Hatch EI. A multiple chemotherapeutic approach to the management of hepatoblastoma. Cancer 1975;35:1083.
127. Evans AE, Land VJ, Newton WA. Combination chemotherapy (vincristine, adriamycin, cyclophosphamide, and 5-fluorouracil) in the treatment of children with malignant hepatoma. Cancer 1982;50:821.
128. Ragab AH, Heyn R, Tefft M, et al. Infants younger than 1 year of age with rhabdomyosarcoma. Cancer 1986;58:2606.
129. King DR, Clatworthy HW Jr. The pediatric patient with sarcoma. Semin Oncol 1981;8:215.
130. Grosfeld JL, Weber TR, Weetman RM, et al. Rhabdomyosarcoma in childhood: analysis of survival in 98 cases. J Pediatr Surg 1983;18:141.
131. Green DM, Jaffe N. Progress and controversy in the treatment of childhood rhabdomyosarcoma. Cancer Treat Rev 1978;5:7.
132. Chung EB, Enzinger FM. Infantile fibrosarcoma. Cancer 1976; 38:729.
133. Soule EH, Pritchard DJ. Fibrosarcoma in infants and children: a review of 110 cases. Cancer 1977;40:1711.
134. Hays DM, Mirabal VQ, Karlan MS. Fibrosarcomas in infants and children. J Pediatr Surg 1970;8:415.
135. Exelby PR, Knappes WH, Huvos AG, et al. Soft tissue fibrosarcoma in children. J Pediatr Surg 1973;8:415.
136. Grier HE, Perez-Atayde AR, Weinstein HJ. Chemotherapy for inoperable infantile fibrosarcoma. Cancer 1985;56:1507.
137. Chung EB, Enzinger FM. Infantile myofibromatosis. Cancer 1981;48:1807.
138. Briselli MF, Soule EH, Gilchrist GS. Congenital fibromatosis: report of 18 cases of solitary and 4 cases of multiple tumors. Mayo Clin Proc 1980;55:554.
139. Kauffman SL, Stout AP. Congenital mesenchymal tumors. Cancer 1965;18:460.
140. Teng P, Warden MJ, Cohn WL. Congenital generalized fibromatosis (renal and skeletal) with complete spontaneous remission. J Pediatr 1963;62:748.
141. Schaffzin EA, Chung SMK, Kaye R. Congenital generalized fibromatosis with complete spontaneous regression: a case report. J Bone Joint Surg [Am] 1972;54:657.
142. Stein R. Chemotherapeutic responses in fibromatosis of the neck. J Pediatr 1977;90:482.
143. Silverman RA. Hemangiomas and vascular malformations. Pediatr Clin North Am 1991;38:811.
144. Mulliken JB, Glowacki J. Hemangiomas and vascular malformations in infants and children: a classification based on endothelial characteristics. Plast Reconstr Surg 1982;69:412.
145. Edgerton MT, Hiebert JM. Vascular and lymphatic tumors in infancy, childhood and adulthood: challenge of diagnosis and treatment. Curr Probl Cancer 1978;2:1.
146. Williams HB. Vascular neoplasms. Clin Plast Surg 1980;7:397.
147. Pereyra R, Andrassy RJ, Mahow GH. Management of massive hepatic hemangiomas in infants and children: a review of 13 cases. Pediatrics 1982;70:254.
148. Assaf A, Nasr A, Johnson T. Corticosteroids in the management of adnexal hemangiomas in infancy and childhood. Ann Ophthalmol 1992;24:12.
149. Padalkar JA, Bapat VS, Phadke MA, et al. Successful treatment of hepatic hemangiomas with corticosteroids. Indian Pediatr 1992;29:769.
150. Park WC, Phillips R. The role of radiation therapy in the management of hemangiomas of the liver. JAMA 1970;212: 1496.
151. Bennett RG, Keller JW, Ditty JF Jr. Hemangiosarcoma subsequent to radiotherapy for a hemangioma in infancy. J Dermatol Surg Oncol 1978;4:881.
152. Schild SE, Buskirk SJ, Frick LM, et al. Radiotherapy for large symptomatic hemangiomas. Int J Radiat Oncol Biol Phys 1991;21:729.
153. Belli L, DeCarlis L, Beati C, et al. Surgical treatment of symptomatic giant hemangiomas of the liver. Surg Gynecol Obstet 1992;174:474.
154. Flint LM, Polk HC. Selective hepatic artery ligation: limitations and failure. J Trauma 1979;19:319.
155. Williams MD, Pearson MH, Thomas FD. Arterial embolisation of a facial haemangioma. Br Dent J 1992;173:102.
156. Carnelli V, Bellini F, Ferrari M. Giant hemangioma with consumption coagulopathy: sustained response to heparin and radiotherapy. [Letter] J Pediatr 1977;91:504.
157. Koerper MA, Addiego JE Jr, Delorimier AA. Use of aspirin and dipyridamole in children with platelet trapping syndromes. J Pediatr 1983;102:311.
158. de-Prost Y, Teillac D, Bodemer C, et al. Successful treatment of Kasabach-Merritt syndrome with pentoxifylline. J Am Acad Dermatol 1991;25:854.
159. Dresse MF, David M, Hume H, et al. Successful treatment of Kasabach-Merritt syndrome with prednisone and epsilon-aminocaproic acid. Pediatr Hematol Oncol 1991;8:329.
160. Lemarchand-Venecie F. Indications for laser in the treatment of capillary hemangioma. J Mal Vasc 1992;17:41.
161. Ezekowitz RA, Mulliken JB, Folkman J. Interferon alfa-2a therapy for life-threatening hemangiomas of infancy. N Engl J Med 1992;326:1456.

162. Falk H, Herbert JT, Edmonds L. Review of four cases of childhood hepatic angiosarcoma: elevated environmental arsenic exposure in one case. Cancer 1981;47:382.
163. Bedos AA, Munson J, Toomey FE. Hemangioendothelioma presenting as posterior mediastinal mass in a child. Cancer 1980;46:801.
164. Osband MEaP C, ed. Histiocytosis X. Hematol Oncol Clin North Am 1987;1.
165. Cassady JR. Current role of radiation therapy in the management of histiocytosis-X. Hematol Oncol Clin North Am 1987;1:123.
166. Starling KA. Chemotherapy of histiocytosis. Am J Pediatr Hematol Oncol 1981;3:157.
167. Starling KA. Chemotherapy for histiocytosis-X. Hematol Oncol Clin North Am 1987;1:119.
168. Glass AG, Miller RW. U.S. mortality from Letterer-Siwe disease 1900. Pediatrics 1968;42:364.
169. Jugberg RC, Kloepfer HW, Oberman HA. Genetic determination of acute disseminated histiocytosis X (Letterer-Siwe syndrome). Pediatrics 1970;45:753.
170. Komp DM, Vietti TJ, Berry DH. Combination chemotherapy in histiocytosis X. Med Pediatr Oncol 1977;3:267.
171. Matus-Ridley M, Raney RB, Thawerani H, et al. Histiocytosis X in children: patterns of disease and results of treatment. Med Pediatr Oncol 1983;11:99.
172. Greenberger JS, Crocker AC, Vawter G. Results of treatment of 127 patients with systemic histiocytosis (Letterer-Siwe syndrome, Schuller-Christian syndrome and multifocal eosinophilic granuloma). Medicine 1981;60:331.
173. Urbano-Marquez A, Estruch R, Fernandez-Huerta JM, et al. Etoposide in the treatment of multifocal eosinophilic granuloma. Cancer Treat Rep 1985;69:238.
174. Ceci A, deTerlizzi M, Colella R, et al. Etoposide in recurrent childhood Langerhans' cell histiocytosis: an Italian cooperative study. Cancer 1988;62:2528.
175. Mahmoud H, Wang WC, Murphy SB. Cyclosporine therapy for advanced Langerhans cell histiocytosis. Blood 1991;77:721.
176. Stoll M, Freund M, Schmid H, et al. Allogeneic bone marrow transplantation for Langerhans' cell histiocytosis. Cancer 1990;66:284.
177. Ringden O, Ahstrom L, Lonnqvist B, et al. Allogeneic bone marrow transplantation in a patient with chemotherapy-resistant progressive histiocytosis X. N Engl J Med 1987;316:733.
178. Richter MP, D'Angio GJ. The role of radiation therapy in the management of children with histiocytosis X. Am J Pediatr Hematol Oncol 1981;3:161.
179. Osband ME, Lipton JM, Lavin P. Histiocytosis-X: demonstration of abnormal immunity, T-cell histamine H2-receptor deficiency, and successful treatment with thymic extract. N Engl J Med 1981;304:146.
180. Farguhar J, Claireaux A. Familial haemophagocytic reticulosis. Arch Dis Child 1952;27:519.
181. MacMahon HE, Bedizel M, Ellis CA. Familial erythrophagocytic lymphohistiocytosis. Pediatrics 1963;32:868.
182. Price DL, Woolsey JE, Rosman NP, et al. Familial lymphohistiocytosis of the nervous system. Arch Neurol 1971;24:270.
183. Akima M, Sumi SM. Neuropathology of familial erythrophagocytic lymphohistiocytosis. Hum Pathol 1984;15:161.
184. Ansbacher LG, Singsen BH, Hosler MW, et al. Familial erythrophagocytic lymphohistiocytosis: an association with serum lipid abnormalities. J Pediatr 1983;102:270.
185. Ladisch S, Ho W, Matheson D, et al. Immunologic and clinical effects of repeated blood exchange in familial erythrophagocytic lymphohistiocytosis. Blood 1982;60:814.
186. Ambrusso DR, Hays T, Zwartjes WJ. Successful treatment of lymphohistiocytic reticulosis with epipodophyllotoxin VP 16-213. Cancer 1980;45:2516.
187. Lilleyman JS. The treatment of familial erythrophagocytic lymphohistiocytosis. Cancer 1980;46:468.
188. Henter JI, Elinder G, Finkel Y, et al. Successful induction with chemotherapy including teniposide in familial erythrophagocytic lymphohistiocytosis. Lancet 1986;13(2):1402.
189. Alvarado CS, Buchanan GR, Kim TH, et al. Use of VP-16-213 in the treatment of familial erythrophagocytic lymphohistiocytosis. Cancer 1986;57:1097.
190. Fischer A, Cerf-Bensussan N, Blanche S. Allogeneic bone marrow transplantation for erythrophagocytic lymphohistiocytosis. J Pediatr 1986;108:267.
191. Hashimoto K, Griffin D, Kohsbaki M. Self-healing reticulohistiocytosis: a clinical, histologic, and ultrastructural study of the fourth case in the literature. Cancer 1982;49:331.
192. Marsh WI, Lew SW, Heath VC, et al. Congenital self-healing histiocytosis-X. Am J Pediatr Hematol Oncol 1983;5:227.
193. deLorimier AA, Harrison MR. Surgical treatment of tumors in the newborn. Am J Pediatr Hematol Oncol 1981;3:271.
194. Littman P, D'Angio GJ. Radiation therapy in the neonate. Am J Pediatr Hematol Oncol 1981;3:279.
195. Pastore G, Antonelli R, Fine W. Late effects of treatment of cancer in infancy. Med Pediatr Oncol 1982;10:369.
196. Siegel SE, Moran RG. Problems in the chemotherapy of cancer in the neonate. Am J Pediatr Hematol Oncol 1981;3:287.
197. Mulhern RK, Kovnar E, Langston J, et al. Long-term survivors of leukemia treated in infancy: factors associated with neuropsychologic status. J Clin Oncol 1992;10:1095.
198. Meadows ATaG-F J. Secondary cancers in pediatric patients: assessing the risks. Contemporary Oncology 1992;2:47.

Neonatology: Pathophysiology and Management of the Newborn, Fourth Edition,
edited by Gordon B. Avery, Mary Ann Fletcher, and Mhairi G. MacDonald.
J.B. Lippincott Company, Philadelphia © 1994.

chapter 55

Dermatologic Conditions

ANDREW M. MARGILETH

Careful assessment of skin in the sick newborn frequently provides clues for a presumptive diagnosis of a primary cutaneous disease, a systemic disease, or both. During the initial examination, an exact dermatologic diagnosis often is difficult to make. The diagnosis evolves, however, by analysis of the descriptive morphology, configuration, and distribution of the skin lesions. Close observation with a bright light and small magnifying glass identifies the type of primary and secondary cutaneous lesions (see the following outline). In the well newborn, there are many skin lesions that are normal and transient but require differentiation from those that are permanent, pathologic, or indicative of underlying conditions. Many of the skin lesions present in neonates require little or no therapy, but, because of their visibility, are of concern to the parents. These conditions are summarized in Table 55-1. The following is an outline of the classification of skin lesions.

- Primary cutaneous lesions
  - Lesions $\leq$ 5 mm
    - Papule
    - Comedo
    - Vesicle
  - Lesions $>$ 5 mm
    - Patch
    - Plaque
    - Nodule (5–20 mm)
    - Tumor
    - Bulla
  - Lesions of varying sizes
    - Pustule
    - Wheal
    - Macule
    - Burrow
    - Telangiectasia
- Secondary skin lesions
  - Atrophy
  - Crusts
  - Erosion
  - Excoriation
  - Fissure
  - Pigmentation
  - Scar
  - Scale
  - Ulcer

Configuration refers to patterning of lesions (*e.g.*, annular, circinate, serpiginous or gyrate, linear, iris, zosteriform, along lines of cleavage, marbled, multiform). Distribution refers to the body area, sites of predilection, and whether symmetric, localized or circumscribed, scattered, generalized, single or multiple, and discrete or confluent. With a good history, including that of family and medications, presence or absence of pruritus, and a descriptive analysis of the lesions, common dermatologic entities are identified. Finally, if the diagnosis is not clear after a short period of observation with a few selected tests, dermatologic consultation is indicated.[1–6]

Skin consists of epidermis, a relatively impermeable membrane, and dermis, which constitutes the

TABLE 55–1
NEONATAL SKIN LESIONS REQUIRING MINIMAL OR NO THERAPY

Lesion	Frequency	Location and Usual Course	Associated Conditions
Hemangioma, macular stain, salmon patch	Caucasian: 75%; black: 60%	Eyelids clear by 6 to 12 mo of age; neck and glabella persist for 5–6 y or longer	Over 36 syndromes[7]
Milia	40% 64%	Cheeks, forehead, nasolabial folds; few weeks to 2 months of age Palate; Epstein pearls	Gorlin and orofaciodigital syndromes[7]
Sebaceous gland hyperplasia	Common in full-term infants	Nose, upper lip, malar areas; clear by 6 months of age	None
Acne neonatorum	Occurs more often in boys than girls	Face, chest, back, groin; papules, comodones, occasionally pustules by 2 to 4 weeks of age, clear by 1 to 2 years of age; kertolytic gel is prescribed for extensive cases	Beckwith–Wiedemann, Apert, and XYY syndromes[7]
Cutis marmorata	Uncommon	Extremities, trunk; fade by adulthood	Adams–Oliver, De Lange, Down, KTW, and Trisomy 18 and 21 syndromes
Harlequin color change	Rare in low-birth-weight infants	Dependent one-half of body, deep red color for 15 to 20 min	None
Miliaria rubra, crystillina	Common in warm environment	Forehead, neck, intertriginous areas; resolve rapidly in cool environment; dry, cool environment is prescribed	Consider secondary infection if pustules occur
Erythema toxicum	50% of full-term infants, less in premature infants	Body except palms and soles; onset 24–28 h of age, resolving in few hours to 10 d of age	Eosinophils in vesicle or pustule, blood eosinophilia 20%
Transient neonatal pustular melanosis	Relatively common	Generalized, including palms and soles; pustules resolve by 5 days of age, hyperpigmented macules resolve by 3 months of age	Pustule aspirate shows predominance of neutrophils
Mongolian spot	Black, oriental, Indian: 90%; Caucasian: 5%	Buttocks, flanks, shoulders, extremities; fades in late infancy to adulthood	Seen in six rare syndromes[7]
Caput succedaneum	Common	Presenting part, usually scalp; resolves by 7 d of age	Prolonged labor
Sucking blisters	Uncommon	Thumb, finger, wrists, lip; resolve in a few days	None
Subcutaneous fat necrosis	Uncommon	Cheeks, buttocks, arms, thighs; begins in the first 2 weeks of age; resolves in weeks to months	Well infant, hypercalcemia[6]
Aplasia cutis congenita	Rare (*i.e.,* 1 per 3000 live births)	Scalp, commonly; trunk, face or proximal extremities with healing in several months, leaving a scar	Cleft palate, lip; absent digits, syndactyly; congenital heart disease; trisomy 13[7]; dystrophic EB
Hemangioma: raised, strawberry, or cavernous	5%–10% neonates, increased in premature infants	Generalized; spontaneous involution 5 to 10 y; steroids prescribed if vital orifice affected, platelet trapping occurs or cardiac failure occurs	More than 15 syndromes[7]

(*continued*)

TABLE 55–1
NEONATAL SKIN LESIONS REQUIRING MINIMAL OR NO THERAPY (*continued*)

Lesion	Frequency	Location and Usual Course	Associated Conditions
Incontinentia pigmenti	Rare; Female–male ratio 9 : 1	Extremities; trunk with vesicles resolves in first 3 months of age to warty linear lesion, then to linear hyperpigmented swirls after 1 year of age	Dental, hair, ocular, CNS, osseous defects occur in 30%
Urticaria pigmentosa, mastocytosis	Rare	Trunk, face, head, extremities as single or multiple lesions; resolve by adolescence	Urtication sign (*i.e.*, Darier); dermatographism
Juvenile xanthogranuloma	Rare	Generalized: head, neck, upper trunk, extremities; spontaneous involution occurs by 6 months to 2 years of age	Ocular, pulmonary, testicular, renal lesions are rare[50]

CNS, central nervous system; EB, epidermolysis bullosa; KTW, Klippel–Trenauney–Weber.

bulk of skin. Dermis consists of minimally cellular fibrous tissue containing collagen and elastic and reticular fibers embedded in an amorphous ground substance that contains blood and lymphatic vessels, neural structures, eccrine and apocrine sweat glands, hair follicles, sebaceous glands, and smooth muscle. The epidermis is an avascular, cellular structure composed chiefly of keratinocytes stratified into five layers.[1–3] Prenatal and postnatal epidermal changes and the functional components of skin are discussed in detail by Solomon and Esterly.[3,5]

PHYSIOLOGIC AND GENETIC VARIATIONS

The appearance of the newborn skin primarily depends on gestational maturation, state of nutrition, racial origin, and amount of vernix caseosa. Activity, distribution and amount of fat, hemoglobin and bilirubin levels, and the type and intensity of available light produce variations in the skin appearance. The premature infant has thin, taut skin, whereas the dysmature infant has loose, wrinkled skin.

KERATINIZATION

The degree of desquamation, part of the keratinization process, varies with maturity, nutritional state, and presence of cutaneous disease. Normally, term infants show little or no desquamation until 1 or 2 days of age; peeling is complete after a few days with no treatment necessary. Desquamation occurs later in premature infants and may be quite severe in very immature infants. Desquamation is abnormal if present at birth but may indicate dysmaturity, intrauterine asphyxia, or, rarely, congenital ichthyosiform dermatosis.

MACULAR HEMANGIOMAS

Macular stains of the nape, eyelids, and glabella are found in 50% of newborns. These salmon patches (*i.e.*, nevus simplex) have diffuse borders and become pinker when the infant cries; most eyelid lesions fade by 1 year of age. The nuchal and glabellar lesions persist longer and may appear transiently in the older child or adult when angered. Unna nevus is a persistent nuchal salmon patch.[1] No therapy is indicated.

CUTIS MARMORATA

Cutis marmorata is a physiologic, generalized marbling effect in infants who become chilled. The netlike pattern is caused by dilation of the capillaries and venules and usually disappears with rewarming. It is uncommon after several months of age unless there is prolonged exposure to low environmental temperatures. Persistent cutis marmorata is frequent in trisomies 18 and 21 and De Lange syndrome.[7] Localized marbling or reticulation that becomes intense with crying or change in temperature is called "cutis marmorata telangiectatica congenita."[8] This vascular ectasia involves both capillaries and veins, and most lesions fade by adulthood.[3] If the condition persists or is extensive, the patient should be evaluated for associated malformations.[7,8]

HARLEQUIN COLOR CHANGE

Harlequin color change is a rare phenomenon observed only in neonates, especially low-birth-weight infants. A sharply demarcated, deep red color develops in the dependent one-half of the body when the infant is side lying, compared to the pale, superior one-half. The color change lasts from 1 to 30 minutes and reverses sides if the infant is rotated to the opposite side. The harlequin sign, observed in well and sick infants, is of no pathologic significance.[1,3]

MILIA

Epidermal inclusion cysts, or milia, are multiple yellow or white, 1-mm papules noted over the cheeks, nasal bridge, forehead, nasolabial folds, hard palate, and alveolar ridges (*i.e.*, Epstein pearls). Epstein pearls, seen in 85% of newborns, usually rupture soon after birth. Milia, observed in 40% of term infants as grouped, noninflamed papules, disappear within a few weeks to 2 months.[1]

SEBACEOUS GLAND HYPERPLASIA

In contrast to milia are innumerable tiny (<0.5 mm) white or yellow spots involving the pilosebaceous follicles of the nose, upper lip, and malar areas. These hyperplastic sebaceous glands, rare in preterm infants, spontaneously become smaller and disappear by 2 to 6 months of age.

ACNE NEONATORUM

This disorder, seen more often in boys, occasionally develops during the first or second postnatal months, particularly in breast-fed infants (Fig. 55-1). Characteristically, erythematous comodones and papules are seen; pustules, nodules, and cystic lesions are rare. Lesions occur over the cheeks primarily, but also on the chin and forehead. Most lesions disappear by 1 or 2 years of age; rarely, they may persist to puberty. Most patients require no therapy except daily cleansing with a mild soap. Petrolatum, baby oils, and lotions should be avoided. Keratolytic agents or 4% benzoyl peroxide gel may be needed for more severe cases well after the neonatal period.[1,4]

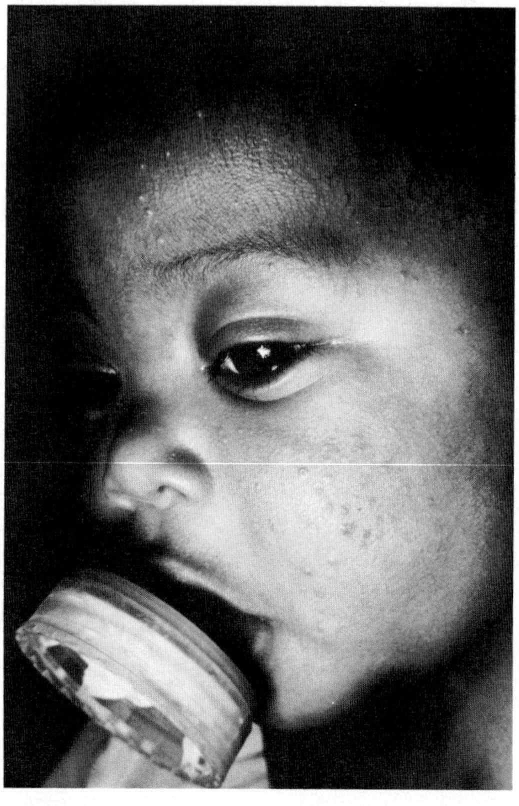

FIG. 55–1. Acne neonatorum of the cheeks is present in a 4-month-old boy; comedones developed at 4 weeks of age. Six miliaria pustulosa lesions are present on the forehead. There was much improvement 1 month after petrolatum was discontinued.

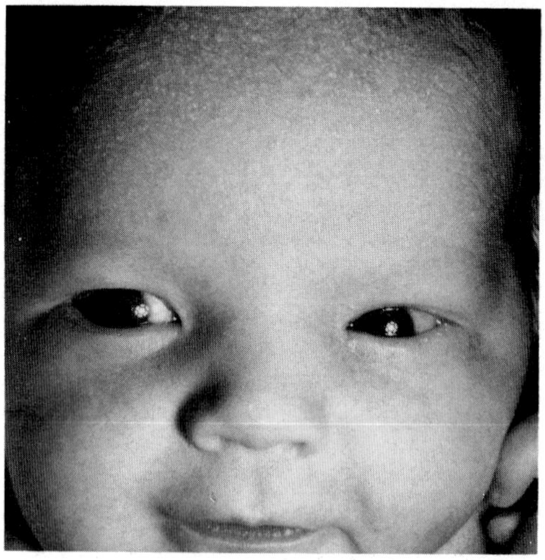

FIG. 55–2. Miliaria crystallina in a 5-day-old infant. Cooling resulted in disappearance of the lesions overnight.

MILIARIA

Retention of sweat as a result of keratinous plugging of eccrine ducts causes four types of miliaria (m.): m. rubrum (*i.e.*, prickly heat), m. crystallina (*i.e.*, sudamina), m. pustulosa, and m. profunda.[1,3,4] The last two conditions are rarely seen in temperate climates. M. rubrum, small groups of erythematous papules and papulovesicles, is observed commonly in infants but rarely in neonates unless environmental temperature and humidity are excessively high. M. crystallina, 1- to 2-mm superficial vesicles that are clear and uninflamed, is observed commonly over the forehead, neck, and intertriginous areas, and occasionally in the diaper area (Fig. 55-2). They may be seen at birth, particularly if there has been maternal fever. The distribution and grouping of vesicles that contain no eosinophils distinguish m. crystallina from erythema toxicum. The lesions disappear rapidly in a cooler environment and reappear in heat and humidity. M. pustulosa, with leukocytic infiltration of the vesicles, is rare but may be distinguished from staphylococcal impetigo by a negative Gram stain or culture and by its rapid resolution in a cool, dry environment.[1]

ERYTHEMA TOXICUM

This benign, self-limiting, perifollicular eruption, observed in 30% to 70% of term infants, usually is seen at birth or shortly thereafter. Its peak incidence is at 24 to 48 hours of life, but it may appear until 1 or 2 weeks of age. The lesion starts as a red macule that quickly becomes smaller and fades as it develops into a firm, 1- to 3-mm white or pale yellow papule or pustule with a small erythematous base (Fig. 55-3). Occasionally, only erythematous macules 3 cm or smaller are seen. These may become confluent, especially over the trunk, but any body area may be involved except the palms and soles. The lesions usually fade spontaneously in a few hours or by age 10 days. Diagnosis can be confirmed by resolution within hours or by a smear of the pustule aspirate showing numerous eosinophils but no bacteria. The etiology is unknown and treatment is unnecessary.[6]

TRANSIENT NEONATAL PUSTULAR MELANOSIS

Transient vesicopustular melanosis or transient pustulosis occurs more often in the healthy newborn than generally is appreciated.[1,5] Three stages of lesions may be observed: noninflammatory pustules, ruptured vesicopustules with a collarette of scale usually surrounding a central hyperpigmented macule (Fig. 55-4), and hyperpigmented macules that may persist for up to 3 months of age. Cultures are sterile; aspirated pus shows neutrophils, rare or no eosinophils, and cellular debris. The pustules, lasting 1 to 5 days, may never be observed because they ruptured before birth or with the first bath, leaving only the collarette or hyperpigmented macule. This dermatosis is more common in dark-skinned infants but occurs in light-skinned infants. It is self-limited and requires no treatment. Differential diagnosis of vesicopustules is discussed later.[1,5,6]

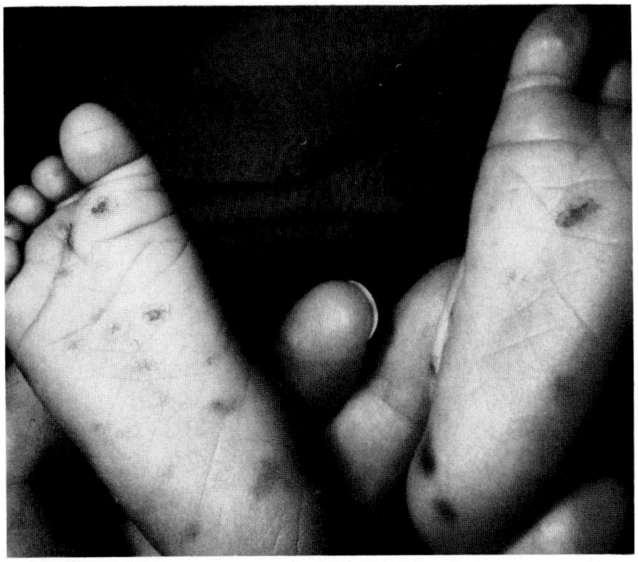

FIG. 55–4. Transient neonatal pustular melanosis in a 6-day-old African-American infant. Vesicles that were noted over the entire body at birth began scaling at 24 hours of age. A few vesicopustules developed. Note collarette of scales surrounding the hyperpigmented macules, which were very prominent by 1 month of age. TORCHES studies were negative.

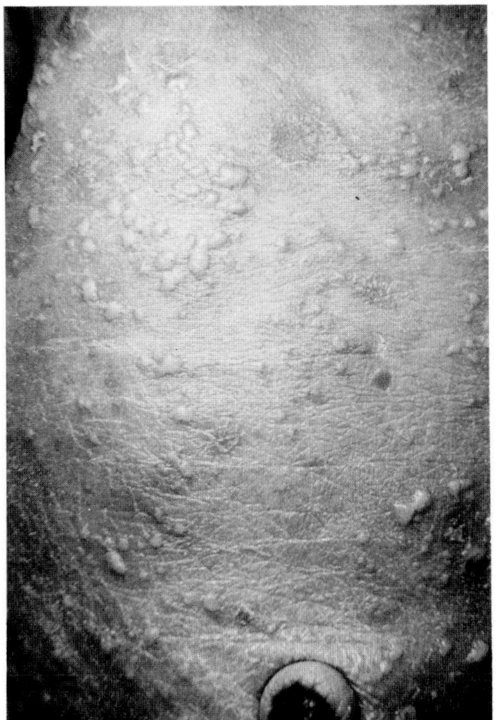

FIG. 55–3. Erythema toxicum in a 12-hour-old healthy full-term infant. At birth, many sterile pustulaes were present and continued to form. Wright stain of aspirate showed numerous eosinophils. The skin cleared spontaneously in 1 week.

PIGMENTARY LESIONS

MONGOLIAN SPOT

Mongolian spot, the most common pigmented lesion seen at birth, is present in 90% of black, Indian, and Oriental infants.[1] It occurs in 5% of Caucasian infants. These large (2–10 cm or more), macular, slate blue or gray lesions, usually seen over the lumbosacral area, also may be observed over buttocks, flanks, shoulders, and extremities. Lesions may be single or multiple and are caused by infiltration of melanocytes deep in the dermis. The spots usually fade during late infancy but may persist into adulthood.[1,6,9]

CAFÉ-AU-LAIT SPOTS

Café-au-lait spots, which are tan or brown macules, are seen occasionally in newborns, may develop during infancy, and are more likely in black infants (120/1000 live births) than Caucasian infants (3/1000).[6,10] Single lesions under 3 cm in length are found in 19% of normal children.[3] An infant with five or fewer café-au-lait spots smaller than 0.5 cm and a negative family history for von Recklinghausen disease probably is normal. Subsequently, if six or more spots larger than 1.5 cm develop, a diagnosis of cutaneous neurofibromatosis, Proteus or Albright syndrome, or tuberous sclerosis should be considered and the patient followed closely.[1,5,6]

MELANOCYTIC NEVI

Melanocytic nevi (*i.e.*, flat, junctional nevi) are pigmented lesions noted in 1% to 2% of neonates.[9] These nevi are brown or black and vary from 0.1 to several centimeters. Usually, very few lesions are present at birth, with their number increasing with age. They may be associated with neurofibromatosis, tuberous sclerosis, bathing trunk nevi, lentiginosis, or xeroderma pigmentosum.[3] Therapy rarely is necessary except that lesions larger than 1.5 cm should be followed closely with measurements and photographs to document any change or dysplasia, particularly if there is a family history of malignant melanoma.[1,5,9]

DIFFUSE HYPERPIGMENTATION

Diffuse hyperpigmentation in the newborn is unusual. The degree and location of hyperpigmentation must be considered in view of the infant's racial and genetic background. Diffuse hyperpigmentation may be caused by congenital Addison disease, nutritional disorders (*e.g.*, pellagra, sprue), hepatitis or biliary atresia, hereditary disorders (*e.g.*, lentiginosis, melanism),[1,3] metabolic disease (*e.g.*, Hartnup disease, porphyria), or be the result of bronze discoloration in Niemann–Pick disease. Androgens may produce hyperpigmentation of the labial folds with clitoral hypertrophy as a result of transplacental passage during pregnancy. Therapy depends on the basic disorder. I observed a newborn boy with slate gray melanosis at birth secondary to maternal malignant melanoma with placental metastases. The mother died 6 weeks postpartum; the infant survived without treatment and was well at 10 years of age. Although his deciduous teeth were brown, his permanent teeth were normal.

HYPOPIGMENTATION

Hypopigmentation, a diffuse or localized loss of pigment in the neonate, may be the result of genetic (*e.g.*, piebaldism, vitiligo, tuberous sclerosis, albinism), metabolic (*e.g.*, phenylketonuria), endocrine (*e.g.*, Addison disease), traumatic, or postinflammatory causes.[1,6,9] The melanocytes may be absent or sparse.

HYPOMELANOSIS OF ITO

Hypomelanosis of Ito, a neurocutaneous syndrome, may be associated with seizures, delayed development, and ocular and musculoskeletal anomalies. The skin lesions resemble those of incontinentia pigmenti, but as a negative image.[1,5,6,9]

ALBINISM

Albinism, an autosomal recessive disorder, occurs in all races. The infant shows markedly reduced pigmentations, yellow or white hair, pink pupils, gray irides, and photophobia with photosensitivity. Nystagmus with reduced vision is common. Small stature, mental retardation, and deafness may occur. Protection from ultraviolet light is necessary to prevent actinic keratoses and squamous cell carcinomas.[1,5,9]

PIEBALDISM OR PARTIAL ALBINISM

Piebaldism, or partial albinism, an autosomal dominant disorder that is present at birth, is detected easily in the dark-skinned infant. Usually amelanotic (*i.e.*, off-white) macules involve the scalp, widow's peak, and forehead, with extension to the base of the nose, chin, trunk, and extremities. Because an isolated white forelock may be the only manifestation, with deafness developing much later, Klein–Waardenburg syndrome must be considered.[1,6,9] Other diagnoses in the newborn are vitiligo, nevus anemicus, Addison disease, and white macules of tuberous sclerosis. Most of these entities may be excluded by the characteristic distribution of the hypomelanotic areas in piebaldism, which contain normal pigmented islands (*i.e.*, 1- to 5-cm macules). Vitiligo (*i.e.*, pure white macules) usually develops after 6 months of age at sites of repeated trauma.[1,5,9] When illuminated with a Wood light, these amelanotic areas exhibit a brilliant whiteness.

NEVUS ACHROMICUS OR DEPIGMENTOSUS

Nevus achromicus or depigmentosus, present at birth, appears as irregularly shaped, long, linear streaks of hypomelanosis that are very small or that may cover one-half of the body (Fig. 55-5). The area of hypopigmentation is uniform in color and usually unilateral. The lesion, when rubbed, shows a normal vasodilation response, in contrast to nevus anemicus, which is unresponsive and remains pale compared to normal adjacent vasodilated skin. Therapy is not necessary for either lesion because each usually occurs in covered areas.[1]

WHITE MACULES

White macules (*i.e.*, leukoderma, hypopigmented spots), detected in 90% of infants with tuberous sclerosis (*i.e.*, epiloia), may be present at birth. These spots may be missed in light-skinned infants unless a Wood lamp is used. The macules are about the size of a thumbprint or mountain ash leaf,[1,5,6] vary in number from 4 to more than 100, usually are seen over the trunk or buttocks, and have a normal physiologic response to stroking. All infants with otherwise explained seizures should be examined carefully for

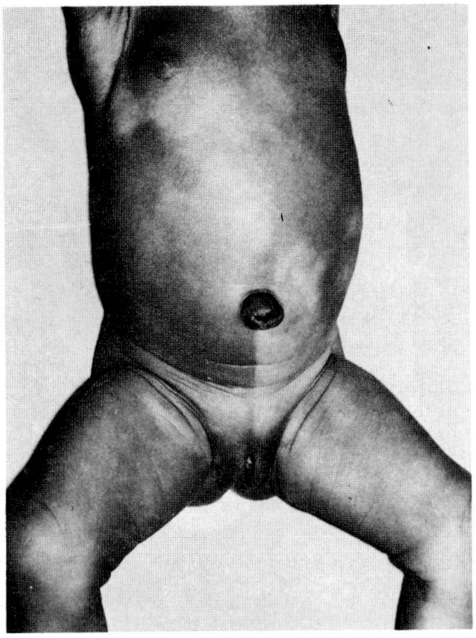

FIG. 55–5. Nevus achromicus of the right chest, left abdomen, and leg in a healthy 3-week-old premature infant. Hypopigmentation was noted at 10 days of age. A normal flare response developed after rubbing. Family history was negative for hypopigmented lesions. (Courtesy of M. Renfield, M.D. and F. Bowen, M.D.)

these macules with a Wood lamp. Most hypopigmented macules seen at birth are not associated with epiloia.[10] In one study, only 1 of 35 hypopigmented macules seen in 4641 newborns was due to tuberous sclerosis.[10] The other macules may be normal or associated with nevus anemicus, neurofibromatosis, or a developing hemangioma.[10] Because other cutaneous features of epiloia[11] (*e.g.*, angiofibromas, shagreen patch, periungual fibroma) take years to develop, careful follow-up is essential.[1,9,10]

TRAUMA

CAPUT SUCCEDANEUM

A diffuse, edematous, occasionally hemorrhagic swelling of the presenting part occurs secondary to compression of local vessels associated with prolonged labor. The scalp, scrotum, labia majora, or an extremity (Fig. 55-6) may be involved. Edema recedes in a few days; ecchymoses, if present, clear in several weeks. No therapy is needed, and sequelae are not reported.[12]

SUCKING BLISTERS

Occasionally, a few intact or ruptured 1-cm bullae may be noted on the thumb, index finger, wrist, or lip where the infant sucked vigorously *in utero*.[6,10] The blisters contain sterile, serous fluid and resolve spontaneously.

SKIN TRAUMA

Abrasions, ulcerations, ecchymoses, lacerations, or areas of pressure necrosis of the presenting part may be seen after prolonged labor, vacuum extraction, application of forceps or scalp electrodes, or fetal blood sampling. Ulcerated areas should be kept clean and dry, especially if a deep ulcer develops from pressure necrosis.[3] If serious drainage occurs, application of water or normal saline dressings, changed every 4 hours, for 1 to 2 days will effectively minimize exudate formation and infection. A povidone–iodine (Betadine) skin cleanser, four times daily followed by application of 2% mupirocin ointment, will be effective for any secondary superficial infection. Subconjunctival hemorrhage or petechiae usually are inconsequential and spontaneously disappear within a few weeks.

FAT NECROSIS

Fat necrosis, an uncommon, sharply circumscribed, indurated subcutaneous nodule or plaque appearing on the extremities, trunk, or buttocks during the first weeks of life, has been attributed to trauma, shock, cold, and asphyxia. It appears most commonly under the area of forceps application if a fat cheek has been compressed against the zygoma. The lesion is nonpitting and hard, may be painful, and have a deep reddish or purplish discoloration. As the lesions resolve, some rarely may undergo liquefaction and appear as a sterile abscess, but should not be drained. All lesions resolve spontaneously over weeks to months. Residual atrophy and scarring are unusual.[1,6]

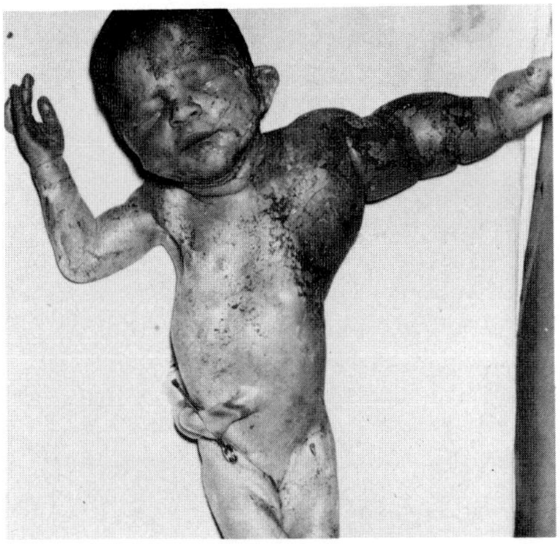

FIG. 55–6. Caput succedaneum edema and ecchymoses of the presenting part in a 1-day-old premature infant. Labor was prolonged; a cesarean section was necessary. Swelling disappeared spontaneously in 1 week; the arm functioned normally.

SCLEREMA NEONATORUM

Sclerema neonatorum more commonly affects the preterm or severely debilitated infant. It may have the same etiology and adipose tissue abnormality in the subcutaneous tissues as noted in fat necrosis.[3] Low environmental temperature alone can produce the injury. A diffuse hardening of subcutaneous tissue develops with cold, stony hard, nonpitting induration. The extremities may be involved at first, but generalized involvement occurs within 3 to 4 days. Most infants are severely ill but, if they survive, the sclerematous changes rarely persist beyond 2 weeks. Differential diagnosis includes edema neonatorum, Milroy and Turner syndromes, and panniculitis.[3] Therapy is based on the underlying systemic disease, restoration of body temperature, and adequate nutrition.[1,6]

DIAPER DERMATITIS

Napkin or diaper dermatitis is a common, transient, erythematous eruption localized to the diaper area. Maceration and scaling are common; eventually, nodular ulcerations develop after improper care. Neonatal skin is more permeable and susceptible to irritation. Predisposing factors are inheritance of a reactive skin with a seborrheic or atopic diathesis; systemic disease such as syphilis, acrodermatitis enteropathica, or Letterer–Siwe disease; activating factors such as occlusive moist heat or retention of sweat; secondary infection caused by pyogenic invaders, viruses, or yeasts; mechanical irritation; contact factors (*e.g.*, retained urine and stool); and parental factors such as overcleaning or inability to carry out proper skin care or therapeutic directions.[1,5,6,13]

CONTACT DIAPER DERMATITIS

Primary irritant or contact dermatitis, a common problem, often is caused by direct application of harsh soaps, detergents, lanolin, and sensitizers (*e.g.*, neomycin, nystatin, parabens, ethylenediamine, sulfur),[1] or is secondary to recurrent diarrhea, especially with alkaline stools. Petrolatum or mineral oil, tolerated in older infants or young black infants, may cause maceration with sweat retention in Caucasian infants. When the intertriginous areas are clear and the eruption involves the mons pubis, scrotum, penis, medial thighs, and buttocks, a clinical diagnosis of contact dermatitis is likely (Fig. 55-7).

Therapy consists of frequent diaper changes; keeping the area clean, dry, and cool; and elimination of the offending irritant (*e.g.*, stool and urine). Impermeable plastic pants foster heat and sweat retention and are to be avoided. In the acute stage, rapid healing will occur if no diapers are used for 24 to 72 hours. Irritation will be diminished by frequent diaper changes and by application of a diaper paste or powder containing zinc oxide. Warm water only or with a mild soap (Dove) should be used for cleansing. Aveeno or starch baths are soothing. Diapers may be loosened and used without plastic pants, and multiple cotton diapers that have been laundered in a mild soap and carefully rinsed with a vinegar solution may be used. Loosely applied paper diapers with wicking materials to keep moisture away from the skin and without added perfumes are effective if changed often enough.

INTERTRIGO

Intertrigo, a symmetric moist eruption in skin folds and creases, is secondary to excessive sweating and close approximation of opposing gluteal or inguinal surfaces. It is managed in the same way as contact diaper dermatitis, with exposure to dry air most helpful. Ointments must be avoided. Because secondary yeast or bacterial infection usually occurs within a few days, cultures or smears should be considered if the eruption persists or in debilitated, hospitalized infants.[1,5,6,13]

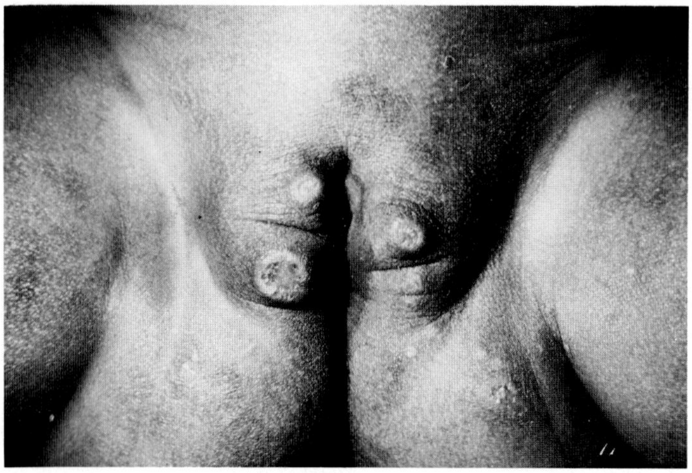

FIG. 55–7. Chronic ulceronodular contact diaper dermatitis and secondary staphylococcal infection in a 1-month-old infant. The rolled edges of the ulcers are characteristic. Note the absence of skin involvement in the thigh folds.

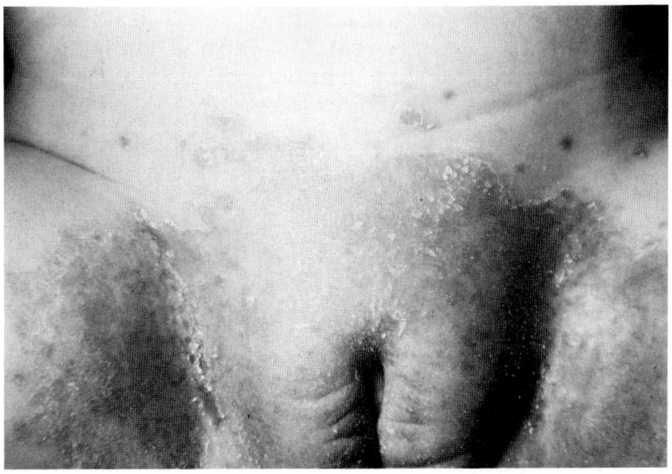

FIG. 55–8. Monilial diaper rash persisted for 3 weeks in a 6-week-old infant. There was no response to nystatin ointment. However, gentian violet, 1% aqueous, applied three times a day for 3 days was effective. Note the presence of satellite lesions.

PRIMARY IRRITANT DIAPER DERMATITIS

Ammonia dermatitis may be caused by urea-splitting bacteria or nonalkaline irritants produced by putrefactive enzymes. Dry erythematous skin resembling a scald is found on the convex surfaces.[13] A pungent ammonia odor invariably is present when the first morning diaper is changed. Frequent changing of diapers and maintenance of dry, clean skin usually is sufficient for clearance but, rarely, feeding D,L-methionine, 0.2 g twice a day for 7 to 10 days may be necessary. Recurrences are unusual. Secondary *Candida* infection may be present.[1,5,6]

MONILIAL DIAPER DERMATITIS

Diaper dermatitis occasionally is caused by or associated with *Candida* species. Over several days, a vesicular eruption becomes confluent to form a moist, bright red, macerated rash. Diagnosis is suspected by the presence of many, 0.5- to 1-cm superficial satellite erosions or moist patches and pustules outside the diaper rash (Fig. 55-8) or perianal eruption. *Candida albicans* can be identified quickly by Gram stain of scrapings. Oral thrush with white plaques over the tongue and soft and hard palates usually is seen after the second week of life, whereas cutaneous lesions may occur at any age. A generalized rash may develop in untreated infants, especially if an endocrinopathy or immunologic deficiency exists or the infant is very premature. Prolonged antibiotic therapy, diabetes mellitus, and excessive sweating are predisposing factors. Simple candidal diaper dermatitis is treated with proper cleansing followed by alternate use of 1% hydrocortisone cream and nystatin powder or cream (100,000 U/g) applied three times a day for 7 to 10 days. When there is failure of nystatin (see Fig. 55-8), 1% aqueous gentian violet, applied three times a day for 3 days, is recommended. A second 3-day course of therapy occasionally is necessary after a 3-day lapse following the initial treatment. It is essential that the diaper area remain clean and dry. Generalized cutaneous and systemic candidal infections are quite rare in infants unless they are immunologically compromised or very premature.[1,6]

SEBORRHEIC DIAPER DERMATITIS

Seborrhea of the diaper area, rarely seen in the absence of scalp or truncal involvement (see Seborrheic Dermatitis), is characterized by patchy redness, fissuring, scaling, and occasional weeping, especially in intertriginous (*i.e.*, gluteal) folds. The scalp and postauricular regions should be examined carefully for an oily, scaly, minimally erythematous eruption. Diagnosis is suspected if scraping the scales and rubbing them between the fingers produce a soapy sensation. The eruption, rarely seen during the first week of life, may become widespread (*i.e.*, truncal) by 1 or 2 months of age. The principal therapy consists of a sulfur–salicylic acid shampoo to the scalp every other night for several weeks. Application of 2% ketoconazole cream to the scalp once daily is an alternative therapy. Application of 1% hydrocortisone cream three times a day for 7 to 14 days to the diaper or other inflamed areas may promote faster healing. If secondary candidal infection exists, 1% aqueous gentian violet applied three times a day for 3 days only is recommended.[4]

SUBACUTE AND CHRONIC SECONDARY DIAPER DERMATITIS

Diaper rash may occur in association with cutaneous or systemic bacterial, viral, or fungal infections; diarrhea; atopic eczema, or prolonged use of fluorinated topical steroids.[1,5,13] Secondary staphylococcal infection superimposed on eczematous diaper dermatitis can produce an erosive nodular eruption (see Fig. 55-7) that can be resistant to local therapy.[3,14] Elimination of the primary irritant and of allergic and physical agents (*e.g.*, cold, heat) at well as use of a systemic antibiotic effective against staphylococci will clear the infection. Hydrocortisone, 1%, in zinc oxide ointment or zinc oxide paste alone will provide protection from irritants in infants with atopic dermatitis. Mild, nonalkaline soaps are necessary to keep the skin clean without irritation. Education of the parent is essential to avoid recurrence.[5,6]

MISCELLANEOUS SKIN LESIONS

REDUNDANT SKIN

Loose skin folds are observed over the neck posteriorly in Turner, Down, and trisomy 13 syndromes. Redundant skin in a more generalized distribution is seen in infants with trisomy 18 and combined immunodeficiency syndrome with dwarfism and alopecia. Dermatomegaly or cutis laxa and cutis hyperelastica (*i.e.*, Ehlers–Danlos syndrome), although rare, must be differentiated. The diagnostic features may not be evident in the neonatal period.[1,3,5–8,15,16]

CONGENITAL FISTULAS

Auricular, branchiogenic, and thyroglossal fistulas and cysts are relatively common and easily detected in the ear, lower lip, and anterolateral neck. Most fistulas may be noted in the neonatal period; cysts develop in later infancy or childhood, particularly, when secondary infection develops. Surgical excision is the definitive treatment.[1]

UMBILICAL ANOMALIES

After the cord has separated, a small (3–7 mm), dull red, dry, velvety granuloma may slowly develop. Purulent exudate caused by secondary infection may occur. Daily application of a silver nitrate stick effectively will cauterize the granuloma and cause it to recede, whereas the rare umbilical polyp (*i.e.*, persistent remnant of the omphalomesenteric duct or urachus) will not. The latter lesions require surgical excision.

APLASIA CUTIS CONGENITA

Congenital absence of skin, not uncommon, may present as a localized, midline posterior scalp defect or as several small or one large defect involving the extremities and occasionally the trunk.[9,16,17] The typical scalp lesion is a 2- to 3-cm, circular, sharply marginated area (Fig. 55-9). At birth, the lesion usually is covered by a smooth membrane that often desquamates, leaving a dry ulcer. These lesions heal slowly over several months by reepithelialization, leaving a hypertrophic (Fig. 55-10) or atrophic scar. Infection is rare. Other malformations, cleft lip and palate, defects of hands and feet, and trisomy 13 may be associated.[1,3,6,7,17]

Extensive congenital defects of the skin present at birth (Fig. 55-11*A)* usually are multiple and heal spontaneously by epithelial growth from the borders. The end result is an acceptable, thin scar (Fig. 55-11*B*). Histologically, these areas show an absence of epidermis, few appendageal structures, and decreased dermal elastic tissue. Infection should be prevented by handling with gloves, local cleaning with Betadine soap, and application of bacitracin or 2% mupirocin ointment two to four times daily. Extensive aplasia cutis may be associated with epidermolysis bullosa (EB).[1,3,6,7,9,16] In either case, skin grafting should be avoided.

HYPOPLASIAS

Focal dermal hypoplasia (*i.e.*, Goltz syndrome) is characterized by linear areas of thinning or absence of dermis with herniation of fat through surrounding

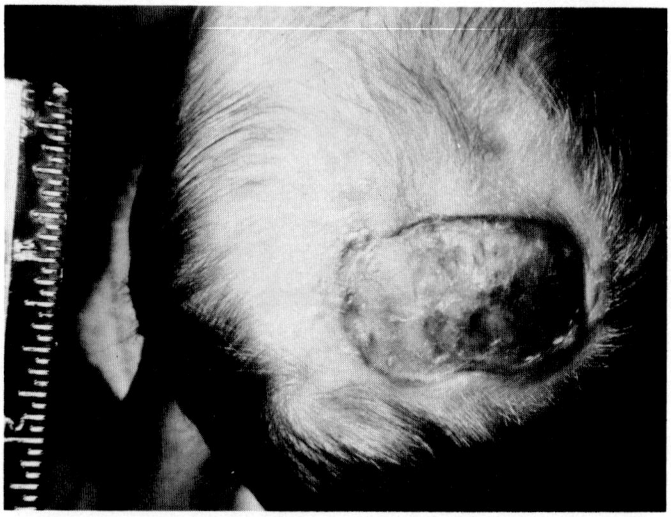

FIG. 55–9. Cutis aplasia of the scalp in a 1-month-old infant with trisomy 13. Healing occurred spontaneous by 4 months of age.

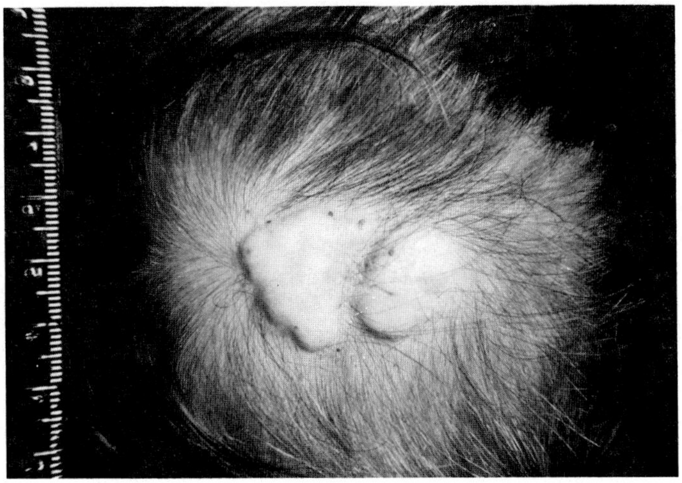

FIG. 55–10. Keloid of the scalp of a normal 1-year-old child who had an isolated posterior scalp defect at birth. A hypertrophic scar developed spontaneously during the first 3 months of life.

skin.[1,5–7,9,16] The areas resemble red or yellowish brown deflated balloons. Atrophic scars, aplasia cutis, telangiectasias, intense whealing after stroking, and red papillomas (*e.g.*, perioral, intraoral, perianal, vulvar) may be found. Additional cutaneous (*e.g.*, alopecia, nail), skeletal, ocular, dental, aural, and mental defects may be present.[3,6,7] Therapy is symptomatic and based on the major findings.

NAIL, SWEAT, AND HAIR DISORDERS

NAIL DISORDERS

Total absence (*i.e.*, anonychia), partial absence, or dysplasia of nails occurs in 25 known disorders.[1,3,5–7,16] Well known entities include anhidrotic ectodermal dysplasia and Apert, Ellis–van Creveld,

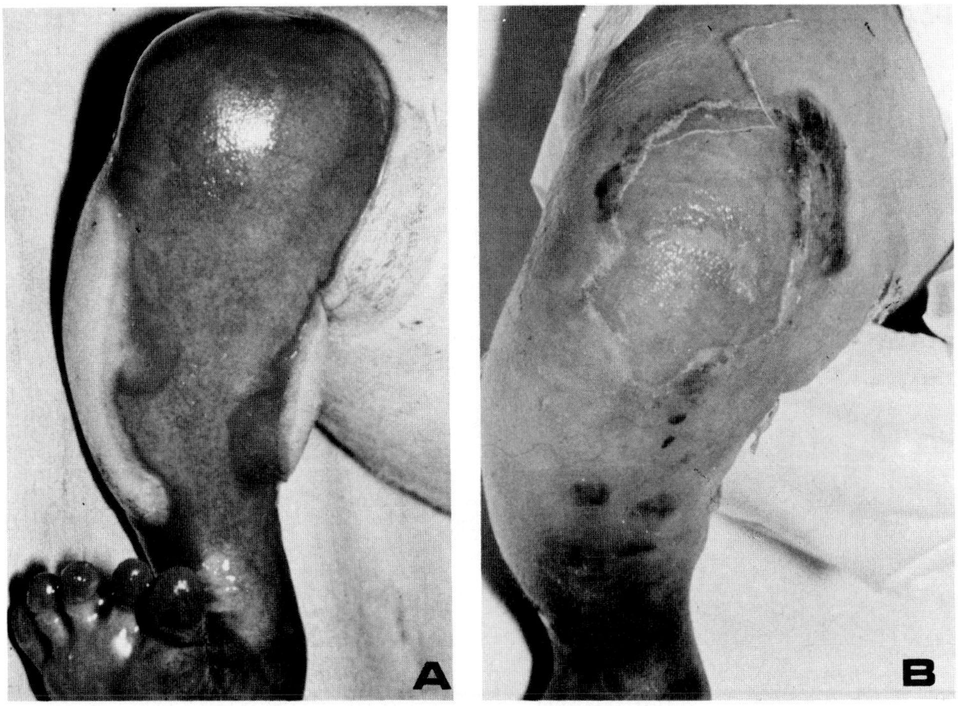

FIG. 55–11. **(A)** Cutis aplasia and epidermolysis bullosa simplex in a 4-day-old infant with absent epidermis of the leg. Note bullae on the toes. **(B)** The same patient with spontaneous healing at 6 weeks of age. (Courtesy of K. A. Gill, Jr., M.D.)

trisomy, and nail–patella syndromes. Many of these conditions will be apparent in the neonatal period; a large number are familial (Fig. 55-12). In general, etiology and pathogenesis are poorly understood; therapy is not available or needed.

HYPERTROPHIC NAILS

Hypertrophic nails, rarely observed in the neonate, may occur as familial onychogryposis, as congenital onychauxis, or in association with congenital hemihypertrophy or the pachyonychia congenita syndrome.[1,3,6,7,16] Treatment is relatively ineffective; amputation may be necessary for restoration of function.

SWEAT DISORDERS

ANHIDROTIC OR HYPOHIDROTIC SWEATING

Anhidrotic (*i.e.*, absent) or hypohidrotic (*i.e.*, decreased) sweating occurs in several disorders.[1,5,6] Anhidrotic ectodermal dysplasia with hypotrichosis and defective dentition is the most striking disorder and may be recognized during early infancy by absence of the eyebrow and eyelashes.[6,16] By 1 year of age, facies are distinctive with frontal bossing, flattened nasal bridge, depressed central face, and absent eyebrows. Alopecia occurs later. The skin is dry, hypopigmented, and thin with prominent vessels. Absence of sweat can be detected after 6 weeks of age by pilocarpine iontophoresis. Hyperpyrexia with fever of undetermined origin, caused by marked heat intolerance, often is the first major clue that brings the infant to the physician's attention. Therapy consists of a cool environment and application of wet towels during warm weather. Deficient lacrimation can be palliated by regular use of artificial tears; a wig will conceal severe alopecia. Genetic counseling is indicated because the disease is inherited in an X-linked recessive fashion; over 90% of patients are boys.[1,7]

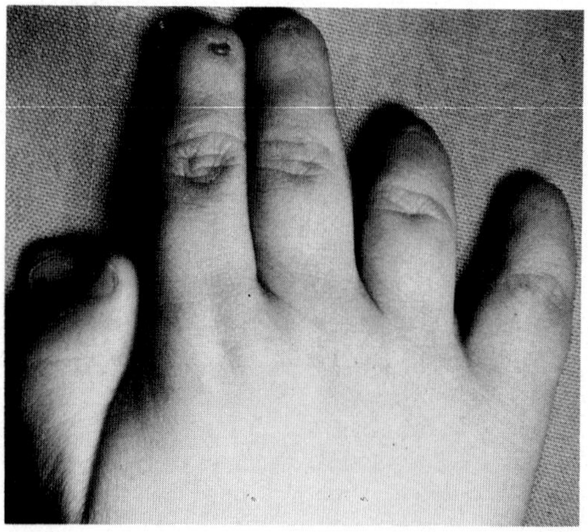

FIG. 55–12. Anonychia and hypoplasia of the nails in an infant who was otherwise normal. Similar nail defects with broad thumbs were present in five siblings and family members for five generations.

HAIR DISORDERS

Hair disorders rarely present as isolated defects.[1,5,6] Hypertrichosis, hypotrichosis, and abnormal morphology (*e.g.*, twisted, ringed, beaded, nodelike hair) usually are not appreciated until after the neonatal period. Exceptions are hypertrichosis of the De Lange syndrome and trisomy 18 and localized hairiness seen in congenital hemihypertrophy and diastematomyelia. Alopecia totalis congenita may occur alone or with hidrotic ectodermal dysplasia. Changes in hair color, caliber, and fragility may suggest a specific diagnosis. The best test is to perform dissecting microscopic examination of the hair shaft. Therapy is based on the specific diagnosis because many systemic disorders are associated with hair disorders.[1,3,5–7,16]

NEVI AND TUMORS

Many nevi and cutaneous tumors are not present at birth but develop during the early months of life. A nevus is a localized, highly differentiated, proliferative malformation arising from keratinocytes, melanocytes, or appendageal (*i.e.*, organoid) or vascular structures. Some dermal and epidermal nevi found in young infants are listed below. The type of nevus is described best by its origin or location, as in the terms melanocytic nevus, sebaceous nevus, and systematized nevus. Rare types also have been described.[1,3,5,16] The following is an outline of the classification of nevi.

- Dermal
  - Melanocytic: nevocellular or pigmented
    - Junctional
    - Intradermal
    - Compound
    - Giant hairy
    - Blue: common and cellular
  - Vascular
  - Connective tissue
    - Solitary nodular calcification
    - Osteoma cutis
  - Nervous tissue
  - Mixed
- Epidermal
  - Keratinocytic
    - Nevus unius lateris
    - Small verrucoid
    - Systematized verrucoid
    - Epidermal nevus syndrome
  - Appendageal (*i.e.*, organoid)
    - Sebaceous
    - Hair follicle
    - Apocrine duct
  - Melanocytic
    - Junction (*i.e.*, flat melanocytic)

MELANOCYTIC NEVI

Junctional, compound, and intradermal nevi rarely are encountered birth. They are classified histologically as follows: in junctional nevi, all melanocytes are above the basement membrane; in compound nevi, all melanocytes are in the epidermis and dermis; and in intradermal nevi, all melanocytes are in the dermis. In one study, pigmented nevi occurred in 2.4% of Caucasian newborns; in another, 1.1% of 4641 newborn infants had these lesions.[10]

BLUE NEVI

Blue nevi in newborns present in two forms. The common Mongolian spot (*i.e.*, cellular dermal melanocytoma) has been discussed.[10] The dermal melanocytoma (*i.e.*, blue nevus) appears rarely at birth as a grayish or steel blue 0.3- to 1.0-cm papule or nodule that grows slowly. Found on the buttocks and upper body, these nevi may be difficult to differentiate clinically from vascular lesions. If diagnosed clinically, routine follow-up is sufficient; otherwise, simple complete elliptic excision with histologic diagnosis is curative.

GIANT HAIRY NEVI

Giant hairy nevi (*i.e.*, congenital raised melanocytic nevi, nevocellular nevi [NCN]), larger than 20 cm, are present at birth in 4 of 4641 newborns[10] and may be found anywhere on the body. Less commonly found lesions on the neck and scalp may be associated with leptomeningeal melanocytosis and epilepsy or signs of focal neurologic abnormalities. Complete excision (Fig. 55-13) with plastic reconstruction should be performed by 15 years of age because the lesions may be associated with a 1% to 10% incidence of malignant melanoma in adults.[1,5,6,9,16] Depilation alone of associated small (<1.5 cm), hairy, intradermal nevi may produce a cosmetically acceptable result. Shave excision and electrodesiccation of hairy nevi in special areas (*e.g.*, eyebrow) may be more desirable than total excision with skin grafting.[1,6,9]

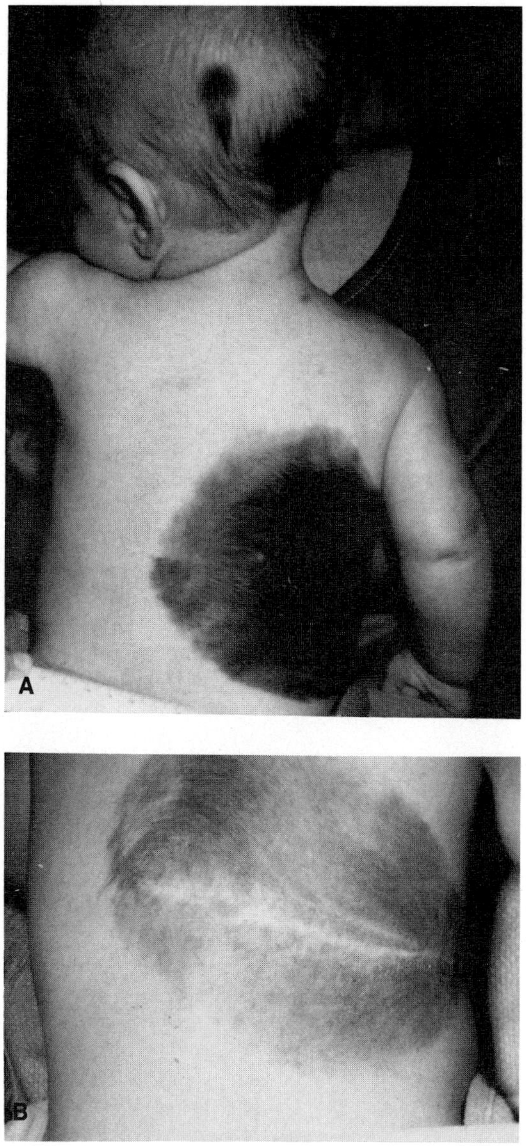

FIG. 55–13. (A) Giant hairy nevus in a 9-week-old healthy infant. Multiple smaller hairy nevi were present. **(B)** Same infant at 20 months of age after first wedge resection of the center of the nevus. Note the much lighter color of the entire nevus. (Courtesy of M. Boyajian, M.D., Childrens National Medical Center, Washington, DC.)

NERVOUS TISSUE NEVI

Nevi of neural origin, found in neurofibromatosis, rarely are observed in the newborn. Occasionally, these nevi may be part of a mixed cutaneous malformation with osseous defects (Fig. 55-14*A*). These congenital lesions may consist of hemangioma or lymphangioma tissue, nevus pigmentosus et pilosus, and plexiform neuromas. Localized hypertrophy with or without elephantiasis of tissues usually is seen; rarely, atrophy of the affected part is observed (Fig. 55-14*B*). In selected cases, surgical resection will improve function and appearance (Fig. 55-15). Fortunately, these lesions change very slowly over many years.[6,9,16]

Malignant skin tumors rarely are observed in the newborn period. Congenital melanoma has been described in one infant; basal cell and squamous cell carcinomas are very rare.[1,5,16,18] The following are congenital skin tumors and cysts:

- dermoids
- digital fibroma
- epithelial cysts
- fibrosarcoma, rhabdomyosarcoma
- lipomas
- mastocytomas

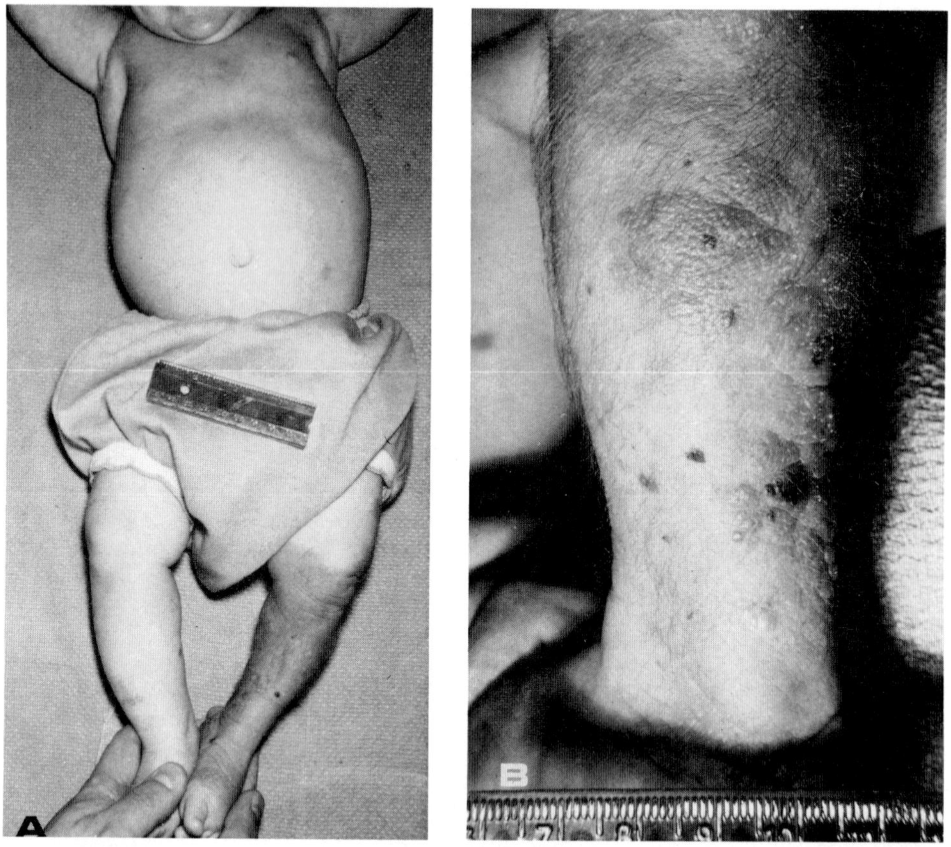

FIG. 55–14. **(A)** Mixed nevus with atrophy of the leg in a 3-month-old child. More than six café-au-lait spots larger than 1.5 cm are present. **(B)** Elements of lymphangioma circumscriptum (*i.e.*, angioma cystica), hairy pigmentation, and shagreen plaques are present.

- neuroblastomas
- neurofibromas
- teratomas
- xanthogranulomas.

Because of concern about malignant potential of congenital nevi, consultation is indicated. Potential precursors of cutaneous melanoma in children include small and giant congenital NCN, which are seen in 1% of newborns,[10,16] and dysplastic melanocytic nevi, which usually are seen during early adolescence.[9] Most small (<15 mm) NCN require no therapy. After a detailed history is obtained, the lesion should be examined carefully with a magnifying lens; it should be palpated and measured accurately. In cosmetically objectionable lesions, a photograph is invaluable for subsequent reference. Repeated assessment of the nevus every 6 to 12 months will help the physician decide whether excisional therapy is needed.[1,16,19] Excision of NCN should be considered in the following situations: for cosmetic reasons, particularly if the lesion is a large hairy nevus; repeated trauma to the nevus with changes in the lesion morphology; changes in the color, size, surface, or borders of the lesion, or if the lesion is pruritic, bleeding, or painful; the lesion appears atypical (*e.g.*, very dark, irregular pigmentation); or there is a positive family history of cutaneous melanoma or dysplastic nevi.[1,9,16] Histopathologic examination of all tissue removed is mandatory. Alper and coworkers noted that most congenital nevi are speckled at the periphery; all 47 nervous tissue nevi found in 4641 newborns showed an increase in skin markings.[10]

EPIDERMAL NEVI

Verrucoid nevi commonly seen in the neonate are local or systematized nevi and nevus unius lateris (Fig. 55-16). The latter lesion consists of linear or spiral, unilateral, hypertrophic papules or warty lesions in a continuous or interrupted pattern in single or multiple sites. They usually are found over the neck, trunk, or an extremity at a single site. Pruritus and inflammation may occur. Rarely, one-half of the body is involved and shows signs identical with those seen in congenital ichthyosiform erythroderma. Widespread linear, systematized, verrucous lesions may involve the oral mucosa, ocular conjunctiva, or

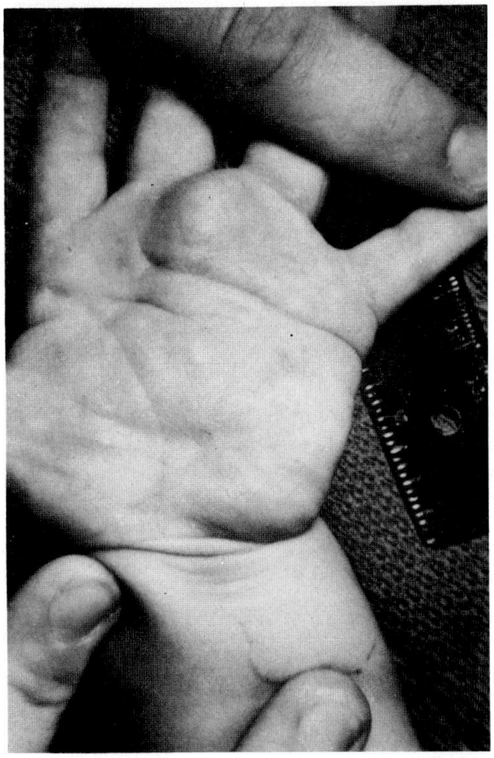

FIG. 55–15. Neurofibroma of the left wrist and hand in an infant. The larger left hand and swelling were noted at 9 months of age. Resection of a painful plexiform neuroma of the palmar area was performed at 2 and 6 years of age, resulting in improved function.

scalp.[1,3,16,18] Cases involving epidermal nevi, skeletal defects, vascular anomalies, and severe mental retardation, convulsions, or both (Fig. 55-17) were designated the epidermal nevus syndrome.[3,18]

Management consists of repeated observation and application of Eucerin or 10% urea cream to soften the lesions. Spontaneous improvement of the nevus unius lateris has been noted. Eventually, the verrucous epidermal nevus should be removed by plastic repair during late childhood.[1,18]

SEBACEOUS NEVI

This lesion, observed in the newborn over the scalp (Fig. 55-18) or forehead, is a discrete yellowish to yellowish brown or pinkish orange, cobblestoned, oval, hairless plaque.[10] It occasionally occurs on the face, ears, or neck. Untreated, these lesions change little, if at all, for years. A few eventually transform into basal cell epitheliomas; therefore, simple excision during late childhood is advised. Juvenile xanthogranuloma and syringocystadenoma papilliferum must be considered differentially in the young infant.[1,5,6,16]

CONGENITAL TUMORS

DERMOIDS

Dermoids (*i.e.,* epidermal inclusion cysts), which present at birth or soon thereafter, are round or ovoid 1- to 10-cm subcutaneous tumors of soft or rubbery

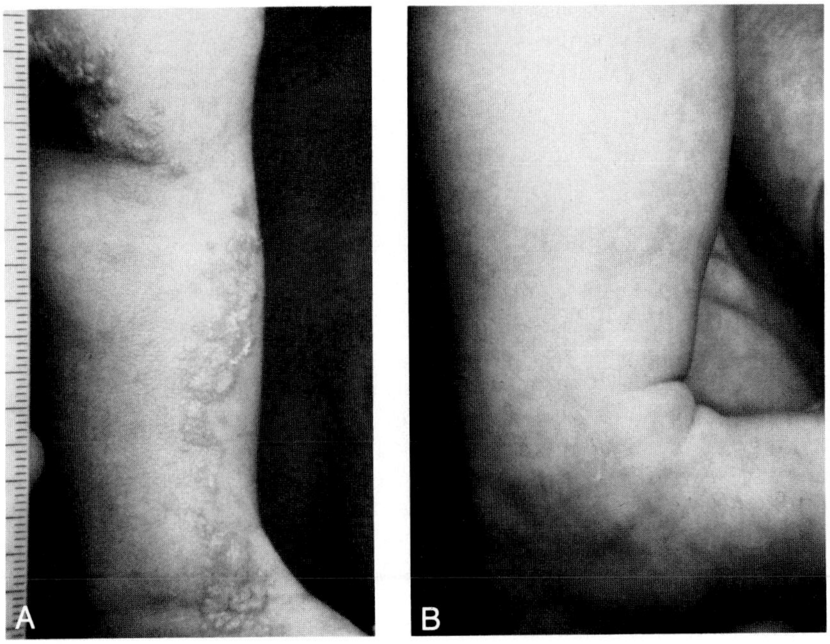

FIG. 55–16. Nevus unius lateris. **(A)** Left leg of a 13-day-old healthy infant with linear hypertrophic papules and warty lesions noted at birth. **(B)** Same infant at 3 months of age had spontaneous clearing of most of the lesions.

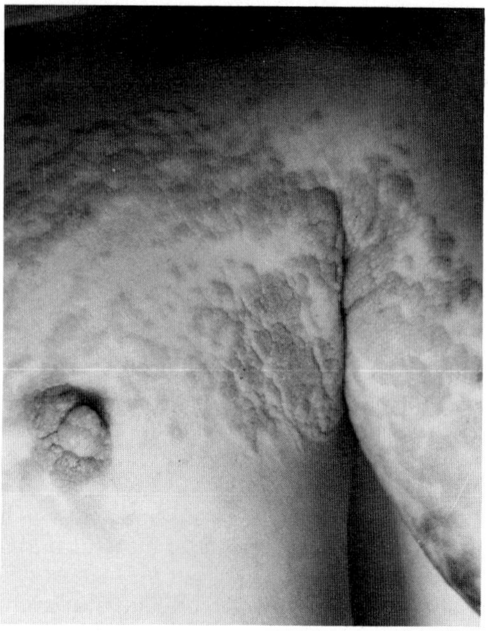

FIG. 55–17. Epidermal nevus syndrome. The left chest of a 5-month-old infant who had a large epidermal nevus that covered the left scalp, forehead, face, and upper chest at birth. Infantile spasms and severe mental retardation occurred at 2 months of age.

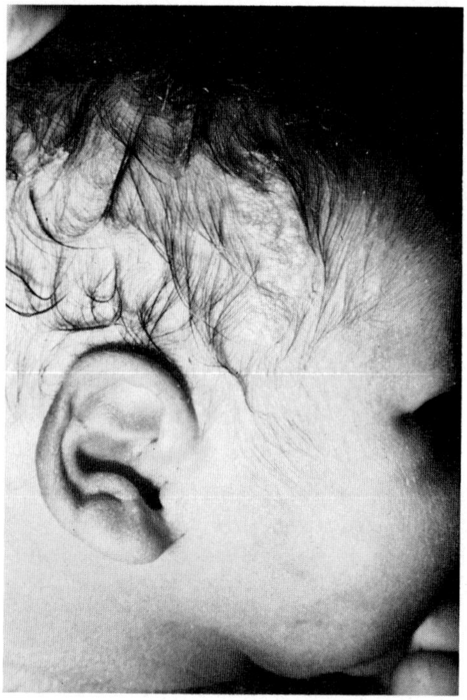

FIG. 55–18. Nevus sebaceous in a newborn infant's scalp. The cobblestone yellowish lesion remained unchanged after several years.

consistency.[20] They are encapsulated and contain sebaceous material and hair and often are located at the outer ends of eyebrows or on the neck, sternum, scrotum, perineal raphe, or sacrum. In one study, they were found in 58% of 775 superficial lumps.[20] Simple surgical excision is effective.[6]

NEUROBLASTOMA

Neuroblastoma, the most common cutaneous cancer at birth, is detected in one third of affected infants by the presence of 5 to 30 small (2–20 mm), bluish or pale blue nontender nodules (Fig. 55-19). Infantile neuroblastoma also may present with cutaneous blanching nodules.[16] Hepatomegaly and a retroperitoneal primary neuroblastoma frequently are present. Prognosis in this age group is excellent (90%) with surgery and chemotherapy.[16]

TERATOMAS

Teratomas present as neck, intraoral, or sacrococcygeal tumors. They are large (3–10 cm), firm, nontender, and fixed to underlying tissue. Multiple calcifications often are seen on radiographs. Epignathi (*i.e.*, intraoral teratomas) contain structures resembling fetal parts (Fig. 55-20). Prompt surgical excision is necessary for functional and cosmetic reasons. After the patient is 5 months of age, these tumors tend to reveal embryonal carcinomatous elements. Recurrences, if they appear, will do so within 2 years after removal. Epulis, a fibrous tumor of the gums, tends to resolve spontaneously.[16]

DEVELOPMENTAL VASCULAR ABNORMALITIES

Angiomas, or vascular nevi, are common cutaneous congenital malformations seen in 10% of infants,[1,21,22] but in only 2% of newborns.[10] Classifications and descriptions of these vascular tumors have been reported.[11,22,23] Two major groups seen in children are the involuting and noninvoluting vascular lesions, which may be flat (*i.e.*, macular or telangiectatic) or raised (*i.e.*, hemangiomatous).[11,21,23] The following is an outline of these abnormalities.

- Macular or telangiectatic nevi (*i.e.*, capillary)
  - Involuting
    - Salmon patch
    - Erythema nuchae
    - Infantile hemangioma
    - Cutis marmorata congenita (*i.e.*, livedo reticularis)
  - Noninvoluting
    - Port-wine nevus (*i.e.*, nevus flammeus)
    - Pyogenic granuloma (*i.e.*, granuloma telangiectaticum)

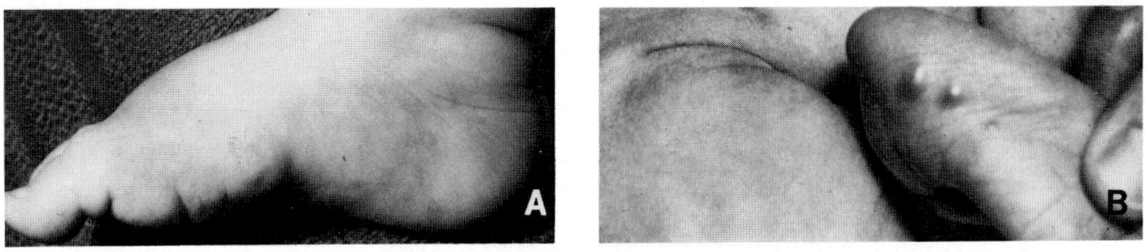

FIG. 55–19. (A) Neuroblastoma. Thirty cutaneous nodules and hepatosplenomegaly occurred in a 1-month-old infant. The nodules regressed after surgical removal of a retroperitoneal neuroblastoma and cyclophosphamide therapy for 1 year. The patient was well at 4 years of age. (Courtesy of S. Leikin, M.D., Childrens National Medical Center, Washington, DC.) **(B)** A 2-month-old infant had 13 violaceous nodules; excision of 8 of the nodules revealed neuroblastoma. No primary tumor was found; no treatment was given. The nodules involuted by 6 months of age; the patient was well at 3 years of age. (Courtesy of J.L. Kennedy, Jr., M.D., Saint Elizabeth Hospital, Boston, MA.)

Angiomatous nevi (*i.e.*, involuting)
- Strawberry (*i.e.*, capillary–endothelial)
- Cavernous–superficial, subcutaneous types
- Mixed capillary–cavernous, combined type
- Hemangioendothelioma
- Giant hemangioma with thrombocytopenia (*i.e.*, Kasabach–Merritt syndrome)

Cutaneous nevi with systemic hemangiomatosis
- Congenital multiple hemangiomatosis
- Phakomatoses
  - Sturge–Weber syndrome
  - Tuberous sclerosis
- Blue rubber bleb nevus

Vascular nevi and cutaneous vascular tumors
- Phlebectasia (*i.e.*, venous cavernous angiectasia)
- Hemangiectatic (*i.e.*, angiectatic) hypertrophy (*i.e.*, Klippel–Trenaunay–Weber syndrome)
- Angiokeratoma circumscriptum
- Mibelli porokeratosis

Vasoformative and noninvoluting lymphangiomas and lymphedema
- Simple lymphangioma
- Lymphangioma circumscriptum
- Cystic lymphangioma or hygroma
- Diffuse cavernous lymphangioma
- Lymphedema, congenital, hereditary

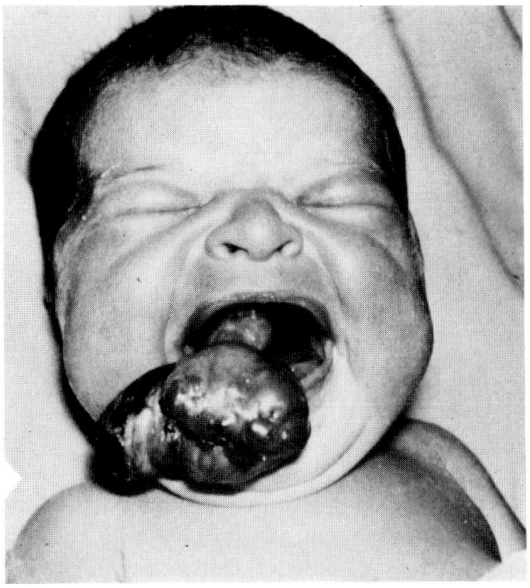

FIG. 55–20. Epignathi arising from a hard palate in a newborn infant. Surgical removal took place at 1 day of age; no recurrence was seen at 1 year of age. (Courtesy of W. Bason, M.D. and M. Museles, M.D.)

Studies of the common involuting types (*i.e.*, erythema nuchae, salmon patch, spider nevi or telangiectases, strawberry, cavernous, mixed strawberry–cavernous) have shown that no active therapy is necessary and that problems occur only when improper intervention is attempted. The natural pattern for the strawberry or cavernous hemangioma is rapid growth (*i.e.*, to double or triple in size) within several weeks or months during early infancy. At birth, the skin usually appears normal or shows a macular lesion that has a pink flush or off-white color. Occasionally, a tumor will be present at birth (Fig. 55-21). By 2 months of age, the strawberry lesion is bright red, or blue if cavernous type, in about 90% of infants. When maximal size is attained, usually between 9 and 12 months of age, the color becomes a dark red.

At this time the hemangioma remains quiescent; its growth rate is the same as that of the infant. By 12 to 18 months, often earlier, spontaneous involution begins. The color gradually fades to a grayish pink; a grayish white hue appears in the center of the lesion and spreads until the whole area becomes white or pink. There is a decrease in tenseness as involution progresses. Although the bulk of the lesion diminishes, the area of discoloration decreases very slowly over several years.

MACULAR STAINS AND TELANGIECTATIC NEVI

Involuting nevi, the salmon patch (*i.e.*, erythema nuchae), and cutis marmorata congenita or livedo reticularis, have been discussed previously.[22]

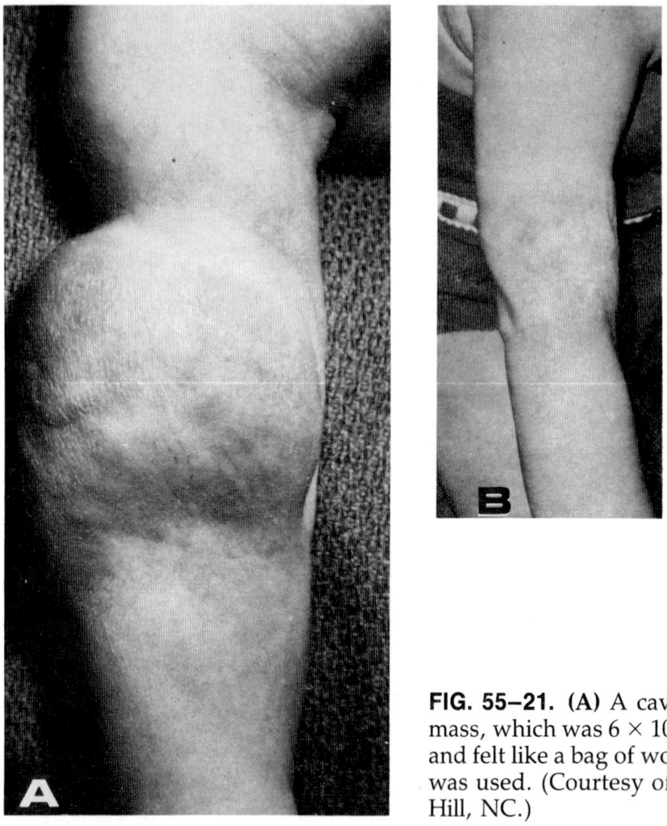

FIG. 55–21. (A) A cavernous hemangioma of the arm in 6-day-old infant. The mass, which was 6 × 10 cm × 1 cm elevated, was compressible (50%) and blanced and felt like a bag of worms. (B) The same patient at 15 months of age; no therapy was used. (Courtesy of E. Kraybill, M.D., University of North Carolina, Chapel Hill, NC.)

NONINVOLUTING NEVI

Noninvoluting nevi, seen less commonly in the newborn, are the port-wine nevus or stain and, rarely, the pyogenic granuloma. Granuloma pyogenicum is a rapidly growing, solitary, small (3–20 mm), dull red, papular lesion that bleeds easily. It is composed of granulation tissue with many capillaries and usually develops after minor skin trauma. Histologic examination is recommended to detect the rare benign juvenile melanoma.

PORT-WINE NEVUS

The port-wine (*i.e.*, nevus flammeus) nevus, which is present at birth, is a capillary angioma consisting of mature, dilated, and congested capillaries directly beneath the epidermis. The lesion is flat and sharply delineated, does not grow in area or size, and blanches minimally. It may be very small (*i.e.*, a few millimeters in diameter) or cover almost one-half of the body. In black infants, these nevi appear jet-black. The characteristic red or reddish purple color intensifies when the infant cries. Unfortunately, facial lesions are common. Involvement of the lower and upper eyelids (*i.e.*, first and second branches of trigeminal nerve) with the presence of convulsions, mental retardation, contralateral hemiplegia, or intracortical calcification suggests the Sturge–Weber syndrome.[1,3,6,7,11,21,24] Patients with upper eyelid port-wine stains alone had no eye or CNS complications.[22] Most port-wine nevi occur as isolated defects.[22] They may occur in trisomy 13, Rubenstein–Taybi, Beckwith–Wiedemann, and Klippel–Trenauney–Weber syndromes.[3,5,6,7,16] In a few children, the lesions may become lighter with age; however, they rarely disappear. A water-repellent cosmetic cream (*e.g.*, Covermark, Retouch) will conceal the mark effectively. Tattooing cannot be recommended because of possible scar formation and inability to match the color of the normal skin properly. Plastic surgical repair may be necessary in the older child because of the development of a verrucous, thickened nodular surface. Laser beam therapy appears to be cosmetically effective.[25,26]

ANGIOMATOUS INVOLUTING NEVI OR RAISED LESIONS

STRAWBERRY HEMANGIOMA

Strawberry hemangioma, or hemangioma simplex, is a capillary hemangioma, usually bright red or purplish red with well defined margins. Rarely present at birth, it usually appears within a few days or weeks as a pink or red macule, resulting from a myriad of tiny capillaries. The lesion enlarges during the first 5 to 6 months. The strawberry nevus blanches incom-

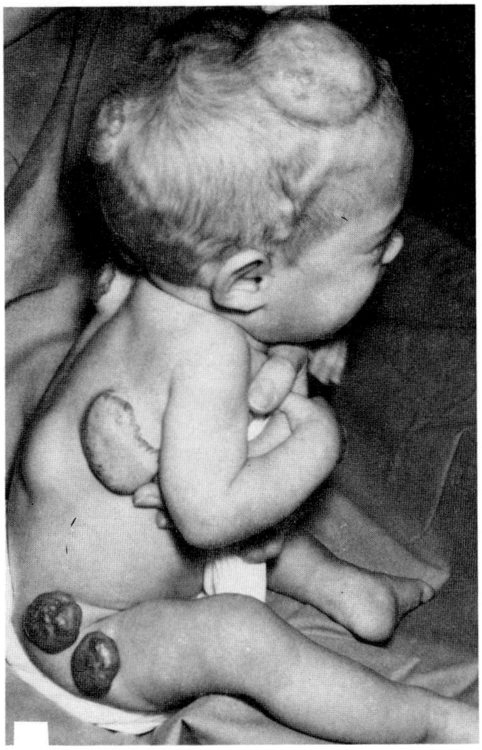

FIG. 55–22. A 7-month-old infant with 21 strawberry, cavernous, and mixed hemangiomas. No lesions were seen until 1 month of age. Between 7 and 8 months of age, one new lesion developed. Nine hemangiomas are visible over the scalp, back, and thigh. By 6 years of age, only three involuting lesions remained; these were gone by 12 years of age.

pletely with pressure, and on palpation is a firm, rubbery mass that compresses minimally. It is found on any part of the cutis and rarely involves mucous membranes. One or two are common; rarely, 20 or 30 lesions may be observed in an infant (Fig. 55-22).

CAVERNOUS HEMANGIOMA

The cavernous hemangioma arises deeper in the dermis, usually with poorly defined borders (see Fig. 55-21*A*), but may be well circumscribed and elevated (see Fig. 55-21*B*). The tumor, composed primarily of large venous channels and vascular lakes lined by mature endothelial cells, usually imparts a reddish blue discoloration to the overlying normal skin. On palpation, these lesions often are cystic and feel like a bag of worms. The swelling usually compresses to one-half of the original size and quickly resumes its usual size on release of pressure. When the infant strains and cries, the tumor often becomes larger and darker blue. The mixed (*i.e.*, combined) hemangioma consists of a cavernous lesion with an overlying strawberry component (Fig. 55-23).

NATURAL COURSE

The natural growth pattern of strawberry, cavernous, and mixed hemangiomas is a noticeable increase in size during the first 3 to 6 months of life, a stationary period of several months during which the hemangioma grows at the same rate as the patient, and then spontaneous involution. Based on the size of the hemangioma at 1 to 3 months, 80% of 420 hemangiomas observed in 308 children grew less than double in size. Six lesions continued to show minimal growth during the second year of observation.[23] About 5% tripled and 2% quadrupled their size. Six lesions continued to show minimal growth during the second year of observation. Because hemangiomas are benign and diagnosis is made easily by careful evaluation and repeated observation, a biopsy is not indicated.[1,3,21] In one series that extended over 20 years, the strawberry, cavernous, and mixed hemangiomas regressed spontaneously and at similar rates during an 8- to 10-year period.[27] By 5 years of age, one-half of these had involuted spontaneously. One infant I ob-

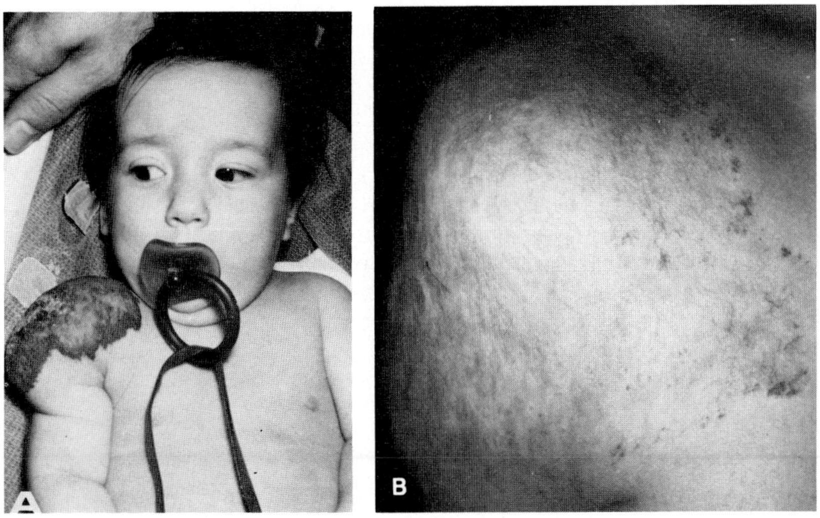

FIG. 55–23. (A) A combined hemangioma in a 4-month-old infant was first noted at 1 month of age. Rapid growth occurred until 2½ months of age. Ulceration developed at 3 months. The volume was 284 cm^3. **(B)** When the patient was 9 years and 10 months of age, the volume was 20 cm^3; this is a spontaneous reduction of 90%. The lesion disappeared by 11.5 years of age.

served had 33 hemangiomas that involuted spontaneously by 3 years of age.[28]

TREATMENT

Those vascular nevi located in exposed areas often cause great parental concern because of their cosmetic impact. Parental anxiety increases as the hemangioma grows and causes deformities, especially in the breast, lip, ear, or eye. Additional concern develops when ulceration or bleeding occurs from trauma, maceration, or infection.

Complications following unnecessary therapy are significant; they occurred in 12 of 20 of my patients treated elsewhere before referral.[28] Radiation and injection therapy caused greater morbidity and resulted in more extensive scarring than did surgery or dry ice. Seven of 19 hemangiomas showed subsequent growth within a few months after therapy. All these lesions involuted spontaneously.

By contrast, complications during spontaneous involution are infrequent. In decreasing frequency, these are ulceration, bleeding, and infection. If necessary, therapy after breakdown includes local saline compresses, cleaning measures, and an antibiotic ointment when indicated. Bleeding and secondary infection appear to be natural processes that are beneficial and hasten spontaneous involution. Residual scarring after complete involution is uncommon and rarely unsightly. Minimal bleeding, that is stopped by direct local pressure, occurs in about 5% of children.

Active treatment rarely is needed and must be determined individually.[11,21,23,25] Observation for sev-

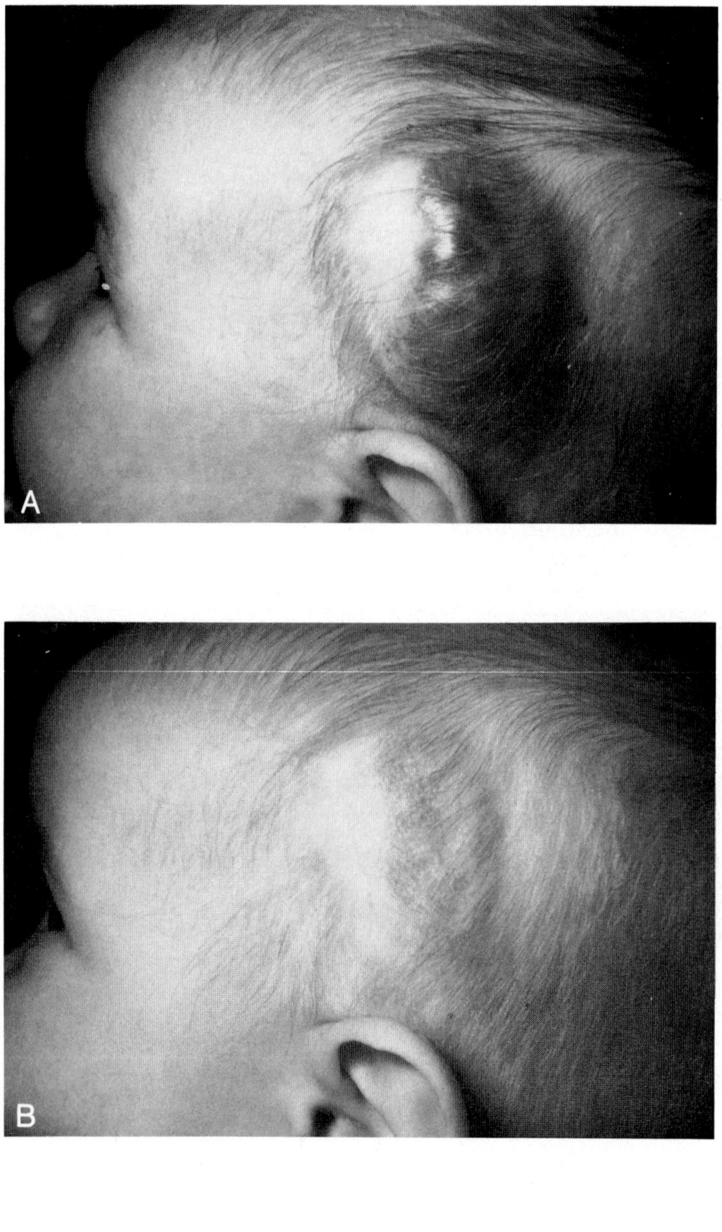

FIG. 55–24. **(A)** A cavernous strawberry hemangioma grew rapidly since birth in a healthy 5-week-old infant; the volume of the lesion was 42 cm^3. **(B)** At 4.5 months of age, the lesion was 90% involuted because of active daily compression and massage by the infant's mother 100 times per day.

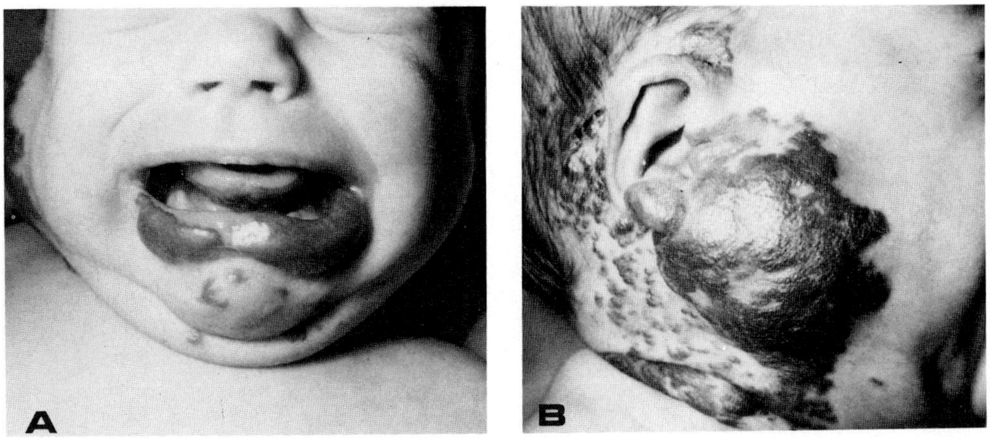

FIG. 55–25. **(A)** Strawberry hemangiomas of the lip and chin. **(B)** A combined dermal and right parotid hemangioma in a 6-week-old infant. The lesions were first noted at 5 days of age and continued to enlarge; new strawberry hemangiomas appeared on the neck and chin.

eral years usually is necessary. Color photographs should be taken of lesions on exposed areas to document the natural pattern of involution for other parents.[28] For the parent who wishes a more active yet conservative treatment, local massage or application of a compression bandage for 11 hours twice daily may be effective (Fig. 55-24).[28,29]

In rare instances in which the diagnosis is uncertain (*e.g.*, atypical growth pattern or no evidence of a vascular lesion), excisional biopsy may be required. In a patient in whom a hemangioma enlarges rapidly (*i.e.*, within a few weeks) and vital structures are compromised (Fig. 55-25) so that tissue destruction results, prednisone may be effective. Prednisone for 3 to 4 weeks was beneficial in 24 of 28 patients with hemangiomas obstructing the nares, auditory canal, or vision.[11,30] If signs of involution (Fig. 55-26) occur after several weeks of daily prednisone, therapy should be continued as alternate-day therapy for an additional 4 weeks. After 8 weeks, the prednisone should be stopped and the lesion observed for recurrence. Regrowth may occur; it was not noted in 26 of my 28 patients (see Fig. 55-26). A second course of prednisone may be effective when necessary. The use of intralesional corticosteroid injections has proved effective in treating capillary hemangiomas of the eyelid; however, visual loss may occur after injection.[31] Plastic surgery may be necessary for redundant tissue persisting after spontaneous regression or in a 5- or 6-year-old child whose lesion has not regressed.

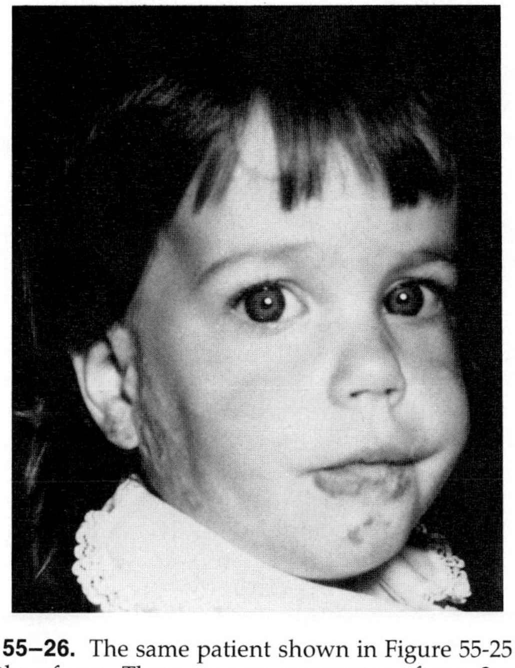

FIG. 55–26. The same patient shown in Figure 55-25 at 18 months of age. There was no recurrence after a 3-month course of prednisone, 10 mg, on alternate days.

Over 150 patients with giant hemangioma with thrombocytopenia (*i.e.*, Kasabach–Merritt syndrome) have been seen during infancy.[1,3,6,16,23] The hemangioma may be as small as 5 to 6 cm or consist of small, multiple hemangiomas involving dermal or internal organs. These hemangiomas usually are cavernous, with most occurring during the first few months of life.[1,5,16,30] Thrombocytopenia with or without hemorrhagic manifestations may be found shortly after birth or appear only after several weeks or months. Sequestration of platelets in the hemangioma has been demonstrated by infusion of chromium-51–tagged platelets and by biopsy studies. The hemangioma itself may suddenly enlarge because of bleeding.

Anemia, splenomegaly, and purpura with or without thrombocytopenia are reported. Therefore, close observation and appropriate hematologic studies are

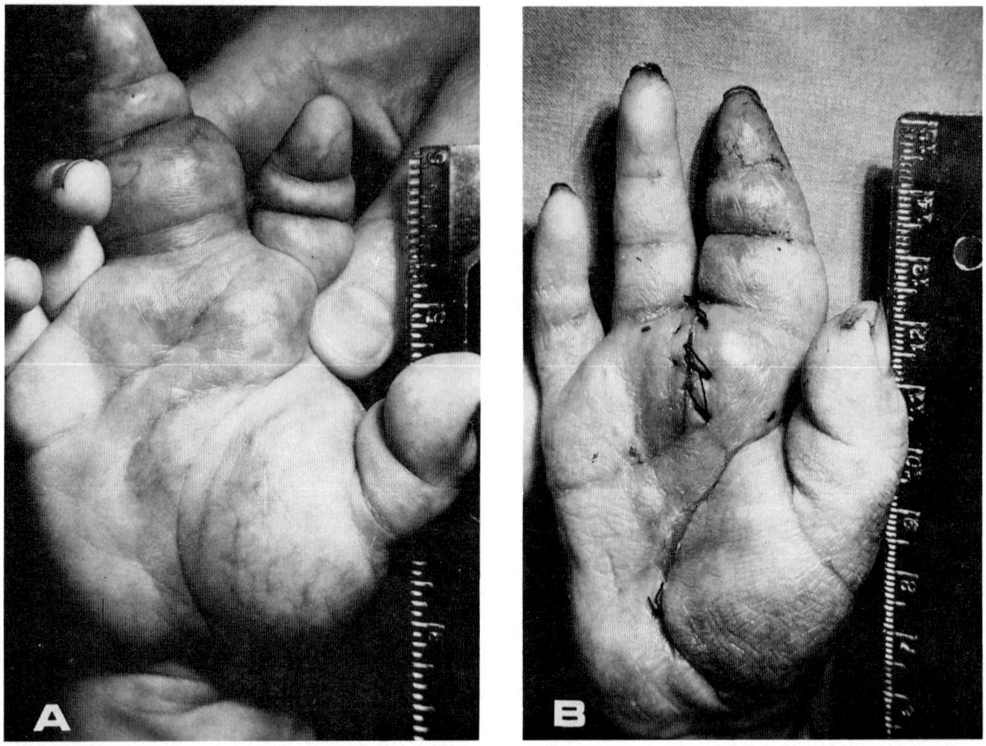

FIG. 55–27. **(A)** Hemangiectatic venous hypertrophy of the hand, arm, and shoulder of a 3-year-old child. The lesion was present at birth and enlarged slowly during the first 6 months of life. There was no growth in the following 2 years, but the hand functioned poorly. **(B)** The same patient at 3.5 years of age, 7 days postamputation of the middle finger. Subsequently, useful function of the hand returned.

indicated. Spontaneous resolution has been reported in a significant number of patients who were treated conservatively or who did not respond to x-ray therapy or splenectomy.[28,30] Prednisone for 1 to 2 months may be effective treatment. If feasible, compression of the tumor by an elastic bandage 10 to 20 hours daily may reduce its size within a few weeks.[28,29] Although x-ray therapy may be effective, the long-term effects are potentially serious.[11] Death may occur from infection or hemorrhage.

CUTANEOUS NEVI WITH SYSTEMIC HEMANGIOMATOSIS

Diffuse neonatal hemangiomatosis, an extremely rare condition, results in an early death in infants from cardiac failure, gastrointestinal hemorrhage, infection, or hydrocephalus from aqueductal compression by hemangioma. Criterion for diagnosis is the recognition of nonmalignant visceral hemangiomas in three or more organ systems; cutaneous hemangiomas in varying numbers (1–100 or more) are found concomitantly.[6,16]

Therapy is supportive. Perhaps oral prednisone in large doses (4–10 mg/kg daily) should be tried initially in these seriously ill infants, whose mean survival time is 71 days. Diffuse neonatal hemangiomatosis should be differentiated from the hamartomatous, Riley, and blue rubber bleb syndromes.[1,3,6,16,21]

OTHER VASCULAR NEVI AND CUTANEOUS VASCULAR TUMORS

Phlebectasia, or venous ectasia, a rare vascular lesion consisting of dilated mature vessels in the dermis and subcutaneous tissues, presents in two forms in the newborn or young infant. Single or multiple tumors resembling cavernous hemangiomas grow slowly and may be associated with hypertrophy of the extremity.[11] I observed three children with neck varicosities and four with unilateral leg or forearm lesions.[23,28] The other form, cutis marmorata telangiectatica with generalized phlebectasia, is apparent at birth and involves underdevelopment of subcutaneous and osseous tissues and other associated anomalies in 50% of patients. In both types, therapy rarely is necessary because steady improvement occurs with growth.[1,3,6,16,21]

Hemangiectatic hypertrophy (*i.e.*, Klippel–Trenaunay–Weber syndrome) of a limb associated with an extensive cutaneous nevus and a developmental hypertrophy of underlying bone and soft structures (*i.e.*, osteohypertrophic varicose nevus) is a rare congenital abnormality. It is seen more frequently in boys than in girls. The three major clinical features—hypertrophy of an extremity, vascular nevus, and venous varicosity—are not necessarily proportionate in extent and severity.[1,16] The nevus may be unilateral and the hypertrophy bilateral; minimal hypertrophy may be associated with an extensive nevus. Varicosity of the superficial veins with deep subcutaneous involvement may be a conspicuous feature noted at birth (Fig. 55-27). The nevus may be flat, strawberry, or cavernous with thickening and deformity of subcutaneous tissues. Occasionally, atrophy of bone, muscle, and soft tissue develops and, in fact, did occur in one of my eight patients. Selective amputation of a grossly malformed digit and orthopaedic measures to prevent limb hypertrophy will improve appearance and function (see Fig. 55-27). When lymphedema is extensive with gross deformity of an extremity, treatment with a sequential linear compression device 8 to 12 hours daily may be helpful.[32] Education of parents in care is essential.[27]

LYMPHANGIOMAS

Tumors of lymphatic origin, less common than hemangiomas, are hamartomatous malformations consisting of dilated lymph channels of various sizes lined by normal endothelium. Of four major types observed, each may be present at birth or develop during infancy or before the age of 5 years.[1,6,16,21,23] Generally, these tumors grow slowly or not at all. Clinical classification is difficult.[33]

Simple lymphangioma, the least common, presents as a solitary, well defined, skin-colored dermal subcutaneous tumor on the face or neck. Mucous membranes rarely are involved. Simple surgical excision usually is satisfactory.

Lymphangioma circumscriptum, observed most commonly, consists of small, thick-walled vesicles in the skin resembling frog spawn (Fig. 55-28). Sites commonly involved are axillary folds, neck, shoulder, proximal limbs (see Fig. 55-28*A*), perineum, tongue, and buccal mucous membrane.[6,10,16,23] Usually localized, such lesions may be extensive. Often a hemangiomatous component is present, including blood-filled vesicles (see Fig. 55-28*B*). Rarely, after several years of observation during which the lesion remains unchanged, the tumor will enlarge suddenly because of spontaneous bleeding or trauma.[11] Spontaneous involution is uncommon, occurring in only 1 of 10 patients in my series. Satisfactory results will follow complete surgical excision, which is difficult but necessary to avoid recurrence.[1,6,16,21,23,33]

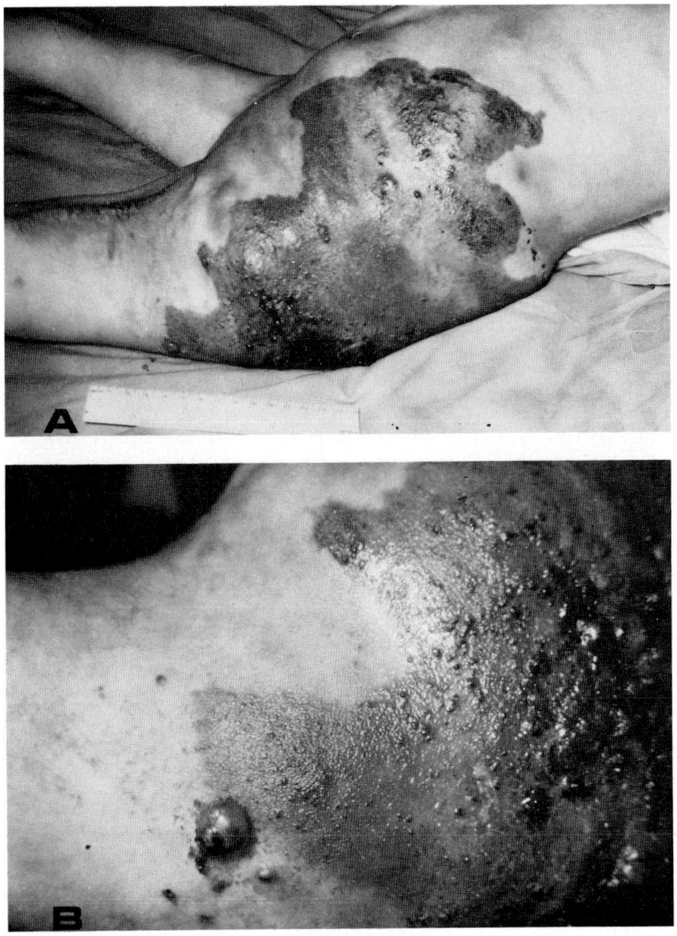

FIG. 55–28. **(A)** A giant hemolymphangioma involving the upper thigh, flank, and retroperitoneal areas was present since birth. Radical extirpation was necessary to drain a staphylococcal abscess within the mass. **(B)** Lymphangioma circumscriptum in the same patient show thick-walled vesicles (*i.e.*, frog spawn) overlying the tumor.

CYSTIC LYMPHANGIOMA, OR HYGROMA

Cystic lymphangioma, or hygroma, occurs most often in the neck (*i.e.*, hygroma colli) and axilla, but it may also occur in inguinal, popliteal, and retroperitoneal regions and as mesenteric cysts. These are usually large unilocular cysts, but they may also be multilocular, especially in the neck. Transillumination will be present unless bleeding occurs. Because these lesions may grow rapidly with infiltration of vessels and nerves, surgical excision should be considered, but surgical results are often unsatisfactory.[33] Spontaneous regression may occur.[1]

DIFFUSE OR CAVERNOUS LYMPHANGIOMAS

Diffuse, or cavernous, lymphangiomas are ill-defined cystic dilatations involving the skin, muscles, mucous membranes, and large areas of the face, trunk, and limbs (elephantiasis lymphangiectatica). Macroglossia and macrocheila[10] may occur because of involvement of the tongue and lips.[1,16,21] Recurrent local infections (pre- and postoperative) are common and will usually respond to specific antibiotic therapy. Surgical excision will effectively remove small lesions, although recurrences are common. Surgical extirpation of more diffuse lesions with multiple procedures is often unsatisfactory.[34,35]

LYMPHEDEMA

Congenital lymphedema occurs in two forms: as primary lymphedema, which mainly involves the lower extremities and occurs mostly in girls; and as Milroy disease (*i.e.*, hereditary lymphedema), which is almost always confined to the legs and feet. In Milroy disease, the edema is firm and the temperature of overlying skin is elevated. Its pathogenesis is unclear; treatment during infancy is unnecessary. In both conditions, upper extremities and genitalia may be involved.[1,3,7,16]

Rarely, chylothorax and chylous ascites may develop in infants with congenital lymphedema. The brawny edema that becomes permanent as progressive tissue fibrosis occurs, may respond to compression therapy 8 to 12 hours daily with a sequential linear compression device.[32] Antibiotics are effective for secondary streptococcal and staphylococcal infections. Reconstructive surgery may be helpful. Chronic recurrent obstructive jaundice with associated cutaneous hemangiomas, lymphatic anomalies, and lymphedema has been reported in several families.[35]

INFECTIONS OF THE SKIN

Blistering disorders in the neonate frequently result from infection of bacterial, fungal, or viral origin. The following is an outline of some of these eruptions.[36]

- Bacterial
  - Impetigo caused by *Staphylococcus* sp., group A streptococci, or group B streptococci
  - *Haemophilus influenzae*
  - *Listeria monocytogenes*
  - *Pseudomonas aeruginosa*
  - *Staphylococcus aureus* causing staphylococcal scalded-skin syndrome (SSSS) or toxic epidermal necrolysis (TEN; *i.e.*, Ritter disease)
- Fungal
  - Cutaneous candidiasis
  - Oral candidiasis (*i.e.*, thrush)
  - Mucocutaneous candidiasis
- Spirochetal
  - Congenital syphilis
  - Lyme disease[37]
- Viral
  - Cytomegalovirus (CMV)
  - Varicella
  - Variola/vaccinia
  - Herpes simplex
  - Herpes zoster

Blistering has not been reported in congenital rubella or toxoplasmosis.[16,37] Maculopapular eruptions, usually without purpura, occur in the neonate as a result of fungal, parasitic, and viral infections. When purpuric or petechial maculopapular eruptions are seen, the clinician must look for bacterial sepsis, hematologic disorders, histiocytosis X, or viral (*e.g.*, rubella) infections.[6] The following is an outline of various nonpurpuric and purpuric or petechial eruptions.

- Nonpurpuric
  - Aspergillosis
  - Coccidiodomycosis
  - Congenital syphilis (purpura may occur)
  - Lyme
  - Molluscum contagiosum
  - Toxoplasmosis (purpura may occur)
  - Warts
- Purpuric or petechial
  - CMV disease
  - Hematologic disorders
  - Histiocytosis X
  - Listeriosis
  - Rubella syndrome
  - Septicemia: group A and B streptococci, gram-negative bacilli

The clinical history and the morphologic characteristics of the cutaneous lesion (*e.g.*, maculopapular, with or without purpura, vesicobullous) suggest the differential diagnosis of a specific eruption.[16,36,37] Although a skin biopsy is simple and clearly delineates the cutaneous level of blister formation[1,3,5] or histologic nature of the eruption, it rarely is necessary. Routine or special cultures (*e.g.*, fungal, viral), stained smears, scraping using 10% KOH solution, or antibody titers, coupled with the history and morphologic findings, provide a diagnosis in most infants.[1,3,6,16,36,37]

VESICOBULLOUS ERUPTIONS

The following is a list of noninfectious disorders that produce vesicobullous eruptions.[16,36]

- acrodermatitis enteropathica
- acropustulosis of infancy
- arthropod-induced blisters (*i.e.*, scabies)
- bullous ichthyosiform erythroderma
- epidermolysis bullosa
- erythema toxicum neonatorum
- erythropoietic porphyria
- graft-*versus*-host disease (GVHD)
- histiocytosis X
- incontinentia pigmenti
- protein C deficiency
- transient neonatal pustular melanosis
- urticaria pigmentosa (*i.e.*, mastocytosis).

Bullous impetigo of the newborn, a superficial vesicopurulent pyoderma involving the stratum corneum, commonly occurs in the neonate and infant and usually is caused by staphylococci. The blisters vary from small vesicles to large, flaccid bullae filled with clear or straw-colored fluid. These rupture quickly and leave a red, moist denuded area (Fig. 55-29). Lesions may be widely dispersed and vary from a few single ones to large denuded areas. Because of thick stratum corneum, blisters over the palms and soles are less likely to rupture. Regional lymphadenopathy is rare unless ecthyma or secondary infection occurs with insect bites, eczema, scabies, herpetic lesions, or varicella.

Coagulase-positive *S. aureus* frequently are cultured on aspiration of bullae. Rarely, β-hemolytic streptococci or a gram-negative bacteria will be isolated. Group A streptococci usually produce omphalitis, paronychia, erysipelas, perianal cellulitis, or sepsis.[1,3,5,6,16,36] Skin abscesses or umbilical lesions can occur as a result of group B streptococci, although this is unusual. Blood cultures should be done if sepsis is suspected. Aseptic technique is essential to prevention in the hospital nursery. Infected infants should be isolated, with universal precautions carefully followed.

Topical therapy consists of cleansing the lesions with povidone–iodine (Betadine) skin cleanser three to four times daily for 5 to 7 days until no new lesions appear. Concomitantly, a bacitracin or 2% mupirocin ointment should be applied locally. For extensive lesions or symptoms compatible with sepsis, systemic antibiotics specific to the isolated organism are indicated.

STAPHYLOCOCCAL SCALDED-SKIN SYNDROME

Staphylococcal scalded-skin syndrome occurs primarily in children younger than 10 years of age, whereas TEN (*i.e.*, Ritter–Lyell disease) seen in adults, appears to be a hypersensitivity disease triggered by drugs, infection, vaccination, and malignancy.[1,5,6,16,36] Staphylococcal scalded-skin syndrome begins with an acute, painful, generalized erythema, followed rapidly by spreading bullous eruption and intraepidermal peeling, which closely resembles scalded skin. The skin is shed in sheets with minimal trauma (*i.e.*, Nikolsky sign). In my series of 46 children with SSSS, 5 infants younger than 6 months of age were observed; 3 had Ritter disease, 2 had bullous impetigo. Characteristically, the skin was tender and edema was noted about the mouth and eyes; low-grade fever (38°C; 101°F) occurred in 56% of 35 children. Within 24 hours of onset, vesicobullae were filled with clear, sterile fluid. Conjunctivitis, often purulent, developed with prominent perioral wrinkling of the skin (Fig. 55-30). Within 1 or 2 days, most bullae ruptured spontaneously with large, red, moist, denuded areas that became dry and tan or bronze. Within 48 hours of onset, the infants were less toxic, and exfoliation with large sheets of epidermis was widespread. Within 3 to 5 days, desquamation involved most of the erythematous areas, and by days 6 to 12, desquamation was complete. Cultures were positive for coagulase-positive *S. aureus*, in all five of infants seen at Childrens National Medical Center.

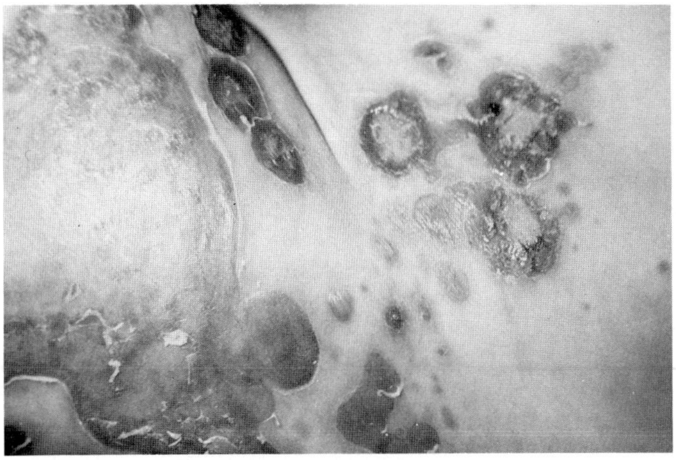

FIG. 55–29. Bullous impetigo in the groin of an infant. Note a collarette of scales around the red, superficial, ruptured pustules caused by *Staphylococcus aureus*.

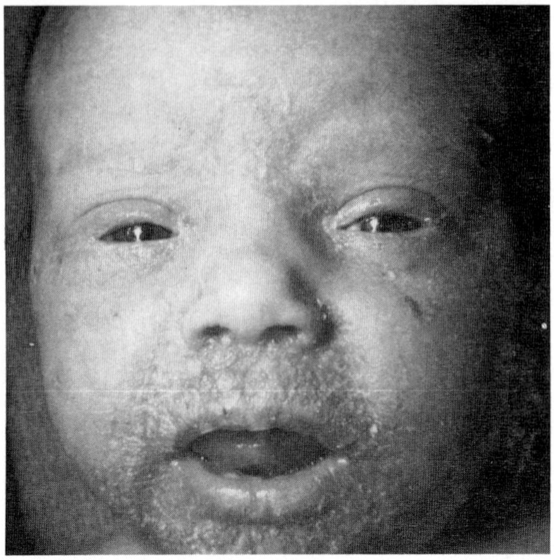

FIG. 55–30. Staphylococcal scaled-skin syndrome. This neonate had fever, exfoliative dermatitis, and positive *Staphylococcus aureus* blood culture for 2 days. Note the intraepidermal peeling with perioral crusting and rhagades of vermillion borders; *S aureus* was cultured from purulent conjunctivitis.

This syndrome includes Ritter disease, scarletiniform eruption, staphylococcal scarlet fever, and bullous impetigo of infancy.[5,6,16,36] The first three disorders have generalized cutaneous involvement; bullous impetigo usually is localized. In each disorder, *S. aureus* can be isolated from the nose, throat, conjunctivae, or skin. Bullae most often are sterile because they result from an exfoliative exotoxin produced by *S. aureus*. The staphylococci usually are phage type 71, group II, and penicillin resistant.

Differential diagnosis may include syphilis, listeriosis, EB, bullous erythema multiforme, and GVHD.[36] Erythema multiforme, extremely rare in young infants, is recognized easily by the typical target or iris lesions. Cultures and smears or dark-field examination would exclude bacterial or spirochetal infection. Family history and close observation over several days should exclude EB. Erythema multiforme major and TEN may be distinguished from the SSSS and acute GVHD by skin biopsy.[6,36]

Management of the rare, mild case of SSSS in an older infant consists of gentle washing of lesions with Betadine skin cleanser three times daily, followed by bacitracin or 2% mupirocin ointment and close observation. Younger infants require hospitalization in reverse isolation and systemic antistaphylococcal antibiotics.[38] Steroids are contraindicated. Fluids, electrolytes, and temperature should be monitored carefully. If denudation is extensive, compresses of sterile water or normal saline, to which 0.1% silver nitrate has been added, are effective. In the healing phase, tepid baths twice daily followed by application of Eucerin cream are effective for dry skin. Sulfacetamide sodium eye drops or ointment is effective for conjunctivitis. Recovery in most cases is complete in 9 or 10 days. Prognosis is excellent for patients younger than 5 years of age; death has been reported in 0% to 7% of cases. One death occurred in 46 of children seen at Childrens National Medical Center.

PHAGEDENIC OR ECTHYEMA-LIKE ULCERS

Phagedenic or ecthyemalike ulcers are small, circumscribed ulcers with black necrotic centers and erythematous areolas complicating preexisting lesions (*e.g.*, varicella, puncture wounds.) Severe debilitating disease, dysgammaglobulinemia, leukemia, or prematurity may be predisposing factors.[16,36] The umbilicus may serve as a portal of entry. Initially, the lesions appear as grouped erythematous opalescent vesicles that rapidly become green, and pustular and hemorrhagic at times. Because tissue is destroyed beyond the epithelium, ecthyma usually is followed by scars. *P. aeruginosa* is most frequently cultured; rarely, *S. aureus*, *β*-streptococci, or *Aeromonas hydrophila* may be isolated. Treatment with systemic ceftazidime and gentamicin should be prompt and vigorous because of the likelihood of severe sepsis.[38] For local lesions, polymyxin B, 0.1% solution in 1% acetic acid, may be useful. Silver nitrate 0.5% soaks also are effective. Soaks are applied locally for 1 to 2 hours, two or three times daily for 7 to 10 days.

If the clinical course is rapidly progressive with associated toxicity and involvement of the fascial planes overlying muscle, necrotizing fasciitis, a severe soft tissue infection, must be considered and treated vigorously.[6,16]

LISTERIOSIS

Listeriosis, caused by *L. monocytogenes*, may produce serious infection (*e.g.*, sepsis, meningitis) or disseminated miliary granulomatosis in the neonate.[3,16,39] A small percentage of infants show gray papules or papulopustules that resemble miliary abscesses at times. These may be widespread or localized to the back, oropharynx, or conjunctiva, where they appear as small, white foci. Occasionally, generalized erythema, maculopapular, or petechial–purpuric eruptions have been reported. The organism may be isolated from the pustule, blood, or spinal fluid. It is a gram-positive bacillus that produces hemolysis on blood agar. Treatment is with systemic penicillin or ampicillin and gentamicin.[38]

FUNGAL INFECTION

Fungal infection of skin in the newborn is uncommon except for candidal vesicopustular diaper rash and thrush. Persistent oral or diaper candidal infection occurs in over 65% of children infected with human immunodeficiency virus (HIV).[39]

PARONYCHIAL INFECTIONS

Paronychial infections, occasionally seen in young infants, are most often secondary to thumbsucking or local injury. Continuous wetness and sucking results in maceration and secondary mixed infection caused by *Candida* species and *S. aureus* or *P. aeruginosa*.[5,6,16] Red, swollen skin at the nail base with purulent discharge suggests a bacterial infection. Exudate rarely is seen with candidal infection. After cultures are taken, a finger cot, partially filled with Betadine ointment or skin cleaner, is taped over the finger for 7 to 10 days. Drainage is facilitated, and infection usually resolves without need for systemic antibiotics or surgical incision. Candidal paronychia usually responds to topical application of nystatin or Lotrimin cream with a cotton applicator to fill the gap between the nail plate and posterior nail fold. The finger must be kept perfectly dry, since *Candida* species thrive in a moist environment.[6,16]

CONGENITAL SYPHILIS

Congenital syphilis, if untreated, will produce a maculopapular or bullous skin eruption in about 50% of infants between 2 and 6 weeks of life.[6] Bullae, and maculopapular or maculosquamous lesions occasionally are seen at birth on the palms and soles; infants with these lesions tend to have a more severe disease. These vesicles are of irregular size and contain a cloudy fluid teeming with spirochetes that can be seen by dark-field examination (Fig. 55-31). When the lesions rupture, the denuded area dries and crusts or macerates if moisture is present. The most common eruption consists of erythematous or copper-colored maculopapular ovoid lesions of the palms and soles, which may spread over the entire body. Mucocutaneous lesions about the mouth, anus, and genitalia, and snuffles with a highly infectious nasal discharge may be the first clinical manifestations of the disease, occurring in one third of infants.[1,6,16] Fissures may

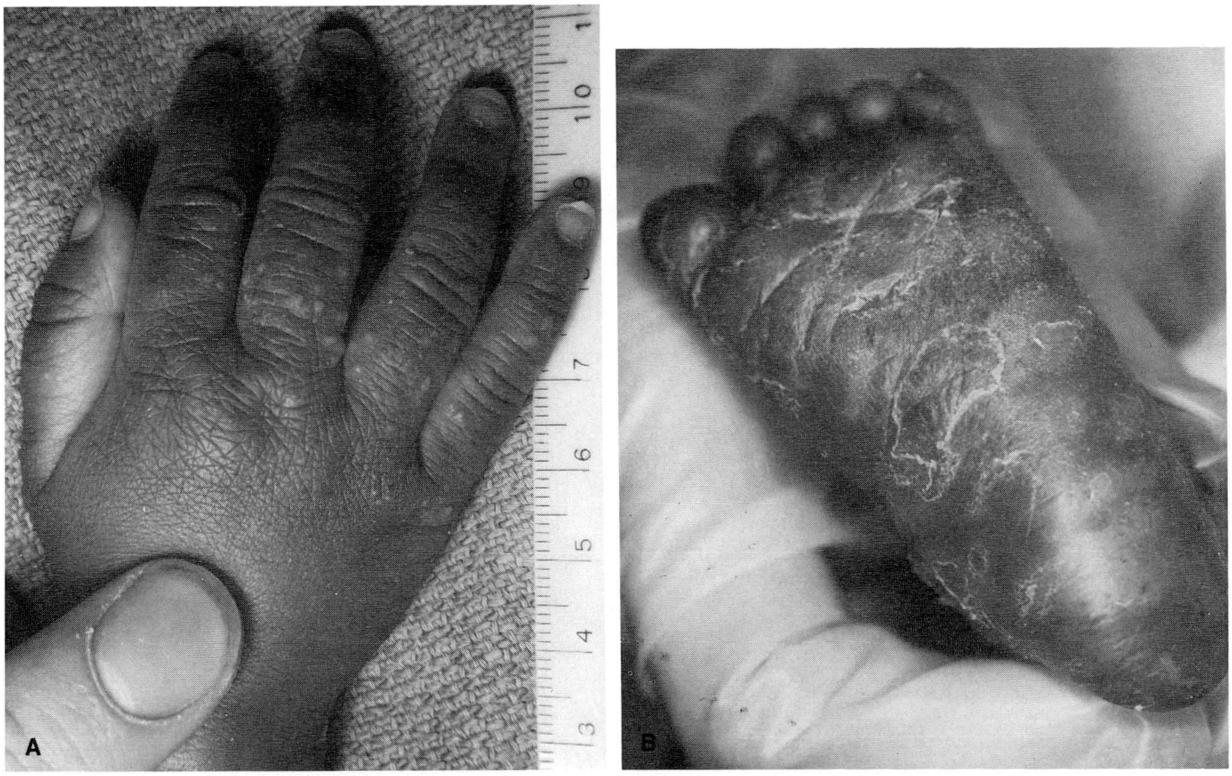

FIG. 55–31. (A) Pustules on both hands and feet in a 4.5-month-old infant who had sniffles and respiratory congestion for 3 weeks, was VDRL positive and had VDRL-positive parents, and showed periosteal new born formation in radiographs of long bones. Dark-field aspirate of pustules showed many spirochetes. **(B)** Full-term girl born at 41 weeks of gestation to a 24-year-old quadripara with a history of drug abuse. Examination of the infant was negative except for marked hepatosplenomegaly and extensive exfoliation of skin, especially palms and soles. RPR was 1:256; CSF FTA 2+. Radiographs of the knees showed new bone periosteal formation of the femurs. Penicillin therapy was effective. (Courtesy of Joseph L. Kennedy, Jr., M.D., Saint Elizabeth Hospital, Boston, MA.)

develop in these moist areas and, on healing, result in fine periorofacial scars (*i.e.*, rhagades). Raised, flat, moist lesions, condylomata lata, may appear at angles of the mouth, nares, or anogenital region. Mucus patches may be seen on the lips, tongue, and palate. If untreated, the skin lesions regress spontaneously in 1 to 3 months, leaving residual hyperpigmentation or hypopigmentation.

The routine VDRL on the mother invariably is positive. If the infant is infected, the serology will be positive in 85% of infants at 1 month of age, 95% at 2 months of age, and 100% by 3 months of age. An infant's serologic titer higher than the maternal titer is diagnostic. Other clinical features are reviewed elsewhere (see Chap. 48).[1,3,6,16] Therapy consists of intramuscular aqueous procaine penicillin, 50,000 units/kg/24 hours in two divided daily doses over 10 to 14 days.[38] Monitoring should continue with the infant having a monthly quantitative titer for 6 months, then every 3 months for a year so that adequate therapeutic response is ensured. Serologic reversal usually is expected in 1 year. An examination of cerebrospinal fluid is recommended before therapy and 12 to 24 months after therapy.[16,38] All physicians should be alert for this disease because of its increased incidence.[1,40,41]

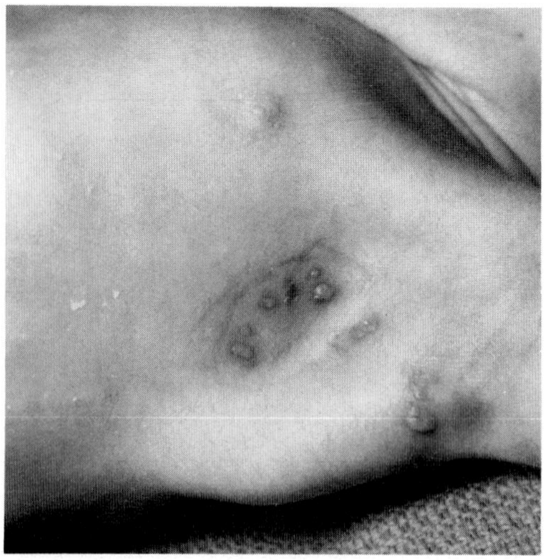

FIG. 55–32. Herpes simplex vesicles in the axilla of a 12-day-old infant with severe type 2 herpes encephalitis of 3 days' duration. The lesions cleared in 12 days. Severe mental retardation developed.

VIRAL EPIDERMAL LESIONS

Viral epidermal lesions usually present in the neonate or young infant with a characteristic morphologic picture.[1,2,9,16] Vesicles are seen in varicella, variola/vaccinia, herpes simplex, and herpes zoster; the virus may be isolated from early lesions. These diseases manifest in unusual and severe forms in infants with acquired immunodeficiency syndrome (AIDS).[1,6,9,16] Multinucleated balloon cells and eosinophilic mononuclear cells may be seen on a Giemsa-stained Tzanck smear from scrapings of the base of a fresh vesicle in the herpes group (*e.g.*, simplex, varicella-zoster).[1,6,16] Rarely, they are detected in the pox group (*e.g.*, variola, vaccinia). Petechial–purpuric lesions occurred in CMV inclusion disease and congenital rubella. Papular eruptions are characteristic of molluscum contagiosum and warts.

HERPESVIRUS HOMINIS SIMPLEX

Herpesvirus hominis simplex infection is one of the most potentially serious viral diseases in infants. Cutaneous lesions are uncommon at birth in the absence of ruptured membranes but develop at any time up to 21 days in 72% of affected infants. Lesions vary from a few scattered depressed scars or a local boggy swelling to one (Fig. 55-32) or many discrete groups of vesicles. A zosteriform distribution may occur. Vesicles may coalesce and become erosive. Cutaneous lesions can recur up to 5 years of age at the original site or in different areas.[16] Concomitantly, erythema multiforme may occur in some infants. Acyclovir should be started as soon as this infection is suspected because the prognosis is guarded.[1,6,16,42,43] Two thirds of infants in whom encephalitis develops either die or live with mental retardation or hemiparesis.[43,44]

VARICELLA-ZOSTER

Varicella-zoster, a rare transplacental infection, is one of the least threatening infections to the fetus and newborn. Varicella occurring in the first 10 days of life probably has been acquired *in utero*, because the incubation period is 10 to 21 days. The vesicular eruption, lesions, and course of disease are identical with the signs of varicella at any age.[37] Although a mortality of 20% has been reported, the course of neonatal varicella has been mild in most patients. In two of my patients, depressed white scars were observed at birth; each mother had varicella during the first trimester. Scars in a zosteriform distribution have been seen.[3,16] Rarely, neonates with congenital varicella will have visceral involvement.[1] Acyclovir may be effective if given within 24 hours of the onset of rash; intravenous Varicella-zoster immune globulin (VZIG) may modify the course of disease if given shortly after exposure.[45]

Vaccinia virus and variola infections rarely are seen in the neonate. Abortion or stillbirth may occur if the mother is vaccinated or maternal variola occurs.[3] Congenital vaccinia may be associated with cutaneous scars, ocular damage, and hypoplastic bony defects.

PETECHIAL, PURPURIC, AND MACULOPAPULAR ERUPTIONS WITH INFECTION

CYTOMEGALOVIRUS INCLUSION DISEASE

Cytomegalovirus inclusion disease usually is recognized in a small-for-dates infant with jaundice, lethargy, pallor, petechiae, or purpura with hepatosplenomegaly and chorioretinitis. Thrombocytopenia accounts for the purpuric lesions. In a few infants, generalized dark blue and magenta papules or nodules occur as a result of collections of extramedullary dermal erythropoiesis. These regress in 2 to 3 weeks, leaving dark red to pale gray macules. Differential diagnosis includes sepsis, toxoplasmosis, rubella, syphilis, and herpes simplex infections. Isolation of CMV from urine or liver biopsy with a rising complement fixation titer will confirm the diagnosis.[1,45] Treatment with intravenous ganciclovir and CMV immune globulin may be beneficial for retinitis, but experience in neonates is limited.[38,45]

RUBELLA

Rubella infection in the neonate produces purpura in 35% of infants. Petechiae and purpura often are seen at birth; new lesions rarely develop after several days of age unless thrombocytopenia is severe. Most lesions have faded by the second week and are gone by 4 to 6 weeks of age. The most unusual cutaneous finding is the blueberry-muffin lesion noted at birth in severely affected infants. These firm, bluish red papules, 2 to 8 mm in diameter, occur over the head, trunk, and extremities. They are caused by dermal erythropoiesis and resolve spontaneously in 3 to 6 weeks, unless death occurs. Cutis marmorata, slate blue discoloration of dependent extremities and capillary flushing, is reported.[1,3] Isolation of these infants from susceptible personnel is mandatory because the virus is excreted for months to years.[6,45] Septicemia caused by streptococci or gram-negative bacilli, toxoplasmosis, CMV, and syphilis should be considered in the differential diagnosis. Therapy is supportive.[45]

MOLLUSCUM CONTAGIOSUM

Molluscum contagiosum, very rarely seen in neonates, is caused by a poxvirus.[1,45] The benign lesions are characterized by discrete, waxy papules with a pink, tan, or ivory hue and central umbilication. Size varies from 1 mm to 1 cm, and lesions are found anywhere. The lesions are self-limiting after 6 to 12 months. Hundreds of lesions should raise suspicion of AIDS. Treatment is not necessary unless new lesions develop by autoinoculation. Treatment consists of removal by curettage or by blistering with 0.7% cantharidin in colloidin, used in minute quantities under an occlusive plastic tape for 12 hours to enhance blister formation.[1,6,16,36] Examination of a curetted plug after clearing debris with 10% KOH will reveal the typical molluscum bodies.

WARTS

Warts, extremely uncommon in the newborn or young infant, are caused by a virus of the papova group. Mucous membrane warts (*i.e.*, condylomata acuminata) occasionally are seen in older infants on moist mucosa of the anus, genitalia, or mouth.[46] A VDRL always should be done.[6] Anogenital warts can be acquired through direct contact with maternal lesions at delivery,[6,45] or by nonsexual contact with family members.[46] The treatment of choice is 20% podophyllin in compound tincture of benzoin, applied carefully to the lesion for 4 to 6 hours and then washed off. Applications are repeated weekly for several weeks.

TOXOPLASMOSIS

Toxoplasmosis, relatively uncommon in neonates, is caused by an intracellular parasite, *Toxoplasma gondii*. It is a transplacental infection with features simulating those found in erythroblastosis fetalis, rubella syndrome, CMV infection, or bacterial sepsis. A generalized maculopapular rash has been seen in 25% of infants, with hepatosplenomegaly, jaundice, fever, and anemia. The rash tends to spare the scalp, palms, and soles and rarely persists longer than 2 weeks. Desquamation and hyperpigmentation have followed severe eruptions.[1] Diagnosis is made by observation of rising titers, measured by the Sabin–Feldman dye test or a fluorescent antibody test to detect fetal IgM antibody to *T. gondii*.[1,45] Therapy is with pyrimethamine and sulfonamides.[1,45]

Both coccidioidomycosis and aspergillosis, extremely rare in the neonate, may produce maculopapular nonspecific eruptions.[1] Vesicopustules have been reported in aspergillosis, and vesicles have occurred in the former disease. Systemic or disseminated disease is more likely in patients with AIDS. Clinical features and therapy with amphotericin B are discussed elsewhere.[1,16,45]

NONINFECTIOUS BLISTERING DISEASES

ACRODERMATITIS ENTEROPATHICA

The classic tetrad of diarrhea, periorofacial vesicobullous dermatitis, alopecia, and apathy is diagnostic of this rare disorder. Acrodermatitis enteropathica usually presents during the first year of life (average age, 2 weeks–9 months) and is characterized by remissions and exacerbations. Premature infants and those with AIDS may have severe disease.[9] Acrodermatitis enteropathica may occur in breast-fed infants.[6] Symmetric vesicopustules, which usually evolve into chronic, persistent, erythematous eczematous patches, may be seen over the trunk and extremities.[1,6,9] Low plasma zinc levels (≤ 65 μg/dL) should establish the diagnosis. Zinc gluconate or sulfate therapy, given two times a day in a dosage of 5 mg/kg/day is very effective and may prevent death.[1,6,9]

TABLE 55–2
NEONATAL EPIDERMOLYSIS BULLOSA

Type	Inheritance
Nonscarring: Intraepidermal and Junctional Separation	
Epidermolysis bullosa simplex, generalized and superficialis	Autosomal dominant
Junctional epidermolysis bullosa letalis	Autosomal recessive
Scarring: Dermolytic Subepidermal Separation	
Dominant dystrophic	Autosomal dominant
Recessive dystrophic (*i.e.*, polydysplastic)	Autosomal recessive

ARTHROPOD-INDUCED BLISTER

Bites and stings, although uncommon in the young infant, may product erythema, blisters, wheals, and rarely a gangrenous slough. Lesions tend to be localized or in a linear arrangement. Spiders (*e.g.*, brown recluse) and scorpions can produce severe reactions locally and systemically.[5,6,16,36] Intense erythema rapidly progresses through a blister, sometimes hemorrhagic, to sloughing of skin. The blister beetle may produce a subepidermal blister. Papular urticaria, caused by flea, fly, mosquito, bedbug, moth, wasp, or bee stings, characteristically develops on the distal extremities in a symmetric pattern. Lesions may become purpuric and occasionally develop over the trunk and face if repeated bites occur. Pruritus with secondary excoriations often is seen in the infant. Local therapy consists of cool tap water compresses or baths, diphenhydramine (Benadryl), 5 to 10 mg/kg/24 hours, and calamine lotion or 1% hydrocortisone cream applied three times a day. Oral steroids rarely are necessary.[1,6,16,36]

Mite infestations (*i.e.*, scabies) may be considered, especially if the parent, sibling, or family pet has a pruritic rash.[1,5,6,16,36] The gray or flesh-colored burrows vary in length up to 1.5 cm and commonly occur on the palms, soles, head, axillae, and neck. Vesicles often appear at the end of the burrow. Because of the intense pruritus, excoriations, eczematous changes, and secondary infection are common. Diagnosis is confirmed by presence of ova, mites, or fecal concretions seen microscopically from scrapings of burrows. Mineral oil is placed on a glass slide and on the tip of a no. 15 scalpel blade. The skin lesion or underside of the fingernail is scraped, and the material obtained is placed back into the drop of oil. A cover slip is applied, and the specimen is examined microscopically.[5,6,16,37] Larvae of *Diptera* sp. may be similarly identified.[1] A very effective treatment for the entire family with scabies is 5% permethrin cream (Elimite). The cream or lotion is applied from the neck down on dry skin for 8 to 14 hours. The skin is then bathed. Parents are advised that itching may persist for several weeks; diphenhydramine (Benadryl), 5 to 10 mg/kg/24 hours, may be needed. A second application of Elimite for 8 hours only may be necessary in 1 week if new burrows, vesicopustules, or papulonodular lesions occur.[1,5,6,16,36] Bacitracin or mupirocin ointment applied three times a day will be effective for secondary infection.

EPIDERMOLYSIS BULLOSA

Pearson has classified this rare hereditary mechanobullous disease into two major subgroups: nonscarring and scarring EB. Five of the subtypes (Table 55-2) may occur at birth or in early infancy.[1,3,5,6,16] The disorder is identified further by location of blister formation in the intraepidermal, junctional, or subepidermal layers produced as a result of minor trauma. At least 17 distinct hereditary types of EB have been described.[6,16,37]

NONSCARRING EPIDERMOLYSIS BULLOSA

Nonscarring EB presents in three forms: epidermolysis bullosa letalis (EBL), which is extremely rare; and epidermolysis bullosa simplex (EBS), in generalized or superficialis forms. Characteristically, in EBS, the legs, feet, and scalp show erosions or peeling skin that heal slowly without scars. Blisters can be produced within a few hours by gentle rubbing, as in most forms of EB. Bullae may contain blood (Fig. 55-33). Pyogenic infection may be prevented by proper skin care and aseptic technique. Protection from minor trauma is essential. Clean, soft cotton or fleece dressings may be helpful over pressure points. Bacitracin or 2% mupirocin ointment should be used after Betadine skin cleanser two or three times daily for secondary infection. Maceration must be avoided. Emollients (*e.g.*, Nivea or Aquaphor cream) will prevent dry skin. Prognosis for EBS is good, with a tendency to improve by adolescence. Education of parents is essential.[6,27,36]

Sheets of epidermis loosen with minimal trauma (*i.e.*, dermal–epidermal separation) in EBL. The oral mucosa is severely affected.[6,16] The resulting moist erosions become infected, ulcerate, and develop vegetating granulomas. Multiorgan involvement, septi-

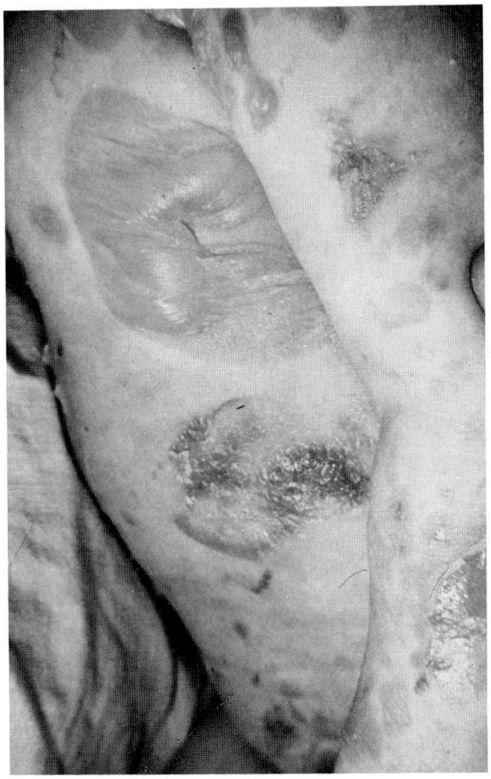

FIG. 55–33. Nonscarring epidermolysis bullosa (EB) in a 4-month-old infant whose sister died in infancy of EB letalis. The vesiculobullae noted at birth recurred often until the patient was 2 years of age, when improvement began. The patient was much improved at 17 years of age.

cemia, growth retardation, and anemia are common.[5,16] The prognosis is poor when large, denuded areas continually develop. In a few patients, lesions heal spontaneously and completely. Treatment is protective, palliative, and supportive, particularly with good nutritional supplements.[6,36] Heat should be avoided; cool water compresses to traumatized skin and air conditioning are helpful. Local and systemic antibiotics are indicated for secondary infection.[1,5,6,16,37]

DOMINANT DYSTROPHIC EPIDERMOLYSIS BULLOSA

Dominant dystrophic EB (*i.e.*, dermolytic bullous dermatosis), seen uncommonly in the newborn, is less severe than the recessive type of scarring EB (see Table 55-2). Lesions usually appear well after birth on the hands, feet, and sacrum secondary to minimal trauma. Nails may be lost, but deforming scars and contractures are infrequent. Mucous membrane lesions occur but are mild. Hypopigmentation and hyperpigmentation with soft, wrinkled scars are observed with healing. Therapy is the same as noted previously for EBS. Disposable diapers should be used. Adhesive tape should never be used on the skin. Once blistering has occurred, lancing the bullae, applying cool wet soaks for 15 minutes, and then applying 2% mupirocin ointment or silver sulfadiazine (Silvadene) cream and Telfa pad dressings encourage wound healing.[5,6,16,36] Silvadene is contraindicated in neonates as long as hyperbilirubinemia remains a threat.[36]

RECESSIVE SCARRING POLYDYSPLASTIC AND DYSTROPHIC EPIDERMOLYSIS BULLOSA

Recessive scarring polydysplastic and dystrophic EB initially appear to be benign in the neonate, except rarely they may present with congenital localized absence of skin (*i.e.*, Bart syndrome; see Fig. 55-11).[16] Eventually, after many months, the toe and finger blisters heal with pseudofusion of the digits and loss of nails (Fig. 55-34*A*). Finally, over several years, the hands and arms become fixed in a flexed position and contractures ensue. A positive family history helps differentiate this type from EBS and dominant scarring EB. Consanguinity has been reported. During early infancy, a skin biopsy to localize depth of blister formation (Fig. 55-34*B*) may help to differentiate the severe scarring and nonscarring types,[2,3,6,16,36] and rule out bullous congenital ichthyosiform erythroderma. Therapy is similar to that for other forms of EB. For large nonhealing erosions, wound dressings (*e.g.*, Vigilon, Second Skin, Duo Derm) may be useful.[6,16,36] Oral phenytoin (Dilantin) therapy has been helpful in some patients with recessive dystrophic EB.[1,16]

ERYTHROPOIETIC PORPHYRIA CONGENITA

This rare autosomal recessive disease, caused by a defect in heme synthesis, may be seen in the newborn. Because of severe photosensitivity, usually in late infancy, burning, pruritus, erythema, and vesicobullous eruptions develop on sun exposure. Ulcerations and secondary infection are common. Scarring and loss of nails, digit, and cartilage of the ears and nose develop later. The urine may be pink or red. When teeth erupt, they are stained pinkish brown and have a red fluorescence under ultraviolet illumination. Systemic and cutaneous manifestations are progressive, and there is a decreased life expectancy. Excess uroporphyrin I and orange-red fluorescence of erythrocytes are diagnostic. Therapy is symptomatic and includes protection from light with application of sunscreen creams and appropriate management of hemolytic anemia and infection.[1,5,16]

INCONTINENTIA PIGMENTI

Incontinentia pigmenti, affecting primarily skin, is an uncommon disorder that is either autosomal or X-linked dominant and prenatally lethal to boys.[1] Extra-

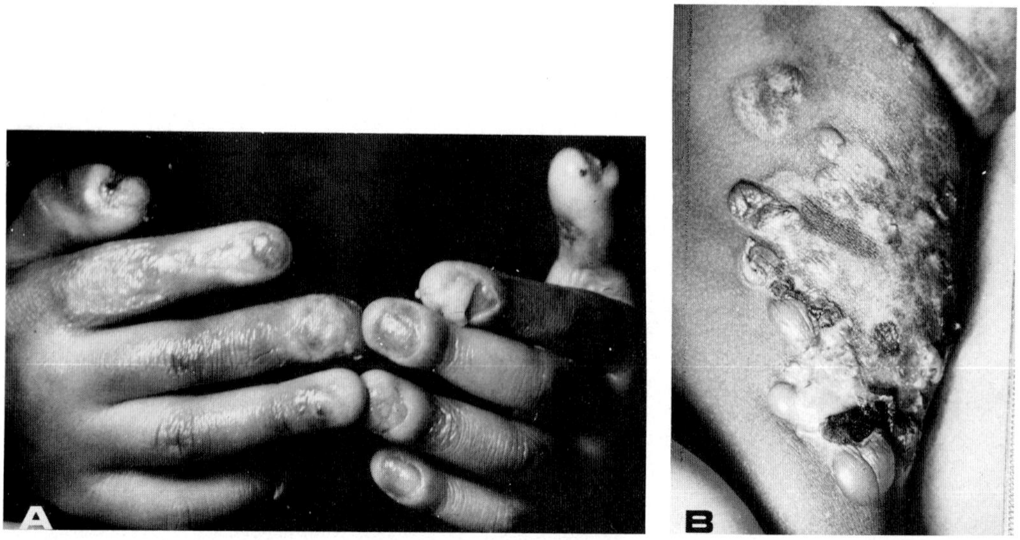

FIG. 55–34. Dystrophic scarring epidermolysis bullosa in a 3.5-year-old boy whose fingernails and toenails were absent at birth. At 1 week of age, recurrent clear and hemorrhagic blisters developed after minor trauma. **(A)** Atrophic scarring of the fingertips occurred. **(B)** The thigh showed blisters and dystrophic scars at 18 months of age.

cutaneous defects of the eyes, central nervous system, teeth, heart, and bones often are seen after the neonatal period and denote the Bloch–Sulzberger syndrome, which occurs in 30% of patients.[1,5,6,7] The girl–boy ratio is 9:1 or greater. At birth or shortly thereafter, inflammatory vesicobullae and papules (Fig. 55-35) erupt in linear crops over the trunk or limbs. After several months, pigmented hypertrophic or verrucous lesions appear that gradually resolve, usually by 1 year of age,[6] and form macular pigmented whorls and brush-stroke lines (Fig. 55-36). These bizarre brown or slate gray macules are diagnostic and should alert the physician to watch for retarded development, microcephaly, seizures, ocular pseudotumors, pegged teeth, and cardiac defects. Eosinophilia (65%) is present during the vesicular stage; the subcorneal vesicles are filled with eosinophils. No therapy is required for the skin. Genetic counseling is advisable.[1,5,6,27] Approximately 50% of patients with incontinentia pigmenti achromians, or hypomelanosis of Ito (see Pigmentary Lesions), have internal abnormalities.[1,5,16]

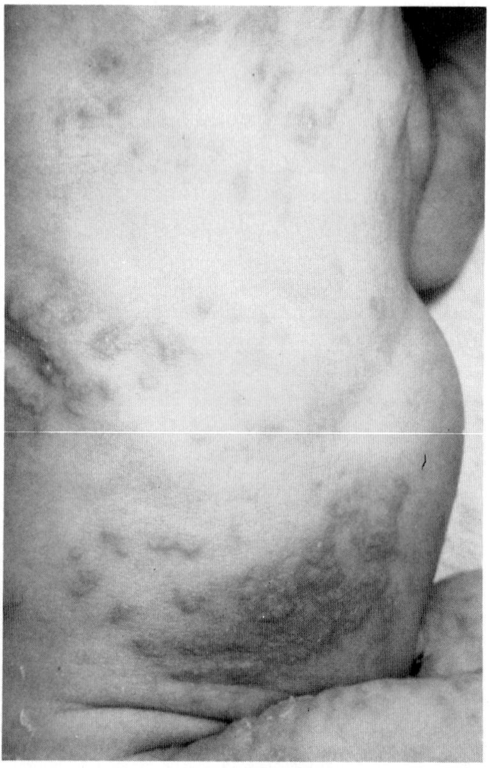

FIG. 55–35. Incontinentia pigmenti in a 1-week-old infant. Erythematous vesicles and papules developed at 4 days of age and progressed to pigmented whorls by 6 months of age. No other defects were present. The mother had similar pigmented linear macules on the thigh.

URTICARIA PIGMENTOSA

CUTANEOUS MASTOCYTOSIS

Cutaneous mastocytosis (*i.e.*, mast cell disease), rarely observed in the newborn, is not uncommon during infancy. In young infants, the lesions may be single or multiple sterile bullae, appearing primarily on the trunk, limbs, or scalp. A single 2- to 6-cm

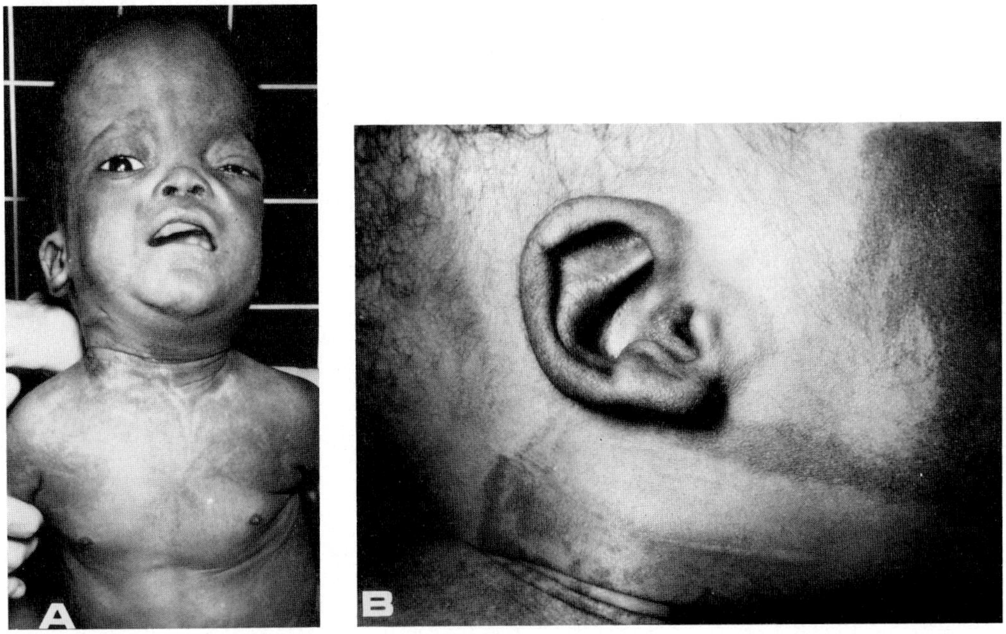

FIG. 55–36. (A) Bloch–Sulzberger syndrome in a 6-month-old infant who demonstrated incontinentia pigmenti, ocular pseudogliomas, mental retardation, hydrocephalus, and heart disease. **(B)** Note the typical pigmented brown brush strokes on the face.

mastocytoma may be seen. In older infants, disseminated maculopapular or nodular eruptions occur. As many as 20 to 400 tan to light brown lesions may develop gradually. Minimal rubbing may produce urtication (*i.e.*, Darier sign; Fig. 55-37) within a few minutes. This reaction is diagnostic, occurring in 90% of patients. Spontaneous resolution of lesions occurs over several years. About 50% persist through puberty, with residual hyperpigmentation.[1,5,6,16,36]

SYSTEMIC MASTOCYTOSIS

Systemic mastocytosis is rare in infants but occurs in about 5% of patients with mastocytosis.[1,5] Diffuse mast cell proliferation occurs in the skin, bone, liver, nodes, spleen, and bone marrow. In addition to presenting with multiple blisters (Fig. 55-38), these infants manifest episodes of flushing, irritability, tachycardia, respiratory distress, hypotension, pruritus, diarrhea, and abdominal pain. Cutaneous biopsy may be diagnostic.[1,6,16,36] Therapy, rarely necessary for cutaneous lesions, is difficult in infants with extensive lesions. Cyproheptadine hydrochloride (Periactin), not to exceed 0.5 mg/kg/24 hours in four divided doses, or diphenhydramine (Benadryl), 5 to 120 mg/kg/24 hours in three or four doses orally, will alleviate pruritus and irritability. Rubbing of skin and hot water must be avoided. Aspirin, codeine, opiates,

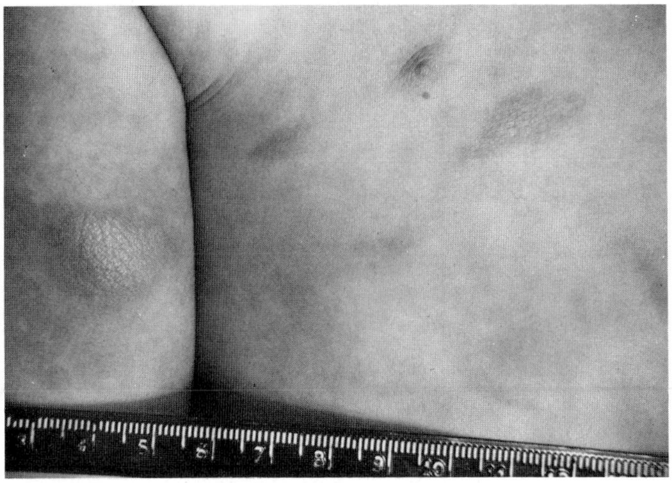

FIG. 55–37. Urticaria pigmentosa (*i.e.*, mastocytosis) in a healthy infant with 30 maculopapular truncal lesions. Note the positive Darier sign on the arm, produced after a similar lesion was stroked ten times.

TABLE 55–3
TYPES OF ICHTHYOSIS IN INFANTS

Condition	Incidence	Age at Onset	Inheritance	Clinical Features	Associated Features
Ichthyosis vulgaris (*i.e.*, ichthyosis simplex)	Common (1 : 250)	Usually after 3 months of life	Autosomal dominant	Scales: fine, branny, white Forehead and cheeks involved Extensor extremities and back involved Flexures always spared Increased palmar and plantar markings	Localized shiny hyperkeratosis of knees and elbows Atopic dermatitis common (50%) Family history positive for atopy Keratosis pilaris common
Sex-linked ichthyosis	Uncommon (1 : 6000)	Birth to 3 months of age	X-linked recessive; female–male transmission	Scales: thick, dark brown, large, tightly adherent Lateral face, neck, and scalp most severely affected Abdomen involved more than back Limbs: total involvement common Flexures variably affected Palms and soles normal	Dirty appearance of scales Only boys affected Occasionally, collodion membrane at birth Deep corneal dystrophy by slit lamp Normal cellular kinetics
Lamellar ichthyosis (*i.e.*, nonbullous congenital ichthyosiform erythroderma)	Rare (1 : 300,000)	Birth (*i.e.*, collodion baby)	Autosomal recessive	Scales: flat, dark, large, coarse Upper face more than lower face Uniform generalized hyperkeratosis of trunk Limbs: generalized involvement Flexures always affected (dry) Palms and soles thickened	Universal erythroderma Prematurity common Collodion membrane possible Harlequin fetus, the most rare and severe Ectropion present and progressive Increased epidermal mitotic
Epidermolytic hyperkeratosis (*e.g.*, bullous congenital ichthyosiform erythroderma, ichthyosis hystrix)	Rare (<1 : 100,000)	Birth to 6 months of age	Autosomal dominant	Scales: hard, verrucous, small Face relatively spared Limbs and trunk variably affected Flexures always affected (moist) Palms and soles usually affected	Variable erythroderma Bullae, recurrent during infancy and childhood Increased epidermal mitotic rate

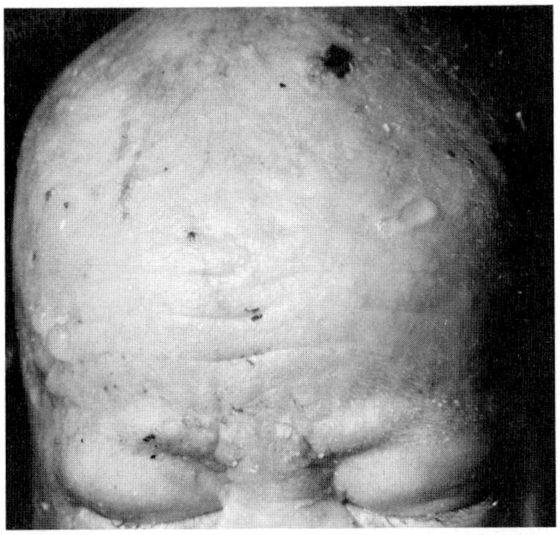

FIG. 55–38. Systemic mastocytosis in a 2-month-old infant. At 2 days of age, bright red macules that urticated and vesiculated with trauma were noted. Episodes of flushing and severe diarrhea occurred. Hepatosplenomegaly, pulmonary infiltrates, and anemia were present. (Courtesy of N. Movassaghi, M.D., Childrens National Medical Center, Washington, DC.)

and procaine are contraindicated because severe reactions may occur after histamine release from mast cell granules. Prognosis is good for cutaneous mastocytosis but poor for systemic mastocytosis.[1,5,6,16]

SCALING DISORDERS

Desquamation of skin occurs in 75% of newborns. It is observed commonly in infants of 40 to 42 weeks of gestation and rarely, if ever, in those under 35 weeks of gestation. Maximum shedding is observed by the end of the first week of life. Differential diagnosis of the scaly infant includes physiologic desquamation, dysmaturity, and the rare ichthyosiform dermatoses. Three of the four major types of ichthyosis (Table 55-3) may be present at birth.[6,16,36] These are gender-linked ichthyosis, nonbullous congenital ichthyosiform erythroderma, and bullous congenital ichthyosiform erythroderma. Ichthyosis vulgaris, the most common and benign form, rarely is observed before the third month. The well known terms "harlequin fetus" and "collodion baby" are descriptive only and not separate types of ichthyosis (see Table 55-3). Very rare syndromes (*e.g.*, Netherton, Sjögren–Larsson, Rud, Conradi, Refsum, Tay) have been reviewed elsewhere.[1,3,5,7,16,36]

X-LINKED ICHTHYOSIS

This relatively mild disorder occurs in boys only; however, in female heterozygotes scaling of the arms and lower legs may be present. In boys, the entire body is involved except palms and soles, midface, and flexural areas. Scales are large, yellow to dark brown, and thick (Fig. 55-39). At birth, the infant may present as a collodion baby or simply as a scaly infant. In one series, 36% were affected at birth; only 6% were unaffected by 3 months of age. Prognosis is good, and therapy (see Management) is simple.

LAMELLAR ICHTHYOSIS OR NONBULLOUS CONGENITAL ICHTHYOSIFORM ERYTHRODERMA

At birth, this autosomal recessive disorder may present in a healthy infant with generalized brilliant erythema or as the rare collodion baby (Fig. 55-40). Desquamation is universal, and with drying, the skin assumes a parchmentlike appearance. In general, these infants do well. After the neonatal period, scales develop that vary from a yellow to brownish black color and eventually form warty excrescences or thick horny plates covering large body areas in childhood. Secondary infection may occur if the skin becomes macerated, especially in intertriginous areas. Prognosis generally is good except for the extremely rare harlequin fetus for whom therapy is ineffective; death usually occurs from sepsis during the neonatal period (Fig. 55-41)[1,3,5,6,16,36]

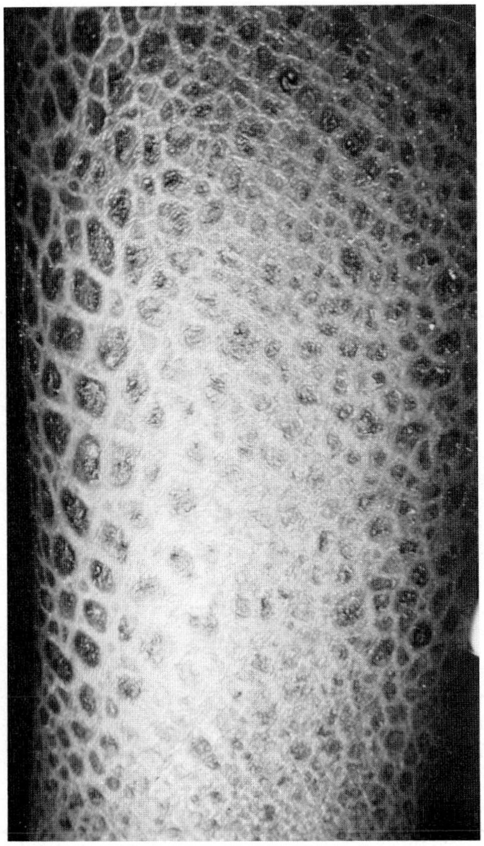

FIG. 55–39. X-linked ichthyosis on the leg of a 5-year-old boy. Five other males in the family were affected. Note the large, thick, dark scales.

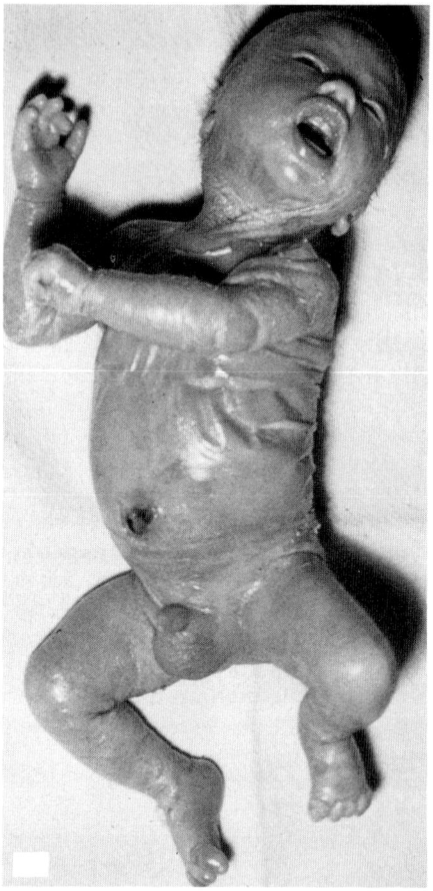

FIG. 55–40. A collodion baby, shortly after birth. By 3 days of age, the yellow collodion membrane peeled and shed in sheets, leaving large, coarse, lamellar scales. The older sister of this infant had dry, minimally scaly, hyperkeratotic skin and a similar appearance at birth.

EPIDERMOLYTIC HYPERKERATOSIS OR BULLOUS CONGENITAL ICHTHYOSIFORM ERYTHRODERMA

Infants born with this disorder have widespread (0.5–30 cm) erythema, and dry, peeling skin. The blisters, commonly appearing in crops during childhood, differentiate this disease from nonbullous congenital ichthyosiform erythroderma. In the newborn, extensive denudation with secondary infection and sepsis occur often because of β-hemolytic streptococci or staphylococci. In older infants, hyperkeratosis may remain generalized or localized to flexural areas. Scales are small, hard, and coarse and shed in large quantities. Normal bacteria in the thickened horny layers produce a putrid odor, as in lamellar ichthyosis. Bacterial population may be decreased with antiseptic baths. It is common to find several affected family members because this is an autosomal dominant disorder.

MANAGEMENT

Management of ichthyosis primarily consists of the continued use of topical lubricants. Daily hydration and lubrication of the skin are essential. One or two baths are given daily, containing a water-dispersible bath oil (*e.g.*, Alpha Keri), followed by application of an ointment or cream (*e.g.*, Eucerin, Aquaphor) several times daily. In severely affected areas, use of 12% ammonium lactate lotion (Lac-Hydrin), lactic or citric acid (5%), or urea (10%–20%) in an ointment base may be effective.[1,5,6,16] It is is most important to avoid detergents and soaps that are drying and irritating. Dry indoor heat should be avoided.

In my experience, oral 13-*cis*-retinoic acid has been

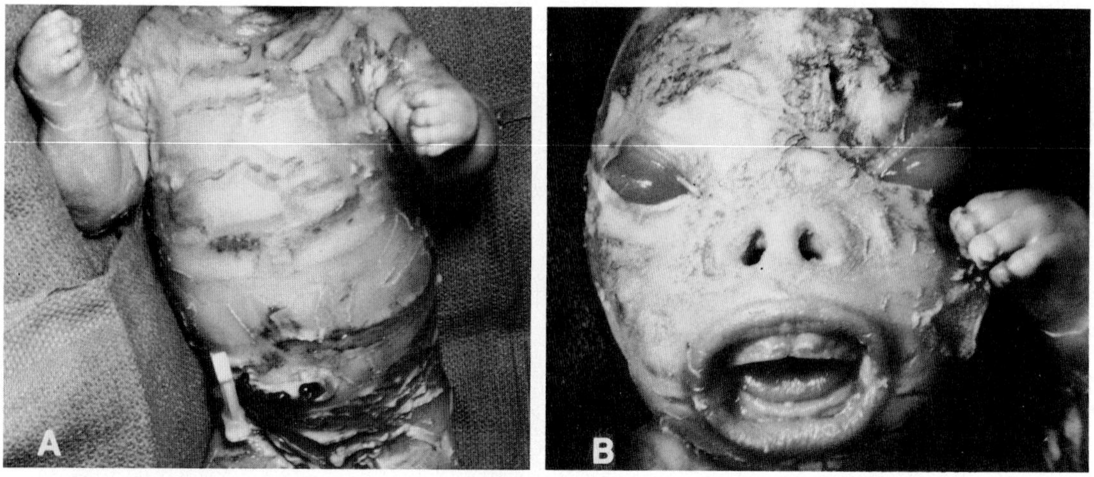

FIG. 55–41. (A, B) Nonbullous ichthyosiform erythroderma is present in a harlequin fetus, 1 day of age, with severe ectropion, eclabium, and fissures; scaling; and deformity of hands, feet, and ears. Death resulted from sepsis and extensive bacterial abscesses at 1 month of age. Patient was the offspring of a primipara, and family history was negative. (Courtesy of A. Fletcher, M.D., Childrens National Medical Center, Washington, DC.)

beneficial to older children with lamellar ichthyosis and epidermolytic hyperkeratosis.[6] Genetic counseling is essential to these patients and their families.[6,16,27,36]

ECZEMA

Eczema, from the Greek *eksein,* meaning to boil out, is a common problem in the infant older than 2 months of age but is much less common in the newborn. Nevertheless, it is such a difficult problem for the infant, mother, and physician and its causes are so varied, that two of the common conditions will be discussed. Several have been reviewed here and elsewhere.[1,3,5,6,16,36] The following is an outline of some of these causes.

- Exogenous
  - Contact primary irritant dermatitis
  - Allergic, contact, or drug dermatitis
  - Infectious eczematoid dermatitis
  - Physical (*e.g.,* light, cold, heat dermatitis)
- Endogenous
  - Atopic infantile dermatitis
  - HIV
  - Ichthyosis
  - Seborrheic dermatitis
  - Systemic diseases
    - Acrodermatitis enteropathica
    - Histidinemia
    - Anhidrotic ectodermal dysplasia
    - Histiocytosis X
    - Leiner disease (*i.e.,* C5 dysfunction)
    - Phenylketonuria
    - Wiskott–Aldrich syndrome
  - Psoriasis

The four phases of eczema usually are seen simultaneously in the same patient. Pruritus, the major symptom, occurs in all phases. Initially, acute erythema proceeds rapidly to microvesicles with weeping. A burst of epidermal mitotic activity leads to scaling, and finally to lichenification (*i.e.,* thickened skin with prominent dermal markings). Hypopigmentation or hyperpigmentation eventually develops. Some exogenous and endogenous types of eczema observed during early infancy have been discussed. Primary irritant diaper dermatitis and infectious eczema, including that caused by physical agents, were discussed earlier. Allergic, contact, and drug dermatitis are extremely rare.[1,3,5,6,16,36]

ATOPIC DERMATITIS

Atopic, or infantile, eczema is the most common type of eczematous eruption after 1 month of age, but its etiology is unknown. Diagnostic features are a healthy child with a highly pruritic, erythematous, oozing, symmetric eruption of the cheeks, extensor surfaces of limbs, and diaper area, and patchy lesions of the scalp and trunk; family history of allergy; rapid response to topical therapy and environmental measures; and recurrent exacerbations with a chronic (1- to 3-year) course. Elimination of possible exogenous causes and continued consideration of other systemic disorders that may be excluded by time, course of the patient's disease, and a few specific tests (*e.g.,* phenylalanine blood test for phenylketonuria) make atopic dermatitis the likely diagnosis. Management consists of skin hydration emollients, topical steroids, and elimination of pruritus.[5,6,16,36]

SEBORRHEIC DERMATITIS

This is the most difficult entity to differentiate from atopic dermatitis. In seborrheic dermatitis, the eruption usually begins on the scalp and is found most often behind the ears and in skin folds of the neck, axillae, and inguinal regions. Diaper area involvement is common. If the eruption becomes generalized, it is known as exfoliative erythroderma or Leiner disease. The scales are greasy, and, with drying, potato-chip scales may develop (Fig. 55-42). Patchy redness with weeping and fissuring may develop. Pruritus is minimal or absent, in contrast to

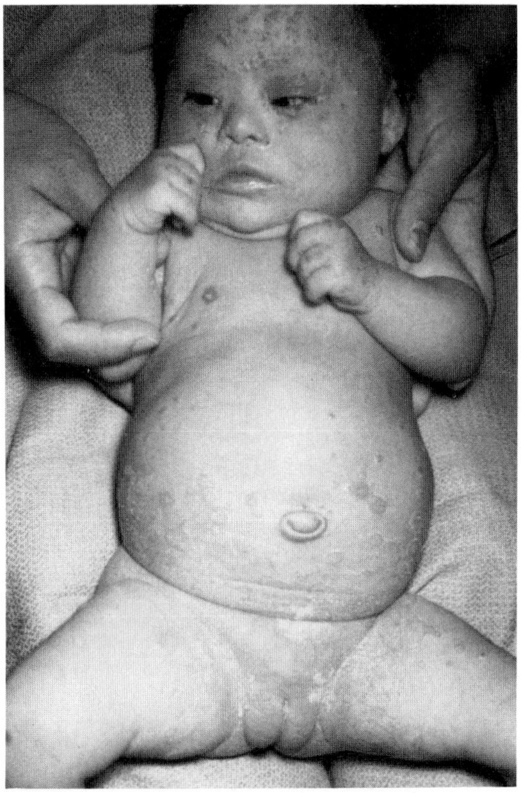

FIG. 55–42. Seborrheic dermatitis and Down syndrome occurred in a 6-week-old, otherwise healthy infant. Diaper rash with secondary monilial infection was present for 1 week; multiple scaly, greasy, crusted lesions involving the body, extremities, and scalp was present for 3 weeks.

atopic dermatitis. Rarely, eczema may occur simultaneously in the same patient. In most infants, several visits with careful observation and assessment of the therapeutic response will decide the proper diagnosis.

Cradle cap and seborrheic dermatitis may be treated with Selsun blue or Sebutone shampoo or 2% ketoconazole cream rubbed into the scalp nightly followed by a neutral baby shampoo in the morning. Five or six courses may be necessary, and then once or twice weekly thereafter. Application of 1% hydrocortisone cream three times daily to inflamed areas may be helpful. This disorder usually clears in a few months; recurrences are rare. Persistent severe atopic or seborrheic dermatitis may be associated with HIV infection.

Management of eczematous dermatoses must be individualized. Detailed written instructions for each infant must be given to nurses or parents to avoid confusion.[27] Environmental factors, clothing, hygiene, and socioeconomic aspects must be reviewed during each visit. The details of management include parental reassurance, elimination of pruritus, topical medications, baths, avoidance of dry heat and skin irritants, and treatment of secondary infections.[1,5,6,16,36]

IDIOPATHIC DERMATOSES

HISTIOCYTOSIS X

The severe Letterer–Siwe variant and the benign, congenital, self-healing reticulohistiocytosis are observed at birth or during the first year of life.[1,6,16] The cutaneous features that may precede systemic signs (*e.g.*, fever, hepatosplenomegaly, lymphadenopathy, anemia) are valuable clues to the diagnosis of the severe form. In my experience, initial lesions usually are papular and scaly and become petechial with or without purpura. Nodular lesions occur in the benign form.[6] An eczematous, seborrheic eruption also is common; however, maculopapules, pustules, and widespread erythema have been observed. The eruption usually occurs over the neck, groin, axillae, and scalp. Skin biopsy will reveal histiocytic infiltration and establish the diagnosis. Topical therapy is limited to emollients or steroid cream or both for eczematous lesions. For the severe form, systemic steroids, alkylating agents, or vincristine are effective.[1,6]

CONNECTIVE TISSUE DISEASES

SCLERODERMA

Scleroderma, from the Greek *skleros* and *derma*, meaning hard skin, is rarely seen in the neonatal period but may develop as local lesions during early infancy. Localized scleroderma occurs in two forms: morphea and linear scleroderma. Morphea develops insidiously as purplish indurated areas of shiny skin surrounded by a lilac border. Lesions may be multiple on the face, trunk, and limbs. Spontaneous resolution occurs in 3 to 5 years and leaves a brown pigmentation.[1,6,16] Linear scleroderma usually involves the scalp, face, or limbs and often coexists with morphea. A particular type of linear scleroderma, the *en coup de sabre*, was so named because of its resemblance to a saber cut. This type shows a linear depressed groove in the frontoparietal region that may extend into the scalp and down to the chin and neck. Progressive atrophy of underlying structures, including the skull, may occur.[27] Plastic surgical excision may be beneficial. One report of good results in 14 patients treated with penicillamine is encouraging; however, side effects may occur.[1,47] Evidence implicating *Borrelia* sp. infection in biopsy tissue is intriguing.[48]

NEONATAL LUPUS ERYTHEMATOSUS

Neonatal lupus erythematosus (NLE) has been reported in newborns of both affected and unaffected mothers. These infants usually are not ill and have a discoid lupus rash (*i.e.*, sharply demarcated, erythematous annular plaques or central atropic macules with peripheral scaling), that is especially predominant over the head, neck, and periorbital areas but rarely extends into the trunk and extremities.[6,16] Biopsy of an active lesion shows histopathologic features of, but is not necessary for diagnosis of, NLE. Very rarely, NLE with systemic involvement occurs in newborns.[6,16,49]

One third of mothers who give birth to infants with NLE have systemic lupus erythematosus. These infants must be followed closely for cardiac involvement (*e.g.*, primarily congenital complete heart block) because the mortality with heart block is significant.[27,49] Otherwise, the prognosis is very good, with most manifestations disappearing by 1 year of age. Transplacental passage of Ro Sjögren syndrome A antigen antibody (ss-ARo) is a diagnostic marker for NLE.[16]

Therapy consists of avoidance of sunlight and physical trauma to the skin and use of sunscreen creams. Topical use of steroid creams is effective for skin lesions.[1,6,16]

JUVENILE XANTHOGRANULOMA

This benign, self-limiting disorder often is seen at birth or shortly thereafter. The typical lesion, often located in the head, neck, upper trunk, or extremities, is a firm, nontender, yellowish brown, orangish brown, or reddish nodule. Size varies from 0.3 to 4 cm in diameter (Fig. 55-43), and from five to ten to several hundred widely scattered or closely grouped lesions may be seen. Biopsy is diagnostic, showing a dense infiltrate of histiocytic cells throughout the dermis in early lesions and Touton giant cells in mature lesions. Spontaneous regression usually occurs within 6 months to 2 years.[1,3,5,6,16,50]

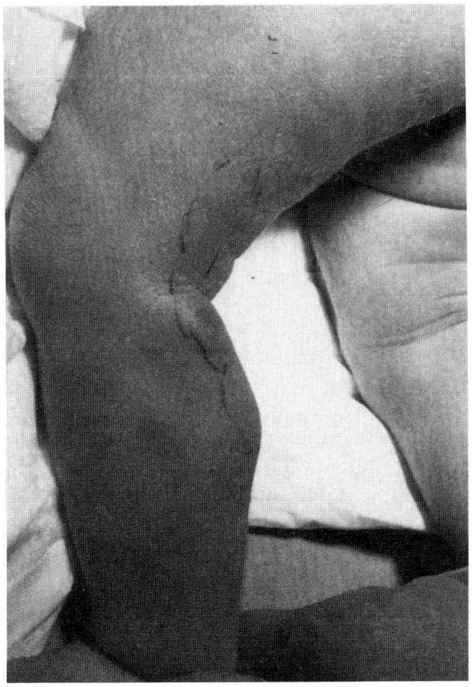

FIG. 55–43. Juvenile xanthogranuloma was noted at birth in a 2-week-old healthy neonate. Six nontender nodules slowly increased in size. Biopsy confirmed the diagnosis. Lesions involuted spontaneously by 15 months of age.

Of major importance is that ocular, pulmonary, testicular, and pericardial lesions may occur. The ocular infiltrates may involve the iris, ciliary body, or orbit and may predate the onset of skin nodules.[50] Before ocular surgery is done, an infant should be examined thoroughly for skin tumors. Thus, a major ophthalmologic procedure may be avoided.

REFERENCES

1. Hurwitz S. Clinical pediatric dermatology. 2nd ed. Philadelphia: WB Saunders, 1981.
2. Weinberg S, Prose NS. Color atlas of pediatric dermatology. New York: McGraw-Hill, 1990.
3. Solomon LM, Esterly NB. Neonatal dermatology. Philadelphia: WB Saunders, 1973.
4. Arndt KA. Manual of dermatologic therapeutics. 4th ed. Boston: Little, Brown & Co., 1989.
5. Esterly NB. The skin. In: Behrman RE, Kliegman RM, Nelson WE, et al, eds. Nelson textbook of pediatrics. Philadelphia: WB Saunders, 1992:1621.
6. Weston WL, Lane AT. Color textbook of pediatric dermatology. St. Louis: Mosby Year Book, 1991.
7. Jones KL, Smith DW. Recognizable patterns of human malformation. 4th ed. Philadelphia: WB Saunders, 1988.
8. Picascia D, Esterly NB. Cutis marmorata telangiectasia congenita: report of 22 cases. J Am Acad Dermatol 1989;20:1098.
9. Prose NS, Williams ML. The skin. In: Rudolph AM, ed. Pediatrics. 19th ed. Norwalk, CT: Appleton & Lange, 1991:882.
10. Alper JC, Holmes LB. The incidence and significance of birthmarks in a cohort of 4,641 newborns. Pediatr Dermatol 1983;1:58.
11. Margileth AM. Developmental vascular abnormalities. Pediatr Clin North Am 1971;18:713.
12. Setzer ES, Webb IB, Cruz AC, et al. Intrauterine positional deformations masquerading as multiple congenital malformations. Am J Dis Child 1984;138:642.
13. Jacobs AH. Eruptions in the diaper area. Pediatr Clin North Am 1978;25:209.
14. Bluestein J, Furner BB, Phillips D. Granuloma gluteale infantum. Pediatr Dermatol 1990;7:196.
15. Agha A, Sakati NO, Higginbottom MC, et al. Two forms of cutis laxa presenting in the newborn period. Acta Paediatr Scand 1978;67:775.
16. Schachner LA, Hansen RC. Pediatric dermatology. New York: Churchill-Livingston, 1988.
17. Frieden IJ. Aplasia cutis congenita: clinical review and proposal for classification. J Am Acad Dermatol 1986;26:646.
18. Hurwitz S. Epidermal nevi and tumors of epidermal origin. Pediatr Clin North Am 1983;30:483.
19. Feins NR, Rubin R, Borger JA. Ambulatory serial excision of giant nevi. J Pediatr Surg 1982;17:851.
20. Knight PJ, Reiner CB. Superficial lumps in children: what, when and why? Pediatrics 1983;72:147.
21. Jacobs AH. Vascular malformations. In: Schachner LA, Hansen RC, eds. Pediatric dermatology. New York: Churchill-Livingston, 1988:1017.
22. Burns AJ, Kaplan LS, Mulliken JB. Is there an association between hemangiomas and syndromes with dysmorphic features? Pediatrics 1991;88:1257.
23. Margileth AM. Cutaneous vascular tumors. Modern Problems in Paediatrics 1975;17:101.
24. Tallman B, Tan OT, Morelli J, et al. Location of port-wine stains and the likelihood of ophthalmic and/or central nervous system complications. Pediatrics 1991;87:323.
25. Mulliken JB. Editorial: a plea for a biologic approach to hemangiomas of infancy. Arch Dermatol 1991;127:243.
26. Ashinoff R, Geronemus RG. Flash-lamp-pumped-pulsed dye laser for port-wine stains in infancy. J Am Acad Dermatol 1991;24:467.
27. Sybert VP. Guide to information for families with inherited skin disorders. Pediatr Dermatol 1990;7:214.
28. Margileth AM. Hemangiomas: a before and after look. Contemporary Pediatrics 1986;3:14.
29. Miller SH, Smith RL, Skochat SJ. Compression treatment of hemangiomas. Plast Reconstr Surg 1976;58:573.
30. Weber TR, Connors RH, Tracy TF Jr, et al. Complex hemangiomas of infants and children. Arch Surg 1990;125:1017.
31. Johns KJ, Chandra SR. Visual loss following intranasal corticosteroid injection. JAMA 1989;261:2413.
32. Goldsmith MF. A granddaughter's distress leads to lymphedema aid. JAMA 1984;251:1002.
33. Hilliard RI, McKendry JBJ, Phillips MJ. Congenital abnormalities of the lymphatic system: a new clinical classification. Pediatrics 1990;86:988.
34. Saijo M, Munro IR, Mancer K. Lymphangioma: longterm follow-up study. Plast Reconstr Surg 1975;56:642.
35. Sharp H, Kruit W. Hereditary lymphedema and obstructive jaundice. J Pediatr 1971;78:491.
36. Williams ML. The skin. In: Rudolph AM, ed. Pediatrics. 19th ed. Norwalk, CT: Appleton & Lange, 1991:875.
37. Weber K, Bratzke HJ, Neubert U, et al. *Borrelia burgdorferi* in a newborn despite oral penicillin for Lyme borreliosis during pregnancy. Pediatr Infect Dis J 1988;7:286.
38. Nelson JD. Pocketbook of pediatrics antimicrobial therapy. vol. 9. Baltimore: Williams & Wilkins, 1991–1992:9.

39. Grossman M. Listeriosis. In: Rudolph AM, ed. Pediatrics. 19th ed. Norwalk, CT: Appleton & Lange, 1991:591.
40. Ricci JM, Fojaco MR, O'Sullivan MJ. Congenital syphilis: the University of Miami/Jackson Memorial Medical Center Experience, 1986–1988. Obstet Gynecol 1989;74:687.
41. Dorfman DH, Glaser JH. Congenital syphilis presenting in infants after the newborn period. N Engl J Med 1990;323:1299.
42. Whitley R, Aroin A, Prober C, et al. A controlled trial comparing vidarabine with acyclovir in neonatal herpes simplex virus infection. N Engl J Med 1991;324:444.
43. Whitley R, Aroin A, Prober C, et al. Predictors of morbidity and mortality in neonates with herpes simplex virus infections. N Engl J Med 1991;324:450.
44. Brown ZA, Benedetti J, Ashley R, et al. Neonatal herpes simplex infection in relation to asymptomatic maternal infection at the time of labor. N Engl J Med 1991;324:1247.
45. Report of the Committee on Infectious Diseases Red Book. 22nd ed. Elk Grove, IL: American Academy of Pediatrics, 1991.
46. Obalek S, Jablonska S, Favre M, et al. Condylomata acuminata in children: frequent association with human papillomaviruses responsible for cutaneous warts. J Am Acad Dermatol 1990; 23:205.
47. Moynahan EJ. Penicillamine in treatment of morphea and keloid in children. Postgrad Med J 1974;50(Suppl):39.
48. Aberer E, Kollegger H, Kristoferitsch W, et al. Neuroborreliosis in morphea and lichen sclerosus et atrophicus. J Am Acad Dermatol 1988;19:820.
49. Laxer RM, Roberts EA, Gross KR, et al. Liver disease in neonatal lupus erythematosus. J Pediatr 1990;116:238.
50. Resnick SD, Woosley J, Azizkhan RG. Giant juvenile xanthogranuloma: exophytic and endophytic variants. Pediatr Dermatol 1990;7:185.

Part Six

Pharmacology

Neonatology: Pathophysiology and Management of the Newborn, Fourth Edition,
edited by Gordon B. Avery, Mary Ann Fletcher, and Mhairi G. MacDonald.
J.B. Lippincott Company, Philadelphia © 1994.

chapter 56

The Use of Therapeutic Drugs

ROBERT M. WARD

The developmental uniqueness of the neonate has tremendous impact on drug therapy. This uniqueness and the potential for dramatic and rapid developmental change shortly after birth defy accurate generalizations, and illustrate the need for age-specific studies in the increasingly premature patients surviving today. These developmental changes affect all aspects of drug action, from absorption and protein binding to receptor interaction and elimination. The impact of these developmental changes on drug action and the use of pharmacokinetics to adjust drug dosages will be outlined, to guide the clinician between the Charybdis of ineffective therapy and the Scylla of drug overdose and toxicity.

PRINCIPLES OF PHARMACOLOGY APPLIED TO NEONATES

FREE-DRUG THEORY AND PROTEIN BINDING

In general, only the nonprotein-bound or free-drug molecules are active (*i.e.*, cross membranes, bind to receptors to exert pharmacologic action, undergo metabolism and excretion).[1–3] In contrast, most clinical drug assays measure both bound and unbound drug. The albumin of term newborns, compared to that of adults, binds less warfarin and sulfonamides but similar amounts of diazepam.[4] For most drugs in premature infants, a greater percentage of the total drug in the circulation is unbound, because both the amount and the binding affinity of circulating proteins are decreased.[5] In the premature neonate, circulating total drug concentrations that are in the therapeutic range for adults or older children may reflect free-drug concentrations that are in a toxic range.[6]

Serum protein binding usually is a rapidly reversible interaction, so that additional drug is released to replace the unbound drug removed by distribution into tissue or by elimination. The rate of release from serum protein binding usually is much faster than the rate of transfer across membranes. Seldom is the rate of release from serum proteins so slow that it limits the availability of drug molecules for transfer across membranes to exert pharmacologic effects. Since the effects of a drug are related to the amount of unbound drug reaching the site of action, some complex situations may be explained only by measurement of the circulating concentrations of free and protein-bound drug.

ABSORPTION

Absorption refers to the transfer of drug from the site of administration into the circulation. The rates of drug absorption are related to several factors, beginning with the route of administration and including the same characteristics that influence transfer of any substance across lipid bilayers: degree of ionization, molecular weight, lipid solubility, and active transport.

ENTERAL

Enteral drug treatment of neonates may not produce reliable and reproducible circulating drug concentrations for a variety of reasons. Although most studies of enteral drug therapy have been conducted in adults, many of the problems of enteral drug administration identified from these studies are likely to occur in neonates.

Intestinal villi and microvilli amplify the surface of the gastrointestinal tract, so that rates of drug absorption are much greater from the intestine than from the stomach. Delayed gastric emptying slows passage of drug into the intestine, which prolongs the absorption phase. Elimination begins during this absorption phase, so that delayed gastric emptying reduces the area under the curve (AUC) for circulating drug concentration. This reduces the desired therapeutic effect for many drugs whose effects are directly proportional to the AUC for concentration over time. Gastroesophageal reflux is common in neonates and often is associated with delayed gastric emptying that may reduce the therapeutic effects of drugs administered orally. Few studies have addressed this aspect of drug treatment of newborns.

Additional problems, unique to the more immature patient, may affect enteral drug treatment of newborns. Neonates, especially premature neonates, malabsorb fat, which may alter enteral drug absorption. Elevated right atrial pressure, leading to passive congestion of hepatic and mesenteric circulations, often reduces enteral drug absorption in adults. Chronic, enteral drug administration often is necessary for treatment of infants with disorders, such as bronchopulmonary dysplasia (BPD) or congestive heart failure, that may increase right atrial pressure and decrease enteral drug absorption. Large doses may be required to achieve the desired therapeutic goals, due to decreased bioavailability. This has been reported for furosemide treatment of an infant with BPD, who required a sixfold higher enteral dose to reach plasma concentrations comparable to a 1 mg/kg dose administered intravenously (IV).[7]

INTRAMUSCULAR

Intramuscular drug absorption is directly proportional to blood flow and the surface area of the collection of drug in the muscle.[8] Although intramuscular drug administration is considered more reliable than enteral, the sick or hypothermic neonate often has poor perfusion of muscle and limited muscle mass. Due to limited amounts of muscle, injections intended for the muscle may enter subcutaneous tissue, from which absorption is slow and unpredictable. Caustic drugs (*e.g.*, phenytoin, *p*H 12) damage surrounding tissues and isolate the dose of drug from blood flow, or precipitate to a chemical form that is absorbed very slowly in what has been described as a depot effect.[9] Intramuscular injection sites in neonates also may leave sterile abscesses that later require surgical repair. In general, prolonged intramuscular administration of drugs in neonates should be avoided.

INTRAVENOUS

Intravenous drug administration is most likely to ensure effective drug therapy in neonates. Although this route of drug treatment is the most reliable, certain problems must be recognized that are unique to neonates. The infusion rate for IV fluids in extremely small neonates is so slow that drug doses injected up the IV tubing away from the patient may not reach the circulation for several hours.[10]

The most reliable method for IV drug administration to neonates uses a separate, small-volume syringe pump and narrow-bore tubing connected to the infusion tubing as close to the patient as possible. Although it is more costly, I prefer filling the syringe with the dose and the narrow-bore tubing with extra drug so that the syringe and tubing, which contains extra drug, may be discarded after the dose is infused, without flushing the tubing. This provides convenient, accurate, safe control of IV drug administration.

DISTRIBUTION

Distribution is the partitioning of drugs from the circulation into various body fluids, organs, and tissues. At equilibrium, this distribution is related to organ blood flow; *p*H and composition of body fluids and tissues; physical and chemical properties of the drug including lipid solubility, polarity, and size; and the extent of binding to plasma and tissue proteins.

Dramatic developmental changes in body composition of newborns influence the distribution of polar and nonpolar drugs within the body. At 26 weeks of gestation, water comprises about 85% of body weight, with less than 1% as fat.[5] By 40 weeks of gestation, the body is approximately 75% water and 15% fat, compared to adults in whom the body is about 65% water and the fat content is variable. The low fat content of the brain of the extremely premature newborn may affect the distribution and effects of centrally active drugs, such as barbiturates and gaseous anesthetics.

METABOLISM

Many drugs require biotransformation to more polar forms before they can be eliminated from the body. Biotransformation reactions are designated phase I, nonsynthetic reactions such as oxidation, reduction, and hydrolysis; or phase II, synthetic or conjugation reactions, such as glucuronidation, sulfation, and acetylation.[11] The liver is the primary site for many of these reactions, but other organs also are involved. Human fetal drug metabolizing pathways at 9 to 22 weeks of gestation vary from 2% to 36% of adult activity, according to the specific enzyme involved.[12] Slow metabolic reactions and decreased elimination function combine to prolong half-life for many drugs, compared to adults. Certain biotransformation reactions, especially those involving certain forms of cytochrome P450, are inducible before birth through maternal exposure to drugs, cigarette smoke, or other inducing agents. After birth, biotransformation reactions may be accelerated or slowed by organ damage, drug interactions, nutrition, or illness. Additional changes in hepatic blood flow, hepatocyte extraction of drugs, protein binding, and biliary function prevent accurate prediction of rates of drug elimination after birth. Dosages often must be adjusted empirically based on therapeutic drug monitoring. Additional study of the extremely immature neonates who survive today, however, will help to provide population kinetics that serve as guidelines for drug dosages.

EXCRETION

Excretion involves elimination of drug from the body by several potential routes, including the biliary tract, lungs, and kidneys. Both unchanged and metabolized forms of drug may be excreted. Glomerular and tubular function are decreased at birth, both in absolute units and after normalization to body mass.[13,14] Glomerular filtration of newborns averages 30% of the adult rate, after normalization to body surface area. Birth accelerates maturation of glomerular filtration through an increase in cardiac output, decreased renal vascular resistance, redistribution of intrarenal blood flow, and changes in the intrinsic function of the glomerular basement membrane. Renal tubular maturation seems to proceed more slowly than glomerular maturation after birth. This produces an imbalance in glomerular and tubular function that persists for several months. Since most low-molecular-weight, unbound molecules are filtered, tubular reabsorption exerts a profound influence on the elimination rate for many drugs. In addition, renal function of newborns may be altered by hypoxemia, nephrotoxic drugs, and underperfusion, which prevent accurate prediction of the rates of drug elimination after birth.

PHARMACOKINETICS

Pharmacokinetics describes the changes in drug concentrations (dC) within the body with time. These concepts are presented in a general overview, to assist the clinician with dose adjustments and practical interpretation of therapeutic drug monitoring.[15–17] The more rigorous mathematical intricacies of pharmacokinetics are covered elsewhere.[18–20] Although a drug may penetrate several body fluids and tissues at different rates, the change in its circulating concentrations usually are used to characterize its kinetics and to guide dosages. The rate of removal of drug from the circulation usually fits either zero-order or first-order exponential mathematical equations. These two types of equations describe two different processes that have important implications for dosage regimes.

RATES AND DISTRIBUTION

ZERO-ORDER KINETICS

When drugs are removed by zero-order rates, a constant amount is removed for each unit of time.[15] These kinetics fit the following equation:

$$uc/dt = -k_0, \qquad \text{(Eq. 56-1)}$$

where uc is the change in concentration, dt is the change in time, and k_0 is the elimination rate constant with units of amount/time. After solving this equation, it has the following form:

$$C = (-k_0)(t). \qquad \text{(Eq. 56-2)}$$

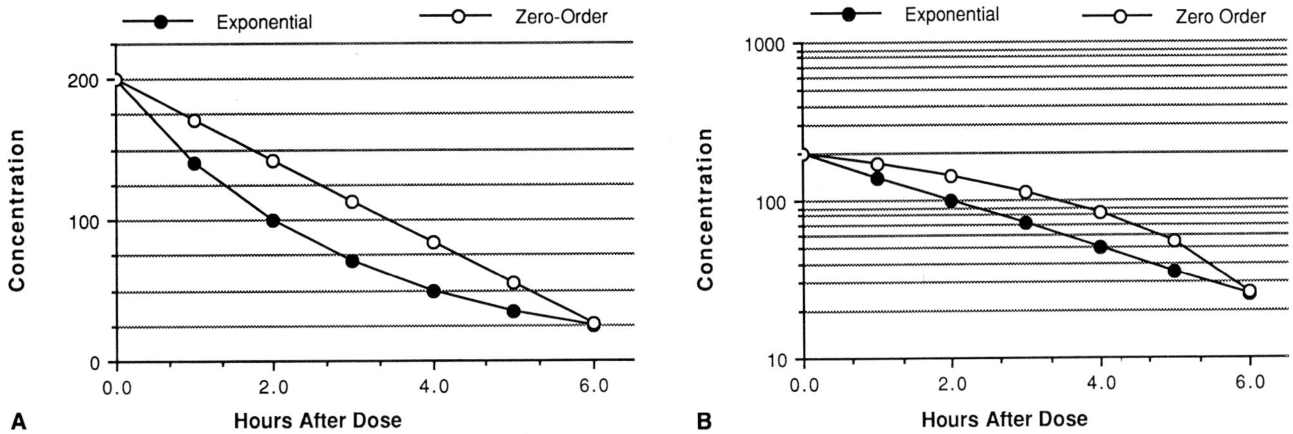

FIG. 56–1. Zero-order kinetics (*open circles*) and first-order exponential kinetics (*closed circles*), showing differences in shapes of lines graphed on **(A)** linear–linear axes and **(B)** linear–logarithmic axes.

TABLE 56–1
DRUGS THAT DEMONSTRATE SATURATION KINETICS WITH THERAPEUTIC DOSES IN NEONATES

Caffeine
Chloramphenicol
Diazepam
Furosemide
Indomethacin
Phenytoin

From Ward RM. Pharmacologic principles and practicalities. In: Taeusch HW, Ballard RA, Avery ME, eds. Schaffer and Avery's diseases of the newborn. 6th ed. Philadelphia: WB Saunders, 1991:285.

Order refers to the power of the exponential term. For example, e^{ϕ} is zero order and $e^{\beta t}$ and $e^{\alpha t}$ are first order. Since the exponent raised to the zero power equals 1, this trivial term usually is omitted. A graph of zero-order change in concentration with time (see Eq. 56-2) on linear–linear axes produces a straight line with a slope of k_0 (Fig. 56-1*A*). When zero-order changes in concentration are graphed on logarithmic–linear (*i.e.*, semilogarithmic) axes, the graph is a curve (Fig. 56-1*B*).

Zero-order kinetics also is referred to as saturation kinetics, because it may occur when excess amounts of drug saturate enzymes or transport systems so that only a constant amount of drug is metabolized or transported per unit of time. This is observed clinically after administration of excess doses, or during dysfunction of the organ of elimination without a decrease of dosage. For drugs exhibiting zero-order kinetics, small increments in dose may cause disproportionately large increments in serum concentrations. Certain drugs frequently administered to newborns exhibit zero-order kinetics at therapeutic doses, and may accumulate to excessive concentrations (Table 56-1).

FIRST-ORDER KINETICS

After absorption into the circulation, most drugs are cleared from the circulation with first-order exponential rates. Exponential clearance indicates that a constant fraction or constant proportion of drug is removed during the same increment of time. Such rates fit exponential equations of the following form:

$$C = Ae^{-k_1 t}, \qquad \text{(Eq. 56-3)}$$

where C is the concentration at a particular time t, A is the starting concentration, which is a constant, and k_1 is the rate constant with units of 1/time. First-order indicates that the exponent is raised to the first power ($-k_1t$ in Eq. 56-3). Second-order processes fit equations with the exponent raised to the second power: for example, $e - k^2$.

First-order exponential equations, such as Equation 56-3, may be solved by taking the natural logarithm of both sides to give Equation 56-4:

$$\ln C = \ln A + -k_1 t. \qquad \text{(Eq. 56-4)}$$

This converts the equation to a form that fits the equation of a straight line. If ln (*i.e.*, natural logarithm) C is graphed *versus* time, the slope is $-k_1$, and the intercept is ln A. If log (*i.e.*, common logarithm) C is graphed *versus* time, the slope is $-k_1/2.303$, since ln x equals 2.303 log x. When graphed on linear–linear axes, exponential rates are curvilinear (see Fig. 56-1*A*), and on semilogarithmic axes, they produce a straight line (see Fig. 56-1*B*).

HALF-LIFE

One of the more familiar exponential rates used clinically is the time for a drug concentration to decrease by one-half with its half-life. Half-life is a first-order kinetic process, since the same proportion or fraction of the drug is removed during equal time periods. At higher concentrations, a greater amount is removed during a single half-life than when the concentration is lower. For example a drug concentration may decrease by 200 from 400 to 200 in one half-life, and decrease by 100 from 200 to 100 in the next half-life (Fig. 56-2).

Half-life can be determined by several methods. If the concentration is converted to the natural logarithm of concentration and graphed over time, as described in Equation 56-4, the slope of this graph is the elimination rate constant, k_1. A minimum of three concentration-time points, in which the concentration decreases at least 50%, are needed to determine the slope accurately. The slope of ln C *versus* t may be calculated easily by least-squares linear regression analysis. Half-life may be calculated from the elimina-

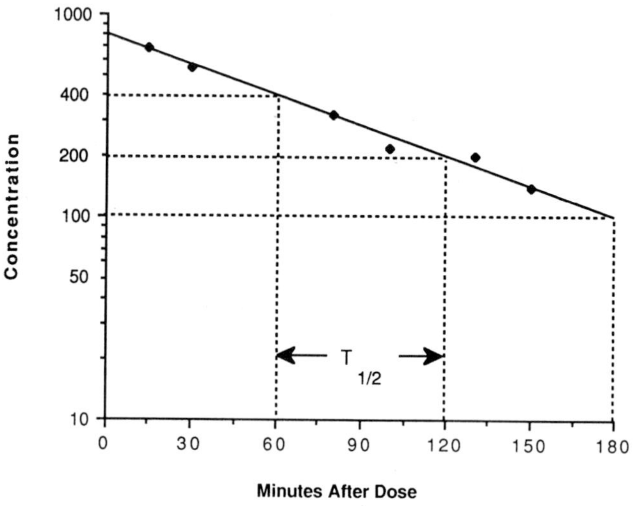

FIG. 56–2. Graph method for estimation of half-life. (From Ward RM. Pharmacologic principles and practicalities. In: Taeusch HW, Ballard RA, Avery ME, eds. Diseases of the newborn. 6th ed. Philadelphia: WB Saunders, 1991:289.)

tion rate constant, k_1 (1/time), as follows:

$$t_{1/2} = \frac{\text{natural logarithm } 2}{k_1} = \frac{0.693}{k_1}. \quad \text{(Eq. 56-5)}$$

Half-life may be determined graphically from a series of drug concentrations graphed on semilogarithmic axes. The best-fit line is determined either visually or by linear regression analysis. The time corresponding to various concentrations then is used to estimate the interval required for the concentration to decrease by one-half. In Figure 56-2, this is illustrated by the times corresponding to concentrations of 400, 200, and 100, estimated by the horizontal broken line intercepts with the concentration line and the intercepts with the time axis indicated by the vertical broken lines. Note that the concentrations decrease by 50% every 60 minutes, so that $t_{1/2}$ equals 60 minutes. The apparent slope of such a semilogarithmic graph $\Delta e/\Delta t$, does not equal k.

FIRST-ORDER SINGLE-COMPARTMENT KINETICS

The number of compartments refers to the number of exponential equations required to describe the observed changes in concentration. Kinetics are described as first-order and single-compartment, if a single first-order exponential equation describes the rate of disappearance of drug from the circulation. This may be judged visually, if a semilogarithmic graph of a series of concentrations fits a single straight line. If the kinetics appear to have two or more slopes, the differences in the slopes should be tested statistically to confirm that more than one slope is present. Noncompartmental (*i.e.*, nonlinear) kinetic analysis determines this automatically.

Although multiple transfers of drug among tissues and body fluids may be occurring, a drug may be viewed as demonstrating first-order, single-compartment kinetics if it distributes rapidly and homogeneously within the circulation from which it is removed through metabolism or excretion. Kinetics may falsely appear to be single-compartment if drug concentrations are not measured quickly enough after IV administration to detect the initial distribution phase.

FIRST-ORDER MULTICOMPARTMENT KINETICS

If drug clearance from the circulation is studied carefully, with measurement of concentration several times within the first 15 to 30 minutes after IV administration as well as during the next several hours, two or more rates of clearance often are detected by a change in slope of a semilogarithmic graph of concentration *versus* time (Fig. 56-3). When two first-order exponential equations are required to describe the clearance of drug from the circulation, the kinetics are designated first-order and two-compartment.[15] Such kinetics are seen commonly for drugs that rapidly distribute out of the plasma phase of the circulation after IV administration. For such drugs, the initial

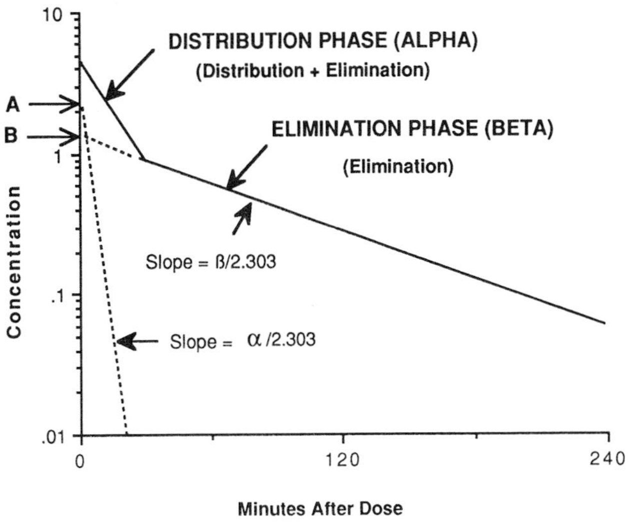

FIG. 56–3. Multicompartment first-order exponential kinetics. (From Ward RM. Pharmacologic principles and practicalities. In: Taeusch HW, Ballard RA, Avery ME, eds. Diseases of the newborn. 6th ed. Philadelphia: WB Saunders, 1991:289.)

rapid decrease in concentration represents both distribution and elimination. After an inflection point in the slope, elimination accounts for most of the change in drug concentration. The rate of distribution can be determined by subtracting the rate of elimination from the initial combined rates of distribution and elimination (see Fig. 56-3)[15]:

$$C = Ae^{-\alpha t} + Be^{-\beta t}. \quad \text{(Eq. 56-6)}$$

In Equation 56-6, C is concentration, A is the concentration at time 0 for the distribution rate represented by the broken line graph, α is the rate constant for distribution, B is the concentration at time 0 for the elimination rate, and β is the rate constant for elimination.

The number and nature of the compartments for the clearance of a drug do not necessarily correspond to specific body fluids or tissues. Seldom are more than three exponential equations required to describe a drug's kinetics.

The most accurate approach to pharmacokinetic analysis relies on equations that do not require assumptions about the number of compartments. These methods of noncompartmental analysis are discussed in textbooks of pharmacokinetics.[19,20] Use of these methods for pharmacokinetic calculations requires sophisticated computer programs that are not generally available at the bedside.

APPARENT VOLUME OF DISTRIBUTION

The apparent volume of distribution (aVD) is a mathematical term that relates the dose to the circulating concentration observed immediately after administration of that dose. It might be viewed as the volume of dilution. The units used to express concentration are amount/volume, and may help to remind the reader of the relation between dose in amount/kg and the aVD in volume/kg that dilutes the dose to produce the concentration:

$$\text{Concentration change (mg/L)} = \frac{\text{Dose (mg/kg)}}{\text{Apparent volume of distribution (L/kg)}}. \quad \text{(Eq. 56-7)}$$

The aVD does not necessarily correspond to a physiologic body fluid or tissue volume, hence the designation of "apparent." For drugs, such as digoxin, that reach much higher concentrations in tissue than in the circulation, aVD may exceed 1.0 L/kg, a physical impossibility. This emphasizes the mathematical nature of aVD.

Knowledge of the aVD is essential for dose adjustments to achieve a desired drug concentration. To facilitate canceling units, concentration has been expressed in the following equations with the unconventional units of milligrams per liter rather than micrograms per milliliter, since they are equivalent.

$$\text{aVD (L/kg)} = \frac{\text{Dose (mg/kg)}}{\text{Concentration postdose (mg/L)} - \text{Concentration predose (mg/L)}}. \quad \text{(Eq. 56-8)}$$

The concentration after drug infusion must be measured after the distribution phase ends, to avoid an overestimation of the peak concentration, which will reduce the aVD inaccurately. For the first dose, the predose concentration is 0.

PHARMACOKINETIC EXAMPLE

A theoretical drug will be used to illustrate the application of the principles outlined above. A drug was administered IV over 5 minutes, in a dose of 10 mg/kg every 24 hours. The following serum concentrations were measured on the third day of treatment: the predose or trough concentration, just before infusing the dose was 3 mg/L; the peak concentration, 30 minutes after the end of the infusion, was 18 mg/L; and the trough just before the next infusion was 4.5 mg/L. These data are used in the following equation:

$$\text{aVD (L/kg)} = \frac{10\ \text{mg/kg}}{18\ \text{mg/L} - 3\ \text{mg/L}} = \frac{10/\text{kg}}{15/\text{L}} = 0.67\ \text{L/kg}. \quad \text{(Eq. 56-9)}$$

The serum concentration decreased from 18 to 9 mg/L, one half-life, and then from 9 to 4.5 mg/L, a second half-life, in 23.5 hours. Thus, the half-life is 23.5 hours/2 half-lives, or 11.75 hours. If the effective peak concentration is 25 mg/L and toxicity occurs when the trough concentration exceeds 10 mg/L, the following dose adjustments can be estimated to reach a concentration of 25 mg/L.

The following equation is used to reach the effective peak concentration of 25 mg/L after the next dose:

$$\text{aVD (L/kg)} = \frac{\text{Dose (mg/kg)}}{\text{Concentration postdose (mg/L)} - \text{Concentration predose (mg/L)}},$$

$$0.67\ \text{L/kg} = \frac{\text{Dose (mg/kg)}}{25\ \text{mg/L} - 4.5\ \text{mg/L}} = \frac{\text{Dose (mg/kg)}}{21.5\ \text{mg/L}},$$

$$\text{Dose (mg/kg)} = 21.5\ \text{mg/L} \times 0.67\ \text{L/kg} = 14.4\ \text{mg/kg}. \quad \text{(Eq. 56-10)}$$

Assuming the aVd and half-life remain unchanged, the dosage change should be tested through two to three more doses to ensure that the peak and trough concentrations do not accumulate to toxic levels with the proposed dosage change. With the dosage change, the next peak concentration will reach 25 mg/L, and the serum concentration will decrease to 12.5 in one half-life and to 6.25 mg/L in the second half-life, which is less than the toxic range. The second dose of 14.4 mg/kg will raise the serum concentration by 21.5 mg/L, from 6.25 to 27.75 mg/L. After two more half-lives, the predose concentration will have decreased to 6.94 mg/L. Even though the higher dose has increased the predose concentration, it still is in a nontoxic range while the peak concentration remains in the therapeutic range.

THERAPEUTIC DRUG MONITORING

Circulating concentrations of drugs should be measured primarily to ensure that the treatment regime achieves concentrations that are effective in clinical situations where drug treatment is critical, response is not immediately apparent (*e.g.*, for culture-proven sepsis), and a good correlation exists between circulating drug concentration and desired effect. Drug concentrations should be measured to avoid toxicity when they clearly correlate with toxicity in newborns (*e.g.*, for chloramphenicol), to verify toxicity when symptoms correspond to a known drug toxicity, or to investigate symptoms that are unexplained by the disease process. Extrapolation of toxic and therapeutic ranges from adults to neonates has led to some recommendations about therapeutic drug monitoring in newborns (*e.g.*, for gentamicin) that are not well supported by subsequent experience.[21]

Several basic requirements must be met to justify therapeutic drug monitoring in newborns and to modify drug treatment accurately based on measured circulating drug concentrations.[22]

Drug analysis using small blood volumes must be accurate.

Circulating drug concentrations must correlate with both effective and toxic pharmacologic effects. This implies that the circulating total (*i.e.*, free plus protein-bound) drug concentration correlates with the free-drug concentration at the site of drug action, such as the drug receptor or tissue site.

The therapeutic index, the concentration range between efficacy and toxicity, should be narrow.

Clinical studies should have established a concentration range for efficacy and toxicity in the population being monitored.

A wide range of pharmacokinetics for the drug being monitored should occur in the population being studied.

In the extremely premature newborn, decreased protein binding may significantly affect therapeutic drug monitoring (see Appendix H-5). Due to unpredictable decreases in protein binding associated with organ dysfunction or immaturity, free-drug concentrations may be much higher than would be predicted from the total drug concentration that usually is measured clinically. Higher percentages of free drug in the newborn may account for signs of toxicity or adequate therapeutic response at paradoxically low total drug concentrations. When available and when therapeutic concentration ranges have been established, as for phenytoin, measurement of free-drug concentrations may be helpful in newborns demonstrating signs of drug toxicity with therapeutic or subtherapeutic circulating total drug concentrations.

Effective drug therapy is measured by response, not by achieving a particular circulating drug concentration. Concentration ranges described as therapeutic are statistical ranges for drug levels that usually are effective and nontoxic. Individual patients may require drug concentrations outside these ranges to achieve optimal drug treatment.

REPETITIVE DOSING AND DRUG ACCUMULATION

During most courses of repetitive drug therapy, the doses are administered before complete elimination of the previous one. This leads to accumulation of drug, with increasing peak and trough concentrations until a steady state concentration (C_{ss}) is reached:

$$C_{ss} = \frac{1}{\text{Clearance}} \times \frac{f \times D}{T}, = \frac{1}{\beta \times aVD_{(area)}} \times \frac{f \times D}{T}, = \frac{1.44 \times t_{1/2\beta}}{aVD_{(area)}} \times \frac{f \times D}{T}. \quad \text{(Eq. 56-11)}$$

In Equation 56-11, f is the fraction of the dose that is absorbed, D is the dose, T is the dosing interval in the same units of time as the elimination half-life ($t_{1/2\beta}$), β is the elimination rate constant, and 1.44 equals 1/0.693 (see Eq. 56-5). The magnitude of the C_{ss} is directly proportional to a ratio of $T/t_{1/2}$ and D.[16]

STEADY STATE

Steady state occurs when the amount of drug eliminated between doses equals the amount of the dose.[17,18] Drug may continue to be removed from the circulation to distribute among tissue and fluid compartments for five or more half-lives, until a complete equilibrium is reached (Table 56-2). Constant peak and trough concentrations after intermittent doses, or constant concentrations during drug infusions, do not prove that a steady state has been achieved. Conversely, at steady state, the peak and trough concentrations are the same after each dose. To prove that a steady state has been reached by strict pharmacokinetic criteria, the amount of drug eliminated by excretion or metabolism/time must equal the amount of drug administered/time. During continuous infusion, the fraction of steady state concentration that has been reached can be calculated in terms of multiples of the drug's half-life. Table 56-2 illustrates this calculation.[16] The effect of dosage changes on drug concentrations during chronic treatment usually should not be rechecked until several half-lives have elapsed, unless elimination is impaired or toxic symptoms occur. Drug concentrations may not need to be checked if symptoms improve.

LOADING DOSE

If the time to reach a constant concentration by continuous or intermittent dosing is too long, a loading dose may be used to reach a higher constant concentration more quickly. This frequently is applied to initial treatment with digoxin, which has a 35- to 69-hour half-life in term neonates and an even longer half-life in preterm newborns.[23] Use of a loading dose produces a higher circulating drug concentration earlier in the therapeutic course, but the equilibration to

TABLE 56–2
FRACTION OF STEADY-STATE CONCENTRATION ACHIEVED DURING CONTINUOUS DRUG INFUSION

Duration of Infusion (Multiples of $t_{1/2}$)	Fraction of Steady-State Level Reached
1	0.500
2	0.750
3	0.875
4	0.938
5	0.969
6	0.984
7	0.992

From Greenblatt DJ, Koch-Weser J. Clinical pharmacokinetics (second part). N Engl J Med 1975;293:964.

reach a true steady state still requires treatment for five or more half-lives. Loading doses must be used cautiously, since they increase the likelihood of drug toxicity, as has been observed with digoxin digitalizing doses.[23]

SPECIAL CONSIDERATIONS FOR NEONATES

INTRAVENOUS ADMINISTRATION

Intravenous administration of drugs is considered the most reliable route. In neonates, especially those who weigh 500 to 1000 g and receive small volumes of IV fluids, IV drug administration may not reliably deliver the dose into the circulation.[10,24] Since IV tubing may contain 12 to 15 mL of fluid and the IV infusion rates for 500- to 1000-g neonates may be 1.5 to 2.5 mL/hour, infusion of a drug into the IV tubing side port 5 cm from the patient will markedly delay drug administration. This may confound therapeutic drug monitoring by causing the peak concentration to be less than the trough, because the dose has not reached the patient. Gould and Roberts estimated that 36% of drug is discarded daily in the neonatal intensive care unit (NICU) with IV tubing changes.[25] Slow delivery of drug to the circulation may prevent the attainment of an adequate peak concentration to enhance drug diffusion into tissue down a concentration gradient. Filters present potential blocks to effective IV drug treatment. Drugs may adsorb to the filter or settle to the bottom of a reservoir in the filter, out of the main flow of the infusing solution.[26]

TABLE 56–3
ESTIMATED DRUG LOSS BY EXCHANGE TRANSFUSION

	Percent Removed	
Drug	Single Volume	Double Volume
Amikacin	7.1	13.8
Ampicillin	7.7	14.7
Carbamazepine	3.7	7.2
Carbenicillin	5.6	10.9
Colistin	18.7	33.9
Diazepam	2.3	4.5
Digoxin*	1.2	2.4
Furosemide	4.9	9.5
Gentamicin	5.2	10.1
Kanamycin	5.6	10.9
Methicillin	10.1	19.1
Oxacillin	19.6	35.4
Penicillin G (crystalline)	6.0	11.6
Penicillin G (procaine)	2.4	4.8
Phenobarbital	6.4	12.3
Phenytoin	3.1	6.2
Theophylline*	17.8	32.4
Tobramycin	10.3	19.6
Vancomycin	5.7	11.0

* Whole blood volume used in calculation.
From Lackner TE. Dose replacement following exchange transfusion. J Pediatr 1982;100:811.

EXCHANGE TRANSFUSION

Because few studies have evaluated the amount of drug actually removed from neonates during an exchange transfusion, theoretical estimates have been developed.[24,27] The amounts removed vary with the individual drug's volume of distribution, rate of distribution, and circulating concentration at the time of the exchange, as well as the volume of blood exchanged and the rate of the exchange (Table 56-3).

CLINICAL TOXICOLOGY

Newborn infants, both full-term and premature, present an alarmingly wide spectrum of susceptibilities to unanticipated, adverse effects from exposure to exogenous chemicals. New drugs, together with unrecognized chemicals ranging from tape remover to plasticizers, are introduced into the care of neonates each year. Prescription drug exposure of the extremely preterm neonate is extensive. In the late 1970s, neonates admitted to a NICU received 1 to 26 drugs, averaging 6.2 drugs per infant.[28] This drug exposure was not innocuous, since 30% of infants in the NICU manifested an adverse drug reaction, of which 15% were considered fatal or life-threatening.[29] Similar drug exposure of newborns was documented in Boston from 1974 to 1977, where infants in the intensive care nursery received more drugs (10.4/patient) than any other hospitalized children.[30]

Several factors increase the susceptibility of newborns and preterm newborns to chemical toxicities. Immaturity of liver and renal function frequently delays drug elimination, which prolongs the exposure of the newborn to a drug and predisposes to drug accumulation during repeated administration. New therapeutic agents often are introduced into treatment of critically ill neonates when all other therapy has failed, although pharmacokinetic data to guide dose and dosing intervals are lacking. Without the guide of pharmacokinetic or concentration–response studies, treatment failure may be considered an indication to increase the dose, rather than the result of administering excess amounts of the drug.[31]

Specific enzyme immaturities of the newborn also may place them at risk. Inadequate function of the glucuronyl transferase system predisposes the newborn to inadequate elimination of chemicals requiring glucuronide conjugation, such as bilirubin. Circulating albumin binds bilirubin at the levels encountered in physiologic jaundice and protects the newborn from bilirubin encephalopathy as long as the blood–brain barrier remains intact.[32,33] Failure to recognize the competition of drugs for bilirubin's albumin-binding sites has led to displacement of bound bilirubin and kernicterus.[34–36]

Large doses of chloramphenicol were associated with unexplained cardiovascular collapse in infants in 1959.[37] That same year, a randomized, controlled study of antibiotics for neonatal sepsis revealed that the groups treated with chloramphenicol alone or in combination had a 60% mortality, threefold higher than neonates receiving no antibiotics.[38] The no-treatment control group, however, showed the same survival as the nonchloramphenicol antibiotic treatment group. Inadequate glucuronide conjugation of chloramphenicol and decreased tubular secretion of conjugated chloramphenicol combined to reduce chloramphenicol elimination and led to accumulation to toxic concentrations.[39] Acute intoxication with high serum chloramphenicol concentrations manifested with jaundice, vomiting, anorexia, respiratory distress, abdominal distention, cyanosis, green stools, lethargy, and ashen color.[38]

The preservative benzyl alcohol has been implicated in a fatal syndrome in premature infants of cardiovascular collapse and death associated with metabolic acidosis, gasping respirations, thrombocytopenia, hepatic and renal failure, and progressive central nervous system (CNS) depression. The minimal intake to produce toxicity was estimated at 130 mg/kg/day.[40] Removal of benzyl alcohol as a preservative in the fluid frequently used to flush IV catheters in neonates essentially has eliminated this problem. Although many nurseries and pharmacies have excluded all solutions and medications containing benzyl alcohol, the major problem seemed to lie with IV solutions and flush solutions. Considering the dose estimated for toxicity, exposure to the small amounts in medications may pose an acceptable risk, which can be estimated from the benzyl alcohol concentration and dosing volume, compared to the benefit of the drug treatment. Propylene glycol, frequently used as a solvent for non–water-soluble drugs, also has been associated with toxicity in neonates.[41,42]

Unintended percutaneous absorption of toxic substances through the permeable skin of neonates has recurred with several substances. This has led to toxicity from methanol,[43] isopropanol,[44] hexachlorophene,[45] iodine-containing topical disinfectants,[46] aniline dye in diapers,[47] and topical antibiotics such as neomycin.[48] Advantageous and disadvantageous transcutaneous drug absorption by newborns has been reviewed.[49] Chemical intoxication of the fetus and newborn has been reviewed in detail.[50]

Inadvertent exposure of the neonate to a variety of chemicals may occur with little notice. Phthalate plasticizers accumulate in the myocardial and gastrointestinal tissue of neonates with umbilical catheters and those who receive blood products.[51] Although phthalates probably produce minimal acute toxicity, they accumulate in tissues and may exert effects that are not recognized. Since the report by Hillman and colleagues,[51] the extent of exposure of NICU patients to plastic products appears to have increased, causing greater exposure to soluble chemicals in the plastic, such as phthalates.

SPECIFIC CLASSES OF DRUGS

ANTIARRHYTHMICS

Treatment of cardiac arrhythmias has improved with better knowledge of the mechanisms of myocardial physiology and new therapeutic agents. Although the transmembrane potential changes for myocardial and conducting cells have been known for years, the exact roles of the various currents produced by inward and outward transport of sodium, potassium, and calcium still are being clarified.[52]

Antiarrhythmic drugs have been classified according to their effects on ion channels, repolarization, receptor interactions, and structure (Table 56-4).[52,53] Such classification systems help with analysis of the effects of individual antiarrhythmic drugs and selection of treatment for specific arrhythmias. Drugs within a given class, however, frequently differ in their effectiveness for an individual patient's arrhythmia. Dosages for drugs used frequently for resuscitation of newborns are listed (see Table 5-5).

The most frequent arrhythmia requiring management in neonates is supraventricular tachycardia (SVT).[54] Some cardiologists recommend synchronized cardioversion as the treatment of choice, since it usually is effective and more rapid in onset than pharmacologic management.[54] Supraventricular tachycardia in patients without Wolff–Parkinson–White syndrome (WPW) often is treated successfully with digitalis, if vagal stimulation is unsuccessful. Digitalis is considered by some cardiologists to be relatively contraindicated in patients with WPW, because it may increase the ventricular response rate and lead to ventricular fibrillation.[55] A review of patients treated for SVT at Texas Children's Hospital revealed no difference in the success rate for treatment of SVT with digitalis among patients with and without WPW.[56]

Adenosine has been used for the treatment of SVT, with moderate success. Adenosine slows spontaneous heart rate, prolongs the PR interval, and decreases the slope of phase 4 repolarization through activation of A_1-purinoceptors coupled to sarcolemmic potassium channels. It has minimal effect on the ventricle. Adenosine's action begins within seconds. With a 9-second half-life, it must be administered as a rapid IV infusion over 5 to 10 seconds. Adenosine treatment may be started with 30 to 40 μg/kg doses, with increases in the dose by 30 to 40 μg/kg every minute until SVT ceases or atrioventricular block occurs.[57,58] Adenosine may precipitate bronchoconstric-

TABLE 56–4
ANTIARRYTHMIC DRUGS BY MECHANISM OF ACTION

Class	Action	Drugs
I.	Sodium channel blockade	
A.	Moderate phase-0 depression and slowed conduction; repolarization usually prolonged	Quinidine, procainamide, disopyramide, moricizine
B.	Minimal phase-0 depression and slowed conduction; repolarization usually shortened	Lidocaine, mexiletine, phenytoin, tocainide
C.	Marked phase-0 depression and slowed conduction; repolarization minimal change	Encainide, flecainide, propafenone
II.	Beta-Adrenergic blockade	Propranolol, acebutolol, esmolol, others
III.	Prolong repolarization	Amiodarone, bretylium, sotalol
IV.	Ca^{++} channel blockade	Verapamil, diltiazem
V.	Digitalis glycosides	Digoxin
VI.	Purinergic agonists	Adenosine

Adapted from Bigger JT, Hoffman BF. Antiarrhythmic drugs. In: Gilman AG, Rall TW, Nies AS, et al, eds. Goodman and Gilman's the pharmacologic basis of therapeutics. 8th ed. New York: Pergamon Press, 1990:847, and Moak JP. Pharmacology and electrophysiology of antiarrhythmic drugs. In: Gillette PC, Garson A Jr, eds. Pediatric arrhythmias: electrophysiology and pacing. Philadelphia: WB Saunders, 1990:43.

tion and wheezing as well as hypotension due to vasodilation.[53] Its short half-life limits its usefulness to the acute treatment of SVT.

Supraventricular tachycardia that has not responded to adenosine may be managed with an infusion of procainamide. Rapid infusion may precipitate hypotension, whereas chronic treatment produces antinuclear antibodies in 50% to 90% of patients associated with a systemic lupus erythematosus–type syndrome.[53] High concentrations of procainamide may depress myocardial contractility and predispose to congestive heart failure. Although more than half of a procainamide dose is excreted unchanged, it is metabolized in the liver to N-acetylprocainamide (NAPA), an active metabolite, although it acts through a different antiarrhythmic mechanism.[52] The rate of acetylation to NAPA involves the N-acetyltransferase enzyme system involved in the metabolism of isoniazid, which segregates into fast and slow acetylators.[59] Both NAPA and procainamide accumulate with renal insufficiency.

Lidocaine primarily blocks the fast inward sodium channel, like other local anesthetic antiarrhythmic drugs.[53] Its effects are much greater on the conducting system and the ventricular muscle than on the atrium. Plasma concentration monitoring is indicated during treatment with lidocaine, since concentrations exceeding 6 μg/mL may produce seizures or respiratory arrest. Drugs known to decrease hepatic blood flow, such as cimetidine, will decrease hepatic clearance of lidocaine and increase concentrations unless the dose is reduced.

Several β-adrenergic blocking drugs are available, but propranolol is the one used most frequently in the treatment of arrhythmias in neonates. It has special pharmacokinetic features that must be considered in its administration. When administered enterally, propranolol is cleared largely through a first-pass extraction by the liver. It is metabolized extensively to 4-hydroxypropranolol, an active metabolite.[60] During repetitive doses, hepatic extraction decreases, and a steady state eventually will be achieved. This occurs at different dosages for different patients, leading to wide variations in plasma concentrations after the same dose. If administered IV, the propranolol dose must be reduced at least tenfold because it bypasses hepatic extraction and produces a dose- and concentration-related decrease in heart rate and cardiac contractility. Propranolol has been used most frequently to treat supraventricular and ventricular arrhythmias. It also has a role in treatment of sinus tachycardia related to hypermetabolic states such as thyrotoxicosis.[53] Data on dosing, kinetics, and efficacy in neonates for other β-adrenergic blocking drugs such as atenolol, nadolol, and esmolol are limited.

Verapamil has been used for treatment of SVT with moderate success, but its use in infants younger than 12 months of age has been discouraged.[61] Due to its negative inotropic activity and ability to decrease sinus function, verapamil should not be used with β-adrenergic blocking drugs in infants and children.[53] They have been used together successfully in adults.

Amiodarone should be reserved for refractory, life-threatening arrhythmias. Although the frequency of side effects is less common in children than in adults, the side effects are frequent and serious.[62,63] Adverse effects have included corneal microdeposits, slate gray pigmentation in sun-exposed areas, skin rashes, hepatic failure, neurologic symptoms, hypothyroidism, and atrioventricular block.[53] Additional side effects have been observed in adults that have not been reported in infants to date. Mason concluded that amiodarone should not be administered to pregnant and nursing women, due to adverse effects and embryotoxicity in animals.[63]

Amiodarone increases the concentration of several

drugs, usually by decreasing clearance and volume of distribution, including digoxin, quinidine, procainamide, phenytoin, and flecainide. Decreased clearance of warfarin by amiodarone may precipitate hemorrhage.

ANTICONVULSANTS

Seizures remain a frequent therapeutic problem for newborns that may be caused by a variety of disorders, such as meningitis, inadequate pyridoxal-5-phosphate binding (*i.e.*, pyridoxine dependency), hypoglycemia, hypocalcemia, inborn errors of metabolism, neonatal abstinence from narcotics, or intracranial hemorrhage.[64] Since treatment differs according to etiology, causes for seizures outside the brain always should be considered and evaluated. Some noncerebral causes of seizures may produce recurrent seizures that require prolonged anticonvulsant drug treatment, in addition to treatment of the primary metabolic or infectious disorder. Since seizures *per se* may harm the brain, treatment should not be delayed.[64]

Phenobarbital remains the mainstay of seizure therapy in neonates.[65] The volume of distribution of phenobarbital has been measured in several studies and averages 0.9 L/kg.[66] Although seizures are controlled in some patients with phenobarbital levels of 15 μg/mL, the minimal effective therapeutic range should be regarded as 20 μg/mL. To maximize efficacy and minimize adverse effects, neonatal seizures should be treated with a single drug to its maximal dose before adding a second drug or changing to a second drug. Using this approach and a maximum dose of 40 mg/kg of phenobarbital, 85% of neonatal seizures could be controlled with phenobarbital alone.[67] The half-life of phenobarbital at birth is prolonged, ranging from 43 to 217 hours.[68] Consequently, daily doses of phenobarbital at birth should be reduced from the previous recommendations of 5 mg/kg/day to 2 mg/kg/day, to avoid accumulation while elimination is quite slow. As clearance increases within the first few weeks after birth, dosages may need to be increased. A good correlation has been demonstrated between plasma and brain concentrations of phenobarbital and phenytoin, so that increasing plasma concentrations should increase the anticonvulsant concentration at the site of action.[66]

The second line of anticonvulsant treatment for neonates usually is phenytoin. It has a similar volume of distribution to phenobarbital and a therapeutic range of 10 to 20 μg/mL.[69] Thus, a loading dose of 10 to 20 mg/kg should be used for phenytoin. To avoid bradycardia and precipitation of the drug, phenytoin (*p*H approximately 12) should be administered slowly into an IV line containing only saline. Intramuscular administration should be avoided, since the drug is caustic to tissues. Chronic phenytoin therapy in infants requires higher doses than originally suspected; dosages range as high as 18 mg/kg/day to maintain concentrations of 8 to 25 μg/mL. This appears to reflect incomplete absorption over time, rather than increased metabolism.[69]

Additional drug therapy beyond phenobarbital and phenytoin sometimes is required to control seizures in the newborn. Diazepam has been used to treat refractory seizures in neonates, but its efficacy is limited by its short duration of action, respiratory depression, prolonged half-life, and metabolism to active metabolites.[70] Another benzodiazepine, lorazepam, in a dose of 0.05 mg/kg has been effective for controlling refractory seizures in neonates with a duration of action up to 24 hours.[70] Inadvertent tenfold overdoses of lorazepam have been tolerated in neonates without hypotension or respiratory depression.* The dose of benzyl alcohol associated with lorazepam treatment is low enough not to represent a risk for toxicity.[50]

Concerns have increased about the effects of long-term phenobarbital treatment on cognitive development. When phenobarbital was compared to placebo in two randomized groups of children treated for 2 years for febrile seizures, the phenobarbital-treated group had significantly lower IQs.[71] In a randomized, crossover trial of three anticonvulsants, phenobarbital produced more impairment of neuropsychological performance than carbamazepine or phenytoin.[72] The American Academy of Pediatrics Committee on Drugs summarized concerns about the cognitive effects of phenobarbital.[73]

The decision to continue or to stop treatment with anticonvulsant medications before discharge from the NICU remains controversial. Scher and Painter suggest that anticonvulsants may be discontinued for infants who show no abnormalities of the brain on imaging studies, have an age-appropriate neurologic examination, and have a normal interictal electroencephalogram.[74] Up to 30% of neonates with seizures later have epilepsy, but frequently the later seizure pattern takes the form of infantile spasms or minor motor seizures that are not very responsive to phenobarbital and phenytoin.[74]

ANTIHYPERTENSIVES

Drug treatment of hypertension in pediatric patients should follow a stepped treatment regime, in which a single drug's effects are optimized before adding another.[75,76] When this approach is extended to the newborn, treatment may begin with diuretics, and centrally acting agents, such as methyldopa, or β-receptor blockers such as propranolol, are added if needed. A vasodilator, such as hydralazine, may be substituted or added to β-adrenergic blockers. Recently, calcium channel blockers such as nifedipine, verapamil, and diltiazem have emerged as effective antihypertensives.[77] Other vasodilators need to be used with a diuretic to avoid fluid retention. Calcium

* Ward RM, personal observation, November 1992.

channel blockers, however, do not cause fluid retention and are roughly equivalent to β-adrenergic antagonists or diuretics for the treatment of hypertension.[77]

Angiotensin-converting enzyme inhibitors (*e.g.*, captopril) have a special role in the treatment of neonatal renovascular hypertension that is caused by markedly elevated renin and angiotensin.[78] Aortic catheters may distribute microemboli to the kidneys, which increase secretion of renin and angiotensin in response to focal underperfusion. Although captopril may be relatively specific treatment for many cases of renovascular hypertension in neonates, dosage adjustments are difficult because it is not dispensed in a suspension. Dosage adjustments require the pharmacy to grind tablets and weigh individual doses, or the parents to formulate tablets into suspensions for each dose. Captopril treatment of neonates should start with doses of 0.01 mg/kg, rather than the earlier recommendations of 0.1 to 0.3 mg/kg/dose, to avoid hypotension and acute renal insufficiency.[79] Doses should be increased daily if hypertension persists. Initial captopril treatment may cause a triphasic reaction of hypotension with renal failure, managed by dose reduction, followed by a rise in blood pressure despite increasing doses above the original dose.[80] At the start of captopril treatment, hypotension is exaggerated in salt- and water-depleted patients.[81] As in adults, captopril may be useful for afterload reduction in the treatment of chronic congestive heart failure in newborns.[81]

Hypertensive emergencies are infrequent in neonates, but can be treated with sodium nitroprusside if renal function is normal or with diazoxide if renal function is inadequate.[76] As observed in older patients, thiocyanate and cyanide may accumulate during sodium nitroprusside treatment, and hyperglycemia may occur with diazoxide infusions.

ANTIMICROBIALS

Patterns of antimicrobial use in neonatology evolve with the changing spectrum of infections and development of new antimicrobial agents. Emergence of neonatal infections with *Staphylococcus epidermidis* resistant to semisynthetic penicillins and aminoglycosides has led to treatment of many neonates with vancomycin.[82] Even though current formulations of vancomycin are much safer than those available 20 years ago, its toxicities are relevant to newborn medicine. Studies suggest a decrease in vancomycin nephrotoxicity, unless administered with aminoglycosides, and in ototoxicity.[83,84] Thrombophlebitis is common, and subcutaneous administration may cause skin necrosis and sloughing. Doses of vancomycin should be infused over at least 1 hour to avoid diffuse histamine release, hypotension, and the red-man syndrome.[85] Vancomycin clearance in premature infants is directly proportional to postconceptional age, body weight, and surface area.[86] To minimize antibiotic pressure selecting for resistant organisms, vancomycin should be reserved for staphylococci that are resistant to nafcillin.

Nafcillin largely has replaced methicillin for the treatment of *Staphylococcus aureus* infections since it has a lower risk of adverse reactions. Nafcillin is eliminated largely through biliary excretion, which may be impaired in neonates with cholestasis related to prolonged hyperalimentation.[87]

Piperacillin provides a broader gram-negative spectrum than ampicillin or carbenicillin.[88] For treatment of *Pseudomonas* sp. infections, piperacillin may be combined with an aminoglycoside to decrease the emergence of resistant organisms.[89] When combined with an aminoglycoside such as gentamicin, piperacillin provides excellent coverage for the aerobic and anaerobic bacteria encountered after intestinal perforation.

Strains of enteric organisms that are resistant to multiple antibiotics are emerging, possibly due to the increased use of cephalosporin antibiotics in NICUs.[90–93] Both *Enterobacter cloacae* and *Enterococcus* sp. are emerging in neonatal patients as multiply resistant organisms that may require treatment with antibiotics that have received little study in neonates such as the monobactam, aztreonam, and the carbapenem, imipenem, that has been combined with cilastatin, a renal dehydropeptidase inhibitor.[93,94] Both of these antibiotics should be used judiciously, with guidance from a specialist in infectious diseases who is familiar with alternative antimicrobials that may be studied more thoroughly in newborns.

Cephalosporins continue to proliferate, and in some clinical settings have replaced gentamicin for gram-negative coverage of neonates receiving initial treatment for presumed sepsis.[91] This is cause for concern, since cephalosporins have been reported to induce antibiotic resistance rapidly from antibiotic pressure.[92,93] Aminoglycosides, first kanamycin and then gentamicin, have been mainstays for treatment of presumed sepsis at birth in neonates, with minimal development of resistant organisms.[95]

Monitoring of aminoglycoside levels involves cost and blood removal that may not be necessary during the first 2 to 3 days of therapy while cultures are pending, unless the patient exhibits overt renal dysfunction.[21] Aminoglycoside monitoring is particularly appropriate to ensure that effective concentrations have been achieved for treatment of proven infections. Gentamicin-induced renal toxicity and ototoxicity are uniquely less frequent in neonates than in adults.[21] For treatment beyond 3 days, or with evidence of renal dysfunction, monitoring of drug levels is indicated because the clearance of aminoglycosides is directly related to the glomerular filtration rate, which is quite immature and variable in premature and sick newborns. The aminoglycosides are examples of very water-soluble drugs, the blood levels of which are influenced significantly by the patient's state of hydration.

Certain cephalosporins have unique properties that fit clinical problems encountered frequently in neonates. Cefuroxime achieves high concentrations in spinal fluid needed for treatment of *Haemophilus influenzae* type B, *Neisseria meningitidis*, and penicillin-sensitive strains of *Streptococcus pneumoniae*.[96] Although ceftazidime usually is active against *Pseudomonas* sp., it should be used with a second antibiotic to avoid emergence of resistant strains. The third-generation cephalosporins, cefoperazone, cefotaxime, and moxalactam, are effective against *Escherichia coli* and *Klebsiella* sp. Nephrotoxicity is minimal, and they diffuse readily into spinal fluid to provide effective treatment of meningitis produced by sensitive organisms. The fact that moxalactam may cause hemorrhage due to decreased platelet aggregation has decreased its use. Diarrhea is a common side effect of broad-spectrum cephalosporin treatment that is seen in children and occasionally in neonates.

ANTIREFLUX MEDICATIONS

The relation of gastroesophageal reflux in newborns to apnea and chronic lung disease remains controversial. Certain infants with BPD clearly reflux, aspirate, and have apnea.[97] Many other infants regurgitate feeds without a clear association with symptoms of chronic lung disease or apnea. Despite the debate, treatment for gastroesophageal reflux in neonates is frequent in NICUs.[97] Euler reported a blinded, placebo-controlled, crossover trial of bethanechol for the treatment of gastroesophageal reflux in 30 infants aged 3 weeks to 12 months.[98] Esophageal manometry revealed low-average lower esophageal sphincter pressure and normal sphincter relaxation before treatment. Bethanechol decreased the number of vomiting episodes and more than doubled the rate of weight gain. Sphincter tone began to increase by 25 minutes after bethanechol administration and reached a maximum 8 minutes later. The effect was then sustained for at least 1 hour and documented for 2 hours in older patients who underwent prolonged manometry. Esophageal *p*H probe testing showed a significant decrease in number and duration of reflux episodes. Other studies have confirmed these observations.[99]

Sondheimer and colleagues, however, found that bethanechol did not improve symptomatic gastroesophageal reflux in infants.[100] In 11 infants, aged 0.5 to 7.5 months, bethanechol improved acid clearance from the esophagus, shortened the episodes of reflux, decreased the total time that the esophageal *p*H was less than 4.0, but did not decrease the frequency of reflux episodes. They suggest that bethanechol is effective by improving esophageal motor function, rather than by increasing lower esophageal sphincter pressure.

As a cholinomimetic, bethanechol may increase bronchial secretions as well as bronchoconstriction. Euler considers reactive airway disease to be a relative contraindication to treatment with bethanechol.[98] Like carbachol, bethanechol stimulates muscles of the urinary tract and the gastrointestinal tract to contract. Cardiovascular side effects are less frequent with bethanechol than with other members of this drug class, methacholine and acetylcholine, that may produce hypotension, flushing, sweating, abdominal cramps, and atrial fibrillation in hyperthyroid patients.

Metoclopramide, a derivative of procainamide with dopamine antagonist properties, originally was administered as a stimulant of gastrointestinal mobility and as an antiemetic.[101] As gastroesophageal reflux gained importance in neonatology, metoclopramide was used for its treatment.[102] Through its cholinergic effects, metoclopramide increases gastric fundal and lower esophageal sphincter tone as well as peristalsis in the esophagus, gastric antrum, and small intestine. Consistent with its central dopamine antagonist activities, it may precipitate extrapyramidal symptoms and stimulate prolactin secretion. Facial spasms, opisthotonos, and oculogyric crisis have been observed in children treated with metoclopramide.[101]

In a trial of metoclopramide for treatment of gastroesophageal reflux in six very-low-birth-weight infants (790–1040 g), gastric residual volumes decreased, feeding tolerance improved, weight gain increased, and intestinal transit time decreased.[102] Discontinuation of the drug caused resumption of symptoms. With a dose of 0.1 mg/kg/day, no dystonic reactions or abnormalities of hematologic or biochemical testing were noted. In a well designed, prospective, blinded, crossover trial, metoclopramide was compared to placebo in 30 infants younger than 1 year of age.[103] In this study, there was a significant placebo effect on symptom scores reported by parents. In a dosage of 0.1 mg/kg/dose four times daily, metoclopramide decreased the length of time that the esophageal *p*H was less than 4.0 without changing the total number of episodes when the *p*H was less than 4, nor the number of prolonged episodes when the *p*H was less than 4. Gastric emptying was unchanged compared to controls, but the percentage of time that the *p*H was less than 4 was significantly decreased. The reduction was modest, from an average of 13.4% to 10.3%. Acid reflux was not eliminated by metoclopramide. No side effects were noted during the study.

Higher doses of metoclopramide may improve its efficacy for treatment of gastroesophageal reflux, but adverse effects are more likely.[104] With dosages of 0.5 mg/kg/day divided into four doses, metoclopramide actually increased the number of reflux episodes and the time during which the esophageal *p*H was less than 4.[105] More important, this dosage was associated with a high frequency of irritability, causing parents to discontinue therapy. At the outset, a large number of parents refused to participate because of prior negative experiences with metoclopramide treatment of their child. Presumably, the increased number of episodes of reflux related to increased irritability.

Thus, there is no single optimal treatment for gastroesophageal reflux. Potentially significant side effects are associated with pharmacologic treatment, and debate persists about the efficacy and indications for drug treatment of gastroesophageal reflux.

BRONCHODILATORS

Bronchodilator treatment of neonates has been controversial because of presumed lack of adequate amounts of bronchiolar smooth muscle to produce bronchoconstriction (see Methylxanthines). Two divergent populations of young infants have been studied, those with wheezing bronchitis and those with BPD following lung disease at birth. In the former population, Lenney and Milner detected no response to inhaled salbutamol (albuterol) in wheezing children younger than 18 months of age.[106] In contrast, pulmonary reactivity to methacholine that could be relieved by inhaled metaproterenol has been demonstrated in a group of normal male infants ranging in age from 3.5 to 14.5 months.[107]

In infants with BPD after mechanical ventilation for hyaline membrane disease, aerosol treatment with isoproterenol markedly improved airway resistance and specific airway conductance at 41 weeks postconceptional age.[108] As would be predicted, a mean increase in heart rate of 27% occurred and was sustained for 15 minutes after administration of the isoproterenol aerosol. Both a β-adrenergic agonist, salbutamol (albuterol), and an anticholinergic, ipratropium bromide, produced bronchodilatation in ventilator-dependent neonates who were progressing into chronic lung disease.[109] These infants, who ranged from 25 to 29 weeks of gestation with birth weights of 560 to 1050 g, demonstrated bronchodilatation as early as 19 days after birth. Others confirmed these findings in ventilator-dependent preterm infants who demonstrated dose-related bronchodilatation to ipratropium alone, and in combination with salbutamol (albuterol), by 18 to 34 days after birth.[110] Salbutamol (albuterol) administered orally also improved lung function in infants with BPD.[111]

When administered to neonates recovering from hyaline membrane disease, isoetharine, a β_2-receptor agonist with limited cardiovascular side effects, decreased total pulmonary resistance in all infants and raised dynamic compliance in 11 of 13.[112] Serial pulmonary function studies in mechanically ventilated premature neonates showed a progressive decrease in forced vital capacity and expiratory flow velocity with postnatal age.[113] Expiratory flow velocity showed a positive response to isoetharine aerosol by 2 weeks postnatal age. The greater the degree of airway reactivity, the longer the infant ultimately required mechanical ventilatory support. Motoyama and colleagues concluded that the initial airway dysfunction was due primarily to reactive airway disease.[113] These serial observations indicate that significant lower airway obstruction may begin by 3 to 4 weeks postnatal age, in preterm infants who remain ventilator dependent. Motoyama and colleagues detected severe reactive airway disease as early as 26 weeks postconception, well before clinical signs of BPD were apparent.[113]

Several issues remain unresolved with regard to bronchodilator therapy of neonates. Dose–response relationships need to be established, but are hindered by uncertainties about how much aerosol actually is delivered to the site of action. Chronic bronchodilator therapy of neonates frequently is administered by aerosol, but might produce a more prolonged effect if administered enterally. More study is needed of the use of antimuscarinic agents in neonates, such as ipratropium, both alone and in combination with β-adrenergic agonists. Improvement in lung function in infants with BPD after treatment with bronchodilators may reflect bronchodilation, improved mucociliary transport, or decreased pulmonary edema.[112]

DIURETICS

Several classes of diuretic drugs are available, including osmotic agents such as mannitol, carbonic anhydrase inhibitors such as acetazolamide, thiazides such as chlorothiazide, high-ceiling or loop diuretics such as furosemide, potassium-sparing diuretics such as spironolactone, and methylxanthines such as theophylline.[114] The last four of these classes are used frequently in the treatment of neonates, both for acute fluid overload and for chronic therapy of BPD and congestive heart failure. Distinct differences in mechanisms of action and potency should guide selection of specific drugs.[115,116]

Thiazides are sulfonamide diuretics whose major action is to block sodium and chloride cotransport in the first portion of the distal tubule, which causes a natriuresis.[114–116] Thiazide-induced diuresis produces a greater loss of sodium and potassium per urine volume than does a diuresis induced by loop diuretics, although only a moderate amount of sodium is excreted.[114] Among diuretics, thiazides are relatively unique in that they decrease the renal excretion of calcium, although magnesium excretion is increased. In high doses, thiazides may inhibit carbonic anhydrase with a potency equal to that of acetazolamide. They also may induce hypoglycemia, hypercholesterolemia, and hypertriglyceridemia.[114] Thiazide elimination occurs through the renal tubular organic acid transport system, and may be inhibited by other organic acids such as probenecid. The diuretic action of thiazides depends on secretion into the renal tubular fluid, so that competitive inhibition of the transport of a thiazide by another organic acid may blunt its diuretic effect.

Spironolactone, the potassium-sparing diuretic most frequently used for treatment of newborns, is a 17-spironolactone steroid that competitively antagonizes mineralocorticoids, predominantly aldosterone.[114,115] Since aldosterone increases sodium reabsorption and potassium secretion, increased aldosterone secretion may be suspected by the ratio of urine sodium to potassium. Similarly, effective antagonism of aldosterone by spironolactone may be detected by an increasing urine sodium to potassium ratio. The appropriate dose of spironolactone relates to the concentration of aldosterone, since it acts through competitive inhibition. Spironolactone is available only for enteral administration and undergoes extensive first-pass hepatic metabolism to an active metabolite, canrenone.

The most serious toxicity of spironolactone is hyperkalemia during cotreatment with potassium supplements.[115] Spironolactone increases calcium excretion and, in older men, has been reported to produce gynecomastia due to an antiandrogen effect. In rats exposed to high doses of spironolactone for prolonged periods, tumors may develop that have not been reported in humans to date.[114] Other side effects include rashes, diarrhea, and vomiting.

Alternate potassium-sparing diuretics that do not work through aldosterone inhibition, such as triamterene and amiloride, rarely are administered to neonates. Their potassium-sparing action probably occurs through inhibition of the electrogenic sodium transport in the distal nephron.[114]

Among the three loop diuretics in clinical use in the United States, bumetanide, ethacrynic acid, and furosemide, furosemide is the best studied in neonates. All three are organic acids, but furosemide and bumetanide are sulfonamides. All three diuretics induce diuresis by inhibiting the chloride pump in the ascending limb of the loop of Henle. Their diuretic effects require secretion into the tubular fluid by the organic acid transport system that may be competitively inhibited by other organic acids such as probenecid.[116,117] Because of these similarities in action, there is almost no reason to use two loop diuretics simultaneously. Patients who are resistant to furosemide, however, may still respond to bumetanide.[115] Loop diuretics produce excretion of dilute urine, with an increase in free-water excretion compared to sodium excretion.[118]

Calcium excretion is increased by furosemide.[115] This contributes to renal parenchymal calcification, nephrolithiasis, and osteopenia during chronic treatment of neonates with furosemide. Cholelithiasis has been observed infrequently during chronic furosemide treatment. Although furosemide is highly protein bound, it appears unlikely that doses administered to neonates produce high enough concentrations to displace bilirubin.[116]

As might be expected for a drug eliminated by renal tubular secretion, the half-life of furosemide in neonates is long and variable, ranging from 4.7 to 44.9 hours.[119] During repetitive dosing, Vert and colleagues demonstrated an inverse relationship between postconceptional age and furosemide half-life. Petersen and colleagues have confirmed this prolonged half-life for furosemide in preterm neonates during the first few weeks after birth.[7] They also noted that some neonates have poor absorption of orally administered furosemide, leading to an inadequate diuretic response. The prolonged half-life does not support the current clinical practice of administering furosemide every 6 to 8 hours in neonates.

The effects of furosemide on lung function, both acutely and chronically, have been studied in neonates with BPD[120] and in neonates recovering from hyaline membrane disease.[121] In patients with BPD, pulmonary compliance improved after a single dose of furosemide. Prolonged treatment, however, improved pulmonary compliance, resistance, and oxygenation without an effect on transcutaneous PCO_2.[120] In a controlled study of preterm neonates recovering from hyaline membrane disease, furosemide improved pulmonary compliance by 2 hours after administration.[121] This improvement persisted for 4 hours and then returned to baseline by 6 hours. Chronic furosemide treatment for 4 days produced a further improvement in alveolar–arterial difference in partial pressure of oxygen ($AaDO_2$).

One prospective, controlled study of newborns has found that furosemide treatment increases the frequency of patent ductus arteriosus, presumably due to the release of prostaglandin (PG) E_2 that accompanies diuresis.[122] Other investigators have administered furosemide with indomethacin to blunt the oliguric response to indomethacin without loss of indomethacin-induced ductal closure.[123] Indomethacin is known to block the natriuretic response to furosemide as well as the increase in renal blood flow that furosemide produces.[124]

Both furosemide and ethacrynic acid may produce ototoxicity.[114] Furosemide-induced hearing loss occurs after large (1000 mg) doses administered IV, especially to patients with renal failure who would be expected to have poor clearance of the drug.[125] This transient ototoxicity correlates with changes in electrolyte concentrations in the middle ear fluids, endolymph and perilymph, that reduce endocochlear potentials.[125] Compared to furosemide, bumetanide caused a similar frequency of adverse effects, except for ototoxicity, which appeared to be less with bumetanide.[126]

Both thiazides and furosemide may produce allergic interstitial nephritis.[114] The most frequent adverse effects associated with treatment of newborns with loop diuretics reflect their actions, and frequently lead to hypochloremic and hypokalemic alkalosis. Electrolyte monitoring is needed at the start of treatment to avoid sodium depletion to serum values less than 120 mEq/L.

Although seldom used as a diuretic, methylxanthines may produce significant diuresis, natriuresis, and choliuresis.[127]

HISTAMINE$_2$ RECEPTOR ANTAGONISTS

The existence of a histamine$_2$ receptor that controls histamine-induced secretion of gastric acid was predicted when classic antihistamines (*i.e.*, histamine$_1$ receptor antagonists such as diphenhydramine) did not block this and other effects of histamine. After synthesis of hundreds of compounds, the first histamine$_2$ receptor antagonist, burimamide, was found to inhibit histamine-induced gastric acid secretion.[128] Histamine$_2$ receptors actively mediate local inflammatory responses, with a lesser effect on cardiac contractility.[129,130] A series of structurally related compounds have been developed to block the histamine$_2$ receptor, including metiamide, cimetidine, ranitidine, and famotidine. The last three of these drugs are used clinically.

Overall, patients report adverse effects more often after treatment with cimetidine than during treatment with ranitidine.[131] Adults report diarrhea, nausea, vomiting, and constipation more often than other adverse effects. The most important adverse effect of cimetidine in newborns is its inhibition of the elimination of numerous drugs cleared by the microsomal oxidation enzyme system, cytochrome P450. Cimetidine, like other drugs with an imidazole structure such as ketoconazole and metronidazole, binds to cytochrome P450 and reduces its activity.[132] Ranitidine, in which the imidazole ring is replaced with a furan ring, binds to liver microsomes and cytochrome P450 with approximately one tenth the affinity of cimetidine.[132] Because of its greater potency and longer duration of effect, ranitidine is administered less frequently than cimetidine. Since ranitidine has at least three to four times the molar potency of cimetidine, it has minimal effects on cytochrome P450 in usual clinical doses.[133,134]

One of the most frequently encountered drug–drug interactions during cimetidine therapy of newborns is its antagonism of theophylline metabolism. Other potential interactions include decreased clearance of propranolol, phenytoin, lidocaine, nifedipine, and niazepam.[132] The elimination of these drugs involves oxidation. Drugs such as lorazepam, which requires conjugation for elimination, are not affected by cimetidine treatment. Cimetidine also decreases hepatic blood flow, which may decrease the elimination of some drugs. The effects of histamine$_2$ receptor antagonists on drugs cleared by low and high hepatic extraction have been discussed in detail.[132]

Little information is available about ranitidine pharmacokinetics and pharmacodynamics in pediatric patients, and these data are extremely limited with respect to the neonate. In children aged 2 to 18 years, ranitidine has been administered in doses of 0.2 mg/kg/hour after a loading dose of 0.6 mg/kg.[135] The bioavailability averages 50% when administered orally.[136] Parenteral dosing at 1.5 mg/kg every 6 hours was significantly more effective than oral dosing at 2 mg/kg every 6 hours for raising gastric *p*H above 4.[136] Ranitidine provided effective treatment for a preterm neonate with a life-threatening upper gastrointestinal hemorrhage after indomethacin.[137] In this preterm newborn, a dose of 0.2 mg/kg/hour produced quite high concentrations with a half-life of approximately 5.5 hours, which is over twice as long as the elimination half-life reported in older children.[135]

Mallet and associates have examined ranitidine kinetics and therapeutic responses of 11 infants with reflux esophagitis or near-miss sudden infant death syndrome.[138] They noted that formula or milk feeding raised gastric *p*H for 2 to 3 hours after the meal. Gastric *p*H could be maintained above 4 as long as the plasma ranitidine concentration remained above 100 ng/mL. Doses were administered 2 hours after meals, every 12 hours.

Famotidine is a relatively new histamine$_2$ antagonist that is not well studied in children and neonates. It does not appear to inhibit oxidative drug metabolism or hepatic blood flow, but its use has been too limited to evaluate efficacy or safety.[139]

INOTROPES

Although inotropy refers to myocardial contractility, inotropic drugs improve cardiac contractility, increase cardiac rate, and alter vascular tone.[140,141] The inotrope should be selected according to the specific cardiovascular disorder to be corrected. Since cardiac output is determined by preload, contractility, and afterload, these pharmacologic properties of various inotropes will be described and may be used to select the optimal drug for a specific clinical situation. Despite frequent administration of inotropes to newborns, they have received limited study in young infants.

Shock occurs when blood flow and oxygen supply are inadequate to meet tissue demands. The same principles apply to the myocardium. Increasing cardiac wall stiffness increases myocardial oxygen consumption, and may decrease flow during diastole. Inotropic drug treatment for the failing heart must balance increasing myocardial oxygen consumption against the increase in cardiac output that provides more oxygenated blood through the coronary circulation to the myocardium. Disproportionate increases in myocardial wall stiffness may impede coronary flow and worsen myocardial ischemia. Similarly, excess peripheral vasodilation may reduce the blood pressure to a level where there is too little pressure to maintain coronary flow during diastole.

The following receptor-mediated cardiovascular responses may be observed during treatment with cardiovascular drugs[141]:

Alpha$_1$: constriction of arterioles and veins; cardiac contractility.
Alpha$_2$: inhibition of presynaptic release of norepinephrine; constriction of selected arterioles.
Beta$_1$: increase in force and rate of cardiac contraction, cardiac conduction velocity, and heart rate.
Beta$_2$: dilation of arterioles, veins, and bronchioles.
Dopaminergic: dilation of arterioles in renal, coronary, and splanchnic circulations.

Specific receptor interactions of inotropic drugs should guide their clinical use (Table 56-5).[141–143] Dosages for drugs used frequently in newborn resuscita-

TABLE 56–5
RELATIVE CARDIOVASCULAR RECEPTOR INTERACTIONS OF INOTROPES

	Receptor					
Catecholamine	α_1	α_2	β_1	β_2	Dopaminergic	Indirect
Dobutamine	1+	0	3+	1+	0	0
Dopamine	0–3+	1+	2+–3+	2+	3+	1+
Epinephrine	2+	2+	3+	3+	0	0
Isoproterenol	0	0	3+	3+	0	0

1, lowest interaction; 4, greatest interaction;
From Zaritsky A, Chernow B. Use of catecholamines in pediatrics. J Pediatr 1984;105:341.

tion are indicated in Table 56-6. Isoproterenol is a direct-acting, potent, pure β-adrenergic agonist whose usefulness is limited by tachycardia and peripheral vasodilation. Tachycardia and diversion of blood flow to the large vasculature in muscle may steal perfusion away from more vital organs and extend myocardial infarction.[144] Isoproterenol is most effective for raising heart rate, for instance in the treatment of complete heart block. Although isoproterenol is a potent inotrope, tachycardia, diversion of blood flow away from the heart, and lowered mean blood pressure limit its usefulness for treatment of cardiovascular collapse.

Epinephrine stimulates all adrenergic receptors directly, but its vascular effects vary among organs, with β_2 stimulation usually exceeding α_1 vasoconstriction.[143] Peripheral vascular resistance usually falls. Blood pressure rises due to increases in cardiac contractility and cardiac output.

Dopamine, the immediate precursor of norepinephrine, is unique among inotropes because it dilates renal, coronary, and mesenteric vascular beds at low doses through activation of the Dp_1-dopaminergic receptors. At high concentrations, its α_1 receptor activity causes vasoconstriction to predominate in all circulations. Although dosages above 20 μg/kg/minute have been described as causing a predominance of vasoconstriction,[140] studies of renal vascular resistance in newborn animals infused with 32 to 50 μg/kg/minute of dopamine have not detected this effect.[145,146] Dopamine exerts some of its effects through release of endogenous norepinephrine, which may become depleted during prolonged infusions.[143] Peripheral infusions of dopamine do not cross the blood–brain barrier to interact with CNS dopamine receptors. Extravasation of dopamine may cause severe ischemic tissue damage, which may be treated by local infiltration of diluted phentolamine.[147]

The dose–response relationship of dopamine has been studied in a small number of hypotensive neonates with hyaline membrane disease who did not respond to volume expansion with 5% albumin.[148] Dopamine doses of 2 μg/kg/minute increased systolic blood pressure alone. With doses of 4 μg/kg/minute, both systolic and diastolic blood pressures increased significantly. At 8 μg/kg/minute, both systolic and diastolic blood pressures increased farther and heart rate increased significantly.

Dobutamine is the product of directed structural manipulation of dopamine and isoproterenol to produce hydroxyphenyl–isobutyl–dopamine (dobutamine), an inotrope designed to increase contractility with a minimum of tachycardia and vasodilation.[149] Initially, dobutamine was thought to possess balanced vascular α_1 and β_2 activities. Later study demonstrated that dobutamine exists in two enantiomorphic forms, with different receptor activities.[150] The (−) isomer is a potent α_1-agonist that increases cardiac contractility, whereas the (+) isomer is a potent α_2-antagonist. The (+) isomer is manyfold more potent for β receptors than the (−) isomer. Overall, dobutamine is more selective for β_1 than for β_2 receptors. With infusions at less than 20 μg/kg/minute, dobutamine increases cardiac output and contractility with minimal changes in peripheral resistance and modest increases in heart rate.[143] In neonates, dosages of 5 and 7.5 μg/kg/minute increased cardiac output without changing heart rate or blood pressure.[151] The lack of vasoconstriction may limit dobutamine's usefulness in patients with severe hypotension, but may be useful in patients with cardiogenic failure in whom cardiac function may worsen with increased afterload.

Digoxin remains a useful drug for the chronic enteral treatment of congestive heart failure. The efficacy of digitalis for the treatment of congestive heart failure varies according to myocardial dynamics.[152] In a study of 21 infants with congestive heart failure due to ventricular septal defects, digoxin improved 12 clinically, but only 6 improved by echocardiographic measurements.[153]

Digoxin toxicity, like efficacy, is not defined by a specific concentration, but by signs and symptoms such as emesis, arrhythmias, or conduction abnormalities, such as complete heart block. Life-threatening arrhythmias due to excessive digitalis concentrations may be treated successfully with antidigoxin Fab antibody fragments.[154]

Therapeutic monitoring of digoxin in newborns has become more complex with the discovery of a circulating endogenous molecule, digoxinlike immuno-

TABLE 56–6
DRUGS USED IN RESUSCITATION OF NEWBORN INFANTS

Drug and Formulation	Final Concentration	Dose (amount/kg)	Dose (mL/kg)	Route
Cardiorespiratory Resuscitation				
Atropine 10.0%	0.1 mg/mL	0.01–0.03 mg/kg; May repeat in 10 min; maximum = 0.04 mg/kg; IT dose is 2–3 times IV dose	0.1–0.2 mL/kg	IV, IT
Bicarbonate 0.5 mEq/mL	0.5 mEq/mL	1–2 mEq/kg; treat measured metabolic acidosis; avoid 1.0 mEq/mL formulation in newborns; maintain adequate ventilation	2–4 mL/kg	IV
Calcium gluconate 10%	100 mg/mL (9.3 mg Ca^{++}/mL)	100–200 mg/kg; extravasation causes tissue necrosis	1–2 mL/kg	IV
Calcium chloride 10%	100 mg/mL (27 mg Ca^{++}/mL	35–70 mg/kg; extravasation causes tissue necrosis	0.35–0.70 mL/kg	IV
Epinephrine 1 : 10,000	0.1 mg/mL	0.01–0.03 mg/kg	0.1–0.3 mL/kg	IV, IT
Glucose 10.0%	100 mg/mL	200–500 mg/kg	2–5 mL/kg	IV
Naloxone 0.4 mg/mL	0.4 mg/mL	0.1 mg/kg; minimum dose for full-term neonate at delivery is 1.25 mL (0.5 mg)	0.25 mL/kg	IV, IT
Antiarrhythmic Treatment				
Adenosine 6 mg/2 mL	3 mg/mL	30–40 μg/kg, rapid IV push; increase dose by 30–40 μg/kg and repeat in 60 sec if no effect until AV block or conversion of SVT	Dilute 0.5 mL and 49.5 mL normal saline Infuse: 1.0–1.3 mL/kg	IV
Direct-current defibrillation		1 Watt-sec/kg; increase by 1 Watt-sec/kg, if unsuccessful		
Lidocaine 2%	20 mg/mL	0.5–1.0 mg/kg; repeat every 5–10 minutes to maximum of five times	Dilute 0.5 mL + 9.5 mL D5W Infuse: 0.5–1.0 mL/kg	IV
Procainamide 100 mg/mL	100 mg/mL	10–15 mg/kg; maximum rate of 0.5 mg/kg/min; slow with impaired myocardial function	Dilute 1 mL + 9 mL D5W Infuse: 1.0–1.5 mL/kg	IV

AV, atrioventricular; IT, intratracheal; SVT, supraventricular tachycardia.
Adapted from Moak JP. Pharmacology and electrophysiology of antiarrhythmic drugs. In: Gillette PC, Garson A Jr, eds. Pediatric arrythmias: electrophysiology and pacing. Philadelphia: WB Saunders, 1990:37; American Academy of Pediatrics Committee on Drugs. Emergency drug doses for infants and children. Pediatrics 1988;81:462; and Roberts RJ. Drug therapeutics in infants. Philadelphia: WB Saunders, 1984.

reactive substance (DLIS), which cross reacts with exogenous digoxin in several radioimmunoassays.[155] Digoxinlike immunoreactive substance is increased in the circulation of newborns, pregnant women, and patients with renal failure. The more premature the newborn, the higher the estimated concentration of digoxin.[156] Between 24 and 28 weeks of gestation, DLIS produced serum digoxin concentrations from 1.6 to 5.3 ng/mL without prior administration of digoxin. Levels of DLIS in the serum of premature newborns rise for several days after birth, and then persist for over 2 weeks. Since DLIS values vary among assays for digoxin, it may be useful to measure serum digoxin for DLIS before initiating digoxin treatment in neonates during the first 2 to 3 weeks after birth.[157]

METHYLXANTHINES

Caffeine and theophylline are administered frequently to preterm neonates. Besides metabolism of the trimethylxanthine, caffeine, to theophylline, a dimethylxanthine, methylation of theophylline to caffeine occurs in preterm newborns, so that both compounds may contribute to the responses observed after administration of either drug to neonates.[158,159]

Theophylline still plays an important role as a bronchodilator for neonates with reactive airway disease, a frequent concomitant of BPD. Few studies have examined the theophylline concentration associated with relief of bronchoconstriction in neonates. In asthmatic children, theophylline concentrations averaging 3.8 μg/mL significantly improve pulmonary function.[160]

Theophylline illustrates the effects of protein binding on interpretation of drug levels in neonates. Cord plasma binds theophylline to a much smaller degree than does adult plasma, so that the total theophylline concentration reported from clinical laboratories for newborns will be associated with a higher free concentration than for adults.[161] Using the average cord blood binding of theophylline observed by Aranda and colleagues, a newborn plasma theophylline concentration of 13.8 μg/mL corresponds to an adult concentration of 20 μg/mL.[161]

Theophylline is metabolized by the hepatic mixed function oxidases, cytochrome P450 enzymes. Its metabolism is increased by inducing agents such as anticonvulsants,[162] and is delayed by influenza[163] or treatment with macrolide antibiotics, such as erythromycin.[164]

The changes in theophylline kinetics during maturation of infants born at gestations of 25 to 30 weeks were studied with stable isotopes.[165] This technique allows more accurate determination of the elimination phase by monitoring concentrations for prolonged periods while continuing administration of the unlabeled medication. Theophylline half-life correlated best with postnatal age, rather than postconceptional age. As would be expected, the theophylline half-life varied inversely with postnatal age as follows:

$$\log t_{1/2}\ (\text{hours}) = 1.72 - 0.00565 \times \text{Postnatal age (days)}. \quad \text{(Eq. 56-12)}$$

Theophylline relaxes the gastroesophageal sphincter of adults and probably has the same effect in newborns. If apnea is due to gastroesophageal reflux, theophylline treatment may worsen this problem. In adults, caffeine produces little effect on lower esophageal sphincter pressure, whereas coffee tends to increase it.[166]

Caffeine is an effective treatment for apnea of prematurity.[167] Apnea was reduced in 18 preterm infants at an average gestation of 27.5 weeks from 13.6 to 2.1 episodes per day by caffeine base, 5 or 10 mg/kg, one to three times per day. Note that caffeine citrate doubles the weight of the administered drug, so that 20 mg/kg is equivalent to 10 mg/kg of caffeine base. Large variability in the elimination rate of caffeine was noted in this original study, with the $t_{1/2}$ ranging from 40.7 to 231 hours. Subsequent pharmacokinetic studies from the same group lead to the current dosing recommendations of 10 mg caffeine base/kg loading dose, followed by 2.5 mg caffeine base/kg/day as a single dose for maintenance treatment.[168] Even full-term infants exposed to caffeine transplacentally have prolonged half-lives, ranging from 31 to 132 hours.[169]

As with theophylline, the half-life of caffeine decreases after birth when studied serially in a group of preterm neonates.[170] The adult values for the half-life were reached at approximately 60 weeks postconception. Effective caffeine concentrations for the treatment of apnea of prematurity range from 5 to 25 μg/mL.[171]

MUSCLE RELAXANTS

Muscle relaxants are administered frequently to neonates during mechanical ventilation and anesthesia for surgical procedures.[172] Nondepolarizing muscle relaxants have become the mainstay for neuromuscular blockade in the NICU. This may relate to hypotension, tachycardia, and bronchoconstriction associated with histamine release by the depolarizing agent, curare.[172] Although pancuronium has been used extensively in treatment of neonates, vecuronium and atracurium, developed as short-acting, nondepolarizing neuromuscular blockers, are being administered to newborns.

Pancuronium bromide has been used successfully for neuromuscular blockade of neonates for many years. When compared to d-tubocurarine in children, pancuronium had a similar onset of action, produced similar changes in heart rate and blood pressure, but had a shorter duration of action.[173] Pancuronium dosage requirements for neonates increase with age after birth, and decrease with prematurity.[174] Treatment during the first week after birth required a dose of 0.03 mg/kg, compared to 0.09 mg/kg by 2 to 4 weeks after birth. Dose reductions were required not only for prematurity, but also for acidosis and hypothermia. Using muscle twitch analysis to detect neuromuscular blockade, others have shown wide variation in pancuronium dose requirements among newborns, with prolongation of blockade by renal insufficiency.[175] Repeated administration of pancuronium to neonates may lead to prolonged neuromuscular blockade, possibly due to its long half-life, which is related to immaturity of liver and renal function.

Atracurium is eliminated by ester hydrolysis and Hoffmann elimination, a nonenzymatic, chemical change.[176] Breakdown products are not pharmacologically active. Metabolites of pancuronium are pharmacologically active. The prolonged duration of action seen after repeated doses of pancuronium is minimal with repeated doses of vecuronium and essentially absent with repeated doses of atracurium. Although vecuronium was developed as a short-acting neuromuscular blocking agent, its effects are much longer in neonates and infants than in children and adolescents.[177] A 100 μg/kg dose maintained neuromuscular blockade by analysis of muscle twitch for more than 58 minutes in infants and 18 minutes in children, aged 3 to 10 years.[177]

In contrast to these two newer agents, pancuronium frequently increases heart rate and blood pressure.[176] Repeated doses of pancuronium may lead to prolonged neuromuscular blockade lasting for several days. Histamine release is negligible after pancuronium and vecuronium, whereas atracurium releases 30% as much histamine as equivalent doses of d-tubocurarine.

Larger doses of pancuronium are required for muscle relaxation in infants, presumably due to a larger volume of distribution. The same observation has been made for atracurium.[176] Vecuronium is cleared by the liver, and is not dependent on renal excretion for termination of its effects. In contrast, renal dysfunction prolongs the half-life of pancuronium. As for vecuronium, impairment of renal function has little effect on the pharmacokinetics of atracurium.

Neuromuscular blockade for several days may produce prolonged muscle weakness. The contribution of drug accumulation at the myoneural junction or alteration of the myoneural junction requires more study. Monitoring of muscle fiber twitch during prolonged paralysis may be helpful for evaluating and avoiding this side effect.

PROSTAGLANDINS AND PROSTAGLANDIN INHIBITORS

During the last 25 years, understanding of the pharmacology and physiology of the eicosanoids has expanded dramatically from PGE_1 and $PGF_{1\alpha}$ to thromboxane and prostacyclin, products of the cyclooxygenase pathway, and leukotrienes, noncyclized products of the lipoxygenase pathway. Better understanding of leukotrienes has helped to account for previously recognized biologic mediators such as slow-reacting substance A, which is the same as leukotriene C. Despite the enormous variety of functions mediated through the eicosanoids, PGE_1 and PGE_2 are the most frequently used eicosanoids in newborn medicine.[178] They have been used primarily to maintain patency of the ductus arteriosus, and occasionally, for pulmonary vasodilation in the treatment of persistent pulmonary hypertension of the newborn (PPHN). The effectiveness of PGE_1 for maintaining ductal patency has been confirmed in various studies, including a multicenter collaborative investigation.[179]

Prostaglandin E_1 usually has been administered only by continuous venous or arterial infusion.[180] Dosages generally have started at 0.1 μg/kg/minute and have been associated with a variety of adverse reactions, including cutaneous vasodilation, edema, hypotension, apnea, fever, irritability, seizures, hypoglycemia, diarrhea, disseminated intravascular coagulation, osteolysis, hypercalcemia, and thrombocytopenia.[180] Starting dosages may be lowered to 0.05 μg/kg/minute and then tapered to 0.01 μg/kg/minute if oxygenation is maintained.[181]

Prolonged treatment with PGE_2 is needed for patients with ductal-dependent cardiac malformations awaiting transplantation. Oral PGE_2 also is effective for maintaining ductal patency and oxygenation.[181] Patients who were changed from the IV to the oral route, however, did have a significant decrease in PaO_2. Oral treatment used doses of 35 to 65 μg/kg/hour, with a slow increase in dosing intervals from 1 to 4 hours during the second and third week of treatment. This is consistent with recent reports of treatment of adults with PGE analogues for healing of ulcers.[182]

Closure of the patent ductus arteriosus with cyclooxygenase inhibitors also is an integral part of neonatal pharmacology. Ductal patency after birth is maintained by PGE_2, the secretion of which is inhibited by rising oxygen tension.[178] Ductal closure was first achieved with oral indomethacin in large dosages (2.5–5 mg/kg).[183] Since that report, indomethacin has been formulated in an IV preparation and used in a multicenter collaborative trial that demonstrated the efficacy of treatment with a 0.2 mg/kg loading dose, followed by 0.1 to 0.25 mg/kg/doses every 12 hours for a total of three doses.[184] This study also illustrated the side effects of cyclooxygenase inhibition in neonates, including oliguria, increased serum creatinine, and transient mild bleeding.

Infants with intracranial hemorrhage were excluded from the collaborative study.[184] Subsequent studies have found that early indomethacin treatment actually decreases the risk of intracranial hemorrhage.[185] When the presence of an intracranial hemorrhage was not a contraindication to indomethacin treatment, it has not been shown to cause extension of intracranial hemorrhages.[186,187] These studies do not indicate that intracranial hemorrhage should be a contraindication for indomethacin treatment, although some physicians follow the approach used in the multicenter collaborative trial and avoid administration of indomethacin to neonates with intracranial hemorrhages.[184]

Developmental changes in the pharmacokinetics of indomethacin have been defined for preterm infants.[188] Lower average indomethacin concentrations were noted in patients who did not sustain ductal closure after treatment with indomethacin. Indomethacin clearance increased with both postnatal age and body weight. A correlation between individual indomethacin levels and ductal closure was not found, however, possibly relating to variation in rates of PGE_2 production among patients.

The optimal length of indomethacin treatment for low-birth-weight neonates has not been settled. After initial treatment with two doses of indomethacin, once-daily doses of indomethacin have been continued for 5 additional days in 22 infants with birth weight under 1500 g.[189] The group that was treated for a sustained period of time had no patent ductus 3 days after ending treatment and fewer intraventricular hemorrhages. The ductus reopened eventually in almost one-half of this group, but at a much older age. Longer courses of indomethacin need more study, but may be more effective for ductal closure.

The neonate who is several weeks old and has a symptomatic patent ductus arteriosus presents a therapeutic dilemma. McCarthy and colleagues reported failure of ductal closure in infants who were 37 to 40 weeks postconceptional age at the time of indomethacin treatment.[190] Efforts to maintain effective indomethacin concentrations in older patients with patent ductus arteriosus, by higher doses administered more frequently, have not ensured ductal closure.[191]

The renal effects of indomethacin in premature infants are quite similar to those observed in symptomatic adults.[192] In premature infants, indomethacin decreases urine flow, glomerular filtration rate, and free-water clearance, which combine to decrease renal electrolyte excretion.[193] Oliguria during indomethacin treatment of premature infants has been improved with dopamine[194] and with furosemide.[121] Seri and colleagues found that dopamine prevented a decrease in urine flow and increased sodium excretion.[194]

The rate of indomethacin infusion has a significant effect on its cardiovascular effects. When indomethacin was infused over 0.2 to 4 minutes, cerebral blood flow velocity decreased 48% to 75%.[195] When indomethacin was infused over 20 minutes, cerebral blood flow velocity was not reduced.[196] A similar reduction in mesenteric blood flow occurs when indomethacin is administered over 20 seconds or less, and this can be prevented by slow infusion over 30 to 35 minutes.[197] It is too early to determine whether the common practice of discontinuation of feeds during indomethacin treatment is unnecessary when doses are administered more slowly.

PULMONARY VASODILATORS

Since the pulmonary vasculature of many neonates is in parallel with the systemic vasculature, through patency of the ductus arteriosus and foramen ovale, an effective pulmonary vasodilator must dilate the pulmonary vasculature more than the systemic vasculature.[198] Among the drugs that have been used, with mixed success, for treatment of PPHN are tolazoline, PGE_1, PGI_2, PGD_2, acetylcholine, isoproterenol, chlorpromazine, and nitroprusside.[199] Although tolazoline has been reported to improve oxygenation in approximately 60% of patients, high mortality persisted, and adverse effects occurred at an unacceptably high rate.[31] Inappropriately high doses of tolazoline, used without the guidance of kinetic studies, may have contributed to the high rate of adverse effects associated with tolazoline treatment.[31] In a study of tolazoline kinetics in newborns, using a low-dose infusion of 0.2 mg/kg/hour, after a 1.0 mg/kg bolus loading dose, prevented accumulation to high concentrations that were potentially toxic.[200]

Prostaglandins, thromboxanes, and leukotrienes may play a significant role in pulmonary vascular control; thus, eicosanoid derivatives or their antagonists are likely to be found effective for reversing neonatal pulmonary vasoconstriction. Newly discovered mediators of pulmonary vasomotor tone also are likely to lead to more effective treatments of pulmonary vasoconstriction in neonates. Platelet activating factor increases pulmonary artery pressure in animal models, and is elevated in patients with PPHN.[201] Endothelium-derived relaxing factor (EDRF) plays a regulatory role in vascular tone in several organs within the body, including the lungs. In rats, EDRF inhibits hypoxic pulmonary vasoconstriction.[202] The pulmonary vascular effects of nitric oxide appear to be identical to those of EDRF,[203] and it shares many of the properties of other nitrovasodilators, such as nitroglycerin and nitroprusside. Endothelium-derived relaxing factor actions are mediated through guanylate cyclase, leading to increased vascular smooth muscle concentrations of cyclic guanosine 3′,5′-monophosphate (cGMP).

RESPIRATORY STIMULANTS

Doxapram has been administered to newborns both IV and orally, to treat apnea that was unresponsive to methylxanthines (see Methylxanthines).[204] Doxapram is a general stimulant of the CNS respiratory center, along with the entire cerebrospinal axis. Originally, doxapram was administered by continuous IV infusion for treatment of apnea of prematurity.[205,206] When administered enterally, doxapram is poorly absorbed, with a ratio of plasma concentration to oral dose of 0.10 to 0.12.[207] Despite poor absorption when administered enterally, doxapram decreases apnea of the newborn.[208] Side effects observed during enteral administration included occult blood in stools, necrotizing enterocolitis, and premature teeth buds. Seizures have been associated with high circulating concentrations, although Alpan and colleagues suggest that the ratio of effective to convulsive concentration is 1 : 70.[206] Seizures have been observed in two neonates treated with doxapram, but these were thought most likely to reflect intraventricular hemorrhages.[205]

STEROIDS

Corticosteroid treatment of neonates with BPD has increased since the initial randomized, double-blind, controlled study of six patients demonstrated clear improvement during treatment with dexamethasone (0.5 mg/kg/day divided into two daily doses).[209] This study used a sequential analysis design to minimize the number of patients needed to test the hypothesis.[210] Although dexamethasone treatment improved respiratory function, prolonged treatment with dexamethasone was associated with a high rate of infections, two of which were fatal.[209] Avery and associates reported that dexamethasone, in the same dose (0.5 mg/kg/day divided into two doses), facilitated weaning of infants with BPD from respirator support and improved dynamic lung compliance.[211] This study has been criticized because it was not blinded, and the investigators recognized that the respirator settings for dexamethasone-treated infants could be decreased despite minimal improvement in blood gases. Infections were not increased in the dexamethasone-treated group. Hypertension was observed in one dexamethasone-treated infant and hyperglycemia was distributed equally between the two groups. Subsequent larger studies have confirmed the efficacy of dexamethasone in a dose of 0.5 mg/kg/day for improving pulmonary function in neonates with BPD.[212,213] Treatment for 42 days shortened the time for weaning from mechanical ventilation and supplemental oxygen, compared to placebo and to treatment for 18 days.[213]

Animal studies raised concerns that prolonged dexamethasone treatment may decrease brain and body growth.[214] In clinical trials, however, Cummings and colleagues noted better neurologic outcome in the 42-day dexamethasone treatment group compared to the 18-day treatment and to placebo group. Harkavy and colleagues observed a higher frequency of hyperglycemia and delayed weight gain in the dexamethasone-treated group. There was no difference in the frequency of hypertension, intracranial hemorrhage, infection, or retinopathy of prematurity (ROP) between dexamethasone-treated and placebo-treated groups.[212]

Dexamethasone treatment of mechanically ventilated neonates improved pulmonary compliance and resistance within 12 hours of starting treatment.[215] Decrease in expiratory resistance was greater than decrease in inspiratory resistance, and was associated with a marked increase in urine output despite keeping fluid intake constant. Oxygen requirement and mean airway pressure also improved.

Certain aspects of dexamethasone pharmacology should be recognized. It is a potent, synthetic, halogenated steroid with a longer half-life than the nonhalogenated steroids, such as hydrocortisone, which more closely resemble endogenous adrenal hormones. Dexamethasone is a pure glucocorticoid, without mineralocorticoid activity and with a potency approximately 30 times that of hydrocortisone.[216] Thus, 0.5 mg/kg/day of dexamethasone is equivalent to 15 mg/kg/day of hydrocortisone. Dexamethasone half-life averages 4.3 hours in children and appears to be longer in newborns, whose plasma concentrations were approximately double those in infants and adults.[217] This compares to cortisol, with a half-life of approximately 1.5 hours.[216]

After 7 days of dexamethasone treatment in a dose of 0.5 mg/kg/day for the last 6 days, resting cortisol values were lower than in the placebo-treated group, indicating suppression of basal pituitary gland secretion of adrenocorticotropic hormone (ACTH).[218] A normal response to ACTH stimulation persisted after 7 days of dexamethasone treatment, indicating continued responsiveness of the adrenal gland to ACTH, which should provide hormonal reserve for periods of stress.[218] This is consistent with the observation that glucocorticoid treatment for longer than 10 days frequently suppresses the pituitary–adrenal axis.[219,220]

The frequent treatment of neonates with potent glucocorticoids in high dosages for longer than 10 days leads to a population of neonates with a suppressed hypothalamic–pituitary–adrenal axis. Adrenal suppression may persist for months, so this population may require tapering of steroids over a prolonged period.[221] During this period, Byyny found that stresses such as surgery or infection require temporary administration of exogenous glucocorticoids at two to three times the maintenance doses (see Chap. 41).[219] In my experience, the general approach for tapering steroids outlined by Byyny is useful for neonates after prolonged treatment with glucocorticoids.[219] The total daily steroid dose is tapered every 3 to 7 days, unless pulmonary function worsens. Endogenous cortisol peaks in the morning, once diurnal variation in adrenal secretion is established after birth. The time of onset of diurnal variation is not clearly established in extremely premature neonates.[222,223] To mimic this, the evening glucocorticoid dose is tapered and a portion of the tapered dose is added to the morning dose until a single morning dose is administered. Tapering of this dose continues every 3 to 7 days. Return of function of the hypothalamic–pituitary–adrenal axis may be evaluated with resting cortisol values and a metyrapone test.[221] Additional studies of the dose response of pulmonary function in patients with BPD to lower doses of glucocorticoids are needed. Personal experience with hydrocortisone for infants exhibiting inadequate secretion of cortisol suggests that much lower doses may be effective.

VITAMIN E

Vitamin E refers to several chemically related compounds, differing in degrees of methylation, desaturation, and oxygen content, classified generically as tocopherols.[224] The oxygen molecules and aromatic ring conjugation allow interconversion between hydroxyl and quinone forms, so that vitamin E functions as an antioxidant. Alpha-tocopherol is the primary, naturally occurring member of this group.

The clinical administration of vitamin E to premature neonates is based on its antioxidant activity, low vitamin E concentrations in many preterm neonates at birth, and animal studies suggesting that vitamin E protects against oxidant injury to the lung and eye. Initial favorable effects of vitamin E on BPD[225] were not confirmed in a subsequent randomized, double-blind study by the same investigators.[226]

For prevention of ROP, a prospective, double-blind, randomized trial reported that 100 mg of vitamin E per day reduced the severity, but not frequency of ROP.[227] Studies of tocopherol in a kitten model of ROP, in doses of 50 to 1000 mg/kg/day, revealed a high frequency of mortality with lethargy, weight loss, and seizures.[228] Livers were enlarged and extensively vacuolated with fat in the vitamin E-treated animals.

In 1984, the Centers for Disease Control and Bodenstein separately described infants with a new symptom complex that included pulmonary deterioration, thrombocytopenia, liver failure, ascites, and renal failure leading to death in some cases.[229,230] These symptoms were attributed to a specific brand of α-tocopherol acetate, E-Ferol, which had begun to be administered IV to prevent oxidant injury to eyes and lungs. This syndrome ceased after the use of E-Ferol was discontinued. It was never completely clear whether the toxicity was due to α-tocopherol, the polysorbate emulsifiers, or an unknown contaminant.[231,232] Sepsis, necrotizing enterocolitis, and intraventricular hemorrhage also have been attributed to treatment of neonates with vitamin E.[224] The Committee on Fetus and Newborn concluded that pharmacologic doses of vitamin E should be regarded as experimental, and not routinely indicated for infants weighing under 1500 g.[233]

Vitamin E concentration data must be viewed in light of the analytic procedure used for its measurement, since colorimetric analyses may detect other substances besides vitamin E, and several isomers may be isolated by liquid chromatography.[234] When administered to rabbits, both organ accumulation and disposition rates differ significantly between vitamin E in the form of α-tocopherol and α-tocopheryl acetate.[235] At serum concentrations close to the upper limits of normal for newborns, significant accumulation of α-tocopherol occurred in the liver and to a lesser extent in the lungs of rabbits. The reported half-lives for vitamin E imply that dosing every 2 to 3 days would be appropriate.[224] The Committee on the Fetus and Newborn recommends 5 to 10 IU of vitamin E per day for preterm infants, provided through supplemented formulas or supplemental vitamins.[236]

DRUG EXCRETION IN BREAST MILK

Over 50% of newborn infants are breast-feeding at the time of discharge.[237] Although almost all drugs and chemicals present in the maternal circulation may enter human milk, the extent of transfer is quite variable. Maternal intake of prescription medications, over-the-counter medications, illicit drugs, and exposure to a multitude of environmental substances may expose the breast-feeding infant to a myriad of chemicals.

The nature of human milk influences its drug content. Human milk has been described as a suspension of fat in a protein–mineral–carbohydrate solution.[238] The lactose secreted in milk is synthesized from glucose by the alveolar cell of the breast, in a process that requires α-lactalbumin. Milk contains a variety of proteins, including α-lactalbumin, lactoferrin albumin, lysozyme, and immunoglobulin A, all of which may bind drugs during transport into milk.[238] The lipid within milk is maintained in the aqueous phase in milkfat globules surrounded by lipoprotein membranes. Milk is isosmotic to plasma, with an average *p*H of 7.2.

Several factors affect drug transfer into milk, including molecular weight, lipid solubility, maternal plasma protein binding, and extent of ionization. These are similar factors to those that influence transfer of molecules across any lipid bilayer membrane. Since milk usually is acidic to maternal plasma, and non–protein-bound, nonionized molecules are free to cross membranes, the Henderson–Hasselbach equation may be used to estimate drug distribution between maternal plasma and milk.[239] This predicts that organic bases ($pK_a > 7.4$) will reach a higher concentration in milk than in maternal serum. Many quantitative studies of human milk drug excretion have estimated that approximately 1% to 2% of a maternal drug dose will appear in milk.[240]

These data on human milk drug excretion have been reviewed and updated with respect to specific recommendations about continuing or discontinuing breast-feeding during specific drug intake by the mother (see Appendix H-1).[237]

ACKNOWLEDGMENT

I thank Carolyn M. Smith for her invaluable assistance in typing and retyping the manuscript.

REFERENCES

1. Koch-Weser J, Sellers EM. Binding of drugs to serum albumin (first of two parts). N Engl J Med 1976;294:311.
2. Svensson CK, Woodruff MN, Lalka D. Influence of protein binding and use of unbound (free) drug concentrations. In: Evans WE, Schentag JJ, Jusko WJ, et al, eds. Applied pharmacokinetics. 2nd ed. Spokane, WA: Applied Therapeutics, 1986:187.
3. Oellerich M. Influence of protein binding commentary. In: Evans WE, Schentag JJ, Jusko WJ, et al, eds. Applied pharmacokinetics. 2nd ed. Spokane, WA: Applied Therapeutics, 1986:220.
4. Brodersen R, Honore B. Drug binding properties of neonatal albumin. Acta Paediatr Scand 1989;78:342.
5. Boreus LO. Principles of pediatric pharmacology. New York: Churchill-Livingston, 1982.
6. Roberts RJ. Pharmacologic principles in therapeutics in infants. In: Drug therapy in infants. Philadelphia: WB Saunders, 1984:3.

7. Peterson RG, Simmons MA, Rumack BH, et al. Pharmacology of furosemide in the premature newborn infant. J Pediatr 1980;97:139.
8. Evans EF, Proctor JD, Fratkin MJ, et al. Blood flow in muscle groups and drug absorption. Clin Pharmacol Ther 1975;17:44.
9. Kostenbauder HB, Rapp RP, McGovren JP, et al. Bioavailability and single-dose pharmacokinetics of intramuscular phenytoin. Clin Pharmacol Ther 1975;18:449.
10. Leff RD, Roberts RJ. Methods for intravenous drug administration in the pediatric patient. J Pediatr 1981;98:631.
11. Ward RM. Pharmacologic principles and practicalities. In: Taeusch HW, Ballard RA, Avery ME, eds. Schaffer and Avery's diseases of the newborn. 6th ed. Philadelphia: WB Saunders, 1991:285.
12. Pelkonen O, Kaltiala EH, Larmi TKI, et al. Comparison of activities of drug-metabolizing enzymes in human fetal and adult livers. Clin Pharmacol Ther 1973;14:840.
13. Aperia A, Broberger O, Elinder G, et al. Postnatal development of renal function in pre-term and full-term neonates. Acta Paediatr Scand 1981;70:183.
14. Engle WD. Evaluation of renal function and acute renal failure in the neonate. Pediatr Clin North Am 1986;33:129.
15. Greenblatt DJ, Koch-Weser J. Clinical pharmacokinetics (first of two parts). N Engl J Med 1975;293:702.
16. Greenblatt DJ, Koch-Weser J. Clinical pharmacokinetics (second of two parts). N Engl J Med 1975;293:964.
17. Roberts RJ. Pharmacokinetics: basic principles and clinical application. In: Drug therapy in infants. Philadelphia: WB Saunders, 1984:13.
18. Notari RE. Principles of pharmacokinetics. In: Biopharmaceutics and clinical pharmacokinetics. 3rd ed. New York: Marcel Dekker, 1980:45.
19. Gibaldi M, Perrier D. Pharmacokinetics. 2nd ed. New York: Marcel Dekker, 1982.
20. Jusko WJ. Guidelines for collection and analysis of pharmacokinetic data. In: Evans WE, Schentag JJ, Jusko WJ, et al, eds. Applied pharmacokinetics. 2nd ed. Spokane, WA: Applied Therapeutics. 1986:9.
21. McCracken GH. Aminoglycoside toxicity in infants and children. Am J Med 1986;80(suppl 6B):172.
22. Spector R, Park GD, Johnson GF, et al. Therapeutic drug monitoring. Clin Pharmacol Ther 1988;43:345.
23. Roberts RJ. Cardiovascular drugs. In: Drug therapy in infants. Philadelphia: WB Saunders, 1984:138.
24. Roberts RJ. Special considerations in drug therapy in infants. In: Drug therapy in infants. Philadelphia: WB Saunders, 1984:25.
25. Gould T, Roberts RJ. Therapeutic problems arising from the use of the intravenous route for drug administration. J Pediatr 1979;95:465.
26. Wagman GH, Bailey JV, Weinstein MJ. Binding of aminoglycoside antibiotics to filtration materials. Antimicrob Agents Chemother 1975;7:316.
27. Lackner TE. Dose replacement following exchange transfusion. J Pediatr 1982;100:811.
28. Aranda JV, Collinge JM, Clarkson S. Epidemiologic aspects of drug utilization in a newborn intensive care unit. Semin Perinatol 1982;6:148.
29. Aranda JV, Portuguez-Malavasi A, Collinge JM, et al. Epidemiology of adverse drug reactions in the newborn. Dev Pharmacol Ther 1982;5:173.
30. Mitchell AA, Goldman P, Shapiro S, et al. Drug utilization and reported adverse reactions in hospitalized children. Am J Epidemiol 1979;110:196.
31. Ward RM. Pharmacology of tolazoline. Clin Perinatol 1984; 11:703.
32. Maisels MJ. Jaundice in the newborn. Pediatr Rev 1982;3:305.
33. Hansen TWR, Bratlid D. Bilirubin and brain toxicity. Acta Paediatr Scand 1986;75:513.
34. Silverman WA, Andersen DH, Blanc WA, et al. A difference in mortality rate and incidence of kernicterus among premature infants allotted to two prophylactic antibacterial regimens. Pediatrics 1956;18:614.
35. Odell GB. The distribution and toxicity of bilirubin. Pediatrics 1970;46:16.
36. Rose AL, Wisniewski H. Acute bilirubin encephalopathy induced with sulfadimethoxine in Gunn rats. J Neuropathol Exp Neurol 1979;38:152.
37. Sutherland JM. Fatal cardiovascular collapse of infants receiving large amounts of chloramphenicol. Am J Dis Child 1959; 97:761.
38. Burns LE, Hodgman JE, Cass AB. Fatal circulatory collapse in premature infants receiving chloramphenicol. N Engl J Med 1959;261:1318.
39. Weiss CF, Glazko AJ, Weston JK. Chloramphenicol in the newborn infant a physiologic explanation of its toxicity when given in excessive doses. N Engl J Med 1960;262:787.
40. Brown WJ, Buist NRM, Gipson HTC. Fatal benzyl alcohol poisoning in a neonatal intensive care unit. Lancet 1982; 1:1250.
41. Glasgow AM, Boeckx RL, Miller MK, et al. Hypersmolality in small infants due to propylene glycol. Pediatrics 1983;72: 353.
42. MacDonald MG, Getson PR, Glasgow AM, et al. Propylene glycol: increased incidence of seizures in low birth weight infants. Pediatrics 1987;79:L622.
43. Wenzl JE, Mills SD, McCall JT. Methanol poisoning in an infant: successful treatment with peritoneal dialysis. Am J Dis Child 1968;116:445.
44. Moss MH. Alcohol-induced hyperglycemia and coma caused by alcohol sponging. Pediatrics 1970;46:445.
45. Shuman RM, Leech RW, Alvord EC Jr. Neurotoxicity of hexachlorophene in humans: II. A clinical pathological study of 46 premature infants. Arch Neurol 1975;32:320.
46. D l'Allemand D, Grüters A, Heidemann P, et al. Iodine-induced alterations of thyroid function in newborn infants after prenatal and perinatal exposure to povidone iodine. J Pediatr 1983;102:935.
47. Fisch RO, Berglund EB, Bridge AG, et al. Methemoglobinemia in a hospital nursery. JAMA 1963;185:760.
48. Morrell P, Hey E, Mackee IW, et al. Deafness in a preterm baby associated with topical antibiotic spray containing neomycin. Lancet 1985;1:1167.
49. Rutter N. Percutaneous drug absorption in the newborn: hazards and uses. Clin Perinatol 1987;14:911.
50. Roberts RJ. Fetal and infant intoxication. In: Drug therapy in infants. Philadelphia: WB Saunders, 1984:322.
51. Hillman LS, Goodwin SL, Sherman WR. Identification and measurement of plasticizer in neonatal tissues after umbilical catheters and blood products. N Engl J Med 1975;292:381.
52. Bigger JT Jr., Hoffman BF. Antiarrhythmic drugs. In: Gilman AG, Rall TW, Nies AS, et al, eds. Goodman and Gilman's the pharmacological basis of therapeutics. 8th ed. New York: Pergamon Press, 1990:840.
53. Moak JP. Pharmacology and electrophysiology of antiarrhythmic drugs. In: Gillette PC, Garson A Jr, eds. Pediatric arrythmias: electrophysiology and pacing. Philadelphia: WB Saunders, 1990:37.
54. Gillette PC, Garson A Jr, Crawford F, et al. Dysrhythmias. In: Adams FH, Emmanouilides GC, Riemenschneider TA, eds. Heart disease in infants, children, and adolescents. 4th ed. Baltimore: Williams & Wilkins, 1989:925.

55. Byrum CJ, Wahl RA, Behrendt DM, et al. Ventricular fibrillation associated with the use of digitalis in the newborn infant with Wolff-Parkinson-White syndrome. J Pediatr 1982;101:400.
56. Ludomirsky A, Garson A Jr. Supraventricular tachycardia. In: Gillette PC, Garson A Jr, eds. Pediatric arrythmias: electrophysiology and pacing. Philadelphia: WB Saunders, 1990:380.
57. Watt AH, Bernard MS, Webster J, et al. Intravenous adenosine in the treatment of supraventricular tachycardia: a dose ranging study and interaction with dipyridamole. Br J Clin Pharmacol 1986;21:227.
58. Clarke B, Rowland E, Barnes PJ, et al. Rapid and safe termination of supraventricular tachycardia in children by adenosine. Lancet 1987;1:299.
59. Reidenberg MM, Drayer DE, Levy M, et al. Polymorphic acetylation of procainamide in man. Clin Pharmacol Ther 1975;17:722.
60. Nies AS, Shand DG. Clinical pharmacology of propranolol. Circulation 1975;52:6.
61. Epstein ML, Kiel EA, Victorica BE. Cardiac decompensation following verapamil therapy in infants with supraventricular tachycardia. Pediatrics 1985;75:737.
62. Garson A, Gillette PC, McVey P, et al. Amiodarone treatment of critical arrhythmias in children and young adults. J Am Coll Cardiol 1984;4:749.
63. Mason JW. Amiodarone. N Engl J Med 1987;316:455.
64. Volpe JJ. Neurology of the newborn. 2nd ed. Philadelphia: WB Saunders, 1987:129.
65. Pellock JM. Efficacy and adverse effects of antiepileptic drugs. Pediatr Clin North Am 1989;36:448.
66. Painter MJ, Pippenger C, Wasterlain C, et al. Phenobarbital and phenytoin in neonatal seizures: metabolism and tissue distribution. Neurology 1981;31:1107.
67. Gal P, Toback J, Boer HR, et al. Efficacy of phenobarbital monotherapy in treatment of neonatal seizures-relationship to blood levels. Neurology 1982;32:1401.
68. Fischer JH, Lockman LA, Zaske D, et al. Phenobarbital maintenance dose requirements in treating neonatal seizures. Neurology 1981;31:1042.
69. Albani M, Wernicke I. Oral phenytoin in infancy: dose requirement, absorption, and elimination. Pediatr Pharmacol 1983;3:229.
70. Deshmukh A, Wittert W, Schnitzler E, et al. Lorazepam in the treatment of refractory neonatal seizures. Am J Dis Child 1986;140:1042.
71. Farwell JR, Lee YJ, Hirtz DG, et al. Phenobarbital for febrile seizures: effects on intelligence and on seizure recurrence. N Engl J Med 1990;322:364.
72. Meador KJ, Loring DW, Huh K, et al. Comparative cognitive effects of anticonvulsants. Neurology 1990;40:391.
73. American Academy of Pediatrics Committee on Drugs. Behavioral and cognitive effects of anticonvulsant therapy. Pediatrics 1985;76:644.
74. Scher MS, Painter MJ. Controversies concerning neonatal seizures. Pediatr Clin North Am 1989;36:281.
75. Sinaiko AR, Mirkin BL. Clinical pharmacology of antihypertensive drugs in children. Pediatr Clin North Am 1978;25:137.
76. Task Force on Blood Pressure Control in Children. Report of the second task force on blood pressure control in children: 1987. Pediatrics 1987;79:1.
77. Inouye IK, Massie BM, Benowitz N, et al. Antihypertensive therapy with diltiazem in comparison with hydrochlorothiazide. Am J Cardiol 1984;53:1588.
78. Bauer SB, Feldman SM, Gellis SS, et al. Neonatal hypertension a complication of umbilical-artery catheterization. N Engl J Med 1975;293:1032.
79. O'Dea RF, Mirkin BL, Alward CT, et al. Treatment of neonatal hypertension with captopril. J Pediatr 1988;113:403.
80. Tack ED, Perlman JM. Renal failure in sick hypertensive premature infants receiving captopril therapy. J Pediatr 1988;112:805.
81. Romankiewicz JA, Brogden RN, Heel RC, et al. Captopril: an update review of its pharmacological properties and therapeutic efficacy in congestive heart failure. Drugs 1983;25:6.
82. Baumgart S, Hall SE, Campos JM, et al. Sepsis with coagulase-negative staphylococci in critically ill newborns. Am J Dis Child 1983;137:461.
83. Wise RI. The vancomycin symposium: summary and comments. Rev Infect Dis 1981;3(Suppl):S293.
84. Sorrell TC, Collignon PJ. A prospective study of adverse reactions associated with vancomycin therapy. J Antimicrob Chemother 1985;16:235.
85. Levy M, Koren G, Dupuis L, et al. Vancomycin-induced red man syndrome. Pediatrics 1990;86:572.
86. Reed MD, Kliegman RM, Weiner JS, et al. The clinical pharmacology of vancomycin in seriously ill preterm infants. Pediatr Res 1987;22:360.
87. Banner W Jr, Gooch WM III, Burckart G, et al. Pharmacokinetics of nafcillin in infants with low birth weights. Antimicrob Agents Chemother 1980;17:691.
88. Placzek M, Whitelaw A, Want S, et al. Piperacillin in early neonatal infection. Arch Dis Child 1983;58:1006.
89. Eichenwald HF. Antimicrobial therapy in infants and children: update 1976–1985: part II. J Pediatr 1985;107:337.
90. Seeberg AH, Tolxdorff-Neutzling RM, Wiedemann B. Chromosomal β-lactamases of *Enterobacter cloacae* are responsible for resistance to third-generation cephalosporins. Antimicrob Agents Chemother 1983;23:918.
91. Snelling S, Hart CA, Cooke RWI. Ceftazidime or gentamicin plus benzylpenicillin in neonates less than forty-eight hours old. J Antimicrob Chemother 1983;12(Suppl A):353.
92. Bryan CS, John JF, Pai MS, et al. Gentamicin vs cefotaxime for therapy of neonatal sepsis. Relationship to drug resistance. Am J Dis Child 1985;139:1086.
93. Tullus K, Burman LG. Ecological impact of ampicillin and cefuroxime in neonatal units. Lancet 1989;1:1405.
94. Jacobs RF. Imipenem-cilastatin: the first thienamycin antibiotic. Pediatr Infect Dis 1986;5:444.
95. Neu HC. Antibiotics in the second half of the 1980s: areas of future development and the effect of new agents on aminoglycoside use. Am J Med 1986;80:195.
96. Eichenwald HF. Antimicrobial therapy in infants and children: update 1976–1985: part I. J Pediatr 1985;107:161.
97. Hampton FJ, MacFadyen UM, Beardsmore CS, et al. Gastrooesophageal reflux and respiratory function in infants with respiratory symptoms. Arch Dis Child 1991;66:848.
98. Euler AR. Use of bethanechol for the treatment of gastroesophageal reflux. J Pediatr 1980;96:321.
99. Strickland AD, Chang JHT. Results of treatment of gastroesophageal reflux with bethanechol. J Pediatr 1983;103:311.
100. Sondheimer JM, Mintz HL, Michaels M. Bethanechol treatment of gastroesophageal reflux in infants: effect on continuous esophageal pH records. J Pediatr 1984;104:128.
101. Schultze-Delrieu K. Metoclopramide. N Engl J Med 1981;305:28.
102. Sankaran K, Yeboah E, Bingham WT, et al. Use of metoclopramide in preterm infants. Dev Pharmacol Ther 1982;5:114.
103. Tolia V, Calhoun J, Kuhns L, et al. Randomized, prospective double blind trial of metoclopramide and placebo for gastroesophageal reflux in infants. J Pediatr 1989;115:141.
104. Hyams JS, Leichter AM, Zanett LO, et al. Effect of metoclo-

pramide on prolonged esophageal pH testing in infants with gastroesophageal reflux. J Pediatr Gastroenterol Nutr 1968; 5:716.
105. Machida HM, Forbes DA, Gall DG, et al. Metoclopramide in gastroesophageal reflux in infancy. J Pediatr 1988;112:483.
106. Lenney W, Milner AD. At what age do bronchodilator drugs work? Arch Dis Child 1978;53:532.
107. Tepper RS. Airway reactivity in infants: a positive response to methacholine and metaproterenol. J Appl Physiol 1987;62: 1155.
108. Kao LC, Warburton D, Platzker ACG, et al. Effect of isoproterenol inhalation on airway resistance in chronic bronchopulmonary dysplasia. Pediatrics 1984;73:509.
109. Wilkie RA, Bryan MH. Effect of bronchodilators on airway resistance in ventilator-dependent neonates with chronic lung disease. J Pediatr 1987;111:278.
110. Brundage KL, Mohsini KG, Froese AB, et al. Bronchodilator response to ipratropium bromide in infants with bronchopulmonary dysplasia. Am Rev Respir Dis 1990;142:1137.
111. Kraemer R, Birrer P, Schöni MH. Dose-response relationships and time course of the response to systemic beta adrenoreceptor agonists in infants with bronchopulmonary disease. Thorax 1988;43:770.
112. Gomez-Del Rio M, Gerhardt T, Hehre D, et al. Effect of a beta-agonist nebulization on lung function in neonates with increased pulmonary resistance. Pediatr Pulmonol 1986;2: 287.
113. Motoyama EK, Fort MD, Klesh KW, et al. Early onset of airway reactivity in premature infants with bronchopulmonary dysplasia. Am Rev Respir Dis 1987;136:50.
114. Weiner IM. Drugs affecting renal function and electrolyte metabolism. In: Gilman AG, Rall TW, Nies AS, et al, eds. Goodman and Gilman's the pharmacological basis of therapeutics. 8th ed. New York: Pergamon Press, 1990;708.
115. Green TP. The pharmacologic basis of diuretic therapy in the newborn. Clin Perinatol 1987;14:951.
116. Chemtob S, Kaplan BS, Sherbotie JR, et al. Pharmacology of diuretics in the newborn. Pediatr Clin North Am 1989;36: 1231.
117. Brater DC. Determinants of the overall response to furosemide: pharmacokinetics and pharmacodynamics. Fed Proc 1983;42:1711.
118. Schrier RW, Lehman D, Zacherle B, et al. Effect of furosemide on free water excretion in edematous patients with hyponatremia. Kidney Int 1973;3:30.
119. Vert P, Broquaire M, Legagneur M, et al. Pharmacokinetics of furosemide in neonates. Eur J Clin Pharmacol 1982;22:39.
120. Engelhardt B, Elliott S, Hazinski TA. Short-and long-term effects of furosemide on lung function in infants with bronchopulmonary dysplasia. J Pediatrics 1986;109:1034.
121. Najak ZD, Harris EM, Lazzara A Jr, et al. Pulmonary effects of furosemide in preterm infants with lung disease. J Pediatr 1983;102:758.
122. Green TP, Thompson TR, Johnson DE, et al. Furosemide promotes patent ductus arteriosus in premature infants with the respiratory-distress syndrome. N Engl J Med 1983;308:743.
123. Yeh TF, Wilks A, Singh J, et al. Furosemide prevents the renal side effects of indomethacin therapy in premature infants with patent ductus arteriosus. J Pediatr 1982;101:433.
124. Brater DC. Resistance to loop diuretics: why it happens and what to do about it. Drugs 1985;30:427.
125. Rybak LP. Furosemide ototoxicity: clinical and experimental aspects. Laryngoscope 1985;94(Part II, Suppl 38):1.
126. Flamenbaum W, Friedman R. Pharmacology, therapeutic efficacy, and adverse effects of bumetanide, a new "loop" diuretic. Pharmacotherapy 1982;2:213.
127. Shannon DC, Gotay F. Effects of theophylline on serum and urine electrolytes in preterm infants with apnea. J Pediatr 1979;94:963.
128. Black JW, Duncan WA, Durant CJ, et al. Definition and antagonism of histamine H_2-receptors. Nature 1972;236:385.
129. Hirschowitz BI. H-2 histamine receptors. Ann Rev Pharmacol Toxicol 1979;19:203.
130. Garrison JC. Histamine, bradykinin, 5-hydroxytryptamine, and their antagonists. In: Gilman AG, Rall TW, Nies AS, et al, eds. Goodman and Gilman's the pharmacological basis of therapeutics. 8th ed. New York: Pergamon Press, 1990:575.
131. Smith K, Crisp C. Clinical comparison of H_2-antagonists. Conn Med 1986;50:815.
132. Powell JR, Donn KH. Histamine H_2-antagonist drug interactions in perspective: mechanistic concepts and clinical implications. Am J Med 1984;77:57.
133. Peterson WL, Richardson CT. Intravenous cimetidine or two regimens of ranitidine to reduce fasting gastric acidity. Ann Intern Med 1986;104:505.
134. Zeldis JB, Friedman LS, Isselbacher KJ. Ranitidine: a new H2-receptor antagonist. N Engl J Med 1983;309:1368.
135. Blumer JL, Rothstein FC, Kaplan BS, et al. Pharmacokinetic determination of ranitidine pharmacodynamics in pediatric ulcer disease. J Pediatr 1985;107:301.
136. Lopez-Herce J, Velasco LA, Codoceo R, et al. Ranitidine prophylaxis in acute gastric mucosal damage in critically ill pediatric patients. Crit Care Med 1988;16:591.
137. Rosenthal M, Miller PW. Ranitidine in the newborn. Arch Dis Child 1988;63:88.
138. Mallet E, Mouterde O, Dubois F, et al. Use of ranitidine in young infants with gastro-oesophageal reflux. Eur J Clin Pharmacol 1989;36:641.
139. Langtry HD, Grant SM, Goa KL. Famotidine an updated review of its pharmacodynamic and pharmacokinetic properties, and therapeutic use in peptic ulcer disease and other allied diseases. Drugs 1989;38:551
140. Driscoll DJ. Use of inotropic and chronotropic agents in neonates. Clin Perinatol 1987;14:931.
141. Lefkowitz RJ, Hoffman BB, Taylor P. Neurohumoral transmission: the autonomic and somatic motor nervous systems. In: Gilman AG, Rall TW, Nies AS, et al, eds. Goodman and Gilman's the pharmacological basis of therapeutics. 8th ed. New York: Pergamon Press, 1990:84.
142. Zaritsky A, Chernow B. Use of catecholamines in pediatrics. J Pediatr 1984;105:341.
143. Hoffman BB, Lefkowitz RJ. Catecholamines and sympathomimetic drugs. In: Gilman AG, Rall TW, Nies AS, et al, eds. Goodman and Gilman's the pharmacological basis of therapeutics. 8th ed. New York: Pergamon Press, 1990:187.
144. Rude RE, Bush LR, Izquierdo C, et al. Effects of inotropic and chronotropic stimuli on acute myocardial ischemic injury: III. Influence of basal heart rate. Am J Cardiol 1984;53:1688.
145. Driscoll DJ, Gillette PC, Lewis RM, et al. Comparative hemodynamic effects of isoproterenol, dopamine, and dobutamine in the newborn dog. Pediatr Res 1979;13:1006.
146. Fiser DH, Fewell JE, Hill DE, et al. Cardiovascular and renal effects of dopamine and dobutamine in healthy, conscious piglets. Crit Care Med 1988;16:340.
147. Siwy BK, Sadove AM. Acute management of dopamine infiltration injury with regitine. Plast Reconstr Surg 1987;80:610.
148. Seri L, Tulassay T, Kiszel J, et al. Cardiovascular response to dopamine in hypotensive preterm neonates with severe hyaline membrane disease. Eur J Pediatr 1984;142:3.
149. Tuttle RR, Mills J. Dobutamine development of a new catecholamine to selectively increase cardiac contractility. Circ Res 1975;36:185.

150. Ruffolo RR Jr, Yaden EL. Vascular effects of the stereoisomers of dobutamine. J Pharmacol Exp Ther 1983;224:46.
151. Martinez AM, Padbury JF, Thio S. Dobutamine pharmacokinetics and cardiovascular responses in critically ill neonates. Pediatr 1992;89:47.
152. Smith TW. Digitalis: mechanism of action and clinical use. N Engl J Med 1988;318:358.
153. Berman W, Yabek SM, Dillon T, et al. Effects of digoxin in infants with a congested circulatory state due to a ventricular septal defect. N Engl J Med 1983;308:363.
154. Smith TW, Butler VP, Haber E, et al. Treatment of life-threatening digitalis intoxication with digoxin-specific Fab antibody fragments: experience in 26 cases. N Engl J Med 1982; 307:1357.
155. Valdes R. Endogenous digoxin-immunoactive factor in human subjects. Fed Proc 1985;44:2800.
156. Seccombe DW, Pudek MR, Whitfield MF, et al. Perinatal changes in a digoxin-like immunoreactive substance. Pediatr Res 1984;18:1097.
157. Koren G, Farine D, Maresky D, et al. Significance of the endogenous digoxin-like substance in infants and mothers. Clin Pharmacol Ther 1984;36:759.
158. Bory C, Baltassat P, Porthault M, et al. Metabolism of theophylline to caffeine in premature newborn infants. J Pediatr 1979;94:988.
159. Bada HS, Khanna NN, Somani SM, et al. Interconversion of theophylline and caffeine in newborn infants. J Pediatr 1979; 94:993.
160. Maselli R, Casal GL, Ellis EF. Pharmacologic effects of intravenously administered aminophylline in asthmatic children. J Pediatr 1970;76:777.
161. Aranda JV, Sitar DS, Parson WD, et al. Pharmacokinetic aspects of theophylline in premature newborns. N Engl J Med 1976;295:413.
162. Marquis J-F, Carruthers SG, Spence JD, et al. Phenytoin-theophylline interaction. N Engl J Med 1982;307:1189.
163. Kraemer MJ, Furukawa CT, Koup JR, et al. Altered theophylline clearance during an influenza B outbreak. Pediatrics 1982;69:476.
164. Prince RA, Wing DS, Weinberger MM, et al. Effect of erythromycin on theophylline kinetics. J Allergy Clin Immunol 1981; 68:427.75.
165. Dothey CI, Tserng K-Y, Kaw S, et al. Maturational changes of theophylline pharmacokinetics in preterm infants. Clin Pharmacol Ther 1989;45:461.
166. Cohen S, Booth GH. Gastric acid secretion and lower-esophageal-sphincter pressure in response to coffee and caffeine. N Engl J Med 1975;293:897.
167. Aranda JV, Gorman W, Bergsteinsson H, et al. Efficacy of caffeine in treatment of apnea in the low-birth-weight infant. J Pediatr 1977;90:467.
168. Aranda JC, Cook CE, Gorman GW, et al. Pharmacokinetic profile of caffeine in the premature newborn with apnea. J Pediatr 1979;94:663.
169. Parsons WD, Neims AH. Prolonged half-life of caffeine in healthy term newborn infants. J Pediatr 1981;98:640.
170. LeGuennec J-H, Billon B, Pare C. Maturational changes of caffeine concentrations and disposition in infancy during maintenance therapy for apnea of prematurity: influence of gestational age, hepatic disease, and breast feeding. Pediatrics 1985;76:834.
171. Roberts RJ. Methyl xanthine therapy: caffeine and theophylline. In: Drug therapy for infants. Philadelphia: WB Saunders, 1984:119.
172. Costarino AT, Polin RA. Neuromuscular relaxants in the neonate. Clin Perinatol 1987;14:965.
173. Bennett EJ, Bowyer DE, Giesecke AH, et al. Pancuronium bromide: a double-blind study in children. Anesth Analg 1973;52:12.
174. Bennett EJ, Ramamurthy S, Dalal FY, et al. Pancuronium and the neonate. Br J Anaesth 1975;47:75.
175. Goudsouzian NG, Crone RK, Todres ID. Recovery from pancuronium blockade in the neonatal intensive care unit. Br J Anaesth 1981;53:1303.
176. Hilgenberg JC. Comparison of the pharmacology of vecuronium and atracurium with that of other currently available muscle relaxants. Anesth Analg 1983;62:524.
177. Meretoja OA. Is vecuronium a long-acting neuromuscular blocking agent in neonates and infants? Br J Anaesth 1989; 62:184.
178. Coceani F, Olley PM. Role of prostaglandins, prostacyclin, and thromboxanes in the control of prenatal patency and postnatal closure of the ductus arteriosus. Semin Perinatol 1980;4:109.
179. Freed MD, Heymann MA, Lewis AB, et al. Prostaglandin E_1 in infants with ductus arteriosus-dependent congenital heart disease. Circulation 1981;64:899.
180. Lewis AB, Takahashi M, Lurie PR. Administration of prostaglandin E_1 in neonates with critical congenital cardiac defects. J Pediatr 1978;93:481.
181. Thanopoulos BD, Andreou A, Frimas C. Prostaglandin E_2 administration in infants with ductus-dependent cyanotic congenital heart disease. Eur J Pediatr 1987;146:279.
182. Monk JP, Clissold SP. Misoprostol: a preliminary review of its pharmacodynamic and pharmacokinetic properties, and therapeutic efficacy in the treatment of peptic ulcer disease. Drugs 1987;33:1.
183. Friedman WF, Hirschklau MJ, Printz MP, et al. Pharmacologic closure of patent ductus arteriosus in the premature infant. N Engl J Med 1976;295:526.
184. Gersony WM, Peckham GJ, Ellison RC, et al. Effects of indomethacin in premature infants with patent ductus arteriosus: result of a national collaborative study. J Pediatr 1983;102: 895.
185. Bandstra ES, Mantalvo BM, Goldberg RN, et al. Prophylactic indomethacin for prevention of intraventricular hemorrhage in premature infants. Pediatrics 1988;82:533.
186. Merritt TA, Bejar R, Corazza M, et al. Clinical trials of intravenous indomethacin for closure of the patent ductus arteriosus. Pediatr Cardiol 1983;4(Suppl II):71.
187. Maher P, Lane B, Ballard R, et al. Does indomethacin cause extension of intracranial hemorrhages? A preliminary study. Pediatrics 1985;75:497.
188. Wiest DB, Pinson JB, Gal PS, et al. Population pharmacokinetics of intravenous indomethacin in neonates with symptomatic patent ductus arteriosus. Clin Pharmacol Ther 1991; 49:550.
189. Rhodes PG, Ferguson MG, Reddy NS, et al. Effects of prolonged versus acute indomethacin therapy in very low birthweight infants with patent ductus arteriosus. Eur J Pediatr 1988;147:481.
190. McCarthy JS, Zies LG, Gelband H. Age-dependent closure of the patent ductus arteriosus by indomethacin. Pediatrics 1978;62:706.
191. Achanti B, Pyati S, Yeh TF. Indomethacin therapy in premature infants of advanced postnatal age. J Perinatol 1987;7:235.
192. Dibona GF. Prostaglandins and nonsteroidal anti-inflammatory drugs: effects on renal hemodynamics. Am J Med 1986;80:(Suppl 1A):12.
193. Cifuentes RF, Olley PM, Balfe JW, et al. Indomethacin and renal function in premature infants with persistent patent ductus arteriosus. J Pediatr 1979;95:583.

194. Seri I, Tulassay T, Kiszel J, et al. The use of dopamine for the prevention of the renal side effects of indomethacin in premature infants with patent ductus arteriosus. Int J Pediatr Nephrol 1984;5:209.
195. Cowan F. Indomethacin, patent ductus arteriosus, and cerebral blood flow. J Pediatr 1986;109:341.
196. Colditz P, Murphy D, Rulfe P, et al. Effect of infusion rate of indomethacin on cerebral vascular responses in premature neonates. Arch Dis Child 1989;64:8.
197. Coombs RC, Morgan MEI, Durbin GM, et al. Gut blood flow velocities in the newborn: effects of patent ductus arteriosus and parenteral indomethacin. Arch Dis Child 1990;65:1067.
198. Ward RM. Persistent pulmonary hypertension. In: Nelson NM, ed. Current therapy in neonatal-perinal medicine-2. Toronto: BC Decker, 1990;331.
199. Kulik TJ, Lock JE. Pulmonary vasodilator therapy in persistent pulmonary hypertension of the newborn. Clin Perinatol 1984;11:693.
200. Ward, RM, Daniel CH, Kendig JW. Oliguria and tolazoline pharmacokinetics in the newborn. Pediatrics 1986;77:307.
201. Caplan MS, Hsueh W, Sun X-M, et al. Circulating plasma platelet activating factor in persistent pulmonary hypertension of the newborn. Am Rev Respir Dis 1990;142:1258.
202. Liu S, Crawley DE, Barnes PJ, et al. Endothelium-derived relaxing factor inhibits hypoxic pulmonary vasoconstriction in rats. Am Rev Respir Dis 1991;143:32.
203. Ignarro LJ, Ross G, Tillisch J. Pharmacology of endothelium-derived nitric oxide and nitrovasodilators. West J Med 1991; 154:51.
204. Peliowski A, Finer NN. A blinded, randomized, placebo-controlled trial to compare theophylline and doxapram for the treatment of apnea of prematurity. J Pediatr 1990;116:648.
205. Barrington KJ, Finer NN, Peters KL, et al. Physiologic effects of doxapram in idiopathic apnea of prematurity. J Pediatr 1986;108:125.
206. Alpan G, Eyal F, Sagi E, et al. Doxapram in the treatment of idiopathic apnea of prematurity unresponsive to aminophylline. J Pediatr 1984;104:634.
207. Bairam A, Akramoff-Gershan L, Beharry K, et al. Gastrointestinal absorption of doxapram in neonates. Am J Perinatol 1991;8:110.
208. Tay-Uyboco J, Kwiatkowski K, Cates DB, et al. Clinical and physiological responses to prolonged nasogastric administration of doxapram for apnea of prematurity. Biol Neonate 1991;59:190.
209. Mammel MC, Johnson DE, Green TP, et al. Control trial of dexamethasone therapy in infants with bronchopulmonary dysplasia. Lancet 1983;1:1356.
210. Ward RM, Green TP. Developmental pharmacology and toxicology: principles of study design and problems of methodology. Pharmacol Ther 1988;36:309.
211. Avery GB, Fletcher AB, Kaplan M, et al. Controlled trial of dexamethasone in respirator-dependent infants with bronchopulmonary dysplasia. Pediatrics 1985;75:106.
212. Harkavy KL, Scanlon JW, Chowdhry PK, et al. Dexamethasone therapy for chronic lung disease in ventilator- and oxygen-dependent infants: a controlled trial. J Pediatr 1989; 115:979.
213. Cummings JJ, D'Eugenio DB, Gross SJ. A controlled trial of dexamethasone in premature infants at high risk for bronchopulmonary dysplasia. N Engl J Med 1989;320:1505.
214. Weichsel ME Jr. The therapeutic use of glucocorticoid hormones in the perinatal period: potential neurological hazards. Ann Neurol 1977;2:364.
215. Gladstone IM, Ehrenkranz RA, Jacobs HC. Pulmonary function tests and fluid balance in neonates with chronic lung disease during dexamethasone treatment. Pediatrics 1989;84: 1072.
216. Haynes RC. Adrenocorticotropic hormone; adrenocortical steroids and their synthetic analogs; inhibitors of the synthesis and actions of the adrenocortical hormones. In: Gilman AG, Rall TW, Nies AS, et al, eds. Goodman and Gilman's the pharmacologic basis of therapeutics, 8th ed. New York: Pergamon Press, 1990:1431.
217. Richter O, Ern B, Reinhardt D, et al. Pharmacokinetics of dexamethasone in children. Pediatr Pharmacol 1983;3:329.
218. Wilson DM, Baldwin RB, Ariagno RL. A randomized, placebo-controlled trial of effects of dexamethasone on hypothalamic-pituitary-adrenal axis in preterm infants. J Pediatr 1988; 113:764.
219. Byyny RL. Withdrawal from glucocorticoid therapy. N Engl J Med 1976;295:30.
220. Chamberlin P, Meyer WJ III. Management of pituitary-adrenal suppression secondary to corticosteroid therapy. Pediatrics 1981;67:245.
221. Alkalay AL, Pomerance JL, Puri AR, et al. Hypothalamic-pituitary-adrenal axis function in very low birth weight infants treated with dexamethasone. Pediatrics 1990;86:204.
222. Onishi S, Miyazawa G, Nishimura Y, et al. Postnatal development of circadian rhythm in serum cortisol levels in children. Pediatrics 1983;72:399.
223. Hindmarsh KW, Tan L, Sankaran K, et al. Diurnal rhythms of cortisol, ACTH, and β-endorphin levels in neonates and adults. West J Med 1989;151:153.
224. Roberts RJ, Knight ME. Pharmacology of vitamin E in the newborn. Clin Perinatol 1987;14:843.
225. Ehrenkranz RA, Bonta BW, Ablow RC, et al. Amelioration of bronchopulmonary dysplasia after vitamin E administration: a preliminary report. N Engl J Med 1978;299:564.
226. Ehrenkranz RA, Ablow RC, Warshaw JB. Prevention of bronchopulmonary dysplasia with vitamin E administration during the acute stages of respiratory distress syndrome. J Pediatr 1979;95:873.
227. Hittner HM, Godio LB, Rudolph AJ, et al. Retrolental fibroplasia: efficacy of vitamin E in a double-blind clinical study of preterm infants. N Engl J Med 1981;305:1365.
228. Phelps DL. Local and systemic reactions to the parenteral administration of vitamin E. Dev Pharmacol Ther 1981;2: 156.
229. Centers for Disease Control. Unusual syndrome with fatalities among premature infants: association with a new intravenous vitamin E product. MMWR 1984;73:387.
230. Bodenstein CJ. Intravenous vitamin E and deaths in the intensive care unit. [Letter] Pediatrics 1984;73:733.
231. Balistreri WF, Farrell MK, Bove KE. Lessons from the E-Ferol tragedy. Pediatrics 1986;78:503.
232. Martone WJ, Williams WW, Mortensen ML, et al. Illness with fatalities in premature infants: association with an intravenous vitamin-E preparation, E-Ferol. Pediatrics 1986;78:591.
233. American Academy of Pediatrics, Committee on Fetus and Newborn. Vitamin E and the prevention of retinopathy of prematurity. Pediatrics 1985;76:315.
234. Howell SK, Wang Y–M. Quantitation of physiological α-tocopherol, metabolites, and related compounds by reversed-phase high-performance liquid chromatography. J Chromatogr 1982;227:174.
235. Knight ME, Roberts RJ. Disposition of intravenously administered pharmacologic doses of vitamin-E in newborn rabbits. J Pediatr 1986;108:145.
236. Committee on Fetus and Newborn. Guidelines for perinatal

care. 2nd ed. Elk Grove Village, IL: American Academy of Pediatrics; Washington, DC: American College of Obstetricians and Gynecologists, 1988:203.

237. American Academy of Pediatrics, Committee on Drugs. Transfer of drugs and other chemicals into human milk. Pediatrics 1989;84:924.

238. Berlin CM Jr. Pharmacologic considerations of drug use in the lactating mother. Obstet Gynecol 1981;58(Suppl):17S.

239. Berlin CM Jr. The excretion of drugs in human milk. Prog Clin Biol Res 1980;36:115.

240. Berlin CM Jr. Drugs and chemicals: exposure of the nursing mother. Pediatr Clin North Am 1989;36:1089.

Neonatology: Pathophysiology and Management of the Newborn, Fourth Edition,
edited by Gordon B. Avery, Mary Ann Fletcher, and Mhairi G. MacDonald.
J.B. Lippincott Company, Philadelphia © 1994.

chapter 57

The Infant of the Drug-Dependent Mother

ENRIQUE M. OSTREA, JR.
JOSE L. LUCENA
MARIA ASUNCION SILVESTRE

The problem of drug abuse has reached epidemic proportions during the past two decades, with increases not only in the number of drug users but also in the types of drugs abused. Equally alarming is the increase in the proportion of drugs users who are women of childbearing age or who are pregnant, since the effects of drugs on the pregnancy and fetus can be significant. In this chapter, the latter will be addressed; existing information in the literature on the maternal, neonatal, and long-term complications in infants of drug use during pregnancy will be consolidated; and a brief historical and epidemiologic perspective on the problem will be given. There will be many instances in which the data presented are conflicting. This reflects the limitations of studies on the human population, because the confounding effects of many factors such as types of drugs used, socioeconomic status, parent education, and the like are difficult to identify accurately and control for.

NARCOTICS

The terms "opiate" or "narcotic" refer to any natural or synthetic drug that has morphinelike pharmacologic actions. The natural opiates include morphine and codeine, whereas the synthetic opiates include heroin, methadone, propoxyphene (Darvon), pentazocine (Talwin), meperidine (Demerol), oxycodone (Percodan, Tylox, Vecodine, Percocet), morphinone (Dilaudid), and fentanyl (Immovar, Sublimaze). Chronic use of narcotics, even in therapeutic doses, results in addiction, which is characterized by psychological as well as physical dependence on the drug.

HISTORY OF NARCOTICS

Opium use probably dates back about 6000 years.[1] One of the earliest references to opiate complications in the perinatal period was made by Hippocrates, who mentioned "uterine suffocation" as possibly secondary to opium use.[2] By the late nineteenth and early twentieth century, reference to the passively addicted neonate is evident from reports describing the diffusion through the placenta and transmission through the breast milk of morphine.[3]

The naturally occurring opiates, morphine and codeine, are derived from the seeds of the unripe poppy plant, *Papaver somniferum*, and were consumed for their narcotic and analgesic properties. Heroin (diacetylmorphine), a semisynthetic opioid, was first introduced in 1874. It became popular because of the rapid onset of its central nervous system (CNS) effects. By 1950, heroin had supplanted morphine as the drug of choice among abusers.[4] It is available illicitly in bags containing up to 40 to 50 mg of the active ingredient, cut or diluted variably with quinine, lactose, starch, lidocaine, or even powdered milk. Methadone was first synthesized in 1945. It is longer-acting than heroin, and can be administered orally. These properties render it the drug of choice for replacement–substitution therapy of heroin addicts undergoing detoxification. Since Dole and Nyswander advocated the use of methadone in maintenance treatment programs,[5] it has become the most widely used and studied opiate in pregnancy.

EPIDEMIOLOGY

A survey in 1985 by the National Institute of Drug Abuse (NIDA) estimated that approximately 23 million people in the United States used illicit drugs. It also was estimated that about 250,000 women were intravenous drug users, predominantly using opiates, and approximately 90% were women of reproductive age.[6] Estimates are that approximately 6000 to 10,000 newborns are born to opiate-addicted women each year.[7]

Almost all narcotic drugs ingested by the female addict during pregnancy cross the placenta and enter the fetal circulation. Thus, the fetus is chronically exposed to these drugs and encounters problems *in utero* and after birth. Although the development of passive addiction to narcotic agents is the most widely known of these fetal complications, other major problems also are encountered (Table 57-1).

ANTENATAL PROBLEMS

Intrauterine asphyxia is perhaps the single greatest risk to the fetus of a drug-dependent woman. This is based on findings within this group of infants of a high incidence of stillbirths, meconium-stained amniotic fluid, fetal distress, low Apgar scores, and neonatal aspiration pneumonia.[8–14] The predisposition of the fetus to asphyxia underscores the need for repeated evaluation of fetal well-being during the course of the pregnancy. Fetal asphyxia in the pregnant addict may be secondary to a number of factors. Studies using methadone in a fetal lamb model suggest that opiates may act directly to affect both quiet and rapid-eye-movement (REM) sleep, resulting in a hyperactive state that causes a 20% increase in fetal oxygen consumption.[15] Sleep disturbances, consisting of more REM and less quiet sleep, have been demonstrated in newborn infants chronically exposed *in utero* to low doses of methadone with or without concomitant heroin usage.[16,17] Another possible cause of fetal asphyxia is fetal withdrawal, which usually coincides with the mother's withdrawal. Since fetal withdrawal can manifest as hyperactivity, this increases the oxygen consumption of the fetus, which, if not adequately compensated for, leads to fetal asphyxia.[18] In a fetal lamb model, withdrawal has been induced in the morphine-exposed lamb fetus by the administration of naloxone, an opiate antagonist. Manifestations included immediate bradycardia associated with transient increases in systolic and diastolic blood pressure, rapid, continuous deep breathing movements, increased total body movements, eye movements and neck tone, and desynchronization of electrocortical activity.[17] The high incidence of preeclampsia, abruptio placentae, and placenta previa in the pregnant addict also predisposes to placental insufficiency and fetal distress.[14]

TABLE 57–1
PERINATAL PROBLEMS ASSOCIATED WITH ABUSE OF NARCOTICS DURING PREGNANCY

Antenatal Problems
Intrauterine asphyxia
Meconium-stained amniotic fluid
Infection
Abruptio placentae or placenta previa
Neonatal Problems
Prematurity
Low birth weight
Small head circumference
Small for gestational age
Low Apgar score
Jaundice
Aspiration pneumonia
Meconium aspiration
Transient tachypnea
Hyaline membrane disease
Congenital malformation
Infection
Thrombocytosis
Neurobehavioral effects
Withdrawal

Meconium-stained amniotic fluid frequently is encountered in the pregnant addict and is a manifestation of fetal distress.[14] Aspiration of meconium during fetal distress may account for the increased frequency of meconium aspiration syndromes seen in these infants.

Intrauterine infection is another risk in the fetus of a drug addict. The life-style of the pregnant addict predisposes her to infection, particularly venereal disease, hepatitis, and acquired immunodeficiency syndrome (AIDS), which also may affect her fetus.[14,19–22] During delivery or before labor, the increased incidence of premature membrane rupture in the pregnant addict further exposes the fetus to the risk of nonspecific infections.[14] Opiates may compromise immune functions through their effect on both cell-mediated and humoral immune responses.[23]

NEONATAL PROBLEMS

PREMATURITY AND LOW BIRTH WEIGHT

Infants born to mothers on heroin have a higher incidence of prematurity, low birth weight, and small head circumference (*i.e.*, between the 3rd and 5th percentile) than drug-free control subjects.[24–27] Birth weights of infants of mothers on methadone programs, on the other hand, have variably been reported as higher[28,29] or lower[26,27] than those infants of untreated pregnant addicts, or not significantly different from the general newborn population.[25] This may reflect the better prenatal care that the women receive while on the program. Studies on pregnant rats exposed to methadone have shown their offspring to have significantly lower body weight, length, head diameter, and organ weight,[30] and impaired brain development[31] and thermoregulation[32] compared to non–methadone-exposed pups.

LOW APGAR SCORE

There is a high incidence of low Apgar score in infants of drug-dependent mothers. This may be related to intrauterine asphyxia or to the effects of narcotics that the mother received before delivery. Not infrequently, the pregnant addict will obtain a heroin fix before entering the hospital, which can depress the infant. Significantly large amounts of morphine have been found in the urine and cord blood of infants born to these women.[29] Caution must be exercised with the use of narcotic antagonists to reverse the respiratory depression in drug-dependent infants, however, because narcotic antagonists also may precipitate an acute withdrawal.

OTHERS

In addition to withdrawal, other problems are seen with increased frequency in the infant of a drug-dependent mother: jaundice, aspiration pneumonia and meconium aspiration, transient tachypnea, hyaline membrane disease, congenital malformations, and infections.[14] These problems are significant because they are the leading causes of death in these infants.

Aspiration pneumonia, hyaline membrane disease, and transient tachypnea are the principal pulmonary problems in the infant of the drug-dependent mother. About 30% of aspiration pneumonia is due to meconium aspiration.[14] Transient tachypnea may be secondary to the inhibitory effects of narcotics on the reflex clearing of fluid by the lungs.[33] The high incidence of hyaline membrane disease among infants of drug-dependent mothers is secondary to prematurity. What has been reported as a protection of premature, drug-dependent infants against hyaline membrane disease is due primarily to the increased incidence of small-for-gestational-age infants in this group.[14,34] Thus, the factors that cause a fetus to be small for gestational age are probably more important determinants of the infant's risk for development of hyaline membrane disease than is the direct action of narcotics (*e.g.*, heroin) in accelerating pulmonary maturation.[35,36,37] Meconium aspiration and hyaline membrane disease account for more than 50% of the deaths among infants of drug-dependent mothers.[14]

In general, the opiates are not believed to be teratogenic to the fetus. Most reports do not show an increase in the frequency of congenital anomalies,[9,13,19,23,38,39] and in one study, although an increased frequency of malformations was found,[14] no consistent pattern of malformation was observed. Animal studies, however, have shown a dose-related teratogenic effect of narcotics on the CNS of the developing hamster, which was blocked by narcotic antagonists.[40]

There is an increased incidence of jaundice in the infants of drug-dependent mothers, which may be related to the high incidence of prematurity in this group.[14] In animals, induction of liver enzymes by morphine has been demonstrated,[41] although the dose of morphine used was exceedingly high (250 mg/kg), a situation unlikely to be paralleled in a clinical setting.

A significant thrombocytosis, occasionally exceeding 1,000,000 platelets per mm^3, has been reported in infants of mothers receiving maintenance doses of 40 to 90 mg of methadone per day. Onset was by the second week of life, with counts remaining high for over 16 weeks. The thrombocytosis, and associated increased circulating platelet aggregates, may play a role in the development of the focal cerebral infarctions and germinal matrix and subarachnoid hemorrhages encountered in postmortem examinations of some of these infants.[42]

Along with the high incidence of infection in the pregnant addict is a correspondingly high incidence of infection in her infant. Although a number of the neonatal infections are nonspecific in nature, such as sepsis, omphalitis, necrotizing enterocolitis, and the enteritides, some of the infections are related to the antenatal life-style and problems of the mother. The latter include hepatitis and venereal diseases (*e.g.*, syphilis, gonorrhea, herpes simplex), group B streptococcal infections, and AIDS.[14,19–22]

NEONATAL NARCOTIC WITHDRAWAL OR ABSTINENCE SYNDROME

The onset of withdrawal usually occurs within the first 72 hours after birth, commonly within the first 24 to 48 hours. In a few instances, the onset may appear soon after birth, if the mother has already begun to experience withdrawal before delivery. Reports of withdrawal occurring after the first or second week may be secondary to withdrawal from other drugs beside the narcotics.[43] Many factors, such as maternal drug dosage, the timing of the last dose before delivery, the character of the labor, the type and amount of anesthesia or analgesia given to the mother, and the maturity and nutritional status of the infant, influence the onset of withdrawal.[29]

Withdrawal in the infant usually peaks by about the third day of postnatal life and subsides by the fifth to seventh day. The duration of withdrawal is related to its severity. When drugs are used to treat the withdrawal, relapse may occur if treatment is discontinued abruptly. The withdrawal manifestations, although they subside within a week, do not completely disappear until about 8 to 16 weeks of age (see Long-Term Outcome).

Neonatal narcotic withdrawal involves the CNS and respiratory, gastrointestinal, vasomotor, and cutaneous systems (Table 57-2).[44]

Central Nervous System Signs. Neurologic signs predominate and appear early. Findings are those of CNS excitability, such as hyperactivity, irritability, tremors, and hypertonicity. Occasionally, fever may accompany these increased neuromuscular activities.

Hyperactivity manifests as almost incessant movements of the extremities. When the infant is supine and unrestrained, movements assume a jerky, purposeless, *en masse* nature, apparently perpetuated by unchecked proprioceptive stimuli. When placed in the prone position, the motor behavior becomes more organized. There are crawling movements, which may actually lead to the infant's displacement from the crib, and other motions such as chin lifting, head movement from side to side, chest elevation, and hand-to-mouth facility. The latter usually quiets the infant, indicating the usefulness of pacifiers.

TABLE 57–2
MANIFESTATIONS OF NEONATAL NARCOTIC WITHDRAWAL

Central Nervous System Signs
Hyperactivity
Hyperirritability—excess crying, high-pitched outcry
Increased muscle tone
Exaggerated reflexes
Tremors
Sneezing, hiccups, yawning
Short, nonquiet sleep
Fever
Respiratory Signs
Tachypnea
Excess secretions
Gastrointestinal Signs
Disorganized, vigorous sucking
Vomiting
Drooling
Sensitive gag
Hyperphagia
Diarrhea
Abdominal cramps (?)
Vasomotor Signs
Stuffy nose
Flushing
Sweating
Sudden, circumoral pallor
Cutaneous Signs
Excoriated buttocks
Facial scratches
Pressure-point abrasions

From Ostrea EM, Chavez CJ, Stryker JS. The care of the drug dependent woman and her infant. Lansing, MI: Michigan Department of Public Health, 1978:30.

Hyperirritability manifests as an almost incessant crying with shrill, high-pitched outcries. The infant's muscle tone is exaggerated; sometimes an opisthotonic position is assumed. This makes the infant hard to hold due to its failure to mold to the body of the holder. Sleep also is disturbed.

Tremors and myoclonic jerks are frequent, and sometimes are sustained. To distinguish from seizures, tremors can be abolished by restraint of the tremulous extremity.

The reflexes of the infant (*i.e.*, Moro, traction response, weight bearing, placing, stepping, crawling, and Landau) all are exaggerated. The infant's response to stimuli, such as sound and light, also is increased disproportionately.

Electroencephalographic (EEG) tracings on the addicted neonate may be abnormal and show high-frequency dysynchronous activity suggestive of CNS irritability.

In premature infants, the neural hyperexcitability is more episodic. The infants appear restless and overactive for short periods and then lapse into periods of lethargy and inactivity. Sustained tremors usually are not seen in premature infants until they mature to a point when sufficient tone is present in the upper and lower extremities.

Respiratory Signs. Infants who are withdrawing tend to be tachypneic, with irregular respirations. Alkalosis due to hyperventilation may result. Fluid loss also may be increased.

Gastrointestinal Signs. The suck of the infant is disorganized and poorly coordinated with swallowing. Consequently, milk frequently drools around the corners of the infant's mouth. The infant appears incessantly hungry, which, when unfulfilled, leads to mounting agitation, persistent crying, hyperactivity, and exhaustion. Proper positioning of the infant to enhance hand-to-mouth facility may be extremely soothing. Vomiting and diarrhea also often are observed. This can lead to dehydration, electrolyte imbalance, and excoriations around the buttocks (see Complications).

Vasomotor Signs. Significant vasomotor instability manifests as stuffy nose, flushing, mottling, sweating, and episodes of sudden, circumoral pallor.

Cutaneous Signs. Because of hyperactivity, facial scratches and abrasions on pressure points may be observed on the infant's skin. Excoriations of the buttocks may occur if diarrhea is present.

It has been shown that neither the infant's gender, race, and Apgar score nor the mother's age, parity, and duration of heroin intake correlate with the severity of the infant's withdrawal.[29] Similarly, manipulation of the environment such as reducing the amount of light or noise in the nursery does not ameliorate the severity of withdrawal in the infants.[29]

Adults experience abdominal cramps, palpitation, nausea, and other discomforts while undergoing withdrawal. It is possible that similar discomforts also are experienced by the infant, and these may nullify any potential benefits from light or noise reduction in the nursery. On the other hand, it has been noted that the severity of the infant's withdrawal correlates significantly with the methadone dose of the mother.[29] Withdrawal in the infant tends to be more intense if the mother has been on more than 20 mg of methadone per day before delivery.

COMPLICATIONS

The complications associated with neonatal drug withdrawal are related to the severity of the withdrawal. Alterations in the serum electrolytes and *p*H and dehydration may occur secondary to vomiting and diarrhea. Weight loss may be profound, not only due to excess fluid losses but also to poor and ineffective oral intake. Aspiration pneumonia may occur, secondary to vomiting and uncoordinated sucking and swallowing. Respiratory alkalosis can result from tachypnea in the infant. In rare cases, convulsions may be observed. It should be noted that convulsions are a rare manifestation of narcotic withdrawal. On the other hand, convulsions are a frequent manifestation of withdrawal from the non-narcotic drugs (see Non-narcotic Abstinence Syndrome).

MORTALITY

The mortality rate among infants born to drug-dependent mothers used to be as high as 50%. With early recognition and treatment of the withdrawal syndrome and prevention of its complications, the mortality from neonatal withdrawal is negligible. Nonetheless, mortality in infants of drug-dependent mothers remains high; in one report, mortality rate was 27 per 1000 live births compared to 12 per 1000 live births in the general population.[14] The causes of death were immaturity (14%), hyaline membrane disease (40%), severe meconium aspiration (23%), and major congenital malformations (23%). Pulmonary problems (*e.g.*, meconium aspiration, hyaline membrane disease) accounted for more than 50% of the deaths.

NEUROBEHAVIORAL ABNORMALITIES

Using the Brazelton Neonatal Assessment Scale, the manifestations of neonatal withdrawal such as hypertonicity, hyperirritability, hyperactivity, and increased hand-to-mouth facility can be demonstrated. Some other fine behavioral abnormalities also are found that could affect early infant–caregiver interactions.[45–48] For instance, congenital addiction seems to affect those behavior systems associated with arousal and those implicated in the early development of mother–infant bonding. Although the addicted infant is more likely to elicit caregiver consolation because he cries more often, he is less easy to cuddle. He also is less readily maintained in an alert state through the course of handling and becomes increasingly less responsive to stimuli, particularly visual stimuli, although auditory evoked responses are better integrated. Since cuddliness, alertness, and visual regard are the primary means by which the infant initiates and maintains social interaction with his caregiver, the impairment of these behavior patterns may have a profound effect on the early infant–caregiver interaction.

LONG-TERM OUTCOME

Persistence of Withdrawal. Infants who manifest narcotic withdrawal may show a persistence of the withdrawal for as long as 8 to 16 weeks.[49] The prolonged manifestations usually are milder than the initial withdrawal, and consist of irritability, tremors, hypertonicity, sneezing, hiccups, and regurgitation. The persistence of withdrawal is related directly to its initial severity; it is more prolonged in those who had severe initial withdrawal. Infants who were treated for withdrawal also show prolonged withdrawal. Thus, drug treatment may ameliorate the manifestations of withdrawal, but does not shorten its duration. It is important that the mother is made aware of the persistence of the infant's withdrawal when the infant is discharged from the nursery. Otherwise, she may become alarmed when the infant continues to manifest some withdrawal at home. The unwarned mother also may misinterpret the infant's irritability as hunger, and overfeed the infant. This can lead to diarrhea and vomiting. The mother also should be instructed on how to reduce the infant's discomfort by swaddling and cuddling the infant. In addition, she should be reassured that the infant's withdrawal will subside eventually without the use of medications. In most instances, the mother who is well informed can cope with the situation successfully.

Child Abuse and Sudden Infant Death Syndrome. The high incidence of child abuse and neglect constitutes one of the serious medical problems in the infant of the drug-addicted woman. Thermal burns, usually cigarette burns, traumatic ecchymoses, and hematoma have been observed in 8% of infants during the first 8 months of life.[44] During the same period, about 8.3% of the infants had to be placed in alternative care because of maternal neglect or abandonment or maternal death. Many factors contribute to the risk of abuse. The persistence of the withdrawal, feeding problems, abnormal sleep patterns, and periods of restlessness in the infant can generate undue tension in the mother, whose tolerance for frustration already is low. Thus, the mother, unable to cope with the situation, may simply withdraw from her infant and avoid any contact or she may abandon or injure the infant. It is therefore important that someone is available at home to help the mother in the care of her child, and that the visiting or public health nurse or the social and protective service workers actively follow up these infants.

There is a fourfold to fivefold increase in the incidence of sudden death syndrome in infants of narcotic-dependent mothers.[50,51] This is observed whether the infant is cared for by the mother or in an extended family or foster care home. The cause is not known, although its occurrence is significantly higher in those infants who had moderate to severe withdrawal after birth.[50]

Growth and Psychomotor Development. At 12 months of age, the growth in terms of weight, head circumference, and length of infants of narcotic-dependent mothers has been observed to fall within the 10th to the 90th percentile on the growth chart. Similarly, the percentage of addicted infants whose growth parameters were below the 10th percentile did not differ significantly from the nonaddict group.[52] At the age of 3 to 6 years, however, some retardation in the weight, length, and head circumference of these infants has been reported.[53–56]

Within the first year of life, the infants of narcotic addicts have been shown to manifest difficulty in regulating their behavior, but otherwise had normal developmental scores.[53–55] A high incidence of transient or minor motor deficits and poor attention span also were observed,[55] as well as a high incidence of otitis media and abnormal eye findings, such as nystagmus.[57] At preschool age, compared to controls (*i.e.*, children at similar environmental risk and sociodemographic background), the addicted children performed less well in terms of perception, short-term memory, and organization, but did just as well on objective tests of activity and attention.[54] Others have reported behavioral abnormalities such as aggressiveness, hyperactivity, high risk for poorer visual coordination, socioemotional problems, and poor school performance.[58]

Results of developmental studies of infants prenatally exposed to methadone have been varied. At 1 month of age, hyperirritable motor responses (*e.g.*, tremulousness, jerkiness, and hypertonia), independent of the infant's general state of alertness or irritability, were demonstrated,[59,60] as well as poor habituation to light and sound stimulation, inconsolability, and poor state control.[60] Infants of well controlled, low-dose methadone-maintained mothers had poorer state control and interactive behavior than the infants of polydrug abusers, who, in turn, performed more poorly than drug-free control subjects.[25] At 3 to 4 months of age, the infants still exhibited hyperactivity, sleep problems, and feeding difficulties, although these problems resolved by 6 months of age.[25]

NON-NARCOTIC HYPNOSEDATIVES

NON-NARCOTIC ABSTINENCE SYNDROME

Infants born to women who have used non-narcotic hypnosedatives during pregnancy (Table 57-3) also manifest addiction and withdrawal from these drugs. The manifestations of non-narcotic withdrawal in the neonate are similar to those of narcotic withdrawal. In a few instances (*e.g.*, with barbiturate withdrawal, with ethchlorvynol withdrawal), hyperphagia has been described as a prominent manifestation.

Although the manifestations of withdrawal from narcotic and non-narcotic drugs are similar, major differences do exist[44]:

In adults, the rate of developing physical dependence to the non-narcotic hypnosedatives does not increase with the drug dose, as it does with narcotics. Rather, prolonged and continuous administration of large and partially incapacitating doses usually are necessary, over months or years, to produce addiction to non-narcotics, especially if the drugs are taken orally. The exception is seen in the newborn infant. Passive addiction in the fetus and infant has been observed even when therapeutic doses of non-narcotic drugs have been used by the mother during pregnancy. Thus, a pregnant woman who is treated with phenobarbital for epilepsy can induce addiction in her fetus, even if she is not addicted to the drug.[43]

The manifestations of the non-narcotic abstinence syndrome more frequently are intense and life-threatening compared to narcotic withdrawal. The occurrence of convulsions also is more frequent in non-narcotic withdrawal.

Most of the withdrawal from narcotics is seen within the first 3 days of postnatal life, due to the relatively short half-life of the narcotics. In contrast, withdrawal from the non-narcotics, such as phenobarbital, may be seen at 7 to 10 days after birth due to the slow clearance of the drug in the infant.

TABLE 57–3
NONNARCOTIC DRUGS

Hypnosedatives
Barbiturate
Nonbarbiturate sedatives and tranquilizers
Bromide
Chloral hydrate
Chlordiazepoxide (Librium)
Diazepam (Valium)
Ethchlorvynol (Placidyl)
Glutethimide (Doriden)
Alcohol
Ethanol

Unlike the narcotics, addiction to many of the non-narcotic hypnosedatives has been induced by physicians because of the mistaken notion that the drugs are nonaddicting.[44]

BARBITURATES

Although barbiturates have been used in clinical medicine for more than 50 years, their addiction potential was recognized only relatively recently. The frequent association in the adult of barbiturate use with alcohol may have contributed to the delayed recognition of the addicting potential of the barbiturates, because of the ability of barbiturates to abolish withdrawal from alcohol.[61,62]

Barbiturates are classified on the basis of the duration of their action as ultrashort, intermediate, and long acting. The intermediate-acting barbiturates are the most frequently abused (*e.g.*, secobarbital [Seconal], pentobarbital [Nembutal], amobarbital [Amytal], butabarbital [Butisol]). The abuse of the long-acting barbiturates (*e.g.*, phenobarbital) is not as common as the abuse of the shorter-acting forms. Phenobarbital, however, is involved most frequently with non-narcotic abstinence in the newborn since it is used frequently for insomnia, for the relief of anxiety, as an anticonvulsant, or for sedation when toxemia of pregnancy occurs.

Passive acquisition by the fetus of physical dependence to barbiturates can occur after prolonged intrauterine exposure to the drug.[43,63] Barbiturates cross the placenta readily, and establish high levels in both the maternal and cord blood. Relatively high levels of barbiturates have been found in the fetal brain, liver, and adrenal glands.[64] The manifestations of barbiturate withdrawal in the neonate are similar, regardless of which barbiturate was used by the mother; however, the onset of withdrawal may differ. Withdrawal typically occurs within a day after birth with intermediate-acting barbiturates,[65] and from 3 to 7 days after birth with the long-acting barbiturates.[45,63]

Barbiturates are metabolized principally by the liver, although a significant portion may be excreted unchanged by the kidney. In adults, up to 30% of the total dose of phenobarbital ingested is excreted unchanged in the urine.[66] The half-life of phenobarbital prenatally administered to infants is almost twice that in the adult, and varies inversely with the extent of the prenatal exposure to phenobarbital.[67]

The signs of withdrawal from barbiturates in neonates are similar to those described in adults. The infants are overactive and restless, with excessive crying, twitching, hyperactive reflexes, and hypertonicity. They also manifest diarrhea, vomiting, and poor sucking ability. When tonic–clonic convulsions occur, the EEG patterns show diffuse, paroxysmal, high-voltage, slow-wave bursts not unlike those seen in adults.[63] A subacute phase of hyperphagia, episodes of prolonged crying, episodic irritability, hyperacusis, and sweating have been described.[45] These manifestations may last from 2 to 6 months.

Recognition of the abstinence syndrome is essential to the adequate management of the infant. An awareness of the possibility of a late onset of withdrawal, especially after exposure to long-acting barbiturates, should alert the clinician to follow these infants closely during the first 2 weeks of life.

BROMIDE AND CHLORAL HYDRATE

Bromides and chloral hydrate were popular hypnosedative drugs for many years, until they gradually were replaced by the barbiturates and other hypnosedative agents. Addiction to chloral hydrate has been described in adults.[68] Many cases of bromide intoxication could have been due partly to chloral hydrate, since combination of the two drugs was not unusual.[68] A withdrawal syndrome and growth retardation have been reported in newborn infants after the use of bromides by the mother during pregnancy.[69,70] In one report, the mother took a large amount of bromide, in the form of Relaxa tablets, to relieve anxiety. The infant was born at term, but was small for gestational age and heavily meconium stained. Soon after birth the infant manifested extreme irritability, a high-pitched cry, and feeding difficulties, which lasted for 9 weeks.[70]

CHLORDIAZEPOXIDE AND DIAZEPAM

Chlordiazepoxide (Librium) and diazepam (Valium) are widely used for their hypnosedative effects. Abuse of these drugs and dependence on them both have been reported in adults. During pregnancy, benzodiazepines cross the placenta with relative ease, resulting in significant levels of the drug in the serum and tissue of the fetus.[71]

An acute withdrawal syndrome from chlordiazepoxide or diazepam has been observed in the newborn infant.[72,73] A presumptive diagnosis of chlordiazepoxide withdrawal was made in a set of twins born to a mother who used chlordiazepoxide, 20 mg per 24 hours, during the second and third trimesters of her pregnancy.[72] The withdrawal occurred on day 21 of life, and consisted of severe irritability and coarse tremors.

Three cases of presumptive neonatal withdrawal from diazepam also have been noted.[73] The onset of symptoms of withdrawal occurred within 2.5 to 6 hours after birth and consisted of tremors, irritability, hypertonicity, vigorous sucking, vomiting, and diarrhea. The dose of diazepam taken by the mother during pregnancy and up to the time of birth ranged from 15 to 20 mg per 24 hours. In all three cases, phenobarbital was effective in controlling the withdrawal in the infant, although the drug had to be administered for a prolonged period (13–25 days).

ETHCHLORVYNOL

Ethchlorvynol (Placidyl) was introduced in 1955 as a nonbarbiturate hypnotic for the treatment of insomnia. Like other nonbarbiturate sedatives, claims were made regarding its nonaddictive property.[74–76] The drug was used to relieve anxiety and as a sleep-inducing medication.[77] Like the barbiturate and the nonbarbiturate sedatives, tolerance to this drug develops with continued use, so that there is a tendency for a person to increase the dose to continue to get the desired effect. Reports of addiction to ethchlorvynol subsequently have been reported.[78–82]

Ethchlorvynol crosses the placenta readily, and studies in animals indicate that the drug achieves rapid equilibration between the maternal and fetal blood. It also can be detected in the chorionic and amniotic fluids.[83]

An abstinence syndrome in a newborn infant due to withdrawal from ethchlorvynol taken by the mother during pregnancy has been reported.[84] Extreme jitteriness, irritability, and hyperphagia were noted in the infant on the second day of life. The mother took the drug (500 mg/24 hours) for 3 months before giving birth. This dose was within the therapeutic range recommended in the adult. The onset of withdrawal in the infant occurred during the second day of life. No convulsions were noted, but the infant had received treatment with phenobarbital from early in the course of the abstinence syndrome.

GLUTETHIMIDE

Glutethimide (Doriden) was first introduced in 1954 as a nonbarbiturate hypnosedative, allegedly free of addicting properties. As was the case with the other nonbarbiturate hypnosedatives, this led to its widespread use, particularly as a substitute drug for the treatment of alcohol addiction.[85] Since that time, there have been numerous reports of acute and sometimes fatal intoxication with the drug in adults, and the occurrence of physical dependence.[86–88]

Glutethimide is structurally related to phenobarbital and to the teratogenic sedative thalidomide. It is metabolized in the liver to a hydroxylated product, as is phenobarbital. There are, however, no reports of teratogenicity after the use of glutethimide during pregnancy.

A possible case of neonatal withdrawal to glutethimide has been observed.[89] The mother was a heroin addict who supplemented her habit with 2 to 3 g of glutethimide three or four times a week to get the desired euphoric effect. Within 8 hours of birth, the infant had shown initial signs of withdrawal from narcotics that were readily controlled with chlorpromazine. On the tenth day of life, however, while receiving a tapered dose of chlorpromazine, the patient suddenly manifested diarrhea, fever, tachypnea, irritability, hypertonicity, and diaphoresis. It was presumed that the unusual recurrence of withdrawal on the tenth day of life may have been secondary to withdrawal from glutethimide.

DIFFERENTIAL DIAGNOSIS

Withdrawal from the narcotic and non-narcotic drugs should be distinguished from entities such as hypoglycemia, hypocalcemia, hypomagnesemia, sepsis, meningitis, subarachnoid hemorrhage, infectious diarrhea, and intestinal obstruction. Blood chemistry, cerebrospinal fluid examination, radiographic examination, and cultures should be performed as indicated by the clinical circumstances.

Infants whose mothers took tricyclic antidepressants and lithium during pregnancy, for psychiatric conditions, may manifest toxicity similar to withdrawal, such as irritability, tachycardia, respiratory distress, sweating, and convulsions.[90–94] Likewise, maternal ingestion of phenothiazines (*e.g.*, chlorpromazine) may induce extrapyramidal dysfunctions in the newborn infant, such as tremors, facial grimacing, increased muscle tone, cogwheel rigidity, increased reflexes, and torticollis, all of which can resemble the withdrawal syndrome.[95,96] The prenatal history and the identification of the metabolites of the offending drug in the infant's serum or urine are necessary to establish the diagnosis.

COCAINE

HISTORY OF COCAINE

The chewing of coca leaves dates back to 3000 B.C. to the Indians in the Andes Mountains of South America, who used coca leaves for various reasons.[97] When the Incas came in contact with these Indians, coca became an integral part of the Incan religion. The Incas believed that the coca leaf was a divine gift of their sun god; thus, its use was restricted to the priests and the privileged classes only. The chewing of coca leaves became widespread when the Spaniards conquered the Incas in the sixteenth century. The use of the coca leaf was promoted among the lower class and slaves, since the Spaniards realized that coca leaf chewing was essential to maintain the working pace of Indians in the mines and other places where conditions were harsh.[97]

In 1659, Nicholas Monardes was the first to write about the use of coca leaves.[97] He or Francisco Pizarro is credited with bringing coca leaves to Europe. In Europe, however, the coca plant essentially was ignored until interest in it was revived in the nineteenth century. The first medical report on coca leaves appeared in 1859 with the writings of Dr. Paolo Mantegazza, an Italian neurologist who referred to the coca leaves as "man's newest weapon against disease." Sigmund Freud was among the first to experiment scientifically with coca. He wrote five papers on coca between 1884 and 1887, and became intrigued with the effects that cocaine had on humans. He used cocaine to cure his colleague, Dr. Ernst Fleischl von Marxow, of his heroin addiction. Unfortunately, Fleischl von Marxow became addicted to cocaine, and therefore became one of the earliest cocaine addicts on record. Dr. Carl Koller in Vienna also was interested in cocaine and delivered a three-page paper on the local anesthetic effects of cocaine for ophthalmologic surgery. The late nineteenth and early twentieth century was a period when serious interest in cocaine developed in the United States. Cocaine was used freely and was incorporated into items such as tonics, ointments, nose powders, wines, and cigarettes. Vin Mariani was a specific brand of wine that was popular for its cocaine content. Coca-Cola was, at first, a patented cocaine-containing medicine that was introduced in 1886. It was advertised as "a valuable brain tonic and cure for all nervous afflictions."[97]

The Pure Food and Drug Act was passed in 1906 and the Harrison Tax (Narcotic) Act in 1914. Cocaine was classified as a narcotic, and from then on cocaine was "driven underground."[97]

EPIDEMIOLOGY

From the household surveys conducted by the National Institute on Drug Abuse, cocaine abuse among women of childbearing age (*i.e.*, between 15 and 44 years of age) was estimated at 3.5% in 1985, 1.7% in 1988, and 0.9% in 1990.[98] Although there appears to be an overall decline in illicit drug use during the periods surveyed, the total number of women of childbearing age who have used illicit drugs remained high (Table 57-4). The prevalence of illicit drug use specifically among pregnant women is more difficult to determine, due to significant underreporting of drug use by these women. One study, based on a survey of predominantly urban hospitals, gave an estimate of drug use among pregnant women as 0.4% to 27%; cocaine use ranged from 0.2% to 17%.[99] Drug detection was obtained by maternal history, urine toxicology, or both. With the use of a more sensitive drug screening method (*i.e.*, meconium drug test), a 44% prevalence of illicit drug use in pregnant women was found, in contrast to 11% by maternal self-report, and 30% of the infants also were positive for cocaine.[100]

TYPES

Cocaine is an alkaloid that is extracted from the leaves of the *Erythroxylon coca* bush. Its chemical name is methylbenzoylecgonine, and it is the only known local anesthetic that is found naturally. The pure cocaine substance was first extracted and identified by a German chemist, Albert Nieman in 1860. The drug is extracted from the leaves of the coca plant by a series of solvent extractions.

Coca paste is the first extraction product of cocaine and contains about 80% cocaine.[101] The paste can be smoked after applying it to tobacco or marijuana. Cocaine hydrochloride is the most common available form of cocaine. In its acid state, cocaine HCl is a white powder that is soluble in water and can be snorted or injected. Cocaine HCl usually is adulterated with starch, glucose, phencyclidine (PCP), heroin, or amphetamines, and its purity ranges from 20% to 80%.[101]

TABLE 57–4
DRUG USE AMONG WOMEN 15 TO 44 YEARS OF AGE

Drug Use	1985	1988	1990
Sample size	3144	3292	3522
Estimated number of women	56,126	59,605	60,064
Any ilicit drug (%)			
Lifetime	50.0	50.5	48.5
Past year	25.4	18.1	17.3
Past month	14.8	8.8	8.0
Marijuana (%)			
Lifetime	43.9	46.6	44.8
Past year	19.0	12.9	13.9
Past month	11.2	6.3	6.5
Cocaine (%)			
Lifetime	14.3	14.3	14.8
Past year	7.6	4.7	3.4*
Past month	3.5	1.7	0.9*

* Significantly different from 1988 data at $p < 0.05$.
Data from the National Household Survey on Drug Abuse, 1985, 1988, 1990.
From Khalsa J, Gfroerer J. Epidemiology and health consequences of drug abuse among pregnant women. Semin Perinatol 1991;15:265.

An alkaloidal base of cocaine can be obtained from cocaine HCl (*i.e.*, free-basing) by alkalizing the aqueous solution of cocaine HCl and then extracting the cocaine alkaloid base using volatile organic solvents, such as ether. The gummy cocaine residue, called rock, has a lower melting point than cocaine HCl and can be smoked using a special pipe. Crack cocaine is the most popular abused form of the drug. Crack cocaine is produced when cocaine HCl is mixed with ammonia, water, and baking soda and heated. The resulting paste, once dried, forms a hard, rocklike substance that can be smoked. The term "crack" is derived from the crackling sound that is produced when crack cocaine is prepared or smoked.

When taken orally, cocaine HCl has a peak effect at between 45 minutes and 90 minutes. Intranasal administration of cocaine (*i.e.*, snorting) has a peak effect in 15 to 30 minutes, and lasts from 60 to 90 minutes. Smoking cocaine (*i.e.*, free-basing) provides the most rapid delivery of the drug to the body. Peak effect is within 60 to 90 seconds, but the high lasts only for about 5 to 10 minutes. The intense high is followed by a down period as the effect wears off. Sometimes, the down period can be so unpleasant that more of the drug is used to reexperience the high, or other drugs are used. Thus, cocaine use not only is associated with, but may even promote the abuse of other drugs.[97]

Cocaine is metabolized by plasma and hepatic esterases into three major water-soluble metabolites, ecgonine methyl ester, benzoylecgonine, and ecgonine. The half-life of the drug in adults depends on the route of administration—an average of 0.6 hour after intravenous administration, 0.9 hour after oral use, and 1.3 hours after intranasal use. The metabolites can be found in the urine 72 hours after administration. In infants, metabolites can be found for up to 2 weeks after administration.[102]

PHARMACOLOGY

The neuropharmacologic effect of cocaine is secondary to its effect on three neurotransmitters: norepinephrine, dopamine, and serotonin.

Cocaine inhibits the reuptake of norepinephrine and dopamine,[103] which accumulate at the synaptic cleft, leading to prolonged stimulation of their corresponding receptors. Therefore, the effects of norepinephrine stimulation (*e.g.*, tachycardia, hypertension, arrhythmia, diaphoresis, tremors) and dopamine stimulation (*e.g.*, increased alertness, euphoria or enhanced feeling of well-being, sexual excitement, heightened energy) are experienced. Cocaine also decreases the uptake of tryptophan, which affects serotonin biosynthesis. A diminished serotonin level is associated with diminished need for sleep, since serotonin regulates the sleep–wake cycle.[101]

ADVERSE EFFECTS ON PREGNANCY

Studies in pregnant sheep have shown that maternal blood pressure becomes elevated within 5 minutes after cocaine infusion,[104–106] coupled with an increase in uterine vascular resistance and decrease in uterine blood flow. Fetal heart rate and blood pressure also increase, but fetal PO_2 and O_2 content decrease as a consequence of the reduced uterine blood flow. Thus, oxygen availability to the fetus is impaired.

The cocaine-induced uterine vasoconstriction does not appear to be mediated solely by an α-adrenergic stimulation because α-adrenergic blockade by phentolamine does not ablate the response. Pregnancy can potentiate the toxic effects of cocaine, since progesterone can increase the α-adrenergic sensitivity of the receptors or delay cocaine metabolism.[106]

At serum levels found in humans, cocaine *per se* has no effect on human and animal umbilical arteries; however, cocaine enhances the umbilical artery vasoconstrictor action of catecholamines and serotonin, presumably by increasing the sensitivity of the α-adrenergic receptors of arterial smooth muscle.[107]

Overall, the cardiovascular effect of cocaine on the maternofetal circulation is maternal hypertension, increase in uterine vascular resistance, decrease in uterine blood flow, decrease in oxygen transport to the fetus, and fetal hypoxemia.

OBSTETRIC EFFECTS

A characteristic profile has been observed in the pregnant woman who abuses cocaine: a multigravid, multiparous, service patient with little to no prenatal care.[100] The life-style of prostitution, with little attention to personal health care, contributes to these attributes. In addition, the pregnant addict generally is of poor health due to poor nutrition and vitamin deficiency, and is at high risk for infection, particularly hepatitis, veneral disease, and AIDS.

Maternal use of cocaine has been associated with a number of obstetric complications (Table 57-5). Spontaneous abortion occurs in 25% to 38% of pregnancies of cocaine-using women.[108–110] The data, however, are inconsistent as to whether the incidence of spontaneous abortion is significantly increased in cocaine users *versus* nonusers.[108]

The rate of stillbirth is five to ten times higher among pregnant women who continue to use cocaine late in the third trimester. This has been ascribed to placental abruptio, fetal hypoxemia, or hemorrhage.[108]

Cocaine use during pregnancy has been associated with up to a tenfold increase in the incidence of abruptio placenta.[108–111] This has been attributed to an increased incidence of hypertension in these women. Other studies, however, do not show an association between cocaine use and placental abruption.[100,112,113] One of these was a study based on a large obstetric

TABLE 57–5
PERINATAL COMPLICATIONS ASSOCIATED WITH COCAINE USE DURING PREGNANCY

Obstetric Effects
Spontaneous abortion
Stillbirth
Uterine ischemia
Abruptio placentae
Premature labor
Precipitous delivery
Meconium-stained amniotic fluid
Neonatal Effects
Fetal distress
Low Apgar score
Prematurity
Low birth weight
Small length and head circumference
Small for gestational age
Congenital malformation
Cerebral infarction
Neurobehavioral effects

population and the use of a more sensitive test to detect widespread cocaine exposure in the infants.[100]

The increased occurrence of premature labor and premature rupture of the membranes has been observed among women who use cocaine.[108,114–116] There is a belief among them that cocaine will shorten the duration of their labor. Although one study has refuted this belief,[117] another has shown a significant decrease in the duration of labor in women who used cocaine compared to nonusers or those who used only opiates during their pregnancy.[100]

There has not been an observed increase in the incidence of amnionitis, abnormal presentation, eclampsia, preeclampsia, or placenta praevia in pregnant women who abuse cocaine.[108]

PLACENTAL TRANSFER

Because of its low molecular weight and high lipid solubility, cocaine can cross the placenta by simple diffusion[110]; however, the fetal concentration of cocaine is only one fourth to one ninth that of the mother. Nonetheless, the elimination of cocaine and its metabolites is much slower in the fetus than in the mother; thus, the risk of cocaine toxicity in the fetus is increased.

EFFECTS ON THE NEONATE

The cocaine-exposed infant is at risk for a number of complications (see Table 57-5).

Cocaine decreases placental perfusion, which leads to poor gas exchange and fetal oxygenation.[104–106] Fetal hypoxemia in turn leads to fetal distress, meconium staining of the amniotic fluid, and low Apgar scores. Meconium staining has been observed in 23% of the births in cocaine-abusing women—approximately twice the incidence among nondrug users.[100,108]

Premature birth has occurred in approximately 25%,[108,114,115,118–122] and intrauterine growth retardation in about 21% of the pregnancies of cocaine users.[110,113,116,119,123] These rates are three to four times higher than in nonusers. Studies also report lower birth weights and smaller body length and head circumference in the infants.[110,111,115,118,119,121,122,124–126] Neonatal complications such as hyaline membrane disease, intraventricular hemorrhage, bronchopulmonary dysplasia, and the like are consequences of prematurity.

Cocaine use during pregnancy has been associated with an increased incidence of the congenital malformations listed in Table 57-6.[108,116,127,128] No specific pattern of organ involvement has been observed;

TABLE 57–6
CONGENITAL MALFORMATIONS REPORTED WITH COCAINE EXPOSURE DURING PREGNANCY

Facial Malformations
Hypertelorism, epicanthal folds, micrognathia
Central Nervous System
Cerebral infarcts and intracranial hemorrhages
Exencephaly, encephalocele
Small head circumference
Enlarged ventricles, thin cortical mantle, absent brain stem
Sensory Malformations
Eye anomalies
Skeletal Malformations
Parietal bone defects, delayed ossification of calvarium
Sacral exostosis
Limb and digit anomalies (*e.g.*, syndactyly, polydactyly, absent digits)
Cardiac Malformations
Atrial and ventricular septal defects, cardiomegaly
Heart murmur
Transposition of great arteries, hypoplastic right heart syndrome
Urogenital Malformations
Cryptorchidism
Horseshoe kidney
Prune-belly syndrome, pseudohermaphroditism, hydronephrosis, renal infarction
Hypospadias
Intestinal Malformations
Ileal atresia, possible bowel infarction
Necrotizing enterocolitis
Other Malformations
Capillary hemangiomata, subgaleal hemotoma
Diaphragmatic hernia
Inguinal hernia
Esophageal atresia

From Church MW, Kaufmann RA, Keenan JA, et al. Effect of prenatal cocaine exposure. In: Watson R, ed. Bichemistry and physiology of substance abuse. vol. 3. Boca Raton, FL: CRC Press 1990:179.

however, polydrug abuse, including alcohol abuse, is not uncommon among cocaine users.[100] Thus, the potential of cocaine alone as a teratogen is difficult to establish in these clinical settings. Nonetheless, studies in the offspring of rats that have received cocaine during pregnancy have shown teratogenic effects such as neural tube defects, skeletal deficits (*e.g.*, camptodactyly, bradydactyly) and hydrocephalus.[108]

In utero cocaine exposure of the human fetus also has been associated with a number of multiorgan effects,[129] listed in Table 57-7. An increased incidence of congenital syphilis and human immunodeficiency virus (HIV) infection in infants also has been observed.[130,131]

Although prenatal exposure to cocaine is associated with problems or complications in the infant, most appear clinically normal at birth.[100] When perinatal problems do occur, they frequently are observed in the group in which the mother admits to the abuse of drugs during pregnancy. Since these women have been shown to be more consistent, heavy users of drugs,[100] it appears that the complications that occur in the infants are related to their heavy exposure to drugs *in utero*. Because most drug-exposed infants appear clinically normal at birth, they will escape detection unless sensitive drug screens are used routinely (see Diagnoses of Drug Exposure) or done selectively on infants who are considered to be at high risk.[100]

TABLE 57–7
REPORTED COMPLICATIONS INVOLVING SPECIFIC ORGAN SYSTEMS IN INFANTS EXPOSED TO COCAINE DURING PREGNANCY

Central Nervous System
Cerebral infarction
Seizures
Cortical atrophy
Porencephaly
Abnormal head ultrasound (*e.g.*, white matter cavities or densities, acute infarct, periventricular–intraventricular hemorrhage, ventricular enlargement)
Periventricular and germinal matrix cysts
Abnormal EEG (*i.e.*, sharp waves and spikes)
Sensory Organs
Abnormal brain stem auditory evoked potential (*i.e.*, prolongation of interpeak latencies and reduction in amplitudes)
Increased auditory startle response
Tortuosity and dilation of iris vessels
Unilateral retinopathy and persistent hyperplastic primary vitreous
Cardiovascular System
Transient tachycardia
Hypertension and diminished stroke volume and cardiac output
Lower minimal heart rate and higher mean maximal heart rate
Respiratory System
Apnea
Periodic breathing
Abnormal fetal breathing
SIDS
Gastrointestinal System
Necrotizing enterocolitis
Genitourinary System
Persistent hyperchloremic, metabolic acidosis

EEG, electroencephalogram; SIDS, sudden infant death syndrome.

NEUROBEHAVIORAL EFFECTS

Neurobehavioral abnormalities have been observed in newborn infants who have been prenatally exposed to cocaine. The infants exhibit tremulousness, irritability, hypertonicity, high-pitched cry, abnormal sleep pattern, and sometimes seizures.[109,110,114,118–120,124] These manifestations are not unlike those seen in opiate withdrawal (see Opiates). It is difficult to separate the overlapping effects of cocaine and opiates, because it is common for the drug-abusing woman to use multiple drugs. However, the CNS manifestations in the cocaine-exposed infants are, in general, significantly milder than those observed for narcotic withdrawal.[116,124] Abnormalities in cardiorespiratory patterns (*e.g.*, increased episodes of apnea, periodic breathing),[132] EEG abnormalities (*e.g.*, bursts of sharp waves and spikes),[113] and abnormal neonatal behavior as assessed by the Brazelton test and other methods (*i.e.*, impairment of orientation and motor and state regulation)[109,132,133] have been described in cocaine-exposed neonates. Again, these same abnormalities also are seen in infants exposed to opiates alone.[134]

Evidence of sensorineural hearing loss has been detected by recording the brain stem auditory evoked potential of rats prenatally exposed to cocaine.[135,136] Similar observations have been found in cocaine-exposed infants that suggest compromised auditory functions.[137] Some studies have demonstrated an increase in the infant's auditory startle response.[126]

LONG-TERM OUTCOME

Long-term neurobehavioral outcome in cocaine-exposed infants has yet to be determined. Disabilities such as attention deficits, difficulties in concentration, abnormal play pattern, difficulties in the performance of unstructured tasks (*i.e.*, tasks that require the child's initiation, goal setting, and follow-through), and flat, apathetic moods have been described.[138–140] As in the opiate-exposed infants, the risk for the sudden infant death syndrome or child abuse in the cocaine-exposed infant is increased.[131] Manifestations of cocaine toxicity, such as extreme irritability, tremors, tachycardia, tachypnea, and hypertension also have been reported in infants and children who were exposed to cocaine either through breast milk[141] or through passive inhalation.[142]

ALCOHOL

The use or abuse of alcohol during pregnancy has serious effects on the fetus and newborn. The adverse effects of alcohol on the offspring have been observed for centuries, although the fetal alcohol syndrome (FAS) was not defined as a medical entity until 1973.[143,144] Children born to alcoholic parents were observed to have a higher than expected incidence of delayed growth and development and of neurologic disorders.[145,146] Since 1973, numerous reports on the mild or severe effects of maternal alcohol use on the fetus and newborn have been reported. Excellent reviews on the subject also have been written.[147–149]

EPIDEMIOLOGY

The prevalence of alcohol use in the population of women at greatest risk for pregnancy is high. The 1985 NIDA Household Survey on Drug Abuse reported that approximately 60.9% of an estimated 56 million women of childbearing age (*i.e.*, 15–44 years of age) had used alcohol in the past month.[150] In 1990, a similar survey reported that approximately 50.8% of an estimated 60 million women of childbearing age had used alcohol in the past month.[151] One study further showed that 64% of all women drank alcohol, 25% drank at least once a week, and 5% had at least 60 drinks a month.[152] It is estimated that 8% to 11% of women of childbearing age are either problem drinkers or alcohol dependent.[153,154]

Most women, however, decrease their drinking during pregnancy. This decrease begins with pregnancy recognition, usually during the first trimester, and continues through the third trimester. In one study, it was noted that 44% of the women reported drinking at least one drink per day before pregnancy. This rate decreased to 37% during the first month, 21% during the second month, and 14% by the end of the third month of the pregnancy. By the third trimester, only 5% of the women reported drinking an average of a drink a day.[155]

METABOLISM AND PLACENTAL TRANSFER

Ethanol is an anxiolytic analgesic with a depressant effect on the CNS.[148] It is absorbed rapidly by diffusion across the mucosa of the stomach (20%) and intestines (80%). The absorption rate is not affected by pregnancy, but blood alcohol levels may be higher in pregnancy.[147] Alcohol usually is cleared from the bloodstream within 1 hour in adults and 2 hours in newborns. Approximately 95% is metabolized by the liver and 5% is eliminated by the kidneys and lungs. Ethanol is metabolized to acetaldehyde, then to acetate. Acetaldehyde is more toxic than ethanol itself.

There is an unimpeded bidirectional placental transfer of ethanol during pregnancy. Fetal ethanol is eliminated by maternal hepatic biotransformation. Ethanol has been detected in amniotic fluid, a reservoir for additional fetal exposure.[148,156]

Ethanol has been implicated in the impairment of normal placental function. It affects or interferes with the transport of amino acids across the placenta to the fetus.[157]

EFFECTS ON PREGNANCY

An increase in the incidence of spontaneous abortion, abruptio placentae, and breech presentation has been observed among women who abuse alcohol during pregnancy.

The incidence of spontaneous abortion among alcoholic pregnant women is high, ranging from 18.8% to 52% of pregnancies.[147] In a large prospective study of 12,127 pregnant women, alcoholic women were found to have a 2.3 times higher incidence of three or more spontaneous abortions than nonalcoholics.[158] The single variable that correlated highly with spontaneous abortion was an extremely heavy episode of drinking during the early first trimester. Other reports, however, do not show an association of alcohol consumption with an increased risk for spontaneous abortions in nonheavy drinkers.[159] Studies in nonhuman primates showed that an increase in spontaneous abortion occurred only when blood alcohol levels reached approximately 200 mg/dL.[160–162]

An increase in the frequency of aneuploidy was found in abortuses of women who consumed two or more drinks per week.[163] Although in mice preovulatory alcohol exposure did not increase the incidence of abortion[164] or aneuploidy,[165] alcohol administration shortly after ovulation resulted in a 7.5% incidence of aneuploidy. Injection shortly after mating also resulted in a 15% incidence of aneuploidy.[166] Alcohol administration to mating female mice 2 hours after ovulation resulted in a significant increase in fetal death associated with aneuploidy. These studies raise the possibility that the high rate of spontaneous abortions among alcoholic women may be due to a single episode of heavy drinking around the time of conception.[167]

An increased risk of stillbirths has not been shown with alcohol use during pregnancy, even among women classified as problem or heavy drinkers.[158,159,168,169] The risk of abruptio placentae is increased, however.[170,171]

Fetal alcohol syndrome is strongly associated with breech presentation. Seventy percent of infants with FAS were breech births.[147] In other studies, 9 of 23 (39%) infants born to heavy drinkers were delivered as breech[172]; however, only 3 of 59 infants of moderate drinkers had breech presentation.[173] Thus, it appears that heavy consumption of alcohol increases the incidence of breech births.

EFFECTS ON THE FETUS

Animal studies have shown that *in utero* alcohol exposure may cause fetal malnutrition and chronic fetal hypoxia by inducing hypoglycemia at high blood alcohol levels.[148] Alcohol decreases adrenergic receptors on the hepatic plasma membrane, resulting in reduced epinephrine-induced stimulation of glycogen phosphorylase activity and interference with carbohydrate metabolism and prenatal and postnatal growth. Low concentrations of somatomedin C and high growth hormone levels have been noted in infants of alcoholic mothers.[174] There also is a reduction in the neurotransmitters in the human brain, as well as a decrease in the myelination process.[175–179]

EFFECTS ON THE NEWBORN INFANT

PREMATURITY

The incidence of prematurity ranges from 46% to 52% in infants with FAS.[179,180] The relationship between alcohol exposure and preterm birth in which FAS is not a factor is not as clear. Several reports indicate increased preterm delivery in alcohol abusers.[181,182] This may be due to an associated increase in congenital anomalies, rather than directly to alcohol itself. Nonetheless, heavy alcohol consumption during pregnancy (*i.e.*, six or more drinks per day) has been associated with an approximately threefold increased risk of preterm delivery.[183,184]

GROWTH AND MORPHOLOGY

Maternal alcohol consumption has been associated with an increased risk for infants with low birth weight and with length and head circumference below the tenth percentile, if the mother's drinking took place during the early first trimester of pregnancy.[149] Similarly, birth weight, length, and head circumference have been reported to be significantly reduced in the offspring of women who drank continuously throughout pregnancy.[185] The low birth weight was influenced both by dose and duration of alcohol exposure. Moderate or light drinking also has been associated with a decrease in the birth weight of the infants.[147] The birth weights, however, are within the range of normal, have no biologic significance, and often cease to achieve statistical significance when other risk factors, such as smoking, are taken into account. On the other hand, there are reports that show no association between alcohol use and the infant's birth weight. In a group of healthy, full-term infants, no growth difference was noted between those exposed and those not exposed to alcohol.[186,187]

Some minor morphologic malformations in the infant have been observed with alcohol use during pregnancy.[154,187–189] In contrast, other reports have failed to demonstrate this.[186,190–192] In a large prospective birth defects study involving 32,870 women, light and moderate drinkers were not found to have an increased rate of malformations in their offspring compared to nondrinkers.[193]

NEWBORN WITHDRAWAL

Withdrawal from alcohol occurs in infants but rarely is noted, since the withdrawal may be confused with narcotic or other drug withdrawal. The withdrawal from ethanol has been described to occur within 12 hours of birth and may manifest as abdominal distention, opisthotonus, convulsions, tremors, hypertonia, apnea, and cyanosis. The infants are irritable, have restless sleep, and engage in exaggerated mouthing behavior.[194,195]

NEUROBEHAVIORAL EFFECTS

Alcohol-exposed infants have been found to habituate less well to aversive stimuli as measured by the Neonatal Behavioral Assessment Scale,[196] exhibit changes in their reflexive behavior, state control, and motor behavior,[186] and have increased irritability[197] and depressed range of state.[198] These effects, however, have not been universally observed.[187,189]

Sleep cycling and arousal have been studied as a measure of neurophysiologic development, integrity, and maturation. Infants of mothers who drank heavily throughout pregnancy showed a greater amount of restless sleep and more bodily movements.[199,200] Electroencephalographic power spectra analyses of the infants showed hypersynchrony of the EEG as well as an increase in the integrated power in all sleep states, particularly with active sleep.[201,202] Electroencephalographic maturation also was affected by maternal binge drinking.[203]

BREAST-FEEDING AND ALCOHOL

Alcohol is distributed into breast milk; however, the amount ingested by the infant is only a small fraction of that consumed by the mother.[147] Short-term alcohol consumption by lactating women has an immediate effect on the odor of their milk and the feeding behavior of their infant.[204] The infants sucked more frequently during the first minute after their mothers had consumed alcohol, but they consumed significantly less milk.

In animal studies, ethanol has been shown to block the secretion of oxytocin, thereby preventing milk ejection.[205] A similar effect was found in normal women.[206] A slight but significant negative effect on motor development as measured by the psychomotor developmental index (PDI) but not on the mental developmental index was observed, using the Bayley scales, in infants who ingested ethanol through breast milk.[207]

LONG-TERM EFFECTS OF PRENATAL ALCOHOL USE

GROWTH

Growth deficits were found in infants at 8 and 18 months of age and were related to alcohol use during the second and third trimesters of pregnancy.[208] These children continued to be smaller in weight, length, and head circumference at 3 years of age, even after controlling for nutrition, current environment, exposure to alcohol during lactation, and other significant covariates. They did not exhibit catch-up growth. Others have found growth retardation at 8 months of age, but not at subsequent evaluations,[209] and significant effects on height and head circumference in children at 6 years of age that were related to alcohol use before pregnancy.[189] On the other hand, other reports found no growth effects at 1 and 2 years of age.[210,211]

BEHAVIORAL AND COGNITIVE EFFECTS

Infants of mothers who drank throughout pregnancy showed less improvement in reflexes and autonomic regulation over the first month of life than infants of women who stopped drinking or who never drank.[212] At 6 to 8 months of age, these infants had significantly lower Bayley mental and motor scores.[213,214] At 13 months of age, infants of women who drank during pregnancy did less well on the mental index and on the verbal comprehension and spoken language cluster scores derived from the Bayley Scales.[210,215] In contrast, Richardson and Day noted that prenatal alcohol use did not significantly predict Bayley mental or motor scores at either 8 or 18 months of age.[216]

Alcohol use during pregnancy was associated negatively with IQ at 4 years of age.[217] At 4 years of age, children who were exposed prenatally to moderate drinking were less attentive and more active during naturalistic observations at home,[218] and were less attentive and had longer reaction times on a vigilance task in a laboratory setting.[219] Prepregnancy alcohol exposure also was related to increased fine motor errors, increased time to correct the errors, and poorer gross motor balance.[220]

Attention, distraction, and reaction time on a continuous performance task at 7 years of age continued to be negatively related to alcohol exposure during pregnancy.[221] Intelligence quotient effects persisted at 7.5 years, with a decrement of 7 IQ points with exposure to more than 1 ounce of alcohol per day during pregnancy.[222] Achievement scores were related to binge drinking before pregnancy.

On the other hand, Fried and Watkinson found that infants exposed to alcohol prenatally evidenced no deficits at 12 months of age.[223] At 24 months of age, they performed more poorly than non–alcohol-exposed controls on the Bayley Mental Scale and the Reynell Language Scale. At 36 months of age, the language development of the exposed children continued to be affected, but at 48 months of age no significant relationships were found.[224]

These inconsistencies regarding the long-term effects of prenatal alcohol exposure on the child's development may lie in the difficulty in separating the teratogenic effects of alcohol from the effects of the disordered environments, both interpersonal and structural, that often accompany alcohol and drug use.[151]

FETAL ALCOHOL SYNDROME

The Fetal Alcohol Study Group of the Research Society on Alcoholism defined three specific criteria for the diagnosis of FAS.[147] An infant must exhibit an abnormality from each category to qualify for a diagnosis of FAS:

- Prenatal or postnatal growth retardation (*i.e.*, weight, length, or head circumference < the 10th percentile when corrected for gestational age)
- CNS involvement, which includes signs of neurologic abnormalities (*e.g.*, irritability in infancy, hyperactivity during childhood), developmental delay, hypotonia or intellectual impairment (*e.g.*, mental retardation)
- Characteristic facial dysmorphology (at least two of the three must be present)
  - Microcephaly (*i.e.*, head circumference < 3rd percentile)
  - Microphthalmia or short palpebral fissures
  - Poorly developed philtrum, thin upper lip (*i.e.*, vermillion border), and flattening of the maxilla.

The presence of some, but not all, of these features is defined as alcohol-related birth defects (ARBD), or fetal alcohol effects.

INCIDENCE

The incidence of FAS in the world is approximately 1.9 per 1000 live births. The reported rate in the United States is 2.2 per 1000 live births.[147] Prevalence estimates vary, depending on geographic location and specific population studied. The highest reported incidence of FAS occurs in the Native American and black population and those with low socioeconomic status. Sokol and colleagues, in a prospective study of 8331 pregnancies, identified 25 cases of FAS.[225] Four significant prenatal risk factors were identified: black race, high parity, percentage drinking days, and positive Michigan Alcoholism Screening Test. In the absence of any of these factors, the probability of a child being afflicted with FAS was 2%; in the presence of all four, the probability was 85.2%.

Among alcohol-abusing women, the incidence of FAS in the world literature is 71 per 1000 live births, and in the United States, from 24 to 42 per 1000 live births.[147] One factor that has been associated with an increase in the risk of FAS is the history of previous siblings with FAS in the family. It has been estimated that the risk of a younger sibling having FAS, given an older sibling diagnosed as having FAS, is increased by 406 times, so that the incidence of FAS occurring in this group is 771 per 1000 live births.[147] Older siblings are not as likely to be severely affected as younger siblings.[147]

Alcohol-Related Birth Defects. Alcohol-related birth defects may account for as many as 5% of all congenital anomalies.[148] Alcohol-related birth defects result from variable dose exposures at variable gestational times, and are offset by the genetic background. These determinants place the fetus at a higher risk for possible adverse outcome. The frequency of ARBD is 3 to 5 per 1000 live births. Table 57-8 shows the various dysmorphic features that may be observed in the infant after prenatal alcohol exposure.

Follow-Up of Infants With Fetal Alcohol Syndrome. Postnatal growth retardation and retarded motor performance are hallmarks of prenatal alcohol exposure, especially of FAS. A 10-year follow-up of the first 11 patients diagnosed to have FAS showed that the children continued to be growth retarded with respect to weight, height, and head circumference. Weight-for-height was especially decreased.[226] Similar observations were noted in a retrospective study of 21 children born to alcoholic women, 10 of whom had features of FAS.[227]

Children with FAS have a multitude of problems that include mental retardation ranging from severe to near normal.[228,229] They may have behavioral prob-

TABLE 57–8
ALCOHOL AND FETAL DYSMORPHOGENESIS

Central Nervous System	
Neurobehavioral	Intellectual impairment (*i.e.,* mild to moderate mental retardation),* low IQ (65–70), hypotonia,† developmental delay, poor coordination, cognitive and sensory deficits, attention deficits, hyperactivity and irritability in infancy, hyperactivity in childhood,† language disabilities and sleep–wake cycle disturbances, electroencephalogram hypersynchrony, delayed or deficient myelination, corpus callosum hypoplasia, echolalia, cerebral palsy
Craniofacial	
Head	Microcephaly,* Dandy–Walker malformation, anencephaly, porencephaly, meningomyelocele, spasmus nutans
Eyes	Ocular retinal tortuosity, ptosis, strabismus, epicanthal folds, myopia, retinal coloboma, astigmatism, steep corneal curvature, anterior chamber anomalies, sensorineural hearing loss
Ears	Poorly formed conchae and posterior rotation of the ear and eustachian tube
Nose	Short, upturned† hypoplastic philtrum*
Mouth	Dental malalignments, small teeth with faulty enamel, retrognathia in infancy* or relative prognathia in adolescence, cleft lip or cleft palate, malocclusions, prominent palatine ridges, thinned upper vermillion,* poor suck reflex
Maxilla	Hypoplastic†
Cardiovascular	
Heart	All cardiac defects (57%), particularly ventricular septal defect, atrial septal defects, murmurs, tetralogy of Fallot, double-outlet right ventricle, dextrocardia, patent ductus arteriosus, and great vessel anomalies
Pulmonary	
Chest	Pectus excavatum, bifid xiphoid
Lungs	Pulmonary atresia, atelectasis, upper respiratory infections
Gastrointestinal	
Abdomen	Inguinal and abdominal hernias, diastasis recti, gastroschisis, hepatic fibrosis, childhood cirrhosis, extrahepatic biliary atresia, hyperbilirubinemia in childhood
Urogenital	
Renal	Hydronephrosis; small rotated kidneys; aplastic, dysplastic, or hypoplastic kidneys; horseshoe kidneys; ureteral duplications; megaloureter, cystic diverticula; vesicovaginal fistula; pyelonephritis
Dermatologic	
Dermatogliphic	Aberrant fingerprint and palmar creases, hemangiomas in one-half of the cases, disproportionately diminished adipose tissue,† abnormal whorls on scalp, hirsutism in infancy, nail hypoplasia, poor proprioception
Orthopaedic	
Skeletal	Polydactyly, radioulnar synostosis, talipes equinovarus, dislocated hip, scoliosis, Klippel–Feil syndrome, limited joint movement, lumbosacral lipoma, shortened fifth digit, syndactyly, camptodactyly, clinodactyly, flexion contractures
Endocrinology	
Congenital	DiGeorge syndrome

* Feature seen in 80% of patients.
† Feature seen in more than 50% of patients.
From Pietrantoni M, Knuppel RA. Alcohol in pregnancy. Clin Perinatol 1991;18:93.

lems, including stereotyped behaviors, irritability, hyperactivity, tremulousness, and hyperdistractibility.[180,229–231] Speech may be delayed or impaired, which may be due partly to hearing impairments.[231–235]

MARIJUANA

Marijuana is the most widely used illicit drug among women of childbearing age in the United States.[151] An extensive historical review of marijuana use is available.[236] Some common terminology pertaining to marijuana follows. Cannabis refers to the crude material from the plant, *Cannabis sativa;* marijuana refers to a mixture of crushed leaves, twigs, seeds, and sometimes flowers of the plant; sinsemilla is a variety of high-potency marijuana originally grown in northern California; and hashish is a resin obtained by pressing, scraping, and shaking the plant in hash oil, to produce a potent extract.[237]

The prevalence of marijuana use in the population of women at greatest risk for pregnancy is high; in 1985, 44% of women aged 15 to 44 years reported that they had used marijuana in their lifetime, although only a small percentage (11.2%) were current users.[150] Of the 56 million women in this age group, 6 million therefore were current marijuana users. In 1990, a similar survey revealed that 44.8% of women in the childbearing age group had used marijuana in their lifetime and 6.5% were current users. Of the estimated 60 million women in this age group, 3.9 million were current marijuana users.[151]

The rate of marijuana use during pregnancy varies widely in different studies. In one study,[238] 42% of women interviewed in their fourth month of pregnancy in an urban setting had used marijuana in the year prior to conception, and 31% reported use during the first trimester. As cited from a number of studies, the prevalence of marijuana use during pregnancy ranged between 10% to 42%.[100,238–243]

Cannabis contains more than 400 chemicals; 61 are unique to cannabis and are referred to collectively as cannabinoids. The primary psychoactive component is δ-9-tetrahydrocannabinol (THC). Other cannabinoids, however, such as cannabidiol and cannabinol, also have biologic activity and potentially can affect the fetus.[244,245]

PLACENTAL TRANSFER

Tetrahydrocannabinol is highly bound to the lipoprotein fraction in the blood. Studies using radiolabeled THC have shown that tissues with high blood flow show a rapid uptake of the drug.[147] Tetrahydrocannabinol crosses the placenta within minutes of administration; however, the placenta may retard THC passage to the fetus. In rats, the placenta contained ten times more radiolabeled THC than fetal serum,[246] and fetal rat THC serum levels were well below the maternal serum levels.[247] In humans, however, the concentrations of THC in maternal and fetal sera essentially are identical.[248]

EFFECTS ON PREGNANCY

Based on the report of a large perinatal center study, no significant differences were observed between marijuana users and control subjects who were matched in terms of alcohol consumption, cigarette use, and family income with regard to several birth outcome measures, such as miscarriage rate, presentation at birth, Apgar status, and the frequency of complications at birth.[249,250]

EFFECTS ON THE FETUS AND NEWBORN INFANT

A significant reduction, 0.8 weeks, was observed in the gestational age of infants of heavy marijuana users (six or more times/week) compared to infants of nonusers.[250] In other studies, 25% of heavy users had premature infants.[251] On the other hand, some studies have not found such an effect of marijuana on gestation.[238,240,252]

Most studies have not reported an increase in the incidence of major or minor malformations in the offspring with prenatal marijuana exposure.[242,252,253] In the few reported cases of malformations, the confounding variables of poor nutrition, little prenatal care, low socioeconomic status, and other factors that may have interacted to produce these abnormalities were not controlled for.[254]

There seems to be an increase in the gender ratio of live male–female offspring in marijuana users. In animals, litters from dams fed 50 mg/kg of THC showed a significant dose-related increase in the proportion of male offspring, ranging from 57% to 61%.[255,256] In a study of women who smoked marijuana during pregnancy, heavy use similarly was associated with a significant increase in male over female births.[240]

Although there are reports to the contrary,[192,242] most studies show no significant relationship between prenatal marijuana use and the infant's birth weight, if appropriate covariates such as socioeconomic status, alcohol, tobacco and other drug use, race, and maternal age are controlled for.[211,238,252] In animal studies, reduced birth weights among the drug-exposed offspring were observed,[247] but appeared to have resulted largely from the reduced maternal food and water intake rather than the effect of the drug.[257]

There is an equivocal relationship between prenatal marijuana use and neurobehavioral outcome of the offspring.[258] Prenatal marijuana exposure has been associated with increased fine tremors in the infant, accompanied by exaggerated and prolonged startles, both spontaneous and in response to mild stimuli;

poorer visual but not auditory stimuli habituation[258]; and decreased ability to regulate state and disrupted sleep patterns.[259] Some reports, however, have found no altered neurobehavioral patterns in marijuana-exposed offspring.[199,240,260]

LONG-TERM OUTCOME

After controlling for confounding variables, prenatal marijuana use was found to be associated with increased infant weight at 12 months and increased height at 24 months of age.[223] One report, however, found no effect on infant growth at 12 months of age.[240] In general, there has been no observed effect of marijuana use on infant motor and mental development at 12 months of age, as determined by the Bayley Scales of Infant Development.[223,240] Women who used marijuana prenatally were less involved with their children at 24 months of age, however, and provided less stimulating home environments. From a preschool sample, no effect of prenatal marijuana use on IQ scores as measured by the Wechsler Preschool and Primary Scale of Intelligence was found at 4 years of age. At 48 months of age, however, memory and verbal outcome were associated negatively with heavy prenatal marijuana use.[223,224,258]

NICOTINE AND SMOKING

Cigarette smoke contains about 4000 chemical compounds. Most of these chemical agents are in the gas phase of cigarette smoke and include carbon monoxide, carbon dioxide, nitrogen oxides, ammonia, hydrogen cyanide, and other compounds. A smaller number of these undesirable compounds are in the particulate phase of cigarette smoke (*i.e.*, nicotine and tar). Tar is what remains after the moisture and nicotine are subtracted. It consists primarily of polycyclic aromatic hydrocarbons (*e.g.*, nitrosamines, aromatic amines, polycyclic hydrocarbons) and numerous other compounds, including metallic ions and radioactive compounds.[261]

ABSORPTION AND METABOLISM

Nicotine is the most studied substance in cigarette smoke, and is considered the compound primarily responsible for the pharmacologic effects of smoking. It is absorbed readily from the lungs, almost with the same efficiency as intravenous administration. Blood nicotine levels vary depending on the amount of nicotine delivered. The amount of nicotine delivered depends on the duration and intensity of inhalation, the number of inhalations per cigarette, the presence or absence of filters, the brand of the cigarette (which affects the composition of the tobacco) how densely the tobacco is packed, and the length of the column of tobacco.[261]

Nicotine is distributed rapidly throughout the body. It reaches the brain within 8 seconds after inhalation. Peak concentrations of nicotine in plasma after a cigarette is smoked are typically 25 to 50 ng/mL. The course of elimination of nicotine is multiexponential. After a single cigarette, concentrations decline rapidly (*i.e.*, over 5–10 minutes), primarily reflecting distribution. After long-term smoking, the elimination half-life of nicotine is approximately 2 hours.[261]

Nicotine is metabolized mainly in the liver but also in the kidneys and lungs. The two main metabolites are cotinine and nicotine-1′-N-oxide. Cotinine has few or no cardiovascular or subjective effects. It is cleared more slowly than nicotine, with a half-life of about 19 hours. Thus, it is a better measure of overall intake than nicotine itself. Nicotine crosses the placenta and also is excreted in the milk of lactating women.[261]

INCIDENCE

Tobacco is widely used by the population of women at greatest risk for pregnancy. The 1985 NIDA Household Survey on Drug Abuse reported that approximately 33.4% of an estimated 56 million women of childbearing age (*i.e.*, 15–44 years of age) had smoked tobacco in the past month.[150] In 1990, a similar survey reported that approximately 29.4% of an estimated 60 million women of childbearing age had smoked tobacco in the past month. Another national survey published in 1990 reported that 32% of Caucasian women aged 20 to 44 years smoked cigarettes regularly at a rate of at least one cigarette per day during the 12 months before they found out they were pregnant.[151] The percentage of smokers in the age range between 20 and 29 years was 37.5%.

The incidence of smoking during pregnancy is still quite high, despite all the warnings and the known health hazards. One study reported that 60.7% of pregnant women continued to smoke during their pregnancy.[262] Of the women who quit smoking while pregnant, 27% relapsed within a month of the delivery, and 52% relapsed within 4 months.

SPONTANEOUS ABORTION

The relationship between cigarette smoking and spontaneous abortion has been documented in both animal and human studies. When other risk factors are controlled, women who smoke cigarettes during pregnancy are 1.2 to 2 times more likely to have a spontaneous abortion than those who do not smoke.[263] The higher rate of abortion was noted in women who smoke one-half of a pack per day compared to nonsmokers. The mechanism for this association has not been identified, although studies support the theory that it may be due to abnormalities in placental development, as well as dysfunction of hormones that sustain pregnancy.[264,265]

PLACENTAL EFFECTS

An increased incidence of placental abruption, and an increase in fetal death due to abruption, were seen among women who smoke more than ten cigarettes per day.[266] Maternal smoking was associated with the finding of decidual necrosis on pathologic examination. Extensive placental calcification occurred significantly more often in smokers than in nonsmokers (46% *versus* 14%).[264] Intervillous blood flow was reported to be reduced acutely during smoking, and for 15 minutes afterward.[265]

APGAR SCORES

Several studies have noted that maternal cigarette smoking during pregnancy is associated with low Apgar scores; however, other risk factors were not controlled for in the analysis.[267] When potentially confounding factors were controlled for, no significant independent association was noted between cigarette smoking and Apgar scores.[268]

PRETERM BIRTH

Maternal smoking has been reported to be a risk factor for preterm labor. The incidence of preterm labor increases with the number of cigarettes smoked per day.[269,270]

SUDDEN INFANT DEATH SYNDROME

Several studies have reported that maternal cigarette smoking significantly increases the likelihood of sudden infant death syndrome.[271] Mothers of victims of sudden infant death syndrome were more likely to smoke cigarettes either during pregnancy or after their baby was born.

FETAL DEATH AND NEONATAL MORTALITY

Two epidemiologic studies noted a significant effect of smoking on late fetal death and neonatal mortality. In one, a greater risk was noted in smokers compared to nonsmokers.[272] Among first-born infants, there was a 25% greater risk for fetal death and neonatal mortality for less than one-pack-per-day smokers and a 56% greater risk for more than one-pack-per-day smokers, compared to the nonsmokers. For second or higher births, a 30% greater risk of late fetal death and neonatal mortality was noted in maternal smokers compared to nonsmokers. Another study noted that maternal smoking had a relative risk for late fetal death of 1.4 and a relative risk for early neonatal mortality of 1.2.[273]

GROWTH AND DEVELOPMENT

Several studies have examined the association between smoking during pregnancy and birth weight. These studies consistently have demonstrated a decrease in birth weight of approximately 200 g, as well as an increased percentage of low-birth-weight (LBW) infants.[270,274] In addition, a dose–response relationship has been demonstrated between the number of cigarettes smoked and both the decrease in birth weight[275] and the percentage of LBW infants.[276] These findings remain consistent when different confounding variables are controlled for. For Caucasian mothers, the incidence of LBW babies ranges from 4.8% for women who do not smoke, to 8% for women who smoke 1 to 10 cigarettes per day, and to 13.4% for women who smoke more than 20 cigarettes per day. For black women, the incidence of LBW babies ranges from 8.3% for women who do not smoke, to 13.5% for women who smoke 1 to 10 cigarettes per day, to 22.7% for women who smoke more than 20 cigarettes per day.[276] One study demonstrated that serum nicotine levels were more strongly correlated with reduced birth weight than with smoking history.[277] This indicates the importance of using biochemical markers in studies of pregnancy outcome.

Studies comparing infant birth weights show that mothers who quit smoking during pregnancy have infants with higher birth weights than do mothers who continue to smoke during pregnancy. The difference in birth weight was highly significant when smoking was stopped by as late as 16 weeks of gestation, compared to persistent smokers. Even stopping after 16 weeks of gestation was found to be associated with infants of significantly higher birth weights than the offspring of persistent smokers.[275]

The nature of the growth deficit, in terms of newborn body composition, was assessed by looking at the anthropometric indices of subcutaneous fat deposition and lean body mass in infants of smokers and nonsmokers. There was no difference between the two groups of infants in any of the skinfold measurements or in the calculated cross-sectional fat area of the upper arm. These results suggest that the reduction in birth weight of infants whose mothers smoke is due primarily to a decrease in the lean body mass of the newborn, whereas deposition of subcutaneous fat is relatively unaffected.[278] Birth weight, length, and head circumference were smaller for infants of smoking mothers.

Various studies assessing the association between cigarette smoking during pregnancy and congenital malformations have shown conflicting results. The British Perinatal Mortality Survey, in a study of 17,418 subjects, demonstrated that maternal smoking was associated with congenital heart defects, even when age, parity, and social class were controlled for.[279] The United States Collaborative Perinatal Project, in a study of 50,282 subjects, did not demonstrate this association.[280] The inconsistency of reports suggests that cigarette smoking *per se* may not be a cause of congenital malformations in infants.

NEUROBEHAVIORAL EFFECTS

Several studies have investigated the impact of cigarette smoking during pregnancy on newborn behavior and on later child development.[281–283] Offspring of mothers who smoked during pregnancy have been observed to perform less well on the Brazelton Neonatal Behavioral Assessment Score in items such as habituating to sound or orienting to a voice, compared to offspring of nonsmoking mothers. Other studies indicate poorer performance with head turning and sucking, lower visual alertness, more crying, tremors and startles, and increased lability of color. Most of the studies, however, do not demonstrate a clinically significant effect on neonatal behavior that can be attributed independently to maternal cigarette smoking alone.

Long-term follow-up evaluation of children's cognitive and developmental functions seems to indicate that when sociodemographic factors are controlled for, children exposed to cigarette smoke *in utero* do less well in tests of cognitive, psychomotor, language, and general academic achievement, including reading and mathematics. Although differences are statistically significant between the two groups, they are small compared to other factors that affect the children's performance.[284–287]

PHENCYCLIDINE

Phencyclidine was first introduced as a dissociative anesthetic in 1957. Despite its wide margin of safety in humans, its clinical use was discontinued after reports of adverse effects that include agitation, confusion, delirium, and persistent hallucinations. Other untoward effects noted with its use were feelings of paranoia, impending death, outbursts of bizarre, agitated, or violent behavior, and a psychosis mimicking schizophrenia. It remains popular as a drug of abuse due to its sedative and hallucinogenic effects, its synthesis from readily available precursors, low cost, and variety of routes of administration. Most users smoke PCP; others sniff or snort the powder, drink the liquid form mixed with lemonade or alcohol, or inject it intravenously.[288–291]

PLACENTAL TRANSFER AND METABOLISM

Placental transfer of PCP has been studied in the pig, mouse, rabbit, and humans. In piglets, serum levels of PCP were ten times higher than in the sow[292,293]; in fetal rabbits, similar high serum levels were found that reached a peak 2 hours after parenteral administration of the drug to the doe.[294] In the mouse, there was almost a tenfold higher concentration of PCP in fetal tissue than in maternal blood,[294] and PCP appeared in the pup's brain as early as 15 minutes after subcutaneous injection to the dam.[289] Phencyclidine also has been detected in amniotic fluid and umbilical cord blood at high concentrations.[295]

Phencyclidine appears rapidly in breast milk, appearing within 15 minutes of maternal administration. By 3 hours, the ratio of levels in milk to those in plasma is approximately ten to one.[294]

Phencyclidine is lipophilic. It is stored in body fat and in the CNS for a prolonged period and is released slowly into the bloodstream. The major routes of elimination involve metabolism of PCP in the liver and excretion in the urine and feces.[296] The half-life of the drug in the body usually is about 3 days, although it has been found in the urine as long as 8 days after last use.[297] The half-life of PCP in the fetus is approximately twice that in the mother.[294]

MODE OF ACTION

Phencyclidine has strong, centrally mediated effects in animals and humans, and influences many different neuronal systems. It inhibits the uptake and increases the release of monoamines in the brain, interacts with cholinergic and serotonergic systems, and antagonizes the neuronal stimulation caused by the excitatory amino acid, N-methyl aspartate.[288] Phencyclidine may produce a general enhancement of neurotransmitter release by blocking voltage-sensitive potassium channels, and thus might act at several different loci.[298]

INCIDENCE

The abuse of PCP first occurred in 1970, peaked in 1979, and then declined by 1981.[299] National surveys, however, since have indicated that PCP abuse is again on the rise, especially in large urban areas.

The prevalence of PCP abuse during pregnancy has not been firmly established, because most reports have come from urban areas and could not be generalized to a national level. Between 1981 and 1982 in Cleveland, 7.5% of 2327 pregnant women gave a history of PCP use, although only 0.8% could be confirmed by maternal urine screening.[300,301] In 1983, a study from Los Angeles reported that 12% of a random sample of 200 newborns had measurable quantities of PCP in their cord blood.[295]

GROWTH AND MORPHOLOGY

Animal studies indicate that maternal weight gain is lower in PCP-exposed mice. The birth weights of exposed pups were approximately 7% lower than those of nonexposed pups.[289] In humans, no significant difference in the birth weight and length and head circumference was observed in PCP-exposed newborns compared to matched controls.[302] In another study, two of five preterm and none of seven term PCP-exposed newborns were small for gestational age. All

12 newborns were normocephalic.[303] In one study, however, intrauterine growth retardation was observed in PCP-exposed newborns that was comparable with cocaine effects.[304]

In both animal and human studies, PCP has not been shown to be teratogenic, and no reports of congenital malformations attributable to PCP have as yet been made.

NEUROBEHAVIORAL EFFECTS

Early case reports of PCP-exposed newborns showed abnormal neurobehavioral findings in the infants. These included irritability, tremors, hypertonicity, poor attention, bizarre eye movements, staring spells, hypertonic ankle reflexes, and depressed grasp and rooting reflexes.[301,302,305] One of the most characteristic features in infants is a sudden and rapid change in level of consciousness, with lethargy alternating with irritability. The behavioral outcome of these newborns has been attributed to PCP intoxication, rather than to withdrawal. The very low threshold of stimulation, coarse, flapping tremors, and rapid changes in state are similar to behavior reported in children and adults intoxicated with PCP.[302]

LONG-TERM OUTCOME

Given the early neurobehavioral changes observed in the PCP-exposed newborn, there is concern whether these will translate into long-term learning and behavioral problems.[303] Unfortunately, there is little available information on this. The Bayley psychomotor and mental development indices of PCP-exposed infants at 3 months of age were not statistically different from those of controls.[302] At 9 and 18 months of age, fine motor development, adaptive or playing behavior, language skills, and personal–social development as determined by the Gesell Developmental Evaluation were within normal range. These findings are consistent with the interpretation that the observed PCP effects on infants at birth result from acute intoxication rather than from morphologic CNS damage.

AMPHETAMINES

The amphetamines are a group of chemically related sympathomimetic amines that have both CNS stimulant and peripheral α and β actions.[306] Since their synthesis in the 1880s, therapeutic uses have included the treatment of exogenous obesity, narcolepsy, hyperkinesis, and depression. There is a very strong abuse potential because of their psychic effects, which include a decreased sense of fatigue, wakefulness, alertness, mood elevation, self-confidence, and often euphoria and elation.

EPIDEMIOLOGY

After initial epidemics of abuse of speed in the 1950s and 1960s, there was a decline in the abuse of amphetamines with the emergence of other drugs of abuse (*e.g.*, heroin, crack cocaine).

Lately, a resurgence of amphetamine use in epidemic proportions has occurred, particularly in Japan and parts of Asia, Hawaii, and areas of the West Coast.

METHAMPHETAMINE

Methamphetamine is the methylated derivative of amphetamine, and is prepared through the reduction of ephedrine or pseudoephedrine. The ease of its synthesis, its availability and affordability, and a prolonged high have made it an increasingly popular drug of abuse. Ice, the smokable form of methamphetamine, is claimed to produce an intense euphoria. High doses may cause aggressive behavior, arrhythmias, severe anxiety, seizures, shock, and death. Chronic use can produce paranoid psychosis.

EFFECTS ON PREGNANCY

Outcomes of pregnancies in 52 self-reported intravenous methamphetamine abusers were studied; these patients used other drugs as well.[307] The infants had significantly lower birth weight, length, and head circumference than infants of non–drug-users. There was no significant difference, however, in the frequency of pregnancy complications such as pregnancy-induced hypertension, peripartal hemorrhage, chorioamnionitis, syphilis, and hepatitis.

No significant increase in the frequency of major congenital anomalies has been associated with methamphetamine use during pregnancy.[307,308]

Higher incidences of prematurity, intrauterine growth retardation, and smaller head circumference have been reported in infants of mothers who abused cocaine and methamphetamine.[309,310] A higher incidence of retroplacental hemorrhage also was noted.[309]

EFFECTS ON NEONATES

An infant of a known amphetamine addict manifested after birth with diaphoresis, episodes of agitation alternating with lassitude, miosis, and vomiting.[311] Infants exposed to both cocaine and methamphetamine were described as having abnormal sleep patterns, tremors, poor feeding, hypertonia, sneezing, a high-pitched cry, frantic fist sucking, tachypnea, loose stools, fever, yawning, hyperreflexia, and excoriation.[309]

LONG-TERM EFFECTS

Long-term, prospective follow-up of 65 children of women who abused amphetamines and also used alcohol and smoked cigarettes during pregnancy revealed that, at 1 year of age, somatic growth was normal, although illness and accident rates were increased.[312] At 4 and 8 years of age, somatic growth and general health still were normal.[313,314]

Developmental screening at 4 years of age, using the Terman Merrill method, revealed significantly lower IQs,[313] but IQ and psychomotor development were within normal limits by 8 years of age.[314] Aggressive behavior and peer-related problems also were noted.[314]

DIAGNOSIS OF DRUG EXPOSURE

METHODS TO DETECT DRUG EXPOSURE IN THE MOTHER AND INFANT

The identification of drug exposure in the mother or her neonate is not easy. Mothers rarely spontaneously admit to the use of drugs, because of fear of the consequences stemming from such an admission. Even with maternal cooperation, information on the type and extent of drug use often is inaccurate.[14] Similarly, many of the drugs to which the fetus is exposed *in utero* do not produce immediate or recognizable effects in neonates.[315] There are a number of methods used to detect prenatal drug exposure.

Methods to detect substance abuse in a pregnant woman or intrauterine drug exposure in a neonate ideally should address not only the types of drug abused, but also the amount, frequency, and duration of drug exposure. Two general methods are used to achieve this: maternal interview and laboratory tests.

MATERNAL INTERVIEW

Maternal interview has the greatest potential for providing comprehensive information on the type, amount, frequency, and duration of drug use. Two types of maternal interview generally are used.

Routine Interview. The routine interview forms an integral part of the obstetric history, which is obtained either prenatally or when a woman is admitted in labor. The accuracy of the data obtained by this method depends on the attention devoted to the interview. Cursory interview often results in underreporting of drug use, whereas the incidence increases threefold to fivefold if a more organized protocol is used.[316] There are many elements inherent to routine history taking that affect its accuracy. Maternal fear of the consequences of admission, underestimation of drug use even by those who admit to the use of drugs, and physical discomfort experienced by the woman, particularly if in labor, all influence the accuracy of her self-report.[14] Under these circumstances, the reporting of drug abuse by the mother can be as low as one fourth of the true incidence.[100]

Structured Interview. A structured interview is a highly organized interview, frequently using a standard questionnaire. Examples of this are the Khavari Alcohol Test,[317,318] or its modification,[24] and the Cahalan Volume Variability Scale.[319] The structured interview is more accurate because more time is spent with the patient and the interview frequently is conducted in a more favorable environment than is the routine interview (*i.e.*, it is not conducted when the mother is in labor). Structured interviews frequently are used as research tools. On the other hand, structured interviews are expensive and time-consuming to conduct, and are not practical for routine clinical use when dealing with patients who present in labor and have received little or no prenatal care.

LABORATORY TESTS

Most of the laboratory tests for drug detection are used simply for screening purposes. Confirmation with the use of another, unrelated procedure usually is needed if results are to withstand further scrutiny. It is apparent that as more confirmatory tests are done, the testing process becomes more expensive. Thus, the extent to which further tests are carried out after the initial screen is determined by the reasons that initiated the test.

Various analytical procedures are used for drug detection: thin-layer chromatography and immunoassays for screening; high-performance liquid chromatography (HPLC), gas chromatography, and gas chromatography–mass spectrometry for confirmation. A good review of the use and limitations of these procedures has been published.[320]

Specimens for Drug Testing

Urine. The testing for drugs in biologic fluids is by far the most common method used to detect drug abuse in a pregnant woman, or intrauterine drug exposure in a neonate. There are several limitations to this method, however. Identification of drugs in biologic fluids will differentiate only those who have been exposed to drugs *versus* those who were not. The test cannot provide information on the amount, frequency, duration, or the time of last drug use. Among the biologic fluids, urine has been most often tested owing to several advantages[321]: urine collection is easy and noninvasive; drug metabolites in urine usually are found in higher concentrations than in serum, as a result of the concentrating ability of the kidneys; large volumes of urine can be collected;

urine is easier to analyze than blood because it usually is devoid of protein and other cellular constituents; the metabolites in urine usually are stable, especially if frozen; and urine is amenable to all of the drug-testing methods described earlier.

There are several drawbacks to the use of urine for testing, however. Foremost is the high rate of false-negative results.[14,322] In the mother, unless collection is watched closely, urine easily can be substituted with a clean specimen. Urine samples can be tampered with by dilution or by the addition of ions, such as salt, which may interfere with the testing methods. Drug metabolites in urine also reflect only very recent use of the drug, so that negative results may occur if the woman abstains from the use of the drug a few days before testing.[321] In the infant, the incidence of false-negative urine tests also is high, ranging from 32% to 63%.[323–325] Urine specimens must be obtained as close to birth as possible to reflect the intrauterine exposure of the infant to drugs. The later after birth urine is collected and tested, the higher is the likelihood of a false-negative test. Collection of the requisite volume of urine for both the screening test and the confirmatory test from an extremely small or very sick infant may prove impossible. The cutoff concentration for positivity used by the laboratory also may influence the detection rate.[326] Recent abstention by the mother from the use of drugs may result in a negative urine test in the infant. The detection rate for drugs in the urine also can improve if a battery rather than a single test is used.[325]

Meconium. A method has been developed for identifying fetal drug exposure by detecting drug metabolites in meconium. The concept behind this method was based on studies in pregnant, morphine-addicted monkeys,[327] and subsequently in rats addicted to morphine and cocaine.[323] These studies showed that a high concentration of drug metabolites is present in the gastrointestinal tract of these fetuses. This observation was interpreted to be a consequence of the following mechanism: the drug is metabolized by the fetal liver into water-soluble conjugates that are then excreted into the bile or urine. In either case, the metabolites accumulate in the fetal intestines, either from bile secretion or from fetal urine, which is swallowed via the amniotic fluid.

Subsequent clinical studies have validated meconium analysis as a reliable drug screen in the newborn infant:

> Meconium obtained from 20 infants of drug-dependent mothers and 5 control infants was analyzed by radioimmunoassay for the metabolites of heroin, cocaine, and cannabinoids.[323] Control stools showed no drug. Meconium from the infants of drug-dependent mothers showed the presence of at least one drug metabolite: 80% of the infants of drug-dependent mothers showed cocaine (range, 0.14–19.91 μg/g in stool); 55% showed morphine (range, 0.41–14.97 μg/g in stool); and 60% showed cannabinoid (range, 0.05–0.67 μg/g in stool). The concentrations of metabolites were highest during the first 2 days; some stools tested positive up to the third day. In contrast, only 37% of the infants had positive results on a urine screen by fluorescent polarization immunoassay method.
>
> Meconium testing was used to determine the prevalence of illicit drug use among pregnant women who delivered in a large, urban, perinatal center.[100] A total of 3010 infants were screened for the metabolites of cocaine, morphine, and cannabinoids in their meconium by radioimmunoassay: 44.3% were positive for metabolites of one of the 3 drugs; 41% were positive for cocaine or morphine; 30.7% were positive for cocaine (15.4% positive for cocaine only); 20.5% were positive for morphine (7.3% positive for morphine only); and 11.5% were positive for cannabinoid (5.2% positive for cannabinoid only). In contrast, only 11.1% of the mothers in the entire population studied admitted to the use of drugs during pregnancy.
>
> The sensitivity of meconium testing is high. The method was compared to drug detection by maternal hair analysis and in-depth interview of the mother.[322,328] In 26 high-risk mothers studied, the abuse of one drug during pregnancy was identified by history in 19 subjects (73%); by meconium analysis in 19 subjects (73.1%); and by hair analysis in 12 of 16 (75%) subjects. Abuse of two or more drugs was identified only in six subjects (23%) by history, as compared to nine subjects (34.6%) by meconium analysis and in eight (50%) by hair analysis. There was 96% concordance for cocaine identification in hair and meconium, and 73% for heroin and cannabinoids. There also was a high correlation between the cocaine concentration in meconium and in hair.[322]

The meconium test has been adapted to other methods of analysis such as gas chromatography–mass spectroscopy and enzyme immunoassay and fluorescence polarization immunoassay. The latter is significant, since it has rendered meconium testing useful for mass screening.[329] Criteria can be established to allow selection of infants for routine meconium drug screening. Infants who are born to women who have used any illicit drug or alcohol in the past or current pregnancies, and walk-in patients or those with no prenatal care are in the highest risk groups for drug exposure.

The validity of meconium testing as a diagnostic tool, as well as its sensitivity and specificity, have been reported by other workers.[330–332]

In summary, meconium is an ideal specimen for drug testing in the newborn infant because its collection is easy and noninvasive; it contains high concentrations of drugs and their metabolites; and drugs may be present in meconium for up to the third day after birth. Meconium testing is sensitive, quantitative, rapid, and amenable to analysis by standard laboratory methods. The test therefore is useful for diagnostic purposes as well as for clinical and epidemiologic research.

Hair. Hair analysis is one of the most recent additions to drug testing.[333] The test is based on the principle that illicit substances and their metabolic products in the patient's blood become incorporated into the hair follicle and grow into the cuticle and hair shaft. The drug, once deposited in the hair shaft, remains for an indefinite period. As the hair grows at the rate of 1 to 2 cm month, the deposited drugs follow the growth of the hair shaft. The section of the hair closest to the scalp is the most recently exposed portion. Sectional analysis can be performed by month to provide information on the duration and time of drug use. The information on the chronicity of drug use makes hair analysis advantageous compared with urine or other body fluid testing. Furthermore, quantitative detection of drugs in hair has been correlated with the amount of drug use in the past.

Hair has been analyzed successfully to detect opiates,[334] cocaine,[335] PCP,[336] methamphetamine, antidepressants, and nicotine.[337] The analytical procedures that have been used include radioimmunoassay,[333] gas chromatography–mass spectroscopy,[338] HPLC,[339] and collisional spectroscopy.[340]

The validity of hair analysis for drug detection has been demonstrated both in the mother[328] and her neonate.[341] Although hair analysis has some exciting potential, there are some significant drawbacks to the use of hair for testing in women.[342] Patients who are not chronic drug users may not be detected by this technique, since drug deposition in hair relies on serum levels during hair growth. The expense of the test mounts with the number of drugs being screened for, and this has limited its usefulness in prenatal clinics. The quantity of hair necessary to perform the drug screen (*i.e.*, a pencil-sized diameter plug of hair from the posterior scalp) may be difficult to collect in some newborns. Use of hair dye, bleach, and other cosmetic agents by the woman may modify the quantity of drug found in hair, but should not totally eliminate its presence because the drug is incorporated into the hair shaft. Some ethnic groups weave hair from other individuals into their own hair, and this creates the potential for false test results. Because of misconceptions about cosmetic effects, some patients may refuse hair testing. Hair can also be passively exposed to drugs that can be smoked (*e.g.*, cocaine, marijuana).

Others. Other types of specimens have been tested for drugs. These include perspiration, nail clippings, menstrual blood, semen, and saliva.[343,344] The use of these specimens for drug detection has been uncommon, however.

TREATMENT

Initial management of the infant is directed to the antenatal and neonatal complications associated with maternal drug abuse such as asphyxia, fetal distress, prematurity, meconium aspiration, and congenital malformation. In addition, the infant should routinely receive serologic tests for syphilis, HIV disease and hepatitis B; be assessed for signs of drug withdrawal; undergo a drug screen; and receive social service referral.

NARCOTIC WITHDRAWAL

The infant of an opiate-dependent mother should be observed closely for withdrawal. The severity of the withdrawal can be assessed by several clinical scoring systems.[345,346] We use a system that evaluates the infant specifically on manifestations that are life-threatening: vomiting, diarrhea, weight loss, irritability, tremors, and tachypnea (Table 57-9). With this system, drugs are used to treat the withdrawal if there is moderate vomiting, diarrhea, or weight loss; or any severe criterion.

Both narcotic and non-narcotic drugs have been used to treat narcotic withdrawal (Table 57-10). Narcotics are preferred, however, since their action is more physiologic for an abstinence state. The neurologic manifestations of withdrawal may be controlled successfully by non-narcotic drugs, but the narcotics are more effective in relieving the non-CNS manifestations (*e.g.*, diarrhea).

Among the narcotic drugs, paregoric, laudanum, and sometimes methadone are used. We prefer to use tincture of opium or laudanum, United States Pharmacopeia (USP) over paregoric, since paregoric contains camphor, a CNS stimulant. Laudanum USP is available in a standard 10% solution, contains 1.0% morphine, and must be used with caution. Laudanum USP must be diluted 25-fold to a concentration of 0.4% to reduce its morphine content to a level equivalent to that present in paregoric. Laudanum USP 0.4% can be given at the same dose as paregoric (*i.e.*, 3–6 drops every 4–6 hours).

The aim of treatment with drugs is to render the infant comfortable, but not obtunded. Thus, the drug should be titrated, starting with the smallest recommended dose and increased accordingly until the desired effect is achieved. Once the infant is asymptomatic, the drug can be tapered slowly until it is completely discontinued. This usually takes from 4 to 6 days. The infant should be observed for a day or two after discontinuance of the drug for possible recurrence of the symptoms (*i.e.*, rebound phenomenon). When the infant is discharged from the nur-

TABLE 57–9
ASSESSMENT OF THE CLINICAL SEVERITY OF NEONATAL NARCOTIC WITHDRAWAL

Symptom	Mild	Moderate	Severe
Vomiting	Spitting up	Extensive vomiting for three successive feedings	Vomiting associated with imbalance of serum electrolytes
Diarrhea	Watery stools < four times per day	Watery stools five to six times per day for 3 days; no electrolyte imbalance	Diarrhea associated with imbalance of serum electrolytes
Weight loss	<10% of birth weight	10%–15% of birth weight	>15%
Irritability	Minimal	Marked but relieved by cuddling or feeding	Unrelieved by cuddling or feeding
Tremors or twitching	Mild tremors when stimulated	Marked tremors or twitching when stimulated	Convulsions
Tachypnea	60–80 breaths/min	80–100 breaths/min	>100 breaths/min; associated with respiratory alkalosis

From Ostrea EM, Chavez CJ, Stryker JS. The care of the drug dependent woman and her infant. Lansing, MI: Michigan Department of Public Health, 1978:33.

sery, the mother should be instructed to anticipate some mild jitteriness and irritability that may persist in the infant for 8 to 16 weeks, depending on the initial severity of the withdrawal.

In view of their hyperirritability, infants manifesting withdrawal should be swaddled, placed in a prone position, and cuddled more often. Swaddling, particularly with the infant's extremities flexed and hands placed in front of its mouth, enhances the infant's hand-to-mouth facility, which is soothing. A similar soothing action can be achieved with a pacifier.

The frequency of diarrhea and vomiting should be noted, and the infant's weight checked at least every 8 hours. Temperature, heart rate, and respiratory rates should be recorded every 4 hours. Laboratory examinations to detect serum electrolyte or *p*H imbalance should be done as indicated.

TABLE 57–10
TREATMENT OF NEONATAL WITHDRAWAL SYNDROME

Drug	Dosage
Paregoric	3–6 drops every 4 to 6 h, PO
Laudanum (0.4%)	3–6 drops every 4 to 6 h, PO
Chlorpromazine	2–3 mg/kg/d every 6 h, PO
Phenobarbital	3–5 mg/kg/d every 6 h, PO

NON-NARCOTIC WITHDRAWAL

A cross reaction exists between the different drugs belonging to the alcohol–hypnosedative group (see Table 57-3). Each drug is therefore effective in treating withdrawal from any of the drugs belonging to this group.[1] Thus, barbiturates can be used to treat withdrawal from nonbarbiturates, including alcohol, or *vice versa*.

The two drugs that have been used commonly during the neonatal period for this purpose are phenobarbital, 3 to 5 mg/kg/day in divided doses every 6 hours, and chlorpromazine, 1 to 2 mg intramuscularly every 8 hours. Chlorpromazine also has been used successfully at a dose of 2 to 3 mg/kg/day in divided doses every 6 hours.[14] Although chlorpromazine does not belong to the group of non-narcotic drugs that can cause withdrawal manifestations, its ability to ameliorate the signs and symptoms of withdrawal may be secondary to its capacity to suppress REM sleep, which is exaggerated during the state of withdrawal.[16]

During the treatment of withdrawal, attention also should be focused on the nutrition and the fluid and electrolyte balance of the infants, particularly if vomiting, diarrhea, hyperpyrexia, and hyperhidrosis occur. Appropriate intravenous fluids may be required to correct deficits or prevent the occurrence of imbalances in some patients.

MATERNAL SUPPORT

The addicted woman has some serious impediments to a successful mothering role. She has meager past mothering experience to rely on; often there is little or no support from a father or husband because frequently she is single, and, finally, the neurobehavioral abnormalities and withdrawal in her infant may hamper the gratifying feedback that she wishes to experience from her infant.

Thus, the mother and child should have early and repeated contacts. A staff member also should have repeated and relatively brief contacts with the mother, to describe the status of the child and to reassure her that, with the disappearance of withdrawal, the infant will feed more vigorously and will respond better to maternal ministrations.

On the other hand, should it be decided that the infant will be placed in a foster care home, it should be remembered that the infant will need human contact for its normal growth and development. As part of its care in the nursery, the child should be stimulated appropriately through frequent handling or fondling by the staff professionals.

BREAST-FEEDING

Most drugs taken by the mother will cross into her breast milk. The concentration of illicit drug in the breast milk will depend on the amount and time of drug intake by the mother. There also is the danger of transmission of HIV through the breast milk. In general, breast-feeding is not recommended if the mother has been shown to abuse drugs continuously during pregnancy or is HIV antibody-positive.

DRUG-ADDICTED WOMEN AS INFANT CAREGIVERS

The ability of the drug-addicted woman to perform her functions as a mother and provide adequate care for her infant has been seriously questioned on many occasions. Frequently, these women have been denied their maternal rights and responsibilities soon after the infant's birth on the basis of their unstable homes, life-styles, and their emotional and psychological weaknesses. Evidence suggests that this practice may be unnecessary and counterproductive in many cases. A study that determined outcome of infants on the basis of the type of caregiver showed that the outcome, measured by growth, development, frequency of medical illnesses, and child abuse, for infants cared for by the mother with the help of a caregiver (*i.e.*, either a husband or relative) was better than the outcome for infants in foster home care.[57] Thus, with proper guidance and supervision, the addict mother may be capable of providing adequate care for her infant, particularly since most of these women desire to fulfill their mothering functions. Similarly, although a high incidence of problems suggestive of child abuse (*e.g.*, cigarette burns, hematoma) were noted in infants who were cared for exclusively by the mother, very few of these complications were noted in infants whose mother had help available. Thus, it is important that when allowing the mother to care for her infant, someone should help her at home to ensure better care and protection of the infant.

SOCIAL SERVICE REFERRAL

All infants of drug-dependent mothers should have a social service referral to assess the adequacy of parenting and care at home. The discharge of the infant to the mother's care is the primary objective, unless serious conditions dictate otherwise. The care of the infant by the mother, with the help of a support person, usually a grandmother or other relative, has, in our experience, been the best arrangement for a favorable outcome for the infant. The discharge of the infant to a person other than the mother (*i.e.*, foster parent) or an agency should be resorted to only when it is apparent that the infant will be neglected, poorly cared for, or abused. Most mothers hesitate to admit to the use of drugs during pregnancy because of fear that their infants will be taken away from them. They should be assured otherwise; in fact, they should be encouraged to be responsible for the primary care of their infants. The social worker and physician also should advise the mother about available medical and social services in the community, such as substance abuse counseling and family planning services.

POTENTIAL CHILD ABUSE

As part of child protection laws that are operative in many states, infants born to drug-dependent mothers are considered as potentially abused and are required by law to be reported to child protection agencies. Many of these agencies require a positive drug screen in the infant before they will take action on the reports. The precautionary measure intended in the referral of the infant to the child protection agencies is useful if the intent is to ensure the adequacy of care of the infant at home. It is when punitive measures are taken against the mother that the outcome may become counterproductive, or even opposite to the original intent.

FOLLOW-UP

The infant of the drug-dependent mother is at risk for many long-term problems. These include child abuse, delays in physical, mental, and motor development, and learning disabilities. The infant also is at risk for ongoing exposure to the drugs in the household as a result of accidental ingestion or passive exposure, particularly to crack cocaine. Follow-up of these infants should be planned not only to assess their medical well-being but to ascertain the occurrence of such complications and to initiate appropriate interventions.

ACKNOWLEDGMENTS

We thank Mr. Raymund Utarnachitt for his help in the preparation of some sections of the manuscript, and Ms. Sara Anderson for her invaluable secretarial help.

REFERENCES

1. Blum RH. A history of opium. In: Blum RH. Society and drugs: I. Social and cultural observations. San Francisco: Jossey-Bass Inc., 1969:45.
2. Martin E. L'opium ses abus, mangeurs et fumerus d'opium morphinomenes. Paris: 1893.
3. Zagon IS. Opioids and development: new lessons from old problems. NIDA Research Monograph Series 1985;60:58.
4. Goodfriend MJ, Shey IA, Klein MD. The effect of maternal narcotic addiction on the newborn. Am J Obstet Gynecol 1956;71:29.
5. Dole VP, Nyswander MA. Medical treatment for diacetylmorphine (heroin) addiction. JAMA 1965;193:646.
6. Finnegan LP, Blake DA, Chappel JN, et al. Drug dependence in pregnancy: clinical management of mother and child. NIDA Research Monograph Series 1979.
7. Edelin, KC, Gurganious L, Golar K, et al. Methadone maintenance in pregnancy: consequences to care and outcome. Obstet Gynecol 1988;71:399.
8. Connaughton JF, Finnegan LP, Schur J, et al. Current concepts in the management of the pregnant opiate addict. Addictive Disease 1975;2:21.
9. Naeye RL, Blanc W, Leblanc W, et al. Fetal complications of maternal heroin addiction: abnormal growth, infections, and episodes of stress. J Pediatr 1973;83:1055.
10. Zelson C. Infant of the addicted mother. N Engl J Med 1973;288:1393.
11. Strauss ME, Andresko M, Stryker JC, et al. Methadone maintenance during pregnancy, birth and neonatal course. Am J Obstet Gynecol 1974;120:895.
12. Kandall SR, Album S, Dreyer E, et al. Differential effects of heroin and morphine on birth weights. Addict Dis 1975;2:347.
13. Little BB, Snell LM, Klein VR, et al. Maternal and fetal effects of heroin addiction during pregnancy. J Reprod Med 1990; 35:159.
14. Ostrea EM, Chavez CJ. Perinatal problems (excluding neonatal withdrawal) in maternal drug addiction: a study of 830 cases. J Pediatr 1979;94:292.
15. Szeto HH. Effects of narcotic drugs on fetal behavioral activity: acute methadone exposure. Am J Obstet Gynecol 1983; 146:211.
16. Dinges DF, Davis MM, Glass P. Fetal exposure to narcotics: neonatal sleep as a measure of nervous system disturbance. Science 1980;209:619.
17. Umans JG, Szeto HH. Precipitated opiate abstinence in utero. Am J Obstet Gynecol 1985;151:441.
18. Zuspan FB, Gumpel JA, Mejia-Zelaya A, et al. Fetal stress from methadone withdrawal. Am J Obstet Gynecol 1975; 122:43.
19. Stone M, Salerno LJ, Green M, et al. Narcotic addiction in pregnancy. Am J Obstet Gynecol 1971;109:716.
20. Finnegan LP. Narcotic dependence in pregnancy. Journal of Psychedelic Drugs 1975;7:299.
21. Perlmutter JF. Heroin addiction and pregnancy. Obstet Gynecol Surv 1974;29:439.
22. Rementeria JL, Lotongkhum K. The fetus of the drug-addicted woman: conception fetal wastage and complications. In: Rementeria JL, ed. Drug abuse in pregnancy and neonatal effects. St. Louis: CV Mosby, 1977:1.
23. Donahoe R. Opiates as immunocompromising drugs: the evidence and possible mechanisms. NIDA Research Monograph Series 1988;90:105.
24. Harper RG, Solish GI, Purow HM, et al. The effect of a methadone treatment program upon pregnant heroin addicts and their newborn infants. Pediatrics 1974;54:300.
25. Chasnoff I, Hatcher R, Burns WJ. Early growth patterns in methadone-addicted infants. Am J Dis Child 1980;134:1049.
26. Chasnoff I, Hatcher R, Burns WJ. Polydrug and methadone addicted newborns: a continuum of impairment. Pediatrics 1982;70:210.
27. Kaltenbach K, Finnegan LP. Children exposed to methadone in utero. Ann NY Acad Sci 1989;562:360.
28. Rosen TS, Johnson. Children of methadone-maintained mothers: follow-up to 18 months of age. J Pediatr 1982; 101:192.
29. Ostrea EM, Chavez CJ, Strauss ME. A study of the factors that influence the severity of neonatal narcotic withdrawal. J Pediatr 1976;88:642.
30. McLaughlin PJ, Zagon IS, White WJ. Perinatal methadone exposure in rats: effects on body and organ development. Biol Neonate 1978;34:48.
31. Zagon IS, McLaughlin PJ. Effect of chronic maternal methadone exposure on perinatal development. Biol Neonate 1977;31:271.
32. Thompson CI, Zagon IS. Long-term thermoregulatory changes following perinatal methadone exposure in rats. Pharmacol Biochem Behav 1980;14:653.
33. Sundell H, Garrot J, Blakenship WJ, et al. Studies on infants with type II respiratory distress syndrome. J Pediatr 1971; 78:754.
34. Glass L, Rajegowda BK, Evans HE. Absence of respiratory distress syndrome in premature infants of heroin-addicted mothers. Lancet 1971;2:685.
35. Gluck L, Kulovich MV. Lecithin/sphingomyelin ratios in amniotic fluid in normal and abnormal pregnancy. Am J Obstet Gynecol 1973;115:539.
36. Taeusch HM Jr, Carson SH, Wang NS, et al. Heroin induction of lung maturation and growth retardation in fetal rabbits. J Pediatr 1973;82:869.
37. Smith BT, Torday JS. Factors affecting lecithin synthesis by fetal lung cells in culture. Pediatr Res 1974;8:848.
38. Rothstein P, Gould JB. Born with a habit: infants of drug-addicted mothers. Pediatr Clin North Am 1974;21:307.
39. Stimmell B, Adams K. Narcotic dependency in pregnancy: methadone maintenance compared to use of street drugs. JAMA 1976;235:1121.
40. Geber WF, Schramm LC. Congenital malformations of the central nervous system produced by narcotic analgesics in the hamster. Am J Obstet Gynecol 1975;123:705.
41. Nathenson G, Cohen M, Litt I, et al. The effect of maternal heroin addiction on neonatal jaundice. J Pediatr 1972;81:899.
42. Burstein Y, Giardina PJV, Rausen AR, et al. Thrombocytosis and increased circulating platelet aggregates in newborn infants of polydrug users. J Pediatr 1979;94:895.
43. Desmond MM, Schwanecke RP, Wilson GS, et al. Maternal barbiturate utilization and neonatal withdrawal symptomatology. J Pediatr 1972;80:190.
44. Ostrea EM, Chavez CJ, Stryker JS. The care of the drug dependent women and her infant. Lansing, MI: Michigan Department of Public Health, 1978:28.

45. Strauss ME, Lessen-Firestone JK, Starr RH, et al. Behavior of narcotic addicted newborns. Child Dev 1975;46:887.
46. Soule AB, Standley K, Cpoans SA, et al. Clinical uses of the Brazelton Neonatal Scale. Pediatrics 1974;54:583.
47. Lodge A, Marcus MM, Ramer CM. Behavioral and electrophysical characteristics of the addicted neonate. Addictive Disease 1975;2:235.
48. Coppolillo HP. Drug impediments to mothering behavior. Addict Dis Int J 1975;2:201.
49. Chavez CJ, Ostrea EM, Strauss ME, et al. Prognosis of infants born to drug dependent mothers: its relation to the severity of the withdrawal during the neonatal period. Pediatr Res 1976;10:328A.
50. Chavez CJ, Ostrea EM, Stryker JS, et al. Sudden infant death syndrome among infants of drug dependent mothers. J Pediatr 1979;95:407.
51. Pierson PS, Howard P, Kleber HD. Sudden deaths in infants born to methadone maintained addicts. JAMA 1972;220:1933.
52. Strauss ME, Starr RH, Ostrea EM, et al. Behavior concomitants of prenatal addiction to narcotics. J Pediatr 1976;89:842.
53. Wilson GS, Desmond MM, Verniaud WW. Early development of infants of heroin addicted mothers. Am J Dis Child 1973;126:457.
54. Wilson, GS, McCreary R, Kean J, et al. The development of preschool children of heroin-addicted mothers: a controlled trial study. Pediatrics 1979;63:135.
55. Wilson GS, Desmond MM, Wait RB. Follow-up of methadone-treated and untreated narcotic-dependent women and their infants: health, developmental and social implications. J Pediatr 1981;98:716.
56. Rosen TS, Johnson HL. Children of methadone-maintained mothers: follow-up to 18 months of age. J Pediatr 1982; 101:192.
57. Chavez CJ, Ostrea EM. Outcome of infants of drug dependent mothers based on the type of caregiver [abstract]. Pediatr Res 1977;11:375A.
58. Herjanic BM, Barredo VH, Herjanic M, et al. Children of heroin addicts. Int J Addict 1979;14:919.
59. Marcus J, Hans SL, Jeremy RJ. Differential motor and state functioning in newborns of women on methadone. Neurobehavioral Toxicology and Teratology 1982;4:459.
60. Jeremy RJ, Bernstein VJ. Dyads at risk: methadone-maintained women and their four-month-old infants. Child Dev 1984;55:1141.
61. Essig CF. Addiction to barbiturate and non barbiturate sedative drugs. Res Publ Assoc Res Nerv Ment Dis 1968;46:188.
62. Isbell H. Addiction to barbiturates and the barbiturate abstinence syndrome. Ann Intern Med 1950;33:108.
63. Bleyer W, Marshall RE. Barbiturate withdrawal syndrome in a passively addicted infant. JAMA 1972;221:185.
64. Ploman L, Persson BH. On the transfer of barbiturates to the human fetus and their accumulation in some of its vital organs. Br J Obstet Gynaecol 1957;64:706.
65. Ostrea EM Jr. Neonatal withdrawal from intrauterine exposure to butalbital. Am J Obstet Gynecol 1982;143:597.
66. Harvey SC. Hypnotics and sedatives: barbiturates. In: Gilman A, Rall TW, Goodman LS, et al, eds. Goodman and Gilman's the pharmacological basis of therapeutics. 8th ed. New York: Pergamon Press, 1990:358.
67. Jalling B, Boreus LO, Kallberg N, et al. Disappearance from the newborn of circulating prenatally administered phenobarbital. Eur J Clin Pharmacol 1973;6:234.
68. Margetts EL. Chloral delirium. Psychiatry 1950;24:278.
69. Opitz JM, Grosse FR, Heneberg B. Congenital effects of bromism. Lancet 1972;1:91.
70. Rossiter EJR, Rendle-Short TJ. Congenital effects of bromism. Lancet 1972;2:705.
71. Erkkola R, Kangas L, Pekkarinen A. The transfer of diazepam across the placenta during labour. Acta Obstet Gynecol Scand 1973;52:167.
72. Athinarayanan P, Pierog SH, Nigam SK, et al. Chlordiazepoxide withdrawal in the neonate. Am J Obstet Gynecol 1976; 124:212.
73. Rementeria JL, Bhatt K. Withdrawal symptoms in neonates from intrauterine exposure to diazepam. J Pediatr 1977;90: 123.
74. Cuthburt KJR. Two hypnotics. Practitioner 1963;190:509.
75. Tsapogas MJC, Modle J, Wheeler T. A comparison between two hypnotics: ethchlorvynol and dichloralphenazone. Br J Clin Pract 1963;17:407.
76. Wood-Walker RB. A clinical evaluation of a nonbarbiturate hypnotic. Ethchlorvynol. Br J Clin Pract 1963;17:201.
77. Garetz FD. Ethchlorvynol: addiction hazard. Minn Med 1969;52:1131.
78. Magness JL. Ethchlorvynol intoxication and severe abstinence reaction. Lancet 1965;1:80.
79. Harenko A. On special traits of acute ethchlorvynol poisoning. Acta Neurol Scand 1967;43:141.
80. Aycrigg JB. Two cases of withdrawal from ethchlorvynol. Am J Psychiatry 1964;120:1201.
81. Flemenbaum A, Gunby B. Ethchlorvynol (placidyl) abuse and withdrawal. Dis Nerv Syst 1971;32:188.
82. Hudson HS, Walker HI. Withdrawal symptoms following ethchlorvynol dependence. Am J Psychiatry 1961;118:361.
83. Hume AS, Williams JM, Douglas BG. Disposition of ethchlorvynol in maternal blood, amniotic fluid and chorionic fluid. J Reprod Med 1971;6:229.
84. Rumack BH, Walravens PA. Neonatal withdrawal following maternal ingestion of ethchlorvynol (Placidyl). Pediatrics 1973;52:714.
85. Sadwin A, Glen RS. Addiction to glutethimide (Doriden). Am J Psychiatry 1958;115:469.
86. Eidelman JR. Doriden intoxication. Mo Med 1956;53:194.
87. Kanter DM. The acute toxicity of Doriden overdosage. Conn Med J 1957;21:314.
88. McBay AJ, Katsas GG. Glutethimide poisoning: a report of four fatal cases. N Engl J Med 1957;257:97.
89. Pildes RS. Neonatal withdrawal symptoms associated with gluthetimide (Doriden) addiction in the mother during pregnancy. Clin Pediatr 1977;16:424.
90. Eggermont E. The adverse influence of imipramine on the adaptation of the newborn infant to extrauterine life. Acta Pediatr Belg 1972;26:197.
91. Sothers J. Lithium toxicity in the newborn. Br Med J 1973;3:233.
92. Tunnessen W. Toxic effects of lithium in newborn infants. J Pediatr 1972;81:804.
93. Webster PAC. Withdrawal symptoms in neonates associated with maternal antidepressant therapy. Lancet 1973;2:318.
94. Wilbanks B. Toxic effects of lithium carbonate in a mother and newborn infant. JAMA 1970;213:865.
95. Hill RM, Desmond MM, Kay JL. Extrapyramidal dysfunction in an infant of a schizophrenic mother. J Pediatr 1966;69: 589.
96. Levy W, Wisniewski K. Chlorpromazine causing extrapyramidal dysfunction in newborn infant of psychotic mother. NY State J Med 1974;74:684.
97. Krug S. Cocaine abuse: historical epidemiologic and clinical perspectives for pediatricians. Adv Pediatr 1989;36:369.
98. Khalsa JH, Gfroerer J. Epidemiology and health consequence

of drug abuse among pregnant women. Semin Perinatol 1991;15:265.
99. Chasnoff IJ, Landress HJ, Barrett ME. The prevalence of illicit drug or alcohol use during pregnancy and discrepancies in mandatory reporting in Pinellas County, Florida. N Engl J Med 1990;322:1202.
100. Ostrea EM, Brady M, Gause S, et al. Drug screening of newborn infants by meconium analysis: a large scale prospective, epidemiologic study. Pediatrics 1992;89:107.
101. Farrar HC, Kearns GL. Cocaine: clinical pharmacology and toxicology. J Pediatr 1989;115:665.
102. Udell B. Crack cocaine: crack vs. cocaine. In: Special Currents: cocaine babies. Columbus, OH: Ross Laboratories, November, 1989:5.
103. Tarr JE, Macklin M. Cocaine. Pediatr Clin North Am 1987; 34:319.
104. Woods JR, Plessinger MA, Clark KE. Effect of cocaine on uterine blood flow and fetal oxygenation. JAMA 1987;257:957.
105. Moore TR, Sorg J, Miller L, et al. Hemodynamic effects of intravenous cocaine on the pregnant ewe and fetus. Am J Obstet Gynecol 1986;155:883.
106. Woods JR, Plessinger MA. Pregnancy increases cardiovascular toxicity to cocaine. Am J Obstet Gynecol 1990;162:529.
107. Cejtin HE, Parsons MT, Wilson L. Cocaine use and its effects on umbilical artery prostacyclin production. Prostaglandins 1990;40:249.
108. Church MW, Kaufmann RA, Keenan JA, et al. Effect of prenatal cocaine exposure. In: Watson R, ed. Biochemistry and physiology of substance abuse. vol. 3. Boca Raton, FL: CRC Press, 1990:179.
109. Chasnoff IJ, Burns WJ, Schnoll SH, et al. Cocaine use in pregnancy. N Engl J Med 1985;313:666.
110. Hadeed AJ, Siegel SR. Maternal cocaine use during pregnancy: effect on the newborn infant. Pediatrics 1989;84:205.
111. Bingol N, Fuchs M, Diaz V, et al. Teratogenicity of cocaine in humans. J Pediatr 1987;110:93.
112. Chouteau M, Namerow PB, Leppert P. The effect of cocaine abuse on birth weight and gestational age. Obstet Gynecol 1988;72:351.
113. Doberczak TM, Shanzer S, Senie RT, et al. Neonatal neurologic and electroencephalographic effects of intrauterine cocaine exposure. J Pediatr 1988;133:354.
114. Neerhof M, MacGregor S, Retzky S, et al. Cocaine abuse during pregnancy: peripartum prevalence and perinatal outcome. Am J Obstet Gynecol 1989;161:633.
115. Cerukuri R, Minkoff H, Feldman J, et al. A cohort study of alkaloidal cocaine ("crack") in pregnancy. Obstet Gynecol 1988;72:147.
116. Fulroth R, Phillips B, Durand D. Perinatal outcome of infants exposed to cocaine and or heroin in utero. Am J Dis Child 1989;143:905.
117. Dombrowski MP, Wolfe HM, Welch RA, et al. Cocaine abuse is associated with abruptio placentae and decreased birth weight, but not shorter labor. Obstet Gynecol 1991;77:139.
118. Little B, Snell L, Klein V, et al. Cocaine abuse during pregnancy: maternal and fetal complications. Obstet Gynecol 1989;73:157.
119. Oro A, Dixon S. Perinatal cocaine and methamphetamine exposure: maternal and neonatal correlates. J Pediatr 1987; 117:571.
120. Chasnoff I, Griffith D, MacGregor S, et al. Temporal patterns of cocaine use in pregnancy. JAMA 1989;261:1741.
121. Leblar P, Parekh A, Naso B, et al. Effects of intrauterine exposure to alkaloidal cocaine (crack). Am J Dis Child 1987; 141:937.
122. Zuckerman B, Frank D, Hingson R, et al. Effects of maternal marijuana and cocaine use on fetal growth. N Engl J Med 1989;320:762.
123. Hume R Jr, O'Donnell K, Stanger C, et al. In utero cocaine exposure: observations of fetal behavioral state may predict neonatal outcome. Am J Obstet Gynecol 1989;161:685.
124. Ryan L, Ehrlich S, Finnegan L. Cocaine abuse in pregnancy: effects on the fetus and newborn. Neurotoxicol Teratol 1987;9:295.
125. Chouteau M, Namerow P, Leppert P. The effects of cocaine abuse on birth weight and gestational age. Obstet Gynecol 1988;72:351.
126. Anday E, Cohen M, Kelly N, et al. Effect of in utero cocaine exposure on startle and its modifications. Dev Pharmacol Ther 1989;12:137.
127. Chasnoff I, Burns K, Burns W. Cocaine use in pregnancy: perinatal morbidity and mortality. Neurotoxicol Teratol 1987; 9:291.
128. Chasnoff I, Chisum G, Kaplan W. Maternal cocaine use and genitourinary tract malformations. Teratology 1988;37:201.
129. Bandstra E, Burkett G. Maternal–fetal and neonatal effects of in utero cocaine exposure. Semin Perinatol 1991;15:288.
130. Michele S, Greenberg Z, Singh T, et al. The association between congenital syphilis and cocaine/crack use in New York City: a case control study. Am J Public Health 1991;81:1316.
131. Minkoff HL, McCalla S, Delke I, et al. The relationship of cocaine use to syphilis and immunodeficiency virus infections among inner city parturient women. Am J Obstet Gynecol 1990;163:521.
132. Chasnoff IJ, Hunt CE, Kletter R, et al. Prenatal cocaine exposure is associated with respiratory pattern abnormalities. Am J Dis Child 1989;143:583.
133. Hume RF Jr, O'Donnell KJ, Stanger CL, et al. In utero cocaine exposure: observations of fetal behavioral state may predict neonatal outcome. Am J Obstet Gynecol 1989;161:685.
134. Ostrea EM Jr, Kresbach P, Knapp DK, et al. Abnormal heart rate tracings and serum creatine phosphokinase in addicted neonates. Neurotoxicol Teratol 1987;9:305.
135. Church MW, Overbeck GW. Prenatal cocaine exposure in the Long-Evans rat: II. Dose-dependent effects on offspring behavior. Neurotoxicol Teratol 1990;12:335.
136. Church MW, Overbeck GW. Prenatal cocaine exposure: sensorineural hearing loss as evidenced by the brainstem auditory evoked potential. Soc Neurosci Abstr 1989;15:253.
137. Salamy A, Eldredge L, Anderson J, et al. Brainstem transmission time in infants exposed to cocaine in utero. J Pediatr 1990;117:627.
138. Hurt H. Medical controversies in evaluation and management of cocaine exposed infants. In: Special Currents: cocaine babies. Columbus, OH: Ross Laboratories, November, 1989:3.
139. Lewis KD, Bennett B, Schmeder NH. The care of infants menaced by cocaine abuse. MCN 1989;14:324.
140. Rodning C, Beckwith L, Howards J. Characteristics of attachment organization and play organization in prenatally drug exposed toddlers. Dev Psychopathol 1990;1:277.
141. Chasnoff I, Lewis DE, Squires L. Cocaine intoxication in a breast fed infant. Pediatrics 1989;80:836.
142. Bateman DA, Heagarty MC. Passive freebase cocaine ('crack') inhalation by infants and children. Am J Dis Child 1989; 143:25.
143. Jones KL, Smith DW. Recognition of the fetal alcohol syndrome in early infancy. Lancet 1973;2:999.
144. Jones KL, Smith DW, Ulleland CN, Streissguth AP. Pattern of malformation in offspring of chronic alcoholic mothers. Lancet 1973;1:1267.

145. Christiaens L, Mizon JP, Delmarie G. Sur la descendance des alcooliques (On the offspring of alcoholics). Ann Pediatr 1960;36:37.
146. Heuyer H, Mises R, Dereux JF. La descendance les alcooliques (The offspring of alcoholics). Nouvelle Press Medicale (Paris) 1957;29:657.
147. Abel EL. Fetal alcohol syndrome. Oradell, NJ: Medical Economics Company, Inc., 1990.
148. Pietrantoni M, Knuppel RA. Alcohol in pregnancy. Clin Perinatol 1991;18:93.
149. Day NL, Richardson GA. Prenatal alcohol exposure: a continuum of effects. Semin Perinatol 1991;15:271.
150. Adams EH, Gfroerer JC, Rouse BA. Epidemiology of substance abuse including alcohol and cigarette smoking. Ann NY Acad Sci 1989;562:14.
151. Khalsa JH, Gfroerer JC. Epidemiology and health consequences of drug abuse among pregnant women. Semin Perinatol 1991;15:265.
152. Hilton ME. The demographic distribution of drinking patterns in 1984. Drug Alcohol Depend 1988;22:37.
153. Kolata GB. Fetal alcohol advisory debated. Science 1981; 214:642.
154. Sokol RJ, Miller SI, Debanne S, et al. The Cleveland NIAAA prospective alcohol-in-pregnancy study: the first year. Neurotoxicol Teratol 1981;3:203.
155. Day NL, Jasperse D, Richardson GA, et al. Prenatal exposure to alcohol: effect on infant growth and morphological characteristics. Pediatrics 1989;84:536.
156. Brien J, Clark D, Smith G, et al. Disposition of acute, multiple-dose ethanol in the near-term pregnant ewe. Am J Obstet Gynecol 1987;157:204.
157. Fisher ES. Selective fetal malnutrition: the fetal alcohol syndrome. J Am Coll Nutr 1988;7:101.
158. Sokol RJ, Miller SI, Reed G. Alcohol abuse during pregnancy: an epidemiologic study. Alcoholism: Clinical and Experimental Research 1980;4:135.
159. Plant M. Women, drinking and pregnancy. London: Tavistock Publications, 1985.
160. Clarren SK. Fetal alcohol syndrome: a new primate model for binge drinking and its relevance to human ethanol teratogenesis. J Pediatr 1982;101:819.
161. Scott WJ, Fradkin R. The effects of prenatal ethanol in cynomolgus monkeys Macaca fascicularis. Teratology 1984;29:49.
162. Altshuler HL, Shippenberg TS. A subhuman primate model for fetal alcohol syndrome research. Neurotoxicol Teratol 1981;3:121.
163. Kline J, Shrout P, Stein Z, et al. Drinking during pregnancy and spontaneous abortion. Lancet 1980;2:176.
164. Machemer L, Lorke D. Experiences with the dominant lethal test in female mice: effects of alkylating agents and artificial sweeteners on pre-ovulatory oocyte stages. Mutat Res 1975;29:209.
165. Koike M. Cytogenetic effects of maternal alcohol uptake on F1 mouse fetuses. Japanese Journal of Hygiene 1985;40:575.
166. Kaufman MH. Ethanol-induced chromosomal abnormalities at conception. Nature 1983;302:258.
167. Washington WJ, Cain KT, Cacheiro NLA, et al. Ethanol-induced late fetal death in mice exposed around the time of fertilization. Mutat Res 1985;147:205.
168. Marbury MC, Linn S, Monson RP, et al. The association of alcohol consumption with outcome of pregnancy. Am J Public Health 1983;73:1165.
169. Prager K, Malin H, Graves C, et al. Maternal smoking and drinking behavior before and during pregnancy. In: Health and prevention profile. Hyattsville, MD: U.S. Department of Health and Human Services, National Center for Health Statistics, 1983:19.
170. National Institute on Alcohol Abuse and Alcoholism. Program strategies for preventing fetal alcohol syndrome and alcohol-related birth defects. Washington, DC: U.S. Department of Health and Human Services, Public Health Service, Alcohol, Drug Abuse, and Mental Health Administration, 1986.
171. Randall CL, Taylor WJ, Walker DW. Ethanol-induced malformations in mice. Alcoholism: Clinical and Experimental Research 1977;1:219.
172. Halliday HC, MacReid M, MacClure G. Results of heavy drinking in pregnancy. Br J Obstet Gynaecol 1982;89:892.
173. Staisey N, Fried P. Relationships between moderate maternal alcohol consumption during pregnancy and infant neurological development. J Stud Alcohol 1983;44:262.
174. Halmesmaki E, Valimaki M, Karonen S. Low somatomedin C and high growth hormone levels in newborns damaged by maternal alcohol abuse. Obstet Gynecol 1989;74:366.
175. Druse MJ, Hoffeig JH. The effect of chronic maternal alcohol consumption on the development of the central nervous system myelin subfractions in rat offspring. Drug Alcohol Depend 1977;2:421.
176. Hoff S. Synaptogenesis in the hippocampal dentae gyrus: effects of in utero ethanol exposure. Brain Res Bull 1988; 21:47.
177. Kennedy LA. The pathogenesis of brain abnormalities in the fetal alcohol syndrome: an intergrading hypothesis. Teratology 1984;29:263.
178. Shoemaker WJ, Baetge G, Azad R, et al. Effects of prenatal alcohol exposure on amine and peptide neurotransmitter systems. Monogr Neural Sci 1983;9:130.
179. Dehaene PH, Crepin G, Delahousse G, et al. Aspects epidemiologiques du syndrome d'alcoolisme foetal: 45 observations en 3 ans (Epidemiological aspects of the foetal alcoholism syndrome: 45 cases). Nouvelle Press Medicale 1981; 10:2639.
180. Ollegard R, Sabel K, Aronsson M, et al. Effects on the child of alcohol abuse during pregnancy: retrospective and prospective studies. Acta Paediatr Scand 1979;275:112.
181. Dehaene PH, Samaille-Villette CH, Samaille P, et al. Le syndrome d'alcoolisme foetal dans le nord de la France (The fetal alcohol syndrome in the north of France). Revue de l'Alcoolisme (Paris) 1977;23:145.
182. Ouellette EM, Rosett HL, Rosman NP, et al. Adverse effects on offspring of maternal alcohol abuse during pregnancy. N Engl J Med 1977;297:528.
183. Wilsnack SC, Klassen AD, Wilsnack RW. Drinking and reproductive dysfunction among women in a 1981 national survey. Alcoholism: Clinical and Experimental Research 1984;8:451.
184. Berkowitz GS. An epidemiologic study of preterm delivery. Am J Epidemiol 1981;113:81.
185. Smith IE, Coles CD, Lancaster J, et al. The effect of volume and duration of prenatal ethanol exposure on neonatal physical and behavioral development. Neurotoxicol Teratol 1986; 8:375.
186. Coles CD, Smith I, Fernhoff PM, et al. Neonatal neurobehavioral characteristics as correlates of maternal alcohol use during gestation. Alcoholism: Clinical and Experimental Research 1985;9:454.
187. Ernhart CB, Wolf AW, Linn PL, et al. Alcohol-related birth defects: syndromal anomalies, intrauterine growth retardation, and neonatal behavioral assessment. Alcoholism: Clinical and Experimental Research 1985;9:447.
188. Hanson J, Streissguth AP, Smith D. The effects of moderate

alcohol consumption during pregnancy on fetal growth and morphogenesis. J Pediatr 1978;92:457.
189. Russell M. Clinical implications of recent research on the fetal alcohol syndrome. Bull NY Acad Med 1991;67:207.
190. Kaminski M, Rumeau C, Schwartz D. Alcohol consumption in pregnant women and the outcome of pregnancy. Alcoholism: Clinical and Experimental Research 1978;2:155.
191. Tennes K, Blackard C. Maternal alcohol consumption, birth weight and minor physical anomalies. Am J Obstet Gynecol 1980;138:774.
192. Hingson R, Alpert J, Day NL, et al. Effects of maternal drinking and marijuana use on fetal growth and development. Pediatrics 1982;70:539.
193. Mills JL, Graubard BI. Is moderate drinking during pregnancy associated with an increased rate of malformations? Pediatrics 1987;80:309.
194. Robe LB, Gromisch DS, Iosub S. Symptoms of neonatal ethanol withdrawal. Currents in Alcoholism 1981;8:485.
195. Coles CD, Smith I, Fernhoff PM, et al. Neonatal ethanol withdrawal: characteristics in clinically normal, nondysmorphic neonates. J Pediatr 1984;105:445.
196. Streissguth A, Barr H, Martin D. Maternal alcohol use and neonatal habituation assessed with the Brazelton Scale. Child Dev 1983;545:1109.
197. Fried PA, Makin JE. Neonatal behavioral correlates of prenatal exposure to marijuana cigarettes and alcohol in a low-risk population. Neurotoxicol Teratol 1987;9:1.
198. Jacobson SW, Fein GG, Jacobson JL, et al. Neonatal correlates of prenatal exposure to smoking, caffeine, and alcohol. Infant Behavior Development 1984;7:253.
199. Richardson GA, Day NL, Taylor P. The effect of prenatal alcohol, marijuana and tobacco exposure on neonatal behavior. Infant Behav Dev 1989;12:199.
200. Rosett H, Snyder P, Sander LW, et al. Effects of maternal drinking on neonate state regulation. Dev Med Child Neurol 1979;21:464.
201. Chernick V, Childiaeva R, Ioffe S. Effects of maternal alcohol intake and smoking on neonatal electroencephalogram and anthropometric measurements. Am J Obstet Gynecol 1983; 146:41.
202. Ioffe S, Childiaeva R, Chernick V. Prolonged effects of maternal alcohol ingestion on the neonatal encephalogram. Pediatrics 1984;74:330.
203. Ioffe S, Chernick, V. Development of the EEG between 30 and 40 weeks gestation in normal and alcohol-exposed infants. Dev Med Child Neurol 1988;30:797.
204. Mennella JA, Beauchamp GK. The transfer of alcohol to human milk. N Engl J Med 1991;325:981.
205. Kiessling KH, Pilstrom L. Effects of ethanol on rat liver: the influence of vitamins, electrolytes and amino acids on the structure and function of mitochondria from rats receiving ethanol. Br J Nutr 1967;21:547.
206. Cobo E. Effect of different doses of ethanol on the milk-ejecting reflex in lactating women. Am J Obstet Gynecol 1973; 115:817.
207. Little RE, Anderson KW, Ervin CH, et al. Maternal alcohol use during breast-feeding and infant mental and motor development at one year. N Engl J Med 1989;321:425.
208. Day NL, Richardson GA, Robles N, et al. Effect of prenatal alcohol exposure on growth and morphology of offspring at 8 months of age. Pediatrics 1990;85:748.
209. Barr HM, Streissguth AP, Martin DC, et al. Infant size at 8 months of age: relationships to maternal use of alcohol, nicotine and caffeine during pregnancy. Pediatrics 1984;74: 336.
210. O'Connor MJ, Brill NJ, Sigman M. Alcohol use in primiparous women older than 30 years of age: relation to infant development. Pediatrics 1986;78:444.
211. Fried, PA, O'Connell CM. A comparison of effects of prenatal exposure to tobacco, alcohol, cannabis and caffeine on birth size and subsequent growth. Neurotoxicol Teratol 1987;9:79.
212. Coles CD, Smith IE, Lancaster JS, et al. Persistence over the first month of neurobehavioral differences in infants exposed to alcohol prenatally. Infant Behav Dev 1987;10:23.
213. Coles CD, Smith IE, Falek A. Prenatal alcohol exposure and infant behavior: immediate effects and implications for later development. In: Bean-Bayog M, ed. Children of alcoholics. New York: Hayworth Press, 1987:87.
214. Streissguth AP, Barr HM, Martin DC, et al. Effects of maternal alcohol, nicotine and caffeine use during pregnancy on infant mental and motor development at eight months. Alcoholism: Clinical and Experimental Research 1980;4:152.
215. Gusella J, Fried P. Effects of maternal social drinking and smoking on offspring at 13 months. Neurotoxicol Teratol 1984;6:13.
216. Richardson GA, Day NL. Prenatal exposure to alcohol, marijuana and tobacco: effect on infant mental and motor development. Presented at the meeting of the Society for Research in Child Development, Seattle, Washington, April 1991.
217. Streissguth AP, Barr HM, Sampson PD, et al. IQ at age 4 in relation to maternal alcohol use and smoking during pregnancy. Dev Psychol 1989;25:3.
218. Landesman-Dwyer S, Ragozin A, Little R. Behavioral correlates of prenatal alcohol exposure: a four-year follow-up study Neurotoxicol Teratol 1981;3:187.
219. Streissguth AP, Martin DC, Barr HM, et al. Intrauterine alcohol and nicotine exposure: attention and reaction time in 4-year-old children. Dev Psychol 1984;20:533.
220. Barr HM, Streissguth AP, Darby BL, et al. Prenatal exposure to alcohol, caffeine, tobacco and aspirin: effects on fine and gross motor performance in 4-year-old children. Dev Psychol 1990;26:339.
221. Streissguth AP, Barr HM, Sampson PD, et al. Attention distraction and reaction time at seven years and prenatal alcohol exposure. Neurotoxicol Teratol 1986;8:717.
222. Streissguth AP, Barr HM, Sampson PD. Moderate prenatal alcohol exposure: effects on child IQ and learning problems at age 7½ years. Alcoholism: Clinical and Experimental Research 1990;14:662.
223. Fried PA, Watkinson B. 12- and 24-month neurobehavioral follow-up of children prenatally exposed to marijuana, cigarettes and alcohol. Neurotoxicol Teratol 1988;10:305.
224. Fried PA, Watkinson B. 36- and 48-month neurobehavioral follow-up of children prenatally exposed to marijuana, cigarettes and alcohol. J Dev Behav Pediatr 1990;11:49.
225. Sokol RJ, Ager J, Martier S, et al. Significant determinants of susceptibility to alcohol teratogenicity. Ann NY Acad Sci 1986;77:87.
226. Streissguth AP, Clarren SK, Jones KL. Natural history of the fetal alcohol syndrome: a ten-year follow-up of eleven patients. Lancet 1985;2:85.
227. Kyllerman M, Aronson M, Sabel KG, et al. Children of alcoholic mothers (growth and motor performance compared to matched controls). Acta Paediatr Scand 1985;70:20.
228. Landesman-Dwyer S. The relationship of children's behavior to maternal alcohol consumption. In: Abel EL, ed. Fetal alcohol syndrome: human studies. vol. 2. Boca Raton, FL: CRC Press, 1982:127.
229. Streissguth AP, Herman C, Smith D. Stability of intelligence in the fetal alcohol syndrome: a preliminary report. Alcoholism: Clinical and Experimental Research 1978;2:165.
230. Shaywitz S, Cohen D, Shaywitz B. Behavior and learning

difficulties in children of normal intelligence born to alcoholic mothers. J Pediatr 1980;96:978.
231. Steinhausen HC, Nestler V, Spohr HL. Development and psychopathology of children with the fetal alcohol syndrome. J Dev Behav Pediatr 1982;3:49.
232. Church MW, Gerkin KP. Hearing disorders in children with fetal alcohol syndrome: findings from case reports. Pediatrics 1988;82:147.
233. Flint EF. Severe childhood deafness in Glasgow, 1965–1979. J Laryngol Otol 1983;97:421.
234. Thiringer K, Kankkunen A, Liden G, et al. Perinatal risk factors in the etiology of hearing loss in preschool children. Dev Med Child Neurol 1984;26:799.
235. Aronson M, Kyllerman M, Sabel KG, et al. Children of alcoholic mothers (developmental, perceptual and behavioral characteristics as compared to matched controls). Acta Paediatr Scand 1985;74:27.
236. Abel EL. Marijuana, the first twelve thousand years. New York: Plenum Press, 1980
237. Marijuana and Health. Report of a study by the Committee of the Institute of Medicine, Division of Health Sciences Policy. Washington, DC: National Academy Press, 1982.
238. Day NL, Richardson, GA. Prenatal marijuana use: epidemiology, methodologic issues, and infant outcome. Clin Perinatol 1991;18:77.
239. Fried PA, Watkinson B, Grant A, et al. Changing patterns of soft drug use during pregnancy: a prospective study. Drug Alcohol Depend 1980;6:323.
240. Tennes K, Avitable N, Blackard C, et al. Marijuana: prenatal and postnatal exposure in the human. NIDA Research Monograph Series 1985;59:48.
241. Kline J, Stein Z, Hutzler M. Cigarettes, alcohol and marijuana: varying associations with birth weight. Int J Epidemiol 1987;16:44.
242. Zuckerman B, Frank D, Hingson R, et al. Effects of maternal marijuana and cocaine use on fetal growth. N Engl J Med 1989;320:762.
243. Greenland S, Richwalds GA, Honda GD. The effects of marijuana use during pregnancy: II. A study in a low risk home-delivery population. Drug Alcohol Depend 1983;11:359.
244. Dewey WL. Cannabinoid pharmacology. Pharmacol Rev 1986;38:151.
245. Martin BR. Cellular effects of cannabinoids. Pharmacol Rev 1986;38:45.
246. Harbison RD, Mantilla-Plata B. Prenatal, toxicity, maternal distribution and placental transfer of tetrahydrocannabinol. J Pharmacol Exp Ther 1972;180:446.
247. Abel EL, Rockwood GA, Riley EP. The effects of early marijuana exposure. In: Riley EP, Vorhees CV, eds. Handbook of behavioral teratology. New York: Plenum Press, 1986:267.
248. Ostrea EM, Subramanian MG, Abel EL. Placental transfer of cannabinoids in humans: comparison between meconium, maternal and cord blood sera. In: Chesner G, Consroe P, Musty R, eds. Marijuana: an international research report: proceedings of the Melbourne Symposium on Cannabis. Series 7. Canberra: Australian Government Publishing Service, 1987:103.
249. Fried PA, Buckingham M, Von Kulmiz P. Marijuana use during pregnancy and perinatal risk factors. Am J Obstet Gynecol 1983;144:22.
250. Fried PA, Watkinson B, Willan A. Marijuana use during pregnancy and decreased length of gestation. Am J Obstet Gynecol 1984;150:23.
251. Gibson GT, Baghurst PA, Colley DP. Maternal alcohol, tobacco and cannabis consumption and the outcome of pregnancy. Aust N Z J Obstet Gynaecol 1983;23:15.
252. Linn S, Schoenbaum S, Monson R, et al. The association of marijuana use with outcome of pregnancy. Am J Public Health 1983;73:1161.
253. O'Connell CM, Fried PA. An investigation of prenatal cannabis exposure and minor physical anomalies in a low risk population. Neurotoxicol Teratol 1984;6:345.
254. Qazi QH, Mariano E, Milman DH, et al. Abnormalities in offspring associated with prenatal marijuana exposure. Dev Pharmacol Ther 1985;8:141.
255. Hutchings DE, Morgan B, Brake SC, et al. Delta-9-tetrahydrocannabinol during pregnancy in the rat: I. Differential effects on maternal nutrition, embryotoxicity and growth in the offspring. Neurotoxicol Teratol 1987;9:39.
256. Morgan B, Brake SC, Hutchings DE, et al. Delta-9-tetrahydrocannabinol during pregnancy in the rat: effects on development of RNA, DNA, and protein in offspring brain. Pharmacol Biochem Behav 1988;31:365.
257. Hutchings DE, Dow-Edwards D. Animal models of opiate, cocaine and cannabis use. Clin Perinatol 1991;18:1.
258. Fried PA. Marijuana use during pregnancy: consequences for the offspring. Semin Perinatol 1991;15:280.
259. Scher MS, Richardson GA, Coble PA, et al. The effects of prenatal alcohol and marijuana exposure: disturbances in neonatal sleep cycling and arousal. Pediatr Res 1988;24:101.
260. Hayes JS, Dreher MC, Nugent JK. Newborn outcomes with maternal marihuana use in Jamaican women. Pediatric Nursing 1988;14:107.
261. Taylor P. Agents acting at the neuromuscular junction and autonomic ganglia: nicotine. In: Gilman A, Goodman LS, Rall TW, et al, eds. Goodman and Gilman's the pharmacologic basis of therapeutics. 8th ed. New York: Pergamon Press, 1990:180.
262. Fingerhut LA, Kleinman JC, Kendrick JS. Smoking before, during and after pregnancy. Am J Public Health 1990;80:541.
263. Kline J, Stein ZA, Susser M. Smoking as a risk factor for spontaneous abortion. N Engl J Med 1977;297:793.
264. Brown HL, Miller JM, Khawli O, et al. Premature placental calcification in maternal cigarette smokers. Obstet Gynecol 1988;71:914.
265. Lehtovirta P, Forss M. The acute effect of smoking on intervillous blood flow of the placenta. Br J Obstet Gynaecol 1978; 85:729.
266. Naeye RL, Harkness WL, Utts J. Abruptio placentae and perinatal death: a prospective study. Am J Obstet Gynecol 1977;128,740.
267. Garn SM, Johnson M, Ridella SA, et al. Effects of maternal cigarette smoking on Apgar scores. Am J Dis Child 1981; 135:503.
268. Hingson R, Gould JR, Morelock S, et al. Maternal cigarette smoking, psychoactive substance use and infant Apgar scores. Am J Obstet Gynecol 1982;144:959.
269. Meyer MB, Tonascia JA. Maternal smoking, pregnancy complications, and perinatal mortality. Am J Obstet Gynecol 1977; 128:494.
270. Wen SW, Goldenberg RL, Cutter GR, et al. Smoking, maternal age, fetal growth, and gestational age at delivery. Am J Obstet Gynecol 1990;162:53.
271. Bergman AB, Wiesner LA. Relationship of passive cigarette smoking to sudden infant death syndrome. Pediatrics 1976;58:665.
272. Kleinman JC, Pierre MB, Madans JS, et al. The effects of maternal smoking on fetal and infant mortality. Am J Epidemiol 1988;127:274.
273. Cnattingius S, Haglund B, Meirik O. Cigarette smoking as risk factor for late fetal and early neonatal death. Br Med J 1988;297:258.

274. Miller HC, Hassanein K. Maternal smoking and fetal growth of full term infants. Pediatr Res 1974;8:960.
275. MacArthur C, Knox EG. Smoking in pregnancy: effects of stopping at different stages. Br J Obstet Gynaecol 1988;95:551.
276. Abel EL. Marijuana, tobacco, alcohol and reproduction. Boca Raton, FL: CRC Press, 1983.
277. Haddow JE, Knight GJ, Palomaki GE, et al. Cigarette consumption and serum cotinine in relation to birth weight. Br J Obstet Gynaecol 1987;94:678.
278. Harrison GG, Ranson RS, Vaugher YE. Association of maternal smoking with body composition of the newborn. Am J Clin Nutr 1983;38:757.
279. Fedick J, Alberman E, Goldstein H. Possible teratogenic effect of cigarette smoking. Nature 1971;231:530.
280. Heinonen OP. Risk factors for congenital heart disease: a prospective study. In: Kelly S, Hook EB, Janerich DT, eds. Birth defects: risks and consequences. New York: Academic Press, 1976:221.
281. Saxton DW. The behavior of infants whose mothers smoke in pregnancy. Early Hum Dev 1978;2:363.
282. Martin JC, Martin DC, Lund C. Maternal alcohol ingestion and cigarette smoking and their effect upon newborn conditioning. Alcoholism: Clinical and Experimental Research 1973;1:243.
283. Landesman-Dwyer S, Keller LS, Streissguth AP. Naturalistic observations of newborns: effects of maternal alcohol intake. Alcoholism: Clinical and Experimental Research 1978;2:171.
284. Woodson EM, DaCosta P, Woodson RH. Maternal smoking and newborn behavior. Presented at the International Conference on Infant Studies, New Haven, Connecticut, 1980.
285. Butler NR, Goldstein H. Smoking in pregnancy and subsequent child development. Br Med J 1973;4:573.
286. Dunn HG, McBurney AK, Ingram S, et al. Maternal cigarette smoking during pregnancy and the child's subsequent development: II. Neurological and intellectual maturation to the age of 6.5 years. Can J Public Health 1977;68:43.
287. Zuckerman B. Marijuana and cigarette smoking during pregnancy: neonatal effects. In: Chasnoff IJ, ed. Drugs, alcohol, pregnancy and parenting. Lancaster, UK: Kluwer Academic Publishers, 1988:73.
288. Johnston M, Evans V, Baigel S. Phencyclidine. Br J Anaesth 1959;31:433.
289. Marwah J, Pitts DK. Psychopharmacology of phencyclidine. NIDA Research Monograph Series 1986;64:127.
290. Fico TA, Vanderwende C. Phencyclidine during pregnancy: behavioral and neurochemical effects in the offspring. Ann NY Acad Sci 1989;562:319.
291. McCarron M. Phencyclidine intoxication. NIDA Research Monograph Series 1986;64:209.
292. Cummings AJ. Transplacental disposition of phencyclidine in the pig. Xenobiotica 1979;9:447.
293. Cooper JE, Cummings AJ, Jones H. The placental transfer of phencyclidine in the pig, plasma levels in the sow and its piglets. J Physiol 1977;267:17.
294. Nicholas JM, Lipshitz J, Schreiber E. Phencyclidine: its transfer across the placenta as well as into breast milk. Am J Obstet Gynecol 1982;143:143.
295. Kaufman KR, Petrucha RA, Pitts FN, et al. Phencyclidine in umbilical cord blood: preliminary data. Am J Psychiatry 1983;140:450.
296. Aniline O, Pitts FN. Phencyclidine (PCP): a review and perspectives. Crit Rev Toxicol 1982;10:145.
297. Domino ET, Wilson AE. Effects of urine acidification on plasma and urine phencyclidine levels in overdosage. Clin Pharmacol Ther 1977;22:421.
298. Blaustein MP, Bartschat DK, Sorensen RG. Phencyclidine (PCP) selectively blocks certain presynaptic potassium channels. NIDA Research Monograph Series 1986;64:37.
299. Crider R. Phencyclidine: changing abuse patterns. NIDA Research Monograph Series 1986;64:163.
300. Golden NL, Kuhnert BR, Sokol RJ, et al. Phencyclidine use during pregnancy. Am J Obstet Gynecol 1984;148:254.
301. Golden NL, Kuhnert BR, Sokol RJ, et al. Neonatal manifestations of maternal phencyclidine exposure. J Perinat Med 1987; 15:185.
302. Chasnoff IJ, Burns WJ, Hatcher RP, et al. Phencyclidine: effects on the fetus and neonate. Dev Pharmacol Ther 1983;6: 404.
303. Howard J, Kropenske V, Tyler R. The long-term effects on neurodevelopment in infants exposed prenatally to PCP. NIDA Research Monograph Series 1986;64:237.
304. Tabor BL, Smith-Wallace T, Yonekura ML. Perinatal outcome associated with PCP versus cocaine use. Am J Drug Alcohol Abuse 1990;16:337.
305. Strauss AA, Modanlou D, Bosu SK. Neonatal manifestations of maternal phencyclidine (PCP) abuse. Pediatrics 1981; 68:550.
306. Hoffman BB, Lefkowitz RJ. Catecholamines and sympathomimetics. In: Gilman AG, Rall TW, Nies AS, et al, eds. Goodman and Gilman's the pharmacological basis of therapeutics. 8th ed. New York: Pergamon Press, 1990:187.
307. Little BB, Snell LM, Gilstrap LC III. Methamphetamine abuse during pregnancy: outcome and fetal effects. Obstet Gynecol 1988;72:541.
308. Milkovich L, Van den Berg BJ. Effects of antenatal exposure to anorectic drugs. Am J Obstet Gynecol 1977;129:637.
309. Oro AS, Dixon SD. Perinatal cocaine and methamphetamine exposure: maternal and neonatal correlates. J Pediatr 1987; 111:571.
310. Dixon SD. Effects of transplacental exposure to cocaine and methamphetamine on the neonate. West J Med 1989;150: 436.
311. Ramer CM. The case history of an infant born to an amphetamine-addicted mother. Clin Pediatr 1974;13:596.
312. Eriksson M, Larsson G, Winbladh B, et al. The influence of amphetamine addiction on pregnancy and the newborn infant. Acta Paediatr Scand 1978;67:95.
313. Billing L, Eriksson M, Steneroth G, et al. Pre-school children of amphetamine-addicted mothers: I. Somatic and psychomotor development. Acta Paediatr Scand 1985;74:179.
314. Eriksson M, Billing L, Steneroth G, et al. Health and development of 8 year-old children whose mother abused amphetamines during pregnancy. Acta Paediatr Scand 1989;78:944.
315. Kandall SR, Gartner LM. Late presentation of drug withdrawal symptoms in newborns. Am J Dis Child 1974;127:58.
316. Chasnoff IJ. Drug use and women: establishing a standard of care. Ann NY Acad Sci 1989;562:208.
317. Khavari K, Farber P. A profile instrument for the quantification and assessment of alcohol consumption. J Stud Alcohol 1978;39:1525.
318. Khavari KA, Douglass FM. The drug use profile (DUP): an instrument for clinical and research evaluations for drug use patterns. Drug Alcohol Depend 1981;8:119.
319. Cahalan D, Cisin I, Crossley H. American drinking practices. Monograph No. 6. New Brunswick, NJ: Rutgers Center of Alcohol Studies, 1969.
320. Ostrea EM Jr, Welch RR. Detection of prenatal drug exposure in the pregnant woman and her newborn infant. Clin Perinatol 1991;18:629.
321. Schonberg SK, Blasinsky M, eds. Substance abuse: a guide for health professionals. American Academy of Pediatrics and Center for Advanced Health Studies, 1988:48.

322. Ostrea EM, Martier S, Welch R, et al. Sensitivity of meconium drug screen in detecting intrauterine drug exposure of infants. Pediatr Res 1990;27:219 A.
323. Ostrea EM, Brady MJ, Parks PM, et al. Drug screening of meconium in infants of drug dependent mothers: an alternative to urine testing. J Pediatr 1989;115:474.
324. Halstead AC, Godolphin W, Lockitch G, et al. Timing of specimens is crucial in urine screening of drug dependent mothers and infants. Clin Biochem 1988;21:59.
325. Osterloh JD, Lee BL. Urine drug screening in mothers and infants. Am J Dis Child 1989;143:791.
326. Hicks, JM, Morales A, Soldin SJ. Drugs of abuse in a pediatric outpatient population. Clin Chem 1990;36:1256.
327. Ostrea EM, Lynn SN, Wayne RH, et al. Tissue distribution of morphine in the newborns of addicted monkeys and humans. Dev Pharmacol Ther 1980;1:163.
328. Welch RR, Martier SS, Ager JW, et al. Radioimmunoassay of hair is a valid technique for determining maternal cocaine abuse. Substance Abuse 1990.
329. Ostrea EM Jr, Yee H, Thrasher S, et al. Adaptation of the meconium test to mass drug screening in the neonate. J Pediatr 1993;122:152.
330. Ostrea EM Jr. Selection criteria for drug screening of infants by the meconium test in a high risk, urban, obstetric population. [abstract] Clin Res 1991;39:717A.
331. Maynard EC, Amuroso LP, Oh W. Meconium for drug testing. Am J Dis Child 1991;145:650.
332. Callahan CM, Grant TM, Phipps BS, et al. Measurement of gestational cocaine exposure: sensitivity of newborn hair, meconium and urine. J Pediatr 1992;120:763.
333. Baumgartner A, Jones P, Black C. Detection of phencyclidine in hair. J Forensic Sci 1981;26:576.
334. Baumgartner A, Jones P, Baumgartner W, et al. Radioimmunoassay of hair for determining opiate abuse histories. J Nucl Med 1979;2:748.
335. Baumgartner W, Black C, Jones P, et al. Radioimmunoassay of cocaine in hair: a concise communication. J Nucl Med 1982;23:790.
336. Baumgartner A, Jones P, Black C. Detection of phencyclidine in hair. J Forensic Sci 1981;26:576.
337. Ishiyama I. Detection of basic drugs (methamphetamine, antidepressants and nicotine) from human hair. J Forensic Sci 1983;28:380.
338. Balabanova S, Homoki J. Determination of cocaine in human hair by gas chromatography/mass spectrometry. Z Rechtsmed 1987;98:235.
339. Marigo M, Tagliaro F, Poiesi C, et al. Determination of morphine in the hair of heroin addicts by high performance liquid chromatography with fluorimetric detection. J Anal Toxicol 1986;10:158.
340. Pelli B, Traldi P, Tagliaro F, et al. Collisional spectroscopy for unequivocal and rapid determination of morphine at ppb level in the hair of heroin addicts. Biomed Environ Mass Spectrom 1987;14:63.
341. Graham K, Koren G, Klein J, et al. Determination of gestational cocaine exposure by hair analysis. JAMA 1989;262: 3328.
342. Bailey DN. Drug screening in an unconventional matrix: hair analysis. JAMA 1989;262:3331.
343. Smith FP, Liu RH. Detection of cocaine metabolites in perspiration stain, menstrual bloodstain and hair. J Forensic Sci 1986;31:1269.
344. Smith FP. Detection of phenobarbital in bloodstains, semen, seminal stains, saliva stains, saliva, perspiration stains and hair. J Forensic Sci 1981;26:582.
345. Finnegan LP. Neonatal abstinence. In: Nelson NM, ed. Current therapy in neonatal perinatal medicine. Philadelphia: BC Decker, 1990:314.
346. Lipsitz PJ. A proposed narcotic withdrawal score for use with newborn infants. Clin Pediatr 1975;14:592.

Neonatology: Pathophysiology and Management of the Newborn, Fourth Edition,
edited by Gordon B. Avery, Mary Ann Fletcher, and Mhairi G. MacDonald.
J.B. Lippincott Company, Philadelphia © 1994.

chapter **58**

Anesthesia and Analgesia

JOHN H. ARNOLD
K. J. S. ANAND

Despite the widespread use of potent analgesic agents in adult patients and older children, it is remarkable that until recently systemic analgesia and sedation were rarely administered to neonates. An analysis of neonatal anesthetic practice published in 1985 revealed that only 23% of preterm infants undergoing patent ductus arteriosus ligation received adequate intraoperative anesthesia.[1] In a retrospective survey of opioid use in a single institution, only 14% of 933 neonates received opioid analgesia after a variety of surgical procedures.[2] Although adequate anesthesia and analgesia were not given to neonates in the past because of the belief that they could not feel pain, there is overwhelming evidence that pain perception and physiologic responses to stress occur in neonates of all gestational ages.[3] It is broadly accepted that anesthesia and analgesia in the neonatal population have important clinical and physiologic consequences and may have long-term psychologic impact. Control of the stress response in the perioperative period may improve the outcome of infants after cardiac surgery.[4,5]

As these data are assimilated and accepted, there is often a discrepancy between the growing understanding of neonatal pain and actual clinical practice. A survey of British pediatric anesthetists found that only 5% routinely prescribed systemic opioids to neonates postoperatively although 80% of the respondents believed that neonates feel pain.[6] There are probably several reasons for the lag in changing clinical practice to match current knowledge, but a crucial element may be the lack of standard guidelines for the use of drugs, doses, and schedules that can be applied to various clinical situations by the practitioner at the bedside.

This chapter reviews the rapidly developing field of neonatal anesthesia and analgesia, summarizes the relevant pharmacokinetic and pharmacodynamic data, and highlights practical considerations for the most commonly used agents.

PAIN PERCEPTION

In addition to the ethical arguments for preventing needless human suffering, the risks and benefits of using anesthesia and analgesia to prevent pain and stress must be physiologically evaluated. Pivotal aspects of this physiologic rationale are based on one question: Does the neonate feel pain?

Components of the pain system may be traced from sensory receptors in the skin to sensory areas in the cerebral cortex and used as a framework to study its development.[3] The density of nociceptive nerve endings in newborn skin, the labeling of specific proteins (*e.g.*, GAP-43) produced by axonal growth cones, the reflex activity and receptive fields of primary afferent neurons, and the development of synapses between primary afferents and interneurons in the dorsal horn of the spinal cord indicate the anatomic and functional maturity of the peripheral pain system during fetal life.[7,8] Cellular and subcellular organization in the dorsal horn, with maturation of primary afferent terminations, occur during later gestation and postnatally.[9,10] In the dorsal horn, various neurotransmitter and neuromodulator substances associated with pain (*e.g.*, substance P, somatostatin, calcitonin gene–related peptide (CGRP), vasoactive intestinal peptide, met-enkephalin, glutamate) appear during early gestation.[11]

Lack of myelination in neonatal nerves or central nerve tracts is offset completely by the shorter interneuronal and neuromuscular distances traveled by the impulse. Quantitative neuroanatomic data show that nociceptive nerve tracts in the spinal cord and CNS undergo complete myelination during the second and third trimesters of gestation.[3] Subcortical foci associated with nociception are characterized by a high density of opioid receptors during the middle of gestation, with a differential reduction in binding capacities during the third trimester.[12] Development of the fetal neocortex begins at 8 weeks of gestation, and by 20 weeks, each cortex has a full complement of 10^9 neurons. Arborization of dendritic processes in the cortical neurons is followed by synaptogenesis with incoming thalamocortical fibers by 24 to 26 weeks of gestation. Functional maturity of the cerebral cortex is suggested by fetal and neonatal electroencephalographic (EEG) patterns, cortical somatosensory evoked potentials, studies of regional cerebral metabolism, early behavioral development, and the specific behavioral responses of neonates to painful stimuli.[3,13]

Endorphinergic cells in the anterior pituitary are responsive to CRF stimulation *in vitro* and show increased β-endorphin production during fetal and neonatal life. Endogenous opioids and other hormones (*e.g.*, catecholamines, steroid hormones, glucagon, growth hormone) are secreted by the human fetus in response to stress, leading to catabolism and other complications.[5,14] Significant changes in cardiovascular parameters, transcutaneous partial pressure of oxygen (PO_2), and palmar sweating have been observed in neonates undergoing painful clinical procedures. These physiologic changes are closely associated with behavioral responses of newborns to pain. Neonatal behavioral responses are characterized by simple motor responses, precise changes in facial expression associated with pain, highly specific patterns of crying activity, and a variety of complex behavioral changes. These neonatal responses suggest integrated emotional and behavioral changes correlated with pain, and they are retained in memory long enough to modify subsequent behavior patterns.[3]

The surgical stress responses of neonates can be inhibited by potent anesthesia, as demonstrated by randomized trials of halothane anesthesia in term neonates, fentanyl anesthesia in preterm neonates, and sufentanil anesthesia in neonates undergoing cardiac surgery.[5,15,16] These results imply that the nociceptive stimuli during surgery are at least partially responsible for the marked stress responses of neonates and are prevented by the provision of adequate anesthesia. In these trials, the reduction in surgical stress responses was associated with significant improvements in clinical outcome, supporting the use of potent anesthetic agents for newborns undergoing surgery.

ANESTHESIA

Anesthesia is classically defined as a drug-induced state that includes analgesia, amnesia, and muscle relaxation. The provision of anesthesia to infants undergoing surgical procedures has undergone a remarkable transition coincident with the development of new intravenous agents and more sophisticated monitoring techniques. As recently as 1985, there was considerable debate about whether neonates feel pain, and sophisticated researchers advocated the use of minimal anesthesia in neonates undergoing surgical procedures, citing the dangers of anesthetic administration to this population.[17–19] Beginning with the landmark paper of Robinson and Gregory, practitioners of neonatal and pediatric anesthesia have proclaimed the importance of providing adequate anesthesia, particularly to ill preterm infants.[20,21] In modern anesthetic practice, adequate anesthetic depth and control of the neonatal stress response can be achieved without undue risk to the infant.

The appropriate anesthetic technique is dictated by the preoperative condition of the patient, the planned surgical procedure, and the skills of the anesthetist. The encounter between the anesthesiologist and the neonate usually occurs in the setting of a surgical emergency, and a general anesthetic with control of the airway is most often the technique of choice. General anesthesia is provided using a combination of inhaled and intravenous agents and muscle relaxants. The inhaled agents include an inorganic gas (*e.g.*, nitrous oxide) and the volatile liquids (*e.g.*, halothane, enflurane isoflurane). Delivery of potent inhaled agents by means of the respiratory system offers a reliable route of administration and excretion with the ability to rapidly alter anesthetic concentrations in the central nervous system.

INHALED ANESTHETICS

Each of the inhaled anesthetic agents has unique effects on the cardiovascular, respiratory, and central nervous systems, which are not exhaustively reviewed here (Table 58-1). The volatile anesthetics produce dose-dependent decreases in mean arterial blood pressure, particularly in premature infants, due to direct myocardial depression and decreases in systemic vascular resistance due to exaggerated depression of the baroreceptor reflex.[22–24] Nitrous oxide produces minimal alterations in myocardial performance or systemic vascular resistance, due in part to direct stimulation of the sympathetic nervous sys-

TABLE 58–1
SYSTEMIC EFFECTS OF INHALED ANESTHETICS

	Myocardial Function	Heart Rate	Systemic Vascular Resistance	Cerebral Blood Flow
Halothane	− −	−	+/−	+ +
Enflurane	−	+	−	+
Isoflurane	−	+ +	− −	+/−*
N_2O	+/−	+/−	+/−	+/−

* In doses < 1.0 minimum alveolar concentration.
++, greatly increased; +, moderately increased; +/− no consistent effect; −, moderately decreased; − − greatly decreased.

tem.[25] However, if combined with a potent volatile agent or opioids, nitrous oxide significantly depresses myocardial contractility.[26] If ventilation is carefully controlled, nitrous oxide has insignificant effects on pulmonary vascular resistance.[27]

All inhaled agents increase the respiratory rate, reduce tidal volume and functional residual capacity, decrease the ventilatory responses to hypoxemia and hypercapnia, and decrease bronchial smooth muscle reactivity. These agents produce a dose-dependent increase in cerebral blood flow despite simultaneous depression of cerebral metabolic oxygen requirement. At high concentrations, isoflurane induces an isoelectric EEG pattern; this property is not shared by the other inhaled anesthetic agents.

Although halothane is most frequently associated with perioperative hepatic dysfunction, other inhaled agents and intravenous anesthetics may result in hepatic necrosis.[28] True halothane-induced hepatitis is a rare event, occurring in approximately 1 of 30,000 patients. It is seen most commonly after repeated administration and is probably mediated by an immune mechanism involving an intermediate oxidative metabolite.[29,30] The inhaled agents produce dose-related decreases in renal blood flow and urine output due to effects on cardiac output and systemic vascular resistance. Fluoride-induced nephrotoxicity is a potential complication of prolonged exposure to the fluorinated hydrocarbons (*e.g.*, enflurane, isoflurane), although it is of practical concern only during prolonged administration of enflurane.[31]

OPIOID ANESTHESIA

Morphine and the synthetic opioids have been a consistent adjunct to the volatile agents throughout the history of anesthesia. High-dose opioids have become the preferred anesthetic technique for cardiac surgical procedures in adults and children.[32,33] The virtues of opioids include minimal effects on myocardial performance, ablation of pulmonary vascular responses to nociceptive stimuli, and preservation of hypoxic pulmonary vasoconstriction.[34–36]

Because of their wide margin of safety in ill infants with congenital heart disease, opioid anesthesia is often effective in ill preterm infants with cardiopulmonary instability undergoing surgical stress. Fentanyl and sufentanil are the most popular agents due to their negligible effect on cardiovascular function, but if combined with other anesthetic agents, these opioids may be associated with significant hemodynamic instability. Morphine anesthesia may increase plasma histamine concentrations and decrease vascular resistance, and it is not recommended as a primary anesthetic for ill neonates.[37]

The elimination half-lives ($T_{1/2}\beta$) of the opioids are significantly prolonged in the neonate (Table 58-2) and may be further prolonged by any compromise of hepatic blood flow.[38–43] Prolonged postoperative respiratory depression may occur if these important pharmacokinetic variables are ignored in the perioperative period.

REGIONAL, NEURAXIAL, AND LOCAL ANESTHESIA

Regional anesthetic techniques have become increasingly popular in the pediatric and neonatal populations.[44] General anesthesia may be associated with an increased incidence of postoperative apnea in the preterm infant.[45] This may be a particularly difficult issue in the day-surgery setting, where former preterm neonates commonly present for minor surgical procedures (*e.g.*, circumcision, herniorrhaphy). It is in this population that regional or local anesthetic techniques may be particularly advantageous; preliminary experience suggests that the use of spinal anes-

TABLE 58–2
ELIMINATION HALF-LIVES OF OPIOIDS

		$T_{1/2}\beta$ (hours)	
Opioid	Relative dose	Neonate	Child
Morphine	0.1 mg	6.8	2.2
Fentanyl	1–5 μg	4.2	3.5
Sufentanil	0.2–1 μg	12.3	2.3
Alfentanil	5–25 μg	8.8	1.4

thesia may reduce the risk of postoperative apnea in former preterm infants.[46]

Spinal anesthesia consists of injection of an anesthetic agent into the subarachnoid space. The technique is easy to perform and safe.[47] The most frequent local anesthetic agents are hyperbaric lidocaine, tetracaine, and bupivacaine. Compared with older children and adults, infants and toddlers require higher doses of local anesthetic and demonstrate a shorter duration of effect. Side-effects of spinal anesthesia, such as dural puncture headaches and hemodynamic compromise, are common in adults but surprisingly uncommon in infants or children.[47,48]

Epidural anesthesia consists of injection of an anesthetic agent into the potential space between the dura mater and the ligamentum flavum by a single injection or repeated injections through an epidural catheter. Although the epidural space can be approached at any level, for most infants, a lumbar or caudal epidural blockade is used. Caudal epidural blockade with bupivacaine is used most frequently for postoperative pain relief after lower abdominal and lower extremity procedures. Caudal anesthesia has been sufficient as the sole anesthetic technique for lower abdominal procedures.[49] Caudal epidural blockade may be used in combination with general anesthesia in infants during abdominal procedures. Rarely, complications result from improper placement of the needle and injection of the anesthetic agent into a vein, the dura, the subarachnoid space, or sacral marrow.

Local anesthetics may be used to block peripheral nerves in infants undergoing limited surgical procedures (*e.g.*, orchiopexy, herniorrhaphy, circumcision). These techniques are simple to perform, have limited complications, and significantly decrease the need for postoperative analgesia.[50–52]

Local anesthetic toxicity is manifested by effects on the cardiovascular system (*e.g.*, myocardial depression, arrhythmias) and the central nervous system (*e.g.*, delirium, seizures).[53,54] In premature infants, the subtle behavioral changes that precede cardiovascular collapse and generalized seizures may be difficult to recognize. The reduced protein binding and prolonged elimination of local anesthetics in this population make the neonate susceptible to toxic effects at lower doses, decreasing the therapeutic index. Careful attention to total administered dose (particularly with field blocks) and monitoring of cardiovascular parameters during the administration of any local anesthetic are essential.

ANALGESIA

OPIOIDS

The provision of adequate analgesia for painful diseases and procedures should be of utmost concern to the neonatologist.[55] Despite widespread misgivings about their potential side-effects, systemic therapy with opioid analgesics remains the mainstay of treatment for severe pain in neonates. The administration of opioids produces profound analgesia and sedation through specific activity on μ_1, δ, and other opioid receptors in the brain and spinal cord.[56]

The dosage and mode of administration of opioids should be carefully titrated to avoid undertreatment of pain or oversedation (Fig. 58-1). Continuous intravenous infusion of opioids provides an effective alternative to intermittent intravenous doses, with constant blood levels and minimal fluctuations in analgesia. All opioids have prolonged half-lives in neonates (see Table 58-2), and continuous infusions can result

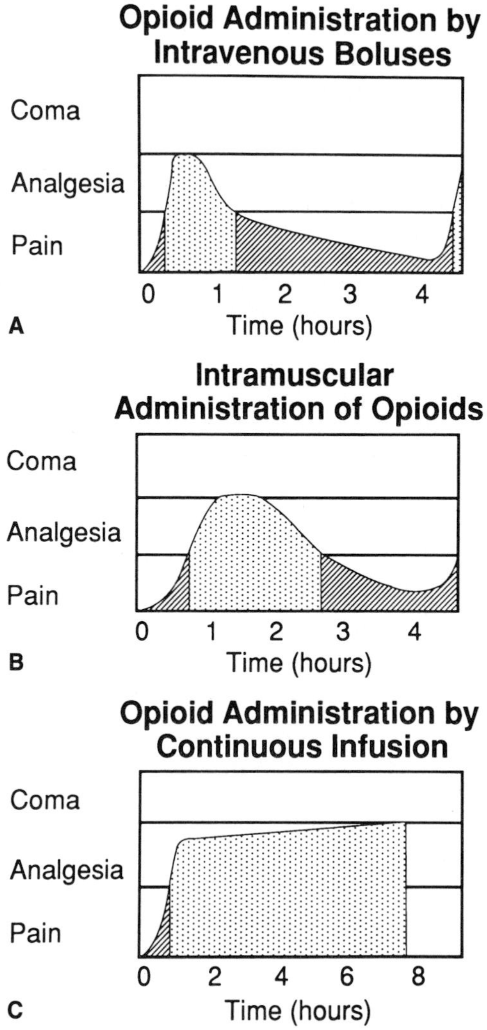

FIG. 58–1. Modes of opioid administration. **(A)** Patients given intermittent intravenous boluses every 4 hours experience deep sedative effects at peak levels after a dose, with prolonged periods of pain between doses. **(B)** Patients given intramuscular injections experience less fluctuation in opioid effects but undergo alternate periods of pain and analgesia. **(C)** Patients receiving continuous infusions of opioids experience constant analgesia but are at risk for a slow build-up in plasma levels resulting in sedation or toxicity. (Adapted from Berde CB. Pediatric postoperative pain management. Pediatr Clin North Am 1989;36:926.)

in a slow accumulation of the drug over time, with high blood levels that may not be considered or detected immediately. Despite this disadvantage, continuous intravenous infusion is ideal for providing a constant level of analgesia if appropriate precautions are observed.

Alternative modes of administration are rarely indicated in neonates. Subcutaneous morphine or transdermal fentanyl are not routinely used in neonates, because precise documentation of their efficacy and safety is not available. The transdermal route may be an attractive future alternative to intravenous infusions in premature neonates, particularly because the permeability of preterm skin is 10^2 to 10^3 times greater than the skin of term neonates.[57] Oral or rectal opioids can be used in the neonate, but only if the same close monitoring provided for intravenous opioid analgesia can be given to these patients. The oral bioavailability of commonly used opioids is listed in Table 58-3, although these data have been derived mostly from older children and adults. The pharmacokinetics of oral opioids have not been studied in neonates, but the onset and duration of action are likely to be delayed, and close monitoring should continue for at least 24 hours after the last dose.

Opioid side-effects include respiratory depression, tolerance and dependence, alterations in chest wall compliance, decreased gastrointestinal motility, and nausea. Exogenously administered opioids may alter endogenous opioid receptor physiology and possibly influence subsequent behavioral development.[12,58,59] However, these agents are probably the most suitable and effective analgesics currently available for treatment of severe pain in neonates.

All opioids produce dose-related respiratory depression characterized by decreased ventilatory and behavioral responses to hypoxemia and hypercarbia. The CO_2 response curve is displaced to the right and resting PCO_2 rises. Clinically, the respiratory rate decreases with an incomplete compensatory increase in tidal volume. It is not widely appreciated that standard doses of morphine (0.1 mg/kg) almost abolish the ventilatory response to hypoxemia. In patients with airway obstruction or atelectasis after surgery, blunting of hypoxic drive can lead to dangerous hypoventilation. Opioid-induced respiratory depression can be reversed with naloxone, but the effect of this drug diminishes within 30 minutes and repeated dosing may be required, particularly after the use of morphine or methadone.[60] It was long believed that newborn infants were more prone to opioid-induced respiratory depression than older children or adults, perhaps because of an immature blood–brain barrier.[61] However, recent data suggest that opioid-induced apnea is less common in neonates than in older infants and children at similar plasma concentrations.[62,63]

Tolerance occurs if there is a reduction in the clinical effects of a drug with repeated administration. The rate of development of tolerance to the analgesic effects of opioids is extremely variable; there is evidence that tolerance may develop more rapidly in the absence of nociceptive stimulation.[64] Dependence is the requirement for continued drug administration to prevent withdrawal symptoms, including agitation, dysphoria, tachycardia, tachypnea, piloerection, nasal congestion, temperature instability, and feeding intolerance. Tolerance and dependence have been

TABLE 58–3
RECOMMENDED DOSAGES AND ORAL–PARENTERAL RATIOS FOR OPIOIDS

Drug	Routes of Administration	Parenteral Dosage (mg/kg)	Frequency (Parenteral)	Oral–Parenteral Ratio	Frequency (Oral/Rectal)
Morphine	IM, IV,* SQ, PO, PR, neuraxial†	0.05–0.2	q 1–2 h IV q 2–4 h IM or SQ	3–6	q 4–6 h‡ q 8–12 h§
Meperidine	IM, IV, SQ, PO	0.5–1.5	q 1–2 h IV q 2–4 h IM or SQ	4	q 4–6 h
Codeine	IM, IV,* SQ, PO	0.5–1.0	q 2–4 h	1.5–2	q 4–6 h
Hydromorphone	IM, IV, SQ, PO, PR	0.02–0.04	q 2–4 h	2–4	q 4–6 h PO q 6–8 h PR
Methadone	IM, IV, SQ, PO	0.05–0.2	q 12–24 h	2	q 24 h
Fentanyl	IM, IV, TM/TD,‖ neuraxial†	0.001–0.005	q 1–2 h		

* IV administration may be associated with significant histamine release and possible hypotension.

† Neuraxial (*i.e.*, epidural, subarachnoid) administration can be performed only by qualified and experienced anesthesiologists.

‡ Pertains to regular oral preparations (*e.g.*, MSIR, Roxanal; tablets and oral solutions).

§ Pertains to slow-release oral or rectal preparations (*e.g.*, MS Contin, Duramorph, Roxanol SR).

‖ Transmucosal/transdermal (TM/TD) preparations have not been standardized for use in full-term or preterm neonates.

described in neonatal and pediatric patients during the therapeutic use of opioids.[65–68] Although tolerance to opioids may appear to develop more rapidly in neonates than at other ages, it is likely that tolerance to the sedative and cardiovascular effects of opioids may precede a tolerance to their analgesic effects.[69] The development of physical dependence is quite variable, and withdrawal symptoms have been observed in infants for whom opioid administration was abruptly discontinued after periods of administration as short as 5 days.[67] Fear of precipitating the abstinence syndrome should not inhibit the appropriate administration of opioids, because withdrawal symptoms can be effectively managed by gradually tapering the opioid dosage over 5 to 7 days (Fig. 58-2).

Dependence is a set of physiologic responses that should be differentiated from addiction, which is a behavioral syndrome of compulsive drug seeking. Addiction is extremely rare in patients of all ages receiving opioids for pain or sedation, and fear of addiction should not affect the appropriate treatment of acute pain or agitation in neonatal intensive care.

Opioids increase airway resistance, and there is much debate about the effect of histamine release on bronchial smooth muscle and whether histamine-releasing agents such as morphine are contraindicated in patients with reactive airway disease.[70] Although intravenous morphine releases greater amounts of histamine than fentanyl, precipitation of bronchospasm has not been reported after the administration of morphine.[37] Intravenous morphine has frequently been employed in patients with severe asthma requiring mechanical ventilation based on evidence that it might inhibit bronchoconstriction and mucous hypersecretion.[71–73]

Chest wall rigidity is a well-described complication of opioid administration and has been documented in patients receiving large doses of fentanyl, sufentanil, or alfentantil.[26,74,75] The administration of 30 μg/kg of fentanyl in tracheostomized patients produced a minor increase in total lung compliance, suggesting that inability to maintain a mask airway during fentanyl administration is due to supraglottic obstruction and not chest wall rigidity.[76,77] Rigidity has occurred at an average dose of 15 to 17 μg/kg of fentanyl.[76,77] There are no data available in term or preterm neonates receiving fentanyl, although clinical experience suggests that chest wall rigidity may occur at lower opioid doses in the neonate. The mechanism that mediates this phenomenon may involve μ_1-opioid receptor modulation of GABA pathways in the spinal cord. Rigidity on induction of anesthesia is avoided by pretreatment with a subrelaxant dose of pancuronium (0.01–0.02 mg/kg) and by slow intravenous infusion of the opioid.[74,78,79]

All opioids delay gastric emptying, decrease intestinal motility, produce nausea by direct stimulation of the chemoreceptor trigger zone, and increase the common bile duct pressure. Impaired absorption of enteral nutrients is undesirable in neonates, and opiate-induced ileus may increase the risk of regurgitation and aspiration of gastric contents. One case report described a newborn given morphine who developed a reversible and nonobstructive dilation of the common hepatic duct that resolved after morphine was discontinued.[80] Although such side-effects are mediated by means of μ_2-opioid receptors, they may occur with high doses of opioids devoid of μ_2-activity (*e.g.*, fentanyl) as a result of nonspecific effects on all opioid receptors.

NONOPIOID AGENTS

There are many nonopioid agents available for the treatment of mild pain or use as adjuvants for decreasing the doses and potential side-effects of opioid drugs. Various other analgesic agents can be used systemically for providing sedation or in combination with regional and topical analgesia to produce effec-

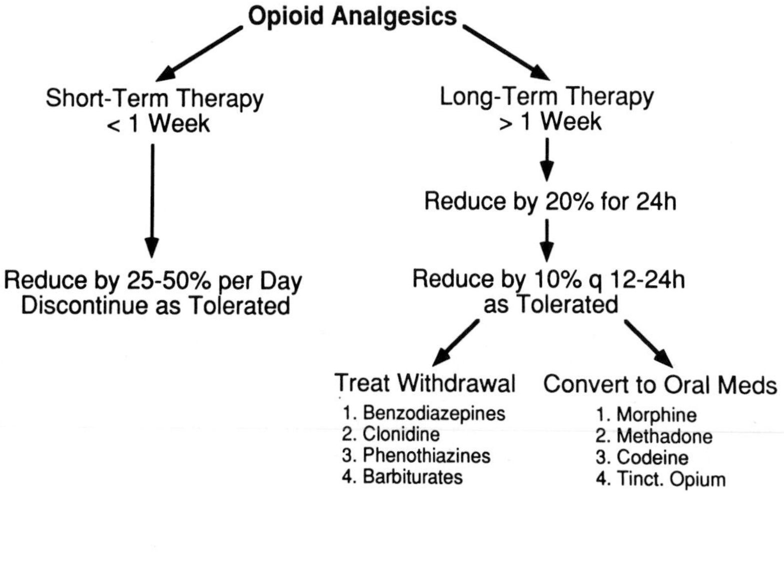

FIG. 58–2. Suggested algorithm for weaning a patient from opioid analgesics after short-term and long-term therapy. These pharmacologic approaches can be applied in conjunction with nonpharmacologic therapies to decrease the duration of therapy for the opioid abstinence syndrome.

tive analgesia while minimizing the side-effects of any single agent.

ACETAMINOPHEN

Acetaminophen (*N*-acetyl-*p*-aminophenol) is used commonly in all age groups as an antipyretic and analgesic. Its use in neonates has been limited by misconceptions about its metabolism and excretion and about its potential for hepatotoxicity. Experimental data and clinical experience have supported the relative safety and analgesic efficacy of acetaminophen in newborn infants, without the significant side-effects on platelet aggregation, the ductus arteriosus, or the gastric mucosa, commonly seen with aspirin or other nonsteroidal antiinflammatory drugs (NSAIDs).[81]

The hepatic metabolism of acetaminophen occurs primarily by sulfation or glucuronidation, but a small fraction is oxidized by the cytochrome P450 mixed-function oxidase system into an arene compound (*i.e.*, a reactive metabolite), which is conjugated with glutathione before excretion.[82,83] In acute toxicity, the hepatic stores of glutathione are depleted rapidly, and this reactive metabolite binds irreversibly to membrane proteins, leading to liver cell necrosis. In the newborn or fetal liver, this metabolic pathway is seven to ten times slower than in the adult liver and occurs well after the development of glutathione synthesis, mediating a protective effect in fetal hepatocytes.[84] These experimental data have been substantiated by the absence of hepatic dysfunction in clinical reports of neonatal poisoning with acetaminophen.[85,86] The clinical use of acetaminophen in term or preterm neonates should not be overly restrained by concerns about its potential hepatotoxicity.

Acetaminophen has many potential advantages as an analgesic in neonates. It has approximately the same analgesic efficacy as 0.5 to 1.0 mg/kg of codeine, and the analgesia is additive to that provided by opioids. It produces no respiratory depression, and tolerance to acetaminophen-induced analgesia has not been reported. It can be given rectally in doses of 20 to 25 mg/kg, avoiding the need for intravenous lines in infants who cannot be given oral medications.

NONSTEROIDAL ANTIINFLAMMATORY DRUGS

The NSAIDs are a group of drugs with many actions, including potent analgesic and antiinflammatory properties. The antiinflammatory effects are mediated through inhibition of prostaglandin synthesis by means of the cyclooxygenase pathway. Several NSAIDs have been used in pediatric patients, although data pertaining to neonates is scarce and comes from uncontrolled clinical reports.[87] Indomethacin and ibuprofen are the most commonly prescribed NSAIDs, but drugs such as ketorolac tromethamine, Tolectin, and Naprosyn are being used with increasing frequency.

The toxicity of NSAIDs limits their potency and clinical usefulness as analgesics.[88] Major toxicity is related to gastrointestinal bleeding, hepatotoxicity, blood dyscrasias, decreased renal and splanchnic perfusion, and severe skin reactions. Because of their chemical diversity, adverse reactions to a particular NSAID does not predict similar reactions to other NSAIDs. Significant advantages include the low incidence of side-effects in judicious analgesic doses (Table 58-4), the absence of respiratory depression or sedative effects, the relatively long duration of analgesia, and the lack of tolerance or potential for abuse.

SEDATION

The goals of sedation in the intensive care unit include analgesia for painful diseases and procedures and compliance with controlled ventilation and routine care. The ideal agent would not have hemodynamic or pulmonary side-effects and would not be associated with the production or accumulation of toxic metabolites. It would have a short duration of action and a high therapeutic index. The wide variety of medications and combinations of agents that have been employed suggests that no single agent meets this ideal standard. Opioids have become exceeding popular due to their relatively high toxic–therapeutic ratio, reported lack of side-effects, and their potent analgesic properties. Although opioids are considered the mainstay of sedation in the intensive care

TABLE 58–4
RECOMMENDED DOSES FOR NONSTEROIDAL ANTIINFLAMMATORY DRUGS

Drug	Dosage (mg/kg)	Routes of Administration	Frequency
Acetaminophen	10–20	PO, PR	q 4–6 h
Aspirin	10–15	PO	q 4 h
Choline-magnesium trisalicylate	10–15	PO	q 6–8 h
Ibuprofen	5–15	PO, PR	q 6–8 h
Naprosyn	5–7	PO	q 8–12 h
Tolectin	5–7	PO	q 8–12 h
Ketorolac tromethamine	0.3–0.6	PO, IM, IV	q 6–8 h

setting, tolerance to their sedating effects may occur rapidly, and adequate sedation for prolonged periods can be ensured only by administration of adjuvant sedative agents.[67,89]

BENZODIAZEPINES

The benzodiazepines have a variety of desirable clinical effects that include hypnosis, anxiolysis, anticonvulsant activity, anterograde amnesia, and muscle relaxation. The amnestic properties of benzodiazepines may be affected by the clinical status of the patient before administration, and in the presence of a painful stimulus, the benzodiazepines may produce hyperalgesia and agitation.[90–92] These problems usually do not occur if benzodiazepines are combined with opioids.

Benzodiazepines act on specific receptors, located mainly in the cerebral cortex, hypothalamus, cerebellum, corpus striatum, and medulla oblongata, that are coupled to GABA receptors by means of a common chloride channel in synaptic membranes.[93] Early pharmacokinetic data showed that the half-life of diazepam and its active metabolites was markedly prolonged in neonates.[94] Diazepam is used commonly for sedation in neonates, with doses of 0.1 to 0.3 mg/kg given every 4 to 6 hours. Doses as high as 50 mg/kg/day have been used to treat neonatal tetanus, with a low incidence of side-effects.[95] Diazepam has no analgesic effects, and it causes respiratory depression and mild hypotension, both of which are potentiated by opioids and other sedatives. Prolonged use may produce tolerance and withdrawal. In preterm neonates, doses as high as 0.5 mg/kg were associated with cardiovascular stability and no alteration in cerebral blood flow.[96]

Lorazepam is five to ten times more potent than diazepam, and in doses of 0.05 to 0.1 mg/kg, therapeutic levels may persist for 24 to 48 hours. Oral administration results in reliable absorption, with maximal plasma concentrations in 2 to 4 hours. Although lorazepam is water insoluble combined with an organic solvent, it is suitable for intramuscular or intravenous injection and causes much less tissue irritation than diazepam.[97] Lorazepam is glucuronidated to form inactive metabolites; its elimination half-life is 10 to 20 hours, but clinical effects may be prolonged because of its pharmacodynamic differences from the other benzodiazepines. The cardiovascular and respiratory effects of lorazepam are similar to those of diazepam. Lorazepam should be used judiciously for sedation in the intensive care setting because of prolonged effects on mental status and respiratory drive.

Midazolam, a water-soluble and shorter-acting benzodiazepine, has been used in neonates requiring sedation, alone or combined with opioid analgesics such as fentanyl. Loading doses of 0.2 mg/kg and continuous infusions of 0.4 μg/kg/minute of midazolam were used in patients weighing as little as 3 kg and provided good sedation without any apparent adverse effects.[98] At the benzodiazepine receptor, midazolam has twice the binding affinity of diazepam and inhibits GABA reuptake. The pharmacokinetics of midazolam in neonates are characterized by rapid redistribution, a plasma clearance of 6.9 mL/kg/minute and an elimination half-life of 6.5 hours, which is significantly longer than the elimination half-life reported for older infants and children.[99,100]

After prolonged intravenous therapy with midazolam, a withdrawal syndrome characterized by agitation, poor visual tracking, constant choreoathetoid and dyskinetic movements of the face, tongue, and limbs, and depression of consciousness in infants has been described.[101–103] Midazolam may be used intermittently as premedication for specific invasive procedures in doses of 0.05 to 0.2 mg/kg or for short-term sedation by continuous infusion (<12 hours) at rates of 25 to 50 μg/kg/hour. The respiratory depression and hypotension caused by benzodiazepines are synergistic with the similar effects of potent opioids. Midazolam and fentanyl given by rapid intravenous injection may cause severe, life-threatening hypotension and cardiorespiratory arrest.[104] This combination should be used with extreme caution in neonates and only with close monitoring in an intensive care unit.

BARBITURATES

Phenobarbital has long been used as an anticonvulsant in newborns and children, although its routine use for sedation has been discouraged because of several drawbacks. Phenobarbital has hyperalgesic effects and may increase the requirement for analgesia, and rapid tolerance to its sedative action invariably occurs.[105] It has a prolonged elimination half-life in neonates (5–6 days), and it may increase the risk of intraventricular hemorrhage in premature neonates.[106,107] Phenobarbital has no specific antagonist, and prolonged use is associated with microsomal induction of hepatic enzymes and with a withdrawal syndrome. Its advantages in neonates include increased bilirubin metabolism, relatively mild cardiovascular and respiratory depression, and familiarity with its usage in preterm and term neonates. In ventilated preterm neonates, the changes in mean arterial pressure and intracranial pressure associated with endotracheal suctioning were blunted with phenobarbital therapy.[108] A neonatal dose–response study found increasing degrees of sedation and feeding difficulties with increasing serum phenobarbital concentrations; these responses were greater in preterm neonates than in term neonates.[109] Loading doses of 5 to 10 mg/kg and maintenance doses of 2.5 mg/kg every 12 hours, given orally or intravenously, are generally used for sedation.

CHLORAL HYDRATE

Chloral hydrate is used frequently as a sedative in doses of 25 to 50 mg/kg or as a hypnotic in doses of 50 to 100 mg/kg for short procedures in neonates and for infants with chronic lung disease.[110] Higher doses may be required after repeated use in neonates because of the slow development of tolerance. The advantages of chloral hydrate include ease of administration (*e.g.*, oral syrup, rectal suppositories), although repeated doses can be irritating to the enteral mucosa); lack of respiratory depression; lack of other side-effects (*e.g.*, emesis, changes in vital signs or behavior) with usual therapeutic doses; and familiarity with its use in newborns and older infants.[111,112] However, an infant who received 165 mg/kg of chloral hydrate over 16 hours developed the toxic reactions of respiratory depression and lethargy.[113] Other reports have documented complications such as direct hyperbilirubinemia, decreased tidal volume, hypertriglyceridemia, acute laryngeal edema, and cardiac arrhythmias (*e.g.*, supraventricular tachycardia) in neonates and infants.[114–118]

The sedative action of chloral hydrate may be mediated by generalized neuronal depression, similar to other halogenated hydrocarbons. A precise mechanism of action is unknown, and there is no specific antagonist. The pharmacokinetics of chloral hydrate are not clearly defined in neonates; onset of clinical effects after oral dosage occurs at 30 minutes, and its duration of action is usually 2 to 4 hours, depending on the exact doses used.

KETAMINE

Ketamine is a dissociative anesthetic that has been used as an induction agent for anesthesia, an analgesic for conscious sedation, a premedication before induction of anesthesia, and a sedative for critically ill patients. There is a broad range of experience with this agent in older patients, but limited experience in infants and newborns.[119,120] Ketamine has been used to provide anesthesia in the spontaneously breathing, nonintubated newborn and causes less neonatal neurobehavioral depression than thiopental after maternal administration for vaginal delivery.[121,122] Ketamine produces reliable serum levels within 1 minute when administered intravenously or within 5 minutes when administered intramuscularly, and it is rapidly redistributed, with awakening occurring in 10 to 15 minutes. In neonates, the elimination half-life is significantly longer than 130 minutes, which has been reported in older children and adults.[123,124] Extensive hepatic biotransformation necessitates higher doses when administered orally or rectally.

Tolerance and hepatic enzyme induction have been demonstrated during chronic administration of ketamine. Cross tolerance with opiates has been demonstrated in animals, but convincing evidence from human studies is lacking.[125,126] The precise site of action of ketamine is unknown, despite suggestions that ketamine may interfere with excitatory transmission by means of *N*-methyl-D-aspartate receptors.[127] The anesthetic effects of ketamine have been attributed to electrophysiologic dissociation between the thalamoneocortical and limbic systems. Other clinical effects at anesthetic plasma concentrations include catalepsy, nystagmus, hypertonicity, and nonpurposeful movements. Ketamine is a potent stimulator of the cardiovascular system, presumably by means of central sympathetic effects and inhibition of catecholamine reuptake.[128] Compared with isoflurane, halothane, and fentanyl, ketamine had the least effects on mean arterial pressure in ill preterm neonates undergoing surgery.[129] Pulmonary vascular resistance does not appear to be altered in infants with or without preexisting pulmonary hypertension.[130] For critically ill patients with moderate hypovolemia, low doses of ketamine (*i.e.*, 0.5–1 mg/kg) are safer than barbiturates as rapid induction agents before tracheal intubation.

SUMMARY

The proper approach to sedation includes an individualized regimen, which ensures analgesia with careful consideration of the important pharmacokinetic and pharmacodynamic differences in the neonatal population. Analgesia and sedation is needed for neonates undergoing stressful or painful procedures required for essential monitoring and therapy in intensive care. Safe and effective techniques are available that can be used in a variety of clinical circumstances. We strongly urge the reader to follow the guidelines proposed by the American Academy of Pediatrics and later endorsed by the American Society of Anesthesiologists:

> . . . local or systemic pharmacologic agents are now available to permit relatively safe administration of anesthesia and analgesia to neonates undergoing surgical procedures, and . . . such administration is indicated according to the usual guidelines. . . . The decision to withhold such medication should be based on the same medical criteria used for older patients.[131,132]

REFERENCES

1. Anand KJ, Aynsley Green A. Metabolic and endocrine effects of surgical ligation of patent ductus arteriosus in the human preterm neonate: are there implications for improvement of postoperative outcome? Mod Probl Pediatr 1985;23:143.
2. Purcell-Jones G, Dormon F, Sumner E. The use of opioids in neonates. A retrospective study of 933 cases. Anaesthesia 1987;42:1316.
3. Anand KJ, Hickey PR. Pain and its effects in the human neonate and fetus. N Engl J Med 1987;317:1321.
4. Anand KJ, Hansen DD, Hickey PR. Hormonal-metabolic stress responses in neonates undergoing cardiac surgery. Anesthesiology 1990;73:661.

5. Anand KJ, Hickey PR. Stress responses and clinical outcome in neonatal cardiac surgery: randomized trial of high dose sufentanil *vs.* halothane-morphine anesthesia. N Engl J Med 1992;326:1.
6. Purcell-Jones G, Dormon F, Sumner E. Paediatric anaesthetists' perceptions of neonatal and infant pain. Pain 1988;33:181.
7. Reynolds ML, Fitzgerald M, Benowitz LI. GAP-43 expression in developing cutaneous and muscle nerves in the rat hind limb. Neuroscience 1991;41:201.
8. Fitzgerald M. A physiological study of the prenatal development of cutaneous sensory inputs to dorsal horn cells in the rat. J Physiol (Lond) 1991;432:473.
9. Rizvi TA, Wadhwa S, Mehra RD, Bijlani V. Ultrastructure of marginal zone during prenatal development of human spinal cord. Exp Brain Res 1986;64:483.
10. Pignatelli D, Ribeiro da Silva A, Coimbra A. Postnatal maturation of primary afferent terminations in the substantia gelatinosa of the rat spinal cord. An electron microscopic study. Brain Res 1989;491:33.
11. Anand KJ, Carr DB. The neuroanatomy, neurophysiology, and neurochemistry of pain, stress, and analgesia in newborns and children. Pediatr Clin North Am 1989;36:795.
12. Kinney HC, Ottoson CK, White WF. Three-dimensional distribution of ^{3}H-naloxone binding to opiate receptors in the human fetal and infant brainstem. J Comp Neurol 1990;291:55.
13. Klimach VJ, Cooke RW. Maturation of the neonatal somatosensory evoked response in preterm infants. Dev Med Child Neurol 1988;30:208.
14. Anand KJ. Hormonal and metabolic functions of neonates and infants undergoing surgery. Curr Opin Cardiol 1986;1:681.
15. Anand KJ, Sippell WG, Schofield NM, Aynsley Green A. Does halothane anaesthesia decrease the metabolic and endocrine stress responses of newborn infants undergoing operation? Br Med J 1988;296:668.
16. Anand KJ, Sippell WG, Aynsley Green A. Randomised trial of fentanyl anaesthesia in preterm babies undergoing surgery: effects on the stress response. Lancet 1987;1:62.
17. Richards T. Can a fetus feel pain? Br Med J 1985;291:1220.
18. Lippmann M, Nelson RJ, Emmanouilides GC, et al. Ligation of patent ductus arteriosus in premature infants. Br J Anaesth 1976;48:365.
19. Shearer MH. Surgery on the paralyzed, unanesthetized newborn. Birth 1986;13:79.
20. Robinson S, Gregory GA. Fentanyl-air-oxygen anesthesia for ligation of patent ductus arteriosus in preterm infants. Anesth Analg 1981;60:331.
21. Yaster M. Analgesia and anesthesia in neonates. J Pediatr 1987;111:394.
22. Friesen RH, Lichtor JL. Cardiovascular effects of inhalation induction with isoflurane in infants. Anesth Analg 1983;62:411.
23. Friesen RH, Lichtor JL. Cardiovascular depression during halothane anesthesia in infants: study of three induction techniques. Anesth Analg 1982;61:42.
24. Gregory GA. The baroresponses of preterm infants during halothane anaesthesia. Can Anaesth Soc J 1982;29:105.
25. Eisele JH, Smith NT. Cardiovascular effects of 40 percent nitrous oxide in man. Anesth Analg 1972;51:956.
26. Lunn JK, Stanley TH, Eisele J, et al. High dose fentanyl anesthesia for coronary artery surgery: plasma fentanyl concentrations and influence of nitrous oxide on cardiovascular responses. Anesth Analg 1979;58:390.
27. Hickey PR, Hansen DD, Strafford M, et al. Pulmonary and systemic hemodynamic effects of nitrous oxide in infants with normal and elevated pulmonary vascular resistance. Anesthesiology 1986;65:374.
28. Shingu K, Eger EI II, Johnson BH, et al. Effect of oxygen concentration, hyperthermia, and choice of vendor on anesthetic-induced hepatic injury in rats. Anesth Analg 1983;62:146.
29. Summary of the National Halothane Study. Possible association between halothane anesthesia and postoperative hepatic necrosis. JAMA 1966;197:775.
30. Hubbard AK, Roth TP, Gandolfi AJ, et al. Halothane hepatitis patients generate an antibody response toward a covalently bound metabolite of halothane. Anesthesiology 1988;68:791.
31. Mazze RI, Calverley RK, Smith NT. Inorganic fluoride nephrotoxicity: prolonged enflurane and halothane anesthesia in volunteers. Anesthesiology 1977;46:265.
32. Bovill JG, Sebel PS, Stanley TH. Opioid analgesics in anesthesia: with special reference to their use in cardiovascular anesthesia. Anesthesiology 1984;61:731.
33. Koren G, Goresky G, Crean P, et al. Pediatric fentanyl dosing based on pharmacokinetics during cardiac surgery. Anesth Analg 1984;63:577.
34. Hickey PR, Hansen DD, Wessel DL, et al. Pulmonary and systemic hemodynamic responses to fentanyl in infants. Anesth Analg 1985;64:483.
35. Hickey PR, Hansen DD, Wessel DL, et al. Blunting of stress responses in the pulmonary circulation of infants by fentanyl. Anesth Analg 1985;64:1137.
36. Bjertnaes L, Hauge A, Kriz M. Hypoxia-induced pulmonary vasoconstriction: effects of fentanyl following different routes of administration. Acta Anaesthesiol Scand 1980;24:53.
37. Rosow CE, Moss J, Philbin DM, Savarese JJ. Histamine release during morphine and fentanyl anesthesia. Anesthesiology 1982;56:93.
38. Lynn AM, Slattery JT. Morphine pharmacokinetics in early infancy. Anesthesiology 1987;66:136.
39. Gauntlett IS, Fisher DM, Hertzka RE, et al. Pharmacokinetics of fentanyl in neonatal humans and lambs: effects of age. Anesthesiology 1988;69:683.
40. Greeley WJ, de Bruijn NP, Davis DP. Sufentanil pharmacokinetics in pediatric cardiovascular patients. Anesth Analg 1987;66:1067.
41. Greeley WJ, de Bruijn NP. Changes in sufentanil pharmacokinetics within the neonatal period. Anesth Analg 1988;67:86.
42. Killian A, Davis PJ, Stiller RL, et al. Influence of gestational age on pharmacokinetics of alfentanil in neonates. Dev Pharmacol Ther 1991;15:82.
43. Mather LE. Clinical pharmacokinetics of fentanyl and its newer derivatives. Clin Pharmacokinet 1983;8:422.
44. Dalens B. Regional anesthesia in children. Anesth Analg 1989;68:654.
45. Liu LM, Cote CJ, Goudsouzian NG, et al. Life-threatening apnea in infants recovering from anesthesia. Anesthesiology 1983;59:506.
46. Welborn LG, Rice LJ, Hannallah RS, et al. Postoperative apnea in former preterm infants: prospective comparison of spinal and general anesthesia. Anesthesiology 1990;72:838.
47. Abajian JC, Mellish RW, Browne AF, et al. Spinal anesthesia for surgery in the high-risk infant. Anesth Analg 1984;63:359.
48. Mahe V, Ecoffey C. Spinal anesthesia with isobaric bupivacaine in infants. Anesthesiology 1988;68:601.
49. Spear RM, Deshpande JK, Maxwell LG. Caudal anesthesia in the awake, high-risk infant. Anesthesiology 1988;69:407.

50. Shandling B, Steward DJ. Regional analgesia for postoperative pain in pediatric outpatient surgery. J Pediatr Surg 1980;15:477.
51. Broadman LM, Hannallah RS, Belman AB, et al. Post-circumcision analgesia—a prospective evaluation of subcutaneous ring block of the penis. Anesthesiology 1987;67:399.
52. Hannallah RS, Broadman LM, Belman AB, et al. Comparison of caudal and ilioinguinal/iliohypogastric nerve blocks for control of post-orchiopexy pain in pediatric ambulatory surgery. Anesthesiology 1987;66:832.
53. Reiz S, Nath S. Cardiotoxicity of local anaesthetic agents. Br J Anaesth 1986;58:736.
54. Scott DB. Toxic effects of local anaesthetic agents on the central nervous system. Br J Anaesth 1986;58:732.
55. Truog R, Anand KJ. Management of pain in the postoperative neonate. Clin Perinatol 1989;16:61.
56. Callahan P, Pasternak GW. Opiates, opioid peptides, and their receptors. J Cardiothorac Anesth 1987;569:576.
57. Barker N, Hadgraft J, Rutter N. Skin permeability in the newborn. J Invest Dermatol 1987;88:409.
58. Hess GD, Zagon IS. Endogenous opioid systems and neural development: ultrastructural studies in the cerebellar cortex of infant and weanling rats. Brain Res Bull 1988;20:473.
59. Bardo MT, Hughes RA. Single-dose tolerance to morphine-induced analgesic and hypoactive effects in infant rats. Dev Psychobiol 1981;14:415.
60. Evans JM, Hogg MIJ, Rosen M. Reversal of narcotic depression in the neonate by naloxone. Br Med J 1976;2:1098.
61. Way WL, Costley EC, Way EL. Respiratory sensitivity of the newborn infant to meperidine and morphine. Clin Pharmacol Ther 1965;6:454.
62. Hertzka RE, Gauntlett IS, Fisher DM, Spellman MJ. Fentanyl-induced ventilatory depression: effects of age. Anesthesiology 1989;70:213.
63. Olkkola KT, Maunuksela E-L, Korpela R, Rosenberg PH. Kinetics and dynamics of postoperative intravenous morphine in children. Clin Pharmacol Ther 1991;44:128.
64. Colpaert FC, Niemegeers CJ, Janssen PA, Maroli AN. The effects of prior fentanyl administration and of pain on fentanyl analgesia: tolerance to and enhancement of narcotic analgesia. J Pharmacol Exp Ther 1980;213:418.
65. Hasday JD, Weintraub M. Propoxyphene in children with iatrogenic morphine dependence. Am J Dis Child 1983;137:745.
66. Miser AW, Chayt KJ, Sandlund JT, et al. Narcotic withdrawal syndrome in young adults after the therapeutic use of opiates. Am J Dis Child 1986;140:603.
67. Arnold JH, Truog RD, Orav EJ, et al. Tolerance and dependence in neonates sedated with fentanyl during extracorporeal membrane oxygenation. Anesthesiology 1990;73:1136.
68. Tobias JD, Schleien CL, Haun SE. Methadone as treatment for iatrogenic narcotic dependency in pediatric intensive care unit patients. Crit Care Med 1990;18:1292.
69. Arnold JH, Truog RD, Scavone JM, Fenton T. Changes in the pharmacodynamic response to fentanyl in neonates during continuous infusion. J Pediatr 1991;119:639.
70. Yasuda I, Hirano T, Yusa T, Satoh M. Tracheal constriction by morphine and by fentanyl in man. Anesthesiology 1978;49:117.
71. Soleymani Y, Weiss NS, Sinnott EC, Goldzier S II. Management of life-threatening asthma in children. A preliminary study of the use of morphine in respiratory failure. Am J Dis Child 1972;123:533.
72. Eschenbacher WL, Bethel RA, Boushey HA, Sheppard D. Morphine sulfate inhibits bronchoconstriction in subjects with mild asthma whose responses are inhibited by atropine. Am Rev Respir Dis 1984;130:363.
73. Rogers DF, Barnes PJ. Opioid inhibition of neurally mediated mucus secretion in human bronchi. Lancet 1989;1:930.
74. Comstock MK, Carter JG, Moyers JR, Stevens WC. Rigidity and hypercarbia associated with high dose fentanyl induction of anesthesia. [Letter]. Anesth Analg 1981;60:362.
75. Kentor ML, Schwalb AJ, Lieberman RW. Rapid high-dose fentanyl induction for CABG. Anesthesiology 1980;53:S95.
76. Scamman FL. Fentanyl-O_2-N_2O rigidity and pulmonary compliance. Anesth Analg 1983;62:332.
77. Hill AB, Nahrwold ML, de Rosayro AM, et al. Prevention of rigidity during fentanyl–oxygen induction of anesthesia. Anesthesiology 1981;55:452.
78. Bailey PL, Wilbrink J, Zwanikken P, et al. Anesthetic induction with fentanyl. Anesth Analg 1985;64:48.
79. Freye E, Hartung E, Buhl R. Lung compliance in man is impaired by the rapid injection of alfentanil. Anaesthetist 1986;35:543.
80. Schlesinger AE, Null DM. Enlarged common hepatic duct secondary to morphine in a neonate. Pediatr Radiol 1988;18:235.
81. Peterson RG. Consequences associated with nonnarcotic analgesics in the fetus and newborn. Fed Proc 1985;44:2309.
82. Levy G, Khanna NN, Soda DM, et al. Pharmacokinetics of acetaminophen in the human neonate: formation of acetaminophen glucuronide and sulfate in relation to plasma bilirubin concentration and D-glucaric acid excretion. Pediatrics 1975;55:818.
83. Miller RP, Roberts RJ, Fischer LJ. Acetaminophen elimination kinetics in neonates, children, and adults. Clin Pharm 1976;19:284.
84. Collins E. Maternal and fetal effects of acetaminophen and salicylates in pregnancy. Obstet Gynecol 1981;58(Suppl):57.
85. Beattie JO, Chen CP, MacDonald TH. Neonatal distalgesic poisoning. Lancet 1981;2:49.
86. Roberts I, Robinson MJ, Mughal MZ, et al. Paracetamol metabolites in the neonate following maternal overdose. Br J Clin Pharm 1984;18:201.
87. Stiehm ER. Nonsteroidal anti-inflammatory drugs in pediatric patients. Am J Dis Child 1988;142:1281.
88. Brogden RN. Nonsteroidal anti-inflammatory analgesics other than salicylates. Drugs 1986;4:27.
89. Norton SJ. Aftereffects of morphine and fentanyl analgesia: a retrospective study. Neonatal Network 1988;7:25.
90. Desai N, Taylor Davies A, Barnett DB. The effects of diazepam and oxprenolol on short term memory in individuals of high and low state anxiety. Br J Clin Pharmacol 1983;15:197.
91. Niv D, Davidovich S, Geller E, Urca G. Analgesic and hyperalgesic effects of midazolam: dependence on route of administration. Anesth Analg 1988;67:1169.
92. Rattan AK, McDonald JS, Tejwani GA. Differential effects of intrathecal midazolam on morphine-induced antinociception in the rat: role of spinal opioid receptors. Anesth Analg 1991;73:124.
93. Reves JG, Fragen RJ, Vinik HR, Greenblatt DJ. Midazolam: pharmacology and uses. Anesthesiology 1985;62:310.
94. Morselli PL, Principi N, Tognoni G. Diazepam elimination in premature and full term infants, and children. J Perinatol 1973;1:133.
95. Tekur U, Gupta A, Tayal G, Agrawal KK. Blood concentrations of diazepam and its metabolites in children and neonates with tetanus. J Pediatr 1983;102:145.
96. Jorch G, Rabe H, Rickers E, et al. Cerebral blood flow velocity

assessed by Doppler technique after intravenous application of diazepam in very low birth weight infants. Dev Pharmacol Ther 1989;14:102.

97. Hegarty JE, Dundee JW. Sequelae after the intravenous injection of three benzodiazepines—diazepam, lorazepam, and flunitrazepam. Br Med J 1977;2:1384.
98. Silvasi DL, Rosen DA, Rosen KR. Continuous intravenous midazolam infusion for sedation in the pediatric intensive care unit. Anesth Analg 1988;67:286.
99. Jacqz-Aigrain E, Wood C, Robieux I. Pharmacokinetics of midazolam in critically ill neonates. Eur J Clin Pharmacol 1990; 39:191.
100. Byatt CM, Lewis LD, Dawling S, Cochrane GM. Accumulation of midazolam after repeated dosage in patients receiving mechanical ventilation in an intensive care unit. Br Med J 1984;289:799.
101. Boisse NR, Quaglietta N, Samoriski GM, Guarino JJ. Tolerance and physical dependence to a short-acting benzodiazepine, midazolam. J Pharmacol Exp Ther 1990;252:1125.
102. McLellan I, Douglas E. Midazolam withdrawal syndrome. Anaesthesia 1991;46:420.
103. Bergman I, Steeves M, Burckart G, Thompson A. Reversible neurologic abnormalities associated with prolonged intravenous midazolam and fentanyl administration. J Pediatr 1991; 119:644.
104. Burtin P, Daoud P, Jacqz-Aigrain E, et al. Hypotension with midazolam and fentanyl in the newborn. Lancet 1991;337:1545.
105. Kissin I, Mason JO, Bradley EL Jr. Morphine and fentanyl interactions with thiopental in relation to movement response to noxious stimulation. Anesth Analg 1986;65:1149.
106. Grasela TH, Donn SM. Neonatal population pharmacokinetics of phenobarbital derived from routine clinical data. Dev Pharmacol Ther 1985;8:374.
107. Kuban KCK, Leviton A, Krishnamoorthy KS. Neonatal intracranial hemorrhage and phenobarbital. Pediatrics 1986;77: 443.
108. Ninan A, O'Donnell M, Hamilton K, et al. Physiologic changes induced by endotracheal instillation and suctioning in critically ill preterm infants with and without sedation. Am J Perinatol 1986;3:94.
109. Gilman JT, Gal P, Duchowny MS, et al. Rapid sequential phenobarbital treatment of neonatal seizures. Pediatrics 1989;83:674.
110. Franck LS. A national survey of the assessment and treatment of pain and agitation in the neonatal intensive care unit. J Obstet Gynecol Neonatal Nurs 1987;16:387.
111. Lees MH, Olsen GD, McGilliard KL, et al. Chloral hydrate and the carbon dioxide chemoreceptor response: a study of puppies and infants. Pediatrics 1982;70:447.
112. Rumm PD, Takao RT, Fox DJ, Atkinson SW. Efficacy of sedation of children with chloral hydrate. South Med J 1990; 83:1040.
113. Laptook AR, Rosenfeld CR. Chloral hydrate toxicity in a preterm infant. Pediatr Pharmacol 1984;4:161.
114. Lambert GH, Muraskas J, Anderson CL, Myers TF. Direct hyperbilirubinemia associated with chloral hydrate administration in the newborn. Pediatrics 1990;86:277.
115. Turner DJ, Morgan SE, Landau LI, LeSouef PN. Methodological aspects of flow-volume studies in infants. Pediatr Pulmonol 1990;8:289.
116. Gonzalez JL, Lambert GH, Muraskas J, Anderson CL. Hypertriglyceridemia in infants with bronchopulmonary dysplasia. [Letter] J Pediatr 1989;115:506.
117. Farber B, Abramow A. Acute laryngeal edema due to chloral hydrate. Isr J Med Sci 1985;21:858.
118. Hirsch IA, Zauder HL. Chloral hydrate: a potential cause of arrhythmias. Anesth Analg 1986;65:691.
119. Reich DL, Silvay G. Ketamine: an update on the first twenty-five years of clinical experience. Can J Anaesth 1989;36:186.
120. Tashiro C, Matsui Y, Nakano S, et al. Respiratory outcome in extremely premature infants following ketamine anaesthesia. Can J Anaesth 1991;38:287.
121. Chatterjee SC, Syed A. Ketamine and infants. [Letter] Anaesthesia 1983;38:1007.
122. Hodgkinson R, Marx GF, Kim SS, Miclat NM. Neonatal neurobehavioral tests following vaginal delivery under ketamine, thiopental, and extradural anesthesia. Anesth Analg 1977;56:548.
123. Grant IS, Nimmo WS, McNicol LR, Clements JA. Ketamine disposition in children and adults. Br J Anaesth 1983;55:1107.
124. Cook DR. Newborn anaesthesia: pharmacological considerations. Can Anaesth Soc J 1986;33:S38.
125. Winters WD, Hance AJ, Cadd GG, et al. Ketamine- and morphine-induced analgesia and catalepsy. I. Tolerance, cross-tolerance, potentiation, residual morphine levels and naloxone action in the rat. J Pharmacol Exp Ther 1988;244:51.
126. Finck AD, Samaniego E, Ngai SH. Morphine tolerance decreases the analgesic effects of ketamine in mice. Anesthesiology 1988;68:397.
127. Thomson AM, West DC, Lodge D. An *N*-methylaspartate receptor-mediated synapse in rat cerebral cortex: a site of action of ketamine. Nature 1985;313:479.
128. Lundy PM, Lockwood PA, Thompson G, Frew R. Differential effects of ketamine isomers on neuronal and extraneuronal catecholamine uptake mechanisms. Anesthesiology 1986;64: 359.
129. Friesen RH, Henry DB. Cardiovascular changes in preterm neonates receiving isoflurane, halothane, fentanyl, and ketamine. Anesthesiology 1986;64:238.
130. Hickey PR, Hansen DD, Cramolini GM, et al. Pulmonary and systemic hemodynamic responses to ketamine in infants with normal and elevated pulmonary vascular resistance. Anesthesiology 1985;62:287.
131. American Academy of Pediatrics, Committee on Fetus and Newborn, Committee on Drugs, Section on Anesthesiology, Section on Surgery. Neonatal anesthesia. Pediatrics 1987; 80:446.
132. American Society of Anesthesiologists. Neonatal anesthesia. ASA Newsletter 1987;51:12.

Part Seven

Beyond the Nursery

Neonatology: Pathophysiology and Management of the Newborn, Fourth Edition,
edited by Gordon B. Avery, Mary Ann Fletcher, and Mhairi G. MacDonald.
J.B. Lippincott Company, Philadelphia © 1994.

chapter 59

Discharge Planning

MAUREEN EDWARDS

Hospitalization of an infant is a significant life stressor for families. Discharge from the hospital may relieve some aspects of the stress while simultaneously intensifying others and creating new concerns. A key factor in making the event as positive and comfortable as possible is effective discharge planning.

The elements of discharge planning for infants vary in complexity, depending on each patient's clinical needs and support systems, the discharge destination, and the community health care providers as well as the interactions among the components. Geography and climate also influence the complexity. No matter how simple any case may be, discharge planning always is multidisciplinary, varying from interaction solely between a parent and primary provider to one involving a legion of disciplines for more complicated health problems. In most hospitals, nursing and social workers have primary responsibility for discharge planning, with physicians advising on specific medical needs. Physicians who see the patients for follow-up visits are in a good position to assess the efficacy of discharge plans retrospectively, so they should be involved actively in the generation of the plans so that they may add that insight. Case managers for third-party payers or managed care providers frequently play an important and directive role as well. If a plan is to be of optimum benefit to the patient, it is important that all players understand their roles and responsibilities and how they affect one another.

To ensure the orderly execution of a timely and workable discharge plan for every patient, hospitals can benefit by developing an organized discharge planning process tailored to their unique operational systems. The organization includes discharge policies, definition of roles and responsibilities for each discipline, directed rounds or meetings, and appropriate documents.[1] Establishing a method of evaluation also helps to identify and correct problems and to improve the process.

DISCHARGE PLANNING FOR THE HEALTHY, FULL-TERM BABY

The key steps in planning for the well baby's discharge are:

1. Verify that the baby is well.
2. Confirm that the family can provide for the basic physical needs of the infant.
3. Ensure that the family is educated in normal infant care and problem identification
4. Specify a plan for continuing health care and parenting support.

Many of the issues in preparing an infant and parents for routine discharge after short-term hospitalization are discussed in Chapter 22.

The emphasis by health care financiers on minimal length of hospital stay hampers the ability of the hospital team to use the postpartum time for teaching infant care to those parents who would benefit from it the most: the teenager with no prenatal care, the first-time parent, and the mother with limited access to community support.[2,3] How much education is needed for any mother–infant pair varies. All hospitals, particularly those with patients of widely diverse socioeconomic and cultural backgrounds, need to address these differences in their educational approaches. Literacy and primary language are important issues to consider in teaching plans, as are factors such as availability of refrigeration, heating, or air conditioning, type of sleeping arrangements, and numbers and ages of other household members. Discharge planning programs for well babies are most effective when they allow a customized approach to planning for the needs of individual families.

After discharge home, families need accessible pediatric care. Parents unaccustomed to preventive health care may be unaware of the importance of well baby care and infant immunization. Identification of a source for health care is an essential part of discharge planning so that there can be transmission of appropriate medical information, arrangements for following unresolved medical issues, and prompt initiation of well baby medical care.

DISCHARGE PLANNING FROM INTENSIVE CARE NURSERIES

Infants may leave the neonatal intensive care unit (NICU) for further care in another unit such as a step-down unit within the same institution, a community nursery, or a chronic care facility or for home. The discharging NICU can be an effective player in the overall discharge plan by adjusting its role, depending on the infant's needs and the expertise of the follow-up health care providers.

TRANSFER TO ANOTHER UNIT

If families are prepared well before their infant is ready for transfer to another unit, the transition goes more smoothly.[4] By discussing this potential graduation early in the hospital course and by giving reminders as the infant's treatment advances, parents can accept the steps as part of a positive progression in the baby's care. Visits by the family to the receiving unit in anticipation of the coming transfer may be helpful. Although families may embrace the progress signaled by transfer of their baby to a less-intensive care situation, they also may feel uncomfortable outside the NICU environment. Addressing these concerns directly minimizes repercussions later.

DISCHARGE TO HOME

Releasing the infant to another unit is relatively simple compared to discharge home. The family's inexperience in caring for fragile infants means each factor must be planned in detail. All the issues addressed in preparing a family for a healthy, full-term infant are just as important when the infant is premature or has been ill. What follows is a discussion of the general factors to be considered in discharge from the NICU. Because of the specialized needs for infants with cardiac or surgical diagnoses, which will not be discussed here, the reader is referred to Chapters 33, 34, and 44.

TIMING OF DISCHARGE

The best timing of discharge home is a balance between the advantages of early discharge and its risks. Early discharge may enhance parent–infant bonding, improve the developmental environment for the infant, decrease exposure to hospital pathogens, and decrease cost of the hospital stay. Discharge too early, however, can result in deterioration of the infant, making readmission necessary and creating additional strain on the family. Whether the family is ready often can be surmised by observing and talking to parents during the hospital stay. If questions arise, formal assessments of family capabilities, including a home evaluation, may be helpful. Although there are no absolute criteria for discharge to home, at a minimum, the needs of the infant and the family's capacity to meet them must agree. For a premature infant, barring preemptive medical conditions, the criteria for the earliest possible discharge include reaching a weight and maturity where he or she can maintain body temperature in an open crib (*i.e.*, at approximately 2000 g and 34 weeks of gestational age); feeding by mouth well enough to grow 20–30 g/day; and having no medical problem requiring hospital management. Smaller, more mature but healthy infants may safely be discharged to an appropriate home environment.[5]

It is vitally important that no major changes be initiated immediately before discharge that could cause deterioration in the infant's condition at home. Such changes would include discontinuation of oxygen or major modifications in diuretics or in feedings.

EDUCATING PARENTS

Teaching routine care to parents of premature or sick infants signals that the baby has become well. Neonatal intensive care units must guard against an understandable tendency to overlook routine instructions in basic infant care, such as formula preparation and bathing, in their desire to communicate to parents the complexities of critical medical matters. Moreover, families of sick infants need additional attention focused on their arrangements for child care, the home environment, and safety.[6]

Although education occurs throughout the nursery stay, individualized teaching intensifies near the time of discharge. In many hospitals, the infant's primary nurse may play the pivotal role in teaching; in others, a discharge planning coordinator may collaborate with the bedside nursing staff. Teaching infant care is accomplished best by the nursing staff most familiar with both the infant and his or her needs and the family and their home care issues.[7,8] Educating families to care for their premature or sick infant requires a structured, documented approach; the instructor must know what topics are applicable and in what depth. To be effective, instruction must be sensitive to the cultural and educational differences among people. Some parents will be unable to read and understand written instructions. For sick infants, it is important that several family members, ideally including the father, are comfortable with the infant's routine and special medical care so that all the burden of home care does not fall solely on the mother.

Parents should prepare for the early days at home by providing as much care to their hospitalized infants as practical. In turn, the hospital staff needs to prepare the infant for a comfortable home routine by replacing a rigid schedule with more flexible feeding and sleeping schedules, and letting the infant sleep at night in darkened areas. Allowing rooming-in before discharge is particularly valuable for families who must be proficient with special medical equipment and procedures by the time the baby goes home.

To prepare for whatever difficulties may develop after discharge, it is helpful for parents to know the range of problems that other similar families have experienced. Ambivalence and fear are common feelings as preparations for discharge are underway; some families may need license to acknowledge these feelings. Parents need to prepare for the temporary changes in life-style that having a fragile infant will impose of them. This may mean adjusting work plans to allow full-time parental supervision, revising child care plans because of special risks of infection, or tolerating the intrusion of technology into family life. Estimating a time frame for these special needs helps families put them into perspective.

FEEDING AND NUTRITION

At 32 weeks of gestational age, healthy preterm infants develop the coordinated suck and swallow necessary to feed comfortably by nipple, but they still may require skilled feeding techniques. Parents need to develop these skills while the infant is hospitalized.

When infants are fed human milk, introducing the breast early stimulates milk production and may enhance breast-feeding. Many women find it too time-consuming and stressful to breast-feed, pump their breasts, and provide that breast milk in a bottle while giving all the other care needed after discharge. Alternative plans should be developed prospectively.

A demand feeding approach generally is recommended for healthy infants, with most infants easily adapting to a flexible feeding schedule at home. Others in whom weight gain or fluid balance is a concern require boundaries and may have little leeway in their feedings. Infants with complex feeding or nutritional difficulties may benefit from gavage feedings, night or full-time continuous feedings, or parenteral nutrition at home, requiring that families learn and practice these special techniques before discharge.

Healthy preterm infants who weigh more than 1800 g and have no laboratory evidence of rickets, low protein, or feeding intolerance may take regular formulas before discharge. Some immature babies need a protein- and calcium-enriched premature formula at home. A source for any special formulas must be identified. Additionally, there needs to be planning for monitoring growth and nutrition. Providing the infant's inpatient growth curves to the follow-up team will assist in tracking growth.

If hypercaloric formula (>20 calories/ounce) is required, the parents need to understand how to make the appropriate mixture from concentrate or powder or by adding glucose polymers or fat. At home, formula usually is made in a 24-hour quantity, so parents need to learn about preparation, sterilization, and storage of the formula and additives.

Premature infants taking unfortified breast milk or regular formulas should receive a daily multivitamin preparation, with fluoride if indicated, because their volume intake is insufficient to provide recommended daily allowances of many vitamins. Special vitamin supplements, such as vitamins E or A, usually discontinued before discharge, may be needed in some instances at home, so there will need to be a specific plan for their use and duration. Most NICU graduates will need iron supplementation, which should be supplied in the easiest, most appropriate dosage form. The physician assessing the infant's iron requirement should plan for 2 to 6 mg/kg of elemental iron, taking into consideration all sources of iron. Iron-fortified formula consumed at 150 to 180 mL/kg/day provides approximately 2 mg/kg of elemental iron.

IMMUNIZATIONS

The American Academy of Pediatrics recommends that premature infants be immunized on the same chronologic age schedule and with the same dosages as their full-term counterparts. Contraindications to immunization are the same for premature or recuperating infants as for other children. Live virus vaccines (*e.g.*, oral polio vaccine) should not be administered in the inpatient setting or to immunocompromised infants, including those receiving corticosteroids. Physicians may choose to defer temporarily the immunization of infants who are still ill or weigh less than 1800 g when they reach 2 months of chronologic age. For infants 60 days of age for whom immunization is indicated, the first course of immunizations should be completed by the time of hospital discharge, with oral polio vaccine given as the infant leaves. Parent information and consent should parallel that recommended by the American Academy of Pediatrics and Centers for Disease Control. Special attention to the maintenance of appropriate immunization history on the inpatient medical record and transmittal to the family and follow-up provider are necessary.

PREDISCHARGE EVALUATIONS

An integral part of discharge planning is a careful review of the infant's medical record to determine the indications for special evaluations, including sensory testing (*e.g.*, hearing, eye examinations) and follow-up of any previously abnormal results. Discussing the evaluation process with parents before testing and informing them of the likely outcomes makes communicating results easier while simultaneously preparing them should a specific concern be uncovered in their child. Because the infant usually is past life-threatening crises by the time of screening, news of additional abnormalities, however minor relative to what the infant has faced, can be very upsetting for families who believed that the worst was behind them; they may feel that they are incapable of coping with anything more.

Infants at risk for retinopathy of prematurity (ROP) require periodic retinal assessments until their retinal vasculature is mature or ROP has resolved. If an infant's retinal vessels are immature at the time of discharge or if ROP is present, there should be arrangements for specific ophthalmologic follow-up to look for potential progression and to detect candidates for therapy.

Almost all NICU graduates will meet criteria for hearing screening (see Chap. 60). Assessments may be done after the infant is in an open crib as long as there is a quiet area available. If done before discharge, not only will results be available to the caretakers but it will mean one less outpatient visit for families. In all series, there are a significant number of false-positive or false-negative results from hearing evaluations in the nursery population. Any infant with abnormal results will need further evaluation, as will any infant clinically suspect for progressive hearing loss.

Many centers recommend neuroimaging for infants who approximate 40 weeks of gestation and who have a history of intraventricular hemorrhage or are at risk for periventricular leukomalacia. If discharged before 38 to 40 weeks of gestational age, arrangements for outpatient testing should be discussed with parents before discharge.

Infants with persistent apnea may be candidates for home monitoring or xanthine therapy. If therapy hinges on results of recorded monitoring (*e.g.*, pneumograms), these tests should be arranged far enough before discharge for results to be available.

Circumcision should be discussed with parents early enough so that, if desired and appropriate, this procedure can be performed in a timely fashion before discharge.

Physical examination done regularly throughout an infant's hospitalization should disclose any abnormalities, but the particular findings often first detected in premature infants nearing discharge include inguinal hernias and murmurs of peripheral pulmonic stenosis or anemia. Neurodevelopmental assessments are most informative when done closest to 40 weeks of gestational age. Performing either a formal developmental assessment or a physical–occupational therapy evaluation provides information to families that allows them to focus on the developmental accomplishments and needs of their child and prepares them for any future developmental interventions.

RESPIRATORY CARE

Many premature or sick infants have continuing respiratory risks at the time of discharge. When apnea of prematurity is an unresolved issue at the time of discharge, home monitoring or xanthine therapy may allow an earlier discharge. Apprising parents of the possibility of home monitoring early in the hospital course allows them to adjust to the concept and focus on necessary educational activities. Teaching parents the appropriate responses for monitor alarms and cardiopulmonary resuscitation takes several days to be most effective, and should not be rushed in a flurry of discharge activity. Clarification of insurance coverage or method of reimbursement for durable medical equipment also should be preplanned. Families ought to notify the local rescue squad, telephone company, and electric utilities that there is a monitored infant in their home. An outside source of medical and technical information to answer parents' questions about the monitor and alarms should be listed in the discharge documents.

Discharge of an infant with persistent pulmonary disease, such as bronchopulmonary dysplasia (BPD), may require the use of medications, special feedings, and respiratory treatment.[9,10] The infant should be stable on the discharge regimen and not in need of frequent laboratory assessments. The continuous administration of oxygen at home may be beneficial to the infant with BPD, but it is a significant undertaking for families. Oxygen is supplied at 100% from liquid oxygen tanks or at lower concentrations from nitrogen extractors. A reliable supply of oxygen in tanks is necessary to back up systems requiring electricity. Parents must be trained to assess the infant's oxygen status visually, by changes in heart rate and other respiratory symptoms, or by oximetry. If an infant is on low levels of oxygen, a brief test of the infant's response to loss of supplemental oxygen helps identify whether he or she needs oximetric monitoring; if he or she is on more than 28% to 30%, he or she should have oximetry available. For infants with abnormal radiographs, providing a copy to the primary physician and to the parents may help when visits to an emergency room or different clinic is necessary. It is important that families are aware that infants with a neonatal history of respiratory problems are at particular risk for deterioration after discharge, so they will seek early medical intervention.

Tracheostomy home care is needed primarily for infants with airway abnormalities or for those requiring home ventilation. Well before discharge, families require training in suctioning and changing the tracheostomy tube, providing humidity, monitoring, and preventing infection. Home ventilator care in conjunction with a tracheostomy is possible only for stable infants with trained, willing parents and extensive community health care supports, often including skilled nursing care.

MEDICATIONS

Before discharge, all medications should be reassessed for need and efficacy. Adjusting dosing schedules to coincide with expected feeding intervals minimizes how often the baby is disturbed. Calculating nutritional supplements of electrolytes for mixing in a 24-hour supply of formula simplifies the preparation and generally is well tolerated by infants who reliably take an anticipated volume. Determination must be made that the appropriate medications for young infants are available in the community and prescriptions provided to the family several days before discharge. Many pharmacies do not compound special dosage forms, nor do they stock specialized pediatric preparations that hospitals use. If a more easily procured product is unacceptable, a plan for how to fill the prescriptions must be made before discharge. A plan to adjust dosages as the infant gains weight or a strategy for letting the infant outgrow the medication should be specified.

If blood tests for drug levels or side effects are indicated, a specific plan for where and how often they are to be done as well as who assumes responsibility for their interpretation must be spelled out.

FOLLOW-UP MEDICAL AND HOME VISITS

The follow-up pediatrician plays the focal role in the infant's continuing care at home. When the family does not have a pediatrician, the discharging physicians should assist the family in selection of a primary care provider based on locale, availability, and experience in caring for infants with complicated medical or developmental problems; insurance participation must be considered as well. Involvement of the follow-up pediatrician before discharge is ideal, but, at the least, careful verbal and written communication can emphasize the essential features of the neonatal hospital course. If the family can meet the pediatrician before discharge, just as they might in a prenatal visit, they will feel more comfortable in transferring their infant's care to someone they have met. There should be a visit to the pediatrician as soon after discharge as feasible.

The primary pediatric care provider or a designated consultant should assist the family in organizing outpatient follow-up visits. Infants commonly leave the hospital with unresolved medical issues and appointments for many medical visits in the first weeks after discharge. These visits may be to general pediatrics, neonatology, child development, ophthalmology, audiology, surgery, or pulmonary medicine. Arranging to have as many of these evaluations as possible before discharge will simplify the schedule. It is important to balance the value of the medical input gained by these visits against the risk of exposing the infant to infections from other patients or even the simple disturbance of the infant's sleep–feeding cycles. Specific appointments for follow-up visits often best are scheduled before discharge to ensure that the infant's necessary evaluations will not be delayed unwittingly.

General pediatric care and patient education usually are provided best by the infant's primary care provider. When many specialists are involved, it must be clear which physician will advise the family on which aspect of care, and that all areas are covered. Families easily can be confused by conflicting advice, so good communication among the family, the primary care physician, and specialists is important.

Home health visits by visiting nurses, respiratory therapists, and other care specialists are helpful in the overall assessment of the infant, education of the family, and fine-tuning of the home care plan. Home visits before discharge may assist in developing realistic plans. It is essential that a limited number of health visitors be involved, their care be coordinated, and their messages be consistent with one another.

Community and social support services should be arranged before discharge whenever possible. Eligible infants should be enrolled in Medicaid, WIC, Social Security, or early intervention programs. Where appropriate, the State Child Protection Service should be apprised of anticipated discharge problems.

REFERENCES

1. Bernbaum JC, Hoffman-Williamson M. Primary care of the preterm infant. St. Louis: CV Mosby, 1991:3.
2. Beck CT. Early postpartum discharge programs in the United States: a literature review and critique. Women Health 1991;17:125.
3. Conrad PD, Wilkening RB, Rosenberg AA. Safety of newborn discharge in less than 36 hours in an indigent population. Am J Dis Child 1989;143:96.
4. Donovan TL, Schmitt R. Discharge planning for neonatal back transfer. Journal of Perinatal and Neonatal Nursing 1991;5:64.
5. Committee on Fetus and Newborn and Committee on Obstetrics. Follow-up care. In: Freeman RK, Poland RL, eds. Guide-

lines for perinatal care. 3rd ed. Elk Grove, IL: American Academy of Pediatrics, American College of Obstetrics, 1992:109.
6. Committee on Injury and Poison Prevention and Committee on Fetus and Newborn. Safe transportation of premature infants. Pediatrics 1991;87:120.
7. Damato EG. Discharge planning from the neonatal intensive care unit. Journal of Perinatal and Neonatal Nursing 1991; 5:43.
8. Baker K, Kuhlmann T, Magliaro BL. Homeward bound. Nurs Clin North Am 1989;24:655.
9. Embon CM. Discharge planning for infants with bronchopulmonary dysplasia. Journal of Perinatal and Neonatal Nursing 1991;5:54.
10. Rodriquez AM, McCutcheon L, Simpser M. Home management of the infant with complex BPD: an alternative to long-term hospitalization. Int Pediatr 1990;5:350.

Neonatology: Pathophysiology and Management of the Newborn, Fourth Edition,
edited by Gordon B. Avery, Mary Ann Fletcher, and Mhairi G. MacDonald.
J.B. Lippincott Company, Philadelphia © 1994.

chapter 60

Medical Care After Discharge

JUDY C. BERNBAUM

Once the high-risk infant is discharged from the hospital, his or her many special care needs do not cease. Although still requiring well-child care, many of these infants have needs that are far from routine. Special attention must be given to their growth and nutrition, immunizations, vision and hearing, and sequelae of illnesses experienced during the neonatal period. Premature infants have more likelihood for long-term sequelae and continuing medical problems than term infants do, but many of the issues discussed specifically about prematurity apply to term infants as well.

EXPECTATIONS OF GROWTH

The growth pattern is a valuable indicator of an infant's well-being. Aberrant growth may reflect the presence of chronic illness, feeding difficulties, inadequate nutrition, or social–emotional difficulties. Preterm infants are at particular risk for growth disorders. Many infants with chronic illness, while at an age when rapid growth is expected, have high caloric requirements but are unable to meet them because they have impaired feeding abilities. It is crucial to monitor nutritional intake closely and to interpret growth rates with a complete understanding of the infant's past history, current problems, and expectations for growth.

Many factors affect the growth of a preterm infant, including gestational age, birth weight, severity of neonatal illness, caloric intake, current illnesses, environmental factors in the home, and heredity. Caloric requirements for a healthy, preterm infant generally exceed those of a term, normal-birth-weight infant, especially during rapid catch-up growth.[1] Chronic illnesses that increase caloric expenditure add to an infant's daily requirements. Malabsorption after necrotizing enterocolitis (NEC) or chronic emesis from gastroesophageal reflux (GER) may impair growth due to increased losses. In contrast, decreased intake may be caused by fatigue, hypoxemia, oral motor dysfunction, or reflux esophagitis. Finally, infants with intrauterine growth retardation caused by congenital infections, chromosomal abnormalities, or other syndromes may never achieve normal growth.

PATTERNS OF GROWTH

When evaluating the growth of a low-birth-weight (LBW) infant, the gestational age should be considered. Growth parameters should be plotted on standard curves according to the infant's adjusted age until approximately 2.5 years of age, when the age difference is insignificant. Various patterns of growth emerge from different groups of patients.

Healthy, LBW, appropriate-for-gestational-age (AGA) infants generally experience catch-up growth during the first 2 years of life, with maximal growth rates between 36 and 40 weeks postconception. Little catch-up growth occurs after 3 years of age. Head circumference usually is the first parameter to demonstrate catch-up growth, and often plots at a higher percentile relative to weight and length. Increases in weight are followed within several weeks by increases in length. Rapid catch-up head growth must be distinguished from pathologic growth associated with hydrocephalus. An imaging study may be indicated if the infant's history or symptoms suggest hydrocephalus. Insufficient brain growth, a head circumference falling more than three standard deviations below the mean, indicates that the infant is at risk for significant developmental disability.

Growth velocities for weight and height vary considerably. Some preterm infants show growth on curves between the 75th and 97th percentiles by 3 months adjusted age, whereas others remain on low curves well beyond the child's first year. It is helpful to evaluate an infant's weight gain in comparison to gains in length. Low weight for length or a decline in all growth parameters suggests inadequate nutrition. Weight percentiles significantly greater than length percentiles indicate obesity. Obesity may occur in a preterm infant whose parents overfeed their previously underweight baby. It is common to see an infant who was formerly failing to thrive rather abruptly become obese when the medical problems resolve but the diet remains high in calories.

Growth of the small-for-gestational-age (SGA) infant is influenced strongly by the cause of the intrauterine growth retardation. Overall, LBW–SGA infants demonstrate less catch-up growth than LBW–AGA infants, but if they do, it starts by 8 to 12 months of adjusted age. Approximately 50% of LBW–SGA infants are below average in weight at 3 years of age, whereas only 15% of LBW–AGA infants remain below average weight at the same age.[2] Symmetric SGA infants with birth head circumference similar in percentile to birth weight are less likely to demonstrate catch-up growth than are those asymmetric SGA infants whose birth head circumference was at a significantly higher percentile than their weight. As with AGA infants, head circumference is normally the first parameter to demonstrate catch-up, followed by weight and then by length.

Because of the wide range of growth that is considered normal during the first several years of life, it is best to analyze trends in growth rather than make assumptions based on single measurements. When abnormalities are noted in growth trends, investigation of the infant's nutritional status during hospitalization, the results of cranial sonography studies, and the status of continuing illnesses should be undertaken to identify a possible cause.

NUTRITIONAL REQUIREMENTS

Traditionally, although somewhat controversial, the goal for preterm infants is to achieve a growth rate approximating the expected fetal growth rate at the same postconceptional age.[1] Since weight gain is suboptimal during acute illness, all efforts should be made to promote catch-up growth once the medical condition is stable. The nutritional needs of the preterm infant during the first few months of life exceed those of a term neonate, but by 40 weeks postconception, if there are no exceptional medical or feeding problems, the dietary needs are similar. Appropriate choices for most preterm infants include breast milk and term infant formulas.[3] Other infants continue to need more highly concentrated formula or fortified breast milk because of increased caloric requirements or dysfunctional feeding. Most infants do not tolerate feedings with caloric densities greater than 30 kcal/ounce. Infants given feedings concentrated beyond 24 kcal/ounce should be monitored for symptoms of intolerance such as vomiting and diarrhea and for hyperosmolar dehydration with insufficient free water. Whole cow milk is poorly tolerated and should be avoided. When caloric additives or concentrated formula are used, care should be taken to maintain an appropriate caloric distribution of nutrients with a ratio among carbohydrates–fats–protein of approximately 40–50–10.

Caloric requirements for adequate growth vary. Healthy preterm infants generally require 110 to 130 kcal/kg/day, but some infants with chronic disease may require up to 200 kcal/kg/day. Caloric intake should be increased as tolerated until weight gain is satisfactory. Caloric requirements needed for catch-up growth can be calculated for infants older than 40 weeks postconceptional age by using the following formula[4]:

$$\text{kcal/kg Required} = 120\ \text{kcal/kg} \times \frac{\text{Ideal weight for actual height}}{\text{Actual weight}}.$$

FEEDING PROBLEMS

Although unusual in term infants, feeding disorders are relatively common in preterm infants. Most feeding problems occur in the neonatal period, but many infants demonstrate recurrent or chronic problems with sucking and swallowing.[5] Unrecognized, these problems may lead to significantly impaired nutritional intake and negatively affect the parent–infant relationship. Infants at risk for development of feeding problems include those with oral feedings delayed during the neonatal period and those with immature oral motor skills related to prematurity. In addition, those with transient neurologic immaturity or more permanent neurologic deficits are at highest risk. Additional risk factors for development of feeding dysfunction include chronic lung disease, tracheostomy, GER, and inconsistent feeding techniques by multiple caregivers.

Oral reflexes that allow normal feeding and protect the airway from aspiration may be hypoactive or hyperactive in preterm infants. Abnormal reflexes such as the tonic bite reflex, abnormal tongue thrust, and hyperactive gag can complicate further any hope for successful and pleasurable feeding. A hyperactive gag is particularly troublesome because the infant may manifest oral hypersensitivity and be unable to tolerate the nipple or spoon on the tongue and resist any oral stimulation. Other causes of hypersensitivity or tactile defensiveness include prolonged intubation and repeated suctioning or passage of nasogastric feeding tubes.

The evaluation of a possible feeding disorder includes a detailed history of feeding behaviors and nutritive intake, a physical examination with assessment of oral motor reflexes, and observation of a feeding. If an infant with chronic lung disease desaturates during feeding, increasing the supplemental oxygen during feeding can improve feeding behavior.[6] Evaluation of the type of nipple and its hole may show that the hole is too small, causing fatigue, or too large, making it difficult to control the flow. Indications for radiologic evaluation include suspected aspiration during feeding or an anatomic abnormality such as a tracheoesophageal fistula.

All of these conditions are amenable to therapy if identified early. Treatment of underlying medical problems often helps ameliorate the feeding problems. A pediatric speech pathologist or occupational therapist trained in feeding techniques can assess an infant and develop an appropriate feeding program once the problem has been defined.

Feeding an infant is normally a relaxing, nurturing act that plays a role in parent–infant bonding. In the presence of a feeding disorder, feedings may become a major source of stress, frustration, and anxiety for the infant, parents, and physicians.

IMMUNIZATIONS

Most preterm infants should receive the same immunizations as the term infant and on similar schedules. Measles, mumps, rubella, *Haemophilus* influenza type B, and hepatitis B vaccines should be given at the same chronologic age as recommended for full-term infants.

DIPHTHERIA, TETANUS, PERTUSSIS

The American Academy of Pediatrics (AAP) recommends that full doses of DTP vaccine be administered to prematurely born infants at the appropriate postnatal (*i.e.*, chronologic) age.[7] A large percentage of preterm infants demonstrate inadequate protection if given a reduced dosage of DTP vaccine at the routine intervals.[7] Fewer side effects occur in preterm infants who receive full-dose vaccine than in their full-term counterparts. The same contraindications to immunizing full-term infants against pertussis apply to preterm infants. Most important, infants with bronchopulmonary dysplasia (BPD) are at highest risk for serious sequelae if they contract pertussis. Therefore, the pertussis component of this vaccine should not be withheld due to their chronic disease. Similarly, the pertussis component should be given to any child with cerebral palsy or other muscle tone abnormalities as long as there is no seizure disorder.

POLIO

The AAP Committee on Immunization Practices recommends that full-dose oral polio vaccine be administered at the appropriate chronologic age, but only after discharge from the hospital. A full course of inactivated polio vaccine, enhanced potency, should be given instead to any child who remains hospitalized beyond 2 months of age, is immunocompromised, or lives with an immunodeficient person.

INFLUENZA

Infants with chronic pulmonary disease (*e.g.*, BPD) or cardiac disease with pulmonary vascular congestion are at high risk for development of serious illness if infected with an influenza virus.[8] Infants with influenza have presented with symptoms of sepsis, apnea, and lower airway disease. To protect vulnerable infants, immunization with influenza vaccine is indicated for household contacts, including siblings, primary caretakers, and home care nurses as well as hospital personnel. For infants older than 6 months of age, two doses of split virus vaccine should be given 1 month apart between October and December, followed by an annual dose. Adults and older siblings with natural immunity or who have received previous immunizations need only one yearly dose.

SPECIALIZED CARE

In addition to routine well-child care, the preterm infant may require specialized follow-up for the monitoring, detection, and management of sequelae from neonatal problems. The remainder of this chapter is devoted to a discussion of these special needs.

RETINOPATHY OF PREMATURITY

Retinopathy of prematurity (ROP; see Chap. 53) is a disorder that interrupts the normal vascularization of the developing retina. Although reported in term infants, ROP is mainly a disease associated with prematurity. The incidence and severity of ROP increase with decreasing gestational age. Most cases of ROP resolve spontaneously, but even with complete resolution, scarring of the retina may occur. Generally, the more severe the disease, the longer it takes for resolution. An infant who has had ROP, however, is at a ten times greater risk for visual sequelae than one who has not.[9]

According to recommendations in the *AAP Guidelines for Perinatal Care,*[1] all infants delivered at less than 35 weeks of gestation or under 1800 g who received oxygen therapy, and all infants younger than 30 weeks of gestational age or weighing less than 1300 g, regardless of oxygen exposure, should have an ophthalmologic examination for ROP. The initial examination should not take place before 4 to 6 weeks in the younger infants because a vitreous haze may interfere with visualization of the retina, and the yield for identifying ROP is low. If only one examination is possible, it should be at 7 to 9 weeks of age to catch the peak period of occurrence. A schedule of follow-up visits is based on the retinal findings. All infants with immature fundi or any stage of ROP require close monitoring until the eyes have matured or the ROP has completely resolved. Thereafter, follow-up to assess for refractive errors should be at 1 year of age, before kindergarten, or earlier for clinical signs. Infants with resolving ROP need careful follow-up because some revert to severe active disease.

Sequelae of ROP depend largely on the extent of retinal scarring. As much as 80% of stage 3 ROP resolves spontaneously without significant scarring, but, even in infants with fully regressed ROP, there may be subtle retinal changes resulting in refractive errors, strabismus, or amblyopia. In addition, an infant left with moderate scarring can experience retinal tears, late retinal detachment, nystagmus, glaucoma, cataracts, vitreous hemorrhage or membranes, and severe scarring that can lead to blindness.[10]

Services for visually impaired children are available on county and state levels. Early identification of a child with visual handicaps to such programs is essential to provide the child and family with the services and resources they need.

HEARING PROBLEMS

The incidence of sensorineural hearing loss in preterm infants is generally reported to be between 1% and 3%.[11,12] Several factors place these infants at particular risk for hearing loss, including hypoxia, hyperbilirubinemia, infections, unstable blood pressure, environmental noise, and ototoxic drugs. According to the Joint Committee on Infant Hearing, infants with any of the criteria listed should receive auditory screening, preferably by brain stem auditory evoked response, before 3 months of age.

The factors that identify neonates (*i.e.*, infants from birth to 28 days of age) who are at risk for sensorineural hearing impairment include the following:

- family history of congenital or delayed onset of sensorineural impairment in childhood
- congenital infection known or suspected to be associated with sensorineural hearing impairment (*e.g.*, toxoplasmosis, syphilis, rubella, cytomegalovirus, herpes)
- craniofacial anomalies (*e.g.*, morphologic abnormalities of the pinna and ear canal, absent philtrum)
- birth weight < 1500 g (3.3 lb)
- hyperbilirubinemia at a level exceeding indication for exchange transfusion
- ototoxic medications including but not limited to the aminoglycosides (*e.g.*, gentamicin, tobramycin, kanamycin, streptomycin), used for more than 5 days, and loop diuretics used in combination with aminoglycosides
- bacterial meningitis
- severe depression at birth, which may include infants with Apgar scores of 0 to 3 at 5 minutes after birth, those who fail to initiate spontaneous respiration by 10 minutes after birth, or those with hypotonia persisting to 2 hours of age
- prolonged mechanical ventilation for longer than 10 days (*e.g.*, persistent pulmonary hypertension)
- stigmata or other findings associated with a syndrome known to include sensorineural hearing loss (*e.g.*, Waardenburg syndrome, Usher syndrome).

Passing an initial hearing screening does not preclude the possibility of a later, acquired hearing loss. Absent or abnormal responses to auditory stimulation, delays in speech development, poor articulation, or inattentiveness should raise the suspicion of a hearing loss that requires a more thorough evaluation. All infants who fail an initial hearing screen should be referred to an audiologist for further testing and intervention. In general, an infant with a sensorineural hearing loss should have a repeat audiologic evaluation performed every 3 months for 1 year after initial diagnosis, every 6 months during the preschool period, and yearly while in school.

In hearing tests, zero-decibel (dB) represents the level at which response to a sound should occur 50% of the time. If sound is not heard at this level, the decibel level is raised until the sound is audible 50% of the time. Responses above 15 dB are indicative of some degree of hearing loss (Table 60-1).

Children with moderate to profound hearing loss are at high risk for delayed onset of language, problems with articulation, language impairment, and alterations in voice quality. Cognitive delays may be encountered due to a loss of auditory input or a lan-

TABLE 60–1
CLASSIFICATION OF HEARING LOSS

Hearing Loss (dB)	Description
0–15	Normal
16–25	Borderline–mild
26–40	Mild
41–55	Mild–moderate
56–70	Moderate–severe
71–90	Severe
91 and above	Profound

guage delay. Behavior problems often are experienced and include inattentiveness, overactive or aggressive behaviors, and immature peer relations.

Hearing aids can be fitted early in infancy to avoid acoustic deprivation. With auditory stimulation being provided, language acquisition may proceed more normally. Along with hearing amplification, language stimulation therapy should be provided.

For those children whose hearing loss cannot be improved by hearing aids, different modes of communication are necessary. These include sign language, alternate methods of gesturing or word spelling, language boards, or computer-assisted communication devices. The latter two methods are particularly useful for a child with cerebral palsy.

NECROTIZING ENTEROCOLITIS

Survivors of NEC, especially those who required surgical intervention, may have problems after discharge. The most common complications include strictures or adhesions and short bowel syndrome (SBS).

Strictures or adhesions of the small or large intestines may develop within 2 weeks to 2 months after the acute episode of NEC. Symptoms of complete or, more commonly, partial intestinal obstruction include vomiting, abdominal distention, constipation or obstipation, or hematochezia. Lower gastrointestinal bleeding may be the only symptom of stricture formation without any obstruction. Intermittent or persistent problems with constipation or obstipation are the more common symptoms that an infant may experience well into the first year of life. Management of significant strictures or adhesions generally involves surgical resection, but those with minimal symptoms may be treated conservatively. Stool softeners are useful in preventing obstipation or constipation.

Short bowel syndrome often results from decreased intestinal length or function. Necrotizing enterocolitis requiring significant bowel resection is one of the most common causes of SBS. The associated symptoms are caused by decreased digestion and absorption of nutrients by a smaller intestinal surface area and a more rapid transit time. Most often, evidence is seen of carbohydrate, protein, fat, vitamin, and mineral malabsorption, and an increase in colonic water secretion. Occasionally, SBS is associated with a decreased enterohepatic circulation and gallstones. The resultant problems of SBS constitute a syndrome of chronic diarrhea, malabsorption, growth retardation, and vitamin and mineral deficiencies.[13] The prognosis of SBS is reasonably good if more than 20 cm of small bowel without an ileocecal valve, or more than 15 cm of small bowel with an ileocecal valve remains after surgery. The existence of complications related to total parenteral nutrition also will affect the child's prognosis.

GASTROESOPHAGEAL REFLUX

Gastroesophageal reflux refers to a condition where gastric contents reflux into the esophagus and cause subtle or overt signs and symptoms. Although it can develop in full-term infants, GER occurs more commonly in preterm infants. Symptoms develop from incompetence of the lower esophageal sphincter. Recurrent, nonprojectile emesis is the most common presenting symptom of GER. Usually, infants vomit within 1 to 2 hours after a feeding. An infant may experience several small-volume emeses after a feeding or only one or two large-volume emeses. Some children, however, have no significant emesis but reflux into the esophagus or mouth and then reswallow. Infants also may present with Sandifer syndrome, a condition in which an infant cranes his or her neck in various directions, attempting to kink the esophagus and reduce the discomfort associated with reflux. An infant with this presentation may be misdiagnosed as having dystonia or a neurologic abnormality.

Failure to thrive or dehydration may result from chronic vomiting. In addition, many of these infants avoid or refuse feedings. They quickly learn to associate feeding with the discomfort of GER and its related esophagitis.

Apnea and bradycardia are complications of GER. Often, GER will worsen if an attempt is made to treat apnea and bradycardia with a methylxanthine because these medications decrease lower esophageal tone. The physician should consider an evaluation for GER in an infant when his or her apnea or bradycardia worsens, fails to respond to traditional therapy, or persists beyond 44 weeks of adjusted age.[14]

Aspiration pneumonia is a serious sequela of GER. If acute in onset, symptoms are overt, so GER-related aspiration is more likely to be suspected and diagnosed. If chronic, unrecognized aspiration may cause or exacerbate underlying reactive airway disease. The possibility of GER should be considered in infants with BPD whose disease worsens or fails to improve even in the absence of other signs and symptoms of GER.[15]

The evaluation of GER should be individualized. A clinical assessment is sufficient if the history and observation of a feeding presents a classic picture of reflux. A technetium-labeled milk scan is helpful to document suspected aspiration. A *p*H–thermistor study is useful to document acid reflux and associated apnea or bradycardia. Because of the high false-positive and false-negative rate, a barium swallow and upper gastrointestinal series are of limited value except in demonstrating associated anatomic abnormalities.[15]

Management of GER depends on the severity of the reflux and its associated symptoms. Simple medical management, successful in 80% of patients, includes thickening formula with cereal, keeping the infant in a semiupright position after meals, and avoiding any increase in abdominal pressure such as placing the infant in an infant seat after meals. Medications may be considered for infants who do not respond to conservative management or who have more severe symptoms. Medications are used to increase lower esophageal sphincter tone and include metoclopramide (Reglan) and bethanecol (Urecholine). Bethanecol should be used with caution in infants with chronic lung disease because it may induce or worsen bronchospasm. Antacids or the histamine$_2$-receptor antagonists, cimetadine or ranitidine, can be used as adjunct therapy to treat or prevent secondary esophagitis.

Surgical management, most often a Nissen fundoplication, is necessary in about 10% of patients with GER. Surgery should be reserved for infants either who fail to respond to medical management or who manifest recurrent pulmonary infections, unremittent apnea, or failure to thrive despite aggressive medical management.

INTRAVENTRICULAR HEMORRHAGE

Intraventricular hemorrhage (IVH) is one of the most serious neurologic events encountered by neonates. It occurs in up to 50% of infants born weighing under 1500 g.[16] There is an inverse relationship between gestational age and the incidence of hemorrhage. With the increase in survival of infants at lower gestational ages, an increase in the number of infants with IVH may be expected as well. Follow-up imaging studies should be performed to demonstrate resolution of hemorrhage and to diagnose any anatomic sequelae. The most common complications of IVH include hemorrhagic infarction, post-hemorrhagic hydrocephalus, porencephalic cyst, periventricular leukomalacia (PVL), and ventriculomegaly without hydrocephalus (*i.e.,* hydrocephalus ex vacuo).

In clinical practice, a common problem is distinguishing the onset of hydrocephalus from catch-up head growth when an infant's head circumference crosses percentiles. Clinically, all premature infants with and without IVH should be monitored with at least monthly measurements of head circumference and documentation of neurodevelopmental progress. If a child has greater than a 2-cm weekly increase in head circumference or demonstrates any symptoms of increased intracranial pressure or a change in neurologic status, hydrocephalus should be considered and evaluated by cranial imaging studies.[2] In general, most ventriculomegaly following IVH occurs within 2 weeks of the initial insult, and radiographic appearance rarely changes after 3 months unless a shunt was required.

Most often, ventriculoperitoneal shunts for hydrocephalus continue to work without complication according to the principle of volume dependence. If complications occur, they usually are caused by mechanical malfunction or infection. Mechanical malfunctions result from disruptions at any point along the shunt apparatus or an obstruction either proximally, along the length of the tubing, or distally within the peritoneum. Signs of malfunction are those related to obstruction and resultant increase in intracranial pressure.

If symptoms suggest malfunction, ultrasonography or computed tomography (CT) scan is recommended to evaluate the size of the ventricles compared to baseline, as is a simple roentgenogram of the entire length of shunt tubing to determine its integrity. Pumping the reservoir, if one is present, should be performed only by a physician familiar with the procedure. The information obtained can help determine the location of a blockage but could be misinterpreted by those unfamiliar with the technique. An obstructed or malfunctioning shunt dictates immediate neurosurgical evaluation.

Symptoms of an infected shunt include signs of increased intraventricular pressure associated with an obstruction plus fever and irritability. Shunt infection results in ventriculitis more often than meningitis. Infection may represent colonization of the apparatus only. Diagnosis is made by performing a needle aspiration of cerebrospinal fluid (CSF) from the reservoir using aseptic technique and obtaining a Gram stain and culture. Treatment usually includes appropriate intravenous antibiotics and removing or externalizing the shunt tubing. If necessary, the shunt tubing can be replaced if it is still necessary once the CSF remains sterile for at least 72 hours.[17]

If a shunt functions properly, follow-up usually is based on the individual neurosurgeon's recommendations. A routine imaging study for baseline usually is obtained when the infant is medically stable before hospital discharge. The clinician following the infant as an outpatient should use the same imaging technique so that a comparison can be made with the baseline study for any change suggestive of an obstruction. If the brain appears normal and no symptoms of obstruction or infection develop, a follow-up scan may be avoided.

PERIVENTRICULAR LEUKOMALACIA

Periventricular leukomalacia is ischemic infarction of the white matter adjacent to the lateral ventricles. A weakening in the integrity of the white matter in this area occurs, followed by either repair or the development of cysts. The reported incidence of PVL in infants with birth weights under 1500 g varies from 2% to 22%.[18–20] Infants at risk for PVL are those whose perinatal course was complicated by severe hypoxia, ischemia, or both. Infants of early gestational age are particularly susceptible to the development of PVL because of their poorly developed cerebral vascular system, especially after sepsis, seizures, meningitis, IVH, cardiorespiratory (CR) arrest, or life-threatening apnea.

In the weeks that follow a major insult leading to

PVL, phagocytosis of the necrotic material occurs with development of fluid-filled, periventricular cysts. Periventricular leukomalacia and, subsequently, the presence and size of cysts can be determined using cranial ultrasonography, CT, or magnetic resonance imaging scan. Resolution of the cysts is highly variable and some never completely resolve.

Beyond the neonatal period, screening for the presence of PVL should be considered in any child with cerebral palsy without an apparent cause.[21] Since there are no symptoms specific for PVL, it can easily be missed during the neonatal period.

If PVL is associated with the loss of vital areas of neural tissue, and formation of cysts greater than 3 mm in diameter, the infant so affected is at increased risk for cerebral palsy, developmental delay, and visual or auditory impairments. If PVL is not associated with residual cysts, few if any sequelae develop. When cysts persist, an infant's motor development is most affected. Cerebral palsy, manifested as moderate-to-severe quadriplegia or diplegia, is reported to develop in 90% to 100% of children with cystic residua after PVL. The intellectual capacities of children with PVL and cyst formation are more variable. Mental retardation is more common in infants with residual cysts, but ranges from mild to severe. If the cysts develop in the occipital region, visual impairment may result.[21]

All infants with PVL, especially with cysts, should be monitored closely for neurodevelopmental sequelae. Periodic cranial imaging studies, preferably head ultrasonography, will determine stability or resolution of the cysts. Parents of infants with PVL should be counseled on the importance of periodic neurodevelopmental assessments for early detection of any sequelae, and intervention when appropriate.

SEIZURES

Seizures during the newborn period may be subtle or overt and may occur singly or repetitively. Diagnosis usually is made while the infant still is hospitalized. Medical staff often document motor activity or behavioral changes consistent with seizure activity that can then be confirmed by electroencephalography (EEG). Although the normal immature cortex has a relatively high seizure threshold, cortical injury enhances the brain's susceptibility to seizures. Most neonatal seizures are provoked by a significant neurologic insult such as intracranial hemorrhage, hypoxic–ischemic encephalopathy (*i.e.*, asphyxia), metabolic disturbances, or central nervous system (CNS) infections.[22]

The primary determinant of the outcome of neonatal seizures is correlated closely with the underlying cause. Infants with relatively harmless conditions such as hypocalcemia do well with appropriate treatment of the underlying disturbance. Those with an intracranial hemorrhage or an anoxic insult experience greater morbidity. Infants with seizures associated with asphyxia that were noted at younger than 24 hours of age have a poorer outcome than those with later onset of seizures.[22] Similarly, those with more severe seizures (*e.g.*, status epilepticus, frequent seizures) fare worse.

The decision to treat seizures with anticonvulsants usually is made early in the evolution of the infant's evaluation. If a transient metabolic abnormality is identified and corrected, seizure activity should cease, usually without anticonvulsant therapy. Recommendations regarding the duration of long-term anticonvulsant therapy for neonatal seizures vary. In some cases, medications may be discontinued before initial hospital discharge. Most often, however, once seizures are well controlled, a seizure-free interval of at least 3 months passes before anticonvulsants are withdrawn. Before making a decision to withdraw medications, the physician should make certain that the infant has no further clinical seizure activity and no epileptiform discharges on EEG. A neurologist should evaluate any infant with seizures that persist, to help in their long-term management.

APNEA AND BRADYCARDIA

Infants may continue to experience episodes of apnea or bradycardia after initial hospital discharge. The incidence of apnea and bradycardia and its chronicity are inversely proportional to the gestational age of the infant and parallel the severity of problems the infant had during the neonatal period. Although CNS immaturity is the most common cause for apnea in term infants, it is important to rule out medical problems that may cause apnea even after hospital discharge. If clinically indicated, the symptomatic infant with apnea should be evaluated for the possibility of underlying anemia,[23] sepsis or meningitis, upper airway obstruction, GER, hypoxia, or bronchospasm as possible inciting causes.

Once it has been determined that no remediable factors exist, a decision should be made whether to monitor a child at home.[24] The need for home CR monitoring with or without medication is determined before hospital discharge based on clinical judgment or results of specialized evaluations. The use of CR monitoring remains somewhat controversial. The 1986 National Institutes of Health Consensus Panel on Apnea, Sudden Infant Death Syndrome (SIDS), and Home Monitoring established medical indications for use of CR monitoring[25]:

- one or more severe apparent life-threatening events requiring vigorous stimulation or mouth-to-mouth resuscitation
- symptomatic premature infants documented by parental report or observation by trained personnel
- documentation of episodes of apnea or increased periodic breathing by means of a thermistor–pneumocardiogram
- siblings in families in which two or more infants have died from SIDS

- infants with diseases such as central hypoventilation.

Alarm settings usually are placed at a low heart rate of 80 beats per minute with a maximum respiratory pause of 20 seconds. These may be changed depending on the infant's age or specific clinical circumstances. In most infants, resting heart rate decreases with increasing age.

Often, preterm infants require either theophylline or caffeine in addition to or in lieu of home monitoring.[26] Unless adjusted as the infant gains weight, the blood level of medication gradually will fall, but it rarely is necessary to recheck levels after discharge as long as apneic episodes are infrequent. If episodes continue or increase in frequency despite therapeutic xanthine levels, an evaluation for other possible causes is indicated.

In most cases, the infant should be allowed to outgrow and discontinue the medication when there are no more episodes of apnea for 2 months either clinically or by CR monitor or pneumogram. If, however, the infant is receiving theophylline as a bronchodilator for BPD, it should not be discontinued until symptoms associated with underlying bronchospasm have resolved. Parents should be counseled as to the signs of toxicity of these and all medications.

Most infants initially requiring methylxanthines may be permitted to outgrow the medication while on CR monitors. Many institutions send infants receiving a methylxanthine alone home with no CR monitor and allow them to outgrow this medication. Once they are at least 40 weeks postconceptional age, true apnea of prematurity should no longer be significant, although some infants have prolonged need for xanthine therapy in the absence of other causes. As infants mature, their resting heart rate decreases. This may result in an increase in frequency of false alarms if the lower alarm limit is too high. If the infant is otherwise healthy and without accompanying apnea, the monitor company should lower the heart rate alarm by 10 beats per minute to as low as 60 to 70 beats per minute. If bradycardia persists when awake, or at less than 60 to 70 beats per minute, further evaluation is warranted.

Once the infant is symptom-free for 2 months, medication most often can be safely stopped. If no subsequent episodes are identified by the monitor, a home pneumocardiogram recording can be performed several days after stopping the medication. If the study indicates a mature breathing pattern, 1 to 2 more months of home monitoring without medication is recommended. If no further episodes are documented, a second home pneumogram recording can help to determine if the monitor can be safely discontinued (Fig. 60-1).

CHRONIC LUNG DISEASE

Bronchopulmonary dysplasia is the most frequently diagnosed chronic lung disease in preterm infants. Usually it develops as a sequel to the acute lung injury experienced during the first few weeks of life. The definition of BPD has changed over the years. A traditional diagnosis covered lung disease resulting from respiratory distress shortly after birth and that required more than 28 days of oxygen exposure with representative findings noted on chest roentgenogram.[27] Since many infants with a gestational age younger than 30 weeks require oxygen for more than 28 days without developing chronic lung disease, however, a more restrictive definition of BPD is lung disease in an infant who requires supplemental oxygen beyond 36 weeks postconceptional age.[6]

Although the diagnosis of BPD is given before initial hospital discharge, some infants with mild or minimal residual lung disease may come to the primary care provider's attention with their first viral respiratory tract infection. Those with more severe disease often will be discharged with medications, nebulizer treatments, and supplemental oxygen. Clinical manifestations are similar to those in the nursery and include tachypnea, tachycardia, retractions, rhonchi, bronchospasm, and poor air movement into the lungs bilaterally. More subtle signs of chronic respiratory distress include poor weight gain, feeding intolerance, decreased activity, and a reduced tolerance of exercise. Medical management of infants with BPD often includes any combination of the following: fluid restriction, diuretic therapy, bronchodilator medications, steroids, and supplemental oxygen, even after initial hospital discharge. These therapies are altered depending on the infant's clinical status and potentially withdrawn as the infant matures and improves. How early withdrawal can begin depends on the severity of lung disease at the time of discharge. Additionally, BPD may continue to worsen after discharge so that infants who tolerated either no medication or lower doses may begin to require aggressive intervention after discharge.

DIURETICS

Most often diuretic therapy supplements fluid restriction in an attempt to decrease the fluid retention typical of BPD. Although rarely initiated after discharge, diuretics require monitoring of oral intake, urine output, weight gain, and, less frequently, electrolytes. Normally, one spot-check of serum electrolytes a few weeks after discharge is sufficient and, if negative, need not be rechecked as long as the infant remains medically stable with no significant dietary changes. Infants can outgrow their diuretic doses if there is no worsening of respiratory distress, evidence of peripheral or pulmonary edema, or clinical signs or symptoms of right ventricular strain or failure.

BRONCHODILATORS

Many infants with BPD are discharged on maintenance bronchodilator medications. Unlike diuretics, these medications may need to be modified and continued as part of an aggressive medical regimen.

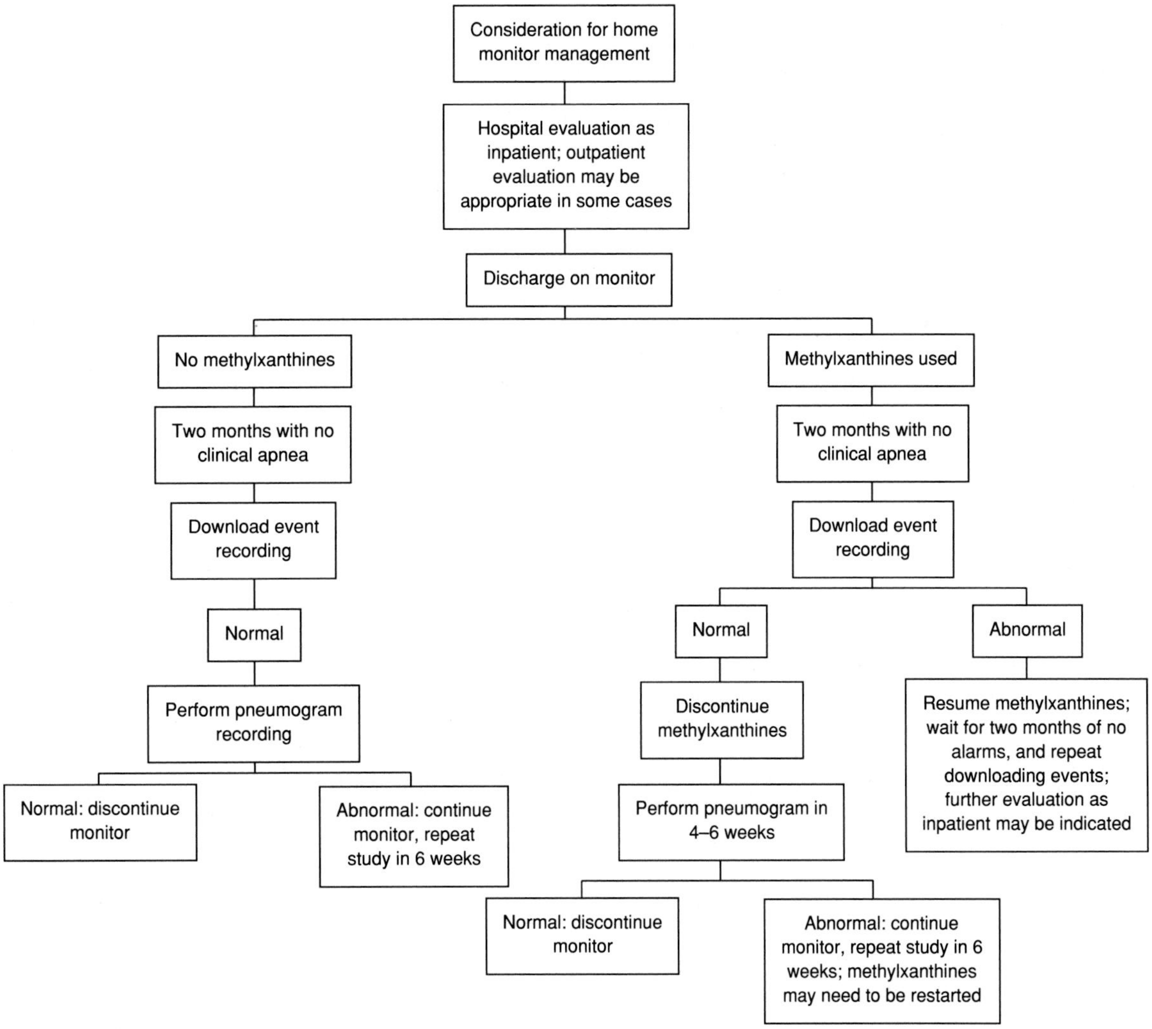

FIG. 60–1. Schema for home monitor management. (From Spitzer AR, Gibson E. Considerations for home monitor management. Clin Perinatol 1992;19:916.)

Bronchodilators are used for outpatient therapy of BPD primarily to help maintain the infant maximally bronchodilated and in a bronchospasm-free state. They are used either as maintenance therapy or during intercurrent illnesses. Although the mechanisms of action of the different medications vary, all cause bronchodilation and relaxation of the smooth muscles of the small airways, allowing better oxygenation and prevention of recurrent bronchospasm. Common bronchodilators used in BPD are described in Appendix H-4.[8]

When xanthines are used as bronchodilators, the dosage needs adjustment for weight gain. This is particularly true if there continues to be a supplemental oxygen requirement or if there is intermittent exacerbation of underlying bronchospasm, tachypnea or increased work of breathing, or a poor activity level. If the infant remains stable or improves, bronchodilators can be weaned by allowing the child to outgrow the medication. Bronchodilators can be withdrawn if there has been adequate weight gain, medical stability, good activity level and continued developmental progress, and no exacerbation of underlying bronchospasm. Usually, weaning is not attempted until the infant is off supplemental oxygen. Bronchodilators may be needed intermittently for acute intercurrent illnesses that precipitate bronchospasm (Table 60-2; see Intercurrent Illnesses).

SUPPLEMENTAL OXYGEN

The decision to continue an infant on supplemental oxygen relates to the severity of underlying lung disease; however, the need for supplemental oxygen should not necessarily interfere with hospital discharge. Some of the more common indications for the use of supplemental oxygen include the following: evidence of desaturation while breathing room air, poor oral feeding due to air hunger, apnea or bradycardia associated with hypoxia, poor growth associ-

TABLE 60–2
EXAMPLES OF MEDICATION CHANGES FOR INFANTS WITH CHRONIC LUNG DISEASE WHO HAVE INCREASED BRONCHOSPASM ASSOCIATED WITH ACUTE ILLNESS

Maintenance Regimen	During Acute Illness With Bronchospasm*
No medication	Add theophylline PO, beta$_2$-agonist, or both†
Theophylline	Add beta$_2$-agonist†
Beta$_2$-agonist	Add theophylline, a second beta$_2$-agonist (by inhalation), or both
Theophylline and beta$_2$-agonist,†	Add a second beta$_2$-agonist (by inhalation) with or without cromolyn inhalation
Theophylline, beta$_2$-agonist,† and cromolyn inhalation	Add a second beta$_2$-agonist† and consider short course of adrenocortical steroid

* Consider subcutaneous epinephrine, beta$_2$-agonist nebulizer treatment in office, or both for immediate stabilization before initiating supplemental therapy. Consider increasing inspired oxygen as needed.
† Beta$_2$-agonist can be given orally or by inhalation.
From Bernbaum JC, Hoffman-Williamson M. Primary care of the preterm infant. St. Louis: Mosby Year Book, 1991:110.

ated with borderline hypoxia, poor exercise tolerance, lethargy, and tachycardia or tachypnea that improves with the use of supplemental oxygen. If possible, it is best to determine the adequacy of oxygenation during sleep, feedings, and periods of activity. Pulse oximetry should indicate saturations of at least 95%. This level of saturation has been shown to result in a significant increase in pulmonary vasodilation, which may preclude the development of pulmonary hypertension and resultant right heart strain.[28] Although many centers begin weaning infants with lower oxygen saturations, studies have shown that infants with chronic lung disease who are optimally oxygenated demonstrate better weight gain, attain corrected age-appropriate milestones more readily, and have fewer intercurrent respiratory illnesses than do infants with lower oxygenation.[6]

Before weaning from supplemental oxygen, the infant's medical stability must be assured, as must adequacy of weight gain, exercise tolerance, and caloric intake. It is preferable to wean a child off oxygen slowly and in a stepwise fashion.[8] A period of several weeks to a month should pass for each step, during which the infant remains medically stable, gains adequate weight, demonstrates good exercise tolerance, and maintains adequate oxygen saturations (Table 60-3). Many home care services can perform intermittent oximetry in the home to assist management. It is easier to wean an infant off oxygen if he or she is kept maximally bronchodilated with supplemental medications. During an illness, it is common to have to increase the amount of supplemental oxygen or to restart it temporarily if the child has weaned recently.

To compensate for increased energy expenditures, the infant with BPD often requires a high caloric intake, between 120 and 150 kcal/kg/day.[29] Increased caloric needs complicated by poor nutritional intake often result in poor growth. Poor nutritional intake in this population may be caused by hypoxemia, anorexia, tachypnea, exercise intolerance, oral motor dysfunction, or GER. In addition, it often is difficult to maximize caloric intake in the face of fluid restriction and intolerance to the exercise of feeding. Caloric intake can be maximized by adding supplements, concentrating formulas, or using isocaloric formulas (Table 60-4).

Even with supplemental calories there are times that growth is not adequate because the infant either tires easily or refuses any additional increased oral intake. It is then that supplemental nasogastric feedings should be considered, to be given either after bottle feedings or continuously during the night. Each method has its own advantages and disadvantages and must be considered within the context of individual family and patient needs. It is crucial to offer sucking opportunities routinely to any child who is tube fed to stimulate the development of the sucking reflex.[5] A feeding therapist may need to begin working early with an infant with BPD and feed-

TABLE 60–3
WEANING A PATIENT FROM SUPPLEMENTAL OXYGEN

Time	Amount of Oxygen per Minute
At hospital discharge	0.5 L at all times
1 month after discharge*	0.5 L during feedings and sleep; 0.25 L when awake
2 months after discharge*	0.25 L at all times
3 months after discharge*	0.25 L during feedings and sleep; room air when awake
4 months after discharge*	Room air at all times

* Assumes clinical stability, appropriate weight gain, and documentation of adquate oxygen saturation. Intervals may vary depending on such criteria.
From Bernbaum JC, Hoffman-Williamson M. Primary care of the preterm infant. St. Louis: Mosby Year Book, 1991:102.

TABLE 60–4
SELECTED CALORIC SUPPLEMENTS

Supplement	Caloric Density	Advantages	Disadvantages
Polycose*	2 kcal/mL	Well tolerated	Low caloric density
Karo syrup*	4 kcal/mL	Well tolerated; readily available; inexpensive	May cause loose stools
Microlipids†	4.5 kcal/mL	Well tolerated	Limited availability; high cost
Medium-chain triglyceride oil†	7.6 kcal/mL	High caloric density; usually well tolerated	May cause diarrhea; does not mix well with formula
Vegetable oil†	9 kcal/mL	Easily available and low cost	Does not mix well with formula
Avocado (pureed; ½ avocado/26 oz formula)‡			
California variety, brown	Adds 7.4 kcal/oz	High caloric density; well tolerated	Season availability; expensive; more preparation needed
Florida variety, green	Adds 5.7 kcal/oz		
Dry baby cereal	10 kcal/Tbsp	Readily available; inexpensive; may help with gastroesophageal reflux	Low caloric density; may cause constipation
Powdered skim milk	27 kcal/Tbsp	Readily available; mixes well with formula	

* Often not used as a supplementation for infants with bronchopulmonary dysplasia, since those infants have been shown to have increased work of breathing when receiving a high-carbohydrate load, compared to those supplemented with fat.
† Use of oil supplements is contraindicated in cases where aspiration is suspected.
‡ May be pureed in large batches and frozen in half-avocado portions.
From Bernbaum JC, Hoffman-Williamson M. Primary care of the preterm infant. St. Louis: Mosby Year Book, 1991:105.

TABLE 60–5
SIGNS AND SYMPTOMS SUGGESTIVE OF LOWER AIRWAY DISEASE

Signs and Symptoms	Likely Causes	Best Treatment
Cough	Underlying bronchospasm	Bronchodilator(s)
	Inflamed and irritated airways	Bronchodilator(s)
	Increased secretions from upper respiratory infection	Consider antihistamine
Tachypnea	Same as for cough	Same as for cough
	Partial obstruction of nasal passages by increased secretions	Suctioning and saline nose drops
	Borderline hypoxia	Consider adding or increasing supplemental oxygen
	Fever	Antipyretics
	Cor pulmonale	Diuretics; digoxin (controversial)
		Treatment directed at improving hypoxia and bronchospasm
Fever	Underlying inflammatory reaction (unlikely to be bacterial etiology); otitis media can often cause respiratory exacerbation	Antipyretics
Wheezing	Underlying bronchospasm and prolonged expiration	Bronchodilators
Desaturation	Poor oxygen exchange because of tachypnea and wheezing	Consider treatments for cough, tachypnea, fever, and wheezing plus supplemental oxygen
Infiltrate on chest roentgenogram	Pneumonia	Consider antibiotic only if certain of diagnosis
	Partial atelectasis common in chronic lung disease	Chest percussion
	Residual chronic changes that were present since time of initial hospital discharge	Supportive treatment only

From Bernbaum JC, Hoffman-Williamson M. Primary care of the preterm infant. St. Louis: Mosby Year Book, 1991:109.

ing difficulties to prevent the poor-quality sucking frequently encountered in these children.

INTERCURRENT ILLNESSES

Bronchospasm with viral or bacterial respiratory illnesses will develop in many infants with BPD (Table 60-5). When the infant is not already on maintenance therapy, bronchodilators can be initiated during acute illnesses. If the infant is on maintenance bronchodilator therapy, synergistic medications can be added during acute exacerbations and withdrawn as the acute symptoms resolve, returning to maintenance therapy. The modes of action of the common bronchodilators and supplemental medications are detailed in Appendix H-4.

Minimizing the exposure of infants with BPD to environmental irritants and communicable diseases will help decrease the frequency of intercurrent episodes of bronchospasm and allow more time for the lung to heal. Some environmental irritants include cigarette or fireplace smoke, pet fur or dander, kerosene heaters, paint, and infectious agents. The less irritation the lung is exposed to, the quicker the recovery process will be.

Rehospitalization is a common occurrence in children with BPD, especially during the first year of life. Parents of these infants should be advised of this possibility before the initial hospital discharge. Every effort should be made to treat intercurrent illnesses and associated bronchospasm on an outpatient basis, but if the infant does not respond readily, hospitalization is appropriate for more aggressive treatment. If, however, the child requires an elective surgical procedure such as a hernia repair, admission should be avoided during epidemics of respiratory-related illnesses.

Managing infants with BPD is clinical challenge for the practicing physician. The many facets of their care require a complete understanding of how their lung disease affects their physical well-being. Fortunately, most of their medical problems occur during the first year or two of life, and improvement can be expected in each subsequent year.

REFERENCES

1. American Academy of Pediatrics and American College of Obstetricians and Gynecologists. AAP guidelines for perinatal care. 2nd ed. Elk Grove Village, IL: American Academy of Pediatrics, 1992.
2. Hack M, Fanaroff AA. Growth patterns in the ICN graduate. In: Ballard RA, ed. Pediatric care of the ICN graduate. Philadelphia: WB Saunders, 1988.
3. Reynolds JW. Nutrition of the low birth weight infant. In: Walker WA, Watkins JB, eds. Nutrition in pediatrics. Boston: Little, Brown & Co., 1985:649.
4. Maclean WC, LeRomana GL, Masse E, et al. Nutritional management of chronic diarrhea and malnutrition: primary reliance on oral feeding. J Pediatr 1980;97:316.
5. Bernbaum JC, Pererra GR, Watkins JB, et al. Non-nutritive sucking during gavage feeding enhances growth and maturation in premature infants. Pediatrics 1983;71:41.
6. Shennan AT, Dunn MS, Ohlsson A, et al. Abnormal pulmonary outcomes in premature infants: prediction from oxygen requirement in the neonatal period. Pediatrics 1988;82:327.
7. Bernbaum JC, Daft AL, Anolik R, et al. Response of preterm infants to routine DTP immunizations. J Pediatr 1985;107:184.
8. Bernbaum J, Hoffman-Williamson M. Primary care of the preterm infant. St. Louis: Mosby Year Book, 1991.
9. Flynn J, Phelps D. Retinopathy of prematurity: problem and challenge. New York: Alan R. Liss, 1988.
10. Cryotherapy for Retinopathy of Prematurity Cooperative Group: multicenter trial of cryotherapy for ROP. Arch Ophthalmol 1988;106:471.
11. Northern J, Gerkin K. New technology in infant hearing screening. Otolaryngol Clin North Am 1989;22:75.
12. American Academy of Pediatrics Joint Committee on Infant Hearing. 1990 position statement. ASHA 1991;33(Suppl 5):3.
13. Cooper A, Floyd TF, Ross AJ, et al. Morbidity and mortality of short-bowel syndrome acquired in infancy: an update. J Pediatr Surg 1984;19:711.
14. Spitzer AR, Boyle JT, Tuchman DM, et al. Awake apnea associated with GE reflux: a specific clinical syndrome. J Pediatr 1984;104:200.
15. Sondheimer JM. Gastroesophageal reflux: update on pathogenesis and diagnosis. Pediatr Clin North Am 1988;35:103.
16. Larroche JC. Intraventricular hemorrhage in the premature neonate. Advances in Perinatal Neurology 1979;1:115.
17. Odio C, McCraken G, Nelson J. CSF shunt infections in pediatrics: a seven year experience. Am J Dis Child 1984;138:1103.
18. Bozynski MEA, Nelson MN, Matalont AS, et al. Cavitary periventricular leukomalacia: incidence and short-term outcome in infants weighing < 1200 grams at birth. Dev Med Child Neurol 1985;85:572.
19. DeVries LS, Regey R, Pennock JM, et al. Ultrasound evolution and later outcome of infants with periventricular densities. Early Hum Dev 1988;16:225.
20. Ford LM, Han K, Steichan J, et al. Very low-birth-weight, preterm infants with or without intracranial hemorrhage. Clin Pediatr 1989;28:302.
21. Graziani LJ, Pasto M, Stanley C, et al. Neonatal neurosonographic correlates of cerebral palsy in preterm infants. Pediatrics 1986;78:88.
22. Clancy RR. Neonatal seizures. In: Stevenson DL, Sunshine P, eds. Fetal and neonatal brain injury: mechanisms, management and the risk of practice. Philadelphia: BC Decker, 1989:123.
23. DeMaio JG, Harris MC, Deuber C, et al. Effect of blood transfusion on apnea frequency in growing premature infants. J Pediatr 1989;114:1039.
24. Spitzer AR, Gibson E. Considerations for home monitor management. Clin Perinatol 1992;19:907.
25. Forster J. The latest word on apnea monitoring. Contemporary Pediatrics 1986;3:77.
26. Bairam A, Boutroy MJ, Badonnel Y, et al. Theophylline versus caffeine: comparative effects in treatment of idiopathic apnea in the preterm infant. J Pediatr 1987;110:636.
27. Avery ME, Tooley WH, Keller JB, et al. Is chronic lung disease in LBW infants preventable? A survey of 8 centers. Pediatrics 1987;79:26.
28. Abman SH, Woolfe RR, Acccurso FJ, et al. Pulmonary vascular response to oxygen in infants with severe BPD. Pediatrics 1985; 75:80.
29. Yeh TF, McClenan DA, Ajayi OA, et al. Metabolic rate and energy balance in infants with BPD. J Pediatr 1989;114:448.

Neonatology: Pathophysiology and Management of the Newborn, Fourth Edition,
edited by Gordon B. Avery, Mary Ann Fletcher, and Mhairi G. MacDonald.
J.B. Lippincott Company, Philadelphia © 1994.

chapter 61

Developmental Outcome

FORREST C. BENNETT

More than 250,000 low-birth-weight infants (LBW; ≤2500 g) are born each year in the United States, constituting approximately 7% of all live births. Of these infants, approximately 50,000 annually are of very low birth weight (VLBW; ≤1500 g), constituting approximately 1.5% of all births. Since the estimated LBW incidence has remained relatively stable over the past 30 years (Fig. 61-1), contemporary reductions in neonatal mortality are steadily increasing the prevalence of biologically vulnerable infants and children in the overall population.[1]

Although much medical, legal, ethical, and economic debate continues to occur over the effects of neonatal intensive care on the long-term developmental status of LBW survivors, most investigators are in agreement that the single clearest outcome of this technically enhanced care has been a dramatic and continuing reduction in neonatal mortality since the early 1960s, particularly for VLBW infants since the mid-1970s (see Fig. 61-1).[2,3] With current standards of practice in the neonatal intensive care unit (NICU), many more LBW, premature infants are surviving to be discharged home after extended hospitalizations than was the case even 5 to 10 years ago. The major factors responsible for this increased survival include the technical ability to provide assisted mechanical ventilation to the smallest of LBW infants, the regionalization of perinatal–neonatal care with greater numbers of maternal transports to and infants born in tertiary centers, and the widespread use of exogenous surfactant.

Remarkable improvements in the birth-weight–specific mortality rates accounted for 90% of the overall decline in neonatal mortality between 1960 and 1980.[4] During these two decades, decreases in the mortality rates of infants weighing between 1500 and 2500 g contributed more than any other weight group because of both greater proportional decreases and higher absolute declines in mortality; however, there has been steady and statistically significant reduction in mortality rates among VLBW infants throughout the last 10 to 15 years. Mortality for infants with birth weights of 1001 to 1500 g has fallen from more than 50% in 1961 to less than 10% today. Moreover, the most substantial improvement of the 1980s over the 1970s in neonatal mortality rates was in the 751- to 1000-g birth weight group, where today's infants have greater than an 80% chance of surviving if they are admitted to an NICU.[5] Finally, in the 1990s, 40% to more than 60% survival for infants between 500 and 750 g birth weight is being accomplished.[6,7] The intact survival of a 380-g infant has been described.[8]

Although survival continues to increase in all LBW categories, the greatest impact of neonatal intensive care technology clearly has been on the smallest, sickest, and most medically fragile infants. The success in achieving these improved survival rates for LBW, premature infants raises obvious concerns about the subsequent development of such vulnerable infants. It mandates an organized neurodevelopmental follow-up approach to carefully and continuously monitor the quality of survival of the NICU graduate.

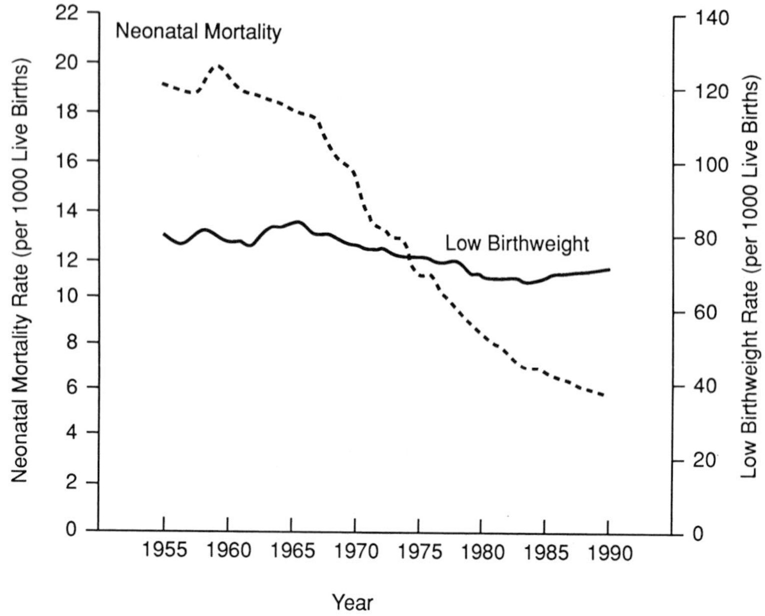

FIG. 61–1. United States annual rates of neonatal mortality and low-birth-weight births from 1955–1990. (Adapted from Lee KS, Paneth N, Gartner LM, et al. Neonatal mortality: an analysis of the recent improvement in the United States. American J of Public Health 1980;70:15.)

ORGANIZATION OF A HIGH-RISK INFANT FOLLOW-UP PROGRAM

OBJECTIVES

There are a number of compelling reasons for conducting longitudinal neurodevelopmental surveillance of survivors of neonatal intensive care. There also are practical problems encountered in providing comprehensive follow-up services. Individual follow-up programs must clearly define their own goals and objectives and then organize their roles and activities accordingly. A community hospital's follow-up efforts likely will be determined by a different set of expectations than those of a university-affiliated tertiary care center. Furthermore, ideal follow-up care in the United States frequently is constrained by limited resources. In general, follow-up programs are designed to meet one or more of the following objectives.

QUALITY CONTROL

Regular, periodic follow-up of a large proportion of survivors can provide one type of audit of an individual NICU's performance. Since intensive care nurseries differ in such critical management areas as neonatal resuscitation, modes of assisted ventilation, treatment of ventriculomegaly, and use of parenteral nutrition, and also in such neonatal outcomes as mortality and prevalence of medical complications (*e.g.*, bronchopulmonary dysplasia [BPD], intracranial hemorrhage), units may wish to compare their neurodevelopmental morbidity with the contemporary experience of similar nurseries.[9] They also may wish to monitor their major disabling morbidities from year to year to detect any significant differences that might accompany further reductions in mortality or the introduction of new intensive care procedures or treatments. It must be recognized that follow-up at 1 or 2 years of age, although providing much useful information about the prevalence of major neurosensory impairment among survivors, is of insufficient duration to identify changes over time in more subtle aspects of brain function such as learning and behavior.

DEVELOPMENTAL SERVICES

Neurodevelopmental follow-up can provide important ongoing subspecialty care to at-risk children and families. Follow-up clinic personnel with a multidisciplinary approach will likely have the most experience and expertise in a given community concerning the unique developmental patterns of LBW, premature infants. In general, the follow-up program will complement and serve as secondary or tertiary developmental consultants to the primary health care providers. The program will encourage and facilitate the establishment of a community-based medical home (*e.g.*, private practitioner, public health clinic) for every medically complex survivor. Experience with biologically and environmentally vulnerable indigent populations, however, suggests that actual provision of primary health care, in addition to evaluation and case management services, may be necessary in some situations to prevent attrition and maintain contact with those children and families at greatest long-term risk.[10] Although the appropriate approach to this issue of role definition is likely to vary with different populations and access to medical care in different settings, it obviously is of fundamental importance to the organization of follow-up clinics and also to the maintenance of mutual trust relationships with the primary care community.

The specific objectives of follow-up neurodevelopmental assessment activities may be grouped conveniently as follows: to provide cautious reassurance to anxious parents; to ensure early identification and intervention for persistent developmental abnormalities; and to recognize the natural history of transient developmental abnormalities and thereby avoid unnecessary, costly interventions. Maintaining an appropriate balance of diagnostic and reassurance functions is one of the greatest challenges for the contemporary high-risk follow-up program.

DEVELOPMENTAL TRAINING

The follow-up clinic provides a marvelous setting for interdisciplinary developmental training. It is a clinical laboratory for the observation of the gradual recovery and normalization over time of most at-risk infants and, in other cases, the gradual evolution of a wide variety of permanent neurodevelopmental dysfunctions. As such, the at-risk population offers a longitudinal training experience that spans the normal–abnormal development continuum. In many pediatric training programs, the follow-up clinic is the sole opportunity for pediatric residents to observe the outcomes of their own intensive care efforts. It would seem virtually impossible for physicians to be informed adequately about the ethical debates and dilemmas surrounding neonatal intensive care without a first-hand follow-up experience. Likewise, other child development professionals (*e.g.*, psychologists, physical therapists, communication disorders specialists) can use the follow-up clinic profitably as a diverse training base, particularly to broaden the range of normative development for their students. Obviously, these training objectives will apply primarily to university-affiliated tertiary care centers, with their numerous and varied trainee availability.

OUTCOME RESEARCH

The university-affiliated follow-up program should be engaged actively in clinical research that contributes to the understanding of the neurodevelopmental and neurobehavioral outcomes of children who experienced neonatal intensive care. These studies may take the form of either descriptive observational reports or clinical trials of specific perinatal–neonatal interventions. For example, the University of Washington's High Risk Infant Follow-Up Program has published studies describing the outcome of infants weighing less than 800 g at birth,[11–13] as well as studies evaluating the utility of procedures such as electronic fetal monitoring of premature labor and delivery,[14] and treatments such as high-frequency mechanical ventilation.[15] Although tremendous variability exists in the target populations, methodologies, and general scientific quality of the accumulated high-risk follow-up research, a growing consensus of valid outcome observations gradually has emerged over the last 25 years, and informative summary conclusions can be synthesized. Even though the ideal, population-based, non–risk-controlled, longitudinal to school age study rarely is accomplished for a variety of practical reasons (*e.g.*, cost, subject mobility, investigator discontinuity), individual follow-up investigations, carefully performed albeit with a limited scope, continue to modify and refine overall knowledge and, in some cases, challenge assumptions.

This is not to say that broad, well funded, collaborative follow-up efforts should not be pursued vigorously on both regional and national, and even international, levels. A recognized need for uniform population descriptions, standardized assessment protocols, common disability definitions, and adequate numbers of pooled subjects still exists. Threats to the interpretability and generalizability of small, local studies include population demographic bias, neonatal treatment differences, attrition of highest-risk (*i.e.*, doubly vulnerable) subjects, and cross-sectional data analysis combining multiple age end points. A great deal has been learned about the short- and long-term prognoses of NICU survivors from hundreds of independent follow-up studies, but much more awaits to be clarified by enhanced research approaches.[16]

PERSONNEL

The size and complexity of the neurodevelopmental follow-up team depend on the scope of the program and the size of the patient population. For example, a level II to III community hospital with primarily developmental service objectives likely will employ a smaller team, follow for a shorter period of time, and administer fewer standardized measures than a university-affiliated tertiary care center with training and research responsibilities. In either case, certain key tasks must be accomplished. Probably the most critical role in terms of maximizing follow-up compliance and minimizing attrition is that of the follow-up coordinator, usually a program nurse. This person is the liaison between the NICU and the follow-up clinic. The nurse coordinator can identify and meet eligible infants and families before they leave the nursery, participate in the discharge conference and transition plans, and, in some cases, make preliminary contact with the family by means of a home visit before the initial follow-up evaluation. This liaison function is particularly important in those programs that conduct high-risk follow-up at a separate site away from the intensive care nursery and in which none of the follow-up personnel is involved actively in the NICU.

Overall program direction is typically provided by a physician or psychologist. This person ultimately is responsible both for meeting the broad programmatic objectives and also for day-to-day operations. The director of a university-affiliated follow-up program frequently must balance competing service, training, and research obligations while eclectically maintaining sufficient funding sources to ensure long-term program viability. The director certainly should be knowledgeable in terms of current follow-up literature and contemporary models of program structure and function.

Other follow-up roles of the interdisciplinary team include the following:

Medical–neurologic assessment: this may be provided by a neonatologist, developmental pediatrician, or child neurologist. In some programs a pediatric nurse practitioner or the nurse coordinator may provide health, nutritional, and behavioral guidance pertaining especially to such issues as feeding, sleeping, temperament, and discipline.

Developmental–intellectual–academic achievement assessment: this often will be performed by a physical therapist during infancy and by a clinical psychologist or psychometrist thereafter. Some tertiary centers may use a neuropsychologist at school age. In some programs, an early childhood educator or infant developmental specialist participates in early assessments.

Neuromotor assessment: this usually will be done by a physical therapist during the first years of life when gross motor concerns are paramount, and then by an occupational therapist during the preschool and school years when fine motor concerns predominate.

Language–speech assessment: in many follow-up programs, this responsibility is assumed by the psychologist. Some programs have the necessary personnel and funding resources to use a communication disorders specialist on a regular basis.

Family assessment: the increasingly important task of evaluating and monitoring the home parenting environment may be performed by a social worker, a clinical nurse specialist, or both. As the number of dysfunctional families in the NICU setting steadily increases because of such prevalent influences as poverty, single parenthood, and prenatal substance abuse, so does the requirement of follow-up programs increase for qualified psychosocial personnel.

Hearing assessment: the adequate ability to assess hearing at any age by a clinical audiologist is imperative for tertiary follow-up programs. Both electrophysiologic and behavioral audiometric procedures should be available.

Visual assessment: a pediatric ophthalmologist should be readily accessible by consultation to the follow-up program, particularly for extremely-low-birth-weight (ELBW; ≤1000 g birth weight) infants.

PATIENT SELECTION

Once again, the goals, objectives, personnel, and resources of an individual follow-up program will combine to determine the proportion and nature of at-risk survivors that can be served. Since it usually is impossible for a program to follow all infants receiving neonatal intensive care, somewhat arbitrary risk criteria generally are established to provide broad follow-up guidelines.[17] In light of the variation and imperfection of assigned risk factors in accurately predicting neurodevelopmental outcome, a follow-up program is wise to adopt a flexible, rather than rigid, approach to the issue of eligibility. In general, a follow-up program will target the smallest and sickest NICU graduates to maximize the likely necessity of its services. Different levels of follow-up priority (*e.g.*, high, medium, low) frequently are used to structure the selection and longitudinal monitoring process. University-affiliated follow-up programs conducting specific clinical research will tailor patient selection according to study requirements.

Common risk criteria for follow-up include the following factors:

VLBW: in smaller programs with limited personnel and resources, the birth weight criterion may, by necessity, be arbitrarily lowered to 1250, 1200, or even 1000 g. This category also generally will incorporate those infants of 32 weeks of gestational age or younger.

Small for gestational age (SGA): most programs strive to include infants whose weight or head circumference at birth was more than two standard deviations below the mean for gestational age.

BPD: programs will vary on the required duration of mechanical ventilation and oxygen administration.

Neuroimaging abnormalities: this criterion typically will include such findings as severe intracranial hemorrhage (*e.g.*, large intraventricular hemorrhage, intraparenchymal hemorrhage), severe ventriculomegaly, or extensive cystic periventricular leukomalacia.

Prolonged seizures or other abnormal neurologic behavior: this would include those infants who continue to demonstrate an atypical neurologic examination at the time of nursery discharge.

Central nervous system infection: the targeted infection may have occurred during the intrauterine, intrapartum, or neonatal time period.

Miscellaneous perinatal–neonatal events of potential neurodevelopmental significance: most programs will prioritize infants who have experienced to a severe degree such complications as asphyxia, hyperbilirubinemia, hypoglycemia, or polycythemia. Specific threshold determinations will vary from program to program. Table 61-1 quantifies the major neurodevelopmental risk as-

TABLE 61–1
RISK FACTORS FOR MAJOR NEUROLOGIC AND COGNITIVE SEQUELAE IN SURVIVING INFANTS REQUIRING NEONATAL INTENSIVE CARE

Birth Weight (g)	Category	Risk Factor (%)
>2500	All admissions	<5
	Respiratory distress syndrome	5
	Postasphyxia seizure	30–50
	Meningitis	30–50
1501–2500	All admissions	10
	Small for gestational age	<10
	Respiratory distress syndrome	<10
	Bronchopulmonary dysplasia	20–30
	Postasphyxia seizure	30–50
	Meningitis	30–50
≤1500	All admissions	10–30
	Appropriate for gestational age, nonventilated	10–15
	Appropriate for gestational age, ventilated	30–40
	Small for gestational age	30–50
	Seizures, decerebrate posture	75–80

From Fitzhardinge PM. Follow-up studies of the high risk newborn. In: Avery GB, ed. Neonatology: pathophysiology and management of the newborn. 2nd ed. Philadelphia: JB Lippincott, 1981:353.

sociated with many of these follow-up inclusion criteria.

Many states use or are developing some type of comprehensive high-risk tracking or screening system to monitor the growth and development of biologically vulnerable infants.[18] In some states (*e.g.*, Iowa, North Carolina, Washington) this broadly based tracking system serves as an initial screen to identify those infants and toddlers who merit complete, tertiary developmental assessment. This coordinated approach to follow-up offers the advantages of tracking many more at-risk infants and families while also increasing the efficiency and appropriate use of the formal follow-up clinic.

CLINIC SCHEDULE

The schedule of evaluations conducted by the University of Washington's High Risk Infant Follow-Up Program is outlined in Table 61-2. This plan is illustrated as an example of a follow-up program with combined clinical service, training, and research objectives. Smaller hospital-based programs without training or research requirements often will be able to meet their clinical needs with different formats, shorter duration of follow-up, and fewer standardized assessments. Basic monitoring concepts applicable to all follow-up programs, however, include special attention to neuromotor development the first year, language and cognitive development the second and third years, school readiness skills between 4 and 5 years of age, and academic achievement during

TABLE 61–2
HIGH-RISK INFANT FOLLOW-UP CLINIC SCHEDULE

Corrected Age	Test
4 mo	BSID
	MAI
	Physical and Neurologic Examination
8 mo*	BSID
	MAI
	Audiologic Evaluation by Visual Reinforcement Audiometry
	Physical and Neurologic Examination
12 mo	BSID
	Physical and Neurologic Examination
24 mo	BSID
	Physical and Neurologic Examination
36 mo	Stanford–Binet Intelligence Scale
	Peabody Picture Vocabulary Test
	Expressive Language Sample
	Physical and Neurologic Examination
4.5 y	Wechsler Preschool and Primary Scale of Intelligence
	Peabody Developmental Motor Scales
	Physical and Neurologic Examination
6 and 8 y	Wechsler Intelligence Scale for Children
	Peabody Individual Achievement Test
	Physical and Neurologic Examination

* Scheduled selectively for those infants with possible neuromotor abnormalities at 4 months of age.

BSID, Bayley Scales of Infant Development; MAI, Movement Assessment of Infants.

the early school years. In addition, attention to family function ideally should be an integral part of each clinic visit. With this developmental sequence of evaluations, timely identification of delays and dysfunctions as well as appropriate referral to community-based intervention services are optimized.[19]

A frequent topic of debate concerns the calculation of assessment age for premature infants.[20] Whereas most follow-up programs plan their clinic visit schedule and score their evaluation measures on the basis of fully corrected age (*i.e.*, chronologic age minus the number of weeks premature), a number of others continue to use unadjusted chronologic age or even, in a few cases, one-half correction (*i.e.*, chronologic age minus one-half the number of weeks premature). The reluctance to use full gestational age correction stems from a concern over the potential artificial inflation of developmental test scores and coincident underuse of early intervention services during the first several years of life. Although these are valid clinical concerns to consider when providing parental feedback and making referral decisions, the weight of the evidence in terms of the neuromaturation of premature infants favors the practice of gestational age correction, at least to 3 years of age, when monitoring the growth and development of NICU survivors.

Regardless of the scheduling mode used, all follow-up personnel must appreciate the imprecisions and variabilities of early developmental assessment. Low-birth-weight, premature infants may demonstrate improving developmental performance during the first years of life as they recover from perinatal–neonatal insults and chronic health impairments (*e.g.*, BPD, necrotizing enterocolitis). Conversely, they also may demonstrate additional developmental dysfunction over time as more subtle disabilities become increasingly apparent and testable. Realizing these patterns of development, health and developmental professionals who work with premature infants and their families must be aware of the hazards implicit in the high-risk concept. Parents may permanently regard their child as vulnerable, once so labeled, and contribute to a self-fulfilling prophecy. There can be an overzealous tendency in well intended follow-up programs to presume the presence of abnormality rather than normality, despite the evidence of more optimistic outcome data to the contrary. In fact, most high-risk infants do not develop the conditions for which they are at increased statistical risk, and there frequently is a poor correlation between the severity of the neonatal course and specific neurodevelopmental outcomes for individual premature infants. There is a need for monitoring of this population with a keen awareness of, but not an expectation of, adverse sequelae. Documented developmental dysfunction certainly should not be ignored, but an initial follow-up posture of cautious optimism is appropriate in most cases.

NEURODEVELOPMENTAL OUTCOME OF LOW-BIRTH-WEIGHT PREMATURE INFANTS

Despite contemporary reductions in LBW morbidity compared to disability rates before the introduction of neonatal intensive care, permanent neurodevelopmental problems are seen in many survivors. Such problems include major neurosensory handicapping conditions, cognitive and language delays, specific neuromotor deficits, neurobehavioral and socioemotional abnormalities, and school dysfunction.[21] Figures 61-2 and 61-3 illustrate mortality and morbidity trends for VLBW and ELBW infants, respectively, in their first 2 years of life, between 1960 and 1985.

MAJOR NEUROSENSORY HANDICAPPING CONDITIONS

The major neurosensory handicapping conditions associated with prematurity are cerebral palsy, particularly of the spastic diplegia type; mental retardation

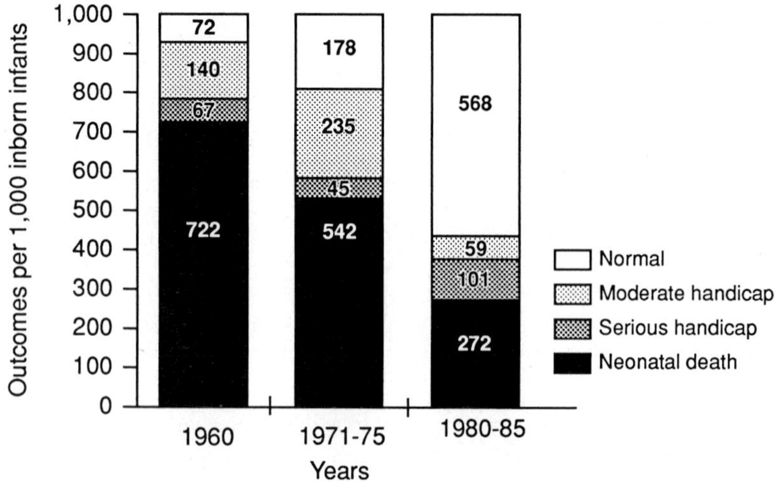

FIG. 61–2. Outcomes for very-low-birth-weight infants (*i.e.*, <1500 g) born in level III hospitals, from 1960–1985. (From Herdman RC, Behney CJ, Wagner JL, et al. Neonatal intensive care for low birthweight infants: costs and effectiveness. Health Technology Case Study 38, Publication OTA-HCS-38. Washington DC: Office of Technology Assessment, Congress of the United States, 1987.)

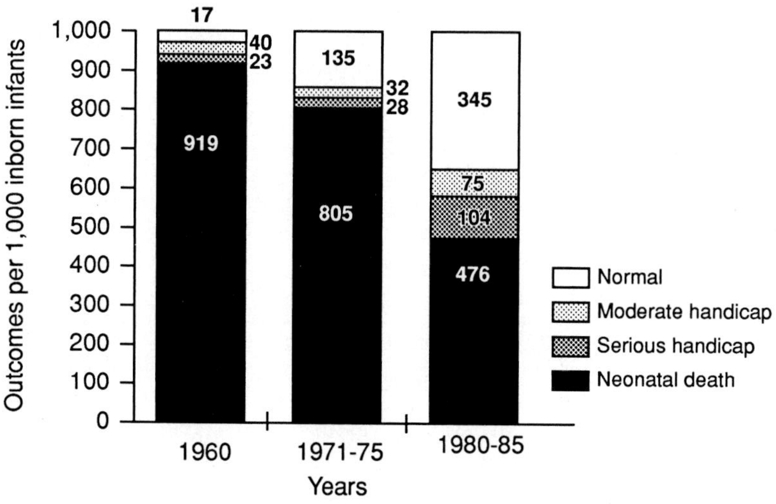

FIG. 61–3. Outcomes for extremely-low-birth-weight infants (*i.e.*, <1000 g) born in level III hospitals from 1960–1985. (From Herdman RC, Behney CJ, Wagner JL, et al. Neonatal intensive care for low birthweight infants: costs and effectiveness. Health Technology Case Study 38, Publication OTA-HCS-38. Washington, DC: Office of Technology Assessment, Congress of the United States, 1987.)

(*i.e.*, intelligence quotient [IQ] more than two standard deviations below the standardized test mean); sensorineural hearing loss; and visual impairment, primarily the consequences of retinopathy of prematurity (ROP).[22] These major developmental disabilities may occur together in the same child and occasionally are complicated by progressive hydrocephalus or a chronic seizure disorder. They usually are clinically apparent by 2 years of age and vary in severity from mild to profound. Children with one or more of these major handicaps generally require special educational programming and individual therapeutic intervention throughout childhood. These conditions occur two to five times more frequently in LBW compared to full-birth-weight (FBW) infants. As a group, their prevalence increases with decreasing birth weight and gestational age; the handicap rate in boys consistently exceeds that in girls.[23] Table 61-3 provides combined prevalence estimates and ranges by birth weight group for these chronic neurosensory impairments. The actual numbers represent a synthesis from reporting tertiary care centers in the United States, Canada, Australia, and Western Europe.

Such major morbidity statistics may be viewed either positively or negatively, or both. On the one hand, the occurrence of these major sequelae is far less than initially predicted at the beginning of the NICU era, and many more nonhandicapped than handicapped survivors (*i.e.*, 7 : 1) are being added to the population.[5] Conversely, epidemiologic investigations appear to document that reductions in LBW major morbidity have not paralleled or kept pace with reductions in LBW mortality, and that the major handicap rate has changed little over the past 15 to 20 years. Actual increases in both the incidence and prevalence of major handicaps among the smallest and sickest survivors have been reported by some.[24,25] Others, however, have reported a stable major morbidity rate over the past decade for infants weighing less than 800 g at birth, a subgroup whose survival has dramatically increased during this time period.[11–13]

TABLE 61–3
LOW-BIRTH-WEIGHT INFANTS WHO SURVIVE WITH ONE OR MORE MAJOR HANDICAPS

Birth Weight (g)	Percent With Major Handicapping Conditions (range)
1501–2500	8 (5–20)
1001–1500	15 (5–30)
≤ 1000	25 (8–40)

CEREBRAL PALSY

Cerebral palsy, of varying types and severities, remains the most prevalent major developmental disability encountered in premature infants; the prevalence in VLBW infants varies between 6% and 10%, and approximately 40% of all children with cerebral palsy were born prematurely (*i.e.*, <37 weeks of gestation).[26] Although both spastic (*i.e.*, pyramidal) and athetoid (*i.e.*, extrapyramidal) types of cerebral palsy may be encountered in NICU graduates, the spastic cerebral palsy syndromes (*i.e.*, diplegia, hemiplegia, and quadriplegia) are the neuromuscular disorders most commonly seen in LBW infants. One specific type, spastic diplegia, in which the legs are much more affected than arms, is so strongly associated with prematurity (*i.e.*, at least two-thirds of all children with this disorder are born before 37 weeks of gestation) that for over a century it has been referred to as "the disease of immaturity."[26a] Figure 61-4 illustrates the relationship between spastic diplegia and gestational age.

Despite the long consistency of the spastic diplegia–prematurity association, the exact etiologic fac-

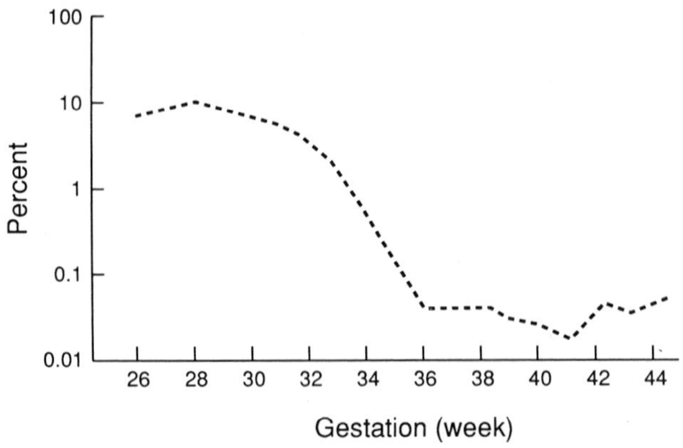

FIG. 61–4. Occurrence of spastic diplegia as related to gestational age.

tors involved often have been elusive and difficult to identify precisely prospectively.[27] Neither the severity of perinatal–neonatal illness nor the presence or the severity of intracranial hemorrhage reliably predict spastic diplegia. Data derived primarily from studies correlating ultrasonographic, neuropathologic, and clinical information led to the conclusion that spastic diplegia is the clinical expression of periventricular leukomalacia and its variants.[28] Periventricular leukomalacia appears to be caused, in large part, by hypoxic–ischemic injury to the periventricular white matter. The demonstration on serial cranial ultrasounds of initial extensive periventricular echodensities followed in days to weeks by large, bilateral cyst formation (*i.e.*, periventricular white matter infarction) is highly predictive (80%–85%) of permanent cerebral palsy, especially the spastic diplegia type.[29,30] Several investigators have implicated prenatal factors (*e.g.*, intrauterine growth retardation) in the etiology of some cases of spastic diplegia. Hagberg has postulated that the complex interaction of prenatal abnormalities (*i.e.*, "fetal deprivation of supply") with perinatal difficulties in the birth process and the adjustment to the extrauterine environment may constitute a common pathogenetic mechanism of spastic diplegia.[31] Accordingly, the etiology of spastic diplegia frequently is multifactorial, and all LBW infants merit close neuromotor monitoring during the first 2 years of life, regardless of the severity of their nursery course.

In contrast, NICU graduates in whom the more severe spastic quadriplegia type of cerebral palsy, in which all four extremities are equally affected, develops often can be predicted better on the basis of specific perinatal or neonatal events, including asphyxia, marked bilateral intraventricular hemorrhage with ventriculomegaly, prolonged neonatal seizures, and central nervous system infection. Although most premature children with spastic diplegia have average or near-average mental abilities, children with spastic quadriplegia are far more likely also to have serious cognitive impairments. Spastic hemiplegia, in which only one side is affected, with the arm usually more than the leg, often is heralded by the ultrasonographic appearance of a unilateral, periventricular hemorrhagic infarction with subsequent cystic transformation that occurs in association with and presumably as a result of substantial asymmetric intraventricular hemorrhage.[28]

Cerebral palsy typically presents over time in a developmental manner. Thus, very early neurologic signs and symptoms may prove to be transient in nature and not indicative of eventual cerebral palsy. Conversely, infants may initially appear asymptomatic with a relatively normal neurologic examination at the time of nursery discharge and even for several months thereafter, particularly in the cases of spastic diplegia and spastic hemiplegia, only to manifest clearly evident cerebral palsy by 1 year of age. Premature infants with evolving cerebral palsy reveal increasing neuromotor abnormalities of muscle tone, movement, posture, and reflex activity, particularly between 6 and 18 months of corrected age, in combination with increasingly delayed motor milestones.

MENTAL RETARDATION

Mental retardation, as defined by a standardized intelligence or developmental quotient consistently more than two standard deviations below the test mean for corrected age, often occurs in conjunction with one or more of the other major handicaps, especially cerebral palsy. In fact, severe mental retardation and severe cerebral palsy share associated perinatal–neonatal risk factors. Evidence suggests some increase in the prevalence of severely multihandicapped children after increased VLBW survival.[25] Mental retardation occurs in 4% to 5% of VLBW infants followed longitudinally to school age. Isolated mental retardation, without cerebral palsy, is a reported consequence of severe BPD, particularly in cases of greatly prolonged duration of mechanical ventilation and oxygen administration.[32]

HEARING IMPAIRMENT

Neonatal intensive care unit graduates are at increased risk for both sensorineural and conductive hearing loss. Although the risk of sensorineural loss sufficient to require hearing aids, special education, and nonvocal communication strategies (60–100 dB) usually is estimated to be 2% to 3% for VLBW infants, some investigators have reported prevalence estimates between 5% and 9% coincident with the increased survival of more vulnerable infants.[33] Exposure to ototoxic drugs, infections, hypoxia–ischemia, and hyperbilirubinemia are among the interacting and cumulative factors contributing to the risk of sensorineural loss. The duration and extent of hyperbilirubinemia in VLBW infants has been examined carefully. DeVries and colleagues found bilirubin levels in excess of 14 mg/dL to be associated with a high risk of deafness in VLBW infants, but not in healthy premature infants with a birth weight greater than 1500 g.[34] Others also have emphasized the potential ototoxicity of hyperbilirubinemia in VLBW infants in combination with hypoxia, acidosis, and prolonged administration of multiple ototoxic medications such as the aminoglycoside antibiotics and furosemide. These investigators conclude that the additive effects of protracted illness plus its associated treatments, independent of specific diagnostic categories, constitute important risk factors for permanent hearing loss in this population.[35]

There is ample evidence that infants of all birth weights who sustain severe persistent pulmonary hypertension of the newborn comprise a particularly high-risk subgroup for sensorineural hearing loss, with prevalence estimates ranging from 20% to 40%.[36] In some cases, the loss is progressive during the first 3 years of life. The exact mechanism of insult remains unclear in this population of infants who typically experience prolonged hypoxia, severe acute and chronic lung disease, and multiple aggressive interventions. Another concern has been the potential deleterious effect of prolonged incubator noise on hearing function. Abramovich and associates found no evidence for this hypothesis in VLBW infants.[37] Many of the risk factors associated with hearing impairment also are associated with cerebral palsy, and these two disabilities often occur together in the same child.

Mild and moderate (25–59 dB) sensorineural hearing losses, sufficient to contribute to delayed language development but compatible with oral communication, also occur with increased frequency (6%–8%) in LBW infants. Previously unrecognized, unilateral sensorineural hearing losses, with adverse language and learning consequences, may become apparent in the older child.[38] A high prevalence (20%–30%) of chronic otitis media with middle ear effusion and fluctuating, conductive hearing loss of greater than 25 dB is reported in LBW, premature infants.[39] Suggested mechanisms for this relationship focus on probable eustachian tube dysfunction initiated by a combination of dolichocephalic head shape, muscular hypotonia, and prolonged nasotracheal intubation.

There have been important advances in the hearing assessment of LBW infants. Two techniques in particular, electrophysiologic auditory brain stem response (ABR) audiometry and behavioral visual reinforcement audiometry, have made early, reliable detection of hearing loss in the NICU graduate clinically feasible. Centers that routinely screen high-risk, LBW infants with ABR before nursery discharge report a false-positive rate of 8% to 10% compared to follow-up testing at 4 months of age.[40] Conversely, the unanticipated appearance of severe sensorineural hearing loss in high-risk survivors of neonatal intensive care after having passed an initial ABR screening test in the newborn period has been reported.[41] It also must be recognized that ABR tests only the high sound frequencies (*i.e.*, 2000 Hz and above) and will not detect hearing losses confined to the lower frequencies. Thus, clinicians must remember that determinations of the adequacy of hearing made only with ABR test data before nursery discharge are subject to error. Visual reinforcement audiometry is an operant conditioning technique that reliably can provide auditory thresholds for infants who are functioning at a developmental age of approximately 6 months or older. It has great utility in the high-risk follow-up clinic.

VISUAL IMPAIRMENT

The major cause of visual loss in LBW infants is retrolental fibroplasia, more recently included under the rubric of ROP. With controlled oxygen administration, ROP was relatively rare until the last decade or so, when significant numbers of extremely premature infants began to survive. The new name, ROP, recognizes that immaturity at birth is the single largest risk factor for this disease. For all practical purposes, this is a disorder of the VLBW infant. Virtually no retinal detachment and little retinal scarring is described in larger premature infants. For the entire VLBW population, current prevalence estimates range from 20% to 25% with early-stage, regressed ROP; 5% to 10% with more advanced-stage, scarred ROP; and 2% to 4% with major visual impairments, including legal blindness, requiring special educational assistance. The distribution of visually impaired infants, however, is skewed heavily toward those weighing 1000 g or less at birth. In these ELBW infants, regressed ROP occurs in 40% to 50% of survivors, scarred ROP in 10% to 25%, and major visual impairments in 5% to 10%. Figure 61-5 shows the overall prevalence of ROP by birth weight.

Alteration of normal retinal vascular development is the hallmark of ROP. Although a great deal of effort has been invested in clinical and animal studies of ROP, an etiologic maze, in which no single factor stands alone, remains.[42] It appears that the embryonic retina of the small premature, developing outside the uterus, is vulnerable to many sources of disturbance that can disrupt orderly differentiation and vascularization. In addition to the well known impact of hyperoxia, it seems that hypoxia, variations in $PaCO_2$, *p*H, retinal oxygen consumption, light exposure, and other factors that affect retinal perfusion all may play a role. A formula for ROP could be: Immaturity (always) + Oxygen (often) + Other Factors (variably) = ROP.[43] Simply stated, the smallest and sickest newborns have the most complications that potentially can impede retinal function, and they also have the most ROP.

Even regressed ROP is associated with an increased risk for refractive errors, amblyopia, and strabismus. "Myopia of prematurity," even without

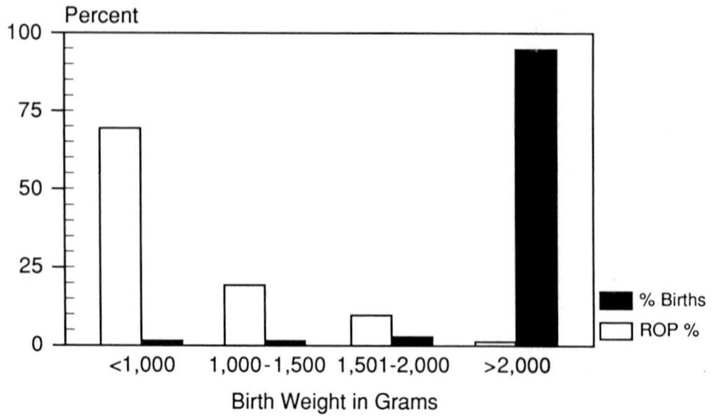

FIG. 61–5. Percentage of retinopathy of prematurity (ROP) by birth weight *versus* proportion of births by birth weight. (From Glass P, Avery GB, Subramanian KNS, et al. Effect of bright light in the hospital nursery on the incidence of retinopathy of prematurity. N Engl J Med 1985;313:401.)

ROP, has been described to occur in approximately one third of surviving ELBW infants.[44] It is considered to be mostly lenticular in origin and to improve slowly, but not completely, throughout childhood, with slight visual acuity differences still apparent in early adulthood. Strabismus may represent an isolated problem or, in some cases, may be an initial indication of a generalized neuromotor problem such as cerebral palsy. Visual and hearing impairments may coexist, and prematurity is the leading cause of children with both handicaps. Monitoring of eye muscle balance and alignment and visual acuity should be part of routine follow-up of the premature infant, particularly during the preschool years. Required interventions may include eye muscle surgery, antisuppression patching, or corrective lenses.

PROGRESSIVE HYDROCEPHALUS

Depending on the reporting center, between 25% and 45% of VLBW infants have neonatal ultrasonographic evidence of intracranial hemorrhage, frequently including intraventricular hemorrhage with ventriculomegaly.[9] Whereas older reports indicated discouragingly high rates of post-hemorrhagic hydrocephalus, recent reports are much more hopeful in describing a very low prevalence (2%–4%) of progressive hydrocephalus requiring ventriculoperitoneal shunting in VLBW infants.[45,46] Serial scanning with cranial ultrasonography has revealed that most cases of early ventriculomegaly either spontaneously resolve or arrest. The necessity of medical intervention (*e.g.*, repeated lumbar puncture, diuresis) to prevent the transition from relatively asymptomatic ventriculomegaly to progressive hydrocephalus remains unclear.

For the infant in whom post-hemorrhagic progressive hydrocephalus does develop, it generally becomes clinically evident between 2 and 8 weeks of age; however, appearance during late infancy occasionally has been reported. Vigilance in measurement of the head circumference at each follow-up examination of the infant is important, and obtaining a cranial ultrasound if head growth becomes substantially out of proportion to the other growth parameters may be indicated. Although the initial months of life are the time when progressive hydrocephalus is most likely to develop in premature infants, it also is the period of time when the normal phenomenon of catch-up head growth in these recovering infants becomes most apparent. Thus, increase in head circumference relative to weight and length usually is an anticipated sign rather than a pathologic one, and such awareness should guide clinical investigative decisions. When progressive hydrocephalus does occur, neurodevelopmental outcome is frequently, although not invariably, abnormal, complicated by one or more of the major handicaps (*e.g.*, cerebral palsy, mental retardation, sensory impairments).[47]

MINOR HANDICAPPING CONDITIONS

Although major handicapping sequelae are by far the easiest to quantify and report, a growing body of long-term follow-up studies clearly indicates that a broad spectrum of cognitive, behavioral, and other minor neurodevelopmental and neurobehavioral sequelae are at least as, if not more, prevalent in surviving LBW, premature infants. These morbidities become increasingly apparent in a variety of clinical manifestations with increasing age, particularly during the first 6 years of life. These early, often subtle, developmental and behavioral delays and differences are not necessarily outgrown, but frequently portend future school dysfunction and may therefore become major impediments to normal academic and social progress. Collectively, these problems often are referred to as the "new morbidity" of prematurity, reflecting their more insidious nature and more recent attention.[22]

Specific types of developmental morbidities described in LBW cohorts include cognitive delays (*i.e.*, lower IQ), speech and language disorders, persistent neuromotor abnormalities, including difficulties with balance and coordination, and perceptual problems. Specific areas of suboptimal behavioral style and performance include neonatal behavior, infant and toddler temperament, emotional maturity, social competence, and selective attention. As with major handicaps, the overall prevalence of these minor sequelae increases with decreasing birth weight and gestational age, and also is greater in male survivors. Prevalence estimates in VLBW infants vary between 15% and 25%. Accordingly, when the 15% to 20% major handicap rate is combined, between 35% and 45% of VLBW survivors demonstrate a residual developmental or behavioral problem that compromises their anticipated function.[48] As with major handicaps, most of the minor developmental morbidities associated with LBW and prematurity also are related to the severity of perinatal–neonatal illness. That is, LBW infants who experience a prolonged hospital course with many medical complications have an increased likelihood of development of some type of developmental dysfunction. Despite the large number of positive group associations in follow-up studies, however, individual developmental outcome remains very difficult to predict prospectively with accuracy in the NICU, and infants with apparently similar neonatal courses may develop remarkably differently.

COGNITIVE AND PERCEPTUAL DEVELOPMENT

Consistent deficits in performance on intelligence measures repeatedly have been observed and reported in LBW, premature children compared to FBW, full-term children.[49,50] Furthermore, these differences in cognitive development already become apparent in the first years of life, and then persist and increase during the preschool and early school years even when the single most powerful predictor of IQ—socioeconomic status—is adequately controlled. In other words, significant deficits in cognitive and perceptual function occur frequently even in middle to upper-middle social class children born prematurely, particularly compared to their full-term peers. This important and academically relevant group difference exists despite the fact that most LBW children will have measured IQs within the average range.[21]

Cognitive developmental differences between premature and full-term infants have been reported in early infancy. Rose investigated the effect of increasing familiarization time on the visual recognition memory of 6- and 12-month-old premature and full-term infants.[51] Whereas the older infants showed evidence of recognition memory after less familiarization time than the younger ones, at both ages premature infants required considerably longer familiarization times (*i.e.*, more practice) than did full-term infants. These results suggest that there are persistent differences between premature and full-term infants throughout at least the first year of life in a very fundamental aspect of cognition, namely, visual information processing.

Because manipulative exploration of objects may be important to the infant's perception and conceptualization of objects, Ruff and colleagues studied this developmental function in both premature and full-term 9-month-old infants by means of coded and scored videotapes.[52] The videotapes were scored for behaviors such as looking, handling, mouthing, turning the object around, transferring the object from hand to hand, and banging. A high-risk subgroup of premature infants based on neonatal complications manipulated the objects significantly less than either the low-risk prematures or the full-term infants. There was a relationship between manipulative exploration at 9 months and later cognitive functioning at 24 months.

Low-birth-weight cognitive deficits have been described from the earliest days of neonatal intensive care and even before. Using a sample of approximately 600 children born in two Edinburgh, Scotland, hospitals in 1953 to 1955, Drillien demonstrated that IQ scores decline with decreasing birth weight in the first 4 years of life.[53] The percentage of children with IQ scores below 80 at 4 years was 29% for those under 4.8 pounds, 13% for those between 4.8 and 5.8 pounds, and 4% for those above 5.8 pounds. Wiener and colleagues, reporting on a sample of 417 8- to 10-year-old LBW children who had been tested with the Wechsler Intelligence Scale for Children, found that the Verbal IQ, which consists of predominantly cognitive and language items, Performance IQ, which consists of predominantly motor–perceptual items, and Full-Scale IQ, which consists of a combination of the Verbal and Performance Scales, all showed increasing impairment with decreasing birth weight even though all subtest means remained within the average range of intelligence.[54] Moreover, approximately twice as large a proportion of LBW children as FBW control children fell into the borderline IQ category (70–84), which usually is associated with special educational needs. Visual–motor–perceptual skills, as measured independently by the Bender Gestalt Test, also varied directly with birth weight. Hunt and colleagues reported the following cognitive outcome proportions in a cohort of 108 VLBW children at 8 years of age: 4.6% had a very low IQ (<70), 13.9% had a low IQ (70–84), and, for those with an IQ greater than 84, 12.0% had language disability, 12.0% had performance disability, 21.4% had visual–motor disability, and 36.1% were apparently normal.[55]

In a Vancouver, British Columbia, study of 501 LBW and 203 FBW children born between 1958 and 1965, the IQ difference between LBW and FBW groups on the Stanford–Binet Intelligence Scale was 9 points at 30 months of age and 15 points at 48 months, even after excluding children with major cerebral deficit or IQ scores under 50 or significant visual problems.[49] In both the Edinburgh and Vancouver studies, the poor functioning of LBW children is convincingly exacerbated in socioeconomically disadvantaged subgroups. Table 61-4 illustrates this interaction of both biologic and environmental risk factors in the determination of measured IQ of the Vancouver study children. At both 2.5 and 4 years of age,

TABLE 61–4
COMPARISON OF INTELLIGENCE QUOTIENT MEANS FOR LOW-BIRTH-WEIGHT CHILDREN *versus* NORMAL-BIRTH-WEIGHT CONTROLS WITHIN SOCIAL CLASS GROUPS

Hollingshead Social Class	Statistic	30 Months of Age		48 Months of Age	
		IQ	Number	IQ	Number
I, II, III	LBW mean ± SD	97.0 ± 15.1	48	99.5 ± 13.7	67
	Control mean ± SD	108.8 ± 8.2	19	118.3 ± 11.4	26
	Difference ± SE	11.8 ± 2.9		18.8 ± 2.8	
	p	<0.001		<0.001	
IV	LBW mean ± SD	91.7 ± 10.7	59	94.3 ± 11.3	100
	Control mean ± SD	102.9 ± 12.6	43	110.0 ± 16.8	58
	Difference ± SE	11.2 ± 2.4		15.7 ± 2.5	
	p	<0.001		<0.001	
V	LBW mean ± SD	89.5 ± 13.9	52	90.6 ± 15.8	79
	Control mean ± SD	96.0 ± 9.7	32	102.3 ± 12.9	42
	Difference ± SE	6.5 ± 2.6		11.7 ± 2.7	
	p	<0.01		<0.001	

LBW, low birth weight; FBW, full birth weight. IQ determined from Stanford–Binet tests.
Adapted from McBurney AK, Eaves LC. Evolution of developmental and psychological test scores. In: Dunn HG, ed. Sequelae of low birthweight: the Vancouver Study. Philadelphia: JB Lippincott, 1986:61.

FBW, highest social class children earned the highest subgroup mean IQ score, whereas LBW, lowest social class children earned the lowest. Both FBW and LBW groups demonstrated an IQ score continuum from the highest social class, which had the highest mean IQ, to the lowest social class, which had the lowest mean IQ, with the FBW subgroup always higher than the LBW regardless of social class; at 4 years of age, even FBW, lowest-social-class children scored higher than their LBW, highest-social-class peers.

LANGUAGE DEVELOPMENT

Communication skills involving auditory and visual perception, the learning and conceptualizing of a verbal symbol system (*i.e.*, language), and the actual production of speech are critical to academic learning and social adjustment. Several investigations have focused exclusively on this important area of development in premature infants. Zarin-Ackerman and colleagues noted both receptive and expressive language deficiencies at 2 years of age in a group of children born as at-risk (*i.e.*, predominantly premature) infants compared to others born as healthy, full-term infants.[56] They emphasized that these deficits could not be a function of social class, which is a major factor influencing language development, since this variable was controlled. In Switzerland, Largo and associates compared 114 premature children to 97 healthy, full-term children throughout the first 5 years of life.[57] Most stages of language development occurred at slightly later ages among the premature children than among those born at term. Birth weight and gestational age were negatively correlated with language development at all ages. Perinatal–neonatal complications also were significantly negatively correlated with the ages at which the stages of language development were reached, and also with final language performance at 5 years of age. There were no significant differences in socioeconomic status between the premature and full-term groups. The particular demographics of this unique study allowed the authors to conclude that biomedical factors exert a considerable effect on the early language development of premature children, and that this effect is greater than previously has been recognized.[57]

Several smaller studies have confirmed the existence of linguistic dysfunctions among premature children, particularly those with complicated neonatal courses.[58,59] Using a wide variety of measures, inferior performance has been reported consistently in receptive language or comprehension, expressive language parameters such as vocabulary and word finding, and speech qualities such as articulation and fluency.

MOTOR DEVELOPMENT

Numerous studies from several continents repeatedly have documented that the neuromotor development of LBW, premature infants during the first 2 years of life is different, more delayed, and generally more worrisome than that of healthy, full-term infants. Not only are premature developmental scores, using such measures as the Bayley Scales of Infant Development, consistently and significantly below those of full-term infants at 12 months of corrected age, but premature motor scores also usually are 10 to 15 points (*i.e.*, practically one standard deviation) below premature mental scores at this age.[60]

This phenomenon of transiently abnormal neuromotor signs in the first years of life was described initially by Drillien, in a 1972 report from Scotland, as "transient dystonia of low birth weight infants."[61] Drillien reported that its prevalence during the first one-half of infancy varied inversely with birth weight, involving approximately 35% of infants weighing 1501 to 2000 g at birth and 60% to 70% of infants weighing 1500 g or less at birth, and that its prevalence also varied directly with perinatal–neonatal complications (*i.e.*, more frequent among sick premature infants). Transient dystonia includes such neurologic findings as increased or decreased muscle tone, diminished volitional movement, retention and accentuation of primitive reflex patterns, delayed appearance of normal infantile automatic reactions, and asymmetric neuromotor development. Because these neuromotor signs also are the very signs seen in infants in whom cerebral palsy is developing, it is not surprising that a reliable diagnosis of cerebral palsy is quite difficult in most premature infants throughout early infancy. As described by Amiel-Tison, however, by 8 to 10 months of corrected age, most LBW infants with transient dystonia are gradually and spontaneously normalizing on examination, whereas those relatively few infants in whom permanent cerebral palsy is developing appear increasingly abnormal.[62] With the knowledge of this common evolution of neuromotor signs, every VLBW infant can be assigned to one of three diagnostic and prognostic groups at 12 months of age: those who were always neurologically normal throughout infancy (25%–30%); those who showed transient dystonia with subsequent normalization (65%–70%); and those with cerebral palsy (5%–10%).

Coolman and colleagues and others have extended these observations to 24 months of age, albeit most neuromotor changes occur in the first year of life.[63] They found that some infants with transient dystonia retained subtle, persistent neuromotor differences that would not be labeled as cerebral palsy but that represented qualitative deviations from the norm. Longitudinal studies indicate that infants who have experienced transient dystonia are far more likely to have language, learning, and behavioral problems (*i.e.*, minimal brain dysfunction) in later childhood than are infants who never demonstrated these abnormalities.[64,65] This would indicate that although transient dystonia largely resolves, these neuromotor signs in early infancy may be predictive markers for later manifestations of central nervous system disorganization.

Differences in the motor development of premature infants throughout the preschool years have been reported. Burns and Bullock found premature children at 5 years of age to be significantly different from their full-term peers in terms of tremulous involuntary hand movements, less competent gross motor ability, and difficulties in postural control and balance.[66] Crowe and associates described ELBW infants as a group to have significantly inferior skills in all motor functions at 4 years of age.[67] Symptomatic intracranial hemorrhage was associated with poorer motor performance.

NEUROBEHAVIORAL DEVELOPMENT

As LBW, premature survivors are assessed more critically and at older ages, a variety of potential behavioral dysfunctions throughout infancy and childhood become evident. Numerous studies have compared the neonatal neurobehavioral performance of LBW infants to that of FBW infants. These studies typically compare premature infants at their corrected age and also tend to use premature infants with relatively uncomplicated neonatal courses. Nevertheless, despite these sampling features that might obscure group differences, premature infants consistently perform less optimally than healthy, full-term infants on these early measures.

Ferrari and colleagues compared low-risk premature infants to healthy, full-term infants using the Brazelton Neonatal Behavioral Assessment Scale.[68] They found the premature infants to be significantly inferior in sensory orientation, regulation of behavioral state (*i.e.*, quiet–active status), and autonomic regulation. Additionally, the clustering of neurobehavioral items was more heterogeneous among premature infants. The authors concluded that prematurity itself is associated with a behavioral repertoire that is different, more variable, and on the average less competent than that of full-term infants.[68] Friedman and colleagues, also comparing low-risk premature infants and healthy, full-term infants, found that the premature infants fussed and cried more, were less soothable, and tended to change behavioral state more frequently.[69] They suggested that these neonatal neurobehavioral differences are potential contributors to suboptimal interaction between premature infants and their caregivers. Aylward and colleagues, in a report from the National Institutes of Health (NIH) Collaborative Study on Antenatal Steroid Therapy, reported significant effects of both gestational age and severity of perinatal–neonatal illness on the neurobehavioral responses of premature infants.[70] Specifically, at 40 weeks of corrected age, premature infants born at younger gestational ages and with greater medical complications demonstrated altered behavior in terms of diminished spontaneous activity and vigor, inability to maintain and modulate responses, and poorer visual orientation capabilities.

A number of more recent studies using a wide variety of electrophysiologic techniques have supported the results of these clinical behavioral investigations. Compared to full-term infants, premature infants have been shown to have delayed maturation of both cortical and brain stem auditory evoked potentials, more variable and labile behavioral state organization as measured by time-lapse videosomnography, and decreased resting heart rate variability and vagal tone (*i.e.*, an indirect measure of overall autonomic nervous system activity).[71–74] Several of these functions, particularly state organization and autonomic regulation, have been related positively to longer-term developmental outcome.[75,76]

Several studies have explored the related behavioral areas of temperament, social interaction and competence, and emotional expression and affect. Most of these studies have examined mother–infant interactions, and there is an overall consensus of findings that indicates an imbalance in LBW, premature dyads compared to FBW, full-term dyads, with LBW infants typically less responsive and low in communicative signaling behavior, and their mothers compensating for this relative inactivity by displaying high levels of stimulating and engaging activity. Investigations of LBW infants with complicated perinatal–neonatal courses have indicated that these infants exhibit high levels of gaze aversion, avoidance of interaction, and low levels of vocalizing and playing.[77–79] Field has reported these interactional differences in depth, and succinctly summarizes the problem: "High risk infants and their parents 'have less fun' than normal infants and their parents during their early interactions together."[80] In a study comparing premature–mother dyads with full-term–mother dyads at approximately 4 months of corrected age, Field found the premature infants to be less alert and attentive, less responsive, less interested in game playing, less contingent, less smiling and content, and more affectively negative and irritable than the matched full-term infants. Correspondingly, the mothers of prematures exhibited fewer happy expressions than the mothers of full-terms, but were more vocal as they attempted to elicit social and communicative responses from their infants.

Crnic and associates[81] and Malatesta and colleagues[82] have replicated and extended these observations throughout the entire first year of life; LBW–FBW differences in expressive behavior and affect were persistent and continued to affect maternal behavior. Malatesta and colleagues emphasized that in their primarily middle to upper-middle social class sample, these differences were seen even in the absence of confounding neonatal medical complications. They speculate that the observed LBW–FBW differences probably are even more pronounced with less advantaged, more stressed, or sicker premature infants. Of long-term importance and concern is the increasing evidence of continuity between early interactional disturbances and later behavioral dysfunctions.

SCHOOL FUNCTION

Finally, as increasing numbers of studies have followed LBW, premature infants into the school years, the full spectrum of these children's learning and behavioral performance is emerging and becoming clearer. Although prevalence estimates of school problems vary between reports, almost all investigators agree that LBW survivors have a distinctly increased risk for school dysfunction in some form.[22] There also is general agreement that although this substantial risk exists independently of socioeconomic status, the combination and interaction of biologic and environmental risks produces an especially worrisome doubly-vulnerable milieu and a highly appropriate target population for early developmental intervention efforts because of the documented importance of psychosocial variables in the ultimate prognosis for LBW, premature infants.[83]

Dunn and colleagues, in one of the most extensive longitudinal follow-up studies published, reported minimal cerebral dysfunction (*i.e.*, minor developmental and behavioral abnormalities) to be the single most prevalent (20%) handicapping syndrome at school age in a population of over 300 LBW, premature children.[84] Furthermore, the authors stress the difficulty in adequately predicting or identifying such dysfunctions before school entry at the age of 5 years.[84] This important group of sequelae consequently is liable to be missed when the outcome of NICU graduates is assessed before that age. Figure 61-6 illustrates this diagnostic evolution and increase in developmental–behavioral problems over time. As in other studies, this study found a disproportionate number of boys compared to girls who experienced school dysfunction and required remedial assistance. This investigation has been continued into adolescence.[85] Although several of the LBW children with earlier problems no longer were demonstrating all of them, an almost equal number of previously unrecognized children had manifested academic and social problems, thus resulting in a relatively stable number of such problems over time. Additionally, whereas behaviors such as overactivity, temper tantrums, and perseveration had greatly subsided, symptoms of neuropsychiatric disturbance, including distractibility, irritability, unhappiness, low frustration tolerance, fears, disobedience, poor motivation, and sleep difficulties, persisted or increased.

Other studies have confirmed these observations in VLBW children at 8 to 15 years of age, and have documented, in such areas as verbal expression, academic achievement, social competence, and emotional maturity, continued problems that cannot be attributed primarily to social class or differences in the quality of parenting.[86,87] Nickel and colleagues evaluated the school performance at a mean age of 10 years of 25 ELBW children who were cared for at a time (1960–1972) when only very premature infants who had little or no neonatal illness survived.[88] Despite an overall mean IQ of 90 (range, 50–141), 16 (64%) of these children had been or currently were in special educational programs. Only seven (28%) were rated by their teachers to be achieving at or above grade level. Arithmetic reasoning, mathematics achievement, reading comprehension, balance, fine motor coordination, and perceptual function were specific and common weaknesses for these children.

In a more recent long-term follow-up study, Klein

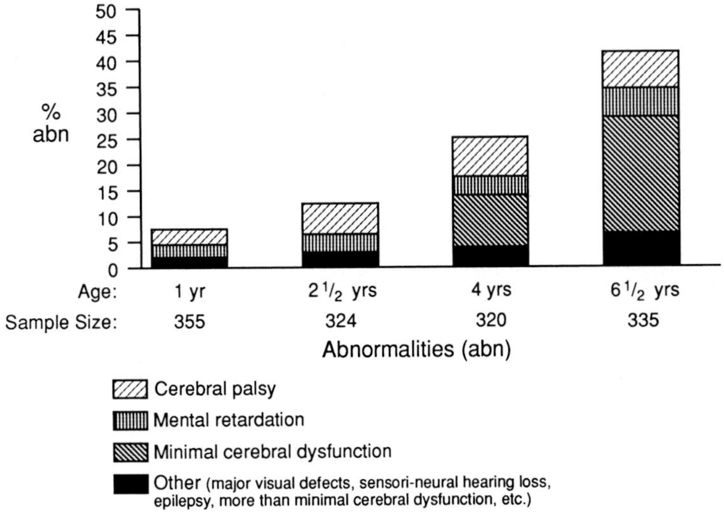

FIG. 61–6. Evolution of developmental dysfunction in low-birth-weight, premature children. (Adapted from Dunn HG, Crichton JV, Grunav RVE, et al. Neurological, psychological and educational sequelae of low birthweight. Brain Dev 1980;2:57.)

and associates compared 65 9-year-old children born in Cleveland, Ohio, in 1976, who were VLBW and who were free of neurologic impairment, to 65 FBW children who had been matched for age, gender, race, and social class on measures of IQ, visual–motor and fine motor abilities, and academic achievement.[89] The following were the major findings:

- VLBW children scored significantly lower than FBW children on tests that measure general intelligence, even though both group means were within the average range.
- VLBW children scored significantly lower than FBW children on tests that measure academic achievement.
- VLBW children had particular deficits in mathematics achievement.
- VLBW children had particular deficits on tests that involve visual or spatial skills.
- These results were independent of social class.

In a similarly controlled and longitudinal New York City study, Ross and colleagues showed that a much higher proportion of 8-year-old VLBW children required special educational interventions (48%) than either FBW children (15%) or the New York State public elementary school population (10%).[90] Very-low-birth-weight children scored significantly lower than FBW children on tests of IQ, verbal ability, academic achievement, and auditory memory. There was an interaction of prematurity and social class on IQ, verbal tests, academic achievement, and attention, with premature children of lower socioeconomic status scoring lowest on these measures.

Although data on the prevalence of behavior problems in older LBW children are quite sparse, it is likely that the prevalence is substantially higher than in FBW children. For example, Escalona found that 30% of a primarily disadvantaged premature sample exhibited major behavior problems before the age of 4 years.[91] The most recent and comprehensive investigation of long-term behavioral function in this population comes from the same Cleveland, Ohio cohort described in terms of academic achievement.[89] Breslau and colleagues compared 65 9-year-old VLBW children to 65 FBW children, matched for age, gender, race, social class, and school, on parents' ratings on the Child Behavior Checklist and teachers' ratings on the Teacher's Report Form.[92] Results from parents and teachers converged on key findings. The major findings were the following:

- VLBW boys manifested significantly more behavioral disturbance and poorer social competence than FBW boys.
- The excess in behavior problems in VLBW boys spanned over a wide range of behavioral domains, including both internalizing (*e.g.*, depressive–anxious) and externalizing (*e.g.*, hyperactive, aggressive, conduct problems) syndromes.
- The effect of VLBW on behavior problems and social adjustment in boys was not a function of IQ.
- These results were independent of social class.

Although VLBW girls did not differ significantly from FBW girls, suggestive trends in the same direction as the boys may indicate that there is an increased risk for behavior problems in both genders, but that these sequelae become evident at an earlier age in boys than in girls.

SPECIFIC PERINATAL–NEONATAL COMPLICATIONS IN HIGH-RISK INFANTS

INTRAUTERINE GROWTH RETARDATION

The SGA infant has a higher mortality rate, a higher incidence of perinatal–neonatal complications, and a higher prevalence of chronic neurologic handicaps than the appropriate-for-gestational-age (AGA) infant of similar gestational age.[93] The diagnosis of SGA is useful in identifying a high-risk population needing careful follow-up; however, the population of

SGA infants is a heterogeneous one with multiple etiologies. Intrauterine growth pattern, associated congenital anomalies, mortality rate, risk of perinatal–neonatal complications, and long-term outcome reflect not only the nature of the insult, but the timing as well. Drillien and colleagues have stressed the need to differentiate early-pregnancy-onset SGA infants, many of whom demonstrate intrinsic defects such as congenital anomalies, from late-pregnancy-onset SGA infants, who may have antenatal histories of placental insufficiency or maternal chronic illness.[64] Long-term developmental prognosis, in terms of major and minor handicaps and school function, is significantly worse for early-pregnancy-onset SGA infants.

Most SGA outcome studies also distinguish between full-term and premature SGA infants because of marked differences in mortality and morbidity rates, both of which are significantly higher for premature SGA infants. For both groups of SGA infants, great variability among outcome studies is the norm, again reflecting the inevitable heterogeneity of the SGA diagnosis. Many studies report that no major neurologic handicap in full-term SGA infants followed from birth. In 96 full-term SGA infants followed to the age of 5 years, Fitzhardinge and Stevens reported only a 1% prevalence of cerebral palsy and a 6% prevalence of seizures.[94] In a cerebral-palsied population in Sweden, full-term SGA infants had a somewhat higher risk for cerebral palsy than full-term AGA infants, but a much lower risk than premature AGA and premature SGA infants.[31] Most full-term SGA infants are of average intelligence, whether tested during the preschool or school years, even though the mean IQ of the SGA population usually has been somewhat lower than that of control groups.[95] Fitzhardinge and Stevens, however, found that, despite average intelligence, 50% of the SGA boys and 36% of the SGA girls were doing poorly in school. One third of the SGA children with IQs above 100 were failing consistently at school. A history of perinatal asphyxia was an important contributing risk factor. Other studies provide good evidence of an increased prevalence of speech and language problems, minor neurologic findings, and attention deficits in this subgroup.[96]

Relatively few studies evaluate the outcome of premature SGA infants, and the results are contradictory. The prevalence of reported handicaps varies from nearly 50% to as low as 10%. Commey and Fitzhardinge found that 15% of premature SGA infants had cerebral palsy at the age of 2 years, twice the prevalence encountered in premature AGA infants.[97] In the Swedish cerebral palsy study, premature SGA infants had the highest risk for cerebral palsy, 15 times greater than full-term AGA infants and significantly more than full-term SGA and premature AGA infants.[31] Commey and Fitzhardinge found a high prevalence of subnormal intelligence in premature SGA infants tested at the age of 2 years. Drillien reported that, in all birth weight subgroups, fewer premature SGA infants were average cognitively, and more had borderline intelligence or mental retardation, especially those born to parents of low socioeconomic status.[98] There is little specific information about school function in this subgroup, but premature SGA infants certainly must be presumed to be at substantial risk in this area as well.

ASPHYXIA

Hypoxic–ischemic brain injury is the single most important neurologic problem occurring in the perinatal period.[99] This variety of brain injury accounts for many, although not the majority, of the severe, nonprogressive neurologic deficits seen in children. This is particularly the case for full-term infants, but also is of etiologic significance for premature infants. The neurodevelopmental deficits of concern are principally the triad of cerebral palsy, mental retardation, and epilepsy, often occurring together in varying degrees. In addition, more subtle developmental and behavioral dysfunctions in the areas of language, fine motor coordination, socioemotional competence, attention, and school learning increasingly are recognized in the relatively few studies designed to investigate these long-term sequelae. The common denominator of this form of brain injury is deprivation of the supply of oxygen to the central nervous system. The developing brain can be deprived of oxygen by two major pathogenetic mechanisms—hypoxemia (*i.e.*, diminished amount of oxygen in the blood supply) or ischemia (*i.e.*, diminished amount of blood perfusing the tissue). These two overlapping mechanisms typically coexist clinically, are virtually impossible to isolate and delineate precisely in the individual infant, and together constitute the basis of the syndrome of asphyxia.[100]

As noted by Paneth and Stark, the fundamental problem in assessing the exact relationship between asphyxia and subsequent neurodevelopmental outcome has been the difficulty in assessing the degree of asphyxia.[101] Various techniques have been used to identify the asphyxiated infant, including the time to initiate spontaneous respiration (>1 minute), the time that positive-pressure ventilation was required to sustain the infant (>1 minute), and the use of the neonatal scoring system developed by Virginia Apgar.[102] This scoring system originally was created to identify infants who were physiologically depressed at birth and who required resuscitative efforts. Although Apgar did not design the scoring system to be used as a tool to predict long-term neurologic status, it has been used by many for correlation with ultimate outcome because of the paucity of alternative asphyxial markers. Fetal scalp blood and umbilical cord blood sampling for *p*H and other acid–base parameters have been recommended as potentially providing more objective perinatal data.

Although the Apgar scoring system is not perfect,

it continues to be the standard by which almost all neonates are evaluated immediately after birth, and, as such, was the perinatal measure used in the NIH National Collaborative Perinatal Project between 1959 and 1966. This multisite prospective study of more than 50,000 pregnant woman and their children remains the largest single resource for investigating the associations between perinatal asphyxia and neurodevelopmental outcome, particularly cerebral palsy. Several main conclusions emerge[103]:

Cerebral palsy does not develop in most (95%) of asphyxiated full-term infants with an Apgar of $\leq$ 3 at 5 minutes.

As the duration of severe asphyxia increases from 5 to 20 minutes, the likelihood of neonatal death or permanent cerebral palsy also increases in parallel fashion; approximately 60% cerebral palsy prevalence exists in full-term survivors with Apgar scores of $\leq$ 3 at 20 minutes.

The more premature the infant, the greater the incidence (*i.e.*, approximately 30% at 28 weeks of gestational age), severity, and mortality associated with perinatal asphyxia.

Most infants in whom cerebral palsy develops were not asphyxiated at birth.

Although perinatal asphyxia, certainly is an important cause of severe psychomotor retardation, especially during the intrapartum period, its relative contribution to these adverse outcomes has, in the past, frequently been overstated. It is estimated that between 10% and 20% of all cases of cerebral palsy are attributable to intrapartum asphyxia. Many of these cases are complicated by mental retardation of variable severity. Freeman and Nelson correctly emphasize the four necessary criteria to link causally intrapartum asphyxia and neurodevelopmental disability in full-term infants[104]:

1. Intrapartum abnormalities (*e.g.*, nonreassuring fetal heart rate patterns, passage of meconium, hemorrhage)
2. Depression at birth (*e.g.*, low Apgar scores, need for resuscitation)
3. Neonatal hypoxic–ischemic encephalopathy (*e.g.*, seizures in the first 48 hours, hypotonia and lethargy, metabolic acidosis, apnea)
4. Anticipated outcomes (*e.g.*, cerebral palsy with associated deficits, not severe mental retardation or epilepsy by themselves).

Outcome studies in full-term infants have identified the neonatal factors most predictive of neurodevelopmental disability after an episode of intrapartum asphyxia. The key predictors include failure to establish spontaneous respiration by 5 minutes, onset of seizures within the first 12 hours and refractory to treatment, prolonged deep encephalopathy (*i.e.*, Sarnat stage 3[105]), failure of the electroencephalogram to normalize by 5 to 7 days, and inability to establish adequate oral feedings by 1 week of age.[106] Fitzhardinge and colleagues described the predictive utility of the computed tomography scan between 1 and 2 weeks after birth.[107] The most ominous findings were diffuse hypodensities throughout both the white and gray matter and extensive intraparenchymal or intraventricular hemorrhage. Byrne and associates reported that 8 months of age appears to be the earliest time at which magnetic resonance imaging findings (*e.g.*, delayed myelination, acquired structural abnormalities) correlate well with later adverse neurodevelopmental outcome in this population.[108] Finally, Robertson and colleagues compared 145 asphyxiated full-term children who had experienced neonatal encephalopathy with a similar number of nonasphyxiated peer children at 8 years of age.[109] The prevalence of major impairment, which included cerebral palsy, mental retardation, epilepsy, cortical blindness, and severe hearing loss, was 16%. Intellectual, visual–motor integration, and receptive vocabulary scores, as well as reading, spelling, and arithmetic grade levels for those children with moderate or severe encephalopathy were significantly below those in the mild encephalopathy or peer comparison groups. Thus, children who survive moderate or severe neonatal asphyxial encephalopathy are at increased risk for both major neurosensory impairment and reduced school performance.

REFERENCES

1. McCormick MC. The contribution of low birthweight to infant mortality and childhood morbidity. N Engl J Med 1985;312:82.
2. Philip AGS, Little GA, Polivy DR, et al. Neonatal mortality risk for the 80s: the importance of birthweight/gestational age groups. Pediatrics 1981;68:122.
3. Paneth N, Kiely JL, Wallenstein S, et al. Newborn intensive care and neonatal mortality in low birthweight infants: a population study. N Engl J Med 1982;307:149.
4. Buehler JW, Kleinman JC, Hogue CJR. Birthweight-specific infant mortality, United States, 1960 and 1980. Public Health Rep 1987;102:151.
5. Herdman RC, Behney CJ, Wagner JL, et al. Neonatal intensive care for low birthweight infants: costs and effectiveness. Health Technology Case Study 38, Publication OTA-HCS-38. Washington, DC: Office of Technology Assessment, 1987.
6. Hack M, Fanaroff AA. Outcomes of extremely low birthweight infants between 1982 and 1988. N Engl J Med 1989;321:1642.
7. Phelps DL, Brown DR, Tung B, et al. 28-day survival rates of 6,676 neonates with birthweights of 1250 grams or less. Pediatrics 1991;87:7.
8. Ginsberg HG, Goldsmith JP, Stedman CM. Intact survival and 20-month follow-up of a 380-gram infant. J Perinatol 1990; 10:330.
9. Hack M, Horbar JD, Malloy MH, et al. Very low birthweight outcomes of the National Institute of Child Health and Human Development Neonatal Network. Pediatrics 1991;87:587.
10. Lasky RE, Tyson JE, Rosenfeld CR, et al. Disappointing follow-up findings for indigent high-risk newborns. Am J Dis Child 1987;147:100.
11. Bennett FC, Robinson NM, Sells CJ. Growth and develop-

ment of infants weighing less than 800 grams at birth. Pediatrics 1983;71:319.
12. Hoffman EL, Bennett FC. Birthweight less than 800 grams: changing outcomes and influences of gender and gestation number. Pediatrics 1990;86:27.
13. LaPine TR, Bennett FC, Jackson JC. Outcome trends of infants weighing less than 800 grams at birth. [abstract] Clin Res 1992;40:8.
14. Shy KK, Luthy DA, Bennett FC, et al. Effects of electronic fetal heart rate monitoring, as compared with periodic auscultation, on the neurologic development of premature infants. N Engl J Med 1990;322:588.
15. The HIFI Study Group. High-frequency oscillatory ventilation compared with conventional intermittent mechanical ventilation in the treatment of respiratory failure in preterm infants: neurodevelopmental status at 16 to 24 months of postterm age. J Pediatr 1990;117:939.
16. Aylward GP, Pfeiffer SI, Wright A, et al. Outcome studies of low birthweight infants published in the last decade: a metaanalysis. J Pediatr 1989;115:515.
17. Blackman J. Warning signals: basic criteria for tracking at-risk infants and toddlers. Washington, DC: National Center for Clinical Infant Programs, 1986.
18. Blackman JA, Hein HA. Iowa's system for screening and tracking high-risk infants. Am J Dis Child 1985;139:826.
19. TeKolste KA, Bennett FC. The high risk infant: transitions in health, development, and family during the first years of life. J Perinatol 1987;7:368.
20. Barrera ME, Rosenbaum PL, Cunningham CE. Corrected and uncorrected Bayley scores: longitudinal developmental patterns in low and high birthweight infants. Infant Behavior and Development 1987;10:337.
21. McCormick MC. Long-term follow-up of infants discharged from neonatal intensive care units. JAMA 1989;261:1767.
22. Bennett FC. Neurodevelopmental outcome in low birthweight infants: the role of developmental intervention. Clinics in Critical Care Medicine 1988;13:221.
23. Brothwood M, Wolke D, Gamsu H, et al. Prognosis of the very low birthweight baby in relation to gender. Arch Dis Child 1986;61:559.
24. Paneth N, Kiely JL, Stein Z, et al. Cerebral palsy and newborn care: III. Estimated prevalence rates of cerebral palsy under differing rates of mortality and impairment of low birthweight infants. Dev Med Child Neurol 1981;23:801.
25. Hagberg B, Hagberg G, Olow I, et al. The changing panorama of cerebral palsy in Sweden: V. The birth year period 1979–82. Acta Paediatr Scand 1989;78:283.
26. Pharoah PO, Cooke T, Cooke RW, et al. Birthweight specific trends in cerebral palsy. Arch Dis Child 1990;65:602.
26a. Freud S. Infantile cerebral paralysis. Russin LA, trans. Coral Gables, FL: University of Miami Press, 1968.
27. Bennett FC, Chandler LS, Robinson NM, et al. Spastic diplegia in premature infants: etiologic and diagnostic considerations. Am J Dis Child 1981;135:732.
28. Volpe JJ. Cognitive deficits in premature infants. N Engl J Med 1991;325:276.
29. Graziani LJ, Pasto M, Stanley C, et al. Neonatal neurosonographic correlates of cerebral palsy in preterm infants. Pediatrics 1986;78:88.
30. Bozynski ME, Nelson MN, Genaze D, et al. Cranial ultrasonography and the prediction of cerebral palsy in infants weighing ≤ 1200 grams at birth. Dev Med Child Neurol 1988;30:342.
31. Hagberg B. Epidemiological and preventive aspects of cerebral palsy and severe mental retardation in Sweden. Eur J Pediatr 1979;130:71.
32. Gibson RL, Jackson JC, Twiggs GA, et al. Bronchopulmonary dysplasia: survival after prolonged mechanical ventilation. Am J Dis Child 1988;142:721.
33. Bradford BC, Baudin J, Conway MJ, et al. Identification of sensory neural hearing loss in very preterm infants by brainstem auditory evoked potentials. Arch Dis Child 1985;60:105.
34. de Vries LS, Lary S, Dubowitz LMS. Relationship of serum bilirubin levels to ototoxicity and deafness in high-risk low birthweight infants. Pediatrics 1985;76:351.
35. Salamy A, Eldredge L, Tooley WH. Neonatal status and hearing loss in high-risk infants. J Pediatr 1989;114:847.
36. Leavitt AM, Watchko JF, Bennett FC, et al. Neurodevelopmental outcome following persistent pulmonary hypertension of the neonate. J Perinatol 1987;7:288.
37. Abramovich SJ, Gregory S, Slemick M, et al. Hearing loss in very low birthweight infants treated with neonatal intensive care. Arch Dis Child 1979;54:421.
38. Bess FH, Tharpe AM. Unilateral hearing impairment in children. Pediatrics 1984;74:206.
39. Thompson G, Folsom R. Hearing assessment of at-risk infants. Clin Pediatr 1981;20:257.
40. Marshall RE, Reichert TJ, Kerley SV, et al. Auditory function in newborn intensive care unit patients revealed by auditory brainstem potentials. J Pediatr 1980;96:731.
41. Nield TA, Schrier S, Ramos AD, et al. Unexpected hearing loss in high-risk infants. Pediatrics 1986;78:417.
42. Avery GB, Glass P. Retinopathy of prematurity: progress report. Pediatr Ann 1988;17:528.
43. Avery GB, Glass P. Retinopathy of prematurity: what causes it? Clin Perinatol 1988;15:917.
44. Scharf J, Zonis S, Zeltzer M. Refraction in premature babies: a prospective study. J Pediatr Ophthalmol Strabismus 1978; 15:48.
45. Camfield PR, Camfield CS, Allen AC, et al. Progressive hydrocephalus in infants with birthweights less than 1500 grams. Arch Neurol 1981;38:653.
46. Shinnar S, Molteni RA, Gammon K, et al. Intraventricular hemorrhage in the premature infant. N Engl J Med 1982; 306:1464.
47. Chaplin ER, Goldstein GW, Myerberg DZ, et al. Posthemorrhagic hydrocephalus in the preterm infant. Pediatrics 1980; 65:901.
48. Saigal S, Rosenbaum P, Stoskopf B, et al. Follow-up of infants 501 to 1500 gm birthweight delivered to residents of a geographically defined region with perinatal intensive care facilities. J Pediatr 1982;100:606.
49. McBurney AK, Eaves LC. Evolution of developmental and psychological test scores. In: Dunn HG, ed. Sequelae of low birthweight: the Vancouver Study. Philadelphia: JB Lippincott, 1986.
50. Hoy EA, Bill JM, Sykes DH. Very low birthweight: a long-term developmental impairment? International Journal of Behavior and Development 1988;11:37.
51. Rose SA. Differential rates of visual information processing in full-term and preterm infants. Child Dev 1983;54:1189.
52. Ruff HA, McCarton C, Kurtzberg D, et al. Preterm infants' manipulative exploration of objects. Child Dev 1984; 55:1166.
53. Drillien CM. The growth and development of the prematurely born infant. Edinburgh: Livingstone, 1964.
54. Wiener G, Rider RV, Oppel WC, et al. Correlates of low birthweight: psychological status at eight to ten years of age. Pediatr Res 1968;2:110.
55. Hunt JV, Cooper BAB, Tooley WH. Very low birthweight infants at 8 and 11 years of age: role of neonatal illness and family status. Pediatrics 1988;82:596.

56. Zarin-Ackerman J, Lewis M, Driscoll JM. Language development in 2-year-old normal and risk infants. Pediatrics 1977; 59:982.
57. Largo RH, Molinari L, Comenale-Pinto L, et al. Language development of term and preterm children during the first five years of life. Dev Med Child Neurol 1986;28:333.
58. Michelsson K, Noronen M. Neurological, psychological and articulatory impairment in five-year-old children with a birthweight of 2000 g or less. Eur J Pediatr 1983;137:96.
59. Hubatch LM, Johnson CJ, Kistler DJ, et al. Early language abilities of high-risk infants. J Speech Hear Disord 1985; 50:195.
60. Bennett FC, Robinson NM, Sells CJ. Hyaline membrane disease, birthweight, and gestational age: effects on development in the first two years. Am J Dis Child 1982;136: 888.
61. Drillien CM. Abnormal neurologic signs in the first year of life in low birthweight infants: possible prognostic significance. Dev Med Child Neurol 1972;14:575.
62. Amiel-Tison C. A method for neurologic evaluation within the first year of life. Curr Probl Pediatr 1976;7:1.
63. Coolman RB, Bennett FC, Sells CJ, et al. Neuromotor development of graduates of the neonatal intensive care unit: patterns encountered in the first two years of life. J Dev Behav Pediatr 1985;6:327.
64. Drillien CM, Thomson AJM, Burgoyne K. Low birthweight children at early school age: a longitudinal study. Dev Med Child Neurol 1980;22:26.
65. Ross G, Lipper EG, Auld PAM. Consistency and change in the development of premature infants weighing less than 1501 grams at birth. Pediatrics 1985;76:885.
66. Burns YR, Bullock MI. Comparison of abilities of preterm and mature born children at 5 years of age. Aust Paediatr J 1985; 21:31.
67. Crowe TK, Deitz JC, Bennett FC, et al. Preschool motor skills of children born prematurely and not diagnosed as having cerebral palsy. J Dev Behav Pediatr 1988;9:189.
68. Ferrari F, Grosoli MV, Fontana G, et al. Neurobehavioral comparison of low-risk preterm and full-term infants at term conceptional age. Dev Med Child Neurol 1983;25:450.
69. Freidman SL, Jacobs BS, Werthmann MW. Preterms of low medical risk: spontaneous behaviors and soothability at expected date of birth. Infant Behavior and Development 1982;5:3.
70. Aylward GP, Hatcher RP, Leavitt LA, et al. Factors affecting neurobehavioral responses of preterm infants at term conceptional age. Child Dev 1984;55:1155.
71. Kurtzberg D, Hilpert PL, Kreuzer JA, et al. Differential maturation of cortical auditory evoked potentials to speech sounds in normal full-term and very low birthweight infants. Dev Med Child Neurol 1984;26:466.
72. Anders TF, Keener M. Developmental coarse of nighttime sleep-wake patterns in full-term and premature infants during the first year of life: I. Sleep 1985;8:173.
73. Fox NA, Porges SW. The relation between neonatal heart period patterns and developmental outcome. Child Dev 1985; 56:28.
74. Kaga K, Hashira S, Marsh RR. Auditory brainstem responses and behavioral responses in preterm infants. Br J Audiol 1986;20:121.
75. Anders TF, Keener M, Kraemer H. Sleep-wake state organization, neonatal assessment and development in premature infants during the first year of life: II. Sleep 1985;8:193.
76. Cohen SE, Parmelee AH, Beckwith L, et al. Cognitive development in preterm infants: birth to eight years. J Dev Behav Pediatr 1986;7:102.
77. DiVitto B, Goldberg S. The effects of newborn medical status on early parent-infant interactions. In: Field TM, ed. Infants born at risk. New York: Spectrum, 1979:311.
78. Field TM. Interaction patterns of preterm and term infants. In: Field TM, ed. Infants born at risk. New York: Spectrum, 1979:333.
79. Watt J. Interaction and development in the first year: I. The effects of prematurity. Early Hum Dev 1986;13:195.
80. Field TM. High-risk infants "have less fun" during early interactions. Topics in Early Childhood Special Education 1983;3(1):77.
81. Crnic KA, Ragozin AS, Greenberg MT, et al. Social interaction and developmental competence of preterm and full-term infants during the first year of life. Child Dev 1983;54: 1199.
82. Malatesta CZ, Grigoryev P, Lamb C, et al. Emotion socialization and expressive development in preterm and full-term infants. Child Dev 1986;57:316.
83. Kopp CB. Risk factors in development. In: Haith MM, Campos JJ, eds. Handbook of child psychology. vol. 2. Infancy and developmental psychobiology. New York: John Wiley & Sons, 1983:1081.
84. Dunn HG, Crichton JU, Grunau RVE, et al. Neurological, psychological and educational sequelae of low birthweight. Brain Dev 1980;2:57.
85. Dunn HG, ed. Sequelae of low birthweight: the Vancouver Study. Clinics in Developmental Medicine 1986;95:96.
86. Wright FH, Blough RR, Chamberlin A, et al. A controlled follow-up study of small prematures born from 1952 through 1956. Am J Dis Child 1972;124:506.
87. Caputo DV, Goldstein KM, Taub HB. The development of prematurely born children through middle childhood. In: Field TM, ed. Infants born at risk. New York: Spectrum, 1979: 219.
88. Nickel RE, Bennett FC, Lamson FN. School performance of children with birthweights of 1000 g or less. Am J Dis Child 1982;136:105.
89. Klein NK, Hack M, Breslau N. Children who were very low birthweight: development and academic achievement at nine years of age. J Dev Behav Pediatr 1989;10:32.
90. Ross G, Lipper EG, Auld PAM. Educational status and school-related abilities of very low birthweight premature children. Pediatrics 1991;88:1125.
91. Escalona SK. Babies at double hazard: early development of infants at biologic and social risk. Pediatrics 1982;70:670.
92. Breslau N, Klein N, Allen L. Very low birthweight: behavioral sequelae at nine years of age. J Am Acad Child Adolesc Psychiatry 1988;27:605.
93. Allen MC. Developmental outcome and follow-up of the small for gestational age infant. Semin Perinatol 1984;8:123.
94. Fitzhardinge PM, Stevens EM. The small-for-date infant: II. Neurological and intellectual sequelae. Pediatrics 1972; 50:50.
95. Westwood M, Kramer MS, Munz D, et al. Growth and development of full-term nonasphyxiated small-for-gestational-age newborns: follow-up through adolescence. Pediatrics 1983; 71:376.
96. Neligan GA, Kolvin I, Scott DM, et al. Born too soon or born too small: a follow-up study to seven years of age. Clinics in Developmental Medicine 1976;61:81.
97. Commey JO, Fitzhardinge PM. Handicap in the preterm small-for-gestational age infant. J Pediatr 1979;94:779.
98. Drillien CM. Aetiology and outcome in low birthweight infants. Dev Med Child Neurol 1972;14:563.
99. Shaywitz BA. The sequelae of hypoxic-ischemic encephalopathy. Semin Perinatol 1987;11:180.

100. Volpe JJ. Perinatal hypoxic-ischemic brain injury. Pediatr Clin North Am 1976;23:383.
101. Paneth N, Stark RI. Cerebral palsy and mental retardation in relation to indicators of perinatal asphyxia: an epidemiologic overview. Am J Obstet Gynecol 1983;147:960.
102. Apgar V, James LS. Further observations on the newborn scoring system. Am J Dis Child 1962;104:419.
103. Nelson KB, Ellenberg JH. Apgar scores as predictors of chronic neurologic disability. Pediatrics 1981;68:36.
104. Freeman JM, Nelson KB. Intrapartum asphyxia and cerebral palsy. Pediatrics 1988;82:240.
105. Sarnat HB, Sarnat MS. Neonatal encephalopathy following fetal distress: a clinical and electroencephalographic study. Arch Neurol 1976;33:696.
106. Finer NN, Robertson CM, Richards RT, et al. Hypoxic–ischemic encephalopathy in term neonates: perinatal factors and outcome. J Pediatr 1981;98:112.
107. Fitzhardinge PM, Flodmark O, Fitz CR, et al. The prognostic value of computed tomography as an adjunct to assessment of the term infant with postasphyxial encephalopathy. J Pediatr 1981;99:777.
108. Byrne P, Welch R, Johnson MA, et al. Serial magnetic resonance imaging in neonatal hypoxic-ischemic encephalopathy. J Pediatr 1990;117:694.
109. Robertson CM, Finer NN, Grace MG. School performance of survivors of neonatal encephalopathy associated with birth asphyxia at term. J Pediatr 1989;114:753.

Appendices

CONTENTS

Neonatology: Pathophysiology and Management of the Newborn, Fourth Edition,
edited by Gordon B. Avery, Mary Ann Fletcher, and Mhairi G. MacDonald.
J.B. Lippincott Company, Philadelphia © 1994.

appendix A

Selected Laboratory Values

These ranges are for guidance only. They are derived from published and unpublished sources and represent measurements taken using different methodologies and varying numbers of subjects. Parametric statistics frequently have been used even when the data are not normally distributed. Readers are advised to obtain reference range information from their local laboratory.

1. BLOOD

APPENDIX A–1a
NORMAL BLOOD CHEMISTRY VALUES, TERM INFANTS*

		Capillary Blood Mean (Range)			
Determination	**Cord Blood Mean (Range)**	1–12 Hours of Age	12–24 Hours of Age	24–48 Hours of Age	48–72 Hours of Age
Sodium (mM/L)	147 (126–166)	143 (124–156)	145 (132–159)	148 (134–160)	149 (139–162)
Potassium (mM/L)	7.8 (5.6–12)	6.4 (5.3–7.3)	6.3 (5.3–8.9)	6 (5.2–7.3)	5.9 (5–7.7)
Chloride (mM/L)	103 (98–110)	101 (90–111)	103 (87–114)	102 (92–114)	103 (93–112)
Calcium (mg/dL)	9.3 (8.2–11.1)	8.4 (7.3–9.2)	7.8 (6.9–9.4)	8 (6.1–9.9)	7.9 (5.9–9.7)
Phosphorus (mg/dL)	5.6 (3.7–8.1)	6.1 (3.5–8.6)	5.7 (2.9–8.1)	5.9 (3–8.7)	5.8 (2.8–7.6)
Blood urea (mg/dL)	29 (21–40)	27 (8–34)	33 (9–63)	32 (13–77)	31 (13–68)
Total protein (g/dL)	6.1 (4.8–7.3)	6.6 (5.6–8.5)	6.6 (5.8–8.2)	6.9 (5.9–8.2)	7.2 (6–8.5)
Glucose (mg/dL)	73 (45–96)	63 (40–97)	63 (42–104)	56 (30–91)	59 (40–90)
Lactic acid (mg/dL)	19.5 (11–30)	14.6 (11–24)	14 (10–23)	14.3 (9–22)	13.5 (7–21)
Lactate (mM/L)†	2–3	2			

* Acharya PT, Payne WW: Arch Dis Child 1965;40:430.
† Daniel SS, Adamsons K Jr, James LS: Pediatrics 1966;37:942. Copyright © American Academy of Pediatrics, 1966.

APPENDIX A–1b
NORMAL BLOOD CHEMISTRY VALUES, LOW-BIRTH-WEIGHT INFANTS, CAPILLARY BLOOD, FIRST DAY

Determination	<1000 g	1001–1500 g	1501–2000 g	2001–2500 g
Sodium (mM/L)	138	133	135	134
Potassium (mM/L)	6.4	6.0	5.4	5.6
Chloride (mM/L)	100	101	105	104
Total CO_2 (mM/L)	19	20	20	20
Urea (mg/dL)	22	21	16	16
Total protein (g/dL)	4.8	4.8	5.2	5.3

Pincus JB, et al. Pediatrics 1956;18:39.

APPENDIX A–1c
BLOOD CHEMISTRY VALUES DURING THE FIRST 7 WEEKS OF LIFE IN PREMATURE INFANTS WITH BIRTH WEIGHTS OF 1500 TO 1750 g

	1 Week of Age			3 Weeks of Age			5 Weeks of Age			7 Weeks of Age		
Determination	Mean	SD	Range	Mean	SD	Range	Mean	SD	Range	Mean	SD	Range
Na (mM/L)	139.6	±3.2	133–146	136.3	±2.9	129–142	136.8	±2.5	133–148	137.2	±1.8	133–142
K (mM/L)	5.6	±0.5	4.6–6.7	5.8	±0.6	4.5–7.1	5.5	±0.6	4.5–6.6	5.7	±0.5	4.6–7.1
Cl (mM/L)	108.2	±3.7	100–117	108.3	±3.9	102–116	107	±3.5	100–115	107	±3.3	101–115
CO_2 (mM/L)	20.3	±2.8	13.8–27.1	18.4	±3.5	12.4–26.2	20.4	±3.4	12.5–26.1	20.6	±3.1	13.7–26.9
Ca (mg/dL)	9.2	±1.1	6.1–11.6	9.6	±0.5	8.1–11	9.4	±0.5	8.6–10.5	9.5	±0.7	8.6–10.8
P (mg/dL)	7.6	±1.1	5.4–10.9	7.5	±0.7	6.2–8.7	7	±0.6	5.6–7.9	6.8	±0.8	4.2–8.2
BUN (mg/dL)	9.3	±5.2	3.1–25.5	13.3	±7.8	2.1–31.4	13.3	±7.1	2–26.5	13.4	±6.7	2.5–30.5
Total protein (g/dL)	5.49	±0.42	4.4–6.26	5.38	±0.48	4.28–6.7	4.98	±0.5	4.14–6.9	4.93	±0.61	4.02–5.86
Albumin (g/dL)	3.85	±0.3	3.28–4.5	3.92	±0.42	3.16–5.26	3.73	±0.34	3.2–4.34	3.89	±0.53	3.4–4.6
Globulin (g/dL)	1.58	±0.33	0.88–2.2	1.44	±0.63	0.62–2.9	1.17	±0.49	0.48–1.48	1.12	±0.33	0.5–2.6
Hemoglobin (g/dL)	17.8	±2.7	11.4–24.8	14.7	±2.1	9–19.4	11.5	±2	7.2–18.6	10	±1.3	7.5–13.9

BUN, blood urea nitrogen; SD, standard deviation.
Adapted from Reichelderfer TJ. Clin Chem 1968;14:272.

APPENDIX A–1d
OTHER SERUM VALUES*

Ammonia nitrogen, newborn	
(μg/dL)	Up to 150
(μM/L)	Up to 107
Amylase (U/L)	5–65
Copper, 0–6 mo (μg/dL)	≤70
Ceruloplasmin (g/L)	0.05–0.18
Zinc (μg/dL)	77–137
Serum enzymes	
Alkaline phosphatase (U/L)	150–400
CPK (U/L)	
1 d	Up to 500
2 d–2 wk	Up to 440
LDH (37°C; U/L)	160–1500
AST, newborn (IU/L)	Up to 54
ALT, newborn (IU/L)	Up to 50
Triglyceride, fasting (mg/dL)	Up to 110
Magnesium (mM/L)	0.75–1.25 (1.5–2.1 mEq/L)
Osmolality (mOsmol/kg)	285–295
Phenylalanine, newborn (mg/dL)	Up to 4
α_1-Antitrypsin (g/L)	2.1–5.0
Vitamin A (retinol; μg/dL)	
0–1 y	20–90
Vitamin E (μg/dL)	5–20
IgG (g/L)	
Birth	5.52–13.8
1–3 mo	1.34–5.49
4–6 mo	0.73–4.34
IgA (g/L)	
Birth	None detected
1–3 mo	≤0.37
4–6 mo	0.40–0.68
IgM (g/L)	
Birth	≤0.31
1–3 mo	0.16–1.24
4–6 mo	0.42–1.40
Transferrin (g/L)	
≤3 mo	2.03–3.60

* Normal values depend on method used.

ALT, alanine aminotransferase, formerly SGPT; AST, aspartate aminotransferase, formerly SGOT; CPK, creatine phosphokinase; LDH, lactate dehydrogenase.

APPENDIX A–1e
AMINO ACID CONCENTRATION IN PLASMA OR SERUM (MICROMOLAR)

Amino Acid	Neonates Mean ± SD	Infants Mean ± SD
Taurine	141 ± 40	
Hydroxyproline	32	
Aspartic acid	8 ± 4	19 ± 2
Threonine	217 ± 21	177 ± 36†
Serine	163 ± 34	131 ± 27
Asparagine and glutamine*	759 ± 136	
Proline	183 ± 32	193 ± 52
Glutamic acid	52 ± 25	
Glycine	343 ± 69	213 ± 35
Alanine	329 ± 55	292 ± 53
Valine	136 ± 39	161 ± 38
Half cystine	62 ± 13	42 ± 9
Methionine	29 ± 8	18 ± 3
Isoleucine	39 ± 8	39 ± 8
Leucine	72 ± 17	77 ± 21
Tyrosine	69 ± 16	54 ± 21
Phenylalanine	78 ± 14	55 ± 10
Ornithine	91 ± 25	50 ± 11
Lysine	200 ± 46	135 ± 28
Histidine	77 ± 16	78 ± 14
Arginine	54 ± 17	62 ± 9
Tryptophan	32 ± 17	
β-Alanine	14.5	

All data obtained by elution chromatography on ion exchange resin columns.

* Stands for asparagine and glutamine as combined amounts.

† Includes asparagine.

SD, standard deviation.

Adapted from Hicks J, Boeckx RL. Pediatric clinical chemistry. Philadelphia: WB Saunders, 1984:684.

2. URINE

APPENDIX A–2
URINARY VALUES

Determination	17-Ketosteroids	17-Hydroxycorticoids	Pregnanetriol
Adrenal Steroids (mg/d)			
Newborn–1 wk	2–2.5	0.05–0.3	0.01
1 wk–3 mo	0.5	0.05–0.5	0.01
3 mo–1 y	0.5	0.1–0.5	0.01

Determination	Values
Electrolytes (Depends on Intake)	
Sodium (mM/L)	18–60
Potassium (mM/L)	10–40
Chloride (mM/kg/d)	1.7–8.5
Bicarbonate (mM/L)	1.5–2
Calcium (mM/kg/d)	<2
Other Urinary Values	
Ammonia (μM/minute/m^2)	
Infants 2–11.5 mo	4–40
Older children	5.9–16.5
Creatinine (mg/kg/d)	
Premature, 2–12 wk	8.3–19.9
Full-term, 1–7 wk	10–15.5
Older child, 2–3 y	6.4–21.9
Glucose (mg/L)	50
Osmolality (infant; mOsm/kg)	50–600
VMA (infant; μg/mg creatinine)	5–19 (<1 mg/24 h)
HVA (μg/mg creatinine)	3–16
Protein	Trace
Urea nitrogen (depends on intake; mg/L)	300–3000
Titratable acidity (μM/minute/m^2)	Minus bicarbonate
Premature	0–12
Term	0–11

HVA, homovanillic acid; VMA, vanillylmandelic acid.
Data from Normal Values for Pediatric Clinical Chemistry, Special Committee on Pediatric Clinical Chemistry, American Association of Clinical Chemists, August, 1974.

3. CEREBROSPINAL FLUID

APPENDIX A–3a
CEREBROSPINAL FLUID EXAMINATION IN HIGH-RISK NEONATES WITHOUT MENINGITIS

Determination	Term	Preterm
WBC count (cells/mm³)		
Number of infants	87	30
Mean	8.2	9.0
Median	5	6
SD	7.1	8.2
Range	0–32	0–29
±2 SD	0–22.4	0–25.4
Percentage PMN	61.3%	57.2%
Protein (mg/dl)		
Number of infants	35	17
Mean	90	115
Range	20–170	65–150
Glucose (mg/dl)		
Number of infants	51	23
Mean	52	50
Range	34–119	24–63
CSF/blood glucose (%)		
Number of infants	51	23
Mean	81	74
Range	44–248	55–105

CSF, cerebrospinal fluid; PMN, polymorphonuclear cells; SD, standard deviation; WBC, leukocyte.
From Sarff LD, et al. Cerebrospinal fluid evaluation in neonates: comparison of high-risk infants with and without meningitis. J Pediatr 1976;88(3):474.

APPENDIX A–3b
COMPARISON OF LEUKOCYTE COUNTS IN CEREBROSPINAL FLUID IN NEONATES WITH OR WITHOUT MENINGITIS

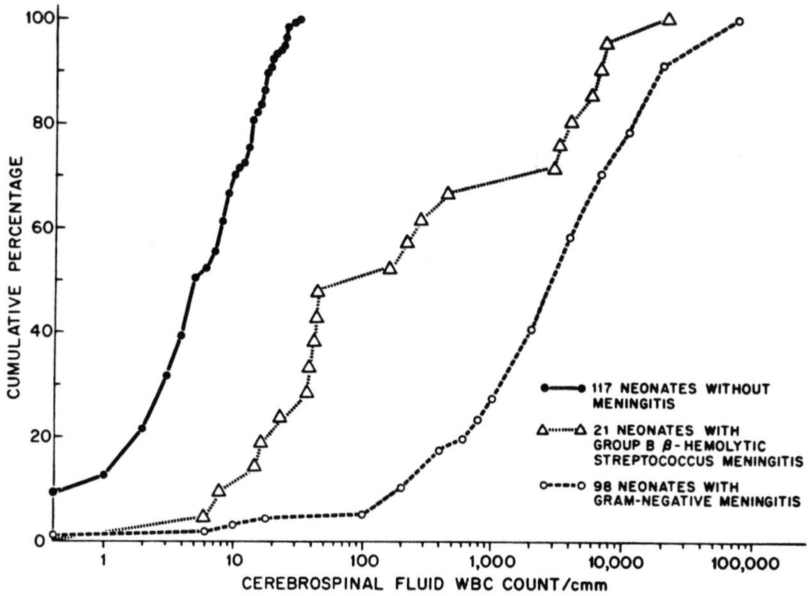

From Sarff LD, et al. Cerebrospinal fluid evaluation in neonates: comparison of high-risk infants with and without meningitis. J Pediatr 1976;88(3):475.

4. ANALYTE UNIT CONVERSION

APPENDIX A–4
SI UNIT CONVERSION TABLE

Analyte	Present Unit	Conversion Factor	SI Unit
Acetaminophen	mg/dL	66.16	μmol/L
Acetoacetic acid	mg/dL	97.95	μmol/L
Adrenocorticotropin	pg/mL	0.2202	pmol/L
Alanine aminotransferase	U/L	1.0	U/L
	Karmen units/mL	0.482	U/L
Albumin	g/dL	10.0	g/L
Aldolase	U/L	1.0	U/L
	Sibley–Lehninger units/mL	0.7440	U/L
Aldosterone (serum)	ng/dL	27.74	pmol/L
Aldosterone (urine)	μg/24 h	2.774	nmol/d
α_1-Antitrypsin	mg/dL	0.01	g/L
α_2-Macroglobulin	mg/dL	0.01	g/L
Aminolevulinic acid	mg/24 h	7.626	μmol/d
Ammonia			
As ammonia	μg/dL	0.5872	μmol/L
As ammonium ion	μg/dL	0.5543	μmol/L
As ammonia nitrogen	μg/dL	0.7139	μmol/L
Amylase	U/L	1.00	U/L
	Somogyi units/dL	1.850	U/L
	Dye units/dL	1.59	U/L
	Street Close units/dL	5.7	U/L
Androstenedione	μg/L	3.492	nmol/L
Aspartate aminotransferase	U/L	1.00	U/L
	Karmen units/mL	0.482	U/L
β-Hydroxybutyric acid	mg/dL	96.05	μmol/L
β_2-Microglobulin (serum)	mg/L	84.75	nmol/L
β_2-Microglobulin (urine)	μg/24 h	0.08475	nmol/d
Bilirubin	mg/dL	17.10	μmol/L
Calcium	mg/dL	0.2495	mmol/L
Calcium, ionized	mEq/L	0.500	mmol/L
Calcium (urine)	mg/24 h	0.02495	mmol/d
Carbon dioxide (total)	mEq/L	1.00	mmol/L
Ceruloplasmin	mg/dL	10.0	mg/L
Chloride	mEq/L	1.00	mmol/L
Cholesterol	mg/dL	0.02586	mmol/L
Chorionic gonadotropin	mIU/mL	1.00	IU/L
Complement, C3	mg/dL	0.01	g/L
Complement, C4	mg/dL	0.01	g/L
Copper (serum)	μg/dL	0.1574	μmol/L
Copper (urine)	μg/24 h	0.01574	μmol/d
Coproporphyrins	μg/24 h	1.527	nmol/d
Cortisol (free, urine)	μg/24 h	2.759	nmol/d
Cortisol (serum)	μg/dL	27.59	nmol/L
Creatine kinase	U/L	1.00	U/L
Creatinine (serum)	mg/dL	88.40	μmol/L
Creatinine (urine)	g/24 h	8.840	mmol/d
Creatinine clearance	mL/min	0.01667	mL/s
Dehydroepiandrosterone	μg/L	3.467	nmol/L
Dehydroepiandrosterone sulfate	ng/mL	0.002714	μmol/L
11-Deoxycortisol	μg/dL	28.86	nmol/L
Diazepam	mg/L	3512	nmol/L
Digoxin	ng/mL	1.281	nmol/L
Epinephrine	pg/mL	5.458	pmol/L
Estradiol	pg/mL	3.671	pmol/L
Estriol (urine)	μg/24 h	3.468	nmol/d

(continued)

APPENDIX A–4
SI UNIT CONVERSION TABLE (*continued*)

Analyte	Present Unit	Conversion Factor	SI Unit
Estrone (plasma)	pg/mL	3.699	pmol/L
Estrone (urine)	μg/24 h	3.699	nmol/d
Ethanol	mg/dL	0.2171	mmol/L
Fat (fecal), as stearic acid	g/24 h	3.515	mmol/d
Ferritin	ng/mL	1.00	μg/L
Folate	ng/mL	2.226	nmol/L
Follicle stimulating hormone	mIU/mL	1.00	IU/L
Galactose	mg/dL	0.05551	mmol/L
γ-Glutamyltransferase	U/L	1.00	U/L
Gases			
PO_2	mm Hg	0.1333	kPa
PCO_2	mm Hg	0.1333	kPa
Gastrin	pg/mL	1	ng/L
Glucose	mg/dL	0.05551	mmol/L
Growth hormone	ng/mL	1.00	μg/L
Haptoglobin	mg/dL	0.01	g/L
Homovanillic acid	mg/24 h	5.489	μmol/d
5-Hydroxyindoleacetic acid	mg/24 h	5.230	μmol/d
17-Hydroxyprogesterone	μg/L	3.026	nmol/L
Immunoglobulins			
IgA	mg/dL	0.01	g/L
IgD	mg/dL	10	mg/L
IgE	U/mL	2.4	μg/L
IgG	mg/dL	0.01	g/L
IgM	mg/dL	0.01	g/L
Insulin	mU/L	7.175	pmol/L
Iron	μg/dL	0.1791	μmol/L
Iron-binding capacity	μg/dL	0.1791	μmol/L
Lactate, as lactic acid	mEq/L	1.00	mmol/L
	mg/dL	0.1110	mmol/L
Lactate dehydrogenase	U/L	1.00	U/L
	Wrobleski units/mL	0.482	U/L
Lipase	U/L	1.00	U/L
	Cherry Crandall units	278	U/L
Lipoproteins			
Low density as cholesterol	mg/dL	0.02586	mmol/L
High density as cholesterol	mg/dL	0.02586	mmol/L
Lithium	mEq/L	1.00	mmol/L
Luteinizing hormone (LH)	mIU/mL	1.00	IU/L
Magnesium	mg/dL	0.4114	mmol/L
	mEq/L	0.500	mmol/L
Metanephrines	mg/24 h	5.458	μmol/d
Methanol	mg/dL	0.3121	mmol/L
Methotrexate	mg/L	2.200	μmol/L
Norepinephrine	pg/mL	0.005911	nmol/L
Osmolality	mOsm/kg	1.00	mmol/kg
Oxalate	mg/24 h	11.11	μmol/d
Pentobarbital	mg/L	4.419	μmol/L
Phenobarbital	mg/L	4.306	μmol/L
Phenytoin	mg/L	3.964	μmol/L
Phosphatase, acid	King Armstrong units/dL	1.77	U/L
	Bodansky units/dL	5.37	U/L
	Kind-King units/dL	1.77	U/L
	Bessey-Lowry-Brock units/dL	16.67	U/L

(continued)

APPENDIX A–4
SI UNIT CONVERSION TABLE (*continued*)

Analyte	Present Unit	Conversion Factor	SI Unit
Phosphatase, alkaline	U/L	1.00	U/L
	Bodansky units/dL	5.37	U/L
	King Armstrong units/dL	7.1	U/L
	Bessey-Lowry-Brock units/dL	16.67	U/L
Phosphate, as inorganic phosphorus	mg/dL	0.3229	mmol/L
Porphobilinogen	mg/24 h	4.420	μmol/d
Potassium	mEq/L	1.00	mmol/L
Pregnanediol	mg/24 h	3.120	μmol/d
Pregnanetriol	mg/24 h	2.972	μmol/d
Primidone	mg/L	4.582	μmol/L
Procainamide	mg/L	4.249	μmol/L
N-Acetylprocainamide	mg/L	3.606	μmol/L
Progesterone	ng/mL	3.180	nmol/L
Prolactin	ng/mL	1.00	μg/L
Propranolol	ng/mL	3.856	nmol/L
Protein (total, cerebrospinal fluid)	mg/dL	0.01	g/L
Protein (total, serum)	g/dL	10.0	g/L
Protein (total, urine)	mg/24 h	0.001	g/d
Protoporphyrin (erythrocyte)	μg/dL	0.0177	μmol/L
Pyruvate, as pyruvic acid	mg/dL	113.6	μmol/L
Quinidine	mg/L	3.082	μmol/L
Renin	ng/mL/h	0.2778	ng/L/s
Salicylate, as salicylic acid	mg/dL	0.07240	mmol/L
Serotonin	μg/dL	0.05675	μmol/L
Sodium	mEq/L	1.00	mmol/L
Testosterone	ng/mL	3.467	nmol/L
Theophylline	mg/L	5.550	μmol/L
Thiocyanate	mg/dL	0.1722	mmol/L
Thiopental	mg/L	4.126	μmol/L
Thyroid stimulating hormone	μU/mL	1.00	mU/L
Thyroxine (T4)	μg/dL	12.87	nmol/L
Thyroxine, free	ng/dL	12.87	pmol/L
Thyroxine binding globulin, as T4	μg/dL	12.87	nmol/L
Transferrin	mg/dL	0.01	g/L
Triglycerides	mg/dL	0.01129	mmol/L
Triiodothyronine (T3)	ng/dL	0.01536	nmol/L
T3 uptake	%	0.01	1
Urate, as uric acid	mg/dL	59.48	μmol/L
Urea nitrogen	mg/dL	0.3570	mmol/L urea
Urobilinogen	mg/24 h	1.693	μmol/d
Uroporphyrin	μg/24 h	1.204	nmol/d
Valproic acid	mg/L	6.934	μmol/L
Vanillylmandelic acid	mg/24 h	5.046	μmol/d
Vitamin A	μg/dL	0.03491	μmol/L
Vitamin B_{12}	ng/dL	7.378	pmol/L
Vitamin D_3 (25-OH-cholecalciferol)	ng/mL	2.496	nmol/L
Vitamin E	mg/dL	23.22	μmol/L
Zinc (serum)	μg/dL	0.1530	μmol/L
Zinc (urine)	μg/24 h	0.0153	μmol/d

Adapted from the SI manual in health care. 2nd ed. Ottawa: Metric Commission of Canada, 1982.

Neonatology: Pathophysiology and Management of the Newborn, Fourth Edition,
edited by Gordon B. Avery, Mary Ann Fletcher, and Mhairi G. MacDonald.
J.B. Lippincott Company, Philadelphia © 1994.

appendix B

Hematologic Values

1. ERYTHROCYTES

APPENDIX B–1a
ERYTHROCYTE VALUES AT VARIOUS AGES: MEAN AND LOWER LIMIT OF NORMAL (±2 SD)

	Hemoglobin (g/dL)		Hematocrit (%)		Erythrocyte Count (RBC × 10^{-6})		MCV (fl)		MCH (pg)		MCHC (g/dL)	
Age	Mean	±2 SD	Mean	±2 SD	Mean	±2 SD	Mean	±2 SD	Mean	±2 SD	Mean	±2 SD
Birth (cord blood)	16.5	13.5	51	42	4.7	3.9	108	98	34	31	33	30
1–3 d (capillary)	18.5	14.5	56	45	5.3	4.0	108	95	34	31	33	29
1 wk	17.5	13.5	54	42	5.1	3.9	107	88	34	28	33	28
2 wk	16.5	12.5	51	39	4.9	3.6	105	86	34	28	33	28
1 mo	14	10	43	31	4.2	3	104	85	34	28	33	29
2 mo	11.5	9	35	28	3.8	2.7	96	77	30	26	33	29
3–6 mo	11.5	9.5	35	29	3.8	3.1	91	74	30	25	33	30
0.5–2 y	12	10.5	36	33	4.5	3.7	78	70	27	23	33	30
2–6 y	12.5	11.5	37	34	4.6	3.9	81	75	27	24	34	31
6–12 y	13.5	11.5	40	35	4.6	4	86	77	29	25	34	31
12–18 y												
Female	14	12	41	36	4.6	4.1	90	78	30	25	34	31
Male	14.5	13	43	37	4.9	4.5	88	78	30	25	34	31
18–49 y												
Female	14	12	41	36	4.6	4	90	80	30	26	34	31
Male	15.5	13.5	47	41	5.2	4.5	90	80	30	26	34	31

These data have been compiled from several sources. Emphasis is placed on studies employing electronic counters and on the selection of populations that are likely to exclude individuals with iron deficiency. The mean ±2 SD can be expected to include 95% of the observations in a normal population.
SD, standard deviation.
From Dallman PR. In: Rudolph A, ed. Pediatrics. 16th ed., New York: Appleton-Century-Crofts, 1977:1111.

APPENDIX B–1b
THE RELATIVE CONCENTRATION OF FETAL HEMOGLOBIN IN INFANTS AND ITS VARIATION WITH AGE

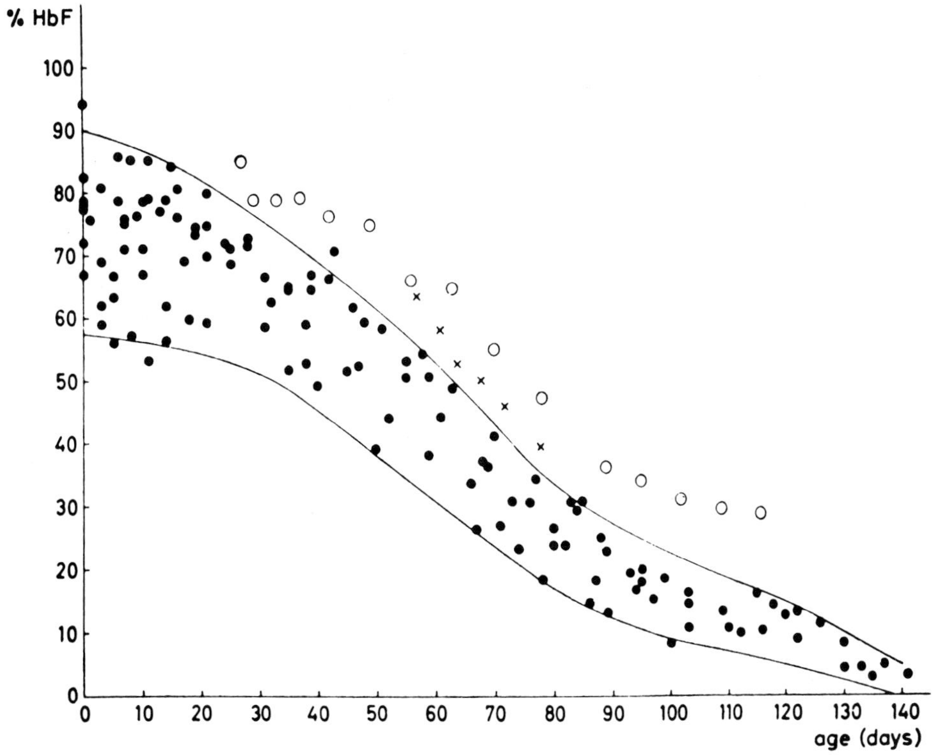

The region between the curved lines contains 120 observations in 17 normal children.
HbF, fetal hemoglobin.
From Garby L, Sjolin S. Acta Paediatr 1962;51:245.

2. LEUKOCYTES

APPENDIX B–2a
THE LEUKOCYTE COUNT AND THE DIFFERENTIAL COUNT DURING THE FIRST 2 WEEKS OF LIFE (number/mm^3)

		Neutrophils						
Age	**Leukocytes**	Total	Segmented	Band	**Eosinophils**	**Basophils**	**Lymphocytes**	**Monocytes**
Birth								
Mean	18,100	11,000	9400	1600	400	100	5500	1050
Range	9,000–30,000	6,000–26,000			20–850	0–640	2,000–11,000	400–3,100
Mean (%)	100	61	52	9	2.2	0.6	31	5.8
7 Days								
Mean	12,200	5500	4700	830	500	50	5000	1100
Range	5,000–21,000	1,500–10,000			70–1100	0–250	2,000–17,000	300–2,700
Mean (%)	100	45	39	6	4.1	0.4	41	9.1
14 Days								
Mean	11,400	4500	3900	630	350	50	5500	1000
Range	5,000–20,000	1,000–9,500			70–1000	0–230	2,000–17,000	200–2,400
Mean (%)	100	40	34	5.5	3.1	0.4	48	8.8

APPENDIX B–2b
TOTAL NEUTROPHIL COUNT IN THE FIRST 60 HOURS OF LIFE

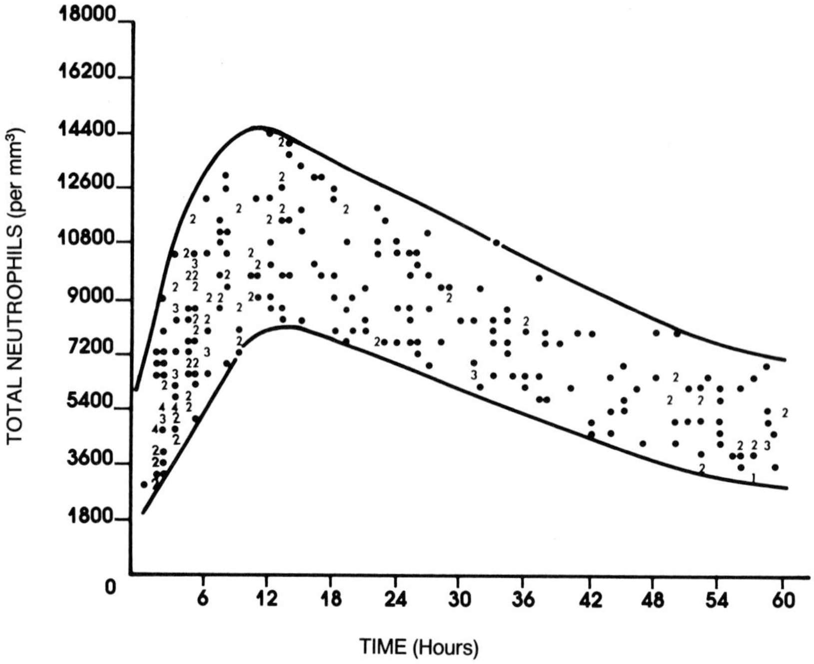

•, Single value; number, number of values at the same point; ———, envelope banding the data.
From Monroe BL, et al. J Pediatr 1979;95:91.

3. PLATELETS

APPENDIX B–3a
VENOUS PLATELET COUNTS* IN NORMAL LOW-BIRTH-WEIGHT INFANTS

Day	Number of Infants	Mean (mm^3)	Range (×10,000)
0	60	203,000	80–356
3	47	207,000	61–335
5	14	233,000	100–502
7	52	319,000	124–678
10	40	399,000	172–680
14	50	386,000	147–670
21	47	388,000	201–720
28	40	384,000	212–625

* Manual method.
From Appleyard WJ, Bunton WA. Biol Neonate 1971;17:30.

APPENDIX B–3b
PLATELET COUNTS IN FULL-TERM INFANTS

	Mean	Range (×1,000)
Cord	200,000	100–280
1 day	192,000	100–260
3 days	213,000	80–320
7 days	248,000	100–300
14 days	252,000	

From Behrman R, ed. Neonatology: diseases of the fetus and infant. St Louis: CV Mosby, 1973.

4. BONE MARROW

APPENDIX B–4
BONE MARROW DIFFERENTIAL COUNTS: MEAN PERCENT CHANGES WITH AGE (RANGE)

	1 Week	1 Month	3 Months	6 Months	12 Months	Adult
Myeloblasts	0.3 (0–1)	1.2 (0.4–1.9)	2.5	0.4	0.7	0.9 (0.75–1.1)
Promyelocytes	1 (0.5–1.5)	1.8 (1–2.5)	4.5	1.6	2.6	1.9 (1.8–2.1)
Myelocytes	1.6 (0.6–2.4)	4.3 (2.5–7.2)	5.4	1.5	4.8	10.5 (2.4–18.7)
Metamyclocytes	2 (0.7–3)	5.5 (3.1–9.1)	6.9	2	6.2	13.4 (3.1–23.8)
Bands	19 (13–23)	22.9 (17–32)	33.2 (14–52)	8.3	15.7	13.9 (7–20)
Segmented neutrophils	23.3 (9.6–39)	22 (8.7–30.2)	5.8 (4–7.6)	8.1 (3.7–11.5)	10.6	13.9 (9.7–14.6)
Eosinophils	1.3 (1–3)	2.9 (1.9–5.3)	6	3.9	3.2	4 (5–7)
Basophils	<0.1 (0–0.2)	<0.1 (0–0.2)	2.5 (0–5)	0.1	0.2	0.2 (0.2–1.8)
Pronormoblasts	1.6 (0.4–2.5)	0.8 (0.4–1.1)	1.3	0.3	0.2	1 (0.2–2.5)
Normoblasts	37.8 (21–54)	19.1 (12–25)	13.9	18.4 (13–24)	10.4	23.4 (19–29)
Lymphocytes	6.1 (3.7–8)	14.5 (9.5–19)	12.1 (4–20)	51	37.2	24.3 (14–28)
Monocytes	5.3 (2–7.3)	5.2 (3–10)	6.8	5	8	6.3 (2–12)
Plasma cells		0.2 (0–0.2)			0.2	0.8 (0.6–0.9)
M : E ratio	1.24	2.91	3.83	1.4	3.83	2.71

From Miller DR, et al. Blood diseases of infancy and childhood. 5th ed. St. Louis: CV Mosby, 1984:27.

See also Rosse C, et al. J Lab Clin Med 1977;89:1225; Mauer AM. Pediatric hematology. New York: McGraw-Hill, 1969; Jandl JH. Blood: textbook of hematology. Boston: Little, Brown & Co., 1987.

5. SERUM IRON AND IRON-BINDING CAPACITY

APPENDIX B–5
VALUES OF SERUM IRON, TOTAL IRON-BINDING CAPACITY, AND TRANSFERRIN SATURATION IN INFANTS DURING THE FIRST YEAR OF LIFE

	0.5 Month of Age	1 Month of Age	2 Months of Age	4 Months of Age	6 Months of Age	9 Months of Age	12 Months of Age
SI (median 95% range)							
μM/L	22 (11–36)	22 (10–31)	16 (3–29)	15 (3–29)	14 (5–24)	15 (6–24)	14 (6–28)
μg/dL	120 (63–201)	125 (58–172)	87 (15–159)	84 (18–164)	77 (28–135)	84 (34–135)	78 (35–155)
TIBC (mean ± SD)							
μM/L	34 ± 8	36 ± 8	44 ± 10	54 ± 7	58 ± 9	61 ± 7	64 ± 7
μg/dL	191 ± 43	199 ± 43	246 ± 55	300 ± 39	321 ± 51	341 ± 42	358 ± 38
S% (median 95% range)	68 (30–99)	63 (35–94)	34 (21–63)	27 (7–53)	23 (10–43)	25 (10–39)	23 (10–47)

These data were obtained from a group of healthy, full-term infants who were born at the Helsinki University Central Hospital. Infants received iron supplementation in formula and cereal throughout the 12-month period. Infants with hemoglobin below 110 g/dl, mean corpuscular volume of red blood cells below 71 μ^3, or serum ferritin below 10 ng/ml were excluded from the study. The 95% range of the transferrin saturation values indicates that the lower limit of normal is about 10% after 4 months of age.

S%, transferrin saturation; SD, standard deviation; SI, serum iron; TIBC, total iron-binding capacity.

From Saarien UM, Siimes MA. J Pediatr 1977;91:876.

6. COAGULATION

APPENDIX B–6a
REFERENCE VALUES FOR COAGULATION TESTS IN HEALTHY PREMATURE INFANTS (30 TO 36 WEEKS OF GESTATION) DURING THE FIRST 6 MONTHS OF LIFE AND IN THE ADULT

Tests	Day 1		Day 5		Day 30		Day 90		Day 180		Adult	
	Mean	Boundaries	Mean	Boundaries	Mean	Boundaries	Mean	Boundaries	Mean	Boundaries	Mean	Boundaries
PT (s)	13.0	(10.6–16.2)*	12.5	(10.0–15.3)*†	11.8	(10.0–13.6)*	12.3	(10.0–14.6)*	12.5	(10.0–15.0)*	12.4	(10.8–13.9)
APTT (s)	53.6	(27.5–79.4)‡	50.5	(26.9–74.1)‡	44.7	(26.9–62.5)	39.5	(28.3–50.7)	37.5	(21.7–53.3)*	33.5	(26.6–40.3)
TCT (s)	24.8	(19.2–30.4)*	24.1	(18.8–29.4)*	24.4	(18.8–29.9)*	25.1	(19.4–30.8)*	26.2	(18.9–31.5)*	25.0	(19.7–30.3)
Fibrinogen (g/L)	2.43	(1.50–3.73)*†‡	2.80	(1.60–4.18)*†‡	2.54	(1.50–4.14)*†	2.46	(1.50–3.52)*†	2.28	(1.50–3.60)†	2.78	(1.56–4.00)
H (u/mL)	0.45	(0.20–0.77)†	0.57	(0.29–0.85)‡	0.57	(0.36–0.95)†‡	0.68	(0.30–1.06)	0.87	(0.51–1.23)	1.08	(0.70–1.46)
V (U/mL)	0.88	(0.41–1.44)*†‡	1.00	(0.46–1.54)	1.02	(0.48–1.56)	0.99	(0.59–1.39)	1.02	(0.58–1.46)	1.06	(0.62–1.50)
VII (U/mL)	0.67	(0.21–1.13)	0.84	(0.30–1.38)	0.83	(0.21–1.45)	0.87	(0.31–1.43)	0.99	(0.47–1.51)*	1.05	(0.67–1.43)
VIII (U/mL)	1.11	(0.50–2.13)*†	1.15	(0.53–2.05)*†‡	1.11	(0.50–1.99)*†‡	1.06	(0.58–1.88)*†‡	0.99	(0.50–1.87)*†‡	0.99	(0.50–1.49)
vWF (U/mL)	1.36	(0.78–2.10)†	1.33	(0.72–2.19)†	1.36	(0.66–2.16)†	1.12	(0.75–1.84)*†	0.98	(0.54–1.58)*†	0.92	(0.50–1.58)
IX (U/mL)	0.35	(0.19–0.65)†‡	0.42	(0.14–0.74)†‡	0.44	(0.13–0.80)†	0.59	(0.25–0.93)	0.81	(0.50–1.20)†	1.09	(0.55–1.63)
X (U/mL)	0.41	(0.11–0.71)	0.51	(0.19–0.83)	0.56	(0.20–0.92)	0.67	(0.35–0.99)	0.77	(0.35–1.19)	1.06	(0.70–1.52)
XI (U/mL)	0.30	(0.08–0.52)†‡	0.41	(0.13–0.69)‡	0.43	(0.15–0.71)‡	0.59	(0.25–0.93)‡	0.78	(0.46–1.10)	0.97	(0.67–1.27)
XII (U/mL)	0.38	(0.10–0.66)‡	0.39	(0.09–0.69)‡	0.43	(0.11–0.75)	0.61	(0.15–1.07)	0.82	(0.22–1.42)	1.08	(0.52–1.64)
PK (U/mL)	0.33	(0.09–0.57)	0.45	(0.26–0.75)†	0.59	(0.31–0.87)	0.79	(0.37–1.21)	0.78	(0.40–1.16)	1.12	(0.62–1.62)
HMWK (U/mL)	0.49	(0.09–0.89)	0.62	(0.24–1.00)‡	0.64	(0.16–1.12)‡	0.78	(0.32–1.24)	0.83	(0.41–1.25)*	0.92	(0.50–1.36)
XIIIa (U/mL)	0.70	(0.32–1.08)	1.01	(0.57–1.45)*	0.99	(0.51–1.47)*	1.13	(0.71–1.55)*	1.13	(0.65–1.61)*	1.05	(0.55–1.55)
XIIIb (U/mL)	0.81	(0.35–1.27)	1.10	(0.68–1.58)*	1.07	(0.57–1.57)*	1.21	(0.75–1.67)	1.15	(0.67–1.63)	0.97	(0.57–1.37)
Plasminogen (CTA, U/mL)	1.70	(1.12–2.48)†‡	1.91	(1.21–2.61)‡	1.81	(1.09–2.53)	2.38	(1.58–3.18)	2.75	(1.91–3.59)‡	3.36	(2.48–4.24)

All factors except fibrinogen and plasminogen are expressed as U/mL, where pooled plasma contains 1.0 U/mL. Plasminogen units are those recommended by the Committee on Thrombolytic Agents (CTA). All values are given as a mean followed by the lower and upper boundaries encompassing 95% of the population. Between 40 and 96 samples were assayed for each value for newborns.

* Values indistinguishable from those of adults.

† Measurements are skewed owing to a disproportionate number of high values. Lower limit which excludes the lower 2.5% of the population is given.

‡ Values different from those of full-term infants.

APTT, activated partial thromboplastin time; H, biotin; HMWK, high-molecular-weight kininogen; PK, pyruvate kinase; PT, prothrombin time; TCT, thrombin clotting time; VIII, factor VIII coagulant; vWF, von Willebrand factor.

From Andrew M, et al. Development of the coagulation system in the healthy premature infant. Blood 1988;72:1653.

APPENDIX B–6b
REFERENCE VALUES FOR COAGULATION INHIBITORS IN HEALTHY PREMATURE INFANTS DURING THE FIRST 6 MONTHS OF LIFE AND IN THE ADULT

	Day 1		Day 5		Day 30		Day 90		Day 180		Adult	
Tests	Mean	Boundaries	Mean	Boundaries	Mean	Boundaries	Mean	Boundaries	Mean	Boundaries	Mean	Boundaries
AT-III (U/mL)	0.38	(0.14–0.62)‡	0.56	(0.30–0.82)*	0.59	(0.37–0.81)‡	0.83	(0.45–1.21)‡	0.90	(0.52–1.28)‡	1.05	(0.79–1.31)
α_2M (U/mL)	1.10	(0.56–1.82)†‡	1.25	(0.71–1.77)*	1.38	(0.72–2.04)	1.80	(1.20–2.66)†	2.09	(1.10–3.21)†	0.86	(0.52–1.20)
α_2AP (U/mL)	0.78	(0.40–1.16)	0.81	(0.49–1.13)*	0.89	(0.55–1.23)‡	1.06	(0.64–1.48)*	1.15	(0.77–1.53)	1.02	(0.68–1.36)
C_1INH (U/mL)	0.65	(0.31–0.99)	0.83	(0.45–1.21)	0.74	(0.40–1.24)†‡	1.14	(0.60–1.68)*	1.40	(0.96–2.04)†	1.01	(0.71–1.31)
α_2AT (U/mL)	0.90	(0.36–1.44)*	0.94	(0.42–1.46)‡	0.76	(0.38–1.12)‡	0.81	(0.49–1.13)*‡	0.82	(0.48–1.16)*	0.93	(0.55–1.31)
HCII (U/mL)	0.32	(0.00–0.60)‡	0.34	(0.00–0.69)*	0.43	(0.15–0.71)	0.61	(0.20–1.11)†	0.89	(0.45–1.40)*†‡	0.96	(0.66–1.26)
Protein C (U/mL)	0.28	(0.12–0.44)*‡	0.31	(0.11–0.51)*	0.37	(0.15–0.59)‡	0.45	(0.23–0.67)‡	0.57	(0.31–0.83)	0.96	(0.64–1.28)
Protein S (U/mL)	0.26	(0.14–0.38)‡	0.37	(0.13–0.61)*	0.56	(0.22–0.90)	0.76	(0.40–1.12)‡	0.82	(0.44–1.20)	0.92	(0.60–1.24)

All values are expressed in U/mL, where pooled plasma contains 1.0 U/mL. All values are given as a mean followed by the lower and upper boundaries encompassing 95% of the population. Between 40 and 75 samples were assayed for each value for newborns.

* Values indistinguishable from those of adults.

† Measurements are skewed owing to a disproportionate number of high values. Lower limit, which excludes the lower 2.5% of the population, is given.

‡ Values different from those of full-term infants.

α_2AP, α_2-antiplasmin; α_2AT, α_2-antitrypsin; α_2M, α_2-macroglobulin; AT-III, antithrombin-III; C_1INH, C_1 esterase inhibitor; HCII, heparin cofactor II.

From Andrew M, et al. Development of the coagulation system in the healthy premature infant. Blood 1988;72:1653.

APPENDIX B–6c
REFERENCE VALUES FOR COAGULATION TESTS IN THE HEALTHY FULL-TERM INFANT DURING THE FIRST 6 MONTHS OF LIFE AND IN THE ADULT

Tests	Day 1	Day 5	Day 30	Day 90	Day 180	Adult
PT (s)	13.0 ± 1.43 (61)*	12.4 ± 1.46 (77)*†	11.8 ± 1.25 (67)*†	11.9 ± 1.15 (62)*	12.3 ± 0.79 (47)*	12.4 ± 0.78 (29)
APTT (s)	42.9 ± 5.80 (61)	42.6 ± 8.62 (76)	40.4 ± 7.42 (67)	37.1 ± 6.52 (62)*	35.5 ± 3.71 (47)*	33.5 ± 3.44 (29)
TCT (s)	23.5 ± 2.38 (58)*	23.1 ± 3.07 (64)†	24.3 ± 2.44 (53)*	25.1 ± 2.32 (52)*	25.5 ± 2.86 (41)*	25.0 ± 2.66 (19)
Fibrinogen (g/L)	2.83 ± 0.58 (61)*	3.12 ± 0.75 (77)*	2.70 ± 0.54 (67)*	2.43 ± 0.68 (60)*†	2.51 ± 0.68 (47)*†	2.78 ± 0.61 (29)
II (U/mL)	0.48 ± 0.11 (61)	0.63 ± 0.15 (76)	0.68 ± 0.17 (67)	0.75 ± 0.15 (62)	0.88 ± 0.14 (47)	1.08 ± 0.19 (29)
V (U/mL)	0.72 ± 0.18 (61)	0.95 ± 0.25 (76)	0.98 ± 0.18 (67)	0.90 ± 0.21 (62)	0.91 ± 0.18 (47)	1.06 ± 0.22 (29)
VII (U/mL)	0.66 ± 0.19 (60)	0.89 ± 0.27 (75)	0.90 ± 0.24 (67)	0.91 ± 0.26 (62)	0.87 ± 0.20 (47)	1.05 ± 0.19 (29)
VIII (U/mL)	1.00 ± 0.39 (60)*†	0.88 ± 0.33 (75)*†	0.91 ± 0.33 (67)*†	0.79 ± 0.23 (62)*†	0.73 ± 0.18 (47)†	0.99 ± 0.25 (29)
vWF (U/mL)	1.53 ± 0.67 (40)†	1.40 ± 0.57 (43)†	1.28 ± 0.59 (40)†	1.18 ± 0.44 (40)†	1.07 ± 0.45 (46)†	0.92 ± 0.33 (29)†
IX (U/mL)	0.53 ± 0.19 (59)	0.53 ± 0.19 (75)	0.51 ± 0.15 (67)	0.67 ± 0.23 (62)	0.86 ± 0.25 (47)	1.09 ± 0.27 (29)
X (U/mL)	0.40 ± 0.14 (60)	0.49 ± 0.15 (76)	0.59 ± 0.14 (67)	0.71 ± 0.18 (62)	0.78 ± 0.20 (47)	1.06 ± 0.23 (29)
XI (U/mL)	0.38 ± 0.14 (60)	0.55 ± 0.16 (74)	0.53 ± 0.13 (67)	0.69 ± 0.14 (62)	0.86 ± 0.24 (47)	0.97 ± 0.15 (29)
XII (U/mL)	0.53 ± 0.20 (60)	0.47 ± 0.18 (75)	0.49 ± 0.16 (67)	0.67 ± 0.21 (62)	0.77 ± 0.19 (47)	1.08 ± 0.28 (29)
PK (U/mL)	0.37 ± 0.16 (45)†	0.48 ± 0.14 (51)	0.57 ± 0.17 (48)	0.73 ± 0.16 (46)	0.86 ± 0.15 (43)	1.12 ± 0.25 (29)
HMWK (U/mL)	0.54 ± 0.24 (47)	0.74 ± 0.28 (63)	0.77 ± 0.22 (50)*	0.82 ± 0.32 (46)*	0.82 ± 0.23 (48)*	0.92 ± 0.22 (29)
XIIIa (U/mL)	0.79 ± 0.26 (44)	0.94 ± 0.25 (49)*	0.93 ± 0.27 (44)*	1.04 ± 0.34 (44)*	1.04 ± 0.29 (41)*	1.05 ± 0.25 (29)
XIIIb (U/mL)	0.76 ± 0.23 (44)	1.06 ± 0.37 (47)*	1.11 ± 0.36 (45)*	1.16 ± 0.34 (44)*	1.10 ± 0.30 (41)*	0.97 ± 0.20 (29)
Plasminogen (CTA, U/mL)	1.95 ± 0.35 (44)	2.17 ± 0.38 (60)	1.98 ± 0.36 (52)	2.48 ± 0.37 (44)	3.01 ± 0.40 (47)	3.36 ± 0.44 (29)

All factors except fibrinogen and plasminogen are expressed as units per milliliter where pooled plasma contains 1.0 U/mL. Plasminogen units are those recommended by the Committee on Thrombolytic Agents (CTA). All values are expressed as mean ±1 standard deviation.

* Values that do not differ statistically from the adult values.

† These measurements are skewed because of a disproportionate number of high values. The lower limit that excludes the lower 2.5th percentile of the population has been given in the respective figures. The lower limit for factor VIII was 0.50 U/mL at all time ponts for the infant.

APTT, activated partial thromboplastin time; HMWK, high-molecular-weight kininogen; PK, pyruvate kinase; PT, prothrombin time; TCT, thrombin clotting time; vWF, von Willebrand factor.

From Andrew M, et al. Development of the human coagulation system in the full-term infant. Blood 1987;70:166.

APPENDIX B–6d
REFERENCE VALUES FOR THE INHIBITION OF COAGULATION IN THE HEALTHY FULL-TERM INFANT DURING THE FIRST 6 MONTHS OF LIFE AND IN THE ADULT

Tests	Day 1	Day 5	Day 30	Day 90	Day 180	Adult
AT-III	0.63 ± 0.12 (58)	0.67 ± 0.13 (74)	0.78 ± 0.15 (66)	0.97 ± 0.12 (60)*	1.04 ± 0.10 (56)*	1.05 ± 0.13 (28)
α_2M	1.39 ± 0.22 (54)	1.48 ± 0.25 (73)	1.50 ± 0.22 (61)	1.76 ± 0.25 (55)	1.91 ± 0.21 (55)	0.86 ± 0.17 (29)
α_2AP	0.85 ± 0.15 (55)	1.00 ± 0.15 (75)*	1.00 ± 0.12 (62)*	1.08 ± 0.16 (55)*	1.11 ± 0.14 (53)*	1.02 ± 0.17 (29)
C_1INH	0.72 ± 0.18 (59)	0.90 ± 0.15 (76)*	0.89 ± 0.21 (63)	1.15 ± 0.22 (55)	1.41 ± 0.26 (55)	1.01 ± 0.15 (29)
α_1AT	0.83 ± 0.22 (57)*	0.89 ± 0.20 (75)*	0.62 ± 0.13 (61)	0.72 ± 0.15 (56)	0.77 ± 0.15 (55)	0.93 ± 0.19 (29)
HCII	0.43 ± 0.25 (56)	0.48 ± 0.24 (72)	0.47 ± 0.20 (58)	0.72 ± 0.37 (58)	1.20 ± 0.35 (55)	0.96 ± 0.15 (29)
Protein C	0.35 ± 0.09 (41)	0.42 ± 0.11 (44)	0.43 ± 0.11 (43)	0.54 ± 0.13 (44)	0.59 ± 0.11 (52)	0.96 ± 0.16 (28)
Protein S	0.36 ± 0.12 (40)	0.50 ± 0.14 (48)	0.63 ± 0.15 (41)	0.86 ± 0.16 (46)*	0.87 ± 0.16 (49)*	0.92 ± 0.16 (29)

All values are expressed in units per milliliter as the mean ±1 standard deviation.

* Values that do not differ statistically from the adult values.

α_2AP, α_2-antiplasmin; α_1AT, α_1-antitrypsin; α_2M, $\alpha_2$macroglobulin; AT-III, antithrombin III; C_1INH, C_1 esterase inhibitor; HCII, heparin cofactor II.

From Andrew M, et al. Development of the coagulation system in the full-term infant. Blood 1987;70:167.

Neonatology: Pathophysiology and Management of the Newborn, Fourth Edition,
edited by Gordon B. Avery, Mary Ann Fletcher, and Mhairi G. MacDonald.
J.B. Lippincott Company, Philadelphia © 1994.

appendix C

Physiologic Values

1. BLOOD PRESSURE AND HYPERTENSION

APPENDIX C–1a
AVERAGE SYSTOLIC, DIASTOLIC, AND MEAN BLOOD PRESSURES DURING THE FIRST 12 HOURS OF LIFE IN NORMAL NEWBORN INFANTS GROUPED ACCORDING TO BIRTH WEIGHT

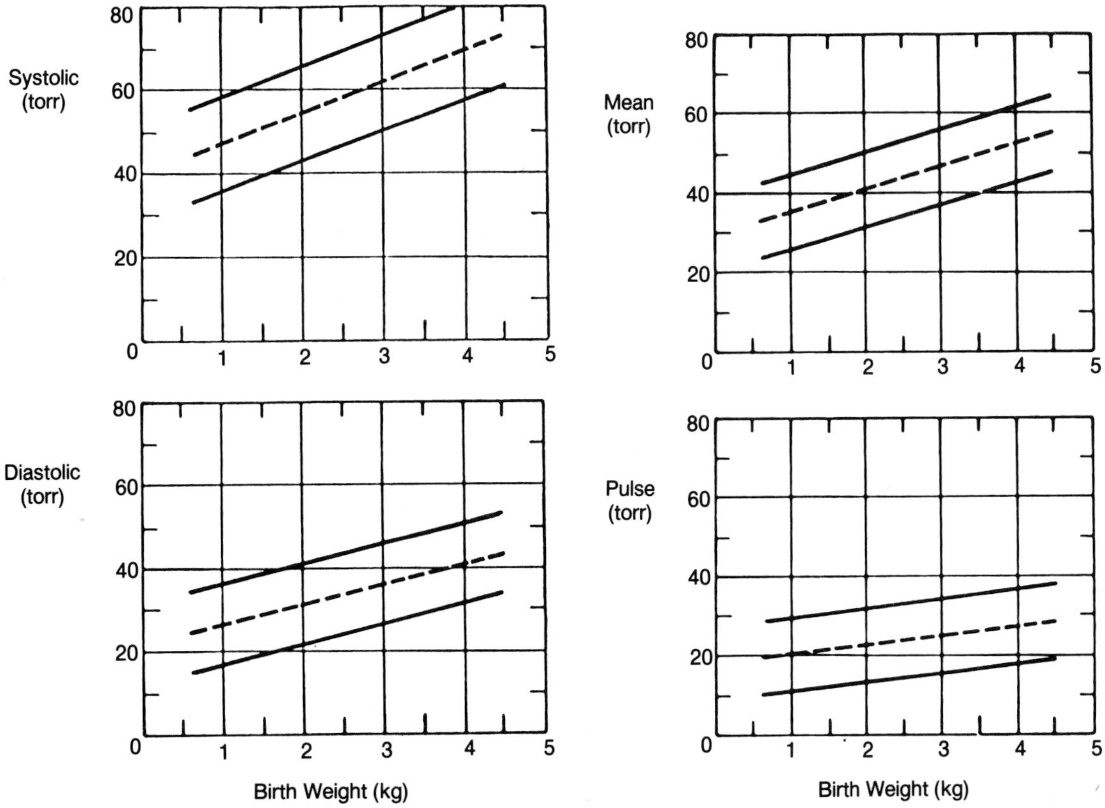

Pressures were obtained by direct measurement through umbilical artery catheter in healthy newborn infants during the first 12 hours of life. Broken lines represent linear regressions; solid lines represent 95% confidence limits.

From Versmold HT, Kitterman JA, Phibbs RH, et al. Aortic blood pressure during the first 12 hours of life in infants with birth weight 610 to 4220 grams. Pediatrics 1981;67(5):611. Copyright © American Academy of Pediatrics, 1981.

APPENDIX C–1b
EVOLUTION OF SYSTOLIC BLOOD PRESSURE DURING THE FIRST MONTH OF LIFE IN PREMATURE INFANTS

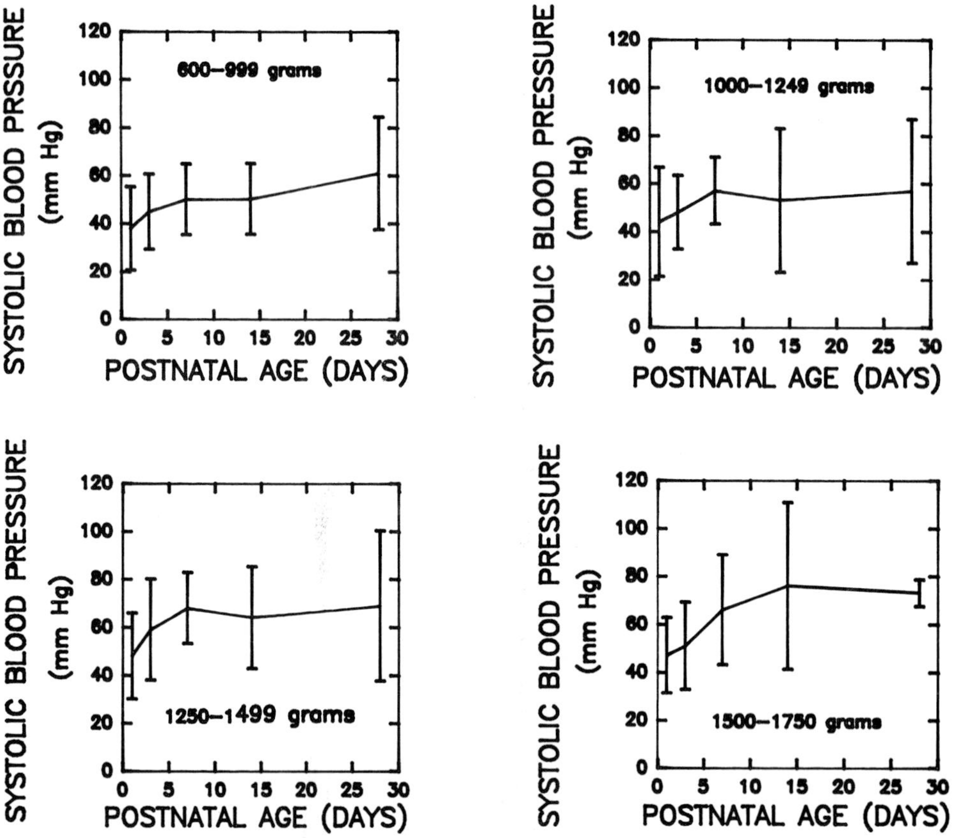

These values were obtained by Doppler or by oscillometric technique (*i.e.*, Dinamap) in "well" infants (*i.e.*, in the absence of respiratory distress syndrome, sepsis, or heart failure. Each point represents the mean ± 2 standard deviations for systolic or diastolic blood pressure from 5 to 18 infants.

Adapted from Ingelfinger J, et al. Pediatr Res 1983;17:319.

APPENDIX C–1c
EVOLUTION OF MEAN BLOOD PRESSURE IN PREMATURE INFANTS

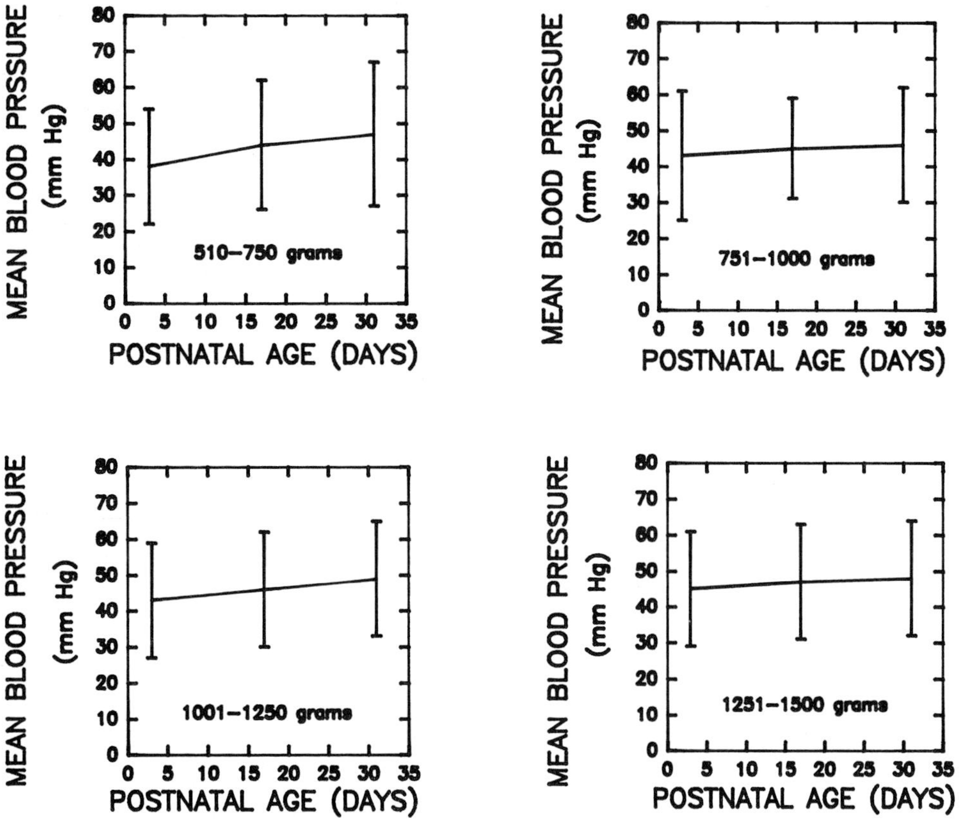

These values were obtained by oscillometric technique (*i.e.*, Dinamap) in 896 infants. Each point represents the mean ± 2 standard deviations. The mean GA in these 4 groups was 25.6, 27.3, 29.0, and 30.3 weeks, respectively.
Adapted from Fanaroff AA, et al. Pediatr Res 1990;27:205.

APPENDIX C–1d
EVOLUTION OF SYSTOLIC BLOOD PRESSURE IN FULL-TERM INFANTS

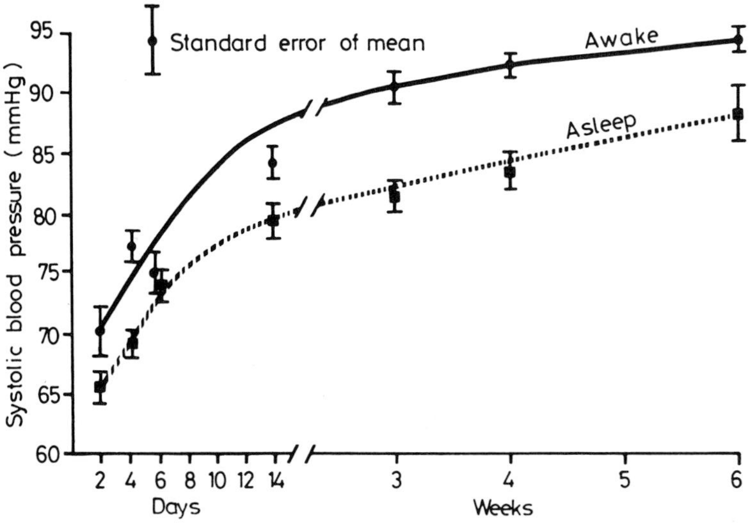

Systolic blood pressure was measured in 99 full-term infants (gestational age ≥ 38 weeks) using a Doppler technique, first in the maternity ward and then at home. Each value was the average of 3 successive measurements. Values represent the mean ± the standard error of mean. Note the difference between the measurements awake (*top*) and asleep (*bottom*).
From Earley A, et al. Arch Dis Child 1980;55:755.

APPENDIX C–1e
CAUSES OF NEONATAL OR INFANTILE HYPERTENSION AND SPECIFIC THERAPY

Diagnosis	Specific Treatment/Approach
Inaccurate Diagnosis	
Agitation, crying, pain, procedure	Local or general anesthesia; consider sedation
Indirect measurement: too small cuff	Cuff width : limb circumference ratio should be 0.45–0.55
Direct measurement: poor transducer calibration	Calibrate routinely
Iatrogenic	
Excessive sodium or fluid intake	Diuretics, fluid restriction, PD, hemofiltration
Aminophylline, theophylline	Hold, check level, decrease dose, consider D/C
Adrenergic agents by mouth, IV, aerosols, or eye drops	Decrease dose, use a more selective agonist, or D/C
Corticosteroids	Decrease dose, consider D/C, or treat symptomatically
Vitamin D	Hold vitamin D, correct hypercalcemia if any
Doxapram	Hold, decrease dose, consider D/C
Pancuronium	Try infusion instead of bolus; use other medication
ECMO	Check fluid intake; induce diuresis
Surgical repair of omphalocele or gastroschisis	Symptomatic therapy
Bronchopulmonary dysplasia	
Pneumothorax (initially)	Most often needs chest tube
Renovascular Hypertension	
Thrombo or embolism of the aorta and/or renal artery	Heparin, urokinase, or PTA, surgery if refractory hypertension
Stenosis or hypoplasia of the renal artery and aorta	Surgery
Segmental Intimal hyperplasia	Surgery
Idiopathic arterial calcification of infancy	Biphosphonate, flunarizin
Intramural hematoma of the renal artery	Surgery
Extrinsic compression: urinoma, hematoma, adrenal hemorrhage	Surgery
Renal vein thrombosis	Surgery if refractory hypertension
Renal	
Acquired	
Acute tubular necrosis, interstitial nephritis	
Renal medullary or cortical necrosis	Surgery if refractory hypertension
Renal tumor: Wilms, congenital mesoblastic nephroma	Chemotherapy and surgery
Postoperative: urinary tract obstruction	Surgery
Neurofibromatosis	
Congenital	
Dysplasia, hypoplasia, glomerular dysgenesis	Surgery if refractory hypertension
Polycystic or multicystic kidney disease	Surgery if refractory hypertension
Cockayne syndrome	
Acquired or congenital	
Urinary tract obstruction	Surgery
Nephrolithiasis, nephrocalcinosis	Replace furosemide by thiazide, if possible
Acute or chronic renal failure	Consider peritoneal dialysis or hemofiltration
Coarctation of the Aorta	Prostaglandin E_1 for initial stabilization; surgery
Neurologic	
Pain	Appropriate pain medicine
Drug withdrawal: narcotics	Phenobarbital, diazepam, paregoric, or methadone
Drug intoxication through placenta or breast milk: cocaine	
Intracranial hypertension	Hyperventilation or surgery
Seizures	Phenobarbital, dilantin, lorazepam.
Familial dysautonomia	

(continued)

APPENDIX C–1e
CAUSES OF NEONATAL OR INFANTILE HYPERTENSION AND SPECIFIC THERAPY (*continued*)

Diagnosis	Specific Treatment/Approach
Endocrine	
Congenital adrenal hyperplasia:	
11β-Hydroxylase deficiency	Cortisol
17α-Hydroxylase deficiency	Cortisol
11β-Hydroxysteroid dehydrogenase deficiency	Cortisol
Dexamethasone-suppressible hyperaldosteronism	Dexamethasone
Primary hyperaldosteronism	Surgery (tumor)
Cushing disease	Surgery (tumor)
Hyperthyroidism	Lugol; propylthiouracil or methimazole
Neural crest tumors	
Neuroblastoma	Radiotherapy, chemotherapy and surgery
Ganglioneuroma, pheochromocytoma	Surgery with several antihypertension medications
Idiopathic	

D/C, discontinue; ECMO: extracorporeal membrane oxygenation; PD, peritoneal dialysis; PTA, plasma thromboplastin antecedent.

APPENDIX C–1f
WORK-UP OF NEONATAL HYPERTENSION

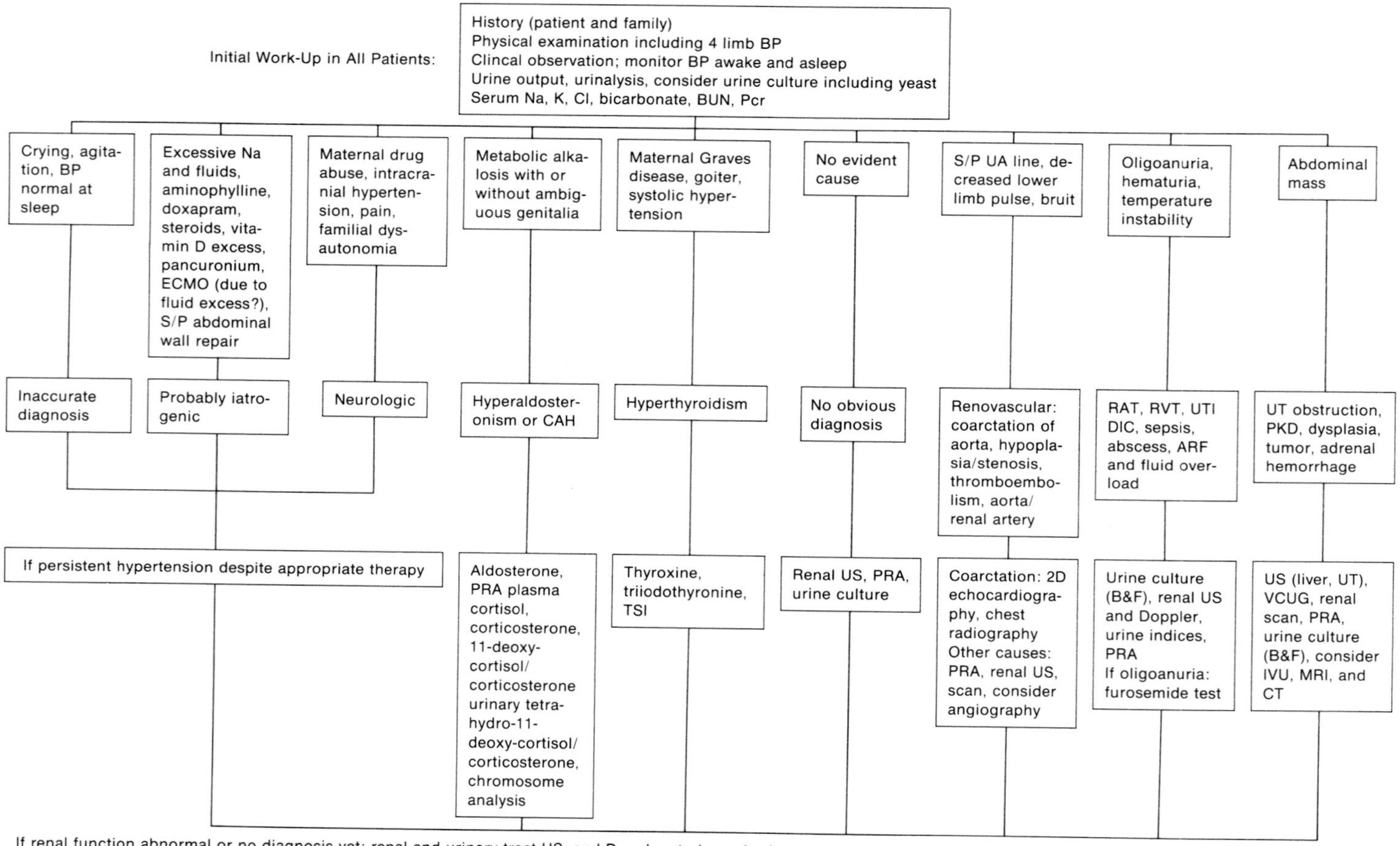

If renal function abnormal or no diagnosis yet: renal and urinary tract US, and Doppler study, and urine culture (B&F).
If no diagnosis yet, consider: plasma aldosterone, PRA, thyroxin, triiodothyronine, urinary catecholamines and metabolites, urine aldosterone, renal vein PRA, long bone radiographs, plain abdomen radiograph, IVU, MRI, CT.
If severe or persistent hypertension: chest radiograph, 2D echocardiography, ECG, eye fundus.

After the initial work-up, the patient should be classified according to the most pertinent features (*top*); this leads to a series of presumptive diagnoses (*middle*) and to further diagnostic tests (*bottom*).

2D, two-dimensional; ARF, acute renal failure; B&F, bacterial and fungal; BP, blood pressure; BUN, blood urea nitrogen; CAH, congenital adrenal hyperplasia; CT, computed tomography; DIC, disseminated intravascular coagulation; ECG, echocardiography; ECMO, extracorporeal membrane oxygenation; IVU, intravenous urography; MRI, magnetic resonance imaging; Pcr, plasma creatinine concentration; PKD, polycystic kidney disease; PRA, plasma renin activity; RAT, renal artery thrombosis; RVT, renal vein thrombosis; S/P, status post; TSI, thyroid stimulating immunoglobulin; UA, umbilical artery; US, ultrasonography; UT, urinary tract; UTI, urinary tract infection; VCUG, voiding cystourethrogram.

2. ACID–BASE STATUS

APPENDIX C–2a
ACID–BASE STATUS

Determination	Sample Site	Birth	1 Hour	3 Hours	24 Hours	2 Days	3 Days
Vigorous Full-Term Infants, Vaginal Delivery							
*p*H	Umbilical artery	7.26					
	Umbilical vein	7.29					
PCO_2 torr	Arterial	54.5	38.8	38.3	33.6	34	35
	Venous	42.8					
O_2 saturation	Arterial	19.8	93.8	94.7	93.2		
	Venous	47.6					
*p*H	Left atrial		7.3	7.34	7.41	7.39 (temporal artery)	7.38 (temporal artery)
CO_2 content, mM/L			20.6	21.9	21.4		
Premature Infants <1250 g							
*p*H	Capillary				7.36	7.35	7.35
PCO_2 torr	Capillary				38	44	37
Premature Infants >1250 g							
*p*H	Capillary				7.39	7.39	7.38
PCO_2 torr	Capillary				38	39	38

Data from Weisbort LM, et al. J Pediatr 1958;52:395 and Bucci E, et al. Biol Neonate 1965;8:81.

APPENDIX C–2b
SIGGAARD-ANDERSEN NOMOGRAM

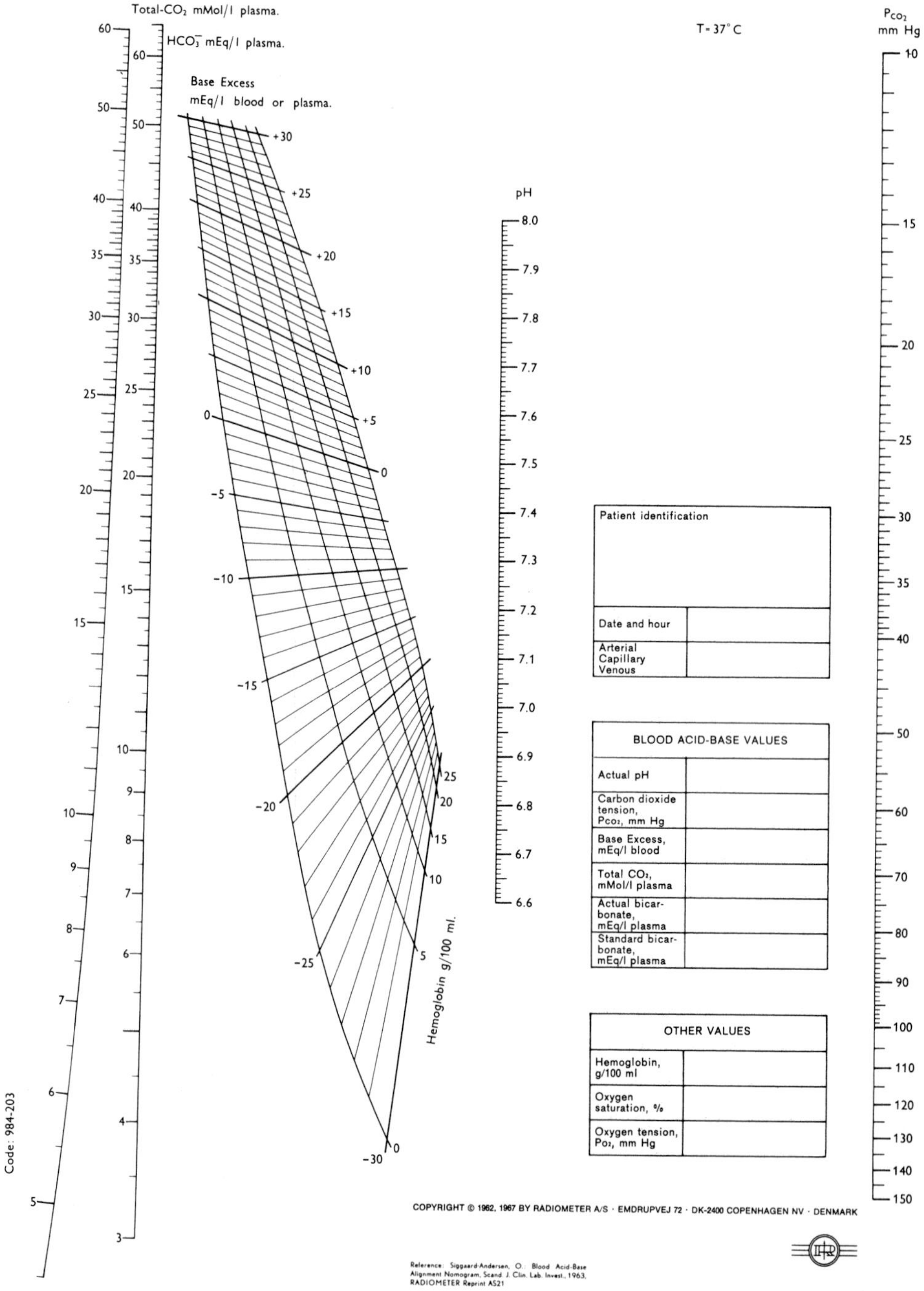

From Siggaard-Anderson O. Blood acid–base alignment nomogram. Scand J Clin Lab Invest 1963; Radiometer reprint AS21.

3. RIGHT-TO-LEFT SHUNT CURVES

APPENDIX C–3
RIGHT-TO-LEFT SHUNT CURVES

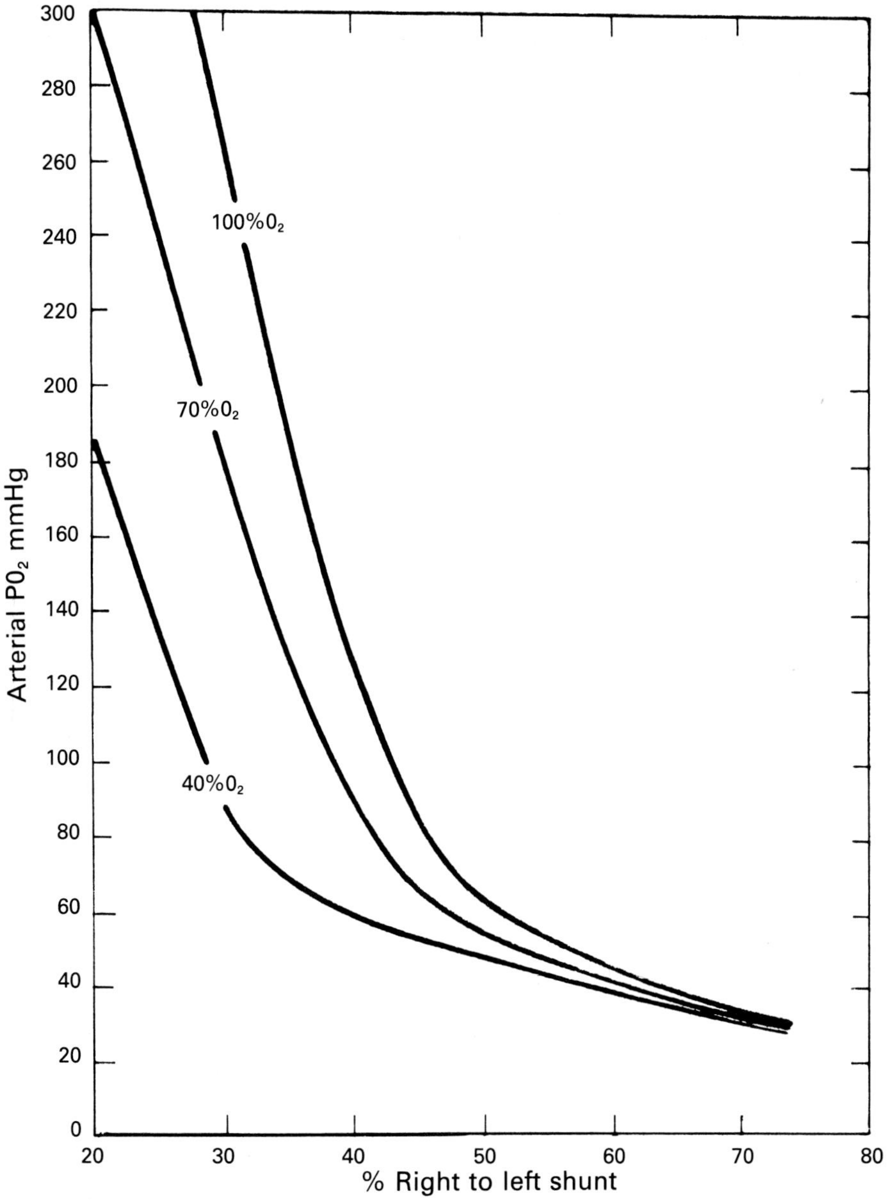

Arterial oxygen tensions at different right-to-left shunts, breathing 40%, 70%, and 100% oxygen. Calculations assumed hemoglobin 16 g/dl, arterial *p*H 7.4, temperature 37°C, constant arteriovenous saturation difference 13.8%, and no change in cardiac output or oxygen consumption.

From Barnett H. Pediatrics. 15th ed. Englewood Cliffs, NJ: Appleton-Century-Crofts, 1972.

4. HEMOGLOBIN–OXYGEN DISSOCIATION CURVES

APPENDIX C–4
OXYGEN DISSOCIATION CURVES OF FETAL AND ADULT HEMOGLOBINS AT A *p*H OF 7.4 AND TEMPERATURE OF 37°C

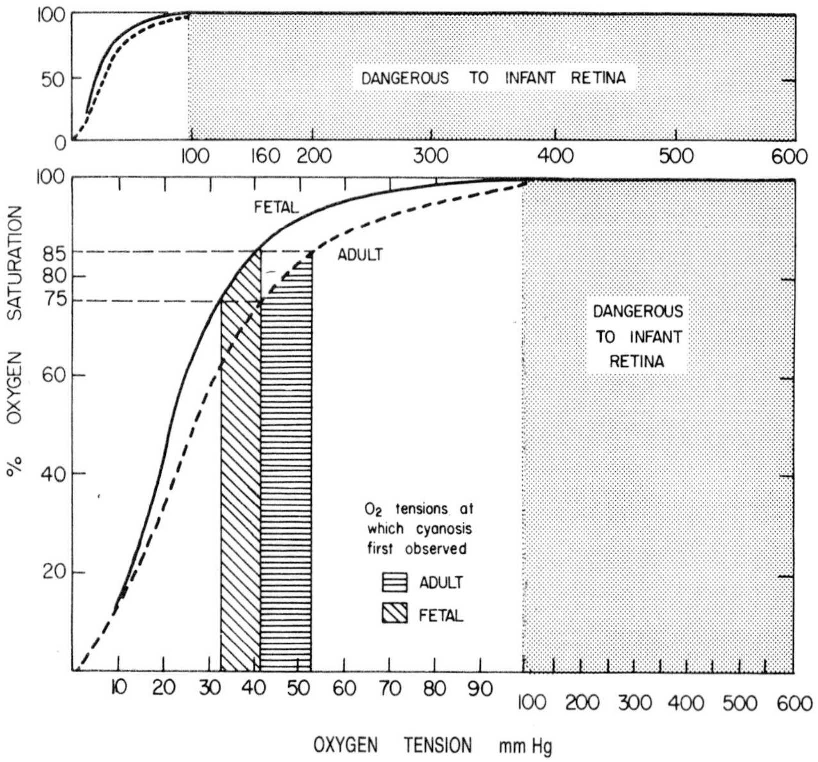

Cyanosis is observed at 5 g unsaturated hemoglobin, which corresponds to different arterial tensions in the adult and the infant.

From Klaus MH, Fanaroff AA. Care of the high risk neonate. Philadelphia: WB Saunders, 1973.

5. BLOOD VOLUMES

APPENDIX C–5
ESTIMATED BLOOD VOLUMES

			Total Blood Volume (mL/kg)	
Age	**Plasma Volume (mL/kg)**	**Erythrocyte Mass (mL/kg)**	From Plasma Volume	From Erythrocyte Mass
Newborn	41.3	43.1	82.1	86.1
	46		78	84.7
1–7 d	51–54		82–86	
		37.9		77.8
1–12 mo	46.1		78.1	
		25.5		72.8
1–3 y	44.4		73.8	
	47.2		81.8	
		24.9		69.1
4–6 y	48.5		80	
	49.6		85.6	
		25.5		67.5
7–9 y	52.2		87.6	
	49		86.1	
		24.3		67.5
10–12 y	51.9		87.6	
	46.2		83.2	
		26.3		67.4
13–15 y	51.2		88.3	
16–18 y	50.1		90.2	
Adult	39–44	25–30	68–88	55–75

From Price DC, Ries C. In: Handmaker H, Lowenstein JM, eds. Nuclear medicine in clinical pediatrics. New York: Society of Nuclear Medicine, 1975.

Neonatology: Pathophysiology and Management of the Newborn, Fourth Edition,
edited by Gordon B. Avery, Mary Ann Fletcher, and Mhairi G. MacDonald.
J.B. Lippincott Company, Philadelphia © 1994.

appendix D

Growth Parameters

1. INTRAUTERINE GROWTH CURVES

APPENDIX D–1
THE COLORADO INTRAUTERINE GROWTH CHARTS

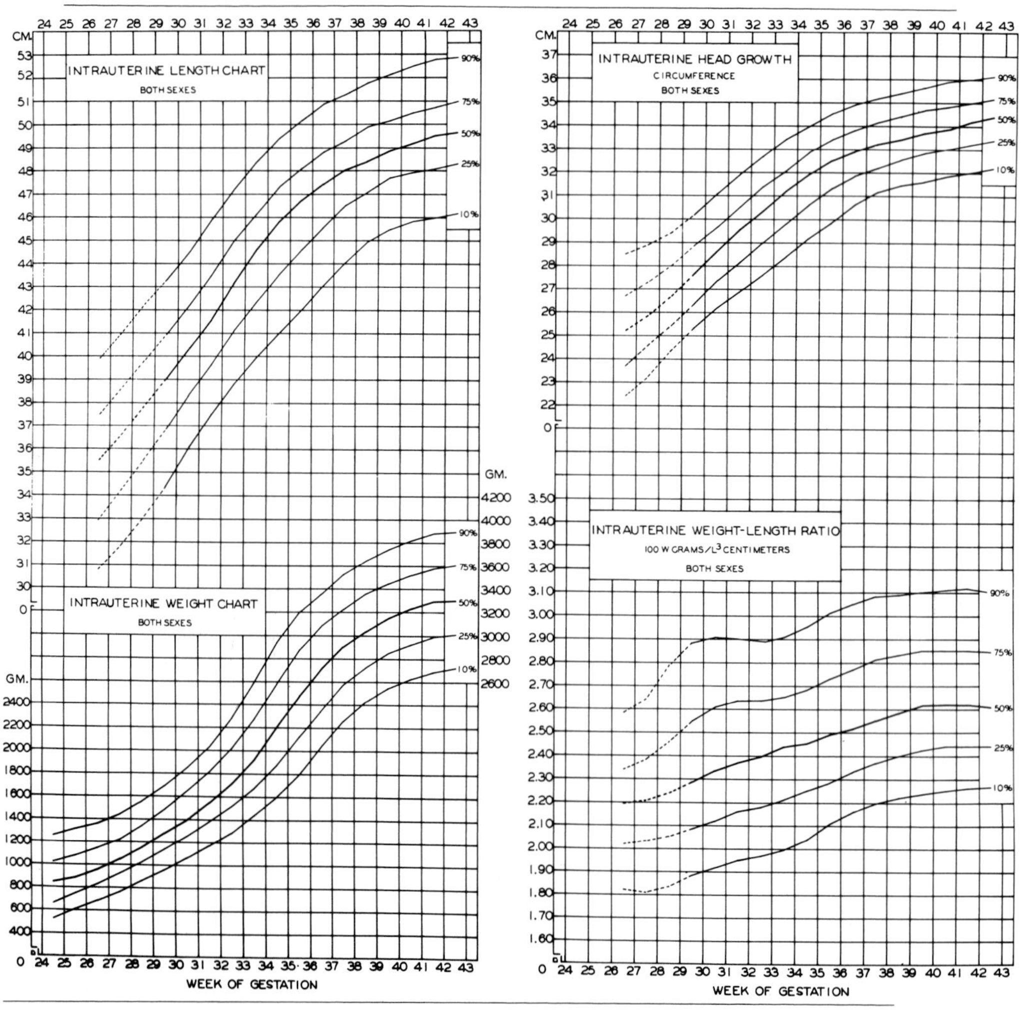

The Colorado curves give percentiles of intrauterine growth for weight, length, and head circumference.

From Lubchenco LO, Hansman C, Boyd E. Pediatrics 1966;37:403. Copyright © American Academy of Pediatrics, 1966.

2. INTRAUTERINE GROWTH CURVES FOR TWINS

APPENDIX D–2a
INTRAUTERINE GROWTH CHARTS FOR MONOCHORIONIC TWINS, BOTH GENDERS

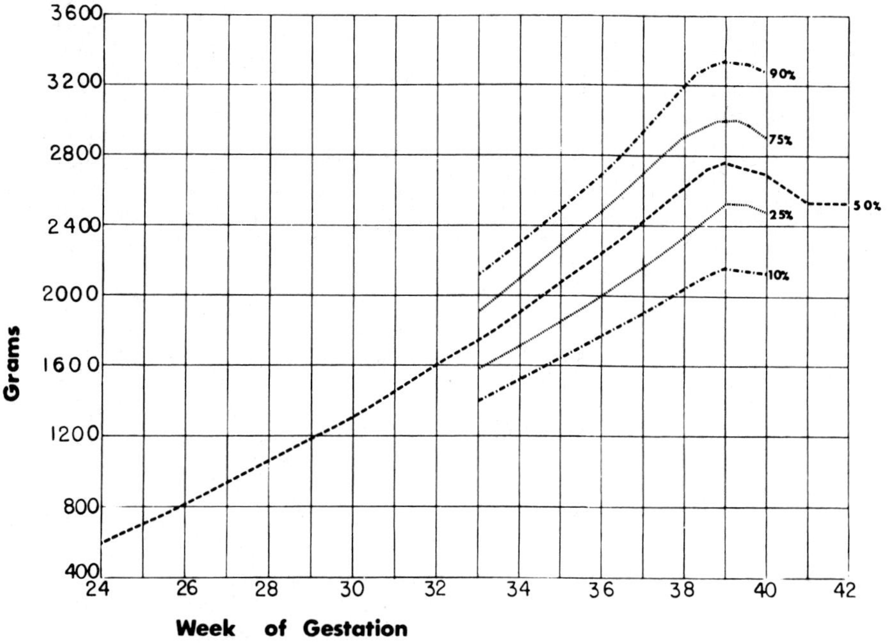

The weights of liveborn monochorionic twins at 24 to 42 weeks gestational ages are graphed as percentages.

From Naeye R, Bernirschke K, Hagstrom J, et al. Pediatrics 1966;37:409. Copyright © American Academy of Pediatrics, 1966.

APPENDIX D–2b
INTRAUTERINE GROWTH CHART FOR DICHORIONIC TWINS, BOTH GENDERS

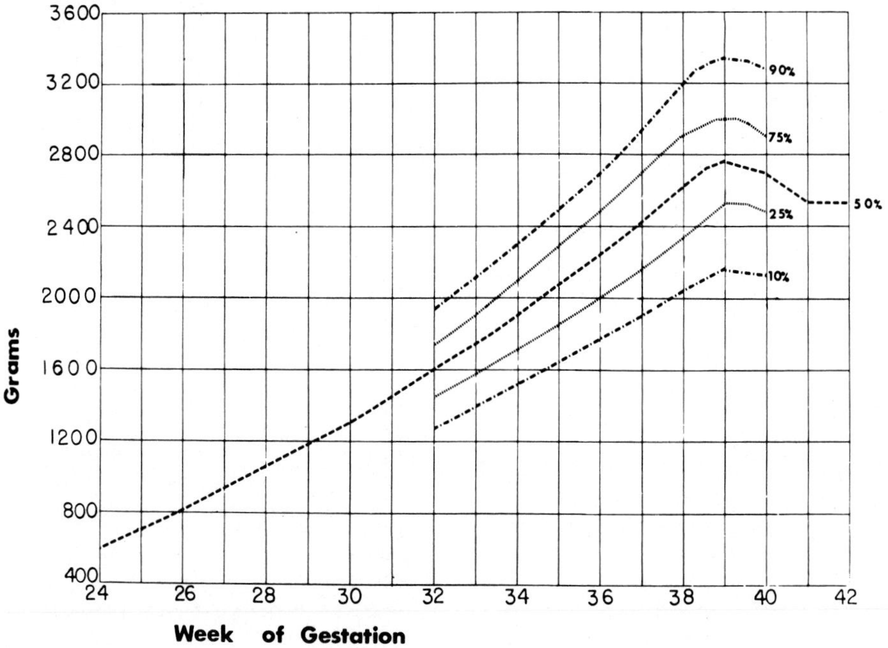

From Naeye R, Bernirschke K, Hagstrom J, et al. Pediatrics 1966;37:409. Copyright © American Academy of Pediatrics, 1966.

3. POSTNATAL GROWTH CURVES FOR FULL-TERM INFANTS

APPENDIX D–3a
POSTNATAL GROWTH CURVES, BOYS

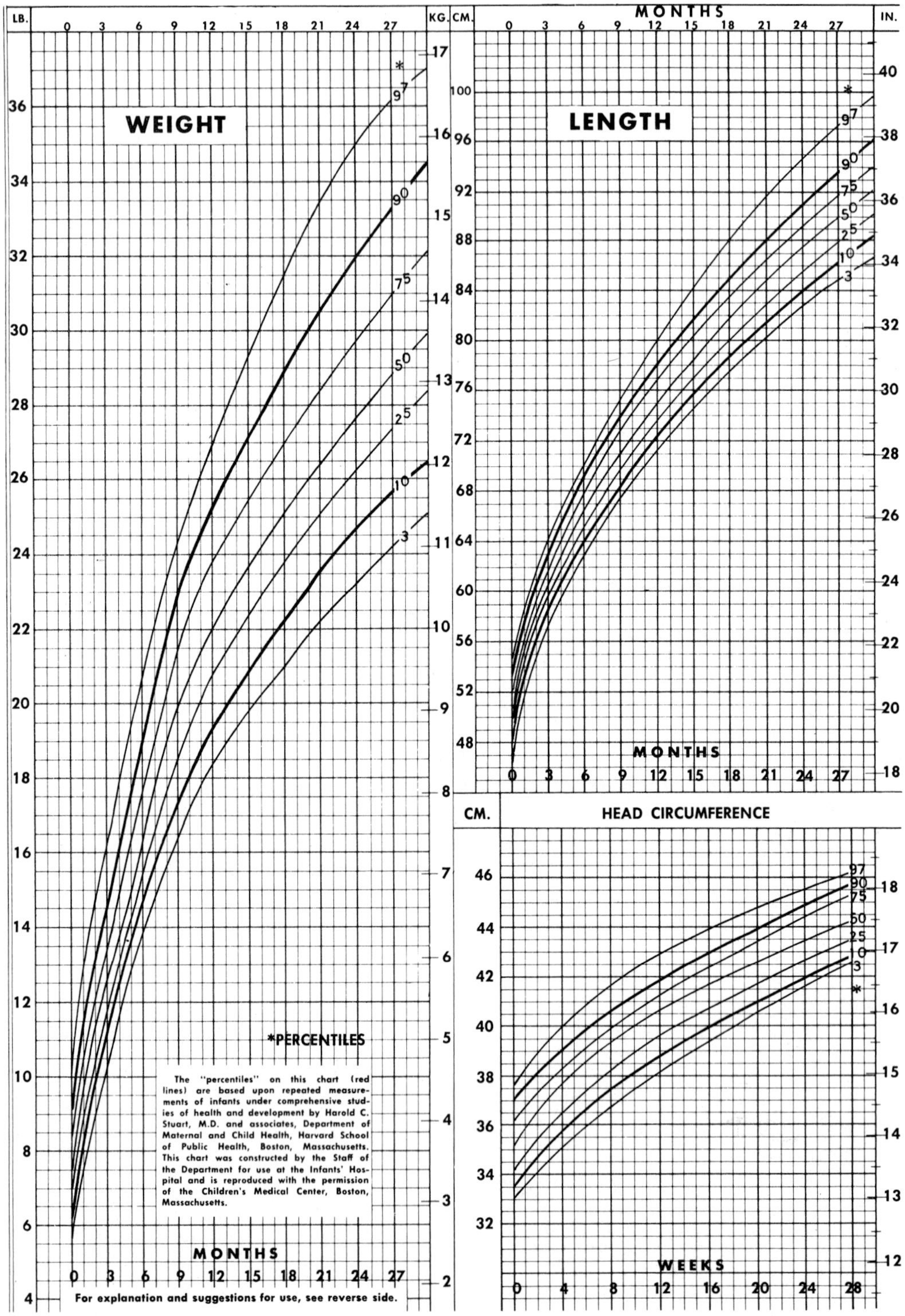
WEIGHT
LB.
KG.
MONTHS
LENGTH
CM.
IN.
HEAD CIRCUMFERENCE
WEEKS
*PERCENTILES
The "percentiles" on this chart (red lines) are based upon repeated measurements of infants under comprehensive studies of health and development by Harold C. Stuart, M.D. and associates, Department of Maternal and Child Health, Harvard School of Public Health, Boston, Massachusetts. This chart was constructed by the Staff of the Department for use at the Infants' Hospital and is reproduced with the permission of the Children's Medical Center, Boston, Massachusetts.
For explanation and suggestions for use, see reverse side.

Courtesy of The Children's Medical Center, Boston, MA.

APPENDIX D–3b
POSTNATAL GROWTH CURVES, GIRLS

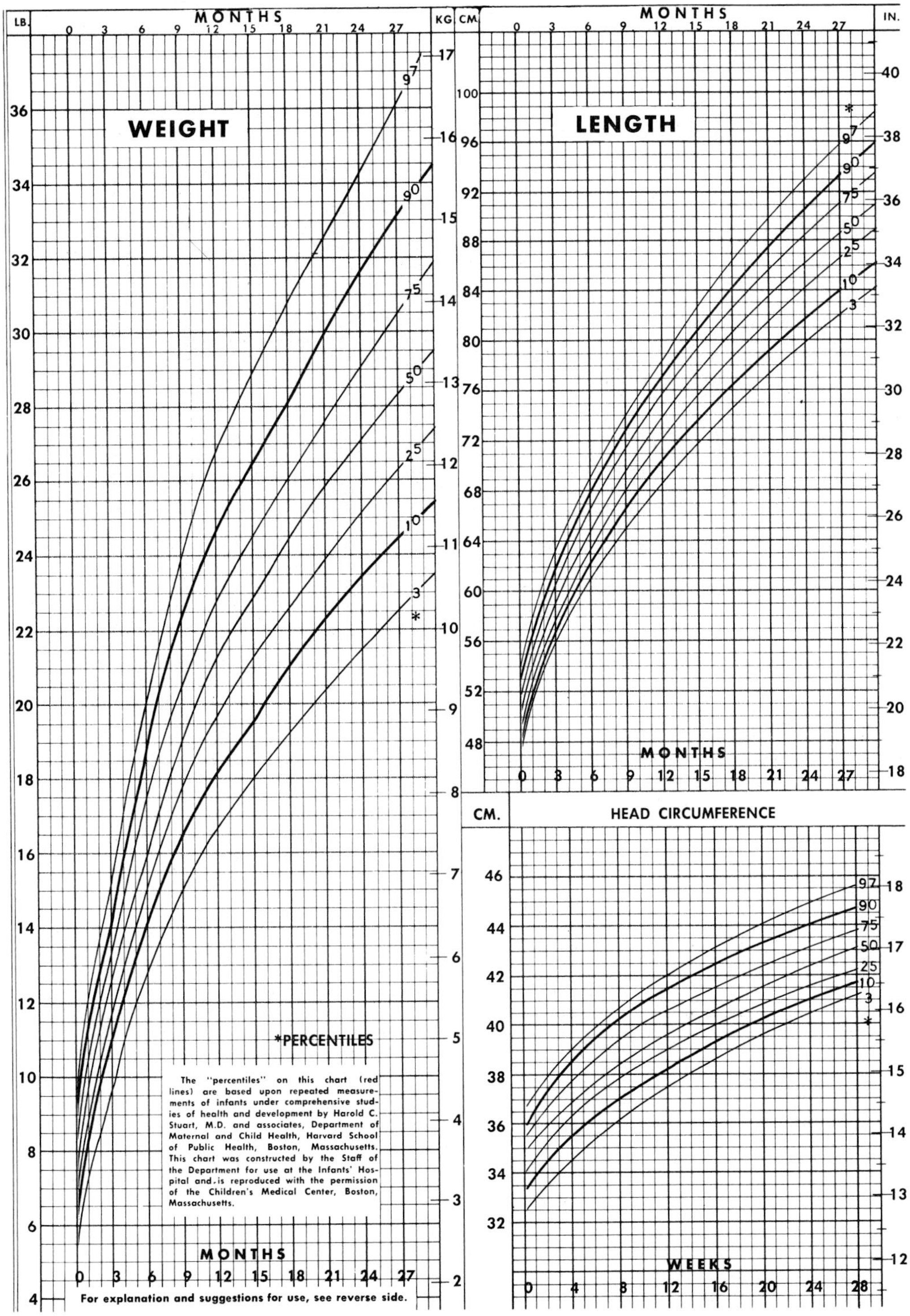
WEIGHT
LENGTH
HEAD CIRCUMFERENCE
MONTHS
WEEKS
LB.
KG
CM.
IN.
*PERCENTILES
The "percentiles" on this chart (red lines) are based upon repeated measurements of infants under comprehensive studies of health and development by Harold C. Stuart, M.D. and associates, Department of Maternal and Child Health, Harvard School of Public Health, Boston, Massachusetts. This chart was constructed by the Staff of the Department for use at the Infants' Hospital and is reproduced with the permission of the Children's Medical Center, Boston, Massachusetts.
For explanation and suggestions for use, see reverse side.

Courtesy of The Children's Medical Center, Boston, MA.

4. HEAD CIRCUMFERENCE

APPENDIX D–4a
HEAD CIRCUMFERENCE, BOYS

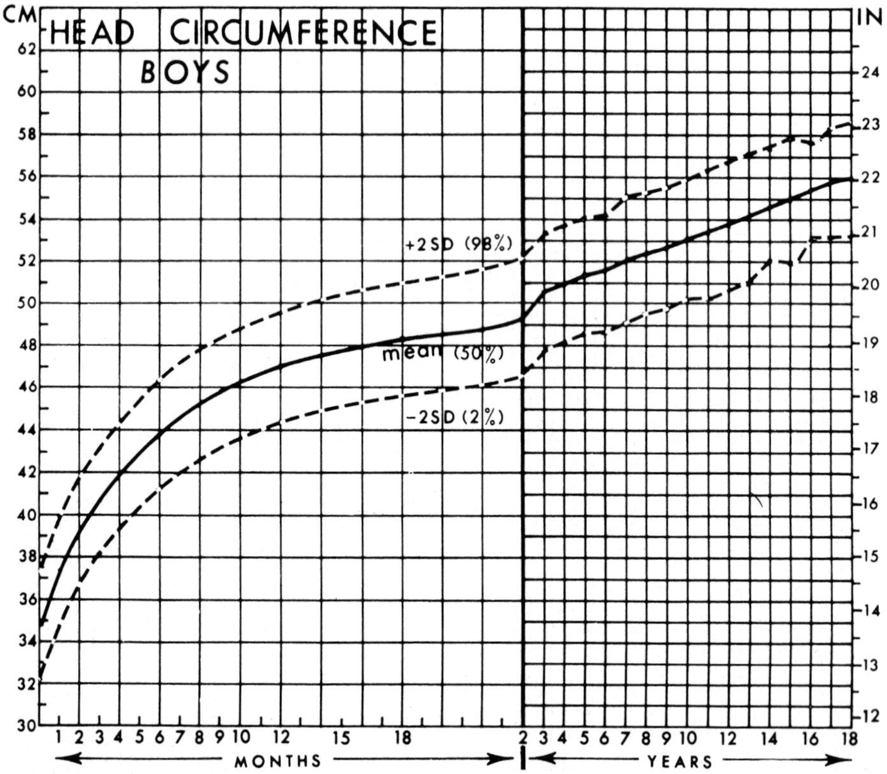

From Nellhaus G. Head circumference from birth to eighteen years: practical composite international and interracial graphs. Pediatrics 1968;41:106.

APPENDIX D–4b
HEAD CIRCUMFERENCE, GIRLS

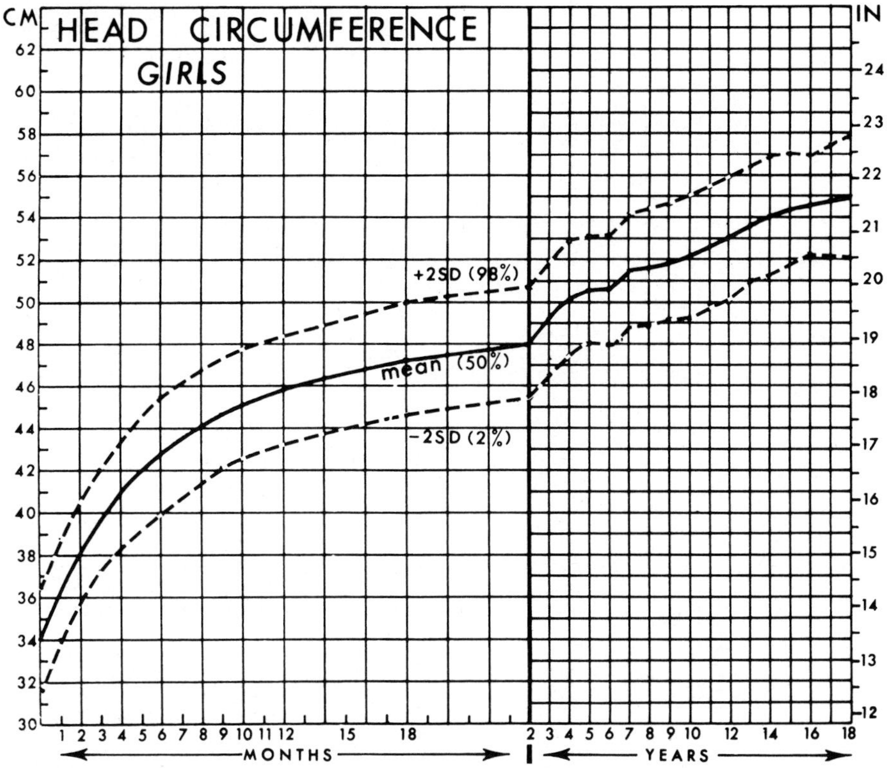

From Nellhaus G. Head circumference from birth to eighteen years: practical composite international and interracial graphs. Pediatrics 1968;41:106.

5. WEIGHT CONVERSION

APPENDIX D–5
CONVERSIONS OF POUNDS AND OUNCES TO GRAMS

Pounds	Ounces															
	0	1	2	3	4	5	6	7	8	9	10	11	12	13	14	15
0		28	57	85	113	142	170	198	227	255	283	312	340	369	397	425
1	454	482	510	539	567	595	624	652	680	709	737	765	794	822	850	879
2	907	936	964	992	1021	1049	1077	1106	1134	1162	1191	1219	1247	1276	1304	1332
3	1361	1389	1417	1446	1474	1503	1531	1559	1588	1616	1644	1673	1701	1729	1758	1786
4	1814	1843	1871	1899	1928	1956	1984	2013	2041	2070	2098	2126	2155	2183	2211	2240
5	2268	2296	2325	2353	2381	2410	2438	2466	2495	2523	2551	2580	2608	2637	2665	2693
6	2722	2750	2778	2807	2835	2863	2892	2920	2948	2977	3005	3033	3062	3090	3118	3147
7	3175	3203	3232	3260	3289	3317	3345	3374	3402	3430	3459	3487	3515	3544	3572	3600
8	3629	3657	3685	3714	3742	3770	3799	3827	3856	3884	3912	3941	3969	3997	4026	4054
9	4082	4111	4139	4167	4196	4224	4252	4281	4309	4337	4366	4394	4423	4451	4479	4508
10	4536	4564	4593	4621	4649	4678	4706	4734	4763	4791	4819	4848	4876	4904	4933	4961
11	4990	5018	5046	5075	5103	5131	5160	5188	5216	5245	5273	5301	5330	5358	5386	5415
12	5443	5471	5500	5528	5557	5585	5613	5642	5670	5698	5727	5755	5783	5812	5840	5868
13	5897	5925	5953	5982	6010	6038	6067	6095	6123	6152	6180	6209	6237	6265	6294	6322
14	6350	6379	6407	6435	6464	6492	6520	6549	6577	6605	6634	6662	6690	6719	6747	6776
15	6804	6832	6860	6889	6917	6945	6973	7002	7030	7059	7087	7115	7144	7172	7201	7228
16	7257	7286	7313	7342	7371	7399	7427	7456	7484	7512	7541	7569	7597	7626	7654	7682
17	7711	7739	7768	7796	7824	7853	7881	7909	7938	7966	7994	8023	8051	8079	8108	8136
18	8165	8192	8221	8249	8278	8306	8335	8363	8391	8420	8448	8476	8504	8533	8561	8590
19	8618	8646	8675	8703	8731	8760	8788	8816	8845	8873	8902	8930	8958	8987	9015	9043
20	9072	9100	9128	9157	9185	9213	9242	9270	9298	9327	9355	9383	9412	9440	9469	9497
21	9525	9554	9582	9610	9639	9667	9695	9724	9752	9780	9809	9837	9865	9894	9922	9950
22	9979	10007	10036	10064	10092	10120	10149	10177	10206	10234	10262	10291	10319	10347	10376	10404

Neonatology: Pathophysiology and Management of the Newborn, Fourth Edition,
edited by Gordon B. Avery, Mary Ann Fletcher, and Mhairi G. MacDonald.
J.B. Lippincott Company, Philadelphia © 1994.

appendix E

Nutritional Values

1. BASIC REQUIREMENTS

APPENDIX E–1
RECOMMENDED DIETARY ALLOWANCES*

Age (years) or Condition	Weight† (kg)	Weight† (lb)	Height† (cm)	Height† (in)	Protein (g)	Fat-Soluble Vitamins: Vitamin A (μg RE)‡	Vitamin D (μg)§	Vitamin E (mg α-TE)‖	Vitamin K (μg)	Water-Soluble Vitamins: Vitamin C (mg)	Thiamin (mg)	Riboflavin (mg)	Niacin (mg NE)#	Vitamin B_6 (mg)	Folate (μg)	Vitamin B_{12} (μg)	Minerals: Calcium (mg)	Phosphorus (mg)	Magnesium (mg)	Iron (mg)	Zinc (mg)	Iodine (μg)	Selenium (μg)
Infants																							
0.0–0.5	6	13	60	24	13	375	7.5	3	5	30	0.3	0.4	5	0.3	25	0.3	400	300	40	6	5	40	10
0.5–1.0	9	20	71	28	14	375	10	4	10	35	0.4	0.5	6	0.6	35	0.5	600	500	60	10	5	50	15
Children																							
1–3	13	29	90	35	16	400	10	6	15	40	0.7	0.8	9	1.0	50	0.7	800	800	80	10	10	70	20
4–6	20	44	112	44	24	500	10	7	20	45	0.9	1.1	12	1.1	75	1.0	800	800	120	10	10	90	20
7–10	28	62	132	52	28	700	10	7	30	45	1.0	1.2	13	1.4	100	1.4	800	800	170	10	10	120	30
Males																							
11–14	45	99	157	62	45	1000	10	10	45	50	1.3	1.5	17	1.7	150	2.0	1200	1200	270	12	15	150	40
15–18	66	145	176	69	59	1000	10	10	65	60	1.5	1.8	20	2.0	200	2.0	1200	1200	400	12	15	150	50
19–24	72	160	177	70	58	1000	10	10	70	60	1.5	1.7	19	2.0	200	2.0	1200	1200	350	10	15	150	70
25–50	79	174	176	70	63	1000	5	10	80	60	1.5	1.7	19	2.0	200	2.0	800	800	350	10	15	150	70
51+	77	170	173	68	63	1000	5	10	80	60	1.2	1.4	15	2.0	200	2.0	800	800	350	10	15	150	70
Females																							
11–14	46	101	157	62	46	800	10	8	45	50	1.1	1.3	15	1.4	150	2.0	1200	1200	280	15	12	150	45
15–18	55	120	163	64	44	800	10	8	55	60	1.1	1.3	15	1.5	180	2.0	1200	1200	300	15	12	150	50
19–24	58	128	164	65	46	800	10	8	60	60	1.1	1.3	15	1.6	180	2.0	1200	1200	280	15	12	150	55
25–50	63	138	163	64	50	800	5	8	65	60	1.1	1.3	15	1.6	180	2.0	800	800	280	15	12	150	55
51+	65	143	160	63	50	800	5	8	65	60	1.0	1.2	13	1.6	180	2.0	800	800	280	10	12	150	55
Pregnant					60	800	10	10	65	70	1.5	1.6	17	2.2	400	2.2	1200	1200	320	30	15	175	65
Lactating																							
First 6 months					65	1300	10	12	65	95	1.6	1.8	20	2.1	280	2.6	1200	1200	355	15	19	200	75
Second 6 months					62	1200	10	11	65	90	1.6	1.7	20	2.1	260	2.6	1200	1200	340	15	16	200	75

* The allowances, expressed as average daily intakes over time, are intended to provide for individual variations among most normal persons as they live in the United States under usual environmental stresses. Diets should be based on a variety of common foods in order to provide other nutrients for which human requirements have been less well defined.

† Weights and heights of reference adults are actual medians for the United States population of the designated ages, as reported by NHANES II. The median weights and heights of those under 19 years of age were taken from Hamill PUV, Drizd TA, Johnson CL, et al. Physical growth: National Center for Health Statistics percentiles. Am J Clin Nutr 1979;32:607. The use of these figures does not imply that the height-to-weight ratios are ideal.

‡ Retinol equivalents. 1 retinal equivalent = 1 μg retinol or 6 μg β-carotene.

§ As cholecalciferol. 10 μg cholecalciferol = 400 IU of vitamin D.

‖ α-Tocopherol equivalents. 1 mg d-α tocopherol = 1 α-TE.

\# Niacin equivalents. 1 NE = 1 mg of niacin or 60 mg of dietary tryptophan.

From Recommended Dietary Allowances. 10th ed. Washington, DC: National Academy Press, 1989.

2. SELECTED VITAMIN AND MINERAL REQUIREMENTS

APPENDIX E–2
ESTIMATED SAFE AND ADEQUATE DAILY DIETARY INTAKES OF SELECTED VITAMINS AND MINERALS

		Vitamins		Trace Elements*				
Category	**Age (years)**	Biotin (μg)	Pantothenic Acid (mg)	Copper (mg)	Manganese (mg)	Fluoride (mg)	Chromium (μg)	Molybdenum (μg)
Infants	0–0.5	10	2	0.4–0.6	0.3–0.6	0.1–0.5	10–40	15–30
	0.5–1	15	3	0.6–0.7	0.6–1.0	0.2–1.0	20–60	20–40
Children and adolescents	1–3	20	3	0.7–1.0	1.0–1.5	0.5–1.5	20–80	25–50
	4–6	25	3–4	1.0–1.5	1.5–2.0	1.0–2.5	30–120	30–75
	7–10	30	4–5	1.0–2.0	2.0–3.0	1.5–2.5	50–200	50–150
	11+	30–100	4–7	1.5–2.5	2.0–5.0	1.5–2.5	50–200	75–250
Adults		30–100	4–7	1.5–3.0	2.0–5.0	1.5–4.0	50–200	75–250

* Since the toxic levels for many trace elements may be only several times usual intakes, the upper levels for the trace elements given in this table should not be habitually exceeded.
From Recommended Dietary Allowances. 10th ed. Washington, DC: National Academy Press, 1989.

3. ENERGY REQUIREMENTS

APPENDIX E–3
MEDIAN HEIGHTS AND WEIGHTS AND RECOMMENDED ENERGY INTAKE

		Weight		Height			Average Energy Allowance (kcal)†		
Category	**Age (years) or Condition**	(kg)	(lb)	(cm)	(in)	**REE* (kcal/day)**	Multiples of REE	Per kg	Per day‡
Infants	0.0–0.5	6	13	60	24	320		108	650
	0.5–1.0	9	20	71	28	500		98	850
Children	1–3	13	29	90	35	740		102	1300
	4–6	20	44	112	44	950		90	1800
	7–10	28	62	132	52	1130		70	2000
Males	11–14	45	99	157	62	1440	1.70	55	2500
	15–18	66	145	176	69	1760	1.67	45	3000
	19–24	72	160	177	70	1780	1.67	40	2900
	25–50	79	174	176	70	1800	1.60	37	2900
	51+	77	170	173	68	1530	1.50	30	2300
Females	11–14	46	101	157	62	1310	1.67	47	2200
	15–18	55	120	163	64	1370	1.60	40	2200
	19–24	58	128	164	65	1350	1.60	38	2200
	25–50	63	138	163	64	1380	1.55	36	2200
	51+	65	143	160	63	1280	1.50	30	1900
Pregnant	First trimester								+0
	Second trimester								+300
	Third trimester								+300
Lactating	First 6 months								+500
	Second 6 months								+500

* Calculation based on the World Health Organization equations, then rounded.
† In the range of light to moderate activity, the coefficient of variation is ±20%.
‡ Figure is rounded.
REE, resting energy expenditure.
From Recommended Dietary Allowances, 10th ed. Washington, DC: National Academy Press, 1989.

4. COMMERCIAL FORMULAS AND FOODS

APPENDIX E–4a
FORMULAS FOR METABOLIC DISORDERS

Intended Use	Product	Manufacturer*
PKU	Lofenalac	Mead Johnson
PKU	Phenyl-Free	Mead Johnson
Infant PKU	PKU 1	Mead Johnson
Childhood PKU	PKU 2	Mead Johnson
Maternal PKU	PKU 3	Mead Johnson
Infant PKU	Analog XP	Ross
Child PKU	Maxamaid XP	Ross
Adult PKU	Maxamaid XP	Ross
MSUD	MSUD	Mead Johnson
Infant MSUD	MSUD 1	Mead Johnson
Childhood MSUD	MSUD 2	Mead Johnson
Infant MSUD	Analog MSUD	Ross
Child MSUD	Maxamaid MSUD	Ross
Adult MSUD	Maximum MSUD	Ross
Tyrosinemia	LowPhenylTyr (3200AB)	Mead Johnson
Infant tyrosinemia	TYR 1	Mead Johnson
Child tyrosinemia	TYR 2	Mead Johnson
Infant tyrosinemia, types I and II	Analog XPHEN, TYR	Ross
Child tyrosinemia	Maxamaid XPHEN, TYR	Ross
Tyrosinemia, Type I	Analog XPHEN, TYR, MET	Ross
Homocystinuria	Low methionine (3200K)	Mead Johnson
Infant homocystinuria	HOM 1	Mead Johnson
Child homocystinuria	HOM 2	Mead Johnson
Homocystinuria	Maxamaid XMET	Ross
Miscellaneous metabolic errors	Protein-Free Powder (80056)	Mead Johnson
Disaccharidase deficiency	Monosaccharide and Disaccharide-Free Diet Powder (3232A)	Mead Johnson
Infant histidinemia	HIST 1	Mead Johnson
Child histidinemia	HIST 2	Mead Johnson
Infant hyperlysinemia	LYS 1	Mead Johnson
Child hyperlysinemia	LYS 2	Mead Johnson
I proprionicacidemia methylmalonicaciduria	OS 1	Mead Johnson
C proprionicacidemia methylmalonicaciduria	OS 2	Mead Johnson
Methylmalanic acidemia	Analog XMET, TYR, MET	Ross
Methylmalanic acidemia or propionic acidemia	Maxamaid XMET, THRE, VAL, ISLEU	Ross
Infant hyperammonemia	UCD 1	Mead Johnson
Child hyperammonemia	UCD 2	Mead Johnson

* Mead Johnson Laboratories, Evansville, IN; Ross Laboratories, Columbus, OH.
MSUD; maple syrup urine disease; PKU, phenylketonuria.

APPENDIX E–4b
COMPOSITION OF FREQUENTLY USED FORMULAS

Formula	Percent Composition				mEq/dL		mg/dL		Type of CHO	Type of Protein	Comments
	cal/dL	Protein	Fat	CHO	Na	K	Ca	P			
Advance	54	2	2.7	5.5	0.8	2.0	51	39	Corn syrup, lactose	Cow, soy*	16 cal/oz
Alimentum	67	1.9	3.8	6.9	1.3	2.1	71	51	Sucrose, tapioca starch	Casein hydrolysate*†	Fat = MCT; safflower, soy
Cow's milk	67	3.5	3.7	4.9	2.1	3.8	17	92	Lactose	Cow	
Enfamil or Enfamil w/Iron	67	1.5	3.6	6.6	0.8	1.7	46	31	Lactose	Cow*	Whey : casein = 60 : 40
Enfamil Premature 24	81	2.3	3.9	8.5	1.3	2.0	133	65	Corn syrup solids	Cow*	Fat = 40% MCT; whey : casein = 60 : 40
Gerber Baby Formula	67	1.5	3.7	7.3	1.0	1.9	51	39	Lactose	Cow*	
Goat milk	67	3.2	4	4.6	2.2	5.1	129	106	Lactose	Goat	Insufficient folate
Good Start	67	1.6	3.4	7.2	0.6	1.6	41	24	Lactose, maltodextrin	Whey*	
Human Milk	77	1.1	4.0	9.5	0.7	1.3	33	14	Lactose	Human	Mature milk
Human Milk Fortifier	3.5/packet	0.2	0.1	0.7	0.1	0.1	22	11	Corn syrup	Whey, casein	Add 1 packet/25 mL human milk
Isomil	67	1.8	3.7	6.8	1.3	1.9	71	51	Corn syrup, sucrose	Soy, methionine*	
Isomil SF	67	1.8	3.7	6.8	1.3	1.9	71	51	Glucose polymers	Soy, methionine*	
I-Soyalac	67	2.1	3.7	6.9	1.2	2.0	69	48	Sucrose, tapioca	Soy, methionine	
Nursoy	67	2.1	3.6	6.9	0.9	1.8	60	42	Sucrose	Soy, methionine*	
Nutramigen	67	1.8	2.5	8.6	1.3	1.8	60	40	Corn syrup solids	Casein hydrolysate*†	
Pregestimil	67	1.8	3.6	6.6	1.1	1.8	63	42	Corn syrup, tapioca	Casein hydrolysate*†	Fat = 40% MCT
Portagen	67	2.2	3.0	7.4	1.5	2	63	47	Corn syrup, sucrose	Na caseinate*	Fat = 88% MCT
Premie SMA24	81	2	4.4	8.6	1.4	2	75	40	Lactose, maltodextrins	Cow*	Whey :casein = 60 : 40; fat = part MCT
ProSobee	67	1.9	3.4	6.4	1.2	1.9	62	40	Corn syrup	Soy, methionine*	
RCF with CHO	67	2	3.6	6.8	1.3	1.9	70	50	None (added separately)	Soy, methionine*	CHO of choice to be added
Similac or Similac w/Iron	67	1.5	3.6	7.2	1	2	51	39	Lactose	Cow*	
Similac PM 60/40	67	1.5	3.8	6.9	0.7	1.5	38	19	Lactose	Whey, casein*	Lactalbumin : casein = 60 : 40; less Na, K
Similac Special Care 24	81	2.2	4.4	8.6	1.7	2.8	144	72	Lactose, glucose polymers	Cow,* whey	Whey : casein = 60 : 40; fat = 50% MCT
Similac Natural Care	81	2.2	4.4	8.6	1.5	2.7	171	85	Lactose, glucose polymers	Cow,* whey	Human milk fortifier; whey : casein = 60 : 40
Soyalac	69	2.2	3.8	6.6	1.4	2.3	63	52	Dextrose, maltose, sucrose	Soy, methionine*	
SMA	67	1.5	3.6	7.2	0.7	1.4	42	28	Lactose	Cow whey, cow*	Lactalbumin : whey = 60 : 40
Tolerex	67	1.4	0.1	15.4	1.4	2	37	37	Glucose, glucose, oligosaccharides	Amino acids	Low fat, low Ca, high CHO

* Taurine and carnitine added.
† Cystine, tyrosine, and tryptophan added.
CHO, carbohydrate; MCT, medium-chain triglycerides.
Data from Ross Laboratories Product Handbook, Mead Johnson Infant Formula Products Nutritional Information, and the Children's Hospital National Medical Center Diet Manual.

APPENDIX E–4c
IRON AND CALORIC CONTENT OF COMMERCIALLY PREPARED STRAINED AND JUNIOR FOODS

Food	Mean Iron Content (mg/100 g)	Caloric Content (kcal/100 g)
Dry Cereals		
1 tbsp = 2.4 g	73.8	378
Mixed 1 : 6 with milk	12.3	110
Cereal With Fruit, Strained Rice	6.6	79
Strained Food		
Juices	0.5	40–72
Fruits	0.2	37–83
Plain vegetables	0.3	25–59
Creamed vegetables	0.3	37–56
Meats	1.5	99–113
Egg yolks	2.6	203
High-meat dinners	0.76	74–85
Soups and dinners	1.4	47–87
Desserts	0.2	60–80
Junior Foods*		
Meat sticks	1.4	185

* Other foods similar to strained foods.

From Pennington, JAT. Bowes and Church's food values of portions commonly used. 16th ed. Philadelphia: JB Lippincott, 1994.

Neonatology: Pathophysiology and Management of the Newborn, Fourth Edition,
edited by Gordon B. Avery, Mary Ann Fletcher, and Mhairi G. MacDonald.
J.B. Lippincott Company, Philadelphia © 1994.

appendix F

Technical Procedures

1. LOCATION OF ABDOMINAL AORTIC BRANCHES

APPENDIX F–1
DISTRIBUTION OF THE MAJOR AORTIC BRANCHES IN FIFTEEN INFANTS

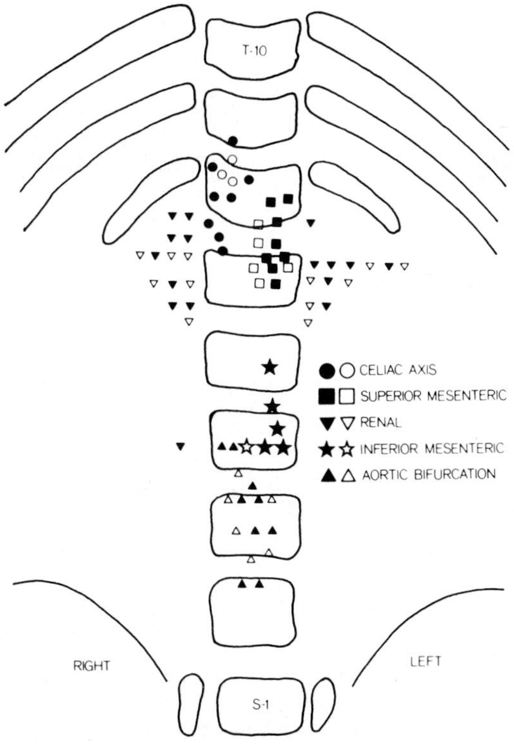

Solid symbols, infants with cardiac and/or renal anomalies; open symbols, infants without these abnormalities.

From Phelps DL, Lachman RS, Leake RD, Oh W. J Pediatr 1972;81:337.

2. PLACEMENT OF UMBILICAL CATHETERS

APPENDIX F–2a
THE LENGTH OF CATHETER INSERTED INTO THE UMBILICAL ARTERY IN ORDER TO REACH THE BIFURCATION OF THE AORTA, THE DIAPHRAGM, OR THE AORTIC VALVES *versus* THE TOTAL BODY LENGTH OF AN INFANT

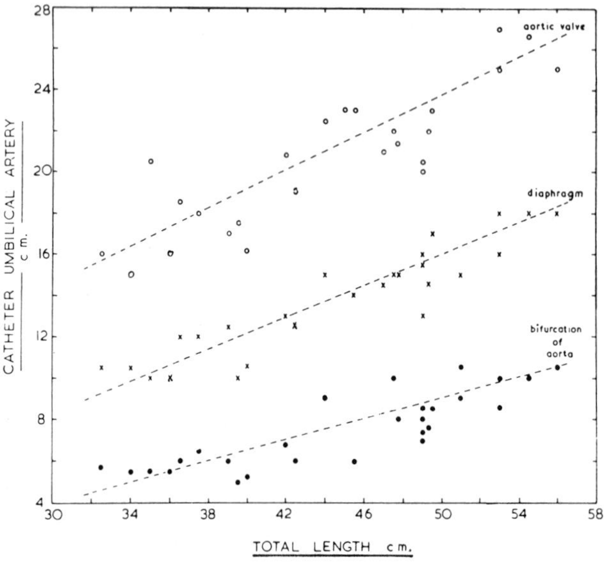

From Dunn PM. Arch Dis Child 1966;41:71.

APPENDIX F–2b
THE LENGTH OF CATHETER INSERTED INTO THE UMBILICAL VEIN IN ORDER TO REACH THE DIAPHRAGM (x) AND THE LEFT ATRIUM (o) *versus* THE SHOULDER–UMBILICUS LENGTH OF AN INFANT

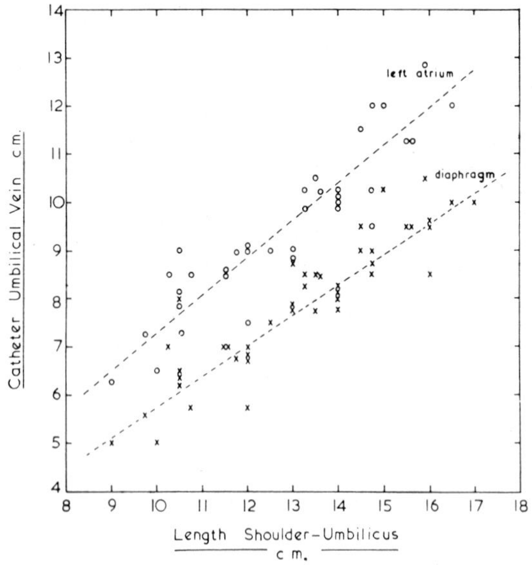

From Dunn PM. Arch Dis Child 1966;41:71.

APPENDIX F–2c
DISTANCE OF CATHETER INSERTION FROM THE UMBILICAL RING FOR L3, L5, AND AORTIC BIFURCATION

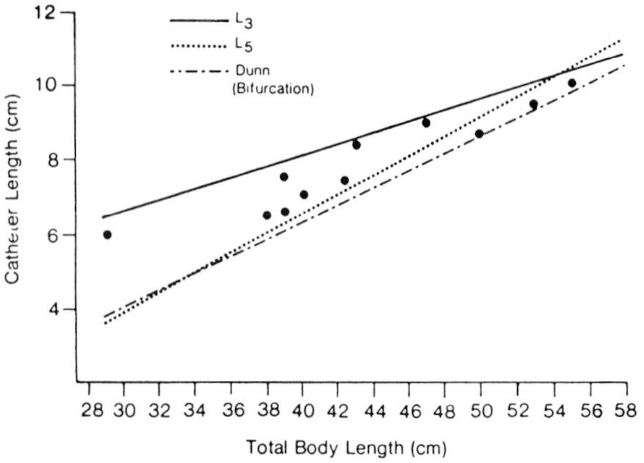

●, catheters positioned at L4.

From Rosenfeld W, Estrada R, Jhaveri R, et al. Evaluation of graphs for insertion of umbilical artery catheters below the diaphragm. J Pediatr 1981;98:628.

APPENDIX F–2d
CATHETER INSERTION TO LEVEL OF T8 USING THE TOTAL BODY LENGTH OF THE INFANT

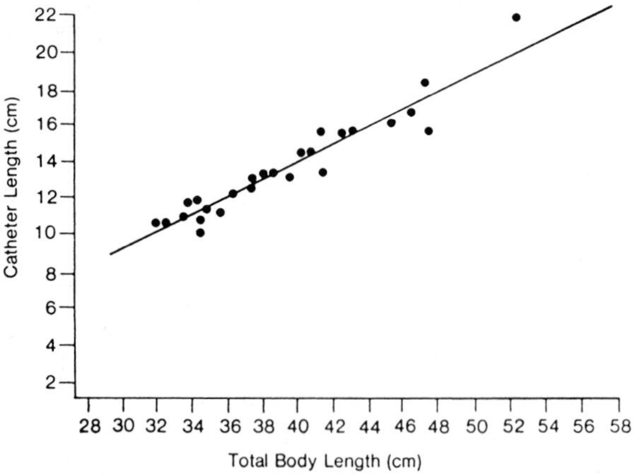

From Rosenfeld W, Biagtan J, Schaeffer H, et al. Evaluation of graphs for insertion of umbilical artery catheters below the diaphragm. J Pediatr 1981;98:628.

APPENDIX F–2e
ESTIMATES OF INSERTIONAL LENGTH OF UMBILICAL CATHETERS BASED ON BIRTH WEIGHT, WITH 95% CONFIDENCE INTERVALS

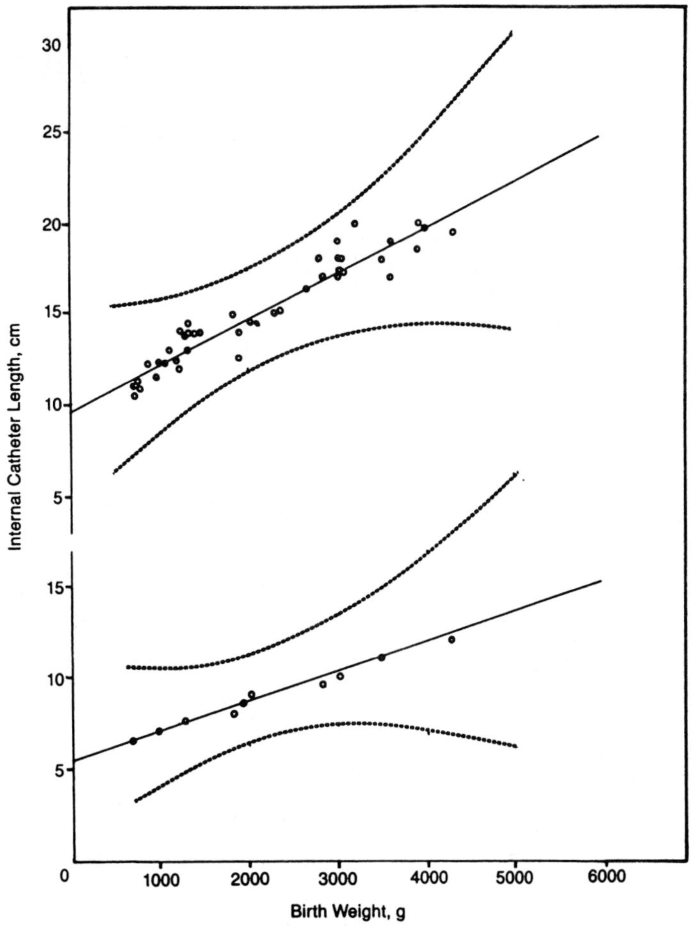

Umbilical artery catheter tip inserted between T6 and T10; umbilical vein catheter tip inserted above diaphragm in inferior vena cava near the right atrium. Modified estimating equations using birth weight (BW) are as follows: umbilical artery length = 2.5 × BW + 9.7 (*top*) and umbilical vein length = 1.5 × BW + 5.6 (*bottom*), where BW is measured in kilograms and lengths in centimeters.
From Shukla H, Ferrara A. Am J Dis Child 1986;140:786.

3. DETERMINING ENDOTRACHEAL TUBE SIZE

APPENDIX F–3
ENDOTRACHEAL TUBE SIZE

	Tube Diameter	
Infant Weight (g)	Inside	Outside
<1000	2.5 mm	12 Fr
1000–1500	3 mm	14 Fr
1500–2200	3.5 mm	16 Fr
2200+	4 mm	18 Fr

4. DETERMINING OROTRACHEAL TUBE SIZE AND LENGTH

APPENDIX F–4
OROTRACHEAL TUBE SIZE AND DISTANCE *versus* BODY WEIGHT

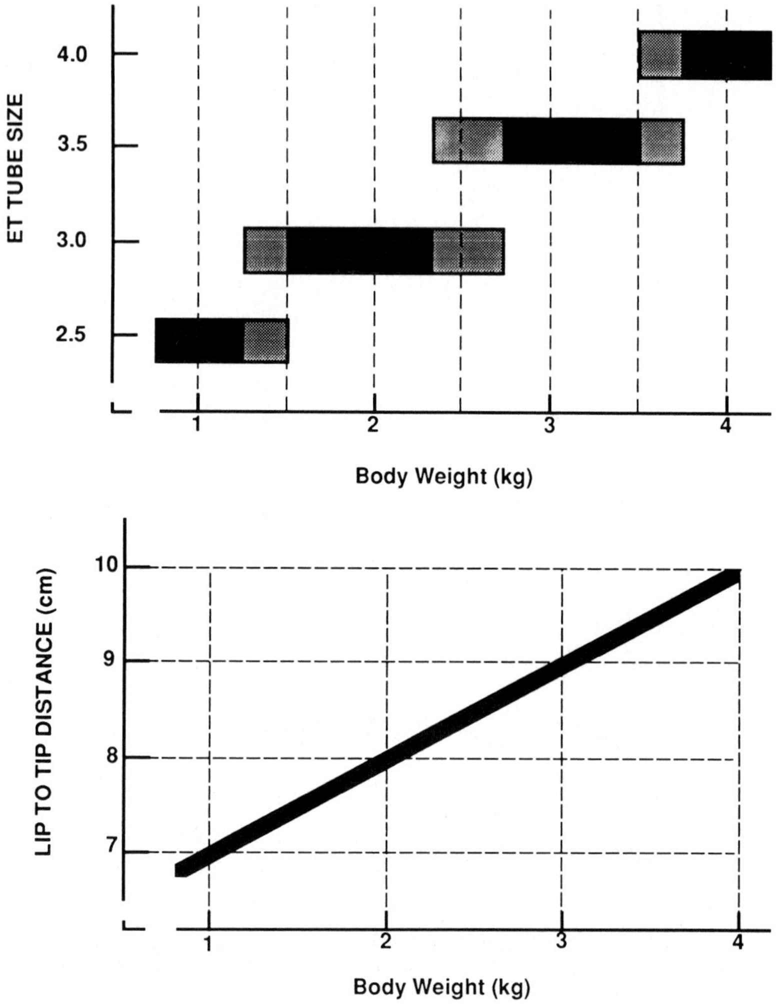

R.H. Phibbs, M.D. 1992

Top: solid bars, usual size of tube to be used for infants of the corresponding birth weight; shaded bars, range of bigger and smaller infants in which that size of tube may be needed on occasion.

Bottom: Distance from the infant's lip to the tip of the tube when the tip is in the midtrachea. Most endotracheal tubes have numbered centimeter marks on the sides indicating the distance to the tip. The appropriate number should be even with the infant's lip.

These are guidelines. There will be some variation among infants.

Neonatology: Pathophysiology and Management of the Newborn, Fourth Edition,
edited by Gordon B. Avery, Mary Ann Fletcher, and Mhairi G. MacDonald.
J.B. Lippincott Company, Philadelphia © 1994.

appendix G

Developmental Screening

APPENDIX G–1 DENVER II DEVELOPMENTAL SCREENING TEST

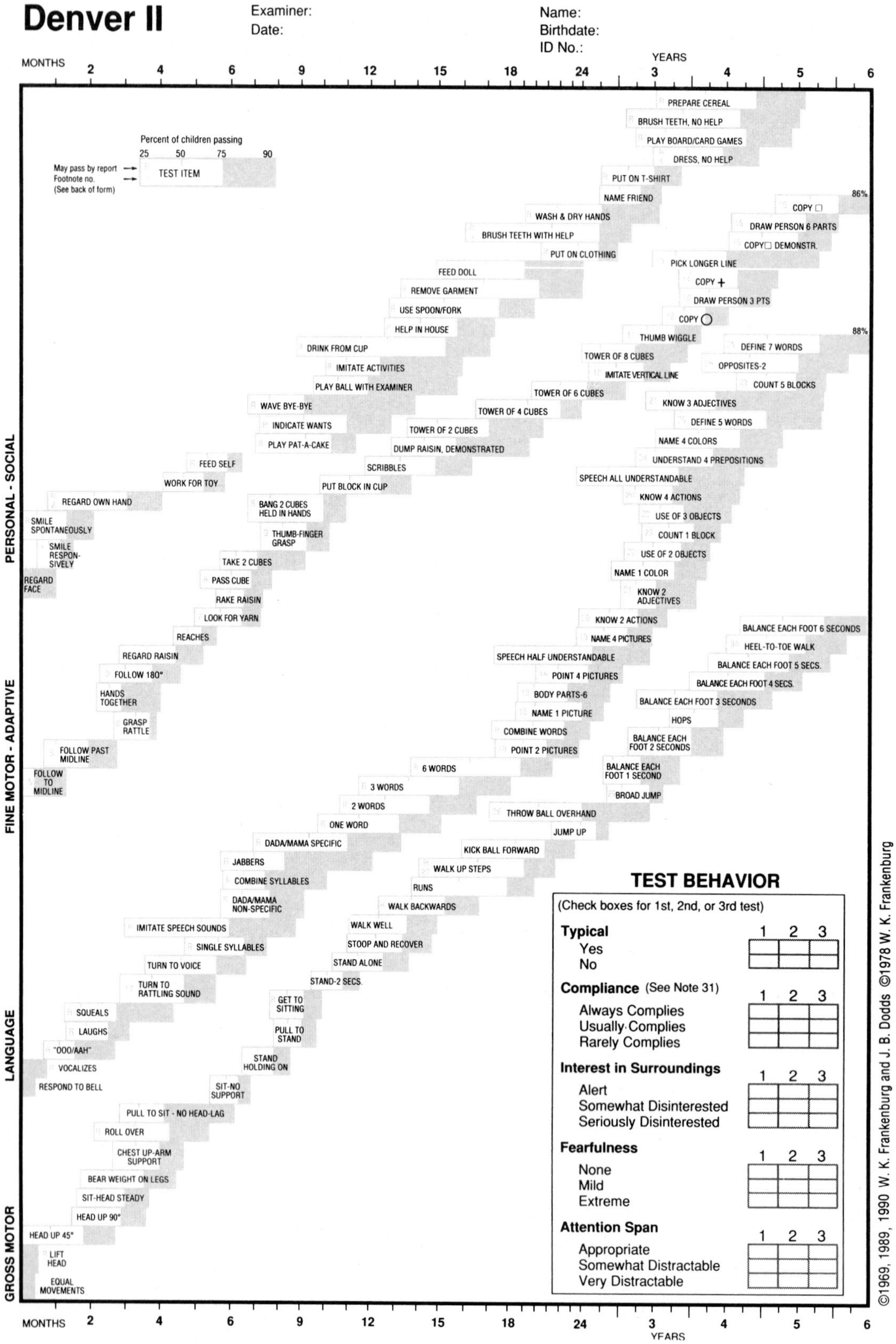

This test should be administered and scored in accordance with the guidelines in the Denver II Technical Manual. Accurate interpretation of the screening results requires consideration of the entire clinical picture. Its purpose is to serve as a screening tool to indicate infants who require further testing. It is not intended to be either diagnostic or predictive.

From Frankenburg WK, Dodds JB. University of Colorado Medical Center and Denver Developmental Materials, Inc.

Neonatology: Pathophysiology and Management of the Newborn, Fourth Edition,
edited by Gordon B. Avery, Mary Ann Fletcher, and Mhairi G. MacDonald.
J.B. Lippincott Company, Philadelphia © 1994.

appendix **H**

Drugs

1. MEDICATIONS IN BREAST MILK

APPENDIX H–1
DRUG PRECAUTIONS DURING BREAST FEEDING

Contraindicated
Bromocriptine
Cyclophosphamide
Cyclosporine
Doxorubicin
Ergotamine
Lithium
Methotrexate
Phenindione

Drugs of Abuse–Contraindicated
Amphetamine
Cocaine
Heroin
Marijuana
Nicotine (smoking)
Phencyclidine (PCP)

Require Temporary Cessation of Breast Feeding
Radiopharmaceuticals
- ^{67}Gallium
- ^{111}Indium
- ^{125}Iodine
- ^{131}Iodine
- Radioactive sodium
- ^{99m}Technetium

Effects Unknown, but of Concern
Antianxiety agents
- Diazepam
- Lorazepam
- Prazepam
- Quazepam

Effects Unknown, but of Concern (*continued*)
Antidepressants
- Amitriptyline
- Amoxapine
- Desipramine
- Dothiepin
- Doxepin
- Imipramine
- Trazodone

Antipsychotics
- Chlorpromazine
- Chlorprothixene
- Haloperidol
- Mesoridazine

Chloramphenicol
Metoclopramide
Metronidazole
Tinidazole

Occasional Significant Effects—
Give With Caution During Breast Feeding
Aspirin
Clemastine
Phenobarbital
Primidone
Salicylazosulfapyridine (Sulfasalazine)

From American Academy of Pediatrics, Committee on Drugs. Transfer of drugs and other chemicals into human milk. Pediatrics 1989;84:924.

2. PHARMACOPOEIA

APPENDIX H–2
PHARMACOPOEIA

Drug	Dose/kg	Route and Frequency	Comments
Acetazolamide	Diuretic, 5 mg Glaucoma, 2–7.5 mg; 5–10 mg when acute	PO, IV; qd–qod PO; q 6–8 h IV; q 6 h	• May cause acidosis, hypokalemia and GI irritation
ACTH (aqueous) corticotropin	0.5 U (0.5 mg)	IV, IM, SC; q 6–8 h	• Steroid complications • IV for diagnostic use only • Glucocorticoids preferred for immunosuppression
Adrenalin (epinephrine) 1 : 10,000	0.1–0.3 mL	SC, IV, ET; repeat in 3–5 min Drip: start at 0.1 μg/kg/min and titrate up	• Intracardiac route should be last resort • Higher dosage is for cardiac resuscitation • Drip for hypotension refractory to dopamine and dobutamine.
Albumin, 5%, 1 g/20 mL	0.5–1 g	IV over 2–4 h	• Contains 0.13–0.16 mEq Na^+/mL • Avoid circulatory overload
Amikacin	<7 d of age <28 wk: 7.5 mg q 24 h 28–34 wk: 7.5 mg q 18 h Term: 7.5 mg q 12 h >7 d of age <28 wk: 7.5 mg q 18 h 28–34 wk: 7.5 mg q 12 h Term: 7.5 mg q 8 h	IM, IV	• Therapeutic levels Peak: 20–30 μg/mL Trough: 5–10 μg/mL • Adjust does with renal impairment • Ototoxicity synergistic with furosemide
Aminophylline	Loading dose: 5 mg Maintenance dose: 2 mg	IV, PO; once IV, PO; q 8–12 h; give first dose 12 h after loading dose	• Therapeutic blood levels Bronchospasm: 10–20 μg/mL Neonatal apnea: 6–15 μg/mL • Monitor caffeine levels in infants of postconceptional age <36 wk • Toxicity: irritability, GI upset, arrhythmias
Ammonium chloride	1–2 mEq	PO, IV (slow infusion)	• For correction of hypochloremic metabolic alkalosis • Gastric irritation • Maximum IV concentration: 0.4 mEq/mL
Amoxicillin	7–13 mg	PO; q 8 h	• Like ampicillin

(*continued*)

APPENDIX H–2
PHARMACOPOEIA (*continued*)

Drug	Dose/kg	Route and Frequency	Comments
Amphotericin B	Test dose: 0.1 mg (up to 1 mg total) Initial dose: 0.25 mg, increase as tolerated in increments of 0.125–0.25 mg Maintenance dose: 0.5–1 mg *Total dose* for disseminated fungal infection: 25–30 mg/kg *Total dose* for catheter-associated nondisseminated disease: 10–15 mg/kg	IV; once followed by initial dose IV; qd over 4–6 h qd qd	• Maximum concentration, 0.1 mg/mL • Monitor electrolytes, renal, hepatic, and hematologic status closely
Ampicillin	Minimum dose: Sepsis, 50 mg Meningitis, 75–100 mg	IM, IV <7 days: q 12 h >7 days: q 8–6 h	• May cause rash, hemolytic anemia, interstitial nephritis, and pseudomembranous colitis
Atracurium	Initial dose: 0.3–0.5 mg Maintenance dose: 0.08–0.1 mg	IV; once q 20–45 min to maintain paralysis	• Hypertension associated with histamine release • Ventilatory rate may need to be adjusted to compensate for loss of spontaneous ventilation • Aminoglycoside antibiotics prolong duration of action • Contains 9 mg benzyl alcohol/mL • Elimination not substantially altered by renal or hepatic dysfunction
Atropine	General: 0.01 mg CPR: 0.01–0.03 mg	PO, SC, IV (maximum: 0.4 mg/dose); may repeat q 4–6 h IV, IT; repeat q 2–5 min by 2–3 prn; maximum dose, 1 mg	• May cause hyperthermia, urinary retention, tachycardia, and elevated WBC count • Antidote: physostigmine
Bacitracin	450 U 350 U 500 U	IM, premies or <2.5 kg; q 12 h IM, term or >2.5 kg; q 8 h IM, term or >2.5 kg; q 12 h	• Use only for treatment of empyema or pneumonia sensitive only to bacitracin • Do not administer IV; severe thrombophlebitis occurs • Nephrotoxic; monitor renal function daily
Bumetanide	0.015–0.1 mg	IV, IM, PO qod-qd Push IV dose over 1–2 min	• 40 times more potent than furosemide • Electrolyte imbalances, dehydration, ototoxicity

(*continued*)

APPENDIX H–2
PHARMACOPOEIA (*continued*)

Drug	Dose/kg	Route and Frequency	Comments
Caffeine base	Loading dose: 10 mg Maintenance dose: 2.5 mg	IV, IM, PO; once IV, IM, PO; qd First maintenance dose 24 h after loading dose	• Therapeutic drug levels: 8–25 μg/mL • CV, neurologic, and GI symptoms rarely appear at levels <50 μg/mL • Doses for caffeine citrate are twice the caffeine base dose
Calcium chloride, 10%, 27 mg Ca/mL	Neonatal hypocalcemia, 75 mg (20 mg Ca) Cardiac arrest, 20 mg (5 mg Ca)	PO; q 6 h IV; slow push q 10 min	• Dilute solution to 2% for PO use • GI irritation • Use IV with extreme caution; severe tissue necrosis may occur • Acidifying effect • Monitor serum Ca levels
Calcium glubionate, 23 mg Ca/mL	Neonatal hypocalcemia, 300 mg (20 mg Ca)	PO; q 6 h	• Give prior to feeds for best absorption • High osmotic load may cause diarrhea • Monitor serum Ca levels
Calcium gluconate, 10%, 9.4 mg Ca/mL	Neonatal hypocalcemia, 200 mg (~20 mg Ca) Cardiac arrest, 100 mg (~10 mg Ca)	IV, PO; q 6–12 h IV; q 10 min	• Bradycardia • Potentiation of digitalis • Extravasation may cause necrosis of subcutaneous tissues • Do not use scalp veins • Precipitates with bicarbonate • Monitor serum Ca levels
Calcium lactate; 13%, Ca	Maintenance dose for hypocalcemia: 75–150 mg (10–20 mg Ca)	PO; q 4–6 h	• GI distress • Tablets do not dissolve in milk
Captopril	0.05–0.1 mg	PO; q 8–6 h	• When diluted in water, use within 15 min • Give 1 h prior to feeding • Adjust dose if renal dysfunction • May cause rash, proteinuria, neutropenia, or hypotension
Carbenicillin	Maintenance dose 75 mg 100 mg	IV, IM <2 kg <7 d: q 8 h >2 kg >7 d: q 6 h	• Hypernatremia • Inhibition of platelet aggregation • Rash • Adjust dose if renal impairment
Cefazolin	20 mg	IV, IM <7 d: q 12 h >7 d: q 8 h	• Adjust dose if renal impairment • Allergic rash • Elevated liver enzymes

(*continued*)

APPENDIX H–2
PHARMACOPOEIA (*continued*)

Drug	Dose/kg	Route and Frequency	Comments
Cefotaxime	50 mg	IV, IM <7 d: q 12 h >7 d: q 8 h	• Good CNS penetration • Adjust dose if renal dysfunction • Positive Coombs test • Elevated BUN • Allergic rash
Ceftazidime	30–50 mg	IV, IM <1200 g 0–4 wk: q 12 h >1200 g <7 d: q 12 h >1200 g >7 d: q 8 h	• Adjust dose if renal impairment • False-positive Coombs test • Allergic rash
Cefuroxime	10–25 mg	IV, IM; q 12 h	• Thrombophlebitis • Pseudomembranous colitis • Transient elevation in BUN and creatinine • Adjust dose if renal failure • Allergic rash
Cephalothin	20 mg	IV, IM <1200 g 0–4 wk: q 12 h >1200 g <7 d: q 12–8 h >1200 g >7 d: q 8–6 h	• Adjust dose if renal dysfunction • False-positive Coombs test • Neutropenia • Nephrotoxic • Allergic rash
Chloral hydrate	Sedative: 10–15 mg Hypnotic: 25–50 mg	PO, PR; q 8 h prn PO, PR; once	• Accumulation of toxic metabolites in prematures • Paradoxical excitement • Use with caution if hepatic or renal impairment • GI irritation • Increased direct and indirect bilirubin levels
Chloramphenicol	25 mg	IV, PO <2 kg: qd >2 kg <7 d: qd >2 kg >7 d: q 12 h	• Therapeutic blood levels: 15–25 μg/mL • Bone marrow suppression • Gray baby syndrome with levels >50 μg/mL • Increases phenytoin level
Chlorpromazine (see Thorazine)			
Chlorothiazide	20 mg	IV, PO; q 12 h	• Use with caution if liver or severe renal disease. • May cause fluid and electrolyte imbalance, hyperbilirubinemia, and hyperglycemia
Cholestyramine	80 mg active resin	PO; tid with feeds	• May cause constipation, diarrhea, malabsorption of fat soluble vitamins and metabolic acidosis • Alters absorption of other drugs; give oral medications 1 h before or 4–6 h after cholestyramine

(*continued*)

APPENDIX H–2
PHARMACOPOEIA (*continued*)

Drug	Dose/kg	Route and Frequency	Comments
Cimetidine	2.5–5 mg	IV, IM, PO; q 6 h	• May cause diarrhea, rash, neutropenia, and gynecomastia • Increases blood levels of theophylline, phenytoin, and other drugs • Decrease dose if renal dysfunction
Clindamycin	5 mg 5–10 mg	IV, IM <2 kg <1 mo: q 12 h >2 kg <1 mo: q 8–6 h >1 mo: q 6 h	• Not indicated in meningitis • GI disturbance • Pseudomembranous colitis (rare in children)
Colistin	2.5 mg	IV, IM <7 days: q 12 h >7 days: q 8 h	• Nephrotoxic
Cortisone	Physiologic replacement: 0.25 mg Antiinflammatory: 1–2.5 mg Stress: 0.5–1 mg	IM; q 24 h IM; q 12–24 h IM during illness or perioperatively	• Slow IM absorption • Risk of infection • Hypertension • Salt retention • Adrenal suppression • Hyperglycemia • Leukocytosis
Curare (see Tubocurarine)			
Dexamethasone*	Bronchopulmonary dysplasia: 0.25 mg Antiinflammatory: 0.025–0.05 mg Airway edema: 0.25 mg	IV, IM, PO; q 12 for 3 days, then 0.15 mg/kg q 12 h for 3 d, then reduce dose by 10% q 3 d to minimum dose of 0.05 mg/kg/dose (can be given as a single daily dose of 0.1 mg/kg); maintain minimum dose for 7 d, then every other day for 7 d IV, IM, PO; q 6–12 h IV, IM, PO; q 6 h prn For extubation: start 24 h prior to extubation and continue for 4–6 doses	• Infection • Hypertension • Salt retention • Adrenal suppression* • Hyperglycemia • Leukocytosis
Dextran-40 (10% solution)	Initial dose: Maximum of 2 g (20 mL) Maintenance dose: Maximum of 1 g (10 mL)	IV; first 24 h IV; daily after first 24 h	• Therapy should not be continued longer than 5 d • Monitor for circulatory overload
Diazepam (Valium)	Status epilepticus: 0.1–0.5 mg	Slow IV push over 3 min; q 15–30 min for 2–3 doses; may repeat again in 4 h to a maximum of 2 mg/kg/24 h	• Hypotension and respiratory depression • Displacement of bilirubin by Na benzoate

(*continued*)

APPENDIX H–2
PHARMACOPOEIA (*continued*)

Drug	Dose/kg	Route and Frequency	Comments
Diazoxide	1–3 mg	IV push; q 5–15 min until BP is controlled, then q4–24 h	• Hyperglycemia • Ketoacidosis • GI irritation • Salt and water retention • Hypotension
Dicloxacillin	3–6 mg	PO; q 6 h	• Give 1 h before or 2 h after feeding • Penicillin sensitivity
Digoxin	TDD oral dose Premie: 20–30 μg Term: 25–30 μg 1–24 mo: 35–60 μg Oral maintenance dose (25% TDD) Premie: 2.5–3.75 μg Term: 3–3.75 μg 1–24 mo: 4–7.5 μg TDD IV, IM dose Premie: 15–25 μg Term: 20–30 μg 1–24 mo: 30–50 μg IV, IM maintenance dose (25% TDD) Premie: 2–3 μg Term: 2.5–3.75 μg 1–24 mo: 3.75–6 μg	Give ½ of the TDD initially, then ¼ of the TDD q 8–24 h in 2 doses q 12 h Same as oral digitalization schedule q 12 h	• Bradycardia • PVCs • Vomiting • Poor feeding • Arrhythmias • Check ECG trace during digitalization and periodically • Adjust dose per clinical response and renal function
Dobutamine	2.5–20 μg/min Maximum dose: 40 μg/min	IV infusion	• Titrate according to patient response • Same precautions as dopamine
Dopamine	2–5 μg/min 5–15 μg/min >20 μg/min Maximum dose: 50 μg/min	IV infusion; mostly dopaminergic effect and some β-adrenergic at higher dose range Mostly β-adrenergic; some dopaminergic at lower dose range and some α-adrenergic at higher dose range Mostly α-adrenergic	• Monitor BP and pulse pressure • Observe for pulmonary hypertension • Tissue necrosis if extravasation occurs • Ectopic beats
Doxapram	Loading dose: 3 mg Maintenance dose: 1–2.5 mg/h	Over 1 h Continuous IV infusion; start at 1 mg/kg/h and titrate up to minimum effective dose	• Maintain therapeutic theophylline or caffeine levels • Taper drug to avoid rebound apneic episodes • Increases oxygen consumption • Hypertension • Tachycardia • Seizures
Edrophonium (see Tensilon)			

(*continued*)

APPENDIX H–2
PHARMACOPOEIA (*continued*)

Drug	Dose/kg	Route and Frequency	Comments
Epinephrine, Racemic (see also Adrenalin)	2.25% aqueous solution *Total dose:* 0.25 mL in 3 mL NS solution	Inhalation via nebulizer over 15 min q 4 h prn	• Tachycardia • Arrhythmias
Erythromycin	10 mg	IV, PO <7 days <1.2 kg: q 12 h >7 days >1.2 kg: q 8 h	• Decreases clearance of theophylline, digoxin, carbamazepine, and others • GI distress
Ethacrynic acid (Edecrin)	0.5–1 mg 0.5–1 mg	IV over 5–10 min; q 24–48 h PO; q 24–48 h	• Na and K depletion • Possible ototoxicity with aminoglycosides • Avoid use in renal failure
Fentanyl	1–3 μg	IV, IM; q 2–4 h prn	• Fewer cardiovascular effects than morpine • Muscle rigidity • Respiratory depressant • Withdrawal
Furosemide (Lasix)	1–2 mg 2–6 mg	IV, IM; q 6–24 h; may increase up to maximum of 6 mg/kg/dose PO; q 6–24 h	• Na and K depletion • Dehydration • Ototoxicity with aminoglycosides
Gentamicin	2.5 mg	IV, IM <28 wk: q 24 h 28–34 wk: q 18 h >34 wk: q 12 h >14 postnatal days: adjust dosing interval up one level	• Renal and eighth nerve toxicity in adults • Serum level should be monitored
Gentian violet	1%, 2% solution	Topically bid–tid	• Messy
Glucagon	0.03–0.1 mg Maximum single dose: 1 mg	IV, IM, SC; may repeat q 20–30 min prn	• Rebound hypoglycemia
Heparin	Initial bolus: 50 U Maintenance: 10–25 U/h Intermittent: 100 U	IV bolus; once Continuous IV infusion IV q 4 h	• Follow clotting time • Protamine sulfate is antidote
Hydralazine (Apresoline)	0.1–0.5 mg 0.2–2 mg	IV, IM; q 4–6 h prn PO; q 6–12 h	• Tachycardia • Hypotension
Hydrocortisone (Solu-Cortef)	Congenital adrenal hyperplasia Initial: 30–36 mg/m$_2$/d Maintenance: 20–25 mg/m$_2$/d Shock Initial: 35–50 mg Maintenance: 12.5–37.5 mg	PO; divided 1/4-dose in A.M. and midday, 1/2-dose at night IV; once IV; q 6 h for 48–72 h	• Infection • Hypertension • Salt and water retention • Adrenal suppresstion • Hyperglycemia
Indomethacin (Indocin)	#1 #2 #3 0.2 mg 0.1 mg 0.1 mg 0.2 mg 0.2 mg 0.2 mg 0.2 mg 0.25 mg 0.25 mg	IV; q 8–12 h in 3 doses <48 h 2–7 d >7 d	• Renal toxicity • Decreased platelet aggregation

(*continued*)

APPENDIX H–2
PHARMACOPOEIA (*continued*)

Drug	Dose/kg	Route and Frequency	Comments
Insulin	Hyperglycemia Initial: 0.1 U Maintenance: 0.02–0.1 U/h Intermittent: 0.1–0.2 U Hyperkalemia: 0.3 U/g of glucose	 IV over 15–20 min Continuous IV infusion SC q 6–12 h IV, with glucose: 500 mg/kg/dose	• Hypoglycemia • Monitor blood glucose and titrate • Hyperglycemic rebound
Isoniazid	10–20 mg	PO, IM; q 24 h	• Vitamin B_6 depletion • Monitor liver function
Isoproterenol (Isuprel)	0.05–0.1 μg/min up to 2 μg/min	IV, slow infusion of diluted solution: 2–10 μg/mL	• Monitor heart rate • Arrhythmia noted with overdose • Hypotension or hypertension
Kanamycin	 7.5 mg 7.5 mg 10 mg 10 mg	IV, IM ≤2 kg and 0–7 d: q 12 h ≤2 kg and >7 d: q 8 h >2 kg and 0–7 d: q 12 h >2 kg and >7 d: q 8 h	• Renal and eighth nerve toxicity • Monitor serum level
Kayexalate	1 g	PO, PR; repeat q 6 h prn	• Hyperosmotic • Follow serum electrolytes
Levothyroxine (T4)	5–8 μg 10–14 μg	IV over 30–60 s; q 24 h (IV dose is 75% of PO dose) PO; q 24 h	• Use with caution in patients on anticoagulants • Monitor serum T4 and TSH.
Lidocaine	0.5–1 mg 10–50 μg/min	IV, intratracheal; repeat q 5–10 min up to a maximum of 5 mg/kg IV infusion (dilute: 2–4 mg/mL)	• Bradycardia • Hypotension • Contraindicated in severe heart block • Therapeutic levels: 1.5–5 mg/mL
Lorazepam (Ativan)	Status epilepticus: 0.05 mg Sedation: 0.03 mg	IV; may repeat twice q 15–20 min IV	• Repiratory depression • Hypotension • Bradycardia
Magnesium sulfate	Hypomagnesemia: 0.2–0.4 mEq	IV, IM q 6 h for 3–4 doses (10% solution)	• Respiratory depression • Hypotension • Monitor serum level
Mannitol	0.25–2 g as 15%–20% solution Oliguria test dose: 0.2 g	IV; once over 2–6 h IV; once over 3–5 min	• Rebound edema • Circulatory overload • Monitor serum osmolality
Meperidine (Demerol)	0.25 mg–1 mg 0.5–1 mg	IV, IM, SC; q 4–6 h prn PO; q 4-6 h prn	• CNS depression • Active metabolite may precipitate seizure • Withdrawal
Methicillin	 Meningitis: 50 mg Other infections: 25 mg	IV, IM ≤2 kg and 0–7 d: q 12 h ≤2 kg and >7 d: q 8 h >2 kg and 0–7 d: q 8 h >2 kg and >7 d: q 6 h	• Penicillin allergy • Interstitial nephritis occurs more often than with other penicillins

(*continued*)

APPENDIX H–2
PHARMACOPOEIA (*continued*)

Drug	Dose/kg	Route and Frequency	Comments
Methyldopa (Aldomet)	2.5–10 mg	PO, IV; q 6–12 h; increase dose gradually	• Hemolytic anemia • Positive Coombs test • Liver damage • Hypotension
Methylene blue	1–2 mg	IV slowly over 5 min (1% solution)	• Reducing agent • May decrease hemoglobin oxygen-carrying capacity
Metoclopramide (Reglan)	0.1 mg	IV, IM, PO; q 6 h	• Extrapyramidal reactions may occur • Use with caution in patients with history of seizures
Metolazone (Zaroxolyn)	0.2 mg	PO; qd or q 12 h	• Monitor electrolytes • May cause metabolic alkalosis • May cause hyperuricemia
Metronidazole (Flagyl)	7.5 mg 7.5 mg 15 mg	IV, <2 kg: q 12 h IV, >2 kg and 0–7 d: q 12 h IV, >2 kg and >7 d: q 12 h	• Effectively penetrates into CSF
Midazolam (Versed)	0.03–0.1 mg	IV, IM; q 2–4 h prn	• Respiratory depression • Hypotension
Morphine sulfate	0.05–0.2 mg	IV, IM, SC; q 2–4 h prn	• Respiratory and CNS depression • Hypotension • Withdrawal • Antidote Narcan (for acute overdose)
Naloxone (Narcan)	0.1 mg	IV, intratracheal; repeat prn	• Recommended dosage strength 0.4 mg/mL
Neomycin	12.5–25 mg	PO; q 6 h	• Follow for renal or ototoxicity
Neostigmine	Myasthenia test: 0.04 mg Treatment 0.01–0.04 mg 0.25–0.3 mg	 IM; once IV, IM, SC; q 2–3 h prn PO, q 3–4 h	• Cholinergic crisis • Antidote: Atropine (0.01–0.04 mg/kg)
Nitroprusside (Nipride)	0.5–6 μg/min	Continuous IV infusion Protect solution from light.	• Hypotension • May have cyanide toxicity (hemoglobin binding) • Tachyphylaxis
Nystatin	100,000–200,000 U total dose	PO; q 6 h	
Oxacillin	 25 mg 33 mg 25 mg 37.5 mg	IV, IM ≤ 2 kg and 0–7 d: q 12 h ≤ 2 kg and >7 d: q 8 h >2 kg and 0–7 d: q 8 h >2 kg and >7 d: q 6 h	• Penicillin allergy • Monitor liver function
Pancuronium (Pavulon)	0.03–0.1 mg	IV; q 1–4 h prn	• Short half-life

(*continued*)

APPENDIX H–2
PHARMACOPOEIA (*continued*)

Drug	Dose/kg	Route and Frequency	Comments
Paraldehyde	0.3 mL (1 g/mL solution) up to a maximum of 5 ml single dose	PR; dilute 1 : 1 with olive oil or mineral oil; may repeat q 4–6 h	• Depression with overdose • Parenteral dosage form no longer available in U.S. • Do not use discolored solution or plastic equipment
Paregoric	Initial: 0.2–0.3 mL total dose Increase by 0.05 mL up to a maximum of 0.7 mL total dose (please note dose is not per kilogram)	PO; q 3–4 h	• Tincture of opium should be diluted 1 : 25 (0.4 mg morphine/mL)
Penicillin G (aqueous)	Meningitis/group B streptococcus: 75,000–100,000 U Other infections: 25,000–50,000 U	IV, IM ≤2 kg and 0–7 d: q 12 h ≤2 kg and >7 d: q 8 h >2 kg and 0–7 d: q 8 h >2 kg and >7 d: q 6 h	• Use the same dosing schedule for either indication; just change dose
Phenobarbital	Status: 15–20 mg Maintenance: 2–3 mg	IM, IV; stat IV, IM, PO; q 12–24 h	• Depression with overdose • Monitor serum level (20–40 μg/mL)
Phenytoin (Dilantin)	Loading dose: 15–20 mg Maintenance dose: 2–5 mg	IV; stat IV, PO; q 8–12 h	• Rapid IV infusion may precipitate cardiovascular collapse • Monitor serum level (10–20 μg/mL)
Piperacillin	50–100 mg 50–75 mg	IV, IM; 0–7 d: q 12 h IV, IM; >7 d: q 6–8 h	• Limited experience in newborn
Polymyxin B (1 mg = 10,000 U)	0.75–1 mg Total dose: 2 mg (children <2 y)	IM, IV infusion over 60–90 min; q 6–8 h Intrathecal: q 24 h for 3–4 d	• Nephrotoxicity • Neurotoxicity • Adjust dose for renal impairment
Prednisone	Antiinflammatory: 0.2–0.5 mg	PO; q 6–12 h	• Infection • Hypertension • Salt and fluid retention • Adrenal suppression • Hyperglycemia
Propranolol (Inderal)	0.01–0.1 mg Maximum single dose: 1 mg Arrhythmia, 0.05–1 mg Hypertension, 0.05–0.5 mg	IV; stat over 10 min PO; q 6–8 h PO; q 6–12 h	• Hypotension • Bronchospasm • Heart block • Atropine for excess bradycardia
Prostaglandin E_1 (PGE_1)	0.05–0.4 μg/min	Continue IV infusion; decrease to lowest dose to maintain response	• Apnea • Fever • Hypotension • Cutaneous vasodilation
Protamine sulfate	1 mg for each 100 U heparin given in past 4 h Maximum single dose: 50 mg	IV; stat	• Hypotension • Bradycardia

(continued)

APPENDIX H–2
PHARMACOPOEIA (*continued*)

Drug	Dose/kg	Route and Frequency	Comments
Pyridoxine (vitamin B_6)	Deficiency: 5–10 mg total dose B_6-dependent seizure Test dose: 50–100 mg total dose Maintenance dose: 50–100 mg total dose	PO, IV, IM; q 24 h IV once PO, IV, IM; q 24 h	
Pyrimethamine (Daraprim)	Toxoplasmosis, load 2 mg Maintenance dose: 1 mg	PO; qd for 3 d PO; qd for 4 wk	• Bone marrow depression • Folic acid deficiency
Quinidine sulfate	4–15 mg Test dose: 2 mg	PO; q 6 h PO once for idiosyncratic reactions	• Hold dose or discontinue if QRS interval ≥ 0.02 s • Contraindicated with AV nodal block
Sodium bicarbonate	1–2 mEq Maximum: 8 mEq/24 h	IV, slow push up to 1 mEq/kg; higher doses slow infusion	• Dilute 1 : 1 with sterile water to produce 0.5 mEq/mL solution • Alkalosis, edema; hyperosmolarity, hypernatremia
Spironolactone (Aldactone)	0.5–1 mg	PO; q 8–12 h	• To be avoided in hyperkalemia • Contraindicated in renal failure
Tensilon (Edrophonium)	Myasthenia gravis test, 0.1 mg single dose	IV; once IM, SC if IV access not possible	• Keep atropine available
THAM (Tromethamine) 0.3 M solution (1 mL = 0.3 mEq; 1 mm = 1 mEq)	1–2 mEq/kg/dose	IV; slow infusion in large vessel, maximum 1 mL/min	• Hypoglycemia • Apnea • Hyperkalemia • Danger of fluid overload
Thorazine (chlorpromazine)	Neonatal abstinence, 0.5–0.75 mg	PO; q 6 h IV, IM if PO not tolerated	• Hypotension • Arrhythmia
Ticarcillin	 75 mg	IV, IM ≤2 kg and 0–7 d: q 12 h ≤2 kg and >7 d: q 8 h >2 kg and 0–7 d: q 8 h >2 kg and >7 d: q 6 h	• Inhibition of platelet aggregation • Hypernatremia
Tobramycin	2.5 mg	IV, IM; <28 wk: q 24 h 28–34 wk: q 18 h >34 wk: q 12 h >14 postnatal days, adjust dosing interval up one level	• Possible renal and eighth nerve toxicity • Monitor serum level

(*continued*)

APPENDIX H–2
PHARMACOPOEIA (*continued*)

Drug	Dose/kg	Route and Frequency	Comments
Tolazoline (Priscoline)	Test dose: 1–2 mg Maintenance dose: 1–2 mg/h	IV; over 10 min Continuous IV infusion through peripheral or central vein that drains into superior vena cava	• Hypotension • GI and pulmonary hemorrhage • For severe hypotension use ephedrine to increase peripheral resistance, not epinephrine or norepinephrine
Tubocurarine (curare)	0.3–0.5 mg	IV; push over 60–90 sec; repeat prn IM; if IV access is not available	• Hypotension • Histamine release • Voluntary muscle paralysis
Vancomycin	Clostridium difficile 10 mg 15 mg 24 mg 18 mg 22.5 mg 15 mg	 PO; q 6 h IV; over 60 min Postconceptual age <28 wk: q 24 h 28–30 wk: q 24 h 31–36 wk: q 12 h or 27 mg/kg q 18 h >37 wk: q 12 h Term and >30 d: q 8 h	 • Ototoxicity • Nephrotoxicity • Thrombophlebitis • Red-man syndrome may occur with rapid IV infusion • Monitor serum level
Vasopressin (Pitressin), aqueous 20 U/mL	Total dose: 0.125–0.5 ml	IM, SC; q 6–8 h	• Fluid overload • Electrolyte imbalance
Vecuronium	Intubation: 0.08–0.15 mg Maintenance dose: 0.01–0.02 mg	IV; may repeat q 1–2 h prn	• No significant cardiovascular effects or histamine release
Vitamin K_1 (phytonadione)	Prevention: 0.5–1 mg total dose Treatment: 1–2 mg total dose	IM; once within 1 h of birth IM, IV, SC, PO; may repeat q day	• Check prothrombin time • Hypotension • Severe reactions resembling anaphylaxis may occur with IV administration

Dosages in this table are single dose per kilogram. Frequency is suggested in the third column but may vary with maturity and rate of metabolism. In most cases, the most conservative dosage is given.

* Consider steroid coverage for period of stress after therapy for bronchopulmonary dysplasia.

ACTH, adrenocorticotropic hormone; AV, atrioventricular; BP, blood pressure; BUN, blood urea nitrogen; CNS, central nervous system; CSF, cerebrospinal fluid; ECG, electrocardiogram; ET, endotracheal; GI, gastrointestinal; IT, intrathecal; NS, normal saline; PO, by mouth; PR, per rectum; prn, as needed; PVC, premature ventricular contraction; SC, subcutaneous; TDD, total digitalizing dose; TSH, thyroid stimulating hormone; WBC, leukocyte.

Reviewed and updated by Luisa Lopez, R. Ph. and Fannie Choy, R.Ph., Senior Clinical Pharmacists (Neonatology), Children's National Medical Center, Washington, DC.

3. ANTIDYSRHYTHMIC AGENTS

APPENDIX H–3
ANTIDYSRHYTHMIC AGENTS

Drug	Currently Commonly Used	Group, Action	Oral Dose	IV Dose	Theraputic Level	Indications	Contraindications	Toxicity
Adenosine	Yes	Purine, increase K conductance, transient AV node conduction block		0.075 mg/kg rapid IV push q 1 min prn, increase in 0.05 mg/kg increments to a maximum dose of 0.15–0.25 mg/kg prn		Rx-Rentry SVT, Dx, atrial flutter		Transient AV block, decreased HR, decreased BP, and flushing
Digoxin	Yes	Glycoside, Na-K ATPase, inhibition, vagotonic	Loading: 20–30 μg/kg divided in 3 doses Maintenance: 3–5 μg/kg/12 h, decrease with renal hepatic dysfunction	80% of oral	0.8–2.0 ng/mL	SVT, atrial flutter	AV block VT, many WPW	AV block, decreased HR, tachydysrhythmias, vomiting, use with caution with renal failure
Quinidine	Yes	IA, Na channel inhibition, decrease conduction, slow repolarization	4–15 mg/kg/6 h, decrease with renal hepatic dysfunction Test dose: 2 mg/kg		2–7 mg/L	SVT, WPW with propranolol, PVC, VT	Long Q–T interval, known sensitivity, IV use, conduction block, myasthenia gravis	Decreased contractility, increased QT, VT, conduction block, vomiting, diarrhea, rash, blood dyscrasias, increased HR with atrial flutter without digoxin, increased digoxin level, decreased digoxin dose by one-half
Procainamide	Yes	IA	2.5–8 mg/kg/4 h	Loading: 2–7 mg/kg over 1 h Infusion: 20–60 μg/kg/min	PA 4–10 mg/L	SVT, WPW, PVC, VT	Conduction block, myasthenia gravis	Similar to quinidine, decreased BP, lupuslike reaction, no effect on digoxin level
Lidocaine	Yes	IB, Na channel inhibition, decrease refractoriness, decrease APD		Bolus: 1 mg/kg/5–10 min Infusion: 20–50 μg/kg/min, decrease with cyanosis, hepatic dysfunction	2–5 mg/L	PVC, VT	Conduction block decreased junctional and ventricular escape rate	CNS reactions, seizures, decrease BP, decreased respiratory drive

Phenytoin	No	IB	2–3 mg/kg/12 h, decrease with hepatic dysfunction	Loading: 10 mg/kg IV push: 1.25 mg/kg q 5 min to a maximum dose of 10–15 mg/kg	10–20 mg/L	PVC, VT, digitalis intoxication	Not FDA approved for VT	CNS reactions, decreased BP, blood dyscrasias, hepatic dysfunction, hypertrichosis, gingival hyperplasia, coarse facies, rash
Flecainide	No	IC, Na channel inhibition, decrease conduction, decrease automaticity	1–2.5 mg/kg/8 h, decrease with renal, hepatic dysfunction		0.2–1.0 mg/L	Refractory life-threatening SVT, PJRT, PVC, VT	Conduction block, hepatic, myocardial dysfunction, not FDA approved for children, SVT	Occasional increased SVT frequency with WPW, increased pacing threshold and conduction block, VT, nausea, decreased contractility
Propranolol	Yes	II, blockade, decrease conduction, increase refractoriness, decrease automaticity	0.3–1.0 mg/kg/6 h, decrease with chronic cyanosis, renal, hepatic dysfunction	0.02–0.10 mg/kg over 20 min		SVT, WPW, PVC, VT, hypertrophic cardiomyopathy, prolonged Q–T interval	Use with verapamil, bronchospasm, conduction block, CHF	Decrease HR, conduction block, bronchospasm, decreased BP, hypoglycemia, depression, decreased cardiac reflexes with anesthesia
Amiodarone	No	III, prolong AP, decrease conduction, decrease automaticity	600–800 mg/1.73 m^2/d	Investigational	1–2 mg/L	Refractory, life-threatening, SVT, VT, recurrent VF	Conduction block, not FDA approved for children	Extremely long half-life, corneal deposits, thyroid and hepatic dysfunction, pulmonary fibrosis may increase conduction block and digoxin and quinidine levels, decreased digosin by ½
Bretylium	No	III, inhibits norepinephrine release		Loading: 5 mg/kg over 15 min Infusion: 20–50 μg/kg/min		Refractory VT, VF	Not FDA approved for children	Transient increased BP, dysrhythmia, then decreased BP
Verapamil	No	IV, Ca channel blockade, decrease conduction, increase refractoriness, decrease automaticity	10 mg/kg/d; decrease with hepatic, renal dysfunction, neuromuscular disease			Refractory SVT, hypertrophic cardiomyopathy, some PVC, VT	IV use, conduction dysfunction, CHF, many WPW propranolol, muscular dystrophy, use with Quinidine	Decreased BP, decreased HR, conduction block, myocardial depression, constipation, may increase digoxin level, decreased digoxin dose by ⅓ to ½
DC cardioversion	Yes	SVT, VT	0.5–1.0 w/kg 1.0–2.0 w/kg					

Continuous echocardiographic monitoring should be done during initiation of antidysrhythmic therapy and with IV administration because of potentialprodysrhythmia and conduction block.

AP, action potential; APD, action potential duration; AV, atrioventricular; BP, blood pressure; CHF, congestive heart failure; CNS, central nervous system; DC, direct current; Dx, diagnosis; FDA, Federal Drug Administration; HR, heart rate; IV, intravenous; PA, procaine amide; PJRT, permanent junctional reciprocating tachycardia; PVC, premature ventricular depolarization; Rx, prescription; SVT; supraventricular tachycardia; VT, ventricular tachycardia; WPW, Wolff–Parkinson–White syndrome.

Courtesy of Flanagan MF and Fyler DC.

4. SUPPLEMENTAL MEDICATIONS FOR CONTROL OF BRONCHOSPASM

APPENDIX H–6
SUPPLEMENTAL MEDICATIONS FOR CONTROL OF BRONCHOSPASM

Name	Chemical Group	Primary Actions	Secondary Actions	Most Common Significant Side-Effects	Route of Administration	Usual Dosage
Atropine	Belladonna alkaloid; antimuscarinic agent	Bronchiolar and bronchial relaxation	Inhibition of secretions in nose, mouth, pharynx, and bronchi	Low dose: slight cardiac slowing, dryness of mouth, and decreased sweating Higher dose: tachycardia, mild pupillary dilatation, and dryness of mouth and thirst	Inhalation	0.1 mg/kg/dose 3 to 4 times/day
Epinephrine	α- β-Adrenergic stimulator	Bronchial smooth muscle relaxation	Vasoconstriction; direct myocardial stimulation	Increased blood pressure Increased heart rate Reduced cutaneous blood flow Occasional cardiac rhythm disturbances Agitation, apprehension, and tremors Headache Emesis	Subcutaneous (rarely inhalation)	0.01 mg/kg/dose of 1 : 1,000 concentration every 20 min × 3 followed by Sus-Phrine if appropriate)
Cromolyn sodium (Intal)		Inhibits release of histamine thus reducing stimulus for bronchospasm		Infrequent and minor and usually from direct irritant effect of medication in powder form Bronchospasm, cough, nasal congestion,and pharyngeal irritation	Inhalation only Nebulizer—younger children Turbo inhaler—older children	20 mg/dose 3 to 4 times/day
Steroids (see Appendix H-2)						

Theophylline	Methylxanthine	Relaxation of smooth muscles	Central nervous system stimulant Cardiac muscle stimulant Diuretic effect Relaxation of smooth muscles	Irritability, restlessness, tremors, seizures (rare) Tachycardia, arrhythmias (rare) Emesis, increased secretion of gastric acid	Oral	10–20 mg/kg/day in 3–4 divided doses (therapeutic blood level 10–18 μg/mL)
Metaproterenol (Alupent)	Selective β_2-adrenergic agonist	Specific relaxation of bronchial smooth muscles (less stimulant effect on heart than other sympathomimetics)	Other β_2- adrenergic effects on smooth muscles of uterus and vascular supply to skeletal muscles	Mild tachycardia, hypertension, restlessness, nausea and vomiting, and rare sweating	Oral Inhalation	1–2 mg/kg/day in 3–4 divided doses 0.1–0.3 cc 5% solution in 2.5 cc of NS q 4–6 h
Terbutaline (Brethaire, Brethine)	Selective β_2-adrenergic agonist	Same as for theophylline and metaproterenol	Same as for theophylline and metaproterenol	Same as for theophylline and metaproterenol	Inhalation	0.5 mg in 2.5 cc NS q 3–4 h
Albuterol (Ventolin, Proventil)	Selective β_2-adrenergic agonist	Same as for theophylline and metaproterenol	Same as for theophylline and metaproterenol	Same as for theophylline and metaproterenol	Oral Inhalation	0.3–0.6 mg/kg/day in 3–4 divided doses 0.15 mg/kg/dose; minimum dose: 0.5 mg in 2 : 5 cc NS q 3–4 h

5. EFFECT OF DRUGS USED IN NEONATOLOGY ON BILIRUBIN–ALBUMIN BINDING

APPENDIX H–5
EFFECT OF DRUGS USED IN NEONATOLOGY ON BILIRUBIN–ALBUMIN BINDING

Agent	δ
Anticonvulsants	
Diazepam	1.00
Phenobarbital	1.04
Phenytoin	1.02
Valproate	1.09
Testing not required: lorazepam	
Antihypertensive Agents	
Diazoxide	?
Testing not required: hydralazine, methyldopa, nitroprusside, reserpine	
Cardiac Drugs	
Lidocaine	1.00
Procainamide	1.00
Testing not required: bretylium tosylate, digoxin, disopyramide, quinidine, verapamil	
Diuretics	
Acetazolamide	1.10
Bumetanide	1.00
Chlorothiazide	1.03
Ethacrynic acid	1.27
Furosemide	1.07
Hydrochlorothiazide	1.04
Testing not required: spironolactone	
Infectious Disease Agents	
Acyclovir	1.00
Amdinocillin	1.00
Ampicillin	1.08
Azlocillin	1.33
Atreonam	1.12
Carbenicillin	1.35
Cefamandole	1.07
Cefazolin	1.17
Cefmenoxime	1.10
Cefmetazole	2.01
Cefonicid	1.71
Cefoperazone	1.18
Ceforanide	1.04
Cefotaxime	1.05
Cefotetan	1.74
Cefoxitin	?
Ceftazidime	1.02
Ceftizoxime	1.03
Ceftriaxone	3.00
Cefuroxime	1.02
Cephalothin	1.03
Cephapirin	1.03
Cephradine	1.02
Infectious Disease Agents (*continued*)	
Chloramphenicol	1.02
Chloroquine	1.00
Cilastatin	1.00
Clindamycin	1.00
Fusidate	1.00
Imipenem	1.00
Lincomycin	1.00
Methicillin	1.17
Metronidazole	1.00
Mezlocillin	1.11
Moxalactam	1.63
Nafcillin	1.05
Oxacillin	1.07
Penicillin G	1.06
Piperacillin	1.03
Polymyxin B	1.00
Quinine	?
Spiramycin	1.00
Streptomycin	1.00
Sulfadiazine	1.18
Sulfamethoxazole	1.69
Sulfisoxazole	2.43
Tazobactam	1.00
Ticarcillin	1.27
Trimethoprim	1.01
Vancomycin	1.01
Vidarabine	1.00
Testing not required: amphotericin B, ciprofloxacin, erythromycin, isoniazid, miconazole, netilmicin, pyrimethamine, tobramycin	
Miscellaneous	
Calcium chloride	1.00
Calcium gluconate	1.00
Calcium lactate	1.00
Carnitine	1.00
Clofibrate	1.00
Diatrizoate	1.24
Indomethacin	1.00
Magnesium sulfate	1.00
Mannitol	1.00
Tin protoporphyrin	?
Tolazoline	1.00
Tromethamine	1.00
Testing not required: bicarbonate, cimetidine, dextran, enalapril, flumecinol, heparin, ketamine, metoclopramide, naloxone, nicardipine, prostaglandin E_1	

(*continued*)

APPENDIX H–5
EFFECT OF DRUGS USED IN NEONATOLOGY ON BILIRUBIN–ALBUMIN BINDING (*continued*)

Agent	δ
Neuromuscular Junction Agents	
Pancuronium	1.01
Testing not required: atracurium besylate, neostigmine, tubocurarine, vecuronium	
Sedative and Analgesic Agents	
Chloral hydrate	1.00
Paraldehyde	1.00
Pentobarbital	1.03
Thiopental	1.04
Testing not required: alfentanil, chlorpromazine, fentanyl, meperidine, midazolam, morphine	
Stimulants	
Aminophylline	1.24
Doxapram	1.00
Sympathetic and Parasympathetic Agents	
Edrophonium chloride	1.00
Testing not required: atropine dobutamine, dopamine, epinephrine, isoproterenol, propranolol	

Drugs are listed according to the category of their use. The symbol δ represents the maximal displacement factor. If δ = 1.2, there is a 20% increase in free-bilirubin concentration following drug administration. Drugs listed as not requiring testing have low protein binding or low mean peak serum concentrations. A question mark indicates that the drug requires testing but that the peroxidase technique is not applicable.

From Robertson A, Carp W, Brodersen R. Bilirubin displacing effect of drugs used in neonatology. Acta Paediatr Scand 1991;80:1119.

Neonatology: Pathophysiology and Management of the Newborn, Fourth Edition,
edited by Gordon B. Avery, Mary Ann Fletcher, and Mhairi G. MacDonald.
J.B. Lippincott Company, Philadelphia © 1994.

appendix I

Renal Anomalies

1. ASSOCIATIONS WITH OTHER STRUCTURAL DEFECTS

APPENDIX I–1
ASSOCIATIONS BETWEEN RENAL–URINARY TRACT ANOMALIES AND OTHER STRUCTURAL DEFECTS

Diagnosis (Mode of Genetic Transmission)	Frequency of Anomalies	Renal Anomalies	Urologic Anomalies	Other Associations
Hereditary Associations				
Acrorenal syndrome, or radial ray aplasia and renal anomalies (AD)	100%	Agenesis, ectopia		Absence of radius and thumb
Acrorenocular syndrome (AD/sporadic)	100%	Malrotation, ectopia	VUR, bladder diverticula	Thumb hypoplasia, preaxial polydactyly, coloboma, ptosis
Acrorenomandibular syndrome (AR)	Frequent	agenesis, ectopia		Split hand/split foot, cataracts, ear and genital anomalies
Adams–Oliver syndrome (AD)	Occasional		Duplicated collecting system	Aplasia cutis congenita, terminal transverse defects of limbs
Alport syndrome (AD, but fully expressed only in males; X-linked)	Frequent	Nephritis: recurrent hematuria		Deafness, cataracts, myopia, lenticonus
Antley–Bixler syndrome (AR?)	Occasional	Displaced kidney, accessory renal artery		Craniosynostosis, choanal atresia, radiohumeral synostosis
Arthrogryposis multiplex congenita with renal and hepatic abnormalities (AR/X-linked?)	100%	Glycosuria, polyuria, nephrocalcinosis hypercalciuria, hyperphosphaturia		Arthrogryposis multiplex congenita, rarefaction of motor neurons in anterior horn, cholestasis, all reported patients died before 4 months of age
Baller–Gerold syndrome, or Craniosynostosis–radial aplasia syndrome (AR)	Occasional	Pelvic kidney		MR (50%), growth deficiency, craniosynostosis, radial aplasia/hypoplasia, CHD
Branchiootoureteral syndrome (AD)	50%	Bifid renal pelvis	Bifid ureters	Preauricular pit/tag, bilateral hearing loss
Campomelic dysplasia (AR)	30%	Usually hydronephrosis, MKD		Bowed tibiae, hypoplastic scapulae, flat facies growth deficiency, CNS disorganization, most die of respiratory failure as neonates or in infancy
Carpenter syndrome (AR)	Occasional		Ureteral dilatation	Acrocephaly, polydactyly–syndactyly of feet, lateral displacement of inner canthi, hypogenitalism
CHILD syndrome (X-linked?, lethal in hemizygotic male)	Occasional	Unilateral agenesis		Unilateral hypomelia, ichthyosis, CHD, mild SGA
COFS syndrome (AR)	Occasional	Agenesis		Neurogenic arthrogryposis, microcephaly, microphthalmia/cataract/blepharophimosis, large ear pinnae, prominent nasal bridge, no growth, usually die before 5 years of age
Cohen syndrome (AR)	Occasional		UPJ obstruction	Hypotonia, obesity, prominent incisors, moderate MR

(*continued*)

APPENDIX I–1
ASSOCIATIONS BETWEEN RENAL–URINARY TRACT ANOMALIES AND OTHER STRUCTURAL DEFECTS (*continued*)

Diagnosis (Mode of Genetic Transmission)	Frequency of Anomalies	Renal Anomalies	Urologic Anomalies	Other Associations
Deal syndrome (AR)	100%	Fanconi syndrome		Ichthyosis, jaundice, musculoskeletal deformities, diarrhea, failure to thrive, death in infancy (larger than 6 months of age
Digitorenocerebral syndrome (AR)	Frequent	Agenesis, hypoplasia, dysplasia		Facial dysmorphism, seizures, malformed fingers and toes
EEC syndrome (AD, variable penetrance)	Occasional	Agenesis, hydronephrosis medullary dysplasia	Ureterocele	Ectrodactyly, ectodermal dysplasia, cleft lip/palate, defective lacrimal duct
Fanconi–pancytopenia syndrome (AR)	Frequent	Hypoplastic/malformed	Hypospadias, ureter duplication	Radial hypoplasia, hyperpigmentation, pancytopenia, short stature, microcephaly, MR
FG syndrome (X-linked R)	Occasional		Dilation	Prominent forehead, hypotonia, MR, imperforate anus
Fraser or cryptophthalmos syndrome (AR)	Frequent	Agenesis or hypoplasia		Cryptophthalmos, ear anomalies, genital anomaly, laryngeal stenosis/atresia, anal atresia, CHD
Frontometaphyseal dysplasia (X-linked, severe in male)	Occasional		Obstruction	Coarse facies, prominent supraorbital ridges, joint limitations, splayed metaphyses
Hereditary renal adysplasia (AD, 50%–90% penetrance)	50%–90%	Unilateral or bilateral agenesis		Potter (oligohydramnios) sequence if bilateral agenesis, uterine anomaly
Jarcho–Levin syndrome, or spondylothoracic dysplasia (AR)	Occasional	Hydronephrosis	Urethral atresia Ureteral obstruction, bilobate bladder	Prominent occiput, short neck, most die in infancy due to lung hypoplasia, short thorax, diminished ribs, vertebral defects, most Puerto Rican origin
Johanson–Blizzard syndrome (AR)	Frequent	Calicectasis, hydronephrosis		Hypoplasia alae nasi, hypothyroidism, deafness
LEOPARD syndrome, or multiple lentigines syndrome (AD)	Occasional	Agenesis or hypoplasia		Lentigines, hypertelorism, deafness, pulmonary stenosis, obstructive cardiomyopathy, mild growth failure, variable expression in individual patient
Lethal multiple pterygium syndrome (AR)	Occasional	Hydronephrosis	Megaureter	SGA, hypertelorism, epicanthal folds, joint contractures, pterygia, early death due to lung hypoplasia
Levy–Hollister syndrome, or lacrimo-auriculo-dento-digital syndrome (AD)	Occasional	Agenesis, nephrosclerosis		Nasolacrimal duct obstruction, ear anomalies, hearing loss, variable anomalies of upper limbs
Melnick–Fraser syndrome, or branchio-oto-renal syndrome (AD)	Frequent	Dysplasia, hypoplasia, agenesis, ectopia		Hearing loss, preauricular pits, anomalous pinna, branchial fistula
Melnick–Needles syndrome (AD?; lethal in male or X-linked)	Occasional	Hydronephrosis	Ureteral stenosis	Prominent eyes, bowing of long bones, ribbonlike ribs
Neu–Laxova syndrome (AR)	Occasional	Agenesis		Microcephaly, lissencephaly, exophthalmos, syndactyly and edema, polyhydramnios, short umbilical cord, early death
Opitz–Frias syndrome, G syndrome, or hypertelorism–hypospadias syndrome (AD)	Occasional	Renal defect	Hypospadias, cryptorchidism, bifid scrotum	Hypertelorism, swallowing difficulties
Perlman syndrome (AR?)		Nephromegaly, nephroblastomatosis	Cryptorchidism, hypospadias	Macrosomia, visceromegaly, polyhydramnios, diaphragmatic hernia, interrupted aortic arch, polysplenia
Rutledge syndrome (AR?)	100%	Oligopapillary renal hypoplasia	Urethral anomalies	Joint contractures, cerebellar hypoplasia, tongue cysts, short limbs, eye and ear anomalies, CHD, gallbladder agenesis
Saethre–Chotzen syndrome (AD)	Occasional	Renal anomaly		Craniosynostosis, brachycephaly, maxillary hypoplasia, abnormal ear, syndactyly
Schinzel–Giedion syndrome (AR)	Frequent	Hydronephrosis	Hydroureter, hypospadias	Severe growth failure, profound MR, midface retraction, cardiac and skeletal anomalies
TAR syndrome (AR)	Occasional	Ectopia, dysplasia	Hypospadias	Thrombocytopenia, granulocytosis, eosinophilia, anemia, radial absence or hypoplasia with thumbs present, CHD
Townes syndrome (AD)	Frequent	Hypoplasia	Ureterovesical reflux, urethral valves	Thumb, ear, and anal anomalies
Weyers oligodactyly syndrome (AR)	Frequent	Bilateral hydronephrosis		Deficient ulnar and fibular rays, oligodactyly

(*continued*)

APPENDIX I–1
ASSOCIATIONS BETWEEN RENAL–URINARY TRACT ANOMALIES AND OTHER STRUCTURAL DEFECTS (*continued*)

Diagnosis (Mode of Genetic Transmission)	Frequency of Anomalies	Renal Anomalies	Urologic Anomalies	Other Associations
Chromosomal Anomalies				
4p− syndrome	Occasional	Agenesis		Hypertelorism, broad or beaked nose, microcephaly, cranial asymmetry, low set ears, dimple, CHD, severe MR, seizures
5p− syndrome, or cri du chat syndrome	Occasional	Agenesis		SGA, slow growth, catlike cry, MR, hypotonia, CHD, microcephaly, downslanting palpebral fissures, hypertelorism, round face, epicanthal folds, strabismus, low set ears
9p− syndrome	Occasional	Hydronephrosis		Craniostenosis, trigonocephaly, upslanting palpebral fissures, hypoplastic supraorbital ridges
13q− syndrome	Occasional	Agenesis or hypoplasia, PKD, hydronephrosis		Microcephaly, high nasal bridge, MR, CHD, hypertelorism, coloboma, microphthalmia, retinoblastoma
18q− syndrome	Occasional	Horseshoe kidney		Poor growth, microcephaly, hypotonia, midfacial hypoplasia, abnormal ears, cleft palate, thumb hypoplasia
Cat-eye syndrome*	Frequent	Horseshoe kidney, agenesis, hydronephrosis		Coloboma of the iris, downslanting palpebral fissures, anal atresia
Partial trisomy 10q syndrome	Frequent			Ptosis, short palpebral fissures, campodactyly, marked MR
Penta X syndrome, or XXXXX syndrome	Occasional	Dysplasia		Microcephaly, growth deficiency, upward slanting palpebral fissures, low nasal bridge, short neck, small hands, clinodactyly of fifth fingers, PDA
Triploidy syndrome	Frequent	Cystic kidney, hydronephrosis, dysplasia		Large placenta and hydatiform changes; poor growth; brain, facies, and cardiac anomalies; syndactyly
Trisomy 4p syndrome	Occasional	Atresia, horseshoe kidney, hypoplasia, hydronephrosis	VUR	Microcephaly, severe MR, hypertonia in infancy, seizures, SGA, bulbous nose, prominent forehead, clinodactyly
Trisomy 8 syndrome, or mosaic syndrome	Occasional	Hydronephrosis, horsehshoe kidney, agenesis	Bifid pelvis	Prominent forehead and ears, deep-set eyes, hypertelorism, micrognathia, MR, CHD, vertebral anomalies, campodactyly
Trisomy 9 mosaic syndrome	Frequent			Joint contractures; heart, CNS, and ear anomalies
Trisomy 9p syndrome	Occasional	Malformations		SGA, macrocephaly, hypertelorism, downslanting palpebral fissures, distal phalangeal hypoplasia, skeletal anomalies
Trisomy 13 syndrome	Occasional	PKD, glomerular cysts, duplication	Ureter duplication, hydroureter	Holoprosencephaly, occipital scalp defect, polydactyly, microphthalmia, narrow hyperconvex fingernails
Trisomy 18 syndrome	Frequent	Horseshoe kidney, ectopic, PKD, hypoplasia or agenesis, duplication	Ureter duplication	Polyhydramnios, single UA, poor growth, prominent occiput, clenched hand
Trisomy 20p syndrome	Occasional	Malformations		Blepharophimosis, brachycephaly, large ears, MR, cubitus valgus, vertebral defects, CHD
Turner syndrome, or XO syndrome	60%	Horseshoe kidney, hypertension	Double or cleft pelvis	Short broad chest, widely spaced nipples, lymphedema, webbed neck, cubitus valgus
Sporadic Associations				
Aniridia–Wilms tumor association†	50%	Bilateral Wilms tumor		Microcephaly, growth deficiency, MR, prominent lips, cataracts, ptosis, nystagmus, ambiguous genitalia
Beckwith–Wiedemann syndrome, or exomphalos–macroglossia–gigantism syndrome	Frequent	Large kidneys, medullary dysplasia	Hypospadias	Omphalocele, macroglossia, gigantism, ear creases, polyhydramnios, prematurity, hypoglycemia, polycythemia, apnea
Caudal dysplasia sequence, or caudal regression sequence	Occasional	Agenesis	Neurogenic bladder	Abnormal vertebrae and lower limbs, neurologic defects, R/O maternal diabetes, imperforate anus

(*continued*)

APPENDIX I–1
ASSOCIATIONS BETWEEN RENAL–URINARY TRACT ANOMALIES AND OTHER STRUCTURAL DEFECTS (*continued*)

Diagnosis (Mode of Genetic Transmission)	Frequency of Anomalies	Renal Anomalies	Urologic Anomalies	Other Associations
CHARGE association	5%	Agenesis, hypoplasia, hydronephrosis, heterotopic kidneys		Coloboma (iris, retina, anophthalmos), CHD, choanal atresia, growth retardation (postnatal), mental deficiency, genital hypoplasia (in males), ear anomalies, deafness
Goldenhar syndrome, facioauriculovertebral spectrum, first and second branchial arch syndrome	Occasional	Renal anomalies		Hemifacial microsomia, hemivertebrae, occasional abnormal ears and eyes, deafness, CHD, MR, SGA
Klippel–Feil syndrome	Frequent	Renal anomalies		Short neck, abnormal cervical vertebrae, deafness, CHD
Laterality sequences				
Ivemark syndrome, or bilateral right-sidedness	Frequent	Renal anomalies		Situs inversus, asplenia, CHD and vessel anomalies,
Bilateral left-sidedness	Occasional	Renal anomalies		Situs inversus, CHD, polysplenia
Meningomyelocele, spina bifida and occult spinal dysraphism sequence	Frequent	Hydronephrosis, UTI, renal failure, horseshoe kidney, hypoplasia, agenesis, ectopia, duplication	Neurogenic bladder	Neurologic defect, hydrocephalus
Megacystis–microcolon–intestinal hypoperistalsis syndrome	100%	Hydronephrosis	Massive bladder distention (100%), VUR	Neonatal bowel obstruction, hypoperistalsis, microcolon, frequently early death
Müllerian aplasia, Rokitansky sequence, or Rokitansky–Kustner–Hauser syndrome	30%–50%	Unilateral renal aplasia, hypoplasia, ectopia	Ureter duplication	Vaginal atresia, rudimentary uterus
MURCS assocation	>50%	Agenesis or ectopia (88%)		Absence of vagina, hypoplasia of uterus, abnormal cervicothoracic vertebrae
Monozygote twinning	Occasional		Exstrophy of the cloaca	Sacrococcygeal teratoma, sirenomelia, VATER, holoprosencephaly, anencephaly
Pallister–Hall syndrome	Frequent	Dysplasia		Hypothalamic hamartoblastoma, hypopituitarism, imperforate anus, polydactyly
Poland anomaly	Occasional	Renal anomaly		Variable unilateral features: absence of pectoralis muscle, upper limb hypoplasia, syndactyly
Potter sequence, or oligohydramnios sequence	100%	Hypoplasia, aplasia, agenesis, PKD, dysplasia	Urethral valves	Amnion nodosum, oligohydramnios, lung hypoplasia, limb malposition, facies compression
Prune-belly syndrome, or early urethral obstruction sequence	100%	Dysplasia, hypoplasia, horseshoe kidney, hydronephrosis	Urethral valves, persistent urachus, bladder agenesis, ectopic ureter	Prune belly, cryptorchidism, abnormal genitalia, Potter GI malformation (anal, hepatobiliary, mesentery, esophageal, pancreas), talipes equinovarus, scoliosis, thorax deformities, cardiac anomalies, iliac vessel compression
Rubinstein–Taybi syndrome	Frequent	Duplication	Ureter duplication	Broad thumbs and toes, hypoplastic maxilla, MR, slanted palpebral fissures
Sirenomelia sequence	Frequent	Agenesis, dysplasia	Bladder agenesis	Fusion of lower limbs, single UA, absence of genitalia except gonads, absence of sacrum and rectum, imperforate anus
Thanatophoric dysplasia	Occasional	Horseshoe kidney, hydronephrosis		Short limbs, flat vertebrae, large cranium, low nasal bridge, severe SGA, hypotonia, polyhydramnios, lung hypoplasia, early death
Tracheal agenesis assocation[‡]	50%	Agenesis, hydronephrosis, dysplasia	Duplication	Laryngeal/tracheal atresia, GI anomalies (*e.g.*, duodenal atresia), CHD, limb reduction defect (*i.e.*, radial hypoplasia),
VATER/VACTERL association	50%–74%	Agenesis, hydronephrosis, cystic dysplasia	Duplication, urethral atresia	TEF, vertebral and anal atresia, CHD, limb anomalies (*i.e.*,radial dysplasia)
Renal Cystic Disease[§]				
Alagille syndrome, or arteriohepatic dysplasia (AD)	Occasional	Cystic tubular dilatations, CRF, tubulointerstitial disease		Facies: deep-set eyes, prominent forehead, cholestasis, PPS, butterfly vertebrae

(*continued*)

APPENDIX I–1
ASSOCIATIONS BETWEEN RENAL–URINARY TRACT ANOMALIES AND OTHER STRUCTURAL DEFECTS (*continued*)

Diagnosis (Mode of Genetic Transmission)	Frequency of Anomalies	Renal Anomalies	Urologic Anomalies	Other Associations
Apert syndrome, or acrocephalosyndactyly (AD; fresh mutation common)	Occasional	MKD, hydronephrosis		Craniosynostosis, midfacial hypoplasia, syndactyly, broad distal phalanx (*i.e.,* thumb and big toe), occasional CHD, GI tract and lung anomalies
Congenital nephrotic syndrome, Finnish type (AR)	100%	CNF, tubular cystic dilatations		Polyhydramnios, elevated α-fetoprotein in amniotic fluid
Cystic hamartomata of lung and kidney	100%	Multilocular cysts		Hamartomatous pulmonary cysts
Dandy–Walker malformation	Occasional	MKD		Congenital hepatic fibrosis
Ehler–Danlos syndrome (AD, AR, X-linked)	Occasional	RTA		Skin and joint hyperextensibility, poor wound healing
Elejalde syndrome (AR)		Cystic dysplasia		Short-limb dwarfism, acrocephaly, polysyndactyly, subcutaneous hypertrophy, cholestasis, pancreatic dysplasia
Ellis–van Creveld syndrome, or chondroectodermal dysplasia (AR)	Occasional	Agenesis, cystic/medullary dysplasia	Epispadias	Short distal extremities, polydactyly, nail hypoplasia CHD (50%), SGA and short eventual stature, cholestasis
Familial juvenile nephronophthisis with hepatic fibrosis (AR)	Frequent	Glomerular cysts		Congenital hepatic fibrosis
Familial renal–retinal dystrophy (AR)	Common	Nephronophthisis–medullary cystic kidney disease		Pigmentary retinal dystrophy
Femoral hypoplasia–unusual facies syndrome		PKD, agenesis	Abnormal collecting system	Femoral hypoplasia, short nose, cleft palate
Fryns syndrome (AR)	50%	MKD, cortical cysts		Facial dysmorphism, microretrognathia, diaphragm defects, lung hypoplasia, neonatal death, bicornuate uterus or scrotum anomaly, distal limb hypoplasia
Glutaric aciduria syndrome, type II, or multiple acyl-coA dehydrogenase deficiency (AR)	Frequent	Cystic dysplasia, ultrastructural anomaly of glomerular basement membrane		Cerebral dysplasia, macrocephaly, facial dysmorphism, fatty liver, genital defects, hypoglycemia, metabolic acidosis
Ivemark syndrome, or renal–hepatic–pancreatic dysplasia (AR)	Frequent	Glomerular cysts, cystic dysplasia		Hepatic and pancreatic dysplasia, occasional splenic anomalies, may be associated with homogenous syndrome (Bernstein)
Jeune asphyxiating thoracic dystrophy (AR)	Frequent	Glomerular sclerosis, tubular cysts, renal failure		Small chest, lung hypoplasia, short limbs, cholestasis
Lowe syndrome, or oculocerebrorenal syndrome (X-linked)	100% (male)	Fanconi syndrome, CRF		Cataracts, mental deficiency, hypotonia
Meckel–Gruber syndrome, or dysencephalia splanchnocystica (AR)	100%	MKD, PKD, dysplasia, hypoplasia		Encephalocele, holoprosencephaly, polydactyly, Potter sequence, cholestasis
Nail–patella syndrome, or hereditary osteoonychodystrophy	Frequent	Proteinuria, hematuria, casts, CRF, PKD	Ureter duplication	Nail dysplasia, patella hypoplasia, iliac spurs
Orofacidigital syndrome, type 1 (D, lethal in male)	Frequent	Glomerular cysts		Oral frenula and clefts, hypoplasia of alae nasi, digital asymmetry
Roberts-SC phocomelia syndrome, hypomelia–hypotrichosis–facial hemangioma syndrome, or pseudothalidomide (AR)	Occasional	MKD, horseshoe kidney		Hypomelia, midfacial defect, cleft palate and lip, severe growth deficiency, cholestasis
Short rib–polydactyly, type I (Saldino–Noonan type)	Frequent	MKD, hypoplastic		Short-limb dwarfism, severe lung hypoplasia, early death, short ribs, with or without polydactyly, CHD, imperforate anus
Short rib–polydactyly syndrome, type II (Majewski type) (AR)	Frequent	Glomerular cysts, focal dilatation of distal tubules		Short-limb dwarfism, severe lung hypoplasia, early death, short ribs, with or without polydactyly, CHD, ambiguous genitalia
Smith–Lemli–Opitz syndrome (AR)	Occasional	MKD		MR, growth retardation, microcephaly, micrognathia, anteverted nostrils, ptosis of eyelids, syndactyly of second–third toes, ambiguous genitalia
Tuberous sclerosis (AD)	50%–80%	Glomerular and tubular cysts (rarely neonatal), angiomyolipomas, CRF		Seizures, skin lesions, tumors
Von Hippel–Lindau syndrome (AD)	Occasional	PKD		Retinal angioma, cerebellar hemangioblastoma

(*continued*)

APPENDIX I–1
ASSOCIATIONS BETWEEN RENAL–URINARY TRACT ANOMALIES AND OTHER STRUCTURAL DEFECTS (*continued*)

Diagnosis (Mode of Genetic Transmission)	Frequency of Anomalies	Renal Anomalies	Urologic Anomalies	Other Associations
Zellweger syndrome, or cerebrohepatorenal syndrome (AR)	100%	Glomerular cysts, albuminuria		Hypotonia, abnormal brain, seizures, flat facies, peroxisomal deficiency, cholestasis
Metabolic Diseases				
Hyperoxaluria type I, or oxalosis (AR)	100%	Nephrocalcinosis/lithiasis, CRF		Anorexia, failure to thrive, vomiting, dehydration and fever, liver failure, acidosis
Galactose-1-phosphate uridyl transferase deficiency, or galactosemia (AR)	Frequent	Fanconi syndrome		Hypoglycemia, anorexia, liver failure, sepsis, cataracts, MR
Hereditary fructose intolerance, fructose-1-phosphate aldolase deficiency (AR)	Frequent	Fanconi syndrome		Hypoglycemia, anorexia, liver failure, failure to thrive
Tyrosinemia type I, tyrosinosis, or hepatorenal tyrosinemia (AR)	Frequent	Famnconi syndrome		Growth failure, cabbagelike odor, vomiting, diarrhea, metabolic acidosis, liver failure, edema, fever
Glycogenosis with Fanconi syndrome, or Fanconi–Bickel syndrome (AR)	100%	Fanconi syndrome		Fever, vomiting, growth failure, rickets, hypoglycemia, hepatomegaly
Cystinosis (AR)	100%	Fanconi syndrome		Light skin and hair, failure to thrive, anorexia, fussiness, episodes of acidosis, dehydration and fever, rickets
Teratogens				
Fetal alcohol syndrome	18%	Renal agenesis, hypoplasia, hydronephrosis	Ureteral duplication	SGA, microcephaly, facial dysmorphism, MR
Fetal hydantoin syndrome	Occasional	Various malformations		Poor growth; microcephaly; craniofacial dysmorphism; brain, limb, and GI anomalies; CHD
Thalidomide embryopathy	Occasional	Various malformations		Phocomelia; polydactyly; syndactyly; hydrocephalus; facial capillary hemangioma; CHD; ear, eye, and GI anomalies
Fetal trimethadione syndrome	Occasional	Various malformations		Poor growth, craniofacial anomalies, CHD
Angiotensin converting enzyme inhibitors	Frequent(?)	Nephron dysgenesis		Hypocalvaria
Congenital Infections				
Congenital syphilis	Occasional	Nephrotic syndrome		Snuffles, meningitis, bone changes
Congenital toxoplasmosis	Rare	Nephrotic syndrome		Microcephaly, deafness, chorioretinitis, SGA
Renal Failure″				
Bardet–Biedl syndrome, or Laurence–Moon–Biedl syndrome (AR)	Frequent	Dysplasia, nephrosclerosis, interstitial scarring, cyst, HTN	Hydroureter	Retinitis pigmentosa, obesity, polydactyly
Drash syndrome, or nephropathy associated with gonadal dysgenesis and Wilms tumor	100%	Glomerulonephritis, interstitial changes, nephrotic syndrome, hematuria, HTN, ESRD, often Wilms tumor		Ambiguous genitalia (often male pseudohermaphroditism)
Fabry syndrome, or angiokeratoma corporis diffusum (X-linked)	Frequent	Proteinuria, hematuria, casts, leukocyturia		Dark nodular angiectases, corneal opacities, seizures, CNS symptoms
Russell–Silver syndrome (AD)	Occasional			Small skeletal asymmetry, small fifth finger, small triangular facies
Williams syndrome	Occasional	Hypertension	Bladder diverticula	Decreased growth, hypercalcemia, subaortic stenosis, prominent lips, hoarse voice

This table has been made by selecting well-defined associations, described in at least 3 patients, in which renal manifestations may develop before 1 year of age.

* Extra chromosome corresponding to segments of chromosome 22.

† May have partial deletion of chromosome 1p.

‡ Overlaps with VATER association.

§ See also trisomy 13 and 18, VATER, cocaine, and other subheadings (*i.e.*, renal dysplasia).

″ See also other headings.

AD, autosomal dominant; AR, autosomal recessive; CHD, congenital heart disease; CHARGE, coloboma, heart disease, atresia of the choanae, retarded mental development and growth, genital hypoplasia, ear anomalies; CHILD, congenital hemidysplasia with ichthyosiform erythroderma and limb defects; COFS, cerebrooculofacioskeletal; CNS; central nervous system; CRF, chronic renal failure; D, dominant; EEC, ectrodactyly–ectodermal dysplasia–clefting; EKG, electrocardiogram; ESRD, end-stage renal disease; GI, gastrointestinal; HTN, hypertension; LEOPARD, lentigenes, EKG anomalies, ocular anomalies, pulmonary stenosis, abnormal genitalia, retardation of growth, and deafness; MKD, multicystic kidney disease; MR, mental retardation; MURCS, Müllerian duct, renal, cervical somite; PDA, patent ductus arteriosus; PKD; polycystic kidney disease; PPS, peripheral pulmonic stenosis; R, recessive; R/O, rule out; RTA, renal tubular acidosis; SGA, small for gestational age; TAR, radial aplasia–thrombocytopenia; TEF, tracheoesophageal fistula; UA, umbilical artery; UPJ, ureteropelvic junction; UTI, urinary tract infection; VACTERL, vertebrae, anus, cardiac, tracheoesophageal, renal, limb; VATER, vertebrae, anus, trachoesophageal, renal; VUR, vesicoureteral reflux.

2. SINGLE SIGNS OF RENAL–URINARY TRACT MALFORMATIONS

APPENDIX I–2
RELATIONSHIP BETWEEN SINGLE SIGNS AND RENAL–URINARY TRACT MALFORMATIONS

Sign	Criteria for Entry Into the Study	Method Used To Detect Renal–Urinary Tract Malformations	Type of Malformations	Minimum Incidence* of Patients With Renal–Urinary Tract Anomalies	Incidence of Patients With Renal–Urinary Tract Anomalies Who Had No Evidence of Other Malformations at Birth
Abnormal Vertebrae					
Kohler, 1982[1]	Abnormal vertebrae or vertebrae	IVU	Agenesis, ectopic, horseshoe kidney, duplication	8/46 (17%)	NA
Macewen, 1972[2]	Congenital scoliosis, without suspicion of neurogenic bladder	IVU	Agenesis, duplication, ectopia, obstruction, VUR, horseshoe kidney	42/231 (18%)	NA
Anorectal Anomalies					
Munn, 1983[3]	Imperforation or atresia	IVU	Agenesis, duplication, VUR, hypospadias, UPJ obstruction, neurogenic bladder	20/28 (71%)	NA
Hoekstra, 1983[4‡]	Congenital anomalies	Autopsy; IVU excess in 3/126	VUR, agenesis, hypoplasia, ectopia, PKD UPJ obstruction, horseshoe kidney, hypospadias	95/150 (63%)	NA
Khuri, 1981[5§]	Imperforate anus and hypospadias	IVU	NA (part of study on hypospadias)	6/13 (46%)	NA
Congenital Diaphragmatic Hernia					
Siebert, 1990[6]	Autopsy	Autopsy	Agenesis, dysplasia or hypoplasia, UPJ/ ureterovesical obstruction	16/27 (59%)	4/16 (25%)
Cunniff, 1990[7]	Chart review	Surgery or autopsy	Agenesis, hydronephrosis, cysts, ectopic or duplicated ureter	5/103 (5%)	0%
Hypospadias					
Khuri, 1981[5]	Hypospadias	IVU in 460/1076	Agenesis, UPJ obstruction, VUR, Wilms, PKD, ectopic kidney, horseshoe kidney	48/1076 (4%)	15/48 (31%)[∥]
Shelton, 1985[8]	Asymptomatic hypospadias	IVU, VCUG	Agenesis, duplication, pelvic kidney, VUR	27/102 (27%)	0%
Pulmonary Hypoplasia					
Page, 1982[9]	Neonatal autopsy	Autopsy	Agenesis, dysgenesis, dysplasia, PKD	16/77 (21%)	NA
Single Umbilical Artery					
Bernischke, 1960[10]	Neonatal	Autopsy or clinical examination	Renal agenesis	1/15 (7%)	0%
Bourne, 1960[11]	Infant autopsy	Autopsy or clinical examination	Renal aplasia, PKD, obstruction	12/113 (11%)	NA
Faierman, 1960[12]	Neonatal autopsy	Autopsy	Hydronephrosis, agenesis, MKD, duplication	7/11 (64%)	0%
Lyon, 1960[13]	Infant	Autopsy or clinical examination	PKD and horseshoe kidney	1/11 (9%)	0%
Little, 1960[14]	Neonatal	Autopsy or clinical examination		0/21 (0%)	
Järvinen, 1962[15]	Neonatal	Autopsy or clinical examination	Renal aplasia	1/15 (7%)	NA
Adler, 1963[16]	Neonatal	Autopsy or clinical examination	PKD, hyplasia ectopia	2/19 (11%)	NA
Feingold, 1964[17]	Neonatal	IVU in 23/29	VUR, obstruction, non visualization at IVU	7/32 (21%)	NA
Gömöri, 1964[18]	Infant	Autopsy or clinical examination	Unilateral renal aplasia and heterolateral duplication	1/11 (8%)	0%

(continued)

APPENDIX I–2
RELATIONSHIP BETWEEN SINGLE SIGNS AND RENAL–URINARY TRACT MALFORMATIONS (*continued*)

Sign	Criteria for Entry Into the Study	Method Used To Detect Renal–Urinary Tract Malformations	Type of Malformations	Minimum Incidence* of Patients With Renal–Urinary Tract Anomalies	Incidence of Patients With Renal–Urinary Tract Anomalies Who Had No Evidence of Other Malformations at Birth
Single Umbilical Artery (*continued*)					
Fujikura, 1964[19]	Neonatal	Autopsy or clinical examination		0/38 (0%)	
Papadatos, 1965[20]	Neonatal	Autopsy or clinical examination	Hypospadias	0/32 (0%)	
Gornicka, 1965[21]	Neonatal	Autopsy or clinical examination		0/14 (0%)	
Peckham, 1965[22]	Neonatal	Autopsy or clinical examination	Renal agenesis (stillborn), urethral stenosis	2/51 (4%)	50%
Froehlich, 1966[23]	Neonatal	Autopsy or follow-up	PKD, renal or bladder aplasia, ectopia, duplication	10/203 (5%)	NA
Rohatgi, 1967[24]	Neonatal	Autopsy or clinical examination		0/7 (0%)	
Hnat, 1967[25]	Neonatal	Autopsy or clinical examination		0/38 (0%)	
Lewenthal, 1967[26]	Infant	Autopsy or clinical examination	PKD	2/50 (4%)	NA
Pereira, 1967[27]	Neonatal	Autopsy or clinical examination	PKD, hypoplasia	2/60 (3%)	NA
Harris, 1968[28]	Neonatal	IVU		0/11 (0%)	
Dellenbach, 1968[29]	Neonatal	Autopsy or clinical examination	PKD, agenesis	2/27 (7%)	0%
Bret, 1968[30]	Neonatal	Autopsy or clinical examination		0/9 (0%)	
Toulouse, 1969[31]	Neonatal	Autopsy or clinical examination		0/5 (0%)	
Mital, 1969[32]	Neonatal	Autopsy or clinical examination		0/37 (0%)	
Kristoffersen, 1969[33]	Neonatal	Autopsy or clinical examination	Cystic or hypoplastic kidney, bladder distention	2/11 (18%)	0%
Jean, 1969[34]	Neonatal	Autopsy or clinical examination	Renal hypoplasia, renal malformation (unspecified)	2/112 (2%)	NA
Muller, 1969[35]	Neonatal or abortion	Autopsy or clinical examination	Bladder exstrophy, unilateral agenesis	1/54 (2%)	0%
Broussard, 1972[36]	Neonatal	Autopsy or clinical examination	Bilateral renal agenesis, VUR	4/45 (9%)	NA
Le Marec, 1972[37]	Neonatal	Autopsy or clinical examination	Horseshoe kidney, bladder exstrophy, PKD, unilateral or bilateral agenesis	4/30 (13%)	0%
Vlietinck, 1972[38]	Neonatal	Autopsy or IVU (19/23)	PKD, pelvis duplication	2/29 (7%)	50%
Zeman, 1972[39]	Neonatal	Autopsy or clinical examination	Urethral valves, diverticulum	2/12 (17%)	NA
Froehlich, 1973[40]	Neonatal or infant autopsy	Autopsy	PKD; kidney, bladder, or urethral agenesis; horseshoe kidney; duplication	10/36 (28%)	0%
Bryan, 1974[41] and 1975[42]	Neonatal	Autopsy or follow-up	PKD, agenesis, absent urethra, horseshoe kidney	8/143 (6%)	0%
Altshuler, 1975[43]	Neonatal	Autopsy or clinical examination	Horseshoe kidney, MKD, obstruction, gastrourinary fistula	4/48 (8%)	25%

(*continued*)

APPENDIX I–2
RELATIONSHIP BETWEEN SINGLE SIGNS AND RENAL–URINARY TRACT MALFORMATIONS (*continued*)

Sign	Criteria for Entry Into the Study	Method Used To Detect Renal–Urinary Tract Malformations	Type of Malformations	Minimum Incidence* of Patients With Renal–Urinary Tract Anomalies		Incidence of Patients With Renal–Urinary Tract Anomalies Who Had No Evidence of Other Malformations at Birth
Mikulandra, 1976[44]	Neonatal	Autopsy or clinical examination		0/20	(0%)	
Tortora, 1984[45]	Prenatal US	Autopsy or clinical examination		0/5	(0%)	
Spontaneous Air Leak Syndrome						
Bashour, 1977[46]	Symptomatic pneumothorax	IVU	Hypoplasia or agenesis, PKD, dysplasia, urethral valves, Potter facies (n = 3)	12/47	(26%)	3/12 (25%)
Supernumerary Nipples						
Mehes, 1979[47]	Neonatal and follow-up (Hungary)	Clinical examination and IVU	Hydronephrosis, major anomalies	8/20	(40%)	8/8 (100%)#
Mehes, 1983[48]	Hospitalized	Clinical examination and IVU	Hydronephrosis, mega-ureter, duplication	9/37	(24%)	NA
Mimouni, 1983[49]	Neonatal (Israel)	Physical examination US (11/42)		0/43	(0%)	0%
Varsano, 1984[50]	ER/pediatric clinic (Israel)	IVU	PKD, hydronephrosis (UPJ obstruction), duplicated ureter, ureteral prolapse	6/26	(23%)	6/6 (100%)**
Robertson, 1986[51]	Neonatal (African-Americans)	US		0/32	(0%)	0%
Hersh, 1987[52]	Genetic/developmental clinic; 10 controls (United States, mostly Caucasian)	US or IVU	MKD, agenesis, hydronephrosis, horseshoe kidney	7/65	(11%)	2/7 (29%)††

* Hypospadias excluded.
† Except for minor anomalies such as pes equinovarus.
‡ Eighty-one of 150 patients in the study had no congenital abnormalities of the other organs (54%).
§ Among patients with first-degree hypospadias, the incidence of upper urinary tract malformations was 1.3%.
‖ Also 3 patients with undescended testes.
\# One patient had epilepsy; two patients had pyloric stenosis.
** One patient had Niemann–Pick disease.
†† Three patients had minor anomalies.
ER, emergency room; IVU, intravenous urography; MKD, multicystic kidney dysplasia; NA, not available; PKD, polycystic kidney disease; UA, umbilical artery; UPJ/UV, ureteropelvic junction–ureterovesical; US, ultrasound; VUR, vesicoureteral reflex.

REFERENCES

1. Kohler R, Dodat H, Charollais Y. Malformations congénitales vertébrales et urinaires. Fréquence de leur association et conduite à tenir. Pédiatrie 1982;37:91.
2. Macewen GD, Winter RB, Hardy JH. Evaluation of kidney anomalies in congenital scoliosis. J Bone Joint Surg 1972; 54:1451.
3. Munn R, Schillinger JF. Urologic abnormalities found with imperforate anus. Urol 1983;21:260.
4. Hoekstra WJ, Scholtmeijer RJ, Molenaar JC, Schreeve RH, Schroeder FH. Urogenital tract abnormalities associated with congenital anorectal anomalies. J Urol 1983;130:962.
5. Khuri FJ, Hardy BE, Churchill BM. Urologic anomalies associated with hypospadias. Urol Clin North Am 1981;8:565.
6. Siebert JR, Benjamin DR, Juul S, Glick PL. Urinary tract anomalies associated with congenital diaphragmatic defects. Am J Med Genet 1990;37:1.
7. Cunniff C, Jones KL, Jones MC. Patterns of malformation in children with congenital diaphragmatic defects. J Pediatr 1990;116:258.
8. Shelton TB, Noe HN. The role of excretory urography in patients with hypospadias. J Urol 1985;134:97.
9. Page DV, Stocker JT. Anomalies associated with pulmonary hypoplasia. Am Rev Resp Dis 1982;125:216.
10. Benirschke K, Bourne GL. The incidence and prognostic implication of congenital absence of one umbilical artery. Am J Obstet Gynecol 1960;79:251.
11. Bourne GL, Benirschke K. Absent umbilical artery. A review of 113 cases. Arch Dis Child 1960;35:534.
12. Faierman E. The significance of one umbilical artery. Arch Dis Child 1960;35:285.
13. Lyon FA. Fetal abnormalities with umbilical cords containing one umbilical artery and one umbilical vein. Obstet Gynecol 1960;16:719.
14. Little WA. Umbilical Artery Aplasia. Obstet Gynecol 1961; 17:695.

15. Järvinen PA, Österlund K, von Numers C. Umbilical artery aplasia. Duodecim 1962;78:937.
16. Adler J, Lewenthal H, Ben-Adereth N. Absence of one umbilical artery and its relationship to congenital malformations. Harefuah 1963;65:286.
17. Feingold M, Fine RN, Ingall D. Intravenous pyelography in infants with single umbilical artery. A preliminary report. N Engl J Med 1964;270:1178.
18. Gömöri VZ, Koller T, Jr. Über das Fehlen einer Arterie in der Nabelschnur. Gynaecologia 1964;157:177.
19. Fujikura T. Single umbilical artery and congenital malformations. Am J Obstet Gynecol 1964;88:829.
20. Papadatos C, Paschos A. Singel umbilical artery and congenital malformations. Obstet Gynecol 1965;3:367.
21. Gornicka Z, Matusiak J, Teczynska T. The significance of single umbilical artery detection in attempts of early disclosure of congenital malformations. Ginekol Polska 1965;36:1261.
22. Peckham CH, Yerushalmy J. Aplasia of one umbilical artery: incidence by race and certain obstetric factors. Obstet Gynecol 1965;26:359.
23. Froehlich LA, Fujikura T. Significance of a single umbilical artery. Am J Obstet Gynecol 1966;94:274.
24. Rohatgi P. Single umbilical artery. J Obstet Gynaecol India 1967;17:718.
25. Hnat RF. The practical importance of the single artery umbilical cord. J Reprod Fertil 1967;14:195.
26. Lewenthal H, Alexander DJ, Ben-Adereth N. Single umbilical artery. A report of 50 cases. Isr J Med Sci 1967;3:899.
27. Pereira JS. Anomalias vascularas del condon umbilical (con espicial consideración a la arteria umbilical única). Rev Obst Gin Venezuela 1967;27:421.
28. Harris RJ, Van Leeuwen G. Single umbilical artery. J Pediatr 1968;72:98.
29. Dellenbach P, Leissner P, Philippe E, Gillet JY, Muller P. Anomalies of the umbilical cord and foetal malformations I. Single umbilical artery, velamentous insertion of the umbilical cord and foetal malformations. Rev Franç Gynécol Obstét 1968;63:603.
30. Bret AJ, Blanchier H. Single umbilical artery. Value of the systematic examination of the placenta. Rev Franç Gynécol Obstét 1968;63:399.
31. Toulouse R, Chevrel ML, Guigores MC, Kerisit J. Artère ombilicale unique. Archiv Méd de L'ouest 1969;1:269.
32. Mital VK, Garg BK, Gupta U. Single umbilical artery-its association with congenital malformations. J Obstet Gynaecol India 1969;19:583
33. Kristoffersen K. The significance of absence of one umbilical artery. Acta Obstet Gyn Scand 1969;48:195.
34. Jean C, Dupré A, Carrier C. L'artère ombilicale unique: etude de 112 observations. Can Med Assoc J 1969;100:1088.
35. Muller G, Dehalleux JM, Trutt B, Philippe E, Dreyfus J, Gandar R. L'artère ombilicale unique-A propos de 54 cas. Bulletin de la Société Royale Belge de Gynécologie Obstét 1969;39: 333.
36. Broussard P, Raudrant D, Picaud JJ, Bonglet C, Dumont M. Artère ombilicale unique. Etude de 45 cas. J Gyn Obst Biol Repr 1972;1:551.
37. Le Marec B, Kerisit J, De Villartay A, Ferrand B, Toulouse R, Seńécal J. A. single umbilical artery. A report on 31 cases. J Gyn Obst Biol Repr 1972;1:825.
38. Vlietinck KF, Thiery M, Orye E, de Clercq A, van Vaerenbergh P. Significance of the single umbilical artery. A clinical, radiological, chromosomal, and dermatoglyphic study. Arch Dis Child 1972;47:639.
39. Zeman V. Aplazie umbilikální artérie. CS Pediatr 1972;27:78.
40. Froehlich LA, Fujikura T. Follow-up of infants with single umbilical artery. Pediatr 1973;52:6.
41. Bryan EM, Kohler HG. The missing umbilical artery. I. Prospective study based on a maternity unit. Arch Dis Child 1974;49:844.
42. Bryan EM, Kohler HG. The missing umbilical artery. II. Paediatric follow-up. Arch Dis Child 1975;50:714.
43. Altshuler G, Tsang RC, Ermocilla R. Single umbilial artery. Correlation of clinical status and umbilical cord histology. Am J Dis Child 1975;129:697.
44. Mikulandra F. Occurrence of aplasia of the umbilical artery in fetuses with intrauterine retardation. Jugosl Ginek Opstet 1976;16:295.
45. Tortora M, Cherevenak FA, Mayden K, Hobbins JC. Antenatal sonographic diagnosis of single umbilical artery. Obstet Gynecol 1984;63:693.
46. Bashour BN, Balfe JW. Urinary tract anomalies in neonates with spontaneous pneumothorax and/or pneumomediastinum. Pediatr 1977;59(Suppl):1048.
47. Méhes K. Association of supernumerary nipples with other anomalies. J Pediatr 1979;95:274.
48. Méhes K. Association of supernumerary nipples with other anomalies (letter). J Pediatr 1983;102:161.
49. Mimouni F, Merlob P, Reisner SH. Occurrence of supernumerary nipples in newborns. Am J Dis Child 1983;137: 952.
50. Varsano IB, Jaber L, Garty BZ, Mukamel MM, Grünebaum M. Urinary tract abnormalities in children with supernumerary nipples. Pediatrics 1984;73:103.
51. Robertson A, Sale P, Sathyanarayan. Lack of association of supernumerary nipples with renal anomalies in black infants. J Pediatr 1986;109:502.
52. Hersh JH, Bloom AS, Cromer AO, Harrison HL, Weisskopf B. Does a supernumerary nipple/renal field defect exist? Am J Dis Child 1987;141:989.

3. CLASSIFICATION OF CYSTIC KIDNEY DISEASE

APPENDIX I–3
CLASSIFICATION OF CYSTIC KIDNEY DISEASE

Genetic Diseases

AR polycystic kidney disease: associated with congenital hepatic fibrosis
AD polycystic kidney disease: associated with central nervous system aneurysms
Juvenile nephronophthisis–medullary cystic disease complex
- Juvenile nephronophthisis with hepatic fibrosis (AR)
- Medullary cystic disease complex (AD)

Glomerulocystic kidney disease:
- AD glomerulocystic kidney disease
- Familial hypoplastic glomerulocystic kidney disease (AD)

Malformation syndromes
- Multicystic kidney disease
  - Apert syndrome, or acrocephalosyndactyly (AD, fresh mutation common)
  - Elejalde syndrome (AR)
  - Ellis–van Creveld syndrome, or chondroectodermal dysplasia (AR)
  - Fryns syndrome (AR)
  - Meckel–Gruber syndrome, or dysencephalia splanchnocystica (AR)
  - Roberts phocomelia, hypomelia–hypotrichosis–facial hemangioma syndrome, or pseudothalidomide syndrome (AR)
  - Short rib–polydactyly syndrome, Saldino–Noonan type (AR)
  - Smith-Lemli-Optiz syndrome (AR)
- Glomerulocystic disease
  - Short rib-polydactyly syndrome, Majewski type (AR)
  - Tuberous sclerosis (AD): glomerular and tubular cysts
  - Zellweger cerebrohepatorenal syndrome (AR)
  - Ivemark syndrome, or renal–hepatic–pancreatic dysplasia (AR): cystic dysplasia
  - Orofaciodigital syndrome, type 1 (D, lethal in male infants)
- Nephronophthisis-medullary cystic disease
  - Familial renal-retinal dystrophy (AR)
- Other
  - Von Hippel–Lindau syndrome (AD)
  - Jeune syndrome, or asphyxiating thoracic dystrophy (AR)
  - Alagille syndrome, or arteriohepatic dysplasia (AD)
  - Trisomy D (13)
  - Trisomy E (18)
  - Ehlers–Danlos syndrome (AD, AR, X-linked)
  - Glutaric aciduria syndrome, type II, or multiple acyl-coA dehydrogenase deficiency (AR)
  - Lowe syndrome, or oculo-cerebro-renal syndrome (X-linked)
  - Nail–patella syndrome, or hereditary osteoonychodystrophy (AD)

Congenital hypernephronic nephromegaly with tubular dysgenesis syndrome (AR)
Congenital nephrotic syndrome, Finnish type, or infantile microcystic disease (AR)

Sporadic and Acquired Diseases

Multicystic kidney disease, or multicystic dysplasia
- Dandy–Walker malformation

Sporadic glomerulocystic kidney disease
Nephron dysgenesis: glomerular or tubular immaturity
Brachymesomelia–renal syndrome (only 1 case described)
Femoral hypoplasia–unusual facies syndrome
Multilocular cystic nephroma, or cystadenoma
Simple cyst (benign)
Medullary sponge kidney (<5% inherited; no renal failure)
Cystic hamartoma of lung and kidney (multilocular cysts)
Acquired renal cystic disease in chronic hemodialysis patients
Caliceal diverticulum, or pyelogenic cyst

AD, autosomal dominant; AR, autosomal recessive; D, dominant.
See Appendix I-1 for description of associated malformations.

INDEX

Note: Page numbers followed by f *indicate figures; those followed by* t *indicate tables.*